PRINCIPLES
AND
PRACTICE OF

Sleep
Medicine

SECTION EDITORS

Michael S. Aldrich
Michael H. Chase
J. Christian Gillin
Christian Guilleminault
Max Hirshkowitz
Mark W. Mahowald
Wallace B. Mendelson
John Orem
R. T. Pivik
Leon Rosenthal
Mark H. Sanders
Fred W. Turek
Frank J. Zorick

PRINCIPLES AND PRACTICE OF

Sleep Medicine

THIRD EDITION

Meir H. Kryger, MD, FRCPC
Director, Sleep Research
St. Boniface General Hospital Research Center
Professor of Medicine
University of Manitoba
Winnipeg, Manitoba, Canada

Thomas Roth, PhD
Head, Division of Sleep Disorders Medicine
Henry Ford Hospital
Clinical Professor of Psychiatry
University of Michigan
Detroit, Michigan

William C. Dement, MD, PhD
Lowell W. and Josephine Q. Berry
Professor of Psychiatry and Behavioral Sciences
and Director, Sleep Disorders Center
Stanford University School of Medicine
Stanford, California

W.B. SAUNDERS COMPANY
A Harcourt Health Sciences Company
Philadelphia London New York St. Louis Sydney Toronto

W.B. SAUNDERS COMPANY
A Harcourt Health Sciences Company

The Curtis Center
Independence Square West
Philadelphia, Pennsylvania 19106

Library of Congress Cataloging-in-Publication Data

Principles and practice of sleep medicine /
[edited by] Meir H. Kryger, Thomas Roth, William C. Dement.—3rd ed.

p.   cm.

Includes bibliographical references and index.

ISBN 0–7216–7670–7

1. Sleep disorders.   2. Sleep.   I. Kryger, Meir H.
II. Roth, T. (Tom).   III. Dement, William C.
[DNLM: 1. Sleep Disorders.   2. Sleep—physiology.
WM 188 P957 2000]

RC547.P75   2000   616.8'498—dc21

DNLM/DLC   99-31929

6/21/00 $145,00 M BC

Acquisitions Editor: Richard Zorab
Developmental Editor: Cathy Carroll
Designer: Marie Gardocky-Clifton
Senior Production Manager: Linda R. Garber
Copy Editor: Amy L. Cannon
Illustration Coordinator: Rita Martello

PRINCIPLES AND PRACTICE OF SLEEP MEDICINE   ISBN 0–7216–7670–7

Printed in the United States of America.

Last digit is the print number: 9   8   7   6   5   4   3   2   1

This book is dedicated to our children:
Shelley, Michael, and Steven
Daniel, Adam, Jonathan, and Andrea
Elizabeth, Catherine, and Nicholas

But the tigers come at night,
With their voices soft as thunder,
As they tear your hope apart,
As they turn your dream to shame.

Blessings on him who first invented sleep.—It covers a man all over, thoughts and all, like a cloak.—It is meat for the hungry, drink for the thirsty, heat for the cold, and cold for the hot.—It makes the shepherd equal to the monarch, and the fool to the wise.—There is but one evil in it, and that is that it resembles death, since between a dead man and a sleeping man there is but little difference.

From DON QUIXOTE
by Saavedra M. de Cervantes

Contributors

Peter Achermann, PhD
Senior Research Associate, Institute of Pharmacology and Toxicology, University of Zurich, Zurich, Switzerland
Sleep Homeostasis and Models of Sleep Regulation

Michael S. Aldrich, MD
Professor of Neurology and Director, Sleep Disorders Center, University of Michigan Medical School, Ann Arbor, Michigan
Stimulants: Efficacy and Adverse Effects; Section Editor: Impact, Presentation, and Diagnosis; Approach to the Patient With Disordered Sleep; Cardinal Manifestations of Sleep Disorders; Parkinsonism; Neurological Monitoring Techniques

Angela Anagnos, MD
Fellow, Stanford University Sleep Clinic, Stanford University Sleep Disorders Center, Stanford, California
Narcolepsy

Amit Anand, MD
Instructor in Medicine, Harvard Medical School; Research Associate, Beth Israel Deaconess Medical Center, Boston, Massachusetts
Cardiorespiratory Changes in Sleep-Disordered Breathing

Sonia Ancoli-Israel, PhD
Professor of Psychiatry, University of California, San Diego; Director, Sleep Disorders Clinic, Veterans Affairs San Diego Healthcare System, San Diego, California
Actigraphy

John Antrobus, PhD
Professor of Psychology and Head, PhD Subprogram in Experimental Cognition/Psychology, The City College of the City University of New York, New York, New York
Theories of Dreaming

Josephine Arendt, BSc, PhD, FRCPath
Professor of Endocrinology, School of Biological Sciences, University of Surrey, Guildford, Surrey, England
Jet Lag and Sleep Disruption

Steven K. Baker, MD
Assistant Professor of Medicine, Pulmonary Division, Center for Circadian Biology and Medicine, Northwestern University Medical School, Chicago, Illinois
Circadian Disorders of the Sleep-Wake Cycle

Claudio Bassetti, MD
Associate Professor, Attending Physician, and Director of Sleep Disorders Center, Neurology Department, University Hospital, Bern, Switzerland
Cerebrovascular Diseases

Ali G. Bassiri, MD
Fellow, Stanford University Sleep Clinic, Stanford University Sleep Disorders Center, Stanford, California
Clinical Features and Evaluation of Obstructive Sleep Apnea-Hypopnea Syndrome

Ruth M. Benca, MD, PhD
Professor, Department of Psychiatry, University of Wisconsin—Madison, Madison, Wisconsin
Mood Disorders; Eating Disorders

Kathleen L. Benson, PhD
Associate Clinical Professor, Department of Psychiatry and Behavioral Sciences, Stanford University School of Medicine, Stanford; Director, Sleep Disorders Program, Veterans Administration Palo Alto Healthcare System, Palo Alto, California
Schizophrenia

Donald L. Bliwise, PhD
Associate Professor, Department of Neurology; Director, Sleep Disorders Center, Wesley Woods Geriatric Hospital, Emory University Medical School, Atlanta, Georgia
Normal Aging; Dementia

Michael H. Bonnet, PhD
Professor of Neurology, Department of Neurology, Wright State University School of Medicine; Director of Sleep Center, Department of Veterans Affairs Medical Center, Dayton, Ohio
Sleep Deprivation

Alexander A. Borbély, MD
Professor of Pharmacology, University of Zurich, Zurich, Switzerland
Sleep Homeostasis and Models of Sleep Regulation

Roger J. Broughton, MD, PhD
Professor of Neurology, University of Ottawa; Medical Director, Sleep Medicine Center, Ottawa Hospital (General Campus), Ottawa, Ontario, Canada
NREM Arousal Parasomnias: Confusional Arousals, Sleep Terrors, and Sleepwalking

Dedra Buchwald, MD
Professor, Department of Internal Medicine, University of Washington School of Medicine; Director, Chronic Fatigue Clinic, Harborview Medical Center, Seattle, Washington
Chronic Fatigue Syndrome and Fibromyalgia

Daniel J. Buysse, MD
Associate Professor of Psychiatry, University of Pittsburgh; University of Pittsburgh Medical Center Health Systems, Pittsburgh, Pennsylvania
Psychometric and Psychiatric Evaluation

Christian Cajochen, PhD
Instructor in Medicine, Harvard Medical School; Associate Neuroscientist, Brigham and Women's Hospital, Boston, Massachusetts
Melatonin in the Regulation of Sleep and Circadian Rhythms

Mary A. Carskadon, PhD
Professor, Psychiatry and Human Behavior, Brown University School of Medicine, Providence; Director of Sleep and Chronobiology Research, E. P. Bradley Hospital, East Providence, Rhode Island
Normal Human Sleep: An Overview; Daytime Sleepiness and Alertness; Monitoring and Staging Human Sleep; Evaluating Sleepiness

Regina C. Casper, MD
Professor, Department of Psychiatry, Stanford University, Palo Alto, California
Eating Disorders

Michael H. Chase, PhD
Professor of Physiology, Department of Physiology, Center for Health Sciences, University of California at Los Angeles School of Medicine, Los Angeles, California
Section Editor: *Sleep Mechanisms; Control of Motoneurons During Sleep*

Ronald D. Chervin, MD, MS
Assistant Professor, Department of Neurology and Sleep Disorders Center, University of Michigan, Ann Arbor, Michigan
Use of Clinical Tools and Tests in Sleep Medicine; Cerebrovascular Diseases

Charles A. Czeisler, PhD, MD
Professor of Medicine, Harvard Medical School; Chief, Circadian, Neuroendocrine and Sleep Disorders Section, Division of Endocrinology, Brigham and Women's Hospital, Boston, Massachusetts
The Human Circadian Timing System and Sleep-Wake Regulation; Melatonin in the Regulation of Sleep and Circadian Rhythms

Joseph De Koninck, PhD
Professor of Psychology and Dean of Graduate Studies, University of Ottawa, Ottawa, Ontario, Canada
Waking Experiences and Dreaming

William C. Dement, MD, PhD
Lowell W. and Josephine Q. Berry Professor of Psychiatry and Behavioral Sciences, Stanford University Medical School; Director, Sleep Disorders Center, Stanford University School of Medicine, Stanford, California
History of Sleep Physiology and Medicine; Normal Human Sleep: An Overview; Daytime Sleepiness and Alertness; Sleep Medicine, Public Policy, and Public Health

David F. Dinges, PhD
Professor of Psychology in Psychiatry, University of Pennsylvania School of Medicine, Philadelphia, Pennsylvania
Circadian Rhythms in Fatigue, Alertness, and Performance; Sleep Medicine, Public Policy, and Public Health

G. William Domhoff, PhD
Professor of Psychology, University of California, Santa Cruz, California
Methods and Measures for the Study of Dream Content

Neil J. Douglas, MD, FRCPE, FRCP
Professor of Respiratory and Sleep Medicine, The University of Edinburgh; Consultant Physician and Director, Sleep Centre, Royal Infirmary, Edinburgh, Scotland
Respiratory Physiology: Control of Ventilation; Asthma; Chronic Obstructive Pulmonary Disease

Sean P. A. Drummond, PhD
Postdoctoral Fellow, Department of Psychiatry, University of California, San Diego; Veterans Administration San Diego Healthcare System, San Diego, California
Medication and Substance Abuse

Jidong Fang MD, PhD
Associate Professor, Department of Veterinary and Comparative Anatomy, Pharmacology and Physiology, Washington State University, Pullman, Washington
Host Defense

Carlo Franzini, MD
Professor of Physiology, Medical School, University of Bologna, Bologna, Italy
Cardiovascular Physiology: The Peripheral Circulation

Charles F. P. George, MD, FRCPC
Associate Professor of Medicine, University of Western Ontario; Director, Sleep Disorders Laboratory, London Health Sciences Centre, London, Ontario, Canada
Hypertension, Ischemic Heart Disease, and Stroke; Neuromuscular Disorders

J. Christian Gillin, MD
Professor of Psychiatry, University of California, San Diego, La Jolla; Staff Psychiatrist, Veterans Affairs San Diego Healthcare System, San Diego, California
Section Editor: *Psychiatric Disorders; Medication and Substance Abuse*

Anne M. Gillis, MD

Professor of Medicine, University of Calgary; Medical Director, Pacing and Electrophysiology, Foothills Hospital, Calgary, Alberta, Canada

Cardiac Arrhythmias

Steven F. Glotzbach, PhD

Consultant, Stanford University Medical Media and Information Technologies, Stanford University Medical Center, Stanford, California

Temperature Regulation

Paul B. Glovinsky, PhD

Adjunct Assistant Professor, Department of Psychology, The City College of New York, New York; Clinical Director, Capital Region Sleep-Wake Disorders Center, Saint Peter's Hospital, Albany, New York

Assessment Techniques for Insomnia

Roger Godbout, PhD

Associate Professor, Université de Montréal, Faculté de Médecine, Département Psychiatrie; Hôpital du Sacré-Coeur de Montréal Centre de Recherches, Montréal, Québec, Canada

Restless Legs Syndrome and Periodic Limb Movement Disorder

Ronald Grunstein, MB, BS, MD, PhD, FRACP

Clinical Associate Professor, Department of Medicine, University of Sydney; Senior Staff Specialist, Centre for Respiratory Failure and Sleep Disorders, Royal Prince Alfred Hospital; Consultant Physician, Sleep Disorders Service, St. Vincent's Clinic, Sydney, Australia

Continuous Positive Airway Pressure for Sleep Breathing Disorders; Endocrine Disorders

Christian Guilleminault, MD

Professor of Psychiatry and Behavioral Sciences and Director of Training, Stanford University Sleep Research Center and Sleep Disorders Center, Stanford University School of Medicine, Stanford, California

Section Editor: *Primary Disorders of Daytime Sleepiness; Narcolepsy; Idiopathic Central Nervous System Hypersomnia; Clinical Features and Evaluation of Sleep Apnea-Hypopnea Syndrome; Surgical Therapy for Obstructive Sleep Apnea-Hypopnea Syndrome;* Section Editor: *Medical and Neurological Disorders*

Martica Hall, PhD

Assistant Professor of Psychiatry, University of Pittsburgh; University of Pittsburgh Medical Center Health Systems, Pittsburgh, Pennsylvania

Psychometric and Psychiatric Evaluation

Ronald M. Harper, PhD

Professor of Neurobiology, University of California at Los Angeles; University of California at Los Angeles Brain Research Institute, Los Angeles, California

Cardiovascular Physiology: Central and Autonomic Regulation

Mary E. Harrington, PhD

Associate Professor, Department of Psychology, Smith College, Northampton, Massachusetts

Anatomy and Physiology of the Mammalian Circadian System

Peter J. Hauri, PhD

Professor, Department of Psychology, Mayo Medical School; Administrative Director, Mayo Sleep Disorders Center, Rochester, Minnesota

Primary Insomnia

H. Craig Heller, PhD

Professor, Department of Biological Sciences, Stanford University, Stanford, California

Temperature Regulation

Max Hirshkowitz, PhD

Associate Professor, Baylor College of Medicine, Department of Psychiatry; Director, Sleep Research Center and Associate Director, Sleep Disorders Center, Veterans Affairs Medical Center, Houston, Texas

Section Editor: *Methodology; Assessment of Sleep-Related Erections; Evaluating Sleepiness; Computers in Sleep Medicine*

J. Allan Hobson, MD

Professor of Psychiatry, Harvard Medical School; Director, Laboratory of Neurophysiology, Massachusetts Mental Health Center, Boston, Massachusetts

Cardiovascular Physiology: Central and Autonomic Regulation

Victor Hoffstein, PhD, MD

Professor of Medicine, University of Toronto; Staff Respirologist and Director, Pulmonary Function Laboratories, St. Michael's Hospital, Toronto, Ontario, Canada

Snoring

Christer Hublin, MD, PhD

Chief Neurologist, Haaga Neurological Research Centre, Helsinki, Finland

Epidemiology of Sleep Disorders

Suzan E. Jaffe, MSN, PhD, ARNP

Assistant Adjunct Professor, University of Miami, Departments of Psychiatry and Nursing, Miami; Consultant, Sleep Disorders Center, Mt. Sinai Medical Center, Miami Beach, Florida

Sleep and Infectious Disease

Barbara E. Jones, PhD

Professor, Department of Neurology and Neurosurgery; Staff, Montreal Neurological Institute, McGill University, Montréal, Québec, Canada

Basic Mechanisms of Sleep-Wake States

Nancy H. Kerr, PhD

Provost and Professor of Psychology, Oglethorpe University, Atlanta, Georgia

Dreaming, Imagery, and Perception

Sat Bir S. Khalsa, PhD
Instructor in Medicine, Harvard Medical School; Associate Neuroscientist, Brigham and Women's Hospital, Boston, Massachusetts
The Human Circadian Timing System and Sleep-Wake Regulation

George F. Koob, PhD
Adjunct Professor, Departments of Psychology and Psychiatry, University of California, San Diego; Professor and Director, Division of Psychopharmacology, Department of Neuropharmacology, The Scripps Research Institute, La Jolla, California
Stimulants: Basic Mechanisms and Pharmacology

Milton Kramer, MD
Clinical Professor of Psychiatry, School of Medicine, Wright State University, Dayton; Volunteer Professor of Psychiatry, University of Cincinnati, College of Medicine, Cincinnati, Ohio
Dreams and Psychopathology

Jean Krieger, MD
Professor of Neurology, Faculté de Médecine, Université Louis Pasteur; Head of Department, Service d'Explorations Fonctionnelles du Système Nerveux et de Pathologie du Sommeil, Hôpitaux Universitaires de Strasbourg, Strasbourg, France
Respiratory Physiology: Breathing in Normal Subjects

James M. Krueger, PhD
Professor, Washington State University College of Veterinary Medicine, Department of Veterinary and Comparative Anatomy, Pharmacology and Physiology, Pullman, Washington
Host Defense

Meir H. Kryger, MD, FRCPC
Director, Sleep Research, St. Boniface General Hospital Research Center; Professor of Medicine, University of Manitoba, Winnipeg, Manitoba, Canada
Management of Obstructive Sleep Apnea-Hypopnea Syndrome: An Overview; Restrictive Lung Disorders; Monitoring Respiratory and Cardiac Function

Leszek Kubin, PhD
Research Associate Professor of Physiology, Department of Animal Biology, School of Veterinary Medicine, University of Pennsylvania, Philadelphia, Pennsylvania
Respiratory Physiology: Central Neural Control

Samuel Kuna, MD
Associate Professor of Medicine, University of Pennsylvania; Associate Professor, Veterans Administration Medical Center, Philadelphia, Pennsylvania
Anatomy and Physiology of Upper Airway Obstruction

Sandrine H. Launois, MD
Instructor in Medicine, Harvard Medical School; Associate Physician, Beth Israel Deaconess Medical Center, Boston, Massachusetts
Cardiorespiratory Changes in Sleep-Disordered Breathing

Gilles J. Lavigne, DMD, MSc, FRCDC
Professor, Facultés Médecine Dentaire et Médecine, Université de Montréal; Centre d'Étude du Sommeil, Hôpital du Sacré-Coeur, Montréal, Québec, Canada
Bruxism

Patrick Leger, MD
Edouard Rist Hospital, Paris, France
Noninvasive Ventilation for Sleep Breathing Disorders

Kasey K. Li, MD, DDS
Associate Director of Sleep Surgery, Stanford Sleep Disorders Clinic and Research Center, Stanford, California
Surgical Therapy for Obstructive Sleep Apnea-Hypopnea Syndrome

Alan A. Lowe, DMD, PhD, FRCDC
Professor and Chair, Division of Orthodontics, Faculty of Dentistry, Vancouver, British Columbia, Canada
Oral Appliances for Sleep Breathing Disorders

Mark W. Mahowald, MD
Professor of Neurology, University of Minnesota; Director, Minnesota Regional Sleep Disorders Center, Hennepin County Medical Center, Minneapolis, Minnesota
Section Editor: *Parasomnias; Epilepsy and Sleep Disorders; REM Sleep Parasomnias; Violent Parasomnias: Forensic Medicine Issues*

Beth A. Malow, MD, MS
Assistant Professor, Department of Neurology, University of Michigan Medical School, Ann Arbor, Michigan
Neurological Monitoring Techniques

Christiane Manzini
Research Assistant, Faculté de Médecine Dentaire, Université de Montréal; Centre d'Étude du Sommeil, Hôpital du Sacré-Coeur, Montréal, Québec, Canada
Bruxism

W. Vaughn McCall, MD, MS
Associate Professor of Psychiatry, Wake Forest University School of Medicine, Winston-Salem, North Carolina
Psychiatric Disorders and Insomnia

Wallace B. Mendelson, MD
Professor of Psychiatry, Medicine, and Clinical Pharmacology and Director, Sleep Research Laboratory, Department of Psychiatry, University of Chicago, Chicago, Illinois
Section Editor: *Pharmacology; Hypnotics: Basic Mechanisms and Pharmacology*

Emmanuel Mignot, MD, PhD
Associate Professor of Psychiatry and Behavioral Sciences and Director, Center for Narcolepsy, Stanford University; Stanford Sleep Disorders Clinic, Stanford, California
Pathophysiology of Narcolepsy

Ralph E. Mistlberger, PhD

Professor, Department of Psychology, Simon Fraser University, Burnaby, British Columbia, Canada

Circadian Rhythms in Mammals: Formal Properties and Environmental Influences; Anatomy and Physiology of the Mammalian Circadian System

Merrill H. Mitler, PhD

Clinical Professor of Psychiatry, University of California, San Diego; Professor, Department of Neuropharmacology, The Scripps Research Institute, La Jolla, California

Stimulants: Efficacy and Adverse Effects; Sleep Medicine, Public Policy, and Public Health; Evaluating Sleepiness

Murray A. Mittleman, MD, DrPH

Assistant Professor of Medicine, Harvard Medical School; Co-Director, Institute for Prevention of Cardiovascular Disease, Beth Israel Deaconess Medical Center, Boston, Massachusetts

Sleep-Related Cardiac Risk

Timothy H. Monk, PhD, DSc

Professor of Psychiatry, University of Pittsburgh School of Medicine; Director, Human Chronobiology Research Program, University of Pittsburgh Medical Center, Western Psychiatric Institute and Clinic, Pittsburgh, Pennsylvania

Shift Work

Jacques Montplaisir, MD, PhD, CRCPc

Professor Titulaire, Faculté de Médecine, Department Psychiatrie, Université de Montréal; Directeur, Hôpital du Sacré-Coeur de Montréal, Centre d'Étude du Sommeil, Montréal, Québec, Canada

Restless Legs Syndrome and Periodic Limb Movement

Constance A. Moore, MD

Associate Professor, Baylor College of Medicine, Department of Psychiatry; Director, Sleep Disorders Center, Veterans Affairs Medical Center, Houston, Texas

Computers in Sleep Medicine

Francisco R. Morales, MD

Research Physiologist, Department of Physiology, University of California at Los Angeles School of Medicine, Center for Health Sciences, Los Angeles, California

Control of Motoneurons During Sleep

Michael W. Naylor, MD

Visiting Associate Professor of Psychiatry, University of Illinois at Chicago Medical Center; Director, Comprehensive Assessment and Response Training System, Department of Psychiatry, University of Illinois at Chicago, Chicago, Illinois

Approach to the Patient With Disordered Sleep

Alain Nicolas, MD, PhD

Medecin, Centre Hospitalier Le Vinatier, Unité Clinique Le Vinatier, Paris, France

Restless Legs Syndrome and Periodic Limb Movement Disorder

Tore A. Nielsen, PhD

Associate Professor, Department of Psychiatry, Université de Montréal; Director, Dream and Nightmare Laboratory, Centre d'Étude du Sommeil, Hôpital du Sacré-Coeur de Montréal, Montréal, Québec, Canada

Dreaming Disorders

Peter D. Nowell, MD

Assistant Professor of Psychiatry, Dartmouth-Hitchcock Medical School, Lebanon, New Hampshire

Psychometric and Psychiatric Evaluation

John Orem, PhD

Department of Physiology, School of Medicine, Texas Tech University, Lubbock, Texas

Section Editor: *Physiology in Sleep; Respiratory Physiology: Central Neural Control*

William C. Orr, PhD

Adjunct Professor of Psychiatry and Behavioral Sciences, University of Oklahoma Health Sciences; President and Chief Executive Officer, Lynn Health Science Institute, Oklahoma City, Oklahoma

Gastrointestinal Physiology; Gastrointestinal Disorders; Gastrointestinal Monitoring Techniques

Pier Luigi Parmeggiani, MD

Professor of Physiology, Department of Human and General Physiology and Faculty of Medicine, University of Bologna, Bologna, Italy

Physiological Regulation in Sleep

Markku Partinen MD, PhD

Docent, Department of Clinical Neurosciences, University of Helsinki; Director, Haaga Neurological Research Center, Helsinki, Finland

Epidemiology of Sleep Disorders

Ralph Pascualy, MD

Director, Sleep Medicine Institute, Swedish Medical Center, Seattle, Washington

Chronic Fatigue Syndrome and Fibromyalgia

Rafael Pelayo, MD

Staff Physician and Head, Stanford University Pediatric Sleep Disorders Clinic, Stanford, California

Idiopathic Central Nervous System Hypersomnia

Lawrence H. Pinto, PhD

Professor and Chair, Department of Neurobiology and Physiology, Northwestern University, Evanston, Illinois

Molecular Genetic Basis for Mammalian Circadian Rhythms

R. T. Pivik, PhD

Professor, Department of Psychiatry and Physiology and School of Psychology, University of Ottawa; Director, Clinical Psychophysiology Laboratory, Ottawa General Hospital, Ottawa, Ontario, Canada

Section Editor: *Psychophysiology of Dreams; Psychophysiology of Dreams*

Nelson B. Powell, MD

Clinical Professor of Psychiatry and Behavioral Sciences and Co-Director, Sleep and Research Center, Stanford University School of Medicine, Stanford, California

Surgical Therapy for Obstructive Sleep Apnea-Hypopnea Syndrome

Allan Rechtschaffen, PhD

Professor Emeritus, University of Chicago, Chicago, Illinois

Monitoring and Staging Human Sleep

John E. Remmers, MD

Professor of Physiology, University of Calgary Health Science Center, Calgary, Alberta, Canada

Anatomy and Physiology of Upper Airway Obstruction

Charles F. Reynolds III, MD

Professor of Psychiatry, Neurology and Neuroscience, University of Pittsburgh; University of Pittsburgh Medical Center Health System, Pittsburgh, Pennsylvania

Psychometric and Psychiatric Evaluation

Dianne Reynolds, MD

Private Practice, Washington, District of Columbia

Psychiatric Disorders and Insomnia

Robert W. Riley, MD, DDS

Associate Clinical Professor of Psychiatry and Behavioral Sciences and Director of Sleep Surgery, Stanford Sleep and Research Center, Stanford University, School of Medicine, Stanford, California

Surgical Therapy for Obstructive Sleep Apnea-Hypopnea Syndrome

Dominique Robert, MD

Professor of Medicine, Claude Bernard University of Lyon; Chief of the Medical Intensive Care and Ventilatory Assistance Division, Croix-Rousse Hospital, Lyon, France

Noninvasive Ventilation for Sleep Breathing Disorders

Richard W. Robinson, MD

Associate Professor of Medicine, Sections of General Internal Medicine and Pulmonary Allergy and Critical Care Medicine, Penn State University College of Medicine, M. S. Hershey Medical Center, Hershey, Pennsylvania

Medications, Sleep, and Breathing

Timothy Roehrs, PhD

Adjunct Professor, Department of Psychology, University of Detroit Mercy; Adjunct Professor, Department of Psychiatry and Department of Psychology, Wayne State University; Director of Research, Sleep Disorders and Research Center, Henry Ford Health System, Detroit, Michigan

Daytime Sleepiness and Alertness; Hypnotics: Efficacy and Adverse Effects; Transient and Short-Term Insomnias

Leon Rosenthal, MD

Adjunct Associate Professor, Wayne State University School of Medicine; Medical Director, Sleep Disorders Center, Henry Ford Hospital, Detroit, Michigan

Section Editor: *Normal Sleep and Its Variations*

Thomas Roth, PhD

Clinical Professor, Department of Psychiatry, University of Michigan, Ann Arbor; Adjunct Professor, Department of Psychiatry, Wayne State University; Chief, Division Head, Sleep Disorders and Research Center and Director of Research Administration, Henry Ford Health System, Detroit, Michigan

Daytime Sleepiness and Alertness; Hypnotics: Efficacy and Adverse Effects; Transient and Short-Term Insomnias

Benjamin Rusak, PhD

Professor, Departments of Psychiatry, Pharmacology, and Psychology, Dalhousie University, Halifax, Nova Scotia, Canada

Circadian Rhythms in Mammals: Formal Properties and Environmental Influences

Mark H. Sanders, MD

Professor of Medicine, University of Pittsburgh School of Medicine; Chief, Pulmonary Sleep Disorders Program, University of Pittsburgh Medical Center; Assistant Chief, Pulmonary Service, Pittsburgh Veterans Affairs Health Care System, Pittsburgh, Pennsylvania

Section Editor: *Sleep Breathing Disorders; Medical Therapy for Obstructive Sleep Apnea-Hypopnea Syndrome*

Carlos H. Schenck, MD

Associate Professor of Psychiatry, University of Minnesota Medical School; Staff Psychiatrist, Minnesota Regional Sleep Disorders Center, Hennepin County Medical Center, Minneapolis, Minnesota

REM Sleep Parasomnias; Violent Parasomnias: Forensic Medicine Issues

Markus H. Schmidt, MD, PhD

Resident, Department of Neurology, Cleveland Clinic Foundation, Cleveland; Ohio Sleep Medicine and Neuroscience Institute, Dublin, Ohio

Sleep-Related Penile Erections

Paula K. Schweitzer, PhD

Associate Director, Unity Sleep Medicine and Research Center, St. Luke's Hospital, Chesterfield, Missouri

Drugs That Disturb Sleep and Wakefulness

Margaret N. Shouse, PhD

Professor, Department of Neurobiology, University of California, Los Angeles, Los Angeles, California

Epilepsy and Sleep Disorders

Jerome M. Siegel, PhD

Department of Psychiatry and Brain Research Institute, University of California at Los Angeles Medical Center, Los Angeles; Chief, Neurobiology Research, Sepulveda Veterans Administration Medical Center, North Hills, California

Brainstem Mechanisms Generating REM Sleep

Debra Skene, BPharm, MSc, PhD

Reader, School of Biological Sciences, University of Surrey, Guildford, Surrey, England

Jet Lag and Sleep Disruption

Arthur J. Spielman, PhD

Professor, Department of Psychology and Director, Sleep Disorders Center, The City College of New York, New York; Associate Director, Sleep Disorders Center, New York Methodist Hospital, Brooklyn, New York

Assessment Techniques for Insomnia

Edward J. Stepanski, PhD

Associate Professor, Department of Psychology, Rush Medical College; Laboratory Director, Sleep Disorders Service and Research Center, Rush-Presbyterian-St. Luke's Medical Center, Chicago, Illinois

Behavioral Therapy for Insomnia

Mircea Steriade, MD, DSc

Professor, Laval University School of Medicine, Québec, Québec, Canada

Brain Electrical Activity and Sensory Processing During Waking and Sleep States

Barbara Stone, BSc

Technical Manager, DERA Centre for Human Sciences, Farnborough, Hampshire, England

Jet Lag and Sleep Disruption

Colin Sullivan, MB, BS, BSc, PhD, FRACP

Professor, Department of Medicine, University of Sydney; Head, Centre for Respiratory Failure and Sleep Disorders, Royal Prince Alfred Hospital, Sydney; Head, David Read Sleep Laboratory, New Children's Hospital, Westmead, New South Wales, Australia

Continuous Positive Airway Pressure for Sleep Breathing Disorders

Jiuan Su Terman, PhD

Research Scientist, New York State Psychiatric Institute, New York, New York

Light Therapy

Michael Terman, PhD

Professor, Department of Psychiatry, College of Physicians and Surgeons, Columbia University; Research Scientist and Director, Clinical Chronobiology, New York State Psychiatric Institute, New York, New York

Light Therapy

Michael J. Thorpy, MD

Associate Professor of Neurology, Albert Einstein College of Medicine; Director, Sleep Disorders Center, Montefiore Medical Center, Bronx, New York

Classification of Sleep Disorders

Irene Tobler, PhD

Professor of Zoology, University of Zurich, Zurich, Switzerland

Phylogeny of Sleep Regulation

Fred W. Turek, PhD

Charles E. and Emma H. Morrison Professor of Biology, Northwestern University, Evanston, Illinois

Section Editor: *Chronobiology; Introduction: Chronobiology; Molecular Genetic Basis for Mammalian Circadian Rhythms; Melatonin in the Regulation of Sleep and Circadian Rhythms;* Section Editor: *Disorders of Chronobiology; Introduction: Disorders of Chronobiology*

Thomas W. Uhde, MD

Professor and Chair, Department of Psychiatry and Behavioral Neurosciences; Professor, Department of Pharmacology; Associate Dean, Research and Graduate Programs, School of Medicine, Wayne State University; Psychiatrist-in-Chief, Detroit Medical Center; President and Chief Executive Officer, Psychiatry and Behavioral Medicine Professionals, University Psychiatric Centers, Detroit, Michigan

Anxiety Disorders

Eve Van Cauter, PhD

Research Associate (Professor), Department of Medicine, University of Chicago, Chicago, Illinois

Endocrine Physiology

Hans P. A. Van Dongen, PhD

Research Assistant Professor of Sleep and Chronobiology in Psychiatry, University of Pennsylvania School of Medicine, Philadelphia, Pennsylvania

Circadian Rhythms in Fatigue, Alertness, and Performance

Richard L. Verrier, PhD

Associate Professor of Medicine, Harvard Medical School; Director, Institute for Prevention of Cardiovascular Disease, Beth Israel Deaconess Medical Center, Boston, Massachusetts

Cardiovascular Physiology: Central and Autonomic Regulation; Sleep-Related Cardiac Risk

Martha Hotz Vitaterna, PhD

Research Associate, Department of Neurobiology, Northwestern University, Evanston, Illinois

Molecular Genetic Basis for Mammalian Circadian Rhythms

James K. Walsh, PhD

Clinical Professor, Department of Psychiatry, St. Louis University Health Sciences Center, St. Louis; Executive Director and Senior Scientist, Unity Sleep Medicine and Research Center, St. Luke's Hospital, Chesterfield, Missouri

Evaluation and Management of Insomnia: An Overview

Arthur Walters, MD

Professor of Neuroscience, Seton Hall University, South Orange; John Fitzgerald Kennedy New Jersey Neuroscience Institute, Edison, New Jersey

Restless Legs Syndrome and Periodic Limb Movement Disorder

J. Catesby Ware, PhD
Professor, Departments of Psychiatry and Behavioral
Medicine, Internal Medicine, Eastern Virginia Medical
School; Director, Sleep Disorders Center, Sentara Norfolk
General Hospital, Norfolk, Virginia
Assessment of Sleep-Related Erections

John V. Weil, MD
Professor of Medicine, Cardiovascular Pulmonary Research
Laboratory, University of Colorado Health Sciences Center,
Denver, Colorado
Respiratory Physiology: Sleep at High Altitudes

J. Woodrow Weiss, MD
Associate Professor of Medicine, Harvard Medical School;
Chief, Division of Pulmonary and Critical Care Medicine,
Beth Israel Deaconess Medical Center, Boston,
Massachusetts
Cardiorespiratory Changes in Sleep-Disordered Breathing

David P. White, MD
Associate Professor of Medicine, Harvard Medical School;
Director, Sleep Disorders Program, Brigham and Women's
Hospital, Boston, Massachusetts
Central Sleep Apnea

Chien-Ming Yang, PhD
Assistant Professor, Institute of Behavioral Medicine,
National Cheng Kung University Medical College, Tainan,
Taiwan
Assessment Techniques for Insomnia

Antonio Zadra, PhD
Assistant Professor, Department of Psychology, Université
de Montréal; Researcher, Dream and Nightmare Laboratory,
Centre d'Étude du Sommeil, Hôpital du Sacré-Coeur de
Montréal, Montréal, Québec, Canada
Dreaming Disorders

Vincent P. Zarcone, Jr, MD
Professor, Department of Psychiatry and Behavioral
Sciences, Stanford University School of Medicine, Stanford;
Staff Psychiatrist, Veterans Administration Palo Alto Health
Care System, Palo Alto, California
Sleep Hygiene; Schizophrenia

Phyllis C. Zee, MD, PhD
Associate Professor of Neurology, Center for Circadian
Biology and Medicine, Northwestern University Medical
School, Chicago, Illinois
Circadian Disorders of the Sleep-Wake Cycle

Harold Zepelin, PhD
Professor Emeritus (Psychology), Oakland University,
Rochester, Michigan
Mammalian Sleep

Frank J. Zorick, MD
Professor, Clinical Medicine and Psychiatry, Medical College
of Ohio, Toledo, Ohio
Section Editor: *Insomnia; Evaluation and Management of
Insomnia: An Overview; Transient and Short-Term Insomnias*

Clifford W. Zwillich, MD
Professor of Medicine and Chief of Medicine, Denver
Veterans Administration Medical Center; Vice Chair,
University of Colorado School of Medicine, Denver,
Colorado
Medications, Sleep, and Breathing

Foreword

It is an honor and a privilege for me to introduce the third edition of this excellent textbook, *Principles and Practice of Sleep Medicine*. It has been 11 years since the editors assembled the first edition of this textbook as a means of providing a comprehensive book on sleep and sleep disorders for the practitioner, student, researcher, and clinician. It is amazing how much revision is required between editions. Throughout the years, this book has gained the reputation of being the primary resource for the field of sleep disorders medicine. This edition comes at a fascinating and challenging time for this discipline and once again promises to become the principal reference for this field. The book approaches the topic with a commitment to accuracy, a utility of information, and a scholarly account of the current state of the science.

It is interesting to note that 30 years ago, much of the information contained in this book did not exist. Since that time, there has been an increased awareness that sleep disorders are indeed a true public health problem. The recognition of the clinical problem and the growth of research, particularly related to the magnitude of the problem and the consequences to society, have been notable. It is now estimated that as many as 40 million Americans and millions of others around the world suffer from some type of sleep disruption or sleep disorder, and the numbers are still increasing. The potential economic costs to society are enormous and touch many facets of our lives, from human health to traffic safety. As impressive is the public outcry for more information on sleep disorders and sleep deprivation and the ensuing demand for more research on its causes and treatments. Research advances over this time have influenced the directions of studies in the basic laboratory as well as in clinical management, and these advances have opened the eyes of the medical community to the importance of sleep to health and productivity. Within this span, sleep disorders—once an experimental venture—have become increasingly recognized and accepted within many spheres of medicine. This is, in part, due to a more thorough understanding of the etiology of common sleep disorders and the introduction of new treatments with the promise of more interventions on the horizon. Today, we can say with confidence that sleep disorders medicine

is a real medical discipline, grounded in science, and worthy of the respect and attention of the entire medical enterprise.

Much has been learned about sleep and sleep disorders in the past 3 decades, and much of this knowledge has resulted from research supported by the National Institutes of Health (NIH). In the past decade alone, sleep research funding at NIH has increased more than 40%, with many institutes demonstrating sizable commitments to sleep research. With the establishment of the National Center on Sleep Disorders Research within the National Heart, Lung and Blood Institute, the information gained through this publicly sponsored research is being communicated and disseminated to the public through public awareness efforts, education campaigns, outreach activities, and broad coordination of public and private activities to translate advances in biomedical research to benefit and improve health care and quality of life for those with sleep disorders. Today, we have more opportunities than ever to translate current knowledge about sleep into better strategies for care. New biomedical technologies are advancing our understanding of disease and health in ways that even a few years ago would have been impossible to predict.

However, much remains to be done to meet the many needs and opportunities of this field. This book reflects, in many ways, the moving focus of research over the past several decades, progressing from clinical observation to systems physiology and now to molecular and cellular neurobiology, genetics, and advanced therapeutics. It is this fundamental bench-to-bedside research effort that provides not only the fuel for this textbook but also the foundation of scientific evidence on which we base all our educational messages.

This book provides an in-depth critical evaluation of the contemporary status of sleep disorders medicine, ranging from the underlying scientific concepts to clinical approaches and the latest technical advances. It capitalizes on the strengths of the multidisciplinary nature of this field by exploring the fundamental physiological and pharmacological mechanisms involved with sleep regulation and homeostasis; the latest advances in chronobiology; important aspects in the identification, evaluation, and management of the patient with disordered sleep; a comprehensive description of the common sleep disorders and their relationship with other medical disorders and conditions; and a detailed accounting of the latest methodological approaches for

---

All material in this Foreword is in the public domain, with the exception of any borrowed figures or tables.

studying and assessing sleep in the laboratory and clinic. Readers should be impressed with how much our understanding of sleep and sleep disorders has been enhanced over these years, how much more solid information is available, and how relevant concepts have become more clear. The book also serves as an invaluable aid to identifying some future research opportunities in this dynamic and growing field.

Finally, it is important to be mindful that during this period of rapid expansion and shifting physician attitudes toward acceptance of sleep disorders, there is an inherent conflict between health care providers and health management. Medical practice is no longer at the sole discretion of individual physicians. More often budget constraints, cost-efficiency considerations, and standard operating procedures dictate treatment plans. In this era of health care delivery, it is critical to have the tools to respond and adapt to this complex medical environment. A textbook such as this, providing the latest science-based evidence, is essential to document the legitimacy of this field of medicine.

In summary, this is a dynamic book that incorporates an authoritative review of the physiology, its de-rangement and resulting clinical manifestations, and the available contemporary therapy. This book surely constitutes a milestone in the history of sleep disorders medicine. I certainly expect that not only those seriously interested in the field of sleep and sleep disorders but also others in related disciplines will find this textbook valuable in their research and clinical practice. The field owes the editors and contributors a great debt of gratitude for this massive undertaking and impressive textbook. As important, the public and patients who suffer from disorders of sleep should benefit greatly from the knowledge, wisdom, insights, and collective clinical experience contained in this book, and they can look forward to the not-too-distant future when further scientific advances will lead to the prevention of sleep disorders. Clearly, the reward will be the well-being of the patients.

JAMES P. KILEY, PhD
Director
Division of Lung Diseases
National Heart, Lung and Blood Institute
National Institutes of Health
Bethesda, Maryland

Preface to the First Edition

Medical disorders related to sleep are obviously not new. Yet the discipline of sleep disorders medicine is in its infancy. There is a large body of knowledge on which to base the discipline of sleep disorders medicine. We hope that this textbook will play a role in the evolution of this field.

Douglas Hofstadter reviewed how ideas and concepts evolve and are transmitted.[1] In 1965, Roger Sperry[2] wrote the following: "Ideas cause ideas and help evolve new ideas. They interact with each other and with other mental forces in the same brain, in neighboring brains, and thanks to global communication, in far distant, foreign brains. And they also interact with the external surroundings to produce *in toto* a burstwise advance in evolution that is far beyond anything to hit the evolutionary scene yet, including the emergence of the living cell." Jacques Monod[3] wrote the following in *Chance and Necessity:* "For a biologist it is tempting to draw a parallel between the evolution of ideas and that of the biosphere. For while the abstract kingdom stands at a yet greater distance above the biosphere than the latter does above the non-living universe, ideas have retained some of the properties of organisms. Like them they tend to perpetuate their structure and to breed; they too can fuse, recombine, segregate their content; indeed they too can evolve, and in this evolution selection must surely play an important role." Hofstadter has called this universe of ideas the ideosphere analogous to the biosphere. The ideosphere's counterpart to the biosphere gene has been called meme by Richard Dawkins.[4] He wrote "just as genes propagate themselves in a gene pool by leaping from body to body via sperm or eggs, so memes propagate themselves in the meme pool by leaping from brain to brain. . . . If a scientist hears or reads about a good idea, he passes it on to his colleagues and students. He mentions it in his articles and his lectures. If the idea catches on it can be said to propagate itself spreading from brain to brain . . . memes should be regarded as living structures, not just metaphorically but technically."

Thus, this texbook represents an attempt to summarize the body of science and ideas that up to now has been transmitted verbally, in articles, and in a few more specialized books. The memes in this volume are drawn from a variety of disciplines, including psychology, psychiatry, neurology, pharmacology, internal

medicine, pediatrics, and the basic biological sciences. That a field evolves from multidisciplinary roots certainly has precedents in medicine. The field of infectious diseases has its roots in microbiology, and its practitioners are expected to know relevant aspects of internal medicine, surgery, gynecology, and pediatrics. Similarly, oncology has its roots in surgery, hematology, and internal medicine, and its practitioners today must also know virology and molecular biology. Patients with sleep problems in the past have "fallen through the cracks." It is not uncommon to see a patient with classic narcolepsy who has seen 5 to 10 specialists before the diagnosis is finally made. There is a clinical need for physicians to know about sleep and its disorders.

Much of the research in the sleep field has been conducted in animals; thus, a review of sleep mechanisms and the basic sciences relating to sleep must include a certain amount of data obtained in experimental animals. Wherever possible, the focus will be on data obtained from humans. In many cases, these are simply not available.

The book is divided into two parts: The first surveys normal sleep, and the second deals with disorders of sleep. Part I reviews sleep in normal humans, sleep in other species, the anatomy and physiology and pharmacology of sleep mechanisms, chronobiology, and the behavior of various organ systems during sleep. It was felt by the editors that an important aspect of the book should be the basic sciences of sleep. The reason for this focus is that the vast majority of medical schools simply do not teach anything about sleep in their curricula, in either the basic sciences years or the clinical years. Thus, the individual interested in clinical sleep disorders will usually not have the basic science grounding that is necessary for the comprehensive understanding of any clinical field.

The editors also decided that sleep in other species would have to be reviewed in some detail for several reasons. First, much of the research in sleep has been done in animals, and we have learned much about human sleep from such studies. Second, sleep researchers who are likely to do pharmacological or neurophysiological research are likely to use experimental animals. Thus, we thought it was necessary to include a detailed overview of nonhuman sleep.

The second part of the book focuses on the clinical

problems most commonly seen by a clinician interested in sleep disorders. No matter what a clinician's primary subspecialty, if he or she is interested in sleep disorders, patients who may have pulmonary problems, psychiatric problems, or neurological problems will be referred. Thus, this section of the book is written by individuals in many medical subspecialties and is aimed at pulmonologists, neurologists, psychiatrists, otolaryngologists, and pediatricians. Some degree of duplication is inevitable in this type of volume. The editors decided that each chapter should be as self-contained as possible, without forcing the reader to go elsewhere in the book from within a chapter.

No field in medicine is static. We are continuously learning to understand new function and dysfunction. The aim of this textbook is to transmit the body of information pertaining to sleep disorders medicine to students, scientists, and clinicians concerned with sleep.

MEIR H. KRYGER, WINNIPEG

THOMAS ROTH, DETROIT

WILLIAM C. DEMENT, STANFORD

1. Hofstadter DR: Chapter 3. *In* Metamagical Themas: Questing for the Essence of Mind and Pattern. Toronto, Bantam Books, 1986.
2. Sperry R: Mind, brain, and humanist values. *In* Platt JR (ed): New Views of the Nature of Man. Chicago, The University of Chicago Press, 1965.
3. Monod J: Chance and Necessity. New York, Vintage Books, 1972.
4. Dawkins R: The Selfish Gene. Oxford, England, Oxford University Press, 1976, p 206.

Preface to the Third Edition

Since the last edition of this volume, there have been many events that have impacted medicine in general and the field of sleep medicine in particular. The editors, in evaluating this changing landscape, have made substantial changes to the organization and content of the book to reflect the needs of the reader and society.

One of the most dramatic events to affect sleep medicine has been the establishment of the Center for Sleep Disorders Research housed in the National Institutes of Health. This event both reaffirmed this important field and highlighted educational and research needs.

A book is a living entity that is continuously changing. The knowledge base keeps growing. Some authors from previous editions have died or retired; in some cases, new authors seemed more appropriate contributors in the judgment of the section editors. Thus, this book is very different from the first edition, published a mere 10 years ago. The number of chapters (not counting pediatrics) has increased from 95 to 110. The number of entirely new chapters (new topic or new author) is 45. New knowledge and new clinical problems have superseded topics that seemed important a decade ago.

In the past 5 years, there have been some cataclysmic changes in the structure of health care delivery throughout the world. Many systems focusing on specialists have changed directions, emphasizing primary care, continuing care, and prevention. Many of the chapters of the book have been changed to reflect these new directions and these issues. An important goal of this edition is for the reader to understand exactly how an expert would manage each sleep problem the practitioner is likely to encounter.

Sleep medicine continues to be a field that is a model of diversity. Practitioners include pulmonologists, neurologists, psychiatrists, psychologists, internists, otolaryngologists, primary caregivers, and dentists. We hope that this new edition appreciates and builds on this diversity. The authors include experts in each of these disciplines.

We have also introduced a new feature in this edition to address the multidisciplinary background of our readership. A short synopsis has been added to some of the basic science chapters to help readers who have no background in that topic. This is an experiment. Let us know what you think. Is this a good idea or a bad idea? Should we apply this to the entire volume in the future?

We recently reread the Preface to the First Edition and were amazed by the prediction by Sperry that we quoted, which talked about the spread of ideas globally. He almost predicted the Internet in 1965 and how ideas would be spread. A dramatic change in the past 5 years has been the acceptance of the Internet as a form of communication. Almost all of the chapters were transmitted from author to section editor to editor by electronic means.

The editors considered very seriously whether this book should be distributed on CD-ROM. The consensus reached on surveying many readers is that reading a book on a computer display is not optimal and certainly much more difficult than reading a printed book.

The pediatric companion volume, *Principles and Practice of Sleep Medicine in the Child*, is a separate book. We surveyed our readers and found that most preferred the books be kept separate. The reason for this is that not many practitioners see both pediatric and adult patients. Most pediatricians felt that they wanted their own book and that they would be uncomfortable with a volume three quarters of whose content would be geared to adult medicine.

All our efforts are geared to presenting an evidenced-based presentation so that ultimately our patients will be better served. Let us know how we are doing.

MEIR H. KRYGER, MD, FRCPC
Winnipeg
Kryger@sleep.umanitoba.ca

THOMAS ROTH, PhD
Detroit
troth1@hfhs.org

WILLIAM C. DEMENT, MD, PhD
Stanford
dement@leland.stanford.edu

Acknowledgments

As in the first and second editions, there were hundreds of people who helped, directly or indirectly, in putting this volume together. They range from our own teachers whose values guided us, to our secretaries and editorial assistants who typed and retyped (and retyped) manuscripts and then photocopied them, to librarians who found articles, to illustrators, and to the editorial and production staff at W.B. Saunders Company. E-mail played an important part in the transfer of text at various stages of production. We thank all the people who made this possible. We do not know the names of all the people who helped and, thus, are sorry that they could not all be listed below. We are especially grateful.

To the section editors, who assembled a magnificent group of authors.

To Zoe Pouliot, who kept track of all the chapters, figures, and permissions and retyped several of the manuscripts and without whose help this book would not have been possible. What an angel!

To Cathy Carroll, Faith Voit, Amy Cannon, Linda R. Garber, and Richard Zorab at W.B. Saunders, who helped nurse the book as it evolved and helped us jump over the hurdles as they appeared.

Abbreviations

The following is a list of abbreviations that appear in the text of *Principles and Practice of Sleep Medicine.*

AC: alternating current
ACE: angiotensin-converting enzyme
ACh: acetylcholine
AChE: acetylcholinesterase
ACTH: adrenocorticotropic hormone
AD: Alzheimer's disease
AHI: apnea-hypopnea index
AHP: after-spike hyperpolarization
AMPT: alpha-methyl-*p*-tyrosine
AMT: alpha-methyltyrosine
AMY: amygdaloid nuclei
AP: angina pectoris
A-P rating: atricial-precocial rating
AS: active sleep
AV: atrioventricular
Av3V: anteroventral portion of the hypothalamus near the third ventricle
AW: wakefulness
BAC: bacterial artificial chromosome
BAEP: brainstem auditory evoked potential
BB: bundle branch
BDZ: benzodiazepine
BEAM: brain electrical activity mapping
BERS: benign epilepsy with rolandic spikes
BMI: body mass index
BMR: basal metabolic rate
BR: baroreceptor
BRAC: basic rest-activity cycle
BUN: blood urea nitrogen
cAMP: cyclic adenosine monophosphate
Canarc-1: canine narcolepsy gene
CC: chronic chorea
β-CCE: β-carboline-3-carboxylic acid—(ethyl ester)
CCHS: congenital central hypoventilation syndrome
β-CCM: β-carboline-3-carboxylic acid—(methyl ester)
CF: cystic fibrosis
cGMP: cyclic guanosine monophosphate
ChAT: choline acetyltransferase

CNS: central nervous system
CNV: contingent negative variation
COAD: chronic obstructive airway disease
COLD: chronic obstructive lung disease
COPD: chronic obstructive pulmonary disease
CPAP: continuous positive airway pressure
CPR: cardiopulmonary resuscitation
CRF: chronic renal failure; corticotropin-releasing factor
CSF: cerebrospinal fluid
CSR: Cheyne-Stokes respiration
CT: computed tomography
CVA: cerebrovascular accident
CVD: cerebrovascular disease
CVS: cardiovascular system
DA: dopamine
DAT: dementia of the Alzheimer type
DBP: diastolic blood pressure
DC: direct current
dClock: the Drosophila ortholog of the mouse Clock gene
DD: constant darkness
5,6-DHT: 5,6-dihydroxytryptamine
5,7-DHT: 5,7-dihydroxytryptamine
DIMS: disorders of initiating and maintaining sleep
DMD: Duchenne's muscular dystrophy
DOES: disorders of excessive sleepiness
DOPAC: dihydroxyphenyl acetic acid
DS: dysautonomia syndrome
DSIP: delta sleep-inducing peptide
DSM-IV: *Diagnostic and Statistical Manual of Mental Disorders, Fourth Edition*
DST: dexamethasone suppression test
DU: duodenal ulcer
ECoG: electrocortical activity; electrocorticogram
EDS: excessive daytime sleepiness
EEG: electroencephalogram
EKG: electrocardiogram
EMG: electromyogram
ENT: ear, nose, and throat
EOG: electro-oculogram
EPSP: excitatory postsynaptic potential
EQ: encephalization quotient

ERP: event-related potential
ERSP: event-related slow-brain potential
EST: electroshock therapy
EWL: evaporative water loss
FECT: food-elicited cataplexy test
FM: frequency modulation
FRC: functional residual capacity
FSH: follicle-stimulating hormone
FTG: gigantocellular tegmental field (fastigial
    tegmental gigantocellular field)
FTL: lateral tegmental field
FTM: magnetocellular tegmental field
GABA: gamma-aminobutyric acid
GER: gastroesophageal reflux
GH: growth hormone
GHB: gamma hydroxybutyrate
GHT: geniculohypothalamic tract
GI: gastrointestinal
GSR: galvanic skin response
H_1: histamine receptor type I
H_2: histamine receptor type II
HA: hyperstriatum acessorium
Hcrtr: hypocretin receptor
5-HIAA: 5-hydroxyindole acetic acid
HLA: human leukocyte antigen
HPA: hypothalamic-pituitary-adrenal [axis]
5-HT: 5-hydroxytryptamine (serotonin)
Hth: hypothalamus
5-HTP: 5-hydroxy-L-tryptophan
L-5HTP: L-5-hydroxytryptophan
HVA: homovanillic acid
ICU: intensive care unit
IgE: immunoglobulin E
IGL: intrageniculate leaflet
IID: interictal discharge
IL-1: interleukin-1
IPPV: intermittent positive-pressure ventilation
IPSP: inhibitory postsynaptic potential
IS: initial segment
ITP: inferior thalamic peduncle
LD: light-dark
LED: light-emitting diode
LES: lower esophageal sphincter
LG: lateral geniculate
LGN: lateral geniculate nucleus
LH: luteinizing hormone
LL: constant light
LOC: left outer canthus
LTMV: long-term mechanical ventilation
LTP: long-term potentiation (of synaptic efficacy)
LTS: low-threshold spike
MAO: monoamine oxidase
MAOI: monoamine oxidase inhibitor
MBF: myocardial blood flow
MEMA: middle ear muscle activity
MHC: major histocompatibility complex
MHPG: 3-methoxy-4-hydroxyphenylglycol

MI: myocardial infarction
MID: multi-infarct (vascularized) dementia
MMC: migrating motor complex
MMPI: Minnesota Multiphasic Personality Inventory
MPA: medroxyprogesterone acetate
mPer1, mPer2: mouse orthologs of Per
mPRF: medial pontine reticular formation
alpha-MPT: alpha-methyl-paratyrosine
MPTP: methylphenyltetrahydropyridine
MR: metabolic rate
MRI: magnetic resonance imaging
MS: multiple sclerosis
alpha-MSH: alpha–melanocyte-stimulating hormone
MSLT: multiple sleep latency test
MVP: mitral valve prolapse
MWT: Maintenance of Wakefulness Test
NA: nucleus ambiguus
NAT: N-acetyltransferase
NE: norepinephrine
NGC: nucleus reticularis gigantocellularis
NINCDS: National Institute of Neurological and
    Communicative Disorders and Stroke
NIPPV: nasal intermittent positive pressure
    ventilation
NPD: nocturnal paroxysmal dystonia
NPPV: noninvasive positive pressure ventilation
NPT: nocturnal penile tumescence
NREM: nonrapid eye movement
NTS: nucleus tractus solitarius
17-OHCS: 17-hydroxycorticosteroid
6-OHDA: 6-hydroxydopamine
18-OH-DOC: 18-hydroxydeoxycorticosterone
OHS: obesity hypoventilation syndrome
OSA: obstructive sleep apnea
OSAHS: obstructive sleep apnea-hypopnea
    syndrome
OSAS: obstructive sleep apnea syndrome
P_{close}: closing pressure (of pharynx)
P_{lumen}: luminal pressure (of pharynx)
P_{mus}: muscle pressure (of pharynx)
PAP: pulmonary artery pressure
PAS: posterior airway space
PCPA: parachlorophenylalanine
PCR: polymerase chain reaction
PCS: postconcussion syndrome
PD: panic disorder; Parkinson's disease
PDC: paroxysmal dystonic choreoathetosis
Per,per: the period gene in Drosophila
PER: the protein product of the per gene
PGO: ponto-geniculo-occipital [spike]
PIP: phasic integrated potential
PKD: paroxysmal kinesigenic dystonia
PLM: periodic limb movement
PLMD: periodic limb movement disorder
PLMS: periodic limb movements in sleep
PMD: pseudohypertrophic muscular dystrophy
PMS: periodic movements during sleep

PND: paroxysmal nocturnal dystonia
POAH: preoptic anterior hypothalamic nuclei
POMC: pro-opiomelanocortin
POMS: Profile of Mood States
Ppa: pulmonary arterial pressure
Ppl: intrapleural pressure
PPP: palatopharyngoplasty
PRC: phase response curve
PS: paradoxical sleep
PSG: polysomnogram
PTT: pulse transit time
PVC: premature ventricular contraction
QS: quiet sleep
QW: quiet wakefulness
RA: rheumatoid arthritis
RAS: reticular activating system
RAST: radioallergosorbent test
RBD: REM behavior disorder
RDC: Research Diagnostic Criteria
RDI: respiratory disturbance index
REM: rapid eye movement
REML: REM latency
RERA: respiratory effort-related arousal
RF: reticular formation
RHT: retinohypothalamic tract
RLS: restless legs syndrome
ROC: right outer canthus
RPC: reticularis pontis caudalis
RPO: reticularis pontis oralis
RV: residual volume
SA: sinoatrial
SAD: seasonal affective disorder
SBP: systolic blood pressure
SC: spinal cord
SCN: suprachiasmatic nucleus
SD: soma-dendritic
SEM: slow eye movement
SHR: spontaneously hypertensive rat
SIDS: sudden infant death syndrome
SNR: substantia nigra pars reticulata
SOREMP: sleep-onset REM period
SPS: sleep-promoting substance
SRRD: sleep-related respiratory disturbance

SSEP: somatosensory evoked potential
SSS: Stanford Sleepiness Scale
SW: slow wave
SWS: slow-wave sleep
SWSD: sleep-wake schedule disorder
T: light-dark cycle of a given periodicity
T&A: tonsillectomy and adenoidectomy
T_a: ambient temperature
T_b: body temperature
T_{br}: brain temperature
T_{hy}: hypothalamic temperature
T_i/T_{TOT}: duty cycle of breathing
T_{rec}: rectal temperature
T_{set}: threshold hypothalamic temperature
T_{sk}: skin temperature
TCA: tricyclic antidepressant
THC: tetrahydrocannabinol
TIB: time in bed
tim: the timeless gene
TIM: the protein product of the tim gene
TLC: total lung capacity
TNZ: thermoneutral zone
TRF: thyrotropin-releasing factor
TS: Tourette's syndrome; total sleep
TSH: thyrotropin
TST: total sleep time
TTX: tetrodotoxin
TWL: transepidermal water loss
UAR: upper airway resistance
UARS: upper airway resistance syndrome
UES: upper esophageal sphincter
UF: uncinate fasciculus
UPPP: uvulopharyngopalatoplasty
UQS: unihemispheric quiet time
V_T/T_I: mean inspiratory flow
VAS: Visual Analogue Scale
VF: ventricular fibrillation
VH: ventral hippocampus
VIP: vasoactive intestinal polypeptide
VM: vasomotor
VS: vigilant sleep
WAFA: wake time after final awakening
WASO: wake time after sleep onset

Abbreviations used in human electrode placement: (see Fig. 100–1)
A detailed description of the Ten Twenty Electrode System is described in Japser HH (Committee Chairman). The Ten Twenty Electrode System: International Federation of Societies for Electroencephalography and Clinical Neurophysiology. Electroenc Clin Neurophysiol. 1958;(2):371–375.

Landmarks
Fp: frontal pole   A "z" (for zero) following a landmark indicates a midline position (eg, F_z, C_z, etc.)
F: frontal
C: central
P: parietal   A *number* following a landmark is used to differentiate left (odd numbers) and right (even
O: occipital   numbers) hemispheres.
A: auricular   The two most commonly used electrode pairs for sleep are C4/A1 and C3/A2.
T: temporal

Contents

Part II
Abnormal Sleep

one

Normal Sleep and Its Variations

Leon Rosenthal

1

History of Sleep Physiology and Medicine

William C. Dement

Interest in sleep and dreams has existed since the dawn of history. Perhaps only love and human conflict have received more attention from poets and writers. Some of the world's greatest thinkers, such as Aristotle, Hippocrates, Freud, and Pavlov, have attempted to explain the physiological and psychological bases of sleep and dreaming. However, it is not the purpose of this chapter to present a scholarly review across the ages about prehistoric, biblical, and Elizabethan thoughts and concerns regarding sleep or the history of man's enthrallment with dreams and nightmares. This has been reviewed by others.[1] What is emphasized here for the benefit of the student and the practitioner is the evolution of the key concepts that define and differentiate sleep research and sleep medicine, crucial discoveries and developments in the formative years

of the field, and those principles and practices that have stood the test of time.

SLEEP AS A PASSIVE STATE

Sleep is the intermediate state between wakefulness and death; wakefulness being regarded as the active state of all the animal and intellectual functions, and death as that of their total suspension.[2(p1)]

The foregoing is the first sentence of _The Philosophy of Sleep,_ a book by Robert MacNish, a member of the faculty of physicians and surgeons of Glasgow; the first American edition was published in 1834 and the Scottish edition somewhat earlier. This sentence exem-

1

plifies the overarching historical dichotomy of sleep research and sleep medicine—sleep as a passive process versus sleep as an active process. Until the discovery of rapid eye movements and the duality of sleep, sleep was universally regarded as an inactive state of the brain; with one or two exceptions, most thinkers regarded sleep as the inevitable result of reduced sensory input with the consequent diminishment of brain activity and the occurrence of sleep. Waking up and being awake were considered a reversal of this process, mainly as a result of bombardment of the brain by stimulation from the environment. No real distinction was seen between sleep and other states of quiescence such as coma, stupor, intoxication, hypnosis, anesthesia, and hibernation. The passive to active historical dichotomy is also given great weight by the modern investigator J. Allan Hobson,[3] whose first sentence of his book *Sleep*, published in 1989, stated "more has been learned about sleep in the past 60 years than in the preceding 6,000." He went on,

> In this short period of time, researchers have discovered that sleep is a dynamic behavior. Not simply the absence of waking, sleep is a special activity of the brain, controlled by elaborate and precise mechanisms.[3(p1)]

Dreams and dreaming were regarded as transient, fleeting interruptions of this quiescent state. Because dreams seem to occur spontaneously and sometimes in response to environmental stimulation (e.g., the well-known alarm clock dreams), the notion of a stimulus that produces the dream was generalized by postulating internal stimulation from the digestive tract or some other internal source. Some anthropologists have suggested that notions of spirituality and the soul arose from primitive people's need to explain how their essence could leave the body temporarily at night in a dream and permanently at death.

In addition to the mere reduction of stimulation, a host of less popular theories were espoused to account for the onset of sleep. Vascular theories were proposed from the notion that the blood left the brain to accumulate in the digestive tract and the opposite that sleep was due to pressure on the brain by blood. Around the turn of this century, various versions of a "hypnotoxin" theory were formulated in which fatigue products, toxins, and the like were accumulated during the day, finally causing sleep, during which they were gradually eliminated. It had, of course, been observed since biblical times that alcohol would induce a sleep-like state. More recently, these observations included other compounds such as opium. It was finally noted that coffee and caffeine had the power to prevent sleep.

The hypnotoxin theory reached its zenith in 1907 when Legendre and Pieron,[4] the French physiologists, did experiments showing that blood serum from sleep-deprived dogs could induce sleep in dogs who were not sleep deprived. The notion of a toxin's causing the brain to sleep has gradually given way to the notion that there are a number of endogenous "sleep factors" that actively induce sleep by specific mechanisms.

In the 1920s, the University of Chicago physiologist Nathaniel Kleitman carried out a series of sleep deprivation studies and made the simple but brilliant observation that individuals who stayed up all night were generally less sleepy and impaired the next morning than in the middle of their sleepless night. Kleitman argued that this observation was incompatible with the notion of a continual buildup of a hypnotoxin in the brain or blood. In addition, he felt that human beings were about as impaired as they would get, that is, very impaired, after about 60 h of wakefulness, and that longer periods of sleep deprivation would produce little additional change. In the 1939 (first) edition of his comprehensive landmark monograph, *Sleep and Wakefulness* Kleitman summed up by saying,

> It is perhaps not sleep that needs to be explained, but wakefulness, and indeed, there may be different kinds of wakefulness at different stages of phylogenetic and ontogenetic development. In spite of sleep being frequently designated as an instinct, or global reaction, an actively initiated process, by excitation or inhibition of cortical or subcortical structures, there is not a single fact about sleep that cannot be equally well interpreted as a let down of the waking activity.[5]

THE ELECTRICAL ACTIVITY OF THE BRAIN

As the 20th century got under way, Camillo Golgi and Santiago Ramón y Cajal had demonstrated that the nervous system was not a mass of fused cells sharing a common cytoplasm but rather a highly intricate network of discrete cells that had a key property of signaling to one another. Luigi Galvani had discovered that the nerve cells of animals produce electricity, and Emil duBois-Reymond and Hermann von Helmholtz found that nerve cells use their electrical capabilities for signaling information to one another. The Scottish physiologist Richard Caton in 1875 demonstrated electrical rhythms in the brains of animals. The centennial of his discovery was commemorated at the 15th annual meeting of the Association for the Psychophysiological Study of Sleep convening at the site of the discovery, Edinburgh, Scotland.

However, it was not until the German psychiatrist Hans Berger[6] recorded electrical activity of the human brain beginning in 1928 and clearly demonstrated differences in these rhythms when subjects were awake or asleep that a real scientific interest commenced. Berger correctly inferred that the signals he recorded, which he called "electroencephalograms," were of brain origin. For the first time, the presence of sleep could be conclusively established without disturbing the sleeper, and more important, sleep could be continuously and quantitatively measured without disturbing the sleeper.

All the major elements of sleep brain wave patterns were described by Harvey, Hobart, Davis, and others[7–9] at Harvard University in a series of extraordinary papers published in 1937, 1938, and 1939. Blake, Gerard, and Kleitman[10, 11] added to this from their studies at the University of Chicago. In the human electroencephalogram (EEG), sleep was characterized by high-amplitude slow waves and spindles, whereas wakefulness was characterized by low-amplitude waves and alpha rhythm. The image of the sleeping brain completely "turned off" gave way to the image of the sleeping brain engaged in slow, synchronized, "idling" neuronal activity. Although it was not widely recognized at the time, these studies were some of the most critical turning points in sleep research. Indeed, Hobson[3] dated the turning point of sleep research to 1928, when Berger began his work on the human EEG. Used today in much the same way as they were in the 1930s, brain wave recordings have been extraordinarily important to sleep research and sleep medicine.

The 1930s also saw one series of investigations that seemed to establish conclusively both the passive theory of sleep and the notion that it occurred in response to reduction of stimulation and activity. These were the investigations of Frederick Bremer,[12, 13] reported in 1935 and 1936. These investigations were made possible by the aforementioned development of EEG. Bremer studied brain wave patterns in two cat preparations. One, which Bremer called *encephale isolé*, was made by a section in the lower part of the medulla. The other, *cerveau isolé*, was made by cutting the midbrain just behind the origin of the oculomotor nerves. The first preparation permitted the study of cortical electrical rhythms under the influence of olfactory, visual, auditory, vestibular, and musculocutaneous impulses; in the second preparation, the field was narrowed practically entirely to the influence of olfactory and visual impulses.

In the first preparation, the brain continued to present manifestations of wakeful activity alternating with phases of sleep as indicated by the EEG. In the second preparation, however, the EEG assumed a definite deep sleep character and remained in this condition. In addition, the eyeballs immediately turned downward with a progressive miosis. Bremer concluded that in sleep there occurs a functional (reversible, of course) deafferentation of the cerebral cortex. The *cerveau isolé* preparation results in a suppression of the incessant influx of nerve impulses, particularly cutaneous and proprioceptive, which are essential for the maintenance of the waking state of the telencephalon. Apparently, olfactory and visual impulses are insufficient to keep the cortex awake. It is probably misleading to assert that physiologists assumed the brain was completely turned off, whatever this metaphor might have meant, because blood flow and, presumably, metabolism continued. However, Bremer and others certainly favored the concept of sleep as a reduction of activity—idling, slow, synchronized, "resting" neuronal activity.

THE ASCENDING RETICULAR SYSTEM

After World War II, insulated, implantable electrodes were developed, and sleep research on animals began in earnest. In 1949, one of the most important and influential studies dealing with sleep and wakefulness, Moruzzi and Magoun's classic paper, "Brain Stem Reticular Formation and Activation of the EEG," was published. These authors concluded that

. . . transitions from sleep to wakefulness or from the less extreme states of relaxation and drowsiness to alertness and attention are all characterized by an apparent breaking up of the synchronization of discharge of the elements of the cerebral cortex, an alteration marked in the EEG by the replacement of high voltage, slow waves with low voltage fast activity.[14(p455)]

High-frequency electrical stimulation through electrodes implanted in the brainstem reticular formation produced EEG activation and behavioral arousal. Thus, EEG activation, wakefulness, and consciousness were at one end of the continuum; sleep, EEG synchronization, and lack of consciousness were at the other end. This view, as can be seen, is hardly different from the statement by MacNish quoted at the beginning of this chapter.

The demonstration by Starzl et al.[15] that sensory collaterals discharge into the reticular formation suggested that a mechanism was present by which sensory stimulation could be transduced into prolonged activation of the brain and sustained wakefulness. By attributing an amplifying and maintaining role to the brainstem core and the conceptual ascending reticular activating system, it was possible to account for the fact that wakefulness outlasts or is occasionally maintained in the absence of sensory stimulation.

Chronic lesions in the brainstem reticular formation produced persisting slow waves in the EEG and immobility. The usual animal for this research was the cat because excellent stereotaxic coordinates had become available.[16] These findings appeared to confirm and extend Bremer's observations. The theory of the reticular activating system was an anatomically based passive theory of sleep or active theory of wakefulness. Figure 1–1 is from the published proceedings of a symposium entitled *Brain Mechanisms and Consciousness* published in 1954 and probably the first genuine neuroscience bestseller.[17] Horace Magoun had extended his studies to the monkey, and the illustration represents the full flowering of the ascending reticular activating system theory.

EARLY OBSERVATIONS OF SLEEP PATHOLOGY

Insomnia has been described since the dawn of history and attributed to many causes, including a recognition of the association of emotional disturbance and sleep disturbance. Scholars and historians have the duty to bestow credit accurately. However, we may note that many discoveries lie fallow for want of a contextual soil in which they may be properly understood and in which they may extend the understanding of more general phenomena. Important early observa-

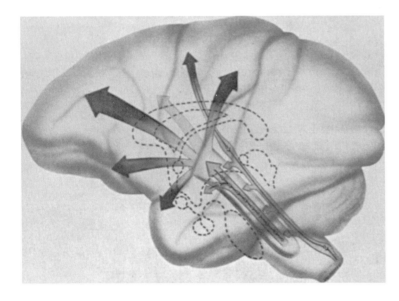

Figure 1–1. Lateral view of the monkey's brain, showing the ascending reticular activating system in the brainstem receiving collaterals from direct afferent paths and projecting primarily to the associational areas of the hemisphere. (From Magoun HW. The ascending reticular system and wakefulness. In: Adrian ED, Bremer F, Jasper HH, eds. Brain Mechanisms and Consciousness. A Symposium Organized by The Council for International Organizations of Medical Sciences, 1954. Courtesy of Charles C Thomas, Publisher, Springfield, Illinois.)

tions were those of von Economo on "sleeping sickness" and of Pavlov, who observed dogs falling asleep during conditioned reflex experiments.

Two early observations stand out with regard to sleep research and sleep medicine. The first is the description in 1880 of narcolepsy by Jean Baptiste Edouard Gélineau (1859–1906), who derived the name narcolepsy from the Greek words *narkosis* (a benumbing) and *lepsis* (to overtake). He was the first to clearly describe the collection of components that constitute the syndrome, although the term *cataplexy* for the emotionally induced muscle weakness was subsequently coined in 1916 by Richard Henneberg.

What might be called the leading sleep disorder of the 20th century, obstructive sleep apnea syndrome, was described in 1836, not by a clinician but by the novelist Charles Dickens. Dickens published a series of papers entitled the "Posthumous Papers of the Pickwick Club" in which he described Joe, the fat boy who was always excessively sleepy. Joe, a loud snorer who was obese and somnolent, may have had right-sided heart failure that led to his being called Young Dropsy. Meir Kryger[18] and Peretz Lavie[19] have published scholarly accounts of many early references to snoring and conditions that were most certainly manifestations of sleep apnea syndrome. Professor Pierre Passouant[20] has provided an account of the life of Gélineau and his landmark description of the narcolepsy syndrome.

SIGMUND FREUD AND THE INTERPRETATION OF DREAMS

By far the most widespread interest in sleep by health professionals was engendered by the theories of Sigmund Freud, specifically about dreams. Of course, the interest was really in dreaming with sleep as the necessary concomitant. Freud developed psychoanalysis, the technique of dream interpretation, as part of his therapeutic approach to emotional and mental problems. As the ascending reticular activating system

concept dominated behavioral neurophysiology, so the psychoanalytic theories about dreams dominated the psychological side of the coin. Dreams were thought to be the guardians of sleep and to occur in response to a disturbance in order to obviate waking up, as exemplified in the classic alarm clock dream. Freud's concept that dreaming discharged instinctual energy led directly to the notion of dreaming as a safety valve of the mind. At the time of the discovery of rapid eye movements during sleep (circa 1952), academic psychiatry was dominated by psychoanalysts, and medical students all over America were interpreting one another's dreams.

From the vantage point of today's world, the dream deprivation studies of the early 1960s, engendered and reified by the belief in psychoanalysis, may be regarded by some as a digression from the mainstream of sleep medicine. On the other hand, because the medical-psychiatric establishment had begun to take dreams seriously, it was also ready to support sleep research fairly generously under the guise of dream research.

CHRONOBIOLOGY

Most, but not all, sleep specialists share the opinion that what has been called chronobiology or the study of biological rhythms is a legitimate part of sleep research and sleep medicine. The 24-h rhythms in the activities of plants and animals have been recognized for centuries. These biological 24-h rhythms were quite reasonably assumed to be a direct consequence of the periodic environmental fluctuation of light and darkness. However, in 1729, Jean Jacques d'Ortous de Mairan described a heliotrope plant that opened its leaves during the day even after de Mairan had moved the plant so that sunlight could not reach it. The plant opened its leaves during the day and folded them for the entire night even though the environment was constant. Thus, the persistence of circadian rhythms in the absence of environmental time cues was first demonstrated. Figure 1–2, which represents de Mairan's original experiment, is reproduced from *The Clocks That Time Us* by Moore-Ede, Sulzman, and Fuller.[21]

Some of the factors that appeared to influence the separate development of chronobiology and sleep research were the following:

1. The long-term studies commonly used in biological rhythm research precluded continuous recording of brain wave activity. Certainly, in the early days, this was far too difficult and not really necessary. Thus, the measurement of wheel-running activity was a convenient and widely used method for demonstrating circadian rhythmicity.
2. The favorite animal of sleep research from the 1930s through the 1970s was the cat, and neither cats nor dogs demonstrate clearly defined circadian activity rhythms. The separation was further maintained by the tendency for chronobiologists to know very little about sleep and for sleep researchers to remain ignorant of such biological clock mysteries as phase response curves, entrainment, and internal desynchronization.

THE DISCOVERY OF REM SLEEP

The discovery or identification of the discrete organismic state known as rapid eye movement (REM) sleep should be distinguished from the discovery that rapid eye movements occur during sleep. The historical threads of the discovery of rapid eye movements can be identified. Nathaniel Kleitman (Fig. 1–3), a professor of physiology at the University of Chicago, had long been interested in cycles of activity and inactivity in infants and in the possibility that this cycle ensured that an infant would have an opportunity to respond to her or his own hunger. He postulated that the times infants awakened to nurse on a self-demand schedule would be integral multiples of a basic rest-activity cycle. The second thread was Kleitman's interest in eye motility as a possible measure of "depth" of sleep. The reasoning for this was that eye movements had a much greater cortical representation than did almost any other observable motor activity and that slow, rolling, or pendular eye movements had been described at the onset of sleep with a gradual slowing and disappearance as sleep "deepened."[22]

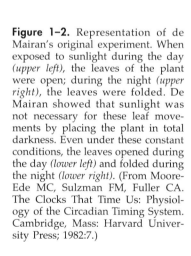
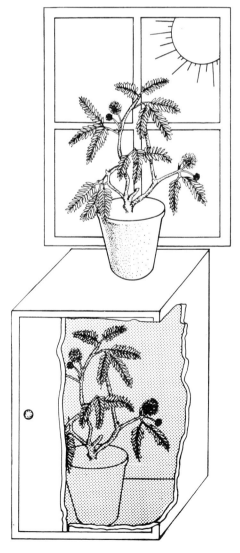
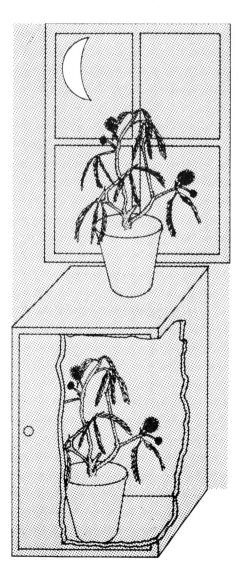

Figure 1–2. Representation of de Mairan's original experiment. When exposed to sunlight during the day *(upper left)*, the leaves of the plant were open; during the night *(upper right)*, the leaves were folded. De Mairan showed that sunlight was not necessary for these leaf movements by placing the plant in total darkness. Even under these constant conditions, the leaves opened during the day *(lower left)* and folded during the night *(lower right)*. (From Moore-Ede MC, Sulzman FM, Fuller CA. The Clocks That Time Us: Physiology of the Circadian Timing System. Cambridge, Mass: Harvard University Press; 1982:7.)

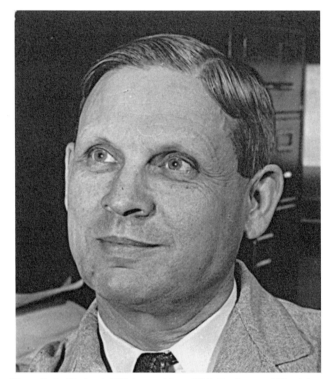

Figure 1–3. Nathaniel Kleitman (circa 1938), Professor of Physiology, University of Chicago, School of Medicine.

In 1951, Kleitman assigned the task of observing eye movement to a graduate student in physiology named Eugene Aserinsky. Watching the closed eyes of sleeping infants was tedious, and Aserinsky soon found that it was easier to designate successive 5-min epochs as "periods of motility" if he observed any movement at all, usually a writhing or twitching of the eyelids, versus "periods of no motility."

After describing an apparent rhythm in eye motility, Kleitman and Aserinsky decided to look for a similar phenomenon in adults. Again, watching the eyes during the day was tedious, and at night was even worse. Casting about, they came upon the method of electro-oculography (EOG) and decided correctly that this would be a good way to measure eye motility continuously and would relieve the human observer of the tedium of direct observations. Some time in the course of recording EOG during sleep, bursts of electrical potential changes were seen that were quite different from the slow movements at sleep onset.

When they were observing infants, Aserinsky and Kleitman had not differentiated slow and rapid movements. However, with the EOG, the different nature of the slow eye movements at sleep onset and the newly discovered rapid motility was obvious. Initially, there was a great deal of concern that these potentials were electrical artifacts. With their presence in the EOG as a signal, however, it was possible to watch the subject's eyes simultaneously, and when this was done, the distinct movement of the eyes beneath the closed lids was extremely easy to see.

At this point, Aserinsky and Kleitman made two assumptions:

1. These eye movements represented a "lightening" of sleep
2. Because they were associated with irregular respiration and accelerated heart rate, they might represent dreaming.

The basic sleep cycle was not identified at this time, primarily because the EOG and other physiological measures, notably EEG, were not recorded continuously but rather by sampling a few minutes of each hour or half hour. The sampling strategy was done to conserve paper (there was no research grant) because there was not a clear reason to record continuously and because it was possible to take a nap between sampling episodes.

Aserinsky and Kleitman initiated a small series of awakenings either when rapid eye movements were present or when rapid eye movements were not present for the purpose of eliciting dream recall. They did not apply sophisticated methods of dream content analysis, but the descriptions of dream content from the two conditions were generally quite different, which made it possible to conclude that rapid eye movements were associated with dreaming. This was, indeed, a breakthrough in sleep research.[23, 24]

The occurrence of the eye movements was quite compatible with the contemporary dream theories that dreams occurred when sleep lightened in order to prevent or delay awakening. In other words, dreaming could still be regarded as the "guardian" of sleep. However, it could no longer be assumed that dreams were fleeting and evanescent.

ALL-NIGHT SLEEP RECORDINGS AND THE BASIC SLEEP CYCLE

The seminal Aserinsky and Kleitman paper was published in 1953. To understand how little attention it attracted, it should be noted that no publications on the subject appeared from any other laboratory until 1959. Staying up at night to study sleep remained an undesirable occupation by anyone's standards. In the early 1950s, most previous research on the EEG patterns of sleep, like most approaches to sleep physiology generally, had either equated short periods of sleep with all sleep or relied on intermittent time sampling during the night. The notion of obtaining continuous records throughout typical nights of sleep would have seemed highly extravagant.

However, motivated by the desire to expand and quantify the description of rapid eye movements, Dement and Kleitman[25] did just this over a total of 126 nights from 33 subjects and, by means of a simplified categorization of EEG patterns, scored the paper recordings in their entirety. When they examined these 126 records, they found that there was a predictable sequence of patterns over the course of the night, such as had been hinted at by Aserinsky's study but entirely overlooked in all previous EEG studies of sleep. Although this sequence of regular variations has been observed tens of thousands of times in hundreds of laboratories, the original description has remained essentially unchanged:

> The usual sequence was that after the onset of sleep, the EEG progressed fairly rapidly to Stage 4, which persisted for varying amounts of time, generally about 30 minutes, and then a lightening took place. While the progression from wakefulness to Stage 4 at the beginning of the cycle was almost invariable through a continuum of change, the lightening was usually abrupt and coincident with a body movement or series of body movements. After the termination of Stage 4, there was generally a short period of Stage 2 or 3 which gave way to Stage 1 and Rapid Eye Movements. When the first eye movement period ended, the EEG again progressed through a continuum of change to Stage 3 or 4 which persisted for a time and then lightened, often abruptly, with body movement to Stage 2 which again gave way to Stage 1 and the second Rapid Eye Movement period.[25(p679)]

Dement and Kleitman found that this cyclical variation of EEG patterns occurred repeatedly throughout the night at intervals of 90 to 100 min from the end of one eye movement period to the end of the next. The regular occurrence of REM periods and dreaming strongly suggested that dreams did not occur in response to chance disturbances.

At the time of these observations, sleep was still considered to be a single state. Dement and Kleitman characterized the EEG during REM periods as "emergent stage 1" as opposed to "descending stage 1" at the onset of sleep. The percentage of the total sleep time occupied by REM sleep was between 20 and 25%, and the periods of REM sleep tended to be shorter in the early cycles of the night. Variations in this picture of all-night sleep have been seen over and over in normal human beings of both genders, in widely varying environments and cultures, and, to all intents and purposes, across the life span.

REM SLEEP IN ANIMALS

The developing knowledge of the nature of sleep with rapid eye movements was in direct opposition to the ascending reticular activating system theory and constituted a paradigmatic crisis. The following observations were crucial:

- Arousal thresholds in human beings were much higher during periods of REM with a low-amplitude, relatively fast (stage 1) EEG pattern than during similar "light sleep" at the onset of sleep.
- Rapid eye movements during sleep were discovered in cats; the concomitant brain wave patterns (low-amplitude, fast) were indistinguishable from active wakefulness.
- By discarding the sampling approach and recording continuously a basic 90-min cycle of sleep without rapid eye movements, alternating with sleep with rapid eye movements, was discovered. The all-night sleep patterns had regular, lawful, predictable patterns of occurrence. Continuous recording that revealed a consistent EEG pattern during an entire period of sleep within which bursts of REM occurred additionally established these as periods of vivid dreaming.
- Observations of motor activity in both human beings and animals revealed the unique occurrence of an active suppression of spinal motor activity.

Thus, sleep consisted not of one state but rather of two distinct organismic states, as different from one another as both were from wakefulness. It had to be conceded that sleep could no longer be thought of as a time of brain inactivity and EEG slowing. By 1960, this fundamental change in our thinking about the nature of sleep was well established; it exists as fact that has not changed in any way since that time.

The discovery of rapid eye movements during sleep in human beings plus the all-night sleep recordings that revealed the regular recurrence of lengthy periods during which rapid eye movements occurred and during which brain wave patterns resembled light sleep prepared the way for the discovery of REM sleep in cats, in spite of the extremely powerful bias that an "activated" EEG could not be associated with sleep. In the first study of cats, maintaining the insulation and, therefore, the integrity of implanted electrodes was not yet solved, so an alternative, small pins in the scalp, was used. With this approach, the waking EEG was totally obscured by the electromyogram from the large temporal muscles of the cat. However, when the cat fell asleep, slow waves could be seen, and the transition to REM sleep was clearly observed because muscle potentials were completely suppressed. One could directly observe the cat's rapid eye movements and also the twitching of the whiskers and paws.

The following note from a more personal account[26] is included to illustrate both the power and the danger of scientific dogma.

> It is very difficult today (circa 1990) to understand and appreciate the exceedingly controversial nature of these findings. I wrote them up, but the paper was nearly impossible to publish because it was completely contradictory to the totally dominant neurophysiological theory of the time. The assertion by me that an activated EEG could be associated with unambiguous sleep was considered to be absurd. As it turned out, previous investigators had observed an activated EEG during sleep in cats,[27, 28] but simply could not believe it and ascribed it to arousing influences during sleep. A colleague who was assisting me was sufficiently skeptical that he preferred I publish the paper as sole author. After four or five rejections, to my everlasting gratitude, Editor-in-Chief Herbert Jasper accepted the paper without revision for publication in Electroencephalography and Clinical Neurophysiology.[29(p23)]

It is notable, however, that the significance of the absence of muscle potentials during the REM periods in the cats was not appreciated. It remained for Michel Jouvet working in Lyon, France, to insist on the importance of electromyographic suppression in his early papers,[30, 31] the first of which was published in 1959. Hodes and Dement began to study the "H" reflex in human beings in 1960, finding complete suppression of reflexes during REM sleep,[32] and Octavio Pompeiano and others in Pisa, Italy, worked out the basic mechanisms of REM atonia in the cat.[33]

THE DUALITY OF SLEEP

Even though the basic nonrapid eye movement (NREM)–REM sleep cycle was well established, the realization that REM sleep was qualitatively different from the remainder of sleep took years to evolve. Jouvet[34] and his colleagues performed an elegant series of investigations on the brainstem mechanisms of sleep that forced the inescapable conclusion that sleep consists of two fundamentally different organismic states. Among his many early contributions were clarification of the role of pontine brainstem systems as the primary anatomic site for REM sleep mechanisms and the clear demonstration that electromyographic activity and muscle tonus are completely suppressed during REM periods and only during REM periods.

The investigations began in 1958 and were carried out during 1959 and 1960. It is now an established fact that atonia is a fundamental characteristic of REM sleep and that it occurs and it is mediated by an active and highly specialized neuronal system. The pioneering microelectrode studies of Edward Evarts[35] in cats and monkeys and observations on cerebral blood flow in the cat by Reivich and Kety[36] provided convincing evidence that the brain during REM sleep is very active. Certain areas of the brain appear to be more active in REM sleep than in wakefulness. By now, the notion of sleep as a passive process was totally demolished, although for many years there was a lingering attitude that NREM sleep was essentially inactive and quiet. By 1960, it was possible to define REM sleep as a completely separate organismic state characterized by cerebral activation, active motor inhibition, and, of course, an association with dreaming. The fundamental duality of sleep was an established fact.

PREMONITIONS OF SLEEP MEDICINE

Sleep research, which emphasized all-night sleep recordings, burgeoned in the 1960s and was the legitimate precursor of sleep medicine and particularly its core clinical test, polysomnography. Much of the research at this time emphasized studies of dreaming and REM sleep and had its roots in a psychoanalytic approach to mental illness, which strongly implicated dreaming in the psychotic process. After sufficient numbers of human all-night sleep recordings had been carried out to demonstrate a highly characteristic "normal" sleep architecture, investigators noted a significantly shortened REM latency in association with endogenous depression.[37] This phenomenon has been intensively investigated ever since. Other important precursors of sleep medicine were

1. Discovery of sleep onset REM periods in patients with narcolepsy.
2. Interest in sleep, epilepsy, and abnormal movement—primarily in France.
3. Introduction of benzodiazepines and the use of sleep laboratory studies in defining hypnotic efficacy.

Sleep-Onset REM Periods and Cataplexy

In 1959, a patient with narcolepsy came to the Mount Sinai Hospital in New York City to see Dr. Charles Fisher. Fisher suggested that a sleep recording might be of interest. Within seconds after he fell asleep, the patient was showing the dramatic, characteristic rapid eye movements as well as sawtooth waves in the EEG. The first paper documenting sleep onset REM periods in a single patient was published in 1960 by Gerald Vogel.[38] In a collaborative study between the University of Chicago and the Mount Sinai Hospital, nine patients were studied, and the important sleep onset REM periods at night were described in a 1963 paper.[39] Subsequent research showed that sleepy patients who did not have cataplexy did not have sleep-onset REM periods (SOREMPs), and those with cataplexy always had SOREMPs.[40] It was clear that the best explanation for cataplexy was the normal motor inhibitory mechanisms of REM sleep occurring in a precocious or abnormal way.

The Narcolepsy Clinic: A False Start

In January 1963, after moving to Stanford University, Dement was eager to test the hypothesis of an association between cataplexy and SOREMPs. However, not a single narcoleptic patient could be identified. A final attempt was made by placing a "want ad," a few words about an inch high, in a daily newspaper, the San Francisco Chronicle. More than 100 people responded! About 50 of these patients were bona fide narcoleptics having both sleepiness and cataplexy.

The response to the ad was a noteworthy event in the development of sleep disorders medicine. With one or two exceptions, none of the narcoleptics had ever been diagnosed correctly. A responsibility for their clinical management had to be assumed for their use in research. The late Dr. Stephen Mitchell, who had completed his neurology training and was entering a psychiatry residency at Stanford University, joined Dement in creating a narcolepsy clinic in 1964, and they were soon managing well over 100 patients. Mostly, this involved seeing the patients at regular intervals and adjusting their medication. Nonetheless, the seeds of the typical sleep disorders clinic were sowed because at least one daytime polygraphic sleep recording was done in all patients to look for the presence of SOREMPs, and patients were questioned exhaustively about their sleep. If possible, an all-night sleep recording was carried out. Unfortunately, most of the patients were unable to pay cash to cover their bills, and insurance companies declared that the recordings of narcoleptic patients were experimental. Because it was unable to generate sufficient income, the clinic was discontinued and most of the patients were referred back to local physicians with instructions about treatment.

European Interest

In Europe, a genuine clinical interest in sleep problems had arisen that achieved its clearest expression in a 1963 symposium held in Paris, organized by Professor H. Fischgold, and published as *La Sommeil de Nuit Normal et Pathologique* in 1965.[41] The greatest clinical emphasis in this symposium was the documentation of sleep-related epileptic seizures and a number of related studies on sleepwalking and night terrors. Investigators from France, Italy, Belgium, Germany, and the Netherlands took part.

Benzodiazepines and Hypnotic Efficacy Studies

Benzodiazepines were introduced in 1960 with the marketing of chlordiazepoxide (Librium). This compound offered a significant advance in terms of safety over the use of barbiturates for the purpose of tranquilizing and sedating. It was quickly followed by diazepam (Valium) and the first benzodiazepine introduced specifically as an hypnotic, flurazepam (Dalmane). Although a number of studies had been done on the effects of drugs on sleep, usually in service of answering theoretical questions, the first use of the sleep laboratory to evaluate sleeping pills was the 1965 study by Oswald and Priest.[42] An important series of studies establishing the role of the sleep laboratory in the evaluation of hypnotic efficacy was carried out by Anthony Kales and his colleagues at University of California, Los Angeles.[43] The group also carried out studies of patients with hypothyroidism, asthma, Parkinson's disease, and somnambulism.[44–47]

The Discovery of Sleep Apnea

One of the most important events in the history of sleep disorders medicine occurred in Europe. Sleep apnea was discovered independently by Gastaut, Tasinari, and Duron[48] in France and Jung and Kuhlo in Germany.[49] Both these groups reported their findings in 1965. As noted earlier, scholars have found references to this phenomenon in many places, but this was the first clear-cut recognition and description that had a direct causal continuity to sleep disorders medicine as we know it today.

These important findings were widely ignored in America. What should have been an almost inevitable discovery by either the otolaryngologic surgery community or pulmonary medicine community did not occur because there was no tradition in either specialty

for observing breathing carefully during sleep. The well-known and frequently cited study of Burwell et al.[50]—although impressive in a literary sense in its evoking of the somnolent boy, Joe, from the "Posthumous Papers of the Pickwick Club"—erred badly in evaluating their somnolent obese patients *only* during waking and attributing the cause of the somnolence to hypercapnea.

The popularity of this paper further reduced the likelihood of discovery of sleep apnea by the pulmonary community. To this day, there is no evidence that hypercapnea causes true somnolence, although, of course, high levels of Pco_2 are associated with impaired cerebral function. Nonetheless, the term *pickwickian* became an instant success as a neologism and may have played a role in stimulating interest in this syndrome by the European neurologists who were also interested in sleep.

A small group of French neurologists who specialized in clinical neurophysiology and electroencephalography were in the vanguard of sleep research. One of the collaborators in the French discovery of sleep apnea, C. Alberto Tassinari, joined the Italian neurologist Elio Lugaresi in Bologna in 1970. These clinical investigators along with Giorgio Coccagna and a host of others over the years performed a crucial series of clinical sleep investigations and, indeed, provided a complete description of the sleep apnea syndrome, including the first observations of the occurrences of sleep apnea in nonobese patients, an account of the cardiovascular correlates, and a clear identification of the importance of snoring and hypersomnolence as diagnostic indicators. These studies are recounted in Lugaresi's book, *Hypersomnia With Periodic Apneas*.[51]

Italian Symposia

In 1967, Henri Gastaut and Elio Lugaresi (Fig. 1–4) organized a symposium, published as *The Abnormalities of Sleep in Man*,[52] which encompassed issues across a

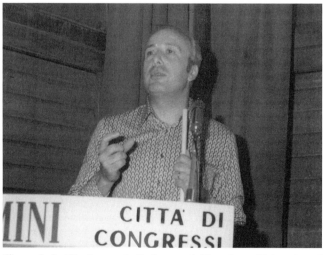

Figure 1–4. Elio Lugaresi, Professor of Neurology, University of Bologna, at the 1972 Rimini Symposium.

full range of pathological sleep in humans. This meeting took place in Bologna, Italy, and the papers presented covered many of what are now major topics in the sleep medicine field: insomnia, sleep apnea, narcolepsy, and periodic leg movements during sleep. It was an epic meeting from the point of view of the clinical investigation of sleep; the only major issues not represented were clear concepts of clinical practice models and clear visions of the high population prevalence of sleep disorders. However, the event that may have finally triggered a serious international interest in sleep apnea syndromes was organized by Lugaresi in 1972 and took place in Rimini, a small resort on the Adriatic coast.[53]

Birth Pangs

In spite of all the clinical research, the clear concept of all-night sleep recordings as a clinical diagnostic test did not emerge unambiguously. It is worth considering the reasons for this failure, partly because they continue to operate today, in altered forms, as impediments to the expansion of the field, and partly to understand the field's long overdue development.

The first important reason was the unprecedented nature of an all-night diagnostic test, particularly if it was conducted on outpatients. The cost of all-night polygraphic recording, in terms of its basic expense, was high enough without adding the cost of hospitalization, which would have legitimized a patient's spending the night in a testing facility, however. To sleep in an outpatient clinic for a diagnostic test was a totally unprecedented, time-intensive, and labor-intensive enterprise and completely in conflict with the image of going to the chemistry laboratory to give a blood sample, breathe into pulmonary function apparatus, undergo a radiographic examination, and so forth.

A second important barrier was the assumed reluctance of nonhospital clinical professionals to work at night. Although medical house staff have numerous experiences with night work, they are generally not enjoyed; further, clinicians seeing patients, then ordering tests, particularly if they had to conduct the tests themselves, could not work 24-h days.

Finally, except for a small number of people, there was no concept that complaints of daytime sleepiness and nocturnal sleep disturbance represented anything of clinical significance. Even narcolepsy, which was by this time fully characterized as an interesting and disabling clinical syndrome requiring sleep recordings for diagnosis, was not recognized in the larger medical community and had too low a prevalence to support the needs of creating a medical subspecialty. A study carried out in 1972 documented a mean of 15 years from onset of the characteristic symptoms of excessive daytime sleepiness and cataplexy to recognition by a clinician, and the study showed a mean of five and one half different physicians consulted throughout the long interval.[54]

THE EVOLUTION OF SLEEP MEDICINE CLINICAL PRACTICE

The practice of sleep medicine evolved in many centers in the 1970s. The development was often a function of the original research interests of the center. The development of the sleep disorders clinic at Stanford University described here is in many ways a microcosm of how sleep medicine evolved throughout the world. The use of patients complaining of insomnia in hypnotic efficacy studies brought the Stanford group closely into relation with many insomnia patients and demolished the notion that the majority of such patients were psychiatric cases. One early question was, How reliable were the descriptions of their sleep by these patients? Here, the classic all-night sleep recording could yield a great deal of information. A second factor was that throughout the second half of the 1960s, research of the Stanford group continued to require managing patients with narcolepsy. As Stanford's reputation for expertise in narcolepsy grew, it found itself receiving referrals for evaluation from physicians all over the United States. Although the identification and treatment of sleep apnea as a frequent cause of severe daytime sleepiness had not occurred, it was clear that a number of patients referred with the presumptive diagnosis of narcolepsy certainly did not possess narcolepsy's two cardinal signs, SOREMPs and cataplexy. True pickwickians were an infrequent referral at this time.

In January 1972, Christian Guilleminault, a French neurologist and psychiatrist, joined the Stanford group. He had extensive knowledge of and experience with the European studies of sleep apnea. Until his arrival, the Stanford group had not routinely used respiratory and cardiac sensors in their all-night sleep studies. Starting in 1972, these measurements became a routine part of the all-night diagnostic test, which was named polysomnography in 1974 by Dr. Jerome Holland, a member of the group. Publicity about narcolepsy and excessive sleepiness resulted in a small flow of referrals to the Stanford sleep clinic, usually with the presumptive diagnosis of narcolepsy. During the first year or two, the goal for the practice was to see at least five new patients per week. To foster financial viability, the group did as much as possible, within ethical limits, to publicize its services. Accordingly, there was also a sprinkling of patients, often self-referred, with chronic insomnia. The diagnosis of obstructive sleep apnea in patients with profound excessive daytime sleepiness was nearly always completely unambiguous.

During 1972, the search for sleep abnormality in patients with sleep-related complaints continued; an attempt was made as well to conceptualize the pathophysiological process both as an entity and as the cause of the presenting symptom. With this approach, a number of phenomena seen during sleep were rapidly linked to the fundamental sleep-related presenting complaints. Toward the end of 1972, the basic concepts and formats of sleep disorders medicine were sculpted to the extent that it was possible to offer a daylong course through Stanford University's Division of Postgraduate Medicine with the title "The Diagnosis and Treatment of Sleep Disorders." The topics covered were normal sleep architecture; the diagnosis and treatment of insomnia with drug-dependent insomnia, pseudoinsomnia, central sleep apnea, and periodic leg movement as diagnostic entities; and the diagnosis and treatment of excessive daytime sleepiness or hypersomnia, with narcolepsy, NREM narcolepsy, and obstructive sleep apnea as diagnostic entities.

The disability and cardiovascular complications of severe sleep apnea were alarming, but at that time, the treatment options were limited to weight loss and chronic tracheostomy. The dramatic results of chronic tracheostomy in ameliorating the symptoms and complications of obstructive sleep apnea had been reported by Lugaresi et al.[55] in 1970. However, the notion of using such a treatment was strongly resisted at the time by the medical community, both at and around the Stanford University sleep clinic. Among the first patients who were referred for investigation of their severe somnolence and eventually had tracheostomy was a 10-year-old boy. The challenges that were met to secure the proper management of this patient are worthy of presenting a personal account by Christian Guilleminault (personal communication, 1990).

CASE HISTORY

Raymond M. was a 10½-year-old boy referred to the Pediatrics clinic in 1971 for evaluation of unexplained hypertension, which had developed progressively over the preceding 6 months. There was a positive family history of high blood pressure, but never so early in life. Raymond was hospitalized and had determination of renin, angiotensin, and aldosterone, renal function studies including contrast radiographs, and extensive cardiac evaluation. All results had been normal except that his blood pressure oscillated between 140–170/90–100. It was noticed that he was somnolent during the daytime and Dr. S. suggested that I see him for this "unrelated" symptom.

I reviewed Raymond's history with his mother. Raymond had been abnormally sleepy "all his life." However, during the past 2 to 3 years, his schoolteachers were complaining that he would fall asleep in class and was at times a "behavioral problem"—not paying attention, hyperactive, aggressive. His mother confirmed that he had been a very loud snorer since he was very young, at least since age 2, perhaps before.

Physical examination revealed an obese boy with a short neck and a very narrow airway. I recommended a sleep evaluation which was accepted. An esophageal balloon and measurement of end tidal CO_2 was added to the usual array. His esophageal pressure reached 80 to 120 cm H_2O, he had values of 6% end tidal CO_2 at end of apnea, apneic events lasted between 25 and 65 sec, and the apnea index was 55. His SaO_2 was frequently below 60%.

I called the pediatric resident and informed him that the sleep problem was serious. I also suggested that the sleep problem might be the cause of the as yet unexplained hyper-

tension. The resident could not make sense of my information and passed it to the attending physician. I was finally asked to present my findings at the pediatric case conference which was led by Dr. S. I came with the recordings, showed the results, and explained why I believed that there was a relationship between the hypertension and the sleep problem. There were a lot of questions. They simply could not believe it. I was asked what treatment I would recommend, and I suggested a tracheostomy. I was asked how many patients had this treatment in the United States, and how many children had ever been treated with tracheostomy. When I had to answer "zero" to both questions, the audience was somewhat shocked. It was decided that such an approach was doubtful at best, and completely unacceptable in a child. However, they did concede that if no improvement was achieved by medical management, Raymond would be reinvestigated including sleep studies.

This was spring 1972. In the fall, he was, if anything, worse in spite of vigorous medical treatment. At the end of 1972, Raymond finally had his tracheostomy. His blood pressure went down to 90/60 within 10 days, and he was no longer sleepy. During the 5 years we were able to follow Raymond, he remained normotensive and alert, but I had to fight continuously to prevent outside doctors from closing his tracheostomy. I don't know what happened to him since.

CHRISTIAN GUILLEMINAULT

In addition to medical skepticism, a major obstacle to the practice of sleep disorders medicine was the retroactive denial of payment by insurance companies, primarily the largest one in the United States. A 3-year period of educational efforts directed toward third-party carriers finally culminated in the recognition of polysomnography as a reimbursable diagnostic test in 1975. Another issue was obtaining state licensure of an outpatient clinic that offered overnight testing for avoidance of the licensing requirements of a hospital for the sleep clinic and its polysomnographic testing bedrooms. This, too, was finally accomplished in 1974.

CLINICAL SIGNIFICANCE OF EXCESSIVE DAYTIME SLEEPINESS

Christian Guilleminault, in a series of studies, had clearly recognized excessive daytime sleepiness as a major presenting complaint and as a pathological phenomenon unto itself.[56] However, it was recognized that methods to quantify this symptom and condition in terms of improvement with treatment were not adequate. The Stanford Sleepiness Scale, developed by Hoddes et al.,[57] was used but clearly did not give reliable results. The problem was not a crisis because patients with severe apnea and overwhelming daytime sleepiness who had tracheostomy were dramatically improved, and the reduction in daytime sleepiness was unambiguous. Nonetheless, documenting the pharmacological treatment of narcolepsy and the objective improvement of sleepiness in less severe sleep apnea patients continued to be a problem.

The apparent lack of interest in daytime sleepiness

by individuals who were unambiguously interested in sleep and devoting their careers to its investigation remains a scientific puzzle. There is no question that the current active investigation of this phenomenon is due to the early interest of sleep disorders specialists. The neglect of sleepiness is all the more difficult to understand because it is now widely recognized that sleepiness and the tendence to fall asleep during the performance of hazardous tasks is one of the most important problems in our society. A number of reasons have been put forward. One is that sleepiness and drowsiness are negative qualities. A second is that the societal failure to confront the issue was fostered by language ambiguities in identifying sleepiness. A third is that the early sleep laboratory studies focused almost exclusively on REM sleep and nighttime operations with little concern for the daytime except for psychopathology. Finally, a fourth is that the focus with regard to sleep deprivation was on performance from the perspective of human factors rather than on sleepiness as representing a homeostatic response to sleep reduction.

An early attempt to develop an objective measure of sleepiness was that of Yoss et al.[58] They observed pupil diameter directly by video monitoring and described changes in sleep deprivation and narcolepsy. Subsequently designated pupillometry, this technique has not been widely accepted. Dr. Mary Carskadon deserves most of the credit for the development of the latter-day standard approach to the measurement of sleepiness called the multiple sleep latency test (MSLT). She noted that subjective ratings of sleepiness made before a sleep recording not infrequently predicted the sleep latency. In spring 1976, she undertook to establish sleep latency as an objective measurement of the state of sleepiness-alertness by measuring sleep tendency before, during, and after 2 days of total sleep deprivation.[59] A protocol was designed for this study that has essentially become the standard protocol for the MSLT. The choices of a 20-min duration of a single test and a 2-h interval between tests were essentially arbitrary and dictated by the practical demands of that study. This test was then formally applied to the evaluation of sleepiness in patients with narcolepsy[60] and, later, in patients with obstructive sleep apnea syndrome (OSAS).[61]

Carskadon and her colleagues then undertook a monumental study of sleepiness in children by following them longitudinally across the 2nd decade of life, which is also the decade of highest risk for the development of narcolepsy. Using the new MSLT measure, she found that 10-year-old children were completely alert in the daytime, but by the time they reached sexual maturity, they were no longer fully alert with the same amount of sleep at night. Results of this remarkable decade of work and other studies are summarized in an important review.[62]

The important advances in thinking that early MSLT research established were

1. Daytime sleepiness and nighttime sleep are an interactive continuum, and the adequacy of nighttime sleep absolutely cannot be understood without a complementary measurement of the level of daytime sleepiness or its antonym, alertness.
2. Excessive sleepiness, also known as impaired alertness, was sleep medicine's most important symptom.

RECENT HISTORY

As the decade of the 1970s drew to a close, the consolidation and formalization of the practice of sleep disorders medicine was largely completed. The American Sleep Disorders Association was formed and provided a home for professionals interested in sleep and, particularly, the diagnosis and treatment of sleep disorders. This organization began as the Association of Sleep Disorders Centers with five members in 1975. The organization then was responsible for the initiation of the scientific journal *Sleep*, and it fostered the setting of standards through center accreditation and an examination for practitioners by which they were designated Accredited Clinical Polysomnographers.

The first international symposium on narcolepsy took place in the French Languedoc in summer 1975, immediately after the Second International Congress of the Association for the Physiological Study of Sleep in Edinburgh. The former meeting, in addition to being scientifically productive, had landmark significance because it produced the first consensus definition of a specific sleep disorder,[63] drafted, revised, and unanimously endorsed by 65 narcoleptologists of international reputation. The first sleep disorders patient volunteer organization, the American Narcolepsy Association, was also formed in 1975. The *ASDC/APSS Diagnostic Classification of Sleep and Arousal Disorders* was published in fall 1979 after 3 years of extraordinary effort by a small group of dedicated individuals who composed the "nosology" committee chaired by Howard Roffwarg.[64]

Before the 1980s, the only effective treatment for severe OSAS was chronic tracheostomy. This highly effective but personally undesirable approach was replaced by two new procedures—one surgical,[65] the other mechanical.[66] The first was uvulopalatopharyngoplasty, which is giving way to more complex and effective approaches. The second is the widely used and highly effective continuous positive nasal airway pressure technique introduced by the Australian pulmonologist Colin Sullivan. The combination of the high prevalence of OSAS and effective treatments fueled a strong expansion of centers and individuals offering the diagnosis and treatment of sleep disorders to patients. The decade of the 1980s was capped by the publication of sleep medicine's first textbook, *Principles and Practice of Sleep Medicine*.[67]

The 1990s saw an acceleration in the acceptance of sleep medicine throughout the world.[68] In the United States, the National Center on Sleep Disorders Research (NCSDR) was established by statute as part of the National Heart, Lung, and Blood Institute of the National Institutes of Health.[69, 70] The mandate of NCSDR is to support research, promote educational activities, and coordinate sleep-related activities throughout various branches of the U.S. government. This initiative led to the development of large research projects dealing with various aspects of sleep disorders and the establishment of awards to develop educational materials at all levels of training.

The 1990s also saw the establishment of the National Sleep Foundation[71] as well as other organizations for patients.[72] This foundation points out to society at large the dangers of sleepiness, and its efforts culminated in National Sleep Awareness Week. As the Internet increases exponentially in size, so do the sleep resources on the Internet,[72, 73] both for physicians and patients and for the public at large. There are numerous World Wide Web sites devoted to sleep and its disorders. The average person today knows a great deal more about sleep and its disorders than the average person at the end of the 1980s.

THE CHALLENGE OF THE FUTURE

Chapter 48 of this volume deals with public policy and public health issues. From today's vantage (circa 2000), the greatest challenge for the future is the cost-effective expansion of sleep medicine so that its benefits will be readily available throughout society. The major barrier to this availability currently is the failure of sleep research and sleep medicine to effectively penetrate the educational system at any level. As a consequence, the majority of individuals remain unaware of important facts of sleep and wakefulness, fundamentals of biological rhythms, and sleep disorders, particularly of the symptoms that suggest a serious pathological process. The management of sleep deprivation and its serious consequences in the workplace, particularly in those industries that maintain sustained operations, is barely addressed.

Finally, the education and training of health professionals and sleep specialists has far to go to reach adequate numbers. Take heart! All of these problems are grand opportunities. Sleep medicine has come into its own. It has made a concern for the health of human beings truly a 24-h enterprise, and it has energized a new effort to reveal the secrets of the healthy and unhealthy sleeping brain.

References

1. Thorpy M. History of sleep and man. In: Thorpy M, Yager J, eds. The Encyclopedia of Sleep and Sleep Disorders. New York, NY: Facts on File; 1991.
2. MacNish R. The Philosophy of Sleep. New York, NY: D Appleton & Co; 1834.
3. Hobson J. Sleep. New York, NY: Scientific American Library; 1989.
4. Legendre R, Pieron H. Le probleme des facteurs du sommeil. Resultats d'injections vasculaires et intracerebrales de liquides insomniques. C R Soc Biol. 1910;68:1077–1079.
5. Kleitman N. Sleep and Wakefulness. Chicago, Ill: University of Chicago Press; 1939.
6. Berger H. Ueber das Elektroenkephalogramm des Menschen. J Psychol Neurol. 1930;40:160–179.
7. Davis H, Davis PA, Loomis AL, et al. Changes in human brain potentials during the onset of sleep. Science. 1937;86:448–450.
8. Davis H, Davis PA, Loomis AL, et al. Human brain potentials during the onset of sleep. J Neurophysiol. 1938;1:24–38.
9. Harvey EN, Loomis AL, Hobart GA. Cerebral states during sleep as studied by human brain potentials. Science. 1937;85:443–444.
10. Blake H, Gerard RW. Brain potentials during sleep. Am J Physiol. 1937;119:692–703.
11. Blake H, Gerard RW, Kleitman N. Factors influencing brain potentials during sleep. J Neurophysiol. 1939;2:48–60.
12. Bremer F. Cerveau "isole" et physiologie du sommeil. C R Soc Biol. 1935;118:1235–1241.
13. Bremer F. Cerveau. Nouvelles recherches sur le mecanisme du sommeil. C R Soc Biol. 1936;122:460–464.
14. Moruzzi G, Magoun H. Brain stem reticular formation and activation of the EEG. Electroencephalogr Clin Neurophysiol. 1949;1:455–473.
15. Starzl TE, Taylor CW, Magoun HW. Collateral afferent excitation of reticular formation of brain stem. J Neurophysiol. 1951;14:479.
16. Jasper H, Ajmone-Marsan C. A Stereotaxic Atlas of the Diencephalon of the Cat. Ottawa, Ontario, Canada: The National Research Council of Canada; 1954.
17. Magoun HW. The ascending reticular system and wakefulness. In: Adrian ED, Bremer F, Jasper HH, eds. Brain Mechanisms and Consciousness. A Symposium Organized by The Council for International Organizations of Medical Sciences. Springfield, Ill: Charles C Thomas; 1954.
18. Kryger MH. Sleep apnea: from the needles of Dionysius to continuous positive airway pressure. Arch Intern Med. 1983;143:2301–2308.
19. Lavie P. Nothing new under the moon. Historical accounts of sleep apnea syndrome. Arch Intern Med. 1986;144:2025–2028.
20. Passouant P. Doctor Gélineau (1828–1906): narcolepsy centennial. Sleep. 1981;3:241–246.
21. Moore-Ede M, Sulzman F, Fuller C. The Clocks That Time Us: Physiology of the Circadian Timing System. Cambridge, Mass: Harvard University Press; 1982.
22. Toni G de. I movimenti pendolari dei bulbi oculari dei bambini durante il sonno fisiologico, ed in alcuni stati morbosi. Pediatria. 1933;41:489–498.
23. Aserinsky E, Kleitman N. Regularly occurring periods of eye motility, and concomitant phenomena, during sleep. Science. 1953;118:273–274.
24. Aserinsky E, Kleitman N. Two types of ocular motility occurring in sleep. J Appl Physiol. 1955;8:11–18.
25. Dement W, Kleitman N. Cyclic variations in EEG during sleep and their relation to eye movements, body motility, and dreaming. Electroencephalogr Clin Neurophysiol. 1957;9:673–690.
26. Dement W. A personal history of sleep disorders medicine. J Clin Neurophysiol. 1990;1:17–47.
27. Derbyshire AJ, Rempel B, Forbes A, et al. The effects of anesthetics on action potentials in the cerebral cortex of the cat. Am J Physiol. 1936;116:577–596.
28. Hess R, Koella WP, Akert K. Cortical and subcortical recordings in natural and artificially induced sleep in cats. Electroencephalogr Clin Neurophysiol. 1953;5:75–90.
29. Dement W. The occurrence of low voltage, fast electroencephalogram patterns during behavioral sleep in the cat. Electroencephalogr Clin Neurophysiol. 1958;10:291–296.
30. Jouvet M, Michel F, Courjon J. Sur un stade d'activite electrique cerebrale rapide au cours du sommeil physiologique. C R Soc Biol. 1959;153:1024–1028.
31. Jouvet M, Mounier D. Effects des lesions de la formation reticulaire pontique sur le sommeil du chat. C R Soc Biol. 1960;154:2301–2305.
32. Hodes R, Dement W. Depression of electrically induced reflexes ("H-reflexes") in man during low voltage EEG "sleep." Electroencephalogr Clin Neurophysiol. 1964;17:617–629.
33. Pompeiano O. Mechanisms responsible for spinal inhibition during desynchronized sleep: experimental study. In: Guilleminault C, Dement WC, Passouant P, eds. Advances in Sleep Research. Vol. 3. Narcolepsy. New York, NY: Spectrum; 1976:411–449.
34. Jouvet M. Recherches sur les structures nerveuses et les meca-

nismes responsales des differentes phases du sommeil physiologique. Arch Ital Biol. 1962;100:125–206.

35. Evarts E. Effects of sleep and waking on spontaneous and evoked discharge of single units in visual cortex. Fed Proc. 1960;4(suppl):828–837.

36. Reivich M, Kety S. Blood flow metabolism couple in brain. In: Plum F, ed. Brain Dysfunction in Metabolic Disorders. New York, NY: Raven Press; 1968:125–140.

37. Kupfer D, Foster F. Interval between onset of sleep and rapid eye movement sleep as an indicator of depression. Lancet. 1972;2:684–686.

38. Vogel G. Studies in psychophysiology of dreams, III: the dream of narcolepsy. Arch Gen Psychiatry. 1960;3:421–428.

39. Rechtschaffen A, Wolpert E, Dement W, et al. Nocturnal sleep of narcoleptics. Electroencephalogr Clin Neurophysiol. 1963;15:599–609.

40. Dement W, Rechtschaffen A, Gulevich G. The nature of the narcoleptic sleep attack. Neurology. 1966;16:18–33.

41. Fischgold H, ed. La Sommeil de Nuit Normal et Pathologique: Etudes Electroencephalographiques. Paris, France: Masson et Cie; 1965.

42. Oswald I, Priest R. Five weeks to escape the sleep pill habit. BMJ. 1965;2:1093–1095.

43. Kales A, Malmstrom EJ, Scharf MB, et al. Psychophysiological and biochemical changes following use and withdrawal of hypnotics. In: Kales A, ed. Sleep: Physiology and Pathology. Philadelphia, Pa: JB Lippincott; 1969:331–343.

44. Kales A, Beall GN, Bajor GF, et al. Sleep studies in asthmatic adults: relationship of attacks to sleep stage and time of night. J Allergy. 1968;41:164–173.

45. Kales A, Heuser G, Jacobson A, et al. All night sleep studies in hypothyroid patients, before and after treatment. J Clin Endocrinol Metab. 1967;27:1593–1599.

46. Kales A, Ansel RD, Markham CH, et al. Sleep in patients with Parkinson's disease and normal subjects prior to and following levodopa administration. Clin Pharmacol Ther. 1971;12:397–406.

47. Kales A, Jacobson A, Paulson NJ, et al. Somnambulism: psychophysiological correlates, I: all-night EEG studies. Arch Gen Psychiatry. 1966;14:586–594.

48. Gastaut H, Tassinari C, Duron B. Etude polygraphique des manifestations épisodiques (hypniques et respiratoires) du syndrome de Pickwick. Rev Neurol. 1965;112:568–579.

49. Jung R, Kuhlo W. Neurophysiological studies of abnormal night sleep and the pickwickian syndrome. Prog Brain Res. 1965;18:140–159.

50. Burwell CS, Robin ED, Whaley RD, et al. Extreme obesity associated with alveolar hypoventilation. A pickwickian syndrome. Am J Med. 1956;21:811–818.

51. Lugaresi E, Coccagna G, Mantovani M. Hypersomnia With Periodic Apneas. New York, NY: Spectrum; 1978.

52. Gastaut H, Lugaresi E, Berti-Ceroni G, et al, eds. The Abnormalities of Sleep in Man. Bologna, Italy: Aulo Gaggi Editore; 1968.

53. Lugaresi E. Organizer symposium: hypersomnia with periodic breathing. Rimini, Italy, May 25–27. Bull Physiopath Resp. 1972;8:967–1292.

54. Dement W, Guilleminault C, Zarcone V, et al. The narcolepsy syndrome. In: Conn H, Conn R, eds. Current Diagnosis. Vol 2. Philadelphia, Pa: WB Saunders Co; 1974.

55. Lugaresi E, Coccagna G, Mantovani M, et al. Effects de la trachéotomie dans les hypersomnies avec respiration périodique. Rev Neurol. 1970;123:267–268.

56. Guilleminault C, Dement W. 235 cases of excessive daytime sleepiness. Diagnosis and tentative classification. J Neurol Sci. 1977;31:13–27.

57. Hoddes E, Zarcone V, Smythe H, et al. Quantification of sleepiness: a new approach. Psychophysiology. 1973;10:431–436.

58. Yoss R, Moyer N, Hollenhorst R. Pupil size and spontaneous pupillary waves associated with alertness, drowsiness, and sleep. Neurology. 1970;20:545–554.

59. Carskadon M, Dement W. Effects of total sleep loss on sleep tendency. Percept Mot Skills. 1979;48:495–506.

60. Richardson G, Carskadon M, Flagg W, et al. Excessive daytime sleepiness in man: multiple sleep latency measurements in narcoleptic and control subjects. Electroencephalogr Clin Neurophysiol. 1978;45:621–627.

61. Dement W, Carskadon M, Richardson G. Excessive daytime sleepiness in the sleep apnea syndromes. In: Guilleminault C, Dement W, eds. Sleep Apnea Syndromes. New York, NY: Alan R Liss; 1978.

62. Carskadon M, Dement W. Daytime sleepiness: qualification of a behavioral state. Neurosci Biobehav Rev. 1987;11:307–317.

63. Guilleminault C, Dement W, Passouant P, eds. Narcolepsy. New York, NY: Spectrum; 1976.

64. Sleep Disorders Classification Committee. Diagnostic classification of sleep and arousal disorders. 1979 first edition. Association of Sleep Disorders Centers and the Association for the Psychophysiological Study of Sleep. Sleep. 1979;2:1–137.

65. Fujita S, Conway W, Zorick F, et al. Surgical correction of anatomic abnormalities in obstructive sleep apnea syndrome: uvulopalatopharyngoplasty. Otolaryngol Head Neck Surg. 1981;89:923–934.

66. Sullivan CE, Issa FG, Berthon-Jones M, et al. Reversal of obstructive sleep apnea by continuous positive airway pressure applied through the nares. Lancet. 1981;1:862–865.

67. Kryger M, Roth T, Dement WC. Principles and Practice of Sleep Medicine. Philadelphia, Pa: WB Saunders Co; 1989.

68. University of California, Los Angeles. This World's Sleep Researchers. Available at: http://bisleep.medsch.ucla.edu/map/world.map.html. Accessed May 17, 1999.

69. Lefant C, Kiley JP. Sleep research: celebration and opportunity. Sleep. 1998;21:665–669.

70. National Heart, Lung, and Blood Institute. Sleep Disorders Information. Available at: http://www.nhlbi.nih.gov/about/ncsdr/index.htm. Accessed January 18, 2000.

71. National Sleep Foundation. Available at: http://www.sleepfoundation.org. Accessed January 18, 2000.

72. Sleep Support Organizations. Available at: http://bisleep.medsch.ucla.edu/htdocs/support.html. Accessed January 18, 2000.

73. Sleep Home Pages. Available at: http://bisleep.medsch.ucla.edu/. Accessed January 18, 2000.

2

Normal Human Sleep: An Overview

Mary A. Carskadon
William C. Dement

SLEEP DEFINITIONS

According to a simple behavioral definition, *sleep* is a reversible behavioral state of perceptual disengagement from and unresponsiveness to the environment. It is also true that sleep is a complex amalgam of physiological and behavioral processes. Sleep is usually (but not necessarily) accompanied by postural recumbency, quiescence, closed eyes, and all the other indicators one commonly associates with sleeping. In the unusual circumstance, other behaviors can occur during sleep. These behaviors may include sleepwalking, sleeptalking, toothgrinding, and other physical activities. Anomalies involving sleep processes also include intrusions of the sleep processes—sleep itself, dream imagery, or muscle weakness—into wakefulness.

Within sleep, two separate states have been defined on the basis of a constellation of physiological parameters. These two states, nonrapid eye movement (NREM) and rapid eye movement (REM), exist in virtually all mammals and birds and are as distinct from one another as each is from wakefulness.

NREM (pronounced non-REM) sleep is conventionally subdivided into four stages, which are relatively precisely, although somewhat arbitrarily, defined along one measurement axis, the electroencephalogram (EEG). The EEG pattern in NREM sleep is commonly described as synchronous, with such characteristic waveforms as sleep spindles, K complexes, and high-voltage slow waves (Fig. 2–1). The four NREM stages (stages 1, 2, 3, and 4) roughly parallel a depth of sleep continuum, with arousal thresholds generally lowest in stage 1 and highest in stage 4 sleep. NREM sleep is usually associated with fragmented mental activity. A shorthand definition of *NREM* is a relatively inactive yet actively regulating brain in a movable body.

REM sleep, by contrast, is defined by EEG activation, muscle atonia, and episodic bursts of rapid eye movements. REM sleep generally is not divided into stages, although tonic and phasic types of REM sleep are often distinguished for certain research purposes. The tonic versus phasic distinction is based on short-lived events that tend to occur in clusters separated by episodes of relative quiescence. In cats, REM sleep phasic activity is epitomized by bursts of ponto-geniculo-occipital (PGO) waves, which are accompanied peripherally by rapid eye movements, twitching of distal muscles, middle ear muscle activity, and other phasic events that correspond to the phasic event markers easily measurable in human beings. As described in Chapter 100, PGO waves are not usually detectable in human beings. Thus, the most commonly used marker of REM sleep phasic activity in human beings is, of course, the bursts of rapid eye movements (Fig. 2–2). The mental activity of human REM sleep is associated with dreaming, based on vivid dream recall reported after approximately 80% of arousals from this state of sleep.[1] Inhibition of spinal motoneurons via

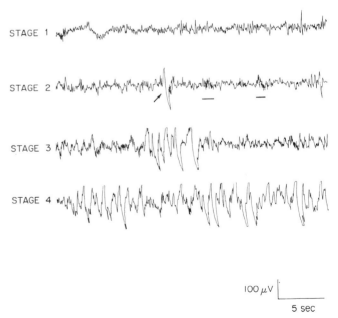

Figure 2–1. The stages of NREM sleep. The four EEG tracings depicted here are from a 19-year-old female volunteer. Each tracing was recorded from a referential lead (C3/A2) recorded on a Grass Instruments Co. Model 7D polygraph with a paper speed of 10 mm/sec, time constant of 0.3 sec, and ½-amplitude high-frequency setting of 30 Hz. On the second tracing, the arrow indicates a K complex, and the underlining shows two sleep spindles.

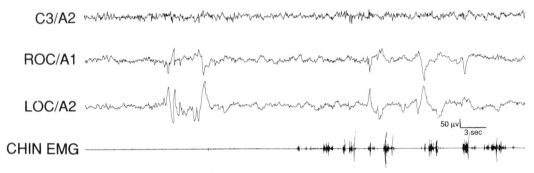

Figure 2–2. Phasic events in human REM sleep. On the left side is a burst of several rapid eye movements (out-of-phase deflections in ROC/A1 and LOC/A2). On the right side, there are additional rapid eye movements as well as twitches on the EMG lead. The interval between eye movement bursts and twitches illustrates tonic REM sleep.

brainstem mechanisms mediates suppression of postural motor tonus in REM sleep. A shorthand definition of *REM sleep*, therefore, is a highly activated brain in a paralyzed body.

SLEEP ONSET

The onset of sleep under normal circumstances in normal adult humans is through NREM sleep. This fundamental principle of normal human sleep reflects a highly reliable finding and is important in considering normal versus pathological sleep. For example, the abnormal entry into sleep via REM is a diagnostic sign in adult patients with narcolepsy.

Definition of Sleep Onset

The precise definition of the onset of sleep has been a topic of debate for many years, primarily because there is not one single measure that is 100% clear-cut 100% of the time. For example, a change in EEG pattern is not always associated with whether a person perceives sleep; yet even when individuals may report that they are still awake, clear behavioral changes can indicate the presence of sleep. To begin a consideration of this issue, let us examine the three basic polysomnographic measures of sleep and how they change with sleep onset. The electrode placements are described in Chapter 100.

Electromyograph

Electromyograph (EMG) levels may show a gradual diminution as sleep approaches, but there is rarely a discrete change that can be pinpointed as sleep onset. Furthermore, the waking level of the EMG, particularly if the individual is relaxed, can be entirely indistinguishable from that of unequivocal sleep (Fig. 2–3).

Electro-Oculogram

As sleep approaches, the electro-oculogram (EOG) shows slow, often asynchronous eye movements (see Fig. 2–3) that generally disappear within several minutes of the EEG changes described next. Occasionally, the onset of these slow eye movements coincides with a person's perceived sleep onset; more often, individuals will report that they are awake.

Electroencephalogram

In the simplest circumstance (see Fig. 2–3), the EEG changes from a pattern of clear rhythmic alpha (8 to 13 cycles per sec [cps]) activity, particularly in the occipital region, to a relatively low-voltage, mixed-frequency pattern (stage 1 sleep). This EEG change generally occurs seconds to minutes after the start of slow eye movements. With regard to introspection, the onset of a stage 1 EEG pattern may or may not coincide with perceived sleep onset. For this reason, a number of investigators require the presence of specific EEG

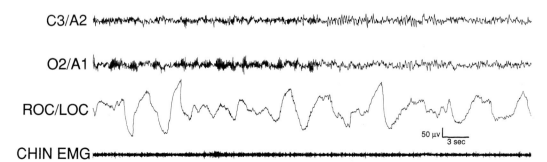

Figure 2–3. The transition from wakefulness to stage 1 sleep. The most marked change is visible on the two EEG channels (C3/A2 and O2/A1), where a clear pattern of rhythmic alpha activity (8 cps) changes to a relatively low-voltage, mixed-frequency pattern at about the middle of the figure. The level of EMG activity does not change markedly. Slow eye movements (ROC/LOC) are present throughout this episode, preceding the EEG change by at least 20 sec. In general, the change in EEG patterns to stage 1 as illustrated here is accepted as the onset of sleep.

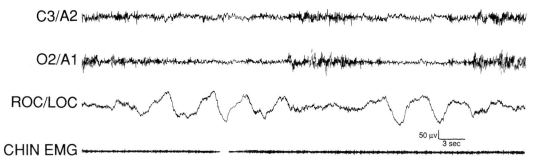

Figure 2–4. A common wake-to-sleep transition pattern. Note that the EEG pattern changes from wake (rhythmic alpha) to stage 1 (relatively low-voltage, mixed-frequency) sleep twice during this attempt to fall asleep.

patterns—the K complex or sleep spindle (i.e., stage 2 sleep)—to acknowledge sleep onset. Even these stage 2 patterns, however, are not unequivocally associated with perceived sleep.[2] A further complication is that sleep onset frequently does not occur all at once, but there may be a wavering of vigilance before "unequivocal" sleep ensues (Fig. 2–4). Thus, it is difficult to accept a single variable as marking sleep onset. As Davis and colleagues wrote many years ago,

> Is "falling asleep" a unitary event? Our observations suggest that it is not. Different functions, such as sensory awareness, memory, self-consciousness, continuity of logical thought, latency of response to a stimulus and alterations in the pattern of brain potentials all go in parallel in a general way, but there are exceptions to every rule.[3(p35)]

Nevertheless, a reasonable consensus exists that the EEG change to stage 1, usually heralded or accompanied by slow eye movements, identifies the transition to sleep, provided that another EEG sleep pattern does not intervene. One may not always be able to pinpoint this transition to the millisecond, but it is usually possible to determine the change reliably within several seconds.

Behavioral Concomitants of Sleep Onset

Given the changes in EEG that accompany the onset of sleep, what are the behavioral correlates of the wake-to-sleep transition? The following material reviews a few common behavioral concomitants of sleep onset. Keep in mind that "different functions may be de-pressed in different sequence and to different degrees in different subjects and on different occasions."[3(p35)]

Simple Behavioral Task

In the first example, volunteers were asked to tap two switches alternately at a steady pace. As shown in Figure 2–5, this simple behavior continues after the onset of slow eye movements and may persist for several seconds after the EEG changes to a stage 1 sleep pattern.[4] The behavior then ceases, usually to recur only after the EEG reverts to a waking pattern. This is an example of what one may think of as the simplest kind of "automatic" behavior pattern.

Visual Response

In the second example, a bright light is placed in front of the subject's eyes. The individual is asked to respond when a light flash is seen by pressing a sensitive microswitch taped to the hand.[5] When the EEG pattern is stage 1 or stage 2 sleep, the response is absent more than 85% of the time. When volunteers are queried afterward, they report that they did not see the light flash, not that they saw the flash but the response was inhibited. This is one example of the perceptual disengagement from the environment that accompanies sleep onset.

Auditory Response

In this example, a series of tones is played over earphones to a subject who is instructed to respond each time a tone is heard. One study of this phenomenon showed that reaction times became longer in prox-

Figure 2–5. Failure to perform a simple behavioral task at the onset of sleep. The volunteer had been deprived of sleep overnight and was required to tap two switches alternately, shown as pen deflections of opposite polarity on the channel labeled SAT. When the EEG (C3/A2) pattern changes to stage 1 sleep, the behavior stops, returning when the EEG pattern reverts to wakefulness. SEMs, slow eye movements. (From Carskadon MA, Dement WC. Effects of total sleep loss on sleep tendency. Percept Mot Skills. 1979;48:495–506. © Perceptual and Motor Skills, 1979.)

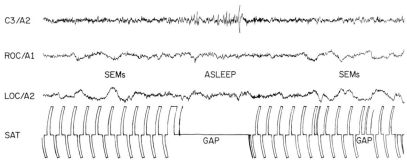

imity to the onset of stage 1 sleep, and responses were absent coincident with a change in EEG to unequivocal sleep.[6] For responses in both visual and auditory modalities, the return of the response after its sleep-related disappearance requires the resumption of a waking EEG pattern.

Response to Meaningful Stimuli

One should not infer from the preceding studies that the mind becomes an impenetrable barrier to sensory input at the onset of sleep. Indeed, one of the earliest modern studies of arousability during sleep showed that sleeping human beings were differentially responsive to auditory stimuli of graded intensity.[7] Another way of illustrating sensory sensitivity is shown in experiments that have assessed discriminant responses during sleep to meaningful versus nonmeaningful stimuli, with meaning supplied in a number of ways and response usually measured as evoked K complexes or arousal. The following are examples.

1. A person tends to have a lower arousal threshold for his or her own name versus someone else's name.[8] In light sleep, for example, one's own name spoken softly will produce an arousal; a similarly applied nonmeaningful stimulus will not. Similarly, a sleeping mother is more likely to hear her own baby's cry than the cry of an unrelated infant.
2. Williams and his colleagues[9] showed that the likelihood of an appropriate response during sleep was improved when an otherwise nonmeaningful stimulus was made meaningful by linking the absence of response to punishment (a loud siren, flashing light, and the threat of an electric shock).

From these examples and others, it seems clear that sensory processing at some level does continue after the onset of sleep.

Hypnic Myoclonia

What other behaviors accompany the onset of sleep? If you awaken and query someone shortly after the stage 1 sleep EEG pattern appears, the individual will generally report the mental experience as one of losing a direct train of thought and of experiencing vague and fragmentary imagery, usually visual.[10] Another fairly common sleep onset experience is hypnic myoclonia, which is experienced as a general or localized muscle contraction very often associated with rather vivid visual imagery. Hypnic myoclonias are not pathological events, although they tend to occur more frequently in association with stress or with unusual or irregular sleep schedules.

The precise nature of hypnic myoclonias is not clearly understood. According to one hypothesis, the onset of sleep in these instances is marked by a dissociation of REM sleep components, wherein a breakthrough of the imagery component of REM sleep (hypnagogic hallucination) occurs in the absence of the REM motor inhibitory component. A response by the individual to the image, therefore, results in a movement or jerk. The increased frequency of these events in association with irregular sleep schedules is consistent with the increased probability of REM sleep occurring at the wake-to-sleep transition under such conditions (see later). Although the usual transition in adult human beings is to NREM sleep, the REM portal into sleep, which is the norm in infancy, may become partially opened under unusual circumstances.

Memory

What happens to memory at the onset of sleep? The transition from wake to sleep tends to produce a memory impairment. One view is that it is as if sleep may close the gate between short-term and long-term memory stores. This phenomenon is best described by the following experiment.[11] During a presleep testing session, word pairs were presented to volunteers over a loudspeaker at 1-min intervals. The subjects were then awakened either 30 sec or 10 min after the onset of sleep (defined as EEG stage 1) and asked to recall those words presented before sleep onset. As illustrated in Figure 2–6, the 30-sec condition was associated with a consistent level of recall from the entire 10 min before sleep onset. (Primacy and recency effects are apparent, although not large.) In the 10-min condition, however, recall paralleled that in the 30-sec group for only the 10 to 4 min before sleep onset and then fell abruptly from that point until sleep onset.

In the 30-sec condition, therefore, both longer term (4 to 10 min) and shorter term (0 to 3 min) memory stores remained accessible. In the 10-min condition, by contrast, words that were in longer term stores (4 to 10 min) before sleep onset were accessible, whereas words that were still in shorter term (0 to 3 min) stores at sleep onset were no longer accessible, that is, had not been consolidated into longer term memory stores. One conclusion of this experiment is that sleep inactivates the transfer of storage from short- to long-term memory. Another interpretation is that encoding of the material before sleep onset is of insufficient strength to allow recall. The precise moment at which this deficit occurs is not known and may be a continuing process, perhaps reflecting anterograde amnesia. Nevertheless, one may infer that if sleep persists for approximately 10 min, memory is lost for the few minutes before sleep. The following experiences represent a few familiar examples of this phenomenon:

1. Inability to grasp the instant of sleep onset in your memory.
2. Forgetting a telephone call that had come in the middle of the night.
3. Forgetting the news you were told when awakened in the night.
4. Not remembering the ringing of your alarm clock.
5. Experiencing morning amnesia for coherent "sleeptalking."
6. Having fleeting dream recall.

Patients suffering from syndromes of excessive sleepiness may experience similar memory problems in the daytime if sleep becomes intrusive.

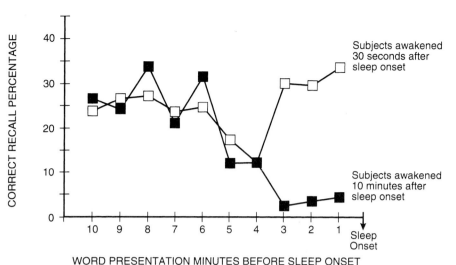

Figure 2–6. Memory is impaired by sleep, as shown by the study results illustrated in this graph. See text for explanation.

PROGRESSION OF SLEEP ACROSS THE NIGHT

Pattern of Sleep in a Normal Young Adult

The simplest description of sleep begins with the ideal case, the normal young adult (Fig. 2–7). In general, no consistent male versus female distinctions have been found in the normal pattern of sleep in young adults. In briefest summary, the normal human adult enters sleep through NREM sleep, REM sleep does not occur until 80 min or longer thereafter, and NREM sleep and REM sleep alternate through the night, with an approximately 90-min cycle. (See Chapter 100 for a full description of sleep stages.)

First Sleep Cycle

The first cycle of sleep in the normal young adult begins with stage 1 sleep, which generally persists for only a few (1 to 7) minutes at the onset of sleep. Sleep is easily discontinued during stage 1 by, for example, softly calling a person's name, touching the person lightly, quietly closing a door, and so forth. Thus, stage

1 sleep is associated with a low arousal threshold. In addition to its role in the initial wake-to-sleep transition, stage 1 sleep occurs as a transitional stage throughout the night. A common sign of severely disrupted sleep is an increase in the amount and percentage of stage 1 sleep.

Stage 2 NREM sleep, signaled by sleep spindles or K complexes in the EEG (see Fig. 2–1), follows this brief episode of stage 1 sleep and continues for about 10 to 25 min. In stage 2 sleep, a more intense stimulus is required to produce arousal. The same stimulus that produced arousal from stage 1 sleep often results in an evoked K complex but no awakening in stage 2 sleep.

As stage 2 sleep progresses, there is a gradual appearance of high-voltage slow wave activity in the EEG. Eventually, this activity meets the criteria[12] for stage 3 NREM sleep, that is, high-voltage ($\geq 75 \mu V$) slow (≤ 2 cps) wave activity accounting for more than 20% but less than 50% of the EEG activity. Stage 3 sleep usually lasts only a few minutes in the first cycle and is transitional to stage 4 as more and more high-voltage slow wave activity occurs. Stage 4 NREM sleep—identified when the high-voltage slow wave activity is more than 50% of the record—generally lasts

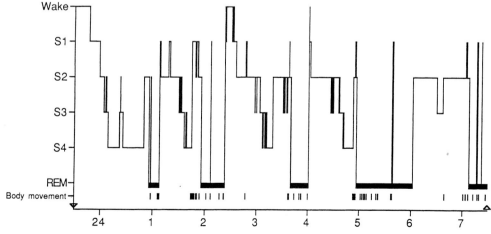

Figure 2–7. The progression of sleep stages across a single night in a normal young adult volunteer is illustrated in this sleep histogram. The text describes the "ideal" or "average" pattern. This histogram was drawn on the basis of a continuous overnight recording of EEG, electro-oculogram, and EMG in a normal 19-year-old man. The record was assessed in 30-sec epochs for the various sleep stages.

about 20 to 40 min in the first cycle. An incrementally larger stimulus is generally required to produce an arousal from stage 3 or 4 sleep than from stage 1 or 2 sleep. (Investigators often refer to the combined stages 3 + 4 sleep as slow-wave sleep [SWS], delta sleep, or deep sleep.)

A series of body movements usually signals an "ascent" to lighter NREM sleep stages. There may be a brief (1- or 2-min) episode of stage 3 sleep, followed by perhaps 5 to 10 min of stage 2 sleep interrupted by body movements preceding the initial REM episode. REM sleep in the first cycle of the night is usually short lived (1 to 5 min). The arousal threshold in this REM episode is variable, as is true for REM sleep throughout the night. Theories to explain the variable arousal threshold of REM sleep have suggested that at times, the individual's selective attention to internal stimuli precludes a response or that the arousal stimulus is incorporated into the ongoing dream story rather than producing an awakening. Certain early experiments examining arousal thresholds in cats found highest thresholds in REM sleep, which was then termed *deep sleep* in this species. Although this terminology is still often used in publications about sleep in animals, it should not be confused with human NREM stage 3 + 4, which is also called *deep sleep*. One should also note that SWS is sometimes used (as is synchronized sleep) as a synonym for all of NREM sleep in other species and is thus distinct from SWS (stages 3 + 4 NREM) in human beings.

NREM–REM Cycle

NREM sleep and REM sleep continue to alternate through the night in cyclical fashion. REM sleep episodes generally become longer across the night. Stages 3 and 4 sleep occupy less time in the second cycle and may disappear altogether from later cycles, as stage 2 sleep expands to occupy the NREM portion of the cycle. The average length of the first NREM–REM sleep cycle is approximately 70 to 100 min; the average length of the second and later cycles is about 90 to 120 min. Across the night, the average period of the NREM–REM cycle is approximately 90 to 110 min.

Distribution of Sleep Stages Across the Night

In the young adult, SWS dominates the NREM portion of the sleep cycle toward the beginning of the night (the first one third); REM sleep tends to be greatest in the last one third of the night. Brief episodes of wakefulness tend to intrude later in the night, generally near REM sleep transitions, and usually do not last long enough to be remembered in the morning. The preferential distribution of REM sleep toward the latter portion of the night in normal human adults is thought to be linked to a circadian oscillator and can be gauged by the oscillation of body temperature.[13, 14] The preferential distribution of SWS toward the beginning of a sleep episode is not thought to be mediated by circadian processes but is linked to the initiation of sleep, the length of prior wakefulness, and the time course of sleep per se.[15]

Length of Sleep

The length of nocturnal sleep is dependent on a great number of factors—of which volitional control is among the most significant in human beings—and it is thus difficult to characterize a "normal" pattern. Most young adults *report* sleeping approximately 7.5 h a night on weekday nights and slightly longer, 8.5 h, on weekend nights. The variability of these figures from person to person and from night to night, however, is quite high. Sleep length also depends on genetic determinants,[16] and one may think of the volitional determinants (staying up late, waking by alarm, and so on) superimposed on the background of a genetic sleep need. The length of sleep is also determined by processes associated with circadian rhythms. Thus, *when* one sleeps helps to determine *how long* one sleeps. In addition, as sleep is extended, the amount of REM sleep increases because REM is dependent on the persistence of sleep into the peak circadian time in order to occur.

Generalizations About Sleep in the Normal Young Adult

A number of general statements can be made regarding sleep in the normal young adult individual who is living on a conventional sleep-wake schedule and who is without sleep complaints:

1. Sleep is entered through NREM.
2. NREM sleep and REM sleep alternate with a period near 90 min.
3. SWS predominates in the first third of the night and is linked to the initiation of sleep.
4. REM sleep predominates in the last third of the night and is linked to the circadian rhythm of body temperature.
5. Wakefulness within sleep usually accounts for less than 5% of the night.
6. Stage 1 sleep generally constitutes about 2 to 5% of sleep.
7. Stage 2 sleep generally constitutes about 45 to 55% of sleep.
8. Stage 3 sleep generally constitutes about 3 to 8% of sleep.
9. Stage 4 sleep generally constitutes about 10 to 15% of sleep.
10. NREM sleep, therefore, is usually 75 to 80% of sleep.
11. REM sleep is usually 20 to 25% of sleep, occurring in four to six discrete episodes.

Factors Modifying Sleep Stage Distribution

Age

The strongest and most consistent factor affecting the pattern of sleep stages across the night is age. The most marked age-related differences in sleep from the patterns described earlier are found in newborn infants. For the 1st year of life, the transition from wake to sleep is often accomplished through REM sleep (called *active sleep* in newborns). The cyclical alternation of NREM–REM sleep is present from birth but has a period of about 50 to 60 min in the newborn compared with about 90 min in the adult. Infants also only gradually acquire a consolidated nocturnal sleep cycle, and the fully developed EEG patterns of the NREM sleep stages are not present at birth but emerge over the first 2 to 6 months of life. When brain structure and function achieve a level that can support high-voltage slow wave EEG activity, NREM stages 3 and 4 sleep become prominent.

SWS is maximal in young children and decreases markedly with age. The SWS of young children is both qualitatively and quantitatively different from that of older adults. For example, it is nearly impossible to wake youngsters in the SWS of the night's first sleep cycle. In one study,[17] a 123-dB tone failed to produce any sign of arousal in a group of children whose mean age was 10 years. There is a similar, although less profound, qualitative difference between SWS occurring in the first and later cycles of the night in a given individual. The quantitative change in SWS may best be seen across adolescence, when SWS decreases by nearly 40% during the 2nd decade, even when length of nocturnal sleep remains constant.[18] Feinberg[19] hypothesized that the age-related decline in nocturnal SWS may parallel loss of cortical synaptic density (Fig. 2–8). By age 60 years, SWS may no longer be present, particularly in men. Women appear to maintain SWS later into life than men do.

REM sleep as a percentage of total sleep is maintained well into healthy old age; the absolute amount of REM sleep at night has been correlated with intellectual functioning[20] and declines markedly in the case of organic brain dysfunctions of the elderly.[21]

Arousals during sleep increase markedly with age, both extended wakenings, of which the individual is aware and can report, and brief and probably unremembered arousals.[22] The latter type of transient arousals may occur with no known correlate but are frequently associated with occult sleep disturbances, such as periodic movements during sleep (PMS) and sleep-related respiratory irregularities, which also become more prevalent in later life.[23, 24]

Perhaps the most notable finding regarding sleep in the elderly is the profound increase in interindividual variability,[25] which thus precludes generalizations such as those made for young adults.

Prior Sleep History

An individual who has experienced sleep loss on one or more nights will show a sleep pattern that favors SWS during recovery (Fig. 2–9). Recovery sleep is also usually prolonged and deeper—that is, having a higher arousal threshold throughout—than basal sleep.

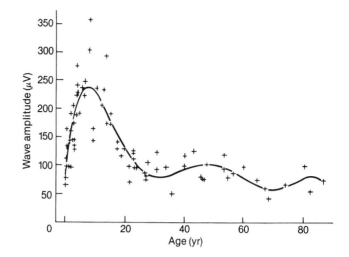

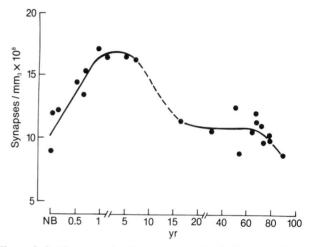

Figure 2–8. These graphs illustrate age-related changes in human EEG amplitude and in cortical synaptic density. Although relatively few data points were used to produce the lower curve, Feinberg[19] suggested that the decline in EEG amplitude during adolescence, which is most remarkable during sleep, is causally linked to a "programmed" thinning of synaptic density in the cortex. (Reprinted from Journal of Psychiatric Research, vol. 17, Feinberg I, Schizophrenia: caused by a fault in programmed synaptic elimination during adolescence?, 319–334, Copyright 1983, with permission from Elsevier Science.)

REM sleep tends to show a rebound on the 2nd or subsequent recovery nights after an episode of sleep loss. Therefore, with total sleep loss, SWS tends to be preferentially recovered compared with REM sleep, which tends to recover only after the recuperation of SWS.

Cases in which an individual is differentially deprived of REM or SWS—either operationally by being awakened each time the sleep pattern occurs, or pharmacologically (see later)—a preferential rebound of that stage of sleep occurs when natural sleep is resumed. This phenomenon has particular relevance in a clinical setting, in which abrupt withdrawal from a therapeutic regimen may result in misleading diagnostic findings (e.g., sleep-onset REM periods [SOREMs] as a result of a REM sleep rebound) or could conceiv-

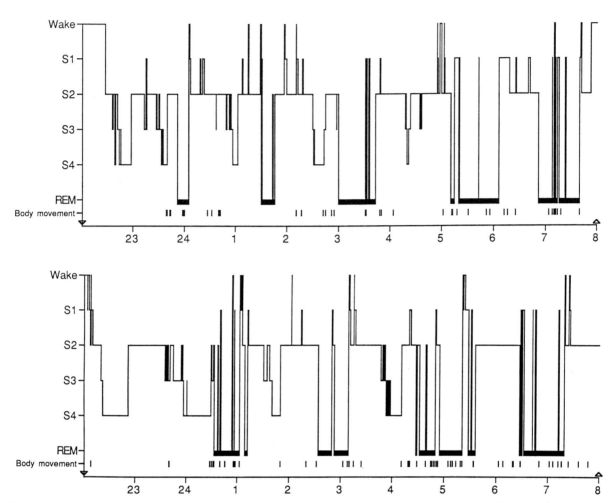

Figure 2–9. The upper histogram shows the baseline sleep pattern of a normal 14-year-old female volunteer. The lower histogram illustrates the sleep pattern in this volunteer for the first recovery night after 38 h without sleep. Note that the amount of stage 4 sleep on the lower graph is greater than on baseline, and the first REM episode is markedly delayed.

ably exacerbate a sleep disorder (e.g., if sleep apneas tend to occur preferentially or with greater intensity in the rebounding stage of sleep)

Chronic restriction of nocturnal sleep, an irregular sleep schedule, or frequent disturbance of nocturnal sleep can result in a peculiar distribution of sleep states, most frequently characterized by premature REM sleep, that is, SOREMPs. Such episodes can be associated with hypnagogic hallucinations, sleep paralysis, or an increased incidence of hypnic myoclonia in individuals with no organic sleep disorder.

Although not strictly related to prior sleep history, the first night of a laboratory sleep evaluation is commonly associated with a disruption of the normal distribution of sleep states, characterized chiefly by a delayed onset of REM sleep.[26] Frequently, this delay takes the form of missing the first REM episode of the night. In other words, the NREM sleep stages progress in a normal fashion, but the first cycle ends with an episode of stage 1 or a brief arousal instead of the expected brief REM episode. In addition, REM sleep episodes are often disrupted, and the total amount of REM sleep

on the first night in the sleep laboratory is also usually reduced from the normal value.

Circadian Rhythms

The circadian phase at which sleep occurs affects the distribution of sleep stages. REM sleep, in particular, occurs with a circadian distribution that peaks in the morning hours coincident with the trough of body temperature.[13, 14] Thus, if sleep onset is delayed until the peak REM phase of the circadian rhythm—that is, the early morning—REM sleep tends to predominate and may even occur at the onset of sleep. This reversal of the normal sleep onset pattern is commonly seen in a normal person who acutely undergoes a phase shift, either as a result of a work shift change or a change resulting from jet travel across a number of time zones. Studies of individuals sleeping in environments free of all cues to time have shown that the timing of sleep onset and the length of sleep occur as a function of circadian phase.[27, 28] In patients whose sleep distribution is examined with reference to the circadian body temperature phase position, it is clear that sleep onset is likeliest to occur on the falling limb of the temperature cycle, although a secondary peak of sleep onsets, corresponding to afternoon napping, also occurs; the offset of sleep occurs most often on the rising limb of the circadian body temperature curve.[29]

Temperature

Extremes of temperature in the sleeping environment tend to disrupt sleep. REM sleep is commonly more sensitive to temperature-related disruption than is NREM sleep. Accumulated evidence from human beings and other species suggests that mammals have only minimal, if any, ability to thermoregulate during REM sleep; in other words, the control of body temperature is virtually poikilothermic in REM sleep.[30] This inability to thermoregulate in REM sleep probably affects the response to temperature extremes and suggests that such conditions are less of a problem early during a night than late, when REM sleep tends to predominate. It should be clear, as well, that sweating or shivering during sleep in response to ambient temperature extremes occurs in NREM sleep and ceases in REM sleep.

Drug Ingestion

The distribution of sleep states and stages is affected by many common drugs, including those typically prescribed in the treatment of sleep disorders as well as those not specifically related to the pharmacotherapy of sleep disorders and those used socially or recreationally. It is unknown whether changes in sleep stage distribution have any relevance to health, illness, or psychological well-being; however, particularly in the context of specific sleep disorders that differentially affect one sleep stage or another, such distinctions may be relevant to diagnosis or treatment. A number of generalizations regarding the effects of certain of the more frequently used compounds on sleep stage distribution follow:

1. Benzodiazepines tend to suppress SWS and have no consistent effect on REM sleep.
2. Tricyclic antidepressants and monoamine oxidase inhibitors (MAOIs) tend to suppress REM sleep. An increased level of motor activity during sleep occurs with certain of these compounds, leading to a pattern of REM sleep without motor inhibition or an increased incidence of PMS.
3. Withdrawal from drugs that selectively suppress a stage of sleep tends to be associated with a rebound of that sleep stage. Thus, acute withdrawal from a benzodiazepine compound is likely to produce an increase of SWS; acute withdrawal from a tricyclic antidepressant or MAOI is likely to produce an increase of REM sleep. In the latter case, this REM rebound could result in abnormal SOREMPs in the absence of an organic sleep disorder, perhaps leading to a false-positive diagnosis of narcolepsy.
4. Acute presleep alcohol intake produces REM suppression early in the night, which is often followed by REM sleep rebound in the latter portion of the night as the alcohol is metabolized.
5. Acute effects of marijuana (tetrahydrocannabinol [THC]) include minimal sleep disruption, characterized by a slight reduction of REM sleep. Chronic ingestion of THC produces a long-term suppression of SWS.[31]

Pathology

Sleep disorders, as well as other nonsleep problems, have an impact on the structure and distribution of sleep. As suggested before, these distinctions appear to be more important in diagnosis and in the consideration of treatments than in any implications about general health or illness resulting from specific sleep stage alterations. Listed are a number of common sleep stage anomalies associated with sleep disorders:

1. *Narcolepsy* is characterized by an abnormally short delay to REM sleep, marked by SOREMPs. This abnormal sleep onset pattern occurs with some consistency, but not exclusively; that is, NREM sleep onset can also occur. Thus, the preferred diagnostic test consists of several opportunities to fall asleep across a day (see Chapter 104). If REM sleep occurs abnormally on two such opportunities, narcolepsy is extremely probable. The occurrence of this abnormal sleep pattern in narcolepsy is thought to be responsible for the rather unusual symptoms of this disorder. In other words, dissociation of components of REM sleep into the waking state results in hypnagogic hallucinations, sleep paralysis, and, most dramatically, cataplexy. Other conditions in which a short REM latency may occur include infancy, in which sleep-onset REM is normal; sleep reversal or jet lag; acute withdrawal from REM-suppressant compounds; chronic restriction or disruption of sleep; and endogenous depression, in which a shortened latency to REM sleep is thought to be a biological marker of this psychiatric entity.[32] Recent reports have indicated a relatively high prevalence of REM onsets in young adults[32a] and in adolescents with early rise times.[32b] In the latter, the REM onsets on morning (8:30 and 10:30 AM) naps were related to a delayed circadian phase as indicated by later onset of melatonin secretion.
2. *Sleep apnea syndromes* may be associated with suppression of SWS or REM sleep, secondary to the sleep-related breathing problem. Suppression of SWS occurs most commonly in children with sleep apnea; REM suppression is more common in adults with sleep apnea syndromes. Successful treatment of this sleep disorder, as with nocturnal continuous positive airway pressure (CPAP), produces huge rebounds of SWS or REM sleep (Fig. 2–10).

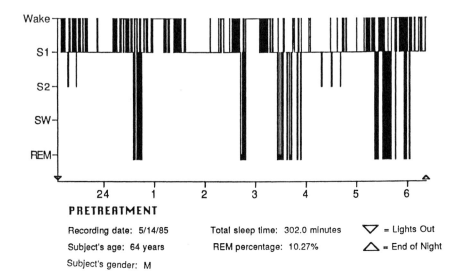

PRETREATMENT

Recording date: 5/14/85	Total sleep time: 302.0 minutes	▽ = Lights Out
Subject's age: 64 years	REM percentage: 10.27%	△ = End of Night
Subject's gender: M		

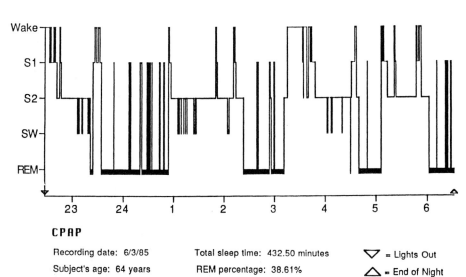

CPAP

Recording date: 6/3/85	Total sleep time: 432.50 minutes	▽ = Lights Out
Subject's age: 64 years	REM percentage: 38.61%	△ = End of Night
Subject's gender: M		

Figure 2-10. These sleep histograms depict the sleep of a 64-year-old male patient with obstructive sleep apnea syndrome. The upper graph shows the sleep pattern before treatment. Note the absence of slow wave (SW) (stage 3 or 4) sleep, the preponderance of stage 1 (S1), and the very frequent disruptions. The lower graph shows the sleep pattern in this patient during the second night of treatment with continuous positive airway pressure (CPAP). Note that sleep is much deeper (more SW) and more consolidated, and REM sleep in particular is abnormally increased. The pretreatment REM percentage of sleep was only 10%, versus nearly 40% with treatment. (Data supplied by G. Nino-Murcia, Stanford University Sleep Disorders Center, Stanford, California.)

3. *Fragmentation of sleep and increased frequency of arousals* occur in association with a number of sleep disorders as well as with medical disorders involving physical pain or discomfort. PMS, sleep apnea syndromes, chronic fibrositis, and so forth may be associated with tens to hundreds of arousals each night. Brief arousals are prominent in such conditions as allergic rhinitis,[33, 34] juvenile rheumatoid arthritis,[35] and Parkinson's disease.[36] In upper airway resistance syndrome (UARS),[37] EEG arousals are important markers because the respiratory signs of UARS are less obvious than in frank obstructive sleep apnea syndrome (OSAS), and only subtle indicators may be available.[38] In specific situations, autonomic changes, such as transient changes of blood pressure,[39] may signify arousals; Lofaso and colleagues[40] indicated that autonomic changes are highly correlated with the extent of EEG arousals. Less well studied is the possibility that sleep fragmentation may be associated with subcortical events not visible in the cortical EEG signal. These disorders also often involve an increase in the absolute amount of and the proportion of stage 1 sleep.

Acknowledgments

We thank Joan Mancuso for preparing the figures and Lisa Donovan for preparing the typescript.

References

1. Dement W, Kleitman N. The relation of eye movements during sleep to dream activity: an objective method for the study of dreaming. J Exp Psychol. 1957;53:339–346.
2. Agnew HW, Webb WB. Measurement of sleep onset by EEG criteria. Am J EEG Technol. 1972;12:127–134.
3. Davis H, Davis PA, Loomis AL, et al. Human brain potentials during the onset of sleep. J Neurophysiol. 1938;1:24–38.
4. Carskadon MA, Dement WC. Effects of total sleep loss on sleep tendency. Percept Mot Skills. 1979;48:495–506.
5. Guilleminault C, Phillips R, Dement WC. A syndrome of hypersomnia with automatic behavior. Electroencephalogr Clin Neurophysiol. 1975;38:403–413.

6. Ogilvie RD, Wilkinson RT. The detection of sleep onset: behavioral and physiological convergence. Psychophysiology. 1984;21:510–520.

7. Williams HL, Hammack JT, Daly RL, et al. Responses to auditory stimulation, sleep loss and the EEG stages of sleep. Electroencephalogr Clin Neurophysiol. 1964;16:269–279.

8. Oswald I, Taylor AM, Treisman M. Discriminative responses to stimulation during human sleep. Brain. 1960;83:440–453.

9. Williams HL, Morlock HC, Morlock JV. Instrumental behavior during sleep. Psychophysiology. 1966;2:208–216.

10. Foulkes D. The Psychology of Sleep. New York, NY: Charles Scribner's Sons; 1966.

11. Wyatt JK, Bootzin RR, Anthony J, et al. Does sleep onset produce retrograde amnesia? Sleep Res. 1992;21:113.

12. Rechtschaffen A, Kales A, eds. A Manual of Standardized Terminology, Techniques and Scoring System for Sleep Stages of Human Subjects. Los Angeles, Calif: UCLA Brain Information Service/Brain Research Institute; 1968.

13. Czeisler CA, Zimmerman JC, Ronda JM, et al. Timing of REM sleep is coupled to the circadian rhythm of body temperature in man. Sleep. 1980;2:329–346.

14. Zulley J. Distribution of REM sleep in entrained 24 hour and free-running sleep-wake cycles. Sleep. 1980;2:377–389.

15. Weitzman ED, Czeisler CA, Zimmerman JC, et al. Timing of REM and stages 3 + 4 sleep during temporal isolation in man. Sleep. 1980;2:391–407.

16. Karacan I, Moore CA. Genetics and human sleep. Psychiatr Ann. 1979;9:11–23.

17. Busby K, Pivik RT. Failure of high intensity auditory stimuli to affect behavioral arousal in children during the first sleep cycle. Pediatr Res. 1983;17:802–805.

18. Carskadon MA, Dement WC. Sleepiness in the normal adolescent. In: Guilleminault C, ed. Sleep and Its Disorders in Children. New York, NY: Raven Press; 1987:53–66.

19. Feinberg I. Schizophrenia: caused by a fault in programmed synaptic elimination during adolescence? J Psychiatr Res. 1983;17:319–334.

20. Prinz P. Sleep patterns in the healthy aged: relationship with intellectual function. J Gerontol. 1977;32:179–186.

21. Prinz PN, Peskind ER, Vitaliano PP, et al. Changes in the sleep and waking EEGs of nondemented and demented elderly subjects. J Am Geriatr Soc. 1982;30:86–93.

22. Carskadon MA, Brown ED, Dement WC. Sleep fragmentation in the elderly: relationship to daytime sleep tendency. Neurobiol Aging. 1982;3:321–327.

23. Ancoli-Israel S, Kripke DF, Mason W, et al. Sleep apnea and nocturnal myoclonus in a senior population. Sleep. 1981;4:349–358.

24. Carskadon MA, Dement WC. Respiration during sleep in the aging human. J Gerontol. 1981;36:420–423.

25. Williams RL, Karacan I, Hursch CJ. EEG of Human Sleep: Clinical Applications. New York, NY: John Wiley & Sons; 1974.

26. Agnew HW, Webb WB, Williams RL. The first-night effect: an EEG study of sleep. Psychophysiology. 1966;2:263–266.

27. Czeisler CA, Weitzman ED, Moore-Ede MC, et al. Human sleep: its duration and organization depend on its circadian phase. Science. 1980;210:1264–1267.

28. Zulley J, Wever R, Aschoff J. The dependence of onset and duration of sleep on the circadian rhythm of rectal temperature. Pflugers Arch. 1981;391:314–318.

29. Strogatz SH. The Mathematical Structure of the Human Sleep-Wake Cycle. New York, NY: Springer-Verlag; 1986.

30. Parmeggiani PL. Temperature regulation during sleep: a study in homeostasis. In: Orem J, Barnes CD, eds. Physiology in Sleep. New York, NY: Academic Press; 1980:98–143.

31. Freemon FR. The effect of chronically administered delta-9-tetrahydrocannabinol upon the polygraphically monitored sleep of normal volunteers. Drug Alcohol Depend. 1982;10:345–353.

32. Kupfer DJ. REM latency: a psychobiologic marker for primary depressive disease. Biol Psychiatry. 1976;11:159–174.

32a. Bishop C, Rosenthal L, Helmus T, et al. The frequency of multiple sleep onset REM periods among subjects with no excessive daytime sleepiness. Sleep. 1996;19:727–730.

32b. Carskadon MA, Wolfson AR, Acebo C, et al. Adolescent sleep patterns, circadian timing, and sleepiness at a transition to early school days. Sleep. 1998;21:871–881.

33. Lavie P, Gertner R, Zomer J, et al. Breathing disorders in sleep associated with "microarousals" in patients with allergic rhinitis. Acta Otolaryngol. 1981;92:529–533.

34. Craig TJ, Teets S, Lehman EB, et al. Nasal congestion secondary to allergic rhinitis as a cause of sleep disturbance and daytime fatigue and the response to topical nasal corticosteroids. J Allergy Clin Immunol. 1998;101:633–637.

35. Zamir G, Press J, Tal A, et al. Sleep fragmentation in children with juvenile rheumatoid arthritis. J Rheumatol. 1998;25:1191–1197.

36. Stocchi F, Barbato L, Nordera G, et al. Sleep disorders in Parkinson's disease. J Neurol. 1998;245(suppl 1):S15–S18.

37. Guilleminault C, Stoohs R, Clerk A, et al. From obstructive sleep apnea syndrome to upper airway resistance syndrome—consistency of daytime sleepiness. Sleep. 1992;15(6 suppl):S13–S16.

38. Hosselet JJ, Norman RG, Ayappa I, et al. Detection of flow limitation with a nasal cannula/pressure transducer system. Am J Respir Crit Care Med. 1998;157:1461–1467.

39. Pitson DJ, Stradling JR. Autonomic markers of arousal during sleep in patients undergoing investigation for obstructive sleep apnoea, their relationship to EEG arousals, respiratory events and subjective sleepiness. J Sleep Res. 1998;7:53–59.

40. Lofaso F, Goldenberg F, Dortho MP, et al. Arterial blood pressure response to transient arousals from NREM sleep in nonapneic snorers with sleep fragmentation. Chest. 1998;11qq3:985–991.

3

Normal Aging

Donald L. Bliwise

As the populations of industrialized societies age, knowledge of defining how sleep is affected by age will assume greater importance. Within the United States, the average current life expectancy of 77 years means that 80% of residents now live to be at least 65; the fastest growing segment of the population is those who are 85 and older. These huge numbers force sleep specialists to confront what is *normal*. Investigators often use the term to connote a variety of meanings. In sleep disorders, frequent confusion occurs because the term is used descriptively, to indicate representativeness, as well as clinically, to indicate absence of disease.

Aging is also subject to semantic confusion. Chronological age has been shown repeatedly only to approximate physiological age. The decline in slow-wave sleep, for example, may occur at a chronological age far earlier than most age-related declines in other biological functions. Some researchers in gerontology have noted that distance from death may be a far better approximation of the aging process, but too few longitudinal sleep studies exist to yield these types of findings.

In addition to the issue of physiological age, subjective age must be considered. Because the practice of sleep disorders medicine in geriatrics relies heavily on the increased self-reports of sleep disturbance seen in aging, subjective appraisal of the older person's symptoms must be considered. Whether an aged person views 75% sleep efficiency as insomnia or merely accepts this as a normal part of aging may depend largely on that individual's perspective on growing old and what that means to him or her. Middelkoop et al.[1] have recently suggested that older people are more likely to perceive themselves as having sleep problems if they have difficulty falling asleep rather than staying asleep, even though the latter continues to be a generally more commonly endorsed symptom. In addition, some have suggested that self-reports of polysomnographically (PSG) measured sleep are inherently less accurate and valid in older relative to younger subjects,[2] although evidence for such age differences in other studies is decidedly mixed and varies according to the variables under consideration or the subject's gender.[3]

Finally, normal aging must be viewed in counterpoint to pathological aging (see Chapter 89). Although the prevalence of dementing illnesses is high in late life, determination of the number of normal elderly persons who may be in incipient stages of dementia has seldom been addressed. Unlike sleep studies in dementia, in which diagnostic procedures have been used typically to rule out causes of reversible dementia, few sleep studies of normal aging rely on extensive diagnostic work to eliminate individuals in the earliest stages of mental impairment.

The point here is not to dismiss all that is known about sleep patterns in normal aging as inadequate but rather to point out the complexities of defining normal aging. Normal aging can never be defined without some arbitrary criteria. In most of the work summarized, sleep is defined in normal aging in humans as those representative sleep characteristics occurring in the presumed nondemented population older than 60 years. It is also important to recognize that the age-dependent alterations in sleep described in the following sections may have minimal relationship to age changes in sleep processes per se and may simply be secondary manifestations of senescence.

INSOMNIA AND ASSOCIATED RISK FACTORS IN OLD AGE

Prevalence, Incidence, and Medical Risk Factors

The prevalence of insomnia in the aged varies across studies, but a recent summary suggested a range of prevalence between 19.0 and 38.4%.[4] In one of the largest surveys of an American population (the Established Populations for Epidemiologic Studies of the Elderly [EPESE] with more than 9000 participants), Foley et al.[4] reported that 29% of the over-65 population had difficulty maintaining sleep. Relative to sleep maintenance, sleep latency is less likely to be problematic for the elderly population with prevalence figures on the order of 10 to 19% typically seen,[4] although Ganguli et al[5] reported a relatively high prevalence of sleep latency problems (36.7%) in a largely rural aged population. In nearly all studies, elderly women have a greater probability of sleep complaints (for review, see reference 6) and sedative-hypnotic use than elderly men (for review, see reference 7). Elderly black individuals generally report fewer sleep complaints than the elderly white population.[8]

Much evidence suggests medical diseases and chronic illness play an important role in much of the poor sleep seen in old age. In fact, when a sufficient number of other causes of poor sleep are taken into account, chronological age may explain little of the observed prevalence in the elderly.[4] Bliwise et al.[6] reported that individuals screened for medical disease and psychiatric history had low prevalence of sleep complaints. Morgan et al.[9, 10] reported that the use of medications (excluding hypnotics) for a variety of health conditions differentiated good and poor sleepers and noted that the number of physician visits and self-ratings of health also distinguished the groups. Gislason and Almqvist[11] reported that when somatic diseases were controlled multivariately, some types of insomnia complaints showed no age-dependent increase, and some even showed a decrease with age. Hanson and Ostergren[12] noted that among a representative sample of 68-year-old men, users of the health care system were more likely to suffer from insomnia.

Finally, Ford and Kamerow's[13] study showed that when individuals with poor sleep accompanying physical illness, medication use, or drug and alcohol use were not included in a definition for insomnia, age-dependent prevalence rates of poor sleep were far less striking than in most previous studies, and, in fact, no age-dependent increase was detected unless insomnia was present on two separate interviews separated by 1 year. More specifically, conditions such as headache, diabetes, and chronic pain have all been shown to have differential impact on the sleep of older subjects.[7, 11, 14-18] Respiratory symptoms (chronic cough, phlegm) in particular appear to frequently be associated with insomnia in the elderly population.[18-20] The effects may be independent from use of respiratory stimulant medication[4, 21] and may not be reflected by spirometry.[20]

Several longitudinal studies examining the incidence (development of new cases) of insomnia over periods of up to 10 years have been reported. Klink et al.[22] have shown that the single best predictor of insomnia continuing longer than 10 years was insomnia at a previous time, although cardiovascular and pulmonary comorbidities conferred risk as well in the over-65 population. Reported remissions were less likely in older subjects than younger.[21] The EPESE data indicated a yearly incidence of insomnia complaints in the aged population of about 5%, with a spontaneous remission rate of about 50% over 3 years.[23] In these data, incident insomnia was related to heart disease, stroke, hip fracture, and new onset depression; spontaneous remission was related to the resolution of depression, physical illness, and physical disability affecting activities of daily living.[23]

Nocturia

An often overlooked cause of nocturnal awakenings in the elderly population is *nocturia*, the voluntary voiding of urine during the night. Some have suggested that older people are simply more susceptible to such events; they are more likely to awaken during the night because of their intrinsic sleep fragmentation, which leads to awareness of the need to void.[24] Several epidemiologic studies have shown that nocturia is common in the aged population. Foley et al.[4] estimated

that the prevalence of middle of the night awakening increases from 28 to 43% if awakenings due to nocturia are included. Middelkoop et al.[1] listed nocturia as by far the most common explanation (cited by 63 to 72%) offered by elderly people as to the cause of their inability to stay asleep.

Nocturia is associated with daytime tiredness and poor sleep.[25-27] Although it is often assumed that nocturnal voiding represents urologic causes, such as benign prostatic hypertrophy in men and decreased urethral resistance in women (secondary to declines in estrogen),[28, 29] the association between symptoms of sleep apnea and nocturia,[30] as well as potential increases in urine output in association with the sleep apnea of the elderly (possibly caused by increased levels of circulating atrial natriuretic peptide [ANP]),[31, 32] suggest a nonurologic basis for nocturia. Sleep apnea might operate to increase urinary urgency primarily by mechanical factors[33] by increasing detrusor pressure secondary to negative intrathoracic pressure. In view of this, it is of interest to note that *nocturnal enuresis* (involuntary voiding during the night) occurs in 2.9% (women) and 1.0% (men) of the elderly community-dwelling population. Nocturnal enuresis is associated with nocturnal shortness of breath and use of multiple pillows for sleep.[34]

Menopause

Menopause may be associated with poor sleep.[15] These changes are thought to reflect endocrine effects and, only secondarily, psychological factors. Among a French cohort of more than 1000 midlife women, subjective sleep disturbance was associated with menopausal status apart from chronologic age.[35] Vasomotor symptoms result in lower sleep efficiency and a higher number of arousals in menopausal women,[36, 37] although the peak incidence of hot flashes occurred before the usual onset of sleep. The possibility that sleep is disturbed perimenopausally apart from vasomotor symptoms has been suggested. Polo-Kantola et al.[38] and others have shown that nocturia may be a better predictor of self-reported sleep disturbance in menopausal women relative to the vasomotor symptoms.[26, 39]

In view of these results, it may not be surprising that some studies have reported that estrogen replacement therapy (ERT), typically initiated for symptoms other than poor sleep, is associated with better quality sleep,[38, 40] whereas other studies do not show improvement or even suggest poorer quality sleep is associated with ERT.[35, 41] Moe et al. have suggested that the improvement in sleep (or lack thereof) seen with ERT may be a function of the extent to which estrogen negatively affects the insulin-like growth factor-1/ growth hormone (IGF-1/GH) axis; higher IGF-1 levels are associated with better quality sleep recorded on PSG.[41-43]

Montplaisir et al.[44] have shown, in a randomized clinical trial, that women receiving ERT plus a natural form of progesterone showed on PSG better sleep than women receiving ERT with a standard progesterone formulation. The effects of menopausal status on snoring and sleep apnea symptoms have been shown to largely be a function of the confounding effects of advancing age and increased body mass index (BMI) occurring menopausally.[45, 46] Similarly, increased nasal resistance was better related to BMI and craniofacial structure than menopausal status,[47] and ERT had no beneficial effect on disordered breathing in sleep in postmenopausal women with sleep apnea.[48]

Factors Intrinsic to Sleep

There are many alterations specific to sleep itself that change in aging (e.g., sleep architecture) (see later). Additionally, factors such as a greater susceptibility to external arousal[49] may predispose the aged person to poor sleep. Putative changes in circadian rhythm amplitude (see later), as evidenced by age-dependent increases in daytime napping and fatigue and, possibly, increased daytime sleep tendency on the multiple sleep latency test (MSLT) or other daytime nap tests,[50–52] may also predispose a person to poor quality of sleep. Simple inactivity and bedrest, so common in the more infirm geriatric population, have been shown to disrupt sleep in younger subjects,[53] and curtailment of daytime napping and bedrest may improve sleep in the elderly.[54] Levels of outdoor light exposure in elderly subjects, although not always significantly less than in younger subjects,[55] have been speculated to predispose elderly subjects to poor sleep; preliminary data suggest bright light as an effective treatment for poor sleep in the elderly.[56] Finally, the role of periodic limb movements (PLMs) in the disturbed sleep of the elderly is highly controversial and is discussed more fully later in this chapter.

Psychological and Psychosocial Factors

Despite the importance of the factors intrinsic to sleep in the widespread poor sleep experienced by elderly people, the role of psychological issues must not be dismissed. Loss of a spouse, a yearly occurrence for 1.6% of elderly men and 3.0% of elderly women in the American population, is a particularly devastating condition associated with depression in many older adults.[57, 58] Recent PSG studies of such geriatric populations who do not have a history of previous depression have shown some of the same findings as geriatric patients with major depressive disorders. Specifically, such patients demonstrated similar low sleep efficiencies (about 72 to 73%).[59] Conversely, bereaved patients with adjustment reactions (subsyndromally depressed) showed PSG characteristics that did not differ[58] or differed only minimally[60] from elderly controls. Factors salient for geriatric populations such as retirement,[61] holocaust trauma,[62] and fear of death in sleep[63] can disrupt sleep, as can anxiety and depression,[64] and there is only mixed evidence that the associations between psychopathology and disturbed sleep, so well

demonstrated in younger patients, are in any way abated in older patients.[65, 66]

Treatment Considerations

The overwhelming message from the aforementioned literature regarding the huge number of potential co-morbidities disrupting sleep in the elderly is that effective insomnia treatment implies that management should first focus on primary medical disease. In practice, of course, the sleep medicine specialist may be asked to offer management apart from such considerations. The following issues should be considered in the elderly.

The prevalence of prescription hypnotic medication use in the elderly population is approximately 10 to 16%,[67, 68] and many elderly people continue to use medications for sleep even when their sleep continues to be disturbed.[4, 19, 69] In one recent study, although both medical and psychological burden predicted hypnotic drug use in the aged, persistent use in the elderly over a period of 6 years was far more related to depression than medical disease.[67] The analysis by Kripke et al.[70] of prescription hypnotic use in 1982 in a study population of 1.1 million Americans showed that higher all-cause and specific-cause mortality were associated with regular use of such medication. In subjects over age 70, these risks were conferred by nightly use, whereas in younger subjects, the risks were apparent at both nightly and more moderate levels of consumption. These results suggest that nonpharmacological alternatives or adjunctive treatments for late-life insomnia should always be considered.

Several nonpharmacological treatments have been shown to improve sleep in the elderly: cognitive behavior therapy,[71, 72] sleep restriction therapy,[54] appropriately timed bright light,[56] exercise (including both strength training and aerobic activity),[73, 74] and passive body heating.[75] Melatonin's utility as a hypnotic is covered in Chapter 31.

Finally, although the poor sleep of old age may have many causes, the possibility exists that poor sleep itself leads to adverse outcomes. For example, poor sleep not only reduces quality of life in older subjects but also several epidemiologic studies examining subjective total sleep times (TSTs) have shown that lower sleep durations were associated with higher rates of all-cause mortality.[76, 77] These findings were not attenuated by age. More recent studies examining the natural history of insomnia complaints[4, 5, 78, 79] and estimated sleep durations[78, 80] did not support these results. Nonetheless, poor sleep may predispose for psychiatric morbidity; at least three longitudinal studies have noted that poor sleep confers a risk for incident depression in older subjects.[13, 23, 81]

SLEEP ARCHITECTURE

Age-dependent changes in sleep architecture have been well described, although not until recently have such data eliminated sleep disordered breathing and PLMs as possible confounding variables in generating such normative data. The presence of even mild forms of such sleep pathology would be expected to contribute to increased levels of stage 1 and lower sleep efficiencies.

Following adaptation to the sleep laboratory or in ambulatory home recordings, elderly subjects in optimal health without sleep pathology typically have sleep efficiencies in the range of 80 to 85%[82–85] and stage 1 in the range of 4 to 10%.[82, 85–87] Gender effects may be apparent; a meta-analysis of PSG data showed that older women sleep somewhat better than older men.[88] This contrasts with the self-report data mentioned earlier in which elderly women typically report more sleep complaints than do elderly men. Spindle counts have been shown to decrease with age.[89]

Although it is generally agreed that transient arousals increase in the elderly population, normative data on brief arousals may prove more difficult to reconcile across laboratories. Boselli et al.[90] have shown that elderly people without sleep apnea and without upper airway resistance (UAR) had approximately 27 arousals per sleep hour, using the American Sleep Disorders Association (ASDA) criteria. Earlier work by Carskadon et al.[91] reported about 23 arousals per hour, despite the fact that these data included some individuals with mild levels of sleep-disordered breathing (SDB), did not exclude for UAR or PLMs, and were scored before the advent of ASDA criteria. Reliable scoring of brief arousals remains a formidable task.[92, 93] Additionally, even among healthy young adults with sleep efficiencies of 90%, arousal rates of 10 per hour may be seen.[94]

The most easily recognized age-related change in a sleep stage is the decrease in slow-wave sleep (SWS) (stage 3 and 4). Studies relying on visual analysis of stages 3 and 4 sleep suggested that these stages occupy approximately 5 to 10% of total sleep in healthy elderly subjects,[83–85, 87] although preliminary data from the Sleep Heart Health Study suggested that figures as high as 18 to 20% may be seen.[86] Additionally, visually scored SWS decreased with advancing age in men but increased with age in women.[86] The precise age at which SWS declines has yet to be determined conclusively, although some studies suggest a decline may be seen by age 20 years (see Maturation and Aging). A computer analysis of delta activity suggested age-dependent declines can be seen when individuals in their 70s are compared with those in their 80s.[95] Another meta-analysis found little evidence of an age-dependent decline in visually scored SWS above age 20 years, although interlaboratory and interscorer differences probably affected these results more than for other visually scored sleep architecture measures.[96] Computer analyses have suggested that the decline in delta is best characterized as a decrease in the amplitude of the slow wave activity (Fig. 3–1), although a slightly higher frequency of delta may be seen as well.[97] Some researchers have proposed that the usual (75 µV) amplitude criterion for delta activity be abolished for old age,[98] thus correcting for the absence of delta by scoring only for frequency. Studies adopting such a definition have effectively eliminated age differences in SWS. The potential merit of such alterations in conventional scoring and recording procedures would be the greater validity of such age-corrected SWS data; however, inasmuch as the functional significance and mechanism of delta activity remains obscure, such normalization procedures remain premature. Some data have suggested that older women have better-preserved SWS than do men,[99] and computer electroencephalographic (EEG) analysis has confirmed this finding.[95] Dijk et al.[100] contended that the gender difference in SWS in the elderly is discernible in younger people as well and predominantly reflects extracerebral factors such as skull thickness.

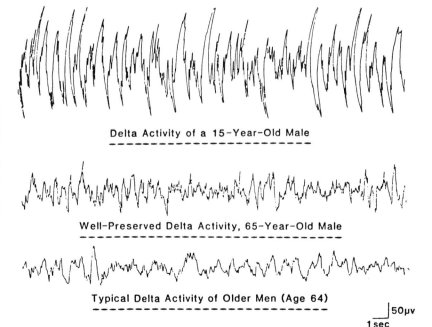

Figure 3–1. Age differences in delta activity. The top tracing shows typically abundant high-amplitude delta in an adolescent. The middle tracing shows particularly well-preserved delta in an older man. Note the marked decrease in amplitude relative to the adolescent. The bottom tracing is a more typical example of delta activity in an older man. Note the number of waves failing to meet the 75-µV amplitude criterion. (From Zepelin H. Normal age related change in sleep. In: Chase MH, Weitzman ED, eds. Sleep Disorders: Basic and Clinical Research. New York, NY: Spectrum; 1983:431–445.)

Delta Activity of a 15-Year-Old Male

Well-Preserved Delta Activity, 65-Year-Old Male

Typical Delta Activity of Older Men (Age 64)

50µv

1 sec

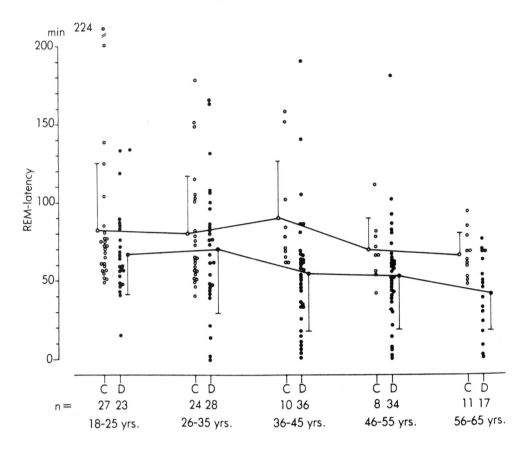

Figure 3–2. Mean, standard deviation, and individual values for REM latency as a function of age in control subjects (C) *(open circles)* and depressed (D) *(closed circles)* patients. REM latency is defined in this study as the time from the first epoch of stage 2 sleep to the first epoch of REM. (From Reiman D, Laver C, Hohagen F, et al. Long term evolution of sleep in depression. In: Smirne S, Franceschi M, Ferini-Strambi L, eds. Sleep and Aging: Proceedings of the Second Milano International Symposium on Sleep, Milano, October 12–14, 1989. Milan, Italy: Masson; 1991:195–204.)

Disagreement exists regarding whether or not the proportion of nocturnal sleep spent in rapid eye movement (REM) sleep (i.e., REM percentage) varies with aging.[101–103] Meta-analysis by Benca et al.[96] showed some evidence of a decline in REM time but a lengthening of the first REM period with aging. Even when age differences are observed, the magnitude of the findings is certainly not impressive. In Sleep Heart Health Study subjects without sleep apnea, for example, REM percentage dropped slightly from about 21% in subjects younger than 60 to about 18% in subjects older than 80 years of age but without the gender effects noted for SWS.[86] Perhaps some of the disagreement across studies involves the fact that REM percentage can be manipulated in a quasi-artificial manner by allowing different lengths of sleep (i.e., adjusting wake-up times). Because the laboratory environment can never mimic a true ad lib sleep situation (unless the studies are performed in a time isolation protocol), REM percentage may simply be an inherently less stable parameter.[104] Suffice it to say that if REM percentage declines with normal aging, the effect is not of sufficient magnitude to overpower these confounds across studies. Gender differences in REM percentage in old age are inconsistent.[88]

Age differences in the duration of nonrapid eye movement (NREM) sleep before the first REM period of the night (REM latency), with older subjects showing shorter latencies than younger subjects, have been shown in some studies of normal and depressed patients,[96, 105, 106] although some find the effect only in the latter[107, 108] (Fig. 3–2). The result may be a function of the decreased stages 3 and 4 sleep within that cycle as a function of aging. One additional possibility in explaining short REM latencies in aged individuals is an age-dependent change in the circadian timing system. Specifically, if the core body temperature (T_b) curve is phase-advanced relative to sleep onset, an early-onset REM might be predicted.

Because some have contended that differences in sleep parameters between normal and depressive patients should be more pronounced in the elderly,[109] several meta-analyses have attempted to examine standardized differences between such groups as a function of age.[96, 110] Results suggested that aged depressive patients showed relatively lower sleep efficiencies than did aged controls and that those differences were more pronounced than in younger patients and controls. Findings with REM parameters (including REM latencies) were somewhat more ambiguous. As a final note on this issue, Vitiello et al.[111] suggested that if elderly normal and depressive patients are recruited from the community rather than by clinical referrals, there are few differences in sleep patterns.

MATURATION AND AGING

The point at which age-dependent decline in delta activity begins has been a subject of controversy. Several studies suggested that the decline begins around age 20 years.[105, 106, 112, 113] Studies using automated analysis showed negative relationships between age and the number of delta zero–crossings[114] and delta amplitude[114, 115] in young adults in their 20s, although a replication by Feinberg et al.[116] found only the former. Delta wave counts showed a 50% reduction when men 21 to 30 years old were compared with men ages 31 to 40 years old.[117] Perhaps even more provocative are results suggesting declines across adolescence per se.[118] Consistent with this are enormous individual differences in visually scored SWS in young adults, even within a highly restricted age range.[119, 120]

Assuming the validity of such age-dependent changes, how can one interpret these results? Such changes may reflect normal maturational processes regarding declining cortical metabolic rate, increasing dendritic pruning, and decreasing cortical synaptic activity.[121] Or such changes may represent an extremely early biomarker of aging within the central nervous system (CNS). This would link aging processes to attainment of reproductive maturity, a model supported by studies in several mammalian species.[122] Evidence of aging at such a young *chronological age* is not nearly as incongruous as it appears when one considers *physiological age*. Human life expectancy before the development of modern civilization was on the order of 20 to 30 years.[123] Declines in delta activity across adolescence may thus be an evolutionary remnant of the initiation of senescent processes.

CHANGES IN SLEEP NEED WITH AGE

One of the common myths regarding aging and sleep is that the need for sleep does not change with age. There are several ways to examine this issue.[124] One approach is simply to look at sleep quotas, the amount of time individuals typically sleep as they age. Although some laboratory studies[105, 125] and some surveys[126, 127] have shown reduced sleep times in the elderly, not all survey data concur[76, 128, 129]; some suggest no change or even increases in sleep times with age (see earlier data on nocturnal awakenings with aging). Some of these studies included napping in their totals, which implies a redistribution of sleep around the 24-h day. If, in fact, net sleep amounts do not change with aging, the need for sleep may be just as strong in old age, but that need may be met differently. Napping in old age, however, cannot simply be equated with unfulfilled sleep need, because both cultural and social factors undoubtedly have a role. Physiological studies of daytime alertness in elderly subjects demonstrated enhanced pupillary miosis[130] and, in some[50–52, 131, 132] but not all studies,[133] enhanced sleepiness on the MSLT or other daytime nap tests, findings that provide some additional support for the notion of a modified expression of sleep need. Nonetheless, the presence of sleep apnea may provide a partial, but not complete, explanation of such increased sleepiness (see later).

Among experimental paradigms, the most frequently used putative manipulation of sleep need in the elderly has been sleep deprivation. Most studies showed increases in TSTs after 36 to 64 h of sleep loss.[134–138] In one study, elderly insomniacs undergoing 64 h of sleep loss showed recovery increases in TST of more than 90 min, which essentially made their postdeprivation sleep equivalent to good-sleeping elderly subjects[138] (Fig. 3–3). However, in another report of 36 h of sleep loss, neither elderly depressives nor demented patients showed such a "re-normalization" of sleep length, although clear, significant increases in TST were noted.[135] Increases in SWS after deprivation have been noted in elderly subjects.[134–138] REM sleep results are more complicated to interpret inasmuch as REM percentage has been reported to increase,[137] decrease,[135] or not change[134, 136] after sleep deprivation. REM latency, however, has been shown to increase after deprivation in both patients with depression and

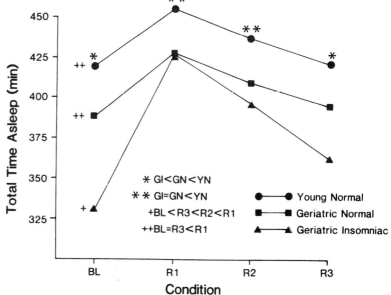

Figure 3–3. Changes in total sleep time after 64 h of sleep deprivation as a function of age. BL, baseline; R1–R3, recovery nights 1–3; YN, young normals; GN, geriatric normals; GI, geriatric insomniacs. Significant group differences are indicated by asterisks, and significant study day differences by plus (+) signs. Note that the effects of sleep deprivation in young and elderly subjects are similar, but age differences in absolute sleep amounts remain. (From Bonnet MH, Rosa RR. Sleep and performance in young adults and older normals and insomniacs during acute sleep loss and recovery. Biol Psychol. 1987;25:153–172.)

with dementia but to decrease in controls,[135] the latter result also noted by Bonnet and Rosa.[138] In a later study of selective REM deprivation, Reynolds et al.[139] noted that during recovery sleep, most REM measures showed predictable patterns of response (greater number of REM periods, higher REM percentage, reduced REM latencies, higher REM density) regardless of diagnostic group, although on the deprivation night some differential diagnostic group interactions were observed.

Taken as a whole, sleep deprivation studies suggest that the fundamental homeostatic response to sleep loss in the elderly is preserved. However, it has been noted that most aspects of sleep architecture are modified only on the 1st night of postdeprivation recovery sleep in elderly subjects, whereas in younger subjects, the effects persist for several additional nights.[134, 138] Age differences in MSLT-defined daytime sleepiness after sleep deprivation[134] also suggest more rapid recovery in this measure as well as in older relative to younger subjects. Furthermore, during sleep deprivation, elderly subjects appear to have fewer microsleep episodes than do younger subjects.[140] When examining performance measures, a number of studies have suggested that older subjects, particularly if they are poor sleepers,[141] appear *less* affected by sleep loss than are younger subjects and return to baseline levels of performance more quickly or at least no more slowly.[134, 138, 142, 143]

These studies indicate that to speak of continued sleep need (or modification thereof) in old age is an overly simplistic concept that is not consistently and unequivocally supported by the existing knowledge base. The results can be variously construed as evidence for an age-dependent decreased need, an unchanged need, an unchanged need but deficient mechanism, or perhaps an alteration in type of need. More recent studies of circadian rhythms in aging also suggest a complex interpretation of altered homeostatic regulation of sleep in the aged (see Circadian Rhythms in Aging).

CIRCADIAN RHYTHMS IN AGING

Besides the changes in sleep mentioned earlier, there are many age-dependent chronobiological changes in physiological functions including body temperature, the endocrine system, and numerous blood constituents. Some have considered the temporal disorganization of physiology to be the fundamental characterization of the aging process.[144] Integration of circadian rhythms depends on the suprachiasmatic nucleus (SCN) of the anterior hypothalamus. Because the SCN is known to deteriorate with age, particularly in women, alteration of circadian rhythms in aging may reflect deterioration at these brain structures.[145, 146]

Several different kinds of studies of humans are used to infer age differences in circadian rhythms. Under *entrained conditions*, individuals maintain their customary sleep-wake schedules and various physiologic parameters are recorded. Although relatively easy to perform, such studies are subject to masking effects,

which can be considered extraneous influences that may effect the key measures (e.g., body temperature) under study. For example, posture, activity, meals, light exposure, and even sleep itself may all effect the body temperature cycle. Alternatively, the *constant routine*, a protocol that controls for all of these factors by having subjects remain in bed in constant low illumination while they are being deprived of sleep and eating small meals every hour, affords a better appreciation of the endogeneous components of circadian rhythms. Finally, *forced desynchrony*, in which subjects live for an extended period—often for a month or more—in a non–24-h light-dark cycle, allows modeling of how circadian and homeostatic components of sleep-wake regulation may interact.

Under entrained conditions, the amplitude of the sleep-wake rhythm declines with age. Similar findings are noted for body temperature[147] (Fig. 3–4) and some hormones and blood constituents,[148] although not necessarily cortisol.[149] Studies of human age differences in simple rest activity amplitude in entrained environments often show conflicting results suggesting both more robust[150] and less robust rhythm[151] amplitude. Some studies have yielded data about possible age-dependent alterations in phase relationships among physiological functions. In parallel with studies suggesting earlier bedtimes and wake-up times with aging, some human studies have shown earlier acrophases for body temperature[147] (Fig. 3–4), thyroid-stimulating hormone,[152] and cortisol.[153] Despite these relatively uniform findings, Monk et al.[154] have published data from a relatively large group of extraordinarily healthy aged subjects (mean ages 77 to 89), which challenge the notion that the body temperature amplitude is decreased in normal aging under entrained conditions. Whether or not these results can be general-

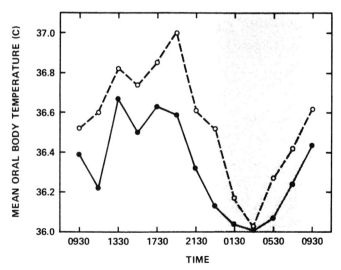

Figure 3–4. Oral temperatures in young *(open circles)* and old *(dark circles)* subjects, showing apparent decreased amplitude and earlier phase in body temperature cycle as a function of aging. Data obtained under entrained conditions. (From Richardson GS, Carskadon MA, Orav EJ. Circadian variation of sleep tendency in elderly and young adult subjects. Sleep. 1982;5[suppl 2]:S82–S94.)

ized remains to be seen because the aged subjects in these studies were exceptionally healthy.

Under the constant routine protocol,[155–160] results regarding age differences in the amplitude of the body temperature rhythm conflict. Findings regarding earlier phase estimates for the body temperature nadir seem somewhat more likely, although these were originally reported to be on the order of 2 h,[155] and more recently, with a sample of nearly 150 subjects of varying ages, age differences in phase estimates were less than 60 minutes.[157] Monk et al.[154] reported no age differences in circadian phase in a constant routine; however, their older group included some atypical subjects with phase estimates occurring in the late morning hours (10 AM to 11 AM), which may have affected the results. An interesting emerging theme from the constant routine studies is that relationships between the habitual timing of morning awakening and the body temperature nadir vary differentially by age. That is, in addition to their relative phase advance, older subjects tend to wake up at a time closer to their temperature minimum[157] a finding similar to that seen in young adult "larks" when compared to "owls."[161] Similar findings were noted by Monk et al. in their study of age differences in morningness-eveningness.[162] The implications of these studies for the elderly are that much of the insomnia due to early morning awakenings seen in human aging reflects not only circadian effects but also homeostatic influences as well.

Somewhat consistent gender differences have been reported for data from both entrained conditions and from constant routines. Older women go to bed at earlier times and/or wake up earlier relative to older men.[163, 164] Additionally, temperature rhythms appear to be phase-advanced in elderly women as well.[154, 164, 165]

Using a forced desynchrony protocol, Haimov and Lavie[166] reported that in a 20-min day (7 min sleep, 13 min awake), maximum sleep propensity showed a predictable phase advance; however, no age differences were apparent for the time of minimum sleep propensity (the so-called forbidden zone). Using a 28-h day (9.33 h of scheduled sleep; 18.67 h of scheduled waking), Czeisler, Dijk, and colleagues[156, 167] reported that older subjects showed a different pattern of sleep in relation to body temperature minimum than younger subjects. When sleep episodes were divided into quintiles and adjusted for the nadir of body temperature, older subjects slept less only on the 4th and 5th quintile of their episodes, regardless of when that sleep episode occurred in relation to the temperature nadir. These results suggest that homeostatic processes may play a larger role in age-dependent phenomena typically ascribed in the past to circadian rhythms. For a more complete review of this topic the reader is directed elsewhere.[168]

Evidence for age-associated decrements in entrainment ability comes from studies of shift work and jet lag, which suggest that older subjects have disproportionate sleep disturbance relative to younger subjects.[169] Experimental studies of phase shifting in humans have shown that elderly subjects, when exposed to a 6-h phase advance, show a similar pattern of recovery of body temperature rhythm amplitude and phase when compared with middle-aged subjects.[170, 171] Shifting of sleep-wake, however, showed a substantially different pattern of recovery between the two age groups. For example, sleep efficiency was severely disrupted throughout a 9-day recovery period in the older subjects and never achieved baseline levels. Recovery of REM sleep (REM percentage) showed a pattern of recovery more closely paralleling the temperature rhythm. These results reiterate that changes in sleep-wake in the aged often attributed to rhythm decrements may be primarily a function of age differences in homeostatic, rather than circadian, factors.

Perhaps as a consequence to such decrements in ability to tolerate phase shifts and minor perturbations in sleep-wake schedule, healthy older subjects may adapt their routines and schedules accordingly. Monk et al. suggested that healthy elderly with good sleep maintain high degrees of regularity in their sleep habits,[162] in their social activities, and in the timing of such things as meals and bathing.[172] Presumably, in homebound, socially impoverished elderly subjects, absence of such zeitgebers may have detrimental effects. Such zeitgebers not only may promote good sleep but also may serve as a protective buffer for psychosocial stressors (e.g., bereavement) in late life.[173, 174] However, the interaction between sleep-wake rhythms and social milieu may be complex. In one study, age was positively correlated with napping regardless of whether the older subject lived alone or with a partner; however, advancing age was correlated (negatively) with bedtime only if the subject lived alone.[175]

Although social factors are obviously important in entraining the sleep-wake rhythm in old age, the powerful effects of illumination as a synchronizing factor should not be underestimated. The role of bright light in the alleviation of sleep maintenance insomnia was demonstrated by Campbell et al.,[56] who showed that 2 h of bright light exposure of approximately 4000 lux administered between 8 and 11 PM (approximately 6 to 8 h before the body temperature minimum) was successful not only in phase-delaying the temperature rhythm but also in decreasing stage 1% and wake time after sleep onset and increasing sleep efficiency.

SLEEP PATHOLOGY

Sleep Apnea (See Also Chapters 71–79)

Prevalence With Aging

The prevalence of snoring clearly increases with age at least up to age 70,[176] although the pathologic significance of snoring per se in old age appears dubious. Data from more than 5000 elderly individuals in the Cardiovascular Health Study suggest that reported snoring (present in 33% of the men and 19% of the women) had few correlates except for alcohol use in men and obesity, diabetes, and arthritis in women.[177] After age 80, snoring prevalence appears to decline.

In clinical case series, the occurrence of breathing

abnormalities in sleep increases with age, at least up to 60 years.[178] In nonclinical elderly populations, a number of cross-sectional studies have shown a relatively high age-associated prevalence of sleep apnea.[179–181] The most comprehensive series of the cross-sectional studies has demonstrated that 24% of the independently living elderly (over 65 years) population, 33% of a similarly aged, acute care inpatient population, and 42% of an elderly nursing home population had an apnea index (AI) of 5 or more.[181, 182] This suggests that tens of millions of people older than 65 years incur some form of disturbed respiration in sleep. Most studies examining sleep apnea in community-based elderly populations show that obstructive, rather than central, events predominate,[183, 184] and sleep apnea continues to be modestly male predominant.[181, 183, 185] Although some longitudinal data imply that the increases in sleep apnea observed in cross-sectional studies may not be confirmed,[186] it seems unlikely that such well-documented age-dependent prevalence would not be confirmed longitudinally, given populations of sufficient size.[187]

Largely on the basis of data comparing sleep apnea in middle-aged and elderly populations, some have posited that sleep apnea actually represents two different conditions: one manifesting itself in middle age (i.e., an age-related disorder) and the other occurring in old age (i.e., an age-dependent condition) (Fig. 3–5).[176, 188] The critical concept here, relevant for geriatrics, is that many diseases show age dependence, that is, the longer one lives, the more likely one is to develop the condition. Preliminary data on sleep apnea from an aged cohort of community volunteers suggests that this is indeed the case. Older members of the cohort were more likely to develop SDB (incidence) over time relative to younger cohort members.[187]

Risk Factors and Mechanisms

The age-dependent component of sleep apnea suggests that many sleep apnea risk factors and their underlying mechanisms might best be modeled as markers of physiologic or biologic age.[189] In this sense, chronologic age may serve only as a proxy for other risk factors which themselves show age dependence. Increased body weight with advancing age is one example. In nonclinical elderly populations, a number of studies show that body weight predicts sleep apnea at least as powerfully as chronologic age.[181, 185, 190] Enhanced upper airway collapsibility has been shown to be related to age[191, 192] and could be related to overall declines of muscular strength and endurance seen with aging both in the skeletal muscles and the genioglossus.[193] To the extent that sleep apnea may involve changes in structure or function of upper airway afferents, age-dependent impairment in vibratory sensation and two-point discrimination have also been described,[194] which might also be relevant to the apnea of old age. In older animals, the pharyngeal muscles appear to have a worse profile for endurance relative to the diaphragm,[195] which would enhance susceptibility to collapse with aging. On the other hand, in humans, Krieger et al.[196] have demonstrated lower endoesophageal pressures generated during apnea episodes in older relative to middle-aged (obstructive) sleep apnea patients, which implies that diaphragmatic fatigue may indeed be likely to occur in aged humans with apnea.

Other putative risk factors for sleep apnea in old age showing age dependence might include factors such as hypothyroidism, declining vital capacity,[187] and altered ventilatory control, and may even include the intrinsic lightening of sleep architecture (decreased SWS and increased sleep fragmentation, see earlier). Figure 3–6 demonstrates the potential role of these markers of physiologic age as risk factors for sleep apnea, as well as potential consequences of the condition.

Outcomes and Consequences

In contrast to the many cross-sectional and intervention studies of sleep apnea and cardiovascular morbid-

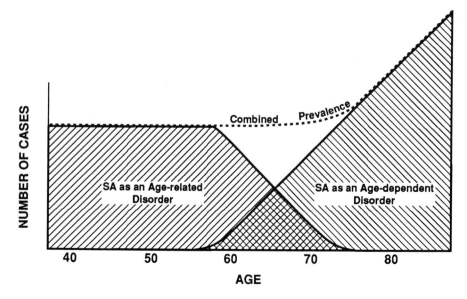

Figure 3–5. Heuristic model suggesting sleep apnea (SA) as both an age-related and an age-dependent condition with potential overlap of distributions in the 60- to 70-year-old age range. Cross-sectionally, note that the number of cases observed may remain high and increase with age, despite a presumed decrease in age-related sleep apnea. See text for a more complete description of evidence in support of such a dual-condition model.

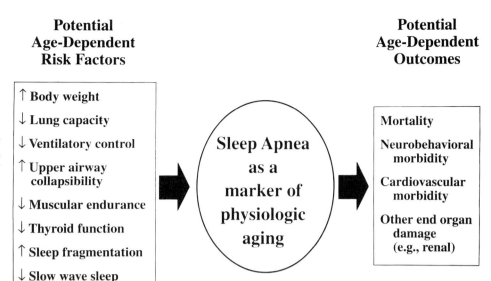

Figure 3–6. Sleep apnea in the elderly as an age-dependent condition with other potential associated age-dependent risk factors and outcomes.

ity in the middle-aged population, only a few studies have specifically examined cardiovascular sequelae in the aged, and findings often conflict. With regard to systemic hypertension, for example, some studies report no association[197]; some report a positive relationship using either daytime, in-clinic measurements[198] or 24-h measurements[199]; others report relationships ultimately confounded by variables such as obesity.[200]

Regarding daytime sleepiness, a critical question remains: to what extent is sleep apnea a predictor of sleepiness in aged populations? The most customary measure of daytime sleepiness, the MSLT, was shown to relate to sleep apnea in a few studies of elderly volunteers,[91] but a larger study could not document this effect.[185] A number of studies have reported MSLT or Maintenance of Wakefulness Test (MWT) findings in clinical populations with sleep apnea.[201–204] Although the focus of these studies was typically on the relative contributions of disturbed sleep and nocturnal hypoxemia to the daytime sleepiness, some age-relevant effects have been reported. In two of these studies, older patients with sleep apnea were shown to be less sleepy relative to younger patients with sleep apnea.[202, 204] In one study, age had no effect,[203] and one study noted greater levels of confirmed MSLT-defined sleepiness in symptomatic elderly clinic patients relative to asymptomatic, age-matched and sex-matched elderly controls.[201] In the largest of these studies (n = 466), Roehrs et al.[202] noted that the most alert sleep apnea patients (who were older) also had fewer breathing disruptions and desaturations during sleep.

Because there is less consensus regarding how to inquire about subjective sleepiness, associations between sleep apnea and questionnaire assessments of somnolence in the elderly are ambiguous.[181, 185] Because studies typically ask about this symptom in a variety of different ways using a variety of time frames, it is difficult to evaluate these data. It may be that more detailed questions provide less ambiguous data. In the San Diego studies of several geriatric populations,[181, 182] responses involving falling asleep at inappropriate

times (e.g., while conversing, by taking an unintended nap) related to various measures of SDB, whereas more global responses regarding daytime sleepiness did not.[181]

Studies examining neuropsychological function in elderly individuals with sleep apnea have suggested some associated impairment, though the role of competing co-morbidities appears to be substantial.[205–207] Some evidence supports the notion of sleep apnea as a potentially reversible dementia in old age.[206]

Obviously, daytime sleepiness and neuropsychological impairment are behavioral measures that imply structural, neurochemical, and/or metabolic change in brain function. Altered cerebrovascular regulation in sleep apnea, particularly relevant for the aged population, is compatible with findings that elderly patients with ischemic stroke have higher rates of sleep apnea than elderly controls,[208] although causality cannot be inferred from such data. These findings are supported by prospective studies of large populations showing associations between ischemic stroke and snoring[209] and hypersomnolence,[80] which were as strong in older as in middle-aged populations. The putative mechanisms involved in producing such events remain uncertain. Studies with transcranial Doppler have variously shown both increased and decreased blood flow velocities during apnea events.[210–212]

Among the sleep apnea outcomes relevant for the aged population, perhaps mortality has engendered the most considerable debate. Some retrospectively collected, nonrandomized clinical trials have suggested that associations between mortality and sleep apnea are, in fact, stronger in the younger, rather than older, clinic populations.[213] Without controlled clinical trials, however, observational cohort studies provide the bulk of the relevant data on this topic. Bliwise et al.[214] reported that an RDI of 10 events per hour or greater was associated with higher rates of 5-year mortality in a community-residing elderly population. However, when other mortality predictors were considered, such as simple chronologic age, the effect disappeared. Mant et al.[215] reported similar results, as did Ancoli-Israel et al.,[216] who found that, by itself, a respiratory disturbance index (RDI) of greater than or equal to 30 events per hour predicted mortality (odds ratio [OR] = 1.5). Elsewhere, we have argued that comparing sleep apnea to chronologic age is probably misleading because, in essence, one is comparing one marker of physiologic age (sleep apnea) against a proxy for all other mortality risks subsumed by chronologic age.[189] Of note was that when Ancoli-Israel et al. excluded chronologic age from the model but continued to include numerous other disease markers, elevated RDI remained a risk factor of borderline significance ($P < .09$). In another study of a clinical population of diverse ages, Lavie et al.[217] presented data suggesting a lower than expected mortality rate in individuals 70 to 79 years of age, but others have interpreted the data differently.[218]

Some of these controversies may be resolved by the ongoing Sleep Heart Health Study (SHHS), which has among its goals the elucidation of the significance of sleep apnea in the aged population. SHHS, which is on target to complete studies on more than 6600 individuals, many of whom will be aged, should afford statistical power to determine to what extent sleep apnea represents a unique marker of physiologic age relative to other mortality risk factors.[219]

Periodic Limb Movements

Relative to sleep apnea, for which at least some evidence has accumulated, vastly less is known about associations between PLMs and morbidity in the elderly. Age-dependent increases in the occurrence of PLMs have been noted cross-sectionally in clinical case series.[178] Unlike sleep apnea, there appears to be no drop in the oldest (e.g., over age 80 years) groups.[220] About 45% of a randomly selected independently living population over 65 years of age meets an arbitrary criterion for the presence of such movements,[220] which makes PLMs a more common pathology than sleep apnea. Youngstedt et al.[221] have noted that over five recording nights in an aged insomnia sample, the mean number of PLMs per movement per hour of sleep was 34.5; 86% of subjects had a mean movement index of greater than 5 events per hour of sleep. The prevalence of PLMs in the elderly is to be contrasted with the prevalence of restless leg syndrome (RLS) in the elderly, which has been estimated at between 18% (for unpleasant leg muscle sensations) to 23% (for bedtime leg restlessness).[222] This fact, together with studies showing a lack of significant associations between PLMs and sleep-wake symptoms (see later), suggests that in many cases, high levels of PLMs in the elderly may represent an incidental finding. PLMs appear to be male predominant, while there is a slight female predominance in selected RLS symptoms.[220, 222]

A number of mechanisms may underlie PLMs in old age. Their distinctive periodic motor output may be related to cycles (20 to 40 sec) in arterial blood pressure,[223] but supraspinal factors represent another possibility. Deficits in central dopaminergic transmission, as evidenced by the successful treatment of PLMs by dopamine agonists as well as lower binding of the D_2 receptor in the basal ganglia of such patients,[224] are likely. Unmedicated elderly patients with advanced stage Parkinson's disease have abundant PLMs.[225] Some alteration in glabellar reflex has been noted in PLMs.[226] At the spinal level, lumbosacral narrowing has been noted in some people with PLMs,[227] which fits with other data suggesting that proprioceptive feedback of limb position may be important in initiation and termination of episodes.[228] Osteoarthritic changes or disk abnormalities, common in the geriatric population, might thus account for some of the high PLMs prevalence in the aged. Systemic factors may also be relevant. Venous insufficiency in the lower limbs has been speculated to relate to PLMs.[229] This could represent a common occurrence in elderly persons, although other data have suggested blood flow is typically increased, not decreased, in the lower limbs during sleep[230] in younger people who presumably had few PLMs. In a retrospective study, high-normal levels of blood urea nitrogen (BUN) were related to PLMs in elderly women[231]; however, a prospective study examining 24-h creatinine clearance in elderly subjects was unable to document any association between renal function and PLMs.[232] More recent data have raised the possibility that iron deficiency, originally noted to be associated with RLS in an early study of patients post-gastrectomy,[233] may be associated with RLS (and by inference, PLMs) in community-residing elderly individuals. More specifically, elderly RLS subjects with serum ferritin levels of lower than 45 mg/ml showed subjective improvement following use of ferrous sulfate.[234] Aged patients did not differ from controls in total iron, suggesting that iron stores may be most critical. Because iron plays a critical role in the structure of the D_2 receptor, this provides further evidence of the importance of central dopaminergic transmission in the PLMs of old age.

The association of sleep-wake symptoms and PLMs in the aged continues to be an area rife with controversy. Although clinical case series suggest PLMs are a major cause of insomnia in old age,[178] much of the apparently high prevalence of PLMs in elderly insomniacs could represent coincidental comorbidity. In one study of 63 elderly insomniacs,[231] 23 demonstrated more than 40 PLMs during sleep, yet only 5 and 8 individuals experienced symptoms of restless legs and leg twitching, respectively. The latter symptom was weakly associated with the presence of PLMs. Other larger studies using elderly persons unselected for sleep-wake complaints have had considerable difficulty showing relationships between PLMs and general nocturnal sleep disturbance or daytime sleepiness,[179, 183, 220] although more specific histories of leg kicking, restless legs symptoms, and difficulty falling back to sleep did relate to PLMs. Given the number of variables examined and the relative strength of the relationships, however, the findings must be considered far from robust. More recently, both Mendelson,[235] who examined PLMs accompanied by EEG-defined arousals, and Youngstedt et al.,[221] who examined PLMs without arousal, failed to find any meaningful associations between such events and sleep-wake symptoms. Although the significance of the movements with arousals for sleep-wake symptomatology remains a case unproven, the possibility that the presence of such movements serves as an early indicator of decreased central dopaminergic transmission and incipient basal ganglia deterioration[224, 225] remains a plausible hypothesis.[236]

The difficulty in demonstrating specific morbidity associated with PLMs in elderly nonclinical populations must be qualified by the relative scarcity of studies examining this feature of sleep (see Sleep Apnea) in old age. In addition, the highly variable nature of PLMs across nights,[221] possibly four times as large as that seen in sleep apnea,[237] makes it likely that any single result will be difficult to replicate. As a case in point, Ancoli-Israel et al.[220] noted that the number of estimated awakenings the morning after a sleep study was the best single symptom correlate of PLMs the previous night in a nonclinical elderly population. The occurrence of clinical presentations of PLMs, often with accompanying dyskinesias and restless legs symptoms in people 60 years old and above, cannot be minimized, but their significance in more mild forms remains uncertain. See Chapter 65 for a more complete discussion of symptomatic PLMs and treatments.

Narcolepsy

Although it has often been assumed that incident cases of narcolepsy decrease with age, data published in 1998 suggest that this may not be the case and, in fact, exacerbation of cataplexy in the aged patient with long-established narcolepsy may not be rare.[238] Such cataplexy may mimic cerebrovascular or cardiac events and may lead to costly and unnecessary diagnostic workups. The recognition of narcolepsy as a phenotypic continuum[239] and the vast underestimation of its prevalence in the general population[240] probably mean that potentially large segments of the population may incur genetic vulnerability to daytime sleepiness in old age.

DAYTIME SLEEPINESS AS A FINAL COMMON OUTCOME IN THE ELDERLY

Given the sundry medical, psychological, sleep-specific, circadian, breathing- or movement-related, and even genetic factors potentially affecting daytime level of arousal in the aged, it is hardly surprising that many older people are behaviorally sleepy and nap during the day. Is sleepiness simply a consequence of poor, discontinuous sleep, or does it reflect specific sleep pathology? Do changes in circadian rhythms or homeostatic regulation account for most of the changes? Perhaps the two most basic questions are

1. What factor or factors best explain the sleepiness of old age?

2. Are these age effects of any functional significance for the health of the elderly person?

Understanding what makes old people sleepy during the day is a complex, multivariate problem. Perhaps the most direct way of studying daytime sleepiness is a case control design in which sleepy and nonsleepy aged individuals are compared on a host of parameters. Results of such work are just emerging and suggest that variables as diverse as sleep apnea, nocturnal pain, sleep-related movement, and depression may all be involved.[241–243a]

Sleepiness during the day is not an inevitable component of aging. Studies of *successful aging* (defined as absence of sleep disorders, psychiatric disorders and medical disease) have shown that elderly people, even well into their 80s, may incur no deficits in daytime alertness on the MSLT.[133] On the other hand, subjective reports of absence of daytime sleepiness must be interpreted with suspicion. This is amply illustrated by the June 1997 Gallup Poll, Sleepiness in America, which demonstrated that, despite showing lower Epworth Sleepiness Scale scores relative to younger people, older people were far more likely to use both over-the-counter and prescription medication to maintain daytime alertness and be more likely to hold the belief that it is normal to feel sleepy during the day.[244]

Data demonstrating the complexity and the potential importance of EDS in the aged population comes from several rigorous epidemiologic studies. In more than 4500 elderly individuals in the Cardiovascular Health Study (CHS), sleepiness (as assessed with the Epworth Sleepiness Scale) was associated with a greater number of nighttime awakenings, nocturnal symptoms of sleep apnea, depression, the presence of congestive heart failure (CHF), use of digitalis and diuretics, limitations in mobility, and absence of sedative and hypnotic use in both men and women.[245] Additionally, black people tended to be sleepier than white people. Within men only, there was some suggestion that sleepiness was also predicted by lower cognitive function (but not brain imaging assessed by magnetic resonance imaging) and certain measures of central obesity, whereas in women, a different set of predictors, such as reduced daily exercise and nasal congestion, were more important. These data imply that a host of specific variables consistent with intrinsic lightening of sleep (nighttime awakenings), specific sleep pathologies (symptoms of sleep apnea, nasal congestion), medical disease burden (CHF), dampening of circadian rhythmicity (bedrest and physical incapacity), psychological issues (depression), and genetics (race, gender) may all contribute to the final common outcome of EDS in the elderly. At least one other study of a large aged population suggested an association between napping and psychomotor test performance,[207] and several prospective studies of populations have suggested that napping is predictive of stroke[80] and mortality.[4, 5, 246] These data imply that EDS in the elderly deserves careful evaluation with full consideration of multiple etiologies.

Regardless of the ultimate causes of daytime sleepiness and the potentially adverse outcomes that may be portended by its presence, an inability to remain awake during the daytime hours undeniably affects the quality of the life for the elderly person.[247] As such, EDS in the older person should constitute an immediate cause of referral. Understanding why a given older patient naps or is excessively sleepy during the day and knowing what treatment regimen to undertake will clearly continue to provide the utmost challenge for sleep medicine specialists.

References

1. Middelkoop HAM, Smilde-van den Doel DA, Neven AK, et al. Subjective sleep characteristics of 1,485 males and females aged 50–93: effects of sex and age, and factors related to self-evaluated quality of sleep. J Gerontol A Biol Sci Med Sci. 1996;51:M108–M115.

2. Buysse DJ, Reynolds CF, Monk TH, et al. Quantification of subjective sleep quality in healthy elderly men and women using the Pittsburgh Sleep Quality Index (PSQI). Sleep. 1991;14:331–338.

3. Webb WB, Schneider-Helmert D. Awakenings: subjective and objective relationships. Percept Mot Skills. 1984;59:63–70.

4. Foley DJ, Monjan AA, Brown SL, et al. Sleep complaints among elderly persons: an epidemiologic study of three communities. Sleep. 1995;18:425–432.

5. Ganguli M, Reynolds CF, Gilby JE. Prevalence and persistence of sleep complaints in a rural older community sample: the MoVIES project. J Am Geriatr Soc. 1996;44:778–784.

6. Bliwise DL, King AC, Harris RB, et al. Prevalence of self-reported poor sleep in a healthy population aged 50–65. Soc Sci Med. 1992;34:49–55.

7. Morgan K. Sleep and Aging: A Research-Based Guide to Sleep in Later Life. Baltimore, Md: The Johns Hopkins University Press; 1987.

8. Blazer DG, Hays JC, Foley DJ. Sleep complaints in older adults: a racial comparison. J Gerontol A Biol Sci Med Sci. 1995;50:M280–M284.

9. Morgan K, Dallosso H, Ebrahim S, et al. Characteristics of subjective insomnia in the elderly living at home. Age Ageing. 1988;17:1–7.

10. Morgan K, Healey DW, Healey PJ. Factors influencing persistent subjective insomnia in old age: a follow-up study of good and poor sleepers aged 65–74. Age Ageing. 1989;18:117–122.

11. Gislason T, Almqvist M. Somatic diseases and sleep complaints. Acta Med Scand. 1987;221:475–481.

12. Hanson BS, Ostergren PO. Different social network and social support characteristics, nervous problems and insomnia: theoretical and methodological aspects on some results from the population study men born in 1914 Malmo, Sweden. Soc Sci Med. 1987;25:849–859.

13. Ford DE, Kamerow DB. Epidemiologic study of sleep disturbances and psychiatric disorders. JAMA. 1989;262:1479–1484.

14. Mant A, Eyland EA. Sleep patterns and problems in elderly general practice attenders: an Australian survey. Community Health Stud. 1988;12:192–199.

15. Ballinger CB. Subjective sleep disturbance at the menopause. J Psychosom Res. 1976;20:509–513.

16. Cook NR, Evans DA, Funkenstein H, et al. Correlates of headache in a population based cohort of elderly. Arch Neurol. 1989;46:1338–1344.

17. Yunus MB, Holt GS, Masi AT, et al. Fibromyalgia syndrome among the elderly: comparison with younger patients. J Am Geriatr Soc. 1988;36:987–995.

18. Gislason T, Reynisdottir H, Kristbjarnarson H, et al. Sleep habits and sleep disturbances among the elderly—an epidemiological survey. J Intern Med. 1993;234:31–39.

19. Maggi S, Langlois JA, Minicuci N, et al. Sleep complaints in community-dwelling older persons: prevalence, associated factors, and reported causes. J Am Geriatr Soc. 1998;46:161–168.

20. Klink ME, Dodge R, Quan SF. The relation of sleep complaints to respiratory symptoms in a general population. Chest. 1994;105:151–154.

21. Dodge R, Cline MG, Quan SF. The natural history of insomnia and its relationship to respiratory symptoms. Arch Intern Med. 1995;155:1797–1800.

22. Klink ME, Quan SF, Kaltenborn WT, et al. Risk factors associated with complaints of insomnia in a general adult population. Arch Intern Med. 1992;152:1634–1637.

23. Monjan AA. Epidemiologic studies of sleep in aging. Paper presented at: 12th Annual Meeting of the Associated Professional Sleep Societies; June 19, 1998; New Orleans, La.

24. Pressman MR, Figueroa WG, Kendrick-Mohamed J, et al. Nocturia: a rarely recognized symptom of sleep apnea and other occult sleep disorders. Arch Intern Med. 1996;156:545–550.

25. Asplund R, Aberg H. Health of the elderly with regard to sleep and nocturnal micturition. Scand J Prim Health Care. 1992;10:98–104.

26. Asplund R, Aberg H. Nocturnal micturition, sleep and well-being in women of ages 40–64 years. Maturitas. 1996;24:73–81.

27. Gentili A, Weiner DK, Kuchibhatla M, et al. Factors that disturb sleep in nursing home residents. Aging (Milano). 1997;9:207–213.

28. Hunter DJW, McKee CM, Black NA, et al. The impact of lower urinary tract symptoms on general health status and on the use of prostatectomy. Qual Life Res. 1995;4:335–341.

29. Kane RL, Ouslander JG, Abrass IB. Essentials of Clinical Geriatrics. New York, NY: McGraw-Hill Book Co; 1984.

30. Ohayon MM, Guilleminault C, Priest RG, et al. Snoring and breathing pauses during sleep: telephone interview survey of a United Kingdom population sample. BMJ. 1997;314:860–863.

31. Umlauf MG, Burgio KL, Shettar S, et al. Nocturia and nocturnal urine production in obstructive sleep apnea. Appl Nurs Res. 1997;10:198–201.

32. Warley ARH, Stradling JR. Abnormal diurnal variation in salt and water excretion in patients with obstructive sleep apnoea. Clin Sci. 1988;74:183–185.

33. Dahlstrand C, Hedner J, Wang YH, et al. Snoring—a common cause of voiding disturbance in elderly men. Lancet. 1996;347:270–271.

34. Burgio KL, Locher JL, Ives DG, et al. Nocturnal enuresis in community-dwelling older adults. J Am Geriatr Soc. 1996;44:139–143.

35. Ledesert B, Ringa V, Breart G. Menopause and perceived health status among the women of the French GAZEL cohort. Maturitas. 1995;20:113–120.

36. Woodward S, Freedman RR. The thermoregulatory effects of menopausal hot flashes on sleep. Sleep. 1994;17:497–501.

37. Woodward S, Freedman RR. Sleep fragmentation in menopausal women with and without hot flashes. Sleep Res. 1995;24:63.

38. Polo-Kantola P, Erkkola R, Helenius H, et al. When does estrogen replacement therapy improve sleep quality? Am J Obstet Gynecol. 1998;178:1002–1009.

39. Kujak J, Young T. The average month-to-month effect of menopausal symptoms on sleep complaints. Sleep Res. 1997;26:403.

40. Assmus JD, Kripke DF. Differences in actigraphy and self-reported sleep quality in women on estrogen replacement therapy. Sleep. 1998;21(suppl):268.

41. Moe KE, Larsen LH, Vitiello MV, et al. Objective and subjective sleep of post-menopausal women: effects of long-term estrogen replacement therapy. Sleep Res. 1997;26:143.

42. Moe KE, Prinz PN, Dulberg EM, et al. IGF-1 and its relationship to delta sleep in healthy older women: role of other anabolic measures and estrogen. Sleep Res. 1994;23:92.

43. Moe KE, Prinz PN, Larsen LH, et al. Growth hormone in post-menopausal women after long-term oral estrogen replacement therapy. J Gerontol A Biol Sci Med Sci. 1998;53:B117–B124.

44. Montplaisir J, Lorrain J, Petit D, et al. Differential effects of two regimens of hormone replacement therapy on sleep in postmenopausal women. Sleep Res. 1997;26:119.

45. Gislason T, Benediktsdottir B, Bjornsson JK, et al. Snoring, hypertension, and the sleep apnea syndrome: an epidemiologic survey of middle-aged women. Chest. 1993;103:1147–1151.

46. Young TB, Zaccaro DJ. Are postmenopausal women at increased risk of sleep-disordered breathing? Am Rev Respir Dis. 1992;145:A866.

47. Carskadon MA, Bearpark HM, Sharkey KM, et al. Effects of menopause and nasal occlusion on breathing during sleep. Am J Respir Crit Care Med. 1997;155:205–210.

48. Cistulli PA, Barnes DJ, Grunstein RR, et al. Effect of short term hormone replacement in the treatment of obstructive sleep apnoea in postmenopausal women. Thorax. 1994;49:699–702.

49. Zepelin H, McDonald CS, Zammit GK. Effects of age on auditory awakening thresholds. J Gerontol. 1984;39:294–300.

50. Carskadon MA, Dement WC. Daytime sleepiness: quantification of a behavioral state. Neurosci Biobehav Rev. 1987;11:307–317.

51. Levine B, Roehrs T, Zorick F, et al. Daytime sleepiness in young adults. Sleep. 1988;11:39–46.

52. Valencia M, Campos RM, Mendez J, et al. Multiple sleep latency test (MSLT) and sleep apnea in aged women. Sleep. 1993;16:114–117.

53. Campbell SS. Duration and placement of sleep in a disentrained environment. Psychophysiology. 1984;21:106–113.

54. Friedman L, Bliwise DL, Yesavage JA, et al. A preliminary study comparing sleep restriction and relaxation treatments for insomnia in older adults. J Gerontol. 1991;46:P1–8.

55. Campbell SS, Kripke DF, Gillin JC, et al. Exposure to light in healthy elderly subjects and Alzheimer's patients. Physiol Behav. 1988;42:141–144.

56. Campbell SS, Dawson D, Anderson MW. Alleviation of sleep maintenance insomnia with timed exposure to bright light. J Am Geriatr Soc. 1993;41:829–836.

57. Breckenridge JN, Gallagher D, Thompson LW, et al. Characteristic depressive symptoms of bereaved elders. J Gerontol. 1986;41:163–168.

58. Pasternak RE, Reynolds CF III, Hoch CC, et al. Sleep in spousally bereaved elders with subsyndromal depressive symptoms. Psychiatry Res. 1992;43:43–53.

59. Reynolds CF III, Hoch CC, Buysse DJ, et al. Electroencephalographic sleep in spousal bereavement and bereavement-related depression of late life. Biol Psychiatry. 1992;31:69–82.

60. Reynolds CF III, Hoch CC, Buysse DJ, et al. Sleep after spousal bereavement: a study of recovery from stress. Biol Psychiatry. 1993;34:791–797.

61. Hoffmann G, Vanderbeke H, De Cock W, et al. The psychophysiological incidences of retirement. 3rd European Congress on Sleep Research, Montpellier 1976. Sleep 1976. Basel, Germany: Karger; 1977:317–320.

62. Rosen J, Reynolds CF, Yeager AL, et al: Sleep disturbances in survivors of the Nazi holocaust. Am J Psychiatry. 1991;148:62–66.

63. Berlin RM: Disturbed sleep in the elderly. Am J Psychiatry. 1989;146:810–811.

64. Morin C, Gramling SE. Sleep patterns and aging: comparison of older adults with and without insomnia complaints. Psychol Aging. 1989;4:290–294.

65. Roehrs T, Lineback W, Zorick F, et al. Relationship of psychopathology to insomnia in the elderly. J Am Geriatr Soc. 1982;30:312–315.

66. Bliwise NG, Bliwise DL, Dement WC. Age and psychopathology in insomnia. Clin Gerontol. 1985;4:3–9.

67. Dealberto MJ, Seeman T, McAvay GJ, et al. Factors related to current and subsequent psychotropic drug use in an elderly cohort. J Clin Epidemiol. 1997;50:357–364.

68. Ohayon MM, Caulet M. Insomnia and psychotropic drug consumption. Prog Neuropsychopharmacol Biol Psychiatry. 1995;19:421–431.

69. Englert S, Linden M. Differences in self-reported sleep complaints in elderly persons living in the community who do or do not take sleep medication. J Clin Psychiatry. 1998;59:137–144.

70. Kripke DF, Klauber MR, Wingard DL, et al. Mortality hazard associated with prescription hypnotics. Biol Psychiatry. 1998;43:687–693.

71. Morin CM, Kowatch RA, Barry T, et al. Cognitive-behavior therapy for late-life insomnia. J Consult Clin Psychol. 1993;61:137–146.

72. Edinger JD, Marsh GR, Hoelscher TJ, et al. A cognitive-behavioral therapy for sleep-maintenance insomnia in older adults. Psychol Aging. 1992;7:282–289.

73. King AC, Oman RF, Brassington GS, et al. Moderate-intensity exercise and self-rated quality of sleep in older adults: a randomized controlled trial. JAMA. 1997;277:32–37.

74. Vitiello MV, Prinz PN, Schwartz RS. Slow wave sleep but not overall sleep quality of healthy older men and women is improved by increased aerobic fitness. Sleep Res. 1994;23:149.

75. Dorsey CM, Lukas SE, Teicher MH, et al. Effects of passive body heating on the sleep of older female insomniacs. J Geriatr Psychiatry Neurol. 1996;9:83–90.

76. Kripke DF, Simons RN, Garfinkel L, et al. Short and long sleep and sleeping pills: is increased mortality associated? Arch Gen Psychiatry. 1979;36:103–116.

77. Wingard DL, Berkman LF, Brand RJ. A multivariate analysis of health-related practices: a nine-year mortality follow-up of the Alameda County study. Am J Epidemiol. 1982;116:765–775.

78. Rumble R, Morgan K. Hypnotics, sleep, and mortality in elderly people. J Am Geriatr Soc. 1992;40:787–791.

79. Althuis MD, Fredman L, Langenberg PW, et al. The relationship between insomnia and mortality among community-dwelling older women. J Am Geriatr Soc. 1998;46:1270–1273.

80. Qureshi AI, Giles WH, Croft JB, et al. Habitual sleep patterns and risk for stroke and coronary heart disease: a 10-year follow-up from NHANES I. Neurology. 1997;48:904–911.

81. Livingston G, Blizard B, Mann A. Does sleep disturbance predict depression in elderly people? A study in inner London. Br J Gen Pract. 1993;43:445–448.

82. McCall WV, Erwin CW, Edinger JD, et al. Ambulatory polysomnography: technical aspects and normative values. J Clin Neurophysiol. 1992;9:68–77.

83. Buysse DJ, Browman KE, Monk TH, et al. Napping and 24-hour sleep/wake patterns in healthy elderly and young adults. J Am Geriatr Soc. 1992;40:779–786.

84. Vitiello MV, Prinz PN, Williams DE, et al. Sleep disturbances in patients with mild-stage Alzheimer's disease. J Gerontol A Biol Sci Med Sci. 1990;45:M131–138.

85. Hirshkowitz M, Moore CA, Hamilton CR III, et al. Polysomnography of adults and elderly: sleep architecture, respiration, and leg movement. J Clin Neurophysiol. 1992;9:56–62.

86. Redline S, Bonekat W, Gottlieb D, et al. Sleep stage distributions in the sleep heart health study (SHHS) cohort. Sleep. 1998;21(suppl):210.

87. Hoch CC, Dew MA, Reynolds CF III, et al. A longitudinal study of laboratory- and diary-based sleep measures in healthy "old old" and "young old" volunteers. Sleep. 1994;17:489–496.

88. Rediehs MH, Reis JS, Creason NS. Sleep in old age: focus on gender differences. Sleep. 1990;13:410–424.

89. Wauquier A. Aging and changes in phasic events during sleep. Physiol Behav. 1993;54:803–806.

90. Boselli M, Parrino L, Smerieri A, et al. Effect of age on EEG arousals in normal sleep. Sleep. 1998;21:351–357.

91. Carskadon MA, Brown ED, Dement WC. Sleep fragmentation in the elderly: relationship to daytime sleep tendency. Neurobiol Aging. 1982;3:321–327.

92. Bliwise DL, Keenan S, Burnburg D, et al. Inter-rater reliability for scoring periodic leg movements in sleep. Sleep. 1991;14:249–251.

93. Drinnan MJ, Murray A, Griffiths CJ, et al. Interobserver variability in recognizing arousal in respiratory sleep disorders. Am J Respir Crit Care Med. 1998;158:358–362.

94. Anderson TW, Waters WF. Frequency of spontaneous, transient arousals in normals, sleep apnea, periodic limb movement disorder and insomnia. Sleep. 1998;21(suppl):76.

95. Reynolds CF, Monk TH, Hoch CC, et al. Electroencephalographic sleep in the healthy "old old": a comparison with the "young old" in visually scored and automated measures. J Gerontol. 1991;46:M39–46.

96. Benca RM, Obermeyer WH, Thisted RA, et al. Sleep and psychiatric disorders: a meta-analysis. Arch Gen Psychiatry. 1992;49:651–668.

97. Feinberg I, Hibi S, Carlson VR. Changes in EEG amplitude during sleep with age. In: Nandy K, Sherwin I, eds. The Aging Brain and Senile Dementia. New York, NY: Plenum Press; 1977:85–98.

98. Webb WB, Dreblow LM. A modified method for scoring slow wave sleep of older subjects. Sleep. 1982;5:195–199.

99. Reynolds CF III, Kupfer DJ, Taska LS, et al. Sleep of healthy seniors: a revisit. Sleep. 1986;8:20–29.

100. Dijk DJ, Beersma DGM, Bloem GM. Sex differences in the sleep

EEG of young adults: visual scoring and spectral analysis. Sleep. 1989;12:500–507.

101. Feinberg I, Koresko RL, Heller N. EEG sleep patterns as a function of normal and pathological aging in man. J Psychiatr Res. 1967;5:107–144.

102. Hayashi Y, Endo S. All-night sleep polygraphic recordings of healthy aged persons: REM and slow wave sleep. Sleep. 1982;5:277–283.

103. Prinz PN. Sleep patterns in the healthy aged: relationship with intellectual function. J Gerontol. 1977;32:179–186.

104. Bliwise DL, Bergmann BM. Individual differences in stages 3 and 4 sleep. Psychophysiology. 1987;34:35–40.

105. Gillin JC, Duncan WC, Murphy DL, et al. Age-related changes in sleep in depressed and normal subjects. Psychiatry Res. 1981;4:73–78.

106. Feinberg I. Changes in sleep cycle patterns with age. J Psychiatr Res. 1974;10:283–306.

107. Giles DE, Roffwarg HP, Rush AJ, et al. Age-adjusted threshold values for reduced REM latency in unipolar depression using ROC analysis. Biol Psychiatry. 1990;27:841–853.

108. Riemann D, Lauer C, Hohagen F, et al. Longterm evolution of sleep in depression. In: Smirne S, Franceschi M, Ferini-Strambi L, eds. Sleep and Ageing. Milano, Italy: Masson; 1991:195–204.

109. Reynolds CF, Kupfer DJ, Houck PR, et al. Reliable discrimination of elderly depressed and demented patients by electroencephalographic sleep data. Arch Gen Psychiatry. 1988;45:258–264.

110. Knowles JB, MacLean AW. Age-related changes in sleep in depressed and healthy subjects: a meta-analysis. Neuropsychopharmacology. 1990;3:251–259.

111. Vitiello MV, Prinz PN, Avery DH, et al. Sleep is undisturbed in elderly, depressed individuals who have not sought health care. Biol Psychiatry. 1990;27:431–440.

112. Williams RL, Karacan I, Hursch CJ. EEG of Human Sleep: Clinical Applications. New York, NY: John Wiley & Sons; 1974.

113. Gaillard JM. Chronic primary insomnia: possible physiopathological involvement of slow wave sleep deficiency. Sleep. 1978;1:133–147.

114. Feinberg I, March JD, Fein G, et al. Period and amplitude analysis of 0.5–3.0 Hz activity in NREM sleep of young adults. Electroencephalogr Clin Neurophysiol. 1978;44:202–213.

115. Bliwise DL. Individual Differences in EEG Delta Activity During Sleep [dissertation]. Chicago, Ill: University of Chicago; 1982.

116. Feinberg I, Fein G, Floyd TC. Period and amplitude analysis of NREM EEG sleep: repeatability of results in young adults. Electroencephalogr Clin Neurophysiol. 1980;48:212–221.

117. Ehlers CL, Kupfer DJ. Effects of age on delta and REM sleep parameters. Electroencephalogr Clin Neurophysiol. 1989;72:118–125.

118. Carskadon MA, Orav EJ, Dement WC. Evolution of sleep and daytime sleepiness in adolescents. In: Guilleminault C, Lugaresi E, eds. Sleep/Wake Disorders: Natural History, Epidemiology and Long-term Evolution. New York, NY: Raven Press; 1983:201–216.

119. Johns MW, Rinsler MG. Sleep and thyroid function: further studies in healthy young men. J Psychosom Res. 1977;21:161–166.

120. Nakazawa I, Kotorii M, Ohshima M, et al. Changes in sleep patterns after sleep deprivation. Folia Psychiatr Neurol Jpn. 1978;32:85–93.

121. Feinberg I, Thode HC, Chugani HT, et al. Gamma distribution model describes maturational curves for delta wave amplitude, cortical metabolic rate and synaptic density. J Theor Biol. 1990;142:149–161.

122. Finch CE. The regulation of physiological changes during mammalian aging. Q Rev Biol. 1976;51:49–83.

123. Laslett P. Societal development and aging. In: Binstock RH, Shanas E, eds. Handbook of Aging and the Social Sciences. New York, NY: Van Nostrand & Reinhold; 1985:199–230.

124. Rechtschaffen A. The function of sleep: methodological issues. In: Drucker-Colin R, Shkurovich M, Sterman MB, eds. The Functions of Sleep. New York, NY: Academic Press; 1979:1–17.

125. Bixler EO, Kales A, Jacoby JA, et al. Nocturnal sleep and wakefulness: effects of age and sex in normal sleepers. Int J Neurosci. 1984;23:33–42.

126. Cirignotta F, Mondini S, Zucconi M, et al. Insomnia: an epidemiological study. Clin Neuropharmacol. 1985;8:S49–S54.

127. Partinen M, Kaprio J, Koskenvuo M, et al. Sleeping habits, sleep quality, and use of sleeping pills: a population study of 31,140 adults in Finland. In: Guilleminault C, Lugaresi E, eds. Sleep/Wake Disorders: Natural History, Epidemiology and Long-term Evolution. New York, NY: Raven Press; 1983:29–35.

128. Tune GS: Sleep and wakefulness in 509 normal human adults. Br J Med Psychol. 1969;42:75–80.

129. Zepelin H. A life span perspective on sleep. In: Mayes A, ed. Sleep Mechanisms and Functions: In Humans and Animals: An Evolutionary Perspective. Wokingham, Berkshire, England: Van Nostrand Reinhold (UK) Co Ltd; 1983:120–160.

130. Pressman MK, DiPhillip MA, Fry JM. Senile miosis: the possible contribution of disordered sleep and daytime sleepiness. J Gerontol. 1986;41:629–634.

131. Bonnet MH, Arand DL. The use of triazolam in older patients with periodic leg movements, fragmented sleep, and daytime sleepiness. J Gerontol. 1990;45:M139–144.

132. Hoch CC, Reynolds CF III, Jennings JR, et al. Daytime sleepiness and performance among healthy 80 and 20 year olds. Neurobiol Aging. 1992;13:353–356.

133. Reynolds CF III, Jennings JR, Hoch CC, et al. Daytime sleepiness in the healthy "old old": a comparison with young adults. J Am Geriatr Soc. 1991;39:957–962.

134. Carskadon MA, Dement WC. Sleep loss in elderly volunteers. Sleep. 1985;8:207–221.

135. Reynolds CF III, Kupfer DJ, Hoch CC, et al. Sleep deprivation as a probe in the elderly. Arch Gen Psychiatry. 1987;44:982–990.

136. Reynolds CF III, Kupfer DJ, Hoch CC, et al. Sleep deprivation in healthy elderly men and women: effects on mood and on sleep during recovery. Sleep. 1986;9:492–501.

137. Bonnet MH. Effect of 64 hours of sleep deprivation upon sleep in geriatric normals and insomniacs. Neurobiol Aging. 1986;7:89–96.

138. Bonnet MH, Rosa RR. Sleep and performance in young adults and older normals and insomniacs during acute sleep loss and recovery. Biol Psychol. 1987;25:153–172.

139. Reynolds CF, Buysse DJ, Kupfer DJ, et al. Rapid eye movement sleep deprivation as a probe in elderly subjects. Arch Gen Psychiatry. 1990;47:1128–1136.

140. Buysse DJ, Monk TH, Jarrett DB, et al. Old and young men have different circadian patterns of "microsleeps" during a constant routine. Sleep Res. 1991;20:445.

141. Bonnet MH. Recovery of performance during sleep following sleep deprivation in older normal and insomniac adult males. Percept Mot Skills. 1985;60:323–334.

142. Bonnet MH. The effect of sleep fragmentation on sleep and performance in younger and older subjects. Neurobiol Aging. 1989;10:21–25.

143. Bonnet MH, Arand DL. Sleep loss in aging. Clin Geriatr Med. 1989;5:405–420.

144. Samis HV. Aging: the loss of temporal organization. Perspect Biol Med. 1968;12:95–102.

145. Swaab DF, Fliers E, Partiman TS. The suprachiasmatic nucleus of the human brain in relation to sex, age and senile dementia. Brain Res. 1985;342:37–44.

146. Hofman MA, Fliers E, Goudsmit E, et al. Morphometric analysis of the suprachiasmatic and paraventricular nuclei in the human brain: sex differences and age-dependent changes. J Anat. 1988;160:127–143.

147. Richardson GS, Carskadon MA, Orav EJ. Circadian variation of sleep tendency in elderly and young adult subjects. Sleep. 1982;5:S82–S94.

148. Casale G, deNicola P. Circadian rhythms in the aged: a review. Arch Gerontol Geriatr. 1984;3:267–284.

149. Colucci CF, D'Alessandro B, Bellastella A, et al. Circadian rhythm of plasma cortisol in the aged. Gerontol Clin (Basel). 1975;17:89–95.

150. Lieberman HR, Wurtman JJ, Teichner MH. Circadian rhythms of activity in healthy young and elderly humans. Neurobiol Aging. 1989;10:259–265.

151. Renfrew JW, Pettigrew KD, Rapoport SI. Motor activity and sleep duration as a function of age in healthy men. Physiol Behav. 1987;41:627–634.

152. Guagnano MT, Angelucci E, Blasioli A, et al. Circadian rhythm in the elderly. Boll Soc Ital Biol Sper. 1986;62:307–313.

153. Sherman B, Wysham C, Pfohl B. Age-related changes in the circadian rhythm of plasma cortisol in man. J Clin Endocrinol Metab. 1985;61:439–443.

154. Monk TH, Buysse DJ, Reynolds CF III, et al. Circadian temperature rhythms of older people. Exp Gerontol. 1995;30:455–474.

155. Czeisler CA, Dumont M, Duffy JF, et al. Association of sleep-wake habits in older people with changes in output of circadian pacemaker. Lancet. 1992;340:933–936.

156. Czeisler CA. Sleep-wake regulation and circadian rhythms. Paper presented at: 11th Annual Meeting, Association of Professional Sleep Societies; June 12, 1997; San Francisco, Calif.

157. Duffy JF, Dijk DJ, Klerman EB, et al. Altered phase relationship between body temperature cycle and habitual awakening in older subjects. Sleep Res. 1997;26:711.

158. Buysse DJ, Monk TH, Reynolds CF III, et al. Patterns of sleep episodes in young and elderly adults during a 36-hour constant routine. Sleep. 1993;16:632–637.

159. Monk TH, Buysse DJ, Reynolds CF III, et al. Subjective alertness rhythms in elderly people. J Biol Rhythms. 1996;11:268–276.

160. Monk TH, Buysse DJ, Reynolds CF III, et al. Circadian rhythms in human performance and mood under constant conditions. J Sleep Res. 1997;6:9–18.

161. Hall EF, Duffy JF, Dijk DJ, et al. Interval between waketime and circadian phase differs between morning and evening types. Sleep Res. 1997;26:716.

162. Monk TH, Reynolds CF III, Buysse DJ, et al. Circadian characteristics of healthy 80-year-olds and their relationship to objectively recorded sleep. J Gerontol. 1991;46:M171–M175.

163. Reyner A, Horne JA. Gender- and age-related differences in sleep determined by home-recorded sleep logs and actimetry from 400 adults. Sleep. 1995;18:127–134.

164. Campbell SS, Gillin JC, Kripke DF, et al. Gender differences in the circadian temperature rhythms of healthy elderly subjects: relationships to sleep quality. Sleep. 1989;12:529–536.

165. Moe KE, Prinz PN, Vitiello MV, et al. Healthy elderly women and men have different entrained circadian temperature rhythms. J Am Geriatr Soc. 1991;39:383–387.

166. Haimov I, Lavie P. Circadian characteristics of sleep propensity function in healthy elderly: a comparison with young adults. Sleep. 1997;20:294–300.

167. Dijk DJ, Duffy JF, Riel E, et al. Altered interaction of circadian and homeostatic aspects of sleep propensity results in awakening at an earlier circadian phase in older people. Sleep Res. 1997;26:710.

168. Bliwise DL. Sleep and circadian rhythm disorders in aging and dementia. In: Turek F, Zee P, eds. Regulation of Sleep and Circadian Rhythms. New York, NY: Marcel Dekker; 1999:487–525.

169. Foret J, Bensimon G, Benoit O, et al. Quality of sleep as a function of age and shift work. Adv Biosci. 1981;30:149–154.

170. Monk TH, Buysse DJ, Reynolds CF III, et al. Inducing jet lag in older people. Exp Gerontol. 1993;28:119–133.

171. Carrier J, Monk TH, Buysse DJ, et al. Inducing a 6-hour phase advance in the elderly: effects on sleep and temperature rhythms. J Sleep Res. 1996;5:99–105.

172. Monk TH, Reynolds CF III, Machen MA, et al. Daily social rhythms in the elderly and their relation to objectively recorded sleep. Sleep. 1992;15:322–329.

173. Dew MA, Reynolds CF III, Monk TH, et al. Psychosocial correlates and sequelae of electroencephalographic sleep in healthy elders. J Gerontol. 1994;49:P8–P18.

174. Prigerson HG, Reynolds CF III, Frank E, et al. Stressful life events, social rhythms, and depressive symptoms among the elderly: an examination of hypothesized causal linkages. Psychiatry Res. 1994;51:33–49.

175. Minors DS, Rabbitt PMA, Worthington H, et al. Variation in meals and sleep-activity patterns in aged subjects: its relevance to circadian rhythm studies. Chronobiol Int. 1989;6:139–146.

176. Bliwise DL. Sleep in normal aging and dementia. Sleep. 1993;16:40–81.

177. Enright PL, Newman AB, Wahl PW, et al. Prevalence and correlates of snoring and observed apneas in 5,201 older adults. Sleep. 1996;19:531–538.

178. Roehrs T, Zorick F, Sicklesteel J, et al. Age-related sleep-wake disorders at a sleep disorders center. J Am Geriatr Soc. 1983;31:364–370.

179. Dickel MJ, Mosko SS. Morbidity cut-offs for sleep apnea and periodic leg movements in predicting subjective complaints in seniors. Sleep. 1990;13:155–166.

180. Krieger J, Turlot JC, Mangin P, et al. Breathing during sleep in normal young and elderly subjects: hypopneas, apneas, and correlated factors. Sleep. 1983;6:108–120.

181. Ancoli-Israel S, Kripke DF, Klauber MR, et al. Sleep-disordered breathing in community-dwelling elderly. Sleep. 1991;14:486–495.

182. Ancoli-Israel S: Epidemiology of sleep disorders. Clin Geriatr Med. 1989;5:347–362.

183. Mosko SS, Dickel MJ, Paul T, et al. Sleep apnea and sleep-related periodic leg movements in community resident seniors. J Am Geriatr Soc. 1988;36:502–508.

184. Ancoli-Israel S, Kripke DF, Mason W. Characteristics of obstructive and central sleep apnea in the elderly: an interim report. Biol Psychiatry. 1987;22:741–750.

185. Phillips BA, Berry DTR, Schmitt FA, et al. Sleep disordered breathing in the healthy elderly: clinically significant? Chest. 1992;101:345–349.

186. Ancoli-Israel S, Kripke DF, Klauber MR, et al. Natural history of sleep disordered breathing in community dwelling elderly. Sleep. 1993;16:S25–S29.

187. Bliwise, DL. Development of sleep disordered breathing and changes in body weight over time in an elderly population. Sleep Res. 1994;23:234.

188. Young T. Sleep-disordered breathing in older adults: is it a condition distinct from that in middle-aged adults? Sleep. 1996;19:529–530.

189. Bliwise DL. Chronologic age, physiologic age and mortality in sleep apnea. Sleep. 1996;19:275–276.

190. Bliwise DL, Feldman DE, Bliwise NG, et al. Risk factors for sleep disordered breathing in heterogeneous geriatric populations. J Am Geriatr Soc. 1987;35:132–141.

191. White DP, Lombard RM, Cadieux RJ, et al. Pharyngeal resistance in normal humans: influence of gender, age and obesity. J Appl Physiol. 1985;58:365–371.

192. Martin SE, Mathur R, Marshall I, et al. The effect of age, sex, obesity and posture on upper airway size. Eur Respir J. 1997;10:2087–2090.

193. Crow HC, Ship JA. Tongue strength and endurance in different aged individuals. J Gerontol A Biol Sci Med Sci. 1996;51:M247–M250.

194. Calhoun KH, Gibson B, Hartley L, et al. Oral sensation and aging. In: Kuna ST, Suratt PM, Remmers JE, eds. Sleep and Respiration in Aging Adults. New York, NY: Elsevier Science; 1991:215–228.

195. Van Lunteren E, Vafaie H, Salomone RJ. Comparative effects of aging on pharyngeal and diaphragm muscles. Respir Physiol. 1995;99:113–125.

196. Krieger J, Sforza E, Boudewijns A, et al. Respiratory effort during obstructive sleep apnea: role of age and sleep state. Chest. 1997;112:875–849.

197. Phillips BA, Berry DTR, Lipke-Molby TC. Sleep-disordered breathing in healthy, aged persons: fifth and final year follow-up. Chest. 1996;110:654–658.

198. Stoohs RA, Gingold J, Cohrs S, et al. Sleep-disordered breathing and systemic hypertension in the older male. J Am Geriatr Soc. 1996;44:1295–1300.

199. Swan GE, Bliwise DL, Carmelli D, et al. Sleep-related breathing disturbance and night time blood pressure variability: prevalence and covariation in older adults. Sleep. 1998;21(suppl):84.

200. Jennum P, Hein HO, Suadicani P, et al. Cardiovascular risk factors in snorers: a cross-sectional study of 3,323 men aged 54 to 74 years: the Copenhagen Male Study. Chest. 1992;102:1371–1376.

201. Berry DTR, Phillips BA, Cook YR, et al. Geriatric sleep apnea syndrome: a preliminary description. J Gerontol. 1990;45:M169–M174.

202. Roehrs T, Zorick F, Wittig R, et al. Predictors of objective level of daytime sleepiness in patients with sleep-related breathing disorders. Chest. 1989;95:1202–1206.

203. Guilleminault C, Partinen M, Quera-Salva MA, et al. Determinants of daytime sleepiness in obstructive sleep apnea. Chest. 1988;94:32–37.

204. Poceta JS, Jeong D, Ho S, et al. Hypoxemia as a determinate of daytime sleepiness in obstructive sleep apnea. Sleep Res. 1990;19:269.

205. Bliwise DL. Neuropsychological function and sleep. Clin Geriatr Med. 1989;5:381–394.

206. Bliwise DL. Is sleep apnea a cause of reversible dementia in old age? J Am Geriatr Soc. 1996;44:1407–1409.

207. Dealberto MJ, Pajot N, Courbon D, et al. Breathing disorders during sleep and cognitive performance in an older community sample: the EVA study. J Am Geriatr Soc. 1996;44:1287–1294.

208. Dyken ME, Somers VK, Yamada T, et al. Investigating the relationship between stroke and obstructive sleep apnea. Stroke. 1996;27:401–407.

209. Koskenvuo M, Kaprio J, Telakivi T, et al. Snoring as risk factor for ischaemic heart disease and stroke in men. BMJ. 1987;294:16–19.

210. Fischer AQ, Chaudhary BA, Taormina MA, et al. Intracranial hemodynamics in sleep apnea. Chest. 1992;102:1402–1406.

211. Balfors EM, Franklin KA. Impairment of cerebral perfusion during obstructive sleep apnea. Am J Respir Crit Care Med. 1994;150:1587–1591.

212. Hajak G, Klingelhorfer J, Schulz-Varszegi M, et al. Sleep apnea syndrome and cerebral hemodynamics. Chest. 1996;110:670–679.

213. He J, Kryger MH, Zorick FJ, et al. Mortality and apnea index in obstructive sleep apnea: experience in 385 male patients. Chest. 1988;94:9–14.

214. Bliwise DL, Bliwise NG, Partinen M, et al. Sleep apnea and mortality in an aged cohort. Am J Public Health. 1988;78:544–547.

215. Mant A, King M, Saunders NA, et al. Four-year follow-up of mortality and sleep-related respiratory disturbance in non-demented seniors. Sleep. 1995;18:433–438.

216. Ancoli-Israel S, Kripke DF, Klauber MR, et al. Morbidity, mortality and sleep-disordered breathing in community dwelling elderly. Sleep. 1996;19:277–282.

217. Lavie P, Herer P, Peled R, et al. Mortality in sleep apnea patients: a multivariate analysis of risk factors. Sleep. 1995;18:149–157.

218. Baltzan M, Suissa S. Mortality in sleep apnea patients: a multivariate analysis of risk factors—a response to Lavie and collaborators. Sleep. 1997;20:377–378.

219. Quan SF, Howard BV, Iber C, et al. The Sleep Heart Health Study: design, rationale, and methods. Sleep. 1997;20:1077–1085.

220. Ancoli-Israel S, Kripke DF, Klauber MR, et al. Periodic limb movements in sleep in community-dwelling elderly. Sleep. 1991;14:496–500.

221. Youngstedt SD, Kripke DF, Klauber MR, et al. Periodic leg movements during sleep and sleep disturbances in elders. J Gerontol A Biol Sci Med Sci. 1998;53:M391–M394.

222. Lavigne GJ, Montplaisir JY. Restless legs syndrome and sleep bruxism: prevalence and association among Canadians. Sleep. 1994;17:739–743.

223. Coccagna G, Mantovani M, Brignani F, et al. Arterial pressure changes during spontaneous sleep in man. Electroencephalogr Clin Neurophysiol. 1971;31:277–281.

224. Staedt J, Stoppe G, Kogler A, et al. Dopamine D_2 receptor alteration in patients with periodic movements in sleep (nocturnal myoclonus). J Neural Transm Gen Sect. 1993;93:71–74.

225. Bliwise DL, Rye DB, Dihenia BH, et al. Periodic leg movements in sleep in elderly patients with parkinsonism. Sleep. 1998;21(suppl):196.

226. Wechsler LR, Stakes JW, Shahani BT, et al. Periodic leg movements of sleep (nocturnal myoclonus): an electrophysiological study. Ann Neurol. 1986;19:168–173.

227. Shafor R. Prevalence of abnormal lumbo-sacral spine imaging in patients with insomnia associated restless legs, periodic movements in sleep. Sleep Res. 1991;20:396.

228. Dzvonik ML, Kripke DF, Klauber M, et al. Body position changes and periodic movements in sleep. Sleep. 1986;9:484–491.

229. Ware JC, Blumoff R, Pittard JT. Peripheral vasoconstriction in patients with sleep related periodic leg movements. Sleep. 1988;11:182–187.

230. Sindrup JH, Kastrup J, Jorgensen B, et al. Nocturnal variations in subcutaneous blood flow rate in lower leg of normal human subjects. Am J Physiol. 1991;260:H480–H485.

231. Bliwise D, Petta D, Seidel W, et al. Periodic leg movements during sleep in the elderly. Arch Gerontol Geriatr. 1985;4:273–281.

232. Bliwise DL, Ingham RH, Date ES, et al. Nerve conduction and creatinine clearance in aged subjects with periodic movements in sleep. J Gerontol. 1989;44:M164–167.

233. Ekbom K. Restless leg syndrome after partial gastrectomy. Acta Neurol Scand. 1966;42:79–89.

234. O'Keeffe ST, Gavin K, Lavan JN. Iron status and restless legs syndrome in the elderly. Age Ageing. 1994;23:200–203.

235. Mendelson WB. Are periodic leg movements associated with clinical sleep disturbance? Sleep. 1996;19:219–223.

236. Rye DB, Bliwise DL. Movement disorders specific to sleep and the nocturnal manifestations of waking movement disorders. In: Watts RL, Koller WC, eds. Movement Disorders: Neurologic Principles and Practice. New York, NY: McGraw-Hill: 1997:687–713.

237. Bliwise DL, Carskadon MA, Dement WC: Nightly variation of periodic leg movements in sleep in the elderly. Arch Gerontol Geriatr. 1988;7:273–279.

238. Rye DB, Dihenia B, Weissman JD, et al. Presentation of narcolepsy after 40. Neurology. 1998;50:459–465.

239. Mignot E, Young T, Lin L, et al. Reduction of REM sleep latency associated with HLA-DQB1*0602 in normal adults. Lancet. 1998;351:727.

240. Hublin C, Partinen M, Kaprio J, et al. Epidemiology of narcolepsy. Sleep. 1994;17:S7–S12.

241. Pack AI, Dinges DF, Gehrman PR, et al. Sleepiness in the elderly, role of sleep apnea: a case control approach. Sleep Res. 1997;26:453.

242. Samuel S, Pack FM, Pack AI, et al. Sleep-wake behaviors of elderly living in residential communities: results from a case-control study of excessive daytime sleepiness. Sleep Res. 1996;25:131.

243. Maislin G, Dinges DF, Pack FM, et al. The use of the geriatric depression scale to exclude depressed subjects in a case-control study of excessive daytime sleepiness. Sleep Res. 1996;25:289.

243a. Maislin G, Dinges DF, Hachadoorian R, et al. A case-control study of sleepiness in the elderly: role of sleep apnea. Sleep. 1999;22(suppl):S102.

244. Gallup Organization. Sleepiness in America. Princeton, NJ: Gallup Organization; June 1997.

245. Whitney CW, Enright PL, Newman AB, et al. Correlates of daytime sleepiness in 4578 elderly persons: the Cardiovascular Health Study. Sleep. 1998;21:27–36.

246. Hays JC, Blazer DG, Foley DJ. Risk of napping: excessive daytime sleepiness and mortality in an older community population. J Am Geriatr Soc. 1996;44:693–698.

247. Schmitt FA, Phillips BA, Cook YR, et al. Self report of sleep symptoms in older adults: correlates of daytime sleepiness and health. Sleep. 1996;19:59–64.

4

Daytime Sleepiness and Alertness

Timothy Roehrs

Mary A. Carskadon

William C. Dement

Thomas Roth

INTRODUCTION

Scientific and clinical attention to sleepiness arose from the recognition of excessive daytime sleepiness (EDS) as a symptom associated with serious life-threatening medical conditions. In the late 1960s, this symptom—which earlier had been ignored, attributed to lifestyle excesses, viewed as a sign of laziness and malingering, or at best, seen as a sign of narcolepsy—began to be seriously studied by scientist-clinicians. Consequently, methods to detect and quantify sleepiness were developed. The result has been a growing scientific literature on the nature of sleepiness and its determinants in clinical populations and in selected populations of healthy volunteers.

EPIDEMIOLOGY AND CLINICAL SIGNIFICANCE OF SLEEPINESS

Sleepiness in Limited Populations

In surveys of relatively small, selected populations, 0.5 to 36% of respondents reported excessive sleepiness. Variations in prevalence depend on the population sampled and the questions asked. Surveys with reported excessive sleepiness rates of less than 3% generally are from earlier studies that focused on hypersomnia.[1–3] In later studies, in which 4 to 9% rates were reported, more specific questions about excessive sleepiness during the day[4, 5] or relative to one's peers[6] were asked. In some surveys, postprandial, or midday, sleepiness was distinguished from sleepiness at other times of the day, a distinction discussed later in regard to the circadian correlates of sleepiness.[7, 8]

Prevalence rates for sleepiness of 15% and greater have been found for specific age groups, such as young adults and elderly people.[9, 10] These survey results are consistent with many smaller laboratory studies using the physiological measure of sleepiness (as described later). Young adults were sleepier, on average, than a comparison group of middle-aged adults, and about 20% of the young adults had mean daily sleep latencies of less than 5 min, a level of sleepiness considered pathological.[11] Healthy elderly also were found to be physiologically sleepier than middle-aged adults.[12] In surveys of the nearly 25% of the work force engaged in shift or night work, complaints of excessive sleepiness during waking hours are more frequent than among day workers,[13] and continuous ambulatory electroencephalographic (EEG) field monitoring has confirmed the sleepiness.[14]

Sleepiness in Representative Populations

Although no representative studies have been done of the U.S. population, several are available of Scandinavian populations. In a study representative of the Finnish population, 11% of women and 7% of men reported daytime sleepiness almost every day.[15] In another survey, representative of a large geographical area in Sweden, 12% of respondents thought their sleep was insufficient.[16] In that survey, insufficient sleep, and not its consequent daytime sleepiness, was the focus of the questions.

Risk Factors for Sleepiness in the Survey Data

The risk factors for sleepiness identified in the various surveys include hours of daily sleep, employment status, marital status, snoring, and depression. Among 26- to 35-year-old members of a large health maintenance organization in Michigan, respondents reported 6.7 h sleep on weekdays and 7.4 h on weekend days, on average.[17] The hours of sleep were inversely related to daytime sleepiness scores on the Sleep-Wake Activity Inventory (SWAI). Both these variables were related to employment and marital status, with full employment and being single predictive of less sleep time and more sleepiness. Self-reported snoring and depression, as measured by a structured diagnostic interview, were also associated with increased sleepiness. In the Finnish study cited earlier, sleepiness was associated with moderate to severe depression and with snoring more than three times per week.[15]

Clinical Significance of Sleepiness

Although the patients at sleep disorders centers are not representative of the general population, they do provide some indications regarding the clinical significance of sleepiness. Their sleep-wake histories directly indicate the serious impact excessive sleepiness has on their lives.[18] Nearly half the patients with excessive sleepiness report automobile accidents; half report occupational accidents, some life threatening; and many have lost jobs because of their sleepiness. In addition, sleepiness is considerably disruptive of family life.[19] An elevated automobile accident rate (i.e., sevenfold) among patients with excessive sleepiness has been verified through driving records obtained from motor vehicle agencies.[20, 21]

Population-based information regarding traffic and industrial accidents also suggests a link between sleepiness and life-threatening events. The highest rate of automobile accidents occurs in the early morning hours, which is notable because the fewest automobiles are on the road during these hours. Also during these early morning hours, the greatest degree of sleepiness is experienced.[22] Long-haul truck drivers have accidents most frequently (even corrected for hours driving before the accident) during the early morning hours, again when sleepiness reaches its zenith.[23]

Workers on the graveyard shift were identified as a particularly sleepy subpopulation. In 24-h ambulatory EEG recordings of sleep and wakefulness, workers (20% in one study) were found to actually fall asleep during the night shift.[14] Not surprisingly, the poorest job performance consistently occurs on the night shift, and the highest rate of industrial accidents is usually found among workers on this shift.[24]

Cognitive function is also impaired by sleepiness. In children, excessive sleepiness has been associated with learning disabilities,[9] and adults with various disorders of excessive sleepiness also have cognitive and memory problems.[25] The memory deficiencies are not specific to a certain sleep disorder but rather specific to the sleepiness associated with the disorder. When treated adequately, sleepiness is rectified and the memory and cognitive deficits similarly improve.[26, 27] Results of sleep deprivation studies in healthy normal patients support the relation between sleepiness and memory deficiency.[28] Even modest reductions of sleep time are associated with cognitive deficiencies.[29]

Sleepiness also depresses arousability to physiological challenges: 24-h sleep deprivation decreases upper airway dilator muscle activity[30] and decreases ventilatory reponses to hypercapnia and hypoxia.[31] In a canine model of sleep apnea, periodic disruption of sleep with acoustic stimuli (i.e., sleep fragmentation, in contrast to sleep deprivation) resulted in lengthened response times to airway occlusion, greater oxygen desaturation, increases in inspiratory pressures, and surges in blood pressure.[32] Depressed physiological responsivity due to sleepiness is clinically significant for patients with sleep apnea and other breathing disorders as they are all exacerbated by sleepiness.

Finally, life expectancy data directly link excessive sleep (not specifically sleepiness) and mortality. A 1976 study found that men and women who reported sleeping more than 10 h a day were about 1.8 times more likely to die prematurely than those sleeping between 7 and 8 h daily.[33] This survey, however, associated hypersomnia and increased mortality and not necessarily EDS, for which the relation is currently unknown.

NATURE OF SLEEPINESS

Physiological Need State

Sleepiness, according to a consensus among sleep researchers and clinicians, is a basic physiological need state.[34] It may be likened to hunger or thirst, which are physiological need states basic to the survival of the individual organism. The presence and intensity of this state can be inferred by how readily sleep onset occurs, how easily sleep is disrupted, and how long sleep endures. Deprivation or restriction of sleep increases sleepiness, and as hunger or thirst are reversible by eating or drinking, sleep reverses sleepiness. In the organism's daily homeostatic economy, severe deprivation states do not normally occur and hence are not routinely responsible for regulating eating, drinking, or sleeping; other factors (i.e., taste, smell, time-of-day, social factors, biological variables) modulate these behaviors before severe deprivation states develop.

The subjective experience of sleepiness and its behavioral indicators (yawning, eye rubbing, nodding) can be reduced under conditions of high motivation, excitement, exercise, and competing needs (e.g., hunger, thirst); that is, physiological sleepiness may not necessarily be manifest. But when physiological sleepiness is most severe or persistent, the ability to reduce its impact on overt behavior wanes. On the other hand, a physiologically alert (*sleepiness* and *alertness* are used as antonyms) person does not experience sleepiness or appear sleepy even in soporific situations. Heavy meals, warm rooms, boring lectures, and the monotony of long-distance automobile driving unmask physiological sleepiness, but they do not cause it.

Within a conventional 24-h sleep and wake schedule, maximum sleepiness ordinarily occurs in the middle of the night when the individual is sleeping, and consequently this sleepiness typically is not experienced or remembered. When forced to be awake in the middle of the night, one experiences loss of energy, fatigue, weariness, difficulty concentrating, and memory lapses. When significant physiological sleepiness (as a result of reduced sleep quantity or quality) intrudes on one's usual waking activities during the day, similar symptoms are experienced.

The specific nature of this physiological need state is unclear. Whether sleepiness is unidimensional, varying only in severity, or multidimensional, varying as to sleep stage or chronicity, has been discussed.[35] And if it is unidimensional, whether or not sleepiness and alertness are at opposite poles of the dimension is also an issue. Earlier, it was noted that sleepiness and alertness are being used as antonyms, which suggests a unipolar state. However, it is possible that sleepiness varies from presence to absence and is distinct from alertness. Pivik noted that sleepiness may be multidimensional, and among the different types of sleepiness he cited are rapid eye movement (REM) versus non-rapid eye movement (NREM) and core versus optional sleepiness.[35] A complete discussion of the heuristic value and evidence to support these distinctions is beyond the scope of this chapter. Nonetheless, the point must be made that these theoretical perspectives may be colored by different measures, experimental demands, populations studied, and subject or patient motivations (i.e., sensitivity to and capacity to counteract sleepiness). Measurement and standardization issues are further discussed in the following section.

Neural Substrates of Sleepiness

The substrates of sleepiness have yet to be determined. It is assumed that sleepiness is a central nervous system (CNS) phenomenon with identifiable neural mechanisms and neurochemical correlates. Various electrophysiological events suggestive of incipient sleep processes appear in behaviorally awake organisms undergoing sleep deprivation. In sleep-deprived animals, ventral hippocampal spike activity, which normally is a characteristic of NREM sleep, increases during behavioral wakefulness and in the absence of the usual changes in cortical EEG results indicative of sleep.[36] Human beings deprived of or restricted from sleep show identifiable microsleep episodes (brief intrusions of EEG indications of sleep) and increased amounts of alpha and theta activity while behaviorally awake.[37, 38] The evidence suggests that these electrophysiological events are indicants of sleepiness.

A limited number of neuroimaging studies, both structural and functional, have suggested specific brain systems that may be involved in sleepiness. Sleep deprivation in young healthy volunteers reduced regional cerebral glucose metabolism, as assessed by positron emission tomography, in thalamic, basal ganglia, and limbic regions of the brain.[39] Functional magnetic resonance imaging (fMRI) after chlorpheniramine (a sedating antihistamine) compared with placebo showed increased frontal and temporal activation.[40] Because fMRI is conducted while the subject is performing cognitive tasks, the authors interpreted the increased brain activation to result from the increased mental effort, due to sleepiness, required to perform the task. Two groups of patients with severe or slight hypersomnia associ-

ated with paramedian thalamic stroke on an MRI showed lesions involving dorso- and centromedial thalamic nuclei, bilateral lesions in the severe group and unilateral in the slight group.[41] As yet, these imaging data are not conclusive. They do suggest it may be possible to identify brain regions and functions that vary with sleepiness. But the nature of the alteration may depend on the behavioral load imposed on the sleepy subject.

The neurochemistry of sleepiness-alertness involves critical and complex issues that have not yet been fully untangled (see Chapters 10, 32, and 34 for a complete discussion). First, a basic issue concerns whether sleepiness-alertness has a neurochemistry specific and unique from that associated with the sleep process, per se. Second, it is not clear whether sleepiness and alertness are controlled by separate neurochemicals or by a single substance or system. Third, the relation of the neurochemistry of sleepiness-alertness to circadian mechanisms has not yet been determined. Given the number of questions, it should be of no surprise that these are areas of active research.

Neurophysiological studies of sleep and wake mechanisms have implicated histamine, serotonin, the catecholamines, and acetycholine in control of sleep and wake, and these neurotransmitters also may play some role in sleepiness-alertness.[42] Other studies have explored a variety of sleep-inducing substances (e.g., peptides and endocrines) as possible sleep regulators, and any of these substances may prove to be a correlate of sleepiness-alertness.[43]

Pharmacological studies provide other interesting hypotheses regarding the neurochemistry of sleepiness-alertness. For example, the benzodiazepines induce sleepiness and facilitate gamma-aminobutyric acid (GABA) function at the GABA receptor complex, thus implicating this important and diffuse inhibitory neurotransmitter.[44] Another example involves histamine, which is now considered to be a CNS neurotransmitter and is thought to have CNS-arousing activity.[45] Antihistamines that penetrate the CNS produce sleepiness.[46]

Stimulant drugs suggest several other transmitters. The mechanism of action of one class of drugs producing psychomotor stimulation and arousal, the amphetamines, is blockade of catecholamine uptake.[47] Another class of stimulants, the methylxanthines, which include caffeine and theophylline, are adenosine receptor antagonists. Adenosine, although not a transmitter in the classic sense, is thought to modulate transmitter activity.[48] Currently available information remains too sketchy for definitive conclusions, and the space here is too limited to discuss all the evidence in detail. Thus, although it is widely held that sleepiness is a physiological state, its physiological substrates are as yet unknown.

ASSESSMENT OF SLEEPINESS
Quantifying Sleepiness

The behavioral signs of sleepiness include yawning, ptosis, reduced activity, lapses in attention, and head nodding. An individual's subjective report of his or her level of sleepiness also can be elicited. As noted earlier, a number of factors such as motivation, stimulation, and competing needs can reduce the behavioral manifestation of sleepiness. Thus, behavioral and subjective indicators do not always accurately reflect physiological sleepiness.

Assessment problems were evident early in research on the daytime consequences of sleep loss. Sleep loss compromises daytime functions; virtually everyone experiences dysphoria and reduced peformance efficiency when not sleeping adequately. But a majority of the tasks used to assess the effects of sleep loss are insensitive.[37] In general, only long and monotonous tasks are reliably sensitive to changes in the quantity and quality of nocturnal sleep. An exception is a 10-min visual vigilance task during which lapses (response times $\geq$500 msec) and declines in the best response times are increasingly observed as sleep is lost, either during total deprivation or cumulatively over nights of restricted bedtimes.[49, 50]

In various measures of mood, including factor analytic scales, visual analogue scales, and scales for specific aspects of mood, subjects have shown increased fatigue or sleepiness with sleep loss. Among the various subjective measures of sleepiness, the Stanford Sleepiness Scale (SSS) is the best validated.[51] Yet clinicians have found that patients may rate themselves alert on the SSS even while they are falling asleep behaviorally.[52] All of these scales are state measures that query individuals about how they feel at the present moment. Another perspective is to view sleepiness behaviorally, as in the likelihood of falling asleep, and thus ask individuals to rate that likelihood in different social circumstances and over longer periods. Two such behavioral rating scales, the Epworth Sleepiness Scale (ESS) and the SWAI, have quite acceptable psychometrics.[53, 54] The ESS has been validated in clinical populations and the SWAI in both clinical and experimental settings. Both ask about falling asleep in settings in which patients typically report falling asleep (e.g., while driving, at church, in social conversation). The time frame over which ratings are to be made is 2 to 4 weeks.

The standard physiological measure of sleepiness, the multiple sleep latency test (MSLT), similarly conceptualizes sleepiness as the likelihood of falling asleep. The MSLT has gained wide acceptance within the field of sleep and sleep disorders as the standard method of quantifying sleepiness.[55] Using standard polysomnographic techniques, this test measures, on repeated opportunities at 2-h intervals throughout the day, the latency to fall asleep while lying in a quiet, dark bedroom. The MSLT is based on the assumption, as outlined earlier, that sleepiness is a physiological need state that leads to an increased tendency to fall asleep. The reliability and validity of this measure have been documented in a variety of experimental and clinical situations.[56] In contrast to tests of performance, motivation does not seem to reduce the impact of sleep loss as measured by the MSLT. After total sleep deprivation, subjects can compensate for impaired per-

formance, but they cannot stay awake long while in bed in a darkened room, even if they are instructed to do so.[57]

An alternative to the MSLT, suggested by some clinical investigators, is the Maintenance of Wakefulness Test (MWT). This test requires that subjects lie in bed or sit in a chair in a darkened room and try to remain awake.[58] Like the MSLT, the measure of ability to remain awake is the latency to sleep onset. The test has not been standardized: there are 20-min and 40-min versions, and the subject is variously sitting upright in a chair, lying in bed, or semirecumbent in bed. The reliability of the MWT has not been established either. One study reported sensitivity to the therapeutic effects of continuous positive airway pressure (CPAP) in patients with sleep apnea,[59] and several studies reported sensitivity to the therapeutic effects of stimulants in narcolepsy.[60]

The rationale for the MWT is that clinically the critical issue for patients is how long wakefulness can be maintained. A basic assumption underlying this rationale, however, may not be valid: it assumes that a set of circumstances can be evaluated in the laboratory that will reflect an individual's probability of staying awake in the real world. Such a circumstance is not likely because environment, motivation, circadian phase, and any competing drive states all affect an individual's tendency to remain awake. Stated simply, an individual crossing a congested intersection at midday is more likely to stay awake than an individual driving on an isolated highway in the middle of the night. The MSLT, on the other hand, addresses the question of the individual's risk of falling asleep by establishing a setting to maximize the likelihood of sleep onset: all factors competing with falling asleep are removed from the test situation. Thus, the MSLT identifies sleep tendency or clinically identifies maximum risk for the patient. Obviously, the actual risk will vary from individual to individual, from hour to hour, and from environment to environment.

Relation of Sleepiness to Behavioral Functioning

Given that the MSLT is a valid and reliable measure of sleepiness, the question arises as to how this measure relates to an individual's capacity to function. Direct correlations of the MSLT with other measures of performance under normal conditions have not been too robust.[61] Several studies have found, however, that when sleepiness is at maximum levels, correlations with performance are high. For example, MSLT scores after sleep deprivation,[62, 63] after administration of sedating antihistamines,[64] and after benzodiazepine administration[65] correlate with measures of performance and even prove to be the most sensitive measure.[65] A recent study relating performance lapses on a vigilance task to the cumulative effects of sleep restriction found a function comparable to that of the MSLT under a similar cumulative sleep restriction[66] (Fig. 4–1). The reason many studies have found weak correlations be-

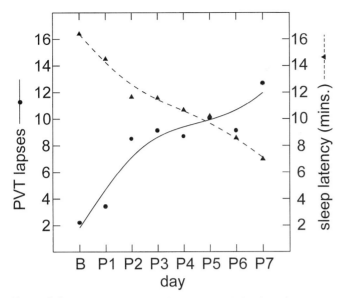

Figure 4–1. Similar functions relating mean daily sleep latency on the multiple sleep latency test (MSLT) and mean daily lapses on the visual psychomotor vigilance test (PVT) to the cumulative effects of sleep restriction (about 5 h bedtime nightly) across 7 consecutive nights (P1 to P7). (From Dinges DF, Pack F, Williams K, et al. Cumulative sleepiness, mood disturbance, and psychomotor vigilance performance decrements during a week of sleep restricted to 4–5 hours per night. Sleep. 1997;20:275.)

tween performance and MSLT at normal or moderate levels of sleepiness is that laboratory performance and MSLT are differentially affected by variables such as age, education, and motivation.

Clinical Assessment of Sleepiness

Assessing the clinical significance of a patient's complaint of excessive sleepiness can be complex for an inexperienced clinician. The assessment depends on two important factors: chronicity and reversibility. Chronicity can be explained simply. Although a healthy normal individual may be acutely sleepy, the patient's sleepiness is persistent and unremitting. As to reversibility, unlike the healthy normal person, increased sleep time may not completely or consistently ameliorate a patient's sleepiness. Patients with excessive sleepiness may not complain of sleepiness per se, but rather its consequences: loss of energy, fatigue, lethargy, weariness, lack of initiative, memory lapses, or difficulty concentrating.

To clarify the patient complaint, it is important to focus on soporific situations in which physiological sleepiness is more likely to be manifest, as was discussed earlier. Such situations might include watching TV, reading, riding in a car, listening to a lecture, or sitting in a warm room. Table 4–1 presents the commonly reported sleep-inducing situations for a large sample of patients with sleep apnea syndrome. After clarifying the complaint, one should ask the patient about the entire day: morning, midday, and evening. In the next section, it will become clear that most adults

experience sleepiness over the midday. However, patients experience sleepiness at other times of the day as well, and often throughout the day. Whenever possible, objective documentation of sleepiness and its severity should be sought. As indicated earlier, the standard and accepted method to document sleepiness objectively is the MSLT.

Guidelines for interpreting the results of the MSLT are available.[55] A number of case series of patients with disorders of excessive sleepiness have now been published with accompanying MSLT data for each diagnostic classification.[67, 68] These data provide the clinician with guidelines for evaluating the clinical significance of a given patient's MSLT results. Although these data cannot be considered norms, a scheme for ranking MSLT scores to indicate degree of pathology has been suggested.[67] An average daily MSLT score of 5 min or fewer suggests pathological sleepiness, a score of more than 5 min but fewer than 10 min is considered a diagnostic gray area, and a score of more than 10 min is considered to be in the normal range. The MSLT results, however, must also be evaluated with respect to the conditions under which the testing was conducted. Standards have been published for administering the MSLT, which must be followed to obtain a valid, interpretable result.[55]

Determinants of Sleepiness

Quantity of Sleep

The degree of daytime sleepiness is directly related to the amount of nocturnal sleep. Partial or total sleep deprivation in healthy normal subjects is followed by increased daytime sleepiness the following day.[69] Therefore, modest nightly sleep restriction accumulates over nights to progressively increase daytime sleepiness and performance lapses (see Fig. 4–1).[70] On the other hand, increased sleep time in healthy normal young adults, by extending bedtime beyond the usual 7 to 8 h per night, produces an increase in alertness (i.e., reduction in sleepiness).[71, 72] Further, the pharmacological extension of sleep time by an average of 1 h in elderly people produces an increase in mean sleep latency on the MSLT (i.e., increased alertness).[73]

Table 4–1. SLEEP-INDUCING SITUATIONS IN APNEA PATIENTS*

Situation	Percentage of Patients
Watching television	91
Reading	85
Riding in a car	71
Attending church	57
Visiting friends and relatives	54
Driving	50
Working	43
Waiting for a red light	32

*n = 384 patients.

Reduced sleep time explains the excessive sleepiness of several patient and nonpatient groups. For example, a subgroup of sleep clinic patients has been identified whose excessive daytime sleepiness can be attributed to chronic insufficient sleep.[74] These patients show objectively documented excessive sleepiness, "normal" nocturnal sleep with unusually high efficiency (time asleep–time in bed), and report about 2 h more sleep on each weekend day than each weekday. Regularizing bedtime and increasing time in bed produces a resolution of their symptoms and normalized MSLT results.[75, 76] The increased sleepiness of healthy young adults also can be attributed to insufficient nocturnal sleep. When the sleepiest 25% of a sample of young adults is given extended time in bed (10 h) for as long as 5 to 14 consecutive nights, their sleepiness is reduced to a level resembling the general population.[71, 72]

Quality of Sleep

Daytime sleepiness also relates to the quality and the continuity of a previous night's sleep. Sleep in patients with a number of sleep disorders is punctuated by frequent, brief arousals of 3 to 15 sec duration. These arousals are characterized by bursts of EEG speeding or alpha activity and, occasionally, transient increases in skeletal muscle tone. Standard scoring rules for transient EEG arousals have been developed.[77] A transient arousal is illustrated in Figure 4–2. These arousals typically do not result in awakening by either Rechtschaffen and Kales sleep staging criteria or behavioral indicators, and the arousals recur in some conditions as often as 1 to 4 times per minute. The arousing stimulus differs in the various disorders and can be identified in some cases (apneas, leg move-

ments, pain) but not in others. Regardless of etiology, the arousals generally do not result in shortened sleep but rather in fragmented or discontinuous sleep, and this fragmentation produces daytime sleepiness.

Correlational evidence suggests a relation between sleep fragmentation and daytime sleepiness. Fragmentation, as indexed by number of brief EEG arousals, number of shifts from other sleep stages to stage 1 sleep or wake, and the percentage of stage 1 sleep, correlates with EDS in various patient groups.[78] Treatment studies also link sleep fragmentation and excessive sleepiness. Patients with sleep apnea syndrome who are successfully treated by surgery (i.e., number of apneas are reduced) show a reduced frequency of arousals from sleep as well as a reduced level of sleepiness, whereas those who do not benefit from the surgery (i.e., apneas remain) show no decrease in arousals or sleepiness, despite improved sleeping oxygenation.[79] Similarly, CPAP, by providing a pneumatic airway splint, reduces breathing disturbances and consequent arousals from sleep and reverses EDS.[80] The reversal of daytime sleepiness following CPAP treatment of sleep apnea syndrome is presented in Figure 4–3.

Experimental fragmentation of the sleep of healthy normal subjects has been produced by inducing arousals with an auditory stimulus. Several studies have shown that subjects awakened at various intervals during the night demonstrate performance decrements and increased sleepiness on the following day.[81, 82] Studies have also fragmented sleep without awakening subjects by terminating the stimulus on EEG signs of arousal rather than on behavioral response. Increased daytime sleepiness (shortened latencies on the MSLT) resulted from nocturnal sleep fragmentation in one study,[83] and in a second study, the recuperative effects (measured as increased latencies on the MSLT) of a

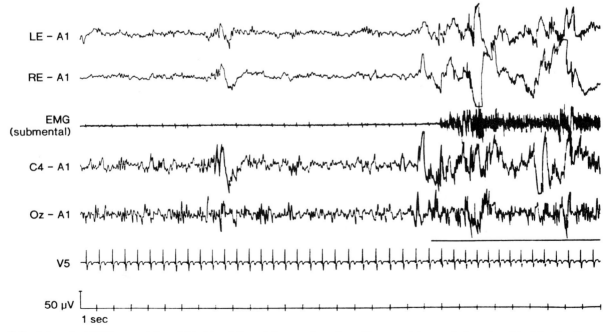

Figure 4–2. A transient EEG arousal (on right side of figure) fragmenting sleep. The preexistence of sleep is evident by the K-complex at second 9 of the epoch preceding the arousal. (From American Sleep Disorders Association. EEG arousals: scoring rules and examples. Sleep. 1992;15:173–184.)

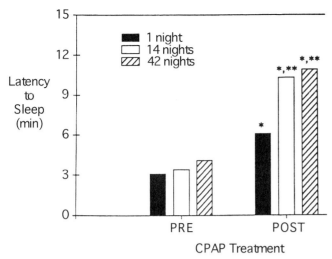

Figure 4–3. Mean daily sleep latency on the multiple sleep latency test (MSLT) in patients with obstructive sleep apnea syndrome before (pre) and after (post) 1, 14 and 42 nights of continuous positive airway pressure (CPAP) treatment. (From Lamphere J, Roehrs T, Wittig R, et al. Recovery of alertness after CPAP in apnea. Chest. 1989;96:1364–1367.)

nap following sleep deprivation were compromised by fragmenting the sleep on the nap.[84]

One population in whom sleep fragmentation is an important determinant of excessive sleepiness is the elderly. Many studies have now shown that even elderly people without sleep complaints show an increased number of apneas and periodic leg movements during sleep.[85, 86] As noted earlier, the elderly as a group are sleepier than other groups.[12] Furthermore, it has been demonstrated that elderly people with the highest frequency of arousal during sleep have the greatest daytime sleepiness.[87]

Circadian Rhythms

A biphasic pattern of objective sleep tendency was observed when healthy normal young adult and elderly subjects were tested every 2 h over a complete 24-h day.[88] During the sleep period (11:30 PM to 8 AM) the latency testing was accomplished by awakening subjects for 15 min and then allowing them to return to sleep. Two troughs of alertness—one during the nocturnal hours (about 2 to 6 AM) and another during the daytime hours (about 2 to 6 PM)—were observed. Figure 4–4 shows the biphasic pattern of sleepiness-alertness.

Other research protocols have yielded similar results. In constant routine studies, where external environmental stimulation is minimized and subjects remain awake, superimposed on the expected increase in self-rated fatigue resulting from the deprivation of sleep is a biphasic circadian rhythmicity of self-rated fatigue similar to that seen for sleepiness.[89] In another constant routine study in which EEG results were continuously monitored, a biphasic pattern of "unintentional sleep" was observed.[90] In studies with sleep scheduled at unusual times, the duration of sleep peri-

ods has been used as an index of the level of sleepiness. A pronounced circadian variation in sleep duration is found with the termination of sleep periods closely related to the biphasic sleep latency function in the studies cited earlier.[91, 92] If individuals are permitted to nap when they are placed in time-free environments, this biphasic pattern becomes quite apparent in the form of a midcycle nap.[93]

This circadian rhythm in sleepiness is part of a circadian system in which many biological processes vary rhythmically over 24 h. The sleepiness rhythm parallels the circadian variation in body temperature, with shortened latencies occurring in conjunction with temperature reductions.[88] But these two functions, sleep latency and body temperature, are not mirror images of each other; the midday body temperature decline is relatively small compared with that of sleep latency. Further, under freerunning conditions, the two functions can be dissociated.[94] However, no other biological rhythm is as closely associated with the circadian rhythm of sleepiness as is body temperature.

Earlier, it was noted that shift workers are unusually sleepy, and jet travelers experience sleepiness acutely in a new time zone. The sleepiness in these two conditions results from the placement of sleep and wakefulness at times that are out of phase with the existing circadian rhythms. Thus, not only is daytime sleep shortened and fragmented but also wakefulness occurs at the peak of sleepiness or trough of alertness. Several studies have shown that pharmacological extension and consolidation of out-of-phase sleep can improve daytime sleepiness[95, 96] (see Chapter 54 for more detail). Yet, the basal circadian rhythm of sleepiness remains, although the overall level of sleepiness has been reduced. In other words, the synchronization of circadian rhythms to the new sleep-wake schedule is not hastened.

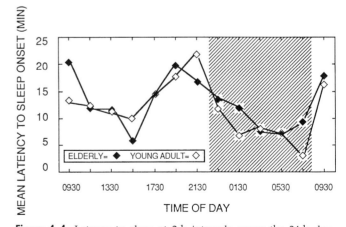

Figure 4–4. Latency to sleep at 2-h intervals across the 24-h day. Testing during the daytime followed standard multiple sleep latency test (MSLT) procedures. During the night, from 11:30 PM to 8:00 AM (shaded area), subjects were awakened every 2 h for 15 min, and latency of return to sleep was measured. Elderly subjects (n=10) were aged 60 to 83 years; young subjects (n=8) were aged 19 to 23 years. (Reprinted from Neuroscience and Biobehavioral Reviews, vol. 11, Carskadon MA, Dement WC, Daytime sleepiness: quantification of a behavioral state, 307–317, Copyright 1987, with permission from Elsevier Science.)

Drugs

Sedating Drug Effects

CNS depressant drugs, as expected, increase sleepiness. The benzodiazepine hypnotics hasten sleep onset at bedtime and shorten the latency to return to sleep after an awakening during the night (which is their therapeutic purpose), as demonstrated by a number of objective studies.[97] Long-acting benzodiazepines continue to shorten sleep latency on the MSLT the day following bedtime administration.[98] Barbiturates also reduce sleep latency at night, and during the following day they continue to produce sedation as measured by performance testing.[99] The common use of barbiturate hypnotics was discontinued before the development of the MSLT, and, consequently, no studies have assessed their daytime sedating effects by MSLT. Finally, ethanol administered during the daytime (9 AM) reduces sleep latency in a dose-related manner as measured by the MSLT.[100, 101]

One of the most commonly reported side effects associated with the use of H_1 antihistamines is daytime sleepiness. Several double-blind, placebo-controlled studies have shown that certain H_1 antihistamines, such as diphenhydramine, increase sleepiness using sleep latency as the objective measure of sleepiness, whereas others, such as terfenadine or loratadine do not.[102, 103] The difference among these compounds relates to their differential CNS penetration and binding. Others of the H_1 antihistamines (e.g., tazifylline) are thought to have a greater peripheral compared with central H_1 affinity, and, consequently, effects on daytime sleep latency are found only at relatively high doses.[103]

Antihypertensives, particularly beta adrenoreceptor blockers, are also reported to produce sedation during the daytime.[104] These CNS effects are thought to be related to the differential liposolubility of the various compounds. However, we are unaware of any studies that directly measure the daytime sleepiness produced by beta blockers; the information is derived from reports of side effects. As noted earlier, it is important to differentiate sleepiness from tiredness or fatigue. Patients may be describing tiredness or fatigue resulting from the drugs' peripheral effects (i.e., lowered cardiac output and blood pressure), not sleepiness, a presumed central effect.

Alerting Drug Effects

Stimulant drugs reduce sleepiness and increase alertness. Amphetamine, methylphenidate, modafinil, and pemoline are used to treat the EDS associated with narcolepsy and some have been studied as medications to maintain alertness and vigilance in normal subjects under conditions of sustained sleep loss (e.g., military operations). Studies in patients with narcolepsy using MSLT or MWT have shown improved alertness with amphetamine, methylphenidate, modafinil, and pemoline.[105, 106] There is dispute as to the extent to which the excessive sleepiness of narcoleptics is reversed and the comparative efficacy of the various drugs. In healthy normal patients restricted or deprived of sleep, both amphetamine and methylphenidate increase alertness on the MSLT and improve psychomotor performance.[107, 108] Caffeine, in doses equivalent to 1 to 3 cups of coffee, reduced daytime sleepiness on the MSLT in normal subjects after 5 h of sleep the previous night.[109]

Influence of Basal Sleepiness

The preexisting level of sleepiness-alertness can interact with a drug to influence the drug's behavioral effect. In other words, a drug's effect may differ when sleepiness is at its maximum compared to its minimum. As noted previously, the basal level of daytime sleepiness can be altered by restricting or extending time in bed[69, 70]; this in turn alters the usual effects of a stimulating versus a sedating drug. A study showed comparable levels of sleepiness-alertness during the day following 5 h in bed and morning (9 AM) caffeine consumption compared to 11 h in bed and morning (9 AM) ethanol ingestion.[110] Follow-up studies explored the dose relations of ethanol's interaction with basal sleepiness.[101] Dose-related differences in daytime sleepiness following ethanol and 8 h of sleep were diminished after even 1 night of 5 h sleep, although the measured levels of ethanol in breath were consistent day to day. In other words, sleepiness enhanced the sedative effects of ethanol. In contrast, caffeine and methylphenidate produced a similar increase in alertness, regardless of the basal level of sleepiness. Clinically, these findings imply, for example, that a sleepy driver with minimal blood ethanol levels may be as dangerous as an alert driver who is legally intoxicated.[111]

Sleep Pathologies

Pathology of the CNS is assumed to be another determinant of daytime sleepiness. An unidentified CNS pathology is thought to cause excessive sleepiness in patients with narcolepsy.[112] Another sleep disorder associated with excessive sleepiness and thought to be due to an unknown pathology of the CNS is idiopathic CNS hypersomnolence.[113] In both conditions, although the pathophysiology has not been definitively established, the excessive sleepiness has been well documented. These two conditions are described in detail in Chapters 60 and 61.

References

1. McGhie A, Russel SM. The subjective assessment of normal sleep patterns. J Ment Sci. 1962;8:642–654.
2. Bixler ED, Kales JD, Soldatos CR, et al. Prevalence of sleep disorders in the Los Angeles metropolitan area. Am J Psychiatry. 1979;136:1257–1262.
3. Ford DE, Kamerow DB. Epidemiologic study of sleep disturbances and psychiatric disorders. JAMA. 1989;262:1479–1484.
4. Billiard M, Alperovitch A, Perot C, et al. Excessive daytime somnolence in young men: prevalence and contributing factors. Sleep. 1987;10:297–305.
5. Lavie P. Sleep habits and sleep disturbances in industrial work-

ers in Israel: main findings and some characteristics of workers complaining of excessive daytime sleepiness. Sleep. 1981;4:147–158.

6. Partinen M. Sleeping habits and sleep disorders of Finnish men before, during, and after military service. Ann Med Milit Fenn. 1982;57(suppl):96.

7. Lugaresi E, Cirignotta F, Zucconi M, et al. Good and poor sleepers: an epidemiological survey of the San Marino population. In: Guilleminault C, Lugaresi E, eds. Sleep/Wake Disorders: Natural History, Epidemiology, and Long-Term Evolution. New York, NY: Raven Press; 1983:2–12.

8. Martikainen K, Hasan J, Uropen H, et al. Daytime sleepiness: a risk factor in community life. Acta Neurol Scand. 1992;86:337–341.

9. Carskadon MA. Patterns of sleep and sleepiness in adolescents. Pediatrician. 1990;17:5–12.

10. Asplund R. Daytime sleepiness and napping amongst the elderly in relation to somatic health and medical treatment. J Intern Med. 1996;239:261–267.

11. Levine B, Roehrs T, Zorick F, et al. Daytime sleepiness in young adults. Sleep. 1988;11:39–46.

12. Dement WC, Carskadon MA. An essay on sleepiness. In: Baldy-Mouliner M, ed. Actualités en Medecine Experimentale. Montpellier, France: Euromed; 1981:47–71.

13. Akerstedt T, Frober JE. Shift work and health—interdisciplinary aspects. In: Rentos PGR, Shepard RD, eds. Shift Work and Health—A Symposium. Washington, DC: NIOSH; 1976:179–197.

14. Torsvall L, Akerstedt T, Gillander K, et al. Sleep on the night shift: 24h EEG monitoring of spontaneous sleep/wake behavior. Psychophysiology. 1989;26:352–358.

15. Hublin C, Kaprio J, Partinen M, et al. Daytime sleepiness in an adult Finnish population. J Intern Med. 1996;239:417–423.

16. Broman JE, Lundh LG, Hetta J. Insufficient sleep in the general population. Neurophysiol Clin. 1996;26:30–39.

17. Breslau N, Roth T, Rosenthal L, et al. Daytime sleepiness: an epidemiological study of young adults. Am J Public Health. 1997;87:1649–1653.

18. Guilleminault C, Carskadon M. Relationship between sleep disorders and daytime complaints. In: Koeller WP, Oevin PW, eds. Sleep 1976. Basel, Switzerland: Karger; 1977:95–100.

19. Broughton R, Ghanem Q, Hishikawa Y, et al. Life effects of narcolepsy in 180 patients from North America, Asia and Europe compared to matched controls. J Can Sci Neurol. 1981;8:299–304.

20. Findley LJ, Unverzagt ME, Suratt PM. Automobile accidents involving patients with obstructive apnea. Am Rev Respir Dis. 1988;138:337–340.

21. Findley LJ, Unverzagt ME, Guchu R, et al. Vigilance and automobile accidents in patients with sleep apnea or narcolepsy. Chest. 1995;108:619–624.

22. Mitler MM, Carskadon MA, Czeisler CA, et al. Catastrophes, sleep, and public policy: consensus report. Sleep. 1988;11:100–109.

23. Mackie RR, Miller JC. Effects of hours of service, regularity of schedules, and cargo loading on truck and bus driver fatigue. Washington, DC: US Government Printing Office;1978. Technical Report 1765-F DOT-HS-5-01142.

24. Folkard S: Shiftwork and performance. In Johnson LC, Tepas DI, Colquhoun WJ, et al, eds. The Twenty-Four Hour Workday: Proceedings of a Symposium on Variations in Work-Sleep Schedules. Washington DC: US Government Printing Office; 1981:347–373. DHHS publication (NIOSH) 81-127.

25. Roehrs TA, Merrion M, Pedrosi B, et al. Neuropsychological function in obstructive sleep apnea syndrome (OSAS) compared to chronic obstructive pulmonary disease (COPD). Sleep. 1995;18:382–388.

26. Aguirre M, Broughton RJ, Stuss D. Does memory impairment exist in narcolepsy-cataplexy? J Clin Exp Neuropsychol. 1985;7:14–24.

27. Bedard MA, Montplaisir J, Malo J, et al. Persistent neuropsychological deficits and vigilance impairment in sleep apnea syndrome after treatment with continuous positive airway pressure (CPAP). J Clin Exp Neuropsychol. 1993;15:330–341.

28. Dinges DF, Kribbs NB. Performing while sleep: effects of experimentally-induced sleepiness. In: Monk T, ed. Sleep, Sleepiness and Performance. New York, NY: John Wiley & Sons; 1991:97–128.

29. Blagrove M, Alexander C, Horne JA. The effects of chronic sleep reduction on the performance of cognitive tasks sensitive to sleep deprivation. Appl Cogn Psychol. 1994;9:21–40.

30. Leiter JC, Knuth SL, Barlett D. The effect of sleep deprivation on activity of the genioglossus muscle. Am Rev Respir Dis. 1985;132:1242–1245.

31. White DP, Douglas NJ, Pickett CK, et al. Sleep deprivation and control of ventilation. Am Rev Respir Dis. 1983;128:984–986.

32. Brooks D, Horner RL, Kimoff RJ, et al. Effect of obstructive sleep apnea versus sleep fragmentation on responses to airway occlusion. Am J Respir Crit Care Med. 1997;155:1609–1617.

33. Kripke DF, Simons NR, Garfinkel L, et al. Short and long sleep and sleeping pills. Is increased mortality associated? Arch Gen Psychiatry. 1979;36:103–116.

34. Carskadon MA, Dement WC. The multiple sleep latency test: what does it measure? Sleep. 1982;5:S67–S72.

35. Pivik RT. The several qualities of sleepiness: psychophysiological considerations. In: Monk T, ed. Sleep, Sleepiness and Performance. New York, NY: John Wiley & Sons; 1991:3–37.

36. Friedman L, Bergmann BM, Rechtschaffen A. Effects of sleep deprivation on sleepiness, sleep intensity, and subsequent sleep in the rat. Sleep. 1979;1:369–391.

37. Webb WB. Sleep deprivation: total, partial and selective. In: Chase MH, ed. The Sleeping Brain. Los Angeles, Calif: BIS/BRS; 1972:323–362.

38. Akerstedt T, Torsvall L, Gillberg M. Sleepiness and shift work: field studies. Sleep. 1982;5:S95–S106.

39. Wu JC, Gillin JC, Buchsbaum MS, et al. The effect of sleep deprivation on cerebral glucose metabolic rate in normal humans assessed with positron emission tomography. Sleep. 1991;14:155–162.

40. Starbuck VN, Kay GG, Platenberg RC. Functional magnetic resonance imaging shows evidence of daytime sleepiness following evening dosing with chlorpheniramine. J Allergy Clin Immunol. 1998:101:408.

41. Lovblad KO, Bassetti C, Mathis J, et al. MRI of paramedian thalamic stroke with sleep disturbance. Neuroradiology. 1997;39:693–698.

42. Monnier M, Gaillard JM. Biochemical regulation of sleep. Experientia. 1980;36:21–24.

43. Inoue S. Sleep substances: their roles and evolution. In: Inoue S, Borbely AA, eds. Endogenous Sleep Substances and Sleep Regulation. Tokyo, Japan: Japan Scientific Societies Press; 1985:3–12.

44. Gallager DW. Benzodiazepines and gamma-aminobutyric acid. Sleep. 1982;5:S3–S11.

45. Pollard H, Schwartz JC. Histamine neuronal pathways and their functions. Trends Neurosci. 1987;10:86–89.

46. Roehrs T, Zwyghuizen-Doorenbos A, Roth T. Sedative effects and plasma concentrations following single doses of triazolam, diphenhydramine, ethanol and placebo. Sleep. 1993;16:301–305.

47. Chiarello RJ, Cole JO. The use of psychostimulants in general psychiatry. Arch Gen Psychiatry. 1987;44:286–295.

48. Dunwiddie TV. The physiological role of adenosine in the central nervous system. Int Rev Neurobiol. 1985;27:63–139.

49. Wilkinson RT, Houghton D. Field test of arousal: a portable reaction timer with data. Hum Factors. 1982;24:487–493.

50. Dinges DF, Orne MT, Whithouse WG, et al. Temporal placement of a nap for alertness: contributions of circadian phase and prior wakefulness. Sleep. 1987;10:313–329.

51. Hoddes E, Zarcone VP, Smythe H. Quantification of sleepiness: a new approach. Psychophysiology. 1973;10:431–436.

52. Dement WC, Carskadon MA, Richardson G. Excessive daytime sleepiness in the sleep apnea syndrome. In: Guilleminault C, Dement WC, eds. Sleep Apnea Syndromes. New York, NY: Alan R Liss; 1978:23–46.

53. Johns MW. Sleepiness in different situations measured by the Epworth Sleepiness Scale. Sleep. 1994;17:703–710.

54. Rosenthal L. The sleep wake activity inventory: a self report measure of daytime sleepiness. Biol Psychiatry. 1993;34:810–820.

55. Carskadon MA, Dement WC, Mitler MM, et al. Guidelines for the multiple sleep latency test (MSLT): a standard measure of sleepiness. Sleep. 1986;9:519–524.

56. Carskadon MA, Dement WC. Nocturnal determinants of daytime sleepiness. Sleep. 1982;5:S73–S81.

57. Hartse KM, Roth T, Zorick FJ. Daytime sleepiness and daytime wakefulness: the effect of instruction. Sleep. 1982;5:S107–S118.

58. Mitler MM, Gujavarty KS, Browman CP. Maintenance of wakefulness test: a polysomnographic technique for evaluating treatment efficacy in patients with excessive somnolence. Electroencephalogr Clin Neurophysiol. 1982;53:658–661.

59. Sangal RB, Thomas L, Mitler MM. Disorders of excessive sleepiness: treatment improves ability to stay awake, but does not reduce sleepiness. Chest. 1992;102:699–703.

60. Mitler MM, Hajdukovic R. Relative efficacy of drugs for the treatment of sleepiness in narcolepsy. Sleep. 1991;14:218–220.

61. Carskadon MA, Harvey K, Dement WC. Acute restriction of nocturnal sleep in children. Percept Mot Skills. 1981;53:103–112.

62. Carskadon MA, Dement WC. Effects of total sleep loss on sleep tendency. Percept Mot Skills. 1977;48:495–506.

63. Carskadon MA, Harvey K, Dement WC. Sleep loss in young adolescents. Sleep. 1981;4:299–312.

64. Nicholson AN, Stone BM. Impaired performance and the tendency to sleep. Eur J Clin Pharmacol. 1986;30:27–32.

65. Roehrs T, Kribbs N, Zorick F, et al. Hypnotic residual effects of benzodiazepines with repeated administration. Sleep. 1986;9:309–316.

66. Dinges DF, Pack F, Williams K, et al. Cumulative sleepiness, mood disturbance, and psychomotor vigilance performance decrements during a week of sleep restricted to 4–5 hours per night. Sleep. 1997;20:267–277.

67. Van den Hoed J, Kraemer H, Guilleminault C, et al. Disorders of excessive somnolence: polygraphic and clinical data for 100 patients. Sleep. 1981;4:23–37.

68. Zorick F, Roehrs T, Koshorek G, et al. Patterns of sleepiness in various disorders of excessive daytime somnolence. Sleep. 1982;5:S165–S174.

69. Carskadon MA, Dement WC. Nocturnal determinants of daytime sleepiness. Sleep. 1982;5:S73–S81.

70. Carskadon MA, Dement WC. Cumulative effects of sleep restriction on daytime sleepiness. Psychophysiology. 1981;18:107–113.

71. Roehrs T, Timms V, Zwyghuizen-Doorenbos A, et al. Sleep extension in sleepy and alert normals. Sleep. 1989;12:449–457.

72. Roehrs T, Shore E, Papineau K, et al. A two-week sleep extension in sleepy normals. Sleep. 1996;19:576–582.

73. Roehrs T, Zorick F, Wittig R, et al. Efficacy of a reduced triazolam dose in elderly insomniacs. Neurobiol Aging. 1985;6:293–296.

74. Roehrs T, Zorick F, Sicklesteel J, et al. Excessive daytime sleepiness associated with insufficient sleep. Sleep. 1983;6:319–325.

75. Wittig R, Zorick F, Roehrs T, et al. Chronically insufficient sleep complicated by an irregular sleep-wake schedule: a case report. Sleep Res. 1984;12:297.

76. Manber R, Bootzin RR, Acebo C, et al. The effects of regularizing sleep-wake schedules on daytime sleepiness. Sleep. 1996;19:432–441.

77. The Atlas Task Force. EEG arousals: scoring rules and examples. Sleep. 1992;15:173–184.

78. Stepanski E, Lamphere J, Badia P, et al. Sleep fragmentation and daytime sleepiness. Sleep. 1984;7:18–26.

79. Zorick F, Roehrs T, Conway W, et al. Effects of uvulopalatopharyngoplasty on the daytime sleepiness associated with sleep apnea syndrome. Bull Eur Physiopathol Respir. 1983;19:600–603.

80. Lamphere J, Roehrs T, Wittig R, et al. Recovery of alertness after CPAP in apnea. Chest. 1989;96:1364–1367.

81. Bonnet MH. The effect of sleep disruption on performance, sleep, and mood. Sleep. 1985;8:11–19.

82. Bonnet MH. Performance and sleepiness as a function of the frequency and placement of sleep disruption. Psychophysiology. 1986;23:263–271.

83. Stepanski E, Lamphere J, Roehrs T, et al. Experimental sleep fragmentation in normal subjects. Int J Neurosci. 1987;33:207–214.

84. Levine B, Roehrs T, Stepanski E, et al. Fragmenting sleep diminishes its recuperative value. Sleep. 1987;10:590–599.

85. Ancoli-Israel S, Kripke D, Mason W, et al. Sleep apnea and nocturnal myoclonus in a senior population. Sleep. 1981;4:349–358.

86. Carskadon MA, Dement WC: Respiration during sleep in the aged human. J Gerontol 1981;36:420–423.

87. Carskadon MA, Brown E, Dement WC. Sleep fragmentation in the elderly: relationship to daytime sleep tendency. Neurobiol Aging. 1982;3:321–327.

88. Richardson GS, Carskadon MA, Orav EJ, et al. Circadian variation of sleep tendency in elderly and young adult subjects. Sleep. 1982;5:S82–S94.

89. Monk TH. Circadian aspects of subjective sleepiness: a behavioral messenger? In: Monk TH, ed. Sleep, Sleepiness and Performance. New York, NY: John Wiley & Sons; 1991:39–63.

90. Carskadon MA, Dement WC. Multiple sleep latency tests during the constant routine. Sleep. 1992;15:393–399.

91. Akerstedt T, Gillberg M. The circadian variation of experimentally displaced sleep. Sleep. 1981;4:159–169.

92. Strogatz SH, Kronauer RE, Czeisler CA. Circadian pacemaker interferes with sleep onset at specific times each day: role in insomnia. Am J Physiol. 1987;253:R172–R178.

93. Zulley J, Campbell SS. Napping behavior during "spontaneous internal desynchronization": sleep remains in synchrony with body temperature. Hum Neurobiol. 1985;4:123–126.

94. Jacklet JW. The neurobiology of circadian rhythm generators. Trends Neurosci. 1985;8:69–73.

95. Seidel WF, Roth T, Roehrs T, et al. Treatment of a 12-hour shift of sleep schedule with benzodiazepines. Science. 1984;22:1262–1264.

96. Nicholson AN, Pascoe PA, Spenser MB, et al. Sleep after transmeridian flights. Lancet. 1986;122:1205–1208.

97. Roth T, Zorick F, Wittig R, et al. Pharmacological and medical considerations in hypnotic use. Sleep. 1982;5:S46–S52.

98. Roth T, Roehrs T. Determinants of residual effects of hypnotics. Accid Anal Prev. 1985;17:291–296.

99. Roth T, Zorick F, Sicklesteel J, Stepanski E. Effects of benzodiazepines on sleep and wakefulness. Br J Clin Pharmacol. 1981;11:31S–35S.

100. Papineau K, Roehrs T, Petrucelli N, et al. Electrophysiological assessment (the multiple sleep latency test) of the biphasic effects of ethanol in humans. Alcohol Clin Exp Res. 1998;22:231–235.

101. Zwyghuizen-Doorenbos A, Roehrs T, Lamphere J, et al. Increased daytime sleepiness enhances ethanol's sedative effects. Neuropsychopharmacology. 1988;1:279–286.

102. Roehrs T, Tietz E, Zorick F, et al. Daytime sleepiness and antihistamines. Sleep. 1984;7:137–141.

103. Nicholson AN, Stone BM. Antihistamines: impaired performance and the tendency to sleep. Eur J Clin Pharmacol. 1986;30:27–32.

104. Conway J, Greenwood DT, Middlemiss DN. Central nervous actions of beta-adrenoreceptor antagonists. Clin Sci Mol Med. 1978;54:119–124.

105. Parkes JD, Fenton GW. Levo (−) amphetamine and dextro (+) amphetamine in the treatment of narcolepsy. J Neural Neurosurg Psychiatry. 1973;36:1076–1081.

106. Mitler MM, Shafor R, Hajdukovich R, et al. Treatment of narcolepsy: objective studies on methylphenidate, pemoline and protriptyline. Sleep. 1986;9:260–264.

107. Newhouse PA, Belenky G, Thomas M, et al. The effects of d-amphetamine on arousal, cognition, and mood after prolonged total sleep deprivation. Neuropsychopharmacology. 1989;2:153–163.

108. Bishop C, Roehrs T, Rosenthal L, et al. Alerting effects of methylphenidate under basal and sleep-deprived conditions. Exp Clin Psychopharmacol. 1997;4:344–352.

109. Karacan I, Booth G, Thornby J, et al. The effect of caffeinated and decaffeinated coffee on nocturnal sleep in young adult males. Sleep Res. 1976;2:64.

110. Lumley M, Roehrs T, Asker D, et al. Ethanol and caffeine effects on daytime sleepiness/alertness. Sleep. 1987;10:306–312.

111. Roehrs T, Beare D, Zorick F, et al. Sleepiness and ethanol effects on simulated driving. Alcohol Clin Exp Res. 1994;18:154–158.

112. Kilduff TS, Bowersox SS, Kaitin KI, et al. Muscarinic cholinergic receptors and the caine model of narcolepsy. Sleep. 1986;9:102–106.

113. American Sleep Disorders Association. International Classification of Sleep Disorders. Lawrence, Kan: Allen Press; 1990.

5

Sleep Deprivation

Michael H. Bonnet

PERSPECTIVE

Historically, sleep deprivation has been used as a major tool in understanding the function of sleep. A broad range of physiological responses and behavioral abilities have been examined after varying periods without sleep, and many relationships have been described. These relationships and the theories they represent are important in their own right, but sleep deprivation is more than a scientific tool. In fact, chronic partial sleep deprivation may be one of the most common unrecognized public health problems. Questionnaire-, sleep log–, and laboratory-based multiple sleep latency test (MSLT) evaluations support the contention that one third or more of the population may be suffering from excessive sleepiness secondary to chronic partial sleep deprivation.[1, 2]

The conscious decision or behavioral imperative to sacrifice sleep has existed since animals first began to sleep. Human beings initially were protected from excessive loss of sleep by having limited vision at night. The advent of electricity, while providing many benefits, has also provided significant challenges to the sleep system.

A study by Wehr and colleagues[3] examined the impact of winter darkness on the sleep of young adults by placing test subjects (Ss) in a laboratory environment that mimicked the natural light-dark cycle of North America in winter months. On the 3 initial nights, Ss slept more than 10 h, probably as recovery from chronic sleep loss. However, during the 4th week, Ss still slept an average of 8.2 h, even though their initial baseline sleep amount was 7.2 h. If one accepts 8.2 h of sleep as the underlying sleep propensity for young adults, questionnaire studies suggest that as many as 86% of young adults have chronically reduced sleep.[1]

This chapter reviews behavioral, physiological, and theoretical implications of sleep deprivation. These effects can also be described as the clinical symptoms of insufficient sleep syndrome (International Classification of Sleep Disorders [ICSD] #307.49-4). Two meta-analyses of areas of sleep deprivation were published in the 1990s.[4, 5] Both analyses indicated that sleep deprivation has a significant impact on psychomotor performance. One meta-analysis of 27 studies concluded that longer periods of sleep loss had increasingly greater impact on performance and that speed of performance rather than accuracy was more affected.[4] The other analysis (of 19 studies) concluded that mood measures were more strongly affected than cognitive tasks, which in turn were more strongly affected than motor tasks.[5] However, in contrast to traditional reviews, the latter meta-analysis suggested, particularly for mood and cognitive tasks, that partial sleep deprivation resulted in larger effects than either short-term or long-term total sleep (TS) loss.[5] This apparent opposite sensitivity may exist because many of the partial sleep deprivation studies reviewed were more recent than the total sleep loss studies and may have used more sensitive tests on subjects biased toward showing an impact of sleep loss (e.g., medical residents who may not have liked working on call).

Studies of sleep deprivation can suffer from some common methodological problems that should be remembered in interpreting them. The most important control issue is that one cannot perform a blinded study. Motivation of both experimenter and subject can have a large impact on results, particularly in the behavioral and subjective domains. Motivation effects are frequently most apparent near the end of studies (at which time performance improvement is sometimes found), but these effects also may account for the difficulty in showing decrements early in periods of sleep loss. Animal studies are probably less open to subject expectation effects, but they may contain additional elements of stress, which may interact with sleep loss itself and therefore may not be directly comparable with stress control conditions. Almost all sleep loss experiments involve more than simple loss of sleep. Maintenance of wakefulness usually includes upright posture, light, movement, cognition, and all the underlying physiological processes implied by these activities. The experimental setting itself is usually far from routine. There are studies that have attempted to control some of these factors during sleep loss, but it is probably impossible to control all of these variables in a single experiment.

Over 1000 studies of sleep deprivation have been published during the past 100 years, and the resulting knowledge database has been remarkably consistent. Current work, however, makes it clear that studies of sleep deprivation will continue to add both theoretical and practical knowledge to the practice of sleep disorders medicine. This chapter includes sections on TS deprivation, partial sleep deprivation, selective sleep stage deprivation, sleep fragmentation, and recovery from sleep deprivation.

TOTAL SLEEP DEPRIVATION

The first published TS loss studies date to 1894 for puppies[6] and 1896 for human beings.[7] The puppy study indicated that prolonged sleep loss in animals could be fatal, an idea dismissed until recent animal studies. The human study, in which a range of physiological and performance measurements was made, remains a model study. For purposes of this review, the effects of TS loss have been divided into behavioral effects, physiological effects, and a separate section on additional animal findings.

BEHAVIORAL EFFECTS

Perhaps the clearest effect of sleep loss is sleepiness, which can be inferred from subjective report, MSLT, electroencephalographic (EEG) change, or simply looking at the face of the participant. The variables that determine the impact of sleep loss have been divided into four categories: sleep-circadian influences; arousal system influences; subject characteristics; and test characteristics. An outline of categories and variables that has grown from the cogent Johnson summary[8] can be found in Table 5–1.

Sleep-Circadian Influences

Sleep deprivation, like nutritional status, is a relative concept. How an individual responds to sleep loss is dependent on the prior sleep amount and distribution. Performance during a period of sleep loss is also directly dependent on the length of time awake and the circadian time. Experiments usually try to control these factors by requiring a "normal" night of sleep before initiation of a sleep loss episode. Data from multiple regression analyses of behavioral and EEG data during sleep loss[9, 10] suggest that time awake accounts for 25 to 30% of the variance in alertness in 64 h of sleep loss,

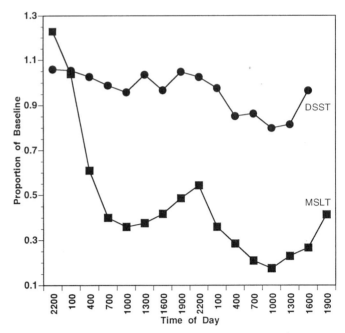

Figure 5–1. Latency to stage 2 sleep *(boxes)* and number of correctly completed symbol substitutions in repeated 5-min test sessions *(dots)* over a 64-h period of sleep deprivation both expressed as a proportion of baseline values. (Data from Bonnet NH, Gomez S, Wirth O, et al. The use of caffeine versus prophylactic naps in sustained performance. Sleep. 1995;18:97–104.)

whereas circadian time accounts for about 6% of the variance.

Using a correlation method, Dinges et al.[11] estimated that about 39% of the variance in a group of psychomotor tests and subjective measures was attributable to prior wakefulness and that about 23% of the variance was associated with circadian time in their 64-h sleep deprivation study. When prophylactic naps of varying length were introduced early in a period of sleep loss, it was found that the prophylactic nap sleep accounted for about 5% of the variance in alertness during the sleep deprivation period. In terms of reducing the effect of sleep loss, the overall effect of increasing the prophylactic nap period was linear for additional sleep amounts ranging up to 8 h in length. Figure 5–1 displays the effects of time awake and the circadian rhythm on objective alertness as measured by the MSLT and ability to complete correct symbol substitutions over 64 h of sleep loss.

Arousal Influences

Environmental and emotional surroundings can have a large impact on the course of a period of sleep loss. In early stages of sleep deprivation, several intervening variables can easily reverse all measurable sleep loss decrements. These influences, which include activity, bright light, noise, temperature, posture, stress, and drugs, have not been specifically ascribed to arousal, but work has shown that independent effects of arousal can actually have a greater impact on standard measures of sleepiness than sleep deprivation.[12]

Table 5–1. DETERMINANTS OF THE IMPACT OF SLEEP LOSS

Sleep and Circadian Influences	Subject Characteristics
Prior sleep amount and distribution	Age
	Personality and psychopathology
Length of time awake	
Circadian time	**Test Characteristics and Types**
Arousal Influences	Length of test
Activity	Knowledge of results
Bright light	Test pacing
Noise	Proficiency level
Temperature	Difficulty or complexity of test
Posture	
Drugs	Short-term memory requirement
Interest	
Motivation	Subjective (versus objective) measures
History of exposure to sleep loss	EEG measures (MSLT)

MSLT, multiple sleep latency test.

Activity

In one study,[12] a 5-min walk immediately preceding MSLT evaluations had a large impact (about 6 min) on MSLT values. The arousal associated with the walk completely masked the impact of a 50% reduction of nocturnal sleep (about a 2-min impact on MSLT). It has been shown that a period of exercise immediately before performing tasks provided transient reversal of some psychomotor[13] and subjective[14] decrements secondary to sleep loss. However, more ambitious studies comparing high activity and low activity continuing over 40 to 64-h periods of sleep deprivation have shown no beneficial effects of exercise on overall performance[15–17] and no differential effects of the exercise on recovery sleep following sleep loss in human beings.[16, 18] These different results are probably a result of the fact that arousing stimuli only act for a discrete period of time that is probably less than 30 min.[12] There may also be a trade off between production of arousal and production of physical fatigue.

Bright Light

It is known that bright light can shift circadian rhythms. Some controversy exists concerning whether bright light can also act as a source of stimulation during sleep loss to help to maintain alertness. One of four studies found that periods of bright light immediately before sleep onset significantly increased sleep latencies.[19] Other studies have found improved night shift performance under bright light conditions.[20–22] However, the contention has been made that bright light administration in the late evening may simply inhibit melatonin, which promotes sleep, or produce a phase shift to give the appearance of improved performance rather than being intrinsically stimulating.[23]

Noise

Noise has complex and occasionally negative effects on the performance of well-rested individuals, but small beneficial effects of noise have been reported in several sleep deprivation paradigms.[24–27] It is generally assumed that noise increases arousal level, and although this may not be beneficial in normal wakefulness, it usually is during sleep loss.

Temperature

Although temperature variation is commonly used as an acute stimulus to maintain alertness, there has been little research on the effects of ambient temperature interacting with sleep loss. One study has shown that heat (92°F) was effective in increasing performance over baseline sleep deprivation levels on a vigilance task for the initial minutes of that test.[28] A 1998 study[29] showed a nonsignificant decrease in subjectively rated sleepiness for about 15 min after a car air conditioner was turned on during simulated driving.

Posture

Despite the lack of direct empirical evidence, the literature[30] and most personal experience supports that contention that it is easier to maintain wakefulness when standing than when sitting and when sitting as compared to lying down. Such differences in alertness could be accounted for by increasing sympathetic nervous system activity, which occurs with these changes in posture.[31]

Drugs

Many drugs have been studied in conjunction with sleep loss. Most studies have examined stimulants, including amphetamine, caffeine, methylphenidate, pemoline, modafinil, nicotine, and cocaine. Amphetamine typically does not improve performance in individuals who have had normal sleep, but positive effects on mood, performance, and alertness have been found following sleep deprivation.[32–34]

In a well-done study, Newhouse et al.[32] administered amphetamine at three doses after 48 h of sleep loss and reported a classic dose-response curve. A 5-mg dose had little effect, but a 10-mg dose improved performance on a serial math test to close to baseline levels from 1.5 to 2.5 h after administration. Return to placebo levels was found 4.5 h after administration. After a 20-mg dose, improved performance was maintained for at least 10.5 h on the math test, and alertness on the MSLT was increased for 7 h. In another study,[35] amphetamine 20 mg was administered at three points during 64 h of sleep loss. Amphetamine (as well as modafinil 300 mg) reliably increased core temperature over a 4-h period, improved subjective alertness for 10 h or more, and improved psychomotor performance over a 6- to 8-h period.

There are several studies of caffeine use during sleep loss. When 300 mg of caffeine was ingested at 11 PM, alertness significantly increased for 7.5 h, as measured by MSLT,[36] and performance improved for 6 h.[37] Repeated use of caffeine in 150 to 300 mg doses was effective in maintaining alertness and performance above placebo levels during 48 h of sleep loss in one study and 44 hours in another.[38, 39] In another study,[40] a single 600-mg dose of caffeine significantly increased alertness as measured by MSLT for about 5 h, although the improvement associated with a single 300-mg dose was not significant.

In a similar design, 20 mg of amphetamine showed greater improvement of MSLT values for about 7 h. The beneficial effect of caffeine (300 mg) during periods of sleep loss was approximately equivalent to that seen after a 3- to 4-h prophylactic nap before the sleep loss period.[36, 39] The combination of a 4-h prophylactic nap followed by 200 mg of caffeine at 1:30 AM and 7:30 AM resulted in significantly improved performance (remaining at baseline levels) compared to the nap alone for 24 h.[41] The combination of naps and caffeine appeared additive[41] and was also superior to the provision of 4 h of nocturnal naps.[42] The combination of 200 mg of caffeine administered at 10 PM and 2 AM and exposure to 2500 lux bright light had no impact above the effect of caffeine alone on the Maintenance of Wakefulness Test (MWT) but did provide significant benefit above caffeine alone on a vigilance task at three time points.[38]

Pemoline (37.5 mg each three times a day) and methylphenidate (10 mg each four times a day) were examined in one 64-h sleep loss study.[43] Pemoline was successful in improving performance on a tapping task during the 1st night of sleep loss, whereas methylphenidate was ineffective in increasing performance or alertness above baseline levels. In another study,[44] sleepiness, as measured by MSLT, was reduced by methylphenidate 10 mg two times a day after baseline and 1 night of sleep deprivation, and performance on reaction time and vigilance tasks was improved after sleep deprivation. Modafinil 200 mg two times a day was shown effective in maintaining MSLT values above placebo levels through 60 h of sleep loss.[45] Modafinil 300 mg was shown to be equivalent to 20 mg of amphetamine in providing increased body temperature, alertness, and psychomotor performance compared to placebo over 64 h of sleep deprivation.[35] Nicotine, infused intravenously at doses of 0.25, 0.37, and 0.5 mg after 48 h of wakefulness, had no significant impact on MSLT or psychomotor performance.[46] Cocaine (96 mg), like amphetamine, did not improve performance in subjects before sleep loss. However, cocaine significantly improved reaction time performance and alertness, as measured by the Profile of Mood States (POMS), after 24 and 48 h of sleep loss.[47]

Studies that have examined alcohol use during sleep loss have come to different conclusions based on the amount of alcohol ingested, the test used, and the time of testing. In one study,[48] Ss were tested on MSLT and simulated driving after 0.6 g/kg alcohol or placebo after normal sleep or 4 h of sleep. There was a significant main effect for condition, and MSLT latencies were respectively 10.7, 6.3, 6.1, and 4.7 min after placebo (normal sleep), placebo (4 h sleep), ethanol (normal sleep), and ethanol (4 h sleep). Similar results were found in the driving simulator. In addition, three simulator "crashes" occurred, all in the reduced sleep with ethanol condition. In another study, the interaction of 4 days of partial sleep deprivation and dose of alcohol was examined.[49] Both increasing alcohol dose and length of partial deprivation increased objective sleepiness, but the lack of a nonalcohol control makes it difficult to determine the contribution of alcohol to the results.

Interest

The propensity of individuals to seek all-night poker games, video games, or battle games attests to the ability of an interesting task to allow individuals to maintain baseline levels of performance for as long as 50 h without sleep.[50] Components of interest have not been empirically quantified, but any variable producing increases in arousal could be included.

Motivation

More work has looked at the effect of motivation than interest level during sleep loss because the same task can usually be examined under low motivation and high motivation conditions. For example, in one study, monetary rewards for "hits" on a vigilance task and "fines" for false alarms[51] resulted in performance being maintained at baseline levels for the first 36 h of sleep loss in the high incentive group. Performance began to decline during the next 24 h but remained significantly better than in the "no incentive" group. However, the incentive was ineffective in maintaining performance at a higher level during the third day of sleep loss. Knowledge of results, for example, the publication of daily test results for everyone to see, was sufficient to remove the effects of 1 night of sleep loss.[52]

In another variation, simply the knowledge that a prolonged episode of sleep deprivation was going to end in a few hours was sufficient incentive for performance to improve by 30% in a group of soldiers.[53] Clearly, the effects of motivation can be significant. However, sleep loss effects themselves are probably based on more than simply motivational effects, as witnessed by the decline in performance on irrelevant tasks such as the completion of crossword puzzles, which had been provided to Ss only as a time filler between required performance tasks.[54]

Repeated Periods of Sleep Loss

Two studies of repeated episodes of sleep loss have agreed that the magnitude of performance loss increases as a function of the number of exposures to sleep loss.[52, 55] Increasingly poor performance may be secondary to decreased motivation or secondary to familiarization with the sleep deprivation paradigm (reduced stress resulting in decreased arousal).

Subject Characteristics

The impact of sleep loss on a given individual is dependent on characteristics that each participant brings to the sleep loss situation. For example, age and personality represent differences in physiological or psychological function that may interact with the sleep loss event.

Age

Age appears to play a relatively minor role in the response of human beings to loss of sleep. Tests of performance and alertness in normal older Ss undergoing sleep loss reveal a decrease in performance and alertness similar to that seen in younger individuals. If anything, older Ss had a smaller decrease in simple reaction time, alertness, and digit symbol substitution ability at nocturnal times during sleep loss[56, 57] than young adults. It frequently has been shown that older individuals perform more poorly than young adults on a broad range of tasks, but this relationship may not be maintained for periods of nocturnal performance or performance during sleep loss. These findings may be explained by the decrease in amplitude of the circadian body temperature curve in older individuals.[56, 58] The same flattened curve that results in lower temperatures and decreased performance during the day also produces elevated temperatures, as compared with young adults, during the night. These elevated temperatures may improve performance at night as they reduce ability to maintain sleep.

Personality and Psychopathology

Mood changes, including increased sleepiness, fatigue, irritability, difficulty concentrating, and disorientation are commonly reported during periods of sleep loss. Perceptual distortions and hallucinations, primarily of a visual nature, occur in up to 80% of normal individuals, depending on work load, visual demands, and length of deprivation.[59] Such misperceptions are normally quite easy to differentiate from the primarily auditory hallucinations of a schizophrenic patient, but normal individuals undergoing sleep loss may express paranoid thoughts. Two percent of 350 individuals sleep deprived for 112 h experienced temporary states resembling acute paranoid schizophrenia.[60] Some predisposition toward psychotic behavior existed in individuals who experienced significant paranoia during sleep loss, and the paranoid behavior tended to become more pronounced during the night with partial recovery during the day and disappearance after recovery sleep. In a review of the area, Johnson concluded, "each subject's response to sleep loss will depend upon his age, physical condition, the stability of his mental health, expectations of those around him, and the support he receives . . . ."[61(p208)]

In view of the commonly reported effects of sleep deprivation, it seems unusual that one would seek to treat depression by sleep deprivation. However, a review of 61 papers involving 1700 depressed patients concluded that TS loss was effective in ameliorating depressive symptoms in 59% of patients.[62] The relationship between sleep and depression is reviewed at more length in Chapter 96. However, because sleep deprivation decreases arousal level in normal Ss (which produces sleepiness), it may also reduce arousal level in hyperaroused depressed patients. Such a reduction in hyperarousal could improve mood, at least until recovery sleep reinstates the pathological level of hyperarousal. If arousal level is the key, however, sleep loss would also be predicted to normalize mood in anxious or other hyperaroused patients.

Test Characteristics and Types

The measured response to sleep deprivation is critically dependent on the characteristics of the test used. Several specific test characteristics common to sensitive psychomotor tests have been identified.[8] Other measures, such as mood scales and the MSLT, are discussed for comparison.

Length of Test

Individuals undergoing sleep loss can usually rally momentarily to perform at their nonsleep-deprived levels, but their ability to maintain that performance decreases as the length of the task increases. For example, subjects attempted significantly fewer addition problems than baseline after 10 min of testing following 1 night of sleep loss, but they reached the same criterion after 6 min of testing following the 2nd night of sleep loss. It took 50 min of testing to show a significant decrease in percentage of correct problems after 1 night of sleep loss and 10 min of testing to reach that criterion after the 2nd night.[63] The common wisdom in sleep loss studies is that performance tests need to be as long as possible and that during short-term sleep loss it is difficult to show reliable differences with almost any test that is shorter than 10 min. Momentary arousal, even as minor as an indication that 5 min remained on a task, was sufficient to reverse 75% of the decrement accumulated over 30 min of testing.[64]

Knowledge of Results

Immediate performance feedback, possibly acting through motivation, has been shown to improve performance during sleep deprivation.[52, 64] Simply not giving knowledge of results to subjects with normal sleep doubled their number of long responses ("gaps") on a serial reaction time test. One night of total sleep loss increased the number of gaps 9.3 times the baseline level, but provision of immediate knowledge of results decreased the number of gaps to 2.3 times the baseline level. The 2.3 times baseline level was approximately the number of gaps seen after normal sleep when knowledge of results was not given.[52]

Test Pacing

Self-paced tasks are usually more resistant to the effects of sleep loss than tasks that are timed or in which items are presented by the experimenter. In a self-paced task, one can concentrate long enough to complete items correctly and not be penalized for lapses in attention that occur between items. When tasks are externally paced, errors occur if items are presented during lapses in attention.

Proficiency Level

Sleep loss is likely to affect newly learned skills more than well-known activities, as long as arousal level remains constant. For example, in a study of the effects of sleep loss on doctors in training, significant performance decrements were found in PGY 1 (1st postgraduate year) surgical residents but not in PGY 2–5 surgical residents.[65]

Difficulty or Complexity

During sleep loss, performance on simple tasks such as monitoring a light on a control panel (on/off) declines less than performance on more complex tasks such as mental subtraction.[66] However, such tasks differ on several dimensions, and a more general way to test the effect of complexity is to examine more similar tasks. Ryman et al.[67] hypothesized that passively worded items on a logical reasoning task were more difficult based on the fact that reaction times to such items were longer before sleep deprivation. However, during sleep deprivation they found that Ss performed at baseline levels on passively constructed items while showing significant performance decline on the active constructions. They interpreted their results as indicating that the passive items themselves increased arousal level and that this was beneficial during sleep loss but not before sleep loss. Task difficulty can also be adjusted by increasing the speed at which the work must be performed. When 2 seconds were allowed to complete mental arithmetic problems, no significant performance decline was found after 2 nights of sleep loss, but when the rate of presentation was increased to 1.25 seconds, significant performance decline was found after sleep loss.[68] Similarly, in short-term memory tests, significant deficits may not be found after sleep loss when the memory load is low but may appear at higher memory loads.[69]

Short-Term Memory

Impairment of immediate recall for elements placed in short-term memory is a classic finding in sleep deprivation studies.[70] Because subjects are usually required to write down each item as presented, the observed decrements, which can usually be seen after 1 night of sleep loss, do not result from impaired sensory registration of items. Observed decrements may be secondary to decreased ability to encode,[71] from an increasing inability to rehearse old items (due to lapses) while the items are being presented, or from a combination of memory effects with reduced ability to respond.

Subjective Versus Objective Measures

Measures of mood such as sleepiness, fatigue, and ability to think or concentrate are inversely correlated with performance and body temperature during sleep loss.[72] Mood changes are some of the earliest noted indicators of sleep loss. As such, a 1 min mood scale may be as sensitive to sleep loss as a longer word memory test but less sensitive than a 50-min vigilance test.[8, 73]

EEG Measures

Clear changes in EEG are seen during sleep loss (see Physiological Effects of Sleep Deprivation, Neurological Changes). A standard test, the MSLT, was developed as an objective measure of sleepiness. The MSLT was validated, in part, by being shown to be sensitive to several types of partial and TS loss.[74, 75] The relatively greater sensitivity of the MSLT as compared with psychomotor tasks can be seen in Figure 5–1, which displays performance changes on the number of symbol substitutions correctly completed in 5-min test periods and MSLT data.[39]

Summary

Tasks most effected by sleep loss are long, monotonous, without feedback, externally paced, newly learned, and have a memory component. One example of a task containing many of these elements is driving. Between 1994 and 1998, more than 20 studies have examined the impact of reduced sleep on various measures of driving ability or safety. One study,[76] for example, found that 49% of medical residents who worked on call and averaged 2.7 h of sleep reported falling asleep at the wheel (90% of the episodes were post-call). The residents also had 67% more citations for moving violations and 82% more car accidents than the control group.[76] Patients with sleepiness secondary to sleep apnea had more accidents both on the road and in simulators, and their driving performance improved after continuous positive airway pressure treatment.[77]

PHYSIOLOGICAL EFFECTS OF SLEEP DEPRIVATION

Physiological changes that occur during sleep loss can be categorized into neurological (including EEG), autonomic, and biochemical changes. Physiological and biochemical effects of sleep deprivation were extensively reviewed by Horne[78] and earlier by Kleitman.[30]

Neurological Changes

Although it is easy to visually identify an individual who has been sleep-deprived and to demonstrate behavioral changes, measurable neurological changes are relatively minor and quickly reversible. In extended sleep loss studies (205 h or more), mild nystagmus, hand tremor, intermittent slurring of speech, and ptosis have been noted.[79] Sluggish corneal reflexes, hyperactive gag reflex, hyperactive deep tendon reflexes, and increased sensitivity to pain were reported[80] after more extensive deprivation. All of these changes immediately reversed after recovery sleep.

Sleep loss is consistently accompanied by characteristic EEG changes. In careful studies, Ss have been required to stand or be involved in tasks in an attempt to stabilize arousal level. Several studies have reported a generally linear decrease in alpha during sleep loss. In one study, Ss were unable to sustain alpha for longer than 10 seconds after 24 h of sleep loss, and ability to sustain alpha continued to decline to 4 to 6 sec after 72 h and 1 to 3 sec after 120 h of sleep loss.[81] After 115 h of sleep loss, eye closure failed to produce alpha activity.[82] In another study, in which individuals were recorded standing with their eyes closed, the percentage of time spent with an alpha pattern in the EEG decreased from 65% in the early deprivation period to about 30% after 100 h of sleep loss.[83] Delta and theta in the waking EEG were increased from 17% and 12% to 38% and 26% of the time, respectively.[83] No change in beta was found.[83] Performance errors during sleep loss were usually accompanied by a slowing of the EEG,[84] which was labeled a *microsleep*. However, during sleep loss, a subject may produce delta waves while speaking and clearly awake.[85]

Although the neurological changes associated with significant sleep loss are relatively minor in normal young adults, sleep loss has repeatedly been shown to be a highly activating stress in individuals suffering seizure disorders. Using a period of sleep loss as a "challenge" to elicit abnormal EEG events is currently a standard neurological test.[86]

Autonomic Changes

In human beings, autonomic changes, even during prolonged periods of sleep loss, are relatively minor. Individual studies may report either increases or decreases in systolic blood pressure, diastolic blood pressure, finger pulse volume, heart rate, respiration rate, and tonic and phasic skin conductance, but the majority of 10 to 15 studies have reported no change in these variables during sleep loss in human beings.[78, 83, 87–90] More recent studies have suggested that sleep loss does result in about a 20% reduction in response to hypoxia and hypercapnia.[91–93] However, these modifications suggest a transient set point change rather than system failure.

Sleep deprivation has been associated with small decreases in forced expiratory volume in 1 second (FEV_1) and forced vital capacity (FVC) in patients with pulmonary disease.[94] Two studies, one in healthy infants[95] and one in adults,[96] have shown more apneic events and longer apneic events after sleep loss. Brooks et al.[97] have shown that apneas become longer as a function of the sleep fragmentation produced by the apneas (as opposed to the respiratory pathology). Several human studies have found a small (0.3 to 0.4°C) overall decrease in body temperature during sleep loss.[7, 82, 98] Effects of sleep loss on the ability to perform exercise are subtle. Animal studies have consistently shown that sleep deprivation decreases spontaneous activity by up to 40%,[99] but most human studies have focused on maximal exercise ability, where large differences as a function of sleep loss are more difficult to demonstrate. For example, one well-done study[100] reported a 7% decrease in maximum oxygen uptake ($\dot{V}O_2max$) during 64 h of sleep loss. This change was not associated with heart rate, respiratory exchange ratio, or blood lactate, which remained unchanged. However, there was a decrease in minute ventilation and hemodilution.[101] Recovery from exercise may be slowed by sleep loss.[102] Studies are evenly divided between claims that the amplitude of the circadian rhythm of temperature is increased, decreased, or unchanged during sleep loss.[78]

One well-done study has shown no sleep deprivation–related changes in whole body metabolism at normal temperatures and in a cold stress situation.[88] These findings in human beings are of particular import because a series of elegant studies in rats has shown that after a week of sleep loss, metabolic levels are greatly increased, increased food consumption is accompanied by significant weight loss, and significant difficulty with thermoregulation is apparent (see Animal Studies). Several studies have examined aspects of brain metabolism in animals during short periods of sleep deprivation. Direct measures of brain metabolic rate were not different after a short period of sleep deprivation,[103] although several related enzymes did differ. Another study indicated that some of the noted differences could have been related to stress rather than sleep deprivation per se.[104]

Biochemical Changes

Several studies (10 or more for some variables) have examined various biochemical changes in human beings during sleep loss. There is generally no significant change in cortisol (73% of studies reported no change in human beings), adrenaline and related compounds (80% of human studies reported no differences), catecholamine output,[88, 105] hematocrit,[87] plasma glucose,[87] creatinine (no difference in 83% of human studies[88, 106], or magnesium[88] during sleep loss. One study imposed an additional cold stress during sleep loss and still failed to find a physiological component due to sleep loss over that seen with cold.[88]

Results from analyses of blood components largely parallel the results found in urine components. None of the adrenal or sex hormones (including cortisol, adrenaline, noradrenaline, luteinizing hormone, follicle-stimulating hormone, variants of testosterone and progesterone) rise during sleep deprivation in human beings.[107, 108] Some of these hormones actually decreased somewhat during sleep loss, perhaps secondary to sleepiness and decreased physiological activation. Thyroid activity, as indexed by thyrotropin, thyroxine, and triiodothyronine was increased, probably secondary to the increased energy requirements of continuous wakefulness.[109] A majority of studies now seem to indicate that melatonin is not increased during sleep deprivation or in recovery sleep.[110] Most studies have concluded that there is no significant change in hematocrit levels,[88] erythrocyte count,[111] or plasma glucose during sleep deprivation in human beings.[87] As would be expected, those hormones such as noradrenaline, prolactin,[112] and growth hormone, which are dependent on sleep for their circadian rhythmicity or appearance, lose their periodic pattern of excretion during sleep loss (see references 113 and 114 for excellent reviews). Several studies have reported rebounds in growth hormone during recovery sleep following sleep loss or slow-wave sleep (SWS) deprivation.[110, 115]

Immune Function

Several human studies have examined various aspects of immune function after varying periods of partial or TS loss, but because parameters measured, time of blood draw, and degree of sleep deprivation vary across studies, simple conclusions are not possible. All of the studies found changes in immune function after sleep loss.[116] Four studies, primarily of partial or short-term total sleep deprivation, found decreases in natural killer cell activity (up to 50%) or numbers.[117] One additional study found a nonsignificant decrease in natural killer cells after 39 h of sleep loss but with an increase after 63 h of sleep loss.[118] Other findings have included decreased proliferation of lymphocytes and granulocytes in response to an antigen[119] and increased proliferative responses to pokeweed mitogen.[120] At a more macroscopic level, one study reported the development of respiratory illness or asthma in three subjects after a 64-h sleep deprivation protocol,[121] whereas another reported no incidence of illness after a similar protocol.[118] In longer studies involving strenuous exercise and other factors along with sleep loss, increased infection rates were reported about 50% of the time.[122]

One animal study has suggested that mice that had been immunized against a respiratory influenza virus responded to that virus as if they had never been immunized only when exposed after sleep loss.[123] However, an extensive study of sleep loss in rats (7 to 49 days) was unable to show significant changes in spleen cell numbers, mitogen responses, or in vivo or in vitro splenic antibody-secreting cell responses[124] (see also Animal Studies).

ANIMAL STUDIES

Modern animal sleep deprivation studies differ from human studies in enough important aspects that they need to be treated separately. Many techniques have been developed to maintain wakefulness in animals, and most of them capitalize on the fact that when an animal falls asleep, muscles relax and the animal takes up more floor space than when sitting or standing awake. As a result, animals are typically placed on a small stationary platform (flower pot technique) or on a slightly larger slowly moving circular platform above water. Recent studies have added continuously computer monitored EEG so that when an experimental animal on one half of a circular platform falls asleep, the platform begins to move and the animal is awakened by either the platform movement or by falling into water below. The computer control of platform movement allows a yoked-control animal to be placed on the other side of a wall that divides the circular platform. The control animal must move when the experimental animal falls asleep because the platform moves (in this sense, number and placement of required movements are controlled from experimental to control animal), but the control animal is free to sleep whenever the experimental animal is awake. In this paradigm, control animals were able to obtain about 72% of their normal sleep, whereas experimental animals obtained about 9% of their previous TS.[125] Reviews of the studies in this area are available.[126, 127] The studies reviewed in this section include both TS loss

studies and some studies that selectively deprived either rapid eye movement (REM) sleep or SWS sleep (see Selective Sleep Deprivation for more details) because reported results were similar.

Overall, rats totally sleep deprived by the moving platform method developed a characteristic appearance including disheveled, clumped fur; skin lesions on tail and paws; and weight loss. The weight loss occurred despite large increases in food intake and with indications that energy expenditure had increased to more than double baseline values. The sleep-deprived rats all died (or were sacrificed at imminent death) within 11 to 22 days of deprivation. On examination, the histology and organs of the sleep-deprived rats differed little from the control rats, who had remained healthy. Sleep-deprived rats did have slightly heavier hearts, kidneys, and adrenals compared to controls, but these effects appeared later than the increased energy expenditure and debilitated appearance.[125] The findings did not appear related to the rats being immersed in water or as a specific result of weight loss.

Other studies examined REM[128] and SWS[129] deprivation in the same methodological paradigm. In both types of selective deprivation, rats developed the same symptoms seen after TS loss and died in 16 to 54 days (REM deprivation) or 23 to 66 days (SWS deprivation). However, both SWS and REM deprivation paradigms included substantial loss of both REM and SWS, despite preservation of 70 to 80% of baseline TS time. The many awakenings required to eliminate SWS or REM sleep probably also caused significant sleep fragmentation, and, as such, these studies could be viewed as sleep fragmentation studies (see Sleep Fragmentation).

In sleep-deprived rats, body temperature declined as much as 2°C during the second half of the deprivation period.[130] Activity increased 23% from baseline levels while energy expenditure doubled, and this finding was not based on reduced efficiency of energy use. Heart rate increased,[128] plasma norepinephrine increased and plasma thyroxine decreased.[130] Increased energy expenditure could not be explained by increased wakefulness alone or by water exposure. It was concluded that the increased energy expenditure was produced in an attempt to maintain body temperature in the face of excessive heat loss during deprivation. The increase in energy expenditure apparently was not mediated by the hypothalamic-pituitary-adrenal system.[130] Another study indicated that the increased energy expenditure was not controlled specifically by norepinephrine, although a catecholamine contribution (through epinephrine when norepinephrine was blocked) could not be ruled out.[131] One study put rats on either a high fat or a high protein diet during sleep deprivation to determine whether the increased calories would prolong survival.[132] Rats with a high fat diet lived about 10 days longer than rats fed a high protein diet and developed a very high metabolism (249% of baseline). In addition, rats on the high fat diet did not develop skin lesions as quickly, and blood changes occurred later (because the rats lived longer). These data were interpreted as showing that some of the symptoms commonly seen in these rats sleep-deprivation studies could have been the result of a continuous demand to degrade protein (causing protein deficiency symptoms). If such were the case, the high fat diet would have provided a significant number of nonprotein calories, which may have delayed inevitable protein synthesis difficulties.

Rechtschaffen[127] identified three possible causes of death in the rats. All rats showed a drop in body temperature of 1°C or more as an indicator of death within 1 or 2 days. One hypothesis, therefore, is that hypothermia is the cause of death. Unfortunately, attenuation of the temperature drop did not improve survival,[133] and more rapid temperature drops did not shorten survival.[134, 135] Another hypothesis, that death was caused by catabolism related to the high metabolic rate, was supported by declines in cell division[136]; decreased survival time in rats with increased metabolic rate from being made hyperthyroid[133]; and increased survival in rats that had less weight loss after being put on a high calorie diet.[132] Nonetheless, rats protected from the catabolic effects by the high calorie diet or being made hypothyroid still died. A third hypothesis advanced by Everson[126] is that prolonged sleep deprivation impairs host defense against otherwise common bacteria. In an initial study, Everson[137] found bacteria in the blood of five of six rats at the point that sleep deprivation led to a rapid drop in body temperature. However, in a follow-up study, Bergmann et al.,[138] while finding bacteremia in 3 of 11 rats early in sleep deprivation, found no evidence of increased life span or bacteremia in 6 rats treated with an antibiotic cocktail during sleep deprivation. This seems to imply that although there may be some breakdown of tissue barriers to microbes late in sleep deprivation in rats, this breakdown is not the cause of many of the common effects and is not the universal cause of death.

Rats that were allowed recovery sleep died within 2 to 6 recovery days if they had had large decreases in body temperature. Rats with less severe decrease in body temperature generally showed complete reversal of the deprivation-associated changes in appearance, temperature, and energy expenditure within 15 days. Immediate, large REM rebounds were found regardless of deprivation type, and modest increases in nonrapid eye movement (NREM) sleep were seen following initial REM rebound.[139] The existence of REM as the deepest stage of sleep and the stage of immediate rebound during recovery is also in contrast to the findings in human studies. The theoretical significance of this difference is unknown.

Other studies of rats and studies of cats, dogs, and rabbits have been relatively consistent in reporting increased food intake (57% of seven reporting studies), weight loss (64% of 14 reporting studies), and increased heart rate (100% of five reporting studies) during long periods of TS deprivation or selective REM deprivation and large predominant REM rebounds during recovery sleep (see review in reference 140). Two older studies (of four older studies reporting) found hypothermia after long periods of sleep loss, and 5 older studies (of some 27) reported death in some animals. It should be remembered, however, that these generalizations have been made from several species deprived under many conditions for periods ranging from 4 to 77 days.

Summary

A great deal is known about general physiological, psychomotor, subjective, and EEG effects of TS loss for periods of up to about 11 days in human beings. Characteristic circadian decreases in alertness and performance accumulating over time are well documented. Physiological changes are relatively minor. TS loss in rats appears to be different from TS loss in people. Although eating is usually increased in human beings during sleep deprivation,[98] changes in heart rate, weight, metabolism, or most biochemical measures have not been reported. Minor decreases in body temperature are frequently noted in human studies, but the animal studies may report increased body temperature early in deprivation and decreased temperature only after long periods of sleep loss. A review of the animal studies[140] suggested that the human and animal studies are not directly comparable because

1. Daily sleep quotients differ
2. Sleep-wake cycle times (the "pressure" to sleep) differ
3. Basal energy expenditure rates differ
4. Life span differs
5. Surface area differs
6. Survival time during other stresses such as starvation differ.

Examination of human versus rat values on each of these parameters indicates that people should tolerate sleep loss more easily than rats. For example, using basal O_2 consumption as a predictor of energy use, people should be able to tolerate 2 to 7 months of TS deprivation before death. It is also likely that all six factors above help insulate human beings against the effects of sleep loss to some extent as compared to rats. If one considers the combined effect of daily sleep quotients, sleep-wake cycle times and basal energy expenditure differences, human beings might be able to tolerate 2 to 10 years of total sleep loss. More recent animal experiments have tried to control stress per se by using yoked controls in the deprivation experiments. However, the animal studies cannot determine whether the interaction of profound sleep loss with stress is responsible for the reported effects. Differences between the human and rat response to sleep loss may be moot because sleep loss of the magnitude apparently required for system failure is unlikely in human beings, and the rat studies indicate that animals even near the brink of death appear to recover completely if allowed to sleep.

PARTIAL SLEEP DEPRIVATION

Partial sleep deprivation refers to nonsleep stage–specific reduction in TS. As such, partial sleep deprivation is certainly the most common form of sleep deprivation seen in the real world. Both acute and chronic studies of partial sleep loss have been performed.

Acute Partial Sleep Deprivation

Many studies have examined the effect of 1 or 2 nights of reduced sleep on performance and sleep variables. Rosenthal et al.[141] found a significant reduction in MSLT in Ss who had been allowed 6 h in bed or 4 h in bed compared to 8 h (respective latencies for 8, 6, and 4 h in bed were 12.4, 8.4, and 7.0 min). In a 1997 study, Dinges et al.[142] reduced sleep to approximately 5 h per night. After 1 night, Ss reported significant increases in sleepiness and performed more poorly on one measure from a reaction time task (slow 10). Wilkinson et al.[143] varied sleep by allowing Ss 0, 1, 2, 3, 5, or 7.5 h in which to sleep. Despite having only six Ss, significant decreases in vigilance performance were found the following day when sleep was reduced below 3 h for 1 night or was set at 5 h for 2 consecutive nights.

Most partial sleep deprivation designs allowing more than 3 h of sleep cause reductions in REM and stage 2 sleep due to the distribution of sleep stages across the night. The acute partial sleep deprivation studies suggest that all stages of sleep except SWS are reduced during sleep restriction.[144] Recovery sleep following a night of sleep reduced to 2 to 4 h may differ little from baseline if the recovery sleep period is held to 8 h.[144] There may be a small increase in TS time and a corresponding decrease in sleep latency.[75] If ad lib sleep is allowed, the increased TS consists primarily of stage 2 and REM.[144]

Chronic Partial Sleep Deprivation

As sleep restriction continues beyond a single night, cumulative effects may be seen depending on the sleep quota allowed on each night. When the time available for sleep was reduced to 6 h for 42 days, differences were not found for any daytime measures.[145] When the time available for sleep was reduced to 5.5 h for 60 days, a decrease in vigilance performance was found in the final 2 weeks of the study.[146] SWS was maintained and moved more toward the beginning of the sleep period, REM was reduced about 25% throughout the study, and REM latencies were reduced by 10 to 30 min. Sleep latency was significantly reduced only during the last week of the study.

In a more recent study,[147] two small groups of Ss had their nightly sleep reduced to about 5.2 h for 3 weeks and a third group had their sleep reduced to 4.3 hours for 6 nights. Significant performance decrements were not found on 20-min vigilance tests. In a study mentioned earlier in which Ss were allowed 5 h of sleep for 7 consecutive nights,[142] cumulative deficits were reported for both subjective and psychomotor performance measures after the 1st night. Over the course of the week, subjective sleepiness continued to increase and performance on a reaction time task continued to decrease in a linear fashion consistent with a slowly accumulating sleep debt. In a similar study, Carskadon and Dement[75] restricted sleep to 5 h per night for 7 consecutive nights. MSLT scores were significantly reduced after the 2nd restriction night and continued a declining trend from baseline values of 17 min (after sleep satiation) to about 7 min after the last night of sleep reduction. The absolute reduction in MSLT latencies across nights in these last two studies is similar. The significant results of these latter two studies suggest that increased test sensitivity and in-laboratory designs have allowed identification of increasingly small decreases in TS as producing significant increases in sleepiness.

In a different experimental paradigm, Ss had their available sleep time shortened in 30-min increments from 8 h until the Ss were unwilling to continue sleep reduction.[148, 149] During the 4 to 6 month course of the stepped reductions, Ss had frequent laboratory sleep and performance evaluations. The mean level of time in bed that both 8-h and 6.5-h baseline sleepers were able to reduce to was 5.0 h. During sleep reduction, Ss reported less difficulty falling asleep and feeling less rested. Ss began to complain of discomfort (fatigue and falling asleep in class and difficulty remaining vigilant while driving) when spending 6 to 6.5 h in bed. Significant performance decline was not found on psychomotor tests, but subjects nonetheless felt impaired. One said,[148(p248)] "I am noticeably less efficient, less energetic; e.g., I can't seem to study as long as I used to, I get discouraged more easily, slightly depressed about overcoming difficulties, very much like I feel when I am sick with a cold."

EEG changes during chronic partial sleep deprivation include reduction in amounts of all sleep stages except SWS. There is a tendency for stage 4 sleep, measured by standard scoring[151] or delta power density,[152] to increase. Nocturnal sleep latency, in agreement with MSLT, was reduced from a mean of 10 min at normal sleep levels to 2 min after 4.5-h sleep periods in the Mullaney et al.[149] study. Webb[151] reported no SWS rebound after 8 nights of 3 h of sleep, but Brunner et al.[152] found an increase in SWS on the 1st recovery night after 4 nights with 4 h of sleep.

The Mullaney et al. study[149] also followed Ss for a year after the experiment proper. The 6.5-h sleepers returned to their baseline sleep levels, but the original 8-h sleepers reported on sleep logs that they were sleeping between 6.1 and 6.4 h per night throughout the 1-year follow-up period.

Summary

The studies of partial sleep loss suggest that functional impairment will appear relatively rapidly with nocturnal sleep periods of 5 h or less. More recent studies, in contrast to the older literature, suggest that decrements from partial sleep loss may be measurable after 6-h sleep lengths[141] and that decrements accumulate across continued partial sleep loss periods.[142]

Occupational Consequences of Partial Sleep Deprivation

Reduced sleep, usually in a chronic sense, is seen in many important groups, including doctors, soldiers, shift workers, mothers, and cross-country truck drivers. Studies of individuals in many of these groups have been performed. Because several more recent studies have examined partial sleep loss in doctors, those studies are reviewed as a relevant applied example.

A number of studies have examined sleep, mood, and performance in doctors at various levels of training. Eleven of 14 studies that examined various types of performance or mood in doctors who had slept an average of 2.6 h compared with recent baseline sleep of 7.1 h found significantly worse performance on at least one test. One study that was unable to demonstrate significant changes in performance after reduced sleep did show that mood as measured by the Profile of Mood States (POMS) was made more negative by sleep reduction.[153] As might be expected, the studies suggest that performance decrement is more likely to be found in doctors with less experience,[65] on reasoning tasks,[154–156] or on nonstimulating tasks.[150] The impact on performance was less noticeable than accompanying changes in mood.[157] House staff were likely to have fallen asleep while driving or at a traffic light and had increased traffic citations and accidents.[76] Studies that did not demonstrate some change in performance did not control the time of testing closely and were performed in small groups of subjects.[153, 158] One study indicated that even the reported baseline sleep amounts in doctors were about an hour reduced from prehospital baseline sleep amounts[155] in the same doctors. This implies that even baseline comparisons in these studies may have included some chronic partial sleep reduction. As expected from the empirical studies, the reduction of sleep to the 3-h range in the applied medical setting is sufficient to demonstrate decline in performance ability. Studies have not examined physician performance from 4 to 6 AM, when it would be predicted that the maximal impact of sleep loss would be found.

Insomnia

Partial sleep deprivation is usually a voluntary choice, but an argument can be made that insomnia is a special case of partial sleep loss. From the partial sleep loss data, one would predict that chronic insomnia would not result in measurable performance decrements unless the insomnia was so severe that TS time was decreased to 5 to 6 h. EEG studies of patients with insomnia suggest that large, consistent reductions of TS time are unusual. As such, most cases of insomnia should not produce a significant sleep debt. Three studies have examined the effects of TS loss on insomniacs to determine if these hypothetically chronically sleep deprived patients were more susceptible to TS loss.[56, 159, 160] The two studies that examined well-defined insomniacs concluded that the sleep loss had no greater impact (and perhaps less impact) on insomniacs than on matched normal sleepers.[56, 160] These data, therefore, do not support the notion that insomniacs generally suffer from chronic partial sleep deprivation.

SELECTIVE SLEEP DEPRIVATION

Selective sleep deprivation experiments attempt to eliminate one or more stages of sleep while having minimal impact on TS time and other sleep stages. An extensive review of selective sleep deprivation was published in 1982.[161] Studies of selective deprivation were originally intended as a means of determining the functional significance of REM or SWS and typically involved the placement of experimental awakenings or arousals at the onset of the forbidden stage of sleep for 1 or more nights. A large number of selective deprivation studies were performed in the years after the discovery of REM sleep to test psychoanalytic theories of dreams and pressure to dream. Early experiments[162, 163] determined that selective deprivation of REM sleep accomplished by the awakening technique resulted in increasingly frequent attempts by Ss to enter REM sleep. For example, in one study, 17 awakenings were required on the 1st night, 42 awakenings were required on the 4th night, and 68 awakenings were required on the 7th night to maintain REM deprivation.[164] Large increases in REM amount were also noted when nondisturbed recovery sleep was allowed. Although these EEG effects were large and easily replicated, the impact of REM deprivation on psychological function or performance has been much more difficult to determine.[161] The studies have generally compared personality measures after REM deprivation with the same measures after a similar amount of sleep disturbance has been performed during NREM sleep. Of some 35 studies reviewed by Pearlman,[161] about 33% reported no significant differences found on any test. Another 14% reported nonspecific or individual difference responses that could not have been statistically tested or would have been nonsignificant if tested. The remaining studies reported a range of findings including "less interpersonally effective"[164]; increased drive behavior (restlessness, hypersexuality, increased appetite) in rats[165]; increased aggression[166]; and increased inspection of sexual areas in pictures in human beings.[167] The lack of frank psychopathology or other consistent findings after REM deprivation decreased identification of REM sleep as necessary to maintain sanity. However, the studies cited have been interpreted as providing some support that REM sleep is a means of discharging drive tension (and therefore serves as a psychoanalytic safety valve). As such, it has been proposed that REM deprivation acts to disinhibit various aggressive, sexual, or eating behavior. However, several other theories of the function of REM sleep were proposed, and a number of REM deprivation studies have been performed as tests of those theories.

Theories of the function of REM sleep include

1. The activation-synthesis hypothesis[168]
2. The catecholamine-restoration hypothesis[169]

3. The cortical homeostasis hypothesis[170]
4. The drive facilitation hypothesis (earlier)
5. The information processing hypothesis
6. The neural growth promotion hypothesis[171]
7. The oculomotor hypothesis[172, 173]
8. The protein synthesis hypothesis
9. The sentinel hypothesis[161, 174, 175]

Only the drive facilitation hypothesis and the information processing hypothesis have had several direct tests in human Ss.

Perhaps the most frequently studied view of REM sleep function has been the proposal that the activated brain associated with REM sleep is involved in memory consolidation, synthesis of new or adaptive information, or arrangement of information into an internal association framework. A number of animal studies have shown that REM sleep increases after learning and that REM deprivation after a learning task results in decreased retention (see reference 175 for review). Unfortunately, the results from human REM deprivation studies have not been as favorable as the results of the animal studies (see reference 176 for review). In human beings, REM deprivation did not impair learning of nonsense syllables or paired associates,[177] although decrements have been shown in some more complex tasks such as retention of stories.[178] The negative human studies in conjunction with the possibility that the results in the animal studies were dependent on the stress of animal sleep deprivation techniques[179] have made some reviewers conclude that the relationship between REM sleep and memory is not of great significance.[98] However, a 1994 human study[180] found improvement in perceptual performance occurred 8 to 10 h after a training session only when REM sleep was allowed in the interim. This study of perceptual learning, rather than retention of memorized material, is consistent with the animal studies and suggests that earlier human studies may have examined the wrong types of task.

In contrast to the large number of studies of selective REM deprivation, there are relatively few studies of selective SWS deprivation. Early studies determined that when stage 4 sleep was selectively deprived in human beings by an arousal procedure, Ss made increasing efforts to enter the stage and had stage 4 rebounds when sleep was not disturbed.[164, 181] In a study specifically comparing the effects of stage 4 and REM sleep deprivation,[164] it was found that subjects required five to seven times as many arousals to deprive them of stage 4 sleep than to deprive them of REM during each night of selective sleep deprivation. Recovery nights following stage 4 sleep deprivation were similar to recovery nights following TS loss: stage 4 increased only on the 1st recovery night and REM, which had not been deprived, increased on recovery nights 2 and 3. In contrast, after REM deprivation, REM sleep was increased throughout 3 recovery nights, but there was no increase of stage 4 sleep on any recovery night.

Daytime performance following selective stage 4– and REM-deprivation conditions in human beings has been tested, but decrements were not found after as many as 7 nights of either stage 4 or REM sleep deprivation.[164, 182] In more extensive studies,[182, 183] the hypothesis that REM or stage 4 sleep might serve a specific recuperative function was tested by performing either selective stage 4 or REM deprivation before[182] or following[183] 2 nights of TS loss. Neither REM nor stage 4 selective sleep stage deprivation before TS loss potentiated the normal effects of the TS loss night. Similarly, performance recovered in subjects at the same rate whether they were allowed to have undisturbed recovery sleep, stage 4–deprived recovery sleep, or REM-deprived recovery sleep following 2 nights of TS loss. It was concluded in these studies that the major predictor of performance during these sleep loss paradigms was the total amount of time spent asleep irrespective of sleep stage parameters. This view led Johnson[184] to conclude that specific sleep stage amounts were not related to daytime waking behavior in normal young adults.

SLEEP FRAGMENTATION

Sleep is a time-based cumulative process that can be impeded both by several types of deprivation and by systematic disturbance. A number of studies have shown that brief repetitive arousals from sleep systematically reduce the restorative power of sleep.

Experimental Sleep Fragmentation

Studies have shown that brief arousals during sleep reduced daytime alertness depending on 1) the frequency of the arousals; 2) the type of arousal; and 3) the age of the subject. When periodic arousals fell at intervals greater than 20 min, no effects on daytime function were seen.[185] Orderly increasing loss of daytime function was found when the period of sleep between arousals was reduced from 20 min to 1 min.[185–190] Any manipulation resulting in frequent changes in ongoing EEG resulted in daytime deficits,[189] but no deficits were seen in a condition composed of frequent passively produced leg movements that did not result in EEG arousals.[191] However, one study of *nonvisible sleep fragmentation*, defined as an increase in heart rate by 4 bpm or blood pressure by 4 mmHg without EEG change in response to tones, showed increased sleepiness on the MSLT about half as great as in a similar study using an EEG arousal criterion.[192] Older Ss were less sensitive to sleep fragmentation than young adults.[190] Results from several studies indicated that effects were dependent on the rate of sleep fragmentation and not on associated changes in EEG sleep stages.[187–189]

Sleep Disorders and Fragmentation

It has been documented for some time that a large percentage of older individuals have frequent brief arousals during sleep, primarily from periodic leg movements or apnea. The number of these brief arousals is significantly correlated with the magnitude of daytime sleepiness in these groups of patients.[193, 194] Further, the sleep disturbance caused by the apnea events themselves results in the production of longer and more pathological apneas.[97] Traditional sleep stage rebounds (see Recovery Sleep) are seen when the pathology is corrected. Following effective treatment of sleep apnea and the corresponding decrease in frequency of arousals during sleep, alertness is improved as measured by either MSLT or reduction in traffic accidents.[77] It is certain that there are many other instances of sleep fragmentation as a component in both medical illnesses (such as fibrositis, intensive care unit syndrome, chronic movement disorders, and chronic pain disorders) and life requirements (infant care, medical residents). Some of these impositions may not reach the critical number of arousal levels required for significant decrements in the apnea patients and sleep fragmentation studies. However, most of these situations are a combination of chronic partial sleep loss and chronic sleep fragmentation, and the combination of these factors clearly has greater impact than either factor in isolation.

RECOVERY SLEEP

Only sleep is required to reverse the effects of sleep deprivation in almost all circumstances.

Performance Effects

Several efforts have been made to assess recovery of performance following sleep deprivation. It is commonly reported that recovery from periods of sleep loss of up to 10 days and nights is rapid and can occur within 1 to 3 nights. Several studies have reported recovery of performance after a single (usually 8 h) night of sleep following anywhere from 40 to 110 hours of continous wakefulness.[15, 16, 70, 195, 196] Taken together, these experiments suggest that an equal amount of sleep is not required to recover from sleep lost. However, sleep deprivation itself was the main concern of these studies and, therefore, recovery was given minimal attention.

A few studies have specifically examined the rate of performance recovery during sleep in young adults, normal older subjects, and insomniacs following 40- and 64-h sleep loss periods.[56, 197] In these studies, participants were awakened from stage 2 sleep for 20-min test batteries approximately every 2 h during baseline and recovery nights. As such, it was possible to follow the time course of return to baseline performance during recovery sleep in the three groups. In normal young adults, reaction time returned to levels not significantly less than baseline after 4 hours of sleep during recovery sleep following 40 h of sleep loss. However, reaction time remained significantly slower than baseline in young adults throughout the 1st night of recovery sleep (including the postsleep morning test) following 64 h of sleep loss. In contrast, reaction time in both older normal sleeper and insomniac groups was significantly slower than baseline at 5:30 AM but had returned to baseline levels by 8:00 AM following the 1st recovery night after 64 h of sleep loss. The young adults not only recovered more slowly from sleep loss on the initial recovery night but also had some decrease in their reaction times that extended into the 2nd recovery night. This result is consistent with data presented by Carskadon and Dement,[198] who found that older subjects had daytime MSLT values at baseline levels following sleep loss and a single night of recovery sleep while shorter-than-normal latencies continued in young adults.

EEG Effects

A large number of studies have reported consistent effects on sleep EEG when totally sleep deprived individuals are finally allowed to sleep. If undisturbed, young adults will typically sleep only 12 to 15 h, even after 264 h of sleep loss.[89] If sleep times are held to 8 h on recovery nights, effects on sleep stages may be seen for 2 or more nights.

The effects of 40 and 64 h of sleep loss on recovery sleep stages during the initial recovery night are summarized in Table 5–2 for normal young adults[18, 74, 199–201] young adult short sleepers[202]; young adult long sleepers[202]; 60- to 80-year-old normal sleepers[198, 203, 204] 60- to 70-year-old chronic insomniacs[203, 205]; and 60- to 80-year-old depressed and demented patients.[206, 207] Table 5–2 presents percentage change from baseline data with an indication of study-to-study variability where the number of studies allowed computation. Table 5–2 is presented as a summary device so that 1) EEG effects of sleep deprivation can be predicted (roughly by multiplying population baseline values by figures presented in Table 5–2; and 2) the potential differential effects of sleep deprivation on EEG recovery sleep as a function of group can be more clearly seen. The results of these several studies indicate that recovery sleep EEG changes that occur as a function of sleep deprivation are remarkably consistent across studies and across several experimental groups including men, women, older subjects, and older insomniacs. Significant deviations from population recovery values are seen primarily in the REM latency changes in depressed and demented patients and in some less robust differences found in small groups of long and short sleepers. These latter findings might be related to differential sleep stage distributions secondary to long or short sleep times.

On the 1st recovery night after TS loss, there is a large increase in SWS over baseline amounts.[87, 205, 208] As would be expected, wake time and stage 1 sleep are usually reduced. Stage 2 and REM sleep may both be decreased on the 1st recovery night following 64 h of sleep loss,[56, 74] at least in young adults, as a function of increased SWS. In older normal sleepers and insomniacs, there is less absolute increase in SWS than in

Table 5–2. EFFECTS OF SLEEP LOSS ON RECOVERY SLEEP STAGES

	Young Adults (SD)	Older Adults (SD)	Depressed	Demented	Short Sleepers	Long Sleepers	64-h Older Normals	64-h Older Insomniacs
Sleep latency	0.38 (0.09)		0.22	0.14				
Wake time	0.44 (0.19)	0.51 (0.11)			0.13	0.48		
Stage 1	0.42 (0.12)	0.59 (0.14)	0.61	0.68	0.98	0.60	0.56	0.52
Stage 2	0.87 (0.10)	0.95 (0.07)	1.06	1.08	1.38	0.99	1.07	1.20
Stage 3	0.98	1.32 (0.25)	1.14	1.16			2.36	3.00
Stage 4	2.40	2.06 (0.45)	1.35	1.12			7.00	5.25
Stage SWS	1.53 (0.11)	1.56 (0.23)	1.23	1.15	1.37	1.52	2.56	3.30
Stage REM	0.89 (0.13)	1.04 (0.09)	0.84	0.78	1.26	1.03	0.26	0.92
Latency to REM	1.01 (0.20)	0.77 (0.20)	2.20	2.00	1.13	1.26	0.35	0.96

The values presented in this table are the mean proportion of baseline levels of the indicated sleep stages for the indicated groups during the 1st sleep recovery night after 1 night of sleep loss 40 h or 64 h (2 nights) where indicated. Where sufficient studies were available, the standard deviation (SD) around the mean percentage is also given. For example, on their recovery night after 1 night of sleep loss, young adults have a sleep latency that is 38 ± 9% of their baseline sleep latency.

SWS, slow wave sleep.

young adults on the 1st recovery night, although the percentage increase in SWS may be as great. As a result of less SWS rebound, there may be no change (geriatric normals) or even an increase in stage 2.[56, 207] Recovery sleep stage changes were generally similar regardless of age (see Table 5–2) except that normal older individuals had a decrease in REM latency during recovery sleep,[198, 203, 207] rather than the increased REM latency common in young adults. It was found that REM latency in the older population was positively correlated with baseline SWS amounts[203, 207] and that sleep onset REM periods occurred in about 20% of those carefully screened normal subjects.[203, 207] These REM changes were interpreted to be the result of decreased pressure for SWS in older human beings. The REM latency findings did not apply to older depressed or demented individuals. REM rebound effects appear to be related to the amount of lost SWS; that is, REM rebound is more likely on an early recovery night when there is less SWS loss as a function of either a shorter period of sleep loss or age.

On the 2nd recovery night following TS loss, SWS amounts approached normal values, and an increase in REM sleep was found in young adults.[74, 209] TS time was still elevated. By the 3rd recovery night, all sleep EEG values approached baseline. In situations in which REM rebounds on the 1st sleep recovery night, sleep EEG values may normalize by the 2nd recovery night. Exceptions to these general rules may include older insomniacs, who have increased TS for at least 3 nights after 64 h of sleep loss[56] and individuals who have had significant selective REM deprivation.

Relationship Between EEG and Psychomotor Performance Recovery Effects

The earliest systematic evaluations of sleep in human beings posited that the recuperative value of sleep was directly related to its depth. The consistent data show that recovery sleep following sleep loss seems to result in return to baseline performance levels after much less sleep than had originally been lost. The parallel increase in SWS during recovery leads to the direct speculation that SWS is somehow implicated in the sleep recovery process. Unfortunately, studies designed to test this hypothesis directly by experimentally varying the amount of SWS during the recovery sleep period or during a sleep fragmentation period have not implicated any sleep stages as central in the recovery process. When either SWS or REM was selectively deprived during the initial recovery night following sleep loss, no difference was found between those groups and a group that was allowed a nondisturbed night of recovery sleep.[183] A study looking at the relationship between systematic sleep fragmentation and the distribution of SWS came to the same conclusion.[188] However, both studies were not designed to look for more subtle effects that might have occurred within the initial recovery night.[183]

Horne[98] postulated that only part of a normal night of sleep is essential (core sleep) and that the remaining sleep exists primarily as a buffer. In one sense, core sleep could be approximately reduced to SWS and REM. In another sense, core sleep could refer to a period of sleep that is not fragmented by arousals or awakenings. Several types of studies suggest that TS time can be reduced somewhat, at least on an acute basis, with statistically minor effects (see Partial Sleep Deprivation). The decreased requirement for essential sleep could by itself explain why recovery sleep following sleep loss does not appear to replace all lost sleep. However, to postulate that portions of a night of sleep are nonessential without being able to describe an explicit relationship based on time asleep or sleep stage makes it difficult to interpret any finding where TS time or sleep stages change. If the restoration that occurs during sleep is viewed as an exponential process instead of a linear process, rapid changes would occur in the initial hours of sleep and increasingly small increments would occur as sleep continues past 5 or 6 hours.[210] These final small changes may not be measurable in typical sleep deprivation studies involving only a few subjects and as a result may give the appearance that the last 1 or 2 h of sleep is less essential.

CONCLUSIONS

The physiological and behavioral effects of partial and TS loss in human beings are consistent and well defined. Unfortunately, several of the consistent findings in human studies do not agree with the findings of animal studies, and the hope that sleep deprivation would serve as the tool to define the function of sleep has not been realized. It is generally agreed that there is a physiological imperative to sleep in human beings and other mammals and that the drive to sleep can be as strong as the drive to breathe. Beyond our applied knowledge of the mechanics of deprivation and response, future work must do the following:

1. Address in more detail the microstructure of the sleep process and its relationship to sleep restoration.
2. Specifically address response differences among species.
3. Comprehend the apparent differences in response to sleep deprivation in normal and depressed human beings.
4. Elucidate the interaction of the sleep system and the arousal system.
5. Ensure that our understanding of the lawful relationship between sleep loss, alertness, and behavior be disseminated for use by government and industry.

Acknowledgments

Supported by the Medical Research Service of the Dayton Department of Veterans Affairs Medical Center and Wright State University, Dayton, Ohio. Literature searches supported by the Sleep-Wake Disorders Research Institute, Dayton, Ohio.

References

1. Bonnet MH, Arand DL. We are chronically sleep deprived. Sleep. 1995;18:908–911.
2. Partinen M. Epidemiology of sleep disorders. In: Kryger MH, Roth T, Dement WC, eds. Principles and Practice of Sleep Medicine. 2nd ed. Philadelphia, Pa: WB Saunders; 1994:437–452.
3. Wehr TA, Moul DE, Barbato G, et al. Conservation of photoperiod-responsive mechanisms in humans. Am J Physiol. 1993;265:R846–R857.
4. Koslowski M, Babkoff H. Meta-analysis of the relationship between total sleep deprivation and performance. Chronobiol Int. 1992;9:132–136.
5. Pilcher JJ, Huffcutt AI. Effects of sleep deprivation on performance: a meta-analysis. Sleep. 1996;19:318–326.
6. Manaceine M. Quelques observations experimentales sur l'influence de l'insomnie absolue. Arch Ital Biol. 1894;21:322–325.
7. Patrick GTW, Gilbert JA. On the effect of loss of sleep. Psychol Rev. 1896;3:469–483.
8. Johnson LC. Sleep deprivation and performance. In: Webb WB, ed. Biological Rhythms, Sleep, and Performance. New York, NY: John Wiley & Sons; 1982:111–142.
9. Rosa RR, Bonnet MH. Predicting nighttime alertness following prophylactic naps. Sleep Res. 1991;20:417.
10. Mikulincer M, Babkoff H, Caspy T, et al. The effects of 72 hours of sleep loss on psychological variables. Br J Psychol. 1989;80:145–162.
11. Van Dongen HPA, Dinges DF. Circadian rhythms in fatigue, alertness, and performance. In: Kryger MH, Roth T, Dement WC, eds. Principles and Practice of Sleep Medicine. 3rd ed. Philadelphia, Pa: WB Saunders; 2000.
12. Bonnet MH, Arand DA. Sleepiness as measured by modified multiple sleep latency testing varies as a function of preceding activity. Sleep. 1998;21:477–483.
13. Wilkinson RT. Sleep deprivation. In: Edholm OG, Bacharach A, eds. The Physiology of Human Survival. New York, NY: Academic Press; 1965:399–430.
14. Leproult R, Van Reeth O, Byrne MM, et al. Sleepiness, performance, and neuroendocrine function during sleep deprivation: effects of exposure to bright light or exercise. J Biol Rhythms. 1997;12:245–258.
15. Lubin A, Hord DJ, Tracy ML, et al. Effects of exercise, bedrest and napping on performance decrement during 40 hours. Psychophysiology. 1976;13:334–339.
16. Webb WB, Agnew HWJ. Effects on performance of high and low energy-expenditure during sleep deprivation. Percept Mot Skills. 1973;37:511–514.
17. Angus RG, Heslegrave RJ, Myles WS. Effects of prolonged sleep deprivation, with and without chronic physical exercise, on mood and performance. Psychophysiology. 1985;22:276–282.
18. Moses J, Lubin A, Naitoh P, et al. Exercise and sleep loss: effects on recovery sleep. Psychophysiology. 1977;14:414–416.
19. Dijk D-J, Cajochen C, Borbely A. Effect of a single 3-hour exposure to bright light on core body temperature and sleep in humans. Neurosci Lett. 1991;121:59–62.
20. Campbell SS, Dawson D. Enhancement of nighttime alertness and performance with bright ambient light. Physiol Behav. 1990;48:317–320.
21. Dawson D, Encel N, Lushington K. Improving adaptation to simulated night shift: timed exposure to bright light versus daytime melatonin administration. Sleep. 1995;18:11–21.
22. Daurat A, Aguirre A, Foret J, et al. Bright light affects alertness and performance rhythms during a 24-h constant routine. Physiol Behav. 1993;53:929–936.
23. Murphy P, Myers B, Badia P, et al. The effects of bright light on daytime sleep latencies. Sleep Res. 1991;20:465.
24. Wilkinson RT. Interaction of noise with knowledge of results and sleep deprivation. J Exp Psychol. 1963;66:332–337.
25. Gunter TC, van der Zande RD, Wiethoff M, et al. Visual selective attention during meaningful noise and after sleep deprivation. Electroencephalogr Clin Neurophysiol Suppl. 1987;40:99–107.
26. Hartley L, Shirley E. Sleep-loss, noise and decisions. Ergonomics. 1977;20:481–489.
27. Tassi P, Nicolas A, Seegmuller C, et al. Interaction of the alerting effect of noise with partial sleep deprivation and circadian rhythmicity of vigilance. Percept Mot Skills. 1993;77:1239–1248.
28. Poulton EC, Edwards RS, Colquhoun WP. The interaction of the loss of a night's sleep with mild heat: task variables. Ergonomics. 1974;17:59–73.
29. Reyner LA, Horne JA. Evaluation of "in-car" countermeasures to sleepiness: cold air and radio. Sleep. 1998;21:46–50.
30. Kleitman N. Sleep and Wakefulness. 2nd ed. Chicago, Ill: University of Chicago Press; 1963.
31. Lindqvist A, Jalonen J, Parviainen P, et al. Effect of posture on spontaneous and thermally stimulated cardiovascular oscillations. Cardiovasc Res. 1990;24:373–380.
32. Newhouse PA, Belenky G, Thomas M, et al. The effects of d-amphetamine on arousal, cognition, and mood after prolonged total sleep deprivation. Neuropsychopharmacology. 1989;2:153–164.
33. Kornetsky C, Mirsky AF, Kessler EK, et al. The effects of dextroamphetamine on behavioral deficits produced by sleep loss in humans. J Pharmacol Exp Ther. 1959;127:46–50.
34. Caldwell JA, Caldwell JL. An in-flight investigation of the efficacy of dextroamphetamine for sustaining helicopter pilot performance. Aviat Space Environ Med. 1997;68:1073–1080.
35. Pigeau R, Naitoh P, Buguet A, et al. Modafinil, d-amphetamine and placebo during 64 hours of sustained mental work, I: effects on mood, fatigue, cognitive performance and body temperature. J Sleep Res. 1995;4:212–228.
36. Walsh JK, Muehlbach MJ, Humm TM, et al. Effect of caffeine on physiological sleep tendency and ability to sustain wakefulness at night. Psychopharmacology. 1990;101:271–273.
37. Borland RG, Rogers AS, Nicholson AN, et al. Performance overnight in shiftworkers operating a day-night schedule. Aviat Space Environ Med. 1986;57:241–249.

38. Wright KP, Badia P, Myers BL, et al. Combination of bright light and caffeine as a countermeasure for impaired alertness and performance during extended sleep deprivation. J Sleep Res. 1997;6:26–35.

39. Bonnet MH, Gomez S, Wirth O, et al. The use of caffeine versus prophylactic naps in sustained performance. Sleep. 1995;18:97–104.

40. Penetar D, McCann U, Thorne D, et al. Caffeine reversal of sleep deprivation effects on alertness and mood. Psychopharmacology. 1993;112:359–365.

41. Bonnet MH, Arand DL. The use of prophylactic naps and caffeine to maintain performance during a continuous operation. Ergonomics. 1994;37:1009–1020.

42. Bonnet MH, Arand DL. The impact of naps and caffeine on extended nocturnal performance. Physiol Behav. 1994;56:103–109.

43. Babkoff H, Kelly TL, Matteson LT, et al. Pemoline and methylphenidate: interaction with mood, sleepiness, and cognitive performance during 64 hours of sleep deprivation. Mil Psychol. 1992;4:235–265.

44. Bishop C, Roehrs T, Rosenthal L, et al. Alerting effects of methylphenidate under basal and sleep-deprived conditions. Exp Clin Psychopharmacol. 1997;5:344–352.

45. Lagarde D, Batejat D, Van Beers P, et al. Interest of modafinil, a new psychostimulant, during a sixty-hour sleep deprivation experiment. Fundam Clin Pharmacol. 1995;9:271–279.

46. Newhouse PA, Penetar DM, Fertig JB, et al. Stimulant drug effects on performance and behavior after prolonged sleep deprivation: a comparison of amphetamine, nicotine, and deprenyl. Mil Psychol. 1992;4:207–233.

47. Fischman MW, Schuster CR. Cocaine effects in sleep-deprived humans. Psychopharmacology. 1980;72:1–8.

48. Roehrs T, Beare D, Zorick F, et al. Sleepiness and ethanol effects on simulated driving. Alcohol Clin Exp Res. 1994;18:154–158.

49. Zwyghuizen-Doorenbos A, Roehrs T, Lamphere J, et al. Increased daytime sleepiness enhances ethanol's sedative effects. Neuropsychopharmacology. 1988;1:279–286.

50. Wilkinson RT. Effects of up to 60 hours' sleep deprivation on different types of work. Ergonomics. 1964;7:175–186.

51. Horne JA, Pettitt AN. High incentive effects on vigilance performance during 72 hours of total sleep deprivation. Acta Psychol. 1985;58:123–139.

52. Wilkinson RT. Interaction of lack of sleep with knowledge of results, repeated testing, and individual differences. J Exp Psychol. 1961;62:263–271.

53. Haslam DR. The incentive effect and sleep deprivation. Sleep. 1983;6:362–368.

54. Bonnet MH, Webb WB. The effect of repetition of relevant and irrelevant tasks over day and night work periods. Ergonomics. 1978;21:999–1005.

55. Webb WB, Levy CM. Effects of spaced and repeated total sleep deprivation. Ergonomics. 1984;27:45–58.

56. Bonnet MH, Rosa RR. Sleep and performance in young adults and older insomniacs and normals during acute sleep loss and recovery. Biol Psychol. 1987;25:153–172.

57. Webb WB. A further analysis of age and sleep deprivation effects. Psychophysiol. 1985;22:156–161.

58. Weitzman ED, Moline ML, Czeisler CA, et al. Chronobiology of aging: temperature, sleep-wake rhythms and entrainment. Neurobiol Aging. 1982;3:299–309.

59. Mullaney DJ, Kripke DF, Fleck PA, et al. Sleep loss and nap effects on sustained continuous performance. Psychophysiology. 1983;20:643–651.

60. Tyler DB. Psychological changes during experimental sleep deprivation. Dis Nerv Syst. 1955;16:293–299.

61. Johnson LC. Physiological and psychological changes following total sleep deprivation. In: Kales A, ed. Sleep Physiology and Pathology. Philadelphia, Pa: JB Lippincott; 1969:206–220.

62. Wu JC, Bunney WE. The biological basis of an antidepressant response to sleep deprivation and relapse: review and hypothesis. Am J Psychiatry. 1990;147:14–21.

63. Donnell JM. Performance decrement as a function of total sleep loss and task duration. Percept Mot Skills. 1969;29:711–714.

64. Steyvers FJJM, Gaillard AWK. The effects of sleep deprivation and incentives on human performance. Psychol Res. 1993;55:64–70.

65. Light AI, Sun JH, McCool C, et al. The effects of acute sleep deprivation on level of resident training. Curr Surg. 1989;46:29–30.

66. Alluisi EA, Coates GD, Morgan BBJ. Effects of temporal stressors on vigilance and information processing. In: Mackie RR, ed. Vigilance: Theory, Operational Performance, and Physiological Correlates. New York, NY: Plenum Press; 1977:361–421.

67. Ryman DH, Naitoh P, Englund CE. Decrements in logical reasoning performance under conditions of sleep loss and physical exercise: the factor of sentence complexity. Percept Mot Skills. 1985;61:1179–1188.

68. Williams HL, Lubin A. Speeded addition and sleep loss. J Exp Psychol. 1967;73:313–317.

69. Babkoff H, Mikulincer M, Caspy T, et al. The topology of performance curves during 72 hours of sleep loss: a memory and search task. Q J Exp Psychol A. 1988;40:737–756.

70. Williams HL, Gieseking CF, Lubin A. Some effects of sleep loss on memory. Percept Mot Skills. 1966;23:1287–1293.

71. Nilsson LG, Backman L, Karlsson T. Priming and cued recall in elderly, alcohol intoxicated and sleep deprived subjects: a case of functionally similar memory deficits. Psychol Med. 1989;19:423–433.

72. Akerstedt T, Froberg JE, Friberg Y, et al. Melatonin excretion, body temperature and subjective arousal during 64 hours of sleep deprivation. Psychoneuroendocrinology. 1979;4:219–225.

73. Moses JM, Lubin A, Naitoh P, et al. Subjective evaluation of the effects of sleep loss: the NPRU mood scale. 1975. Unpublished paper.

74. Carskadon MA, Dement WC. Effects of total sleep loss on sleep tendency. Percept Mot Skills. 1979;48:495–506.

75. Carskadon MA, Dement WC. Cumulative effects of sleep restriction on daytime sleepines. Psychophysiology. 1981;18:107–113.

76. Marcus CL, Loughlin GM. Effect of sleep deprivation on driving safety in housestaff. Sleep. 1996;19:763–766.

77. Cassel W, Ploch T, Becker C, et al. Risk of traffic accidents in patients with sleep-disordered breathing: reduction with nasal CPAP. Eur Respir J. 1996;9:2606–2611.

78. Horne JA. A review of the biological effects of total sleep deprivation in man. Biol Psychol. 1978;7:55–102.

79. Kollar EJ, Namerow N, Pasnau RO, et al. Neurological findings during prolonged sleep deprivation. Neurology. 1968;18:836–840.

80. Ross JJ. Neurological findings after prolonged sleep deprivation. Arch Neurol. 1965;12:399–403.

81. Rodin EA, Luby ED, Gottlieb JS. The EEG during prolonged experimental sleep deprivation. Electroencephalogr Clin Neurophysiol. 1962;14:544–551.

82. Naitoh P, Kales A, Kollar EJ, et al. Electroencephalographic activity after prolonged sleep loss. Electroencephalogr Clin Neurophysiol. 1969;27:2–11.

83. Naitoh P, Pasnau RO, Kollar EJ. Psychophysiological changes after prolonged deprivation of sleep. Biol Psychiatry. 1971;3:309–320.

84. Williams HL, Granda AM, Jones RC, et al. EEG frequency and finger pulse volume as predictors of reaction time during sleep loss. Electroencephalogr Clin Neurophysiol. 1962;14:64–70.

85. Blake H, Gerard RW, Kleitman N. Factors influencing brain potentials during sleep. J Neurophysiol. 1939;2:48–60.

86. Pratt KL, Matteson RH, Weckers NJ, et al. EEG activation of epileptics following sleep deprivation. Electroencephalogr Clin Neurophysiol. 1968;24:11–15.

87. Kollar EJ, Slater GG, Palmer JO, et al. Stress in subjects undergoing sleep deprivation. Psychosom Med. 1966;28:101–113.

88. Fiorica V, Higgins EA, Iampietro PF, et al. Physiological responses of men during sleep deprivation. J Appl Physiol. 1968;24:167–176.

89. Johnson LC, Slye ES, Dement WC. Electroencephalographic and autonomic activity during and after prolonged sleep deprivation. Psychosom Med. 1965;27:415–423.

90. Ax A, Luby ED. Autonomic responses to sleep deprivation. Arch Gen Psychiatry. 1961;4:55–59.

91. Cooper KR, Phillips BA. Effect of short-term sleep loss on breathing. J Appl Physiol. 1982;53:855–858.

92. Schiffman PL, Trontell MC, Mazar MF, et al. Sleep deprivation

decreases ventilatory response to CO_2 but not load compensation. Chest. 1983;84:695–698.

93. White DP, Douglas NJ, Pickett CK, et al. Sleep deprivation and the control of ventilation. Am Rev Respir Dis. 1983;128:984–986.

94. Phillips BA, Cooper KR, Burke TV. The effect of sleep loss on breathing in chronic obstructive pulmonary disease. Chest. 1987;91:29–32.

95. Canet E, Gaultier C, D'Allest AM, et al. Effects of sleep deprivation on respiratory events during sleep in healthy infants. J Appl Physiol. 1989;66:1158–1163.

96. Persson HE, Svanborg E. Sleep deprivation worsens obstructive sleep apnea. Comparison between diurnal and nocturnal polysomnography. Chest. 1996;109:645–650.

97. Brooks D, Horner RL, Kimoff RJ, et al. Effect of obstructive sleep apnea versus sleep fragmentation on responses to airway occlusion. Am J Respir Crit Care Med. 1997;155:1609–1617.

98. Horne J. Why We Sleep. New York, NY: Oxford University Press; 1987:1–319.

99. Tobler I, Sigg H. Long-term motor activity recording of dogs and the effect of sleep deprivation. Experientia. 1986;42:987–991.

100. Plyley MJ, Shephard RJ, Davis GM, et al. Sleep deprivation and cardiorespiratory function. Influence of intermittent submaximal exercise. Eur J Appl Physiol. 1987;56:338–344.

101. Goodman JM, Plyley MJ, Hart LE, et al. Moderate exercise and hemodilution during sleep deprivation. Aviat Space Environ Med. 1990;61:139–144.

102. McMurray RG, Brown CF. The effect of sleep loss on high intensity exercise and recovery. Aviat Space Environ Med. 1984;55:1031–1035.

103. Van Den Noort S, Brine K. Effect of sleep on brain labile phosphates and metabolic rate. Am J Physiol. 1970;218:1434–1439.

104. Mendelson W, Guthrie RD, Guynn R, et al. Rapid eye movement (REM) sleep deprivation, stress and intermediary metabolism. J Neurochem. 1974;22:1157–1159.

105. Froberg JE. Twenty-four-hour patterns in human performance, subjective and physiological variables and differences between morning and evening active subjects. Biol Psychol. 1977;5:119–134.

106. Kant GJ, Genser SG, Thorne DR, et al. Effects of 72 hour sleep deprivation on urinary cortisol and indices of metabolism. Sleep. 1984;7:142–146.

107. Akerstedt T, Palmblad J, de la Torre B, et al. Adrenocortical and gonadal steroids during sleep deprivation. Sleep. 1980;3:23–30.

108. Palmblad J, Akerstedt T, Froberg J, et al. Thyroid and adrenomedullary reactions during sleep deprivation. Acta Endocrinol (Copenh). 1979;90:233–239.

109. Gary KA, Winokur A, Douglas SD, et al. Total sleep deprivation and the thyroid axis: effects of sleep and waking activity. Aviat Space Environ Med. 1996;67:513–519.

110. von Treuer K, Norman TR, Armstrong SM. Overnight human plasma melatonin, cortisol, prolactin, TSH, under conditions of normal sleep, sleep deprivation, and sleep recovery. J Pineal Res. 1996;20:7–14.

111. Frank G, Halberg F, Harner R, et al. Circadian periodicity, adrenal corticosteroids, and the EEG of normal man. J Psychiatr Res. 1966;4:73–86.

112. Beck U. Hormonal secretion during sleep in man. Modification of growth hormone and prolactin secretion by interruption and selective deprivation of sleep. Int J Neurol. 1981;15:17–29.

113. Akerstedt T. Altered sleep-wake patterns and circadian rhythms. Acta Physiol Scand Suppl. 1979;469:1–48.

114. Parker DC, Rossman LG, Kripke DF, et al. Endocrine rhythms across sleep-wake cycles in normal young men under basal conditions. In: Orem J, Barnes CD, eds. Physiology in Sleep. New York, NY: Academic Press; 1980:146–180.

115. Sassin JF, Parker DC, Johnson LC, et al. Effects of slow wave sleep deprivation on human growth hormone release in sleep: preliminary study. Life Sci. 1969;8:1299–1307.

116. Dinges DF, Douglas SD, Hamarman S, et al. Sleep deprivation and human immune function. Adv Neuroimmunology. 1995;5:97–110.

117. Irwin M, McClintick J, Costlow C, et al. Partial night sleep deprivation reduces natural killer and cellular immune responses in humans. FASEB J. 1996;10:643–653.

118. Dinges DF, Douglas SD, Zaugg L, et al. Leukocytosis and natural killer cell function parallel neurobehavioral fatigue induced by 64 hours of sleep deprivation. J Clin Invest. 1994;93:1930–1939.

119. Palmblad J, Petrini B, Wasserman J, et al. Lymphocyte and granulocyte reactions during sleep deprivation. Psychosom Med. 1979;41:273–278.

120. Moldofsky H, Lue FA, Davidson JR, et al. Effects of sleep deprivation on human immune functions. FASEB J. 1989;3:1972–1977.

121. Moldofsky H. Central nervous system and peripheral immune functions and the sleep-wake system. J Psychiatry Neurosci. 1994;19:368–374.

122. Boyum A, Wiik P, Gustavsson E, et al. The effect of strenuous exercise, calorie deficiency and sleep deprivation on white blood cells, plasma immunoglobulins and cytokines. Scand J Immunol. 1996;43:228–235.

123. Brown R, Pang G, Husband AJ, et al. Suppression of immunity to influenza virus infection in the respiratory tract following sleep disturbance. Reg Immunol. 1989;2:321–325.

124. Benca RM, Kushida CA, Everson CA, et al. Sleep deprivation in the rat, VII: immune function. Sleep. 1989;12:47–52.

125. Everson CA, Bergmann BM, Rechtschaffen A. Sleep deprivation in the rat, III: total sleep deprivation. Sleep. 1989;12:13–21.

126. Everson CA. Functional consequences of sustained sleep deprivation in the rat. Behav Brain Res. 1995;69:43–54.

127. Rechtschaffen A, Bergmann BM. Sleep deprivation in the rat by the disk-over-water method. Behav Brain Res. 1995;69:55–63.

128. Kushida CA, Bergmann BM, Rechtschaffen A. Sleep deprivation in the rat, IV: paradoxical sleep deprivation. Sleep. 1989;12:22–30.

129. Gilliland MA, Bergmann BM, Rechtschaffen A. Sleep deprivation in the rat, VIII: high EEG amplitude sleep deprivation. Sleep. 1989;12:53–59.

130. Bergmann BM, Everson CA, Kushida CA, et al. Sleep deprivation in the rat, V: energy use and medication. Sleep. 1989;12:31–41.

131. Pilcher JJ, Bergmann BM, Fang VS, et al. Sleep deprivation in the rat, XI: the effect of guanethidine-induced sympathetic blockade on the sleep deprivation syndrome. Sleep. 1990;13:218–231.

132. Everson CA, Wehr TA. Nutritional and metabolic adaptations to prolonged sleep deprivation in the rat. Am J Physiol. 1993;264:R376–R387.

133. Bergmann BM, Gilliland MA, Balzano S, et al. Sleep deprivation in the rat, XIX: effects of thyroxine administration. Sleep. 1995;18:317–324.

134. Feng PF, Bergmann BM, Rechtschaffen A. Sleep deprivation in rats with preoptic/anterior hypothalamic lesions. Brain Res. 1995;703:93–99.

135. Pilcher JJ, Bergmann BM, Refetoff S, et al. Sleep deprivation in the rat, XIII: the effect of hypothyroidism on sleep deprivation symptoms. Sleep. 1991;14:201–210.

136. Kushida CA, Everson CA, Suthipinittharm P, et al. Sleep deprivation in the rat, VI: skin changes. Sleep. 1989;12:42–46.

137. Everson CA. Sustained sleep deprivation impairs host defense. Am J Physiol. 1993;265:R1148–R1154.

138. Bergmann BM, Gilliland MA, Feng PF, et al. Are physiological effects of sleep deprivation in the rat mediated by bacterial invasion? Sleep. 1996;19:554–562.

139. Everson CA, Gilliland MA, Kushida CA, et al. Sleep deprivation in the rat, IX: recovery. Sleep. 1989;12:60–67.

140. Rechtschaffen A, Bergmann BM, Everson CA, et al. Sleep deprivation in the rat, X: integration and discussion of the findings. Sleep. 1989;12:68–87.

141. Rosenthal L, Roehrs TA, Rosen A, et al. Level of sleepiness and total sleep time following various time in bed conditions. Sleep. 1993;16:226–232.

142. Dinges DF, Pack F, Williams K, et al. Cumulative sleepiness, mood disturbance, and psychomotor vigilance performance decrements during a week of sleep restricted to 4–5 hours per night. Sleep. 1997;20:267–277.

143. Wilkinson RT, Edwards RS, Haines E. Performance following a night of reduced sleep. Psychonomic Sci. 1966;5:471–472.

144. Webb WB, Agnew HWJ. The effects on subsequent sleep of an acute restriction of sleep length. Psychophysiology. 1975;12:367–370.

145. Horne JA, Wilkinson S. Chronic sleep reduction: daytime vigilance performance and EEG measures of sleepiness, with particular reference to "practice" effects. Psychophysiology. 1985;22:69–78.

146. Webb WB, Agnew HWJ. The effects of a chronic limitation of sleep length. Psychophysiology. 1974;11:265–274.

147. Blagrove M, Alexander C, Horne JA. The effects of chronic sleep reduction on the performance of cognitive tasks sensitive to sleep deprivation. Appl Cogn Psychol. 1995;9:21–40.

148. Friedmann J, Globus G, Huntley A, et al. Performance and mood during and after gradual sleep reduction. Psychophysiology. 1977;14:245–250.

149. Mullaney DJ, Johnson LC, Naitoh JP, et al. Sleep during and after gradual sleep reduction. Psychophysiology. 1977;14:237–244.

150. Friedman RC, Bigger JT, Kornfeld DS. The intern and sleep loss. N Engl J Med. 1971;285:201–203.

151. Webb WB, Agnew HWJ. Sleep: effects of a restricted regime. Science. 1965;150:1745–1747.

152. Brunner DP, Dijk DJ, Borbely AA. Repeated partial sleep deprivation progressively changes the EEG during sleep and wakefulness. Sleep. 1993;16:100–113.

153. Engel W, Seime R, Powell V, et al. Clinical performance of interns after being on call. South Med J. 1987;80:761–763.

154. Hawkins MR, Vichick DA, Silsby HD, et al. Sleep and nutritional deprivation and performance of house officers. J Med Educ. 1985;60:530–535.

155. Poulton EC, Hunt GM, Carpenter A, et al. The performance of junior hospital doctors following reduced sleep and long hours of work. Ergonomics. 1978;21:279–295.

156. Beatty J, Ahern SK, Katz R. Sleep deprivation and the vigilance of anesthesiologists during simulated surgery. In: Mackie RR, ed. Vigilance: Theory, Operational Performance, and Physiological Correlates. New York, NY: Plenum Press; 1977:511–527.

157. Friedman RC, Kornfeld DS, Bigger TJ. Psychological problems associated with sleep deprivation in interns. J Med Educ. 1973;48:436–441.

158. Reznick RK, Folse JR. Effect of sleep deprivation on the performance of surgical residents. Am J Surg. 1987;154:520–525.

159. Williams HL, Williams CL. Nocturnal EEG profiles and performance. Psychophysiology. 1966;3:164–175.

160. Stepanski E, Zorick F, Peters M, et al. Effects of sleep deprivation on alertness in chronic insomnia. Sleep Res. 1990;19:297.

161. Pearlman CA. Sleep structure variation and performance. In: Webb WB, ed. Biological Rhythms, Sleep, and Performance. New York, NY: John Wiley & Sons; 1982:143–173.

162. Dement WC. The effect of dream deprivation. Science. 1960;131:1705–1707.

163. Dement WC, Fisher C. Experimental interference with the sleep cycle. Can Psychiatry Assoc J. 1963;8:400–405.

164. Agnew HWJ, Webb WB, Williams RL. Comparison of stage 4 and 1—REM sleep deprivation. Percept Mot Skills. 1967;24:851–858.

165. Clemens SR, Dement WC. Effect of REM sleep deprivation on psychological functioning. J Nerv Ment Dis. 1967;144:485–491.

166. Puca FM, Livrea P, Genco S, et al. REM sleep deprivation in normal humans. Changes in anxiety, depression and aggressiveness, and HVA and 5-HIAA levels in the lumbar cerebrospinal fluid. Boll Soc Ital Biol Sper. 1976;52:782–787.

167. Zarcone V, de la Penna A, Dement WC. Heightened sexual interest and sleep disturbance. Percept Mot Skills. 1974;39:1135–1141.

168. Hobson JA, McCarley RW. The brain as a dream state generator: an activation-synthesis hypothesis of the dream process. Am J Psychiatry. 1977;134:1335–1348.

169. Stern WC, Morgane PJ. Theoretical view of REM sleep function: maintenance of catecholamine systems in the central nervous system. Behav Biol. 1974;11:1–32.

170. Ephron HS, Carrington P. Rapid eye movement sleep and cortical homeostasis. Psychol Rev. 1966;73:500–526.

171. Roffwarg HP, Muzio J, Dement WC. Ontogenetic development of the human sleep-dream cycle. Science. 1966;152:604–619.

172. Berger RJ. Occulomotor control: a possible function for REM sleep. Psychol Rev. 1969;76:144–164.

173. Herman JH, Roffwarg HP, Rosenmann CJ, et al. Binocular depth perception following REM deprivation or awake state visual deprivation. Psychophysiology. 1980;17:236–242.

174. Snyder F. Towards an evolutionary theory of dreaming. Am J Psychiatry. 1966;123:126–136.

175. Pearlman CA. REM sleep and information processing: evidence from animal studies. Neurosci Biobehav Rev. 1979;3:57–68.

176. McGrath MJ, Cohen DB. REM sleep facilitation of adaptive waking behavior: a review of the literature. Psychol Bull. 1978;85:24–57.

177. Greenberg R, Pearlman C. Cutting the REM nerve: an approach to the adaptive role of REM sleep. Perspect Biol Med. 1974;17:513–521.

178. Tilley AJ, Empson JA. REM sleep and memory consolidation. Biol Psychol. 1978;6:293–300.

179. Oniani TN, Lortkipanidze ND, Mgaloblishvili MM, et al. Neurophysiological analysis of paradoxical sleep deprivation. In: Oniani T, ed. Neurobiology of Sleep-Wakefulness Cycle. Tbilisi, USSR: Metsniereba; 1988:19–43.

180. Karni A, Tanne D, Rubenstein BS, et al. Dependence on REM sleep of overnight improvement of a perceptual skill. Science. 1994;265:679–682.

181. Agnew HW, Webb WB, Williams RL. The effects of stage four sleep deprivation. Electroencephalogr Clin Neurophysiol. 1964;17:68–70.

182. Johnson LC, Naitoh P, Moses JM, et al. Interaction of REM deprivation and stage 4 deprivation with total sleep loss: experiment 2. Psychophysiology. 1974;11:147–159.

183. Lubin A, Moses JM, Johnson LC, et al. The recuperative effects of REM sleep and stage 4 sleep on human performance after complete sleep loss: experiment I. Psychophysiology. 1974;11:133–146.

184. Johnson LC. Are stages of sleep related to waking behavior? Am Scientist. 1973;61:326–338.

185. Bonnet MH. Infrequent periodic sleep disruption: effects on sleep, performance and mood. Physiol Behav. 1989;45:1049–1055.

186. Bonnet MH. Effect of sleep disruption on sleep, performance, and mood. Sleep. 1985;8:11–19.

187. Bonnet MH. Performance and sleepiness as a function of frequency and placement of sleep disruption. Psychophysiology. 1986;23:263–271.

188. Bonnet MH. Performance and sleepiness following moderate sleep disruption and slow wave sleep deprivation. Physiol Behav. 1986;37:915–918.

189. Bonnet MH. Sleep restoration as a function of periodic awakening, movement, or electroencephalographic change. Sleep. 1987;10:364–373.

190. Bonnet MH. The effect of sleep fragmentation on sleep and performance in younger and older people. Neurobiol Aging. 1989;10:21–25.

191. Bonnet MH. Sleep disruption by mechanical leg jerk and periodic awakening and its effect on sleep, performance and mood. Paper presented at: Association of Sleep Disorders Centers Meeting; 1984; Dallas, Tex.

192. Martin SE, Wraith PK, Deary IJ, et al. The effect of nonvisible sleep fragmentation on daytime function. Am J Respir Crit Care Med. 1997;155:1596–1601.

193. Carskadon MA, Brown ED, Dement WC. Sleep fragmentation in the elderly: relationship to daytime sleep tendency. Neurobiol Aging. 1982;3:321–327.

194. Stepanski E, Lamphere J, Badia P, et al. Sleep fragmentation and daytime sleepiness. Sleep. 1984;7:18–26.

195. Fenz WD, Graig JG. Autonomic arousal and performance during sixty hours of sleep deprivation. Percept Mot Skills. 1972;34:543–553.

196. Williams HL, Lubin A, Goodnow JJ. Impaired performance with sleep loss. Psychol Monographs. 1959;73(14)(Whole No. 484):1–26.

197. Rosa RR, Bonnet MH, Warm JS. Recovery of performance during sleep following sleep deprivation. Psychophysiology. 1983;20:152–159.

198. Carskadon MA, Dement WC. Sleep loss in elderly volunteers. Sleep. 1985;8:207–221.

199. Bonnet MH. The effect of varying prophylactic naps on performance, alertness and mood throughout a 52-hour continuous operation. Sleep. 1991;14:307–315.

200. Borbely AA, Baumann F, Brandeis D, et al. Sleep deprivation: effect on sleep stages and EEG power density in man. Electroencephalogr Clin Neurophysiol. 1981;51:483–495.

201. Nakazawa Y, Kotorii M, Ohshima M, et al. Changes in sleep pattern after sleep deprivation. Folia Psychiatr Neurol Jpn. 1978;32:85–93.

202. Benoit O, Foret J, Bouard G, et al. Habitual sleep length and patterns of recovery sleep after 24 hour and 36 hour sleep deprivation. Electroencephalogr Clin Neurophysiol. 1980;50:477–485.

203. Bonnet MH. Effect of 64 hours of sleep deprivation upon sleep in geriatric normals and insomniacs. Neurobiol Aging. 1986;7:89–96.

204. Reynolds CF, Kupfer DJ, Hoch CC, et al. Sleep deprivation in healthy elderly men and women: effects on mood and on sleep during recovery. Sleep. 1986;9:492–501.

205. Bonnet MH, Arand DL. Sleep loss in aging. Clin Geriatr Med. 1989;5:405–420.

206. Reynolds CF, Kupfer DJ, Hoch CC, et al. Sleep deprivation effects in older endogenous depressed patients. Psychiatry Res. 1987;21:95–109.

207. Reynolds CF, Kupfer DJ, Hoch CC, et al. Sleep deprivation as a probe in the elderly. Arch Gen Psychiatry. 1987;44:982–990.

208. Berger RJ, Oswald I. Effects of sleep deprivation on behavior, subsequent sleep, and dreaming. J Ment Sci. 1962;108:457–465.

209. Kales A, Tan T, Kollar EJ, et al. Sleep patterns following 205 hours of sleep deprivation. Psychosom Med. 1970;32:189–200.

210. Jewett ME, Dijk D, Kronauer RE, et al. Dose-response relationship between sleep duration and human psychomotor vigilance and subjective alertness. Sleep. 1999;22:171–180.

6

Phylogeny of Sleep Regulation

Irene Tobler

Tracing the evolution of sleep to its origins is an important approach that can provide clues to its functions. Sleep studies have centered on the presence of sleep and its stages in the higher vertebrates (birds and reptiles), but only a few studies have investigated sleep in the lower vertebrates (amphibians and fish). Behavioral sleep has been identified in many nonmammalian species, but the electroencephalogram correlates commonly used to define sleep in mammals and birds have not been identified in reptiles, amphibians, and fish.

Studies of mammals have revealed that sleep is finely regulated. Thus, a constant daily quota of sleep is maintained through a balance between sleep duration and intensity. Slow-wave activity in nonrapid eye movement sleep may serve as the measure of sleep intensity, but other measures including motor activity, arousal threshold, and heart rate can serve as indicators to document compensatory mechanisms after sleep deprivation. Such regulatory mechanisms indicate that there is a need for sleep and therefore it must have an adaptive value.

The search for the stages underlying sleep regulation is a major aim in sleep research. Several studies investigating sleep in animals that do not necessarily meet the electrophysiological criteria for the definition of sleep have shown that compensation occurs after sleep deprivation or rest deprivation in lower vertebrates (reptiles and fish) and invertebrates (scorpions, cockroaches, and Drosophila). *These more simple animals can be useful for investigating basic mechanisms of compensatory activity at the molecular and genetic level and thereby provide clues to the functions of sleep.*

It is remarkable that the function of sleep is still unknown. The study of sleep in animals is likely to yield insights into its origins and functional significance because animals represent different stages of evolution. Whether sleep, in its complexity as it has been described for mammalian species, is a unique phenomenon present only in the most highly evolved vertebrates—the homeothermic mammals and birds—or is present in simpler form in the poikilothermic, lower vertebrates and perhaps even in invertebrates, needs to be clarified. In simpler organisms, in which more genetic information is available, documenting a sleep-like state provides the possibility of investigating the molecular regulation of this state and of searching for similar states in more evolved species.

Following sleep deprivation (SD), there is a compensatory rebound in several variables that has led to the suggestion that the homeostatic property that is typical for sleep in mammals might be included in a broader definition of sleep.[1] These sleep regulatory mechanisms allow the maintenance of a relatively constant daily amount of sleep when faced with alterations in the opportunity to sleep.

SLEEP REGULATION IN MAMMALS

Sleep Duration and Intensity of Sleep

A homeostatic component of sleep regulation has been demonstrated in many mammals from several orders. The maintenance of a constant quota for sleep is attained by balancing between sleep duration and sleep intensity. After extended waking, depending on the duration of the deprivation, nonrapid eye movement (NREM) sleep and rapid eye movement (REM) sleep are enhanced. The most striking feature manifested early during recovery sleep is the remarkable increase of electroencephalographic (EEG) slow waves. This was first demonstrated in the rabbit[2] and then extensively documented in the rat.[3, 4] Varying the duration of SD showed that the increase in slow wave activity (SWA, mean EEG power density approximately 0.75 to 4.0 Hz) is a function of the duration of prior waking (rat, see references 5 and 6; cat, see references 7 through 9; human beings, see Chapter 29). Studies in inbred laboratory mice also showed such a relationship[10] (Fig. 6–1), paving the way to investigate the underlying mechanisms at the genetic level. The notion that slow wave activity reflects NREM sleep intensity[3, 4] is supported by the higher arousal threshold during NREM sleep with high amounts of slow waves (cat, see reference 11; rat, see references 12 and 13). Although there is already an increase in SWA after 3 h of SD in the rat, sleep duration (and REM sleep) are only increased after at least 6 h of enforced waking.[5, 6, 14] The increase in sleep duration is larger when recovery from SD begins in the circadian phase of predominant waking, whereas the enhancement of SWA is less dependent on circadian factors.[15]

The question remains, is the waking state per se or are some specific aspects of waking responsible for the increase in SWA? Because SD was performed by forced locomotion in some experiments, the influence of this procedure was examined by varying the rotation rate

SLOW-WAVE ACTIVITY AS A FUNCTION OF PRIOR WAKING DURATION IN TWO MOUSE STRAINS

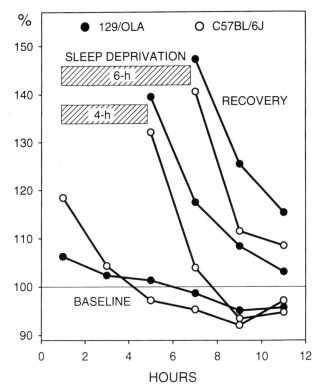

Figure 6–1. Effect of 4-h and 6-h sleep deprivation (SD) on slow-wave activity (mean EEG power density 0.75 to 4.0 Hz) in NREM sleep in two inbred mouse strains (129/OLA and C57BL/6J). Mean hourly values (n = 5–7) expressed as percentage of the 12-h baseline value. A significant increase of slow wave activity during recovery compared with the corresponding interval in baseline was observed after 4-h SD, for the first two intervals in both strains, after 6-h SD for all intervals in C57BL/6, and after interval one in 129/OLA ($P < 0.05$; paired t test). Total sleep time and REM sleep were not affected.

of the sleep deprivation cylinder[3, 4] and allowing the animal to engage in voluntary running activity.[16] No major effect on the slow wave part of NREM sleep was found. In both the rat[17] and the Syrian hamster,[18] SD by forced locomotion and by gentle handling affected sleep in similar ways. Finally, a major stress effect on SWA appears to be unlikely because the forced locomotion procedure did not entail a significant increase in the level of plasma corticosterone,[19] and the expression pattern of genes was similar after spontaneous wakefulness lasting 3 h and 3-h enforced SD.[19a] Moreover, in mice, SWA was increased after spontaneous, undisturbed bouts of waking.[19b] Therefore, neither motor activity nor stress is crucial for promoting SWA. The possibility that the increased brain metabolism during waking is a critical variable is improbable because the changes of SWA induced by SD performed both in a warm environment and at room temperature were similar, even though brain temperature was higher in the warm deprivation condition.[14]

The compensation in sleep after sleep loss can be taken as an indication of regulatory mechanisms with

a possible adaptive function. Under natural conditions, animals need to be vigilant and avoid long bouts of sleep. But, if the benefits of sleep are needed as well, a recovery from the sleep deficit can occur not only by prolonging sleep, which may interfere with other waking behaviors, but also by intensifying sleep.

Slow Wave Activity

Because EEG SWA is determined by the prior sleep and waking history, a prominent 24-h rhythm of sleep should be associated with high initial SWA values in the main sleep period and a prominent decline as the need for sleep dissipates (Fig. 6–2). This relationship can be observed in nocturnal rodents (e.g., rat and hamster) in which SWA is high at light onset. In the diurnal chipmunk[20] and in human beings, whose main sleep period is in the dark, the highest values are at the beginning of the dark period. The overall progressive SWA decline, despite the intermittent waking bouts that are typical for most mammals, reveals the presence of a stable, continuous process underlying the sleep-wake pattern. In animals that exhibit only a small preference for sleep in the light period, such as the rabbit and the guinea pig, only a minor decline of SWA was seen[21, 22] (see Fig. 6–2). This relationship between the sleep-wake pattern and SWA is also evident in experiments in the rat and Djungarian hamster in which the photoperiod is changed. The total amount of sleep was unchanged, but sleep was redistributed according to the new light-dark ratio, and the time course of SWA followed the new sleep-wake pattern.[23, 24] Using a quantitative simulation of NREM sleep homeostasis in the rat and two mouse strains, the biphasic time course of SWA during baseline, its initial increase after SD, and the subsequent prolonged negative rebound was reproduced[19b, 25] (see Chapter 29).

There are large differences in the magnitude of the SWA increase among various rodents, rabbits, the cat and human beings, and even within mouse strains. Simulations showed that the dynamics of Process S in the rat and mouse, reflected by the time constants of its increase and decrease, was faster than in human beings[19b, 25] (see Chapter 29), and preliminary simulations of SWA in the guinea pig showed that larger time constants of Process S are needed in this species than in the rat.[26] An alternative interpretation is that the guinea pigs live at a higher level of Process S, which then increases only to a smaller extent after SD than in the rat and mouse. Similarly, the remarkable difference of approximately 40% in the increase of SWA after 4 h of SD in two relatively small rodents, the Djungarian hamster and inbred mice[27, 28] (see Fig. 6–1, Fig. 6–3) may reflect different levels of Process S in these species during baseline. Such an interpretation is supported by the different magnitude of the SWA response to SD in human long and short sleepers.[30]

A compensatory increase of EEG variables after prolonged wakefulness has been described not only for human beings and rodents but also for several other mammals, including two nonhuman primates: Rhesus

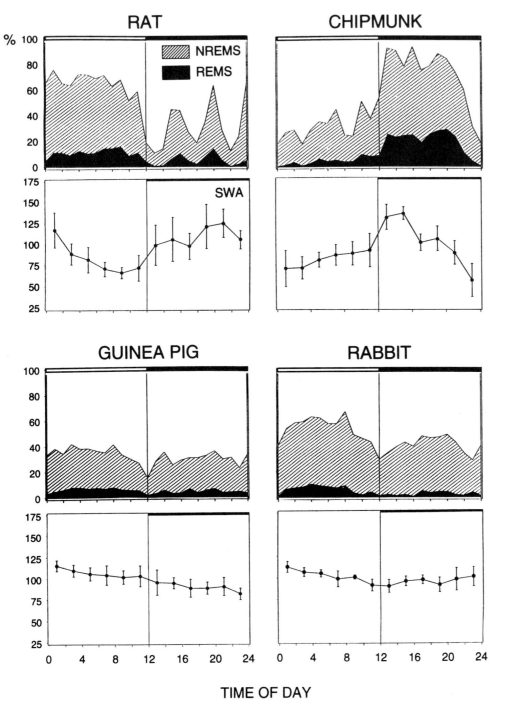

Figure 6–2. Vigilance state distribution and slow wave activity (SWA, mean EEG power density 0.75 to 4.0 Hz or 1.0 to 2.0 Hz for chipmunk) in species with a marked (rat and chipmunk, n = 6 and 7) or minor (guinea pig and rabbit, n = 9 and 7) preference for sleep in the light or the dark period. Mean hourly values of REM sleep (REMS), NREM sleep (NREMS), and waking (white area). SWA is expressed as a percentage of the mean 24-h value. Note the decrease of SWA in the course of the main 12-h sleep period and its absence when there is no preference for sleep in either phase.

monkey and Macaque mulatta.[31, 32] Among the carnivores, the cat has been extensively investigated after SD,[7–9, 31, 33, 34] and in dogs, an increase of slow waves was found after 12-h SD.[35]

Is REM Sleep Homeostatically Regulated?

There is extensive literature on the regulation of REM sleep in many mammalian species, including cat,[36–38] dog, rat, mouse and cow, but it has not been addressed from a phylogenetic point of view. Although

there is a compensatory increase of REM sleep after total SD and selective REM sleep deprivation, there is as yet little indication that REM sleep may also have an intensity dimension. However, in the rat[17, 39] and rabbit,[21] the enhancement of theta activity during REM sleep following 24 h of SD could reflect an increase in REM sleep intensity.

Circadian Versus Homeostatic Aspects of Sleep Regulation

There are several lines of evidence from animal experiments to indicate that the homeostatic (Process S)

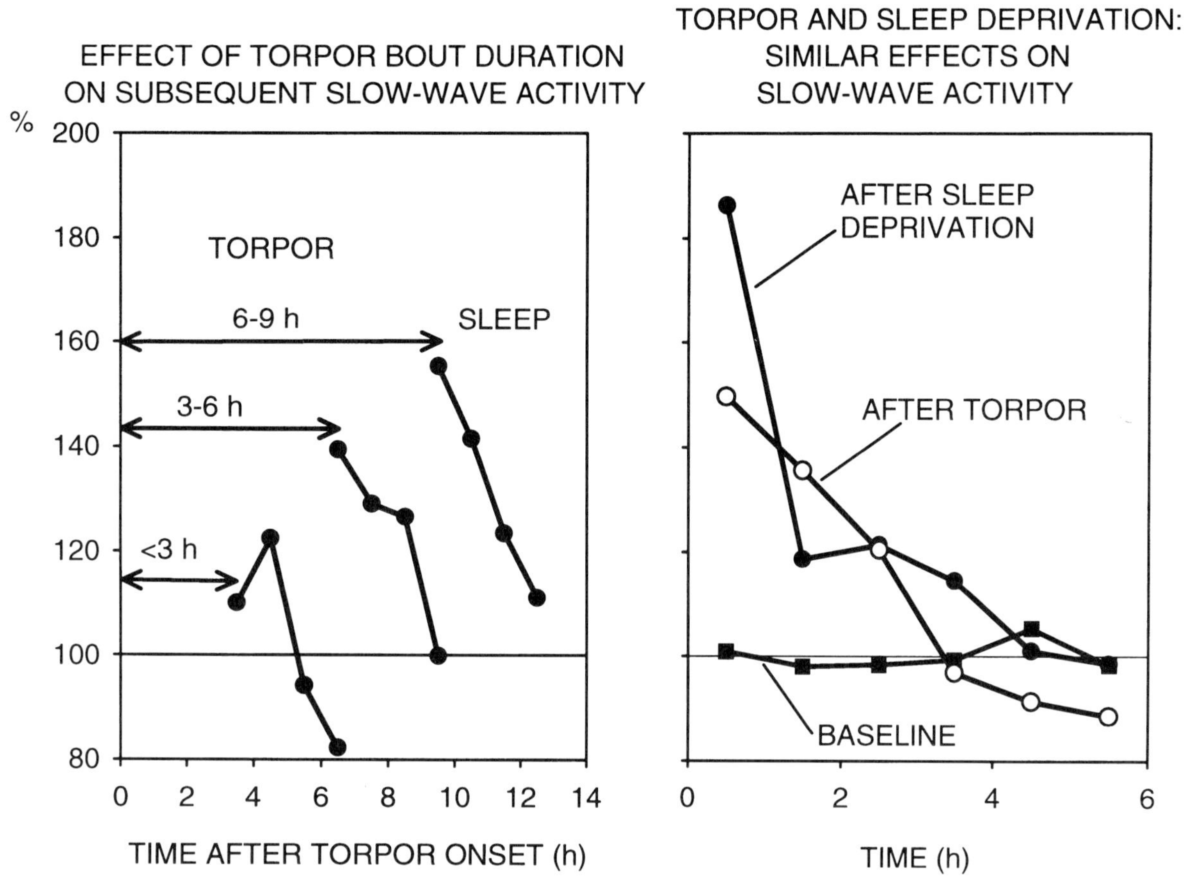

EFFECT OF TORPOR BOUT DURATION ON SUBSEQUENT SLOW-WAVE ACTIVITY

TORPOR AND SLEEP DEPRIVATION: SIMILAR EFFECTS ON SLOW-WAVE ACTIVITY

Figure 6–3. Time course of slow wave activity (SWA, mean EEG power density 0.75 to 4.0 Hz) in NREM sleep during sleep after torpor episodes of different durations (< 3 h, 3 to 6 h, and 6 to 9 h; *left*) and during baseline, recovery from 4-h sleep deprivation and after torpor (mean torpor duration = 4.8 ± 0.3 h SEM). *Left*, mean hourly values (n = 3, 8, and 5 for < 3 h, 3 to 6 h, and 6 to 9 h, respectively). A linear correlation between torpor bout duration and increase in SWA was significant (n = 16, $r^2 = 0.38$, $P = 0.011$). Moreover, a saturating exponential function resulted in a better fit (the r^2 was larger, 0.62; $P < 0.05$).[60] *Right*, mean hourly values (n = 8). All three recordings were performed in a short photoperiod, light = 8 h, dark = 16 h, at 16 to 18°C. The first 3 h after torpor and sleep deprivation differed significantly from baseline ($P < 0.05$; paired t test).

and circadian (Process C) facets of sleep regulation (see Chapter 29) are mediated by separate processes. A conflict can be created between the two tendencies in the rat by ending a 24-h SD period either at the onset or in the middle of the dark period, which is the circadian period in which waking predominates.[3, 15] SWA shows a rebound in two stages: an immediate increase followed by waking and a second, delayed increase at light onset. The effects of 4-h SD performed at two different phases of the light-dark cycle in cats, which show a minor circadian sleep-wake modulation,[7, 34] also depended on the circadian phase at which recovery was allowed.[7]

The circadian facet of sleep regulation can be disrupted by lesions of the suprachiasmatic nuclei.[40–42] The arrhythmic rats were subjected to 24-h SD to test their ability to compensate for sleep loss. Both SWA in NREM sleep and the amount of REM sleep were increased. Conversely, SD affected neither the phase nor the period of the free-running rest-activity rhythm of intact rats.[43, 44] These results indicate that the homeostatic component of sleep regulation is morphologically and functionally distinct from the circadian component.

This conclusion is supported by the results obtained in species that do not have a natural, distinct preference for sleep in a particular circadian phase, such as the guinea pig, rabbit, and some strains of mice[21, 45, 45a] (see Fig. 6–2). After 6-h SD in guinea pigs, SWA was enhanced during recovery to a similar extent, independent of whether SD occurred in the light or dark period.[46]

Special Features

Herbivores: Cows and Horses

The investigation of sleep regulation in herbivores is important because they include species with large bodies and brain weights (see Chapter 7), and ruminants have the capacity to ruminate during sleep. The effects of SD have been investigated in three species. The prevention of recumbency in cows for 14 to 22 h per day for 2 to 4 weeks, primarily resulted in REM sleep deprivation, although NREM sleep and drowsiness were also reduced (for drowsiness, see Chapter 7).[47] The chronic sleep loss was partially compensated by intensifying NREM sleep at the cost of drowsiness. During recovery, both NREM sleep and REM sleep were increased. Similarly, in ponies recorded in a stall and outdoors, NREM sleep was reduced at the cost of drowsiness when they were exposed to the more disturbed conditions outdoors.[48] A donkey sleep deprived for 48 h showed an increase in sleep during recovery.[49] Therefore, sleep seems to be also regulated in herbivores. Because EEG spectral analysis of the vigilance states is lacking, the question of whether herbivores have an intensity component in NREM sleep is still open.

Unihemispheric Sleep and Sleep Deprivation in Dolphins

Aquatic mammals belonging to the orders cetacea, pinnipedia, and sirenia, have developed one of the most interesting sleep specializations. They engage in episodes of unihemispheric "deep" sleep (i.e., with a predominance of delta waves), which may last from minutes to several hours, while the other hemisphere exhibits an EEG resembling waking (see Chapter 7). This specialization provides a unique possibility to investigate sleep regulation. Keeping bottlenose dolphins awake for 35 to 72 h resulted in an increase in delta sleep in three of the six dolphins, and in an early study, a more regular alternation of deep sleep between the brain hemispheres was found during recovery.[50] Thus, slow waves in NREM sleep also seem to represent sleep intensity in dolphins. The crucial question then was whether it is feasible to sleep deprive a single brain hemisphere and whether this would elicit unilateral compensation. SD of one hemisphere attained by disturbing dolphins only when the EEG of one hemisphere was synchronized, and leaving them undisturbed when slow waves were present in the other hemisphere resulted in a larger compensation of delta sleep in the deprived hemisphere during recovery in seven of the nine deprivations.[50] Although there are several theories regarding the function of this specialization, the data show that sleep, as defined by EEG criteria, does not necessarily have to encompass the entire brain. It follows that sleep may be a local phenomenon leading to recuperation of those regions that were most active during waking (see Chapter 29).

Sleep and Hibernation

The investigation of hibernation and daily torpor, which are considered to be processes homologous to sleep (for a review, see reference 51), can contribute to the understanding of sleep. Hibernation and daily torpor are specializations that constitute the most effective ways to reduce energy requirements in endothermic animals. During hibernation, body temperature is lowered to approximately 5°C or less for several months,[52] with short (less than 24 h) euthermic interruptions.[53, 54] In daily torpor, temperature is lowered to approximately 15 to 20°C for several hours during the circadian rest period.[55] Such episodes also occur in some birds (e.g., hummingbird).[56]

It is puzzling that animals arouse regularly from hibernation, even though the energetic costs of the arousals are high and lead to a reduced energetic benefit.[54] Moreover, the animals arouse from hibernation and go to sleep. Paradoxically, it was found in three species of ground squirrels that the initial values of SWA during euthermia are high and decline progressively, resembling the time course after SD,[53, 57, 58] and long hibernation bouts are followed by higher initial levels of SWA than short ones. This led to the hypothesis that during hibernation, animals may be "sleep deprived"[53, 58]; in other words, hibernation, especially at low temperatures, is not compatible with restorative processes potentially occurring during sleep.

The relation between the torpid state, the subsequent arousal, and SD was investigated in the Djungarian hamster (Phodopus sungorus sungorus), in which days with torpor alternating with days at euthermic levels can be compared. During euthermia, as in the hibernating ground squirrels, the initial value of SWA in NREM sleep was high and followed by a progressive decline.[59] The increase in SWA was compared to recovery from 4-h SD in conditions resembling summer and winter.[23, 27] The time course of SWA in NREM sleep during recovery closely resembled the pattern after torpor (see Fig. 6–3, left). Moreover, the initial level of SWA was higher after long torpor bouts compared with short bouts[60] (see Fig. 6–3, right), which resembled the increase after differing lengths of SD documented for other species. A saturating exponential curve resulted in a better fit between the duration of torpor and the initial SWA values than a straight line.[60] Therefore, the increase in sleep pressure indeed follows similar kinetics as its increase during SD (e.g., rat[25] but at a slower rate (see Fig. 6–3), supporting the hypothesis that during hypothermia, animals incur an SD that is recovered by returning to euthermia.[53, 58] It remains to be clarified whether or not the return to euthermia during hibernation and after daily torpor is driven by the need to recover (i.e., it may be triggered by the accumulation of Process S).

Other Measures for Sleep Regulation

Sleep is apparently regulated relative to an internal reference level. Usually EEG spectral parameters, especially SWA, serve as indicators of these regulatory processes in mammals. However, other variables are also affected, such as sleep state continuity and motor activity.

Sleep continuity in the rat was enhanced after 24-h SD.[61] The frequency of short wake episodes (of shorter duration than 32 sec) was reduced, leading to a consolidation of sleep states. In similar experiments in the rat and other rodents (guinea pigs, laboratory mice), the number of brief awakenings decreased in parallel with the increase of SWA.[10, 22, 24, 61a] The inverse relationship of these variables led to the hypothesis that brief awakenings may represent a behavioral correlate of sleep intensity.[24] This finding may also contribute to the reduced NREM-REM sleep cycle length variability in the rat[61] and bottlenose dolphin,[50] and the shortening of the length of the sleep cycle, the increase in its regularity, and the duration of single-cell activity discharge cycle in brain stem dorsal raphe nucleus in the cat[62] after SD.

The decrease of motor activity after SD in human beings[63] can be observed in several other mammals. In dogs subjected to SD, motor activity assessed continuously using a portable activity monitor attached to the collar was reduced by 40% during recovery.[64] Similarly, motor activity was reduced to 84% of baseline when recovery from SD coincided with dark onset in the rat.[3] Thus, motor activity is an easily measured variable that can serve to investigate sleep regulation in animals in which invasive EEG interventions are not possible, or in nonmammalian species in which sleep cannot be defined by electrophysiological measures.

SLEEP REGULATION IN NONMAMMALIAN VERTEBRATES

Birds

The investigation of sleep regulation in birds is important because its presence may clarify whether sleep regulation is related to homeothermy. For some birds, three vigilance states could be distinguished by spectral analysis of the EEG. But in contrast to mammals, in which NREM sleep power density values in the low frequency range (0.25 to 6.0 Hz) exceed those of REM sleep and waking by approximately one order of magnitude, in birds, the differences between the sleep stages are smaller.[65, 66] SWA in NREM sleep in pigeons did not decline in the course of the dark period, the main sleep period of these birds.[66] Moreover, SWA was not affected by SD.[65, 66] In this respect, SWA in the pigeon seems to differ from mammals and may not reflect sleep intensity. More studies in birds are needed to clarify this issue.

Despite the lack of a mammalian homology of the intensity dimension within NREM sleep in birds, several variables are affected by 24-h SD (Fig. 6–4). Sleep duration, the amount of REM sleep, and electro-oculographic (EOG) activity in waking and in NREM sleep are increased during recovery.[66] Furthermore, in Barbary doves, the behavioral parameter of eye-blinking frequency was substantially decreased after 3- to 36-h SD achieved by exposing the animals to a ferret on a leash.[67] Moreover, the level of vigilance estimated by the blinking frequency depended on the length of SD. These findings indicate a need to compensate for sleep

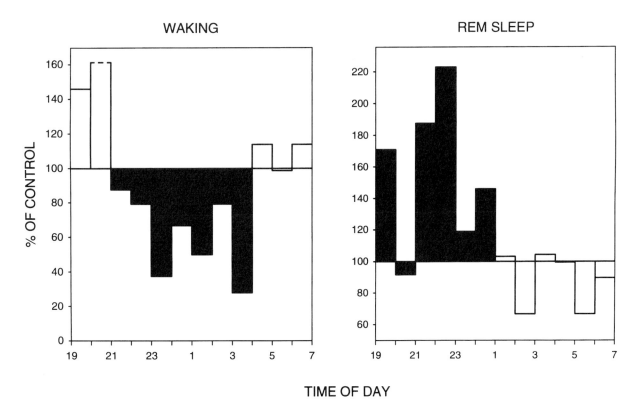

SLEEP REGULATION IN THE PIGEON

WAKING

REM SLEEP

TIME OF DAY

Figure 6–4. Effect of 24-h sleep deprivation ending at dark onset on waking and REM sleep in pigeons. Hourly mean values (n = 4) expressed as percentage of the corresponding interval of the control day for the 12-h dark period. The black bars indicate the 7-h and 6-h interval for which waking and REM sleep were significantly below or above control, respectively ($P < 0.05$, paired t test). Initially, after the end of deprivation, the birds were very active. (Modified from *Journal of Comparative Physiology. A, Sensory, Neural, and Behavioral Physiology [Berlin]*, Sleep and EEG spectra in pigeon *(Columbia livia)* under baseline conditions and after sleep deprivation, Tobler I, Borbély AA, vol 163, 729–738, 1988, Copyright © Springer-Verlag GmbH & Co. KG.)

loss. There is a trade-off between the benefits of frequent eye blinking (i.e., optimizing predator detection by increasing vigilance) and sleep with few interruptions.[67, 68] The results imply that the birds benefitted from sleep with closed eyes, and that those benefits are reduced during SD.

Reptiles

Sleep in reptiles differs in many ways from sleep in mammals. Considerable diversity in the appearance of high-voltage slow waves (sharp waves and spikes) superimposed on the waking and sleeping EEG has been reported. It has been suggested that this type of EEG activity may be a precursor or correlate of the slow waves associated with sleep in mammals.[69] The pertinent question is, therefore, whether these EEG phenomena change as a function of prior waking, indicating the reptile's need for sleep.

In the early 1970s, Flanigan performed a unique set of SD experiments in species belonging to several orders: (crocodilian *[Caiman sclerops]*; chelonian, box turtle *[Terrapene carolina]* and red-footed tortoise *[Geochelone carbonaria]*; and Squamata iguanid lizards, green iguana *[Iguana iguana]* and spiny-tailed lizard, also called black lizard *[Ctenosaura pectinata]*.[29] Depending on the species, 24 to 48 h of stimulation was performed by stroking, handling, or gently tugging the animal's leash when it showed signs of behavioral sleep. In turtles, more stimulations were required toward the last hours of SD, and the iguanas became increasingly limp. Such behavior was especially evident when the animals were picked up and handled and was only seen during the enforced waking, supporting the notion of an accumulating need for sleep. Several variables showed an apparent compensatory rebound. The latency to behavioral sleep was decreased and the duration and overall amount of behavioral sleep increased. Furthermore, the occurrence of EEG spikes, which predominate during behavioral sleep, were markedly enhanced in all the species after the deprivation. The arousal threshold to electrical stimulation of either the EOG or electrocardiogram (EKG) electrodes was higher during recovery.

Therefore, reptilian EEG spikes and sharp waves may reflect sleep intensity and appear to reflect processes that occur during sleep, which must be compensated for when waking is prolonged. Their increase after prolonged wakefulness, just as slow waves in mammals, suggests that they also have a functional similarity.

Amphibians and Fish

Compensatory mechanisms after SD have not been investigated in amphibians and only in two studies in fish. Although there are many signs of behavioral sleep in fish, the concomitant electrophysiological changes are difficult to determine and remain unclear. Thus, the effect of rest deprivation has been confined to behavioral measures.[70] Activation of carp for up to 96 h by continuous illumination was followed by a decreased latency to sleep behavior during the reinstatement of the dark period,[71] and in perch, the activation induced by exposure to 6 and 12 h of light during the habitual rest period (i.e., the dark period), resulted in an increase of resting behavior during recovery.[70] The effect depended on the length of the light exposure, confirming the notion that homeostatic mechanisms may also be involved in the regulation of rest in fish.

SLEEP REGULATION IN INVERTEBRATES

Sleep in mammals has a circadian and a homeostatic component. A circadian rest-activity cycle has been well documented in invertebrates, and many, especially arthropods, meet the behavioral criteria for sleep.[29, 72, 72a] In addition, there seem to be aspects of rest in invertebrates that are homeostatically regulated. The evidence stems from three invertebrate species: two cockroaches and the scorpion.

The resting state was prevented for 3 h at the end of the daily rest period (we predicted that a compensatory increase of rest would best be manifested at the time of habitual activity) in cockroaches (*Leucophea maderae*,[73] *Blaberus giganteus*,[74] and *Periplaneta australasiae* [K. Sly and R. Brown, PhD, unpublished data, October 1994]). Rest was increased after this rest deprivation (Fig. 6–5), while the control experiment, in which the insects were

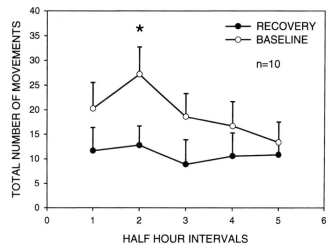

COCKROACH *Periplaneta australasiae* EFFECTS OF 3-H REST DEPRIVATION

Figure 6–5. Effects of 3-h rest deprivation in the cockroach, *Periplaneta australasiae*, on motor activity. The curves represent mean 30-min values ± SEM (n = 10) of the baseline day and recovery after rest deprivation. Rest deprivation was performed 3 h before dark onset by gently shaking the cage when motor activity was absent. The presence or absence of movements in 30 sec epochs was scored on the basis of video recordings. A significant decrease of movements was present after the deprivation (ANOVA, $P < 0.009$; *$P < 0.05$, paired t test). (Modified from K. Sly and R. Brown, PhD, unpublished data, October 1994.)

only removed from their home cages for 3 h, elicited a smaller and shorter lasting decrease of activity. These data were interpreted as a compensatory reaction to the rest deficit.[73] In a more refined approach, behavior was scored as "rest" and "activity," and rest was subdivided based on the position of the head, abdomen, and antennae in order to clarify whether substates could be characterized by different thresholds of arousal. In one of the nine behavioral states, characterized by a horizontal body axis with the antennae touching the substrate, the arousal threshold was significantly higher than in all other states. After disturbing the cockroaches for an entire 12-h dark period, it was the behavioral state mentioned earlier that showed a tendency to be increased in duration and frequency after the rest deprivation; however, locomotion was also increased.[74]

The rest deprivation studies were extended to another arthropod, the scorpion (*Heterometrus longimanus, Heterometrus spinnifer,* and *Pandinus imperator*). The scorpion was chosen because it belongs to the oldest living arthropod group (marine scorpions can be traced back to the Silurian period of about 400 million years ago). The 24-h pattern of activity and, on the basis of the reaction to a vibration stimulus, an intermediate "alert" state and a "rest" state were obtained. Deprivation of the rest state for 12 h elicited an initial rise of activity and a significant increase in the resting state[75] (Fig. 6–6).

OUTLOOK

Compensation for the loss of sleep has been found in many mammals, and similar phenomena were described in birds, reptiles, fish, and some invertebrates. In natural environments, there are many disturbances that may prevent animals from obtaining their normal quota of sleep. It seems that various animals have developed mechanisms to compensate for the loss of sleep. This is an important indication that there is a benefit of sleep that is reduced during SD and that seems to be indispensable.

Rest behavior may be a state from which sleep evolved. A more detailed characterization of rest in different classes of animals contributes to clarifying the origin of sleep and helps to identify the unique properties of sleep in comparison to rest. The comparison of sleep, which is a well-defined state in mammals and birds, and rest, a ubiquitous state in lower vertebrates and invertebrates, shows an important common feature: both sleep and rest are not mere functions of the circadian rest-activity rhythm but are determined by additional regulatory mechanisms. Both sleep and rest deprivation elicit compensatory responses. This regulatory property of sleep can be used to examine rest in a broad range of animals that, due to the absence of EEG criteria, are not considered to manifest sleep. The effects of rest deprivation in invertebrates are, in some aspects, analogous to the compensation of sleep after SD in mammals. Elementary properties of sleep

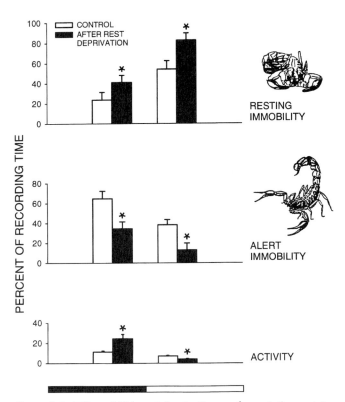

EFFECT OF REST DEPRIVATION

Figure 6–6. Effect of 12-h rest deprivation on three vigilance states in the scorpion. Mean values ± SEM (n = 7) for the 12-h intervals of the control day and after rest deprivation (*$P < 0.05$, Wilcoxon matched pairs signed rank test; differences between control and recovery.) Light-dark conditions are indicated by the white and black bar at the bottom of the figure.

may be found that will allow the investigation of the underlying mechanisms in less complex organisms.

It is probable that many genes are involved in the control of sleep and circadian rhythms. The development of gene technology[75a] has led, in mice, to the identification of a circadian clock gene[76, 77] and the localization of genomic regions involved in their sleep.[78, 78a] In rats, gene technology has brought about the recognition of changes in gene expression at sleep-waking transitions during the sleep-wake cycle (see references 79, 79a, and 80). Although these technologies allow the application of genetics to complex systems such as those encountered in mammals, the use of simpler systems should provide an interesting parallel avenue to solve the involvement of genes in sleep regulation. For example, the extensive knowledge of genes in drosophila will allow investigation of the mechanisms underlying the effects of rest deprivation.

Acknowledgments

This work was supported by the Swiss National Science Foundation. The author thanks Drs. P. Achermann, A. Borbély, T. Deboer, and H. Driver for their comments.

References

1. Tobler I. Evolution of the sleep process: a phylogenetic approach. Exp Brain Res. 1984(suppl 8):207–226.

2. Pappenheimer JR, Koski G, Fencl V, et al. Extraction of sleep-promoting factor S from cerebrospinal fluid and from brains of sleep-deprived animals. J Neurophysiol 1975;38:1299–1311.

3. Borbély AA, Neuhaus HU. Sleep-deprivation: effects on sleep and EEG in the rat. J Comp Physiol [A]. 1979;133:71–87.

4. Friedman L, Bergmann BM, Rechtschaffen A. Effects of sleep deprivation on sleepiness, sleep intensity, and subsequent sleep in the rat. Sleep. 1979;1:369–391.

5. Tobler I, Borbély AA. Sleep EEG in the rat as a function of prior waking. Electroencephalogr Clin Neurophysiol. 1986;64:74–76.

6. Tobler I, Borbély AA. The effect of 3-h and 6-h sleep deprivation on sleep and EEG spectra of the rat. Behav Brain Res. 1990;36:73–78.

7. Lancel M, van Riezen H, Glatt A. Effects of circadian phase and duration of sleep deprivation on sleep and EEG power spectra in the cat. Brain Res. 1991;548:206–214.

8. Lucas EA. Effects of five to seven days of sleep deprivation produced by electrical stimulation of the midbrain reticular formation. Exp Neurol. 1975;49:554–568.

9. Ursin R. Differential effect of sleep deprivation on the two slow wave sleep stages in the cat. Acta Physiol Scand. 1971;83:352–361.

10. Tobler I, Gaus SE, Deboer T, et al. Altered circadian activity rhythms and sleep in mice devoid of prion protein. Nature. 1996;380:639–642.

11. Grahnstedt S, Ursin R. Awakening thresholds for electrical brain stimulation in five sleep-waking stages in the cat. Electroencephalogr Clin Neurophysiol. 1980;48:222–229.

12. Frederickson CJ, Rechtschaffen A. Effects of sleep deprivation on awakening thresholds and sensory evoked potentials in the rat. Sleep. 1978;1:69–82.

13. Neckelmann D, Ursin R. Sleep stages and EEG power spectrum in relation to acoustical stimulus arousal threshold in the rat. Sleep. 1993;16:467–477.

14. Tobler I, Franken P, Gao B, et al. Sleep deprivation in the rat at different ambient temperatures: effect on sleep, EEG spectra and brain temperature. Arch Ital Biol. 1994;132:39–52.

15. Trachsel L, Tobler I, Borbély AA. Sleep regulation in rats: effects of sleep deprivation, light, and circadian phase. Am J Physiol. 1986;251:R1037–R1044.

16. Hanagasioglu M, Borbély AA. Effect of voluntary locomotor activity on sleep in the rat. Behav Brain Res. 1982;4:359–368.

17. Franken P, Dijk DJ, Tobler I, et al. Sleep deprivation in rats: effects on EEG power spectra, vigilance states, and cortical temperature. Am J Physiol. 1991;261:R198–R208.

18. Tobler I, Jaggi K. Sleep and EEG spectra in the Syrian hamster (Mesocricetus auratus) under baseline conditions and following sleep deprivation. J Comp Physiol [A]. 1987;161:449–459.

19. Tobler I, Murison R, Ursin R, et al. The effect of sleep deprivation and recovery sleep on plasma corticosterone in the rat. Neurosci Lett. 1983;35:297–300.

19a. Cirelli C, Tononi G. Differences in brain gene expression between sleep and waking as revealed by mRNA differential display and cDNA microarray technology. J Sleep Res. 1999; 8(suppl 1):44–52.

19b. Huber R, Deboer T, Tobler I. Sleep and dynamics of sleep EEG in three mouse strains: effects of sleep deprivation and simulations. Brain Res. In press.

20. Dijk DJ, Daan S. Sleep EEG spectral analysis in a diurnal rodent: Eutamias sibiricus. J Comp Physiol [A]. 1989;165:205–215.

21. Tobler I, Franken P, Scherschlicht R. Sleep and EEG spectra in the rabbit under baseline conditions and following sleep deprivation. Physiol Behav. 1990;48:121–129.

22. Tobler I, Franken P, Jaggi K. Vigilance states, EEG spectra, and cortical temperature in the guinea pig. Am J Physiol. 1993;264:R1125–R1132.

23. Deboer T, Tobler I. Vigilance state episodes and cortical temperature in the Djungarian hamster: the influence of photoperiod and ambient temperature. Pflugers Arch. 1997;433:230–237.

24. Franken P, Tobler I, Borbély AA. Varying photoperiod in the laboratory rat: profound effect on 24-h sleep pattern but no effect on sleep homeostasis. Am J Physiol. 1995;269:R691–R701.

25. Franken P, Tobler I, Borbély AA. Sleep homeostasis in the rat: simulation of the time course of EEG slow-wave activity [published erratum appears in Neurosci Lett. 1991;132:279]. Neurosci Lett. 1991;130:141–144.

26. Tobler I, Franken P, Trachsel L, et al. Models of sleep regulation in mammals. J Sleep Res. 1992;1:125–127.

27. Deboer T, Franken P, Tobler I. Sleep and cortical temperature in the Djungarian hamster under baseline conditions and after sleep deprivation. J Comp Physiol [A]. 1994;174:145–155.

28. Tobler I, Deboer T, Fischer M. Sleep and sleep regulation in normal and prion protein-deficient mice. J Neurosci. 1997;17:1869–1879.

29. Flanigan WFJ. Sleep and wakefulness in Iguanid lizards, Ctenosaura pectinata and Iguana iguana. Brain Behav Evol. 1973;8:401–436.

30. Aeschbach D, Cajochen C, Landolt HP, et al. Homeostatic sleep regulation in habitual short sleepers and long sleepers. Am J Physiol. 1996;270:R41–R53.

31. Berger R J, Meier GW. The effects of selective deprivation of states of sleep in the developing monkey. Psychophysiology. 1966;2:354–371.

32. Pegram GV, Reite ML, Stephens LM, et al. Prolonged sleep deprivation in the monkey: effects on sleep patterns, brain temperature, and performance. In: Primate Electrophysiology, Particularly Related to Sleep. Holloman, Air Force Base, NM: 6571st Aeromedical Research Laboratory; 1969:51–53. Report ARL-TR-69-5.

33. Kiyono S, Kawamoto T, Sakakura H, et al. Effects of sleep deprivation upon the paradoxical phase of sleep in cats. Electroencephalogr Clin Neurophysiol. 1965;19:34–40.

34. Tobler I, Scherschlicht R. Sleep and EEG slow-wave activity in the domestic cat: effect of sleep deprivation. Behav Brain Res. 1990;37:109–118.

35. Takahashi Y, Ebihara S, Nakamura Y, et al. Temporal distributions of delta wave sleep and REM sleep during recovery sleep after 12-hour forced wakefulness in dogs: similarity to human sleep. Neurosci Lett. 1978;10:329–334.

36. Jouvet D, Vimont P, Delorme F, et al. Etude de la privation sélective de la phase paradoxale de sommeil chez le Chat. C R Soc Biol. 1964;4:756–759.

37. Siegel J, Gordon TP. Paradoxical sleep: deprivation in the cat. Science. 1965;148:978–980.

38. Jouvet M. Paradoxical sleep mechanisms. Sleep. 1994;17:S77–S83.

39. Borbély AA, Tobler I, Hanagasioglu M. Effect of sleep deprivation on sleep and EEG power spectra in the rat. Behav Brain Res. 1984;14:171–182.

40. Mistlberger RE, Bergmann BM, Waldenar W, et al. Recovery sleep following sleep deprivation in intact and suprachiasmatic nuclei-lesioned rats. Sleep. 1983;6:217–233.

41. Tobler I, Borbély AA, Groos G. The effect of sleep deprivation on sleep in rats with suprachiasmatic lesions. Neurosci Lett. 1983;42:49–54.

42. Trachsel L, Edgar DM, Seidel WF, et al. Sleep homeostasis in suprachiasmatic nuclei-lesioned rats: effects of sleep deprivation and triazolam administration. Brain Res. 1992;589:253–261.

43. Beersma DGM, Daan S, Dijk DJ. Sleep intensity and timing: a model for their circadian control. In: Carpenter GA, ed. Some Mathematical Questions in Biology: Circadian Rhythms. Providence, RI: American Mathematical Society; 1987:39–62. Lectures on Mathematics in the Life Sciences; vol 19.

44. Borbély AA. Sleep regulation: circadian rhythm and homeostasis. Curr Top Neuroendocrinol. 1982;1:83–103.

45. Pellet J, Béraud G. Organisation nycthémérale de la veille et du sommeil chez le cobaye (Cavia porcellus). Comparaisons interspécifiques avec le rat et le chat. Physiol Behav. 1967;2:131–137.

45a. Franken P, Malafosse A, Tafti M. Genetic determinants of sleep regulation in inbred mice. Sleep. 1999;22:155–169.

46. Tobler I, Franken P. Sleep homeostasis in the guinea pig: similar response to sleep deprivation in the light and dark period. Neurosci Lett. 1993;164:105–108.

47. Ruckebusch Y. Sleep deprivation in cattle. Brain Res. 1974;78:495–499.

48. Ruckebusch Y. The hypnogram as an index of adaptation of farm animals to changes in their environment. Appl Anim Ethol. 1975;2:3–18.

49. Ruckebusch Y. Un problème controversé: la perte de vigilance chez le cheval et la vache au cours du sommeil. Cah Med Vet. 1970;39:210–225.

50. Oleksenko AI, Mukhametov LM, Polyakova IG, et al. Unihemi-

spheric sleep deprivation in bottlenose dolphins. J Sleep Res. 1992;1:40–4.

51. Kilduff TS, Krilowicz B, Milsom WK, et al. Sleep and mammalian hibernation: homologous adaptations and homologous processes? Sleep. 1993;16:372–386.

52. Barnes BM. Freeze avoidance in a mammal: body temperatures below 0°C in an arctic hibernator. Science. 1989;244:1593–1595.

53. Daan S, Barnes BM, Strijkstra AM. Warming up for sleep? Ground squirrels sleep during arousal from hibernation. Neurosci Lett. 1991;128:265–268.

54. Wang LCH. Energetic and field aspects of mammalian torpor: the Richardson's ground squirrel. In: Wang LCH, Hudson JW, eds. Strategies in the Cold. New York, NY: Academic Press; 1978:109–145.

55. Heldmaier G, Steinlechner S. Seasonal pattern and energetics of short daily torpor in the Djungarian hamster, Phodopus sungorus. Oecologia. 1981;48:265–270.

56. Hainsworth FR. Regulation of oxygen consumption and body temperature during torpor in a hummingbird, Eulampis jugularis. Science. 1970;168:368–369.

57. Strijkstra AM, Daan S. Sleep during arousal episodes as a function of prior torpor duration in hibernating European ground squirrels. J Sleep Res. 1997;6:36–43.

58. Trachsel L, Edgar DM, Heller HC. Are ground squirrels sleep deprived during hibernation? Am J Physiol. 1991;260:R1123–R1129.

59. Deboer T, Tobler I. Sleep EEG after daily torpor in the Djungarian hamster: similarity to the effects of sleep deprivation. Neurosci Lett. 1994;166:35–38.

60. Deboer T, Tobler I. Natural hypothermia and sleep deprivation: common effects on recovery sleep in the Djungarian hamster. Am J Physiol. 1996;271:R1364–R1371.

61. Trachsel L, Tobler I, Achermann P, et al. Sleep continuity and the REM-nonREM cycle in the rat under baseline conditions and after sleep deprivation. Physiol Behav. 1991;49:575–580.

61a. Trachsel L, Tobler I, Borbély AA. Electroencephalogram analysis of non-rapid eye movement sleep in rats. Am J Physiol. 1988;255:R27–R37.

62. Lydic R, McCarley RW, Hobson JA. Forced activity alters sleep cycle periodicity and dorsal raphe discharge rhythm. Am J Physiol. 1984;247:R135–R145.

63. Naitoh P, Muzet A, Johnson LC, et al. Body movements during sleep after sleep loss. Psychophysiology. 1973;10:363–368.

64. Tobler I, Sigg H. Long-term motor activity recording of dogs and the effect of sleep deprivation. Experientia. 1986;42:987–991.

65. Berger RJ, Phillips NH. Constant light suppresses sleep and circadian rhythms in pigeons without consequent sleep rebound in darkness. Am J Physiol. 1994;267:R945–R952.

66. Tobler I, Borbély AA. Sleep and EEG spectra in the pigeon (Columba livia) under baseline conditions and after sleep deprivation. J Comp Physiol [A]. 1988;163:729–738.

67. Lendrem DW. Sleeping and vigilance in birds, II: an experimental study of the Barbary dove (Streptopelia risoria). Anim Behav. 1984;32:243–248.

68. Lendrem DW. Sleeping and vigilance in birds. In: Koella WP, ed. Sleep 1982. Basel, Switzerland: Karger; 1983:134–138.

69. Hartse KM, Rechtschaffen A. The effect of amphetamine, nembutal, alpha-methyl-tyrosine, and parachlorophenylalanine on the sleep-related spike activity of the tortoise, geochelone carbonaria, and on the cat ventral hippocampus spike. Brain Behav Evol. 1982;21:199–222.

70. Tobler I, Borbély AA. Effect of rest deprivation on motor activity of fish. J Comp Physiol [A]. 1985;157:817–822.

71. Shapiro CM, Hepburn HR. Sleep in a schooling fish, Tilapia mossambica. Physiol Behav. 1976;16:613–615.

72. Piéron H. Le problème physiologique du sommeil. Paris, France: Masson; 1913.

72a. Kaiser W, Steiner-Kaiser J. Neuronal correlates of sleep, wakefulness and arousal in a diurnal insect. Nature. 1983;301:707–709.

73. Tobler I. Effect of forced locomotion on the rest-activity cycle of the cockroach. Behav Brain Res. 1983;8:351–360.

74. Tobler I, Neuner-Jehle M. 24-h variation of vigilance in the cockroach Blaberus giganteus. J Sleep Res. 1992;1:231–239.

75. Tobler I, Stalder J. Rest in the scorpion—a sleep-like state? J Comp Physiol [A]. 1988; 163:227–235.

75a. Schibler U, Tafti M. Molecular approaches towards the isolation of sleep-related genes. J Sleep Res. 1999;8(suppl 1):1–10.

76. Antoch MP, Song EJ, Chang AM, et al. Functional identification of the mouse circadian clock gene by transgenic BAC rescue. Cell. 1997;89:655–667.

77. Hotz Vitaterna M, King DP, Chang AM, et al. Mutagenesis and mapping of a mouse gene, clock, essential for circadian behavior. Science. 1994;264:719–725.

78. Tafti M, Franken P, Kitahama K, et al. Localization of candidate genomic regions influencing paradoxical sleep in mice. Neuroreport. 1997;8:3755–3758.

78a. Tafti M, Chollet D, Valatx J-L, Franken P. Quantitative trait loci approach to the genetics of sleep in recombinant inbred mice. J Sleep Res. 1999;8:Suppl. 1, 37–43.

79. Tononi G, Cirelli C, Pompeiano M. Changes in gene expression during the sleep-waking cycle: a new view of activating systems. Arch Ital Biol. 1995;134:21–37.

80. Ledoux L, Sastre JP, Buda C, et al. Alterations in C-fos expression after different experimental procedures of sleep deprivation in the cat. Brain Res. 1996;735:108–118.

7

Mammalian Sleep

Harold Zepelin

Knowledge about sleep comes primarily from research on mammalian species whose daily sleep quotas range from 3 to 19 h, with rapid eye movement (REM) sleep occupying 10 to 50% of this time. Findings of REM sleep or elements of it in monotremes has filled a gap in its evolutionary history. In the opinion of some writers, this suggests that REM was inherited from reptiles, although the absence of REM in living reptiles casts doubt on this view.

The function of sleep remains controversial. On one hand, restorative theories hold that brain processes during sleep sustain waking behavior (e.g., visual function, learning). On the other hand, the negative correlation of sleep quotas with body size across species suggests that sleep is a state of enforced rest most urgent in species with low energy reserves. Because most of the variance in sleep quotas remains unaccounted for statistically, supplementary theories are in order.

There are strikingly strong correlations of REM sleep quotas with degree of maturity at birth, that is, higher quotas in large litters of altricial species born with a low percentage of adult brain weight after short gestation periods, as opposed to low REM quotas in precocial species. Given its other fetal characteristics (e.g., lapse of thermoregulation), REM may be a carryover from fetal life.

Most of the available knowledge about sleep comes from the study of mammals. Human beings, cats, and rats have been the most frequent subjects of sleep research, but about 100 other species have also been studied. There are at least two published reports about the daily sleep of mammalian species for every such report pertaining to other classes.[1] This not only makes for mammal-centeredness in thinking about sleep but also affords the opportunity for extensive interspecies comparisons that can shed light on the purpose of sleep, which is still without adequate explanation. This chapter considers relevant theories in the light of available findings.

Despite their relative abundance, the mammalian data represent less than 3% of roughly 4000 extant species. It is safe, however, to assume that all mammals sleep. The belief that some do not (e.g., prey, because of a need for constant vigilance, or shrews, because of incessant foraging) has been superseded by systematic observations. Sleep in some species and in some circumstances may be postponable for long periods, or it may simply be difficult to recognize, as in the ever-swimming, blind Indus dolphin, whose sleep occurs in periods measured in seconds as it contends with strong river currents.[2]

SLEEP CRITERIA

Sleep can usually be identified by sustained quiescence in a species-specific posture accompanied by reduced responsiveness to external stimuli, but a definition of mammalian sleep requires the additional criteria of (1) quick reversibility to the wakeful condition and (2) characteristic changes in the electroencephalogram (EEG). Quick reversibility distinguishes sleep from coma and hypothermic states (e.g., hibernation). With only minor exceptions, EEG changes reliably confirm sleep-related change in behavior and brain activity. Probably another fundamental criterion of sleep, although not yet systematically documented in many species, is its spontaneous occurrence with endogenous periodicity that is essentially independent of other bodily needs and of environmental cues, including variations in ambient temperature. This sets sleep apart from hibernation, torpor, and estivation, which are related to variations of temperature and availability of food and water.

These definitional criteria are fulfilled with notable interspecies variation. Quiescence does not necessarily mean immobility; for example, some cetaceans reportedly swim while sleeping.[3] In terrestrial mammals, lateral and sternoabdominal recumbency with eyes closed are the postures most commonly associated with sleep, but there are striking variations (Figs. 7–1 and 7–2). The horse and the elephant, for example, sleep some while standing. Some species (e.g., cattle) sleep some of the time with eyes open. Choice of sleeping site is an element of species-specific sleep behavior and varies with mode of life and social organization. Burrows, caves, and trees are common sites because of the safety they afford, but some species (e.g., the zebra) sleep in the open and rely on the presence of vigilant conspecifics for protection.[4–7] Ritualistic presleep activity is characteristic of some species, ranging from the dog's circling of a chosen spot to the construction of a nest each evening by the great apes. This justifies the description of sleep as appetitive, instinctive behavior. The timing of daily sleep varies with the species and in each case is complementary to the activity pattern, which may be diurnal, nocturnal, crepuscular, or ar-

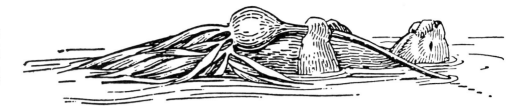

Figure 7–1. Sea otter sleeping "moored" to a float of algae. (From Bourliere F. The Natural History of Mammals. 3rd ed. New York, NY: Alfred A Knopf; 1967:68.)

rhythmic. Sleep in some species consequently tends to be concentrated in a single period each day, whereas in others, it is distributed across two or more periods. Species also vary in the degree of responsiveness to external stimuli during sleep, some awakening more readily than others.[8, 9]

Sleep onset in mammals is associated with the slowing of EEG activity and the rising of EEG amplitude, followed in most species by the appearance of spindling activity, and in all cases culminating in sustained slow activity at relatively high amplitude. Spindling and slow waves are the hallmarks of mammalian quiet or nonrapid eye movement (NREM) sleep (also called slow-wave sleep).[10, 11]

In some species, however, the distinction between wakefulness and sleep is not always clear-cut. Especially in carnivores, ungulates, and insectivores, there are frequent or protracted periods when spindles or slow EEG components appear sporadically against background activity that may not be clearly different from that of wakefulness. This characterizes the state commonly described as drowsiness. Whether such periods should be classified as wakefulness or sleep is an unsettled question.[12]

Spindling activity varies from species to species; it occurs over a wide range of amplitudes and at a variety of frequencies (e.g., 2 to 5 Hz in dogs, 6 to 7 Hz in the sloth, 8 to 11 Hz in the opossum, 12 to 16 Hz in primates). Slow wave activity (0.5 to 4 Hz) is more concentrated at lower frequencies in some species (human beings) than in others (rats), with considerable interspecies variation in its amplitude, which ranges roughly from 75 to 400 μV. In most primates (as in human beings), the density of slow wave activity fluctuates in a manner that allows visual subdivision of NREM sleep into as many as four stages. Two such stages are easily discernible in cetaceans, in some carnivores, and, surprisingly, also in the mole.[11, 13, 14] In other mammals, subdivision into stages may be difficult but is attainable with computerized, electronic analyses of EEG activity. It appears that the differentiation of the sleep EEG varies with neocortical endowment, but a firm conclusion awaits more detailed information on relationships of EEG morphology to brain structure.

Another characteristic of mammalian sleep is its homeostatic self-regulation, which keeps the amount and depth of sleep in equilibrium with prior wakefulness. Sleep loss creates a debt that is repaid, in part, by some lengthening of subsequent sleep and, in addition, by the intensification of slow wave activity, as indicated by its increased amplitude and density[15] (see Chapter 6).

Mammalian sleep, as is well known, also includes paradoxical sleep (PS) or REM sleep, which is distinguished by desynchronized, low-amplitude EEG activity in association with eye movements, twitching of the extremities, and postural atonia. Eye movements vary in prominence and may even be absent, as in the mole. Detectability of atonia also varies. Rhythmic theta activity (4 to 8 Hz) originating in the hippocampus is a reliable indicator of PS in animals with implanted epidural electrodes. Other striking features of PS are ponto-geniculo-occipital (PGO) spikes, cardiorespiratory irregularity, inhibited thermoregulatory responsiveness, and a relatively high arousal threshold.[16] In all species, PS is at its height in early life, either in the fetus or in the neonate. It is initially the predominant state, for example, occupying 90% of the kitten's first 10 days of life and perhaps even more time in the infant rat.[17] By virtue of this pattern, PS can be considered ontogenetically primitive sleep. As quiet sleep and wakefulness emerge with maturation, PS time is reduced.

The alternation of quiet sleep with periods of REM constitutes the sleep cycle, also know as the NREM-REM or REM-NREM cycle, which can be considered the basic organizational unit of mammalian sleep. Duration of the cycle varies widely from species to species, as do daily sleep quotas and the percentage of sleep time occupied by REM. The cyclic organization of sleep is a characteristic shared by mammals and birds, which also share the same behavioral and EEG criteria of sleep that apply to mammals. Notable differences in birds compared with mammals are a lack of stage differentiation in NREM sleep and the absence of spindling. Because relatively little is known about

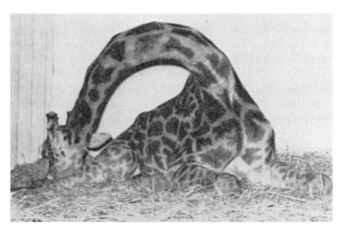

Figure 7–2. Giraffe in a zoo, presumably in paradoxical sleep. (From Immelman K, Gebbing H. Schlaf bei Giraffiden. Z Tierpsychol. 1962;19:84–92.)

avian sleep physiology, other unsuspected differences from mammalian sleep may exist. On the basis of current knowledge, however, what chiefly distinguishes avian from mammalian sleep is the much lower percentage of REM in birds (about 5% of sleep time, on the average, as opposed to 15 to 30% in mammals), much briefer REM periods (often less than 10 sec), and correspondingly short sleep cycles.

EVOLUTIONARY HISTORY

The essential similarity of sleep in birds and mammals commands attention as a likely clue to its history and function.[18] The sleep cycle first appears in evolutionary history in association with *endothermy*, which is the maintenance of a high, constant body temperature by metabolic means, as found only in birds and mammals, enabling them to occupy nocturnal niches and survive in cold climates. The alternation between REM and NREM states has yet to be explained, but it is likely that the cycle evolved independently (in parallel) in birds and mammals or in their immediate forbears (the extinct dinosaurs and mammal-like reptiles) (Figure 7–3). Inheritance from a common ancestor is ruled out by the difference in lines of descent from the rep-

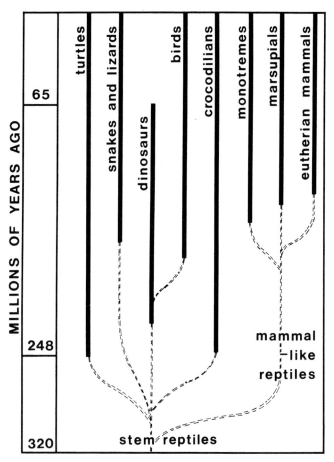

Figure 7–3. Temporal relationships and lines of descent for birds, mammals, and reptiles. Solid lines indicate availability of fossil record; dotted lines indicate still uncertain relationships.

tiles. Research on living reptiles has not produced convincing evidence of sleep organization suggesting a cycle, but repeated, independent evolution of sleep cycles in birds and in mammals is not an extravagant conjecture. It is generally accepted that endothermy, the four-chambered heart, and powered flight all evolved independently in birds and mammals and that eyes evolved more than 40 times in the animal kingdom.[19, 20] Just as the prior existence of light-sensitive cells was the basis for evolution of the eye, and just as behavioral thermoregulation and hypothalamic temperature sensitivity were forerunners of endothermy,[21] sleep phenomena in reptiles must have been the matrix for further evolution.

Discussions of mammalian sleep typically consider quiet sleep and PS to be states that evolved separately at different points in time. Belief that the emergence of PS was relatively recent has been encouraged by its reported absence (although quiet sleep is present) in the Australian short-nosed echidna,[22] one of the three surviving *monotremes* (egg-laying mammals) who diverged early from the main paths of mammalian evolution (see Fig. 7–3). It may seem that some characteristic of the echidna (mode of reproduction, fossorial adaptation, or low body temperature) obviates the need for PS and explains its absence, but this is not the case. The presence of PS in birds shows that it is not related to viviparity. PS is clearly present in other fossorial mammals (e.g., the mole) and in other species with very low body temperature (e.g., the sloth).

Need for qualification of the belief that PS is absent in the echidna is indicated, however, by a finding that, at some times when the echidna's EEG indicates quiet sleep, there are bursts of neuronal activity in its brainstem similar to activity characteristic of REM sleep in therian mammals.[23] This is said to indicate that REM and NREM sleep did not evolve sequentially but as a differentiation of a primitive state which held the seeds of both sleep states. Furthermore, there now is unequivocal evidence of REM sleep in another of the three surviving monotremes, the platypus, occupying 6 to 8 h per day (more than in any other mammal) and accompanied by eye movements, atonia, twitching, and an elevated response threshold, as generally found in mammalian PS, although with EEG voltage at a level characteristic of quiet sleep in eutherian mammals.[24, 25] It has consequently been suggested that REM sleep is of reptilian origin, a view that is questionable in the absence of convincing evidence of REM sleep in any living reptiles.

Complicating speculation about the history of PS are reports of its absence in the bottle-nosed dolphin and the common porpoise, which cannot be considered primitive mammals.[3, 26, 27] Most NREM sleep in these species is unihemispheric, consisting of synchronized, slow activity in one cerebral hemisphere and desynchronized activity characteristic of wakefulness in the other. Sleep signs are sometimes present simultaneously in both hemispheres, but there is no bilateral high-amplitude (delta) sleep. This sleep organization seems necessary to guarantee respiratory function.[28] It has been suggested that PS is also absent on this account, although it is present in the northern fur seal[29] and the manatee,[30] both of whom also have unihemispheric sleep. Other reports make it advisable to reserve judgment regarding the absence of PS in any cetaceans. Its possible presence in the bottle-nosed dolphin is suggested by a report of quiescent hanging behavior in captive animals whose slow drifting was accompanied by eye movements, twitching, and penile erections that are characteristic of PS.[31] Similar behavior has been reported in the killer whale[32] and the Pacific white-sided dolphin.[33] EEG recordings from the pilot whale have reportedly given evidence of brief incidents of PS as judged primarily by trunk muscle atonia.[34]

COMPARATIVE THEORIES

The emerging evolutionary perspective has undermined the previously dominant influence of common-sensical restorative theory, which holds that sleep is for relief of bodily or cerebral deficits caused by waking activity. Restorative theory cannot readily explain the dramatic interspecies variation in daily mammalian sleep quotas (Table 7–1). (For a comprehensive compilation, see *Principles and Practice of Sleep Medicine*, first edition, pages 39–41. See also references 35 through 38). Inspired by this variation, comparative theories have been advanced as alternatives. Guided by an assumption that sleep varies with complexity of the brain, some of these assert that sleep has cerebral functions. PS has attracted interest in this respect because of its cerebral activation. For example, taking note of instinctive behaviors (e.g., rage) released during PS in cats whose postural atonia is surgically abolished,

Jouvet[39] suggested that PS evolved for daily reprogramming of innate behaviors to preserve them in species that rely chiefly on learning. This view is attractive as an explanation for the absence of PS in reptiles and its meagerness in birds, who rely heavily on instinctive behaviors. On the other hand, if the theory is correct, PS quotas should be greatest in mammals with the most learning ability (e.g., primates), but as can be judged by the data in Table 7–1, this is not the case.

Berger,[40] in his oculomotor innervation hypothesis, also suggested a cerebral role for REM sleep, namely, that it is linked with binocularly coordinated eye movement as required for stereopsis, found only in mammals. In this view, REM activation in early life provides stimulation for maturation of the oculomotor system; later, such stimulation keeps the system in readiness for waking activity. In support of this view, Berger pointed to the prominence of REM sleep in species with a high percentage of partial decussation of optic nerve fibers at the chiasma (e.g., human beings, cats) and low REM percentages in species with little or no decussation (e.g., guinea pigs, rabbits). Because of numerous exceptions to this pattern, however, including the presence of REM in avian and mammalian species with little or no eye movement, the theory is not convincing.[41]

In what can be called the eraser theory of REM sleep, Crick and Mitchison have treated its reported absence in the echidna as evidence that it amounts to a mechanism for *reverse learning*, in which stimulation of the forebrain weakens the synaptic strength of undesirable "parasitic modes" of neuronal activity, thus fine-tuning the brain's operation.[42] The echidna, it is said, gets by without REM sleep because its surprisingly large neocortex makes reverse learning unnecessary. If true, an inverse relationship between size of neocortex and REM sleep quotas is to be expected in other species, but supportive data are lacking.[43] Furthermore, although the echidna's neocortex by some measures is unexpectedly large, its specialness is much in doubt because it is among the most primitive in terms of neuronal structure.[44]

ENERGY CONSERVATION

A major alternative to restorative theory is the view that mammalian sleep is for energy conservation, as suggested by its association with endothermy. Two versions of this view are frequently mistaken to be the same. One of these, advocated by Berger and coworkers, holds that sleep is for reduction of energy expenditure below the level attainable by rest alone. Interdependence of quiet sleep and endothermy is inferred from their concurrent maturation in mammalian infancy and the uninterrupted operation of thermoregulatory processes during quiet sleep at a reduced temperature level.[45, 46] The inhibition of thermoregulation during PS (see Chapter 22) is considered evidence that PS is a vestige of a reptilian state of ectothermic inactivity. An energy-conserving role for quiet sleep seems to be suggested by the similarity of its EEG activity to

Table 7–1. DAILY SLEEP QUOTAS IN A SAMPLE OF MAMMALIAN SPECIES

Species	Total Daily Sleep Time* (h)	Daily REM Time (h)
Echidna	8.5	?
Platypus	14.0	7.0
Opossum	18.0	5.0
Koala	14.5	?
Mole	8.5	2.0
Bat	19.0	3.0
Baboon	9.5	1.0
Humans	8.0	2.0
Armadillo	17.0	3.0
Rabbit	8.0	1.0
Rat	13.0	2.5
Hamster	14.0	3.0
Dolphin	10.0	?
Seal	6.0	1.5
Guinea pig	9.5	1.0
Cat	12.5	3.0
Ferret	14.5	6.0
Horse	3.0	0.5
Elephant	4.0	?
Giraffe	4.5	0.5

*Total daily sleep time includes daily REM time.
Values are rounded to the half hour and exclude drowsiness. Some
    values are averages for two or more members of the same genus.
?, reported absence of REM sleep or uncertainty.

that of shallow torpor, by entrance into hibernation from quiet sleep, and by a circannual rhythm of sleep in hibernators, its maxima coinciding with the hibernation season. The general conclusion drawn is that quiet sleep, torpor, and hibernation are related dormant states with a common purpose.[47]

This conclusion is questionable. Sleep may have merely a permissive role with respect to hibernation, without sharing of mechanisms or function. This is indicated by the upsurge and intensification of slow wave activity directly following bouts of torpor or hibernation, suggesting compensation for loss of sleep during those bouts.[48, 49] Above all is the question of whether reduction of metabolic rate is sufficient as the raison d'etre for sleep. At most, sleep could effect a metabolic saving of about 15%.[50] Taking into account the effects of body movement and arousals, the overnight saving in human beings is more likely to be only 5 to 11%.[51-53] A 200-lb person expends about 80 calories per hour while asleep. Sitting quietly awake, the same person would use 95 calories. The saving effected by 8 h of uninterrupted sleep would be 120 calories—the equivalent of a cup of low-fat milk or one frankfurter bun. If this is all that sleep accomplishes, it would have to be judged an inefficient if not a remarkably wasteful process.

Correlational Findings

The second version of energy conservation theory considers the reduction of metabolic rate during sleep of minor importance. The principal contribution of sleep (with no qualification regarding PS) is held to be the enforcement of rest so as to set a limit on activity and energy expenditure. This view emerged from Zepelin and Rechtschaffen's[35] comparative study of sleep parameters, potential life span, and other constitutional variables in 53 mammalian species. The study assessed a long-standing belief that species with high daily sleep quotas have relatively long potential life spans because they benefit from lowered metabolism during sleep. The contrary proved to be the case: long-sleeping species typically are short-lived. They also tend to be small

in size and high in basal or resting metabolic rate per unit of body weight. There was an impressive correlation (0.63) between sleep quotas and metabolic rate. Together with knowledge that the metabolic cost of physical activity varies inversely with body size[54] and that daily food requirements relative to body size are disproportionately high in small mammals,[55] the finding on metabolic rate led to the conclusion that sleep sets a limit on energy expenditure to the extent necessary to balance a species' energy budget.

A shift to emphasis on total energy expenditure (as opposed to metabolic rate) proved necessary, however. Experimental studies failed to find expected effects on daily sleep time in rats whose metabolic rates were elevated by administration of thyroxine.[56, 57] It became apparent that the Zepelin-Rechtschaffen study relied unduly on estimates of weight-specific metabolic rate given by the Kleiber equation as the -0.25 power of body weight. Metabolic rate had thus been confounded with body weight, and its role was consequently exaggerated. The lingering influence of this error is apparent in the importance that Berger and coworkers attach to metabolic rate, as noted previously.

Table 7–2 summarizes relevant correlations found in updated analyses of EEG and behavioral sleep data for 85 taxa (species or genera), with missing data for some taxa in each analysis. Despite recent revisions in the sleep data (Asian elephant,[58] giraffe[59]), added data for newly studied species (koala,[60] ferret[61]), and some adjustments and expansion of the data for constitutional variables, the results are quite similar to previous findings. Previous and present correlations of body weight, brain weight, and encephalization quotient with total daily sleep time and cycle length are virtually identical. Consistency was somewhat less for correlations of metabolic rate and the correlations of PS measures. Correlations of quiet sleep time differed most from previous findings. This was because the present analyses made no adjustment of sleep quotas for drowsiness.

With body weight and brain weight partialed out in a reduced sample with complete data (N = 55), sleep time correlated negatively with metabolic rate (r = $-.30$; P <.05). This indicates a secondary trend in the data with respect to metabolic rate; there are some

Table 7–2. CORRELATIONS BETWEEN SLEEP PARAMETERS AND CONSTITUTIONAL VARIABLES

Constitutional Variables	Total Daily Sleep Time (h)	Quiet Sleep Time (h)	Paradoxical Sleep Time (h)	Paradoxical Sleep %	Cycle Length
Body weight	−.53*	−.53*	−.45*	−.12	.83*
	(85)	(65)	(65)	(65)	(33)
Brain weight	−.55*	−.48*	−.52*	−.25	.89*
	(71)	(56)	(54)	(56)	(32)
Metabolic rate	33†	.30‡	.13	−.09	−.82*
	(65)	(51)	(50)	(50)	(29)
Encephalization quotient	−.17	−.10	−.20†	−.30‡	.52†
	(69)	(55)	(53)	(55)	(32)

Common logarithmic transformations were used for the constitutional variables. Log (1 + X) transformations were used for paradoxical sleep values. Number of cases per coefficient is in parentheses.
*P < .001
†P < .01
‡P < .05

species with high sleep quotas and low metabolic rates, a condition traceable to energy-deficient diets.[62] An outstanding example is the endangered koala (see Table 7–1), whose diet consists of rare types of eucalyptus leaves with low nutritional value.[63] Other examples are edentates (e.g., the sloth) and armadillos. Such species cannot afford high activity levels. Their extended sleep seems necessary to ease metabolic pressure and is consistent with a role for sleep in energy conservation.

Analyses of partial correlations found, as in previous research, that brain weight and cycle length were positively correlated independently of body weight (r = .64; P <.001), but body weight and cycle length did not correlate independently, thus leaving brain weight alone as a likely determinant of cycle length. Brain weight and body weight both failed to correlate with sleep time independently of each other, as was found in a previous set of analyses.[64] It therefore seems best to consider the correlations of sleep time with brain weight and body weight, without distinction between them, as consequences of *body size*. Multiple regression analysis showed that brain weight and body weight together (i.e. body size) could account for 31% of the variance in sleep time.

Findings similar to those discussed earlier were obtained by Elgar et al.[37, 38] in a study based solely on electrographic sleep data for 69 species with family as the unit of analysis. Agreement between the two sets of findings is important because the choice of families as the taxonomic level for analysis guards against possible inflation of sample size owing to similarities between species with shared phylogenetic backgrounds. A possible consequence of analyses at the family level was the reported finding that, with data for human beings removed, cycle length and brain weight failed to correlate independently of body weight. There is no justification, however, for the exclusion of human data; therefore, the reported result is not meaningful. An updated, exhaustive analysis based on families would be in order, but impeding such analysis are numerous gaps in the available data, especially in behavioral studies.

The correlational findings underwrite the view that sleep occurs to enforce rest and keep energy expenditure at an affordable level. There may be less pressure for sleep in large species because of their greater energy reserves. The proportion of fat to body mass increases with size, ranging from less than 5% in the smallest mammals up to 25 to 30% in species weighing 1000 kg.[55] As body size increases, the ratio of surface to body mass decreases and thickness of fur increases. Large mammals consequently have lower *thermal conductance* (flow of heat to the environment) and wider thermoneutral zones. This lessens requirements for active heat production to maintain body temperature. Lindstedt and Boyce,[65] as illustrated by Figure 7–4, have shown that *fasting endurance* (survival time) at thermoneutrality is a function of body size, and the size advantage is accentuated in the cold. Even at thermoneutrality, as Figure 7–4 shows, survival time is short for small species. Many are frequently only hours away from death by starvation. They may require more

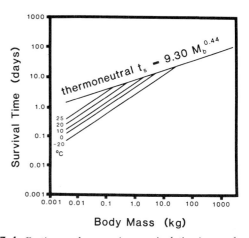

Figure 7–4. Fasting endurance (or survival time) as a function of body size for mammals. The top line represents survival time at thermoneutral ambient temperature, where $t_s = 9.30M_b^{0.44}$. Steeper lines represent survival times at elevated metabolism induced by cold. (From Lindstedt SL, Boyce MS. Seasonality, fasting endurance, and body size in mammals. Am Nat. 1985;125:873–878. © The University of Chicago Press. All rights reserved.)

sleep to avoid exhaustion of energy reserves. Also consistent with an energy conservation role are the relatively high sleep quotas that all mammals have early in the maturational period, when energy must be channeled into growth.

This version of energy conservation theory befits the requirements of endothermy, which is not only for thermoregulation alone but also for increased aerobic capacity required for sustained running, climbing, and other vigorous activities. A mammal's basal energy requirement is at least five times that of an ectotherm similar in size and body temperature.[66] This theory is also in accord with findings on prolonged sleep deprivation in rats. With ultimately fatal consequences, the rats suffered from increased metabolism, as shown by weight loss in spite of increased food intake, along with reduced body temperature in spite of increased metabolic rate. Prolonged deprivation of REM sleep alone has similar effects.[67–69] These findings indicate an indispensable role for sleep in energy regulation, as suggested by the relationships of sleep quotas and constitutional variables. The convergence here of experimental and correlational findings is theoretically promising.

Immobilization Theory

Because correlational findings in support of energy conservation theory fall short of explaining even half of the variance in sleep quotas, the way is open for other viewpoints. Restorative theories having failed to explain species differences, behavioral theories have come to the fore, expanding the concept of sleep as a state of enforced rest. It is suggested, for example, that large mammals sleep relatively little because they require extra time for foraging.[70] A related view is that the function of sleep amounts to *adaptive nonresponding*,[36, 70] meaning that it prevents activity

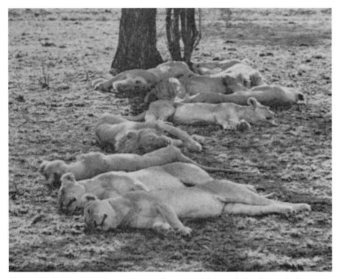

Figure 7–5. Nine African lions share a ribbon of shade and sleep in the heat of day. (From Schaller GB. *Life with the King of Beasts.* National Geographic. 1969;135:494–519. By permission of Dr. George B. Schaller. © 1969 National Geographic Society. All rights reserved.)

(e.g., foraging) when it would be dangerous or inefficient, and it blocks harmful reactions that might occur in an animal merely resting but aware of ongoing events. Meddis elaborated, "The benefits of sleep depend upon the species. For some the conservation of energy is most valuable, for others, the protection from predation . . . for others, the timing element."[36(p54)] In effect, however, such theory is untestable, for there will always be some need that sleep can be said to meet. Filling spare time, can be considered a function of sleep. But how much spare time does a species have? With circular reasoning it is argued that time sleep is a measure of spare time (Fig. 7–5).

Judging the correlational evidence too weak to justify the theory that sleep is for energy conservation, Rechtschaffen[71] argued that sleep must be for some purpose other than rest. This judgment seems arbitrary. What is the minimum correlation required to underwrite the theory? The correlation undoubtedly would be higher if costs of activity and temperature regulation were included. Rechtschaffen holds that if not for the still-to-be-identified function of sleep (which, he suspects, is at the molecular level), simple rest could take its place and would be more advantageous. He paints a picture of sleep (as enforced rest) occurring at inopportune times, for example, during foraging or in the face of predatory threat. He overlooks the well-established knowledge that predation is synchronized with the activity of prey, not with their sleep. Cats catch mice that are up and about, hyenas and lions prey on active wildebeest, and wolves prey on active moose and caribou.[72–74] Rechtschaffen speculated that the asserted benefit of sleep should be obtainable simply by resting. This is wishful theorizing, imagining that mammals could stay awake and at rest for long periods despite their built-in reactivity to events in the environment.

An argument against the view that sleep is for en-

ergy conservation enforced by rest is the reported continuous movement of dolphins while asleep.[3] This is considered evidence of some sleep function other than enforced rest. Doubt on this point arises, however, from an earlier report by Mukhametov and coworkers[75] that dolphins became practically immobile irrespective of unilateral or bilateral EEG synchronization. Another report on dolphins' sleep mentioned their rest on the tank bottom and at the surface.[76] Kovalzon[77] described dolphins during periods of unilateral EEG synchronization as "suspended floating almost immobile," which certainly qualifies as rest.

Enforced rest, if not the primary purpose of sleep, is clearly indispensable for its function.

ECOLOGICAL INFLUENCES: THE ALTRICIAL-PRECOCIAL DIMENSION

It is often assumed that species differences in sleep reflect environmental influences, but this is not readily apparent. Probably the clearest case of an ecologically determined characteristic is the unihemispheric sleep found in some marine mammals. Drowsiness in some species seems to have an ecological basis. Its prominence in ungulates (e.g., the horse) may be a compromise between sleep and alertness to predatory threat. On the other hand, there is no simple explanation for the prominent drowsiness of carnivores (e.g., the cat), which seems like purposeless fraying of sleep.

Predation is the ecological variable that has attracted most interest. Because of the scarcity of data on the extent to which individual species are subject to predation or have suffered from it in their evolutionary past, judgments of its influence are open to question. Findings by Allison and Cicchetti,[70] however, raised the possibility that PS quotas are reduced by predatory threat because the elevation of sensory thresholds during PS puts prey at a disadvantage.

Relatively neglected in ecological theorizing about sleep is the role of species differences in reproductive strategies and life histories. Adaptation to the environment occurs not only through fine-tuning of physical and behavioral characteristics but also through changes in the number of offspring and the timing of their maturation. Interspecies variation in sleep may be secondary to such adaptations. Commanding attention in this respect is the variation of REM sleep with maturational variables as illustrated in Figures 7–6 and 7–7.

In *precocial species*, that is, those born fairly mature (e.g., the guinea pig, sheep) the REM percentage at birth is low and near the adult level. In *altricial species*, that is, those born immature (e.g., the rat, the cat) the REM percentage is initially high and remains relatively high even after maturation.[17] Also indicative of influence by maturational timing is the inverse correlation of REM quotas with gestation time.[35, 37]

Previous findings of correlation between daily REM time and degree of maturity at birth were confirmed with expanded data for up to 65 viviparous species or genera (echidna and platypus excluded). For eutherian mammals, the four-point altricial-precocial (A-P) rat-

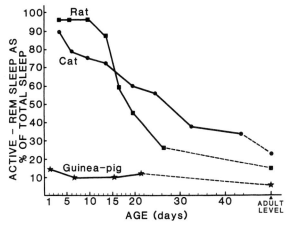

Figure 7–6. Maturational changes in REM sleep as a percentage of total sleep time in two altricial species (rat and cat) and a precocial species (guinea pig). (Reprinted by permission of John Wiley & Sons, Inc. from Jouvet-Mounier D, Astic L, Lacote D. Ontogenesis of the states of sleep in rat, cat, and guinea pig during the first postnatal month. Dev Psychobiol. 1970;2:216–239. Copyright © 1970 John Wiley & Sons.)

Table 7–3. ALTRICIAL-PRECOCIAL SCALE FOR NEONATES OF VIVIPAROUS SPECIES

Scale Value	Description
1	Eyes closed; naked; rolls; sometimes can cling (1.5: fur shows)
2	Eyes barely closed or just open; furred; crawls well (2.5: eyes open; can cling)
3	Eyes open; furred; can stand
4	Eyes open; furred; can walk and follow or swim

Intermediate scale values (e.g., 2.8) were assigned to some species.

ings were assigned previously by an expert mammalogist without knowledge of the sleep data (Table 7–3). For this analysis, the author gave marsupials a rating of "1" based on the criteria of the scale. The results, shown in Table 7–4, were independent of body weight and brain weight and differed from previous findings chiefly in terms of a significant correlation in the present research between the PS percentage and gestation period. It is noteworthy that in the four marsupial species, the two with the shortest gestation periods had PS quotas and percentages radically higher than the others, the highest in the entire sample. The absence or minimal presence of PS in cetaceans is understandable on the basis of their extreme precociality.

These analyses also found a correlation of .49 (P <.001) between daily quotas of PS and quiet sleep. In the 49 species with complete data, this correlation with body weight and brain weight partialed out was .28 (P <.05). These results are consistent with the view that PS provides endogenous stimulation to the brain to promote recovery from sleep.[78]

The striking relationships between REM quotas and neonatal characteristics give no clear indication of the maturational events that are responsible. If one adopts Parmeggiani's[79] view that REM physiology is under rhombencephalic regulation as opposed to hypothala-

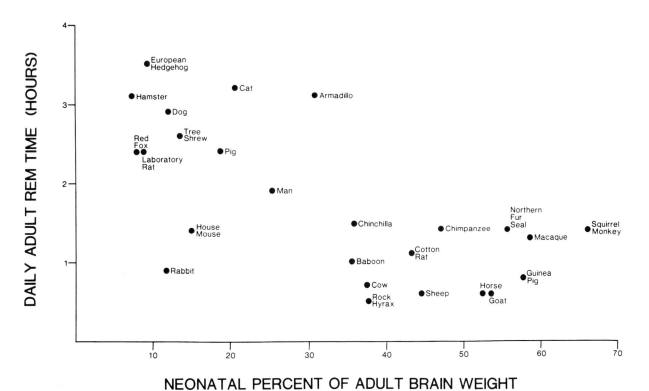

Figure 7–7. Daily REM time in adult mammals as a function of neonatal maturity represented by the percentage of adult brain weight in neonates of the same species.

Table 7–4. CORRELATIONS OF PARADOXICAL SLEEP PARAMETERS WITH MEASURES OF NEONATAL MATURITY AND REPRODUCTIVE VARIABLES

Measures of Neonatal Maturity and Reproductive Variables	Paradoxical Sleep Time (h)	Paradoxical Sleep %
Altricial-precocial rating	−.66* (65)	−.45† (64)
Neonatal brain weight (%)	−.61* (27)	−.55† (27)
Gestation period	.63* (60)	−.39† (59)
Litter size	.51* (63)	.41† (62)

To minimize skewness, common logarithmic transformations were used for gestation period and litter size. Log (1 + X) transformations were used for paradoxical sleep values. Number of cases per coefficient is in parentheses.
*$P < .001$
†$P < .01$

mic regulation in the rest of sleep, then maturation of the hypothalamus may be the critical factor. Given the apparent ontogenetic primacy of REM sleep plus the expression of fetal characteristics (lapse of thermoregulation, respiratory irregularity, and twitching) in REM sleep during maturity, REM appears to be a carryover from fetal life. The difference between mammals and birds in the representation of REM may well be explained by unidentified differences between them in maturational timing.

The association of REM with altriciality takes on added significance with the realization that reptiles are strictly precocial and that altriciality evolved in birds and mammals in conjunction with endothermy. Evolutionary theorists agree that the metabolic cost of endothermy favored altriciality, which meant the birth of exothermic rather than endothermic young. One view is that altriciality reduced the energy requirements for maturation by placing reliance on parental body heat for temperature regulation in the young, allowing their food to be channeled primarily into growth.[80] Another view is that altriciality mainly allowed greater flexibility in meeting energy requirements by shortening gestation and incubation periods, putting off much of the expense of propagation until after birth, thus splitting the expense between parents, both of whom could then forage for the young.[81] Precociality in some mammals evolved as a later adaptation.

Rather than outright inheritance from reptiles, as the finding of REM sleep in the platypus has suggested to some writers, REM seems to be part of the evolution of endothermy, which distinguishes mammals from reptiles. It is simultaneously part of the transition from the strict precociality of reptiles. The limited indications of REM features in the echidna are evidence of this transitional origin as opposed to straightforward inheritance from reptilian forebears.

SUMMARY

Evolutionary history suggests that mammalian sleep developed in association with endothermy, paralleling a similar development of sleep in birds. Consistent with this impression are several clusters of correlated variables that must also be taken into account in theorizing about the function of sleep. One is the correlation of daily mammalian sleep quotas with body weight and weight-specific metabolic rate, indicating greater requirements of sleep in species with low energy reserves. Another is the correlation of REM sleep parameters with A-P status, gestation time, and litter size, indicating the influence of maturational timetables on the prominence of REM and suggesting that REM is a byproduct of altriciality and endothermy. Less clearly related to endothermy is the positive correlation of the NREM-REM cycle length with brain weight, a relationship that is also apparent in the increase of cycle length with maturation in mammals. Because cortical acetylcholine content and cholinesterase activity correlate highly with mammalian brain weight,[82] cholinergic mechanisms known to influence cycle length are probably its operative link with brain weight.[83] The cycle can be described as the alternation of an endothermic with an ectothermic state, each reflecting a different stage of brain development.

Acknowledgments

Thanks to Cathleen S. Zepelin for artwork and assistance with data analysis and to Beverly Darrenkamp for preparing the manuscript.

References

1. Campbell SS, Tobler I: Animal sleep: a review of sleep duration across phylogeny. Neurosci Biobehav Rev. 1984;8:269–300.
2. Pilleri G. The blind Indus dolphin, *Platanista indi.* Endeavour. 1979;3:48–56.
3. Mukhametov LM. Sleep in marine mammals. Exp Brain Res. 1984;8(suppl):227–238.
4. Bourliere F. The Natural History of Mammals. 3rd ed. New York, NY: Alfred A Knopf; 1967.
5. Hediger H. Comparative observations on sleep. Proc R Soc Med. 1969;62:1–4.
6. Hediger H. The biology of natural sleep in animals. Experientia. 1980;36:13–16.
7. Moss C. Portraits in the Wild. Boston, Mass: Houghton Mifflin; 1975.
8. Van Twyver H. Sleep patterns in five rodent species. Physiol Behav. 1969;4:901–905.
9. Zepelin H. Sleep in the jaguar and the tapir: a prey-predator contrast. Psychophysiology. 1970;7:306.
10. Rechtschaffen A, Kales A. A Manual for Standardized Terminology, Techniques, and Scoring System for Sleep Stages of Human Subjects. Washington, DC: Public Health Service, US Government Printing Office; 1968.
11. Ursin R. The two stages of slow wave sleep in the cat and their relation to REM sleep. Brain Res. 1968;11:347–356.
12. Allison T. Comparative and evolutionary aspects of sleep. In: Chase MH, ed. The Sleeping Brain. Los Angeles, Calif: Brain Information Service; 1972:1–57.
13. Mukhametov LM, Supin AY. EEG study of different behavioral states in free-moving dolphin. *Tursiops truncatus* [in Russian]. Zh Vyssh Nerv Deiat. 1975;25:396–401.
14. Allison T, Van Twyver H. Sleep in the moles, *Scalopus aquaticus* and *Condylura cristata.* Exp Neurol. 1970;27:564–578.

15. Borbély AA, Tobler I. Homeostatic and circadian principles in sleep regulation in the rat. In: McGinty DJ, ed. Brain Mechanisms of Sleep. New York, NY: Raven Press; 1985:35–44.

16. McGinty DJ, Siegel JM. Sleep states. In: Satinoff E, Teitelbaum P, eds. Motivation. New York, NY: Plenum Press; 1983:105–181. Handbook of Behavioral Neurobiology, vol 6.

17. Jouvet-Mounier D, Astic L, Lacote D. Ontogenesis of the states of sleep in rat, cat, and guinea pig during the first postnatal month. Dev Psychobiol. 1968;2:216–239.

18. Allison T, Van Twyver H. The evolution of sleep. Nat Hist. 1970;79:56–65.

19. Heath JE. The origins of thermoregulation. In: Drake ET, ed. Evolution and Environment. New Haven, Conn: Yale University Press; 1968.

20. Mayr E. The Growth of Biological Thought: Diversity, Evolution, and Inheritance. Cambridge, Mass: Belknap Press; 1982.

21. Richards SA. Temperature Regulation. London, England: Wykeham Publications; 1973.

22. Allison T, Van Twyver H, Goff WR. Electrophysiological studies of the echidna, Tachyglossus aculeatus, I: waking and sleep. Arch Ital Biol. 1972;110:145–184.

23. Siegel JM, Manger PR, Nienhuis R, et al. The echidna Tachyglossus aculeatus combines REM and non-REM aspects in a single sleep state. J Neurosci. 1996;16:3500–3506.

24. Siegel JM. Monotremes and the evolution of REM sleep. SRS Bull. 1997;4:31–32.

25. Siegel JM, Manger PR, Nienhuis R, et al. Sleep in the platypus. Neuroscience. 1999;91:391–400.

26. Mukhametov LM, Supin AY. EEG study of different behavioral states in free-moving dolphin. Tursiops truncatus [in Russian]. Zh Vyssh Nerv Deiat. 1975;25:396–401.

27. Mukhametov LM, Poliakova IG. EEG investigation of sleep in porpoises, Phocoena phocoena [in Russian]. Zh Vyssh Nerv Deiat. 1981;3:333–339.

28. Mukhametov LM, Supin AY, Polyakova IG. Interhemispheric asymmetry of the electroencephalographic sleep patterns in dolphins. Brain Res. 1977;124:581–584.

29. Mukhametov LM, Liamin OI, Poliakova IG. Sleep and wakefulness in Callorhinus ursinus [in Russian]. Zh Vyssh Nerv Deiat. 1984;34:465–471.

30. Mukkhametov LM, et al. Sleep and wakefulness in an Amazonian manatee. In: Horne JA, ed. Sleep '90: Proceedings of the Tenth European Congress on Sleep Research, Strasbourg, France, 1990 May 20–25. Bochum, Germany: Pontenagel Press; 1990:119–122.

31. Flanigan WJ Jr. Nocturnal behavior of captive small cetaceans, I: the bottlenosed porpoise, Tursiops trancatus. Sleep Res. 1974;3:84.

32. Flanigan WF Jr. More nocturnal observations of captive small cetaceans, I: the killer whale, Orcinus orca. Sleep Res. 1975;4:139.

33. Flanigan WJ Jr. More nocturnal observations of captive small cetaceans, II: the Pacific white-sided dolphin, Lagenorhynchus obliquidens. Sleep Res. 1975;4:140.

34. Shurley JT, Serafetinides EA, Brooks RE, et al: Sleep in cetaceans, I: the pilot whale (Globicephala scammoni). Psychophysiology. 1969;6:230.

35. Zepelin H, Rechtschaffen A. Mammalian sleep, longevity, and energy metabolism. Brain Behav Evol. 1974;10:425–470.

36. Meddis R. The Sleep Instinct. London, England: Routledge and Kegan Paul; 1977:54.

37. Elgar MA, Pagel MD, Harvey PH, et al: Sleep in mammals. Anim Behav. 1988;36:1407–1419.

38. Elgar MA, Pagel MD, Harvey PH, et al: Sources of variation in mammalian sleep. Anim Behav. 1990;40:991–994.

39. Jouvet M. The function of dreaming: a neurophysiologist's point of view. In: Gazzaniga MS, Blakemore C, eds. Handbook of Psychobiology. New York, NY: Academic Press; 1975:499–527.

40. Berger RJ. Oculomotor control: a possible function of REM sleep. Psychol Rev. 1969;76:144–164.

41. Van Twyver H. Sleep in primitive mammals. In: Chase M, ed. The Sleeping Brain. Los Angeles, Calif: Brain Information Service; 1972:19–21.

42. Crick F, Mitchison G. The function of dream sleep. Nature. 1983;304:111–114.

43. Zepelin H. Encephalization and species differences in REM sleep: a test of the Crick-Mitchison theory. Sleep Res. 1985;14:85.

44. Pirlot P, Nelson J. Volumetric analyses of monotreme brains. Aust J Zool. 1978;20:171–179.

45. Berger RJ. Bioenergetic functions of sleep and activity rhythms and their possible relevance to aging. Fed Proc. 1975;34:97–102.

46. Glotzbach SF, Heller HC. Central nervous regulation of body temperature during sleep. Science. 1976;194:537–539.

47. Walker JM, Berger RJ. Sleep as an adaptation for energy conservation functionally related to hibernation and shallow torpor. Prog Brain Res. 1980;53:255–278.

48. Deboer T, Tobler, I. Sleep EEG after daily torpor in the Djungarian hamster: similarity to the effects of sleep deprivation. Neurosci Lett. 1994;166:35–38.

49. Trachsel L, Edgar DM, Heller HC. Are ground squirrels sleep-deprived during hibernation? Am J Physiol. 1991;R1123–R1129.

50. Shapiro CM, Goll CC, Cohen GR, et al. Heat production during sleep. J Appl Physiol. 1984;56:671–677.

51. Ravussin E, Lillioja S, Anderson TE, et al. Determinants of 24-hour energy expenditure in man. Methods and results using a respiratory chamber. J Clin Invest. 1986;78:1568–1578.

52. Garby L, Kurzer MS, Lammert O, et al. Energy expenditure during sleep in men and women: evaporative and sensible heat losses. Hum Nutr Clin Nutr. 1987;41:225–233.

53. Goldberg GR, Prentice AM, Davies HL, et al. Overnight and basal metabolic rates in men and women. Eur J Clin Nutr. 1988;42:137–144.

54. Schmidt-Nielsen K. Locomotion: energy cost of swimming, flying, and running. Science. 1972;177:222–228.

55. Calder WA III. Size, Function, and Life History. Cambridge, Mass: Harvard University Press; 1984.

56. Eastman CI, Rechtschaffen A. Effect of thyroxine on sleep in the rat. Sleep. 1979;2:215–232.

57. Carpenter AC, Timiras PS. Sleep organization in hypo- and hyperthyroid rats. Neuroendocrinology. 1982;34:438–443.

58. Tobler I. Behavioral sleep in the Asian elephant in captivity. Sleep. 1992;15:1–12.

59. Tobler I, Schwierin B. Behavioural sleep in the giraffe (Giraffa camelopardalis) in a zoological garden. J Sleep Res. 1996;5:21–32.

60. Nagy KA, Martin RW. Field metabolic rate, water flux, food consumption, and time budget of koalas, Phascolarctos cinereus, in Victoria. Aust J Zool. 1985;33:655–665.

61. Marks GA, Shaffery JP. A preliminary study of sleep in the ferret, Mustela putorius furo: a carnivore with an extremely high proportion of REM sleep. Sleep. 1996;19:83–93.

62. McNab BK. The influence of food habits on the energetics of eutherian mammals. Ecol Monogr. 1986;56:1–19.

63. Lee A, Martin R. Life in the slow lane. Nat Hist. 1990;8:34–42.

64. Zepelin H. Mammalian sleep, metabolic rate, and body size. Sleep Res. 1986;15:62.

65. Lindstedt SL, Boyce MS. Seasonality, fasting endurance, and body size in mammals. Am Naturalist. 1985;125:873–878.

66. Bennett AF, Ruben JA. Endothermy and activity in vertebrates. Science. 1979;206:649–654.

67. Rechtschaffen A, Gilliland MA, Bergmann BM, et al. Physiological correlates of prolonged sleep deprivation in rats. Science. 1983;221:182–184.

68. Rechtschaffen A, Bergmann BM, Everson CA, et al. Sleep deprivation in the rat, X: integration and discussion of the findings. Sleep. 1989;12:68–87.

69. Rechtschaffen A, Bergmann BM. Sleep deprivation in the rat by the disk-over-eater method. Behav Brain Res. 1995;69:55–63.

70. Allison T, Cicchetti DV. Sleep in mammals: ecological and constitutional correlates. Science. 1976;194:732–734.

71. Rechtschaffen A. Current perspectives on the function of sleep. Perspect Biol Med. 1998;41:359–390.

72. Curio E. The Ethology of Predation. New York, NY: Springer-Verlag; 1976.

73. Mech LD. The Wolves of Isle Royale. Washington, DC: National Park Service, US Government Printing Office; 1966.

74. Daan S. Adaptive daily strategies in behavior. In: Aschoff J, ed. Handbook of Behavioral Neurobiology. New York, NY: Plenum Press; 1981:275–298.

75. Mukhametov LM, Supin AY, Polyakova IG. Interhemispheric asymmetry of the electroencephalographic sleep patterns in dolphins. Brain Res. 1977;134:581–584.

76. McCormick JG. Relationship of sleep, respiration, and anesthesia in the porpoise: a preliminary report. Proc Natl Acad U S A. 1969;62:697–703.

77. Kovalzon VM. Brain temperature variations and ECoG in free-swimming bottlenosed dolphin. Sleep. Basel, Switzerland: Karger; 1976:239–241.

78. Vertes RP. A life-sustaining function for REM sleep: a theory. Neurosci Biobehav Rev. 1986;10:371–376.

79. Parmeggiani PL. Regulation of physiological functions during sleep in mammals. Experientia. 1982;38:1405–1408.

80. Hopson JA. Endothermy, small size, and the origin of mammalian reproduction. Am Naturalist. 1973;107:446–452.

81. Case TJ. Endothermy and parental care in the terrestrial vertebrates. Am Naturalist. 1978;112:861–874.

82. Tower DB, Elliott KAC. Activity of acetylcholine system in cerebral cortex of carious unanesthetized mammals. Am J Physiol. 1952;168:747–759.

83. Sitaram N, Moore AM, Gillin JC. Experimental acceleration and slowing of REM sleep ultradian rhythm by cholinergic agonist and antagonist. Nature. 1978;274:490–492.

two

Sleep Mechanisms

Michael H. Chase

8

Brain Electrical Activity and Sensory Processing During Waking and Sleep States

Mircea Steriade

Different types of brain rhythms characterize wakefulness, nonrapid eye movement (NREM), and rapid eye movement (REM) sleep. There are changes in excitability of cortical and thalamic neurons during shifts between these states of vigilance.

Two main points should be emphasized with regard to brain oscillations. (1) The newly discovered slow sleep oscillation (0.6 to 0.9 Hz), first described in intracellular recordings from animals and also described during natural NREM sleep of both cats and human beings, has the virtue of entraining other sleep oscillations (spindles and delta waves) in complex wave sequences. This is due to the synchronous firing of neocortical neurons whose discharges trigger thalamic circuits. Thus, the neocortex and thalamus constitute a unified oscillatory machine. The best example is the fact that K-complexes, a major grapho-element of NREM sleep, have the same pattern and rhythmicity as the slow cortical oscillation, and they are followed by a short sequence of spindle waves due to setting into action of thalamic neuronal circuits. (2) The activation of brain electrical activity during waking and REM sleep is associated with short-scale synchronization of fast (20 to 50 Hz) waves over the cerebral cortex as well as among cortical areas and related thalamic nuclei. Thus, the notion of desynchronization, long used to define activated states, becomes obsolete and should be replaced with the term EEG activation.

The first relay station where blockade of synaptic transmission is observed during the period of falling asleep is the thalamus. The synaptic transmission in thalamocortical systems is enhanced during both waking and REM sleep, as compared with NREM sleep. During wakefulness, inhibitory periods are shorter than during NREM sleep but very effective. This provides a mechanism for selection of relevant input signals, as required during an adaptive state.

The states of wakefulness and sleep are characterized by a set of three cardinal physiological correlates: brain wave activity (electroencephalogram [EEG]), eye movements, and muscle tone. This chapter addresses (1) the morphological substrates and cellular bases of spontaneous EEG rhythms and (2) the responses elicited by sensory inputs, as changed during the two basic cerebral conditions of resting and active behavioral states.

In the initial sections of this chapter, the basic mechanisms underlying high-amplitude synchronized EEG oscillations during sleep and the neuronal substrates of EEG changes when the state of the brain shifts from sleep to arousal are discussed. Work has revealed a series of intrinsic electrophysiological properties of neurons that have an important role in the patterning of various EEG oscillations.[1] However, the synchronous activation of a *neuronal ensemble* (or network) requires a mechanism for coordination of the individual oscillations. The determining role of neuronal networks involved in the genesis of sleep oscillations and in their disruption on arousal is discussed with emphasis on EEG slow, delta, and spindle rhythms.

In the second half of this chapter, the dependency of sensory synaptic transmission on the behavioral state of vigilance is analyzed. On one hand, data indicate that blockade of afferent information at sleep onset takes place within the thalamus. On the other hand, the enhanced excitability of thalamic and cortical neurons on arousal and during dreaming sleep is due to a series of brainstem modulatory systems. The actions of those systems on responses to external stimuli during the waking state and the events associated with the internally generated brain activation during dreaming sleep are discussed.

PRELIMINARY DEFINITIONS

The resting state of quiet sleep is easily distinguishable from both wakefulness and rapid eye movement (REM) sleep by high-amplitude and synchronous EEG rhythms. Synchronization is a state in which two or more oscillators display the same frequency owing to mutual or unilateral influences. From an EEG point of view, the notion of synchronization supposes the coactivation of a large number of neurons whose summated synaptic events as well as intrinsic currents are sufficiently large to be recorded with gross electrodes. The systems that synchronize (or unite) the activity of single neurons into ensembles (or networks) may be viewed as single or multiple pacemakers. In the case of a unique pacemaker of a given EEG rhythm, a postulated group of neurons that are homogeneous morphologically and use the same chemical transmitters display signs of rhythmicity, even disconnected from their major inputs, and establish the necessary connections to secure the spread of rhythmicity toward follower elements, and rhythmicity is abolished in the target structures when the pacemaker is destroyed. If rhythms were induced by virtue of inhibitory connections between the pacemaker and satellite systems, *inverse* (or reciprocal) images would be expected to occur in pacemaking and target neurons. In the case of multiple (or distributed) pacemakers, the rhythms may start in any of them as a function of activity in various afferent systems; lesioning any part does not prevent rhythmicity in others, and the rhythms do not beat necessarily in a synchronous manner.

Desynchronization during waking and REM sleep means the disruption of high-amplitude and synchronous EEG waves and the replacement of low-frequency oscillations by fast rhythms with usually lower amplitude.[2] However, the spontaneously occurring fast rhythms (20 to 50 Hz) during brain-active states are synchronized over some distances within the cortex[3] as well as among cortical areas and related thalamic nuclei.[4, 5] Therefore, it is better to use the term *activation*[2] than *desynchronization* to designate the electrical activity during waking and REM sleep. The paradox that a similar EEG activity characterizes two states of vigilance that are commonly regarded as extreme poles of the wake-sleep cycle suggests that, with regard to brain cellular activities, waking and REM sleep are closer than it is usually believed and both are opposed to EEG-synchronized sleep. Indeed, data discussed in this chapter indicate that thalamic and cortical neurons similarly display an increased excitability during both waking and REM sleep. This brain state is called *activation*, a term used at the cellular level and implying a readiness of neuronal networks of the cerebrum to receive afferent information and to ensure quick responses. As such, the notion of activation refers to the response readiness of brain neurons either to stimuli from the outside world (as in waking) or to internal drives (as in REM sleep), whether or not an overt motor response is generated. Hence, both waking and REM sleep are regarded as brain-activated states, in spite of illogical thought and largely suppressed motor output in REM sleep.

Activation was initially viewed as a globally energizing system of the brain, originating in the brainstem reticular formation.[2, 6] Because both processes of excitation and sculpturing inhibition are present in complex integrative tasks of the alert state, one should include inhibition in the process of activation.[7] Later, it was expected that with an increased level of activation on awakening, both excitatory and inhibitory components of brain responses would increase. Instead, a series of experiments during the 1960s and 1970s reported results suggesting that the increased excitability of thalamic neurons on arousal is due to a global blockade of inhibitory effects acting on them. This embarrassing conclusion was derived from the earlier zeitgeist that viewed the thalamic reticular nucleus as the only source of thalamic inhibition, as well as from the lack of evidence, during that time, of a significant proportion of inhibitory elements intrinsic to each thalamic nucleus.[8]

Since 1980, it has been clear that 20 to 30% of neurons in all major thalamic nuclei of cats and primates operate on a local basis and use gamma-aminobutyric acid (GABA), a potent inhibitory synaptic transmitter. In the section on processing of sensory information, the evidence is further discussed that activation processes in thalamocortical systems involve a direct excitation from the brainstem reticular core, associated with the blockade of long-lasting and cyclic inhibitory potentials that are not only involved in EEG synchronizing patterns but also accompanied by preservation and even enhancement of shorter lasting inhibitory influences, which result in an increased receptive field specificity and orientation selectivity.

CELLULAR BASES OF SYNCHRONOUS OSCILLATIONS AND ACTIVATION PATTERN IN THALAMOCORTICAL SYSTEMS

Low-Frequency (Less Than 15 Hz) Oscillations in Corticothalamic Networks During Resting Sleep

Three types of oscillations characterize the state of resting sleep: spindles (7 to 14 Hz), delta (1 to 4 Hz),

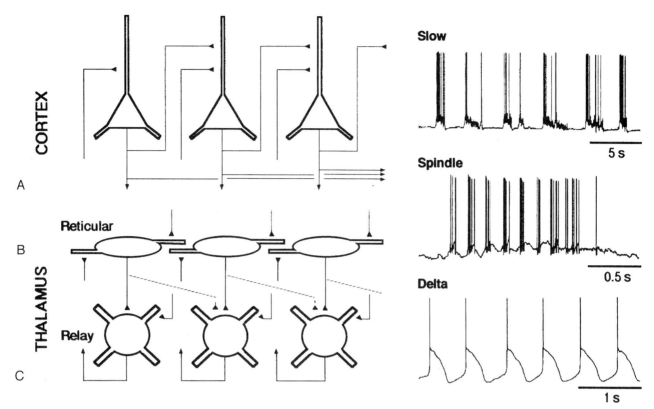

Figure 8–1. *A*, Building blocks of corticothalamic networks and different types of sleep oscillations generated by excitatory glutamatergic neocortical; *B*, inhibitory GABA reticular thalamic neurons; and *C*, excitatory glutamatergic thalamocortical or relay neurons. The direction of axons is indicated by arrows. Short- and long-scale intracortical pathways are illustrated. Divergent axons of thalamic reticular neurons are shown as broken lines. Note the different time calibrations in intracellular traces showing the cortical slow oscillation (~0.3 Hz), the spindles in thalamic reticular neuron (~7 Hz) and the intrinsic, clock-like delta rhythm of thalamocortical neuron (~1.5 Hz). These oscillations might be generated at each of these levels, even after disconnection from afferent inputs. However, in the intact brain, these structures are interacting and their rhythms are combined within complex wave sequences. (From Steriade M, Contreras D, Amzica F. Synchronized sleep oscillations and their paroxysmal developments. Trends Neurosci. 1994;17:199–209.)

and slow oscillation (less than 1 Hz).[9] Each of these rhythms originates through intrinsic neuronal properties and network operations in the thalamus and neocortex, even after isolation of these structures (Fig. 8–1). However, in an intact brain, there are no pure rhythms because thalamus and neocortex are interconnected and the cortical slow oscillation has the virtue of grouping different sleep rhythms into complex wave sequences.[10, 11] For didactic purposes, I describe each of the three major sleep oscillations separately.

Spindle Oscillation. Spindles appear during early stages of sleep (Fig. 8–2). *Spindles* are waxing and waning waves at 7 to 14 Hz, grouped in sequences that last 1 to 2 sec and that recur periodically with a slow rhythm of 0.1 to 0.3 Hz (see Fig. 8–2). Both of these rhythms (7 to 14 Hz and 0.2 to 0.5 Hz) should be considered in defining spindle activity. Spindles are generated in the thalamus, but the cerebral cortex plays a major role in their synchronization and virtually simultaneous appearance over widespread thalamic and cortical areas.[12]

The rostral pole of GABAergic thalamic reticular nuclear complex can generate spindle rhythmicity even after disconnection from dorsal thalamic nuclei and cerebral cortex,[13] due to connections among thalamic reticular neurons. The crucial role played by the thala-

mic reticular nucleus in the generation of sleep spindles is also demonstrated by abolition of spindling in target thalamocortical systems after disconnection from the reticular nucleus.[14] Spindles result from repetitive spike-bursts in GABAergic reticular cells that produce rhythmic inhibitory postsynaptic potentials (IPSPs) in thalamocortical neurons, leading to postinhibitory rebound spike-bursts that are transferred to cortex and produce excitatory postsynaptic potentials (EPSPs) in cortical cells, occasionally leading to action potentials (Fig. 8–3).

As thalamocortical neurons spend much of their sleep time during spindle-related IPSPs, there is a powerful inhibition of incoming messages in their route to the cerebral cortex. Recording field potentials evoked by stimulation of prethalamic axons (a method that permits the monitoring of the presynaptic deflection reflecting the magnitude of the afferent volley, together with the synaptically relayed, thalamically generated waves) reveals that the thalamus is the first station where afferent signals are completely blocked from the very onset of sleep (Fig. 8–4). This obliteration of synaptic transmission in the thalamus leads to the deafferentation of the cerebral cortex, a prerequisite for the process of falling asleep. More recently, intracellular recordings from thalamic and cortical neurons have

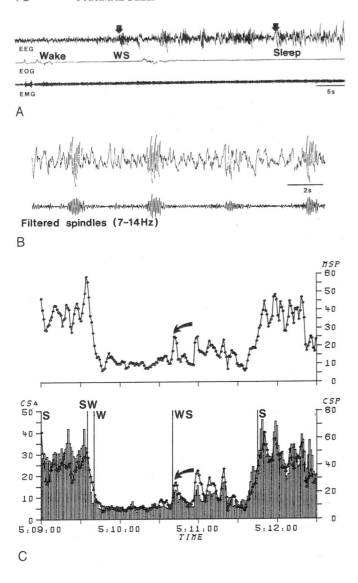

Figure 8–2. Electrographic criteria of wake-sleep states and characteristics of spindle rhythmicity. *A,* Behaving cat with chronically implanted electrodes. Electroencephalogram (EEG) from the anterior part (pericruciate areas) of the neocortical surface, electrooculogram (EOG), and electromyogram (EMG) of neck muscles. Spindle oscillations appear during the transitional period between waking and sleep (WS). *B,* Thalamic spindles in a *cerveau isolé* cat with an intercollicular transection. Top trace shows the field electrical activity recorded by means of a microelectrode in the rostral intralaminar (central lateral) nucleus; bottom trace shows spindle waves (filtered from 7 to 14 Hz) from the same period. Note that sequences of spindle waves recur periodically with a slow rhythm. *C,* Normalized amplitudes (ordinates) of simultaneously recorded focal spindle waves in the reticular thalamic nucleus (MSP, *top line—circle trace*), cortical spindle waves (CSP, *bottom line—circle trace*), and cortical slow waves (CSΔ, bottom bar graph) in a behaving cat. Spindles are filtered 7 to 14 Hz; slow waves are filtered 0.5 to 4 Hz. Abscissa indicates real time (h, min, sec). S, EEG-synchronized sleep; W, waking; SW and WS, transitional periods from S to W and from W to S, respectively. Note desynchronization with decreased wave amplitudes on awakening (SW and W); rhythmic sequences of spindles (recurring with a period of about 8 to 10 sec) in both thalamic and cortical recordings beginning with drowsiness (WS); and increased amplitudes of both spindles and slow waves beginning with S. (Modified from Steriade M, Domich L, Oakson G. Reticularis thalami neurons revisited: activity changes during shifts in states of vigilance. J Neurosci. 1986;6:68–81; and Paré D, Steriade M, Deschênes M, et al. Physiological properties of anterior thalamic nuclei, a group devoid of inputs from the reticular thalamic nucleus. J Neurophysiol. 1987;57:1669–1685.)

shown that, because of their hyperpolarization during sleep, thalamocortical cells do not transfer to cortex signals from prethalamic relay station, whereas the internal (corticocortical and corticothalamic) dialogue of the brain may be maintained during sleep.[15]

Delta Oscillation. The delta oscillation appears during later sleep stages (see Fig. 8–2) and has two components. The cortical one survives complete thalamectomy,[11, 16] and the spectral content in the delta band (1 to 4 Hz) results, at least partially, from the shape and duration of the K-complex[17] (see later). The other stereotypical clock-like component is generated in the thalamus and results from the hyperpolarization-activated interplay between two intrinsic currents of thalamocortical (relay) neurons (see bottom right trace in Fig. 8–1). Although this rhythm is also seen in thalamic slices after blockage of synaptic transmission,[18, 19] its appearance at the level of local field potentials and cortical EEG is possible because corticothalamic volleys synchronize thalamocortical cells through the action of inhibitory thalamic reticular neurons[20] that fulfill two requirements: they set the membrane potential of relay cells at the required level of hyperpolarization for the generation of delta oscillation, and they have distributed projections to the dorsal thalamus, thus synchronizing various relay cells.

As delta oscillation appears at a more hyperpolarized level of membrane potential in thalamocortical neurons than spindles,[20] the two sleep oscillations are incompatible in single cells. These intracellular data from anesthetized preparations are supported by results obtained in naturally sleeping animals and human beings, showing that thalamic spindles are maximal at sleep onset and decrease thereafter, whereas thalamic delta waves increase gradually during resting sleep. Thus, with increasing hyperpolarization of thalamocortical cells during resting sleep, due to the progressive diminished firing rates of cholinergic and other types of brainstem-thalamic activating neurons,[21] the incidence and amplitude of spindles are largely diminished during deep sleep stages. On the other hand, the reappearance of spindles toward the end of resting sleep[22] is attributable to a relative depolarization of thalamocortical cells, due to the increased firing

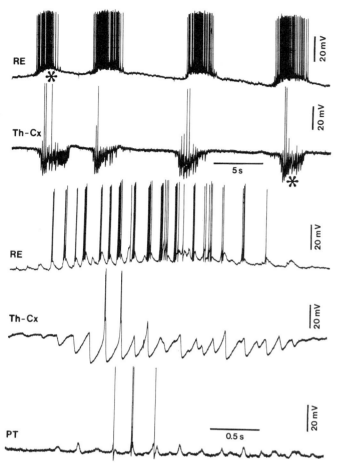

Figure 8–3. Cellular bases of spindling in thalamocortical systems. Intracellular aspects of spindle oscillations in reticular thalamic (RE), thalamocortical (Th-Cx; from the ventrolateral nucleus), and pyramidal tract (PT; from the precruciate gyrus) neurons of a cat under barbiturate anesthesia. The spindle sequences marked by asterisks in the top traces of RE and Th-Cx neurons are depicted below at higher speed. Note that spindle oscillations and rhythmic spike-bursts develop on a slowly growing and decaying depolarization in the RE neuron; on the contrary, rhythmic hyperpolarizations, occasionally interrupted by LTSs, underlie spindles in the Th-Cx cell. (Adapted from Steriade M, Deschênes M. Intrathalamic and brainstem-thalamic networks involved in resting and alert states. In: Bentivoglio M, Spreajico R, eds. Thalamic Mechanisms. Amsterdam, Netherlands: Elsevier; 1988:37–62.)

rates of brainstem-thalamic reticular neurons that display precursor increased rates of spontaneous firing, 30 to 60 sec before the onset of REM sleep.[23]

Slow Oscillation. The slow oscillation has a frequency peak at 0.7 to 0.8 Hz in cats under ketamine-xylazine anesthesia,[24] as well as during natural sleep in cats[3, 5, 17, 22] and in human beings.[17, 25] The cortical nature of the slow oscillation was demonstrated by its survival in the cerebral cortex after thalamectomy,[11] its absence in the thalamus of decorticated animals,[26] and the disruption of its long-range synchronization after disconnection of intracortical synaptic linkages.[27]

Intracellular analyses of the slow oscillation showed that cortical neurons throughout layers II to VI (many of them with physiologically identified thalamic or callosal input projections) displayed a spontaneous oscillation consisting of prolonged depolarizing and hyper-

polarizing components[10] (Fig. 8–5A). All major cellular classes in the cerebral cortex, as identified by electrophysiological characteristics and intracellular staining, display the slow oscillation: regular-spiking and intrinsically bursting cells, as well as local-circuit inhibitory basket cells.[24] Both long-axoned and short-axoned cells exhibit similar relations with the EEG components of the slow oscillation: during the depth-positive EEG wave, cortical neurons are hyperpolarized, whereas during the sharp depth-negative EEG deflection, cortical neurons are depolarized. The long-lasting depolarization of the slow oscillation consists of EPSPs, fast prepotentials (FPPs), and fast IPSPs reflecting the action of synaptically coupled GABAergic local-circuit cortical cells. Data also indicated that the depolarizing component is made up of both N-methyl-D-aspartate (NMDA)-mediated synaptic excitatory events and a voltage-dependent persistent sodium current $g_{Na(p)}$.[10] The long-lasting hyperpolarization, interrupting the depolarizing envelopes, is a combination of a $g_{K(Ca)}$ and disfacilitation in the corticothalamic network. The disfacilitation mechanism is supported by measuring the membrane input resistance (R_{in}), showing that R_{in} is highest during the long-lasting hyperpolarizing component of the slow oscillation.[28]

The spectacular similarity between all types of cortical neurons and EEG waveforms raised the question of mechanisms underlying these synchronization processes. Dual intracellular recordings in vivo revealed that the overt synchronization of EEG patterns is associated with the simultaneous hyperpolarizations in cortical neurons.[24, 27]

The neuronal synchronization also implicates thala-

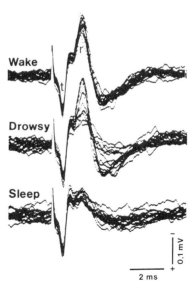

Figure 8–4. Blockade of synaptic transmission in the thalamus at sleep onset in a behaving cat. Field potentials evoked in the ventrolateral thalamic nucleus by stimulation of the cerebellothalamic pathway. The evoked response consists of a presynaptic (tract, *t*) component and a monosynaptically relayed *(r)* wave. Note the progressively diminished amplitude of the *r* wave during drowsiness, up to its complete obliteration during EEG-synchronized sleep, in spite of lack of changes in the afferent volley monitored by the *t* component. (M. Steriade, unpublished data, 1988.)

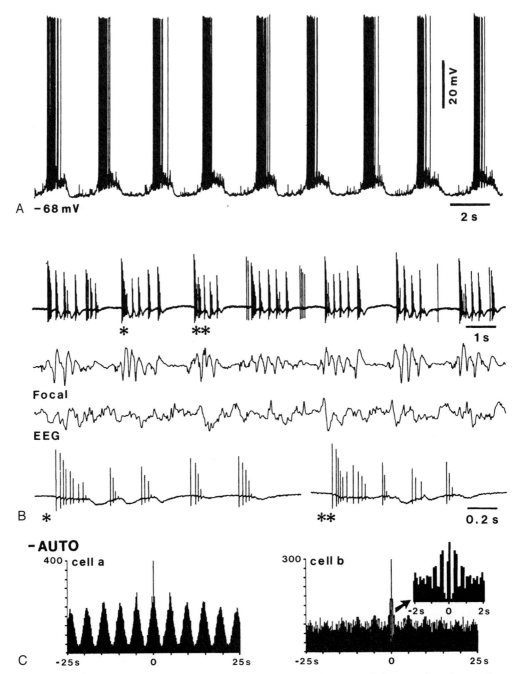

Figure 8–5. The slow sleep oscillation and the delta oscillations are distinct activities. Intracellular recordings in acutely prepared cats under urethane anesthesia. *A*, Intracellular recording of cortical motor area 4 neuron shows slow oscillation at ~0.35 Hz. *B*, Extra(juxta)cellular recording of bursting neuron from cortical association area 7, together with focal slow waves (through the same microelectrode) and EEG. Parts indicated by one (*) or two (**) asterisks are expanded below. Note sequences of delta waves (3 to 4 Hz) grouped by slow oscillation (~0.4 Hz). *C*, Autocorrelograms of two cells (a and b) recorded from cortical area 4 showing the slow oscillation (~0.2 Hz) and delta rhythmicity (~2.5 Hz, inset in cell b). (Modified from Steriade M, Nuñez A, Amzica F. Intracellular analysis of relations between the slow (<1 Hz) neocortical oscillation and other sleep rhythms of the electroencephalogram. J Neurosci. 1993;13:3266–3283.)

mic neurons. Remarkably, GABAergic thalamic reticular cells (identified by their peculiar bursting pattern and cortically elicited spindle-like depolarizing oscillations), whose intrinsic electrophysiological properties are quite different from those of neocortical cells, exhibit patterns of the slow sleep oscillation, with prolonged depolarizations interrupted by prolonged hyperpolarizations, that are very similar to those of cortical neurons. The depolarizing component of the

cortically generated slow oscillation is transmitted to thalamic reticular neurons at which level it triggers rhythmic spike-bursts and, consequently, is reflected in thalamocortical cells as rhythmic IPSPs leading to rebound spike-bursts.[24, 26] This is the mechanism underlying the brief sequence of EEG spindles that follows every cycle of the slow oscillation (see third cycle of slow oscillation in the top trace of Fig. 8–6*A*). Distinct from the prolonged, waxing-and-waning pattern of

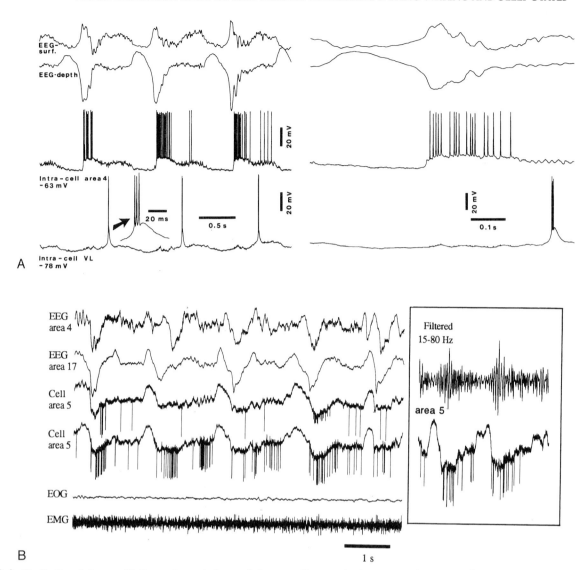

Figure 8–6. Similarity of slow oscillation patterns in intracellular recordings under ketamine-xylazine anesthesia and extracellular recordings in chronically implanted, naturally sleeping cats. *A*, the slow oscillation (~0.9 Hz) in dual intracellular recordings from regular-spiking neuron in cortical area 4 and thalamocortical (TC) neuron in ventrolateral (VL) nucleus. Cat under ketamine-xylazine anesthesia. Arrow points to a low-threshold spike-burst. An expanded cycle is shown at right. Note: (1) depth-positive (upward) EEG waves are associated with hyperpolarization of cortical and thalamic cells, whereas the sharp depth-negativities are associated with depolarization and action potentials in cortical cell, while the thalamic neuron displays a rebound spike-burst with a delay of 150–200 ms; (2) brief sequence of EEG spindles after the depth-negative sharp deflection (third cycle of slow oscillation); and (3) fast depolarizing waves (40 to 50 Hz) in cortical neuron during the sustained depolarization. *B*, chronically implanted, naturally sleeping cat. Six traces depict depth-EEG from motor (precruciate) area 4; depth-EEG from visual area 17; unit discharges and slow focal potentials from association area 5 in the anterior suprasylvian gyrus and similar recording from an adjacent focus (2 mm apart) in area 5; electro-oculogram (EOG); and electromyogram (EMG). Right part in slow-wave sleep panel shows reduction, up to disappearance, of fast rhythms (filtered 15 to 80 Hz) during the prolonged depth-positive wave of the slow oscillation that, in intracellular recordings *(A)*, is associated with hyperpolarization of cortical and thalamic neurons. (Modified from Steriade M. Synchronized activities of coupled oscillators in the cerebral cortex and thalamus at different levels of vigilance. Cerebr Cortex. 1997;7:583–604.)

spindle oscillations in animals decorticated or under barbiturate anesthesia, when cortical neurons display reduced spontaneous activities, the spindles triggered by the corticothalamic volley of the slow oscillation under ketamine-xylazine anesthesia are much shorter. This is due to the fact that the synchronous excitation of corticothalamic neurons during the slow oscillation entrain, right from the start, a great population of neurons implicated in the genesis of spindles within a thalamic territory, thus explaining the absence of an initial waxing process.

Thus, although the systematization of sleep rhythms into three categories (spindles, delta, slow) may be useful for didactic purposes, in brain-intact animals and human beings *the sleep oscillations are not seen in isolation but are grouped by the cortically generated slow oscillation.* The coalescence of the slow and spindle oscillations is especially visible during light sleep.[22] However, spindling is not the only sleep rhythm that is modulated and grouped by the cortical slow oscillation. The intrinsically generated delta rhythm of thalamocortical cells is influenced by the slow oscillation because the rhythmic depolarizing corticothalamic drives increase the membrane conductance of thalamocortical cells and prevent the interplay between the intrinsic currents I_h and I_t,[18, 19] thus periodically dampening the slow oscillation.[29] As to the other component of delta waves, which is generated intracortically after thalamectomy (see earlier), the frequency band of 1 to 4 Hz in the power spectrum during late stages of resting sleep results, at least partially, from the shape of the depth-negative (depolarizing) component of the slow oscillation (0.3 to 0.4 sec), which represents the K-complex.[17] Typical delta waves, at a frequency of 2 to 4 Hz, generated by both regular-spiking and intrinsically bursting cortical neurons, are grouped within sequences recurring with the slow rhythm[11] (see Fig. 8–5B–C). And, in human sleep EEG, sequential mean amplitudes of delta waves show their periodic recurrence with the rhythm of slow oscillation.[10] That delta and slow oscillation represent two distinct phenomena in human sleep EEG was recently demonstrated by showing differences in the dynamics between the slow and the delta oscillations, as the latter declines in activity from the first to the second NREM sleep episode, whereas the former does not.[25]

As the slow oscillation was first described intracellularly under different anesthetics, the similarity between these cellular patterns and those observed during natural sleep was validated in extracellular recordings from chronically implanted, unanesthetized animals. Under these conditions, the depth-positive waves are accompanied by silenced firing (due to cells' hyperpolarizations), whereas depth-negative sharp deflections are associated with brisk firing[3] (see Fig. 8–6B).

Independent experiments from two laboratories[17, 25] have demonstrated the presence of the slow oscillation in human sleep. In our study,[17] during stage 2, scalp recordings showed a prevalent peak (0.8 Hz) within the frequency range of the slow oscillation as well as a minor mode around 15 Hz reflecting spindle waves (Fig. 8–7). The power spectrum revealed a major peak around 1 Hz, which became evident from stage 2 and continued throughout resting sleep. These data invite

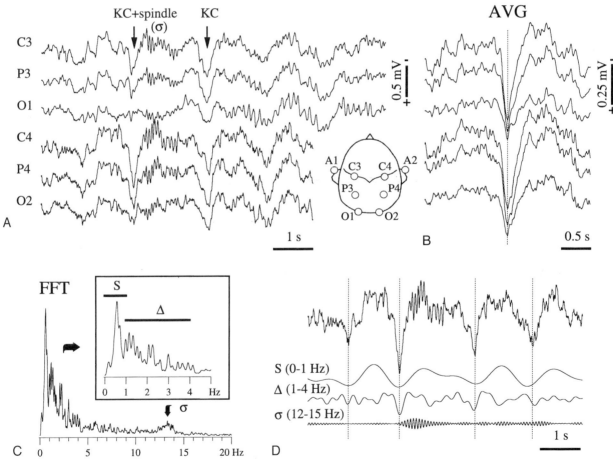

Figure 8–7. K-complexes (KCs) result from slow oscillation in human sleep. Resting sleep EEG of a normal human subject. Scalp monopolar recordings with respect to the contralateral ear (figurine). A, Short episode from a stage 3 period of sleep. The two arrows point to a KC followed by a spindle (σ) and to an isolated KC. The two KCs are embedded into a slow oscillation of ~0.6 Hz. Note the synchrony of the KCs in all recorded sites and their amplitude diminution in the occipital area. B, Average of 50 KCs aligned on the positive peak of the upper channel (*vertical dotted line*). C, Frequency decomposition of the C3 lead (upper trace) into three frequency bands: slow (S, 0 to 1 Hz), delta (Δ, 1 to 4 Hz), and sigma (σ, 12 to 15 Hz). It is shown that the KC results from a combination of slow and delta waves. D, Power spectrum of the C3 lead for a period of 80 sec of stable stage 3 activity containing the one depicted in panel A. The three frequency bands considered in panel C are clearly represented in the power spectrum. Moreover, the slow (S) activity displays a high peak, distinct from the ones of the delta activity. (Modified from Amzica F, Steriade M. The K-complex: its slow (<1 Hz) rhythmicity and relation to delta waves. Neurology. 1997;49:952–959.)

human sleep researchers to consider the two types of oscillatory activities below 4 Hz (delta, 1 to 4 Hz; slow, less than 1 Hz) and, accordingly, to analyze their results by taking into account the distinctness of these two oscillations.[25]

Brainstem-Thalamic Circuits Involved in Brain Activation and Fast Oscillations (20 to 50 Hz) During Waking and REM Sleep

That the brainstem reticular formation has a role in the blockade of low-frequency EEG rhythms is known from early experiments showing that periodic spindle sequences appear on the EEG after transections at the collicular level[30] and that both spindles and slow waves are readily erased by high-frequency electrical stimulation of the upper brainstem reticular core.[2] The role of brainstem monoaminergic aggregates, particularly the locus coeruleus, in the tonic EEG desynchronization that characterizes waking and REM sleep can be discarded because bilateral lesions of the locus coeruleus, with a consequent 85 to 95% depletion of cortical norepinephrine, result in control values of EEG activation immediately after recovery from surgery.[31] The firing features of both locus coeruleus and dorsal raphe are opposite in waking and REM sleep, with virtual neuronal silence during the latter state,[21] which clearly contrasts with the similar EEG patterns during these two behavioral states.

Because the replacement of synchronized EEG waves during sleep by EEG activation on natural states of arousal or REM sleep is associated with facilitation of synaptic transmission through major relay thalamic nuclei, these potentiating effects awaited the clarification of the underlying pathways. Moreover, because acetylcholine (ACh) blockers antagonize some components of brainstem-thalamic influences, the morphological search for these projections should be combined with the immunohistochemical identification of their cholinergic nature. Evidence of such projections to the thalamus after injections of retrograde tracers within the limits of distinct thalamic nuclei is now available for all sensory, motor, associational, reticular, limbic, and intralaminar thalamic nuclei in the cat,[32–34] as well as for associational nuclei in the monkey.[34] All major sensory (visual, auditory, and somesthetic) thalamic nuclei and the ventrolateral nucleus, which is specifically related to the motor cortex, receive fewer than 10% of their brainstem reticular afferents from noncholinergic neurons located in the rostral midbrain reticular formation; they receive 85 to 95% of their brainstem reticular innervation from a region at the midbrain-pontine junction, where two cholinergic nuclear groups are maximally developed. Of the total number of neurons that were retrogradely labeled in these two cholinergic brainstem (pedunculopontine, or peribrachial, and laterodorsal tegmental) nuclei after tracer injections in various thalamic nuclei, 70 to 85% were also identified as cholinergic by concurrent visualization of choline acetyltransferase immunoreactivity. Three to eight times more brainstem reticular cells were found to project toward associational thalamic nuclei and to those nuclear groups that have widespread cortical projections. The more important brainstem projections to the associational and diffusely projecting thalamic nuclei are accounted for by massive projections from noncholinergic brainstem neurons whose synaptic transmitters (peptides, glutamate) remain to be identified.

At their targets, the brainstem-thalamic projections underlie two distinct effects, which represent the main components of activation processes in thalamocortical systems: (1) a direct excitation of thalamocortical, and (2) an inhibition of thalamic reticular neurons, thus disinhibiting thalamocortical neurons and blocking spindle oscillations.

Stimulation of the rostral brainstem reticular formation elicits monosynaptic excitation of thalamocortical neurons (see reference 1 for a review). Earlier studies conducted on preparations under barbiturate anesthesia have concluded that midbrain reticular stimulation indirectly enhances the synaptic transmission of thalamocortical cells through a process of disinhibition. It is now established that small doses (2 mg/kg) of barbiturate block the direct excitatory effect of either brainstem reticular stimulation[35] or ACh application[36] on thalamocortical neurons. In fact, intracellular recordings in unanesthetized animals show that midbrain reticular stimulation in the region of the cholinergic peribrachial nucleus directly depolarizes thalamocortical neurons.[37] The early depolarization is nicotinic in nature, and it starts at latencies compatible with monosynaptic excitation, whereas the late-depolarizing component has a long latency and a long duration[35] (Fig. 8–8). The prolonged depolarizing response of thalamocortical cells to brainstem cholinergic stimulation is associated with EEG activation reaction having a similar time course (see Fig. 8–8A) and is accompanied by an increase in neuronal excitability (see Fig. 8–8B).[35] The association between a prolonged depolarization and an increase in excitability provides the necessary mechanism for the shift from the sleepy state of the closed brain to the activated state characterized by tonic firing and enhanced synaptic responsiveness. The long-lasting depolarization is blocked by scopolamine, a muscarinic antagonist.[35] In those cases in which scopolamine does not succeed in completely blocking the prolonged depolarizing response, other transmitters are probably involved. Peptides (and among them substance P) are co-localized in some cholinergic brainstem reticular neurons.

In addition to direct excitation of thalamocortical neurons, brainstem reticular stimulation blocks the spindle-related, rhythmic hyperpolarizing episodes in those neurons (Fig. 8–9A). This finding is due to the blockade of spindle oscillations at the site of their genesis, the reticular thalamic nucleus[38] (Fig. 8–9B). The effect of stimulating the brainstem peribrachial cholinergic nucleus on intracellularly recorded reticular thalamic neurons is a dual one and consists of two direct and opposed components: a short depolarization and a long-lasting hyperpolarization.[38] The hyperpolarization

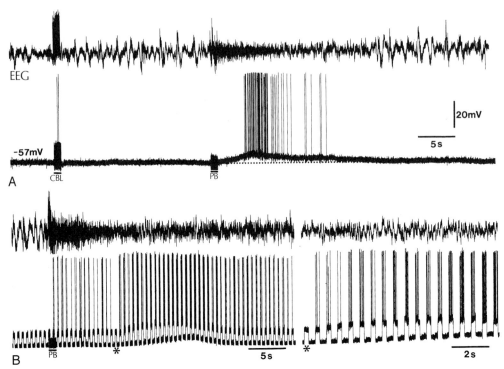

Figure 8–8. Stimulation of the mesopontine cholinergic peribrachial (PB) area induces long-lasting depolarization associated with increased input resistance in the thalamocortical ventrolateral cell. These cellular events are accompanied by desynchronization of ipsilateral EEG. *A,* Comparison between the effects of stimulating contralateral the deep cerebellar nuclei (CBL) and ipsilateral PB area to determine whether the effects of PB stimulation are due to activation of PB perikarya or to passing cerebellothalamic axons (for both CBL and PB, stimulation was 1-sec pulse-train at 30 Hz). Note the similar time course of membrane depolarization and EEG desynchronization in response to PB stimulation. *B,* Membrane conductance tested by injecting depolarizing current pulses. Note the 30% increase in the pulse amplitude riding on a 4-mV depolarization. The part indicated by the asterisk on the left is also depicted at higher speed on the right. (From Curró Dossi R, Paré D, Steriade M. Short-lasting nicotinic and long-lasting muscarinic depolarizing responses of thalamocortical neurons to stimulation of mesopontine cholinergic nuclei. J Neurophysiol. 1991;65:393–406.)

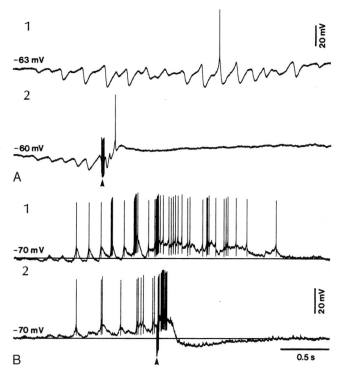

Figure 8–9. The obliteration of sleep spindles in the thalamocortical systems during arousal is produced by their disruption at the very site of genesis, the thalamic reticular nucleus, pacemaker of spindles. Intracellularly recorded spindle sequences in a lateral geniculate neuron *(A)* and a perigeniculate (reticular) thalamic neuron *(B)* of cat. The blockade of spindles in the relay thalamocortical neuron results from the disruption of spindles in the thalamic reticular nucleus where this sleep oscillation is generated. (Modified. Reprinted from Neuroscience, vol 31, Hu B, Steriade M, Deschênes M, The effects of brainstem peribrachial simulation on perigeniculate neurons: the blockage of spindle waves, 1–12, Copyright 1989, with permission from Elsevier Science.)

prevents the occurrence of spindle oscillations and effectively blocks ongoing spindle sequences that normally develop in thalamic reticular cells on a depolarizing envelope (see Fig. 8–9B). The blockade of spindles by hyperpolarization of reticular thalamic neurons is a muscarinic effect because it is blocked by atropine. This hyperpolarization is associated with a marked conductance increase, probably to K ions.[39] In contrast, the early depolarization is not affected by cholinergic antagonists, and after the blockade of the hyperpolarizing component by atropine, it lasts for 200 msec.

The powerful hyperpolarization elicited by brainstem cholinergic fibers acts on the generalized thalamic inhibition produced by GABAergic thalamic reticular neurons but is quite different from the action exerted by the same system on the other class of thalamic GABAergic neurons, namely, the short-axoned cells intrinsic to each other nucleus. Indirect evidence, discussed in the next section, shows that local inhibitory processes related to discriminatory tasks and attributable to short-axoned interneurons are, in fact, enhanced during natural arousal, brainstem reticular stimulation, or ACh application.

The dampening effect of the brainstem reticular cholinergic system on spindle genesis is consistent with data relating the activity of thalamically projecting midbrain reticular neurons to the appearance of EEG spindles at sleep onset (reviewed in references 1 and 21). Midbrain reticular neurons with antidromically identified projections to the intralaminar thalamus significantly decrease their firing rates during the transitional wake-to-sleep period and reliably slow or completely arrest their discharges about 1 sec before the onset of spindle sequences in repeated transitions from EEG-desynchronized to EEG-synchronized epochs (Fig. 8–10). The withdrawal of tonic brainstem reticular discharges is probably an effective factor for spindle genesis at two thalamic targets: it creates the hyperpolarization by disfacilitation in thalamocortical neurons (see earlier), and it removes the source of muscarinic hyperpolarization at the level of thalamic reticular neurons, the spindle pacemaker.

The tonic activating role of the upper brainstem reticular neurons in the EEG activation during waking is synergic with the role played by thalamically projecting medullary reticular neurons in the EEG activation during REM sleep.[40] This additional source of EEG activation is required because the destruction of the midbrain reticular formation was found to be much more efficient in impairing EEG activation during waking than during REM sleep. Bulbar reticular neurons (antidromically identified as projecting to thalamic nuclei that, in turn, send axons to widespread cortical areas) significantly increase their firing rates about 30 to 60 sec before the first sign of EEG activation during transition from EEG-synchronized to REM sleep.[40]

The mechanism of cholinergic activation of the cerebral cortex is less clear. The cortical ACh output increases after brainstem reticular stimulation and during both EEG-activated states of arousal and REM sleep (reviewed in reference 41). As discussed earlier, the brainstem reticular cholinergic system plays a decisive role in activation processes in the thalamus, but thalamocortical neurons use aspartate or glutamate, not ACh, as synaptic transmitters. There is now evidence of direct projections from the upper brainstem reticular core to cholinergic nuclei of the basal forebrain,[42, 43] which are known to have widespread cortical projections. These data indicate that in addition to the noncholinergic thalamocortical activation, the cholinergic activation of the cerebral cortex is produced by basal forebrain neurons driven by brainstem reticular neurons. Another circuit involves the projection from cholinergic and noncholinergic (GABAergic) basal forebrain neurons located in the substantia innominata and diagonal band nuclei toward a few thalamic nuclear groups, most importantly to the rostral pole of the reticular thalamic complex.[44] The indirect influence of brainstem reticular systems on the synchronizing spindle pacemaker, the reticular thalamic neurons, an influence mediated by basal forebrain neurons, remains to be explored electrophysiologically.

As mentioned earlier, the reason we call the EEG pattern during waking and REM sleep *activated* and avoid the term *desynchronized* is the occurrence of spontaneous fast (20 to 50 Hz) oscillations that, far from being desynchronized, are coherent within intracortical, intrathalamic, and corticothalamic neuronal networks[3, 5] (Fig. 8–11). These oscillations are often termed *gamma* and are distinguished from beta oscillations at lower frequencies; however, fast oscillations can double their frequencies during periods as short as 0.5 to 1 sec,[3] without obvious relations with changes in behavioral state. The recent interest in fast brain oscillations was aroused by claims about their possible significance in focused attention and in phenomena of binding different features of an object into a global percept.[45] Spatially localized, coherent fast oscillations are present on the background electrical activity, without necessarily requiring optimal sensory stimuli, during all states of vigilance, including resting sleep.[3, 5] The fast oscillations depend on the depolarization of thalamic and cortical neurons,[3, 5] which occurs transiently (but predictably) during given phases of slow sleep oscillation and continuously during behavioral states with tonically increased brain excitability, waking, and REM sleep. Far from being exclusively generated in the cerebral cortex, the fast oscillations also occur in thalamic neurons and are synchronized within corticothalamic networks (see Fig. 8–11).[46]

PROCESSING OF SENSORY INFORMATION

Briefly, the synaptic transmission of sensory information through the thalamus and the cerebral cortex is enhanced during the states of waking and REM sleep, compared with EEG-synchronized sleep. The obliteration of synaptic transmission occurs in the thalamus at the first EEG signs of drowsiness, before overt behavioral manifestations of sleep, and despite the unchanged magnitude of the incoming volley (see Fig. 8–4). During wakefulness, enhanced synaptic excitabil-

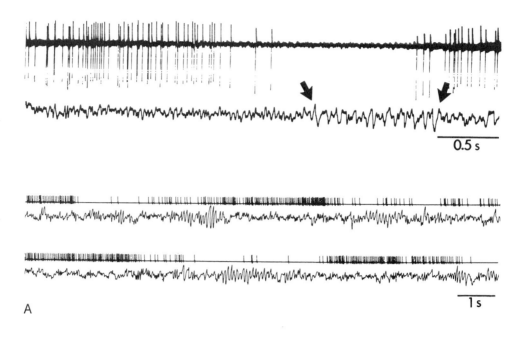

A

0.5 s

1 s

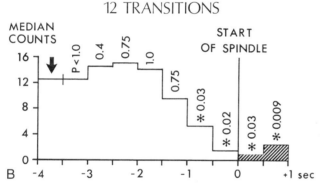

12 TRANSITIONS

MEDIAN
COUNTS

START
OF SPINDLE

B

Figure 8–10. Midbrain reticular neurons decrease discharge rates in advance of EEG spindles during a transitional state from waking (W) to sleep (S) in the cat. *A*, Neuron antidromically identified as projecting to the caudal intralaminar thalamic nuclei. Top two traces depict original spikes and EEG waves simultaneously displayed on the oscilloscope. Note the decreased firing rate, leading to neuronal silence, before the first spindle sequence *(between arrows)* during transition from W to S. Bottom traces depict the same activities during repeated EEG desynchronization-synchronization transitions (polygraphic recordings). *B*, Twelve transitions of unit firing with respect to the start of EEG spindle (time 0). Arrow indicates the level of discharge (median rate) during W. Asterisks mark bins with significant ($P < .05$) decrease in firing rate compared with median rate during W. A significantly decreased firing rate occurred 1 sec before spindle onset. (Adapted from Steriade M. The excitatory-inhibitory response sequence in thalamic and neocortical cells: state-related changes and regulatory systems. In: Edelman GM, Gall WE, Cowan WM, eds. Dynamic Aspects of Neocortical Function. New York, NY: Wiley-Interscience; 1984:107–157.)

ity of thalamocortical systems is accompanied by an increased efficacy of the inhibitory sculpturing of afferent information. This section discusses data from extracellular and intracellular studies on animals and from scalp recordings in human beings related to excitatory and inhibitory processes of sensory processing during alertness to external stimuli in waking, during the resting state of EEG-synchronized sleep, and during the dreaming state of REM sleep.

Enhanced Excitability

One of the best (and the simplest) methods for investigating state-dependent changes in information processes of thalamic nuclei and cortical areas is the

use of field (mass) potentials evoked by stimulation of afferent pathways. This method has the advantages of monitoring the earliest and rapid deflection that reflects the activity in the presynaptic axons and of ascertaining whether the fluctuations in synaptically evoked components of thalamic or cortical response are dependent on parallel modifications in the incoming volley (see Fig. 8–4). In detailed analyses of animals, stimuli applied to central pathways (prethalamic fibers, in the case of thalamic responses) are highly artificial and abnormally synchronous. Nonetheless, such central stimuli have the advantage of avoiding unknown alterations at multiple intercalated synapses when peripheral stimulation is employed. For an evaluation of this old method of centrally evoked field potentials and its use in long-term processes of plasticity, short-term

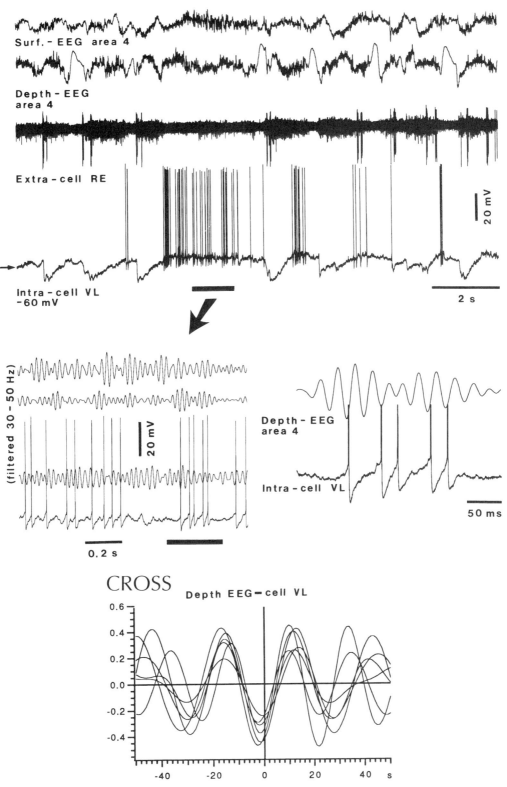

Figure 8–11. Brief episodes of tonic activation are accompanied by sustained and correlated fast rhythms (40 Hz) in cortex and intracellularly recorded thalamocortical (TC) cell. Cat under ketamine and xylazine anesthesia. *Top left,* Four traces represent simultaneous recording of surface- and depth-EEG from precruciate area 4, intracellular activity of TC neuron from the ventrolateral (VL) nucleus, and extracellular discharges of rostrolateral thalamic reticular (RE) neuron. EEG, VL, and RE cells display a slow oscillation (0.7 to 0.8 Hz) consisting of long-lasting, depth-positive EEG waves, leading to sharp depth-negative EEG potentials, related to the initiation of biphasic, long-lasting inhibitory postsynaptic potentials in VL cell. The period from activated epoch is expanded below *(arrow),* with filtered (30 to 50 Hz) activities from surface- and depth-EEG as well as from local field potentials from RE nucleus (picked up by the same microelectrode that served for recording of unitary discharges), and with intracellular activity of VL neuron. Part marked by *horizontal bar* is further expanded at right to show close temporal relations, at ~40 Hz, between the action potentials in VL neuron and depth-negative waves in cortical EEG. CROSS (cross-correlation) is taken from a period of activity without action potentials in VL cell and shows clear-cut relation, with opposition of phase, between depth-EEG and intracellularly recorded VL neuron. (Modified from Steriade M, Contreras D, Amzica F, et al. Synchronization of fast (30–40 Hz) spontaneous oscillations in intrathalamic and thalamocortical networks. J Neurosci. 1996;16:2788–2808.)

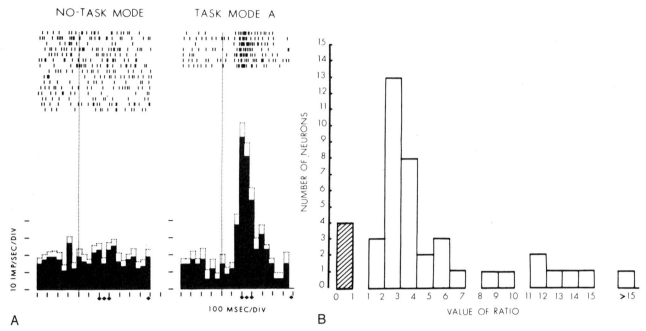

Figure 8–12. Facilitation of the monkey's parietal visual neurons by attentive fixation. *A,* Comparison of responses of parietal light-sensitive neurons to visual stimuli in no-task and task modes (absence of responses during no-task mode compared with strong responses in task mode). Summing histograms: standard error of mean calculated for each bin of the histograms; value shown by dotted line. Corresponding bin pairs within the histograms tested for significant differences (*t* test; bin pairs marked with diamonds differed at 5 level of significance). Overall responses in no-task and task states were compared in the following way. The rate of impulse discharges in the prestimulus period was subtracted from that in the poststimulus period for each trial, and populations of remainders were tested for significant differences (*P* < .05 required) and used to form a facilitation ratio for each neuron. Ratios for neurons with significant differences plotted in *B.* Facilitation ratio is that of the net increment in response evoked by a light stimulus in a state of interested fixation over that evoked by a physically identical and retinotopically similar stimulus delivered in no-task or the intertrial states. Fifty-one neurons showed ratios of > 1:1 and, of these, the difference was significant at 5 level (*t* test) for 38; values plotted in histogram. The ratio was fractional for four neurons indicated to the left; for them, the response was significantly greater in no-task state than during interested fixation. (Adapted from Mountcastle VB, Andersen RA, Motter BO The influence of attentive fixation upon the excitability of the light-sensitive neurons of the posterior parietal cortex. J Neurosci. 1981;1:1218–1235.)

changes during wake and sleep states, and experiments on selective attention and motor set, see the monograph by Evarts et al.[47]

Diffuse Brain Activation in Arousal and REM Sleep. The amplitude of the monosynaptically evoked wave of thalamic and cortical field response is greatly increased both during EEG-desynchronized behavioral states (waking and REM sleep) in chronic experiments and on brainstem reticular stimulation in acutely prepared animals. These changes are observed in all sensory and motor thalamocortical systems. The synaptically relayed component progressively diminishes in amplitude from the onset of EEG synchronization during drowsiness and is completely obliterated during EEG-synchronized sleep, in spite of the unchanged amplitude of the presynaptic component (see Fig. 8–4). *This finding indicates that the thalamus is the first relay station where afferent information is blocked at sleep onset.* Indeed, the excitability of somatosensory cuneothalamic brainstem neurons does not change from waking to EEG-synchronized sleep.[48] The blockade of synaptic transmission through the thalamus prevents the cerebral cortex from elaborating a response and is a necessary deafferentation prelude for falling asleep.

Besides a parallel increase in spontaneous and evoked discharges during EEG-desynchronized states, another picture emerged when a reduction in spontaneous discharges of cortical neurons on awakening was observed in conjunction with an enhanced probability of their responses to afferent stimulation. Thus, the majority of visual cortex neurons reduce their background firing on arousal, simultaneously increasing their responses to optimally oriented moving slits of light.[49] Even when both spontaneous and sensory-evoked discharges are reduced during waking, the ratio of evoked to spontaneous activity becomes higher, which thus indicates a higher signal-to-noise ratio.[50]

These results are explained in the light of data on the action of various modulatory systems. The locus coeruleus acts as an enabling device by suppressing weak inputs and enhancing strong inputs, thus increasing the efficiency of feature extraction from sensory information and switching emphasis from one set of inputs to another.[51] The underlying mechanism of the effects induced by stimulating the locus coeruleus or by iontophoretic application of norepinephrine is a hyperpolarization that accounts for the depressed spontaneous discharges, associated with an increase in input resistance that explains the increased responsiveness to incoming volleys.[52] The association between membrane hyperpolarization and the blockade of after-spike-hyperpolarization is a decisive factor in preventing neuronal activation to weak stimuli while enhancing responses to stimuli that overcome inhibition.

Selective Attention. The effects of general arousal can be dissociated from those related to selective attention and initiation of movements. In the experiments conducted by Mountcastle and colleagues,[53] the monkey is in three types of behavioral conditions: a *no-trial state*, that is, a quiescent state of waking with no involvement in behavioral tasks; a *trial state*, that is, a condition of attentive fixation on a target when the animal is engaged in a dimming detection task; and an *intertrial state*, which alternates with the trial state. Although the low degree of responsiveness of parietal cortex visual cells in the intertrial state is virtually equal to that in the no-trial state, the same light-sensitive neurons display a significantly increased excitability during the task mode (Fig. 8–12). The conclusion is that the enhanced responsiveness does not merely occur with changes in general arousal but is more specifically related to the directed attention to the target light. Other studies on the somatosensory cortex of behaving primates have also shown that the response of single neurons increases when the monkey "attends" to the part of the body that is to receive the stimulus.[54] These results are in keeping with data from scalp recordings in human beings, discussed later.

In human beings, sensory information processing can be studied by recording from intact scalp electrical signals as small as 0.1 μV, which are resolved by using computer averaging techniques. A warning stimulus elicits a slow negative potential shift termed *contingent negative variation* and is followed by an imperative stimulus that evokes an event-related potential. The scalp-recorded, event-related potential consists of a series of components designated by their polarities and peak latencies. In the somatosensory system, all event-related potential components up to and including P14 (a positive wave with 14 msec peak latency) are generated below the thalamus. The first cortical component is the negative wave N20 followed by at least five intracortical components with linger latencies.[55] Although the early components reflecting transmission up to and through the thalamus are unchanged under attentional manipulations, the amplitudes of P40, N60, and especially P100 and P300 components are increased when the subject is instructed to attend to an infrequent somesthetic stimulus (e.g., to the left thumb) designated as target and to press a button as quickly as possible (with the right index finger) for each such target[56] (Fig. 8–13). Desmedt and colleagues proposed

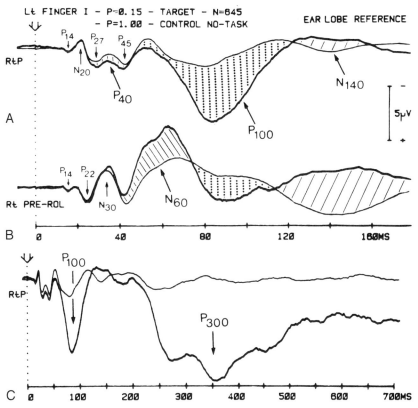

Figure 8–13. Cognitive components in the somatosensory evoked potential (SEP) of a human to electrical stimuli delivered to the left thumb. The thicker SEP traces are averaged in runs when the thumb stimuli are infrequent (*P* = .15) targets to which the subject has to respond by pressing a microswitch with the right index finger. Thicker traces were obtained by asking the computer to redraw three times the same trace with an appropriate vertical shift. These SEPs are superimposed on control SEPs averaged in other runs of the same experiment when identical thumb stimuli are delivered alone (*P* = 1.0) at the same intervals and not mixed with any other stimuli. *A*, Right parietal (R + P) scalp derivation. *B*, Right prerolandic (R + PRE-ROL) scalp derivation. *C*, Same trace as *A* displayed on a slower time base. Yoked ear lobes served as reference. The vertical dotted line on the left side indicates the time of delivery of the thumb stimulus. The small arrows identify standard early SEP components, namely, the P14 far field, the parietal N20-P27-P45, and the prerolandic P22–N30. Cognitive components identified through divergence of the superimposed traces are indicated by the following symbols: P40 (vertical lines), N60 (oblique lines), P100 *(vertical rows of dots)*, N140 *(widely spaced oblique lines)*. Vertical calibration: 5 μV. Horizontal calibration in milliseconds. Negativity of the active scalp electrode registers upward in all traces. (From Desmedt JE, Huy NT, Bourguet M. The cognitive P40, N60 and P100 components of somatosensory evoked potentials and the earliest electrical signs of sensory processing in man. Electroencephalogr Clin Neurophysiol. 1983;56:272–282.)

that P100 might index the identification of input signals and that P300 reflects the nonspecific postdecision closure. Similarly, the earliest component of the visual cortical response is little affected by psychological variables, whereas subsequent rhythmic waves (which probably reflect intracortical information processing) are selectively enhanced during attention.[57, 58]

Circuits Underlying Phasic Events in Alertness and REM Sleep. There are at least two neuronal circuits that are probably involved in phasic processes induced by external sensory stimuli during arousal and in phasic events triggered by brain-stored information during REM sleep.

One of these circuits comprises the GABAergic neurons of substantia nigra pars reticulata (SNr) and their follower elements in the superior colliculus, peribrachial zone of the upper brainstem reticular formation, and various thalamic nuclei. Novel sensory stimuli that trigger orienting reactions are accompanied by a decrease in the discharge rate of SNr neurons,[59] with the consequence of the release from tonic inhibition and increased firing in their superior collicular targets, eventually leading (through collicular projections to pontine oculomotor nuclei) to eye movement saccades toward the signal. The decrease in firing rates of GABAergic SNr neurons on sensory stimuli is interpreted as resulting from direct inhibitory inputs arising in GABAergic caudate neurons, which receive projections from some fields in the upper brainstem reticular core, medial and intralaminar thalamic nuclei, and widespread cortical areas.[60] All of these structures are the sites of profuse collateralization of sensory pathways. In addition, reciprocal projections link the pars reticulata and pars compacta of the substantia nigra with the cholinergic peribrachial (or pedunculopontine) nucleus of the midbrain-pontine junction.

Therefore, an alerting stimulus would have access to two distinct systems. The first one is the SNr-colliculopontine circuit responsible for the phasic shift of gaze involved in the orienting behavior. The relative hyperpolarization of premotor pontine reticular neurons during the alert state[61] is a favorable condition that underlies their Ca^{2+}-dependent, low-threshold spike and superimposed spike-bursts, which are operational in driving oculomotor neurons. The second system consists of the brainstem peribrachial and thalamic targets of SNr that are disinhibited during the periods of silenced firing in SNr on sensory stimulation. The direct disinhibition of thalamic neurons with widespread cortical projections and depolarizing actions on the superficial cortical layer (such as the cells in the ventromedial thalamic nucleus[62]), together with the secondary brainstem-thalamic activation, is crucial in the EEG activating reaction induced by an alerting stimulus.

Other intrabrainstem and brainstem-thalamic circuits generate the PGO waves that are the physiological correlate of the internal activation of the brain during REM sleep, "the stuff that dreams are made off." PGO waves are sharp field potentials, generally recorded in the visual thalamic (lateral geniculate [LG]) nucleus, where they appear in clusters of up to six waves, closely related to the time occurrence and the

direction of eye movement saccades. For example, rightward eye movements are correlated with predominantly right LG waves.[63] Although the original term indicated their presence in the visual pathway, PGO waves largely transcend this sensory system and are disseminated in many thalamic nuclei and in the corresponding cortical areas outside the visual cortex. This widespread distribution of PGO waves is explained by the generalized thalamic projections of PGO generators, and the cholinergic neurons of peribrachial and laterodorsal tegmental nuclei located at the junction of the midbrain and pontine reticular formation. Indeed, peribrachial and some laterodorsal tegmental neurons with antidromically identified projections to various thalamic nuclei discharge spike-bursts reliably precede the PGO waves.[21, 64-66] PGO waves can also be triggered by stimulating the upper brainstem core when the animal is in REM sleep, which thus suggests a selective gate opening of internal sensory activation during this behavioral state.

How are PGO waves generated? The input sources of the peribrachial, laterodorsal tegmental, and adjacent areas in the upper brainstem reticular formation are in the spinal cord, bulbopontine reticular core, posterior and anterior hypothalamic areas, and cerebral cortex, to mention only some. It is likely that initiation of impulses in the PGO generators can be triggered by any of the mentioned inputs through a mechanism that should conceivably lead to a postinhibitory rebound excitation because high-frequency spike-bursts are the signature of PGO-on peribrachial neurons. The peribrachial neurons can then be regarded as the final link in the brainstem-thalamic path that generates PGO waves in thalamocortical systems. Because these phenomena occur in REM sleep when the brain is disconnected from peripheral sensory gates, and because the content of oneiric behavior may relate to past experience, hypothalamic and forebrain structures (which are hypothesized to store some of the emotionally charged information) may be most effective in driving the PGO brainstem neuronal generators.

Sculpturing Inhibition

During waking, the increased response readiness of thalamocortical and corticofugal neurons is accompanied by fine inhibitory sculpturing, which provides input selection and output tuning, the necessary requirements for an adaptive state. There are few investigations concerning the inhibitory processes of thalamic and cortical neurons during REM sleep. A detailed comparative picture of feedforward and feedback inhibition during waking and REM sleep should be obtained in future studies. Such an analysis could differentiate, at the cellular level, these two brain-activated states, which are otherwise indistinguishable regarding their EEG-desynchronized activity and the enhanced probability of thalamic and cortical responses to synaptic and antidromic volleys.

The general conclusion of data discussed in the following is that the inhibitory processes in thalamocortical and corticofugal cells are more effective but much shorter in duration during wakefulness, compared with EEG-synchronized sleep. By inference, the progenitors of short-duration inhibitory events involved in discriminatory tasks would be potentiated during the waking state.

In the thalamus, there are two GABAergic cell types: the reticular neurons, which are leading elements of oscillatory activity during EEG-synchronized sleep, and the short-axoned neurons, which are hypothesized to generate local (intraglomerular) inhibitory processes, which would be effective in input selection during the waking state. Only the reticular neurons were directly investigated during sleep and arousal, brainstem reticular stimulation, and ACh application, both in vivo and in vitro. As yet, there is no available study of state-related alterations in the activity of formally identified inhibitory local-circuit thalamic neurons. To complicate the matter, axonal terminals of thalamic reticular neurons contact local-circuit thalamic neurons.[67] The functional significance of this finding is the inhibition exerted by one GABAergic cell type on the other, with the consequence of disinhibition of GABAergic local-circuit cells after disconnection from the thalamic reticular thalamic nucleus.[14, 68] This complex circuit and its consequences on the target thalamocortical neurons at various levels of vigilance are yet unknown. The tremendous variety of local-circuit cortical neurons also remains unexplored with regard to their inhibitory actions across the sleep-waking cycle.

In what follows, the experimental evidence on inhibitory processes of thalamocortical and corticofugal neurons—as changed during states of vigilance—is discussed, and state-dependent changes in the activity of inhibitory elements are inferred. The earlier idea of a general disinhibition on arousal has evolved and was replaced by the concept of a differential action exerted by brainstem modulatory systems, consisting of the blockade of generalized cyclic inhibition (which underlies spindle genesis) and the preservation or even enhancement of local inhibition involved in discriminatory processes.[1, 69] The first type of brainstem-induced cholinergic inhibition that is operational in the blockade of spindles at their site of genesis, the thalamic reticular nucleus, was discussed previously in the section, Cellular Bases of Synchronous Oscillations and Activation Patterns in Thalamocortical Systems. Data on enhanced inhibitory actions related to input specificity are summarized in the following.

However efficiently midbrain reticular stimulation in acute experiments and natural arousal in behaving animals block cyclic, long-lasting inhibitions in thalamocortical neurons, neither of these conditions does eliminate the early, shorter-lasting inhibitory phase.[70] This result was obtained with both extracellular and intracellular recordings and can be related to the improvement of receptive field specificity and orientation selectivity of visual thalamic neurons on arousal.[49] The effect of brainstem reticular stimulation or natural arousal is mainly cholinergic in nature. Indeed, whereas the ACh effect on thalamic reticular neurons is inhibitory and effective in blocking the generalized

inhibition, the same transmitter induces an improvement of receptive field function.[71, 72] This result suggests an ACh-induced potentiation of inhibitory local-circuit thalamic neurons.[73]

The results on inhibitory processes in corticofugal neurons are basically similar to those reported for thalamocortical neurons. Prolonged and cyclic inhibitory periods during behavioral EEG-synchronized sleep develop into significantly shorter but efficient periods of inhibition during wakefulness. The preservation of an initial, short-lasting (20 to 30 msec) inhibitory phase on arousal was reported for both spontaneous and evoked activities of corticospinal neurons.[70]

These data on the facilitatory effects of brainstem reticular stimulation and natural arousal on short-range specific inhibition are congruent with those of the iontophoretic applications of ACh on cortical neurons. The increased discrimination applies to receptive field specificity as well as to orientation and direction selectivity.

The common conclusion of these studies on thalamic and cortical inhibitory processes related to discrimination functions is that during waking, deep but short inhibition provides a mechanism subserving an accurate discrimination of incoming messages, a fine control of performances, and a faithful following of rapidly recurring activity.

Acknowledgments

This work was supported by grants from the Medical Research Council of Canada, National Sciences and Engineering Research Council of Canada, and Human Frontier Science Program.

References

1. Steriade M, Llinás R. The functional states of the thalamus and the associated neuronal interplay. Physiol Rev. 1988;68:649–742.
2. Moruzzi G, Magoun HW. Brain stem reticular formation and activation of the EEG. Electroencephalogr Clin Neurophysiol. 1949;1:455–473.
3. Steriade M, Amzica F, Contreras D. Synchronization of fast (30–40 Hz) spontaneous cortical rhythms during brain activation. J Neurosci. 1996;16:392–417.
4. Llinás R, Ribary U. Coherent 40-Hz oscillation characterizes dream state in humans. Proc Nat Acad Sci U S A. 1993;90:2078–2081.
5. Steriade M, Contreras D, Amzica F, et al. Synchronization of fast (30–40 Hz) spontaneous oscillations in intrathalamic and thalamocortical networks. J Neurosci. 1996;16:2788–2808.
6. Moruzzi G. The sleep-waking cycle. Ergebn Physiol. 1972;64:1–165.
7. Jasper HH. Recent advances in our understanding of the ascending activities of the reticular system. In: Jasper HH, Proctor LD, Knighton RS, et al, eds. Reticular Formation of the Brain. Boston, Mass: Little Brown & Co; 1958:319–331.
8. Jones EG. Thalamus. New York, NY: Plenum Press; 1985.
9. Steriade M. Cellular substrates of brain rhythms. In: Niedermeyer E, Lopes da Silva F, eds. Electroencephalography: Basic Principles, Clinical Applications and Related Fields. Baltimore, Md: Williams & Wilkins; 1998:28–75.
10. Steriade M, Nuñez A, Amzica F. A novel slow (<1 Hz) oscillation of neocortical neurons in vivo: depolarizing and hyperpolarizing components. J Neurosci. 1993;13:3252–3265.
11. Steriade M, Nuñez A, Amzica F. Intracellular analysis of relations between the slow (<1 Hz) neocortical oscillation and other sleep rhythms of the electroencephalogram. J Neurosci. 1993;13:3266–3283.

12. Contreras D, Destexhe A, Sejnowski TJ, et al. Control of spatio-temporal coherence of a thalamic oscillation by corticothalamic feedback. Science. 1996;274:771–774.

13. Steriade M, Domich L, Oakson G, et al. The deafferented reticularis thalami nucleus generates spindle rhythmicity. J Neurophysiol. 1987;57:260–273.

14. Steriade M, Deschênes M, Domich L, et al. Abolition of spindle oscillations in thalamic neurons disconnected from nucleus reticularis thalami. J Neurophysiol. 1985;54:1473–1497.

15. Timofeev I, Contreras D, Steriade M. Synaptic responsiveness of cortical and thalamic neurones during various phases of slow sleep oscillation in cat. J Physiol (Lond). 1996;494:265–278.

16. Villablanca J. Role of the thalamus in sleep control: sleep-wakefulness studies in chronic diencephalic and athalamic cats. In: Petre-Quadens O, Schlag J, eds. Basic Sleep Mechanisms. New York, NY: Academic Press; 1974:51–81.

17. Amzica F, Steriade M. The K-complex: its slow (<1 Hz) rhythmicity and relation to delta waves. Neurology. 1997;49:952–959.

18. Leresche N, Jassik-Gerschenfeld D, Haby M, et al. Pacemaker-like and other types of spontaneous membrane potential oscillations of thalamocortical cells. Neurosci Lett. 1990;113:72–77.

19. McCormick DA, Pape HC. Properties of a hyperpolarization-activated cation current and its role in rhythmic oscillation in thalamic relay neurones. J Physiol (Lond). 1990;431:291–318.

20. Steriade M, Curró Dossi R, Nuñez A. Network modulation of a slow intrinsic oscillation of cat thalamocortical neurons implicated in sleep delta waves: cortical potentiation and brainstem cholinergic suppression. J Neurosci. 1991;11:200–217.

21. Steriade M, McCarley RW. Brainstem Control of Wakefulness and Sleep. New York, NY: Plenum Press; 1990.

22. Steriade M, Amzica F. Coalescence of sleep rhythms and their chronology in corticothalamic networks. Sleep Res Online [serial online]. 1998;1:1–10. Available at: http://www.sro.org/1998/Steriade/1/. Accessed November 25, 1999.

23. Steriade M, Datta S, Paré D, et al. Neuronal activities in brainstem cholinergic nuclei related to tonic activation processes in thalamocortical systems. J Neurosci. 1990;10:2541–2559.

24. Contreras D, Steriade M. Cellular basis of EEG slow rhythms: a study of dynamic corticothalamic relationships. J Neurosci. 1995;15:604–622.

25. Achermann P, Borbély AA. Low-frequency (<1 Hz) oscillations in the human sleep EEG. Neuroscience. 1997;81:213–222.

26. Timofeev I, Steriade M. Low-frequency rhythms in the thalamus of intact-cortex and decorticated cats. J Neurophysiol. 1996;76:4152–4168.

27. Amzica F, Steriade M. Disconnection of intracortical synaptic linkages disrupts synchronization of a slow oscillation. J Neurosci. 1995;15:4658–4677.

28. Contreras D, Timofeev I, Steriade M. Mechanisms of long-lasting hyperpolarizations underlying slow sleep oscillations in cat corticothalamic networks. J Physiol (Lond). 1996;494:251–264.

29. Steriade M, Contreras D, Curró Dossi R, et al. The slow (<1 Hz) oscillation in reticular thalamic and thalamocortical neurons: scenario of sleep rhythm generation in interacting thalamic and neocortical networks. J Neurosci. 1993;13:3284–3299.

30. Bremer F. Cerveau "isolé" et physiologie du sommeil. C R Soc Biol (Paris). 1935;118:1235–1241.

31. Jones BE, Harper ST, Halaris AE. Effects of locus coeruleus lesions upon cerebral monoamine content, sleep-wakefulness states and the response to amphetamine in the cat. Brain Res. 1977;124:473–496.

32. Paré D, Smith Y, Parent A, et al. Projections of brainstem core cholinergic and non-cholinergic neurons of cat to intralaminar and reticular thalamic nuclei. Neuroscience. 1988;25:69–86.

33. Smith Y, Paré D, Deschênes M, et al. Cholinergic and non-cholinergic projections from the upper brainstem core to the visual thalamus in the cat. Exp Brain Res. 1988;70:166–180.

34. Steriade M, Paré D, Parent A, et al. Projections of cholinergic and non-cholinergic neurons of the brainstem core to relay and associational thalamic nuclei in the cat and macaque monkey. Neuroscience. 1988;25:47–67.

35. Curró Dossi R, Paré D, Steriade M. Short-lasting nicotinic and long-lasting muscarinic depolarizing responses of thalamocortical neurons to stimulation of mesopontine cholinergic nuclei. J Neurophysiol. 1991;65:393–406.

36. Eysel UT, Pape HC, Van Schayck R. Excitatory and differential disinhibitory actions of acetylcholine in the lateral geniculate nucleus of the cat. J Physiol (Lond). 1986;370:233–254.

37. Steriade M, Deschênes M. Intrathalamic and brainstem-thalamic networks involved in resting and alert states. In: Bentivoglio M, Spreafico R, eds. Cellular Thalamic Mechanisms. Amsterdam, Netherlands: Elsevier; 1988:51–76.

38. Hu B, Steriade M, Deschênes M. The effects of brainstem peribrachial stimulation on reticular thalamic neurons: the blockage of spindle waves. Neuroscience. 1989;31:1–12.

39. McCormick DA, Prince DA. Acetylcholine induces burst firing in thalamic reticular neurones by activating a K+ conductance. Nature. 1986;319:147–165.

40. Steriade M, Sakai K, Jouvet M. Bulbothalamic neurons related to thalamocortical activation processes during paradoxical sleep. Exp Brain Res. 1984;54:463–475.

41. Krnjevic K. Chemical nature of synaptic transmission in vertebrates. Physiol Rev. 1974;54:418–540.

42. Jones BE, Beaudet A. Retrograde labeling of neurons in the brain stem following injections of (^{3}H)choline into the forebrain of the rat. Exp Brain Res. 1987;65:437–448.

43. Woolf NJ, Butcher LL. Cholinergic systems in the rat brain, III: projections from the pontomesencephalic tegmentum to the thalamus, tectum, basal ganglia and basal forebrain. Brain Res Bull. 1986;16:603–637.

44. Steriade M, Parent A, Paré D, et al. Cholinergic and non-cholinergic neurons of cat basal forebrain project to reticular and mediodorsal thalamic nuclei. Brain Res. 1987;408:372–376.

45. Singer W. Synchronization of cortical activity and its putative role in information processing and learning. Ann Rev Physiol. 1993;55:349–374.

46. Steriade M. Synchronized activities of coupled oscillators in the cerebral cortex and thalamus at different levels of vigilance. Cereb Cortex. 1997;7:583–604.

47. Evarts EV, Shinoda Y, Wise SP. Neurophysiological Approaches to Higher Brain Functions. New York, NY: John Wiley & Sons; 1984.

48. Carli G, Diete-Spiff K, Pompeiano O. Presynaptic and postsynaptic inhibition of transmission of somatic afferent volleys through the cuneate nucleus during sleep. Arch Ital Biol. 1967;105:52–82.

49. Livingstone MS, Hubel DH. Effects of sleep and arousal on the processing of visual information in the cat. Nature. 1981;291:554–561.

50. Evarts EV. Photically evoked responses in visual cortex units during sleep and waking. J Neurophysiol. 1963;26:229–248.

51. Foote SL, Bloom FE, Aston-Jones G. Nucleus locus coeruleus: new evidence of anatomical and physiological specificity. Physiol Rev. 1983;63:844–914.

52. Madison DV, Nicoll RA. Actions of noradrenaline recorded intracellularly in rat hippocampal CA1 pyramidal neurones, in vitro. J Physiol (Lond). 1986;72:221–244.

53. Mountcastle VB, Andersen RA, Motter BC. The influence of attentive fixation upon the excitability of the light-sensitive neurons of the posterior parietal cortex. J Neurosci. 1981;1:1218–1235.

54. Hyvärinen J, Poranen A, Jokinen Y. Influence of attentive behavior on neuronal responses to vibration in primary somatosensory cortex of the monkey. J Neurophysiol. 1980;43:870–882.

55. Desmedt JE, Bourguet M. Color imaging of parietal and frontal somatosensory potential fields evoked by stimulation of median or posterior tibial nerve in man. Electroencephalogr Clin Neurophysiol. 1985;62:1–17.

56. Desmedt JE, Huy NT, Bourguet M. The cognitive P40, N60 and P100 components of somatosensory evoked potentials and the earliest electrical signs of sensory processing in man. Electroencephalogr Clin Neurophysiol. 1983;56:272–282.

57. Jung R. Neuronal integration in the visual cortex and its significance for visual information. In: Rosenblith WA, ed. Sensory Communication. New York, NY: John Wiley & Sons; 1961:627–674.

58. MacKay DM, Jeffreys DA. Visually evoked potentials and visual perception in man. In: Jung R, ed. Handbook of Sensory Physiology. Vol 7/3/B. Berlin, Germany: Springer; 1973:647–678.

59. Hikosaka O, Wurtz RH. Visual and oculomotor function of monkey substantia nigra pars reticulata, IV: relation of substantia nigra to superior colliculus. J Neurophysiol. 1983;49:1285–1301.

60. Graybiel AM, Ragsdale CW. Fiber connections of the basal ganglia. In: Cuenod M, Kreutzberg GW, Bloom FR, eds. Development and Chemical Specificity of Neurons. Amsterdam, Netherlands: Elsevier;1979:239–283.

61. Ito K, McCarley RW. Alterations in membrane potential and excitability of cat medial pontine reticular formation neurons during changes in naturally occurring sleep-wake states. Brain Res. 1984;292:169–175.

62. Glenn LL, Hada J, Roy JP, et al. Anterograde tracer and field potential analysis of the neocortical layer I projection from nucleus ventralis medialis of the thalamus in cat. Neuroscience. 1982;7:1861–1877.

63. Nelson JP, McCarley RW, Hobson JA. REM sleep burst neurons, PGO waves, and eye movement information. J Neurophysiol. 1983;50:784–797.

64. Hobson JA, Steriade M. Neuronal basis of behavioral state control. In: Mountcastle V, Bloom FE, eds. Handbook of Physiology. Vol 4. Bethesda, Md: American Physiological Society; 1986:701–823.

65. Sakai K. Anatomical and physiological basis of paradoxical sleep. In: McGinty DA, Morrison A, Drucker-Colin R, et al, eds. Brain Mechanisms of Sleep. New York, NY: Raven; 1985:111–137.

66. Steriade M, Paré D, Datta S, et al. Different cellular types in mesopontine cholinergic nuclei related to ponto-geniculo-occipital waves. J Neurosci. 1990;10:2560–2579.

67. Liu XB, Warren RA, Jones EG. Synaptic distribution of afferents from reticular nucleus in ventroposterior nucleus of cat thalamus. J Comp Neurol. 1995;352:187–202.

68. Steriade M, Domich L, Oakson G. Reticularis thalamic neurons revisited: activity changes during shifts in states of vigilance. J Neurosci. 1986;6:68–81.

69. Steriade M, Jones EG, McCormick DA. Organisation and Function. Oxford, England: Elsevier; 1997. Thalamus; vol 1.

70. Steriade M, Deschênes M. Inhibitory processes and interneuronal apparatus in motor cortex during sleep and waking, II: recurrent and afferent inhibition of pyramidal tract neurons. J Neurophysiol. 1974;37:1093–1113.

71. Sillito AM, Kemp JA. Cholinergic modulation of the functional organization of the cat visual cortex. Brain Res. 1983;289:143–155.

72. Sillito AM, Kemp JA, Berardi N. The cholinergic influence on the function of the cat dorsal lateral geniculate nucleus (dLGN). Brain Res. 1983;280:299–307.

73. Curró Dossi R, Paré D, Steriade M. Various types of inhibitory postsynaptic potentials in anterior thalamic cells are differentially altered by stimulation of laterodorsal tegmental cholinergic nucleus. Neuroscience. 1992;47:279–289.

9

Brainstem Mechanisms Generating REM Sleep

Jerome M. Siegel

Rapid eye movement (REM) sleep was first identified by its most obvious behavior: rapid eye movements during sleep. In most adult mammals the electroencephalogram (EEG) of the neocortex is low in voltage during REM sleep. The hippocampus has regular high-voltage theta waves throughout REM sleep.

The key brain structure for generating REM sleep is the brainstem, particularly the pons and adjacent portions of the midbrain. These areas contain cells that are maximally active in REM sleep, called REM-on cells, and cells that are minimally active in REM sleep, called REM-off cells. Subgroups of REM-on cells use the transmitter gamma-aminobutyric acid (GABA), acetylcholine, glutamate, or glycine. Subgroups of brainstem REM-off cells use the transmitter norepinephrine, epinephrine, or serotonin. It is likely that interactions between REM-on and REM-off cells control the key phenomena of REM sleep.

Destruction of the entire area of midbrain and pons responsible for REM sleep generation can prevent the occurrence of this state. Damage to portions of the brainstem can cause abnormalities in certain aspects of REM sleep. Of particular interest are manipulations that affect the regulation of muscle tone within REM sleep. Lesions in the pons and medulla cause REM sleep to occur without the normal loss of muscle tone. In REM sleep without atonia animals exhibit locomotor activity, appear to attack imaginary objects, and execute other motor programs during a state that otherwise resembles REM sleep. This syndrome may have some commonalties with the REM sleep behavior disorder seen in humans. Stimulation of portions of the REM sleep–controlling area of the pons can produce a loss of muscle tone in waking. This phenomenon may have some relevance to cataplexy, *the loss of muscle tone seen in narcoleptics, as well as to the muscle tone reductions that underlie sleep apnea.*

The functions of REM sleep remain unknown. However, it is likely that these functions will emerge in studies of the effects of REM sleep on neuronal structure and metabolism.

REM (rapid eye movement) sleep is the state in which our most vivid dreams occur. For this reason the elucidation of its function has been the goal of some of the greatest ancient and modern thinkers. The modern era of sleep research, resulting from the physiological identification of the REM sleep state in man and animals, has added a new dimension to this search. Although modern sleep researchers have offered additional, physiologically based theories of REM sleep function, the adaptive function of this state remains unclear. However, tremendous progress has been made since the 1960s in understanding the mechanism producing REM sleep. Because function and mechanism questions ultimately merge, it seems likely that the further exploration of the physiology of REM sleep will, within the next few decades, produce an answer to the age-old question of the function of the "dream state."

WHAT IS REM SLEEP?

REM sleep has also been called *paradoxical sleep, desynchronized sleep, active sleep,* and *dream sleep.* Each of these terms reflects a slightly different emphasis on what its essential, defining features are. In most cases this is merely a semantic issue. However, when one studies a "new" species, works with young or brain-injured animals, or is limited to surface electroencephalogram (EEG) electrodes, the question of definition becomes critical.

In intact, adult humans, REM sleep is identified by the simultaneous presence of a relatively low-voltage (sometimes termed *desynchronized*) cortical EEG, an absence of activity in the antigravity muscles (atonia), and periodic bursts of rapid eye movements.

The REM bursts are often accompanied by changes in respiration and by phasic muscle activity (i.e., twitching of the distal somatic musculature and face). In human infants and in many young animals, *active sleep*—the ontogenetic precursor of the REM sleep state—is not accompanied by a low-voltage cortical EEG or by muscle atonia. In these young animals, it is identified by the muscle twitches and eye movements that recur periodically during sleep.

Studies with deep electrodes have established that whereas the EEG of the neocortex is low in voltage during the REM sleep state, the EEG of the hippocampus is increased in size at a 4- to 10-Hz (theta) frequency (Fig. 9–1, *top*). Theta rhythm is produced by the pyramidal cells of CA1, in the dentate gyrus,[1] and

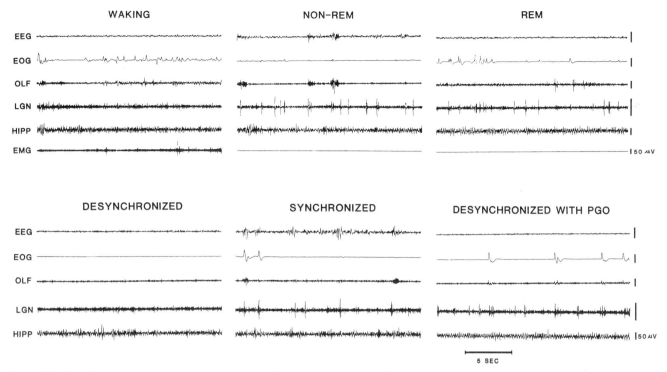

Figure 9–1. *Top,* Polygraph tracings of states seen in the intact cat. *Bottom,* States seen in the forebrain 4 days after transection at the pontomedullary junction. EEG, sensorimotor electroencephalogram; EOG, electro-oculogram; OLF, olfactory bulb; LGN, lateral geniculate nucleus; HIPP, hippocampus; EMG, dorsal neck electromyogram. (From Siegel JM, Nienhuis R, Tomaszewski KS. REM sleep signs rostral to chronic transections at the pontomedullary junction. Neurosci Lett. 1984; 45:241–246.)

in the medial entorhinal cortex.[2] High-voltage hippocampal theta waves can also be observed in active waking, particularly during certain classes of movements, at times when neocortical EEG is low voltage.[3] Another subcortically observed phenomenon characteristic of REM sleep is the ponto-geniculo-occipital (PGO) spike. These waves, which are generated in the pons,[4] propagate rostrally through pathways in the vicinity of the brachium conjunctivum[5, 6] and project through the lateral geniculate and other thalamic nuclei[7] to the cortex. PGO spikes are one of several phasic events of REM sleep. Among the most significant of these phasic events are eye movements, changes in respiration,[8] and irregularities of heart rate.[9]

One phenomenon that is unique to REM sleep is the total loss of activity in the antigravity musculature.[4] In most animals, only the diaphragm and extraocular muscles retain their tone during REM sleep. Although muscle tone may also be reduced in nonrapid eye movement (NREM) sleep, only in REM sleep is tone consistently absent. The atonia of REM sleep may be interrupted by muscle twitches, which accompany bursts of PGO spikes and eye movements.

All of the above-mentioned EEG and electromyographic (EMG) phenomena can be readily explained in terms of changes in neuronal activity. Thus, the low-voltage neocortical EEG results from the asynchronous activity of thalamocortical projection neurons (see Chapter 8). The high-voltage EEG of NREM sleep results from synchronized rhythmical activity in adjacent cortical neurons, at approximately the frequency observed in surface electrodes. Unit activity *rate* does not

change in all cortical regions from NREM sleep to REM sleep, but the *pattern* changes dramatically.[10]

Hippocampal unit activity shows the reverse pattern. In REM sleep, hippocampal, dentate, and entorhinal units become highly synchronized due to inputs from cholinergic and gamma-aminobutyric acid–ergic (GABAergic) cells in the medial septal nucleus.[11–13] This results in the high-voltage 4- to 8-Hz signal recorded across the pyramidal layers.

The loss of activity in antigravity muscles results from a cessation of discharge in the motoneurons supplying these muscles. Intracellular recordings have demonstrated that this cessation is due to a hyperpolarization of the motoneurons. This hyperpolarization is thought to result from the release of glycine onto the motoneurons (see Chapter 11). In addition to active hyperpolarization, a disfacilitation of motoneurons may also occur in REM sleep. Neurons containing serotonin and norepinephrine innervate motoneurons and depolarize (facilitate) them. A loss of serotonergic facilitation in REM sleep may make a major contribution to the REM sleep–related reduction of muscle tone in the hypoglossal nucleus.[14] Aminergic facilitation may have a role in the control of tone in other muscle groups.[15]

WHERE IS REM SLEEP GENERATED?

A powerful technique for localizing function is to divide the brain in half and ask, Which half has the function of interest? If this question can be clearly answered, one can repeat the process, continuing the "half split technique" until the critical area is localized. One might suspect that since brain systems are so thoroughly interconnected, any major subdivision of the brain would so disorganize brain function that REM sleep–like activity would not be present in either half. This is clearly not the case. To an astounding degree, the REM sleep generator mechanisms can survive disconnection from well over 95% of the rest of the central nervous system. Conversely, destruction of a small portion of the brainstem can permanently prevent REM sleep. This characteristic of REM sleep has been demonstrated repeatedly in a number of lesion and transection studies, and has allowed us to achieve a relatively precise localization of the neurons critical to this state.

Transection Studies

One can cut through the midbrain in the coronal plane, so as to separate the brainstem from diencephalic and telencephalic structures. Animals with such lesions can survive for weeks or months. These animals manifest a striking dissociation between states in the forebrain and brainstem as defined by polygraph recording; by transecting the neuraxis, two independent generators of behavioral state are created, one in front of and one behind the transection. When transections are placed at levels A or B in Figure 9–2, all the brainstem signs of REM sleep can be recorded *caudal to the*

cut. Thus, atonia, rapid eye movements, and PGO spike bursts, as well as an REM sleep–like activation of reticular formation units, occur in a regular ultradian rhythm.[4, 16, 17]

A striking phenomenon is that the amount of REM sleep seen after such transections is a function of central temperature. Reducing the body temperature of the pontine cat (i.e., the cat with transections at level A or B in Fig. 9–2) produces a progressive increase in REM sleep. REM sleep constitutes less that 10% of the time at a body temperature of 36°C and 80% at a temperature of 23°C.[18]

The *cerebral cortex* of animals with transections at levels A and B shows both high- and low-voltage states that alternate spontaneously.[19] No PGO spikes are seen in the forebrain. No eye movements or variation in pupil diameter linked to EEG states occurs, because all of the extraocular motor nuclei and the Edinger-Westphal nuclei, controlling pupil diameter, are behind the cut.

REM sleep is present caudal to midbrain transections and absent rostral to such transections. Therefore, one may conclude that structures rostral to the midbrain are not required for REM sleep and that structures caudal to the midbrain are sufficient to generate REM sleep.

Transection at the junction of the spinal cord and medulla (Fig. 9–2, level C) does not prevent the features of REM sleep from occurring rostral to the cut.[19, 20] Atonia in muscles innervated by spinal motoneurons

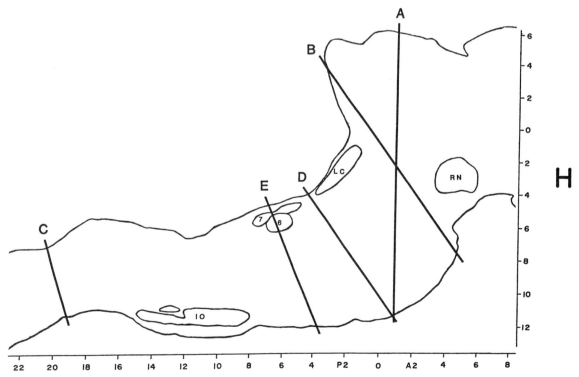

Figure 9–2. Outline of a sagittal section of the brainstem of the cat drawn from level L=1.6 of the Berman atlas[36] indicating the level of key brainstem transection studies. RN, Red nucleus; LC, locus coeruleus; 6, abducens nucleus; 7, genu of the facial nerve; IO, inferior olive. H (horizontal) and A-P (anterior-posterior) scales are drawn from the atlas. (From Siegel JM. Pontomedullary interactions in the generation of REM sleep. In: McGinty DJ, Drucker-Colin R, Morrison A, et al, eds. Brain Mechanisms of Sleep. New York, NY: Raven Press; 1985:157–174.)

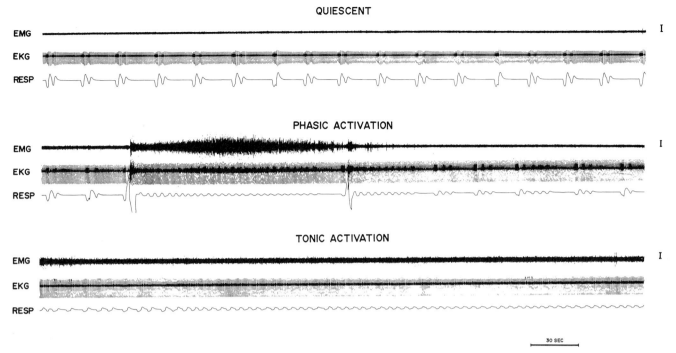

Figure 9–3. States seen in the chronic medullary cat. Note the absence of periods of atonia. EKG, electrocardiogram; EMG, electromyogram; RESP, thoracic strain gauge. Calibration, 50 µV. (From Siegel JM, Tomaszewski KS, Nienhuis R. Behavioral states in the chronic medullary and mid-pontine cat. Electroencephalogr Clin Neurophysiol. 1986;63:274–288.)

is, of course, disrupted by the lesion. Transection of the spinal cord at the midthoracic level in the otherwise intact animal produces the Schiff-Sherrington phenomenon, which interferes with atonia generation, although REM sleep is otherwise normal.[21] Thus, whereas spinal mechanisms interact with rostral structures in the generation of REM sleep atonia, they are not essential to the generation of the REM sleep state itself.

> From the earlier text, we may conclude that structures caudal to the midbrain and rostral to the spinal cord are necessary and sufficient for REM sleep.

This technique has been carried one step further by transecting between the medulla and the pons and maintaining the animals for extended periods to allow the fullest possible recovery from the transection.[22, 23] As was the case with pontine sections, the brain regions rostral and caudal to the cut produce independent, physiologically defined states. The medulla cycles regularly between an activated state and a quiescent state.[23] The activated state is characterized by high levels of muscle tone, similar to those seen in active waking, and by accelerated respiration and heart rate. The quiescent state is characterized by lower levels of muscle tone, resembling those seen in NREM sleep, and by slow, regular respiration. Periods of muscle atonia are never seen (Fig. 9–3). Neuronal activity in the medial medulla during the quiescent state resembles that seen in this region in NREM sleep, that is, it is slow and regular. Neuronal activity during the activated state increases as it does in waking in the intact animal. However, medial medullary neurons do not show the characteristic burst-pause discharge pattern

seen in REM sleep. Therefore, the medulla and spinal cord, disconnected from rostral structures, show spontaneous variations in level of arousal but do not show the medullary signs of REM sleep.

> Structures caudal to the pons are not sufficient to generate REM sleep.

A very different picture is seen in rostral structures after transection between the pons and medulla[22] (Fig. 9–2, level E). Three states can be distinguished rostral to the transection (see Fig. 9–1, bottom). The first is a high-voltage EEG state without PGO spikes, resembling NREM sleep. The second is a low-voltage state without PGO spikes, resembling waking. The third state is a low-voltage state with PGO spikes. The PGO activity occurs in irregular bursts and as isolated spikes in a manner similar to that seen in REM sleep. Midbrain reticular units show irregular burst-pause patterns of discharge in conjunction with this third state, as they do in REM sleep[24] (Fig. 9–4). There are, however, significant differences between this state and the REM sleep state seen in intact animals. In transected animals, the state of PGO spike bursts with low-voltage EEG may last for hours, compared to a maximum of 20 to 30 min for REM sleep in intact cats. Furthermore, rapid eye movements do not consistently accompany the PGO bursts of this state.

Partial transections of the brainstem at approximately this same level produce somewhat different phenomena.[25] Transections of the medial portion of the brainstem reticular formation (up to 5 mm lateral to the midline) produce animals that are capable of thermoregulation,[26] unlike animals with complete transec-

POST–TRANSECTION
DAY 11

UNIT ACTIVITY DURING PGO

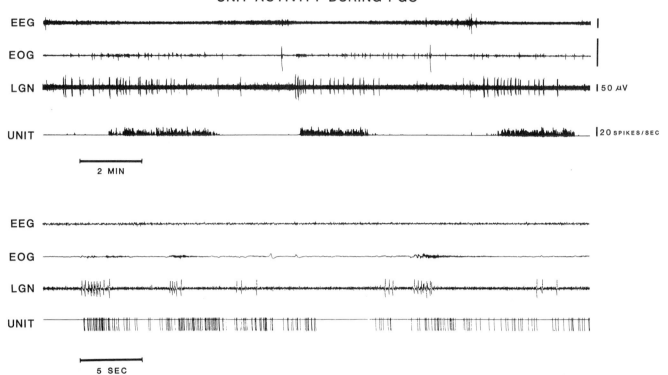

Figure 9–4. Midbrain unit: electroencephalographic (EEG), electro-oculographic (EOG), and lateral geniculate nucleus (LGN) activity rostral to chronic transections at the pontomedullary junction. In the upper portion of the figure, the unit channel displays the output of an integrating digital counter resetting at 1-sec intervals. In the lower portion, one pulse is produced for each spike by a window discriminator. (From Siegel JM. Pontomedullary interactions in the generation of REM sleep. In: McGinty DJ, Drucker-Colin R, Morrison A, et al, eds. Brain Mechanisms of Sleep. New York, NY: Raven Press; 1985:157–174.)

tions. In these animals, PGO spikes with EEG desynchrony (as in REM sleep) are seen in a state with motor activation that behaviorally resembles waking. Responsiveness to the environment is maintained, distinguishing this state from normal REM sleep, whereas the presence of PGO spikes and spike bursts distinguishes this state from normal waking.

From the above one can see that when the pons and caudal midbrain are connected to mid- and forebrain structures, some signs of REM sleep are seen in these rostral structures. When the pons and caudal midbrain are connected to the medulla and spinal cord, as in the midbrain decerebrate animal, the defining signs of REM sleep are seen in caudal structures.

One can then transect through the middle of the pons (Fig. 9–2, level D) and again ask the question, Which side has REM sleep?[22, 27] After this transection, the caudal pons and medulla cycle between the aroused and quiescent states seen in the medullary animal.[28] No atonia or other signs of REM sleep are present. The forebrain EEG shows low-voltage, waking-like states and high-voltage, NREM sleep–like states. Eye movements that can be used to help identify sleep-wake states in the forebrain are limited to those

that can be generated by the oculomotor nucleus. This is because the abducens nucleus is caudal to the cut (the trochlear nucleus and nerve are usually damaged by such a transection). The EEG of the forebrain shows an irregular alternation of high-voltage and low-voltage states. However, the low-voltage states are not accompanied by spontaneous rapid eye movements. During low-voltage states, vertical pursuit eye movements and changes in pupil diameter can be evoked by external visual stimuli. However, the stereotyped pattern of spontaneous rapid eye movements with myosis (constriction of the pupil) that characterizes REM sleep is not present.[29] The low-voltage state seen in the rostral portion of these preparations resembles waking.

The high-voltage state in the forebrain may be accompanied by PGO spikes and PGO spike bursts. However, midbrain unit activity is greatly *decreased* at these times, directly the opposite of the pattern seen in REM sleep in the intact animal and in animals transected at the pontomedullary junction. PGO spikes do not occur in the low-voltage state. Therefore, with this midpontine transection we have reached the limit of the transection technique. The major defining characteristics of the REM sleep state are absent on both sides of the transection, even in chronically maintained animals, although some aspects of REM sleep are present.

Although the foregoing indicates that the caudal pons and adjacent midbrain are necessary for the generation of REM sleep–like states in both rostral and caudal structures, one may ask if this region is in and of itself sufficient to generate the mesopontine aspects of REM sleep. One can monitor REM sleep signs after transecting *both* rostral and caudal to the pons, producing an isolated "pons-caudal midbrain" preparation[30] (see Fig. 9–2, levels B and E). In this case, the pons generates periodic episodes of rapid eye movements and PGO spikes in a pattern which, in the intact animal, is seen only in REM sleep. Neuronal activity has not been monitored in this preparation. However, the presence of PGO spikes and rapid eye movements in a REM sleep–like pattern is impressive evidence of the pontine control of these basic aspects of REM sleep.

> From the previous text, we can conclude that the pons and the caudal midbrain region are both necessary and sufficient to generate some of the basic phenomena of REM sleep.

Pontine Anatomy and Nomenclature

Several different systems for naming the nuclei of the brainstem reticular formation (RF) have been developed. Different physiologists have employed different naming systems in describing their work, resulting in much unnecessary confusion and controversy. I briefly review some of the major naming systems applied to the brainstem and how they relate to each other. I then present the results of studies attempting to further localize REM sleep–generating functions within the pons and caudal midbrain reticular formation.

The simplest nomenclature system divides the brainstem RF into the midbrain, pontine, and medullary regions. On the ventral surface of the human brainstem there is universal agreement on the meaning of these terms. The cerebral peduncles define the midbrain; the basilar pons defines the pons. The medulla is the region between the pons and the spinal cord, its caudal boundary being defined by the decussation of the pyramidal tracts and the appearance of the C1 ventral root. Dorsally, the caudal limit of the inferior colliculus defines the caudal boundary of the midbrain. The dorsal boundary between the pons and the medulla, a critical point for descriptions of REM sleep–generating mechanisms, is less clearly defined. In the human brain, the dorsal pons is commonly considered to include the abducens nucleus, the vestibular and cochlear nuclei, the facial nucleus, and all adjacent reticular nuclei.[31] The medulla encompasses the regions caudal to these landmarks. This usage has not been consistently followed in the cat. In some studies in the cat, the abducens nucleus has been considered to mark the caudalmost portion of the pons, with the vestibular, cochlear, and facial nuclei considered to be in the medulla. Therefore, it is critical to describe where the area of interest is located with respect to the abducens and caudal cranial nerve nuclei, rather than using the terms *pons* or *medulla*. Even less clear is the boundary between the *medial* and *lateral* reticular formations. There is no landmark to divide the RF in this way. Common usage in the cat is to reserve the term "medial" for the region from the midline to 2 mm lateral to the midline.

An alternate nomenclature system, going from rostral to caudal, divides the core of the brainstem RF, into the midbrain RF, nucleus reticularis pontis oralis (RPO), nucleus reticularis pontis caudalis (RPC), and nucleus gigantocellularis (NGC) of the medulla. As used by Brodal,[32] the RPO begins at the rostral limit of the pons and is devoid of giant cells. The RPC is immediately caudal to the RPO and contains giant cells. There is no cranial nerve landmark defining the boundary between these nuclei. However, one of the most widely used atlases of the cat brainstem[33] places the junction at the level of the dorsal tegmental nucleus. The uncertainty over the definition of the RPO can be seen in the conflicting descriptions given by different authors working with the cat brain. The Snider and Niemer[33] atlas has the rostral boundary of RPO at 2.5 mm anterior to stereotactic zero, while Carli and Zanchetti[34] give it as 1.0 mm anterior to zero, and the Reinoso-Suarez[35] atlas has the rostral boundary at 2.0 mm posterior to zero. The junction of the RPC and NGC is at the level of the abducens nucleus, although this usage is also not universally followed. The caudal limit of the NGC is at the most rostral extension of the hypoglossal nucleus.

A third system for subdividing the RF was originated by Berman.[36] This nomenclature replaces the term *nucleus* with *field*. Thus, the terms *gigantocellular tegmental field* (FTG), *lateral tegmental field* (FTL), and *magnocellular tegmental field* (FTM) were coined. This nomenclature has only been defined for the cat, and these terms *do not correspond* to either of the terminologies described above. The FTG comprises the medial portions of the RPC and the rostral tip of the NGC. Most of its area is *not* coincident with the NGC, with which it is often confused. The FTL runs all the way from the most caudal portions of the medulla to the RPC. The FTM refers to the ventral portion of the NGC.

As research has focused on portions of the RF adjacent to the locus coeruleus nucleus, a more detailed anatomical nomenclature has come into use to describe this region.[37] The locus coeruleus proper is within the clearly defined central gray region. Immediately ventral and somewhat lateral to the caudal locus coeruleus is a region termed the *nucleus subcoeruleus*.[37] Ventral to the locus coeruleus and dorsomedial to the subcoeruleus is the locus coeruleus α. The term *peri–locus coeruleus* α has been coined to describe regions ventral to the locus coeruleus α.[38]

Much of the confusion in the literature about REM sleep–generating mechanisms has resulted from the inconsistent use of these various terminologies. Indeed, the only reliable way to evaluate and integrate new findings is to carefully inspect the actual histology or refer to atlas coordinates.[33, 36] In this chapter, I have brought together findings from a number of laboratories, and mapped them all on the Berman[36] cat atlas plates for comparison (see Figs. 9–2, 9–5, 9–7, 9–9, 9–11, 9–12, and 9–13).

Lesion Studies

In an attempt to further localize the neurons generating REM sleep, a number of investigators have damaged portions of the pons and caudal midbrain within the region defined as critical by transection studies. The first comprehensive study of this problem[34] found that electrolytic lesions that destroyed the bulk of the RPO permanently eliminated REM sleep. Further work has confirmed this finding while providing a greater localization of the critical neurons. Following the development of techniques that permitted the localization of catecholamine neurons, much research interest was focused on the noradrenergic locus coeruleus, dorsal to the region identified by Carli and Zanchetti. Although Carli and Zanchetti had concluded that locus coeruleus lesions did not block REM sleep, a study by Jouvet and Delorme[39] found that lesions of this structure did prevent REM sleep. This was disputed in further investigations.[40, 41] Depletion of norepinephrine and relatively selective destruction of norepinephrine neurons with 6-hydroxydopamine also did not prevent

REM sleep.[42] Thus, the consensus of subsequent studies, in agreement with the original findings of Carli and Zanchetti, is that the norepinephrine cells of the locus coeruleus are not critical for REM sleep.

There has been some uncertainty regarding the laterality of the region critical for REM sleep. Carli and Zanchetti's[34] lesions that blocked REM sleep included both medial and lateral RPO. One study suggested that the medial RF (i.e., within 2 mm of the midline in the cat) was critical.[43] However, further studies by the same group and by the Lyon group have concluded that the lateral rather than the medial regions of RPO are critical[44-46] (Fig. 9–5). This small region might be critical either because it contains the somas of cells involved in REM sleep generation, or because major axonal pathways traverse this region. These possibilities can be distinguished by using the cytotoxin kainic acid to remove cells in this region. Using these techniques, it was found that extensive lesions of RPO disrupted REM sleep even with minimal axonal damage. The loss of REM sleep produced by the lesions was proportional to the number of cholinergic cells removed, but was

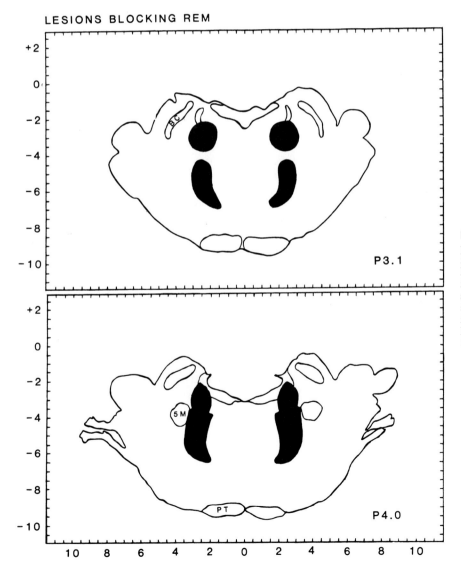

LESIONS BLOCKING REM

Figure 9–5. Pontine lesions producing a complete suppression of REM sleep. (Redrawn from Brain Research, vol 229, Sastre JP, Sakai H, Jouvet M, Are the gigantocellular tegmental field neurons responsible for paradoxical sleep? 147–161, Copyright 1981, with permission from Elsevier Science; coordinates derived from Berman AL. The Brain Stem of the Cat. Madison, Wisc: University of Wisconsin Press; 1968.)

not related to the number of noradrenergic cells lost.[46] Therefore, cholinergic and perhaps other cell types yet to be identified within this region are critical.

To summarize, the lateral region (L2–4 in the cat) of the RPO, ventral to the locus coeruleus, is the brain region most critical for REM sleep.

Unit Recording Studies

Guided by the lesion data, researchers have recorded from the pons to observe the activity of neuronal elements that might be involved in REM sleep generation.

Medial Pontine Reticular Cells

A number of studies have focused on the medial pontine region first implicated in REM sleep control by lesion studies. Cells in this area were found to have very high discharge rates in REM sleep but were silent or had relatively low discharge rates in NREM sleep.[47, 48] In cats that were well adapted to the head restraint employed in the recording sessions, medial pontine reticular cells have little activity in waking, discharging at rates comparable to those seen in NREM sleep.[47] However, in freely moving cats, virtually all medial pontine RF cells discharge in waking at rates comparable to mean REM sleep rates.[49, 50] Discharge rates during REM sleep are positively correlated with active waking rates.[51] Studies in the awake, freely moving animal have revealed that most medial reticular cells discharge maximally in conjunction with a directionally specific movement of either the head, neck, eyes, limbs, or facial musculature.[22, 52] One would expect centrally commanded skeletal movements (whose expression in REM sleep is blocked by motoneuron hyperpolarization) to accompany the REM bursts and muscle twitches of REM sleep. Thus, the apparent "selectivity" of discharge in medial reticular cells for REM sleep in cats adapted to head restraint can be seen as a consequence of the reduction in waking motor activity caused by the restraint, rather than indicating any selective role for these cells in REM sleep control.[53] This conclusion was confirmed by studies showing no disruption of REM sleep when cytotoxins were injected into this region. Even though this manipulation removed almost all cells in the medial pontine FTG region, REM sleep was not disturbed, appearing in normal amounts within 24 h of the lesion.[44, 45] However, these lesions did greatly reduce head movement.[54]

Lateral Pontine and Medial Medullary Reticular Cells

A different picture has emerged in unit recordings from the lateral pontine and the medial medullary reticular formation. Many cells in these regions have discharge profiles similar to those seen in the medial pontine regions. However, these areas also contain a population of cells that discharge at a high rate

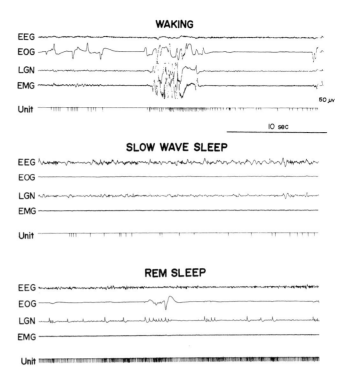

Figure 9–6. Activity of medullary "REM sleep-on" cell. Note the tonic activity during REM sleep. In waking, activity is generally absent even during vigorous movement. However, some activity is seen during movements involving head lowering and postural relaxation. (From Siegel JM, Wheeler RL, McGinty DJ. Activity of medullary reticular formation neurons in the unrestrained cat during waking and sleep. Brain Res. 1979;179:49–60.)

throughout REM sleep and that have little or no activity in NREM sleep.[55–58] In waking, these cells are generally silent, even during vigorous movement; however, some become active during head lowering and related postural changes that involve reductions of tone in a number of muscles[56] (Fig. 9–6). The pontine REM sleep-on cells are distributed throughout the lateral region implicated by lesion studies in REM sleep control[58, 59] (Fig. 9–7). This distribution is significant because it indicates that the critical lesion removes the somas of cells that are selectively active in REM sleep. Unit recording studies have found that whereas some of the REM sleep-on cells may release acetylcholine, many are not cholinergic.[55, 58, 60] However, it is likely that most respond to acetylcholine (i.e., are cholinoceptive). The medullary REM sleep-on cells are located in an area receiving projections from the pontine REM sleep-on region.[61] The neurochemistry of this medial medullary region is discussed next. It is likely that many of the medial medullary and pontine REM sleep-on cells use amino acid transmitters, such as glycine or GABA, as well as peptides.

Noradrenergic Cells of the Locus Coeruleus Complex and Serotonergic Cells of the Raphe System

Cells in both of these regions have a similar discharge pattern during the sleep-waking cycle. During

REM ON CELLS

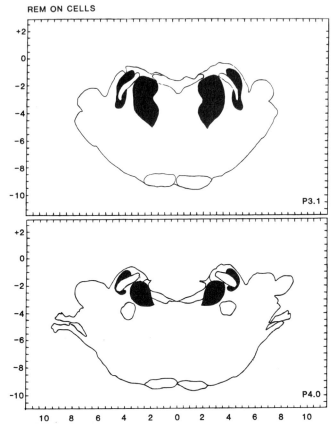

Figure 9–7. Location of pontine "REM sleep-on" cells. (Redrawn from Sakai K. Some anatomical and physiological properties of pontomesencephalic tegmental neurons with special reference to the PGO waves and postural atonia during paradoxical sleep in the cat. In: Hobson JA, Brazier MAB, eds. The Reticular Formation Revisited. New York, NY: Raven Press; 1980:427–447; and from Brain Research Bulletin, vol 18, Shiromani PJ, Armstrong DM, Bruce G, et al, Relation of pontine choline acetyltransferase immunoreactive neurons with cells which increase discharge during REM sleep, 447–455, Copyright 1987, with permission from Elsevier Science.)

waking, discharge is regular (Fig. 9–8), in contrast to the movement-related burst-pause discharge pattern seen in most medial reticular neurons. During the initial stages of NREM sleep, norepinephrine- and serotonin-containing cells slow slightly. During the *transition to REM sleep* (defined in the cat as the time at which PGO spikes begin appearing), discharge in both serotonergic and noradrenergic cells slows dramatically. During REM sleep, these cells have their lowest discharge rates and many are completely silent.[62–65] The slowing of discharge in these cells in NREM sleep suggests that reduced release of serotonin or norepinephrine plays a permissive role in the initiation of NREM sleep.[66, 67] However, as mentioned above, lesion studies have shown that destruction of locus coeruleus neurons does not prevent or cause substantial increases in REM sleep. The minimal discharge rate of these cells in REM sleep suggests some role in the "gating" of aspects of REM sleep. When we discuss PGO spike control below, we review the very impressive evidence that serotonergic cells regulate PGO spikes. The role of

serotonergic and noradrenergic cells in facilitation of muscle tone is discussed under Muscle Atonia, later. The possible relation of the cessation of activity in locus coeruleus and raphe cells to the function of REM sleep is discussed in the conclusion to this chapter.

The tonic discharge of aminergic cells in waking, and even in some circumstances in vitro, suggests that active inhibition is involved in their cessation of activity in REM sleep. We have found that the release of GABA, an inhibitory amino acid, is increased in both the raphe and the locus coeruleus nuclei during REM sleep.[68, 69] Microinjection of the GABA agonist muscimol into the serotonergic raphe nucleus increases REM sleep amounts, indicating that the cessation of discharge in aminergic neurons can facilitate REM sleep.[68] Electrophysiological studies show that locus coeruleus neurons are tonically inhibited by GABA during sleep.[70] Studies using the labeling of *c-fos*, a transcription regulator whose expression is often increased when cells discharge more rapidly, show increased labeling of some cholinergic cells in REM sleep.[71] There is also substantial labeling of noncholinergic cells.[71a, 72] Further studies are needed to determine if the labeled cells contain GABA, glutamate, peptides, or other transmitters.

Figure 9–9 presents maps summarizing current knowledge about the localization of REM sleep-off cells. Figure 9–10 summarizes current findings on the localization of cholinergic and catecholaminergic neurons within the pons.

We can describe the present state of our knowledge

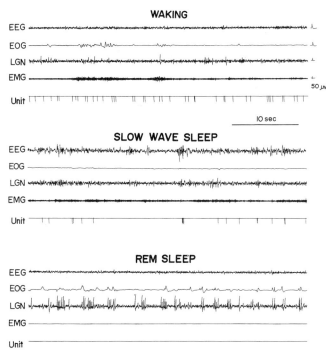

Figure 9–8. Activity of a "REM sleep-off" cell recorded in the locus coeruleus. (From Siegel JM. REM sleep control mechanisms: evidence from lesion and unit recording studies. In: Mayes A, ed. Sleep Mechanisms and Functions. New York, NY: Van Nostrand Reinhold; 1983.)

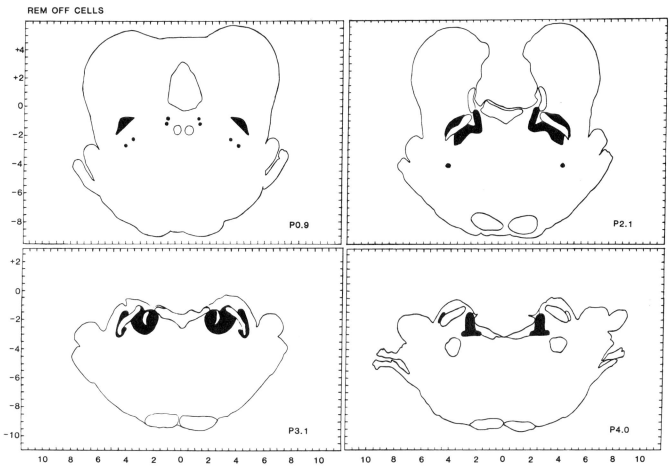

Figure 9–9. Location of "REM sleep-off" cells. (Redrawn from Sakai K. Some anatomical and physiological properties of pontomesencephalic tegmental neurons with special reference to the PGO waves and postural atonia during paradoxical sleep in the cat. In: Hobson JA, Brazier MAB, eds. The Reticular Formation Revisited. New York, NY: Raven Press; 1980:427–447.)

about the localization of mechanisms generating REM sleep as follows. Transection studies have determined that the caudal midbrain and the pons are sufficient to generate much of the phenomenology of REM sleep. Lesion studies have identified a region in the caudal midbrain and the pontine tegmentum, corresponding to lateral portions of the RPO and the region immediately ventral to the locus coeruleus, which is required for REM sleep. Unit recording studies have found a population of cells within this region that are selectively active in REM sleep. It does not appear that this small region is sufficient for REM sleep generation, in the same sense that the suprachiasmatic nucleus is sufficient to generate a circadian signal.[73] Nevertheless, it has become clear that much of the mechanism that drives this very complex behavioral state is localized to the RPO nucleus of the pons and caudal midbrain.

It should be emphasized that in the intact animal many brain regions distant from the pons actively participate in the control of the REM sleep state. Obviously the phenomenology of REM sleep, such as muscle atonia, cortical desynchrony, rapid eye movements, alteration of sensory thresholds, and autonomic changes, requires the recruitment of many brain systems. What is not always appreciated is the subtler role of non-

brainstem systems in shaping the structure of REM sleep. While the decerebrate animal has the basic brainstem physiology of REM sleep, closer inspection reveals substantial differences between the 'REM sleep' of the isolated brainstem and the REM sleep of the intact animal. PGO spikes and associated eye movements in the decerebrate animal come in regular alternating clusters, distinct from the irregular pattern seen in the intact animal.[4, 74] Removal of the cerebellum, while not blocking REM sleep, alters the amplitude of PGO activity.[75, 76] Lesions of the frontal cortex alter the amplitude and the pattern of spiking.[75] PGO spikes are tightly coupled to the eye movements of REM sleep, which in humans are correlated with dream imagery. Stimulation of the amygdala increases REM sleep in cats.[77] The amygdala is the forebrain area most intensely activated in normal, human REM sleep.[78] Therefore, one must not view the rest of the brain as merely a passive responder to a REM sleep state generated in the pons and caudal midbrain. Instead, present evidence suggests a dynamic interaction between the forebrain and the pons in molding the structure and timing of PGO spikes and the other "phasic" events of REM sleep and, in all likelihood, the dream imagery of REM sleep.

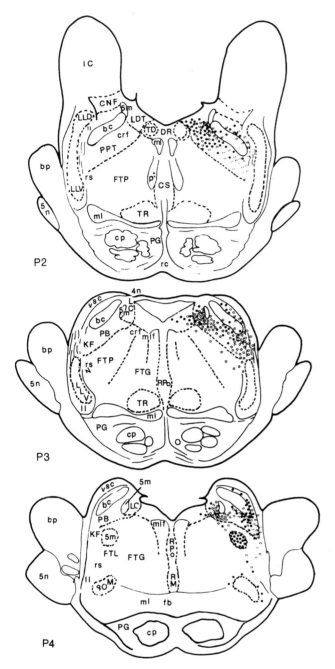

Figure 9–10. Closed circles indicate location of CHAT containing (presumably cholinergic) neurons and open circles the location of tyrosine hydroxylase-containing (presumably noradrenergic) cells in the pons: 4n, 5n, fourth, fifth nerves; 5m, mesencephalic tract of the trigeminal nucleus; BC, brachium conjunctivum; BP, brachium pontis; CNF, cuneiform nucleus; cp, cerebral peduncle; crf, central reticular fasciculus; CS, central superior nucleus; DR, dorsal raphe; FTG, gigantocellular tegmental field; FTL, lateral tegmental field; FTP, paralemniscal tegmental field; IC, inferior colliculus; KF, Kölliker-Fuse nucleus; LDT, laterodorsal tegmental nucleus; LC, locus ceruleus; LLD, LLV, dorsal and ventral nuclei of the lateral lemniscus; ml, medial lemniscus; MLF, medial longitudinal fasciculus; PB, parabrachial nucleus; PPT, pedunculopontine nucleus; PG, pontine gray; RPo, raphe pontis nucleus; rs, rubrospinal nucleus; SO, superior olive: TD, dorsal tegmental nucleus; TR, tegmental reticular nucleus; vsc, ventral spinal cerebellar tract. (From Jones BE, Beaudet A. Distribution of acetylcholine and catecholamine neurons in the cat brain stem. J Comp Neurol. 1987;261:15–32. Reprinted by permission of Wiley-Liss, a division of John Wiley & Sons, Inc.)

DISSOCIATION OF REM SLEEP COMPONENTS

Experimental manipulations and pathological states allow us to further localize and analyze the mechanisms generating REM sleep. Lesion studies have demonstrated that PGO spikes, atonia, and EEG desynchrony can be individually dissociated from the REM sleep state. Conversely, stimulation studies have demonstrated that each of these phenomena can be separately evoked.

Muscle Atonia

REM Sleep Without Atonia

Pontine lesions can produce the syndrome of REM sleep without atonia.[39, 79] The critical lesions for producing this effect are much smaller than those required to block the REM sleep state (Fig. 9–11). Animals with these lesions have relatively normal NREM sleep. During sleep they have periods of low-voltage EEG, rapid eye movements, myosis, and PGO spikes, as seen in normal REM sleep. However, muscle tone is present throughout these periods. Depending on the exact placement of the lesion,[80] the animal's motor activity during this state will range from a slight raising of the head, to elaborate displays of exploratory and aggressive behaviors. The animal remains generally unresponsive to the environment and can be "awakened" by strong stimulation. With incomplete lesions, one may often see a partial syndrome of REM sleep with muscle tone interrupted by periods of atonia, gradually progressing to REM sleep periods with complete atonia over a period of several weeks. These findings leave

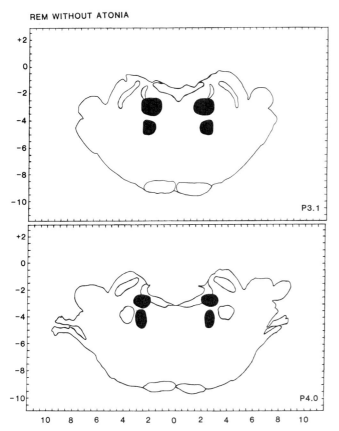

REM WITHOUT ATONIA

P3.1

P4.0

Figure 9–11. Location of lesions producing REM sleep without atonia. (Redrawn from Sakai K. Some anatomical and physiological properties of pontomesencephalic tegmental neurons with special reference to the PGO waves and postural atonia during paradoxical sleep in the cat. In: Hobson JA, Brazier MAB, eds. The Reticular Formation Revisited. New York, NY: Raven Press; 1980:427–447.)

little doubt that REM sleep without atonia is a variant of the normal REM sleep state.

The same syndrome can be produced by lesions of the medial medulla.[81] This finding supports the hypothesis that the output of the atonia systems in the pons is relayed in these regions of the medulla, on its way to the spinal motoneurons. A population of slowly conducting reticulospinal neurons in the nucleus magnocellularis is activated by stimulation that inhibits muscle tone. These neurons may form part of the "final common path" for brainstem atonia.[82]

Atonia Without REM Sleep

Muscle tone can not only be suppressed by stimulation of the medial medulla but also by stimulation of a number of pontine and midbrain areas. These include the ventrally located tegmental reticular fields of the pons, the dorsally located pedunculopontine nuclei,[83] and, most rostrally, the retrorubral nuclei[84] (Fig. 9–12). The systems producing muscle tone suppression constitute a widespread brainstem network.

A loss of muscle tone can be evoked by injection of the cholinergic agonist carbachol or the cholinesterase inhibitor physostigmine into the pons. The region of the RPO where injection produces the most immediate

and complete loss of tone corresponds very well to the region which, when lesioned, results in REM sleep without atonia (Fig. 9–13). Depending on the exact injection site, carbachol may evoke only atonia of the skeletal muscles without the other signs of REM sleep. The animal may demonstrate perception of the outside environment by visually tracking stimuli with its extraocular muscles.[84, 85] Larger injections or injections at other pontine sites can produce the full REM sleep pattern.[87–94] During spontaneous REM sleep, acetylcholine release is increased in the RPO region.[95, 96] Muscarinic receptors are responsible for the cholinergic induction of REM sleep signs in the pons, with M2, M3, and other "non-M1" receptors being particularly important.[97–100] Cholinergic cells in the pons also synthesize nitric oxide, and microinjection of nitric oxide agonists into the pons increases REM sleep amounts, whereas antagonists suppress REM sleep.[101] The neurons critical for inducing REM sleep also respond to local microinjections of nerve growth factor.[102] Injection of glutamate at pontine sites where cholinergic agonists are effective also produces atonia[103] and REM sleep.[104]

> Thus a coordinated release of glutamate, acetylcholine, nitric oxide, and other transmitters into the dorsal pons (nucleus RPO) can trigger REM sleep or, depending on injection site and agonist dosage, just produce muscle atonia.

A second area in which chemical stimulation can elicit atonia is the medial medulla. Magoun and Rhines[105] first reported that electrical stimulation of this area in the decerebrate cat produces an immediate loss of muscle tone. Glutamate stimulation of the nucleus magnocellularis, the rostral portion of the area identified by Magoun and Rhines, will trigger atonia[103] (Fig. 9–14). During REM sleep, glutamate release is increased in this region.[106] Although glutamate stimulation was effective in the nucleus magnocellularis, acetylcholine stimulation was not. Acetylcholine release is not elevated in this region during REM sleep.[107] However, the situation is reversed in caudal portions of the medial medulla, corresponding to the nucleus paramedianus. Here acetylcholine injection produces a suppression of muscle tone, whereas glutamate does not. Acetylcholine release is elevated in the nucleus paramedianus during REM sleep,[107] but glutamate release is not.[106] Both the nucleus paramedianus and the cholinoceptive regions of the dorsolateral pons were found to receive a projection from cholinergic neurons in the pedunculopontine nucleus of the pons. This region and medullary cholinergic cells are the main sources of the acetylcholine released in the nucleus paramedianus and the dorsal pons in REM sleep.[108–111]

We investigated the nature of the receptor responsible for the suppression of muscle tone after glutamate microinjection. We found that non-NMDA (N-methyl-D-aspartate) glutamate receptors mediated muscle tone suppression in both the pons and the medial medulla.[112] When NMDA glutamate agonists were microinjected at sites where non-NMDA agonists produced atonia, motor excitation and locomotion were

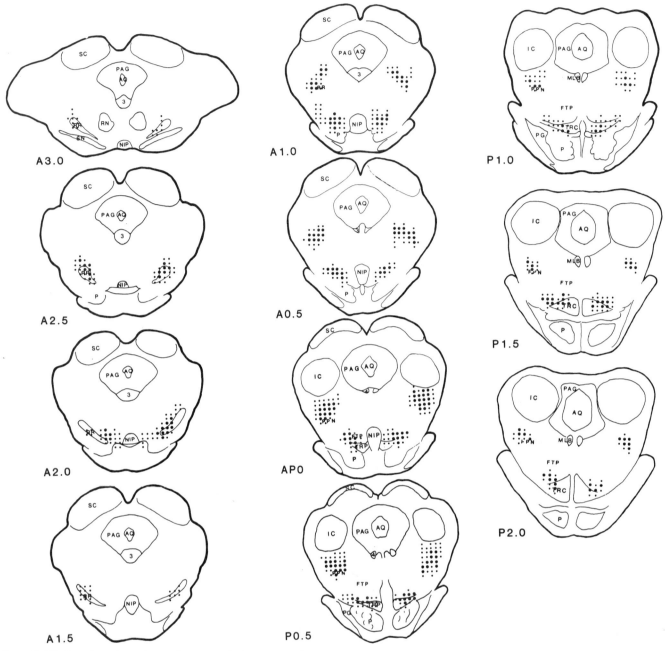

Figure 9–12. Location of pontine and mesencephalic regions whose electrical stimulation produces suppression of muscle tone. Large dots indicate points at which stimulation produces more than 70% inhibition of muscle tone. Widespread pontine and midbrain regions can produce suppression of muscle tone. 4, trochlear nucleus; AQ, aqueduct; IC, inferior colliculus; FTP, paralemniscal tegmental field; MLB, medial longitudinal bundle; NIP, interpeduncular nucleus; P, pyramidal tract; PAG, periaqueductal gray; PG, pontine gray; PPN, pedunculopontine tegmental nucleus; RD, red nucleus; RR, retrorubral nucleus; SC, superior colliculus; SN, substantia nigra; TRC, TRN (tegmental reticular nucleus), central division; TRP, TRN, pericentral division. (From Lai YY, Siegel JM. Muscle tone suppression and stepping produced by stimulation of midbrain and rostral pontine reticular formation. J Neurosci. 1990;10:2727–2734.)

evoked. These opposite effects of the two types of glutamate receptors provide a mechanism for the "paradoxical" motor phenomena of REM sleep: the combination of rapid eye movements and phasic twitching, with the suppression of muscle tone. We hypothesize that release of glutamate in REM sleep activates both receptor types simultaneously, producing the muscle tone suppression of REM sleep and at the same time the motor activation manifested as twitching and rapid

eye movements.[84, 112] Whereas medullary stimulation in the decerebrate cat can produce loss of muscle tone, identical stimulation in the intact animal usually increases muscle tone.[113] Thus, the forebrain in the normal animal seems to contain mechanisms that produce a net inhibition of the brainstem atonia control mechanism. Furthermore, although animals with transections at the midbrain produce atonia when stimulated in the medulla, acute and chronic transection at the pon-

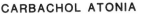

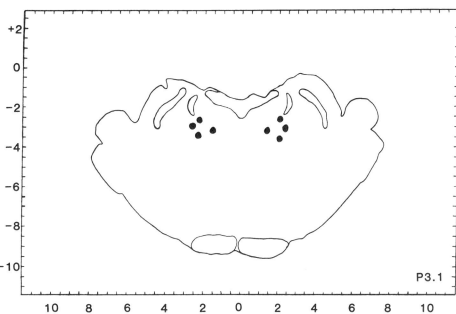

Figure 9–13. Location of pontine sites producing atonia at the shortest latency after carbachol microinjection. (Redrawn from Katayama Y, DeWitt DS, Becker DP, et al. Behavioral evidence for cholinoceptive pontine inhibitory area: descending control of spinal motor output and sensory input. Brain Res. 1984; 296:241–262.)

tomedullary junction greatly reduces atonia elicited by medullary stimulation[22, 81a, 82]; that is, if the pons is removed, the medulla does not readily produce muscle atonia. This indicates that the atonia system is not a simple "one way" descending pathway. In summary, the transection level strongly modulates the effect of medullary activation on muscle atonia. In the intact animal there are mechanisms in the pons and the medulla which contribute to atonia, and mechanisms in the forebrain which block atonia.

In addition to transection level, blood pressure also modulates the tendency toward atonia. Medullary stimulation that produces atonia will produce muscle excitation when blood pressure is lowered by as little as 10 to 20 mmHg.[114]

Cataplexy

Cataplexy, a symptom of narcolepsy, is the sudden loss of muscle tone during active waking, usually triggered by strong emotions or physical activity. Physiologically, it is similar to the "atonia without REM sleep" state mentioned above. Narcoleptic patients are aware of their environment and have a clear memory of all aspects of the cataplexy episode. It is reasonable to hypothesize that one or more of the mechanisms that have been identified as promoting or inhibiting atonia are malfunctioning in narcolepsy. The result is that a stimulus that elicits a strong emotional response, producing arousal in an intact individual, produces cataplexy in the individual with narcolepsy. Cholinergic mechanisms seem to play an important role in cataplexy, as they do in experimental atonia. Physostigmine, a cholinesterase inhibitor, increases cataplexy in narcoleptic dogs, while atropine blocks spontaneously occurring cataplexy in these animals.[115] Narcoleptic dogs have increased numbers of cholinergic receptors in the pons and the medial medulla. Receptors are increased at the same sites where stimulation is effective in producing atonia in the decerebrate preparation.[116] In summary, we can hypothesize that a hypersensitivity of cholinoceptive cells in the pons or the medial medulla, or both, is a factor contributing to cataplectic attacks.

In the narcoleptic dog, we can study the state of cataplexy at the neuronal level. Surprisingly, most brainstem neurons do not behave in a similar way in cataplexy and REM sleep. Whereas most brainstem neurons in the pontine and the medullary RF increase activity during REM sleep, most decrease activity during cataplexy.[117] A specialized group of cells within the nucleus magnocellularis of the medial medulla has selective elevations of discharge rate in both REM sleep and cataplexy.[117] All REM sleep-off (presumably noradrenergic) cells in the locus coeruleus cease discharge immediately prior to and throughout cataplexy episodes.[118]

Locus coeruleus cells receive a massive projection from the hypocretin (also known as orexin) system whose cell bodies are in the lateral hypothalamus. Canine narcolepsy is linked to a mutation of the gene coding for the hypocretin-2 receptor, leading to diminished action of hypocretin in several brain areas.[117a] The loss of function in the hypocretin system reduces activity in the locus coeruleus and possibly in other monoaminergic and cholinergic cell populations. The reduced tonic activation of locus coeruleus can explain cataplexy, linked to loss of locus coeruleus activity. Reduced tonic activation of cholinergic cell populations, which are involved in maintaining cortical arousal, is a possible explanation for the sleepiness that characterizes narcolepsy.[118a]

Both REM sleep and cataplexy are accompanied by a loss of muscle tone. However, awareness of the envi-

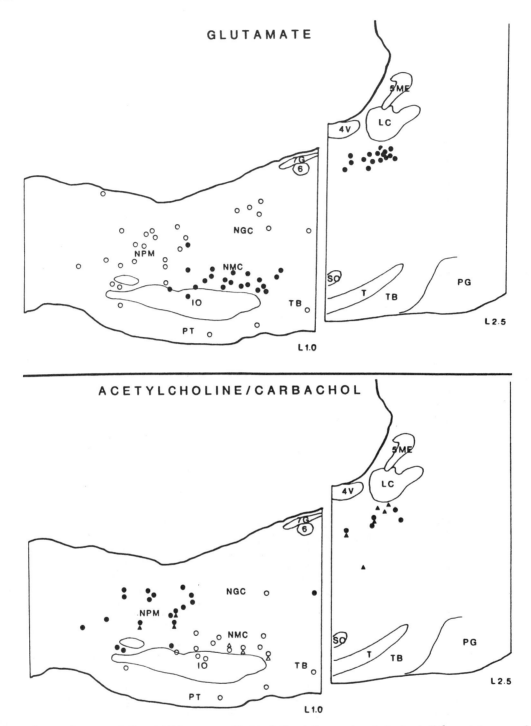

Figure 9–14. Sagittal map of pontomedullary inhibitory areas. Electrical stimulation produced atonia at all the points mapped. All electrically defined inhibitory sites were microinjected with glutamate or cholinergic agonists. Filled symbols represent points at which microinjections decreased muscle tone (to less than 30% of baseline values or to complete atonia). Open circles indicate points at which injections increased or produced no change in baseline values. Glutamate injections are shown at the top, acetylcholine (ACh) and carbachol (Carb) injections at the bottom. At the bottom, circles and triangles represent ACh and Carb injections, respectively. 4V, fourth ventricle; 5ME, mesencephalic trigeminal tract; 6, abducens nucleus; 7G, genu of the facial nerve; IO, inferior olivary nucleus; LC, locus coeruleus nucleus, NGC, nucleus gigantocellularis; NMC, nucleus magnocellularis; NPM, nucleus paramedianus; PG, pontine gray; PT, pyramid tract; SO, superior olivary nucleus; T, nucleus of the trapezoid body; TB, trapezoid body. (From Lai YY, Siegel JM. Medullary regions mediating atonia. J Neurosci. 1988;8:4790–4796.)

ronment is preserved in cataplexy. The complete cessation of discharge in locus coeruleus (and medial reticular) cells during cataplexy suggests that the activity of these cells is more tightly linked to muscle tone than to awareness of the environment. Consistent with this behavioral correlation is work showing that the release of norepinephrine from locus coeruleus cells facilitates motoneurons (reviewed in reference 118).

Individual noradrenergic locus coeruleus cells can have both descending projections to the spinal cord and ascending projections to widespread regions of the cortex. In addition to their relation to muscle activity, the tonic activity of locus coeruleus cells also modulates forebrain activity. Damage to the locus coeruleus increases metabolic rate[119] and prevents cortical expression of the *c-fos* gene.[120] Stimulation of the locus coeruleus decreases glucose consumption and increases *c-fos* expression.[121, 122] Therefore the reduction in locus coeruleus discharge in REM sleep is likely to cause an increase in cortical metabolism[123] and a decrease in *c-fos* expression. One may speculate that locus coeruleus activity serves to integrate descending motor control with forebrain sensorimotor control systems.

Thus, two elements of REM sleep, cessation of locus coeruleus discharge and increased activity of nucleus magnocellularis cells, contribute to cataplexy. The cessation of discharge in medial reticular cells, seen in cataplexy but not in REM sleep, may also contribute to the reduced motor activity of cataplexy.

Cataplectic attacks are preceded by a marked increase in heart rate.[124] Systemic blood pressure is not affected during spontaneous attacks, although increases in blood pressure will trigger cataplectic attacks in narcoleptic dogs. In summary, changes in circulatory control appear to play a role in the triggering of cataplectic attacks, just as they do in determining the response to medullary stimulation. The means by which the brainstem systems responsible for cataplexy are triggered is not completely understood. However, it is likely that forebrain degeneration[125] releases the brainstem circuits responsible for loss of muscle tone.

Figure 9–15 summarizes the current state of our knowledge about the anatomical relation of sites where carbachol produces atonia, the location of REM sleep-on and REM sleep-off cells, and lesions blocking REM sleep.

Ponto-Geniculo-Occipital Spikes

PGO spikes accompany the eye movements and many of the other phasic motor and sensory events of REM sleep. They occur during a period of phasically enhanced excitability within REM sleep.[126] Similar potentials can be elicited in waking by intense auditory stimulation that elicit orienting.[127, 128] Transection studies have localized the generator mechanisms responsible for this activity. Transections at the level of the abducens nucleus (see Fig. 9–1) allow PGO spikes to occur in a relatively normal pattern and amplitude distribution in the forebrain, rostral to the transection.[24] Transections and lesions a few millimeters rostral to this level completely block forebrain PGO spikes.[129] Lesions of the peribrachial region (the region around the superior cerebellar peduncle or brachium conjunctivum) can produce REM sleep without PGO waves or rapid eye movements (Fig. 9–16). Lesions that spare the peribrachial regions but damage more ventrome-

dial areas of the pons produce REM sleep without atonia, but with large numbers of PGO waves and rapid eye movements[28] (see Fig. 9–16).

PGO waves can be generated in the absence of other REM sleep phenomena by cholinergic stimulation of the pons.[130] The best sites for this stimulation are in the peribrachial region. Unit activity studies have identified the cellular elements involved in PGO waves generation. They are localized to the reticular regions around the superior cerebellar peduncle (peribrachial region) and the area below the locus coeruleus.[83, 101, 131–136] Many of these cells are cholinergic. They have a characteristic short burst of activity before each ipsilateral PGO wave and project to the thalamus.

Serotonin inhibits PGO waves. Serotonin depletion with parachlorophenylalanine produces continuous PGO activity in all behavioral states.[137] Lesions of the serotonergic dorsal raphe or small cuts lateral to the raphe also produce a release of PGO activity.[138] In vitro studies have shown that serotonin blocks the burst-firing mode of *PGO cells* by hyperpolarizing them.[139] In the transition from NREM to REM sleep the cessation of activity in serotonergic cells allows the PGO cells to begin discharging in bursts, generating PGO waves.

In summary, PGO waves are generated by cholinergic neurons in the peribrachial region which project rostrally. They are inhibited by serotonergic neurons of the raphe system.

Electroencephalographic Desynchrony in the Neocortex and Hippocampal Theta Waves

A single mechanism appears to be responsible for generating the EEG voltage reduction seen in REM sleep and waking (relative to the high-voltage EEG of NREM sleep). Likewise, hippocampal theta waves are indistinguishable in waking and REM sleep. Both hippocampal theta waves and EEG desynchrony can exist in the forebrain disconnected from the pons.[140] This is in contrast to PGO waves, which do not occur in the forebrain after disconnection of the pons.

Hippocampal theta waves are normally continuous during REM sleep. During periods of PGO spike bursts and associated phasic activity, the theta wave frequency increases. Rats deprived of REM sleep can have REM sleep episodes even when heavily atropinized. Under these conditions the tonic theta waves of REM sleep are abolished.[3] However, the theta waves that accompany bursts of phasic motor activity are still present. In a similar way, neocortical desynchrony, which is normally present throughout most of REM sleep, is absent in the atropinized rat and cat.[141] Instead, brief periods of EEG desynchrony are present only in conjunction with bursts of phasic activity. Therefore, it has been concluded that both the tonic EEG desynchrony and the tonic hippocampal theta waves that accompany REM sleep are generated by cholinergic mechanisms. The phasic EEG desynchrony and hippocampal theta waves accompanying movement and phasic activity in REM sleep have been attributed to a

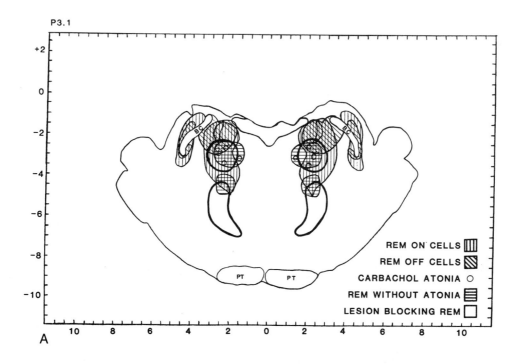

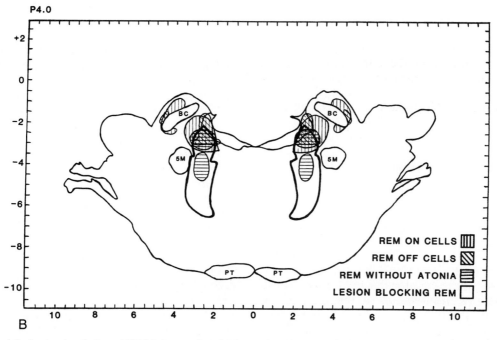

Figure 9–15. *A* and *B*, Anatomic relation of "REM sleep-on" and "sleep-off" cells, carbachol-induced atonia sites, lesions blocking atonia but not preventing REM sleep, and lesions completely blocking REM sleep. The inhibitory regions shown in Figure 9–12 are not plotted. (From Siegel JM, Rogawski MA. A function for REM sleep: regulation of noradrenergic receptor sensitivity. Brain Res. 1988;13:213–233.)

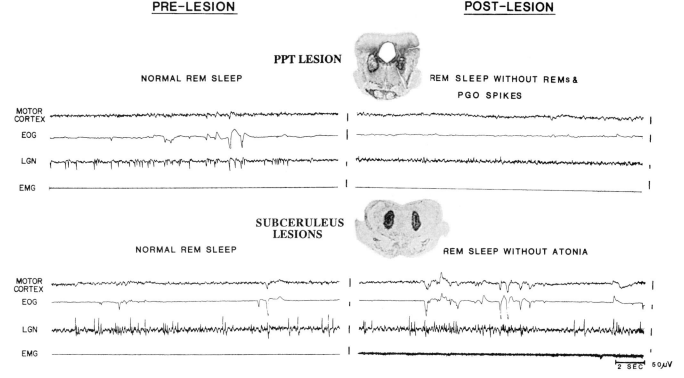

Figure 9–16. Twenty-second polygraph tracings of REM sleep before and after lesions, together with a coronal section through the center of the pontine lesions. EEG voltage reduction of REM sleep (recorded from motor cortex) was present after both lesions. *Top*, Radiofrequency lesions of the pedunculopontine region diminished ponto-geniculo-occipital (PGO) spikes and eye movement bursts during REM sleep. *Bottom*, Lesions in the region ventral to the locus coeruleus produced REM sleep without atonia without any diminution of PGO spike or REM frequency. (Reprinted from Brain Research, vol 571, Shouse MN, Siegel JM, Pontine regulation of REM sleep components in cats: integrity of the pedunculopontine tegmentum [PPT] is important for phasic events but unnecessary for atonia during REM sleep, 50–63, Copyright 1992, with permission from Elsevier Science.)

noncholinergic mechanism.[3] Theta waves can be triggered by electrical stimulation of the brainstem reticular formation. The best brainstem site for elicitation of hippocampal theta waves is in the pontine RF at the level of the RPO,[13] that is, at the same level at which cholinergic stimulation is most effective in triggering REM sleep and lesions are most effective in blocking REM sleep. The control of EEG changes in sleep and waking is discussed in greater detail in Chapters 8 and 10.

A SYNTHESIS OF FINDINGS ON REM SLEEP CONTROL MECHANISMS

Are There Executive Neurons?

We have seen that there are brainstem neurons that discharge during each ipsilateral PGO spike. There are also cells that are tonically active in REM sleep, but are silent at other times. These neurons may be related to the atonia or other tonic aspects of REM sleep. Still other cell groups are tonically active during both waking and REM sleep and may be related to EEG control. But is there a cell group that serves to coordinate all of the phenomenology of REM sleep, which triggers other cell groups producing each of the defining signs of this

state? It is unclear whether such an "executive" cell group exists. While this coordinating property may or may not be manifest within the activity of individual neurons, it is clear that an "executive system" of neurons for the triggering and maintenance of REM sleep resides in the lateral pons and adjacent midbrain. This system may be comprised of an interacting population of cells, each of which is primarily tied to one or more of the physiological aspects of REM sleep, but none of which is, in and of itself, sufficient to trigger the state. The anatomical discreteness of such cell populations is evident in the dissociation of REM sleep signs that can be revealed by stimulation and lesion studies. Conversely, the synaptic linkage of these populations is evident in the fact that such dissociations never occur in the undisturbed animal and only rarely occur in disease, as in narcolepsy.

What Is the Function of REM Sleep?

Whether the triggering of REM sleep is manifest in a group of executive neurons or in an executive system, these cells must be fulfilling some biological function. Although our knowledge of the mechanism has increased enormously, the question of function remains in the realm of speculation, in stark contrast to that of other behavioral activities occupying substantially smaller amounts of time. While this difficult question remains unanswered, I offer the following speculation.

The changes in brain unit activity during REM sleep should provide a clue to its function. We have described two kinds of unit activity unique to REM sleep: REM sleep-on and REM sleep-off cells. REM sleep-off cells in the raphe system appear to have an important role in the gating of PGO spikes. REM sleep-off cells in the locus coeruleus and raphe system may have a role in the maintenance of muscle tone in waking. Histaminergic cells of the posterior hypothalamus are also "off" in REM sleep (and in NREM sleep). Whereas monoaminergic cells are important in shaping the phenomena of REM sleep, the lesions that eliminate REM sleep are centered on the locations of the REM sleep-on cells, not the REM sleep-off cells. The number of REM-off cells appears to be much greater than the number of REM-on cells. The cessation of activity in the aminergic cells may not only be important in the modulation of REM sleep components but may also be significant for the function of REM sleep. Specifically, I propose that this periodic cessation of discharge prevents desensitization of aminergic receptors, which are continuously activated in waking.[142] Desensitization would reduce the effectiveness of these transmitters. Experimental support for this concept comes from studies of pontine activity during REM sleep deprivation. Deprivation greatly reduces the amplitude of a noradrenergic-mediated inhibition normally seen in the pons after auditory stimulation.[143] REM sleep deprivation produces a slowing of presumably noradrenergic cells of the dorsolateral pons,[144] though serotonergic REM sleep-off cells may speed up under similar conditions.[145] This slowing of noradrenergic cells may be responsible for some of the symptoms of sleep deprivation, because norepinephrine release has been shown to increase the signal-to-noise ratio of information processing in a number of brain regions.[142] Receptor assays directed at testing this hypothesis have produced both supportive and contradictory findings.[142, 146]

The other major neuronal phenomenon of REM sleep is the burst discharge and elevated discharge rate in a majority of brainstem and forebrain systems.[10, 22, 48, 147] This burst discharge, synchronized in adjacent cells,[148] underlies the rapid eye movements and twitches that characterize this state. It is dramatically different from the slow regular discharge pattern seen in these same cells during NREM sleep. Does this transmitter release desensitize certain groups of receptors? Does it function to potentiate neuronal circuits? Does it have a role in maintaining intracellular homeostasis? These questions remain unanswered.

Acknowledgments

Supported by the Medical Research Service of the Veterans Administration and PHS grants NS14610, HL41370, HL60296, and HL/MH/HD/AR/NS59594.

References

1. Robinson TE. Hippocampal rhythmic slow activity (RSA; Theta): a critical analysis of selected studies and discussion of possible species-differences. Brain Res Rev. 1980;2:69–101.

2. Mitchell SJ, Ranck JB Jr. Generation of theta rhythm in medial entorhinal cortex of freely moving rats. Brain Res. 1980;189:49–66.

3. Vanderwolf CH, Robinson TE. Reticulo-cortical activity and behavior: a critique of the arousal theory and a new synthesis. Behav Brain Sci. 1981;4:459–514.

4. Jouvet M. Recherches sur les structures nerveuses et les mécanismes responsables des différentes phases du sommeil physiologique. Arch Ital Biol. 1962;100:125–206.

5. Laurent JP, Guerrero FA. Reversible suppression of ponto-geniculo-occipital waves by localized cooling during paradoxical sleep in cats. Exp Neurol. 1975;49:356–369.

6. Sakai K, Petitjean F, Jouvet M. Effects of ponto-mesencephalic lesions and electrical stimulation upon PGO waves and EMPs in unanesthetized cats. Electroencephalogr Clin Neurophysiol. 1976;41:49–63.

7. Hobson JA, Alexander J, Frederickson CJ. The effect of lateral geniculate lesions on phasic electrical activity of the cortex during desynchronized sleep in the cat. Brain Res. 1969;14:607–621.

8. Orem J. Neuronal mechanisms of respiration in REM sleep. Sleep 1980;3:251–267.

9. Baust W, Holzbach E, Zechlin O. Phasic changes in heart rate and respiration correlated with PGO-spike activity during REM sleep. Pflugers Arch. 1972;331:113–123.

10. Evarts EV. Temporal pattern of discharge of pyramidal tract neurons during sleep and waking in the monkey. J Neurophysiol. 1964;27:152–171.

11. Buzsaki G. Functions for interneuronal nets in the hippocampus. Can J Physiol Pharmacol. 1997;75:508–515.

12. Petsche H, Stumpf C, Gogolak G. The significance of the rabbit's septum as a relay between the midbrain and the hippocampus, I: the control of hippocampus arousal activity by the septum. Electroencephalogr Clin Neurophysiol. 1962;14:202–211.

13. Vertes RP, Kocsis B. Brainstem-diencephalo-septohippocampal systems controlling the theta rhythm of the hippocampus. Neuroscience. 1997;81:893–926.

14. Kubin L, Tojima H, Reignier C, et al. Interaction of serotonergic excitatory drive to hypoglossal motoneurons with carbachol-induced, REM sleep-like atonia. Sleep. 1996;19:187–195.

15. Lai YY, Strahlendorf HK, Fung SJ, et al. The actions of two monoamines on spinal motoneurons from stimulation of the locus coeruleus in the cat. Brain Res. 1989;484:268–272.

16. Pompeiano O, Hoshino K. Tonic inhibition of dorsal pontine neurons during the postural atonia produced by an anticholinesterase in the decerebrate cat. Arch Ital Biol. 1976;114:310–340.

17. Villablanca J. The electrocorticogram in the chronic cerveau isolé cat. Electroencephalogr Clin Neurophysiol. 1965;19:576–586.

18. Jouvet M, Buda C, Debilly G, et al. La température centrale est le facteur principal de régulation du sommeil paradoxal chez le chat pontique. C R Acad Sci III. 1988;306:69–73.

19. Adey WR, Bors E, Porter RW. EEG sleep patterns after high cervical lesions in man. Arch Neurol. 1968;19:377–383.

20. Puizillout JJ, Ternaux, JP, Foutz, AS, et al. Les stades de sommeil de la préparation "encéphale isolé," I: déclenchement des pointes ponto-génico-occipitales et du sommeil phasique à ondes lentes. Role des noyaux du raphé. Electroencephalogr Clin Neurophysiol. 1974;37:561–576.

21. Morrison AR, Bowker RM. A caudal source of cervical and forelimb inhibition during sleep. Exp Neurol. 1971;33:684–692.

22. Siegel JM, Nienhuis R, Tomaszewski KS. Rostral brainstem contributes to medullary inhibition of muscle tone. Brain Res. 1983;268:344–348.

23. Siegel JM, Tomaszewski KS, Nienhuis R. Behavioral states in the chronic medullary and mid-pontine cat. Electroencephalogr Clin Neurophysiol. 1986;63:274–288.

24. Siegel JM, Nienhuis R, Tomaszewski KS. REM sleep signs rostral to chronic transections at the pontomedullary junction. Neurosci Lett. 1984;45:241–246.

25. Jones BE, Pare M, Beaudet A. Retrograde labeling of neurons in the brain stem following injections of [3H] choline into the rat spinal cord. Neuroscience. 1986;18:901–916.

26. Vanni-Mercier G, Sakai K, Lin JS, et al. Carbachol microinjections in the mediodorsal pontine tegmentum are unable to

induce paradoxical sleep after caudal pontine and prebulbar transections in the cat. Neurosci Lett. 1991;130:41–45.

27. Siegel JM. Pontomedullary interactions in the generation of REM sleep. In: McGinty DJ, Drucker-Colin R, Morrison A, et al, eds. Brain Mechanisms of Sleep. New York, NY: Raven Press; 1985:157–174.

28. Shouse MN, Siegel JM. Pontine regulation of REM sleep components in cats: integrity of the pedunculopontine tegmentum (PPT) is important for phasic events but unnecessary for atonia during REM sleep. Brain Res. 1992;571:50–63.

29. Batini C, Moruzzi G, Palestini M, et al. Persistent patterns of wakefulness in the pretrigeminal midpontine preparation. Science. 1958;128:30–32.

30. Matsuzaki M. Differential effects of sodium butyrate and physostigmine upon the activities of para-sleep in acute brain stem preparations. Brain Res. 1969;13:247–265.

31. Crosby C, Humphrey T, Lauer EW. Correlative Anatomy of the Nervous System. New York, NY: Macmillan; 1962.

32. Brodal A. Neurological Anatomy in Relation to Clinical Medicine. London, England: Oxford University Press; 1969.

33. Snider RS, Niemer WT. A Stereotaxic Atlas of the Cat Brain. Chicago, Ill: University of Chicago Press; 1961.

34. Carli G, Zanchetti A. A study of pontine lesions suppressing deep sleep in the cat. Arch Ital Biol. 1965;103:725–750.

35. Reinoso-Suarez F. Topographischer Hirnatlas der Katze, für experimental-physiologische Untersuchungen. Darmstadt, Germany: Merck; 1961.

36. Berman AL. The Brain Stem of the Cat. Madison, Wisc: University of Wisconsin Press; 1968.

37. Taber E. The cytoarchitecture of the brain stem of the cat, I: brain stem nuclei of cat. J Comp Neurol. 1961;116:27–70.

38. Sakai K. Anatomical and physiological basis of paradoxical sleep. In: McGinty DJ, Drucker-Colin R, Morrison A, et al, eds. Brain Mechanisms of Sleep. New York, NY: Raven Press; 1985:111–138.

39. Jouvet, M. and Delorme, F. Locus coeruleus et sommeil paradoxal. C R Seances Soc Biol Fils. 1965;159:895–899.

40. Jones BE. Neuroanatomical and neurochemical substrates of mechanisms underlying paradoxical sleep. In: McGinty DJ, Drucker-Colin R, Morrison A, et al, eds. Brain Mechanisms of Sleep. New York, NY: Raven Press; 1985:139–156.

41. Monmaur P, Delacour J. Effets de la lésion bilaterale du tegmentum pontique dorsolateral sur l'activité theta hippocampique au cours du sommeil paradoxal chez le rat. C R Acad Sci III. 1978;286:761–764.

42. Laguzzi RF, Adrien J, Bourgoin S, et al. Effects of intraventricular injection of 6-hydroxydopamine in the developing kitten, 1: on the sleep-waking cycles. Brain Res. 1979;160:445–459.

43. Jones BE. Elimination of paradoxical sleep by lesions of the pontine gigantocellular tegmental field in the cat. Neurosci Lett. 1979;13:285–293.

44. Drucker-Colin R, Pedraza, JGB. Kainic acid lesions of gigantocellular tegmental field (FTG) neurons does not abolish REM sleep. Brain Res. 1983;272:387–391.

45. Sastre JP, Sakai K, Jouvet M. Are the gigantocellular tegmental field neurons responsible for paradoxical sleep? Brain Res. 1981;229:147–161.

46. Webster HH, Jones BE. Neurotoxic lesions of the dorsolateral pontomesencephalic tegmentum-cholinergic cell area in the cat, II: effects upon sleep-waking states. Brain Res. 1988;458:285–302.

47. Hobson JA, McCarley RW, Pivik T, et al. Selective firing by cat pontine brain stem neurons in desynchronized sleep. J Neurophysiol. 1974;37:497–511.

48. Huttenlocher PR. Evoked and spontaneous activity in single units of medial brain stem during natural sleep and waking. J Neurophysiol. 1961;24:451–468.

49. Siegel JM, McGinty DJ. Pontine reticular formation neurons: relationship of discharge to motor activity. Science. 1977;196:678–680.

50. Siegel JM, McGinty DJ, Breedlove SM. Sleep and waking activity of pontine gigantocellular field neurons. Exp Neurol. 1977;56:553–573.

51. Siegel JM, Behavioral relations of medullary reticular formation cells. Exp Neurol. 1979;65:691–698.

52. Siegel JM, Tomaszewski KS. Behavioral organization of reticular formation: studies in the unrestrained cat, I: cells related to axial, limb, eye, and other movements. J Neurophysiol. 1983;50:696–716.

53. Siegel JM, Behavioral functions of the reticular formation. Brain Res Rev. 1979;1:69–105.

54. Suzuki SS, Siegel JM, Wu MF. Role of pontomedullary reticular formation neurons in horizontal head movements: an ibotenic acid lesion study in the cat. Brain Res. 1989;484:78–93.

55. Netick A, Orem J, Dement W. Neuronal activity specific to REM sleep and its relationship to breathing. Brain Res. 1977;120:197–207.

56. Siegel JM, Wheeler RL, McGinty DJ. Activity of medullary reticular formation neurons in the unrestrained cat during waking and sleep. Brain Res. 1979;179:49–60.

57. El Mansari M, Sakai K, Jouvet M. Responses of presumed cholinergic mesopontine tegmental neurons to carbachol microinjections in freely moving cats. Exp Brain Res. 1990;83:115–123.

58. Shiromani PJ, Armstrong DM, Bruce G, et al. Relation of pontine choline acetyltransferase immunoreactive neurons with cells which increase discharge during REM sleep. Brain Res Bull. 1987;18:447–455.

59. Sakai K. Some anatomical and physiological properties of ponto-mesencephalic tegmental neurons with special reference to the PGO waves and postural atonia during paradoxical sleep in the cat. In: Hobson JA, Brazier MA, eds. The Reticular Formation Revisited. New York, NY: Raven Press; 1980:427–447.

60. Sakai K, Koyama Y. Are there cholinergic and non-cholinergic paradoxical sleep-on neurons in the pons? Neuroreport. 1996;7:2449–2453.

61. Sakai K, Sastre JP, Salvert D, et al. Tegmentoreticular projections with special reference to the muscular atonia during paradoxical sleep in the cat: an HRP study. Brain Res. 1979;176:233–254.

62. Aston-Jones G, Bloom FE. Activity of norepinephrine-containing locus coeruleus neurons in behaving rats anticipates fluctuations in the sleep-waking cycle. J Neurosci. 1981;1:876–886.

63. Hobson JA, McCarley RW, Nelson JP. Location and spike-train characteristics of cells in anterodorsal pons having selective decreases in firing rat during desynchronized sleep. J Neurophysiol. 1983;50:770–783.

64. McGinty DJ, Harper RM. Dorsal raphe neurons: depression of firing during sleep in cats. Brain Res. 1976;101:569–575.

65. Jacobs BL, Heym J, Trulson ME. Behavioral and physiological correlates of brain serotoninergic unit activity. J Physiol Paris. 1981;77:431–436.

66. Semba K. Aminergic and cholinergic afferents to REM sleep inducing regions of the pontine reticular formation in the rat. J Comp Neurol. 1993;330:543–556.

67. Horner RL, Sanford LD, Annis DA, et al. Serotonin at the laterodorsal tegmental nucleus suppresses rapid-eye-movement sleep in freely behaving rats. J Neurosci. 1997;17:7541–7552.

68. Nitz D, Siegel JM. GABA release in the dorsal raphe nucleus: role of the control of REM sleep. Am J Physiol. 1997;273:R451–R455.

69. Nitz D, Siegel JM. GABA release in the cat locus coeruleus as a function of permanently isolated forebrain of the cat. Brain Res Bull. 1977;2:93–100.

70. Gervasoni D, Darraca L, Fort P, et al. Electrophysiological evidence that noradrenergic neurons of the rat locus coeruleus are tonically inhibited by GABA during sleep. Eur J Neurosci. 1998;10:964–970.

71. Shiromani PJ, Winston S, McCarley RW. Pontine cholinergic neurons show Fos-like immunoreactivity associated with cholinergically induced REM sleep. Mol Brain Res. 1996;38:77–84.

71a. Maloney K, Mainville L, Jones B. Differential c-Fos expression in cholinergic, monoaminergic, and GABAergic cell groups of the pontomesencephalic tegmentum after paradoxical sleep deprivation and recovery. J Neurosci. 1999;19:3057–3072.

72. Yamuy J, Mancillas JR, Morales F, et al. C-fos expression in the pons and medulla of the cat during carbachol induced active sleep. J Neurosci. 1993;13:2703–2718.

73. Kawamura H, Inouye ST. Circadian rhythm in a hypothalamic island containing the suprachiasmatic nucleus. In: Suda M, Hayaishi O, Nakagawa H, eds. Biological Rhythms and Their Central Mechanism. Amsterdam, Netherlands: Elsevier/North Holland Biomedical Press; 1979:335–341.

74. Hoshino K, Pompeiano O, Magherini PC, et al. Oscillatory activity of pontine neurons related to the regular occurrence of REM bursts in the decerebrate cat. Brain Res. 1976;116:125–130.

75. Gadea-Ciria M. Tele-encephalic versus cerebellar control upon ponto-geniculo-occipital waves during paradoxical sleep in the cat. Experientia. 1976;32:889–890.

76. Morrison AR, Bowker RM. The biological significance of PGO spikes in the sleeping cat. Acta Neurobiol Exp. 1975;35:821–840.

77. Calvo JM, Simon-Arceo K, Fernandez-Mas R. Prolonged enhancement of REM sleep produced by carbachol microinjection into the amygdala. Neuroreport. 1996;7:577–580.

78. Maquet P, Peters JM, Aerts J, et al. Functional neuroanatomy of human rapid-eye-movement sleep and dreaming. Nature. 1996;383:163–166.

79. Henley K, Morrison AR. A re-evaluation of the effects of lesions of the pontine tegmentum and locus coeruleus on phenomena of paradoxical sleep in the cat. Acta Neurobiol Exp. 1974;34:215–232.

80. Hendricks JC, Morrison AR, Mann GL. Different behaviors during paradoxical sleep without atonia depend on pontine lesion site. Brain Res. 1982;239:81–105.

81. Schenkel E, Siegel JM. REM sleep without atonia after lesions of the medial medulla. Neurosci Lett. 1989;98:159–165.

81a. Kohyama J, Lai YY, Siegel JM. Inactivation of the pons blocks medullary-induced muscle tone suppression in the decerebrate cat. Sleep 1998;21:695–700.

82. Kohyama J, Lai YY, Siegel JM. Conduction velocity of the reticulospinal system mediating muscle tone suppression. J Neurophysiol. 1998;80:1839–1851.

83. Rye D. Contributions of the pedunculopontine region to normal and altered REM sleep. Sleep. 1997;20:757–788.

84. Lai YY, Siegel JM. Muscle tone suppression and stepping produced by stimulation of midbrain and rostral pontine reticular formation. J Neurosci. 1990;10:2727–2738.

85. Mitler MM, Dement WC. Cataplectic-like behavior in cats after microinjection of carbachol in the pontine reticular formation. Brain Res. 1974;68:335–343.

86. Katayama Y, De Witt DS, Becker DP, et al. Behavioral evidence for cholinoceptive pontine inhibitory area: descending control of spinal motor output and sensory input. Brain Res. 1984;296:241–262.

87. Baxter BL. Induction of both emotional behavior and a novel form of REM sleep by chemical stimulation applied to cat mesencephalon. Exp Neurol. 1969;23:220–229.

88. George R, Haslett WL, Jenden DJ. A cholinergic mechanism in the brainstem reticular formation: induction of paradoxical sleep. Int J Neuropharmacol. 1964;3:541–552.

89. Van Dongen PAM, Broekkamp CLE, Cools AR. Atonia after carbachol microinjections near the locus coeruleus in cats. Pharmacol Biochem Behav. 1978;8:527–532.

90. Amatruda TT, Black DA, McCarley RW, et al. Sleep cycle control and cholinergic mechanisms: differential effects of carbachol injections at pontine brainstem sites. Brain Res. 1975;98:501–515.

91. Baghdoyan HA, Rodrigo-Angulo ML, McCarley RW, et al. Site-specific enhancement and suppression of desynchronized sleep signs following cholinergic stimulation of three brain stem regions. Brain Res. 1984;306:39–52.

92. Shiromani P, Siegel JM, Tomaszewski KS, et al. Alterations in blood pressure and REM sleep after pontine carbachol microinfusion. Exp Neurol. 1986;91:285–292.

93. Vanni-Mercier G, Sakai K, Lin JS, et al. Mapping of cholinoceptive brainstem structures responsible for the generation of paradoxical sleep in the cat. Arch Ital Biol. 1989;127:133–164.

94. Garzon M, Deandres I, Reinoso-Suarez F. Sleep patterns after carbachol delivery in the ventral oral pontine tegmentum of the cat. Neuroscience. 1998;83:1137–1144.

95. Kodama T, Takahashi T, Honda Y. Enhancement of acetylcholine release during paradoxical sleep in the dorsal tegmental field of the cat brain stem. Neurosci Lett. 1990;114:277–282.

96. Leonard TO, Lydic R. Pontine nitric oxide modulates acetylcholine release, rapid eye movement sleep generation, and respiratory rate. J Neurosci. 1997;17:774–785.

97. Velazquez-Moctezuma J, Shalauta M, Gillin JC, et al. Cholinergic antagonists and REM sleep generation. Brain Res. 1991;543:175–179.

98. Imeri L, Bianchi S, Angeli P, et al. Selective blockade of different brain stem muscarinic receptor subtypes: effects on the sleep-wake cycle. Brain Res. 1994;636:68–72.

99. Baghdoyan HA. Location and quantification of muscarinic receptor subtypes in rat pons: implications for REM sleep generation. Am J Physiol. 1997;273:R896–904.

100. Sakai K, Onoe H. Critical role for M3 muscarinic receptors in paradoxical sleep generation in the cat. Eur J Neurosci. 1997;9:415–423.

101. Datta S, Patterson EH, Siwek DF. Endogenous and exogenous nitric oxide in the pedunculopontine tegmentum induces sleep. Synapse. 1997;27:69–78.

102. Yamuy J, Morales FR, Chase M. Induction of rapid eye movement by the microinjection of nerve growth factor into the pontine reticular formation of the cat. Neuroscience. 1995;66:9–13.

103. Lai YY, Siegel JM. Medullary regions mediating atonia. J Neurosci. 1988;8:4790–4796.

104. Onoe H, Sakai K. Kainate receptors: a novel mechanism in paradoxical sleep generation. Neuroreport. 1995;6:353–356.

105. Magoun HW, Rhines R. An inhibitory mechanism in the bulbur reticular formation. J Neurophysiol. 1946;9:165–171.

106. Kodama T, Lai YY, Siegel JM. Enhanced glutamate release during REM sleep in the rostromedial medulla as measured by in vivo microdialysis. Brain Res. 1998;780:178–181.

107. Kodama T, Lai YY, Siegel JM. Enhancement of acetylcholine release during REM sleep in the caudomedial medulla as measured by in vivo microdialysis. Brain Res. 1992;580:348–350.

108. Mitani A, Ito K, Hallanger A, et al. Cholinergic projections from the laterodorsal and pedunculopontine tegmental nuclei to the pontine gigantocellular tegmental field in the cat. Brain Res. 1988;451:397–402.

109. Shiromani PJ, Armstrong DM, Gillin JC. Cholinergic neurons from the dorsolateral pons project to the medial pons: a WGA-HRP and choline acetyltransferase immunohistochemical study. Neurosci Lett. 1988;95:19–23.

110. Shiromani PJ, Lai YY, Siegel JM. Descending projections from the dorsolateral pontine tegmentum to the paramedian reticular nucleus of the caudal medulla in the cat. Brain Res. 1990;517:224–228.

111. Sherriff FE, Henderson Z. The paragigantocellular nucleus of the ventral medulla: a secondary source of cholinergic innervation of rat brainstem nuclei. Brain Res. 1994;636:119–125.

112. Lai YY, Siegel JM. Ponto-medullary glutamate receptors mediating locomotion and muscle tone suppression. J Neurosci. 1991;11:2931–2937.

113. Sprague JM, Chambers WW. Regulation of posture in intact and decerebrate cat, I: cerebellum, reticular formation, vestibular nuclei. J Neurophysiol. 1953;16:451–463.

114. Lai YY, Siegel JM, Wilson WJ. Effect of blood pressure on changes in muscle tone produced by stimulation of the medial medulla. Am J Physiol. 1987;252:H1249–H1257.

115. Baker TL, Dement WC. Canine narcolepsy-cataplexy syndrome: evidence for an inherited monoaminergic-cholinergic imbalance. In McGinty DJ, Drucker-Colin R, Morrison A, et al, eds. Brain Mechanisms of Sleep. New York, NY: Raven Press; 1985:199–234.

116. Kilduff TS, Bowersox SS, Kaitin KI, et al. Muscarinic cholinergic receptors and the canine model of narcolepsy. Sleep. 1986;9:102–106.

117. Siegel JM, Nienhuis R, Fahringer H, et al. Neuronal activity in narcolepsy: identification of cataplexy related cells in the medial medulla. Science. 1991;262:1315–1318.

117a. Siegel JM. Narcolepsy: a key role for hypocretins (orexins). Cell. 1999;98:409–412.

118. Wu MF, Gulyani S, Yao E, et al. Locus coeruleus neurons: cessation of activity during cataplexy. Neuroscience. 1999;91:1389–1399.

118a. Siegel JM. Narcolepsy. Sci Am. 2000;282:76–81.

119. Schwartz W. 6-Hydroxydopamine lesions of rat locus coeruleus alter brain glucose consumption, as measured by the 2-deoxy-d-[14,C]glucose tracer technique. Neurosci Lett. 1978;7:141–150.

120. Cirelli C, Pompeiano M, Tononi G. Neuronal gene expression in the waking state: a role for the locus coeruleus. Science. 1996;274:1211–1217.

121. Abraham W, Delanoy R, Dunn A, et al. Locus coeruleus stimula-

tion decreases deoxyglucose uptake in ipsilateral mouse cerebral cortex. Brain Res. 1979;172:387–392.

122. Stone EA, Zhang Y, Carr KD. Massive activation of c-fos after mechanical stimulation of the locus coeruleus. Brain Res Bull. 1994;36:77–80.

123. Everson CA, Smith CB, Sokoloff L. Effects of prolonged sleep deprivation on local rates of cerebral energy metabolism in freely moving rats. J Neurosci. 1994;14:6769–6778.

124. Siegel JM, Tomaszewski KS, Fahringer H, et al. Heart rate and blood pressure changes during sleep-waking cycles and cataplexy in narcoleptic dogs. Am J Physiol 1989;256:H111–H119.

125. Siegel JM, Nienhuis R, Gulyani S, et al. Neuronal degeneration in canine narcolepsy. J Neuroscience. 1999;19:248–257.

126. Wu MF, Siegel JM. Facilitation of the acoustic startle reflex by ponto-geniculo-occipital waves: effects of PCPA. Brain Res. 1990;532:237–241.

127. Wu MF, Mallick BN, Siegel JM. Lateral geniculate spikes, muscle atonia and startle response elicited by auditory stimuli as a function of stimulus parameters and arousal state. Brain Res. 1989;499:7–17.

128. Sanford LD, Morrison AR, Ball WA, et al. The amplitude of elicited PGO waves: a correlate of orienting. Electroencephalogr Clin Neurophysiol. 1993;86:438–445.

129. Laurent JP, Cespuglio R, Jouvet M. Délimitation des voies ascendants de l'activité ponto-géniculo-occipitale chez le chat. Brain Res. 1974;65:29–52.

130. Baghdoyan HA, Rodrigo-Angulo ML, McCarley RW, et al. A neuroanatomical gradient in the pontine tegmentum for the cholinoceptive induction of desynchronized sleep signs. Brain Res. 1987;414:245–261.

131. Datta S, Patterson EH, Siwek DF. Endogenous and exogenous nitric oxide in the pedunculopontine tegmentum induces sleep. Synapse. 1997;27:69–78.

132. Saito H, Sakai K, Jouvet M. Discharge patterns of the nucleus parabrachialis lateralis neurons of the cat during sleep and waking. Brain Res. 1977;134:59–72.

133. McCarley RW, Nelson JP, Hobson JA. Ponto-geniculo-occipital (PGO) burst neurons: correlative evidence for neuronal generators of PGO waves. Science. 1978;201:269–272.

134. Sakai K, El Mansari M, Jouvet M. Inhibition by carbachol microinjections of presumptive cholinergic PGO sleep-on neurons in freely moving cats. Brain Res. 1990;527:213–223.

135. Steriade M, Datta S, Pare D, et al. Neuronal activities in brainstem cholinergic nuclei related to tonic activation processes in thalamocortical systems. J Neurosci 1990;10:2541–2559.

136. Steriade M, Pare D, Datt S, et al. Different cellular types in mesopontine cholinergic nuclei related to ponto-geniculo-occipital waves. J Neurosci. 1990;10:2560–2579.

137. Cohen HB, Dement WC, Barchas JD. Effects of chlorpromazine on sleep in cats pretreated with para-chlorophenylalanine. Brain Res. 1973;53:363–371.

138. Simon RP, Gershon MD, Brooks DC. The role of the raphe nuclei in the regulation of ponto-geniculo-occipital wave activity. Brain Res. 1973;58:313–330.

139. Luebke JJ, Greene RW, Semba K, et al. Serotonin hyperpolarizes cholinergic low-threshold burst neurons in the rat laterodorsal tegmental nucleus in vitro. Proc Natl Acad Sci U S A. 1992;89:743–747.

140. Olmstead CE, Villablanca JR. Hippocampal theta rhythm persists in the permanently isolated forebrain of the cat. Brain Res Bull. 1977;2:93–100.

141. Henriksen SJ, Jacobs BL, Dement WC. Dependence of REM sleep PGO waves on cholinergic mechanisms. Brain Res. 1972;48:412–416.

142. Siegel JM, Rogawski MA. A function for REM sleep: regulation of noradrenergic receptor sensitivity. Brain Res Rev. 1988;13:213–233.

143. Mallick BN, Fahringer H, Wu MF, et al. REM sleep deprivation reduces auditory evoked inhibition of dorsolateral pontine neurons. Brain Res. 1991;552:333–337.

144. Mallick BN, Siegel JM, Fahringer H. Changes in pontine unit activity with REM sleep deprivation. Brain Res. 1989;515:94–98.

145. Gardner JP, Fornal CA, Jacobs BL. Effects of sleep deprivation on serotonergic neuronal activity in the dorsal raphe nucleus of the freely moving cat. Neuropsychopharmacology. 1997;17:72–81.

146. Tsai L, Bergman B, Perry B, et al. Effects of chronic total sleep deprivation on central noradrenergic receptors in rat brain. Brain Res. 1993;602:221–227.

147. Hobson JA, McCarley RW. Neuronal Activity in Sleep 1969–1974. Los Angeles, Calif: Brain Information Service; 1977.

148. Siegel JM, Nienhuis R, Wheller RL, et al. Discharge pattern of reticular formation unit pairs in waking and REM sleep. Exp Neurol. 1981;74:875–891.

10

Basic Mechanisms of Sleep-Wake States

Barbara E. Jones

A state of wakefulness is maintained by neurons within the brainstem reticular formation, which in turn excite neurons in the nonspecific thalamo-cortical projection system along a dorsal pathway and in the posterior hypothalamus and basal forebrain along a ventral pathway. The thalamocortical, hypothalamocortical, and basalocortical projections serve to activate the cerebral cortex in turn in a long-lasting and widespread manner, stimulating high-frequency activity (low-voltage fast activity on electroencephalography [EEG]). The major population of neurons comprising the ascending reticular activating system use glutamate as a neurotransmitter. Other contributing pontomesencephalic tegmental neurons use acetylcholine. In addition, locus ceruleus neurons containing norepinephrine project in a diffuse manner from the brainstem to the entire forebrain, including directly to the cerebral cortex, and thereby also serve to stimulate and maintain cortical activation. Similarly, posterior hypothalamic neurons containing histamine project diffusely to the forebrain and cortex. Although the thalamocortical projection system uses glutamate as neurotransmitter, the basalocortical system primarily uses acetylcholine. In addition to the smaller neurotransmitter molecules, neurons in these activating systems also contain and often co-localize peptides, including substance P, vasoactive intestinal peptide, and neurotensin, that serve to enhance and/or prolong their excitatory influences.

For sleep, a shift from sympathetic to parasympathetic regulation occurs, and activating systems must be dampened. Neurons in the solitary tract nuclei and in the anterior hypothalamus and preoptic region, constituting parasympathetic control centers, are particularly important in these processes. Inhibition of activating systems is probably effected by particular gamma-aminobutyric acid–ergic neurons, which may be relatively selectively active during slow-wave sleep. Shutting off the brainstem, hypothalamic, and basal forebrain systems leads to disfacilitation and hyperpolarization of thalamocortical systems, which consequently shift the mode of operation from fast, tonic discharge to slow, burst discharge, reflected as spindle and slow wave activity in the EEG. Certain peptides, such as somatostatin and corticostatin, are colocalized with gamma-aminobutyric acid in particular neurons and may enhance and prolong the inhibition of the activating systems in the initiation and maintenance of slow-wave sleep.

Since the 1930s, the basic mechanisms of sleep-wake states have been studied through an interdisciplinary approach that includes neurophysiology, neuroanatomy, and neurochemistry. In early studies, lesions and stimulation were used to identify brain regions and neuronal systems that are involved in the generation and maintenance of wakefulness and sleep. Such experimental studies in animals were also important for the elucidation of the neuroanatomical substrates of coma or sleep perturbation that occur in association with brain lesions in human beings. Neurophysiological research has involved the recording of single neurons in the brain to discriminate putative wake- and sleep-generating neurons and to clarify the cellular mechanisms of sleep-wake state generation. Since the early 1960s, research has focused on the involvement of chemical neurotransmitters and the neurons containing those chemicals in the generation of sleep and wakefulness.

Through this search, what was initially considered to be a unitary process of sleep emerged as a dual process consisting of two distinct states: slow-wave sleep and paradoxical (or rapid eye movement [REM]) sleep. Although normally dependent on the prior occurrence of slow-wave sleep, paradoxical sleep involves mechanisms and neural systems different than those involved in slow-wave sleep. In the following historical consideration of basic mechanisms, the term *sleep* refers in a general manner to total sleep regarding research before 1960 and, more specifically, to slow-wave sleep in reviews of more contemporary research. In the treatment of contemporary knowledge of the basic mechanisms of sleep-wake states, this chapter deals with the particular mechanisms of slow-wave sleep, and other chapters focus on the specific mechanisms of paradoxical sleep. The following review is presented with a historical progression and parallel subdivision according to the different techniques and approaches applied in different periods.

NEURONAL SYSTEMS IMPLICATED IN SLEEP-WAKE STATE GENERATION

The Activating System

Identification of an Activating System. In the early 1900s, many physiologists, including, notably, Kleitman, believed that wakefulness and consciousness were maintained by ongoing sensory input to the brain.[1] Bremer[2] showed that in the *cerveau isolé,* in which the cerebrum was separated from the brainstem by a complete transection in front of the midbrain, physiological signs of wakefulness were lacking, whereas those of sleep, typified by slow waves on the cerebral cortex along with pupillary miosis, were prominent. This lack of wakeful signs was interpreted at the time as being due to the interruption of sensory inputs from the body and head to the cerebrum. In the 1940s, Moruzzi and Magoun questioned this interpretation and demonstrated that the most important input for the maintenance of waking, which was interrupted by these transections, was not from somatosensory pathways but rather from the reticular formation of the brainstem. To prove this point, first they demonstrated that electrical stimulation of the brainstem reticular core, and not of the sensory pathways, produced long-lasting and widespread cortical activation marked by the replacement of cortical slow wave activity with fast activity[3] (Fig. 10–1). Second, they showed that lesions of the reticular formation, but not of the sensory pathways, produced a loss of cortical activation that was replaced by cortical slow wave activity and behavioral immobility as in a comatose state.[4] Lesions with the most marked and permanent effect were located in the more rostral end of the reticular formation in the oral pontine and midbrain tegmentum and extended into the posterior hypothalamus and subthalamus, where the ascending impulses from the reticular formation were found to pass into the forebrain (see Fig. 10–1).[4–6] By electrophysiological and subsequently neuroanatomical techniques, it was learned that the neurons of the reticular formation receive collateral input from visceral, somatic, and special sensory systems and that they in turn send long ascending projections into the forebrain via a dorsal pathway to thalamic nuclei and a ventral pathway to and through the hypothalamus, subthalamus, and ventral thalamus up to the level of the basal forebrain (see Fig. 10–1).[7–11] The ascending reticular activating system thus was identified as a neuronal system—located in the core of the brainstem, recipient to collaterals from sensory inputs, and giving rise to long ascending forebrain projections—that was necessary and sufficient for the tonic maintenance of the cortical activation and behavioral arousal of wakefulness.

In human clinical studies, neurologists in the 20th century also noted certain cases of patients with somnolence and coma due to lesions of the midbrain and posterior diencephalon.[12, 13] In the early part of the century, von Economo[14] carefully studied the neuroanatomical correlates of symptoms in "encephalitis lethargica" and concluded that a "sleep-regulating center" was present within the midbrain and diencephalon.[14] He conceived of this center as composed of antagonistic parts: a waking part and a sleeping part. On the basis of the location of lesions in cases characterized by somnolence, he posited that the waking part was localized in the rostral midbrain tegmentum and caudal diencephalon. Since these early observations, multi-

ple clinical cases of somnolence, stupor, and coma resulting in a loss of consciousness have been studied and reported to be associated with lesions in the oral pontine and midbrain tegmentum or posterior hypothalamus and subthalamus.[15–18]

With smaller and more localized lesions in the midbrain and caudal diencephalon, a dissociation between the cortical activation and behavioral arousal of wakefulness was subsequently noted in both experimental animals and patients with somnolence and coma. Thus, in animals, lesions of the central midbrain tegmentum were found to produce a deficiency in cortical activation without preventing behavioral responsiveness to sensory stimulation.[19] However, lesions of the ventral tegmentum and hypothalamus were found to produce a state of behavioral somnolence and unresponsiveness, without a loss of cortical activation and alerting. Similar clinical symptoms had previously been noted in human beings and were referred to as *akinesia* and *akinetic mutism.*[18] It thus appeared that two different systems control cortical activation and behavioral arousal.

The existence of a cortical activating system was substantiated by multiple studies conducted in various species of experimental animals throughout the 1940s and 1950s.[6] However, further investigation in the 1960s and 1970s indicated that in the chronic course, the brainstem reticular formation was not absolutely necessary for wakefulness because cortical activation could eventually recover given sufficient time after lesions or transections through the brainstem.[6, 20–22] In fact, when large lesions of the midbrain reticular formation were performed in stages, allowing recovery after each partial lesion, they did not result in coma and were instead followed by total recovery.[23] This recovery could be explained by a certain amount of regeneration and plasticity that are now known to occur in the central nervous system. The recovery must also be interpreted as a manifestation of the function of other activating systems contained within the forebrain. In fact, the conclusion was reached by Villablanca in 1965[22] that electroencephalographic (EEG) desynchronization is an autochthonous phenomenon of the forebrain.[22]

By using both electrophysiological and lesion techniques, physiologists showed that the tonic activating influence of the reticular formation is transmitted to the cerebral cortex via a dorsal relay through the thalamus and via a ventral, extrathalamic relay through the hypothalamus up to the basal forebrain.[11] Within the thalamus, the ventromedial, intralaminar, and midline nuclei were found to project in a widespread manner to the cortex and were shown by high-frequency electrical stimulation to be capable of activating the entire cerebral cortex (see Fig. 10–1).[11, 24–26] The nonspecific thalamocortical system appears to depend on the tonic drive from the reticular formation for this activation. Ablation of the thalamus leads to a temporary loss of cortical activation in animals; however, in the chronic course, cortical activation returns.[27] In patients with bilateral paramedian thalamic lesions, a "dearousal" or "subwakefulness" syndrome was noted, with the possibility for such individuals to perform adequately

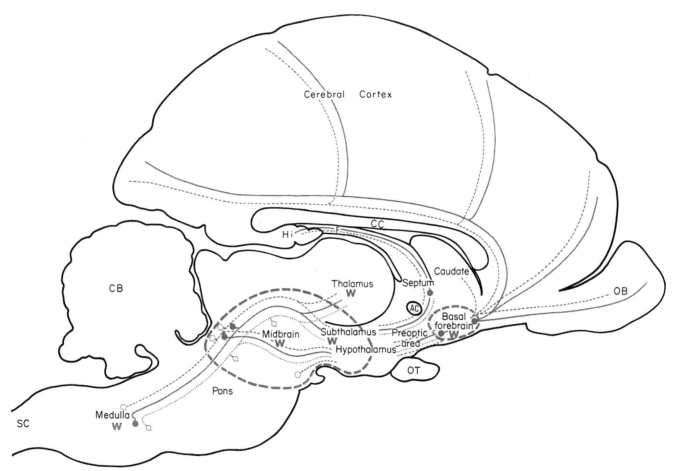

Figure 10–1. Mechanisms generating wakefulness. Schematic depiction of lateral, sagittal (S ~ 2.5 mm from midline) section of the cat brain representing neuronal systems implicated in the generation and maintenance of wakefulness. Outlined areas represent the regions in the brainstem (oral pontine and midbrain reticular formation) and caudal diencephalon (posterior hypothalamus, subthalamus, and ventral thalamus) and in the basal forebrain where large lesions are associated with a chronic decrease or loss of cortical activation and behavioral activity and responsiveness indicative of wakefulness. Although lesions of the central midbrain tegmentum primarily affect cortical activation, lesions of the ventral midbrain tegmentum predominantly alter behavioral arousal. Points marked with W (waking) indicate regions where high-rate electrical stimulation produces cortical activation and arousal and where neurons manifest a higher rate of spontaneous activity during wakefulness than during slow-wave sleep (including the ventral medullary, central pontine, and midbrain reticular formation; the ventral, intralaminar, and midline-medial thalamic nuclei; the posterior subthalamus and hypothalamus; and the basal forebrain). Diamond-shaped symbols represent the neurons of the reticular formation; dotted lines indicate their major ascending projections into the forebrain, which proceed along two major routes. The dorsal route terminates in the nonspecific thalamic nuclei, which in turn project in a widespread manner to the cerebral cortex. The ventral route passes through and terminates in the subthalamus and hypothalamus and continues into the basal forebrain and septum, where neurons in turn project in a widespread manner to the cerebral cortex and hippocampus. Open circles represent catecholaminergic neurons of the lower brainstem and locus coeruleus (dorsal pons), which contain norepinephrine, and of the substantia nigra and ventral tegmental area (ventral midbrain), which contain dopamine. The noradrenergic neurons are mainly implicated in processes of cortical activation and project (dashed lines) directly and diffusely to the cerebral cortex, as well as to the subcortical way stations. The dopaminergic neurons are predominantly implicated in processes of behavioral activity and responsiveness and project (dashed lines) heavily into the basal ganglia and frontal cortex. Solid circles represent acetylcholine-containing neurons of the brainstem reticular formation (including the laterodorsal and pedunculopontine tegmental nuclei in the dorsal pons and midbrain) and basal forebrain (substantia innominata, diagonal band nuclei, and septum). Cholinergic neurons are implicated in cortical activation and from the brainstem project (solid lines) predominantly to subcortical way stations, including the thalamus, subthalamus, hypothalamus, and basal forebrain and septum. The cholinergic basal forebrain neurons project (solid lines) in a widespread manner to the cerebral cortex and hippocampus. Not shown are other neuronal systems implicated in wakefulness, including histaminergic neurons in the posterior hypothalamus, which also project directly to the cerebral cortex. Glutamatergic neurons comprise the projection neurons of the reticular formation, thalamus, and cerebral cortex and thus are critical at all levels in processes of cortical activation and wakefulness. Multiple peptides, such as substance P, coricotropin-releasing factor, thyrotropin-releasing factor, vasoactive intestinal polypeptide, and neurotensin, may be involved in wakefulness and often are co-localized with one of the other primary neurotransmitters, such as norepinephrine or acetylcholine. The neuronal systems implicated in the maintenance of wakefulness may be involved in primary processes of sensory transmission and attention, motor response and activity, and orthosympathetic and neuroendocrine (particularly adrenocorticotropic hormone and thyrotropin-releasing hormone) responses and regulation, by which they may also enhance and prolong vigilance and arousal. AC, anterior commissure; CB, cerebellum; CC, corpus callosum; F, fornix; Hi, hippocampus; OB, olfactory bulb; OT, optic tract; SC, spinal cord. (Schematic diagrams drawn by reference to Berman AL. The Brain Stem of the Cat: A Cytoarchitectonic Atlas With Stereotaxic Coordinates. Madison, Wisc: University of Wisconsin Press; 1968; and Berman AL, Jones EG. The Thalamus and Basal Telencephalon of the Cat: A Cytoarchitectonic Atlas With Stereotaxic Coordinates. Madison, Wisc: University of Wisconsin Press; 1982.)

on tasks.[28] In animals with complete thalamic ablation, cortical desynchronization could still be elicited by stimulation of the midbrain reticular formation, which indicated that another, alternate extrathalamic route and relay to the cortex existed.[11] Demonstrated electrophysiologically in the 1950's, this pathway was identified through the use of neuroanatomical techniques only in the 1970's.[29] It originates from neurons located within the posterior hypothalamus, subthalamus, and basal forebrain (substantia innominata or nucleus basalis of Meynert, nuclei of the diagnonal band, and septum), which project in a widespread manner to the entire cortical mantle.[29–31] High-frequency electrical stimulation through these regions can produce widespread cortical activation (see Fig. 10–1).[11] In early studies, electrolytic lesions or transections destroying cells and fiber systems in the posterior hypothalamus and subthalamus were known to produce severe coma, thought at the time by some to be primarily due to destruction of ascending reticular pathways.[6] However, like Ranson[32] and Hess,[33] Nauta[34] attributed particular importance to the posterior hypothalamus as an orthosympathetic and waking center and even envisaged the possibility of a direct projection to the cortex from hypothalamic neurons. Neurotoxic lesions destroying nerve cell bodies and not nerve fibers of the posterior hypothalamus have been shown to decrease wakefulness[35] and thus to confirm the importance of hypothalamic neurons for this state. Lesions of cells in the basal forebrain, which project to the cortex, have also been found to be associated with a loss of cortical activation of wakefulness (see Fig. 10–1).[36, 37] The activating system must be enlarged to include the reticular formation of the brainstem and the posterior hypothalamus-subthalamus and basal forebrain, which receive ascending input from the reticular formation[7] and project in turn to the cerebral cortex.[30, 31] These forebrain systems also appear to be able to maintain cortical activation of the forebrain in the long-term absence of input from the brainstem reticular formation.

Single-Unit Recording of Wake-Active Neurons. In recording from neurons through the brain, neurophysiologists have found that the majority of cells are more active (i.e., have a higher spontaneous rate of firing) during wakefulness than during slow-wave sleep.[38–41] In the midbrain reticular formation, neurons that project forward into the forebrain have been found to have a tonic high rate of discharge in association with cortical activation and to decrease their rate of firing before the onset of cortical slow wave activity (see Fig. 10–1).[26] These neurons project forward onto nonspecific thalamocortical projection neurons, which are activated by the midbrain reticular neurons. The thalamic neurons also manifest a tonic high rate of firing during wakefulness and, via projections to widespread cortical areas, activate the large cortical projection neurons, which in turn fire at a high sustained rate during activation. Neurons that lie within the trajectory of the ventral, extrathalamic pathway and cortical relay, through the lateral hypothalamus and basal forebrain, have also been found to have a higher rate of firing during wakefulness than during slow-wave sleep (see Fig. 10–1).[42–46]

Sleep-Generating Systems

Identification of Sleep-Generating Systems. After acceptance in the 1940s and 1950s of the existence of an activating system, many physiologists believed that sleep was the result of fatigue and a decrease in activity of this system, thus representing a passive deactivation.[6] However, in experimental studies that used transections through the brainstem, it was found that sleep could be diminished to indicate that active sleep-inducing structures must also be present in the brain. Batini and colleagues[47] thus showed that transections of the brainstem behind the oral pontine tegmentum resulted in total insomnia; these results indicated that sleep-generating structures were located in the lower brainstem.

In support of this notion, slow-wave sleep has been reported to be diminished or absent in patients with lesions in the pons or medulla.[48–50] These cases show a predominance of alpha activity on the EEG, typical of waking, even though behavioral alertness and responsiveness are lacking in what has been referred to as an *alpha coma*.

Cortical synchronization indicative of slow-wave sleep could be produced in an awake animal preparation through low-frequency electrical stimulation of the medullary reticular formation, particularly the dorsal reticular formation and the solitary tract nucleus (Fig. 10–2).[51] Lesions of the dorsal reticular formation and solitary tract nucleus produced desynchronization of the EEG in a sleeping preparation.[52] Collectively, these results indicated the existence of neurons in the dorsal medullary reticular formation and the nucleus of the solitary tract that could generate sleep. The mechanism was hypothesized to involve inhibition of the rostrally located neurons of the ascending reticular activating system, although a direct synchronogenic influence on forebrain systems was also considered a possibility.

The solitary tract nucleus, of which stimulation induces sleep, receives afferent fibers from the vagus and glossopharyngeal nerves. Ascending projections from the solitary tract nucleus and dorsolateral medullary reticular formation were originally traced through the lateral and dorsal tegmentum and periventricular gray up to the level of the rostral pons and midbrain.[53] Here, fibers were found to terminate in the parabrachial nuclei, which in turn project rostrally into the thalamus, hypothalamus, preoptic area, amygdala, and orbitofrontal cortex, regions commonly belonging to the viscerolimbic forebrain. A direct projection from the solitary tract nucleus was subsequently demonstrated to all of these forebrain structures, except the cortex (see Fig. 10–2).[54] From these neuroanatomical data, it appeared that the predominant effect of the solitary tract nucleus does not occur via the reticular activating system but instead occurs via limbic forebrain structures, which also are implicated in sleep generation, as well as in autonomic regulation.

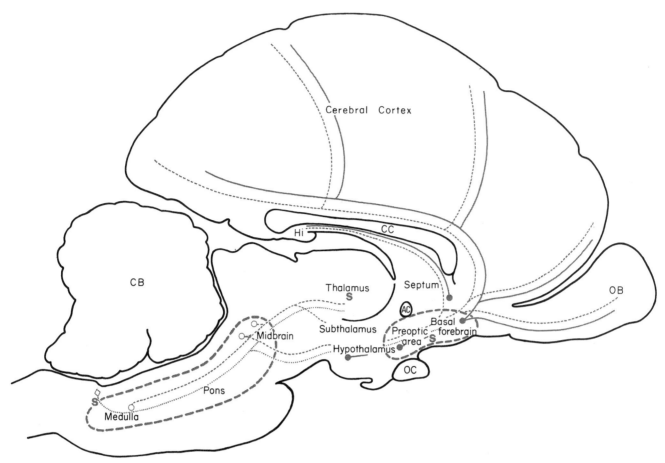

Figure 10–2. Mechanisms generating slow-wave sleep. Schematic depiction of paramedian, sagittal (S ~ 1.0 mm from midline) section of the cat brain representing neuronal systems implicated in the generation and maintenance of slow-wave sleep. Outlined areas represent the regions in the brainstem (raphe nuclei) and forebrain (anterior hypothalamus, preoptic area, and basal forebrain) where large lesions are associated with a chronic decrease or loss of slow wave sleep. Points marked with S (slow-wave sleep) indicate regions where low-frequency electrical stimulation produces cortical synchrony and behavioral sleep and where particular neurons manifest a higher rate of spontaneous activity (or typical burst-pause pattern of activity) during slow-wave sleep than during waking (including the solitary tract nucleus, nonspecific thalamic nuclei, and anterior hypothalamus-preoptic area and basal forebrain). Diamond-shaped symbols represent neurons of the solitary tract nucleus and adjacent tegmentum, implicated in slow-wave sleep regulation, which project (dotted lines) forward into the viscero limbic forebrain. Open circles represent serotonin neurons of the brainstem raphe nuclei, which may facilitate the onset of slow wave sleep and which project forward into the rostral tegmentum, thalamus, subthalamus, hypothalamus, and basal forebrain and from the midbrain directly to the cerebral cortex and hippocampus. Solid circles represent GABAergic neurons of the hypothalamus and basal forebrain-septum, which project (solid lines) in a widespread manner to the cerebral cortex and hippocampus. GABAergic neurons are also located in the thalamic reticular nucleus and cerebral cortex, where they play important roles in spindling and slow waves of slow-wave sleep. Not shown are other neuronal systems or factors implicated in slow-wave sleep, including adenosine. Multiple peptides, such as the opiates, alpha-melanocyte-stimulating hormone, somatostatin or cortistatin, and growth hormone–releasing hormone, may be involved in slow-wave sleep generation and often are co-localized with one of the other primary neurotransmitters, such as serotonin or GABA. The neuronal systems implicated in the maintenance of slow-wave sleep may be involved in primary processes of sensory inhibition and analgesia, behavioral inhibition, and parasympathetic and neuroendocrine (notably growth hormone) responses and regulation, by which they may also facilitate the onset and maintenance of slow-wave sleep. AC, anterior commissure; CB, cerebellum; CC, corpus callosum; Hi, hippocampus; OB, olfactory bulb; OC, optic chiasm. (Schematic diagrams drawn by reference to Berman AL. The Brain Stem of the Cat: A Cytoarchitectonic Atlas With Stereotaxic Coordinates. Madison, Wisc: University of Wisconsin Press; 1968; and Berman AL, Jones EG. The Thalamus and Basal Telencephalon of the Cat: A Cytoarchitectonic Atlas With Stereotaxic Coordinates. Madison, Wisc: University of Wisconsin Press; 1982.)

From the original studies of Bremer[2] using the *cerveau isolé* preparation, it had been known that synchronogenic structures must also be located in the forebrain. Cortical slow wave activity occurs continuously in these preparations, in which the brainstem influence has been suddenly removed. In experimental studies that use electrical stimulation, synchronous cortical activity could be driven or recruited by low-frequency stimulation of the midline thalamus.[55] In chronic preparations, prolonged thalamic stimulation was shown by Akert and colleagues[56] to induce natural sleep, as defined by both behavioral and EEG criteria (see Fig. 10–2), findings that lead to the conclusion that the thalamus is the head ganglion of sleep.[56] Such a conclusion has been supported in patients with *fatal familial insomnia*, which is reportedly associated with selective degeneration of thalamic nuclei.[57] However, experimental lesion studies in animals have shown that although the thalamus is necessary for the production of cortical spindles, it is not necessary for the generation of cortical slow waves and behavioral sleep, which persist after its complete ablation.[27]

Early in the 1900s, von Economo[14] noted that in some cases of "encephalitis lethargica," insomnia was the prominent symptom, and in these cases, lesions were centered in the anterior hypothalamus. He posited that a sleep center was located in the anterior hypothalamus, which would be in opposition to, as well as normally in balance with, the waking center in the posterior hypothalamus. Nauta[34] later experimentally confirmed the existence of a sleep facilitatory region in the anterior hypothalamus and preoptic area through the use of knife cuts. Hess[58, 59] demonstrated that electrical stimulation of this area could elicit behavioral suppression along with autonomic changes consonant with sleep. Neurons in this anterior region were posited to exert an inhibitory influence on the neurons of the ascending reticular activating system, a notion to be later proved with neurophysiological studies.

Electrical stimulation of the preoptic area and basal forebrain was subsequently shown in the 1960s by Sterman and Clemente[60] to lead to drowsiness and behavioral and EEG sleep (see Fig. 10–2). Conversely, they found that large lesions of these areas led to an elimination of or a decrease in sleep and a disruption of the sleep cycle (see Fig. 10–2).[61] The importance of the anterior hypothalamus, preoptic area, and basal forebrain, in addition to the lower brainstem, in the generation of sleep appeared to be clear.

However, Villablanca and colleagues[62] were to show that these structures were not sufficient for slow-wave sleep and that the basal ganglia and cerebral cortex may also contribute to sleep onset and maintenance. They found that animals without neocortex and striatum (thus called *diencephalic cats*) but with intact sleep-inducing structures of both the lower brainstem and the anterior diencephalon did not show a normal sleep cycle but instead showed a large decrease in slow-wave sleep. Although some damage to basal forebrain structures may have occurred in these preparations to explain the decrease in sleep, the results nevertheless suggested that the basal ganglia and the cerebral cortex also may have a role in sleep induction or maintenance, normally in balance with sleep-suppressing influences of the caudal diencephalon and rostral brainstem. Electrical stimulation of both the caudate nucleus and the orbitofrontal cortex had been shown to produce cortical synchrony and behavioral sleep.[63] Bilateral lesions of the frontal cortex resulted in a permanent moderate reduction in sleep, whereas lesions of the caudate nuclei led to a temporary decrease in sleep.[64] Other lesion studies indicated that the orbitofrontal cortex is particularly important in the generation of slow wave activity and behavioral sleep.[65] Evidence thus suggested that neurons in the orbitofrontal cortex, together with those in basal forebrain, preoptic area, and anterior hypothalamus, constitute a forebrain sleep-inducing system.

From neuroanatomical and neurophysiological studies, several principles were to emerge concerning the linkage of forebrain sleep-inducing systems with the limbic system and the interaction of this larger system with the brainstem activating system. From early neuroanatomical studies, neurons in the preoptic area and anterior hypothalamus were known to be interconnected with limbic forebrain structures, including, notably, the septum, amygdala, and orbitofrontal cortex, and to send descending projections to the limbic midbrain region, in what Nauta[66] termed the limbic forebrain-midbrain circuit. This descending projection extended into medial structures including the central gray and raphe nuclei but also terminated laterally in the midbrain reticular formation.[66–68] Electrical stimulation of the basal forebrain was shown to disrupt ongoing activity in midbrain reticular neurons, supporting the hypothesis that sleep-generating neurons in the forebrain may act in part by antagonizing neurons of the ascending reticular activating system.[69, 70] Connections of the forebrain limbic regions with lower brainstem autonomic centers were also apparent. Neurons in the anterior hypothalamus project directly to the solitary tract nucleus and adjacent region in the medulla, sending fibers through, as well as to, the parabrachial nuclei in the pons.[71] The orbitofrontal cortex also projects directly to the solitary tract nucleus, in addition to supplying an important input to the preoptic area, anterior hypothalamus, and parabrachial nuclei.[72] These forebrain and lower brainstem structures thus appear, through their interconnections, to form a system that is known to play an important role in visceral reflexes, in addition to having the capacity to influence sleep. The importance of visceral regulatory mechanisms to sleep regulation was originally proposed years ago by Hess and Nauta, both of whom emphasized the anatomical overlap between centers involved in regulation of the autonomic system and those involved in the sleep-wake cycle.[33, 59] It was noted that an overlap existed between sleep and parasympathetic centers in the anterior hypothalamus-preoptic area, where stimulation can elicit both behavioral and EEG signs of sleep and, in parallel, elicit a decrease in blood pressure, heart rate, and pupillary miosis. Conversely, an overlap is evident between waking and orthosympathetic centers in the posterior hypothalamus and midbrain reticular formation, where stimulation elicits behavioral arousal and cortical activation and, in parallel, elicits an increase in blood pressure, heart rate, and pupillary mydriasis.

Single-Unit Recording of Sleep-Active Neurons. Neurons that increase their rate of firing during slow-wave sleep are in the minority within the brain and particularly in the brainstem.[40, 41] In the region of the solitary tract nucleus, however, a number of neurons have been found to be more active during slow-wave sleep than during waking (see Fig. 10–2), although whether their increase in activity precedes sleep, which would suggest a role in the generation of sleep, is not certain.[73] Such sleep-related cells are intermingled with cells in the same area that show a higher rate of spontaneous activity during wakefulness.

It came as a surprise to early electrophysiologists to find that neurons in the cerebral cortex are active during slow-wave sleep and actually discharge in a bursting pattern.[74] However, because of long pauses between bursts, this burst-pause pattern of discharge is actually associated with a decrease in the average spike rate in both the cortex and thalamus during slow-wave sleep, a pattern that may allow relative rest for the thalamocortical system during this state. The bursting activity occurs first in association with spindles that are generated in the thalamus and driven by the neurons of the thalamic reticular nucleus.[75] As shown by Steriade and colleagues,[75] these cells manifest particular intrinsic properties that allow them to oscillate at a frequency identical to that of thalamocortical sleep spindles and to drive, in turn, the thalamocortical projection neurons that they innervate. Through intrinsic properties of the thalamic relay neurons and of cortical projection neurons, other slow oscillations that characterize slow-wave sleep EEG activity are also carried through the thalamocortical network.[76]

Neurons that increase their overall rate of discharge during slow-wave sleep compared with during waking were found in the anterior hypothalamus and preoptic area, as well as in the amygdala (see Fig. 10–2).[40, 43, 77] Sleep-active neurons were also found by Szymusiak and McGinty[45] to be distributed among wake-active cells in the basal forebrain (including the substantia innominata and nucleus of the horizontal limb of the diagonal band) (see Fig. 10–2).

CHEMICALS IMPLICATED IN SLEEP-WAKE STATES

In the early part of the 1900s, Pieron[78] introduced the concept of a chemical factor that would accumulate in the brain during waking and eventually generate sleep. He also provided experimental evidence for this concept by showing that transfer of cerebrospinal fluid (CSF) from sleep-deprived animals to non-deprived animals would cause the latter to sleep. This concept lay dormant for many years, in the absence of adequate techniques and knowledge to pursue the identification of such a hypnogenic factor.

With the development of increasingly sensitive biochemical techniques throughout the 1950s and 1960s, it was discovered that chemical neurotransmitters, previously identified in the peripheral nervous system, were also contained in the central nervous system. Drugs shown to act on these chemicals were found to have profound effects on sleep-wake states, suggesting that these neurotransmitters are normally involved in the generation of these states. After the development of histochemical techniques that permitted the localization of certain neurotransmitters to specific neurons, a direct approach to the study of the importance of chemically specific neuronal systems in sleep-wake states was made possible. This approach led by Jouvet in the 1960s[79] introduced the concept that sleep and waking may be generated by specific neurotransmitters contained within specific neuronal systems with widespread projections through the brain. With the localization of monoamines and acetylcholine to neurons in the reticular formation and the delineation of widespread projections from these neurons to the central nervous system, the monoamine- and acetylcholine-containing neurons were early, prime candidates for such state-generating systems. Other small amino acid neurotransmitters and large peptide neuroactive substances also have been localized to both local and more widespread projecting neuronal systems, as well as shown to have short-to long-duration actions. Thus, chemicals of different molecular size may function as neurotransmitters, neuromodulators, or neurohormones through local, widespread, or diffuse projections to provide the possibility for short- to long-accumulating and-acting molecules that could participate collectively in the generation, elaboration, and maintenance of the sleep-wake cycle.

CHEMICALS IMPLICATED IN WAKING

Neurotransmitters or Neuromodulators and Wakefulness. *Catecholamines* were first shown to be involved in arousal and wakefulness in the 1950s and 1960s in early pharmacological studies.[79, 80] Reserpine, which produces a state of inactivity and tranquilization, was discovered to act through depletion of the monamines. This tranquilization could be reversed by administration of the catecholamine precursor L-dihydroxyphenylalanine (L-dopa). The precursor administered by itself also stimulated a strong and long-lasting arousal and cortical activation.[81] Amphetamines known to produce an intense behavioral arousal and prolonged vigilance, associated with cortical activation, were also discovered to act through the catecholamines, that is, through the release of dopamine and norepinephrine. Cocaine also acts on metabolism of catecholamines by blocking their inactivation through reuptake. Drugs that inhibit monoamine oxidase prevent the enzymatic catabolism of monoamines, and those, such as pheniprazine and tranylcypromine, that appear to act predominantly on the catabolism of catecholamines cause an intense and prolonged arousal. Similarly, experimentally administered drugs that inhibit catechol O-methyltransferase and block catabolism of catecholamines produce a prolongation and intensification of waking, which can be extreme if combined with L-dopa.[81] Conversely, wakefulness is decreased after inhibition of catecholamine synthesis with α-methyl-p-tyrosine, which inhibits tyrosine hydroxylase or FLA-63 (bis [4-methyl-1-homopiperazinyl-thiocarbonyl] disulfide), which inhibits dopamine-β-hydroxylase.[79, 82]

Histochemical studies in the 1960s revealed that catecholamine perikarya were located in the brainstem reticular formation and in regions of the oral pontine and mesencephalic tegmentum classically known to be important to the maintenance of wakefulness (see Fig. 10–1).[83] The dopamine and norepinephrine-containing neurons had distinctly different distributions and projections such as to suggest different functional roles. Dopamine-containing neurons are localized in the substantia nigra and ventral tegmental area in the midbrain and scattered through the posterior hypothalamus and subthalamus. The dopaminergic neurons of the substantia nigra project forward through the lateral hypothalamus into the neostriatum, to which they provide a dense innervation (see Fig. 10–1).[84] Together with those of the ventral tegmental area, these dopaminergic neurons also innervate the basal forebrain, nucleus accumbens, septum, amygdala, and frontal cortex. Through these efferent projections, the midbrain dopaminergic neurons may modulate activity in motor and limbic systems.[85] The norepinephrine-containing neurons are found in the pontine and medullary reticular formation.[86] The largest cluster of noradrenergic neurons, giving rise to ascending projections, is in the locus coeruleus nucleus in the dorsolateral pontine tegmentum. Noradrenergic neurons of the locus coeruleus project in a diffuse manner to the entire forebrain, along pathways and terminal areas that overlap to a certain extent with those of the reticular formation but that most uniquely also include all areas of the cerebral cortex (see Fig. 10–1).[87] Other noradrenergic or adrenergic neurons are scattered through the ventrolateral pontine and medullary tegmentum and in the dorsomedial medulla.[88, 89] Collectively, the noradrenergic and adrenergic brainstem neurons provide an innervation to the entire forebrain, brainstem, and spinal cord and thus can directly modulate activity throughout the central nervous system, including the cerebral cortex.

Lesions of the dopamine-containing perikarya in the ventral tegmental area and substantia nigra in the cat were found to produce a state of behavioral unresponsiveness and immobility or akinesia (see Fig. 10–1).[79, 90] With lesions limited to the ventral midbrain tegmentum, this behaviorally comatose state was not associated with a decrease in cortical activation of wakefulness. On the other hand, lesions of the central midbrain tegmentum, where the ascending noradrenergic fibers pass, produced a severe decrease in cortical activation of wakefulness (see Fig. 10–1).[90, 91] In these animals, behavioral responses to stimulation could be elicited along with cortical activation; however, behavioral somnolence associated with moderately slow EEG activity characteristic of stage 1 sleep was in evidence the majority of time when the animals were not stimulated. The results of these physiological studies together with those of the neuroanatomical studies suggested that dopaminergic neurons of the substantia nigra and ventral tegmental area, which project to the striatum and frontal cortex, play an important role in behavioral arousal, whereas noradrenergic neurons of the locus coeruleus and brainstem, which project diffusely to the forebrain, including the cortex, play an integral role in cortical activation.

Clinical studies have provided evidence for the respective involvement of dopaminergic and noradrenergic neurons in conditions of akinesia and coma. Cases of akinesia and akinetic mutism often involve lesions of the ventral midbrain tegmentum or ventral posterior hypothalamus, where dopaminergic perikarya and pathways are located respectively[18, 92] Similarly, advanced cases of parkinsonism associated with severe akinesia have been found to involve extensive degeneration of dopaminergic neurons in the midbrain and depletion of dopamine in the striatum.[93] Such akinesia can be improved by treatment with L-dopa. Truly somnolent comas marked by a loss of cortical activation (*hypo-éveil* or *a-éveil*) occur with lesions of the mesencephalic reticular formation, through which the ascending noradrenergic pathways course.[92] Improvement in comatose states due to cerebral lesions has been reported after the administration of the catecholamine precursor L-dopa.[94]

Recovery from destruction of catecholaminergic neurons has been found to occur spontaneously in animals. The recovery of motor function, however, after substantia nigra lesions was shown to depend on intact dopaminergic neurons, which are capable of compensation, plasticity, and regeneration.[95] In such cases, functional recovery can occur if more than 5% of the dopaminergic nigrostriatal projection is left intact by the lesion. With such plasticity, severe long-term deficits may be rare and difficult to detect. Indeed, selective lesions of catecholaminergic neurons by intraventricular administration of 6-hydroxydopamine were found to have small to minimal transient effects on spontaneous motor activity and cortical activation of wakefulness.[82, 96] Moreover, localized thermolytic lesions of the noradrenergic locus coeruleus neurons in the oral pontine tegmentum did not produce the significant loss of wakefulness or alter cortical activation in the manner that midbrain lesions of ascending pathways had been found to do.[82, 91] On the other hand, reversible cooling of the locus ceruleus has been found to produce sleep in a waking animal, and electrical stimulation has been found to produce arousal in a sleeping animal.[97] These results indicate that collectively, catecholaminergic neurons normally enhance and prolong wakefulness but may not be essential for behavioral arousal and cortical activation because they represent components of larger and thus partially redundant neuronal systems.

Single-unit recording and neurotransmitter release studies have substantiated the role of catecholaminergic neurons in arousal processes (see Fig. 10–1). Presumed dopaminergic neurons in the substantia nigra and ventral tegmental area have a low basal rate of discharge that is similar across sleep-wake states, but they do increase their discharge and tend to fire in bursts of action potentials in association with significant sensory stimulation, purposive movements, or behavioral arousal.[98, 99] Presumed noradrenergic locus coeruleus neurons are most active during attentive, highly aroused, or stressful waking situations and otherwise show a regular, slow rate of spontaneous activity during quiet waking.[100, 101] They progressively decrease their rate of discharge during slow-wave sleep and virtually cease firing during paradoxical sleep. The release of dopamine and norepinephrine is greatest during the waking state and greatest in association with behavioral arousal.[102, 103]

The postsynaptic effect of the catecholamines differs from that originally described for the classic neurotransmitters because they do not act on receptors that directly gate ion channels (ionotropic) but instead stimulate second messengers (metabotropic). As in the periphery, central adrenergic receptors (alpha and beta) and dopaminergic receptors are associated with relatively long-lasting changes in target cells, which may include changes in their response to other neurotransmitters. According to such actions, catecholamines have been considered neuromodulators more than neurotransmitters. In the thalamus and cortex, stimulation of adrenergic receptors results in a depolarization and excitation of the projection neurons and a switch from a burst discharge typical of slow-wave sleep to a tonic discharge typical of waking.[104] Recently, a new drug, modafinil, that enhances and prolongs wakefulness in humans and animals but does not elicit behavioral excitation like that produced by amphetamine was found to act on postsynaptic adrenergic receptors (and not dopaminergic receptors) and to not act on presynaptic sites like amphetamine, which increases release of both norepinephrine and dopamine.[105, 106] These pharmacological results further substantiate the notion that norepinephrine and adrenergic receptors appear to be particularly important in stimulating and maintaining activating processes in thalamocortical systems, whereas dopaminergic systems are potent in stimulating behavioral arousal. Via projections that are long and widespread to diffuse and via slow modulatory actions on other systems, catecholamine-containing neurons may collectively stimulate, enhance, or prolong a waking, attentive, and aroused state of the animal.

Acetylcholine was known to be important for vigilance and cortical activation during waking based on pharmacological evidence from the 1950s and 1960s.[79, 107] Atropine or belladonna, which acts by blocking muscarinic cholinergic receptors, was well known to decrease vigilance. This deficit was shown in animals to be due to the appearance of slow wave activity on the cerebral cortex that persisted even during spontaneous movement in what was thus described as a dissociation between EEG and behavior. Conversely, neostigmine, which inhibits the catabolic enzyme acetylcholinesterase and thus prolongs the postsynaptic action of acetylcholine, was shown to enhance vigilance, in association with prolonged cortical activation. Cholinergic agonists, of either muscarinic or nicotinic type, thus including tobacco, have also long been known to elicit, enhance, or prolong vigilance and cortical fast activity. Acetylcholine thus appeared to play an important role in cortical activation, independent of waking behavior, and thus potentially during both waking and paradoxical sleep.[108]

Histochemical studies aimed at the identification of neurons containing acetylcholine were first attempted in the 1960s by localizing cells containing the degradative enzyme for acetylcholine, acetylcholinesterase. Although some of the major central cholinergic pathways were correctly delineated with this approach by Shute and Lewis,[109] the acetylcholine-containing neurons and their projections were only definitively identified with immunohistochemical staining of the synthetic enzyme for acetylcholine, choline acetyltransferase in the 1980s.[110] Two major groups of cholinergic neurons giving rise to forebrain and cortical projections have been identified (see Fig. 10–1). One is located in the oral pontine-caudal mesencephalic reticular formation (in the laterodorsal and pedunculopontine tegmental nuclei) and gives rise to projections into the forebrain, particularly to the medial-intralaminar thalamic nuclei but also to a lesser degree to the lateral hypothalamus and basal forebrain. Another is made up of cholinergic neurons located within the basal forebrain (nucleus basalis, substantia innominata, nuclei of the horizontal and vertical limbs of the diagonal band, and septum), which project in a widespread manner to the entire cerebral cortical mantle. The latter cells appeared to serve as the ventral, extrathalamic relay from the brainstem reticular formation to the cerebral cortex.

Lesions of the midbrain reticular formation, which diminish or eliminate cortical activation, as the early physiologists demonstrated, would have destroyed the pontomesencephalic cholinergic neurons and/or their ascending pathways going to the forebrain (see Fig. 10–1). Thus, as Shute and Lewis[109] had correctly posited, these cholinergic neurons would represent an important component of the ascending reticular activating system. However, more discrete neurotoxic lesions of a majority of the pontomesencephalic cholinergic neurons were not found to produce any notable deficit in cortical activation or decrease in the waking state.[111] These cholinergic cells thus must be considered to represent only one component of the ascending reticular activating system of the brainstem.

Lesions of the cholinergic neurons in the basal forebrain have been reported to produce alterations in cortical activity that are similar to those seen after atropine administration, that is, slowing of cortical activity and loss of vigilance (see Fig. 10–1).[36, 37] Such lesions have, however, also been reported to affect slow-wave sleep.[61, 112] The latter effects could be due to the destruction of intermingled or differentially distributed sleep-active cells, which would not likely contain acetylcholine. Pharmacological inhibition or inactivation of the cholinergic cells by local microinjections of chemical agents clearly diminishes the high-frequency cortical activity (gamma) that characterizes cortical activation as evident in aroused, attentive awake states and in paradoxical sleep.[113] These results confirm that the cholinergic neurons of the basal forebrain are very important for cortical activation.

Clinical investigations have demonstrated that Alzheimer's disease may be associated with a loss of cholinergic innervation of the cerebral cortex and degeneration of cholinergic neurons of the basal forebrain.[114, 115] This dementia is characterized by a diffuse slowing of cortical activity,[116–118] which could be explained by the degeneration of an activating system. However, in later stages of the disease, sleep is also greatly perturbed and marked by a loss of stages 3 and 4, as well as an absence of spindles and a decrease in REM sleep. Such general disruption of the EEG and sleep cycle probably reflects the diffuse degeneration and neurofibrillary changes of neurons in the cortex, as well as such changes documented in the basal forebrain and brainstem reticular formation and thus concerning multiple neuronal cell populations.[119, 120]

Single-unit recordings of neurons located in the region of the pontomesencephalic cholinergic neurons have revealed that a majority of these cells manifest a higher rate of firing during waking than during slow-wave sleep (and often an even higher rate during paradoxical sleep) (see Fig. 10–1).[121] Recordings in the region of the basal forebrain cholinergic neurons also show that the majority of these cells are most active during waking (and paradoxical sleep) compared with during slow-wave sleep (see Fig. 10–1).[42] Intermingled with the wake-active cells, however, are other cells that are most active during slow-wave sleep.[45] It remains to be determined which neurotransmitter is contained within each of these different cell types.

Studies of the release of acetylcholine in both the thalamus and cortex indicate that the brainstem and basal forebrain cholinergic neurons are indeed most active in association with cortical activation across the sleep-wake cycle.[122, 123] Acetylcholine release from the cerebral cortex has been found to be highest in association with both spontaneous cortical activation during waking or paradoxical sleep and that induced by electrical stimulation of the midbrain reticular formation.[122, 124, 125] It is greatly decreased in association with slow wave activity in natural sleep or anesthetized states.

Acetylcholine may act on muscarinic or nicotinic receptors within the central nervous system. Muscarinic receptors are associated through second-messenger systems (metabotropic) with slow and prolonged postsynaptic actions that are predominantly excitatory in nature, although some are inhibitory. Nicotinic receptors are associated by a direct link to ion channels (ionotropic) with fast postsynaptic excitatory actions. The application of acetylcholine to the cerebral cortex was shown by Krnjevic[126] to produce a prolonged excitation, which is characteristic of a slow neuromodulatory action mediated by muscarinic receptors. The slow depolarization of cortical pyramidal cells results in a shift in their mode of firing from a burst discharge associated with cortical slow waves to a tonic discharge associated with cortical fast activity.[104, 127] By such a modulatory synaptic action of acetylcholine and via widespread projections from the brainstem into the forebrain and from the basal forebrain to all cortical regions, cholinergic neurons may exert a tonic facilitatory influence on transmission and activity in the brain to promote cortical activation during both wakefulness and paradoxical sleep.

Histamine has long been assumed to play a role in waking given the well known sedative action of antihistaminergic drugs. Intraventricular administration of histamine was also shown to have an arousing effect.[128] Immunohistochemical studies have found that histamine-containing neurons are located in the posterior hypothalamus,[129] the region where in early experimental and clinical studies, lesions had been shown to be associated with coma or a decrease in wakefulness (see Fig. 10–1). Neurotoxic lesions, selective to cell bodies and sparing fibers of passage, have also been shown to produce a decrease in wakefulness and an increase in both slow-wave and paradoxical sleep.[35] Neurons in this area project to the cortex and may receive input from neurons of the brainstem reticular formation.[129, 130]

Similarly located neurons have been shown to be most active in association with the cortical activation of wakefulness.[45] Histamine acts on second-messenger–linked receptors, which are generally excitatory and produce a depolarization and resulting tonic discharge in thalamic and cortical projection neurons, as typically associated with waking, fast cortical activity.[104] Like norepinephrine, histamine thus would promote cortical activation during wakefulness.

Glutamate, the major excitatory neurotransmitter, is recognized as playing a fundamental role in neural activity of the waking brain. Glutamate agonists produce seizures. Some glutamate receptor antagonists (e.g., ketamine) are used as sedatives or anesthetic agents.[131] Glutamate is found in high concentrations in the large neurons of the brainstem reticular formation and likely represents the primary neurotransmitter of the ascending reticular activating system.[8] It is also contained in the projection neurons of the thalamus and cerebral cortex.[132] Glutamate is released from the cerebral cortex in highest quantities in association with cortical activation of spontaneous wakefulness or that evoked by stimulation of the midbrain reticular formation.[133] Glutamate acts on different postsynaptic receptors, including both ionotropic (kainate, AMPA [alpha-amino-hydroxymethyl-isoxazole proprionic acid], and NMDA [*N*-methyl-D-aspartate]) and metabotropic (*t*-ACPD [trans-aminocyclo-pentane-dicarboxylic acid]) receptors, which are all excitatory but are associated with different durations of excitation and induced patterns of discharge. Stimulation of the different receptors is commonly associated with increased spiking in thalamic and cortical neurons.[104] However, the stimulation of NMDA receptors can induce a burst discharge in many cells that has been implicated in the burst discharge of pyramidal cells during slow-wave sleep.[134] Thus, glutamate, which is contained in the reticular neurons of the brainstem activating system and in the majority of the projection neurons in the forebrain, is critical for cortical activation and a waking, responsive state. In addition, different glutamate receptors may be activated during slow-wave sleep in association with a burst mode of discharge.

Cerebrospinal Fluid-Borne Factors, Peptides, and Wakefulness. *Wake-promoting factors* are suspected of being present in the CSF because wakefulness and activity have been produced in recipient animals after the extraction of CSF from waking host animals.[135–137] It has long been suspected that such factors would be peptides, although other chemicals, such as the catecholamines, have been shown to accumulate in the CSF and to vary according to a circadian rhythm.

Peptides have been tested for wake- or sleep-promoting effects by intraventricular administration. Although it had been suspected that peptides may be released into the CSF and may diffuse widely by this route, they are known to be contained in neuronal systems with widespread projections that would permit such diffuse actions via chemical neurotransmission. The intraventricular route of administration for peptides, therefore, may or may not mimic physiological routes of action or reach physiological sites of effect for these factors. Peptides are often co-localized with other smaller molecule neurotransmitters, although they may be differentially released from the same nerve terminals as a function of different levels of neuronal activity. Neuroactive peptides act on second-messenger–linked receptors to produce relatively long-duration postsynaptic effects, some of which serve only to modulate the effects of other neurotransmitters or neuromodulators. One of the peptides that has the effect of slightly increasing the duration of waking when introduced into the CSF is *substance P.*[138] It may be significant that substance P has been co-localized with choline acetyltransferase in the cholinergic neurons of the pontomesencephalic tegmentum.[139] *Corticotropin-releasing factor* and *thyrotropin-releasing factor* have also been shown, after intraventricular administration, to produce a behavioral arousal associated with prolonged cortical activation and an antagonism of pentobarbital-induced sleep.[140–142] Corticotropin-releasing factor is also co-localized with choline acetyltransferase within pontomesencephalic cholinergic neurons.[143] When administered intraventricularly in small doses, *vasoactive intestinal peptide* has been associated with an increase in waking with cortical activation but appears to induce paradoxical sleep with cortical activation in larger doses.[144] In addition to being present in several subcortical systems,[145] vasoactive intestinal peptide has been co-localized with choline acetyltransferase in cortical neurons in the rat.[146] It is possible that vasoactive intestinal peptide, like acetylcholine, may have a role in the cortical activation that occurs during wakefulness and paradoxical sleep. Finally, *neurotensin*, which is contained in neurons distributed throughout the brain but includes neurons projecting to the basal forebrain, can stimulate cortical activation marked by high-frequency (gamma) activity when injected into the region of the cholinergic basal forebrain neurons.[147, 148] Such activation induced relatively selectively through the cholinergic system can be associated with wakefulness and paradoxical sleep.

Wake-Promoting Blood-Borne Factors. *Epinephrine,* which is normally released in the blood by the adrenal medulla, was shown through intraveneous administration in early pharmacological studies to produce cortical activation in a sleeping animal preparation.[52] The results of multiple studies suggested that peripherally circulating epinephrine released through sympathetic discharge could act centrally via the reticular activating system to produce cortical activation and wakefulness. Only later was it learned that epinephrine does not cross the blood-brain barrier. However, epinephrine and other blood-borne substances could act on the specialized circumventricular organs that lie outside the blood-brain barrier and within regions thought to be important in the sleep-wake cycle and in autonomic and neuroendocrine regulation, such as the area postrema in the medulla and the median eminence and organum vasculosum in the hypothalamus.

Histamine, which is produced in peripheral tissues, was shown to produce an arousing effect in rabbits when administered intravenously.[128] Furthermore, higher concentrations of histamine have been measured in the blood of aroused (through stimulation of the midbrain reticular formation) versus sleeping rabbits, which suggests its participation as a neurohumoral factor in the regulation of wakefulness and arousal. Like epinephrine, it must have its effect via regions of the brain that are outside the blood-brain barrier.

The action of peripheral chemical factors, which may include pituitary hormones such as *corticotropin* and *thyrotropin*, may permit the reinforcement of or alteration in centrally generated states. In addition, steroid hormones, such as the glucocorticoids secreted by the adrenal cortex, readily enter the brain and act directly via specific receptors on multiple neurons, through which they may also enhance arousal. Plasma *cortisol* has a very marked circadian rhythm as measured in human beings, reaching a nadir during slow-wave sleep in the night and then increasing in the early morning before sunrise and awakening, likely reflecting a hormonal preparatory mechanism for the waking state.[149]

CHEMICALS IMPLICATED IN SLOW-WAVE SLEEP

Neurotransmitters or Neuromodulators and Slow-Wave Sleep. *Serotonin* (5-hydroxytryptamine, [5-HTP]) appeared in the early pharmacological studies of the 1950s to have a possible role in sleep-wake states that would be opposite the role of catecholamines because the tranquilization produced through depletion of monoamines with reserpine was not reversed with subsequent administration of the serotonin precursor 5-hydroxy-L-tryptophan (5-HTP), as it was with the catecholamine precursor L-dopa.[80] Monoamine oxidase inhibitors that primarily block serotonin catabolism, such as pargyline and nialamide, were shown to enhance and prolong slow-wave sleep. Conversely, parachlorophenylalanine, which prevents the synthesis of serotonin by blocking the enzyme tryptophan hydroxylase, was shown to lead to insomnia, which could be reversed by the administration of small amounts of the serotonin precursor 5-HTP, which bypasses tryptophan hydroxylase.

In the 1960s, histochemical studies using the histofluorescent technique localized serotonin to raphe neurons within the brainstem,[83] suggesting the possibility to Jouvet[79] that the serotonin raphe nuclei may compose part of the brainstem slow-wave sleep system (see Fig. 10–2). According to the name, these nuclei are located on the midline through the brainstem and extend from the medulla into the pons and midbrain. Serotonin raphe neurons provide a diffuse innervation to the brain and spinal cord, the rostrally located (dorsal and central superior) raphe nuclei projecting mainly forward into the forebrain (including the thalamus, hypothalamus, basal forebrain, and all cortical areas), and the caudally located (magnus, pallidus, and obscurus) nuclei projecting mainly caudally into the spinal cord.[150]

Lesions of the raphe serotonin nuclei were shown

by Jouvet and associates[79] to produce total insomnia in the cat (see Fig. 10–2). Subtotal lesions involving the medullary, pontine, or midbrain raphe nuclei were associated with varying decreases in sleep, but the amount of slow-wave sleep was correlated with the percentage of destruction of the raphe nuclei and the percentage of depletion of serotonin in the forebrain. These results suggested that serotonin raphe neurons constitute an integral component of a brainstem sleep-generating system, which lies within the midline midbrain, pontine, and medullary raphe nuclei, as well as in the dorsolateral medullary region of the solitary tract nucleus.

Clinical cases of insomnia due to cerebral lesions have been found to be associated with lesions located in the region of the caudal midbrain and pontine tegmentum and particularly involving the midline raphe nuclei at these levels.[48, 49, 92] In one case of extreme insomnia (or *agrypnie* in a patient with *chorée fibrillarie de Morvan*), the administration of the serotonin precursor 5-HTP was found to restore natural slow-wave sleep.[151]

Recovery from the insomnia produced by raphe lesions has since been found to occur in animals, particularly after lesions produced by serotonin-selective neurotoxins 5,6-dihydroxytryptamine, and 5,7-dihydroxytryptamine.[82, 152] Similarly, recovery from the insomnia produced by pharmacological depletion of serotonin was demonstrated in prolonged long-term studies. It thus appeared that serotonin was not necessary for slow-wave sleep.

Further demonstrating the lack of a critical role of serotonergic neurons in the maintenance of sleep, single-unit recording subsequently revealed that presumed serotonergic raphe neurons actually decreased their rate of firing with the onset and for the duration of slow-wave sleep, to cease firing in paradoxical sleep.[153] These single-unit recording data were supported by results from biochemical studies of serotonin release, which was found to be lower during slow-wave sleep and paradoxical sleep than during wakefulness.[154] On the basis of these results, it was concluded that serotonergic neurons did not play an essential role in sleep maintenance.

Given the overwhelming evidence indicating that serotonin could normally facilitate sleep onset, it appeared that serotonergic neurons must exert an influence during waking that could facilitate sleep onset. Experiments applying electrical stimulation to raphe nuclei had in fact shown that although sleep is not produced by such stimulation, behavioral inhibition and sensory modulation and analgesia are produced.[155–157] Serotonin thus could act by attenuating other systems that normally stimulate cortical activation and arousal. In this regard, serotonin has recently been shown to have an inhibitory action on cholinergic neurons in both the pontomesencephalic tegmentum and basal forebrain.[158, 159] Microinjections of serotonin into the basal forebrain lead to decreases in cortical high-frequency (gamma) EEG activity, suggesting that serotonin may attenuate cortical activation and be associated with either a quiet waking state or an initiation

of slow-wave sleep.[113] Jouvet[160, 161] has also hypothesized that serotonin neurons may be responsible for the synthesis and accumulation of sleep factors during waking in neurons of the anterior hypothalamus. In sum, serotonin may prepare the brain and organism for slow-wave sleep during waking by attenuating activating systems and possibly stimulating accumulation of other sleep factors.

Serotonin acts on multiple receptors, which include second-messenger–linked receptors but also ionotropic receptors and which thus range from long- to fast-acting with inhibitory as well as excitatory effects on different postsynaptic cells.[162] The pharmacological effects of selective serotonin receptor agonists or antagonists on EEG activity and sleep have to date not been clearly interpretable, as is perhaps not surprising given the variety of receptors on diverse projection as well as interneuronal cell populations. It is certainly significant, nevertheless, that the ionotropic excitatory postsynaptic receptor (5-HT$_3$) is found mainly on gamma-aminobutyric acid (GABA)–ergic interneurons within the cortex and forebrain[163] and that the major inhibitory postsynaptic receptor (5-HT$_{1A}$) is found on many projection neurons and notably on the cholinergic basal forebrain neurons, which are hyperpolarized and inhibited by serotonin through this receptor.[158] Serotonin thus may act through concerted activation of multiple different receptors on different cell types to attenuate cortical activation and thus facilitate the initiation of slow-wave sleep.

Adenosine, the nucleoside, has long been thought to play a role in slow-wave sleep since the discovery that caffeine (methylxanthine), which acts as a stimulant, blocks adenosine receptors.[164] It has been shown that adenosine analogs can increase slow-wave sleep and cortical slow wave activity and that this increase can be prevented by the administration of caffeine.[165–167]

Adenosine is found in high concentrations in particular neurons from which it may be released as a neurotransmitter,[168] but it is also present in the extracellular space as a degradation product of adenosine triphosphate (ATP), which is packaged and released by many, including acetylcholine-containing, synaptic vesicles.[169] Adenosine is also transported out of cells when production of adenosine monophosphate (AMP) is increased during the formation of ATP from two molecules of adenosine diphosphate (ADP), as occurs as a consequence of energy demand.[170]

Although extracellular concentrations of adenosine in the brain are higher during waking than during slow-wave sleep, the concentrations appear to increase progressively with prolonged waking and to decrease progressively with subsequent sleep, such as to suggest a cumulative extracellular increase in what could be a fatigue-like and sleep-inducing factor in the brain.[171, 172]

Adenosine acts as a neuromodulator through second-messenger–linked postsynaptic receptors to inhibit neuronal discharge but also through other receptors to block neurotransmitter release from nerve terminals. It thus suppresses transmission at excitatory synapses in the brain and periphery.[173, 174] It inhibits cholinergic neurons in the brainstem and basal forebrain.[175] In the thalamus and cortex, it hyperpolarizes projection neurons and can facilitate the burst discharge that underlies the slow wave activity of slow-wave sleep.[176] Adenosine thus could function in the brain, as it has been shown to do in the body, as a factor that accumulates with continuous activity and acts to protect cells from damage that could result from excess activity.[170] In the brain, its action could be associated with the specialized burst discharge within thalamocortical circuits that underlies slow-wave sleep.[177]

GABA, the amino acid that is the major inhibitory neurotransmitter in the brain, has long been thought to have a role in sleep. The major sedative and hypnotic agents, benzodiazepines, are known to act by enhancing the postsynaptic action of GABA through binding to GABA receptors.[178] Pentobarbital and many other anesthetic agents are also known to act by enhancing GABA receptor–mediated synaptic currents.[179] Drugs that enhance GABA levels in the brain through inhibition of its catabolism (via GABA transaminase) also increase slow-wave sleep to a certain extent.[178, 180]

Interestingly, in human beings diagnosed with *idiopathic recurring stupor,* an endogenous benzodiazepine-like factor ("endozepine") has been identified in the CSF and found to be present in elevated levels in association with stuporous episodes.[181] The stupor could also be reversed with a benzodiazepine antagonist.

GABA-synthesizing neurons (containing the synthetic enzyme glutamic acid decarboxylase) are distributed through the brainstem, diencephalon, and forebrain and represent both interneurons and projection neurons.[182] In the brainstem reticular formation, relatively small GABAergic neurons are intermingled with larger glutamatergic projection neurons of the ascending reticular activating system and thus appear to have the capacity by local projections to inhibit the glutamatergic neurons of the ascending reticular activating system.[8] The neurons of the thalamic reticular nucleus that generate thalamocortical spindles[183] contain GABA and thus simultaneously inhibit and pace thalamocortical relay neurons by inhibitory postsynaptic potentials. This inhibition of the thalamus, the afferent gateway to the cerebral cortex, is fundamental to slow-wave sleep.[184] GABAergic neurons are distributed through the anterior hypothalamus-preoptic area and basal forebrain, and some give rise to descending projections to the posterior hypothalamus, where they could inhibit neurons of the activating system located there.[185, 186] A cluster of GABAergic neurons in the ventrolateral preoptic region that appear to be activated (as evident by c-Fos expression) during sleep were also found to give rise to descending projections to the posterior hypothalamus.[187] GABA release in the posterior hypothalamus has been found to be significantly higher during slow-wave sleep than during waking (or paradoxical sleep).[188] There also are GABAergic neurons in the hypothalamus and basal forebrain that give rise to long ascending projections to the cortex (see Fig. 10–2).[189–191] It is possible that these GABAergic neurons may correspond to long-projecting sleep-active cells recorded in these regions.[192] The release of GABA from

the cortex was shown by Jasper[133] to be highest in association with cortical slow waves of natural sleep or that following lesions of the midbrain reticular formation. GABA is also contained within interneurons of the cerebral cortex that were once shown to be more active during slow-wave sleep than waking.[41] GABAergic interneurons and projection neurons, however, are certainly active during waking in all regions of the brain and can also be important in pacing both fast and slow activity in the cortex. It would thus be most likely that particular GABAergic cells may be active during sleep, that particular GABAergic receptors may be activated during sleep, or both. Moreover, larger amounts of GABA, which could potentially diffuse to more receptors, could be released in association with the burst mode of discharge by GABAergic reticularis neurons in the thalamus during slow-wave sleep.

GABA acts on two types of receptors—one ($GABA_A$) that is linked directly to the chloride ion channel (and is the one that is modulated by benzodiazepines and pentobarbital), and another ($GABA_B$) that acts through second-messenger systems to modulate different ion channels (K^+ and Ca^{2+}).[193] Although both receptors are generally associated with inhibition, the action of the first ($GABA_A$) is very rapid, whereas that of the second ($GABA_B$) is slow and prolonged and includes attenuation of neurotransmitter release as well as neuronal spiking. In the thalamocortical system, both $GABA_A$ and $GABA_B$ receptors participate in the hyperpolarization associated with spindling and slow waves.[194, 195] The $GABA_A$ agonist THIP (tetra hydro isoxazolo pyridine) has recently been shown to enhance slow-wave sleep and slow wave activity in human beings.[196] The enhancement of slow wave activity and sleep clinically shown to be produced by gamma-hydroxybutyrate may well be mediated through $GABA_B$ receptors.[197–199] In sum, it is clear that GABAergic transmission is fundamentally involved in the induction and maintenance of slow-wave sleep—first, by inhibition of activating systems, and second, by initiating, pacing, and sustaining the thalamocortical burst discharge that underlies spindling and slow wave activity. This involvement must entail, however, selective activity of particular GABAergic neurons or different discharge of GABAergic neurons and resulting selective or prolonged activation of particular GABAergic receptors.

Cerebrospinal Fluid-Borne Factors, Peptides, and Slow-Wave Sleep. *Sleep-inducing factors* (as previously noted) were originally posited by Pieron[78] to accumulate within the brain and CSF. Over the past 25 years, the presence of such factors has been confirmed.[135–137, 160, 200] CSF or brain extract removed from a sleep-deprived animal or from an animal in the sleep-intense part of the cycle has been shown to promote sleep when it is injected into the ventricles of a normal animal, even during the awake, active period of the day. Identification of the sleep-promoting factors, however, has proved to be more difficult and remains controversial.

During the 1970s, it was discovered that neuroactive *peptides* are present in neurons of the central nervous system and could be released from nerve terminals.

Accordingly, it appeared that certain peptides could act as sleep-promoting factors within particular neuronal systems and/or by release and diffusion into the CSF. Attempted isolation of sleep factors from the CSF has not yet yielded any one unequivocal substance or peptide, although many candidates have been proposed and tested with ambiguous results. The testing of known peptides through intraventricular administration has revealed several peptides (enumerated below) that have an effect on sleep, and knowledge of the localization and projections of the peptide-containing neurons has allowed certain preliminary speculations to be made regarding the potential importance of these substances in sleep.

Opiate peptides have long been suspected of influencing sleep-wake states, in view of the sensory anesthesia, behavioral stupor, and associated EEG synchrony produced by the synthetic opiate analog morphine.[201] Administered intraventricularly, opiate peptides also produce anesthesia, akinesia, and EEG hypersynchrony,[202] but they do not appear to induce or increase physiological slow-wave sleep.[203] This negative effect may simply be due to the fact that opiate peptides normally act within specific neuronal circuits and not by release and diffusion through the CSF. The endogeneous opiate peptides, including enkephalin, endorphin, and dynorphin, have all been shown to have a role in sensory modulation and analgesia,[204] that could be important in the onset and maintenance of sleep. These peptides thus could be involved in attenuation of systems that normally stimulate arousal and waking. *Enkephalin* is contained in neurons that are widely distributed through the brain, including the cerebral cortex, and in neurons within regions involved in slow-wave sleep, including the solitary tract nucleus, the preoptic area, and the raphe, where it is co-localized with serotonin.[205] The locus coeruleus noradrenergic neurons, which stimulate waking, are known to be potently inhibited by opiates and to receive enkephalinergic afferents; local delivery of opiates results in a decrease in waking and enhancement of natural slow-wave sleep.[206] Derived from pro-opiomelanocortin, *beta-endorphin* is contained in neurons located in the arcuate region of the hypothalamus that give rise to widespread projections, which are particularly dense in the periventricular regions of the hypothalamus and preoptic area.[207] Other pro-opiomelanocortin–beta-endorphin cells are located in the nucleus of the solitary tract. Also derived from pro-opiomelanocortin and contained in neurons of the arcuate and solitary tracts, *alpha-melanocyte-stimulating hormone* (αMSH) may have sleep-inducing properties. It was found that intraventricular administration of desacetyl-αMSH produced a significant increase of slow-wave sleep.[208] It is particularly interesting that cells containing αMSH, which lack other pro-opiomelanocortin–derived peptides, have been identified in the lateral hypothalamus and zona incerta and have been found to project to the entire cortical mantle[209] in a diffuse projection system that could provide an anatomical substrate for widespread cortical modulation, which would occur in the generation of slow-wave sleep.

Somatostatin, administered intraventricularly, produces analgesia, akinesia, and a depression of EEG activity.[202] Not clearly involved in sleep, it was nevertheless originally believed to act as a central nervous system depressant because it can increase barbiturate-induced anesthesia.[140] Although distributed within multiple systems in the brain, somatostatin-containing neurons are located in the solitary tract nucleus and raphe nuclei.[210] Furthermore, somatostatin is co-localized with GABA in certain neuronal systems, including, notably, neurons of the thalamic reticular nucleus and a proportion of cortical interneurons.[210, 211] Like GABA, somatostatin has been found to have primarily inhibitory effects on central neurons and to reduce strychnine-induced seizures.[140] Like other peptides, it acts on second-messenger–linked receptors that are inhibitory to neuronal discharge and to neurotransmitter release from nerve terminals. Recently, a peptide named *cortistatin*, which is structurally similar to somatostatin and found in the cerebral cortex, was also found to suppress neuronal activity and to antagonize the effects of acetylcholine on cortical neurons. In addition, this peptide was found to induce slow waves in the cortex.[212] Because peptides are often co-localized with other smaller neurotransmitters and because somatostatin and cortistatin appear to be commonly co-localized with GABA,[213] it is possible that they are coreleased with the smaller inhibitory neurotransmitter. Moreover, peptides may be released particularly in association with bursting discharge of neurons,[214] which would occur in the thalamocortical system during slow-wave sleep, where and when somatostatin or cortistatin could be co-released with GABA and thus further sustain conditions for slow wave activity.

Growth hormone–releasing factor, which is produced by neurons in the hypothalamus,[215] from which it stimulates the release of growth hormone from the pituitary, also appears to have slow-wave sleep–inducing properties by acting on neurons in the anterior hypothalamus-preoptic area.[141] Its release would accordingly facilitate slow-wave sleep at the same time that it would stimulate the surge in growth hormone release from the pituitary that occurs during slow-wave sleep in the early part of the night in human beings. It should be noted that within these specific systems in the hypothalamus, somatostatin acts to suppress growth hormone release and thereby can also decrease slow-wave sleep.[216]

Other substances, including serotonin, that are not peptides and have sleep-inducing effects can be found in the CSF. *Prostaglandin D₂*, which is synthesized in brain (predominantly by glia) with a circadian fluctuation that is parallel to the sleep-wake cycle, has been shown to induce sleep in rats when it is administered in small amounts into the third ventricle.[217] Cytokines, most particularly, *interleukins*, which are now known to be synthesized in the brain (predominantly by glia), also produce sleep and enhance slow-wave activity when injected into the ventricles.[218–220] Most recently, a brain lipid called *cerebrodiene* has been isolated from the CSF of sleep-deprived cats that induced physiological sleep when injected into the ventricles of rats.[221, 222]

It thus appears that in addition to neuropeptides that are released by specific neurons, other substances, which may be synthesized by glia as well as neurons and released by nonexocytotic mechanisms from these cells, may participate in facilitating slow-wave sleep. Whether such substances accumulate in the CSF and thereby diffuse through the entire brain to exert their effects remains to be established.

Blood-Borne Factors and Slow-Wave Sleep. Presumably derived from blood platelets, *serotonin* in the blood could act in specialized regions of the brain located outside the blood-brain barrier to facilitate the onset of sleep. This possibility is suggested by the finding that local application of serotonin in the area postrema produced slow-wave sleep.[223]

Insulin, which is naturally secreted by the pancreatic islets in response to glucose, has been shown to have marked slow-wave sleep–inducing effects when it is administered intravenously in normal and insulin-depleted rats.[224] It is suggested that the accumulation of insulin during the active, hyperphagic waking periods would lead to the subsequent induction of sleep. Insulin receptors have been found in the brain within circumventricular organs located outside the blood-brain barrier and in nearby nuclei, notably in the basal hypothalamus and solitary tract, paravagal region.[225] Because the intraventricular administration of insulin has also been shown to induce sleep, it is suggested that its sleep-inducing action would be directly on the brain.

Cholecystokinin is a hormone that is released in the gut after food ingestion and suppresses further food intake. This so-called satiety hormone also promotes rest and may induce slow-wave sleep.[226] Another gut hormone, *bombesin,* which is also released after food ingestion, increases slow-wave sleep when it is administered peripherally.[227] These peripheral hormones that are in part responsible for postprandial satiety thus may also contribute to postprandial induction of rest and sleep, either by indirect action via vagal afferents to the solitary tract nucleus or by direct action on circumventricular organs located outside the blood-brain barrier.

Muramyl peptides also originate in the gut from intestinal bacteria and have been shown to have sleep-inducing properties.[226] Like other bacteria and viruses, they stimulate synthesis and release of cytokines, partiuclarly *interleukins,* that promote slow-wave sleep.[218] Sleep may thus be facilitated through hormones and other peptides that are released from the gut or from the immune system in response to exogenous substances.

Delta sleep–inducing peptide was identified and isolated by Monnier and colleagues[228] in the blood of rabbits during slow-wave sleep produced by low-frequency thalamic stimulation.[227] It was shown to induce sleep when injected into the blood or CSF of recipient rabbits. Although conflicting reports have appeared regarding the sleep-inducing effects of delta sleep–inducing peptide in various species, confirmation of an increase in slow-wave sleep has been obtained in mice after intraperitoneal administration of delta sleep–inducing peptide, an increase comparable to that obtained after intraperitoneal administration of sleep-promoting substance isolated from brain tissue.[200] Whether a similar peripheral and central peptide exists, where the peripheral substances are produced, and how they reach relevant receptors in the brain remain to be elucidated.

It appears that as in the regulation of waking, blood-borne substances can have an influence on the central sleep-generating systems, in part via the circumventricular organs by which they all have access to the brain. Included in these factors would accordingly also be certain pituitary hormones, such as *growth hormone* and *prolactin,* which are released maximally during slow-wave sleep[226] and also may influence sleep.

CONCLUSIONS

Neurophysiological and Neuroanatomical Results

Although early experimental lesions clearly indicated that particular regions of the brain were critical for the generation and maintenance of wakefulness or sleep and thus were particularly important in clinical cases involving lesions of these areas, they offered only clues about where integral neuronal systems would be located. First, early electrolytic lesions destroyed large areas of tissue. In fact, from these studies and subsequent ones using more refined techniques, it has become evident that a major loss of states is the result of sudden, massive damage to the brain, as occurs in clinical cases of infarct or hemorrhage. Slower and more limited disease processes are not often associated with the loss of a state or can be followed by recovery, as has been evident experimentally by staged lesions. Second, early electrolytic lesions destroyed both neuronal perikarya and fibers and, as such, revealed the localization of major ascending or descending pathways as well as cells critically involved in states. Thus, for example, the localization of the critical ascending reticular activating system to the rostral midbrain and caudal diencephalon must be attributed in part to the localization of the ascending reticular pathway from all brainstem reticular cells in these areas, in addition to the cell soma in these regions. More discrete perikaryal lesions with neurotoxins at any level of the reticular formation have not been associated with such dramatic and permanent changes.

However, what has emerged from these early studies and their sequelae is that the neuronal systems that govern the cyclic alternation between waking and sleep are contained within the isodendritic core of the brain that extends from the medulla through the brainstem and hypothalamus up into the basal forebrain. No structure within this core is uniquely or monolithically involved in the control of one state. Instead, as was first suggested by differential effects of low-frequency versus high-frequency electrical stimulation of the reticular core and subsequently indicated by single-unit recording of sleep-active in addition to wake-active neurons within the reticular core, different neurons within the same structure or field of cells are important sleep versus waking. Despite such an intermingling of sleep-active and wake-active neurons, a differential concentration of such cells may exist in different regions. It appears that neurons mainly involved in maintaining activation are concentrated within the oral pontine and midbrain central tegmentum and posterior hypothalamus, whereas cells that exert an important sleep-promoting influence are concentrated within the midline brainstem and dorsolateral medullary reticular formation and the anterior hypothalamus-preoptic area, with possible intermingling of the two in the basal forebrain. Just as cells with different activity profiles and primary functional involvements are codistributed in such fields, cells with different projections, including ascending versus descending, are intermingled in the same fields and may modulate forebrain and spinal activities, respectively, during the sleep-wake cycle.

Neurochemical Results

Just as cells with different activities and projections are interdigitated within the reticular core, so cells containing different neuroactive chemicals are intermingled through the same regions. It is possible that the specificity of action derives from the neurotransmitter released, as well as from the activity and projections of the neurons. Although such a behavioral specificity may not apply to the small amino acid neurotransmitters that are contained and act within multiple local-circuit neurons, it may apply to the amine (more appropriately called) neuromodulators, including catecholamines, acetylcholine, histamine, and serotonin, which are contained within restricted neuronal aggregates located in the reticular core and have widespread projections to the forebrain and spinal cord. Such systems may simultaneously bias or modify the mode of activity of entire populations of neurons within the central nervous system. Moreover, molecules of larger peptides may also function as neuromodulators or even neurohormones that may be responsible for even longer-lasting alterations in neuronal function that would underlie the sleep-wake states and cycle. However, to date, no single chemical neurotransmitter, neuromodulator, or neurohormone has been identified that is necessary or sufficient for the generation and maintenance of sleep or waking. Instead, multiple factors and systems are involved in the onset and maintenance of these states.

Overview of Sleep-Wake Mechanisms

Wakefulness is initiated and reinforced by particular visceral, somatic, and special sensory input, which is transmitted fairly directly to special cortical areas but also, more important for wakefulness, via collaterals to the brainstem reticular formation, extending from the medulla to the midbrain, in which visceral, somatic, auditory, vestibular, and visual sensory collaterals proliferate. This system overlaps extensively with orthosympathetic systems in the brainstem and caudal hypothalamus. Activation is transmitted into the forebrain and cortex via the nonspecific thalamocortical projection system and via the subthalamus, hypothalamus, and basal forebrain, where cortically projecting cells are also located. Olfactory sensory input may also influence activation by collateral transmission through the basal forebrain neurons. Within this isodendritic core, particular neurons that are distributed through the brainstem, hypothalamus, and basal forebrain are activated more or less during waking, depending on sensory input from internal and external milieus; however, they appear to remain tonically active at some level during this state, regardless of sensory input, according to an autochthonous rhythm. This activating system is essential for the maintenance of wakefulness and cortical activation indicative of that state. Within this system of cells are located catecholaminergic and cholinergic neurons, which are tonically active during wakefulness and which, via particularly long and widespread forebrain projections, may modulate the activity of the subcortical and cortical neurons and circuits to facilitate tonic fast discharge in thalamocortical systems. Histamine-containing neurons located in the posterior hypothalamus may also contribute via long projections to this modulation. The predominant neurotransmitter of neurons of the reticular activating system, as well as thalamic and cortical projection neurons, is glutamate, the excitatory amino acid that is essential for activity in these systems. Certain neuropeptides, contained in neurons with relatively long and widespread projections and also co-localized with catecholamines or acetylcholine, such as substance P, corticotropin-releasing factor, thyrotropin-releasing factor, vasoactive intestinal peptide, and neurotensin, may enhance and prolong such actions to promote activation. Certain factors carried in the blood, including epinephrine, histamine, and some peptides, can serve to reinforce the central state of arousal.

Aided by a decrease in certain types of sensory input and facilitated by an increase in other types of somatic and visceral sensory input, such as warmth and satiation, sleep-inducing neurons become active and promote cortical slow wave activity by damping the cyclic activity of reticular activating neurons and directly modulating activity through the forebrain. Sleep-inducing neurons are concentrated in the lower brainstem reticular formation and solitary tract nucleus and in the rostral hypothalamus, preoptic area, and basal forebrain, extensively overlapping with autonomic, particularly parasympathetic, regulatory systems. Cortical slow wave activity evolves from a change in pattern of discharge of cortical and thalamic neurons from tonic and fast to bursting at a slow rate with intervening pauses. Serotonin-containing neurons of the raphe may be important in dampening certain sensory input and attenuating cortical activation in the initiation of slow-wave sleep. Adenosine may be a factor that accumulates during waking and could promote slow bursting discharge in thalamocortical systems. Critical for spindling and slow waves is the activity of GABAergic neurons located within the thalamic reticular nucleus. GABAergic neurons in many other regions, including the reticular formation, hypothalamus, and basal forebrain, also may be important for inhibiting neurons involved in cortical activation. GABAergic interneurons in the cortex and perhaps also long-projecting neurons located in the hypothalamus and basal forebrain that project to the cortex may be important for initiating and maintaining slow-wave sleep. Multiple neuropeptide-containing neurons are located in the brainstem and hypothalamic-basal forebrain regions and may, via release onto other neurons or into the CSF, alter activity and transmission through the forebrain. Certain peptides, somatostatin and cortistatin, are co-localized with GABA in neurons within the thalamus and cortex. The sleep-promoting substances of the CSF remain to be identified; however, several known peptides, including the opiates, αMSH, and cortistatin have been shown to have certain sleep-inducing properties therein. Peripheral factors, such as serotonin, insulin, gut hormones, cytokines, and sleep peptides, may also influence the sleep-wake cycle and facilitate sleep.

In summary, many of the chemical and neuronal substrates of the sleep-wake states have been identified and characterized according to their activity and transmission. Many other chemical neuroactive substances await discovery and, as components of multifarious systems, hold promise for important roles in the generation of waking and sleep.

Acknowledgments

The author would like to thank Alain Beaudet and Edmund Cape for their helpful comments on the manuscript, Beverley Lindsay for her secretarial assitance, Lynda Mainville for her technical assistance, and Margo Oelstzschner and Marcus Arts for their assistance with the illustrations. Laboratory research of BEJ has been supported by the Medical Research Council of Canada.

References

1. Kleitman N, Camille N. Studies on the physiology of sleep, VI. the behavior of decorticated dogs. Am J Physiol. 1932;100:474.
2. Bremer F. Cerveau "isolé" et physiologie du sommeil. C R Soc Biol (Paris). 1929;102:1235.
3. Moruzzi G, Magoun HW. Brain stem reticular formation and activation of the EEG. Electroencephalogr Clin Neurophysiol. 1949;1:455.
4. Lindsley DB, Schreiner LH, Knowles WB, et al. Behavioral and EEG changes following chronic brain stem lesions. Electroencephalogr Clin Neurophysiol. 1950;2:483.
5. French JD, Magoun HW. Effects of chronic lesions in central cephalic brain stem of monkeys. Arch Neurol Psychiatr. 1952;68:591.
6. Moruzzi G. The sleep-waking cycle. Ergeb Physiol. 1972;64:1.
7. Dempsey EW, Morison RS, Morison BR. Some afferent diencephalic pathways related to cortical potentials in the cat. Am J Physiol. 1941;131:718.
8. Jones BE. Reticular formation: cytoarchitecture, transmitters and projections. In: Paxinos G, ed. The Rat Nervous System. New South Wales, Australia: Academic Press Australia; 1995:155.
9. Nauta WJH, Kuypers HGJM. Some ascending pathways in the brain stem reticular formation. In: Jasper HH, Proctor LD, Knighton RS, et al, eds. Reticular Formation of the Brain. Boston, Mass: Little, Brown & Co; 1958:3.
10. Scheibel ME, Scheibel AB. Structural substrates for integrative patterns in the brain stem reticular core. In: Jasper HH, Proctor LD, Knighton RS, et al, eds. Reticular Formation of the Brain. Boston, Mass: Little, Brown & Co; 1958:31.
11. Starzl TE, Taylor CW, Magoun HW. Ascending conduction in reticular activating system, with special reference to the diencephalon. J Neurophysiol. 1951;14:461.
12. Gayet M. Affection encephalique (encephalite diffuse probable). Arch Physiol Norm Pathol. 1875;2:341.
13. Mauthner L. Zur Pathologie und Physiologie des Schlafes nebst Bermerkungen ueber die "Nona." Wien Klin Wochenschr. 1890;40:961.
14. von Economo C. Encephalitis Lethargica: Its Sequelae and Treatment. London, England: Oxford University Press; 1931.
15. Cairns H. Disturbances of consciousness with lesions of the brain-stem and diencephalon. Brain. 1952;75:109.
16. Castaigne P, Escourolle R. Etude topographique des lesions anatomiques dans les hypersomnies. Rev Neurol. 1967;116:547.
17. Facon E, Steriade M, Wertheim N. Hypersomnie prolongee engendree par des lesions bilaterales du systeme activateur medial: le syndrome thrombotique de la bifurcation du tronc basilaire. Rev Neurol. 1958;98:117.
18. Plum F, Posner JB. The Diagnosis of Stupor and Coma. Philadelphia, Pa: FA Davis; 1980.
19. Feldman SM, Waller HJ. Dissociation of electrocortical activation and behavioural arousal. Nature. 1962;196:1320.
20. McGinty DJ. Somnolence, recovery and hyposomnia following ventro-medial diencephalic lesions in the rat. Electroencephalogr Clin Neurophysiol. 1969;26:70.
21. Slosarska M, Zernicki B. Chronic pretrigeminal and cerveau isole cats. Acta Neurobiol Exp. 1973;33:811.
22. Villablanca J. The electrocorticogram in the chronic cerveau isolé cat. Electroencephalog Clin Neurophysiol. 1965;19:576.
23. Adametz JH. Rate of recovery of functioning in cats with rostral reticular lesions. J Neurosurg. 1959;16:85.
24. Jasper H. Diffuse projection systems: the integrative action of the thalamic reticular system. Electroencephalogr Clin Neurophysiol. 1949;1:405.
25. Monnier M, Kalberer M, Krupp P. Functional antagonism between diffuse reticular and intralaminary recruiting projections in the medial thalamus. Exp Neurol. 1960;2:271.
26. Steriade M. Mechanisms underlying cortical activation: neuronal organization and properties of the midbrain reticular core and intralaminar thalamic nuclei. In: Pompeiano O, Ajmone Marsan C, eds. Brain Mechanisms and Perceptual Awareness. New York, NY: Raven Press; 1981:327.
27. Villablance J, Salinas-Zeballos ME. Sleep-wakefulness, EEG and behavioral studies of chronic cats without the thalamus: the "athalamic" cat. Arch Ital Biol. 1972;110:383.
28. Guilleminault, C Quera-Salva M-A, Goldberg MP. Pseudo-hypersomnia and pre-sleep behaviour with bilateral paramedian thalamic lesions. Brain. 1993;116:1549.
29. Kievit J, Kuypers HGJM. Basal forebrain and hypothalamic connections to frontal and parietal cortex in the rhesus monkey. Science. 1975;187:660.
30. Saper CB. Organization of cerebral cortical afferent systems in the rat, I: magnocellular basal nucleus. J Comput Neurol. 1984;222:313.
31. Saper CB. Organization of cerebral cortical afferent systems in the rat, II: hypothalamocortical projections. J Comput Neurol. 1985;237:21.
32. Ranson SW. Somnolence caused by hypothalamic lesions in the monkey. Arch Neurol Psychiatr. 1939;41:1.
33. Hess WR. The Functional Organization of the Diencephalon. New York, NY: Grune & Stratton; 1957.
34. Nauta WJH. Hypothalamic regulation of sleep in rats: an experimental study. J Neurophysiol. 1946;9:285.
35. Sallanon M, Sakai K, Buda C, et al. Augmentation du sommeil paradoxal, induite par l'injection d'acide ibotenique dans l'hypothalamus ventrolateral posterior, chez le chat. C R Acad Sci Paris. 1986;303:175.
36. Lo Conte G, Casamenti F, Bigi V, et al. Effect of magnocellular forebrain nuclei lesions on acetylcholine output from the cerebral cortex, electrocorticogram and behaviour. Arch Ital Biol. 1982;120:176.
37. Stewart DJ, MacFabe DF, Vanderwolf CH. Cholinergic activation

of the electrocorticogram: role of the substantia innominata and effects of atropine and quinuclidinyl benzilate. Brain Res. 1984;322:219.

38. Kasamatsu T. Spontaneous unitary discharges of the mesencephalic reticular formation during sleep and wakefulness in normal and chronically blinded cats. Brain Res. 1969;14:506.

39. Manohar S, Noda H, Ross Adey W. Behavior of mesencephalic reticular neurons in sleep and wakefulness. Exp Neurol. 1972;34:140.

40. McGinty DJ, Harper RM, Fairbanks MK. Neuronal unit activity and the control of sleep states. In: Weitzman ED, ed. Advances in Sleep Research. New York, NY: Spectrum Publications; 1974:173.

41. Steriade M, Hobson JA. Neuronal activity during the sleep-waking cycle. Progr Neurobiol. 1976;6:155.

42. Detari L, Juhasz G, Kukorelli T. Firing properties of cat basal forebrain neurones during sleep-wakefulness cycle. Electroencephalogr Clin Neurophysiol. 1984;58:362.

43. Findlay ALR, Hayward JN. Spontaneous activity of single neurones in the hypothalamus of rabbits during sleep and waking. J Physiol. 1969;201:237.

44. Oomura Y, Ooyama H, Naka F, et al. Some stochastical patterns of single unit discharges in the cat hypothalamus under chronic conditions. Ann NY Acad Sci. 1969;157:666.

45. Szymusiak R, McGinty D. Sleep-related neuronal discharge in the basal forebrain of cats. Brain Res. 1986;370:82.

46. Vanni-Mercier G, Sakai K, Jouvet M: Neurones specifiques de l'eveil dans l'hypothalamus posterieur. C R Acad Sci (Paris). 1984;298(III):195.

47. Batini C, Moruzzi G, Palestini M, et al. Effects of complete pontine transections of the sleep-wakefulness rhythm: the mid-pontine pretrigeminal preparation. Arch Ital Biol. 1959;97:1.

48. Freemon FR, Salinas-Garcia RF, Ward JW. Sleep patterns in a patient with a brain stem infarction involving the raphe nucleus. Electroencephalogr Clin Neurophysiol. 1974;36:657.

49. Markand ON, Dyken ML. Sleep abnormalities in patients with brain stem lesions. Neurology. 1976;26:769.

50. Westmoreland BF, Klass DW, Sharbrough FW, et al. Alpha-coma. Arch Neurol. 1975;32:713.

51. Magnes J, Moruzzi G, Pompeiano O. Synchronization of the EEG produced by low-frequency electrical stimulation of the region of the solitary tract. Arch Ital Biol. 1961;99:33.

52. Bonvallet M, Dell P, Hiebel G. Tonus sympathique et activite electrique corticale. Electroencephalogr Clin Neurophysiol. 1954;6:119.

53. Norgren R. Projections from the nucleus of the solitary tract in the rat. Neuroscience. 1978;3:207.

54. Ricardo JA, Koh ET. Anatomical evidence of direct projections from the nucleus of the solitary tract to the hypothalamus, amygdala, and other forebrain structures in the rat. Brain Res. 1978;153:1.

55. Morison RS, Dempsey EW. A study of thalamo-cortical relations. Am J Physiol. 1942;135:281.

56. Akert K, Koella WP, Hess RJ. Sleep produced by electrical stimulation of the thalamus. Am J Physiol. 1952;168:260.

57. Lugaresi E, Medori R, Montagna P, et al. Fatal familial insomnia and dysautonomia with selective degeneration of thalamic nuclei. N Engl J Med. 1986;315:997.

58. Hess WR. Le sommeil. C R Soc Biol. 1931;107:1333.

59. Hess WR. Diencephalon: Autonomic and Extrapyramidal Functions. New York, NY: Grune & Stratton; 1954.

60. Sterman MB, Clemente CD. Forebrain inhibitory mechanisms: sleep patterns induced by basal forebrain stimulation in the behaving cat. Exp Neurol. 1962;6:103.

61. McGinty DJ, Sterman MB. Sleep suppression after basal forebrain lesions in the cat. Science. 1968;160:1253.

62. Villablanca J, Marcus R. Sleep-wakefulness, EEG and behavioral studies of chronic cats without neocortex and striaatum: the "diencephalic" cat. Arch Ital Biol. 1972;110:348.

63. Penaloza-Rojas JH, Elterman M, Olmos N. Sleep induced by cortical stimulation. Exp Neurol. 1964;10:140.

64. Villablanca JR, Marcus RJ, Olmstead CE. Effects of caudate nuclei or frontal cortex ablations in cats, II: sleep-wakefulness, EEG, and motor activity. Exp Neurol. 1976;53:31.

65. Jouvet M. Recherches sur les structures nerveuses et les meca-

nismes responsables des differentes phases du sommeil physiologique. Arch Ital Biol. 1962;100:125.

66. Nauta WJ, Haymaker W. Hypothalamic nuclei and fiber connections. In: Haymaker W, Andersoon E, Nauta WJH, eds. The Hypothalamus. Springfield, Ill: CC Thomas: 1969:136.

67. Swanson LW. An autoradiographic study of the efferent connections of the preoptic region in the rat. J Comput Neurol. 1976;167:227.

68. Swanson LW, Cowan WM. The connections of the septal region in the rat. J Comput Neurol. 1979;186:621.

69. Lineberry CG, Siegel J. EEG synchronization, behavioral inhibition, and mesencephalic unit effects produced by stimulation of orbital cortex, basal forebrain and caudate nucleus. Brain Res. 1971;34:143.

70. Siegel J, Wang RY. Electroencephalographic, behavioral, and single-unit effects produced by stimulation of forebrain inhibitory structures in cats. Exp Neurol. 1974;42:28.

71. Ricardo JA. Hypothalamic pathways involved in metabolic regulatory functions, as identified by track-tracing methods. In: Szabo AJ, ed. Advances in Metabolic Disorders. New York, NY: Academic Press; 1983:1.

72. van der Kooy D, Koda LY, McGinty JF, et al. The organization of projections from the cortex, amygdala, and hypothalamus to the nucleus of the solitary tract in rat. J Comp Neurol. 1984;224:1.

73. Eguchi K, Satoh T. Characterization of the neurons in the region of solitary tract nucleus during sleep. Physiol Behav. 1980;24:99.

74. Evarts EV. Temporal patterns of discharge of pyramidal tract neurons during sleep and waking in the monkey. J Neurophysiol. 1964;27:152.

75. Steriade M, Llinas RR. The functional states of the thalamus and the associated neuronal interplay. Physiol Rev. 1988;68:649.

76. Steriade M, Contreras D, Amzica F. Synchronized sleep oscillations and their paroxysmal developments. Trends Neurosci. 1994;17:199.

77. Jacobs BL, McGinty DJ. Amygdala unit activity during sleep and wakefulness. Exp Neurol. 1971;33:1.

78. Pieron H. Le Probleme Physiologique du Sommeil. Paris, France: Masson; 1913.

79. Jouvet M. The role of monoamines and acetylcholine-containing neurons in the regulation of the sleep-waking cycle. Ergeb Physiol. 1972;64:165.

80. Carlsson A, Lindqvist M, Magnusson T. 3,4-Dihydroxyphenylalanine and 5-hydroxytryptophan as reserpine antagonists. Nature. 1957;180:1200.

81. Jones BE. The respective involvement of noradrenaline and its deaminated metabolites in waking and paradoxical sleep: a neuropharmacological model. Brain Res. 1972;39:121.

82. Jacobs BL, Jones BE. The role of central monoamine and acetylcholine systems in sleep-wakefulness states: mediation or modulation. In: Butcher LL, ed. Cholinergic-Monoaminergic Interactions in the Brain. New York, NY: Academic Press; 1978:271.

83. Dahlstrom A, Fuxe K. Evidence for the existence of monoamine-containing neurons in the central nervous system, I: demonstration of monoamines in the cell bodies of brain stem neurons. Acta Physiol Scand. 1964;62:1.

84. Bjorklund A, Lindvall O. Dopamine-containing systems in the CNS. In: Bjorklund A, Hokfelt T, eds. Handbook of Chemical Neuroanatomy. Vol 2. Classical Transmitters in the CNS, Part I. Amsterdam, Netherlands: Elsevier; 1984:55.

85. Nauta WJH, Domesick VB. Crossroads of limbic and striatal circuitry: hypothalamo-nigral connectioons. Limbic Mechanisms. 1978;75.

86. Moore RY, Card JP. Noradrenaline-containing neuron systems. In: Bjorklund A, Hokfelt T, eds. Handbook of Chemical Neuroanatomy. Vol 2. Classical Transmitters in the CNS, Part I. Amsterdam, Netherlands: Elsevier; 1984:123.

87. Jones BE, Yang T-Z. The efferent projections from the reticular formation and the locus coeruleus studied by anterograde and retrograde axonal transport in the rat. J Comp Neurol. 1985;242:56.

88. Hokfelt T, Johansson O, Goldstein M. Central catecholamine neurons as revealed by immunohistochemistry with special reference to adrenaline neurons. In: Bjorklund A, Hokfelt T, eds. Handbook of Chemical Neuroanatomy. Vol 2. Classical Trans-

mitters in the CNS, Part I. Amsterdam, Netherlands: Elsevier; 1984:157.

89. Hokfelt T, Martensson R, Bjorklund A, et al. Distributional maps of tyrosine-hydroxylase-immunoreactive neurons in the rat brain. In: Bjorklund A, Hokfelt T, eds. Handbook of Chemical Neuroanatomy. Vol 2. Classical Transmitters in the CNS, Part I. Amsterdam: Elsevier; 1984:277.

90. Jones BE, Bobillier P, Pin C, et al. The effect of lesions of catecholamine-containing neurons upon monoamine content of the brain and EEG and behavioral waking in the cat. Brain Res. 1973;58:157.

91. Jones BE, Harper ST, Halaris AE. Effects of locus coeruleus lesions upon cerebral monoamine content, sleep-wakefulness states and the response to amphetamine. Brain Res. 1977;124:473.

92. Schott B, Michel D, Mouret J, et al. Monoamines et regulation de la vigilance, II: syndromes lesionnels du systeme nerveux central. Rev Neurol. 1972;127:157.

93. Bernheimer H, Birkmayer W, Hornykiewicz O, et al. Brain dopamine and the syndromes of Parkinson and Huntington. J Neurol Sci. 1973;20:415.

94. Di Rocco C, Maira G, Meglio M, et al. L-dopa treatment of comatose states due to cerebral lesions. J Neurosurg Sci. 1974;18:169.

95. Stricker EM, Zigmond MJ. Recovery of function following damage to central catecholamine-containing neurons: a neurohemical model for the lateral hypothalamic sydrome. In: Sprague JM, Epstein AN, eds. Prog Psychobiol Physiol Psychol. New York, NY: Academic Press; 1975:121.

96. Laguzzi R, Petitjean F, Pujol JF, et al. Effets de l'injection intraventriculaire de 6-hydroxydopamine, II: sur le cycle veille-sommeils du chat. Brain Res. 1972;48:295.

97. Cespuglio R, Gomez ME, Faradji H, et al. Alterations in the sleep-waking cycle induced by cooling of the locus coeruleus area. Electroencephalogr Clin Neurophysiol. 1982;54:570.

98. Jacobs BL. Overview of the activity of brain monoaminergic neurons across the sleep-wake cycle. In: Wauquier A, Monti JM, Gaillard JM, et al, eds. Sleep: Neurotransmitters and Neuromodulators. New York, NY: Raven Press; 1985:1.

99. Ljungberg T, Apicella P, Schultz W. Responses of monkey dopamine neurons during learning of behavioral reactions. J Neurophysiol. 1992;67:145.

100. Jacobs BL. Single unit activity of locus coeruleus neurons in behaving animals. Progr Neurobiol. 1986;27:183.

101. Steriade M, Hobson JA. Neuronal activity during the sleep-waking cycle. Prog Neurobiol. 1976;6:155.

102. Kalen P, Rosegren E, Lindvall O, et al. Hippocampal noradrenaline and serotonin release over 24 hours as measured by the dialysis technique in freely moving rats: correlation to behavioural activity state, effect of handling and tail-pinch. Eur J Neurosci. 1989;1:181.

103. Trulson ME. Simultaneous recording of substantia nigra neurons and voltammetric release of dopamine in the caudate of behaving cats. Brain Res Bull. 1985;15:221.

104. McCormick DA. Neurotransmitter actions in the thalamus and cerebral cortex and their role in neuromodulation of thalamocortical activity. Progr Neurobiol. 1992;39:337.

105. Broughton RJ, Fleming JA, George CF, et al. Randomized, double-blind, placebo-controlled crossover trial of modafinil in the treatment of excessive daytime sleepiness in narcolepsy. Neurology. 1997;49:444.

106. Lin JS, Roussel B, Akaoka H, et al. Role of catecholamines in the modafinil and amphetamine induced wakefulness, a comparative pharmacological study in the cat. Brain Res. 1992;591:319.

107. Domino EF, Yamamoto K, Dren AT. Role of cholinergic mechanisms in states of wakefulness and sleep. Progr Brain Res. 1968;28:113.

108. Jones BE. The organization of central cholinergic systems and their functional importance in sleep-waking states. In: Cuello AC, ed. Cholinergic Function and Dysfunction, Progress in Brain Research. Vol 98. Amsterdam, Netherlands: Elsevier; 1993:61.

109. Shute CCD, Lewis PR. The ascending cholinergic reticular system: neocortical, olfactory and subcortical projections. Brain. 1967;90:497.

110. Mesulam M-M, Mufson EJ, Wainer BH, et al. Central cholinergic pathways in the rat: an overview based on an alternative nomenclature (Ch1-Ch6). Neuroscience. 1983;10:1185.

111. Webster HH, Jones BE. Neurotoxic lesions of the dorsolateral pontomesencephalic tegmentum-cholinergic cell area in the cat, II: effects upon sleep-waking states. Brain Res. 1988;458:285.

112. Szymusiak R, McGinty D. Sleep suppression following kainic acid-induced lesions of the basal forebrain. Exp Neurol. 1986;94:598.

113. Cape EG, Jones BE. Differential modulation of high frequency gamma electroencephalogram activity and sleep-wake state by noradrenaline and serotonin microinjections into the region of cholinergic basalis neurons. J Neurosci. 1998;18:2653.

114. Davies P, Moloney AJF. Selective loss of central cholinergic neurones in Alzheimer's disease. Lancet. 1976;2:1403.

115. Rossor MN, Garrett NJ, Johnson AL, et al. A post-mortem study of the cholinergic and GABA systems in senile dementia. Brain. 1982;105:313.

116. Gordon EB, Sim M. The E.E.G. in presenile dementia. J Neurol Neurosurg Psychiatr. 1967;30:285.

117. Johannesson G, Brun A, Gustafson I, et al. EEG in presenile dementia related to cerebral blood flow and autopsy findings. Acta Neurol Scand. 1977;56:89.

118. Prinz PN, Peskind ER, Vitaliano PP, et al. Changes in the sleep and waking EEGs of nondemented and demented elderly subjects. J Am Geriatr Soc. 1982;30:86.

119. Hirano A, Zimmerman HM. Alzheimer's neurofibrillary changes. Arch Neurol. 1962;7:227.

120. Ishii T. Distribution of Alzheimer's neurofibrillary changes in the brain stem and hypothalamus of senile dementia. Acta Neuropathol. 1966;6:181.

121. El Mansari M, Sakai M, Jouvet M. Unitary characteristics of presumptive cholinergic tegmental neurons during the sleep-waking cycle in freely moving cats. Exp Brain Res. 1989;76:519.

122. Marrosu F, Portas C, Mascia S, et al. Microdialysis measurement of cortical and hippocampal acetylcholine release during sleep-wake cycle in freely moving cats. Brain Res. 1995;671:329.

123. Williams JA, Comisarow J, Day J, et al. State-dependent release of acetylcholine in rat thalamus measured by in vivo microdialysis. J Neurosci. 1994;14:5236.

124. Casamenti F, Deffenu G, Abbamondi AL, et al. Changes in cortical acetylcholine output induced by modulation of the nucleus basalis. Brain Res Bull. 1986;16:689.

125. Celesia GG, Jasper HH. Acetylcholine released from cerebral cortex in relation to state of activation. Neurology. 1966;16:1053.

126. Krnjevic K. Chemical transmission and cortical arousal. Anesthesiology. 1967;28:100.

127. Metherate R, Cox CL, Ashe JH. Cellular bases of neocortical activation: modulation of neural oscillations by the nucleus basalis and endogenous acetylcholine. J Neurosci. 1992;12:4701.

128. Monnier M, Sauer R, Hatt AM. The activating effect of histamine on the central nervous system. Int Rev Neurobiol. 1970;12:265.

129. Steinbusch HWM, Mulder AH. Immunohistochemical localization of histamine in neurons and mast cells in the rat brain. In: Bjorklund A, Hokfelt T, Kuhar MJ, eds. Handbook of Chemical Neuroanatomy. Vol 3. Classical Transmitters in the CNS, Part II. Amsterdam, Netherlands: Elsevier; 1984:126.

130. Sakai K. Neurons responsible for paradoxical sleep. In: Wauquier A, Gaillard JM, Monti JM, et al, eds. Sleep: Neurotransmitters and Neuromodulators. New York, NY: Raven Press; 1985:29.

131. Mayer ML, Westbrook GL. The physiology of excitatory amino acids in the vertebrate central nervous system. Progr Neurobiol. 1987;28:197.

132. Ottersen OP, Storm-Mathisen J. Neurons containing or accumulating transmitter amino acids. In: Bjorklund A, Hokfelt T, Kuhar MJ, eds. Handbook of Chemical Neuroanatomy. Vol 3, Classical Transmitters and Transmitter Receptors in the CNS, Part II. Amsterdam, Netherlands: Elsevier; 1984:141.

133. Jasper HH, Khan RT, Elliott KAC. Amino acids released from the cerebral cortex in relation to its state of activation. Science. 1965;147:1448.

134. Armstrong-James M, Fox K. Evidence for a specific role for cortical NMDA receptors in slow wave sleep. Brain Res. 1988;451:189.

135. Fencl V, Koski G, Pappenheimer JR. Factors in cerebrospinal fluid from goats that affect sleep and activity in rats. J Physiol. 1971;216:565.

136. Sachs J, Ungar J, Waser PG, et al. Factors in cerebrospinal fluid affecting motor activity in the rat. Neurosci Lett. 1976;2:83.

137. Ursin R. Endogenous sleep factors. Exp Brain Res. 1984; 8(suppl):118.

138. Riou F, Cespuglio R, Jouvet M. Endogenous peptides and sleep in the rat, I: peptides decreasing paradoxical sleep. Neuropeptides. 1982;2:243.

139. Vincent SR, Satoh K, Armstrong DM, et al. Substance P in the ascending cholinergic reticular system. Nature. 1983;306:688.

140. Brown M, Vale W. Central nervous system effects of hypothalamic peptides. Endocrinology. 1975;96:1333.

141. Ehlers C, Reed TK, Henriksen SJ. Effects of corticotropin-releasing factor and growth hormone-releasing factor on sleep and activity in rats. Neuroendocrinology. 1986;42:467.

142. Imaki T, Shibasaki T, Masuda A, et al. The antagonistic effect of corticotropin-releasing factor on pentobarbital in rats. Brain Res. 1986;383:323.

143. Vincent SR, Satoh K, Armstrong DM, et al. Neuropeptides and NADPH-diaphorase activity in the ascending cholinergic reticular system of the rat. Neuroscience. 1986;17:167.

144. Riou F, Cespuglio R, Jouvet M. Endogenous peptides and sleep in the rat, III: the hypnogenic properties of vasoactive intestinal polypeptide. Neuropeptides. 1982;2:265.

145. Abrams GM, Nilaver G, Zimmerman EA. VIP-containing neurons. In: Bjorklund A, Hokfelt T, eds. Handbook of Chemical Neuroanatomy. Vol 4, GABA and Neuropeptides in the CNS, Part I. Amsterdam, Netherlands: Elsevier; 1985:335.

146. Eckenstein F, Baughman RW. Two types of cholinergic innervation in cortex, one co-localized with vasoactive intestinal polypeptide. Nature. 1984;309:153.

147. Cape EG, Alonso A, Beaudet A, et al. Neurotensin micro-injections into the basal forebrain promote cortical activation associated with the states of wake and PS in the rat. Soc Neurosci Abstr. 1996;22:149.

148. Morin AJ, Tajani M, Jones BE, et al. Neurotensinergic innervation of cholinergic neurons in the rat basal forebrain: a light microscopic study with three-dimensional reconstruction. J Chem Neuroanat. 1996;10:147.

149. Weitzman ED, Zimmerman JC, Czeiler CA, et al. Cortisol secretion is inhibited during sleep in normal men. J Clin Endocrinol Metab. 1983;56:352.

150. Steinbusch HWM. Serotonin-immunoreactive neurons and their projections in the CNS. In: Bjorklund A, Hokfelt T, eds. Handbook of Chemical Neuroanatomy. Vol 3. Classical Transmitters in the CNS, Part II. Amsterdam, Netherlands: Elsevier; 1984:68.

151. Fischer-Perroudon C, Mouret J, Jouvet M. Sur un cas d'agrypnie (4 mois sans sommeil) au cours d'une maladie de Morvan: effet favorable du 5-hydroxytryptophane. Electroencephalogr Clin Neurophysiol. 1974;36:1.

152. Froment J-L, Petitjean F, Bertrand N, et al. Effets de l'injection intracérébrale de 5,6-hydroxytryptamine sur les monoamines cérébrales et les états de sommeil du chat. Brain Res. 1974;67:405.

153. McGinty D, Harper RM. Dorsal raphe neurons: depression of firing during sleep in cats. Brain Res. 1976;101:569.

154. Puizillout JJ, Gaudin-Chazal G, Daszuta A, et al. Release of endogenous serotonin from "encephale isolé" cats. J Physiol (Paris). 1979;75:531.

155. Fields HL, Basbaum AI. Brain stem control of spinal pain transmission neurons. Annu Rev Physiol. 1978;40:193.

156. Jacobs BL. Electrophysiological and behavioral effects of electrical stimulation of the raphe nuclei in cats. Physiol Behav. 1973;11:489.

157. Siegel J, Brownstein RA. Stimulation to N. raphe dorsalis, central gray and hypothalamus: inhibitory and aversive effects. Physiol Behav. 1975;14:431.

158. Khateb A, Fort P, Alonso A, et al. Pharmacological and immuno-histochemical evidence for a serotonergic input to cholinergic nucleus basalis neurons. Eur J Neurosci. 1993;5:541.

159. Luebke JI, Greene RW, Semba K, et al. Serotonin hyperpolarizes cholinergic low-threshold burst neurons in the rat laterodorsal tegmental nucleus in vitro. Proc Natl Acad Sci U S A. 1992;89:743.

160. Jouvet M. Neuromediateurs et facteurs hypnogenes. Rev. Neurol (Paris). 1984;140:389.

161. Sallanon M, Buda C, Janin M, et al. Implication of serotonin in sleep mechanisms: induction, facilitation? In: Wauquier A, Monti JM, Gaillard JM, et al, eds. Sleep: Neurotransmitters and Neuromodulators. New York, NY: Raven Press; 1985:136.

162. Bobker DH, Williams JT. Ion conductances affected by 5-HT receptor subtypes in mammalian neurons. Trends Neurosci. 1990;13:169.

163. Morales M, Bloom FE. The 5-HT$_3$ receptor is present in different subpopulations of GABAergic neurons in the rat telencephalon. J Neurosci. 1997;17:3157.

164. Radulovacki M, Virus RM, Djuricic-Nedelson M, et al. Adenosine and adenosine analogs: effects on sleep in rats. In: McGinty DJ, Morrison A, Drucker-Colin R, et al, eds. Brain Mechanisms of Sleep. New York, NY: Raven Press; 1985:235.

165. Benington JH, Kodali SK, Heller HC. Stimulation of A$_1$ adenosine receptors mimics the electroencephalographic effects of sleep deprivation. Brain Res. 1995;692:79.

166. Radulovacki M, Virus RM. Purine, 1-methylisoguanosine and pyrimidine compounds and sleep. In: Wauquier A, Monti JM, Gaillard JM, et al, eds. Sleep: Neurotransmitters and neuromodulators. New York, NY: Raven Press; 1985:221.

167. Ticho SR, Radulovacki M. Role of adenosine in sleep and temperature regulation in the preoptic area of rats. Pharmacol Biochem Behav. 1991;40:33.

168. Braas KM, Newby AC, Wilson VS, et al. Adenosine-containing neurons in the brain localized by immunocytochemistry. J Neurosci. 1986;6:1952.

169. Smith DO. Sources of adenosine released during neuromuscular transmission in the rat. J Physiol. 1991;432:343.

170. Newby AC. Adenosine and the concept of "retaliatory metabolites." Trends Biol Sci. 1984;9:42.

171. Huston JP, Haas HL, Boix F, et al. Extracellular adenosine levels in neostriatum and hippocampus during rest and activity periods of rats. Neuroscience. 1996;73:99.

172. Porkka-Heiskanen T, Strecker RE, Thakkar M, et al. Adenosine: a mediator of the sleep-inducing effects of prolonged wakefulness. Science. 1997;276:1265.

173. Dolphin A, Archer E. An adenosine agonist inhibits and a cyclic AMP analogue enhances the release of glutamate but not GABA from slices of rat dentate gyrus. Neurosci Lett. 1983;43:49.

174. Smith DO, Lu Z. Adenosine derived from hydrolysis of presynaptically released ATP inhibits neuromuscular transmission in the rat. Neurosci Lett. 1991;122:171.

175. Rainnie DG, Grunze HCR, McCarley RW, et al. Adenosine inhibition of mesopontine cholinergic neurons: implications for EEG arousal. Science. 1994;263:689.

176. Pape H-C. Adenosine promotes burst activity in guinea-pig geniculocortical neurones through two different ionic mechanisms. J Physiol. 1992;447:729.

177. Benington JH, Heller HC. Restoration of brain energy metabolim as the function of sleep. Progr Neurobiol. 1995;45:347.

178. Mendelson WB. GABA-benzodiazepine receptor-chloride ionophore complex: implications for the pharmacology of sleep. In: Wauquier A, Monti JM, Gaillard JM, et al, eds. Sleep: Neurotransmitters and Neuromodulators. New York, NY: Raven Press; 1985:229.

179. Nicoll RA. Pentobarbital: differential postsynaptic actions on sympathetic ganglion cells. Science. 1978;199:451.

180. Scherschlicht R. Role for GABA in the control of the sleep-wakefulness cycle. In: Wauquier A, Monti JM, Gaillard JM, et al, eds. Sleep: Neurotransmitters and Neuromodulators. New York, NY: Raven Press; 1985:237.

181. Rothstein JD, Guidotti A, Tinuper P, et al. Endogenous benzodiazepine receptor ligands in idiopathic recurring stupor. Lancet. 1992;340:1002.

182. Mugnaini E, Oertel WH. An atlas of the distribution of GABAergic neurons and terminals. In: Bjorklund A, Hokfelt T, eds. Handbook of Chemical Neuroanatomy. Vol 4: GABA and Neuropeptides in the CNS, Part I. Amsterdam, Netherlands: Elsevier; 1985:436.

183. Steriade M, Deschenes M. The thalamus as a neuronal oscillator. Brain Res Rev. 1984;8:1.

184. Hofle N, Paus T, Reutens D, et al. Regional cerebral blood flow

changes as a function of delta and spindle activity during slow wave sleep in humans. J Neurosci. 1997;17:4800.

185. Gritti I, Mainville L, Jones BE. Codistribution of GABA- with acetylcholine-synthesizing neurons in the basal forebrain of the rat. J Comput Neurol. 1993;329:438.

186. Gritti I, Mainville L, Jones BE. Projections of GABAergic and cholinergic basal forebrain and GABAergic preoptic-anterior hypothalamic neurons to the posterior lateral hypothalamus of the rat. J Comput Neurol. 1994;339:251.

187. Sherin JE, Shiromani PJ, McCarley RW, et al. Activation of ventrolateral preoptic neurons during sleep. Science. 1996;271:216.

188. Nitz D, Siegel JM. GABA release in posterior hypothalamus across sleep-wake cycle. Am J Physiol. 1996;271:R1707.

189. Fisher RS, Buchwald NA, Hull CD, et al. GABAergic basal forebrain neurons project to the neocortex: the localization of glutamic acid decarboxylase and choline acetyltransferase in feline corticopetal neurons. J Comput Neurol. 1988;272:489.

190. Gritti I, Mainville L, Mancia M, et al. GABAergic and other non-cholinergic basal forebrain neurons project together with cholinergic neurons to meso- and iso-cortex in the rat. J Comput Neurol. 1997;383:163.

191. Vincent SR, Hokfelt T, Skirboll LR, et al. Hypothalamic gamma-aminobutyric acid neurons project to the neocortex. Science. 1983;220:1309.

192. Szymusiak R, McGinty D. Sleep-waking discharge of basal forebrain projection neurons in cats. Brain Res Bull. 1989;22:423.

193. Bowery N. $GABA_B$ receptors and their significance in mammalian pharmacology. Trends Pharmacol. 1989;101:401.

194. Crunelli V, Leresche N. A role for $GABA_B$ receptors in excitation and inhibition of thalamocortical cells. Trends Neurosci. 1991;14:16.

195. von Krosigk M, Bal T, McCormick DA. Cellular mechanisms of a synchronized oscillation in the thalamus. Science. 1993;261:361.

196. Faulhaber J, Steiger A, Lancel M. The $GABA_A$ agonist THIP produces slow wave sleep and reduces spindling activity in NREM sleep in humans. Psychopharmacology. 1997;130:285.

197. Lapierre O, Montplaisir J, Lamarre M, et al. The effect of gamma-hydroxybutyrate on nocturnal and diurnal sleep of normal subjects: further considerations on REM sleep-triggering mechanisms. Sleep. 1990;13:24.

198. Williams SR, Turner JP, Crunelli V. Gamma-hydroxybutyrate promotes oscillatory activity of rat and cat thalamocortical neurons by a tonic $GABA_B$ receptor-mediated hyperpolarization. Neuroscience. 1995;66:135.

199. Yamada Y, Yamamoto J, Fujiki A, et al. Effect of butyrolactone and gamma-hydroxybutyrate on the EEG and sleep cycle in man. Electroencephalogr Clin Neurophysiol. 1967;22:558.

200. Nagasaki H, Kitahama K, Valatx J-L, et al. Sleep-promoting effect of the sleep-promoting substance (SPS) and delta sleep-inducing peptide (DSIP) in the mouse. Brain Res. 1980;192:276.

201. Bronzino JD, Kelly ML, Cordova C, et al. Amplitude and spectral quantification of the effects of morphine. Electroencephalogr Clin Neurophysiol. 1982;53:14.

202. Havlicek V, Friesen HG. Comparison of behavioral effects of somatostatin and beta-endorphin in animals. In: Collu R, Ducharme JR, Barbeau A, et al, eds. Central Nervous System Effects of Hypothalamic Hormones and Other Peptides. New York, NY: Raven Press; 1979:381.

203. Riou F, Cespuglio R, Jouvet M. Endogenous peptides and sleep in the rat, II: peptides without significant effect on the sleep-waking cycle. Neuropeptides. 1982;2:255.

204. Basbaum AI, Fields HL. Endogeneous pain control systems: brainstem spinal pathways and endorphin circuitry. Annu Rev Neurosci. 1984;7:309.

205. Petrusz P, Merchenthaler I, Maderdrut JL. Distribution of enkephalin-containing neurons in the central nervous system. In: Bjorklund A, Hokfelt T, eds. Handbook of Chemical Neuroanatomy. Vol 4. GABA and Neuropeptides in the CNS, Part I. Amsterdam, Netherlands: Elsevier; 1985:273.

206. Garzon M, Tejero S, Beneitez AM, et al. Opiate microinjections in the locus coeruleus area of the cat enhance slow wave sleep. Neuropeptides. 1995;29:229.

207. Khachaturian H, Lewis ME, Tsou K, et al. β-Endorphin, α-MSH, ACTH, and related peptides. In: Bjorklund A, Hokfelt T, eds. Handbook of Chemical Neuroanatomy. Vol 4. GABA and Neuropeptides in the CNS, Part I. Amsterdam, Netherlands: Elsevier; 1985:216.

208. Chastrette N, Cespuglio R. Influence of proopiomelanocortin-derived peptides on the sleep-waking cycle of the rat. Neurosci Lett. 1985;62:365.

209. Saper CB, Akil H, Watson SJ. Lateral hypothalamic innervation of the cerebral cortex: immunoreactive staining for a peptide resembling but immunochemically distinct from pituitary/arcuate α-melanocyte stimulating hormone. Brain Res Bull. 1986;16:107.

210. Johansson O, Hokfelt T, Elde RP. Immunohistochemical distribution of somatostatin-like immunoreactivity in the central nervous system of the adult rat. Neuroscience. 1984;13:265.

211. Schmechel D, Vickrey B, Fitzpatrick D, et al. GABAergic neurons of mammalian cerebral cortex: widespread subclass defined by somatostatin content. Neurosci Lett. 1984;47:227.

212. de Lecea L, Criado JR, Prospero-Garcia O, et al. A cortical neuropeptide with neuronal depressant and sleep-modulating properties. Nature. 1996;381:242.

213. de Lecea L, del Rio JA, Criado JR, et al. Cortistatin is expressed in a distinct subset of cortical interneurons. J Neurosci. 1997;17:5868.

214. Hokfelt T. Neuropeptides in perspective: the last ten years. Neuron. 1991;7:867.

215. Sawchenko PE, Swanson LW, Rivier J, et al. The distribution of glowth hormone-releasing factor (GRF) immunoreactivity in the central nervous system of the rat: an immunohistochemical study using antisera directed against rat hypothalamic CRF. J Comput Neurol. 1985;237:100.

216. Beranek L, Obal F, Taishi P, et al. Changes in rat sleep after single and repeated injections of the long-acting somatostatin analog octreotide. Am J Physiol. 1997;273:R1484.

217. Ueno R, Honda K, Inoue S, et al. Prostaglandin D_2, a cerebral sleep-inducing substance in rats. Proc Natl Acad Sci U S A. 1983;80:1735.

218. Krueger JM, Takahashi S, Kapas L, et al. Cytokines in sleep regulation. Adv Neuroimmunol. 1995;5:171.

219. Krueger JM, Walter J, Dinarello CA, et al. Sleep-promoting effects of an endogenous pyrogen (interleukin-1). Am J Physiol. 1984;246:R994.

220. Tobler I, Borbely AA, Shwyzer M, et al. Interleukin-1 derived from astrocytes enhances slow wave activity in sleep EEG of the rat. Eur J Pharmacol. 1984;104:191.

221. Cravatt BF, Prospero-Garcia O, Siuzdak G, et al. Chemical characterization of a family of brain lipids that induce sleep. Science. 1995;268:1506.

222. Lerner RA, Siuzdak G, Prospero-Garcia O, et al. Cerebrodiene: a brain lipid isolated from sleep-deprived cats. Proc Natl Acad Sci U S A. 1994;91:9505.

223. Bronzino JD, Morgane PJ, Stern WC. EEG synchronization following application of serotonin to area postrema. Am J Physiol. 1972;223:376.

224. Dangiur J, Nicolaidis S. Feeding, metabolism and sleep: Peripheral and central mechanisms. In: McGinty DJ, Morrison A, Druker-Colin R, et al, eds. Brain Mechanisms of Sleep. New York, NY: Raven Press; 1985:322.

225. van Houten M, Posner BI, Kopriwa BM, et al. Insulin-binding sites in the rat brain: in vivo localization. Endocrinology. 1979;105:666.

226. Kapas L, Obal F, Krueger JM. Humoral regulation of sleep. Int Rev. Neurobiol. 1993;35:131.

227. de Saint Hilaire-Kafi A, Gibbs J, Nicolaidis S. Satiety and sleep: the effects of bombesin. Brain Res. 1989;478:152.

228. Monnier M, Dudler L, Gachter R, et al. Delta sleep-inducing peptide (DSIP): EEG and motor activity in rabbits following intravenous administration. Neurosci Lett. 1977;6:9.

11

Control of Motoneurons During Sleep

Michael H. Chase
Francisco R. Morales

During nonrapid eye movement (NREM) sleep, there is a slight decrease in somatic muscle activity compared with that during wakefulness. During REM sleep, there is a dramatic reduction in ongoing muscle activity to the extent that even background muscle tone is abolished. This occurs because the motoneurons that innervate muscle fibers are actively inhibited. The inhibitory neurotransmitter is glycine.

During REM sleep, however, there also are brief periods of muscle contraction (the "twitches and jerks"), which usually take place during periods of rapid eye movements. These contractions occur due to excitatory processes (postsynaptic potentials) that impinge on motoneurons. Interestingly, even during these periods of excitatory potentials, motoneurons continue to be inhibited by glycine. Thus, throughout REM sleep, there is tonic inhibition of motoneurons, as well as phasically occurring brief periods of motoneuron excitation.

There are various sleep disorders that involve abnormal patterns of motor inhibition, excitation, or both; these include cataplexy, restless leg syndrome, REM sleep behavior disorder, and sleep apnea, among others. These disorders occur in part, or in whole, because of the abnormal expression of the mechanisms, which are described above, that control muscle activity during REM sleep.

In human beings, the passage from wakefulness to sleep is accompanied by a decrease in the degree of contraction of muscle fibers—that is, there is a decrease in muscle tone.[1, 2] One of the first investigators to describe this reduction in muscle tone was Pakhomov,[3] who used a complex hydrodynamic system of tubes to measure the tonus of the flexors of the fingers. Atonia, or the complete lack of tone of somatic muscles, was subsequently found to occur in human beings during the state of active (i.e., rapid eye movement [REM]) sleep.[1] In 1959, Jouvet and co-workers[4] observed atonia of the neck muscles of the cat during active sleep. In human beings and cats, as well as in many other species,[1, 5] there is a decrease in muscle tone during quiet (i.e., nonrapid eye movement [NREM]) sleep and atonia during active sleep. In this chapter, we describe the neural mechanisms that produce hypotonia during quiet sleep and atonia during active sleep.

In the somatic motor system, the alpha motoneuron is defined unambiguously: it is any nerve cell with an axon terminating on skeletal muscle fibers. The significance of motoneurons resides in the fact that they are the principal access of the nervous system to skeletal muscles. Sherrington stressed this point by referring to motoneurons as the final common pathway.[6]

The axon of a motoneuron gives off several terminals, each one innervating a muscle fiber. The motoneuron and the muscle fibers it supplies form a *motor unit*. It is truly a functional unit because all of the muscle fibers supplied by a single motoneuron contract simultaneously.

Command signals, which take the form of trains of action potentials, travel from the initial segment of the motor axon, where they originate, along the motor axon to muscle fibers. Most, but not all, muscles are constantly active when we are awake, especially when we maintain a posture or perform a movement. Their *tone* is due to the asynchronous, sustained firing of motoneurons.

All conscious or reflex commands to initiate or suppress movements are eventually directed to motoneurons. (Unless otherwise specified, all references to motoneurons are to alpha, rather than to gamma, motoneurons.) Activation of motoneurons leads to muscle contraction, and inhibition of motoneurons results in muscle atonia.

It is thought that motoneurons generate action potentials, which they use to initiate muscle contraction by changing the permeability of their cell membrane so ions can diffuse down preestablished electrochemical gradients. The suppression of motoneuron activity is achieved by a change in membrane permeability to certain ions (e.g., Cl^- and K^+). Instead of determining permeability changes themselves, their electrical consequences are directly measured with an intracellularly located recording microelectrode.

Before 1978,[7] all intracellular studies of motoneurons in all animals used acute techniques that required immobilization of the animal and, in most cases, artificial

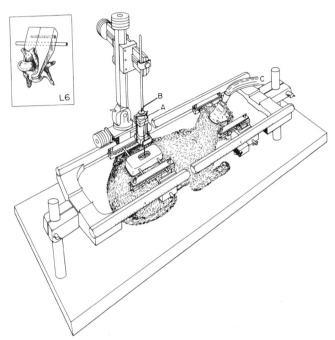

Figure 11–1. Diagram of the chronic cat preparation used to record intracellularly from spinal cord motoneurons. The intracellular electrode carrier is shown with a micropipette (A) being lowered by a microdrive (B) through a hole in the dorsal lamina of L5 in order to record from cells in the ventral horn (L7-S1 motonuclei). C is a cable connecting permanently placed electrodes with stimulating and recording equipment. Inset depicts one of the clamp and bar configurations used to immobilize the vertebral column. (Reprinted from Physiology and Behavior, vol 27, Morales FR, Chase MH, Intracellular recording from spinal cord motoneurons in the chronic cat, 355–362, Copyright 1981, with permission from Elsevier Science.)

grative systems is differentially modulated during these states, especially during the background behaviors of sleep and wakefulness.[8] Moreover, certain phenomena are present during only one state of sleep or wakefulness and are nonexistent throughout the other states.[9]

Consequently, to examine the modulation of membrane potential and synaptic activity during the behaviors of sleep and wakefulness, we developed experimental techniques for intracellular recording from antidromically identified motoneurons that are located in the brainstem and lumbar spinal cord. The preparation is the intact, unanesthetized, undrugged, normally respiring cat; the techniques that are used are illustrated in Figures 11–1 and 11–2. These techniques have also been used for intracellular recording from brainstem reticular neurons.[10]

Because the immediate pre–motor neural circuitry and neurotransmitters that control motoneurons bear the ultimate responsibility for the control of motor tone, this chapter is limited to a discussion of the specific factors that excite and inhibit motoneurons during sleep and wakefulness. At the end of this chapter, the suprasegmental sites and mechanisms that in turn control these controllers are briefly discussed. Unless otherwise specified, the work presented in this chapter represents data obtained from brainstem and spinal cord motoneurons that were reviewed in references 9 and 11 through 14.

BASIC PATTERNS OF MUSCLE ACTIVITY DURING SLEEP

There is a gradual decline in muscle tone (i.e., *hypotonia*) during quiet sleep compared with that during wakefulness. During active sleep, there is a strikingly potent tonic suppression of muscle activity, which often

respiration and either anesthesia, decerebration, or spinal transection. However, it is necessary to study neuronal processes during naturally occurring behavioral states because the activity of sensory, motor, and inte-

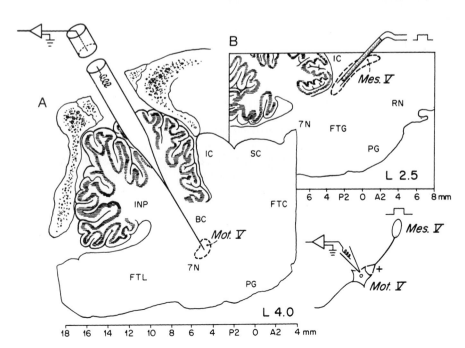

Figure 11–2. Sagittal sections of the brainstem showing the relationship between various brainstem structures and the intracellular micropipette in the motor V nucleus. The recording and stimulating electrodes are drawn approximately to scale. Inset (*B*) shows the anatomic and electrophysiological relationship between the mesencephalic V nucleus and the motor V nucleus. 7N, facial nerve; BC, brachium conjunctivum; FTC, central tegmental field; FTG, giganto-cellular tegmental field; FTL, lateral tegmental field; IC, inferior colliculus; INP, nucleus interpositus; PG, pontine gray; RN, red nucleus; SC, superior colliculus. (From Chase MH, Chandler SH, Nakamura Y. Intracellular determination of membrane potential of trigeminal motoneurons during sleep, and wakefulness. J Neurophysiol. 1980;44:349–358.)

culminates in the complete loss of muscle tone, or *atonia*. In addition, a number of specific patterns of somatomotor suppression occur within the state of active sleep, such as at the onset of active sleep, during REM periods, and during NREM periods. Some of these patterns of suppression operate in conjunction with the concurrent excitation of motoneurons, whose discharge results in myoclonic twitches and jerks.

The two basic mechanisms that may be responsible for the suppression of muscle tone during active sleep are postsynaptic inhibition and disfacilitation (i.e., a reduction in the discharge of tonically active presynaptic excitatory neurons). The two mechanisms may operate continuously, be superimposed on each other at certain times, or act individually for restricted periods. Because measurements of disfacilitation are only indirect in intracellular recording from motoneurons and to keep our focus centered on the final common executor, the motoneuron, we directed our attention to an exploration of the extent to which postsynaptic inhibition during active sleep could account for muscle atonia and postsynaptic excitation for myoclonic activity. These processes were explored through examination of the state dependence of motoneuron membrane properties and the action potentials and synaptic activity of brainstem and spinal cord motoneurons in the chronic, unanesthetized, undrugged cat during spontaneously occurring episodes of sleep and wakefulness.

MODULATION OF THE RESTING MEMBRANE POTENTIAL OF MOTONEURONS DURING SLEEP

In the resting state, the membrane potential of a motoneuron is determined by the unequal concentration of ions inside and outside the cell and the differential permeability of its membrane to diverse ions, principally K^+, Na^+, and Cl^-. Experimentally, an initial membrane potential is recorded when the cell is first penetrated with an intracellularly directed microelectrode. A final determination of the resting membrane potential is obtained by taking, as a reference, the voltage recorded by the microelectrode when it is immediately withdrawn from the cell and is located juxtacellularly. Generally, when a neuron is hyperpolarized, it is relatively less excitable; when it depolarizes, it is more excitable.

TRANSITIONS BETWEEN WAKEFULNESS AND QUIET SLEEP

When cats are awake and resting quietly (i.e., drowsy), passage into quiet sleep is accompanied by either a slight increase or no discernible change in the level of the membrane potential of the motoneuron. When the animal is alert or actively moving or when the tonic electromyographic activity is at a high level, the subsequent transition to quiet sleep is accompanied by an increase in the level of membrane polarization—hyperpolarization. However, in most cases, the membrane potential level remains relatively constant because quiet wakefulness or drowsiness usually is the forerunner of quiet sleep.

The transition from quiet sleep to aroused wakefulness is accompanied by membrane depolarization (Fig. 11–3). The degree of depolarization is usually correlated with the level of arousal, as indicated in the initial 15-sec period of wakefulness in Figure 11–3 and the subsequent 15-sec epoch, in which there occurred an increase in neck muscle activity and membrane depolarization.

TRANSITION FROM QUIET SLEEP TO ACTIVE SLEEP

Motoneurons are hyperpolarized during active sleep compared with quiet sleep (Fig. 11–4). The degree of

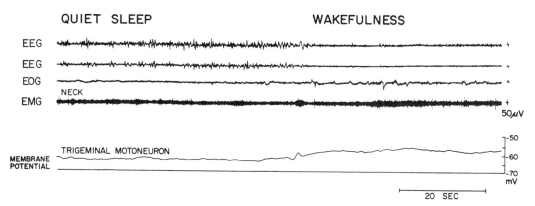

Figure 11–3. Intracellular recording from a trigeminal jaw-closer motoneuron: change in membrane potential during quiet sleep compared with wakefulness. When an extended period of quiet sleep was followed by sustained wakefulness, membrane depolarization occurred. The degree of depolarization was positively correlated with the level of arousal and muscular activity, as portrayed in the middle of the figure when a brief increase in neck EMG activity was correlated with a time-locked decrease in membrane polarization. Membrane potential band pass on polygraphic record: DC to 0.1 Hz. Other polygraphic traces are the same as in Figure 11–4: EEG trace, marginal cortex. EEG, electroencephalogram; EMG, electromyogram; EOG, electro-oculogram. (From Chase MH, Chandler SH, Nakamura Y. Intracellular determination of membrane potential of trigeminal motoneurons during sleep and wakefulness. J Neurophysiol. 1980;44:349–358.)

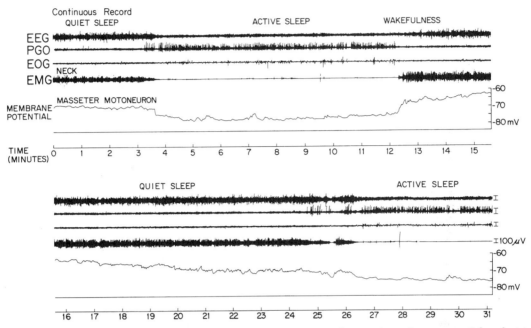

Figure 11–4. Intracellular recording from a trigeminal jaw-closer motoneuron: correlation of membrane potential and state changes. The membrane potential increased rather abruptly at 3.5 min in conjunction with the decrease in neck muscle tone and transition from quiet to active sleep. At 12.5 min, the membrane depolarized and the animal awakened. After the animal passed into quiet sleep again, a brief, aborted episode of active sleep occurred at 25.5 min that was accompanied by a phasic period of hyperpolarization. A minute later, the animal once again entered active sleep, and the membrane potential increased. EEG trace, marginal cortex, membrane potential band pass on polygraphic record, DC to 0.1 Hz. EEG, electroencephalogram; EMG, electromyogram; EOG, electro-oculogram; PGO, ponto-geniculo-occipital potential. (From Chase MH, Chandler SH, Nakamura Y: Intracellular determination of membrane potential of trigeminal motoneurons during sleep and wakefulness. J Neurophysiol. 1980;44:349–358.)

hyperpolarization varies from 2 to 10 mV; its development parallels the various ways in which active sleep emerges from quiet sleep. For example, although the onset of active sleep is demarcated by electroencephalographic desynchronization and a reduction in muscle tone, these indices are not always present at the same time, and either may precede the other as the animal enters the active sleep state. Moreover, electroencephalographic desynchronization and electromyographic suppression (see Fig. 11–4, 3- to 4-min time marks) often are correlated with each other and with membrane hyperpolarization, whereas at other times, hyperpolarization continues to develop beyond the period of the initial onset of electromyographic suppression (see Fig. 11–4, 26- to 27-min time marks). When the muscle units innervated by the recorded motoneurons are monitored, a perfect correlation is observed between the discharge of a motoneuron and the action potentials of individual muscle fibers (Fig. 11–5).

TRANSITION FROM ACTIVE SLEEP TO WAKEFULNESS

When cats awake from active sleep, the membrane potential rapidly depolarizes (see Fig. 11–4, 12- to 13-min and 25- to 26-min time marks). The degree of depolarization is equal to or exceeds the level maintained during the preceding episode of quiet sleep.

In summary, these data demonstrate that the membrane potential is strongly hyperpolarized during ac-

tive sleep compared with during quiet sleep and wakefulness and, in contrast, that it is only slightly hyperpolarized or remains at the same potential level when quiet sleep is compared with wakefulness.

ACTION POTENTIAL, RHEOBASE, AND INPUT RESISTANCE OF MOTONEURONS DURING SLEEP

Action Potential

Under natural conditions, motoneurons generate action potentials as the result of a summation of currents generated at synapses on their soma or dendrites. All synaptic currents are integrated in the region of the initial segment of the axon, which is the most excitable portion of the motoneuron. If the voltage drop produced by electrical currents is above a certain threshold level, an action potential is triggered—first in the initial segment and second in the soma. Consequently, motoneuron action potentials exhibit two basic components—the initial segment (IS) and somadendritic (SD) spikes—that reflect activity in these two regions of the cell.[15]

Spontaneous Action Potentials. Changes in behavioral state are reflected by variations in the frequency of action potential activity. This finding is evident in masseter motoneurons, which normally present a high level of tonic activity during wakefulness; the sus-

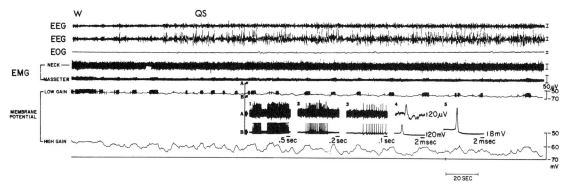

Figure 11-5. Intracellular recording from a masseter motoneuron. This illustrates the gradual increase in membrane potential and decrease in spike occurrence as the animal changed its behavioral state from wakefulness to quiet sleep. An oscilloscopic picture of the activity of an individual masseter motor unit is shown in the inset, which portrays the time-locked relationship between each motoneuron spike potential and an action potential of a masseter muscle unit at increasing faster time bases (A and B, 1–4). In 5, the motoneuron spike is presented at higher gain (spike amplitude, 40 mV). Membrane potential band pass on polygraphic record: low gain, DC to 35 Hz; high gain, DC to 0.5 Hz. Top EEG trace, frontal cortex; bottom EEG trace, marginal cortex. EEG, electroencephalogram; EMG, electromyogram; EOG, electro-oculogram. (From Chase MH, Chandler SH, Nakamura Y. Intracellular determination of membrane potential of trigeminal motoneurons during sleep and wakefulness. J Neurophysiol. 1980;44:349–358.)

tained discharge of wakefulness first decreases during quiet sleep and then is replaced by brief bursts of spikes (see Fig. 11–5).

As the animal changes state from quiet sleep to active sleep, there is an accompanying cessation of spontaneous spike activity (Fig. 11–6). During active sleep, isolated or short bursts of spike potentials are occasionally observed in conjunction with facial twitches and rapid eye movements.

Induced Antidromic Action Potentials. The interval between the IS and SD spikes, which is referred to as the IS-SD delay, is lengthened when the animal enters active sleep, which indicates that motoneuron excitability is depressed during this state. During bursts of rapid eye movements, the IS-SD delay is further prolonged, and there are phasic changes in the peak amplitude of the antidromic spike. These variations in IS and SD spikes are indirect evidence of an increase in

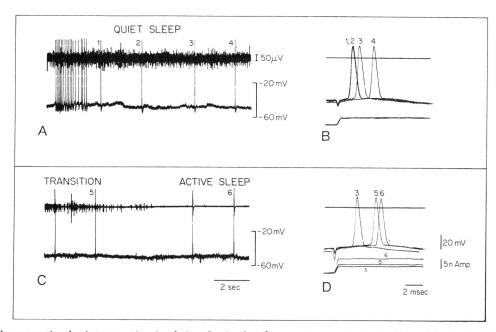

Figure 11-6. Spike generation by intrasomatic stimulation. In *A*, after the spontaneous burst of spike activity in the initial portion of the record had receded, four consecutive threshold determinations were performed during quiet sleep using currents of 4 nA with a duration of 20 msec. Note that membrane potential fluctuations present during quiet sleep were accompanied by changes only in the latency of the direct spikes (*B*). *C* and *D* show an increase in threshold that commenced in the transition period (5) after quiet sleep and was most pronounced during active sleep (6). In *D*, the increase is shown for spikes obtained during quiet sleep (3), the transition period (5), and active sleep (6). During active sleep, a threshold increase of 100% was observed. Note that both the overshoot and the absolute amplitude of the direct spike were smaller during active sleep than during quiet sleep. These reductions in spike size began during the transition period. The lower traces in *B* and *D* reflect the intrasomatic depolarizing current. The heavy line crossing the spike tips represents zero voltage obtained when the electrode was withdrawn from the motoneuron. Upper traces in *A* and *C* are the EMG recordings. (From Morales FR, Chase MH. Postsynaptic control of lumbar motoneuron excitability during active sleep in the chronic cat. Brain Res. 1981;225:279–295.)

conductance of the soma membrane, which is the basis for postsynaptic inhibition.[16, 17]

Rheobase

The rheobase is operationally defined as the minimal electrical current that is necessary to elicit an action potential when current is injected into a cell. In considering the effectiveness of an intracellularly applied current pulse in inducing an action potential, attention must be paid not only to the strength of the current but also to the time during which it is allowed to flow through the cell. By choosing different voltages as well as pulse durations, a strength-duration curve can be developed that relates these two factors insofar as the effective level of stimulation is concerned, thereby providing an index of the intrinsic excitability of the neuron.

Rheobasic currents during quiet sleep are comparable to those during wakefulness, whereas they are 80% greater in active sleep than in quiet sleep. An example of the increase in rheobasic current during active sleep compared with that during quiet sleep is given (see Fig. 11–6). These data indicate a dramatic decrease in cellular excitability during active sleep. Although an elevated rheobase is always accompanied by hyperpolarization, hyperpolarization alone cannot completely account for the increase in rheobase currents. An analysis of the data from rheobasic determinations and input resistance indicates that current flow is "shunted" by an increase in membrane conductance during active sleep; moreover, both hyperpolarization and increased conductance appear to contribute to the observed increase in rheobasic current.

Input Resistance

The manner in which a neuron responds to injected subthreshold or synaptic currents is related to its input resistance. This basic electrotonic characteristic of motor cells depends, in turn, principally on the specific resistivity of the cell membrane, as well as on its area and the geometric characteristics of the dendritic tree.[15]

There is no dramatic difference in motoneuron input resistance when quiet sleep is compared with wakefulness. During active sleep, there is a striking (44%) decrease in input resistance. During active sleep, when rapid eye movements occur, there are frequent phasic decreases in the voltage drop produced by the same current, which indicates a continuously fluctuating motoneuron input resistance.

INDUCED ORTHODROMIC EXCITATORY POSTSYNAPTIC POTENTIALS DURING SLEEP

The amplitude of the Ia monosynaptic excitatory postsynaptic potential (EPSP) is smaller during active

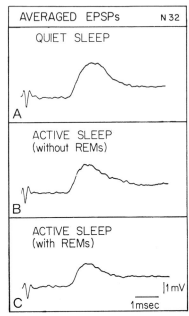

Figure 11–7. Averaged excitatory postsynaptic potential (EPSP) activity (n = 32) during quiet sleep (*A*), active sleep without rapid eye movements (REMs) (*B*), and active sleep with REMs (*C*). Note the decrease in amplitude when active sleep without REMs is compared with quiet sleep and a further decrease during active sleep with REMs. The averaged peak amplitude decreased 19% during active sleep without REMs and 37% during active sleep with REMs. Peripheral nerve (common peroneal) stimulation: 0.5 V, 0.3 msec. (From Morales FR, Chase MH. Postsynaptic control of lumbar motoneuron excitability during active sleep in the chronic cat. Brain Res. 1981;225:279–295.)

sleep than during quiet sleep (Fig. 11–7). The fact that in active sleep there is a decrease in excitability and an increase in membrane conductance, together with motoneuron hyperpolarization, clearly indicates that the EPSP amplitude is depressed by a mechanism of postsynaptic inhibition.[18, 19] Phasic periods of additional suppression of EPSP amplitude are present during intense bursts of rapid eye movements in active sleep (see Fig. 11–7). These periods are generally accompanied by further hyperpolarization of the postsynaptic membrane and a greater increase in motoneuron conductance. It is evident that phasic enhancements of postsynaptic inhibitory processes act to decrease the size of EPSPs during REM periods.

In summary, the data emerging from analyses of the action potential, rheobase, input resistance, and Ia monosynaptic EPSPs of motoneurons indicate that postsynaptic inhibition is the principal, and probably sufficient, mechanism responsible for atonia of the somatic musculature during active sleep.

SYNAPTIC POTENTIALS RESPONSIBLE FOR POSTSYNAPTIC INHIBITION DURING ACTIVE SLEEP

The preceding section describes the data that indicate motoneurons are subjected to postsynaptic inhibition during active sleep. Because the synapse is the

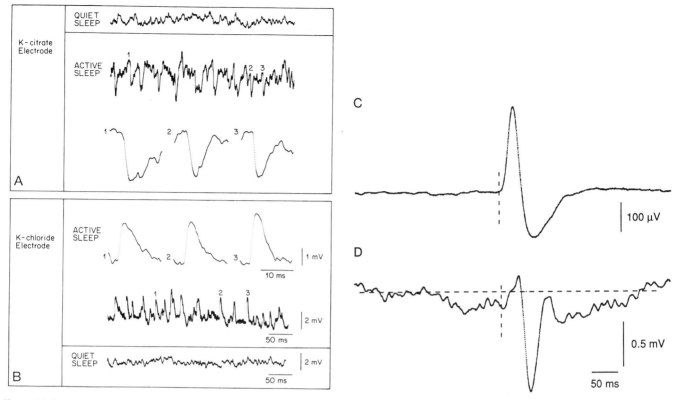

Figure 11–8. *A* and *B*, Representative recordings from two different motoneurons during quiet sleep and active sleep using microelectrodes filled with two different electrolyte solutions. *A*, K-citrate electrode. During active sleep, hyperpolarizing potentials were easily distinguishable. Potentials labeled 1 to 3 are shown in an expanded format. Their 10 to 90% amplitude rise times, measured from the digitized record, were 1.4, 1.6, and 1 msec, respectively. *B*, K-chloride electrode. Recordings were maintained for 6 min during quiet sleep without any retention current. A hyperpolarizing current of 10 nA was passed for 45 sec during quiet sleep approximately 1 min before the animal entered into active sleep. The quiet sleep recording of the membrane potential was obtained after current injection had ceased. The active sleep record of the membrane potential revealed the advent of high-frequency depolarizing potentials. In *B*, 1 to 3 are potentials shown in greater detail; their 10 to 90% rise times were 0.95, 1.05, and 1 msec, respectively. Depolarizing potentials like these were never observed during recording with K-citrate electrodes; they are interpreted as being reversed inhibitory potentials. Calibration signals are identical for the two cells. Both records are from sciatic motoneurons. Antidromic action potentials: *A*, 72 mV; *B*, 75 mV. (From Morales FR, Chase MH: Repetitive synaptic potentials responsible for inhibition of spinal cord motoneurons during active sleep. Exp Neurol 78:471–476, 1982.)

C and *D*, Changes in motoneuron membrane potential in conjunction with ipsilateral primary PGO waves. *C* and *D* are averages of 50 PGO waves and the corresponding motoneuron membrane potential. In this example, the changes in motoneuron membrane potential that were present in conjunction with PGO waves were the ponto-geniculo-occipital inhibitory postsynaptic potential (PGO-IPSP), the pre-PGO hyperpolarization, and a succession of IPSPs that followed the PGO-IPSP (see text). The vertical dotted line marks the foot of the PGO wave, and the horizontal dotted line in *D* marks the baseline of the motoneuron membrane potential. (Reprinted with permission from López-Rodríguez F, Chase MH, et al. PGO-related potentials in lumbar motoneurons during active sleep. J Neurophysiol. 1992;68:109–116.)

point of contact and the site of communication for postsynaptic inhibition, a study of synaptic transmission is central to an understanding of motor control during sleep. In an effort to further elucidate the bases for motoneuron inhibition during active sleep, we analyzed the spontaneous inhibitory postsynaptic potential (IPSP) activity in high-gain intracellular recordings obtained from motoneurons during active sleep, as well as during quiet sleep and wakefulness.

COMPARISON OF SPONTANEOUS INHIBITORY POSTSYNAPTIC POTENTIALS DURING SLEEP AND WAKEFULNESS

During wakefulness and quiet sleep, intracellular records of motoneurons reveal relatively few spontane-

ous IPSPs. However, during active sleep, a great increase occurs in the number of spontaneous IPSPs (Fig. 11–8*A* and *B*). Even more manifest is the development of large-amplitude active sleep-specific IPSPs that are *unique* to this state. The amplitude and time course of these active sleep-specific IPSPs differentiate them from the smaller potentials impinging on the same motoneurons during quiet sleep as well as during active sleep. These large-amplitude active sleep-specific IPSPs are more readily reversed by the iontophoretic injection of chloride ions than are the smaller potentials, a finding that indicates that the responsible synapses are situated closer to the soma region; therefore, they are strategically located to facilitate the suppression of motoneuron activity.

Because the atonia of active sleep is generalized to flexor and extensor muscles,[2] it was expected that every motoneuron innervating hindlimb muscles would show a significant increase in inhibitory activity during active sleep. We therefore compared the IPSP rate within recordings obtained from the same motoneuron during consecutive behavioral states. This comparison was accomplished by an analysis of the interpotential intervals of IPSPs during quiet sleep, the initial period of active sleep, and the NREM periods of active sleep. The interpotential intervals were significantly shorter during both the initial period of active sleep and the NREM periods of the same active sleep episode than during the preceding quiet sleep episode. It appears as if all motoneurons within pools whose neurons project to flexors as well as extensors receive an increase in inhibitory synaptic input during active sleep.

The occurrence of small-amplitude IPSPs during wakefulness and quiet sleep, albeit of relatively low frequency, was an unpredicted finding, of which the functional significance is unknown. These potentials may reflect the inhibitory control of motoneuron activity that is required to maintain limb position and postural adjustments, and thus they may not be related primarily to motor inhibition vis-á-vis sleep physiology. On the other hand, the increase in IPSP frequency observed in all motoneurons during active sleep was found to be the result not only of the appearance of large-amplitude active sleep-specific IPSPs but also of an increase in the number of small-amplitude IPSPs. Therefore, it is possible that the inhibitory system that generates the small IPSPs of active sleep, which undoubtedly contribute to motoneuron inhibition during this state, also functions, albeit to a much lesser degree, during wakefulness and quiet sleep.

It is clear, however, that there is a unique set of inhibitory synapses that generate the active sleep-specific IPSPs, which are activated only during active sleep. In turn, this observation implies the existence of a group of inhibitory interneurons that are driven to discharge, selectively, during active sleep. New evidence gathered with the use of immunohistochemical techniques (see later) supports the hypothesis that rather than being short-axoned cells located in the spinal cord, active sleep inhibitory interneurons are mainly situated in the brainstem and that their long projecting axons end directly on spinal motoneurons.[20] For brainstem motoneurons, the inhibitory interneurons that generate active sleep-specific IPSPs are, without doubt, located in the brainstem. Regardless of the location of the interneurons that give rise to the active sleep-specific IPSPs, we suggest that these IPSPs represent the final synaptic expression of a supraspinal inhibitory system that is responsible for promoting the suppression of motoneuron activity and the development of atonia during active sleep.

In association with periods of rapid eye movements during active sleep, phasic enhancement of the postsynaptic inhibition occurs that is directed to motoneurons.[13, 21] In addition, in relation to ponto-geniculo-occipital (PGO) activity, there are inhibitory potentials that arise in the membrane potential of both spinal cord and trigeminal motoneurons; these inhibitory changes are reflected in the appearance of a complex pattern of motoneuron hyperpolarization that is centered around PGO waves (see Fig. 11–8D). It is clear

that a postsynaptic inhibitory process that suppresses motoneuron excitability tonically during active sleep also entails episodes of phasic enhancement during REM periods and PGO waves that further suppresses the excitability of motoneurons during active sleep.

EXCITATORY CONTROL OF MOTONEURONS DURING ACTIVE SLEEP

Postsynaptic inhibition is one of the principal synaptic processes affecting motoneurons during the REM periods of active sleep. In fact, all of the inhibitory phenomena that are described in the previous sections are not only present but also enhanced during REM periods, including the frequency and amplitude of the active sleep-specific IPSPs (Fig. 11–9). How, then, could there be twitches and jerks of the eyes and limbs during REM periods? The answer is simple because most REM periods are accompanied not only by increased motoneuron inhibition but also by strikingly potent motor excitatory drives (Figs. 11–10 and 11–11).

The excitatory drives that impinge on motoneurons during REM periods of active sleep are reflected in

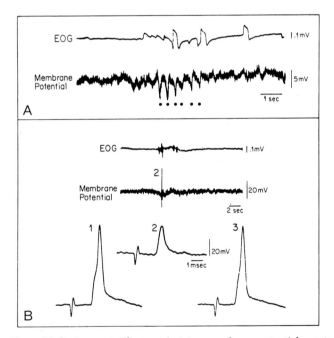

Figure 11–9. Summated hyperpolarizing membrane potential events (A) and blockade of antidromic action potential (B) during active sleep accompanied by periods of rapid eye movements. In A, hyperpolarizing events arise (the most evident indicated by dots) that are composed of repetitively occurring inhibitory synaptic potentials. In B, an antidromic spike was induced immediately before (1) and after (3) a burst of rapid eye movements. When the antidromic action potential coincided with the period of hyperpolarizing potentials, the soma-dendritic spike was blocked and only the initial segment spike was present (2). Data are unfiltered; records were obtained from a peroneal motoneuron in A (resting membrane potential: −65 mV) and from a tibial motoneuron in B (resting membrane potential: −72 mV). (From Chase MH, Morales FR. Phasic changes in motoneuron membrane potential during REM periods of active sleep. Neurosci Lett. 1982;34:177–182.)

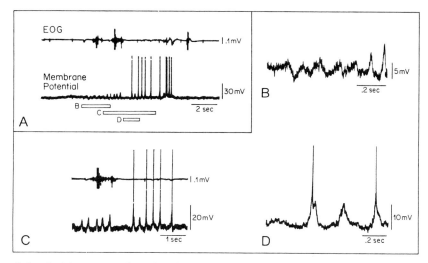

Figure 11–10. *A,* Summated depolarizing potentials and spike activity in conjunction with active sleep periods of rapid eye movements. During the first burst of eye movements, phasic hyperpolarizing events arose (*B*). In conjunction with the second burst of eye movements, there was a series of rhythmic depolarizing shifts (*C*). Action potentials occurred during the third episode of eye movements; they were also present during the interval between the second and third bursts of ocular activity. The recordings over the bars in *A* are presented at a faster sweep speed and greater magnification in *B, C,* and *D*. In *D,* note that spikes arise from the first and third depolarizing shifts, whereas the second does not reach threshold. The action potentials in *C* and *D* are truncated owing to the high gain of the records. Data are unfiltered; records were obtained from a tibial motoneuron (resting membrane potential: −70 mV). (From Chase MH, Morales FP. Phasic changes in motoneuron membrane potential during REM periods of active sleep. Neurosci Lett. 1982;34:177–182.)

depolarizing and spike potentials. This pattern of activity is illustrated in Figure 11–10A. During the second cluster of eye movements in this REM episode, there are depolarizing shifts in potential (Fig. 11–10B to D); subthreshold depolarizing potentials and action potentials are also present. These patterns of activation probably reflect descending excitatory activity emanating from supraspinal systems.[2, 22]

In contrast to the gradual depolarization that precedes neuronal discharge during wakefulness (Fig. 11–11A, A), in most instances during active sleep, there is an initial hyperpolarization that is followed immediately by a depolarization shift and action potential generation (Fig. 11–11A, B). These depolarization shifts in membrane potential appear to be the result of cumulative EPSP activity rather than to reflect a process of disinhibition, for the following reasons. First, examination of high-gain, high-speed records reveals that each depolarization consists of the summation of wavelets whose form is comparable to that of previously described EPSPs.[23] Second, the depolarizing potentials remain, even though inhibitory processes are reversed by the intracellular injection of chloride ions.

From time to time for reasons that remain unknown, during the REM periods of active sleep, excitatory drives overpower inhibitory drives, motoneurons discharge, and the muscle fibers that they innervate contract. It appears as if, at these times, there is an increase in excitatory drives that is actually accompanied by an increase in inhibitory drives; momentarily, the excitatory drives predominate and motoneurons discharge (see Figs. 11–10 and 11–11A). When motoneurons do discharge during the REM periods of active sleep, their activity, as well as the resultant contraction of the muscles that they innervate, is unlike that occurring during

any other state. Movements are abrupt, twitchy and jerky, and without apparent purpose.

The coactivation of synaptic drives with opposite functions appears, from a functional perspective, to be paradoxical. However, some rationality may be ascribed to each of these processes when they are examined individually. For example, the inhibitory input that is present during active sleep may reflect a need to suppress contraction of the somatic musculature to protect the organism at a time when it is blind and unconscious. Although we do not understand the function of the REM periods of active sleep (and perhaps the rapid eye movements themselves are only an easily observable indicator of a more basic process), we do know that during these periods, most populations of cortical and subcortical cells discharge at rates that often exceed those that occur during wakefulness.[8] In fact, the activity of practically all motor pathways, including those whose discharge results in movements during wakefulness, is greatly enhanced in an apparently random manner during active sleep (compared with quiet sleep) and, even more strikingly, during the REM periods of active sleep.[8, 22, 24] It is possible that episodes of motoneuron spike potentials that result in myoclonic activity during REM periods may have no specific functional significance but may simply reflect the status of a highly activated nervous system whose motor facilitatory pathways are discharging at extremely high rates. It is also possible that myoclonic activity represents brief episodes of an otherwise integrated behavior that is suppressed by the presence of motor inhibition. Evidently, there is a need during all REM periods for a compensatory increase in motor inhibition to prevent movements (integrated or random) that would otherwise ensue during the activation of motor facilitatory systems.

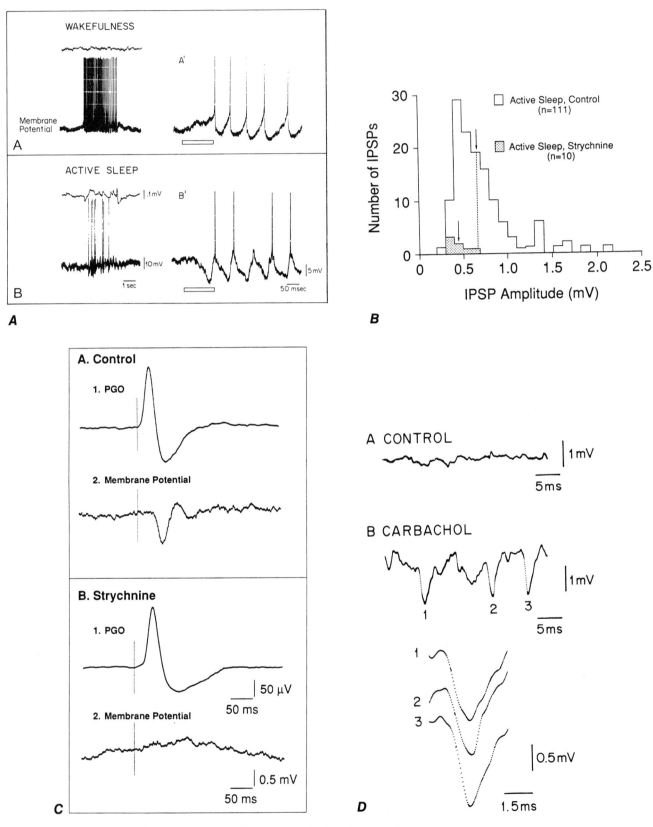

Figure 11-11. *See legend on opposite page*

NEUROTRANSMITTERS MEDIATING THE INHIBITORY SYNAPTIC CONTROL OF MOTONEURONS DURING ACTIVE SLEEP

This section focuses on an investigation of the neurotransmitters that mediate the unique inhibitory potentials that are responsible, at least in part, for the postsynaptic inhibition of motoneurons during active sleep.

In previous studies that were performed on acutely anesthetized or decerebrate cats, microiontophoretic experiments have convincingly demonstrated that strychnine antagonizes the postsynaptic inhibitory actions of alpha- and beta-amino acids, such as glycine and beta-alanine. Indeed, it is generally accepted that glycine is the major inhibitory transmitter at the level of the spinal cord.[25-27] Studies conducted in acute preparations have also indicated that picrotoxin and bicuculline are effective antagonists for the postsynaptic inhibitory actions of gamma-amino acids (e.g., gamma-aminobutyric acid).[26, 28-30]

In studies,[31, 32] the neurotransmitter antagonists strychnine, picrotoxin, and bicuculline were microiontophoretically administered adjacent to the cell body of spinal cord motoneurons while intracellular records were obtained during naturally occurring episodes of sleep and wakefulness.

In these studies, it was determined that the active sleep-specific IPSPs were either diminished in amplitude or abolished after the microiontophoretic application of strychnine (see Fig. 11–11B). This finding suggests, on the basis of the documented actions of strychnine, that the neurotransmitter mediating this IPSP activity is glycine or a glycinergic substance. Neither picrotoxin nor bicuculline, when released microiontophoretically near the somas of individual motoneurons, was effective in suppressing the large-amplitude IPSPs of active sleep. Thus, glycine, but not gamma-aminobutyric acid, appears to be the principal postsynaptic inhibitory neurotransmitter responsible for muscle atonia during active sleep. By applying strychnine juxtacellularly through microiontophoresis, we determined that the PGO-related IPSPs are mediated by glycinergic synapses (see Fig. 11–11C). We have postulated that the same inhibitory neurons that tonically inhibit motoneurons during active sleep are phasically activated during PGO waves and provide for the phasic enhancement of postsynaptic inhibition that occurs during the phasic events of active sleep. By blocking the PGO-related IPSPs with strychnine, we unmasked a depolarizing potential, which underscores the complexity of motor control that takes place during active sleep, especially during the phasic events of this state.

In a new series of pharmacological experiments, we applied antagonists of excitatory amino acids juxtacellularly. The broad-spectrum antagonist kyurenic acid completely abolished the phasic depolarizing events that occur during the REM periods of active sleep. The N-methyl-D-aspartate blocker argipressin did not affect these events; therefore, we conclude that the excitatory motor events during REM are mediated by pathways that use an amino acid such as glutamate as their neurotransmitter and that their action is mediated by non–N-methyl-D-aspartate receptors.[33, 34]

PHARMACOLOGICAL MODELS OF ACTIVE SLEEP

Since the work of George and colleagues,[35] it has been known that the injection of cholinergic drugs into the brainstem may induce a state that closely resembles active sleep (see, for example, Baghdoyan et al.[36]).

Figure 11–11. *A,* Action potential generation during wakefulness (A) and a REM period of active sleep (B). Gradual membrane depolarization (bar in A') preceded the development of action potentials during wakefulness, whereas a strong hyperpolarizing drive was evident during a comparable period of active sleep (bar in B'). This difference was also observed before the subsequent generation of each action potential during this REM episode. Action potentials in A' and B' are truncated owing to the high gain of the recording. Resting membrane potentials are −58 mV in A and −63 mV in B. Data are unfiltered; records were obtained from a single tibial motoneuron (From Chase MH, Morales FP. Phasic changes in motoneuron membrane potential during REM periods of active sleep. Neurosci Lett. 1982;34:177–182.)

B, Distribution of the amplitudes of spontaneous IPSPs recorded during active sleep from the same lumbar motoneuron before (*open histogram*) and after the microiontophoretic ejection of strychnine (*dotted histogram*). *Arrows* indicate the median value of each IPSP population. Note that before strychnine, 50% of the potentials were larger in amplitude than the largest potential that was detected following the microiontophoretic ejection of strychnine (10 mM, 250 nA, 2.75 min). (Reprinted with permission from Chase MH, Soja PJ, Morales FP. Evidence that glycine mediates the postsynaptic potentials that inhibit lumbar motoneurons during the atonia of active sleep. J Neurosci. 1989;9:743–751.)

C, Averaged PGO waves and the membrane potential in lumbar motoneurons recorded in two different cats before (control) (A) and following strychnine injection (B). The vertical bars are positioned at the foot of the averaged PGO waves. After the injection of strychnine, the PGO-related IPSP was no longer present; instead, a long depolarizing potential occurred (see text for details). (Reprinted with permission from López-Rodríguez F, Morales FR, Soja PJ, et al. Suppression of the PGO-related lumbar motoneuron IPSP by strychnine. Brain Res. 1990; 535:331–334.)

D, High-gain intracellular recordings obtained from a single hindlimb motoneuron during precarbachol control conditions (A) and 26 min after carbachol microinjection into the pontine reticular formation (B). Following carbachol microinjection, hyperpolarizing potentials were easily distinguishable. Potentials labeled 1 to 3 are shown in an expanded format. These recordings were obtained by employing a KCl-filled microelectrode. A 5nA-depolarizing current was injected to displace the membrane potential away from the equilibrium potential; this procedure facilitated the observation of these potentials and, in addition, avoided shifting the equilibrium potential to a depolarized value by the retention of Cl ions. The waveforms of these potentials were remarkably similar to those that appear exclusively during active sleep in intact animals under natural conditions (compare, for example, the potentials illustrated in this figure with those of Fig. 2A in Morales and associates[48]). (Reprinted with permission from Morales FR, Engelhardt JK, Soja PJ, et al. Motoneuron properties during motor inhibition produced by microinjection of carbachol into the pontine reticular formation of the decerebrate cat. J Neurophysiol. 1987;57:1118–1129.)

In the decerebrate cat, we demonstrated that carbachol induces a complete abolition of somatomotor rigidity. The mechanisms of this cholinergically induced motor suppression appear to be the same as those that are activated during active sleep (see, for example, Fig. 11–11D). The acute decerebrate animal, in which motor suppression is induced by injecting cholinergic substances into the pons, has been used by us and other researchers to explore the synaptic network responsible for the atonia of active sleep and to study the mechanisms of motor suppression of respiratory muscles.[37–40]

Carbachol effects may also be observed in the alpha-chloralose–anesthetized cat. This preparation is being used intensively to study networks of neurons, of which the activity underlies the physiological components of active sleep.[41, 42] In this preparation, we obtained evidence that makes it very unlikely that Ib inhibitory spinal cord neurons, which are glycinergic inhibitory interneurons, are responsible for the inhibition of motoneurons during active sleep.[43] Previously, we rejected the possibility that Renshaw cells inhibit motoneurons during active sleep (paradoxically, Renshaw cells are themselves *inhibited* during active sleep).[38] The work of Takakusaki and associates[40] suggests that Ia inhibitory interneurons also do not participate in this process. Entire populations of spinal inhibitory interneurons are known to not be responsible for the characteristic atonia of active sleep that affects spinal cord musculature.

SUPRASEGMENTAL CONTROL OF MOTONEURON INHIBITION DURING ACTIVE SLEEP

The existence of active sleep-specific IPSPs reflects the activity of supraspinal centers that, directly or indirectly, activate inhibitory interneurons, which, in turn, discharge selectively during active sleep. We know that some of the neuronal elements that control motor inhi-

bition during active sleep are situated caudal to the anterior border of the mesencephalon because a midbrain transection does not eliminate intermittent periods of motor suppression and correlated epiphenomena during this state (see Chapter 9). On the other hand, after a transection caudal to the medulla, facial muscles continue to be subjected to inhibition during active sleep, whereas limb and trunk musculature is unaffected by changes in the animal's state. Thus, a critical neuronal population responsible for somatomotor inhibition during active sleep must be located within the confines of the lower brainstem. These inhibitory interneurons are the last link in a suprasegmental inhibitory system that controls somatomotor outflow in a state-dependent manner.

Recent evidence appears to corroborate an early postulate by Chase,[44] wherein neurons within the nucleus pontis oralis excite, during active sleep, neurons of the inhibitory region of Magoun and Rhines,[45] which in turn promote the motor inhibition of active sleep. Interestingly, new evidence is emanating from the use of immunocytochemical techniques rather than from the use of classic electrophysiological procedures. The first immunohistochemical technique used the detection of the nuclear protein Fos, which is synthesized during certain patterns of neuronal activity. Immunodetection was performed in brainstem slices of cats that had been sacrificed immediately after 2 hours of continuous active sleep induced by the pontine administration of carbachol.[46]

In the ventral region of the medial medullary reticular formation, medial to the facial motor nucleus and laterally to the inferior olive, active sleep-carbachol cats exhibited, bilaterally, a great number of Fos-labeled cells (see Fig. 11–12).[46] The region occupied by these cells corresponded, as postulated, to the inhibitory region of Magoun and Rhines.[45] The second immunocytochemical technique consisted of the retrograde labeling of interneurons by using the subunit B of cholera toxin, which was injected into the trigeminal motor

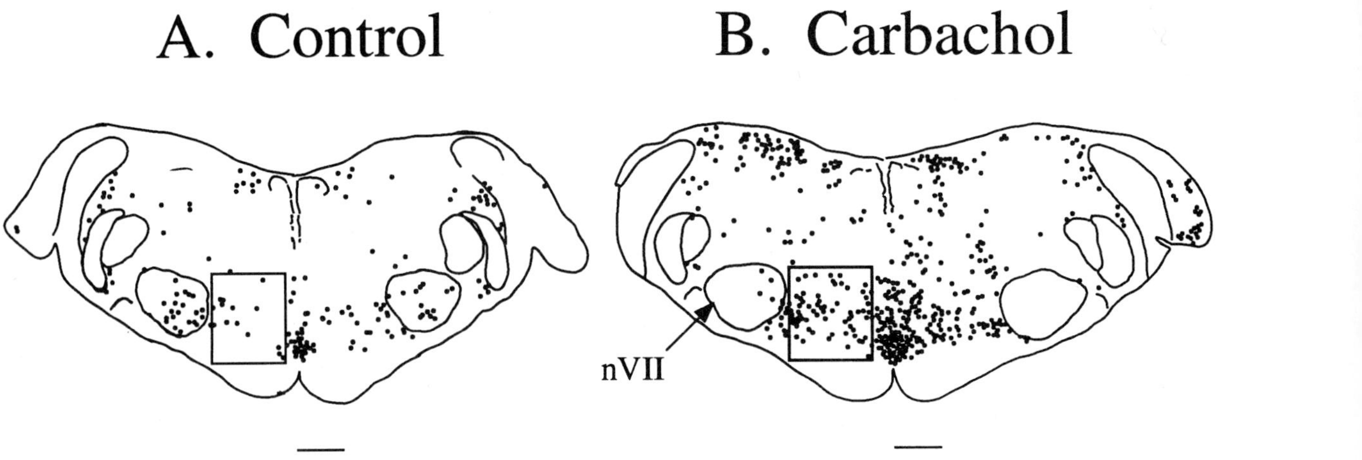

A. Control   B. Carbachol

nVII

Figure 11–12. Distribution of Fos + neurons in the medulla at the level of the facial nucleus of a control (*left*) and an AS-carbachol (*right*) cat. Each dot represents one Fos-labeled neuron. The region that contains double-labeled, Fos +, and cholera toxin + neurons is indicated by the square. (Modified from Yamuy J, Mancillas JR, Morales, FR, Chase MH. C-fos expression in the pons and medulla of the cat during carbachol-induced active sleep. J Neurosci. 1993;13:2703–2718.)

pool.[47] This technique permitted the identification, among all neurons that were activated during active sleep-carbachol, of interneurons that directly innervate the motor nuclei. The most salient result of the combined use of the above-mentioned techniques was the discovery of a subset of neurons in the ventral medulla that were activated during active sleep-carbachol and that also innervate antigravitatory motor nuclei. An important objective of these studies was the identification of the neurotransmitters and neuromodulators used by these neurons, which we believe are inhibitory pre–motor neurons that are responsible for the atonia of active sleep. These interneurons release glycine, which produces the postsynaptic inhibition of motoneurons. The result is the suppression of motoneuron discharge, leading to the profound atonia of the skeletal musculature, which is the key characteristic of the state of active sleep.

CONCLUSIONS

In summary, postsynaptic inhibition is a principal process that is responsible not only for the atonia of the somatic musculature during active sleep but also for the phasic episodes of decreased motoneuron excitability that accompany bursts of rapid eye movements during this state. These postsynaptic processes are dependent on the presence of active sleep-specific IPSPs, which are apparently mediated by glycine. The phasic excitation of motoneurons during REM periods is due to EPSPs, which, when present, encounter a motoneuron already subjected to enhanced postsynaptic inhibition.

From the perspective of motoneurons, active sleep can be characterized as a state abundant in the availability of strikingly potent patterns of postsynaptic inhibition and, during REM periods, by enhanced excitation and enhanced inhibition. The site of origin of these inhibitory drives encompasses the ventromedial medulla. It has also been suggested that this and adjacent regions may, in turn, be activated by more rostrally located nuclei, such as the pontine nucleus pontis oralis. Resolution of the location and mechanisms of action of the supramedullary control of premotor neurons constitutes a major goal of future experiments.

References

1. Kleitman N. Sleep and Wakefulness. Chicago, Ill: The University of Chicago Press; 1963.
2. Pompeiano O. The neurophysiological mechanisms of the postural and motor events during desynchronized sleep. Res Publ Assoc Nerv Ment Dis. 1967;45:351–423.
3. Pakhomov AN. A new method of measuring and recording muscle tonus, and its application to the study of the physiology of sleep in man. Fiziol Zh SSSR. 1947;33:245–254.
4. Jouvet M, Michel F, Courjon J. Sur en stade d'activité électrique cerébrale rapide au cours du sommeil physiologique. C R Soc Biol (Paris). 1959;153:1024–1028.
5. Chase MH, ed. The Sleeping Brain. Perspectives in the Brain Sciences. Vol 1. Los Angeles, Calif: Brain Information Service/ Brain Research Institute, UCLA; 1972.
6. Sherrington CS. The Integrative Action of the Nervous System. New Haven, Conn: Yale University Press; 1906.
7. Nakamura Y, Goldberg LJ, Chandler SH, et al. Intracellular analysis of trigeminal motoneuron activity during sleep in the cat. Science. 1978;199:204–207.
8. Steriade M, Hobson JA. Neuronal activity during the sleep-waking cycle. Prog Neurobiol. 1976;6:155–376.
9. Chase MH. The motor functions of the reticular formation are multifaceted and state-determined. In: Hobson JM, Brazier MAB, eds. Reticular Formation Revisited. New York, NY: Raven Press; 1980:449–472.
10. Chase MH, Enomoto S, Murakami T, et al. Intracellular potential of medullary reticular neurons during sleep and wakefulness. Exp Neurol. 1981;71:226–233.
11. Chase MH. Synaptic mechanisms and circuitry involved in motoneuron control during sleep. In: Bradley RJ, ed. International Review of Neurobiology. Vol 24. New York, NY: Academic Press; 1983:213–258.
12. Chase MH, Morales FR. Phasic changes in motoneuron membrane potential during REM periods of active sleep. Neurosci Lett. 1982;34:177–182.
13. Chase MH, Morales FR. Subthreshold excitatory activity and motoneuron discharge during REM periods of active sleep. Science. 1983;221:1195–1198.
14. Morales FR, Boxer P, Chase MH. Behavioral state-specific inhibitory postsynaptic potentials impinge on cat lumbar motoneurons during active sleep. Exp Neurol. 1988;100:583–595.
15. Burke RE, Rudomin P. Spinal neurons and synapses. In: Kandel ER, ed. Handbook of Physiology. The Nervous System. Bethesda, Md: American Physiological Society; 1977:877–944.
16. Brock LG, Coombs JS, Eccles JC. Intracellular recording from antidromically activated motoneurons. J Physiol (Lond). 1953;122:429–461.
17. Llinas R, Terzuolo CA. Mechanisms of supraspinal actions upon spinal cord activities. Reticular inhibitory mechanisms on alpha-extensor motoneurons. J Neurophysiol. 1964;287:579–591.
18. Cook WA Jr, Cangiano A. Presynaptic and postsynaptic inhibition of spinal motoneurons. J Neurophysiol. 1972;35:389–403.
19. Curtis DR, Eccles JC. The time courses of excitatory and inhibitory synaptic actions. J Physiol (Lond). 1959;145:529–546.
20. Holstege JC. The ventro-medial medullary projections to spinal motoneurons: ultrastructure, transmitters and functional aspects. Prog Brain Res. 1996;107:159–181.
21. Chase MH, Morales FR. Postsynaptic mechanisms responsible for motor inhibition during active sleep. In: Chase MH, Weitzman E, eds. Sleep Disorders: Basic and Clinical Research. New York, NY: Spectrum Publications; 1983:71–94.
22. Marchiafava PL, Pompeiano O. Pyramidal influences on spinal cord during desynchronized sleep. Arch Ital Biol. 1964;102:500–529.
23. Burke RE. Composite nature of the monosynaptic excitatory postsynaptic potential. J Neurophysiol. 1967;30:1114–1137.
24. Evarts EV. Temporal patterns of discharge of pyramidal tract neurons during sleep and waking in the monkey. J Neurophysiol. 1964;27:152–171.
25. Curtis DR, Johnston GAR. Amino acid transmitters in the mammalian central nervous system. Ergeb Physiol. 1974;69:97–188.
26. Davidoff RA, Hackmann JE. GABA presynaptic actions. In: Rogawski MA, Barker JL, eds. Neurotransmitter Action in the Vertebrate Nervous System. New York, NY: Plenum Press; 1985:3–32.
27. Young AB, McDonald RL. Glycine as a spinal neurotransmitter. In: Davidoff RA, ed. Handbook of the Spinal Cord. Vol 1. Pharmacology. New York, NY: Marcel Dekker; 1983:1–43.
28. Curtis DR, Hosli L, Johnston GAR, et al. The hyperpolarization of spinal motoneurons by glycine and related amino acids. Exp Brain Res. 1968;5:235–258.
29. Krnjevic K, Puil E, Werman R. Bicuculline, benzyl penicillin and inhibitory amino acids in the spinal cord of the cat. Can J Physiol Pharmacol. 1976;55:670–680.
30. Nistri A. Spinal cord pharmacology of GABA and chemically related amino acids. In: Davidoff RA, ed. Handbook of the Spinal Cord. Vol 1. Pharmacology. New York, NY: Marcel Dekker; 1983:45–104.
31. Chase MH, Soja PJ, Finch DM. Pharmacological evidence of postsynaptic factors involved in the suppression of the masse-

teric reflex during active sleep. In: Chase MH, McGinty DJ, Crane G, eds. Sleep Research. Vol 15. Los Angeles, Calif: Brain Information Service/Brain Research Institute, UCLA; 1986:3.

32. Soja PJ, Morales FR, Chase MH. Effect of picrotoxin and bicuculline on the waveform characteristics of spontaneous IPSPs involved in motoneuron inhibition during active sleep. Soc Neurosci Abst. 1986;12:154.

33. Soja PJ, López-Rodríguez F, Morales FR, et al. A non-NMDA excitatory amino acid mediates subthreshold synaptic activity influencing cat lumbar motoneurons during quiet and active sleep. Physiologist. 1988;31:A26.

34. Soja PJ, López-Rodríguez F, Morales FR, et al. Depolarizing synaptic events influencing cat lumbar motoneurons during rapid eye movement episodes of active sleep are blocked by kyurenic acid. Soc Neurosci Abstr. 1988;14:941.

35. George R, Hasiett WL, Jenden DJ. A cholinergic mechanism in the brainstem reticular formation: induction of paradoxical sleep. Int J Neuropharmacol. 1964;3:541–552.

36. Baghdoyan HA, Lydic R, Callaway CW, et al. The carbachol-induced enhancement of desynchronized sleep signs is dose-dependent and antagonized by centrally administered atropine. Neuropsychopharmacology. 1989;2:67–79.

37. Kubin L, Kimura H, Tojima H, et al. Suppression of hypoglossal motoneurons during the carbachol-induced atonia of REM sleep is not caused by fast synaptic inhibition. Brain Res. 1993;611:300–312.

38. Morales FR, Engelhardt JK, Pereda AE, et al. Renshaw cells are inactive during motor inhibition elicited by the pontine microinjection of carbachol. Neurosci Lett. 1988;86:289–295.

39. Morales FR, Engelhardt JK, Soja PJ, et al. Motoneuron properties during motor inhibition produced by microinjection of carbachol into the pontine reticular formation of the decerebrate cat. J Neurophysiol. 1987;57:1118–1129.

40. Takakusaki K, Ohta Y, Mori S. Single medullary reticulospinal neurons exert postsynaptic inhibitory effects via inhibitory interneurons upon alpha-motoneurons innervating cat hindlimb muscle. Exp Brain Res. 1989;74:11–23.

41. López-Rodríguez F, Kohlmeier K, Morales FR, et al. Muscle atonia can be generated by carbachol in cats anesthetized with α-chloralose. Brain Res. 1995;699:201–207.

42. Xi M-C, Liu R-H, Yamuy J, et al. Electrophysiological properties of lumbar motoneurons in the α-chloralose-anesthetized cat during carbachol-induced motor inhibition. J Neurophysiol. 1997;78:129–136.

43. Xi M-C, Yamuy J, Liu R-H, et al. Dorsal spinocerebellar tract neurons are not subjected to postsynaptic inhibition during carbachol-induced motor inhibition. J Neurophysiol. 1997;78:137–144.

44. Chase MH. A model of central neural processes controlling motor behavior during active sleep and wakefulness. In: Desiraju T, ed. Mechanisms in Transmission for Signals for Conscious Behavior. Amsterdam, Netherlands: Elsevier; 1976:99–121.

45. Magoun HW, Rhines R. An inhibitory mechanism in the bulbar reticular formation. J Neurophysiol. 1946;9:165–171.

46. Yamuy J, Mancillas JR, Morales FR, et al. C-fos expression in the pons and medulla of the cat during carbachol-induced active sleep. J Neurosci. 1993;13:2703–2718.

47. Morales FR, Sampogna, S, Yamuy J, et al. Premotor trigeminal interneurons activated during carbachol-induced active sleep. Soc Neurosci Abstr. 1996;22:690.

48. Morales FR, Chase MH. Repetitive synaptic potentials responsible for inhibition of spinal cord motoneurons during active sleep. Exp Neurol. 1982;78:471–476.

three

Physiology in Sleep

John Orem

12

Physiological Regulation in Sleep

Pier Luigi Parmeggiani

The ultradian wake-sleep cycle is the basic temporal module of physiological regulation underlying the behavioral continuum. The behavioral states of the cycle depend on permutations in the functional dominance of phylogenetically different structures of the encephalon.

The functional similarity of physiological events during nonrapid eye movement (NREM) sleep in different species and the variety and variability of such events during REM sleep within and between species are the characteristic differences between NREM and REM sleep, respectively.

The basic somatic features of NREM sleep are the assumption of a thermoregulatory posture and a decrease in antigravitary muscle activity. The basic somatic features of REM sleep are muscle atonia, rapid eye movements, and myoclonic twitches. The basic autonomic feature of NREM sleep is the functional prevalence of parasympathetic influences associated with quiescence of sympathetic activity. The basic autonomic feature of REM sleep is the great variability in sympathetic activity associated with phasic changes in tonic parasympathetic discharge.

In all species, the somatic and visceral phenomena of NREM sleep are indicative of closed-loop operations, automatically maintaining homeostasis at a lower level of energy expenditure compared with quiet wakefulness. In contrast, the somatic and visceral phenomena of REM sleep are characterized in all species by the greatest variability as a result of open-loop operations of central origin impairing the homeostasis of physiological functions (poikilostasis).

In the context of this chapter, the term *physiological regulation* refers to the nervous control mechanisms of the entire somatic and visceral activity, which is defined here as the "behavior" of the organism. Several are the criteria that may be used for a general classification of the behavioral phenomena characterizing the ultradian wake-sleep cycle[1] (Table 12–1). In any case, this cycle is a nonreducible functional module to identify whatever behavioral principles of physiological regulation are sequentially operative across the behavioral continuum, notwithstanding circadian variations of physiological activity.[2] The cycle consists of the single sequence of at least three behavioral states, which may be called quiet wakefulness (QW), nonrapid eye movement (NREM) sleep, and REM sleep. To consider further subdivisions of sleep behavior as well as the multifarious behavioral state of active wakefulness (AW) would be outside the general scope intended for this chapter.

A powerful conceptual tool to facilitate understanding of physiological regulation is *homeostasis*,[3] which can be experimentally tested across the behavioral continuum by studying stimulus-response relationships in physiological functions at different levels of integration.[4, 5] Mechanistically, physiological homeostasis is effected by feedforward and feedback operations that predictively and reactively minimize[6] the influences of internal and external disturbances on the organism. This means that it is necessary to verify whether effector activity either maintains (*homeostasis*) or impairs (*poikilostasis*) the stability—within what is

Table 12–1. CLASSIFICATION OF BEHAVIORAL STATES OF THE ULTRADIAN WAKE-SLEEP CYCLE

Criteria	QW	NREMS	REMS
Bioelectrical	Desynchronized	Synchronized	Desynchronized
Ethological	Appetitive (somatic)	Appetitive (visceral)	Consummatory (somatic + visceral)
Hierarchical	Prosencephalic	Diencephalic	Rhombencephalic
Operational	Closed-loop	Closed-loop	Open-loop
Teleological	Homeostatic	Homeostatic	Poikilostatic

From Parmeggiani PL. Behavioral phenomenology of sleep [somatic and vegetative]. Experientia [Basel]. 1980;36:6–11.
NREMS, nonrapid eye movement sleep; QW, quiet wakefulness; REMS, rapid eye movement sleep.

conventionally called a "normal range"—of the "fundamental" variables of the interstitial and cellular compartments (e.g., temperature, pH, water volume, electrolytes, osmolality, nutrients, oxygen, carbon dioxide, and so on) that underlie cellular survival. However, the homeostasis of such variables is the eventual result of continuous adjustments of "instrumental" variables (e.g., heart rate, stroke volume, cardiac output, vascular resistance, blood pressure, ventilation, muscle force, and so on) that are directly affected by the activity of somatic and visceral effectors. It is worth stressing that studies on single variables provide no sound basis for any inference of the behavioral principles of physiological regulation. As Hess[7] pointed out, "It is essential that the data are interrelated and woven into a theoretical fabric." In this respect, the intensive study of the bioelectrical and behavioral (somatic and visceral) aspects of sleep has shown that the principle of homeostatic regulation of physiological functions, conceived by Bernard[8] and formulated by Cannon,[3] does not apply to all behavioral states.[1]

HOMEOSTATIC VERSUS POIKILOSTATIC REGULATION IN SLEEP

In this section, only a short survey of experimental results is presented, and the interested reader is referred to other chapters for further details.

Somatic Behavior

The somatic repertory from QW to NREM sleep displays the appetitive features of an instinct that consists of the search for a safe and thermally comfortable ecological niche and the preparation of the body for the natural sleep posture.[9] NREM sleep is characterized by the cessation of goal-directed motor activity, the assumption of a thermoregulatory posture, and a decrease in antigravitary muscle activity. During REM sleep,[10, 11] muscle atonia, myoclonic twitches, and rapid eye movements are clear signs of a substantial change in motor innervation with respect to NREM sleep but have no apparent functional purpose.[1]

Thermoregulatory Function

In mammals, homeothermy is controlled by hypothalamic-preoptic integrative mechanisms that drive subordinate brainstem and spinal somatic and visceral mechanisms eliciting thermoregulatory effector responses.[12]

The thermoregulatory responses to ambient thermal loads are present during NREM sleep and absent or depressed during REM sleep.[4, 5, 13–15] For example, the cat's posture clearly varies in relation to ambient temperature during NREM sleep, whereas the drop in postural muscle tone during REM sleep is unrelated to ambient temperature.[16] Moreover, notwithstanding a positive (warm) thermal load, tachypnea in the cat[17] and heat exchanger vasodilation in the cat,[18] rabbit,[19] and rat[20] disappear and sweating in human beings[21–28] decreases during the episode of REM sleep. Likewise, under a negative (cold) thermal load, shivering in the cat[17] and armadillo[29–31]; heat exchanger vasoconstriction in the cat,[18] rabbit,[19] and rat[20]; and piloerection in the cat[32] are suppressed during the REM episode. Moreover, the cold-defense function of brown fat is altered in rats.[33]

Thermoregulatory responses elicited by positive and negative thermal loads applied directly to the thermosensitive hypothalamic-preoptic region are dependent on the behavioral state. In the cat, warming elicits tachypnea[34, 35] and heat exchanger vasodilation[18] during NREM sleep but has no such effects during REM sleep. Likewise, in the kangaroo rat[36, 37] and marmot,[38] cooling increases oxygen consumption and metabolic heat production during NREM sleep, whereas it is ineffective during REM sleep. A crucial proof of the behavioral state–dependent changes in the function of the hypothalamic-preoptic thermostat has been provided by experiments of direct thermal stimulation of hypothalamic-preoptic thermosensitive neurons across behavioral states in the cat[39–44] and kangaroo rat.[45] The change in thermosensitivity of the majority of such neurons parallels that in thermoregulatory responses to central thermal loads during both NREM and REM sleep. Moreover, an indirect proof of this is the disappearance of shivering during REM sleep in a cold ambience in cats with pontine lesions producing REM sleep without muscle atonia. The result shows that the pontine inhibitory mechanisms eliciting muscle atonia in the normal animal do not underlie the suppression of this thermoregulatory response.[32, 46]

In conclusion, experimental evidence shows that during NREM sleep, thermoregulatory mechanisms are operative as they are in QW, albeit for some state-dependent differences in the threshold and gain of effector responses to thermal loads.[23, 37, 47] The other difference with respect to QW is that in NREM sleep, body and hypothalamic temperatures are downregulated together with energy expenditure.[48–51]

The events during REM sleep are not simply the result of state-dependent changes in the threshold and gain of the different thermoregulatory responses. From the quantitative point of view, REM sleep is characterized by effector activity that not only is functionally inconsistent with the aim of temperature regulation but also lacks any proportional relationship with the intensity of the thermal stimulus. The result is that the temperature of the body changes according to its thermal inertia, as one would expect in a poikilothermic organism.[52, 53]

Circulatory Function

NREM sleep is characterized by a downregulation of cardiovascular activity of variable intensity depending on the species and its previous level in QW. A decrease in arterial blood pressure occurs in the cat[54] but is lacking in the rabbit[55] and is found less consistently in the rat.[56–58] Of the cardiac variables influencing cardiac output, namely, heart rate and stroke volume, the first is moderately decreased,[54, 59] whereas the latter is practically unchanged in cats.[54] There is a significant decrease in heart rate in rats,[57, 58] but the decrease is not statistically significant in rabbits.[55] In humans, a tonic decrease in arterial blood pressure is observed,[60–64] although it has varying intensity in different individuals.[64a] Baroreceptor reflex sensitivity is increased in human beings.[65] With respect to the vascular conductance, a slight increase occurs in the skin, mesenteric, iliac, and renal beds in the cat[54] and in the skin bed in the rabbit[19] and human beings.[66, 67] On the whole, the cardiovascular changes in NREM sleep are consistent with the changes in respiration and thermoregulation in a condition of postural and motor quiescence.

Different phenomena characterize REM sleep in both animals and human beings. According to some, arterial blood pressure falls markedly in cats as a result of a pronounced bradycardia associated with a practically unchanged stroke volume and an increase in total vascular conductance: the increase in vascular conductance in the skin, mesenteric, and renal beds prevails over the decrease in conductance of the hindlimb muscle vasculature.[54, 68] However, according to others,[69] a slight fall in arterial blood pressure was not consistently detected in cats. In addition, other studies[70, 71] showed that the bradycardia and hypotension observed in cats during REM sleep may be a long-lasting effect from surgical preparation of the animal for the experiment. Thereafter, heart rate and arterial blood pressure are higher in REM sleep than in NREM sleep. This cardiovascular condition appears to depend on forebrain influences.[72] In the rabbit,[55, 73] rat,[56–58] and human beings,[60, 61, 63, 64] arterial blood pressure increases from NREM to REM sleep, but the rise is not always related to consistent changes in the primary variables, (i.e., heart rate and vascular conductance).[60, 62] In the

rabbit, renal and fat vascular conductances appear to be decreased during REM sleep.[55] The poor correlation between regional and systemic variables shows that the central integration of cardiovascular functions is altered in REM sleep. As a result, the regional distribution of blood flow is remarkably modified in comparison with NREM sleep.[13]

The variability of heart rate and arterial blood pressure is an important feature of REM sleep in the cat,[74, 75] rat,[56–58] rabbit,[73] and human beings.[60, 61, 63] It is in general loosely associated with bursts of rapid eye movements, myoclonic twitches, and, probably more often, breathing irregularities. However, such variability is not only the direct result of central changes in the regulation of the autonomic outflow[76, 77]; these changes also activate indirectly a number of feedback loops by affecting the peripherally controlled variables.[59] Therefore, the interaction between the central variability of visceral control during REM sleep and the central effects of activated reflexes are main factors in the generation of REM sleep instability of cardiovascular regulation. The importance of such an interaction is also shown by studies in anesthetized[78] and awake[79] cats showing that the central generator underlying the rhythmicity of synchronized cardiac sympathetic nerve activity is subject to reflex modulation by baroreceptor inputs.

In cats, arterial blood pressure during REM sleep is buffered by sinoaortic reflexes.[69, 75] After sinoaortic denervation, arterial blood pressure is mildly increased during wakefulness, decreases to slightly more than that which occurs in normal animals during NREM sleep, but decreases sharply during REM sleep. This decrease in some REM episodes may produce brain ischemia as revealed by the flattening of the electroencephalogram, motor convulsions, and arousal.[75] The marked drop in arterial blood pressure after sinoaortic denervation depends on the greater vasodilation in the splanchnic vascular bed and the reversal of vasoconstriction to vasodilation in the hindlimb muscles.[54, 80] Selective removal of either baroreceptor or chemoreceptor afferents showed that the arterial hypotension of REM sleep is buffered in the cat primarily by chemoreceptor reflexes because baroreceptor reflexes are depressed in this species.[54, 81, 82] In the rat, the baroreceptor reflexes are more effective than those in the cat in buffering REM sleep hypotension because arterial blood pressure increases during REM sleep, whereas in baroreceptor-denervated rats, hypotension, as occurs in the cat, is observed.[56–58] However, the role of baroreceptors in REM sleep is still problematic due to long-lasting effects from the surgical preparation of animals for the experiment.[70, 71] Also, the results of baroreceptor studies in human beings suggest caution in this respect because reflex sensitivity may either increase[61] or decrease[65] in REM sleep. Nevertheless, when the results are taken together, it appears likely that circulation in different species is affected by similar central influences in REM sleep, although the eventual pattern of change in cardiovascular variables also depends on species-specific differences in the operation of feedback loops[83] and autoregulation.[83a]

With respect to the control of brain integrative centers on brainstem cardiovascular regulation,[84-87] thermoregulatory vasomotion elicited by direct thermal stimulation of the hypothalamic-preoptic region during NREM sleep is suppressed during REM sleep in cats[18] according to the reduced responsiveness of hypothalamic-preoptic thermosensitive neurons.[40, 42-45] Moreover, a depression in telencephalic (amygdala, orbital frontal cortex) control over cardiovascular activity has been observed in cats during REM sleep.[88]

Respiratory Function

Conspicuous changes occur in the regulation of breathing across the behavioral states of sleep.[89, 90] The transition from wakefulness to NREM sleep is characterized by the inactivation of the "wakefulness" (telencephalic) control mechanism and the release of the automatic control mechanism.[91-99] This transition (stages 1 and 2 of NREM sleep in human beings) is characterized by breathing instability[64, 100-105] and the appearance of respiratory and circulatory periodic phenomena.[100, 106, 107] Regular breathing sets in with deep NREM sleep (stages 3 and 4 in human beings) when breathing is driven by the automatic control mechanism. The rate decreases and the tidal volume increases slightly; however, ventilation decreases in both human beings[106, 108, 109] and animals[97, 99] according to the metabolic rate. A concomitant increase in alveolar CO_2 partial pressure in human beings[106, 109] and animals[99, 110] and in arterial CO_2 partial pressure in human beings[108, 111] and cats[112] associated with a decrease in alveolar and arterial O_2 partial pressure in human beings[113] and cats[112] has been observed. Airway resistance is increased.[113, 114] These changes in respiratory variables are in agreement with a state of rest at low energy expenditure. Although the operation of the automatic control mechanism appears to be downregulated, it maintains compensatory physiological responses. Respiratory chemosensitivity to CO_2 is only moderately reduced,[106, 108, 113, 115, 116] whereas the hypoxic response is unaffected in human beings[117] and in dogs.[118] Moreover, pulmonary inflation and deflation reflexes are active during NREM sleep in both human infants[119] and animals.[99, 120] The responses to a mechanical respiratory load (airway occlusion, inspiration from a rigid container) are also practically identical to those observed during wakefulness,[121] thus showing that proprioceptive reflexes of the intercostal muscles are normal during NREM sleep.

The phenomena of REM sleep point to a profound alteration in the activity of the automatic control mechanism of respiration. In fact, the respiratory rhythm in human beings and animals is very irregular,[10, 64, 100, 122-124] with the average frequency being increased or decreased with respect to the rate attained during NREM sleep in eupnea or polypnea, respectively.[47, 89, 125] The respiratory activity of the intercostal muscles is diminished in cats and lambs[47, 126-128]; in human infants, this depression may even produce paradoxical chest collapse during inspiration.[129] However, ventilation increases in human beings[106, 119, 130-133] and dogs,[134] mostly

in temporal relation to myoclonic twitches.[97, 110] During REM sleep, alveolar ventilation may also be variable as shown by either a decrease[99, 106, 110] or no change[112, 131, 135] in alveolar CO_2 partial pressure. It is important to stress that such disturbances are of central origin as they persist after vagotomy,[99, 135, 136] sectioning of the spinal cord at T1–2,[137, 138] afferent denervation of the mid-thoracic chest wall,[98] denervation of the carotid and aortic chemoreceptors and baroreceptors,[112] hypercapnia[134] and hypoxia.[118] Upper airway resistance increases in human beings and cats[114, 139, 140] and respiratory load compensation is irregular and weak in human beings[133, 141-143] and lambs[126] during REM sleep. The alteration of the automatic control mechanism of respiration during REM sleep is also shown by other phenomena. In dogs and human infants, respiratory responses to hypercapnia are depressed,[134, 144] while those to hypoxia are unchanged.[118, 130, 131] Pulmonary deflation and inflation reflexes persist in the opossum, although they are more variable than during NREM sleep.[120] In contrast, the inflation reflex is practically abolished during REM sleep in dogs[99] and human infants.[119]

Depressed hypothalamic-preoptic influence on respiration during REM sleep as compared to NREM sleep was shown by means of either thermal[34, 35] or electrical[145] direct stimulation of this diencephalic region. Moreover, a depression in telencephalic (amygdala, orbital frontal cortex) control on respiration was shown in cats during REM sleep.[146]

CONCLUSIONS

A basic difference between NREM sleep and REM sleep is the functional similarity of the former in different species and the functional variety and variability of the latter within and between species.

In NREM sleep, the changes in visceral regulation are consistent with somatic quiescence, as are the functional prevalence of the parasympathetic over the sympathetic activity, the lowering of metabolic heat production (decrease in muscle tone and heart and breathing rates) and body temperature (vasodilation of heat exchangers, sweating). Moreover, all somatic and visceral regulatory responses to endogenous and exogenous disturbances may be activated during NREM sleep to maintain homeostasis. In conclusion, the phenomenic stereotype of NREM sleep across mammalian species appears to be the coherent result of a common phylogenetic trend to develop a pattern of integrated automatic regulation resulting in the minimization of energy expenditure. Mechanistically, the regulation of physiological functions during this stage of sleep is led essentially by diencephalic structures, as shown particularly by the persistence of normal homeothermic regulation.

Concerning REM sleep, it is difficult to establish a rational foundation of the observed functional phenomena in terms of a centrally integrated regulation. Their physiological aim escapes a teleological explanation in behavioral terms. Remarkably, cause-effect relationships existing between variables during QW and NREM sleep are suppressed during REM sleep, yet the loss of the specific effects of stimuli during REM sleep is not associated with a loss of their nonspecific arousing influences. The arousal effect, however, requires a much higher stimulus intensity compared with that which normally elicits the specific regulatory response. Thus, REM sleep is characterized by the disintegration of a homeostatic physiological equilibrium bringing about effector responses of great instability that are primarily of central origin but secondarily complicated by local autoregulation, altered reflex activity, or both. Mechanistically, the leading neural structures in REM sleep are rhombencephalic, as shown by the occurrence of REM sleep phenomena in brainstem preparations.[11, 147] However, the physiological variability appears to depend not only on autochthonous activities of the brainstem but also on changes in the functional relationship between the former and the forebrain. The concept of release, as first proposed by Hughlings Jackson in 1884, appears to apply, for example, to the alteration of functions, such as temperature, cardiovascular, and breathing regulation during REM sleep in normal animals. In general, it may be assumed that a critical integrative instability would develop during REM sleep as a result of the impaired homeostatic function of high integration levels. Mechanistically, this instability may be considered to result from a loss of the balance between descending excitatory and inhibitory influences of diencephalic (hypothalamic) and telencephalic structures during REM sleep.[148] In contrast, in QW and NREM sleep, such influences would keep the activity of brainstem and spinal somatic and visceral reflex centers within the range imposed by set point–dependent integrative operations underlying the maintenance of homeostasis.

The impairment of homeostatic control in REM sleep is more dramatic and evident in a function, such as temperature regulation in furry animals, that depends on effector mechanisms strictly subordinated to regulatory structures of the diencephalon (hypothalamus). In functions characterized by more widely distributed control mechanisms, such as circulation and respiration, the features of functional impairment are rather more complex as a result of the persistence of more or less efficient reflex regulation or peripheral autoregulation. Nevertheless, it is evident that functional changes in REM sleep depend essentially on the suppression of a highly integrated homeostatic regulation that is operative in NREM sleep. In comparison with REM sleep, volitional and instinctive drives during AW may also impose a load on or interfere with homeostatic mechanisms at central and/or effector levels to overwhelm their regulatory power.[149] However, such homeostatic mechanisms are still operative and capable of reestablishing the functional equilibrium that so well characterizes QW and NREM sleep. In all species, the somatic and visceral phenomena of NREM sleep are indicative of closed-loop operations, automatically maintaining homeostasis at a lower level of energy expenditure compared with QW. The operative principle is, however, unchanged, which would imply the

Table 12–2. BEHAVIORAL PRINCIPLES OF PHYSIOLOGICAL REGULATION

State	Homeostatic	Poikilostatic
AW	Tonic and phasic	Tonic (volitional and instinctive drives)
QW	Tonic and phasic	
NREMS	Tonic and phasic	
REMS	Phasic	Tonic and phasic

Data from Parmeggiani PL. The autonomic nervous system in sleep. In: Kryger MH, Roth T, Dement WC, eds. Principles and Practice of Sleep Medicine. 2nd ed. Philadelphia, Pa: WB Saunders; 1994:194–203.
Tonic (integrative) and phasic (reflex) nervous control mechanisms in closed-loop (homeostatic) or open-loop (poikilostatic) operation modality. AW, active wakefulness; NREMS, nonrapid eye movement sleep; QW, quiet wakefulness; REMS, rapid eye movement sleep.

utilization of the parasympathetic and sympathetic divisions of the autonomic nervous system for homeostatic regulation. In contrast, the somatic and visceral activity of REM sleep is characterized in all species by the greatest variability as a result of nonhomeostatic (open-loop) operations.[1] The differences in state-dependent physiological regulation disclosed with the help of the criterion of homeostasis[1, 4, 5] emphasize the critical role of diencephalic structures in the generation of the somatic and visceral phenomena of the ultradian wake-sleep cycle.[150] These concepts are summarized in Table 12–2.

From the viewpoint of physiological regulation, the behavioral state acquires a temporal dimension firmly based on the experimental testing of a consistent stability of the regulation principle (Fig. 12–1). This concept addresses the problem of the mechanisms underlying not only each behavioral state but also their orderly temporal sequence in the ultradian wake-sleep cycle. An important question is how static regulatory differences between states are achieved in so many somatic and visceral processes characterized by very different temporal courses.[151] Probably, only large-scale changes in neuronal relationships provide the critical functional mass to produce and maintain such differences. From this viewpoint, each behavioral state would require a specific pattern of functional organization of the encephalon. This approach entails the suggestion that apparent complexity is ultimately organized simplicity, which may be schematically represented with the help of a model (Table 12–3). Such a model can be conceived from the perspective of the morphological and functional organization of the central nervous system as brought about by phylogenetic and ontogenetic processes.[5, 77, 152] In other words, behavioral states appear as functional landmarks of the discontinuous development of the mammalian encephalon through successive superimpositions of increasingly complex integrative levels. The model points out the importance of interaction processes within the whole central nervous system abating reductionist emphasis on the role of discrete and specific mechanisms underlying single somatic or visceral events of behavioral states. According to the

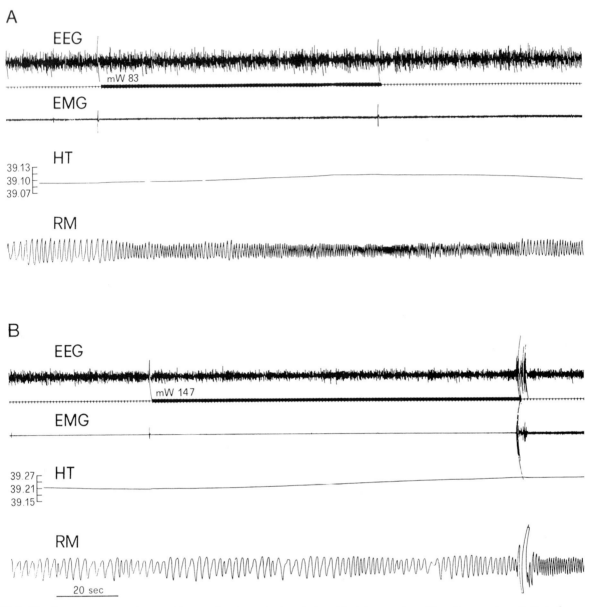

Figure 12–1. Respiratory responses to preoptic warming in a cat at neutral ambient temperature. Preoptic warming elicits tachypnea during nonrapid eye movement (NREM) sleep *(A)* and is ineffective during REM sleep *(B)*. Note that tachypnea starts immediately on awaking. EEG, electroencephalogram; EMG, neck muscle electrogram; HT, hypothalamic temperature (recorded 5 mm behind the heating electrodes); RM, respiratory movements; mW, milliwatt. (Reprinted from Brain Research, vol 52, Parmeggiani PL, Franzini C, Lenzi P, et al, Threshold of respiratory responses to preoptic heating during sleep in freely moving cats, 189–201, Copyright 1973, with permission from Elsevier Science.)

Table 12–3. PERMUTATIONS IN FUNCTIONAL HIERARCHICAL ARRAYS

		FHA					
RANK	MHA	QW	NREMS	REMS	?	?	?
I	T	T	D	R	T	R	D
II	D	D	R	T	R	D	T
III	R	R	T	D	D	T	R

Data from Parmeggiani PL. Regulation of physiological functions during sleep in mammals. Experientia [Basel]. 1982;38:1405–1408; and Parmeggiani PL. The autonomic nervous system in sleep. In: Kryger MH, Roth T, Dement WC, eds. Principles and Practice of Sleep Medicine. 2nd ed. Philadelphia, Pa: WB Saunders; 1994:194–203.

D, diencephalon; FHA, functional hierarchical array; MHA, morphological hierarchical array; NREMS, nonrapid eye movement sleep; QW, quiet wakefulness; R, rhombencephalon; REMS, rapid eye movement sleep; T, telencephalon; ?, abnormal or prohibited behavioral states.

model, the evolution of wake-sleep states in mammals broadly features a stepwise functional regression, which, in a reverse fashion, attains the successive functional levels of the phylogenetic development of the encephalon through the loss of the hierarchical coherence between its morphological and functional organization.[5, 77, 152] In particular, the morphological organization is taken as an invariant reference for the changes (hierarchical permutations) occurring in the functional relationships among phylogenetically different structures of the encephalon during the ultradian wake-sleep cycle. Mechanisms that could explain such hierarchical permutations are still unknown, although the diffuse influences on neuron populations exerted by monoaminergic and peptidergic regulatory systems of the encephalon[153, 154] may be taken into consideration.

In conclusion, although many aspects of physiological regulation in sleep deserve further study, the foregoing analysis foreshadows an important consequence regarding medical practice—namely, that sleep entails a "physiological risk."[155–157]

Acknowledgments

The author is indebted to Dr. John Orem for helpful advice and to Dr. Christine A. Jones for editing the English.

References

1. Parmeggiani PL. Behavioral phenomenology of sleep (somatic and vegetative). Experientia (Basel). 1980;36:6–11.
2. Burgess HJ, Trinder J, Kim Y, et al. Sleep and circadian influences on cardiac autonomic nervous system activity. Am J Physiol. 1997;273:H1761–H1768.
3. Cannon WB. Organization for physiological homeostasis. Physiol Rev. 1929;9:399–431.
4. Parmeggiani PL. Temperature regulation during sleep: a study in homeostasis. In: Orem J, Barnes CD, eds. Physiology in Sleep: Research Topics in Physiology. Vol 3. New York, NY: Academic Press; 1980:97–143.
5. Parmeggiani PL. Thermoregulation during sleep from the viewpoint of homeostasis. In: Lydic R, Biebuyck JF, eds. Clinical Physiology of Sleep. Bethesda, Md: American Physiological Society; 1988:159–169.
6. Moore-Ede MC. Physiology of the circadian timing system: predictive versus reactive homeostasis. Am J Physiol. 1986;250:R737–R752.
7. Hess WR. Sleep as a phenomenon of the integral organism. In: Akert K, Bally C, Schadé JP, eds. Progress in Brain Research, 18. Sleep Mechanisms. Amsterdam, Netherlands: Elsevier; 1965:3–8.
8. Bernard C. Leçons sur les Phenomenes de la Vie Communs aux Animaux et aux Végétaux. Paris, France: Muséum; 1878–1879.
9. Parmeggiani PL. Telencephalo-diencephalic aspects of sleep mechanisms. Brain Res. 1968;7:350–359.
10. Aserinsky E, Kleitman N. Regularly occurring periods of eye motility and concomitant phenomena, during sleep. Science. 1953;118:273–274.
11. Jouvet M. Recherches sur les structures nerveuses et les mécanismes responsables des différentes phases du sommeil physiologique. Arch Ital Biol. 1962;100:125–206.
12. Satinoff E. Neural organization and evolution of thermal regulation in mammals. Science. 1978;201:16–22.
13. Cianci T, Zoccoli G, Lenzi P, et al. Loss of integrative control of peripheral circulation during desynchronized sleep. Am J Physiol. 1991;261:R373–R377.
14. Heller HC, Glotzbach SF. Thermoregulation during sleep and hibernation. In: Robertshaw D, ed. Environmental Physiology, II. Vol 15. Baltimore, Md: University Park Press; 1977:147–188.
15. Heller HC, Glotzbach SF. Thermoregulation and sleep. In: Eberhardt RC, Shitzer A, eds. Heat transfer in biological systems: analysis and application. New York, NY: Plenum Press; 1985:107–134.
16. Parmeggiani PL, Rabini C. Sleep and environmental temperature. Arch Ital Biol. 1970;108:369–387.
17. Parmeggiani PL, Rabini C. Shivering and panting during sleep. Brain Res. 1967;6:789–791.
18. Parmeggiani PL, Zamboni G, Cianci T, et al. Absence of thermoregulatory vasomotor responses during fast wave sleep in cats. Electroencephalogr Clin Neurophysiol. 1977;42:372–380.
19. Franzini C, Cianci T, Lenzi P, et al. Neural control of vasomotion in rabbit ear is impaired during desynchronized sleep. Am J Physiol. 1982;243:R142–R146.
20. Alföldi P, Rubicsek G, Cserni G, et al. Brain and core temperatures and peripheral vasomotion during sleep and wakefulness at various ambient temperatures in the rat. Pflugers Arch. 1990;417:336–341.
21. Amoros C, Sagot JC, Libert JP, et al. Sweat gland response to local heating during sleep in man. J Physiol Paris. 1986;81:209–215.
22. Ogawa T, Satoh T, Takagi K. Sweating during night sleep. Jpn J Physiol. 1967;17:135–148.
23. Sagot JC, Amoros C, Candas V, et al. Sweating responses and body temperatures during nocturnal sleep in humans. Am J Physiol. 1987;252:R462–R470.
24. Satoh T, Ogawa T, Takagi K. Sweating during daytime sleep. Jpn J Physiol. 1965;15:523–531.
25. Libert JP, Candas V, Muzet A, et al. Thermoregulatory adjustments to thermal transients during slow wave sleep and REM sleep in man. J Physiol Paris. 1982;78:251–257.
26. Shapiro CM, Moore AT, Mitchell D, et al. How well does man thermoregulate during sleep? Experientia (Basel). 1974;30:1279–1281.
27. Takagi K: Sweating during sleep. In: Hardy JD, Gagge AP, Stolwijk JAJ, eds. Physiological and Behavioral Temperature Regulation. Springfield, Ill: Thomas; 1970:669–675.
28. Henane R, Buguet A, Roussel B, et al. Variations in evaporation and body temperature during sleep in man. J Appl Physiol. 1977;42:50–55.
29. Prudom AE, Klemm WR. Electrographic correlates of sleep behavior in a primitive mammal, the armadillo Dasypus novemcinctus. Physiol Behav. 1973;10:275–282.
30. Van Twyver H, Allison T. Sleep in the armadillo Dasypus novemcinctus at moderate and low ambient temperatures. Brain Behav Evol. 1974;9:107–120.
31. Affanni JM, Lisogorsky E, Scaravilli AM. Sleep in the giant South American armadillo Priodontes giganteus (Edentata, Mammalia). Experientia (Basel). 1972;28:1046–1047.
32. Hendricks JC. Absence of shivering in the cat during paradoxical sleep without atonia. Exp Neurol. 1982;75:700–710.
33. Calasso M, Zantedeschi E, Parmeggiani PL. Cold-defense function of brown adipose tissue during sleep. Am J Physiol. 1993;265:R1060–R1064.
34. Parmeggiani PL, Franzini C, Lenzi P. Respiratory frequency as a function of preoptic temperature during sleep. Brain Res. 1976;111:253–260.
35. Parmeggiani PL, Franzini C, Lenzi P, et al. Threshold of respiratory responses to preoptic heating during sleep in freely moving cats. Brain Res. 1973;52:189–201.
36. Glotzbach SF, Heller HC. CNS regulation of metabolic rate in the kangaroo rat Dipodomys ingens. Am J Physiol. 1975;228:1880–1886.
37. Glotzbach SF, Heller HC. Central nervous regulation of body temperature during sleep. Science. 1976;194:537–539.
38. Florant GL, Turner BM, Heller HC. Temperature regulation during wakefulness, sleep, and hibernation in marmots. Am J Physiol. 1978;235:R82–R88.
39. Alam MN, McGinty D, Szymusiak R. Neuronal discharge of preoptic/anterior hypothalamic thermosensitive neurons: relation to NREM sleep. Am J Physiol. 1995;269:R1240–R1249.
40. Alam MN, McGinty D, Szymusiak R. Preoptic/anterior hypothalamic neurons: thermosensitivity in rapid eye movement sleep. Am J Physiol. 1995;269:R1250–R1257.
41. Cevolani D, Parmeggiani PL. Responses of extrahypothalamic neurons to short temperature transients during the ultradian wake-sleep cycle. Brain Res Bull. 1995;37:227–232.

42. Parmeggiani PL, Azzaroni A, Cevolani D, et al. Responses of anterior hypothalamic-preoptic neurons to direct thermal stimulation during wakefulness and sleep. Brain Res. 1983;269:382–385.

43. Parmeggiani PL, Azzaroni A, Cevolani D, et al. Polygraphic study of anterior hypothalamic-preoptic neuron thermosensitivity during sleep. Electroencephalogr Clin Neurophysiol. 1986;63:289–295.

44. Parmeggiani PL, Cevolani D, Azzaroni A, et al. Thermosensitivity of anterior hypothalamic-preoptic neurons during the waking-sleeping cycle: a study in brain functional states. Brain Res. 1987;415:79–89.

45. Glotzbach SF, Heller HC. Changes in the thermal characteristics of hypothalamic neurons during sleep and wakefulness. Brain Res. 1984;309:17–26.

46. Kanosue K, Zhang Y-H, Yanase-Fujiwara M, et al. Hypothalamic network for thermoregulatory shivering. Am J Physiol. 1994;267:R275–R282.

47. Parmeggiani PL, Sabattini L. Electromyographic aspects of postural, respiratory and thermoregulatory mechanisms in sleeping cats. Electroencephalogr Clin Neurophysiol. 1972;33:1–13.

48. Berger RJ. Bioenergetic functions of sleep and activity rhythms and their possible relevance to aging. Fed Proc. 1975;34:97–102.

49. Brebbia DR, Altshuler KZ. Oxygen consumption rate and electroencephalographic stage of sleep. Science. 1965;150:1621–1622.

50. Roussel B, Bittel J. Thermogenesis and thermolysis during sleeping and waking in the rat. Pflugers Arch. 1979;382:225–231.

51. Webb P, Hiestand M. Sleep metabolism and age. J Appl Physiol 1975;38:257–262.

52. Parmeggiani PL, Franzini C, Lenzi P, et al. Inguinal subcutaneous temperature changes in cats sleeping at different environmental temperatures. Brain Res. 1971;33:397–404.

53. Walker JM, Walker LE, Harris DV, et al. Cessation of thermoregulation during REM sleep in the pocket mouse. Am J Physiol. 1983;244:R114–R118.

54. Mancia G, Zanchetti A. Cardiovascular regulation during sleep. In: Orem J, Barnes CD, eds. Physiology in Sleep: Research Topics in Physiology. Vol 3. New York, NY: Academic Press; 1980:1–55.

55. Lenzi P, Cianci T, Guidalotti PL, et al. Brain circulation during sleep and its relation to extracerebral hemodynamics. Brain Res. 1987;415:14–20.

56. Junqueira LF Jr, Krieger EM. Blood pressure and sleep in the rat in normotension and in neurogenic hypertension. J Physiol (Lond). 1976;259:725–735.

57. Lacombe J, Nosjean A, Meunier JM, et al. Computer analysis of cardiovascular changes during sleep-wake cycle in Sprague-Dawley rats. Am J Physiol. 1988;254:H217–H222.

58. Meunier JM, Nosjean A, Lacombe J, et al. Cardiovascular changes during the sleep-wake cycle in spontaneous hypertensive rats and in their genetically normotensive precursors. Pflugers Arch. 1988;411:195–199.

59. Baust W, Bohnert B. The regulation of heart rate during sleep. Exp Brain Res. 1969;7:169–180.

60. Coccagna G, Mantovani M, Lugaresi E. Arterial pressure changes during spontaneous sleep in man. Electroencephalogr Clin Neurophysiol. 1971;31:277–281.

61. Jones JV, Sleight P, Smyth HS. Haemodynamic changes during sleep in man. In: Ganten D, Pfaff D, eds. Sleep: Current Topics in Endocrinology. New York, NY: Academic Press; 1982:213–272.

62. Khatri IM, Freis ED. Hemodynamic changes during sleep. J Appl Physiol. 1967;22:867–873.

63. Scharf SM. Influence of sleep state and breathing on cardiovascular function. In: Saunders NA, Sullivan CE, eds. Sleep and Breathing. Vol 21. New York, NY: Dekker; 1984:221–239.

64. Snyder F, Hobson JA, Morrison DF, et al. Changes in respiration, heart rate, and systolic blood pressure in human sleep. J Appl Physiol. 1964;19:417–422.

64a. Mancia G. Autonomic modulation of the cardiovascular system during sleep. N Engl J Med. 1993;328:347–349.

65. Conway J, Boon N, Jones JV, et al. Involvement of the baroreceptor reflexes in the changes in blood pressure with sleep and mental arousal. Hypertension. 1983;5:746–748.

66. Noll G, Elam M, Kunimoto M, et al. Skin sympathetic nerve activity and effector function during sleep in humans. Acta Physiol Scand. 1994;151:319–329.

67. Sindrup JH, Kastrup J, Madsen PL, et al. Nocturnal variations in human lower leg subcutaneous blood flow related to sleep stages. J Appl Physiol. 1992;73:1246–1252.

68. Baccelli G, Albertini R, Mancia G, et al. Central and reflex regulation of sympathetic vasoconstrictor activity of limb muscle during desynchronized sleep in the cat. Circ Res. 1974;35:625–635.

69. Iwamura Y, Uchino Y, Ozawa S, et al. Spontaneous and reflex discharge of a sympathetic nerve during "para-sleep" in decerebrate cat. Brain Res. 1969;16:359–367.

70. Sei H, Morita Y, Morita H, et al. Long-term profiles of sleep-related hemodynamic changes in the postoperative chronic cat. Physiol Behav. 1989;46:499–500.

71. Sei H, Sakai K, Kanamori N, et al. Long-term variations of arterial blood pressure during sleep in freely moving cats. Physiol Behav. 1994;55:673–679.

72. Kanamori N, Sakai K, Sei H, et al. Effects of decerebration on blood pressure during paradoxical sleep in cats. Brain Res Bull. 1995;378:545–549.

73. Dufour R, Court L. Le débit cérébral sanguin au cours du sommeil paradoxal du lapin. Arch Ital Biol. 1977;115:57–76.

74. Gassel MM, Ghelarducci B, Marchiafava PL, et al. Phasic changes in blood pressure and heart rate during the rapid eye movement episodes of desynchronized sleep in unrestrained cats. Arch Ital Biol. 1964;102:530–544.

75. Guazzi M, Zanchetti A. Blood pressure and heart rate during natural sleep of the cat and their regulation by carotid sinus and aortic reflexes. Arch Ital Biol. 1965;103:789–817.

76. Franzini C. The control of peripheral circulation during sleep. In: Mancia M, Marini G, eds. The Diencephalon and Sleep. New York, NY: Raven Press; 1990:343–353.

77. Parmeggiani PL. The autonomic nervous system in sleep. In: Kryger MH, Roth T, Dement WC, eds. Principles and Practice of Sleep Medicine. 2nd ed. Philadelphia, Pa: WB Saunders; 1994:194–203.

78. Gebber GL, Barman SM, Kocsis B. Coherence of medullary unit activity and sympathetic nerve discharge. Am J Physiol. 1990;259:R561–R571.

79. Ninomiya I, Akiyama T, Nishiura N. Mechanism of cardiac-related synchronized cardiac sympathetic nerve activity in awake cats. Am J Physiol. 1990;259:R499–R506.

80. Baccelli G, Albertini R, Mancia G, et al. Control of regional circulation by the sino-aortic reflexes during desynchronized sleep in the cat. Cardiovasc Res. 1978;12:523–528.

81. Guazzi M, Baccelli G, Zanchetti A. Reflex chemoceptive regulation of arterial pressure during natural sleep in the cat. Am J Physiol. 1968;214:969–978.

82. Knuepfer MM, Stumpf H, Stock G. Baroreceptor sensitivity during desynchronized sleep. Exp Neurol. 1986;92:323–334.

83. Gilmore JP, Tomomatsu E. Comparison of carotid sinus baroreceptors in dogs, cats, monkeys, and rabbits. Am J Physiol. 1984;247:R52–R56.

83a. Cowley AW Jr, Hinojosa-Laborde C, Barber BJ, et al. Short-term autoregulation of systemic blood flow and cardiac output. News Physiologic Sci. 1989;4:219–225.

84. Behbehani MM, Da Costa G. Properties of a projection pathway from the medial preoptic nucleus to the midbrain periaqueductal gray of the rat and its role in the regulation of cardiovascular function. Brain Res. 1996;740:141–150.

85. Hirasawa M, Nishihara M, Takahashi M. The rostral ventrolateral medulla mediates suppression of the circulatory system by the ventromedial nucleus of the hypothalamus. Brain Res. 1996;724:186–190.

86. Hosoya Y, Sugiura Y, Okado N, et al. Descending input from the hypothalamic paraventricular nucleus to sympathetic preganglionic neurons in the rat. Exp Brain Res. 1991;85:10–20.

87. Kanouse K, Yanase-Fujiwara M, Hosono T. Hypothalamic network for thermoregulatory vasomotor control. Am J Physiol. 1994;267:R283–R288.

88. Frysinger RC, Marks JD, Trelease RB, et al. Sleep states attenuate the pressor response to central amygdala stimulation. Exp Neurol. 1984;83:604–617.

89. Parmeggiani PL. Integrative aspects of hypothalamic influences on respiratory brainstem mechanisms during wakefulness and sleep. In: Von Euler C, Lagerkrantz H, eds. Central Nervous

Control Mechanisms in Breathing. Oxford, England: Pergamon Press; 1979:53–68.

90. Phillipson EA, Bowes G. Control of breathing during sleep. In: Cherniack NS, Widdicombbe JG, eds. Handbook of Physiology, Section III. The Respiratory System. Bethesda, Md: American Physiological Society; 1986:642–689.

91. Fink BR. Influence of cerebral activity in wakefulness on regulation of breathing. J Appl Physiol. 1961;16:15–20.

92. Lydic R, Orem J. Respiratory neurons of the pneumotaxic center during sleep and wakefulness. Neurosci Lett. 1979;15:187–192.

93. Mitchell RA, Berger AJ. Neural regulation of respiration. Am Rev Respir Dis. 1975;111:206–224.

94. Netick A, Foutz AS. Respiratory activity and sleep-wakefulness in the deafferented, paralyzed cat. Sleep. 1980;3:1–12.

95. Orem J. Neuronal mechanisms of respiration in REM sleep. Sleep. 1980;3:251–267.

96. Orem J, Montplaisir J, Dement WC. Changes in the activity of respiratory neurons during sleep. Brain Res. 1974;82:309–315.

97. Orem J, Netick A, Dement WC. Breathing during sleep and wakefulness in the cat. Respir Physiol. 1977;30:265–289.

98. Phillipson EA. Regulation of breathing during sleep. Am Rev Respir Dis. 1977;115(suppl):217–224.

99. Phillipson EA, Murphy E, Kozar LF. Regulation of respiration in sleeping dogs. J Appl Physiol. 1976;40:688–693.

100. Duron B. La fonction respiratoire pendant le sommeil physiologique. Bull Physiopathol Respir (Nancy). 1972;8:1031–1057.

101. Gillam PMS. Patterns of respiration in human beings at rest and during sleep. Bull Physiopathol Respir (Nancy). 1972;8:1059–1070.

102. Reite M, Jackson D, Cahoon RL, et al. Sleep physiology at high altitude. Electroencephalogr Clin Neurophysiol. 1975;38:463–471.

103. Specht H, Fruhmann G. Incidence of periodic breathing in 2000 subjects without pulmonary or neurological disease. Bull Physiopathol Respir (Nancy). 1972;8:1075.

104. Trinder J, Whitworth F, Kay A, et al. Respiratory instability during sleep onset. J Appl Physiol. 1992;73:2462–2469.

105. Webb P. Periodic breathing during sleep. J Appl Physiol. 1974;37:899–903.

106. Bülow K. Respiration and wakefulness in man. Acta Physiol Scand 1963;59(suppl 209):1–110.

107. Lugaresi E, Coccagna G, Mantovani M, et al. Some periodic phenomena arising during drowsiness and sleep in man. Electroencephalogr Clin Neurophysiol. 1972;32:701–705.

108. Birchfield RI, Sieker HO, Heyman A. Alterations in respiratory function during natural sleep. J Lab Clin Med. 1959;54:216–222.

109. Bülow K, Ingvar DH. Respiration and state of wakefulness in normals, studied by spirography, capnography and EEG. Acta Physiol Scand. 1961;51:230–238.

110. Wurtz RH, O'Flaerty JJ. Physiological correlates of steady potential shifts during sleep and wakefulness, 1: sensitivity of the steady potential to alterations in carbon dioxide. Electroencephalogr Clin Neurophysiol. 1967;22:30–42.

111. Birchfield RI, Sieker HO, Heyman A. Alterations in blood gases during natural sleep and narcolepsy. Neurology. 1958;8:107–112.

112. Guazzi M, Freis ED. Sinoaortic reflexes and arterial pH, P_{O_2} and P_{CO_2} in wakefulness and sleep. Am J Physiol. 1969;217:1623–1627.

113. Robin ED, Whaley RD, Crump GH, et al. Alveolar gas tension, pulmonary ventilation and blood pH during physiological sleep in normal subjects. J Clin Invest. 1958;37:981–989.

114. Orem J, Netick A, Dement WC. Increased upper airway resistance to breathing during sleep in the cat. Electroencephalogr Clin Neurophysiol. 1977;43:14–22.

115. Bellville JW, Howland WS, Seed JC, et al. The effect of sleep on the respiratory response to carbon dioxide. Anesthesiology. 1959;20:628–634.

116. Reed DJ, Kellogg RH. Changes in respiratory response to CO_2 during natural sleep at sea level and at altitude. J Appl Physiol. 1958;13:325–330.

117. Reed DJ, Kellogg RH. Effect of sleep on hypoxic stimulation of breathing at sea level and altitude. J Appl Physiol. 1960;15:1130–1134.

118. Phillipson EA, Sullivan CE, Read DJC, et al. Ventilatory and waking responses to hypoxia in sleeping dogs. J Appl Physiol. 1978;44:512–520.

119. Finer NN, Abroms IF, Taeusch HW Jr. Ventilation and sleep state in the new born infants. J Pediatr. 1976;89:100–108.

120. Farber JP, Marlow TA. Pulmonary reflexes and breathing pattern during sleep in the opossum. Respir Physiol. 1976;27:73–86.

121. Phillipson EA, Kozar LF, Murphy E. Respiratory load compensation in awake and sleeping dogs. J Appl Physiol. 1976;40:895–902.

122. Aserinsky E. Periodic respiratory pattern occurring in conjunction with eye movements during sleep. Science. 1965;150:763–766.

123. Orem J. Respiratory neurons and sleep. In: Kryger MH, Roth T, Dement WC, eds. Principles and Practice of Sleep Medicine. 2nd ed. Philadelphia, Pa: WB Saunders; 1994:177–193.

124. Phillipson EA. Respiratory adaptations in sleep. Annu Rev Physiol. 1978;40:133–156.

125. Parmeggiani PL. Regulation of the activity of respiratory muscles during sleep. In: Fitzgerald RS, Gautier H, Lahiri S, eds. Advances in Experimental Medicine and Biology. New York, NY: Plenum Press; 1978:47–57.

126. Henderson-Smart DJ, Read DJC. Depression of intercostal and abdominal muscle activity and vulnerability to asphyxia during active sleep in the newborn. In: Guilleminault C, Dement WC, eds. Sleep Apnea Syndromes. Kroc Foundation Series. New York, NY: Alan R Liss; 1978:93–117.

127. Islas-Marroquin J. L'activité des muscles respiratoires pendant les différentes phases du sommeil physiologiques chez le chat. Arch Sci Physiol. 1966;20:219–231.

128. Duron B. Activité électrique spontanée des muscles intercostaux et de diaphragme chez l'animal chronique. J Physiol Paris. 1969;61(suppl 2):282–283.

129. Tusiewicz K, Moldofsky H, Bryan AC. Mechanics of the rib cage and diaphragm during sleep. J Appl Physiol. 1977;43:600–602.

130. Bolton DPG, Herman S. Ventilation and sleep state in the newborn. J Physiol (Lond). 1974;240:67–77.

131. Fagenholz SA, O'Connell K, Shannon DC. Chemoreceptor function and sleep state in apnea. Pediatrics. 1976;58:31–36.

132. Hathorn MKS. The rate and depth of breathing in new-born infants in different sleep states. J Physiol (Lond). 1974;243:101–113.

133. Purcell M. Response in the newborn to raised upper airway resistance. Arch Dis Child. 1976;51:602–607.

134. Phillipson EA, Kozar LF, Rebuck AS, et al. Ventilatory and waking responses to CO_2 in sleeping dogs. Am Rev Respir Dis. 1977;115:251–259.

135. Remmers JE, Bartlett D Jr, Putnam MD. Changes in the respiratory cycle associated with sleep. Respir Physiol. 1976;28:227–238.

136. Dawes GS, Fox HE, Leduc BM, et al. Respiratory movements and rapid eye movement sleep in the foetal lamb. J Physiol (Lond). 1972;220:119–143.

137. Puizillout JJ, Ternaux JP, Foutz AS, et al. Les stades de sommeil chez la préparation "encéphale isolé," 1: déclenchement des pointes ponto-géniculo-occipitales et du sommeil phasique à ondes lentes. Role des noyaux du raphé. Electroencephalogr Clin Neurophysiol. 1974;37:561–576.

138. Thach BT, Abroms IF, Frantz ID, et al. REM sleep breathing pattern without intercostal muscle influence. Fed Proc. 1977;36:445.

139. Henke KG, Dempsey JA, Badr MS, et al. Effect of sleep-induced increases in upper airway resistance on respiratory muscle activity. J Appl Physiol. 1991;70:158–168.

140. Wiegand L, Zwillich CW, Wiegand D, et al. Changes in upper airway muscle activation and ventilation during phasic REM sleep in normal men. J Appl Physiol. 1991;71:488–497.

141. Frantz ID, Adler SM, Abroms IF, et al. Respiratory responses to airway occlusion in infants: sleep state and maturation. J Appl Physiol. 1976;41:634–638.

142. Henke KG, Badr MS, Skatrud JB, et al. Load compensation and respiratory muscle function during sleep. J Appl Physiol. 1992;72:1221–1234.

143. Knill R, Andrews W, Bryan AC, et al. Respiratory load compensation in infants. J Appl Physiol. 1976;40:357–361.

144. Bryan HM, Hagan R, Gulston G, et al. CO_2 response and sleep state in infants. Clin Res. 1976;24:A689.

145. Parmeggiani PL, Calasso M, Cianci T. Respiratory effects of preoptic-anterior hypothalamic electrical stimulation during sleep in cats. Sleep. 1981;4:71–82.

146. Marks JD, Frysinger RC, Harper RM. State-dependent respiratory depression elicited by stimulation of the orbital frontal cortex. Exp Neurol. 1987;95:714–729.

147. Futuro-Neto HA, Coote JH. Changes in sympathetic activity to heart and blood vessels during desynchronized sleep. Brain Res. 1982;252:259–268.

148. Parmeggiani PL, Franzini C. On the functional significance of subcortical single unit activity during sleep. Electroencephalogr Clin Neurophysiol. 1973;34:495–508.

149. Spyer KM. Central nervous mechanisms contributing to cardiovascular control. J Physiol (Lond). 1994;474:1–19.

150. Parmeggiani PL. Interaction between sleep and thermoregulation: an aspect of the control of behavioral states. Sleep. 1987;10:426–435.

151. Dworkin BR. Learning and Physiological Regulation. Chicago, Ill: University of Chicago Press; 1993.

152. Parmeggiani PL. Regulation of physiological functions during sleep in mammals. Experientia (Basel). 1982;38:1405–1408.

153. Hobson JA. Homeostasis and heteroplasticity: functional significance of behavioral state sequences. In: Lydic R, Biebuyck JF, eds. Clinical physiology of sleep. Bethesda, Md: American Physiological Society; 1988:199–220.

154. Siegel JM, Rogawski MA. A function of REM sleep: regulation of nonadrenergic receptor sensitivity. Brain Res Rev. 1988;13:213–233.

155. Shapiro CMT. Health risks associated with autonomic nervous system malfunction. In: Peter JH, Penzel T, Podszus T, et al (eds). Sleep and Health Risk. Berlin, Germany: Springer-Verlag; 1991:124–136.

156. Parmeggiani PL. Physiological risks during sleep. In: Peter JH, Penzel T, Podszus T, et al, eds. Sleep and Health Risk. Berlin, Germany: Springer-Verlag; 1991:119–123.

157. Dickerson LW, Huang AH, Nearing BD, et al. Primary coronary vasodilation associated with pauses in heart rhythm during sleep. Am J Physiol. 1993;264:R186–R196.

13

Cardiovascular Physiology: Central and Autonomic Regulation

Richard L. Verrier

Ronald M. Harper

J. Allan Hobson

During a typical night's sleep, a broad spectrum of autonomic patterns unfolds that provides both respite and taxation of the cardiovascular system. The effects are consequences of carefully orchestrated changes in central nervous system physiology as the brain periodically reexcites itself during rapid eye movement (REM) sleep from the relative tranquility of nonrapid eye movement (NREM) sleep.

Because of the close neurohumoral coupling between the central structures and cardiorespiratory system, there is a dynamic fluctuation in critical variables including heart rhythm, arterial blood pressure, coronary artery blood flow, and ventilation. NREM sleep is associated with relative autonomic stability and functional coordination between respiration, pumping action of the heart, and maintenance of arterial blood pressure. During REM sleep, there are remarkable surges in cardiac-bound sympathetic and parasympathetic activity, resulting in significant surges and pauses in heart rhythm. These occur in association with alterations in pontogeniculo-occipital activity and theta rhythm. Whereas the perturbations in autonomic nervous system activity are well tolerated in normal individuals, those with heart disease may be at particular risk during REM sleep. The stress on the system has the potential for triggering life-threatening arrhythmias and myocardial infarction. During NREM sleep in the severely compromised heart, there is a potential for hypotension, which can in turn impair delivery to stenotic coronary vessels. In both states, the coexistence of coronary disease and apnea is associated with heightened risk, as the challenge of dual control of the respiratory and cardiovascular systems may be overwhelming.

Through the course of a typical night's sleep, a broad spectrum of autonomic patterns unfolds which provides both respite and taxation of the cardiovascular system. These effects are consequences of carefully orchestrated changes in central nervous system (CNS) physiology as the brain periodically re-excites itself

during rapid eye movement (REM) sleep from the relative tranquility of nonrapid eye movement (NREM) sleep. Affective states associated with dreaming can also contribute to the nocturnal tumult of autonomic nervous system activity. The main goal of this chapter is to provide insights into the central and peripheral nervous system mechanisms which regulate cardiovascular function during sleep. Particular attention is focused on the impact on cardiac electrical stability and coronary artery blood flow because these factors are critical in triggering life-threatening cardiac arrhythmias and myocardial infarction in individuals with heart disease (see Chapter 84). The annual toll of sleep-related cardiac events is an estimated 20% of myocardial infarctions (or 250,000) and 15% of sudden cardiac deaths (or 38,000) in the United States. Attention is also directed toward cardiovascular function in infants, particularly as perturbations in regulation of this system during the nocturnal period may be an important factor in the sudden infant death syndrome (SIDS).

PHYSIOLOGY OF SLEEP AND NEURAL CONTROL OF CARDIOVASCULAR FUNCTION

The brain's dynamic changes in state during sleep are coordinated by the pons, basal forebrain areas, and other subcortical structures. The main neurotransmitters involved are norepinephrine, serotonin, and acetylcholine.[1-5] It is interesting, and probably significant, that the neuronal populations that produce and distribute these three neuromodulators throughout the brain together constitute the central representation of the sympathetic and parasympathetic subdivisions of the autonomic nervous system. The two aminergic neuronal subgroups (in the locus coeruleus and raphe nuclei) are most active in waking but become progressively less active in NREM sleep and virtually cease

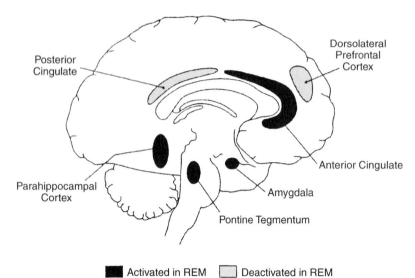

Posterior
Cingulate

Dorsolateral
Prefrontal
Cortex

Parahippocampal
Cortex

Anterior Cingulate

Amygdala

Pontine Tegmentum

■ Activated in REM   □ Deactivated in REM

Figure 13–1. Schematic sagittal view of the human brain showing those areas of relative regional brain activation and deactivation in REM sleep compared with waking and/or NREM sleep as reported in two or more of the three positron emission tomography studies published to date.[25-27] Only those areas which could readily be matched between two or more studies are illustrated here. Considerably more extensive areas of activation and deactivation are reported in the individual studies. The depicted areas are most realistically viewed as representative portions of larger central nervous system areas subserving similar functions (e.g., limbic-related cortex, ascending activation pathways, and multimodal association cortex). (From Hobson JA, Stickgold R, Pace-Schott EF. The neuropsychology of REM sleep dreaming. Neuroreport. 1998;9:R1–R14.)

firing in REM sleep, whereas the cholinergic neurons (in the dorsolateral tegumental and pedunculopontine nuclei) are active in both waking and REM sleep. The net effect is a highly differentiated brain chemistry across the three states (Fig. 13–1). In waking, both systems are active; in NREM sleep both systems are less active; and in REM sleep the cholinergic system acts alone. The functional consequences of this differentiation remain to be elucidated both centrally and in the periphery.[6] The electroencephalographic (EEG) patterns and changes in autonomic and somatic activity elicited by sleep are complex and subserve many functions, and it is clear that sleep is essential to cardiorespiratory homeostasis.

NREM sleep, the initial stage, is characterized by a period of relative autonomic stability, with vagus nerve dominance and heightened baroreceptor gain. During NREM sleep, a near sinusoidal modulation of heart rate variation occurs due to a coupling with respiratory activity and cardiorespiratory centers in the brain and results in what is termed *normal respiratory sinus arrhythmia*. During inspiration, heart rate accelerates

briefly to accommodate increased venous return, resulting in increased cardiac output, while during expiration a progressive slowing in rate ensues. This normal sinus variability in heart rate, particularly during NREM sleep, is generally indicative of cardiac health, whereas the absence of intrinsic variability has been associated with cardiac pathology and advancing age. For example, it has been shown that the loss of heart rate variability is associated with heightened risk for myocardial infarction and life-threatening arrhythmias.[7] Reduced heart rate variation at the respiratory frequency is also observed in infants who later succumb to SIDS (Fig. 13–2) and is also a characteristic of infants afflicted with congenital central hypoventilation syndrome, a condition in which the drive to breathe is lost during sleep.[8] The common denominator of cardiac risk associated with depressed heart rate variability appears to be loss of normal vagus nerve function.

The reflexive cardiovascular changes during breathing manifested as cyclical heart rate variation also have a converse relationship, as transient elevation of arterial blood pressure results in a slowing, cessation, or

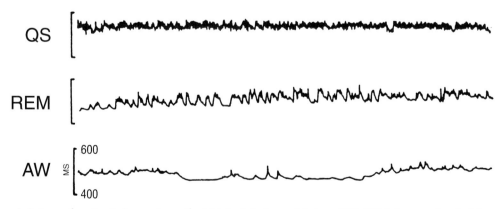

QS

REM

AW

600

MS

400

Figure 13–2. Intervals between heartbeats from a 4-month-old infant during quiet sleep (QS), REM sleep, and wakefulness (AW). The y-axis represents time (in milliseconds) between successive heartbeats. Note rapid modulation of intervals during quiet sleep contributed by respiratory variation. Note also lower frequency modulation during REM sleep and epochs of sustained rapid rate during wakefulness. (From Harper RM, Frysinger RC, Zhang J, et al. Cardiac and respiratory interactions maintaining homeostasis during sleep. In: Lydic R, Biebuyck JF, eds. Clinical Physiology of Sleep. Bethesda, Md: American Physiological Society; 1988.)

diminution of breathing efforts. This effect is enhanced during sleep,[9] when even small reductions in arterial blood pressure increase respiratory rates.[10, 11] These breathing pauses and increased rates apparently serve as compensatory mechanisms to normalize arterial blood pressure. Absence of these normal breathing pauses, and diminished breathing variation, as well as the reductions in respiratory-induced heart rate variation described above, are a characteristic of infants who later succumb to SIDS[12] and may hint at a failure of compensatory mechanisms underlying the syndrome. Obstructive sleep apnea in children is accompanied by exaggerated heart rate variation.[13]

Sympathetic nerve activity appears to be relatively stable during NREM sleep and its cardiovascular input is reduced by more than half from wakefulness to stage 4 of NREM sleep.[14] These findings in normal humans appear to be at variance with those of Baust and Bohnert,[15] who suggested that sympathetic nerve activity was not reduced during sleep in cats. This conclusion was highly inferential because direct nerve recordings were not performed and heart rate following vagotomy and stellectomy was used as the sole indicator of neural autonomic activity during sleep. These investigators, however, employed acute cervical vagotomy, which could have artificially increased sympathetic tone by denervating aortic baroreceptors and by causing physical discomfort. Cervical vagotomy also disrupts the pulmonary inflation reflex by interrupting a major afferent component of respiratory control.

In general, the autonomic stability of NREM sleep, with hypotension, bradycardia, and reductions in cardiac output and systemic vascular resistance, provide a relatively salutary neurohumoral background during which the heart has an opportunity for metabolic restoration.[16] The bradycardias appear to be due mainly to an increase in vagus nerve activity, whereas the hypotension is primarily attributable to a reduction in sympathetic vasomotor tone.[17] During transitions from NREM to REM sleep, bursts of vagus nerve activity may result in pauses in heart rhythm and frank asystole.[18]

At approximately 90-min intervals, REM sleep is initiated, due to increased activity in the brainstem reticular formation, resulting in a major shift in the modulatory chemistry of the brain. REM sleep, in subserving brain neurochemical functions and behavioral adaptations, can disrupt cardiorespiratory homeostasis.[19] The brain's increased excitability during REM sleep can result in major surges in cardiac sympathetic nerve activity to the coronary and skeletal muscular vessels accompanied by muscular twitching and in decreased blood flow to the renal and splanchnic beds. The CNS operates with reduced baroreceptor gain. Heart rate is strikingly variable, with marked episodes of tachycardia and bradycardia.[20, 21] The autonomic instability observed in the periphery is correlated in time with intense bursts of discharge by cholinoreceptive pontine neurones, and the central release of acetylcholine is markedly increased. Cardiac efferent vagus nerve tone is generally suppressed during REM sleep,[16] and breathing patterns are highly irregular and can

lead to oxygen reduction, particularly in patients with pulmonary or cardiac disease.[19] The neurons activating the principal diaphragmatic respiratory muscles normally escape the generalized inhibition,[22] although accessory and upper airway muscles diminish activity.[23] This loss of activity is especially marked in infant thoracic and abdominal muscles during REM sleep.[24] During sleep apnea, there may be cessation of central activity or peripheral obstruction several hundred times each night, with the potential for dire consequences for the cardiorespiratory system.

CARDIORESPIRATORY INTERACTIONS

Central Mechanisms

The integration of the cardiorespiratory systems during sleep is achieved at several levels in the neuraxis. Commonly overlooked is the role of structures above the brainstem. This oversight probably results from the assumption that because respiratory patterning is presumed to be automatic during sleep, there would be no functional adaptation to suprapontine structures. However, several suprapontine as well as pontine mechanisms have the capability of altering cardiorespiratory patterns during both sleep and wakefulness.

The importance of the pontine brainstem in REM sleep activation has recently been documented by positron emission tomography imaging studies of REM sleep dreaming, which document preferential activation of the limbic and paralimbic regions of the forebrain in REM sleep compared with waking or with NREM sleep.[25–27] Specifically, Maquet et al.[25] determined that both amygdalae and anterior cingulate cortex were activated along with the pontine tegmentum. The cortical areas activated in REM sleep are richly innervated by afferents from the amygdala. A number of structures within the limbic system have been implicated in mediating aspects of emotion, including the central nucleus of the amygdala and the anterior geniculate gyrus (Fig. 13–3). The orbital frontal cortex, portions of the hippocampal formation, and hypothalamic structures are frequently included among forebrain structures participating in affective behavior. The central nucleus of the amygdala is strategically positioned to regulate cardiac and respiratory functioning of affective behavior, because it projects extensively to the parabrachial pons and the nucleus of the solitary tract, the dorsal motor nucleus, and the periaqueductal gray region. Portions of the amygdala, hippocampal formation, and frontal and insular cortex all participate in mediating transient arterial blood pressure elevation elicited by cold pressor challenges or Valsalva maneuvers, as indicated by functional magnetic resonance.[28] Lateralization of the sympathetic and parasympathetic branches of the autonomic nervous system within the insular cortex has been demonstrated.[29] These findings are important for sleep studies, in light of the propensity for seizure discharge to be expressed preferentially

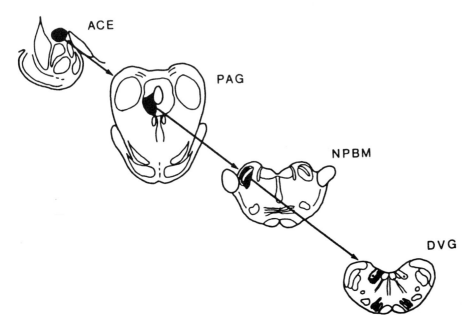

Figure 13–3. Schematic diagram of descending projections from central nucleus of amygdala (ACE) to periaqueductal gray (PAG)region, nucleus parabrachialis medialis (NPBM), and dorsal vagal group (DVG), which includes the dorsal motor nucleus of the vagus and the nucleus of the solitary tract. (From Harper RM, Frysinger RC, Zhang J, et al. Cardiac and respiratory interactions maintaining homeostasis during sleep. In: Lydic R, Biebuyck JF, eds. Clinical Physiology of Sleep. Bethesda, Md: American Physiological Society; 1988.)

during sleep states. Seizure discharge can exert profound influences on arterial blood pressure and heart rate,[30] and a unilateral seizure focus could trigger unique autonomic responses. The complexity of interconnections between cortical and subcortical structures carries significant import for cardiorespiratory control.

Cardiorespiratory Homeostasis

An important consideration in preserving circulatory homeostasis during sleep is coordinating control over two distinct types of systems: the respiratory, essential for oxygen exchange; and the cardiovascular, for blood transport. The difficult balancing act of regulating two motor systems, one which supplies somatic musculature (i.e., diaphragmatic, intercostal, abdominal, and upper airway musculature) and the other involving regulation of autonomic pathways (to the heart and vasculature), is a formidable task during sleep. This challenge is particularly daunting in individuals who have diseased respiratory or cardiovascular systems, particularly in the form of apnea or heart failure, or in infants, whose developing control systems may become compromised. Activity of the respiratory neurons to the somatic musculature varies greatly between sleep states, as does the regularity of heart rhythm. Because of the close coupling between the cardiorespiratory systems, dysfunction in one system can lead to significant failure in the other.

Important affective influences operate during sleep and exert a profound influence on cardiorespiratory patterns. Both negative and positive affective states particularly associated with visual imagery occur primarily during REM sleep. These states have the potential to generate tachycardia, polypnea, sweating, and dramatic elevations in arterial blood pressure secondary to intense autonomic activity. The intensity of the emotional states achieved during dreaming may be as

strong as or stronger than those experienced during wakefulness, and thus to the extent that behavioral stress is an acute risk factor for sudden cardiac death,[31] it is reasonable to hypothesize that dreaming may be capable of precipitating life-threatening arrhythmias.

An important issue for homeostasis is maintenance of perfusion of vital organs through appropriate arterial blood pressure control. As noted earlier, respiratory mechanisms are recruited to support cardiovascular action by assisting venous return and by reflexly altering cardiac rate. REM sleep induces a near paralysis of accessory respiratory muscles and "releases" descending forebrain influences on brainstem control regions.[32, 33] Those reorganizations of control during REM sleep have the potential to interfere substantially with compensatory breathing mechanisms that assist arterial blood pressure management and to remove protective forebrain influences on hypo- or hypertension.

The interactions between breathing and arterial blood pressure have important implications for treatment of hypertension in patients with obstructive sleep apnea. Treatments which resolve apnea, such as continuous positive airway pressure, have the potential to reduce arterial blood pressure immediately. If therapy for hypertension includes antihypertensive agents, the combination of treatments may induce serious hypotension.

The control of arterial blood pressure during sleep is of particular interest to those examining potential mechanisms of failure in SIDS. Several reports indicate that the final sequence in SIDS may be the result of failure in cardiac rhythm.[34] Specifically, bradycardia and hypotension, rather than an initial breathing cessation, characterize the final event.[35, 36] There may be antecedent tachycardia for up to 3 d. The terminal events in SIDS are similar to the two stages of shock, namely, an initial sympathoexcitation followed by a sudden, centrally triggered sympathoinhibition and bradycardia, leading to a life-threatening fall in arterial blood pressure. Some monitored SIDS cases show a near total loss of arterial blood pressure within a minute of onset of the fatal event. Apparently, the inadequate compensatory mechanisms displayed prior to the fatal event by infants at risk for SIDS fail to provide sufficient support. Because SIDS bears a temporal relationship to sleep,[37] some interaction of state and compensatory mechanisms is suspected.

The prone sleeping position contributes to an enhanced risk for SIDS and possibly derives from vestibular and cerebellar contributions to arterial blood pressure control.[38] Vestibular mechanisms assist mediation of arterial blood pressure to rapid postural changes, and static stimuli, such as stimuli from the prone versus supine position, directly modify heart rate. Lesions of the cerebellar fastigial nucleus result in ineffective compensatory responses to hypotension.[39] Sleep effects on vestibular systems must be considered in examination of arterial blood pressure control mechanisms.

SLEEP STATE–DEPENDENT CHANGES IN HEART RHYTHM

Recent evidence supports the conclusion that the pronounced changes in heart rate occurring during REM sleep and transitions between sleep states are attributable to distinct mechanisms associated with specific brain sites, rather than representing a continuum of autonomic change.

Heart Rate Surges

Several investigators have reported REM-induced increases in heart rate in experimental animals.[15, 17, 20, 40-44] The first heart rate response to be fully characterized involved an abrupt, though transitory, 35 to 37% increase in rate which is concentrated during phasic REM, is followed by a baroreceptor-mediated deceleration, and is abolished by interruption of sympathetic neural input to the heart[41-43] (Fig. 13–4). The phenomenon, observed in canines, differs from that observed by Baust and Bohnert[15] in felines in that the heart rate increase observed is more marked and is not dependent on withdrawal of parasympathetic nerve activity. An increased frequency of heart rate surges was observed during periods of REM sleep marked by phasic eye movements.[15, 20, 43]

A second, distinct REM sleep state–dependent heart rate surge attributable to the primary involvement of CNS activation is attended by a concomitant, conspicuous increase in hippocampal theta frequency, ponto-geniculo-occipital (PGO) activity, and eye movements.[44]

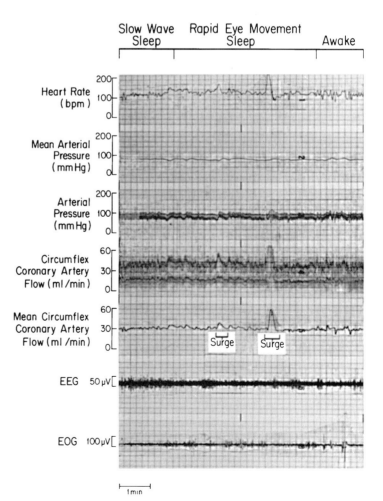

Figure 13–4. Effects of NREM sleep, REM sleep, and quiet wakefulness on heart rate, phasic and mean arterial blood pressure, phasic and mean left circumflex coronary flow, electroencephalogram (EEG), and electro-oculogram (EOG) in the dog. Sleep spindles are evident during NREM sleep, eye movements during REM sleep, and grosser eye movements on awakening. Surges in heart rate and coronary flow occur during REM sleep. (From Kirby DA, Verrier RL. Differential effects of sleep stage on coronary hemodynamic function. Am J Physiol. 1989;256:H1378–1383.)

This increase in theta frequency was observed in cats, the species in which the appearance of theta waves is characteristic of arousal, orienting activity, alertness, and REM sleep, when they are strongly associated with PGO activity and eye movements.[44–48] Observations of PGO activity during sleep associated with heart rate phenomena of any type have been documented only infrequently. Baust and colleagues[40] found only a relatively minor, baseline rate-dependent, variable response in heart rate to PGO activity in cats during REM sleep. Alterations in centrally induced autonomic activity constitute the most likely basis for the abrupt accelerations in heart rate during REM sleep. Plausible peripheral mechanisms include an increase in sympathetic nerve activity or a diminution of vagus nerve tone, either alone or in combination. Our finding that cardioselective beta-adrenergic blockade with atenolol markedly reduced the phenomenon suggests that the REM sleep–induced surges are primarily mediated by bursting of cardiac sympathetic efferent fiber activity, which directly affects heart rate.

Heart Rhythm Pauses

A complementary finding to centrally mediated heart rate surges is the observation in cats of a primary, abrupt deceleration in heart rhythm which occurs predominantly during tonic REM sleep and is not associated with any preceding or subsequent change in heart rate or arterial blood pressure[49] (Fig. 13–5). The involvement of the vagus nerve appears to be directly initiated by central influences, as there is no antecedent or subsequent change in resting heart rate or arterial blood pressure. The primary involvement of CNS activation is demonstrated by the consistent, antecedent abrupt cessation of PGO activity and concomitant interruption of hippocampal theta rhythm. In normal human volunteers, Taylor and colleagues[50] observed heart rate decelerations during REM sleep which preceded eye movement bursts by 3 sec and suggested that the phenomenon reflects an orienting response at the onset of dreaming. How these changes in CNS activity lead to the tonic REM sleep–induced increase in vagus nerve tone to suppress sinus node activity remains unknown. Notwithstanding extensive studies of the physiological and anatomical basis for PGO activity, little is known about the conductivity and functional relationship to heart rhythm control during sleep.

The most likely basis for the abrupt deceleration in heart rate during tonic REM sleep is a change in the centrally induced pattern of autonomic activity to the heart. This could be the result of a decrease in sympathetic nerve activity, or an enhancement of vagus nerve tone, either alone or in combination. We found that cardioselective beta$_1$-adrenergic blockade with atenolol did not affect the incidence or magnitude of decelerations, but muscarinic blockade with glycopyrrolate completely abolished the phenomenon. These observations suggest that the tonic REM sleep–induced decelerations are primarily mediated by bursting of cardiac vagus nerve efferent fiber activity. It is well-known that enhanced vagal activity can abruptly and markedly affect the sinus node firing rate.[51] Because beta-adrenergic blockade exerted no effect on the frequency or magnitude of decelerations, it does not appear that withdrawal of cardiac sympathetic tone is an important factor in the observed rate changes. Respiratory interplay is not an essential component of the deceleration, as the phenomenon often occurred in the absence of a temporal association with inspiratory effort.

This primary pause phenomenon appears to be distinct from the baroreceptor-mediated reductions in heart rate, in which heart rhythm pauses almost invariably followed accelerations in rate and elevation in

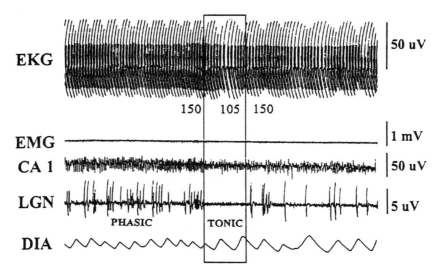

Figure 13–5. Representative polygraphic recording of a primary heart rate deceleration during tonic REM sleep. During this deceleration, heart rate decreased from 150 to 105 bpm, or 30%. The deceleration occurred during a period devoid of ponto-geniculo-occipital (PGO) spikes in the lateral geniculate nucleus (LGN) or theta rhythm in the hippocampal (CA 1) leads. The deceleration is not a respiratory arrhythmia, as it is independent of diaphragmatic (DIA) movement. The abrupt decreases in amplitude of hippocampal theta (CA 1), PGO waves (LGN), and respiratory amplitude and rate (DIA) are typical of transitions from phasic to tonic REM. EKG, electrocardiogram, EMG, electromyogram. (From Verrier RL, Lau RT, Wallooppillai U, et al. Primary vagally mediated decelerations in heart rate during tonic rapid eye movement sleep in cats. Am J Physiol. 1998;43:R1136–1141.)

POST-ASYSTOLE CBF SURGE
DURING INTERRUPTION OF SWS
BY EEG DESYNCHRONIZATION

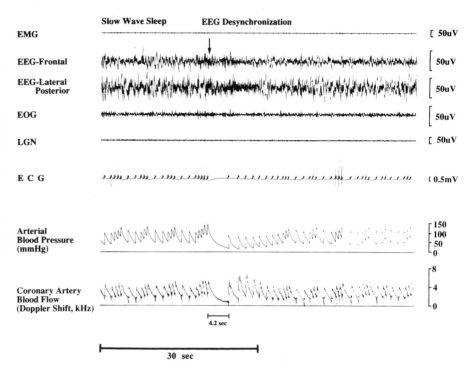

Figure 13–6. Coronary blood flow (CBF) surge during deep NREM sleep interrupted by electroencephalographic (EEG) desynchronization. This response pattern is common and appears to represent a brief, low-grade arousal. The 4.2-sec pause in heart rhythm was followed by a brief increase of 46% in average peak CBF and a decrease of 49% in the heart rate–systolic blood pressure product. ECG, electrocardiogram; EEG, electroencephalogram; EMG, electromyogram; EOG, electro-oculogram; LGN, lateral geniculate nucleus field potential recordings. (From Dickerson LW, Huang AH, Nearing BD, et al. Primary coronary vasodilation associated with pauses in heart rhythm during sleep. Am J Physiol. 1993; 264:R186–196.)

arterial blood pressure[18] (Fig. 13–6). This second group of heart rhythm pauses was observed in canines and occurs mainly during the transition from slow-wave sleep to desynchronized sleep and more frequently during phasic REM than tonic REM sleep. They persist from 1 to 8 sec and are followed by dramatic increases in coronary blood flow averaging 30% and ranging up to 84%, which are independent of metabolic activity of the heart as reflected in heart rate–blood pressure product. An intense burst of vagus nerve activity appears to produce the phenomenon because the pauses developed against a background of marked respiratory sinus arrhythmia, varying degrees of heart block with non-conducted P waves, and low heart rate, and could be emulated by electrical stimulation of the vagus nerve. The REM sleep–related decelerations reported by Baust and Bohnert in their classic study[15] were also heralded by rate accelerations and were therefore likely to have been part of a reflex response. Guilleminault and colleagues[52] documented similar pauses in young adults.

CORONARY BLOOD FLOW
REGULATION DURING SLEEP

Striking changes in coronary blood flow occur during REM and sleep-state transitions.[18, 41–43, 53] Vatner and co-workers[53] used baboons to study the effects of the sleep-wake cycle on coronary function. During the nocturnal period, when the animals were judged to be asleep by behavioral indicators, coronary artery blood flow fluctuated by as much as twofold. The periodic oscillations in blood flow were not associated with alterations in heart rate or arterial blood pressure and occurred while the animals remained motionless with eyes closed. Since the baboons were not instrumented for EEG recordings, no information was obtained regarding sleep stage, nor was the mechanism for the coronary blood flow surge defined.

Concomitant with heart rate, surges of REM sleep observed in canines[41–43] described above were remarkable, episodic surges in coronary blood flow with corresponding decreases in coronary vascular resistance. These phenomena occurred predominantly during periods of REM sleep marked by intense phasic activity, as defined by the frequency of eye movements.[43] There were no significant changes in mean arterial blood pressure. Heart rate was elevated during the flow surges, suggesting an increase in cardiac metabolic activity as the basis for the coronary vasodilation. In fact, the close coupling between rate-pressure product, an index of metabolic demand, and the magnitude of the flow surges indicates that the surges do not constitute a state of myocardial hyperperfusion. These surges in coronary blood flow appeared to be due to enhanced adrenergic discharge, because they were abolished by bilateral stellectomy, and not to nonspecific effects of somatic activity or respiratory fluctuations.

During severe coronary artery stenosis, with baseline flow reduced by 60%, phasic decreases in coronary arterial blood flow, rather than increases, were observed during REM sleep coincident with these heart rate surges[42] (Fig. 13–7). The increase in adrenergic discharge could lead to a coronary blood flow decrement by at least two possible mechanisms. The first is by the stimulation of alpha-adrenergic receptors on

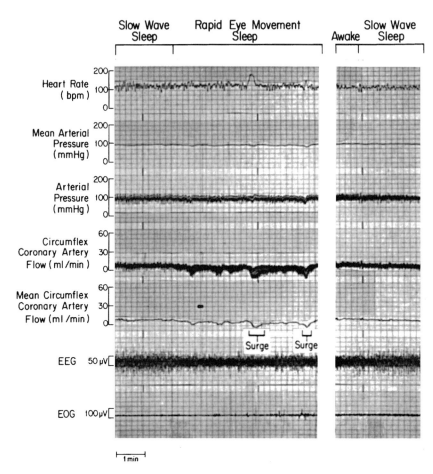

Figure 13–7. Effects of sleep stage on heart rate, mean and phasic arterial blood pressures, and mean and phasic left circumflex coronary artery blood flow in a typical dog during stenosis. Note phasic decreases in coronary flow occurring during heart rate surges while the dog is in REM sleep. EEG, electroencephalogram; EOG, electro-oculogram. (Reprinted from Physiology and Behavior, Volume 45, Kirby DA, Verrier RL, Differential effects of sleep stage on coronary hemodynamic function during stenosis, 1017–1020, Copyright 1989, with permission from Elsevier Science.)

the coronary vascular smooth muscle. Such an effect, however, could be only transitory, as alpha-adrenergic stimulation results in brief (10 to 15 sec) coronary constriction, even during sympathetic nerve stimulation in anesthetized animals[54] or during intense arousal associated with aversive behavioral conditioning.[55] The second possibility of REM-induced reduction in coronary flow during stenosis is mechanical, namely a decrease in diastolic coronary perfusion time due to the surges in heart rate. In support of this explanation, we found a strong correlation ($r^2 = .96$) between the magnitude of the increase in heart rate and the decrease in coronary blood flow.[42] The link between REM-induced changes in heart rate and the occurrence of myocardial ischemia in patients with advanced coronary artery disease is consistent with the clinical experience of Nowlin and co-workers.[56]

IMPACT OF SLEEP ON ARRHYTHMOGENESIS DURING MYOCARDIAL ISCHEMIA AND INFARCTION

Central Nervous System Sites Influencing Cardiac Electrical Stability

Because sleep ultimately exerts its influence on cardiac vulnerability through alterations in activity of the central and peripheral autonomic nervous systems, it is worthwhile to summarize the state of our knowledge with respect to neural control of cardiac electrophysiological and coronary hemodynamic function. Two major concepts have surfaced from extensive investigation of CNS-induced cardiac arrhythmias. The first is that triggering of arrhythmias by the CNS is not only the consequence of intense activation of the autonomic nervous system but is also a function of the specific neural pattern elicited. Thus, the balance in cardiac input from either limb of the autonomic nervous system and their interaction must be considered.

The second pivotal concept is that triggering of arrhythmias by CNS activity may also depend on several intermediary mechanisms. These include direct effects of neurotransmitters on the myocardium and its specialized conducting system and changes in myocardial perfusion due to alterations in coronary vasomotor tone, enhanced platelet aggregability, or both. The net influence on the heart thus depends upon a complex interplay between the specific neural pattern elicited and the underlying cardiac pathology.

Over 80 years ago Levy[57] demonstrated that ventricular tachyarrhythmias can be elicited in normal animals by stimulating specific areas in the brain. This finding was subsequently confirmed in several species. Hockman and colleagues,[58] using stereotactic techniques, demonstrated that cerebral stimulation and hypothalamic activation evoked a spectrum of ventricular arrhythmias. The posterior hypothalamus is an important locus of centrally induced arrhythmias. Stimulation of this structure increased tenfold the incidence of ventricular fibrillation elicited experimentally by occlusion of the coronary artery.[59] This enhanced vulnerability was linked to increased sympathetic nerve activity, because beta-adrenergic receptor blockade, but not vagotomy, prevented it. These findings are consistent with clinical reports that cerebrovascular disease, and particularly intracranial hemorrhage, can elicit significant cardiac repolarization abnormalities and life-threatening arrhythmias.[60, 61] Cryogenic blockade of the thalamic gating mechanism or its output from the frontal cortex to the brainstem[62] and of the amygdala[63] delayed or prevented the occurrence of ventricular fibrillation during stress in pigs. Thus, these distinct pathways within the CNS appear to play a critical role in mediating arrhythmogenesis due to intense behavioral arousal.

Arrhythmias also ensue immediately upon cessation of diencephalic or hypothalamic stimulation, but these required intact vagi and stellate ganglia.[64, 65] The likely electrophysiological basis for such post-CNS stimulation arrhythmias is the loss of rate-overdrive suppression of ectopic activity. This phenomenon occurs when the vagus nerve regains its activity following cessation of centrally induced adrenergic stimulation. Accordingly, the enhanced automaticity induced by adrenergic stimulation of ventricular pacemakers is exposed when vagus nerve tone is restored and slows the sinus rate.[65] Although these arrhythmias may be dramatic in appearance, as they include ventricular tachycardias, they rarely degenerate into ventricular fibrillation.[66] Their occurrence, however, is the basis for the widely held view that dual autonomic activation is highly conducive to arrhythmias, but this proarrhythmic effect has been erroneously interpreted as profibrillatory.

The protective influence of beta-adrenergic receptor blockade against cardiac arrhythmias may result in part from blockade of central beta-adrenergic receptors. Parker and co-workers[67] have shown that intracerebroventricular administration of subsystemic doses of *l*-propranolol but not *d*-propranolol significantly reduced the incidence of ventricular fibrillation during combined left anterior descending coronary artery occlusion and behavioral stress in the pig. Surprisingly, intravenous administration of even a relatively high dose of *l*-propranolol was ineffectual. The latter result may relate in part to a species dependence because, unlike canines, pigs do not show a suppression of ischemia-induced arrhythmias in response to beta blockade.[68] It was proposed that the centrally mediated protective effect of beta blockade is due to a decrease in sympathetic nerve activity and in plasma norepinephrine concentration.[67, 69, 70] Importantly, whereas central actions of beta-adrenergic receptor blockers may play an important role in reducing susceptibility to ventricular fibrillation during acute myocardial ischemia, they are unlikely to constitute the sole mechanisms. This conclusion derives from the finding that beta blockers prevent the profibrillatory effect of direct stimulation of peripheral sympathetic structures such as the stellate ganglia.[71] It is noteworthy that the three beta blockers that have long-term effects on mortality, namely, propranolol, timolol, and metoprolol, are all lipophilic,[72] whereas the long-term effects of beta blockers that are less lipophilic have not been as extensively studied. Thus, it remains to be established whether the protective effect reflects a fundamental pharmacological difference or is related to study design. Finally, it is quite possible that, in the long term, the differences in efficacy of agents based on lipophilicity are offset by diffusion of the agent across the blood-brain barrier. These considerations are also important as beta blockers are widely employed in cardiac patients, and it is essential to understand their action as they affect both sleep structure and cardiac electrophysiological function. There is evidence to suggest that beta blockers that cross the blood-brain barrier have the potential for significant perturbations of sleep continuity.[73]

Autonomic Factors in Arrhythmogenesis During Sleep

The concept that NREM sleep is generally salutary with respect to ventricular arrhythmogenesis is consistent with extensive studies of neurocardiac interactions and clinical experience. This concept, in part, relates to the profound activation of the vagus nerve which occurs during the NREM state, and which reduces heart rate, increases cardiac electrical stability, and reduces rate-pressure product, an indicator of cardiac metabolic activity. The last consideration is important as it can lead to an improved supply-demand relationship in stenotic coronary artery segments. However, hypotension in the setting of severe coronary disease or acute myocardial infarction can lead to myocardial ischemia because of inadequate coronary perfusion pressure,[73a] and this set of circumstances, in turn, can provoke arrhythmias and myocardial infarction.[16, 74, 75, 75a, 75b] (See Chapter 84.) The abrupt increases in vagus nerve tone that can occur during periods of REM or sleep-state transitions can result in significant pauses in heart rhythm, bradyarrhythmias, and, potentially, triggered activity, a mechanism of the lethal cardiac arrhythmia torsades de pointes. Patients with the long Q–T syndrome who have the type 3 phenotype are more prone to experience torsades de pointes at night rather than during stress or exercise, as the classic picture. Tonic control of the vagus nerves over the caliber of the epicardial coronary vessels[76] could be an important factor in dynamic regulation of coronary resistance as a function of the sleep-wake cycle. An important question is whether tonic vagus nerve activity exerts a protective or a deleterious influence on myocardial perfusion and arrhythmogenesis in individuals with atherosclerotic disease. Nocturnal surges in vagus nerve activity could precipitate myocardial ischemia and arrhythmias as a result of coronary vasoconstriction rather than dilation in atherosclerotic segments because of impaired release of endothelium-derived relaxing factor.[77]

REM sleep, because of the attendant surges in autonomic activity and in heart rate, has the potential for triggering ventricular arrhythmias.[78, 78a] The striking variability of heart rate and breathing pattern can have a significant impact on cardiovascular functioning, as is evident in the development of ischemia and arrhythmias in patients whose myocardium is compromised (see Chapter 84). Indeed, the only clinical studies in which sleep staging has been employed have identified REM as the state in which arrhythmias occurred.[16, 79–81] The increase in sympathetic nerve activity that occurs at the onset of REM sleep[14] provides a potent stimulus for ventricular tachyarrhythmias because of the arrhythmogenic influence of neurally released catecholamines. Sympathetic nerve activation by stimulation of central[57–59, 64, 65] or peripheral adrenergic structures,[71, 82] infusion of catecholamines,[83] or imposition of behavioral stress[31] can increase cardiac vulnerability in the normal and ischemic heart.[78] These profibrillatory influences are substantially blunted by beta-adrenergic receptor blockade.[84] A wide variety of supraventricular arrhythmias can also be induced by autonomic activation.[66]

A striking surge in sympathetic nerve activity occurs within minutes of left anterior descending coronary artery occlusion.[85] The enhancement in sympathetic activity is associated with a marked increase in susceptibility to ventricular fibrillation, as evidenced by the spontaneous occurrence of the arrhythmia,[86] a reduction in ventricular fibrillation threshold,[85] and increased T-wave alternans magnitude, a new marker of vulnerability to cardiac arrhythmias.[86–88] Upon reperfusion, a second peak in vulnerability occurs, probably due to liberation of ischemic byproducts from the myocardium.[85, 87, 89] Stellectomy obtunds the surge in vulnerability to ventricular fibrillation during occlusion but enhances its magnitude during reperfusion. These observations are in agreement with the findings that adrenergic factors are pivotal during ischemia and that stellectomy enhances reactive hyperemia during reperfusion.[85] The net effect is a greater release of profibrillatory ischemic byproducts.

Enhanced sympathetic nerve activity increases cardiac vulnerability in the normal and ischemic heart by complex mechanisms. The major indirect effects include an impaired oxygen supply-demand ratio due to increased cardiac metabolic activity and coronary vasoconstriction, particularly in vessels with injured endothelium and in the context of altered preload and afterload.[90] The direct profibrillatory effects on cardiac electrophysiological function are attributable to derangements in impulse formation, conduction, or both.[66] Increased levels of catecholamines activate beta-adrenergic receptors which in turn alter adenylate cyclase activity and intracellular calcium flux. These actions are probably mediated by the cyclic nucleotide and protein kinase regulatory cascade, which can alter spatial heterogeneity of calcium transients and consequently increase dispersion of repolarization. The net influence is an increase in susceptibility to ventricular fibrillation.[55, 91] Conversely, reduction of cardiac sympathetic drive by stellectomy has proved to be antifibrillatory.

Notwithstanding the evidence that presumptive autonomic factors have the potential for significantly altering susceptibility to arrhythmias, the observation that the heart rate surges of REM sleep conduce to myocardial ischemia, and the epidemiological data in humans on the extent of sleep-induced cardiac events,[92] there is a paucity of information regarding the effects of myocardial infarction on sleep state. Ventricular ectopic activity but not ventricular fibrillation has been documented during NREM sleep in pigs following myocardial infarction.[93] This pattern may be attributable to slowing of heart rate and increased vagus nerve activity during NREM sleep, conditions which can inhibit the normal overdrive suppression of ventricular rhythms by sinoatrial node pacemaker activity and result in firing of latent ventricular pacemakers and triggered activity. Snisarenko[94] found significant elevations in heart rate in both the acute (4 to 10 d) and subacute (3 to 12 months) periods following myocardial infarction in a feline model. In the acute period, these effects were accompanied by increased wakefulness, decreased heart rate variability, and severely disordered sleep. In the intervening weeks, sleep quality recovered fully until, in the subacute period, beta blockade with propranolol led to renewed, pronounced disturbances in sleep structure, with increased wakefulness, reduction in REM sleep, and prolongation of stages 1 and 2 of NREM sleep. He attributed these results to reflex activation of adrenergic, noradrenergic, and dopaminergic nerves in several brain structures following coronary artery ligation.[95]

SUMMARY AND CONCLUSIONS

Sleep states exert a major impact on cardiorespiratory function. This is a direct consequence of the significant variations in brain states which occur in the normal cycling between NREM and REM sleep. Because of the close neurohumoral coupling between central structures and the cardiorespiratory system, dynamic fluctuations in critical variables occur, including heart rhythm, arterial blood pressure, coronary artery blood flow, and ventilation. NREM sleep is associated with relative autonomic stability and a functional coordination among respiration, the pumping action of the heart, and maintenance of arterial blood pressure. During REM sleep, remarkable surges in both sympathetic and parasympathetic nerve activity emerge, resulting in significant surges and pauses in heart rhythm. These occur in association with alterations in PGO activity and hippocampal theta rhythm. Whereas these perturbations in autonomic nervous system activity are well tolerated in normal people, those with heart disease may be at particular risk during REM sleep, as the stress on the system has the potential for triggering life-threatening arrhythmias and myocardial ischemia and infarction.[56, 75, 78a] During NREM sleep, in the severely compromised heart, a potential for hypotension exists that can, in turn, impair blood flow through stenotic coronary vessels to trigger ischemia or infarction.[16, 73a, 74, 75, 75a, 75b] Coordination of cardiorespiratory control is especially pivotal in infancy, when developmental immaturity can compromise function and pose special risks. Throughout sleep, the coexistence of coronary disease and apnea is associated with heightened risk[96] due to the challenge of dual control of the respiratory and cardiovascular systems.

Acknowledgments

Supported by grants HL50078 and HL22418 from the National Heart, Lung, and Blood Institute, ES 08129 from the National Institutes of Environmental Health; and MH-13923 from the National Institutes of Mental Health, National Institutes of Health, Bethesda, Md. Additional support was provided by the Mind-Body Network of the John D. and Catherine T. MacArthur Foundation.

References

1. Lydic R, Baghdoyan HA. The neurobiology of rapid-eye-movement sleep. In: Saunders NA, Sullivan CE, eds. Sleep and Breathing. Lung Biology in Health and Disease. Vol 71. New York, NY: Marcel Dekker; 1994.
2. Kodama T, Lai YY, Siegel JM. Enhancement of acetylcholine release during REM sleep in the caudomedial medulla as measured by in vivo microdialysis. Brain Res. 1992;580:348–350.
3. Baghdoyan HA, Carlson BX, Roth MT. Pharmacological characterization of muscarinic cholinergic receptors in cat pons and cortex. Pharmacology. 1994;48:77–85.
4. Gilbert KA, Lydic R. Pontine cholinergic reticular mechanisms cause state-dependent changes in the discharge of parabrachial neurons. Am J Physiol. 1994;266:R136–150.
5. Lopez-Rodriguez F, Kohlmeier K, Morales FR, et al. State dependency of the effects of microinjection of cholinergic drugs into the nucleus pontis oralis. Brain Res. 1994;649:271–281.
6. Hobson JA, Stickgold R, Pace-Schott EF. The neuropsychology of REM sleep dreaming. Neuroreport. 1998;9:R1–14.
7. Task Force of the European Society of Cardiology and the North American Society of Pacing and Electrophysiology. Heart rate variability: standards of measurement, physiological interpretation and clinical use. Circulation. 1996;93:1043–1065.
8. Woo MS, Woo MA, Gozal D, et al. Heart rate variability in congenital central hypoventilation syndrome. Pediatr Res. 1992;31:291–296.
9. Trelease RB, Sieck GC, Marks JD, et al. Respiratory inhibition induced by transient hypertension during sleep. Exp Neurol. 1985;90:173–186.
10. Ohtake PJ, Jennings DB. Ventilation is stimulated by small reductions in arterial pressure in the awake dog. J Appl Physiol. 1992;73:1549–1557.
11. Harper RM, Gozal D, Forster HV, et al. Imaging of ventral medullary surface activity during blood pressure challenges in awake and anesthetized goats. Am J Physiol. 1996;39:R182–191.
12. Schechtman VL, Harper RM, Wilson AJ, et al. Sleep apnea in infants who succumb to the sudden infant death syndrome. Pediatrics. 1991;87:841–846.
13. Aljadeff G, Gozal D, Schechtman VL, et al. Heart rate variability in children with obstructive sleep apnea. Sleep. 1997;20:151–157.
14. Somers VK, Dyken ME, Mark AL, et al. Sympathetic nerve activity during sleep in normal subjects. N Engl J Med. 1993;328:303–307.
15. Baust W, Bohnert B. The regulation of heart rate during sleep. Exp Brain Res. 1969;7:169–180.
16. Mancia G. Autonomic modulation of the cardiovascular system during sleep. N Engl J Med. 1993;328:347–349.
17. Baccelli G, Guazzi M, Mancia G, et al. Neural and non-neural mechanisms influencing circulation during sleep. Nature. 1969;223:184–185.
18. Dickerson LW, Huang AH, Nearing BD, et al. Primary coronary vasodilation associated with pauses in heart rhythm during sleep. Am J Physiol. 1993;264:R186–196.
19. Harper RM, Frysinger RC, Zhang J, et al. Cardiac and respiratory interactions maintaining homeostasis during sleep. In: Lydic R,

Biebuyck JF, eds. Clinical Physiology of Sleep. Bethesda, Md: American Physiological Society; 1988.
20. Gassel MM, Ghelarducci B, Marchiafava PL, et al. Phasic changes in blood pressure and heart rate during the rapid eye movement episodes of desynchronized sleep in unrestrained cats. Arch Ital Biol. 1964;102:530–544.
21. Snyder F, Hobson JA, Morrison DF, et al. Changes in respiration, heart rate, and systolic blood pressure in human sleep. J Appl Physiol. 1964;19:417–422.
22. Lydic R, Baghdoyan HA. Microdialysis of cat pons reveals enhanced acetylcholine release during state-dependent respiratory depression. Am J Physiol. 1991;261:R766–770.
23. Sauerland EK, Harper RM. The human tongue during sleep: electromyographic activity of the genioglossus muscle. Exo Neurol. 1976;51:160–170.
24. Henderson-Smart DJ, Read DJC. Reduced lung volume during behavioral active sleep in the newborn. J Appl Physiol. 1979;46:1081–1085.
25. Maquet P, Peters J, Aerts J, et al. Functional neuroanatomy of human rapid-eye-movement sleep and dreaming. Nature. 1996;383:163–166.
26. Braun AR, Balkin TJ, Wesenten NJ, et al. Regional cerebral blood flow throughout the sleep-wake cycle. An H2(15)O PET study. Brain. 1997;120:1173–1197.
27. Nofzinger EA, Mintun MA, Wiseman M, et al. Forebrain activation in REM sleep: an FDG PET study. Brain Res. 1997;770:192–201.
28. Harper RM, Bandler R, Spriggs D, et al. Lateralized and widespread brain activation during transient blood pressure elevation revealed by magnetic resonance imaging. J Comp Neurol. In press.
29. Oppenheimer SM, Gelb A, Girvin JP, et al. Cardiovascular effects of human insular cortex stimulation. Neurology. 1992;42:1727–1732.
30. Frysinger RC, Harper RM, Hackel RJ. State-dependent cardiac and respiratory changes associated with complex partial epilepsy. In: Engel J Jr, Ojemann GA, Lüders HO, eds. Fundamental Mechanisms of Human Brain Function. New York, NY: Raven Press; 1987:219–226.
31. Verrier RL, Mittleman MA. Life-threatening cardiovascular consequences of anger in patients with coronary heart disease. Cardiol Clin. 1996;14:289–307.
32. Parmegianni PL, Franzini C, Lenzi P. Respiratory frequency as a function of preoptic temperature during sleep. Brain Res. 1976;111:253–260.
33. Frysinger RC, Marks JD, Trelease RB, et al. Sleep states attenuate the pressor response to central amygdala stimulation. Exp Neurol. 1984;83:604–617.
34. Schwartz PJ, Stramba-Badiale M, Segantini A, et al. Prolongation of the QT interval and the sudden infant death syndrome. N Engl J Med. 1998;338:1709–1714.
35. Meny RG, Carroll JL, Carbone MT, et al. Cardiorespiratory recordings from infants dying suddenly and unexpectedly at home. Pediatrics. 1994;93:43–49.
36. Harper RM, Bandler R. Finding the failure mechanism in the sudden infant death syndrome. Nat Med. 1998;4:157–158.
37. Beckwith JB. Pathology discussion. In: Bergman AB, Beckwith FB, Ray CG, eds. Sudden Infant Death Syndrome: Proceedings of the Second International Conference on Causes of Sudden Death in Infants. Seattle, Wash: University of Washington Press; 1970:120–122.
38. Yates BJ. Vestibular influences on the autonomic nervous system. Ann N Y Acad Sci. 1996:781:458–473.
39. Chen CH, Williams JL, Lutherer LO. Cerebellar lesions alter autonomic responses to transient isovolaemic changes in arterial pressure in anaesthetized cats. Clin Auton Res. 1994;4:263–272.
40. Baust W, Holzbach E, Zechlin O. Phasic changes in heart rate and respiration correlated with PGO-spike activity during REM sleep. Pflugers Arch. 1972;331:113–123.
41. Kirby DA, Verrier RL. Differential effects of sleep stage on coronary hemodynamic function. Am J Physiol. 1989;256:H1378–1383.
42. Kirby DA, Verrier RL. Differential effects of sleep stage on coronary hemodynamic function during stenosis. Physiol Behav. 1989;45:1017–1020.
43. Dickerson LW, Huang AH, Thurnher MM, et al. Relationship

between coronary hemodynamic changes and the phasic events of rapid eye movement sleep. Sleep. 1993;16:550–557.

44. Rowe K, Moreno R, Lau RT, et al. Heart rate surges during REM sleep are associated with theta rhythm and PGO activity in the cat. Am J Physiol. 1999;277:R843–R849.

45. Sakai K, Sano K, Iwahara S. Eye movements and hippocampal theta activity in cats. Electroencephalogr Clin Neurophysiol. 1973;34:547–549.

46. Kemp IR, Kaada BR. The relation of hippocampal theta activity to arousal, attentive behaviour and somato-motor movements in unrestrained cats. Brain Res. 1975;95:323–342.

47. Lerma J, Garcia-Austt E. Hippocampal theta rhythm during paradoxical sleep. Effects of afferent stimuli and phase relationships with phasic events. Electroencephalogr Clin Neurophysiol. 1985;60:46–54.

48. Sei H, Morita Y. Acceleration of EEG theta wave precedes the phasic surge of arterial pressure during REM sleep in the rat. Neuroreport. 1996;7:3059–3062.

49. Verrier RL, Lau RT, Wallooppillai U, et al. Primary vagally mediated decelerations in heart rate during tonic rapid eye movement sleep in cats. Am J Physiol. 1998;43:R1136–1141.

50. Taylor WB, Moldofsky H, Furedy JJ. Heart rate deceleration in REM sleep: an orienting reaction interpretation. Psychophysiology. 1985;22:110–115.

51. Pappano AJ. Modulation of the heartbeat by the vagus nerve. In: Zipes DP, Jalife J, eds. Cardiac Electrophysiology: From Cell to Bedside. Philadelphia, Pa: WB Saunders; 1995:411–422.

52. Guilleminault CP, Pool P, Motta J, et al. Sinus arrest during REM sleep in young adults. N Engl J Med. 1984;311:1006–1010.

53. Vatner SF, Franklin D, Higgins CB, et al. Coronary dynamics in unrestrained conscious baboons. Am J Physiol. 1971;221:1396–1401.

54. Feigl EO. Coronary physiology. Physiol Rev. 1983;63:1–205.

55. Billman GE, Randall DC. Mechanisms mediating the coronary vascular response to behavioral stress in the dog. Circ Res. 1981;48:214–223.

56. Nowlin JB, Troyer WG Jr, Collins WS, et al. The association of nocturnal angina pectoris with dreaming. Ann Intern Med. 1965;63:1040–1046.

57. Levy AG. The exciting causes of ventricular fibrillation in animals under chloroform anesthesia. Heart. 1912;4:319–378.

58. Hockman CH, Mauck HP, Hoff EC. ECG changes resulting from cerebral stimulation, II: a spectrum of ventricular arrhythmias of sympathetic origin. Am Heart J. 1966;71:695–700.

59. Verrier RL, Calvert A, Lown B. Effect of posterior hypothalamic stimulation on the ventricular fibrillation threshold. Am J Physiol. 1975;228:923–927.

60. Cropp GJ, Manning GW. Electrocardiographic changes simulating myocardial ischemia and infarction associated with spontaneous intracranial hemorrhage. Circulation. 1960;22:25–38.

61. Hugenholtz PG. Electrocardiographic abnormalities in cerebral disorders: report of six cases and review of the literature. Am Heart J. 1962;63:451–461.

62. Skinner JE, Reed JC. Blockade of frontocortical–brain stem pathway prevents ventricular fibrillation of ischemic heart. Am J Physiol. 1981;240:H156–163.

63. Carpeggiani C, Landisman C, Montaron M-F, et al. Cryoblockade in limbic brain (amygdala) prevents or delays ventricular fibrillation after coronary artery occlusion in psychologically stressed pigs. Circ Res. 1992;70:600–606.

64. Korteweg GCJ, Boeles JTF, Ten Cate J. Influence of stimulation of some subcortical areas on electrocardiogram. J Neurophysiol. 1957;20:100–107.

65. Manning JW, Cotten M de V. Mechanism of cardiac arrhythmias induced by diencephalic stimulation. Am J Physiol. 1962;203:1120–1124.

66. Janse MJ, Wit AL. Electrophysiological mechanism of ventricular arrhythmias resulting from myocardial ischemia and infarction. Physiol Rev. 1989;69:1049–1169.

67. Parker GW, Michael LH, Hartley CJ, et al. Central beta-adrenergic mechanisms may modulate ischemic ventricular fibrillation in pigs. Circ Res. 1990;66:259–270.

68. Benfey BG, Elfellah MS, Ogilvie RI, et al. Antiarrhythmic effects of prazosin and propranolol during coronary artery occlusion and reperfusion in dogs and pigs. Br J Pharmacol. 1984;82:717–725.

69. Lewis PJ, Haeusler G. Reduction in sympathetic nervous activity as a mechanism for the hypotensive action of propranolol. Nature. 1975;256:440.

70. Privitera PJ, Webb JG, Walle T. Effect of centrally administered propranolol on plasma renin activity, plasma norepinephrine, and arterial pressure. Eur J Pharmacol. 1979;54:51–60.

71. Schwartz PJ, Zaza A, et al. The effect of antiarrhythmic drugs on life-threatening arrhythmias induced by the interaction between acute myocardial ischemia and sympathetic hyperactivity. Am Heart J. 1985;109:937–948.

72. Hjalmarson A, Olsson G. Myocardial infarction. Effects of beta-blockade. Circulation. 1991;84 (suppl 6):VI-101–107.

73. Kostis JB, Rosen RC. Central nervous system effects of beta-adrenergic blocking drugs: the role of ancillary properties. Circulation. 1987;75:204–212.

73a. Patel DJ, Knight CJ, Holdright DR, et al. Pathophysiology of transient myocardial ischemia in acute coronary syndromes. Characterization by continuous ST-segment monitoring. Circulation. 1997;95:1185–1192.

74. Broughton R, Baron R. Sleep patterns in the intensive care unit and on the ward after acute myocardial infarction. Electroencephalogr Clin Neurophysiol. 1978;45:348–360.

75. Deedwania PC. Increased demand versus reduced supply and the circadian variations in ambulatory myocardial ischemia. Therapeutic implications [editorial]. Circulation. 1993;88:328–331.

75a. Kleiman NS, Schechtman KB, Young PM, et al. Lack of diurnal variation in the onset of non–Q-wave infarction. Circulation. 1990;81:548–555.

75b. Tsuda M, Hayashi H, Kanematsu K, et al. Comparison between diurnal distribution of onset of infarction in patients with acute myocardial infarction and circadian variation of blood pressure in patients with coronary artery disease. Clin Cardiol. 1993;16:543–547.

76. Kovach JA, Gottdiener JS, Verrier RL. Vagal modulation of epicardial coronary artery size in dogs. A two-dimensional intravascular ultrasound study. Circulation. 1995;92:2291–2298.

77. Ludmer PL, Selwyn AP, Shook TL, et al. Paradoxical vasoconstriction induced by acetylcholine in atherosclerotic arteries. N Engl J Med. 1986;315:1046–1051.

78. Lown B, Verrier RL. Neural activity and ventricular fibrillation. N Engl J Med. 1976;294:1165–1170.

78a. Andrews TC, Fenton T, Toyosaki N, et al. Subsets of ambulatory myocardial ischemia based on heart rate activity: circadian distribution and response to anti-ischemic medication. Circulation. 1993;88:92–100.

79. Smith R, Johnson L, Rothfeld D, et al. Sleep and cardiac arrhythmias. Arch Intern Med. 1972;130:751–753.

80. Rosenblatt G, Hartman E, Zwilling GR. Cardiac irritability during sleep and dreaming. J Psychosom. 1973;17:129–134.

81. Otsuka K, Yanaga T, Ichimaru Y, et al. Sleep and night-type arrhythmias. Jpn Heart J. 1982;23:479–486.

82. Verrier RL, Thompson PL, Lown B. Ventricular vulnerability during sympathetic stimulation: Role of heart rate and blood pressure. Cardiovasc Res. 1974;8:602–610.

83. Han J, Moe GK. Nonuniform recovery of excitability in ventricular muscle. Circ Res. 1964;14:44–60.

84. Verrier RL, Kovach JA. Primary role of beta-adrenergic receptors in arrhythmogenesis during sympathetic nervous system activation. In: Podrid PJ, Kowey PR, eds. Cardiac Arrhythmias: Mechanism, Diagnosis and Management. Baltimore, Md: Williams & Wilkins; 1995.

85. Lombardi F, Verrier RL, Lown B. Relationship between sympathetic neural activity, coronary dynamics, and vulnerability to ventricular fibrillation during myocardial ischemia and reperfusion. Am Heart J. 1983;105:958–965.

86. Nearing BD, Oesterle SN, Verrier RL. Quantification of ischaemia-induced vulnerability by precordial T-wave alternans analysis in dog and human. Cardiovasc Res. 1994;28:1440–1449.

87. Nearing BD, Huang AH, Verrier RL. Dynamic tracking of cardiac vulnerability by complex demodulation of the T-wave. Science. 1991;252:437–440.

88. Verrier RL, Nearing BD. T-wave alternans as a harbinger of ischemia-induced sudden cardiac death. In: Zipes DP, Jalife J, eds. Cardiac Electrophysiology: From Cell to Bedside. Philadelphia, Pa: WB Saunders; 1995.

89. Verrier RL, Hagestad EL. Mechanisms involved in reperfusion arrhythmias. Eur Heart J. 1986;7(suppl A):13–22.
90. Verrier RL. Autonomic modulation of arrhythmias in animal models. In: Rosen MR, Wit AL, Janse MJ, eds. Cardiac Electrophysiology: A Textbook in Honor of Brian Hoffman. New York, NY: Futura Press; 1990.
91. Levy MN. Role of calcium in arrhythmogenesis. Circulation. 1989;80:4-23–30.
92. Lavery CE, Mittleman MA, Cohen MC, et al. Nonuniform nighttime distribution of acute cardiac events: a possible effect of sleep states. Circulation. 1997;96:3321–3327.
93. Skinner JE, Mohr DN, Kellaway P. Sleep-stage regulation of ventricular arrhythmias in the unanesthetized pig. Circ Res. 1975;37:342–349.
94. Snisarenko AA. Cardiac rhythm in cats during physiological sleep in experimental myocardial infarction and beta-adrenergic receptor blockade. Cor Vasa. 1986;38:306–314.
95. Sole MJ, Hussain MN, Lixfeld W. Activation of brain catecholaminergic neurons by cardiac vagal afferents during acute myocardial ischemia in the rat. Circ Res. 1980;47:166–172.
96. Hung J, Whitford EG, Parsons RW, et al. Association of sleep apnoea with myocardial infarction in men. Lancet. 1990;336:261–264.

Cardiovascular Physiology: The Peripheral Circulation

Carlo Franzini

The modest changes in peripheral circulation during non-rapid eye movement (NREM) sleep contrast with the sharp modifications characteristic of rapid eye movement (REM) sleep. During REM sleep, cerebral blood flow changes respond to the functional logic of the organ (flow-metabolism coupling). In contrast, changes in other peripheral beds respond to a sum of central (sympathovagal balance) and peripheral (local activity) changes that are sleep dependent and may contrast with the functional logic of the organs (thermoregulatory, excretory, absorptive). Likewise, cerebral circulation during REM sleep shares the regulatory mechanisms of other brain-activated states, whereas the disrupted integrated control on the remaining peripheral beds is unique to REM sleep. This disruption has no effect under physiological conditions, but may represent a risk factor in pathophysiological conditions when the control of peripheral resistances is an indispensable adaptive mechanism (e.g., in chronic heart failure).

The regulation of physiological systems changes with state—wakefulness, nonrapid eye movement (NREM) sleep and rapid eye movement (REM) sleep.[1] This has been demonstrated in studies of thermoregulation[2] and respiration.[3] The control of circulation during sleep is complex because the changes may reflect the interaction of both the matching of blood flow (BF) to the functional activity of the perfused organ and the change in sleep state.

The sleep process primarily involves the brain, and changes in cerebral activity are the primary events of sleep. When the brain switches its activity from NREM to REM sleep, cerebral blood flow (CBF) changes to match the change in function. In contrast, when circulatory changes occur in other organs they may depend primarily on the sleep-state transition rather than respond to the function of these organs. In other words, whereas brain blood flow changes during sleep are tied to the function of the organ, this may not always be the case for blood flow changes in other vascular beds.

SLEEP-DEPENDENT CHANGES IN CEREBRAL CIRCULATION

The brain circulation during sleep has been the focus of many studies, with the assumption that its under-standing might shed light on the elusive issue of sleep function. A review of the literature before 1990[4] listed more than 80 papers, employing many different techniques. The main conclusions were the following:

1. CBF mostly decreases during NREM sleep with respect to wakefulness, and rises again markedly in REM sleep.
2. The connection between changes in synaptic activity, metabolism, and BF is well established.
3. CBF fluctuations result from changes in vascular resistance whose mechanisms remain to be clarified.
4. CBF fluctuations are mainly independent of systemic hemodynamic changes, particularly the redistribution of BF in other peripheral beds.

More recently, positron emission tomography (PET) and Doppler flowmetry studies have shed light on the spatial and temporal dimension of CBF changes during sleep.

Regional Cerebral Blood Flow Changes During Sleep

Maquet et al.[5] found an increased regional BF during REM sleep in pontine tegmentum, dorsal mesencephalon, thalamic nuclei, amygdala, anterior cingulate, and entorhinal cortex. They interpreted these focal activations as bearing on different aspects of REM sleep neuro- and psychophysiology; that is, the centrencephalic (brainstem, thalamus, basal forebrain) origin of the state, its autonomic phenomenology, and its participation in memory consolidation. A companion study from the same group examined the "Functional Neuroanatomy of Human Slow Wave Sleep."[6] A significant negative correlation was found between the occurrence of NREM sleep and regional CBF in central core structures (pons, mesencephalon, thalamus). A negative correlation has been also reported[7] between sigma (spindle) and delta activity and regional flow in the brainstem reticular formation, cerebellum, and thalamus, whereas at cortical level, both positive and negative correlations of CBF with delta activity were demonstrated. Principal component analysis also indicates decreased thalamic perfusion in NREM sleep.[8] These studies extend to human beings the evidence of a reduced metabolic cost of synchronizing modes of operation in the thalamocortical circuitry which was first shown by measurements of brain glucose uptake in other species (see reference 4); the central role of the thalamus in the genesis of cortical synchronous activity is well established[9] and is confirmed by studies on sleep pathology (e.g., fatal familial insomnia[10, 11]).

Braun et al.[12] measured CBF during wakefulness before and after sleep, and during NREM and REM sleep. Regional CBF in centrencephalic regions decreased during NREM sleep and increased during REM sleep; at a cortical level, heteromodal frontoparietal association cortices were deactivated during both NREM and REM sleep. This deactivation "may be a defining characteristic of sleep itself that involves the highest integrative processes of the brain"; its uniformity across sleep states might relate, in very general terms, to the fact that important features of sleep mental activity are shared by both NREM and REM sleep.[11, 13, 14] The reported BF changes in central core structures agree in essence with those found in other studies[5–8]; in contrast, greater variability across studies is apparent in cortical CBF data. Although a stereotyped circulatory and metabolic pattern links specific brain structures (brainstem, thalamus) during the sleep cycle, differences in cortical activation often ascribed to differences in the species studied or methods used might well result from interindividual or even intraindividual variability intrinsic to the single REM sleep episode.

In addition, Braun et al. reported significantly lower CBF values during postsleep wakefulness than during presleep wakefulness; the effect was more pronounced in cortical and limbic structures.[12] The sleep process might thus reset the circulatory and metabolic activity of the brain to a lower level, in accordance with a "restorative" function of sleep (see later).

BF increments in subcortical and brainstem structures also occur in fetal sheep during the low voltage electrocortical state corresponding to REM sleep.[15–17] Cortical BF is variously reported to be unchanged,[15] or not significantly[17] or significantly[16] increased; this may reflect the different timing of maturational changes in cortical vs. subcortical structures before birth.

Spinal cord BF[16, 18, 19] also increases in REM sleep. The similar trend of BF changes in brain and spinal cord indicates that the sleep process involves a modulation of the activity in the entire central nervous system (CNS). Direct data on spinal cord metabolism during sleep are still lacking.

Finally, cerebral blood perfusion during sleep may change not only quantitatively but also qualitatively. On the basis of local brain temperature changes, Azzaroni and Parmeggiani suggested a carotid-vertebral shift in the quotas of CBF during REM sleep.[20–22]

Time Course of Cerebral Blood Flow Changes During Sleep

Continuous recording of CBF changes during sleep with Doppler probes was instrumental in addressing the following issues: (1) the relationship between tonic and phasic cerebral perfusion changes during sleep; (2) the temporal sequence of CBF and sleep-state modifications; (3) the CBF time course during the night, and the comparison between pre- and postsleep wakefulness levels.

1. In lambs, REM sleep is accompanied by a tonic increase in CBF and by superimposed phasic BF transients.[23, 24] The analysis of the temporal relationship between cerebral perfusion pressure and CBF changes indicates that a fall in vascular resistance is the primary event which both underlies the tonic CBF increment and initiates the phasic CBF surges associated with transient blood pressure (BP) increases.

2. In rats, laser Doppler probes connected to an optical fiber were stereotaxically implanted in the hippocampus[25, 26] and basal forebrain,[27] and relative increments in BF were recorded in the transition from NREM to REM sleep. However, the issue of the temporal relationship between circulatory and sleep-state changes remains unsolved: an early,[27] simultaneous,[26] or late[25] CBF change has been described with respect to the onset of the REM sleep episode. In fetal sheep[28] a thermal clearance study reported CBF increments following by 24 sec the transition from NREM to REM sleep, and previous studies with the same technique reported BF changes preceding or concomitant with EEG changes.[4] Regional differences in brain activation and BF rise with respect to the global state change might explain the different latencies reported.

3. In human adults[29–33] CBF fluctuates from NREM to REM sleep within the same cycle, but decreases tonically throughout the night, and there are lower values in postsleep wakefulness compared to presleep wakefulness (Fig 14–1); this corresponds to results obtained with PET[12] and reinforces the hypothesis of a "restorative" sleep function.

Regulation of Cerebral Circulation During the Sleep-Wake Cycle

The regulation of cerebral circulation aims on the one hand to finely match BF to the metabolic needs of brain activity at a regional level (*flow-metabolism coupling*), whereas on the other hand, it protects the brain from systemic challenges (PaO$_2$, PaCO$_2$, pH changes, *chemical regulation*; BP fluctuations, *autoregulation*).

Flow-Metabolism Coupling

Blood flow, O$_2$ consumption, and glucose uptake undergo similar changes in the brain in different conditions of active wakefulness (sensory stimulation,[34] selective attention[35]) quiet wakefulness,[36] and sleep (NREM and REM sleep[4, 37]).

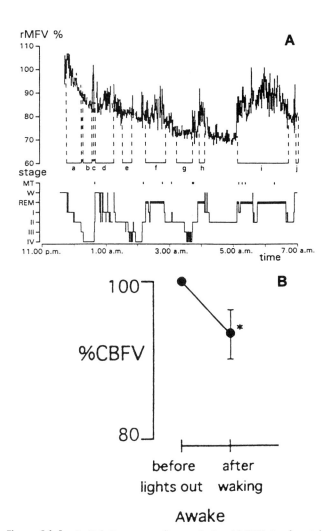

Figure 14–1. *A,* Relative mean flow velocity (rMFV) in the right middle cerebral artery and sleep profile of one normal volunteer. (a) Progressive MFV reduction during NREM sleep; (b) continuous MFV reduction during slow-wave sleep (SWS); (c, j) movement artifact; (d) reduced MFV during nightime awakening; (e, g) constant mean level of MFV during changes from sleep stage 2 to SWS; (f, h, i) rapid increase in MFV during REM sleep. MT, movement; W, wakefulness. (From Hajak G, Klingelhofer J, Schulz-Varszegi M, et al. Relationship between blood flow velocities and cerebral electrical activity in sleep. Sleep. 1994; 17:11–19.) rMFV can be considered a qualitative index of cerebral perfusion based on the assumption of minimal caliber changes in large cerebral arteries in physiological conditions in human beings. A steady overall decrease in cerebral perfusion occurs during sleep, interrupted by pulsatile increments corresponding to each REM sleep episode. *B,* Percent cerebral blood flow velocity (CBFV) changes (means ± SEM) for six subjects in the awake period before and after sleep. After sleep CBFV was 6.6% lower than before sleep (*P<.05). (Modified from Electroencephalography and Clinical Neurophysiology, vol 102, Kubayama T, Hori A, Sato T, et al. Changes in cerebral blood flow velocity in healthy young men during overnight sleep and while awake, 125–131, Copyright 1997, with permission from Elsevier Science.)

In fetal lambs[38, 39] during low-voltage fast activity (REM sleep equivalent) both O_2 and glucose consumption increase, but cerebral glucose uptake exceeds O_2 uptake. The increased glucose/O_2 quotient indicates a modest but significant anaerobic component in brain metabolism; this might be common to brain-activated states (see reference 34) and not specific to REM sleep. Madsen,[36] however, calculated that when CBF values

during REM sleep are corrected for $PaCO_2$ changes, the cerebral metabolic rate for O_2 ($CMRO_2$) remains coupled to CBF and the cerebral metabolic rate for glucose (CMR_{glu}), suggesting an aerobic glucose utilization. The occurrence of anaerobic glycolysis during REM sleep therefore remains to be proved. Comparison of presleep and postsleep brain glucose and O_2 metabolism[40] showed a greater decrease in glucose than in O_2 utilization. Reduced metabolism, reduced flow,[12, 29–32] and reduced anaerobic glycolysis all agree with the "restorative" function of sleep. Wu et al.,[41] however, found no differences in mean cerebral glucose utilization during wakefulness before and after sleep deprivation. This discrepancy should be resolved, because it is central to the issue of a "recovery" function of sleep.

Finally, near infrared spectroscopy (NIRS) has been used in human beings to assess changes in O_2 saturation during sleep[42, 43]; the transition from NREM to REM sleep is accompanied by an increase in oxygenated hemoglobin. Because NIRS measurements mostly reflect the oxygenation level in venous blood, this confirms the decreased arteriovenous (A-V) O_2 difference previously reported in various species (see reference 4).

In conclusion, CMR_{glu} and $CMRO_2$ increase during REM sleep; therefore, both glucose and O_2 might act as mediators between metabolic and circulatory changes. However, the low extraction coefficient of glucose is inconsistent with the idea that it might couple flow and metabolism. On the other hand, the decreased $(A-V)O_2$ difference in REM sleep indicated that the longitudinal O_2 gradient in the capillaries is reduced, so that a steeper transcapillary gradient is available to overcome the high resistance to O_2 diffusion from plasma to interstitium. This favors O_2 delivery. In addition, studies on brain microcirculation during sleep[44–46] indicate that no capillary recruitment accompanies the sleep-wake cycle. In the absence of capillary recruitment (relative constancy of the endothelial surface area), the CBF increase during REM sleep is essential to maintaining the driving force for outward O_2 diffusion. Taken together, these data suggest that O_2 could be the coupling factor between cerebral activity and perfusion during the REM sleep.[47]

Chemical Regulation

In NREM sleep a slight hypercapnia develops (2 to 3 mmHg). This counteracts the circulatory effects of the decreased cerebral metabolic rate and accounts for the small increase in CBF in some species (e.g., goat[48]). $PaCO_2$ becomes an important determinant of CBF changes during sleep in pathological conditions (e.g., sleep apnea[49, 50]).

Autoregulation

Autoregulation has been shown to operate during sleep: in lambs cerebral vasodilation in response to acute hypotension occurs in all behavioral states (wakefulness, NREM and REM sleep[51]). The independence of CBF from systemic hemodynamics is further supported by the lack of correlation between BF increments in the brain and BF changes in the external carotid bed[52] or in other peripheral circulations (kidney, muscle, skin, splanchnic)[53]: CBF is not affected by the redistribution of regional flows occurring in REM sleep.

Conclusions and Implications for Future Research

The main conclusions from the reviewed data can be summarized as follows:

1. A stereotyped pattern of CBF and metabolic changes has been demonstrated during sleep in the central core of brainstem-thalamic structures with decrements in NREM and increments in REM sleep.[5, 6, 12] In contrast, greater fluctuations characterize the cortical circulatory and metabolic pattern; this may result from interindividual variability in small sample populations. Alternatively, it might be a true feature of cortical activation, especially during REM sleep, and even intraindividual activation variability might become apparent when longitudinal studies in the same subject become methodologically feasible. In general terms, associative cortices seem to be more affected by sleep than primary sensory areas (see references 6, 8, 12).
2. The low metabolic cost of the synchronizing mode of operation in the thalamocortical circuits is now well established.[5–8, 12]
3. An overall reduction of CBF (and presumably metabolism) occurs during the night, with postsleep values significantly lower than presleep values.[12, 29–33] Points 1 and 2 finally bring solid experimental evidence to the long-held view of a "restorative" function of sleep.
4. The study of brain microcirculation during sleep has just started.[44] It should shed light on the molecular traffic across the blood-brain barrier during sleep, separating the quota that is common to all activation-deactivation processes in the brain from that which might be specific to the sleep process. This brings us to the main problem that should be addressed by future research in this field: is there a circulatory or metabolic pattern in the brain that identifies the sleep process, or does the same pattern emerge when the activation of the brain is physiologically or pathophysiologically modulated?[35] The reviewed studies on general cerebral brain metabolism and BF raised the curtain on brain activity during sleep. This was a major step forward: we now see the stage, but the actors are still not there, and we can only speculate on their true identity. They might not be specific circulatory or metabolic events (global or regional brain BF or energy metabolism) but, instead, specific modalities of neural network operation, synchronous (NREM sleep) or random (REM sleep).
5. Flow-metabolism coupling currently appears to be the principal mechanism controlling CBF changes during sleep. The other two regulatory

mechanisms (chemical regulation, autoregulation) may be involved in adjusting CBF during sleep in pathophysiological conditions (hypercapnia, hypotension).

SLEEP-DEPENDENT CHANGES IN EXTRACEREBRAL CIRCULATION

The evidence reviewed in this section results from experiments on different animal species (rat, rabbit, cat, dog, pig, sheep, human beings) in which BF was measured with flowmeters or with radioactive microspheres.

Cutaneous Circulation

In the transition from wakefulness to NREM sleep a decrease in set-point temperature is responsible for thermolytic cutaneous vasodilation.[54–57] In REM sleep, on the other hand, skin BF changes result from the hindrance of thermoregulatory cutaneous vasomotion[2]: (1) in a cold environment a BF increment results from the drop in neurogenic vasoconstriction; (2) in a warm environment a BF reduction may result from a decrease in BP[57] or from a drop in neurogenic vasodilation.[54, 55]

Because the regulation of cutaneous BF depends mainly on neural vasomotor activity, the above data support a general paradigm: the sleep-dependent BF change in the different vascular beds correlates with the relative weight of their neural control.

Renal Circulation

The few existing studies on renal circulation during sleep indicate that kidney BF is not state dependent.[58–60] When, however, renal vasoconstriction is an integrated part of the overall thermoregulatory vasomotor response to a thermal load, it wanes in REM sleep like any other thermoregulatory effector response[2]; BF increases accordingly.[61]

Splanchnic Circulation

No significant BF changes occur in the splanchnic territory during sleep.[62, 63] In liver the constancy of total BF depends on a precise mixing of its arterial and portal components: an increase in hepatic arterial flow is compensated by a decrease in portal flow, and vice versa. This entails a significant negative correlation between arterial and portal flow during wakefulness and NREM sleep; in REM sleep the disappearance of this correlation[62] is an example of random *perturbations* (breathing irregularities, changes in abdominal pressure, cardiovascular variability) interfering with a finely tuned regulatory mechanism.

Muscle Circulation

Muscle BF does not change significantly in the transition from wakefulness to NREM sleep; in REM sleep it decreases in red fibers, while increasing, decreasing, or remaining unchanged in white fibers according to the species (rabbit,[64] cat,[65] rat,[66] respectively).

REM sleep entails both an increase in sympathetic tone to muscle blood vessels[67–73] and specific changes in muscle activity (atonia and twitches). The cumulative effect of the following factors determines BF changes in the two muscle fiber populations: (1) differences in basal BF in NREM sleep, which is high in red and low in white fibers; (2) vasodilator influences (local metabolic factors secondary to twitching activity); and (3) vasoconstrictor influences (both neural and local metabolic factors, secondary to atonia). Slight quantitative differences in the same vasodilator and vasoconstrictor mechanisms, acting on different levels of basal BF, may underlie the reported differences according to species and fiber type. Thus, muscle circulation exemplifies the complex way sleep affects vascular conductances both directly (via neural vasomotion changes) and indirectly (via activity changes).

Coronary Circulation

In the dog, left coronary BF decreases significantly from wakefulness to NREM sleep and increases in REM sleep.[74] During phasic REM sleep, BF surges are coupled with episodes of sinus tachycardia, suggesting that local metabolic control is responsible for reduced coronary vascular resistance.[75] However, in the transition from NREM to REM sleep, an increase in coronary BF follows a pause in heart rhythm. This increase in flow without a corresponding increase in cardiac metabolic activity has been attributed to neurogenic cholinergic vasodilation.[76] The sympathetic nervous system triggers the sequence of increased heart rate (HR) causing increased metabolism, which in turn leads to an increased flow. Both tachycardia and BF surges are eliminated by bilateral stellectomy.[74] In contrast, when a marked stenosis is induced by cuff inflation in the left circumflex coronary artery, increases in HR in REM sleep are accompanied by a decrease in coronary BF. A reduced diastolic perfusion time may account for the flow decrement.[77]

The above data stress the complex role of sympathovagal interactions in determining cardiac activity and coronary circulation changes during REM sleep. However, no coherent unitary picture emerged from the few existing experiments of stimulation,[78] lesion,[74, 78] and recording[79, 80] of autonomic nerves to the heart during sleep.

Integrated Vasomotor Patterns

The circulatory system has control mechanisms hierarchically organized in levels of increasing complexity. At the hypothalamic level, the higher integrative control of autonomic functions can interfere with the physiological control of the sleep cycle.[81] According to this model, the need to maintain an integrated autonomic pattern can hinder the natural progression from NREM to REM sleep, and, conversely, the entrance into REM sleep can disrupt the operating autonomic pattern. The model can be tested by applying a stimulus, for example, a thermal load or hemorrhage, that requires a complex cardiovascular response (compensatory distribution of regional flows).

The conflict arising between the maintenance of an adequate vasomotor pattern and the occurrence of REM sleep has been shown in experiments where the intensity of vasoconstrictor sympathetic outflow was manipulated by abdominal cooling or ligature of the common carotid arteries. The higher vasomotor tone caused by these manipulations hinders the transition from NREM to REM sleep, and therefore positively correlates with the length of the NREM sleep episode.[82] Moreover, it has been shown that BP variability during REM sleep decreases at low ambient temperature (T_a)[83] (Fig. 14–2). The wide range of fluctuations of physio-

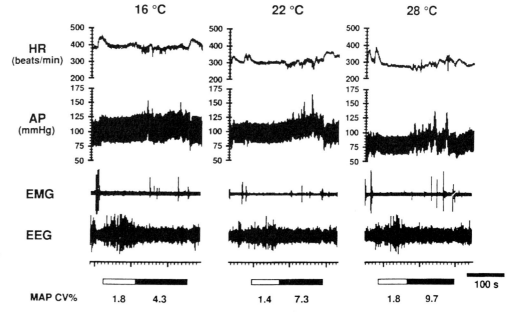

Figure 14–2. Representative computer-assisted digital recordings showing changes in heart rate (HR), arterial pressure (AP), electromyogram (EMG), and electroencephalogram (EEG) during successive NREM (indicated by horizontal open columns at bottom) and REM (indicated by horizontal closed columns at bottom) sleep at three ambient temperatures. MAP CV%, coefficient of variation of mean arterial pressure. The MAP CV% decreased as the ambient temperature was lowered. (From Sei H, Morita Y. Effect of ambient temperature on arterial pressure variability during sleep in the rat. J Sleep Res. 1996;5:37–41.)

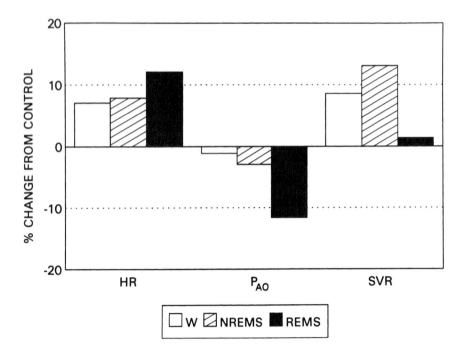

Figure 14–3. Percent change from control values of cardiovascular variables following 10 ml/kg hemorrhage during wakefulness (W), NREM sleep (NREMS), and REM sleep (REMS). In REM sleep, the hemorrhage is not compensated by an increase in vascular resistance, with a consequent fall in blood pressure. HR, heart rate; P_{AO}, aortic blood pressure; SVR, systemic vascular resistance. (Modified from Fewell JE, Williams BJ, Hill DE. Behavioral state influences the cardiovascular response to hemorrhage in lambs. J Dev Physiol. 1984; 6:339–348.)

logical variables is a distinguishing feature of REM sleep. The homeostatic control mechanism entrained by the thermal load may prevent attainment of the full-blown REM sleep episode at low T_a, thus reducing spontaneous variability. Conversely, integrated control mechanisms may fail during REM sleep. (1) After hemorrhage,[84] the adaptive increase in peripheral vascular resistance is absent during REM sleep (Fig. 14–3). This cannot depend on baroreflex impairment, because the tachycardic response to hemorrhage is greater during REM sleep than during NREM sleep or wakefulness. (2) Exposure to a cold environment entails an adaptive increase in cardiac output during wakefulness and NREM sleep but not during REM sleep.[85] As far as the peripheral circulation is concerned,[61] the same thermoregulatory vasomotor adjustments occur in wakefulness and in NREM sleep. At low T_a, vasoconstriction of splanchnic and renal beds and of A-V anastomoses

accompanies muscle vasodilation (coupled with shivering thermogenesis). At high T_a, opening of A-V anastomoses entails compensatory vasoconstriction in the splanchnic and renal beds. This BF redistribution abates in REM sleep and, as a consequence, flow is reduced in previously vasodilated beds and increased in previously vasoconstricted beds. The compensatory modulation of peripheral resistances in response to a thermal load is lost (Fig. 14–4).

Another vasomotor pattern, namely, the gradient of muscle vasoconstriction, increasing from superficial to deeper layers and corresponding to the reduction of the inner thermoregulated "core" in a cold environment, is similarly lost during REM sleep.[86]

This experimental evidence can be referred to the following paradigm: REM sleep occurs when the responsible brainstem structures are freed from hypothalamic homeostatic control. This release is hindered by

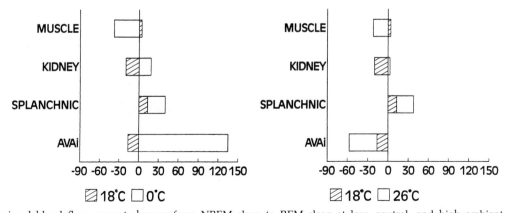

Figure 14–4. Regional blood flow percent changes from NREM sleep to REM sleep at low, neutral, and high ambient temperature (T_a). Regional blood flow changes when entering REM sleep are not stereotyped because they are determined by the disappearance of the adaptive vasomotor pattern preexisting in NREM sleep and different at differing T_a. AVAi, index of arteriovenous anastomotic flow. (Modified from Cianci T, Zoccoli G, Lenzi P, et al. Loss of integrative control of peripheral circulation during desynchronized sleep. Am J Physiol. 1991;261:R373–377.)

homeostatic challenges.[87] The release in turn results from an impairment of hypothalamic integrative activity during REM sleep. The hypothalamus is unresponsive to both thermal[88] and electrical[89] stimulation, and recordings of hypothalamic neurons show that cellular thermosensitivity is attenuated or abolished[90, 91]: the deficit at a central level entails the disorganization of complex adaptive vasomotor patterns at the periphery.

Control Mechanisms of the Extracerebral Circulation During the Wake-Sleep Cycle

Autonomic nervous system activity is a central issue in sleep physiology (see references 81, 92 for reviews). In recent years, two techniques, namely, spectral analysis of HR and BP variability in human beings and other species, and sympathetic nerve activity recordings in human beings, have prompted a series of new studies. The results of these investigations and their congruence with previous reports are considered later.

Spectral Analysis of Heart Rate and Blood Pressure Variability

A new approach to the study of cardiovascular control mechanisms came from the appreciation that oscillations in HR and BP result both from central commands and from the feedback operation of the regulatory loops. The frequency content of these fluctuations can be assessed by spectral analysis[93, 94] and can reflect changes in autonomic control of cardiac and vascular muscle cells.

In HR power spectra, the low-frequency (LF) band (less than 0.15 Hz) has been associated with the modulation of sympathetic outflow, while the high-frequency (HF) band (greater than 0.15 Hz) has been associated with the modulation of parasympathetic outflow.[95] The vast majority of spectral analysis studies during sleep focused on HR spectra. Extrapolation of these results to the autonomic nervous system in general requires the assumption of a uniform "sympathetic tone." However, the concept of a uniform sympathetic tone has been challenged,[96] and regional differences have been demonstrated during sleep[68] (Fig. 14–5). On the other hand, BP power spectra, like BP, are affected by changes in both cardiac output and peripheral resistance. For the above reasons, inferences about the nervous control of peripheral circulation drawn from spectral analysis data can overlook differences in autonomic output to the heart and to discrete peripheral beds. An exception occurs in specific pathophysiological conditions where a global increase in sympathetic tone may arise (e.g., sleep apnea[97]; fatal familial insomnia[98, 99]; see also later).

Studies of HR power spectra during sleep[100–106] report reasonably concordant results: during NREM sleep the LF ("sympathetic") component decreases and the HF ("parasympathetic") component increases compared to wakefulness levels. During REM sleep both the LF and the HF components return toward the wakefulness levels; overshoots and undershoots have been described, to maximal values of the LF components[101, 105] and to zero value of the HF components[101, 106] respectively. The shift in HR precedes electroencephalographic (EEG) changes by several minutes,[102] except for sleep onset when the increase in parasympathetic activity does not anticipate sleep.[107] The contribution of sympathetic and parasympathetic efferent activity to LF and HF power spectra, respectively, has been confirmed during sleep by experiments using selective pharmacological blockade (propranolol, atropine).[106]

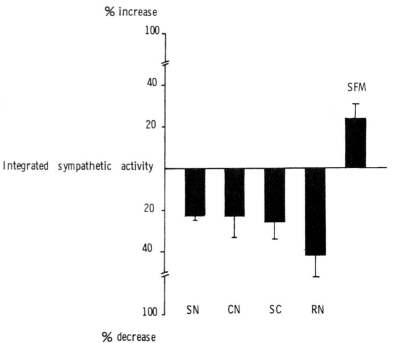

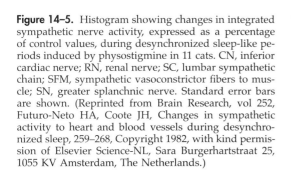

Figure 14–5. Histogram showing changes in integrated sympathetic nerve activity, expressed as a percentage of control values, during desynchronized sleep-like periods induced by physostigmine in 11 cats. CN, inferior cardiac nerve; RN, renal nerve; SC, lumbar sympathetic chain; SFM, sympathetic vasoconstrictor fibers to muscle; SN, greater splanchnic nerve. Standard error bars are shown. (Reprinted from Brain Research, vol 252, Futuro-Neto HA, Coote JH, Changes in sympathetic activity to heart and blood vessels during desynchronized sleep, 259–268, Copyright 1982, with kind permission of Elsevier Science-NL, Sara Burgerhartstraat 25, 1055 KV Amsterdam, The Netherlands.)

Few studies have measured BP power spectra during sleep. In human beings,[103] the LF component decreases and the HF component increases during NREM sleep compared to wakefulness. In REM sleep only the HF component returns toward the waking levels, while the LF component remains low. This contrasts with the increment of the LF components of HR variability and indicates that cardiac and vasomotor sympathetic activity differ during REM sleep. In the cat, the LF component was found to prevail during REM sleep.[108]

Continuous 24-h recordings of HR and BP in human beings outside the laboratory setting show that, by and large, power spectra related to sympathetic control decrease during the night, while power spectra related to parasympathetic activity increase.[109, 110] However, more complex circadian patterns have been described,[111] casting doubt on reductive interpretations of power spectra changes.

Sympathetic Nerve Activity Recordings

Multiunit recordings of sympathetic nerve vasomotor activity during sleep have been obtained both in cats and in human beings. In renal nerves of the normal[112, 113] and decerebrate[68] cat, and in splanchnic nerves of the decerebrate cat,[68] sympathetic vasomotor activity decreases during REM sleep; muscle nerve sympathetic vasomotor activity (MNSA) increases during REM sleep in the decerebrate cat.[68]

In human beings, MNSA decreases during NREM sleep and increases during REM sleep.[69–73] Cutaneous vasodilator activity is unchanged from wakefulness to NREM sleep, but increases in REM sleep.[56]

The above data favor differential sympathetic efferent control, and do not support the idea of a global sympathetic tone during REM sleep (see references 96, 114). Moreover, given the multiple hierarchic controls on the autonomic effector, a strict correspondence in efferent-effector activity is often lacking.[96] This is well exemplified in the control of muscle circulation during REM sleep: BF may increase, decrease, or remain unchanged in white fibers[64–66] in the face of a stereotyped increase in MNSA.

Sleep apnea patients show a high level of MNSA during wakefulness and further increases during sleep. Therefore, in this disorder there is disruption of the sleep state–related profile of MNSA. It remains to be ascertained whether the increase in MNSA in sleep in these patients reflects an increase in overall "sympathetic vasomotor tone" or whether regional differences do remain.[115–117]

CONCLUSIONS AND PATHOPHYSIOLOGICAL IMPLICATIONS

An apparent contradiction emerges from the reviewed data: during REM sleep major modifications in autonomic control entail relatively modest changes at the effector level of vascular smooth muscle. This re-

flects the redundancy of local and neural reflex control of peripheral circulation. However, studies investigating integrated vasomotor patterns show that when a complex adaptive adjustment is required in response to a perturbation (thermal[61]; volemic[84]), a regulatory deficit is evident in REM sleep. In pathophysiological conditions where the overall redistribution of peripheral BF is an indispensable adaptive mechanism (e.g., in chronic heart failure), patients may face two equally risky alternatives: (1) progression into REM sleep is hindered by the increased compensatory vasoconstriction resulting from hypoxia (cf. reference 118), thus contributing to selective sleep deprivation and the disruption of sleep architecture[119, 120], and (2) progression into REM sleep may result in pathological cardiovascular events due to the loss of the adaptive pattern of peripheral vasoconstriction.[121, 122]

Acknowledgments

This work was supported by the National Research Council in Rome. The author thanks Professors P. Lenzi and P.L. Parmeggiani and Dr. G. Zoccoli for their comments on the manuscript. Drs. E. Andreoli and G. Zoccoli also helped generously with references and figures.

References

1. Parmeggiani PL. Behavioral phenomenology of sleep (somatic and vegetative). Experientia. 1980;36:6–11.
2. Parmeggiani PL. Temperature regulation during sleep: a study in homeostasis. In: Orem J, Barnes CD, eds. Physiology in Sleep. New York, NY: Academic Press; 1980:97–143.
3. Phillipson EA, Bowes G. Control of breathing during sleep. In: Cherniack NS, Widdicombe JG, eds. The Respiratory System. Control of Breathing. Bethesda, Md: American Physiological Society, 1986:649–689.
4. Franzini C. Brain metabolism and blood flow during sleep. J Sleep Res. 1992;1:3–16.
5. Maquet P, Péters J-M, Aerts J, et al. Functional neuroanatomy of human rapid-eye-movement sleep and dreaming. Nature. 1996;383:163–166.
6. Maquet P, Degueldre C, Delfiore G, et al. Functional neuroanatomy of human slow wave sleep. J Neurosci. 1997;17:2807–2812.
7. Hofle N, Paus T, Reutens D, et al. Regional cerebral blood flow changes as a function of delta and spindle activity during slow wave sleep in humans. J Neurosci. 1997;17:4800–4808.
8. Andersson JLR, Onoe H, Hetta J, et al. Brain networks affected by synchronized sleep visualized by positron emission tomography. J Cereb Blood Flow Metab. 1998;18:701–715.
9. Steriade M, Contreras D, Amzica F. Synchronized sleep oscillations and their paroxysmal developments. Trends Neurosci. 1994;17:199–208.
10. Lugaresi E, Medori R, Montagna M, et al. Fatal familial insomnia and dysautonomia with selective degeneration of thalamic nuclei. N Engl J Med. 1986;315:997–1003.
11. Perani D, Cortelli P, Lucignani G, et al. [18F] FDG PET in fatal familial insomnia: the functional effects of thalamic lesions. Neurology. 1993;43:2565–2569.
12. Braun AR, Balkin TJ, Wesensten NJ, et al. Regional cerebral blood flow throughout the sleep-wake cycle. An H₂¹⁵O study. Brain. 1997;120:1173–1197.
13. Bosinelli M. Mind and consciousness during sleep. Behav Brain Res. 1995;69:195–201.
14. Cicogna P, Cavallero C, Bosinelli M. Cognitive aspects of mental activity during sleep. Am J Psychol. 1991;104:413–415.
15. Jensen A, Bamford OS, Dawes GS, et al. Changes in organ blood flow between high and low voltage electrocortical activity in fetal sheep. J Dev Physiol. 1986;8:187–194.
16. Rankin JHG, Landauer M, Tian Q, et al. Ovine fetal electrocorti-

cal activity and regional blood flow. J Dev Physiol. 1987;9:537–542.

17. Richardson BS, Caetano H, Homan J, et al. Regional brain blood flow in the ovine fetus during transition to the low-voltage electrocortical state. Dev Brain Res. 1994;81:10–16.

18. Lenzi P, Cianci T, Guidalotti PL, et al. Regional spinal cord blood flow during sleep-waking cycle in rabbit. Am J Physiol. 1986;251:H957–960.

19. Zoccoli G, Bach V, Nardo B, et al. Spinal cord blood flow changes during the sleep-wake cycle in rat. Neurosci Lett. 1993;163:173–176.

20. Azzaroni A, Parmeggiani PL. Mechanisms underlying hypothalamic temperature changes during sleep in mammals. Brain Res. 1993;632:136–142.

21. Azzaroni A, Parmeggiani PL. Postural and sympathetic influences on brain cooling during the ultradian wake-sleep cycle. Brain Res. 1995;671:78–82.

22. Parmeggiani PL. Brain cooling across the wake-sleep behavioral states in homeothermic species: an analysis of the underlying physiological mechanisms. Rev Neurosci. 1995;6:353–363.

23. Franzini C, Walker A, Grant D, et al. The cerebral circulation during active sleep: tonic and phasic vasomotor changes. J Sleep Res. 1998;7(supp 2):92.

24. Grant DA, Franzini C, Wild J, et al. Continuous measurement of blood flow in the superior sagittal sinus of the lamb. Am J Physiol. 1995;269:R274–279.

25. Osborne PG. Hippocampal and striatal blood flow during behavior in rats: chronic laser Doppler flowmetry study. Physiol Behav. 1997;61:485–492.

26. Seno H, Sano A, Maita Y. Cerebral local blood flow with a laser-Doppler flowmetry in rat sleep. Tokushima J Exp Med. 1995;42:1–4.

27. Gerashenko D, Matsumura H. Continuous recording of brain regional circulation during sleep/wake state transitions in rats. Am J Physiol. 1996;270:R855–863.

28. Abrams RM, Gerhardt KJ, Burchfield DJ. Behavioral state transition and local cerebral blood flow in fetal sheep. J Dev Physiol. 1991;15:283–288.

29. Droste DW, Berger W, Schler E, et al. Middle cerebral artery blood flow velocity in healthy persons during wakefulness and sleep: a transcranial Doppler study. Sleep. 1993;16:603–609.

30. Fischer AQ, Taormina MA, Akhtar B, et al. The effect of sleep on intracranial hemodynamics: a transcranial Doppler study. J Child Neurol. 1991;6:155–158.

31. Hajak G, Klingelhofer J, Schulz-Varszegi M, et al. Relationship between blood flow velocities and cerebral electrical activity in sleep. Sleep. 1994;17:11–19.

32. Klingelhofer J, Hajak G, Matzander G, et al. Dynamics of cerebral blood flow velocities during normal human sleep. Clin Neurol Neurosurg. 1995;97:142–148.

33. Kuboyama T, Hori A, Sato T, et al. Changes in cerebral blood flow velocity in healthy young men during overnight sleep and while awake. Electroencephalogr Clin Neurophysiol. 1997;102:125–131.

34. Fox PT, Raichle ME, Mintun MA, et al. Nonoxidative glucose consumption during focal physiologic neural activity. Science. 1988;241:462–464.

35. Madsen PL, Hasselbach SG, Hageman LP, et al. Persistent resetting of the cerebral oxygen/glucose uptake ratio by brain activation: evidence obtained with the Kety-Schmidt technique. J Cereb Blood Flow Metab. 1995;15:485–491.

36. Madsen PL. Blood flow and oxygen uptake in the human brain during various states of sleep and wakefulness. Acta Neurol Scand. 1993;88(suppl 148):1–27.

37. Madsen PL, Vorstrup S. Cerebral blood flow and metabolism during sleep. Cerebrovasc Brain Metab Rev. 1991;3:281–296.

38. Chao CR, Hohimer AR, Bissonnette JM. The effect of electrocortical state on cerebral carbohydrate metabolism in fetal sheep. Dev Brain Res. 1989;49:1–5.

39. Clapp JF, Szeto HH, Abrams R, et al. Physiological variability and fetal electrocortical activity. Am J Obstet Gynecol. 1980;136:1045–1050.

40. Boyle PJ, Scott JC, Krentz AJ, et al. Diminished brain glucose metabolism is a significant determinant for failing rates of systemic glucose utilization during sleep in normal humans. J Clin Invest. 1994;93:529–535.

41. Wu JC, Gillin JC, Buchsbaum MS, et al. The effect of sleep deprivation on cerebral glucose metabolic rate in normal humans assessed with positron emission tomography. Sleep. 1991;14:155–162.

42. Hoshi Y, Mizukami S, Tamura M. Dynamic features of hemodynamic and metabolic changes in the human brain during all-night sleep as revealed by near-infrared spectroscopy. Brain Res. 1994;652:257–262.

43. Onoe H, Watanabe V, Tamura M, et al. REM-sleep associated hemoglobin oxygenation in the monkey forebrain studied using near-infrared spectrophotometry. Neurosci Lett. 1991;129:209–213.

44. Zoccoli G, Lucchi ML, Andreoli E, et al. Brain capillary perfusion during sleep. J Cereb Blood Flow Metab. 1996;16:1312–1318.

45. Zoccoli G, Lucchi ML, Andreoli E, et al. Brain capillary perfusion during sleep in the spontaneously hypertensive rat. J Sleep Res. 1996;5(suppl 1):514.

46. Zoccoli G, Lucchi ML, Andreoli E, et al. Density of perfused brain capillaries in the aged rat. Exp Brain Res [serial online]. 21 September 1999; DOI 10.1007/s002219900219. Available at: http://linkspringer.de/link/service/journals/00221/contents/99/00219/. Accessed October 20, 1999.

47. Lenzi P, Zoccoli G, Walker AM, et al. Cerebral blood flow regulation in REM sleep: a model for flow-metabolism coupling. Arch Ital Biol. 1999;137:165–179.

48. Santiago TV, Guerra E, Neubauer JA, et al. Correlation between ventilation and brain blood flow during sleep. J Clin Invest. 1984;73:497–506.

49. Hajak G, Klingelhofer J, Schulz-Varszegi M, et al. Sleep apnea syndrome and cerebral hemodynamics. Chest. 1996;110:670–679.

50. Siebler M, Nachtmann A. Cerebral hemodynamics in obstructive sleep apnea. Chest. 1993;103:1118–1119.

51. Grant DA, Franzini C, Wild J, et al. Cerebral circulation in sleep: vasodilatory response to cerebral hypotension. J Cereb Blood Flow Metab. 1998;18:639–645.

52. Zoccoli G, Bach V, Cianci T, et al. Brain blood flow and extracerebral carotid circulation during sleep in rat. Brain Res. 1994;641:46–50.

53. Lenzi P, Cianci T, Guidalotti PL, et al. Brain circulation during sleep and its relation to extracerebral hemodynamics. Brain Res. 1987;415:14–20.

54. Alfoldi P, Rubicsek G, Cserni G, et al. Brain and core temperatures and peripheral vasomotion during sleep and wakefulness at various ambient temperatures in the rat. Pflugers Arch. 1990;417:336–341.

55. Franzini C, Lenzi P, Cianci T, et al. Neural control of vasomotion in rabbit ear is impaired during desynchronized sleep. Am J Physiol. 1982;243:R142–146.

56. Noll G, Elam M, Kunimoto M, et al. Skin sympathetic nerve activity and effector function during sleep in humans. Acta Physiol Scand. 1994;151:319–329.

57. Parmeggiani PL, Zamboni G, Cianci T, et al. Absence of thermoregulatory vasomotor responses during fast wave sleep in cats. Electroencephalogr Clin Neurophysiol. 1997;42:372–380.

58. Braaksma MA, Vos J, Dassel ACM, et al. Urine production rate and renal blood flow in near-term ovine fetus are not related to high and low voltage electrocortical activity. Pediatr Res. 1998;43:121–125.

59. Mancia G, Baccelli G, Zanchetti A. Regulation of renal circulation during behavioral changes in the cat. Am J Physiol. 1974;227:536–542.

60. Oosterhof H, Lander M, Aanoudse JG. Behavioral states and Doppler velocimetry of the renal artery in the near term human fetus. Early Hum Dev. 1993;33:183–189.

61. Cianci T, Zoccoli G, Lenzi P, et al. Loss of integrative control of peripheral circulation during desynchronized sleep. Am J Physiol. 1991;261:R373–377.

62. Cianci T, Zoccoli G, Lenzi P, et al. Regional splanchnic blood flow during sleep in the rabbit. Pflugers Arch. 1990;415:594–597.

63. Mancia G, Adams DB, Baccelli G, et al. Regional blood flows during desynchronized sleep in the cat. Experientia. 1969;25:48–49.

64. Lenzi P, Cianci T, Leonardi GS, et al. Muscle blood flow changes during sleep as a function of fibre type composition. Exp Brain Res. 1989;74:549–554.

65. Reis DJ, Moorhead D, Wooten GF. Differential regulation of blood flow to red and white muscle in sleep and defense behavior. Am J Physiol. 1969;217:541–546.

66. Zoccoli G, Lalatta Costerbosa G, Bach V, et al. Muscle blood flow during the sleep-wake cycle in the rat. J Sleep Res. 1994;3(suppl 1):283.

67. Baccelli G, Albertini R, Mancia G, et al. Central and reflex regulation of sympathetic vasoconstrictor activity to limb muscles during desynchronized sleep in the cat. Circ Res. 1974;35:625–635.

68. Futuro-Neto HA, Coote JH. Changes in sympathetic activity to heart and blood vessels during desynchronized sleep. Brain Res. 1982;252:259–268.

69. Hornyak M, Cejnar M, Elam M, et al. Sympathetic muscle nerve activity during sleep in man. Brain. 1991;114:1281–1295.

70. Okada H, Iwase S, Mano T, et al. Changes in muscle sympathetic nerve activity during sleep in humans. Neurology. 1991;41:1961–1966.

71. Shimizu T, Takahashi Y, Suzuki K, et al. Muscle nerve sympathetic activity during sleep and its change with arousal response. J Sleep Res. 1992;1:178–185.

72. Somers VK, Dyken ME, Mark AL, et al. Sympathetic-nerve activity during sleep in normal subjects. N Engl J Med. 1993;328:303–307.

73. Takeuchi S, Iwase S, Mano T, et al. Sleep-related changes in human muscle and skin sympathetic activities. J Autonom Nerv Syst. 1994;47:121–129.

74. Kirby DA, Verrier RL. Differential effects of sleep stage on coronary hemodynamic function. Am J Physiol. 1989; 256:H1378–1383.

75. Dickerson LW, Huang AH, Thurnher MM, et al. Relationship between coronary hemodynamic changes and the phasic events of REM sleep. Sleep. 1993;16:550–557.

76. Dickerson LW, Huang AH, Nearing BD, et al. Primary coronary vasodilation associated with pauses in heart rhythm during sleep. Am J Physiol. 1993;264:R186–196.

77. Kirby DA, Verrier RL. Differential effects of sleep stage on coronary hemodynamic function during stenosis. Physiol Behav. 1989;45:1017–1020.

78. Baust W, Bohnert B. The regulation of heart rate during sleep. Exp Brain Res. 1969;7:169–180.

79. Leichnetz GR. Relationship of spontaneous vagal activity to wakefulness and sleep in the cat. Exp Neurol. 1972;35:194–210.

80. Varbanova A, Nikolov N, Doneshka P. Fluctuations in the vagal and sympathetic tone connected with the circadian cycle and the sleep-wakefulness cycle. Agressologie. 1974;16:23–33.

81. Parmeggiani PL. The autonomic nervous system in sleep. In: Kryger MH, Roth T, Dement WC, eds. Principles and Practice of Sleep Medicine. Philadelphia, Pa: WB Saunders; 1994:194–203.

82. Azzaroni A, Parmeggiani PL. Synchronized sleep duration is related to tonic vasoconstriction of thermoregulatory heat exchanges. J Sleep Res. 1995;4:41–47.

83. Sei H, Morita Y. Effect of ambient temperature on arterial pressure variability during sleep in the rat. J Sleep Res. 1996;5:37–41.

84. Fewell JE, Williams BJ, Hill DE. Behavioral state influences the cardiovascular response to hemorrhage in lambs. J Dev Physiol. 1984;6:339–348.

85. Berger PJ, Horner RSC, Walker AM. Cardio-respiratory response to cool ambient temperature differs with sleep state in neonatal lambs. J Physiol. 1989;412:351–363.

86. Zoccoli G, Cianci T, Lenzi P, et al. Shivering during sleep: relationship between muscle blood flow and fiber type composition. Experientia. 1992;48:228–230.

87. Parmeggiani PL. Telencephalo-diencephalic aspects of sleep mechanisms. Brain Res. 1968;7:350–359.

88. Parmeggiani PL, Franzini C, Lenzi P, et al. Threshold of respiratory responses to preoptic heating during sleep in free moving cats. Brain Res. 1973;52:189–201.

89. Parmeggiani PL, Calasso M, Cianci T. Respiratory effects of preoptic-anterior hypothalamic electrical stimulation during sleep in cats. Sleep. 1980;4:71–82.

90. Glotzbach SF, Heller HC. Changes in the thermal characteristics of hypothalamic neurons during sleep and wakefulness. Brain Res. 1984;309:17–26.

91. Parmeggiani PL, Azzaroni A, Cevolani D, et al. Responses of anterior hypothalamic-preoptic neurons to direct thermal stimulation during wakefulness and sleep. Brain Res. 1983;269:382–385.

92. Parmeggiani PL, Morrison AR. Alterations in autonomic functions during sleep. In: Loewy AD, Spyer KM, eds. Central Regulation of Autonomic Functions. Oxford, England: Oxford University Press; 1990:367–386.

93. Akselrod S, Gordon D, Ubel FA, et al. Power spectrum analysis of heart rate fluctuation: a quantitative probe of beat-to-beat cardiovascular control. Science. 1981;213:220–222.

94. Parati G, Saul JP, Di Rienzo M, et al. Spectral analysis of blood pressure and heart rate variability in evaluating cardiovascular regulation. A critical appraisal. Hypertension. 1995;25:1276–1286.

95. Malliani A, Pagani M, Lombardi F, et al. Cardiovascular neural regulation explored in the frequency domain. Circulation. 1991;84:482–492.

96. Wallin GB, Elam M. Insights from intraneural recordings of sympathetic nerve traffic in humans. News Physiol Sci. 1994;9:203–207.

97. Fletcher EC. Sympathetic activity and blood pressure in the sleep apnea syndrome. Respiration. 1997;64(suppl 1):22–28.

98. Cortelli P, Pierangeli G, Parchi G, et al. Power spectral analysis reveals sympathetic hyperactivity as an early feature of fatal familial insomnia (FFI). Neurology. 1994;44(suppl 2): A363.

99. Cortelli P, Pierangeli G, Provini F, et al. Blood pressure rhythms in sleep disorders and dysautonomia. Ann N Y Acad Sci. 1996;783:204–221.

100. Baharav A, Kotagal S, Gibbons V, et al. Fluctuations in autonomic nervous activity during sleep displayed by power spectrum analysis of heart rate variability. Neurology. 1995;45:1183–1187.

101. Berlad I, Shiltner A, Ben-Haim S, et al. Power spectrum analysis and heart rate variability in stage 4 and REM sleep: evidence for state-specific changes in autonomic dominance. J Sleep Res. 1993;2:88–90.

102. Bonnet MH, Arand DL. Heart rate variability: sleep stage, time of night, arousal influences. Electroencephalogr Clin Neurophysiol. 1997;102:390–396.

103. van de Borne P, Nguyen H, Biston P, et al. Effects of wake and sleep stages on the 24-h autonomic control of blood pressure and heart rate in recumbent men. Am J Physiol. 1994;266:H548–554.

104. Vanoli E, Adamson PB, Ba-Lin MBH, et al. Heart rate variability during specific sleep stages. A comparison of healthy subjects with patients after myocardial infarction. Circulation. 1995;91:1918–1922.

105. Vaughn BV, Quint SR, Messenheimer JA, et al. Heart period variability in sleep. Electroencephalogr Clin Neurophysiol. 1995;94:155–162.

106. Zemaityte D, Varoneckas G, Sokolov E. Heart rhythm control during sleep. Psychophysiology. 1984;21:279–289.

107. Burgess HJ, Trinder J, Kim Y. Cardiac parasympathetic nervous system activity does not increase in anticipation of sleep. J Sleep Res. 1996;5:83–89.

108. Kanamori N, Sakai K, Sei H, et al. Power spectral analysis of blood pressure fluctuations during sleep in normal and decerebrate cat. Arch Ital Biol. 1994;132:105–115.

109. Di Rienzo M, Castiglioni P, Mancia G, et al. 24h sequential spectral analysis of arterial blood pressure and pulse interval in free-moving subjects. IEE Trans Biomed Eng. 1989;36:1066–1075.

110. Furlan R, Guzzetti S, Crivellaro W, et al. Continuous 24-hour assessment of the neural regulation of systemic arterial pressure and RR variabilities in ambulant subjects. Circulation. 1990;81:537–547.

111. Parati G, Castiglioni P, Di Rienzo M, et al. Sequential spectral analysis of 24-hour blood pressure and pulse interval in humans. Hypertension. 1990;16:414–421.

112. Baust W, Weidinger H, Kirchner F. Sympathetic activity during natural sleep and arousal. Arch Ital Biol. 1968;106:379–390.

113. Reiner PD. Correlational analysis of central neuronal activity and sympathetic tone in behaving cats. Brain Res. 1986;378:86–96.

114. Mancia G. Autonomic modulation of the cardiovascular system during sleep. N Engl J Med. 1993;328:347–349.

115. Shimizu T, Takahashi Y, Kogawa S, et al. Muscle sympathetic

nerve activity during apneic episodes in patients with obstructive sleep apnea syndrome. Electroencephalogr Clin Neurophysiol. 1994;93:345–352.

116. Shimizu T, Takahashi Y, Kogawa S, et al. Muscle sympathetic nerve activity during central, mixed and obstructive apnea: are there any differences? Psychiatr Clin Neurosci. 1997;51:397–403.

117. Somers VK, Dyken ME, Clary MP, et al. Sympathetic neural mechanisms in obstructive sleep apnea. J Clin Invest. 1995;96:1897–1904.

118. Yamashiro H, Kryger MH. Review: sleep in heart failure. Sleep. 1993;16:513–523.

119. Hanly PJ, Millar TW, Steljes DG, et al. Respiration and abnormal sleep in patients with congestive heart failure. Chest. 1989;96:480–488.

120. Schafer H, Koehler U, Ploch T, et al. Sleep-related myocardial ischemia and sleep structure in patients with obstructive sleep apnea and coronary heart disease. Chest. 1997;111:387–393.

121. Cassano GB, Maggini C, Guazzelli M. Nocturnal angina and sleep. Prog Neuropsychopharmacol. 1981;5:99–104.

122. Nowlin JB, Troyer WG, Collins WS, et al. The association of nocturnal angina pectoris with dreaming. Ann Intern Med. 1965;63:1040–1046.

Respiratory Physiology: Central Neural Control

John Orem

Leszek Kubin

The medulla and pons contain respiratory neurons that are essential for breathing. In nonrapid eye movement sleep, tonic drives to respiratory neurons are reduced. Tonic drives arise from the reticular formation, from widespread areas of the nervous system that are important for behavioral control of breathing in wakefulness, or from aminergic systems known to be less active in sleep.

In rapid eye movement sleep, there are both inhibitory and excitatory effects on respiratory neurons. The former are related to the atonia of that state, and, in the case of hypoglossal motoneurons, are caused by the loss of excitatory serotonergic input. Excitatory effects, of unknown origins, include activation of inspiratory and expiratory medullary neurons that are important elements of the respiratory oscillator.

Breathing disorders in sleep include obstructive and central sleep apnea. The pathophysiology of these disorders derives in part from the mechanisms described in this chapter.

This chapter discusses the neural control of breathing in sleep and wakefulness and begins with a review of the brainstem respiratory systems.[1]

BRAINSTEM RESPIRATORY NEURONS IN REDUCED OR ANESTHETIZED ANIMALS*

The caudal brainstem has been recognized as the site for the generation of respiration since the early 19th century, when Legallois demonstrated that breathing

*This section, Brainstem Respiratory Neurons in Reduced or Anesthetized Animals, is modified from the corresponding section of the chapter by Orem J, Dick T. Brainstem respiratory neurons and their control during various behaviors. In: Klemm WR, Vertes RP, eds. Brainstem Mechanisms of Behavior. Copyright © 1990 John Wiley & Sons. Reprinted by permission of John Wiley & Sons, Inc.

persisted despite removal of the neuraxis rostral to the medulla oblongata.[2, 3] Several medullary areas contain neurons that either discharge in phase with respiration or tonically drive the cells that produce breathing: the dorsal respiratory group, the ventral respiratory group, the Bötzinger complex, and chemosensitive neurons near the ventral medullary surface. In addition, the pontine respiratory group plays an important role in shaping the pattern of the respiratory motor output.

Dorsal Respiratory Group

The dorsal respiratory group corresponds to the ventrolateral nucleus of tractus solitarius (NTS).[4–7] This nucleus contains neurons whose discharge frequency increases progressively during inspiration. There are other patterns of respiratory activity in the dorsal respiratory group, but these are less common. The dorsal respiratory group receives projections from vagal slowly adapting pulmonary stretch receptors.[8] Three subclasses of dorsal respiratory cells have been defined in the cat on the basis of their response to inflation of the lungs.[9–12] Inspiratory Iα cells are inhibited, just as is breathing; inspiratory Iβ cells are excited paradoxically; and a third subclass, pump cells, are driven entirely by pulmonary stretch receptor afferents.[13] These afferents excite Iβ and pump cells monosynaptically.[11, 14] Both Iα and Iβ cells project to the spinal cord[15–17] and synapse directly on phrenic and intercostal motoneurons.[16, 18] Pump cells project to the ipsilateral and contralateral medial subnuclei of the NTS and to multiple locations within the ventral respiratory group, including the Bötzinger complex.[19, 20]

In addition to the ventrolateral portion of the NTS containing inspiratory neurons, several other subnuclei of the NTS receive vagal afferents from the lungs, bronchi, trachea and larynx[8, 19, 21–24] (see Kubin and Davies[25] for a review). Inspiratory neurons and pump cells have been recorded in the medial and dorsal subnuclei of the NTS.[19, 26] These subnuclei also receive axons from glossopharyngeal sensory neurons that innervate the carotid body,[27, 28] and from laryngeal afferents.[10, 21]

Ventral Respiratory Group and Bötzinger Complex

The ventral respiratory group is a column of cells that extends from the retrofacial nucleus to the first cervical segment and consists of the Bötzinger complex, nucleus ambiguus, and nucleus retroambigualis.[2–6, 29–32] The rostral nucleus ambiguus and the Bötzinger complex contain nonvagal respiratory neurons with many different patterns of respiratory activity. The nucleus retroambigualis contains both inspiratory and expiratory cell types. These neurons may coexist as clusters (see in Merrill,[32] Figure 4) but inspiratory neurons predominate in the rostral part, whereas expiratory neurons predominate at the caudal end.

The striated muscles of the upper airway are innervated by motoneurons of the trigeminal, facial, and hypoglossal nuclei as well as those of the nucleus ambiguus.[33] There is a rostrocaudal somatotopic organization across and within these nuclei: facial motoneurons innervate alae nasi,[34] and nucleus ambiguus motoneurons innervate the pharynx and larynx. Vagal motoneurons innervating the pharynx are located more rostrally in the nucleus ambiguus than are those innervating the larynx.[35, 36]

There are several subtypes of inspiratory neurons in the nucleus retroambigualis.[37–39] They are classified according to their firing patterns and axonal projections. Inspiratory cells with early-onset and augmenting activity may be either propriobulbar cells (i.e., cells with axons remaining in the brainstem) or bulbospinal cells, or they may be vagal motoneurons. Inspiratory neurons with an early-onset, decrementing firing pattern are propriobulbar and project extensively to the contralateral ventral respiratory group.[37] Neurons that discharge a short burst of action potentials late in inspiration and cease firing shortly after inspiration has terminated (late inspiratory neurons) are found in both the dorsal and ventral respiratory groups and are propriobulbar cells. A subset of these cells may play a role in terminating inspiration.[40] There also are cells with an early-expiratory, decrementing pattern of activity, which is referred to as postinspiratory. They are propriobulbar and have inhibitory connections to inspiratory and late expiratory neurons of the ventral respiratory group and to vagal expiratory motoneurons.[41–43] These cells do not excite motoneurons; thus, postinspiratory activity recorded in some upper airway muscles arises from another source. Finally, cells with inspiratory activity patterns are found in the medullary reticular formation between the dorsal and the ventral respiratory group.[44] Some of those cells have spinal axons reaching phrenic motoneurons and medullary axonal ramifications within the hypoglossal motor nucleus. These cells are the first physiologically identified source of inspiratory drive to upper airway, in this case hypoglossal, motoneurons.

Additional cell types with activity related to respiration have been recorded rostrally, ventromedial to the retrofacial nucleus, in an area referred to as the Bötzinger complex. Of those, cells with augmenting expiratory activity have widespread inhibitory connections at both the brainstem and spinal cord levels.[45–47] Another group of cells, generating a preinspiratory burst, are localized in the area just caudal to the Bötzinger complex.[48] These cells are similar to those recorded in the corresponding region of the neonatal rat brainstem in vitro (see below) and make synaptic connections with other cells within the medulla. They may be important elements of the respiratory rhythm–generating network.[49]

Ventral Medullary Surface

The ventral medullary surface has three chemosensitive zones.[50] The use of topical anesthetic agents or cold blockade of these zones eliminates respiratory responses to changes in the pH of the cerebrospinal fluid.[51, 52] Although these chemosensitive areas have been located, the identity of the underlying sensing elements has not been established.[52]

Focal cooling in the region of nucleus paragigantocellularis lateralis causes apnea.[53] Cells near the ventral medullary surface in the in vitro neonatal rat brainstem preparation generate an endogenous respiratory rhythm and are excited by a decrease in pH.[55–61] Comparable cells in adult cats may be localized ventral to the facial nucleus, rostral to the nucleus paragigantocellularis lateralis and Bötzinger complex, and near catecholaminergic cells that project to the spinal cord and synapse with preganglionic sympathetic cells in the intermediolateral cell column.[30, 62]

In contrast to the studies in which the central respiratory chemosensitivity was localized to regions adjacent to the ventral medullary surface, several studies have demonstrated that cells in the NTS,[63] in the medial medulla,[64] or throughout many sites within the pontomedullary reticular formation[65–67] are excited by CO_2. Thus, central respiratory chemosensitivity probably is not limited to the ventral medullary surface.

Pontine Respiratory Group

The pontine respiratory group, which is the pneumotaxic center of Lumsden, is located in the rostral dorsolateral pons and consists of two subnuclei of the parabrachial region: nucleus parabrachialis medialis and the Kölliker-Fuse nucleus. Cells within the pontine respiratory group exhibit inspiratory, expiratory, and phase-spanning activities. The parabrachial nuclei receive input from autonomic and somatic sensory systems and from forebrain structures related to emotional behavior.[68] The pontine respiratory group projects rostrally and caudally.

The pontine respiratory group is not necessary for the generation of respiration because breathing remains rhythmic after separation of the pontine respiratory group from the medulla[69] and because anesthetic agents that attenuate pontine respiratory activity do not prevent breathing.[70] Nevertheless, evidence supports a role for the pontine respiratory group in the processing of vagal afferent input and in determining the duration of the inspiratory and expiratory phases.[2, 71, 72] These functions may be performed by both respiratory- and non–respiratory modulated pontine neurons.[73] One model of the respiratory rhythmogenesis portrays pontine respiratory group neurons synapsing with medullary postinspiratory neurons to affect expiratory phase duration.[74]

Models for the Generation of Respiration

An underlying goal in identifying respiratory neurons and their interconnections is to determine how the respiratory rhythm is generated.[3] There are network[74–78] and pacemaker[79–82] models of the rhythm generator.

Pacemaker models are based on evidence that some cells generate bursts of activity in a respiratory pattern in the absence of synaptic inputs. This evidence is strongest in the in vitro neonatal rat brainstem preparation. In the mature nervous system, however, respiratory cells with pacemaker properties are probably embedded in a network of respiratory neurons that imposes its own rhythm on the pacemakers *(hybrid model).*[83]

Network models depend on interconnections among groups of neurons with distinct properties and activity patterns. The neuronal types incorporated in most such models include early inspiratory, augmenting inspiratory, decrementing inspiratory, late inspiratory, postinspiratory, augmenting expiratory, and expiratory-inspiratory phase–spanning cells. Network models account for the different patterns of activity by postulating specific synaptic relations (excitatory and inhibitory) among the neurons. The models also assume that tonic excitatory inputs to the cells that are parts of the network derive from the reticular formation and central and peripheral chemoreceptors. Reciprocal inhibitory connections among the network cells active in different portions of the respiratory cycle are essential for network theories of respiratory rhythmogenesis.

RESPIRATORY NEURONS IN THE UNANESTHETIZED, INTACT ANIMAL

Some studies have reported respiratory neurons throughout the brainstem,[98–102] but these results have been challenged by the demonstration that the detection methods used to obtain them are faulty.[103] It is certain that respiratory neurons are concentrated in the groups (dorsal, ventral, and pontine) defined by studies of reduced and anesthetized animals.[84–94] In addition, respiratory-related neurons have been recorded in the amygdala, the anterior cingulate gyrus, the orbital frontal cortex, and the mesencephalic central gray.[68, 95–97] There are many respiratory neurons in the intact unanesthetized animal that have a low η^2 value[89]; that is, the relationship of their discharge to breathing is weak and variable. These weakly modulated cells are especially sensitive to changes in the sleep-wake state.

ACTIVITY OF RESPIRATORY NEURONS IN NONRAPID EYE MOVEMENT SLEEP

Medullary Respiratory Neuronal Activity

There is a decrease in medullary respiratory activity in nonrapid eye movement (NREM) sleep[84, 90, 104, 105] (Fig. 15–1). The neurons affected are from the ventral and dorsal respiratory groups and from the hypoglossal nucleus. Some cells are affected more than others. Cells with high η^2 values are little affected, whereas cells with low η^2 values are affected greatly by NREM

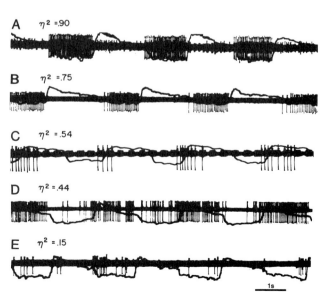

Figure 15–1. Medullary respiratory neurons recorded in intact, unanesthetized cats during NREM sleep. Respiration recorded by pneumotachography; downward deflections signal inspiration. *A–E,* Respiratory cells with differing η^2 values. (Modified from Orem J, Dick T. Consistency and signal strength of respiratory neuronal activity. J Neurophysiol. 1983;50:1098–1107.)

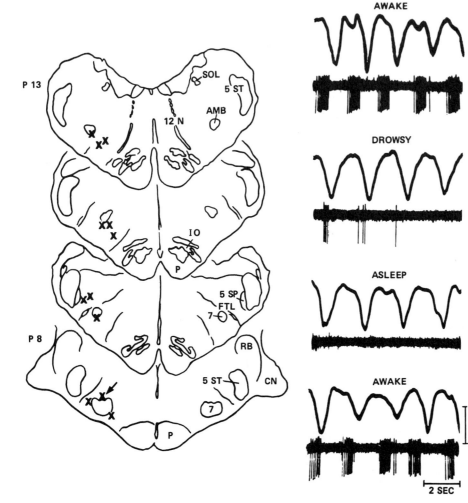

Figure 15–2. The activity of a sleep-sensitive respiratory neuron, and the locations of it and others like it. AMB, Nucleus ambiguus; CN, cochlear nucleus; FTL, lateral tegmental field; IO, inferior olive; P, pyramidal tract; RB, restiform body; SOL, solitary tract; 5 SP, nucleus of the spinal tract of V; 5 ST, spinal tract of V; 7, facial nucleus; 12 N, hypoglossal nerve. (From Orem J, Montplaisir J, Dement W. Changes in the activity of respiratory neurones during sleep. Brain Res. 1974;82:309–315.)

sleep (Figs. 15–2 through 15–4). This indicates that sleep affects primarily neurons that receive larger proportions of nonrespiratory afference (i.e., those with lower η^2 values). In support of this, iontophoresis of glutamate onto silent and sleep-sensitive respiratory neurons can induce a respiratory activity pattern during sleep.[105] This indicates that respiratory-modulated inputs to these cells are preserved in sleep and that these inputs are amplified or depressed by state-dependent tonic inputs.

Pontine, Mesencephalic, and Telencephalic Respiratory Neuronal Activities

Pontine parabrachial respiratory-modulated neurons demonstrate changes in firing rate when the animal enters NREM sleep, but increases and decreases in activity are observed with a similar prevalence, with, on average, a minimal decrease.[93, 94, 106, 107] One study has found that respiratory activity in the pons is weak even in wakefulness and that with sleep there are few consistent changes across the population of pontine respiratory. The functional significance of these and other results showing state-related changes in the activity of respiratory cells in the amygdala, anterior cingu-

late gyrus, orbital frontal cortex, and mesencephalic central gray[68, 95–97] is not known.

SLEEP-DEPENDENT CHANGES IN TONIC INPUTS TO THE RESPIRATORY SYSTEM

Tonic inputs to the respiratory system are apparently much affected by changes in state of consciousness. There are many regions of the central nervous system that provide nonrespiratory (tonic) input to the respiratory system. Those considered in the following three sections are (1) the brainstem reticular formation, (2) the collection of higher structures that exert behavioral control on the respiratory system, and (3) the aminergic brainstem nuclei. One common feature of these three systems is that they provide central respiratory neurons and respiratory motoneurons with various forms of excitation during wakefulness that can be collectively described as the wakefulness stimulus for breathing.

Reticular Activation

Stimulation of the reticular formation excites the respiratory system.[109–119] Midbrain reticular stimulation

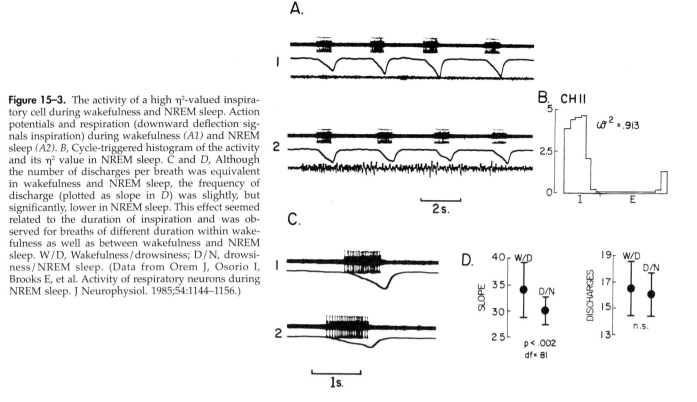

A.

B. CH II

$\eta^2 = .913$

C.

2s.

1s.

D.

SLOPE

W/D

D/N

p < .002
df = 81

DISCHARGES

W/D

D/N

n.s.

Figure 15–3. The activity of a high η^2-valued inspiratory cell during wakefulness and NREM sleep. Action potentials and respiration (downward deflection signals inspiration) during wakefulness *(A1)* and NREM sleep *(A2)*. B, Cycle-triggered histogram of the activity and its η^2 value in NREM sleep. C and D, Although the number of discharges per breath was equivalent in wakefulness and NREM sleep, the frequency of discharge (plotted as slope in *D*) was slightly, but significantly, lower in NREM sleep. This effect seemed related to the duration of inspiration and was observed for breaths of different duration within wakefulness as well as between wakefulness and NREM sleep. W/D, Wakefulness/drowsiness; D/N, drowsiness/NREM sleep. (Data from Orem J, Osorio I, Brooks E, et al. Activity of respiratory neurons during NREM sleep. J Neurophysiol. 1985;54:1144–1156.)

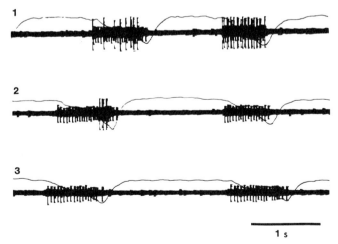

Figure 15–4. Activity of a low η^2-valued (large action potentials) and a high η^2-valued (small action potentials) cell during wakefulness (1), drowsiness (2), and NREM sleep (3). Activity of the low η^2-valued cell varied from breath to breath in wakefulness and drowsiness and was absent in sleep. The discharge rate of the high η^2-valued cell decreased slightly in sleep. Respiration recorded by pneumotachography. Downward deflections signal inspiration. (From Orem J, Osorio I, Brooks E, et al. Activity of respiratory neurons during NREM sleep. J Neurophysiol. 1985;54:1144–1156.)

causes a reduction in the duration of expiration and an increased rate of rise and amplitude of phrenic nerve activity.[116] It also causes an increase in laryngeal abductor activity[118]—converting it from patterns characteristic of NREM sleep to those of wakefulness, and, like wakefulness, reticular stimulation preferentially facilitates the activity of the muscles of the extrathoracic airway rather than the muscles of the diaphragm.[118] Respiratory activation declines slowly after the cessation of reticular stimulation.[116, 117]

Respiratory afterdischarge,[120] an enhancement of respiratory activity after a period of application of an excitatory stimulus, is a reflection of reticular activation. It can last for 1 to 5 min in the cat after a strong compression of a hindlimb muscle or stimulation of the carotid sinus nerve containing afferents from arterial chemoreceptors. Afterdischarge is a central phenomenon requiring only the pontomedullary brainstem (i.e., it occurs in decerebrate and cerebellectomized preparations), and it does not depend on, but rather affects, circuits that produce the respiratory rhythm. The neurotransmitters involved in afterdischarge are not known: cats pretreated with antiserotonergic agents (methysergide, parachlorophenylalanine, and 5,7-dihydroxytryptamine), dopamine-norepinephrine antagonists (alpha-methyltyrosine and haloperidol), and the endorphin antagonist naloxone have afterdischarges equivalent to those of unpretreated animals.

Behavioral Control

Behavioral control of breathing may be *reflexive*, as occurs in sneezing, coughing, vomiting, and eructation, or *voluntary* (or learned), as occurs during speaking, breath holding, and playing a wind instrument. These behavioral acts require the integration of nonrespiratory inputs into circuits of the respiratory oscillator. Behavioral respiratory acts generally occur only in wakefulness. For example, mechanical and chemical

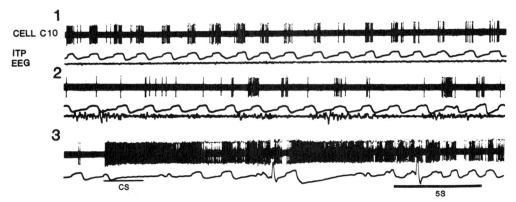

Figure 15–5. A low η^2-valued (0.30) inspiratory cell that was activated when inspiration was stopped behaviorally. 1, Spontaneous activity of the cell during wakefulness; top trace, action potentials of the cell; middle trace, intratracheal pressure, negative pressures (inspiration) indicated by upward deflections; lower trace, electroencephalogram. 2, Activity of the cell during drowsiness and NREM sleep. Note that it is not obviously respiratory in these states. 3, Intense activation of the cell during and after the behavioral inhibition of inspiration elicited by the conditioning stimuli (CS). (Modified from Orem J. Behavioral inspiratory inhibition: inactivated and activated respiratory cells. J Neurophysiol. 1989;62:1069–1078.)

stimulation of the larynx[121] and bronchopulmonary stimulation[122] cause coughing in wakefulness but not in sleep.[123] In human beings, wakefulness, although not sufficient, is necessary for respiratory control from supramedullary structures.[124] The concept has emerged, therefore, that the wakefulness enables, or facilitates, various behavioral and reflexive influences that collectively stimulate the respiratory system.

The list of structures that can control brainstem and spinal respiratory neurons is long and includes structures from all levels of the neuraxis. For example, hypothalamic control occurs in relation to temperature regulation and locomotion,[125] and telencephalic structures can control breathing—a control exerted presumably in relation to emotional and volitional acts.[124, 126] The central nucleus of the amygdala, the anterior cingulate gyrus, the orbital frontal cortex, and the central gray contain cells that have state-dependent respiratory activity.[68, 95–97] Stimulation or inactivation of limbic,[96, 97, 126, 127] subcortical,[128, 129] and cerebellar[130, 131] structures can influence the respiratory system.

The site of behavioral control within the respiratory neuraxis varies depending on the behavioral act[132–147] (Figs. 15–5 and 15–6).

Aminergic Systems

Serotonin (5-hydroxytryptamine [5-HT])- and norepinephrine-containing neurons of the brainstem may play a role in sleep-related changes in breathing because of a dependence of their activity on the sleep-wake state and their known effects on central respiratory neurons and respiratory motoneurons. The activity of the neurons belonging to these two aminergic systems is highest during active wakefulness, declines as the animal enters NREM sleep, and is minimal during REM sleep.[148–150] Both 5-HT[151–156] and norepinephrine[157–160] have excitatory effects on motoneurons, including those innervating the upper airway and respiratory pump muscles. Antagonists of the excitatory effects of 5-HT reduce the spontaneous activity of hypoglossal motoneurons, thus showing the presence of an endogenous serotonergic excitatory drive.[153] Data from a reduced carbachol model of REM sleep–like atonia (described below) reveal that a withdrawal of this drive is associated with decreased activity of hypoglossal motoneurons and decrements in extracellular levels of 5-HT in the hypoglossal nucleus region (Fig. 15–7).[161–163] Thus, 5-HT acting on upper airway

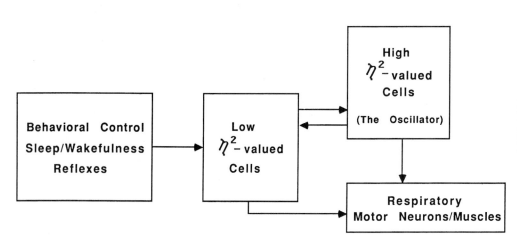

Figure 15–6. Schema illustrating hypothesized relations among nonrespiratory inputs, high and low η^2-valued cells, and respiratory motor neurons.

motoneurons during wakefulness may represent an important neurochemical substrate of the wakefulness stimulus. The magnitude of the excitatory effect of 5-HT on different groups of upper airway motoneurons varies, however, and this may relate, at least in part, to different magnitudes of the suppressant effects of sleep on different upper airway muscles.[164]

In contrast to its excitatory effects in motoneurons, 5-HT has predominantly an inhibitory effect on central respiratory neurons.[152, 165–167] Because serotonergic neurons become silent during REM sleep, this may explain, at least in part, why the activity of respiratory neurons increases during REM sleep. From this, it also follows that 5-HT may exert opposite effects at motoneuronal and respiratory premotoneuronal levels. In different pools of respiratory motoneurons, the relative magnitude of the respiratory drive provided by central respiratory neurons and the tonic drive resulting from a direct excitatory effect of 5-HT may vary. Quantitative differences in this regard among different pools of respiratory motoneurons may help explain why during sleep the level of activity increases in some, but decreases in other, respiratory muscles.

Norepinephrine is also predominantly excitatory to motoneurons but inhibitory at the level of medullary respiratory neurons.[168] However, tonic endogenous noradrenergic effects have not been demonstrated, so far, in the respiratory system during wakefulness. Locus ceruleus neurons, which are often regarded as typical of norepinephrine-containing brainstem neurons, have highly phasic patterns of activity and are prefer-entially excited by peripheral stimuli that are perceived as novel or stressful.[169] Thus, by extrapolation from the behavior of these neurons, noradrenergic effects on breathing may be phasic and particularly relevant during states of emotional or sensory stimulation during wakefulness.

ACTIVITY OF RESPIRATORY NEURONS IN REM SLEEP

Characteristics of Breathing in REM Sleep

Defining characteristics of REM sleep include cortical desynchronization, hippocampal theta rhythm, muscle atonia, ponto-geniculo-occipital (PGO) waves,[170–174] rapid eye movements, and muscle twitches. In the respiratory system, during REM sleep, the frequency of breathing increases to rates often exceeding those in wakefulness.[175] However, peak inspiratory airflow rates are about 15% less than those in NREM sleep or wakefulness. In cats[176] and adolescent human beings,[177] but not in rats,[178] atonia of the intercostal muscles reduces or eliminates costal breathing in REM sleep. Many upper airway respiratory muscles are also atonic or hypotonic.[118, 179, 180] Both apneas and hyperpneas occur as the extremes of very irregular breathing. Ventilatory responses to chemical stimuli and other respiratory reflexes are impaired during phasic REM activity,[181] and laryngeal and diaphragmatic responses to occlusions are inconsistent and variable.[182]

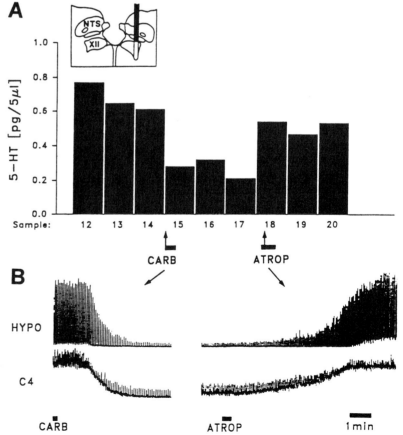

Figure 15–7. Extracellular level of 5-hydroxytryptamine (5-HT) is reduced in the region of the hypoglossal motor nucleus (XII) during the REM sleep–like atonia produced by pontine injection of carbachol. *A*, 5-HT level, as determined by microdialysis, in samples of the dialysate collected in successive 20-min intervals from the XII nucleus in a decerebrate, paralyzed, and artificially ventilated cat. At the end of collection of sample 14, carbachol was injected into the pons and produced a suppression of postural activity and respiratory activity in the XII nerve (*B*). One hour and three samples later, pontine microinjection of atropine terminated the atonia. The level of 5-HT decreased in association with the onset of the atonia and subsequently increased when the atonia was terminated. The inset shows the location of the dialysis probe in this experiment (XII, hypoglossal motor nucleus; NTS, nucleus tractus solitarius). *B*, Moving averages of activities recorded from the XII nerve (HYPO) and a cervical nerve branch innervating dorsal neck muscles (C4) at times of the transition into and out of the carbachol-induced atonia. The bars attached to the marker arrows in *A* show the position of the records shown in *B* relative to the histogram showing the changes in 5-HT level. (Modified from Brain Research, Vol 645, Kubin L, Reignier C, Tojima H, et al, Changes in serotonin level in the hypoglossal nucleus region during the carbachol-induced atonia, 291–302, Copyright 1994, with permission from Elsevier Science.)

The variable breathing pattern of REM sleep does not depend on variations in chemoreceptor,[183] vagal,[184–186] or thoracic[186, 187] afferent activity. Irregular breathing during REM sleep is seen in the neonate[188] and during spontaneously occurring REM sleep–like state in the pontine animal.[189]

Respiratory Neuronal Activity in REM Sleep in the Intact, Unanesthetized Animal

Variability in the Breathing Pattern. An outstanding feature of respiratory neuronal activity in REM sleep is its great variability. There is a good correspondence between the activity of some ventral respiratory group neurons and irregular respiration.[84, 190] This indicates that the irregularities of breathing in REM sleep are, at least in part, mediated by brainstem respiratory neurons.

The source of the extreme variability in breathing in REM sleep has been the subject of studies that, as noted, found it does not depend on variations in chemoreceptor, vagal, thoracic, or suprapontine influences. However, PGO wave activity and the activity of brainstem respiratory neurons covary: greater neuronal activity is associated with periods of greater PGO activity.[190] These relationships suggest that the respiratory activity in the medulla is influenced by nonrespiratory processes peculiar to REM sleep. In addition, fractionations, which are intermittent inhibitions of diaphragmatic activity, are sometimes associated with bursts of PGO waves and rapid eye movements[85, 191, 192] (Figs. 15–8 and 15–9).

The irregular breathing pattern of REM sleep was believed, early on, to be related to the content of the dream. Accordingly, apneas were thought to occur because the dreamer held his or her breath, and tachypneas were thought to occur because of the dreamed excitement or exertion.[193] This idea persists in current control theories of breathing in sleep and wakefulness.[194] An abstract reports that a cat trained to inhibit inspiration in response to a conditioning stimulus performed this response capably in REM sleep.[195] This finding indicates that in this state, the necessary sensory information can be transmitted centrally and appropriately interpreted to produce a behavioral response within the respiratory system. This may be relevant for the occurrence of breathing irregularities characteristic of REM sleep because respiratory irregularities are related to phasic events of REM sleep,[196] and because phasic events are associated with the motor activation shown by cats with pontine lesions resulting in REM sleep without muscle atonia.[197, 198] This association may indicate that the irregular breathing pattern is the result of activation of behavioral mechanisms.

Increased Respiratory Activity in REM Sleep. With few exceptions, cells throughout the nervous system are more active in REM sleep than in NREM sleep. This generalized activation in REM sleep includes also some parts of the respiratory system. For example, the rate of breathing is higher in that state, some respiratory neurons are more active than in NREM sleep,[190]

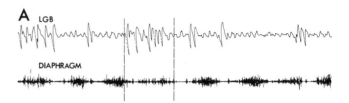

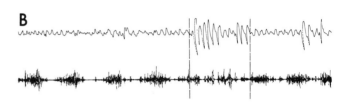

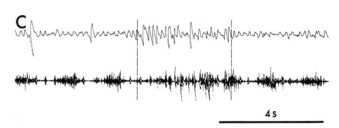

Figure 15–8. Three episodes of diaphragmatic and ponto-geniculo-occipital (PGO) activity recorded from the same cat in the same REM period, illustrating the tendency for bursting PGO activity to fractionate diaphragmatic activity. Bursts are denoted by vertical lines. LGB, lateral geniculate body. (Republished with permission of the American Sleep Disorders Association, 6301 Bandel Road, Suite 101, Rochester, MN 55901. *Neuronal Mechanisms of Respiration in REM Sleep* (figure), J. Orem, *Sleep*, 1980, Vol. 3. Reproduced by permission of the publisher via Copyright Clearance Center, Inc.)

and diaphragmatic activity may have a greater rate of rise.[201]

Medullary respiratory neurons activated in REM sleep include augmenting and late inspiratory cells[200] (Fig. 15–10) and some augmenting expiratory cells.[202] This finding suggests that the various forms of respiratory depression in REM sleep (hypotonia of upper airway and intercostal muscles) do not result from a disfacilitation of respiratory motoneurons secondary to inactivation of brainstem respiratory neurons (see Kubin et al.[199]).

Some augmenting expiratory neurons are active during even the very short expirations that occur during periods of irregular and rapid breathing in REM sleep.[202] Therefore, fractionations, or brief interruptions of diaphragmatic bursts, may not be caused by phasic inhibition of phrenic motoneurons[85]; instead, they may represent the extreme of very rapid breathing produced by the respiratory oscillator in REM sleep.

Similar to medullary respiratory neurons, many, but not all, pontine parabrachial respiratory neurons show prominent increases in activity during REM sleep.[94, 108] Similar changes occur in non–respiratory-modulated cells in this region.[94, 107] Cells showing increases or decreases in activity during natural REM sleep show the same type of change during the REM sleep–like

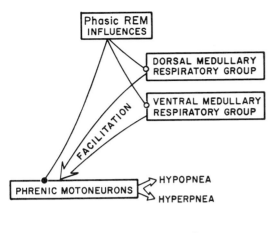

Figure 15–9. A model of opposing phasic REM sleep influences. The model proposes that there are excitatory phasic REM influences on both the dorsal and ventral medullary respiratory group—influences that are, in turn, relayed to phrenic motor neurons. However, there are also phasic REM inhibitory influences that bypass the medullary cells. The result of these antagonistic influences may be either hypopnea or hypernea, depending on their relative weights. (Republished with permission of the American Sleep Disorders Association, 6301 Bandel Road, Suite 101, Rochester, MN 55901. *Neuronal Mechanisms of Respiration in REM Sleep* (figure), J. Orem, *Sleep*, 1980, Vol. 3. Reproduced by permission of the publisher via Copyright Clearance Center, Inc.)

state produced by pontine injections of carbachol in a chronically instrumented, intact animal.[106, 107]

The excitation of central respiratory neurons in REM sleep may arise from nonrespiratory and state-specific excitatory drives. Its function may be to oppose the increased airway resistance and increased chest wall compliance that result from the atonia of that state.

CARBACHOL MODEL OF BREATHING IN REM SLEEP

The characteristic signs of REM sleep (e.g., cortical desynchronization, hippocampal theta rhythm, muscle atonia, PGO waves, rapid eye movements, muscle twitches) depend on, or at least can be controlled from, the rostral brainstem.[203–207]

Mesopontine cholinergic mechanisms play a critical role in the activation and orchestration of these distributed executive systems into the unified state of REM sleep.[208–210] Microinjections of cholinergic agonists (e.g., carbachol, bethanechol, neostigmine) into the dorsal pontine reticular formation induce a REM sleep–like state that includes major hallmarks of the natural REM sleep (e.g., see George et al.,[211] Mitler and Dement,[212] and Baghdoyan et al.[213]). In the cat, the site at which carbachol is effective is discrete and localized ventral to the locus ceruleus,[214, 215] whereas in the rat, the effective sites are more widely distributed within the reticular formation of the rostral pons and caudal midbrain,[216, 217] and the enhancement of REM sleep is less powerful.[218] In both cats and rats, individual signs of REM sleep such as postural atonia, theta rhythm, or PGO waves can be produced from wider or other (or both) regions of the pons and midbrain.[206, 207, 212, 214, 219] Increases in acetylcholine release occur during natural REM sleep in the pontine region sensitive to carbachol,[220] and lesions of the laterodorsal tegmental and pedunculopontine tegmental nuclei, two major pontine groups of cholinergic cells, disrupt REM sleep.[221] Thus, the executive systems that produce the characteristics of REM sleep are localized within the mesopontine tegmentum and are cholinergic and cholinoceptive.

The ability to produce a REM sleep–like state, or its individual signs, by pontine injections of carbachol

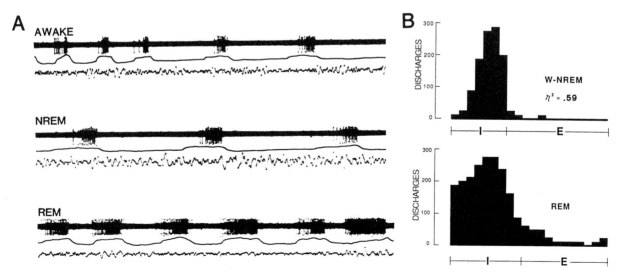

Figure 15–10. Increased and advanced activity of a late inspiratory neuron in REM sleep. *A*, The cell discharges during the last part of inspiration in wakefulness and NREM sleep but is active throughout inspiration during REM sleep. Traces from top to bottom for each section are the action potentials, intratracheal pressure (inspiration is signaled by an upward deflection), and the electroencephalogram. *B*, Cycle-triggered histograms constructed from 50 breaths in wakefulness-NREM sleep and REM sleep. (Modified from Orem J. The activity of late respiratory cells during the behavioral inhibition of inspiration. Brain Res. 1988;458:224–230.)

has been used to study the mechanisms of respiratory changes characteristic of REM sleep in chronically instrumented cats,[222, 223] decerebrate cats,[224-226] decerebrate rats,[217] and urethane-anesthetized rats.[227] The results show that the pattern of the depression of activity in respiratory pump and upper airway muscles after carbachol is similar to that reported during normal REM sleep.[222, 224, 226] However, the respiratory rate is in most cases reduced and regular in contrast to natural REM sleep, where it is highly variable and, on average, accelerated. To explain this difference, Kimura et al.[224] proposed that breathing irregularities may be caused by rapidly changing levels of endogenous acetylcholine in the pons that are likely to occur during natural REM sleep but cannot be adequately mimicked by carbachol microinjections. Such an interpretation is consistent with early reports that irregular breathing is present during the REM sleep–like state occurring spontaneously in the pontine animal.[189]

Suprapontine structures may be necessary for an increase in respiratory rate during REM sleep.[227] In anesthetized rats, pontine carbachol sometimes evokes cortical desynchronization and sometimes does not. When the former, but not the latter, occurs, the respiratory rate increases (Fig. 15–11).

The depressant effects of the carbachol-induced state

are more powerfully expressed in some respiratory motor outputs than in others: phrenic, inspiratory intercostal, and recurrent laryngeal nerve activities are less depressed than are hypoglossal, vagal pharyngeal, and expiratory intercostal nerve activities.[224, 226] These differences in the magnitude of the suppression may be the result of the loss of tonic (nonrespiratory) influences that vary in importance for the different respiratory nerves. Some support for this idea can be gleaned from Figure 2 of Kimura et al.,[224, p. 2283] which shows considerable nonrespiratory (tonic) activity in the hypoglossal nerves but not in the phrenic and inspiratory intercostal nerves. Similarly, in decerebrate rats, pontine carbachol strongly suppresses the tonic, but not the phasic inspiratory, component of the activity recorded from intercostal muscles.[217]

In the decerebrate cat carbachol model, the atonia of hypoglossal motoneurons is not caused by inhibition mediated by amino acids such as glycine or gamma-aminobutyric acid.[228] Instead, there is a withdrawal of serotonergic excitatory influences (discussed previously and in Kubin et al.[229]). These results are supported by the demonstration that antagonism of serotonergic excitatory effects during wakefulness strongly reduced the activity of genihyoid and sternohyoid muscles in the English bulldog, whereas the diaphrag-

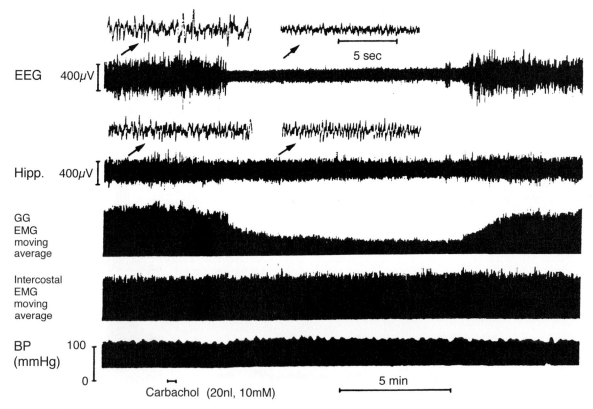

Figure 15–11. Pontine injections of carbachol can produce a complex set of REM sleep–like phenomena in urethane-anesthetized, spontaneously breathing rats. In this example, at the time of slow-wave cortical electroencephalographic (EEG) and desynchronized hippocampal activity, carbachol was injected at the marker and produced EEG desynchronization, theta rhythm in the hippocampus, suppression of the genioglossal muscle activity, and a small increase in blood pressure. The inspiratory-modulated activity of the intercostal muscles was unchanged, as is typical of natural REM sleep in rats. The insets above the cortical and hippocampal EEG signals show 30× expanded segments of the main traces taken from periods before and after pontine carbachol, as marked by arrows. The respiratory rate increased during this response to carbachol from 47 to 52 breaths/min. (Modified from Neuroscience, vol 93, Horner RL, Kubin L, Pontine carbachol elicits multiple REM sleep-like neural events in urethane-anesthetized rats, 215–226, Copyright 1999, with permission from Elsevier Science.)

matic activity was much less affected.[230] It remains to be determined the extent to which these findings can be generalized to other upper airway muscles and applied to natural REM sleep.

CONCLUSIONS

In NREM sleep, respiration is controlled by an automatic system driven by chemical stimuli. There is a class of respiratory neurons in the medulla that seems to be the core of this automatic system. These neurons are quintessentially respiratory, and they are little affected by NREM sleep. These cells (cells with high η^2 values) produce consistent respiratory activity and are relatively insensitive to nonrespiratory influences. There are other respiratory cells that are less ideally respiratory; these cells (cells with low η^2 values) produce weak or inconsistent respiratory signals and are affected greatly by NREM sleep and by various nonrespiratory influences. The contribution of the latter cells to shaping of the respiratory motor output needs more study, but it seems clear that it is unevenly distributed among different respiratory motor outputs (e.g., respiratory pump and upper airway muscles).

The diversity of brainstem respiratory neurons has led to the concept that the effect of sleep on brainstem respiratory activity is proportional to the amount of nonrespiratory component in that activity. The corollary is that the wakefulness stimulus for breathing is nonrespiratory in form and affects some respiratory neurons more than others.

Many structures may send nonrespiratory information to medullary respiratory neurons; these include the reticular formation, the raphe nuclei, and the complex of central nervous system structures involved in behavioral control. Other less-investigated, nonrespiratory motor systems may also provide inputs to the respiratory system in wakefulness as part of a bracing of the muscular system for movement.

Medullary respiratory neurons have extremely variable behavior in REM sleep—behavior that can in large part account for the irregular breathing of that state. It is also known that medullary respiratory activity in REM sleep is influenced by at least one type of phasic REM sleep event, the PGO wave, a finding clearly indicating nonrespiratory and state-specific influences on the respiratory system in REM sleep. There are both excitatory and suppressant influences on the respiratory system in REM sleep. Work with the carbachol model shows that the latter results, at least in part, from the loss of serotonergic excitation of respiratory motoneurons. Work in the intact unanesthetized animals shows that the central respiratory drive, although erratic, is often increased in REM sleep. The source of this excitation is not known.

Acknowledgments

This work was made possible by grants HL21257 (to J.O.) and HL47600 and HL42236 (to L.K.) from the National Heart, Lung, and Blood Institute of the National Institutes of Health.

References

1. Orem J, Dick T. Brainstem respiratory neurons and their control during various behaviors. In: Klemm WR, Vertes RP, eds. Brainstem Mechanisms of Behavior. New York, NY: John Wiley & Sons; 1990:383–406.
2. von Euler C. Brain stem mechanisms for generation and control of breathing pattern. In: Cherniack NS, Widdicombe JG, eds. Handbook of Physiology. Control of Breathing; vol 2. Bethesda, Md: American Physiological Society; 1986:1–67.
3. Feldman JL. Neurophysiology of breathing in mammals. In: Bloom FE, ed. Handbook of Physiology. The Nervous System; vol 4. Bethesda, Md: American Physiological Society; 1986:463–524.
4. Berger AJ, Mitchell RA, Severinghaus JW. Medical progress: regulation of respiration. N Engl J Med. 1977;297(pt 1):92–97.
5. Berger AJ, Mitchell RA, Severinghaus JW. Medical progress: regulation of respiration. N Engl J Med. 1977;297(pt 2):138–143.
6. Berger AJ, Mitchell RA, Severinghaus JW. Medical progress: regulation of respiration. N Engl J Med. 1977;297(pt 3):194–201.
7. de Castro D, Lipski J, Kanjhan R. Electrophysiological study of dorsal respiratory neurons in the medulla oblongata of the rat. Brain Res. 1994;639:49–56.
8. Berger AJ, Averill DB. Projection of single pulmonary stretch receptors to solitary tract region. J Neurophysiol. 1983;49:819–830.
9. von Baumgarten R, Kanzow E. The interaction of two types of inspiratory neurons in the region of the tractus solitarius of the cat. Arch Ital Biol. 1958;96:361–373.
10. Berger AJ. Dorsal respiratory group neurons in the medulla of the cat: spinal projections, responses to lung inflation and superior laryngeal nerve stimulation. Brain Res. 1977;135:231–254.
11. Berger AJ, Dick TE. Connectivity of slowly adapting pulmonary stretch receptors with dorsal medullary respiratory neurons. J Neurophysiol. 1987;58:1259–1274.
12. Cohen MI, Feldman JL. Discharge properties of dorsal medullary inspiratory neurons: relation to pulmonary afferent and phrenic efferent discharge. J Neurophysiol. 1984;51:753–776.
13. Cohen MI, Feldman JL. Models of respiratory phase-switching. Fed Proc. 1977;36:2367–2374.
14. Backman SB, Anders C, Ballantyne D, et al. Evidence for a monosynaptic connection between slowly adapting pulmonary stretch receptor afferents and inspiratory beta neurones. Pflugers Arch. 1984;402:129–136.
15. Dick TE, Viana F, Berger AJ. Electrophysiological determination of the axonal projections of single dorsal respiratory group neurons to the cervical spinal cord of cat. Brain Res. 1988;454:31–39.
16. Duffin J, Lipski J. Monosynaptic excitation of thoracic motoneurones by inspiratory neurones of the nucleus tractus solitarius in the cat. J Physiol (Lond). 1987;390:415–431.
17. Hilaire G, Monteau R. Connexions entre les neurones inspiratoires bulbaires et les motoneurones phréniques et intercostaux. J Physiol Paris. 1976;72:987–1000.
18. Lipski J, Kubin L, Jodkowski J. Synaptic action of R_β neurons on phrenic motoneurons studied with spike-triggered averaging. Brain Res. 1983;288:105–118.
19. Davies RO, Kubin L, Pack AI. Pulmonary stretch receptor relay neurones of the cat: location and contralateral medullary projections. J Physiol (Lond). 1987;383:571–585.
20. Ezure K, Tanaka I. Pump neurons of the nucleus of the solitary tract project widely to the medulla. Neurosci Lett. 1996;215:123–126.
21. Kalia M, Mesulam M-M. Brain stem projections of sensory and motor components of the vagus complex in the cat, II: laryngeal, tracheobronchial, pulmonary, cardiac, and gastrointestinal branches. J Comp Neurol. 1980;193:467–508.
22. Davies RO, Kubin L. Projection of pulmonary rapidly adapting receptors to the medulla of the cat: an antidromic mapping study. J Physiol (Lond). 1986;373:63–86.
23. Kalia M, Richter D. Rapidly adapting pulmonary receptor afferents, I: arborization in the nucleus of the tractus solitarius. J Comp Neurol. 1988;274:560–573.
24. Kubin L, Kimura H, Davies RO. The medullary projections of

afferent bronchopulmonary C fibres in the cat as shown by antidromic mapping. J Physiol (Lond). 1991;435:207–228.

25. Kubin L, Davies RO. Central pathways of pulmonary and airway vagal afferents. In: Dempsey JA, Pack AI, eds. Regulation of Breathing. New York, NY: Marcel Dekker; 1994:219–284.

26. Pantaleo T, Corda M. Respiration-related neurons in the medial nuclear complex of the solitary tract of the cat. Respir Physiol. 1986;64:135–148.

27. Berger AJ. Distribution of carotid sinus nerve afferent fibers to solitary tract nuclei of the cat using transganglionic transport of horseradish peroxidase. Neurosci Lett. 1979;14:153–158.

28. Claps A, Torrealba F. The carotid body connections: a WGA-HRP study in the cat. Brain Res. 1988;455:123–133.

29. Ellenberger HH, Feldman JL. Monosynaptic transmission of respiratory drive to phrenic motoneurons from brainstem bulbospinal neurons in rats. J Comp Neurol. 1988;269:47–57.

30. Feldman JL, Ellenberger HH. Central coordination of respiratory and cardiovascular control in mammals. Annu Rev Physiol. 1988;50:593–606.

31. Kalia MP. Anatomical organization of central respiratory neurons. Annu Rev Physiol. 1981;43:105–120.

32. Merrill EG. The lateral respiratory neurones of the medulla: their associations with nucleus ambiguus, nucleus retroambigualis, the spinal accessory nucleus and the spinal cord. Brain Res. 1970;24:11–28.

33. Iscoe SD. Central control of the upper airway. In: Mathew OP, Sant' Ambrogio G, eds. Respiratory Function of the Upper Airway. New York, NY: Marcel Dekker; 1988:125–192.

34. Bystrzycka EK, Nail BS. The source of the respiratory drive to nasolabialis motoneurones in the rabbit: a HRP study. Brain Res. 1983;266:183–191.

35. Davis PJ, Nail BS. On the location and size of laryngeal motoneurons in the cat and rabbit. J Comp Neurol. 1984;230:13–32.

36. Yoshida Y, Mitsumasu T, Mivazaki T, et al. Distribution of motoneurons in the brain stem of monkeys, innervating the larynx. Brain Res Bull. 1984;13:413–419.

37. Merrill EG. Finding a respiratory function for the medullary respiratory neurons. In: Bellairs R, Gray EG, eds. Essays on the Nervous System. Oxford, England: Clarendon Press; 1974:451–486.

38. Smith JC, Feldman JL. Discharge patterns of medullary respiratory neurons in mammalian brainstem in vitro. Soc Neurosci Abstr. 1988;14:1060.

39. Smith JC, Liu G, Feldman JL. Medullary respiratory neuron populations in neonatal rat brainstem-spinal cord in vitro. FASEB J. 1988;2:A509.

40. Cohen MI, Huang W-X, Barnhardt R, et al. Timing of medullary late-inspiratory neuron discharges: vagal afferent effects indicate possible off-switch function. J Neurophysiol. 1993;69:1784–1787.

41. Richter DW, Ballantyne D, Remmers JE. The differential organization of medullary postinspiratory activities. Pflugers Arch. 1987;410:420–427.

42. Ezure K, Manabe M. Decrementing expiratory neurons of the Bötzinger complex, II: direct inhibitory synaptic linkage with ventral respiratory group neurons. Exp Brain Res. 1988;72:159–166.

43. Ezure K, Manabe M, Otake K. Excitation and inhibition of medullary inspiratory neurons by two types of burst inspiratory neurons in the cat. Neurosci Lett. 1989;104:303–308.

44. Ono T, Ishiwata Y, Inaba N, et al. Hypoglossal premotor neurons with rhythmical inspiratory-related activity in the cat: localization and projection to the phrenic nucleus. Exp Brain Res. 1994;98:1–12.

45. Merrill EG, Lipski J, Kubin L, et al. Origin of the expiratory inhibition of nucleus tractus solitarius inspiratory neurons. Brain Res. 1983;263:43–50.

46. Jiang C, Lipski J. Extensive monosynaptic inhibition of ventral respiratory group neurons by augmenting neurons in the Bötzinger complex in the cat. Exp Brain Res. 1990;81:639–648.

47. Merrill EG, Fedorko L. Monosynaptic inhibition of phrenic motoneurons: a long descending projection from Bötzinger neurons. J Neurosci. 1984;4:2350–2353.

48. Schwarzacher SW, Smith JC, Richter DW. Pre-Bötzinger complex in the cat. J Neurophysiol. 1995;73:1452–1461.

49. Smith JC, Ellenberger HH, Ballanyi K, et al. Pre-Bötzinger complex: brainstem region that may generate respiratory rhythm in mammals. Science. 1991;254:726–729.

50. Mitchell RA, Loeschcke HH, Massion WH, et al. Respiratory responses mediated through superficial chemosensitive areas on the medulla. J Appl Physiol. 1963;18:523–533.

51. Cherniack NS, von Euler C, Homma I, et al. Graded changes in central chemoreceptor input by local temperature changes on the ventral surface of medulla. J Physiol (Lond). 1979;287:191–211.

52. Millhorn DE. Neural respiratory and circulatory interaction during chemoreceptor stimulation and cooling of ventral medulla in cats. J Physiol (Lond). 1986;370:217–231.

53. Budzinska K, von Euler C, Kao FF, et al. Effects of graded focal cold block in rostral areas of the medulla. Acta Physiol Scand. 1985;124:329–340.

54. Suzue T. Respiratory rhythm generation in the in vitro brain stem-spinal cord preparation of the neonatal rat. J Physiol (Lond). 1984;354:173–183.

55. Smith JC, Feldman JL. Central respiratory pattern generation studied in an in vitro mammalian brainstem-spinal cord preparation. In: Sieck GE, Gandevia SC, Cameron WE, eds. Respiratory Muscles and Their Neuromotor Control. New York, NY: Alan R Liss; 1987:27–36.

56. Smith JC, Feldman JL. In vitro brain stem-spinal cord preparations for study of motor systems for mammalian respiration and locomotion. J Neurosci Methods. 1987;21:321–333.

57. Onimaru H, Homma I. Respiratory rhythm generator neurons in medulla of brainstem-spinal cord preparation from newborn rat. Brain Res. 1987;403:380–384.

58. Onimaru H, Arata A, Homma I. Localization of respiratory rhythm-generating neurons in the medulla of brainstem-spinal cord preparations from newborn rats. Neurosci Lett. 1987;78:151–155.

59. Onimaru H, Arata A, Homma I. Primary respiratory rhythm generator in the medulla of brainstem-spinal cord preparation from newborn rat. Brain Res. 1988;445:314–324.

60. Onimaru H, Arata A, Homma I. Intrinsic burst generation of preinspiratory neurons in the medulla of brainstem-spinal cord preparations isolated from newborn rats. Exp Brain Res. 1995;106:57–68.

61. Onimaru H, Arata A, Homma I. Firing properties of respiratory rhythm generating neurons in the absence of synaptic transmission in rat medulla in vitro. Exp Brain Res. 1989;76:530–536.

62. Connelly CA, Ellenberger HH, Feldman JL. Respiratory activity in retrotrapezoid nucleus in cat. Am J Physiol. 1990;258:L33–L44.

63. Dean JB, Lawing WL, Millhorn DE. CO_2 decreases membrane conductance and depolarizes neurons in the nucleus tractus solitarii. Exp Brain Res. 1989;76:656–661.

64. Richerson GB. Response to CO_2 of neurons in the rostral ventral medulla in vitro. J Neurophysiol. 1995;73:933–944.

65. Coates EL, Li A, Nattie EE. Widespread sites of brain stem ventilatory chemoreceptors. J Appl Physiol. 1993;75:5–14.

66. Nattie EE, Li A. Retrotrapezoid nucleus lesions decrease phrenic activity and CO_2 sensitivity in rats. Respir Physiol. 1994;97:63–77.

67. Kita I, Sakamoto M, Arita H. Adrenergic cell group in rostral ventrolateral medulla of cat: its correlation with central chemoreceptors. Neurosci Res. 1994;20:265–274.

68. Frysinger RC, Zhang J, Harper RM. Cardiovascular and respiratory relationships with neuronal discharge in the central nucleus of the amygdala during sleep-waking states. Sleep. 1988;11:317–322.

69. Lumsden T. Observations on the respiratory centres in the cat. J Physiol (Lond). 1923;57:153–160.

70. Bianchi AL, Barillot D Jr. Effects of anesthesia on activity patterns of respiratory neurones. Adv Exp Med Biol. 1978;99:17–22.

71. Cohen MI, Feldman JL. Central mechanisms controlling expiratory duration. Adv Exp Med Biol. 1978;99:369–382.

72. Knox CK. Reflex and central mechanisms controlling expiratory duration. In: von Euler C, Lagercrantz H, eds. Central Nervous Control Mechanisms in Breathing. New York, NY: Pergamon Press; 1979:203–216.

73. Dick TE, Bellingham MC, Richter DW. Pontine respiratory neurons in anesthetized cats. Brain Res. 1994;636:259–269.

74. Richter DW, Ballantyne D, Remmers JE. How is the respiratory rhythm generated? A model. News Physiol Sci. 1986;1:109–112.

75. Richter DW. Generation and maintenance of the respiratory rhythm. J Exp Biol. 1982;100:93–107.

76. Ezure K. Synaptic connections between medullary respiratory neurons and considerations on the genesis of respiratory rhythm. Progr Neurobiol. 1990;35:429–450.

77. Duffin J. A model of respiratory rhythm generation. Neuroreport. 1991;2:623–626.

78. Rybak IA, Paton JFR, Schwaber JS. Modeling neural mechanisms for genesis of respiratory rhythm and pattern, II: network models of the central respiratory pattern generator. J Neurophysiol. 1997;77:2007–2026.

79. Feldman JL, Smith JC. Cellular mechanisms underlying modulation of breathing pattern in mammals. Ann N Y Acad Sci. 1989;536:114–130.

80. Dekin MS, Getting PA. In vitro characterization of neurons in the ventral part of the nucleus tractus solitarius, II: ionic basis for repetitive firing patterns. J Neurophysiol. 1987;58:215–229.

81. Dekin MS, Getting PA, Johnson SM. In vitro characterization of neurons in the ventral part of the nucleus tractus solitarius, I: identification of neuronal types and repetitive firing properties. J Neurophysiol. 1987;58:195–214.

82. Dekin MS, Richerson GB, Getting PA. Thyrotropin-releasing hormone induces rhythmic bursting in neurons of the nucleus tractus solitarius. Science. 1985;229:67–69.

83. Feldman JL, Smith JC, Ellenberger HH, et al. Neurogenesis of respiratory rhythm and pattern: emerging concepts. Am J Physiol 1990;259:R879–R886.

84. Orem J, Montplaisir J, Dement W. Changes in the activity of respiratory neurones during sleep. Brain Res. 1974;82:309–315.

85. Orem J. Neuronal mechanisms of respiration in REM sleep. Sleep. 1980;3:251–267.

86. Orem J. Inspiratory neurons that are activated when inspiration is inhibited behaviorally. Neurosci Lett. 1987;83:282–286.

87. Orem J. The activity of late inspiratory cells during the behavioral inhibition of inspiration. Brain Res. 1988;458:224–230.

88. Orem J. Behavioral inspiratory inhibition: inactivated and activated respiratory cells. J Neurophysiol. 1989;62:1069–1078.

89. Orem J, Dick T. Consistency and signal strength of respiratory neuronal activity. J Neurophysiol. 1983;50:1098–1107.

90. Orem J, Osorio I, Brooks E, et al. Activity of respiratory neurons during NREM sleep. J Neurophysiol. 1985;54:1144–1156.

91. Orem J, Netick A. Behavioral control of breathing in the cat. Brain Res. 1986;366:238–253.

92. Orem J, Brooks EG. The activity of retrofacial expiratory cells during behavioral respiratory responses and active expiration. Brain Res. 1986;374:409–412.

93. Lydic R, Orem J. Respiratory neurons of the pneumotaxic center during sleep and wakefulness. Neurosci Lett. 1979;15:187–192.

94. Sieck GE, Harper RM. Pneumotaxic area neuronal discharge during sleep-waking states in the cat. Exp Neurol. 1980;67:79–102.

95. Frysinger RC, Harper RM. Cardiac and respiratory relationships with neural discharge in the anterior cingulate cortex during sleep-waking states. Exp Neurol. 1986;94:247–263.

96. Harper RM, Frysinger RC, Terreberry RR, et al. Suprapontine control of respiratory activity. In: Sieck GE, Gandevia SC, Cameron WE, eds. Respiratory Muscles and Their Neuromotor Control. New York, NY: Alan R Liss; 1987:93–101.

97. Zhang J, Harper RM, Frysinger RC. Respiratory modulation of neuronal discharge in the central nucleus of the amygdala during sleep and waking states. Exp Neurol. 1986;91:193–207.

98. Bertrand F, Hugelin A, Vibert JF. Quantitative study of anatomical distribution of respiratory related neurons in the pons. Exp Brain Res. 1973;16:383–399.

99. Vibert JF, Bertrand F, Denavit-Saubié M, et al. Discharge patterns of bulbo-pontine respiratory unit populations in cat. Brain Res. 1976;114:211–225.

100. Vibert JF, Bertrand F, Denavit-Saubié M, et al. Three dimensional representation of bulbo-pontine respiratory networks architecture from unit density maps. Brain Res. 1976;114:227–244.

101. Caille D, Vibert JF, Bertrand F, et al. Pentobarbone effects on respiration related units: selective depression of bulbopontine reticular neurones. Respir Physiol. 1979;36:201–216.

102. Vibert JF, Caille D, Bertrand F, et al. Ascending projection from the respiratory centre to mesencephalon and diencephalon. Neurosci Lett. 1979;11:29–33.

103. Netick A, Orem J. Erroneous classification of neuronal activity by the respiratory modulation index. Neurosci Lett. 1981;21:301–306.

104. Puizillout JJ, Ternaux JP. Variations d'activités toniques, phasiques et respiratoires au niveau bulbaire pendant l'endormement de la préparation encéphale isolé. Brain Res. 1974;66:67–83.

105. Foutz AS, Boudinot E, Morin-Surin M-P, et al. Excitability of "silent" respiratory neurons during sleep-waking states: an iontophoretic study in undrugged chronic cats. Brain Res. 1987;171:135–141.

106. Gilbert KA, Lydic R. Parabrachial neuron discharge in the cat is altered during the carbachol-induced REM sleep-like state (DCarb). Neurosci Lett. 1990;120:241–244.

107. Gilbert KA, Lydic R. Pontine cholinergic reticular mechanisms cause state-dependent changes in the discharge of parabrachial neurons. Am J Physiol. 1994; 266:R136–R150.

108. Dick TE, Orem JM. Pontine respiratory neurons in unanesthetized cats. Soc Neurosci Abstr. 1997;23:725.

109. Ferrier D. The Functions of the Brain. London: Smith, Edler; 1876:323.

110. Martin HN. The normal respiratory movements of the frog, and the influence upon its respiratory centre of stimulation of the optic lobes. J Physiol (Lond). 1878;1:131–170.

111. Martin HN, Booker WD. The influence of stimulation of the midbrain upon the respiratory rhythm of the mammal. J Physiol (Lond). 1878;1:370–376.

112. Ranson SW, Kabat H, Magoun HW. Autonomic responses to electrical stimulation of hypothalamus, preoptic region and septum. Arch Neurol. Psych. 1935;33:467–477.

113. Kabat H. Electrical stimulation of points in the forebrain and midbrain: the resultant alterations in respiration. J Comp Neurol. 1936;64:187–208.

114. Baxter DW, Olszewski J. Respiratory responses evoked by electrical stimulation of pons and mesencephalon. J Neurophysiol. 1955;18:276–287.

115. Hugelin A, Cohen MI. The reticular activating system and respiratory regulation in the cat. Ann N Y Acad Sci. 1963;109:586–603.

116. Cohen MI, Hugelin A. Suprapontine reticular control of intrinsic respiratory mechanisms. Arch Ital Biol. 1965;103:317–334.

117. Trouth CO, Loeschke HH, Berndt J. Topography of the respiratory responses to electrical stimulation of the medulla oblongata. Pflugers Arch. 1973;339:153–170.

118. Orem J, Lydic R. Upper airway function during sleep and wakefulness: experimental studies on normal and anesthetized cats. Sleep. 1978;1:49–68.

119. Orem J, Lydic R, Norris P. Experimental control of the diaphragm and laryngeal abductor muscles by brain stem arousal systems. Respir Physiol. 1979;38:203–221.

120. Eldridge FL, Millhorn DE. Oscillation, gating, and memory in the respiratory control system. In: Cherniack NS, Widdicombe JG, eds. Handbook of Physiology. Control of Breathing; vol 2. Bethesda, Md: American Physiological Society; 1986:93–114.

121. Sullivan CE, Kozar LE, Murphy E, et al. Arousal, ventilatory, and airway responses to bronchopulmonary stimulation in sleeping dogs. J Appl Physiol. 1978;45:681–689.

122. Sullivan CE, Zamel N, Kozar LE, et al. Regulation of airway smooth muscle tone in sleeping dogs. Am Rev Respir Dis. 1979;119:87–99.

123. Anderson CA, Dick TE, Orem J. Respiratory responses to tracheobronchial stimulation during sleep and wakefulness in the adult cat. Sleep. 1996;19:472–478.

124. Plum F, Leigh RJ. Abnormalities of central mechanisms. In: Hornhein TF, ed. Regulation of Breathing. Part 2. New York, NY: Marcel Dekker; 1981:989–1067.

125. Eldridge FL, Millhorn DE, Waldrop TG. Exercise hyperpnea and locomotion: parallel activation from the hypothalamus. Science. 1981;211:844–846.

126. Reis DJ, McHugh PR. Hypoxia as a cause of bradycardia during amygdala stimulation in monkey. J Appl Physiol. 1968;214:601–610.

127. Harper RM, Frysinger RC. Suprapontine mechanisms underlying cardiorespiratory regulation: implications for the sudden infant death syndrome. In: Harper RM, Hoffman HJ, eds. Sudden Infant Death Syndrome: Risk Factors and Basic Mechanisms. New York, NY: PMA Publishing; 1988:399–414.

128. Bassal M, Bianchi AL. Effets de la stimulation des structures nerveuses centrales sur les activites respiratoires efferentes chez le chat, II: responses a la stimulation sous corticale. J Physiol Paris. 1981;77:754–777.

129. Bassal M, Bianchi AL. Dussardier M. Effets de la stimulation des structures nerveuses centrales sur l'activite des neurones respiratoires chez le chat. J Physiol Paris. 1981;77:779–795.

130. Lutherer LO, Williams JL. Stimulating fastigial nucleus pressor region elicits patterned respiratory responses. Am J Physiol. 1986;250:R418–R426.

131. Williams JL, Robinson PJ, Lutherer LO. Inhibitory effects of cerebellar lesions on respiration in the spontaneously breathing, anesthetized cat. Brain Res. 1986;399:224–231.

132. Price WH, Batsel HL. Respiratory neurons participating in sneeze and in response to resistance to expiration. Exp Neurol. 1970;29:554–570.

133. Batsel HL, Lines AJ Jr. Neural mechanisms of sneeze. Am J Physiol. 1975;229:770–776.

134. Fukuda H, Fukai K. Postural change and straining induced by distension of the rectum, vagina and urinary bladder of decerebrate dogs. Brain Res. 1986;380:276–286.

135. Fukuda H, Fukai K. Location of the reflex centre for straining elicited by activation of pelvic afferent fibres of decerebrate dogs. Brain Res. 1986;380:287–296.

136. Fukuda H, Fukai K. Ascending and descending pathways of reflex straining in the dog. Jpn J Physiol. 1986;36:905–920.

137. Fukuda H, Fukai K. Discharges of bulbar respiratory neurons during rhythmic straining evoked by activation of pelvic afferent fibers in dogs. Brain Res. 1988;449:157–166.

138. Miller AD, Tan LK, Suzuki I. I. Control of abdominal and expiratory intercostal muscle activity during vomiting: role of ventral respiratory group expiratory neurons. J Neurophysiol. 1987;57:1854–1866.

139. Jodkowski JS, Berger AJ. Influences from laryngeal afferents on expiratory bulbospinal neurons and motoneurons. J Appl Physiol. 1988;64:1337–1345.

140. Remmers JE, Richter DW, Ballantyne D, et al. Reflex prolongation of stage I of expiration. Pflugers Arch. 1986;407:190–198.

141. Richter DW, Ballantyne D, Remmers JE. The differential organization of medullary post-inspiratory activities. Pflugers Arch. 1987;410:420–427.

142. Altshuler SM, Davies RO, Pack AI. Role of medullary inspiratory neurons in the control of the diaphragm during gastrointestinal reflexes. J Physiol (Lond). 1987;391:289–298.

143. Bianchi AL, Grélot L. Converse motor output of inspiratory bulbospinal premotoneurones during vomiting. Neurosci Lett. 1989;104:298–302.

144. Plum F. Neurological integration of behavioral and metabolic control of breathing. In: Porter R, ed. Breathing: Hering-Breuer Centenary Symposium. London, England: Churchill; 1970:159–175.

145. Meyer JS, Herndon RM. Bilateral infarction of the pyramidal tract in man. Neurology. 1962;12:637–642.

146. Mitchell RA, Berger AJ. Neural regulation of respiration. Am Rev Respir Dis. 1975;111:206–224.

147. Lipski J, Bektas A, Porter R. Short latency inputs to phrenic motoneurones from the sensorimotor cortex in the cat. Exp Brain Res. 1986;61:280–290.

148. Trulson ME, Trulson VM. Activity of nucleus raphe pallidus neurons across the sleep-waking cycle in freely moving cats. Brain Res. 1982;237:232–237.

149. Heym J, Steinfels GF, Jacobs BL. Activity of serotonin-containing neurons in the nucleus raphe pallidus of freely moving cats. Brain Res. 1982;251:259–276.

150. Aston-Jones G, Bloom FE. Activity of norepinephrine-containing locus coeruleus neurons in behaving rats anticipates fluctuations in the sleep-waking cycle. J Neurosci. 1981;1:876–886.

151. Schmid K, Böhmer G, Merkelbach S. Serotonergic control of phrenic motoneuronal activity at the level of the spinal cord of the rabbit. Neurosci Lett. 1990;116:204–209.

152. Arita H, Ochiishi M. Opposing effects of 5-hydroxytryptamine on two types of medullary inspiratory neurons with distinct firing patterns. J Neurophysiol. 1991;66:285–292.

153. Kubin L, Tojima H, Davies RO, et al. Serotonergic excitatory drive to hypoglossal motoneurons in the decerebrate cat. Neurosci Lett. 1992;139:243–248.

154. Ribeiro-do-Valle LE, Metzler CW, Jacobs BL. Facilitation of masseter EMG and masseteric (jaw-closure) reflex by serotonin in behaving cats. Brain Res. 1991;550:197–204.

155. Lindsay AD, Feldman JL. Modulation of respiratory activity of neonatal rat phrenic motoneurones by serotonin. J Physiol (Lond). 1993;461:213–233.

156. Al-Zubaidy ZA, Erickson RL, Greer JJ. Serotonergic and noradrenergic effects on respiratory neural discharge in the medullary slice preparation of neonatal rats. Pflugers Arch. 1996;431:942–949.

157. Nishimura Y, Muramatsu M, Asahara T, et al. Electrophysiological properties and their modulation by norepinephrine in the ambiguus neurons of the guinea pig. Brain Res. 1995;702:213–222.

158. Funk GD, Smith JC, Feldman JL. Development of thyrotropin-releasing hormone and norepinephrine potentiation of inspiratory-related hypoglossal motoneuron discharge in neonatal and juvenile mice in vitro. J Neurophysiol. 1994;72:2538–2541.

159. Parkis MA, Bayliss DA, Berger AJ. Actions of norepinephrine on rat hypoglossal motoneurons. J Neurophysiol. 1995;74:1911–1919.

160. Johnson SM, Smith JC, Feldman JL. Modulation of respiratory rhythm in vitro: role of $G_{i/o}$ protein-mediated mechanisms. J Appl Physiol. 1996;80:2120–2133.

161. Kubin L, Reignier C, Tojima H, et al. Changes in serotonin level in the hypoglossal nucleus region during the carbachol-induced atonia. Brain Res. 1994;645:291–302.

162. Woch G, Davies RO, Pack AI, et al. Behavior of raphe cells projecting to the dorsomedial medulla during carbachol-induced atonia in the cat. J Physiol (Lond). 1996;490:745–758.

163. Kubin L, Tojima H, Reignier C, et al. Interaction of serotonergic excitatory drive to hypoglossal motoneurons with carbachol-induced, REM sleep-like atonia. Sleep. 1996;19:187–195.

164. Fenik V, Kubin L, Okabe S, et al. Differential sensitivity of laryngeal and pharyngeal motoneurons to iontophoretic application of serotonin. Neuroscience. 1997;81:873–885.

165. Lalley PM. The excitability and rhythm of medullary respiratory neurons in the cat are altered by the serotonin receptor agonist 5-methoxy-N,N,dimethyltryptamine. Brain Res. 1994;648:87–98.

166. Lalley PM, Bischoff AM, Richter DW. 5-HT-1A receptor-mediated modulation of medullary expiratory neurons in the cat. J Physiol (Lond). 1994;476:117–130.

167. Rampin O, Pierrefiche O, Denavit-Saubié M. Effects of serotonin and substance P on bulbar respiratory neurons in vivo. Brain Res. 1993;622:185–193.

168. Champagnat J, Denavit-Saubié M, Henry JL, et al. Catecholaminergic depressant effects on bulbar respiratory mechanisms. Brain Res. 1979;160:57–68.

169. Aston-Jones G, Rajkowski J, Kubiak P, et al. Role of the locus coeruleus in emotonal activation. Progr Brain Res. 1996;107:379–402.

170. Jouvet M, Michel E. Correlations electromyographiques du sommeil chez le chat decortique et mesencephalique chronique. C R Soc Biol (Paris). 1959;153:422–426.

171. Bizzi E, Brooks DC. Functional connections between pontine reticular formation and lateral geniculate nucleus during deep sleep. Arch Ital Biol. 1963;101:666–680.

172. Brooks DC, Bizzi E. Brain stem electrical activity during deep sleep. Arch Ital Biol. 1963;101:648–665.

173. Mikiten T, Neibyl P, Hendley C. EEG desynchronization during behavioral sleep associated with spike discharges from the thalamus of the cat [abstract]. Fed Proc. 1961;20:327.

174. Gadea-Ciria M. Etudes des latences entre les activites ponto-

geniculo-occipitale au niveau de pont des noyaux genicules lateraux et des muscles droits externes chez le chat. C R Soc Biol (Paris). 1972;166:634–639.

175. Orem JA, Netick A, Dement WC. Breathing during sleep and wakefulness in the cat. Respir Physiol. 1977;30:265–289.

176. Parmeggiani PL, Sabattini L. Electromyographic aspects of postural, respiratory and thermoregulatory mechanisms in sleeping cats. Electroencephalogr Clin Neurophysiol. 1972;33:1–13.

177. Tabachnik E, Muller NS, Bryan AC, et al. Changes in ventilation and chest wall mechanics during sleep in normal adolescents. J Appl Physiol Respir Environ Exerc Physiol. 1981;51:557–564.

178. Megirian D, Pollard MJ, Sherrey JH. The labile respiratory activity of ribcage muscles of the rat during sleep. J Physiol (Lond). 1987;389:99–110.

179. Sauerland EK, Harper RM. The human tongue during sleep: electromyographic activity of the genioglossus muscle. Exp Neurol. 1976;51:160–170.

180. Remmers JE, deGroot WJ, Crump CH, et al. Pathogenesis of upper airway occlusions during sleep. J Appl Physiol. 1978;44:931–938.

181. Sullivan CE. Breathing in sleep. In: Orem J, Barnes CD, eds. Physiology in Sleep. New York, NY: Academic Press; 1980:213–272.

182. Orem J, Dick T, Norris P. Laryngeal and diaphragmatic responses to airway occlusion in sleep and wakefulness. Electroencephalogr Clin Neurophysiol. 1980;50:151–164.

183. Gauzzi M, Freis ED. Sino-aortic reflexes pH, PO_2, and PCO_2 in wakefulness and sleep. Am J Physiol. 1969;217:1623–1627.

184. Dawes GS, Fox HE, Leduc BM, et al. Respiratory movements and rapid eye movement sleep in the foetal lamb. J Physiol (Lond). 1972;220:119–143.

185. Remmers JE, Bartlett D Jr, Putnam MD. Changes in the respiratory cycle associated with sleep. Respir Physiol. 1976;28:227–238.

186. Foutz AS, Netick A, Dement WC. Sleep state effects on breathing after spinal cord section and vagotomy in the cat. Respir Physiol. 1979;37:89–100.

187. Netick A, Foutz AS. Respiratory activity and sleep-wakefulness in the deafferented paralyzed cat. Sleep. 1980;3:1–12.

188. Roffwarg HP, Munio JN, Dement WC. Ontogenetic development of the human sleep-dream cycle. Science. 1966;152:604–619.

189. Jouvet M. Recherches sur les structures nerveuses et les mecanismes responsables des differentes phases du sommeil physiologique. Arch Ital Biol. 1962;100:125–206.

190. Orem J. Medullary respiratory neuron activity: relationship to tonic and phasic REM sleep. J Appl Physiol Respir Environ Exerc Physiol. 1980;48:54–65.

191. Kline LR, Hendricks JC, Davies RO, et al. Control of activity of the diaphragm in rapid-eye-movement sleep. J Appl Physiol. 1986;61:1293–1300.

192. Kline LR, Hendricks JC, Silage DA, et al. Startle-evoked changes in diaphragmatic activity during wakefulness and sleep. J Appl Physiol. 1990;68:166–173.

193. Dement W, Wolpert EA. The relation of eye movements, body mobility, and external stimuli to dream content. J Exp Psychol. 1958;55:543–553.

194. Phillipson EA. Control of breathing during sleep. Am Rev Respir Dis. 1978;118:909–939.

195. Trotter R, Orem J. Behavioral inhibition of inspiration during REM sleep [abstract]. The Second International Symposium on Sleep and Respiration; League City, Tex; 1991.

196. Spreng LF, Johnson LC, Lubin A. Autonomic correlates of eye movement bursts during stage REM sleep. Psychophysiology. 1968;4:311–323.

197. Sastre JP, Jouvet M. Le comportement onirique du chat. Physiol Behav. 1979;22:979–989.

198. Hendricks JC, Morrison AR, Mann GL. Different behaviors during paradoxical sleep without atonia depend on pontine lesion site. Brain Res. 1982;239:81–105.

199. Kubin L, Kimura H, Tojima H, et al. Behavior of VRG neurons during the atonia of REM sleep induced by pontine carbachol in decerebrate cats. Brain Res. 1992;592:91–100.

200. Orem J. Central respiratory activity in rapid eye movement sleep: augmenting and late inspiratory cells. Sleep. 1994;17:665–673.

201. Orem J, Anderson CA. Diaphragmatic activity during REM sleep in the adult cat. J Appl Physiol. 1996;81:751–760.

202. Orem J. Augmenting expiratory neuronal activity in sleep and wakefulness and in relation to duration of expiration. J Appl Physiol. 1998;85:1260–1266.

203. Vertes RP. Brainstem mechanisms of slow-wave sleep and REM sleep. In: Kleem WR, Vertes RP, eds. Brainstem Mechanisms of Behavior. New York, NY: John Wiley & Sons; 1990:535–583.

204. Vertes RP, Kinney GG, Kocsis B, et al. Pharmacological suppression of the median raphe nucleus with serotonin 1A agonists, 8-OH-DPAT and buspirone, produces hippocampal theta rhythm in the rat. Neuroscience. 1994;60:441–451.

205. Monmaur P, Ayadi K, Breton P. Hippocampal EEG responses induced by carbachol and atropine infusions into the septum and the hippocampus in the urethane-anaesthetized rat. Brain Res. 1993;631:317–324.

206. Datta S, Calvo JM, Quattrochi J, et al. Cholinergic microstimulation of the peribrachial nucleus in the cat, I: immediate and prolonged increases in ponto-geniculo-occipital waves. Arch Ital Biol. 1992;130:263–284.

207. Vertes RP, Colm LV, Fortin WJ, et al. Brainstem sites for the carbachol elicitation of the hippocampal theta rhythm in the rat. Exp Brain Res. 1993;96:419–429.

208. Jouvet M. The role of monoamines and acetylcholine-containing neurons in the regulation of the sleep-waking cycle. Ergeb Physiol. 1972;64:166–307.

209. Steriade M, McCarley RW, eds. Brainstem Control of Wakefulness and Sleep. New York, NY: Plenum; 1990.

210. Jones BE. Paradoxical sleep and its chemical/structural substrates in the brain. Neuroscience. 1991;40:637–656.

211. George R, Haslett WL, Jenden DJ. A cholinergic mechanism in the brainstem reticular formation: induction of paradoxical sleep. Int J Neuropharmacol. 1964;3:541–552.

212. Mitler MM, Dement WC. Cataleptic-like behavior in cats after micro-injections of carbachol in pontine reticular formation. Brain Res. 1974;68:335–343.

213. Baghdoyan HA, Rodrigo-Angulo ML, McCarley RW, et al. Site-specific enhancement and suppression of desynchronized sleep signs following cholinergic stimulation of three brainstem regions. Brain Res. 1984;306:39–52.

214. Vanni-Mercier G, Sakai K, Lin JS, et al. Mapping of cholinoceptive brainstem structures responsible for the generation of paradoxical sleep in the cat. Arch Ital Biol. 1989;127:133–164.

215. Yamamoto K, Mamelak AN, Quattrochi JJ, et al. A cholinoceptive desynchronized sleep induction zone in the anterodorsal pontine tegmentum: locus of the sensitive region. Neuroscience. 1990;39:279–293.

216. Bourgin P, Escourrou P, Gaultier C, et al. Induction of rapid eye movement sleep by carbachol infusion into the pontine reticular formation in the rat. Neuroreport. 1995;6:532–536.

217. Taguchi O, Kubin L, Pack AI. Evocation of postural atonia and respiratory depression by pontine carbachol in the decerebrate rat. Brain Res. 1992;595:107–115.

218. Deurveilher S, Hars B, Hennevin E. Pontine microinjection of carbachol does not reliably enhance paradoxical sleep in rats. Sleep. 1997;20:593–607.

219. Datta S. Cellular basis of pontine ponto-geniculo-occipital wave generation and modulation. Cell Mol Neurobiol. 1997;17:341–365.

220. Kodama T, Takahashi Y, Honda Y. Enhancement of acetylcholine release during paradoxical sleep in the dorsal tegmental field of the cat brainstem. Neurosci Lett. 1990;114:277–282.

221. Webster HH, Jones BE. Neurotoxic lesions of the dorsolateral pontomesencephalic tegmentum-cholinergic cell area in the cat, II: effects upon sleep-waking states. Brain Res. 1988;458:285–302.

222. Lydic R, Baghdoyan HA, Zwillich CW. State-dependent hypotonia in posterior cricoarytenoid muscles of the larynx caused by cholinoceptive reticular mechanisms. FASEB J 1989;3:1625–1631.

223. Lydic R, Baghdoyan HA. Cholinoceptive pontine reticular mechanisms cause state-dependent respiratory changes in the cat. Neurosci Lett. 1989;102:211–216.

224. Kimura H, Kubin L, Davies RO, et al. Cholinergic stimulation of the pons depresses respiration in decerebrate cats. J Appl Physiol. 1990;69:2280–2289.

225. Tojima H, Kubin L, Kimura H, et al. Spontaneous ventilation and respiratory motor output during carbachol-induced atonia of REM sleep in the decerebrate cat. Sleep. 1992;15:404–414.

226. Fenik V, Davies RO, Pack AI, et al. Differential suppression of upper airway motor activity during carbachol-induced, REM sleep-like atonia. Am J Physiol. 1998;275(4 pt 2): R1013–R1024.

227. Horner RL, Kubin L. Pontine carbachol elicits multiple REM sleep-like neural events in urethane-anesthetized rats. Neuroscience. 1999;93:215–226.

228. Kubin L, Kimura H, Tojima H, et al. Suppression of hypoglossal motoneurons during the carbachol-induced atonia of REM sleep is not caused by fast synaptic inhibition. Brain Res. 1993;611:300–312.

229. Kubin L, Davies RO, Pack AI. Control of upper airway motoneurons during REM sleep. News Physiol Sci. 1998;13:91–97.

230. Veasey SC, Panckeri KA, Hoffman EA, et al. The effect of serotonin antagonists in an animal model of sleep-disordered breathing. Am Rev Respir Crit Care Med. 1996;153:776–786.

Respiratory Physiology: Control of Ventilation

Neil J. Douglas

Breathing during wakefulness is controlled by a number of factors including voluntary and behavioral elements; chemical factors, including low oxygen levels; high carbon dioxide levels and acidosis, as well as mechanical signals from the lung and chest wall. During sleep there is loss of voluntary control and a decrease in the usual ventilatory response to both low oxygen and high carbon dioxide levels. Both the hypoxemic and hypercapnic responses are most depressed in rapid eye movement (REM) sleep.

These blunted ventilatory responses during sleep are clinically important. They permit the marked hypoxemia that occurs during REM sleep in patients with lung or chest wall disease. It may also be important in the pathogenesis of upper airway obstruction during sleep and particularly in the failure to arouse rapidly during apneas.

Sleep alters both breathing pattern and respiratory responses to many external stimuli.[1] These changes permit the development of sleep-related hypoxemia in patients with respiratory disease and may contribute to the pathogenesis of apneas in patients with sleep apnea syndrome. This chapter reviews the control of ventilation in adults during sleep and its relevance to these clinical problems.

Many respiratory problems during sleep are related to an abnormal control of ventilation. There is much known about the control of breathing during wakefulness, but less is known about how breathing is controlled in the sleeping normal person or in a patient with a sleep disorder. The major goal of the respiratory control system is a homeostatic one, to keep blood gases in a range so that the metabolic functions of the body remain normal.

OVERVIEW OF CONTROL OF BREATHING

The respiratory muscles do not have a built-in pacemaker, as does the heart. These muscles receive impulses from the medulla from a region that has been called the *respiratory center, respiratory oscillator, respiratory signal generator*, and *respiratory pacemaker*. For breathing to change as physiological conditions change, the respiratory center receives and responds to three general types of information: chemical information (from chemoreceptors responding to PaO_2, $PaCO_2$, and pH), mechanical information (from receptors in the lung and chest wall), and behavioral information (from higher cortical centers). The aspects of awake control that may have impact on control of breathing during sleep are briefly reviewed below, and in more detail elsewhere.[1a]

Chemical Information

The carotid body senses PaO_2, which sends impulses to the medulla via the ninth cranial nerve. Ventilation usually increases only when PaO_2 is less than 60 mmHg. When PaO_2 drops acutely below 30 to 40 mmHg, the medulla may be depressed by the hypoxemia and thus ventilation may decrease. CO_2 is sensed in both the carotid body and a region of the medulla called the *central chemoreceptor*. As $PaCO_2$ increases, there is a brisk linear increase in ventilation. Drugs that depress central nervous system function may profoundly depress chemical drives to breathe.

Mechanical Information

In the presence of lung diseases or changes in the load of the respiratory system, receptors in the lung and chest wall send impulses to the medulla. Those in the lung are the best understood: the receptors respond to irritation, inflation (stretch), deflation, and congestion of blood vessels. The information from these sensors travels centrally via the vagus nerve. The major result of stimulating these sensors is to shorten inspiration and reduce tidal volume to cause a rapid, shallow breathing pattern.

Information From Higher Central Nervous System Centers

The respiratory system is used for many nonbreathing functions (e.g., singing, laughing, crying, and speaking) that are directed by higher brain centers. The efferent pathways involved in these activities may actually bypass the respiratory center in the medulla; thus, these nonrespiratory activities can override the metabolic homeostatic function of the respiratory control system. It appears that just as abnormal chemistry may increase the drive to breathe, there is a respiratory drive linked to wakefulness. As one sleeps, arouses, and dreams, there may be dramatic changes in the information from higher central nervous system (CNS) centers.

HYPOXIC VENTILATORY RESPONSE DURING SLEEP

Adult Human Beings. The ventilatory response to hypoxia falls during sleep in adult human beings[1-4] (Fig. 16–1). The hypoxic ventilatory response was lower during nonrapid eye movement (NREM) sleep than during wakefulness in the studies in which the subjects were exclusively or mostly men,[1, 2] but the responses were similar in wakefulness and NREM sleep in the studies in which women predominated.[3-5] It is not clear why there is such a difference between the genders in the effect of sleep on the hypoxic ventilatory response. Comparison of the results in men and women (Fig. 16–2) shows that the major gender difference is in the levels of ventilatory drives during wakefulness, which are much higher in men than in women.[4]

The hypoxic ventilatory response during rapid eye movement (REM) sleep is lower than in NREM sleep in both men and women.[1-4] The hypoxic ventilatory response during REM sleep was remarkably similar in all three directly comparable studies[1, 2, 4]: about 0.4 liter/min/percentage SaO2 (see Fig. 16–2).

Adult Animals. The isocapnic hypoxic ventilatory response has been found to be unchanged[6] or decreased[7] during sleep in tracheostomized dogs and decreased during sleep in goats.[8]

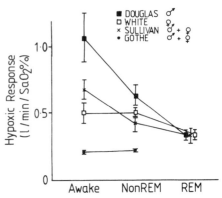

Figure 16–2. Comparison of hypoxic ventilatory responses in different sleep stages in four studies[1, 3, 5] indicating the unchanged responses in NREM sleep in women, and the similarity of responses in REM sleep in all studies.

HYPERCAPNIC VENTILATORY RESPONSE DURING SLEEP

Adult Human Beings. The hypercapnic ventilatory response is depressed during sleep in adult human beings (Fig. 16–3). Studies performed in either electroencephalogram-documented[9-12] or presumed[13-15] NREM sleep showed that the slope of the ventilation-CO2 response line falls during NREM sleep, compared with wakefulness. Two large studies[10, 11] suggested that the decrease in response from wakefulness to NREM sleep is approximately 50%. Although Bülow[10] reported lower responses in stages 3 and 4 sleep than in stage 2 sleep, later researchers[11, 16] found no such difference. In fact, Bülow did not apply statistics, and his data indicate considerable overlap (see Figs. 21, 26, and 27 in reference 10). Indeed, no separation is evident until high CO2 levels are reached when the number of data points is small.

NREM sleep does not significantly change the position of the ventilation-CO2 response line, as assessed by the rebreathing technique with extrapolation of the

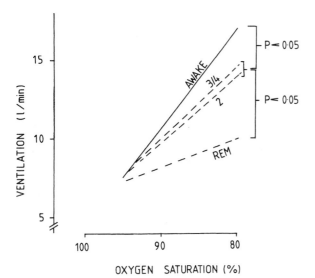

Figure 16–1. Mean relationship between expired ventilation and decreasing O2 saturation in the different sleep stages in 12 subjects, 6 male[1] and 6 female[4] (From Douglas NJ. Control of ventilation during sleep. Clin Chest Med. 1985;6:563.)

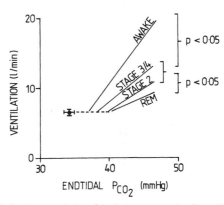

Figure 16–3. Mean relationship between expired ventilation and increasing end-tidal PCO2 in 12 subjects, 6 male and 6 female, indicating the mean + SE resting ventilation-CO2 set-point during wakefulness. (From Douglas NJ. Control of ventilation during sleep. Clin Chest Med. 1985;6:563. [Redrawn from Douglas NJ, White DP, Weil JV, et al. Hypercapnic ventilatory response in sleeping adults. American Review of Respiratory Disease, vol 126, 758–762. Official Journal of the American Thoracic Society. © American Lung Association.])

CO_2 response line to the intercept at zero ventilation.[11, 16] However, as the slope of the response line decreases during NREM sleep, the CO_2 increment between the awake resting ventilatory set-point and the ventilatory response line is increased significantly during NREM sleep[10, 11] (see Fig. 16–3).

Berthon-Jones and Sullivan[16] found that women did not change the hypercapnic ventilatory response from wakefulness to NREM sleep, a result consistent with the finding by Davis et al.[17] of higher ventilatory responses during sleep in women than in men. In contrast, neither Douglas et al.[11] nor Gothe et al.[18] identified any difference between the genders in any stage. Three groups have measured the hypercapnic ventilatory response during REM sleep in adults. Douglas et al.[11] found that in 10 of 12 subjects, the hypercapnic response was lowest in REM sleep, compared with either wakefulness or NREM sleep. The mean hypercapnic ventilatory response during REM sleep was 28% of the level during wakefulness (see Fig. 16–3). These authors were unable to accurately define the position of the hypercapnic ventilatory response line because some responses during REM sleep had negative slopes. Berthon-Jones and Sullivan[16] and White[19] found a tendency for the lowest responses to occur during REM sleep.

Adult Animals. As in adult human beings, the hypercapnic ventilatory response is lower in NREM sleep than in wakefulness in dogs[20, 21] and cats,[22] with a further drop in response from NREM to REM sleep.[20–23] Sullivan and colleagues[21] found that the hypercapnic ventilatory response was lower in phasic than in tonic REM sleep in dogs.

Ventilatory Response to Chemical Stimuli: Conclusions

There appear to be genuine gender and species differences in the effect of sleep on the hypoxic ventilatory response. Although there are no major species differences in the effect of sleep on the hypercapnic ventilatory response, there may be gender differences. In human adults, both responses are reduced during sleep and are at their lowest during REM sleep.

ADDED RESISTANCE AND AIRWAY OCCLUSION DURING SLEEP

Adult Human Beings. Sleep modifies the ventilatory response to added inspiratory resistance.[24–27] All studies agree that NREM sleep blunts the respiratory timing response to added resistance,[24–27, 28] with some reporting a net effect on ventilation as well.[25, 27, 28] In adults with asthma, the ventilatory response to induced bronchoconstriction is not modified by sleep.[29] Issa and Sullivan[30] reported that, in response to airway occlusion, there was a progressive increase in respiratory effort during NREM sleep and rapid, shallow breathing during REM sleep.

Animals. In both dogs[31, 32] and cats,[22] ventilatory compensation for added loads is maintained during NREM sleep at the level found in wakefulness. However, when the respiratory system is further stressed by combining resistive loading with hypercapnia, the ventilatory and airway occlusion responses to loading are found to be impaired during both NREM and REM sleep.[22]

Conclusions

It is not yet clear precisely what effect increased airflow resistance has on ventilation during sleep, particularly during REM sleep, in adults.

AROUSAL RESPONSES

Isocapnic Hypoxia

In normal subjects, isocapnic hypoxia is a poor stimulus to arousal (Fig. 16–4), with many subjects remaining asleep with SaO_2 as low as 70%[1, 2, 5] and no difference between NREM and REM sleep in arousal threshold. Conversely, the arousal sensitivity to hypoxia is decreased in REM sleep in patients having obstructive sleep apnea with asphyxial hypoxia,[33] in dogs with isocapnic hypoxia,[6, 7] and in cats with hypocapnic hypoxia.[34] Carotid body denervation reduces arousal sensitivity in dogs[7] but does not alter the arousal threshold in cats.[34]

Hypercapnia

Hypercapnia also produces arousal at variable levels[3, 9, 11] but awakens most subjects before the end-tidal CO_2 has risen by 15 mmHg above the level in wakefulness.[3, 9–11] Berthon-Jones and Sullivan[16] reported arousal thresholds up to 6 mmHg higher in slow-wave sleep than in either stage 2 or REM sleep in male but not in female subjects, whereas Douglas and associates[11] found no gender or sleep stage-related differences. Hypoxia increases the sensitivity to CO_2 arousal.[35]

Added Resistance

Human beings tend to arouse from sleep following either the addition of an inspiratory resistance[26] or the occlusion of inspiration.[30] Added inspiratory resistance was found to produce a similar percentage increase in arousal frequency in stages 2 and 3-4 and REM sleep.[24] However, the arousal frequency during control sleep periods was lowest in stage 3-4 sleep and remained significantly lower during slow-wave sleep than in REM sleep after the addition of inspiratory resistance[22, 23] (Fig. 16–5).

Arousal from REM sleep after airway occlusion[30, 36] is far more rapid than arousal from NREM sleep (Fig. 16–6), whereas patients with obstructive apneas have longer apneas during REM sleep. Upper airway recep-

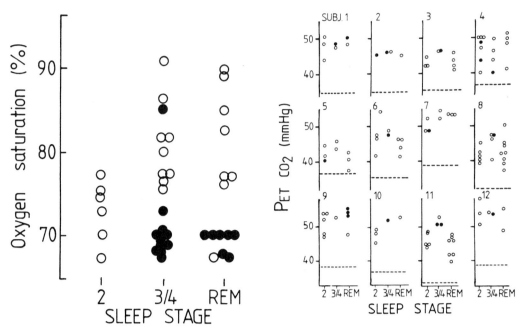

Figure 16–4. Arousal responses to hypoxia and hypercapnia[11] in different sleep stages, indicating whether the subjects remained asleep *(solid circles)* or aroused *(open circles)*. The hypoxic responses are total data for 9 subjects; the hypercapnic plots are for each of 12 individuals, 6 female (1–6) and 6 male (7–12), indicating with the dotted line mean $P_{ET}CO_2$ in wakefulness in each subject. (From Douglas NJ. Control of ventilation during sleep. Clin Chest Med. 1985;6:563.)

tors would be exposed to respiratory pressure changes in normal people with airway occlusion but not in patients with sleep apnea, but why these upper airway receptors should be more effective in REM sleep than in NREM sleep is unclear.

Arousal response to chemostimulation was found to occur at a similar level of ventilation regardless of stimulus.[16] The final common pathway for arousal from sleep after hypoxia, hypercapnia, or increased resistance may actually be the level of ventilatory effort.[37] This is compatible with the observation that patients with upper airway resistance syndrome tend to awaken at relatively reproducible levels of pleural pressure and that this arousal occurs without the development of either significant hypoxemia or significant hypercapnia.

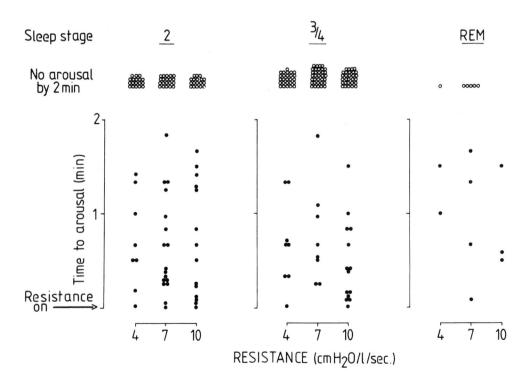

Figure 16–5. Timing of arousal after application of inspiratory resistance of 4, 7, or 10 cm $H_2O/1/s$ in stages 2 and 3–4 and REM sleep. Those occasions in which arousal occurred within 2 min of addition of resistance are indicated by solid circles, and those in which arousal did not occur within 2 min by open circles. (From Gugger M, Molloy J, Gould GA, et al. Ventilatory and arousal responses to added inspiratory resistance during sleep. American Review of Respiratory Disease, vol 140, 1301–1307. Official Journal of the American Thoracic Society. © American Lung Association.)

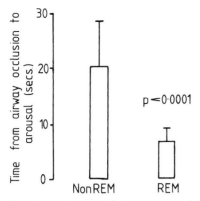

Figure 16–6. Time from airway occlusion to arousal (mean + SD) in 12 subjects, showing that arousal from REM sleep is faster than that from NREM sleepy.[30] (From Douglas NJ. Control of ventilation during sleep. Clin Chest Med. 1985;6:563.)

Bronchial Irritation

Sleep suppresses the cough response to inhaled irritants in human beings,[38] dogs[39] and cats,[40] with cough occurring only after arousal. Similarly, in patients with chronic bronchitis and emphysema, cough is suppressed during sleep.[41] There is no difference between NREM and REM sleep in the arousal response to inhaled citric acid in human beings,[38] but in dogs, the arousal responses both to instilled water and to inhaled citric acid are markedly depressed during REM sleep.[42]

Ventilatory Response to Arousal

The converse of considering which elements of respiration cause arousal is examining the effect of arousal on ventilation. Awakening from sleep, whatever the arousing response, leads to an increase in ventilation,[43, 44] just as sleep onset is associated with a decrease in ventilation.

CONTROL OF BREATHING RHYTHM DURING SLEEP

Spontaneously occurring breathing irregularities during sleep are reviewed in Chapter 17, but a few points are relevant to this chapter.

Human Beings. Bülow[10] found that the subjects who had the most irregular breathing during NREM sleep had the greatest CO_2 tolerance between the awake ventilation-CO_2 set-point and their CO_2 response line. This CO_2 control laxity at sleep onset may be important in the pathogenesis of breathing irregularities, which are common at this time.[10, 45] The induction of hypocapnia either alone or in conjunction with hypoxia can induce irregular breathing in normal subjects during NREM sleep[46] and may lead to occlusive apneas, especially when an inspiratory resistance is added.[47] After airway occlusion in NREM sleep, ventilatory overshoot may occur, especially in those with high hypercapnic ventilatory responses,[12] and this could contribute to respira-tory instability during sleep. During REM sleep, irregular breathing is the norm in adults, and neither isocapnic hypoxia nor hypercapnia regularize this pattern.[1, 11]

Animals. Spontaneous irregular breathing is uncommon in NREM sleep in mature animals. In REM sleep, irregular breathing is universal and is not regularized by hypoxia,[6] hyperoxia,[39] hypercapnia,[21] metabolic alkalosis,[39] carotid body resection,[48] or vagotomy,[49, 50] and indeed respiratory irregularity may increase after vagotomy.[50]

UPPER AIRWAY OPENING MUSCLES DURING SLEEP

In cats, the activity of upper airway opening muscles decreases during NREM sleep, with a further marked reduction during REM sleep.[51] During wakefulness, the activity of these muscles parallels that of the diaphragm during respiratory stimulation with either hypoxia or hypercapnia.[51, 52] Both genioglossal[53] and palatal muscle[53, 54] tone decreased during sleep in normal human beings. However, there have as yet been no studies of the effect of chemostimulation on these muscles during sleep in adults.

FACTORS INFLUENCING RESPIRATORY CONTROL DURING SLEEP

Mechanisms that are likely to contribute to decreased ventilatory responses during sleep include the following.

Decreased Basal Metabolic Rate

Basal metabolic rate falls during sleep, with no major difference in the levels in the different sleep stages.[55, 56] Both ventilation and ventilatory responses are reduced when metabolic rate falls,[57] although the sensor for this is unclear. The decreased basal metabolic rate during sleep is probably a factor in the decreased chemosensitivity during sleep but cannot explain the further reduction in ventilatory response from NREM to REM sleep.

Cerebral Blood Flow– Metabolism Relationship

Brain blood flow increases during sleep.[58–61] The 4 to 25% increase in brain blood flow in slow-wave sleep compared with wakefulness is explicable on the basis of the mild hypercapnia that results from hypoventilation.[60] Brain blood flow increases markedly during REM sleep; this increase was as large as 80% in one study.[59] In goats, Santiago et al.[60] found a 26% increase in brain blood flow during REM sleep and found this to be greater than could be explained by the increase in CO_2. They also found that brain metabolism in REM sleep was similar to that in wakefulness. This increase in the brain blood flow–brain metabolism ratio would depress central chemoreceptor activity during REM sleep and might be a factor in reducing ventilatory responses during REM sleep. However, in human beings, Madsen and colleagues[62] reported that changes in cerebral blood flow paralleled changes in cerebral oxygen metabolism during both slow-wave and REM sleep.

Neurological Changes During Sleep

Cortical activity can influence breathing, with mental concentration increasing both ventilation[63] and ventilatory responses.[10] It seems probable that the hypoventilation and decreased responses to chemical and mechanical stimuli in NREM sleep partially reflect the loss of the "wakefulness" drive to ventilation.[64]

During REM sleep, sensory and motor functions are impaired. There is both presynaptic and postsynaptic inhibition of afferent neurons,[65] which results in raised arousal thresholds to external stimuli,[66] and postsynaptic inhibition of motoneurons,[67] which produces the postural hypotonia typical of REM sleep.[68] This combination of decreased sensory and motor function probably contributes to the marked impairment of ventilatory responses during REM sleep.

It has been suggested that the irregular breathing and impaired ventilatory responses during REM sleep result from alteration of the control of ventilation by behavioral factors.[64] However, evidence suggests that chemical stimuli are the most important ones during REM sleep in people.[69] Furthermore, at least in cats,[51] there seems to be a positive correlation between the activity of some medullary respiratory neurons during REM sleep with pontine-generated discharges termed ponto-geniculo-occipital (PGO) waves. PGO waves are one of the basic electrophysiological phenomena of REM sleep, and thus the dysrhythmic nature of breathing in REM sleep may relate directly to the dysrhythmic nature of REM sleep itself. This is supported by the observation that tidal volume is closely related to the density of eye movements during REM sleep in human beings.[70]

Neuromechanical Factors

Chest-Abdominal Movement. It has been suggested that decreased ventilatory responses in REM sleep result from hypotonia of the intercostal muscles. Although there is no doubt that chest movement and the intercostal electromyogram (EMG) are decreased during REM sleep as compared with NREM sleep, the studies that have included measurements during wakefulness show that chest movement contributes a similar proportion to tidal volume in wakefulness and in REM sleep.[71–73] Clearly, further EMG studies are required, as are studies on the contribution of the chest

to ventilation during the different components of REM sleep.[74]

Reduced Functional Residual Capacity. Functional residual capacity is decreased during REM sleep.[75] Although this might contribute to the hypoxia in REM sleep, it is unlikely to contribute to the decreased ventilatory responses because volume reduction usually increases these responses.[76]

Increased Airflow Resistance. Airflow resistance increases during sleep. The increase is maximal in NREM sleep in human beings,[77, 78] although in cats, resistance seems to be highest during REM sleep.[52] This increased resistance is due to hypotonia of the upper airway opening muscles during sleep. Some of the diminution in ventilatory responses between wakefulness and NREM sleep may be due to changes in upper airway resistance because the occlusion pressure response to hypercapnia is well maintained during NREM sleep.[19] The study[79] that looked at the threshold CO_2 level for respiratory muscle activation in intubated subjects in whom upper airways resistance was thus kept constant suggested that there are sleep stage–related differences in the neuromuscular response to CO_2. The CO_2 level at which respiratory muscle augmentation occurred rose significantly from wakefulness to NREM sleep. The occlusion pressure response to hypercapnia is markedly reduced during REM sleep,[19] which indicates diminution of neuromuscular function.

MECHANISM OF REDUCTION IN VENTILATORY RESPONSES: CONCLUSIONS

It is not possible with our current knowledge to apportion causes for the decrease in ventilatory responses during sleep. It seems likely that the major cause for the decrease in ventilatory responses during NREM sleep is loss of the wakefulness drive to breathe coupled with the decrease in metabolic rate and increase in airflow resistance. The further reduction during REM sleep is likely to result from altered CNS function during REM sleep.

CLINICAL SEQUELAE OF ABNORMAL VENTILATORY RESPONSES

The impaired ventilatory responses permit the development of hypoventilation during sleep and of sleep-related hypoxemia in patients with hypoxic chronic bronchitis and emphysema[80–82] and other respiratory diseases that cause hypoxia.[83, 84] In all of these conditions, the hypoxia is most marked in REM sleep, when the ventilatory responses are at their lowest.

The impaired ventilatory responses during sleep may be accompanied by a decrease in the response of the upper airway opening muscles to chemostimulation during sleep—although this has not been tested—and both factors may be important in the initiation and continuation of apneas. The remarkable insensitivity to external stimuli during sleep allows patients with all of these conditions to develop clinically significant hypoxia and hypercapnia before arousal occurs.

Paradoxically, enhanced ventilatory responses may be present in some patients, which may destabilize ventilation and lead to periodic breathing.[85] This may be an important factor in the development of Cheyne-Stokes respiration in left ventricular heart failure.[86]

References

1. Douglas NJ, White DP, Weil JV, et al. Hypoxic ventilatory response decreases during sleep in normal men. Am Rev Respir Dis. 1982;125:286–289.
1a. Caruana-Montaldo B, Gleeson K, Zwillich CW. The control of breathing in clinical practice. Chest. 2000;117:205–225.
2. Berthon-Jones M, Sullivan CE. Ventilatory and arousal responses to hypoxia in sleeping humans. Am Rev Respir Dis. 1982;125:632–639.
3. Hedemark LL, Kronenberg RS. Ventilatory and heart rate responses to hypoxia and hypercapnia during sleep in adults. J Appl Physiol. 1982;53:307–312.
4. White DP, Douglas NJ, Pickett CK, et al. Hypoxic ventilatory response during sleep in normal women. Am Rev Respir Dis. 1982;126:530–533.
5. Gothe B, Goldman MD, Cherniack NS, et al. Effect of progressive hypoxia on breathing during sleep. Am Rev Respir Dis. 1982;126:97–102.
6. Phillipson EA, Sullivan CE, Read DJC, et al. Ventilatory and waking responses to hypoxia in sleeping dogs. J Appl Physiol. 1978;44:512–520.
7. Bowes G, Townsend ER, Kozar LF, et al. Effect of carotid body denervation on arousal response to hypoxia in sleeping dogs. J Appl Physiol. 1981;51:40–45.
8. Santiago TV, Scardella AT, Edelman NH. Determinants of the ventilatory response to hypoxia during sleep. Am Rev Respir Dis. 1984;130:179–182.
9. Birchfield RI, Sieker HO, Heyman A. Alterations in respiratory function during natural sleep. J Lab Clin Med. 1959;54:216–222.
10. Bülow K. Respiration and wakefulness in man. Acta Physiol Scand. 1963;59(suppl 209):1–110.
11. Douglas NJ, White DP, Weil JV, et al. Hypercapnic ventilatory response in sleeping adults. Am Rev Respir Dis. 1982;126:758–762.
12. Gleeson K, Zwillich CW, White DP. Chemosensitivity and the ventilatory response to airflow obstruction during sleep. J Appl Physiol. 1989;67:1630–1637.
13. Magnussen G. Studies on the Respiration During Sleep. A Contribution to the Physiology of the Sleep Function. London, England: H.K. Lewis; 1944.
14. Ostergaard T. The excitability of the respiratory centre during sleep and during Evipan anaesthesia. Acta Physiol Scand. 1944;8:1–15.
15. Robin ED, Whaley RD, Crump CH, et al. Alveolar gas tensions, pulmonary ventilation and blood pH during physiological sleep in normal subjects. J Clin Invest. 1958;37:981–989.
16. Berthon-Jones M, Sullivan CE. Ventilation and arousal responses to hypercapnia in normal sleeping adults. J Appl Physiol. 1984;57:59–67.
17. Davis JN, Loh L, Nodal J, et al. Effects of sleep on the pattern of CO_2 stimulated breathing in males and females. Adv Exp Med Biol. 1978;99:79–83.
18. Gothe B, Altose MD, Goldman MD, et al. Effect of quiet sleep on resting and CO_2-stimulated breathing in humans. J Appl Physiol. 1981;50:724–730.
19. White DP. Occlusion pressure and ventilation during sleep in normal humans. J Appl Physiol. 1986;61:1279–1287.
20. Phillipson EA, Kozar LF, Rebuck AS, et al. Ventilatory and waking responses to CO_2 in sleeping dogs. Am Rev Respir Dis. 1977;115:251–259.

21. Sullivan CE, Murphy E, Kozar LF, et al. Ventilatory responses to CO_2 and lung inflation in tonic versus phasic REM sleep. J Appl Physiol. 1979;47:1304–1310.
22. Santiago TV, Sinha AK, Edelman NH. Respiratory flow-resistive load compensation during sleep. Am Rev Respir Dis. 1981;123:382–387.
23. Netick A, Dugger WJ, Symmons RA. Ventilatory response to hypercapnia during sleep and wakefulness in cats. J Appl Physiol. 1984;56:1347–1354.
24. Gugger M, Molloy J, Gould GA, et al. Ventilatory and arousal responses to added inspiratory resistance during sleep. Am Rev Respir Dis. 1989;140:1301–1307.
25. Hudgel DW, Mulholland M, Hendricks C. Neuromuscular and mechanical responses to inspiratory resistive loading during sleep. J Appl Physiol. 1987; 63:603–608.
26. Iber C, Berssenbrugge A, Skatrud JB, et al. Ventilatory adaptations to resistive loading during wakefulness and non-REM sleep. J Appl Physiol. 1982;52:607–614.
27. Wiegand L, Zwillich CW, White DP. Sleep and the ventilatory response to resistive loading in normal men. J Appl Physiol. 1988;64:1186–1195.
28. Gora J, Kay A, Colrain IM, et al. Load compensation as a function of state during sleep onset. J Appl Physiol. 1998;84:2123–2131.
29. Ballard RD, Tan WC, Kelly PL, et al. Effect of sleep and sleep deprivation on ventilatory response to bronchoconstriction. J Appl Physiol. 1990;69:490–497.
30. Issa FG, Sullivan CE. Arousal and breathing responses to airway occlusion in healthy sleeping adults. J Appl Physiol. 1983;55:1113–1119.
31. Bowes G, Kozar LF, Andrey SM, et al. Ventilatory responses to inspiratory flow-resistive loads in awake and sleeping dogs. J Appl Physiol. 1983;54:1550–1557.
32. Phillipson EA, Kozar LF, Murphy E. Respiratory load compensation in awake and sleeping dogs. J Appl Physiol. 1976;40:895–902.
33. Sullivan CE, Issa FG. Pathophysiological mechanisms in obstructive sleep apnea. Sleep. 1980;3:235–246.
34. Neubauer J, Santiago TV, Edelman NH. Hypoxic arousal in intact and carotid chemodenervated sleeping cats. J Appl Physiol. 1981;51:1294–1299.
35. Gothe B, Cherniack NS, Williams L. Effect of hypoxia on ventilatory and arousal responses to CO_2 during non-REM sleep with and without flurazepam in young adults. Sleep. 1986;9:24–37.
36. Gugger M, Bogershausen S, Schaffler L. Arousal response to added inspiratory resistance during REM and non-REM sleep in normal subjects. Thorax. 1993;48:125–129.
37. Gleeson K, Zwillich CW, White DP. The influence of increasing ventilatory effort on arousal from sleep. Am Rev Respir Dis. 1990;142:295–300.
38. Jamal K, McMahon G, Edgell G, et al. Cough and arousal responses to inhaled citric acid in sleeping humans [abstract]. Am Rev Respir Dis. 1983;127(suppl):237.
39. Sullivan CE, Kozar LF, Murphy E, et al. Primary role of respiratory afferents in sustaining breathing rhythms. J Appl Physiol. 1978;45:11–17.
40. Anderson CA, Dicke TE, Orem J. Respiratory responses to tracheobronchial stimulation during sleep and wakefulness in the adult cat. Sleep. 1996;19:472–478.
41. Power JT, Stewart IC, Connaughton JJ, et al. Nocturnal cough in patients with chronic bronchitis and emphysema. Am Rev Respir Dis. 1984;130:999–1001.
42. Sullivan CE, Kozar LF, Murphy E, et al. Arousal, ventilatory and airway responses to bronchopulmonary stimulation in sleeping dogs. J Appl Physiol. 1979;47:17–25.
43. Badr MS, Morgan BJ, Finn L, et al. Ventilatory response to induced auditory arousal during non REM sleep. Sleep. 1997;20:707–714.
44. Carley DW, Applebaum R, Basner RC, et al. Respiratory and arousal responses to acoustic stimulation. Chest. 1997;112:1567–1571.
45. Douglas NJ, White DP, Pickett CK, et al. Respiration during sleep in normal man. Thorax. 1982;37:840–844.
46. Skatrud JB, Dempsey JA. Interaction of sleep state and chemical stimuli in sustaining rhythmic ventilation. J Appl Physiol. 1983;55:813–822.
47. Onal E, Burrows DL, Hart RH, et al. Induction of periodic breath-

ing during sleep causes upper airway obstruction in humans. J Appl Physiol. 1986;61:1438–1443.

48. Guazzi M, Freis ED. Sinoaortic reflexes and arterial pH, PO_2 and PCO_2 in wakefulness and sleep. Am J Physiol. 1969;217:1623–1627.

49. Phillipson EA, Murphy E, Kozar LF. Regulation of respiration in sleeping dogs. J Appl Physiol. 1976;40:688–693.

50. Remmers JE, Bartlett D, Putnam MD. Changes in the respiratory cycle associated with sleep. Respir Physiol. 1976;28:227–238.

51. Orem J. Medullary respiratory neuron activity. Relationship to tonic and phasic REM sleep. J Appl Physiol. 1980;48:54–65.

52. Orem J, Netick A, Dement WC. Increased upper airway resistance to breathing during sleep in the cat. Electroencephalogr Clin Neurophysiol. 1977;43:14–22.

53. Mezzanote WS, Tangel DJ, White DP. Influence of sleep onset on upper airway muscle activity in apnea patients versus normal controls. Am J Respir Crit Care Med. 1996;153:1880–1887.

54. Tangel DJ, Mezzanote WS, White DP. Influence of sleep on tensor palatini EMG and upper airways resistance in normal man. J Appl Physiol. 1991;70:2574–2581.

55. Brebbia DR, Altshuler KZ. Oxygen consumption rate and electro-encephalographic stage of sleep. Science. 1965;150:1621–1623.

56. White DP, Weil JV, Zwillich CK. Metabolic rate and breathing during sleep. J Appl Physiol. 1985;59:384–391.

57. Zwillich C, Sahn S, Weil J. Effects of hyper-metabolism on ventilation and chemosensitivity. J Clin Invest. 1977;60:900–906.

58. Mangold R, Sokoloff K, Conner E, et al. The effects of sleep and lack of sleep on the cerebral circulation and metabolism of normal young men. J Clin Invest. 1955;34:1092–1100.

59. Reivich M, Isaacs G, Evarts E, et al. The effect of slow wave sleep and REM sleep on regional cerebral blood flow in cats. J Neurochem. 1968;15:301–306.

60. Santiago TV, Guerra E, Neubauer JA, et al. Correlation between ventilation and brain blood flow during sleep. J Clin Invest. 1984;73:497–506.

61. Townsend RE, Prinz PN, Obrist WD. Human cerebral blood flow during sleep and waking. J Appl Physiol. 1973;35:620–625.

62. Madsen PL, Schmidt JF, Wildschiodtz G, et al. Cerebral O_2 metabolism and cerebral blood flow in humans during deep and rapid-eye movement sleep. J Appl Physiol. 1991;70:2597–2601.

63. Asmussen E. Regulation of respiration: "the black box." Acta Physiol Scand. 1977;99:85–90.

64. Phillipson EA. Control of breathing during sleep. Am Rev Respir Dis. 1978;118:909–939.

65. Pompeiano O. Mechanisms of sensorimotor integration during sleep. Prog Physiol Psychol. 1973;3:1–179.

66. Steriade M, Hobson JA. Neuronal activity during the sleep-waking cycle. Prog Neurobiol. 1976;6:155–376.

67. Nakamura Y, Goldberg LJ, Chandler SH, et al. Intra-cellular analysis of trigeminal motor neuron activity during sleep in the cat. Science. 1978;199:204–207.

68. Pompeiano O. The control of posture and movements during REM sleep: neurophysiological and neurochemical mechanisms. Acta Astronautica. 1975;2:225–239.

69. Meza S, Giannouli E, Younes M. Control of breathing during sleep assessed by proportional assist ventilation. J Appl Physiol. 1998;84:3–12.

70. Gould GA, Gugger M, Molloy J, et al. Breathing pattern and eye movement density during REM sleep in man. Am Rev Respir Dis. 1988;138:874–877.

71. Mortola JP, Anch AM. Chest configuration in supine man: wakefulness and sleep. Respir Physiol. 1978;35:201–213.

72. Stradling JR, Chadwick GA, Frew AJ. Changes in ventilation and its components in normal subjects during sleep. Thorax. 1985;40:364–370.

73. Tabachnik E, Muller NL, Bryan AC, et al. Changes in ventilation and chest wall mechanics during sleep in normal adults. J Appl Physiol. 1981;51:557–564.

74. Millman RP, Knight H, Chung DC, et al. Changes in compartmental ventilation in association with eye movements during REM sleep. J Appl Physiol. 1988;65:1196–1202.

75. Hudgel DW, Devadatta P. Decrease in functional residual capacity during sleep in normal humans. J Appl Physiol. 1984;57:1319–1322.

76. Cherniack NS, Stanley NN, Tuteur PG, et al. Effect of lung volume changes on respiratory drive during hypoxia and hypercapnia. J Appl Physiol. 1973;35:635–641.

77. Hudgel DW, Martin RJ, Johnson B, et al. Mechanics of the respiratory system and breathing pattern during sleep in normal humans. J Appl Physiol. 1984;56:133–137.

78. Lopes JM, Tabachnik E, Muller NL, et al. Total airway resistance and respiratory muscle activity during sleep. J Appl Physiol. 1983;54:773–777.

79. Ingrassia TS III, Nelson SB, Harris CD, et al. Influence of sleep state on carbon dioxide responsiveness: a study of the unloaded respiratory pump in man. Am Rev Respir Dis. 1991;144:1125–1129.

80. Douglas NJ, Calverley PMA, Leggett RJE, et al. Transient hypoxaemia during sleep in chronic bronchitis and emphysema. Lancet. 1979;1:1–4.

81. Fleetham JA, Mezon B, West P, et al. Chemical control of ventilation and sleep arterial oxygen desaturation in patients with COPD. Am Rev Respir Dis. 1980;122:583–589.

82. Koo KW, Sax DS, Snider GL. Arterial blood gases and pH during sleep in chronic obstructive pulmonary disease. Am J Med. 1975;58:663–670.

83. Mezon BL, West P, Israels J, et al. Sleep breathing abnormalities in kyphoscoliosis. Am Rev Respir Dis. 1980;122:617–621.

84. Muller NL, Francis PW, Gurwitz D, et al. Mechanism of hemoglobin desaturation during rapid-eye-movement sleep in normal subjects and in patients with cystic fibrosis. Am Rev Respir Dis. 1980;121:463–469.

85. Cherniack NS. Apnea and periodic breathing during sleep. N Engl J Med. 1999;341:985–987.

86. Javaheri S. A mechanism of central sleep apnea in patients with heart failure. N Engl J Med. 1999;341:949–954.

Respiratory Physiology: Breathing in Normal Subjects

Jean Krieger

Sleep is associated with definite changes in respiratory function in normal human beings. Whether these changes serve a specific function remains unclear and will probably not be clarified before the functions of sleep itself are better understood.

Drowsiness or unsteady nonrapid eye movement (NREM) sleep is characterized in many subjects by a regularly oscillating periodic breathing resulting in swings in Po_2 and Pco_2, with an overall moderate decrease in ventilation. These oscillations seem to be mainly due to sleep instability during this stage, and the natural tendency of breathing regulation to be unstable probably aggravates this situation.

In steady NREM sleep, there occurs a regular pattern of breathing with more pronounced hypoventilation than during drowsiness. This hypoventilation seems to be due to a combination of decreased ventilatory drive and a sleep-related defective compensation of an increased upper airway resistance. Ventilatory mechanics do not seem to be impaired during NREM sleep.

Rapid eye movement (REM) sleep is characterized by erratic, shallow breathing with irregularities both in amplitude and in frequency synchronous to REM bursts that are most probably of central origin and related to REM sleep processes. Hypoxemia equal to or greater than that during NREM sleep seems mainly to result from hypoventilation.

This chapter describes changes in spontaneous breathing during sleep in normal subjects and discusses possible mechanisms for these changes. This topic has become important because of the recognition of sleep breathing disorders.[1-8]

In sleep physiology as a whole, and of respiration during sleep in particular, a general, clearly established finding is that most major functions differ in nonrapid eye movement (NREM) and rapid eye movement (REM) sleep (see reference 9 for a review). Therefore, respiration during sleep in normal human beings is reviewed separately for these two sleep states.

Ventilation performs various secondary functions, such as speech and laughter in human beings and thermoregulation in animals. For this reason, control systems and especially central nervous control systems are likely to be different in human beings and in animals. In animal studies, the upper airways are usually bypassed in experiments; ventilation may then be altered during sleep because changes in upper airway resistance have a crucial role in breathing during sleep. Thus, in this chapter, reference to animal data is seldom made, whether they are used to replace missing human data or as sources for interpreting observations made in human beings.

THE DEFINITION OF NORMALITY

The criteria of normality, whatever the field considered, depend on the methods used to assess the absence of abnormality. Thus, it is clear that the composition of groups selected as "normal" will reflect these criteria and that their variability may result in variability in the observations made. The difficulty in establishing criteria for reference groups is probably of particular importance in the area of breathing during sleep, because breathing abnormalities during sleep have been related to such common conditions as male gender, increased age, excess weight, and snoring.

It must be kept in mind that respiratory measurement devices may alter breathing during sleep in at least two ways: (1) by direct effects on respiration, and (2) by effects on sleep and especially on sleep stability, which may in turn affect breathing stability.

NREM SLEEP

The four stages of NREM sleep are characterized by progressively slower electroencephalographic (EEG) activity associated with transients (spindles and K complexes) in stages 2 and 3. Usually, NREM sleep is divided into light sleep (stages 1 and 2) and slow-wave sleep (stages 3 and 4). When breathing during sleep is considered, it is more convenient to separate unsteady and steady sleep. At sleep onset, deep slow-wave sleep is not attained immediately, but rather the level of vigilance oscillates from arousal to stages 1 and 2 for several minutes or tens of minutes before steady sleep in stage 2 and then stage 3 to 4 is reached. Thus, unsteady NREM sleep includes stage 1 and short periods of stage 2 interrupted by arousals, and steady NREM sleep includes stable stage 2 and stages 3 and 4.

Unsteady NREM Sleep

The irregularity of breathing at sleep onset struck early authors who studied breathing during sleep.[10, 11] The irregularity was not random, however, but consisted of a regular waxing and waning of breathing amplitude. Thus, it was called periodic breathing *(periodische Athmung)*.[10]

Periodic breathing at sleep onset and during drowsiness was later observed by many authors, but the most comprehensive study was that of Bülow.[12] *Periodic breathing* is defined as oscillations in breathing amplitude, which regularly decreases and increases. However, this definition is rather elastic, for the oscillations may be of low amplitude, resulting in alternating hyperventilation and hypoventilation, or of large amplitude, including apneas at the nadir of the oscillations. During the oscillations in amplitude, there are few if any changes in respiratory rate.[13] Different studies report the incidence of periodic breathing at sleep onset ranging from 40 to 80% of normal subjects. This variability may be related to the elastic definition of periodic breathing. Another possible explanation is the age of the subjects studied, because it has been suggested that the frequency of periodic breathing increases with age,[14, 15] although this age relationship is not universally observed.[12] The pattern of periodic breathing (Fig. 17-1) resembles either Cheyne-Stokes respiration, with a progressive decrease and progressive increase in breathing amplitude before the apnea or hypopnea,[12, 15, 16] or Biot's breathing, with a progressive decrease in amplitude and then a brisk increase after the apnea, the first or second breath on breathing resumption being of maximal amplitude.[12, 17]

The wavelength of periodic breathing is usually between 60 and 90 sec[12] but has been found to range from 30 sec[18] to 120 sec.[15] The duration of the apnea itself ranges from 10 sec[19, 20] to 40 sec[12, 15, 17] or more.[14] The apneas observed during drowsiness in normal subjects are generally of the central type,[13] meaning that the interruption (or decrease) of airflow is concomitant with an interruption (or decrease) of respiratory effort. However, obstructive apneas, during which respiratory effort persists during the respiratory arrest, may occasionally be seen.[14]

Simultaneous EEG recordings have shown that the variations in breathing amplitude parallel variations in the level of vigilance.[12, 21] The highest ventilatory levels are recorded during wakefulness or arousal; the progressive decrease in breathing amplitude is synchronous to falling asleep. Resumption of breathing, if it is sudden, usually corresponds to an arousal with reappearance of EEG alpha activity.

The duration of periodic breathing at sleep onset varies in length; it lasts from 10 to 20 min[12] up to 60 min.[15, 16] Periodic breathing persists as long as sleep oscillates between arousal and stage 1 or 2; it disappears when stable stage 2 or deeper sleep is reached.[12] Because the respiratory system is controlled by negative feedback, it is prone to instability, the more so that the feedback loop gain (including the controller gain and the controlled system gain) or the delay between a change and its detection is high. An artificially increased controlled system gain induces periodic breathing in normal subjects; periodic breathing was more likely to occur in males who had higher ventilatory responses to hypercapnia, an index of controller gain.[22] Because hypoxia induces an increase in the controller gain, this may be the mechanism of hypoxia-induced periodic breathing during sleep. Other theories have been proposed to explain the periodic breathing observed at sleep onset.[3, 23] Breathing instability at sleep onset would result from the combination of two factors: (1) the set-point of regulation of ventilation is different in wakefulness and sleep, with a higher PCO_2 level and a lower ventilation during sleep; and (2) sleep onset is not immediate but rather oscillates between arousal, stage 1 sleep, and stage 2 sleep before stable stage 2 and then stages 3 and 4 sleep are reached. Thus, falling asleep results in decreased ventilation and a higher PCO_2 adjusted to the sleep set-point; on subsequent arousal, the increased PCO_2, above the wakefulness set-point constitutes an error signal that provokes hyperventilation until the wakefulness set-point is reached. When the subject subsequently falls asleep, the level of PCO_2 will in turn be below the sleep set-point, with resultant hypoventilation and so forth until stable sleep is reached.

According to this theory, breathing at sleep onset should be more unstable when (1) sleep is more unsta-

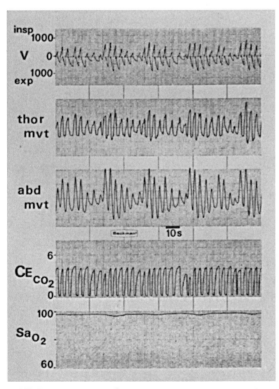

Figure 17-1. Typical breathing pattern during unsteady NREM sleep. $CECO_2$, CO_2 concentration (%) in the face mask; insp, inspiration; exp, expiration; SaO_2, oxygen saturation (%); thor mvt, abd mvt, thoracic and abdominal movements; V, ventilatory volumes (ml) obtained from a pneumotachograph attached to a face mask. (From Krieger J. Breathing during sleep in normal subjects. Clin Chest Med. 1985;6:577-594.)

ble and the changes from arousal to sleep are sudden, (2) the difference between the wakefulness and sleep set-points is greater, and (3) the ventilatory response to chemical stimuli is greater. These implications are in agreement with Bülow's observations.[12]

In other cases, especially in younger healthy subjects, respiratory instability at sleep onset is aperiodic.[12, 24, 25] In those cases, the dependence of ventilatory instability on sleep-wake state has also been demonstrated[25]; the magnitude of sleep state–related fluctuations in ventilation increases over the sleep-onset period due to chemical amplification of sleep-state effects, and to nonchemical factors.[26]

The waking state per se appears to stimulate breathing by a poorly understood mechanism. That this respiratory *wakefulness stimulus* is of crucial importance in sustaining breathing rhythmicity when chemical stimuli are reduced is suggested by posthyperventilation apnea, the occurrence of which is facilitated by falling asleep.[27–29] A threshold level of P_{CO_2} below which sleep apnea appears has been demonstrated.[23] Because of a delay between blood gas changes and the chemoreceptor response, hypercapnia and hypoxia can occur during periodic breathing. Models have shown that once hypoxia occurs during sleep, the intrinsic respiratory control mechanisms lead to breathing instability.[30–32] These models, although they fail to account for the initial disturbance resulting in the hypoxia that initiates periodic breathing, show that periodic breathing, once established, tends to be self-maintained. However, hypoxia does not have a key role in periodic breathing at sea level because periodic breathing is not suppressed by hyperoxic conditions.[12, 17] Because hypoxia and hypercapnia are arousal stimuli,[33] sleep instability is further aggravated. Thus, sleep instability and intrinsic respiratory control mechanisms together create a vicious circle of breathing instability at sleep onset (for a review of the mechanisms of breathing instability at sleep onset, see reference 34). The increase in upper airway resistance related to sleep (see later) and the associated increase in respiratory effort probably contribute to this instability, because partial occlusion of the upper airways in normal subjects has been shown to produce central and obstructive apneas during sleep.[35] The information from the lungs to the centers does not seem to have a major role, because there is no difference in the occurrence of hypopneas and apneas or periodic breathing between patients with heart-lung transplants and age-matched controls.[36] Stable sleep can be reached only if this vicious circle is somehow broken. It is likely that dampening systems more probably neurogenic than chemical in nature have a major role in allowing ventilation and sleep to reach a steady state.

Once instability is established, obstructive apneas may occur as a consequence of the different response of diaphragm and upper airway muscles to chemical stimuli.[37] A similar mechanism has been proposed to explain obstructive sleep apneas in sleep apnea syndromes, which suggests that these syndromes could result from an exaggeration of normal periodic breathing at sleep onset.[38] However, in normal subjects, audi-

tory-induced arousals, although followed by transient hyperpnea, do not induce secondary hypopnea or apnea.[39]

Thus, breathing at sleep onset is physiologically unstable, but the magnitude of the instability is variable, ranging from small fluctuations in breathing amplitude, which result in increased indices of variability during light NREM sleep stages,[40, 41] to severe periodic breathing with repeated apneas. The extremes of this range overlap with what may be called sleep apnea syndromes in regard to both duration and frequency of apneas.

Because of the instability of ventilation during light NREM sleep, these periods have often been disregarded in studies of ventilatory parameters during sleep, so that little is known about them. On average, ventilation decreases and P_{CO_2} increases during periodic breathing.[12] In addition, there is oscillation in Sa_{O_2} (see Fig. 17–1); however, the extent of these Sa_{O_2} oscillations is not clear.

During periods of stage 1 sleep devoid of periodic breathing, minute ventilation decreases to a level intermediate between that of wakefulness and stage 2 sleep[23]; alveolar P_{CO_2} then increases by a mean of about 1 mmHg.[23]

Steady NREM Sleep

Ventilation

During steady NREM sleep, breathing is remarkably regular in both amplitude and frequency,[12, 16, 20, 42, 43] resulting in the lowest indices of variability of all sleep stages[12, 40] (Fig. 17–2). There is a decrease in minute ventilation during steady slow-wave sleep, compared with wakefulness, although in some reports the changes are not statistically significant. The decrease in minute ventilation ranges from 0.4 to 1.5 liters/min.

When all available data are averaged, the decrease in minute ventilation is about 13% of the wakefulness value in sleep stage 2 and about 15% in stage 3 to 4 (Fig. 17–3).[43a] Thus, ventilation appears to decrease progressively from stage 1 to stage 4,[44] which suggests that the decrease is not merely the consequence of the suppression of a wakefulness stimulus for breathing. It could be related to a progressive decrease in metabolic rate[45] with deepening of sleep, a possibility that is, however, contradicted by the progressive increase in P_{CO_2} with deepening of NREM sleep.[12] Thus, it is more likely that the decrease in minute ventilation during NREM sleep is linked to active sleep mechanisms.

It is unclear whether the decrease in minute ventilation is due to a decrease in tidal volume or in respiratory frequency or in both. Most studies report a decrease in tidal volume that averages 16% in stage 2 and 18.5% in stage 3 to 4 (see Fig. 17–3). Generally, the greater the wakefulness tidal volume and the more invasive the respiratory device, the greater the decrease in sleep tidal volume, which suggests that nonadaptation to the experimental conditions may have a role. In terms of minute ventilation, the decrease in tidal vol-

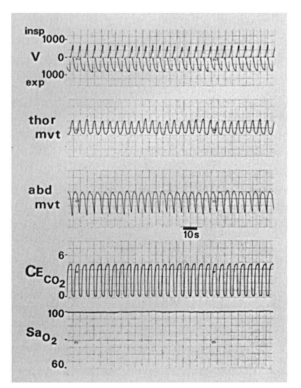

Figure 17-2. Typical breathing pattern during steady NREM sleep. Abbreviations as in Figure 17-1. (From Krieger J. Breathing during sleep in normal subjects. Clin Chest Med. 1985;6:577-594.)

ume is aggravated or partially compensated for by a decrease or an increase in respiratory rate, depending on the study considered, but on average, changes in respiratory rate are minimal (see Fig. 17-3).

The changes in ventilation observed during NREM sleep in human beings are different from those observed in animals,[6] in which the decrease in minute ventilation is due to a decrease in respiratory rate incompletely compensated for by an increase in tidal volume. This fact emphasizes why the greatest care must be used in extrapolating results from animals to humans beings.

Respiratory timing has been less often analyzed during NREM sleep than have minute ventilation and tidal volume. Inspiratory and expiratory durations have been found to change diversely during sleep, compared with wakefulness.[24, 41, 46-48] As a result, the duty cycle of breathing (T_I/T_{TOT}) has been seen to increase,[13, 49] to not change,[24, 47] or to decrease.[46] None of these changes were statistically significant, which suggests that the fluctuations occur at random. In all of these studies, the mean inspiratory flow (V_I/T_I) decreased; the reduction ranged from 0.02 to 0.50 liter/sec.

Conclusion. Quantitative studies show that ventilation during steady NREM sleep is lower than during wakefulness, and the deeper the NREM sleep stages, the lower the ventilation. Mean inspiratory flow is decreased, whereas there are no consistent changes in inspiratory duration and cycle duration; the result is a decreased tidal volume.

Rib Cage and Abdominal Contributions

Most studies of the thoracic and abdominal contributions to breathing during sleep report an increased rib cage contribution.[10, 43, 47, 48, 50-53] This increase involves mainly lateral expansion of the rib cage.[51]

The increase in rib cage contribution to tidal volume is accompanied by an increase in the respiratory electromyographic (EMG) activity of the intercostal muscles,[19, 48, 54] diaphragmatic respiratory activity being a little increased[48] or unchanged[54, 55] (but decreased when alveolar P_{CO_2} is maintained at a constant level).[56] The increased thoracoabdominal muscle activity results in increased esophageal pressure swings.[54] The contradiction between increased EMG activity and decreased flow rate suggests either impaired muscular efficiency or increased airway resistance.[19, 54] Impaired muscular efficiency is unlikely because of the observation that transdiaphragmatic pressure is increased with no change in diaphragmatic activity.[54]

Upper Airway Resistance

Contrary to early studies,[16] a large increase (230%) has been shown to occur in total airway resistance.[54]

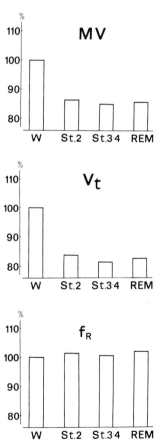

Figure 17-3. Changes in respiratory parameters during sleep. St. 2, stage 2; St. 3-4, stages 3 and 4 of NREM sleep; REM, rapid eye movement sleep. The data are computed from references 12, 41, 43a, 46-48, 50, 54, 69, 82, 84, and 138 as the average percentage of the wakefulness (W) value of minute ventilation (MV: 7.17 liter•min^{-1}), tidal volume (VT 471 ml), and respiratory frequency (fr: 15.4 c•min^{-1}).

The resistance of the upper airway (above the retro-epiglottic space) increases more than twofold during NREM sleep,[24, 57, 58] while the elastic or flow-resistive properties of the lung are not altered.[24] The site of the increased resistance is palatal or hypopharyngeal.[59]

The finding of an increased upper airway resistance during sleep is in keeping with changes in the EMG activity of upper airway muscles during sleep. Using transcutaneous recordings of suprahyoid and infrahyoid muscles, Berger[60] observed a continual discrete decrease in the EMG activity of "laryngeal" muscles from wakefulness to stage 2 sleep. Because of the possible implications of the changes in upper airway muscle activity in the mechanism of the upper airway obstruction during sleep apnea, many muscles have been investigated more specifically during sleep by use of wire electrodes. Two aspects of muscle activity must be considered: the phasic activity, which occurs periodically, in phase with a component of the respiratory cycle, generally inspiration; and the tonic activity, which is the background activity on which phasic activity is superimposed.[61] Whereas the regulation of phasic activity is clearly related to respiratory regulation, the regulation of the tonic background is probably more or less independent of respiratory regulation and more related to the general muscle tone. Sleep-related changes in phasic activity are different in the various muscles investigated: unchanged in the geniohyoid,[62] increased in the genioglossus,[63] and decreased in the posterior cricoarytenoid.[64] The changes in tonic activity are more consistent, because it was found to decrease in the tensor veli palatini,[65] the genioglossus,[66] the geniohyoid,[62] and the posterior cricoarytenoid,[64] but it was found to be unchanged in the genioglossus in other studies.[65, 67] It is noteworthy that the decrease in tonic activity of the tensor veli palatini was correlated with the increase in nasopharyngeal resistance.[65] The contrast between the decreased EMG activity of upper airway muscles and the increased or maintained activity of intercostal and diaphragmatic muscles suggests different neural control of these muscle groups.

In addition to decreased EMG activity of dilating muscles, the decrease in lung volume that occurs during NREM sleep[68, 69] probably concurs to increase upper airway resistance during sleep, because it has been shown that lung inflation decreases upper airway resistance.[70] The thoracic volume dependence of upper airway resistance does not seem to be mediated by a decrease in upper airway muscle activity.[71]

The resulting increase in upper airway resistance has a role in the decrease in ventilation during sleep. During wakefulness, an added external inspiratory resistance similar in magnitude to the increase in upper airway resistance observed during NREM sleep results in decreased mean inspiratory flow compensated for by changes in respiratory timing (increased inspiratory time and decreased expiratory time), which results in an increased tidal volume. Despite a decreased respiratory rate, minute ventilation is maintained, but at the expense of increased respiratory work.[72] The ability to maintain minute ventilation is reduced during NREM sleep, because the mouth occlusion pressure, a measure of the respiratory drive, which is markedly increased during wakefulness, is unchanged during NREM sleep under these loading conditions.[50] An acute resistive load of about 20 cm H_2O/liter/sec (i.e., in the order of magnitude of the change in upper airway resistance during NREM sleep) has more effects on ventilation than during wakefulness[50, 73, 74]; after sustained loading of 12 cm H_2O/liter/sec, tidal volume and minute ventilation returned to baseline values.[73] However, a lower load of 4, 7, and 10 cm H_2O/liter/sec decreased tidal volume and minute ventilation similarly during wakefulness and NREM sleep.[75]

The effect of increased upper airway resistance on ventilation during sleep is further demonstrated by the effects of preventing the physiological increase in upper airway resistance with nasal continuous positive airway pressure (CPAP), which is followed by an increase in ventilation, even when end-tidal $PaCO_2$ is held constant,[76] a finding that was not confirmed in another similar work[77] in which CPAP did not correct the sleep-related decrease in ventilation and increase in end-tidal PCO_2, although total pulmonary resistance returned to wake values. However, in this latter study, the subjects were selected for the absence of obesity and of snoring, and the sleep-related increase in pulmonary resistance was much less. Thus, it can be concluded that increased upper airway resistance is one factor contributing to decreased ventilation during sleep, especially when the increase in upper airway resistance is large. Recent data show that changes in upper airway resistance contribute to the decrease in ventilation early in sleep onset, whereas during stable NREM sleep, larger increases in upper airway resistance are compensated for, so that ventilation decreases less than upper airway resistance increases.[78] Data from otherwise normal laryngectomized subjects show that increased upper airway resistance during sleep is not the only factor of decreased ventilation and CO_2 retention.[79]

In addition, a decreased respiratory drive has also been demonstrated: mouth occlusion pressure decreases during NREM sleep[80]; furthermore, when compared at equal alveolar CO_2 levels, the EMG activities of intercostal and diaphragmatic muscles are lower during NREM sleep than during wakefulness.[81] Thus, the mechanisms of decreased ventilation during sleep involve both a decrease in ventilatory drive and an impaired efficacy of the respiratory pump due to increased upper airway resistance.

Arterial Blood Gases

Alveolar ventilation also decreases during NREM sleep, as reflected by higher alveolar and arterial PCO_2. Alveolar and arterial PCO_2 values increase by 3 to 7 mmHg during NREM sleep.[12, 16, 20, 28, 42, 46, 82, 83] A few studies found increases of 2 mmHg or less or no change.[13, 23, 84, 85]

The reduction in alveolar ventilation decreases alveolar and arterial O_2 (ranging from 3.5 to 9.4 mmHg)[16, 84] and SaO_2 (2% or less).[16, 82, 86] These changes occur despite a reduced metabolic rate reflected by 10 to 20% decreases of O_2 consumption and CO_2 production.[12, 16, 45, 87–91]

Pulmonary Arterial Pressure

Pulmonary arterial pressures have rarely been investigated during sleep in normal subjects. During light NREM sleep, periodic oscillations of pulmonary arterial pressure with a period of 20 to 30 sec occurred in one of three subjects[18]; they occurred even during regular, steady breathing. On average, both diastolic and systolic pulmonary arterial pressures increased by 4 to 5 mmHg during NREM sleep.[20]

Effects of Arousal

Induced transient arousal from NREM sleep (a brief change in EEG without awakening) results in an increase in EMG activity of the diaphragm (150% of wake level) and of upper airway dilating muscles (levator veli palatini, 250%; genioglossus, 150%),[92] together with an increase in maximum inspiratory flow and tidal volume (160%) and a decrease in upper airway resistance,[93, 94] but auditory stimuli without EEG arousal cause no change in ventilation.[94]

REM SLEEP

Ventilation

When Aserinsky and Kleitman[95] first described a hitherto unidentified sleep stage characterized by low-voltage EEG activity and regularly occurring periods of ocular motility, they mentioned, among other associated periodic phenomena, an increased respiratory frequency. This sleep stage was called REM sleep and was identified as the stage during which dreams occur. Later, breathing during REM sleep was described as irregular (Fig. 17–4). The irregularity consists of sudden changes in both respiratory amplitude and frequency,[12, 19, 48, 55, 96–99] at times interrupted by central apneas lasting 10 to 30 sec,[19, 44, 100] and is different from the regular periodic breathing at sleep onset. The breathing irregularities do not occur at random but are linked to bursts of rapid eye movements.[12, 101–103] The first eye movement of a REM burst is associated with a sudden decrease in breathing amplitude, followed by a progressive increase even when the REM burst is prolonged.[101, 103] Although it was first considered to be part of the emotional reaction to the dream content,[98] Aserinsky[101] later ascribed this breathing pattern to REM sleep processes per se. In animals, this irregular pattern persists during hypoxia, hypercapnia, and metabolic alkalosis, as well as after vagotomy and chemodenervation.[6] For these reasons, it has been suggested that the breathing pattern is not dependent on chemical regulation processes but is produced by activation of the behavioral respiratory control system by REM sleep processes.[3] Nevertheless, ventilation over prolonged periods (i.e., 3 to 25 min) was found to be highly correlated with O_2 consumption and CO_2 production in REM sleep, as well as in NREM sleep,[45] which indicates that the chemical regulation of ventilation is not abolished in REM sleep.

Quantitative measurements of ventilation in REM

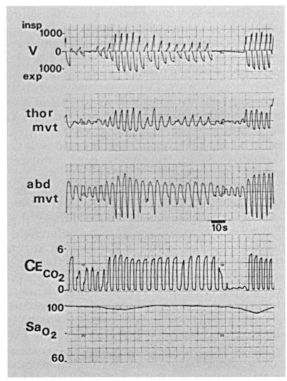

Figure 17–4. Typical breathing pattern during REM sleep. Abbreviations as in Figure 17–1.

sleep in normal subjects show a variable decrease in minute ventilation, compared with that in wakefulness. However, the comparison with NREM ventilation reveals discrepancies: minute ventilation in REM sleep has been found to be increased,[12, 45, 48] slightly decreased,[24, 41, 44, 47] markedly decreased,[84] or unchanged; in addition to the same methodological problems as in NREM sleep, these discrepancies may be due to differences in the choice of the REM sleep period selected for analysis because minute ventilation is lower during phasic REM sleep, when REM bursts are abundant, than during tonic REM sleep, when REM bursts are absent.[49] In addition, body movements, which frequently occur during REM sleep, may alter both the level of ventilation and the calibration of indirect measurement of ventilatory flow.[104] Parallel to reported discrepancies in minute ventilation changes, tidal volume changes also vary. Tidal volume has been found to be decreased,[24] unchanged,[44, 48, 84] or increased[54] in REM sleep, compared with NREM sleep, and the respiratory frequency was either slightly increased[24, 48, 84] or slightly decreased.[44, 54] V_I/T_I has been described as unchanged[24] or increased.[13] All these studies, however, report an unchanged T_I/T_{TOT}. Thus, the available data on breathing during REM sleep in normal human beings are somewhat discordant. Nevertheless, when all available data are averaged, minute ventilation, tidal volume, and respiratory rate during REM sleep differ little from those observed in NREM sleep (see Fig. 17–3).

Rib Cage and Abdominal Contributions

In contrast to the increased rib cage contribution to breathing during NREM sleep, the rib cage contribution during REM sleep is found to be decreased[13, 19] owing to a marked reduction in intercostal muscle activity[13, 35, 105] or to be unchanged.[47] Diaphragmatic activity, both tonic and phasic inspiratory[48, 54, 55] or only phasic,[86] is increased. In addition, even though paradoxical thoracoabdominal movements are not observed, thoracic and abdominal displacements are not exactly in phase.[19] Despite the increase in diaphragmatic activity, transdiaphragmatic pressure is decreased, which implies impaired muscle efficiency.[54] The decreased intercostal EMG activity is attributed to the REM-related supraspinal inhibition of the alpha motoneuron drive and the specific depression of fusimotor function.[95] Because the diaphragm's fusorial innervation is quite low, this muscle is relatively spared from the depressive effects described.[106]

Upper Airway Resistance

Airway resistance measurements during REM sleep are also contradictory. Total airway resistance was said to be lower during REM sleep than during NREM sleep, with large individual variations; but on average, airway resistance in REM sleep is similar to that of awake humans.[107] In contrast, other studies show an increase in upper airway resistance during REM sleep that is approximately the same as in NREM sleep,[24] or intermediate between wakefulness and NREM sleep,[57] while the lower airway resistance is unchanged.[24] The upper airway resistance would be expected to be highest during REM sleep, because the muscular atonia of the upper airway is maximal during this sleep stage,[60, 66, 108] but it has been much less investigated than during NREM sleep.

Arterial Blood Gases

In contrast to the abundant literature concerning changes in oxygenation during REM sleep in patients with chronic obstructive pulmonary disease, data on oxygenation during REM sleep in normal subjects are surprisingly few. Some studies on blood oxygenation during sleep report an unchanged O_2 level during REM sleep, compared with NREM sleep,[48, 105] whereas others give lower values in REM than in NREM sleep.[49, 86] REM values are always reported as lower than wakefulness values, including both a sustained[86] drop and further transient drops in SaO_2 in conjunction with REM-related hypoventilation.[86, 101] CO_2 is even more difficult to evaluate during REM sleep. End-tidal PCO_2 does not yield an approximation of alveolar PCO_2 because end-expiratory plateaus are seldom reached during the rapid, shallow breathing pattern characteristic of REM sleep. Because arterial values have been only occasionally measured during sleep in normal subjects, the lack of reliable information on PCO_2 is probably a cause of the controversy with respect to the mechanisms of hypoxemia during REM sleep. Some authors argue that no sustained hypoventilation can be demonstrated and instead incriminate impaired lung mechanics.[86, 109] According to these hypotheses, loss of intercostal and, to a lesser extent, diaphragmatic tonic activity results in a decreased baseline position of rib cage and

Table 17-1. SUMMARY OF BREATHING PATTERNS DURING SLEEP IN NORMAL SUBJECTS

Breathing Pattern	Type of Sleep
Periodic	Unsteady NREM sleep
Regular	Steady NREM sleep
Mostly regular	"Tonic" REM sleep
Irregular; central apneas common	"Phase" REM sleep

abdomen and thus in a decreased functional residual capacity, which leads to airway closure in the dependent lung regions and a consequent ventilation-perfusion mismatch. However, the measured decrease in functional residual capacity is too low, both in REM and in NREM sleep, to be likely to produce a significant ventilation-perfusion mismatch, at least in normal subjects.[69] Thus, it seems probable that the hypoxemia observed during REM sleep is due to hypoventilation.

CONCLUSIONS

Drowsiness or unsteady NREM sleep is characterized in many subjects by a regularly oscillating periodic breathing resulting in swings in PO_2 and PCO_2, with an overall moderate decrease in ventilation (Table 17-1). These oscillations seem to be mainly due to sleep instability during this stage, and the natural tendency of breathing regulation to be unstable probably aggravates this situation.

In steady NREM sleep, there occurs a regular pattern of breathing with more pronounced hypoventilation than during drowsiness. This hypoventilation seems to be due to a combination of decreased ventilatory drive and a sleep-related defective compensation of an increased upper airway resistance. Ventilatory mechanics do not seem to be impaired during NREM sleep.

REM sleep is characterized by erratic, shallow breathing with irregularities both in amplitude and in frequency synchronous to REM bursts that are most probably of central origin and related to REM sleep processes. Hypoxemia equal to or greater than that during NREM sleep seems mainly to result from hypoventilation.

RESPIRATION-RELATED EVENTS DURING SLEEP

Snoring

Snoring is reviewed in greater detail in Chapter 70. In a survey of 4713 people, it was found that 41% of men and 28% of women were occasional or habitual snorers.[110] After the age of 60 years, the figure rises to 60% of men and 40% of women. This high frequency, confirmed by other studies,[111-113] may explain why snoring is considered to be normal, annoying only to the snorer's bedroom partner, who usually calls for treatment for the snorer.

Snoring may be more than an acoustic nuisance[114];

systemic hypertension, cardiac dysfunction, angina pectoris, and cerebral infarction are more frequent among habitual snorers,[110, 111, 113, 115–117] even when the data are corrected for the effects of increased age, male sex, and obesity, which are more frequent among snorers[110, 117, 118] and are factors contributing to these diseases. The link between blood pressure and snoring seems to be close; Robin[119] had a patient who knew his blood pressure had increased when he was told he snored more heavily. The immediate rise in systemic blood pressure during snoring has been confirmed by polygraphic recordings.[120]

However, because sleep apnea syndromes are frequent in otherwise asymptomatic snorers (30 to 50%),[51, 121] it is not clear whether these diseases (hypertension, angina pectoris, and cerebral infarction) are a consequence of snoring by itself or of the associated obstructive sleep apnea syndrome. Nevertheless, even in nonapneic snorers, the resistance of the upper airways during sleep increases more than in nonsnorers,[58] with resultant distortion of the rib cage, which might cause an increase in respiratory work or hypoventilation during sleep.[122] That snoring is by itself a factor contributing to hypoxemia is further demonstrated by the effects of nasal CPAP on patients with sleep apnea: the elimination of snoring by an increase in the applied pressure is regularly accompanied by an increase in oxyhemoglobin saturation. Snoring may be considered to be part of a continuum including normal, silent, unobstructed breathing; occasional snoring; habitual snoring with occasional obstructive sleep apneas; and, finally, an overt[107, 114, 123] obstructive sleep apnea syndrome. However, the male-to-female ratio of snoring, which is roughly 2:1, is fairly different from the male-to-female ratio of the obstructive sleep apnea syndrome, which is 9:1; this suggests that the link between obstructive sleep apnea and snoring is not as close as postulated.

Sighs

Sighs are deep breaths with higher-than-average tidal volumes. The function of the sigh during wakefulness is to open collapsed alveoli and hence to increase the pulmonary compliance and functional residual capacity,[124] thus preventing atelectasis. Sighing during sleep may thus be of crucial importance. Among normal sleeping subjects, wide intersubject variability was reported, ranging from 1 to 25 sighs per night.[125] Sighs occur in all sleep stages, including REM sleep, but with a higher frequency in light NREM sleep. Sighs are also often associated with arousals. Finally, sighs are often followed by apneas, hypoventilation, or a decreased respiratory frequency.[13, 81]

FACTORS INFLUENCING BREATHING IN SLEEPING NORMAL SUBJECTS

Gender

None of the sleep studies, including quantitative measurement of breathing parameters, demonstrates a significant difference between genders with respect to changes in minute ventilation, tidal volume, or respiratory rate. However, the increase in upper airway resistance is much more important in men than in women.[126] It has been suggested that female hormones have a significant effect on the upper dilator muscles, peaking during the luteal phase, lower during the follicular phase, and lowest in postmenopause.[126a] A gender-related difference is also suggested by a greater frequency of episodes of O_2 desaturation during both NREM and REM sleep in normal men compared with normal women.[14] Yet, a greater frequency of disordered breathing has not been confirmed by other studies.[44, 127] Because increased frequencies of desaturation episodes are also associated with excess weight, it was suggested that the male predominance of desaturation episodes during sleep could be an artifact resulting from poor body weight matching between gender groups.[127]

Age

Owing to maturational differences in the central nervous system and muscle and osteochondral structures, the problems of respiration during sleep in newborns, infants, and children are different from those in adults. Adolescents' breathing patterns during sleep closely resemble those of young adults.[13] Tabachnik et al.,[48] however, noticed less marked O_2 desaturation during REM sleep in the adolescents they studied; they attributed this to the lower closing capacity in adolescents, which results in less ventilation-perfusion mismatching because of the decrease in the functional residual capacity during REM sleep. In young adults of both sexes, no nocturnal desaturation was observed either.[40, 128]

Studies of breathing during sleep in normal adults have demonstrated more periodic breathing[15] and episodes of O_2 desaturation among older subjects. Several investigations have focused specifically on ventilation during sleep in subjects older than 55 years of age who were in good health and had no sleep or respiratory complaints[122, 127, 129–132] or in randomly selected older subjects.[133] Despite a variability among studies concerning the definition of sleep-related breathing disorders, there was striking agreement that among these normal subjects, 30 to 60% fulfilled the generally accepted criterion of sleep apnea syndrome—more than five apneas or episodes of sleep-disordered breathing per hour of sleep. Only one study found fewer than 2% of older subjects fulfilling this criterion.[134] However, in this study, snorers had been excluded, even when they were otherwise healthy. Given the high frequency of snorers, especially among older subjects, the sample studied was not representative of the general population of normal older subjects. This bias might explain the difference with respect to other studies.

Apneas in older sleeping subjects are of both the central and obstructive type.[44, 130, 132, 133] The mean number and duration of apneas are not different in older subjects having more than five apneas per hour of sleep and in subjects diagnosed as having obstructive sleep apnea syndrome.[129] In addition, they closely resemble typical patients with sleep apnea with respect to the number and depth of desaturation episodes.[130] This close similarity raises the important question of why sleep apneas in older subjects may have little effect on health. Not only did most of these subjects exhibit none of the symptoms associated with sleep apnea syndrome but also their future does not seem to be jeopardized by sleep apneas.[54, 127]

The underlying mechanisms of sleep apneas in normal older subjects remain uncertain. No clear relationship to body weight, increased awake airway resistance, or chemoreceptor responses has been demonstrated.[130] Speculations include altered endocrine function, use of alcohol and hypnotic drugs,[130] and an aggravation of normal periodic breathing.[41, 44] Physiological periodic breathing at sleep onset may be aggravated by larger differences between the wakefulness and sleep ventilation set-points, higher controller gain, increased circulatory delay from the lung to the chemoreceptors, or increased sleep instability.

The decrease in minute ventilation from wakefulness to sleep does not differ between older subjects with and without high sleep apnea indices or between older and younger subjects,[44] which suggests that the difference in the ventilation set-points between wakefulness and sleep is not increased in older subjects with sleep apneas. The ventilatory response to chemical stimuli is not greater in these subjects.[130] A delayed circulatory time is not likely to occur in healthy older subjects, in whom blood velocity should be slightly increased owing to stiffening of the arterial walls. Decrease in deep slow-wave sleep stages and more awakening with increasing age have been demonstrated.[81, 135–137] It has been suggested that a primary increase in sleep instability in older subjects could be a factor leading to increased breathing instability, which results in apneas of both the central and obstructive type.[41, 44] This hypothesis is in keeping with the predominance of sleep-disordered breathing in older subjects during light slow-wave sleep, and it is in keeping with the fact that the frequency of periodic breathing in younger subjects is similar to the frequency of high rates of apneas in older subjects. Furthermore, an increased rate of apneas could be merely a consequence of increased sleep instability due to the invasiveness of sleep recording techniques and the spontaneous fragility of sleep in older subjects. This hypothesis would explain the absence of repercussions of sleep-disordered breathing on the health of these subjects.

Aside from sleep-disordered breathing episodes, the ventilatory parameters in sleeping older subjects have been little investigated. Only Krieger et al.[129] and Shore et al.[41] have analyzed minute ventilation, tidal volume, and respiratory frequency quantitatively. They found a decrease in minute ventilation during steady NREM sleep similar in magnitude to that found in younger subjects.[44] It resulted from a smaller tidal volume despite a slightly higher ventilatory frequency.[129]

In middle-aged normal subjects, the occurrence of sleep-disordered breathing was intermediate between younger and older subjects, but the change in minute ventilation, tidal volume, and respiratory rate was of the same order of magnitude.[138]

Pregnancy

Because of a reduced functional residual capacity and residual volume, as well as a reduced cardiac output in the supine position, pregnant women could be exposed to more severe hypoxemia during sleep. A study of breathing during sleep in women at 36 weeks of gestation and postpartum did not show more severe hypoxemia during pregnancy. Indeed, hypopneas and apneas were less frequent during pregnancy, probably owing to the respiratory stimulatory effects of progesterone.[139] However, these results, involving only normal women, may perhaps not be extended to pathological conditions of pregnancy. (See also Chapter 82.)

Drugs

Many drugs probably interfere with breathing during sleep.[140] This topic is covered in more detail in Chapter 69. The effects of alcohol on ventilation in awake subjects are either depressive or stimulatory[141, 142]; those on basic ventilatory parameters during sleep have not been studied. In a group of 20 asymptomatic men aged 20 to 65 years, alcohol significantly increased the number of apneas and the number of episodes of desaturation occurring in conjunction with, as well as independently of, episodes of hypoventilation; the mean duration of hypopneas and apneas was increased.[143] These effects of alcohol are observed in men,[87] but not in women (even postmenopausal ones).[144] Similar effects of alcohol on obstructive sleep apneas have been shown in the sleep apnea syndrome.[145, 146] Even though the type of apnea—central or obstructive—was not specified,[143] one may speculate that alcohol exerts its deleterious effect on breathing during sleep through its depressive effects on upper airway muscle activity,[147] with resultant increased pharyngeal resistance. This opinion is reinforced by the observation that alcohol induces or aggravates snoring,[145] which results from an imbalance between an increased airflow and decreased upper airway tone. The alcohol-induced lengthening of apneas may be due to its depressive effects on arousal systems[143, 148] given that arousal probably has a key role in protective respiratory mechanisms during sleep.[33] These mechanisms, however, do not explain the aggravating effects of alcohol on desaturation episodes unrelated to obvious hypoventilation.

Benzodiazepines have effects on sleep apneas[105, 122, 149] and on snoring[150] similar to those of alcohol in normal subjects. These effects may be due to the depressive respiratory effects of benzodiazepines[122]; however, the same mechanisms as those suggested for alcohol—namely, upper airway muscle hypotonia and arousal depressant effects—may be involved in the effects of benzodiazepines on breathing during sleep.

Deleterious effects of alcohol and benzodiazepines are not observed in all subjects studied, which raises the question of whether the subjects sensitive to these drugs, even though asymptomatic, are normal or whether they should be considered as having latent sleep apnea syndromes revealed by these drugs. The effects of alcohol and benzodiazepines, both of which are widely used, and their possible combination or potentiation may be hazardous. Sleep-disordered breathing may be one of the mechanisms of the reduced longevity associated with the use of these drugs.[151, 152]

CONCLUSIONS

Sleep is associated with definite changes in respiratory function in normal humans. Whether these changes serve a specific function remains unclear and will probably not be clarified before the functions of sleep itself are better understood.

Ventilation during sleep appears to be fragile, being prone to instability, upper airway obstruction, hypoventilation, and ventilation-perfusion mismatch, thus jeopardizing the homeostatic function of CO_2 output and O_2 uptake that it is supposed to serve.

Although the other automatic homeostatic functions are executed by the autonomic nervous system (an important exception being the thermoregulatory function), ventilation, in addition to its homeostatic function, is also under voluntary control by the conscious nervous system. Voluntarily controlled ventilation gives rise to a conflict when consciousness is periodically abolished and motor control is subjected to central nervous system influences specific to sleep. This conflict is incompletely solved in humans. A possible solution would be to sleep like dolphins: alternately and independently with either cerebral hemisphere.[153]

Acknowledgments

I wish to thank Marie-Rose Boh and Véronique Fehr for secretarial assistance.

References

1. Fitzgerald R, Gautier H, Lahiri S. The Regulation of Respiration During Sleep and Anesthesia. New York, NY: Plenum; 1978.
2. Krieger J. Breathing during sleep in normal subjects. Clin Chest Med. 1985;6:577–594.
3. Phillipson EA. Control of breathing during sleep. Am Rev Respir Dis. 1978;118:909–939.
4. Remmers JE. Effects of sleep on control of breathing. Int Rev Physiol. 1981;23:111–147.
5. Saunders NA, Sullivan CE, eds. Sleep and Breathing. New York, NY: Marcel Dekker; 1984.
6. Sullivan CE. Breathing in sleep. In: Orem J, Barnes CD, eds. Physiology in Sleep. New York, NY: Academic Press; 1980:214–272.
7. Goldman MD, Gaultier C, Escourrou P, et al. The thorax pump during sleep: An overview of respiratory muscle function with emphasis on aspects of measurement. In: Saunders NA, Sullivan CE, eds. Sleep and Breathing. New York, NY: Marcel Dekker; 1994:209–238.
8. Gothe B, vanLuteren E, Dick TE. The influence of sleep on respiratory muscle function: Interaction between upper airway and chest wall muscles. In: Saunders NA, Sullivan CE, eds. Sleep and Breathing. New York, NY: Marcel Dekker; 1994:239–256.
9. Orem J, Barnes CD, eds. Physiology in Sleep. New York, NY: Academic Press; 1980.
10. Mosso A. Periodische Athmung and Luxusathmung. Arch Physiol. 1886;(suppl):37–116.
11. Mosso A. Über die gegenseitigen Beziehungen der Bauch- und Brustathmung. In: DuBois Reymond E, ed. Archiv für Physiologie. Leipzig, Germany; 1878:441–468.
12. Bülow K. Respiration and wakefulness in man. Acta Physiol Scand Suppl. 1963;209:1–110.
13. Duron B, Andrag C, Laval P. Ventilation pulmonaire globale, CO_2 alvéolaire et consommation d'oxygène au cours du sommeil normal. C R Seances Soc Biol Fil. 1968;162:139–145.
14. Block AJ, Boysen PG, Wynne JW, et al. Sleep apnea, hypopnea and oxygen desaturation in normal subjects: a strong male predominance. N Engl J Med. 1979;300:513–517.
15. Webb P. Periodic breathing during sleep. J Appl Physiol. 1974;37:899–903.
16. Rist KE, Daubenspeck JA, McGovern JF. Effects of non-REM sleep upon respiratory drive and the respiratory pump in humans. Respir Physiol. 1986;63:241–256.
17. Haab P, Ramel F, Fleisch A. La respiration périodique lors de l'assoupissement. J Physiol. 1957;49:190–194.
18. Lugaresi E, Coccagna G, Mantovani M, et al. Some periodic phenomena arising during drowsiness and sleep in man. Electroencephalogr Clin Neurophysiol. 1972;32:701–705.
19. Duron B, Tassinari CA, Gastaut H. Analyse spirographique et électromyographique de la respiration au cours du sommeil contrôlé par l'EEG chez l'homme normal. Rev Neurol (Paris). 1966;115:562–574.
20. Lugaresi E, Coccagna G, Farnetti P, et al. Snoring. Electroencephalogr Clin Neurophysiol. 1975;39:59–64.
21. de Groen JHM. Influence of diffuse brain stimulation (DBS) on human sleep, II: sleep-induced periodic breathing with apnea. Electroencephalogr Clin Neurophysiol. 1979;46:696–701.
22. Chapman KR, Bruce EN, Gothe B, et al. Possible mechanisms of periodic breathing during sleep. J Appl Physiol. 1988;64:1000–1008.
23. Bülow K, Ingvar D. Respiration and state of wakefulness in normals, studied by spirography, capnography and EEG. Acta Physiol Scand. 1961;51:230–238.
24. Hudgel DW, Martin RJ, Johnson B, et al. Mechanics of respiratory system and breathing pattern during sleep in normal humans. J Appl Physiol. 1984;56:133–137.
25. Trinder J, VanBeveren JA, Smith P, et al. Correlation between ventilation and EEG-defined arousal during sleep onset in young subjects. J Appl Physiol. 1997;83:2005–2011.
26. Dunai J, Wilkinson M, Trinder J. Interaction of chemical and state effects on ventilation during sleep onset. J Appl Physiol. 1996;81:2235–2243.
27. Finck BR. Influence of cerebral activity in wakefulness on regulation of breathing. J Appl Physiol. 1961;16:15–20.
28. Mangin P, Krieger J, Kurtz D. Apnea following hyperventilation in man. J Neurol Sci. 1982;57:67–82.
29. Plum F, Brown HW, Snoep E. Neurologic significance of posthyperventilation apnea. JAMA. 1962;181:1050–1055.
30. Cherniack NS. Respiratory dysrhythmias during sleep. N Engl J Med. 1981;305:325–330.
31. Khoo MC, Kronauer RE, Strohl KP, et al. Factors inducing periodic breathing in humans: a general model. J Appl Physiol. 1982;53:644–659.
32. Longobardo GS, Gothe B, Goldman MD, et al. Sleep apnea considered as a control system instability. Respir Physiol. 1982;50:311–333.
33. Phillipson EA, Sullivan CE. Arousal: the forgotten response to ventilatory stimuli [editorial]. Am Rev Respir Dis. 1978;118:807–809.
34. Dempsey JA, Smith CA, Harms CA, et al. Sleep-induced breathing instability—state of the art review. Sleep. 1996;19:236–247.
35. Lavie P, Fischer N, Zomer J, et al. The effects of partial and complete mechanical occlusion of the nasal passages on sleep structure and breathing in sleep. Acta Otolaryngol. 1983;95:161–166.
36. Sanders MH, Costantino JP, Owens GR, et al. Breathing during

wakefulness and sleep after human heart-lung transplantation. Am Rev Respir Dis. 1989;140:45–51.

37. Cherniack NS, Longobardo GS, Gothe B, et al. Interactive effects of central and obstructive apnea. Adv Physiol Sci. 1981;10:553–560.

38. Önal E, Lopata M. Periodic breathing and the pathogenesis of occlusive sleep apneas. Am Rev Respir Dis. 1982;126:676–680.

39. Badr MS, Morgan BJ, Finn L, et al. Ventilatory response to induced auditory arousals during NREM sleep. Sleep. 1997;20:707–714.

40. Acres JC, Sweatman P, West P, et al. Breathing during sleep in parents of sudden infant death syndrome victims. Am Rev Respir Dis. 1982;125:163–166.

41. Shore ET, Millman RP, Silage DA, et al. Ventilatory and arousal patterns during sleep in normal young and elderly subjects. J Appl Physiol. 1985;59:1607–1615.

42. Magnussen G. Studies on the Respiration During Sleep: A Contribution to the Physiology of the Sleep Function. London, England: HK Lewis; 1944.

43. Reed CI, Kleitman N. Studies of the physiology of sleep. The effect of sleep on respiration. Am J Physiol. 1926;75:600–608.

43a. Skatrud JB, Dempsey JA. Airway resistance and respiratory muscle function in snorers during NREM sleep. J Appl Physiol. 1985;59:328–335.

44. Krieger J, Mangin P, Kurtz D. Incidence of sleep disordered breathing in normal younger and older subjects. Correspondence analysis of related factors. In: Sleep 1982: Sixth European Congress on Sleep Research. Basel, Switzerland: Karger; 1983:308–311.

45. White DP, Weil JV Zwillich CW. Metabolic rate and breathing during sleep. J Appl Physiol. 1985;59:384–391.

46. Gothe B, Altose MD, Goldman MD, et al. Effect of quiet sleep on resting and CO_2 stimulated breathing in humans. J Appl Physiol. 1981;50:724–730.

47. Stradling JR, Chadwick GT, Frew AJ. Changes in ventilation and its components in normal subjects during sleep. Thorax. 1985;40:364–370.

48. Tabachnik E, Muller NL, Bryan AC, et al. Changes in ventilation and chest wall mechanics during sleep in normal adolescents. J Appl Physiol. 1981;51:557–564.

49. Douglas NJ. Control of breathing during sleep. Clin Sci. 1984;67:465–472.

50. Iber C, Berssenbrugge A, Skatrud JB, et al. Ventilatory adaptations to resistive loading during wakefulness and non-REM sleep. J Appl Physiol. 1982;52:607–614.

51. Miles LE, Guilleminault C, Smith LE, et al. Patients who complain only of loud snoring often have significant obstructive sleep apnea. Sleep Res. 1983;12:265.

52. Naifeh KH, Kamiya J. The nature of respiratory changes associated with sleep onset. Sleep. 1981;4:49–59.

53. O'Flaherty JJ, Sant'Ambrogio G, Mognoni P, et al. Rib cage and abdomen diaphragm contribution to ventilation during sleep in man. Arch Physiol. 1973;70:78–80.

54. Lopes JM, Tabachnik E, Muller NL, et al. Total airway resistance and respiratory muscle activity during sleep. J Appl Physiol. 1983;54:773–777.

55. Tusiewicz K, Moldofsky H, Bryan AC, et al. Mechanics of the rib cage and diaphragm during sleep. J Appl Physiol. 1977;43:600–602.

56. Robin ED, Whaley RD, Crump CC, et al. Alveolar gas tensions, pulmonary ventilation and blood pH during physiological sleep in normal subjects. J Clin Invest. 1958;37:981–989.

57. Wiegand DA, Latz B, Zwillich CW, et al. Geniohyoid muscle activity in normal men during wakefulness and sleep. J Appl Physiol. 1990;69:1262–1269.

58. Miljeteig H, Hirschberg A, Cole P, et al. Pharyngeal airflow during sleep. Acta Otolaryngol (Stockh). 1995;115:99–105.

59. Hudgel DW, Hendricks C. Palate and hypopharynx sites of inspiratory narrowing of the upper airway during sleep. Am Rev Respir Dis. 1988;138:1542–1547.

60. Berger RJ. Tonus of extrinsic laryngeal muscles during sleep and dreaming. Science. 1961;134:840.

61. Tangel DJ, Mezzanotte WS, Sandberg EJ, et al. Influences of NREM sleep on the activity of tonic vs inspiratory phasic muscles in normal men. J Appl Physiol. 1992;73:1058–1066.

62. Wiegand DA, Latz B, Zwillich CW, et al. Upper airway resistance and geniohyoid muscle activity in normal men during wakefulness and sleep. J Appl Physiol. 1990;69:1252–1261.

63. Basner RC, Ringler J, Schwartzstein RM, et al. Phasic electromyographic activity of the genioglossus increases in normals during slow-wave sleep. Respir Physiol. 1991;83:189–200.

64. Kuna ST, Smickley JS, Insalaco G. Posterior cricoarytenoid muscle activity during wakefulness and sleep in normal adults. J Appl Physiol. 1990;68:1746–1754.

65. Tangel DJ, Mezzanotte WS, White DP. Influence of sleep on tensor palatini EMG and upper airway resistance in normal men. J Appl Physiol. 1991;70:2574–2581.

66. Harper RM, Sauerland EK. The role of the tongue in sleep apnea. In: Guilleminault C, Dement WC, eds. Sleep Apnea Syndromes. New York, NY: Alan R Liss; 1978:219–234.

67. Sauerland EK, Harper RM. The human tongue during sleep: electromyographic activity of the genioglossus muscle. Exp Neurol. 1976;51:160–170.

68. Ballard RD, Irvin CG, Martin RJ, et al. Influence of sleep on lung volume in asthmatic patients and normal subjects. J Appl Physiol. 1990;68:2034–2041.

69. Hudgel DW, Devadatta P. Decrease in functional residual capacity during sleep in normal humans. J Appl Physiol. 1984;57:1319–1322.

70. Begle RL, Badr S, Skatrud JB, et al. Effect of lung inflation on pulmonary resistance during NREM sleep. Am Rev Respir Dis. 1990;141:854–860.

71. Aronson RM, Carley DW, Önal E, et al. Upper airway muscle activity and the thoracic volume dependence of upper airway resistance. J Appl Physiol. 1991;70:430–438.

72. Daubenspeck JA. Influence of small mechanical loads on variability of breathing pattern. J Appl Physiol. 1981;50:299–306.

73. Badr MS, Skatrud JB, Dempsey JA, et al. Effect of mechanical loading on expiratory and inspiratory muscle activity during NREM sleep. J Appl Physiol. 1990;68:1195–1202.

74. Hudgel DW, Mulholland M, Hendricks C. Neuromuscular and mechanical responses to inspiratory resistive loading during sleep. J Appl Physiol. 1987;63:603–608.

75. Gugger M, Molloy J, Gould GA, et al. Ventilatory and arousal responses to added inspiratory resistance during sleep. Am Rev Respir Dis. 1989;140:1301–1307.

76. Henke KG, Dempsey JA, Kowitz JM, et al. Effects of sleep-induced increases in upper airway resistance on ventilation. J Appl Physiol. 1990;69:617–624.

77. Morrell MJ, Harty HR, Adams L, et al. Changes in total pulmonary resistance and P_{CO_2} between wakefulness and sleep in normal human subjects. J Appl Physiol. 1995;78:1339–1349.

78. Kay A, Trinder J, Kim Y. Progressive changes in airway resistance during sleep. J Appl Physiol. 1996;81:282–292.

79. Morrell MJ, Harty HR, Adams L, et al. Breathing during wakefulness and NREM sleep in humans without an upper airway. J Appl Physiol. 1996;81:274–281.

80. Kawata K, Kotakehara Y, Hosaka K, et al. Airway occlusion pressure during sleep in normal adolescents. Sleep Res. 1983;12:70.

81. Agnew HW, Webb WB, Williams RL. Sleep patterns in late middle age males: an EEG study. Electroencephalogr Clin Neurophysiol. 1967;23:168–171.

82. Birchfield RI, Sieker HD, Heyman A. Alterations in respiratory function during natural sleep. J Lab Clin Med. 1959;54:216–222.

83. Ostergaard T. The excitability of the respiratory centre during sleep and during Evipan anaesthesia. Acta Physiol Scand. 1944;8:1–15.

84. Douglas NJ, White DP, Pickett CK, et al. Respiration during sleep in normal man. Thorax. 1982;37:840–844.

85. Duron B. La fonction respiratoire pendant le sommeil physiologique. Bull Eur Physiopathol Respir. 1972;8:1031–1057.

86. Muller NL, Francis PW, Gurwitz D, et al. Mechanism of hemoglobin desaturation during REM sleep in normal subjects and in patients with cystic fibrosis. Am Rev Respir Dis. 1980;121:463–469.

87. Block AJ, Hellard DW, Slayton PC. Effect of alcohol ingestion on breathing and oxygenation during sleep. Analysis of the influence of age and sex. Am J Med. 1986;80:595–600.

88. Goll CC, Shapiro CM. Oxygen consumption during sleep. J Physiol. 1981;313:35P–36P.

89. Ryan T, Mlynczak S, Erickson T, et al. Oxygen consumption during sleep: influence of sleep stage and time of night. Sleep. 1989;12:201–210.

90. Shapiro CM, Goll CC, Cohen GR, et al. Heat production during sleep. J Appl Physiol. 1984;56:671–677.

91. Webb P, Hiestand M. Sleep metabolism and age. J Appl Physiol. 1974;38:257–267.

92. Carlson DM, Carley DW, Onal E, et al. Acoustically induced cortical arousal increases phasic pharyngeal muscle and diaphragmatic EMG in NREM sleep. J Appl Physiol. 1994;76:1553–1559.

93. Khoo MCK, Koh SSW, Shin JJW, et al. Ventilatory dynamics during transient arousal from NREM sleep: implications for respiratory control stability. J Appl Physiol. 1996;80:1475–1484.

94. Badr MS, Morgan BJ, Finn L, et al. Ventilatory response to induced auditory arousals during NREM sleep. Sleep. 1997;20:707–714.

95. Aserinsky E, Kleitman N. Regularly occurring periods of eye motility and concurrent phenomena during sleep. Science. 1953;118:273–274.

96. Goodenough DR, Witkin HA, Koulack D, et al. The effects of stress films on respiration and eye movement activity during REM-sleep. Psychophysiology. 1975;12:313–320.

97. Rohmer F, Schaff G, Collard M, et al. La motilité spontanée, la fréquence cardiaque et la fréquence respiratoire au cours du sommeil chez l'homme normal. In: Fischgold M. Le Sommeil de Nuit Normal et Pathologique. Paris, France: Masson & Cie; 1965:192–205.

98. Snyder F, Hobson JA, Morrison DF, et al. Changes in respiration, heart rate and systolic blood pressure in human sleep. J Appl Physiol. 1964;19:417–422.

99. Spreng LF, Johnson CL, Lubin A. Autonomic correlates of eye movement bursts during stage REM sleep. Psychophysiology. 1968;4:311–323.

100. Guilleminault C. State of the art: sleep and control of breathing. Chest. 1978;73:2935–2953.

101. Aserinsky E. Periodic respiratory pattern occurring in conjunction with eye movements during sleep. Science. 1965;150:763–766.

102. Gould GA, Gugger M, Molloy J, et al. Breathing pattern and eye movement density during REM sleep in humans. Am Rev Respir Dis. 1988;138:874–877.

103. Schmidt-Nowara W, Snyder MJ. A quantitative analysis of the relationship between REM and breathing in normal man. Sleep Res. 1983;12:75.

104. Zimmermann PV, Connellan SJ, Middleton MC, et al. Postural changes in rib cage and abdominal volume-motion coefficients and their effect on the calibration of a respiratory inductance plethysmograph. Am Rev Respir Dis. 1983;127:209–214.

105. Dolly FR, Block AJ. Effect of flurazepam on sleep-disordered breathing and nocturnal oxygen desaturation in asymptomatic subjects. Am J Med. 1982;73:239–243.

106. Parmeggiani PL, Sabattini L. Electromyographic aspect of postural respiratory and thermoregulatory mechanisms in sleeping cats. Clin Neurophysiol. 1972;33:1–13.

107. Lugaresi E, Cirignotta F, Coccagna G, et al. Some epidemiological data on snoring and cardiocirculatory disturbances. Sleep. 1980;3:221–224.

108. Sauerland EK, Orr WC, Hairston LE. EMG patterns of oropharyngeal muscles during respiration in wakefulness and sleep. Electromyogr Clin Neurophysiol. 1981;21:307–316.

109. Bryan AC, Muller NL. Lung mechanics and gas exchange during sleep. Sleep. 1980;3:401–406.

110. Lugaresi E, Coccagna G, Cirignotta F, et al. Breathing during sleep in man in normal and pathological conditions. In: Fitzgerald R, Gautier H, Lahiri S, eds. The Regulation of Respiration During Sleep and Anesthesia. New York, NY: Plenum; 1978:35–45.

111. Jennum P, Schultz-Larsen K, Wildschiodtz G. Snoring as a medical risk factor, I: Relation to arterial blood pressure, weight and use of antihypertensive medicine. Sleep Res. 1985;14:170.

112. Norton PG, Dunn EV. Snoring as a risk factor for disease. Br Med J. 1985;291:630–632.

113. Partinen M, Palomaki H. Snoring and cerebral infarction. Lancet. 1985;2:325–326.

114. Block AJ. Is snoring a risk factor? Chest. 1981;80:525–526.

115. Koskenvuo M, Kapro J, Partinen M, et al. Snoring as a risk factor for hypertension and angina pectoris. Lancet. 1985;1:893–896.

116. Norton PG, Dunn EV, Haight JSJ. Snoring in adults: some epidemiologic aspects. Can Med Assoc J. 1983;128:674–675.

117. Partinen M, Kaprio J, Koskenvuo M, et al. Snoring and hypertension: a cross-sectional study on 12,808 Finns aged 24–65 years. Sleep Res. 1983;12:273.

118. Cohn MA, Weiss B. An estimate of the prevalence and significance of snoring. Sleep Res. 1983;22:233.

119. Robin IG. Snoring. Proc R Soc Lond B Biol Sci. 1968;61:575–582.

120. Lugaresi E, Coccagna G, Cirignotta F. Snoring and its clinical implications. In: Guilleminault C, Dement WC, eds. Sleep Apnea Syndromes. New York, NY: Alan R Liss; 1978:13–21.

121. Miles LE, Simmons FB. Evaluation of 190 patients with loud and disruptive snoring. Sleep Res. 1984;13:154.

122. Carskadon MA, Dement WC. Respiration during sleep in the aged human. J Gerontol. 1981;36:420–423.

123. Lugaresi E, Mondini S, Zucconi M, et al. Staging of heavy snorer's disease. A proposal. Bull Eur Physiopathol Respir. 1983;19:590–594.

124. Feris BG, Pollard DS. Effect of deep and quiet breathing on pulmonary compliance in man. J Clin Invest. 1960;39:143.

125. Perez-Padilla R, West P, Kryger MH. Sighs during sleep in adult humans. Sleep. 1983;6:234–243.

126. Trinder J, Kay A, Kleiman J, et al. Gender differences in airway resistance during sleep. J Appl Physiol. 1997;83:1986–1997.

126a. Manber R, Armitage R. Sex, steroids, and sleep: a review. Sleep. 1999;22:540–555.

127. Catterall JR, Calverley PMA, Shapiro CM, et al. Breathing and oxygenation during sleep are similar in normal men and normal women. Am Rev Respir Dis. 1985;132:86–88.

128. Gimeno F, Peset R. Changes in oxygen saturation and heart frequency during sleep in young normal subjects. Thorax. 1984;39:673–675.

129. Krieger J, Mangin P, Kurtz D. Les modifications respiratoires au cours du sommeil du sujet âge normal. Rev Electroencephalogr Neurophysiol Clin. 1980;10:177–185.

130. McGinty D, Littner M, Beahm E, et al. Sleep related breathing disorders in older men: a search for underlying mechanisms. Neurobiol Aging. 1982;3:337–350.

131. Smallwood RG, Vitiello MV, Giblin EC, et al. Sleep apnea: relationship to age, sex and Alzheimer's dementia. Sleep. 1983;6:16–22.

132. Smyth M, Giblin EC, Lee K. Prevalence of apneas and oxygen desaturation during sleep in healthy older men. Sleep Res. 1981;10:118.

133. Ancoli-Israel S, Kripke DF, Mason W. Prevalence of sleep apnea and PMS in seniors: an update. Sleep Res. 1983;12:221.

134. Bixler EO, Kales A, Cadieux R, et al. Sleep apneic activity in older healthy subjects. J Appl Physiol. 1985;58:1597–1601.

135. Feinberg I, Carlson VR. Sleep variables as a function of age in man. Arch Gen Psychiatry. 1968;18:239–250.

136. Garma L, Bouard G. Les éveils nocturnes en fonction de l'âge. Rev Neurol (Paris). 1981;137:667–692.

137. Kales A, Wilson T, Kales JD, et al. Measurements of all-night sleep in normal elderly persons: effects of aging. J Am Geriatr Soc. 1967;15:405–414.

138. Krieger J. Maglasiu N, Sforza E, et al. Breathing during sleep in normal middle-aged subjects. Sleep. 1990;13:143–154.

139. Brownell LG, West P, Kryger MH. Breathing during sleep in normal pregnant women. Annu Rev Respir Dis. 1986;133:38–41.

140. Read DJ, Jeffery HE. Some neurochemical influences on breathing. In: Saunders NA, Sullivan CE, eds. Sleep and Breathing. New York, NY: Marcel Dekker; 1984:201–220.

141. Johnstone RE, Reier CE. Acute respiratory effects of ethanol in man. Clin Pharmacol Ther. 1973;14:501–508.

142. Zilm DH. Ethanol-induced spontaneous and evoked EEG, heart rate and respiration rate changes in man. Clin Toxicol. 1981;18:549–563.

143. Taasan V, Block AJ, Boysen P, et al. Alcohol increases sleep apnea and oxygen desaturation in asymptomatic men. Am J Med. 1981;71:240–245.

144. Block AJ, Hellard DW, Slayton PC. Minimal effect of alcohol ingestion on breathing during the sleep of postmenopausal women. Chest. 1985;88:181–184.

145. Issa FG, Sullivan CE. Alcohol, snoring and sleep apnea. J Neurol Neurosurg Psychiatry. 1982;45:353–359.
146. Scrima L, Broudy M, Nay KN, et al. Increased severity of obstructive sleep apnea after bedtime alcohol ingestion: diagnostic potential and proposed mechanism of action. Sleep. 1982;5:318–328.
147. Krol RC, Knuth SL, Bartlett D. Selective reduction of genioglossal muscle activity by alcohol in normal human subjects. Am Rev Respir Dis. 1984;129:247–250.
148. Berry RB, Bonnet MH, Light RW. Effect of ethanol on the arousal response to airway occlusion during sleep in normal subjects. Am Rev Respir Dis. 1992;145:445–452.
149. Mendelson WB, Garnett D, Gillin JC. Flurazepam-induced sleep apnea syndrome in a patient with insomnia and mild sleep-related respiratory changes. J Nerv Ment Dis. 1981;169:261–264.
150. Cirignotta F, Mondini S, Zucconi M, et al. Snoring and sleep apnea: effects of lorazepam and mazindol evaluated by means of snoring and sleep apnea monitoring. Bull Eur Physiopathol Respir. 1982;18:113P–134P.
151. Kripke DF, Garfinkel L. Excess nocturnal deaths related to sleeping pill and tranquilizer use. Lancet. 1984;1:99.
152. Kripke DF, Simons NR, Garfinkel L, et al. Short and long sleep and sleeping pills. Is increased mortality associated? Arch Gen Psychiatry. 1979;36:103–116.
153. Mukhametov LM. Sleep in marine mammals. Exp Brain Res. 1984;8(suppl):227–238.

18

Respiratory Physiology: Sleep at High Altitudes

John V. Weil

Sleep disturbance is a frequent feature of acute ascent to high altitude The symptom is frequent awakening with a sense of suffocation. Objective observations indicate that sleep at altitude is associated with periodic breathing and frequent awakenings but relatively little change in total sleep time. Sleep stages are generally shifted from deeper toward lighter sleep stages.

Periodic breathing at altitude seems to reflect the respiratory dilemma of acute altitude ascent in which the stimulatory effects of hypoxia are opposed by the inhibitory action of hypocapnic alkalosis. The outcome is respiratory oscillation. Hypocapnic alkalosis induces apnea, which in turn lessens alkalotic inhibition and augments hypoxic stimulation. This triggers hyperpnea, which lessens respiratory stimulation by decreasing hypoxia and increasing alkalosis, leading to recurrent apnea. The occurrence of apnea with lessening of ventilatory stimuli is enhanced during sleep.

On balance, the poor subjective sleep quality of sleep seems to reflect the fragmentation of sleep by frequent arousals linked to the marked changes in respiratory pattern of periodic breathing. Arousals commonly occur at the transition from the end of apnea to the onset of hyperpnea. Subsequent acclimatization to altitude is associated with lessening of periodic breathing and better-quality sleep.

The most common treatment is prophylactic administration of acetazolamide, an inhibitor of carbonic anhydrase, which likely works by reducing alkalotic ventilatory inhibition. The results of recent studies suggest that benzodiazepines may improve sleep quality without apparent adverse effects.

Sleep disturbance is a common cause of discomfort among the constellation of symptoms after ascent to high altitude. Subjectively, the sensation is that of a restless or sleepless night. Individuals commonly experience awakening from sleep with a feeling of suffocation, taking a deep breath, feeling much improved, and falling back to sleep. This sleep disturbance is generally viewed as part of a broader group of altitude-induced symptoms, often called *acute mountain sickness* (AMS), manifested as loss of appetite, nausea, vomiting, decreased mental acuity, insomnia, and, in rare cases, coma. In this chapter, a few general, relevant aspects of acute physiological adjustment to high altitude are briefly summarized; the characteristics of the sleep disturbance of altitude, its pathogenesis, and therapeutic interventions are then reviewed. Although much of the focus is on sleep after acute ascent to high altitude, alterations in sleep during long-term altitude exposure are also briefly mentioned.

PHYSIOLOGICAL ADJUSTMENT TO HIGH ALTITUDE

Primary among the changes in physical environment that attend the ascent to altitude is a decrease in barometric pressure such that although the fractional concentration of O_2 is similar to that at sea level, O_2 tension—the product of fractional concentration and barometric pressure—is reduced (Fig. 18–1). This decreased O_2 tension of ambient air presents a threat to arterial and tissue oxygenation and elicits a series of responses that may act to minimize tissue hypoxia. These consist of early increases in ventilation and cardiac output and, during more prolonged exposure, rises in circulating red cell concentration and changes in peripheral tissue, including increased spatial density of capillaries and mitochondria.

INCREASED VENTILATION

Probably the earliest and best studied and one of the most important of these responses is increased ventilation, which acts to minimize the extent of alveolar hypoxia and arterial hypoxemia in the face of a decrease in ambient O_2 tension. The magnitude of the ventilatory response increases with increasing altitude but, in addition, at a fixed altitude varies considerably among individuals. This variability may in part reflect intrinsic, interindividual differences in the strength of the basal (preascent) ventilatory response to hypoxia.[1] In addition, ventilation progressively increases over several days after ascent to high altitude. This gradual increase occurs despite the fact that the increasing ventilation is lessening hypoxia—the presumed stimulus to breathing. This is the phenomenon of ventilatory acclimatization to high altitude, which is manifested as a progressive decrease in arterial P_{CO_2} (Pa_{CO_2}) with

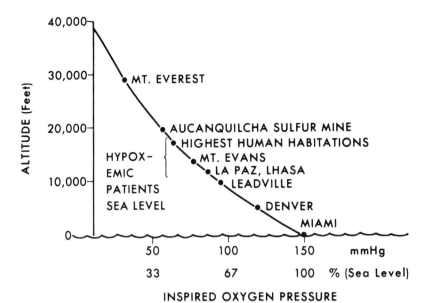

Figure 18–1. Relationship between altitude and inspired O₂ pressure. (From Kryger MH. Pathophysiology of Respiration. Copyright © 1981. John Wiley & Sons. Reprinted by permission of John Wiley & Sons, Inc.)

increasing ventilation over several days. Although the mechanism of acclimatization is debated, studies in human beings and animals suggest that increased hypoxic sensitivity of the carotid body may be a major contributor.[2–4] In any case, it is during the early phase of altitude adjustment, shortly after ascent, that sleep disturbances appear to be most marked; they tend to improve during the period of acclimatization.

SLEEP DISTURBANCES

Acute exposure to hypoxemia leads to a host of features that suggest impaired neural function (Fig. 18–2). Given the prominence of insomnia as a complaint at high altitude, it is surprising that sleep at altitude has been relatively little studied. Some of the earliest work reported in 1970 concerned observations of subjects working in Antarctica, where a combination of geographic elevation and terrestrial spin produces decreased barometric pressure ranging from 485 to 525 mmHg, equivalent to moderately high altitude. The men stationed there experienced a sleep disturbance termed *polar red-eye*, and electroencephalographic studies showed major disruption of sleep with a marked decrease in slow-wave sleep (stages 3 and 4).[5] Although these changes were ascribed to hypobaric hypoxia, the effects of isolation and disturbances of light-dark cycle that are typical in subjects living at the South Pole clouded their interpretation.

As research at low altitude began to elucidate the close links between breathing and sleep and to show

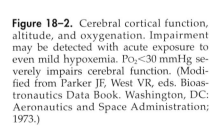

Figure 18–2. Cerebral cortical function, altitude, and oxygenation. Impairment may be detected with acute exposure to even mild hypoxemia. PO₂<30 mmHg severely impairs cerebral function. (Modified from Parker JF, West VR, eds. Bioastronautics Data Book. Washington, DC: Aeronautics and Space Administration; 1973.)

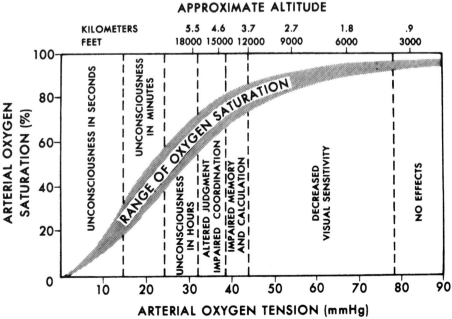

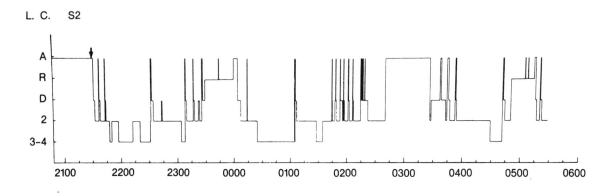

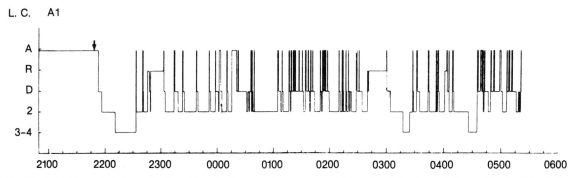

Figure 18–3. All-night sleep plots for a single subject during a night at sea level *(above)* and the first night at altitude *(below)*. Time in hours is plotted on the horizontal axis—lights out occurred at the small vertical arrow in each plot. Sleep stage is shown on the vertical axis: A, stage 1 sleep; 2, stage 2 sleep; 3–4, stages 3 and 4 sleep combined. Sleep at high altitude was associated with increased fragmentation by frequent awakenings and a reduction in stage 3/4 sleep. (Reprinted from Electroencephalography and Clinical Neurophysiology, vol 38, Reite M, Jackson D, Cahoon RL, et al, Sleep physiology at high altitude, 463–471, Copyright 1975, with permission from Elsevier Science.)

that sleep disruption was often closely linked to changes in respiratory rhythm, such as occurs in sleep apnea, studies were performed at high altitude with simultaneous monitoring of sleep state and respiratory pattern. Reite et al.[6] studied normal subjects at sea level and during a stay of several days on the summit of Pike's Peak (4300 m). On the initial night after ascent, most subjects exhibited periodic breathing that was present during roughly half the time asleep but varied among subjects from 0% to 93%. Sleep was characterized by significant decreases in stages 3 and 4, with an increased number of arousals (Fig. 18–3). In most but not all subjects who initially showed periodic breathing, this tended to decrease over subsequent nights with a decreased number of arousals. Although there was a trend toward more wakefulness, the duration of sleep (total sleep time) was not significantly reduced compared with that at sea level.

Although most of these subjects complained of difficulty in sleeping, this could not be related to abbreviated sleep, which was of normal duration, but rather seemed associated with an increased number of arousals. These were synchronous to the transition from termination of apnea to onset of hyperpnea and thus were similar in some respects to the arousal seen in sleep apnea syndromes at low altitude. Although this suggests that periodic breathing, frequent awakenings, and poor-quality sleep are mechanistically interrelated, there must be some reservation about this because increased awakenings in one subject occurred in the absence of periodic breathing[6] and because oxygen administration abolishes periodic breathing but not the increased frequency of arousal.[6–9]

Poor subjective quality of sleep at altitude might also reflect altitude-associated changes in sleep stage distribution. Miller and Horvath[10] studied subjects at simulated altitude after ascent in the evening immediately before sleep with descent the next morning after awakening, so only the nights were spent at a hypobaric level of 493 mmHg, equivalent to an elevation of about 3500 m. They found, under these conditions, an increase in light sleep (stage 1) with a decrease in stage 2 sleep. Total sleep time was unchanged, but there was a significant increase in time spent awake. Another relatively consistent alteration in sleep at altitude is the relative paucity of deeper stages (3 and 4) of nonrapid eye movement (NREM) sleep after ascent with an increase in light, stage 1, sleep.[6–8] There seems to be no consistent change in the amount of REM sleep, which is variably found to be either unchanged[6, 8] or to increase and decrease[9, 11] at altitude.

As mentioned earlier, total sleep time is remarkably preserved in the face of the disruptive effect of periodic breathing. Perhaps this paradox is explained by the frequent but largely unstudied observation that ascent to altitude induces sleepiness, which is consistent, prompt, and often profound. Although this is often presumed to be due to hypoxia, a recent study suggests a marked proclivity of human subjects to fall asleep quickly after brief voluntary hyperventilation at sea level, pointing to a potential role of hypocapnia.[12] Regardless of its cause, the hypnotic effect of altitude could contribute to the maintenance of total sleep duration.

Thus, sleep after ascent to high altitude is characterized by poor subjective quality, with periodic breathing and frequent awakening being the most impressive objective findings. Sleep is nearly normal in duration, with more time spent awake and in stage 1 and less time spent in deep sleep (stages 3 and 4). The amount of REM sleep may be either unchanged[6, 8] or decreased.[13] The increased awakenings seem temporally related to periodic breathing, commonly occurring at the transition from apnea to hyperpnea, pointing to a likely contribution of disturbed respiratory rhythm to sleep disturbance at altitude. The disparity between subjective evaluation of sleep quality and objective findings of normal sleep duration likely reflects the importance of sleep continuity in the apparent subjective quality of sleep and suggests that sleep fragmentation despite normal cumulative duration might produce the impression of sleeplessness.[6, 14]

PERIODIC BREATHING

Occurrence

In the mid-19th century, Cheyne and Stokes[15] described the crescendo-decrescendo breathing pattern in cardiac patients that now bears their names. That periodic breathing is frequent during sleep in normal individuals at high altitude was observed shortly thereafter by Tyndall in 1857, by Egli-Sinclair and Mosso in 1893 and 1894, and by Douglas et al.[16] in 1913[15] and continues to be a consistent finding in current studies of sleep after ascent to high altitude.[6, 10, 17–20] In general, the respiratory dysrhythmia of sleep at altitude seems different from usual sleep apnea at low altitude because of the machinery-like periodicity of the high-altitude respiratory pattern (Fig. 18–4), which contrasts with the erratic, disorganized pattern of most low-altitude sleep apnea. Thus, the high-altitude pattern is nicely described by the term *periodic breathing*, or *Cheyne-Stokes respiration*, which most often occurs at low altitude in patients with heart failure (see Chapters 71 and 86) or with central nervous system disorders.

The temporal pattern of periodic breathing and its linkage to sleep stages show some night-to-night variation and considerable intersubject differences,[6, 8, 9, 11, 19, 21–24] yet on balance, periodicity is usually evident early in sleep and during light stages. Indeed, in some subjects, periodic breathing occurs in wakefulness, especially during periods of drowsiness.[25–27] The pattern, as mentioned, generally has the classic crescendo-descrescendo, Cheyne-Stokes morphology but with a relatively short cycle length ranging from 12 to 34 sec, which progressively shortens with increasing altitude.[28–30] This differs from the longer cycles of 40 to 90 sec in patients with heart failure.[31] The most obvious aspect of this periodic oscillation is the magnitude of respiratory depth (tidal volume), with a less obvious change in breathing frequency. However, there are subtle, but parallel, variations in frequency that produce a reinforcing effect on ventilatory oscillation.[28] As with periodic breathing at sea level, periodicity at altitude is often initiated by movement or a deeper breath with a transient increase in hypocapnia. Periodicity at altitude is also most prevalent in light, stage 1 or 2 sleep. Although deeper stages of NREM sleep are relatively rare after acute ascent, the propensity to periodic breathing seems much reduced at these times. The most striking influence of sleep stage on periodic breathing is the observation in most,[6, 8, 21] but not all,[7, 9] studies that REM sleep promptly and consistently terminates periodicity and restores regular breathing.

Ventilation and oxygenation fall below waking values during sleep at altitude to a similar degree as that occurring at sea level.[4] However, the important difference is that at altitude, basal, awake oxygenation and P_{CO_2} are lower and thus closer to critical thresholds (Fig. 18–5). Oxygen tensions fall closer to the descending limb of the dissociation curve where values are associated with desaturation and are nearer the threshold for stimulation of ventilation. Similarly, CO_2 tensions fall to values nearer the dog leg below which CO_2 loses its ventilatory stimulus potential. As a result, small variations in gas tensions have much greater effects on ventilation under such conditions.

It seems likely that the respiratory pauses in sleep at altitude are of central origin. These are usually unassociated with snoring or other noises suggestive of obstruction and are accompanied by an absence of rib cage and abdominal activity,[7, 8, 17, 19, 32] which suggests a nonobstructive cause, and there is no association with the usual risk factors for obstruction, such as obesity. However, at low altitude, some narrowing of the upper airway is probably common with all apneas, most of which are "mixed" with associated central and obstructive features.[33, 34] This is likely a reflection of the phasic "respiratory" nature of many upper airway muscles such that loss of drive reduces activation of both classic inspiratory muscles and those responsible for maintenance of upper airway patency. Thus, increased upper airway resistance may contribute to periodic breathing at altitude, but likely plays only a minor role.

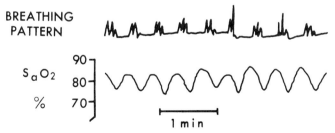

BREATHING PATTERN

S_aO_2 %   90 80 70

1 min

Figure 18–4. Breathing pattern and arterial oxygenation in a normal subject during sleep at high altitude (4300 m). Such a pattern is seen throughout much of sleep in most individuals after ascent. There is characteristic monotonously repetitive, machinery-like periodic alternation of apnea and repetitive clusters of hyperpneic breaths. (From Weil JV, Kryger MH, Scoggin CH. Sleep and breathing at high altitude. In: Sleep Apnea Syndromes. New York, NY: Alan R Liss; 1978:119–136.)

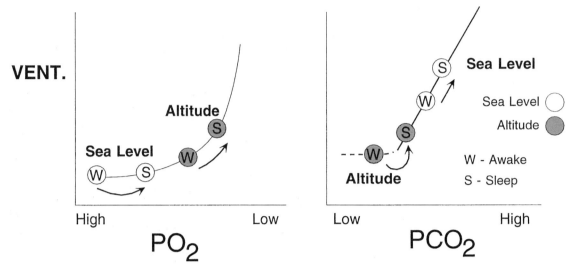

Figure 18–5. A schematic illustration of the relationship of blood gases to ventilatory responses during wakefulness and sleep at low and high altitude. At altitude, during wakefulness (W), arterial oxygen tensions move lower toward the steeper portion of the response hypoxic ventilatory response curve—an effect that is augmented during sleep (S). Hyperventilation causes arterial CO_2 tensions during wakefulness and sleep to decrease and move closer to the dog leg of the CO_2 response curve where the ventilatory response to PCO_2 is greatly reduced. The result is that during sleep at high altitude, small changes in either PO_2 or PCO_2 produce much greater changes in ventilation than at low altitude. This sets the stage for respiratory instability.

As mentioned, sleep disturbance and periodic breathing seem to be most pronounced during the first few nights after altitude ascent, with a tendency toward more regular breathing on subsequent nights. However, several studies describe the persistence of periodic breathing throughout sleep after 10 days to 5 weeks at high altitude.[19, 32, 35]

Mechanisms

In the early 1900s, ingenious, deceptively simple experiments by Douglas and Haldane[26] and Douglas et al.[36] at low altitude explored the physiological mechanisms of periodic breathing and highlighted the importance of both hypoxia and hypocapnia. They were aware that during wakefulness, breathing was characterized by intrinsic momentum, a "flywheel" effect that caused breathing to continue despite brief hypocapnia. They also showed that respiratory periodicity could be readily induced in normal subjects by intense, sustained voluntary hyperventilation with room air, which produced apnea followed by Cheyne-Stokes respiration. When they produced hyperventilation with an O_2-enriched gas, they found that this induced only apnea, indicating the importance of hypoxia in the induction of periodicity. They also demonstrated the specific role of phasic hypoxia through the application of dead space containing the CO_2 absorber, soda lime, which produced rebreathing-induced hypoxia without the usual attendant hypercapnia. When the resulting progressive hyperpnea produced an increase in tidal volume sufficient to bring in "fresh air" replete with O_2, the resolution of hypoxia produced apnea followed by recurrent rebreathing-induced hypoxia and perpetuation of the cycle. Similarly, the addition of simple tubular dead space led to phasic hypercapnia and res-

piratory periodicity. Their findings pointed to the combined roles of hypocapnia, which initiates apnea, and hypoxia, which stimulates hyperpnea, in the genesis of periodic breathing.

That similar principles apply at high altitude is suggested by findings that the administration of O_2 or CO_2 abolishes periodic breathing.[6, 17, 22, 32] Interpretation of the physiological mechanism of this effect has been unclear. Specifically, the relative importance of correction of hypoxia, hypocapnia, and alkalosis remains uncertain because maneuvers such as O_2 administration improve oxygenation but also reduce ventilation, leading to a rise in $PaCO_2$ and a lessening of alkalosis. Similarly, the administration of CO_2 corrects respiratory alkalosis but also increases ventilation and improves oxygenation.

Despite this difficulty, considerable evidence suggests that although hypoxia may be contributory, hypocapnic alkalosis may have a particularly important role. First, respiratory alkalosis is typical in patients with classic Cheyne-Stokes respiration at low altitude[37] and occurs in normal subjects in whom apneas during sleep have been noted to occur after transient episodes of decreased end-tidal PCO_2 and presumed increase in blood pH.[25] Important studies by Sullivan et al.[38] demonstrated that the withdrawal of classic stimuli to breathing through the administration of O_2, induction of metabolic alkalosis, or blockade of vagal afferents led to little change in respiratory rhythm during wakefulness but to profound pauses and slowing of breathing in sleep. This echoes the suggestion of Douglas and Haldane[27] and Douglas et al.[36] that wakefulness acts in some fashion to sustain respiratory rhythm even in the absence of classic extrinsic stimuli but that during sleep, the maintenance of respiratory rhythm becomes critically dependent on such stimulation. Hyperventilation thus seems to be an excellent way to induce a

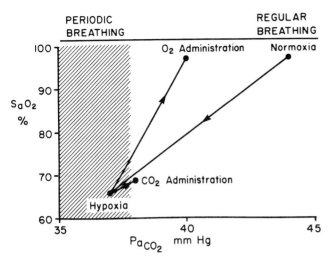

Figure 18–6. Relationship of respiratory pattern to $PaCO_2$ and SaO_2. This figure is a schematic representation of data of Berssenbrugge et al.[17] and demonstrates that reduction in PCO_2 is a critical determinant of periodic breathing in normal human subjects during hypoxia. Even a small increase in PCO_2 after administration of either O_2 or CO_2 restores normal breathing. This effect seems largely independent of changes in SaO_2. (From Weil JV. Sleep at high altitude. Clin Chest Med. 1985;6:615–621.)

respiratory pause in sleep because it simultaneously induces hyperoxia and withdrawal of hydrogen ion–CO_2 stimulation. Indeed, posthyperventilation apnea, which is variable in occurrence in wakefulness[39] but consistently found in sleep, likely is an example of such a relationship.[40] Indeed, Bulow[25] suggests that a stable and slightly elevated PCO_2 is necessary for stable rhythmic breathing during low-altitude sleep.

The critical role of hypocapnic alkalosis in periodic breathing in sleep at altitude is clearly evident in the study of Berssenbrugge et al.,[17] in which it was shown that periodic breathing in NREM sleep at simulated altitude (barometric pressure of 455 mmHg) was abolished by O_2 administration, which was associated with increases in both SaO_2 and $PaCO_2$. However, they also showed that periodic breathing was abolished by a selective increase in $PaCO_2$. This was achieved through the administration of low levels of CO_2 with the addition of nitrogen to prevent the increase in SaO_2 that would be anticipated due to the stimulation of ventilation by a rising $PaCO_2$. They noted in one subject that in NREM sleep, the appearance of periodic breathing during the induction of hypoxia was temporally related more closely to the fall in end-tidal CO_2 than to the decrease in PO_2. Similarly, they showed that breathing was regular in NREM sleep in hypoxia when CO_2 was added to maintain isocapnia. However, when CO_2 administration was terminated, periodic breathing occurred when end-tidal CO_2 fell, although the extent of hypoxia remained constant. Furthermore, Skatrud and Dempsey[40] showed that apneas could be consistently produced at low altitude in NREM sleep through the induction of hypocapnia with passive positive-pressure hyperventilation against a background of either hypoxia or hyperoxia. Apnea tended to occur when the end-tidal CO_2 was lowered 1 to 3 mmHg below levels

observed during wakefulness. Thus, hypoxia alone seems insufficient to produce periodic breathing, for which a fall in PCO_2, perhaps below some apneic threshold, seems important (Fig. 18–6). Indeed, apneas at low altitude frequently follow sighs or breaths of increased tidal volume with a drop in PCO_2,[25] and a breath of increased tidal volume with decreased end-tidal PCO_2 often triggers periodic breathing at altitude.[17, 32]

Thus, these findings collectively point to a critical role of hypocapnic alkalosis in the generation of apnea and periodic breathing during sleep at high altitude. Observations—both new and old—suggest a pathophysiological sequence as illustrated in Figure 18–7, in which hypoxia-induced hyperventilation leads to hypocapnic alkalosis, induces apnea during sleep. Apnea leads to enhanced ventilatory stimulation by increasing hypoxemia and lessening hypocapnic alkalosis, which promotes subsequent hyperpnea and arousal. The ensuing increase in ventilation lessens hypoxia and restores hypocapnic alkalosis, promoting the recurrence of apnea.

Although most experimental interventions have tested the role of hypocapnia, which is easily reversed by the administration of CO_2, this also reverses alkalosis, which may be of greater importance than hypocapnia. This view is supported by the observations described later, which show the resolution of periodic breathing during acclimatization and its prevention by the use of inhibitors of carbonic anhydrase. In both instances, hypocapnia is accentuated while alkalosis is reduced.

The importance of hypocapnia in the genesis of periodic breathing suggests, in turn, a role for the strength of the ventilatory response to the hypoxia of high altitude, which is the primary cause of hyperventilation and hypocapnia after ascent. In a study of healthy

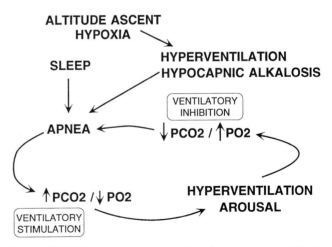

Figure 18–7. Schematic summary of mechanisms responsible for periodic breathing during sleep at altitude. Altitude-induced hypoxia stimulates increased ventilation. The resulting hypocapnic alkalosis together with the effects of sleep promotes apnea. During apnea, increasing hypoxemia and lessening of hypocapnic alkalosis stimulates resumption of ventilation and arousal. This augments oxygenation and lessens hypocapnic alkalosis, permitting recurrence of apnea.

subjects after an acute ascent to high altitude, it was found that the extent of periodic breathing varied considerably among individuals and was most frequent in those subjects with the highest ventilatory responses to both hypoxia and hypercapnia.[4] Although the extent of periodic breathing was not correlated with the stable, baseline value of P_{CO_2}, its apparent relationship to the magnitude of ventilatory drives is consistent with the view that the development of phasic hypocapnia resulting from a brisk ventilatory response to transient hypoxemia during sleep may have been a factor in the development of apnea (periodic breathing) at high altitude. Several subsequent studies have reaffirmed the association of high hypoxic ventilatory responses and periodic breathing in sleep at a high altitude (Fig. 18–8),[17, 19, 22, 24, 32, 35] although some have found no such relationship.[30, 41] Because a steeper slope of ventilatory response to hypercapnia might imply a greater inhibitory action of hypocapnia, there might be a relationship of hypercapnic response to periodic breathing. Two studies suggest such a relationship,[4, 19] but this is less consistent than the correlation with hypoxic response.

It is also apparent that the extent of periodic breathing shows a progressive decline over successive nights at altitude,[4] which suggests that the process of ventilatory acclimatization to altitude may act in some fashion to decrease the tendency toward periodic breathing. This is in some respects paradoxical because the increased hypoxic ventilatory response associated with acclimatization would be expected to produce increased periodic breathing as indicated before. However, an overriding factor may be that acclimatization acts to lessen the inhibitory effects of respiratory alkalosis on ventilation and thus reduces the absolute value of Pa_{CO_2} required to produce an apnea (apneic threshold) (Fig. 18–9).

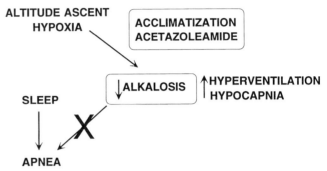

Figure 18–9. Schematic representation of potential mechanisms by which acclimatization and carbonic anhydrase inhibitors decrease periodic breathing during sleep at high altitude. Both resolve hypocapnic alkalosis but augment hyperventilation and hypocapnia. This suggests that alkalosis may be more important than hypocapnia in the genesis of periodic breathing.

Several theoretical models have been suggested to explain respiratory instability on the basis of chemical feedback aspects of ventilatory control.[42, 43] Periodic breathing is predicted in circumstances in which there are delays in information transfer, increased controller gain, or decreased system damping. Typically, these theories emphasize the role of the curvilinear peripheral chemoreceptor response to hypoxia, for which the slope (gain) increases in hypoxia. Such models predict the emergence of periodic breathing during sleep at high altitude, in which the gain of the curvilinear hypoxic response is increased by low PO_2 and the contribution to drive of the linear CO_2–hydrogen ion response is diminished by hypocapnic alkalosis. These theoretical considerations, as well as many of the earlier experimental studies, suggested that both hypoxia and hypocapnia were important in the development of periodic breathing. However, the induction of periodic breathing and apnea by hypocapnia independent of the level of oxygenation suggests that a drop in P_{CO_2} below an apneic threshold, relative to basal P_{CO_2} values, is of critical importance in the initiation of an apnea. Hypoxia may largely act to terminate an apnea and initiate subsequent hyperpnea with resultant hypocapnia, leading to the perpetuating pattern typical of periodic breathing.

Consequences of Periodic Breathing

Sleep fragmentation by frequent awakenings is an important likely byproduct of periodic breathing, which is, in turn, a contributor to the subjective sense of poor-quality sleep. As mentioned, arousals occur in close synchrony to apnea termination—so closely that it is unclear whether arousal stimulates resumption of breathing or the reverse occurs (resumption of breathing causes arousal). It also is unclear whether arousal is triggered by chemosensory response to apnea-induced asphyxia, by mechanical stimuli, or by central command signals associated with the abrupt resumption of breathing. Observations at low altitude suggest that apnea-associated arousals correlate poorly with chemi-

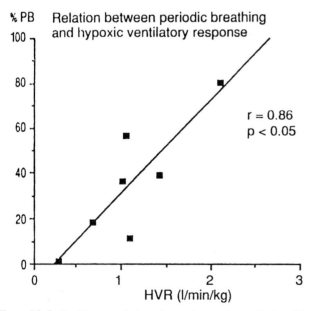

Figure 18–8. Positive correlation of prevalence of periodic breathing in sleep at 6542 m and hypoxic ventilatory response. (From Goldenberg F, Richalet JP, Onnen I, et al. Sleep apneas and high altitude newcomers. Int J Sports Med. 1992;13:S34–S36.)

cal variables but have a consistent relationship to mechanical stimuli, suggesting linkage to the resumption of ventilatory effort rather than to blood chemistry.[44] Regardless of the precise cause of arousal, it seems likely that the awakening or lightening of sleep stage makes an important contribution to periodicity by reversing the respiratory depressant influence of sleep and enhancing the postapneic hyperpnea. Although periodic breathing may contribute to the generation of arousals, this relationship is variable and probably accounts for only a portion of the excess frequency of awakenings at altitude. As mentioned, a clear dissociation is seen with O_2 administration, which abolishes periodic breathing but fails to prevent arousals.[6] Factors responsible for this residual excess remain unknown.

The net influence of periodic breathing on average ventilation in sleep at altitude is incompletely understood. Although it has been suggested that the respiratory pauses may exaggerate nocturnal hypoxemia,[45] most studies show little effect on average ventilation. Indeed, when a difference is found, there appears to be better ventilation and oxygenation during periodic than during nonperiodic breathing and a lesser incidence of symptoms of altitude adaptation that are linked to relative hypoventilation.[8, 19, 24] The association of periodic breathing with better ventilation may reflect the association of periodicity with increased chemosensitivity, with the latter setting the level of overall ventilation and with periodic breathing appearing as a byproduct. It may also be that periodic breathing is mechanically and energetically efficient. Theoretical analysis suggests that the high tidal volumes of the hyperpneic phase enhance relative alveolar versus dead space ventilation and that apneas conserve respiratory muscle work. Modeling suggests that optimal oxygenation, at least "pressure cost," is produced by clusters of two to four large breaths separated by apneas.[28, 46] Such a pattern might be especially efficient at an altitude at which decreased air density reduces the respiratory pressure cost.

Relationship of Sleep Disturbance and Periodic Breathing to Altitude Syndromes. In susceptible individuals, rapid altitude ascent is associated with two well-recognized syndromes of acute altitude maladaptation: AMS and high-altitude pulmonary edema (HAPE). Although both are most common in the early post ascent period when sleep disturbance and respiratory periodicity are also most pronounced, most studies find that periodic breathing in sleep is not correlated with the development of these syndromes. Indeed, in subjects with these disorders, periodic breathing tends to be replaced by an irregular, nonperiodic pattern (Fig. 18–10).[7, 24] However, in one study, periodic breathing was found to be more frequent in those with HAPE than in those with AMS or in control subjects.[47] This may have been due to exaggerated hypoxemia and hypocapnia in the former group. As mentioned, periodic breathing may be either a marker of or perhaps a cause of increased net ventilation and oxygenation, which reduces the likelihood or severity of these maladaptive syndromes.

TREATMENT

The treatment of or prophylaxis for periodic breathing and related sleep disturbance at high altitude is similar to that commonly used for control of the daytime syndrome of AMS. Staged, gradual ascent to altitude is an effective way to prevent or blunt sleep-related symptoms, but it may be inconvenient. Pharmacological approaches are also useful and include inhibitors of carbonic anhydrase, benzodiazepines, stimulators of peripheral chemosensitivity, and progestational agents.

Carbonic Anhydrase Inhibitors. Acetazolamide is

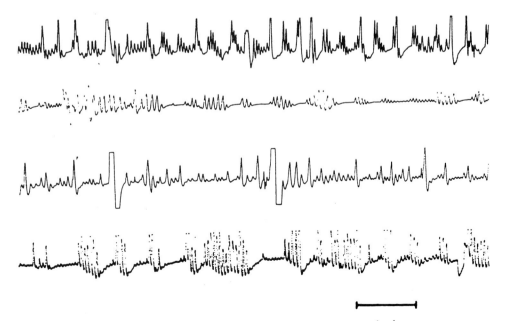

Figure 18–10. Irregular, nonperiodic, breathing during sleep at 2850 m in four subjects susceptible to high altitude pulmonary edema. (From Fujimoto K, Matsuzawa Y, Hirai K, et al. Irregular nocturnal breathing patterns high attitude in subjects susceptible to high-altitude pulmonary edema (HAPE): a preliminary study. Aviat Space Environ Med. 1989; 60:786–791.)

1 min

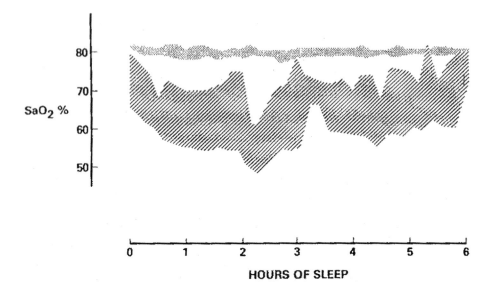

Figure 18–11. Average arterial oxygenation in a sleeping subject at altitude (5360 m) without *(lower hatched area)* and with *(upper)* acetazolamide. Treatment raised and stabilized arterial oxygen saturation. (From Sutton JR, Houston CS, Mansell AL, et al. Effect of acetazolamide on hypoxemia during sleep at high altitude. N Engl J Med. 1979;301:1329–1331. Copyright © 1979, Massachusetts Medical Society. All rights reserved.)

the most common and best studied agent used for amelioration of sleep disturbance at altitude; it has the advantage of also reducing symptoms of AMS.[48–50] This class of agents produces marked reductions in periodic breathing in sleep with higher and less oscillatory SaO_2 (Fig. 18–11).[21, 51] In two studies of sleep at altitude, acetazolamide markedly improved both the mean level and the stability of arterial oxygenation during sleep and reduced the proportion of sleep time during which periodic breathing occurred by roughly 50%[20, 21] (Fig. 18–12). Awakenings that occur more frequently in sleep at high altitude are reduced and subjective and objective sleep quality is improved with augmentation of stage 2 sleep and decreased wakefulness.[52]

The primary action of these agents is thought to be the blockade of enzymatic hydration of CO_2 to carbonic

acid with consequent induction of a bicarbonate diuresis and metabolic acidosis. Blockade of carbonic anhydrase could also promote the accumulation of CO_2 in tissue, which might be responsible for the increase in cerebral blood flow induced by the intravenous administration of acetazolamide,[53] and could stimulate central chemoreceptors. However, these central effects are minimal or absent with the relatively low doses used for symptom reduction at altitude,[54] and selective agents with action limited to the kidney seem as effective as acetazolamide in reducing periodic breathing.[55] Thus, the main mechanism of action is most likely the renal tubular effect with induction of systemic metabolic acidosis. It may be that reduction in periodicity is in part due to lessening of hypoxemia secondary to stimulation of ventilation by acidosis, but carbonic anhydrase inhibitors have a similar use in eliminating central apneas at low altitude[56, 57] where hypoxemia is not a likely factor, suggesting that induction of acidosis, with possible lowering of the apneic threshold, is the major contribution.

These agents raise ventilation with improved oxygenation and greater hypocapnia during wakefulness and sleep at altitude,[48, 49] suggesting an effect on ventilatory control. Although hypoxic ventilatory responses are shifted upward (higher ventilation at all points), the steepness of the relationship is unchanged, indicating no potentiation of hypoxic sensitivity.[21, 51, 55, 58] Effects on the hypercapnic response are variable, and for uncertain reasons, findings differ for progressive versus steady-state measurements.[55] Overall, the findings suggest that these agents act primarily on the kidney to produce a metabolic acidosis, which drives ventilation without any clear effect on peripheral or central chemoreceptor sensitivity.

In some respects, these agents have an action similar to that of CO_2 administration, which also dramatically reduces periodic breathing at altitude.[17, 40] However, the analogy is not simple, because CO_2 administration raises $PaCO_2$ and acetazolamide lowers it, but tissue PCO_2 probably increases under both conditions—in the

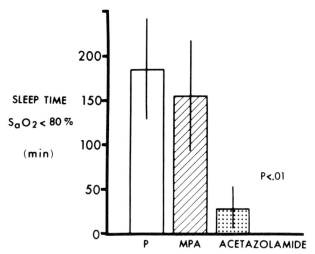

Figure 18–12. Length of time during which SaO_2 is below 80% is used as an arbitrary index of the duration of severe hypoxemia. This was slightly and nonsignificantly reduced by medroxyprogesterone acetate (MPA), whereas acetazolamide led to marked improvement. (From Weil JV, Kryger MH, Scoggin CH. Sleep and breathing at high altitude. In: Sleep Apnea Syndromes. New York, NY: Alan R Liss; 1978:119–136.)

case of acetazolamide because blockade of carbonic anhydrase impedes the transfer of CO_2 from tissues to blood with a consequent rise in tissue P_{CO_2}. An alternative possibility is that reduction in periodic breathing reflects a decrease in blood pH produced by both CO_2 inhalation and acetazolamide administration. Because acidosis is generally considered to potentiate ventilatory responsiveness to hypoxia, this might be a potential mechanism of action of acetazolamide to improve ventilation during wakefulness and sleep at altitude, but as mentioned, the drug fails to increase the gain of the ventilatory response to hypoxia.[21, 28] The resolution of the apparent paradox wherein an agent that increases hypocapnia and should exaggerate periodic breathing but has the opposite effect suggests that the apneic threshold may be a pH rather than a P_{CO_2} threshold. Although alkalosis and hypocapnia are typically coexistent at altitude, their dissociation by carbonic anhydrase inhibition points to a dominant role of pH. The use of low-dose or renal-selective inhibition suggests that it is blood pH rather that local tissue pH that is most important in hyperventilation-induced apnea.

Benzodiazepines. These agents can substantially reduce hypoxic ventilatory responses[59] and were once thought to be hazardous in respiratory disorders of sleep. However, recent evidence suggests that in low doses they are relatively safe in such situations and seem to produce no increase in sleep disordered breathing in the elderly[60] or in nonselected patients with apnea.[61] In sleeping patients with chronic obstructive pulmonary disease, there is no clear increase in apnea or hypopnea or worsening of hypoxemia,[62, 63] and little or no adverse effect is seen in patients with obstructive apnea.[64] In patients with heart failure, temazepam decreased microarousals and improved daytime alertness with no change in the extent of periodic breathing or oxygenation in sleep.[65]

Two studies suggest the safety and usefulness of these agents in the sleep disturbance of high altitude.[7, 13] Shortened latency, decreased arousals, increased sleep efficiency, increased REM, and subjectively better sleep were evident with low-dose temazepam.[13] These were not accompanied by any clear changes in the prevalence of periodic breathing effects and augmented the favorable action of acetazolamide. A benzodiazepine also was said to slightly reduce periodicity, augment slow-wave sleep, and reduce wakefulness during acclimatization but not in early nights after ascent.[7]

Almitrine. This agent, which stimulates the carotid body and augments hypoxic ventilatory responses, augments arterial oxygenation during sleep but increases respiratory periodicity.[35] These effects would be expected to decrease the continuity and subjective quality of sleep, but this has not been directly studied.

Other Agents. Progestational agents such as medroxyprogesterone acetate substantially reduce periodic breathing with little change in oxygenation in sojourners[21] but have greater effects on oxygenation in long-term residents with chronic mountain sickness.[18]

Whether other agents that are used to treat HAPE, such as calcium channel blockers and glucocorticoids, affect breathing, oxygenation, and symptoms related to sleep remains unknown.

Sleep at High Altitude After Long-Term Adaptation

Little is known about sleep and breathing in normal long-term residents of high altitude, although Kryger et al.[66] reported some data. In residents of Leadville, Colorado (3100 m), normal subjects have sleep duration and distribution of stages comparable to those in subjects at lower altitude, but no direct comparisons were made. Although little or no prolonged sleep apnea was noted in such subjects, the majority did have various kinds of respiratory dysrhythmia, typically an undulant oscillation in depth of breathing without true apnea and associated with swings in SaO_2 (Fig. 18–13). Because these subjects were middle-aged men, in whom respiratory dysrhythmias are known to be common during sleep at low altitude, it is unclear to what extent the breathing in sleep at chronic high altitude truly differs from that at sea level. It is possible that arterial desaturation induced by high altitude shifts SaO_2 during sleep to the steeper portion of the dissociation curve and thereby amplifies the influence of ventilatory dysrhythmia on SaO_2. Ventilatory and SaO_2 oscillations similar to those observed by Kryger et al.[66] have also been described at high altitude by Lahiri et al.[32] in Sherpas native to high altitude but not in Sherpas native to low altitude. Although a loss of hypoxic ventilatory response during wakefulness has been observed in natives of Leadville[67] and in Sherpas native to high altitude,[68] it is unclear whether this is related to respiratory dysrhythmia and hypoxemia in highlanders during sleep at altitude. However, improvement in hypoxemia during wakefulness and sleep in

Figure 18–13. Breathing pattern and arterial oxygenation in a subject with chronic mountain polycythemia during sleep at his native altitude of 3100 m. The breathing pattern consists of an undulating depth of breathing with oscillation of SaO_2. (Republished with permission of the American Sleep Disorders Association, 6301 Bandel Road, Suite 101, Rochester, MN 55901. Figure, M. Kryger, R. Glas, D. Jackson, Sleep, 1976, Vol 1. Reproduced by permission of the publisher via Copyright Clearance Center, Inc.)

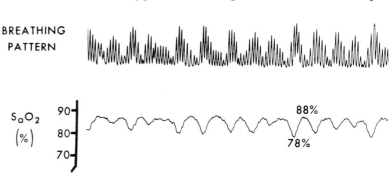

long-term residents at high altitude with use of the ventilatory stimulant medroxyprogesterone acetate suggests that decreased ventilatory drive may have a permissive role.[66, 69]

CONCLUSIONS

The sensation of disrupted sleep after ascent to high altitude is associated with frequent awakenings, which in part probably reflect sleep disruption due to respiratory dysrhythmia typically consisting of monotonously repetitive periodic breathing. This dysrhythmia seems to arise from the combined effects of hypocapnic alkalosis, which leads to suppression of respiratory effort in NREM sleep, and hypoxia, which stimulates the termination of apnea and the occurrence of hyperpnea with consequent hypocapnia, leading to perpetuation of periodicity. Sleep disruption and periodic breathing decrease with time at altitude but may also be considerably reduced by pretreatment with acetazolamide, which may act by correction of alkalosis. In long-term residents of high altitude, less-distinctive, undulating respiratory dysrhythmias are described, with unstable and decreased arterial oxygenation.

References

1. Moore LG, Harrison GL, McCullough RE, et al. Low acute hypoxic ventilatory response and hypoxic depression in acute altitude sickness. J Appl Physiol. 1986;60:1407–1412.
2. Nielsen AM, Bisgard GE, Vidruk EH. Carotid chemoreceptor activity during acute and sustained hypoxia in goats. J Appl Physiol. 1988;65:1796–1802.
3. Weil J. Ventilatory control at high altitude. In: Cherniack NS, Widdicombe JG, eds. Handbook of Physiology: The Respiratory System II. Bethesda, Md: American Physiological Society; 1986.
4. White, DP, Gleeson K, Pickett CK, et al. Altitude acclimatization: influence on periodic breathing and chemoresponsiveness during sleep. J Appl Physiol. 1987;63:401–412.
5. Joern AT, Shurley JT, Brooks RE, et al. Short-term changes in sleep patterns on arrival at the South Polar Plateau. Arch Intern Med. 1970;125:649–654.
6. Reite M, Jackson D, Cahoon RL, et al. Sleep physiology at high altitude. Electroencephalogr Clin Neurophysiol. 1975;38:463–471.
7. Goldenberg F, Richalet JP, Onnen I, et al. Sleep apneas and high altitude newcomers. Int Sports Med. 1992;13:S34–S36.
8. Normand H, Barragan M, Benoit O, et al. Periodic breathing and O_2 saturation in relation to sleep stages at high altitude. Aviat Space Environ Med. 1990;61:229–235.
9. Mizuno K, Asano K, Okudaira N. Sleep and respiration under acute hypobaric hypoxia. Jpn Physiol. 1993;43:161–175.
10. Miller JC, Horvath SM. Sleep at altitude. Aviat Space Environ Med. 1977;48:615–620.
11. Anholm JD, Powles AC, Downey RD, et al. Operation Everest II: arterial oxygen saturation and sleep at extreme simulated altitude. Am Rev Respir Dis. 1992;145(4pt 1):817–826.
12. Ohi M, Chin K, Hirai M, et al. Oxygen desaturation following voluntary hyperventilation in normal subjects. Am J Respir Crit Care Med. 1994;149(3 pt 1):731–738.
13. Nicholson AN, Smith PA, Stone BM, et al. Altitude insomnia: studies during an expedition to the Himalayas. Sleep. 1988;11:354–361.
14. Bonnet MH. Performance and sleepiness as a function of frequency and placement of sleep disruption. Psychophysiology. 1986;23:263–271.
15. Ward M. Periodic respiration: a short historical note. Ann Coll Surg Engl. 1973;52:330–334.
16. Douglas C, Haldane J, Henderson Y, et al. Physiological observations made of Pikes Peak, Colorado, with special reference to adaptation to low barometric pressures. Phil Trans R Soc Lond. 1913;203:185–381.
17. Berssenbrugge A, Dempsey J, Iber C, et al. Mechanisms of hypoxia-induced periodic breathing during sleep in humans. J Physiol. 1983;343:507–526.
18. Kryger M, McCullough RE, Collins D, et al. Treatment of excessive polycythemia of high altitude with respiratory stimulant drugs. Am Rev Respir Dis. 1978;117:455–464.
19. Masuyama S, Kohchiyama S, Shinozaki T, et al. Periodic breathing at high altitude and ventilatory responses to O_2 and CO_2. Jpn J Physiol. 1989;39:523–535.
20. Sutton JR, Houston CS, Mansell AL, et al. Effect of acetazolamide on hypoxemia during sleep at high altitude. N Engl J Med. 1979;301:1329–1331.
21. Weil JV, Kryger MH, Scoggin CH. Sleep and breathing at high altitude. In: Guilleminault C, Dement WC, eds. Sleep Apnea Syndromes. New York, NY: Alan R Liss; 1978:119–136.
22. Lahiri S, Barnard P. Role of arterial chemoreflex in breathing during sleep at high altitude. Progr Clin Biol Res. 1983;136:75–85.
23. Lahiri S, Data PG. Chemosensitivity and regulation of ventilation during sleep at high altitudes. Int J Sports Med. 1992;13:S31–S33.
24. Fujimoto K, Matsuzawa Y, Hirai K, et al. Irregular nocturnal breathing patterns high altitude in subjects susceptible to high-altitude pulmonary edema (HAPE): a preliminary study. Aviat Space Environ Med. 1989;60:786–791.
25. Bulow K. Respiration and wakefulness in man. Acta Physiol Scand. 1963;59:1–110.
26. Douglas C, Haldane J. The causes of periodic or Cheyne-Stokes breathing. J Physiol. 1909;38:401–419.
27. Douglas CG, Haldane JS. The regulation of normal breathing. J Physiol. 1909;38:420–440.
28. Brusil PJ, Waggener TB, Kronauer RE, et al. Methods for identifying respiratory oscillations disclose altitude effects. J Appl Physiol. Respir Environ Exerc Physiol. 1980;48:545–556.
29. Waggener TB, Brusil PJ, Kronauer RE, et al. Strength and cycle time of high-altitude ventilatory patterns in unacclimatized humans. J Appl Physiol Respir Environ Exerc Physiol. 1984;56:576–581.
30. West JB, Peters R Jr, Aksnes G, et al. Nocturnal periodic breathing at altitudes of 6,300 and 8,050 m. J Appl Physiol. 1986;61:280–287.
31. Naughton M, Benard D, Tam A, et al. Role of hyperventilation in the pathogenesis of central sleep apneas in patients with congestive heart failure [see comments]. Am Rev Respir Dis. 1993;148:330–338.
32. Lahiri S, Maret K, Sherpa MG. Dependence of high altitude sleep apnea on ventilatory sensitivity to hypoxia. Respir Physiol. 1983;52:281–301.
33. Fletcher EC. Recurrence of sleep apnea syndrome following tracheostomy: a shift from obstructive to central apnea. Chest. 1989;95:205–209.
34. Badr MS, Toiber F, Skatrud JB, et al. Pharyngeal narrowing/occlusion during central sleep apnea. J Appl Physiol. 1995;78:1806–1815.
35. Hackett PH, Roach RC, Harrison GL, et al. Respiratory stimulants and sleep periodic breathing at high altitude: almitrine versus acetazolamide. Am Rev Respir Dis. 1987;135:896–898.
36. Douglas CG, Haldane JS, Henderson Y, et al. The physiological effects of low atmospheric pressures as observed on Pike's Peak, Colorado. J Physiol. 1912;85:65–67.
37. Gotoh F, Meyer JS, Takagi Y. Cerebral venous and arterial blood gases during Cheyne-Stokes respiration. Am J Med. 1969;47:534–545.
38. Sullivan C, Kosar L, Murphy E, et al. Primary role of respiratory afferents in sustaining breathing rhythm. J Appl Physiol. 1978;45:11–17.
39. Tawadrous FD, Eldridge FL. Posthyperventilation breathing patterns after active hyperventilation in man. J Appl Physiol. 1974;37:353–356.
40. Skatrud JB, Dempsey JA. Interaction of sleep state and chemical stimuli in sustaining rhythmic ventilation. J Appl Physiol Respir Environ Exerc Physiol. 1983;55:813–822.
41. Powels AC, Sutton JR, Gray GW, et al. Sleep hypoxemia at altitude: its relationship to acute mountain sickness and ventila-

tory responsiveness to hypoxia and hypercapnia. In: Folinsbee LJ, ed. Environmental Stress: Individual Human Adaptations. New York, NY: Academic Press; 1978:373–381.

42. Cherniack N, Gothe B, Strohl K. Mechanisms for recurrent apneas at altitude. High Altitude Man. 1984;129–140.

43. Khoo MC, Kronauer RE, Strohl KP, et al. Factors inducing periodic breathing in humans: a general model. J Appl Physiol Respir Environ Exerc Physiol. 1982;53:644–659.

44. Berry RB, Gleeson K. Respiratory arousal from sleep: mechanisms and significance. Sleep. 1997;20:654–675.

45. Milledge JS. The ventilatory response to hypoxia: how much is good for a mountaineer? Postgrad Med J. 1987;63:169–172.

46. Ghazanshahi SD, Khoo MC. Optimal ventilatory patterns in periodic breathing. Ann Biomed Eng. 1993;21:517–530.

47. Eichenberger U, Weiss E, Riemann D, et al. Nocturnal periodic breathing and the development of acute high altitude illness. Am J Respir Crit Care Med. 1996;154(6 pt 1):1748–1754.

48. Cain SM, Dunn JD. Low doses of acetazolamide to aid accommodation of men to altitude. J Appl Physiol. 1966;21:1195–1200.

49. Forwand SA, Landowne M, Follansbee JN, et al. Effect of acetazolamide on acute mountain sickness. N Engl J Med. 1968;279:839–845.

50. Hackett PH, Rennie D. The incidence, importance, and prophylaxis of acute mountain sickness. Lancet. 1976;2:1149–1155.

51. Sutton JR, Gray GW, Houston CS, et al. Effects of duration at altitude and acetazolamide on ventilation and oxygenation during sleep. Sleep. 1980;3:455–464.

52. Nicholson AN, Stone BM. Hypnotics and transient insomnia. Acta Psych Scand Suppl. 1986;332:55–59.

53. Hauge A, Nicolaysen G, Thoresen M. Acute effects of acetazolamide on cerebral blood flow in man. Acta Physiol Scand. 1983;117:233–239.

54. Huang SY, McCullough RE, McCullough RG, et al. Usual clinical dose of acetazolamide does not alter cerebral blood. Respir Physiol. 1988;72:315–326.

55. Swenson ER, Leatham KL, Roach RC, et al. Renal carbonic anhydrase inhibition reduces high altitude sleep periodic breathing. Respir Physiol. 1991;86:333–343.

56. White DP, Zwillich CW, Pickett CK, et al. Central sleep apnea: improvement with acetazolamide therapy. Arch Intern Med. 1982;142:1816–1819.

57. DeBacker WA, Verbraecken J, Willemen M, et al. Central apnea index decreases after prolonged treatment with acetazolamide. Am J Respir Crit Care Med. 1995;151:87–91.

58. Bashir Y, Kann M, Stradling JR. The effect of acetazolamide on hypercapnic and eucapnic/poikilocapnic hypoxic ventilatory responses in normal subjects. Pulmon Pharmacol. 1990;3:151–154.

59. Lakshminarayan S, Sahn SA, Hudson LD, et al. Effect of diazepam on ventilatory responses. Clin Pharmacol Ther. 1976;20:178–183.

60. Camacho ME, Morin CM. The effect of temazepam on respiration in elderly insomniacs with mild sleep apnea. Sleep. 1995;18:644–645.

61. Hoijer U, Hedner J, Ejnell H, et al. Nitrazepam in patients with sleep apnoea: a double-blind placebo-controlled study. Eur Respir J. 1994;7:2011–2015.

62. Gentil B, Tehindrazanarivelo A, Lienhart A, et al. Respiratory effects of midazolam in patients with obstructive sleep apnea syndromes. Ann Fran Anes Reanim. 1994;13:275–279.

63. Steens RD, Pouliot Z, Millar TW, et al. Effects of zolidem and triazolam on sleep and respiration in mild to moderate chronic obstructive pulmonary disease. Sleep. 1993;16:318–326.

64. Berry RB, Kouchi K, Bower J, et al. Triazolam in patients with obstructive apnea. Am J Respir Crit Care Med. 1995;151:450–454.

65. Biberdorf DJ, Steens R, Miller TW, et al. Benzodiazepines in congestive heart failure: effects of temazepam on arousability and Cheyne-Stokes respiration. Sleep. 1993;16:529–538.

66. Kryger M, Glas R, Jackson D, et al. Impaired oxygenation during sleep in excessive polycythemia of high altitude: improvement with respiratory stimulation. Sleep. 1978;1:3–17.

67. Weil JV, Byrne-Quinn E, Sodal IE, et al. Acquired attenuation of chemoreceptor function in chronically hypoxic man at high altitude. J Clin Invest. 1971;50:186–195.

68. Hackett PH, Reeves JT, Reeves CD, et al. Control of breathing in Sherpas at low and high altitude. J Appl Physiol Respir Environ Exerc Physiol. 1980;49:374–379.

69. Kryger M, Weil J, Grover R. Chronic mountain polycythemia: a disorder of the regulation of breathing during sleep? Chest. 1978;73(2 suppl):303–304.

19

Host Defense

James M. Krueger

Jidong Fang

During the onset of infection, excess sleepiness is often experienced. Although this phenomenon was noted by Hippocrates, it was not until the 1980s that sleep over the course of an infection was measured. Changes in sleep induced by microbes appear to be one facet of the acute phase response. Typically, soon after infectious challenge, animals exhibit excess nonrapid eye movement (NREM) sleep and decreased rapid eye movement (REM) sleep. The exact time course of sleep responses depends upon the infectious agent used, the route of administration, and the time of day the infectious challenge is given.

There is a common perception that sleep loss can render one vulnerable to infection. Many studies have combined sleep deprivation with measurement of one or more parameters of the immune response. Very few studies have combined sleep deprivation with infectious challenge. After sleep deprivation, several immune system parameters do, in fact, change, for example, natural killer cell activity. Further, after prolonged (2 to 3 weeks) sleep deprivation, rats become septicemic. Currently it appears that small amounts of sleep loss may help host defenses, whereas prolonged sleep loss is devastating.

The molecular mechanisms responsible for the changes in sleep associated with infection and changes in the immune system induced by sleep are beginning to be understood. It appears that during infection there is an amplification of a sleep-regulatory biochemical cascade. This chain of events includes well-known immune response modifiers such as interleukin-1, tumor necrosis factor, prostaglandins, nitric oxide, and adenosine. All these substances are involved in physiological sleep regulation.

There is, to date, little direct evidence showing that sleep per se aids in recuperative processes. It likely does, but it is difficult to directly test this notion.

Most people have experienced the intense desire to sleep that often occurs at the onset of infection. Further, many have received the advice from loving parents and grandparents that one should get plenty of rest to prevent or recover from infectious disease. These experiences suggest a connection between sleep and host defense systems. Indeed, Hippocrates, Aristotle, and many others of our predecessors acknowledged such a relationship. It is thus somewhat surprising that modern science and medicine have only, within the

past 10 years, systematically investigated whether sleep has anything to do with host defense systems. Chapter 92 reviews clinical aspects of specific infections. In this chapter, four questions related to this issue are addressed:

1. Does sleep change after infectious challenge?
2. Does sleep loss affect immune function?
3. Do the sleep and immune systems share regulatory molecules?
4. Does sleep per se aid in recuperative processes?

Clear affirmative answers are at hand for questions 1, 2, and 3, and the evidence thus far is consistent with a role for sleep in recuperation.

SLEEP IS GREATLY ALTERED AFTER INFECTIOUS CHALLENGE

Viral Challenge

Viral diseases that cause central nervous system lesions or inflammation can affect sleep. In von Economo's seminal paper,[1] he correlated the location of viral-induced brain lesions with changes in sleep patterns. This work led to the concept that sleep was an active process, that is, not simply the withdrawal of sensory stimuli, and to the idea that there was some degree of localization of neural networks regulating sleep. Despite the importance of this work, many years passed before the direct effects of viral infections on sleep were experimentally determined. During the early stages of HIV infections, before the onset of AIDS, patients have excess stage 4 nonrapid eye movement (NREM) sleep during the latter half of the night.[2-5] Another central nervous system viral disease, rabies, is also associated with disrupted sleep.[6, 7] In these diseases, as was the case with von Economo's virus, it is difficult to distinguish whether the effects of the viral infection on sleep are direct or whether they result from viral-induced lesions. Viral pathogenic mechanisms have also been implicated in several conditions that involve sleep disorders; the list includes mononucleosis,[8] sudden infant death syndrome,[9] and chronic fatigue syndrome[10] (reviewed in reference 11). However, the direct involvement of viruses in the sleep disorders associated with these syndromes has not been investigated.

Influenza virus, a virus that localizes to the respiratory tract during the early stage of disease, has been used in several sleep investigations. Smith,[12] at the British Cold Unit, reported that low doses of influenza in human beings induce excess behavioral sleep and cognitive dysfunction; these symptoms appear after low viral doses that fail to induce the better-known characteristics of the acute phase response such as fever. However, polysomnography was not used in his study. More recently, animal studies of influenza virus infections have clearly shown that sleep is profoundly affected by infectious challenge. In a rabbit model, intravenous injections of influenza virus are associated with large increases in NREM sleep lasting 6 to 10 h.[13] However, in rabbits, influenza virus can only undergo a partial replication and therefore the disease is limited because new viruses cannot be formed. (The partial replication of the virus allows double-stranded viral RNA to be formed; the importance of double-stranded RNA in viral pathogenic mechanisms is explained below.)

Another animal model, influenza-infected mice, is more applicable to human beings because in mice this virus can fully replicate. Mice challenged intranasally with influenza virus display profound increases in NREM sleep lasting 3 d or more while rapid eye movement (REM) sleep is inhibited[14–16] (Fig. 19–1). These sleep responses are much attenuated if the viral infection is confined to the upper airway.[16] If the initial viral challenge is limited to the upper airway, it takes about a week for the virus to move down the respiratory tract; by then the animals are able to mount an effective immune response. Different strains of mice respond differentially to viral challenge. Very large changes in sleep are observed in Swiss-Webster[14] and C57BL/6[15] strains, whereas influenza-induced sleep responses in BALB/c mice are much attenuated. This difference may be due to the reduced ability of BALB/c mice[15] to produce cytokines; below we provide evidence that cytokines are involved in physiological sleep regulation and in the sleep responses induced by infectious challenge.

The mechanism by which viruses induce sleep responses seems to involve viral double-stranded RNA induction of cytokines such as interferon and interleukin-1 (IL-1). Influenza virus is a negative-sense single-stranded RNA virus; when it infects a cell it forms the positive-sense RNA strand, which can anneal to the negative-sense strand to form double-stranded RNA. Viral double-stranded RNA can be extracted from lungs of infected mice[17] and from supernates of cells infected in culture.[18] If rabbits are given the viral double-stranded RNA extracted from mouse lungs, they exhibit sleep responses similar to those observed after injection of viable virus; RNA from healthy lungs has no effect on sleep.[17] Similar responses are observed if rabbits are given the synthetic double-stranded RNA, polyriboinosinic:polyribocytidylic (poly I:C), but not if given the corresponding single strands of poly I and poly C.[19] Similarly, rabbits given short double-stranded

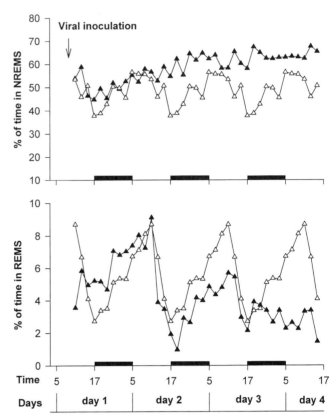

Figure 19–1. Influenza virus challenge induces prolonged increases in NREM sleep *(top panel)* and decreases in REM sleep *(bottom panel)* in mice. Data are from reference 16. Filled triangles represent data collected after viral inoculation. Open triangles represent the averaged baseline data collected over a 3-d period just prior to viral inoculation. Horizontal dark bars show lights-off periods for each experimental day.

oligomers corresponding to a portion of influenza gene segment 3 also exhibit large increases in NREM sleep.[20] Rabbits do not respond if given the single-stranded oligomers. Rabbits challenged with viable virus or poly I:C have increased plasma antiviral activity that occurs concomitantly with the changes in sleep.[13] The antiviral activity is attributed to interferon-α and other cytokines. Injection of interferon-α into rabbits also induces sleep responses similar to those induced by virus, poly I:C, or the double-stranded oligomers.[21–25] The role of other cytokines in sleep regulation is discussed below at length.

Bacterial Challenge

Sleep responses are also observed after bacterial challenge. Indeed, results obtained after challenging rabbits with the gram-positive bacterium *Staphylococcus aureus* were the first to suggest that NREM sleep responses formed part of the acute phase response.[26] In those experiments, rabbits were given *S. aureus* intravenously to induce septicemia; within a few hours of the inoculation large excesses in NREM sleep were observed. Associated with the increase in NREM sleep were increases in amplitude of electroencephalographic

(EEG) slow waves. EEG slow wave (0.5 to 4.0 Hz) amplitudes are thought to be indicative of the intensity of NREM sleep.[27] This initial phase of increased duration and intensity of NREM sleep lasted about 20 h; it was followed by a more prolonged phase of decreased duration of NREM sleep and decreased EEG slow wave amplitudes.[26] During both phases of the NREM sleep changes, REM sleep was inhibited and animals were febrile. Other changes characteristic of the acute phase response, for example, fibrinogenemia and neutrophilia, occurred concurrently with the changes in sleep.

In subsequent studies in which gram-negative bacteria and other routes of administration were used, a similar general pattern of biphasic NREM sleep responses and REM sleep inhibition was observed (reviewed in reference 11). However, the timing of sleep responses depends upon both the bacterial species and the route of administration. For example, after intravenous administration of *Escherichia coli*, NREM sleep responses are rapid in onset but the excess NREM sleep phase lasts only 4 to 6 h.[28] The subsequent phase of reduced NREM sleep and reduced amplitude of EEG slow waves is sustained for relatively long periods. In contrast, if the gram-negative bacterium *Pasteurella multocida* is given intranasally, a different time course of sleep responses is observed.[29] In this case, the increased NREM sleep responses occur after a longer latency and the magnitude of the increases in NREM sleep is less than the effects of this pathogen given by other routes of administration.[29] *P. multocida* is a natural pathogen in rabbits.

Much is known about how bacteria induce sleep responses. Unlike viruses, bacterial replication is not necessary; thus, injection of killed bacteria or purified bacterial cell walls induces excess NREM sleep, enhances EEG slow waves, and inhibits REM sleep (reviewed in references 11 and 30). Bacteria and bacteria cell walls are phagocytized by macrophages. Macrophages will kill bacteria and digest their cell walls and secret low-molecular-weight soluble components derived from these cell walls into the surrounding medium.[31–33] Some of these cell wall–derived substances are biologically active, being effective stimulants of host defense systems and somnogenic (reviewed in reference 34). This process is thought to provide a mechanism whereby the host can amplify its defenses. For example, muramyl peptides are the monomeric building blocks of bacterial peptidoglycan. Macrophages release muramyl peptides if given bacterial cell walls, and the released substances are somnogenic.[31] The sleep-promoting activity of muramyl peptides is dependent upon their chemical structure. For example, *N*-acetyl-muramyl-L-alanyl-D-isoglutamine (or MDP-LD for muramyl dipeptide) is somnogenic,[34–38] whereas the stereoisomers MDP-LL and MPD-DD are not. Many muramyl peptides are also immune adjuvants and pyrogenic, although the structural requirements for these biological activities are distinct from those required for sleep-promoting activity (reviewed in reference 11).

Muramyl peptides were first implicated in sleep regulation after a disaccharide-tetrapeptide, *N*-acetyl-glucosaminyl-1, 6 anhydro-*N*-acetyl-muramyl-alanyl-glutamyl-diaminopimelyl-alanine, isolated from brain and urine, was shown to be somnogenic.[39] Muramyl peptides are not believed to be synthesized by mammals because there are no known synthetic pathways in mammals for muramic acid or diaminopimelic acid. Nonetheless, muramyl peptides are readily available to mammals. The intestinal lumen contains large amounts of bacteria and we are constantly challenged by bacteria. As mentioned above, once entering the body, bacteria are phagocytized and digested and somnogenic muramyl peptides are released in the process. This mechanism is viewed as operating at a low basal rate under normal conditions and amplified greatly during infection. It is also likely involved in sleep responses induced by sleep deprivation and excess food intake (see later). Furthermore, reduction of bacterial populations in the gut is associated with a reduction of sleep.[40, 41]

Another bacterial cell wall product that could be involved in sleep responses induced by gram-negative bacteria is endotoxin or lipopolysaccharide. Endotoxin and its biologically active moiety, lipid A, are somnogenic in animals and human beings[42, 43] (reviewed in reference 11). Sleep responses induced by endotoxin are distinct from those induced by muramyl peptides. Muramyl peptides are somnogenic over a wide dose range and are relatively nontoxic in the sense that very large doses, for example, for MDP, 10,000 times the minimal somnogenic dose, are not lethal. In contrast, the somnogenic dose range of endotoxin is more restricted and small increases in doses above the threshold somnogenic dose, about tenfold, can induce shock. Modification of the lipid A structure alters somnogenic activity, for example, conversion of diphosphoryl lipid A to monophosphoryl lipid A reduces its somnogenicity.[43] Like double-stranded RNA, endotoxin and muramyl peptides induce production of a wide variety of cytokines and hormones. Some of these substances are involved in physiological sleep regulation and the amplified sleep responses observed during infection are believed to be manifestations of the amplification of the production of these substances (see below).

Other microbes, for example, fungal organisms such as *Candida albicans* or protozoans such as *Trypanosoma brucei brucei*, also have the capacity to induce sleep responses. Some of these microbial-induced sleep responses are quite interesting. Trypanosomiasis in rabbits is associated with recurrent bouts of enhanced NREM sleep occurring about every 7 days. Trypanosomes undergo antigenic variations in the host; the proliferating new antigenic variants stimulate the host immune response and such periods are accompanied by excess NREM sleep.[44] Like bacteria and viruses, fungi and protozoans have the capacity to enhance cytokine production by the host.

In summary, infectious challenge is associated with profound changes in sleep. These microbial-induced sleep responses are now considered part of the acute phase response and like the other components of this response, sleep may be adaptive.

SLEEP LOSS AFFECTS IMMUNE FUNCTION

Answering the question of whether sleep loss affects immune function is difficult to answer. For example, what measurement should one use to assess immune function? The important question is whether sleep loss renders the animal more vulnerable to infectious challenge, tumor formation, or inflammation. (We already know that sleep loss renders one more vulnerable to accidental injury.) Unfortunately, only a very few studies have directly measured host outcomes; instead the approach most often used is to pick one or more parameters associated with the immune system, for example, natural killer cell activity or plasma cytokine levels, and determine whether they change after sleep deprivation. Often such results leave the reader uninformed as to whether the outcome is adverse or beneficial for the host. In addition, it is very difficult in sleep deprivation studies to isolate sleep loss per se as the independent variable. Sleep deprivation is usually associated with stress, increased locomotor activity, changes in feeding patterns, hormonal changes, and changes in body temperature. Each of these variables is known to affect immune function. Despite these limitations, a picture is emerging that suggests that sleep loss does indeed influence the immune system. Paradoxically, it may be that short-term sleep deprivation may enhance host defenses, whereas long-term sleep loss is devastating.

Most people are under the impression that sleep loss renders one more vulnerable to infection. Yet in human experimental studies of sleep deprivation there has been a failure to demonstrate an increased incidence of infection. Most of these studies are limited: often healthy young volunteers are used, environmental conditions are unchallenging, and the deprivation periods are short. Some animal studies, in which short-term sleep deprivation is used, are consistent with the human studies. Toth et al.[45] challenged rabbits with *E. coli* before or after 4 h of sleep deprivation; they concluded that sleep deprivation failed to exacerbate the *E. coli*–induced clinical illness. In rats partially deprived of sleep for several days and challenged with a subdermal allogenic carcinoma, Bergmann et al.[46] concluded that host defenses were improved by sleep deprivation because rats deprived of sleep had smaller tumors than those in control animals. In contrast, Brown et al.[47] deprived mice of sleep for 7 h that were immunized against influenza virus, then rechallenged the mice with influenza virus. The sleep-deprived mice, but not the immunized control mice, failed to clear the virus from their lungs. These results strongly suggest that sleep loss is detrimental to host defenses. However, in a similar study by Renegar et al.,[48] sleep loss failed to alter preexisting mucosal and humoral immunity in either young or senescent mice.

The effects of long-term sleep deprivation on host defenses are more striking. If rats obtain only about 20% of their normal sleep, after a period of 2 to 3 weeks they die. Yoked control rats, which manage to keep about 80% of their normal sleep during the depri-

vation period, survive. Everson[49] showed that the experimental rats, but not the yoked controls, develop septicemia. These results were replicated by another group using the same sleep-deprivation protocol.[50] Bacteria cultured from the blood were primarily facultative anaerobes indigenous to the host and environment. Similar opportunistic infections plague patients with suppressed immune systems. Everson's results clearly suggest that host defenses are compromised by long-term sleep loss. One source of possible invading microbes is bacterial translocation across the gut wall. In another study, after only a few days of partial sleep deprivation, viable bacteria could be cultured from mesenteric lymph nodes, although the blood of these animals remained sterile.[51] In another model of sleep deprivation in which rats were placed on a small pedestal in a pool of water, Landis et al.[52] obtained similar results. After 72 h of REM sleep loss, they could culture bacteria from mesenteric lymph nodes. These results suggest that sleep loss likely amplifies the normally occurring process of gut permeability to bacteria and bacterial products. As discussed below, food intake also affects gut permeability to bacteria and bacterial products[53] and also affects sleep. Small amounts of bacterial cell wall products such as endotoxin and peptidoglycan "prime" immunocytes and could thereby render them more effective for nonspecific host defenses (reviewed in reference 54). Thus, perhaps under appropriate experimental conditions, a small amount of sleep loss is associated with more effective priming, whereas after more prolonged sleep loss the host is overwhelmed by microbial challenge.

Regardless of such speculation, an independent literature clearly indicates that sleep loss is associated with changes in parameters normally associated with the immune response. Cytokines, such as interferon, IL-1, and tumor necrosis factor (TNF), are well known for their roles as immune response modifiers. These substances are affected by sleep deprivation. More than 20 years ago, Palmblad et al.[55] showed that after sleep deprivation, the ability of lymphocytes to produce interferon is enhanced. More recently, many laboratories have obtained similar results. For example, Yamasu et al.[56] showed that sleep deprivation enhances TNF production in streptococcal-stimulated white blood cells; other stressors, unlike sleep deprivation, fail to prime for systemic production of TNF. Uthgenannt et al.[57] showed that sleep loss increases the ability of endotoxin-stimulated monocytes to produce TNF. Similarly, Hohagen et al.[58] showed that the ability of cultures of whole blood to produce IL-1β and interferon-α in response to endotoxin is maximal at the time of sleep onset. Moldofsky et al.,[59] showed that in human beings, sleep deprivation leads to enhanced nocturnal plasma levels of IL-1-like activity. In rabbits, Opp and Krueger[60] reached a similar conclusion.

There are several reports that in normal people plasma levels of cytokines are related to the sleep-wake cycle. Moldofsky et al.[61] first described such relationships in human beings, showing that IL-1 activity was related to the onset of slow-wave sleep. Darko et al.[62] showed that plasma levels of TNF vary in phase with EEG slow wave amplitudes. Gudewill et al.[63] and Covelli et al.[64] also described a temporal relationship between sleep and IL-1β activity. Some disease states that are associated with sleep disorders result in disruption of circulating cytokine levels. The circadian rhythm of TNF release is disturbed in obstructive sleep apnea syndrome patients,[65] although in these patients, IL-1 was not disturbed. Vgontzas et al.[66] described elevated TNF levels in sleep apneics and narcoleptic patients compared with controls; this group also failed to show changes in IL-1 in these populations of patients. In contrast, patients with acute psychoses have higher plasma levels of IL-1β; reduced sleep in these patients is the likely reason for the increase in their IL-1β levels.[67]

Other facets of the immune response are also linked to sleep. Over 25 years ago, Casey et al.[68] demonstrated altered antigen uptake after sleep deprivation. Palmblad et al.[69] showed a decrease in lymphocyte DNA synthesis after 48 h of sleep deprivation and in an earlier study[55] a decrease in phagocytosis after 72 h of sleep deprivation. Moldofsky et al.[59] described sleep deprivation–induced changes in mitogen responses. Circulating immune complexes fall during sleep and rise again just before getting out of bed.[70] Renegar et al.[71] showed that in mice, sleep deprivation reduces immunoglobulin G (IgG) catabolism, resulting in elevated IgG levels. In contrast, Benca et al.[72] failed to show an effect of sleep deprivation on spleen cell counts, lymphocyte proliferation, or plaque-forming cell responses to antigens in rats. In an extensive elegant study of human beings deprived of sleep for 64 h, Dinges et al.[73] also failed to show an effect of sleep deprivation on proliferative responses to mitogens. However, they did show a depression of CD4, CD16, CD56, and CD57 lymphocytes after one night of sleep loss, although CD56 and CD57 lymphocytes increased after two nights of sleep loss. Born et al.[74] also showed that a night of sustained wakefulness reduced counts of all lymphocyte subsets measured. Finally, Brown et al.[75] showed that 8 h of sleep deprivation suppressed the secondary antibody response to sheep red blood cells in rats.

Changes in natural killer cell activity in conjunction with sleep and sleep loss have been measured by several laboratories. In several studies, natural killer cell activity decreased after sleep deprivation.[59, 76, 77] In contrast, Born et al.[74] and Dinges et al.[73] reported increased natural killer cell activity after sleep deprivation. In normal men and women, natural killer cell activity may decrease with sleep.[78] However, insomnia is associated with a reduction of natural killer cell activity.[79] It is likely that circulating natural killer cell activity, as well as natural killer cell activity in a variety of tissue compartments, is sensitive to sleep although the exact tissue distribution of natural killer cell activity is likely dependent upon the specific experimental conditions.

SLEEP-REGULATORY MECHANISM AND THE IMMUNE SYSTEM SHARE REGULATORY MOLECULES

There are numerous associations between the nervous and immune systems, for example, neuronal innervation of lymphoid organs and endocrines such as growth hormone, prolactin, and glucocorticoids has the capacity to affect both sleep and immunocytes. There is another class of substances called cytokines, which act as autocrines and exocrines and are well characterized as immune response modifiers (reviewed in references 11 and 80). Two of these cytokines are also well characterized as being involved in physiological NREM sleep regulation: IL-1β (reviewed in reference 81) and TNF-α (reviewed in reference 82). The evidence for the involvement of IL-1β and TNF-α in NREM sleep regulation and in the sleep responses to infectious challenge is briefly reviewed here.

In addition to being immunocyte products whose production is amplified by viral and bacterial products, both IL-1β and TNF-α are found in normal brain. Both IL-1β messenger RNA (mRNA)[83] and TNF-α mRNA[84] have diurnal rhythms in the brain with the highest values being associated with periods of maximum sleep (Fig. 19–2). TNF protein levels also have a sleep-associated diurnal rhythm in several brain areas[85] and IL-1 cerebrospinal fluid (CSF) levels vary with the sleep-wake cycle.[86] Both IL-1β and TNF-α belong to larger functional families of molecules (reviewed in reference 81). All of the IL-1–associated and TNF-associated molecules are constitutively expressed in normal brain.

Administration of either IL-1β or TNF-α (and IL-1α and TNF-β as well) promotes NREM sleep[87–94] (reviewed in reference 11). The excessive NREM sleep occurring after either IL-1β[87, 88] or TNF-α[95, 96] appears to be physiological in the sense that sleep remains episodic, sleep cycle length remains normal, and sleep is readily reversible if the animals are disturbed. Further, if IL-1β or TNF-α is given either intracerebroventricularly (ICV) or intravenously, sleep intensity, as measured by the amplitude of EEG delta waves, is greater. The effects of IL-1 on sleep depend upon dose and the time of day it is given; low doses of IL-1β promote NREM sleep, whereas high doses inhibit NREM sleep.[91, 92]

The inhibition of either IL-1β[97] or TNF-α[98] inhibits spontaneous NREM sleep. Thus, if one administers anti-IL-1 antibodies, anti-TNF antibodies, the soluble IL-1 receptor, the soluble TNF receptor, peptide fragments of the IL-1 or TNF soluble receptor, or the IL-1 receptor antagonist, spontaneous NREM sleep is reduced (reviewed in references 11, 81, 82, and 99). Further, if one gives animals substances that inhibit either the production or actions of IL-1 or TNF, sleep is inhibited. Alpha-melanocyte–stimulating hormone,[100] corticotropin-releasing hormone,[101] prostaglandin E2,[102] IL-4,[103] IL-10,[104] and glucocorticoids, all of which inhibit IL-1 or TNF, or both, all inhibit spontaneous NREM sleep (reviewed in reference 11). Finally, knockout strains of mice that lack either the type I IL-1 receptor[105] or the 55-kD TNF receptor[94] sleep less than strain controls.

Sleep deprivation, excessive food intake, and acute mild increases in ambient temperature (T_a) are effective somnogens. The somnogenic actions of each of these manipulations are associated with enhanced production of either IL-1 or TNF. After sleep deprivation,

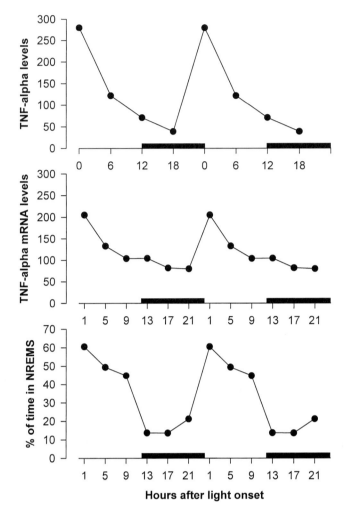

Figure 19–2. In rats, tumor necrosis factor (TNF) bioactivity *(top panel)* and TNF-α messenger RNA (mRNA) *(middle panel)* have diurnal rhythms. Peak levels of these substances occur at the beginning of daylight hours; during that period duration of nonrapid eye movement (NREM) sleep is maximal in rats (lower panel). Horizontal dark bars indicate the lights-off period; rats are nocturnal animals, and thus sleep less during the night. Data were taken from three papers.[60, 84, 85] *Top graph,* values are picograms of TNF per gram of tissue; *middle graph,* values are relative densities of stained bands imaged from electrophoresis gels; *bottom graph,* values are percent of time spent in NREM sleep in 3-h time blocks.

brain levels of IL-1β mRNA increase.[106, 107] The NREM sleep rebound that would normally occur after sleep deprivation is greatly attenuated if either IL-1 or TNF is blocked using antibodies or soluble receptors.[97, 108] In human beings[59] and rabbits,[60] IL-1 plasma levels increase during sleep deprivation. The normal circadian rhythm of plasma levels of TNF are disrupted in sleep apneic patients.[65, 66] Although the somnogenic effects of sleep deprivation seem to involve both IL-1 and TNF, the enhanced NREM sleep associated with mild increases in T_a involves TNF[109] but not IL-1.[110]

Excessive food intake induces enhanced liver and brain production of IL-1β mRNA and the increased brain IL-1β mRNA is dependent on vagal afferent activity induced by liver IL-1β. Thus, rats presented with palatable food (cafeteria diet) display excess NREM sleep[111] and increased IL-1β mRNA levels in liver and brain.[112] The cafeteria diet–induced NREM sleep responses are blocked by vagotomy.[111] Similarly, intraperitoneal IL-1β induces excess NREM sleep and increased IL-1β mRNA in liver and brain; both effects are also lost if animals are vagotomized.[113] Vagal-associated paraganglia in the liver have IL-1 receptors[114] and hepatoportal injection of IL-1β induces vagal afferent activity.[115]

The actions of cafeteria diet–feeding on NREM sleep and liver and brain production of IL-1 represent physiological change, yet they likely involve the actions of bacterial cell wall products. Gut permeability to bacteria and bacterial products is influenced by dietary factors[53] and the gram-negative bacteria cell wall product, endotoxin, is a normal constituent of portal blood.[116] Endotoxin stimulates IL-1 production in the liver and elsewhere. Other bacterial cell wall products, for example, muramyl peptides, also have the capacity to stimulate IL-1 and TNF production (reviewed in reference 11). Muramyl peptides also cross the intestinal wall into blood. NREM sleep responses induced by muramyl dipeptide are attenuated if animals are pretreated with either blockers of IL-1[117] or TNF.[118] As mentioned above, prolonged sleep deprivation results in bacteremia; it thus seems likely that the interaction of those bacteria with liver macrophages results in the amplification of the physiological processes that are also associated with excessive food intake. Other forms of infection also likely interact with these processes resulting in the excess sleep associated with infection (see above).

The molecular steps by which IL-1 and TNF induce sleep are beginning to be understood, although there is yet much to learn about them. IL-1 and TNF act within a cascade of events that include parallel interacting pathways (Fig. 19–3). For example, both IL-1 and TNF stimulate nuclear factor kappa B (NFκB) production. NFκB is a DNA-binding protein involved in transcription. Other somnogenic cytokines, such as acidic fibroblast growth factor, epidermal growth factor, and nerve growth factor, also stimulate NFκB production. In contrast, several substances that inhibit NFκB activation, for example, IL-4, IL-10, and glucocorticoids, all inhibit spontaneous sleep. NFκB promotes IL-1 and TNF production and thus forms a positive feedback loop; such a mechanism could be involved in the amplification of signals promoting sleep. Sleep deprivation is associated with the activation of NFκB in the cerebral cortex.[119]

Several NFκB downstream events also play a role in sleep regulation. Thus inducible nitric oxide synthase DNA has several NFκB enhancer elements. Inhibition of nitric oxide synthase inhibits sleep,[120, 121] whereas nitric oxide donors promote sleep.[122, 123] Adenosine, another substance implicated in sleep regulation,[124] augments IL-1β–induced nitric oxide synthase production[125]; adenosine also induces astrocytes to produce nitric oxide.[126] Activation of NFκB also promotes IL-2 production; IL-2 promotes sleep in rats.[23]

Growth hormone–releasing hormone (GHRH) is likely involved in IL-1 promotion of NREM sleep.

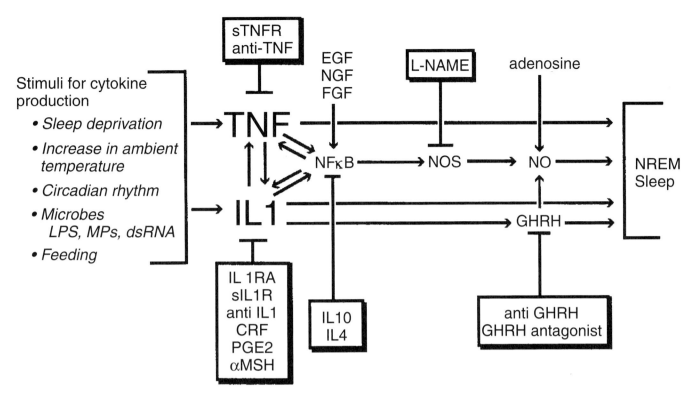

Figure 19–3. Interleukin-1β (IL-1β) and tumor necrosis factor-α (TNF-α) are part of a cascade of events that include several other endogenous somnogenic substances and sleep-inhibitory substances. Substances in boxes inhibit nonrapid eye movement (NREM) sleep and inhibit either the production or the action of substances in the somnogenic pathways. Inhibition of any one step does not result in complete sleep loss; animals likely compensate for the loss of any one step by relying on parallel somnogenic pathways. Such redundant pathways provide stability to the sleep-regulatory system, as well as alternative mechanisms by which a variety of sleep-promoting or sleep-inhibitory stimuli may affect sleep. Our current knowledge of the biochemical events involved in sleep regulation is much more complicated than that shown here. For example, we know that IL-1-β via nuclear factor kappa B (NFκB) induces cyclooxygenase, an enzyme involved in prostaglandin D₂ production; prostaglandin D₂ is involved in physiological sleep regulation. anti-IL-1, anti-IL-1 antibody; anti-TNF, anti-TNF antibody; CRF, corticotropin-releasing hormone; dsRNA, double-stranded RNA; EGF, epidermal growth factor; FGF, fibroblast growth factor; GHRH, growth hormone–releasing hormone; IL1RA, IL-1 receptor antagonist; L-NAME, an arginine analogue; LPS, lipopolysaccharide; MPs, muramyl peptides; αMSH, alpha-melanocyte–stimulating hormone; NFκB: nuclear factor kappa B; NGF, nerve growth factor; NOS, nitric oxide synthase; PGE₂, prostaglandin E₂; sILIR, soluble IL-1 receptor; sTNFR, soluble TNF receptor; ⟶ indicates stimulation; ⟞ indicates inhibition.

There is an independent literature implicating GHRH in sleep regulation (reviewed in reference 127). Administration of GHRH promotes NREM sleep[128–131] and inhibition of GHRH inhibits spontaneous NREM sleep.[132, 133] Hypothalamic GHRH mRNA varies with the sleep-wake cycle[134] and sleep deprivation enhances GHRH mRNA in the hypothalamus.[135] Microinjection of GHRH into the basal forebrain enhances NREM sleep.[136] In contrast, microinjection of a GHRH antagonist inhibits NREM sleep.[137] IL-1 induces growth hormone release; this action is mediated via hypothalamic GHRH.[138] If animals are pretreated with anti-GHRH antibodies and then given IL-1β, IL-1β–induced growth hormone release and increased NREM sleep are blocked,[139] thereby suggesting that GHRH forms part of the IL-1 somnogenic pathway. The somnogenic actions of GHRH may also involve nitric oxide; GHRH-induced GH release involves nitric oxide.[140]

IL-1β and TNF-α also interact with a variety of neurotransmitter systems; the list includes serotonin, acetylcholine, gamma-aminobutyric acid, histamine,

and dopamine (reviewed in references 11, 80, 81, 82). However, little is known about the specificity of these interactions for sleep although there are some promising investigations. For example, Imeri et al.[141] showed that depletion of brain serotonin blocks muramyl dipeptide–induced NREM sleep responses and attenuates IL-1–induced sleep responses. In another report, that group directly measured medial preoptic serotonin metabolism after IL-1 treatment and concluded that serotonergic activation could play a role in mediating the effects of IL-1 on sleep.[142]

In summary, sleep regulatory mechanisms and the immune system share regulatory molecules. The best characterized are IL-1 and TNF. These substances are involved in physiological NREM sleep regulation and are key players in the development of the acute phase response induced by infectious agents. During the initial response to infectious challenge, these proinflammatory cytokines are upregulated and thereby amplify physiological sleep mechanisms leading to the acute phase sleep response.

SLEEP MAY AID RECUPERATIVE PROCESSES

Although physicians have always prescribed bed rest to aid in recuperation from bouts of infectious diseases and other maladies, there is, as yet, no direct evidence that sleep per se aids in recuperation. Nevertheless, physicians will continue to prescribe bed rest; often this is just what the patient wishes to do. It seems likely that such advice is beneficial. The only evidence relevant to this issue that we are aware of is consistent with the notion that sleep aids in recuperation. After infectious challenge, animals that have robust NREM sleep responses have a higher probability of survival than animals that fail to exhibit NREM sleep responses.[143] Although this evidence is strictly correlative, it behooves those of us interested in sleep and sleep disorders to investigate this a little further. Perhaps our grandmothers' folk wisdom of the preventive and curative attributes of sleep is correct.

Acknowledgments

This work was suggested, in part, by grants from the National Institutes of Health, NS-25378, NS-27250, NS-31453, and HD 36520.

References

1. Von Economo C. Sleep as a problem of localization. J Nerv Ment Dis. 1930;71:249–259.
2. Norman SE, Chediak AD, Kiel M, et al. Sleep disturbances in HIV-infected homosexual men. AIDS. 1990;4:775–781.
3. Norman SE, Chediak AD, Freeman C, et al. Sleep disturbances in men with asymptomatic human immunodeficiency (HIV) infection. Sleep. 1992;15:150–155.
4. White JL, Darko DF, Brown SJ, et al. Early central nervous system response to HIF infection: sleep distortion and cognitive-motor decrements. AIDS. 1995;9:1043–1050.
5. Kubicki S, Henkes H, Terstegge K, et al. AIDS related sleep disturbances—a preliminary report. In: Kubicki ST, Henkes H, Bienzle U, et al, eds. HIV and the Nervous System. New York, NY: Fischer; 1988:97–105.
6. Gourmelon P, Biet D, Clarencon D, et al. Sleep alterations in experimental street rabies virus infection occur in the absence of major EEG abnormalities. Brain Res. 1991;554:159–165.
7. Gourmelon P, Biet D, Court L, et al. Electrophysiological and sleep alterations in experimental mouse rabies. Brain Res. 1986;398:128–140.
8. Guilleminault C, Mondini S. Mononucleosis and chronic daytime sleepiness: a long-term follow-up study. Arch Intern Med. 1986;146:1333–1335.
9. Hoffman HJ, Damus K, Hillman L, et al. Risk factors for SIDS: results of the National Institute of Child Health and Human Development SIDS cooperative epidemiological study. Ann N Y Acad Sci. 1988;533:13–30.
10. Komaroff AL. Chronic fatigue syndromes: Relationships to chronic viral infections. J Virol Methods. 1988;21:3–10.
11. Krueger JM, Majde JA. Microbial products and cytokines in sleep and fever regulation. Crit Rev Immunol. 1994;14:355–379.
12. Smith A. Sleep, colds, and performance. In: Broughton RJ, Ogilvie RD, eds. Sleep, Arousal and Performance. Boston, Mass: Birkhäuser; 1992:233–242.
13. Kimura-Takeuchi M, Majde JA, Toth LA, et al. Influenza virus–induced changes in rabbit sleep and acute phase responses. Am J Physiol. 1992;263:R1115–1121.
14. Fang J, Sanborn CK, Renegar KB, et al. Influenza viral infections enhance sleep in mice. Proc Soc Exp Biol Med. 1995;210:242–252.
15. Toth LA, Rehg JE, Webster RG. Strain differences in sleep and

16. Fang J, Tooley D, Gatewood C, et al. Differential effects of total and upper airway influenza viral infection on sleep in mice. Sleep. 1996;19:337–342.
17. Majde JA, Brown RK, Jones MW, et al. Detection of toxic viral-associated double-stranded RNA (dsRNA) in influenza-infected lung. Microb Pathog. 1991;10:105–115.
18. Majde JA, Guha-Thakurta N, Chen Z, et al. Spontaneous release of stable viral double-stranded RNA into the extracellular medium by influenza virus–infected MDCK epithelial cells: implications for the viral acute phase response. Arch Virol. 1998;143:2371–2380.
19. Krueger JM, Majde JA, Blatteis CM, et al. Polyriboinosinic:polyribocytidylic acid (poly I:C) enhances rabbit slow-wave sleep. Am J Physiol. 1988;255:R748–755.
20. Bredow S, Fang J, Guha-Thakurta N, et al. Synthesis of an influenza double-stranded RNA-oligomer that induces fever and sleep in rabbits. Sleep Res. 1995;24A:101.
21. Krueger JM, Dinarello CA, Shoham S, et al. Interferon alpha-2 enhances slow-wave sleep in rabbits. Int J Immunopharmacol. 1987;9:23–30.
22. Birmanns B, Saphier D, Abramsky O. Alpha-interferon modifies cortical EEG activity: dose-dependence and antagonism by naloxone. J Neurol Sci. 1990;100:22–26.
23. DeSarro GB, Masuda Y, Ascioti C, et al. Behavioral and ECoG spectrum changes induced by intracerebral infusion of interferons and interleukin-2 in rats are antagonized by naloxone. Neuropharmacology. 1990;29:167–179.
24. Reite M, Landenslager M, Jones J, et al. Interferon decreases REMS latency. Biol Psychiatry. 1987;22:104–107.
25. Kimura M, Majde JA, Toth LA, et al. Somnogenic effects of rabbit and human recombinant interferons in rabbits. Am J Physiol. 1994;267:R53–61.
26. Toth LA, Krueger JM. Alterations in sleep during Staphylococcus aureus infection in rabbits. Infect Immun. 1988;56:1785–1791.
27. Borbély AA, Tobler I. Endogenous sleep-promoting substances and sleep regulation. Physiol Rev. 1989;69:605–670.
28. Toth LA, Krueger JM. Effects of microbial challenge on sleep in rabbits. FASEB J. 1989;3:2062–2066.
29. Toth LA, Krueger JM. Somnogenic, pyrogenic and hematologic effects of experimental pasteurellosis in rabbits. Am J Physiol. 1990;258:R536–542.
30. Johannsen L, Toth LA, Rosenthal RS, et al. Somnogenic, pyrogenic and hematologic effects of bacterial peptidoglycan. Am J Physiol. 1990;259:R182–186.
31. Johannsen L, Wecke J, Obál F Jr, et al. Macrophages produce somnogenic and pyrogenic muramyl peptides during digestion of staphylococci. Am J Physiol. 1991;260:R126–133.
32. Vermeulon MW, Grey GR. Processing of Bacillus subtilis peptidoglycan by a mouse macrophage cell line. Infect Immun. 1984;46:476–483.
33. Smialowicz RJ, Schwab JH. Processing of streptococcal cell walls by rat macrophages and human monocytes in vitro. Infect Immun. 1977;17:591–598.
34. Masek K. Immunopharmacology of muramyl peptides. Fed Proc. 1986;45:2549–2551.
35. Inoué S, Honda K, Komoda Y, et al. Differential sleep-promoting effects of five sleep substances nocturnally infused in unrestrained rats. Proc Natl Acad Sci U S A. 1984;81:6240–6242.
36. Meltzer LT, Serpa, KA, Moos WH. Evaluation in rats of the somnogenic, pyrogenic and central nervous system depressant effects of muramyl dipeptide. Psychopharmacology. 1989;99:103–108.
37. Krueger JM, Walter J, Karnovsky ML, et al. Muramyl peptides. Variation of somnogenic activity with structure. J Exp Med. 1984;159:68–76.
38. Krueger JM, Pappenheimer JR, Karnovsky ML. Sleep-promoting effects of muramyl peptides. Proc Natl Acad Sci U S A. 1982;79:6102–6106.
39. Krueger JM, Karnovsky ML, Martin SA, et al. Peptidoglycans as promoters of slow-wave sleep, II: somnogenic and pyrogenic activities of some naturally occurring muramyl peptides: correlations with mass spectrometric structure determination. J Biol Chem. 1984;259:12659–12662.

40. Brown R, Price RJ, King MG, et al. Are antibiotic effects on sleep behavior in the rat due to modulation of gut bacteria? Physiol Behav. 1990;48:561–565.

41. Rhee YH, Kim HI. The correlation between sleeping-time and numerical range in intestinal normal flora in psychiatric insomnia patients. Bull Natl Sci Chungbuk Natl Univ. 1987;1:159–172.

42. Krueger JM, Kubillus S, Shoham S, et al. Enhancement of slow-wave sleep by endotoxin and lipid A. Am J Physiol. 1986;251:R591–597.

43. Cady AB, Kotani S, Shiba T, et al. Somnogenic activities of synthetic lipid A. Infect Immun. 1989;57:396–403.

44. Toth LA, Tolley EA, Broady R, et al. Sleep during experimental trypanosomiasis in rabbits. Proc Soc Exp Biol Med. 1994;205:174–181.

45. Toth LA, Opp MR, Mao L. Somnogenic effects of sleep deprivation and Escherichia coli inoculation in rabbits. J Sleep Res. 1995;4:30–40.

46. Bergmann BM, Rechtschaffen A, Gilliland MA, et al. Effect of extended sleep deprivation on tumor growth in rats. Am J Physiol. 1996;271:R1460–1464.

47. Brown R, Pang G, Husband AJ, et al. Suppression of immunity to influenza virus infection in the respiratory tract following sleep disturbance. Reg Immunol. 1989;2:321–325.

48. Renegar KB, Floyd RA, Krueger JM. Effects of short-term sleep deprivation on murine immunity to influenza virus in young adult and senescent mice. Sleep. 1998;21:241–248.

49. Everson CA. Sustained sleep deprivation impairs host defense. Am J Physiol. 1993;265:R1148–1154.

50. Gilliland MA, Feng PF, Shaw P, et al. Bacterial growth during short-term sleep deprivation in rats. Sleep Res. 1994;23:413.

51. Everson CA, Toth LA. Abnormal control of viable bacteria in body tissues during sleep deprivation in rats. Sleep Res. 1997;26:613.

52. Landis C, Pollack S, Helton WS. Microbial translocation and NK cell cytotoxicity in female rats sleep deprived on small platforms. Sleep Res. 1997;26:619.

53. Deitch EA. Bacterial translocation: the influence of dietary variables. Gut. 1994;35:S23–27.

54. Pabst MJ, Beranova-Giorgianni S, Krueger JM. Effects of muramyl peptides on macrophages, monokines, and sleep. Neuroimmunomodulation. 1999;6:261–283.

55. Palmblad J, Cantell K, Strander H, et al. Stressor exposure and immunological response in man: interferon producing capacity and phagocytosis. Psychosom Res. 1976;20:193–199.

56. Yamasu K, Shimada Y, Sakaizumi M, et al. Activation of the systemic production of tumor necrosis factor after exposure to acute stress. Eur Cytokine Net. 1992;3:391–398.

57. Uthgenannt D, Schoolmann D, Pietrowsky R, et al. Effects of sleep on the production of cytokines in humans. Psychosom Med. 1995;57:97–104.

58. Hohagen F, Timmer J, Weyerbrock A, et al. Cytokine production during sleep and wakefulness and its relationship to cortisol in healthy humans. Neuropsychobiology. 1993;28:9–16.

59. Moldofsky H, Lue FA, Davidson JR, et al. Effects of sleep deprivation on human immune functions. FASEB J. 1989;3:1972–1977.

60. Opp MR, Krueger JM. Anti-interleukin-1β reduces sleep and sleep rebound after sleep deprivation in rats. Am J Physiol. 1994;266:R688–695.

61. Moldofsky H, Lue FA, Eisen J, et al. The relationship of interleukin-1 and immune functions to sleep in humans. Psychosom Med. 1986;48:309–318.

62. Darko DF, Miller JC, Gallen C, et al. Sleep electroencephalogram delta frequency amplitude, night plasma levels of tumor necrosis factor α and human immunodeficiency virus infection. Proc Natl Acad Sci U S A. 1995;92:12080–12086.

63. Gudewill S, Pollmacher T, Vedder H, et al. Nocturnal plasma levels of cytokines in healthy men. Eur Arch Psychiatry Clin Neurosci. 1992;242:53–56.

64. Covelli V, D'Andrea L, Savastano S, et al. Interleukin-1 beta plasma secretion during diurnal spontaneous and induced sleeping in healthy volunteers. Acta Neurol (Napoli). 1994;16:79–86.

65. Entzian P, Linnemann K, Schlaak M, et al. Obstructive sleep apnea syndrome and circadian rhythms of hormones and cytokines. Am J Respir Crit Care Med. 1996;153:1080–1086.

66. Vgontzas AN, Papanicolaou DA, Bixler EO, et al. Elevation of plasma cytokines in disorders of excessive daytime sleepiness: role of sleep disturbance and obesity. J Clin Endocrinol Metab. 1997;82:1313–1316.

67. Appelberg B, Katila H, Rimon R. Plasma interleukin-1 beta and sleep architecture in schizophrenia and other nonaffective psychoses. Psychom Med. 1997;59:529–532.

68. Casey FB, Eisenberg J, Peterson D, et al. Altered antigen uptake and distribution due to exposure to extreme environmental temperatures or sleep deprivation. Reticuloendothelial Soc J. 1974;15:87–90.

69. Palmblad J, Petrini B, Wasserman J, et al. Lymphocyte and granulocyte reactions during sleep deprivation. Psychosom Med. 1979;41:273–278.

70. Isenberg DA, Crisp AJ, Morrow WJ, et al. Variation in circulating immune complex levels with diet, exercise, and sleep: a comparison between normal controls and patients with systemic lupus erythematosus. Ann Rheum Dis. 1981;40:466–469.

71. Renegar KB, Floyd R, Krueger JM. Effect of sleep deprivation on serum influenza-specific IgG. Sleep. 1998;21:19–24.

72. Benca RM, Kushida CA, Everson CA, et al. Sleep deprivation in the rat, VII: immune function. Sleep. 1989;12:47–52.

73. Dinges DF, Douglas SD, Zaugg L, et al. Leukocytosis and natural killer cell function parallel neurobehavioral fatigue induced by 64 hours of sleep deprivation. J Clin Invest. 1994;93:1930–1939.

74. Born J, Lange T, Hansen K, et al. Effects of sleep and circadian rhythm on human circulating immune cells. J Immunol. 1997;158:4454–4464.

75. Brown R, Price RJ, King MG, et al. Interleukin-1β and muramyl dipeptide can prevent decreased antibody response associated with sleep deprivation. Brain Behav Immun. 1989;3:320–330.

76. Irwin M, McClintick J, Costlow C, et al. Partial night sleep deprivation reduces natural killer and cellular immune responses in humans. FASEB J. 1996; 10:643–653.

77. Irwin M, Mascovich A, Gillin JC, et al. Partial sleep deprivation reduces natural killer cell activity in humans. Psychosom Med. 1994;56:493–498.

78. Moldofsky H, Lue FA, Davidson J, et al. Comparison of sleep-wake circadian immune functions in women vs men. Sleep Res. 1989;18:431.

79. Irwin M, Smith TL, Gillin JC. Electroencephalographic sleep and natural killer activity in depressed patients and control subject. Pschosom Med. 1992;54:10–21.

80. Plata-Salaman CR. Immunoregulators in the nervous system. Neurosci Biobehav Rev. 1991;15:185–215.

81. Krueger JM, Fang J. Cytokines in sleep regulation. In: Hayaishi O, Inoue S, eds. Sleep and Sleep Disorders: From Molecule to Behavior. San Deigo, Calif: Academic Press; 1997:261–277.

82. Krueger JM, Fang J, Taishi P, et al. Sleep: a physiological role for IL-1 beta and TFN-alpha. Ann N Y Acad Sci. 1998;856:148–159.

83. Taishi P, Bredow S, Guha-Thakurta N, et al. Diurnal variations of interleukin-1β mRNA and β-actin mRNA in rat brain. J Neuroimmunol. 1997;75:69–74.

84. Bredow S, Taishi P, Guha-Thakurta N, et al. Diurnal variations of tumor necrosis factor-α mRNA and α-tubulin mRNA in rat brain. J Neuroimmunomodulation. 1997;4:84–90.

85. Floyd RA, Krueger JM. Diurnal variations of TNFα in the rat brain. Neuroreport. 1997;8:915–918.

86. Lue FA, Bail M, Jephthah-Ochola J, et al. Sleep and cerebrospinal fluid interleukin-1-like activity in the cat. Int J Neurosci. 1988;42:179–183.

87. Krueger JM, Walter J, Dinarello CA, et al. Sleep-promoting effects of endogenous pyrogen (interleukin 1). Am J Physiol. 1984;246:R994–999.

88. Tobler I, Borbély AA, Schwyzer M, et al. Interleukin-1 derived from astrocytes enhances slow-wave activity in sleep EEG of the rat. Eur J Pharmacol. 1984;104:191–192.

89. Susic V, Totic S. "Recovery" function of sleep: effects of purified human interleukin-1 on the sleep and febrile response of cats. Metab Brain Dis. 1989;4:73–80.

90. Friedman EM, Boinski S, Coe CL. Interleukin-1 induces sleep-like behavior and alters sleep structure in juvenile rhesus macaques. Am J Primatol. 1995;35:145–152.

91. Opp MR, Obál F Jr, Krueger JM. Interleukin 1 alters rat sleep:

temporal and dose-related effects. Am J Physiol. 1991;260:R52–58.

92. Lancel M, Mathias S, Faulhaber J, et al. Effect of interleukin-1 beta on EEG power density during sleep depends on circadian phase. Am J Physiol. 1996;270:R830–835.

93. Hansen MK, Krueger JM. Subdiaphragmatic vagotomy blocks the sleep and fever-promoting effects of interleukin-1β. Am J Physiol. 1997;42:R1246–1253.

94. Fang J, Wang Y, Krueger JM. Mice lacking the TNF 55-kD receptor fail to sleep more after TNFα treatment. J Neurosci. 1997;17:5949–5955.

95. Shoham S, Davenne D, Cady AB, et al. Recombinant tumor necrosis factor and interleukin-1 enhance slow-wave sleep. Am J Physiol. 1987;253:R142–149.

96. Kapás L, Hong L, Cady AB, et al. Somnogenic, pyrogenic, and anorectic activities of tumor necrosis factor α (TNFα), and TNFα fragments. Am J Physiol. 1992;263:R708–715.

97. Opp MR, Krueger JM. Interleukin-1 antibodies reduce NREMS and attenuate NREMS rebound after sleep deprivation in the rabbit. Sleep Res. 1992;21:323.

98. Takahashi S, Tooley D, Kapás J, et al. Inhibition of tumor necrosis factor suppresses sleep in rabbits. Pflugers Arch. 1995; 431:155–160.

99. Takahashi S, Kapás L, Seyer JM, et al. Inhibition of tumor necrosis factor attenuates physiological sleep in rabbits. Neuroreport. 1996;7:642–646.

100. Opp MR, Obál F Jr, Krueger JM. Effects of α-MSH on sleep, behavior, and brain temperature: Interactions with IL1. Am J Physiol. 1988;255:R914–922.

101. Opp M, Obál F Jr, Krueger JM. Corticotropin-releasing factor attenuates interleukin 1-induced sleep and fever in rabbits. Am J Physiol. 1989;257:R528–535.

102. Krueger JM, Kapás L, Opp MR, et al. Prostaglandins E₂ and D₂ have little effect on rabbit sleep. Physiol Behav. 1992;51:481–485.

103. Kushikata T, Fang J, Wang Y, et al. Interleukin-4 attenuates spontaneous sleep in rabbits. Soc Neurosci Abst. 1997;23:792.

104. Opp MR, Smith EM, Hughes TK Jr. Interleukin-10 (cytokine synthesis inhibitory factor) acts in the central nervous system of rats to reduce sleep. J Neuroimmunol. 1995;60:165–168.

105. Fang J, Wang Y, Krueger JM. The effects of interleukin-1β on sleep are mediated by the type I receptor. Am J Physiol. 1998;274:R655–660.

106. Mackiewicz M, Sollars PJ, Ogilvie MD, et al. Modulation of IL-1β gene expression in the rat CNS during sleep deprivation. Neuroreport. 1996;7:529–533.

107. Taishi P, Chen Z, Obál F Jr, et al. Sleep-associated changes in interleukin-1beta mRNA in the brain. J Interferon Cytokine Res. 1998;18:793–798.

108. Takahashi S, Fang J, Kapás L, et al. Inhibition of brain interleukin-1 attenuates sleep rebound after sleep deprivation in rabbits. Am J Physiol. 1997;42:R677–682.

109. Takahashi S, Krueger JM. Inhibition of tumor necrosis factor prevents warming-induced sleep responses in rabbits. Am J Physiol. 1997;41:R1325–1329.

110. Kushikata T, Takahashi S, Wang Y, et al. An interleukin-1 receptor fragment blocks ambient temperature–induced increases in brain temperature but not sleep in rabbits. Neurosci Lett. 1998;244:125–128.

111. Hansen M, Kapás L, Fang J, et al. Cafeteria diet–induced sleep is blocked by subdiaphragmatic vagotomy in rats. Am J Physiol. 1998;274:R168–174.

112. Hansen MK, Taishi P, Chen Z, et al. Cafeteria-feeding induces interleukin-1β mRNA expression in rat liver and brain. Am J Physiol. 1998;274:R1734–1739.

113. Hansen MK, Taishi P, Chen Z, et al. Vagotomy blocks the induction of interleukin-1β mRNA in the brain of rats in response to systemic interleukin-1β. J Neurosci. 1998;18:2247–2253.

114. Goehler LE, Relton JK, Dripps D, et al. Vagal paraganglia bind biotinylated interleukin-1 receptor antagonist: a possible mechanism for immune-to-brain communication. Brain Res Bull. 1997;43:357–364.

115. Niijima A. The afferent discharges from sensors for interleukin-1β in the hepatoportal system in the anesthetized rat. J Auton Nerv Syst. 1996;61:287–291.

116. Jacob AI, Goldberg PK, Bloom N, et al. Endotoxin and bacteria in portal blood. Gastroenterology. 1977;72:1268–1270.

117. Takahashi S, Kapás L, Fang J, et al. An interleukin-1 receptor fragment inhibits spontaneous sleep and muramyl dipeptide-induced sleep in rabbits. Am J Physiol. 1996;271:R101–108.

118. Takahashi S, Kapás L, Krueger JM. A tumor necrosis factor (TNF) receptor fragment attenuates TNF-α and muramyl dipeptide–induced sleep and fever in rabbits. J Sleep Res. 1996;5:106–114.

119. Chen Z, Fang J, Gardi J, et al. Sleep-deprivation induces activation of nuclear factor-κB. Soc Neurosci Abst. 1997;23:792.

120. Kapás L, Fang J, Krueger JM. Inhibition of nitric oxide synthesis inhibits rat sleep. Brain Res. 1994;664:189–196.

121. Kapás L, Shibata M, Kimura M, et al. Inhibition of nitric oxide synthesis suppresses sleep in rabbits. Am J Physiol. 1994;266:R151–157.

122. Kapás L, Krueger JM. Nitric oxide donors SIN-1 and SNAP promote non-rapid eye movement sleep in rats. Brain Res Bull. 1996;41:293–298.

123. Datta S, Patterson EH, Siwek DF. Endogenous and exogenous nitric oxide in the pedunculopontine tegmentum induces sleep. Synapse. 1997;27:69–78.

124. Houston JP, Haas HL, Boix F, et al. Extracellular adenosine levels in neostriatum and hippocampus during rest and activity periods of rats. Neuroscience. 1996;73:99–107.

125. Seo HG, Fujii J, Asahi M, et al. Roles of purine nucleotides and adenosine in enhancing NOS II gene expression in interleukin-1 beta–stimulated rat vascular smooth muscle cells. Free Radic Res. 1997;26:409–413.

126. Janigro D, Wender R. Ransom G, et al. Adenosine-induced release of nitric oxide from cortical astrocytes. Neuroreport. 1996;7:1640–1643.

127. Krueger JM, Obál F Jr. Sleep factors In: Saunders NA, Sullivan CE, eds. Sleep and Breathing. New York, NY: Marcel Dekker, Inc; 1994:79–112.

128. Obál F Jr, Opp M, Cady AB, et al. Growth hormone-releasing factor enhances sleep in rats and rabbits. Am J Physiol. 1988;255:R310–316.

129. Steiger A, Guldner J, Hemmeter U, Rothe B, Wiedemann K, Hosboer F. Effects of growth hormone–releasing hormone and somatostatin on sleep EEG and nocturnal hormone secretion in male controls. Neuroendocrinology. 1992;56:566–573.

130. Kerkhofs M, van Cauter E, van Onderberghen A, et al. Growth hormone releasing hormone (GHRH) has sleep promoting effects in man. Am J Physiol. 1993;264:E594–598.

131. Nistico G, DeSarro GB, Bagetta G, et al. Behavioral and electrocortical spectrum power effects of growth hormone releasing factor in rats. Neuropharmacology. 1987;26:75–78.

132. Obál F Jr, Payne L, Kapás L, et al. Inhibition of growth hormone–releasing factor suppresses both sleep and growth hormone secretion in the rat. Brain Res. 1991;557:149–153.

133. Obál F Jr, Payne L, Opp MR, et al. Antibodies to growth hormone–releasing hormone suppress sleep and prevent enhancement of sleep after sleep deprivation. Am J Physiol. 1993;263:R1078–1085.

134. Bredow SP, Taishi P, Obál F Jr, et al. Hypothalamic growth hormone–releasing hormone (GHRH) mRNA varies across the day in rats. Neuroreport. 1996;7:2501–2505.

135. Toppila J, Alanko L, Asikainen M, et al. Sleep deprivation increases somatostatin and growth hormone–releasing hormone messenger RNA in the rat hypothalamus. J Sleep Res. 1997;6:171–178.

136. Zhang J, Obál F Jr, Fang J, et al. Non-rapid eye movement sleep (NREMS) was enhanced by microinjection of growth hormone releasing hormone (GHRH) into the preoptic area in rats. Soc Neurosci Abst. 1997;23:1067.

137. Zhang J, Obál F Jr, Zheng T, et al. Intrapreoptic microinjection of GHRH or its antagonist alters sleep in rats. J Neurosci. 1999;19:2187–2194.

138. Payne LC, Obál F Jr, Opp MR, et al. Stimulation and inhibition of growth hormone secretion by interleukin-1β: the involvement of growth hormone-releasing hormone. Neuroendocrinology. 1992;56:118–123.

139. Obál F Jr, Fang J, Payne LC, et al. Growth hormone releasing hormone (GHRH) mediates the sleep promoting activity of interleukin-1 (IL1) in rats. Neuroendocrinology. 1995;61:559–565.

140. Tene-Sempere M, Pinilla C, Gonzalez D, et al. Involvement of

endogenous nitric oxide in the control of pituitary responsiveness to different elicitors of growth hormone release in
prepubertal rats. Neuroendocrinology. 1996;64:146–152.

141. Imeri L, Bianchi S, Mancia M. Muramyl dipeptide and IL1
effects on sleep and brain temperature following inhibition of
serotonin synthesis. Am J Physiol. 1997;273:R1663–1668.

142. Gemma C, Imeri L, Grazia De Simoni M, et al. Interleukin-1
induces changes in sleep, brain temperature, and serotonergic
metabolism. Am J Physiol. 1997;272:R601–606.

143. Toth LA, Tolley EA, Krueger JM. Sleep as a prognostic indicator
during infectious disease in rabbits. Proc Soc Exp Biol Med.
1993;203:179–192.

20

Endocrine Physiology

Eve Van Cauter

Sleep exerts important modulatory effects on most components of the endocrine system. The secretion of growth hormone (GH) and prolactin (PRL) is markedly increased during sleep, whereas the release of cortisol and thyrotropin (TSH) is inhibited. Conversely, awakenings interrupting sleep inhibit nocturnal GH and PRL secretions and are associated with increased cortisol and TSH concentrations. Modulatory effects of sleep on endocrine release are not limited to the hormones of the hypothalamic-pituitary axes; these effects are also observed for the hormones controlling water and electrolyte balance and carbohydrate metabolism. Sleep loss and decreased sleep quality are associated with disturbances of hormonal secretion and metabolism, which may be of clinical relevance. Findings suggest that part of the constellation of hormonal and metabolic alterations that characterize normal aging may reflect the deterioration of sleep quality. There is good evidence that obstructive sleep apnea contributes to or exacerbates the metabolic syndrome that is highly prevalent in this condition. Strategies to reverse decrements in sleep quality may have beneficial effects on endocrine and metabolic function.

MODULATION OF ENDOCRINE FUNCTION BY SLEEP-WAKE HOMEOSTASIS AND CIRCADIAN RHYTHMICITY

In normal adults, reproducible changes of essentially all hormonal and metabolic variables occur during sleep and around wake-sleep and sleep-wake transitions. These daily events reflect the interaction of circadian rhythmicity and sleep-wake homeostasis (see Chapters 28 and 29). Thus, the dual control of sleep timing and quality by circadian processes (i.e., process C) and sleep-wake homeostasis (i.e., process S) is readily reflected in the modulatory effects exerted by sleep on endocrine and metabolic function. The relative contributions of circadian timing compared with homeostatic control in the regulation of the temporal organization of hormonal release vary from one endocrine axis to another. Similarly, modulatory effects of the transitions between wake and sleep (and vice versa) and between nonrapid eye movement (NREM) and rapid eye movement (REM) stages also vary from one hormone to the other.

The impact of sleep on endocrine function and metabolism has been studied extensively in the human being, probably because methods of measurement, including repeated blood sampling at frequent time intervals, sensitive assays of blood constituents, and polysomnographic (PSG) sleep recordings, are more readily available for people than for laboratory animals. Human sleep is normally consolidated in a single 6- to 9-h period, whereas other mammals generally sleep in several fragmented periods. The detection of hormonal changes during sleep is thus hindered by the short duration of the sleep cycle in laboratory species. Possibly because of the consolidation of the sleep period, the wake-sleep and sleep-wake transitions in the human being are associated with hormonal and metabolic changes that are more marked than those in other mammals.

To differentiate between effects of circadian rhythmicity and those subserving sleep-wake homeostasis, experimental strategies taking advantage of the fact that the circadian pacemaker takes several days to adjust to a large sudden shift of sleep-wake and light-dark cycles (as occur in jet lag and shift work) have been used. Such strategies allow for the effects of circadian modulation to be observed in the absence of sleep and for the effects of sleep to be observed at an abnormal circadian time. Figure 20–1 illustrates mean profiles of plasma growth hormone (GH), plasma cortisol, plasma prolactin (PRL), and plasma thyrotropin (TSH) observed in normal subjects who were studied before and during an abrupt 12-h delay of the sleep-wake and dark-light cycles. To eliminate the effects of feeding, fasting, and postural changes, the subjects remain recumbent throughout the study, and the normal meal schedule was replaced by intravenous glucose infusion at a constant rate.[1] As shown in Figure 20–1, this drastic manipulation of sleep had only modest effects on the wave shape of the cortisol profile, in sharp contrast with the immediate shift of the GH and PRL rhythms that followed the shift of the sleep-wake cycle. The temporal organization of TSH secretion appears equally influenced by circadian and sleep-dependent processes. Indeed, the evening elevation of TSH levels occurs well before sleep onset and has been shown to reflect circadian phase. During sleep, an inhibitory process prevents TSH concentrations from further rising. Consequently, in the absence of sleep, the nocturnal TSH elevation is markedly amplified as shown in the lower panel of Figure 20–1.[2]

This chapter describes the interactions between

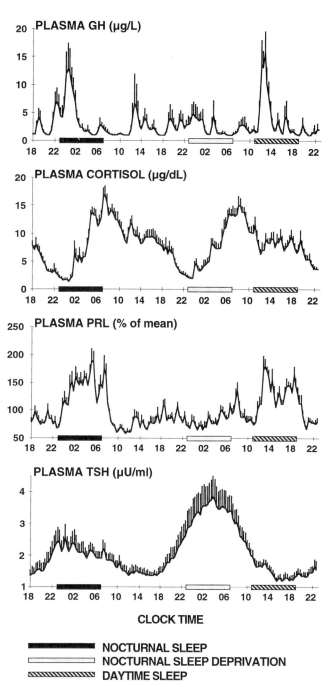

Figure 20–1. *From top to bottom*: mean 24-h profiles of plasma growth hormone (GH), cortisol, prolactin (PRL), and thyrotropin (TSH) in a group of eight normal young men (20 to 27 y) studied during a 53-h period including 8 h of nocturnal sleep, 28 h of sleep deprivation, and 8 h of daytime sleep. The vertical bars at each time point represent the standard error of the mean (SEM). The black bars represent the sleep periods. The open bar represents the period of nocturnal sleep deprivation. The dashed bar represents the period of daytime sleep. Shifted sleep was associated with an immediate shift of GH and PRL release. In contrast, the secretory profiles of cortisol and TSH remained synchronized to circadian time. (Adapted from Van Cauter E, Spiegel K. Circadian and sleep control of endocrine secretions. In: Turek FW, Zee PC, eds. Neurobiology of Sleep and Circadian Rhythms. New York, NY: Marcel Dekker; 1999.)

sleep and endocrine release in the hypothalamic-pituitary axes, hormonal control of body fluid balance and glucose regulation, and the relationships between alterations of sleep in normal aging and obstructive sleep apnea (OSA) and disturbances of endocrine and metabolic function.

INTERACTIONS BETWEEN SLEEP AND THE GROWTH HORMONE AXIS

Pituitary release of GH is stimulated by hypothalamic GH-releasing hormone (GHRH) and inhibited by somatostatin. Both mechanisms are involved in the control of GH secretion during sleep. Although sleep clearly involves major stimulatory effects on GH secretion, as described later, the hormones of the somatotropic axis appear, in turn, involved in sleep regulation.

In normal adult subjects, the 24-h profile of plasma GH levels consists of stable low levels abruptly interrupted by bursts of secretion. Already in the late 1960s it was recognized that the most reproducible GH pulse occurs shortly after sleep onset.[3–9] In men, the sleep-onset GH pulse is generally the largest, and often the only, secretory pulse observed over the 24-h span. In women, daytime GH pulses are more frequent, and the sleep-associated pulse, although still present in the vast majority of individual profiles, does not account for the majority of the 24-h secretory output.

Sleep onset elicits a pulse in GH secretion whether sleep is advanced, delayed, or interrupted and reinitiated. The mean GH profile shown in Figure 20–1 illustrates the maintenance of this relationship in subjects who underwent a 12-h delay shift of the sleep-wake cycle. A pulse of GH secretion following sleep onset has been observed in subjects submitted to a variety of manipulations of the sleep-wake cycle in the laboratory (reviewed in reference 10). In real life conditions, a study of night workers indicated that the main GH secretory episode still occurred during the first half of the sleep period.[11]

Although the beginning of the sleep period clearly involves a major physiological stimulus for human GH secretion, there is also evidence for the existence of a circadian modulation. The late evening and the early part of the night appear to represent a period of increased propensity for GH secretion, even in the absence of sleep.[11–15] A study using repeated injections of GHRH at 3-h intervals clearly demonstrated a diurnal variation in peak GH response, reflecting a diurnal rhythm in somatostatinergic tone.[16] Because elevated GH responses were already apparent in the early evening, well before sleep onset, this diurnal variation is likely to be controlled by circadian rhythmicity.

Well documented studies published in the late 1960s concurred in indicating that there is a consistent relationship between the appearance of delta waves in the EEG and elevated GH concentrations.[5–7, 17] These findings were confirmed and extended in later reports that examined GH secretory rates, rather than plasma

GH levels.[13, 18] Using this approach, a study with 30-sec sampling of plasma GH during sleep indicated that maximal GH release occurs within minutes of the onset of slow wave sleep (SWS).[18] Furthermore, in studies examining GH secretion in normal young men of similar height and weight, it was found that approximately 70% of GH pulses during sleep occurred during SWS and that there was a quantitative correlation between the amount of GH secreted during these pulses and the duration of the SW episode.[13]

Additional evidence for the existence of a robust relationship between SW activity and increased GH release has been obtained in studies using pharmacological stimulation of SWS.[19, 20] Reliable stimulation of SWS in normal subjects has been obtained with oral administration of low doses of gamma hydroxybutyrate (GHB), a metabolite of gamma-aminobutyric acid (GABA) that is used as an investigational drug for the treatment of narcolepsy, as well as with ritanserin, a selective 5-hydroxytryptamine (5-HT2) receptor antagonist. Figure 20–2 depicts the profiles of delta power and GH secretory rates in a subject who received either placebo *(left panels)* or 3 g GHB *(right panels)*. The stimulation of delta power induced by GHB is associated with a marked increase in GH secretion. Across all subjects and all studies, there was an excellent correlation between increases in the amount of stage 4 sleep following GHB administration and corresponding increases in GH secretion during the same period.[20] In an independent study, administration of ritanserin was also found to result in parallel and highly correlated small amplitude increases of delta wave activity and nocturnal GH release.[19]

PLACEBO   3 g GHB

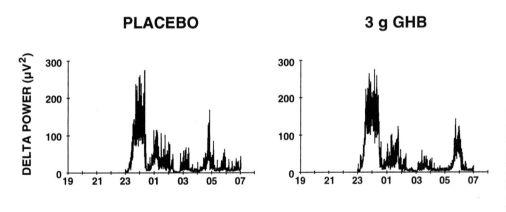

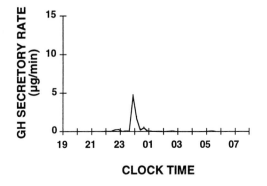

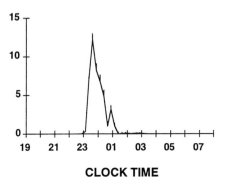

Figure 20–2. Individual profiles of delta power (spectral power in the 0.5 to 3.5 Hz band, *top panels*) and growth hormone (GH) secretory rates from a normal young man sampled at 15-mm intervals after ingestion of either placebo or a 3 g dose of gamma-hydroxybutyrate (GHB) at bedtime. Note the increase in delta power and the concomitant increase in GH secretion under GHB treatment. (Data from Van Cauter E, Plat L, Scharf M, et al. Simultaneous stimulation of slow-wave sleep and growth hormone secretion by gamma-hydroxybutyrate in normal young men. J Clin Invest. 1997; 100:745–753.)

Nevertheless, the relationship between SW activity and GH secretion is not one-to-one. Nocturnal GH secretion can occur in the absence of SWS,[21] and approximately one third of the SW periods are not associated with detectable GH secretion. Selective partial SW stage deprivation does not necessarily suppress or delay the sleep-onset GH pulse.[22] Marked rises in GH secretion before the onset of sleep have been reported by several investigators.[21, 23, 24] Because GH secretion is also under inhibitory control by somatostatin, variability of somatostatinergic tone may cause a dissociation between SWS and nocturnal GH release. The short-term negative feedback inhibition exerted by GH on its own secretion may also explain observations of an absent GH pulse during the first SW period, when a secretory pulse occurred before sleep onset. Such pre-sleep GH pulses are likely to reflect a circadian rhythm in propensity to secrete GH, independent of the occurrence of sleep.[16]

Although robust stimulatory mechanisms clearly activate GH secretion during NREM sleep, awakenings interrupting sleep have an inhibitory effect. In a study in which GH secretion was stimulated by the injection of GHRH at the beginning of the sleep period, it was found that whenever sleep was interrupted by a spontaneous awakening, the ongoing GH secretion was abruptly suppressed.[25] This inhibitory effect of awakenings on the GH response to GHRH was further demonstrated in a study in which sleeping subjects who had received a GHRH injection were awakened 30 min after the injection and then allowed to reinitiate sleep 30 min later.[26] A marked inhibition of the GH response was observed shortly after the awakening. These findings indicate that sleep fragmentation generally decreases nocturnal GH secretion. The inhibitory effect of nocturnal awakenings on GH secretion could be mediated by an increase in somatostatin release

INTERACTIONS BETWEEN SLEEP AND THE CORTICOTROPIC AXIS

Activity of the corticotropic axis—a neuroendocrine system associated with behavioral activation—may be measured peripherally via plasma levels of the pituitary hormone adenocorticotropin (ACTH) and of the adrenal hormone directly controlled by ACTH stimulation, cortisol. The plasma levels of these hormones decline from an early morning maximum throughout the daytime and are near the lower limit of most assays in the late evening and early part of the sleep period. Thus, sleep is normally initiated when corticotropic activity is quiescent. Reactivation of ACTH and cortisol secretion occurs abruptly a few hours before the usual waking time. The mean cortisol profile shown in Figure 20–1 illustrate the remarkable persistence of this diurnal variation when sleep is manipulated. Indeed, the overall waveshape of the profile is not markedly affected by the absence of sleep or the presence of sleep at an abnormal time of day. Studies using similar experimental designs have therefore indicated that the 24-h periodicity of corticotropic activity is primarily controlled by circadian rhythmicity. Nevertheless, modulatory effects of the sleep or wake condition have been clearly demonstrated. Indeed, a number of studies have indicated that sleep onset is reliably associated with a short-term inhibition of cortisol secretion,[1, 22, 27, 28] although this effect may not be detectable when sleep is initiated at the time of the daily maximum of corticotropic activity, that is, in the morning.[29] Under normal conditions, because cortisol secretion is already quiescent in the late evening, this inhibitory effect of sleep (which appears to be related to SW stages[30–32]) results in a prolongation of the quiescent period. Therefore, under conditions of sleep deprivation, the nadir of cortisol secretion is less pronounced and occurs earlier than under normal conditions of nocturnal sleep. Conversely, awakening at the end of the sleep period is consistently followed by a pulse of cortisol secretion.[1, 33, 34] During sleep deprivation, these rapid effects of sleep onset and sleep offset on corticotropic activity are obviously absent, and, as may be seen in the profiles shown in Figure 20–1, the nadir of cortisol levels is higher than during nocturnal sleep (because of the absence of the inhibitory effects of the first hours of sleep), and the morning acrophase is lower (because of the absence of the stimulating effects of morning awakening). Overall, the amplitude of the rhythm is reduced by approximately 15% during sleep deprivation as compared to normal conditions.

Several studies have shown that awakenings interrupting the sleep period consistently trigger pulses of cortisol secretion.[30, 33, 35] In an analysis of cortisol profiles during daytime sleep, it was observed that 92% of awakenings interrupting sleep coincided with or were followed within 20 min by a significant cortisol pulse.[35] A study involving continuous experimentally induced arousals during sleep suggested that feedback inhibition of corticotropic activity is less effective during sleep than during wake.[33] Sleep fragmentation, as occurs in aging,[36] is thus associated with alterations of nocturnal corticotropic activity.

In addition to the immediate modulatory effects of sleep-wake transitions on cortisol levels, even partial nocturnal sleep deprivation appears to affect corticotropic activity on the following evening.[37] Figure 20–3 summarizes the results from a study involving two groups of normal young men studied before, during, and after a night of normal sleep or of total sleep deprivation. In the groups who were sleep deprived, in contrast to the group who had a normal sleep period, evening cortisol levels were significantly higher on the day following sleep deprivation than on the previous day at the same time. Sleep loss thus appears to delay the normal return to evening quiescence of the corticotropic axis. This endocrine alteration is remarkably similar to that occurring in normal aging, where increases in evening cortisol levels of similar magnitude are consistently observed.

THE THYROID AXIS DURING SLEEP AND SLEEP DEPRIVATION

Daytime levels of plasma TSH are low and relatively stable and are followed by a rapid elevation starting

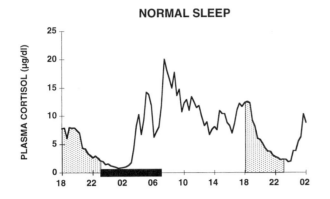

NORMAL SLEEP

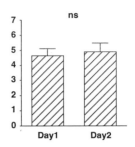

Mean Evening Cortisol Level (µg/dl)

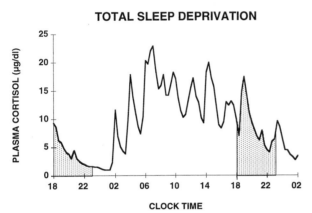

TOTAL SLEEP DEPRIVATION

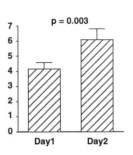

CLOCK TIME

Figure 20–3. Mean profiles of plasma cortisol from two groups of normal young subjects studied during a 32-h period with normal sleep (bedtimes: 23:00 to 07:00, *top*) or total sleep deprivation (*bottom*). The black bar represents the sleep period. The shaded areas highlight cortisol levels during the time interval 18:00 to 23:00 on day 1 and on day 2. Mean cortisol levels for the same time period before and after normal sleep (*top*) and before and after total sleep deprivation (*bottom*) are shown for the two groups on the right panels. One night of sleep loss thus results in increased cortisol levels on the following evening. (Data from Leproult R, Copinschi G, Boxton O, et al. Sleep loss results in an elevation of cortisol levels the next evening. Sleep. 1997;20:865–870.)

in the early evening and culminating in a nocturnal maximum occurring around the beginning of the sleep period.[38, 39] The later part of sleep is associated with a progressive decline in TSH levels, and daytime values resume shortly after morning awakening. The first 24 h of the study illustrated in the lower panel of Figure 20–1 are typical of the diurnal TSH rhythm. Because the nocturnal rise of TSH occurs well before the time of sleep onset, it is believed to reflect a circadian effect. However, a marked effect of sleep on TSH secretion may be evidenced during sleep deprivation (clearly seen in the lower panel of Figure 20–1), when nocturnal TSH secretion is increased by as much as 200% over the levels observed during nocturnal sleep. Thus, sleep exerts an inhibitory influence on TSH secretions, and sleep deprivation relieves this inhibition.[39, 40] Interestingly, when sleep occurs during daytime hours, TSH secretion is not suppressed significantly below normal daytime levels. Thus, the inhibitory effect of sleep on TSH secretion appears to be operative when the nighttime elevation has taken place, indicating once again the interaction of the effects of circadian time and the effects of sleep. When the depth of sleep at the habitual time is increased by prior sleep deprivation, the noctur-

nal TSH rise is more markedly inhibited, suggesting that SWS is probably the primary determinant of the sleep-associated fall.[39] Indeed, analyses of concomitant TSH profiles and sleep parameters has revealed a consistent association between descending slopes of TSH concentrations and SW stages and the existence of a negative cross-correlation between TSH fluctuations and relative spectral power in the delta range.[41, 42] Awakenings interrupting nocturnal sleep appear to relieve the inhibition of TSH and are consistently associated with a short-term TSH elevation.

Circadian and sleep-related variations in thyroid hormones have been difficult to demonstrate, probably because these hormones are bound to serum proteins and thus their peripheral concentrations are affected by diurnal variations in hemodilution caused by postural changes. However, under conditions of sleep deprivation, the increased amplitude of the TSH rhythm may result in a detectable increase in plasma triiodothyronine (T_3) levels, paralleling the nocturnal TSH rise.[43] If sleep deprivation is prolonged for a 2nd night, the nocturnal rise of TSH is markedly diminished as compared with that occurring during the 1st night.[43, 44] It is likely that, following the first night of sleep deprivation, the elevated thyroid hormone levels, which persist during the daytime period because of the prolonged half-life of these hormones, limit the subsequent TSH rise at the beginning of the next nighttime period. A well-documented study involving 64 h of sleep deprivation demonstrated a more than 50% increase in the T_3 level measured at 11 PM across the study period without significant change in the concomitant thyroxin (T_4) concentration.[45] During the 2nd night of sleep deprivation, a nocturnal increase in both T_3 and T_4 levels was observed, contrasting with the decreases seen during normal sleep.[45] These data suggest that prolonged sleep loss may be associated with an upregulation of the thyroid axis.

The fact that the inhibitory effects of sleep on TSH secretion are time dependent may cause, under specific circumstances, elevations of plasma TSH levels that reflect the misalignment of sleep and circadian timing. An example is shown in Figure 20–4, which shows the mean profiles of plasma TSH and T_3 levels observed in a group of normal young men in the course of adaptation to simulated jet lag, achieved by an abrupt 8-h advance of the sleep-dark period.[46] In the course of adaptation to this 8-h advance shift, TSH levels increased progressively because daytime sleep failed to inhibit TSH and nighttime wakefulness was associated with large circadian-dependent TSH elevations. As a result, mean TSH levels following awakening from the second shifted sleep period were more than twofold higher than during the same time interval following normal nocturnal sleep. This overall elevation of TSH levels was paralleled by a small increase in T_3 concentrations.[46] This study demonstrated that the subjective discomfort and fatigue often referred to as *jet lag syndrome* are associated not only with a desynchronization of bodily rhythms but also with a prolonged elevation of a hormonal concentration in the peripheral circulation.

INTERACTIONS BETWEEN SLEEP AND PROLACTIN SECRETION

The major role of sleep in stimulating PRL secretion has been recognized for more than 3 decades. Under normal conditions, PRL levels are minimal around noon, increase modestly during the afternoon, and then undergo a major nocturnal elevation starting shortly after sleep onset and culminate around mid-sleep. Decreased dopaminergic inhibition of PRL during sleep is likely to be the primary mechanism underlying this nocturnal PRL elevation. In adults of both genders, the nocturnal maximum corresponds to an average increase of more than 200% above the minimum level.[47–49] Morning awakenings and awakenings interrupting sleep are consistently associated with a rapid inhibition of PRL secretion.[48, 49]

Studies of the PRL profile during daytime naps or after shifts of the sleep period have consistently demonstrated that sleep onset, irrespective of the time of day, has a stimulatory effect on PRL release. This is well illustrated by the profiles shown in Figure 20–1, in which elevated PRL levels occur both during nocturnal sleep and during daytime recovery sleep, whereas the nocturnal period of sleep deprivation was not associated with an increase in PRL concentrations. However, sleep is not the sole factor responsible for the nocturnal elevation of PRL concentrations. Indeed, a number of experiments involving abrupt advances or delays of sleep times have shown that the sleep-related rise of PRL may still be present, although with a reduced amplitude, when sleep does not occur at the normal nocturnal time and that maximal stimulation is observed only when sleep and circadian effects are superimposed.[48–50] The sleep-independent circadian component of PRL secretion is expressed as a progressive increase across the late afternoon and the hours preceding the usual bedtime and is much more pronounced in women than in men.[49]

Because of the marked effect that sleep onset has on PRL release, several studies have examined the possible relationship between pulsatile PRL release during sleep and the alternation of REM and NREM stages. Although early reports were discordant,[51, 52] more recent studies characterizing sleep structure using power spectral analysis of the electroencephalogram (EEG)

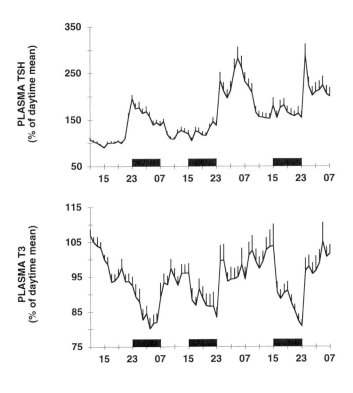

CLOCK TIME

Figure 20–4. Mean (and standard error of the mean) profiles of plasma thyrotropin (TSH) and plasma T_3 from eight normal young men who were submitted to an 8-h advance of the sleep-wake and dark-light cycles (from 23:00 to 07:00 and to 15:00 to 23:00). Black bars indicate bedtime periods. Under these simulated advanced jet lag conditions, both TSH and T_3 increased during the course of adaptation. (Data from Hirschfeld U, Moreno-Reyes R, Akseki E, et al. Progressive elevation of plasma thyrotropin during adaptation to simulated jet lag: effects of treatment with bright lights or zolpidem. J Clin Endocrinol Metab. 1996;81:3270–3277.)

revealed a close temporal association between increased prolactin secretion and delta wave activity.[53] Conversely, awakenings inhibit nocturnal PRL release.[53] Thus, fragmented sleep generally is associated with lower nocturnal prolactin levels.

Benzodiazepine as well as nonbenzodiazepine hypnotics taken at bedtime may cause an increase in the nocturnal PRL rise, resulting in concentrations near the pathological range for part of the night.[54, 55] The upper panels of Figure 20–5 illustrate the effects of bedtime oral administration of triazolam (0.5 mg) compared with placebo on the 24-h PRL profiles obtained in a group of six normal men. Sleep-related PRL release was enhanced by triazolam ingested and, in some subjects, the PRL concentrations during the early part of the night were nearly threefold higher (although still in the physiological range) than with placebo.[54] The lower panels of Figure 20–5 show the similar effects of zolpidem (10 mg) in eight normal women.[55] Neither triazolam nor zolpidem had any effect on the 24-h profiles of cortisol, melatonin, or GH.

There is rapidly accumulating evidence from studies in rats and rabbits that PRL is involved in the humoral regulation of sleep.[56] The primary effect is a stimulation

of REM sleep, which may be observed 1 to 2 h post-treatment. This stimulatory effect of PRL on REM sleep depends on time of day because it is only observed during the light (i.e., inactive) period, and this effect may be exerted by PRL released centrally rather than by pituitary PRL. There are no direct studies of the effects of PRL on sleep in the human being, although one study has used injections of vasoactive intestinal polypeptide to stimulate endogenous PRL secretion and has reported an enhancement of REM sleep. A role for PRL in the circadian regulation of REM sleep propensity has been hypothesized.[56] However, there is also evidence for an involvement of PRL in SWS regulation. In particular, SWS is enhanced in patients with hyperprolactinemia.[57]

SLEEP AND GLUCOSE REGULATION

The consolidation of human sleep in a single 7- to 9-h period implies that an extended period of fast must be maintained overnight. A large number of studies have sampled levels of glucose and insulin in subjects sleeping in the laboratory and have observed that,

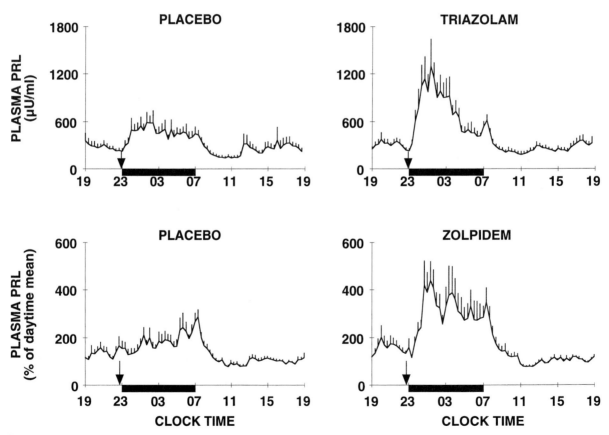

Figure 20–5. Effects of commonly used hypnotics on the 24-h profile of plasma, prolactin (PRL) in normal young subjects. Data are mean + standard error of the mean. Samples were collected at 15 to 20 min intervals. Sleep was polygraphically recorded. *Top*, effects of bedtime administration of triazolam (0.5 mg). *Bottom*, effects of bedtime administration of zolpidem (10 mg). Both benzodiazepine and nonbenzodiazepine hypnotics cause transient hyperprolactinemia during the early part of sleep. (Data from Copinschi G, Van Onderbergen A, L'Hermite-Balériaux M, et al. Effects of the short-acting benzodiazepine triazolam taken at bedtime, on circadian and sleep-related hormonal profiles in normal men. Sleep. 1990;13:232–244; Copinschi G, Akseki E, Moreno-Reyes R, et al. Effects of bedtime administration of zolpidem on circadian and sleep-related hormonal profiles in normal women. Sleep. 1995;18:417–424; and Van Cauter E, Spiegel K. Circadian and sleep control of endocrine secretions. In: Turek FW, Zee PC, eds. Neurobiology of Sleep and Circadian Rhythms. New York, NY: Marcel Dekker; 1999.)

despite the prolonged fasting condition, glucose levels remain stable or fall only minimally across the night.[58-64] In contrast, if subjects are awake and fasting in a recumbent position, in the absence of any physical activity, glucose levels fall by an average of 0.5 to 1.0 mmol/liter (± 10 to 20 mg/dl) over a 12-h period.[65] Thus, a number of mechanisms operative during nocturnal sleep (reviewed later) must intervene to maintain stable glucose levels during the overnight fast.

Experimental protocols allowing for the study of nighttime glucose tolerance during sleep without awakening the subjects include constant intravenous glucose infusion and continuous enteral nutrition. Confounding effects of food ingestion and prolonged fasting are avoided by replacing the normal caloric intake with a constant input, thereby creating a steady-state condition with levels of glucose and insulin secretion within the physiological range. Sleep has been polysomnographically recorded under both conditions and normal sleep parameters observed following a period of habituation to the laboratory procedures. Thus, both constant glucose infusion and continuous enteral nutrition offer the possibility of examining glucose tolerance during the sleep state, although under conditions that are clearly artificial. In particular, prolonged glucose infusion results in a marked inhibition of endogenous glucose production. Both experimental conditions have been used in extended studies in normal subjects[66-68] and have concurred in demonstrating a marked decrease in glucose tolerance during nocturnal sleep (Fig. 20-6). Despite the differences in the mode and nature of caloric intake, the glucose profiles observed in both conditions are remarkably similar and showed that glucose tolerance is markedly decreased during nocturnal sleep. Indeed, when individual profiles were analyzed, the overall increase in plasma glucose ranged from 20 to 30%, despite the maintenance of rigorously constant rates of caloric intake. Maximum levels occur around the middle of the sleep period. During the later part of the night (i.e., at the time of the so-called *dawn phenomenon*), glucose tolerance begins to improve, and glucose levels progressively decrease toward morning values. The mechanisms underlying these robust variations in set-point of glucose regulation across nocturnal sleep are different in early sleep and late sleep, respectively.

Under conditions of constant glucose infusion, the decrease in glucose tolerance during the first half of the sleep period is reflected in a robust increase in plasma glucose, which is followed by a more than 50% increase in insulin secretion. Under these conditions, the major underlying cause of the glucose increase is decreased glucose utilization. It is estimated that about two thirds of the fall in glucose utilization during sleep is due to a decrease in brain glucose metabolism[69] related to the predominance of SW stages, which are associated with a 30 to 40% reduction in cerebral glucose metabolism as compared to the waking state. The last third would then reflect decreased peripheral utilization. Diminished muscle tone during sleep and rapid anti-insulin–like effects of the sleep-onset GH pulse[70]

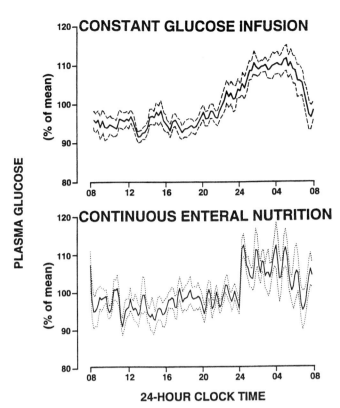

Figure 20–6. 24-h pattern of blood glucose changes in response to constant glucose infusion and continuous enteral nutrition in normal young adults. At each time point, the mean glucose level is shown with the standard error of the mean. Despite the fact that carbohydrate intake was constant throughout the study period, blood glucose levels increased markedly during the nighttime period. (Data from Van Cauter E, Desir D, Decoster C, et al. Nocturnal decrease in glucose tolerance during constant glucose infusion. J Clin Endocrinol Metab. 1989;69:604–611; Simon C, Brandenberger G, Saini J, et al. Slow oscillations of plasma glucose and insulin secretion rate are amplified during sleep in humans under continuous enteral nutrition. Sleep. 1994;17:333–338; and Van Cauter E, Polonsky KS, Scheen AJ. Roles of circadian rhythmicity and sleep in human glucose regulation. Endocr Rev. 1997;18:716–738.)

are both likely to contribute to decreased peripheral glucose uptake.

Under conditions of constant glucose infusion, during the later part of the sleep period, glucose levels and insulin secretion decrease to return to presleep values, and this decrease appears to be partially due to the increase in wake and REM stages.[71] Indeed, glucose utilization during these REM and wake stages is higher than during NREM stages.[69, 72-75] In addition, several other factors may also contribute to the decline of glucose levels during late sleep. These include the hypoglycemic activity of previously secreted insulin during early sleep, the increased insulin-independent glucose disposal due to transient mild hyperglycemia, and the quiescence of GH secretion and thus the rapid attenuation of the short-term inhibitory effects of this hormone on tissue glucose uptake. Finally, the later part of the night appears to be associated with increased insulin sensitivity, reflecting a delayed effect of low cortisol levels during the evening and early part of the night.[76]

HORMONES CONTROLLING HYDROMINERAL BALANCE DURING SLEEP

Water and salt homeostasis is under the combined control of the posterior pituitary, the renin-angiotensin-aldosterone system, and the atrial natriuretic peptide. Urine flow and electrolyte excretion are higher during the day than during the night, and this variation partly reflects circadian modulation. In addition to this 24-h rhythmicity, urine flow and osmolarity oscillate with the REM-NREM cycle. REM sleep is associated with decreasing urine flow and increasing osmolarity. During the 1990s, a series of elegant studies began to elucidate the endocrine control of the ultradian oscillations in hydromineral balance.[77]

Vasopressin release is pulsatile but without apparent relationship to sleep stages.[77] Levels of atrial natriuretic peptide are relatively stable and do not show fluctuations related to the sleep-wake or REM-NREM cycles.[78] Whether the levels of plasma atrial natriuretic peptide exhibit a circadian variation is still a matter of controversy.[78] A close relationship between the beginning of REM episodes and decreased activity has been consistently observed for plasma renin activity.[77, 79–81] Figure 20–7 illustrates the 24-h rhythm of plasma renin activity in a subject studied during a normal sleep-wake cycle (top) and in a subject studied following a shift of the sleep period (bottom). A remarkable synchronization between decreased plasma renin activity and REM stages is apparent during both sleep periods.[82] This relationship was confirmed in studies with selective REM sleep deprivation in normal subjects.[83] Increases in plasma renin activity parallel increases in SW EEG activity.[84] In conditions of abnormal sleep architecture (e.g., narcolepsy, sleeping sickness), the temporal pattern of plasma renin activity faithfully reflects the disturbances of the REM-NREM cycle.[77] The increased release of renin during sleep is associated with elevated levels of plasma aldosterone.[85]

AGE-RELATED SLEEP ALTERATIONS: IMPLICATIONS FOR ENDOCRINE FUNCTION

Normal aging is associated with pronounced age-related alterations in sleep quality, which consist primarily of a marked reduction of SWS (stages 3 and 4), a reduction in REM stages, and an increase in the number and duration of awakenings interrupting sleep (see Chapter 3). There is increasing evidence that these alterations in sleep quality result in disturbances of endocrine function, raising the hypothesis that some of the hormonal and metabolic hallmarks of aging partly reflect the deterioration of sleep quality.

Several studies have shown that decreases in

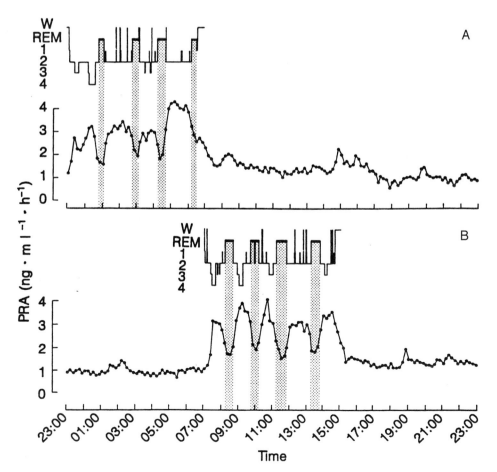

Figure 20–7. 24-h profiles of plasma renin activity sampled at 10-min intervals in a healthy individual. *A*, nocturnal sleep from 23:00 to 07:00. *B*, daytime sleep from 07:00 to 15:00 after a night of total sleep deprivation. The temporal distribution of stages wake (W); REM; 1, 2, 3, and 4 are shown above the hormonal values. The oscillations of plasma renin activity are synchronized to the REM-NREM cycle during sleep. (From Brandenberger G, Follenius M, Goichot B, et al. Twenty-four hour profiles of plasma renin activity in relation to the sleep-wake cycle. J Hypertens. 1994;12:277–283.)

amount of SWS occur rapidly in adulthood (30 to 40 years of age) and precede the appearance of significant sleep fragmentation or declines in REM sleep. A retrospective analysis of sleep and concomitant profiles of plasma GH from over 100 normal healthy men, ages 18 to 83 years, showed that the impact of aging on GH release occurred with a similar chronology characterized by major decrements from early adulthood to mid-life (E.V.C., R. Leproult, L. Plat, unpublished data, 1999). The statistical analysis further indicated that reduced amounts of SWS, and not age per se, may be the primary cause of reduced GH secretion in mid-life and late life. The observation that, in older adults, levels of insulin-like growth factor (IGF-1), the hormone secreted by the liver in response to stimulation by GH, are correlated with the amounts of SWS,[86] is consistent with this finding. Although the clinical implications of decreased SWS are still unclear, the relative GH deficiency of the elderly is associated with increased fat tissue and abdominal obesity, reduced muscle mass and strength, and reduced exercise capacity.[87-89] The persistence of a consistent relationship between SWS and GH secretion in older men suggests that drugs that reliably stimulate SWS in older adults may represent a novel strategy for GH replacement therapy.

In contrast to the rapid decline of SWS and GH secretion from young adulthood to mid-life, the impact of age on REM sleep and sleep fragmentation does not become apparent until later in life. Aging is associated with an elevation of evening cortisol levels, which follows the same chronology (i.e. no alteration until mid-life and then a steady rise from mid-life to old age). Analysis of variance indicates that this inability to achieve or maintain the quiescence of the corticotropic axis in aging partly reflects the loss of REM sleep in old age. Both animal and human studies have indicated that deleterious effects of HPA hyperactivity are more pronounced at the time of the trough of the rhythm than at the time of the peak.[90, 91] Therefore, modest elevations in evening cortisol levels could facilitate the development of central and peripheral disturbances associated with glucocorticoid excess, such as memory deficits and insulin resistance,[90, 92] and further promote sleep fragmentation. Indeed, several studies have demonstrated that elevated corticosteroid levels result in increased propensity for awakenings.[93, 94]

A nearly 50% dampening of the nocturnal PRL elevation is evident in healthy elderly subjects.[95] This diminished nocturnal rise in aging is associated with a decrease in the amplitude of the nocturnal secretory pulses.[96] Whether this age-related endocrine alteration partly reflects the increased number of awakenings (which inhibit PRL release) and decreased amounts of deep NREM stages (which stimulate PRL release) remains to be determined.

HORMONAL FUNCTION AND METABOLISM IN OBSTRUCTIVE SLEEP APNEA

A few studies have examined nocturnal hormonal release in patients with OSA before and after treat-

ment.[97-99] As expected, the nocturnal release of the two pituitary hormones that are markedly dependent on sleep (i.e., GH and PRL), is decreased in untreated apneic subjects. Because adult patients with OSA are frequently obese, the low overnight GH levels could reflect the hyposomatotropism of obesity, rather than result from the shallow and fragmented nature of their sleep. However, two studies that have examined the nocturnal GH profile before and after treatment with continuous positive airway pressure (CPAP) have demonstrated that treatment of OSA resulted in a clear increase in the amount of GH secreted during the first few hours of sleep[97, 99] as illustrated in Figure 20–8. In children, surgical correction of OSA may restore GH secretion and normal growth rate.[98] The effects of CPAP treatment on overnight prolactin secretion were less clear than those seen for GH.[100] Indeed, the total amount of PRL secreted during the sleep period was not modified by CPAP treatment, but the frequency of PRL pulses was restored to values similar to those observed in normal subjects.

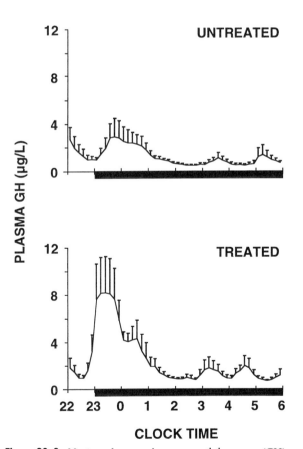

PATIENTS WITH SLEEP APNEA

Figure 20–8. Nocturnal mean plasma growth hormone (GH) profiles before *(top)* and after *(bottom)* continuous positive airway pressure treatment. Treatment was associated with a clear increase in nocturnal GH release. (Data from Saini J, Krieger J, Brandenberger G, et al. Continuous positive airway pressure treatment: effects on growth hormone, insulin and glucose profiles in obstructive sleep apnea patients. Horm Metab Res. 1993;25:375–381.)

The increased urine and sodium excretion and the decreased activity of the renin-angiotensin system of patients with OSA also appears to be partially caused by sleep fragmentation. Indeed, the normal relationship between REM-NREM cyclicity and oscillations of plasma renin activity, which are disturbed in these patients, can be restored by CPAP treatment, which in turn contributes to the normalization of urine and sodium outputs.[101]

The frequent association of OSA with central obesity, insulin resistance, and diabetes has prompted studies of the possible role of OSA per se in the pathogenesis of these metabolic syndromes. Evidence for an association between the apnea-hypopnea index (AHI) and fasting insulin levels, independent of the degree of obesity, was reported in a study of 261 men referred to a sleep laboratory for symptoms of sleep-disordered breathing.[102] Analysis of epidemiological data[103] showing an association between elevated fasting insulin levels and a high likelihood for OSA (as inferred from self-reported loud snoring and observed breathing pauses), after adjustment for body fat distribution and other potential confounds, were consistent with these findings. Furthermore, CPAP treatment of severely obese adults with significant OSA has been shown to improve insulin sensitivity as estimated during a hyperinsulinemic euglycemic clamp.[104] Thus, it appears that OSA may, in itself, cause alterations in glucose regulation, which in turn contribute to the development of insulin resistance and glucose intolerance.

Thus, the limited number of studies that have examined endocrine function and metabolism in patients with OSA have clearly indicated that this sleep disorder is associated with endocrine and metabolic abnormalities, which can be partially corrected by treating the sleep disorder.

CONCLUSION

Sleep exerts important modulatory effects on most components of the endocrine system. Sleep loss and alterations of sleep quality are associated with disturbances of hormonal secretion and metabolism, which may be of clinical relevance. Findings suggest that part of the constellation of hormonal and metabolic alterations that characterize normal aging may reflect the deterioration of sleep quality. In OSA, there is good evidence that the sleep disorder contributes to or exacerbates the metabolic syndrome, which is highly prevalent in this condition. Strategies to reverse decrements in sleep quality may have beneficial effects on endocrine and metabolic function.

References

1. Van Cauter E, Blackman JD, Roland D, et al. Modulation of glucose regulation and insulin secretion by circadian rhythmicity and sleep. J Clin Invest. 1991;88:934–942.
2. Van Cauter E. Hormones and sleep. In: Kales A, ed. The Pharmacology of Sleep. Berlin, Germany: Springer Verlag; 1995:279–306.
3. Quabbe H, Schilling E, Helge H. Pattern of growth hormone secretion during a 24-hour fast in normal adults. J Clin Endocrinol Metab. 1966;26:1173–1177.
4. Hunter WM, Rigal WM. The diurnal pattern of plasma growth hormone concentration in children and adolescents. J Endocrinol. 1966;34:147–153.
5. Takahashi Y, Kipnis DM, Daughaday WH. Growth hormone secretion during sleep. J Clin Invest. 1968;47:2079–2090.
6. Sassin JF, Parker DC, Mace JW, et al. Human growth hormone release: relation to slow-wave sleep and sleep-waking cycles. Science. 1969;165:513–515.
7. Honda Y, Takahashi K, Takahashi S, et al. Growth hormone secretion during nocturnal sleep in normal subjects. J Clin Endocrinol Metab. 1969;29:20–29.
8. Sassin J, Frantz A, Weitzman E, et al. Human prolactin: 24-hour pattern with increased release during sleep. Science. 1972;177:1205–1207.
9. Sassin J, Frantz A, Kapen S, et al. The nocturnal rise of human prolactin is dependent on sleep. J Clin Endocrinol Metab. 1973;37:436–440.
10. Van Cauter E, Plat L, Copinschi G. Interrelations between sleep and the somatotropic axis. Sleep. 1998;21:553–566.
11. Weibel L, Spiegel K, Gronfier C, et al. Twenty-four-hour melatonin and core body temperature rhythms: their adaptation in night workers. Am J Physiol. 1997;272:R948–R954.
12. Aschoff J. Circadian rhythms: general features and endocrinological aspects. In: Krieger DT, ed. Endocrine Rhythms. New York, NY: Raven Press; 1979:1–61.
13. Van Cauter E, Kerkhofs M, Caufriez A, et al. A quantitative estimation of GH secretion in normal man: reproducibility and relation to sleep and time of day. J Clin Endocrinol Metab. 1992;74:1441–1450.
14. Mullington J, Hermann D, Holsboer F, et al. Age-dependent suppression of nocturnal growth hormone levels during sleep deprivation. Neuroendocrinology. 1996;64:233–241.
15. Seifritz E, Hemmeter U, Trachsel L, et al. Effects of flumazenil on recovery sleep and hormonal secretion after sleep deprivation in male controls. Psychopharmacology (Berl). 1995;120:449–456.
16. Jaffe C, Turgeon D, DeMott Friberg R, et al. Nocturnal augmentation of growth hormone (GH) secretion is preserved during repetitive bolus administration of GH-releasing hormone: potential involvement of endogenous somatostatin—a clinical research center study. J Clin Endocrinol Metab. 1995;80:3321–3326.
17. Parker DC, Sassin JF, Mace JW, et al. Human growth hormone release during sleep: electroencephalographic correlations. J Clin Endocrinol Metab. 1969;29:871–874.
18. Holl RW, Hartmann ML, Veldhuis JD, et al. Thirty-second sampling of plasma growth hormone in man: correlation with sleep stages. J Clin Endocrinol Metab. 1991;72:854–861.
19. Gronfier C, Luthringer R, Follenius M, et al. A quantitative evaluation of the relationships between growth hormone secretion and delta wave electroencephalographic activity during normal sleep and after enrichment in delta waves. Sleep. 1996;19:817–824.
20. Van Cauter E, Plat L, Scharf M, et al. Simultaneous stimulation of slow-wave sleep and growth hormone secretion by gamma-hydroxybutyrate in normal young men. J Clin Invest. 1997;100:745–753.
21. Jarrett DB, Greenhouse JB, Miewald JM, et al. A reexamination of the relationship between growth hormone secretion and slow wave sleep using delta wave analysis. Biol Psychiatry. 1990;27:497–509.
22. Born J, Muth S, Fehm HL. The significance of sleep onset and slow wave sleep for nocturnal release of growth hormone (GH) and cortisol. Psychoneuroendocrinology. 1988;13:233–243.
23. Mendlewicz J, Linkowski P, Kerkhofs M, et al. Diurnal hypersecretion of growth hormone in depression. J Clin Endocrinol Metab. 1985;60:505–512.
24. Steiger A, Herth T, Holsboer F. Sleep-electroencephalography and the secretion of cortisol and growth hormone in normal controls. Acta Endocrinol. 1987;116:36–42.
25. Van Cauter E, Caufriez A, Kerkhofs M, et al. Sleep, awakenings and insulin-like growth factor I modulate the growth hormone secretory response to growth hormone-releasing hormone. J Clin Endocrinol Metab. 1992;74:1451–1459.

26. Spath-Schwalbe E, Hundenborn C, Kern W, et al. Nocturnal wakefulness inhibits growth hormone (GH)–releasing hormone-induced GH secretion. J Clin Endocrinol Metab. 1995;80:214–219.

27. Weitzman ED, Zimmerman JC, Czeisler CA, et al. Cortisol secretion is inhibited during sleep in normal man. J Clin Endocrinol Metab. 1983;56:352–358.

28. Spath-Schwalbe E, Uthgenannt D, Voget G, et al. Corticotropin-releasing hormone-induced adrenocorticotropin and cortisol secretion depends on sleep and wakefulness. J Clin Endocrinol Metab. 1993;77:1170–1173.

29. Weibel L, Follenius M, Spiegel K, et al. Comparative effect of night and daytime sleep on the 24-hour cortisol secretory profile. Sleep. 1995;18:549–556.

30. Follenius M, Brandenberger G, Bardasept J, et al. Nocturnal cortisol release in relation to sleep structure. Sleep. 1992;15:21–27.

31. Gronfier C, Luthringer R, Follenius M, et al. Temporal relationships between pulsatile cortisol secretion and electroencephalographic activity during sleep in man. Electroencephalogr Clin Neurophysiol. 1997;103:405–408.

32. Bierwolf C, Struve K, Marshall L, et al. Slow wave sleep drives inhibition of pituitary-adrenal secretion in humans. J Neuroendocrinol. 1997;9:479–484.

33. Spath-Schwalbe E, Gofferje M, Kern W, et al. Sleep disruption alters nocturnal ACTH and cortisol secretory patterns. Biol Psychiatry. 1991;29:575–584.

34. Pruessner JC, Wolf OT, Hellhammer DH, et al. Free cortisol levels after awakening: a reliable biological marker for the assessment of adrenocortical activity. Life Sci. 1997;61:2539–2549.

35. Van Cauter E, van Coevorden A, Blackman JD. Modulation of neuroendocrine release by sleep and circadian rhythmicity. In: Yen SSC, Vale W, eds. Advances in Neuroendocrine Regulation of Reproduction. Norwell, Mass: Serono Symposia USA; 1990:113–122

36. Bliwise DL. Normal aging. In: Kryger MH, Roth T, Dement WC, eds. Principles and Practice of Sleep Medicine. Philadelphia, Pa: WB Saunders; 1994:26–39.

37. Leproult R, Copinschi G, Buxton O, et al. Sleep loss results in an elevation of cortisol levels the next evening. Sleep. 1997;20:865–870.

38. Veldhuis JD, Iranmanesh A, Johnson ML, et al. Twenty-four-hour rhythms in plasma concentrations of adenohypophyseal hormones are generated by distinct amplitude and/or frequency modulation of underlying pituitary secretory bursts. J Clin Endocrinol Metab. 1990;71:1616–1623.

39. Brabant G, Prank K, Ranft U, et al. Physiological regulation of circadian and pulsatile thyrotropin secretion in normal man and woman. J Clin Endocrinol Metab. 1990;70:403–409.

40. Parker DC, Rossman LG, Pekary AE, et al. Effect of 64-hour sleep deprivation on the circadian waveform of thyrotropin (TSH): further evidence of sleep-related inhibition of TSH release. J Clin Endocrinol Metab. 1987;64:157–161.

41. Goichot B, Brandenberger G, Saini J, et al. Nocturnal plasma thyrotropin variations are related to slow-wave sleep. J Sleep Res. 1992;1:186–190.

42. Gronfier C, Luthringer R, Follenius M, et al. Temporal link between plasma thyrotropin levels and electroencephalographic activity in man. Neurosci Lett. 1995;200:97–100.

43. Van Cauter E, Turek FW. Endocrine and other biological rhythms. In: DeGroot LJ, ed. Endocrinology. Philadelphia, Pa: WB Saunders; 1995:2487–2548.

44. Allan JS, Czeisler CA. Persistence of the circadian thyrotropin rhythm under constant conditions and after light-induced shifts of circadian phase. J Clin Endocrinol Metab. 1994;79:508–512.

45. Gary KA, Winokur A, Douglas SD, et al. Total sleep deprivation and the thyroid axis: effects of sleep and waking activity. Aviat Space Environ Med. 1996;67:513–519.

46. Hirschfeld U, Moreno-Reyes R, Akseki E, et al. Progressive elevation of plasma thyrotropin during adaptation to simulated jet lag: effects of treatment with bright light or zolpidem. J Clin Endocrinol Metab. 1996;81:3270–3277.

47. Van Cauter E, L'Hermite M, Copinschi G, et al. Quantitative analysis of spontaneous variations of plasma prolactin in normal man. Am J Physiol. 1981;241:E355–E363.

48. Spiegel K, Follenius M, Simon C, et al. Prolactin secretion and sleep. Sleep. 1994;17:20–27.

49. Waldstreicher J, Duffy JF, Brown EN, et al. Gender differences in the temporal organization of prolactin (PRL) secretion: evidence for a sleep-independent circadian rhythm of circulating PRL levels—a Clinical Research Center study. J Clin Endocrinol Metab. 1996;81:1483–1487.

50. Désir D, Van Cauter E, L'Hermite M, et al. Effects of "jet lag" on hormonal patterns, III: demonstration of an intrinsic circadian rhythmicity in plasma prolactin. J Clin Endocrinol Metab. 1982;55:849–857.

51. Parker DC, Rossman LG, Vanderlaan EF. Relation of sleep-entrained human prolactin release to REM–nonREM cycles. J Clin Endocrinol Metab. 1974;38:646–651.

52. Van Cauter E, Desir D, Refetoff S, et al. The relationship between episodic variations of plasma prolactin and REM–non-REM cyclicity is an artifact. J Clin Endocrinol Metab. 1982;54:70–75.

53. Spiegel K, Luthringer R, Follenius M, et al. Temporal relationship between prolactin secretion and slow-wave electroencephalographic activity during sleep. Sleep. 1995;18:543–548.

54. Copinschi G, Van Onderbergen A, L'Hermite-Balériaux M, et al. Effects of the short-acting benzodiazepine triazolam, taken at bedtime, on circadian and sleep-related hormonal profiles in normal men. Sleep. 1990;13:232–244.

55. Copinschi G, Akseki E, Moreno-Reyes R, et al. Effects of bedtime administration of zolpidem on circadian and sleep-related hormonal profiles in normal women. Sleep. 1995;18:417–424.

56. Roky R, Obal F, Valatx JL, et al. Prolactin and rapid eye movement sleep regulation. Sleep. 1995;18:536–542.

57. Frieboes RM, Murck H, Stalla GK, et al. Enhanced slow-wave sleep in patients with hyperprolactinemia. J Clin Endocrinol Metab. 1998;83:2706–2710.

58. Mauras N, Blizzard RM, Link K, et al. Augmentation of growth hormone secretion during puberty: evidence for a pulse amplitude-modulated phenomenon. J Clin Endocrinol Metab. 1987;64:596–601.

59. Polonsky KS, Given BD, Van Cauter E. Twenty-four-hour profiles and pulsatile patterns of insulin secretion in normal and obese subjects. J Clin Invest. 1988;81:442–448.

60. Levy I, Recasens A, Casamitjana R, et al. Nocturnal insulin and C-peptide rhythms in normal subjects. Diabetes Care. 1987;10:148–151.

61. Clore JN, Nestler JE, Blackard WG. Sleep-associated fall in glucose disposal and hepatic glucose output in normal humans. Diabetes. 1989;38:285–290.

62. Simon C, Brandenberger G, Follenius M. Absence of the dawn phenomenon in normal subjects. J Clin Endocrinol Metab. 1988;67:203–205.

63. Garvey WT, Olefsky JM, Rubenstein AH, et al. Day-long integrated serum insulin and C-peptide profiles in patients with NIDDM. Diabetes. 1988;37:590–599.

64. Kern W, Offenheuser S, Fehm HL. Entrainment of ultradian oscillations in the secretion of insulin and glucagon to the nonREM/REM sleep rhythm in humans. J Clin Endocrinol Metab. 1996; 81:1541–1547.

65. Van Cauter E, Polonsky KS, Scheen AJ. Roles of circadian rhythmicity and sleep in human glucose regulation. Endocr Rev. 1997;18:716–738.

66. Simon C, Brandenberger G, Follenius M. Ultradian oscillations of plasma glucose, insulin, and C-peptide in man during continuous enteral nutrition. J Clin Endocrinol Metab. 1987;64:669–674.

67. Van Cauter E, Desir D, Decoster C, et al. Nocturnal decrease in glucose tolerance during constant glucose infusion. J Clin Endocrinol Metab. 1989;69:604–611.

68. Simon C, Brandenberger G, Saini J, et al. Slow oscillations of plasma glucose and insulin secretion rate are amplified during sleep in humans under continuous enteral nutrition. Sleep. 1994;17:333–338.

69. Boyle PJ, Scott JC, Krentz AJ, et al. Diminished brain glucose metabolism is a significant determinant for falling rates of systemic glucose utilization during sleep in normal humans. J Clin Invest. 1994;93:529–535.

70. Møller N, Jorgensen JOL, Schmitz O, et al. Effects of a growth

hormone pulse on total and forearm substrate fluxes in humans. Am J Physiol. 1990; 258:E86–E91.

71. Scheen AJ, Byrne MM, Plat L, et al. Relationships between sleep quality and glucose regulation in normal humans. Am J Physiol. 1996;271:E261–E270.

72. Buchsbaum MS, Gillin JC, Wu J, et al. Regional cerebral glucose metabolic rate in human sleep assessed by positron emission tomography. Life Sci. 1989;45:1349–1356.

73. Maquet P, Dive D, Salmon E, et al. Cerebral glucose utilization during sleep-wake cycle in man determined by positron emission tomography and [18F]2-fluoro-2-deoxy-D-glucose method. Brain Res. 1990;513:136–143.

74. Maquet P, Dive D, Salmon E, et al. Cerebral glucose utilization during stage 2 sleep in man. Brain Res. 1992;571:149–153.

75. Maquet P. Postron emission tomography studies of sleep and sleep disorders. J Neurol. 1997;244(suppl 1):S23–28.

76. Plat L, Byrne MM, Sturis J, et al. Effects of morning cortisol elevation on insulin secretion and glucose regulation in humans. Am J Physiol. 1996;270:E36–E42.

77. Brandenberger G, Charloux A, Grongier C, et al. Ultradian rhythms in hydromineral hormones. Horm Res. 1998;49:131–135.

78. Follenius M, Brandenberger G, Saini J. Lack of diurnal rhythm in plasma atrial natriuretic peptide. Life Sci. 1992;51:143–149.

79. Portaluppi F, Bagni B, Degli UB, et al. Circadian rhythms of atrial natriuretic peptide, renin, aldosterone, cortisol, blood pressure, and heart rate in normal and hypertensive subjects. J Hypertens. 1990;8:85–95.

80. Brandenberger G, Krauth MO, Ehrhart J, et al. Modulation of episodic renin release during sleep in humans. Hypertension. 1990;15:370–375.

81. Brandenberger G, Follenius M, Muzet A, et al. Ultradian oscillations in plasma renin activity: their relationship to meals and sleep stages. J Clin Endocrinol Metab. 1985;61:280–284.

82. Brandenberger G, Follenius M, Goichot B, et al. Twenty-four hour profiles of plasma renin activity in relation to the sleep-wake cycle. J Hypertens. 1994;12:277–283.

83. Brandenberger G, Follenius M, Simon C, et al. Nocturnal oscillations in plasma renin activity and REM-NREM sleep cycles in man: a common regulatory mechanism? Sleep. 1988;11:242–250.

84. Luthringer R, Brandenberger G, Schaltenbrand N, et al. Slow wave electroencephalographic activity parallels renin oscillations during sleep in humans. Electroencepalogr Clin Neurophysiol. 1995;95:318–322.

85. Charloux A, Gronfier C, Lonsdorfer-Wolf E, et al. Aldosterone release during the sleep-wake cycle in humans. Am J Physiol. 1998;276:E43–E49.

86. Prinz P, Moe K, Dulberg E, et al. Higher plasma IGF-1 levels are associated with increased delta sleep in healthy older men. J Gerontol. 1995;50A:M222–M226.

87. Cuneo R, Salomon F, McGauley G, et al. The growth hormone deficiency syndrome in adults. Clin Endocrinol. 1992;37:387–397.

88. Corpas E, Harman SM, Blackman MR. Human growth hormone and human aging. Endocr Rev. 1993;14:20–39.

89. Rosen T, Hansson T, Granhed H, et al. Reduced bone mineral content in adult patients with growth hormone deficiency. Acta Endocrinol. 1993;129:201–206.

90. Dallman MF, Strack AL, Akana SF, et al. Feast and famine: critical role of glucocorticoids with insulin in daily energy flow. Front Neuroendocrinol. 1993;14:303–347.

91. Plat L, Leproult R, L'Hermite-Balériaux M, et al. Metabolic effects of short-term elevations of plasma cortisol are more pronounced in the evening than in the morning. J Clin Endocrinol Metab. 1999;84:3082–3092.

92. McEwen BS, Sapolsky RM. Stress and cognitive function. Curr Opin Neurobiol. 1995;5:205–216.

93. Holsboer F, von Bardelein U, Steiger A. Effects of intravenous corticotropin-releasing hormone upon sleep-related growth hormone surge and sleep EEG in man. Neuroendocrinology. 1988;48:32–38.

94. Born J, Späth-Schwalbe E, Schwakenhofer H, et al. Influences of corticotropin-releasing hormone, adrenocorticotropin, and cortisol on sleep in normal man. J Clin Endocrinol Metab. 1989;68:904–911.

95. van Coevorden A, Mockel J, Laurent E, et al. Neuroendocrine rhythms and sleep in aging. Am J Physiol. 1991;260:E651–E661.

96. Greenspan SL, Klibanski A, Rowe JW, et al. Age alters pulsatile prolactin release: influence of dopaminergic inhibition. Am J Physiol. 1990;258:E799–E804.

97. Cooper BG, White JES, Ashworth LA, et al. Hormonal and metabolic profiles in subjects with obstructive sleep apnea syndrome and the effects of nasal continuous positive airway pressure (CPAP) treatment. Sleep. 1995;18:172–179.

98. Goldstein SJ, Wu RHK, Thorpy MJ, et al. Reversibility of deficient sleep entrained growth hormone secretion in a boy with achondroplasia and obstructive sleep apnea. Acta Endocrinol. 1987;116:95–101.

99. Saini J, Krieger J, Brandenberger G, et al. Continuous positive airway pressure treatment: effects on growth hormone, insulin and glucose profiles in obstructive sleep apnea patients. Horm Metab Res. 1993;25:375–381.

100. Spiegel K, Follenius M, Krieger J, et al. Prolactin secretion during sleep in obstructive sleep apnea patients. J Sleep Res. 1995;4:56–62.

101. Brandenberger G. Hydromineral hormones during sleep and wakefulness. Sleep Res. 1991;20A:186.

102. Strohl KP, Novak RD, Singer W, et al. Insulin levels, blood pressure and sleep apnea. Sleep. 1994;17:614–618.

103. Grunstein RR, Stenlof K, Hedner J, et al. Impact of obstructive sleep apnea and sleepiness on metabolic and cardiovascular factors in the Swedish Obese Subjects (SOS) Study. Int J Obes Relat Metab Disord. 1995;19:410–418.

104. Brooks B, Cistulli PA, Borkman M, et al. Obstructive sleep apnea in obese noninsulin-dependent diabetic patients: effects of continuous positive airway pressure treatment on insulin responsiveness. J Clin Endocrinol Metab. 1994;79:1681–1685.

21

Gastrointestinal Physiology

William C. Orr

The gastrointestinal system is regulated by both the autonomic nervous system (ANS) and the enteric nervous system (ENS), a complex network of neurons located within the entire luminal gastrointestinal tract.

Esophageal peristalsis is largely regulated by the ENS and, to a much lesser extent, by vagal input. There is a diminution in peristaltic amplitude and a substantial decrease in the swallowing rate and concomitant prolongation of esophageal acid clearance during sleep. Transient lower esophageal sphincter relaxations have been shown to be decreased during sleep.

The basic myoelectric activity of the stomach is regulated by a gastric pacemaker that emits a basic electrical rhythm of approximately three cycles per minute and forms the basis for the production of gastric contractile activity. There is also periodic electrical spike activity associated with gastric contractions. There is, in normal individuals, a peak in acid secretion occurring at approximately midnight, whereas patients with duodenal ulcer disease have increased acid secretion throughout the circadian cycle unrelated to sleep stage.

Intestinal motility is largely composed of the cyclic (every 90 min) occurrence of a sequence of contractions, the migrating motor complex (MMC), which is regulated almost completely by the ENS. This activity is not correlated with rapid eye movement sleep. With sleep, the MMC cycle becomes shorter. During sleep, the colon is relatively quiescent. The high amplitude peristaltic contractions are associated with defecation. Anal rectal functioning, on the other hand, has an endogenous oscillation that is most evident during sleep, resulting in primarily retrograde propagation. This likely serves a protective function against the involuntary loss of stool during sleep.

A description of the normal physiology of any organ system rarely includes the normal alterations of that system during sleep. It would seem inappropriate that nearly one third of the functioning time of an organ system would be ignored in describing its functioning. Profound alterations have been documented during sleep in describing normal physiology, yet these changes do not become part of the litany in describing normal physiology. Sleep-related, or *circadian* changes, have been most commonly addressed in describing blood pressure and the definition of hypertension, but this has not been accomplished with either the description of or clinical application of sleep-related changes in gastrointestinal (GI) physiology. This can be largely attributed to the inaccessibility of the luminal GI tract to easy measurement. Monitoring any of the basic functions of the GI system requires invading an office, which is an unpleasant experience and one that would generally be assumed to be disruptive of normal sleep.

The functioning of the luminal GI tract (to which this review is confined) reflects the final common pathway of a complex interaction of the central nervous system (CNS) with both the ANS and ENS. The latter is a complex neuronal network that is woven throughout the subserosal layers of the luminal GI tract. The ENS provides an autonomous source of GI motor activity. The movement through the GI tract is controlled and regulated by the ENS and ANS, and the interaction of these two influences ultimately determines that appropriate movement, at an appropriate rate, occurs throughout the passage from mouth to anus.[1]

Alterations in GI functioning during sleep appear to be quite different depending on the particular organ studied and its function within the GI system. For example, spontaneous esophageal function is markedly reduced during sleep because there is no need for this organ to function except in the event of food being transmitted from the upper esophageal area. This rarely occurs without volitional swallowing, which is diminished significantly during sleep.[2] On the other hand, rectal motor activity persists during sleep, which appears to be a mechanism necessary to preserve continence during sleep.[3]

The ultimate description of GI functioning and its complex physiology requires that autonomic and central control be separated from the intrinsic control generated by the ENS. Because sleep essentially represents a state of reversible decortication, the study of GI motor functioning during sleep allows an assessment of autonomous activity without higher cortical influence. Thus, the study of GI motility during sleep allows the separation of CNS and ENS processes and a more clear understanding of what has been referred to as the *brain-gut access.*

HISTORICAL ASPECTS

Interest in GI physiology during sleep preceded the development of sophisticated techniques for monitoring GI function by well over 50 years. For example, Friedenwald,[4] in 1906, described the secretory function of the stomach during sleep and reported that it was not appreciably altered. In 1924, Johnson and Washeim[5] reported a decrease in the volume of gastric juice secreted during sleep, and, in addition, they reported an increase in the acidity of the gastric juice. Henning and Norpoth[6] measured acidity hourly during sleep, and they reported that sleep was associated with a cessation of acid secretion and that only in patients with gastric ulcers did there appear to be continuous acid secretion. These results were confirmed nearly 20 years later.[7]

In 1915, Luckhardt[8] described the inhibition of gastric motility during periods of sleep, which, from his description, sounded remarkably like rapid eye movement (REM) sleep. His observations were made in dogs and were described in association with sonorous respiration (snoring?), irregular breathing, movements of the forelimbs and hindlimbs, and occasional "abortive yelps." Luckhardt stated, "I assumed that the dog was experiencing during sleep a form of cerebral excitation akin to or identical with the dreaming state in man."[8]

A few years later, in 1922, Wada[9] reported an extensive study of hunger and its relation to gastric and somatic activity by use of simultaneous records of gastric contractions and body movements during sleep. Gastric contractions were reported that were often associated with body movements and reports of dreaming. The techniques used in these studies were obviously somewhat crude, but it is clear that interest in GI function during sleep was not a development of the more modern era of sleep investigation.

GASTRIC FUNCTION

Acid Secretion

Gastric acid secretion has been shown to exhibit a clear circadian rhythm, which was initially described by Sandweiss et al.[10] It remained, however, for Moore and Englert to provide a definitive description of the circadian oscillation of gastric acid secretion in normal subjects.[11] These investigators described a peak in acid secretion occurring generally between 10 PM and 2 AM while confirming already established data that indicated that basal acid secretion in the waking state is minimal in the absence of meal stimulation. Similar results have been described in patients who have duodenal ulcer (DU) disease with levels of acid secretion markedly enhanced throughout the circadian cycle.[12, 13] It is clear from these results that there is an endogenous circadian rhythm of unstimulated basal acid secretion, but it is not clear that this is specifically altered in any way by sleep.

Initial interest in the role of sleep in gastric acid production was stimulated by the work of the eminent University of Chicago surgeon Dr. Lester Dragstedt.[14]

An interest in the pathogenesis of DU disease and the possible role of nocturnal gastric acid secretion in this process was further stimulated by studies by Levin et al.[12, 15] They analyzed hourly samples of acid secretion in both normal subjects and patients with DU

disease, and they identified nearly continuous acid secretion throughout the night in normal volunteers. They described a considerable degree of night-to-night and subject-to-subject variation. In contrast to the normal subjects, there were increases in both volume and acid concentration during sleep in patients with DU disease. Although emphasizing night-to-night variation, they found that the patients with DU disease who tended to be high secreters were consistently high, and those who were low secreters were consistently low. These studies paved the way for more extensive investigations into the role of nocturnal acid secretion in the pathogenesis of DU disease. This study is at variance with the study by Sandweiss et al.,[10] which did not find a substantial difference in nocturnal acid secretion between normal subjects and patients with DU. These discrepant results may be due to varying degrees of ulcer activity in the patients studied. As previously noted, perhaps the most influential work in nocturnal gastric acid secretion has been done by Dragstedt.[14] Using hourly collections of overnight acid secretion in normal subjects and in patients with DU disease, he reported that the nocturnal acid secretion in patients with DU disease is 3 to 20 times greater than that in his normal subjects. He reported that this greater secretion was abolished by vagotomy, which invariably produced prompt ulcer healing. These data were interpreted to be strong evidence in favor of a "nervous" origin for DU disease.

The decade of the 1950s ushered in the "golden age" of sleep investigation. The realization that sleep is not a unitary, passive state of consciousness focused considerable interest on its unique physiology. The first study to describe gastric acid secretion during conditions of polysomnographic (PSG) monitoring was reported in 1960 by Reichsman et al.[16] Using relatively crude determinations of stages of sleep, they found no correlation between gastric acid secretion and sleep stages in normal subjects. A subsequent study by Armstrong et al.[17] reported the rather startling finding of a hypersecretion of acid during REM sleep in patients with DU disease. Both of these studies suffered from a major methodological flaw in that they used drugs to induce sleep. Another problem in these studies was the relatively small data sample per subject, in most cases only a single night. Earlier studies documented the considerable night-to-night variability in acid secretion. Thus, studying a patient or a normal volunteer for a single night with a nasogastric tube would undoubtedly result in numerous awakenings and generally poor sleep, with correspondingly more variable acid secretion.

Stacher et al.[18] studied gastric acid secretion in a group of normal volunteers during PSG monitored natural sleep. They reported no significant differences in acid secretion during the nonrapid eye movement (NREM) stages of sleep; however, they reported that REM sleep was associated with an inhibition of acid secretion. This study, although avoiding the use of drugs to induce sleep, used a rather cumbersome technique for determining acid output. It was measured by an intragastric titration from a telemetric pH capsule and involved numerous disruptions in the patients' sleep. Thus, although it was natural sleep, it was by no means uninterrupted or spontaneous sleep.

The variability of these results and the various methodological problems of previous studies prompted a concurrent study of both normal subjects and patients with DU disease. Orr et al.[19] studied five normal volunteers and five patients with DU disease, and each subject was studied for 5 consecutive nights in the sleep laboratory. The study involved continuous aspiration of gastric contents divided into 20-min aliquots for gastric analysis as well as complete PSG monitoring for the determination of sleep stages. In addition, serum gastrin levels were assessed at 20-min intervals throughout the study. The results did not reveal any significant correlation between the sleep stage (REM vs. NREM) and acid concentration or total acid secretion. Furthermore, there was no relationship between any of these variables and serum gastrin levels. These data did show, however, that the patients with DU failed to inhibit acid secretion during the first 2 h of sleep, which was consistent with the previously reported studies by Levin et al.,[12] which suggested that acid secretion is poorly inhibited during sleep in patients with DU disease.

In conclusion, the data would support the presence of a clear-cut circadian rhythm in basal acid secretion, with a peak occurring in the early part of the normal sleep interval. However, there are no definitive data at the present time that would suggest a major effect of sleep stages on this process. If one conclusion can be drawn from the various studies that have been done assessing gastric acid secretion during sleep it would be that acid secretion is extremely variable from night to night and from person to person, and for this reason definitive conclusions require numerous replications across and within a large number of subjects and patients. The extremely demanding logistics of sleep studies, as well as the obvious aversive aspects of numerous nasal intubations to study participants, make the acquisition of such data exceedingly difficult.

MOTOR FUNCTION

The motor function of the stomach serves to empty solids and liquids into the duodenum at an appropriate rate and pH. The stomach is functionally divided into two sections: the fundus of the stomach functions primarily to control liquid emptying into the duodenum, whereas the antrum controls emptying of solids.[20] Because liquids and solids are handled differently by the stomach, the regulation of gastric emptying is correspondingly complicated, involving intrinsic regulation of motor activity as well as specific alterations associated with the ingestion of liquids and solids. Thus, although gastric emptying itself can be regarded as the final common pathway reflecting the motor activity of the stomach, one must keep in mind that the processes of liquid and solid emptying are regulated by quite different mechanisms.

There have been many reports of gastric motility during sleep, with sometimes contradictory results. Inhibition of gastric motility during sleep was documented in a study by Scantlebury et al.,[21] in which they implicated the "dream mechanism" as a part of this inhibitory process. A cortical inhibitory mechanism acting through the splanchnic nerve is the postulated mechanism of this inhibition. Nearly 30 years later, using somewhat more sophisticated measurement techniques, Bloom et al.[22] found that gastric motility was enhanced during sleep, compared with waking. Baust and Rohrwasser[23] studied gastric motility during PSG monitored sleep, and they also described a marked enhancement in gastric motility during sleep, but their findings were restricted to REM sleep. Only a year later, a decrease in gastric motility during REM sleep was reported.[24] No consistent findings concerning alterations by sleep stage were noted in a study in unanesthetized and unrestrained cats.[25]

Hall et al.[26] reported data on gastric emptying during sleep. This study required the patient to sleep with a nasogastric tube through which 750 ml of 10% glucose was administered. After 30 min, the gastric contents were aspirated, and the residual volume was determined. Aspiration was followed by a washout meal of 150 ml of saline. This process was done during the presleep waking interval, during NREM and REM sleep, and during postsleep waking. These data suggested a more rapid gastric emptying during REM sleep and a slower emptying during the postsleep waking state. The emptying of a hypertonic solution is controlled by vagally mediated osmoreceptors in the duodenum. These data, therefore, would suggest a possible anticholinergic action during REM and a cholinergic process during the postsleep waking state. These data represent only an approximation of the alterations in gastric emptying during sleep because these measurement techniques are relatively crude, and gastric emptying is a complex process.

Dubois et al.[27] have described a technique that permits the simultaneous assessment of acid secretion, water secretion, and the fractional rate of emptying. These techniques have been applied to the assessment of gastric functioning during sleep; the results indicate that in normal subjects, acid secretion, water secretion, and the fractional rate of emptying all showed significant decrements during sleep.[28] There did not appear to be any differences between REM and NREM sleep, but all of these measures demonstrated a significant difference between presleep waking and REM sleep. Data obtained by use of radionuclide emptying assessments suggest that this difference may be a circadian, rather than a sleep-dependent, effect. Studies by Goo et al.[29] have shown a marked delay in gastric emptying of solids in the evening, compared with the morning.

Gastric motor functioning is characterized by an endogenous electrical cycle generated by the gastric smooth muscle. The electrical rhythm is generated by a pacemaker located in the proximal portion of the greater curvature of the stomach.[30] The electrical cycle occurs at a frequency of approximately three per minute and represents the precursor to contractile activity of the stomach, which allows movement of gastric contents to the antrum and subsequent emptying into the duodenum.

The gastric electrical rhythm can be measured by surface electrodes placed in the periumbilical area. The identification of this basic motor function of the stomach requires highly sophisticated measurement, digital filtering, and spectral analysis to describe the parameters of this oscillation.[31] The noninvasive measurement of the gastric electrical rhythm is called *electrogastrography* (EGG). The progressive sophistication of the measurement and analytic techniques has allowed a reliable noninvasive technique to measure an important function of the GI system.

The sophisticated analysis of gastric electrical activity has documented three fundamental characteristics of this electrical rhythm that determine its normal activity. First, the power in the frequency band is approximately three per minute. This is essentially a method of quantifying the extent to which the wave approximates a sinusoidal rhythm, and the power reflects the peak-to-peak amplitude of the cycle. Second, more sophisticated techniques devised by Chen and colleagues[32] have allowed a minute-by-minute characterization of the cycle. This has permitted other parameters to describe the normal function of the gastric electrical rhythm. For example, 1-min segments can be analyzed for 15 to 20 min and the percentage of 1-min segments in which the peak amplitude is located at the dominant frequency can be calculated. Normal is approximately 70% or greater. Third, this technique of 1-min segmental analysis, termed *the running spectrum*, also allows determination of the instability coefficient, which describes the variability of the center frequency of the cycle. A larger coefficient means greater instability of the endogenous oscillation.

It has been generally thought that the gastric electrical rhythm is a product of the endogenous functioning of the gastric electrical pacemaker and that it is generally without influence from the CNS. However, sleep studies from our laboratory have challenged this traditional belief. Initially, our studies have shown a significant decline in the power in the three-per-minute cycle during NREM sleep.[33] There is a significant recovery of this toward the waking state during REM sleep. Further preliminary data from our laboratory have used running spectral analysis to describe a profound instability in the functioning of the basic electrical cycle during NREM sleep.[34] These two studies clearly suggest that NREM sleep is associated with a marked alteration or destabilization of the basic gastric electrical rhythm. It might be concluded from these results that higher cortical input or a degree of CNS arousal must be present in order to stabilize and promote normal gastric functioning and consequently normal gastric emptying.

It would seem clear from the results described that definitive statements concerning the alteration of gastric motor function and gastric emptying during sleep or specific sleep stages cannot be made. It would have to be concluded that gastric motor function appears to be retarded during sleep, but it is not clear whether this is specifically the result of altered gastric emptying attributable to sleep per se or whether this is simply a natural circadian rhythm independent of sleep.

SWALLOWING AND ESOPHAGEAL FUNCTION

Interest in esophageal function during sleep was stimulated by 24-h esophageal pH studies, which documented the important role of nocturnal gastroesophageal reflux (GER) in the pathogenesis of reflux esophagitis.[35] GER may occur in normal people even while upright and awake. This occurrence was identified primarily postprandially in normal subjects and was associated with multiple episodes of reflux that were relatively rapidly (in less than 5 min) neutralized. Studies by these investigators and others have documented that in normal individuals, sleep is relatively free of episodes of GER.[2, 36] However, when reflux does occur during sleep, it is associated with a marked prolongation in the acid clearance time. Data from these studies suggest that the prolongation in acid clearance during sleep is due to several factors. First, and perhaps most important, there is a delay in the conscious response to acid in the esophagus during sleep, and studies from our laboratory have documented that an arousal response almost invariably precedes the initiation of swallowing.[2, 37]

In fact, a relatively predictable and inverse relationship has been described between the acid clearance time and the amount of time the individual spends awake during the acid clearance interval. That is, if an individual responds with an awakening and subsequent swallowing when acid is infused in the distal esophagus during sleep, clearance is substantially faster than if an individual has a prolonged latency to the initial arousal response.[2, 37] Another important aspect of complete neutralization of the acidic distal esophagus is salivary flow. Helm et al.[38] demonstrated the importance of saliva in the final neutralization of the acidic esophagus. This finding is important because it has been shown that salivary flow stops completely with the onset of sleep, which would therefore substantially retard the acid neutralization.[39]

It is well known that swallowing initiates the acid clearance process, and, in general, swallowing is considered a volitional act. Thus, one would expect that it would be substantially depressed during altered states of consciousness, such as sleep. Studies by Lear et al.[40] and Lichter and Muir[41] have clearly confirmed this supposition by showing a significant diminution in swallowing frequency during sleep. Although the state of sleep certainly depresses the frequency of swallows, it appears that swallowing is usually associated with a brief arousal response.[2, 42] Studies on normal volunteers suggest that even though the swallowing frequency is substantially diminished during sleep, peristalsis appears to be completely normal.[2] This includes primary peristalsis, which is initiated by a swallow, and secondary peristalsis, which is not preceded by a swallow. However, in a study of cats, Anderson et al.[43] noted that, although swallowing frequencies diminished during sleep as noted in human beings, peristaltic amplitudes are hypotonic during REM sleep. Thus, it can be concluded that alterations in esophageal acid clearance during sleep would be primarily the result of two factors: decreased swallowing frequency and absence of salivary flow.

A study has addressed the issue of esophageal function during sleep and has clearly shown that esophageal motor activity is sleep stage dependent.[44] This study showed that the frequency of primary contractions in the esophagus (peristaltic contractions preceded by a swallow) diminish progressively from stage 1 to stage 4 sleep. Of interest is the fact that secondary peristaltic contractions (spontaneous contractions) showed a similar decline from waking to stage 4 sleep but showed a significant recovery during REM sleep. This suggests that spontaneous, or secondary, esophageal peristaltic contractions are perhaps more influenced by the endogenous level of CNS arousal. As has been described in previous studies, this study identified long periods of nocturnal esophageal motor quiescence with apparently random bursts of contractions.[45, 46] In contrast to a previous study, secondary peristaltic contractions during sleep were noted to be of diminished amplitude and shorter duration when compared with primary contractions.[2, 44] In addition, primary peristaltic contractions appeared to be of higher amplitude during sleep than during waking. This supports the notion that primary and secondary contractions may be controlled by different mechanisms and that waking CNS influences may inhibit primary peristaltic contractions. It would appear from these data that studying esophageal function during sleep allows a clearer understanding of central, peripheral, and enteric nervous system mechanisms controlling esophageal function.

The actual mechanism of GER during sleep has been addressed in an elegant study by Dent et al.[42] Via a specially designed monitoring device, the lower esophageal sphincter pressure was continuously monitored during sleep. In addition, a pH probe was placed in the distal esophagus to identify episodes of GER. They determined that the majority of episodes of reflux occurred in association with a spontaneous decline in the lower esophageal sphincter pressure to close to the intragastric pressure. This pressure decline creates a common cavity between the stomach and the esophagus, and because there is a 5-mmHg pressure gradient between the stomach and the midesophagus, this would create a situation particularly conducive to the reflux of gastric contents into the esophagus. The majority of these episodes were associated with a brief arousal response, although they were identified in some cases without movement. Other reflux events were noted to occur when the lower esophageal sphincter pressure was clearly above the intragastric baseline, thereby creating a pressure barrier to reflux. Under these circumstances, reflux occurs mechanically, by the creation of intraabdominal pressure that is sufficient to overcome the pressure barrier in the lower esophageal sphincter. Thus, reflux could occur under these circumstances during transient arousals from sleep associated with positional change, coughing, or swallowing.

The upper esophageal sphincter, created primarily by the cricopharyngeal muscle, serves as an additional protective barrier to prevent the aspiration of noxious material into the lungs. The upper esophageal sphincter is tonically contracted, and a pressure of between 40 and 80 mmHg usually exists within this sphincter. Swallowing induces a reflex relaxation to allow the positioning of food and liquids in the upper esophagus, where the normal peristaltic mechanism transports these materials into the stomach. The tonic contraction of the upper esophageal sphincter therefore prevents the ingestion of material into the esophagus with a previous volitional swallow. A study has documented relatively little change in the functioning of the upper esophageal sphincter during sleep, including REM sleep.[47] Only a modest decline in the resting pressure was noted. This observation is somewhat surprising because the cricopharyngeal muscle is a skeletal muscle, and if this finding can be verified, it would be one of the few skeletal muscles in the body that does not show a substantial inhibition during REM sleep. Obviously, persisting tone in the upper esophageal sphincter during REM sleep is advantageous because it protects the lungs from the aspiration of gastric contents. It should be pointed out that the subjects slept relatively poorly during this study, and, before any particular importance is ascribed to these findings, they should be replicated.

INTESTINAL MOTILITY

The primary functions of the small and large intestine are transport and absorption. These functions are intimately related in that, for example, rapid transit through the colon results in poor absorption and loose, watery stools, whereas slow transit results in increased water absorption, slow transit of fecal material to the rectum, and the clinical consequence of infrequent defecation and complaints of constipation. Alterations in the motor function of the lower bowel are evident from clinical phenomena, such as the occurrence of nocturnal diarrhea in diabetics and nocturnal fecal incontinence, which is commonly noted in patients with ileoanal anastomosis.[48]

The accessibility of the motility of the GI tract to monitoring decreases with distance from the oral cavity. The earliest attempts at measurement were purely observational. Cannon,[49] for example, fluoroscopically observed the progress of food through the intestines of the cat. Similar observational techniques were employed by subsequent investigators to describe the differences in intestinal motility during waking and sleep.[50, 51] These individuals exteriorized a small section of dog intestine and determined via visual observation that motility was relatively unaffected by sleep. In 1926, a similar fluoroscopic observation of exteriorized human intestine was made.[52] In agreement with the animal studies, these observations reported no change in intestinal motility during sleep.

Prolonged monitoring of the large and small bowel by use of a variety of sophisticated techniques, including telemetry, implanted microelectrodes, and suction electrodes, has allowed a more comprehensive description of intestinal motor activity. On the basis of these studies, tonic activity in the stomach and small bowel has been described as a basic electrical rhythm and as more phasic phenomena, such as the *migrating motor complex* (MMC), which is a wave of intestinal contraction beginning in the stomach and proceeding through the colon. The MMC consists of a dependent pattern of interdigestive motor phenomena. Subsequent to food ingestion there is an interval of motor quiescence termed *phase I*. This is followed by a period of somewhat random contractions throughout the small bowel and this is called *phase II*. Phase III describes a coordinated peristaltic burst of contractile activity that proceeds distally throughout the small bowel. Food ingestion establishes a pattern of vigorous contraction throughout the distal stomach and small bowel. If no food enters the stomach, the MMC cycle has a period of about 90 min.[53]

In a more recent study by Soffer and colleagues,[53] the activity of the MMC subsequent to a meal was assessed during waking and during subsequent sleep. In addition, they assessed the behavior of a variety of regulatory peptides. They concluded that postprandial intestinal motor activity was substantially altered by sleep, primarily a reduction in the fed pattern of intestinal motility. Because there was little appreciable alteration in peptide levels, the authors concluded that the alteration in small bowel motility was most likely neurally mediated. The authors noted that responses were similar to those described after vagotomy in the waking state. This suggests that reduced levels of arousal result in diminished vagal modulation of the ENS.

Archer et al.[54] described jejunal motor activity in 20 normal subjects during sleeping and waking and found no difference in the incidence of motor complexes. Thompson and Wingate[55] found that sleep prolonged the interval between motor complexes in the small intestine. A subsequent study by the same group revealed a sleep-related diminution in the number of contractions of a specific type in the jejunum.[56] These changes were also seen in patients with DU and vagotomies as well as in normal subjects, which suggests that this phenomenon is independent of vagal control and unaffected by duodenal disease. Finch et al.[57] addressed the issue of the alteration of the MMC during sleep. Their results showed a statistically significant relationship between REM sleep and the onset of MMCs originating in the duodenum.[57] Kumar et al.[58] described an obvious circadian rhythm in the propagation of the MMC, with the slowest velocities occurring during sleep. This finding appears to be the effect of a circadian rhythm rather than a true modulation by sleep. These results have been confirmed by Kellow et al.,[59] who also noted that the esophageal involvement in the MMC was decreased during sleep, with a corresponding tendency for MMCs to originate in the jejunum at night. Kumar et al.[60] examined the relationship between the MMC cycle and REM sleep. They found

that during sleep, there was a significant reduction in the MMC cycle length as well as the duration of phase II of the MMC. The MMCs were distributed equally between REM and NREM sleep with no obvious alteration in the parameters of the MMC by sleep stage. These data give evidence of alteration in periodic activity in the gut during sleep, but they are also consistent with the notion that the two cycles (i.e., MMCs and REM sleep) are independent. The same group of investigators have examined how the presence or absence of food in the GI tract alters small bowel motility during sleep.[61] A late evening meal restored phase II activity of the MMC, which is normally absent during sleep. These MMC changes during the sleeping interval have been substantially confirmed by subsequent ambulatory studies but without the benefit of PSG.[62, 63]

Sleep, intestinal motility, and symptoms of abdominal pain have been studied in patients with irritable bowel syndrome. Kellow et al.[64] found striking differences between sleeping and waking small bowel motor activity. The marked increase in contractility seen in the daytime is notably absent during sleep. In a related study, Kellow et al.[65] noted that propulsive clusters of small bowel motility were somewhat enhanced in the daytime in patients with irritable bowel syndrome, and this distinguished them from controls. Patients often had pain associated with these propulsive contractions, but there was no difference in small bowel activity between patients with irritable bowel syndrome and controls during sleep. Interestingly, Kumar et al.[66] have described an increase in REM sleep in patients with irritable bowel syndrome. They have proposed that this is evidence of a CNS abnormality in patients with this complex, enigmatic disorder.

With the development of more sophisticated electronic measuring and recording techniques, more accurate measures of intestinal motility have been possible in both animals and human beings. Unfortunately, these studies have produced results that conflict with those noted earlier from direct observation. Decreases in small intestinal motility during sleep were reported in two separate studies conducted 20 years apart.[67, 68] Specific duodenal recordings in human beings have been conflicting, showing no change in one instance and an increase in duodenal motility during sleep in another.[22, 69]

A different approach to duodenal recording was employed by Spire and Tassinari,[70] who recorded duodenal electromyographic (EMG) activity during various stages of sleep. They found an inhibition of duodenal EMG activity during REM sleep and an increase in activity with changes from one sleep phase to another. In a subsequent study, a decrease in duodenal EMG activity during sleep was described by the same group.[71] They also noted an activity rhythm of 80 to 120 min per cycle that was impervious to the changes associated with the sleep-waking cycle.

EFFECT OF INTESTINAL MOTILITY ON SLEEP

Although this chapter has concentrated on the effects of sleep on GI motility, there have been some fascinating studies addressing the issue of how intestinal motility may affect sleep. A practical and provocative thought concerning this issue relates to the familiar experience of postprandial somnolence. There is some question about whether it actually exists. These thoughts raise the issue of whether there may be changes in the GI system with food ingestion that could produce a hypnotic effect. Along these lines, an intriguing observation was made by Alverez[72] in 1920. He noted that distention of a jejunal balloon caused his human subject to drop off to sleep.[72] The hypnotic effects of afferent intestinal stimulation have also been documented in animal studies. Perhaps the most notable work was reported by Kukorelli and Juhasz,[73] who induced cortical synchronization in cats by both mechanical and electrical stimulation of the small bowel. These results were interpreted to be the effect of rapidly adapting phasic afferent fibers from the small intestine carried to the CNS via the splanchnic nerve. These data strongly suggest the existence of a hypnogenic effect of luminal distention.

In a subsequent study, these same investigators reported an increase in the duration of slow-wave sleep and an increase in the number of episodes of paradoxical sleep in cats subjected to low-level intestinal stimulation.[74] The authors also acknowledged the possible hypnogenic role of intestinal hormones such as cholecystokinin, and they cited a study by Rubenstein and Sonnenschein[75] in which administration of intestinal hormones produced a pronounced increase in paradoxical sleep episodes. The final common pathway of the afferent stimulation from the intestinal tract would presumably result in an increase in sleepiness subsequent to either luminal distention or hormonal secretion postprandially. In a fascinating study concerning neuronal processing during sleep, Pigarev[76] showed that neurons in the visual cortex, which usually respond to visual stimulation in the waking state, are activated during sleep by electrical stimulation of the stomach and small bowel.

In an attempt to document the presence of postprandial sleepiness objectively, a study was undertaken to measure sleep onset latency both with and without a prior meal.[77] Statistically, the results of this test did not support the presence of documentable postprandial sleepiness in 16 normal volunteers. However, it was obvious from these results that there was a small group of individuals in whom there was clearly a substantial decrease in the sleep onset latency after ingestion of a meal. This phenomenon seems to be affected by many variables: the volume of the meal, the meal constituents, and the circadian cycle of the individual. In a follow-up study, Orr and colleagues[78] tested the hypothesis that afferent stimulation from the gastric antrum would enhance postprandial sleepiness. This was tested by comparing an equal volume distention of the stomach with water to an equal caloric solid meal and liquid meal. Sleep onset latency was determined subsequent to each of these conditions. Because antral stimulation results from the digestion of a solid meal, sleep onset latency should be shorter subsequent to the consumption of the solid meal. This was confirmed in

this study in that the sleep onset latency after the solid meal was significantly shorter than the equal volume water condition. These results are compatible with the animal studies cited earlier and lend further support to the notion that contraction of the lumen of the GI tract produces afferent stimulation, which induces drowsiness.

COLONIC AND ANORECTAL FUNCTION

As noted, the colon has two main functions: transport and absorption. These are critically determined by the motor activity of the colon, which determines the rate of transport and, therefore, indirectly, the rate of absorption from the colonic lumen. Thus, alterations in colonic motility will have significant consequences in terms of transit through the colon and water absorption and ultimately clinical consequences such as constipation and diarrhea.

Adler et al.[79] described a decrease in colonic function during sleep. These results have been confirmed by two other studies that included measurements of the transverse, descending, and sigmoid colon.[80, 81] In the study by Narducci et al.,[81] a clear inhibition of colonic motility index is evident during sleep in the transverse, descending, and sigmoid colon segments, with a marked increase in activity on awakening. Certainly, this explains the common urge to defecate on awakening in the morning. Neither of these studies attempted to document sleep with standard PSG. However, in a study by Furukawa et al.,[82] colonic activity from cecum to rectum was monitored continuously for 32 h, and sleep was monitored via PSG. This study again noted a rather marked decrease in colonic motor activity during sleep, but it also described an interesting abolition in propagating waves during slow-wave sleep. During REM sleep, the frequency of propagating events rose substantially. Other studies do not provide evidence for any significant change in colonic motility or variability in the rectosigmoid colon during sleep.[83, 84] However, a study of colonic myoelectrical activity in the human being suggested a decrease in spike activity during sleep.[85] Again, this study does not determine whether the results are accounted for on the basis of true physiological sleep or simply reflect a circadian variation in colonic activity independent of sleep.

Collectively, these studies would suggest an inhibition of colonic contractile and myoelectric activity during sleep, and other studies have documented the fact that there is diminished colonic tone during sleep.[86] Resumption of the waking state, and consequently increased CNS arousal, would suggest two different effects on colonic motility. First, it appears that spontaneous awakening does induce high amplitude peristaltic contractions as described by Narducci and noted earlier, and this appears to be somewhat different than colonic motor activity induced by a sudden awakening from sleep. In a study by Bassotti et al.,[87] sudden awakening from sleep induced a pattern of segmental colonic contractions, rather than the propagating high amplitude peristaltic contractions noted in the study by Narducci and colleagues. These data are of considerable interest in that they demonstrate not only the influence of higher cortical functions on colonic motility but also the fact that these functions can affect the colon in rather subtle ways in terms of the induction of different patterns of colonic motility.

The striated muscle of the anal canal was evaluated during sleep in a 1953 study that included EEG documentation of sleep.[88] These investigators described a marked reduction in EMG activity during sleep. They concluded that this muscle is under voluntary control. In a study by Orkin et al.,[89] anal canal pressure was measured continuously during sleep, but without PSG monitoring. The results indicated a decrease in the minute-to-minute variation and the amplitude of spontaneous decreases in anal canal pressure during sleep. The structures of the rectum and anal canal are vital in maintaining normal bowel continence and ensuring normal defecation. In general, normal defecation is associated with sensory responses to rectal distention and appropriate motor responses of the muscles of the anal canal. These responses would include a contraction of the external anal sphincter and a transient decrease in the internal anal sphincter pressure associated with rectal distention. It is thought that the high resting basal pressure in the internal anal sphincter of the anal canal, as well as the response of the external anal sphincter to rectal distention, is critical in maintaining continence.

For assessment of the effect of sleep on these anorectal sensorimotor responses, 10 normal volunteers were studied during sleep with an anorectal probe in place. This probe permits the transient distention of the rectum via a rectal balloon while the responses of the internal and external anal sphincters can be simultaneously monitored.[90] This study documented a marked decrease—and, in most subjects, an abolition—of the external anal sphincter response to rectal distention. The internal anal sphincter response remained unaltered. In addition, there was no evidence of an arousal response with up to 50 ml of rectal distention during sleep. The normal threshold of response in the waking state is approximately 10 ml. These results confirm that the external anal sphincter response to rectal distention is most likely a learned response, whereas the internal anal sphincter response is clearly a reflex response to rectal distention because it persists during sleep. It also raises certain clinical questions with regard to the phenomenon of nocturnal diarrhea and the maintenance of fecal continence during sleep. In an ambulatory study of anorectal functioning, Kumar et al.[91] demonstrated that external anal sphincter contractions occurred periodically during sleep, and these periodic bursts of activity were followed by motor quiescence. These spontaneous contractions were associated with a rise in the anal canal pressure, but internal anal sphincter contractions were shown to occur independently of external anal sphincter activity.[91] The *sampling reflex*, which is a spontaneous relaxation of the internal anal sphincter, occurred frequently in the waking state but was markedly reduced during sleep.

A study by Rao and colleagues[3] has shed light on intrinsic anal-rectal functioning, which is altered during sleep. They confirmed the presence of an endogenous oscillation in rectal motor activity, and they have specifically noted that these bursts of cyclic rectal motor activity occupied approximately 44% of the overall recording time at night. They described the incidence of this motor activity to be nearly twofold greater at night than during the daytime. Of particular importance is the finding that the majority of contractions were propagated in a retrograde direction. Other studies have shown that rectal motor activity is not altered by REM sleep.[89] Studies by Ferrara[92] and Enck[93] and their respective colleagues have both shown that anal canal pressure is decreased during sleep. However, of particular interest is the fact that the study by Ferrara et al.[92] showed that even though there was a diminution in anal canal pressure during sleep, anal canal pressure was always greater than rectal pressure even in the presence of cyclic rectal motor activity.

These studies collectively shed important light on the mechanisms of rectal continence during sleep. There appear to be at least two mechanisms that prevent the passive escape of rectal contents during sleep. First, rectal motor activity increases substantially during sleep, but the propagation is retrograde rather than anterograde. Furthermore, these physiologic studies have shown that, even under the circumstances of periodic rectal contractions, the anal canal pressure is consistently above that of the rectum. Both of these mechanisms would tend to protect against rectal leakage during sleep, and alterations in these mechanisms would explain loss of rectal continence during sleep in individuals with diabetes or who have undergone ileal-anal anastomosis.

CONCLUSIONS

This chapter has described a variety of basic findings concerning the GI system and sleep. It is evident that there are marked alterations in the GI system during sleep, and these have numerous consequences in terms of normal digestive processes as well as digestive disease (reviewed in Chapter 94). Our understanding of the modulation of GI function by sleep has increased, and this has occurred in concert with substantially more sophisticated techniques for the measurement of smooth muscle functioning. Clearly, the past 50 years have shown a marked increase in interest in sleep and GI physiology, and this will undoubtedly continue as the importance of sleep physiology and pathophysiology is further revealed.

References

1. Champion MC, Orr WC, eds. Evolving Concepts in Gastrointestinal Motility. Oxford, England: Blackwell Science; 1996.
2. Orr WC, Johnson LF, Robinson MG. The effect of sleep on swallowing, esophageal peristalsis, and acid clearance. Gastroenterology. 1984;86:814–819.

3. Rao SS, Welcher K. Periodic rectal motor activity: the intrinsic colonic gatekeeper? Am J Gastroenterol. 1996;91:890–897.

4. Friedenwald J. On the influence of rest, exercise and sleep on gastric digestion. Am J Med. 1906;1:249–255.

5. Johnson RL, Washeim H. Studies in gastric secretion. Am J Physiol. 1924;70:247–253.

6. Henning N, Norpoth L. Die Magensekretion waehrend des Schlafes. Dtsch Arch Klin Med. 1932;172:558–562.

7. Banche M. La secrezione gastric notturna durante il sonno. Minerva Med. 1950;1:428–434.

8. Luckhardt AB. Contributions to the physiology of the empty stomach. Am J Physiol. 1915;39:330–333.

9. Wada T. Experimental study of hunger in its relation to activity. Arch Psychol. 1922;8:1–65.

10. Sandweiss DJ, Friedman HF, Sugarman MH, et al. Nocturnal gastric secretion. Gastroenterology. 1946;1:38–54.

11. Moore JG, Englert E. Circadian rhythm of gastric acid secretion in man. Nature. 1970;226:1261–1262.

12. Levin E, Kirsner JB, Palmer WL, et al. A comparison of the nocturnal gastric secretion in patients with duodenal ulcer and in normal individuals. Gastroenterology. 1948;10:952–964.

13. Feldman M, Richardson CT. Total 24-hour gastric acid secretion in patients with duodenal ulcer: comparison with normal subjects and effects of cimetidine and parietal cell vagotomy. Gastroenterology. 1986;90:540–544.

14. Dragstedt LR. A concept of the etiology of gastric and duodenal ulcers. Gastroenterology. 1956;30:208–220.

15. Levin E, Kirsner JB, Palmer WL, et al. The variability and periodicity of the nocturnal gastric secretion in normal individuals. Gastroenterology. 1948;10:939–951.

16. Reichsman F, Cohen J, Colwill J, et al. Natural and histamine-induced gastric secretion during waking and sleeping states. Psychosom Med. 1960;1:14–24.

17. Armstrong RH, Burnap D, Jacobson A, et al. Dreams and acid secretions in duodenal ulcer patients. New Physician. 1965;33:241–243.

18. Stacher G, Presslich B, Starker H. Gastric acid secretion and sleep stages during natural night sleep. Gastroenterology. 1975;68:1449–1455.

19. Orr WC, Hall WH, Stahl ML, et al. Sleep patterns and gastric acid secretion in duodenal ulcer disease. Arch Intern Med. 1976;136:655–660.

20. Dubois A, Castell DO. Abnormal gastric emptying response to pentagastrin in duodenal ulcer disease. Dig Dis Sci. 1981;26:292.

21. Scantlebury RE, Frick HL, Patterson TL. The effect of normal and hypnotically induced dreams on the gastric hunger movements of man. J Appl Physiol. 1942;26:682–691.

22. Bloom PB, Ross DL, Stunkard AJ, et al. Gastric and duodenal motility, food intake and hunger measured in man during a 24-hour period. Dig Dis Sci. 1970;15:719–725.

23. Baust W, Rohrwasser W. Das Verhalten von pH und Motilitat des Megens in naturlichen Schlaf des Menschen. Pflugers Arch. 1969;305:229–240.

24. Yaryura-Tobias HA, Hutcheson JS, White L. Relationship between stages of sleep and gastric motility. Behav Neuropsychiatry. 1970;2:22–24.

25. Fujitani Y, Hosogai M. Circadian rhythm of electrical activity and motility of the stomach in cats and their relation to sleep-wakefulness states. Tohoku J Exp Med. 1983;141:275–285.

26. Hall WH, Orr WC, Stahl ML. Gastric function during sleep. In: Brooks FP, Evers PW, eds. Nerves and the Gut. Thorofare, NJ: Slack; 1977:495–502.

27. Dubois A, Van Eerdewegh P, Gardner JD. Gastric emptying and secretion in Zollinger-Ellison syndrome. J Clin Invest. 1977;59:255.

28. Orr WC, Dubois A, Stahl ML, et al. Gastric function during sleep. Sleep Res. 1978;7:72.

29. Goo RH, Moore JG, Greenburg E, et al. Circadian variation in gastric emptying of meals in humans. Gastroenterology. 1987;93:515–518.

30. Chen JZ, McCallum RW, Familoni BO. Validity of the cutaneous electrogastrogram. Chen JZ, McCallum RW, eds. Electrogastrography: Principles and Applications. New York, NY: Raven Press; 1994:103–125.

31. Chen JZ, McCallum RW, Smout AJPM, et al. Acquisition and analysis of electrogastrographic data. Chen JZ, McCallum RW, eds. Electrogastrography: Principles and Applications. New York, NY: Raven Press; 1994:3–30.

32. Chen JZ, McCallum RW, Lin Z. Comparison of three running spectral analysis methods. Chen JZ, McCallum RW, eds. Electrogastrography: Principles and Applications. New York, NY: Raven Press; 1994:75–99.

33. Orr WC, Crowell MD, Lin B, et al. Sleep and gastric function in irritable bowel syndrome: derailing the brain-gut axis. Gut. 41:20.

34. Elsenbruch S, Harnish MJ, Orr WC, et al. Disruption of normal gastric myoelectric functioning by sleep. Sleep. 1999;22:453–458.

35. Johnson LF, DeMeester TR. Twenty-four-hour pH monitoring of the distal esophagus: A quantitative measure of gastroesophageal reflux. Am J Gastroenterol. 1974;62:325–332.

36. DeMeester TR, Johnson LF, Joseph CJ, et al. Patterns of gastroesophageal reflux in health and disease. Ann Surg. 1976;184:459–470.

37. Orr WC, Robinson MG, Johnson LF. Acid clearing during sleep in patients with esophagitis and controls. Dig Dis Sci. 1981;26:423.

38. Helm JF, Dodds WJ, Hogan WJ, et al. Acid neutralizing capacity of human saliva. Gastroenterology. 1982;83:69–74.

39. Schneyer LH, Pigman W, Hanahan L, et al. Rate of flow of human parotid, sublingual, and submaxillary secretions during sleep. J Dent Res. 1956;35:109–114.

40. Lear CSC, Flanagan JB Jr, Moorees CFA. The frequency of deglutition in man. Arch Oral Biol. 1965;10:83–96.

41. Lichter J, Muir RC. The pattern of swallowing during sleep. Electroencephalogr Clin Neurophysiol. 1975;38:427–432.

42. Dent J, Dodds WJ, Friedman RH, et al. Mechanism of gastroesophageal reflux in recumbent asymptomatic human subjects. J Clin Invest. 1980;65:256–257.

43. Anderson CA, Dick TE, Orem J. Swallowing in sleep and wakefulness in adult cats. Sleep. 1995;18:325–329.

44. Castiglione F, Emde C, Armstrong D, et al. Nocturnal oesophageal motor activity is dependent on sleep stage. Gut. 1993;34:1653–1659.

45. Armstrong D, Emde C, Bumm R, et al. Twenty-four-hour pattern of esophageal motility in asymptomatic volunteers. Dig Dis Sci. 1990;35:1659.

46. Smout AJPM, Breedijk M, van der Zouw C, et al. Physiological gastroesophageal reflux and esophageal motor activity studied with a new system for 24-hour recording and automated analysis. Dig Dis Sci. 1989;34:1659.

47. Kahrilas PJ, Dodds WJ, Dent J, et al. Effect of sleep, spontaneous gastroesophageal reflux, and a meal on upper esophageal sphincter pressure in normal human volunteers. Gastroenterology. 1987;92:466–467.

48. Metcalf AM, Dozois RR, Kelly KA, et al. Ileal J pouch-anal anastomosis: clinical outcome. Ann Surg. 1985;202:735–739.

49. Cannon WB. The movements of the intestine studied by means of the roentgen rays. Am J Physiol. 1902;6:275–276.

50. Barcroft J, Robinson CS. A study of some factors influencing intestinal movements. Am J Physiol. 1929;67:211–220.

51. Douglas DM, Mann FG. An experimental study of the rhythmic contractions in the small intestine of the dog. Am J Dig Dis. 1977;6:318–322.

52. Hines LE, Mead HCA. Peristalsis in a loop of small intestine. Arch Intern Med. 1926;38:539.

53. Soffer EE, Adrian TE, Launspach J, et al. Meal-induced secretion of gastrointestinal regulatory peptides is not affected by sleep. Neurogastroenterol Motil. 1997;9:7–12.

54. Archer L, Benson MJ, Green WJ, et al. Radiotelemetric measurement of normal human small bowel motor activity during prolonged fasting. J Physiol. 1979;296:53.

55. Thompson DG, Wingate DL. Characterisation of interdigestive and digestive motor activity in the normal human jejunum. Gut. 1979;20:A943.

56. Ritchie HD, Thompson DG, Wingate DL. Diurnal variation in human jejunal fasting motor activity. In: Proceedings of the American Physiological Society; March 1980; 54–55.

57. Finch P, Ingram D, Henstridge J, et al. The relationship of sleep stage to the migrating gastrointestinal complex of man. In: Christensen J, ed. Gastrointestinal Motility. New York, NY: Raven Press; 1980: 261–265.

58. Kumar D, Wingate D, Ruckebusch Y. Circadian variation in the

propagation velocity of the migrating motor complex. Gastroenterology. 1986;91:926–930.

59. Kellow JE, Borody TJ, Phillips SF, et al. Human interdigestive motility: variations in patterns from esophagus to colon. Gastroenterology. 1986;91:386–395.

60. Kumar D, Idzikowski C, Wingate DL, et al. Relationship between enteric migrating motor complex and the sleep cycle. Am J Physiol. 1990;259(6pt1):G983–G940.

61. Kumar D, Soffer EE, Wingate DL, et al. Modulation of the duration of human postprandial motor activity by sleep. Am J Physiol. 1989;256(5pt1):G851–G855.

62. Wilson P, Perdikis G, Hinder RA, et al. Prolonged ambulatory antroduodenal manometry in humans. Am J Gastroenterol. 1994;89:1489–1495.

63. Wilmer A, Andrioli A, Coremans G, et al. Ambulatory small Intestinal manometry. Detailed comparison of duodenal and jejunal motor activity in healthy man. Dig Dis Sci. 1997;42:1618–1627.

64. Kellow JE, Gill RC, Wingate DL. Prolonged ambulant recordings of small bowel motility demonstrate abnormalities in the irritable bowel syndrome. Gastroenterology. 1990;98:1208–1218.

65. Kellow JE, Phillips SF. Altered small bowel motility in irritable bowel syndrome is correlated with symptoms. Gastroenterology. 1987;92:1885–1893.

66. Kumar D, Thompson PD, Wingate DL, et al. Abnormal REM sleep in the irritable bowel syndrome. Gastroenterology. 1992;103:12–17.

67. Helm JD, Kramer P, MacDonald RM, et al. Changes in motility of the human small intestine during sleep. Gastroenterology. 1948;10:135–137.

68. Sadler HH, Orten AU. The complementary relationship between the emotional state and the function of the ileum in a human subject. Am J Psychiatry. 1968;124:1377–1381.

69. Bloom PB, Ross DL, Stunkard AJ, et al. Gastric and duodenal motility, food intake and hunger measured in man during a 24-hour period. Dig Dis Sci. 1970;15:719–725.

70. Spire JP, Tassinari CA. Duodenal EMG activity during sleep. Electroencephalogr Clin Neurophysiol. 1971;31:179–183.

71. Tassinari CA, Coccagna G, Mantovani M, et al. Duodenal EMG activity during sleep in man. In: Jovanovic UJ, ed. The Nature of Sleep. Stuttgart, Germany: Gustav Fischer Verlag; 1973.

72. Alverez WC. Physiologic studies on the motor activities of the stomach and bowel in man. Am J Physiol. 1920;88:658–660.

73. Kukorelli T, Juhasz G. Sleep induced by intestinal stimulation in cats. Physiol Behav. 1976;19:355–358.

74. Juhasz G, Kukorelli T. Modifications of visceral evoked potentials during sleep in cats. Act Nerv Super (Praha). 1977;19:212–214.

75. Rubenstein EH, Sonnenschein RR. Sleep cycles and feeding behavior in the cat: role of gastrointestinal hormones. Acta Cient Venez. 1971;22:125–128.

76. Pigarev IN. Neurons of visual cortex respond to visceral stimulation during slow wave sleep. Neuroscience. 1994;62:1237–1243.

77. Stahl ML, Orr WC, Bollinger C. Postprandial sleepiness: objective documentation via polysomnography. Sleep. 1983;6:29–35.

78. Orr WC, Shadid G, Harnish MJ, et al. Meal composition and its effect on postprandial sleepiness. Physiol Behav. 1997;62:709–712.

79. Adler HF, Atkinson AJ, Ivy AC. A study of the motility of the human colon: an explanation of dyssynergia of the colon, or of the unstable colon. Am J Dig Dis. 1941;8:197–202.

80. Rosenblum MJ, Cummins AJ. The effect of sleep and of Amytal on the motor activity of the human sigmoid colon. Gastroenterology. 1954;27:445–450.

81. Narducci F, Bassotti G, Gaburri M, et al. Twenty four hour manometric recording of colonic motor activity in healthy man. Gut. 1987;28:17–25.

82. Furukawa V, Cook IJ, Panagopoulos V, et al. Relationship between sleep patterns and human colonic motor patterns. Gastroenterology. 1991;100(pt 2):A444. Gastroenterology. 1994;107:1372–1381.

83. Kerlin P, Zinsmeister A, Phillips S. Motor responses to food of the ileum, proximal colon, and distal colon of healthy humans. Gastroenterology. 1983;84:762–770.

84. Posey EL, Bargen JA. Observations of normal and abnormal human intestinal motor function. Am J Med Sci. 1951;221:10–20.

85. Frexinos J, Bueno L, Fioramonti J. Diurnal changes in myoelectric spiking activity of the human colon. Gastroenterology. 1985;88:1104–1110.

86. Steadman CJ, Phillips SF, Camilleri M, et al. Variations of muscle tone in the human colon. Gastroenterology. 1991;101:24.

87. Bassotti G, Bucaneve G, Betti C, et al. Sudden awakening from sleep: effects on proximal and distal colonic contractile activity in humans. Eur J Gastroenterol Hepatol. 1990;2:6.

88. Floyd WF, Walls EW. Electromyography of the sphincter and externus in man. J Physiol. 1953;122:599–609.

89. Orkin BA, Hanson RB, Kelly KA, et al. Human anal motility while fasting, after feeding, and during sleep. Gastroenterology. 1991;100:1016–1023.

90. Whitehead WE, Orr WC, Engel BT, et al. External anal sphincter response to rectal distention: learned response or reflex. Psychophysiology. 1981;19:57–62.

91. Kumar D, Waldron D, Williams NS, et al. Prolonged anorectal manometry and external anal sphincter electromyography in ambulant human subjects. Dig Dis Sci. 1990;35:641–648.

92. Ferrara A, Pemberton JH, Levin KE, et al. Relationship between anal canal tone and rectal motor activity. Dis Colon Rectum. 1993;36:337–342.

93. Enck P, Eggers E, Koletzko S, et al. Spontaneous variation of anal "resting" pressure in healthy humans. Am J Physiol. 1991;261:G823–G826.

22

Temperature Regulation

Steven F. Glotzbach
H. Craig Heller

The regulation of body temperature is controlled by the autonomic nervous system which uses many sources of information to generate specific thermoregulatory responses, including evaporative water loss (e.g., sweating, panting), metabolic sleep production (e.g, shivering), and changes in thermal conductivity across the skin by vasomotor adjustments. Characteristics of thermoregulatory control vary significantly between states of sleep and wakefulness, and with time of day. Human studies have shown changes in thermoregulatory responses with vigilance state changes, and animal studies have shown changes in the central nervous system (CNS) feedback sensitivity controlling thermoregulatory responses with state changes. Thus the regulation of body temperature is modulated by the circadian system and by sleep control mechanisms.

Body temperature is regulated at a lower level during nonrapid eye movement (NREM) sleep than during wakefulness, but thermoregulation is mostly suspended during rapid eye movement (REM) sleep. In addition to vigilance states determining the characteristics of the thermoregulatory system, body temperature and the thermal environment are important determinants of sleep architecture. The relationships between sleep and thermoregulatory homeostasis have important implications for a variety of clinical problems, ranging from sudden infant death syndrome (SIDS) to sleep disorders associated with the uncoupling of normally phase-linked circadian rhythms of sleep and body temperature.

The regulation of body temperature (T_b) is remarkably precise in spite of large changes in metabolic heat production and in the exchange of thermal energy between the body and the environment. Thermal balance, the matching of heat loss and heat gain so that T_b remains constant, is achieved by the variable activation of a number of effector mechanisms, including evaporative water loss due to sweating or panting, metabolic heat production due to shivering or nonshivering thermogenesis, changes in thermal conductivity across the skin due to vasomotor adjustments, and thermoregulatory behavior (such as changes in posture). These effector mechanisms are controlled by the autonomic nervous system, which uses a variety of sources of information to generate command signals for specific effectors. Thermoregulatory responses are dependent upon a number of other factors such as skin temperature, time of day, and vigilance state.

The effects of arousal state transitions on thermoregulatory effector responses are due largely to changes in characteristics of a hierarchically, multilevel, central nervous system (CNS) "thermostat," dominated by integrative properties of certain hypothalamic nuclei. Conversely, changes in the thermal environment have powerful effects on arousal state transitions and the distribution of arousal states. In humans and other mammals, the sleep phase of the daily rest-activity cycle is associated with decreases in metabolic rate (MR) and T_b. In addition, the onset of sleep at any time of day tends to result in declines in MR (reviewed in references 1–5). These observations raise a number of questions crucial to an understanding of the relationship between sleep and homeostasis, which have important implications for a variety of clinical problems ranging from sudden infant death syndrome (SIDS) to sleep disorders associated with the uncoupling of normally phase-linked circadian rhythms of sleep and T_b.

First, is the decline in MR and T_b at the onset of sleep simply due to decreased motor and digestive activity or is it a regulated lowering of metabolism or T_b, or both? Second, are the daily cycles of MR and T_b due to direct influences of sleep control mechanisms or are they due to circadian rhythms which are normally phase-locked to the sleep-activity rhythm, or both? Third, if alterations in T_b and thermoregulatory effectors are due to sleep control mechanisms, are they linked to specific sleep states? Finally, how do changes in body and ambient temperatures influence arousal state distributions? We focus on human studies wherever possible in this chapter to address these questions, to review what is known about the relationship between temperature, temperature regulation, and arousal state control, and to discuss directions for further research and clinical applications in these areas.

Some of the conclusions reached in this chapter are: (1) thermoregulation is influenced both by sleep and circadian factors; (2) T_b is regulated at a lower level during nonrapid eye movement (NREM) sleep than during wakefulness (AW); (3) during rapid eye movement (REM) sleep, there is a marked inhibition of thermoregulation; (4) T_b and the thermal environment are important determinants of arousal state distribution; and (5) the relationship between sleep and temperature may be applicable to the understanding and treatment of a variety of clinical sleep disorders.

METABOLISM DECREASES DURING SLEEP RELATIVE TO WAKEFULNESS

The decline in MR during sleep cannot be simply a consequence of decreased motor and digestive activity because it occurs in fasted subjects, patients on total bed rest, and even in paralyzed humans.[4] Also, the daily decline in MR cannot be due entirely to sleep because it occurs in subjects deprived of sleep.[6–8] Clearly, both sleep and circadian factors influence MR. The mechanisms underlying these separate influences are discussed later in conjunction with information on regulation of T_b, but first, changes in MR specific to electroencephalographically defined arousal states are discussed.

A number of studies on rats have shown that MR (as measured by heat production) is lower in NREM sleep than in AW and lower in REM sleep than in NREM sleep.[9–11] These relationships hold at ambient temperatures ranging from high thermoneutrality (35°C) to considerably below thermoneutrality (15°C), where *thermoneutrality* is defined as the ambient temperature (T_a) range within which MR is minimal. Metabolic heat production in nonhuman mammals during sleep decreases 5 to 29% from waking levels.[12]

In humans, the mean drop in metabolism reported in different studies between AW and the sleep minima is on the order of 5 to 17%.[13–17] It should be emphasized that there is considerable intersubject variability in many of these studies. Moreover, metabolic differences between waking and sleep increase at ambient temperatures below thermoneutrality.[5] For example, Palca et al.[16] reported a 40% drop in oxygen consumption during sleep in a naked subject at $T_a = 21°C$. An explanation for this T_a effect of lowering of MR during sleep is based on the lowering of regulated T_b during sleep, which is discussed later. The reduction in regulated T_b is less likely to be reflected in a decrease in MR when the animal or human being is under thermoneutral conditions.

Data on MR in sleeping humans as a function of arousal state are distinctly different from those of animal studies. The pioneering study of Brebbia and Altshuler[18] showed higher metabolism in REM sleep than in NREM sleep stages 3 and 4. This result has been confirmed,[16, 19, 20] but other studies have revealed no difference in MR when comparing REM sleep and NREM sleep episodes.[15, 17, 21] Studies that address this question must take into account circadian effects on MR when comparing MR in different sleep states. For example, in one study,[16] MR in REM sleep was significantly higher than NREM sleep when contiguous episodes were analyzed, but there was no significant difference between REM sleep and NREM sleep when data across the entire night were pooled. Another critical variable is T_a; there is a tendency for the difference between MRs measured in REM sleep and NREM sleep to be greater at lower T_a.[19]

Therefore, in adult humans, MR either shows no change or is elevated in REM sleep compared to NREM sleep; in contrast, results from animal studies show a clear *decrease* in MR in REM sleep compared to NREM sleep. A probable explanation for the human-nonhuman difference in direction of change in MR between REM sleep and NREM sleep is the large contribution of brain metabolism to total MR in humans, and the increase in cerebral blood flow and brain metabolism in humans during REM sleep.[22–25] As shown in this review, the drop in MR between AW and NREM sleep seen in all mammals is due primarily to alterations in the thermoregulatory system between these two states.

THERMOREGULATORY RESPONSES ARE HIGHLY SLEEP STATE DEPENDENT

Even before the use of electroencephalography (EEG), changes in T_b and thermoregulatory responses at sleep onset in humans suggested that T_b is actively regulated at a lower level in sleep than during AW. Day's observation[26] that declines in rectal temperatures of napping children were coincident with increased evaporative water loss and elevated skin temperatures at sleep onset provided strong evidence of a readjustment of the thermoregulatory system coincident with sleep. Decreases in rectal temperature or increases in skin temperature have been reported routinely at the onset of sleep in adult humans sleeping in neutral or cool environments.[27–29] In neutral or warm environments, an increase in sweat rate has been observed at sleep onset.[30, 31] Studies on humans and animals in which sleep and AW were measured with standard electrophysiological montages have extended earlier observations on the changes in thermoregulatory control during NREM sleep, compared to AW, and have produced evidence that thermoregulation is disturbed during REM sleep.

It is commonly observed in animal studies that brain temperature (T_{br}) falls during NREM sleep, compared to AW, but increases in REM sleep relative to NREM sleep (see references 4, 32 for extensive reviews). Changes in T_{br} can be influenced by (1) changes in the temperature of the blood perfusing the brain, (2) changes in cerebral metabolism, and (3) changes in cerebral blood flow.[33–35] Changes in blood flow during NREM sleep reflect thermoregulatory vasomotor adjustments and depend on the T_a. In contrast, REM sleep appears to be a state in which changes in regional blood flow indicate a disruption in thermal homeostasis; the direction of change in blood flow depends solely on the prevailing vasomotor state in NREM sleep. Vasodilated vascular beds showed decreased blood flow and constricted beds showed increased flow in REM sleep, compared to NREM sleep.[36, 37]

Thermoregulatory responses to changes in peripheral or core body temperatures in animal studies show qualitatively different responses in NREM compared to REM sleep. At high T_a, panting increases in cats and pigeons in NREM sleep, compared with AW, which suggests that the increase in heat loss in NREM sleep results from a decrease in the set-point for heat loss responses at sleep onset.[38, 39] In contrast, transitions from NREM sleep to REM sleep are characterized by a disruption of ongoing thermoregulation. Panting is inhibited in REM sleep,[32, 39, 40] although panting mechanisms continue to operate during REM sleep in cats at high T_a, and the degree of panting is proportional to the heat load.[41] Shivering is present during NREM sleep at low T_a, but in REM sleep, ongoing shivering ceases.[9, 40, 42-44] In addition, the temperature of rat interscapular brown adipose tissue increases during cold exposure in NREM sleep, but decreases in REM sleep.[45]

Thermoregulatory responses in people are markedly inhibited during REM sleep. Shivering during sleep in cool environments is confined to NREM sleep stages 1 and 2 and is not seen in NREM sleep stages 3 or 4 or during REM sleep.[19, 46] It is not known whether the thresholds for shivering are lowered during these latter stages or whether the stimulus to shiver is arousing, thus decreasing those states. Evidence from skin and body temperature measurements in subjects selected for their ability to sleep in the cold has been interpreted as suggesting that some aspects of thermoregulatory control may remain intact during REM sleep.[16]

Disruption of thermal effector mechanisms in REM sleep is not limited to heat production; reduction of sweating during REM sleep in subjects in neutral or warm T_a indicates impairment of heat loss effector mechanisms as well.[47-49] The sharp declines in sweat rate associated with REM sleep often precede the onset of REM sleep by 2 to 3 min, consistent with the finding that some REM sleep processes precede electrophysiologically defined REM sleep. Measurements of sweating from subjects at a warm T_a show that evaporative water loss declines sharply at the onset of REM sleep, reaches minimal levels in REM sleep, and rises sharply at the termination of REM sleep.[47-49] Cessation of sweating and increases in skin temperature were accompanied by elevations in rectal temperature of 0.2°C.[49] Evaporative water loss measured from sweat capsules placed on the chest of subjects sleeping in warm environments demonstrated a sleep-dependent change in evaporative water loss; the sweat rate was higher in NREM sleep stages 3 and 4 than in NREM sleep stages 1 and 2, and lowest in REM sleep.[50, 51]

Buguet et al.[52] measured thermoregulatory adjustments during sleep in a patient with anhidrotic dysplasia, a congenital syndrome in which sweat glands are absent. Compared to a control subject, in whom sweating in a warm environment (32.2°C) decreased during REM sleep and T_b decreased during the night, the patient showed no sleep state–dependent change in evaporative water loss and had minimal changes in T_b. Despite the fact that increased convective and radiative heat loss avenues were potentially available by virtue of a higher mean skin temperature, the patient exhibited disturbed sleep as indicated by increased AW and sleep stage 1, less REM sleep, and more state transitions compared to the control subject.

Although evaporative water loss reaches basal levels in REM sleep in subjects sleeping in a warm environment, increases in sweat rate occur during the phasic events of REM sleep, such as during bursts of rapid eye movements.[47] This finding raises the possibility that increases in evaporative water loss during REM sleep may be psychogenic (related to dream content) and not thermoregulatory. Alternatively, inhibition impinging on the thermoregulatory system may be released briefly during the phasic events of REM sleep.

It has been observed that mean T_b was positively correlated with T_a in REM sleep (but not during stage 4 NREM sleep) during heat exposure, which indicates that changes in T_b occur passively in REM sleep in relation to the heat load.[53]

The studies cited in this discussion support the concept that thermoregulatory mechanisms are intact in NREM sleep and inhibited in REM sleep. However, results from numerous studies of changes in skin and body temperatures during REM sleep are extremely variable and do not always support this general conclusion.

In evaluating these studies, it is necessary to keep in mind that changes in blood pressure, blood flow, and peripheral vasomotor tone are under the influence of several systems interacting independently of or in concert with thermoregulation.[54] For example, skin temperature changes are influenced by heat transfer from the skin surface as well as convective and conductive transfer of heat to the surface from deeper tissues. The methods and sites of attaching thermistors and thermocouples to the skin and the amount of insulating covers are important variables that may affect experimental results.

AMBIENT AND BODY TEMPERATURES PROFOUNDLY INFLUENCE SLEEP STRUCTURE

Ambient Temperature

Because thermoregulatory abilities differ with arousal state, one might expect thermal stress to elicit arousal or a shift in the distribution of sleep states. Indeed, environmental temperature has a prominent influence on both the amount and distribution of arousal states. Therefore, accurate comparisons of both interspecies and intraspecies sleep state distributions require information on the thermal environment *and* the thermal neutral zones of the subjects. Parmeggiani and colleagues[40, 55] first showed in cats that total sleep time (TST) is maximal within the thermoneutral zone (TNZ) and decreases above and below the TNZ. Moreover, the NREM sleep-to-REM sleep ratio increases as T_a deviates from thermoneutrality, which is due primarily to a reduction in the number of epochs of REM sleep. These results have been subsequently confirmed and extended in several animal models.[56-62] A key observation in the study of Alfoldi et al.[62] was that the temperature effects on sleep were more prominent during the light phase compared with the dark phase of the diurnal cycle. These results underscore the importance of considering time-of-day effects on the relationship between temperature and sleep, which can be ascertained only by recordings that are substantially longer than a few hours.

REM sleep is influenced by peripheral temperature even within thermoneutrality. When both oxygen consumption and sleep distribution were measured in rats at T_a between 23 and 33°C, NREM sleep did not vary between $T_a = 23$ to 31°C and MR was constant between 25 and 31°C. However, the amount of REM sleep varied significantly in this range, peaking at $T_a = 29$°C.[10] A marked depression of REM sleep occurred at $T_a = 33$°C. Previous work on rats showed a maximum REM sleep propensity at a T_a closer to 33°C than to 29°C.[56, 57] The reasons for these discrepancies are not clear but could be due to differences in heat tolerance, weight, or acclimation of the animals. Another important finding is that slow wave delta activity increases after relatively small elevations in ambient[63] and hypothalamic temperatures,[64] even when there is no significant change in the overall percentage of NREM sleep.

The studies just described were all conducted at constant T_a, but acute changes in the thermal environment *during* NREM sleep can also influence the subsequent distribution of AW and sleep. In rats sleeping at ambient temperatures above (34°C), or below (23°C), thermoneutrality showed increased transitions into REM sleep if T_a was changed *toward* thermoneutrality during sleep. In contrast, if T_a was changed *away* from thermoneutrality, transitions into REM sleep were fewer, while transitions to AW increased, compared with control rats sleeping at $T_a = 29$°C.[65]

The influence of T_a on sleep state distribution has been studied in humans.[16, 46, 53, 66–69] In a cold environment, there was an increase in AW, sleep latency, and movement time, and the decrease in sleep time was due mostly to decreased REM sleep and stage 2 NREM sleep.[46, 67] However, Palca et al.[16] reported that subjects selected for their claimed ability to sleep in the cold showed an increase in AW and a decrease in NREM sleep stage 2 but no decrease in REM sleep when tested at a cold (21°C) vs. a neutral (29°C) T_a.

Increased AW and reductions in both REM sleep and NREM sleep are seen during nocturnal sleep in warm environments.[53, 68] When subjects were exposed to a range of ambient temperatures, TST, NREM sleep stages 3 and 4, and REM sleep were maximum at thermoneutrality ($T_a = 29$°C), and progressively decreased as T_a deviated from thermoneutrality. REM sleep duration also peaked in the thermoneutral zone, significantly decreasing outside of thermoneutrality.[66]

Fragmentation of sleep seen during the night at high temperatures can result in changes in sleep measures during recovery sleep. Libert et al.[70] recorded changes in sleep before, during, and after continuous (24 h), multiday exposure of subjects to a warm (35°C) environment. Although sleep was more fragmented at the warm T_a as manifested by decreased TST and increased AW, there were no differences in the amount of delta sleep or REM sleep between the baseline (20°C) and experimental conditions. TST and stage 3 NREM sleep increased, and the number of epochs of AW and the number of transient arousals in REM sleep decreased

in recovery sleep only. In a follow-up study,[71] the combined influences of heat and noise on sleep organiza-onfirmed that heat exposure significantly increased the number of transient arousals without clear changes in the overall amounts of slow-wave sleep (SWS) and REM sleep. Heat was more potent as a disrupter of sleep than was noise, and the disturbing effects of heat and noise were more prominent during the last third of the night. Finally, thermal stimulation *during* REM sleep was more likely to lead to a state change, especially in response to cooling, compared to NREM sleep.[72]

In summary, results from animal and human studies have shown that T_a is an important determinant of both the quantity and quality of sleep. TST is maximum in thermoneutrality and decreases above and below the TNZ. REM sleep appears to be more sensitive than NREM sleep to deviations of air temperature outside of thermoneutrality. Because of the decrease in sleep efficiency in the elderly, more work needs to be done investigating how the relationship between T_a and sleep organization changes with age. For example, in both young and aged cats, sleep was disrupted as T_a decreased (range 35 to 5°C), although transient arousals in NREM sleep were significantly higher in the aged group at temperature extremes.[73]

BODY TEMPERATURE

The relationship between the duration of sleep, REM sleep propensity, and the phase of the T_b rhythm at sleep onset has been the focus of much work and will be discussed further in the following section on circadian rhythms of T_b and sleep. Here, results from other studies showing the correlation between T_b and sleep parameters are reviewed. Exercise and passive heating of subjects have been used to examine the influence of elevated T_b on sleep. In one study,[74] trained subjects ran on a treadmill or were passively heated in a warm-water tank during the afternoon such that core temperature rose 2°C above resting levels. Both passive heating and high-intensity exercise increased NREM sleep stages 3 and 4 and had no effect on REM sleep. These effects appeared to be due primarily to the influence of core temperature on sleep. This conclusion was further substantiated by recordings of sleep parameters after exercise with and without body cooling.[75] When the normal rise in core temperature of about 2°C during exercise was limited to 1°C by facilitating heat loss during running, nocturnal sleep parameters did not differ from baseline recordings. Horne and Reid[76] later measured the effects of passive heating (to increase core temperature 1.8°C) vs. immersion in cooler water (which caused no change in T_b) on sleep in both fit and unfit subjects. Whereas the neutral condition caused no change in sleep parameters, passive heating in both groups of subjects resulted in an increase of both sleepiness at bedtime and stage 4 sleep. REM sleep decreased slightly, especially in the first REM sleep period.

Further studies have investigated the temporal relationship of imposed core temperature changes on sleep parameters in adult humans. Horne and Shackell[77] speculated that larger "doses" of heating are needed to increase SWS as the time between heating and bedtime increases. Circadian influences may play a role, however, because heatings given at 7.5 vs. 2.5 h before bedtime are at different phases in the circadian temperature rhythm. Pretreatment of the subjects with aspirin (600 mg) at the time of a "late" heating (2.5 h before bedtime) neutralized the increase in SWS, even though the T_b rise *during the heating* was the same in the aspirin-treated and experimental groups. Unfortunately, T_b measurements were not available during the sleep period. These authors speculate that aspirin blocks the heating-induced rise in brain prostaglandin levels, which have been shown to increase NREM sleep in rodents. Of interest is the fact that prostaglandin synthesis inhibitors damp the core temperature rhythm in rats by reducing the nocturnal rise in T_b,[78] which led Horne and Shackell to speculate that the circadian rise in the threshold hypothalamic temperature (T_{set}) may be mediated by prostaglandins.

Bunnell et al.[79] also measured the relationship between passive body heating in the morning, afternoon, early evening, and late evening (immersion in water at 41°C for 1 h) and subsequent sleep changes. Increases in SWS delta activity were seen only following the evening heating periods. A recent study suggests that passive heating by a hot bath prior to bedtime may be useful in ameliorating insomnia in the elderly.[80]

Shapiro et al.[81] also noted changes in sleep following 4-h exposure to 15, 25, 35, or 45°C T_a ending 90 min before bedtime. The young male subjects, who slept at ambient temperatures of 19 to 26°C, had significantly reduced AW and increased SWS after exposure to environments of 35 and 45°C; REM sleep was highest after exposure to the thermoneutral (25°C) T_a.

Some question exists as to whether SWS parameters are related more to the T_b at sleep onset,[82] or to the rate of fall in T_b following sleep onset.[83] To address the question, Jordan et al.[84] repeated earlier passive heating protocols with the important addition of measuring rectal temperature *during the sleep period*. These investigators found that passive heating resulted in a sustained elevation of rectal temperature of about 0.2°C, compared with controls, throughout the night. In addition, both REM sleep and NREM sleep were significantly increased during the first part of the night in this study, and thus increases in NREM sleep were not due to a suppression of REM sleep. Finally, the increase in NREM sleep during the first 150 min of the sleep period could not be accounted for by the rate of change of T_b, which did not differ significantly from control subjects. These authors concluded that the amount of delta sleep is a function of the level of T_b at sleep onset, in agreement with previous studies by Berger et al.[82] Some recent studies have implicated the dynamics of T_b decline in the timing of sleep onset.[85, 86]

It seems clear that body heating before bedtime increases NREM sleep, but how does body heating *during* the sleep period influence sleep? To investigate this question, the core temperatures of subjects were elevated during the late part of the night when REM sleep propensity is high, stage 4 propensity is low, and T_b is normally at its circadian nadir.[87] Contrary to the expectation that body heating would suppress REM sleep when heating took place at the normal temperature nadir, REM sleep parameters following the 2.5°C elevation in core temperature did not change, but NREM sleep stages 2 through 4 increased significantly in the fourth NREM sleep cycle. Despite the differences in the timing and the duration of heating in this study and those that manipulated T_b before sleep onset, similar effects on sleep were obtained. Another observation that suggests a causative association between body warming and delta sleep is that the occurrence of hot flashes in menopausal women during sleep is correlated with increased stage 4 sleep.[88]

A more specific, albeit complicated, example of the effect of T_b on sleep comes from studies of fever. In 1968, Karacan et al.[89] reported that fever had specific effects on nocturnal sleep, including an increase in AW and stage 1 NREM sleep and dramatic decreases in both REM sleep and stage 4 NREM sleep. Because administration of a pyrogen in some individuals did not alter body temperature or sleep, it was concluded that the effects of the pyrogens on sleep were not due to the pyrogens per se, but rather to the ensuing rise in T_b. In apparent support of this view, daytime administration of aspirin (600 mg) to healthy subjects resulted in a 12% reduction in stage 4 NREM sleep,[90] and this reduction in SWS was linked to a small (0.1 to 0.2°C) decrease in oral temperature seen 3 h before sleep onset.[91]

The relationship between sleep and fever has been examined in more detail in the rat.[92] In this multiday study, the effects of a fungal infection on T_b and diurnal variations in sleep distribution were studied at two ambient temperatures. Fevers resulted in a short-term attenuation of the diurnal NREM sleep rhythm and an elimination of the REM sleep and T_b rhythms. At both 20 and 30°C T_a, NREM sleep increased more during lights-off, owing primarily to an increase in the number of NREM sleep bouts. Changes in REM sleep were more complex. Although REM sleep decreased during lights-on and increased during lights-off, the total amount of REM sleep increased at $T_a = 20$°C and decreased at $T_a = 30$°C, contrary to the usual relationship between T_a and REM sleep seen in previous studies. An important conclusion from these studies is that fever may result in changes in the diurnal organization of sleep.

Studies[93–95] have further characterized changes in sleep in rabbits in response to the administration of cytokines, and the associated effects on immune system function (see reference 96 for a review). Human endogenous pyrogen (interleukin-1 or IL-1) leads to a dose-dependent increase in NREM sleep concomitant with a rise in T_b, but IL-1 still increases sleep after administration of the antipyretic anisomycin, which prevents IL-1 from elevating T_b. Therefore, the somnogenic effect of IL-1 is not secondary to its pyrogenic activity. In addition, IL-1 infusion is accompanied by an increase in the amplitude of delta EEG activity and a decrease in the amount of REM sleep, although the T_{br} changes that normally occur at sleep state transitions were not modified by the IL-1 in these febrile rabbits. Similar results have been obtained with muramyl peptides.[94] Despite the close links between sleep and thermoregulatory processes, there are a variety of studies that suggest that the response of these two control systems to various biochemical agents can be uncoupled. For example, studies of the effects of putative somnogens and pyrogens on sleep and temperature have revealed that administration of many of these agents results in an increase in NREM sleep, a decrease in REM sleep, and an increase in core temperature.[97, 98] However, in most cases the sleep and temperature effects are temporally displaced, dose dependent, and dependent upon the site and mode of injection, and time of day.[97, 99–101] In addition, some cytokines are pyrogenic without increasing sleep.[102]

Future studies that attempt to determine the efficacy of putative somnogenic agents or which involve any pharmacological manipulations of sleep must continue to evaluate changes in sleep parameters resulting from temperature variations secondary to the drug treatment. An example that clearly illustrates this principle is shown in a study of the effects of phentolamine on sleep in rats[103]; administration of this alpha-adrenergic substance resulted in decreases in REM sleep and T_b. When changes in body temperature were minimized by testing rats in a warm (32°C) rather than a cool (20°C) T_a, "drug" effects disappeared. A comprehensive inventory of the effects of drugs and a wide variety of biochemical agents on T_b is available[104–111] and should be of general interest to all sleep researchers.

In conclusion, both ambient and core temperatures have prominent influences on sleep parameters. As discussed in the next section, sleep is influenced both by thermal sensation and by indirect effects operating through the thermoregulatory system (thermoregulatory drive). Moreover, thermal sensation and thermoregulatory drive are interactive. The intensity of a thermal sensation is a function of whether actual T_b is above or below the "set-points" of the thermoregulatory system. For proper evaluation of the diverse literature on effects of temperature on sleep, it is essential to understand the properties of the thermoregulatory system.

INTERACTIONS BETWEEN SLEEP STATES AND CENTRAL NERVOUS SYSTEM REGULATION OF BODY TEMPERATURE

The systems properties underlying thermoregulatory integration in mammals have been investigated extensively. In general, a dominant source of feedback information in this system is the temperature of the preoptic anterior hypothalamic nuclei (POAH). A common technique for studying the thermoregulatory system in animals is to use chronically implanted, water-perfused, stainless steel thermodes placed around the POAH to manipulate hypothalamic temperature (T_{hy}) while simultaneously measuring effector responses such as metabolic heat production or evaporative water loss. In this way hypothalamic thermosensitivity can be quantitatively described in terms of thermoregulatory responses that alter thermal balance. For example, by heating and cooling the POAH of a resting mammal a T_{hy} can be identified above which the MR remains at basal levels and below which metabolic heat production increases with further cooling. This T_{hy} can then be defined as the threshold T_{hy} or T_{set} for the metabolic heat production response, and the slope of the response curve below T_{set} represents the gain for this response. Threshold hypothalamic temperature for thermoregulatory responses are sensitive to changes in skin and other body temperatures. It is not clear, however, whether thermoafferent information is integrated in the POAH, as has been generally assumed,[112] or lower in the neural axis, as more recent research suggests.[113]

Direct thermal stimulation of the POAH, which evokes strong thermoregulatory responses in unanesthetized animals, provides quantitative evidence for changes in thermoregulation during sleep. In a series of experiments in which T_{hy} was manipulated by chronically implanted water-perfused thermodes during sleep and AW,[114] both the gain and threshold of the metabolic heat production response decreased in NREM sleep, compared to AW, suggesting a CNS mechanism to account for the changes in body temperatures and thermoregulatory responses associated with the transition from AW to NREM sleep. Moreover, metabolic responses to thermal manipulation of the POAH were absent during REM sleep, explaining the inhibition of thermoregulatory responses during this state.

The lack of POAH thermosensitivity during REM sleep could be due to descending inhibition of effector systems, inhibition of afferent thermal information, or inhibition of POAH integrative circuits. Hendricks[115] showed that the inhibition of thermogenesis during REM sleep could not be simply attributed to the descending motor inhibition characteristic of REM sleep. Lesions of the pontine tegmentum result in "REM sleep without atonia." In cats with such lesions, however, shivering is absent in the cold during REM sleep even though the motor neurons that would mediate shivering were experimentally disinhibited. Further work demonstrated that such pontine lesions render cats more sensitive to thermal loads in AW, and that the absence of shivering in animals during REM sleep without atonia cannot be ascribed to an overall decrease in the threshold for heat gain responses due to lesions.[116] Therefore the inhibition of thermoregulatory control during REM sleep must involve an inhibition of thermal afferent or central thermoregulatory mechanisms. However, in contrast to the results on control of shivering, studies of panting in response to high (35°C) ambient temperatures resulted in panting occurring during 90% of REM sleep episodes in animals with pontine tegmental lesions, compared with 52% of REM sleep episodes in control animals.[41] The mechanisms by which pontine tegmental lesions decrease thresholds for panting in REM sleep and, more generally, the differential manifestation of different effectors (shivering, panting, sweating) in REM sleep remain unexplained.

The separate and combined effects of hypothalamic and peripheral temperature manipulations on arousal state distributions[58] were assessed to see whether skin temperature influences arousal directly, or does so through the thermoregulatory system. Water-perfused thermodes around the POAH were used to disassociate thermoregulatory drive from peripheral thermal stimulation. By first knowing the T_{set} for the metabolic heat production response at each T_a used in the study, we were then able to manipulate T_{hy} to maintain the same difference between T_{hy} and T_{set} (thermoregulatory drive) regardless of T_a. The question was whether distributions of arousal states would follow peripheral temperature or thermoregulatory drive. The results were that TST was a function of thermoregulatory drive. In other words, the animal in a cold environment had a TST equal to that seen in a warm environment if T_{hy} was warmed to reduce thermoregulatory drive, and hence the cold stimulus to the skin had no effect on TST other than its effect through the thermoregulatory system. Reciprocally, the TST of animals in warm environments was reduced by mild cooling of the POAH. The distribution of NREM sleep and REM sleep, however, was not a simple function of thermoregulatory drive. Either central or peripheral thermal stimulation characteristic of non-neutral conditions caused a reduction of the REM/NREM sleep ratio regardless of thermoregulatory drive, a result that has been confirmed in the pigeon,[117] where spinal temperature provides primary feedback modulating thermoregulatory and arousal state control. These results argue for a direct effect of thermal afferents on mechanisms regulating NREM-REM sleep transitions in addition to the indirect influence of those afferents on AW-NREM sleep transitions via the thermoregulatory system.

The neural mechanisms underlying the interaction of sleep and thermoregulation may involve many areas of the CNS and are the focus of work in several laboratories.[118–124] Cholinergic mechanisms may be particularly important in regulating the control of sleep and body temperature in the POAH; injection of the cholinergic agonist carbachol into the POAH results in increased arousal and a decrease in brain temperature.[125, 126] Recent single-unit studies[123, 124, 127–130] have extended earlier observations that POAH and extrahypothalamic neuronal thermosensitivity is suppressed in REM sleep.[118, 120, 124] The majority of warm-sensitive neurons in the hypothalamus increase spontaneous discharge during the transition from AW to NREM sleep, while cold-sensitive neurons decrease firing rate. In addition, changes in thermosensitivity paralleled changes in spontaneous firing rates, such that cells that showed an increased firing rate in NREM sleep relative to AW displayed an increase in thermosensitivity as well.[127] These results suggested that warm-sensitive POAH neurons play a key role in the regulation of NREM sleep.[127, 128] Other data have shown that warm-sensitive

neurons may be less prone to lose thermosensitivity during REM, compared with cold-sensitive neurons.[129]

The interpretation of results from these single-unit studies in defining specific thermal neural networks involved in the modulation of sleep remains controversial. First, it is difficult to assign a role for a neuron in thermoregulatory control on the basis of its thermosensitivity. For example, highly warm-sensitive neurons have been found in the hypothalamus of the unanesthetized duck, even though thermal stimulation of this area fails to evoke the same types of responses seen in mammals.[131] Additionally, it can be argued that warm-sensitivity, or, more specifically, a positive thermal coefficient, should be expected on the basis of biophysical properties. Moreover, firing rates and thermosensitivities of hypothalamic neurons recorded in anesthetized preparations or in in vitro preparations have been, as a whole, much higher than in studies using unanesthetized preparations. Thus, despite the compelling evidence about the role of the POAH as a key site for both the regulation of T_b and arousal state control, the specific neuronal basis for the integration and interaction of sleep and thermoregulation remains elusive. The possible roles of temperature-insensitive neurons (which typically constitute about 70 to 80% of all POAH cells studied) and neurons which respond to changes in the rate or magnitude of variations in temperature with changes in discharge pattern need to be considered.

In conclusion, sleep has a strong influence on homeostatic regulation of T_b, and conversely, temperature influences sleep through both the direct effects of thermal stimuli on centers controlling sleep and AW and indirect effects through the thermoregulatory system. A challenging area for future investigations will be to characterize the neuronal networks at the POAH and at extrahypothalamic levels which mediate the interaction between sleep and thermoregulatory control. In this regard, examining the functional roles of the brainstem in thermoregulation and arousal state control and the connections of these nuclei with the POAH are important.[113, 122, 132–135]

DEVELOPMENTAL STUDIES OF SLEEP AND THERMOREGULATION

This chapter has focused so far on the strong interactions between thermoregulation and sleep control in adult humans and other mammalian species. There is also substantial descriptive information on temperature and sleep in developing infants. In the normal infant, thermoregulatory effector mechanisms are operating within the first weeks of life. As incubator air temperature is changed from 36.6 to 37.6°C for a 3-d-old infant, a clear threshold for the onset of sweating is seen; the resulting response reaches six times above the basal level.[136] Newborn infants appear to retain some thermoregulatory ability during REM; cool T_a results in an increase in nonshivering thermogenesis or body movements, and exposure to warm T_a results in an increase in evaporative water loss.[137] However, thermoregulatory responses are not seen in all infants in REM, and there appears to be a large individual variation in thermoregulatory responses. Full-term infants show a decrease in rectal temperature during the transition from REM to NREM, but no significant change in rectal temperature was noted in preterm infants.[138]

Sleeping position and environment have been shown to influence T_b, thermoregulation and breathing in infants.[139–142] Term infants sleeping prone have lower rates of heat loss than infants sleeping supine,[141] and as a result infants sleeping in nonprone positions achieved significantly lower rectal temperatures during the night. Nonprone sleeping infants also had increased nocturnal movements and could uncover their limbs more in comparison with infants sleeping.[142] In addition, infants sleeping with a parent had rectal temperatures 0.1°C higher during the course of the night than did infants sleeping alone, controlling for sleeping position and thermal environment.[141] Skadberg and Markestad[139] showed that term infants at 2.5 to 5.0 months of age sleeping prone had fewer arousals and body movements and higher heart rates and skin temperatures during both REM sleep and NREM sleep compared with infants sleeping supine. All of these studies indicate that sleeping position alters a number of interdependent physiological regulatory systems.

A number of studies have provided compelling evidence that temperature may be an important factor in SIDS, which has been temporally linked to periods of sleep.[143] Seasonal variations in the occurrence of SIDS indicate that environmental temperature may be correlated with the incidence of SIDS.[144–146] More specifically, high room temperature, high humidity, and inadequate ventilation in combination with excessive clothing and overbundling have been linked with hyperthermia and subsequent death in infants.[147–153] Some of the major epidemiological risk factors for SIDS, such as bottle-feeding, parental smoking, and high room temperatures, are correlated with increased nocturnal rectal temperatures in full-term infants.[154] Hyperthermia in young infants may lead to SIDS in which there are no convulsions or signs of struggle, whereas febrile convulsions resulting from increased T_b tend to occur after the peak age range for the occurrence of SIDS.[147] Depending on the specific environmental conditions, many infant deaths associated with increases in T_b could therefore go undetected as skin or rectal temperature cools rapidly after death.

Temperature and sleep state both have prominent modulatory influences on respiratory control systems, providing another set of potential interactions that could predispose infants to SIDS. The effect of thermal stimuli on breathing occurs early in development; fetal warming coincides with increased apnea in fetal lambs.[155] Daily et al.[156] and Perlstein et al.[157] found that small elevations in ambient and skin temperatures were associated with marked increases in apnea in premature infants. Steinschneider[158] also observed that term infants had more apnea in a warm laboratory environment. It is not known if this is due primarily to a direct modulation of respiration by temperature or instead to changes in distribution of arousal states.

Overbundling of infants can create conditions that are the equivalent of central or peripheral warming and could promote increased sleep, and excessive REM sleep in particular. At the onset of sleep, the regulated decline in T_b is preceded by falls in hypothalamic thresholds for heat loss and heat production responses. In an overbundled infant in warm surroundings where passive heat loss is at a minimum, the core temperature may not be able to follow the fall in the set-points for thermoregulatory responses at sleep onset. An immediate consequence would be vasodilation, thus warming the skin. The combination of warm skin and high core temperature (relative to set-points) could enhance both NREM and REM sleep propensity. In one scenario, increased apnea in concert with reduced central respiratory chemosensitivity associated with REM sleep[159] may increase infant vulnerability to SIDS.

Temperature may influence obstructive events as well as central apneas. Mild increases in core temperature have been associated with decreased respiratory system stability in full-term infants during REM sleep,[160] and hyperthermia in dogs has been associated with changes in laryngeal musculature facilitating upper airway obstruction.[161] POAH warming during sleep in kittens demonstrated age-related maturation of respiratory responses to heating in quiet sleep (QS) but not active sleep (AS).[162]

Sleep disturbances are commonly reported during the minor illnesses that precede many SIDS events. Sleep deprivation in infants resulted in an increase in TST[163] and in the frequency of apneic events[164] during recovery sleep. Of particular interest is the fact that short-term sleep deprivation caused a pronounced increase in the number and duration of obstructive apneas during REM sleep. Because of the prominent effects of temperature on sleep and breathing, it is important to evaluate any possible synergistic effects of temperature and sleep deprivation on sleep architecture, breathing, and arousal.

The study of the interactions of regulatory systems through development is complicated by the fact that the underlying systems are developing in parallel, which means the interactions are changing. In addition, both sleep control and thermoregulation are influenced by the circadian system, which is also developing in parallel. However, recent work on neonatal rats has produced some new insights into the development of the underlying regulatory systems and their interactions. The development of sleep and circadian rhythms has been the subject of an extensive review,[165] so here we shall only offer brief summaries and examine interactions with the thermoregulatory system. What makes this subject so important are the implications that it has for understanding the cause of SIDS.

The first complication in studying the relationships between sleep and temperature in the neonate is the lack of certainty as to the relationships between neonatal vigilance states and those of the adult. The vigilance states of neonatal rats, like those of neonatal human beings, cannot easily be distinguished by EEG criteria. Instead we classify neonatal vigilance states as waking (periods during which the neonate is obviously responsive to its environment and displays coordinated behavior), AS (periods when the neonate is not responsive to its environment, displays uncoordinated phasic behavior such as muscle twitches, and has variable heart and respiratory rates), and QS (periods when the neonate is not responsive to the environment, is quiescent with regular respiration and heart rates). It has been assumed that AS is a premature form of REM sleep and that QS is a premature form of NREM sleep. Studies on neonatal rats cast doubt on these assumptions, however. First, when slow waves first appear in the EEG they are actually more likely to occur in AS than in QS, and the first EEG manifestations of REM sleep seem to lag behind the appearance of EEG slow waves.[166] In addition, pharmacological treatments that are highly disruptive to REM sleep have no effect on the expression of AS.[167] Since spinal cord transections do not eliminate the phasic muscle activity that is the basis for scoring active sleep,[168] it has been proposed that neonatal sleep is really an undifferentiated brain state from which NREM and REM sleep emerge, and the difference between AS and QS is the occurrence in AS of uncontrolled spinal reflexes.[166]

In the neonatal rat, EEG slow waves are the first electrographic manifestation of the vigilance state. They first appear between postnatal day (P) 10 and 11. For the next week the EEG slow wave activity (SWA) increases continuously in amount and in magnitude.[166] Circadian modulation of vigilance state begins to be manifest around P16 and is well established by P20,[169] and the ability of the neonate to maintain a constant T_b when exposed to room temperature without its dam is apparent on about P18 (unpublished data). Therefore, between the period of time from P10 to P24, it is not surprising that there are major changes occurring in the interactions between sleep and temperature.

One study examined the effect of T_a on neonatal sleep by exposing rat pups to different but constant ambient temperatures for 2-h recording periods. Pups were between 12 and 20 d of age. The conclusion was that sleep structure was influenced by the thermal environment but the intensity of SWA was not. In this study AS and REM sleep were combined because it is not possible to clearly differentiate them at any specific time in development. The percentage of total recording time made up of AS and REM sleep was maximal at 33 to 35°C and decreased at higher and lower ambient temperatures. The higher ambient temperatures appeared to be disruptive of sleep in the older pups in that sleep bout lengths decreased while sleep bout numbers increased.[170] In another study rat pups of various ages were exposed to an increase in T_a during the middle hour of 3-h recording periods. The results were quite different from the study at constant ambient temperatures and were markedly age-specific. The P16 to P18 pups showed large increases in the percentage of SWS and SWA during and following the rise in T_a. These studies on neonatal rats show that we must be careful in interpreting the effects of temperature on sleep during development because of the changes that are occurring in the underlying regulatory systems. For our considerations of SIDS, it is important to recognize

that there may be times during development that represent windows of vulnerability because of the changing nature of influences of temperature on various aspects of sleep.

CIRCADIAN MODULATION OF SLEEP AND THERMOREGULATION

In addition to the variations in body temperatures and thermoregulatory responses associated with stages of sleep and AW, there are daily cycles in the properties of the thermoregulatory system that are independent of arousal states. These daily changes in the thermoregulatory system and consequent changes in T_b are under control of the circadian system, which also influences the organization of vigilance states (see Chapter 25). The daily core temperature rhythm is not a simple consequence of the daily activity cycle; paralyzed, bedridden subjects, as well as normal subjects kept inactive in bed, show continuing cycles of T_b independent of levels of muscular activity.[171] Moreover, daily fluctuations in T_b are primarily due to changes in thermal conductance rather than changes in heat production.[172, 173] The magnitude of the sleep-related declines in T_b, which are considered "masking" components of the circadian T_b rhythm, depend on the phase of the T_b rhythm and are maximal (~0.5°C) on the descending phase.[2, 174] Daily fluctuations in temperature continue during sleep deprivation[7, 8, 171] and specific thermoregulatory responses in awake subjects vary with a daily rhythm.[175, 176] One study partitioning circadian vs. sleep influences on central thermoregulatory feedback sensitivity showed that the spinal temperature thresholds for both shivering and thermal polypnea in pigeons were lower during the subjective night than during the subjective day in awake birds, and sleep caused an additional and equal decline in these thresholds.[39] In studies on rats, multiple regression analysis was used to determine the relative influence of sleep occurrence and the circadian system on the daily changes in T_b. The conclusion was that 84% of the daily change in T_b is due to sleep-wake transitions and 16% is due to circadian influence.[177] This dominance of vigilance state over circadian modulation on T_b changes as seen in the rat does not apply to other species. In fact, in the nonhibernating ground squirrel, the circadian modulation of T_b appears far greater than the sleep-related changes (unpublished data). Even though the strength of the circadian rhythm of T_b may differ between species, it is common in mammals and may result in direct thermal influences on sleep.

The daily rhythm of temperature in humans has strong influences on both the timing and duration of sleep. In environments devoid of time cues, the sleep-wake and T_b cycles can uncouple and free-run with different circadian periodicities.[175, 178–180] Under such conditions the voluntary bedtime and sleep onset is most likely to occur near the T_b nadir.[179] When one uncoupled subject went to bed near his T_b minimum, waking usually occurred on the rising phase of his T_b rhythm, 7.8 h later. If, on the other hand, he went to bed at his T_b maximum, he still woke up on the rising phase and his sleep time averaged 14.4 h. This relationship between duration of sleep and the phase of the T_b rhythm when sleep onset occurs was confirmed on 10 desynchronized subjects.[178] The influence of the phase of the T_b cycle on sleep propensity was also determined in an experiment in which subjects were placed on a cycle of 2 h of activity and 1 h of imposed bed rest.[180] If bed rest coincided with the decline or near the nadir of T_b, sleep propensity and especially REM sleep propensity were maximal. However, when bed rest occurred near the rising phase of the T_b rhythm, sleep was disturbed and REM sleep was absent. The timing and duration of minor sleep periods, or naps, also depend on the phase of the T_b cycle in free-running subjects. Naps occurring at temperature minima were shorter than major sleep periods, but longer than naps occurring halfway between minima.[181]

In free-running subjects with desynchronized cycles of T_b and bed rest activity, sleep parameters correlated with the T_b cycle and not with length of prior AW. A very strong influence of T_b on REM sleep is especially evident. REM sleep latency was shortest, REM sleep episode duration was longest, and the amount of REM sleep was greatest at the T_b minimum.[180] Results obtained from subjects entrained to a normal 24-h day but sleep-deprived for varying lengths of time before being permitted to sleep ad lib, beginning at different points in the T_b cycle, have also shown that sleep parameters were more influenced by phase of the T_b cycle at bedtime than by length of prior AW.[182] Several human studies suggest that sleep propensity[183] and REM sleep propensity may have a bimodal distribution in relation to the T_b cycle.[179, 180, 184] A plot of REM sleep propensity as a function of phase of the T_b cycle in subjects under a normal sleep schedule showed two distinct peaks in the occurrence of REM sleep across nights; one occurred at about 20 min and another at about 100 min after the temperature minimum.[184] In summary, the daily T_b rhythm and the characteristics of thermoregulatory responses depend on both circadian and sleep-related influences. But in turn, circadian changes in T_b influence the expression of vigilance states. Although T_b has a strong influence on sleep architecture, it should be emphasized that the timing, duration, and quality of sleep result from the interaction of many factors.

The interaction of sleep and T_b rhythms has important implications for several clinical and applied problems. As discussed previously, changes in the coincident timing of core temperature and sleep resulting from a change in the phase relationship of these rhythms has prominent effects on sleep propensity and sleep architecture. Such uncoupling between T_b and sleep may contribute to disorders of initiating and maintaining sleep (DIMS). DIMS resulting from jet lag and shift work are related to changes in the phase angle between scheduled sleep and the circadian rhythm, as reflected in T_b changes. As a result of shift work or jet lag, scheduled bedtime can occur in the evening "wake maintenance" zone, about 8 h before the T_b minimum, where it is extremely difficult to initiate sleep.[183] Sleep-onset insomniacs were found to have a core temperature rhythm that was phase-delayed several hours compared to normal subjects, placing their bedtimes within what the T_b rhythm would indicate to be the wake-maintenance zone.[185] Sleep *length* is also reduced in the day sleep of nightshift workers, the premature awakenings being correlated with the high or rising phase of the T_b cycle.[186] Treatment for these DIMS and for sleep disturbances resulting from primary affective disorders has included manipulation of sleep-wake scheduling[187] and photic stimulation to entrain the circadian rhythm,[188-191] and involves a phase shift of the temperature rhythm relative to sleep. Photic stimulation has a direct and immediate effect on temperature, and this effect appears to be mediated by the retinohypothalamic tract.[192, 193]

The T_b rhythms of the elderly[194, 195] have been characterized by increased nocturnal T_b minima or a decrease in rhythm amplitude. These changes in T_b rhythms may be related to the alterations of sleep timing and quality that occur in the elderly, such as increases in AW, decreases in stages 3, 4, and REM sleep, and in women, an association of shorter TST, sleep quality, and earlier rising times with the phase advance of the acrophase.[196] Studies examining sex differences in sleep and T_b rhythms suggest that the acrophase in elderly women is phase-advanced about an hour, and the amplitude is higher relative to age-matched males.[196, 197]

The T_b rhythms of depressed patients[198–200] are often characterized by increased nocturnal T_b minima. The reduced REM sleep latency typically reported in many depressed patients was correlated with a higher nocturnal mean temperature and a higher T_b at sleep onset.[200] However, this reduced REM sleep latency was not a simple consequence of a phase advance of the core temperature rhythm. As pointed out by Avery et al.,[200] adequate consideration of age and sex effects in studies of sleep and depression is essential when comparing different studies. Further work is necessary to determine whether sleep disturbances in depression (decreased SWS and short REM sleep latency) are secondary to alterations in thermoregulatory control, or if the reduced amplitude of the T_b rhythm reflects increased nocturnal AW, sleep fragmentation, or other modifications in sleep patterns.

In evaluating the causes and possible treatments of sleep disturbances associated with changes in the phase relationship or amplitude of the core T_b rhythm relative to sleep, it will be important to understand if T_b modulates sleep independently of circadian control mechanisms. Conversely, it is possible that disrupted sleep alters the core T_b rhythm. It must be remembered that while both circadian rhythm and temperature per se are important determinants of sleep propensity, these parameters act in concert with other physiological processes to influence sleep timing and architecture.[201]

DOES SLEEP HAVE THERMOREGULATORY FUNCTIONS?

We have reviewed a large body of research that describes the influences of arousal states on thermoregulation and, conversely, the influences of central and peripheral thermal conditions on sleep structure. In summary, T_b is regulated at a lower level during NREM sleep than during AW, and this regulatory shift is in addition to circadian changes in T_b. Thermoregulation is severely inhibited during REM sleep. Non-neutral thermal environments foster AW and NREM sleep, due both to thermal sensation and to thermoregulatory error signals. Even within thermoneutrality, temperature influences sleep structure with REM sleep being maximum at the upper end of the thermoneutral zone. Given these strong interactions between temperature, thermoregulation, and sleep, a diversity of hypotheses have been advanced about the thermoregulatory functions of sleep.

One of the first hypotheses was that NREM sleep has the primary function of energy conservation.[5, 20] This view is supported by the downregulation of body temperature during NREM sleep, by the coincidence of sleep and hypometabolism,[12] and by the fact that shallow torpor and deep hibernation, clear adaptations for energy conservation, are evolutionary extensions of NREM sleep.[203] Endothermy is metabolically expensive, so its evolution was probably accompanied by selective pressures favoring hypometabolism during daily periods of inactivity. Many birds and mammals that occupy certain ecological niches where energy conservation is highly adaptive may show more sleep than do many other species. Many species, however, do not seem to be under heavy selection to conserve energy, yet sleep is also an essential aspect of their lives. Thus, whereas the energy conservation hypothesis fits well into an evolutionary scenario for NREM sleep and for explaining some specialized adaptive extensions of NREM sleep, it seems unreasonable to expect that whole-body energy conservation is the major and obligatory general function of mammalian sleep.

A more recent hypothesis proposes that NREM sleep is a thermoregulatory adaptation to counter heat loads built up during AW.[121] Support for this hypothesis, as for the energy conservation hypothesis, is circumstantial. There is an anatomical coincidence between thermoregulatory controls and hypnogenic functions in the basal forebrain, and as described earlier in this chapter, gentle warming of the POAH and basal forebrain induces sleep. Furthermore, raising body temperature during the active period, either passively or through exercise, increases NREM sleep during the subsequent inactive period.[76, 77] The "heat loss function of sleep" hypothesis is interesting, but it ignores the time constant for changes in body heat content. Small to medium-sized animals, such as those used in sleep research, can dissipate enormous heat loads in minutes unless they are held at high ambient temperatures. If sleep were primarily a heat loss adaptation, large animals should sleep more than small animals, and whereas the time course for changes in body heat content and sleep might be organized on a daily basis for an animal the size of an elephant, it would not be in a mouse, which can alter its body heat content in only a few minutes. The hypothesis would also predict that animals in cold climates would sleep less than animals

in warm climates, and that whole-body cooling or hypothalamic cooling would reduce sleep need or substitute for sleep. There is no evidence to support these hypotheses.

The extensive experiments of Rechtschaffen and colleagues on the effects of long-term sleep deprivation suggest that sleep is essential to heat production rather than heat loss.[204–206] Prior to death, chronically sleep-deprived rats become extremely hypothermic and behaviorally select very high ambient temperatures, although the cause of this thermoregulatory abnormality is not known. The deficit is probably in cellular mechanisms responsible for basal MR rather than a deficit in nervous system control, but this issue cannot be resolved until metabolic and thermoregulatory data are obtained on chronically sleep-deprived animals. It is unlikely, however, that the thermoregulatory abnormalities that appear only after at least a week of sleep deprivation are reflections of a sleep-specific thermoregulatory function that occurs in the time frame of the daily cycle of sleep and activity.

Thomas Wehr[207] proposed that a function of REM sleep is to warm the CNS. He stated that his argument was largely circumstantial, based on such observations as the fact that (1) in most studies brain metabolism and T_{br} have been seen to rise at the transition from NREM to REM sleep, and (2) REM sleep is accompanied by a variety of heat-producing events such as rapid eye movements and muscle twitches. He also noted that in humans more REM sleep occurs later in the rest period when the T_b is at its lowest levels. The adaptive rationale that Wehr put forward is that brain warming during REM sleep enables animals to sleep at low ambient temperatures without T_{br} falling to levels that would compromise ability to arouse periodically or in response to external stimuli. There are, however, a number of facts that run counter to this brain-warming hypothesis: (1) the thermoregulatory system is relatively unresponsive during REM sleep; (2) there is not more REM sleep in smaller animals or in animals that live in cold climates; (3) REM sleep is inhibited by low ambient and low body temperatures; and (4) in small animals sleeping in the cold, T_{br} falls during REM sleep.

Although at this time we believe there is no convincing evidence to support a thermoregulatory function for sleep, there are two related areas of sleep research that may be leading toward deeper understanding of sleep function. The first of these areas is the study of sleep homeostasis and the underlying neurochemical mechanisms, which indicates that a function of NREM sleep is the restoration of cerebral energy reserves.[208] The rationale for this hypothesis is that the most reliable quantitative relationship between prior wake duration and a sleep parameter is the amount of activity in the NREM sleep EEG in the 0.5- to 4.5-Hz range—delta activity or delta power.[209] Findings that adenosine agonists selective for the adenosine A1 receptor produce increases in delta power that resemble the increases seen after sleep deprivation suggest that adenosine is the feedback molecule that controls the relationship between delta power and prior wake duration. Since adenosine release by neurons and other cells is tightly coupled to the energy charge (adenosine triphosphate–adenosine monophosphate ratio) of the cells, it seems that cerebral energy compromise during AW could influence the intensity of subsequent NREM sleep. The major energy supply for the brain is blood glucose, but the brain does have a small energy reserve in the form of glial glycogen. The adenosine hypothesis of sleep homeostasis draws a relationship between regional depletion of cerebral glycogen reserves during AW that leads to transient declines in cell energy charge, producing increases in extracellular adenosine. It is possible to see in this hypothesis a mechanism whereby higher body and hence brain temperatures could promote sleep. The metabolism of most cells increases with temperature, and therefore higher brain temperatures could contribute to reductions in brain energy charge with concomitant increases in extracellular adenosine. Thus, although conservation of whole-body energy may not be a general function of sleep, the restoration of brain energy reserves may be a function of sleep that could also offer some explanation for thermal effects on NREM sleep.

The second area of sleep research that may hold clues to sleep function is one specialized case where sleep really does have a thermoregulatory function: mammalian hibernation. It is a reasonable hypothesis that hibernation evolved in species exposed to seasonal food scarcity. In such species, natural selection would have favored the decreased body temperature and therefore decreased metabolism that is associated with sleep. Animals in deep hibernation are considered to be in almost continuous NREM sleep that lasts many days. It was therefore surprising when EEG recordings revealed that following arousal from deep hibernation at low temperatures, animals displayed large amounts of NREM sleep with exceptionally high delta power.[210, 211] These animals behaved as if they were extremely sleep-deprived. The suggestion was put forward that although the very low brain and body temperatures during hibernation result in significant energy conservation, they blocked the biochemical mechanisms of sleep restoration, whatever those restorative mechanisms were. It was proposed that the hibernator had to arouse periodically from deep hibernation to get the benefits of euthermic sleep. It was shown that the brain temperature during hibernation, rather than the duration of the hibernation bout, was the predominant factor determining the posthibernation sleep bout length.[212] There was no intense EEG delta power following bouts of hibernation at high ambient temperatures, which prevented T_{br} from falling below 20°C. However, recent studies of this phenomenon have demonstrated that this sleep response of hibernators following arousal is not a reflection of normal sleep homeostasis. If the animals are sleep-deprived immediately following the return to euthermia from a bout of hibernation, they no longer display the enhanced delta power when permitted to sleep.[213, 214] The restorative process has apparently occurred without the occurrence of NREM sleep. Nevertheless, it is still possible that the effects of low temperature on the

hibernator's brain results in a deficit that has to be restored, and that the restoration process is normally associated with NREM sleep.

Hypotheses such as those briefly described in this section have resulted in many interesting investigations that contribute to our understanding, yet none has successfully produced a convincing function for sleep. It should not be disappointing that a clear thermoregulatory function of sleep has not been documented. There is no a priori reason to expect such a function to exist. Many homeostatic systems are altered as a function of sleep, yet we do not suppose that sleep is a respiratory, a cardiovascular, or a feeding adaptation. Sleep is a multifactoral phenomenon. Through its global effects on activity and the nervous system, sleep produces effects in many aspects of the organization of physiology and behavior. It is even possible that temperature-sensitive neurons in the POAH are involved in sleep control, as proposed by Szymusiak and Satinoff,[121] yet those same neurons are not necessarily the same as those involved in thermoregulation. Anatomical and functional coincidences between sleep and thermoregulation are enticing, but they are not evidence that a *primary* function of sleep is a thermoregulatory one. Clearly, however, there are strong interactions between thermoregulation and arousal state control, and it is important to understand these interactions. Many compounds or other interventions known to influence sleep may be acting indirectly through their effects on thermoregulation, as has been demonstrated in one case by Kent and Satinoff,[103] and therefore the actions of such compounds or interventions may not lead to insights about neurochemical mechanisms governing sleep control. Conversely, however, understanding thermal influences on sleep may lead to nonpharmacological means of alleviating certain disorders of sleep such as DIMS and the risk of SIDS.

References

1. Aschoff J. Circadian rhythm of activity and of body temperature. In: Hardy JD, Gagge AP, Stolwijk JAJ, eds. Physiological and Behavioral Temperature Regulation. Springfield, Ill: Charles C Thomas; 1970:905–919.
2. Gillberg M, Akerstedt T. Body temperature and sleep at different times of day. Sleep. 1982;5:378–388.
3. Heller HC, Glotzbach SF. Thermoregulation during sleep and hibernation. Int Rev Physiol. 1977;15:147–187.
4. Heller HC, Glotzbach SF. Thermoregulation and sleep. In: Shitzer A, Eberhart RC, eds. Heat Transfer in Medicine and Biology: Analysis and Applications. New York, NY: Plenum Press; 1985:107–134.
5. Berger RJ, Phillips NH. Comparative physiology of sleep, thermoregulation and metabolism from the perspective of energy conservation. In: Issa FG, Suratt PM, Remmers JE, eds. Sleep and Respiration. New York, NY: Wiley-Liss; 1990:41–52.
6. Kleitman N. Studies of the physiology of sleep, I: the effects of prolonged sleeplessness on man. Am J Physiol. 1923;66:67–72.
7. Kreider MB. Effects of sleep deprivation on body temperature. Fed Proc. 1961;20:214.
8. Timbal J, Colin J, Boutelier C, et al. Bilan thermique en ambience contrôlée pendent 24 heures. Pflugers Arch. 1972;335:97–108.
9. Roussel B, Bittel J. Thermogenesis and thermolysis during sleeping and waking in the rat. Pflugers Arch. 1979;382:225–231.
10. Szymusiak R, Satinoff E. Maximal REM sleep time defines a

narrower thermoneutral zone than does minimal metabolic rate. Physiol Behav. 1981;26:687–690.

11. Schmidek WR, Zachariassen KE, Hammel HT. Total calorimetric measurements in the rat: influences of the sleep-wakefulness cycle and of the environmental temperature. Brain Res. 1983;288:261–271.

12. Heller HC. Sleep and hypometabolism. Can J Zool. 1988;66:61–69.

13. Garby L, Kurzer MS, Lammert O, et al. Energy expenditure during sleep in men and women: evaporative and sensible heat losses. Hum Nutr Clin Nutr. 1987;41:225–233.

14. Goll CC, Shapiro CM. Oxygen consumption during sleep. J Physiol (Lond). 1981;313:35–36P.

15. White DP, Weil JV, Zwillich CW. Metabolic rate and breathing during sleep. J Appl Physiol. 1985;59:384–391.

16. Palca JW, Walker JM, Berger RJ. Thermoregulation, metabolism, and stages of sleep in cold-exposed men. J Appl Physiol. 1986;61:940–947.

17. Ryan T, Mlynczak S, Erickson T, et al. Oxygen consumption during sleep: influence of sleep stage and time of night. Sleep. 1989;12:201–210.

18. Brebbia DR, Altshuler KZ. Oxygen consumption rate and electroencephalographic stage of sleep. Science. 1965;150:1621–1623.

19. Haskell EH, Palca JW, Walker JM, et al. Metabolism and thermoregulation during stages of sleep in humans exposed to heat and cold. J Appl Physiol. 1981;51:948–954.

20. Shapiro CM, Goll CC, Cohen GR, et al. Heat production during sleep. J Appl Physiol. 1984;56:671–677.

21. Webb P, Hiestand M. Sleep metabolism and age. J Appl Physiol. 1975;38:257–262.

22. Ingvar DH, Rosen I, Johannesson G. EEG related to cerebral metabolism and blood flow. Pharmacopsychiatry. 1979;12:200–209.

23. Reivich M. Blood flow metabolism couple in the brain. In: Plum F, ed. Brain Dysfunction in Metabolic Disorders. New York, NY: Raven Press; 1974:125–140.

24. Sakai F, Meyer JS, Karacan I, et al. Normal human sleep: regional cerebral hemodynamics. Ann Neurol. 1980;7:471–478.

25. Townsend RE, Prinz PN, Obrist WD. Human cerebral blood flow during sleep and waking. J Appl Physiol. 1973;35:620–625.

26. Day R. Regulation of body temperature during sleep. Am J Dis Child. 1941;61:734–746.

27. Scholander PF, Hammel HT, Hart JS, et al. Cold adaptation in Australian Aborigines. J Appl Physiol. 1958;13:211–218.

28. Kreider MB, Iampietro PF. Oxygen consumption and body temperature during sleep in cold environments. J Appl Physiol. 1958;14:765–767.

29. Kreider MB, Buskirk ER, Bass DE. Oxygen consumption and body temperatures during the night. J Appl Physiol. 1958;12:361–366.

30. Geschickter EH, Andrews PA, Bullard RW. Nocturnal body temperature regulation in man: a rationale for sweating in sleep. J Appl Physiol. 1966;21:623–630.

31. Satoh T, Ogawa T, Takagi K. Sweating during daytime sleep. Jpn J Physiol. 1965;15:523–531.

32. Parmeggiani PL. Temperature regulation during sleep: A study in homeostasis. In: Orem J, Barnes CD, eds. Physiology in Sleep. New York, NY: Academic Press; 1980:97–143.

33. Baker MA, Hayward JN. Autonomic basis for the rise in brain temperature during paradoxical sleep. Science. 1967;157:1586–1588.

34. Parmeggiani PL, Zamboni G, Cianci T, et al. Absence of thermoregulatory vasomotor responses during fast wave sleep in cats. Electroencephalogr Clin Neurophysiol. 1977;42:372–380.

35. Franzini C, Cianci T, Lenzi P, et al. Neural control of vasomotion in rabbit ear is impaired during desynchronized sleep. Am J Physiol. 1982;243:R142–146.

36. Franzini C. The control of peripheral circulation during sleep. In: Mancia M, Marini G, eds. The Diencephalon and Sleep. New York, NY: Raven Press; 1990:343–353.

37. Tachibana S. Relation between hypothalamic heat production and intra- and extracranial circulatory factors. Brain Res. 1969;16:405–416.

38. Parmeggiani PL, Sabattini L. Electromyographic aspects of postural, respiratory and thermoregulatory mechanisms in sleeping cats. Electroencephalogr Clin Neurophysiol. 1972;33:1–13.

39. Heller HC, Graf R, Rautenberg W. Circadian and arousal state influences on thermoregulation in the pigeon. Am J Physiol. 1983;245:R321–328.

40. Parmeggiani PL, Rabini C. Sleep and environmental temperature. Arch Ital Biol. 1970;108:369–387.

41. Amini-Sereshki L, Morrison AR. Release of heat-loss responses in paradoxical sleep by thermal loads and by pontine tegmental lesions in cats. Brain Res. 1988;450:9–17.

42. Parmeggiani PL, Rabini C. Shivering and panting during sleep. Brain Res. 1967;6:789–791.

43. Nicol SC, Maskrey M. Thermoregulation, respiration, and sleep in the Tasmanian Devil, Sarcophilus harrisii (Marsupialia: Dasyuridae). J Comp Physiol. 1980;140:241–248.

44. van Twyver H, Allison T. Sleep in the armadillo Dasypus novemcinctus at moderate and low ambient temperatures. Brain Behav Evol. 1974;9:107–120.

45. Calasso M, Zantedeschi E, Parmeggiani PL. Cold-defense function of brown adipose tissue during sleep. Am J Physiol. 1993;265(5 pt 2):R1060–1064.

46. Buguet AG, Livingstone SD, Reed LD. Skin temperature changes in paradoxical sleep in man in the cold. Aviat Space Environ Med. 1979;50:567–570.

47. Takagi K. Sweating during sleep. In: Hardy JD, Gagge AP, Stolwijk JAJ, eds. Physiological and Behavioral Temperature Regulation. Springfield, Ill: Charles C Thomas; 1970:669–675.

48. Shapiro CM, Moore AT, Mitchell D, et al. How well does man thermoregulate during sleep? Experientia. 1974;30:1279–1281.

49. Henane R, Buguet A, Roussel B, et al. Variations in evaporation and body temperatures during sleep in man. J Appl Physiol. 1977;42:50–55.

50. Libert JP, Candas V, Muzet A, et al. Thermoregulatory adjustments to thermal transients during slow wave sleep and REM sleep in man. J Physiol Paris. 1982;78:251–257.

51. Sagot JC, Amoros C, Candas V, et al. Sweating responses and body temperatures during nocturnal sleep in humans. Am J Physiol. 1987;252:R462–470.

52. Buguet A, Bittel J, Gati R, et al. Thermal exchanges during sleep in anhidrotic ectodermal dysplasia. Eur J Appl Physiol. 1990;59:454–459.

53. Lenzi P, Libert JP, Cianci T, et al. Comparative aspects of the interaction between sleep and thermoregulation. In: Horne J, ed. Sleep '90. Bochum, Germany: Pontenagel Press; 1990:388–390.

54. Johnson JM. Non-thermoregulatory control of human skin blood flow. J Appl Physiol. 1986;61:1613–1622.

55. Parmeggiani PL, Rabini C, Cattalani M. Sleep phases at low environmental temperature. Arch Sci Biol (Bologna). 1969;53:277–290.

56. Schmidek WR, Hoshino K, Schmidek M, et al. Influence of environmental temperature on the sleep-wakefulness cycle in the rat. Physiol Behav. 1972;8:363–371.

57. Valatx JL, Roussel B, Cure M. Sleep and cerebral temperature in rat during chronic heat exposure. Brain Res. 1973;55:107–122.

58. Sakaguchi S, Glotzbach SF, Heller HC. Influence of hypothalamic and ambient temperatures on sleep in kangaroo rats. Am J Physiol. 1979;237:R80–88.

59. Roussel B, Turrillot P, Kitahama K. Effect of ambient temperature on the sleep-waking cycle in two strains of mice. Brain Res. 1984;294:67–73.

60. Sichieri R, Schmidek WR. Influence of ambient temperature on the sleep-wakefulness cycle in the golden hamster. Physiol Behav. 1984;33:871–877.

61. Rosenthal MS, Vogel G. Prolonged temperature increase produces prolonged REM sleep increase in the rat. Sleep Res. 1991;20A:513.

62. Alfoldi P, Rubicsek G, Cserni G, et al. Brain and core temperatures and peripheral vasomotion during sleep and wakefulness at various temperatures in the rat. Pflugers Arch. 1990;417:336–341.

63. Gao BO, Franken P, Tobler I, et al. Effect of elevated ambient temperature on sleep, EEG spectra, and brain temperature in the rat. Am J Physiol. 1995;268(6 pt 2):R1365–373.

64. McGinty D; Szymusiak R; Thomson D. Preoptic/anterior hypothalamic warming increases EEG delta frequency activity within non-rapid eye movement sleep. Brain Res. 1994;667:273–277.

65. Szymusiak R, Satinoff E, Schallert T, et al. Brief skin temperature

changes towards thermoneutrality trigger REM sleep in rats. Physiol Behav. 1980;25:305–311.

66. Haskell EH, Palca JW, Walker JM, et al. The effects of high and low ambient temperatures on human sleep stages. Electroencephalogr Clin Neurophysiol. 1981;51:494–501.

67. Buguet AC, Livingstone SD, Reed LD, et al. EEG patterns and body temperatures in man during sleep in arctic winter nights. Int J Biometeorol. 1976;20:61–69.

68. Karacan I, Thornby JI, Anch AM, et al. Effects of high ambient temperature on sleep in young men. Aviat Space Environ Med. 1978;49:855–860.

69. Sewitch DE, Kittrell EM, Kupfer DJ, et al. Body temperature and sleep architecture in response to a mild cold stress in women. Physiol Behav. 1986;36:951–957.

70. Libert JP, Di NJ, Fukuda H, et al. Effect of continuous heat exposure on sleep stages in humans. Sleep. 1988;11:195–209.

71. Libert JP, Bach V, Johnson LC, et al. Relative and combined effects of heat and noise exposure on sleep in humans. Sleep. 1991;14:24–31.

72. Candas V, Libert JP, Muzet A. Heating and cooling stimulations during SWS and REM sleep in man. J Therm Biol. 1982;7:155–158.

73. Bowersox SS, Dement WC, Glotzbach SF. The influence of ambient temperature on sleep characteristics in the aged cat. Brain Res. 1988;457:200–203.

74. Horne JA, Staff LH. Exercise and sleep: body-heating effects. Sleep. 1983;6:36–46.

75. Horne JA, Moore VJ. Sleep EEG effects of exercise with and without additional body cooling. Electroencephalogr Clin Neurophysiol. 1985;60:33–38.

76. Horne JA, Reid AJ. Night-time sleep EEG changes following body heating in a warm bath. Electroencephalogr Clin Neurophysiol. 1985;60:154–157.

77. Horne JA, Shackell BS. Slow wave sleep elevations after body heating: proximity to sleep and effects of aspirin. Sleep. 1987;10:383–392.

78. Scales WE, Kluger MJ. Effect of antipyretic drugs on circadian rhythm of body temperature of rats. Am J Physiol. 1987;253:R306–313.

79. Bunnell DE, Agnew JA, Horvath SM, et al. Passive body heating and sleep: Influence of proximity to sleep. Sleep. 1988;11:210–219.

80. Dorsey CM, Lukas SE, Teicher MH, et al. Effects of passive body heating on the sleep of older female insomniacs. J Geriatr Psychiatry Neurol. 1996;9:83–90.

81. Shapiro CM, Allan M, Driver H, et al. Thermal load alters sleep. Biol Psychiatry. 1989;26:736–740.

82. Berger RJ, Palca JW, Walker JM, et al. Correlations between body temperatures, metabolic rate and slow wave sleep in humans. Neurosci Lett. 1988;86:230–234.

83. Sewitch DE. Slow wave sleep deficiency insomnia: a problem in thermodownregulation at sleep onset. Psychophysiology. 1987;24:200–215.

84. Jordan J, Montgomery I, Trinder J. The effect of afternoon body heating on body temperature and slow wave sleep. Psychophysiology. 1990;27:560–566.

85. Murphy JP; Campbell SS. Nighttime drop in body temperature: a physiological trigger for sleep onset? Sleep. 1997;20:505–511.

86. Campbell SS; Broughton RJ. Rapid decline in body temperature before sleep: fluffing the physiological pillow? Chronobiol Int. 1994;11:126–131.

87. Bunnell DE, Horvath SM. Effects of body heating during sleep interruption. Sleep. 1985;8:274–282.

88. Woodward S, Freedman RR. The thermoregulatory effects of menopausal hot flashes on sleep. Sleep. 1994;17:497–501.

89. Karacan I, Wolff SM, Williams RL, et al. The effects of fever on sleep and dream patterns. Psychosomatics. 1968;9:331–339.

90. Horne JA, Percival JE, Traynor JR. Aspirin and human sleep. Electroencephalogr Clin Neurophysiol. 1980;49:409–413.

91. Horne JA. Aspirin and nonfebrile waking oral temperature in healthy men and women: links with SWS changes? Sleep. 1989;12:516–521.

92. Kent S, Price M, Satinoff E. Fever alters characteristics of sleep in rats. Physiol Behav. 1988;44:709–715.

93. Krueger JM, Walter J, Dinarello CA, et al. Sleep-promoting effects of endogenous pyrogen (interleukin-1). Am J Physiol. 1984;246:R994–999.

94. Krueger JM, Kubillus S, Shoham S, et al. Enhancement of slow-wave sleep by endotoxin and lipid A. Am J Physiol. 1986;R251:R591–597.

95. Walter J, Davenne D, Shoham S, et al. Brain temperature changes coupled to sleep states persist during interleukin 1-enhanced sleep. Am J Physiol. 1986;250:R96–103.

96. Krueger JM, Majde, JA. Cytokines and sleep. Int Arch Allergy Immunol. 1995;106:97–100.

97. Krueger JM, Karnovsky ML. Sleep and the immune response. Ann N Y Acad Sci. 1987;496:510–516.

98. Krueger JM, Majde JA. Sleep as a host defense: its regulation by microbial products and cytokines. Clin Immunol Immunopathol. 1990;57:188–199.

99. Walter JS, Meyers P, Krueger JM. Microinjection of interleukin-1 into brain: separation of sleep and fever responses. Physiol Behav. 1989;45:169–176.

100. Opp MR, Obal FJ, Krueger JM. Interleukin 1 alters rat sleep: temporal and dose-related effects. Am J Physiol. 1991;260:R52–58.

101. Onoe H, Ueno R, Fujita I, et al. Prostaglandin D2, a cerebral sleep-inducing substance in monkeys. Proc Natl Acad Sci U S A. 1988;85:4082–4086.

102. Opp M, Obal FJ, Cady AB, et al. Interleukin-6 is pyrogenic but not somnogenic. Physiol Behav. 1989;45:1069–1072.

103. Kent S, Satinoff E. Influence of ambient temperature on sleep and body temperature after phentolamine in rats. Brain Res. 1990;511:227–233.

104. Clark WG. Changes in body temperature after administration of amino acids peptides, dopamine, neuroleptics and related agents. Neurosci Biobehav Rev. 1979;3:179–231.

105. Clark WG, Clark YL. Changes in body temperature after administration of adrenergic and serotonergic agents and related drugs including antidepressants. Neurosci Biobehav Rev. 1980;4:281–375.

106. Clark WG, Clark YL. Changes in body temperature after administration of acetylcholine, histamine, morphine, prostaglandins and related agents. Neurosci Biobehav Rev. 1980;4:175–240.

107. Clark WG, Clark YL. Changes in body temperature after administration of antipyretics, LSD, delta 9-THC, CNS depressants and stimulants, hormones, inorganic ions, gases, 2,4-DNP and miscellaneous agents. Neurosci Biobehav Rev. 1981;5:1–136.

108. Clark WG, Lipton JM. Changes in body temperature after administration of amino acids, peptides, dopamine, neuroleptics and related agents: II. Neurosci Biobehav Rev. 1985;9:299–371.

109. Clark WG, Lipton JM. Changes in body temperature after administration of acetylcholine, histamine, morphine, prostaglandins and related agents: II. Neurosci Biobehav Rev. 1985;9:479–552.

110. Clark WG, Lipton JM. Changes in body temperature after administration of adrenergic and serotonergic agents and related drugs including antidepressants: II. Neurosci Biobehav Rev. 1986;10:153–220.

111. Clark WG. Changes in body temperature after administration of antipyretics, LSD, delta 9-THC and related agents: II. Neurosci Biobehav Rev. 1987;11:35–96.

112. Hammel HT, Heller HC, Sharp FR. Probing the rostral brainstem of anesthetized, unanesthetized, and exercising dogs and of hibernating and euthermic ground squirrels. Fed Proc. 1973;32:1588–1597.

113. Berner NJ, Heller HC. Does the preoptic anterior hypothalamus receive thermoafferent information? Am J Physiol. 1998;274(1 pt 2):R9–18.

114. Glotzbach SF, Heller HC. Central nervous regulation of body temperature during sleep. Science. 1976;194:537–539.

115. Hendricks JC. Absence of shivering in the cat during paradoxical sleep without atonia. Exp Neurol. 1982;75:700–710.

116. Amini-Sereshki L, Morrison AR. Effects of pontine tegmental lesions that induce paradoxical sleep without atonia on thermoregulation in cats during wakefulness. Brain Res. 1986;384:23–28.

117. Graf R, Heller HC, Sakaguchi S, et al. Influence of spinal and hypothalamic warming on metabolism and sleep in pigeons. Am J Physiol. 1987;252:R661–667.

118. Glotzbach SF, Heller HC. Changes in the thermal characteristics of hypothalamic neurons during sleep and wakefulness. Brain Res. 1984;309:17–26.

119. Heller HC, Glotzbach SF. Interrelation between sleep and temperature regulation. In: Obal F, Benedek G, eds. Advances in Physiological Sciences 18: Environmental Physiology. New York, NY: Pergamon Press; 1981:121–128.

120. Parmeggiani PL, Cevolani D, Azzaroni A, et al. Thermosensitivity of anterior hypothalamic-preoptic neurons during the waking-sleeping cycle: a study in brain functional states. Brain Res. 1987;415:79–89.

121. Szymusiak RS, Satinoff E. Thermal influences on basal forebrain hypnogenic mechanisms. In: McGinty DJ, Drucker-Colin R, Morrison A, et al, eds. Brain Mechanisms of Sleep. New York, NY: Raven Press; 1985:301–319.

122. Grahn DA, Radeke CM, Heller HC. Arousal state vs. temperature effects on neuronal activity in subcoeruleus area. Am J Physiol. 1989;256:R840–849.

123. Alam MN, McGinty D, Szymusiak R. Thermosensitive neurons of the diagonal band in rats: relation to wakefulness and non-rapid eye movement sleep. Brain Res. 1997;752:81–89.

124. Cevolani D, Parmeggiani PL. Responses of extrahypothalamic neurons to short temperature transients during the ultradian wake-sleep cycle. Brain Res Bull. 1995;37:227–232.

125. Mallick BN, Joseph MM. Role of cholinergic inputs to the medial preoptic area in regulation of sleep-wakefulness and body temperature in freely moving rats. Brain Res. 1997;750:311–317.

126. Imeri L, Bianchi S, Angeli P, et al. Stimulation of cholinergic receptors in the medial preoptic area affects sleep and cortical temperature. Am J Physiol. 1995;269(2 pt 2):R294–299.

127. Alam MN, McGinty D, Szymusiak R. Preoptic/anterior hypothalamic neurons: thermosensitivity in wakefulness and non rapid eye movement sleep. Brain Res. 1996;718:76–82.

128. Alam MN, McGinty D, Szymusiak R. Neuronal discharge of preoptic/anterior hypothalamic thermosensitive neurons: relation to NREM sleep. Am J Physiol. 1995;269(5 pt 2):R1240–1249.

129. Alam MN, McGinty D, Szymusiak R. Preoptic/anterior hypothalamic neurons: thermosensitivity in rapid eye movement sleep. Am J Physiol. 1995;269(5 pt 2):R1250–1257.

130. Alam N, Szymusiak R, McGinty D. Local preoptic/anterior hypothalamic warming alters spontaneous and evoked neuronal activity in the magno-cellular basal forebrain. Brain Res. 1995;696:221–230.

131. Simon E, Hammel HT, Oksche A. Thermosensitivity of single units in the hypothalamus of the conscious Pekin duck. J Neurobiol. 1977;8:523–535.

132. McGinty D, Szymusiak R. Keeping cool: a hypothesis about the mechanisms and functions of slow-wave sleep. Trends Neurosci. 1990;13:480–487.

133. Denoyer M, Sallanon M, Buda C, et al. The posterior hypothalamus is responsible for the increase of brain temperature during paradoxical sleep. Exp Brain Res. 1991;84:326–334.

134. Denoyer M, Sallanon M, Buda C, et al. Neurotoxic lesion of the mesencephalic reticular formation and/or the posterior hypothalamus does not alter waking in the cat. Brain Res. 1991;539:287–303.

135. Sallanon M, Denoyer M, Kitahama K, et al. Long-lasting insomnia induced by preoptic neuron lesions and its transient reversal by muscimol injection into the posterior hypothalamus in the cat. Neuroscience. 1989;32:669–683.

136. Harpin VA, Rutter N. Sweating in preterm babies. J Pediatr. 1982;100:614–618.

137. Bach V, Bouferrache B, Kremp O, et al. Regulation of sleep and body temperature in response to exposure to cool and warm environments in neonates. Pediatrics. 1994;93:789–796.

138. Scher MS, Dokianakis SG, Sun M, et al. Rectal temperature changes during sleep state transitions in term and preterm neonates at postconceptional term ages. Pediatr Neurol. 1994;10:191–194.

139. Skadberg BT, Markestad T. Behaviour and physiological responses during prone and supine sleep in early infancy. Arch Dis Child. 1997;76:320–324.

140. Tuffnell CS, Petersen SA, Wailoo MP. Prone sleeping infants have a reduced ability to lose heat. Early Hum Dev. 1995;43:109–116.

141. Tuffnell CS, Petersen SA, Wailoo MP. Higher rectal temperatures in co-sleeping infants. Arch Dis Child. 1996;75:249–250.

142. North RG, Petersen SA, Wailoo MP. Lower body temperature in sleeping supine infants. Arch Dis Child. 1995;72:340–342.

143. Glotzbach SF, Ariagno RL, Harper RM. Sleep and sudden infant death syndrome. In: Ferber R, Kryger M, eds. Principles and Practice of Sleep Medicine in the Child. 2nd ed. Philadelphia, Pa: WB Saunders; 1995:231–244.

144. Beal S, Porter C. Sudden infant death syndrome related to climate. Acta Paediatr Scand. 1991;80:278–287.

145. Murphy MF, Campbell MJ. Sudden infant death syndrome and environmental temperature: an analysis using vital statistics. J Epidemiol Community Health. 1987;41:63–71.

146. Nelson EA, Taylor BJ. Climatic and social associations with postneonatal mortality rates within New Zealand. N Z Med J. 1988;101:443–446.

147. Sunderland R, Emery JL. Febrile convulsions and cot death. Lancet. 1981;2:176–178.

148. Stanton AN. Sudden infant death. Overheating and cot death. Lancet. 1984;2:1199–1201.

149. Bass M, Kravath RE, Glass L. Death-scene investigation in sudden infant death. N Engl J Med. 1986;315:100–105.

150. Bacon CJ. Overheating in infancy. Arch Dis Child. 1983;58:673–674.

151. Nelson EA, Taylor BJ, Weatherall IL. Sleeping position and infant bedding may predispose to hyperthermia and the sudden infant death syndrome. Lancet. 1989;1:199–201.

152. Kinmonth AL. Review of the epidemiology of sudden infant death syndrome and its relationship to temperature regulation. Br J Gen Pract. 1990;40:161–163.

153. Tuohy PG, Tuohy RJ. The overnight thermal environment of infants. N Z Med J. 1990;103:36–38.

154. Tuffnell CS, Petersen SA, Wailoo MP. Factors affecting rectal temperature in infancy. Arch Dis Child. 1995;73:443–446.

155. Moss IR, Mautone AJ, Scarpelli EM. Effect of temperature on regulation of breathing and sleep/wake state in fetal lambs. J Appl Physiol. 1983;54:536–543.

156. Daily WJR, Klaus M, Meyer HBP. Apnea in premature infants: monitoring, incidence, heart rate changes, and an effect of environmental temperature. Pediatrics. 1969;43:510–518.

157. Perlstein PH, Edwards NK, Sutherland JM. Apnea in premature infants and incubator-air-temperature changes. N Engl J Med. 1970;282:461–466.

158. Steinschneider A. Prolonged apnea and the sudden infant death syndrome: clinical and laboratory observations. Pediatrics. 1972;50:646–654.

159. Read DJC, Jeffries H. Many paths to asphyxial death in SIDS: a search for underlying defects. In: Tildon JT, Roeder LM, Steinschneider A, eds. Sudden Infant Death Syndrome. New York, NY: Academic Press; 1983:183–200.

160. Gautier C, Canet E, Berterottiere D. Is REM sleep a period at risk after stress in healthy infants? IEEE Eng Med Biol Soc. 1990;12:2029–2030.

161. Haraguchi S, Fung RQ, Sasaki CT. Effect of hyperthermia on the laryngeal closure reflex: implications in the sudden infant death syndrome. Ann Otol Rhinol Laryngol. 1983;92:24–28.

162. Schechtman VL, Ni H, Glotzbach SF, et al. Sleep state effects on nonpanting breathing during preoptic/anterior hypothalamic warming in cats and kittens. Sleep. 1997;20:1–10.

163. Anders TF, Roffwarg HP. The effects of selective interruption and deprivation of sleep in the human newborn. Dev Psychobiol. 1973;6:77–89.

164. Canet E, Gaultier C, D'Allest AM, et al. Effects of sleep deprivation on respiratory events during sleep in healthy infants. J Appl Physiol. 1989;66:1158–1163.

165. Davis F, Frank MG, Heller HC. Ontogeny of sleep and circadian rhythms. In: Turek F, Zee P, eds. Neurobiology of Sleep and Circadian Rhythms. New York, NY: Marcel Dekker; 1999:19–79.

166. Frank MG, Heller HC. The development of REM and slow wave sleep in the rat. Am J Physiol. 1997;272:R1792–R1799.

167. Frank MG, Page J, Heller HC. The effects of REM-sleep inhibiting drugs in neonatal rats: evidence for a distinction between neonatal active sleep and REM sleep. Brain Res. 1997;778:64–72.

168. Blumberg MS, Lucas DE. Dual mechanisms of twitching during sleep in neonatal rats. Behav Neurosci. 1994;108:1196–1202.

169. Frank MG, Heller HC. Development of diurnal organization of slow wave sleep and EEG slow wave activity in the rat. Am J Physiol. 1997;273:R472–R478.

170. Morrissette RN, Heller HC. The effects of temperature on sleep in the developing rat. Am J Physiol. 1998;274:R1087–1093.

171. Kleitman N. Sleep and Wakefulness. 2nd ed. Chicago, Ill: University of Chicago Press; 1963.

172. Aschoff J, Heise A. Thermal conductance in man: its dependence on time of day and ambient temperature. Adv Clin Physiol. 1972;20:334–348.

173. Smith RE. Circadian variations in human thermoregulatory responses. J Appl Physiol. 1969;26:554–560.

174. Mills JN, Minors DS, Waterhouse JM. The effect of sleep upon human circadian rhythms. Chronobiologia. 1978;5:14–27.

175. Wever R. The circadian multi-oscillator system of man. Int J Chronobiol. 1975;3:19–55.

176. Wenger CB, Roberts MF, Stolwijk JAJ, et al. Nocturnal lowering of thresholds for sweating and vasodilation. J Appl Physiol. 1976;41:15–19.

177. Franken P, Tobler I, Borbely AA. Sleep and waking have a major effect on the 24 hr rhythm of cortical temperature in the rat. J Biol Rhythms. 1992;7:341–352.

178. Zulley J, Wever R, Aschoff J. The dependence of onset and duration of sleep on the circadian rhythm of rectal temperature. Pflugers Arch. 1981;391:314–318.

179. Czeisler CA, Weitzman ED, Moore EM, et al. Human sleep: its duration and organization depend on its circadian phase. Science. 1980;210:1264–1267.

180. Czeisler CA, Zimmerman JC, Ronda JM, et al. Timing of REM sleep is coupled to the circadian rhythm of body temperature in man. Sleep. 1980;2:329–346.

181. Campbell SS, Zulley J. Circasemidian distribution of human sleep/wake patterns during disentrainment. Sleep Res. 1985;14:291.

182. Akerstedt T, Gillberg M. The circadian variation of experimentally displaced sleep. Sleep. 1981;4:159–169.

183. Strogatz SH, Kronauer RE, Czeisler CA. Circadian pacemaker interferes with sleep onset at specific times each day: role in insomnia. Am J Physiol. 1987;253:R172–178.

184. Carman GJ, Mealey L, Thompson ST, et al. Patterns in the distribution of REM sleep in normal human sleep. Sleep. 1984;7:347–355.

185. Morris M, Lack L, Dawson D. Sleep-onset insomniacs have delayed temperature rhythms. Sleep. 1990;13:1–14.

186. Akerstedt T, Gillberg M. Displacement of the sleep period and sleep deprivation. Implications for shift work. Hum Neurobiol. 1982;1:163–171.

187. Czeisler CA, Richardson GS, Coleman RM, et al. Chronotherapy: resetting the circadian clocks of patients with delayed sleep phase insomnia. Sleep. 1981;4:1–21.

188. Czeisler CA, Allan JS, Strogatz SH, et al. Bright light resets the human circadian pacemaker independent of the timing of the sleep-wake cycle. Science. 1986;233:667–671.

189. Lewy AJ, Sack RL, Miller LS, et al. Antidepressant and circadian phase-shifting effects of light. Science. 1987;235:352–354.

190. Sack RL, Lewy AJ, Miller LS, et al. Effects of morning versus evening bright light exposure on REM latency. Biol Psychiatry. 1986;21:402–405.

191. Czeisler CA, Kronauer RE, Allan JS. Bright light induction of strong (Type 0) resetting of the human circadian pacemaker. Science. 1989;244:1328–1333.

192. Dijk DJ, Cajochen C, Borbely AA. Effect of a single 3-hour exposure to bright light on core body temperature and sleep in humans. Neurosci Lett. 1991;121:59–62.

193. Drennan M, Kripke DF, Gillin JC. Bright light can delay human temperature rhythm independent of sleep. Am J Physiol. 1989;257:R136–141.

194. Vitiello MV, Smallwood RG, Avery DH, et al. Circadian temperature rhythms in young adult and aged men. Neurobiol Aging. 1986;7:97–100.

195. Weitzman ED, Moline ML, Czeisler CA, et al. Chronobiology of aging: temperature, sleep-wake rhythms and entrainment. Neurobiol Aging. 1982;3:299–309.

196. Campbell SS, Gillin JC, Kripke DF, et al. Gender differences in the circadian temperature rhythms of healthy elderly subjects: relationships to sleep quality. Sleep. 1989;12:529–536.

197. Moe KE, Prinz PN, Vitiello MV, et al. Healthy elderly women and men have different entrained circadian temperature rhythms. J Am Geriatr Soc. 1991;39:383–387.

198. Avery DH, Wildschiodtz G, Rafaelsen OJ. Nocturnal temperature in affective disorder. J Affect Disord. 1982;4:61–71.

199. Souetre E, Salvati E, Wehr TA, et al. Twenty-four-hour profiles of body temperature and plasma TSH in bipolar patients during depression and during remission and in normal control subjects. Am J Psychiatry. 1988;145:1133–1137.

200. Avery DH, Wildschiodtz G, Smallwood RG, et al. REM latency and core temperature relationships in primary depression. Acta Psychiatr Scand. 1986;74:269–280.

201. Borbely AA. A two process model of sleep regulation. Hum Neurobiol. 1982;1:195–204.

202. Berger RJ. Bioenergetic functions of sleep and activity rhythms and their possible relevance to aging. Fed Proc. 1975;34:97–102.

203. Berger RJ. Slow wave sleep, shallow torpor and hibernation: homologous states of diminished metabolism and body temperature. Biol Psychol. 1984;19:305–326.

204. Bergmann BM, Everson CA, Kushida CA, et al. Sleep deprivation in the rat, V: energy use and mediation. Sleep. 1989;12:31–41.

205. Prete FR, Bergmann BM, Holtzman P, et al. Sleep deprivation in the rat, 12: effect on ambient temperature choice. Sleep. 1991;14:109–115.

206. Shaw PJ, Bergmann BM, Rechtschaffen A. Effects of paradoxical sleep deprivation on thermoregulation in the rat. Sleep. 1998;21:7–17.

207. Wehr TA. A brain-warming function for REM sleep. Neurosci Biobehav Rev. 1992;16:379–397.

208. Benington JH, Heller HC. Restoration of brain energy metabolism as the function of sleep. Prog Neurobiol. 1995;45:347–360.

209. Endo T, Roth C, Landolt HP, et al. Selective REM sleep deprivation in humans: effects on sleep and sleep EEG. Am J Physiol. 1998;274(4 pt 2):R1186–1194.

210. Trachsel L, Edgar DM, Heller HC. Are ground squirrels sleep deprived during hibernation? Am J Physiol. 1991;260:R1123–R1129.

211. Daan S, Barnes BM, Strijkstra AM. Warming up for sleep? Ground squirrels sleep during arousals from hibernation. Neurosci Lett. 1991;128:265–268.

212. Larkin JE, Heller HC. Temperature sensitivity of sleep homeostasis during hibernation in the golden-mantled ground squirrel. Am J Physiol. 1996;270:R777–R784.

213. Larkin JE, Heller HC. The disappearing slow wave activity of hibernators. Sleep Res [serial online]. 1998;1:96. Available at: http://www.Sro.org/1998/Larkin/96. Accessed September 15, 1999.

214. Strijkstra AM, Daan S. Dissimilarity of slow-wave activity enhancement by torpor and sleep deprivation in a hibernator. Am J Physiol. 1998;275:R1110–R1117.

23

Sleep-Related Penile Erections

Markus H. Schmidt

Penile erections are a characteristic phenomenon of paradoxical sleep (PS) or rapid eye movement (REM) sleep. Although the neural mechanisms of other classic PS-related events, such as muscle atonia, rapid eye movements, and cortical activation, are well studied, the neural control of penile erections during PS has been explored only recently. A new animal model for sleep-related erection research in freely behaving rats has provided insights.

The spinal control of penile erections is characterized by a complex interplay among parasympathetic, somatic motor, and sympathetic components. Although the supraspinal control is less well understood, numerous structures from the medulla to the telencephalon have been implicated in erectile mechanisms, including the medial preoptic area, which plays an essential role in copulatory behavior. Advances in erectile neurophysiology suggest that penile erections involve a descending oxytocinergic excitation of the spinal erection generator from the hypothalamic paraventricular nucleus (PVN) and the removal of a descending serotonergic inhibition from the medullary nucleus paragigantocellularis (nPGi).

The executive mechanisms of PS, as well as the subsystems that generate its tonic and phasic phenomena, are located in the pedunculopontine tegmentum and rostral medulla. Although these brainstem structures are sufficient for the generation of PS and its classic phenomena, the brainstem is not sufficient for the generation of PS-related erections as demonstrated by brainstem transection experiments. An essential role of the forebrain in PS-related erectile control is confirmed by lesion experiments of the preoptic area. Neurotoxic lesions of the lateral preoptic area (LPOA) severely disrupt PS-related erections while leaving waking-state erections intact, suggesting that the higher central mechanisms of erections are context-specific. Similar lesions of the medial preoptic area have only minimal effects on sleep-related or waking-state erectile activity. Although it does not project to the spinal cord, the LPOA may modulate the spinal erection generator during PS through its relay connections with the PVN and nPGi. Finally, sleep-related erections appear to be androgen sensitive because such erections are diminished in pathologically or experimentally induced hypogonadal states. Since its discovery more than 3 decades ago, numerous hypotheses and assumptions regarding PS-related erectile mechanisms have been postulated and are reviewed in this chapter. Clinical implications and directions for future research also are discussed.

Penile erection cycles during sleep were first described in the early 1940s,[1] more than a decade before the discovery of paradoxical sleep (PS) or rapid eye movement (REM) sleep. These sleep-related erections (SREs) in human beings were found to occur at 85-min intervals and to last about 25 min each.[1] Following the discovery of PS, several authors hypothesized that erections in sleep may coincide with PS because the cyclicity and duration of these two phenomena are virtually identical. Fisher et al.[2] and Karacan et al.[3] later demonstrated a strong temporal association between the occurrence of penile erections and PS.

Penile tumescence cycles in sleep occur in all normal healthy males from early infancy, through adulthood, and into old age.[4] Similar clitoral erection cycles and increases in vaginal blood flow during PS have been described in females.[5–7] Although these erection cycles occur during dream sleep, PS erectile activity is not related to dream content.[8, 9] Because of the consistent, involuntary, and autonomic nature of penile tumescence in sleep, SRE testing has been used as a clinical tool to differentiate "psychogenic" from "organic" impotence.

In addition to penile erections, PS is characterized by other classic tonic and phasic phenomena, including cortical desynchronization, rapid eye movements, ponto-geniculo-occipital (PGO) spikes, and a general muscle atonia. The executive mechanisms of PS and the neural subsystems generating its classic tonic and phasic events have been relatively well elucidated. In contrast, the neural mechanisms of PS-related erections, until recently, were not investigated, primarily because an animal model was not available for recording penile erections across behavioral states.

NEUROPHYSIOLOGY OF "WAKING-STATE" PENILE ERECTIONS

Anatomy and Hemodynamics

The penis is composed of two separate erectile tissue systems, the paired corpora cavernosa of the penis (CCP) and the single corpus spongiosum of the penis (CSP), which envelops the urethra. At the proximal portions, or base, of these erectile tissues, the paired CCP separate to form the crura of the CCP, which lie along the lateral border of the ischiopubic rami. In contrast, the most proximal portion of the CSP, known as the bulb of the CSP, lies between the two crura. The ischiocavernosus (IC) and bulbospongiosus (BS) muscles are located at the base of the penis and are closely associated with these two separate erectile tissue systems.

The erectile tissues are composed of a framework of smooth muscle bundles that, in the flaccid state, form collapsed vascular spaces known as cavernous sinuses.[10] Blood is restricted from entering these vascular spaces when the penis is flaccid. With appropriate autonomic and local control during tumescence (see later), blood enters the cavernous sinuses following a relaxation of the smooth muscle cells within the arteries and trabecular framework.[11] The penis becomes engorged and erect as blood expands the spongy erectile tissue. Reflex IC and BS muscle contractions subsequently compress the crura and bulb, respectively. Repetitive and phasic contractions of these perineal muscles appear to augment rigidity by producing intracavernous and intraspongious pressure peaks in excess of the systolic arterial blood pressure.[12–16]

Spinal Control

The neural control of penile erections involves the complex interplay of parasympathetic, sympathetic, and somatic components. These neural elements comprise what has been referred to as the *spinal generator* or *spinal pacemaker* controlling penile erections, in that erections may still occur after the removal of all descending input from higher brain structures. Indeed, because reflex-induced erections are facilitated by spinal transection[17] or spinal block,[18] it has long been assumed that the brain exhibits a tonic descending inhibition on this spinal generator.

Penile tumescence traditionally is viewed as a parasympathetic phenomenon causing vasodilation of the supplying arteries and relaxation of smooth muscle cells within the erectile tissues.[19] Release of acetylcholine and nitric oxide appear to play a major role in this local, vasodilatory process,[19–22] in part by stimulating the formation of cyclic guanosine monophosphate (GMP).[23] The first oral medication for the treatment of erectile dysfunction, sildenafil (Viagra), is thought to act at the end organ level by preventing the inactivation of cyclic GMP through an inhibition of its deactivating enzyme phosphodiesterase.[23]

Rigidity is augmented by an additional somatic motor component involving reflex skeletal muscle contractions of the IC and BS muscles.[13, 24] In contrast, detumescence and the maintenance of the flaccid state is under primarily sympathetic control involving the release of norepinephrine, causing vasoconstriction of the supplying arteries via alpha$_2$ receptors and contraction of smooth muscles within the erectile tissues via alpha$_1$ receptors.[19, 25] Finally, although proerectile mechanisms may involve parasympathetic control, more recent data suggest that a decrease in sympathetic activity may also play an important role in penile tumescence.[26, 27]

Parasympathetic supply to the penis originates in the pelvic nerve,[28, 29] whose preganglionic neurons are located in the sacral parasympathetic nucleus within S2 to S4 spinal cord segments (Fig. 23–1).[30] The puden-dal nerve carries the somatic motor supply to the IC and BS muscles. The motoneurons of these muscles are located in Onuf's nucleus in the ventral horn at levels S2 to S4 of the spinal cord (see Fig. 23–1).[24, 31, 32] These motoneurons are noted by their extensive, androgen-dependent, dendritic arborizations,[33–35] which may play a role in the bilateral synchronization of IC and BS muscle bursts during penile erections.[36]

Much of the sympathetic innervation to the penis originates in the hypogastric nerve (see Fig. 23–1). Preganglionic sympathetic neurons are located primarily in the dorsal commissural nucleus and the intermediolateral columns of T11–L2 spinal cord segments.[37, 38] Although the hypogastric nerve carries much of the sympathetic innervation, sympathetic fibers are also found in the pelvic and pudendal nerves.[24, 29]

The pelvic and hypogastric nerves join at the pelvic plexus on the lateral aspect of the rectum to form the cavernous nerve, which innervates the penis (see Fig. 23–1). Preganglionic parasympathetic fibers from the pelvic nerve synapse onto their postganglionic counterparts at this level. The cavernous nerve, therefore, carries postganglionic sympathetic and parasympathetic innervation to the penis.[39]

Afferent sensory fibers from the glans penis and surrounding skin travel through the dorsal nerve of the penis to join the pudendal nerve trunk. These sensory fibers innervate the spinal cord through the dorsal root ganglia of S2–S4 spinal cord segments.[40]

Supraspinal Control

Although the spinal control of penile erections has been relatively well elucidated, supraspinal mechanisms remain poorly understood. Many structures within the brain have been implicated in the control of either copulatory behavior or penile erections. Some of these structures, including the nucleus accumbens,[41, 42] hippocampus,[43, 44] septum,[45, 46] and midbrain central tegmental field,[47, 48] are considered to be potential candidates in reproductive mechanisms but will not be examined in this review because their roles in erection neurophysiology are unclear.

The Medial Preoptic Area and Dopaminergic Mechanisms

The medial preoptic area (MPOA) has long been implicated in the neural control of reproductive physiology. Bilateral electrolytic[49–51] or neurotoxic[52] lesions of the MPOA eliminate copulatory behavior in every species examined to date.[53] In contrast, electrical or chemical stimulation of the MPOA has been shown to augment copulatory behavior,[54, 55] to increase intracavernous pressure in anesthetized rats,[56] and to remove a descending inhibition of penile reflexes.[57] Unit recordings of this structure demonstrate increases in unit activity associated with specific copulatory events.[58, 59] Moreover, c-fos expression in the MPOA has been found to increase following copulation in both male[60, 61] and female[62] rats.

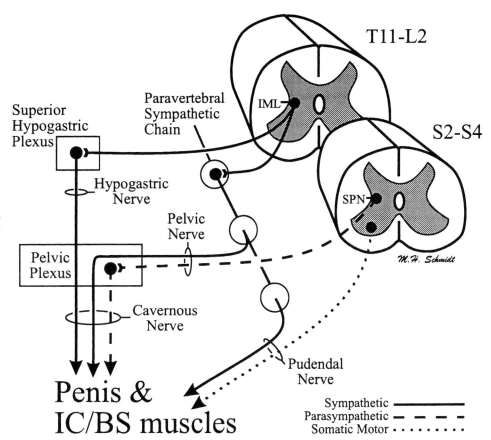

Figure 23–1. A schematic diagram demonstrating spinal erectile mechanisms, including parasympathetic, sympathetic, and somatic motor components. The somatic sensory afferents from the penis and surrounding skin are not depicted in this figure. See text for a detailed explanation. BS, bulbospongiosus; IC, ischiocavernosus; IML, intermediolateral cell column; SPN, sacral parasympathetic nucleus.

Dopaminergic mechanisms appear to play an important role in the afferent modulation of the MPOA. Indeed, dopamine has long been known to play an important role in erectile mechanisms because the systemic administration of dopaminergic agonists, such as apomorphine, induce penile erections.[53, 63] Sexual activity in the male rat is associated with increased concentrations of dopamine in the MPOA.[64] Microinjections of dopaminergic agonists into the MPOA have been shown to facilitate penile reflexes[65, 66] and copulation[67] in this species. In contrast, the administration of dopaminergic antagonists into the MPOA impairs copulatory behavior, penile reflexes, and sexual motivation.[68] Although the source of dopaminergic modulation of the MPOA remains unknown, the incertohypothalamic dopaminergic system has been postulated to play such a role.[65, 68, 69] Finally, the efferent projections of the MPOA related to copulatory mechanisms remain poorly understood because it does not project to the spinal cord.

The MPOA has been hypothesized to play a role in the integration of information from other forebrain structures related to reproductive physiology. For example, the olfactory bulb,[70–72] amygdala[48, 73, 74] and bed nucleus of the stria terminalis (BNST)[75–77] are all implicated in copulatory mechanisms because lesioning of these structures disrupts sexual behavior. A general working hypothesis traditionally has been that the amygdala transmits olfactory and other limbic, copulatory-related input to the BNST through strial and nonstrial pathways.[53, 78] The MPOA is thought to receive, integrate, and transmit information arising from the BNST and amygdala.[51, 53] More recent data suggest that the MPOA is critical for copulatory behavior but is not essential for noncopulatory or noncontact erections because such erections are maintained following MPOA lesions.[77]

The Nucleus Paragigantocellularis and a Descending Serotonergic Inhibition

Serotonin (5-HT) plays an inhibitory role in the production of penile erections, and data suggest that this inhibition occurs at the spinal level. Reflexive erections in awake rats are facilitated by the selective depletion of 5-HT in the lower lumbar spinal cord following local intrathecal application of the 5-HT neurotoxin 5,7-dihydroxytryptamine (5,7-DHT).[79] In contrast, intrathecal application of 5-HT at the lumbar level inhibits reflex-induced erections in rats during general anesthesia following upper spinal cord transection.[80] Reflexive erections can be induced under general anesthesia by urethral stimulation. This reflex, termed the *urethrogenital reflex*, is seen only after complete spinal transection above the lower thoracic level,[81, 82] indicating the presence of a tonic descending inhibition in the intact animal. The 5-HT–induced inhibition of this urethrogenital reflex in spinally transected rats is prevented by the systemic administration of methysergide, a general 5-HT receptor antagonist, given 5 to 20 min before the intrathecal 5-HT.[80]

The nucleus paragigantocellularis (nPGi) has been

postulated to be a major supraspinal source of descending 5-HT erectile inhibition. Electrolytic or neurotoxic lesions with kainic acid of the rostral juxtafacial nPGi remove a tonic descending inhibition of penile erections during general anesthesia comparable to spinal transection.[83] More recent investigators have found that lesions of the nPGi facilitate both mating behavior[84] and reflex-induced erections in the intact unanesthetized rat.[85] Finally, neuronal tracing studies indicate that the nPGi projects to spinal autonomic structures innervating the penis[80, 86–88] and that a majority of these neurons within the nPGi contain 5-HT as their neurotransmitter.[80]

The involvement of medullary 5-HT structures in the excitation of the sympathetic nervous system[89–91] suggests that the descending 5-HT inhibition of penile erections may be mediated, in part, through its sympathoexcitatory function. Microiontophoretic application of 5-HT[92–94] or substance P,[95] which is co-localized in many serotonergic projections from the ventromedial medulla,[96] cause a concentration-dependent membrane depolarization of many sympathetic preganglionic neurons in the thoracolumbar spinal cord. Initial investigations showing an inhibitory role of raphé stimulation on sympathetic activity[97] may be due to the heterogeneity of this and other serotonergic brainstem structures. For example, sympathetic-related neurons in medullary raphé nuclei include nonserotonergic sympathoexcitatory and nonserotonergic sympathoinhibitory neurons that are influenced by baroreceptor reflexes.[90, 91] Other raphé serotonergic neurons appear to exhibit a tonic discharge activity not related to baroreceptor input, which has been postulated to influence the excitability of sympathetic preganglionic neurons.[90]

The Paraventricular Nucleus and a Descending Oxytocinergic Excitation

Is the simple removal of descending inhibition sufficient for the production of penile erections? This appears unlikely because spinal transection, spinal block, and nPGi lesioning do not, in isolation, produce penile erections.[18, 81] Excitatory input from peripheral sensory reflex activation or from higher brain structures appears necessary.

A candidate for such an excitatory role is a descending oxytocinergic excitation from the hypothalamic paraventricular nucleus (PVN). Intracerebroventricular (ICV) injection of oxytocin induces penile erections and yawning in rats.[98–100] In contrast, ICV injection of [Arg[8]] vasopressin, which differs from oxytocin by only two amino acids, is unable to induce such an effect.[100] Oxytocin-induced penile erections are prevented by ICV injections of d(CH$_2$)$_5$Tyr(Me)-[Orn[8]]vasotocin, an oxytocin antagonist.[101] Finally, stimulation of the PVN with excitatory amino acids induces penile erection and yawning,[102, 103] and this effect is inhibited by systemic administration of an oxytocin antagonist.[102]

Neuroanatomical evidence is consistent with the hypothesis that oxytocinergic neurons within the PVN may play a proerectile role through its descending connections with the spinal erection generator. Immunohistochemical data demonstrate the presence of oxytocin-stained fibers in primarily autonomic areas of the spinal cord.[104, 105] Neuronal tracing studies indicate a strong projection from the parvocellular PVN to spinal autonomic structures[106–108] and to ventral horn motoneurons in the lumbar spinal cord, which innervate the IC and BS muscles of the penis.[109–111] Electrophysiological data also suggest that oxytocin may potentially exert its effect on penile erections through its influence on the autonomic nervous system. For example, both electrical stimulation of the PVN and the microiontophoretic application of oxytocin onto spinal autonomic structures inhibit the firing of many sympathetic preganglionic neurons in the spinal cord.[112, 113] In addition, similar microinjections of an oxytocin agonist into parasympathetic structures, such as the dorsal vagal complex, can cause excitation of these parasympathetic preganglionic neurons.[114] Although the effects of oxytocin agonists on parasympathetic preganglionic neurons in the sacral spinal cord remain to be explored, the PVN may theoretically play a proerectile role by simultaneously inhibiting sympathetic preganglionic neurons while stimulating parasympathetic preganglionic neurons at the spinal level.

An Integrated Model on the Neural Control of Penile Erections

Penile erections are generated in different contexts and perhaps, as hypothesized, by different neural mechanisms.[27] For example, reflexive erections may be induced by tactile stimulation of the penis involving a direct reflex activation of the spinal generator without input from supraspinal structures. Moreover, psychogenic erections induced by memory or fantasy may involve higher central mechanisms that are different from penile erections induced by auditory, visual, or chemosensory input.[27] Stimulation of the hippocampus induces penile erections,[44] and one may speculate that the hippocampus and cortex may play a role in penile tumescence generated from memory and fantasy, whereas the olfactory bulbs and amygdala may be more involved in erectile mechanisms induced by olfactory cues.

The MPOA, as well as its functional association with the medial amygdala and BNST, has been one of the most investigated forebrain regions in reproductive physiology. Because few of these structures project to the spinal cord, the mechanisms by which the MPOA and related structures are able to influence the spinal generator controlling erections is unknown.

This author hypothesizes that the missing link between these forebrain structures and descending erectile control may reside in a "final common path" characterized by a descending oxytocinergic excitation from the PVN and a descending 5-HT inhibition from the nPGi (Fig. 23–2). It still remains to be determined how the various forebrain structures involved in context-specific erectile control may tap into this final common path from brain to spinal cord. A neural model of PS erectile control involving the final common path shown in Figure 23–2 is discussed next.

Hypothalamus

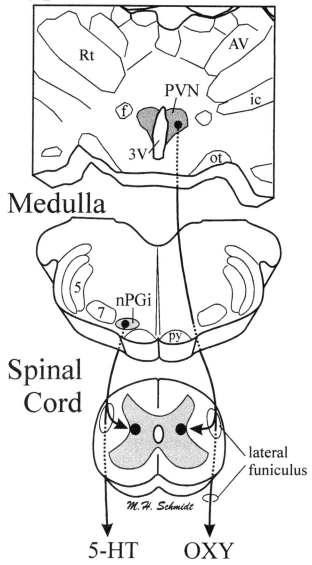

Figure 23–2. A potential final common path from brain to spinal cord in the descending control of the spinal erection generator. Serotonergic (5-HT) neurons in the medullary nucleus paragigantocellularis (nPGi) may exert an inhibitory effect on penile erection generation by stimulating sympathetic preganglionic neurons in the thoracolumbar spinal cord (*arrow* in spinal cord). Oxytocinergic (OXY) neurons in the hypothalamic paraventricular nucleus (PVN), on the other hand, may play a proerectile role in erectile mechanisms through a descending inhibition of sympathetic preganglionic neurons (*arrow* in spinal cord), as well as a simultaneous excitation of parasympathetic preganglionic neurons in the sacral spinal cord. See text for a detailed explanation. AV, anteroventral thalamic nucleus; f, fornix; ic, internal capsule; ot, optic tract; py, pyramid; Rt, reticular thalamic nucleus; 3V, third ventricle; 5, spinal trigeminal nucleus; 7, facial nucleus.

ANIMAL MODEL FOR SLEEP-RELATED ERECTION RESEARCH

In order to elucidate SRE mechanisms, an animal model is essential. Although several early abstracts or anecdotal accounts reported erections visually observed

during sleep in several nonhuman mammals,[115, 116] these reports did not adequately clarify whether such erections in nonhumans are simply occasional random events during sleep or if they are consistently associated with a specific sleep state. Indeed, a method of chronic penile erection recording in common laboratory animals such as the rat was not available. Previous animal erection data relied on visual observation or acute recording conditions under general anesthesia.

A method of chronic penile erection monitoring in freely behaving rats has now been developed, involving pressure monitoring within the erectile tissues as shown in Figure 23–3 and electromyography (EMG) of the IC and BS muscles.[117, 118] Pressure monitoring within the erectile tissues without perineal muscle activity in freely moving rats has been reported by others.[119, 120] Validation of this technique, which can be used for animal SRE research, demonstrates that erectile tissue pressure monitoring with perineal muscle activity both quantitatively and qualitatively records erectile events across behavioral states.[117, 118]

This new technique definitively revealed for the first time that PS-related erections occur in nonhuman mammals.[118] PS erectile events in the rat are associated with an increase in baseline erectile tissue pressure and, concurrent with BS muscle bursts, suprasystolic CSP pressure peaks similar to visually confirmed erections during wakefulness and reflex induction (Fig. 23–4).[117, 118] PS-related erections are found in approximately 30% of all PS phases in the rat, compared to 80 to 95% of PS phases in the human being.[2] Moreover, longer PS episodes are more likely to exhibit an erectile event.[118] Erectile activity in the rat is characterized by approximately 11 erections per hour of PS, 4 erections per hour of wakefulness, and a virtual absence of erec-

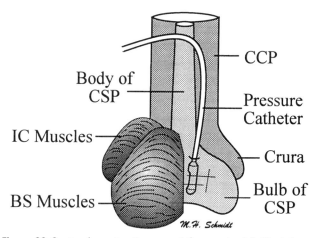

Figure 23–3. A schematic diagram of the proximal half of the rat penis demonstrating a method of chronic erectile tissue pressure monitoring. The ischiocavernosus (IC) and bulbospongiosus (BS) muscles have been removed on one side to expose the underlying erectile tissues. A microtip pressure transducer (outside diameter 1.2 mm) is implanted into the bulb of the corpus spongiosum of the penis (CSP) according to a method previously described.[117] Although not shown, the IC and BS muscles are implanted for perineal muscle recordings with bipolar Teflon-coated hook electrodes (0.002 inch uncoated diameter, multistranded stainless steel wire, AM-Systems) as described by Holmes et al.[155]

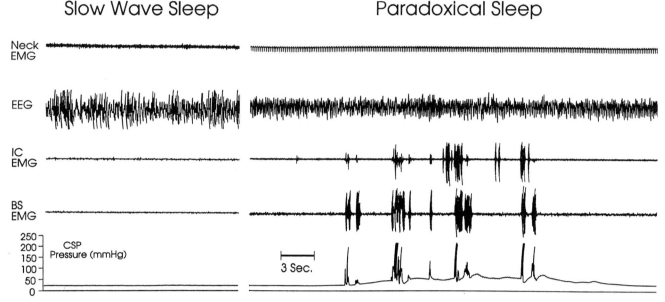

Figure 23–4. Slow-wave sleep is characterized by an absence of erectile events. Specifically, corpus spongiosum of the penis (CSP) pressures remain stable generally below 25 mmHg, and there is an absence of ischiocavernosus (IC) and bulbospongiosus (BS) muscle bursts during high-amplitude slow waves. Paradoxical sleep, on the other hand, is associated with significant erectile activity, characterized by increases in baseline CSP pressure to 50 to 70 mmHg and, concurrent with BS muscle bursts, large CSP pressure peaks that saturate the polygraph pens at 220 mmHg. (From Schmidt MH, Valatx JL, Schmidt HS, et al. Experimental evidence of penile erections during paradoxical sleep in the rat. Neuroreport. 1994;5:561–564.

tions during slow-wave sleep (SWS). Although the average PS erectile duration (mean 11 ± 7 seconds) generally is much shorter than the associated PS episode, this erectile event duration during PS corresponds to that typically observed during either coital or noncoital erections for this species.[117, 119] Finally, no obvious relationships between erectile events and phasic PS phenomena such as rapid eye movements were observed in the rat. These findings in the rat establish a new animal model for SRE research.

NEUROPHYSIOLOGY OF PARADOXICAL SLEEP–RELATED ERECTIONS

The neural mechanisms of penile tumescence in sleep have been investigated only recently. Our previous understanding of SRE neurophysiology was largely speculative and came entirely from human data. Moreover, the etiologies of organic impotence, as defined by clinical SRE criteria, have focused on the end-organ level. Although it is well documented that SREs may be adversely affected by diabetes,[121, 122] depression,[9] cardiovascular disease,[123] and hypogonadal states,[124] potential neurogenic contributions to erectile dysfunction in these disease states are poorly understood. For example, diabetic impotence, generally presumed to be secondary to peripheral vascular or autonomic abnormalities, has been suggested to include a central dysregulation even before peripheral abnormalities are apparent.[121] Elucidation of both sleep-related and waking-state erectile mechanisms is essential for

the eventual diagnosis and treatment of potential supraspinal neurogenic etiologies of impotence.

Numerous assumptions and speculations concerning PS erectile control have been postulated since their discovery in the mid-1960s. An early publication suggested that the neural mechanisms of both PS and PS-related erections are not completely interdependent, given the variable onset of tumescence relative to PS and the occasional occurrence of erections during SWS.[125] Schmidt et al.[118] also speculated that PS mechanisms are not always linked functionally to the neural systems controlling tumescence because erections are observed in only 30% of PS episodes in the rat[118] and 80 to 95% of PS episodes in the human being,[2, 3] unlike other tonic and phasic events such as muscle atonia and rapid eye movements, which occur during every PS episode.

Many authors have speculated about the role of the autonomic nervous system (ANS) in the control of SREs because the pattern of ANS activity during PS changes with respect to SWS and wakefulness. Relative to SWS, PS is associated with a general increase in parasympathetic activity and a decrease in sympathetic tone.[126] It has thus long been assumed that tumescence during PS is the result of these associated autonomic changes.[9] The role of the ANS in PS erectile control, however, is unknown and is complicated by the great variability in activity of the two autonomic divisions both within and among species, as well as by phasic alterations in autonomic activity during PS, which may have variable effects (parasympathetic vs. sympathetic), depending on the effector organ involved.[126]

It is commonly assumed that PS-related erections result from a decrease in descending erectile inhibition.[19, 118, 127] Reflex activation of local spinal erectile mechanisms are thought to be associated with this disinhibition. The source of this assumption may reside historically in the clinical appeal of SRE testing in that "psychogenic" impotence is characterized by normally occurring erections during sleep when psychological inhibitory influences are minimized. Although it is well established that the spinal generator controlling erections is under a tonic descending inhibition during wakefulness,[17, 18] the level of inhibitory control during sleep remains to be explored. Finally, it is unknown if the simple removal of a descending inhibition is sufficient for the production of penile erection. Given the many structures from the brainstem reticular core to cortex that become active during PS, several authors have suggested that SRE control also may involve a descending activation or excitation.[9]

Androgens and Sleep-Related Erections

Androgens have long been thought to play a role in SRE neurophysiology. Testosterone administration can augment SREs in hypogonadal men,[128] whereas terminating testosterone replacement in such patients decreases the number of tumescence episodes, maximum penile circumference, and total tumescence time during sleep.[129] Administration of testosterone in normal healthy males augments penile rigidity during PS but has no effect on the frequency of erections or circumference changes.[130] Antiandrogens such as medroxyprogesterone acetate (MPA) given to patients for deviant sexual behavior adversely affected SREs in several case studies.[131, 132] Finally, the luteinizing hormone releasing hormone agonist, leuprolide acetate, causes a severe reduction in serum testosterone levels, and, when administered to normal eugonadal men, it is associated with a significant decrease in total tumescence time during sleep.[124]

Although the above data appear compelling and the role of androgens in sexual desire, interest, and motivation is well documented,[133, 134] the role of androgens in SRE physiology is unclear for several reasons. First, hypogonadal men show a reduction in SREs as described earlier, yet exhibit normal erections in terms of latency and intensity (rigidity) compared to eugonadal men when watching erotic films.[135] This finding has led to speculation that PS-related erections are "androgen dependent," whereas visually induced erections are "androgen-independent" and that these context-specific erections may be mediated by different neurophysiological mechanisms.[27, 135, 136] Second, although erections during sleep have been called androgen dependent, they may more appropriately be termed *androgen sensitive*.[27] Androgen deficiency may adversely affect erections during sleep as described, but such erections generally persist and, even in hypogonadal men, often remain within the normal range.[129] Third, the role of androgens in SREs is complicated further by the existence of such erections in infants[4] in the face of undetectable testosterone levels. Indeed, young children exhibit more total SRE activity than adults.[4]

Finally, the mechanism by which androgens may affect SREs currently is unknown. Because the frequency, duration, and magnitude of penile tumescence in sleep do not change when varying serum testosterone levels within the normal range,[137] it has been hypothesized that the integrity of such erections depends on a low threshold of serum testosterone level.[124] Others have hypothesized that the effects of androgen on SREs may be mediated noradrenergically.[136]

Spinal Cord Transections

SREs are commonly thought to be disrupted by spinal cord injury as described in two early abstract publications.[138, 139] Although human data is limited, experiments in rats confirmed that midthoracic spinal transections virtually eliminate PS-related erections.[140, 141] Moreover, any residual erectile activity observed during sleep after spinal cord transection occurs at random during SWS and PS, suggesting intermittent reflex activation. Sleep-wake parameters, in contrast, remain unchanged postlesion. The data clearly demonstrate that an intact spinal cord above the midthoracic level is critical for the integrity of PS erectile activity. It remains to be determined what PS erectile activity would remain following transections below the thoracolumbar level, leaving sympathetic innervation from the brain to the penis intact.

Brainstem Transections

The pons and rostral medulla contain the neural elements responsible for the various tonic and phasic phenomena characteristic of PS, including cortical desynchronization,[142, 143] rapid eye movements,[144] PGO spikes,[144, 145] and muscle atonia.[146, 147] Schmidt et al.[140, 141] transected the rostral mesencephalon in the rat (Fig. 23–5) to determine if the brainstem is sufficient to generate PS-related erections, as it is sufficient to generate these other tonic and phasic events. Although PS persists posttransection in all rats, as seen by the rhythmic appearance of rapid eye movements and muscle atonia, penile erections during PS are severely dis-

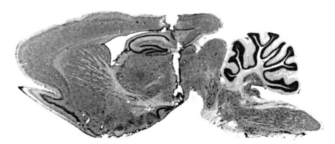

Figure 23–5. A photomicrograph of a sagittal section of the brain stained with cresyl violet demonstrating a typical mesencephalic transection at the level of the rostral superior colliculus. (From Schmidt MH, Sakai K, Valatx JL, et al. The effects of spinal or mesencephalic transections on sleep-related erections and ex-copula penile reflexes in the rat. Sleep. 1999;22:409–418.)

rupted in a cerveau isolé preparation (Fig. 23–6). These data suggest that although brainstem PS mechanisms persist in a cerveau isolé rat, neural structures rostral to the transection, as in the forebrain, are necessary for the production of PS-related erections.

A tonic descending erectile inhibition appears to be enhanced following mesencephalic transection.[141] Spinal transection facilitates reflexive erections as seen by the significantly shorter latency to reflex induction relative to pretransection controls.[17, 18, 141] Mesencephalic transection, on the other hand, significantly increases the latency to reflex induction,[141] suggesting that the descending inhibition following mesencephalic transection not only remains intact but also may be enhanced posttransection. These data suggest that the forebrain may play a role in erectile mechanisms at least in part through an inhibition of tonic brainstem inhibitory mechanisms. Such a disinhibitory role of the forebrain has been postulated by others.[57]

Forebrain Lesions

How does the forebrain control penile tumescence in sleep? As discussed earlier, numerous structures such as the MPOA, amygdala, BNST, and PVN have been implicated in reproductive physiology and, therefore, are potential forebrain candidates in PS erectile mechanisms.

The preoptic area may be a primary candidate in this regard given its dual role in both reproductive physiology and sleep generation. The role of the preoptic area as a "sleep center" is supported by numerous stimulation, lesion, and unit recording studies.[148] Moreover, an investigation has identified a set of neurons in this region that exhibit a specific unitary activity during PS.[149] Finally, the MPOA has been identified to contain androgen-sensitive neurons important for reproductive physiology,[150, 151] and, as noted earlier, SREs are thought to be androgen sensitive.

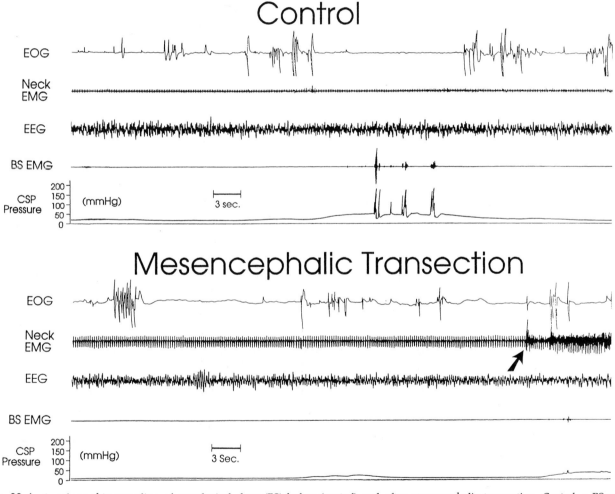

Figure 23–6. A polygraphic recording of paradoxical sleep (PS) before (*control*) and after mesencephalic transection. *Control*, a PS-related erectile event in the intact rat characterized by an increase in baseline corpus spongiosum of the penis (CSP) pressure and, with bulbospongiosus (BS) muscle bursts, large pressure peaks. *Mesencephalic Transection*, a PS episode following mesencephalic transection in the same rat. Note the simultaneous appearance of rapid eye movements in the electro-oculogram (EOG) and muscle atonia in the neck EMG, which defines PS in the cerveau isolé rat. The *arrow* marks the end of the PS episode with a return of neck EMG activity. Activity seen in the neck EMG during the PS episode is EKG artifact on an otherwise atonic baseline. Although PS was found to persist following mesencephalic transection, PS erectile activity was severely disrupted, as seen by the absence of CSP pressure changes or BS muscle bursts. (From Schmidt MH, Sakai K, Valatx JL, et al. The effects of spinal or mesencephalic transections on sleep-related erections and ex-copula penile reflexes in the rat. Sleep. 1999;22:409–418.)

A series of cytotoxic lesions with ibotenic acid of the preoptic area suggest that this region plays an important role in PS erectile control[152] (M.H.S. et al, unpublished data, 1999). Lesions of the lateral preoptic area (LPOA), as in the lateral preoptic (LP) and medial preoptic–lateral preoptic (MP-LP) groups in Figure 23–7, cause a severe and significant reduction in PS-related erections. In contrast, lesions of the entire rostrocaudal extent of the MPOA, as in the MP group in Figure 23–7, have no significant effects on SRE or waking-state erectile activity. Because the total PS duration, average PS episode duration, and number of PS phases did not significantly change postlesion in all groups, the decrease in PS erectile activity cannot be attributed to a disruption in PS architecture. Interestingly, the total number of erections during wakefulness, as well as the number of erections per hour of wakefulness, were only minimally affected in all groups. These data confirm an essential role of the forebrain in PS erectile control, as was originally suggested from the brainstem transection experiments, and they identify a new region in erection neurophysiology.

THEORETICAL CONCLUSIONS

The executive structures of PS are located in the brainstem, as well as the subsystems that generate the classic tonic and phasic events of this sleep state. Although PS persists following mesencephalic transections or even following the complete removal of all neural elements rostral to the pons, an intact LPOA appears critical for the production of PS-related erections. Waking-state erections, however, appear minimally affected by LPOA lesioning. These findings raise

several salient questions regarding SRE neurophysiology.

First, what is the role of the brainstem, if any, in the direct descending control of PS-related erections? Although results from mesencephalic transections suggest that the brainstem is not sufficient for PS erectile generation, the data do not exclude a potential role of the brainstem in the direct descending control of PS-related erections. As described earlier, a major source of tonic descending inhibition of the spinal erection generator is located in the brainstem nPGi and involves 5-HT as a neurotransmitter. It is well established that brainstem serotonergic neurons generally cease firing during PS (PS-off neurons).[153] One may speculate, therefore, that a decrease in serotonergic inhibition from the brainstem could play an important role in the production of PS erectile activity.

How does the LPOA modulate the spinal erection generator during PS since it does not project to the spinal cord? As shown in Figure 23–2, a potential "final common path" has been elucidated in erectile mechanisms, characterized by a descending oxytocinergic excitation from the PVN and the removal of a descending serotonergic inhibition from the nPGi. Microinjections of the anterograde tracer *phaseolus vulgaris* leucoagglutinin into the LPOA demonstrates a strong projection from the LPOA to both the PVN and nPGi (M.H.S. et al, unpublished data, 1999). As shown in Figure 23–8, M.H.S. et al. (unpublished data, 1999) hypothesized that the LPOA may play a role in sleep-related erectile control through its relay connections with the PVN and nPGi. The source of ascending modulation of the LPOA from brainstem PS executive structures, however, remains to be explored. Moreover, the neurotransmitter within the LPOA involved in efferent PS erectile control is un-

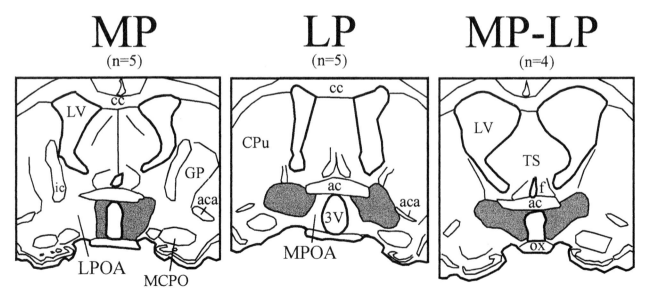

Figure 23–7. Three groups of rats with bilateral neurotoxic lesions of the preoptic area were identified. *MP*, cytotoxic lesions were generally restricted to the medial preoptic area (MPOA). *LP*, bilateral lesions involved the lateral preoptic area (LPOA) while leaving the MPOA intact. *MP-LP*, neurotoxic lesions were more extensive in this group, involving both the MPOA and LPOA. ac, anterior commissure; aca, anterior commissure, anterior part; cc, corpus callosum; CPu, caudate putamen; f, fornix; GP, globus pallidus; ic, internal capsule; LP, lateral preoptic; LV, lateral ventricle; MCPO, magnocellular preoptic nucleus; MP, medial preoptic; MP-LP, medial preoptic-lateral preoptic; ox, optic chiasm; TS, triangular septal nucleus. (From M.H.S., J.L. Valatx, K. Sakai, et al, unpublished data, 1999.)

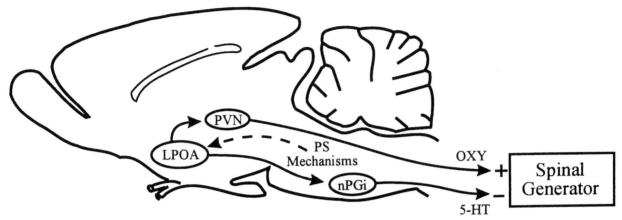

Figure 23–8. A model of the neural control of sleep-related penile erections. The lateral preoptic area (LPOA) may play a role in paradoxical sleep (PS) erectile mechanisms by modulating a final common path from brain to spinal cord. The injection of an anterograde tracer into the LPOA demonstrates a strong projection to the paraventricular nucleus (PVN) and nucleus paragigantocellularis (nPGi) (see text). The PVN and nPGi play an important role in descending excitation (+) and inhibition (−), respectively, of the spinal erection generator and may comprise a final common path in descending erectile control (see Fig. 23–2). The ascending modulation of the LPOA from brainstem PS executive mechanisms remains to be explored. OXY, oxytocin; 5-HT, serotonin. (From M.H.S., J.L. Valatx, K. Sakai, et al. unpublished data, 1999.)

known and would be purely a matter of speculation given the marked heterogeneity of this forebrain region.

Are sleep-related and waking-state erections generated by different neural mechanisms? LPOA lesioning, for example, selectively disrupts tumescence in sleep with only minimal effects on erectile activity during wakefulness (M.H.S. et al, unpublished data, 1999).[152] In addition, hypogonadal states adversely affect SREs yet have little effect on erections induced by visual erotic stimulation during wakefulness.[135] The answer to this question is further complicated by data suggesting that neural mechanisms of waking-state erections may be context-specific.[27] That is, not all waking-state erections may be created equally. For example, lesions of the BNST severely disrupt noncontact erections in male rats when in the vicinity of receptive females but cause only moderate deficits in copulation.[77] Similar lesions of the MPOA, in contrast, disrupt copulation yet leave noncontact erections intact.[77] Moreover, erections may be induced reflexively by stimulating the external genitalia without descending input from supraspinal structures. As noted earlier, stimulation of the hippocampus produces an erection,[44] and one may speculate that the hippocampus and cortex may be involved in psychogenic erections generated from memory or fantasy. The amygdala and olfactory bulbs, on the other hand, may be more involved in erections induced by olfactory stimuli.[53] The various forebrain structures involved in context-specific erectile control may possibly exert their influence on spinal mechanisms by modulating a final common pathway from brain to spinal cord. Our data give further support to the hypothesis that context-specific erections, such as those generated during sleep, may involve specialized higher central mechanisms.

Finally, the function of penile tumescence in sleep remains an enigma. One may speculate that repetitive nocturnal erections from infancy to old age potentially play a role in both the development and maintenance of erectile neural circuitry from the end-organ to supraspinal levels, as well as perhaps in the daily "exercise" of skeletal perineal muscles essential for penile rigidity. Given the unpredictable nature of mating opportunities for many species, it is tempting to hypothesize that daily SRE activity since birth would confer a reproductive advantage in generating an erection relative to a competing male who may have never produced a penile erection before his first sexual encounter.

Although more than half a century has past since the discovery of erection cycles during sleep, the neural mechanisms of such erections have only begun to be explored. Advancements in peripheral mechanisms have seen the development of the first oral medication for erectile dysfunction (i.e., sildenafil), which is hypothesized to exert its effect at the end organ level.[23] Continued research is required to elucidate potential central mechanisms of human erectile dysfunction. For example, supraspinal etiologies of psychogenic impotence remain to be investigated. The hypothesis that context-specific erections may involve specialized higher central mechanisms would suggest that impotent men with normal SREs may suffer from context-specific "organic impotence." The notion of context-specific erectile failure is further highlighted by a small population of patients who appear to have normal erections during wakefulness yet exhibit diminished erectile activity during sleep.[124, 154] Central contributions to erectile dysfunction in common disease entities, such as diabetes, which has numerous peripheral consequences, are also poorly understood. These examples underscore the need to explore both central and peripheral etiologies of erectile failure. The development of an animal model for SRE research may stimulate much needed basic and applied SRE research and help develop new directions for treatment alternatives of erectile dysfunction.

Acknowledgments

Research was supported in part by INSERM U52, CNRS URA 1195, Claude Bernard University, Ohio Sleep Medicine Institute, and the Medical College of Ohio. Special thanks are given to Helmut S. Schmidt for introducing me to the field of sleep and for his ongoing input and critical review of this manuscript, to the laboratory of Professor Michel Jouvet for providing invaluable support for much of the research presented in this chapter, and to Kevin McKenna for his review of portions of the chapter.

References

1. Ohlmeyer P, Brilmayer H, Hüllstrung H. Periodische Vorgänge im schlaf. Pflugers Arch. 1944;248:559–560.
2. Fisher C, Gross J, Zuch J. Cycles of penile erection synchronous with dreaming (REM) sleep. Arch Gen Psychiatry. 1965;12:29–45.
3. Karacan I, Goodenough DR, Shapiro A, et al. Erection cycle during sleep in relation to dream anxiety. Arch Gen Psychiatry. 1966;15:183–189.
4. Karacan I, Salis PJ, Thornby JI, et al. The ontogeny of nocturnal penile tumescence. Waking Sleep. 1976;1:27–44.
5. Cohen HD, Shapiro A. Vaginal blood flow during sleep. Assoc Profess Sleep Soc. 1970;7:338.
6. Karacan I, Rosenbloom AL, Williams RL. The clitoral erection cycle during sleep. Assoc Profess Sleep Soc. 1970;7:338.
7. Fisher C, Cohen HD, Schiavi RC, et al. Patterns of female sexual arousal during sleep and waking: vaginal thermo-conductance studies. Arch Sex Behav. 1983;12:97–122.
8. Karacan I. The Effect of Exciting Presleep Events on Dream Reporting and Penile Erections During Sleep [dissertation]. Brooklyn, NY: Downstate Medical Center, State University of New York; 1965.
9. Hirshkowitz M, Moore CA. Sleep-related erectile activity. Neurol Clin. 1996;14:721–737.
10. Goldstein AMB, Padma-Nathan H. The microarchitecture of the intracavernosal smooth muscle and the cavernosal fibrous skeleton. J Urol. 1990;144:1144–1146.
11. Aboseif SR, Lue TF. Hemodynamics of penile erection. Urol Clin North Am. 1988;15:1–7.
12. Lavoisier P, Courtois F, Barres D, et al. Correlation between intracavernous pressure and contraction of the ischiocavernosus muscle in man. J Urol. 1986;136:936–939.
13. Schmidt MH, Schmidt HS. The ischiocavernosus and bulbospongiosus muscles in mammalian penile rigidity. Sleep. 1993;16:171–183.
14. Beckett SD, Walker DF, Hudson RS, et al. Corpus spongiosum penis pressure and penile muscle activity in the stallion during coitus. Am J Vet Res. 1975;36:431–433.
15. Blaivas JG, O'Donnell TF, Gottlieb P, et al. Measurement of bulbocavernosus reflex latency time as part of a comprehensive evaluation of impotence. In: Zorgniotti AW, Rossi G, eds. Vasculogenic Impotence. Springfield, Ill: Charles C Thomas; 1980:49–64.
16. Purohit RC, Beckett SD. Penile pressures and muscle activity associated with erection and ejaculation in the dog. Am J Physiol. 1976;231:1343–1348.
17. Sachs BD, Garinello LD. Spinal pacemaker controlling sexual reflexes in male rats. Brain Res. 1979;171:152–156.
18. Sachs BD, Bitran D. Spinal block reveals roles for brain and spinal cord in the mediation of reflexive penile erections in rats. Brain Res. 1990;528:99–108.
19. Giuliano FA, Rampin O, Benoit G, et al. Neural control of penile erection. Urol Clin North Am. 1995;22:747–766.
20. Trigo-Rocha F, Aronson WJ, Hohenfellner M, et al. Nitric oxide and cGMP: mediators of pelvic nerve-stimulated erection in dogs. Am J Physiol. 1993;264:H419–H422.
21. Schirar A, Giuliano F, Rampin O, et al. A large proportion of pelvic neurons innervating the corpora cavernosa of the rat penis exhibit NADPH-diaphorase activity. Cell Tissue Res. 1994;278:517–525.
22. Wang R, Domer FR, Sikka SC, et al. Nitric oxide mediates penile erection in cats. J Urol. 1994;151:234–237.
23. Goldstein I, Lue TF, Padma-Nathan H, et al. Oral sildenafil in the treatment of erectile dysfunction. N Engl J Med. 1998;338:1397–1404.
24. McKenna KE, Nadelhaft I. The organization of the pudendal nerve in the male and female rat. J Comp Neurol. 1986;248:532–549.
25. Junemann K-P, Persson-Junemann C, Lue TF, et al. Neurophysiological aspects of penile erection: the role of the sympathetic nervous system. Br J Urol. 1989;64:84–92.
26. Courtois FJ, MacDougall JC, Sachs BD. Erectile mechanism in paraplegia. Physiol Behav. 1993;53:721–726.
27. Sachs BD. Placing erection in context: the reflexogenic-psychogenic dichotomy reconsidered. Neurosci Biobehav Rev. 1995;19:211–224.
28. Nadelhaft I, de Groat WC, Morgan C. Location and morphology of parasympathetic preganglionic neurons in the sacral spinal cord of the cat revealed by retrograde axonal transport of horseradish peroxidase. J Comp Neurol. 1980;193:265–281.
29. Hulsebosch CE, Coggeshall RE. An analysis of the axon populations in the nerves to the pelvic viscera in the rat. J Comp Neurol. 1982;211:1–10.
30. Nadelhaft I, Booth AM. The location and morphology of preganglionic neurons and the distribution of visceral afferents from the rat pelvic nerve: a horseradish peroxidase study. J Comp Neurol. 1984;226:238–245.
31. Ueyama T, Mizuno N, Nomura S, et al. Central distribution of afferent and efferent components of the pudendal nerve in cat. J Comp Neurol. 1984;222:38–46.
32. Roppolo JR, Nadelhaft I, de Groat WC. The organization of pudendal motoneurons and primary afferent projections in the spinal cord of the rhesus monkey revealed by horseradish peroxidase. J Comp Neurol. 1985;234:475–488.
33. Kurtz EM, Sengelaub DR, Arnold AP. Androgens regulate the dendritic length of mammalian motoneurons in adulthood. Science. 1986;232:395–398.
34. Sasaki M, Arnold AP. Androgenic regulation of dendritic trees of motoneurons in the spinal nucleus of the bulbocavernosus: reconstruction after intracellular iontophoresis of horseradish peroxidase. J Comp Neurol. 1991;308:11–27.
35. Hodges LL, Jordan CL, Breedlove SM. Hormone-sensitive periods for the control of motoneuron number and soma size in the dorsolateral nucleus of the rat spinal cord. Brain Res. 1993;602:187–190.
36. Rose RD, Collins WF. Crossing dendrites may be a substrate for synchronized activation of penile motoneurons. Brain Res. 1985;337:373–377.
37. Hancock MB, Peveto CA. A preganglionic autonomic nucleus in the dorsal gray commissure of the lumbar spinal cord of the rat. J Comp Neurol. 1979;183:65–72.
38. Nadelhaft I, McKenna KE. Sexual dimorphism in sympathetic preganglionic neurons of the rat hypogastric nerve. J Comp Neurol. 1987;256:308–315.
39. Steers WD, Mallory B, de Groat WC. Electrophysiological study of neural activity in penile nerve of the rat. Am J Physiol. 1988;254:R989–R1000.
40. Taylor DCM, Korf H-W, Pierau F-K. Distribution of sensory neurones of the pudendal nerve in the dorsal root ganglia and their projection to the spinal cord. Cell Tissue Res. 1982;226:555–564.
41. Louilot A, Gonzalez-Mora JL, Guadalupe T, et al. Sex-related olfactory stimuli induce a selective increase in dopamine release in the nucleus accumbens of male rats. A voltammetric study. Brain Res. 1991;553:313–317.
42. Mas M, Gonzalez-Mora JL, Louilot A, et al. Increased dopamine release in the nucleus accumbens of copulating male rats as evidenced by in vivo voltammetry. Neurosci Lett. 1990;110:303–308.
43. Smock T, Arnold S, Albeck D, et al. A peptidergic circuit for reproductive behavior. Brain Res. 1992;598:138–142.
44. Chen K-K, Chan JYH, Chang LS, et al. Elicitation of penile erection following activation of the hippocampal formation in the rat. Neurosci Lett. 1992;141:218–222.
45. Maeda N, Matsuoka N, Yamaguchi I. Possible involvement of the septo-hippocampal cholinergic and raphe-hippocampal serotonergic activations in the penile erection induced by fenfluramine in rats. Brain Res. 1994;652:181–189.

46. Linke R, Schwegler H, Boldyreva M. Cholinergic and GABAergic septo-hippocampal projection neurons in mice; a retrograde tracing study combined with double immunocytochemistry for choline acetyltransferase and parvalbumin. Brain Res. 1994;653:73–80.

47. Hansen S, Köhler C, Ross SB. On the role of the dorsal mesenchephalic tegmentum in the control of masculine sexual behavior in the rat: effects of electrolytic lesions, ibotenic acid and DSP4. Brain Res. 1982;240:311–320.

48. Shimura T, Shimokochi M. Modification of male rat copulatory behavior by lateral midbrain stimulation. Physiol Behav. 1991;50:989–994.

49. Ginton A, Merari A. Long range effects of MPOA lesion on mating behavior in the male rat. Brain Res. 1977;120:158–163.

50. Lisk RD. Copulatory activity of the male rat following placement of preoptic-anterior hypothalamic lesions. Exp Brain Res. 1968;5:306–313.

51. Kondo Y, Arai Y. Functional association between the medial amygdala and the medial preoptic area in regulation of mating behavior in the male rat. Physiol Behav. 1995;57:69–73.

52. Hansen S, Köhler C, Goldstein M, et al. Effects of ibotenic acid-induced neuronal degeneration in the medial preoptic area and the lateral hypothalamic area on sexual behavior in the male rat. Brain Res. 1982;239:213–232.

53. Sachs BD, Meisel RL. The physiology of male sexual behavior. In: Knobil E, Neill J, eds. The Physiology of Reproduction. New York, NY: Raven Press; 1988:1393–1485.

54. Merari A, Ginton A. Characteristics of exaggerated sexual behavior induced by electrical stimulation of the medial preoptic area in male rats. Brain Res. 1975;86:97–108.

55. Perachio AA, Marr LD, Alexander M. Sexual behavior in male rhesus monkeys elicited by electrical stimulation of preoptic and hypothalamic areas. Brain Res. 1979;177:127–144.

56. Giuliano F, Rampin O, Brown K, et al. Stimulation of the medial preoptic area of the hypothalamus in the rat elicits increases in intracavernous pressure. Neurosci Lett. 1996;209:1–4.

57. Marson L, McKenna KE. Stimulation of the hypothalamus initiates the urethrogenital reflex in male rats. Brain Res. 1994;638:103–108.

58. Shimura T, Yamamoto T, Shimokochi M. The medial preoptic area is involved in both sexual arousal and performance in male rats: re-evaluation of neuron activity in freely moving animals. Brain Res. 1994;640:215–222.

59. Oomura Y, Yoshimatsu H, Aou S. Medial preoptic and hypothalamic neuronal activity during sexual behavior of the male monkey. Brain Res. 1983;266:340–343.

60. Baum MJ, Everett BJ. Increased expression of c-fos in the medial preoptic area after mating in male rats: role of afferent inputs from the medial amygdala and midbrain central tegmental field. Neuroscience. 1992;50:627–646.

61. Robertson GS, Pfaus JG, Atkinson LJ, et al. Sexual behavior increases c-fos expression in the forebrain of the male rat. Brain Res. 1991;564:352–357.

62. Erskine MS. Mating-induced increases in FOS protein in preoptic area and medial amygdala of cycling female rats. Brain Res Bull. 1993;32:447–451.

63. Sachs BD, Akasofu K, McEldowney SS. Effects of copulation on apomorphine-induced erection in rats. Pharmacol Biochem Behav. 1994;48:423–428.

64. Mas M, Rodriguez del Castillo A, Guerra M, et al. Neurochemical correlates of male sexual behavior. Physiol Behav. 1987;41:341–345.

65. Pehek EA, Thompson JT, Hull EM. The effects of intracranial administration of the dopamine agonist apomorphine on penile reflexes and seminal emission in the rat. Brain Res. 1989;500:325–332.

66. Hull EM, Eaton RC, Markowski VP, et al. Opposite influence of medial preoptic D1 and D2 receptors on genital reflexes: implications for copulation. Life Sci. 1992;51:1705–1713.

67. Markowski VP, Eaton RC, Lumley LA, et al. A D1 agonist in the MPOA facilitates copulation in male rats. Pharmacol Biochem Behav. 1994;47:483–486.

68. Warner RK, Thompson JT, Markowski VP, et al. Microinjection of the dopamine antagonist cis-flupenthixol into the MPOA impairs copulation, penile reflexes and sexual motivation in male rats. Brain Res. 1991;540:177–182.

69. Bitran D, Hull EM, Holmes GM, et al. Regulation of male rat copulatory behavior by preoptic incertohypothalamic dopamine neurons. Brain Res Bull. 1988;20:323–331.

70. Fernandez-Fewell GD, Meredith M. Facilitation of mating behavior in male hamsters by LHRH and AcLHRH5-10: interaction with the vomeronasal system. Physiol Behav. 1995;57:213–221.

71. Wang L, Hull EM. Tail pinch induces sexual behavior in olfactory bulbectomized male rats. Physiol Behav. 1980;24:211–215.

72. Meisel RL, Lumia AR, Sachs BD. Effects of olfactory bulb removal and flank shock on copulation in male rats. Physiol Behav. 1980;25:383–387.

73. De Jonge FH, Oldenburger WP, Louwerse AL, et al. Changes in male copulatory behavior after sexual exciting stimuli: effects of medial amygdala lesions. Physiol Behav. 1992;52:327–332.

74. Wood RI, Coolen LM. Integration of chemosensory and hormonal cues is essential for sexual behaviour in the male Syrian hamster: role of the medial amygdaloid nucleus. Neuroscience. 1997;78:1027–1035.

75. Valcourt RJ, Sachs BD. Penile reflexes and copulatory behavior in male rats following lesions in the bed nucleus of the stria terminalis. Brain Res Bull. 1979;4:131–133.

76. Emery DE, Sachs BD. Copulatory behavior in male rats with lesions in the bed nucleus of the stria terminalis. Physiol Behav. 1976;17:803–806.

77. Liu YC, Salamone JD, Sachs BD. Lesions in medial preoptic area and bed nucleus of stria terminalis: differential effects on copulatory behavior and noncontact erection in male rats. J Neurosci. 1997;17:5245–5253.

78. Lehman MN, Winans SS. Evidence for a ventral non-strial pathway from the amygdala to the bed nucleus of the stria terminalis in the male golden hamster. Brain Res. 1983;268:139–146.

79. Marson L, McKenna KE. Serotonergic neurotoxic lesions facilitate male sexual reflexes. Pharmacol Biochem Behav. 1994;47:883–888.

80. Marson L, McKenna KE. A role for 5-hydroxytryptamine in descending inhibition of spinal sexual reflexes. Exp Brain Res. 1992;88:313–320.

81. McKenna KE, Chung SK, McVary KT. A model for the study of sexual function in anesthetized male and female rats. Am J Physiol. 1991;261:R1276–R1285.

82. Chung SK, McVary KT, McKenna KE. Sexual reflexes in male and female rats. Neurosci Lett. 1988;94:343–348.

83. Marson L, McKenna KE. The identification of a brainstem site controlling spinal sexual reflexes in male rats. Brain Res. 1990;515:303–308.

84. Yells DP, Hendricks SE, Prendergast MA. Lesions of the nucleus paragigantocellularis: effects on mating behavior in male rats. Brain Res. 1992;596:73–79.

85. Marson L, List MS, McKenna KE. Lesions of the nucleus paragigantocellularis alter ex copula penile reflexes. Brain Res. 1992;592:187–192.

86. Skagerberg G, Bjorklund A. Topographic principles in the spinal projections of serotonergic and non-serotonergic brainstem neurons in the rat. Neuroscience. 1985;15:445–480.

87. Loewy AD, McKellar S. Serotonergic projections from the ventral medulla to the intermediolateral cell column in the rat. Brain Res. 1981;211:146–152.

88. Marson L, Platt KB, McKenna KE. Central nervous system innervation of the penis as revealed by the transneuronal transport of pseudorabies virus. Neuroscience. 1993;55:263–280.

89. Laskey W, Polosa C. Characteristics of the sympathetic preganglionic neuron and its synaptic input. Prog Neurobiol. 1988;31:47–84.

90. McCall RB, Clement ME. Identification of serotonergic and sympathetic neurons in medullary raphe nuclei. Brain Res. 1989;477:172–182.

91. Morrison SF, Gebber GL. Raphe neurons with sympathetic-related activity: baroreceptor responses and spinal connections. Am J Physiol. 1984;246:R338–R348.

92. Ma RC, Dun NJ. Excitation of lateral horn neurons of the neonatal rat spinal cord by 5-hydroxytryptamine. Dev Brain Res. 1986;24:89–98.

93. Coote JH, Macleod VH, Fleetwood-Walker S, et al. The response of individual sympathetic preganglionic neurones to microelec-

trophoretically applied endogenous monoamines. Brain Res. 1981;215:135–145.

94. McCall RB. Serotonergic excitation of sympathetic preganglionic neurons: a microiontophoretic study. Brain Res. 1983;289:121–127.

95. Gilbey MP, McKenna KE, Schramm LP. Effects of substance P on sympathetic preganglionic neurones. Neurosci Lett. 1983;41:157–159.

96. Sasek CA, Wessendorf MW, Helke CJ. Evidence for co-existence of thyrotropin-releasing hormone, substance P and serotonin in ventral medullary neurons that project to the intermediolateral cell column in the rat. Neuroscience. 1990;35:105–119.

97. Gilbey MP, Coote JH, Macleod VH, et al. Inhibition of sympathetic activity by stimulating in the raphe nuclei and the role of 5-hydroxytryptamine in this effect. Brain Res. 1981;226:131–142.

98. Melis MR, Mauri A, Argiolas A. Apomorphine- and oxytocin-induced penile erection and yawning: role of sexual steroids. Soc Neurosci Abstr. 1992;18:356.

99. Argiolas A, Stancampiano R, Melis MR. Apomorphine-, oxytocin- and ACTH-induced penile erection and yawning: role of excitatory amino acids. Soc Neurosci Abstr. 1992;18:356.

100. Argiolas A, Melis MR, Gessa GL. Oxytocin: an extremely potent inducer of penile erection and yawning in male rats. Eur J Pharmacol. 1986;130:265–272.

101. Argiolas A, Melis MR, Vargiu L, et al. d(CH2)5Tyr(Me)-[Orn8]-vasotocin, a potent oxytocin antagonist, antagonizes penile erection and yawning induced by oxytocin and apomorphine, but not by ACTH-(1-24). Eur J Pharmacol. 1987;134:221–224.

102. Melis MR, Stancampiano R, Argiolas A. Penile erection and yawning induced by paraventricular NMDA injection in male rats are mediated by oxytocin. Pharmacol Biochem Behav. 1994;48:203–207.

103. Melis MR, Stancampiano R, Argiolas A. Nitric oxide synthase inhibitors prevent N-methyl-D-aspartic acid-induced penile erection and yawning in male rats. Neurosci Lett. 1994;179:9–12.

104. Valiquette G, Haldar J, Abrams GM, et al. Extrahypothalamic neurohypophysial peptides in the rat central nervous system. Brain Res. 1985;331:176–179.

105. Swanson LW, McKellar S. The distribution of oxytocin- and neurophysin-stained fibers in the spinal cord of the rat and monkey. J Comp Neurol. 1979;188:87–106.

106. Luiten PGM, ter Horst GJ, Karst H, et al. The course of paraventricular hypothalamic efferents to autonomic structures in medulla and spinal cord. Brain Res. 1985;392:374–378.

107. Ono T, Nishino H, Sasaka K, et al. Paraventricular nucleus connections to spinal cord and pituitary. Neurosci Lett. 1978;10:141–146.

108. Saper CB, Loewy AD, Swanson LW, et al. Direct hypothalamo-autonomic connections. Brain Res. 1976;117:305–312.

109. Wagner CK, Clemens LG. Projections of the paraventricular nucleus of the hypothalamus to the sexually dimorphic lumbosacral region of the spinal cord. Brain Res. 1991;539:254–262.

110. Shen P, Arnold AP, Micevych PE. Supraspinal projections to the ventromedial lumbar spinal cord in adult male rats. J Comp Neurol. 1990;300:263–272.

111. Holstege G, Tan J. Supraspinal control of motoneurons innervating the striated muscles of the pelvic floor including urethral and anal sphincters in the cat. Brain. 1987;110:1323–1344.

112. Gilbey MP, Coote JH, Fleetwood-Walker S, et al. The influence of the paraventriculo-spinal pathway and oxytocin and vasopressin on sympathetic preganglionic neurones. Brain Res. 1982;251:283–290.

113. Kannan H, Nijima A, Yamashita H. Effects of stimulation of the hypothalamic paraventricular nucleus on blood pressure and renal sympathetic nerve activity. Brian Res Bull. 1988;20:779–783.

114. Tolchard S, Ingram CD. Electrophysiological actions of oxytocin in dorsal vagal complex of the female rat in vitro: changing responsiveness during the oestrous cycle and after steroid treatment. Brain Res. 1993;609:21–28.

115. Pearson OP. Reproduction in the shrew (blarina brevicaudasay). Am J Anat. 1944;75:39–93.

116. Snyder F. The REM state in a living fossil. Palo Alto, Calif: Association for the Psychophysiological Study of Sleep; 1964.

117. Schmidt MH, Valatx JL, Sakai K, et al. Corpus spongiosum

118. Schmidt MH, Valatx JL, Schmidt HS, et al. Experimental evidence of penile erections during paradoxical sleep in the rat. Neuroreport. 1994;5:561–564.

119. Giuliano F, Bernabe J, Rampin O, et al. Telemetric monitoring of intracavernous pressure in freely moving rats during copulation. J Urol. 1994;152:1271–1274.

120. Bernabe J, Rampin O, Giuliano F, et al. Intracavernous pressure changes during reflexive penile erections in the rat. Physiol Behav. 1995;57:837–841.

121. Nofzinger EA, Schmidt HS. An exploration of central dysregulation of erectile function as a contributing cause of diabetic impotence. J Nerv Mental Dis. 1990;178:90–95.

122. Schiavi RC, Stimmel BB, Mandeli J, et al. Diabetes, sleep disorders, and male sexual function. Biol Psychiatry. 1993;34:171–177.

123. Rosen RC, Weiner DN. Cardiovascular disease and sleep-related erections. J Psychosom Res. 1997;42:517–530.

124. Hirshkowitz M, Moore CA, O'Connor S, et al. Androgens and sleep-related erections. J Psychosom Res. 1997;42:541–546.

125. Karacan I, Hursch CJ, Williams RL, et al. Some characteristics of nocturnal penile tumescence in young adults. Arch Gen Psychiatry. 1972;26:351–356.

126. Parmeggiani PL. The autonomic nervous system in sleep. In: Kryger MH, Roth R, Dement WC, eds. Principles and Practice of Sleep Medicine. Philadelphia, Pa: WB Saunders; 1994:194–203.

127. Fisher C, Schiavi R, Lear H, et al. The assessment of nocturnal REM erection in the differential diagnosis of sexual impotence. J Sex Marital Ther. 1975;1:277–289.

128. O'Carroll R, Shapiro C, Bancroft J. Androgens, behaviour and nocturnal erection in hypogonadal men: the effects of varying the replacement dose. Clin Endocrinol. 1985;23:527–538.

129. Cunningham GR, Hirshkowitz M, Korenman SG, et al. Testosterone replacement therapy and sleep-related erections in hypogonadal men. J Clin Endocrinol Metab. 1990;70:792–797.

130. Carani C, Scuteri A, Marrama P, et al. The effects of testosterone administration and visual erotic stimuli on nocturnal penile tumescence in normal men. Horm Behav. 1990;24:435–441.

131. Cooper AJ, Cernovsky Z. The effects of cyproterone acetate on sleeping and waking penile erections in pedophiles: possible implications for treatment. J Psychiatry. 1992;37:33–39.

132. Cooper AJ, Losztyn S, Russell NC, et al. Medroxyprogesterone acetate, nocturnal penile tumescence, laboratory arousal, and sexual acting out in a male with schizophrenia. Arch Sex Behav. 1990;19:361–372.

133. Schiavi RC, White D, Mandeli J, et al. Effect of testosterone administration on sexual behavior and mood in men with erectile dysfunction. Arch Sex Behav. 1997;26:231–241.

134. Skakkebaek NE, Bancroft J, Davidson DW, et al. Androgen replacement with oral testosterone undecanoate in hypogonadal men: a double-blind controlled study. Clin Endocrinol. 1981;14:49–61.

135. Carani C, Bancroft J, Granata A, et al. Testosterone and erectile function, nocturnal penile tumescence and rigidity, and erectile response to visual erotic stimuli in hypogonadal men. Psychopharmacology. 1992;17:647–654.

136. Bancroft J. Are the effects of androgens on male sexuality noradrenergically mediated? Some consideration of the human. Neurosci Biobehav Rev. 1995;19:325–330.

137. Buena F, Swerdloff RS, Steiner BS, et al. Sexual function does not change when serum testosterone levels are pharmacologically varied within the normal range. Fertil Steril. 1993;59:1118–1123.

138. Karacan I, Dervent A, Salis PJ, et al. Spinal cord injuries and NPT. Sleep Res. 1978;7:261.

139. Karacan I, Dimitrijevic M, Lauber A, et al. Nocturnal penile tumescence (NPT) and sleep stages in patients with spinal cord injuries. Sleep Res. 1977;6:52.

140. Schmidt MH, Sakai K, Valatx JL, et al. The deficiency of penile erections during paradoxical sleep in the rat following spinal or mesencephalic brainstem transections. Sleep Res. 1994;23:34.

141. Schmidt MH, Sakai K, Valatx JL, et al. The effects of spinal or mesencephalic transections on sleep-related erections and excopula penile reflexes in the rat. Sleep. 1999;22:409–418.

142. Steriade M, Sakai K, Jouvet M. Bulbo-thalamic neurons related to thalamocortical activation processes during paradoxical sleep. Exp Brain Res. 1984;54:463–475.

143. Jones BE. Paradoxical sleep and its chemical/structural sub-strates in the brain. Neuroscience. 1991;40:637–656.

144. Siegel JM. Brainstem mechanisms generating REM sleep. In: Kryger MH, Roth T, Dement WC, eds. Principles and Practice of Sleep Medicine. 2nd ed. Philadelphia, Pa: WB Saunders; 1994:125–144.

145. Sakai K, Jouvet M. Brain stem PGO-on cells projecting directly to the cat dorsal lateral geniculate nucleus. Brain Res. 1980;194:500–505.

146. Holmes CJ, Jones BE. Importance of cholinergic, GABAergic, serotonergic and other neurons in the medial medullary reticular formation for sleep-wake states studied by cytotoxic lesions in the cat. Neuroscience. 1994;62:1179–1200.

147. Sakai K, Sastre JP, Kanamori N, et al. State-specific neurons in the ponto-medullary reticular formation with special reference to the postural atonia during paradoxical sleep in the cat. In: Pompeiano O, Marsan A, eds. Brain Mechanisms and Perceptual Awareness. New York, NY: Raven Press; 1981:405–429.

148. Jones BE. Basic mechanisms of sleep-wake states. In: Kryger MH, Roth T, Dement WC, eds. Principles and Practice of Sleep Medicine. 2nd ed. Philadelphia, Pa: WB Saunders; 1994:145–162.

149. Koyama Y, Hayaishi O. Firing of neurons in the preoptic/anterior hypothalamic areas in rat: its possible involvement in slow wave sleep and paradoxical sleep. Neurosci Res. 1994;19:31–38.

150. Anderson RH, Fleming DE, Rhees RW, et al. Relationships between sexual activity, plasma testosterone, and the volume of the sexually dimorphic nucleus of the preoptic area in prenatally stressed and non-stressed rats. Brain Res. 1986;370:1–10.

151. Cherry JA, Tobet SA, DeVoogd TJ, et al. Effects of sex and androgen treatment on dendritic dimensions of neurons in the sexually dimorphic preoptic/anterior hypothalamic area of male and female ferrets. J Comp Neurol. 1992;323:577–585.

152. Schmidt MH, Valatx JL, Sakai K, et al. The basal forebrain and the control of sleep-related penile erections: evidence from cytotoxic lesions in the rat. Sleep Res. 1996;25:25.

153. Sakai K. Neurons responsible for paradoxical sleep. In: Wauquier A, Gaillard JM, Monti JM, et al., eds. Sleep: Neurotransmitters and Neuromodulators. New York, NY: Raven Press; 1985:29–42.

154. Fisher C, Schiavi RC, Edwards A, et al. Evaluation of nocturnal penile tumescence in the differential diagnosis of sexual impotence. Arch Gen Psychiatry. 1979;36:431–437.

155. Holmes G, Chapple W, Leipheimer R, et al. Electromyographic analysis of male rat perineal muscles during copulation and reflexive erections. Physiol Behav. 1991;49:1235–1246.

four

Chronobiology

Fred W. Turek

Introduction to Chronobiology: Sleep and the Circadian Clock

Fred W. Turek

One of the distinguishing characteristics of sleep in animals as diverse as insects, fish, and mammals is that the timing of sleep and wake is, for the vast majority of species, rigidly confined to certain times of the day or night. As detailed in a number of chapters in this section, the master biological clock regulating the timing of sleep and wake in mammals also regulates most, if not all, 24-h (i.e., circadian) behavioral, physiological, and biochemical rhythms. Since the discovery, in 1972, that destruction of the bilaterally paired suprachiasmatic nuclei (SCN) of the hypothalamus in rats leads to the loss of circadian rhythmicity (i.e., leads to arrhythmicity) of different rhythms,[1,2] the SCN has been the focus of much of the attention of investigators who are interested in the neural basis for the generation of circadian rhythms in mammals (Chapter 26). Indeed, it is a relatively simple and straightforward task to write a review on the neural basis for the generation of circadian rhythms as compared to writing a similar review on the neural mechanisms involved in the generation of sleep and wake (Section 2, Sleep Mechanisms).

During the course of evolution, the control of circadian rhythms has become more and more centralized. Thus, in the fruit fly, *Drosophila*, many "pieces" (e.g., wing, leg, brain) can generate 24-h rhythms and be entrained by the light-dark cycle in vitro,[3] and in lower vertebrates, the generation of 24-h rhythms seems to be under the control of a number of neural or endocrine circadian clocks.[3a] In contrast, in mammals the SCN serves as the master pacemaker for generating circadian rhythms.[4]

Certainly, there is great complexity in the input and output pathways, but at the core, the actual circadian generating system appears to be localized to a few thousand cells in the central nervous system. This simplicity of location is one of the reasons why molecular and genetic approaches have been so successful in the past few years in uncovering the basic mechanisms involved in the entrainment and generation of circadian rhythm.[5] A second major reason for the advances in understanding the molecular and genetic basis for circadian rhythmicity (Chapter 27) has been the overriding assumption in the field that the same basic mechanisms underlying rhythmicity would be the same throughout the animal, and perhaps plant, kingdom. This grand assumption was based, in part, on the finding that many of the formal properties of circadian clock systems were similar in organisms as diverse as fungi, flies, birds, and primates (Chapter 25). This guiding assumption has proved to be correct as evidenced by papers that have uncovered common genetic and molecular elements of the circadian clock of flies and mice and human beings (Chapter 27).

From a historical perspective, it is interesting to note that the assumption that common genetic and molecular elements would underlie circadian rhythmicity throughout at least the animal kingdom was continued even after the discovery of the central role played by the SCN in the generation of circadian rhythms in mammals. That is, even when it was clear that mammalian rhythms depended on a complex neural structure that surely would have no homolog in flies, it was still assumed that at some fundamental level there would be common mechanisms. We now know this assumption to be true: even though the neural structures that ultimately regulate rhythmicity are vastly different and have evolved separately over millions of years, the basic properties at the cellular level have amazing similarities between vertebrates and invertebrates.[6] Only time will tell whether studying the molecular and genetic basis for sleep in *Drosophila* or other lower organisms will shed light on the cellular and molecular core for sleep regulation.

As reviewed by Borbély in this section (Chapter 29), the timing of sleep and wake is a function of both the circadian clock (process C) and a homeostatic process that defines a "need" for sleep that is dependent on the previous times of sleep and wake (process S). Although the expression of many 24-h rhythms may be primarily under the control of the circadian clock in the SCN, many rhythms are largely dependent on whether the organism is asleep or awake, regardless of the circadian clock time.[7] Undoubtedly, the expression of most rhythms at the behavioral, physiological, and biochemical levels are regulated by the integration of inputs from the circadian clock and the sleep-wake state of the animal. Indeed, it can be argued that the entire temporal organization of an organism represents some combined effect of circadian clock inputs and the sleep-wake state of the organism. Thus, the circadian and sleep control centers have evolved together to ensure that the timing of internal events relative to one another and to the external environment are coordinated in such a fashion to maximize the survival of the species.

A recurrent theme throughout many of the chapters in this section is that there are many indications that the circadian clock and sleep-wake centers are indeed linked in more ways than simply the SCN signaling the rest of the brain when to sleep and when to wake. At the behavioral level, there is evidence demonstrating that when animals are active or aroused during the normal sleep time or when they are forced to be inactive during times of normal high activity, phase shifts in the central circadian clock are induced (Chapter 25). At the anatomical level, many of the areas of the brain that relay internal and external information to the SCN (e.g., thalamus, raphe nuclei) and receive afferent inputs from the SCN (Chapter 26) also play important roles in the regulation of sleep and wake states. Findings are also establishing links between the circadian clock and sleep-wake systems at the genetic and molecular levels. A mutation in the first circadian clock gene to be cloned in a mammal, called *Clock*,

leads to changes not only in the timing of sleep and wake but also in the proportion of sleep and wake in any given cycle.[8]

Interestingly, although a great deal is known about the anatomical connections between the various areas of the brain that are involved in sleep regulation (Chapters 9 and 10), little is known about the functional anatomy of how the circadian clock in the SCN regulates the timing of sleep. This lack of information about such an obvious link between the circadian clock and sleep centers is perhaps due to the fact that much of the early work in defining the neural substrate for sleep regulation was performed in the cat, an organism that does not show a pronounced 24-h sleep-wake cycle. Thus, there was little reason to look for the anatomical and physiological connections between the circadian clock and sleep regulatory centers because the model organism for sleep regulation did not lead investigators in that direction. In addition, the focused attention of circadian researchers on the entrainment and generation of 24-h rhythms resulted in little attention being paid to how the output signals from the SCN regulate overt rhythms, including the sleep-wake cycle.[9] Unraveling the linkages between the circadian and sleep-wake systems at the cellular as well as system levels should lead to a better understanding of the fundamental mechanisms underlying these highly integrated systems.

References

1. Valentinuzzi VS, Scarbrough K, Takahashi JS, Takahashi JS, et al. Effects of aging on the circadian rhythm of wheel-running activity in C57BL/6 mice. Am J Physiol. 1997;273: R1957–R1964.
2. Penev PD, Zee PC, Turek FW. Quantitative analysis of the age-related fragmentation of hamster 24-h activity rhythms. Am J Physiol. 1997;273: R2132–R2137.
3. Plautz JD, Kaneko M, Hall JC, et al. Independent photoreceptive circadian clocks throughout *Drosophila*. Science. 1997:278;1632–1635.
3a. Cassone VM. The pineal gland and avian circadian organization: the neuroendocrine loop. In: Moller P, Penet P, eds. Advances in Pineal Research. London, England: John Libbey; 1994:31–40.
4. Klein DC, Moore RY, Reppert SM, eds. Suprachiasmatic Nucleus: The Mind's Clock. New York, NY: Oxford University Press; 1991.
5. Takahashi JS. Molecular neurobiology and genetics of circadian rhythms in mammals. Annu Rev Neurosci. 1995;18:531–553.
6. Dunlap J. Circadian rhythms. An end in the beginning. Science. 1998;280:1548–1549.
7. Van Cauter E, Turek FW. Endocrine and other biological rhythms. In: De Groot L, ed. Endocrinology 1995. 3rd ed. Philadelphia, PA: WB Saunders; 1995:2487–2548.
8. Naylor E, Vitaterna MH, Takahashi JT, et al. Sleep in the *Clock* mutant mouse. Sleep. 1998;21(suppl 9):69E.
9. Turek FW. Introduction, Circadian SCN outputs. In: Klein DC, Moore RY, Reppert SM, eds. Suprachiasmatic Nucleus: The Mind's Clock. New York, NY: Oxford University Press; 1991:191–196.

25

Circadian Rhythms in Mammals: Formal Properties and Environmental Influences

Ralph E. Mistlberger

Benjamin Rusak

Circadian rhythms are ~24-h cycles of behavior and physiology that are generated by one or more internal biological clocks (pacemakers). These rhythms persist with near 24-h periods (cycle lengths) in time-free environments, but normally they are synchronized to the 24-h day by environmental stimuli (zeitgebers). The process of synchronization (entrainment) involves daily, stimulus-induced phase shifts that compensate for the difference between the intrinsic period of the pacemaker and the period of the environmental cycle. Light is the dominant zeitgeber for most species and can induce phase shifts that vary in magnitude and direction depending on the circadian phase of exposure.

Circadian rhythms in some species can also be shifted and entrained by stimuli other than light, such as exercise, social stimuli, temperature, or feeding. These so-called nonphotic zeitgebers may in some cases engage a circadian pacemaker system separate from that affected by light. Interactions between photic and nonphotic zeitgebers are complex; for example, light and exercise, depending on their relative timing and magnitude, may be synergistic or mutually inhibitory in effecting phase shifts.

During development, overt rhythms in most physiological systems may not emerge for weeks or months postnatally, even though the underlying circadian pacemaker is likely entrained prenatally. During aging, circadian rhythms exhibit changes in period, amplitude, and response to zeitgebers, which may disrupt circadian temporal organization. These changes may underlie age-related declines in physiological functioning, including sleep regulation.

THE NATURE OF CIRCADIAN RHYTHMS

Most behavioral and physiological processes are characterized by a temporal structure that matches the 24-h day-night cycle. A familiar experience that people have of this daily cyclicity is in their patterns of sleep and wakefulness. A similar 24-h time frame constrains a myriad of functions, including endocrine secretions, body temperature regulation, sensory processing, and cognitive performance.[1] The existence of these rhythms was historically ascribed to the environmental cues associated with the solar day. As early as 1729, however, it was reported that the daily movements of plant leaves do not depend on exposure to the day-night cycle. Many studies have since confirmed that daily rhythms in a great variety of species, including human beings, persist under constant environmental conditions[2] (Figs. 25–1, 25–2, and 25–3).

The persistence of daily rhythms in constant conditions suggests that they are generated by an internal, self-sustaining, clock-like mechanism. These persisting rhythms are referred to as free-running and usually have a periodicity (the time required for one complete cycle), that is approximately, but not exactly, 24 h; thus, the designation *circadian* (about a day). When rats, for example, are studied in temporal isolation, in the absence of any environmental cycles, they continue to show a daily rest-activity cycle. However, under these constant environmental conditions, spontaneous daily activity onsets become separated by about 24.5 h rather than 24 h; the "free-running" rat wakes up to run a little later each "day" (see Fig. 25–2). The period (τ) of the free-running rest-activity cycle varies among species (see Figs. 25–1, 25–2, and 25–3), ranging typically from 23 h to 26 h, and can be modified by factors such as ambient light intensity, behavioral factors, hormones, and aging (reviewed below and in Chapter 26).

The fact that their periods differ slightly from 24 h provides strong evidence that circadian rhythms are truly internally generated and are not responses to subtle 24-h time cues associated with the solar day. In fact, individuals of the same species recorded in adjacent cages generally display slightly different circadian periodicities, and thus their rhythms gradually drift apart in time, despite sharing a common environment. Other evidence for endogenous generation of circadian rhythms includes the facts that they develop normally in successive generations of organisms kept in constant light or dark,[3, 4] and that they can be modified by

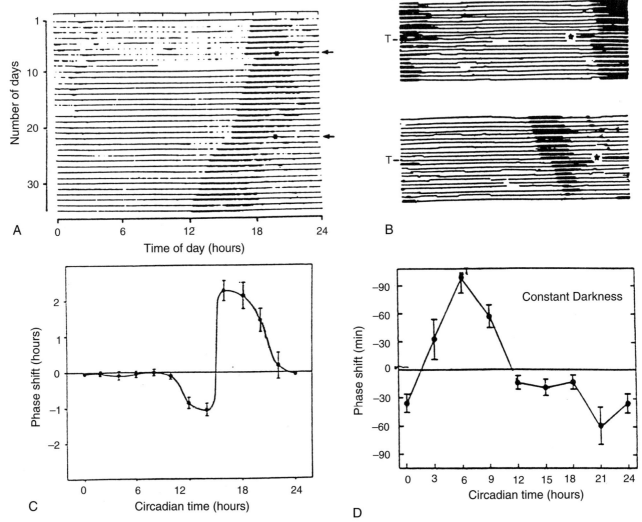

Figure 25–1. *A,* Event record of hamster wheel-running activity in constant darkness (DD). Each line represents 24 h, with time reading left to right and successive days aligned top to bottom. Each revolution of the running wheel caused a single vertical deflection of the event record pen, producing a solid dark line during continuous running. In this chart, the onset of continuous running began earlier each day, that is, the time of the free-running rhythm was less than 24 h. A 15-min light pulse (indicated by stars on the days marked by arrows), which was presented several hours after the beginning of the daily running phase, caused the rhythm to shift to a later time on subsequent days, that is, the rhythm was phase-delayed. The second light pulse, indicated by the second arrow, was presented near the end of the daily running phase. It produced a shift in the opposite direction, causing activity to begin and end earlier on subsequent days, that is, a phase-advance shift. *B,* The phase response curve to light for a group of hamsters summarizes the relationship between the time at which a light pulse is presented and the direction and magnitude of the phase shift produced. To construct this curve, the period of the circadian rhythm, usually different from 24 h, is first normalized to a 24-h time scale, referred to on the abscissa as circadian time (CT, i.e., the daily rhythm is divided into 24 equal segments, each representing one circadian hour). For nocturnal rodents, CT12 is, by convention, the time when running activity begins. When a light pulse is presented around CT12, a delay phase shift of 1 h occurs on average. This is indicated on the ordinate by −1. The largest delay shifts occur at about CT13–14. The largest advance shifts (positive sign) occur at about CT16–18. No significant phase shift occurs when light pulses are presented from CT0–10, which is the hamsters' daily rest phase. This daily rhythm of sensitivity to light causes the pacemaker to entrain to the light-dark (LD) cycle at whatever phase relation produces a net daily phase shift (a combination of delays in the evening and advances in the morning) that precisely offsets the difference between pacemaker period and the period of the LD cycle. *C,* Event records from two hamsters recorded in DD. At the time marked by the stars, the animals received 2.5 mg of triazolam (systemic injection). Injections during the inactive phase induced phase advances, whereas injections during the active phase usually induced phase delays, as summarized in the phase response curve for the group (*D*). Triazolam also triggered a bout of wheel-running lasting several hours. If the animal is prevented from running by confinement, phase shifts usually do not occur. Larger phase advances, on the order of 3 h, can be produced by placing hamsters into novel running wheels for 2 to 3 h. (*A* reprinted from Science. Takahashi JS, Zatz M. Regulation of circadian rhythmicity. Science. 1982;2178:1104–1111.)

internal timing device maintains a correct phase relation to the environment.

This mechanism must also be capable of compensating for the continuous seasonal changes in day-night ratio that characterize temperate zone habitats. Even a precise 24-h clock will not time behavior appropriately throughout the year unless it can track the movement of relevant phases of the day-night cycle. To achieve the appropriate timing of behavior, circadian clocks must (1) adjust their periods each cycle to compensate for the difference between their intrinsic periods (typically not equal to 24 h) and the 24-h environmental day and (2) become synchronized in such a way that the overt rhythms occur at the appropriate daily phases (which may require seasonal adjustments of phase). This process of period and phase control of an oscillator by an environmental cycle is known as *entrainment*. Environmental cycles that can entrain circadian oscillations are termed *zeitgebers* (from the German "time givers").

As might be expected, light is a virtually universal zeitgeber for the circadian rhythms displayed by most organisms, from single-celled protists through mammals. The mechanism by which light entrains circadian rhythms has been investigated by assessing the effects of discrete applications of light on circadian rhythms free-running in constant darkness (DD).[7] Brief light pulses cause phase shifts of free-running rhythms, the magnitude and direction of which depend on when within the circadian cycle the light pulse is presented (see Fig. 25–1A). This phase dependence of light effects is illustrated graphically by plotting the size and direction of the phase shift against the circadian phase of light presentation, producing a *phase response curve* (PRC) for light (see Fig. 25–1B).

Light pulses presented at the beginning of the "subjective night" (the daily active period in nocturnal species and daily rest period in diurnal species) produce phase delays, whereas pulses presented toward the end of the subjective night produce phase advances. During most of the subjective day, light pulses have relatively little effect, resulting in a so-called dead zone on the PRC. A phase delay means that the onset of the next "subjective day" (rest time in nocturnal species, activity time in diurnal species) begins and then ends later than usual, whereas a phase advance means that the subjective day begins and then ends earlier than usual.

A phase shift can be conceptualized as the result of light inducing a brief acceleration or slowing of the underlying circadian clock, thus causing the overt rest-activity rhythm that it drives to be permanently displaced forward or backward in time. However, a shift in phase is also seen in some models as part of a more complex response to a stimulus, involving simultaneous alterations in the amplitude and phase of the underlying oscillator's motion.[8, 9]

Sensitivity of circadian pacemakers to ambient light has also been studied under constant conditions. When the intensity of constant illumination is altered, the free-running τ of most organisms changes. Aschoff[3] summarized these changes and observed that the direction of τ change as constant illumination intensity in-

creases is opposite in most diurnal (day-active) versus nocturnal (night-active) species. While this rule is not universally applicable, for many nocturnal species the free-running τ lengthens as intensity increases, while it shortens for diurnal species. Other, coordinated features of daily rhythms (the duration and amount of activity) also change in parallel to the changes in τ. These features have been summarized as the "circadian rules."[3]

The shape of the PRC for light pulses suggests that entrainment may be accomplished by a combination of phase delays in the evening and advances in the morning, producing a net daily shift equal to the difference between the period of the circadian pacemaker and 24 h. The bidirectionality of the PRC may serve several functions. It can stabilize entrainment in spite of variability in light exposure and spontaneous τ, and it confers the flexibility that allows continued entrainment when endocrine changes, aging, or other factors alter the τ of the pacemaker.

The intrinsic τ of an oscillator and its phase response characteristics should determine whether it will entrain to a light-dark (LD) cycle of a given periodicity (T). Entrainment will occur only in those cases in which the difference between τ and T does not exceed the maximal phase shifts that can be induced by exposure to available light. In practice, these "limits-to-entrainment" are somewhat flexible. Depending on the species studied, entrainment may fail if the LD cycle is abruptly changed from 24 h to less than 22 h or greater than 26 h. However, these limits can be extended if the LD cycle is changed gradually. This phenomenon appears to involve gradual modification of the intrinsic circadian τ by exposure to altered LD cycles.

When released to DD after entrainment to an LD cycle with a long period, the expressed free-running rhythm tends to have a slightly longer τ than usual. Conversely, when released from a short-period LD cycle, τ is correspondingly shorter than usual. These so-called aftereffects, which can persist for many weeks, suggest that entrainment limits are flexible because the intrinsic τ of the circadian clock can be modified by experience. Thus, each organism should be seen as capable of expressing a (narrow) range of endogenous periodicities, depending on both current and previous environmental conditions.

Intrinsic periodicity and PRC shape also determine the phase relation that circadian rhythms will assume with respect to the entraining LD cycle. Stable entrainment will occur at whatever phase produces the photic stimulation that generates the net phase shift necessary to offset the difference between τ and T. The PRCs for nocturnal rodents show maximal phase delays several hours after the beginning of the subjective night (a phase defined by activity onset). Rodents with very short τ will entrain stably when light exposure extends into this delay portion of the circadian cycle; the daily activity period will thus tend to begin somewhat before lights-off. The occurrence of activity onset in anticipation of dusk is designated a positive phase relation. When τ is greater than T, the phase relation between lights-off and activity onset is usually negative, resulting in light exposure of the sensitive phase that yields advance phase shifts. The parallel entrainment differences that define human beings as "early birds" or "night owls" probably reflect in part individual differences in the intrinsic periodicities of our circadian clocks or the shapes of our PRCs.

If differential effects of light exposure at two circadian phases (dawn and dusk) account for entrainment under naturally occurring, Temperate Zone photoperiods (i.e., LD cycles with about 8 to 16 h of light), then it should be possible to entrain an organism to a photoperiod involving only two light pulses in each 24-h cycle, separated by about 8 to 16 h. Stable entrainment under such "skeleton" photoperiods has been documented in several species and appears to be similar in most respects to entrainment under a full photoperiod.[10] In fact, studies of nocturnal rodents in seminatural environments indicate that brief exposure to light at dawn or dusk may fully account for entrainment in these species.[11] Entrainment mechanisms have not been studied as thoroughly in diurnal mammals, which differ from nocturnal species in that they are exposed to light for long durations each day. PRCs to light pulses have been obtained for a few diurnal mammals that are qualitatively similar to those for nocturnal rodents,[12] but other diurnal rodents have been reported to show very different responses to brief light pulses than do nocturnal species.[13, 14] Thus, the applicability of models derived from nocturnal rodents to all diurnal species is uncertain, and it is likely that exposure to light for many hours during the day also plays a role in entrainment that has not yet been well defined.

A PRC to light has been produced for human beings. Other studies demonstrate that human beings may be entrained by strictly imposed 24-h LD cycles during temporal isolation studies and can be acutely phase-shifted by changes in light exposure independently of changes in their sleep-wake schedules. These studies are described in greater detail in Chapter 28.

Nonphotic Entrainment

Masking and Entrainment

Environmental stimuli can have diverse effects on rhythmical physiological and behavioral processes. For example, in rats, 24-h LD cycles entrain the circadian rhythm of activity of the pineal enzyme serotonin N-acetyltransferase to peak at night. However, light also directly suppresses N-acetyltransferase activity when it is elevated during the night.[15] This photosuppressive effect may be viewed as "masking" the true phase of the oscillator generating the N-acetyltransferase rhythm; light can impose low levels of enzyme activity during the night when the circadian clock is specifying high levels. Similarly, locomotor activity in nocturnal rodents is suppressed by light (negative masking of activity) and facilitated by dark (positive masking of activity).[16] Rapid eye movement (REM) sleep in rats is triggered by light-to-dark transitions independently of LD entrainment of the circadian sleep-wake cycle.[17]

These masking effects present interpretive difficulties in evaluating whether a periodic environmental signal functions as a true zeitgeber. A periodic signal may entrain a behavioral or physiological rhythm, in which case it is functioning as a zeitgeber, or it may directly impose a rhythm without affecting an underlying oscillator, in which case it is functioning only as a masking stimulus. The criteria for distinguishing masking from entrainment are based on the properties of oscillator entrainment discussed in relation to photic cycles.

- An entrained rhythm should follow an environmental cycle over only a limited range of environmental periods.
- The phase relation between an entrained rhythm and an environmental cycle should vary depending on the values of τ and T.
- This phase relation should be re-established if the environmental cycle is abruptly shifted. If the rhythm is a direct response to the environmental cycle, shifting will be immediate. If, instead, it reflects entrainment of an underlying oscillator, several "transient" cycles may be evident before the prior phase relation is re-established. The number of transient cycles would presumably reflect the maximal daily phase shifts of the oscillator that can be induced by the zeitgeber.
- The rhythm should persist (free-run) in the absence of the periodic stimulus, just as photically entrained rhythms persist in constant lighting conditions, and the initial phase of the free-run should reflect the apparent phase of the rhythm during entrainment.

As reviewed in the following sections, several nonphotic stimuli have been identified that meet these criteria and can therefore be said to entrain circadian rhythms.

Scheduled Feeding

Rats provided with food for only a few hours each day at a fixed time show changes in locomotor activity, body temperature, and other physiological variables that anticipate the daily mealtime.[18] These anticipatory responses begin to emerge within several days of scheduled feeding, and appear to be generated independently of photically entrained rhythms. If the meal is provided in the middle of the light period, rats will continue to express their usual activity at night in addition to premeal anticipatory activity during the day (see Fig. 25–2A). If the photic cycle is replaced by constant light (LL) or DD, photically entrained rest-activity rhythms will free-run; however, premeal activity will continue to occur precisely every 24 h if meal presentation continues on this schedule (see Fig. 25–2B). It is common, then, to observe two circadian activity components in food-restricted rats in LL, one component free-running with a period slightly different from 24 h, and a second, food-anticipatory component with a period of exactly 24 h.

Several models have been proposed to account for

the emergence of food-anticipatory activity rhythms.[18] Most findings, however, are parsimoniously explained by the hypothesis that anticipatory activity is generated by a circadian oscillator mechanism entrained by food availability:

- Anticipatory responses do not emerge when the period of the food cycle is outside a broad circadian range of about 22 to 33 h.[19]
- The phase relation between anticipatory activity onset and mealtime becomes increasingly positive as the period of the feeding cycle is lengthened and less positive as it is shortened.[20]
- Phase-shifting the feeding time is usually followed by gradual rather than immediate shifts of the activity peak to resynchronize to the mealtime.[21]
- When the period of the food availability cycle is abruptly shortened or lengthened from 24 to 22 or 30 h, the meal-synchronized rhythm may dissociate from feeding time and free-run for many cycles.[19]
- When food is made freely available, the control exerted by these oscillators over behavior diminishes, resulting in a loss of overt activity related to the former mealtime. However, when the rat is subsequently food-deprived for several days, it once again becomes active at a circadian phase previously associated with feeding time[22] (see Fig. 25–2A).

Taken together, these observations provide strong evidence that a self-sustained oscillator is involved in generating meal-anticipatory activity, and indicate that its influence on behavior is gated by the animal's motivational state. Other studies show that rats can utilize food-entrainable oscillators to discriminate time of day, which may enable them to anticipate multiple feeding times and link these with multiple feeding places.[23] Anticipation of multiple meals may also be facilitated by a two-oscillator structure of the food-entrainable circadian mechanism.[24] As elaborated in Chapter 26, these food-entrainable oscillators are anatomically distinct from the circadian pacemaker that mediates photic entrainment.

The stimuli associated with food acquisition and ingestion that provide the timing signals necessary to entrain these oscillators are not well characterized. Rats can anticipate meals of any nutrient composition provided that these meals represent a significant contribution to daily caloric intake.[25, 26] Similar results have been obtained in studies examining the ability of specific nutrients to shift food-anticipatory rhythms.[27] Observations of anticipatory behaviors to restricted schedules of water[28] and salt[29] access suggest that the range of effective stimuli may extend to any motivationally significant resource for which a rat must forage.

The use of separate pacemakers to mediate food and light entrainment in rats confers flexibility on the circadian organization of their behavior, and permits anticipation of a stable window of food availability at any time of day, without necessarily altering the phase of photically entrained activity rhythms. However, in some circumstances, feeding schedules can also affect the rest of the circadian system. Restricted feeding schedules occasionally entrain the entire circadian system in rats and other species maintained under LL, and can induce an apparent phase advance of nocturnal activity in rats fed during the middle of the light period of an LD cycle.[30–33] However, these effects are not observed consistently, and, as will be discussed in the next section, they may reflect coupling forces exerted by anticipatory activity, rather than by food intake or a separate food-entrainable oscillator, on the circadian pacemaker that mediates photic entrainment. Food anticipation has been demonstrated in several species,[34–36] but apart from rats, only in hamsters and mice have the appropriate studies been done to confirm mediation by separate food-entrainable oscillators.[32, 37, 38]

Temperature

Free-running rhythms in a variety of poikilothermic species can be entrained by 24-h cycles of ambient temperature.[39] However, responses of homeothermic animals to temperature cycles are more variable. In some species, temperature cycles failed to entrain various circadian rhythms,[40, 41] whereas in other species, including squirrel monkeys,[42] pig-tailed macaques,[43] rats, and a marsupial mouse,[44] temperature cycles have clear entrainment effects.

The mechanism by which temperature entrains circadian rhythms is unclear. In homeothermic species, it would seem unlikely to involve a direct effect on circadian oscillators because brain temperature is homeostatically protected, although in at least one mammalian species variations in core temperature are associated with modulations of free-running rhythms.[45] One possibility is that temperature cycles directly modulate sleep or wake states, facilitating sleep at some ambient temperatures and inhibiting it at others. The neural and endocrine correlates of the sleep-wake states, and the obvious changes in food and water intake, activity, and light exposure they entail, may in turn have phase-modulating feedback effects on circadian oscillators. Conceivably, any stimulus that has potent effects on behavioral state may ultimately have significance as a circadian zeitgeber (see below).

Activity and Arousal States

In an early description of the circadian rules, Aschoff[3] noted that the relation between light intensity and τ might be mediated by changes in arousal states, since constant bright light both lengthens τ and suppresses activity in nocturnal rodents. A later study provided some support for the idea that metabolism, arousal, or some correlate affected the circadian pacemaker, in that the free-running τ of activity rhythms (measured as general locomotor activity using photocell interruptions) was longer in hamsters with access to running wheels.[46] More recent studies indicate that this effect is weak in hamsters, but is robust in rats and mice; τ shortens when wheels are available, and lengthens when wheels are subsequently locked.[47, 48]

Evidently, some correlate of spontaneous, clock-regulated wheel-running activity provides a feedback signal that alters the rate at which the circadian pacemaker cycles.

The effects of behavior or attendant arousal on functional properties of the circadian pacemaker were not widely recognized until the late 1980s, when a series of studies demonstrated unequivocally that acutely stimulated behavioral activity can reliably induce large phase shifts in hamsters (see Fig. 25–3), and, if repeated on a daily basis, can entrain free-running rhythms in hamsters, rats, and mice (Fig. 25–4). The earliest of these studies showed that hamsters could be phase-shifted or entrained simply by changing their litter or cages,[49] or by the opportunity for a 30-min daily bout of foraging activity in an open field, despite little or no eating at that time.[50] More robust phase shifts were obtained by confining hamsters to novel running wheels for 2 to 3 h, a procedure that has been widely used to characterize the formal properties of phase shifts induced by a nonphotic stimulus. Hamsters typi-

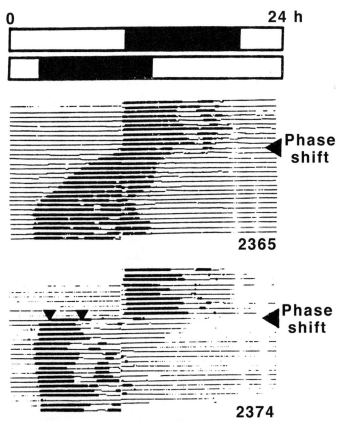

0   **24 h**

►**Phase shift**

2365

◄**Phase shift**

2374

Figure 25–4. Event records of wheel-running from two hamsters maintained in a 14:10 light-dark (LD) cycle. On the days indicated by the triangle, the LD cycle was phase-advanced by 8 h, that is, the dark period began 8 h early. The hamster in the top chart took about 10 d to resynchronize to the shifted LD cycle, which is typical for hamsters. The hamster in the lower chart was transferred to a novel running wheel for 3 h at the beginning of the new time of dark onset on the day of the LD shift. This hamster resynchronized to the shifted LD cycle in 1 d. Acceleration of re-entrainment is dependent on running in the novel wheel. (Modified from Mrosovsky N, Salmon PA. A behavioural method for accelerating re-entrainment of rhythms to new light-dark cycles. Nature. 1987;330:372–373.)

cally exhibit constant wheel-running activity in the novel cage, and exhibit phase shifts of up to 3 h.[51] Studies of temporal sensitivity show that phase advances occur to wheel-running induced in the mid–subjective day (when the hamster is usually inactive) and phase delays to wheel-running induced in the subjective night (see Fig. 25–2B). If repeated at the same time each day, this procedure can entrain free-running rhythms in hamsters maintained in LL.[49, 51] These effects appear to be a response to wheel-running; if running is prevented in the novel cage, phase shifts are usually not observed. Dose-response studies indicate that 3-h activity bouts are more potent than 1- to 2-h bouts, and that maximal phase shifts are reliably induced if the number of revolutions in a 17-cm wheel exceed about 5000 in 3 h.[52] Even larger phase shifts (8 to 12 h) have been observed in hamsters running in wheels for the first time.[53]

The PRC for induced wheel-running is somewhat similar in shape to the PRC generated by exposing hamsters for several hours to periods of darkness ("dark pulses") while they are housed in LL.[54] Dark pulses of 3- to 6-h duration during the mid–subjective day also stimulate wheel-running; if running is prevented by restraint during dark exposure, no phase shift occurs.[55, 56] Although other interpretations are possible, these results suggest that the effects of dark pulses on hamsters are mediated largely by increased activity. Other stimuli that produce similar phase shifts when applied during the mid–subjective day to rodents, such as triazolam or morphine injections, cold exposure, and refeeding after a single bout of food deprivation, also appear to do so by virtue of triggering increases in activity.[56–60]

An alternative interpretation is that hamsters phase-shift in response to arousing stimuli because they are awakened at a circadian phase when they would normally be asleep. Wheel-running may be strongly correlated with phase shifting because it promotes arousal, and when animals do not run, they may not stay awake. In support of this idea, we have demonstrated in Syrian hamsters that 3 h of sleep deprivation by gentle handling, with minimal locomotor activation, fully mimics the phase advancing effect of continuous running for 3 h in the middle of the sleep phase.[60a]

The conclusion that "nonphotic" stimuli phase-shift because they induce activity or arousal is clearly not universally applicable to all stimuli, nor to all species. Dark pulses, for example, phase-shift sparrows even though darkness inhibits their activity,[61] and dark pulses are very effective at shifting rhythms in plants[62] or pineal cells cultured in vitro,[63] where the issue of mediation by arousal or activity is not relevant. The benzodiazepine triazolam phase-shifts monkeys, even though it sedates them.[64] Injections of another benzodiazepine, chlordiazepoxide, induce phase shifts in hamsters similar to those caused by triazolam, but unlike those induced by triazolam, these are not blocked by physical restraint.[65] Central injections of serotonin,[66] neuropeptide Y,[67] muscimol,[68] or saline (only late in the subjective day)[69] can all induce dark pulse-like phase advance shifts in hamsters, but these are also not dependent on the expression of activity. Some of these pharmacological manipulations may directly mimic or activate the central consequences of increased activity.

The adaptive significance of the phase-shifting effects of stimulated activity or arousal in hamsters is unclear, but it may represent a mechanism for modulating circadian activity patterns in response to biologically important events related, for example, to social or sexual interactions.[70] The potential practical applications of this phenomenon are, however, considerable. For example, a single 3-h bout of appropriately scheduled wheel activity in hamsters can greatly accelerate re-entrainment to a shifted LD cycle[71] (see Fig. 25–4) and repeated daily bouts can alter the phase of entrainment to an LD cycle.[72] Scheduled activity may thus represent a potent tool for manipulating human circadian rhythms to remedy acute disorders associated with travel across time zones and with shift work. The first studies on human beings have recently been reported, and these indicate that rhythms in human beings can be shifted or entrained by exercise or some nonphotic correlate.[73–75] Observations of partial or complete entrainment to scheduled activity or arousal in other diurnal[76] and nocturnal species[77–79] suggest that this feature of the mammalian circadian system may be quite general.

Social Cues

Social cues are known to phase-shift, entrain, or modify the period of free-running rhythms in several species, including sparrows,[80] rat pups,[81] beavers,[82] degus,[76] and human beings[83]; however, they are not universally effective. Rodents housed individually in adjacent cages typically do not become mutually synchronized despite auditory, olfactory, and visual contact; and blind and sighted hamsters housed in the same cage may fail to become mutually entrained.[84] Blind human beings may also display free-running sleep-wake and other rhythms despite exposure to the social cues of a 24-h society.[85] The mechanisms by which social cues influence circadian timing are not known, but effects on arousal states are probably a necessary, if not sufficient, component of this mechanism.

Interactions Between Photic and Nonphotic Zeitgebers

The striking effects of spontaneous activity on free-running τ in rats and mice, and of induced activity on phase in free-running hamsters, suggest that the steady-state, entrained phase of circadian rhythms may reflect integration of photic and nonphotic stimuli. Effects of spontaneous activity levels on the phase of photic entrainment have not yet been thoroughly documented, although preliminary analyses indicate that a high level of activity early in the active phase is associated with a more advanced phase of entrainment in mice (R.E.M. and M.M. Holmes, unpublished data, 1999). This effect is consistent with earlier findings that

τ in free-running mice is shortened by access to a running wheel or when running is concentrated early in the active phase.[47]

A number of studies, nearly all using hamsters as subjects, have examined whether activity induced each day at a particular phase of the LD cycle can alter entrainment to lighting cycles. Some of these studies have obtained results suggesting that photic and nonphotic inputs combine linearly, in accordance with their respective PRCs. For example, activity or arousal induced in the middle of the light period by triazolam injections, wheel confinement, social or sexual stimuli, or restricted feeding can advance the phase of nocturnal activity onset,[30, 70, 72, 86, 87] whereas activity induced late in the subjective night can delay the phase of activity onset.[72, 88]

Other results, however, indicate that under some circumstances, photic and nonphotic stimuli may combine nonlinearly and produce phase changes that are not predictable from separate analyses of the photic and nonphotic PRCs. Two studies have shown that activity induced in the middle of the light period can in some cases significantly delay, rather than advance, nocturnal activity onset.[88, 89] This apparent delay may reflect splitting of the activity rhythm into two components, one that delays with respect to dark onset, and another that advances and aligns with the midday wheel-running session.

Another set of studies has examined the interactive effects of single pulses of photic and nonphotic stimuli in combination. The results again suggest complex, nonlinear interactions. Phase advances induced by an activity bout in the mid–subjective day can be blocked by a subsequent light pulse, although the light pulse alone at that time produces no phase shift.[90, 91] Phase advances induced by a light pulse in the late subjective night can be significantly attenuated by an overlapping 45-min bout of induced running, a stimulus that is inadequate on its own to cause a significant shift at this phase.[92, 93] This inhibitory effect of activity on photic shifts appears to be phase dependent; activity early in the night does not attenuate phase delays to light.[92] In scorpions, the phase shift response to light pulses is apparently entirely dependent on whether the scorpion is active during the light pulse.[94]

Finally, at least one study has reported evidence that photic and nonphotic stimuli might in some instances show nonlinear synergy rather than mutual inhibition. Acceleration of re-entrainment to a 7-h phase advance of the LD cycle by a single 3-h bout of activity induced at the onset of the new dark period was somewhat greater than that predicted by summing the phase advances induced by the light and activity stimuli given alone.[71, 95] The analysis of the rules of interaction between photic and nonphotic zeitgebers is at an early stage. It will likely be facilitated by physiological studies of interactions among the neural inputs to the circadian pacemaker that are thought to mediate photic and nonphotic zeitgeber inputs (see Chapter 26).

Although manipulations of activity necessarily affect sleep and waking, the scant evidence, until recently, indicated that sleep deprivation in rats and hamsters does not induce phase shifts.[96, 97] However, the lack of phase shifting in the hamster study may have been because the deprivations were conducted with the lights on. In our more recent study, large phase shifts were induced when deprivations were conducted with the lights off.[60a] Despite the lack of phase shifting to sleep deprivation alone in the initial studies, sleep deprivations as short as 6 h significantly attenuated the phase-delaying effect of light pulses early in the subjective night.[97] Short, intense bouts of wheel-running or stress do not inhibit photic shifting at this phase[92] (R.E.M. and S.V. Sinclair, unpublished data, 1997), but the contributions of slow, continuous activity and heightened arousal to this effect of sleep deprivation need to be more fully examined. Nonetheless, the results do suggest that sleep loss accompanying jet travel or shift work rotation may affect the response of the pacemaker to shifted photic zeitgebers.

The study of nonphotic effects on circadian rhythms in the past decade has produced a number of surprising discoveries, one of which is the report that a neutral, nonphotic stimulus can acquire phase-shifting properties by repeated pairing with light pulses. An air disturbance created by a fan that reliably preceded a daily, phase-shifting light pulse was reported to acquire the capacity to induce a phase shift similar to that induced by light in rats.[98] While attempts to replicate this finding using modified conditions in our laboratories have not been successful in either rats or hamsters (de Groot and Rusak, unpublished observations; R.E.M. et al., unpublished data, 1997), it remains possible that both current and previous exposure to nonphotic stimuli can modify photic entrainment processes. Further research will be needed to define the limits of the conditions under which such phenomena are manifest.

DEVELOPMENT AND AGING OF CIRCADIAN RHYTHMS

Assessment of biological rhythmicity across the life span presents many methodological and interpretive challenges. Despite these challenges, a valid cross-species generalization is that circadian rhythms in behavioral, physiological, or neural functions are first evident prenatally, stabilize and entrain to LD cycles within the first few weeks (e.g., in rodents) or months (e.g., in human beings) postnatally, and may exhibit changes in phase, period, amplitude, and response to zeitgebers in old age, with considerable variability within and among species.

In rodents, behavioral rhythmicity is not apparent before the second week postnatally.[99] However, extrapolation to prenatal life of the phase at which behavioral and physiological rhythms emerge indicates that the circadian pacemaker is functioning at or before birth in rats, hamsters, and mice.[100–102] 2-Deoxyglucose autoradiography has been used to confirm that the circadian pacemaker, which is located in the hypothalamic suprachiasmatic nucleus (SCN; see Chapter 26), ex-

presses a daily rhythm of glucose metabolism as early as day 19 of gestation,[103] 2 to 3 d before birth and prior to significant synaptogenesis in the SCN.[104] Although the fetal pacemaker lacks most input and output pathways, its metabolic rhythm is synchronized to the dam by a mechanism that involves pacemaker sensitivity to endogenous dopamine and maternal melatonin.[81] Postnatally, the pacemaker becomes sensitive to photic stimuli during days 2 to 6, at which time it loses sensitivity to dopamine.[105] Maternal coordination of the fetus in utero ensures that when the pacemaker becomes coupled to effector systems for behavior and physiology postnatally, the emerging rhythms in these functions are appropriately phased with respect to the day-night cycle, and to rhythms of the dam (e.g., see reference 106).

Studies of the human fetus in utero have revealed daily variations in fetal motility, heart rate, and other variables by 20 to 22 weeks' gestation.[107, 108] Although these rhythms may be driven directly by maternal factors, evidence for circadian periodicities of various functions in premature infants suggests that human beings can generate rhythms endogenously as early as 30 weeks' gestation.[109] Neonates tracked over the first year of life exhibit a gradual emergence of circadian rhythmicity, which initially may appear to free-run, but which generally becomes synchronized to the day-night cycle within 2 to 3 months.[110, 111] The conditions under which infants are maintained (e.g., on demand vs. scheduled feeding) can greatly influence the temporal organization of sleep-wake states (reviewed in reference 112). The extent to which maturation of masking and entrainment processes contribute to the appearance of synchronized rhythms early in life is unknown.

Poor sleep is a primary concern of the aged, and deterioration of circadian organization may be a significant contributing factor. The most widely observed change in circadian rhythmicity with age is a decrease in the amplitude of a variety of rhythms, including activity, temperature, and sleep-wake, under entrained and free-running conditions.[113] However, a reduced rhythm amplitude is difficult to interpret, and could reflect changes in intrinsic properties of the pacemaker (e.g., coupling among a population of cellular oscillators), or changes upstream or downstream from the molecular machinery of the circadian clock. Changes upstream from the pacemaker may include reductions in sensitivity to photic or nonphotic stimuli. There is evidence that phase shifts to light at low intensities are reduced in aged rodents, but that responses to saturating intensities are greatly enhanced, at least at the transition point between delays and advances on the photic PRC.[114] These effects are consistent with a reduced sensitivity to light at the receptor level, and reduced amplitude of oscillation at the pacemaker level. Phase-shift responses to nonphotic stimuli (e.g., triazolam injections) have also been reported to be reduced in aged rodents,[115] although this may to some extent be due to a reduced running response to the drug in old animals.[116]

Daily rhythms of sleep in human beings are commonly viewed as "fragmented," with less sleep at night and more napping during the day.[117] A reduced amplitude of circadian rhythms has been reported in entrained and free-running human beings in many but not all studies.[113, 118] Failure to observe differences between young and old subjects in some samples may reflect individual differences and illustrate the limitations of cross-sectional studies, because these of necessity include only survivors in the advanced age groups, whose circadian mechanisms may differ from those of others in the cohort.

Another commonly observed effect of aging in rodents and human beings is an advanced phase of entrainment to the day-night cycle.[113, 119] An advanced phase is consistent with reports that free-running τ is shorter in aged subjects. This effect is consistently evident in studies employing extended longitudinal designs.[120, 121] In some species, τ may lengthen with age (e.g., canaries[122]). Detection of τ changes may depend on the use of sufficiently aged subjects (many studies have used middle-aged subjects), on the duration of recording (aftereffects of previous photoperiods may obscure age-related changes) and on the recording method. In rats and mice, for example, wheel-running activity shortens τ and is significantly attenuated with age. Changes in τ due to pacemaker aging might thus be obscured by τ changes accompanying the reduction of feedback signals from behavior, arousal, hormones, or other factors.

It has been suggested that loss of temporal order may be a cause rather than merely a symptom of aging.[123] In aged rodents, loss of circadian rhythmicity is predictive of impending death,[124] and extended exposure to lighting schedules at the limits of entrainment can reduce life span in some invertebrate species.[125, 126] Although loss of rhythmicity by experimental ablation of the circadian pacemaker does not appear to greatly affect survival of ground squirrels in their natural habitat,[127] effects on mean and maximal life span are unknown. The empirical database is insufficient to draw strong conclusions about the role of the circadian system in normal aging.

CONCLUSION

This overview of the environmental and behavioral events that can affect circadian organization suggests that a wide variety of stimuli may ultimately affect rhythms by altering one of two (i.e., photic and nonphotic) regulatory mechanisms at the cellular level. This view may be too simplistic, however. It is possible that there are many independent routes by which environmental cues can affect circadian rhythms. Resolving this issue will depend on developing a detailed physiological description of the mechanisms by which relevant stimuli impinge on the pacemaker. A review of this physiological analysis is the subject of Chapter 26.

References

1. Moore-Ede MC, Sulzman FM, Fuller CA. The Clocks That Time Us. Cambridge, Mass: Harvard University Press; 1982.

2. Rusak B. Vertebrate behavioural rhythms. In: Aschoff J, ed. Handbook of Behavioural Neurobiology. New York, NY: Plenum; 1980:182–214.

3. Aschoff J. Exogenous and endogenous components in circadian rhythms. Cold Spring Harbor Symp Quant Biol. 1960;25:11–26.

4. Davis FC, Menaker M. Development of the mouse circadian pacemaker: independence from environmental cycles. J Comp Physiol. 1981;143:527–539.

5. Bunning E. The Physiological Clock. New York, NY: Springer-Verlag; 1973.

6. Pittendrigh CS, Bruce VG. An oscillator model of biological clocks. In: Rudnick D, ed. Rhythmic and Synthetic Processes in Growth. Princeton, NJ: Princeton University Press; 1957:39–107.

7. DeCoursey PJ. Daily light sensitivity rhythm in a rodent. Science. 1960;131:33–35.

8. Winfree A. Unclocklike behaviour of biological clocks. Nature. 1975;253:315–319.

9. Jewett ME, Kronauer RE, Czeisler CA. Phase-amplitude resetting of the human circadian pacemaker via bright light: a further analysis. J Biol Rhythms. 1994;9:295–314.

10. Pittendrigh CS, Daan S. A functional analysis of circadian pacemakers in nocturnal rodents; IV: entrainment: pacemaker as clock. J Comp Physiol [A]. 1976;106:291–331.

11. DeCoursey PJ. Circadian photoentrainment: parameters of phase delaying. J Biol Rhythms. 1986;1:171–186.

12. Pohl H. Characteristics and variability in entrainment of circadian rhythms to light in diurnal rodents. In: Aschoff J, Daan S, Groos G, eds. Vertebrate Circadian Systems. New York, NY: Springer-Verlag; 1982:339–346.

13. Lee TM, Labyak SE. P.-Free-running rhythms and light- and dark-pulse phase response curves for diurnal *Octodon degus* (Rodentia). Am J Physiol. 1997;273:R278–286.

14. Abe H, Honma S, Shinohara K, et al. Circadian modulation in photic induction of Fos-like immunoreactivity in the suprachiasmatic nucleus cells of diurnal chipmunk, *Eutamias asiaticus*. J Comp Physiol [A]. 1995;176:159–167.

15. Klein D, Weller J. Rapid light-induced decrease in pineal serotonin N-acetyltransferase activity. Science. 1972;177:532–533.

16. Aschoff J, Daan S, Honma KI. Zeitgebers, entrainment and masking: some unsettled questions. In: Aschoff J, Daan S, Groos G, eds. Vertebrate Circadian Systems. New York, NY: Springer-Verlag; 1982:13–24.

17. Rechtschaffen A, Dates R, Tobias M, et al. The effects of lights-off stimulation on the distribution of paradoxical sleep in the rat. Commun Behav Biol. 1969;3:93–99.

18. Mistlberger RE. Circadian food anticipatory activity: formal models and physiological mechanisms. Neurosci Biobehav Rev. 1994;18:1–25.

19. Stephan FK. Limits of entrainment to periodic feeding in rats with suprachiasmatic lesions. J Comp Physiol [A]. 1981;143:401–410.

20. Aschoff J, von Goetz C, Honma KI. Restricted feeding in rats: effects of varying feeding cycles. Z Tierpsychol. 1983;63:91–111.

21. Stephan FK. Phase shifts of circadian rhythms in activity entrained to food access. Physiol Behav. 1984;32:663–671.

22. Coleman GJ, Harper S, Clarke JD, et al. Evidence for a separate meal-associated oscillator in the rat. Physiol Behav. 1982;29:107–115.

23. Mistlberger RE, de Groot MH, Bossert JM, et al. Discrimination of circadian phase in intact and SCN ablated rats. Brain Res. 1996;739:12–18.

24. Stephan FK. Forced dissociation of activity entrained to T cycles of food access in rats with suprachiasmatic lesions. J Biol Rhythms. 1989;4:467–479.

25. Mistlberger RE, Rusak B. Palatable daily meals entrain anticipatory activity rhythms in free-feeding rats: dependence on meal size and nutrient content. Physiol Behav. 1987;41:219–226.

26. Mistlberger RE, Houpt TA, Moore-Ede MC. Food-anticipatory rhythms under 24h schedules of limited access to single macronutrients. J Biol Rhythms. 1990;5:35–46.

27. Stephan FK. Calories affect zeitgeber properties of the feeding entrained circadian oscillator. Physiol Behav. 1997;62:995–1002.

28. Mistlberger RE. Anticipatory activity rhythms under daily schedules of water access in the rat. J Biol Rhythms. 1992;7:149–160.

29. Rosenwasser AM, Schulkin J, Adler NT. Anticipatory appetitive behavior of adrenalectomized rats under circadian salt-access schedules. Anim Learn Behav. 1988;16:324–329.

30. Challet E, Pevet P, Viviens-Roels B, et al. Phase advanced daily rhythms of melatonin, body temperature, and locomotor activity in food-restricted rats fed during daytime. J Biol Rhythms. 1997;12:65–79.

31. Kennedy G, Coleman GJ, Armstrong S. Restricted feeding entrains circadian wheel-running activity rhythms of the kowari. Am J Physiol. 1991;261:R819–R827.

32. Marchant EG, Mistlberger RE. Anticipation and entrainment to feeding time in intact and SCN-ablated C57B1/6j mice. Brain Res. 1997;765:273–282.

33. Stephan FK. The role of period and phase in interactions between feeding- and light-entrainable circadian rhythms. Physiol Behav. 1986;36:151–158.

34. Boulos Z, Frim DM, Dewey LK, et al. Effects of restricted feeding schedules on circadian organization in squirrel monkeys. Physiol Behav. 1989;45:507–515.

35. O'Reilly H, Armstrong S, Coleman GJ. Restricted feeding and circadian activity rhythms of a predatory marsupial, Dasyuroides byrnei. Physiol Behav. 1986;38:471–476.

36. Zielinski W. Circadian rhythms of small carnivores and the effects of restricted feed on daily rhythms. Physiol Behav. 1986;38:613–620.

37. Abe H, Rusak B. Anticipatory activity and entrainment of circadian rhythms in Syrian hamsters exposed to restricted palatable diets. Am J Physiol. 1992;263:R116–R124.

38. Mistlberger RE. Circadian properties of anticipatory activity to restricted water access in suprachiasmatic-ablated hamsters. Am J Physiol. 1992;264:R22–R29.

39. Sweeney B, Hastings J. Effects of temperature upon diurnal rhythms. Cold Spring Harbor Symp Quant Biol. 1960;25:87–104.

40. Hoffman K. Die relative Wirksamkeit von Zeitgebern. Oecologia. 1969;3:184–206.

41. Stewart MC, Reeder WG. Temperature and light synchronization experiments with circadian activity in two color forms of the rock pocket mouse. Physiol Zool. 1968;41:149–156.

42. Aschoff J, Tokura H. Circadian activity rhythms in squirrel monkeys: entrainment by temperature cycles. J Biol Rhythms. 1986;1:91–100.

43. Tokura H, Aschoff J. Effects of temperature on the circadian rhythm of pig-tailed macaques, Macaca nemestrina. Am J Physiol. 1983;245:R800–R804.

44. Francis A, Coleman GJ. Ambient temperature cycles entrain the free-running circadian rhythms of the stripe-faced dunnart. J Comp Physiol [A]. 1990;167:357–362.

45. Lee TM, Holmes WG, Zucker I. Temperature dependence of circadian rhythms in golden-mantled ground squirrels. J Biol Rhythms. 1990;5:25–34.

46. Aschoff J, Figala J, Poppel E. Circadian rhythms of locomotor activity in the golden hamster measured with two different techniques. J Comp Physiol Psychol. 1973;85:20–28.

47. Edgar DM, Martin C, Dement WC. Activity feedback to the mammalian circadian pacemaker: influence on observed measures of rhythm period length. J Biol Rhythms. 1991;6:185–199.

48. Yamada N, Shimoda K, Ohi S, et al. Free-access to a running wheel shortens the period of free-running rhythms in blinded rats. Physiol Behav. 1988;42:87–91.

49. Mrosovsky N. Phase-response curves for social entrainment. J Comp Physiol [A]. 1988;162:35–46.

50. Rusak B, Mistlberger RE, Losier B, et al. Daily hoarding opportunity entrains the pacemaker for hamster activity rhythms. J Comp Physiol [A]. 1988;164:165–171.

51. Reebs SG, Mrosovsky N. Effects of induced wheel running on the circadian activity rhythms of Syrian hamsters: entrainment and phase-response curve. J Biol Rhythms. 1989;4:39–48.

52. Bobrzynska KJ, Mrosovsky N. Phase shifting by novelty-induced running: activity dose-response curves at different circadian times. J Comp Physiol [A]. 1998;182:251–258.

53. Gannon RL, Rea MA. Twelve-hour phase shifts in hamster circadian rhythms elicited by voluntary wheel running. J Biol Rhythms. 1995;10:196–210.

54. Boulos Z, Rusak B. Circadian phase response curve for dark pulses in the hamster. J Comp Physiol. 1982;146:411–417.

55. Reebs SG, Lavery RJ, Mrosovsky N. Running activity mediates the phase-advancing effects of dark pulses on hamster circadian rhythms. J Comp Physiol [A]. 1989;165:811–818.

56. Van Reeth O, Turek FW. Stimulated activity mediates phase shifts in the hamster circadian clock induced by dark pulses or benzodiazepines. Nature. 1989;339:49–51.

57. Marchant EG, Mistlberger RE. Morphine phase shifts circadian rhythms in mice: role of behavioral activation. Neuroreport. 1996;7:209–212.

58. Mistlberger RE, Marchant EG, Sinclair SV. Nonphotic phase shifting and the motivation to run: cold exposure re-examined. J Biol Rhythms. 1996;11:208–215.

59. Mistlberger RE, Sinclair SV, Marchant EG, et al. Circadian phase shifts to food deprivation and refeeding in the Syrian hamster are mediated by running activity. Physiol Behav. 1997;61:273–278.

60. Mrosovsky N, Salmon P. Triazolam and phase-shifting acceleration re-evaluated. Chronobiol Int. 1990;7:35–41.

60a. Mistlberger RE, Antle MC, Dane L, et al. Sleep deprivation resets the circadian clock in the Syrian hamster. Soc Neurosci Abstr. 1999;25:1614.

61. Binkley S, Mosher K. Direct and circadian control of sparrow behaviour by light and dark. Physiol Behav. 1985;35:785–798.

62. Sundarajan KS. Phase relations between the circadian leaf movement rhythm and its zeitgeber within the range of entrainment in the cotton plant, Gossypium hirsutum L. J Interdiscipl Cycle Res. 1984;15:155–162.

63. Zatz M, Mullen D, Moskal JR. Photoendocrine transduction in cultured chick pineal cells: effects of light, dark, and potassium on the melatonin rhythm. Brain Res. 1988;438:199–215.

64. Mistlberger RE, Houpt TA, Moore-Ede MC. The benzodiazepine triazolam phase-shifts circadian activity rhythms in a diurnal primate, the squirrel monkey (Saimiri sciureus). Neurosci Lett. 1991;124:27–30.

65. Biello S, Mrosovsky N. Nest box restriction does not block phase advances to the benzodiazepine chlordiazepoxide at CT5. Soc Res Biol Rhythms. 1992;3:169.

66. Bobrzynska KJ, Godfrey MH, Mrosovsky N. Serotonergic stimulation and nonphotic phase-shifting in hamsters. Physiol Behav. 1996;59:221–230.

67. Albers HE, Ferris C. Neuropeptide Y: role in the light-dark cycle entrainment of hamster rhythms. Neurosci Lett. 1984;50:163–168.

68. Smith RD, Inoue SI, Turek FW. Central administration of muscimol phase-shift the mammalian circadian clock. J Comp Physiol [A]. 1989;164:805–814.

69. Hastings MH, Mead SM, Vinlacheruvu RR, et al. Non-photic phase shifting of the circadian activity rhythm of Syrian hamsters: the relative potency of arousal and melatonin. Brain Res. 1992;591:20–26.

70. Honrado G, Mrosovsky N. Interaction between periodic socio-sexual cues and light-dark cycles in controlling the phasing of activity rhythms in golden hamsters. Ethol Ecol Evol. 1992;3:221–231.

71. Mrosovsky N, Salmon P. A behavioural method for accelerating re-entrainment of rhythms to new light-dark cycles. Nature. 1987;330:372–373.

72. Mistlberger RE. Scheduled daily exercise or feeding alters the phase of photic entrainment in Syrian hamsters. Physiol Behav. 1991;50:1257–1260.

73. Buxton OM, Frank SA, L'Hermite-Baleriaux M, et al. Roles of intensity and duration of nocturnal exercise in causing phase delays of human circadian rhythms. Am J Physiol. 1997;273:E536–542.

74. Eastman CI, Hoese EK, Youngstedt SD, et al. Phase-shifting human circadian rhythms with exercise during the night shift. Physiol Behav. 1996;58:1287–1291.

75. Klerman EB, Rimmer DW, Dijk D-J, et al. Nonphotic entrainment of the human circadian pacemaker. Am J Physiol. 1998;274(4 pt 2);R991–R996.

76. Goel N, Lee TM. Social cues modulate free-running circadian activity rhythms in the diurnal rodent, Octoden degus. Am J Physiol. 1997;42:R797–804.

77. Edgar DM, Dement WC. Regularly scheduled voluntary exercise synchronizes the mouse circadian clock. Am J Physiol. 1992;261:R928–R933.

78. Marchant EG, Mistlberger RE. Entrainment and phase shifting of circadian rhythms in mice by forced treadmill running. Physiol Behav. 1996;60:657–663.

79. Mistlberger RE. Effects of daily schedules of forced activity on free-running rhythms in the rat. J Biol Rhythms. 1991;6:71–80.

80. Menaker M, Eskin A. Entrainment of circadian rhythms by sound in *Passer domesticus.* Science. 1966;154:1579–1581.

81. Reppert SM. Interaction between the circadian clocks of mother and fetus. Ciba Found Symp. 1995;183:198–211.

82. Bovet J, Oertli E. Free-running circadian activity rhythms in free-living beaver (*Castor canadensis*). J Comp Physiol [A]. 1974;92:1–10.

83. Wever RA. The Circadian System of Man: Results of Experiments Under Temporal Isolation. New York, NY: Springer-Verlag; 1979.

84. Refinetti R, Nelson DE, Menaker M. Social stimuli fail to act as entraining agents of circadian rhythms in the golden hamster. J Comp Physiol [A]. 1992;170:181–187.

85. Miles LEM, Raynal DM, Wilson MA. Blind man living in normal society has circadian rhythms of 249 hours. Science. 1977;198:421–423.

86. Reebs SG, St-Coeur J. After-effects of scheduled daily exercise on free-running circadian period in Syrian hamsters. Physiol Behav. 1994;55:1113–1117.

87. Van Reeth O, Turek FW. Daily injections of triazolam induce long-term changes in hamster circadian period. Am Phys Soc. 1990;R514–R519.

88. Sinclair SV, Mistlberger RE. Scheduled activity reorganizes circadian phase of Syrian hamsters under full and skeleton photoperiods. Behav Brain Res. 1997;87:121–137.

89. Mrosovsky N, Janik D. Behavioral decoupling of circadian rhythms. J Biol Rhythms. 1993;8:57–65.

90. Joy J, Turek FW. Combined effects on the circadian clock of agents with different phase-response curves: phase-shifting effects of triazolam and light. J Biol Rhythms. 1992;7:51–63.

91. Mrosovsky N. Double pulse experiments with nonphotic and photic phase-shifting stimuli. J Biol Rhythms. 1991;6:167–179.

92. Mistlberger RE, Antle MC. Behavioral inhibition of light-induced circadian phase resetting is phase and serotonin dependent. Brain Res. 1998;786:31–38.

93. Ralph MR, Mrosovsky N. Behavioral inhibition of circadian responses to light. J Biol Rhythms. 1992;7:353–360.

94. Hohmann W, Michel S, Fleisnner G. Locomotor activity and light pulses as competing zeitgeber stimuli in the scorpion circadian system. Soc Res Biol Rhythms. 1990;2:52.

95. Reebs SG, Mrosovsky N. Large phase-shifts of circadian rhythms caused by induced running in a re-entrainment paradigm: the role of pulse duration and light. J Comp Physiol [A]. 1989;165:819–825.

96. Borbely AA. Sleep regulation: circadian rhythm and homeostasis. Curr Top Neuroendocrinol. 1982;1:83–103.

97. Mistlberger RE, Landry G, Marchant EG. Sleep deprivation can attenuate light-induced phase shifts of circadian rhythms in hamsters. Neurosci Lett. 1997;238:5–8.

98. Amir S, Stewart J. Resetting of the circadian clock by a conditioned stimulus. Nature. 1996;379:542–545.

99. Reppert SM. Circadian rhythms: basic aspects and pediatric implications. In: Styne DM, ed. Current Concepts in Pediatric Endocrinology. Amsterdam, Netherlands: Elsevier; 1987:91–125.

100. Davis FC, Gorski RA. Development of hamster circadian rhythms, II: prenatal entrainment of the pacemaker. J Biol Rhythms. 1986;1:77–89.

101. Deguchi T. Ontogenesis of a biological clock for serotonin: acetyl coenzyme A *N*-acetyltransferase in the pineal gland of rat. Proc Nat Acad Sci U S A. 1975;72:2914–2920.

102. Weaver DR, Reppert SM. Maternal-fetal communication of circadian phase in a precocious rodent, the spiny mouse. Am J Physiol. 1987;253:E401–407.

103. Reppert SM, Schwartz WJ. Maternal coordination of the fetal biological clock in utero. Science. 1983;220:969–971.

104. Moore RY, Shibata S, Bernstein ME. Developmental anatomy of the circadian system. In: Reppert SM, ed. Development of Circadian Rhythmicity and Photoperiodism in Mammals. Ithaca, NY: Perinatology Press; 1989:1–23.

105. Weaver DR, Reppert SM. Definition of the developmental transition from dopaminergic to photic regulation of c-fos gene expression in the rat suprachiasmatic nucleus. Mol Brain Res. 1995;33:136–148.

106. Hudson R, Distel H. Temporal pattern of suckling in rabbit pups: a model of circadian synchrony between mother and young. In: Reppert SM, ed. Development of Circadian Rhythmicity and Photoperiodism in Mammals. Ithaca, NY: Perinatal Press; 1989:83–102.

107. De Vries JIP, Visser GHA, Mulder EJH, et al. Diurnal and other variations in fetal movement and heart rate patterns at 20 and 22 weeks. Early Hum Dev. 1987;15:333–348.

108. Honnebier MBOM, Swaab DF, Mirmiran M. Diurnal rhythmicity during early human development. In: Reppert SM, ed. Development of Circadian Rhythmicity and Photoperiodism in Mammals. Ithaca, NY: Perinatal Press; 1989:221–243.

109. Mirmiran M, Lunshof S. Perinatal development of human circadian rhythms. Prog Brain Res. 1996;111:217–225.

110. Kleitman N, Engelmann TG. Sleep characteristics of infants. J Appl Psychol. 1953;6:269–282.

111. Recio J, Miguez JM, Buxton OM, et al. E. Synchronizing circadian rhythms in early infancy. Med Hypotheses. 1997;49:229–234.

112. Reppert SM, Rivkees SA. Development of human circadian rhythms: implications for health and disease. In: Reppert SM, ed. Development of Circadian Rhythms and Photoperiodism in Mammals. Ithaca, NY: Perinatal Press; 1989:245–259.

113. Myers BL, Badia P. Changes in circadian rhythms and sleep quality with aging: mechanisms and interventions. Neurosci Biobehav Rev. 1995;19:553–571.

114. Turek FW, Penev P, Zhang Y, et al. Alterations in the circadian system in advanced age. Ciba Found Symp. 1995;183:212–234.

115. Van Reeth O, Zhand Y, Zee P, et al. Aging alters feedback effects of the activity: rest cycle on the circadian clock. Am J Physiol. 1992;263:R981–R986.

116. Mrosovsky N, Biello SM. Nonphotic phase shifting in the old and the cold. Chronobiol Int. 1994;11:232–252.

117. Miles LE, Dement WC. Sleep and aging. Sleep. 1980;3:119–220.

118. Monk TH, Buysse DJ, Reynolds CF, et al. Circadian temperature rhythms of older people. Exp Gerontol. 1995;30:455–474.

119. Czeisler CA, Dumont M, Duffy JF, et al. Association of sleep-wake habits in older people with changes in the output of circadian pacemaker. Lancet. 1992;340:933–936.

120. Pittendrigh CS, Daan S. Circadian oscillations in rodents: a systematic increase in their frequency with age. Science. 1974;186:548–550.

121. Reitveld WJ, Ruis J, Buijs P. The effect of aging on the circadian control of food intake in the rat. J Interdiscpl Cycle Res. 1988;19:289–295.

122. Pohl H. Does aging affect the period of the circadian pacemaker in invertebrates? Naturwissenschaften. 1993;80:478–481.

123. Samis HV. Aging: the loss of temporal organization. Perspect Biol Med. 1968;12:95–102.

124. Wax TM, Goodrick CL. Nearness to death and wheel running behavior in mice. Exp Gerontol. 1978;13:233–236.

125. Hayes DK, Cawley DM, Halberg F, et al. Survival of the codling moth, the pink bollworm, and the tobacco budworm after 90° phase shifts at varied regular intervals throughout the life span. Shift Work and Health: A Symposium. Washington, DC: US Department of Health, Education and Welfare; 1976:48–50.

126. Pittendrigh CS, Minis D. Circadian systems: longevity as a function of circadian resonance in *Drosophila melanogaster.* Proc Natl Acad Sci U S A. 1972;69:1537–1539.

127. DeCoursey PJ, Krulus JR, Mele G, et al. Circadian performance of suprachiasmatic nuclei (SCN)–lesioned antelope group squirrels in a desert enclosure. Physiol Behav. 1997;62:1099–1108.

Anatomy and Physiology of the Mammalian Circadian System

Mary E. Harrington
Ralph E. Mistlberger

The suprachiasmatic nucleus (SCN) of the hypothalamus is of central importance in the generation and entrainment of mammalian circadian rhythms. On the basis of lesion studies conducted more than 25 years ago, the SCN was identified as a putative pacemaker for mammalian circadian rhythms. Many subsequent studies confirmed that SCN ablation disrupts a wide variety of daily rhythms, that this structure can maintain a circadian rhythm in vitro, and that transplantation of the SCN transfers circadian rhythmicity. These observations led to the hypothesis that the SCN functions as a major circadian pacemaker in mammals. Several putative neurotransmitters are important in both photic and nonphotic entrainment pathways, with excitatory amino acids being critical in photic entrainment and both serotonin and neuropeptide Y playing leading roles in mediation of nonphotic entrainment. There are points of interaction between these pathways, with most studies indicating antagonistic effects. For example, light reduces the effects of neuropeptide Y on circadian clock phase; conversely, neuropeptide Y reduces the effects of light. The SCN sends efferents largely to nearby hypothalamic structures and may also control some rhythms via humoral signals. Hormones can modulate circadian rhythms, in some cases providing feedback regulation. Although the current emphasis is on the SCN, it is best viewed as a dominant pacemaker that controls the outputs of many systems, some of which are also circadian oscillators.

BACKGROUND

The general properties of the mammalian circadian system are described in Chapter 25. The goal of this chapter is to review the anatomical structures in mammals that play a role in circadian rhythm generation and entrainment and to discuss the functions of various neurochemicals and hormones in these processes. The focus of this review is the suprachiasmatic nucleus (SCN) of the anterior hypothalamus and its afferent and efferent projections. On the basis of lesion studies conducted more than 25 years ago, the SCN was identified as a putative pacemaker for mammalian circadian rhythms. Many subsequent studies confirmed that SCN ablation disrupts a wide variety of daily rhythms.

These observations led to the hypothesis that the SCN functions as a major circadian pacemaker in mammals, a hypothesis that has been confirmed by a variety of studies using many different approaches.

This chapter examines the roles of several putative neurotransmitters in both photic and nonphotic entrainment pathways, mechanisms for interactions between pathways, the organization of SCN efferents, and the role of hormones in circadian organization. Finally, the structure of the mammalian circadian system is assessed on the basis of both the functional properties discussed in Chapter 25 and the physiological evidence reviewed below.

IDENTIFICATION OF THE SUPRACHIASMATIC NUCLEI PACEMAKER

The localization of biological clocks within several invertebrate species, birds, and mammals has done much to stimulate research in circadian physiology. Evidence is reviewed here that a circadian pacemaker exists in the hypothalamus of mammals; the reader is referred to previous reviews for details on identified invertebrate[1, 2] and avian circadian pacemakers.[1, 3, 4]

The first systematic attempt to localize the circadian pacemaker in mammals was made by Richter[5] in a series of lesion and dissection experiments using rats. Circadian activity rhythms were found to persist after the removal of various endocrine organs or focal destruction of many brain areas but were abolished by large lesions placed ventromedially in the hypothalamus. The critical cell group within this region was subsequently identified by later studies to be the SCN, located in the hypothalamus immediately dorsal to the optic chiasm. A retinal projection terminating in the SCN was identified by autoradiography[6]; and ablation of the SCN had the dramatic effect of eliminating circadian rhythms altogether.[7, 8] Loss of circadian rhythmicity in rodents after SCN destruction has since been confirmed for many variables, including sleep-wake (Fig. 26–1), temperature, activity, corticosterone secretion, heart rate, and pineal N-acetyltransferase.[9] Early

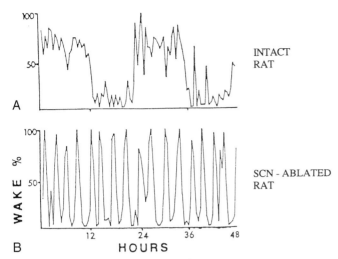

Figure 26–1. Percentage of polygraphically recorded wake time in each 30-min bin over 48 consecutive hours in two adult male rats recorded in constant dim light. *A* is from an intact control rat and illustrates a typical 24-h circadian rhythm of sleep-wake time. *B* is from a rat with complete ablation of the SCN. The 24-h rhythm of sleep-wake time was completely lost. This particular rat shows prominent ultradian rhythms in the 3- to 4-h range. SCN, suprachiasmatic nuclei. (Modified. Republished with permission of the American Sleep Disorders Association, 6301 Bandel Road, Suite 101, Rochester, MN 55501. Figure, R.E. Mistlberger, B.M. Bergmann, A. Rechtschaffen, Sleep, 1987, vol 10. Reproduced by permission of the publisher via Copyright Clearance Center Inc.)

studies indicated that SCN ablation alters the temporal distribution, but not the mean level, of most homeostatically regulated variables. Recent studies have demonstrated significant changes in the regulation of sleep and arousal after SCN destruction.[10] The suggestion that the SCN plays a role in promoting arousal is supported by evidence of the difficulty in sustaining alertness in people with hypothalamic damage that likely involves the SCN.[11]

A pacemaker role for the SCN cannot be established on the basis of lesion studies alone. To establish this function requires a convergence of evidence from a number of approaches that demonstrate, first, that the SCN oscillates independently with a circadian period and, second, that their intrinsic periodicity sets the phase and period for numerous overt rhythms (i.e., that they act as a pacemaker for the circadian system).

The evidence that the SCN contains an independent circadian clock mechanism is diverse and convincing, coming from both in vivo and in vitro studies. The metabolic activity of the SCN, as measured by uptake of 2-deoxyglucose (2-DG) in vivo, shows a high-amplitude circadian rhythm.[12] Neural activity within the SCN, recorded in freely behaving rats, oscillates in phase with the metabolic rhythm, peaking during the subjective day for both nocturnal and diurnal animals.[13–15] Because these findings are subject to the criticism that extrinsic input could still be conferring rhythmicity on SCN cells, other evidence is needed to establish the existence of independent circadian clock mechanisms in SCN cells.

This evidence was provided by studies showing that SCN neurons continue to generate a circadian rhythm of neurophysiological activity, of vasopressin (VP) secretion, and of rhythmic 2-DG uptake when maintained in an in vitro hypothalamic slice preparation.[15, 16] These VP rhythms were shown to persist for several days in vitro,[17] as, subsequently, were rhythms of spontaneous electrical activity.[15, 18] Individual SCN neurons can express circadian rhythms in firing. Dissociated SCN cells cultured on a microelectrode plate showed circadian rhythms in firing that persisted for weeks[19] (Fig. 26–2) with an average period predicted from the strain of animal chosen.[20] Oscillations in VP and vasoactive intestinal polypeptide (VIP) release have been measured from the SCN in culture by several investigators. The work by Shinohara et al.[21] is particularly interesting in that the culture conditions were shown to have dramatic effects. In cultures without mitotic inhibitors, the two rhythms were locked in phase with each other. After the addition of mitotic inhibitors to slow glial growth, the rhythms became uncoupled, with the VP rhythm expressing a rhythm with a longer period than the VIP rhythm. This topic continues to be explored, with the hope that some understanding may be gained of the mechanisms by which SCN neurons are coupled to each other.

The strongest evidence that the SCN functions as a circadian pacemaker, imposing a rhythm on other structures, is provided by studies demonstrating recovery of circadian rhythms in arrhythmic rodents with SCN lesions through the use of intracerebral transplantations of fetal neural tissue containing the SCN.[22, 23] The restored rhythm period is determined by the genotype of the donor brain; this was shown in studies using hamsters of a mutant strain (tau mutants) with free-running periods of either 20 or 22 h (in homozygotes and heterozygotes, respectively), whereas wild-type hamsters have periods near 24 h.[24] When transplants were performed using both mutant and wild-type hamsters, the period expressed was that characteristic of the donor genotype rather than that of the SCN-ablated host[24] (Fig. 26–3). Similarly, the species-characteristic period of the donor SCN tissue emerged when cross-species transplants were used to restore rhythms in rodents.[25] These results show that the transplants do not serve a permissive function for surviving pacemaker neurons in the host but actually function as the pacemaker mechanism. The transplant data, in combination with the electrophysiological, metabolic, and lesion results, confirm the presence of a circadian pacemaker within the SCN that exerts widespread influence on the timing of behavioral and physiological processes.

PHYSIOLOGY OF SUPRACHIASMATIC NUCLEI CELLS

Neurons of the SCN show slow, generally irregular firing rates.[26] Although early work investigated the usefulness of classifying cells on the basis of their firing pattern (e.g., irregular, regular, bursting), the system for classification was not standardized. A recent study[27] uses an objective and quantitative method to demon-

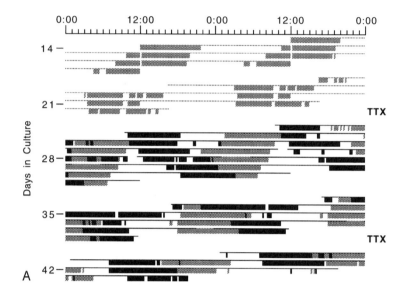

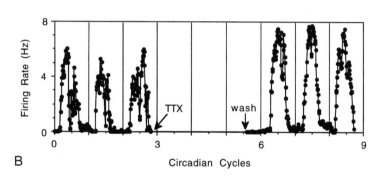

Figure 26–2. Recordings of circadian firing patterns of SCN neurons cultured on multielectrode plates. *A*, Two SCN cells from the same culture (dark versus light bars) were recorded for several weeks. Successive days are plotted top to bottom, with the time of day plotted left to right. Each row is extended to 48 h, duplicating data in the next row, so that patterns crossing midnight can be appreciated. Bars show when the firing rate was above the mean value for that row. The absence of a thin line indicates a gap in the data collection. The second and fourth gaps in the record occur when tetrodotoxin (TTX) was applied for 2.5 days, reversibly blocking all action potentials. Circadian rhythms resumed after tetrodotoxin treatment with unperturbed phase. *B*, Representation of the firing pattern of the one SCN cell before and after tetrodotoxin treatment, showing that the recovered rhythm is in phase with the pretreatment rhythm. SCN, suprachiasmatic nuclei (From Welsh DK, Logothetis DE, Meister M, et al. Individual neurons dissociated from rat suprachiasmatic nucleus express independently phased circadian firing rhythms. Neuron. 1995;14:697–706.)

strate several classes of firing patterns within a population of SCN neurons. Although the regularity of firing of individual cells depends largely on the average firing rate, even when firing rate is taken into account, differences in firing pattern can be observed.[27] The cluster of cells that can adopt bursting patterns of firing are particularly interesting because they show extensive axon collaterals and thus have the potential of affecting many other SCN neurons.[27] An even more striking characteristic than firing pattern is the overall daily variation in firing rate, such that cells reach a peak firing rate once per circadian cycle. The cellular changes that underlie this daily change in firing rate are not understood.

Examination of membrane properties of SCN neurons has not yet provided major clues as to the unique character of these cells as circadian clocks.[26] Synaptic activity appears to be attributable to gamma-aminobutyric acid (GABA)-ergic (inhibitory) and glutamatergic (excitatory) inputs.[28] Infusions of tetrodotoxin (a sodium channel blocker) do abolish the expression of circadian rhythms[29] but do not alter the ability of the clock to keep time.[19, 29] Although treatment with tetrodotoxin does not always totally abolish synaptic activity, this can be accomplished with application of appropriate GABA and glutamate receptor blockers.[28]

A prominent circadian rhythm is observed in glucose utilization,[12] which continues expression at a reduced level even during tetrodotoxin treatment.[16] Levels of intracellular ATP show circadian variation in the SCN.[30] Varied glucose levels in the bathing medium of the SCN in vitro alter clock output (time of peak firing rate) but do not reset the clock.[31] The results of the latter study suggest that metabolic rhythms of SCN cells may underlie the rhythm in electrical excitability. Several types of K⁺ channels that were inhibited by intracellular ATP were observed in SCN neurons, and a K⁺ channel blocker altered the time of peak firing rate, suggesting that the effects of glucose described above may occur via action on K⁺ channel activity.[31]

It is not yet clear whether the clock resides in the neurons, the glia, or both.[32] For example, a circadian rhythm in glial immunoreactivity is observed in the SCN, and disruption of glial function disrupts the rhythm in neural firing.[32] Further research will be needed to clarify the relative roles of these cell types and the methods by which SCN neurons remain coupled.

CHEMICAL NEUROANATOMY OF THE SUPRACHIASMATIC NUCLEI

Neurons in the SCN contain a variety of neurochemicals in addition to those already discussed.[33] Cells

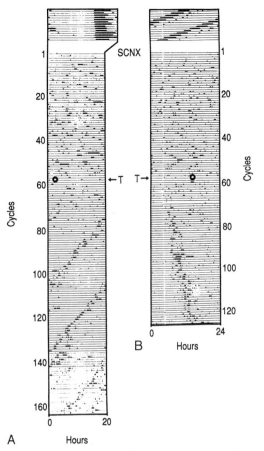

Figure 26–3. Event records of wheel-running activity of *A*, a wild-type Syrian hamster, and *B*, a homozygous tau mutant hamster. The wild-type hamster displays a free-running activity rhythm with a period of 24.05 h in constant darkness (DD), typical for this species. The free-running period of the tau mutant hamster is 21.07 h. Both hamsters received SCN ablations and became arrhythmic. The wild-type hamster then received, at the time marked by the open circle, an SCN transplant from a tau mutant embryo, and the tau mutant received a transplant from a wild-type embryo. Within 2 weeks, a circadian rhythm was restored in each animal but with a free-running period characteristic of the donor, not the host, hamster. SCN, suprachiasmatic nuclei. (From Ralph MR, Foster RG, Davis FC, et al. Transplanted suprachiasmatic nucleus determines circadian period. Science. 1990;247:975–978.)

in the ventrolateral SCN are immunoreactive for VIP, peptide histidine isoleucine, and gastrin-releasing peptide. Dorsomedial SCN cells label with markers for VP, neurophysin, and somatostatin. All of these peptides can be observed to label fibers leaving the SCN as well as fibers forming synaptic connections within the SCN. Most SCN cells appear to contain GABA, and a small population of substance P–immunoreactive cells has been described in the central part of the hamster SCN. Some SCN cells contain vgf, a substance linked to photic responses,[34] whereas calbindin may actually be a marker for SCN cells important for output of locomotor activity rhythms.[35]

The chemical neuroanatomy of the SCN is dynamic. In general, neurochemicals synthesized in ventral SCN cells respond to photic stimuli but do not cycle under constant conditions, whereas neurochemicals synthesized in dorsal SCN cells show endogenous rhythms but do not respond to changes in light.[36] Long-term exposure to short photoperiods decreases the number of cholecystokinin-immunoreactive neurons and increases VIP immunoreactivity in the SCN.[37, 38] Ultrastructural changes are observed in the rat SCN after exposure to constant illumination or constant darkness[39] and in the rabbit after coitus.[40] In human beings, a reduction in SCN volume and cell number is observed with age and in dementia.[41] Although SCN volume and cell number do not appear to differ in general between populations of men and women,[41] the SCN in homosexual men was reported to be twice as large as the SCN in a reference group of men of unknown sexual orientation.[42]

ENTRAINMENT PATHWAYS

Neural Basis of Photic Entrainment

In mammals, photic entrainment is thought to be largely mediated by retinal photoreceptors; blind mammals are generally unresponsive to light-dark cycles.[43] This may seem a trivial observation, but in birds and lizards, photoreceptors in the brain exist that are sufficient to permit photic entrainment. Light intensity, duration of the light pulse, and the spectral characteristics of the light determine the magnitude of a phase shift at any specific circadian phase. The identity of the mammalian photoreceptor mediating entrainment is not yet certain.[44] Light may also act via an extraretinal site in human beings because light applied to the skin was able to alter the phase of several circadian rhythms in one study.[45]

Approximately one third of SCN cells are photically responsive.[26] Cells that are both light activated and light suppressed respond to changing illumination with changes in firing rates, so for a range of light intensities, they can be said to code light intensity.[26] The thresholds for SCN photic responses, rhythm phase shifting, and photic suppression of pineal melatonin in nocturnal rodents are relatively high compared with thresholds for other visual functions.[46] Human circadian rhythms can be shifted by room lights of 180 lux.[47, 48]

The SCN receives direct retinal input via the retinohypothalamic tract (RHT). The neurotransmitter of the RHT probably is an excitatory amino acid.[49] Optic nerve stimulation can cause the release of [³H]glutamate and [³H]asparate in the rat SCN brain slice preparation. Excitatory postsynaptic potentials evoked by stimulation of the optic nerve in the rat or guinea pig SCN in vivo can be blocked by excitatory amino acid receptor antagonists. Both N-methyl-D-aspartate (NMDA) and non-NMDA receptors appear to be involved in mediating photic input to the circadian system. It is likely that a rapidly acting non-NMDA glutamate receptor mediates partial depolarization of cell membranes, which, in turn, releases the voltage-dependent Mg^{2+} block and permits subsequent activation of NMDA-regulated channels. Light-induced phase shifts of activity rhythms in hamsters are reduced by injec-

Table 26–1. SUMMARY OF SUPRACHIASMATIC NUCLEUS AFFERENTS INVOLVED IN PHOTIC AND NONPHOTIC ENTRAINMENT

Source	Associated Neurochemicals
Photic	
Retina	Excitatory amino acids (e.g., glutamate), PACAP, substance P
Tuberomammillary complex	Histamine
Pretectum	?
Parabigeminal nucleus, pedunculopontine tegmentum, substantia innominata, septum, diagonal bands of Broca	Acetylcholine
Nonphotic	
Intergeniculate leaflet, ventral lateral geniculate nucleus	Neuropeptide Y, GABA, Met-enkephalin
Median raphe	Serotonin

GABA, gamma-aminobutyric acid; PACAP, pituitary adenylate cyclase–activating peptide; ?, associated neurochemical is unknown.

tions of either NMDA antagonists or non-NMDA antagonists.[49] NMDA microinjections in the area of the SCN produce phase shifts in activity rhythms that simulate the phase-shifting effects of light pulses.[50] Other neurotransmitters implicated in the RHT include substance P[51] and pituitary adenylate cyclase–activating peptide (PACAP)[52] (Table 26–1).

Neurochemicals from areas of the brain other than the retina may also cause photic shifts. Histamine is a neurotransmitter implicated in the control of sleep and arousal.[53, 54] Histaminergic input to the SCN may arise from the tuberomammillary complex in the posterior basal hypothalamus.[55] Application of histamine to the in vitro SCN phase shifts the rhythm in firing rate in a manner similar to light,[56] possibly via potentiation of glutamatergic NMDA receptors.[57] In agreement with previous published accounts,[58] administration of histamine (1 mmol) in early subjective night did not phase shift the circadian clock (S.M. Biello, personal communication). As histamine's potentiation for the NMDA receptor has an inverted-U shape, two lower doses of histamine at CT 14 were tried. Although no significant phase shifts were seen when the dose was lowered to 100 μmol, phase shifts to histamine were seen in early subjective night when the dose was decreased further to 100 nmol. When this lower dose of histamine was administered to hamsters in late subjective night, phase advances were seen. Thus, at certain doses, histamine can phase shift the clock in a manner similar to light in vivo.

It has been reported that the cholinergic agonist carbachol can induce phase shifts that resemble those caused by light.[59] However, other researchers found that the similarity extends to only some circadian phases and not others.[60, 61] Cholinergic mechanisms may not be tied to a single entrainment route, but they may have a role in modulating several kinds of inputs to the circadian system. The SCN receives cholinergic inputs from several forebrain and brainstem regions.[62] Cholinergic forebrain neurons projecting to the SCN

arise from the substantia innominata, septum, and diagonal bands of Broca. Brainstem projections to the SCN arise from the parabigeminal nucleus and pedunculopontine tegmentum.

Other input pathways to the SCN are less well studied. Input from the pretectal nuclei[63] overlaps with geniculohypothalamic tract (GHT) terminal fields. The paraventricular nucleus of the thalamus provides input distributed to all areas of the SCN, whereas areas of the hypothalamus and limbic system provide input to dorsal SCN areas.[64]

Neural Basis of Nonphotic Entrainment

Nonphotic influences on pacemaker phase appear to be mediated by the GHT and serotonergic pathways (see Table 26–1). As reviewed in Chapter 25, in hamsters, a bout of wheel running triggered by confinement to a novel running wheel or by injection of the benzodiazepine triazolam during the middle of the subjective day can induce phase advance shifts of up to 3 h. Daily treadmill running can entrain circadian rhythms (see Chapter 25). The critical stimulus is not well understood, and the term *nonphotic* is used to refer to these stimuli. The results of numerous studies have identified locomotor activity as a strong correlate or critical stimulus for nonphotic phase shifting. However, a study demonstrated that the phase-shifting effects of 3 h of running in hamsters can be mimicked by 3 h of sleep deprivation induced by gentle handling, with minimal locomotor activation.[64a] This new study provides direct evidence that intense "exercise" is not necessary for nonphotic phase shifts and that arousal, at least during the usual sleep phase, provides endogenous cues sufficient to induce large phase shifts. Although melatonin can produce phase shifts in a pattern somewhat similar to nonphotic stimuli (see Chapter 31), most current research focuses on geniculohypothalamic and serotonergic inputs as possible mediators of nonphotic phase shifting.

The GHT originates largely from cells in the intergeniculate leaflet (IGL), a thin lamina of cells between the dorsal and ventral lateral geniculate nuclei in the thalamus (for a review, see Harrington[65]). Cells in the IGL receive inputs from several areas and have reciprocal connections with many of the areas that provide input, as well as projecting to the superior colliculus, accessory optic system, and pineal (Fig. 26–4).[65] The GHT projection to the SCN is associated with several neurotransmitters; the best studied of these is neuropeptide Y (NPY), which is found in many geniculate neurons projecting to the SCN. GABA, Met-enkephalin,[65] and orphanin-FQ[66] may also be contained in neurons contributing to the GHT. Ablation of the IGL can eliminate novel wheel-induced phase shifts, although this result is in some cases confounded by a reduction in the running response to the stimulus.[67, 68] However, IGL lesions in mice prevent entrainment to daily scheduled treadmill running without interfering with treadmill running.[69] IGL lesions also prevent phase advances induced by other nonphotic stimuli.[70, 71]

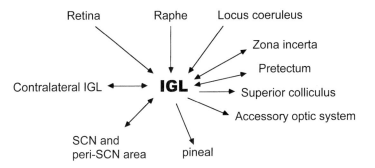

Figure 26–4. Summary of the major anatomical connections of the IGL. IGL, intergeniculate leaflet; SCN, suprachiasmatic nuclei. (From data summarized in Harrington.[65])

Other evidence beyond the lesion studies that the IGL mediates nonphotic phase shifting (reviewed in Harrington[65]) includes observations that electrical stimulation of the IGL or microinjection of NPY into the SCN in vivo can cause phase shifts similar to those induced by novel wheel running. NPY can also phase shift circadian rhythms of SCN neural activity, recorded in vitro, with a phase response profile similar to the nonphotic shifts induced in vivo. Finally, phase shifts induced by wheel running can be blocked in vivo by microinjection of antiserum to NPY into the SCN area, indicating a critical role for this peptide in mediating this function of the GHT.[72] NPY appears to phase shift rhythms via the Y2 receptor,[73, 74] although other effects of NPY on the circadian system may be mediated by other receptors.[75]

Another set of observations suggests that the brainstem raphe nuclei may also contribute to nonphotic entrainment (see review in Miller et al.[76]). The raphe nuclei provide a major projection to the SCN that includes a substantial serotonergic component.[33] In hamsters, serotonergic cells in the median raphe nucleus project to the SCN, whereas serotonergic cells in the dorsal raphe nucleus project to the IGL.[77] Neural activity within the raphe nuclei is strongly correlated with behavioral state and is maximal during periods of activity and arousal.[78] Serotonin levels in the SCN correlate positively with motor activity in rats and have been shown to increase acutely during wheel running induced in the midsubjective day in hamsters.[76] Serotonin (5-hydroxytryptamine [5-HT]) and 5-HT$_{1a/7}$ receptor agonists can phase shift circadian rhythms of neural activity in the rat SCN in vitro, inducing phase advances if applied during the mid–subjective day similar to other nonphotic stimuli.[76] In vivo, the general 5-HT agonist quipazine can phase shift circadian rhythms in rats, and a 5-HT$_{1a/7}$ agonist can induce similar shifts in hamsters.[76, 79, 80] Neurotoxic lesions of serotonergic inputs in mice prevent entrainment to daily running schedules, whether the running is voluntary or forced by treadmill.[81, 82]

Despite this convergence of supporting evidence for a serotonin hypothesis of nonphotic entrainment, there are discordant findings that require resolution. For example, neurotoxic lesions of serotonergic inputs to the SCN can attenuate phase shift responses to nonphotic stimuli, but these results are potentially confounded by reductions in the induced running response, and other studies using neurotoxic lesions in hamsters report normal nonphotic phase shifting.[83] Antagonists to 5-HT$_{1a/7}$ receptors fail to attenuate activity-induced phase advances in hamsters.[84] At present, the exact role of the serotonergic input in mediating nonphotic phase shifts is uncertain.

Interactions Between Photic and Nonphotic Stimuli

The two major neural pathways implicated in nonphotic entrainment arise from areas with direct retinal input (Fig. 26–5); thus, it perhaps is not surprising that behavioral studies indicate that photic and nonphotic zeitgebers may interact in complex ways (reviewed in Chapter 25).

At some points in the circadian cycle, photic and nonphotic stimuli appear to be mutually inhibitory. Light can inhibit phase shifts to nonphotic stimuli (see Chapter 25). This finding is consistent with evidence that glutamate can block phase shifts to NPY in vitro,[18] that light reduces phase shifts to NPY in vivo,[85] and that a light pulse can block phase advances to 5-HT injections in vivo.[76] Phase advance shifts in response to light can be inhibited by wheel running or by NPY microinjections to the SCN area[86, 87] and can be potentiated by anti-NPY microinjections,[88] whereas phase delays to light pulses in vivo are not attenuated by either NPY or wheel running.[87, 89] Phase delay and advance shifts induced by the RHT transmitter glutamate are

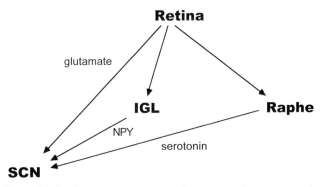

Figure 26–5. The retina projects to the SCN and projects to the IGL and raphe, which in turn project to the SCN. Major identified neurochemicals associated with each input to the SCN are noted. IGL, intergeniculate leaflet; NPY, neuropeptide Y; SCN, suprachiasmatic nuclei.

blocked by co-application of NPY.[18] Serotonin agonists can also reduce behavioral phase shifts to light.[76] Lesions of serotonergic or geniculate afferents to the SCN potentiate phase delay shift responses to light.[90, 91] The likelihood that 5-HT contributes to behavioral inhibition of photic phase shifting is supported by the recent observation that behavioral inhibition of advance shifts can be prevented with a general 5-HT antagonist.[89] Collectively, these findings indicate that both 5-HT and NPY afferents to the SCN can inhibit the phase-shifting effects of light and that light can inhibit their effects.

Cells in the IGL receive direct retinal input from a population of retinal ganglion cells overlapping with those projecting to the SCN. The majority of cells in the IGL show a sustained increase in firing rate when the eye is illuminated and appear to code changes in light intensity, at least through the ranges of light intensity associated with twilight, as reviewed in Harrington.[65] A large proportion of geniculate cells identified as projecting to the SCN share these characteristics. Some cells in the IGL code only increasing light intensities; after prolonged light adaptation, their firing rates drop, and they no longer code for changes in light intensity.[92, 93, 93a] and some raphe neurons appear to reciprocate with a projection to the retina (K. Fite, personal communication). Neither the GHT nor the raphe input is necessary for photic entrainment. It is not clear whether the GHT or raphe inputs are sufficient for photic entrainment because selective ablation of the primary photic pathway to the SCN, the RHT, is difficult to achieve. Knife cuts ventral to the hamster SCN can block photic entrainment, but such cuts may also damage ganglion cells projecting to the geniculate or raphe or may damage other fibers innervating the SCN.[65] Destruction of the cells of origin of the GHT changes photic responsiveness of the circadian system, with effects including decreased phase advances to light pulses, altered responses of circadian rhythms to continuous lighting, and loss of entrainment to "skeleton photoperiods" of several short light pulses each day.[65, 93b] Loss of the serotonergic input to the SCN alters activity onset and may alter other parameters of photic entrainment.[76]

Signal Transduction of Photic and Nonphotic Phase Shifts

Given the current information, we can model how a light pulse might induce a phase shift in the subjective night (see Miller et al.[76] and Golombek and Ralph[94] for reviews; Table 26–2). A light pulse probably induces release of an excitatory amino acid transmitter from retinal terminals in the SCN, as noted above. This transmitter activates non-NMDA receptors, depolarizing the cell. The depolarization is sufficient to remove the Mg^{2+} block of the NMDA receptor, allowing the excitatory amino acid transmitter to open NMDA receptors. Influx of calcium via NMDA receptors probably has several effects. Activation of calmodulin and, thus, calmodulin kinases may allow phosphorylation

Table 26–2. SUMMARY OF SIGNAL TRANSDUCTION PATHWAYS USED BY PHOTIC AND NONPHOTIC ENTRAINMENT PATHWAYS

	Transmitter		
	Photic	Nonphotic	
	Glutamate	NPY	Serotonin
Receptor(s)	NMDA and non-NMDA	Y2	5-HT$_{1a/7}$
Second messengers	Nitric oxide, cGMP	?	cAMP
Kinase	Protein kinase G	Protein kinase C	Protein kinase A
Requires protein synthesis?	Yes	No	?

cGMP, cyclic adenosine monophosphate; NMDA, *N*-methyl-D-aspartate; NPY, neuropeptide Y; ?, unknown.

of cyclic AMP (cAMP) response element–binding protein (CREB). Once CREB is phosphorylated, it binds to cAMP response element sites on various promoter sites on genes, most notably providing activation of immediate-early genes such as c-*fos* and perhaps other genes (see Chapter 27). This gene activation may lead to further gene regulation and, somehow, a shift in the clock phase. Calmodulin activation probably has a second major effect—activating nitric oxide synthase, which then produces nitric oxide from L-arginine. An increase in nitric oxide may directly activate guanylate cyclase, increasing levels of cGMP and then protein kinase G to potentially activate another signaling cascade. Because nitric oxide is a gas that can diffuse out of the cell and into neighboring cells, this may serve as a cell-to-cell coupling signal.

A nonphotic stimulus that induces phase shifts in the subjective day may act via a different mechanism, although this has been less thoroughly researched (see Table 26–2). The peptide or transmitter inducing this shift probably opens K^+ channels,[95–97] thus hyperpolarizing the cell, and also activates either protein kinase C (in the case of NPY[98] or melatonin[99]) or protein kinase A (in the case of serotonergic agonists[76]). Both events appear to be necessary and sufficient for clock resetting by serotonergic agonists,[95] whereas membrane hyperpolarization may not be critical for phase shifts to melatonin[100] or NPY.[96] Nitric oxide may again serve as the coupling signal,[101] although this has not yet been thoroughly investigated.

A circadian rhythm in membrane potential may underlie the cellular physiology of clock neurons; this could give rise to the circadian rhythm in firing rate described above. Given the strong underlying circadian rhythm, the effects of a substance on clock cell physiology are dependent on the time of day of application. It is worth noting that substances that induce phase shifts similar to light, and thus reset the clock only in the subjective night, generally are depolarizing agents. Conversely, substances that are associated with phase shifts in the subjective day generally are hyperpolarizing. We do not yet know whether effects on membrane potential are necessary or sufficient for phase shifting.

An underlying circadian rhythm in protein synthesis may explain why photic and nonphotic phase shifts vary in their mechanism. Photic phase shifts appear to be accompanied by an increase in gene expression and to rely on protein synthesis.[102] Synthesis of transcriptional activators or of clock proteins themselves might alter the timing of a clock that depends on cyclic protein production and degradation. Nonphotic phase shifts could, conversely, act through decreased gene expression or increased protein degradation. Although limited data are available, both decreased gene expression (see Prosser et al.[103] and Mikkelsen et al.[104]) and independence from protein synthesis[96] are implicated in nonphotic pathways.

Given the different nature of the signal transduction cascades underlying photic and nonphotic phase shifts, it perhaps is not surprising that these two input pathways can interact and generally act to oppose the effects of each other. Although the cellular nature of this interaction is not yet well understood, the phenomenon is well established and should be taken into account when considering the design of phase-shifting therapies.

OUTPUT PATHWAYS OF THE SUPRACHIASMATIC NUCLEI

Efferents from the SCN consist of four major projections, as described by Watts and Swanson.[105] One group of fibers leaves the SCN and travels dorsally. Many of these fibers, forming the majority of all SCN efferents, terminate in the area ventral to the paraventricular nucleus of the hypothalamus. Cells in this sub–paraventricular nucleus area project to many of the other regions receiving direct SCN efferent projections, and they have been hypothesized to function as an "amplifier" for SCN efferent signals.[105] Other terminal zones of this dorsal projection are in the paraventricular nucleus of the thalamus, the dorsomedial hypothalamic nucleus, and the posterior hypothalamic nucleus (Fig. 26–6).

The dorsal efferent pathway has been shown to be critical for photoperiodic responses in hamsters and for diurnal surges in luteinizing hormone and prolactin in rats but not for circadian activity rhythms.[106, 107] Several studies indicate that information from the SCN is conveyed via the hypothalamic paraventricular nucleus through a multisynaptic projection to regulate pineal gland function.[108, 109] Other studies suggest that SCN efferents to corticotropin-releasing factor–containing cells in the hypothalamic paraventricular nucleus, to the dorsomedial hypothalamus, and possibly to other hypothalamic sites regulate daily rhythms of adrenal corticosterone secretion.[110]

A second set of SCN efferents terminates in nuclei rostral to the SCN: the medial preoptic area, the anteroventral periventricular nucleus, the lateral septum, the bed nucleus of the stria terminalis, the parataenial nucleus, and rostral parts of the paraventricular nucleus of the thalamus. This efferent pathway appears important for some hormonal rhythms.[111, 112] A third set

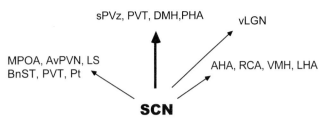

Figure 26–6. Efferent projections from the suprachiasmatic nuclei (SCN). The major group of fibers leaves the SCN and travels dorsally to the sub–paraventricular zone (sPVz), the paraventricular nucleus of the thalamus (PVT), the dorsomedial hypothalamic nucleus (DMH), and the posterior hypothalamic area (PHA). A second set of SCN efferents terminates in nuclei rostral to the SCN: the medial preoptic area (MPOA), the anteroventral periventricular nucleus (AvPVN), the lateral septum (LS), the bed nucleus of the stria terminalis (BnST), the parataenial nucleus (Pt), and rostral parts of the paraventricular nucleus of the thalamus (PVT). A third set of efferent fibers runs caudally from the SCN to terminate in the anterior hypothalamic area (AHA), the retrochiasmatic area (RCA), the ventromedial hypothalamus (VMH), and the lateral hypothalamus (LHA). Finally, a few fibers from the SCN appear to travel dorsal to the optic tracts to terminate in the ventral lateral geniculate nucleus (vLGN).

of efferent fibers runs caudally from the SCN to terminate in the anterior hypothalamic area, the retrochiasmatic area, the ventromedial hypothalamus, and the lateral hypothalamus. Finally, a few fibers from the SCN appear to travel dorsal to the optic tracts to terminate in the ventral lateral geniculate nucleus.

The physiology of SCN efferent projections is poorly understood. SCN firing rates, which presumably reflect their efferent signals, are high during the subjective day in both nocturnal and diurnal species.[15] These results suggest that a common circadian timing signal is transformed at an unidentified effector level into signals that regulate physiological processes in a species-characteristic manner. The infusion of tetrodotoxin into the SCN reversibly blocks expression of overt circadian rhythms,[29] indicating that action potentials may be necessary for circadian clock output. A study using neural grafts encapsulated in polymer, allowing only humoral signals and no neural fiber outgrowth, has challenged this conclusion,[113] indicating that at least activity rhythms may be driven by a humoral signal from the SCN.

HORMONAL EFFECTS ON THE CIRCADIAN SYSTEM

There is growing evidence that hormones have a regulatory influence on circadian rhythms that may be related to modulation of coupling relations among oscillators and between oscillators and driven processes. Richter[5] indicated that endocrine glands and their hormonal secretions are not essential to circadian organization, but other studies reveal that many hormones do affect circadian rhythms. Daily running activity in female rats and hamsters varies with the phase of the estrous cycle. On the day of proestrus, when estradiol secretion is maximal, running activity begins earlier and is more intense.[114] Ovariectomy abolishes this effect and is associated with a later time for activity onset during photic entrainment. Chronic estradiol treatment produces an earlier time of activity onset in entrained conditions and a shorter free-running period in constant conditions,[115] even in blind animals. Period shortening in response to estradiol is not observed in male or neonatally androgenized female hamsters.[116] Estradiol thus appears to regulate the timing of activity onset in female rodents by modulating the periodicity of a circadian system that is sexually differentiated by previous hormonal exposure.

Steroid hormones also modulate circadian timing in male rodents. Free-running rhythm periods in male mice are lengthened by castration and shortened by chronic testosterone treatment.[117] Gonadal regression in hamsters, which occurs in response to short day lengths characteristic of the winter season, is associated with reduced testosterone secretion and unstable daily activity onsets.[118] Male voles show a marked seasonal variation in the phasing of activity rhythms, which appears to be related to gonadal function.[119] Castration increases diurnal and dawn/dusk (crepuscular) activity and decreases nocturnal activity. Testosterone implants reduce crepuscular activity and increase nocturnal activity. Splitting of activity rhythms into two components has been observed in female hamsters in response to reduced estrogen,[120] which suggests that gonadal hormones may generally modulate coupling relations among circadian oscillators.

Circadian effects of other hormones have also been established. Removal of the pituitary,[116] partial thyroidectomy,[121] and treatment with an antithyroid drug[122] all lengthen the period of free-running activity rhythms in hamsters. Dexamethasone, a synthetic corticoid, can phase shift rat circadian rhythms in a phase-dependent fashion.[123] In squirrel monkeys, cortisol controls the phase of renal excretory rhythms.[124] Because these excretory rhythms appear to be intrinsic to the kidney, cortisol may be viewed as a coupling link between a circadian mechanism in the brain regulating corticotropin rhythms and a circadian mechanism in the kidney responsible for excretory rhythms. Although apparently not essential to the rhythm-generating mechanism, endocrine signals nevertheless appear to have a significant role in communication within the circadian system.

The hormone most closely linked to the circadian system is melatonin. Melatonin is secreted by the pineal gland of most vertebrates,[125] and the pineal functions as a circadian oscillator and has an important role in the regulation of circadian rhythms in birds as well as other vertebrate classes.[3] Melatonin may act by helping to synchronize a more or less loosely coupled system of central oscillators, many presumably in the SCN; this topic is reviewed in Chapter 31.

The effects of endocrine secretions on properties of circadian rhythms may be mediated by hormone binding within the SCN neurons or by hormonal effects on locomotor activity or other behaviors. For example, lengthening of circadian period by ovariectomy does not occur in rats that do not have access to running wheels, indicating that the reduction in running activity after ovariectomy is responsible for period modulation.[126] Whether changes in behavior mediate other effects of hormones on circadian function remains to be established.

STRUCTURE OF THE PACEMAKER SYSTEM

Although the SCN is acknowledged to have a major role in mammalian circadian organization, the circadian system clearly consists of more than a single pacemaker driving a number of overt rhythms. Activity rhythms with ultradian periods (much shorter than 24 h) are observed after damage to the SCN.[127] These results have been interpreted to mean that there are oscillators outside the SCN that are normally synchronized by efferent signals from the dominant pacemaker in the SCN. In the absence of the SCN or another external synchronizing agent, the oscillators fail to couple or achieve only weak and unstable coupling, thereby generating ultradian or arrhythmic activity patterns. An alternative interpretation put forth is that the SCN may function to impose a restrictive gate, allowing only the expression of subordinate oscillators during particular phases.

When hamsters are maintained in constant light for many weeks or months, "splitting" of the free-running activity rhythms is frequently observed. During splitting, the daily activity rhythm dissociates into two components that free-run with different periodicities before stabilizing 180 degrees out of phase. This finding is commonly interpreted to mean that the activity rhythm is generated by at least two primary oscillators with two stable coupling modes 180 degrees apart. Given that circadian activity rhythms represent the synchronizing or gating actions of a primary pacemaker in the SCN on subordinate oscillators outside the SCN, the splitting phenomenon further suggests that this primary pacemaker is itself composed of at least two and perhaps a population of dissociable oscillatory units.

These conceptions of the role of the SCN as a dominant pacemaker are challenged by reports that some circadian rhythms survive SCN ablation, which implies a separate circadian pacemaker mechanism located outside the SCN. For example, circadian functions that survive SCN ablation in rats and hamsters include a circadian rhythm of visual sensitivity[128] and the rhythms of anticipatory activity associated with daily mealtimes under food restriction schedules.[129] The visual sensitivity rhythm could be generated by a circadian timing system in the retina.[130] The neural substrates of meal-associated anticipatory rhythms are as yet unspecified. Arrhythmic, SCN-ablated rats will generate activity rhythms with near-circadian periods if they are given drinking water containing methamphetamine,[131] and the neural substrate underlying this effect is unknown.

Analyses of meal timing and time estimations in internally desynchronized humans have supported the idea that rest-activity and temperature rhythms are generated by separate circadian timing mechanisms.[132, 133] The phenomenon of internal desynchronization in humans should be distinguished from splitting in rodents because during splitting, the circadian rhythms of temperature and rest-activity remain in synchrony. Splitting demonstrates that more than one oscillator drives a single rhythm, whereas internal desynchronization suggests that different rhythms may be driven by different oscillators.

In summary, there is clear evidence in mammals for a hierarchical system of circadian oscillators involving at least one dominant and probably a complex pacemaker in the SCN and a set of subordinate oscillators outside the SCN. The nature of the relations among these elements is less certain. A similarly complex, multioscillatory organization is indicated in *Drosophila*,[134, 135] in which clock genes have been shown to continue to express circadian cycles in a multitude of body parts.[135] Understanding how the dominant pacemaker is able to control all of these apparently subordinate oscillators is a major challenge for the future.

Acknowledgments

We thank Eric Bittman, Adam Hall, Roselle Hoffmaster, and Ben Rusak for comments on earlier versions of the manuscript.

References

1. Rosenwasser AM. Behavioral neurobiology of circadian pacemakers: a comparative approach. Prog Psychobiol Physiol Psych. 1988;13:155–226.
2. Block GD, Khalsa SBS, McMahon DG, et al. Biological clocks in the retina: cellular mechanisms of biological timekeeping. Int Rev Cytol. 1993;143:83–144.
3. Gwinner E, Hau M, Heigl S. Melatonin: generation and modulation of avian circadian rhythms. Brain Res Bull. 1997;44:439–444.
4. Takahashi JS, Murakami N, Nikaido SS, et al. The avian pineal, a vertebrate model system of the circadian oscillator: cellular regulation of circadian rhythms by light, second messengers, and macromolecular synthesis. Recent Prog Horm Res. 1989;45:279–348.
5. Richter CP. Sleep and activity: their relation to the 24 hour clock. In: Kety S, Evarts E, Williams H, eds. Sleep and Altered States of Consciousness. Baltimore, Md: Williams & Wilkins; 1967:8–28.
6. Moore RY, Lenn NJ. A retinohypothalamic projection in the rat. J Comp Neurol. 1972;146:1–14.
7. Moore RY, Eichler VB. Loss of circadian adrenal corticosterone rhythms following suprachiasmatic lesion in the rat. Brain Res. 1972;42:201–206.
8. Stephen FK, Zucker I. Circadian rhythms in drinking behavior and locomotor activity of rats are eliminated by hypothalamic lesions. Proc Natl Acad Sci U S A. 1972; 69:1583–1586.
9. Rusak B, Zucker I. Neural regulation of circadian rhythms. Physiol Rev. 1979;59:449–526.
10. Edgar DM, Dement WC, Fuller CA. Effect of SCN lesions on sleep in squirrel monkeys: evidence for opponent processes in sleep-wake regulation. J Neurosci. 1993;13:1065–1079.
11. Cohen RA, Albers HE. Disruption of human circadian and cognitive regulation following a discrete hypothalamic lesion: a case study. Neurology. 1991;41:726–729.
12. Schwartz WJ. SCN metabolic activity in vivo. In: Klein DC, Moore, RY, Reppert SM, eds. Suprachiasmatic Nucleus: The Mind's Clock. New York, NY: Oxford University Press; 1991:144–156.
13. Inouye ST, Kawamura H. Persistence of circadian rhythmicity in a mammalian hypothalamic "island" containing the supra-

chiasmatic nucleus. Proc Natl Acad Sci U S A. 1979;76:5962–5966.
14. Meijer JH. Circadian rhythm in light response in suprachiasmatic nucleus neurons of freely moving rats. Brain Res. 1996;741:352–355.
15. Gillette MU. SCN electrophysiology in vitro: rhythmic activity and endogenous clock properties. In: Klein DC, Moore, RY, Reppert SM, eds. Suprachlasmatic Nucleus: The Mind's Clock. New York, NY: Oxford University Press; 1991:125–143.
16. Newman GG. SCN metabolic activity in vitro. In: Klein DC, Moore RY, Reppert SM, eds. Suprachiasmatic Nucleus: The Mind's Clock. New York, NY: Oxford University Press; 1991:157–176.
17. Murakami N, Takamure M, Takahashi K, et al. Long-term cultured neurons from rat suprachiasmatic nucleus retain the capacity for circadian oscillation of vasopressin release. Brain Res. 1991;545:347–350.
18. Biello SM, Golombek DA, Harrington ME. Neuropeptide Y and glutamate block each other's phase shifts in the suprachiasmatic nucleus in vitro. Neuroscience. 1997;77:1049–1057.
19. Welsh DK, Logothetis DE, Meister M, et al. Individual neurons dissociated from rat suprachiasmatic nucleus express independently phased circadian firing rhythms. Neuron. 1995;14:697–706.
20. Liu C, Weaver DR, Strogatz SH, et al. Cellular construction of a circadian clock: period determination in the suprachiasmatic nuclei. Cell. 1997;91:855–860.
21. Shinohara K, Honma S, Katsuno Y, et al. Two distinct oscillators in the rat suprachiasmatic nucleus in vitro. Proc Natl Acad Sci U S A. 1995;92:7396–7400.
22. DeCoursey PJ, Buggy J. Restoration of circadian locomotor activity in arrhythmic hamsters by fetal SCN transplants. Comp Endocrinol. 1988;7:49–54.
23. Lehman MN, Silver R, Bittman EL. Anatomy of suprachiasmatic nucleus grafts. In: Klein DC, Moore RY, Reppert SM, eds. Suprachiasmatic Nucleus: The Mind's Clock. New York, NY: Oxford University Press; 1991:349–374.
24. Ralph MR, Foster RG, Davis FC, et al. Transplanted suprachiasmatic nucleus determines circadian period. Science. 1990;247:975–978.
25. Sollars PJ, Kimble DP, Pickard GE. Restoration of circadian behavior by anterior hypothalamic heterografts. J Neurosci. 1995;15:2109–2122.
26. Meijer JH, Rietveld WJ. Neurophysiology of the SCN circadian pacemaker in rodents. Physiol Rev. 1989;69:671–707.
27. Pennartz CM, De Jeu MT, Geurtsen AM, et al. Electrophysiological and morphological heterogeneity of neurons in slices of rat suprachiasmatic nucleus. J Physiol (Lond). 1998;506:775–793.
28. Strecker GJ, Wuarin JP, Dudek FE. GABAA-mediated local synaptic pathways connect neurons in the rat suprachiasmatic nucleus. J Neurophysiol. 1997;78:2217–2220.
29. Schwartz WJ, Gross RA, Morton MT. The suprachiasmatic nuclei contain a tetrodotoxin-resistant circadian pacemaker. Proc Natl Acad Sci U S A. 1987;84:1695–1698.
30. Yamazaki S, Ishida Y, Inouye ST. Circadian rhythms of adenosine triphosphate contents in the suprachiasmatic nucleus, anterior hypothalamic area and caudate putamen of the rat: negative correlation with electrical activity. Brain Res. 1994;664:237–240.
31. Hall AC, Hoffmaster RM, Stern EL, et al. Suprachiasmatic nucleus neurons are glucose sensitive. J Biol Rhythms. 1997;12:388–400.
32. Serviere J, Lavialle M. Astrocytes in the mammalian circadian clock: putative roles. Progr Brain Res. 1996;111:57–73.
33. Moore RY. Chemical neuroanatomy of the mammalian circadian system. In: Redfern PH, Lammer B, eds. Handbook of Experimental Pharmacology, Vol 125. Physiology and Pharmacology of Biological Rhythms. Berlin, Germany: Springer-Verlag; 1997:79–93.
34. Wisor JP, Takahashi JS. Regulation of the vgf gene in the golden hamster suprachiasmatic nucleus by light and by the circadian clock. J Comp Neurol. 1997;378:229–238.
35. Silver R, Romero MT, Besmer HR, et al. Calbindin-D28K cells in the hamster SCN express light-induced Fos. Neuroreport. 1996;7:1224–1228.
36. Inouye ST. Circadian rhythms of neuropeptides in the suprachiasmatic nucleus. Progr Brain Res. 1996;111:75–90.

37. Reuss S. Photoperiod effects on bombesin- and cholecystokinin-like immunoreactivity in the suprachiasmatic nuclei of the Djungarian hamster (*Phodopus sungorus*). Neurosci Lett. 1991;128:13–16.

38. Pevet P, Pitrosky B, Vuillez P, et al. The suprachiasmastic nucleus: the biological clock of all seasons. Progr Brain Res. 1996;111:369–384.

39. Guldner FH, Ingham CA. Plasticity in synaptic appositions of optic nerve afferents under different lighting conditions. Neurosci Lett. 1979;14:235–240.

40. Clattenburg RE, Singh RP, Montemurro DG. Post-coital ultrastructural changes in neurons of the suprachiasmatic nucleus of the rabbit. Z Zellforsch. 1972;125:448–459.

41. Swaab DF, Fliers E, Partiman TS. The suprachiasmatic nucleus of the human brain in relation to sex, age and senile dementia. Brain Res. 1985;342:37–44.

42. Swaab DF, Hofman MA. An enlarged suprachiasmatic nucleus in homosexual men. Brain Res. 1990;537:141–148.

43. Nelson RJ, Zucker I. Absence of extraocular photoreception in diurnal and nocturnal rodents exposed to direct sunlight. Comp Biochem Physiol. 1981;69:145–148.

44. Roenneberg T, Foster RG. Twilight times: light and the circadian system. Photochem Photobiol. 1997;66:549–561.

45. Campbell SS, Murphy PJ. Extraocular circadian phototransduction in humans. Science. 1998;279:396–399.

46. Nelson DE, Takahashi JS. Comparison of visual sensitivity for suppression of pineal melatonin and circadian phase-shifting in the golden hamster. Brain Res. 1991;554:272–277.

47. Boivin DB, Duffy JF, Kronauer RE, et al. Dose-response relationships for resetting of human circadian clock by light. Nature. 1996;379:540–542.

48. Jewett ME, Rimmer DW, Duffy JF, et al. Human circadian pacemaker is sensitive to light throughout subjective day without evidence of transients. Am J Physiol. 1997;273:R1800–R1809.

49. Ebling FJ. The role of glutamate in the photic regulation of the suprachiasmatic nucleus. Progr Neurobiol. 1996;50:109–132.

50. Mintz EM, Albers HE. Microinjection of NMDA into the SCN region mimics the phase shifting effect of light in hamsters. Brain Res. 1997;758:245–249.

51. Takatsuji K, Senba E, Mantyh PW, et al. A relationship between substance P receptor and retinal fibers in the rat suprachiasmatic nucleus. Brain Res. 1995;698:53–61.

52. Hannibal J, Ding JM, Chen D, et al. Pituitary adenylate cyclase-activating peptide (PACAP) in the retinohypothalamic tract: a potential daytime regulator of the biological clock. J Neurosci. 1997;17:2637–2644.

53. Sherin JE, Shiromani PJ, McCarley RW, et al. Activation of ventrolateral preoptic neurons during sleep. Science. 1996;271:216–219.

54. Wada H, Inagaki N, Itowi N, et al. Histaminergic neuron system in the brain: distribution and possible functions. Brain Res Bull. 1991;27:367–370.

55. Panula P, Pirvola U, Auvinen S, et al. Histamine-immunoreactive nerve fibers in the rat brain. Neuroscience. 1989;28:585–610.

56. Cote NK, Harrington ME. Histamine phase shifts the circadian clock in a manner similar to light. Brain Res. 1993;613:149–151.

57. Meyer JL, Hall AC, Harrington ME. Histamine phase shifts the hamster circadian pacemaker via an NMDA dependent mechanism. J Biol Rhythms. 1998;13:288–295.

58. Scott G, Piggins HD, Semba K, et al. Actions of histamine in the suprachiasmatic nucleus of the syrian hamster. Brain Res. 1998;783:1–9.

59. Earnest DJ, Turek FW. Neurochemical basis for the photic control of circadian rhythms and seasonal reproductive cycles: role for acetylcholine. Proc Natl Acad Sci U S A. 1985;82:4277–4281.

60. Meijer JH, van der Zee EA, Dietz M. The effects of intraventricular carbachol injections on the freerunning activity rhythm of the hamster. J Biol Rhythms. 1988;4:1–16.

61. Wee BEF, Turek FW. Carbachol phase shifts the circadian rhythm of locomotor activity in the Djungarian hamster. Brain Res. 1989;505:209–214.

62. Bina KG, Rusak B, Semba K. Localization of cholinergic neurons in the forebrain and brainstem that project to the suprachiasmatic nucleus of the hypothalamus in rat. J Comp Neurol. 1993;335:295–307.

63. Mikkelsen JD, Vrang N. A direct pretectosuprachiasmatic projection in the rat. Neuroscience. 1994;62:497–505.

64. Moga MM, Moore RY. Organization of neural inputs to the suprachiasmatic nucleus in the rat. J Comp Neurol. 1997;389:508–534.

64a. Mistlberger RE, Antle MC, Dane L, et al. Sleep deprivation resets the circadian clock in the Syrian hamster. Soc Neurosci Abstr. 1999;25:1614.

65. Harrington ME. The ventral lateral geniculate nucleus and the intergeniculate leaflet: interrelated structures in the visual and circadian systems. Neurosci Biobehav Rev. 1997;21:705–727.

66. Allen CN, Jiang ZG, Nelson CS, et al. Orphanin-FQ (OFQ) modulates the circadian timing of the suprachiasmatic nucleus (SCN). Soc Neurosci Abstr. 1997;23:511.

67. Johnson RF, Smale L, Moore RY, et al. Lateral geniculate lesions block circadian phase-shift responses to a benzodiazepine. Proc Natl Acad Sci U S A. 1988;85:5301–5304.

68. Janik D, Mrosovsky N. Intergeniculate leaflet lesions and behaviorally-induced shifts of circadian rhythms. Brain Res. 1994;651:174–182.

69. Marchant EG, Watson NV, Mistlberger RE. Both neuropeptide Y and serotonin are necessary for entrainment of circadian rhythms in mice by daily treadmill running schedules, J Neurosci. 1997;17:7974–7987.

70. Challet E, Pevet P, Malan A. Intergeniculate leaflet lesion and daily rhythms in food-restricted rats fed during daytime. Neurosci Lett. 1996;216:214–218.

71. Maywood ES, Smith E, Hall SJ, et al. A thalamic contribution to arousal-induced, non-photic entrainment of the circadian clock of the Syrian hamster. Eur J Neurosci. 1997;9:1739–1747.

72. Biello SM, Janik D, Mrosovsky N. Neuropeptide Y and behaviorally induced phase shifts. Neuroscience. 1994;62:273–279.

73. Golombek DA, Biello SM, Rendon RA, et al. Neuropeptide Y phase shifts the circadian clock in vitro via a Y2 receptor. Neuroreport. 1996;7:1315–1319.

74. Huhman KL, Gillespie CF, Marvel CL, et al. Neuropeptide Y phase shifts circadian rhythms in vivo via a Y2 receptor. Neuroreport. 1996;7:1249–1252.

75. Harrington ME, Hoque S. NPY opposes PACAP phase shifts via receptors different from those involved in NPY phase shifts. Neuroreport. 1997;8:2677–2680.

76. Miller JD, Morin LP, Schwartz WJ, et al. New insights into the mammalian circadian clock. Sleep. 1996;19:641–667.

77. Meyer-Bernstein EL, Morin LP. Differential serotonergic innervation of the suprachiasmatic nucleus and the intergeniculate leaflet and its role in circadian rhythm modulation. J Neurosci. 1996;16:2097–2111.

78. Jacobs BL, Azmitia EC. Structure and function of the brain serotonin system. Physiol Rev. 1992;72:165–229.

79. Bobrzynska KJ, Godfrey MH, Mrosovsky N. Serotonergic stimulation and nonphotic phase-shifting in hamsters. Physiol Behav. 1996;59:221–230.

80. Mintz EM, Gillespie CF, Marvel CL, et al. Serotonergic regulation of circadian rhythms in Syrian hamsters. Neuroscience. 1997;79:563–569.

81. Edgar DM, Reid MS, Dement WC. Serotonergic afferents mediate activity-dependent entrainment of the mouse circadian clock. Am J Physiol. 1997;273:R265–R269.

82. Marchant EG, Watson NV, Mistlberger RE. Both neuropeptide Y and serotonin are necessary for entrainment of circadian rhythms in mice by daily treadmill running schedules. J Neurosci. 1997;17:7974–7987.

83. Bobrzynska KJ, Vrang N, Mrosovsky N. Persistence of nonphotic phase shifts in hamsters after serotonin depletion in the suprachiasmatic nucleus. Brain Res. 1996;741:205–214.

84. Antle MC, Marchant EG, Chubaty P, et al. Serotonin antagonists and agonists fail to modulate activity-induced phase shifts of circadian rhythms in syrian hamsters. Soc Neurosci Abstr. 1997;23:240.

85. Biello SM, Mrosovsky NM. Blocking the phase-shifting effect of neuropeptide Y with light. Proc R Soc Lond Biol Sci. 1995;259:179–187.

86. Ralph MR, Mrosovsky N. Behavioral inhibition of circadian responses to light. J Biol Rhythms. 1992;7:353–359.

87. Weber ET, Rea MA. Neuropeptide Y blocks light-induced phase

advances but not delays of the circadian activity rhythm in hamsters. Neurosci Lett. 1997;231:159–162.

88. Biello SM. Enhanced photic phase shifting after treatment with antiserum to neuropeptide Y. Brain Res. 1995;673:25–29.

89. Mistlberger RE, Antle MC. Behavioral inhibition of light-induced circadian phase resetting is phase and serotonin dependent. Brain Res. 1998;786:31–38.

90. Bradbury MJ, Dement WC, Edgar DM. Serotonin-containing fibers in the suprachiasmatic hypothalamus attenuate light-induced phase delays in mice. Brain Res. 1997;768:125–134.

91. Pickard GE, Ralph MR, Menaker M. The intergeniculate leaflet partially mediates effects of light on circadian rhythms. J Biol Rhythms. 1987;2:35–56.

92. Foote WE, Taber-Pierce E, Edwards L. Evidence for retinal projection to the midbrain raphe in the cat. Brain Res. 1978;156:135–140.

93. Shen H, Semba K. A direct retinal projection to the dorsal raphe nucleus in the rat. Brain Res. 1994;635:159–168.

93a. Fite KV, Janusonis S, Foote W, et al. Retinal afferents to the dorsal raphe nucleus in rats and mongolian gerbils. J Comp Neurol. In press.

93b. Edelstein K, Amir S. The role of the intergeniculate leaflet in entrainment of circadian rhythms to a skeleton photoperiod. J Neurosci. 1999;19:372–380.

94. Golombek DA, Ralph MR. Let there be light: signal transduction in a mammalian circadian system. Braz J Med Biol Res. 1996;29:131–140.

95. Prosser RA, Heller HC, Miller JD. Serotonergic phase advances of the mammalian circadian clock involve protein kinase A and K⁺ channel opening. Brain Res. 1994;644:67–73.

96. Hall AC, Earle-Cruickshanks G, Harrington ME. Role of membrane conductances and protein synthesis in subjective day phase advances of the hamster circadian clock by neuropeptide Y. Eur J Neurosci. 1999;11:1–9.

97. Jiang ZG, Nelson CS, Allen CN. Melatonin activates an outward current and inhibits Ih in rat suprachiasmatic nucleus neurons. Brain Res. 1995;687:125–132.

98. Biello SM, Golombek DA, Schak KM, et al. Circadian phase shifts to neuropeptide Y in vitro: cellular communication and signal transduction. J Neurosci. 1997;17:8468–8475.

99. McArthur AJ, Hunt AE, Gillette MU. Melatonin action and signal transduction in the rat suprachiasmatic circadian clock: activation of protein kinase C at dusk and dawn. Endocrinology. 1997;138:627–634.

100. Liu C, Weaver DR, Jin X, et al. Molecular dissection of two distinct actions of melatonin on the suprachiasmatic circadian clock. Neuron. 1997;19:91–102.

101. Starkey SJ. Melatonin and 5-hydroxytryptamine phase-advance the rat circadian clock by activation of nitric oxide synthesis. Neurosci Lett. 1996;211:199–202.

102. Zhang Y, Takahashi JS, Turek FW. Critical period for cycloheximide blockade of light-induced phase advances of the circadian locomotor activity rhythm in golden hamsters. Brain Res. 1996;740:285–290.

103. Prosser RA, Macdonald ES, Heller HC. c-fos mRNA in the suprachiasmatic nuclei in vitro shows a circadian rhythm and responds to a serotonergic agonist. Mol Brain Res. 1994;25:151–156.

104. Mikkelsen JD, Vrang N, Mrosovsky N. Expression of Fos in the circadian system following nonphotic stimulation. Brain Res Bull. 1998;47:367–376.

105. Watts AG, Swanson LW. Efferent projections of the suprachiasmatic nucleus, II: studies using retrograde transport of fluorescent dyes and simultaneous peptide immunohistochemistry in the rat. J Comp Neurol. 1987;258:230–252.

106. Eskes GA, Rusak B. Horizontal knife cuts in the suprachiasmatic area prevent hamster gonadal responses to photoperiod. Neurosci Lett. 1985;61:261–266.

107. Nunez AA, Brown MH, Youngstrom TG. Hypothalamic circuits involved in the regulation of seasonal and circadian rhythms in male golden hamsters. Brain Res Bull. 1985;15:149–153.

108. Vrang N, Mikkelsen JD, Larsen PJ. Direct link from the suprachiasmatic nucleus to hypothalamic neurons projecting to the spinal cord: a combined tracing study using cholera toxin subunit B and Phaseolus vulgaris-leucoagglutinin. Brain Res Bull. 1997;44:671–680.

109. Klein DC, Smoot R, Weller JL. Lesions of the paraventricular nucleus area of the hypothalamus disrupt the suprachiasmatic–spinal cord circuit in the melatonin generating system. Brain Res Bull. 1983;10:647–651.

110. Buijs RM. The anatomical basis for the expression of circadian rhythms: the efferent projections of the suprachiasmatic nucleus. Progr Brain Res. 1996;111:229–240.

111. van der Beek EM, Wiegant VM, van Oudheusden HJ, et al. Synaptic contacts between gonadotropin-releasing hormone-containing fibers and neurons in the suprachiasmatic nucleus and perichiasmatic area: an anatomical substrate for feedback regulation? Brain Res. 1997;755:101–111.

112. de la Iglesia HO, Blaustein JD, Bittman EL. The suprachiasmatic area in the female hamster projects to neurons containing estrogen receptors and GnRH. Neuroreport. 1995;6:1715–1722.

113. Silver R, LeSauter J, Tresco PA, et al. A diffusible coupling signal from the transplanted suprachiasmatic nucleus controlling circadian locomotor rhythms. Nature. 1996;382:810–813.

114. Zucker I. Hormones and hamster circadian organization. In: Suda M, Hayaishi O, Nakagawa H, eds. Biological Rhythms and Their Central Mechanism. New York, NY: Elsevier; 1979:369–382.

115. Morin LP, Fitzgerald KM, Zucker I. Estradiol shortens the period of hamster circadian rhythms. Science. 1977;196:305–307.

116. Zucker I, Fitzgerald KM, Morin LP. Sex differentiation of the circadian system in the golden hamster. Am J Physiol. 1980;238:R97–R101.

117. Daan S, Damassa D, Pittendrigh CS, et al. An effect of castration and testosterone replacement on circadian pacemaker in mice (Mus musculus). Proc Natl Acad Sci U S A. 1975;72:3744–3747.

118. Ellis GB, Turek FW. Changes in locomotor activity associated with the photoperiodic response of the testes in male golden hamsters. J Comp Physiol. 1979;132:277–274.

119. Rowsemitt CN. Seasonal variations in activity rhythms of male voles: mediation by gonadal hormones. Physiol Behav. 1986;37:797–803.

120. Morin LP. Effect of ovarian hormones on synchrony of hamster circadian rhythms. Physiol Behav. 1980;24:741–749.

121. Beasley LJ, Nelson RJ. Thyroid gland influences the period of hamster circadian oscillation. Experientia. 1982;28:870–871.

122. Morin LP, Gavin ML, Ottenweller JE. Propylthiouracil causes phase delays and circadian period lengthening in male and female hamsters. Am J Physiol. 1986;250:R151–R160.

123. Horseman ND, Ehret CF. Glucocorticosteroid injection is a circadian zeitgeber in the laboratory rat. Am J Physiol. 1982;243:R373–R378.

124. Moore-Ede MC, Schmelzer-WS, Kass DA, et al. Cortisol mediated synchronization of circadian rhythm in urinary potassium excretion. Am J Physiol. 1977;233:R230–R238.

125. Reiter RJ. Pineal melatonin: cell biology of its synthesis and of its physiological interactions. Endocr Rev. 1991;12:151–180.

126. de Elvira Ruiz MC, Persaud R, Coen CW. Use of running wheels regulates the effects of the ovaries on circadian rhythms. Physiol Behav. 1992;52:277–284.

127. Rusak B. The role of suprachiasmatic nuclei in the generation of circadian rhythms in the golden hamster, Mesocricetus auratus. J Comp Physiol. 1977;118:145–146.

128. Terman M, Terman J. A circadian pacemaker for visual sensitivity? Ann N Y Acad Sci. 1985;453:147–161.

129. Mistlberger RE. Circadian food-anticipatory activity: formal models and physiological mechanisms. Neurosci Biobehav Rev. 1994;18:171–195.

130. Tosini G, Menaker M. Circadian rhythms in cultured mammalian retina. Science. 1996;272:419–421.

131. Honma S, Honma K-I, Hiroshige T. Methamphetamine induced locomotor rhythm entrains to restricted daily feeding in SCN lesioned rats. Physiol Behav. 1991;49:787–795.

132. Aschoff J. On the perception of time during prolonged temporal isolation. Hum Neurobiol. 1985;4:41–52.

133. Aschoff J, von Goetz C, Wildgruber C, et al. Meal timing in humans during temporal isolation without time cues. J Biol Rhythms. 1986;1:151–162.

134. Helfrich-Forster C. Drosophila rhythms: from brain to behavior. Semin Cell Dev Biol. 1996;7:791–802.

135. Plautz JD, Kaneko M, Hall JC, et al. Independent photoreceptive circadian clocks throughout Drosophila. Science. 1997;278:1632–1635.

Molecular Genetic Basis for Mammalian Circadian Rhythms

Lawrence H. Pinto
Martha Hotz Vitaterna
Fred W. Turek

The molecular mechanisms that generate circadian rhythms in mammals are in the central circadian pacemaker, which is located in the hypothalamic suprachiasmatic nucleus (SCN). The ability to generate circadian rhythms is a property of individual neurons within the SCN, and the components of the cellular circadian oscillator appear to involve a relatively small number of genes and their protein products. To date, the known molecular components of the oscillator have been identified either by the approach of induced mutagenesis or by their interaction with a component identified by mutagenesis.

Four proteins have been identified that participate in an oscillatory pattern of activity within individual neurons of the SCN. The CLOCK and BMAL1 proteins form a heterodimer that activates the transcription of two other circadian genes, tim *and* per. *The protein products of these genes, TIM and PER, form a heterodimer that migrates to the nucleus of the neuron and attenuates the ability of the CLOCK-BMAL1 heterodimer to activate the transcription of the* tim *and* per *genes, thus completing the loop of oscillatory signaling. Still other genes encode proteins that are involved in bringing signals to the circadian oscillator and in transmitting signals from the oscillator to other parts of the brain.*

Over the past few decades, remarkable progress has been made in elucidating the physiological substrates that underlie the generation of 24-h rhythms in mammals. Such rhythms are now known to be generated by a "master" biological clock located in the bilaterally paired suprachiasmatic nuclei (SCN) of the hypothalamus.[1] These nuclei appear to be responsible for regulating all behavioral, physiological, and biochemical 24-h rhythms. Indeed, a few thousand cells in the SCN are ultimately responsible for regulating the temporal organization in billions of cells in the body. Under constant environmental conditions devoid of any time-giving cues, the rhythms regulated by this clock have a period of about 24 h, and therefore are referred to as *circadian* (i.e., about a day) rhythms. The topic of this chapter is the genes expressed in the SCN and the proteins they encode, which are responsible daily for this rhythmicity.

INDIVIDUAL NEURONS OF THE SUPRACHIASMATIC NUCLEUS ARE KEY TO CIRCADIAN FUNCTION

Several lines of evidence point to the SCN as the site of the circadian oscillator. Surgical isolation of the SCN with a Halasz knife, designed to allow preservation of the nearby neuronal tissue, removes circadian oscillations in the plasma concentration of cortisol[2] and in locomotion and drinking.[3] These oscillations are independent of inputs from the eye,[2] although an autonomous circadian clock has been demonstrated to exist within the eye that controls, among other functions, the shedding of rod outer segment disks.[4] Normal circadian rhythms can be restored to an SCN-lesioned animal by transplantation of fetal SCN tissue but not by transplantation of fetal tissue from other regions of the brain.[5] An abnormally short circadian period can be imposed on an SCN-lesioned animal by the transplantation of fetal tissue from the SCN of the tau mutant animal (described later) with an abnormally short period.[6] Thus, several lines of evidence point to the SCN as the site driving or controlling circadian behavior for mammals.

There are several ways in which the neurons of the SCN might produce oscillatory activity. One way would be for the individual neurons to have intrinsic oscillatory behavior. Alternatively, no one neuron may possess oscillatory behavior, but rather the ensemble of neurons oscillates because of the intrinsic properties and connections of the ensemble. Several lines of evidence point to the oscillations being intrinsic to individual SCN neurons. Blockade of action potentials by injection of tetrodotoxin into the SCN does not stop the circadian oscillator, although blockade does prevent inputs and outputs from being transmitted to and from the SCN.[7] In addition, synaptogenesis in the SCN occurs after the development of circadian rhythms.[8] These two findings demonstrate that the oscillations do not depend on communication between SCN neurons. Indeed, the periods of individual SCN cells studied in slices vary widely, and the circadian period of an animal appears to reflect the mean of the periods of many SCN neurons.[9] Finally, individual, dissociated SCN neurons in culture demonstrate oscillations with periods that differ from cell to cell, indicating that these neurons possess an intrinsic oscillatory mechanism.[10] The remainder of this chapter focuses on the mechanism by which individual cells generate activity that oscillates with a period of about 1 day.

PROTEIN SYNTHESIS DRIVES THE CIRCADIAN OSCILLATOR

How do individual SCN neurons generate rhythmic activity with a period of about 1 day? Many pacemaker neurons generate oscillatory activity, such as rhythmic patterns of action potentials, and these relatively rapid oscillations can be explained by the concerted action of a small number of ion channels. However, the much slower oscillations of the individual SCN neurons are not likely to involve the same mechanisms. Indeed, it appears that the synthesis of proteins by each SCN neuron is central to the mechanism for the generation of 24-h rhythms. The initial evidence for this is that application of protein synthesis inhibitors in the region of the SCN shifts the circadian phase of activity of animals by an amount and in a direction that depends on the time at which the inhibition is imposed.[11, 12] A similar shift in the phase of vasopressin release from explanted SCN also results from inhibition of protein synthesis.[13] Thus, protein synthesis is central to the generation of circadian oscillations.

THE per GENE OF THE CIRCADIAN CLOCK

The first gene that encodes a clock component, per, was discovered in 1971 in Drosophila using an approach that is applicable to the discovery of genes that affect sleep. This approach, forward genetics, consists of inducing random mutations in the genome, usually by chemical mutagenesis, and detecting those mutations that affect the process of interest by screening with a carefully crafted screening test. This approach has the advantage that no assumptions are made about the nature of the genes or gene products involved, but the screening test must be based on an aspect of the phenotype, which is reflective of the fundamental properties of the system. An example is the endogenous period of the activity rhythm, rather than amount or distribution of activity.

Three alleles of the per gene were identified by the process of mutagenesis and screening. These alleles had no apparent rhythm in eclosion (emergence from the pupal case) or locomotion, or had either long (e.g., 29 h) or short (e.g., 19 h) periods for the rhythms of eclosion and locomotor activity.[14] It is important to note that the finding of three alleles with three different phenotypes made it possible to have confidence in the conclusion that the per gene encodes a protein that is a clock component. Had only an arrhythmic mutant been found, then the alternative explanation could be proposed that the lack of circadian behavior was secondary to another primary defect that did not lie in a clock component. It should be noted that the approach of mutagenesis and screening has also been successful in identifying circadian clock genes in the bread mold Neurospora crassa.[15] More recently, mutagenesis screens have identified clock mutants in plants[16] and cyanobacteria.[17] However, because no mammalian orthologs of these genes have been found, a discussion of these important findings is outside the scope of this review.

Further support for the importance of the per gene as a central circadian clock component was the rescue of the mutant phenotype after introduction of the wild-type allele of the per gene into mutant animals.[18, 19] The mRNA transcript encoded by the per gene was shown to oscillate in level in a circadian fashion[20] as a result of transcriptional regulation,[21] and the levels of the PER protein were shown to lag behind the per mRNA levels.[22] In fact, shifts in the circadian phase can be evoked by the induction of PER protein under the control of a noncircadian promoter.[23] Thus, many lines of evidence indicate that the per gene encodes a protein that is a clock component. Two homologs of the per gene, mPer1 and mPer2, have been identified in the mouse, and the levels of their mRNA have also been shown to oscillate with a circadian period.[24–27]

How is the level of the PER protein regulated by the circadian clock? The first hint came from the identification of the timeless gene tim, which, when mutated, produces abnormal circadian rhythms in Drosophila.[28] The levels of the mRNA encoded by the tim gene oscillate with a time course that is indistinguishable from those of per mRNA.[29] The levels of the TIM protein lag behind those of tim mRNA by several hours,[30] similar to the finding with per mRNA and PER protein. The PER and TIM proteins form heterodimers[31] that are transported to the nucleus.[32] The finding that the heterodimer is transported to the nucleus suggested that it might be involved in the regulation of transcription of the per or tim genes. Indeed, experiments have shown that the transcription of the per and tim genes is repressed by the PER-TIM protein heterodimer.[33] This finding is important because it demonstrates that the production of mRNA encoded by a clock component gene, the delayed accumulation of the encoded protein, and later feedback to the clock gene's promoter in the nucleus, are able to explain the basic features of the circadian clock. However, a detailed explanation of how this happens is only possible after describing the mammalian Clock gene and the interactions of its protein product with other molecular components of the mammalian circadian clock.

THE MAMMALIAN Clock GENE

Because no mammalian orthologs to Drosophila circadian clock genes had been identified by the early 1990s and no other genes in mammals had been identified as even possible candidate circadian clock genes in genetically accessible organisms, we applied the forward genetic approach in mice in an effort to identify the first circadian clock genes in mammals. We used C57BL/6J mice. Wild-type C57BL/6J mice show robust entrainment to a light-dark (LD) cycle and have a circadian period between 23.6 and 23.8 h under free-running conditions in constant darkness (DD) (Fig. 27–

1). In a screen for dominant or semidominant mutations of more than 300 mice, we found 1 animal that had a free-running period of about 24.8 h, more than 6 SD longer than the mean.[34] In the homozygous condition, this mutation results in a dramatic lengthening of the period to about 28 h, which is usually followed by the eventual loss of circadian rhythmicity (i.e., *arrhythmicity*) after about 1 to 3 weeks in DD. The affected

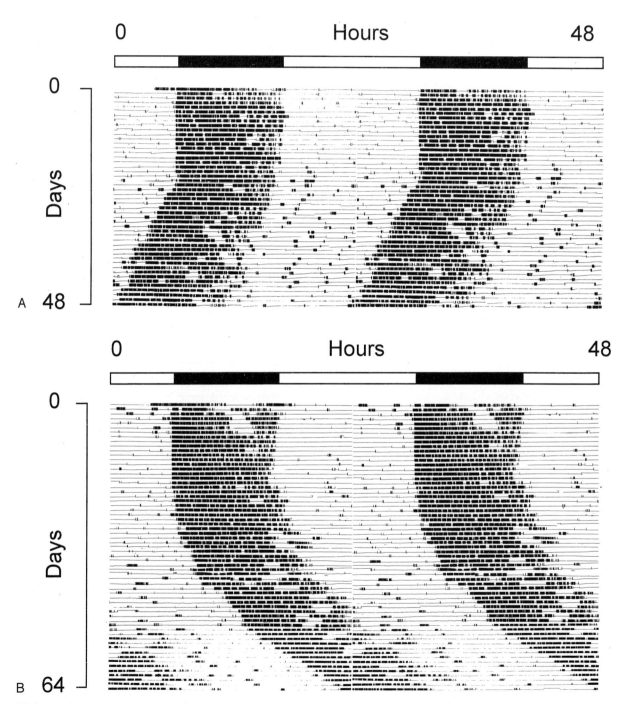

Figure 27-1. Activity records of mice. Each record is double-plotted according to convention so that each day's data are presented both to the right and beneath the day preceding. Times of wheel-running activity are indicated by black. On days 1 through 19, mice were maintained under the light-dark cycle indicated by the bar above each record. Mice were then transferred to continuous darkness by allowing lights to go out at the usual time but remain off through the remaining days of data collection shown. *A*, activity record of a normal C57BL/6J mouse, with a free-running period of approximately 23.7 h. *B*, activity record of the founder *Clock* mutant mouse, with a free-running period that lengthened over time to approximately 24.8 h.

gene was mapped to mouse chromosome 5 and named *Clock*. We have cloned the *Clock* gene by a combination of genetic rescue and positional cloning techniques.

The first step in positional cloning of the *Clock* gene was to obtain a high resolution map of the region of chromosome 5, near the gene. This was done using test crosses that produced more than 2000 meioses and allowed us to identify a set of three bacterial artificial chromosome (BAC) vectors that contained the *Clock* gene in a 250 kilobase (kb) region of the chromosome.[35] To identify the BAC that contained the *Clock* gene, we used the principle of rescue of the phenotype, similar in principle to the rescue experiments that were first carried out in *Drosophila* to identify the *per* gene. Transgenic mice in which each of several BACs were integrated into the genome were produced and assayed for circadian phenotype. We found that if one of the BACs of length 140 kb was incorporated, a wild-type circadian period was produced in transgenic *Clock* mutant mice. In littermate mice that possessed the wild-type allele at the *Clock* locus, the period was shorter than for nontransgenic wild-type mice.[36] However, no alteration of phenotype was found after incorporation of either of the other two BACs. After narrowing down the region of the *Clock* gene to 140 kb, candidate genes were identified within the region by comparison of the sequence of the region with that of cDNAs that are expressed in the SCN. This approach found one candidate gene, which was sequenced in wild-type and *Clock* mutant animals and found to contain a point mutation that caused exon skipping in *Clock* mutant tissues.[37] The *Clock* gene encodes a transcriptional regulatory protein having a basic helix-loop-helix DNA-binding domain, a PAS dimerization domain (PAS, named for *per*, *Arnt*, and *Sim*, the first genes identified with this domain) and a glutamine-rich activation domain. The mutant form of the CLOCK protein lacks a portion of the activation domain found in wild-type protein, and thus, although it is capable of protein dimerization, transcriptional activation is diminished or lost. *Clock* mRNA is expressed in the SCN as well as other tissues, but it has not been found to oscillate in a circadian fashion.[37]

INTERACTIONS OF THE CLOCK PROTEIN WITH THE *per* GENE

The presence of the PAS dimerization domain in CLOCK protein suggested that it may form a heterodimer similar to that of PER-TIM.[38] A screen for potential partners for the CLOCK protein using the yeast two hybrid system revealed that a protein of unknown function, BMAL1, was able to dimerize with the CLOCK protein.[39] Next, the ability of this heterodimer to regulate transcription was tested using a reporter construct based on the upstream regulatory elements of the *per* gene. The *per* gene of *Drosophila* contains an upstream regulatory element, the "clock control region" within which is contained a nucleic acid sequence needed for positive regulation of transcription, the E-box element (CACGTG).[40] CLOCK-BMAL1 heterodimers were found to activate transcription of the *mPer* gene in a process that requires binding to the E-box element.[39] However, CLOCK Δ19 mutant protein was not able to activate transcription, consistent with the finding that exon 19, which is skipped in *Clock* mutant animals,[37] is necessary for transactivation. Thus, CLOCK protein interacts with the regulatory regions of the *per* gene to allow transcription of the *per* mRNA and eventual translation of PER protein. A similar activation of transcription of the *tim* gene by the CLOCK-BMAL1 heterodimer also occurs.[33] However, this positive regulation alone will not produce an oscillation in *per* mRNA levels, which are known to be responsible for the oscillation in PER protein levels.[21]

What is needed to complete our understanding of how circadian oscillations occur is a negative regulatory component to the circadian oscillator. This component has been identified in experiments using a luciferase reporter assay. In this assay, the luminescent luciferase protein was expressed under the control of the promoter regions of the *Drosophila per* and *tim* genes. It was found that the fly homolog of *Clock*, *dClock*,[41] was capable of driving expression of luciferase[33] in cells that have high endogenous levels of the *Drosophila* homolog of BMAL1, dBMAL1. The effect of the PER-TIM heterodimer on the ability of the dCLOCK-dBMAL1 heterodimer to drive the transcription of the *per* and *tim* genes was tested by co-transfecting the encoding genes into the cells that expressed the luciferase reporter gene. Indeed, it was found that the expression of both the *per* and *tim* genes were reduced by their own protein products. This negative feedback has been found for a mammalian heterodimer consisting of orthologs of the TIMELESS and mPER1 proteins.[42]

A WORKING MODEL FOR THE CIRCADIAN OSCILLATOR

The experiments described earlier point to a model in which the following steps occur in order to generate the core oscillations of protein levels that control the circadian clock.[33]

1. The key element is that transcription of the *per* and *tim* genes are enhanced by the binding of the CLOCK-BMAL1 heterodimer to their promoter regions, but this enhancement is itself diminished by inhibition from the PER-TIM heterodimer.
2. In the absence of the PER-TIM heterodimer, the CLOCK-BMAL1 complex drives expression of the *per* and *tim* genes, causing an accumulation of the PER-TIM heterodimer.
3. The accumulation of the PER-TIM heterodimer is followed by its translocation to the nucleus.
4. In the nucleus, the PER-TIM heterodimer inhibits the enhancement of transcription caused by CLOCK-BMAL1.
5. mRNA levels for *per* and *tim* will now fall, resulting in a decrease in their protein products, relieving their inhibition and allowing CLOCK-BMAL1 to initiate a new round of synthesis.

Although other genes may also play a central role in the molecular machinery that comprises the cellular circadian clock, it is now clear that at least four of the circadian clock genes have been identified in mammals. These four genes and their gene products interact in a fashion that would allow circadian oscillation. There are remarkable similarities between the function of these genes in fruit flies and mice.

THE *tau* AND *Wheels* MUTATIONS

The *tau* and *Wheels* mutations should be considered because they are mammalian mutations that affect circadian period: one encodes a protein that is probably a clock component, whereas the other probably does not. The *tau* mutation of the hamster arose spontaneously in laboratory stock.[43] The mutation is semidominant and shortens the period from 24 to 22 h in heterozygotes, and from 24 to 20 h in homozygotes. This mutation has been of great importance for several reasons.

1. The mutation predated the *Clock* mutation and demonstrated that single gene mutations could profoundly alter the circadian clock in mammals, just as in flies and *Neurospora*.
2. *Tau* mutants display several other physiological phenotypes such as alteration of the responses of males to photoperiod length[44] and effects of the estrous cycles in females.[45]
3. The evidence that the SCN is indeed the site of the circadian oscillator (see earlier) was demonstrated unequivocally using manipulations that employed the *tau* mutation.

These manipulations also gave rise to the evidence necessary to conclude that the *tau* mutation encodes a protein that is a clock component. Unfortunately, the genetic tools needed for cloning this important and interesting gene are not available for the hamster.

The *Wheels* mutation of the mouse was identified in a screen similar to that described for the *Clock* mutation. The mutation is semidominant, and in heterozygotes the period is reduced from 24.2 to 23.3 h.[46] Unfortunately, the mutation is homozygous lethal, unlike any known clock component genes, and the development of the inner ear of heterozygotes is disrupted.[47] Thus, the circadian changes are probably secondary to the other abnormalities,[47] and the gene does not encode a protein that is a clock component.

GENES THAT CONTROL CIRCADIAN INPUTS AND OUTPUTS

The induction of a number of immediate early genes and a number of signal-transduction events seems to be involved in mediating the light-evoked alteration of circadian behavior that is mediated by signals transmitted to the SCN through the retinohypothalamic tract (reviewed in reference 48). However, these genes are not thought to be clock component proteins. Light re-

sults in the rapid degradation of the TIM protein and thus in the degradation of the PER-TIM heterodimer through a mechanism that is not yet fully understood.[49, 50] The cryptochromes have been shown to have a modulatory effect on the response to light in mice[51] and *Drosophila*.[52, 53] In addition, several genes have been identified in *Drosophila* that result in alterations in one but not all circadian behaviors and are thus thought to be circadian output genes. One such gene, *Drosophila lark*, produces arrhythmic eclosion but does not alter locomotor activity.[54] Mutation of a second gene, DCO, results in abnormal locomotor activity rhythm but leaves intact the rhythm of the PER protein.[55] No genes have been reported in mammals which when mutated alter only a single circadian behavior.

SLEEP IN *Clock* MUTANT ANIMALS

Although total destruction of the SCN in rats affects the timing of the sleep-wake cycle, it does not affect the total amount of sleep or the need for recovery sleep following sleep deprivation.[56–58] These results have been interpreted to indicate that the circadian regulation of the sleep-wake cycle (known as process C) does not influence the homeostatic drive for sleep (known as process S), which is thought to be dependent on the duration of prior wake and sleep times.[59] However, we have found that homozygous *Clock* mutant animals spend more time awake and less time in both NREM and REM sleep as compared to wild-type animals under both LD and DD conditions.[60] Thus, a genetic alteration in circadian clock function also appears to influence the need for sleep, raising the possibility that the circadian clock may influence not only the timing of sleep and wake but also process S itself. This hypothesis is compatible with the finding that SCN-lesioned squirrel monkeys spend much more time asleep than controls, suggesting that the SCN may produce an "activating" factor that influences the need for sleep.[61]

Knowing that *Clock* was a circadian clock gene led directly to the discovery of a second clock gene, *Bmal1*, which encodes the *Clock* dimerization partner BMAL1. The finding that a mutation in the *Clock* gene can influence the amount of sleep raises the possibility that animals with circadian clock mutations will help in the discovery of other genes that regulate sleep. Thus, finding genes that regulate process C may lead indirectly to genes regulating process S. A second approach that can be taken to discover novel genes involved in the regulation of sleep would be to screen directly for alterations in sleep phenotype in the offspring of mutagenized animals as we did to identify the *Clock* gene in mice. Furthermore, the structure of the circadian clock genes and their protein products and the functional interactions among them are similar in fruit flies and mice. This similarity suggests that the molecular mechanisms that control temporal organization are highly conserved across evolutionary time. If such conservation also occurs in the need for "sleep" at the molecular-cellular level, then the identification of genes regulating sleep in *Drosophila* may lead directly to mammalian sleep genes.

CIRCADIAN CLOCK GENES IN HUMANS

Although no specific gene has been clearly identified as a component of the molecular circadian clock in human beings, the discovery of circadian clock genes in mice indicates it is only a matter of time before these or other genes are identified as components of the human circadian timepiece. A number of laboratories are attempting to use linkage analysis to identify such genes in small pedigrees of families with specific circadian disorders such as advanced sleep phase syndrome or delayed sleep phase syndrome. Such an approach is expected to uncover altered alleles for clock genes that have been identified in lower organisms or lead to the discovery of genes that regulate circadian rhythmicity in human beings. In addition, because human orthologs of the murine clock genes have been identified on a basis of sequence similarity, it is now possible to determine the allelic variability of these genes in the human population and to determine if this variability is associated with any specific circadian phenotype. Katzenberg et al.[61a] reported that subjects carrying one copy of a specific allele of *Clock* had a significantly lower mean Horne-Ostberg score, indicating that these subjects tended to have a "eveningness" preference. The results indicate that human diurnal preference is associated with the *Clock* gene.

Disorders of circadian temporal organization come in two general varieties: those imposed by the lifestyle of the individual (e.g., jet lag and shift work), and those that arise from endogenous alterations in normal rhythmicity.[62, 63] Elucidating the genetic basis of human circadian rhythmicity holds the promise for new therapeutic approaches for both the "voluntary" and the "involuntary" disruption of normal circadian function. It will also be of great interest, both from a scientific as well as a medical perspective, to determine if the expression of human clock genes is altered under various pathophysiological conditions or in advanced age. The effects of aging are of particular interest because it has been associated with abnormal circadian time-keeping.[64]

CONCLUSIONS

The core circadian oscillator is autonomous to individual neurons of the SCN and is the result of the daily oscillation in the levels of several clock component proteins. The basis for this oscillation is that the levels of the heterodimeric proteins PER-TIM alter the rate of transcription of their own genes. This alteration is achieved by inhibition of the enhancement of transcription that results from binding of the CLOCK-BMAL1 heterodimer to the E-box element of the promoter region of the *per* and *tim* genes. It is of interest that all but one of these genes were identified by the process of forward genetics, in which mutations were induced in the genome randomly, and those mutations that specifically affect the circadian oscillator were identified with carefully crafted screens. Now that these clock-component proteins have been identified, it will be easier to find the proteins that serve the input and output pathways of the circadian oscillator and to identify the components that are out of order in disease states that affect circadian rhythms. It is fortuitous that the unraveling of the molecular basis for circadian rhythmicity is occurring at a time when the general public is becoming aware of the importance of normal circadian time-keeping for human health, safety, performance, and productivity.

Acknowledgments

We are grateful to Drs. Joseph S. Takahashi, William Dove, and Alexandra Shedlovsky for thoughtful discussions throughout the course of this work. Supported by NIH R01HL/MH59598 and the National Science Foundation Center for Biological Timing.

References

1. Klein DC, Moore RY, Reppert SM. Suprachiasmatic Nucleus: The Mind's Clock. New York, NY: Oxford University Press; 1991.
2. Moore RY, Eichler VB. Loss of a circadian adrenal corticosterone rhythm following suprachiasmatic lesions in the rat. Brain Res. 1972;42:201–206.
3. Stephan FK, Zucker I. Circadian rhythms in drinking behavior and locomotor activity of rats are eliminated by hypothalamic lesions. Proc Natl Acad Sci U S A. 1972;69:1583–1586.
4. Tosini G, Menaker M. Circadian rhythms in cultured mammalian retina. Science. 1996;272:419–421.
5. Lehman MN, Silver R, Gladstone WR, et al. Circadian rhythmicity restored by neural transplant. Immunocytochemical characterization of the graft and its integration with the host brain. J Neurosci. 1987;7:1626–1638.
6. Ralph MR, Foster RG, Davis FC, et al. Transplanted suprachiasmatic nucleus determines circadian period. Science. 1990;247:975–978.
7. Schwartz WJ, Gross RA, Morton MT. The suprachiasmatic nuclei contain a tetrodotoxin-resistant circadian pacemaker. Proc Natl Acad Sci U S A. 1987;84:1694–1698.
8. Moore RY, Bernstein ME. Synaptogenesis in the rat suprachiasmatic nucleus demonstrated by electron microscopy and synapsin I immunoreactivity. J Neurosci. 1989;9:2151–2162.
9. Liu C, Weaver DR, Strogatz SH, et al. Cellular construction of a circadian clock: period determination in the suprachiasmatic nuclei. Cell. 1997;91:855–860.
10. Welsh DK, Logothetis DE, Meister M, et al. Individual neurons dissociated from rat suprachiasmatic nucleus express independently phased circadian firing rhythms. Neuron. 1995;14:697–706.
11. Takahashi JS. Molecular neurobiology and genetics of circadian rhythms in mammals. Annu Rev Neurosci. 1995;18:531–553.
12. Inouye SIT, Takahashi JS, Wollnik F, et al. Inhibitor of protein synthesis phase shifts a circadian pacemaker in the mammalian SCN. Am J Physiol. 1988;255:R1055–R1058.
13. Watanabe K, Katagai T, Ishida N, et al. Anisomycin reduces phase shifts of circadian pacemaker in primary cultures of rat suprachiasmatic nucleus. Brain Res. 1995;684:179–184.
14. Konopka RJ, Benzer S. Clock mutants of *Drosophila melanogaster*. Proc Natl Acad Sci U S A. 1971;68:2112–2116.
15. Dunlap JC. Genetics and molecular analysis of circadian rhythms. Annu Rev Genet. 1996;30:579–601.
16. Millar AJ, Carre IA, Strayer CA, et al. Circadian clock mutants in *Arabidopsis* identified by luciferase imaging. Science. 1995;267:1161–1163.
17. Kondo T, Tsinoremas NF, Golden SS, et al. Circadian clock mutants of cyanobacteria. Science. 1994;266:1233–1236.

18. Bargiello TA, Jackson FR, Young MW. Restoration of circadian behavioural rhythms by gene transfer in *Drosophila*. Nature. 1984;312:752–754.

19. Zehring WA, Wheeler DA, Reddy P, et al. P-element transformation with period locus DNA restores rhythmicity to mutant, arrhythmic *Drosophila melanogaster*. Cell. 1984;39(2 pt 1):369–376.

20. Hardin PE, Hall JC, Rosbash M. Feedback of the *Drosophila* period gene product on circadian cycling of its messenger RNA levels. Nature. 1990;343:536–540.

21. Hardin PE, Hall JC, Rosbash M. Circadian oscillations in period gene mRNA levels are transcriptionally regulated. Proc Natl Acad Sci U S A. 1992;89:11711–11715.

22. Edery I, Zwiebel LJ, Dembinska ME, et al. Temporal phosphorylation of the *Drosophila* period protein. Proc Natl Acad Sci U S A. 1994;91:2260–2264.

23. Edery I, Rutila JE, Rosbash M. Phase shifting of the circadian clock by induction of the *Drosophila* period protein. Science. 1994;263:237–240.

24. Albrecht U, Sun ZS, Eichele G, et al. A differential response of two putative mammalian circadian regulators, mPer1 and mPer2, to light. Cell. 1997;91:1055–1064.

25. Shearman LP, Zylka MJ, Weaver DR, et al. Two period homologs: circadian expression and photic regulation in the suprachiasmatic nuclei. Neuron. 1997;19:1261–1269.

26. Sun ZS, Albrecht U, Zhuchenko O, et al. RIGUI, a putative mammalian ortholog of the *Drosophila* period gene. Cell. 1997;90:1003–1011.

27. Tei H, Okamura H, Shigeyoshi Y, et al. Circadian oscillation of a mammalian homologue of the *Drosophila* period gene. Nature. 1997;389:512–516.

28. Sehgal A, Price JL, Man B, et al. Loss of circadian behavioral rhythms and per RNA oscillations in the *Drosophila* mutant timeless. Science. 1994;263:1603–1606.

29. Sehgal A, Rothenfluh-Hilfiker A, Hunter-Ensor M, et al. Rhythmic expression of timeless: a basis for promoting circadian cycles in period gene autoregulation. Science. 1995;270:808–810.

30. Hunter-Ensor M, Ousley A, Sehgal A. Regulation of the *Drosophila* protein timeless suggests a mechanism for resetting the circadian clock by light. Cell. 1996;84:677–685.

31. Gekakis N, Saez L, Delahaye-Brown AM, et al. Isolation of timeless by PER protein interaction: defective interaction between timeless protein and long-period mutant PERL. Science. 1995;270:811–815.

32. Saez L, Young MW. Regulation of nuclear entry of the *Drosophila* clock proteins period and timeless. Neuron. 1996;17:911–920.

33. Darlington TK, Wager-Smith K, Ceriani MF, et al. Closing the circadian loop: CLOCK-induced transcription of its own inhibitors per and tim. Science. 1998;280:1599–1603.

34. Vitaterna MH, King DP, Chang AM, et al. Mutagenesis and mapping of a mouse gene, Clock, essential for circadian behavior. Science. 1994;264:719–725.

35. King DP, Vitaterna MH, Chang AM, et al. The mouse Clock mutation behaves as an antimorph and maps within the W19H deletion, distal of Kit. Genetics. 1997;146:1049–1060.

36. Antoch MP, Song EJ, Chang AM, et al. Functional identification of the mouse circadian Clock gene by transgenic BAC rescue. Cell. 1997;89:655–667.

37. King DP, Zhao Y, Sangoram AM, et al. Positional cloning of the mouse circadian clock gene. Cell. 1997;89:641–653.

38. Huang ZJ, Edery I, Rosbash M. PAS is a dimerization domain common to *Drosophila* period and several transcription factors. Nature. 1993;364:259–262.

39. Gekakis N, Staknis D, Nguyen HB, et al. Role of the CLOCK protein in the mammalian circadian mechanism. Science. 1998;280:1564–1569.

40. Hao H, Allen DL, Hardin PE. A circadian enhancer mediates PER-dependent mRNA cycling in *Drosophila melanogaster*. Mol Cell Biol. 1997;17:3687–3693.

41. Allada R, White NE, So WV, et al. A mutant *Drosophila* homolog of mammalian Clock disrupts circadian rhythms and transcription of period and timeless. Cell. 1998;93:791–804.

42. Sangoram AM, Saez L, Antoch MP, et al. Mammalian circadian autoregulatory loop: a timeless ortholog and mPer1 interact and negatively regulate CLOCK-BMAL1-induced transcription. Neuron. 1998;21:1101–1113.

43. Ralph MR, Menaker M. A mutation of the circadian system in golden hamsters. Science. 1988;241:1225–1227.

44. Shimomura K, Menaker M. Light-induced phase shifts in tau mutant hamsters. J Biol Rhythms. 1994;9:97–110.

45. Refinetti R, Menaker M. Evidence for separate control of estrous and circadian periodicity in the golden hamster. Neurobiol Learn Mem. 1992;58:27–36.

46. Pickard GE, Sollars PJ, Rinchik EM, et al. Mutagenesis and behavioral screening for altered circadian activity identifies the mouse mutant, Wheels. Brain Res. 1995;705:255–266.

47. Nolan PM, Sollars PJ, Bohne BA, et al. Heterozygosity mapping of partially congenic lines: mapping of a semidominant neurological mutation, Wheels (Whl), on mouse chromosome 4. Genetics. 1995;140:245–254.

48. Kornhauser JM, Mayo KE, Takahashi JS. Light, immediate-early genes, and circadian rhythms. Behav Genet. 1996;26:221–240.

49. Myers MP, Wager-Smith K, Rothenfluh-Hilfiker A, et al. Light-induced degradation of TIMELESS and entrainment of the *Drosophila* circadian clock. Science. 1996;271:1736–1740.

50. Zeng H, Qian Z, Myers MP, et al. A light-entrainment mechanism for the *Drosophila* circadian clock. Nature. 1996;380:129–135.

51. Thresher RJ, Vitaterna MH, Miyamoto Y, et al. Role of mouse cryptochrome blue-light photoreceptor in circadian photoresponses. Science. 1998;282:1490–1494.

52. Emery P, So WV, Kaneko M, et al. Cry, a *Drosophila* clock and light-regulated cryptochrome, is a major contributor to circadian rhythm resetting and photosensitivity. Cell. 1998;95:669–679.

53. Stanewsky R, Kaneko M, Emery P, et al. The cry-b mutation identifies cryptochrome as a circadian photoreceptor in *Drosophila*. Cell. 1998;95:681–692.

54. Newby LM, Jackson FR. A new biological rhythm mutant of *Drosophila melanogaster* that identifies a gene with an essential embryonic function. Genetics. 1993;135:1077–1090.

55. Majercak J, Kalderon D, Edery I. *Drosophila melanogaster* deficient in protein kinase A manifests behavior-specific arrhythmia but normal clock function. Mol Cell Biol. 1997;17:5915–5922.

56. Mistlberger RE, Bergmann BM, Waldenar W, et al. Recovery sleep following sleep deprivation in intact and suprachiasmatic nuclei-lesioned rats. Sleep. 1983;6:217–233.

57. Tobler I, Borbely AA, Groos G. The effect of sleep deprivation on sleep in rats with suprachiasmatic lesions. Neurosci Lett. 1983;42:49–54.

58. Trachsel L, Edgar DM, Seidel WF, et al. Sleep homeostasis in suprachiasmatic nuclei-lesioned rats: effects of sleep deprivation and triazolam administration. Brain Res. 1992;589:253–261.

59. Daan S, Beersma DG, Borbely AA. Timing of human sleep: recovery process gated by a circadian pacemaker. Am J Physiol. 1984;246(2 pt 2):R161–R183.

60. Naylor E, Vitaterna MH, Takahashi JS, et al. Sleep in the *Clock* mutant mouse. Sleep. 1998;21(suppl):069E.

61. Edgar DM, Dement WC, Fuller CA. Effect of SCN lesions on sleep in squirrel monkeys: evidence for opponent processes in sleep-wake regulation. J Neurosci. 1993;13:1065–1079.

61a. Katzenberg D, Young T, Finn L, et al. A CLOCK polymorphism associated with human diurnal preference. Sleep. 1998;21:569–576.

62. Turek FW, Pénev P, Zhang Y, et al. Alterations in circadian system in advanced age. In: Circadian Clocks and Their Adjustment. London, England: Pitman Press; 1994:212–234.

63. Czeisler C, Cajochen C, Turek FW, eds. Role of Melatonin in the Regulation of Sleep and Circadian Rhythms. Philadelphia, Pa: WB Saunders; 1999.

64. Baker SK, Zee PC. Circadian disorders of the sleep-wake cycle. In: Kryger MH, Roth T, Dement WC, eds. Principles and Practice of Sleep Medicine. 3rd ed. Philadelphia, Pa: WB Saunders; 2000.

28

The Human Circadian Timing System and Sleep-Wake Regulation

Charles A. Czeisler
Sat Bir S. Khalsa

The human circadian timing system includes the circadian pacemaker (or biological clock), the inputs that affect the pacemaker, and the outputs of the pacemaker, which are the circadian rhythms apparent in many physiological variables such as hormone levels, neurobehavioral performance, and the propensity, timing, and internal structure of sleep.

As in animals, the dominant synchronizing input to the human circadian pacemaker is environmental light. Phase response curves characterizing the phase-dependent effects of light stimuli in resetting the pacemaker have indicated that bright light is a potent synchronizing agent in human beings. It is clear that even low levels of lighting, typical of indoor artificial illumination, can also significantly influence the timing of the circadian pacemaker.

In human subjects who are synchronized to the 24-h day and are on a normal sleep-wake schedule, the temporal profile of each of the different circadian rhythms exhibits a characteristic fingerprint. Observed rhythms are influenced by a number of factors, including the timing of the sleep-wake state, the phase and amplitude of the endogenous circadian pacemaker, and responses evoked by changes in posture, exercise, emotional state, and environmental lighting. With the use of laboratory protocols such as the constant routine and forced desynchrony protocols, it has been possible to distinguish the relative contributions of sleep and the circadian pacemaker. This has permitted the construction of schema that describe the temporal interplay of the circadian pacemaker and the sleep homeostatic drive and how it accounts for maintained wakefulness and neurobehavioral performance throughout the day and for consolidated sleep throughout the night.

Unlike animals, human beings in modern society can choose to modify their exposure to light by using artificial illumination (or transmeridian travel), and to change the timing of their intended sleep episodes, as is the case for shift work or jet lag. When these changes have a negative impact on the delicate temporal balance between the circadian pacemaker and homeostatic sleep drive, decrements in physiological functioning, neurobehavioral performance, and sleep result.

The circadian pacemaker (or biological clock) is phylogenetically ubiquitous, having been found in nearly all species examined from prokaryotes to human beings.[1, 2] Circadian pacemakers have several defining characteristics, including (1) rhythmicity that is endogenous to the organism and persists independent of periodic changes in the external environment, (2) a period that is very close to 24 h (hence, the term *circadian* from *circa* meaning "about" and *dies* referring to a "day"), and (3) a timing or phase relative to the time of day that can be modified or reset by environmental inputs.[1, 3–5] The purpose of this chapter is to provide an overview of the human circadian timing system, which includes the pacemaker with its inputs and outputs, and to describe how this pacemaker interacts with sleep-wake regulatory processes to influence many physiological variables, including hormone levels, neurobehavioral performance, and the propensity, timing, and internal structure of sleep. From this perspective, it is important to consider the relative influence of episodic and daily recurring behaviors, including the occurrence of sleep itself, on these physiological variables relative to that of the endogenous circadian pacemaker.

IDENTIFICATION OF THE MAMMALIAN CIRCADIAN PACEMAKER

Localization

In mammals, the suprachiasmatic nucleus in the hypothalamus serves as the central neural pacemaker of the circadian timing system. Based on an assembly of carefully taken patient histories that were characterized by disruptions of the timing of the sleep-wake cycle (e.g., insomnia, reversal of the sleep-wake schedule), Fulton and Bailey[6] postulated in 1929 that there was a region in the anterior hypothalamus that appeared to regulate not the occurrence of sleep itself but rather the timing of sleep within the 24-h day. It was not until 1972 that the suprachiasmatic nucleus (SCN) of the anterior hypothalamus was identified as the site of the mammalian circadian pacemaker,[7, 8] and research in mammals has established without a doubt that the SCN is a principal source of endogenous rhythmicity.[9–12]

Role as Pacemaker

Transplantation studies have provided convincing evidence for the role of the SCN as a central pacemaker, rather than simply an associated component or output of the pacemaker.[12, 13] Using a mutant strain of hamsters with an abnormal circadian period of 20 h,[14] Ralph et al. cross-transplanted the SCN between mutant and wild-type animals.[12] After the transplantation of 1 mm^3 of this brain tissue, the rest-activity cycle of the wild-type animals exhibited the circadian period of the mutant animals, and vice versa. The results of this experiment further suggested that neural connections might not be required for the pacemaker to control behavior because this new pacemaker-driven activity was established within 3 or 4 days of the transplantation, presumably too short of a time in which to reestablish all of the neural connections. The hypothesis that a neurohumoral factor plays a key role in communicating temporal information to the organism has since been borne out by experiments in which SCN tissue was transplanted within a semipermeable membrane (through which neural connections cannot be reestablished) and remained capable of generating circadian rhythmicity of the behavioral rest-activity cycle in the host animal.[15] The suggestion that a humoral factor may participate in circadian regulation was reinforced by a report that treatment of cultured rat fibroblasts with a serum shock induces circadian expression of various genes.[16]

INFLUENCE OF SLEEP AND CIRCADIAN RHYTHMS ON HUMAN PHYSIOLOGY

The discovery of the functional role of the SCN as a central circadian pacemaker set the stage for understanding how a central circadian pacemaker was driving the daily fluctuations in a whole array of physiological functions. In human beings who are synchronized to the 24-h day and are on a normal sleep-wake schedule, a wide variety of physiological variables undergo a prominent daily variation[17–23] (reviewed in Van Cauter and Turek[24]) (Fig. 28–1, left). Core body temperature is lowest and melatonin levels (not shown) are highest[19, 24, 25] during night sleep. Cortisol is low at the time of habitual sleep onset, but then it is high at the habitual morning wake time.[23–28] The temporal profile of each of these different parameters during entrainment to the 24-h day exhibits a characteristic fingerprint that is the result of a combination of drives from the timing of the sleep-wake state, the

endogenous circadian pacemaker, and responses evoked by other factors such as posture, mood, exercise, and environmental lighting.[23–38]

In an effort to isolate the circadian pacemaker–driven component of a diurnal temporal profile from the effects of sleep-wake state, behavior, posture, periodic environmental stimuli, and so on, the constant routine protocol originally proposed by Mills et al.[39] was refined and extended.[40–42] In the constant routine used in our laboratory, subjects undergo continuous enforced wakefulness throughout the day and night in a constant posture at a constant level of activity and in a constant, relatively dim level of ambient room illumination.[40–42] Under such constant routine conditions, the temporal profiles of many physiological variables are significantly altered, and it becomes possible to isolate the component of these rhythms that is driven by the endogenous circadian pacemaker from the components that reflect changes in the sleep-wake state, posture, or the periodic external environment.

It has long been recognized that there is a drop in body temperature during sleep.[43–45] In comparing the profile of core body temperature recorded from individuals on a normal sleep-wake schedule with that in constant routine conditions (see Fig. 28–1, right), it is apparent that the sleep episode itself (including the associated change in posture, light intensity, and activity level) generates a drop in body temperature relative to wakefulness[32, 34, 35, 45–49] Therefore, on a normal sleep-wake schedule, the sleep episode–induced drop in temperature combines with the circadian-induced decline in body temperature (which exhibits a nadir during the latter half of the habitual nocturnal sleep episode) to yield a larger apparent amplitude than that of the endogenous circadian component alone (as measured on the constant routine). Urine volume is an example of another variable that exhibits a robust oscillation under constant routine conditions but also is influenced by sleep-wake state.[19, 40]

Rhythmicity in some variables appears to be nearly independent of sleep-wake state. The temporal profile of the hormone melatonin is relatively unchanged whether an individual is asleep or awake all night on a constant routine,[50] although posture has been reported to influence melatonin secretion.[37, 50, 51] The temporal profile of the hormone cortisol is also relatively unchanged whether an individual sleeps on his or her habitual schedule or remains awake all night, although plasma cortisol concentrations can be suppressed if sleep onset occurs at the crest of the cortisol rhythm rather than at the nadir, as it does under normal conditions.[28]

A number of other hormones are very sensitive to sleep-wake state. Sleep opposes the circadian rhythm regulating thyroid-stimulating hormone (TSH), inhibiting the endogenous circadian rhythm of TSH release, which would otherwise peak in the middle of the night.[20, 23–26, 52–54] Under entrained conditions, that nocturnal peak is blunted by the timing of sleep so that TSH levels reach the highest level just before sleep onset and continue to be suppressed during the remainder of the sleep episode. This inhibitory effect of

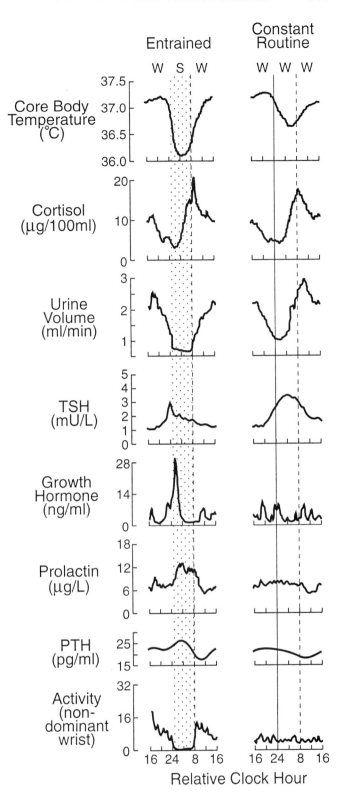

Figure 28–1. Temporal profiles of an array of physiological and behavioral variables from subjects studied under baseline conditions while maintaining a regular schedule of nocturnal sleep (shaded area) and daytime wakefulness at their habitual times (*left*) compared with profiles from those subjects under constant routine conditions while maintaining a schedule of continuous wakefulness in a constant semirecumbent posture (*right*). Vertical dashed line indicates habitual wake time during the week before study, during which subjects were required to maintain a regular sleep-wake schedule. All data are from normal young adult men 18 to 30 years old studied under similar conditions. For a given variable, data in the left panel are from the same subjects as data in the right panel; however, not all variables were monitored in the same subjects. Activity data were measured using a wrist actigraph (Vitalog Monitoring Inc., Redwood City, Calif) worn on the nondominant wrist. TSH, thyroid stimulating hormone; PTH, parathyroid hormone. (TSH data from Allan JS, Czeisler CA. Persistence of the circadian thyrotropin rhythm under constant conditions and after light-induced shifts of circadian phase. J Clin Endocrinol Metab. 1994;79:508–512, © The Endocrine Society; prolactin data from Waldstreicher J, Duffy JF, Brown EN, et al. Gender differences in the temporal organization of prolactin (PRL) secretion: evidence for a sleep-independent circadian rhythm of circulating PRL levels—a clinical research center study. J Clin Endocrinol Metab. 1996; 81:1483–1487, © The Endocrine Society; PTH data from El Hajj Fuleihan G, Klerman EB, Brown EN, et al. Parathyroid hormone circadian rhythm is truly endogenous. J Clin Endocrinol Metab. 1997;82:281–286, © The Endocrine Society.)

sleep on TSH secretion has been closely associated with both slow-wave sleep[55] and relative delta power in the sleep EEG.[56] Growth hormone,[23, 24, 26, 54, 57–60] prolactin,[21, 23, 24, 26, 54, 61–68] and parathyroid hormone[22, 26, 64, 69–71] all show a prominent sleep-dependent increase in levels. For growth hormone, this sleep-related increase has been associated with both slow-wave sleep[57] and rela-

tive delta power of the sleep electroencephalogram (EEG),[60] whereas for prolactin, such associations have been a matter of considerable controversy.[61, 68, 72]

In a series of elegant studies carried out by Brandenberger and colleagues,[23, 73, 74] it has been shown that ultradian variations in the release of renin from the kidney—a key factor in blood pressure control—are very closely linked to the timing of the rapid eye movement (REM)–nonrapid eye movement (NREM) sleep cycle. This association remains evident even among patients with disturbed sleep, whose plasma renin profiles reflect pathological changes in sleep structure.[23] Increased relative delta power in the sleep EEG was associated with increased levels of plasma renin activity, whereas decreased slow wave activity was associated with a decrease in plasma renin activity.[75]

In 1979, Aschoff[76] pointed out that there is some evidence for an endogenously rhythmic component even among "sleep-dependent" hormones, particularly with respect to the magnitude of the response evoked by sleep. In fact, with use of the constant routine protocol, it has been shown that in the absence of sleep, prolactin and parathyroid hormone also have an endogenous circadian component that exhibits a low point a few hours after the habitual wake time.[21, 22]

The effects of the interaction between sleep-dependent and circadian factors on these hormones may have significant importance when the sleep-wake schedule is not synchronized with the circadian pacemaker. In the case of shift workers who must acutely remain awake on the first night shift, for example, one would expect a substantial increase in TSH release relative to that secreted under normal sleep-wake conditions during entrainment (see Fig. 28–1). On the other hand, these shift workers would be deprived of their normally higher levels of growth hormone, prolactin, and parathyroid hormone during the waking night.[53, 77] Such alterations in the profiles of a variety of hormones have been documented in laboratory studies of night shift workers.[77]

Circadian Variation of Alertness and Neurobehavioral Performance

The circadian pacemaker has a significant influence on a variety of neurobehavioral and cognitive functions.[78–89] Under constant routine conditions, subjects display a circadian variation in short-term memory, cognitive performance, alertness, and EEG and oculomotor activity that is closely and tightly coupled to the timing of the body temperature rhythm[90, 91, 91a] (Fig. 28–2). During the constant routine, these cognitive functions tend to be at their nadir at a clock time that is 1 to 3 h after the habitual wake time. However, because subjects are undergoing prolonged wakefulness during the constant routine, the profiles of these variables are determined not only by the drive from the circadian pacemaker but also by a contribution from the consequences of sleep deprivation. This is discussed more extensively later in this chapter.

EFFECTS OF LIGHT ON HUMAN CIRCADIAN RHYTHMS

A biological clock is useful only if it can be set appropriately to local time. The primary synchronizing agent for circadian systems in a wide array of species,

including human beings, is the environmental light-dark cycle.[3, 4, 19, 20, 25, 26, 40, 42, 92, 93] In mammals, the retino-hypothalamic tract (RHT) conveys information on environmental illumination between the retina and the circadian pacemaker in the SCN.[94, 95] This pathway is sufficient for appropriate entrainment of the circadian pacemaker. A neural output pathway of the SCN passes through the intermediolateral cell column of the upper thoracic spinal cord and through the superior cervical ganglion and then provides sympathetic input into the pineal gland.[96, 97]

Photic Suppression of Melatonin Secretion

The neural pathway from the SCN to the pineal provides for the regulation of the pineal output of melatonin by the SCN.[98] The release of this hormone is inhibited by retinal exposure to light by that circuitous pathway from the eye to the pineal.[99, 100] This inhibition of melatonin by light in human beings[36, 101] can therefore be used as an assay for the functional input of light into the circadian system,[102] as first suggested by Reppert.[103]

The nocturnal increase in melatonin is illustrated in Figure 28–3, top, for a normally sighted subject on a constant routine.[102] During a second peak of melatonin on the next night, a bright light stimulus yielded an acute suppression of melatonin levels, which returned to elevated nighttime levels after the light exposure was terminated. In Figure 28–3, bottom, the bright light–induced suppression of melatonin occurred even in an individual who is totally blind and who has no conscious light perception, no pupillary light reflexes, and a negative electroretinogram. This was not the case in all such blind individuals. The loss of conscious light perception is not necessarily indicative of the loss of photic input to the circadian timing system.[102, 104] In fact, there are two distinct visual systems: one for visual perception and a separate circadian visual system for the purpose of detecting environmental illuminance levels and synchronizing the circadian pacemaker in the SCN.[105–110]

Human Phase Response Curves to Light

In circadian biology, the phase response curve (PRC) is used to fully characterize the synchronizing effects of light on a circadian pacemaker.[3, 42, 111, 112] To construct a PRC,[24] discrete light stimuli are applied systematically over the entire circadian cycle, and the magnitudes of the light-induced phase shifts are then plotted as a function of circadian phase at which the organism is exposed to the stimuli. In experiments in human beings, the constant routine has been applied to estimate the initial circadian phase of the pacemaker. In such studies,[42, 113–116] a light stimulus consisting of either a single 5-h exposure to bright light (approximately 10,000 lux) or three consecutive 5-h exposures was applied centered at a discrete circadian phase. After the light stimulus, another constant routine was applied to

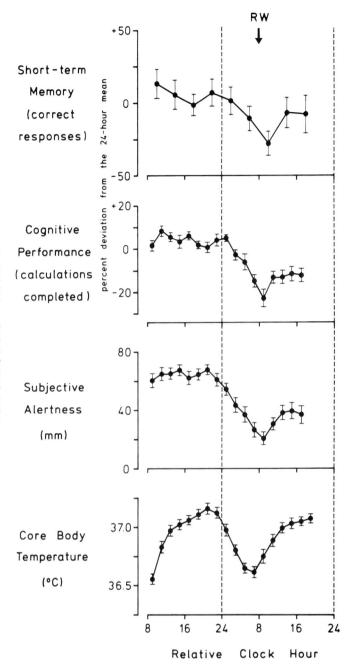

Figure 28–2. Daily patterns of short-term memory, cognitive performance, subjective alertness (mm), and core body temperature (°C) averaged across 18 subjects during a 36-h constant routine. Data collection times are normalized with respect to each subject's regular wake time (assigned a reference value of 8:00 AM and indicated by the downward arrow). The extent to which memory and performance scores deviated from the subject's 24-h mean is averaged across subjects. These data are expressed as the percentage by which these absolute deviations differed from the subjects' overall 24-h mean score (assigned a reference value of zero). Each point is the centered mean (±SEM) of all determinations made across a 2-h interval for performance, alertness, and temperature and across a 4-h interval for short-term memory. (From Johnson MP, Duffy JF, Dijk D-J, et al. Short-term memory, alertness and performance: a reappraisal of their relationship to body temperature. J Sleep Res. 1992;1:24–29.)

evaluate the final circadian phase. The difference in phase between the initial and final constant routines therefore represented the light-induced phase shift. Subsequently, the full range of circadian phases was tested to complete the full PRC.

All circadian systems exhibit a characteristic photic PRC in which the largest light-induced phase shifts are generated in the subjective night of the circadian cycle. Phase delays are generated to light stimuli in the late subjective day/early subjective night, and phase advances are generated in the late subjective night/early subjective day.[3] Figure 28–4 illustrates two PRCs to light stimuli from the studies in human beings described above.[113] Figure 28–4, left, shows the PRC to a single pulse of light. In human beings, phase advances

were observed in response to bright light pulses centered after the fitted minimum of the core body temperature cycle, which occurred on average about 2.3 h before the habitual wake time.[117] Phase delays were observed when light was applied before the fitted minimum of the core body temperature cycle. The human PRC to a single light pulse[113, 118, 119] exhibited the classic pattern of light PRCs observed in many organisms,[3] including both phase advances and phase delays, notwithstanding an early report suggesting that the phase-resetting responses of human beings were largely limited to phase advances.[120] The PRC to three consecutive pulses of light in Figure 28–4, right, shows a distinctly different pattern in which much larger phase shifts were observed.[42] As the strength of the drive increased,

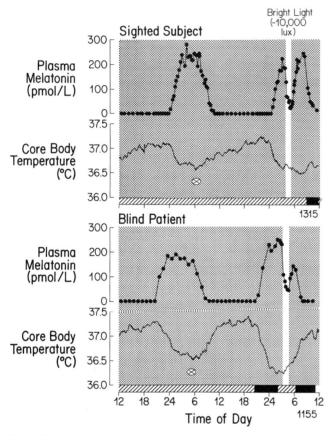

Figure 28–3. Melatonin-suppression test in a healthy sighted subject (*top*) and a blind patient (*bottom*). In each, plasma melatonin (*top* traces) and temperature (*bottom* traces) were measured repeatedly during a constant routine (hatched bar) and subsequent episode or episodes of sleep (solid bars). The light intensity was approximately 10 to 15 lux during the constant routines, less than approximately 0.02 lux during the sleep episodes, and approximately 10,000 lux during 90 to 100 min of exposure to bright light (open columns) 22 to 23 h after the initial fitted temperature minimum (encircled Xs). In both subjects, plasma melatonin concentrations decreased markedly in response to bright light and then increased after the return to dim light. (From Czeisler CA, Shanahan TL, Klerman EB, et al. Suppression of melatonin secretion in some blind patients by exposure to bright light. N Engl J Med. 1995;332:6–11. Copyright © 1995 Massachusetts Medical Society. All rights reserved.)

in this case from 1 day of exposure to 3 consecutive days of exposure to the bright light stimulus, the amount of resetting achieved increased from several hours (after one pulse of light) to up to 12 h (after three consecutive pulses of light).[113, 121–123] This characteristic of weak and strong resetting has also been reported for circadian systems in a number of other organisms, although strong resetting has not yet been shown in all circadian systems.[124–126]

Detailed analysis of the three-pulse PRC in human beings has revealed another significant feature of the human circadian pacemaker. In most nocturnal species, the circadian pacemaker is relatively insensitive to light applied during the subjective day, and this time segment has consequently been termed the *dead zone* for responsiveness to light. However, the subjective day portion of the three-pulse PRC illustrated in Figure 28–5 reveals that the human circadian pacemaker is responsive to light throughout the subjective day.[116] This characteristic of the human PRC has also been reported for other species, especially diurnal ones,[3, 127] and suggests that it is possible to shift the phase of the human circadian pacemaker not just during the night but also in the morning and the late afternoon/evening with appropriate light intensities. This has important clinical implications for the use of phototherapy to reset circadian phase in, for example, delayed or advanced sleep phase syndrome.

Photic Resetting of the Pineal Melatonin Rhythm

Because circadian rhythms are expressed in many physiological and neurobehavioral variables, the phase of the pacemaker can be determined by using any of these variables as a marker. In human beings, the core body temperature rhythm has often been a preferred marker of circadian phase because it can provide an accurate representation of the characteristics of the underlying pacemaker under certain conditions.[128] However, melatonin has also been shown to be an accurate circadian marker.[19, 50, 129, 130] Melatonin is less heavily influenced by sleep and posture than is the core body temperature rhythm.[37, 50] Furthermore, it has been shown in human beings to reflect the phase of the underlying pacemaker after light-induced phase shifts as well as does the endogenous component of the core body temperature rhythm measured during a constant routine.[19, 50a] Both of these rhythms shift by an equivalent amount regardless of whether the rhythm is shifted to an earlier or to a later hour.[50, 50a] Such studies have demonstrated that the endogenous circadian melatonin rhythm can be reset to any desired phase within 2 to 3 days by properly timed light exposure.[50a, 130] Furthermore, photic stimuli designed to suppress the amplitude of the endogenous circadian temperature cycle also lead to suppression of the amplitude of the endogenous circadian melatonin rhythm.[50a, 130]

The use of the rhythm in melatonin levels as a circadian marker has additional practical advantages. The demonstrated melatonin rhythm in human saliva,[131] which correlates well with the rhythm in plasma,[132–135] together with advances in melatonin assay techniques are making it possible to evaluate circadian phase in patients or research subjects in a relatively noninvasive manner.[133, 136–139]

Human Dose-Response Curve to Circadian Phase-Resetting Effects of Light

As described, the degree of light-induced phase shift is dependent on the intensity of the light stimulus and the number of consecutive days of exposure. Three consecutive daily pulses of light can generate a larger phase shift than does a single light pulse (see Fig. 28–4). This intensity relationship also applies to the brightness or illuminance level of the light to which the retina is exposed. After 5-h, three-cycle bright light

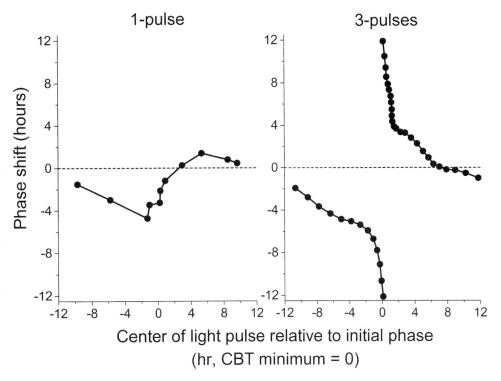

Figure 28–4. Comparison of results of one- and three-pulse phase response curve experiments in human subjects. Phase shift in hours is plotted for a light pulse centered at different times relative to the initial endogenous circadian phase of the fitted core body temperature (CBT) minimum. Symbols are smoothed data points. (See text for further details.) (Adapted from Jewett ME, Kronauer RE, Czeisler CA. Phase-amplitude resetting of the human circadian pacemaker via bright light: a further analysis. J Biol Rhythms. vol 9, issue 3–4, pp 295–314, copyright © 1994 by Sage Publications, Inc. Reprinted by permission of Sage Publications, Inc.)

stimuli of different light intensities applied at a circadian phase known to generate a phase advance, a gradual increase in the resetting response is seen as the intensity increases from approximately 180 lux to almost approximately 10,000 lux.[114] The light intensity versus resetting response relationship is nonlinear (Fig. 28–6),[114] but it is fit very well by a mathematical model developed by Kronauer[140] and recently refined by Jewett and Kronauer.[141]

What also is very significant in these data is that even low levels of light (~180 lux) have a significant phase-shifting effect. Because approximately 180 lux is

in the range of intensity of ordinary room lighting, this has enormous practical significance. It has been reported that human beings are exposed to bright light for a relatively short time each day.[142–144] In modern industrialized societies, human beings are typically exposed to ordinary indoor room light for a greater number of hours each day than they are to bright light. This predominance of exposure to ordinary room light probably has a greater impact on our circadian system than the few minutes to which we are typically exposed to bright light each day.

The simple schema in Figure 28–7 illustrates the

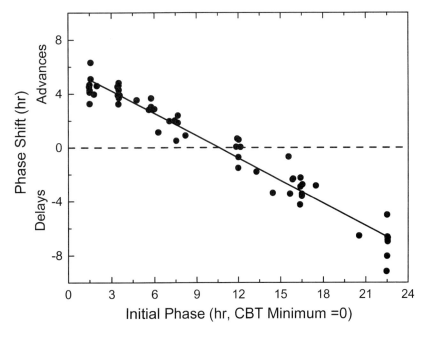

Figure 28–5. The subjective day segment of the phase response curve to a stimulus of three consecutive 5-h pulses of bright light. Initial phase is the number of hours after the fitted minimum of the endogenous core body temperature (CBT) rhythm at which the center of the light stimulus occurred. Phase shift is the difference between the time of the prestimulus and poststimulus temperature minima. A regression line has been fitted to the data points. CBT, core body temperature; PRC, phase response curve. (Adapted from Jewett ME, Rimmer DW, Duffy JF, et al. The human circadian pacemaker is sensitive to light throughout subjective day without evidence of transients. Am J Physiol. 1997; 273:R1800–R1809.)

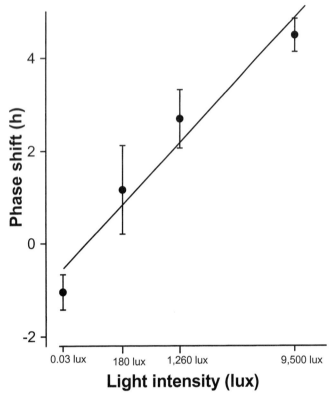

Figure 28–6. Dose-response curve of the phase-shifting effect of three consecutive daily cycles of a 5-h retinal light exposure. The ordinate represents the phase shift observed between the first and second constant routines in each group of subjects. The abscissa represents the light intensity (lux) plotted on a cube root scale. By convention, positive phase shifts represent phase advances, and negative phase shifts represent phase delays. Group averages ($\pm$SEM) are represented by closed circles and vertical error bars, respectively. A linear regression model was applied to the individual phase shifts to evaluate the relationship between the cube root of light intensity and its phase-shifting effects (oblique straight line) (df, 1, 29; $r = 0.742$, $P < .001$). (Reprinted by permission from *Nature,* Boivin DB, Duffy JF, Kronauer RE, et al. Dose-response relationships for resetting of human circadian clock by light. Nature. 1996;379:540–542, copyright 1996 Macmillan Magazines Ltd.)

influence of the circadian pacemaker and the sleep-wake state on the various physiological variables and the influence of light input via the eye to the circadian pacemaker. The feedback loop from the sleep-wake state back to the eye in this schema represents the effects of exposure to the environmental light cycle because the sleeping state in human beings is usually associated with eyelid closure and self-selected exposure to darkness as achieved by drawing window shades and switching off artificial light sources, whereas the waking state in human beings is usually associated with opening of the eyelids and retinal light exposure via self-selected use of artificial light or self-selected exposure to outdoor light during waking hours. Under the conditions of a strict sleep-wake and light exposure schedule, the timing of the pacemaker will be consistent from day to day. However, if sleep were to be initiated late or terminated early or a waking episode were to occur within a sleep episode, the associated light exposure may reset the pacemaker.

This association between waking and light exposure, together with the fact that low levels of light intensity can exert a significant resetting effect on the pacemaker, is not only relevant on a practical level for routine sleep-wake scheduling; it also has significant implications for interpreting the results of early human circadian rhythm studies, especially those involving the study of human behavior in the absence of periodic environmental synchronizers for extended durations.

NONPHOTIC CIRCADIAN PHASE RESETTING

Although light is recognized as the predominant resetting agent, studies in animals have suggested that the timing of activity itself may have an effect on the circadian pacemaker.[145–149] Van Cauter and associates reported that exercise may exert a resetting effect on the human circadian system.[150, 151] Although early reports suggested that social interaction and the sleep-wake schedule were capable of directly influencing the circadian pacemaker,[18, 47, 152–154] it is now believed that the predominant entraining agent for human beings is light.[92, 93] A study in which the effect of inverting the sleep-wake schedule for 3 days was examined revealed no change in the phase of the human circadian pacemaker without concomitant bright light exposure.[115] Therefore, any effect of nonphotic synchronizers associ-

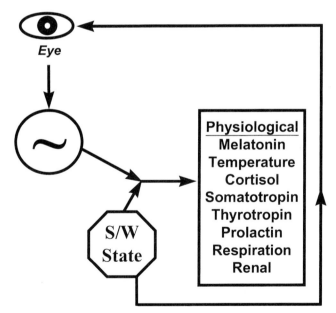

Figure 28–7. Schema illustrating the influence of both the circadian pacemaker (circle with oscillator symbol) and sleep-wake state (octagon) on a number of physiological variables. Under normal conditions, the circadian pacemaker and sleep-wake state each influence these variables; the relative contribution and nature of the interaction (i.e., synergistic or oppositional) of each depends on the variable observed. Also illustrated is the influence of the environmental illumination on the human circadian clock via the eye and the influence of the sleep-wake state in determining the timing of this illumination via both behavioral action (i.e., switching off artificial indoor room lights and drawing bedroom window shades at bedtime, and eyelid closure during sleep and eyelid opening during waking).

ated with inversion of the sleep-wake schedule in human beings must be weaker than that of the environmental light-dark cycle. However, recent studies of blind subjects indicate that some of them can be entrained to the 24-h day in the absence of circadian photoreception[102, 104, 155] and can even reset to an earlier hour,[156] indicating that nonphotic synchronizers may exert a significant resetting effect, even if weaker than light.

INVESTIGATING CIRCADIAN AND SLEEP-WAKE–DEPENDENT MODULATION

The Kleitman Protocol: Separation From 24-h Environmental and Behavioral Cues

Nathaniel Kleitman was the first investigator to conduct an experiment in which human beings were studied in the absence of periodic cues in the external environment[81] (Fig. 28–8). The core body temperature records from one of the two human subjects he studied

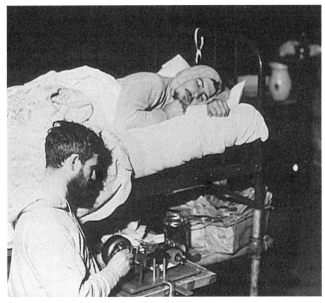

Figure 28–8. Professor Nathaniel Kleitman (*left*) attends to experimental equipment, while fellow research subject Bruce Richardson lays in bed deep within Mammoth Cave in Kentucky, where, for the first time, human subjects were studied while shielded from periodic environmental changes on the earth's surface. The two pioneers lived on an imposed 28-h sleep-wake schedule in these quarters from June 4 to July 6, 1938, in an effort to approximate uniform environmental and behavioral conditions, free from the influence of the earth's 24-h day. In a 60-foot-wide chamber free from any external environmental sounds, the temperature remained at 54°F, humidity approached complete vapor saturation, and darkness was absolute when the artificial light used during waking hours was shut off. The Mammoth Cave Hotel provided daily meals, which were consumed on awakening and after the seventh and thirteenth hour of each 19-h waking day. (Photo courtesy of National Park Service, Mammoth Cave National Park, Mammoth, Ky; description adapted from Kleitman N. Sleep and Wakefulness. Chicago: University of Chicago Press; 1963:178–179. © 1963 by the University of Chicago. All rights reserved.)

in Mammoth Cave, Kentucky, in 1938 during a 28-h imposed sleep-wake schedule are compared with laboratory data collected at the University of Chicago from the same subject living on a 24-h routine[81] (Fig. 28–9). On the 24-h schedule, there were seven cycles of the body temperature rhythm, as would be expected over the course of a 1-week recording (Fig. 28–9, bottom). On the imposed 28-h schedule, there also were seven cycles of the body temperature rhythm, although there were only six sleep-wake cycles over the course of the week (Fig. 28–9, top). Despite the confounding effect of sleep itself on the core body temperature (as noted, see Fig. 28–1), this experimental protocol was still capable of separating the influence of the timing of the sleep-wake schedule from that of the circadian pacemaker—at least in this subject. This imposed desynchrony between the sleep-wake schedule and the output of the circadian pacemaker driving the temperature rhythm occurs under conditions in which the non–24-h sleep-wake schedule is outside the range of entrainment or range of capture of the circadian system. This protocol has been termed the *forced desynchrony protocol* and is an extremely useful tool for evaluating the influence of the circadian pacemaker on many physiological variables because it allows separation of the confounding effect of the sleep-wake schedule from the output of the endogenous circadian pacemaker[81, 157, 158] Figure 28–10 illustrates a raster plot of a forced desynchrony experiment incorporating core body temperature and wakefulness data for a subject living on a 28-h day in a laboratory and shielded from external time cues.[159] The waking episodes in this protocol are 18 h 40 min long, followed by sleep episodes of 9 h 20 min. Core body temperature exhibited a period of 24.3 h in this subject and therefore was desynchronized from both the 24-h day and the timing of the imposed 28-h sleep-wake schedule.

Separating Circadian and Sleep-Wake–Dependent Modulation Via the Kleitman Protocol

The constant routine protocol does not allow for a complete and unconfounded separation of the circadian and homeostatic influences on neurobehavioral and physiological variables. However, in the Kleitman forced desynchrony protocol, sleep and wakefulness are distributed much more evenly over the entire circadian cycle during the course of the experiment. It is thus possible to average data either over successive circadian cycles or over successive sleep-wake episodes and to thereby separate these two components. This averaging serves to isolate the circadian profile of the variable of interest by removing the contribution of the confounding sleep-wake–dependent contribution in the averaging process. Conversely, the temporal profile of the sleep-wake–dependent profile can be isolated from the confounding circadian influence. This averaging process is similar to that of cortical evoked potential recordings that effectively subtract background

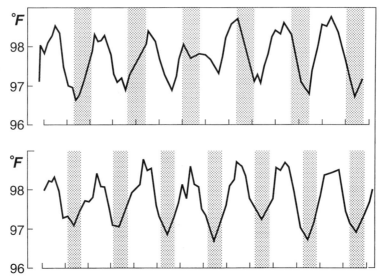

Figure 28–9. Weekly body temperature rhythms of a subject under two different routines of sleep and wakefulness. *Top,* Data from subject K on a 28-hour daily routine consisting of 19 h of wakefulness and 9 h of sleep during Professor Nathaniel Kleitman's historic forced desynchrony protocol carried out in Mammoth Cave, Ky. *Bottom,* Laboratory data recorded at the University of Chicago from subject K on a customary daily 24-h routine consisting of 17 h of wakefulness and 7 h of sleep. Shaded areas represent time spent in bed, attempting to sleep. *Top,* Data based on the last 3 weeks of data collected in Mammoth Cave. *Bottom,* Data based on 5 weeks of following the 24-h routine of living. Each weekly record shows seven body-temperature waves, within the minima in the shaded areas on the customary 24-h routine, but not on the artificial 28-h sleep-wakefulness schedule. In the subject shown, the endogenous circadian temperature cycle maintained a near–24-h oscillation, despite the 28-h day length to which the subject's sleep-wake cycle was scheduled. However, it was reported that temperature data from subject R (not shown) was able to adapt to this non–24-h routine. Such adaptation has not been observed in more recent forced desynchrony studies. Interindividual differences in the strength of the endogenous vs. the evoked component of the body temperature rhythm may account for what appeared to be circadian adaptation observed during the forced desynchrony conducted in subject R of Kleitman's pioneering experiment. (Figure and parts of legend adapted from Kleitman N. Sleep and Wakefulness. Chicago: University of Chicago Press; 1963. © 1963 by the University of Chicago. All rights reserved.)

noise that is not temporally related to the evoked response.[160]

Neurobehavioral Functions

To fully understand and predict the time course of neurobehavioral function, it is necessary to recognize the influence of sleep-wake state on what has been termed a *sleep homeostat* driving neurobehavioral functions. This becomes apparent when one examines these variables during a longer course of sleep deprivation in which more than one circadian cycle has elapsed.[85, 86, 90, 91] The cyclic contribution of the circadian pacemaker in influencing alertness and performance is superimposed on an overall decline in function during the course of the experiment. Schema and mathematical models that incorporate both the homeostatic and circadian influences in the regulation of sleep and wakefulness have been constructed, evaluated, and modified.[91, 161–169]

With use of a 28-h forced desynchrony protocol, the temporal profiles of cognitive performance and subjective alertness as a function of circadian phase and as a function of time in the scheduled day have been determined[90, 170, 171] (Fig. 28–11). The data suggest that the overall magnitudes of the circadian and wake-dependent drives are similar during the course of a typical waking day. From the timing of the circadian and sleep-dependent profiles, it is possible to qualita-

tively reconstruct the separate contributions from each toward the maintenance of alertness and performance over the course of the normal waking day (see Fig. 28–11). In the first half of the day after wake time, there is little homeostatic sleep drive because it has just been discharged by the prior sleep episode, so both alertness and cognitive performance are high. In the latter half of the waking episode, when the homeostatic sleep drive would otherwise cause alertness and cognitive performance to decline, the circadian drive becomes elevated, opposes that decline in alertness and performance, and thereby sustains a high, stable level of alertness throughout the normal waking day.

Sleep and Wakefulness

Similar dynamics apply for reconstruction of the respective circadian and homeostatic contributions to sleep and wakefulness.[172] From the raster plot of the forced desynchrony experiment shown in Figure 28–10, it is apparent that almost all wakefulness within a scheduled sleep episode occurs when the subject's sleep episode is not in phase with the body temperature nadir. This observation was first quantified by Kleitman, based on his data recorded in Mammoth Cave.[81] Averaging polysomnographically recorded sleep data for a number of subjects on the forced desynchrony protocol with respect to all circadian cycles and all sleep episodes of the protocol yields the data

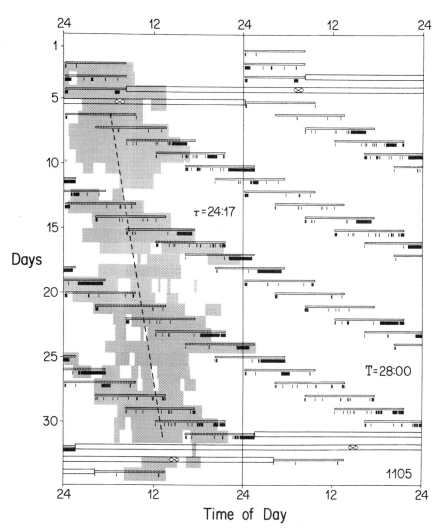

Figure 28–10. Double plot of the 28-h forced desynchrony protocol. Successive days are plotted both next to and beneath each other. Scheduled sleep episodes (open narrow bars), polysomnographically determined wakefulness within each sleep episode (black tick marks below the narrow open bars), and intervals during which core body temperature was below the mean (stippled area) are indicated. An intrinsic temperature cycle period of 24.3 h from the data of this subject was estimated by a nonparametric spectral analysis of the core body temperature data during the forced desynchrony part of the protocol. The phase of the minimum of the circadian temperature rhythm, as estimated by this nonparametric spectral analysis, is indicated by the broken line. The minimum of the endogenous circadian rhythm of core body temperature as unmasked by a 40-h constant routine protocol is indicated by an encircled X. (Reprinted from Neuroscience Letters, vol 166, Dijk D-J, Czeisler CA, Paradoxical timing of the circadian rhythm of sleep propensity serves to consolidate sleep and wakefulness in humans, 63–68, Copyright 1994, with permission from Elsevier Science.)

in Figure 28–12A that show the temporal profiles of wakefulness as a function of circadian phase and time in the sleep episode, respectively.[159] The circadian contribution to wakefulness is robust and exhibits a minimum centered coincident with the core body temperature minimum (compare Fig. 28–12, A and F). A maximum in circadian wake propensity occurs at 180 degrees (about 12 h later in the late afternoon on a normal sleep-wake schedule). The sleep-dependent contribution exhibits an increasing profile over the course of the sleep episode, with the greatest propensity to waking near the end of the sleep episode. A qualitative reconstruction of these contributions suggests that the homeostatic sleep drive is greatest at sleep onset and facilitates sleep in the first half of the night. In the latter half of the sleep episode, as the homeostatic drive declines, the circadian drive for sleep becomes greatest, thus maintaining elevated sleep drive through the end of the sleep episode. Together, these two components act to generate consolidated sleep throughout the night.

The three-dimensional representation in Figure 28–13 combines the temporal profiles of circadian and sleep-dependent drives to further illustrate their respective contributions in maintaining the appropriate

sleep drive on a normal sleep-wake schedule.[159] The dashed line in this figure begins on the horizontal axis at the circadian phase consistent with habitual nocturnal sleep onset. This track then takes a diagonal direction as both circadian phase and length of time in the sleep episode elapse. Under normal conditions, a consolidated bout of sleep is maintained with very little wakefulness during the sleep episode by following this track and avoiding the two peaks of wakefulness in this three-dimensional representation. However, if sleep were to be initiated in the early morning hours (as is the case for a shift worker after the first night shift), the diagonal track would progress directly into the mountain of wakefulness in the latter half of this intended sleep episode, and a high percentage of time would be spent in wakefulness, notwithstanding prior sleep deprivation.

The circadian and sleep-wake modulations of sleep-wake propensity and neurobehavioral function are shown simply in the schema in Figure 28–14. Experimental evidence indicates that a simple additive model is not adequate to account for variations observed in alertness and cognitive performance data.[78, 89, 91, 170, 173, 174] In fact, there is relatively little circadian variation in various waking neurobehavioral measures in the

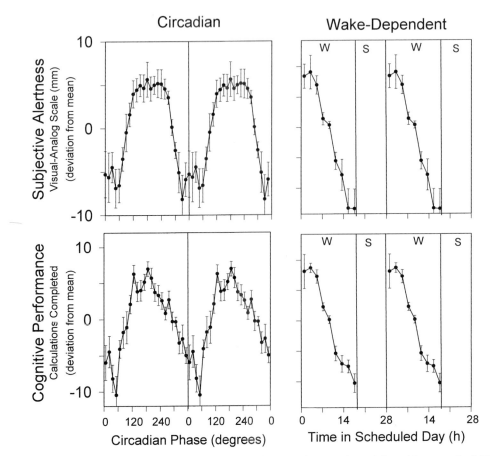

Figure 28–11. Circadian and wake-dependent average variations of subjective alertness (*top:* eight subjects, total of 6142 observations) and cognitive performance (*bottom:* nine subjects, total of 2277 observations) as assessed in the 28-h forced desynchrony protocol. Data are expressed as deviations from each subject's mean value during the forced desynchrony protocol. Data from each subject were first averaged per bin, and then bin values were averaged across subjects. Vertical bars indicate ±1 SEM. *Left,* Circadian component; data were averaged by phase of the endogenous component of the core body temperature rhythm, derived from the intrinsic period of each subject, with the minimum of the educed waveform of the core temperature rhythm assigned a reference value of 0 degrees. *Right,* Wake-dependent component; data were averaged with reference to the rest-activity cycle, at the imposed period of 28 h. W, the scheduled 18.67-h waking episode; S, the scheduled 9.33-h rest episode. (From Czeisler CA, Dijk D-J, Duffy JF. Entrained phase of the circadian pacemaker serves to stabilize alertness and performance throughout the habitual waking day. In: Ogilvie RD, Harsh JR, eds. Sleep Onset: Normal and Abnormal Processes. Washington, DC: American Psychological Association; 1994:89–110. Copyright © 1994 by the American Psychological Association. Reprinted with permission.)

first few hours of wakefulness when averaged across all circadian phases, and the circadian contribution increases as a function of the number of hours awake, suggesting that the homeostatic and circadian drives are not independent.[170] These data suggest that there is a nonadditive interaction between the homeostatic and circadian systems that drive alertness and cognitive performance.[91, 173]

Internal Sleep Structure

It has long been recognized that REM sleep propensity varies with circadian phase.[175] Studies in which nap opportunities were evenly distributed throughout day and night every 1.5 to 3 h were the first to establish the REM sleep propensity rhythm in a protocol that did not involve concomitant variations in prior wake length.[176–178] It was then shown that REM sleep latency, the rate of REM sleep accumulation, REM episode du-

ration, and REM sleep propensity all varied with the phase of the endogenous circadian temperature cycle in free-running subjects whose self-selected rest-activity cycle spontaneously desynchronized from the timing of the endogenous circadian temperature cycle.[178, 179] The peak of the endogenous circadian rhythm in REM sleep propensity found in these free-running desynchronized subjects was just after the nadir of the endogenous component of the circadian temperature cycle, coincident with the circadian peak of sleepiness and sleep propensity.[178] Furthermore, during such spontaneous desynchrony, when free-running subjects selected to go to bed near the peak of the REM sleep propensity rhythm, they usually exhibited sleep-onset REM episodes[178, 179]—an otherwise rare phenomenon normally diagnostic of narcolepsy. Interestingly, under these conditions, the density of rapid eye movements per minute of REM sleep exhibits a sleep-dependent variation that appears to be dissociated from the REM sleep propensity rhythm itself.[180]

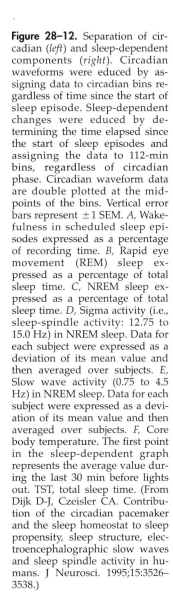

Figure 28–12. Separation of circadian (*left*) and sleep-dependent components (*right*). Circadian waveforms were educed by assigning data to circadian bins regardless of time since the start of sleep episode. Sleep-dependent changes were educed by determining the time elapsed since the start of sleep episodes and assigning the data to 112-min bins, regardless of circadian phase. Circadian waveform data are double plotted at the midpoints of the bins. Vertical error bars represent ±1 SEM. *A*, Wakefulness in scheduled sleep episodes expressed as a percentage of recording time. *B*, Rapid eye movement (REM) sleep expressed as a percentage of total sleep time. *C*, NREM sleep expressed as a percentage of total sleep time. *D*, Sigma activity (i.e., sleep-spindle activity: 12.75 to 15.0 Hz) in NREM sleep. Data for each subject were expressed as a deviation of its mean value and then averaged over subjects. *E*, Slow wave activity (0.75 to 4.5 Hz) in NREM sleep. Data for each subject were expressed as a deviation of its mean value and then averaged over subjects. *F*, Core body temperature. The first point in the sleep-dependent graph represents the average value during the last 30 min before lights out. TST, total sleep time. (From Dijk D-J, Czeisler CA. Contribution of the circadian pacemaker and the sleep homeostat to sleep propensity, sleep structure, electroencephalographic slow waves and sleep spindle activity in humans. J Neurosci. 1995;15:3526–3538.)

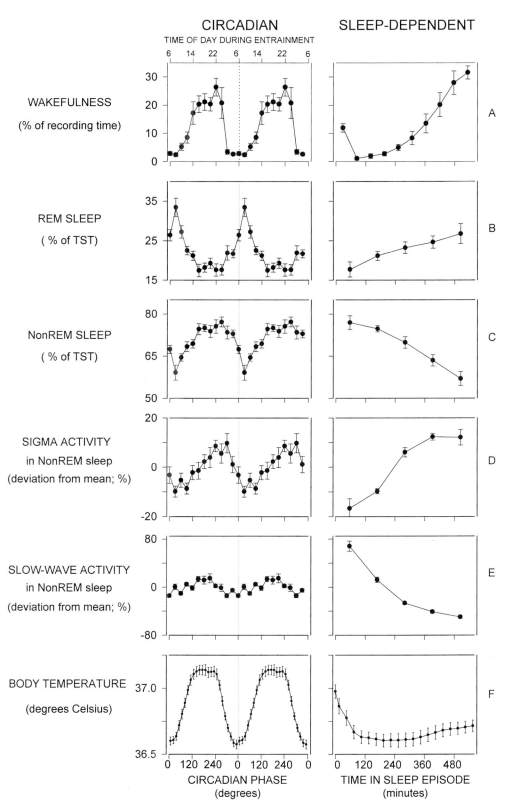

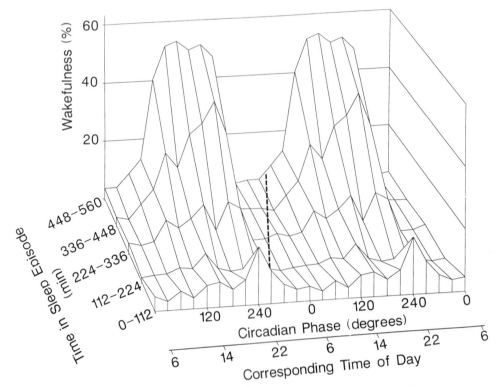

Figure 28–13. Quasi–three-dimensional plot of wakefulness within scheduled sleep episodes, circadian phase, and time elapsed since start of sleep episode. Data were assigned to 12 circadian-phase bins (30 degrees each) and 5 time-since-start-of-the-sleep-episode bins (112 min each). Each point represents wakefulness expressed as percentage of recording time in a bin. Thus, the data point at 0 to 112 min, 0 degrees represents wakefulness within the first 112-min sleep episodes that occurred within the circadian phase interval of −15.0 to 15.0 degrees. To facilitate interpretation of the data, clock times that would correspond approximately to the circadian phase of the core body temperature rhythm under entrained conditions are indicated. The dashed line represents the trajectory of circadian phase and time elapsed since the start of scheduled sleep episodes, corresponding to that trajectory that occurs during a nocturnal sleep episode under entrained conditions. (Reprinted from Neuroscience Letters, vol 166, Dijk D-J, Czeisler CA, Paradoxical timing of the circadian rhythm of sleep propensity serves to consolidate sleep and wakefulness in humans, 63–68, Copyright 1994, with permission from Elsevier Science.)

These findings on the timing of the circadian REM sleep propensity rhythm have since been confirmed and extended with the use of polysomnography data from subjects studied in the forced desynchrony protocol[49] (see Fig. 28–12). Because sleep episodes in the forced desynchrony protocol always begin after a fixed duration of enforced wakefulness, the results were much less subject to the confounding effects of system-

atic variations in prior wake durations characteristic of spontaneous desynchrony. Furthermore, because subjects were scheduled to remain in bed for a fixed interval on the forced desynchrony protocol, the results were not confounded by self-selected termination of the sleep episode, although the circadian variations in sleep efficiency (see Fig. 28–12A) prevent complete elimination of this confounding factor. Nevertheless, under such conditions, the two-fold circadian variation in REM sleep propensity was again found to peak just after the nadir in the endogenous circadian component of the body temperature rhythm (see Fig. 28–12B). Moreover, on average, this was found to be the case within each fifth of the scheduled sleep episode, notwithstanding the average sleep-dependent increase in REM sleep propensity. A sleep-dependent increase in REM sleep propensity that was not dependent on circadian phase was also quantified (see Fig. 28–12). A significant nonadditive interaction between circadian phase and time since the start of the sleep episode was found based on the REM sleep data collected during forced desynchrony.[49]

Using the forced desynchrony protocol, significant and substantial circadian and sleep-dependent variations in NREM sleep propensity were also observed, whereas the robust sleep-dependent decline in slow

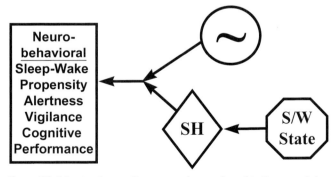

Figure 28–14. A schema illustrating the combined influence of the circadian clock and sleep-wake (S/W) state on neurobehavioral variables (sleep-wake propensity, alertness, vigilance, and cognitive performance). The sleep-wake state influence is illustrated via the intermediary of the sleep homeostat (SH).

wave activity was associated with only a small but statistically significant variation of slow wave activity as a function of circadian phase[49] (see Fig. 28–12). Similar circadian variations in internal sleep structure have been documented in a blind patient whose circadian pacemaker was not synchronized to the 24-h day despite his maintenance of a very regular sleep-wake schedule for decades.[181] Such blind patients are, in essence, living in society on the biological equivalent of a forced desynchrony protocol because the 24-h day is outside the range of entrainment of their circadian pacemaker.

More recently, quantitative analysis of the sleep EEG has revealed circadian variations in the EEG activity during both NREM and REM sleep,[182] with low-frequency sleep spindle activity in NREM sleep paralleling the endogenous circadian melatonin rhythm (see also Fig. 28–12). Overall, these data indicate that the timing and internal sleep structure of sleep are profoundly dependent on an interaction between robust circadian and homeostatic regulatory factors, with circadian factors predominant in the regulation of REM sleep and sleep-dependent factors predominant in the regulation of slow-wave sleep.

Potential Feedback Pathways

As is typical of physiological regulatory systems, feedback pathways play a significant role in this system. The neurobehavioral variables influenced by the circadian pacemaker and the sleep homeostat can influence the sleep-wake state via the influence of wakefulness and sleep propensity on determination of sleep and wake times. For example, a sleep episode is more likely to be initiated after a rise in sleep propensity to a high level during an extended waking episode, and a sleep episode is more likely to be terminated after a decline in sleep propensity to a low level over the course of a sleep episode. This influence on behavior, in turn, influences the level of the sleep homeostat and, due to associated changes in light exposure and activity, may affect the phase, amplitude, or both of the circadian pacemaker.

There may be another important feedback pathway in this system. Studies demonstrating that melatonin receptors can be found on cells within the human SCN have drawn attention to a potential feedback pathway from the pineal gland to the SCN via the circulating hormone melatonin.[183–185] Several physiological studies have suggested that exogenous melatonin may exert a phase-resetting effect on the human circadian pacemaker, and both a PRC and dose-dependent phase shifting have been reported. However, none of these studies have thoroughly controlled for retinal light exposure, confounding interpretation of the results. There has also been a great interest in the potential efficacy of melatonin as a hypnotic agent; however, the reliability and degree of both of these effects remain to be fully established (see Chapter 31).

Examination of the temporal profile of endogenous melatonin secretion during the forced desynchrony protocol reveals that the daily circadian increase in melatonin levels is coincident with a decrease in wakefulness[182] (Fig. 28–15). As researchers have suggested, this melatonin rise may open a gate that allows sleep to occur.[186–188] Taken as a whole, these data provide suggestive evidence that there may be feedback from the pineal gland back to both the circadian pacemaker and to neurobehavioral variables involved in regulating the sleep-wake state.[189] It is likely that other physiological parameters may also have an impact on the sleep-regulating mechanisms; for example, there has been some evidence suggesting an effect of growth hormone[190–192] and changes in body temperature[193, 194] on sleep.

Intrinsic Period of the Human Circadian Pacemaker

Numerous studies have been performed in the absence of environmental synchronizers in human beings, and based on these studies, it was initially concluded that the average period of the human circadian pace-

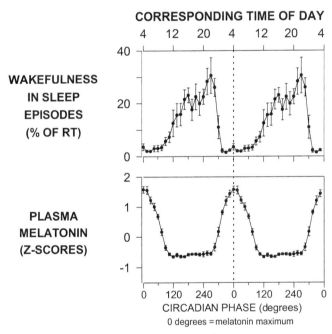

Figure 28–15. Phase relationships between the endogenous circadian rhythms of wakefulness and plasma melatonin as assessed during a forced desynchrony protocol. Data are plotted against circadian phase of the plasma melatonin rhythm (0 degrees on the lower abscissa scale corresponds to the fitted melatonin maximum). To facilitate comparison with the entrained conditions, the upper abscissa scale indicates the approximate clock time corresponding to the circadian melatonin rhythm during the first day of the forced desynchrony protocol (i.e., immediately on release from entrainment). Plasma melatonin data are expressed as Z-scores to correct for interindividual differences in mean values. Wakefulness is expressed as a percentage of recording time (RT). Data are double plotted (i.e., all data plotted left from the dashed vertical line are repeated to the right of this vertical line). (Adapted from Dijk D-J, Shanahan TL, Duffy JF, et al. Variation of electroencephalographic activity during non-rapid eye movement and rapid eye movement sleep with phase of circadian melatonin rhythm in humans. J Physiol [Lond]. 1997;505[3]:851–858.)

maker was 25 h.[18, 27, 35, 47, 128, 195–199] However, many of the early experiments designed to evaluate the characteristics of the human circadian system incorporated self-selected exposure to ordinary room light. These experiments, which had been performed deep within caves and in special laboratories shielded from periodic cues from the external environment, had a common theme in the protocols in which the subjects were permitted to illuminate their living quarters when they were awake and to switch off the lighting when they were asleep, because these experiments were predicated on the strongly entrenched belief that ordinary room light had no effect on the human circadian system.[152, 154] The results of these studies were therefore systematically compromised by the effects of this light exposure.[92, 93, 200] Recognition of this confounding effect of room light on prior attempts to estimate circadian period using a protocol involving self-selected timing of sleep in darkness and wakefulness in artificial room light led to the new suggested use of Kleitman's forced desynchrony protocol to assess the intrinsic period of the human circadian pacemaker.[201, 202] In fact, using simulations based on Kronauer's mathematical model of the effect of light on the circadian system, it was found that under conditions in which room lighting was self-selected, the observed period of the circadian temperature rhythm would be 25 h even when an actual circadian input period of 24.1 to 24.2 h was used in the simulations.[200] Subsequent studies using the forced desynchrony protocol have been performed controlling the intensity of background illumination and the timing of the exposure to the light-dark cycle. Using this forced desynchrony protocol with subjects living in dim light (~10 to 15 lux) on either a 28- or 20-h schedule, the average intrinsic period of the circadian pacemaker has been estimated to be much closer to 24 h, with an average period of 24.2 h[203, 204, 204a] rather than 25 h (see Fig. 28–10). This holds true for all of the circadian markers tested: core body temperature, melatonin and cortisol. This value for the period of the human circadian pacemaker is also consistent with the results of other recent studies performed under a variety of differing protocols in adolescents and young and older adults.[205–208, 208a]

MOLECULAR BASIS OF CIRCADIAN PERIODICITY

Research in molecular biology within the discipline of circadian rhythms has a long and distinguished history that began with the identification of organisms with mutant circadian period phenotypes. After the identification of organisms displaying discrete differences in the characteristics of their circadian rhythmicity, the underlying genetic basis of these phenotypes was identified. These studies suggest the possibility that a regulator of circadian pacemakers is conserved across a broad array of animal species.[209] Identification of the transcripts and proteins associated with clock genes, the feedback interactions between them, and the influence of light on these elements has

permitted the construction of feedback loop models describing the underlying circadian pacemaker mechanism in *Drosophila*, *Neurospora*, and mammals.[209–218]

Studies with human twins have suggested that there may be a genetic influence on the circadian timing system.[219–223] In human beings, it has also been observed that the intrinsic period of the circadian pacemaker is related to the entrained phase of the core body temperature cycle, which in turn is closely coupled to self-selected sleep-wake times.[223a] Subjects exhibiting a longer period tend to have the entrained minimum of their core body temperature occur at a later time under conditions of a normal sleep-wake schedule. This relationship has previously been reported in studies in animals.[24, 224, 225] There is a tendency in some people to retire early in the evening and to arise early in the morning when they feel at their best performance. Conversely, there are others who tend to stay up late at night when they feel they are performing best and to awaken late in the morning. The appearance of these traits of "morningness" and "eveningness"[226–229] may represent an influence of genetic variation in the intrinsic period of the human circadian pacemaker, which has also been found to be related to circadian period.[223a] This is supported by the recent identification of familial inheritance of advanced sleep phase syndrome.[229a]

AGING AND CIRCADIAN SLEEP-WAKE REGULATION

The process of aging is another factor that has a pervasive influence on many aspects of the circadian and sleep-wake regulating system.[230–242] The prevalence of disrupted sleep complaints is much greater in older people than it is in young people. In fact, of persons in the United States who are older than 65 years, 57% complain of at least one chronic sleep problem, 43% complain of difficulty initiating or maintaining sleep, and 19% complain of awakening too early in the morning.[243] A key question in examining the basis for this is the extent to which the circadian pacemaker or the sleep homeostat may play a role in these age-related changes.

In experiments using a constant routine protocol, young subjects tended to have the minima of their core body temperature later than healthy elderly subjects and to exhibit a higher amplitude of their core body temperature rhythm (Fig. 28–16).[117, 232] However, in forced desynchrony experiments with healthy young and elderly subjects, the circadian period was not observed to be different between these two groups.[203, 204a] Although this does not rule out the possibility that circadian period may differ in older people with compromised health or sleep disorders, it does suggest that a change in period is not a necessary consequence of aging. The results from the forced desynchrony study confirmed those of the earlier constant routine study showing that older subjects have their circadian phase set to an earlier hour and exhibit a lower amplitude of the body temperature and melatonin rhythms.[244] More importantly, other results from this study suggest that

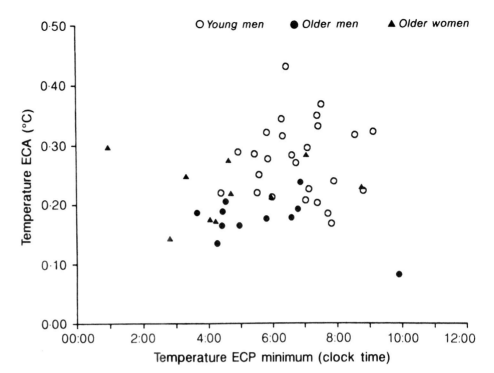

Figure 28–16. Endogenous circadian amplitude (ECA) versus endogenous circadian phase (ECP) of the core body temperature rhythm during a constant routine in 27 young men (18 to 31 years) and 21 older subjects (65 to 85 years; 11 men and 10 women). (From Czeisler CA, Dumont M, Duffy JF, et al. Association of sleep-wake habits in older people with changes in output of circadian pacemaker. Lancet. 1992;340 [8825]:933–936, © by The Lancet Ltd., 1992.)

young subjects are able to sleep over a much wider range of circadian phases than are elderly subjects, and that elderly subjects wake up at an earlier internal circadian phase.[117, 244–246] This waking at an earlier phase may also explain why their circadian system is shifted to an earlier hour, because if they wake up spontaneously at an earlier circadian phase, they are going to be exposed to light at an earlier hour, which will, in turn, reset their pacemaker to an earlier hour and essentially exacerbate this problem.

INFLUENCE OF SOCIETAL FACTORS

The independent self-selection of sleep and wake times in human beings is another important factor in the sleep-regulatory system. Although the circadian and homeostatic drives for sleep exert an influence on the choice of sleep and wake times via a feedback pathway, societal factors often are an overriding influence. This is in stark contrast to animal behavior, in which independent self-selection does not appear to contribute significantly and the observed times of activity and sleep are predictable enough to be used as a marker of the time of day. Human beings, especially since the advent of alarm clocks and artificial lighting, can and do override the signals from the circadian and sleep-wake regulating system and freely decide to stay awake because of job or school requirements or even for recreational and social events. One of the consequences of this is that human beings may be more sleep deprived than their ancestors and exhibit self-determined sleep and wake schedules.[62, 247, 248] The long-term consequences of this recent trend in industrialized society are unknown; however, recent studies have indicated that the modern consolidated sleep episode

shows significant differences from that observed under more naturalistic conditions in which the sleep episode is determined by the longer length of darkness in the natural environment during winter.[62, 249] The most conspicuous example of this self-selection is the phenomenon of rotating shift work, when the choice is made to work in direct opposition to the modulation of the circadian and homeostatic regulatory systems at the cost of internal temporal dissociation, fragmented sleep and impaired wakefulness. Therefore, in any realistic model of the human circadian and sleep-wake regulating system, this environmental/societal factor must be recognized.

CONCLUSIONS

An overall schema of the entire system can be assembled and updated to incorporate the feedback pathway of neurobehavioral variables on the sleep-wake state and the putative feedback pathways from melatonin and other physiological variables onto the circadian pacemaker and neurobehavioral function (Fig. 28–17). This schema also incorporates the global influence of environmental, social, behavioral, genetic, pharmacological, and age factors on all elements of this system. Another addition to this final schema relates to the clear decrements in neurobehavioral performance and alertness that immediately follow the transition from sleep to waking, a phenomenon called *sleep inertia*. The time course of this underappreciated phenomenon has been characterized, and it has been demonstrated that sleep inertia persists for as long as several hours after a long sleep episode.[91, 169, 250, 251] This schema incorporates much of what is known concerning the role of the circadian pacemaker in the regulation of sleep. It is not

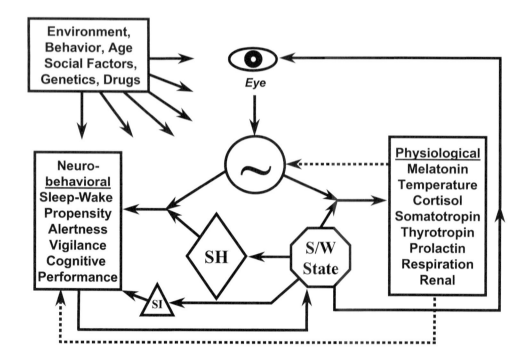

Figure 28–17. An overall schema coalescing those from Figures 28–7 and 28–14. The potential influence of physiological variables (e.g., melatonin, body temperature) on neurobehavioral variables or the circadian clock is indicated by the dashed arrows, the feedback influence of neurobehavioral variables on sleep-wake state is indicated by a solid arrow, and the influence of sleep-wake state on neurobehavioral variables through sleep inertia (SI) is indicated by solid arrows. The global influence of environment, behavior, age, social factors, genetics, and drugs on virtually all elements contributing to sleep-wake regulation is also represented. SH, sleep homeostat; S/W, sleep-wake.

intended to be a complete representation of the factors involved in the system regulating sleep because that would be beyond the scope of this chapter. Nevertheless, the strength of this schema is that it serves as a useful tool in understanding the interplay between the circadian and homeostatic drives and perhaps as a useful framework from which future scientific inquiry can be initiated.

The complexity of the interactions of the circadian pacemaker and the sleep homeostat to regulate the sleep-wake cycle should not be underestimated. Furthermore, it is important to understand the difficulty in separating these two processes functionally. Under ordinary circumstances, in which individuals are sleeping during the night in darkness and are awake during the day in daylight, it is not possible to distinguish the relative contributions of the sleep homeostat from that of the circadian pacemaker to a given recurrent daily characteristic, symptom, or disorder of sleep or wakefulness (e.g., narcolepsy, delayed sleep phase syndrome). The occurrence of a pathological event, such as a nocturnal seizure, at the same time each night may be driven by the circadian pacemaker, the sleep homeostat, a specific sleep stage, or some combination of these processes. It is currently possible, although difficult, to experimentally dissociate these factors for research purposes (e.g., using either the forced desynchrony protocol in human subjects or suprachiasmatic lesions in animal studies). Although clinically feasible techniques, such as the use of dim-light salivary melatonin onset, may provide limited information about circadian phase, a routine complete clinical assessment of whether a disorder is circadian or homeostat-dependent awaits the results of continued basic and clinical research.

Acknowledgments

We give special thanks to Drs. David Dinges, Megan Jewett, and Derk-Jan Dijk for reviewing the manuscript. The research conducted by the Circadian Neuroendocrine and Sleep Disorders Section was supported by grants NIA-1-R01-AG06072, NIA-P01-AG09975, and NIA-1-U01-12642 from the National Institute on Aging; grant NIMH-1-R01-MH45130 from the National Institute of Mental Health; grant R01-HL52992 from the National Heart, Lung, and Blood Institute; grants NAG9-524 and NAG5-3952 from the National Aeronautics and Space Administration; the National Aeronautics and Space Administration through the NASA Cooperative Agreement NCC 9-58 with the National Space Biomedical Research Institute; grants F49620-95-1-0388 and F49620-97-1-0246 from the United States Air Force Office of Scientific Research; and General Clinical Research Center grant NCRR-GCRC-MO1-RR02635 from the National Center for Research Resources and by the Brigham and Women's Hospital. Dr. Khalsa was supported by senior National Research Service Award fellowship F33-HL09588 from the National Heart, Lung, and Blood Institute.

References

1. Edmunds LN Jr. Cellular and Molecular Bases of Biological Clocks: Models and Mechanisms for Circadian Timekeeping. New York, NY: Springer-Verlag; 1988.
2. Johnson CH, Golden SS, Ishiura M, et al. Circadian clocks in prokaryotes. Mol Microbiol. 1996;21:5–11.
3. Johnson CH. An Atlas of Phase Response Curves for Circadian and Circatidal Rhythms. Nashville, Tenn: Department of Biology, Vanderbilt University; 1990.
4. Pittendrigh CS. Circadian systems: entrainment. In: Aschoff J, ed. Handbook of Behavioral Biology: Biological Rhythms. New York, NY: Plenum Press; 1981:95–124.
5. Pittendrigh CS. Circadian systems: general perspective. In: Aschoff J, ed. Handbook of Behavioral Biology: Biological Rhythms. New York, NY: Plenum Press; 1981:57–80.
6. Fulton JF, Bailey P. Tumors in the region of the third ventricle: their diagnosis and relation to pathological sleep. J Nerv Ment Dis. 1929;69:1–25, 145–164.
7. Moore RY, Eichler VB. Loss of a circadian adrenal corticosterone rhythm following suprachiasmatic lesions in the rat. Brain Res. 1972;42:201–206.
8. Stephan FK, Zucker I. Circadian rhythms in drinking behavior and locomotor activity of rats are eliminated by hypothalamic lesions. Proc Natl Acad Sci U S A. 1972;69:1583–1586.
9. Miller JD, Morin LP, Schwartz WJ, et al. New insights into the mammalian circadian clock. Sleep. 1996;19:641–667.

10. Moore RY. Circadian rhythms: basic neurobiology and clinical applications. Annu Rev Med. 1997;48:253–266.

11. Reuss S. Components and connections of the circadian timing system in mammals. Cell Tissue Res. 1996;285:353–378.

12. Ralph MR, Foster RG, Davis FC, et al. Transplanted suprachiasmatic nucleus determines circadian period. Science. 1990; 247:975–978.

13. Lehman MN, Silver R, Gladstone WR, et al. Circadian rhythmicity restored by neural transplant: immunocytochemical characterization of the graft and its integration with the host brain. J Neurosci. 1987;7:1626–1638.

14. Ralph MR, Menaker M. A mutation of the circadian system in golden hamsters. Science. 1988;241:1225–1227.

15. Silver R, Lesauter J, Tresco PA, et al. A diffusible coupling signal from transplanted suprachiasmatic nucleus controlling circadian locomotor rhythms. Nature. 1996;382:810–813.

16. Balsalobre A, Damiola F, Schibler U. A serum shock induces circadian gene expression in mammalian tissue culture cells. Cell. 1998;93:929–937.

17. Weitzman ED, Boyar RM, Kapen S, et al. The relationship of sleep and sleep stages to neuroendocrine secretion and biological rhythms in man. Recent Prog Horm Res. 1975;31:399–441.

18. Aschoff J, Wever R. The circadian system of man. In: Aschoff J, ed. Biological Rhythms: Handbook of Behavioral Neurobiology. New York, NY: Plenum Press; 1981:311–331.

19. Shanahan TL, Czeisler CA. Light exposure induces equivalent phase shifts of the endogenous circadian rhythms of circulating plasma melatonin and core body temperature in men. J Clin Endocrinol Metab. 1991;73:227–235.

20. Allan JS, Czeisler CA. Persistence of the circadian thyrotropin rhythm under constant conditions and after light-induced shifts of circadian phase. J Clin Endocrinol Metab. 1994;79:508–512.

21. Waldstreicher J, Duffy JF, Brown EN, et al. Gender differences in the temporal organization of prolactin (PRL) secretion: evidence for a sleep-independent circadian rhythm of circulating PRL levels—a clinical research center study. J Clin Endocrinol Metab. 1996;81:1483–1487.

22. El Hajj Fuleihan G, Klerman EB, Brown EN, et al. Parathyroid hormone circadian rhythm is truly endogenous. J Clin Endocrinol Metab. 1997;82:281–286.

23. Brandenberger G, Gronfier C, Weibel L, et al. Modulatory role of sleep on hormonal pulsatility. In: Hayaishi O, Inoue S, eds. Sleep and Sleep Disorders: From Molecule to Behavior. Tokyo, Japan: Academic Press; 1997:195–208.

24. Van Cauter E, Turek FW. Endocrine and other biological rhythms. In: DeGroot LJ, ed. Endocrinology. Philadelphia, Pa: WB Saunders; 1995:2487–2548.

25. Leproult R, Van Reeth O, Byrne MM, et al. Sleepiness, performance, and neuroendocrine function during sleep deprivation: effects of exposure to bright light or exercise. J Biol Rhythms. 1997;12:245–258.

26. Czeisler CA, Klerman EB. Circadian and sleep-dependent regulation of hormone release in humans. Rec Progr Horm Res. 1999;54.

27. Weitzman ED, Czeisler CA, Moore-Ede MC. Sleep-wake, neuroendocrine and body temperature circadian rhythms under entrained and non-entrained (free-running) conditions in man. In: Suda M, Hayaishi O, Nakagawa H, eds. Biological Rhythms and Their Central Mechanism. Amsterdam, The Netherlands: Elsevier/North-Holland Press; 1979:199–227.

28. Weitzman ED, Zimmerman JC, Czeisler CA, et al. Cortisol secretion is inhibited during sleep in normal man. J Clin Endocrinol Metab. 1983;56:352–358.

29. Aschoff J. Exogenous and endogenous components in circadian rhythms. Cold Spring Harbor Symp Quant Biol. 1960;25:11–28.

30. Folkard S, Minors DS, Waterhouse JM. "Demasking" the temperature rhythm after simulated time zone transitions. J Biol Rhythms. 1991;6:81–91.

31. Minors DS, Waterhouse JM. Masking in humans: the problem and some attempts to solve it. Chronobiol Int. 1989;6:29–53.

32. Minors DS, Waterhouse JM, Åkerstedt T. The effect of the timing, quality and quantity of sleep upon the depression (masking) of body temperature on an irregular sleep/wake schedule. J Sleep Res. 1994;3:45–51.

33. Czeisler CA, Moore-Ede MC, Regestein QR, et al. Episodic 24-hour cortisol secretory patterns in patients awaiting elective cardiac surgery. J Clin Endocrinol Metab. 1976;42:273–283.

34. Czeisler CA. Human Circadian Physiology: Internal Organization of Temperature, Sleep-Wake, and Neuroendocrine Rhythms Monitored in an Environment Free of Time Cues [dissertation]. Stanford, Calif: Stanford University; 1978.

35. Wever RA. The Circadian System of Man: Results of Experiments under Temporal Isolation. New York, NY: Springer-Verlag; 1979.

36. Lewy AJ, Wehr TA, Goodwin FK, et al. Light suppresses melatonin secretion in humans. Science. 1980;210:1267–1269.

37. Deacon S, Arendt J. Posture influences melatonin concentrations in plasma and saliva in humans. Neurosci Lett. 1994;167:191–194.

38. Monteleone P, Maj M, Fusco M, et al. Physical exercise at night blunts the nocturnal increase of plasma melatonin levels in healthy humans. Life Sci. 1990;47:1989–1995.

39. Mills JN, Minors DS, Waterhouse JM. Adaptation to abrupt time shifts of the oscillator[s] controlling human circadian rhythms. J Physiol (Lond). 1978;285:455–470.

40. Czeisler CA, Johnson MP, Duffy JF, et al. Exposure to bright light and darkness to treat physiologic maladaptation to night work. N Engl J Med. 1990;322:1253–1259.

41. Duffy JF. Constant routine. In: Carskadon MA, ed. Encyclopedia of Sleep and Dreaming. New York, NY: Macmillan; 1993:134–136.

42. Czeisler CA, Kronauer RE, Allan JS, et al. Bright light induction of strong (type 0) resetting of the human circadian pacemaker. Science. 1989;244:1328–1333.

43. Hunter J. Of the heat of animals and vegetables. Philos Trans R Soc Lond. 1778;68:7–49.

44. Benedict FG. Studies in body-temperature, I: influence of the inversion of the daily routine; the temperature of night-workers. Am J Physiol. 1904;11:145–169.

45. Kleitman N, Doktorsky A. Studies on the physiology of sleep, VII: the effect of the position of the body and of sleep on rectal temperature in man. Am J Physiol. 1933;104:340–343.

46. Mills JN, Minors DS, Waterhouse JM. The effect of sleep upon human circadian rhythms. Chronobiologia. 1978;5:14–27.

47. Aschoff J, Wever R. Human circadian rhythms: a multioscillatory system. Fed Proc. 1976;35:2326–2332.

48. Zulley J, Wever RA. Interaction between the sleep-wake cycle and the rhythm of rectal temperature. In: Aschoff J, Daan S, Groos G, eds. Vertebrate Circadian Systems. Berlin, Germany: Springer-Verlag; 1982:253–261.

49. Dijk D-J, Czeisler CA. Contribution of the circadian pacemaker and the sleep homeostat to sleep propensity, sleep structure, electroencephalographic slow waves and sleep spindle activity in humans. J Neurosci. 1995;15:3526–3538.

50. Shanahan TL. Circadian Physiology and the Plasma Melatonin Rhythm in Humans [dissertation]. Boston, Mass: Harvard Medical School; 1995.

50a. Shanahan TL, Kronauer RE, Duffy JF, et al. Melatonin rhythm observed throughout a three-cycle bright-light stimulus designed to reset the human circadian pacemaker. J Biol Rhythms. 1999;14:237–253.

51. Deacon SJ, Arendt J, English J. Posture: a possible masking factor of the melatonin circadian rhythm. In: Touitou Y, Arendt J, Pévet P, eds. Melatonin and the Pineal Gland—From Basic Science to Clinical Application. New York, NY: Elsevier Science Publishers; 1993:387–390.

52. Brabant G, Prank K, Ranft U, et al. Physiological regulation of circadian and pulsatile thyrotropin secretion in normal man and woman. J Clin Endocrinol Metab. 1990;70:403–409.

53. Goichot B, Weibel L, Chapotot F, et al. Effect of the shift of the sleep-wake cycle on three robust endocrine markers of the circadian clock. Am J Physiol. 1998;275:E243–E248.

54. Baumgartner A, Dietzel M, Saletu B, et al. Influence of partial sleep deprivation on the secretion of thyrotropin, thyroid hormones, growth hormone, prolactin, luteinizing hormone, follicle stimulating hormone, and estradiol in healthy young women. Psychiatry Res. 1993;48:153–178.

55. Goichot B, Brandenberger G, Saini J, et al. Nocturnal plasma thyrotropin variations are related to slow-wave sleep. J Sleep Res. 1992;1:186–190.

56. Gronfier C, Luthringer R, Follenius M, et al. Temporal link between plasma thyrotropin levels and electroencephalographic activity in man. Neurosci Lett. 1995;200:97–100.

57. Holl RW, Hartman MI, Veldhuis JD, et al. Thirty-second sampling of plasma growth hormone in man: correlation with sleep stages. J Clin Endocrinol Metab. 1991;72:854–861.

58. Van Cauter E, Kerkhofs M, Caufriez A, et al. A quantitative estimation of growth hormone secretion in normal man: reproducibility and relation to sleep and time of day. J Clin Endocrinol Metab. 1992;74:1441–1450.

59. Winer LM, Shaw MA, Baumann G. Basal plasma growth hormone levels in man: new evidence for rhythmicity of growth hormone secretion. J Clin Endocrinol Metab. 1990;70:1678–1686.

60. Gronfier C, Luthringer R, Follenius M, et al. A quantitative evaluation of the relationships between growth hormone secretion and delta wave electroencephalographic activity during normal sleep and after enrichment in delta waves. Sleep. 1996;19:817–824.

61. Van Cauter E, Desir D, Refetoff S, et al. The relationship between episodic variations of plasma prolactin and REM–nonREM cyclicity is an artifact. J Clin Endocrinol Metab. 1982;54:70–75.

62. Wehr TA, Moul DE, Barbato G, et al. Conservation of photoperiod-responsive mechanisms in humans. Am J Physiol. 1993;265:R846–R857.

63. Logue FC, Fraser WD, O'Reilly DS, et al. The circadian rhythm of intact parathyroid hormone: temporal correlation with prolactin secretion in normal men. J Clin Endocrinol Metab. 1990;71:1556–1560.

64. Logue FC, Fraser WD, O'Reilly DS, et al. Sleep shift dissociates the nocturnal peaks of parathyroid hormone, nephrogenous cyclic adenosine monophosphate, and prolactin in normal men. J Clin Endocrinol Metab. 1992;75:25–29.

65. Miyatake A, Morimoto Y, Oishi T, et al. Circadian rhythm of serum testosterone and its relation to sleep: comparison with the variation in serum luteinizing hormone, prolactin, and cortisol in normal men. J Clin Endocrinol Metab. 1980;51:1365–1371.

66. Veldhuis JD, Johnson ML. Operating characteristics of the hypothalamo-pituitary-gonadal axis in men: circadian, ultradian, and pulsatile release of prolactin and its temporal coupling with luteinizing hormone. J Clin Endocrinol Metab. 1988;67:116–123.

67. Spiegel K, Follenius M, Simon C, et al. Prolactin secretion and sleep. Sleep. 1994;17:20–27.

68. Spiegel K, Luthringer R, Follenius M, et al. Temporal relationship between prolactin secretion and slow-wave electroencephalic activity during sleep. Sleep. 1995;18:543–548.

69. Nielsen HK, Laurberg P, Brixen K, et al. Relations between diurnal variations in serum osteocalcin, cortisol, parathyroid hormone, and ionized calcium in normal individuals. Acta Endocrinol (Copenh). 1991;124:391–398.

70. Chapotot F, Gronfier C, Spiegel K, et al. Relationships between intact parathyroid hormone 24-hour profiles, sleep-wake cycle, and sleep electroencephalographic activity in man. J Clin Endocrinol Metab. 1996;81:3759–3765.

71. Fraser WD, Logue FC, Christie JP, et al. Alteration of the circadian rhythm of intact parathyroid hormone following a 96-hour fast. Clin Endocrinol (Oxf). 1994;40:523–528.

72. Parker DC, Rossman LG, Vanderlaan EF. Relation of sleep-entrained human prolactin release to REM-nonREM cycles. J Clin Endocrinol Metab. 1974;38:646–651.

73. Brandenberger G, Follenius M, Muzet A, et al. Ultradian oscillations in plasma renin activity: their relationships to meals and sleep stages. J Clin Endocrinol Metab. 1985;61:280–284.

74. Brandenberger G, Follenius M, Simon C, et al. Nocturnal oscillations in plasma renin activity and REM-NREM sleep cycles in humans: a common regulatory mechanism? Sleep. 1988;11:242–250.

75. Luthringer R, Brandenberger G, Schaltenbrand N, et al. Slow wave electroencephalic activity parallels renin oscillations during sleep in humans. Electroencephalogr Clin Neurophysiol. 1995;95:318–322.

76. Aschoff J. Circadian rhythms: general features and endocrinological aspects. In: Krieger DT, ed. Endocrine Rhythms. New York, NY: Raven Press; 1979:1–62.

77. Weibel L, Brandenberger G. Disturbances in hormonal profiles of night workers during their usual sleep and work times. J Biol Rhythms. 1998;13:202–208.

78. Babkoff H, Mikulincer M, Caspy T, et al: The topology of performance curves during 72 hours of sleep loss: a memory and search task. Q J Exp Psychol. 1988;40A:737–756.

79. Folkard S, Hume KI, Minors DS, et al. Independence of the circadian rhythm in alertness from the sleep/wake cycle. Nature. 1985;313:678–679.

80. Folkard S, Wever RA, Wildgruber CM. Multi-oscillatory control of circadian rhythms in human performance. Nature. 1983;305:223–226.

81. Kleitman N. Sleep and Wakefulness. Chicago, Ill: University of Chicago Press; 1963.

82. Monk TH, Buysse DJ, Reynolds CF III, et al. Circadian rhythms in human performance and mood under constant conditions. J Sleep Res. 1977;6:9–18.

83. Fröberg JE, Karlsson CG, Levi L, et al. Circadian rhythms of catecholamine excretion, shooting range performance and self-ratings of fatigue during sleep deprivation. Biol Psychol. 1975;2:175–188.

84. Åkerstedt TA, Fröberg JE, Friberg Y, et al. Melatonin excretion, body temperature and subjective arousal during 64 hours of sleep deprivation. Psychoneuroendocrinology. 1979;4:219–225.

85. Dinges DF, Orne MT, Whitehouse WG, et al. Temporal placement of a nap for alertness: contributions of circadian phase and prior wakefulness. Sleep. 1987;10:313–329.

86. Åkerstedt T. Sleepiness as a consequence of shift work. Sleep. 1988;11:17–34.

87. Åkerstedt T, Gillberg M, Wetterberg L. The circadian covariation of fatigue and urinary melatonin. Biol Psychiatry. 1982;17:547–554.

88. Babkoff H, Caspy T, Mikulincer M. Subjective sleepiness ratings: the effects of sleep deprivation, circadian rhythmicity and cognitive performance. Sleep. 1991;14:534–539.

89. Boivin DB, Czeisler CA, Dijk D-J, et al. Complex interaction of the sleep-wake cycle and circadian phase modulates mood in healthy subjects. Arch Gen Psychiatry. 1997;54:145–152.

90. Johnson MP, Duffy JF, Dijk D-J, et al. Short-term memory, alertness and performance: a reappraisal of their relationship to body temperature. J Sleep Res. 1992;1:24–29.

91. Jewett ME. Models of Circadian and Homeostatic Regulation of Human Performance and Alertness [dissertation]. Boston, Mass: Harvard University; 1997.

91a. Cajochen C, Khalsa SBS, Wyatt JK, et al. EEG and ocular correlates of circadian melatonin phase and human performance decrements during sleep loss. Am J Physiol. 1999;277:R640–R649.

92. Czeisler CA. The effect of light on the human circadian pacemaker. In: Waterhouse JM, ed. Circadian Clocks and Their Adjustment. Chichester, West Sussex, England (Ciba Foundation Symposium 183): John Wiley & Sons; 1995:254–302.

93. Czeisler CA, Wright KP Jr. Influence of light on circadian rhythmicity in humans. In: Turek FW, Zee PC, eds. Neurobiology of Sleep and Circadian Rhythms. New York, NY: Marcel Dekker; 1998.

94. Moore RY, Lenn NJ. A retinohypothalamic projection in the rat. J Comp Neurol. 1972;146:1–9.

95. Moore RY. Organization of the mammalian circadian system. In: Waterhouse JM, ed. Circadian Clocks and Their Adjustment. Chichester, West Sussex, England (Ciba Foundation Symposium 183): John Wiley & Sons; 1994:88–99.

96. Watts AG. The efferent projections of the suprachiasmatic nucleus: anatomical insights into the control of circadian rhythms. In: Klein DC, Moore RY, Reppert SM, eds. Suprachiasmatic Nucleus: The Mind's Clock. New York, NY: Oxford University Press; 1991:77–106.

97. Klein DC, Moore RY, Reppert SM. Suprachiasmatic Nucleus: The Mind's Clock. New York, NY: Oxford University Press; 1991.

98. Illnerová H. The suprachiasmatic nucleus and rhythmic pineal melatonin production. In: Klein DC, Moore RY, Reppert SM, eds. Suprachiasmatic Nucleus: The Mind's Clock. New York, NY: Oxford University Press; 1991:197–216.

99. Wurtman RJ, Axelrod J, Phillips LS. Melatonin synthesis in the pineal gland: control by light. Science. 1963;142:1071–1073.

100. McIntyre IM, Norman TR, Burrows GD, et al. Human melatonin suppression by light is intensity dependent. J Pineal Res. 1989;6:149–156.

101. Wetterberg L. Melatonin in humans: physiological and clinical studies. J Neural Transm. 1978;13:289–310.

102. Czeisler CA, Shanahan TL, Klerman EB, et al. Suppression of melatonin secretion in some blind patients by exposure to bright light. N Engl J Med. 1995;332:6–11.

103. Reppert SM. Circadian rhythms: basic aspects and pediatric implications. In: Styne DM, Brook CGD, eds. Current Concepts in Pediatric Endocrinology. Amsterdam, The Netherlands: Elsevier; 1987:91–119.

104. Sack RL, Lewy AJ, Blood ML, et al. Circadian rhythm abnormalities in totally blind people: incidence and clinical significance. J Clin Endocrinol Metab. 1992;75:127–134.

105. Provencio I, Wong S, Lederman AB, et al. Visual and circadian responses to light in aged retinally degenerate (rd) mice. Vision Res. 1994;34:1799–1806.

106. Cooper HM, Herbin M, Nevo E. Ocular regression conceals adaptive progression of the visual system in a blind subterranean mammal. Nature. 1993;361:156–159.

107. Takahashi JS, DeCoursey PJ, Bauman L, et al. Spectral sensitivity of a novel photoreceptive system mediating entrainment of mammalian circadian rhythms. Nature. 1984;308:186–188.

108. Moore RY, Speh JC, Card JP. The retinohypothalamic tract originates from a distinct subset of retinal ganglion cells. J Comp Neurol. 1995;352:351–366.

109. Provencio I, Cooper HC, Foster FG. Retinal projections in mice with inherited retinal degeneration: implications for circadian photoentrainment. J Comp Neurol. 1998;395:417–439.

110. Moore RY. Vision without sight. N Engl J Med. 1995;332:54–55.

111. Hastings JW, Sweeney BM. A persistent diurnal rhythm of luminescence in Gonyaulax polyedra. Biol Bull. 1958;115:440–458.

112. Johnson CH. Phase response curves: What can they tell us about circadian clocks? In: Hiroshige T, Honma K, eds. Circadian Clocks from Cell to Human. Sapporo, Japan: Hokkaido University Press; 1992:209–249.

113. Jewett ME, Kronauer RE, Czeisler CA. Phase/amplitude resetting of the human circadian pacemaker via bright light: a further analysis. J Biol Rhythms. 1994;9:295–314.

114. Boivin DB, Duffy JF, Kronauer RE, et al. Dose-response relationships for resetting of human circadian clock by light. Nature. 1996;379:540–542.

115. Duffy JF, Kronauer RE, Czeisler CA. Phase-shifting human circadian rhythms: influence of sleep timing, social contact and light exposure. J Physiol (Lond). 1996;495:289–297.

116. Jewett ME, Rimmer DW, Duffy JF, et al. The human circadian pacemaker is sensitive to light throughout subjective day without evidence of transients. Am J Physiol. 1997;273:R1800–R1809.

117. Duffy JF, Dijk D-J, Klerman EB, et al. Later endogenous circadian temperature nadir relative to an earlier waketime in older people. Am J Physiol. 1998;275:R1478–R1487.

118. Dawson D, Lack L, Morris M. Phase resetting of the human circadian pacemaker with use of a single pulse of bright light. Chronobiol Int. 1993;10:94–102.

119. Minors DS, Waterhouse JM, Wirz-Justice A. A human phase-response curve to light. Neurosci Lett. 1991;133:36–40.

120. Honma K, Honma S. A human phase response curve for bright light pulses. Jpn J Psychiatry Neurol. 1988;42:167–168.

121. Beersma DGM, Daan S. Strong or weak phase resetting by light pulses in humans? J Biol Rhythms. 1993;8:340–347.

122. Kronauer RE, Jewett ME, Czeisler CA. Commentary: the human circadian response to light—strong and weak resetting. J Biol Rhythms. 1993;8:351–360.

123. Lakin-Thomas PL. Commentary: strong or weak phase resetting by light pulses in humans? J Biol Rhythms. 1993;8:348–350.

124. Jewett ME, Kronauer RE, Czeisler CA. Light-induced suppression of endogenous circadian amplitude in humans. Nature. 1991;350:59–62.

125. Winfree AT. The Geometry of Biological Time. New York, NY: Springer-Verlag; 1980.

126. Winfree AT. The Timing of Biological Clocks. New York, NY: Scientific American; 1987.

127. Pohl H. Characteristics and variability in entrainment of circadian rhythms to light in diurnal rodents. In: Aschoff J, Daan S,

Groos GA, eds. Vertebrate Circadian Systems: Structure and Physiology. Berlin, Germany: Springer-Verlag; 1982:339–346.

128. Aschoff J. Human circadian rhythms in activity, body temperature and other functions. Life Sci Space Res. 1967;5:159–173.

129. Lewy AJ, Sack RL. The dim light melatonin onset as a marker for circadian phase position. Chronobiol Int. 1989;6:93–102.

130. Shanahan TL, Zeitzer JM, Czeisler CA. Resetting the melatonin rhythm with light in humans. J Biol Rhythms. 1997;12:556–567.

131. Vakkuri O. Diurnal rhythm of melatonin in human saliva. Acta Physiol Scand. 1985;124:409–412.

132. Kennaway DJ, Voultsios A. Circadian rhythm of free melatonin in human plasma. J Clin Endocrinol Metab. 1998;83:1013–1015.

133. Voultsios A, Kennaway DJ, Dawson D. Salivary melatonin as a circadian phase marker: validation and comparison to plasma melatonin. J Biol Rhythms. 1997;12:457–466.

134. McIntyre IM, Norman TR, Burrows GD, et al. Melatonin rhythm in human plasma and saliva. J Pineal Res. 1987;4:177–183.

135. Nowak R, McMillen IC, Redman J, et al. The correlation between serum and salivary melatonin concentrations and urinary 6-hydroxymelatonin sulphate excretion rates: two non-invasive techniques for monitoring human circadian rhythmicity. Clin Endocrinol. 1987;27:445–452.

136. Nagtegaal E, Peeters T, Swart W, et al. Correlation between concentrations of melatonin in saliva and serum in patients with delayed sleep phase syndrome. Ther Drug Monit. 1998;20:181–183.

137. Leibenluft E, Feldman-Naim S, Turner EH, et al. Salivary and plasma measures of dim light melatonin onset (DLMO) in patients with rapid cycling bipolar disorder. Biol Psychiatry. 1996;40:731–735.

138. Carskadon M, Acebo C, Richardson GS, et al. An approach to studying circadian rhythms of adolescent humans. J Biol Rhythms. 1997;12:278–289.

139. Wirz-Justice A, Graw P, Krauchi K, et al. "Natural" light treatment of seasonal affective disorder. J Affect Disord. 1996;37:109–120.

140. Kronauer RE. A quantitative model for the effects of light on the amplitude and phase of the deep circadian pacemaker, based on human data. In: Horne J, ed. Sleep '90: Proceedings of the Tenth European Congress on Sleep Research. Dusseldorf, Germany: Pontenagel Press; 1990:306–309.

141. Jewett ME, Kronauer RE. Refinement of a limit cycle oscillator model of the effects of light on the human circadian pacemaker. J Theor Biol. 1998;192:455–465.

142. Cole RJ, Kripke DF, Wisbey J, et al. Seasonal variation in human illumination exposure at two different latitudes. J Biol Rhythms. 1995;10:324–334.

143. Okudaira N, Kripke DF, Webster JB. Naturalistic studies of human light exposure. Am J Physiol. 1983;245:R613–R615.

144. Hébert M, Dumont M, Paquet J. Seasonal and diurnal patterns of human illumination under natural conditions. Chronobiol Int. 1998;15:59–70.

145. Mrosovsky N. Locomotor activity and non-photic influences on circadian clocks. Biol Rev. 1996;71:343–372.

146. Van Reeth O, Turek FW. Stimulated activity mediates phase shifts in the hamster circadian clock induced by dark pulses or benzodiazepines. Nature. 1989;339:49–51.

147. Edgar DM, Dement WC. Regularly scheduled voluntary exercise synchronizes the mouse circadian clock. Am J Physiol. 1991;261:R928–R933.

148. Edgar DM, Martin CE, Dement WC. Activity feedback to the mammalian circadian pacemaker: influence on observed measures of rhythm period length. J Biol Rhythms. 1991;6:185–199.

149. Wickland CR, Turek FW. Phase-shifting effects of acute increases in activity on circadian locomotor rhythms in hamsters. Am J Physiol. 1991;261:R1109–R1117.

150. Van Reeth O, Sturis J, Byrne MM, et al. Nocturnal exercise phase delays circadian rhythms of melatonin and thyrotropin secretion in normal men. Am J Physiol. 1994;266:E964–E974.

151. Van Cauter E, Sturis J, Byrne MM, et al. Preliminary studies on the immediate phase-shifting effects of light and exercise on the human circadian clock. J Biol Rhythms. 1993;8:S99–S108.

152. Aschoff J, Fatranská M, Giedke H, et al. Human circadian rhythms in continuous darkness: entrainment by social cues. Science. 1971;171:213–215.

153. Aschoff J, Hoffmann K, Pohl H, et al. Re-entrainment of circadian rhythms after phase-shifts of the zeitgeber. Chronobiologia. 1975;2:23–78.

154. Wever R. Zur Zeitgeber-Stärke eines Licht-Dunkel-Wechsels für die circadiane Periodik des Menschen. Eur J Physiol. 1970;321:133–142.

155. Lockley SW, Skene D-J, Arendt J, et al. Relationship between melatonin rhythms and visual loss in the blind. J Clin Endocrinol Metab. 1997;82:3763–3770.

156. Klerman EB, Rimmer DW, Dijk D-J, et al. Nonphotic entrainment of the human circadian pacemaker. Am J Physiol. 1998;43:R991–R996.

157. Kleitman N, Jackson DP. Body temperature and performance under different routines. J Appl Physiol. 1950;3:309–328.

158. Kleitman N, Kleitman E. Effect of non-twenty-four-hour routines of living in oral temperature and heart rate. J Appl Physiol. 1953;6:283–291.

159. Dijk D-J, Czeisler CA. Paradoxical timing of the circadian rhythm of sleep propensity serves to consolidate sleep and wakefulness in humans. Neurosci Lett. 1994;166:63–68.

160. Chiappa KH. Evoked Potentials in Clinical Medicine. Philadelphia, Pa: Lippincott-Raven; 1997.

161. Edgar DM, Dement WC, Fuller CA. Effect of SCN lesions on sleep in squirrel monkeys: evidence for opponent processes in sleep-wake regulation. J Neurosci. 1993;13:1065–1079.

162. Borbély AA, Achermann P. Concepts and models of sleep regulation: an overview. J Sleep Res. 1992;1:63–79.

163. Beersma DGM, Daan S, Dijk D-J. Sleep intensity and timing: a model for their circadian control. Lect Math Life Sci. 1987;19:39–62.

164. Borbély AA. A two process model of sleep regulation. Hum Neurobiol. 1982;1:195–204.

165. Borbély AA, Achermann P, Trachsel L, et al. Sleep initiation and initial sleep intensity: interaction of homeostatic and circadian mechanisms. J Biol Rhythms. 1989;4:149–160.

166. Daan S, Beersma DGM, Borbély AA. Timing of human sleep: recovery process gated by a circadian pacemaker. Am J Physiol. 1984;246:R161–R178.

167. Babkoff H, Caspy T, Mikulincer M, et al. Monotonic and rhythmic influences: a challenge for sleep deprivation research. Psychol Bull. 1991;109:411–428.

168. Åkerstedt T, Folkard S. Predicting duration of sleep from the three process model of regulation of alertness. Occup Environ Med. 1996;53:136–141.

169. Folkard S, Åkerstedt T. A three-process model of the regulation of alertness-sleepiness. In: Broughton RJ, Ogilvie RD, eds. Sleep, Arousal, and Performance. Boston, Mass: Birkhäuser; 1992:11–26.

170. Dijk D-J, Duffy JF, Czeisler CA. Circadian and sleep/wake dependent aspects of subjective alertness and cognitive performance. J Sleep Res. 1992; 1:112–117.

171. Czeisler CA, Dijk D-J, Duffy JF. Entrained phase of the circadian pacemaker serves to stabilize alertness and performance throughout the habitual waking day. In: Ogilvie RD, Harsh JR, eds. Sleep Onset: Normal and Abnormal Processes. Washington, DC: American Psychological Association; 1994:89–110.

172. Czeisler CA, Dijk D-J. Human circadian physiology and sleep-wake regulation. In: Takahashi JS, Turek FW, Moore RY, eds. Handbook of Behavioral Neurobiology: Circadian Clocks. New York, NY: Plenum; 1998.

173. Jewett ME, Dijk D-J, Kronauer RE, et al. Homeostatic and circadian components of subjective alertness interact in a non-additive manner during 48 hours of sleep deprivation. J Sleep Res. 1996;5:101.

174. Wyatt JK, Dijk D-J, Ronda JM, et al. Interaction of circadian and sleep/wake homeostatic-processes modulate psychomotor vigilance test (PVT) performance. Sleep Res. 1997;26:759.

175. Czeisler CA, Guilleminault C. REM Sleep: Its Temporal Distribution. New York, NY: Raven Press; 1980.

176. Carskadon MA, Dement WC. Sleep studies on a 90-minute day. Electroencephalogr Clin Neurophysiol. 1975;39:145–155.

177. Weitzman ED, Nogeire C, Perlow M, et al. Effects of a prolonged 3-hour sleep-wake cycle on sleep stages, plasma cortisol, growth hormone, and body temperature in man. J Clin Endocrinol Metab. 1974;38:1018–1030.

178. Czeisler CA, Zimmerman JC, Ronda JM, et al. Timing of REM sleep is coupled to the circadian rhythm of body temperature in man. Sleep. 1980;2:329–346.

179. Czeisler CA, Weitzman ED, Moore-Ede MC, et al. Human sleep: its duration and organization depend on its circadian phase. Science. 1980;210:1264–1267.

180. Zimmerman JC, Czeisler CA, Laxminarayan S, et al. REM density is disassociated from REM sleep timing during free-running sleep episodes. Sleep. 1980;2:409–415.

181. Klein T, Martens H, Dijk D-J, et al. Chronic non-24-hour circadian rhythm sleep disorder in a blind man with a regular 24-hour sleep-wake schedule. Sleep. 1993;16:333–343.

182. Dijk D-J, Shanahan TL, Duffy JF, et al. Variation of electroencephalographic activity during nonREM and REM sleep with phase of circadian melatonin rhythm in humans. J Physiol (Lond). 1997;505.3:851–858.

183. Weaver DR, Stehle JH, Stopa EG, et al. Melatonin receptors in human hypothalamus and pituitary: implications for circadian and reproductive responses to melatonin. J Clin Endocrinol Metab. 1993;76:295–301.

184. Reppert SM, Weaver DR, Rivkees SA, et al. Putative melatonin receptors in a human biological clock. Science. 1988;242:78–81.

185. Liu C, Weaver DR, Jin X, et al. Molecular dissection of two distinct actions of melatonin on the suprachiasmatic circadian clock. Neuron. 1997;19:91–102.

186. Lavie P. Melatonin: role in gating nocturnal rise in sleep propensity. J Biol Rhythms. 1997;12:657–665.

187. Shochat T, Luboshitzky R, Lavie P. Nocturnal melatonin onset is phase locked to the primary sleep gate. Am J Physiol. 1997;273:R364–R370.

188. Tzischinsky O, Shlitner A, Lavie P. The association between the nocturnal sleep gate and nocturnal onset of urinary 6-sulfatoxymelatonin. J Biol Rhythms. 1993;8:199–209.

189. Dawson D, van den Heuvel CJ. Integrating the actions of melatonin on human physiology. Ann Med. 1998;30:95–102.

190. Wu RH, Thorpy MJ. Effect of growth hormone treatment on sleep EEGs in growth hormone-deficient children. Sleep. 1988;11:425–429.

191. Mendelson WB, Slater S, Gold P, et al. The effect of growth hormone administration on human sleep: a dose-response study. Biol Psychiatry. 1980;15:613–618.

192. Astrom C, Trojaborg W. Effect of growth hormone on human sleep energy. Clin Endocrinol (Oxf). 1992;36:241–245.

193. Jordan J, Montgomery I, Trinder J. The effect of afternoon body heating on body temperature and slow wave sleep. Psychophysiology. 1990;27:560–566.

194. Dorsey CM, Lukas S, Teicher MH, et al. Effects of passive body heating on the sleep of older female insomniacs. J Geriatr Psychiatry Neurol. 1996;9:83–90.

195. Aschoff J, Wever R. Spontanperiodik des Menschen bei Ausschluss aller Zeitgeber. Die Naturwissenschaften. 1962;49:337–342.

196. Mills JN. Circadian rhythms during and after three months in solitude underground. J Physiol (Lond). 1964;174:217–231.

197. Webb WB, Agnew HW Jr. Sleep and waking in a time-free environment. Aerospace Med. 1974;45:617–622.

198. Findley JD, Mailer BM, Brady JV. A long term study of human performance in a continuously programmed experimental environment. Space Research Laboratory Technical Report Series. College Park, Md: University of Maryland; 1963.

199. Siffre M. Beyond Time. New York, NY: McGraw-Hill; 1964.

200. Klerman EB, Dijk D-J, Kronauer RE, et al. Simulations of effects of light on the human circadian pacemaker: implications for assessment of intrinsic period. Am J Physiol. 1996;270:R271–R282.

201. Czeisler CA, Allan JS, Kronauer RE. A method to assess the intrinsic period of the endogenous circadian oscillator. Sleep Res. 1986;15:266–266.

202. Czeisler CA, Allan JS, Kronauer RE. A method for assaying the effects of therapeutic agents on the period of the endogenous circadian pacemaker in man. In: Montplaisir J, Godbout R, eds. Sleep and Biological Rhythms: Basic Mechanisms and Applications to Psychiatry. New York, NY: Oxford University Press; 1990:87–98.

203. Czeisler CA, Duffy JF, Shanahan TL, et al. Reassessment of the

intrinsic period (t) of the human circadian pacemaker in young and older subjects. Sleep Res. 1995;24A:505.

204. Shanahan TL, Emens JS, Czeisler CA. Estimation of the intrinsic period of the human circadian pacemaker during forced desynchrony using the daily melatonin pattern. Sleep Res. 1994;23:511.

204a. Czeisler CA, Duffy JF, Shanahan TL, et al. Stability, precision, and near 24-hour period of the human circadian pacemaker. Science. 1999;284:2177–2181.

205. Campbell SS, Dawson D, Zulley J. When the human circadian system is caught napping: evidence for endogenous rhythms close to 24 hours. Sleep. 1993;16:638–640.

206. Middleton B, Arendt J, Stone BM. Complex effects of melatonin on human circadian rhythms in constant dim light. J Biol Rhythms. 1997;12:467–477.

207. Middleton B, Arendt J, Stone BM. Human circadian rhythms in constant dim light (8 lux) with knowledge of clock time. J Sleep Res. 1996;5:69–76.

208. Hiddinga AE, Beersma DGM, van den Hoofdakker RH. Endogenous and exogenous components in the circadian variation of core body temperature in humans. J Sleep Res. 1997;6:156–163.

208a. Carskadon MA, Labyak SE, Acebo C, et al. Intrinsic circadian period of adolescent humans measured in conditions of forced desynchrony. Neurosci Lett. 1999;260:129–132.

209. Dunlap JC. An end in the beginning. Science. 1998;280:1548.

210. Roenneberg T, Merrow M. Molecular circadian oscillators: an alternative hypothesis. J Biol Rhythms. 1998;13:167–179.

211. Leloup JC, Goldbeter A. A model for circadian rhythms in *Drosophila* incorporating the formation of a complex between the PER and TIM proteins. J Biol Rhythms. 1998;13:70–87.

212. Darlington TK, Wager-Smith K, Ceriani MF, et al. Closing the circadian loop: CLOCK-induced transcription of its own inhibitors *per* and *tim*. Science. 1998;280:1599–1603.

213. Gekakis N, Staknis D, Nguyen HB, et al. Role of CLOCK protein in the mammalian circadian mechanism. Science. 1998; 280:1564–1569.

214. Carter DA, Murphy D. Circadian rhythms and autoregulatory transcription loops: going round in circles? Mol Cell Endocrinol. 1996;124:1–5.

215. Young DM. The *Drosophila* genes *timeless* and *period* collaborate to promote cycles of gene expression composing a circadian pacemaker. Prog Brain Res. 1996;111:29–39.

216. Rosato E, Piccin A, Kyriacou CP. Circadian rhythms: from behavior to molecules. Biofeed Self-Reg. 1997;19:1075–1082.

217. Dunlap JC, Loros JJ, Merrow M, et al. The genetic and molecular dissection of a prototypic circadian system. Prog Brain Res. 1996;111:11–27.

218. Dunlap JC. Genetic and molecular analysis of circadian rhythms. Annu Rev Genet. 1996;30:579–601.

219. Linkowski P, Spiegel K, Kerkhofs M, et al. Genetic and environmental influences on prolactin secretion during wake and during sleep. Am J Physiol. 1998;274:E909–E919.

220. Linkowski P. Genetic influences on EEG sleep and the human circadian clock: a twin study. Pharmacopsychiatry. 1994;27:7–10.

221. Linkowski P, Van Onderbergen A, Kerkhof G, et al. Twin study of the 24-h cortisol profile: evidence for genetic control of the human circadian clock. Am J Physiol. 1993;264:E173–E181.

222. Degaute JP, Van Cauter E, Van de Borne P, et al. Twenty-four-hour blood pressure and heart rate profiles in humans: a twin study. Hypertension. 1994;23:244–253.

223. Fukuda K. Twins under shift work: a case study of sleep log data. Percept Mot Skills. 1997;84:931–937.

223a. Duffy JF, Rimmer DW, Silva EJ, et al. Correlation of intrinsic circadian period with morningness-eveningness in young men. Sleep. 1999;22:S92.

224. Hoffmann K. Zur beziehung zwischen phasenlage und spontanfrequenz bei der endogenen tagesperiodik. Z Naturforsch. 1963; 18:154–157.

225. Pittendrigh CS, Daan S. A functional analysis of circadian pacemakers in nocturnal rodents, IV: entrainment: pacemaker as clock. J Comp Physiol [A]. 1976;106:291–331.

226. Kerkhof GA, van Dongen HPA. Morning-type and evening-type individuals differ in the phase position of their endogenous circadian oscillator. Neurosci Lett. 1996;218:153–156.

227. Duffy JF, Dijk D-J, Hall EF, et al. Relationship of endogenous circadian melatonin and temperature rhythms to self-reported preference for morning or evening activity in young and older people. J Investig Med. 1999;47:141–150.

228. Lacoste V, Wetterberg L. Individual variations of rhythms in morning and evening types with special emphasis on seasonal differences. In: Wetterberg L, ed. Light and Biological Rhythms in Man. Oxford, England: Pergamon Press; 1993:287–304.

229. Horne JA, Östberg O. Individual differences in human circadian rhythms. Biol Psychol. 1977;5:179–190.

229a. Jones CR, Campbell SS, Zone SE, et al. Familial advanced sleep-phase syndrome: a short-period circadian rhythm variant in humans. Nature Med. 1999;5:1062–1065.

230. Campbell SS, Murphy PJ. Relationships between sleep and body temperature in middle-aged and older subjects. J Am Geriatr Soc. 1998;46:458–462.

231. Copinschi G, Van Cauter E. Effects of ageing on modulation of hormonal secretions by sleep and circadian rhythmicity. Horm Res. 1995;43:20–24.

232. Czeisler CA, Dumont M, Duffy JF, et al. Association of sleep-wake habits in older people with changes in output of circadian pacemaker. Lancet. 1992;340:933–936.

233. Davis FC, Viswanathan N. Stability of circadian timing with age in Syrian hamsters. Am J Physiol. 1998;275:R960–R968.

234. Van Cauter E, Leproult R, Kupfer DJ. Effects of gender and age on the levels and circadian rhythmicity of plasma cortisol. J Clin Endocrinol Metab. 1996;81:2468–2473.

235. Kramer CJ, Hofman WF, Kerkhof GA. Circadian rhythmicity and performance in healthy aging. J Sleep Res. 1996;5:112.

236. Touitou Y, Bogdan A, Haus E, et al. Modifications of circadian and circannual rhythms with aging. Exp Gerontol. 1997;32:603–614.

237. Myers BL, Badia P. Changes in circadian rhythms and sleep quality with aging: mechanisms and interventions. Neurosci Biobehav Rev. 1995;19:553–571.

238. Bliwise DL. Review: sleep in normal aging and dementia. Sleep. 1993;16:40–81.

239. Haimov I, Lavie P. Circadian characteristics of sleep propensity function in healthy elderly: a comparison with young adults. Sleep. 1997;20:294–300.

240. Monk TH, Buysse DJ, Reynolds CF III, et al. Subjective alertness rhythms in elderly people. J Biol Rhythms. 1996;11:268–276.

241. Monk TH, Buysse DJ, Reynolds CF III, et al. Circadian temperature rhythms of older people. Exp Gerontol. 1995;30:455–474.

242. Turek FW, Penev P, Zhang Y, et al. Alterations in the circadian system in advanced age. Ciba Found Symp. 1995;183:212–226.

243. Foley DJ, Monjan AA, Brown SL, et al. Sleep complaints among elderly persons: an epidemiologic study of three communities. Sleep. 1995;18:425–432.

244. Duffy JF, Dijk D-J, Klerman EB, et al. Altered phase relationship between body temperature cycle and habitual awakening in older subjects. Sleep Res. 1997;26:711.

245. Dijk D-J, Duffy JF, Riel E, et al. Aging and the circadian and homeostatic regulation of human sleep during scheduled desynchrony of rest, melatonin and temperature rhythms. J Physiol (Lond). 1999;516:611–627.

246. Duffy JF, Dijk D-J, Czeisler CA. Subjective assessment of early awakening in young and older subjects during forced desynchrony. Sleep Res. 1996;25:546.

247. Harrison Y, Horne JA. Should we be taking more sleep? Sleep. 1995;18:901–907.

248. Dement WC, Mitler MM. It's time to wake up to the importance of sleep disorders. JAMA. 1993;269:1548–1550.

249. Wehr TA, Giesen HA, Moul DE, et al. Suppression of men's responses to seasonal changes in day length by modern artificial lighting. Am J Physiol. 1995;269:R173–R178.

250. Achermann P, Werth E, Dijk D-J, et al. Time course of sleep inertia after nighttime and daytime sleep episodes. Arch Ital Biol. 1995;134:109–119.

251. Jewett ME, Wyatt JK, Ritz-DeCecco AR, et al. Time course of sleep inertia dissipation in human performance and alertness. J Sleep Res. 1999;8:1–8.

29

Sleep Homeostasis and Models of Sleep Regulation

Alexander A. Borbély

Peter Achermann

The level of electroencephalographic (EEG) slow wave activity (SWA) is determined by the duration of prior sleep and waking. SWA is a marker of nonrapid eye movement (NREM) sleep intensity and may serve as an indicator of NREM sleep homeostasis. Power in the range of sleep spindles (spindle frequency activity, SFA) shows in part an inverse relationship to SWA. This observation can be accounted for by neurophysiological data. Thalamocortical neurons exhibit oscillations in the range of sleep spindles at an intermediate level of hyperpolarization (corresponding to superficial NREM sleep), and slow oscillations at a high level of hyperpolarization (corresponding to deep NREM sleep). Although the homeostatic NREM sleep process is largely independent of circadian factors, it interacts with the circadian rhythm of sleep propensity.

The two-process model of sleep regulation is based on the homeostatic process S and the circadian process C. Advanced versions of its homeostatic part can simulate the SWA pattern for a variety of experimental schedules. Essential aspects of the model have been validated by results from forced desynchrony protocols. Other models include the two-oscillator model, the reciprocal interaction models, and combined models. The incorporation of rapid eye movement (REM) sleep homeostasis is still at an early stage.

There is recent evidence for a local, use-dependent facet of sleep regulation. This concept is derived from unihemispheric sleep experiments in marine mammals, and from studies revealing specific regional effects in the sleep EEG of humans. The modeling approach could be extended to local sleep.

Three basic processes underlie sleep regulation: (1) a homeostatic process determined by sleep and waking; (2) a circadian process, a clock-like mechanism defining the alternation of periods with high and low sleep propensity and being basically independent of sleep and waking; and (3) an ultradian process occurring within sleep and represented by the alternation of the two basic sleep states—nonrapid eye movement (NREM) sleep and rapid eye movement (REM) sleep. This chapter focuses on "sleep homeostasis." Homeostasis has been defined as "the coordinated physiological processes which maintain most of the steady states in the organism."[1] The term *sleep homeostasis*[2] refers to the sleep-wake–dependent aspect of sleep regulation, as homeostatic mechanisms counteract deviations from an average "reference level" of sleep. They augment sleep propensity when sleep is curtailed or absent, and they reduce sleep propensity in response to excess sleep.

The interest in modeling the processes underlying sleep regulation has increased over the past decade. In the research briefing report of the Institute of Medicine,[3] a panel of leading North American experts in basic sleep research recommended that "the homeostatic and circadian influences need to be integrated into a single functional model that can describe both the timing of sleep and its quality." Models help delineate the processes involved in the regulation of sleep and thereby offer a conceptual framework for the analysis of existing and new data.

HOMEOSTATIC REGULATION OF SLEEP

Electroencephalographic Slow Wave Activity: A Physiological Indicator of NREM Sleep Homeostasis

Slow-Wave Sleep and Slow Wave Activity. NREM sleep is not a homogeneous substate of sleep, but can be subdivided according to the predominance of electroencephalographic (EEG) slow wave activity (SWA). The percentage of slow waves (frequency, 0 to 2 Hz; minimum peak-to-peak value, 75 μV) is the major criterion for scoring human NREM sleep into the stages 2, 3, or 4.[4] Stages 3 and 4 are commonly referred to as slow-wave sleep (SWS). However, the conventional sleep scoring method is inadequate for a quantitative analysis, because the sleep stages are based on rather general and arbitrary criteria. Presently, EEG parameters can be assessed by computer-aided methods of signal analysis. One of the most important functional EEG parameters will be referred to as "slow wave activity." It is equivalent to "delta activity" and encompasses components of the EEG signal in the frequency range of approximately 0.5 to 4.5 Hz as obtained by spectral analysis (e.g., see reference 5).

Slow Oscillations (Less Than 1 Hz). Recently, a novel low-frequency component with a mean peak value of 0.7 to 0.8 Hz was identified in the power spectrum of NREM sleep.[6, 7] Its frequency corresponded to the 0.7- to 0.9-Hz oscillation that has been reported in the sleeping cat[8] (see: Relationship to Neurophysiology). This slow component had been obscured in previous studies of the human sleep EEG owing to the attenuating effect of EEG amplifiers in the low-frequency range. The typical decline in delta activity from the first to the second NREM sleep episode was not present at frequencies below 2 Hz. Periodicity at even lower frequencies was identified. Thus the occurrence of sleep spindle activity showed a 4-sec periodicity[6, 9] and slow waves tended to recur at 20- to 30-sec intervals.[6]

Slow Waves and Sleep Intensity. It was recognized as early as 1937 that sleep intensity is reflected by the predominance of slow waves in the sleep EEG.[10] Subsequent studies confirmed that the responsiveness to stimuli decreases as EEG slow waves become more predominant.[11] Under physiological conditions, this EEG parameter can be regarded therefore as an indicator of "sleep depth" or "sleep intensity." This statement applies not only to human beings but also to animals.

Global Time Course of Slow Wave Activity During Sleep. Figure 29–1 illustrates the conventionally scored sleep stages and SWA of a young subject. Note that SWS provides a rough indication of the prevalence of SWA. However, this EEG parameter shows a rather continuous rise from sleep onset to stage 4, a change that is only grossly reflected by the stepwise transitions of the sleep stages. In general, the measure derived directly from the EEG signal shows the variations of the NREM-REM sleep cycle and the fluctuations within NREM sleep episodes in much greater detail than the sleep profile. Moreover, the EEG parameter lends itself to a quantitative analysis from which inferences can be made regarding the underlying processes.

It is a plausible assumption that "sleep need" is high during the initial part of the sleep episode and gradually declines with the progression of sleep. In

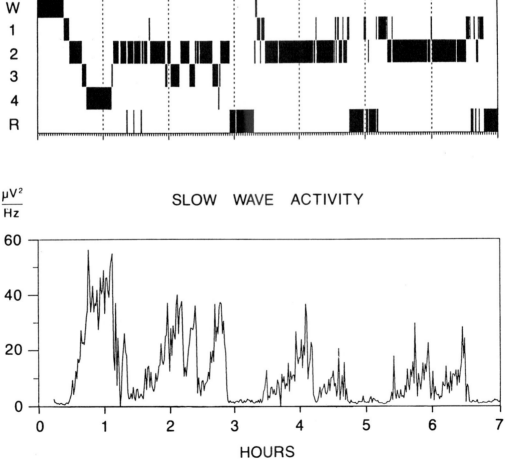

Figure 29–1. Sleep stages and slow wave activity. Sleep stages were scored for 30-sec epochs, slow wave activity (i.e., mean power density in the 0.75- to 4.5-Hz band) was calculated for 1-min epochs. (Modified from Achermann P, Borbély AA. Dynamics of EEG slow wave activity during physiological sleep and after administration of benzodiazepine hypnotics. Hum Neurobiol. 1987;6:203–210.)

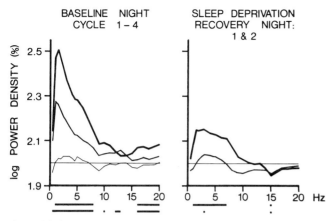

Figure 29–2. *Left,* Changes of relative spectral power density over the first four NREM-REM sleep cycles of a baseline night (N = 8; curves for consecutive cycles indicated by decreasing thickness of lines). In each frequency bin the data are expressed relative to the value in the fourth cycle (100%; horizontal line). *Right,* Effect of sleep deprivation (40.5 h waking) on spectra of the sleep electroencephalogram. In each bin, the values of the first two recovery nights are plotted relative to the baseline night (100%). The upper and lower horizontal bars below the abscissa indicate for the left part significant differences between cycle 1 and 2, and between cycle 2 and 3, respectively, and for the right part between recovery 1 and baseline, and between recovery 2 and baseline, respectively. (Modified from Borbély AA, Baumann F, Brandeis D, et al. Sleep deprivation: effect on sleep stages and EEG power density in man. Electroencephalogr Clin Neurophysiol. 1981;51:483–493.)

accordance with this notion, it has been reported in early studies that both the arousal threshold and the predominance of slow waves in the EEG were high in the initial part of sleep and then progressively decreased.[10] Thus SWS, the high-intensity part of NREM sleep, appeared to be a good candidate for a physiological indicator of sleep homeostasis. The predominance of SWS in the early part of the sleep episode was confirmed in subsequent studies.[11–13]

All-night spectral analysis of the sleep EEG made it possible to quantify SWA and to delineate its time course during sleep.[5] Its mean value per cycle plotted for consecutive NREM-REM sleep cycles showed a monotonic decline over the first three cycles.

Figure 29–2 (left) shows the changes of mean EEG power density over four cycles for the frequency range between 0.25 and 20 Hz. The values of each bin are expressed relative to the reference level of cycle 4 (100%). Note that although the largest changes occur in the low delta range, they encompass frequencies up to the theta band.

Nap Studies. The analysis of daytime naps is useful for assessing the level of SWA after various durations of waking. The observation that the naps taken later in the day contained more SWS than naps taken early in the day[14] has been recently confirmed.[15] In a detailed study of daytime naps scheduled at 2-h intervals throughout the day, direct evidence for a monotonic rise of SWA was obtained.[16–18]

If naps reverse the rising trend of slow wave propensity, a reduction of SWA in the subsequent nighttime sleep can be expected. This prediction was borne out by the results of several experiments.[19–24] When the

duration of nighttime sleep was shortened, SWA in a subsequent morning nap was enhanced.[25, 26]

Effect of Sleep Deprivation. It has been repeatedly shown that partial or total sleep deprivation gives rise to increased SWS in the recovery night (see reference 27 for a review of the older literature). Webb and Agnew[13] presented compelling evidence that SWS increases as a function of prior waking. The quantitative assessment of SWA by all-night spectral analysis revealed that a night without sleep (i.e., 40.5 h of wakefulness) resulted in an enhancement of this EEG parameter during recovery sleep.[5] Figure 29–2 (right) illustrates the changes of power density in the two recovery nights relative to the baseline level (100%). In the first recovery night, the largest increase was present in the low delta range, the part of the spectrum undergoing the largest changes in the course of baseline sleep (see Fig. 29–2, left).

Figure 29–3 depicts the global trend as well as the ultradian dynamics of SWA over successive NREM-REM sleep cycles. The prolongation of the waking period causes a prominent rise of SWA during recovery sleep. A declining trend over three to four cycles is evident in both records. Note that the peaks are at a steady low level during last four cycles of recovery sleep.

The enhancement of SWA by sleep deprivation was confirmed in several studies[28, 29] (for references before 1992, see reference 30). The extent of the increase was shown to be a function of the duration of prior waking.[18, 31]

Intranight Rebound After Selective Slow Wave Deprivation. The propensity of SWA does not necessarily steeply decline during sleep but may persist at an elevated level if the occurrence of SWS is prevented. Thus a slow wave suppression by acoustic stimuli during the first 3 h of sleep resulted in a prominent rise of SWA after discontinuation of the stimuli[32] (see also reference 33 for a related study). In another study, daytime sleep episodes with and without SWS deprivation were compared.[34] The experimental suppression of SWS during an interval corresponding to 90% of the undisturbed episode resulted in an increased accumulation of SWS and an extension of sleep duration. Taken together, the results indicate that slow waves are not merely an epiphenomenon of sleep but reflect major sleep-regulating mechanisms.

Ultradian Dynamics of Slow Wave Activity and Spindle Frequency Activity

Buildup of Slow Wave Activity Within NREM Sleep Episodes. Not only the mean level and the peak of SWA is determined by the duration of prior waking and sleep but also the rise rate within single NREM sleep episodes.[35–37] It is evident from Figures 29–3 and 29–4 that the rise rate of SWA decreases over the first three episodes both under baseline conditions and during recovery from sleep deprivation. In addition, the effect of prolonged waking manifests itself in a steeper

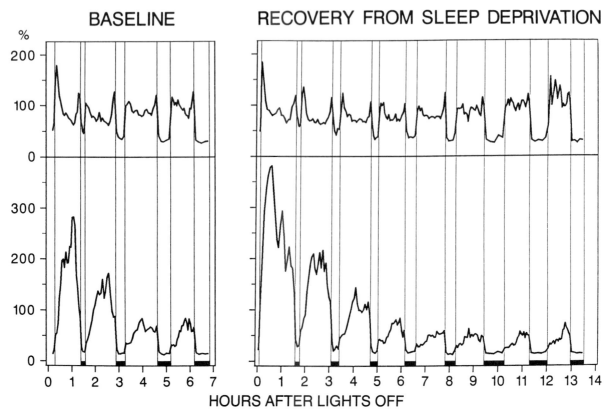

Figure 29–3. Time course of slow wave activity (power density in the 0.75- to 4.5-Hz band; lower curves) and activity in the spindle frequency range (13.25- to 15.0-Hz; upper curves) recorded under baseline conditions and after sleep deprivation (36 h of wakefulness). The NREM sleep episodes were divided into 20 equal parts, the REM sleep episode into five equal parts. The curves represent mean percentile values (N = 8 except for cycle 8 of recovery sleep where N = 6) and have been expressed relative to the mean slow wave activity level in baseline NREM sleep (100%). The mean timing of REM sleep episodes is delimited by vertical lines and horizontal bars above the abscissa. (Reanalysis of the data from Dijk DJ, Brunner DP, Borbély AA. Time course of EEG power density during long sleep in humans. Am J Physiol. 1990;258:R650–651, by D. Aeschbach.)

buildup (of SWA) within the episodes[28, 29, 37] (see Fig. 29–4).

Slow Wave Activity and Spindle Frequency Activity. The term *spindle frequency activity* (SFA) is used to denote the power density in the frequency range of sleep spindles (12 to 15 Hz). There is a close correspondence between this measure and measures based on the occurrence of sleep spindles.[28]

The time courses of SWA and SFA differ in several respects. The global declining trend of SWA is not present in the spindle frequency range. Within NREM sleep episodes, SFA shows a bimodal pattern with an initial and a terminal peak. This gives rise to a U-shaped curve within the episode and a partly inverse relationship to SWA[28, 38–43] (see Fig. 29–3). This inverse relationship becomes less prominent with age.[44] Within the 12- to 15-Hz range, low-frequency (12 to 13 Hz) and high-frequency (14 to 15 Hz) activity exhibited opposite circadian variations.[40, 45, 46] These results support the notion that there are at least two different types of spindles (see also references 47 through 50).

Sleep spindles in the 13- to 14-Hz band are remarkable because of their high intrahemispheric and interhemispheric coherence.[51, 52] This raises the question whether this episodic, high-coherence activity is of functional significance for sleep and whether sleep

spindles may represent carrier frequencies upon which some relevant information is modulated (see reference 51 for a further discussion).

Relationship to Neurophysiology. In recent years it has become increasingly evident that the typical oscillations in the sleep EEG are closely associated with cellular changes at the level of thalamic and cortical neurons.[53–58] The progressive hyperpolarization of thalamocortical neurons that occurs during the progression from waking to deep NREM sleep[59] results in fluctuations in the membrane potential, which are initially in the frequency range of sleep spindles and then in the range of delta waves.[53, 54, 56, 60] Synchronized oscillations appear to arise from the progressive recruitment of neurons, and their spontaneous cessation from a hyperpolarization-activated cation conductance.[61] The oscillations at the neuronal level are associated with corresponding changes in the EEG. The progressive hyperpolarization of thalamocortical neurons after sleep onset[59] provides an explanation for the predominance of SFA in the initial phases of NREM sleep, which give way to slow waves as sleep progresses.[28, 38] These changes occur more rapidly when sleep pressure is high[28, 29, 39] and are retarded when sleep pressure is reduced.[24]

In 1993 a new type of slow oscillation was reported

to occur in the thalamocortical system.[53-55] Its frequency (less than 1 Hz) was lower than that of the delta rhythm (1 to 4 Hz). This slow oscillation originating in cortical networks consisted of rhythmical depolarizing components separated by prolonged (0.2 to 0.8 sec) hyperpolarizations,[55] which grouped the thalamically generated spindles and the delta waves in slowly recurring sequences.[53, 55, 62] Long-lasting hyperpolarizations were associated with prolonged depth positive waves in the cortical EEG. Recently, a novel low-frequency component with a mean peak value of 0.7 to 0.8 Hz was identified in the power spectrum of NREM sleep.[6, 7] Its frequency corresponded to the 0.7- to 0.9-Hz oscillation that has been reported in the sleeping cat.[8] The important role of gamma oscillations in sleep is increasingly recognized and is studied both at the level of neurons[7, 8, 63] and the EEG.[64-66] Taken together, the new developments indicate that not only the sleep-related changes but also the mechanisms underlying sleep homeostasis will be open for investigation at the cellular level.

NREM vs REM Sleep Homeostasis

Effect of NREM Sleep Pressure on REM Sleep Homeostasis. During recovery from total sleep deprivation, SWS and EEG SWA exhibit an immediate rebound, whereas the increase in REM sleep is delayed to subsequent nights or is not present at all. Selective REM sleep deprivation augments "REM sleep pressure," which is manifested by the increasing number of interventions required to prevent REM sleep episodes (for the older literature, see references in Borbély[27]). However, the occurrence of a REM sleep rebound during recovery sleep is either inconsistent[67] or smaller than expected on the basis of the deficit.[68] This may suggest that REM sleep is not as finely regulated as SWS. However, this notion is contradicted by recent partial sleep deprivation studies. A REM sleep deprivation in the first 5 h of sleep induced a REM sleep rebound in the subsequent 2.25 h.[69] A curtailment of sleep duration during 2 or 4 nights, which induced a substantial REM sleep deficit, was followed by a REM sleep rebound in the 2 recovery nights.[70, 71] In these experiments, the REM sleep rebound occurred at a time when slow wave pressure was either low at the end of sleep[69] or was much less increased than "REM sleep pressure."[70, 71] These results also suggest that REM sleep is finely regulated but that the manifestation of REM sleep homeostasis is hampered by an elevated slow wave pressure.

Effect of REM Sleep Pressure on the REM Sleep EEG. An electrophysiological indicator of an intensity dimension of human REM sleep, comparable to SWA in NREM sleep, has not been identified. The density of rapid eye movements is not associated with REM sleep pressure[72] but is inversely related to slow wave propensity.[24, 29, 73-75] In a recent selective REM sleep experiment, power in the alpha band was reduced in the REM sleep EEG during recovery sleep.[68, 68a] This effect was most pronounced in the first recovery night and then gradually subsided. A progressive and persistent attenuation of alpha activity in REM sleep has been ob-

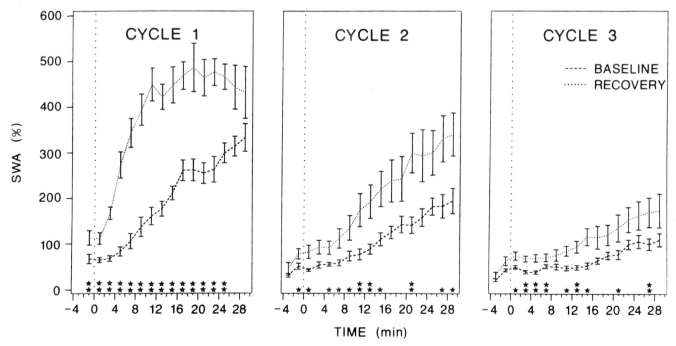

Figure 29–4. Buildup of slow wave activity (power density in the 0.75- to 4.5-Hz range) during the first 30 min of NREM sleep episodes 1, 2, and 3 for baseline conditions and after sleep deprivation (36 h of wakefulness). The data are expressed relative to the mean slow wave activity in the baseline sleep episode (100%). Mean values with standard errors (N = 9). Interrupted vertical lines delineate beginning of NREM sleep episode. Asterisks indicate significant differences between baseline and recovery nights (*P <.05; **P <.01; paired t-test on log-transformed values). (From Dijk DJ, Brunner DP, Borbély AA. Time course of EEG power density during long sleep in humans. Am J Physiol. 1990; 258:R650–651.)

served previously during recovery from total sleep deprivation,[5] as well as in a 4-day partial sleep deprivation protocol that induced a preferential deficit in REM sleep.[71] Therefore, alpha activity in REM sleep seems to be inversely related to REM sleep pressure. This conclusion is supported by a forced desynchrony study where the circadian rhythm of alpha activity in REM sleep and the REM sleep fraction of total sleep showed an inverse relationship.[46]

Effect of REM Sleep Pressure on the NREM Sleep EEG. In accordance with the notion of a mutual inhibitory interaction of the factors controlling SWA and REM sleep,[27] not only REM sleep is inhibited by "slow wave pressure," but also SWA by REM sleep pressure. Thus there was a significant reduction in the low-frequency activity of the NREM sleep EEG during selective REM sleep deprivation,[69] an observation that was also made in a recent animal experiment.[76] Also, the rise in REM sleep pressure induced by partial sleep deprivation suppressed the typical low-delta peak in the NREM sleep spectrum.[70, 71] However, this effect was not seen after selective REM sleep deprivation.[68]

Independence and Interactions of Homeostatic and Circadian Processes

There is evidence that homeostatic and circadian facets of sleep regulation can be independently manipulated and therefore may be controlled by separate mechanisms. Thus, throughout a 72-h sleep deprivation period, the subjective alertness ratings continued to show a prominent circadian rhythm.[77] Conversely, in a study in which the phase of the circadian process (as indexed by body temperature and plasma melatonin) was shifted by bright light in the morning, the time course of SWA remained unaffected.[78]

A powerful experimental paradigm is the forced desynchrony schedule in which the homeostatic and circadian facet of sleep can be separately analyzed. In this protocol, subjects were scheduled to a 28-h sleep-wake cycle.[45, 46, 79] During one third of the cycle the lights were off and the subjects were encouraged to sleep. Because under these experimental conditions the free-running circadian rhythm has a period of 24.18 h,[80] the sleep episodes occurred at different circadian phases. The data showed that sleep propensity was at the maximum when the circadian rhythm of rectal temperature was at the minimum. Sleep propensity gradually decreased on the rising limb of the rectal temperature rhythm and reached the minimum 16 h after the temperature minimum. This phase corresponds to the habitual bedtime under entrained conditions. When sleep was initiated at this phase, sleep continuity was high. In contrast, poor sleep continuity was observed when sleep was initiated after the temperature minimum.

The analysis of the data showed that SWA was determined mainly by homeostatic (i.e., sleep-waking dependent) factors, whereas the REM/NREM sleep ratio depended on both homeostatic and circadian factors. Furthermore, a previously postulated sleep-related inhibition of REM sleep[27] was confirmed by the results of the forced desynchrony study. Not only was the timing of sleep shown to be governed by the interaction of a homeostatic and a circadian process, but also the changes in daytime vigilance.

MODELS OF SLEEP REGULATION

Models help delineate the processes involved in the regulation of sleep and thereby offer a conceptual framework for the analysis of existing and new data. A synopsis of the major models discussed in this chapter is provided in Table 29–1 (see also references 30, 81, and 81a).

Two-Process Model and Related Models

The relationship between SWS and the duration of prior waking has been documented by Webb and Agnew[13] and placed into a theoretical framework by Feinberg.[82] The two-process model, originally proposed to account for sleep regulation in the rat,[2, 83] postulates that a homeostatic process (process S) rises during waking and declines during sleep, and interacts with a circadian process (process C) that is independent of sleep and waking (Fig. 29–5A). The time course of the homeostatic variable S was derived from EEG SWA. Various aspects of human sleep regulation were addressed in a qualitative version of the two-process model.[27] An elaborated, quantitative version of the model was established in which process S varied between an upper and a lower threshold that are both modulated by a single circadian process[84, 85] (Fig. 29–5B). This model was able to account for such diverse phenomena as recovery from sleep deprivation, circadian phase dependence of sleep duration, sleep during shift work, sleep fragmentation during continuous bed rest, and internal desynchronization in the absence of time cues.[85]

The two-process model triggered numerous experimental studies to test its predictions and was recently used to predict the response of habitual short and long sleepers to sleep deprivation.[29] It was concluded that short sleepers live under a higher NREM sleep pressure than long sleepers, and that the two groups do not differ with respect to the homeostatic regulatory mechanisms.

In a later version of the model (proposed by Beersma et al.[16] and Dijk et al.[32] and formalized by Achermann and Borbély[86]) it is the change of S, and not its level, which is proportional to the momentary SWA. The elaborated model addressed not only the global changes of SWA as represented by process S, but also the changes within NREM sleep episodes. The magnitude of the intranight rebound after selective SWS deprivation in the first 3 h of sleep was in accordance with the prediction.[86]

A further elaborated version of the model was subjected to an optimization procedure.[87] In general, a close fit was obtained between the simulated and em-

Table 29–1. MODELS OF SLEEP REGULATION AND CIRCADIAN RHYTHMS

Designation	Assumption	Description/Comment
Two-Process (S-C) Model and Related Models		
Two-process model[27, 84, 85, 89, 91]	Sleep propensity in humans is determined by a homeostatic process S and circadian process C; the interaction of S and C determines the timing of sleep and waking	Time course of S is derived from EEG slow wave activity; phase position and shape (skewed sine wave) of C are derived from sleep duration data obtained at various times of the 24-h cycle
Model of ultradian variation of slow wave activity[86–88, 122]	Derived from the two-process model; the level of S determines the buildup rate and the saturation level of slow wave activity within NREM sleep episodes	In contrast to the original two-process model, the change of S, not the level of S, corresponds to slow wave activity; a REM sleep oscillator triggers the decline of slow wave activity prior to REM sleep
Three-process model of the regulation of sleepiness and alertness[123–127]	Sleepiness and alertness are simulated by the combined action of a homeostatic process, a circadian process, and sleep inertia (process W); extension to performance, sleep latency, and sleep length	Parameters are derived from rated sleepiness during sleep-wake manipulations; time constant of the homeostatic process is similar to process S in the two-process model[85]; alertness nomogram for sleep-related safety risks
Rhythmostat model of the timing of sleep[128]	Modification of two-process model: the homeostatic process undergoes a circadian modulation	In contrast to the original two-process model, slow wave activity may increase during sleep and decrease during wakefulness; there are also differences with respect to the effects of naps
Two-Oscillator (x-y) and Related Models		
Original x-y model: predominant effect of light on y[95]	Two Van der Pol oscillators x and y affecting each other by "velocity"-type coupling; larger effect of x on y than y on x	"Strong" (x) circadian oscillator controlling core body temperature, REM sleep, cortisol; "weak" (y) circadian oscillator controlling the sleep-wake cycle
Revised x-y model: predominant effect of light on x[129, 130, 130a]	Van der Pol oscillator for x; cumulative effect of light; circadian modulation of sensitivity to light	Simulation of light effects on the human circadian pacemaker
Thermoregulatory model of sleep control[131, 132]	A thermoregulatory feedback control mechanism with modulation by two circadian oscillators; homeostatic features of sleep rhythm are generated by integration of heat load during waking	Simulations under entrained conditions of biphasic sleepiness pattern, timing of sleep, and sleep deprivation
Reciprocal Interaction Models of the NREM-REM Sleep Cycle		
Reciprocal interaction model[96]	NREM-REM sleep cycle generated by two coupled cell populations in the brainstem with self-excitatory and self-inhibitory connections according to the Lotka-Volterra model	Simulation of data: discharge rate of cholinergic FTG (or LDT and PPT) cells in cat; the role of postulated cell populations in the control of REM sleep, and their interactions have undergone revisions[97, 133]
Limit cycle reciprocal interaction model: original version[98, 99]	NREM-REM sleep cycle generated by the reciprocal interaction of two coupled cell populations (REM-on and REM-off)	Main features of previous model are maintained, but assumption of a stable limit cycle oscillation that is independent of initial conditions; introduction of a circadian term, which determines mode of approach to the limit cycle
Limit cycle reciprocal interaction model: extended versions[100]	As above; incorporation of sleep homeostasis and arousal events	Assumption of first-order decay dynamics for the arousal system; arousal as a stochastic process

EEG, electroencephalogram; FTG, gigantocellular tegmental field; LDT, laterodorsal tegmental nucleus; PPT, pedunculopontine tegmental nucleus.

pirical SWA data and their time course (see Fig. 29–5C). In particular, the occurrence of late SWA peaks during extended sleep could be simulated. The simulations demonstrated that the model can account in quantitative terms for empirical data and predict the changes induced by the prolongation of waking or sleep. This version of the model was recently used to simulate the dynamics of SWA in an experimental protocol with an early evening nap[24] and the effect of changes in REM sleep latency on the time course of SWA.[88]

It had been already mentioned that the forced de-synchrony protocol allows assessment of the interactions between the homeostatic (sleep-waking dependent) and circadian (sleep-waking independent) facets of sleep regulation and thereby testing of the essential parts of the two-process model. In accordance with its basic assumption, SWA, the marker of process S, was shown to be determined largely by homeostatic factors, whereas the REM sleep fraction of sleep was determined by both homeostatic and circadian factors.[45] This result corresponds to the propositions of the initial version of the model.[27] Also, the postulated sleep-re-

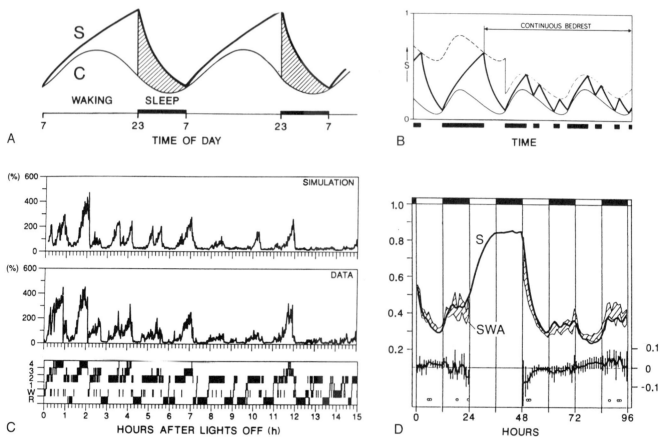

Figure 29–5. Two-process model of sleep regulation. *A,* Time course of homeostatic process S and circadian process C. S rises during waking and declines during sleep. The intersection of S and C defines time of wake-up. (Modified from Borbély AA. A two process model of sleep regulation. Hum Neurobiol. 1982;1:195–204.) *B,* Quantitative two-threshold version of the two-process model. Process S oscillates between upper and lower thresholds that are modulated by the circadian process C and determine the times of onset and termination of sleep, respectively. Due to the reduced arousal level, the upper threshold is lowered in a continuous bed rest schedule, giving rise to a polyphasic sleep-wake cycle. (From Daan S, Beersma DGM, Borbély AA. Timing of human sleep: recovery process gated by a circadian pacemaker. Am J Physiol. 1984;246:R161–178.) *C,* Simulated slow wave activity (*top*), empirical slow-wave activity (*middle*), and sleep stages (*bottom*) of an extended sleep episode. Empirical and simulated values of slow wave activity were standardized with respect to the mean value of the first 7 h of sleep. Values are plotted for 1-min intervals. (Modified from Brain Research Bulletin, Vol 31, Achermann P, Dijk DJ, Brunner DP, et al. A model of human sleep homeostasis based on EEG slow-wave activity: quantitative comparison of data and simulations. 97–113, Copyright 1993, with permission from Elsevier Science.) *D,* Process S and empirical slow wave activity (SWA; 0.75 to 4.0 Hz) in the rat. Simulated process S (continuous line) and confidence interval (95%; n = 9) of slow wave activity in nonrapid eye movement sleep (hatched area) are superimposed for a 96-h period (baseline day, 24-h sleep deprivation, 2 recovery days). Lower curve shows mean differences (±2 SEM) between the linearly transformed SWA and S. SWA was expressed as a percentage of the mean baseline value (100%) and then linearly transformed. The ordinate denotes units of S. Intervals in which SWA and the simulation differed significantly from each other are indicated by circles below the difference curve (P <.05; two-tailed paired *t*-test). Black horizontal bars on top delineate the 12-h dark periods. (Modified from Franken P, Tobler I, Borbély AA. Sleep homeostasis in the rat: simulation of the time course of EEG slow-wave activity [published erratum appeared in Neurosci Lett. 1991;132:279]. Neurosci Lett. 1991;130:141–144.)

lated inhibition of REM sleep was confirmed by the results of the forced desynchrony study. Finally, the data analysis showed that not only the timing of sleep but also the changes in daytime vigilance are governed by the interaction of processes S and C, as simulated by Daan et al.[85] The rising homeostatic sleep pressure during waking seems to be compensated by the declining circadian sleep propensity.[85, 89–91] Conversely, during sleep the rising circadian sleep propensity may serve to counteract the declining homeostatic sleep pressure, thereby ensuring the maintenance of sleep.[79]

Although the two-process model originated from animal data,[2, 83] it was elaborated for human sleep. A quantitative simulation of NREM homeostasis was performed in the rat[92, 93] (see Fig. 29–5D). SWA determined in nine rats for consecutive 8-sec epochs of a 24-h baseline period, a 24-h sleep deprivation period, and a 48-h recovery period[94] served as the database for the simulation. As in the original human version of the model, process S was assumed to decrease exponentially in NREM sleep, and increase according to a saturating exponential function in waking. Unlike in the human model, an increase of S was assumed to occur also in REM sleep. After optimizing the initial value of S as well as its time constants, a close fit was obtained between the hourly mean values of SWA in NREM sleep and process S. In particular, the typical changes of SWA such as its biphasic time course during baseline, its initial increase after sleep deprivation, and the subsequent prolonged negative rebound could be reproduced.

Two-Oscillator Model

A model based on the two circadian oscillators x and y has been proposed by Kronauer et al.[95] The model attempted to describe general features of the circadian system rather than focus specifically on the regulation of sleep and waking. The main problem with the different versions of the two-oscillator model is that the homeostatic aspect of sleep regulation is not addressed, and that additional assumptions are required to account for the effects of sleep deprivation.

Reciprocal Interaction Models

Reciprocal interaction models account for the cyclical alternation of NREM sleep and REM sleep. A distinctive feature of this class of models is that they evolved from neurophysiological data obtained in animals.[96] Although the original anatomical and physiological assumptions had to be modified,[97] the postulate that the NREM-REM sleep cycle is generated by the reciprocal interaction of two neuronal systems has been maintained. The original proposition of a Lotka-Volterra type of interaction was later transposed to humans, and further elaborated into the limit cycle reciprocal interaction model.[98–100]

Combined Models

Attempts were made to integrate various concepts into a combined model. Achermann and Borbély[101] regarded the models of various authors as "modules," which were linked into a combined model. Although its properties need to be further examined, the first simulations showed that it is feasible to incorporate homeostatic, circadian, and ultradian factors regulating nighttime sleep and daytime sleep propensity in a single model. Similarly, in the most recent extension of the limit cycle reciprocal interaction model,[100] homeostatic, circadian, and ultradian processes have been combined.

PERSPECTIVES

Processes and Models

The main characteristics of the homeostatic and the circadian facet of sleep regulation are summarized in Table 29–2. The major difference consists in the dependence of the former on prior sleep and waking, and in the sleep-wake–independent property of the latter. Sleep intensity of NREM sleep as indicated by SWA is the hallmark of a homeostatically regulated process, whereas the REM sleep fraction of sleep, as well as total sleep time, is the factor that is markedly influenced by the circadian phase. Nevertheless, the latter are also subject to a homeostatic regulation. The brain site in which the sleep-related circadian rhythms are generated is known to be the suprachiasmatic nuclei. By contrast, the neurobiological substrate of sleep homeostasis is still unknown. Neither the brain sites nor the mechanisms underlying homeostatic sleep regulation have been specified. Although this chapter deals with sleep regulation, it is pertinent to mention that a homeostatic process is reflected also in the waking EEG. Thus power in the theta and alpha range was shown to be enhanced after total[102] or partial sleep deprivation.[71] The rise in power during sustained wakefulness in a constant routine protocol occurred according to a saturating exponential function.[103]

Whereas models have focused on NREM sleep homeostasis, on the interaction of NREM and REM sleep, and on the circadian oscillator, REM sleep homeostasis has been largely ignored. In the context of a recent selective REM sleep deprivation experiment,[68] two salient observations were made, which were difficult to reconcile. On the one hand, REM sleep deprivation necessitated a dramatic rise in the frequency of interventions during the night to prevent this sleep state. On the other hand, there was a modest rise in the number of interventions across the three consecutive deprivation nights and the 40% REM sleep rebound in

Table 29–2. HOMEOSTATIC AND CIRCADIAN FACETS OF SLEEP REGULATION

	Homeostatic	Circadian
Influence of prior sleep and waking	Yes	No
Influence of the circadian phase	No	Yes
Sleep parameters most prominently affected	NREM sleep intensity (physiological correlate: EEG slow wave activity)	REM sleep fraction of sleep cycle; total sleep time
Nonsleep correlates	Unknown	Core body temperature; plasma level of certain hormones (e.g., melatonin, cortisol)
Regulatory structure in the brain	Not yet identified	Suprachiasmatic nuclei
Effect of lesioning the suprachiasmatic nuclei	Still operational	Disrupted
Effect of scheduled intensive light exposure in humans	Time course of slow wave activity not affected	Evidence for phase shift

EEG, electroencephalogram.

the first recovery night did by no means compensate for the amount of REM sleep lost. Two hypotheses were advanced. In the first, it is assumed that the homeostatic drive is strong, which is reflected by the dramatic rise in interventions during the deprivation nights. Waking may in part substitute for REM sleep, thereby accounting for the moderate night-to-night increase in interventions and the small REM sleep rebound. According to the second hypothesis, the homeostatic drive for REM sleep is weak and the rising trend in the number of interventions is attributed to circadian factors as well as to a sleep-dependent disinhibition of REM sleep propensity. This hypothesis could explain the limited savings from one night to the other as well as the modest rebound. Franken[104] proposed, on the basis of animal studies, that the initiation and maintenance of REM sleep could be controlled by separate processes and that the former may be accounted for by a rise in REM sleep propensity during NREM sleep, as postulated by Benington and Heller.[105] Further experiments are required to resolve this issue.

In conclusion, models help delineate the regulating processes underlying such a complex and little-understood phenomenon as sleep, and thereby offer a conceptual framework for the analysis of existing and new data. The major models have already inspired a considerable number of experiments. This approach has become particularly attractive by the possibility of using quantitative physiological measures in human beings for testing the predictions of a model. Thus EEG SWA represents the key parameter in the investigation of NREM sleep homeostasis, while the "unmasked" core body temperature and plasma melatonin are valuable indicators of the circadian process. Another positive feature of the modeling approach is the fact that the regulatory processes postulated are not restricted to a single species but probably represent basic mechanisms that are typical of mammalian sleep.[106]

Sleep: A Local, Use-Dependent Brain Phenomenon?

Recently, the question arose whether sleep represents a global or a local brain process. The observations that the dolphin does not exhibit deep SWS in both hemispheres simultaneously, and that the selective deprivation of unihemispheric sleep gives rise to a unihemispheric SWS rebound[107] shows that the sleep process is not necessarily present in the entire brain. There is recent evidence from studies in monkeys that the process of falling asleep may not occur synchronously in the entire brain.[108] Two hypotheses were advanced which imply that regional increases in neuronal activity and metabolic demand during wakefulness may result in selective changes in EEG synchronization of these neuronal populations during NREM sleep.[109, 110] Benington and Heller[110] proposed that adenosine, which is released upon increased metabolic demand via facilitated transport by neurons and glia cells throughout the central nervous system (CNS), promotes slow EEG potentials. Thus a use-dependent,

local mechanism would underlie the sleep deprivation–induced changes in the sleep EEG. There is evidence from microdialysis studies that the adenosine level in the brain rises during waking and declines during sleep.[111]

The tenet of a local, use-dependent increase of sleep intensity was tested by investigating whether a local activation of a particular brain region during wakefulness affects the EEG recorded from the same site during sleep.[112] An intermittent vibratory stimulus was applied to the left or right hand during the 6-h period prior to sleep to activate the contralateral somatosensory cortex. Stimulation of the right (dominant) hand resulted in a shift of power in NREM sleep EEG toward the left hemisphere. This effect was most prominent in the delta range, was limited to the first hour of sleep, and was restricted to the central derivation situated over the somatosensory cortex (Fig. 29–6, right). Finally, a recent topographical study revealed a sleep-dependent hyperfrontality of SWA, which varies in the course of sleep.[47, 48] Thus in the initial two NREM sleep episodes, the power in the 2-Hz band was dominant at the frontal derivation, whereas in the second part of sleep the anteroposterior gradient vanished (Fig. 29–6, left). Recent experiments have shown that a sleep deficit impairs primarily high-level cognitive skills, which depend on frontal lobe function.[113, 114] Patients with lesions of the prefrontal cortex suffer from deficits that include distraction by irrelevant stimuli, diminished word fluency, flat intonation of speech, impaired divergent thinking, apathy, and childish humor.[115] Subjects foregoing sleep exhibit similar symptoms. Therefore, it may be more than a coincidence that the prevalence of slow waves is maximal at frontal EEG derivations in the initial part of sleep. This finding is consistent with the notion that the sleep process may occur in a topographically graded manner by involving preferentially those neuronal populations that have been most activated during waking. It could be speculated that the progressive anteroposterior shift in power in the low-frequency range reflects a high "need of recovery" in frontal parts of the cortex, which seem to exhibit the largest activity during wakefulness.[116] In the framework of the two-process model, the results may indicate that process S declines in the anterior region of the brain at a steeper rate than in posterior regions and that therefore the homeostatic NREM sleep-regulating process may exhibit regional differences. Experiments involving a specific manipulation of daytime activity are required to test this possibility.

Neurochemical and Genetic Facets

This chapter has focused on the homeostatic mechanisms of sleep derived largely from EEG variables and which gave rise to models describing the regulatory aspects. It is evident, however, that sleep homeostasis must have a neurochemical substrate and that possibly genetic mechanisms may be causally involved. The putative implication of adenosine has been mentioned. Another promising lead is the association of growth

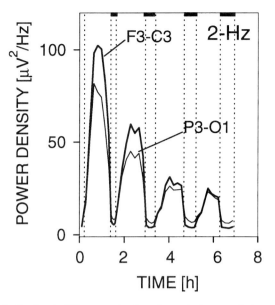
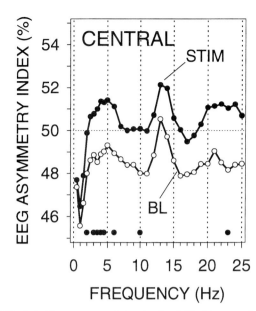

Figure 29–6. Regional differences in the sleep electroencephalogram (EEG). *Left,* Slow wave activity in the 2-Hz bin recorded from the frontocentral (F3-C3; *thick line*) and the parieto-occipital (P3-O1; thin line) derivation. Power density at the anterior site is higher in the first two NREM sleep episodes, but the difference vanishes in the last two episodes. Mean values (N = 20 subjects; 34 nights). Individual NREM sleep episodes were subdivided into seven equal intervals, REM sleep episodes into four intervals, and the time between lights-off and sleep onset was represented as one interval. Data were aligned with respect to sleep onset (cycle 1) or with respect to the first occurrence of stage 2 after a REM sleep episode (cycles 2–4). REM sleep is indicated by horizontal black bars at the top. (Modified from Werth E, Achermann P, Borbély AA. Brain topography of the human sleep EEG: antero-posterior shifts of spectral power. Neuroreport. 1996;8:123–127.) *Right,* Interhemispheric asymmetry index (100* [power in the left derivation]/[power in left and right derivation]) of the central derivation in NREM sleep during the first hour of sleep. An index larger than 50% indicates that power under baseline condition (BL) and after right-hand stimulation (STIM) is larger in the left hemisphere than in the right hemisphere. Circles above the abscissa indicate significant differences from baseline (paired *t*-test, *P* <.05). (Adapted from Kattler H, Dijk DJ, Borbély AA. Effect of unilateral somatosensory stimulation prior to sleep on the sleep EEG in humans. J Sleep Res. 1994;3:159–164.)

hormone (GH) release with SWS, and the evidence that the activation of GH–releasing hormone (GHRH) controls both these factors.[117] Pharmacological agents acting as GH secretagogues (e.g., gamma-hydroxybutyrate[118] and ritanserin[119]) enhance SWA. The question to be resolved is whether it is the homeostatic sleep–regulating mechanism itself that is affected by these agents.

Another approach to uncovering the basic substrates of sleep is derived from the observation that the activity of neuromodulatory systems, which project diffusely to the reticular formation subsides during sleep and that thereby the pathways mediating the phosphorylation of transcription factors and the induction of immediate early genes become ineffective.[120] This change may represent an essential cellular signature of sleep (see reference 120). A link to energy metabolism is suggested by the recent finding that the level of mitochondrial messenger RNAs (mRNAs) that are transcribed and translated into subunits of respiratory enzymes is considerably higher during waking than during sleep.[121] In conclusion, the identification of cellular and genetic correlates of sleep regulation may open the possibility of performing in vitro experiments (i.e., brain slices or cell cultures) to investigate the basic mechanisms of sleep.

Acknowledgments

This work was supported by the Swiss National Science Foundation. The comments of Dr. Irene Tobler and the assistance of Ms. Yvonne Maeder are gratefully acknowledged.

References

1. Cannon WB. The Wisdom of the Body. New York: NY, WW Norton; 1939.
2. Borbély AA. Sleep: Circadian rhythm versus recovery process. In: Koukkou M, Lehmann D, Angst J, eds. Functional States of the Brain: Their Determinants. Amsterdam, Netherlands: Elsevier; 1980:151–161.
3. Basic Sleep Research. Research Briefing. Division of Health Sciences Policy, Institute of Medicine. Washington, DC: National Academy Press; 1990.
4. Rechtschaffen A, Kales A, eds. A Manual of Standardized Terminology, Techniques and Scoring System for Sleep Stages of Human Subjects. Bethesda, Md: National Institutes of Health; 1968.
5. Borbély AA, Baumann F, Brandeis D, et al. Sleep deprivation: effect on sleep stages and EEG power density in man. Electroencephalogr Clin Neurophysiol. 1981;51:483–493.
6. Achermann P, Borbély AA. Low-frequency (<1 Hz) oscillations in the human sleep EEG. Neuroscience. 1997;81:213–222.
7. Amzica F, Steriade M. The K-complex—its slow (<1-Hz) rhythmicity and relation to delta waves. Neurology. 1997;49:952–959.
8. Steriade M, Amzica F, Contreras D. Synchronization of fast (30–40 Hz) spontaneous cortical rhythms during brain activation. J Neurosci. 1996;16:392–417.
9. Evans BM, Richardson NE. Demonstration of a 3-5 s periodicity between the spindle bursts in NREM sleep in man. J Sleep Res. 1995;4:196–197.
10. Blake H, Gerard RW. Brain potentials during sleep. Am J Physiol. 1937;119:692–703.
11. Williams HL, Hammack JT, Daly RL, et al. Responses to auditory stimulation, sleep loss and the EEG stages of sleep. Electroencephalogr Clin Neurophysiol. 1964;16:269–279.
12. Dement W, Kleitman N. Cyclic variations in EEG during sleep and their relation to eye movements, body motility, and dreaming. Electroencephalogr Clin Neurophysiol. 1957;9:673–690.

13. Webb WB, Agnew HW Jr. Stage 4 sleep: influence of time course variables. Science. 1971;174:1354–1356.
14. Maron L, Rechtschaffen A, Wolpert EA. Sleep cycle during napping. Arch Gen Psychiatry. 1964;11:503–507.
15. Knowles JB, Coulter M, Wahnon S, et al. Variation in process S: effects on sleep continuity and architecture. Sleep. 1990;13:97–107.
16. Beersma DGM, Daan S, Dijk DJ. Sleep intensity and timing: A model for their circadian control. In: Carpenter GA, ed. Some Mathematical Questions in Biology—Circadian Rhythms. Lectures on Mathematics in the Life Sciences. Vol. 19. Providence, RI: The American Mathematical Society; 1987:39–62.
17. Dijk DJ, Beersma DGM, Daan S. EEG power density during nap sleep: reflection of an hourglass measuring the duration of prior wakefulness. J Biol Rhythms. 1987;2:207–219.
18. Dijk DJ. EEG slow waves and sleep spindles: windows on the sleeping brain. Behav Brain Res. 1995;69:109–116.
19. Karacan I, Williams RL, Finley WW, et al. The effects of naps on nocturnal sleep: Influence on the need for stage-1 REM and stage 4 sleep. Biol Psychiatry. 1970;2:391–399.
20. Feinberg I, Maloney T, March JD. Precise conservation of NREM period 1 (NREMP1) delta across naps and nocturnal sleep: implications for REM latency and NREM/REM alternation. Sleep. 1992;15:400–403.
21. Feinberg I, March JD, Floyd TC, et al. Homeostatic changes during post-nap sleep maintain baseline levels of delta EEG. Electroencephalogr Clin Neurophysiol. 1985;61:134–137.
22. Daan S, Beersma DGM, Dijk DJ, et al. Kinetics of an hourglass component involved in the regulation of human sleep and wakefulness. In: Hekkens WTJM, Kerkhof GA, Rietveld WJ, eds. Trends in Chronobiology: Advances in the Biosciences. Vol. 73. Oxford, England: Pergamon Press; 1988:183–193.
23. Knowles JB, MacLean AW, Brunet D, et al. Nap-induced changes in the time course of process S. Effects on nocturnal slow wave activity. In: Horne J, ed. Sleep '90. Bochum, Germany: Pontenagel Press; 1990:68–70.
24. Werth E, Dijk DJ, Achermann P, et al. Dynamics of the sleep EEG after an early evening nap: experimental data and simulations. Am J Physiol. 1996;271:R501–510.
25. Åkerstedt T, Gillberg M. Sleep duration and the power spectral density of the EEG. Electroencephalogr Clin Neurophysiol. 1986;64:119–122.
26. Gillberg M, Åkerstedt T. The dynamics of the first sleep cycle. Sleep. 1991;14:147–154.
27. Borbély AA. A two process model of sleep regulation. Hum Neurobiol. 1982;1:195–204.
28. Dijk DJ, Hayes B, Czeisler CA. Dynamics of electroencephalographic sleep spindles and slow wave activity in men: effect of sleep deprivation. Brain Res. 1993;626:190–199.
29. Aeschbach D, Cajochen C, Landolt HP, Borbély AA. Homeostatic sleep regulation in habitual short sleepers and long sleepers. Am J Physiol. 1996;270:R41–53.
30. Borbély AA, Achermann P. Concepts and models of sleep regulation: an overview. J Sleep Res. 1992;1:63–79.
31. Dijk DJ, Brunner DP, Beersma DGM, et al. Electroencephalogram power density and slow wave sleep as a function of prior waking and circadian phase. Sleep. 1990;13:430–440.
32. Dijk DJ, Beersma DGM, Daan S, et al. Quantitative analysis of the effects of slow wave sleep deprivation during the first 3 h of sleep on subsequent EEG power density. Eur Arch Psychiatry Clin Neurol. 1987;236:323–328.
33. Dijk DJ, Beersma DGM. Effects of SWS deprivation on subsequent EEG power density and spontaneous sleep duration. Electroencephalogr Clin Neurophysiol. 1989;72:312–320.
34. Gillberg M, Anderzén I, Åkerstedt T. Recovery within day-time sleep after slow wave sleep suppression. Electroencephalogr Clin Neurophysiol. 1991;78:267–273.
35. Sinha AK, Smythe H, Zarcone VP, et al. Human sleep-electroencephalogram: a damped oscillatory phenomenon. J Theor Biol. 1972;35:387–293.
36. Achermann P, Borbély AA. Dynamics of EEG slow wave activity during physiological sleep and after administration of benzodiazepine hypnotics. Hum Neurobiol. 1987;6:203–210.
37. Dijk DJ, Brunner DP, Borbély AA. Time course of EEG power density during long sleep in humans. Am J Physiol. 1990;258:R650–661.
38. Aeschbach D, Borbély AA. All-night dynamics of the human sleep EEG. J Sleep Res. 1993;2:70–81.
39. Aeschbach D, Dijk DJ, Trachsel L, et al. Dynamics of slow-wave activity and spindle frequency activity in the human sleep EEG: effect of midazolam and zopiclone. Neuropsychopharmacology. 1994;11:237–244.
40. Aeschbach D, Dijk DJ, Borbély AA. Dynamics of EEG spindle frequency activity during extended sleep in humans: relationship to slow-wave activity and time of day. Brain Res. 1997;748:131–136.
41. Uchida S, Maloney T, March JD, et al. Sigma 12–15 Hz and delta 0.3–3 Hz EEG oscillate reciprocally within NREM sleep. Brain Res Bull. 1991;27:93–96.
42. Uchida S, Atsumi Y, Kojima T. Dynamic relationships between sleep spindles and delta waves during a NREM period. Brain Res Bull. 1994;33:351–355.
43. Merica H, Blois R. Relationship between the time courses of power in the frequency bands of human sleep EEG. Neurophysiol Clin. 1997;27:116–128.
44. Landolt HP, Dijk DJ, Achermann P, et al. Effect of age on the sleep EEG: slow-wave activity and spindle frequency activity in young and middle-aged men. Brain Res. 1996;738:205–212.
45. Dijk DJ, Czeisler CA. Contribution of the circadian pacemaker and the sleep homeostat to sleep propensity, sleep structure, electroencephalographic slow waves, and sleep spindle activity in humans. J Neurosci. 1995;15:3526–3538.
46. Dijk DJ, Shanahan TL, Duffy JF, et al. Variation of electroencephalographic activity during non-rapid eye movement and rapid eye movement sleep with phase of circadian melatonin rhythm in humans. J Physiol. 1997;505:851–858.
47. Werth E, Achermann P, Borbély AA. Brain topography of the human sleep EEG: antero-posterior shifts of spectral power. Neuroreport. 1996;8:123–127.
48. Werth E, Achermann P, Borbély AA. Fronto-occipital EEG power gradients in human sleep. J Sleep Res. 1997;6:102–112.
49. Werth E, Achermann P, Dijk DJ, et al. Spindle frequency activity in the sleep EEG: individual differences and topographical distribution. Electroencephalogr Clin Neurophysiol. 1997;103:535–542.
50. Zeitlhofer J, Gruber G, Anderer P, et al. Topographic distribution of sleep spindles in young healthy subjects. J Sleep Res. 1997;6:149–155.
51. Achermann P, Borbély AA. Coherence analysis of the human sleep electroencephalogram. Neuroscience. 1998;85:1195–1208.
52. Achermann P, Borbély AA. Temporal evolution of coherence and power in the human sleep electroencephalogram. J Sleep Res. 1998;7(suppl 1):36–41.
53. Steriade M, Nuñez A, Amzica F. Intracellular analysis of relations between the slow (<1 Hz) neocortical oscillation and other sleep rhythms of the electroencephalogram. J Neurosci. 1993;13:3266–3283.
54. Steriade M, Nuñez A, Amzica F. A novel slow (<1 Hz) oscillation of neocortical neurons in vivo: depolarizing and hyperpolarizing components. J Neurosci. 1993;13:3252–3265.
55. Steriade M, Contreras D, Curro Dossi R, et al. The slow (<1 Hz) oscillation in reticular thalamic and thalamocortical neurons: scenario of sleep rhythm generation in interacting thalamic and neocortical networks. J Neurosci. 1993;13:3284–3299.
56. Steriade M, Contreras D, Amzica F. Synchronized sleep oscillations and their paroxysmal developments. Trends Neurosci. 1994;17:199–208.
57. McCormick DA, Bal T. Sleep and arousal: thalamocortical mechanisms. Annu Rev Neurosci. 1997;20:185–215.
58. Steriade M, McCormick DA, Sejnowski TJ. Thalamocortical oscillations in the sleeping and aroused brain. Science. 1993;262:679–685.
59. Hirsch JC, Fourment A, Marc ME. Sleep-related variations of membrane potential in the lateral geniculate body relay neurons of the cat. Brain Res. 1983;259:308–312.
60. Contreras D, Timofeev I, Steriade M. Mechanisms of long-lasting hyperpolarizations underlying slow sleep oscillations in cat corticothalamic networks. J Physiol. 1996;494:251–264.
61. Bal T, McCormick DA. What stops synchronized thalamocortical oscillations. Neuron. 1996;17:297–308.
62. Steriade M, Amzica F. Slow sleep oscillation, rhythmic K-com-

plexes, and their paroxysmal developments. J Sleep Res. 1998;7(suppl 1):30–35.

63. Steriade M. Synchronized activities of coupled oscillators in the cerebral cortex and thalamus at different levels of vigilance. Cereb Cortex. 1997;7:583–604.

64. Llinás R, Ribary U. Coherent 40-Hz oscillation characterizes dream state in humans. Proc Natl Acad Sci U S A. 1993;90:2078–2081.

65. Franken P, Dijk DJ, Tobler I, et al. High-frequency components of the rat electrocorticogram are modulated by the vigilance states. Neurosci Lett. 1994;167:89–92.

66. Maloney KJ, Cape EG, Gotman J, et al. High-frequency gamma electroencephalogram activity in association with sleep-wake states and spontaneous behaviors in the rat. Neuroscience. 1997;76:541–555.

67. Cartwright RD, Monroe LJ, Palmer C. Individual differences in response to REM deprivation. Arch Gen Psychiatry. 1967;16:297–303.

68. Endo T, Roth C, Landolt HP, et al. Selective REM sleep deprivation in humans: effects on sleep and sleep EEG. Am J Physiol. 1998;274:R1186–1194.

68a. Roth C, Achermann P, Borbély AA. Alpha activity in the human REM sleep EEG: topography and effect of REM sleep deprivation. Clin Neurophysiol. 1999;110:632–635.

69. Beersma DGM, Dijk DJ, Blok CGH, et al. REM sleep deprivation during 5 hours leads to an immediate REM sleep rebound and to suppression of non-REM sleep intensity. Electroencephalogr Clin Neurophysiol. 1990;76:114–122.

70. Brunner DP, Dijk DJ, Tobler I, et al. Effect of partial sleep deprivation on sleep stages and EEG power spectra: Evidence for non-REM and REM sleep homeostasis. Electroencephalogr Clin Neurophysiol. 1990;75:492–499.

71. Brunner DP, Dijk DJ, Borbély AA. Repeated partial sleep deprivation progressively changes in EEG during sleep and wakefulness. Sleep. 1993;16:100–113.

72. Antonioli M, Solano L, Torre A, et al. Independence of REM density from other REM sleep parameters before and after REM deprivation. Sleep. 1981;4:221–225.

73. Borbély AA, Wirz-Justice A. Sleep, sleep deprivation and depression. A hypothesis derived from a model of sleep regulation. Hum Neurobiol. 1982;1:205–210.

74. Feinberg I, Floyd TC, March JD. Effects of sleep loss on delta (0.3-3 Hz) EEG and eye movement density: new observations and hypotheses. Electroencephalogr Clin Neurophysiol. 1987;67:217–221.

75. Barbato G, Barker C, Bender C, et al. Extended sleep in humans in 14 hour nights (LD 10:14): relationship between REM density and spontaneous awakening. Electroencephalogr Clin Neurophysiol. 1994;90:291–297.

76. Endo T, Schwierin B, Borbély AA, et al. Selective and total sleep deprivation: effect on the sleep EEG in the rat. Psychiatry Res. 1997;66:97–110.

77. Åkerstedt T, Fröberg JE. Psychophysiological circadian rhythms in women during 72 h of sleep deprivation. Waking Sleeping. 1977;1:387–394.

78. Dijk DJ, Beersma DGM, Daan S, et al. Bright morning light advances the human circadian system without affecting NREM sleep homeostasis. Am J Physiol. 1989;256:R106–111.

79. Dijk DJ, Czeisler CA. Paradoxical timing of the circadian rhythm of sleep propensity serves to consolidate sleep and wakefulness in humans. Neurosci Lett. 1994;166:63–68.

80. Czeisler CA, Duffy JF, Shanahan TL, et al. Stability, precision, and near-24-hour period of the human circadian pacemaker. Science. 1999;284:2177–2181.

81. Beersma DGM. Models of human sleep regulation. Sleep Med. Rev. 1998;2:31–43.

81a. Borbély AA, Achermann P. Sleep homeostasis and models of sleep regulation. J Biol Rhythms. In press.

82. Feinberg I. Changes in sleep cycle patterns with age. J Psychiatr Res 1974;10:283–306.

83. Borbély AA. Sleep regulation: circadian rhythm and homeostasis. Curr Top Neuroendocrinol. 1982;1:83–103.

84. Daan S, Beersma D. Circadian gating of human sleep-wake cycles. In: Moore-Ede MC, Czeisler CA, eds. Mathematical Models of the Circadian Sleep-Wake Cycle. New York, NY: Raven Press; 1984:129–155.

85. Daan S, Beersma DGM, Borbély AA. Timing of human sleep: recovery process gated by a circadian pacemaker. Am J Physiol. 1984;246:R161–178.

86. Achermann P, Borbély AA. Simulation of human sleep: ultradian dynamics of electroencephalographic slow-wave activity. J Biol Rhythms. 1990;5:141–157.

87. Achermann P, Dijk DJ, Brunner DP, et al. A model of human sleep homeostasis based on EEG slow-wave activity: quantitative comparison of data and simulations. Brain Res Bull. 1993;31:97–113.

88. Beersma DGM, Achermann P. Changes of sleep EEG slow-wave activity in response to sleep manipulations: to what extent are they related to changes in REM sleep latency? J Sleep Res. 1995;4:23–29.

89. Borbély AA, Achermann P, Trachsel L, et al. Sleep initiation and initial sleep intensity: interactions of homeostatic and circadian mechanisms. J Biol Rhythms. 1989;4:149–160.

90. Edgar DM, Dement WC, Fuller CA. Effect of SCN lesions on sleep in squirrel monkeys: evidence for opponent processes in sleep-wake regulation. J Neurosci. 1993;13:1065–1079.

91. Achermann P, Borbély AA. Simulation of daytime vigilance by the additive interaction of a homeostatic and a circadian process. Biol Cybern. 1994;71:115–121.

92. Franken P, Tobler I, Borbély AA. Sleep homeostasis in the rat: simulation of the time course of EEG slow-wave activity [published erratum appeared in Neurosci Lett. 1991;132:279]. Neurosci Lett. 1991;130:141–144.

93. Franken P, Tobler I, Borbély AA. Sleep and waking have a major effect on the 24-hr rhythm of cortical temperature in the rat. J Biol Rhythms. 1992;7:341–352.

94. Franken P, Dijk DJ, Tobler I, et al. Sleep deprivation in rats: effects on EEG power spectra, vigilance states, and cortical temperature. Am J Physiol. 1991;261:R198–208.

95. Kronauer RE, Czeisler CA, Pilato SF, et al. Mathematical model of the human circadian system with two interacting oscillators. Am J Physiol. 1982;242:R3–R17.

96. McCarley RW, Hobson JA. Neuronal excitability modulation over the sleep cycle: a structural and mathematical model. Science 1975;189:58–60.

97. McCarley RW, Massaquoi SG. Neurobiological structure of the revised limit cycle reciprocal interaction model of REM cycle control. J Sleep Res. 1992;1:132–137.

98. McCarley RW, Massaquoi SG. A limit cycle mathematical model of the REM sleep oscillator system. Am J Physiol. 1986;251:R1011–1029.

99. Massaquoi S, McCarley R. Resetting the REM sleep oscillator. In: Horne J, ed. Sleep '90. Bochum, Germany: Pontenagel Press; 1990:301–305.

100. Massaquoi SG, McCarley RW. Extension of the limit cycle reciprocal interaction model of REM cycle control. An integrated sleep control model. J Sleep Res. 1992;1:138–143.

101. Achermann P, Borbély AA. Combining different models of sleep regulation. J Sleep Res. 1992;1:144–147.

102. Torsvall L, Åkerstedt T. Sleepiness on the job: continuously measured EEG changes in train drivers. Electroencephalogr Clin Neurophysiol. 1987;66:502–511.

103. Cajochen C, Brunner DP, Kräuchi K, et al. Power density in theta/alpha frequencies of the waking EEG progressively increases during sustained wakefulness. Sleep. 1995;18:890–894.

104. Franken P. REM sleep regulation in the rat. Sleep Res. 1995;24A:433.

105. Benington JH, Heller HC. Does the function of REM sleep concern non-REM sleep or waking? Prog Neurobiol. 1994;44:433–449.

106. Tobler I, Franken P, Trachsel L, et al. Models of sleep regulation in mammals. J Sleep Res. 1992;1:125–127.

107. Oleksenko AI, Mukhametov LM, Polyakova IG, et al. Unihemispheric sleep deprivation in bottlenose dolphins. J Sleep Res. 1992;1:40–44.

108. Pigarev IN, Nothdurft HC, Kastner S. Evidence for asynchronous development of sleep in cortical areas. Neuroreport. 1997;8:2557–2560.

109. Krueger JM, Obál F Jr. A neuronal group theory of sleep function. J Sleep Res. 1993;2:63–69.

110. Benington JH, Heller HC. Restoration of brain energy metabolism as the function of sleep. Prog Neurobiol. 1995;45:347–360.

111. Porkka-Heiskanen T, Strecker RE, Thakkar M, et al. Adenosine: a mediator of the sleep-inducing effects of prolonged wakefulness. Science. 1997;276:1265–1268.

112. Kattler H, Dijk DJ, Borbély AA. Effect of unilateral somatosensory stimulation prior to sleep on the sleep EEG in humans. J Sleep Res. 1994;3:159–164.

113. Harrison Y, Horne JA. Sleep loss affects frontal lobe function, as shown in complex "real world" tasks. Sleep Res. 1996;25:467.

114. Harrison Y, Horne JA. Sleep deprivation affects speech. Sleep. 1997;20:871–877.

115. Horne JA. Human sleep, sleep loss and behaviour. Implications for the prefrontal cortex and psychiatric disorder. Br J Psychiatry. 1993;162:413–419.

116. Horne JA. Why We Sleep: The Functions of Sleep in Humans and Other Mammals. New York, NY: Oxford University Press; 1988.

117. Van Cauter E, Copinschi G. Interactions between growth hormone secretion and sleep. In: Smith RG, Thorner MO, eds. Human Growth Hormone: Research and Clinical Practice. Totowa, NJ: Humana Press; 2000.

118. Van Cauter E, Plat L, Scharf MB, et al. Simultaneous stimulation of slow-wave sleep and growth hormone secretion by gamma-hydroxybutyrate in normal young men. J Clin Invest. 1997;100:745–753.

119. Gronfier C, Luthringer R, Follenius M, et al. A quantitative evaluation of the relationships between growth hormone secretion and delta wave electroencephalographic activity during normal sleep and after enrichment in delta waves. Sleep. 1996;19:817–824.

120. Cirelli C, Pompeiano M, Tononi G. Neuronal gene expression in the waking state: a role for the locus coeruleus. Science. 1996;274:1211–1215.

121. Cirelli C, Tononi G. Differences in gene expression between sleep and waking as revealed by mRNA differential display. Mol Brain Res. 1998;56:293–305.

122. Achermann P, Beersma DGM, Borbély AA. The two-process model: ultradian dynamics of sleep. In: Horne JA, ed. Sleep '90. Bochum, Germany: Pontenagel Press; 1990:296–300.

123. Folkard S, Åkerstedt T. Towards a model for the prediction of alertness and/or fatigue on different sleep/wake schedules. In: Oginski A. Pokorski J, Rutenfranz J, eds. Contemporary Advances in Shiftwork Research. Kraków, Poland: Medical Academy, 1987:231–240.

124. Folkard S, Åkerstedt T. A three-process model of the regulation of alertness-sleepiness. In: Broughton RJ, Ogilvie RD, eds. Sleep, Arousal, and Performance. A Tribute to Bob Wilkinson. Boston, Mass.: Birkhäuser; 1992:11–26.

125. Åkerstedt T, Folkard S. Predicting sleep latency from the three-process model of alertness regulation. Psychophysiology. 1996;33:385–389.

126. Åkerstedt T, Folkard S. Predicting duration of sleep from the three process model of regulation of alertness. Occup Environ Med. 1996;53:136–141.

127. Åkerstedt T, Folkard S. The three-process model of alertness and its extension to performance, sleep latency, and sleep length. Chronobiol Int. 1997;14:115–123.

128. Putilov AA. Timing of sleep modelling: circadian modulation of the homeostatic process. Biol Rhythm Res. 1995;26:1–19.

129. Kronauer RE. A quantitative model for the effects of light on the amplitude and phase of the deep circadian pacemaker, based on human data. In: Horne J, ed. Sleep '90. Bochum, Germany: Pontenagel Press; 1990:306–309.

130. Klerman EB, Dijk DJ, Kronauer RE, et al. Simulations of light effects on the human circadian pacemaker: implications for assessment of intrinsic period. Am J Physiol. 1996;270:R271–282.

130a. Jewett ME, Kronauer RE. Refinement of a limit cycle oscillator model of the effects of light on the human circadian pacemaker. J Theor Biol. 1998;192:455–465.

131. Nakao M, McGinty D, Szymusiak R, et al. A thermoregulatory model of sleep control. Jpn J Physiol. 1995;45:291–309.

132. Nakao M, McGinty D, Szymusiak R, et al. Dynamical features of thermoregulatory model of sleep control. Jpn J Physiol. 1995;45:311–326.

133. Hobson JA, Lydic R, Baghdoyan HA. Evolving concepts of sleep cycle generation. From brain centers to neuronal populations. Behav Brain Sci. 1986;9:371–448.

30

Circadian Rhythms in Fatigue, Alertness, and Performance

Hans P. A. Van Dongen

David F. Dinges

The biological clock, located in the suprachiasmatic nuclei of the hypothalamus, endogenously regulates our hour-to-hour waking behavior, as reflected in fatigue, alertness, and cognitive performance. As a consequence, a circadian rhythm can be detected in almost all neurobehavioral variables. This phenomenon explains why people are more alert in the afternoon than early in the morning or late at night, even if they had enough sleep beforehand. A variety of factors (e.g., practice effects, motivational factors, background noise) can exert masking influences on the circadian profile of neurobehavioral functions. Masking refers to the evoked effects of these noncircadian factors on the measurements of circadian rhythmicity. Some of these factors may be difficult to control, so that it is important to study the circadian rhythmicity of neurobehavioral functions under strictly controlled laboratory conditions.

Even if all masking influences are controlled, however, measurements of the endogenous circadian rhythmicity in fatigue, alertness, and cognitive performance are still confounded by the interaction of the biological clock with the homeostatic regulation of sleep. Furthermore, it can be argued that some masking influences (e.g., sensory stimulation, body movement) are an integral part of the system regulating waking neurobehavioral functions, and therefore controlling them does not necessarily eliminate their effects. A more thorough understanding of their interactions with the circadian rhythmicity in neurobehavioral functions is needed to accurately predict and prevent the occurrence of performance deficits, which may reach dangerous levels leading to accidents.

Both wakefulness and sleep are modulated by an endogenous regulating system, the biological clock, located in the suprachiasmatic nuclei of the hypothalamus. The impact of the biological clock goes beyond compelling the body to fall asleep and to wake up again. The biological clock also modulates our hour-to-hour waking behavior, as reflected in fatigue, alertness, and performance, generating circadian rhythmicity in almost all neurobehavioral variables.

Before focusing on circadian rhythmicity in waking functions, it is appropriate to give a brief description of the three variables mentioned in the title of this chapter. In the literature, various definitions of fatigue, alertness, and performance can be found (e.g., see references 1, 2) and differences of opinion exist about their meaning. For the purposes of this chapter, the term *performance* comprises cognitive functions ranging in complexity from simple psychomotor reaction time, to logical reasoning, working memory, and complex executive functions. By *alertness* is meant selective attention, vigilance, and attentional control (after reference 3). *Fatigue* refers to subjective reports of loss of desire or ability to continue performing. Additionally, *subjective sleepiness* is used here for subjective reports of sleepiness or the desire to sleep.

The meanings of fatigue and subjective sleepiness given above express the relationship that exists between alertness and performance during wakefulness on the one hand and sleep on the other hand. The interaction of the circadian and sleep-wake systems in regulating fatigue, alertness, and performance is described in the second part of this chapter. It is important to note that this chapter does not cover sleep propensity,[4, 5] but rather focuses on circadian regulation in effortful performance and its corresponding subjective states.

CIRCADIAN RHYTHMICITY

Subjective Measures of Fatigue and Alertness

Many techniques are available for the detection of circadian rhythmicity in neurobehavioral variables. Successful results have been reported in studies with a wide array of subjective measures of alertness and fatigue. These have been obtained with, for instance, visual analogue scales (VAS)[6] and Likert-type rating scales such as the Stanford Sleepiness Scale (SSS),[7] the Karolinska Sleepiness Scale (KSS),[8] the Activation-Deactivation Adjective Check List (AD-ACL),[9] and the Profile of Mood States (POMS).[10] Subjective measures of fatigue and alertness in particular are vulnerable to numerous confounding influences, however, which can *mask* their distinct circadian rhythmicity. Masking is a critical concept to understand when considering the assessment of circadian rhythms in neurobehavioral variables. Masking refers to the evoked effects of noncircadian factors on the measurements of circadian rhythmicity. The *context* in which such measurements are taken (i.e., the environmental and experimental conditions) is a major source of masking effects. Masking can both obscure a circadian rhythm, or create the appearance of a circadian rhythm. Masking factors may include the following: demand characteristics of the experiment,[11] distractions by irrelevant stimuli,[12] boredom and motivational factors,[13-15] stress,[16] food intake,[17] posture,[18] ambient temperature,[14] background noise,[19] lighting conditions,[20] and drug intake (e.g., caffeine).

Physical and mental activity can be masking factors as well, as illustrated in Figure 30–1, where the effects

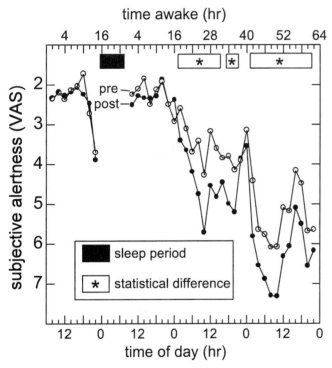

Figure 30–1. Average subjective alertness ratings (visual analogue scale, VAS) in 24 healthy adults during 64 h of wakefulness following 8 h of sleep *(black bar)* from 11:30 PM until 7:30 AM. In this experiment subjects were tested on a 35-min performance and mood neurobehavioral battery every 2 h when awake. Alertness ratings are shown for two conditions: (1) ratings made just before each 35-min performance test bout *(open circles)*; (2) ratings made directly after each 35-min performance test bout *(closed circles)*. No graphical or statistical differences between prebout and postbout alertness ratings were evident during the 16-h baseline day, or during the first 16 h of wakefulness in the sleep deprivation period. However, for most of the time from 2 AM on the first night awake, until 10 PM after 62 h awake, postbout alertness ratings were statistically significantly (P ≤.05) lower than prebout ratings (times involving statistically significant differences are shown with boxes containing asterisks atop the graph). Only near the circadian peak in body temperature (i.e., from 8 PM hours until 10 PM) did these prebout vs. postbout differences disappear during sleep deprivation. Such data highlight the masking effects of ambulation, conversation, and other activity-based factors on subjective ratings of alertness, and the circadian rhythm therein, once there is a heightened pressure for sleep.

of performance tests on subjective estimates of alertness become apparent at certain circadian phases during sleep deprivation. In this example, subjects reported feeling less alert after being challenged to perform. This suggests that prior activity can influence subjective estimates, and that it can contaminate circadian effects if not properly controlled when measuring circadian rhythmicity in subjective states.

Prior wakefulness and sleep can also be considered masking factors when it comes to observing circadian rhythmicity in neurobehavioral variables. Sleep and sleep loss have large effects on alertness and performance. These issues are illustrated in the second half of the chapter. Despite potential masking factors and their interactions, subjective scales have been used to index circadian rhythmicity, by applying them repeatedly across the day under carefully controlled conditions.[21, 22]

Performance Measures

Rather than relying on subjective measures, many studies of circadian rhythms have relied on objective performance measures. For example, studies have employed search-and-detection tasks[23, 24] and simple and choice reaction time tasks[25] to obtain objective measures of circadian variation in performance. Typically, the speed and the accuracy of responses to a series of repetitive stimuli are analyzed.

There are many performance outputs that have been conceptually distinguished, including simple sorting,[26] logical reasoning,[27] memory access,[28] and more complex activities such as school performance[29] and meter reading accuracy.[30] Various tasks have been used to study circadian variation in these different aspects of performance. A number of studies have concluded that different tasks[31, 32] and different task parameters[33-35] may yield different peak phases of circadian rhythmicity. This has led to the speculation that there are many different circadian rhythms and many different clock mechanisms controlling them.[36, 37] Under strictly controlled laboratory conditions, however, most of the intertask differences disappear.[38, 39] As illustrated in Figure 30–2, it can generally be stated that under such conditions, the circadian rhythms of cognitive and psychomotor performance covary with subjective sleepiness. Furthermore, these rhythms mimic the circadian rhythm of core body temperature, which has been demonstrated to be a good marker of the biological clock. Roughly, high and low body temperature values correspond to good and poor performance, respectively.[39-41]

The Midafternoon Dip

In addition to the circadian covariation of neurobehavioral variables with core body temperature, in some individuals there appears to be a short-term dip in these variables in the afternoon that has been referred to as the midafternoon, siesta, postlunch, or postpran-

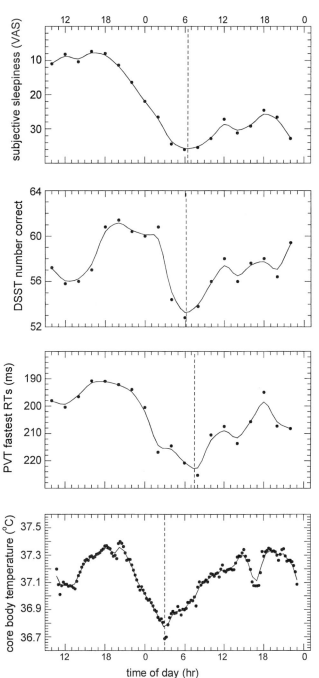

Figure 30–2. Circadian covariation of changes in subjective sleepiness, as assessed by a reversed visual analogue scale (VAS); in cognitive performance, as assessed by the digit symbol substitution task (DSST); in 10% fastest reaction times (RTs), as assessed by the psychomotor vigilance task (PVT); and in core body temperature (CBT), as assessed by means of a rectal probe. Data are the mean values from five subjects who remained awake in dim light, in bed, in a constant routine protocol, for 36 consecutive hours (a distance-weighted least-squares function was fitted to each variable). The circadian trough is evident in each variable (marked by vertical broken lines). A phase difference is also apparent, such that all three neurobehavioral variables had their average minimum between 3.0 and 4.5 h after the time of the body temperature minimum. This phase delay in neurobehavioral functions relative to CBT has been observed in many protocols, but remains unexplained. While body temperature reflects predominantly the endogenous circadian clock, neurobehavioral functions also are affected by the homeostatic pressure for sleep, which escalates with time awake, and which may contribute to the phase delay through interaction with the circadian clock. This explanation is not universally supported by the available data, but at the very least such data make it necessary to correct the common misconception that performance and alertness are worst at the body temperature minimum. In reality they are often worse after the time of the CBT minimum. Neurobehavioral functions generally do show the circadian decline at night as observed in CBT, but they appear to continue their decline after CBT has begun to rise, making the subsequent 2- to 6-h period (i.e., clock time approximately 6 AM to 10 AM) a zone of maximum vulnerability to loss of alertness and performance failure.

dial dip (even though it appears to have no relationship to food intake). This dip has been observed in field studies (e.g., see reference 30) and in controlled laboratory experiments (e.g., see reference 42). However, it is not consistently found (e.g., see references 43, 44).

The most compelling evidence for the existence of a midafternoon dip comes from studies on sleep propensity[45, 46] and on the timing of daytime naps.[47] Yet, there is little evidence for a consistent midafternoon dip in performance measures. Consequently, the phenomenon of a midafternoon increase in sleep propensity that does not necessarily express itself in performance deficits is poorly understood, and its relation-

ship to the biological clock remains unknown. Field studies of human performance have been used as evidence for the existence of a midafternoon dip in performance,[48] but such data cannot be used as positive evidence owing to the uncontrolled influence of differential amounts of activity by varying numbers of people over time (i.e., exposure), which may confound these studies.

The Practice Effect and Other Artifacts

A problem that limits the reliability of task performance for the assessment of circadian rhythmicity in alertness and fatigue is the well-known practice effect. This is illustrated in Figure 30–3, which shows cognitive performance improving across three consecutive days. The practice effect is difficult to distinguish from the circadian rhythm, but this dilemma might be circumvented by testing subjects in different orders across times of day. The practice effect is then balanced out by averaging over subjects. This assumes that the practice effect and the circadian rhythm are additive and have the same relationship in every subject. Since this assumption is often untested, it remains unclear whether practice effects on cognitive tests can be averaged out. A better way to deal with this problem is by training subjects to asymptotic performance levels before attempting to assess circadian rhythmicity.

Practice effects are not the only masking factors that may conceal, accentuate, or otherwise distort circadian rhythmicity in task results. Many of the same variables that serve to mask circadian rhythmicity in subjective estimates of fatigue and alertness also can mask circadian variation in performance. The effects of masking can vary from changes in the range of circadian variation to changes in the shape of the circadian curve; even total concealment of the circadian rhythm is possible (see Fig. 30–3, where sleep prevents measurement of nocturnal performance and the practice effect obscures measurement of diurnal performance). Thus, it is not easy to extract meaningful information about the amplitude (i.e., magnitude) and the phase (i.e., timing) of the circadian rhythm in performance measures without an understanding of the masking effects that influence these variables.

In comparison to subjective alertness and fatigue, circadian rhythmicity in cognitive performance is more complicated to assess. Not only is performance often affected by learning, aptitude, and other masking factors (e.g., lighting, background noise, as listed above) but it is also affected by the parallelism of the various brain processes that regulate performance. As an example, it has been reported that subjects may change their performance strategy on a task by invoking subvocalization, in a rhythmical, circadian pattern.[49] This example illustrates that it can be difficult to distinguish the circadian rhythm in task performance per se from that of corresponding changes in performance strategy. The same applies to compensatory effort (i.e., increased effort to keep up performance). Furthermore, the effect of compensatory effort may be enhanced if subjects are informed about their results during a performance task.

Electroencephalographic Measures

The circadian rhythm in task performance is believed to reflect functional changes in the brain. The electroencephalogram (EEG) and brain potentials associated with the reaction to a stimulus, which are called evoked potentials or event-related potentials (ERPs), have been used as a measure of alertness. In order to average out the background EEG, many ERP measurements must be taken (i.e., many stimuli must be offered) consecutively. Therefore, ERPs are usually recorded during repetitive search-and-detection and reaction time tasks. Diurnal changes in the amplitude and the location of ERP waves have been interpreted as reflecting circadian variations in alertness.[50, 51] Hemispheric differences have been detected,[52] suggesting separate circadian rhythms for the left and right hemisphere. However, masking from a variety of sources presents a problem in the interpretation of such ERP data (e.g., see reference 53).

Circadian variations in alertness have also been associated with changes in the background EEG during wakefulness. The amount of alpha activity (i.e., EEG activity in the frequency band from 8 to 12 Hz) in the resting EEG with eyes held either open or closed (to avoid artifacts from blinking) is thought to be related to the level of alertness.[54] Unfortunately, difficulties in the recording, analysis, and interpretation of the alpha band[55] and other EEG frequency bands[56] have substantially limited its usefulness. Furthermore, it has been shown that significant effects in the EEG occur primarily when alertness is much lower than what is normally encountered at the trough of circadian variation, as when subjects are sleep-deprived.[8, 57] This has also been reported for slow-rolling eye movements (SEMs) in the

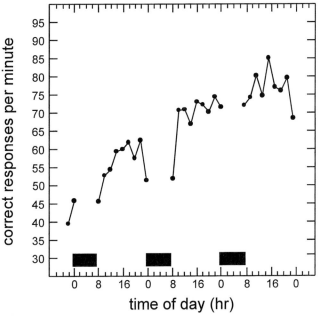

Figure 30–3. Average cognitive throughput performance for 29 healthy adult subjects tested every 2 h from 7:30 AM until 11:30 PM each day, during a 3-d period in which they were allowed up to 8 h of sleep per night *(black bars)*. The performance task was the serial addition/subtraction test, which is a part of the Walter Reed performance assessment battery.[88] In this task, subjects were presented with a rapid sequence of two single digits (0–9) followed by an operator (plus or minus), and they were to enter only the least-significant single digit of the algebraic sum, unless the result was negative, in which case 10 was to be added to the answer. Note the substantial learning curve (i.e., practice effect) across days, resulting in a doubling of the mean correct responses within 23 trials. This learning effect dominates the performance profile, obscuring circadian changes from 7:30 AM to 11:30 PM within any single day. Such practice effects "contaminate" nearly all tasks that involve mental operations.

electro-oculogram (EOG), which have been used as an electrophysiological measure of alertness as well.[8]

Another way in which the EEG has been used is to measure the latency with which subjects fall asleep (i.e., sleep propensity) at various times of day. These sleep latency tests include the Multiple Sleep Latency Test (MSLT) and the Maintenance of Wakefulness Test (MWT), as well as many variations of these paradigms. The sleep latency tests have been well documented to be sensitive to sleep loss and pathological conditions, and are covered elsewhere in this book.

Interindividual Differences

Interindividual differences in circadian amplitude, circadian phase, and mean performance level are reported throughout the literature. Occasionally, interindividual differences in the circadian period (τ) have been reported as well (e.g., see reference 58), but it should be emphasized that under normal entrained circumstances τ equals 24 h.

Morningness/eveningness (i.e., the tendency to be an early "lark" or a late "owl") is the most substantial source of interindividual variation. Morning- and evening-type individuals differ endogenously in the circadian phase of their biological clock.[59] This is echoed in the diurnal course of their neurobehavioral variables (as reviewed in references 60, 61). Some people are consistently at their best in the morning, whereas others are more alert and perform better in the evening. There is reason to believe that this difference in circadian phase preference and its reflection in neurobehavioral functions is a more or less enduring trait. To the extent that this is the case, it may be seen as a phenotypical aspect of the circadian rhythmicity in human beings.

Other, less substantial sources of interindividual variation in the circadian rhythmicity of alertness and performance include personality (e.g., introversion/extraversion) and age. No consistent relevance of gender has been reported.

CIRCADIAN RHYTHMICITY INTERACTS WITH SLEEP AND WAKEFULNESS

Sleep Deprivation

Considerable research effort has been put into *unmasking* the circadian rhythm, that is, eliminating sources of extraneous variance in order to expose the "pure" circadian rhythm in variables, including alertness and performance. In particular, the constant routine procedure[62] and its modifications are generally regarded as the gold standard for measuring circadian rhythmicity. By keeping subjects awake with a fixed posture in a constant laboratory environment for at least 24 h, circadian rhythms in a host of physiological and neurobehavioral variables can be recorded (see Fig. 30–2). Indeed, for body temperature, the circadian rhythm is believed to be free of masking effects.

However, masking factors can differ greatly among variables. In particular, when neurobehavioral variables are considered, the elimination of sleep (i.e., sleep deprivation) and the stimuli delivered to sustain wakefulness can constitute masking factors. In fact, in constant routine experiments these masking effects have become evident in subjective measures of alertness and fatigue.[57, 59, 63] Figure 30–2 shows the somewhat reduced values for subjective alertness, and cognitive and psychomotor performance after 30 h awake in the constant routine, as compared to the values of these variables 24 h earlier (i.e., at the same circadian phase but without sleep deprivation).

Typically, superimposed on the circadian rhythm in a given variable there is also a progressive change that is associated with the time spent awake (e.g., see reference 64). When total sleep deprivation is continued for several days (whether in a constant routine procedure or an experimental design involving ambulation), the detrimental effects on alertness and performance grow, and although the circadian process can thus be exposed, it is overlaid on an almost linear change reflecting increasing homeostatic pressure for sleep (e.g., see references 65, 66). This is illustrated in Figure 30–4 for performance lapses on a psychomotor vigilance task.

Sleep-Wake Regulation

The circadian modulation of alertness and performance that appears to be superimposed on monotonic changes during sleep deprivation has prompted efforts to mathematically model the processes involved. The two-process model of sleep-wake regulation[67, 68] has been applied to the understanding of the temporal profile of neurobehavioral functioning across days of sleep deprivation. The model consists of a *homeostatic* process (process S) and a *circadian* process (process C), which combine to determine the timing of the onset and offset of sleep. The homeostatic process represents the drive for sleep that increases during wakefulness (as can be felt when wakefulness is maintained beyond the habitual bedtime into the night) and decreases during sleep (symbolizing the neurobehavioral recovery obtained from sleep). When the "homeostat" increases above a certain level, sleep is triggered; when it decreases below a lower level, wakefulness is invoked. The circadian process represents the daily oscillatory component in the drive for sleep and wakefulness. In particular, it has been suggested that the circadian system actively promotes wakefulness more so than sleep,[69] although this hypothesis is not universally accepted. The circadian drive for wakefulness is experienced, for example, as the spontaneously enhanced alertness in the early evening, even after a sleepless night.

Homeostatic and circadian processes do more than determine the timing of sleep. They interact to determine waking neurobehavioral alertness as expressed

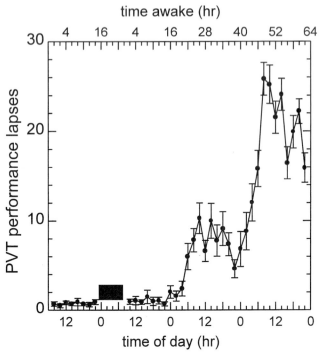

Figure 30–4. Average (with SEM) frequency of performance lapses (reaction times longer than 500 ms) on the 10-min psychomotor vigilance task (PVT) in 24 healthy adults during 64 h of wakefulness following 8 h of sleep *(black bar)* from 11:30 PM until 7:30 AM. In this experiment subjects were tested on a 35-min performance and mood neurobehavioral battery that included the PVT every 2 h when awake. As is evident in the figure, there is no circadian variation in PVT lapses during the 16-h baseline day, or during the first 16 h of wakefulness in the sleep deprivation period, because lapses are relatively rare events within this range of wakefulness duration and during this largely diurnal portion of the circadian cycle (i.e., from 7:30 AM until 11:30 PM). However, from 18 h awake (i.e., at 2:00 AM on the first sleepless night) to 62 h awake (i.e., at 10 PM before the third sleepless night) PVT lapses are clearly evident, indicating a substantial increase in neurobehavioral dysfunction. From 18 to 62 h of waking, there appears to be a circadian modulation of lapsing within days, superimposed on an almost linear increase in lapses across days. This interaction makes it difficult to estimate the relative contributions of the circadian versus homeostatic influences within and between each 24-h period. Mathematical deconvolution of the two influences, even if statistically sound, does not resolve this problem owing to potential nonlinearities of the interaction. Nevertheless, it is interesting that all neurobehavioral performance and subjective variables that show circadian variation also respond to sleep loss, and vice versa, and that the combined effect of the two processes typically takes the form of a rough staircase function as seen in this figure (see Fig. 30–1).

in fatigue and performance.[70] This is clearly seen in sustained sleep deprivation experiments (see Figs. 30–1 and 30–4). Consequently, for fatigue, alertness, and performance (unlike body temperature), sleep and sleeplessness are not only masking factors but also dynamic biological forces that interact with the circadian system.

The forced desynchrony protocol (e.g., see references 71, 72) is a sophisticated experimental procedure for studying the interaction of the circadian and homeostatic processes.[38, 44, 73] In such a protocol, a subject stays in an isolated laboratory in which the times for sleep and waking are scheduled to deviate from the normal 24-h day (e.g., 20- or 28-h days have been used), to such an extent that the subject's biological clock is unable to synchronize to this schedule. The subject experiences two distinct influences simultaneously: the schedule of predetermined sleep and waking times (i.e., time awake), which represents the homeostatic system; and the rhythm of the subject's unsynchronized (i.e., free-running) circadian system. Neurobehavioral variables can be recorded when the subject is in the waking periods of the schedule. By folding the data over either the free-running circadian rhythm or the imposed sleep-wake cycle, the other component can be balanced out (e.g., see reference 74). Thus, insight is gained into the separate effects of the circadian rhythm and the wake duration (i.e., homeostatic drive for sleep) on the recorded variables.

Not surprisingly, it has been observed in forced desynchrony studies that both the circadian and homeostatic processes influence fatigue, alertness, and performance. The interaction of the two seems to be oppositional during natural diurnal wake periods (from about 7 AM until 11 PM), such that a relatively stable level of alertness and performance can be maintained throughout the day.[44] This may explain why often in studies of alertness and performance, very little temporal variation is seen during the waking portion of the day.

Forced desynchrony studies have shown that the interaction of the homeostatic and circadian processes is complex and nonlinear. Therefore, the separation of circadian and homeostatic influences on neurobehavioral variables in studies involving sleep deprivation presents a conceptual and mathematical problem.[75] It is difficult to quantify the relative importance of the two influences on neurobehavioral functions, and it is likely that their relative contributions may vary among subjects (e.g., see reference 76) and across different experimental conditions. In this sense the relative contribution of the circadian system may be inestimable.

Very Short Artificial Days

The importance of taking into account sleep-wake rhythmicity when studying alertness and performance has led to the design of paradigms with very short artificial (i.e., ultradian) days, which seek to redistribute the opportunities for sleep and wakefulness across the natural 24-h day, to sample waking behavior across the circadian cycle without significantly curtailing the total amount of sleep allowed. Studies have been performed with the "90-min day" schedule,[77] which alternately allows subjects to sleep for 30 min and forces them to stay awake for 60 min, and with the "7- to 13-min sleep-waking" schedule,[5] which alternately allows subjects to sleep for 7 min and forces them to stay awake for 13 min. With respect to objective measures, studies with very short days have primarily focused on sleep propensity rather than performance, alertness, and fatigue. However, subjective sleepiness scores have been recorded in both the 90-min day schedule[77] and the 7- to 13-min sleep-waking schedule.[78] Surprisingly,

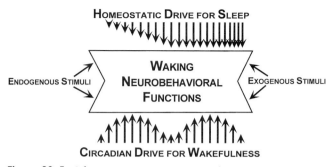

Figure 30–5. Schematic representation of the speculative oppositional interplay of circadian and homeostatic drives in the regulation of alertness, performance, and related neurobehavioral functions. This representation was inspired by a number of theoretical conceptualizations, but it does not necessarily reflect their authors' original intentions. These include the two-process model of sleep-wake regulation[67] and the opponent-process model of sleep-wake regulation[69]; the two- and three-process models of the endogenous neurobiological regulation of subjective sleepiness[70, 81] and of performance and alertness[38, 89]; and by a study of the effects of postural, environmental, cognitive, and social stimulation (masking) on neurobehavioral functions at different circadian phases during sleep deprivation[90]. The schematic is necessarily simplified (e.g., an additional factor, *sleep inertia*, is subsumed under the homeostatic drive for sleep). As represented in the figure, the *homeostatic* drive for sleep, which involves continuous time awake and loss of sleep (or disruption of the recovery function of sleep), decreases waking neurobehavioral performance and alertness (and increases fatigue and subjective sleepiness) as it accumulates over time. Unlike the circadian component, which is limited by its amplitude, the homeostatic drive for sleep can accumulate far beyond the levels typically encountered in a 24-h day (illustrated by the increasing density of downward arrows). The neurobiology of the cumulative homeostatic pressure is unknown. In opposition to this downward influence on performance and alertness is the endogenous *circadian* rhythmicity of the biological clock, which, through its promotion of wakefulness, modulates the enhancement of performance and alertness. Although the neurobiology of the biological clock is increasingly elucidated, the ways in which it controls the drive for wakefulness and enhances alertness are still unknown. The improvement in waking neurobehavioral functions by the circadian drive is an oscillatory output with some phases involving robust opposition to the homeostatic drive, although the phase of the lowest circadian opposition may involve a complete absence of the circadian drive for wakefulness. Critical modulators of neurobehavioral functions other than the sleep and circadian drives are subsumed in the schematic under the broad categories of *endogenous* and *exogenous* stimulation. Although common in the real world, these factors are considered masking factors in most laboratory experiments. They can include endogenous (e.g., anxiety) or exogenous (e.g., environmental cues) wake-promoting processes that oppose the homeostatic drive for sleep. Alternatively, they can include endogenous (e.g., narcolepsy) or exogenous (e.g., rhythmical motion) sleep-promoting processes that oppose the circadian drive for wakefulness either directly, or indirectly by exposing the previously countered sleep drive[4, 91]. The neurobiological underpinnings of these exogenous and endogenous processes are undoubtedly diverse, and few of their interactions with the circadian and homeostatic systems have been studied systematically.

after 24 h of 7- to 13-min sleep-waking cycles, the level of subjective sleepiness is elevated with respect to the initial level 24 h earlier (this does not seem to be the case in the 90-min day schedule). Thus, at least from the standpoint of subjective sleepiness, the sleep obtained across 24 h during the 7- to 13-min sleep-waking schedule may not have the same recovery potential as natural nighttime sleep.

Performance was assessed in one experiment employing the 7- to 13-min sleep-waking schedule[79]. A clear circadian rhythm emerged for the response time on a choice reaction time task. Furthermore, a movement time component was recorded, which showed a circadian rhythm as well, but also an overall gradual increase over time. This may reflect a growing homeostatic "pressure" across the artificial days. This study shows that even in paradigms with very short artificial days, it is difficult to separate the circadian and homeostatic influences on neurobehavioral functions.

Another problem that may be expected to interfere with the assessment of alertness and performance in these studies, is *sleep inertia*. This is the performance impairment and the feeling of disorientation experienced immediately after waking up[80]. In the three-process model of alertness[81], which is a recent expansion of the two-process model of sleep-wake regulation, sleep inertia is the third process, called process W. Sleep inertia affects alertness and performance on every artificial day of a study with very short days. There are some indications that the other two processes of the three-process model of alertness (i.e., processes C and S) may interact with the sleep inertia to vary its impact across artificial days[82], which complicates making corrections for its effect.

CONCLUSION

Figure 30–5 schematically shows how the circadian drive for wakefulness, the homeostatic drive for sleep, and various endogenous and exogenous masking factors simultaneously affect neurobehavioral functioning. When alertness and performance are considered, masking factors cannot be regarded as mere undesirable influences that should be ignored or controlled. Rather, they are an integral part of the regulation of neurobehavioral functions. Manipulation of these endogenous and exogenous stimuli may affect the circadian and homeostatic systems via interactions which cannot yet be accurately quantified.

Thorough understanding of circadian rhythmicity in neurobehavioral functions is important when either the sleep-wake rhythm is displaced, as is the case with night work[83, 84] or when the circadian rhythm is displaced, as is the case after transmeridian flights[85]. In such situations the circadian and homeostatic systems interact to decrease alertness and performance. In fact, performance deficits and fatigue may reach dangerous levels, inducing opportunities for accidents[86, 87].

References

1. Thayer RE. Toward a psychological theory of multidimensional activation (arousal). Motiv Emot. 1978;2:1–34.
2. Moldofsky H. Evaluation of daytime sleepiness. Clin Chest Med. 1992;13:417–425.
3. Parasuraman R. The attentive brain: issues and prospects. In: Parasuraman R. ed. The Attentive Brain. Cambridge, Mass: MIT Press; 1998:3–15.
4. Carskadon MA, Dement WC. The multiple sleep latency test: what does it measure? Sleep. 1982;5:S67–S72.
5. Lavie P. The 24-hour sleep propensity function (SPF): practical

and theoretical implications. In: Monk TH, ed. Sleep, Sleepiness and Performance. Chichester, England: John Wiley & Sons; 1991:65–93.

6. Monk TH, Embrey DE. A visual analogue scale technique to measure global vigor and affect. Psychiatry Res. 1989;27:89–99.

7. Hoddes E, Zarcone V, Smythe H, et al. Quantification of sleepiness: a new approach. Psychophysiology. 1973;10:431–436.

8. Åkerstedt T, Gillberg M. Subjective and objective sleepiness in the active individual. Int J Neurosci. 1990;52:29–37.

9. Thayer RE. Factor analytic and reliability studies on the Activation-Deactivation Adjective Check List. Psychol Rep. 1978;42:747–756.

10. McNair DM, Lorr M, Druppleman LF. EITS Manual for the Profile of Mood States. San Diego, Calif: Educational and Industrial Test Services; 1971.

11. Orne MT. On the social psychology of the psychological experiment: with particular reference to demand characteristics and their implications. Am Psychol. 1962;17:776–783.

12. Landström U, Englund K, Nordström B, et al. Laboratory studies of a sound system that maintains wakefulness. Percept Mot Skills. 1998;86:147–161.

13. Minors DS, Waterhouse JM. Circadian rhythm amplitude—is it related to rhythm adjustment and/or worker motivation? Ergonomics. 1983;26:229–241.

14. Mavjee V, Horne JA. Boredom effects on sleepiness/alertness in the early afternoon vs. early evening and interactions with warm ambient temperature. Br J Psychol. 1994;85:317–333.

15. Hayashi M, Minami S, Hori T. Masking effect of motivation on ultradian rhythm. Percept Mot Skills. 1998;86:127–136.

16. Orr WC, Hoffman HJ, Hegge FW. The assessment of time-dependent changes in human performance. Chronobiologia. 1976;3:293–205.

17. Paz A, Berry EM. Effect of meal composition on alertness and performance of hospital night-shift workers. Ann Nutr Metab. 1997;41:291–298.

18. Kräuchi K, Cajochen C, Wirz-Justice A. A relationship between heat loss and sleepiness: effects of postural change and melatonin administration. J Appl Physiol. 1997;83:134–139.

19. Landström U, Lindblom-Häggqvist S, Löfstedt P. Low frequency noise in lorries and correlated effects on drivers. J Low Frequency Noise Vibr. 1988;7:104–109.

20. Leproult R, Van Reeth O, Byrne MM, et al. Sleepiness, performance, and neuroendocrine function during sleep deprivation: effects of exposure to bright light or exercise. J Biol Rhythms. 1997;12:245–258.

21. Monk TH, Leng VC, Folkard S, et al. Circadian rhythms in subjective alertness and core body temperature. Chronobiologia. 1983;10:49–55.

22. Babkoff H, Caspy T, Mikulincer M. Subjective sleepiness ratings: the effects of sleep deprivation, circadian rhythmicity and cognitive performance. Sleep. 1991;14:534–539.

23. Colquhoun WP. Circadian variations in mental efficiency. In: Colquhoun WP, ed. Biological Rhythms in Human Performance. London, England: Academic Press, 1971:39–107.

24. Monk TH. Temporal effects in visual search. In: Clare JN, Sinclair MA, eds. Search and the Human Observer, London, England: Taylor & Francis; 1979:30–39.

25. Kleitman N. Sleep and Wakefulness. Chicago, Ill: University of Chicago Press; 1963.

26. Kleitman N. Diurnal variation in performance. Am J Physiol. 1933;104:449–456.

27. Folkard S. Diurnal variation in logical reasoning. Br J Psychol. 1975;66:1–8.

28. Folkard S, Monk TH. Circadian rhythms in human memory. Br J Psychol. 1980;71:295–307.

29. Laird DA. Relative performance of college students as conditioned by time of day and day of week. J Exp Psychol. 1925;8:50–63.

30. Bjerner B, Holm A, Swensson A. Diurnal variation in mental performance: a study of three-shift workers. Br J Ind Med. 1955;12:103–110.

31. Hockey GRJ, Colquhoun WP. Diurnal variation in human performance: a review. In: Colquhoun WP, ed. Aspects of Human Efficiency: Diurnal Rhythm and Loss of Sleep. London, England: English Universities Press; 1972:1–23.

32. Gillooly PB, Smolensky MH, Albright DL, et al. Circadian variation in human performance evaluated by the Walter Reed performance assessment battery. Chronobiol Int. 1990;7:143–153.

33. Mullin J, Corcoran DW. Interaction of task amplitude with circadian variation in auditory vigilance performance. Ergonomics. 1977;20:193–200.

34. Monk TH, Leng VC. Time of day effects in simple repetitive tasks: some possible mechanisms. Acta Psychol. 1982;51:207–221.

35. Kirkcaldy BD. Performance and circadian rhythms. Eur J Appl Physiol. 1984;52:375–379.

36. Folkard S, Wever RA, Wildgruber CM. Multi-oscillatory control of circadian rhythms in human performance. Nature. 1983;305:223–226.

37. Monk TH, Weitzman ED, Fookson JE, et al. Task variables determine which biological clock controls circadian rhythms in human performance. Nature. 1983;304:543–545.

38. Johnson MP, Duffy JF, Dijk D-J et al. Short-term memory, alertness and performance: a reappraisal of their relationship to body temperature. J Sleep Res. 1992;1:24–29.

39. Monk TH, Buysse DJ, Reynolds CF III, et al. Circadian rhythms in human performance and mood under constant conditions. J Sleep Res. 1997;6:9–18.

40. Kleitman N, Jackson DP. Body temperature and performance under different routines. J Appl Physiol. 1950;51:309–328.

41. Blake MJF. Time of day effects on performance in a range of tasks. Psychonomic Sci. 1967;9:349–350.

42. Monk TH, Buysse DJ, Reynolds CF III, et al. Circadian determinants of the postlunch dip in performance. Chronobiol Int. 1996;13:123–133.

43. Folkard S. Diurnal variation. In: Hockey GRJ, ed. Stress and Fatigue in Human Performance. New York, NY: John Wiley & Sons; 1983:245–272.

44. Dijk D-J, Duffy JF, Czeisler CA. Circadian and sleep/wake dependent aspects of subjective alertness and cognitive performance. J Sleep Res. 1992;1:112–117.

45. Richardson GS, Carskadon MA, Flagg W, et al. Excessive daytime sleepiness in man: multiple sleep latency measurement in narcoleptic and control subjects. Electroencephalogr Clin Neurophysiol. 1978;45:621–627.

46. Lavie P. To nap, perchance to sleep—ultradian aspects of napping. In: Dinges DF, Broughton RJ, eds. Sleep and Alertness: Chronobiological, Behavioral, and Medical Aspects of Napping. New York, NY: Raven Press; 1989:99–120.

47. Dinges DF. Nap patterns and effects in human adults. In: Dinges DF, Broughton RJ, eds. Sleep and Alertness: Chronobiological, Behavioral and Medical Aspects of Napping. New York, NY: Raven Press; 1989:171–204.

48. Mitler MM, Mitler JC. Methods of testing for sleeplessness. Behav Med. 1996;21:171–183.

49. Folkard S, Monk TH. Time of day and processing strategy in free recall. Q J Exp Psychol. 1979;31:461–475.

50. Münte T-F, Heinze H-J, Kunkel H, et al. Human event-related potentials and circadian variations in arousal level. Prog Clin Biol Res. 1987;227B:429–437.

51. Stolz G, Aschoff JC, Born J, et al. VEP, physiological and psychological circadian variations in humans. J Neurol. 1988;235:308–313.

52. Corbera X, Grau C, Vendrell P. Diurnal oscillations in hemispheric performance. J Clin Exp Neuropsychol. 1993;15:300–310.

53. Geisler MW, Polich J. P300 and time of day: circadian rhythms, food intake, and body temperature. Biol Psychol. 1990;31:117–136.

54. Bjerner B. Alpha depression and lowered pulse rate during delayed actions in a serial reaction test. Acta Physiol Scand Suppl. 1949;19:65.

55. Gale A, Harpham B, Lucas B. Time of day and the EEG: some negative results. Psychonomic Sci. 1972;28:269–271.

56. Jones D, Gale A, Smallbone A. Short-term recall of nine-digit strings and the EEG. Br J Psychol. 1979;70:97–119.

57. Cajochen C, Brunner DP, Kräuchi K, et al. Power density in theta/alpha frequencies of the waking EEG progressively increases during sustained wakefulness. Sleep. 1995;18:890–894.

58. Frazier TW, Rummel JA, Lipscomb HS. Circadian variability in vigilance performance. Aerospace Med. 1968;39:383–385.

59. Kerkhof GA, Van Dongen HPA. Morning-type and evening-type

individuals differ in the phase position of their endogenous circadian oscillator. Neurosci Lett. 1996;218:153–156.

60. Kerkhof GA. Inter-individual differences in the human circadian system: a review. Biol Psychol. 1985;20:83–112.

61. Van Dongen HPA. Inter- and Intra-Individual Differences in Circadian Phase. Leiden, Netherlands: Leiden University; 1998.

62. Mills JN, Minors DS, Waterhouse JM. Adaptation to abrupt time shifts of the oscillator(s) controlling human circadian rhythms. J Physiol. 1978;285:455–470.

63. Monk TH, Carrier J. Speed of mental processing in the middle of the night. Sleep. 1997;20:399–401.

64. Åkerstedt T, Gillberg M, Wetterberg L. The circadian covariation of fatigue and urinary melatonin. Biol Psychiatry. 1982;17:547–554.

65. Bohlin G, Kjellberg A. Self-reported arousal during sleep deprivation and its relation to performance and physiological variables. Scand J Psychol. 1973;14:78–86.

66. Horne JA, Anderson NR, Wilkinson RT. Effects of sleep deprivation on signal detection measures of vigilance: implications for sleep function. Sleep. 1983;6:347–358.

67. Borbély AA. A two-process model of sleep regulation. Hum Neurobiol. 1982;1:195–204.

68. Daan S, Beersma DGM, Borbély AA. Timing of human sleep: recovery process gated by a circadian pacemaker. Am J Physiol. 1984;246:R161–R178.

69. Edgar DM, Dement WC, Fuller CA. Effect of SCN lesions on sleep in squirrel monkeys: evidence for opponent processes in sleep-wake regulation. J Neurosci. 1993;13:1065–1079.

70. Folkard S, Åkerstedt T. Towards the prediction of alertness on abnormal sleep/wake schedules. In: Coblentz A, ed. Vigilance and Performance in Automated Systems. Dordrecht, Netherlands: Kluwer Academic Publishers; 1989:287–296.

71. Kleitman N, Kleitman E. Effect of non–twenty-four-hour routines of living on oral temperature and heart rate. J Appl Physiol. 1953;6:283–291.

72. Dijk D-J, Czeisler CA. Paradoxical timing of the circadian rhythm of sleep propensity serves to consolidate sleep and wakefulness in humans. Neurosci Lett. 1994;166:63–68.

73. Monk TH, Moline ML, Fookson JE, et al. Circadian determinants of subjective alertness. J Biol Rhythms. 1989;4:393–404.

74. Hiddinga AE, Beersma DGM, Hagedoorn M. On the circadian organization of core body temperature. Sleep-Wake Res Neth. 1995;6:43–46.

75. Babkoff H, Mikulincer M, Caspy T, et al. Selected problems of analysis and interpretation of the effects of sleep deprivation on temperature and performance rhythms. Ann N Y Acad Sci. 1992;658:93–110.

76. Lenné MG, Triggs TJ, Redman JR. Interactive effects of sleep deprivation, time of day, and driving experience on a driving task. Sleep. 1998;21:38–44.

77. Carskadon MA, Dement WC. Sleepiness and sleep state on a 90-min schedule. Psychophysiology. 1977;14:127–133.

78. Lavie P. Modelling sleep propensity—a need for rethinking. J Sleep Res. 1:99–102, 1992.

79. Lavie P, Gopher D, Wollman M. Thirty-six hour correspondence between performance and sleepiness cycles. Psychophysiology. 1987;24:430–438.

80. Dinges DF. Are you awake? Cognitive performance and reverie during the hypnopompic state. In: Bootzin RR, Kihlstrom J, Schacter DL, eds. Sleep and Cognition. Washington, DC: American Psychological Association; 1990:159–175.

81. Åkerstedt T, Folkard S. The three-process model of alertness and its extension to performance, sleep latency, and sleep length. Chronobiol Int. 1997;14:115–123.

82. Wilkinson RT, Stretton M. Performance after awakening at different times of night. Psychonomic Sci. 1971;23:283–285.

83. Freivalds A, Chaffin DB, Langolf GD. Quantification of human performance circadian rhythms. Am Ind Hyg Assoc J. 1983;44:643–648.

84. Folkard S, Totterdell P, Minors D, et al. Dissecting circadian performance rhythms: implications for shiftwork. Ergonomics. 1993;36:283–288.

85. Wegmann HM, Klein KE. Jet-lag and aircrew scheduling. In: Folkard S, Monk TH, eds. Hours of Work. Temporal Factors in Work-Scheduling. Chichester, England: John Wiley & Sons, 1985:263–276.

86. Mitler MM, Carskadon MA, Czeisler CA, et al. Catastrophes, sleep, and public policy: consensus report. Sleep. 1988;11:100–109.

87. Dinges DF. An overview of sleepiness and accidents. J Sleep Res. 1995;4:4–14.

88. Thorne DR, Genser SG, Sing GC, et al. The Walter Reed performance assessment battery. Neurobehav Toxicol Teratol. 1985;7:415–418.

89. Jewett ME. Models of Circadian and Homeostatic Regulation of Human Performance and Alertness. Cambridge, Mass: Harvard University; 1997.

90. Dijkman M, Sachs N, Levine E, et al. Effects of reduced stimulation on neurobehavioral alertness depend on circadian phase during human sleep deprivation. Sleep Res. 1997;26:265.

91. Dinges DF. The nature of sleepiness: causes, contexts, and consequences. In: Stunkard AJ, Baum A, eds. Eating, Sleeping, and Sex. Hillsdale, NJ: Lawrence Erlbaum Associates; 1989:147–179.

31

Melatonin in the Regulation of Sleep and Circadian Rhythms

Charles A. Czeisler

Christian Cajochen

Fred W. Turek

The pineal hormone melatonin is secreted primarily during the hours of darkness in all mammalian species. Melatonin can be thought of as a neuroendocrine transducer of the light-dark cycle. In human beings, high levels of melatonin are present in the bloodstream during the normal time of sleep at night and low levels are present during the waking day. The fact that the endogenous melatonin rhythm, driven by the suprachiasmatic nuclei, exhibits a close temporal association with the endogenous circadian component of the sleep propensity rhythm[1] (see Fig. 15 in Chapter 28), coupled with reports that treatment with exogenous melatonin can have sleep-promoting and phase-shifting effects (for a review, see Czeisler and Turek[2]), has led to the hypothesis that melatonin could be useful in the treatment of insomnia and the readjustment of daily rhythms. The purpose of this chapter is to summarize the present state of the scientific literature with respect to the use of melatonin for these purposes.

During their lifetime, most people will likely experience brief, if not prolonged, bouts of insomnia (i.e., subjective complaints of poor-quality sleep due to perceived difficulty in falling or remaining asleep), which may be associated with daytime sleepiness and decrements in mental and physical performance. Insomnia is likely to occur when individuals voluntarily choose to alter the timing of their sleep-wake schedule; this can be due to rapid travel across time zones, inducing what is known as the *jet lag syndrome*, or to shift work schedules that require work at their usual sleep time, leaving only their usual wake time for sleep. A second type of insomnia occurs "involuntarily" when for many different reasons, which may involve anxiety, illness, age, the care of babies, genetic predisposition, diet, alcohol, the sleep environment, and other factors, it is difficult to sleep during the desired normal sleep time.

The sleep-wake cycle is regulated primarily by two processes (see Chapter 28). One process, referred to as the *circadian component,* involves an internal near–24-h clock (i.e., the circadian clock) that regulates the timing

of sleep. The second process, referred to as the *homeostatic component,* is dependent on the duration of prior wakefulness and the quality and duration of sleep during previous sleep episodes. Thus, an effective agent for the treatment of insomnia or jet lag would be one that could (1) induce sleep when the homeostatic drive to sleep is insufficient to induce or maintain normal sleep (i.e., a *hypnotic* agent), (2) inhibit the drive for wakefulness emanating from the circadian pacemaker during the wake-propensity phase of the cycle (i.e., a *chronohypnotic* agent), or (3) induce phase shifts in the circadian clock regulating the sleep-wake cycle such that the circadian phase of increased sleep propensity occurs at a new, desired time (i.e., a *chronobiotic* agent). The evidence that melatonin can act as a hypnotic, a chronohypnotic, and/or a chronobiotic and the significance of this evidence for the use of melatonin to treat insomnia or jet lag are described.

USE OF MELATONIN AS A SLEEP-PROMOTING AGENT

An ideal hypnotic may be thought of as a substance that effectively induces sleep during both short- and long-term use. An efficacious hypnotic is one that induces or maintains sleep, or both. Much of the evidence that treatment with melatonin can have sleep-promoting properties has come from studies on normal volunteers to whom melatonin was administered either (1) just before scheduled naps during the normal wake time (when endogenous melatonin levels are very low) or (2) several hours before the subjects' habitual bedtimes, during the circadian wake-maintenance zone[3, 4] that occurs just before the nocturnal rise of endogenous melatonin levels (see Fig. 15 in Chapter 28) (for reviews, see references 5 to 10).

Subjective Sleepiness and Sleep Initiation

There is a general consensus in the literature that melatonin in doses ranging from 0.3 to 80 mg has somnogenic properties when ingested throughout the biological day, that is, during the entire phase in which endogenous melatonin levels are low.[5, 7, 9, 11–13] In fact, even when a low (0.3 mg) dose of melatonin was administered 1 h before sleep episodes scheduled to begin at the peak of the circadian wake propensity rhythm, several hours before habitual bedtime, sleep latency was significantly shortened.[14] Due to the high individual variability in the pharmacokinetics of melatonin, it is difficult to determine which of the aforementioned doses induces physiological or supraphysiological levels in a particular individual. In young subjects without sleep complaints, *daytime* melatonin administration increased self-rated sleepiness and improved sleep initiation as indexed by a reduction in polysomnographically measured sleep latency. This effect was dose dependent and paralleled by hypothermia.[12, 15–17] Therefore, some investigators have suggested that melatonin-induced hypothermia may underlie a sleep-promoting action.[11, 12, 17, 18]

In contrast, studies on the effects of melatonin administered near the time of the habitual nocturnal sleep episode (and thus near the time of rising endogenous melatonin levels) have not yielded consistent results. Melatonin (5 mg) administered to healthy volunteers at 8:40 PM significantly enhanced subjective sleepiness and also reduced sleep latency in the following sleep episode, which started at midnight.[19] In a study designed to investigate the effects of experimentally induced insomnia, 80 mg of melatonin ingested at 9:00 PM decreased sleep latency in the following sleep episode, which started 1.5 h later.[20] In contrast, when melatonin (1 and 5 mg) was administered later in the evening at 10:45 PM, 15 min before the lights were turned off, no reduction in sleep latency has been observed.[21]

Sleep Consolidation

In studies investigating the effects of *daytime* melatonin administration, the scheduled sleep durations have generally been short naps. For example, when subjects were not sleep deprived before a 2-h nap, melatonin (3 and 6 mg) increased the amount of total sleep time in polygraphically recorded sleep episodes.[13, 22] However, this effect appears to have resulted primarily from a decrease in sleep latency during this short nap. To assess the effects of exogenous melatonin on sleep consolidation, experiments are required in which sleep episode durations are scheduled to last sufficiently long (4 to 9 h). Improved sleep efficiency during the last hour of a 4-h daytime nap was reported by Hughes and Badia.[12] In this study, melatonin was administered orally in three different doses (1, 10, or 40 mg) at 8:00 PM to young healthy volunteers.

There is only one study that reported an increase in *nighttime* sleep efficiency when melatonin (80 mg) was administered before the nocturnal sleep episode in subjects sleeping at their habitual times in an artificial insomnia paradigm involving exposure to ambient street noise during the scheduled sleep time.[20] No ef-

fects on nighttime sleep consolidation have been reported in studies using lower melatonin doses. Negative effects on sleep consolidation at the very end of the nocturnal sleep episode (i.e., earlier awakening or earlier sleep offset) have been reported in a protocol in which melatonin (0.05 to 5 mg) was administered 7 h before habitual bedtime and sleep was assessed by the use of questionnaires.[16] In a study using polysomnographic recording, such an earlier offset of sleep was not observed on the first night after the administration of 5 mg of melatonin 5 h before habitual bedtime.[23] Interestingly, in this latter study, an earlier offset of sleep was observed during the second night, 29 h after melatonin administration.

Sleep Structure

A number of studies have investigated the effects of melatonin on sleep structure (i.e., the contribution of rapid eye movement [REM] sleep and nonrapid eye movement [NREM] sleep to total sleep time). In general, in response to melatonin administration, it was found that either REM sleep duration was not affected or an increase was observed. After melatonin (5 mg) administration either 5 or 3 h before nocturnal sleep, the first REM sleep episode was markedly lengthened.[19, 23] These effects are consistent with earlier experiments in which higher doses of melatonin were administered (for a review, see Zhdanova and Wurtman[10]). However, the increase in REM sleep was observed primarily during *nocturnal* sleep.

A number of studies have reported the suppression of slow-wave sleep (stages 3 and 4 of NREM sleep) after melatonin ingestion in doses of 1 to 250 mg[12, 24]; a tendency for reduced slow-wave sleep was also reported after 0.3 mg of melatonin.[14] This effect has been observed primarily in daytime sleep when melatonin was administered close to the beginning of the scheduled sleep episode.

Sleep Electroencephalography

Quantitative analysis of the sleep electroencephalogram (EEG) based on the fast Fourier transform has revealed that 5 mg of melatonin given shortly before a daytime sleep episode suppresses low EEG components and increases EEG activity in the sleep-spindle frequency range.[25] These effects are short lasting and are only moderate. The effects of melatonin on sleep-stage–specific EEG spectra during daytime sleep were replicated by Nave et al.,[22] and both research groups noted that the effects of melatonin are, to some extent, similar to the changes induced by benzodiazepine hypnotics. However, the effects of melatonin on sleep EEG spectra could not be blocked by flumazenil, which may indicate that the effects are not mediated by the gamma-aminobutyric acid$_A$ receptor complex.

The effects of melatonin on the sleep EEG are short lasting and were not observed when melatonin (5 mg) was administered 5 h before the nocturnal sleep episode,[23] even though melatonin levels were pharmacologically high at the time of sleep onset.

Implications

Melatonin is a natural hormone that partially fits the definition of a hypnotic because it induces sleepiness and facilitates and can maintain sleep. Unlike the benzodiazepine hypnotics, melatonin is not a tranquilizer in the classic sense or a sedative drug, and there is little evidence for any anxiolytic characteristics. Some have even considered melatonin to be a *soporific* (to make drowsy, sleepy, preparing for sleep) rather than a hypnotic per se.[26] This may be because the hypnotic effects of melatonin are time dependent, showing stronger efficacy during the daytime. Evidence from studies in both animals[27] and human beings[28, 29] that the circadian pacemaker promotes wakefulness at certain times of day, together with evidence that mammalian suprachiasmatic nuclei (SCN) neuronal firing is inhibited by SCN Mel_{1a} receptor–specific melatonin binding,[30] has led to the hypothesis that melatonin may act to facilitate sleep by inhibiting the circadian drive for waking that emanates from the SCN.[7, 9, 31] If this hypothesis proves to be correct, we propose that it would be more appropriate to classify the action of melatonin as a chronohypnotic, rather than simply a hypnotic.

Of course, if the sleep-promoting action of melatonin were indeed stronger during daytime sleep episodes, when endogenous melatonin levels are low, than during nighttime sleep episodes, when endogenous melatonin levels are normally higher, this could limit the clinical usefulness of melatonin as a sleeping pill. There has been no reported evidence, for example, that nighttime melatonin administration increases subsequent daytime alertness, which is a major goal of therapy. However, if insomniacs or even a subset of insomniacs prove to be melatonin deficient, as has been reported,[32, 33] then there would at least be a rationale for nocturnal melatonin administration. However, a recent study in age-related sleep-maintenance insomniacs failed to show a correlation between melatonin levels and sleep. Furthermore, low melatonin-producing insomniacs did not preferentially respond to melatonin replacement.[34]

In fact, surprisingly few attempts have been made to determine the effects of melatonin as a hypnotic in persons with insomnia. Indeed, only three reports in the literature have examined the effects of melatonin on sleep in chronic insomniacs younger than 65. In one study involving treatment with supraphysiological doses of melatonin (75 mg orally) for 14 consecutive days, there was a significant increase in the subjective assessment of total sleep time and daytime alertness.[35] In contrast, in a double-blind, placebo-controlled trial of 15 patients with psychophysiological insomnia, 5 mg of melatonin administered at 8:00 PM did not improve subjective estimates of bedtime, sleep onset time, estimated total sleep and wake times, sleep quality, or estimates of next-day function.[36] However, there were no objective polysomnographic sleep recordings to verify the self-reports in either study. A third study in which sleep was polysomnographically recorded[37] failed to find any effects on the onset or duration of sleep or on mood or alertness the day after treatment with a single low dose of melatonin (1 or 5 mg orally). However, the insomniacs studied had unusually high sleep efficiencies before the treatment.

Three studies in which motor activity of the wrist was used as an outcome variable have reported that elderly subjects complaining of insomnia have reduced motor activity at night after treatment with both high and low doses of melatonin just before bedtime.[38–40] This has raised the hope that melatonin administration may prove to be effective in the treatment of disrupted sleep in the elderly. The potential use of melatonin for treating sleep-wake disorders in the elderly is in fact a particularly attractive hypothesis because disturbed sleep becomes more prevalent with age.[41–43] Furthermore, as noted above, it has been reported that melatonin levels may be significantly lower in elderly insomniac patients than in age-matched control subjects.[39] However, a recent study using polysomnographic recording to investigate three different melatonin replacement delivery strategies in a group of patients with age-related sleep-maintenance insomnia reported that none of the treatments improved total sleep time, sleep efficiency, or wake after sleep onset, whereas sleep latency was reduced and paralleled by hypothermia.[34] This randomized, double-blind, placebo-controlled trial with an adequate sample size did not confirm the hypothesis that melatonin has positive sleep-maintaining effects or daytime alertness-enhancing effects in elderly insomniacs. Overall, there are no positive polysomnographic data to document the improvement with melatonin of sleep maintenance insomnia comparable to the demonstrated efficacy of the short-acting benzodiazepines.[44]

Most of the studies that have examined the effects of melatonin for the treatment of jet lag (after real or simulated phase shifts in the time structure of the external environment) have assessed the effects of treatment on subjective well-being or on the phase of circadian rhythms (see next section). Even in studies that have examined the effects of melatonin on sleep in a real or simulated jet lag paradigm, the measures of sleepiness have always been subjectively evaluated.[45–49] Although it has been suggested that the major effects of melatonin for alleviating the adverse effects of jet lag are due to the improvement in sleep, objective measures of the effect of melatonin on sleep under jet lag conditions have yet to be measured. There clearly is a need for randomized, double-blind, placebo-controlled trials on the possible sleep-inducing effects of melatonin in human beings after traveling rapidly across time zones before any firm conclusions can be made about the effects of melatonin on sleep under such conditions.

USE OF MELATONIN AS A CHRONOBIOTIC

A *chronobiotic* is defined as a chemical substance capable of therapeutically reentraining short-term dissociated or long term desynchronized circadian rhythms or prophylactically preventing their disruption after an environmental insult.[50] It has been known for a number of years that treatment with melatonin in a variety of animal species can induce phase shifts and entrain the circadian clock underlying the expression of multiple 24-h rhythms (for a review, see Redman[51]). In addition, melatonin is a major entraining signal for the circadian systems of fetal and neonatal mammals (for a review, see Davis[52]). Daily exposure to circulating melatonin allows fetuses to be synchronized with each other and with their mother long before they are able to perceive directly the environmental light-dark cycle on their own. Overall, the animal literature does support a role of melatonin as a chronobiotic. The next concern is whether melatonin administration can entrain circadian rhythms or shift circadian phase in human beings.

Entrainment

In nearly all eukaryotic organisms studied, periodic environmental stimuli normally synchronize (or entrain) the non–24-h intrinsic period of endogenous circadian rhythms to a period of exactly 24 h. In contrast to the periodic light-dark cycle—which is the primary signal by which the human circadian pacemaker is synchronized—melatonin obviously does not represent a periodic environmental stimulus. However, melatonin feeds back onto melatonin receptors in the SCN,[53] the brain site of the circadian clock, and therefore may play an important role in modulating the synchronizing effects of the light-dark cycle or in attenuating the postulated SCN-dependent alerting mechanism in human beings. Because the fetal pacemaker also expresses melatonin-binding sites, it is likely to be a target for maternal melatonin, which entrains the developing mammalian circadian pacemaker.

It has recently been reported that exogenous melatonin administration can entrain free-running rhythms to the 24-h day in some blind adults.[54, 55] In addition, melatonin was able to stabilize sleep-wake timing even in those blind people whose circadian system is not entrained to the 24-h day. (For a review, see Arendt.[56]) The therapeutic effectiveness of melatonin administration in nonentrained blind people is thus probably due to its acute chronohypnotic effects on sleep, whereas the therapeutic effectiveness of melatonin administration in those blind people who are entrained is probably due to its chronobiotic effect. Data from sighted individuals studied by Arendt et al.[57] indicated that when normally sighted subjects are studied in very dim light, daily melatonin administration alone has weak *zeitgeber* (synchronizing) effects, perhaps accounting for the variability in its efficacy as a chronobiotic in the blind.[54, 55]

Phase Shifting

The findings that the human SCN contains a high concentration of melatonin receptors[54] and that melatonin exerts circadian actions at the SCN in vitro[58] support the possibility that melatonin may have direct phase-shifting effects on the human circadian clock. There are intriguing reports that a single or repeated daily treatment with a near-physiological dose of melatonin can induce phase delays or phase advances in human circadian rhythms, with the direction for the phase shift dependent on the time of administration.[59, 60] This has led to a number of hypotheses regarding the possible use of melatonin for treating disorders of circadian timekeeping, including those related to insomnia and jet lag. Unfortunately, the melatonin rhythm itself, rather than an independent marker of the output of the human circadian pacemaker, was used to assess the phase shifts reportedly elicited in response to melatonin administration in those trials. Furthermore, light exposure, known to exert a phase-shifting effect on the human circadian pacemaker, which is an order of magnitude more powerful than that reported for melatonin, was not controlled in those resetting trials; however, in a recent double-blind, placebo-controlled, crossover study in which subjects were studied under dim light (less than 10 lux) and constant posture conditions, a single melatonin dose (5 mg) administered at 6:00 PM induced an advance of the circadian nocturnal decline in core body temperature, heart rate, and the dim light melatonin onset as assessed on the second day (more than 24 h) after melatonin administration.[61] In the same study, an earlier offset of sleep was observed in the second night after melatonin administration. Because this sleep episode was initiated 29 h after melatonin administration, these effects have been interpreted as reflecting a phase advance of the circadian timing system similar to the effects of bright light exposure in the morning hours.[23] Some evidence that exogenous melatonin can also induce a phase shift in an another circadian-regulated variable, the hormone cortisol, comes from a double-blind controlled study in which the effects of melatonin administration on pituitary hormone secretion were investigated. Ten male volunteers received 5 mg of melatonin or placebo orally for 4 consecutive days at 5:00 PM. Serum cortisol was measured over the 24-h period after the last dose of melatonin. After melatonin administration, the recorded peak in cortisol concentrations occurred at 6:00 AM and at 8:00 AM after placebo.[62] However, whether this reflects a phase advance in the circadian rhythm of serum cortisol induced by the melatonin administration lacks a confounding interpretation because light exposure—which itself can shift human cortisol rhythms[63]—was not controlled in the study.

To our knowledge, there is only one randomized, double-blind, placebo-controlled trial under controlled light conditions that investigated the capacity melatonin to induce phase delays. The authors report dose-dependent phase delays in the onset of melatonin secretion after the administration of melatonin at 7:00 AM in doses between 0.05 and 5 mg.[64] However, the mechanisms controlling the offset of melatonin secretion were less sensitive to an exogenous melatonin stimulus.

Implications

There is evidence that melatonin administration alone is able to elicit phase advances in circadian rhythm markers other than its own endogenous rhythm. However, the phase-resetting effects of the light-dark cycle are more powerful than those observed so far for melatonin. The phase-resetting effects of melatonin appear to be insufficient to induce entrainment reliably in human beings but may be considered as an adjuvant or a stabilizing factor. There is some positive evidence for such effects. For the chronobiotic properties of melatonin to be useful in the treatment of insomnia, the underlying cause of the insomnia would need to be due to an abnormal timing of sleep with respect to circadian phase. Such abnormal timing occurs in what is know as the *delayed sleep phase syndrome* (DSPS), in which sleep occurs at a delayed clock time relative to the light-dark cycle, and social, economic, and family demands (see Chapter 52).[65] Although originally described in adults,[66] DSPS often begins in childhood and is relatively common among adolescents.[67, 68] In the first use of melatonin in patients with DSPS, it was found that when administered 5 h before sleep onset for a period of 4 weeks, melatonin (5 mg orally) advanced sleep onset and wake times compared with placebo.[69] Although the sample size in this study was small (N = 8), a similar study, another small sample size (N = 7) produced similar results.[70] A recent study with a larger sample size confirmed the result of the first placebo-controlled study[69] in showing that melatonin induces an advance in sleep onset in patients with DSPS.[71] These initial studies indicate that melatonin may be an effective treatment for this specific sleep disorder. However, as reported for the blind, the therapeutic effectiveness of melatonin administration in the patient with DSPS may also be due to its acute sleep-promoting effects.

In contrast to the timing of sleep in DSPS, one of the most common sleep complaints in the elderly is that the timing of sleep onset or offset is advanced.[72] In principle, if melatonin could be used to phase delay the circadian clock timing the sleep-wake cycle, it could perhaps normalize the timing of sleep in elderly insomniacs who have an advanced circadian cycle; however, to date, no such studies have been reported. Furthermore, the evidence that melatonin has phase-delaying effects in human beings is based on a very small number of data points,[73] and these few delays were observed in response to melatonin administered in the morning hours. Thus, treatment of elderly people who have a phase-advanced sleep-wake cycle with melatonin in the early morning hours might be counterproductive if it were to also act as a hypnotic at wake time. There clearly are many issues that relate to the appropriate timing of melatonin treatment for its use in insomnia associated with alterations in the timing of the sleep-wake cycle in the elderly that need to be addressed in large clinical trails before any recommendations can be made for its use in the elderly.

A number of studies have attempted to use melatonin to alleviate the perceived effects of jet lag (primarily sleep disturbances) under both placebo-controlled and uncontrolled conditions (see also Chapter 50). Indeed, one laboratory has reported that in a population of 474 subjects taking melatonin versus 112 subjects taking placebo, there is an overall 50% reduction in self-related jet lag, and it was hypothesized that at least part of the beneficial effects of melatonin for jet lag may be due to a phase-shifting effect.[46, 59, 74] However, the largest double-blind, placebo-controlled randomized clinical study conducted to date has failed to confirm the efficacy of melatonin in the treatment of jet lag, with no improvement in self-reported jet lag symptoms and no evidence of an effect on reported sleep onset, time of awakening, and hours slept or napping.[75] Even if these discrepancies are favorably resolved, such subjective data alone provide little evidence about the mechanism by which the positive subjective effect occurs. In fact, objective assessment of circadian phase markers or of sleep efficiency was not conducted in most jet lag studies, and it is not clear whether the beneficial effect evident from the subjective data was due to a hypnotic, chronohypnotic, or chronobiotic effect of melatonin. Nevertheless, based on the reported phase-response curve to melatonin, elaborate timetables have been developed to advise travelers when they should take melatonin after eastward and westward travel over different numbers of time zones.[74] One difficulty in using melatonin for jet lag is that its use as a chronobiotic may require administration at times when it will have undesired hypnotic properties.[46, 74, 76]

Although it has become routine for researchers to assume that melatonin can reduce the number of days it takes endogenous circadian rhythms, including the sleep-wake cycle, to re-entrain after rapid travel across time zones,[46] there is very little evidence that under jet lag conditions treatment with melatonin does indeed have phase-shifting effects on objectively measured phase markers of human circadian rhythms that are under control of the central circadian clock. In one study that involved a simulated 9-h time shift, melatonin treatment was found to enhance the resynchronization speed of some, but not all, hormone and electrolyte secretion rhythms that were monitored.[77] However, the authors of that study concluded that the enhanced synchronization of rhythms was not sufficiently enough to warrant the use of melatonin as a phase-shifting agent for alleviation of the effects of jet lag.

CONCLUSIONS

Data from studies in human beings indicate that melatonin has sleep-inducing properties that are less consistent when near the evening endogenous melatonin rise. There also is evidence that melatonin may induce phase shifts in human circadian rhythms. If this were the case, melatonin could be useful for the treatment of insomnia and jet lag. Indeed, the combined circadian and hypnotic effects of melatonin would make it an attractive candidate for the treatment of sleep disorders related to inappropriate circadian timing. Carefully controlled clinical trials that focus on the possible beneficial effects of melatonin on specific sleep disorders are urgently needed. Furthermore, issues that relate to dose of melatonin, method of delivery, time of delivery, pharmacological profile, and so on should be examined because they are relevant to specific sleep disorders. Given the hypothesized hypnotic and phase-shifting effects of melatonin, it is clear that self-medication with this hormone could potentially exacerbate the adverse effects associated with insomnia. More importantly, the chronic use of melatonin cannot be justified for any sleep disorder at this time because neither the therapeutic nor the potential toxic effects of long-term use of this hormone, which has profound effects on the reproductive system of other mammals, are known.[78] Unfortunately, melatonin has been released for public use in the United States by the Food and Drug Administration and is available on an over-the-counter basis nationwide and in many other countries before controlled studies of its safety and efficacy have been carried out. A spate of books and magazine articles with many misstatements of fact and irresponsible conclusions, together with the release of melatonin, has led the U.S. public to presume that melatonin has been adequately tested for safety and clinical efficacy. No other hormone is available in the United States without a prescription, yet melatonin is being consumed nightly by millions of Americans in amounts that cause blood levels of the hormone to exceed those found naturally by more than 1000%. By releasing this hormone as a so-called food supplement, the Food and Drug Administration is conducting a large-scale uncontrolled clinical trial of the toxicity of this hormone; it may be up to epidemiologists to piece together the long-term consequences of this trial.

Acknowledgments

We thank Dr. Rod J. Hughes for helpful comments on the manuscript. This work was supported in part by grants from the National Institute on Aging (NIA-P01-AG09975 and NIA-1-U01-12642), the National Aeronautics and Space Administration (NAG9-524 and NAG5-3952), and the National Aeronautics and Space Administration through the NASA Cooperative Agreement NCC 9-58 with the National Space Biomedical Research Institute. Christian Cajochen was supported by a Swiss National Science Foundation postdoctoral fellowship (823A-046640). Some portions of a white paper entitled "Is Melatonin a Treatment for Insomnia and Jet Lag?" by C. A. Czeisler and F. W. Turek and published by the National Sleep Foundation are included here with permission from the publisher.

References

1. Dijk DJ, Shanahan TL, Duffy JF, et al. Variation of electroencephalographic activity during non-rapid eye movement and rapid eye movement sleep with phase of circadian melatonin rhythm in humans. J Physiol (Lond). 1997;505:851–858.
2. Czeisler C, Turek FW. Melatonin, sleep and circadian rhythms: current progress and controversies. J Biol Rhythms. 1997;12:710.
3. Lavie P. Ultrashort sleep-waking schedule III: "gates" and "forbidden zones" for sleep. Electroencephalogr Clin Neurophysiol. 1986;63:414–425.
4. Strogatz SH, Kronauer RE, Czeisler CA. Circadian pacemaker interferes with sleep onset at specific times each day: role in insomnia. Am J Physiol. 1987;253:R172–R178.
5. Cajochen C, Kräuchi K, Wirz-Justice A. The acute soporific action

of daytime melatonin administration: effects on the EEG during wakefulness and subjective alertness. J Biol Rhythms. 1997;12:636–643.
6. Dijk D-J, Cajochen C. Melatonin and the circadian regulation of sleep initiation, consolidation, structure and the sleep EEG. J Biol Rhythms. 1997;12:627–635.
7. Lavie P. Melatonin: role in gating nocturnal rise in sleep propensity. J Biol Rhythms. 1997;12:657–665.
8. Mendelson WB. Efficacy of melatonin as a hypnotic agent. J Biol Rhythms. 1997;12:651–656.
9. Sack RL, Hughes RJ, Edgar DM, et al. Sleep-promoting effects of melatonin: at what dose, in whom, under what conditions, and by what mechanisms? Sleep. 1997;20:908–915.
10. Zhdanova IV, Wurtman RJ. Efficacy of melatonin as a sleep-promoting agent. J Biol Rhythms. 1997;12:644–650.
11. Dawson D, Encel N. Melatonin and sleep in humans. J Pineal Res. 1993;15:1–12.
12. Hughes RJ, Badia P. Sleep-promoting and hypothermic effects of daytime melatonin administration in humans. Sleep. 1997;20:124–131.
13. Nave R, Peled R, Lavie P. Melatonin improves evening napping. Eur J Pharmacol. 1995;275:213–216.
14. Zhdanova IV, Wurtman RJ, Morabito C, et al. Effects of low oral doses of melatonin, given 2–4 hours before habitual bedtime, on sleep in normal young humans. Sleep. 1996;19:423–431.
15. Dollins AB, Zhdanova IV, Wurtman RJ, et al. Effect of inducing nocturnal serum melatonin concentrations in daytime on sleep, mood, body temperature, and performance. Proc Natl Acad Sci U S A. 1994;91:1824–1828.
16. Deacon S, Arendt J. Melatonin-induced temperature suppression and its acute phase-shifting effects correlate in a dose-dependent manner in humans. Brain Res. 1995;688:77–85.
17. Kräuchi K, Cajochen C, Wirz-Justice A. A relationship between heat loss and sleepiness: effects of postural change and melatonin administration. J Appl Physiol. 1997;83:134–139.
18. Badia P, Myers BL, Murphy PJ. Melatonin and thermoregulation. In: Reiter R, Yu HS, eds: Melatonin: Biosynthesis, Physiological Effects, and Clinical Application. Boca Raton, Fla: CRC Press; 1992:349–364.
19. Cajochen C, Kräuchi K, Danilenko KV, et al. Evening administration of melatonin and bright light: interactions on the EEG during sleep and wakefulness. J Sleep Res. 1998;7:145–157.
20. Waldhauser F, Saletu B, Trinchard-Lugan I. Sleep laboratory investigations on hypnotic properties of melatonin. Psychopharmacology. 1990;100:222–226.
21. James SP, Mendelson WB, Sack DA, et al. The effect of melatonin on normal sleep. Neuropsychopharmacology. 1987;1:41–44.
22. Nave R, Herer P, Haimov I, et al. Hypnotic and hypothermic effects of melatonin on daytime sleep in humans: lack of antagonism by flumazenil. Neurosci Lett. 1996;214:123–126.
23. Cajochen C, Kräuchi K, Möri D, et al. Melatonin and S-20098 increase REM sleep propensity and the wake-up tendency without modifying NREM-sleep homeostasis. Am J Physiol. 1997;272:R1189–R1196.
24. Anton-Tay F, Diaz JL, Fernandez-Guardiola A. On the effect of melatonin upon human brains: its possible therapeutic implications. Life Sci. 1971;10:841–850.
25. Dijk D-J, Roth C, Landolt H-P, et al. Melatonin effect on daytime sleep in men: suppression of EEG low frequency activity and enhancement of spindle frequency activity. Neurosci Lett. 1995;201:13–16.
26. Wirz-Justice A, Armstrong SM. Melatonin: nature's soporific? J Sleep Res. 1996;5:137–141.
27. Edgar DM, Dement WC, Fuller CA. Effect of SCN lesions on sleep in squirrel monkeys: evidence for opponent processes in sleep-wake regulation. J Neurosci. 1993;13:1065–1079.
28. Dijk DJ, Czeisler CA. Contribution of the circadian pacemaker and the sleep homeostat to sleep propensity, sleep structure, electroencephalographic slow waves, and sleep spindle activity in humans. J Neurosci. 1995;15:3526–3538.
29. Dijk DJ, Czeisler CA. Paradoxical timing of the circadian rhythm of sleep propensity serves to consolidate sleep and wakefulness in humans. Neurosci Lett. 1994;166:63–68.
30. Liu C, Weaver DR, Jin X, et al. Molecular dissection of two distinct actions of melatonin on the suprachiasmatic circadian clock. Neuron. 1997;19:91–102.

31. Barinaga M. How jet-lag hormone does double duty in the brain. Science. 1997;277:480.
32. Haimov I, Laudon M, Zisapel N, et al. Sleep disorders and melatonin rhythms in elderly people. Br Med J. 1994;309:167.
33. Hajak G, Rodenbeck A, Staedt J, et al. Nocturnal plasma melatonin levels in patients suffering from chronic primary insomnia. J Pineal Res. 1995;19:116–122.
34. Hughes RJ, Sack RL, Lewy AJ. The role of melatonin and circadian phase in age-related sleep-maintenance insomnia: assessment in a clinical trial of melatonin replacement. Sleep. 1998;21:52–68.
35. MacFarlane JG, Cleghorn JM, Brown GM, et al. The effects of exogenous melatonin on the total sleep time and daytime alertness of chronic insomniacs: a preliminary study. Biol Psychol. 1991;30:371–376.
36. Ellis CM, Lemmens G, Parkes JD. Melatonin and insomnia. J Sleep Res. 1996;5:61–65.
37. James SP, Sack DA, Rosenthal NE, et al. Melatonin administration in insomnia. Neuropsychopharmacology. 1990;3:19–23.
38. Garfinkel D, Laudon M, Nof D, et al. Improvement of sleep quality in elderly people by controlled-release melatonin. Lancet. 1995;346:541–544.
39. Haimov I, Lavie P. Potential of melatonin replacement therapy in older patients with sleep disorders. Drugs Aging. 1995;7:75–78.
40. Wurtman RJ, Zhdanova I. Improvement of sleep quality by melatonin. Lancet. 1995;346:1491.
41. Bliwise DL. Normal aging. In: Kryger MH, Roth T, Dement WC, eds. Principles and Practices of Sleep Medicine. 2nd ed. Philadelphia, Pa: WB Saunders; 1994:26–39.
42. Dement WC, Miles L, Carskadon M. "White paper" on sleep and aging. J Am Geriatr Soc. 1982;30:25–50.
43. Prinz PN. Sleep and sleep disorders in older adults. J Clin Neurophysiol. 1995;12:139–146.
44. Roth T, Richardson G. Commentary: is melatonin administration an effective hypnotic? J Biol Rhythms. 1997;12:666–669.
45. Arendt J, Aldhous M, English J, et al. Some effects of jet-lag and their alleviation by melatonin. Ergonomics. 1987;30:1379–1393.
46. Arendt J, Deacon S, English J, et al. Melatonin and adjustment to phase shift. J Sleep Res. 1995;4:74–79.
47. Claustrat B, Brun J, David M, et al. Melatonin and jet lag: confirmatory result using a simplified protocol. Biol Psych. 1992;32:705–711.
48. Deacon S, Arendt J. Adapting to phase shifts, II: effects of melatonin and conflicting light treatment. Physiol Behav. 1996;59:675–682.
49. Petrie K, Dawson AG, Thompson L, et al. A double-blind trial of melatonin as a treatment for jet lag in international cabin crew. Biol Psychol. 1993;33:526–530.
50. Short RV, Armstrong SM. Method for minimizing disturbances in circadian rhythms and bodily performance and function. Australia Patent Application PG 4737; 1984.
51. Redman JR. Circadian entrainment and phase shifting in mammals with melatonin. J Biol Rhythms. 1997;12:581–587.
52. Davis FC. Melatonin: role in development. J Biol Rhythms. 1997;12:498–508.
53. Reppert SM, Weaver DR, Rivkees SA, et al. Putative melatonin receptors in a human biological clock. Science. 1988;242:78–81.
54. Sack RL, Brandes RL, Lewy AJ. Totally blind people with free-running circadian rhythms can be normally entrained with melatonin. Sleep Res Online. 1999;2(suppl 1):624.
55. Skene DJ, Lockley SW, Arendt J. Melatonin entrains the free-running circadian rhythms of some blind subjects. Sleep Res Online. 1999;2(suppl 1):725.
56. Arendt J. Safety of melatonin in long-term use. J Biol Rhythms. 1997;12:673–681.
57. Arendt J, Skene DJ, Middleton B, et al. Efficacy of melatonin treatment in jet lag, shift work, and blindness. J Biol Rhythms. 1997;12:604–617.
58. Gillette MU, McArthur AJ. Circadian actions of melatonin at the suprachiasmatic nucleus. Behav Brain Res. 1996;73:135–139.
59. Lewy AJ, Sack RL, Blood ML, et al. Melatonin marks circadian phase position and resets the endogenous circadian pacemaker in humans. In: Ciba Foundation Symposium 183: Circadian Clocks and Their Adjustments. Chichester, England: John Wiley & Sons; 1995.
60. Zaidan R, Geoffriau M, Brun J, et al. Melatonin is able to influence its secretion in humans: description of a phase-response curve. Neuroendocrinology. 1994;60:105–112.
61. Kräuchi K, Cajochen C, Möri D, et al. Early evening melatonin and S-20098 advance circadian phase and nocturnal regulation of core body temperature. Am J Physiol. 1997;272:R1178–R1188.
62. Kostoglou-Athanassiou I, Treacher DF, Wheeler MJ, et al. Melatonin administration and pituitary hormone secretion. Clin Endocrinol (Oxf). 1998;48:31–37.
63. Boivin D, Czeisler CA. Resetting of circadian melatonin and cortisol rhythms in humans by ordinary room light. Neuroreport. 1998;9:779–782.
64. Deacon S, English J, Arendt J. Sensitivity of the human circadian pacemaker to melatonin timed phase delay: a dose response study. Chronobiol Int Abstr. 1997;14(suppl 1):41.
65. Parkes JD. Melatonin and sleep. In: Fraschini F, Reiter RJ, Stankov B, eds. The Pineal Gland and Its Hormones: Fundamentals and Clinical Perspectives. New York, NY: Plenum Press; 1995:183–197.
66. Weitzman ED, Czeisler CA, Coleman RM, et al. Delayed sleep phase insomnia: a chronobiologic disorder associated with sleep onset insomnia. Arch Gen Psych. 1981;38:737–746.
67. Thorpy MJ, Korman E, Spielman AJ, et al. Delayed sleep phase syndrome in adolescents. J Adolesc Health Care. 1988;9:22–27.
68. Pelayo RP, Thorpy MJ, Glovinsky P. Prevalence of delayed sleep phase syndrome among adolescents. Sleep Res. 1988;17:391.
69. Dahlitz M, Alvarez B, Vignau J, et al. Delayed sleep phase syndrome response to melatonin. Lancet. 1991;337:1121–1124.
70. Oldani A, Ferini-Strambi L, Zucconi M, et al. Melatonin and delayed sleep phase syndrome: ambulatory polygraphic evaluation. Neuroreport. 1994;6:132–134.
71. Nagtegaal JE, Kerkhof GA, Smits MG, et al. Delayed sleep phase syndrome: a placebo-controlled cross-over study on the effects of melatonin administered five hours before the individual dim light melatonin onset. J Sleep Res. 1998;7:135–143.
72. van Coevorden A, Mockel J, Laurent E, et al. Neuroendocrine rhythms and sleep in aging. Am J Physiol. 1991;260:E651–E661.
73. Lewy AJ, Ahmed S, Jackson JML, et al. Melatonin shifts human circadian rhythms according to a phase-response curve. Chronobiol Int. 1992;9:380–392.
74. Arendt J, Aldhous M, Marks V. Alleviation of jet lag by melatonin: preliminary results of controlled double blind trial. Br Med J. 1986;292:1170.
75. Spitzer RL, Terman M, Malt U, et al. Failure of melatonin to affect jet lag in a randomized double-blind trial. Soc Light Treatment Biol Rhythms Abstr. 1997;9:1.
76. Lino A, Silvy S, Condorelli L, et al. Melatonin and jet lag: treatment schedule. Biol Psych. 1993;34:587.
77. Samel A, Wegmann HM, Vejvoda M, et al. Influence of melatonin treatment on human circadian rhythmicity before and after a simulated 9-hr time shift. J Biol Rhythms. 1991;6:235–248.
78. Reiter RJ. Melatonin and human reproduction. Ann Med. 1998;30:103–108.

five

Pharmacology

Wallace B. Mendelson

32

Hypnotics: Basic Mechanisms and Pharmacology

Wallace B. Mendelson

At the time of this writing, the clinically used sedative-hypnotics in the United States include five benzodiazepines ("Valium-like" compounds) available in both prescription and generic forms and two nonbenzodiazepines (zolpidem and zaleplon) available as prescription agents (Table 32–1). Zopiclone, a nonbenzodiazepine, although not available in the United States, is used in many countries. Hypnotics represent a large market in the United States, involving approximately 18.4 million prescriptions, the value of which, in 1997, was approximately $441 million (data from IMS America, Inc.). Older hypnotics, such as barbiturates, were used substantially less, with approximately 3.9 million prescriptions with a market value of $16.9 million (data from IMS America, Inc.). In addition, there were approximately 60.2 million packages* of nonprescription hypnotics bought in 1997 (data from Information Resources, Inc). These included agents sold specifically for sleep, with a market value of approximately $93.1 million; combination analgesic and sleep aids, with an approximate market value of $168.4 million; and melatonin, the market value of which was approximately $50 million (data from Information Resources, Inc).

Although in one sense, the amount of prescription hypnotics sounds large, to put it in perspective, the total market for benzodiazepines used primarily as anxiolytics was $692 million, and for antidepressants, it was almost $5 billion during the same period (data from IMS America, Inc). Indeed, one could make a case that in the population at large, prescription hypnotics are taken relatively infrequently by insomniacs. In one survey of more than 7000 enrollees in five large health maintenance organizations (HMOs),[1] patients with insomnia were divided into those with only sleep complaints (level 1) and those who believed that their sleep difficulties had an adverse effect on their daytime functioning (level 2). The percentage of level 1 insomniacs taking prescription and nonprescription hypnotics was 5.5% and 11.2%; comparable values for level 2 insomniacs were 11.6% and 21.4%, respectively. Many

---

*Number of nonprescription hypnotic packages for 1997 estimated using 52 weeks of data ending 12 October 1997. For sleeping remedies and combination analgesic-sleep aids, a volume equates to a package. For melatonin, volume data are reported in increments of 10 pills. To convert a volume to a package, the volume data was divided by 5 to represent a bottle of 50 pills. Thus the amounts consumed would be sleeping remedies, 18.8 million packages; total combination analgesic and sleep aids, 30.6 million packages; melatonin, 10.1 million (bottle of 50 pills).

Table 32–1. SEDATIVE-HYPNOTIC MARKET IN THE UNITED STATES: SEDATIVE NONBARBITURATES

Trade Name	Generic Equivalent
Ambien	Zolpidem tartrate
Dalmane	Flurazepam HCl
Doral	Quazepam
Halcion	Triazolam
ProSom	Estazolam
Restoril	Temazepam
Sonata	Zaleplon

patients, of course, receive other classes of prescription drugs given for purposes of helping sleep. One study of primary care patients in an HMO indicated that 13% of insomniacs who were not considered to have affective disorder were receiving antidepressant medications.[2] Many people also self-medicate with alcohol; a telephone survey of approximately 1000 representative adults in the general population found that 10% had done so in the past year.[3] In general, this widespread practice should be discouraged. It exposes the patient to the risk of ethanol dependence and is also relatively ineffective. Although orally administered ethanol has some sleep-inducing properties, it often promotes sleep disturbance as the night progresses.[4]

MECHANISM OF ACTION

When the benzodiazepines first gained prominence in the 1960s, most theories of how they might act were inherited from previous studies of ethanol and barbiturates and involved possible alterations in membrane phospholipid integrity and energy metabolism. With the discovery of the benzodiazepine receptor (now generally referred to as the gamma-aminobutyric acid-A [GABA_A]-benzodiazepine receptor complex) in the late 1970s, attention was focused on the possibility that the pharmacologic effects of these compounds results from their saturable, stereospecific binding to a specific recognition site.[5, 6] The receptor complex is part of a group of ligand-gated ion channel complexes that also includes glycine, serotonin type 3, neuronal nicotinic acetylcholine, and other receptors.[7] It is functionally comprised of three moieties: a benzodiazepine recognition site, a GABA_A recognition site, and a chloride ionophore. Molecular cloning studies indicate that, structurally, it is composed of at least five different glycoprotein subunits (Fig. 32–1), each of which may have multiple isoforms.[8] Two particular combinations of isoforms that are often noted are the type I configuration (alpha 1, beta 2, gamma 2) and type II (alpha 3, beta 2, gamma 2). Most traditional benzodiazepine hypnotics bind to both types. Some of the newer non-

benzodiazepine agents, including zolpidem and zaleplon, bind with relatively greater specificity to the type I receptor. Whether this selective binding translates into more specific pharmacologic properties is not certain.

The end result of a benzodiazepine agonist binding to its specific site is that, as an outcome of a complex interaction with the GABA recognition site, the flow of negatively charged chloride ions into the neuron is enhanced, changing the postsynaptic membrane potential and altering input resistance such that the postsynaptic neuron is less likely to achieve an action potential. One of the intriguing features of this view is that it provides a beginning for understanding a longstanding puzzle—how hypnotic medications of many different pharmacologic classes may have relatively similar effects on the process of inducing sleep. Indeed, the newer nonbenzodiazepine agents such as zolpidem and zaleplon bind to a subclass of benzodiazepine recognition sites, ethanol has profound effects on chloride channel function,[4] and barbiturates bind to a distinct site.[9] Barbiturates, for instance, may cause chloride channels to open for prolonged periods,[10] whereas benzodiazepines may increase the frequency of opening of these channels.[11] Similarly, the active metabolite of chloral hydrate[7] and the anesthetic propofol[12] modulate GABA_A receptor function. Several lines of evidence have also suggested that the hypnotic effects of benzodiazepines may also involve presynaptic effects mediated by alterations in potential-dependent calcium channel activity.[13]

The original characterization of the receptor complex indicated that it mediates the anxiolytic, muscle relaxant, and anticonvulsant effects of benzodiazepines.[5, 6] That it also mediates the sleep-inducing effects was demonstrated in a series of studies showing, for instance, that some beta-carboline compounds that act as receptor inverse agonists induce increased wakefulness and at low doses block sleep induction by benzodiazepines,[13] and that the binding of benzodiazepines is stereospecific, such that an enantiomeric form (the "B_10" compounds) have opposite effects, one inducing sleep and the other promoting wakefulness.[4, 13]

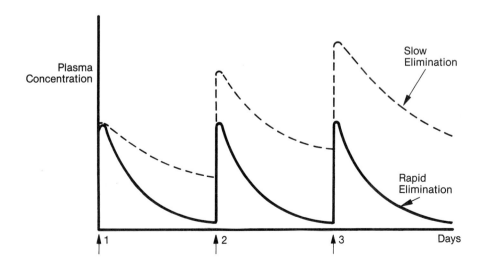

Figure 32–1. A hypnotic with a relatively long elimination half life (e.g., greater than 24 h) accumulates during nightly use, in contrast to an agent with relatively short elimination half-life (e.g., 6 h).

In contrast to the growing understanding of the interaction of benzodiazepine agonists at a molecular level, the anatomic sites at which they act to induce sleep has been more poorly understood. The most parsimonious view would be that hypnotics act at loci thought to be important in sleep regulation on the basis of lesion or stimulation studies (a general review of the neuroanatomy of sleep is found in Chapter 10). Using that approach, Mendelson and Martin[14] microinjected triazolam into a number of such sites. One of the most striking findings was how, in many areas, injections produced no effect on sleep (e.g., the locus coeruleus, the gigantocellular tegmental fields, the basomedial nucleus of the amygdala), or actually enhanced wakefulness (the dorsal raphe nuclei). In contrast, injections into the medial preoptic area (MPA) of the anterior hypothalamus consistently enhanced sleep, an anatomically specific effect insofar as injections into nearby structures (the lateral preoptic area, the horizontal limb of the diagonal band of Broca,[14] the ventrolateral preoptic area[14a]) had no effect. The basal forebrain and anterior hypothalamus have long been thought to play an important role in sleep regulation.

The MPA is a complex structure that receives afferents from many areas in the forebrain and brainstem. Among these are projections from various areas of the hypothalamus, as well as serotonergic fibers from the dorsal raphe nuclei and noradrenergic projections.[15] Cell bodies and fibers of different parts cross-react in immunohistochemical studies with a number of neurotransmitters such as substance P and neuropeptide Y.[16] Push-pull cannula studies have reported release of catecholamines, GABA, and glutamate.[17] GABA is uniformly distributed throughout the hypothalamus, and its synthetic enzyme is found in high concentrations in the preoptic area.[18] GABA$_A$-benzodiazepine receptors appear in significant concentrations here,[19] suggesting that benzodiazepines might inhibit neuronal activity. The preoptic area also contains cells that are responsive to temperature, osmolarity, glucose, and steroids[20] and receives afferents from various sensory systems.[15] The basal forebrain contains neurons that increase firing during nonrapid eye movement (NREM) sleep compared to waking (*sleep active neurons*), although higher concentrations are found in the lateral preoptic area and diagonal band of Broca.[21] There are also neurons that selectively increase or decrease firing rates during rapid eye movement (REM) sleep and NREM sleep.[22] The preoptic area in general, and the MPA in particular, appears to have a role in coordinating various systems involved in reproductive and homeostatic functions.[23] Given the bidirectional interactions of sleep with cardiovascular, thermoregulatory, endocrine, and sensory systems,[24] it seems likely that the preoptic area might be involved in coordinating sleep with other systems. It may be, then, that the preoptic area is among the loci at which benzodiazepine agonists act to induce sleep. Subsequent studies have also indicated that microinjections of pentobarbital,[25] ethanol,[26] and adenosine[27] into the MPA enhance sleep. Indeed, looking at a somewhat broader area, adenosine has been shown to accumulate extracellularly in the basal forebrain cho-

linergic region,[28] which in turn has efferents to cortical and thalamic systems involved in arousal. It has been suggested that alteration of functioning of this cholinergic area may be the mechanism by which the propensity to sleep is enhanced by prolonged wakefulness. Similarly, it may be that possible sleep-promoting effects of antihistamines and some antidepressants (many of which have significant anticholinergic properties) might be mediated by alterations of cholinergic neurons in the basal forebrain. In summary, the manner in which hypnotics may function to induce sleep is not fully elucidated, but a number of findings suggest that the basal forebrain–anterior hypothalamus is among the crucial areas to consider.

Moving from the neuroanatomic to the clinical level, less is understood about the mechanism by which hypnotics act. One approach raises the possibility that, among their actions, they alter the *perception* of sleep and wakefulness.[29] This notion grew out of the classical observation by Rechtschaffen[30] that poor sleepers, when experimentally awakened early in stage 2 sleep, tend to report that they had been awake, whereas good sleepers tend to report that they had been asleep. Later studies by Mendelson[31, 32] replicated this process and demonstrated that after administration of triazolam or zolpidem, insomniacs were more likely to report that they believed they had been asleep. In contrast, when zolpidem was given to normal subjects, this effect was not evident.[33] One interpretation of these data is that hypnotics such as triazolam and zolpidem may correct a misperception of sleep in insomniacs, such that their experience of whether they are awake or asleep becomes more like that of good sleepers.

PHARMACOKINETICS

Benzodiazepines

With the possible exception of temazepam, the benzodiazepines used as hypnotics are rapidly and completely absorbed, with peak plasma levels in 1.0 to 1.5 h. Some, notably flurazepam, are detectable primarily only in the form of their active metabolites, and many display kinetics that reflect enterohepatic circulation.[34] Generally, oral administration is more reliable and complete than after intramuscular injection. Although there is significant protein binding, there are few or no cases in which displacement of other protein-bound drugs is clinically relevant. Most are lipophilic and rapidly enter the central nervous system (CNS), where concentrations reflect unbound drug in plasma. Whereas the older, longer-acting agents are metabolized to active compounds, the shorter-acting agents such as triazolam are broken down into inactive substances (Table 32–2). The elimination half-lives vary widely, from the relatively short-acting triazolam to intermediate agents such as temazepam to long-acting substances such as flurazepam (see Table 32–2). As is discussed in Chapter 33, accumulation of the longer elimination half-life agents taken nightly has significant bearing on one major clinical issue—the appearance of

Table 32–2. PHARMACOKINETIC PROPERTIES AND DOSAGES OF SOME HYPNOTIC DRUGS USED IN THE TREATMENT OF INSOMNIA

	$T_{1/2}$ (h)	Pharmacologically Active Metabolites	Dosage (mg)
Benzodiazepines*			
Quazepam	48–120	Desalkyl-flurazepam	7.5–15
Flurazepam	48–120	Desalkyl-flurazepam	15–30
Triazolam	2–6	None	0.125–0.25
Estazolam	8–24	None	1–2
Temazepam†	8–20	None	15–30
Loprazolam‡	4.6–11.4	None	1–2
Flunitrazepam‡	10.7–20.3	None	0.5–1
Lormetazepam‡	7.9–11.4	None	1–2
Nitrazepam‡	25–35	None	5–10
Nonbenzodiazepines			
Zolpidem	1.5–2.4		5–10 (age > 65 y) 10–20 (age < 65 y)
Zopiclone‡	5–6		3.75 (age > 65 y) 7.5 (age < 65 y)
Zaleplon	1	None	5 (age > 65 y) 5–10 (age < 65 y)

*Citations for kinetic information on benzodiazepines are found in reference 37.
†Originally formulated as a hard capsule in the United States; concerns with kinetics and efficacy led to reformulation of the preparation to a soft gelatin capsule with comparable characteristics of other marketed benzodiazepines of its class.[35, 36]
‡Not available in the United States.

daytime residual sedation (Fig. 32–2). Because of the lipophilicity, many are rapidly redistributed, which may play as important a role in the decline in CNS effects as the metabolism. Another implication of the high lipophilicity is that the volume of distribution is often increased in the elderly, resulting in an increased half-life. Most are broken down by hepatic microsomal systems and excreted as conjugated glucuronides. There is no stimulation of the microsomal systems and hence no enhancement of the rate of breakdown of other drugs that undergo the same metabolic processes. Their own metabolism may be inhibited by some compounds, such as cimetidine, and some steroids and may be accelerated in smokers.

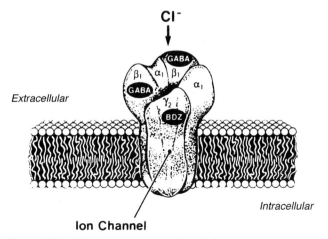

Figure 32–2. Schematic representation of the gamma-aminobutyric acid-$_A$–benzodiazepine receptor complex. (From American Journal of Psychiatry, vol 148, 162, 1991. Copyright 1991, the American Psychiatric Association. Reprinted by permission.)

Zolpidem

Zolpidem, an imidazopyridine compound with relative selectivity for the type-I GABA$_A$-benzodiazepine receptor, is rapidly absorbed. Due to first-pass metabolism, it has a bioavailability of 67% after oral administration of doses up to 20 mg.[38] Peak concentrations are reached after 1.6 h. Total protein binding is approximately 92%. Absorption is slightly decreased when taken on a full stomach. It has no pharmacologically active metabolites and is eliminated primarily by renal excretion.

Zopiclone

Zopiclone, which is not on the market in the United States, is a cyclopyrrolone that acts not only at the GABA$_A$-benzodiazepine receptor complex but also possibly at a different binding domain than benzodiazepines or by producing different conformational changes than the benzodiazepines.[39] It is rapidly absorbed, with peak plasma concentrations occurring in 0.5 to 2 h.[39] Bioavailability is about 80%, implying that the first pass effect is relatively small.[40] It is lipophilic and enters rapidly into the CNS. Protein binding is approximately 45%. It has two major metabolites: the N-oxide, which has lower pharmacologic activity, and the inactive N-desmethyl derivative, which along with various minor metabolites, is excreted primarily by the kidneys and lungs.[39]

Zaleplon

A pyrazolopyrimidine that binds selectively to the benzodiazepine-1 receptor, zaleplon is rapidly absorbed after oral administration, with peak concentrations being reached in 1 h, and has an elimination half-life of approximately 1 h. Protein binding is approximately 60%. It is rapidly metabolized to inactive forms, with approximately 71% of labeled compound recovered in the urine and 17% in the feces. Recommendations for administration in the United States include immediately before bedtime or after the patient has gone to bed and has experienced difficulty falling asleep. In the latter case, it should be taken at least 4 h before time of arising, in order to avoid any possible memory difficulties.

PHARMACOLOGICAL PROPERTIES

Although the hypnotic benzodiazepines are given for purposes of aiding sleep, they share a spectrum of pharmacological properties with agents given as daytime sedatives or anxiolytics. Indeed, some authors have suggested that the designation of some benzodiazepines as hypnotics is as much a marketing as it has been a pharmacological decision. Some of their effects are anxiolytic, myorelaxant, and anticonvulsant. Many, particularly the longer-acting agents, have mild respiratory depressant properties,[41, 42] which are much less evident in shorter-acting agents.[43] There is even some limited evidence that triazolam may improve sleep-disturbed respiration in central sleep apnea,[44] although whether this is related to direct respiratory effects or secondary to decreasing the number of arousals during sleep is not clear. Even for the longer-acting agents, however, respiratory depression is much milder than those of older nonbenzodiazepines such as the barbiturates. In practical terms, there is no significant effect in patients with normal ventilation, although it may become evident in patients with compromised respiration such as chronic obstructive pulmonary disease (COPD) or unrecognized sleep-disordered breathing. In general, adverse reactions are relatively rare and mild. One review of 3 years' experience in a 1000-bed teaching hospital found the median rate of reported adverse events to be 0.01% (1 in 10,000) doses administered and ran as high as 0.05%.[25] The rate for triazolam was 0.02%.

Unlike older hypnotics such as the barbiturates, the hypnotic benzodiazepines are relatively benign in overdose when taken alone by a medically healthy individual. They may be toxic, however, when taken in combination with other CNS depressants such as alcohol, and because a significant portion of overdoses involve a combination of drugs,[45] it is wise to treat them as potentially toxic or even lethal agents. In practice, this translates into being conscious of the possibility that a patient seeking help for sleep disturbance may be suffering from unrecognized depressive illness, and if it is present, initiating appropriate antidepressant therapy. In most cases, the preceding generalizations in this section apply to zolpidem as well. There is some evidence from animal studies that zolpidem possesses a greater separation of hypnotic and sedative doses. It has been reported to have no respiratory depressant

properties up to doses of 10 mg and to exhibit mild inhibition of mean inspiratory drive at 20 mg.[46] Zopiclone in therapeutic doses appears to have no significant effect on sleep-disordered breathing in COPD patients.[47]

EFFECTS ON SLEEP

Polysomnographic studies of benzodiazepines indicate that, consistent with their clinical effects, sleep latency and wake time after sleep onset are generally reduced, and total sleep time is increased.[4] As with barbiturates and ethanol, spindle activity may be increased. REM sleep time may be reduced mildly, in contrast to the potent REM suppression induced by barbiturates. In the early years after the introduction of benzodiazepines into the U.S. market, much was made of this observation, which was interpreted to mean that they somehow produced a more "natural" sleep. With hindsight, many investigators recognize that the psychological effects of REM deprivation are much less clear than originally thought and that, indeed, in the case of depressed patients, REM deprivation may even be therapeutic (see Chapter 96); whether having only mild REM suppressant properties translates into some clinical advantage seems uncertain. The benzodiazepines are, however, in contrast to the barbiturates, potent suppressors of slow-wave sleep. The same dilemma that arises in terms of REM sleep appears once again; because the function of slow-wave sleep remains unknown, the clinical significance of pharmacologically suppressing this stage remains uncertain. The nonbenzodiazepine zolpidem shares with the benzodiazepines the mild effects on REM sleep but in contrast does not alter slow-wave sleep, which may even increase toward more expected values in some insomniacs with low baseline levels. Zaleplon has been reported to have minimal or no effects on total REM or slow wave sleep.

Clinical efficacy studies indicate that virtually all of these agents potently improve polysomnographic measures of sleep and result in better subjective ratings of sleep quality during short-term use. One of the few distinctions among the benzodiazepines is that the longer-acting agents such as flurazepam may not have as much effectiveness on sleep latency until the 2nd night of administration.[48] One concern that was initially raised in terms of the short-acting agents such as triazolam was the possibility that the relatively rapid metabolism might lead to disturbed sleep after several hours; later studies analyzing awakening in the latter part of the night have generally found no evidence that this is the case.[49, 50]

One still unsettled issue is the rate at which tolerance develops to the clinically used hypnotics. The common clinical lore has traditionally been that these agents lose their effectiveness after 2 or 3 weeks' administration. More recently, a number of investigators have questioned this view. Although the data are less clear for benzodiazepines, a number of studies reviewed[81] have shown minimal or no tolerance to zolpidem in nightly use for 6 months or longer, and in one case a preliminary study indicated no loss of effectiveness during 1 y of administration of zaleplon. The evaluation of this question is difficult, however, due to the powerful effect of study design (parallel or sequential treatment with placebo) and outcome measure (polysomnographic or self-report) on the results. There are also minimal data available on the effectiveness of intermittent administration and on combined pharmacological and nonpharmacological therapy.

Acknowledgement

This work was partially supported by National Institutes of Health grant 1KO7HL03640.

References

1. Hatoum HT, Kania CM, Kong SX, et al. Prevalence of insomnia: a survey of the enrollees at five managed care organizations. Am J Manag Care. 1998;4:79–86.
2. Simon GE, VonKorff M. Prevalence, burden, and treatment of insomnia in primary care. Am J Psychiatry. 1997;154:1417–1423.
3. National Sleep Foundation. 1998 Omnibus Sleep in America Poll. Washington, DC: National Sleep Foundation; 1998.
4. Mendelson WB. Human Sleep: Research and Clinical Care. New York, NY: Plenum Press; 1987:1–436.
5. Mohler H, Okada T. Benzodiazepine receptor: demonstration in the central nervous system. Science. 1977;198:849–851.
6. Squires RF, Braestrup C. Benzodiazepine receptors in rat brain. Nature. 1977;266:732–734.
7. Krasowski MD, Finn SE, Ye Q, et al. Trichloroethanol modulation of recombinant GABA-A, glycine, and GABA p1 receptors. J Pharmacol Exp Ther. 1998;934–942.
8. Whiting PJ, McKernan RM, Wager-Srdar SA. Structure and pharmacology of vertebrate GABA-A receptor subtypes. Int Rev Neurobiol. 1995;38:95–138.
9. Harrison N, Mendelson W, de Wit H. Barbiturates. In: Psychopharmacology: 4th Generation of Progress. In press.
10. Macdonald RL, Rogers CJ, Twman RE. Barbiturate regulation of kinetic properties of the GABA-A receptor channel of mouse spinal neurones in culture. J Physiol. 1989;417:483–500.
11. Study RE, Barker JL. Diazepam and (-)pentobarbital: fluctuation analysis reveals different mechanisms for potentiation of gamma-aminobutyric acid responses in cultured neurons. Proc Natl Acad Sci U S A. 1981;78:7180–7184.
12. Krasowski MD, O'Shea SM, Rick CEM, et al. Alpha subunit isoform influences GABA-A receptor modulation by propofol. Neuropharmacology. 1997;36:941–949.
13. Mendelson WB. Neuropharmacology of sleep induction by benzodiazepines. Crit Rev Neurobiol. 1992;6:221–232.
14. Mendelson WB, Martin JV. Characterization of the hypnotic effects of triazolam microinjections into the medial preoptic area. Life Sci. 1992;50:1117–1128.
14a. Mendelson WB. Effects of microinjection of triazolam into the ventrolateral preoptic area on sleep in the rat. Life Sci. In press.
15. Simerly RB, Swanson LW. The organization of neural inputs to the medial preoptic nucleus of the rat. J Comp Neurol. 1985;246:312–342.
16. Simerly RB, Gorski RA, Swanson LW. Neurotransmitter specificity of cell and fibers in the medial preoptic nucleus: an immunohistochemical study in the rat. J Comp Neurol. 1986;246:343–363.
17. Demling J, Fuchs E, Baumert M, et al. Preoptic catecholamine, GABA, and glutamate release in ovariectomized estrogen-primed rats utilizing a push-pull cannula technique. Neuroendocrinology. 1985;41:212–218.
18. Tappaz ML, Brownstein MJ, Kopin IJ. Glutamate decarboxylase (GAD) and gamma-aminobutyric acid (GABA) in discrete nuclei of hypothalamus and substantia nigra. Brain Res. 1977;125:109–121.
19. Unnerstall JR, Niehoff DL, Kuhar MJ, et al. Quantitative receptor autoradiography using 3H-ultrofilm: application to multiple benzodiazepine receptors. J Neurosci. 1982;6:59–73.
20. Boulant JA, Silva NL. Neuronal sensitivities in preoptic tissue slices: interactions among homeostatic systems. Brain Res Bull. 1988;20:871–878.
21. Szymusiak R, McGinty DJ. Sleep-related neuronal discharge in the basal forebrain of cats. Brain Res Bull. 1986;370:82–92.
22. Koyama Y, Hayaishi O. Firing of neurons in the preoptic/anterior hypothalamic areas in rat: its possible involvement in slow wave sleep and paradoxical sleep. Neurosci Res. 1994;19:31–38.
23. Simerly RB, Swanson LW. The organization of neural inputs to the medial preoptic nucleus of the rat. J Comp Neurol. 1986;246:312–342.
24. McGinty D. Brain mechanisms of sleep. In: McGinty D, Morrison A, Drucker-Colin R, et al, eds. Brain Mechanisms of Sleep. New York, NY: Raven Press; 1985:361–384.
25. Mendelson WB, Thompson C, Franko T. Adverse reactions to sedative/hypnotics: three years' experience. Sleep. 1996;19:702–706.
26. Ticho SR, Stojanovic M, Lekovic G, et al. Effects of ethanol injection to the preoptic area on sleep and temperature in rats. Alcohol. 1992;9:275–278.
27. Ticho SR, Radulovacki M. Role of adenosine in sleep and temperature regulation in the preoptic area of rats. Pharmacol Biochem Behav. 1991;40:33–40.
28. Porkka-Heiskanen T, Strecker RE, Thakkar M, et al. Adenosine: a mediator of the sleep-inducing effects of prolonged wakefulness. Science. 1997;276:1265–1268.
29. Mendelson WB. Clinical neuropharmacology of sleep. Neurol Clin. 1990;8:153–160.
30. Rechtschaffen A. Polygraphic aspects of insomnia. In: Gastaut H, Lugaresi L, Berti G, et al, eds. The abnormalities of sleep in man. Bologna, Italy: Gaggi; 1968:109–125.
31. Mendelson WB. Pharmacologic alteration of the perception of being awake or asleep. Sleep. 1993;16:641–646.
32. Mendelson WB. Effects of flurazepam and zolpidem on the perception of sleep in insomniacs. Sleep. 1995;18:92–96.
33. Mendelson WB. Effects of flurazepam and zolpidem in the perception of sleep in normal volunteers. Sleep. 1995;18:88–91.
34. Hobbs WR, Rall TW, Verdoorn TA. Hypnotics and sedatives: ethanol. In: Hardman JG, Limbird LE, Molinoff PB, et al, eds. The Pharmacological Basis of Therapeutics. New York, NY: McGraw-Hill; 1996:361–396.
35. Roehrs T, Vogel G, Vogel F, et al. Dose effects of temazepam tablets on sleep. Drugs Exp Clin Res. 1986; 12:693–699.
36. Physicians' Desk Reference. Montvale, NJ: Medical Economics; 1998.
37. Maczaj M. Pharmacological treatment of insomnia. Drugs. 1993;45:44–45.
38. Langtry HD, Benfield P. Zolpidem: a review of its pharmacodynamic and pharmacokinetic properties and therapeutic potential. Drugs. 1990;40:291–313.
39. Noble S, Langtry HD, Lamb HM. Zopiclone: an update of its pharmacology, clinical efficacy and tolerability in the treatment of insomnia. Drugs. 1998;55:277–302.
40. Hindmarch I. Zopiclone monograph. Manchester, England: Adis Press; 1990:1–68.
41. Rudolf M, Geddes DM, Turner JA, et al. Depression of central respiratory drive by nitrazepam. Thorax. 1978;33:97–100.
42. Dolly FR, Block AJ. Effect of flurazepam on sleep-disordered breathing and nocturnal oxygen desaturation in asymptomatic patients. Am J Med. 1982;73:239–243.
43. Mendelson WB. Drugs which alter sleep and sleep-related respiration. In: Kuna ST, ed. Sleep and Respiration in Aging Adults. New York, NY: Elsevier Science; 1991:49–54.
44. Bonnet MH, Dexter JR, Arand DL. The effect of triazolam on arousal and respiration in central sleep apnea patients. Sleep. 1990;13:31–41.
45. Mendelson WB, Rich CR. Sedatives and suicide: the San Diego study. Acta Psychiatr Scand. 1993;88:337–341.
46. Cohn MA. Effects of zolpidem, codeine phosphate and placebo on respiration. A double-blind, crossover study in volunteers. Drug Saf. 1993;9:312–319.
47. Muir JF, Defouilloy C, Broussier P, et al. Incidence of zopiclone

vs placebo on sleep-disordered breathing in COPD patients. Rev Respir Dis. 1988;13:12–14.

48. Kripke DF, Hauri P, Ancoli-Israel S, et al. Sleep evaluation in chronic insomniacs during 14-day use of flurazepam and midazolam. J Clin Psychopharmacol. 1990;10:32S–43S.

49. Roehrs T, Zorick F, Wittig R, et al. Efficacy of a reduced triazolam dose in elderly insomniacs. Neurobiol Aging. 1985;6:293–296.

50. Kales A, Bixler EO, Vela-Bueno A, et al. Comparison of short and long half-life benzodiazepine hypnotics: triazolam and quazepam. Clin Pharmacol Ther. 1986;49:378–386.

33

Hypnotics: Efficacy and Adverse Effects

Timothy Roehrs
Thomas Roth

A variety of drugs have been shown to possess sedative-hypnotic effects, but such demonstrations do not necessarily indicate their hypnotic efficacy. Hypnotic efficacy is the capacity of a drug to induce and maintain sleep in people with disturbed sleep, either from a chronic insomnia condition or a transient challenge to their sleep. This definition emphasizes both the target population and the extent of effects on sleep; the issues surrounding what defines insomnia and how hypnotic efficacy is measured are discussed in this chapter. Hypnotic efficacy can and should be distinguished from *chronobiotic efficacy*, which is the ability and degree of circadian phase–shifting properties. Such an agent would only be effective for a subset of insomnia patients (i.e., those with a circadian rhythm disorder) or at a specific time of day (i.e., for day sleep in shift work). A *chronobiotic* is an agent that is used to treat a specific subtype of insomnia, and it directly corrects the underlying problem. In contrast, hypnotics improve insomnia regardless of etiology but are symptomatic treatments. Hypnotic effectiveness also implies that the dose range for hypnotic effects relative to the dose range for side effects has been well defined for a given drug. The clinical use of hypnotics always involves balancing benefits and risks, and dose is critical to this ratio. Increased dosage is a major predictor of side effects, but rarely does it lead to greater hypnotic efficacy. Thus, this chapter also discusses the range and the clinical significance of the various side effects associated with hypnotics.

DEFINITION OF INSOMNIA

Insomnia is a complaint either of difficulties initiating and maintaining sleep or of nonrestorative and nonrefreshing sleep. Most experts also understand insomnia as involving an accompanying complaint of daytime difficulty attributed to the poor sleep, although the specific nature of the daytime consequences may differ among patients.[1] Insomnia differs in its etiology and expression; a discussion of the variety of etiologies and expressions of insomnia is beyond the scope of this chapter (see Chapters 53–56). Critical to

this chapter is the issue of what insomnia really is: the subjective complaint alone or objective evidence of disturbed sleep and daytime impairment? And in regard to hypnotic efficacy, is it resolution of the complaints or objective evidence of increased and consolidated sleep and improved daytime function? Controversy exists as to whether or not patients with insomnia complaints and response to hypnotics differ from controls in any polysomnographic (PSG) measures of sleep and daytime function. One large study reported extensive overlap in PSG measures of sleep between insomnia patients and normals.[1] Other PSG studies have shown clear differences in the sleep of insomnia patients and normal subjects and even differences among patients with differing insomnia etiologies.[2] But systematic impairment of daytime function in insomniacs has been difficult to demonstrate. Regardless, both PSG and patient assessments are required by the U.S. Food and Drug Administration and by other pharmaceutical regulatory agencies in demonstrating hypnotic efficacy.[1] Yet daytime assessments are not typically required.

DRUGS OF CHOICE FOR INSOMNIA TREATMENT

The drug class of choice for the symptomatic treatment of insomnia is the benzodiazepine receptor agonist.[3, 4] The class name is derived from the generally recognized mechanism of these drugs (see Chapter 32). All the drugs of this class occupy benzodiazepine receptors on the gamma-aminobutyric acid (GABA) receptor complex, with receptor occupation opening ion channels and facilitating GABA inhibition.[5] Some of these drugs have a benzodiazepine chemical structure and others do not.

The benzodiazepine receptor agonists are preferred as hypnotics for several clear reasons. Compared to other drug classes they are safe; that is, the margin of safety or therapeutic index (i.e., the effective dose relative to lethal dose) is wide.[6] For example, barbiturates have margins of safety on the order of two to four times the effective dose, whereas for benzodiazepine receptor agonists, the margin of safety can be as great as 100. Also, tolerance to the hypnotic effects of benzodiazepine receptor agonists does not develop rapidly as it does with other drugs in this category.[4] Tolerance to the hypnotic effects of barbiturates can develop within days, while studies have shown continued hypnotic effects of benzodiazepine receptor agonists for at least 6 weeks of nightly use.[4]

Efficacy of the Benzodiazepine Receptor Agonists

Sleep Induction and Maintenance. In assessing sleep induction–maintenance with PSG, minutes to sleep onset, minutes of wakefulness after sleep onset, minutes of total sleep, minutes of stage 1 sleep, and frequency of brief EEG arousals have all been used.[1] In patient assessments, morning questionnaires that ask about ease of sleep onset and quality and quantity of sleep are used. Intermediate in cost is *actigraphy,* the monitoring of motor activity with wrist-worn sensors; it too has been used with some success to document hypnotic efficacy.

Many studies have shown the efficacy of benzodiazepine receptor agonists using PSG and questionnaires.[3, 4] All have been shown to reduce minutes to sleep onset, reduce wakefulness after sleep onset, increase sleep time, and reduce the amount of stage 1 sleep. These effects have been shown in patients with chronic insomnia and in individuals experiencing transient sleep problems.[7] The drugs do differ somewhat in their pharmacokinetics profiles and metabolic pathways (see Chapter 32). Most have a rapid onset of effect and thus effectively induce sleep, and all the short- and intermediate-acting drugs sufficiently maintain sleep for the usual 7 to 8 h. Those that are long-acting or have long-acting metabolites have the potential to produce residual sedation the following day (see later for a discussion of residual sedation).

Sleep Staging. The relative effects of benzodiazepine receptor agonists on sleep stages compared to other drug classes (i.e., alcohol, barbiturates, opiates) and the specific differential sleep stage effects of various agents within the benzodiazepine receptor agonist class are often cited as providing an advantage to a particular drug.[8] The clinical significance of any specific sleep stage alteration, with the exception of stage 1 reduction, is unknown. Alcohol, barbiturates, and opiates are rapid eye movement (REM)-suppressing agents to which tolerance to the REM-suppressing effect develops rapidly.[9] When drug use is discontinued, increased amounts of REM sleep, termed *REM rebound,* are found. REM suppression and rebound is usually not found with clinical doses of the benzodiazepine receptor agonists. On the other hand, the most consistent REM-suppressing drugs are the antidepressants, and tolerance to their REM suppression does not develop. It has been argued that the antidepressant efficacy of these drugs is mediated by their REM suppression.[9] Among the benzodiazepine receptor agonists, the benzodiazepines themselves suppress stage 3-4 sleep, whereas the nonbenzodiazepine members of that class

do not.[10] Some have argued that there is a special benefit to these newer nonbenzodiazepines in that the sleep induced is more natural (i.e., includes stage 3-4 sleep). Again, the significance of drug-induced changes in stage 3-4 sleep is not known. Further, certain sleep disorders, such as somnambulism and night terrors, are specifically associated with stage 3-4 sleep, and suppression of stage 3-4 sleep may play a therapeutic role in these cases.

Daytime Function. Insomnia, as indicated earlier, is defined as a sleep problem with consequent daytime impairment. Thus, one should be able to demonstrate the insomnia-related impairment and a subsequent improvement with the increased sleep. Yet few studies have shown systematic daytime impairment in insomnia and improvement with increased sleep time. One interesting finding is the observation that some patients with insomnia differ from normal subjects in sleepiness compared with alertness as measured by the multiple sleep latency test (MSLT). Rather than showing greater daytime sleepiness as might be expected given the reduced sleep times of these middle-age insomnia patients, they had longer daytime sleep latencies (as they do at night) than did age-matched normal subjects. This finding has been interpreted as reflecting a persisting state of *hypervigilance,*[11] which is an inability to relax and fall asleep. In contrast, a study done in elderly patients using the MSLT to assess improvement in daytime function showed increased daytime alertness resulting from increased sleep time.[12] Although that study did not include age-matched controls, other studies have shown that elderly people, as a group, have poorer nighttime sleep and are sleepier during the daytime on the MSLT than those in middle-age.[13] In part, then, the difficulty in finding systematic daytime impairment in insomnia, noted earlier, may be due to differing etiologies of the insomnia. In the elderly, the sleep problems are often associated with primary sleep disorders, and in younger patients, they are associated with behavioral and psychiatric problems.[14] The daytime consequences associated with the insomnias may also display different characteristics (i.e., sleepiness vs. hypervigilance). That is true of transient insomnia. In a study of transient insomnia associated with jet lag, the prophylactic use of hypnotics resulted in prevention of the daytime impairment shown in the placebo condition.[15]

Adverse Effects

Residual Effects. Many of the side effects associated with benzodiazepine receptor agonists are mediated by their primary pharmacological activity, sedation.[16] The residual sedation mentioned earlier is merely a prolongation of the hypnotic effect of the drug into the daytime and results in adverse reactions such as hangover, drowsy feelings, sleepiness, and impairment in psychomotor performance. Residual sedation is determined by the duration of drug activity, which in turn is determined by the half-life and dose of the drug. Many studies, using the MSLT and performance assessments, have shown differences in residual effects between short- and long-acting drugs and between different doses of the same drug.

Amnestic Effects. Another side effect that, in part, is related to the sedative effects of hypnotics is anterograde amnesia. Anterograde amnesia is memory failure for information presented after consumption of the drug. It is associated with all hypnotics, including all the benzodiazepine receptor agonists, alcohol, and barbiturates. The extent of amnesia is related to the plasma concentration of the drug. That is, the proximity of information input to peak plasma concentration determines the degree of amnesia, and higher doses, which increase plasma concentration, are associated with greater amnesia.[17, 18] Furthermore, maintaining wakefulness for 10 to 15 min after presentation of memory material, rather than allowing a drug-induced rapid sleep onset, attenuates the amnesia.[19]

Discontinuation Effects. The most frequently cited discontinuation effect of benzodiazepine receptor agonists is rebound insomnia. Sleep is worsened relative to the patient's baseline for 1 to 2 nights after discontinuing several previous nights of hypnotic use. Rebound insomnia can occur even on discontinuation of short-term hypnotic use[20] and does not increase in severity with the number of repeated nights of use, at least in the short-term. Rebound insomnia occurs after high doses of *all* short- and intermediate-acting benzodiazepine receptor agonists. It does not occur with long-acting drugs because of the gradual decline in plasma concentration that is inherent to the pharmacology of such drugs. Similarly, it can be minimized in short- and intermediate-acting drugs by gradually tapering the dose. Importantly, it usually can be avoided by initially using the lowest effective dose.

One must differentiate rebound insomnia from recrudescence and from a withdrawal syndrome. *Recrudescence* is a return of the original symptom at its original severity that does not disappear with time. A *withdrawal syndrome* is the addition of new symptoms, which last weeks rather than days. *Rebound insomnia* is the brief (i.e., 1 to 2 nights) exacerbation of the original symptom. It does not reflect the presence of physical dependence and does not increase the likelihood of hypnotic self-administration and behavioral dependence.[18] Patient expectancies can also play a role in the experience of rebound insomnia. Discontinuing placebo pills, that is, stopping pill-taking per se, has been found to produce a sleep disturbance.[21]

Dependence Liability. In long-term use, there is concern regarding addiction. The epidemiological data indicate that the majority of patients use hypnotics for 2 weeks or less.[22] A percentage of individuals use them nightly on a chronic basis but with no dose escalation. Whether this pattern of use reflects addiction (i.e., physical or behavioral dependence) is unknown. Although there are reports of physical dependence at therapeutic doses in long-term daytime use, no such study of long-term hypnotic use has been done. Daytime studies of the reinforcing effects of these drugs indicate that they have a low behavioral dependence liability.[23] Studies of their behavioral dependence liability in the context of their use as hypnotics have come to a similar conclusion.[21, 24] Hypnotic self-administration in insomniacs is therapy-seeking behavior in that it does not lead to short-term dose escalation and does not generalize to daytime use (i.e. does not occur outside of the therapeutic context), and the rate of self-administration varies as a function of the nature and severity of the sleep problem.

Special Considerations

Elderly. Those drugs that are primarily metabolized by conjugation are potentially safer for aged patients or patients with liver disease (see Chapter 32).[25] The characteristic pharmacokinetics of oxidated drugs are altered in elderly people and in patients with liver disease by increasing the area under the plasma concentration curve. For some drugs this alteration occurs by increasing the peak plasma concentration (e.g., triazolam) and for others by extending the duration of action (e.g., flurazepam).

INDICATIONS FOR PHARMACOTHERAPY

The present consensus regarding the use of hypnotics in the symptomatic treatment of insomnia is that benzodiazepine receptor agonists are the appropriate choice for transient and short-term insomnia and that the duration of nightly use should be limited (i.e., 4 weeks or less).[7] Transient insomnia, such as the 1st night in a new sleep environment or the shifting sleep schedule required in shift work and jet lag, are considered a primary indication for hypnotic pharmacotherapy.[3, 4] Any stress-related insomnia of a short-term nature is also considered an appropriate indication for pharmacotherapy. Usually, these insomnia patients report a previous history of normal sleep, and once the transient or stressful event has resolved, the patients return to their normal sleep patterns. The acute use of hypnotics in transient and short-term insomnia may prevent development of persistent psychophysiologic insomnia. Such an insomnia is considered a conditioned insomnia with either cognitive or physiological (i.e., peripheral and central arousal) components or both. It is believed that transient and short-term insomnia can develop into persistent psychophysiological insomnia. In a persistent psychophysiological insomnia there usually is little daytime anxiety, but the anxiety and arousal are specifically focused on the ability to sleep and on the sleep environment. Unless there is additional need for daytime anxiolysis, in which long-acting drugs might be appropriate, for the symptomatic treatment of transient and short-term insomnia, a short- or intermediate-acting drug should be chosen.

Although short-term drug use in chronic insomniacs is indicated, there is controversy as to whether long-term pharmacotherapy in chronic insomnia is ever indicated. Some sleep disorder specialists advise long-term use in an insomnia associated with restless leg syndrome (RLS), periodic limb movements (PLMs), central sleep apnea, and chronic medical conditions.[26] The studies of the efficacy of benzodiazepine receptor agonists in patients with RLS and PLMs have shown they improve sleep. But they are symptomatic treatment: they do not remove the leg paresthesias or leg movements; they suppress the EEG arousals associated with the movements.[27] In apnea-associated insomnia treatment, one must differentiate central sleep apnea from obstructive sleep apnea-hypopnea syndrome (OSAHS) where any central nervous system (CNS) depressant drug is contraindicated. Differentiation of central sleep apnea and OSAHS requires a sleep disorders evaluation. Some would also suggest that long-term hypnotic use is appropriate as an adjunct in insomnia associated with various chronic medical diseases.[26] All of these chronic insomnias (i.e., RLS, PLMs, central sleep apnea, OSAHS, and chronic medical conditions) are more likely to occur in elderly patients.

CONTRAINDICATIONS TO TREATMENT

As to the contraindications for pharmacotherapy, it is believed that patients with a history of alcoholism or drug abuse should not receive these drugs in outpatient settings.[26] They are also contraindicated for pregnant women; the teratogenic effects of all psychoactive drugs is a matter of concern. People who may be required to awaken in the middle of the night and perform duties should avoid any CNS depressant drugs. All hypnotics disrupt cognitive and motor function for the duration of the sedative activity of the drug. One should be cautious in people who drink large quantities of alcohol and in elderly people. Alcohol is known to have additive effects with hypnotics, and the wide margin of safety described earlier is narrowed considerably with the addition of alcohol. In the elderly, as noted earlier, the pharmacokinetics of certain benzodiazepine receptor agonists are changed, producing either higher peak concentrations or longer durations of activity, in both cases resulting in greater area under the plasma concentration curve.

Frequently, other drug classes are inappropriately chosen for insomnia pharmacotherapy. Sometimes histamine receptor type 1 (H$_1$) antihistamines are used as hypnotics, either by prescription or as over the counter (OTC) sleeping aids. The primary active ingredient in most OTC sleeping aids is an H$_1$ antihistamine. Although studies have shown that H$_1$ antihistamines do increase sleepiness in healthy normal individuals, no studies have clearly established the dose range over which hypnotic effects in people with insomnia might be found.[28] Low-dose antidepressants have also been used as hypnotics. It is the sedating side effect of the drug that is being sought.[29] However, the antidepressants have cardiotoxic side effects and anticholinergic side effects that make this class of drugs a poor choice as a hypnotic in the absence of a clinical depression. In clinical depression, a frequent symptom is insomnia; typically, it is a sleep maintenance insomnia.[29] The ap-

propriate treatment for an insomnia associated with depression is a sedating antidepressant at standard antidepressant doses. When treating depression with a sedating antidepressant at standard antidepressant doses, the insomnia generally resolves within the 1st week of treatment, even before the depressed state has improved.[29]

TREATMENT GUIDELINES

Depending on the presumptive diagnosis, hypnotic pharmacotherapy can be considered as part of the treatment plan. The list of conditions for which hypnotic pharmacotherapy is appropriate was discussed earlier. The specific drug should be carefully chosen by the clinician to fit the patient, considering the pharmacokinetics of the drug and the patient characteristics (e.g., age, diseases). The dose and treatment regimen should be carefully prescribed, agreed to by the patient, and monitored by the clinician. The hypnotic should only be taken as agreed upon or when needed. The dose should be the lowest clinically indicated dose, and that dose should be used for a short period of time (3 to 5 nights) before the clinician and patient jointly determine its effectiveness. Then the dose can be adjusted as appropriate. Patients should not be allowed to self-initiate a dose escalation. This only reinforces obsessional thinking regarding sleep, the number of pills to be taken, and whether or not to arise in the middle of the night to take additional pills. There are both pharmacological and behavioral considerations associated with the middle-of-the-night administration of medications. Pharmacologically, it is possible that a middle-of-the-night administration will produce daytime residual sedation, which was discussed earlier. With the exception of midazolam and zaleplon, all medications need to be taken before going to bed. These two medications are ultra–short-acting and have been evaluated in middle-of-the-night protocols (i.e., medication is administered with 5 h or less bedtime remaining) and have been found to improve sleep in the remaining bedtime while avoiding residual effects the next morning.[30, 31] Behaviorally, middle-of-the-night administration can be thought of as rescue medication. If a particular behavioral treatment fails on a given night, the middle-of-the-night medication serves as a rescue, thereby enabling the patient to avoid frustration with the behavioral treatment. Thus, in cases of sleep maintenance insomnia characterized only by a middle-of-the-night awakening, or in cases of intermittent sleep-onset insomnia, and the selection of an ultra–short-acting medication, a middle-of-the-night administration can be considered.

There is disagreement due to the absence of systematic information as to whether the prescription should be nightly (i.e., at bedtime [hs]), or intermittently (i.e., every 2nd or 3rd night). It seems clear that the prescription should not be "as needed" because this schedule, as noted earlier, can reinforce the patient's belief that he or she is unable to sleep without medication. The goal of hs treatment is to provide the patient who has a conditioned insomnia with a 2- to 3-week period of consistently good nightly sleep, during which the patient's conditioned arousal to the sleep environment or cognitions regarding his or her inability to sleep can be extinguished. The intent behind the use of an intermittent schedule is to avoid the possibility of tolerance development in patients being treated chronically. But as noted earlier, no study has systematically determined the extent to which tolerance, physical dependence, and behavioral dependence develop in chronic treatment of patients with properly diagnosed and treated insomnia. No study has determined whether nightly or intermittent treatment is more likely to have an adverse outcome and which specific insomnia diagnoses are appropriate and which are inappropriate. The point can be made that even with a clinician-prescribed intermittent treatment schedule, perceptions regarding an inability to sleep may be reinforced.

Acknowledgments

Supported by National Institutes of Health (NIAAA) grant R01 AA07147 and (NIDA) grant R01 DA05086.

References

1. Roth T, Roehrs TA, Vogel GW, et al. Evaluation of hypnotic medications. In: Prien RF, Robinson DS, eds. Clinical Evaluation of Psychotropic Drugs, Principles and Guidelines. New York, NY: Raven Press; 1995:579–592.
2. Zorick F, Kribbs N, Roehrs T, et al. Polysomnographic and MMPI characteristics of patients with insomnia. In: Hindmarch I, Ott H, Roth T, eds. Sleep, Benzodiazepines, and Performance. Heidelberg, Germany: Springer-Verlag; 1984:165–172.
3. National Institute of Mental Health, Consensus Development Conference. Drugs and insomnia: the use of medications to promote sleep. JAMA. 1984;251:2410–2414.
4. American Psychiatric Association Task Force on Benzodiazepine Dependency. Benzodiazepine Dependence, Toxicity, and Abuse. Washington, DC: American Psychiatric Association; 1990.
5. Haefely W. Benzodiazepine receptor and ligands: structural and functional differences. In: Hindmarch I, Beaumont G, Grandon S, eds. Benzodiazepines: Current Concepts. New York, NY: Wiley; 1990:1–18.
6. Greenblatt DJ, Shader RI. Benzodiazepines in Clinical Practice. New York, NY: Raven Press; 1974.
7. Gillin JC, Byerley WF. The diagnosis and management of insomnia. N Engl J Med. 1990;322:239–248.
8. Roth T, Zorick F, Wittig R, et al. Pharmacological and medical considerations in hypnotic use. Sleep. 1982;5:S46–S52.
9. Vogel GW, Buffenstein A, Minter K, et al. Drug effects on REM sleep and on endogenous depression. Neurosci Biobehav Rev. 1990;14:49–63.
10. Monti JM. Concluding remarks: toward a third generation of hypnotics. In: Sauvanet JP, Langer SZ, Morselli PL, eds. Imidazopyridines in Sleep Disorders: A Novel Experimental and Therapeutic Approach. New York, NY: Raven Press; 1990:363–368.
11. Stepanski E, Zorick FJ, Roehrs TA, et al. Daytime alertness in patients with chronic insomnia compared with asymptomatic control subjects. Sleep. 1988;11:39–46.
12. Roehrs T, Zorick F, Wittig R, et al. Efficacy of a reduced triazolam dose in elderly insomniacs. Neurobiol Aging. 1985;6:293–296.
13. Miles LE, Dement WC. Sleep and aging. Sleep. 1982;3:119–220.
14. Roehrs T, Zorick F, Sicklesteel J, et al. Age-related sleep-wake disorders at a sleep disorder center. J Am Geriatr Soc. 1983;31:364–370.
15. Seidel W, Roth T, Roehrs T, et al. Treatment of a 12-hour shift of sleep schedule with benzodiazepines. Science. 1984;224:1262–1264.
16. Roth T, Roehrs T. Issues in the use of benzodiazepine therapy. J Clin Psychiatry. 1992;53:S14–S18.
17. Roth T, Roehrs TA, Stepanski EJ, et al. Hypnotics and behavior. Am J Med. 1990;88:43S–46S.
18. Greenblatt D, Harmatz JS, Shapiro L, et al. Sensitivity to triazolam in elderly. N Engl J Med. 1991;324:1691–1698.
19. Roehrs T, Zorick F, Sicklesteel J, et al. Effects of hypnotics on memory. J Clin Psychopharmacol. 1983;3:310–313.
20. Roehrs T, Vogel G, Roth T. Rebound insomnia: its determinants and significance. Am J Med. 1990;88:39S–42S.
21. Roehrs T, Merlotti L, Zorick F, et al. Rebound insomnia and hypnotic self administration. Psychopharmacology. 1992;107:480–484.
22. Mellinger GD, Balter MB, Uhlenhuth EH. Insomnia and its treatment. Arch Gen Psychiatry. 1985;42:225–232.
23. Griffiths RR, Roache JD. Abuse liability of benzodiazepines: a review of human studies evaluating subjective and/or reinforcing effects. In: Smith DE, Wesson DR, eds. The benzodiazepines: current standards for medical practice. Hingman, Mass: MTP Press; 1985:209–225.
24. Roehrs T, Pedrosi B, Rosentha L, et al. Hypnotic self administration and dose escalation. Psychopharmacology. 1996;127:150–154.
25. Roehrs T, Roth T. Drugs, sleep disorders, and aging. Clin Geriatr Med. 1989;5:395–404.
26. Stepanski E, Zorick F, Roth T. Pharmacotherapy of insomnia. In: Hauri PJ, ed. Case Studies in Insomnia. New York, NY: Plenum Publishing; 1991:115–129.
27. Roth T, Roehrs T, Zorick F. Pharmacological treatment of sleep disorders. In: Williams RL, Karacan IU, Moore CC, eds. Sleep Disorders: Diagnosis and Treatment. New York, NY: John Wiley & Sons; 1988:373–395.
28. Roth T, Roehrs T, Koshorek G, et al. Sedative effects of antihistamines. J Allergy Clin Immunol. 1987;80:94–98.
29. Benca RM. Mood disorders. In: Kryger MH, Roth T, Dement WC, eds. Principles and Practice of Sleep Medicine. Philadelphia, Pa: WB Saunders; 1994:899–913.
30. Roth T, Hauri P, Zorick F, et al. The effects of midazolam and temazepam on sleep and performance when administered in the middle of the night. J Clin Psychopharm. 1985;5:66–69.
31. Danjou P, Paty I, Fruncillo R, et al. A comparison of the residual effects of zaleplon and zolpidem following administration 5 to 2 hrs before awakening. Br J Clin Pharmacol. 1999;48:367–374.

34

Stimulants: Basic Mechanisms and Pharmacology

George F. Koob

Psychomotor stimulants are drugs that produce a behavioral activation usually accompanied by increases in arousal, motor activity, and alertness. There are two major classes of psychomotor stimulants: (1) those that act as sympathomimetics, either directly or indirectly, such as cocaine and amphetamine (Table 34–1), and (2) those that are not sympathomimetics. The term *sympathomimetic* derives originally from the description of the mechanism of action of these drugs. Sympathomimetics mimic the action of the sympathetic nervous system when it is activated. Indeed, the term *sympathin* was originally used to describe the hormone norepinephrine found in the central nervous system (CNS).[1–3] Thus, sympathomimetic drugs mimic the actions of norepinephrine in the autonomic system and neuropharmacologically either directly or indirectly activate monoamine receptors (see later). Nonsympathomimetics (see Table 34–1) act via different neuropharmacological mechanisms altogether.

COCAINE, AMPHETAMINE, METHYLPHENIDATE

Pharmacokinetics

Cocaine is derived from the coca plant (*Erythroxylon coca*) and has a long history as a stimulant. It has been used for centuries in tonics and other preparations to allay fatigue and treat a large variety of ailments (for reviews, see references 4 and 5). Cocaine was once a component of Coca Cola, and its extract (sans cocaine) is still an ingredient. Freud briefly advocated its use to treat a variety of disorders, including psychiatric disorders and drug addiction[6] but quickly lost his enthusiasm after observing his first cocaine psychosis (see reference 7 for a review of Freud's writings on cocaine), and cocaine has been involved in more than one epidemic of drug abuse in the United States.[8]

Amphetamines were synthesized originally as possible alternative drugs for the treatment of asthma and were the principal component of the original benzedrine inhaler.[9] They were used (and still are used) by the military as antifatigue indications, and they are currently legally available for medical use as adjuncts for short-term weight control, in attention-deficit hyperactivity disorder, and in narcolepsy.

Most indirect sympathomimetic compounds share a common molecular structure: a benzene ring with an ethylamine side chain. Amphetamine differs from the parent compound, β-phenethylamine, by the addition of a methyl group, whereas methamphetamine has two additional methyl groups. Methylphenidate and cocaine are structurally similar. Figure 34–1 presents the molecular structures of five stimulants (methylphenidate, dextroamphetamine, methamphetamine, mazindol, and pemoline) commonly used for the treatment of narcolepsy, along with the molecular structure of cocaine, a naturally occurring alkaloid found in the leaves of *E. coca*.[10]

Both cocaine and amphetamine produce increases in systolic and diastolic blood pressure. In human beings, a dose of 10 mg of dextroamphetamine intravenously produces an increase in blood pressure equal to that produced with a dose of 32 mg of intravenous cocaine.[11] Cocaine and amphetamine also stimulate heart rate,[11] but amphetamine may cause less of an effect than one would expect based on other physiological measures because of a reflex slowing of heart rate. These drugs also produce bronchial dilation and pupillary dilation, as well as decreases in glandular secretions, all effects observed after activation of the sympathetic nervous system.

Table 34–1. PSYCHOMOTOR STIMULANT DRUGS

Direct Sympathomimetics	*Nonsympathomimetics*
Isoproterenol	Caffeine
Epinephrine	Nicotine
Norepinephrine	Scopolamine
Phenylephrine	Strychnine
Phenylpropanolamine	Pentylenetetrazol
Apomorphine	Modafinil
Indirect Sympathomimetics	
Amphetamine	
Methamphetamine	
Cocaine	
Methylphenidate	
Phenmetrazine	
Pipradrol	
Tyramine	
Pemoline	

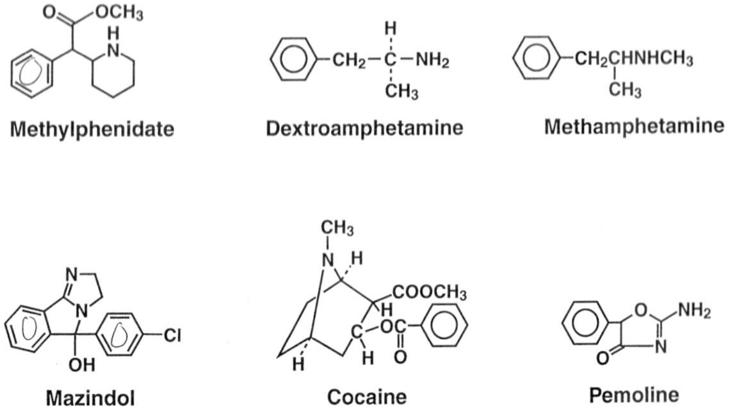

Figure 34–1. The molecular structures of methylphenidate, dextroamphetamine, methamphetamine, mazindol, and pemoline, which are drugs commonly used for the treatment of narcolepsy. The molecular structure of cocaine, a naturally occurring alkaloid found in the leaves of *Erythroxylum coca*, is shown for comparison (bottom center). (Redrawn from USP Dictionary of USAN and International Drug Names. Rockville, Md: United States Pharmacopeia Convention; 1998.)

The mechanism of action of these autonomic effects of indirect sympathomimetics such as amphetamines and cocaine has long been known. Both drugs indirectly cause the release of norepinephrine and epinephrine by blocking both reuptake and potentiating release.[12, 13] Chronic postganglionic adrenergic denervation, or treatment with reserpine, which dramatically depletes tissue stores of catecholamines, abolishes the autonomic effects of amphetamine, establishing that these effects are due to an indirect sympathomimetic action.[14]

Amphetamines and cocaine are powerful stimulants of the CNS. This analeptic action is characterized by increased wakefulness, alertness, decreased sense of fatigue, elevations of mood and euphoria, increased motor activity and talkativeness, and increased performance in some tasks and athletic situations. These CNS effects are more pronounced by three to fourfold in the dextro-isomer of amphetamine. With methamphetamine at low doses, these CNS effects are more pronounced than the autonomic effects, presumably due to its increased lipophilicity which allows it to readily cross the blood-brain barrier.[10]

The nature of stimulant effects of cocaine and amphetamines depends on the route of administration. Intravenous or inhaled freebase preparations produce marked, intense, pleasurable sensations characterized as a "rush" that has been likened to sexual orgasm and is thought to be a powerful motivation for the abuse of these drugs. Intravenous doses producing these subjective effects are approximately 8 to 16 mg of cocaine and 10 mg of dextroamphetamine.[11] Smoked cocaine in the freebase form has absorption characteristics similar to intravenous administration, and 50 mg of freebase produce cardiovascular effects approximately equivalent to 32 mg of cocaine administered intravenously.[15]

Intranasal doses of 20 to 30 mg of cocaine also produce euphoria, increased confidence and talkativeness, a sense of well-being, and fatigue reduction for approximately 30 min. Cocaine has less powerful effects administered orally, presumably due to a markedly slower absorption. Indeed, South American Indians have used for centuries an oral coca leaf preparation combined with ash to promote absorption. This use was effective as a stimulant to reduce fatigue and hunger and is not characterized by any obvious untoward physical or psychic effects.[16]

Intranasal or oral administration of dextroamphetamine in the dose range of 2.5 to 15 mg produces stimulant effects similar to cocaine. Subjects report feelings of alertness, energetic vitality, confident assertiveness, and a decrease in appetite and fatigue. Intranasal absorption is faster with more intense effects than oral administration, and the stimulant effects of amphetamines last considerably longer than cocaine (up to 4 to 6 h).

Amphetamine is metabolized in the liver via deamination to phenylacetone and ultimately oxidized to benzoic acid, then excreted as glucoroxide or glycine conjugates.[17] However, in normal pH, approximately 30% is excreted unchanged, accounting for a significant portion of its removal. Amphetamine has a relatively long half-life of approximately 12 h, but because it has a pK_a of 9.9, that half-life can be extended with an alkaline urine to over 16 h and shortened to 8 h with acid urine.[18] Methamphetamine has a pK_a and renal excretion similar to amphetamine. Cocaine is rapidly metabolized to benzoylecgonine and ergonine methylester; less than 10% is excreted unchanged in the urine. The half-life of cocaine ranges from 48 to 75 min.[19] Methylphenidate has a half-life of 2 to 4 h and is rapidly de-esterized to ritalinic acid which is inactive and excreted in the urine. This accounts for over 80% of the removal of methylphenidate.[20]

Behavioral Pharmacology

Amphetamines in the dose ranges described above produce stimulant effects. Beneficial effects reported include increased stimulation, improved coordination, increased strength and endurance, and increased mental and physical activation, with mood changes of boldness, elation, and friendliness.[21] However, the most dramatic effects of amphetamines have been observed in situations of fatigue and boredom. These drugs can both remove the subjective sensation of fatigue and can prolong physical performance for long periods.[22–25] Amphetamines also enhance performance in simple motor and cognitive tasks, including measures of reaction time, speed, attention, and performance.[26, 27] Amphetamines can also significantly improve athletic performance by slight amounts (0.5 to 4.0%), and these small percent improvements may be sufficient to be significant in competitive situations.[25]

Amphetamines can also impair performance of the well-functioning, motivated subject,[28] and there is little evidence to suggest that amphetamines can enhance intellectual functioning in complex tasks or tests of intelligence.[27] In fact, there is evidence that methamphetamine failed to improve performance on a complex attention task, even though methamphetamine did increase the rate at which a visual display was scanned.[29] Also, hyperactive children treated with methylphenidate showed impairment in performance of the Wisconsin Card Sorting Test that suggested an overfocusing of behavior.[30] An inverted U-shaped relationship between performance and dose of stimulant that is related to the complexity of the task has been hypothesized.[25] This inverted U-shaped function may reflect the observation that as the dose of stimulant increases, behavior becomes progressively more constricted and repetitive, resulting in both cognitive and behavioral perseveration (see later).

Other acute actions of amphetamines include a decrease in appetite, for which these drugs have been used therapeutically and to which rapid tolerance develops.[31] Amphetamines and methylphenidate also produce decreases in sleepiness, increased latency to fall asleep, increased latency to the onset of rapid eye movement (REM) sleep, and a reduction in the proportion of REM sleep,[32–34] and these drugs are effective treatments for narcolepsy.[35, 36] Amphetamines also improve attention in attention-deficit hyperactivity disorder, and decrease the hyperactivity observed in children with this disorder.[37–39]

Finally, amphetamines and cocaine have long been touted as aphrodisiacs and often have been reported to heighten sexual interest and prolong orgasm. In some instances, such delays in ejaculation have led to "marathon" bouts of intercourse lasting for hours and probably reflect some of the behavioral psychopathological effects produced by these drugs (see Behavioral Pathology later). Systematic studies of the effects of amphetamines on sexual behavior show that in amphetamine users, amphetamine use can dramatically heighten preexisting sexual tension, but can also lead to significant decreases in sexual interest with prolonged use of the drugs.[5]

Behavioral Pathology

High doses of amphetamines and cocaine can lead to significant behavioral pathological activity. Amphetamine abusers can persist in repetitive thoughts or acts for hours. These behaviors can include repetitively cleaning the home or an item such as a car, bathing in a tub all day, elaborately sorting small objects, or endlessly dismantling or putting back together items such as clocks or radios. Such behavior was termed *punding* by Rylander[40] and was well described as "organized, goal-directed but meaningless activity." This behavior is also called stereotyped behavior and can also be defined as "integrated behavioral sequences that ac-

quire a stereotyped character, being performed at an increasing rate in a repetitive manner."[41] Stereotyped behavior is observed in many animal species.[42, 43] Monkeys will pick at their skin, exhibit mouth and tongue movements, and stare; rats will sniff intensely in one location; pigeons will repetitively peck at one location on a stimulus display.

Further experimental and theoretical analysis of stereotyped behavior led to insights into the nature and behavioral mechanism of action of amphetamine-like drugs.[44] Lyon and Robbins[44] hypothesized that as the dose of amphetamine increases, the repetition rate of all motor activities increases with the result that the organism will exhibit "increases in response rates within a decreasing number of response categories." This type of analysis makes a number of predictions. Complex behavioral chains or behaviors are the first to be eliminated as the response categories decrease. Behaviors capable of repetition without long pauses then dominate, and shorter and shorter response sequences result. As a result, high rates of responding in operant situations decrease and locomotor activity decreases[45, 46] (Fig. 34–2). Thus, the classic inverted U-shaped dose–response function relating amphetamines and locomotor activity (or any other high-rate behavior) may reflect the competitive nature of that activity and stereotyped behavior.[30]

Extending this analysis from actual overt motor effects to the actions of these drugs on cognitive function leads also to possible understanding of how amphetamines produce paranoid ideation and psychosis. Amphetamines are well documented to produce paranoid psychotic episodes in individuals abusing chronically, or even taking large doses acutely.[5] In a study of otherwise healthy volunteers, repetitive oral administration of 5 to 10 mg of dextroamphetamine produced paranoid delusions, often with blunted affect in all subjects when a cumulative dose range of 55 to 75 mg was obtained.[47] This paranoid psychosis induced by stimulants in its severest form can produce actual physical toxicity where subjects believe that bugs under their skin need to be gouged out ("crank bugs"). This stereotyped behavior and psychosis associated with high-dose use of stimulants may also contribute to the cycle of abuse associated with these drugs.

Tolerance and Dependence

Tolerance can be defined as a given drug producing a decreasing effect with repeated dosing or when larger doses must be administered to produce the same effect.[48, 49] Tolerance to psychomotor stimulants is differential. In human beings, rapid tolerance develops to the anorexic effects and the lethal effects of amphetamine and cocaine.[5, 50] No tolerance or changes in sensitivity of behavioral responses was observed after repeated daily oral doses of dextroamphetamine 10 mg.[51] Similarly, no tolerance developed to the subjective "high" after 10 mg of methamphetamine, but tolerance did develop to the cardiovascular effects with repeated daily dosing.[52] Some acute tolerance appears to de-

A General Theory Concerning Amphetamine Effects

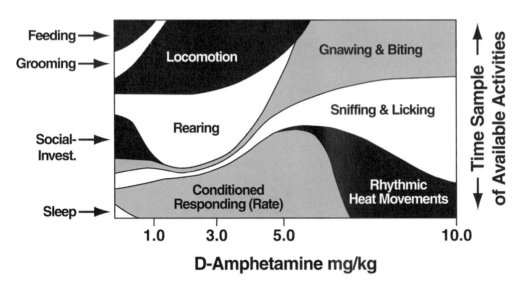

Figure 34–2. Schematic drawing depicting the relative distribution of varying behavioral activities within a given time sample relative to increasing doses of dextroamphetamine. Note that as the dose increases, the number of activities decreases, but the rate of behavior within a given behavioral activity increases. (Redrawn from Lyon M, Robbins TW. The action of central nervous stimulant drugs: a general theory concerning amphetamine effects. In: Essman WB, Valzelli L, eds. Current Developments in Psychopharmacology. Vol 2. New York, NY: Spectrum; 1975:79–163.)

velop to the cardiovascular effects of cocaine even over a 4-h infusion period.[53] Subjective, behavioral, and cardiovascular effects declined after sequential oral doses of dextroamphetamine despite substantial plasma levels, also suggesting acute tolerance.[54] Tolerance does not develop to the stereotyped behavior and psychosis induced by stimulants, and in fact these behavioral effects appear to show an increase with repeated administration or sensitization.[55] Similar results have been observed in animal studies, with tolerance developing to the anorexic and lethal effects of amphetamine but not to the stereotyped behavior.[56]

Amphetamine and cocaine have high abuse potential and are now well documented to produce substance dependence (addiction) by most modern definitions.[57] Although most users (85%) do not become addicted to the drug,[58] clinical observations indicate that controlled use often shifts to more compulsive use, either when there is increased access to the drug or when a more rapid route of administration is used. The abuse cycle with amphetamines and cocaine follows a particular pattern where euphoria, dysphoria, paranoia, and psychosis represent successive stages, either within a single smoking episode with high dosages or within a chronic pattern of use with lower dosages. Compulsive use results in an exaggeration of the binge stage where a user characteristically readministers the drug every 10 min for up to 7 days but usually averaging 12 h. Following a binge, the abstinence syndrome has been characterized by an exaggeration of the dysphoria stage and consists of major decreases in mood and motivation, including limited interest in the environment and a limited ability to experience pleasure, as well as strong drug craving that persists for weeks and months in an outpatient setting.[57] Inpatient studies have documented similar but less intense negative ef-

fective symptoms and craving, suggesting an important role for environmental conditioning in the abstinence syndrome.[59]

Neuropharmacology

Indirect sympathomimetics, such as amphetamine, methylphenidate, and cocaine, are known to act neuropharmacologically to enhance the amount of monoamines available within the synaptic cleft of monoamine synapses in the CNS.[12, 13, 60–63] Amphetamine, methylphenidate, and cocaine block the reuptake and also enhance release of norepinephrine, dopamine, and serotonin in the CNS.[12, 13, 61–65] (Fig. 34–3). Amphetamine is also a weak monoamine oxidase inhibitor.[66] However, the primary neuropharmacological action responsible for its psychomotor stimulant effects appears to be on the dopamine systems in the CNS (see Fig. 34–3).

The brain dopamine systems can be divided into two major pathways that originate in the midbrain and project to the forebrain and appear to be responsible for different aspects of psychomotor stimulant actions (Fig. 34–4). The mesocorticolimbic dopamine system originates in the ventral tegmental area and projects to the ventral forebrain, including the nucleus accumbens, olfactory tubercle, septum, and frontal cortex; the nigrostriatal dopamine system arises primarily in the substantia nigra and projects to the corpus striatum.

The midbrain dopamine systems have long been associated with motor function and response initiation. Degeneration or destruction of the nigrostriatal and mesolimbic dopamine systems together result in the severe motor disturbances of Parkinson's disease, including tremor, dystonic involuntary movements, and akinesia.[67] Large bilateral lesions of the midbrain dopa-

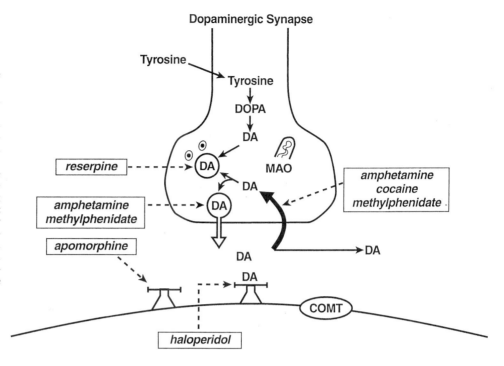

Figure 34–3. Schematic drawing of a hypothetical monoamine synapse, the dopaminergic synapse. Illustrated are the sites for the sympathomimetic actions of the drugs discussed in this chapter. Amphetamine both blocks reuptake and enhances dopamine release. Cocaine predominantly blocks reuptake. Reserpine blocks reuptake of amine into the storage vesicles, effectively depleting amine stores. A variety of different drugs can directly access the receptor as agonists (apomorphine) or antagonists (haloperidol). COMT, Catechol-O-methyltransferase; DA, dopamine; DOPA, 3,4-dihydroxy-phenylalanine; MAO, monoamine oxidase.

mine system using a selective neurotoxin for dopamine, 6-hydroxydopamine, can reproduce many of these deficits. Rats become akinetic to the point of aphagia and adipsia and will die unless intubated.[68] These rats also have severe deficits in learning a conditioned avoidance task, and these deficits can be reversed with levodopa (L-dopa) treatment.[69]

Destruction of the mesocorticolimbic dopamine system, separately, with the neurotoxin 6-hydroxydopamine blocks amphetamine- and cocaine-stimulated lo-

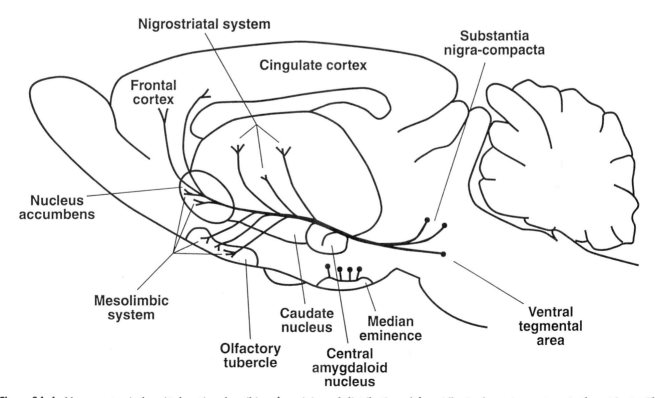

Figure 34–4. Neuroanatomical sagittal section describing the origin and distribution of the midbrain dopamine systems in the rat brain. The nigrostriatal dopamine system originates in the substantia nigra and projects to the caudate putamen. The mesocorticolimbic dopamine system originates in the ventral tegmental area and projects to the nucleus accumbens, olfactory tubercle, amygdala, and frontal cortex.

comotor activity.[70, 71] Similar neurotoxin-selective lesions of the mesocorticolimbic dopamine system block the reinforcing effects of cocaine.[72–74] Rats trained to self-administer cocaine or amphetamine intravenously and subjected to a 6-hydroxydopamine lesion to the nucleus accumbens show an extinction-like response pattern and a long-lasting decrease in responding. Similar effects have been observed following microinjection of selective dopamine antagonists into the region of the nucleus accumbens.[75]

At the cellular level, electrophysiological recordings in animals during intravenous cocaine self-administration have identified several types of neurons that respond in the nucleus accumbens in a manner time-locked to drug infusion and reinforcement. These results suggest that at the cellular level the integration of reinforcement and motivation for cocaine are indeed occurring at the level of the nucleus accumbens.[76–80] One group of neurons shows anticipatory neuronal responses and may be part of an initiation or trigger mechanism. Another group appears to fire post cocaine and may represent a direct reinforcement effect. A third group of neurons appears to have its firing positively correlated with the interinfusion interval of cocaine linking it to the initiation of the next response.[79] Interestingly, the neurons that fire in response to cocaine reinforcement do not fire to cocaine-only probes, but do fire to stimuli paired with cocaine delivery (tone-houselight probes),[81] suggesting that at least a subset of nucleus accumbens neurons may be involved in mediating conditioned responses associated with cocaine reinforcement.

In contrast, disruption of function in the nigrostriatal system, separately, blocks the stereotyped behavior associated with administration of high doses of dextroamphetamine.[71, 82, 83] When 6-hydroxydopamine lesions are restricted to the striatum itself,[84] such lesions block the intense, restricted, repetitive behavior produced by high doses of amphetamine, and this results in intense locomotor activity. Such striatal lesions do not block the reinforcing effects of cocaine. More recently, subregions of the corpus striatum have been implicated in the stereotyped behavior produced by amphetamine.[85] Amphetamine injected into the ventrolateral striatum of rats produced licking, biting, and self-gnawing to the exclusion of other psychomotor behaviors. Thus, the terminal regions of the nigrostriatal and mesocorticolimbic dopamine systems appear to mediate different aspects of psychomotor stimulant actions that can have significant implications for the behavioral effects and psychopathological activity associated with stimulant abuse (Fig. 34–5).

At the molecular level, several different dopamine receptors have been identified both by pharmacological and molecular biological techniques.[86] Five dopamine receptor subtypes have been cloned,[87, 90] and selective ligands exist for three of them (D1, D2, and D3). There is also some evidence to support the hypothesis of differential functional actions on psychostimulant effects for the D1 and D2 dopamine receptors at the behavioral level. Low doses of the selective D1 dopamine receptor antagonist SCH 23390 potently block

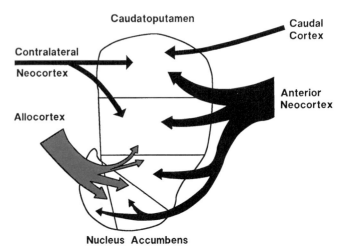

Figure 34–5. Schematic drawing depicting the afferent and efferent connections of the basal ganglia, including both the dorsal and ventral striatum in the context of their functional roles for the action of the indirect sympathomimetic psychomotor stimulants. The nigrostriatal dopamine system is largely responsible for the stereotyped behavior associated with high-dose stimulant use. The mesocorticolimbic dopamine system appears to be responsible for both the locomotor activating and reinforcing effects of these drugs. Note that the predominant cortical influence on the terminal projections of these two dopamine systems is neocortical for the dorsal striatum and allocortical for the ventral striatum.

amphetamine-induced locomotion[91] and intravenous cocaine self-administration,[92] while similar effects were observed with low doses of D2 antagonists. However, low doses of D2 antagonists and not D1 antagonists are effective in impairing responding in a reaction time task particularly sensitive to disruption of nigrostriatal function.[93] Also, the D3 receptor subtype appears to be restricted in its distribution to the terminal projections of the mesocorticolimbic dopamine system.[94] D3 agonists dose-dependently facilitate cocaine self-administration and their potency correlates highly with their potency to activate D3 receptor transduction mechanisms.[95, 96] In contrast, although D3 antagonists do block cocaine self-administration, their effectiveness has yet to be correlated with a selective D3 over D2 action.

Molecular biological techniques combined with a molecular genetic approach have provided a selective deletion of the genes for expression of different dopamine receptor subtypes and the dopamine transporter.[97, 98] To date, D1, D2, D3, D4, D5, and dopamine transporter knockout mice exist and have been subjected to challenges with psychomotor stimulants.[97–99a]

D1 knockout mice show no response to D1 agonists or antagonists and show a blunted response to the locomotor activating effects of cocaine and amphetamine.[99] D2 knockout mice have severe motor deficits and blunted responses to psychostimulants and opiates,[100, 101] and D3 and D4 knockout mice show hyperactivity but no blunting of psychostimulant activity, and, in some cases, supersensitivity to psychostimulants.[102] Dopamine transporter mice are dramatically hyperactive, but also show a blunted response to psychostimulants.[98]

Although developmental factors must be taken into account for the compensation or overcompensation, it is clear that the D1 and D2 receptors, and dopamine transporter, appear to play an important role in the actions of psychomotor stimulants. Knockouts of other monoamine system receptors will provide insights into the role of serotonin and norepinephrine in psychostimulant actions. However, conditional knockouts, where developmental factors are eliminated, may be required to more precisely delineate the functional roles of the molecular entities within the dopamine system. There may also be some differential sensitivity of the dopamine receptors of the mesocorticolimbic and nigrostriatal dopamine systems to the effects of psychostimulants based on differential actions at the different dopamine receptor subtypes.

A recent exciting development has been the identification of a brain neuropeptide orexin (hypocretin) that appears to have a role in modulating arousal and the sleep-wake cycle and may be a potential site for the action of modafanil.[102a] Cell bodies containing orexin are located exclusively in the hypothalamus, and orexin immunoreactivity has been localized to the lateral hypothalamus, inferior colliculus, superior colliculus, and brainstem. Orexin knockout mice present a phenotype very similar to that of human narcolepsy patients, and modafanil activates the orexin neurons.[102b] In addition, positional cloning studies have revealed that the autosomal recessive mutation responsible for canine narcolepsy is disruption of the hypocretin (orexin) receptor-2 gene (Hcrtr2).[102c] These results suggest a novel substrate and mechanism for narcolepsy and suggest a new neuropharmacological domain for pursuit of understanding the mechanism of this sleep disorder.

MODAFINIL AND PEMOLINE

Modafinil is a CNS stimulant currently being used abroad and approved in 1999 in the United States and Canada for the treatment of narcolepsy (for review, see references 103, 104). Randomized, placebo-controlled studies in narcolepsy patients by Fry[103] showed that modafinil at 200 and 400 mg doses resulted in significantly reduced mean scores of sleepiness, increased wakefulness, and increased latency to sleep. These results occurred with only subjectively mild to moderate side effects being reported, with headache being the most severe.[105] Unlike conventional psychostimulants such as cocaine and amphetamine, the waking effect of modafinil is not followed by rebound somnolence in the cat[106] or rat,[107] which suggests that modafinil induces wakefulness through mechanisms that are distinct from traditional psychostimulants. Though the specific mechanism of action of modafinil is not yet known, modafinil has alpha$_1$-noradrenergic agonist properties and may have a mechanism of action different from that of classic indirect sympathomimetics such as amphetamine. Modafinil produces locomotor activation in mice at doses 10 times higher than those of dextroamphetamine. These stimulant effects were not blocked by D1 or D2 dopamine receptor antagonists or by blockade of tyrosine hydroxylase activity, suggesting that modafinil has a locomotor activating effect completely different from that of dextroamphetamine.[108] Modafinil, however, substitutes for cocaine in drug discrimination and was self-administered by rhesus monkeys, but in these tests modafinil was 200 times less potent than dextroamphetamine.[109] One pharmacological study found that modafinil increased c-Fos immunoreactivity in the suprachiasmatic nucleus but had no effect on c-Fos immunoreactivity in the frontal cortex, striatum, lateral habenula, supraoptic nucleus, and the basolateral nucleus of the amygdala, areas that were all increased by amphetamine.[110] Also, in vivo microdialysis studies in the rat have shown that modafinil 30 to 100 mg/kg, intraperitoneally increases glutamate release in the ventromedial and ventrolateral thalamus and hippocampal formation[111] and decreases gamma-aminobutyric acid (GABA) release in the medial preoptic area and posterior hypothalamus.[112] These effects were hypothesized to reflect an action on the serotonergic 5-HT3 (5-hydroxytryptamine) receptor because modafinil's effect on GABA was partially blocked by a 5-HT3 antagonist.

Pemoline also is a CNS stimulant currently in clinical trials in the United States and being used abroad for the treatment of narcolepsy and daytime somnolence (for review, see reference 103). Studies have shown that at doses of 30, 60, and 90 mg, pemoline significantly lengthens daytime sleep latencies,[113, 114] improves attention,[114] improves performance on cognitive tasks,[115] and increases wakefulness during nocturnal sleep.[114] It is less effective than methylphenidate, dextroamphetamine, or methamphetamine, however, at controlling somnolence.[36, 116] Pemoline produces stereotyped behavior in the rat and acts as an indirect dopamine agonist.[117, 118] It inhibits catecholamine uptake in the hypothalamus and dopamine uptake in the corpus striatum.[118, 119]

SUMMARY

Significant advances have been made in our understanding of the mechanism of action of psychomotor stimulant drugs, from the behavioral, neuropharmacological, and molecular perspectives. Challenges for the future include exciting new avenues for research at the molecular, cellular, and system levels of analysis. Still unknown are exactly what differential roles different dopamine receptor subtypes may play in psychomotor stimulant actions, particularly the D3 and D4 receptor subtypes for which highly selective ligands have yet to be discovered. There are wide gaps in our knowledge of the neurophysiological mechanisms that translate the neuropharmacological actions of the behavioral actions of these drugs. Several co-neurotransmitters have been identified in the mesocorticolimbic dopamine system such as neurotensin and cholecystokinin, and their functional role has yet to be delineated. Finally, a major reevaluation of the neuroanatomical connections within the basal forebrain has given rise to the possibility that a hierarchical circuitry may exist in the afferents and efferents of the basal forebrain that may ultimately define the functional significance of the mesocorticolimbic and nigrostriatal dopamine systems and their role in psychomotor stimulant action. Recent evidence suggests that the basal forebrain interface between the limbic and extrapyramidal motor systems may be composed of separate neural circuits, a striatopallidal circuit and ventral striatal–medial pallidal circuits that form the extended amygdala.[121] How these circuits are modulated by the dopamine afferents and what implication this has for the actions of psychomotor stimulants is an important area for future research.

Acknowledgments

This is publication number 11521-NP from The Scripps Research Institute. The author would like to thank Mike Arends for his assistance with manuscript preparation.

References

1. Cannon WB, Rosenblueth A. Studies on conditions of activity in endocrine organs XXIX sympathin E and sympathin I. Am J Physiol. 1933;104:557–574.
2. von Euler US. A specific sympathomimetic ergone in adrenergic nerve fibres (sympathin) and its relations to adrenaline and noradrenaline. Acta Physiol Scand. 1947;12:73–97.
3. Vogt M. The concentration of sympathin in different parts of the central nervous system under normal conditions and after the administration. J Physiol (Lond). 1954;123:451–481.
4. Haddad LM. 1978: cocaine in perspective. J Am Coll Emerg Physicians. 1979;8:374–376.
5. Angrist B, Sudilovsky A. Central nervous system stimulants: historical aspects and clinical effects. In: Iversen LL, Iversen SD, Snyder SH, eds. Handbook of Psychopharmacology. Vol 11. New York, NY: Plenum; 1976:99–165.
6. Freud S. Über Coca. Centralbl Gesamte Ther. 1884;2:289–314.
7. Byck R. Cocaine Papers by Sigmund Freud. New York, NY: Stonehill; 1974.
8. Byck R. Cocaine use and research: three histories. In: Fisher S, Raskin A, Uhlenhuth EH, eds. Cocaine: Clinical and Biobehavioral Aspects. New York, NY: Oxford University Press; 1987.
9. Benzedrine. Report of the Council on Pharmacy and Chemistry. JAMA. 1933;101:1315.
10. USP Dictionary of USAN and International Drug Names. Rockville, Md: United States Pharmacopeia Convention; 1998.
11. Fischman MW, Schuster CR. Cocaine self-administration in humans. Fed Proc. 1982;41:241–246.
12. Iversen LL. Catecholamine uptake processes. Br Med Bull. 1973;29:130–135.
13. Ferris RM, Tank FLM, Maxwell RA. A comparison of the capacities of isomers of amphetamine, deoxypipradol and methylphenidate to inhibit the uptake of tritiated catecholamines into rat cerebral cortex slices, synaptosomal preparations of rat cerebral cortex, hypothalmus and striatum and into adrenergic nerves of rabbit aorta. J Pharmacol Exp Ther. 1972;181:407–416.
14. Trendelenberg U, Muskus A, Fleming WW, et al. Modification by reserpine of the action of sympathomimetic amines in spinal cats: a classification of sympathomimetic amines. J Pharmacol Exp Ther. 1962;138:170–180.
15. Foltin RW, Fischman MW, Nestadt G, et al. Demonstration of naturalistic methods for cocaine smoking by human volunteers. Drug Alcohol Depend. 1990;26:145–154.
16. Siegel RK. New patterns of cocaine use: changing doses and routes. In: Kozel NJ, Adams EH, eds. Cocaine Use in America: Epidemiologic and Clinical Perspectives. NIDA Research Monograph 61. Rockville, Md: National Institute on Drug Abuse; 1985;204–220.
17. Dring LC, Smith RL, Williams RT. The fate of amphetamine in man and other animals. J Pharm Pharmacol. 1966;18:402–405.
18. Davis JM, Kopin IJ, Lemberger L, et al. Effects of urinary pH on amphetamine metabolism. Ann N Y Acad Sci. 1971;179:493–501.
19. Wilkinson P, Van Dyke C, Jatlow P, et al. Intranasal and oral cocaine kinetics. Clin Pharmacol Ther. 1980;27:386–394.
20. Faraj BA, Israili ZH, Perel JM, et al. Metabolism and disposition of methylphenidate-14 C: studies in man and animals. J Pharmacol Exp Ther. 1974;191:535–547.
21. Smith CM, Beecher HK. Amphetamine, secobarbital, and athletic performance, II: subjective evaluations of performance, mood states and physical states. JAMA. 1960;172:1502–1514.
22. Heyrodt H, Weissenstein H. Über Steigerung körperlicher Leistungsfähigkeit durch Pervitin. Arch Exp Pathol Pharmakol. 1940;195:273–275.
23. Cuthbertson DP, Knox JAC. The effects of analeptics on the fatigued subject. J Physiol. 1947;106:42–58.
24. Kornetsky C, Mirsky AF, Kessler EK, et al. The effects of dextroamphetamine on behavioral deficits produced by sleep loss in humans. J Pharmacol Exp Ther. 1959;127:46–50.
25. Laties VG, Weiss B. The amphetamine margin in sports. Fed Proc. 1981;40:2689–2692.
26. Smith GM, Beecher HK. Amphetamine sulfate and athletic performance, I: objective effects. JAMA. 1959;170:542–557.
27. Weiss B, Laties VG. Enhancement of human performance by caffeine and the amphetamines. Pharmacol Rev. 1962;14:1–36.
28. Kornetsky C. Effects of meprobamate, phenobarbital and dextroamphetamine on reaction time and learning in man. J Pharmacol Exp Ther. 1958;123:216–219.
29. Mohs RC, Tinklenberg JR, Roth WT, et al. Methamphetamine and diphenhydramine effects on the rate of cognitive processing. Psychopharmacology. 1978;59:13–19.
30. Robbins TW, Sahakian BJ. "Paradoxical" effects of psychomotor stimulant drugs in hyperactive children from the standpoint of behavioural pharmacology. Neuropharmacology. 1979;18:931–950.
31. Penick SB. Amphetamines on obesity. Semin Psychiatry. 1969;1:144–162.
32. Oswald I. Drugs and sleep. Pharmacol Rev. 1968;20:273–303.
33. Rechtschaffen A, Maron L. The effect of amphetamine on the sleep cycle. Electroencephalogr Clin Neurophysiol. 1964;16:438–445.
34. Baekeland F. The effect of methylphenidate on the sleep cycle in man. Psychopharmacologia. 1966;10:179–183.
35. Prinzmetal M, Bloomberg W. Use of benzedrine for the treatment of narcolepsy. JAMA. 1935;105:2051–2054.
36. Mitler MM, Hajdukovic R, Erman M, et al. Narcolepsy. J Clin Neurophysiol. 1990;7:93–118.
37. Bradley C. The behavior of children receiving benzedrine. Am J Psychiatry. 1937;94:577–585.
38. Lambert NM, Windmiller M, Sandoval J, et al. Hyperactive children and the efficacy of psychoactive drugs as a treatment intervention. Am J Orthopsychiatry. 1976;46:335–352.
39. Huey LY. Attention deficit disorders. In: Judd LL, Groves PM, eds. Psychological Foundations of Clinical Psychiatry. Vol 4. New York, NY: BasicBooks; 1986:1–31.
40. Rylander G. Stereotype behaviour in man following amphetamine abuse. In: Baker SBC, ed. The Correlation of Adverse Effects in Man With Observations in Animals. Amsterdam, Netherlands: Excerpta Medica; 1971:28–31.
41. Randrup A, Munkvad I. Biochemical, anatomical and psychological investigations of stereotyped behavior induced by amphetamines. In: Costa E, Garattini S, eds. International Symposium on Amphetamines and Related Compounds. New York, NY: Raven Press; 1970:695–713.
42. Ellinwood EH Jr, Sudilovsky A, Nelson L. Evolving behavior in the clinical and experimental amphetamine (model) psychosis. Am J Psychiatry. 1973;130:1088–1093.
43. Randrup A, Munkvad I. Stereotyped activities produced by amphetamine in several animal species and man. Psychopharmacologia. 1967;11:300–310.
44. Lyon M, Robbins TW. The action of central nervous system stimulant drugs: a general theory concerning amphetamine effects. In: Essman WB, Valzelli L, eds. Current Developments in Psychopharmacology. Vol 2. New York, NY: Spectrum; 1975:79–163.
45. Segal DS. Behavioral characterization of d- and 1-amphetamine: Neurochemical implications. Science. 1975;190:475–477.

46. Rapoport JL, Buchsbaum MS, Weingartner H, et al. Dextroamphetamine, its cognitive and behavioral effects in normal and hyperactive boys and normal men. Arch Gen Psychiatry. 1980;37:933–943.

47. Griffith J, Oates JA, Cavanaugh JH. Paranoid episodes induced by drug. JAMA. 1968;205:39.

48. Jaffe JH. Drug addiction and drug abuse. In: Gilman AG, Goodman LS, Rall TW, eds. Goodman and Gilman's The Pharmacological Basis of Therapeutics. 7th ed. New York, NY: Macmillan; 1985:522–573.

49. Jaffe JH. Drug addiction and drug use. In: Goodman A, Gilman AG, Rall TW, et al, eds. Goodman and Gilman's The Pharmacological Basis of Therapeutics. 8th ed. New York, NY: Pergamon Press; 1990:522–573.

50. Hoffman BB, Lefkowitz RJ. Catecholamines and sympathomimetic drugs. In: Goodman A, Gilman A, Rall TW, et al, eds. Goodman and Gilman's The Pharmacological Basis of Therapeutics. 8th ed. New York, NY: Pergamon Press; 1990:187–220.

51. Johanson CE, Kilgore K, Uhlenhuth EH. Assessment of dependence potential of drugs in humans using multiple indices. Psychopharmacology (Berl). 1983;81:144–149.

52. Perez-Reyes M, White WR, McDonald SA, et al. Clinical effects of daily methamphetamine administration. Clin Neuropharmacol. 1991;14:352–358.

53. Ambre JJ, Belknap SM, Nelson J, et al. Acute tolerance to cocaine in humans. Clin Pharmacol Ther. 1988;44:1–8.

54. Angrist B, Corwin J, Bartlik B, Cooper T. Early pharmacokinetics and clinical effects of oral d-amphetamine in normal subjects. Biol Psychiatry. 1987;22:1357–1368.

55. Post RM, Weiss SRB, Fontana D, et al. Conditioned sensitization to the psychomotor stimulant cocaine. Ann N Y Acad Sci. 1992;654:386–399.

56. Lewander T. Effect of chronic treatment with central stimulants on brain monoamines and some behavioral and physiological functions in rats, guinea pigs, and rabbits. In: Usdin E, ed. Neuropsychopharmacology of Monoamines and Their Regulatory Enzymes. New York, NY: Raven Press; 1974:221–239.

57. Gawin FH, Ellinwood EH Jr. Cocaine and other stimulants: actions, abuse, and treatment. N Engl J Med. 1988;318:1173–1182.

58. Anthony JC, Warner LA, Kessler RC. Comparative epidemiology of dependence on tobacco, alcohol, controlled substances, and inhalants: basic findings from the National Comorbidity Survey. Exp Clin Psychopharmacol. 1994;2:244–268.

59. Weddington WW, Brown BS, Haertzen CA, et al. Changes in mood, craving, and sleep during short-term abstinence reported by male cocaine addicts: a controlled, residential study. Arch Gen Psychiatry. 1990;47:861–868.

60. Iversen SD, Fray PJ. Brain catecholamines in relation to affect. In: Beckman AL, ed. Neural Basis of Behavior. New York, NY: SP Medical and Scientific Books; 1982:229–269.

61. Taylor D, Ho BT. Comparison of inhibition of monoamine uptake by cocaine, methylphenidate and amphetamine. Res Commun Chem Pathol Pharmacol. 1978;21:67–75.

62. Glowinski J, Axelrod J. Effects of drugs on the uptake, release and metabolism of 3H-norepinephrine in the rat brain. J Pharmacol Exp Ther. 1965;149:43–49.

63. Raiteri M, Bertollini A, Angelini F, et al. d-Amphetamine as a releaser or reuptake inhibitor of biogenic amines in synaptosomes. Eur J Pharmacol. 1975;34:189–195.

64. Chiueh CC, Moore KE. Blockade by reserpine of methylphenidate-induced release of brain dopamine. J Pharmacol Exp Ther. 1975;193:559–563.

65. Moore KE, Chiueh CC, Zeldes G. Release of neurotransmitters from the brain in vivo by amphetamine, methylphenidate, and cocaine. In: Ellinwood EH Jr, Kilbey MM, eds. Cocaine and Other Stimulants. New York, NY: Plenum Press; 1977.

66. Robinson JB. Stereoselectivity and isoenzyme selectivity of monoamine oxidase inhibitors: enantiomers of amphetamine, N-methylamphetamine, and deprenyl. Biochem Pharmacol. 1985;34:4105–4108.

67. De Long MR. Primate models of movement disorders of basal ganglia origin. Trends Neurosci. 1990;13:281–285.

68. Ungerstedt U. Adipsia and aphagia after 6-hydroxydopamine-induced degeneration of the nigro-striatal dopamine system. Acta Physiol Scand Suppl 1971;367:95–122.

69. Zis AP, Fibiger HC, Phillips AG. Reversal by L-dopa of impaired learning due to destruction of the dopaminergic nigro-neostriatal projection. Science. 1974;185:960–962.

70. Joyce EM, Koob GF. Amphetamine-, scopolamine- and caffeine-induced locomotor activity following 6-hydroxydopamine lesions of the mesolimbic dopamine system. Psychopharmacology. 1981;73:311–313.

71. Kelly PH, Iversen SD. Selective 6-OHDA-induced destruction of mesolimbic dopamine neurons: abolition of psychostimulant-induced locomotor activity in rats. Eur J Pharmacol. 1976;40:45–56.

72. Roberts DCS, Koob GF, Klonoff P, et al. Extinction and recovery of cocaine self-administration following 6-hydroxydopamine lesions of the nucleus accumbens. Pharmacol Biochem Behav. 1980;12:781–787.

73. Lyness WH, Friedle NM, Moore KE. Destruction of dopaminergic nerve terminals in nucleus accumbens: effect of d-amphetamine self-administration. Pharmacol Biochem Behav. 1979;11:553–536.

74. Koob GF, Vaccarino FJ, Amalric M, et al. Positive reinforcement properties of drugs: search for neural substrates. In: Engel J, Oreland L, eds. Brain Reward Systems and Abuse. New York, NY: Raven Press; 1987:35–50.

75. Pijnenburg AJJ, Woodruff GN, Van Rossum JM. Antagonism of apomorphine and d-amphetamine-induced stereotyped behavior by injection of low doses of haloperidol into the caudate nucleus and the nucleus accumbens. Psychopharmacologia. 1986;45:61–65.

76. Carelli RM, Deadwyler SA. A comparison of nucleus accumbens neuronal firing patterns during cocaine self-administration and water reinforcement in rats. J Neurosci. 1994;14:7735–7746.

77. Carelli RM, King VC, Hampson RE, et al. Firing patterns of nucleus accumbens neurons during cocaine self-administration in rats. Brain Res. 1993;626:14–22.

78. Chang JY, Sawyer SF, Lee R-S, et al. Electrophysiological and pharmacological evidence for the role of the nucleus accumbens in cocaine self-administration in freely moving rats. J Neurosci. 1994;14:1224–1244.

79. Peoples LL, West MO. Phasic firing of single neurons in the rat nucleus accumbens correlated with the timing of intravenous cocaine self-administration. J Neurosci. 1996;16:3459–3473.

80. Peoples LL, Uzwiak AJ, Gee F, et al. Operant behavior during sessions of intravenous cocaine infusion is necessary and sufficient for phasic firing of single nucleus accumbens neurons. Brain Res. 1997;757:280–284.

81. Carelli RM, Deadwyler SA. Dual factors controlling activity of nucleus accumbens cell-firing during cocaine self-administration. Synapse. 1996;24:308–311.

82. Creese I, Iversen SD. A role of forebrain dopamine systems in amphetamine-induced stereotyped behavior in the rat. Psychopharmacology. 1974;39:345–357.

83. Iversen SD. Brain dopamine system and behavior. In: Iversen LL, Iversen SD, Snyder SH, eds. Handbook of Psychopharmacology. Vol 8. New York, NY: Plenum Press; 1977:334–384.

84. Koob GF, Simon H, Herman JP, et al. Neuroleptic-like disruption of the conditioned avoidance response requires destruction of both the mesolimbic and nigrostriatal dopamine systems. Brain Res. 1984;303:319–329.

85. Kelley AE, Gauthier AM, Lang CG. Amphetamine microinjections into distinct striatal subregions cause dissociable effects on motor and ingestive behavior. Behav Brain Res. 1989;35:27–39.

86. Kebabian JW, Calne DB. Multiple receptors for dopamine. Nature. 1979;277:93–96.

87. Monsma FJ, Mahan LC, McVittie LD, et al. Molecular cloning and expression of a D1 dopamine receptor linked to adenylyl cyclase activation. Proc Natl Acad Sci U S A. 1990;87:6723–6727.

88. Sokoloff P, Giros B, Martres M-P, et al. Molecular cloning and characterization of a novel dopamine receptor (D3) as a target for neuroleptics. Nature. 1990;347:146–151.

89. Van Tol HHM, Bunzow JR, Guan HC, et al. Cloning of the gene for a human dopamine D4 receptor with high affinity for the antipsychotic clozapine. Nature. 1991;350:610–614.

90. Sunahara RK, Guan HC, O'Dowd BF, et al. Cloning of the gene for a human dopamine D5 receptor with higher affinity for dopamine than D1. Nature. 1991;350:614–619.

91. Amalric M, Koob GF. Functionally selective neurochemical afferents and efferents of the mesocorticolimbic and nigrostriatal dopamine system. In: Arbuthnott GW, Emson PC, eds. Chemical Signalling in the Basal Ganglia. Amsterdam, Netherlands: Elsevier; 1993:209–226.

92. Koob GF, Le HT, Creese I. The D-1 dopamine receptor antagonist SCH 23390 increases cocaine self-administration in the rat. Neurosci Lett. 1987;79:315–320.

93. Amalric MA, Berhow M, Polis I, et al. Selective effects of low dose D2 dopamine receptor antagonism in a reaction time task in rats. Neuropsychopharmacology. 1993;8:195–200.

94. Levesque D, Diaz J, Pilon C, et al. Identification, characterization, and localization of the dopamine D3 receptor in rat brain using 7-[3H] hydroxy-N,N,-di-N-propyl-2-aminotetralin. Proc Natl Acad Sci U S A. 1992;89:8155–8159.

95. Caine SB, Koob GF. Modulation of cocaine self-administration in the rat through D-3 dopamine receptors. Science. 1993;260:1814–1816.

96. Caine SB, Koob GF, Parsons LH, et al. D3 receptor test in vitro predicts decreased cocaine self-administration in rats. Neuroreport. 1997;8:2373–2377.

97. Xu M, Hu X-T, Cooper DC, et al. Elimination of cocaine-induced hyperactivity and dopamine-mediated neurophysiological effects in dopamine D1 receptor mutant mice. Cell. 1994;79:945–955.

98. Giros B, Jaber M, Jones SR, et al. Hyperlocomotion and indifference to cocaine and amphetamine in mice lacking the dopamine transporter. Nature. 1996;379:606–612.

99. Xu M, Moratalla R, Gold LH, et al. Dopamine D1 receptor mutant mice are deficient in striatal expression of dynorphin and in dopamine-mediated behavioral responses. Cell. 1994;79:729–742.

99a. Hollon TR, Gleason TC, Grinberg A, et al. Generation of D5 dopamine receptor-deficient mice by gene targeting. Soc Neurosci Abstr. 1998;24:594.

100. Baik JH, Picetti R, Saiardi A, et al. Parkinsonian-like locomotor impairment in mice lacking dopamine D-2 receptors. Nature. 1995;377:424–428.

101. Maldonado R, Saiardi A, Valverde O, et al. Absence of opiate rewarding effects in mice lacking dopamine D-2 receptors. Nature. 1997;388:586–589.

102. Rubinstein M, Phillips T, Bunzow JR, et al. Mice lacking dopamine D-4 receptors are supersensitive to ethanol, cocaine, and methamphetamine. Cell. 1997;90:991–1001.

102a. Hagan JJ, Leslie RA, Patel S, et al. Orexin A activates locus coeruleus cell firing and increases arousal in the rat. Proc Natl Acad Sci U S A. 1999;96:10911–10916.

102b. Chemelli RM, Willie JT, Sinton CM, et al. Narcolepsy in orexin knockout mice: molecular genetics of sleep regulation. Cell. 1999;98:437–451.

102c. Lin L, Faraco J, Li R, et al. The sleep disorder canine narcolepsy is caused by a mutation in the hypocretin (orexin) receptor 2 gene. Cell. 1999;98:365–376.

103. Fry JM. Treatment modalities for narcolepsy. Neurology. 1998;50:S43–S48.

104. Green PM, Stillman MJ. Narcolepsy: Signs, symptoms, differential diagnosis, and management. Arch Fam Med. 1998;7:474–478.

105. US Modafinil in Narcolepsy Multicenter Study Group. Randomized trial of modafinil for the treatment of pathological somnolence in narcolepsy. Ann Neurol. 1998;43:88–97.

106. Lin JS, Roussel B, Akaoka H, et al. Role of catecholamines in the modafinil and amphetamine-induced wakefulness, a comparative pharmacological study in the cat. Brain Res. 1992;591:319–336.

107. Edgar DM, Seiel WF. Modafinil induces wakefulness without intensifying motor activity or subsequent rebound hypersomnolence in the rat. J Pharmacol Exp Ther. 1997;283:757–769.

108. Simon P, Hemet C, Ramassamy C, et al. Non-amphetaminic mechanism of stimulant locomotor effect of modafinil in mice. Eur J Neuropsychopharmacol. 1995;5:509–514.

109. Gold LH, Balster RL. Evaluation of the cocaine-like discriminative stimulus effects and reinforcing effects of modafinil. Psychopharmacology. 1996;126:286–292.

110. Engber TM, Koury EJ, Dennis SA, et al. Differential patterns of regional c-Fos induction in the rat brain by amphetamine and the novel wakefulness-promoting agent modafinil. Neurosci Lett. 1998;241:95–98.

111. Ferraro L, Antonelli T, O'Connor WT, et al. The antinarcoleptic drug modafinil increases glutamate release in thalamic areas and hippocampus. Neuroreport. 1997;8:2883–2887.

112. Ferraro L, Tanganelli S, O'Connor WT, et al. The vigilance-promoting drug modafinil decreases GABA release in the medial preoptic area and in the posterior hypothalamus of the awake rat: possible involvement of the serotonergic 5-HT3 receptor. Neurosci Lett. 1996;220:5–8.

113. Mitler MM, Hajdukovic R. Relative efficacy of drugs for the treatment of sleepiness in narcolepsy. Sleep. 1991;14:218–220.

114. Nicholson AN, Pascoe PA. Dopaminergic transmission and the sleep-wakefulness continuum in man. Neuropharmacology. 1990;29:411–417.

115. Mitler MM, Shafor R, Hajdukovic R, et al. Treatment of narcolepsy: Objective studies on methylphenidate, pemoline, and protriptyline. Sleep. 1986;9:260–264.

116. Mitler MM. Evaluation of treatment with stimulants in narcolepsy. Sleep. 1994; 17(suppl 8):S103–S106.

117. Mueller K, Nyhan WL. Pharmacologic control of pemoline-induced self-injurious behavior in rats. Pharmacol Biochem Behav. 1982;16:957–963.

118. Molina VA, Orsingher OA. Effects of Mg-pemoline on the central catecholaminergic system. Arch Int Pharmacodyn Ther. 1981;251:66–79.

119. Ramirez A, Vial H, Barailler J, et al. Effects of levophacetoperane, pemoline, fenozolone, and centrophenoxine on catecholamines and serotonin uptake in various parts of the rat brain. C R Acad Sci III. 1978;187:53–56.

35

Stimulants: Efficacy and Adverse Effects

Merrill M. Mitler
Michael S. Aldrich

Psychomotor stimulants produce behavioral activation and increased arousal, motor activity, and alertness. Psychomotor stimulants are divided into three classes: (1) direct acting sympathomimetics, such as the alpha$_1$-adrenergic stimulant phenylephrine; (2) indirect acting sympathomimetics, such as methylphenidate, amphetamine, mazindol, and pemoline; and (3) stimulants that are not sympathomimetics and have different mechanisms of action, such as caffeine. The pharmacology of sympathomimetics is reviewed in Chapter 34. This chapter focuses on the clinical use of sympathomimetics with predominantly indirect action. However, some stimulants have both direct and indirect actions.[1, 2]

HISTORY

Psychostimulants have been used for centuries in tonics and other preparations to allay fatigue and treat a variety of ailments (for reviews, see references 3,4). Coffee, along with leaves of sage or rosemary, was prescribed as early as 1672 for disorders associated with sleepiness. The Indians of Peru and Bolivia used cocaine, a crystalline alkaloid derived from the leaves of the coca plant, for pleasure and to increase stamina. From 1886 to 1905, cocaine was an ingredient in Coca-Cola. The medicinal use of cocaine was advocated by Freud.[5] However, cocaine's profound potential for abuse and addiction soon limited the role of this stimulant in modern medicine.

In general, the central nervous system (CNS) stimulant drugs now prescribed by sleep specialists for the control of sleepiness were introduced into the market for weight loss or the treatment of attention-deficit hyperactivity disorder. In sleep medicine the principal indications for treatment with a stimulant are narcolepsy and idiopathic CNS hypersomnia. Occasionally, stimulants are prescribed for the sleepiness associated with jet lag. Additionally, patients with sleep apnea who continue to have disabling sleepiness despite treatment of airway obstruction during sleep may receive stimulant therapy.

Few stimulant drugs (e.g., dextroamphetamine and methylphenidate) have Food and Drug Administration (FDA) approval for the indication of narcolepsy. Amphetamine, racemic β-phenylisopropylamine, is a powerful CNS stimulant which was first used in the 1930s as a bronchodilator, respiratory stimulant, and analeptic. Several preparations of amphetamine have been developed as oral preparations which vary in terms of the concentration of the dextro-isomer and whether a phosphate or sulfate salt is used. Methylphenidate, a piperidine derivative, was introduced in the 1950s as a milder stimulant. Pemoline, an oxazolidine compound, was later introduced as a mild CNS stimulant. Mazindol, an imidazoline derivative, is another mild stimulant marketed as an appetite suppressant. Modafinil, (2-[(diphenylmethyl)sulfinyl] acetamide) is a racemic compound unrelated to the amphetamines or other CNS stimulants. Modafinil began to appear on the world market for the indication of narcolepsy and CNS hypersomnia in the early 1990s.

STIMULANTS AND NARCOLEPSY

In 1931, Doyle and Daniels[6] and Janota[7] described the use of ephedrine to treat sleepiness. After 1956, methylphenidate came into broad use as suggested by Yoss and Daly.[8] Since the 1970s, the use of stimulants has been modified by the introduction of rapid eye movement (REM)–suppressing antidepressants to treat cataplexy and the reintroduction of psychological and sleep hygiene advice.

The treatment of narcolepsy underwent a dramatic change with the introduction of ephedrine. Despite its clinically noteworthy efficacy, it was soon apparent that side effects, incomplete patient acceptance, rapid development of tolerance, and cost limited its usefulness. In 1935, Prinzmetal and Bloomberg[9] suggested that amphetamine sulfate would be appropriate treatment for narcolepsy because of its close relationship to ephedrine and epinephrine, its low toxicity and low cost, its prolonged action, and its lack of pronounced sympathomimetic side effects. In their first report, nine patients noted complete relief from sleep attacks and practically complete relief from cataplexy. They noted that insomnia and restlessness were potential problems and that the medication should not be given late in the day. They recommended 10 mg doses initially with a gradual increase until an optimal effect was obtained. Subsequent reports described the benefits of dextroamphetamine[10] and methamphetamine,[11] and the use of up to 80 mg of amphetamine sulfate to achieve control of sleepiness.[12] By 1949, amphetamines, in one or another of the several oral preparations as a phosphate or sulfate, had become the treatment of choice for excessive sleepiness, with a typical initial treatment of 10 mg three times a day, followed by gradual increases until sleepiness was controlled.

Side effects of amphetamines were noted soon after their introduction. In 1937 Shapiro[13] noted that 2 of 15 patients treated with amphetamine sulfate experienced side effects. Young and Scoville[14] noted psychotic symptoms in three narcoleptic patients and suggested that amphetamine sulfate may have "precipitated the psychotic reaction" in two of them; the patients showed "a great apprehension" amounting to panic, confusion, and bewilderment. By 1949 there were at least four reports of an association between narcolepsy and paranoid psychosis (further reviewed in reference 15).

In the 1950s, Daly and Yoss, who introduced methylphenidate as a treatment for narcolepsy, reported their experience in using daily doses of methylphenidate ranging from 20 to 200 mg.[8, 16] As their patients were assessed before polysomnography was developed and sleep apnea was discovered, their series and other early series of narcoleptic patients may have included patients with other sleep disorders. The use of high doses of methylphenidate may have been partly motivated by the report of Yoss and Daly[16] of reversal of pupillographic abnormalities in narcoleptic patients by methylphenidate 120 mg/d. For patients who did not respond well to methylphenidate, Yoss subsequently recommended methamphetamine up to 40 mg/d. In Daly and Yoss's 1974 summary[17] of their experience, they advocated that patients be given initial trials of low to moderate dosages of methamphetamine or methylphenidate with gradual increases in doses to as much as 200 mg of either drug if needed to control sleep attacks.

Although numerous disorders and diseases lead to excessive somnolence,[18] multicenter surveys based on standardized diagnostic techniques and criteria[19, 20] indicate that more than 80% of patients who present with this symptom have sleep apnea, narcolepsy, idiopathic hypersomnia, or insufficient sleep.[21, 22] While the sleepiness associated with sleep apnea resolves or improves with effective treatment of the apnea, and that associated with insufficient sleep syndrome improves with increased amounts of sleep, narcolepsy and idiopathic hypersomnia are chronic CNS disorders, and the sleepiness caused by these two conditions can only be treated symptomatically with behavioral and pharmacological interventions.

For many patients with these disorders, controlling excessive sleepiness is critically important to allow adequate functioning at home, while driving, or in the workplace. Furthermore, sleepiness and fatigue, stem-

ming either from sleep disorders or from sleep deprivation, create major safety problems.[23] However, psychomotor stimulants, the primary treatments for sleepiness associated with these disorders, have significant potential for abuse and side effects. Thus, clinicians must weigh the patient's need for adequate treatment and the personal and social risks of inadequate treatment against the potential for side effects and abuse.

CLINICAL STUDIES OF STIMULANT DRUGS

Criteria of Response to Stimulant Medications

The initial evaluations of the effectiveness of stimulants for the treatment of sleepiness and sleep attacks in narcolepsy were based on clinical assessment.[6, 7, 9, 10] Yoss and colleagues, the first to apply pupillography[24] to the assessment of sleepiness, measured pupil diameter and stability of pupil diameter to evaluate the response of individual patients to alerting drugs.[25, 26] More recently, the multiple sleep latency test (MSLT)[27] and the Maintenance of Wakefulness Test (MWT) (see Chapter 104)[28] have been used to assess sleepiness in a variety of sleep disorders[29] and to evaluate pharmacotherapeutic efficacy.[30–36] Because the average MSLT or MWT sleep latency can be regarded as a single numerical measure of sleep tendency, some determinations of the relative efficacy of pharmacotherapeutic agents have been calculated.[37]

Published Data

In one of the first clinical reports of a series of narcoleptic patients, 84% had a good to excellent response to methylphenidate; 60 to 80 mg/d was the usual dose required by those who obtained an excellent result.[16] This and subsequent clinical reports and clinical trials of a number of medications are summarized in Table 35–1. Most studies report substantial improvements in 65 to 85% of subjects. Clinical trials have demonstrated significant improvements in sleep tendency assessed by the MSLT or MWT for dextroamphetamine, methylphenidate, modafinil, and pemoline.[37]

Idiopathic hypersomnia has not been studied as extensively as narcolepsy and there are few controlled studies that objectively evaluate the efficacy of any pharmacological or nonpharmacological treatment for idiopathic hypersomnia. The sleepiness of idiopathic hypersomnia appears to respond in substantially the same manner to stimulant drugs as does the sleepiness of narcolepsy.[38] In one series, 15 of 21 patients (71%) with idiopathic hypersomnia had a good subjective response to stimulants.[39]

Relative Efficacy of Stimulants

Some clinicians believe that stimulants vary in the degree to which they control sleepiness. On the basis

Table 35–1. EFFICACY OF STIMULANTS FOR TREATMENT OF SLEEPINESS IN NARCOLEPSY

Reference (Year)	Type of Study	N	Medications	Daily Dose (mg)	Efficacy	Side Effects
Daly and Yoss (1956)[16]	Case series	25	Methylphenidate	40–240	Good–excellent in 84%	Nervousness and tremulousness (35%); anorexia (22%); insomnia (17%); palpitations (3%)
Yoss and Daly (1959)[8]	Case series	60	Methylphenidate	40–80*	Good–excellent in 68%	
Parkes et al. (1975)[45]	Case series	63	Dextroamphetamine	5–150	Moderate–good in 73%	Side effects—73%: irritability (49%); headache (48%); palpitations (24%); jitteriness (24%); muscle jerks (22%); insomnia (11%); dyskinesias (5%); hallucinations (3%); psychosis (1.6%)
Honda et al. (1960)[123]	Case series	80	Methamphetamine Methylphenidate Dextroamphetamine	5–15 20–80	Disappearance of sleep attacks	Disturbed nocturnal sleep
Mitler et al. (1993)[36]	Sleep laboratory	8	Methamphetamine	20–60	Improved by MSLT	
Mitler et al. (1990)[30]	Sleep laboratory	13	Methylphenidate	10–60	Improved by MWT	
	Sleep laboratory	5	Dextroamphetamine	30–60	Improved by MWT	
	Sleep laboratory	14	Pemoline	19–113	Improved by MWT at 113 mg	Side effects in fewer than 10%
Laffont et al. (1987)[124]	Placebo-controlled clinical trial	19†	Modafinil	200	Decrease of sleep attacks	Side effects in fewer than 10%
Bastuji and Jovvet (1988)[96]	Clinical trial	42‡	Modafinil	200–500	Improvement in 71% with narcolepsy; in 83% with idiopathic hypersomnia	
Broughton et al. (1997)[42]	Placebo-controlled, crossover clinical trial	75	Modafinil	200–400	Improved, by MWT clinical and self-report criteria	Side effects not significantly different from placebo
US Modafinil in Narcolepsy Multicenter Study Group (1998)[43]	Placebo-controlled, parallel groups clinical trial	283	Modafinil	200–400	Improved, by MSLT, MWT clinical and self-report criteria	Side effects not significantly different from placebo
US Modafinil in Narcolepsy Multicenter Study Group (1998)[125]	Placebo-controlled, parallel groups clinical trial	271	Modafinil	200–400	Improved, by MSLT, MWT clinical and self-report criteria	Side effects not significantly different from placebo
Alvarez et al. (1991)[94]	Clinical retrospective review	41	Mazindol	1–16	Moderate–good in 78%	39%—mainly gastrointestinal
Schindler et al. (1985)[47]	Placebo-controlled clinical trial	20	Dextroamphetamine Mazindol Fencamfamin	10–30 4 60	Sleep attacks reduced by 36–52%	Side effects similar to placebo
Roselaar et al. (1987)[50]	Clinical trial	7	Selegiline	20–30	Sleep attacks reduced by 30%	Similar to dextroamphetamine
Saletu et al. (1989)[126]	Placebo-controlled clinical trial	10§	Modafinil Dextroamphetamine	100–200 10–20		Disturbed nocturnal sleep with dextroamphetamine but not with modafinil

*One patient took 300 mg.
†Twelve patients with narcolepsy; seven with idiopathic hypersomnia.
‡Twenty-four patients with narcolepsy; 18 with idiopathic hypersomnia.
§Elderly non-narcoleptic patients.
MSLT, multiple sleep latency test; MWT, Maintenance of Wakefulness Test.

of available publications, it is impossible to measure objectively the relative efficacy of stimulants. Among the most important problems hampering quantitative comparisons of stimulants are the following: (1) investigators have used different outcome measures (e.g., clinical assessment, MSLT, MWT, etc.); (2) among published reports, subject samples varied widely in the baseline level of sleepiness; (3) some investigators have studied multiple doses, thereby providing a basis for estimating the dose-response curve, while others have not; (4) there is little correlation between oral doses and blood levels of methylphenidate and probably of other stimulants.[40] One approach to the relative efficacy problem employed a normalization technique on published data from a number of possible pharmacotherapies for narcolepsy.[37] Clinical trials for the following drugs were reviewed: codeine, gamma-hydroxybutyrate, ritanserin, viloxazine, pemoline, modafinil, protriptyline, dextroamphetamine, and methylphenidate. The greatest effect of each drug, as measured by mean MSLT or MWT sleep latency, was normalized in terms of the degree to which narcoleptic patients treated with the drug approached normal values. Later, employing this same normalization technique, Mitler et al.[41] focused on the following treatment and testing conditions because the published articles reported both statistically significant efficacy and what was judged to be clinically meaningful therapeutic effects: pemoline 112.5 mg using the MWT[30]; modafinil 200 and 400 mg using the MWT[42, 43]; dextroamphetamine 60 mg using the MWT[30]; methylphenidate 60 mg using the MWT[30]; and methamphetamine 40 to 60 mg using the MSLT.[36] Sleep latencies measured during drug-free baseline and appropriate treatment phases of each study were then expressed as a percentage of published values for normal subjects[30] for either the MSLT (13.4 min) or the MWT (18.9 min). The results are summarized in Figure 35–1. The lighter bars represent mean sleep latency observed during baseline conditions and the darker bars represent mean sleep latency observed during treatment.

Quantitative comparisons of these treatments cannot be made with this normalization technique. There are also other important limitations: (1) only the single endpoint of percent change in average sleep latency was considered. Other important endpoints not considered are the number of subjects who did respond vs. the number who did not, subjective alertness, and psychomotor performance; (2) due to the small number of subjects, no interdrug statistical tests were performed. For quantitative assessment of the relative efficacy of stimulants, parallel groups, placebo-controlled designs are necessary. For example, in one parallel group's study of modafinil vs. dextroamphetamine, there were no statistically significant differences between the efficacy of the two active drugs.[44] More such studies are needed.

The data in Figure 35–1 are useful for establishing a framework within which a patient's treatment response can be viewed. Limitations notwithstanding, one can appreciate that each drug did produce a clinically significant change above baseline toward normal levels. Dextroamphetamine, methamphetamine, and methyl-

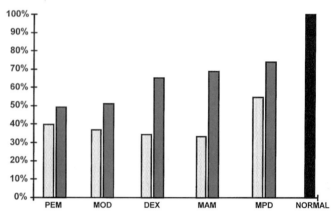

Figure 35–1. Relative efficacy of stimulant drugs commonly used to treat narcolepsy must be estimated on a post hoc basis (see text). The lightest shading denotes baseline sleep latencies on either the multiple sleep latency test (MSLT) or Maintenance of Wakefulness Test (MWT) expressed in terms of percentage of normal levels (13.4 min for the MSLT and 18.9 for the MWT); the darker shading denotes values observed at the highest dose of each drug evaluted. See text for methods. DEX, dextroamphetamine; MAM, methamphetamine; MOD, modafinil; MPD, methylphenidate; PEM, pemoline.

phenidate brought measurements above 60% of normal levels. Modafinil brought patients to about 51% of normal levels. The largest change from baseline occurred with methamphetamine.[36] In the study of methylphenidate,[30] although baseline levels were greater than 50% of normal, measures during treatment were closest to normal levels. The drugs studied in these trials did not, however, normalize sleepiness and it is not possible to predict whether treatment with higher doses of these drugs would normalize sleepiness. Clinicians treat individual patients based on their particular therapeutic needs and abilities to tolerate side effects. Nevertheless, some narcoleptic patients report satisfactory control of sleepiness with doses of stimulants higher than the usually recommended range.

Unwanted Effects of Stimulants

Side Effects

When used in the treatment of narcolepsy or other conditions, stimulants commonly produce side effects, including irritability, talkativeness, and sympathomimetic side effects such as sweating, particularly at higher doses. The reported frequency of side effects of stimulants in clinical practice and in clinical trials varies from 0 to 73% (see Table 35–1); the extreme variation reflects, at least in part, differences in method of determining side effects and the definition of a side effect. Common side effects include headaches, irritability, nervousness or tremulousness, anorexia, insomnia, gastrointestinal complaints, dyskinesias, and palpitations.[8, 45, 46] In one series of 100 patients, 10% discontinued stimulants due to failure to respond, tolerance, or side effects.[45] However, in a different series of 20 narcoleptics, dextroamphetamine 10 to 30 mg/d caused no increase in side-effects compared with baseline.[47]

Disturbed nocturnal sleep documented with polysomnography occurred in eight narcoleptics given methamphetamine 20 to 60 mg/d for 4 d[36] and Regestein et al.[48] noted their clinical impression that doses of dextroamphetamine or methylphenidate above 50 to 60 mg/d interfere with sleep. Stimulants do not appear to cause a clinically significant increase in blood pressure at commonly used doses in normotensive individuals.[8, 45, 49] Side effects may be less frequent with modafinil than with amphetamines (see Table 35–1) whereas side effects with selegiline 20 to 30 mg/d are comparable to dextroamphetamine in similar dose.[50] Pemoline use has been associated with hepatocellular liver damage[51–54]; the mechanism appears to be idiosyncratic and metabolic rather than immunologic.[55]

Psychosis and hallucinations are rare in narcoleptics treated with stimulants.[48, 56] In four series totaling 243 patients, there were two cases of amphetamine psychosis, two of hallucinations, and three of addiction.[45, 57–59] Although there are no data in narcoleptics indicating that the incidence of hallucinations and psychosis differs with different stimulants, some authors suggest that the incidence of side effects is less with methylphenidate than with dextroamphetamine.[60, 61]

The likelihood of psychosis or hallucinations induced by stimulants is increased in patients with coexisting or preexisting psychiatric conditions.[14, 62–65] The risk of psychiatric complications is probably greater at higher doses.

Cardiac and vascular complications of stimulants have been reported only rarely in narcoleptics. Three patients in one series had strokes while on amphetamines,[45] but this incidence may not have been above baseline. Among narcoleptic patients, there are isolated case reports of cardiomyopathy after treatment with amphetamine 100 mg/d for 7 years and ischemic colitis after treatment with dextroamphetamine 30 mg/d.[66, 67] A narcoleptic patient who took more than 200 mg/d of methylphenidate for several years developed diminished peripheral pulses and symptoms suggestive of peripheral vascular occlusive disease; symptoms improved after stimulants were discontinued (M.S. Aldrich, personal communication, 1997). These complications must be assessed in light of the many narcoleptic patients who have taken stimulants on a regular basis for decades, often into the 7th or 8th decade of life, without developing cardiovascular disturbances. While some clinicians consider hypertension to be a contraindication to stimulant therapy, there are no systematic studies indicating that stimulants prescribed to reduce sleepiness aggravate preexisting hypertension. Our experience suggests that well-controlled hypertension is not exacerbated by moderate doses of stimulants.

A three- to sevenfold increase in amphetamine content in breast milk compared to plasma in a nursing mother with narcolepsy[68] suggests that amphetamines should be used cautiously or not at all in nursing mothers.

Pemoline has been associated with elevated liver enzymes and rarely with hepatic failure. Liver functions should therefore be monitored before and during therapy. Given the potential for serious side effects, the role of pemoline in the treatment of sleepiness is thus problematic. Because of these concerns, pemoline has been withdrawn from the market in Canada.

Abuse

Amphetamines and related compounds have high abuse potential and can produce dependence. While most users (more than 90%) do not become addicted, controlled use may become compulsive use, especially when the drug is readily available or when a rapid route of administration is used. A sequence of euphoria, dysphoria, paranoia, and psychosis can occur after a single exposure to a high dose or with chronic exposure to low doses. During a binge, the user characteristically administers the drug repeatedly for up to several days. Following a binge, there is the crash: extreme exhaustion, often with depression, anxiety, and an intense desire to sleep. The subsequent withdrawal phase is characterized by apathy, anhedonia, and strong drug craving. Episodic craving gradually diminishes over weeks and months.

Sustained use of high doses of amphetamines and related compounds can lead to cognitive and behavioral disorders. In healthy volunteers, repetitive oral administration of 5 to 10 mg of dextroamphetamine produces paranoid delusions, often with blunted affect, after a cumulative dose of 55 to 75 mg.[69] In amphetamine abusers, paranoid psychosis can lead to physical toxicity associated, for example, with the belief that bugs under the skin ("crank bugs") need to be gouged out. Amphetamine abusers can persist in repetitive thoughts or organized, goal-directed but meaningless activity[70] such as repetitive cleaning, elaborate sorting of small objects, or endless disassembly and reassembly of such items as clocks and radios. These stereotyped behavioral sequences[71] are also observed in animal species.[72, 73] For example, monkeys pick at their skin, exhibit mouth and tongue movements, and stare; rats sniff intensely in one location; pigeons repetitively peck at one location on a stimulus display. Lyon and Robbins[74] hypothesized that as the dose of amphetamines increases, the repetition rate of motor activities increases with the result that the organism exhibits "increases in response rates within a decreasing number of response categories." As a result, complex behaviors are eliminated as the response categories decrease. Behaviors capable of repetition without long pauses dominate, and shorter and shorter response sequences result. High rates of responding in operant situations decrease and locomotor activity decreases.[75, 76] Thus, the observation that amphetamine produces an inverted U-shaped dose response in locomotor activity may be due to the competitive nature of locomotor activity and the emergence of stereotyped behavior.[77] Similar effects on cognition may contribute to paranoid ideation and psychosis.

A variety of complications can occur with intravenous, intranasal, or oral amphetamine or methamphetamine abuse (see Table 35–1); in one case brain hemorrhage followed a single oral dose of 20 mg of amphetamine.[78–92] In young adults, the relative risk of stroke is estimated to be 6.5 times greater for drug abusers compared to nonabusers,[84] with amphetamines implicated in a substantial proportion of young drug abusers with stroke.[84, 85] Although complications are probably more common after intravenous use of large quantities of stimulants, catastrophic cerebrovascular events may follow oral or inhalational use of relatively modest drug doses. In many cases the actual doses ingested are unknown because of the use of "street" drugs. Despite the potential for disastrous complications, long-term stimulant abuse does not appear to cause permanent major intellectual and neuropsychological dysfunction.[93]

Tolerance

Although tolerance can develop to many of the effects of stimulants, the clinical significance of tolerance to alerting effects is uncertain. In narcoleptic patients, tolerance to alerting effects appears to occur with variable frequency. In one review, 10 of 100 patients had discontinued stimulants due to failure to respond, tolerance, or side effects, and 31 others had required doubling of dosage over a 1-year period for the same control of symptoms.[45] Passouant and Billiard[59] observed tolerance in 11 of 50 narcoleptics taking stimulants, and tolerance occurred in 14 of 41 patients treated with mazindol up to 16 mg/d.[94] While Parkes[56] concluded that tolerance to central stimulant effects develops in 30 to 40% of subjects after a few days or weeks of repeated intake, others observed no tolerance in 106 narcoleptic patients treated with methylphenidate for up to several years,[95] in 42 patients treated with modafinil 200 to 500 mg/d for up to 3 years,[96] nor in 12 narcoleptic patients treated for 6 months with levoamphetamine or dextroamphetamine.[97]

Tolerance to stimulants appears to be more likely with high doses.[60, 98–100] Among six patients who had increased their intake of dextroamphetamine to more than 100 mg/d because of an increase in sleep attacks and cataplexy, "the increased amphetamine intake did not help them in any way."[57] With lower doses, none worsened and three improved. In one study, three of four patients with minimal or no clinical benefit took methylphenidate 160 to 240 mg/d, whereas none of 21 patients with good to excellent responses took more than 140 mg/d.[16]

There is little evidence that the incidence of tolerance and side effects is less in narcoleptic patients than in others taking comparable doses,[101] that the tolerance reported by some patients is an effect of inadequate nocturnal sleep rather than true tolerance,[25] and that tolerance and other side effects are less likely to occur with methylphenidate than with dextroamphetamine.[17, 60]

Dealing With Specific Situations

Use of Stimulants in Children

Side effects of stimulants in children with narcolepsy have not been studied in detail; much of the available data concern the use of stimulants for children with attention-deficit hyperactivity disorder. The potential side effect of greatest concern is growth retardation.[102] For example, deficits in weight gain and height increase may occur after treatment of attention-deficit hyperactivity disorder with pemoline, dextroamphetamine, or methylphenidate.[103–106] However, these deficits may be reversed during summers off medication,[107, 108] and there is little or no evidence of long-term effects on growth. In one of the few studies noting an effect on growth lasting as long as 4 years, the growth-suppressant effect of methylphenidate accounted for just 2% of the variance in final height.[105] The effects of methylphenidate on growth in prepubertal children appear not to extend into adolescence,[109] and in one study the adult height of treated children was not different from the height of controls or national norms.[110] A 1989 review concluded that there is no evidence that stimulants affect adult height in children with attention-deficit hyperactivity disorder.[111] Other side effects of stimulants in the treatment of children with attention-deficit hyperactivity disorder—anorexia and insomnia—are usually transient and diminish with continued treatment.[106]

In children with attention-deficit hyperactivity disorder, methylphenidate treatment does not appear to lead to emotional maladjustment, delinquency, cognitive deficits, or reduced academic performance.[112] Tics can occur in children taking stimulants,[111] but in a review of 1000 children taking stimulants for up to 10 years, Eichlseder[113] concluded that long-term stimulant treatment is safe in children.

Thus, it seems likely that the incidence and severity of side effects and the overall safety of stimulants are similar in children with narcolepsy and children with attention-deficit hyperactivity disorder at comparable dosing levels. Typical initial doses of stimulants for attention-deficit hyperactivity disorder are methylphenidate 0.3 mg/kg, dextroamphetamine 0.15 mg/kg, or pemoline 37.5 mg, followed by dose titration to achieve optimal effects.[111] The safety in narcoleptic children of higher doses than those currently recommended for attention-deficit hyperactivity disorder (e.g., methylphenidate 60 mg/d) is unknown.

Use of Stimulants in Pregnancy

The risk of teratogenicity with commonly used stimulants is uncertain because well-controlled studies of stimulant use by pregnant women are unavailable. Based on limited evidence, the estimated risk associated with use during pregnancy is shown in Table 35–2. Given the uncertainties, the benefits for any given patient must be weighed carefully against the potential risks. For many patients, it may be advisable to reduce or discontinue stimulants during attempts at conception and for the duration of pregnancy. The efficacy of commonly used stimulants for treatment of narcolepsy during pregnancy is probably similar to efficacy at other times.

Stimulants in Sustained Military Operations

Amphetamines and other stimulants temporarily reduce many of the effects of sleep loss on attention and

Table 35–2. RISKS IN PREGNANCY OF DRUGS USED TO TREAT NARCOLEPSY

Methylphenidate—not categorized*	Dextroamphetamine—pregnancy category C rating	Mazindol—pregnancy category C rating
Modafinil—pregnancy category C rating	Methamphetamine—pregnancy category C rating	Pemoline—pregnancy category B rating

The FDA has established five categories (A, B, C, D, and X) to indicate a drug's potential for causing teratogenicity.[130, 131] Pregnancy category A means controlled studies have shown no risk to the human fetus in the first trimester and the possibility of fetal harm appears remote; B—animal studies indicate no fetal risk and there are no controlled studies in humans; C—animal studies have shown teratogenic or embryocidal effects and there are no controlled studies in humans; D—there is evidence of risk to human fetuses but benefits may make risks acceptable; X—studies in animals or humans have demonstrated fetal abnormalities and the risks outweigh any possible benefit. This table presents the most conservative ratings given by either the manufacturer's package insert or Briggs et al.[131] for methylphenidate, dextroamphetamine, methamphetamine, mazindol, and pemoline. Thus, there appear to be no well-controlled studies of stimulant use on pregnant women. While the efficacy of stimulants for the treatment of narcolepsy during pregnancy is probably similar to efficacy at other times, commonly used stimulants vary with respect to their pregnancy rating category, with most falling in category C. Pemoline is the only commonly used stimulant with a category B rating. Because the potential for teratogenicity is unknown, the benefits for any given patient must be weighed carefully against the potential risks. For many patients, it may be advisable to reduce or discontinue stimulants during attempts at conception and for the duration of pregnancy.

*Methylphenidate is not categorized but has the following warning in the U.S. product labeling under "Usage in Pregnancy": "Adequate animal reproduction studies to establish safe use of Ritalin during pregnancy have not been conducted. Therefore, until more information is available, Ritalin should not be prescribed for women of childbearing age, unless, in the opinion of the physician, the potential benefits outweigh the possible risks."

performance.[114] In military operations during World War II, pilots and other members of the allied forces were issued dextroamphetamine to reduce the effects of fatigue during sustained operations. During the 1991 Persian Gulf War, United Nations forces were issued modafinil for the same purpose (S. Lubin, personal communication, 1992). Although there are few controlled studies, in a study of U.S. Army helicopter pilots engaged in flight simulation after prolonged periods of wakefulness, dextroamphetamine 10 mg, in comparison with placebo, improved aviator simulator control on descents and turns. Performance was facilitated most noticeably after 22, 26, and 34 h of continuous wakefulness. Alertness was sustained significantly by dextroamphetamine—there was reduced slow-wave electroencephalographic (EEG) activity and improved rating of vigor and fatigue. No adverse behavioral or physiological effects were observed.[115, 116]

Use of Stimulants for Sleepiness Due to Insufficient Sleep: Is There a Role?

Insufficient sleep, beyond the military situation, arises in many circumstances. Common among these circumstances are jet lag, shift work, and the residual sleepiness of patients treated for sleep apnea. Under such circumstances and in the interest of patient or public safety, the physician may consider prescribing a stimulant to be used on a limited basis and with periodic supervision. This use of stimulants is problematic for many physicians and active debate continues. The key points of this debate center on the relative importance of the potential for abuse and dependency vs. the benefits of pharmacologically assisted alertness. The demand for stimulants in these circumstances is likely to increase as our society continues to depend upon 24-h operations in the manufacturing, transportation, and service industries.

Establishing the Proper Dose

The physician should consider the following points in establishing the proper dose of a stimulant drug and structuring a management plan.

1. Education. Clarify the goals of treatment, side effects, risks, and benefits. This process will involve discussions with the patient and, perhaps, the patient's spouse or companions. Normal alertness throughout the day may not be attainable in many patients, because of drug side effects, work schedules, and other idiosyncratic circumstances.
2. Begin with a low to moderate dose of a stimulant or wake-promoting agent and match the drug and dosage to the patient. Initially, this process should be guided by regular (e.g., weekly) contact with the patient. For patients starting on stimulants, evaluate after 3 to 4 weeks, then again in 2 to 3 months. Once the dose is stable, see the patient every 6 to 12 months. Under circumstances where the patient's safety or the safety of others depends on adequate control of excessive somnolence, laboratory confirmation of therapeutic efficacy with the MSLT or MWT is helpful. Such laboratory documentation may not be possible in certain healthcare settings.
3. Emphasize sleep hygiene; consider naps.
4. Adjust dosages based on clinical information. Narcolepsy and idiopathic hypersomnia are generally stable conditions that do not progressively worsen. For a patient who has been on a stable dose for some time (years) and now appears to require more, consider other possible causes of increased sleepiness such as the following:
   A. Interval development of sleep apnea (a common scenario in our experience).
   B. Change in schedule (such as a new work shift causing less sleep at night).
   C. Change in life situation (such as a new baby causing sleep disruption) or a new job that requires greater vigilance.
   D. Stress, anxiety, depression.
   E. Unrealistic expectations.
   Thus, evaluation should include a detailed history covering the above possibilities as well as a review of the sleep schedule and napping. If dose increases are necessary, they should be made systematically with regular patient contacts.
5. Recommend counseling and long-term support.

Available evidence suggests that patients tend to take less, not more, of their prescribed stimulant.[117] While the reasons for such noncompliance are undoubtedly complex and incompletely understood, it is important that the patient understand the long-term nature of his or her condition and the benefits that can be obtained with regular use of stimulant medications.

Discontinuation of Stimulant Medication

There are no systematic studies of the advantages and disadvantages of abrupt discontinuation vs. gradual dose reduction before discontinuation. However, practitioners have found few problems with abrupt discontinuation for patients taking a stimulant drug within the dose ranges discussed in this chapter. The consequences of abrupt discontinuation include a return of symptoms of excessive sleepiness and lethargy. Some patients who can remember the severity of their symptoms prior to pharmacotherapy with stimulants may report that, for some days after discontinuation, sleepiness was more profound than before stimulant therapy began. Marked hypotension or hypotensive sequelae such as fainting have not been reported with abrupt discontinuation of stimulant therapy. However, in patients taking higher doses of a stimulant (e.g., over 100 mg dextroamphetamine per day), it is wise, before abrupt discontinuation, to successively reduce the daily dose by half every 3 to 7 days until reaching the highest dose range recommended by the manufacturer.

Changing Stimulant Drugs

For most patients, abrupt replacement of one stimulant with another should present few problems. However, as discussed above, for patients taking high doses of stimulant medications, a gradual weaning period may be called for.

In cases in which a change in medications is prompted by specific side effects attributed to the current medication or in cases in which there is concern about potential side effects of a new medication, arranging for a drug-free period of 3 to 7 days can help clarify which effects are attributable to which drug. However, the literature does not suggest that one CNS stimulant (e.g., amphetamine) is more likely to produce side effects than another (e.g., methylphenidate). So, for example, if concern about cardiac side effects is a major source of anxiety, then cardiac evaluation is indicated for reassurance. If a patient is having palpitations or other cardiac symptoms, the dose should be reduced and a cardiac evaluation obtained.

Combining Stimulants

There are no systematic studies of treatment with more than one stimulant at a time. Some patients report satisfactory management with combinations such as methylphenidate and pemoline, using pemoline for long-lasting effects and small doses of methylphenidate as needed. However, the most common initial approach is to develop a single stimulant medication regimen.

Combining Antidepressants With Stimulants

In patients who require treatment for cataplexy, as well as treatment for excessive sleepiness, it is usually best to select a nonsedating antidepressant agent as an anticataplectic agent (e.g., protriptyline or fluoxetine). Both the stimulant and the anticataplectic drug may be taken in the morning with possible additional dosing of a stimulant throughout the day. It is rarely necessary to divide the dose of any antidepressant when it is used as an anticataplectic agent. If a sedating antidepressant is selected (e.g., imipramine or amitriptyline), this drug should be taken at bedtime.

Diversity of Current Practices

Stimulants, however prescribed, represent only part of a comprehensive therapeutic approach to excessive somnolence. Sound sleep hygiene, attention to other substances and drugs that may disrupt the sleep-wake cycle, and periodic reassessment of symptom severity and of the need for and adequacy of treatment modalities are other important aspects of management.

Current practices in the use of stimulants vary considerably. Although the only stimulants approved through 1997 by the FDA for use in narcolepsy are dextroamphetamine and methylphenidate at dosages of 5 to 60 mg/d, substantial numbers of narcoleptic patients take methylphenidate or dextroamphetamine at doses above 60 mg or take other medications, particularly pemoline and methamphetamine.[118] Mazindol, modafinil (approved in 1999 in the United States for the treatment of narcolepsy), and protriptyline are also used. The criteria used to determine stimulant dose, the maximum acceptable dose, the frequency and clinical significance of tolerance, and the need for drug holidays are areas of debate.

Many clinicians recommend methylphenidate as the preferred initial treatment for daytime sleepiness.[8, 60, 119] Methylphenidate is marketed for the indications of attention-deficit disorders and narcolepsy and comes in 5, 10, and 20 mg tablets as well as a 20 mg sustained release formulation. Peak bioavailability of methylphenidate is reached in about 2 h and in about 4 h for the sustained release formulation. Several authorities recommend doses of methylphenidate, as well as amphetamines, that are consistent with the manufacturers' package inserts (Table 35–3), often along with daytime naps[46, 56, 119–122] and avoidance of evening doses of stimulants.[8, 46] A number of clinicians prescribe stimulants in combination, such as a single dose of pemoline in the morning plus small doses of methylphenidate as needed throughout the day.[46] Some authorities add the proviso that doses of methylphenidate 60 mg/d or dextroamphetamine 60 mg/d should usually not be exceeded,[119] whereas others recommend methylphenidate doses of up to 80 mg/d or more (see Table 35–3). Methamphetamine is recommended by some authori-

Table 35–3. PUBLISHED RECOMMENDATIONS OF STIMULANT DOSAGES FOR TREATMENT OF NARCOLEPSY

Medication	Daily Dose Range (mg)	References
Methylphenidate (Ritalin)	Up to 60	46, 48, 56, 97–100, 119–122, 127, 128
Methylphenidate (Ritalin)	Up to 80	8, 16, 25, 61, 101, 122, 123, 128, 129
	Occasional use of up to 100–300	
	Up to 40–60 in children	
Dextroamphetamine (Adderall, Biphetamine)	Up to 60	
Methamphetamine (Desoxyn)	5–15	25, 36, 123
	25–100	
Pemoline (Cylert)	100	46
Mazindol (Mazanor, Sanorex)	2–8	56
Levo-amphetamine (not available in the United States)	20–60	97
Fencamfamin (Reactivan) (not available in the United States)	20–30	56
Modafinil (Provigil, Modiodal, Alertec)	200–400	42, 43, 125

ties as first-line treatment (see Table 35–3), by others as an alternative for patients who do not respond to methylphenidate,[17, 25] and by still others as a last resort.[46, 101]

Another factor that probably influences clinical practice is whether or not a stimulant drug has been placed on Schedule II by the Drug Enforcement Agency. In 10 of the most populous states of the United States, the dispensation of Schedule II drugs requires a special triplicate prescription and throughout the United States prescription amounts and refills of Schedule II drugs are limited. Thus, regardless of their efficacy, non-Schedule II drugs such as pemoline and mazindol may be preferentially prescribed.

Modafinil, introduced to the world market in 1995 for the indication of narcolepsy and idiopathic hypersomnia, comes in 100 mg and 200 mg tablets and appears to reach peak bioavailability in about 2 h. The typical dosage for narcolepsy is 200 to 400 mg in a single morning dose. Physicians often recommend taking modafinil in divided doses with an early-morning and a midafternoon administration. Recommendation for medications are summarized in Table 35–3.

Although many authorities recommend temporary withdrawal of medications or reduction of dose for 1 to 28 d if tolerance develops, that is, drug holidays,[56, 100, 120, 121] this recommendation appears to be based on clinical experience. There are no published studies demonstrating the efficacy of drug holidays.

The criteria for determining drug dose vary. Many authorities recommend a goal of obtaining maximal alertness at selected times of the day, for example, during work or school hours and while driving, and using scheduled naps to help maintain alertness. Others recommend a goal of maximal or "normal" alertness throughout conventional waking hours. Unfortunately, available data indicate that although daytime sleep episodes can be reduced in most, they cannot be completely abolished in all patients.

CONCLUSIONS

The potentially disabling symptom of sleepiness occurs in narcolepsy, idiopathic CNS hypersomnia, and sleep deprivation. Sleepiness may be treated with psychomotor stimulants. Such drugs produce behavioral activation and increased wakefulness, enhanced alertness, decreased sense of fatigue, elevations of mood, and increased performance. Treatment of excessive sleepiness associated with narcolepsy or idiopathic hypersomnia with psychomotor stimulants is indicated when sustained alertness is necessary for individual or public safety. Stimulant medications improve daytime alertness in 65 to 85% of narcoleptic patients; in 15 to 35%, improvement of alertness is minimal because of lack of efficacy, side effects, or other factors. Tolerance to stimulants is variable depending on the effect observed, dose, and other factors. Side effects (headaches, nervousness, anxiety, palpitations, and insomnia) are common, dose-related, and may require discontinuation of therapy. There is no evidence that stimulant use in young narcoleptic patients causes growth failure or cognitive dysfunction. As the risk for teratogenicity associated with stimulant use is uncertain, use of these drugs generally should be avoided in pregnancy unless the benefits associated with their use are likely to outweigh the risks. There is no evidence that narcoleptic patients are more prone to complications associated with stimulant use than other individuals. Severe psychiatric complications are rare with amphetamine use in narcolepsy, but they are more likely to occur with high doses and in patients with coexisting psychiatric illness. Although the safety and added efficacy of doses higher than those recommended by the manufacturers of stimulant drugs are not well established with controlled clinical trials, some patients obtain added benefit with higher doses without ill effects. When cataplexy and related symptoms are clinical problems, concomitant treatment is often implemented with a REM sleep–suppressing antidepressant drug. There are no data from controlled studies to indicate that daytime naps and drug holidays reduce tolerance to, or increase the efficacy of, stimulants.

Acknowledgments

This chapter is based in part on a review of the literature done by a task force (see reference 41).

References

1. Weiner N. Norepinephrine, epinephrine, and the sympathomimetic amines. In: Gilman AG, Goodman LS, Rall TW, et al, eds. Pharmacological Basis of Therapeutics. New York, NY: Macmillan; 1985:145–180.
2. Zaimis E. Vasopressor drugs and catecholamines. Anesthesiology. 1968;29:732–762.
3. Haddad LM. 1978: Cocaine in perspective. J Am Coll Emers Physicians 1979;8:374–376.
4. Angrist B, Sudilovsky A. Central nervous system stimulants: Historical aspects and clinical effects. In: Iversen LL, Iversen SD, Snyder SH, eds. Handbook of Psychopharmacology. Vol 11. New York: Plenum; 1976:99–165.
5. Byck R. Cocaine Papers by Sigmund Freud. New York, NY: Stonehill; 1974.
6. Doyle JB, Daniels LE. Symptomatic treatment for narcolepsy. JAMA. 1931;96:1370–1372.
7. Janota O. Symptomatische Behandlung der pathologischen Schlafsucht, besonders der Narkolepsie. Med Klin. 1931;27:278–281.
8. Yoss RE, Daly DD. Treatment of narcolepsy with Ritalin. Neurology. 1959;9:171–173.
9. Prinzmetal M, Bloomberg W. Use of benzedrine for the treatment of narcolepsy. JAMA. 1935;105:2051–2054.
10. Prinzmetal M, Alles GA. The central nervous system stimulant effects of dextro-amphetamine sulphate. Am J Med Sci. 1940;200:665–673.
11. Eaton LM. Treatment of narcolepsy with desoxyephedrine hydrochloride. Proc Staff Meet Mayo Clin. 1943;7:262–264.
12. Brock S, Wiesel B. The narcoleptic-cataplectic syndrome—and excessive and dissociated reaction of the sleep mechanism—accompanying mental states. J Nerv Ment Dis. 1941;94:700–712.
13. Shapiro MJ. Benzedrine in the treatment of narcolepsy. Minn Med. 1937;1:28–31.
14. Young D, Scoville WB. Paranoid psychosis in narcolepsy and the possible danger of benzedrine treatment. Med Clin North Am. 1938;22:637–646.
15. Sours JA. Narcolepsy and other disturbances in the sleep waking rhythm: a study of 115 cases with review of the literature. J Nerv Ment Dis. 1963;137:525–542.
16. Yoss RE, Daly DD. Treatment of narcolepsy with Ritalin. Neurology. 1959;9:171–173.
17. Daly D, Yoss R. Narcolepsy. In: Magnus O, Lorentz de Haas A, eds. The Epilepsies. Amsterdam, Netherlands: North Holland; 1974:836–852. Handbook of Clinical Neurology; Vol 15.
18. International Classification of Sleep Disorders, Revised: Diagnostic and Coding Manual. Rochester, Minn: American Sleep Disorders Association; 1997.
19. Guilleminault C. Sleeping and Waking Disorders. Indications and Techniques. Menlo Park, Calif: Addison-Wesley; 1982.
20. Sleep Disorders Classification Committee. Association of Sleep Disorders Centers. Diagnostic Classification of Sleep and Arousal Disorders. Sleep. 1979;2:1–137.
21. Coleman RM, Roffwarg HP, Kennedy SJ, et al. Sleep-wake disorders based on a polysomnographic diagnosis. A national cooperative study. JAMA. 1982;247:997–1003.
22. Coleman RM. Diagnosis, treatment, and follow-up of about 8,000 sleep/wake disorder patients. In: Guilleminault C, Lugaresi E, eds. Sleep/Wake Disorders: Natural History, Epidemiology, and Long-Term Evolution. New York, NY: Raven Press; 1983:87–98.
23. Mitler MM, Erman M, Hajdukovic R. The treatment of excessive somnolence with stimulant drugs. Sleep. 1993;16:203–206.
24. Lowenstein O, Loewenfeld I. Eletronic pupillography—a new instrument and some clinical applications. Arch Opthalmol. 1958;59:352–363.
25. Yoss RE. Treatment of narcolepsy. Mod Treatment. 1969;6:1263–1274.
26. Yoss RE, Moyer NJ, Ogle KN. The pupillogram and narcolepsy. A method to measure decreased levels of wakefulness. Neurol. 1969;19:921–928.
27. Richardson GS, Carskadon MA, Flagg W, et al. Excessive daytime sleepiness in man: multiple sleep latency measurement in narcoleptic and control subjects. Electroencephalogr Clin Neurophysiol. 1978;45:621–627.
28. Mitler MM, Gujavarty KS, Browman CP. Maintenance of wakefulness test: a polysomnographic technique for evaluation treatment efficacy in patients with excessive somnolence. Electroencephalogr Clin Neurophysiol. 1982;53:658–661.
29. Thorpy MJ. Report from the American Sleep Disorders Association. The clinical use of the multiple sleep latency test. Sleep. 1992;15:268–276.
30. Mitler MM, Hajdukovic R, Erman M, et al. Narcolepsy. J Clin Neurophysiol. 1990;7:93–118.
31. Scrima L, Hartman PG, Johnson FH, et al. Effects of gamma-hydroxybutyrate (GHB) on sleep of narcolepsy patients: a double blind study. Sleep. 1990;13:479–490.
32. Fry JM, Pressman MR, DiPhillipo MA, et al. Treatment of narcolepsy with codeine. Sleep. 1986;9:269–274.
33. Scrima L, Hartman PG, Johnson FH, et al. Effects of gamma-hydroxybutyrate (GHB) on multiple sleep latency test (MSLT) in narcolepsy patients: a long term study. Sleep Res. 1990;19:288.
34. Godbout R, Poirier G, Montplaisir J. New treatments for narcolepsy (viloxazine). In: Diego S, ed. Narcolepsy 3rd International Symposium. Wilmington, DE: ICI Pharma; 1988:79–81.
35. Lammers GJ, Arends J, Declerk AC, et al. Ritanserin, a 5-HT2 receptor blocker, as add-on treatment in narcolepsy. Sleep. 1991;14:130–132.
36. Mitler MM, Hajdukovic R, Erman MK. Treatment of narcolepsy with methamphetamine. Sleep. 1993;16:306–317.
37. Mitler MM, Hajdukovic R. Relative efficacy of drugs for the treatment of sleepiness in narcolepsy. Sleep. 1991;14:218–220.
38. Guilleminault C, Pelayo R. Idiopathic central nervous system hypersomnia. In: Kryger MH, Roth T, Dement WC, eds. Principles and Practice of Sleep Medicine. Philadephia, Pa: WB Saunders; 2000.
39. Bassetti C, Aldrich MS. Idiopathic hypersomnia. A series of 42 patients. Brain. 1997;120:1423–1435.
40. Gualtieri CT, Wargin W, Kanoy R, et al. Clinical studies of methylphenidate serum levels in children and adults. J Am Acad Child Psychiatry. 1982;21:19–26.
41. Mitler MM, Aldrich MS, Koob GF, et al. Narcolepsy and its treatment with stimulants. ASDA standards of practice. Sleep. 1994;17:352–371.
42. Broughton RJ, Fleming JA, George CF, et al. Randomized, double-blind, placebo-controlled crossover trial of modafinil in the treatment of excessive daytime sleepiness in narcolepsy. Neurology. 1997;49:444–451.
43. US Modafinil in Narcolepsy Multicenter Study Group. Randomized trial of modafinil for the treatment of pathological somnolence in narcolepsy. Ann Neurol. 1998;43:88–97.
44. Pigeau R, Naitoh P, Buguet A, et al. Modafinil, d-amphetamine and placebo during 64 hours of sustained mental work, I: effects on mood, fatigue, cognitive performance and body temperature. J Sleep Res. 1995;4:212–228.
45. Parkes JD, Baraitser M, Marsden CD, et al. Natural history, symptoms and treatment of the narcoleptic syndrome. Acta Neurol Scand. 1975;52:337–353.
46. Honda Y. Clinical features of narcolepsy. In: Honda T, Juji T, eds. HLA in Narcolepsy. Berlin, Germany: Springer-Verlag; 1988:24–57.
47. Shindler J, Schachter M, Brincat S, et al. Amphetamine, mazindol and fencamfamin in narcolepsy. Br Med J. 1985;290:1167–1170.
48. Regestein QR, Reich P, Mufson MJ. Narcolepsy: an initial clinical approach. J Clin Psychiatry. 1983;44:166–172.
49. Simpson LL. The effects of behavioral stimulant doses of amphetamine on blood pressure. Arch Gen Psychiatry. 1976;33:691–695.
50. Roselaar SE, Langdon N, Lock CB, et al. Selegiline in narcolepsy. Sleep. 1987;10:491–495.
51. Tolman KG, Freston JW, Berenson MM, et al. Hepatotoxicity due to pemoline. Report of two cases. Digestion. 1973;9:532–539.
52. Elitsur Y. Pemoline (Cylert)-induced hepatotoxicity [letter]. J Pediatr Gastroent Nutr. 1990;11:143.
53. Pratt DS, Dubois RS. Hepatotoxicity due to pemoline (Cylert): a report of two cases. J Pediatr Gastroent Nutr. 1990;10:239–241.
54. Jaffe SL. Pemoline and liver function [letter]. J Am Acad Child Adolesc Psychiatry. 1989;28:457–458.

55. Nehra A, Mullick F, Ishak KG, et al. Pemoline-associated hepatic injury. Gastroenterology. 1990;99:1517–1519.

56. Parkes JD. Sleep and Its Disorders. Philadelphia, PA: WB Saunders; 1985.

57. Guilleminault C, Carskadon M, Dement WC. On the treatment of rapid eye movement narcolepsy. Arch Neurol. 1974;30:90–93.

58. Akimoto H, Honda Y, Takahashi Y. Pharmacotherapy in narcolepsy. Dis Nerv Syst. 1960;21:704–706.

59. Passouant P, Billiard M. Evolution of narcolepsy with age. In: Guilleminault C, Dement WC, Passouant P, eds. Narcolepsy. New York, NY: Spectrum; 1976:179–196.

60. Billiard M. Narcolepsy. Clinical features and aetiology. Ann Clin Res. 1985;17:220–226.

61. Yoss RE, Daly DD. Narcolepsy. Med Clin North Am. 1960;44:953–968.

62. Cadieux RJ, Kales JD, Kales A, et al. Pharmacologic and psychotherapeutic issues in coexistent paranoid schizophrenia and narcolepsy: a case report. J Clin Psychiatry. 1985;46:191–193.

63. Leong GB, Shaner AL, Silva JA. Narcolepsy, paranoid psychosis and analeptic abuse. Psychiatr J Univ Ottawa. 1989;14:481–483.

64. Pfefferbaum A, Berger PA. Narcolepsy, paranoid psychosis, and tardive dyskinesia: a pharmacological dilemma. J Nerv Ment Dis. 1977;164:293–297.

65. Schrader G, Hicks EP. Narcolepsy, paranoid psychosis, major depression and tardive dyskinesia. J Nerv Ment Dis. 1984;172:439–441.

66. Smith HJ, Roche AH, Jausch MF, et al. Cardiomyopathy associated with amphetamine administration. Am Heart J. 1976;91:792–797.

67. Beyer KL, Bickel JT, Butt JH. Ischemic colitis associated with amphetamine use. J Clin Gastroenterol. 1991;13:198–201.

68. Steiner E, Villen T, Halberg M, et al. Amphetamine secretion in breast milk. Eur J Clin Pharmacol. 1984;27:123–124.

69. Griffith J, Oates JA, Cavanaugh JH. Paranoid episodes induced by drug. JAMA. 1968;205:39.

70. Rylander G. Stereotype behaviour in man following amphetamine abuse. In: De SB, Baker C, eds. The Correlation of Adverse Effects in Man With Observations in Animals. Amsterdam, Netherlands: Excerpta Medica; 1971:28–31.

71. Randrup A, Munkvad I. Biochemical, anatomical and psychological investigations of stereotyped behavior induced by amphetamines. In: Costa E, Garattini S, eds. Amphetamines and Related Compounds. New York, NY: Raven Press; 1970:695–713.

72. Ellinwood EH Jr, Sudilovsky A, Nelson LM. Evolving behavior in the clinical and experimental amphetamine (model) psychosis. Am J Psychiatry. 1973;130:1088–1093.

73. Randrup A, Munkvad I. Stereotyped activities produced by amphetamine in several animal species and man. Psychopharmacologia. 1967;11:300–310.

74. Lyon M, Robbins TW. The action of central nervous system stimulant drugs: A general theory concerning amphetamine effects. In: Essman W, Valzelli L, eds. Current Developments in Psychopharmacology. Vol 2. New York, NY: Spectrum; 1975:79–163.

75. Segal DS. Behavioral characterization of d- and l-amphetamine: neurochemical implications. Science. 1975;190:475–477.

76. Rapoport JL, Buchsbaum MS, Weingartner H, et al. Dextroamphetamine, its cognitive and behavioral effects in normal and hyperactive boys and men. Arch Gen Psychiatry. 1980;37:933–943.

77. Robbins TW, Sahakian BJ. "Paradoxical" effects of psychomotor stimulant drugs in hyperactive children from the standpoint of behavioural pharmacology. Neuropharmacology. 1979; 18:931–950.

78. Alldredge BK, Lowenstein DH, Simon RP. Seizures associated with recreational drug abuse. Neurology. 1989;39:1037–1039.

79. Conci F, D'Angelo V, Tampieri D, et al. Intracerebral hemorrhage and angiographic beading following amphetamine abuse. Ital J Neurol Sci. 1988;9:77–81.

80. Harrington H, Heller HA, Dawson D, et al. Intracerebral hemorrhage and oral amphetamine. Arch Neurol. 1983;40:503–507.

81. Olsen ER. Intracranial hemorrhage and amphetamine usage. Review of the effects of amphetamines on the central nervous system. Angiology. 1977;28:464–471.

82. Rothrock JF, Rubenstein R, Lyden PD. Ischemic stroke associated with methamphetamine inhalation. Neurology. 1988; 38:589–592.

83. Margolis MT, Newton TH. Methamphetamine ("speed") arteritis. Neuroradiology. 1971;2:179–182.

84. Kaku DA, Lowenstein DH. Emergence of recreational drug abuse as a major risk factor for stroke in young adults. Ann Intern Med. 1991;113:821–827.

85. Grant I, Mohns L. Chronic cerebral effects of alcohol and drug abuse. Int J Addict. 1975;10:883–920.

86. Michel R, Adams AP. Acute amphetamine abuse. Problems during general anaesthesia for neurosurgery. Anaesthesia. 1979;34:1016–1019.

87. O'Neill ME, Arnolda LF, Coles DM, et al. Acute amphetamine cardiomyopathy in a drug addict. Clin Cardiol. 1983;6:189–191.

88. Packe GE, Garton MJ, Jennings K. Acute myocardial infarction caused by intravenous amphetamine abuse. Br Heart J. 1990;64:23–24.

89. Stafford CR, Bogdanoff BM, Green L, et al. Mononeuropathy multiplex as a complication of amphetamine angiitis. Neurology. 1975;25:570–572.

90. Foley RJ, Kapatkin K, Verani R, et al. Amphetamine-induced acute renal failure. South Med J. 1984;77:258–260.

91. Rifkin SI. Amphetamine-induced angiitis leading to renal failure. South Med J. 1977;70:108–109.

92. Terada Y, Shinohara S, Matui N, et al. Amphetamine-induced myoglobinuric acute renal failure. Jpn J Med. 1988;27:305–308.

93. Bruhn P, Maage N. Intellectual and neuropsychological functions in young men with heavy and long-term patterns of drug abuse. Am J Psychiatry. 1975;132–397–401.

94. Alvarez B, Dahlitz M, Grimshaw J, et al. Mazindol in long-term treatment of narcolepsy. Lancet. 1991;337:1293–1294.

95. Honda Y, Hishikawa Y, Takahashi Y. Long-term treatment of narcolepsy with Ritalin (methylphenidate). Curr Ther Res. 1979;25:288–298.

96. Bastuji H, Jouvet M. Successful treatment of idiopathic hypersomnia and narcolepsy with modafinil. Prog Neuropsychopharmacol Biol Psychiatry. 1988;12:695–700.

97. Parkes JD, Fenton GW. Levo(-)amphetamine and dextro(+)amphetamine in the treatment of narcolepsy. J Neurol Neurosurg Psychiatry. 1973;36:1076–1081.

98. Zarcone VP. Narcolepsy. N Engl J Med. 1973;288:1156–1166.

99. Dement WC, Carskadon MA, Guilleminault C, et al. Narcolepsy. Diagnosis and treatment. Prim Care. 1976;3:609–623.

100. Thorpy MJ, Goswami M. Treatment of narcolepsy. In: Thorpy MJ, ed. Handbook of Sleep Disorders. New York, NY: Marcel Dekker; 1990:235–258.

101. Soldatos CR, Kales A, Cadieux RJ. Treatment of sleep disorders, II: narcolepsy. In: Rational Drug Therapy. Bethesda, Md: American Society for Pharmacology and Experimental Therapeutics, 1983;17:1–7.

102. Croche AF, Lipman RS, Overall JE, et al. The effects of stimulant medication on the growth of hyperkinetic children. Pediatrics. 1979;63:847–850.

103. Friedmann N, Thomas J, Carr R, et al. Effect on growth in pemoline-treated children with attention deficit disorder. Am J Dis Child. 1981;135:329–332.

104. Satterfield JH, Cantwell DP, Schell A, et al. Growth of hyperactive children treated with methylphenidate. Arch Gen Psychiatry. 1979;36:212–217.

105. Mattes JA, Gittelman R. Growth of hyperactive children on maintenance regimen of methylphenidate. Arch Gen Psychiatry. 1983;40:317–321.

106. Golinko BE. Side effects of dextroamphetamine and methylphenidate in hyperactive children—a brief review. Prog Neuropsychopharmacol Biol Psychiatry. 1984;8:1–8.

107. Klein RG, Landa B, Mattes JA, et al. Methylphenidate and growth in hyperactive children. A controlled withdrawal study. Arch Gen Psychiatry. 1988;45:1127–1130.

108. Safer DJ, Allen RP, Barr E. Growth rebound after termination of stimulant drugs. J Pediatr. 1975;86:113–116.

109. Vincent J, Varley CK, Leger P. Effects of methylphenidate on early adolescent growth. Am J Psychiatry. 1990;147:501–502.

110. Klein RG, Mannuzza S. Hyperactive boys almost grown up, III: methylphenidate effects on ultimate height. Arch Gen Psychiatry. 1988;45:1131–1134.

111. Stevenson RD, Wolraich ML. Stimulant medication therapy in the treatment of children with attention deficit hyperactivity disorder. Pediatr Clin North Am. 1989;36:1183–1197.

112. Weiss G, Kruger E, Danielson U, et al. Effects of long-term treatment of hyperactive children with methylphenidate. Can Med Assoc J. 1975;112:159–165.

113. Eichlseder W. Ten years experience with 1,000 hyperactive children in a private practice. Pediatrics. 1985;76:176–184.

114. Weiner N. Norepinephrine, epinephrine, and the sympathomimetic amines. In: Gilman AG, Goodman LS, Gilman A, eds. Goodman and Gilman's The Pharmacological Basis of Therapeutics. New York, NY: Macmillan; 1980:138–175.

115. Caldwell JA, Caldwell JL, Crowley JS, et al. Sustaining helicopter pilot performance with Dexedrine during periods of sleep deprivation. Aviat Space Environ Med. 1995;66:930–937.

116. Caldwell JA Jr. Effects of operationally effective doses of dextroamphetamine on heart rates and blood pressures of army aviators. Mil Med. 1996;161:673–678.

117. Rogers AE, Aldrich MS, Berrios AM, et al. Compliance with stimulant medications in patients with narcolepsy. Sleep. 1997;20:28–33.

118. American Narcolepsy Association. Medication survey results. The Eye Opener. January 1992;1–3.

119. Kales A, Vela-Bueno A, Kales JD. Sleep disorders: sleep apnea and narcolepsy. Ann Intern Med. 1987;106:434–443.

120. Aldrich MS. Narcolepsy. Engl J Med. 1990;323:389–394.

121. Mitler MM, Nelson S, Hajdukovic R. Narcolepsy. Diagnosis, treatment, and management. Psychiatr Clin North Am. 1987;10:593–606.

122. Richardson JW, Fredrickson PA, Lin S-C. Narcolepsy update. Mayo Clin Proc. 1990;65:991–998.

123. Honda Y, Akimoto H, Takahashi Y. Pharmacotherapy in narcolepsy. Dis Nerv Sys. 1960;21:1–3.

124. Laffont F, Cathala HP, Kohler F. Effect of modafinil on narcolepsy and idiopathic hypersomnia. Sleep Res. 1987;16:377.

125. US Modafinil in Narcolepsy Multicenter Study Group. Modafinil administration and withdrawal in narcolepsy patients with excessive daytime somnolence. Neurology. In press.

126. Saletu B, Frey R, Krupka M, et al. Differential effects of a new central adrenergic agonist modafinil and d-amphetamine on sleep and early morning behavior in elderlies. Arzneimittelforschung. 1989;39:1268–1273.

127. Dahl RE. The pharmacologic treatment of sleep disorders. Psychiatr Clin North Am. 1992;15:161–178.

128. Yoss RE, Daly DD. On the treatment of narcolepsy. Med Clin North Am. 1968;52:781–787.

129. Yoss RE, Daly DD. Narcolepsy in children. Pediatrics. 1960;25:1025–1033.

130. U.S. Food and Drug Administration. Pregnancy categories for prescription drugs. FDA Drug Bull. 1982;12:24–25.

131. Briggs GG, Freeman RK, Yaffe SJ. Drugs in Pregnancy and Lactation: A Reference Guide to Fetal and Neonatal Risk. Baltimore, Md: Williams & Wilkins; 1990.

36

Drugs That Disturb Sleep and Wakefulness

Paula K. Schweitzer

Numerous prescription drugs act within the central nervous system (CNS) and have the potential to affect sleep or daytime functioning. Insomnia, sleepiness, sedation, and fatigue are some of the listed side effects of many prescription and over-the-counter medications. Although such side effects can be problematic, they may not occur in all patients, their severity can vary considerably, and in some situations failure to provide treatment may be more disruptive of sleep or wakefulness than these side effects. In some instances, the desired action of a drug (e.g., sedation to treat insomnia or stimulation to treat sleepiness) becomes an undesirable action when the effect carries over into daytime or nighttime hours, respectively. In other cases, the desired action of a drug may be produced by effects at specific receptor sites and undesired actions occur because of concomitant effects at other receptor sites (e.g., tricyclic antidepressants, which have effects on 5-hydroxytryptamine [5-HT], norepinephrine, and dopamine, as well as effects on histamine and acetylcholine). In addition, undesired actions (e.g., unwanted sedation) may be the result of a discontinuation or withdrawal effect (i.e., a reflection of declining plasma levels after a period of stimulation such as might occur with the use of caffeine). Thus, understanding the mechanisms of action as well as the pharmacokinetics of a drug can help determine when a desired action might become an undesired action or when desired actions may be accompanied by undesirable actions. A review of the pharmacology of all drugs discussed is beyond the scope of this chapter, but limited information is presented when it adds to an understanding of the objective and subjective clinical data. References are provided for more extensive pharmacological review.

This chapter reviews commonly used drugs that disturb sleep or waking function. Hypnotics and stimulant medications (including caffeine), as well as drugs of abuse (including alcohol and nicotine), are discussed in Chapters 32 to 35. See also Chapter 69 for a review of drugs that may affect sleep-disordered breathing. The text is organized by drug type and subdivided by drug class and, in some cases, by the individual drug. When relevant, the effects of the disorder under treatment on sleep and waking function are briefly summarized. Presentation of the effects of drugs on sleep and wakefulness proceeds in the following order and is based on (1) subjective data, including clinical trials; (2) polysomnographic (PSG) data, with a focus on measures relevant to sleep disruption (sleep latency [SL], total sleep time [TST], frequency of awakenings), generally excluding changes in sleep stages; (3) objective data on sleepiness/alertness (primarily multiple sleep latency test [MSLT] data); and (4) objective performance data. In many cases, there are few PSG or MSLT data available. In general, sleep data are not presented if the drugs under review do not disturb sleep. Conversely, waking data typically are not presented for drugs that do not adversely affect alertness or performance. Drug withdrawal effects are not addressed.

A summary of the relevant literature and a comparison of the drugs are difficult because methodological differences abound and, often, research is limited. Among the most important methodological issues are composition of the subject population, presence or absence of placebo and/or positive control drugs, and dose, timing, and duration of treatment. Sleep itself, as well as drug pharmacokinetics, is influenced by age and sex; thus, it is difficult to generalize from studies that are often conducted on young healthy male individuals. Moreover, healthy individuals may respond differently than the population for whom treatment is intended. Furthermore, the treatment population may already have impaired sleep or poor cognitive performance. These factors make the issue of the use of positive controls and placebo controls quite important. Finally, it must be remembered that many patients take a variety of drugs in combination, which may affect one another. Little research has been conducted on drug combinations.

ANTIDEPRESSANT AGENTS

Antidepressant drugs can both improve and disturb sleep, as well as have effects on waking function. Evaluation of the effects of these drugs on sleep and wakefulness is complicated by the fact that many individuals with depression typically have disturbed sleep[1, 2] as well as daytime complaints such as fatigue, sleepiness, somatic complaints, and decreased cognitive and psychomotor functioning.[3-6] In addition, PSG evidence of disturbed nocturnal sleep does not always correlate with the subjective reports of patients and is not related to the efficacy of these drugs in the treatment of depression.

The first-generation antidepressants (tricyclics [TCAs] and monoamine oxidase inhibitors [MAOIs]) have multiple mechanisms of action, some of which are believed to mediate the antidepressant response (e.g., via effects on serotonin, norepinephrine, and/or dopamine) and others that mediate side effects such as sedation (via histamine blockade), dry mouth (via cholinergic blockade), orthostatic hypotension (alpha adrenergic receptors), and so on. During the past 10 to 15 years, a number of new antidepressants that are more receptor specific have been developed; these compounds include the selective serotonin reuptake inhibi-

tors (SSRIs) and other drugs such as trazodone (a 5-HT$_2$ antagonist), bupropion (dopamine and norepinephrine reuptake inhibitor), venlafaxine (5-HT and norepinephrine uptake inhibitor), and so on. For a review of their pharmacology and a comparison of their side effects, see references 7 through 12.

Although most of these drugs (Tables 36–1 and 36–2) decrease rapid eye movement (REM) sleep, and some of these drugs have effects on slow-wave sleep (SWS), only measures associated with sleep disruption are reported because the focus of this chapter is on clinically relevant disruption of sleep or wakefulness. The PSG effects of many of these drugs are reviewed in Obermeyer and Benca[13] and Buysse.[14] Performance effects are also reviewed in a number of articles.[14–18]

Table 36–1. EFFECTS OF ANTIDEPRESSANTS ON SLEEP AND WAKING BEHAVIOR (TRICYCLIC ANTIDEPRESSANTS, MONOAMINE OXIDASE INHIBITORS, AND SELECTIVE SEROTONIN REUPTAKE INHIBITORS)

Class and Drug	Primary Neurotransmitter or Receptor Activity	Subjective Data (Placebo-Corrected %)	PSG Data	Performance and MSLT Data
TCAs (Amitriptyline, doxepin, imipramine, trimipramine, clomipramine, desipramine, nortriptyline, protriptyline)	Norepinephrine, 5-hydroxytryptamine uptake inhibition; acetylcholine, H$_1$, H$_2$ blockade; inhibition of fast sodium channels	Improve sleep; may be sedating during the daytime but effects may lessen with time; doxepin, trimipramine, amitriptyline, and imipramine more sedating than others	Generally ↑ TST, ↓ W, but not universally	Most data on amitriptyline and imipramine: generally ↓ ↓ cognitive and psychomotor performance, at least with acute use in normal subjects, but some evidence that effects lessen with time; decrements may be more likely in elderly; effects on depressed patients are variable; no MSLT data
MAOIs (Classic: phenelzine, tranylcypromine Selective, reversible: moclobemide, brofaromine)	Inhibit MAO enzymes that metabolize norepinephrine, 5-hydroxytryptamine, dopamine	May ↑ daytime sleepiness because of ↓ TST, but generally not considered sedating during the day	Generally ↑ W, ↓ TST	Some evidence of improved performance; no MSLT data
SSRIs	5-Hydroxytryptamine uptake inhibition	May worsen sleep; few daytime complaints	Generally ↑ W, ↓ TST	No effect or mild ↑ performance; no MSLT data
Fluoxetine		Insomnia in 5–9%; daytime sedation in 5–6%, up to 21%	↓ TST, ↑ W, ↑ S1; ↑ SEMs	Generally no change or mild ↑ performance; no MSLT data
Paroxetine		Subjective ratings show improved sleep but in clinical trials insomnia reported in 8–14% and daytime sedation in ~2–21%	↑ W, ↓ TST, ↑ S1, ↑ SL	Mild ↑ performance; no MSLT data
Sertraline		Insomnia in ~7–16%; daytime sedation in ~7–13%	No published studies	Mild ↑ performance
Fluvoxamine		Ratings show no sedation; clinical trials show sedation in ~14–26% and insomnia in ~10–15%	↓ TST, ↑ W, ↑ S1; ↑ SL	No impairment in performance; no MSLT data
Citalopram		Insomnia	No change in TST, W	No impairment in performance; no MSLT data

H, histamine; MAO, monoamine oxidase; MAOI, monoamine oxidase inhibitor; MSLT, multiple sleep latency test; PSG, polysomnographic; S1, stage 1; SEM, slow eye movement; SL, sleep latency; SSRI, selective serotonin reuptake inhibitor; TCA, tricyclic antidepressant, TST, total sleep time; W, wake.

Table 36–2. EFFECTS OF ANTIDEPRESSANTS ON SLEEP AND WAKING BEHAVIOR (OTHER THAN TRICYLIC ANTIDEPRESSANTS, MONOAMINE OXIDASE INHIBITORS, AND SELECTIVE SEROTONIN REUPTAKE INHIBITORS)

Drug	Primary Neurotransmitter/ Receptor Activity	Subjective Data (Placebo-Corrected %)	PSG Data	Performance and MSLT Data
Trazodone	5-HT$_2$ blockade; 5-HT$_1$ blockade; alpha$_1$, H$_1$ blockade	Improved sleep; daytime sedation (15–49%)	Variable, may ↑ TST, ↓ SL	Limited data; ↓ performance in one study on elderly; no MSLT data
Nefazodone	5-HT$_2$, 5-HT$_1$ blockade; alpha$_1$, H$_1$ blockade	Dose-dependent daytime sedation (6–24%)	Variable, may ↑ TST, ↓ W	↑ Performance in 1 study; no impairment of driving, some impairment of cognition and memory, especially with ↑ dose or duration; may be "alerting" after single dose but not repeated dosing; two MSLT studies: ↑ SL
Venlafaxine	5-HT, NE uptake inhibition; also weakly affects dopamine uptake	Insomnia in ~8%; sedation in ~13–31%	↓ TST, ↑ W	↑ Performance in normal subjects; no MSLT data
Mirtazapine	5-HT$_2$, 5-HT$_3$ blockade; alpha$_2$, H$_1$ blockade	Improved sleep; daytime sedation (9–52%; more in U.S. than Europe, perhaps due to dose)	↑ TST, ↓ SL, ↓ S1	Minimal data, may ↓ performance acutely; no MSLT data
Bupropion	Dopamine uptake inhibition; NE uptake inhibition	Insomnia in ~5–19%	Minimal data	Minimal data; generally no impairment
Maprotiline	NE uptake inhibition; H$_1$ blockade	Sedating	Minimal data	Minimal data, no impairment?
Amoxapine	5-HT$_2$ blockade; NE uptake inhibition; H$_1$, alpha$_1$ blockade	Sedating	Minimal data	Insufficient data
Mianserin (not available in the United States)	5-HT$_2$, alpha$_1$, alpha$_2$, H$_1$ blockade	Sedating	↑ TST in depressed patients	Impairs performance

H, histamine; 5-HT, 5-hydroxytryptamine; MSLT, multiple sleep latency test; NE, norepinephrine; PSG, polysomnographic; S1, stage 1; SL, sleep latency; TST, total sleep time; W, wake.

Tricyclic Antidepressants

Sedation, which is frequently reported with the use of TCAs, is more commonly noted with amitriptyline, doxepin, imipramine, and trimipramine (the tertiary amines) than with desipramine, nortriptyline, and protriptyline (the secondary amines). TCAs generally improve PSG sleep in normal individuals and in some depressed patients. These drugs may worsen insomnia in some depressed patients by increasing the frequency of periodic limb movements during sleep (PLMs).[19] However, the relationship between TCAs and PLMs has not been conclusively demonstrated. There are no studies that objectively evaluate daytime sleepiness. However, performance impairment has been objectively demonstrated for many of the TCAs, most notably amitriptyline and imipramine, in both normal subjects and depressed patients. Single doses appear to be more likely to cause impairment than repeated doses over 1 to 2 weeks; however, in at least one study of healthy volunteers, a high degree of performance impairment persisted for at least 14 days of daily administration of 37.5 mg amitriptyline.[20] In another study on healthy individuals,[21] minor performance impairment was noted to persist for 7 days after daily ingestion of imipramine. In this study, driving performance was markedly impaired after the first 50-mg dose of imipramine, but this impairment, although still present, had significantly diminished by the end of 1 week of daily dosing. Both of these studies used doses lower than those typically prescribed for depression.

Monoamine Oxidase Inhibitors

MAOIs inhibit the action of MAO enzymes, which metabolize serotonin, norepinephrine, and dopamine. The classic MAOIs (e.g., isocarboxacid, phenelzine, tranylcypromine) irreversibly inhibit both MAOA and MAOB enzymes. Insomnia and daytime sedation are commonly reported side effects (up to 62% and 42% of patients, respectively),[22] but there are no placebo-controlled studies. The most impressive PSG finding is a marked decrease in REM sleep, including almost complete abolishment of REM in some patients. TST is also decreased.[23, 24] Although MSLT studies are lacking, actigraphic monitoring in a small group of patients confirmed periods of decreased daytime activity coincident with reported episodes of napping,[25] possibly associated with poor nighttime sleep. Cognitive and psychomotor performances do not appear to be influenced by the classic MAOIs, but data are limited.[26–28]

Unlike the classic MAOIs, the newer MAOIs reversibly and selectively inhibit the MAOA enzyme, apparently resulting in fewer severe adverse effects. Drugs of this type include moclobemide, befloxatone, and brofaromine. Sleep disturbance is commonly reported in clinical trials of these drugs, with a reported incidence of up to 67%,[29, 30] but these studies lack a placebo control. PSG data suggest that the degree of sleep disturbance may be dependent on both duration of treatment and dosage.[31, 32] A study on brofaromine demonstrated increased wake during sleep (compared with baseline) for up to 4 weeks of treatment.[24]

Moclobemide may enhance cognitive function in young[33] and older[34, 35] depressed outpatients. In the latter study,[35] an imipramine-treated group failed to show similar improvement. Changes in event-related potentials after 42 days of treatment with moclobemide also suggest a positive effect in cognitive functioning.[36] In psychomotor performance studies of healthy subjects, moclobemide, brofaromine, and befloxatone generally do not differ from placebo, whereas trazodone, mianserin, doxepin, and amitriptyline result in decreased performance.[37–40]

Selective Serotonin Reuptake Inhibitors

Clinical trials of SSRIs show placebo-adjusted rates of insomnia ranging from 5 to 19% in depressed patients, with rates generally similar among the different drugs.[9, 41, 42] Pooled data from several placebo-controlled fixed-dose studies of fluoxetine show the incidence of insomnia to be dose dependent.[43] In these studies, the placebo-adjusted incidence of insomnia was 5 to 9%, emerged within the first weeks of treatment, and remained at steady levels for up to 46 weeks of treatment. Sedation has also been reported in a number of clinical trials of SSRIs, more commonly with fluvoxamine (up to 26% of patients) and paroxetine (up to 24%).[9, 41, 44] PSG studies show that fluoxetine decreases TST and increases wake time and stage 1 in both normal subjects during single-night studies with doses of 20 to 60 mg[45] and depressed patients with doses of 20 to 80 mg for up to 1 year.[46–48] Fluoxetine has also been associated with PLMs[49] and the presence of prominent slow eye movements in nonrapid eye movement (NREM) sleep,[49, 50] the significance of which is unknown. Paroxetine (15 to 30 mg) decreases TST and increases awakenings in normal subjects with 1- to 2-day dosing.[51–53] There also is evidence of increased awakenings and sleep fragmentation after 5 weeks of paroxetine treatment in depressed inpatients, although TST was slightly increased and patients reported improved subjective sleep quality (lack of a placebo control group makes interpretation of the latter difficult).[54] Fluvoxamine has had similar effects on the sleep architecture of depressed patients.[55] Citalopram produced the typical decrease in REM sleep but no changes in SL or TST during 5 weeks of treatment in one study of depressed patients.[56]

There are no MSLT studies or other direct measures of daytime sleepiness and alertness for these drugs. SSRIs generally do not negatively affect daytime performance or cognitive functioning and may actually improve functioning in some patients.[17, 18]

Other Antidepressants

Trazodone

Drowsiness is the most commonly reported adverse effect in clinical trials with trazodone,[57, 58] with placebo-adjusted rates ranging from 5% to more than 45% of patients.[57, 59, 60] In a study of healthy young volunteers, daytime trazodone doses of 100 to 200 mg resulted in marked subjective sleepiness that persisted for the 2 weeks of therapy.[20] Significant daytime sedation has also been reported in depressed individuals taking trazodone for apparent fluoxetine-associated insomnia.[61]

Objective measures of daytime sleepiness are lacking; however, trazodone has been shown to impair performance on a number of psychomotor and memory tasks in healthy individuals in both single- and multiple-dose studies.[15, 37, 57, 62] There is some suggestion that trazodone may not impair performance or memory in depressed individuals,[63, 64] although these studies lack a positive control.

Nefazodone

Nefazodone is structurally related to trazodone but is a much less potent alpha$_1$ blocker and has no affinity for H$_1$ receptors.[65] Nevertheless, drowsiness is one of its major side effects, with placebo-adjusted incidence rates ranging from approximately 6 to 24% and dependent on dose.[10, 65–67]

One study in normal individuals demonstrated an increase in MSLT mean latency (i.e., decreased sleepiness) after 16 days of nefazodone treatment.[68] A second study of healthy adult and elderly subjects also showed increased daytime SL after a single dose of nefazodone in a modified MSLT protocol, although this effect had disappeared by day 7 of treatment.[21] Cognitive and performance studies generally show no impairment or even slight improvement in psychomotor performance and memory in middle-aged and elderly normal subjects.[21, 69] There are no studies of this drug on daytime alertness or performance in depressed patients.

Venlafaxine

Venlafaxine inhibits reuptake of both norepinephrine and serotonin. Insomnia has been reported by 4 to 18% of patients taking venlafaxine,[60, 66, 70] whereas somnolence occurs in a dose-dependent manner in approximately 12 to 31% of patients (placebo-adjusted rates).[60, 65, 66, 70, 71] In normal subjects, 75 to 150 mg of venlafaxine administered for 4 consecutive days produced increased wake and stage 1; in addition, in six of the eight subjects, frequent PLMs (more than 25 per h) were noted.[72] In a double-blind, parallel placebo-controlled study of depressed inpatients treated for 1 month, venlafaxine (maximum dose, 225 mg/day) increased PSG-recorded wake after sleep onset by approximately 30 min compared with placebo.[73] There are no studies that objectively evaluate daytime sleepiness and alertness. Single doses of venlafaxine improved performance and cognitive function in a double-blind placebo-controlled study in normal subjects, particularly 6 to 8 h after dosing.[74]

Mirtazapine

Mirtazapine is described as a noradrenergic and specific serotonergic antidepressant. It also has high affinity for the H_1 receptor, which likely accounts for its sedating effects. Sedation has been reported in up to 52% (placebo-adjusted rate) of patients in clinical trials and was the major reason for drug discontinuation in controlled studies.[10, 17, 70, 75, 76] In comparative studies with other antidepressants, the incidence of sedation with mirtazapine was similar to that of trazodone[77] and amitriptyline.[78] The incidence of reported sedation appears much higher in U.S. (54%) than in European (23%) clinical trials possibly because higher initial doses such as those used in the European trials (15 to 20 mg versus 5 to 10 mg in U.S. studies) produce increased noradrenergic activation counteracting the antihistaminic effect, which may be more prominent at lower doses.[79] (The recommended initial dosage is 15 mg/day with an effective dose range of 15 to 45 mg.) Performance impairment was noted acutely on a number of tests within 6 hours of drug administration.[80] MSLT data are lacking, as are longer-term performance studies.

Bupropion

Bupropion, which inhibits the uptake of dopamine and norepinephrine, is associated with insomnia in 5 to 19% of patients in clinical trials.[9, 81] In a PSG study of seven depressed patients, after 4 weeks of treatment, bupropion did not affect SL or TST but did decrease REM latency and increase REM percent.[82] Bupropion is not generally associated with cognitive or psychomotor performance impairment.[37]

Miscellaneous Antidepressants (Amoxapine, Maprotiline, Mianserin)

Amoxapine, a dibenzoxazepine tricyclic, and maprotiline and mianserin, both tetracyclic compounds (the latter is not yet available in the United States), have sedative profiles similar to that of the TCAs, likely because of their high affinity for H_1 receptors.[7, 83] Amoxapine and maprotiline are not commonly used because of other serious side effects, namely seizures in the case of maprotiline, and dopamine-blocking side effects with amoxapine. There are no studies objectively measuring sleepiness. There appears to be little cognitive impairment with maprotiline,[33] although minimal data are available. In healthy individuals, mianserin impaired driving and tracking performance,[84] as well as reaction time and other psychomotor measures.[15, 37]

Lithium

Lithium, which is used primarily in the treatment of manic-depressive illness, is subjectively associated with improved nocturnal sleep and increased daytime sleepiness, at least initially.[13, 85] Sleep disturbance is a prominent feature of mania and similar polysomnographically to that observed in major depression.[86] There are no objective studies evaluating the effect of lithium on daytime sleepiness. In healthy volunteers, lithium administered for 1 to 3 weeks produced cognitive and psychomotor deficits, including prolonged reaction times, decreased vigilance, and impairment of semantic reasoning.[87, 88] Similar deficits have been shown in psychiatric patients taking lithium for periods of time ranging from 2 weeks to longer than 3 months,[89, 90] although it is difficult to determine whether the deficits seen in the patient population are caused by the medication or their psychiatric illness. In the study by Hatcher et al.,[90] a comparison group of healthy subjects taking lithium for at least 3 months did not show the same psychomotor deficits as did the patient group. As age, severity of disease, or lithium concentration increases, so does the degree of cognitive deficit in patients on long-term lithium.[91]

ANTIPSYCHOTIC AGENTS

Evaluation of the effects of antipsychotic medications is complicated by difficulty with sleep onset, sleep maintenance,[92] and cognitive impairment in schizophrenia.[93] Reported findings such as decreased SWS, decreased REM latency, and increased REM density may reflect prior neuroleptic treatment rather than the pathophysiology of the disorder.[92, 94]

Sedation is a common side effect of the traditional antipsychotics, although extrapyramidal symptoms (EPS) and tardive dyskinesia may be more troublesome.[95] However, the incidence of sedation varies considerably among drugs, probably as a function of variation in affinity for cholinergic and histaminic receptors as well as blockade of alpha$_1$ adrenoreceptors.[96] Among the older neuroleptics, chlorpromazine and thioridazine tend to be more sedating than haloperidol.[95, 96] The newer agents (clozapine, risperidone, olanzapine, sertindole, and quetiapine) have unique pharmacological profiles.[97] Risperidone, sertindole, and quetiapine are dopamine (D_2), serotonin, and norepinephrine (alpha$_1$) antagonists, whereas clozapine and olanzapine also bind to cholinergic, histaminergic, and D_1 receptors. These newer drugs are much less likely to produce EPS. Clinical studies show a high incidence of sedation with clozapine (with transient sedation reported by 54% of patients, persistent sedation by 46%, and sedation requiring drug discontinuation by 24%).[98-100] Sedation is reported much less frequently with risperidone, olanzapine, sertindole, and quetiapine[97, 101-104] and is generally not a significant problem in long-term treatment for most patients.[95] There are no MSLT or other studies that objectively evaluate daytime sleepiness.

Although neuroleptics cause cognitive impairment in normal subjects,[105-107] these drugs in patient populations either have no demonstrable effect[93, 108-110] or may actually improve cognitive function.[93, 111-114] Clozapine, in particular, despite its significant sedation, has been associated with improvement in various aspects of cognitive function in schizophrenic patients.[115-117]

ANXIOLYTIC AGENTS

Benzodiazepines

Benzodiazepines (BZDs), which are used to treat anxiety, are also sometimes used for their sleep-inducing effects. It is not surprising that the most common side effect of these drugs is sedation.[85, 118-120] In a placebo-controlled study of normal subjects, daytime administration of alprazolam and diazepam produced decreased SLs as measured by MSLT on both day 1 and day 7 of treatment, with alprazolam producing greater sleepiness than diazepam on the first day of treatment.[121] Performance impairment, including impairment of actual driving performance,[122, 123] is common with BZDs in studies of normal subjects and patient groups for treatment periods of up to 3 weeks, particularly at higher doses.[85, 124, 125] Well-controlled studies are needed to determine whether longer-term use of BZD anxiolytics results in tolerance to these performance-impairing effects and whether there are differential effects between younger and older individuals.

Buspirone

Buspirone does not have the hypnotic, anticonvulsant, and muscle relaxant properties of the BZDs.[119] The anxiolytic efficacy of buspirone is similar to that of the BZDs, but its onset of action is much slower, requiring up to 3 to 4 weeks.[119, 126, 127] This delay in onset of action as well as the possibility that patients may inappropriately equate subjective feelings of sedation with efficacy may partially account for decreased use of this drug compared with BZD use in the treatment of anxiety. Although its mechanism of action is unknown, buspirone appears to act primarily as a 5-HT$_{1A}$ partial agonist but also appears to have some effect on dopamine (D$_2$) receptors.[19, 126, 128] It has no affinity for the BZD receptors and does not affect gamma-aminobutyric acid binding.[126, 129] In clinical studies of anxious patients, buspirone was comparable to placebo in the frequency of subjective reports of sedation.[130] In non–placebo-controlled clinical trials, reports of sleepiness or drowsiness were much more frequent with diazepam (34 to 45%), chlorazepate (26 to 33%), alprazolam (43 to 45%), and lorazepam (58 to 65%) than with buspirone (8 to 16%), despite similar efficacy.[120, 130, 131]

In a study of 12 chronic insomniacs, alertness as measured by MSLT was not impaired by 20 mg/day buspirone in divided doses over a 3-day period.[132] In addition, the effects of buspirone on quantitative electroencephalography were indistinguishable from placebo.[133] Compared with BZD anxiolytics, buspirone appears to have few negative effects on psychomotor, cognitive, or driving performance in healthy volunteers receiving short-term treatment or patients treated for up to 4 weeks.[119, 122, 127, 132]

CARDIOVASCULAR DRUGS

There are numerous reviews on the effects of cardiovascular drugs, particularly antihypertensive medications, on sleep and waking function.[85, 134-141] This section will focus primarily on antihypertensive medication because of their widespread use (including use for heart failure or arrhythmias) and because many have CNS side effects associated with sleep-waking function. In addition, a number of different classes of antihypertensive agents are available; these data are summarized in Table 36–3.

Antihypertensive Agents

Beta Antagonists

Information on pharmacological characteristics of beta antagonists relevant to CNS sleep-waking function is given in Table 36–4. CNS side effects that have been reported to occur with beta blockers include tiredness, fatigue, insomnia, nightmares and vivid dreams, depression, mental confusion, and psychomotor impairment.[134, 135] Both age of the patient and dose contribute to the frequency of side effects, which may diminish with time. The incidence of sleep disturbance has been reported to be 2 to 4.3%.[141, 142] In general, sleep disturbance appears to be more common with the lipophilic drugs (e.g., propranolol) than with the hydrophilic drugs (e.g., atenolol) in both subjective reports[134, 135, 143] and PSG studies.[135, 144-146] The data are not straightforward, however. Pindolol, which is less lipophilic than propranolol, appears to be more disruptive of sleep.[134] Even atenolol, the most hydrophilic of the beta blockers, has been shown to increase total wake time, at least acutely, in normal subjects.[147] Thus, although lipophilicity may be the primary determinant of the CNS effects of these drugs, other factors are also likely involved, such as the relative affinity for beta$_2$ or 5-HT receptors,[137, 138] plasma catecholamine levels, molecule-specific structural details,[148] plasma concentration,[137] or the degree of melatonin suppression.[149, 150]

Complaints of tiredness, fatigue, and daytime sleepiness may be the consequences of disturbed nocturnal sleep or a direct action of the drugs themselves. There are no studies that have differentially evaluated these

Table 36–3. EFFECTS OF ANTIHYPERTENSIVE DRUGS ON SLEEP AND WAKING BEHAVIOR

Drug Class	Example	Subjective Data	Polysomnographic Data	Performance Data
Beta antagonists	Propranolol, metoprolol, atenolol (see Table 36–4)	Insomnia, nightmares more common with lipophilic drugs	Lipophilic drugs more likely to ↑ W, TWT, S1, ↓ REM, but plasma concentration, receptor selectivity, and other factors may also be important in determining the degree of sleep disruption	Few consistent effects, but many methodological problems in these studies
Alpha₂ agonists	Clonidine	Sedation, mental slowing, ↓ concentration; nightmares	↓ REM; ↑ TST acutely in normal subjects; ↓ TST in hypertensives	No impairment (one study)
	Methyldopa	Sedation; insomnia, nightmares; reports of poor workplace performance and lower QOL	↑ REM; ↑ TST	Memory impairment
Catecholamine depleters	Reserpine	Sedation, insomnia, nightmares, depression, difficulty concentrating	↑ REM; ↑ stage shifts	No studies
Beta antagonists with alpha₁-blocking activity	Carvedilol, labetalol	Fatigue, somnolence, insomnia	No studies	No studies
Calcium antagonists	Verapamil, nifedipine, diltiazam, amlodipine, felopidine, nisoldipine	One report of increased agitation with nifedipine	No PSG studies; one report of increased alpha in waking EEG with nifedipine	No studies
Angiotensin-converting enzyme inhibitors	Captopril, cilazapril	No negative effects on sleep; improvement in QOL	No disturbance	Improved psychomotor performance
Angiotensin II receptor antagonists	Losartan	Rare insomnia	No studies	No studies
Alpha₁ antagonists	Prazosin, terazosin, doxazosin	Transiently sedating?	No studies in human beings	Prazosin: no change in performance (one study)
Vasodilators	Hydralazine	? Anxiety, depression, insomnia	No studies	Hydralazine; no change in performance (one study)
Diuretics	HCTZ, chlorthalidone, indapamide	Central nervous system effects unlikely; one report of subjective-rated worsening of work performance; one report of improved sleep with indapamide	No studies	No evidence of impairment
5-Hydroxytryptamine₂ antagonists (not yet available in the United States)	Ketanserin (acts peripherally)	Fatigue, insomnia	↑ SWS, ↓ REM, no effects on SL or TST	No studies
	Ritanserin (blocks central receptors)	No negative effects reported		
Imidazoline agonists (not yet available in the United States)	Moxonidine, rilmenidine	Rare sedation with low doses; increased sedation with higher doses but less than with clonidine	No studies	Little effect on psychomotor performance; slight decrements in vigilance and memory

HCTZ, hydrochlorothiazide; QOL, quality of life; REM, rapid eye movement; SL, sleep latency; SWS, slow-wave sleep; TST, total sleep time; TWT, total wake time; W, wake.

Table 36–4. SELECTED PHARMACOLOGICAL CHARACTERISTICS OF BETA ANTAGONISTS

Drug	Lipid Solubility	Selectivity*	Relative Affinity for 5-Hydroxy-tryptamine Receptors*
Propranolol	High	None	High
Timolol	High	None	High
Pindolol	Moderate	None	High
Bisoprolol	Moderate	Beta$_1$	Low
Metoprolol	Moderate	Beta$_1$	Low
Acebutolol	Moderate	Beta$_1$	Low
Nadolol	Low	None	High
Sotalol	Low	Beta$_1$	Low
Atenolol	Low	Beta$_1$	Low

*Beta$_1$ receptors are located primarily in cardiac muscle; beta$_2$ receptors are located primarily in bronchial and vascular musculature. The nonselective beta-blocking agents have higher affinity for 5-hydroxytryptamine receptors.[331]

hypotheses, nor are there published reports using the MSLT or other measures to objectively evaluate daytime sleepiness in either normal subjects or hypertensive patients.

Reviews on the effects of beta blockers on cognitive and psychomotor performance[134, 139–141] indicate that these drugs produce few consistent neuropsychological deficits. In a review of 55 studies on neuropsychological effects of beta blockers, Dimsdale et al.[139] concluded that beta blockers improved cognitive function in 16% of subjects, worsened it in 17%, and caused no change in 67%, with no significant difference between lipophilic and nonlipophilic drugs. Decrements in performance appear to be more likely to occur with more complex cognitive or psychomotor tasks and have been reported more often with lipophilic beta blockers than with hydrophilic drugs, although results are not always consistent. Deficits in cognitive function may be more likely with older than with younger patients.[151]

Alpha$_2$ Agonists

Sedation is the most common side effect of both clonidine and methyldopa, occurring in 30 to 75% of patients, but the severity apparently diminishes with time.[142, 152] There also are some reports of insomnia and nightmares.[142] In a double-blind, placebo-controlled crossover study, hypertensive men aged 31 to 59 years who were given 0.1–0.3 mg of clonidine b.i.d. showed significantly decreased TST (320.1 minutes) compared with placebo (366.9 minutes) after 3 months of use.[151] Normal subjects, however, given clonidine acutely showed increases in TST.[153] No MSLT studies exist to objectively quantify daytime sedation. However, one study of a single morning dose of clonidine in young normal subjects demonstrated microsleeps in six of eight subjects despite efforts of study personnel to keep them awake.[154] In that study, subjective ratings of sleepiness were also higher with clonidine compared with placebo. Few well-controlled studies exist that

evaluate the effects of these drugs on performance. Verbal memory impairment[155] and poorer workplace performance[156] have been reported in patients receiving methyldopa.

Beta Antagonists With Alpha$_1$-Blocking Activity

The newer beta-blocking drugs, which also have vasodilating properties (e.g., carvedilol, labetalol), have been associated with fatigue and somnolence (3 to 11% of patients taking labetalol and 1 to 4% of patients taking carvedilol). Insomnia has occasionally been reported.[157, 158] Objective studies of sleep, sleepiness and alertness, and performance are lacking.

5-Hydroxytryptamine$_2$ Antagonists

Ketanserin, which is not yet available in the United States, is a selective 5-HT$_2$ antagonist that acts primarily at peripheral sites; it also has affinity for alpha$_1$ adrenoreceptors, histamine H$_1$ receptors, and dopamine receptors.[129] After 1 to 3 months of use, ketanserin was more frequently associated with fatigue (11%) than was propranolol (6%).[159] There are no published PSG, MSLT, or performance studies.

Ritanserin, which blocks central 5-HT$_2$ receptors, has not been associated with subjective reports of insomnia or fatigue. Ritanserin increases SWS in normal subjects,[160] poor sleepers,[161] dysthymic patients,[162] and narcoleptics[163] without affecting SL or TST. The addition of ritanserin to the usual medication in patients with narcolepsy did not affect MSLT latency.[163] No performance studies exist.

Other Antihypertensives

The remaining drugs used for the control of hypertension (and listed in Table 36–3) generally have few negative effects on sleep or wakefulness, although there are limited objective data for some of these drugs. The new angiotensin receptor antagonist losartan is rarely associated with insomnia.[164] The imidazoline agonists moxonidine and rilmenidine, which are not yet available in the United States, belong to a new class of centrally active antihypertensives with greater selectivity for the imidazoline receptor relative to the alpha$_2$ adrenoreceptor, which theoretically results in fewer central adverse effects while maintaining central antihypertensive properties.[165] In comparison with clonidine in clinical studies, both rilmenidine[166] and moxonidine[167] have had a much lower incidence of sedation. There is some evidence of slightly increased incidence of sedation at higher doses.[152, 164, 165]

The alpha$_1$ antagonists (e.g., prazosin, terazosin) are sometimes associated with transient sedation.[136] There are no reports of sleep disturbance or wake dysfunction with the calcium channel blockers (e.g., verapamil, nifedipine); however, these drugs decrease the effectiveness of hypnotics and potentiate the effects of stimulants, at least in studies in animals.[136] Angiotensin-converting enzyme inhibitors (e.g., captopril, cilazapril)

Table 36–5. EFFECTS OF HYPOLIPIDEMIC DRUGS ON SLEEP AND WAKING BEHAVIOR

Drug	U.S. Trade Name	Subjective Data	Polysomnographic Data	Performance Data
Pravastatin	Pravachol	No effects	No changes	No negative effects
Simvastatin	Zocor	Insomnia per case reports	No changes	No data
Lovastatin	Mevacor	Insomnia per case reports	Conflicting results; some evidence for increased wake and stage 1	Conflicting results
Fluvastatin	Lescol	No effects	No data	No data
Cholestyramine	Questran	Insomnia at rate of 1.3% in clinical trials	No data	No data
Gemfibrozil	Lopid	Reports of sleepiness	No data	No data
Clofibrate	Atromid	Fatigue, drowsiness	No data	No data
Colestipol	Colestid	Infrequent insomnia	No data	No data

reportedly have a low incidence of central side effects. Patients on captopril were less likely to feel tired or sleepy at work compared with patients on propranolol or methyldopa during 24 weeks of therapy.[168] In addition, drowsiness and ability to concentrate improved in patients who switched from a beta blocker to captopril.[169] Vasodilators (e.g., hydralazine) and diuretics do not appear to disrupt sleep,[142, 170] although one might expect more frequent awakenings for micturition with diuretics.

Among the above drugs, PSG data exist only for the angiotensin-converting enzyme inhibitors. In healthy individuals, PSG-recorded sleep was not affected by 14-day administration of cilazapril compared with the positive control, metoprolol, which produced increased awakenings.[171]

There are no objective evaluations of daytime sleepiness for these drugs, but they do not appear to negatively affect daytime function. Patients treated with captopril for 24 weeks demonstrated improvement in quality of life and cognitive function compared with patients treated with methyldopa or propranolol.[156] Studies on prazosin[172] and hydralazine[173] show no change in performance. Although performance impairment appears unlikely with diuretics, there is one report showing worsened scores on indices of subject-rated work performance and general well-being.[174] The imidazoline agonists do not appear to negatively affect

psychomotor performance,[175] although there may be minor decrements in vigilance and memory.[176]

Hypolipidemic Drugs

The effects of hypolipidemic drugs on sleep and waking behavior are summarized in Table 36–5. Lovastatin has been associated with subjective reports of insomnia.[177, 178] However, placebo-controlled clinical trials of lovastatin, simvastatin, and pravastatin have generally failed to show increased sleep disturbance.[179–181] PSG evidence of sleep disruption is conflicting as well.[182–185] In the study by Roth et al.,[183] performance decrements were demonstrated with lovastatin even though nocturnal sleep and daytime sleep tendency (measured by MSLT) were not affected.

Antiarrhythmic Drugs

Subjective data on antiarrhythmic drugs are summarized in Table 36–6. Fatigue is the most common CNS complaint of patients taking these drugs, with placebo-adjusted incidence from clinical trials generally ranging from 0 to 10%,[129, 178, 186] except for the beta antagonists, for which rates may be higher (see separate section on these drugs). There are little objective data available.

Table 36–6. EFFECTS OF ANTIARRHYTHMIC DRUGS ON SLEEP AND WAKING BEHAVIOR

Class*	Drug	Common U.S. Trade Name	Subjective Data†
IA	Disopyramide	Norpace	Fatigue in 3–10%
	Procainamide	Procanbid	None reported
	Quinidine	Quinaglute	Fatigue in 2.9%
1B	Mexiletine	Mexitil	Drowsiness in 7%; insomnia, memory impairment
	Moricizine	Ethmozine	Fatigue in 0.5%
	Tocainide	Tonocard	Fatigue in 0.8–2%
IC	Flecainide	Tambocor	Fatigue in 5–10%; insomnia in 1–3%
	Propafenone	Rythmol	None reported
II	Beta antagonists	Various	See Table 36–3 and section on beta antagonists in text
III	Amiodarone	Cordarone	Fatigue in 5–10%; nightmares, insomnia in 1–3%
IV	Diltiazem	Cardizem	Fatigue in 10%; insomnia, abnormal dreams, sleepiness
	Verapamil	Calan	Fatigue in 2%

*Vaughan Williams classification.
†Percentages indicate placebo-adjusted rates from clinical trials.

HISTAMINE₁ ANTAGONISTS

The effects of H_1 antihistamines (Tables 36–7 and 36–8) on subjective and objective sleepiness and performance are well reviewed in a number of articles.[188–193] The first-generation H_1 antihistamines are lipophilic and easily cross the blood-brain barrier. In addition, these drugs demonstrate poor receptor selectivity as characterized by antagonism of muscarinic cholinergic, alpha-adrenergic, and tryptaminergic receptors. The second-generation H_1 antihistamines are large hydrophilic molecules and do not easily penetrate the CNS; they have high affinity for H_1 receptors and little affinity for other amine receptors.[194]

Sedation is a primary side effect of first-generation H_1 antihistamines.[188, 189, 190] These drugs have been associated with occupational injuries[195] and fatal traffic accidents.[196] In contrast, the second-generation H_1 antihistamines do not appear to be sedating and are much less likely to impair performance.

MSLT studies in normal subjects[197–199] and atopic individuals[200] generally confirm that diphenhydramine, hydroxyzine, and triprolidine are sedating (at least with acute use), whereas cetirizine, loratadine, and terfenadine are not. Cetirizine, however, has essentially been classified as sedating by the Food and Drug Administration.[191, 201] Indeed, there are a number of studies (primarily studies using high doses of cetirizine or cetirizine in combination with alcohol) that suggest cetirizine, which is a metabolite of hydroxyzine, is not completely without sedating effects.[202–204] However, a number of well-controlled studies with objective evaluations of sleepiness and performance indicate that cetirizine in recommended doses of 5 to 10 mg does not differ from placebo.[199, 204–207]

Controlled studies that evaluate psychomotor skills, memory and cognition, attention, visual processing, and actual driving performance generally confirm the performance-impairing properties of the older drugs (the majority of studies are on diphenhydramine, hydroxyzine, chlorpheniramine, and triprolidine) and the performance-sparing properties of the newer compounds (the majority of studies are on cetirizine, loratadine and terfenadine, but there are some reports on acrivastine, astemizole, and fexofenadine). For example, in a study of actual driving performance,[208] 6 of 10 subjects who took chlorpheniramine were unable to complete the 2.5-h test, whereas all subjects who ingested terfenadine or placebo successfully completed the test. Triprolidine was similarly shown to impair driving performance, but terfenadine did not.[209] The driving impairment produced by 5 to 10 mg of triprolidine controlled-release formulation was shown to be similar to that produced by blood alcohol concentrations of 0.5 to 1.0 mg/ml.[210] In contrast to cetirizine and loratadine, hydroxyzine and diphenhydramine have been shown to impair vigilance and psychomotor performance.[197, 199, 200, 211] A review[212] of studies with both positive and placebo controls concluded that the risk of performance impairment was minimal and similar for astemizole, cetirizine, terfenadine, azatadine, and loratadine (all second-generation compounds), whereas the risk of impairment was significantly higher for the first-generation drugs, with triprolidine offering the highest risk, followed by diphenhydramine, clemastine, and chlorpheniramine.

Although all except one[200] of the MSLT studies on antihistamines were conducted on normal adults, performance studies have been done on a broader population, including children and atopic and normal adults. Although there are methodological difficulties in studying affected patient populations, such studies are essential because they represent the primary users of the drugs and responses may be different from those of normal subjects. In fact, drug-induced sedation and performance impairment may be more important in patients whose clinical symptomatology may disturb their nocturnal sleep[213] or affect daytime behavior. Untreated children[214] and adults[215, 216] with allergic rhinitis perform more poorly on learning and vigilance tasks than do normal control subjects. In the study on children, 2 weeks of diphenhydramine therapy impaired learning to an even greater extent, whereas 2 weeks of loratadine improved performance although not to the level seen in normal subjects.[214] On the other hand, adults treated with acrivastine plus pseudoephedrine learned as well as did normal subjects, although treatment with diphenhydramine similarly worsened performance compared with no treatment.[215] In general, studies on atopic individuals confirm the sedating and performance-impairing effects of the older antihistamines in contrast to the newer compounds.

There are insufficient data to make definitive conclusions about whether tolerance develops to the sedating effects of antihistamines. The most convincing evidence for the development of tolerance is a study on atopic individuals who demonstrated decreased MSLT latencies and poorer simulated assembly line performance during the first day of treatment with diphenhydramine (compared with placebo and cetirizine) but not

Table 36–7. COMMON FIRST-GENERATION H_1 ANTAGONISTS

Generic Name	U.S. Trade Name	Comments
Azatadine	Trinalin	Available only in combination with pseudoephedrine
Brompheniramine	Dimetane	
Clemastine	Tavist	
Chlorpheniramine	Chlor-Trimeton	
Cyproheptadine	Periactin	
Diphenhydramine	Benadryl	Main ingredient in many over-the-counter sleep aids
Hydroxyzine	Atarax, Vistaril	
Promethazine	Phenergan	
Triprolidine	Actifed, Actidil	Available in combination with pseudoephedrine in United States; appears to be the most sedating of this group

Table 36–8. SECOND-GENERATION H_1 ANTAGONISTS

Generic Name	U.S. Trade Name	Comments
Acrivastine	Semprex-D	Metabolite of triprolidine; available in combination with pseudoephedrine; short-acting (half-life of 1.4 h)
Astemizole	Hismanal	Onset of action within 2 days; peak efficacy in 4 days; prolonged duration of action; may take 4 weeks to reach steady state; cardiovascular complications have been reported in combinations with other drugs; taken off market by manufacturer
Azelastine	Astelin	Available in United States only as nasal spray
Cetirizine	Zyrtec	Metabolite of hydroxyzine; may be sedating in high doses; may potentiate the sedating effect of alcohol; the only H_1 blocker not metabolized by the hepatic cytochrome P-450 system
Fexofenadine	Allegra	Active metabolite of terfenadine; lacks the adverse cardiac complications of the parent compound
Loratadine	Claritin	Structurally related to azatadine; chemically similar to imipramine
Terfenadine	Seldane	Taken off market by manufacturer; cardiovascular complications reported in combination with other drugs

during the third day of treatment.[200] The remainder of placebo-controlled studies (all on normal subjects) that use therapeutic dosing regimens show less impairment in performance or subjective sedation after 3 to 5 days compared with the first or second day,[210, 217–219] but performance was still poorer than that with placebo.

HISTAMINE$_2$ ANTAGONISTS

H_2 antagonists (e.g., cimetidine, ranitidine, famotidine, and nizatidine) are unlikely to significantly impair CNS function because these compounds do not easily cross the blood-brain barrier, although there is some evidence of CNS penetration.[220] The package inserts for these drugs refer to CNS effects, including insomnia and somnolence, generally occurring in less than 2% of individuals involved in clinical trials. Although such side effects may be infrequent, they are apparently reproducible in susceptible individuals.[221] Moreover, the nature of these side effects and the widespread use of H_2 antagonists suggest that physicians should be aware of their potential occurrence. Side effects have been most frequently reported with cimetidine, possibly because it has been on the market longer than any of the other compounds.[222] In addition, cimetidine slows the clearance of some BZDs, which may make carryover effects of hypnotics more of a problem. Similarly, cimetidine has been shown to increase levels of theophylline, carbamazapine, and beta blockers with resultant increases in the CNS effects of these drugs. Ranitidine has produced some of the same effects, although not to the extent seen with cimetidine.[223, 224]

One crossover study comparing 1-week administration of cimetidine, famotidine, raniditine, and placebo in normal subjects reported no differences in nocturnal sleep or daytime MSLT latencies, although cimetidine produced a slight increase in subjective estimates of sleepiness.[225] This study is weakened by the lack of a positive control but, more importantly, by the fact that on placebo, these subjects were quite sleepy (mean SL, 6.6 min). H_2 antagonists do not appear to affect psychomotor performance.[226, 227] However, because H_2 antagonists are widely used, often in combination with other drugs and frequently in older individuals, addi-

tional data are needed to determine the extent of their CNS effects in specific populations and situations. For example, both cimetidine[228] and ranitidine[229] administered in conventional doses have been associated with an increased incidence of lethargy, somnolence, and confusion in patients with renal impairment. In addition, BZD-produced impairment of psychomotor and cognitive function was significantly prolonged with concomitant administration of cimetidine and was somewhat prolonged with concomitant administration of ranitidine in healthy volunteers.[230]

CORTICOSTEROIDS

Corticosteroids are widely believed to disrupt sleep, but the results of objective studies are inconsistent, making conclusions for all drugs in this class difficult. Differences in receptor affinities between synthetic and endogenous corticosteroids, dosage, methodological issues associated with the study of patient populations (e.g., lack of baseline assessment and influence of the concurrent illness on sleep and behavior), and the variety of organ systems affected by corticosteroids, as well as the variety of side effects reported,[231–233] all contribute to this confusion.

In patient populations, corticosteroids have frequently been associated with sleep disturbance. Approximately 50% of patients treated with prednisone for optic neuritis reported sleep disturbance compared with 20% on placebo.[234] Parent ratings of sleep disturbance increased when steroids were added to the chemotherapy regimen of children with leukemia[235] or other types of cancer.[236] Insomnia has also been reported more frequently in patients with asthma receiving steroid medications.[237, 238] In addition, numerous anecdotal and case reports exist implicating systemic corticosteroid use with insomnia. Behavioral observations of 12 normal subjects given 80 mg prednisone q.d. for 5 days showed decreased sleep in 25% and mild hypomania in 67%.[239] Inhaled glucocorticoids do not appear to have the same negative effects,[240] but there have been case reports of hyperactivity, insomnia, and psychosis with these drugs as well.

The most consistent effect of corticosteroids on PSG-recorded sleep in normal subjects is a marked decrease in REM sleep.[241–244] Although less consistent, there is good evidence for increased wake during the night with cortisol, dexamethasone, and prednisone.[241, 242, 245] Hydrocortisone appears to increase SWS,[243] whereas dexamethasone does not.[245] Aldosterone (the major mineralocorticoid) appears to have no effect on sleep architecture.[242] Dexamethasone, administered before bedtime, resulted in increased daytime alertness the next day as measured with MSLT.[244]

A literature review revealed only one performance study on these compounds. In that placebo-controlled study, 80 mg prednisone q.d. given to 11 normal subjects for 5 days produced increased frequency of errors of commission in a verbal memory task.[246]

THEOPHYLLINE

Theophylline, a respiratory stimulant and bronchodilator, is chemically related to caffeine. Peak plasma concentration is generally reached within 2 h, but the half-life varies by preparation and is typically shorter in children (3.5 h) and longer in adults (8 to 9 h).[129] Absorption is apparently lower at night than in the morning[247] and may be greatly affected by food.[248]

Disturbed sleep is a common complaint among patients taking theophylline. In a prospective study, asthma patients treated with theophylline were more likely to complain of sleep maintenance difficulty (55%) than were patients treated with other asthma medications (31%),[249] and in a retrospective study of treated patients with asthma, 46% of whom complained of insomnia, only theophylline or corticosteroid therapy was associated with the complaint of insomnia.[237] The majority of studies that purport that theophylline does not adversely affect sleep are limited by the lack of a placebo group or condition[250–252] or other methodological difficulties such as a high dropout rate secondary to side effects or noncompliance with study medication[253] or the poor baseline sleep of the patients studied.[251, 252, 254]

Theophylline, administered for up to 3 weeks, has been shown to disturb PSG-recorded sleep in normal subjects,[255, 256] asthmatics,[257, 258] children with cystic fibrosis,[259] and patients with chronic obstructive pulmonary disease.[260, 261]

There are few well-controlled studies that evaluate the effect of theophylline on cognitive performance. In a double-blind study, asthmatic children were more likely to exhibit behavioral or attentional problems when receiving sustained-release theophylline for 4 weeks than when on placebo.[262] However, a meta-analysis of 12 studies of theophylline did not indicate any impairment in cognition or behavior.[263] Furthermore, academic achievement did not differ between 72 asthmatics who were treated with theophylline and siblings without asthma.[264]

ANTIPARKINSONIAN DRUGS

Patients with Parkinson's disease have multiple complaints relating to sleep, including insomnia, hypersomnia, fatigue, and, in some cases, vivid dreaming or nightmares.[265–269] These complaints may be the result of the degenerative processes associated with the disease; accompanying symptoms such as nighttime stiffness, pain, difficulty in turning, and nocturia; or the medications used for treatment. PSG studies confirm prolonged SLs and increased awakenings in untreated patients.[270–272] Dopamine replacement (e.g., levodopa, levodopa-carbidopa combinations) is the primary treatment for Parkinson's disease. Other drugs include selegiline (an MAOB inhibitor), dopamine agonists (e.g., pergolide, bromocriptine), amantadine (a presynaptic releasing agent), and anticholinergic drugs (e.g., trihexyphenidyl, benztropine, biperiden).

Sleep-related complaints have been reported in up to 75% of patients receiving levodopa.[273] The effects of levodopa on sleep appear to be related to dose, timing, and duration of drug administration, as well as to disease severity.[268, 274] Actigraphic,[266] PSG,[272, 275] and subjective[276] studies indicate that low doses tend to improve sleep, whereas higher doses are likely to disrupt sleep, particularly when administered in the evening. In more severely affected patients, drug-related improvement in Parkinson's symptoms may outweigh the sleep-disrupting effects of the drug, resulting in an improvement in sleep overall.[266]

The effects on sleep of the remaining drugs used to treat Parkinson's disease are less well studied, but the data are generally similar to those with dopamine. Insomnia has been reported in 10 to 32% of patients taking selegiline,[277] which preferentially oxidizes dopamine and phenylethylamine and is metabolized to L-methamphetamine and L-amphetamine. As with levodopa, low doses of selegeline are less likely to worsen sleep than are higher doses.[278, 279] Forty-two percent of patients taking pergolide reported insomnia.[280] One crossover study of six patients demonstrated equivalent PSG-recorded sleep with either bromocriptine or levodopa.[281] Fourteen percent of patients receiving amantadine, either alone or in combination with other medications, reported insomnia.[282]

Cognitive and motor deficits are common in Parkinson's disease. Only anticholinergic drugs have been demonstrated to produce worsening of cognitive function, primarily in the areas of memory function.[283–287] Such impairment is more common in older patients and is reversible with discontinuation of medication.[285] Behavioral symptoms that may affect cognitive function, such as hallucinations, delusions, confusion, mania, and anxiety, have been reported in 15 to 30% of patients treated with dopaminergic agents.[288]

ANTIEPILEPTIC AGENTS

Patients with epilepsy frequently complain of daytime fatigue and sleepiness[289–291] and occasionally complain of disturbed nocturnal sleep.[292] In addition, cognitive deficits have been reported to be common in these patients.[291, 293, 294] These problems may result from sleep disruption secondary to seizures or interictal electroencephalographic activity, as well as from effects of antiepileptic drugs.

There are many antiepileptic drugs available for use, including a number of medications recently approved, primarily for use as adjunctive therapy.[295] Findings regarding the effects of these medications are summarized in Table 36–9. The mechanisms of action and pharmacokinetics of antiepileptic drugs are beyond the scope of this chapter but are reviewed in several publications.[296–298]

Subjectively, sedation is one of the most common adverse effects of the older antiepileptic drugs, particularly phenobarbital.[290, 298–300] Sedation is typically dose dependent and more likely to be experienced acutely, with some tolerance developing with chronic use. The incidence of sedation with the older antiepileptic drugs is unclear because there are few placebo-controlled studies. The frequency of sedation has been reported to be as high as 70% with acute use of phenobarbital, 42% with carbamazepine and valproate, and 33% with phenytoin and primidone. In a prospective study of 509 patients treated with a variety of older anticonvulsant medications for more than 3 months, somnolence was the most common complaint (10%) and was most frequently associated with the use of phenobarbital or primidone.[290] Among the newer antiepileptic drugs, the incidence of reported sedation in placebo-controlled clinical trials is 5 to 15% for gabapentin, lamotrigine, vigabatrin, and zonisamide and 15 to 27% for topira-

mate and generally more prevalent during the initial treatment.[291, 298, 301, 302] The incidence of sedation with tiagabine was no different from that for placebo in placebo-controlled studies, but it was 25% in open-label, long-term studies.[303] Both sedation and insomnia have been reported with felbamate.[304, 305] These newer drugs have been studied primarily as "add-on" treatment for ethical reasons. Insufficient comparative data exist to permit firm conclusions regarding the relative sedation among these newer drugs as well as in comparison with older antiepileptic drugs.[306] PSG studies of established antiepileptic drugs generally show these drugs to produce shorter SLs and increased TST.[307–309] There are no PSG studies on the newer antiepileptic drugs.

There are several objective studies of the effects of these drugs on daytime sleepiness but none with a placebo control. Patients treated with phenoparbital[310] or carbamazepine[311, 312] had lower mean MSLT latencies than did normal control subjects. In a 6-min test of ability to maintain wakefulness, patients receiving chronic stable doses of carbamazepine, phenytoin, phenobarbital, or valproate demonstrated increased duration of drowsiness (100.7 sec) compared with healthy control subjects (12.0 sec) and untreated patients with epilepsy (0.8 sec).[300]

Numerous methodological problems make the eval-

Table 36–9. EFFECTS OF ANTIEPILEPTIC DRUGS ON SLEEP AND WAKING BEHAVIOR

Drug	U.S. Trade Name	Subjective Data*	PSG Data	MSLT Data	Cognitive and Performance Data
Established Antiepileptic Drugs					
Benzodiazepines	e.g., Klonopin, Valium	Sedation	See Chapters 32 and 33 on hypnotics	See Chapters 32 and 33 on hypnotics	See Chapters 32 and 33 on hypnotics
Carbamazepine	Tegretol	Sedation	? ↓ SL, ? ↑ TST	↓ SL	Mild impairment
Ethosuximide	Zarontin	Sedation	↑ stage 1	No data	No data
Phenobarbital	Phenobarbital	Sedation	↓ SL, ↓ No. of W, ↑ TST	↓ SL	Significant impairment
Phenytoin	Dilantin	Sedation	↓ SL	No data	Moderate impairment
Primidone	Mysoline	Sedation	↓ SL	No data	No data
Valproic acid	Depakene	Sedation	↑ TST, ↓ No. of W	No negative effect	Mild impairment
Newer Antiepileptic Drugs					
Felbamate	Felbatol	Insomnia in 10%, sedation in 12%	No data	No data	No data
Fosphenytoin	Cerebyx	Sedation	No data	No data	No data
Gabapentin	Neurontin	Sedation in 5–15%	No data	No data	No impairment as add-on therapy
Lamotrigine	Lamictal	Sedation in 4–13%; insomnia in 4%	No data	No data	No data
Tiagabine	Gabitril	Sedation in 0–5%; up to 25% in open-label studies	No data	No data	No impairment as add-on-therapy; improved performance when patients switched from other medications to tiagabine alone
Topiramate	Topamax	Sedation in 15–27%	No data	No data	No data
Vigabatrin	Sabril	Sedation in 7–12%	No effects	No change as add-on to carbamazepine	No impairment as add-on therapy
Zonisamide	Not available in the United States	Sedation in 9–13%	No data	No data	No data

*Placebo-adjusted incidence of sedation listed for the new antiepileptic drugs; placebo-adjusted rates are not available for the older drugs.
MSLT, multiple sleep latency test; PSG, polysomnographic; SL, sleep latency; TST, total sleep time; W, wake.

uation of the effects of antiepileptic drugs on cognitive function difficult. These difficulties notwithstanding, cognitive impairment appears to be more common with phenobarbital than with other drugs, more common when multiple medications are used, and more common in children than in adults. Phenobarbital and phenytoin have most frequently been associated with impaired neuropsychological function, particularly in the areas of short-term memory, concentration, and attention.[293, 310, 313] Carbamazepine and valproate appear to be less impairing.[314] Gabapentin,[315] vigabatrin,[316] and tiagabine[317] used as "add-on" therapy were no different from placebo in tests of cognitive and psychomotor function. Patients who were changed from other antiepileptic agents to tiagabine alone demonstrated improvements in mental ability.[317]

PSEUDOEPHEDRINE AND PHENYLPROPANOLAMINE

Pseudoephedrine and phenylpropanolamine share the pharmacological properties of ephedrine but have less-potent CNS-stimulating effects.[129] These drugs are used extensively as nasal decongestants and are available in a wide variety of over-the-counter cold preparations; phenylpropanolamine is also available in over-the-counter diet aids. Although similar in chemical structure to amphetamine, phenylpropanolamine is much less lipophilic and thus has much less potent CNS effects. Phenylpropanolamine, however, has been reported to increase plasma caffeine levels,[318] possibly adding to the stimulant effect of caffeine. These drugs have been reported to cause insomnia.[319-321] In one study, 27% of patients given 120 mg of extended-release pseudoephedrine for 2 weeks for the treatment of allergic or vasomotor rhinitis complained of insomnia. In a PSG study, the administration of pseudoephedrine in the evening (as part of either a 60-mg q.i.d. or sustained-release 120-mg b.i.d. dosing regimen) produced increased wake time during sleep compared with the morning administration of a once-daily controlled-release formulation (240 mg).[322] Further objective evaluation of dosage, timing, and duration of treatment of these drugs would be useful.

ANORECTIC AGENTS

Dexfenfluramine has been associated with subjective reports of disturbed nocturnal sleep[323] and with daytime complaints of drowsiness (placebo-adjusted incidence of 9%)[324] in patients treated for obesity. In normal subjects, dexfenfluramine caused a dose-related decrease in sleep efficiency.[325] Phentermine, which stimulates the release of dopamine and norepinephrine, has been associated with subjective reports of insomnia.[326] Fenfluramine (which stimulates the release of serotonin), on the other hand, has been associated with subjective sedation.[327] Morning administration of fenfluramine in obese[328] and depressed[329] patients decreased SWS the next night but had no effects on other sleep

variables. Fenfluramine, and sometimes dexfenfluramine, has been combined with phentermine as "fenphen" therapy. Both fenfluramine and dexfenfluramine were removed from the market in September 1997 after reports of valvular heart disease. Sibutramine, a serotonin and nonepinephrine reuptake inhibitor not yet approved for the U.S. market, has also been associated with insomnia in clinical trials.[330]

Acknowledgments

The author thanks James K. Walsh, PhD, for guidance in the development of the manuscript and especially for critical review of earlier drafts. I also thank Gihan A. Kader, MD, for her expertise in preparation of the antiparkinsonian and antiepileptic drug sections of the manuscript.

References

1. Reynolds CF III, Kupfer DJ. Sleep research in affective illness: state of the art circa 1987. Sleep. 1987;10:199–215.
2. Benca RM, Obermeyer WH, Thisted RA, et al. Sleep and psychiatric disorders: a meta-analysis. Arch Gen Psychiatry. 1992;49:651–668.
3. Claghorn JL, Mathew RJ, Weinman ML, et al. Daytime sleepiness in depression. J Clin Psychiatry. 1981;42:342–343.
4. Siegfried K. Cognitive symptoms in late-life depression and their treatment. J Affect Disord. 1985;(suppl 1):533–540.
5. Newman AB, Enright PL, Manolio TA, et al. Sleep disturbance, psychosocial correlates, and cardiovascular disease in 5201 older adults: the Cardiovascular Health Study. J Am Geriatr Soc. 1997;45:1–7.
6. Paradiso S, Lamberty GJ, Garvey MJ, et al. Cognitive impairment in the euthymic phase of chronic unipolar depression. Nerv Ment Dis. 1997;185:748–754.
7. Frazer A. Pharmacology of antidepressants. J Clin Psychopharmacol. 1997;17(suppl 1):2S–18S.
8. Preskorn SH. Pharmacokinetics of antidepressants: why and how they are relevant to treatment. J Clin Psychiatry. 1993;54(suppl):14–34.
9. Preskorn SH. Comparison of the tolerability of bupropion, fluoxetine, imipramine, nefazodone, paroxetine, sertraline, and venlafaxine. J Clin Psychiatry. 1995;56(suppl 6):12–21.
10. Cohen LJ. Rational drug use in the treatment of depression. Pharmacotherapy. 1997;17:45–61.
11. Richelson E. The pharmacology of antidepressants at the synapse: focus on newer compounds. J Clin Psychiatry. 1994;55(suppl A):34–39.
12. Fulton B, Benfield P. Moclobemide: an update of its pharmacological properties and therapeutic use. Drugs. 1996;52:450–474.
13. Obermeyer WH, Benca RM. Effects of drugs on sleep. Neurol Clin. 1996;14:827–840.
14. Buysse D. Drugs affecting sleep, sleepiness, and performance. In: Monk TH, ed. Sleep, Sleepiness and Performance. New York, NY: John Wiley & Sons; 1991:249–306.
15. Volz H-P, Sturm Y. Antidepressant drugs and psychomotor performance. Neuropsychobiology. 1995;31:146–155.
16. Smiley A. Effects of minor tranquilizers and antidepressants on psychomotor performance. J Clin Psychiatry. 1987;48(suppl):22–28.
17. O'Hanlon JF. Antidepressant therapy and behavioural competence. Br J Clin Pract. 1996;50:381–385.
18. Oxman TE. Antidepressants and cognitive impairment in the elderly. J Clin Psychiatry. 1996;57:38–44.
19. Ware JC, Brown FU, Moorad PJ Jr, et al. Nocturnal myoclonus and tricyclic antidepressants. Sleep Res. 1984;13:72.
20. Sakulsripong M, Curran HV, Lader M. Does tolerance develop to the sedative and amnesic effects of antidepressants? A comparison of amitriptyline, trazodone and placebo. Eur J Clin Pharmacol. 1991;40:43–48.
21. Van Laar MW, van Williigenburg APP, Volkerts ER. Acute and subchronic effects of nefazodone and imipramine on highway

driving, cognitive functions, and daytime sleepiness in healthy adult and elderly subjects. J Clin Psychopharmacol. 1995;15:30–40.

22. Remick RA, Froese C, Keller FD. Common side effects associated with monoamine oxidase inhibitors. Prog Neuropsychopharmacol Biol Psychiatry. 1989;13:497–504.

23. Kupfer DJ, Bowers MB Jr. REM sleep and central monoamine oxidase inhibition. Psychopharmacologia. 1972;27:183–190.

24. Nolen WA, Haffmans PMJ, Bouvy PF, et al. Monoamine oxidase inhibitors in resistant major depression: a double-blind comparison of brofaromine and tranylcypromine in patients resistant to tricyclic antidepressants. J Affect Disord. 1993;28:189–197.

25. Teicher MH, Cohen BM, Baldessarini RJ, et al. Severe daytime somnolence in patients treated with an MAOI. Am J Psychiatry. 1988;145:1552–1556.

26. Knegtering H, Eijck M, Huijsman A. Effects of antidepressants on cognitive functioning of elderly patients: a review. Drugs Aging. 1994;5:192–199.

27. Georgortas A, Reisberg B, Ferris S. First results on the effects of MAO inhibitor on cognitive functioning in elderly depressed patients. Arch Gerontol Geriatr. 1983;2:249–254.

28. Raskin A, Friedman AS, Dimascio A. Effects of chlorpromazine, imipramine, diazepam and phenelzine on psychomotor and cognitive skills of depressed patients. Psychopharmacol Bull. 1983;19:649–652.

29. Laux G, Classen W, Sofie E, et al. Clinical, biochemical and psychometric findings with the new MAO-A-inhibitors moclobemide and brofaromine in patients with major depressive disorder. J Neural Transm Suppl. 1990;32:189–195.

30. Volz H-P, Faltus F, Magyar I, et al. Brofaromine in treatment-resistant depressed patients: a comparative trial versus tranylcypromine. J Affect Disord. 1994;30:209–217.

31. Monti JM, Alterwain P, Monti D. The effects of moclobemide on nocturnal sleep of depressed patients. J Affect Disord. 1990;20:201–208.

32. Minot R, Luthringer R, Macher JP. Effect of moclobemide on the psychophysiology of sleep/wake cycles: a neuroelectrophysiological study of depressed patients administered with moclobemide. Int Clin Psychopharmacol. 1993;7:181–189.

33. Allain H, Lieury A, Brunet-Bourgin F, et al. Antidepressants and cognition: comparative effects of moclobemide, viloxazine and maprotiline. Psychopharmacology. 1992;106:S56–S61.

34. Pancheri P, Delle Chiaie R, Donnini M, et al. Effects of moclobemide on depressive symptoms and cognitive performance in a geriatric population: a controlled comparative study versus imipramine. Clin Neuropharmacol. 1994;17(suppl 1):S58–S73.

35. Roth M, Mountjoy CQ, Amrein R, and the International Collaborative Study Group. Moclobemide in elderly patients with cognitive decline and depression: an international double-blind, placebo-controlled trial. Br J Psychiatry. 1996;168:149–157.

36. Galderisi S, Mucci A, Bucci P, et al. Influence of moclobemide on cognitive functions of nine depressed patients: pilot trial with neurophysiological and neuropsychological indices. Neuropsychobiology. 1996;33:48–54.

37. Hindmarch I, Kerr J. Behavioural toxicity of antidepressants with particular reference to moclobemide. Psychopharmacology. 1992;106:S49–S55.

38. Tiller JWG. Antidepressants, alcohol and psychomotor performance. Acta Psychiatr Scand. 1990;(suppl 360):13–17.

39. Ramaekers JG, van Veggel LM, O'Hanlon JF. A cross-study comparison of the effects of moclobemide and brofaromine on actual driving performance and estimated sleep. Clin Neuropharmacol. 1994;17(suppl 1):S9–S18.

40. Warot D, Berlin I, Patat A, et al. Effects of befloxatone, a reversible selective monoamine oxidase-A inhibitor, on psychomotor function and memory in healthy subjects. J Clin Pharmacol. 1996;36:942–950.

41. Grimsley SR, Jann MW. Paroxetine, sertraline, and fluvoxamine: new selective serotonin reuptake inhibitors. Clin Pharm. 1992;11:930–957.

42. Bech P, Ciadella P. Citalopram in depression: meta-analysis of intended and unintended effects. Int Clin Psychopharmacol. 1992;6(suppl 5):45–54.

43. Cooper GL. The safety of fluoxetine: An update. Br J Psychiatry. 1988;153(suppl 3):77–86.

44. Rickels K, Schweizer E. Clinical overview of serotonin reuptake inhibitors. J Clin Psychiatry. 1990;51(suppl B):9–12.

45. Nicholson AN, Pascoe PA. Studies on the modulation of the sleep-wakefulness continuum in man by fluoxetine, a 5-HT uptake inhibitor. Neuropharmacology. 1988;27:597–602.

46. Ciapparelli A, Dani A, Figura A, et al. The effects of fluoxetine (FL) on sleep pattern: a clinical and all-night EEG study in patients with major depression. J Sleep Res. 1992;1:41.

47. Hendrickse WA, Roffwarg HP, Graennemann BD, et al. The effects of fluoxetine on the polysomnogram of depressed outpatients: a pilot study. Neuropsychopharmacology. 1994;10:85–91.

48. Kerkhofs M, Rielaert C, de Maertelaer V, et al. Fluoxetine in major depression: efficacy, safety and effects on sleep polygraphic variables. Int Clin Psychopharmacol. 1990;5:253–260.

49. Dorsey CM, Lukas SE, Cunningham SL. Fluoxetine-induced sleep disturbance in depressed patients. Neuropsychopharmacology. 1996;14:437–442.

50. Schenck, CH, Mahowald MW, Kim SW, et al. Prominent eye movements during NREM sleep and REM sleep behavior disorder associated with fluoxetine treatment of depression and obsessive-compulsive disorder. Sleep. 1992;15:226–235.

51. Oswald I, Adam K. Effects of paroxetine on human sleep. Br J Clin Pharmacol. 1986;22:97–99.

52. Saletu B, Frey R, Krupka M, et al. Sleep laboratory studies on the single-dose effects of serotonin reuptake inhibitors paroxetine and fluoxetine on human sleep and awakening qualities. Sleep. 1991;14:439–447.

53. Sharpley AL, Williamson DJ, Attenburrow MEJ, et al. The effects of paroxetine and nefazodone on sleep: a placebo controlled trial. Psychopharmacology. 1996;126:50–54.

54. Staner L, Kerkhofs M, Detroux D, et al. Acute, subchronic and withdrawal sleep EEG changes during treatment with paroxetine and amitriptyline: a double-blind randomized trial in major depression. Sleep. 1995;18:470–477.

55. Kupfer DJ, Perel JM, Pollock BG, et al. Fluvoxamine versus desipramine: comparative polysomnographic effects. Biol Psychiatry. 1991;29:23–40.

56. van Bemmel AL, van den Hoofdakker RH, Beersma DG, et al. Changes in sleep polygraphic variables and clinical state in depressed patients during treatment with citalopram. Psychopharmacology. 1993;113:225–230.

57. Haria M, Fitton A, McTavish D. Trazodone: a review of its pharmacology, therapeutic use in depression and therapeutic potential in other disorders. Drugs Aging. 1994;4:331–355.

58. Rawls WN. Trazodone. Drug Intell Clin Pharm. 1982;16:7–13.

59. Beasley CM, Dornseif BE, Pultz JA, et al. Fluoxetine versus trazodone: efficacy and activating-sedating effects. J Clin Psychiatry. 1991;52:294–299.

60. Cunningham LA, Borison RL, Carman JS, et al. A comparison of venlafaxine, trazodone, and placebo in major depression. J Clin Psychopharmacol. 1994;14:99–106.

61. Metz A, Shader RI. Adverse interactions encountered when using trazodone to treat insomnia associated with fluoxetine. Int Clin Psychopharmacol. 1990;5:191–194.

62. Curran HV, Sakulsripong M, Lader M. Antidepressants and human memory: an investigation of four drugs with different sedative and anticholinergic profiles. Psychopharmacology. 1988;95:520–527.

63. Fudge JL, Perry PJ, Garvey MJ, et al. A comparison of the effect of fluoxetine and trazodone on the cognitive functioning of depressed outpatients. J Affect Disord. 1990;18:275–280.

64. Botros WA, Ankier SI, McManus IC, et al. Clinical assessment and performance tasks in depression: a comparison of amitriptyline and trazodone. Br J Psychiatry. 1989;155:479–482.

65. Goldberg RJ. Antidepressant use in the elderly: current status of nefazodone, venlafaxine and moclobemide. Drugs Aging. 1997;11:119–131.

66. Augustin BG, Cold JA, Jann MW. Venlafaxine and nefazodone, two pharmacologically distinct antidepressants. Pharmacotherapy. 1997;17:511–530.

67. Robinson DS, Roberts DL, Smith JM, et al. The safety profile of nefazodone. J Clin Psychiatry. 1996;57(suppl 2):31–38.

68. Vogel G, Cohen J, Mullis D, et al. Nefazodone and REM sleep: how do antidepressant drugs decrease REM sleep? Sleep. 1998;21:70–77.

69. Frewer LJ, Lader M. The effects of nefazodone, imipramine, and placebo, alone and combined with alcohol, in normal subjects. Int Clin Psychopharmacol. 1993;8:13–20.

70. Nelson JC. Safety and tolerability of the new antidepressants. J Clin Psychiatry. 1997;58(suppl 6):26–31.

71. Rudolph RL, Fabre LF, Feighner JP, et al. A randomized, placebo-controlled, dose-response trial of venlafaxine hydrochloride in the treatment of major depression. J Clin Psychiatry. 1998;59:116–122.

72. Salin-Pascual RJ, Galicia-Polo L, Drucker-Colin R. Sleep changes after 4 consecutive days of venlafaxine administration in normal volunteers. J Clin Psychiatry. 1997;58:348–350.

73. Luthringer R, Toussaint M, Schaltenbrand N, et al. A double-blind, placebo-controlled evaluation of the effects of orally administered venlafaxine on sleep in inpatients with major depression. Psychopharmacol Bull. 1996;32:637–646.

74. Saletu B, Grunberger J, Anderer P, et al. Pharmacodynamics of venlafaxine evaluated by EEG brain mapping, psychometry and psychophysiology. Br J Clin Pharmacol. 1992;33:589–601.

75. Smith WT, Glaudin V, Panagides J, et al. Mirtazapine vs. amitriptyline vs. placebo in the treatment of major depressive disorder. Psychopharmacology Bull. 1990;20:191–196.

76. Nutt D. Mirtazapine: pharmacology in relation to adverse effects. Acta Psychiatr Scand Suppl. 1997;391:31–37.

77. Halikas JA. Org 3770 (mirtazapine) versus trazodone: a placebo controlled trial in depressed elderly patients. Hum Psychopharmacol. 1995;10:S125–S133.

78. Montgomery SA. Safety of mirtazapine: a review. Int Clin Psychopharmacol. 1995;10(suppl 4):37–45.

79. Stimmel GL, Dopheide JA, Stahl SM. Mirtazapine: an antidepressant with noradrenergic and specific serotonergic effects. Pharmacotherapy. 1997;17:10–21.

80. Mattila M, Mattila MJ, Vrijmoed-de M, et al. Actions and interactions of psychotropic drugs on human performance and mood: single doses of ORG 3770, amitriptyline, and diazepam. Pharmacol Toxicol. 1989;65:81–88.

81. Andrews JM, Nemeroff CB. Contemporary management of depression. Am J Med. 1994;97(suppl 6A):24S–32S.

82. Nofzinger EA, Reynolds CF, Thase ME, et al. REM sleep enhancement by bupropion in depressed men. Am J Psychiatry. 1995;152:274–276.

83. Hayes PE, Kristoff CA. Adverse reactions to five new antidepressants. Clin Pharmacy. 1986;5:471–480.

84. Raemakers JG, Swijgman, O'Hanlon JF. Effects of moclobemide and mianserin on highway driving, psychometric performance and subjective parameters, relative to placebo. Psychopharmacology. 1992;106(suppl):S62–S67.

85. Buysse DJ. Drugs affecting sleep, sleepiness and performance. In: Monk TH, ed. Sleep, Sleepiness, and Performance. New York, NY: John Wiley & Sons; 1991:249–306.

86. Hudson JK, Lipinski JF, Keck PE, et al. Polysomnographic characteristics of young manic patients: comparison with unipolar depressed patients and normal control subjects. Arch Gen Psychiatry. 1992;49:378–383.

87. Linnoila M, Rudorfer MV, Dubryoski KV, et al. Effects of one-week lithium treatment on skilled performance, information processing, and mood in healthy volunteers. J Clin Psychopharmacol. 1986;6:356–359.

88. Judd LL, Hubbard B, Janowsky DS, et al. The effect of lithium carbonate on the cognitive functions of normal subjects. Arch Gen Psychiatry. 1977;34:355–357.

89. Squire LR, Judd, LL, Janowsky DS, et al. Effects of lithium carbonate on memory and other cognitive functions. Am J Psychiatry. 1980;137:1042–1046.

90. Hatcher S, Sims R, Thompson D. The effects of chronic lithium treatment on psychomotor performance related to driving. Br J Psychiatry. 1990;157:275–27.

91. Kocsis JH, Shaw ED, Stokes PE, et al. Neuropsychologic effects of lithium discontinuation. J Clin Psychopharmacol. 1993;13:268–275.

92. Lauer CJ, Schreiber W, Pollmacher T, et al. Sleep in schizophrenia: a polysomnographic study on drug-naive patients. Neuropsychopharmacology. 1997;16:51–60.

93. Mortimer AM. Cognitive function in schizophrenia: do neuroleptics make a difference? Pharmacol Biochem Behav. 1997;56:789–795.

94. Wetter TC, Lauer CL, Gillich G, et al. The electroencephalographic sleep pattern in schizophrenic patients treated with clozapine or classical antipsychotic drugs. J Psychiatr Res. 1996;30:411–419.

95. Casey DE. The relationship of pharmacology to side effects. J Clin Psychiatry. 1997;58(suppl 10):55–62.

96. Gerlach J, Peacock L. New antipsychotics: the present status. Int Clin Psychopharmacol. 1995;10(suppl 3):39–48.

97. Casey DE. Side effect profiles of new antipsychotic agents. J Clin Psychiatry. 1996;57(suppl 11):40–45.

98. Trosch RM, Friedman JH, Lannon MC, et al. Clozapine for the treatment-resistant schizophrenic: a double-blind comparison with chloropromazine. Arch Gen Psychiatry. 1988;45:789–796.

99. Fitton A, Heel RC. Clozapine: a review of its pharmacological properties and therapeutic use in schizophrenia. Drugs. 1990;40:722–747.

100. Fleischhacker WW, Hummer M, Kurz M, et al. Clozapine dose in the United States and Europe: implications for therapeutic and adverse effects. J Clin Psychiatry. 1994;55(suppl B):78–81.

101. Marder SR, Meibach RC. Risperidone in the treatment of schizophrenia. Am J Psychiatry. 1994;151:825–835.

102. Beasley CM, Tollefson G, Tran P, et al. Olanzapine versus placebo and haloperidol: acute phase results of the North American double-blind olanzapine trial. Neuropsychopharmacology. 1996;14:111–123.

103. van Kammen DP, McEvoy JP, Targum S, et al. A randomized, controlled, dose-ranging trial of sertindole in patients with schizophrenia. Psychopharmacology. 1996;124:168–175.

104. Small JG, Hirsch SR, Arvanitis LA, et al, and the Seroquel Study Group. Quetiapine in patients with schizophrenia: a high- and low-dose double-blind comparison with placebo. Arch Gen Psychiatry. 1997;54:549–557.

105. Peretti CS, Danion JM, Dauffmann-Muller, F, et al. Effects of haloperidol and amisulpride on motor and cognitive skill learning in healthy volunteers. Psychopharmacology. 1997;131:329–338.

106. Vitiello B, Martin A, Hill J, et al. Cognitive and behavioral effects of cholinergic, dopaminergic, and serotonergic blockade in humans. Neuropsychopharmacology. 1997;16:15–24.

107. McClelland GR, Cooper SM, Pilgrim AJ. A comparison of the central nervous system effects of haloperidol, chlorpromazine and sulpiride in normal volunteers. Br J Clin Pharmacol. 1990;30:795–803.

108. Cassens G, Inglis AK, Appelbaum PS, et al. Neuroleptics: effects on neuropsychological function in chronic schizophrenic patients. Schizophr Bull. 1990;16:477–499.

109. Medalia A, Gold JM, Merriam A. The effects of neuroleptics on neuropsychological test results of schizophrenics. Arch Clin Neuropsychol. 1988;3:249–271.

110. Spohn HE, Strauss ME. Relation of neuroleptic and anticholinergic medications to cognitive functions in schizophrenia. J Abnorm Psychol. 1989;98:367–380.

111. Goldberg TE, Weinberger DR. Effects of neuroleptic medications on the cognition of patients with schizophrenia: a review of recent studies. J Clin Psychiatry. 1996;57(suppl 9):62–65.

112. Stip E, Lussier I. The effect of risperidone on cognition in patients with schizophrenia. Can J Psychiatry 1996;41(suppl 2):S35–S40.

113. Earle-Boyer EA, Serper MR, Davidson M, et al. Continuous performance tests in schizophrenic patients: stimulus and medication effects on performance. Psychiatry Res. 1991;37:47–56.

114. Gallhofer B, Bauer U, Lis S, et al. Cognitive dysfunction in schizophrenia: comparison of treatment with atypical antipsychotic agents and conventional neuroleptic drugs. Eur Neuropsychopharmacol. 1996;6(suppl 2):S13–S20.

115. Buchanan RW, Holstein C, Breier A. The comparative efficacy and long-term effect of clozapine treatment on neuropsychological test performance. Biol Psychiatry. 1994;36:717–725.

116. Lee MA, Thompson PA, Meltzer HY. Effects of clozapine on cognitive function in schizophrenia. J Clin Psychiatry. 1994;55(suppl B):82–87.

117. Fujii DE, Ahmed I, Jokumsen M, et al. The effects of clozapine on cognitive functioning in treatment-resistant schizophrenic patients. J Neuropsychiatry Clin Neurosci. 1997;9:240–245.

118. Ashton H. The effect of drugs on sleep. In: Cooper R, ed. Sleep. London, England: Chapman and Hall Medical; 1994:175–211.

119. Goa KL, Ward A. Buspirone: a preliminary review of its pharmacological properties and therapeutic efficacy as an anxiolytic. Drugs. 1986;32:114–129.

120. Schnabel T. Evaluation of the safety and side effects of antianxiety agents. Am J Med. 1987;82(suppl 5a):7–13.

121. Seidel WF, Cohen SA, Wilson I, et al. Effects of alprazolam and diazepam on the daytime sleepiness of non-anxious subjects. Psychopharmacology. 1985;87:194–197.

122. van Laar, MW, Volkerts ER, van Willigenburg APP. Therapeutic effects and effects on actual driving performance of chronically administered buspirone and diazepam in anxious outpatients. J Clin Psychopharmacol. 1992;12:86–95.

123. O'Hanlon JF, Vermeeren A, Uiterwijk MMC, et al. Anxiolytics' effects on the actual driving performance of patients and healthy volunteers in a standardized test. Neuropsychobiology. 1995;31:81–88.

124. Smiley A. Effect of minor tranquilizers and antidepressants on psychomotor performance. J Clin Psychiatry. 1987;48(suppl):22–28.

125. Pomara N, Tun H, DaSilva D, et al. The acute and chronic performance effects of alprazolam and lorazepam in the elderly: relationship to duration of treatment and self-rated sedation. Psychopharmacol Bull. 1998;34:139–153.

126. Eison AS, Temple DL. Buspirone: review of its pharmacology and current perspectives on its mechanism of action. Am J Med. 1986;80(suppl 3):61–68.

127. O'Hanlon JF. Review of buspirone's effect on human performance and related variables. Eur Neuropsychopharmacol. 1991;1:489–501.

128. Jann MW. Buspirone: an update on a unique anxiolytic agent. Pharmacotherapy. 1988;8:100–116.

129. Hardman JG, Limbird LE, Molinoff PB, et al. Goodman and Gilman's The Pharmacological Basis of Therapeutics. 9th ed. New York, NY: McGraw-Hill; 1996.

130. Newton RE, Casten GP, Alms DR, et al. The side effect profile of buspirone in comparison to active controls and placebo. J Clin Psychiatry. 1982;43:100–102.

131. Cohn JB, Wilcox CS. Low-sedation potential of buspirone compared with alprazolam and lorazepam in the treatment of anxious patients: a double-blind study. J Clin Psychiatry. 1986;47:409–412.

132. Seidel WF, Cohen SA, Bliwise NG, et al. Buspirone: an anxiolytic without sedative effect. Psychopharmacology. 1985;87:371–373.

133. Greenblatt DJ, Harmatz JS, Gouthro TA, et al. Distinguishing a benzodiazepine agonist (triazolam) from a nonagonist anxiolytic (buspirone) by electroencephalography: kinetic-dynamic studies. Clin Pharmacol Ther. 1994;56:100–111.

134. Rosen RC, Kostis JB. Biobehavioral sequellae associated with adrenergic-inhibiting antihypertensive agents: a critical review. Health Psychol. 1985;4:579–604.

135. McAinsh J, Cruickshank JM. Beta-blockers and central nervous system side effects. Pharmacology. 1990;46:163–197.

136. Monti J. Minireview: disturbances of sleep and wakefulness associated with the use of antihypertensive agents. Life Sci. 1987;41:1979–1988.

137. Dahlof C, Dimenas E, Kendall M, et al. Quality of life in cardiovascular diseases: emphasis on β-blocker treatment. Circulation. 1991;84(suppl 6):VI108–VI118.

138. Yamada Y, Shibuya F, Hamada J, et al. Prediction of sleep disorders induced by β-adrenergic receptor blocking agents based on receptor occupancy. J Pharmacokinet Biopharm. 1995;23:131–145.

139. Dimsdale J, Newton R, Joist T. Neuropsychologic side effects of beta blockers. Arch Int Med. 1989;149:514–525.

140. Muldoon MF, Manuck SB, Shapiro AP, et al. Neurobehavioral effects of antihypertensive medications. J Hypertens. 1991;9:549–555.

141. Gleiter CH, Deckert J. Adverse CNS-effects of beta-adrenoceptor blockers. Pharmacopsychiatry. 1996;29:201–211.

142. Paykel ES, Fleminger R, Watson JP. Psychiatric side effects of antihypertensive drugs other than reserpine. J Clin Psychopharmacol. 1982;2:14–39.

143. Conant J, Engler R, Janowsky D, et al. Central nervous system side effects of β-adrenergic blocking agents with high and low lipid solubility. J Cardiovasc Pharmacol. 1989;13:656–661.

144. Kostis JB, Rosen RC. Central nervous system effects of β-adrenergic-blocking drugs: the role of ancillary properties. Circulation. 1987;75:204–212.

145. Betts TA, Alford C. Beta-blockers and sleep: a controlled trial. Eur J Clin Pharmacol. 1988;28(suppl):65–68.

146. Bender W, Greil W, Ruther E, et al. Effects of the beta-adrenoceptor blocking agent sotalol on CNS: sleep, EEG, and psychophysiological parameters. J Clin Pharmacol. 1979:505–512.

147. van den Heuvel C, Reid K, Dawson D. Effect of atenolol on nocturnal sleep and temperature in young men: reversal by pharmacological doses of melatonin. Physiol Behav. 1997;61:795–802.

148. Drayer ED. Lipophilicity, hydrophilicity, and the central nervous system side effects of beta blockers. Pharmacotherapy. 1987;7:87–91.

149. Dawson D, Encel N. Melatonin and sleep in humans. J Pineal Res. 1993;14:234–256.

150. Brismar K, Hylander B, Eliasson K, et al. Melatonin secretion related to side-effects of β-blockers from the central nervous system. Acta Med Scand. 1988;223:525–530.

151. Kostis JB, Rosen RC, Holzer BC, et al. CNS side effects of centrally-active antihypertensive agents: a prospective, placebo-controlled study of sleep, mood state, and cognitive and sexual function in hypertensive males. Psychopharmacology. 1990;102:163–170.

152. Webster J, Koch H-F. Aspects of tolerability of centrally acting antihypertensive drugs. J Cardiovasc Pharmacol. 1996;27(suppl 3):S49–S54.

153. Kanno O, Clarenbach P. Effects of clonidine and yohimbine on sleep in man: polygraphic study and EEG analysis by normalized slope descriptors. Electroencephalogr Clin Neurophysiol. 1985;60:478–484.

154. Carskadon MA, Cavallo A, Rosekind MR. Sleepiness and nap sleep following a morning dose of clonidine. Sleep. 1989;12:338–344.

155. Solomon S, Hotchkiss E, Saravary M, et al. Impairment of memory function by antihypertensive medication. Arch Gen Psychiatry. 1983;40:1109–1112.

156. Croog SH, Levine S, Testa MA, et al. The effects of antihypertensive therapy on the quality of life. N Engl J Med. 1986;314:1657–1664.

157. Pearce CJ, Wallin JD. Labetalol and other agents that block both alpha- and beta-adrenergic receptors. Cleve Clin J Med. 1994;61:59–69.

158. Dunn CJ, Lea AP, Wagstaff AJ. Carvedilol: a reappraisal of its pharmacological properties and therapeutic use in cardiovascular disorders. Drugs. 1997;54:161–185.

159. Staessen J, Fagard R, Lijnen P, et al. Double-blind comparison of ketanserin and propranolol in hypertensive patients. J Cardiovasc Pharmacol. 1988;12:718–725.

160. Idzikowski C, Mills FJ, James RJ. A dose-response study examining the effects of ritanserin on human slow wave sleep. Br J Clin Pharmacol. 1991;31:193–196.

161. Adam K, Oswald I. Effects of repeated ritanserin on middle-aged poor sleepers. Psychopharmacology. 1989;99:219–221.

162. Paiva T, Arriaga F, Wauquier A, et al. Effects of ritanserin on sleep disturbances of dysthymic patients. Psychopharmacology. 1988;96:395–399.

163. Lammers GJ, Arends J, Declerck AC, et al. Ritanserin, a 5-HT2 receptor blocker, as add-on treatment in narcolepsy. Sleep. 1991;14:130–132.

164. Reid JL. New therapeutic agents for hypertension. Br J Clin Pharmacol. 1996;42:37–41.

165. Yu A, Frishman WH. Imidazoline receptor agonist drugs: a new approach to the treatment of systemic hypertension. J Clin Pharmacol. 1996;36:98–111.

166. Fillastre JP, Letac B, Galiniere F, et al. A multicenter double-blind comparative study of rilmenidine and clonidine in 333 hypertensive patients. Am J Cardiol. 1988;61(suppl):81D–85D.

167. Planitz V. Comparison of moxonidine and clonidine HCl in treating patients with hypertension. J Clin Pharmacol. 1984;27:46–51.

168. Levine S, Croog SH, Sudilovsky A, et al. Effects of antihypertensive medications on vitality and well-being. J Fam Pract. 1987;25:357–363.

169. Paran E, Anson O, Neumann L. The effects of replacing beta-blockers with an angiotensin converting enzyme inhibitor on the quality of life of hypertensive patients. Am J Hypertens. 1996;9:1206–1213.

170. Weit MR, Flack JM, Applegate WB. Tolerability, safety, and quality of life and hypertensive therapy: the case for low-dose diuretics. Am J Med. 1996;101(suppl 3A):83S–92S.

171. Dietrich B, Herrmann WM. Influence of cilazapril on memory functions and sleep behaviour in comparison with metoprolol and placebo in healthy subjects. Br J Clin Pharmacol. 1989;27(suppl 2):249S–261S.

172. Goldstein G, Materson BJ, Cushman WC, et al. Treatment of hypertension in the elderly, II: cognitive and behavioral function. Hypertension. 1990;15:361–369.

173. Lasser NL, Nash J, Lasser VI, et al. Effects of antihypertensive therapy on blood pressure control, cognition, and reactivity. Am J Med. 1989;86(suppl 1B):98–103.

174. Williams GH, Croog SH, Levine S, et al. Impact of antihypertensive therapy on quality of life: effect of hydrochlorothiazide. J Hypertens. 1987;5(suppl 1):S29–S35.

175. Harron DWG, Hasson B, Regan M, et al. Effects of rilmenidine and clonidine on the electroencephalogram, saccadic eye movements, and psychomotor function. J Cardiovasc Pharmacol. 1995;26(suppl 2):S48–S54.

176. Wesnes K, Simpson PM, Jansson B, et al. Moxonidine and cognitive function: interactions with moclobemide and lorazepam. Eur J Clin Pharmacol. 1997;52:351–358.

177. Tobert JA, Shear CL, Chremos AN, et al. Clinical experience with lovastatin. Am J Cardiol. 1990;65:23–26.

178. Rosenson RS, Goranson NL. Lovastatin-associated sleep and mood disturbances. Am J Med. 1993;95:548–549.

179. Bradford RH, Shear CL, Chremos AN, et al. Expanded Clinical Evaluation of Lovastatin (EXCEL) study results, I: efficacy in modifying plasma lipoproteins and adverse event profile in 8245 patients with moderate hypercholesterolemia. Arch Intern Med. 1991;151:43–49.

180. Santanello NC, Barber BL, Applegate WB, et al. Effect of pharmacologic lipid lowering on health-related quality of life in older persons: results from the Cholesterol Reduction in Seniors Program (CRISP) pilot study. J Am Geriatric Soc. 1997;45:8–14.

181. Keech AC, Armitage JM, Wallendszus KR, et al. Absence of effects of prolonged simvastatin therapy on nocturnal sleep in a large randomized placebo-controlled study. Br J Clin Pharmacol. 1996;42:483–490.

182. Vgontzas AN, Kales A, Bixler EO, et al. Effects of lovastatin and pravastatin on sleep efficiency and sleep stages. Clin Pharmacol Ther. 1991;50:730–737.

183. Roth T, Richardson GR, Sullivan JP, et al. Comparative effects of pravastatin and lovastatin on nighttime sleep and daytime performance. Clin Cardiol. 1992;15:426–432.

184. Kostis JB, Rosen RB, Wilson AC. Central nervous system effects of HMG CoA reductase on sleep and cognitive performance in patients with hypercholesterolemia. J Clin Pharmacol. 1994;34:989–996.

185. Eckernas SA, Roos BE, Kvidal P, et al. The effects of simvastatin and pravastatin on objective and subjective measures of nocturnal sleep: a comparison of two structurally different HMG CoA reductase inhibitors in patients with primary moderate hypercholesterolaemia. Br J Clin Pharmacol. 1993;35:284–289.

186. Kruyer WB, Hickman JR Jr. Medication-induced performance decrements: cardiovascular medications. J Occup Med. 1990;32:342–349.

187. Michelson EL, Dreifus LS. Newer antiarrhythmic drugs: cardiovascular pharmacotherapy II. Med Clin North Am. 1988;72:275–319.

188. Estelle F, Simons R. H_1-receptor antagonists: comparative tolerability and safety. Drug Safety. 1994;10:350–380.

189. Passalacqua G, Bousquet J, Bachert C, et al. The clinical safety of H_1-receptor antagonists: an EAACI position paper. Allergy. 1996;51:666–675.

190. Meltzer EO. Performance effects of antihistamines. J Allergy Clin Immunol. 1990;86:613–619.

191. Nolen TM. Sedative effects of antihistamines: safety, performance, learning, and quality of life. Clin Ther. 1997;19:39–55.

192. Rombaut NEI, Hindmarch I. Psychometric aspects of antihistamines: a review. Hum Psychopharmacol. 1994;9:157–169.

193. White JN, Rumbold GR. Behavioural effects of histamine and its antagonists: a review. Psychopharmacology. 1988;95:1–14.

194. Gonzales MA, Estes KS. Pharmacokinetic overview of oral second-generation H1 antihistamines. Int J Clin Pharmacol Ther. 1998;36:292–300.

195. Gilmore TM, Alexander BH, Mueller BA, et al. Occupational injuries and medication use. Am J Indust Med. 1996;30:234–239.

196. Starmer G. Antihistamines and highway safety. Accid Anal Prev. 1985;17:311–317.

197. Roth T, Roehrs T, Koshorek G, et al. Sedative effects of antihistamines. J Allergy Clin Immunol. 1987;80:94–98.

198. Roehrs TA, Tietz EI, Zorick FJ, et al. Daytime sleepiness and antihistamines. Sleep. 1984;7:137–141.

199. Seidel WF, Cohen S, Bliwise NG, et al. Cetirizine effects on objective measures of daytime sleepiness and performance. Ann Allergy. 1987;59:58–62.

200. Schweitzer PK, Muehlbach MJ, Walsh JK. Sleepiness and performance during three-day administration of cetirizine or diphenhydramine. J Allergy Clin Immunol. 1994;94:716–724.

201. Donnelly F, Rihoux JP, DeVos C. Sedative effects of antihistamines: safety, performance, learning, and quality of life. Clin Ther. 1998;20:365–372.

202. Simons FER, Fraser TG, Reggin JD, et al. Comparison of the central nervous system effects produced by six H_1-receptor antagonists. Clin Exp Allergy. 1996;26:1092–1097.

203. Falliers CJ, Brandon ML, Buchman E, et al. Double-blind comparison of cetirizine and placebo in the treatment of seasonal rhinitis. Ann Allergy. 1991;66:257–262.

204. Ramaekers JG, Uiterwijk MM, O'Hanlon JF. Effects of loratadine and cetirizine on actual driving and psychometric test performance, and EEG during driving. Eur J Clin Pharmacol. 1992;42:363–369.

205. Gengo FM, Gabos C. Antihistamines, drowsiness, and psychomotor impairment: central nervous system effect of cetirizine. Ann Allergy. 1987;59:53–57.

206. Gengo FM, Manning C. A review of the effects of antihistamines on mental processes related to automobile driving. J Allergy Clin Immunol. 1990;86:1034–1039.

207. Spencer CM, Faulds D, Peters DH. Cetirizine: a reappraisal of its pharmacological properties and therapeutic use in selected allergic disorders. Drugs. 1993;46:1055–1080.

208. Aso T, Sakai Y. Effects of terfenadine on actual driving performance. Jpn J Clin Pharmacol Ther. 1988;19:681–688.

209. Betts T, Markham D, Debenham S, et al. Effects of two antihistamine drugs on actual driving performance. Br Med J. 1984;288:281–282.

210. O'Hanlon JF, Ramaekers JG. Antihistamines effects on actual driving performance in a standardized test: a summary of Dutch experience, 1989–94. Allergy. 1995;50:234–242.

211. Walsh JK, Muehlbach MJ, Schweitzer PK. Simulated assembly line performance following ingestion of cetirizine or hydroxyzine. Ann Allergy. 1992;69:195–200.

212. Hindmarch I. Psychometric aspects of antihistamines. Allergy. 1990;50:48–54.

213. Dahl RE, Bernheisel-Broadbent J, Scanlon-Holdford S, et al. Sleep disturbances in children with atopic dermatitis. Arch Pediatr Adolesc Med. 1995;149:856–860.

214. Vuurman EF, van Veggel LM, Uiterwijk MM, et al. Seasonal allergic rhinitis and antihistamine effects on children's learning. Ann Allergy. 1993;71:121–126.

215. Vuurman EFPM, van Veggel LMA, Sanders RL, et al. Effects of Semprex-D and diphenhydramine on learning in young adults with seasonal rhinitis. Ann Allergy Asthma Immunol. 1996;76:247–252.

216. Spaeth J, Klimek L, Mosges R. Sedation in allergic rhinitis is caused by the condition and not by antihistamine treatment. Allergy. 1996;51:893–906.

217. Goetz DW, Jacobson JM, Murnane JE, et al. Prolongation of simple and choice reaction time in a double-blind comparison of twice-daily hydroxyzine versus terfenadine. J Allergy Clin Immunol. 1989;84:316–322.

218. Volkerts ER, van Willigenburg APP, van Laar MW, et al. Does cetirizine belong to the new generation of antihistamines? An investigation into its acute and subchronic effects on highway driving, psychometric test performance and daytime sleepiness. Hum Psychopharmacol. 1992;7:227–238.

219. Kay GG, Berman B, Mockoviak SH, et al. Initial and steady-state effects of diphenhydramine and loratadine on sedation, cognition, mood, and psychomotor performance. Arch Intern Med. 1997;157:2350–2356.

220. Jonsson KA, Eriksson SE, Kagevi I, et al. No detectable concentrations of oxmetidine but measurable concentrations of cimetidine in cerebrospinal fluid (CSF) during multiple dose treatment. Br J Clin Pharmacol. 1984;17:781–782.

221. Berlin RG. Effects of H2-receptor antagonists on the central nervous system. Drug Dev Res. 1989;17:97–108.

222. Penston J, Wormsley KG. Adverse reactions and interactions with H2-receptor antagonists. Med Toxicol. 1986;1:192–216.

223. Lipsy RJ, Fennerty B, Fagan T. Clinical review of histamine2 receptor antagonists. Arch Intern Med. 1990;150:745–751.

224. Smith S, Dendall M. Ranitidine versus cimetidine: a comparison of their potential to cause clinically important drug interactions. Clin Pharmacokinet. 1988;15:44–56.

225. Orr WC, Duke JC, Imes NK, et al. Comparative effects of H2-receptor antagonists on subjective and objective assessments of sleep. Aliment Pharmacol Ther. 1994;8:203–207.

226. Nicholson AN, Stome BM. The H2-antagonists, cimetidine and ranitidine: studies on performance. Eur J Clin Pharmacol. 1984;26:579–582.

227. Theofilopoulos N, Szabadi E, Bradshaw CM. Comparison of the effects of ranitidine, cimetidine, and thioridazine on psychomotor functions in healthy volunteers. Br J Clin Pharmacol. 1984;18:135–144.

228. Schentag JJ. Cimetidine-associated mental confusion: further studies in 36 severely ill patients. Ther Drug Monit. 1980;78:791–795.

229. Slugg PH, Haug MT III, Pippenger CE. Ranitidine pharmacokinetics and adverse central nervous system reactions. Arch Intern Med. 1992;152:2325–2329.

230. Sanders LD, Whitehead C, Gildersleve CD, et al. Interaction of H2-receptor antagonists and benzodiazepine sedation. Anaesthesia. 1993;48:286–292.

231. Gallant C, Kenny P. Oral glucocorticoids and their complications. J Am Acad Dermatol. 1986;14:161–177.

232. Searle JP, Compton MR. Side-effects of corticosteroid agents. Med J Aust. 1986;144:139–142.

233. Ling MH, Perry PJ, Tsuang MT. Side effects of corticosteroid therapy: psychiatric aspects. Arch Gen Psychiatry. 1981;38:471–477.

234. Chrousos GA, Kattah JC, Beck RW, et al, and the Optic Neuritis Study Group. Side effects of glucocorticoid treatment: experience of the optic neuritis treatment trial. JAMA. 1993;269:2110–2112.

235. Drigan R, Spirito A, Gelber RD. Behavioral effects of corticosteroids in children with acute lymphoblastic leukemia. Med Pediatric Oncol. 1992;20:13–21.

236. Harris JC, Carel CA, Rosenberg LA, et al. Intermittent high does corticosteroid treatment in childhood cancer: behavioral and emotional consequences. J Am Acad Child Adolesc Psychiatry. 1988;27:720–725.

237. Bailey WC, Richards JM, Manzella BA, et al. Characteristics and correlates of asthma in a university clinic population. Chest. 1990;98:821–828.

238. Estrada De La Riva G. Psychic and somatic changes observed in allergic children after prolonged steroid therapy. South Med J. 1958;51:865–868.

239. Wolkowitz OM, Rubinow D, Doran AR, et al. Prednisone effects on neurochemistry and behavior: preliminary findings. Arch Gen Psychiatry. 1990;47:963–968.

240. Check WA, Kaliner MA. Pharmacology and pharmacokinetics of topical corticosteroid derivatives used for asthma therapy. Am Rev Respir Dis. 1990;141:S44–S51.

241. Gillin JC, Jacobs LS, Fram DH, et al. Acute effect of a glucocorticoid on normal human sleep. Nature. 1972;237:398–399.

242. Born J, Zwick A, Roth G, et al. Differential effects of hydrocortisone, flucortolone, and aldosterone on nocturnal sleep in humans. Acta Endocrinol. 1987;116:129–137.

243. Fehm HL, Benkowitsch R, Kern W, et al. Influences of corticosteroids, dexamethasone and hydrocortisone on sleep in humans. Neuropsychobiology. 1986;16:198–204.

244. Rosenthal L, Folkerts M, Helmus T, et al. Administration of dexamethasone and its effects on sleep and daytime alertness. Sleep Res. 1995;24:58.

245. Born J, DeKloet ER, Wenz H, et al. Gluco- and antimineralocorticoid effects on human sleep: a role of central corticosteroid receptors. Am J Physiol. 1991;260:E183–E188.

246. Wolkowitz OM, Reus VI, Weingartner H, et al. Cognitive effects of corticosteroids. Am J Psychiatry. 1990;147:1297–1303.

247. Scott PH, Tabachnik E, MacLeod S, et al. Sustained release theophylline for childhood asthma: evidence for circadian variation of theophylline pharmacokinetics. J Pediatr. 1981;99:476–479.

248. Hendeles L, Massanari M, Weinberger M. Update on the pharmacodynamics and pharmacokinetics of theophylline. Chest. 1985;88(suppl):103S–111S.

249. Janson C, Gislason T, Boman G, et al. Sleep disturbances in patients with asthma. Respir Med. 1990;84:37–42.

250. Avital A, Steljes DG, Pasterkamp H, et al. Sleep quality in children with asthma treated with theophylline or chromolyn sodium. J Pediatr. 1991;119:979–984.

251. Zwillich CW, Neagley SR, Cicutto L, et al. Nocturnal asthma therapy: inhaled bitolterol versus sustained-release theophylline. Am Rev Respir Dis. 1989;139:470–474.

252. Man GCW, Chapman KR, Ali SH, et al. Sleep quality and nocturnal respiratory function with once-daily theophylline (Uniphyl) and inhaled salbutamol in patients with COPD. Chest. 1996;110:648–653.

253. Fitzpatrick MF, Engleman HM, Boellert F, et al. Effect of therapeutic theophylline levels on the sleep quality and daytime cognitive performance of normal subjects. Am Rev Respir Dis. 1992;145:1355–1358.

254. Berry RB, Desa MM, Branum JP, et al. Effect of theophylline on sleep and sleep-disordered breathing in patients with chronic obstructive pulmonary disease. Am Rev Respir Dis. 1991;143:245–250.

255. Kaplan J, Fredrickson PA, Renaux SA, et al. Theophylline effect on sleep in normal subjects. Chest. 1993;103:193–195.

256. Janson C, Gislason T, Almqvist M, et al. Theophylline disturbs sleep mainly in caffeine-sensitive persons. Pulm Pharmacol. 1989;2:125–129.

257. Richardt D, Driver HS. An evaluative study of the short-term effects of once-daily, sustained-release theophylline on sleep in nocturnal asthmatics. S Afr Med J. 1996;86:803–804.

258. Rhind GB, Connaughton JJ, McFie J, et al. Sustained release choline theophyllinate in nocturnal asthma. Br Med J. 1985;291:1605–1607.

259. Avital A, Sanchez I, Holbrow J, et al. Effect of theophylline on lung function tests, sleep quality, and nighttime SaO2 in children with cystic fibrosis. Am Rev Respir Dis. 1991;144:1245–1249.

260. Mulloy E, McNicholas WT. Theophylline improves gas exchange during rest, exercise, and sleep in severe chronic obstructive pulmonary disease. Am Rev Respir Dis. 1993;148:1030–1036.

261. Fleetham JA, Fera T, Edgell G, et al. The effect of theophylline therapy on sleep disorders in COPD patients. Am Rev Respir Dis. 1983;127:85.

262. Rachelefsky GS, Wo J, Adelson J, et al. Behavior abnormalities and poor school performance due to oral theophylline use. Pediatrics. 1986;78:1133–1138.

263. Stein MA, Krasowski M, Leventhal BL, et al. Behavioral and cognitive effects of methylxanthines: a meta-analysis of theophylline and caffeine. Arch Pediatr Adolesc Med. 1996;150:284–288.

264. Lindgren S, Lokshin B, Stronmquist A, et al. Does asthma or treatment with theophylline limit children's academic performance? N Engl J Med. 1992;327:926–930.

265. van Hilten JJ, Weggeman M, van der Velde EA, et al. Sleep, excessive daytime sleepiness and fatigue in Parkinson's disease. J Neural Transm. 1993;5:235–244.

266. van Hilten B, Hoff JI, Middelkoop MA, et al. Sleep disruption in Parkinson's disease. Arch Neurol. 1994;51:922–928.

267. Stocchi F, Barbato L, Nordera G, et al. Sleep disorders in Parkinson's disease. J Neurol. 1998;245(suppl 1):S15–S18.

268. Partinen M. Sleep disorder related to Parkinson's disease. J Neurol. 1997;244(suppl 1):S3–S6.

269. Scharf B, Moskovitz C, Lupton MD, et al. Dream phenomena induced by chronic levodopa therapy. J Neural Transm. 1978;43:143–151.

270. Kales A, Ansel RD, Markham CH, et al. Sleep in patients with Parkinson's disease and normal subjects prior to and following levodopa administration. Clin Pharmacol Ther. 1971;12:397–406.

271. Bergonzi P, Chiurulla C, Gambi D, et al. L-dopa plus dopa-decarboxylase inhibitor. Acta Neurol Belg. 1975;75:5–10.

272. Askenasy JJM, Yahr MD. Reversal of sleep disturbance in Parkinson's disease by antiparkinson therapy. Neurology. 1985;35:527–532.

273. Nausieda PA, Glantz R, Weber S, et al. Psychiatric complications of levodopa therapy of Parkinson's disease. Adv Neurol. 1984;40:271–277.

274. Nausieda PA, Weiner WJ, Kaplan LR, et al. Sleep disruption in the course of chronic levodopa therapy: an early feature of the levodopa psychosis. Clin Neuropharmacol. 1982;5:183–194.

275. Bergozi P, Chiuruula C, Cianchetti C, et al. Clinical pharmacology as an approach to the study of biochemical sleep mechanisms: the action of L-dopa. Confin Neurol. 1974;36:5–22.

276. Leeman AL, O'Neill CJA, Nicholson PW, et al. Parkinson's disease in the elderly: response to and optimal spacing of night time dosing with levodopa. Br J Clin Pharmacol. 1987;24:637–643.

277. Chrisp P, Mammen GJ, Sorkin EM. Selegiline. A review of its pharmacology, symptomatic benefits and protective potential in Parkinson's disease. Drugs Aging. 1991;1:228–248.

278. Stern GM, Lees AJ, Sandler M. Recent observations on the clinical pharmacology of (−)deprenyl. J Neural Transm. 1978;43:245–251.

279. Lavie P, Wajsbort J, Youdim MBH. Deprenyl does not cause insomnia in parkinsonian patients. Commun Psychopharmacol. 1980;4:303–307.

280. Jeanty P, van den Kerchove M, Lowenthal A, et al. Pergolide therapy in Parkinson's disease. J Neurol. 1984;231:148–152.

281. Vardi J, Glaubman H, Rabey J, et al. EEG sleep patterns in parkinsonian patients treated with bromocryptine and L-dopa: a comparative study. J Neural Transm. 1979;45:307–316.

282. Schwab RS, Poskanzer DC, England AC, et al. Amantadine in Parkinson's disease: review of more than two years' experience. JAMA. 1972;222:792–795.

283. Cooper JA, Sagar HJ, Doherty SM, et al. Different effects of dopaminergic and anticholinergic therapies on cognitive and motor function in Parkinson's disease. Brain. 1992;115:1701–1725.

284. Meco G, Casacchia M, Lazzari R, et al. Mental impairment in Parkinson's disease: the role of anticholinergic drugs. Acta Psychiatr Belg. 1984;84:325–334.

285. Nishiyama K, Sugishita M, Kurisaki H, et al. Reversible memory disturbance and intelligence impairment induced by long-term anticholinergic therapy. Intern Med. 1998;37:514–518.

286. Saint-Cyr JA, Tayler AE, Lang AE. Neuropsychological and psychiatric side effects in the treatment of Parkinson's disease. Neurology. 1993;43(suppl 6):S47–S52.

287. Kieburtz K, McDermott M, Como P, et al, and the Parkinson Study Group. The effect of deprenyl and tocopherol on cognitive performance in early untreated Parkinson's disease. Neurology. 1994;44:1756–1759.

288. Cumming JL. Behavioral complications of drug treatment of Parkinson's disease. J Am Geriatr Soc. 1991;39:708–716.

289. Malow BA, Bowes RJ, Lix X. Predictors of sleepiness in epilepsy patients. Sleep. 1997;20:1105–1110.

290. Collaborative Group for Epidemiology of Epilepsy. Adverse reactions to antiepileptic drugs: a multicenter survey of clinical practice. Epilepsia. 1986;27:323–330.

291. Wallace SJ. A comparative review of the adverse effects of anticonvulsants in children with epilepsy. Drug Safety. 1996;15:378–393.

292. Hoeppner JB, Garron DC, Cartwright RD. Self-reported sleep disorder symptoms in epilepsy. Epilepsia. 1984;25:434–437.

293. Committee on Drugs. Behavioral and cognitive effects of anticonvulsant therapy. Pediatrics. 1985;76:644–647.

294. Binnie CD. Cognitive impairment: is it inevitable? Seizure. 1994;3(suppl A):17–21.

295. Bazil CW, Pedley TA. Advances in the medical treatment of epilepsy. Annu Rev Med. 1998;49:135–162.

296. Blum DE. New drugs for persons with epilepsy. In: French J, Leppik I, Dichter MA, eds. Antiepileptic Drug Development: Advances in Neurology. Philadelphia, PA: Lippincott-Raven; 1998:57–87.

297. Ferrendelli JA. Pharmacology of antiepileptic drugs. Epilepsia. 1987;28(suppl 3):S14–S16.

298. Rogvi-Hansen B, Gram L. Adverse effects of established and new antiepileptic drugs: an attempted comparison. Pharmacol Ther. 1995;68:425–434.

299. Brodie MJ, Dichter MA. Established antiepileptic drugs. Seizure. 1997;6:159–174.

300. Salinsky MC, Oken BS, Binder LM. Assessment of drowsiness in epilepsy patients receiving chronic antiepileptic drug therapy. Epilepsia. 1996;37:181–187.

301. Leppik IE. Antiepileptic drugs in development: prospects for the near future. Epilepsia. 1994;35(suppl 4):S29–S40.

302. Chadwick D, Leiderman DB, Sauermann W, et al. Gabapentin in generalized seizures. Epilepsy Res. 1996;25:191–197.

303. Leppik IE. Tiagabine: the safety landscape. Epilepsia. 1995;36(suppl 6):S10–S13.

304. Ketter TA, Malow BA, Flamini R, et al. Felbamate monotherapy has stimulant-like effects in patients with epilepsy. Epilepsy Res. 1996;23:129–137.

305. Wagner ML. Felbamate: a new antiepileptic drug. Am J Hosp Pharm. 1994;51:1657–1666.

306. Marson AG, Kadir ZA, Hutton JL, et al. The new antiepileptic drugs: a systematic review of their efficacy and tolerability. Epilepsia. 1997;38:859–880.

307. Wolf P, Roeder-Wanner UU, Brede M, et al. Influences of antiepileptic drugs on sleep. In: da Silva AM, Binnie CD, Meinardi H, eds. Biorhythms and Epilepsy. New York, NY: Raven Press; 1985:137–153.

308. Declerck AC, Wauquier A. Influence of antiepileptic drugs on sleep patterns. Epilepsy Res Suppl. 1991;2:153–163.

309. Roeder-Wanner UU, Noachter S, Wolf P. Response of polygraphic sleep to phenytoin treatment for epilepsy: a longitudinal study of immediate, short- and long-term effects. Acta Neurol Scand. 1987;76:157–167.

310. Palm L, Anderson H, Elmqvist D, et al. Daytime sleep tendency before and after discontinuation of antiepileptic drugs in preadolescent children with epilepsy. Epilepsia. 1992;33:687–691.

311. Bonnani E, Massetani R, Galli R, et al. A quantitative study of daytime sleepiness induced by carbamazepine and add-on vigabatrin in epileptic patients. Acta Neurol Scand. 1997;95:193–196.

312. Manni R, Ratti MT, Perucca E, et al. A multiparametric investigation of daytime sleepiness and psychomotor function in epileptic patients treated with phenobarbital and sodium valproate: a comparative controlled study. Electroencephalogr Clin Neurophysiol. 1993;86:322–328.

313. Vining EP. Cognitive dysfunction associated with antiepileptic drug therapy. Epilepsia. 1987;28(suppl 2):S18–S22.

314. Nichols ME, Meador KJ, Loring DW. Neuropsychological effects of antiepileptic drugs: a current perspective. Clin Neuropharmacol. 1993;16:471–484.

315. Leach JP, Girvan J, Paul A, et al. Gabapentin and cognition: a double-blind, dose ranging, placebo controlled study in refractory epilepsy. J Neurol Neurosurg Psychiatry. 1997;62:372–376.

316. Provinciali L, Bartolini M, Mari F, et al. Influence of vigabatrin on cognitive performances and behaviour in patients with drug-resistant epilepsy. Acta Neurol Scand. 1996;94:12–18.

317. Adkins JC, Noble S. Tiagabine. A review of its pharmacodynamic and pharmacokinetic properties and therapeutic potential in the management of epilepsy. Drugs. 1998;55:437–460.

318. Lake CR, Rosenberg DB, Gallant S, et al. Phenylpropanolamine increases plasma caffeine levels. Clin Pharmacol Ther. 1990;47:675–685.

319. Bye CE, Hill HM, Hughes DTD, et al. A comparison of blood levels of L (+)-pseudoephedrine following different formulations and their relation to cardiovascular and subjective effects in man. Eur J Clin Pharmacol. 1975;8:47–53.

320. Empey DW, Medder KT. Nasal decongestants. Drugs. 1981;21:438–443.

321. Bertrand B, Jamart J, Arendt C. Cetirizine and pseudoephedrine retard alone and in combination in the treatment of perennial allergic rhinitis: a double-blind multicentre study. Rhinology. 1996;34:91–96.

322. Rombaut NEI, Alford C, Hindmarch I. Effects of oral administration of different formulations of pseudoephedrine on day- and night-time CNS activity. Med Sci Res. 1989;17:831–833.

323. Bever KA, Perry PJ. Dexfenfluramine hydrochloride: an anorexigenic agent. Am J Health Syst Pharm. 1997;54:2059–2072.

324. Guy-Grand B, Apfelbaum M, Crepaldi G, et al. International trial of long-term dexfenfluramine in obesity. Lancet. 1989;2:1142–1145.

325. Wiegand M, Bossert S, Kinney R, et al. Effect of dexfenfluramine on sleep in healthy subjects. Psychopharmacology. 1991;105:213–218.

326. Groenewoud G, Schall R, Hundt HK, et al. Steady-state pharmacokinetics of phentermine extended-release capsules. Int J Clin Pharmacol Ther Toxicol. 1993;31:368–372.

327. Griffith JD, Nutt JG, Jasinski DR. A comparison of fenfluramine and amphetamine in man. Clin Pharmacol Ther. 1975;18:563–570.

328. Oswald I, Jones HS, Mannerheim JE. Effects of two slimming drugs on sleep. Br Med J. 1968;1:797–799.

329. Myers JE, Buysse DJ, Thase ME, et al. The effects of fenfluramine on sleep and prolactin in depressed inpatients: a comparison of potential indices of brain serotonergic responsivity. Biol Psychiatry. 1993;34:753–758.

330. Lean ME. Sibutramine: a review of clinical efficacy. Int J Obes Relat Metab Disord. 1997;21(suppl 1):S30–S36.

331. Middlemiss DN, Blakeborough L, Leather SR. Direct evidence for an interaction of β-adrenergic blockers with the 5-HT receptor. Nature. 1977;267:289–290.

six

Psychobiology and Dreaming

R. T. Pivik

Methods and Measures for the Study of Dream Content

G. William Domhoff

The systematic study of dream content has led to many interesting and useful findings concerning developmental changes, gender differences, cross-cultural similarities and differences, consistency in what individuals dream about over decades, and the continuity between dream content and waking thought. Such findings lay the groundwork for future studies of psychopathology in dream content.[1-5]

This chapter focuses on the methods, measures, and strategies of data analysis that have generated the many findings alluded to in the opening paragraph. It discusses the advantages and disadvantages of (1) four methods for collecting dream reports, (2) four methods of content analysis, and (3) several approaches to data analysis. It concludes with the presentation of several dream content indicators that might prove useful in the future in understanding psychopathology through dreams.

METHODS FOR COLLECTING DREAM REPORTS

There are four sources of dream reports, the sleep laboratory, the psychotherapy relationship, personal dream journals, and reports written down on anonymous forms in group settings, of which the classroom is the most typical. These four sources provide both *dream series* (two or more dreams from an individual) and *dream sets* (a collection of single dream reports from the members of any given group).

Questionnaires asking people if they think they dream about one or another topic are not considered here because they are not a method of collecting dream reports. Such questionnaires ask for opinions that in fact relate to personality style and cultural beliefs concerning dreams. In four different samples, for example, subjects said they dreamt most frequently about friendliness, secondly about sexuality, and least often about aggression,[6] but representative samples of dream content with similar college student populations show that aggression is the most frequent social interaction in dream reports, followed by friendliness, and—at a very distant third—sexuality.[5, 7, 8] Because there is little or no correlation between snap judgments on questionnaires and dream content, such questionnaires cannot be used as substitutes for dream reports.

There are several factors that may influence the content of the dream report regardless of which collection method is used. They include the instructions given to the dreamer for making the report, the nature of the interpersonal situation if the report is verbal, and the degree of anonymity available to the subject.[1] These and other problems can be mitigated, if not eliminated, by collecting dream reports with a standardized interview protocol or written form and using subjects whose participation is voluntary. Anonymity also is useful when possible, although it is not as crucial as might be thought because most people feel little personal responsibility for their dreams and are therefore willing to report unusual themes and elements.[4, 9] One of the most important safeguards against some of the problems having to do with report quality is a large sample size, which serves to minimize the effects of inadequate or confabulated reports.

Sleep Laboratories

Sleep laboratories provide the opportunity for collecting a large representative sample of a person's dream life under controlled conditions. Awakenings during rapid eye movement (REM) periods or from nonrapid eye movement (NREM) periods late in the sleep period maximize the probability of recall, making it possible to collect as many as four or five dream narratives in a single night.[10] The collection of dreams in the sleep laboratory from those who say they seldom or never dream is only one of the many ways that laboratory studies expanded the horizon for those who study dream content.[11–12]

Studies of dream reports collected in the laboratory suggest that dream content does not differ greatly from early to late in the sleep period.[13–17] Although one careful study of five subjects found there were more references to the past in later REM periods,[18] the finding was not replicated in a larger study.[16] Similarly, even though NREM and REM reports do not differ greatly when report length is held constant, it is also the case that many NREM reports are shorter or more "thoughtlike."[19–21]

Nor do dream reports collected in laboratory settings differ greatly, if at all, from those written down by the same subjects at home.[9, 17, 22–24] To the degree that there are differences, there may be less aggression and sexuality in laboratory-collected reports,[16, 25] but as just noted, sexuality is relatively infrequent in nonlaboratory reports, appearing in 12% of young men's dreams and 4% of young women's dreams in a normative sample based on 500 male and 500 female reports.[5] Furthermore, the magnitude of the statistically significant differences—that is, the *effect size*—is small except in the case of physical aggression, which is more frequent in dreams collected at home.[22]

A major problem with the laboratory collection of dream reports is that it is an expensive and time-consuming process. The sleep laboratory is especially difficult to use in an era when there is little if any outside funding for dream research.[26] If this state of affairs continues, then laboratory studies may have made their greatest contribution to content studies for the time being by

1. Documenting the frequency and regularity of dreaming
2. Demonstrating the relative imperviousness of dreams to either external or internal stimuli
3. Providing a normative context for judging the representativeness of dream samples collected outside the sleep laboratory

Psychotherapy Relationship

The psychotherapy relationship is a long-standing source of dream reports. Such reports have the virtue of rich accompanying biographical and fantasy material. They provide the occasion for the creation of dream journals that include dreams reported in therapy as well as those written down outside of therapy. However, not all psychotherapists make use of dreams, and only Jungian analysts regularly encourage their patients to keep a dream journal. Moreover, patients are a small and unrepresentative sample of the population. Consequently, little use has been made of this method in systematic studies. It is most commonly used in individual case studies involving extended analyses of one or two dreams.

Dream Journals

Dream journals are a third source of dream reports. The best-known dream journals are those discussed by Jungian analysts,[27] but journals kept for personal, artistic, or intellectual reasons have been studied with great profit as well.[28, 29] Dream journals are a form of personal document long recognized in psychology as having the potential for providing insights into personality.[30, 31] They are nonreactive archival sources that have not been influenced by the purposes of the investigators who analyze them. Conclusions drawn from nonreactive archival data are considered most impressive when they are based on a diversity of archives likely to have different types of potential biases.[32] Dream journals have been extremely valuable in establishing the considerable consistency in what people dream about, whatever the purposes of the journal writer.[4]

For all their potential usefulness, dream journals are not without their drawbacks. Even after showing initial willingness, some people may not want to provide dreams for scientific scrutiny. Journals may have gaps or omissions. The journal writer may not be willing to reply to inferences about his or her personal life based on a blind analysis of the journal's contents. Dream journals, therefore, are best used selectively and in the context of other dream samples.

Classrooms and Other Group Settings

The most objective and structured context for the efficient and inexpensive collection of large samples of dream reports is the classroom, where reports can be written by anonymous subjects who reveal only their age and gender.[33] The main drawback of this method is that it is usually not possible to collect much personality or cognitive information about the people providing the dream reports.

The classroom collection of dream reports has led to a focus on the Most Recent Dream a person can remember—a report that can be obtained in any setting in which people can spare 15 to 20 min, such as convention halls, conferences, waiting rooms, and classrooms. In this approach, people are simply asked to provide their gender, age, and "the last dream you remember having, whether it was last night, last week, or last month."[4(p310)] It primes for recency by asking subjects to report the date the dream occurred. The date of recall not only primes for recency in an attempt to eliminate atypical recurrent dreams and nightmares but also allows investigators to eliminate dreams said to have occurred months or years earlier if they desire. The Most Recent Dream technique leads to samples that match the normative findings created by Hall and Van de Castle's coding system.[4, 5] In addition, the results with 12- to 13-year-old preadolescents are similar in some respects to those from laboratory dream reports for this age group.[34] Finally, the legitimacy of the Most Recent Dream approach has been enhanced by the findings mentioned earlier about the similarities between dream reports collected in the sleep laboratory and at home from the same subjects.[9, 17, 22–24]

METHODS FOR ANALYZING DREAM CONTENT

The four general methods for analyzing dream content include

1. Collecting free associations
2. Finding metaphoric meaning
3. Searching for repeated themes
4. Conducting quantitative analyses using either rating systems or nominal (discrete) categories

Whatever method is used, the content analyst should know nothing about the dreamer to guard against the well-known tendency to read expectations into the dream reports. Such "blind analyses," when combined with predictions about the waking thoughts and behaviors of the individual or group under study, are the best scientific alternative in a situation where experiments have restricted usefulness. It is also essential to remove any preparatory remarks, side comments, or interpretations by the dreamer from transcripts or written reports before they are given to those who will analyze them.

Free-Association Method

The free-association method, introduced into the study of dreams by Freud, consists of instructing dreamers to say whatever comes into their minds about each element of the dream without censoring their thoughts.[35] The method, which is theoretically neutral and can be used by non-Freudians, often reveals the day-to-day events incorporated into the dream—the "day residue"—and the emotional concerns of the dreamer. However, in the psychotherapy setting, it is difficult to demonstrate that the free associations actually explain the dream because so much else is known about the dreamer that could be playing a role in constructing a "meaning" for the dream.

The most extensive attempt to use free associations in dream studies outside a clinical setting is presented, along with a complex system for coding both the dreams and the free associations, in Foulkes' *The Grammar of Dreams*.[36] However, Foulkes later noted that "extensive experience in association gathering" convinced him of its "inherent arbitrariness."[26(p617)] Moreover, two studies 40 years apart found that free associations do not improve a blind personality assessment if the assessors are working with a dream series from an individual; that is, the assessors who had free associations along with the dream series did not do any better than those who had only the dream series.[37, 38] Thus, the free-association method seems tied to the clinical setting on the one hand and not necessary if a dream series is available on the other.

Metaphoric Analysis

Symbolic interpretations are used as a supplement to free associations in the analysis of dreams in psychotherapy settings and in some studies of lengthy dream journals. Such symbolic interpretations are perhaps now more appropriately thought of as metaphoric analysis because there is some evidence that dream symbolism may be based in the large system of conceptual metaphors that is universally understood and used in Western civilization.[39–42] For example, in a study of the sexual symbols said by Freud to be present in dreams, Hall[43] found that all of them are used as sexual slang in the English language according to Partridge's *A Dictionary of Slang and Unconventional English*.[44]

Similarly, it can be shown that the *functional symbols* identified by Jungians, that is, symbols that are said to stand for parts of the mind or the mind as a whole, are all based on common metaphors. For example, the equation of "psyche" and "house" in Jungian theory is based on the conceptual metaphor "the mind is a container." The general use of myths in Jungian and neo-Freudian theory to understand aspects of dreams is also a form of metaphoric analysis.

There are several problems with metaphoric analyses, starting with the fact that there is as yet no systematic evidence of how many dreams are metaphoric in nature. It also may be the case that more than one metaphor might plausibly be applied to some dreams. Moreover, it might be that dreams, if they are metaphoric, often rely on personal metaphors based on past experiences.[45] Some of these problems can be overcome in a study of a dream series because the repetition of elements can lead to a strong argument for applying one or another conceptual metaphor, but metaphoric analysis as a rigorous and systematic approach remains undeveloped.[43, 46]

Thematic Analysis

A third method of dream analysis, the thematic method, shades off from metaphoric analysis. It involves repeatedly reading through a dream series to see if one or more themes emerge. Sometimes the search is made easier by the presence of one or more *spotlight* dreams that seem to contain the theme or themes in an obvious fashion.[47] One study concluded that six themes appeared with regularity over a period of 50 years in a dream series consisting of 649 dreams; these six themes accounted for at least part of the content in about 70% of the dreams.[48]

Although it may be a little easier to reach common agreement on the presence of themes than it is in the case of metaphors, there is still considerable room for disagreement among investigators. The method also suffers from the fact that the findings tend to be unique to each dreamer, allowing little opportunity for generalizations across dreamers. Finally, thematic analyses tend to be general. They do not go far in terms of detailed statements about dream content that can be tested on new dream samples.

Quantitative Approaches

Dissatisfaction with the reliability and generalizability of free-associative, metaphoric, and thematic methods of studying dream content led to quantitative approaches called *content analysis*. The major task in content analysis is the creation of carefully defined categories that lead to the same results when used by different investigators and that yield findings that relate to other variables. There are no pat formulas for creating good categories. Usually, it is a matter of trial and error after deep immersion in the material to be analyzed. There are two major issues in formulating categories for the analysis of dream content. Should they be hierarchical or nominal in their level of measurement? Should they be theoretical or empirical in nature? These two questions lead to the possibility of four different types of scales, and in fact all four types have been employed in dream research.[49, 50]

Hierarchical vs. Nominal Scales

Hierarchical scales assume that a characteristic or element can be ranked or weighed. For example, there can be degrees of emotionality, distortion, or vividness in a dream report. In measurement terms, a hierarchical scale is *ordinal* if it is only possible to rank elements from high to low, *equal interval* if all points on the scale are equally distant from each other, and *ratio* if it has an exact zero point (such as weight does). Although a few theoretical scales have assigned "weights" to different elements, making them equal interval scales, most hierarchical scales in dream research have been ordinal ones, resting on the more modest assumption that "more" or "less" is the most that can be judged in a dream report.

Nominal scales, on the other hand, are nonhierarchical. They simply record the presence or absence of a characteristic or element in the dream report. "Male" and "female," for example, are nominal categories, that is, they are *discrete* categories that allow simply for the comparison of frequencies.

Rating scales of an ordinal nature have been employed with great benefit in a wide variety of useful studies, the most important of which are the longitudinal and cross-sectional studies of children's dream reports by Foulkes and his co-workers.[2, 51, 52] Their scales made it possible to show dramatic changes in dream content from primarily single, static images without the dreamer present in children under age 6, to stories with temporal sequences of action and the dreamer as an active participant in the dream by age 8. Generally speaking, rating scales are useful for characteristics of dream reports that have degrees of intensity in waking life, such as activity level or emotionality, or that are without specific content, such as clarity of visual imagery.

Nevertheless, there are drawbacks to the use of rating scales in the study of dream content. First, it is difficult to establish reliability for some scales, especially those that call for subtle judgments such as the degree of distortion or bizarreness present in the overall dream report. Second, a general rating does not make full use of the potential information present in the dream report. An overall "unusualness" or "bizarreness" rating, for example, does not record the fact that in one case the unusualness is due to a metamorphosis, in another to a distorted setting, and in still another to impossible actions and activities.[53, 54]

Third, and most important, some rating scales rest on untenable psychological assumptions when they assign numbers to social interactions such as aggression or friendliness. In the case of aggression, for example, one coding system assigns a score of "4" to a murder and a "1" to an angry remark, but the summation of such codings implies that four angry remarks are equal to one murder. Such examples could be multiplied, but the point is that there is no psychologically defensible way to rate many of the events that occur in dreams.[5, 49, 50, 55]

Nominal scales do not suffer from the same weaknesses that many rating scales do. Higher reliabilities can be obtained because discrete scales usually can be more clearly defined and do not require the subtle judgments that rating scales often do. No information is lost because numerous categories are elaborated. They do not harbor the questionable psychological assumptions within ratings, such as those assigned to different kinds of aggressions. Instead, to continue with the example of aggression, each type of aggression can be put into a separate category, and then a general aggression category can be created that simply presents the sum total of all types of aggressions.

The main problem with coding systems based on nominal categories is that they may or may not lead to findings of psychological relevance and theoretical interest. Moreover, they are more labor-intensive than rating systems. It takes longer to learn a full set of nominal categories and to apply them to a series or set of dreams than is the case with most rating systems.

Theoretical vs. Empirical Categories

Theoretical scales are those derived from one or another theory of personality. *Empirical scales* are defined as scales not derived from any particular theory; they are based on a common-sense or trial-and-error organization of the elements that appear in a dream.

Theoretical scales are far more difficult to construct and validate than empirical ones. Their construction requires a deep understanding of both the theory being used and the nature of dream content to make them useful. The results with theoretical scales to date have not been encouraging enough for new investigators to make use of them in many instances.[4]

By contrast, a variety of empirical scales, both hierarchical and nominal, have been useful in the study of dream content, and some have been employed by several different investigators. Most such scales contain categories for vividness, degree of distortion or bizarreness, characters, emotions, and the activities and interactions of the characters. A factor analysis of the codings of 100 REM dream reports on several different empirical scales found five important dimensions within these seemingly diverse scales.[56] All codings were done by the original authors of the scale or their close associates. The five factors are

1. Dream-like quality (vivid fantasy, imagination, distortion)
2. Hostility and anxiety
3. Motivation to self-improvement (assertiveness, successful striving)
4. Sex
5. Activity level

The set of nominal categories developed by Hall and Van de Castle[5] is the most comprehensive and widely used empirical system of content analysis. Its original 10 general categories include characters, social interactions, activities, misfortunes and good fortunes, successes and failures, emotions, settings and objects, descriptive elements, elements from the past, and food and eating. A way of measuring dramatic intensity and an unusual elements scale were added later.[16] The reliability of coding for this system is good. It includes norms for young men and women that have been replicated several times and that do not differ (except perhaps on aggression) from what has been found with older adults. The system has been used by investigators in Canada, Europe, India, and Japan, and on dream reports collected by anthropologists in small traditional societies.[4] It is this system that has provided the best evidence for consistency over months and years in the dreams in lengthy dream journals. However, to expect consistency in comparisons of two samples of five dream reports each that were collected several weeks apart, as Bernstein and Belicki do, is not reasonable.[4, 6]

In addition, as Van de Castle has shown, it is possible to combine two or more nominal categories to create new indicators that are "quasi-theoretical" in nature.[55] For example, the separate codings for the initiation of friendly interactions and the instigation of aggressive encounters could be combined to create an indicator of "assertiveness." Similarly, personal misfortunes, failures, and victim status in aggressive interactions can be used to create an indicator of a negative self-concept. In fact, one team of investigators found that Beck and Hurvich's Masochism Scale, which has never been validated for actual masochism, is encom-passed by the three categories in the self-negativity index.[57, 58] Then too, a high score on Krohn and Mayman's Object Relations Scale, which requires difficult ratings of the level of maturity in interpersonal interactions, has been shown to be a combination of friendly interactions, nonphysical activities, and an absence of physical aggressions[59] (G. W. Domhoff, PhD, unpublished data). In addition, the Hall and Van de Castle system encompasses the five main dimensions found in Hauri's factor analytic study of several empirical scale.[56]

The Hall and Van de Castle system is readily available anywhere in the world on a Website that includes the complete coding rules, samples of coded dream reports, norms, and new findings.[60] Schneider and Domhoff have determined the sample sizes needed for good studies with this system by drawing subsamples from the dream reports used in creating Hall and Van de Castle's male norms and from lengthy dream journals. It takes 100 to 125 Most Recent Dreams to approximate the Hall–Van de Castle norms and 75 to 100 reports to approximate the results from along dream series.[4]

STRATEGIES OF DATA ANALYSIS

Once metaphors or themes have been located, ratings made, or frequencies for nominal categories tabulated, two main issues arise relating to data analysis.

Intensity

The first issue is how to determine degrees of *intensity* for any given content element. In other words, how can it be decided whether there is lesser or greater saliency for the dimensions or categories being analyzed? The resolution of this issue is built into rating scales: the higher the rating, the greater the intensity. For metaphoric, thematic, and nominal content categories, the best way to handle this issue is to assume that *frequency* is an *indicator* of intensity, that is, the more appearances of a given metaphor or theme, or the higher the frequency in a nominal category, then the greater the intensity or saliency. This is the only assumption underlying the Hall and Van de Castle system, and it has been supported in numerous studies showing that high or low frequencies in specific content categories correlate with greater or lesser concern for the corresponding thought or behavior in waking life.[4, 5]

Unit of Analysis

The second main issue in analyzing dream content data is determining the *unit of analysis*, that is, the standardized baseline against which comparisons with other groups or individuals are going to be made. For example, the unit of analysis in most studies is simply the dream report as a whole: the sum total of ratings (or frequencies in nominal categories) is divided by the total number of dream reports. There are, however, serious problems with using the dream report as the unit of analysis.

Most crucially, the length of dream reports can vary greatly from group to group or person to person. This is a problem because longer reports are likely to have more of most things in them, although one study showed that the relationship is not monotonic for all types of categories.[61] Hall and Van de Castle found that women's dream reports tend to be about 8% longer than men's, so a failure to correct for dream length can produce many spurious gender differences.[5] The failure to correct for dream length is a problem for both rating scales and nominal categories. For example, a frequently used theoretical scale for rating "primary process" in dream content, which is based on degrees of distortion and improbabilities, correlates .60 with the length of the dream report.[62] Any positive relationship between measures of creativity and primary process in dream content often disappears when there is a control for length through partial correlations.[63, 64] Similarly, correction for dream length eliminates gender differences in several of Hall and Van de Castle's nominal categories.

But length is not the only problem that makes the dream report a questionable unit of analysis. Dream reports also can vary in their number of characters even if they are of the same length, which means that there is more likelihood of social interactions in some dreams than others. Once again, there is a gender difference on this issue: there is a greater "density" of characters in women's dream reports, an interesting finding in and of itself, but one that should be taken into account in analyzing social interactions.[49, 50]

There are a number of ways to correct for the length problem. They include the elimination of dream reports that are below or above specific word counts, or using the average number of lines per dream report as the unit of analysis. When rating scales are used, eliminating short and long reports is probably the best solution. However, the ideal solution with nominal categories is to use various kinds of percentages and ratios based on the nominal categories themselves. For example, the percentage of characters in a dream report that are animals (all animals divided by total characters) is completely independent of report length or character density, effectively dealing with two problems at the same time. Such an approach makes it unnecessary to throw out dream reports or use a cumbersome unit of analysis such as average lines—or words—per dream report. The findings are also readily communicated and understood. For example the "animal percentage" declines from 30 to 40% in young children to 4 to 6% in adulthood and is higher in small traditional societies than it is in modern nations.[4]

The likely dependence of social interactions on the number of characters can be handled in the same way by using ratios. Thus, dividing all aggressions by all characters produces an aggressions per character (A/C) index. This ratio can be figured for each of the eight categories of aggression in the Hall and Van de Castle system and for the dreamer's interactions with specific characters or types of characters in the dream reports (e.g., father, mother, men, women). In a similar fashion, dividing all friendly interactions by all characters creates a friendly interactions per character (F/C) ratio, and dividing all sexual interactions by all characters creates a sexual interactions per character (S/C) ratio.

The use of percentages and ratios has one further advantage: they lend themselves to a simple but powerful statistical treatment of the data when two groups are being compared or an individual is being compared to normative findings. In these types of comparisons, a test of the significance of differences between proportions provides the same result as a chi-square test, and the percentage differences are equivalent to both the Pearson r and two measures of effect size.[4]

Within the Hall and Van de Castle system, there are numerous such indicators, most of which are provided instantaneously when codings are entered into an Excel 5 spreadsheet available on the content analysis Website.[60] Tables and bar graphs displaying the results in comparison to Hall and Van de Castle's norms are also part of the spreadsheet, along with significance levels, confidence intervals, and effect sizes.

The "At Least One" Method

Because coding is labor intensive, it is time consuming to code samples with many hundreds or thousands of dream reports in them. Fortunately, with such large samples it can be almost as useful to determine the simple presence or absence of any given category. This allows investigators to calculate what percentage of the dream reports in a large set or series have "at least one" instance of the category. In the Hall and Van de Castle system, there is "at least one" norm for several content categories, including aggression, friendliness, sexuality, misfortune, success, failure, and food or eating. Most of these "at least one" categories are part of the aforementioned Excel 5 spreadsheet. To give one example of the power of this approach, an "at least one" analysis of aggression and sexuality in 3256 dreams reports from a young male's dream journal for 1981 to 1989 and 1994 to 1995 showed consistency in the findings from year to year.[65]

The one drawback with this method is that it does not control for dream length, which means that reports of less than 50 or more than 300 words should not be used in making comparisons with the Hall and Van de Castle norms. However, no such screening for length is necessary if the comparison is with other dream reports in a long dream series.

Potential Psychopathology Measures

There have been numerous attempts to develop indicators of psychopathology in dream content for a wide variety of illnesses, but the results have been meager and often contradictory.[66, 67] Not least among the problems has been the application of global rating scales calling for subtle judgments to dream reports of widely varying lengths. Dream reports from schizophrenic and depressed patients usually are especially brief and lacking in content.[68–70] (See Chapters 42 and 66 for a more extensive treatment of dream content and psychopathology.) Despite the methodological problems within this literature, it seems relatively clear that there are unlikely to be any forms of dream content that are specific to one or another kind of psychopathology. Average people seem to have every kind of dream content that patients do; once again, the difference is in how frequently different characters, social interactions, and activities appear.

Perhaps the most consistent finding with mental patient populations is the simple lack of friends in their dreams.[71, 72] Instead, the characters in mental patients' dream reports tend to be family members or strangers in varying combinations. Nor are there as many friendly interactions in patients' dreams. This brings a slightly different approach to the friendliness issue because there may or may not be friendly interactions with people described as friends, and there can be friendly interactions with family members and strangers. Table 37–1 presents a comparison of 104 dream reports from 20 male schizophrenics with the Hall and Van de Castle male norms, revealing a low friends percentage, F/C ratio, and percentage of dream reports with at least one friendly interaction.

Beyond a few specific indicators, different forms of psychopathology in dreams may turn out to be best identified by patterns of indicators. Moreover, these patterns may involve indicators that do not immediately spring to mind when thinking of psychopathology. For example, a comparison of dreams from teenagers who scored high and low on Krohn and Mayman's Object Relations Scale suggested that a low physical activities percentage (physical activities divided by all activities) characterizes the mature group, which means they are talking and thinking more in their dreams than their less mature counterparts[59] (G. W. Domhoff, PhD, unpublished data). The percentage of dreams with at least one striving attempt by the dreamer and the *self-negativity percentage* (based on personal failures, misfortunes, and victim status in aggressive interactions) may turn out to be useful, as suggested by the small study of schizophrenics presented in Table 37–1. Thus, psychopathology scales might be created in the same way the MMPI was, by simply seeing which indicators among the many that are tried actually distinguish patient groups from each other and control groups. However, it should be emphasized that large sample sizes (at least 75 to 100 dreams from each individual patient or 100 to 125 Most Recent Dreams from any given patient group) would be crucial to the success of such an effort.

CONCLUSION

Three general findings emerged from the systematic study of dream content in the 20th century. First, the dream reports of groups of people from around the world were more similar than they were different on such indicators as the percentage of male and female

Table 37–1. DREAM REPORTS: A COMPARISON OF MALE SCHIZOPHRENICS WITH MALE NORMS

	Schizophrenics (%)	Male Norms (%)	h	p
Characters				
Male/female percentage	58	67	−.20	.021*
Friends percentage	20	31	−.25	.002†
Family percentage	27	12	+.39	.000†
Animal percentage	23	06	+.51	.000†
Social Interaction Percentages				
Befriender percentage	53	50	+.06	.487
Aggressor percentage	56	40	+.33	.000†
Physical aggression percentage	60	50	+.20	.120
Social Interaction Ratios				
F/C index	.11	.21	−.30	.000†
A/C index	.37	.34	+.06	.458
Self-Concept Percentages				
Self-negativity percentage	82	69	+.29	.035*
Bodily misfortunes percentage	35	29	+.13	.482
Dreams With at Least One				
Aggression	47	47	−.01	.941
Friendliness	17	38	−.47	.000†
Sexuality	18	12	+.19	.075
Misfortunate	29	36	−.15	.163
Striving	08	26	−.50	.000†

*Significant at the .05 level.
†Significant at the .01 level.
A/C, aggressions per character; F/C, friendly interactions per character.

characters, the higher ratio of aggression to friendliness, the higher ratio of misfortune to good fortune, and the higher ratio of negative emotions to positive emotions. Second, there are impressive consistencies in long dream series from individuals. Third, there are intriguing individual differences in any group of dreamers.[1, 4, 28]

This chapter shows that new methods for collecting and analyzing dream reports, some available on the Internet,[73] make it possible to refine and extend these general findings. For example, patients coming to a wide range of clinics could be asked for a Most Recent Dream or screened for the presence or absence of a dream journal and then asked for another Most Recent Dream after varying periods of medication or psychotherapy. Moreover, nominal content categories and the "at least one" method make it possible to deal with databases of any size in a rigorous way, and spreadsheets have made data analysis faster and more accurate. Large-scale studies of dream content can contribute to the study of dream meaning and add another dimension to sleep-disorder and mental-health clinics.

References

1. Winget C, Kramer M. Dimensions of dreams. Gainesville, Fla: University of Florida Press; 1979.
2. Foulkes D. Children's Dreams. New York, NY: Wiley; 1982.
3. Foulkes D. Dreaming: A Cognitive-Psychological Analysis. Hillsdale, NJ: Lawrence Erlbaum Associates; 1985.
4. Domhoff GW. Finding Meaning in Dreams: A Quantitative Approach. New York, NY: Plenum Publishing; 1996.
5. Hall CS, Van de Castle R. The Content Analysis of Dreams. New York, NY: Appleton-Century-Crofts; 1966.
6. Bernstein D, Belicki C. Assessing dreams through self-report questionnaires: relations with past research and personality. Dreaming. 1995;5:13–27.
7. Hall CS, Domhoff GW, Blick K, et al. The dreams of college men and women in 1950 and 1980: a comparison of dream contents and sex differences. Sleep. 1982;5:188–194.
8. Tonay V. California women and their dreams: a historical and sub-cultural comparison of dream content. Imag Cog Pers. 1990–91;10:83–97.
9. Foulkes D. Home and laboratory dreams: four empirical studies and a conceptual reevaluation. Sleep. 1979;2:233–251.
10. Foulkes D. The Psychology of Sleep. New York, NY: Charles Scribner's Sons; 1966.
11. Goodenough D, Shapiro A, Holden M, et al. A comparison of "dreamers" and "nondreamers." J Abnorm Soc Psychol. 1959;59:295–302.
12. Butler S, Watson R. Individual differences in memory for dreams: the role of cognitive skills. Percept Mot Skills. 1985;53:841–864.
13. Dement W, Wolpert E. Relationships in the manifest content of dreams occurring in the same night. J Nerv Ment Dis. 1958;126:568–578.
14. Trosman H, Rechtschaffen A, Offenkrantz W, et al. Studies in the psychophysiology of dreams, IV: relations among dreams in sequence. Arch Gen Psychiatry. 1960;3:602–607.
15. Domhoff GW, Kamiya J. Problems in dream content study with objective indicators, III: changes in dream content throughout the night. Arch Gen Psychiatry. 1964;11:529–532.
16. Hall CS. Studies of Dreams Collected in the Laboratory and at Home. Santa Cruz, Calif: Institute of Dream Research Monograph Series (No. 1); 1966.
17. Strauch I, Meier B. In Search of Dreams: Results of Experimental Dream Research. Albany, NY: State University of New York Press; 1996.
18. Verdone P. Temporal reference of manifest dream content. Percept Mot Skills. 1965;20:1253–1268.
19. Foulkes D. Dream reports from different states of sleep. J Abnorm Soc Psychol. 1962;65:14–25.
20. Foulkes D, Schmidt M. Temporal sequence and unit composition in dream reports from different stages of sleep. Sleep. 1983;6:265–280.
21. Antrobus J. REM and NREM sleep reports: comparisons of word frequencies by cognitive classes. Psychophysiology. 1983;20:562–568.
22. Domhoff GW, Schneider A. Much ado about very little: the small effect sizes when home and laboratory collected dreams are compared. Dreaming. 1999;9:139–151.
23. Weisz R, Foulkes D. Home and laboratory dreams collected under uniform sampling conditions. Psychophysiology. 1970;6:588–596.
24. Bose VS. Dream Content Transformations: An Empirical Study of Freud's Secondary Revision Hypothesis [dissertation]. Waltair, India: Andhra University; 1982.
25. Domhoff GW, Kamiya J. Problems in dream content study with objective indicators, I: a comparison of home and laboratory dream reports. Arch Gen Psychiatry. 1964;11:519–524.
26. Foulkes D. Dream research: 1953–1993. Sleep. 1996;19:609–624.
27. Jung C. Dreams. Princeton, NJ: Princeton University Press; 1974.
28. Smith M, Hall CS. An investigation of regression in a long dream series. J Gerontol. 1964;19:66–71.
29. Hobson J. The Dreaming Brain. New York, NY: Basic Books; 1988.
30. Allport G. The Use of Personal Documents in Psychological Science. New York, NY: Social Science Research Council; 1942.
31. Baldwin A. Personal structure analysis: a statistical method for investigating the single personality. J Abnorm Soc Psychol. 1942;37:163–183.
32. Webb E, Campbell D, Schwartz R, et al. Nonreactive Measures in the Social Sciences. 2nd ed. Chicago, Ill: Rand McNally; 1981.
33. Hall CS. What people dream about. Sci Am. 1951,184:60–63.
34. Avila-White D, Schneider A, Domhoff, GW. The most recent dreams of 12–13 year-old boys and girls: a methodological contribution to the study of dream content. Dreaming. 1999;9:163–171.
35. Freud S. The Interpretation of Dreams: The Standard Edition of the Complete, Psychological Works of Sigmund Freud. Vols 4 and 5. London, England: Hogarth Press, 1900.
36. Foulkes D. A Grammar of Dreams. New York, NY: Basic Books; 1978.
37. Reis W. A Comparison of the Interpretation of Dream Series With and Without Free Association [dissertation]. Case Western Reserve University; 1951.
38. Popp G, Luborsky L, Crits-Cristoph P. The parallel of the CCRT from therapy narratives with the CCRT from dreams. In: Luborsky L, Crits-Christoph P, eds. Understanding Transference. New York, NY: Basic Books; 1992.
39. Lakoff G, Johnson M. Metaphors We Live By. Chicago, Ill: University of Chicago Press; 1980.
40. Lakoff G. Women, Fire, and Dangerous Things. Chicago, Ill: University of Chicago Press; 1987.
41. States B. The Rhetoric of Dreams. Ithaca, NY: Cornell University Press; 1987.
42. Lakoff G, Turner M. More Than Cool Reason. Chicago, Ill: University of Chicago Press; 1989.
43. Hall CS. A cognitive theory of dream symbols. J Gen Psychol. 1953;48:169–186.
44. Partridge E. A Dictionary of Slang and Unconventional English. 8th ed. London, England: Routledge & Kegan Paul; 1984.
45. Kramer M, Schoen L, Kinney L. Nightmares in Vietnam veterans. J Am Acad Psychoanal. 1987;15:67–81.
46. Lakoff G. How metaphor structures dreams. Dreaming. 1993;3:77–98.
47. Hall CS. Diagnosing personality by the analysis of dreams. J Abnorm Soc Psychol. 1947;42:68–79.
48. Domhoff GW. The repetition of dreams and dream elements: a possible clue to a function of dreams. In: Moffitt A, Kramer M, Hoffman R, eds. The Functions of Dreams. Albany, NY: State University of New York Press; 1993.
49. Hall CS. Content analysis of dreams: categories, units, and norms. In: Gerbner G, ed. The Analysis of Communication Content. New York, NY: Wiley; 1969:147–158.
50. Hall CS. Normative dream content studies. In: Kramer M, ed. Dream Psychology and the New Biology of Dreaming. Springfield, Ill: Charles C Thomas; 1969:175–184.

51. Foulkes D. Children's dreaming. In: Foulkes D, Cavallero C, eds. Dreaming as Cognition. New York, NY: Harvester Wheatsheaf; 1993.

52. Foulkes D, Hollifield M, Sullivan B, et al. REM dreaming and cognitive skills at ages 5-8: a cross-sectional study. Int J Behav Develop. 1990;13:447–465.

53. Reinsel R, Antrobus J, Wollman M. Bizarreness in dreams and waking fantasy. In: Antrobus J, Bertini M, eds. The Neuropsychology of Sleep and Dreaming. Hillsdale, NJ: Lawrence Erlbaum Associates; 1992:157–184.

54. Revonsuo A, Salmivalli C. A content analysis of bizarre elements in dreams. Dreaming. 1995;5:169–87.

55. Van de Castle R. Problems in applying methodology of content analysis. In: Kramer M, Dream Psychology and the New Biology of Dreaming. Springfield, Ill: Charles C Thomas; 1969:185–197.

56. Hauri P. Categorization of sleep mental activity for psychophysiological studies. In: Lairy G, Salzarulo P, eds. The Experimental Study of Sleep: Methodological Problems. New York, NY: Elsevier Scientific; 1975:271–281.

57. Clark J, Trinder J, Kramer M, et al. An approach to the content analysis of dream scales. In: Chase M, Stern W, Walter P, eds. Sleep Research. Los Angeles, Calif: Brain Research Institute, UCLA; 1972;1:118.

58. Beck AT, Hurvich MS. Psychological correlates of depression, I: frequency of "masochistic" dream content in a private practice sampling. Psychosom Med. 1959;21:50–55.

59. Krohn A, Mayman M. Object relations in dreams and projective tests. Bull Menninger Clin. 1974;38:445–466.

60. Schneider A, Domhoff GW. The Quantitative Study of Dreams. Available at: http://psych.ucsc.edu/dreams/DreamSAT/index.html. Accessed December 1999.

61. Trinder J, Kramer M, Riechers M, et al. The effect of dream length on dream content. Psychophysiology. 1970;7:33.

62. Auld F, Goldenberg G, Weiss J. Measurement of primary process thinking in dream reports. J Pers Soc Psychol. 1968;8:418–426.

63. Wood J, Sebba D, Domino G. Do creative people have more bizarre dreams? A reconsideration. Imag Cog Pers. 1989–90;9:3–16.

64. Livingston G, Levin R. The effects of dream length on the relationship between primary process in dreams and creativity. Dreaming. 1991;1:301–309.

65. Domhoff GW, Schneider A. New rationales and methods for quantitative dream research outside the laboratory. Sleep. 1998;21:398–404.

66. Kramer M. Manifest dream content in normal and psychopathologic states. Arch Gen Psychiatry. 1970;22:149–159.

67. Kramer M, Roth T. Dreams in psychopathology. In: Wolman B, ed. Handbook of Dreams. New York, NY: Van Nostrand Reinhold; 1979:361–367.

68. Kramer M, Roth T. Comparison of dream content in laboratory dream reports of schizophrenic and depressive patient groups. Compr Psychiatry. 1973;14:325–329.

69. Barrett D, Loeffler M. Comparison of dream content of depressed vs. nondepressed dreamers. Psychol Rep. 1992;70:403–407.

70. Armitage R, Rochlen A, Fitch T, et al. Dream recall and major depression: a preliminary report. Dreaming. 1995;5:189–198.

71. Hall CS. A comparison of the dreams of four groups of hospitalized mental patients with each other and with a normal population. J Nerv Ment Dis. 1966;143:135–139.

72. Maharaj N. An Investigation Into the Content and Structure of Schizophrenic Dreams [dissertation]. Leiden, Netherlands: Leiden University; 1997.

73. Resources for Scientists. Available at: http://psych.ucsc.edu/dreams/resources.html. Accessed December 1999.

38

Theories of Dreaming

John Antrobus

From the beginning of written human inquiry, people have proposed conjectures and theories about dreaming, its origin and causes, its meanings, and its function. Long before cognitive psychology existed as a field of inquiry, people assumed that the unusual character of dreaming sleep called for a special stand-alone theory. Implicit in this assumption is the view that waking imagery and thought *are* well understood and that dreaming is the last theoretical frontier to conquer. But intimate familiarity with our mentation does not a theory make—even of waking imagery and thought. Although cognitive theories and models are becoming increasingly broad in their reach and more precise in the detail of their microstructure, comprehensive models of waking thought and imagery are still in their infancy. The most powerful neurocognitive theories depend on experimental procedures where the time separating stimulus and response are of the order of 1000 msec. As the interval increases, the precision and predictability of the models decrease. When imagery and thought are so far removed from the influence of external stimuli as to appear spontaneous, as is the case with dreaming, their characteristics can be predicted only weakly, if at all. For this reason, theories that make claims about the meaning and neurocognitive and motivational attributes of such imagery and thought, whether daydreaming or night dreaming. are difficult to either support or disconfirm, and strong claims based on such theories should be regarded with reservation.

Because dreaming, a cognitive process that occurs during sleep, is produced by some part of the same neural hardware and makes use of some of the same stored memories that accomplish waking mentation, it is reasonable to regard dreaming as a modified form of waking cognitive, affective, and neurophysiological processes. From this perspective, a theory of dreaming must not be a stand-alone theory but rather part of a more comprehensive theory of neurocognitive processes. This heavy dependence on neighboring domains, especially the social, cognitive, and neurosciences, is not only desirable but also essential to the construction of a strong account of dreaming processes. Dreaming is a neurostate-dependent cognitive process in which sometimes dramatic deviations from the characteristics of waking mentation are produced by the cerebral cortex as a consequence of quasirhythmic changes in subcortical processes.

Across history, theories of dreaming have been heavily dependent on concurrent theories in related domains. Theories of the spirit world were replaced with rational theories by Aristotle and with unconscious drive–related theories by Plato and then later expanded on by Freud[1] and the psychoanalysts; cognitive association theories were put forth by European psychologists around the 1900s. With the discovery of the strong association between reported dreaming and stage 1 electroencephalographic (EEG) rapid eye movement (REM) sleep by Aserinsky and Kleitman,[2] an intensive international research effort was made to account for dreaming by mapping its features to an array of psychophysiological processes (peripheral physiological measures). The implicit assumption here was that the relation between these psychophysiological variables and human experience was invariant across waking and sleep states so that waking psychophysiology could conveniently inform the psychophysiology of dreaming.

Unfortunately, the assumption is false. Not only is spontaneous electrodermal activity, the marker of emotional reactivity in the *waking* state, more active in stage 4 EEG sleep,[3] where the sleeper's reported experience is severely impoverished, but the EEG of the most dreamlike periods of sleep (i.e., REM sleep) is remarkably similar to that of waking![2] Although measurement of the cognitive attributes of sleep mentation became more sophisticated during this period of research, the search for a better understanding of the dreaming process through its physiological correlates was not well rewarded.

Neurophysiological studies of sleep in animals, particularly by Hobson and McCarley,[4] suggested a basis for how subcortical processes might account for dreaming in the cerebral cortex, and Ellman et al.[5] showed how the subcortical reward system of Olds[6] might account for the motivational characteristics of dreaming. A new level of precision in the construction of neurocognitive dreaming theory is possible because of the rapid development of brain imaging procedures and computational neural network models that take the hand-waving vagueness out of the earlier theories. This work has brought us to a point where the basic outlines of a theory of dreaming, as a state-dependent component of a general theory of perception and cognition, are beginning to emerge.

HISTORICAL ASPECTS

Theories of dreaming have addressed three questions. The first and most sustained preoccupation has been with the meaning of the dream. The second, more contemporary question concerns how the dream experience is produced, and the third question concerns the function or purpose of the dreaming process.

The Meaning of Dreams

The earliest question has concerned the *meaning* of the dream episode. When the dreams were thought to have a supernatural origin, the question of meaning was the message of the supernatural source. As the source became recognized as the dreamer, the question of meaning changed to the message that one portion of the mental apparatus was attempting to communicate with another part. In his *The Interpretation of Dreams*, Freud[1] proposed that the dream represented unconscious cognitive processes driven by biological, particularly sexual, drives. The conflict between these drives and learned societal constraints tended to produce a variety of classes of psychopathology. Freud assumed that the psychopathology could be treated by helping his patient to understand the sources of the conflict. For Freud and his followers, then, interpretation of the dream meant identification of the specific unconscious conflicts portrayed by what Freud called the manifest, or literal, characteristics of the dream report.

There was little interest within the psychoanalytical community in subjecting Freud's assumptions about dreaming to an empirical test. Nevertheless, when the discovery of REM dreaming was reported[2] and psychoanalytical students felt pressure from other medical specialties to ground their procedures in empirical research, there was a brief period in which several of the psychoanalytical assumptions about dreaming were put to test. Foulkes et al.,[7] however, found no support for the predicted relations between psychosexual stages of development and dream content.

Theories of dream interpretation assume that dreamed objects and events are associates of significant objects and events in the dreamer's waking life. The task of interpreting the dream is one of reconstructing the dreamer's associative sequence to determine its origin. Unfortunately, because this associative process has not been studied systematically, we can only speculate about the process of dream interpretation. Interpreters assume that the manifest reported characteristics of the dream are created in response to higher-order drives and conflicts. Psychoanalysts assume that this associative sequence may be quite complex, so the dream item may be removed from its source by several steps. They implicitly assume that these motivations and meanings can be recovered by associating *backward* from the reported dream events, implicitly assuming that the waking associative processes are at least somewhat similar to the forward association processes of the dream reporter while asleep. Furthermore, dream interpreters make extensive use of biographical, behavioral, and personal life situation information of the dream reporter, so it is

impossible to determine how much of any "dream interpretation" is based on the dream alone.

One very ambitious study attempted to test this associative model by comparing dream reports after a dramatic presleep stimulus: before sleep, the subjects were shown a movie of tribal circumcision known for its ability to arouse sexual conflict. To analyze their dream report data, the experimenters systematically identified associates of many subjects to the dreamed objects and events, but neither the dreamed objects or their associates—removed by one or more steps from the dream report—matched the circumcision movie better than a travelog control film. Unfortunately, despite years of data analysis, the study was never published.[8]

Study of the effect of presleep stimulus influence on dream content continued, but the emphasis shifted from psychoanalytical theory to the broader class of stressors. Again, little effect was observed with stressor movies; even patients awaiting surgery showed no direct or remote associations to cutting or surgery before or after their operations.[9] On the other hand, severe traumatic stress, such as that experienced by soldiers in battle, frequently produced alterations in dream content and affect as well as sleep architecture.[10] One can certainly interpret such terror dreams reliably in the sense that two interpreters can agree on their origin; however, this reliability of interpretation does not appear to extend to the less dramatic events in life, which are the typical domains of dream interpretation. Clearly, if dream interpretation is not reliable, the interpretations cannot be valid. Despite the lack of empirical evidence that supports any interpretation of a dream, most of us have been impressed at one time or another by an impression that a particular event that we have dreamed must have been produced by an associative process that was initiated by a particular recent life experience. In this limited sense, we have proposed an interpretation of our dream. Whether our sense of confidence about this interpretation is based on some systematic regularities in associative processes during dreaming sleep or whether our subjective impression is an illusion is impossible to determine in the individual case. Until better theories and empirical tests are carried out, dream interpretations and the theories on which these assumptions are based must be regarded with skepticism.

How Dreams Are Produced

This second question of how dreams are produced has been addressed from cognitive, neurophysiological, and computational neurocognitive perspectives. Neurophysiological studies have emphasized the alteration of the functional architecture of the dreaming, relative to the waking, brain, that is, the spatial location in the brain of neural events that are associated with dreaming. In this section, I try to integrate the contributions of these diverse sources to produce a working model of dreaming sleep. As stated, such a model of dreaming sleep is necessarily heavily dependent on models acquired in the waking state where it is easier to collect accurate cognitive and neurophysiological data.

Some of the most useful cognitive research in this regard has been the "incorporation" studies in which auditory or tactile stimuli are presented during REM sleep, and the stimulus features compared with the features of a dream are reported about 30 sec later.[11] Almost everyone has had the experience on awakening from sleep that some object or event in one's dream was rather similar to a *concurrent* external stimulus event such as a telephone bell or automobile alarm. In these instances, the dream seemed to incorporate some feature of a concurrent external stimulus rather than perceiving it as an external event that is independent of the dream. The discovery of a strong association between REM sleep and dreaming[2] allowed this incorporation phenomenon to be studied experimentally (i.e., by locating the dream in time, the EEG marker improved the efficiency of cognitive experiments on dreaming). It changed the source of mentation reports from the morning after to seconds after the occurrence of the dream. Studies delivering auditory stimuli, such as bells and buzzers or light flashes and fine sprays of water, to sleepers in REM sleep have found strong associations between stimulus and dream features in 20 to 40% of the trials.[12, 13] For example, in the context of a dream of acting on stage, a spray of water was experienced as rain coming through the ceiling; in the context of sitting in one's living room, a ringing doorbell was experienced as a telephone ring—without interruption of the ongoing dreams.[11]

A remarkable but overlooked characteristic of dreams that incorporate features of external stimuli is the speed and ingenious fit of the incorporations into the meaning and imagery context of the ongoing dream. Dement[11] reported that in response to a fine spray of water, one dreamer complained that his children, with whom he had been playing, must have spilled his glass of water on him. Like other incorporations, this plausible interpretation of the spray was accomplished by the sleeping mind-brain within a few seconds. The previous example in which the dreamer watched the actress in front of him open her umbrella in response to rain coming through the ceiling is somewhat bizarre, but it is difficult to imagine how a waking individual could create a more acceptable response to the same stimulus. The inference to be drawn from these and many comparable examples is that the mind-brain in REM sleep is able to integrate new features in a seamless fashion, from external or internal sources, with the prior event sequence schemata of the current dream. This integration of schemata not only is novel but also is automatic in the sense that it does not require the attentional processes that we typically attribute to such a creative product.

To accomplish this schema construction quickly, some parts of the mind-brain must be quite active, perhaps as active as in the waking state. The work of Hobson and McCarley[4] on pontine and cortical structures of the cat during waking and REM and NREM sleep provided new neurophysiological evidence for the assumption that the brain is in an activated state

in REM sleep. They proposed that the cerebral cortex receives widespread activation from the ascending reticular activating system in REM sleep similar to that in waking. The primary difference is that incoming afferent information and outgoing efferent information are strongly inhibited during REM sleep. This means that aside from some incorporations of the features of concurrent external stimuli, the visual images of dreaming are produced as responses to some form of memorial processing within the isolated brain. Some parts of the brain are making imagined "perceptual" responses to stimuli produced in the same or other parts of the same isolated brain. As we all know from our experience, these visual images are accepted as authentic percepts. The motor cortex often issues motor commands, such as to run or to talk, in response to these images, but because of spinal inhibition, the commands cannot be executed by the motor system, the expected proprioceptive feedback does not occur, and the sleeper experiences motor paralysis.

PONTO-GENICULO-OCCIPITAL AND RAPID EYE MOVEMENT BURSTS: THEIR RELATION TO VISUAL IMAGERY

The respiratory, cardiac, and oculomotor systems that produce REM bursts, however, are exempt from motor inhibition. REM bursts are strongly correlated with ponto-geniculo-occipital (PGO) spikes. Hobson and McCarley[4] claimed that this PGO system is independent of cortical, and therefore free of cognitive, control during REM sleep. They propose that the pontine generator is the source of the information from which the dream is created. They state that PGO activity is random and that the cortex interprets the timing and direction of eye movement (EM) information in the PGO spikes post hoc so as to incorporate, or to "synthesize," it into the ongoing dream. This assumption is supported by the observation that visual imagery immediately following REM bursts is more vivid than imagery further removed in time from the last REM burst.[14, 15] Although this study uses a new method of assessing the effect of REM bursts on mentation, it has been evaluated in only one subject and must be tested on a larger sample. A detailed review of all studies of the REM burst effect by Pivik[16] found no reliable effects of any kind. Moreover, the fact that visual imagery persists throughout long intervals of the REM period when there are no EMs, and therefore no PGO bursts, is clearly at variance with the claim that dreaming is a synthesis of information in the PGO burst; therefore, PGO bursts cannot be the information source for the dream.

In the waking state, the many competing and interacting sources of EM control are sorted out in the frontal eye fields of the cortex, which in turn direct the pontine nuclei that drive the oculomotor system. Antrobus[17] argued that when the frontal cortex is sufficiently active within the REM period, the frontal eye fields retain this control and thereby account for the commonly observed correspondences between imagery and EM direction in REM sleep. He suggested that the apparently random EM activity of REM bursts is a visual "stutter" caused by the failure of the frontal eye field movement command to produce the visual feedback to the retina that is expected because it always occurs in waking visual search. Because the image cannot be found by moving the eyes in the imagined spatial location of the object, dreamers may report that they are unable to find a previously imaged object.

Waking saccades function to position poorly resolved off-fovea images onto the fovea, which are then mapped onto the calcarine region of the visual cortex. Because the REM sleep visual image does not originate in the external environment, the saccade cannot return the anticipated improved image to the visual cortex. In the absence of this visual feedback from the calcarine region to the frontal cortex, the oculomotor system should repeat its command to the pons with increased frequency and intensity, resulting in large PGO feedback to the frontal cortex as well as afferents to the oculomotor system that produces the REM bursts. Support for this model is provided by Hong et al.[18] in a study with positron emission tomography (PET) that showed that the frontal eye field regions were indeed activated during rapid EM within REM sleep.

If the REM bursts associated with PGO bursts are the consequence of feedback failure, the PGO bursts are, by definition, not random events and the two theories of dreaming that rest on the randomness assumption lose their basis. Hobson and McCarley[4] have argued that dreaming is an interpretation of PGO activity and that because the activity is random and originates in the subcortical centers, the dream cannot be attributed to cognitive or motivational sources. Taking the random feature pontine generator model for granted and given that gridlock in very active, artificial neural networks can be eliminated by random activity. Crick and Mitchison[19] have proposed that the PGO spikes in dreaming sleep are a memory-clearing or -resetting process. If the PGO randomness assumption is false, then both of these models of dreaming fall.

Nevertheless, as stated, the assumptions by Hobson and McCarley[4] that the production of dream imagery is dependent on an activated brain and that this activation is controlled by periodic pontine activation (i.e., in REM sleep) are fundamental components of any theory of dreaming. Later, we discuss how the widespread cortical activation picture of their activation-synthesis model is being revised or replaced by increasingly precise topographical images of the sleeping brain that permit a finer mapping of dream features onto activated regions of the cortex. First, we discuss how the dream might produce imaginal sequences in the absence of sensory input. To obtain some insight into how the brain might do that, we further examine the stimulus incorporation studies in which, despite the high sensory thresholds of REM sleep, some features of external stimuli are incorporated into the ongoing dream.

Although the theoretical implication of the incorporation studies was profound, at the time of their publication they spoke to no particular theory of dreaming. It was assumed that a stimulus was first perceived or recognized and then its features were somehow extracted and that these features were somehow incorporated into the dream image. It has been the subsequent development of cognitive psychology, computational models of cognition, and cognitive neuroscience that make it possible to interpret the incorporation studies and to appreciate their contribution to a plausible outline of a theory of dreaming.

COMPUTATIONAL MODELS: NEURAL NETWORKS

Connectionist models are based on the assumption that traditional features—those we can consciously identify and name—are learned as part of a longer sequence that starts with *microfeatures*, which are the smallest units of neural network models and are not cognitively penetrable, and moves through increasingly abstract feature-detecting neural networks, leading to networks that recognize, spatially locate, name, and determine the meaning of the object or event that possesses the features.[20] The features of an external stimulus presented during REM sleep may be recognized even though the entire object or event is not. The development of computational neural network models in 1986[21] demonstrated that when a feature is represented by a cluster of interrelated neural units, it requires the activation of only a few units in the cluster to activate the entire feature cluster. Similarly, activation of only a few features of an object or event may be sufficient to fully activate all of the feature clusters that express that object or event. For example, in the waking world, one can fully recognize one's mother or friend from just a few fragmentary features of voice or face. And it may require only two neighboring dark regions that locate a person's eyes for one to perceive a face. Moreover, contexts can behave in the same fashion as features, so a set of activated stimulus features may activate different object or event clusters depending on which context feature cluster is activated.[21] For example, in the context of "kitchen," a "sink" may activate "stove," but in a "bathroom" context, it could elicit "bathtub."

Furthermore, because the smallest units of neural network models, microfeatures, are smaller than features, the units can be combined to form novel features, objects, and events. A *novel* object is an emergent person schema created as a consequence of the joint activation of a cluster of featural schema that do not normally co-occur but in this situation the microfeatures have a sufficient shared history, expressed as shared connections, to accomplish a seamless fit among the participating features. For example, "flat surface" may be experienced as "table top," but if it is "irregularly shaped," the dreamer may conclude that he or she is "at the circus," where such shapes are more common. Alternately, in the visual context of an imaginary *visual vista*, the experience of "weightlessness" produced by the absence of proprioceptive feedback from pressure receptors as well as the REM sleep activity in the vestibular nuclei may be integrated in the novel emergent schema of "flying on a carpet."

NOVELTY OF IMAGE FEATURES

The implications for a theory of dreaming are clear and powerful. One of the greatest challenges for a theory of dreaming has been to account not only for the vividness of the objects imaged in the absence of external stimuli but also for the ability of the mind-brain to produce novel objects and event sequences. The novel objects may be bizarre from a waking perspective, but they are integrated with one another in such a seamless fashion that their reality is taken for granted by the dreamer. Computational neural network models offer a plausible theory of how these novel objects and events can be produced in dreaming sleep.[22]

There are, of course, constraints on novelty within the dream. For example, faces in dreams are never portrayed with inverted noses and although carpets may fly like airplanes, they do not fly in reverse. Neural networks nicely simulate these constraints. Models of the constraints necessary to simulate behavior in the waking state show that they are largely a function of experience, that is, perceptual learning. The more highly learned the regularities, the less likely are they, during dreaming, to be modified in novel ways. Computational simulations of neuropathological cognition show that alteration of brain architecture can also alter the character of these constraints. Alterations in functional brain architecture have long been thought to be responsible for the novel and bizarre character of dreamed objects and events. Success in simulating the precise patterns of dream novelty and bizarreness provides a demanding test for future theories of dreaming.

Traditional theories of dreaming, as mentioned, implicitly assume that the origins of the image sequence are higher-order meanings and motivational states that direct lower-order visual imagery processes to construct imaginal objects and event sequences that represent the higher-order states and processes. Working with this assumption, Hinton et al.[23] constructed a wake-sleep neural network model in which the "higher" end of the network can reconstruct its input; that is, the higher-level representation of objects and events must be able to reproduce the images (i.e., sensory-like percepts) from which they were derived. Similarly, an abstract representation of an expected event should be able to direct the construction of an image that fits the more abstract representation. As discussed earlier, we do not know at this time whether the higher-level cognitive processes that appear to drive the frontal eye fields and EMs are able to successfully supervise the image-constructing processes in the extrastriate cortex.

This top-down conception of Hinton et al.[23] seems to assume that the processing sequence and neural pathways of normal waking perception do not operate during dreaming, but it is reasonable to assume that dreaming is accomplished by some modified form of these perceptual pathways and processes. Recent computational and spatial neurocognitive models of perceptual and dreaming processes suggest that many characteristics of dreaming can be simulated as bottom-up perception-like processes operating within a closed system. These directional processes have not been well studied. Detailed empirical research is needed to determine whether one or both of these models operate during dreaming sleep.

In waking perception, clusters of neurons within each cortical region "interpret" the information they receive from subcortical sources in the contexts of their own prior state and the states of neighboring cortical regions that represent meanings and goal structures. The clusters in any region represent a very large number of potential attractor states, of which each constitutes a local interpretation of the input to the region. Local attractors compete with their neighbors to form larger, more general attractors that in turn represent solutions to inputs across different modalities and internal contexts. In waking perception, the attractor states may be initiated by external information, information from neighboring regions, or even by quasirandom neural activity. Attractor states vary in their strength primarily on the basis of the frequency with which they have been activated in the past. In one person's visual processing system, this strength might constitute a bias to see "eyes" rather than "buttons"; at high levels of motivation, the motor system might be biased to "run" rather than "fight." In a field of such attractors, even random input will move toward one attractor state or another. In this sense, even if neural activity were random, it would soon become a pattern of some kind.

If attractors can be activated by random activity, they can also be activated by weak patterns. For example, two dark spots in the extrastriate cortex have a high probability of being identified as a "pair of eyes" in the parietal cortex and the "eyes" in turn as a "face" or a "person" by another region. The implication of such attractor models for dreaming theory is that the attractor states that have been learned during waking perception can be activated by weak or quasirandom input. Accordingly, attractors distributed across different cortical regions representing the shape, color, movement, location, and functional significance of a particular image may be produced in the absence either of patterned input from the retina or from top-down instructions from higher-order cortical regions.

Supporting evidence for this conception comes from neural network simulations and from stimulus incorporation studies that depend on the fact that the brain is not a completely closed system during REM sleep. Using a recurrent back propagation neural network to simulate this aspect of dreaming, Antrobus[22] showed that any random input has some similarity to previously learned patterns so a random input is typically recognized as some variation of its most similar attractor. Moreover, if that attractor pattern occurs in a temporal sequence of patterns that the system has

IMAGINAL SEQUENCES

The lifelike experience of novel perceptual-like *sequences* characteristic of longer dreams cannot be explained by a model that simply interprets static forms generated in the visual cortex. Antrobus[23, 24] argued that the ability of the mind-brain to produce the sequences of dream events is possible because anticipation is a fundamental characteristic of waking perception. With each new waking percept, the cognitive system updates its projections for both perceptual input and motor responses. That sequences are a characteristic of dreams suggests that much of this sequence-generating capability is intact in dreaming sleep. As discussed earlier in connection with EMs and the absence of visual feedback, sequencing models may be divided into perceptual and motor segments, and the absence of the feedback component in the imaginary dreaming environment suggests that sequences are most vulnerable to disruption at that point, but more sophisticated sleep mentation reports are needed to render a more precise version of this model than that provided by Antrobus.[22]

THEORETICAL CONSEQUENCES OF DREAMING: REM SLEEP MISMATCH

Because the characteristics of dreamed objects and events differ from those of waking thought, one goal of a neurocognitive theory of dreaming should be to map the distinctive cognitive and motivational characteristics of dreaming sleep onto the distinctive characteristics of the sleeping brain. Because REM sleep mentation reports are distinctly more dream-like than nonrapid eye movement (NREM) reports, matched by sleeper and time of night,[25] theorists wrongly tend to assume that dreaming is unique to REM sleep and that all REM sleep mentation is as wildly bizarre and visually vivid as the dreams we remember on awakening in the morning. These assumptions encourage neurophysiologists to assume that the brain state of REM sleep is equivalent to the brain state of dreaming. Contrary to this simple conception, however, these assumptions are not supported by data.

Early-night REM reports are decidedly brief and rarely bizarre. The long, dramatic, visually vivid, bizarre, and memorable dreams that are the hallmark of dreaming typically come from the late portion of the sleep period, particularly when we sleep beyond our accustomed waking hour.[26] It is in these late-morning REM dreams that speech and auditory imagery appear and sleepers sometimes report the ability to control the course of their lucid dream.[27] Although late REM remains consistently more dream-like than late NREM mentation, late NREM imagery and thought demonstrate all the characteristics of REM mentation, al-

though in a weaker form. Mild stressors may have an effect similar to that of sleeping late.[10] Sleepers with low awakening thresholds have more dream-like reports regardless of sleep stage.[28] These observations have profound significance for neurocognitive theories of dreaming.

If the cognitive characteristics of dreaming can be produced during later-morning NREM sleep, then dreaming cannot be ascribed to neurophysiological characteristics that are unique to REM sleep. That both REM and NREM mentations become more dream-like as sleep persists into the period where the rising edge of the diurnal sleep-wake rhythm supplies activation to the cortex through the ascending-reticular activating system, the same system that activates the cortex during REM sleep,[29] suggests that as long as afferent input to the cortex is inhibited, activation of this cortical system is sufficient to account for the cognitive characteristics of both REM and late-morning NREM dreaming.[29] Furthermore, the most dramatic characteristics of dreaming—namely, bizarre combinations of visual features and meanings, speech imagery, and lucid dreaming—tend to occur primarily in late-morning REM dreams, so that they seem to require the joint effect of the two biological activation rhythms. This finding is based on only one experiment and should, of course, be further studied.

DISTRIBUTION OF BRAIN ACTIVITY IN REM SLEEP

Braun et al.[30, 31] are the only cognitive neuroscientists to acknowledge the possibility that the pattern of cortical activation during REM sleep might interact with time of night, and they recommend that in future PET studies, the time of night be evaluated systematically. They have provided the best available picture of differences in patterns of cortical activation across waking, REM, and NREM sleep. Supporting the results of previous PET studies,[18] they showed that the occipital cortices are significantly more active in REM than in NREM sleep. They found, moreover, that this occipital activation was confined to extrastriate regions and that extrastriate activation was associated with a significant reduction in the activation of the striate cortices, including the calcarine regions, that are essential to waking visual perception. The low level of striate activation parallels the inhibition of afferent transmission in the optic nerve during REM sleep reported by Pompeiano.[32] Extrastriate activation was accompanied by activation of the anterior ventral object processing and dorsal spatial processing—the "what" and "where" pathways. This neural activation pattern maps nicely onto the bottom-up cognitive visual imagery model described above.

Although both expressive and receptive auditory imagery are rare in REM sleep, dreamers commonly report that imaged characters are talking about specific topics[33] (i.e., the meaning of speech is produced without the accompanying auditory speech imagery). Increases in activation that were observed in the secondary regions of the postrolandic auditory cortices during REM[29] may fit this pattern, but more detailed subject-by-subject mapping of waking onto REM auditory and speech patterns is required to make a precise interpretation of the REM sleep patterns.

Reduced activation of the dorsolateral prefrontal and lateral orbital cortices in both REM and NREM sleep[30, 31] is consonant with the sleeper's inability in REM sleep to create the visual images that are fully consonant with their larger context and meaning. This inability to relate the visual image to the long-term memories in the association cortices presumably leaves the dreamer with little basis to question the validity of the image and to accept it as a sensory percept. Only on waking does the information that enables the dreamer to identify the dream as an hallucination become accessible.

The relation of dreaming to drives, goals, and motivational structures is central to many theories of dreaming. Two classes of assumptions of these theories have received some empirical examination. Using a stimulus incorporation procedure during REM sleep, Hoelscher et al.[34] have shown that compared with a set of personally neutral stimuli, dreamers are more likely to incorporate stimuli that represent their personal concerns. On the negative side, the presleep circumcision film mentioned previously and the surgical studies[9] failed to induce any measurable effect on samples of dream content. In fairness to the theory, however, because no motivational state persists unchanged throughout an entire day, it may be unreasonable to expect the cognitive responses to a stressor to persist with sufficient strength to show up in every dream report over an entire night.

Neurophysiological research provides substantial evidence in the waking state of elevated activity in subcortical and cortical centers that participate in drive and motivational processes. Ellman et al.[5] detailed a complex relationship between REM sleep, the locus ceruleus, and neighboring subcortical, self-stimulation pleasure centers. Maquel et al.[35] showed that the limbic structures of the brain, which participate in motivational and emotional behavior in the waking state, are activated in REM sleep. Braun et al.[30, 31] replicated this observation and demonstrated the activation of the limbic projections of the extrastriate cortices in REM sleep, thereby suggesting that the dreamer is able to evaluate the relation of REM images to goals and motives. Activation of limbic structures in REM sleep does not imply, however, that REM dreams are characterized by the full range of characteristics of waking emotional experience.

Although dramatic affect is popularly thought to accompany dreams, the *experience* of emotion during REM dreaming is in fact rare until the late morning or when a dreamer, during what in the waking state would be a stressful episode, struggles out of REM sleep into wakefulness. This pattern suggests that the properties of the REM process inhibit some of the components that are necessary to an integrated emotional experience and that this integration is accomplished only as the sleeper moves toward waking. Certainly in the case of the most intense sleep experience of all, the night terror, which occurs primarily in stage 4, the physiological indices of waking emotional experience are absolutely quiet during the sleeping portion of the terror and become suddenly and intensively reactive only as the subject awakens from the terror.

The motivational states and processes that are heavily dependent on the limbic system are a prime subject of attempts to interpret the dream. Because we know almost nothing about whether these limbic processes are capable of a top-down influence on the image-generating processes in the extrastriate cortices, whether they respond to the bottom-up imaginal activity initiated in the occipital cortices, or both, interpreters have little basis for inferring motivational states from reported images. A more plausible role for limbic processes is the *efferent* leg of the dream. Because of the high salience of dream images, we tend to ignore dreamers' often determined efforts to react to the hallucinated images. When an unidentified person appears, the dreamer typically attempts to escape by running away. When an imaged object or person disappears, the dreamer often goes on a sustained search for the lost item. Limbic process might well be implicated in both of these imaged efforts even though they elicit no visual images. If such imaged reactions are similar to those the dreamer uses in waking life, then some interpretation of the responses might have validity. On the other hand, imaged motor acts such as the common experience of becoming paralyzed or "stuck in the mud" are probably due to the spinal inhibition of motor efferent and proprioceptive afferent activity in REM sleep rather than to arrested personal development as some dream interpreters confidently claim.

BIZARRENESS

Many plausible hypotheses for the bizarreness of dreams have been proposed, most of them based on some presumed random biological process, but none has passed an empirical test. The most compelling hypothesis, proposed by Hobson and McCarley,[4] assumes that PGO spikes are a random event sequence, originating in the pons, with sufficient neural power to interrupt ongoing mentation in the cortex and thereby produce the abrupt changes of scene that constitute the most common form of bizarreness. Although empirical research has failed to support an association between bizarre dream events and PGO activity, whether measured by periorbital potentials or REM bursts,[16, 36] Hobson[37] continues to affirm this hypothesis.

The problem with finding the causal antecedents of bizarreness lies in part with the erroneous assumption that dreaming is exclusively a REM sleep experience. Antrobus et al.[26] found that bizarreness increased substantially as the dreamer approached the morning. Less common types of bizarre mentation, namely incongruous images and identities such as "it was my brother, but he was a girl," occurred almost exclusively in very late morning REM dreams. They suggested that the combination of the activating phases of the 90-min

REM-NREM and the 24-h wake-sleep cycles creates the state that most supports bizarre mentation. First, a feature or event cannot be bizarre by itself; it can be improbable only in some context. The dreamer therefore must be able to experience multiple features and events and hold them in working memory for some elements to be bizarre in the context of others. This in turn demands a higher level of cortical activation, probably frontal, than normally occurs in early REM sleep, where dreams may be static images with few features.

How can one dream of dining with an uncle if he is long deceased or of carrying a set of false teeth if they are too large to fit any mouth? The fundamental picture here is that the image or event generated in one cortical location either cannot suppress unrelated or incongruous images or states in neighboring cortical regions that would typically be incompatible in the waking state or is similarly unable to activate those brain regions that possess the information that would in the waking state render the image compatible with the individual's memory bases. Several lines of evidence support both of these conceptions. First, Braun et al.[30, 31] showed that although some sensory regions are activated in REM sleep, the frontoparietal associations areas that in the waking state play a major role in integrating sensory information from different sources, are deactivated. The authors suggest that this dissociation is furthered by "a partial or fragmented activation of the corticostriatal-thalamocortical association circuitry."[31(p1193)] Such fragmentation would permit the visual-spatial, occipital, and parietal cortices—exclusive of the striate cortex—sufficient independence from the meaning-generating frontal cortex to produce visual image sequences that are independent of whatever meaning the dreamer has attributed to the concurrent dream.

Evidence for the effect of disconnection of perceptual pathways on perceptual recognition is provided by damaging one of the pathways in a neural network model of perception. Damage to the neural network pathway model simulated the characteristics of deep dyslexia in human beings, and these characteristics are similar to some of the bizarre properties of dreaming. The computational model showed that when dual brain pathways collaborate in a recognition process, neither learns to carry out the recognition process to the high level of accuracy that they achieve when they are trained to do the job independently.[38] When one pathway is then damaged or inactivated, the remaining pathway is able to produce only an approximation of accurate perception. Thus, when the direct grapheme-to-auditory naming route is damaged and a printed word can be named only through the word meaning route, *apricot* may be called *peach*. A comparable disconnection error in REM sleep might account for the bizarre report in which the dreamer "saw" the visual image of a "girl" but knew that it was his or her brother. I am suggesting that one source of bizarreness in REM sleep dreaming may be that the cortical pathways that do produce dream objects and event sequences are handicapped by the inactivation of some

of the pathways that normally share the production effort in the waking state.

Although these explanations seem plausible, they wrongly imply that when waking imagery and thought are produced in the same quiet, dark environment as that of sleep, they are free of bizarreness. Studies of waking mentation elicited in such laboratory environments, however, show that the most common form of bizarreness—abrupt shifts in scene—is even more common in waking than in REM sleep mentation.[36] This finding does not establish that scene changes in waking and REM sleep mentation have the same antecedents. Continuity of waking thought may be largely a function of the continuity of external stimuli, but the instability of waking mentation sequences suggests that we cannot assume that shifts in REM imagery are due to processes that are unique to that neurophysiological state.[39] To isolate the necessary and sufficient conditions for the occurrence of abrupt imaginal scene changes, waking control conditions must be used in both cognitive and neurophysiological experiments.

The contribution of neurophysiological studies in animals to the understanding of dreaming is mixed. The original contribution of Hobson and McCarley[4] was invaluable for the details it provided in comparing the activated brain during waking and dreaming sleep. The erroneous assumption, however, that REM sleep is a sufficient state for the creation of the dramatic features of dreaming encouraged neurophysiologists to assume that any neurophysiological characteristic that distinguishes REM from NREM sleep in the cat constitutes an explanation of some characteristic of human dreaming. The assumption that PGO spikes are the source of the dream experience as well as the cause of bizarreness is a case in point. Because of the technical character of the supporting data for these hypotheses, they tend to be viewed less critically by the popular press than are studies that actually measure the characteristics of dream reports. The improved access to PET and other human brain imaging techniques that are compatible with sleep and the willingness to study the effect of sleep time[30] should free us from dependence on animal models. The brain maps have the advantage that they can be compared directly with cognitive and conative activity in the waking human being. This translation process is dependent on a number of untested assumptions; these also must be ultimately examined with concurrent measures of sleep mentation. The power of the brain imaging studies, however, is demonstrated by their ability to generate new hypotheses about the dream process, such as the consequences of the disconnected regions of the cortex, the hippocampus, and limbic system in REM sleep and the unique characteristics of REM sleep dreaming.

Measurement of the characteristics of sleep imagery and thought must also improve. Because of their dependency on word reports, mentation studies implicitly assume that the relation between image and name is invariant across sleep and waking, but the frequent use in dream reports of qualifiers such as "sort of" and "something like" suggests that the verbal dream report provides a description of the features of sleep mentation that is far from accurate and complete. As an alternative to the verbal report, Rechtshaffen and Buchigani[40] suggested that the awakened dreamers match their imagery to photographs that were systematically altered across such dimensions as brightness, clarity, figure-ground contrast, and hue. Antrobus et al.[26] used magnitude estimation procedures to scale several of these dimensions. This photo-scaling procedure is highly informative and should be extended to other mentation characteristics such as form and image sequence. Many of the imaginal characteristics of REM, and even NREM, dreaming persist into the waking state, which implies, of course, that some characteristics of dreaming can be studied in the waking state and again emphasizes the need to use appropriate waking control states to isolate the characteristics of dreaming that are truly unique to different biological sleep states.

THE FUNCTION OF DREAMING

The third question, the function of dreaming, has been addressed in several theories.[19, 40, 41] Crick and Mitchison[19] proposed that dreaming has a memory clearing function, whereas Winson[41] suggested that it is part of a memory consolidation process—the late stage of learning. The social, personal, and motivation attributes of dream content have led several theorists to suggest that dreaming is a learning process with a personal problem-solving emphasis.[40] Within this group, some emphasize a conflict resolution role; among these, Kramer et al.[30] emphasized a mood-regulatory function. With the exception of the Crick and Mitchison proposal, there is some cognitive evidence that supports each of these hypotheses.

The function question may be defined in several ways. In the narrow sense, it implies functions that are unique to dreaming; in the broad sense, it includes processes that are shared by other states, such as daydreaming. In both of these cases, the functions attributed to the cognitive-affective properties of dreaming are confounded with a host of other correlated functions, such as the restorative benefits of physical rest or motor inactivity. Some of these confounds, such as restorative processes, are shared with other stages or periods of sleep; others, such as memory consolidation and problem solving, are shared with wakefulness.

The difficulty of coping with these confounds was first noted after the famous dream/REM deprivation study of Dement,[42] in which REM period–deprived participants compensated for the loss of REM sleep by making up the lost dreaming, or REM sleep, time on subsequent nights. With increasing deprivation, several participants showed signs of mild mental aberration. Dement's colleague, Fisher, interpreted these symptoms as support for the theory that the function of dreaming was to prevent insanity by experiencing hallucinations in the protected or safe circumstances of dreaming sleep (i.e., REM sleep).[43] By depriving a person of dreaming, psychotic behavior might spill over into the waking state. The evidence persuaded several

New York surgeons to delay early-morning surgery so as to avoid interference with the patient's late REM period. However, Zarcone et al.[44] found no evidence that REM deprived schizophrenics increased their cognitive pathololegy in the waking state. The "spillover" metaphor was subsequently examined by Arkin et al.,[45] who compared the effect of stage 1 REM deprivation on stage 2 mentation, using stage 2 deprivation as a control condition. They found no evidence that the deprivation of that part of sleep at which dreaming is most intense (i.e., REM sleep) produced an increase in dream-like mentation in NREM sleep. This lack of spillover into stage 2 mentation suggested that the compensatory REM sleep effect after REM deprivation was due to something other than dream deprivation. In reviewing research that examined the spillover effect of dream deprivation onto the waking state, Lewin and Singer[46] found little evidence of any strong effect.

The conclusion most consonant with the many proposals on the functional value of dreaming is that the statistical dimensionality of the proposed theories, corrected for confounds suggested by other theories, is so high that the theories simply cannot be tested with existing data sets. The biocognitive processes that accomplish dreaming and make its magnitude strongest in REM sleep are, like the subcortical reward processes described by Ellman et al.,[5] processes that appear to support a number of essential adaptive functions for human beings and other mammalian organisms. Not only do we not have a precise account of the biocognitive processes that carry out dreaming, but we also do not possess a complete description of the other adaptive functions, such as memory consolidation and problem solving, that might share in the use of these biocognitive processes. It seems premature, therefore, to make any claims at this point about the function of dreaming.

CONCLUSIONS

The grand personality and psychopathological theories of dream origin and dream interpretation of earlier times have given way since the 1950s to more-detailed neurocognitive models of specific dream characteristics. These models, like previous ones, are heavily indebted to theory and research on subhuman species and on waking neurocognitive processes. The rapidly improving quality and availablity of brain imaging technology, particularly of high-resolution PET scans during human sleep, have substantially improved the neurocognitive basis for our understanding of waking thought and imagery. A good theory of dreaming, however, requires that the cognitive side of the theory be as strongly based on empirical measures as the biological side. The results of many studies that make inferences about the neurophysiological basis of dreaming provide the impression that the authors' personal dreaming experiences form the primary basis of their conceptions of the characteristics of dreaming and that they assume that all of these characteristics are unique attributes of REM sleep processes. A good theory cannot be better than the quality of the data that it attempts to explain. The explanatory power of future theories of dreaming will depend on the quality of cognitive and biological observations and on the neurocognitive, computational models that link the two.

References

1. Freud S. The interpretation of dreams. In: Strachey J, ed. and trans. The Standard Edition of the Complete Psychological Works of Sigmund Freud. London, England: Hogarth Press; 1953:147–159.
2. Aserinsky E, Kleitman N. Regularly occurring periods of ocular motility occurring during sleep. Science. 1953;118:273–274.
3. Johnson LC, Lubin A. Spontaneous electrodermal activity during waking and sleeping. Psychophysiology. 1966;3:8–17.
4. Hobson JA, McCarley RW. The brain as a dream state generator: an activation-synthesis hypothesis of the dream process. Am J Psychiatry. 1977;134:1335–1348.
5. Ellman SJ, Spielman AJ, Lipschutz-Brach L. REM deprivation update. In: Ellman S, Antrobus JS, eds. The Mind in Sleep. 2nd ed. New York, NY: Wiley Interscience; 1991:329–376.
6. Olds J. Hypothalamic substrates of reward. Physiol Rev. 1962;42:554–604.
7. Foulkes D, Pivik T, Steadman HE, et al. Dreams of the male child: an EEG study. J Abnorm Psych. 1967;72:457–467.
8. Witkin HA. Presleep experiences and dreams. In: Fisher J, Berger L, eds. The Meaning of Dreams: Recent Insights From the Laboratory. Vol 3. Sacramento, Calif: Dept of Mental Hygiene; 1969:1–37.
9. Breger L, Hunter I, Lane RW. The effect of stress on dreams. New York, NY: International Universities Press; 1971.
10. Kramer M, Schoen L, Kinney L. The dream experience in dream disturbed Vietnam veterans. In: Vanderkolk B, ed. Post Traumatic Stress Disorders: Psychological and Biological Sequellae. Washington, DC: American Psychiatric Press; 1984.
11. Dement W. The Physiology of Dreaming [dissertation]. Chicago, Ill: University of Chicago; 1958.
12. Foulkes D. The Psychology of Sleep. New York, NY: Scribners; 1966.
13. Arkin AM, Antrobus JS. The effects of external stimuli applied prior to and during sleep on sleep experience. In: Ellman S, Antrobus JS, eds. The Mind in Sleep. 2nd ed. New York, NY: Wiley Interscience; 1991:265–307.
14. Hong CC, Potkin SG, Antrobus JS, et al. REM sleep eye movement counts correlate with visual imagery in dreaming: a pilot study. Psychophysiology. 1997;34:377–381.
15. Hong C, Potkin SG, Antrobus JS, et al. Data analysis based on a sliding 2 min window, scaled by time since the last REM burst. Unpublished data. 1996.
16. Pivik RT. Tonic states and phasic events in relation to sleep mentation. In: Ellman S, Antrobus JS, eds. The Mind in Sleep. 2nd ed. New York, NY: Wiley Interscience; 1991:214–247.
17. Antrobus J. The neurocognition of sleep mentation: phasic and tonic REM sleep. In: Bootzin RR, Kihlstrom JF, Schacter DL, eds. Sleep and Cognition. Washington, DC: American Psychological Association; 1990:1–24.
18. Hong CH, Gillian JC, Dow BM, et al. Localized and lateralized cerebral glucose metabolism associated with eye movements during REM sleep and wakefulness: a positron emission tomography (PET) study. Sleep. 1995;18:570–580.
19. Crick F, Mitchison G, REM sleep and neural nets. J Mind Behav. 1996;7:229–250.
20. McClelland JL, McNaughton BL, O'Reilly RC. Why there are complementary learning systems in the hippocampus and neocortex: insights from the success and failures of connectionist models of learning and memory. Psychol Rev. 1995;102:419–457.
21. Rumelhart DE, Smolensky P, McClelland JL, et al. Schemata and sequential thought processes in PDP models. In: Rumelhart DE, McClelland JL, eds. Parallel Distributed Processing. Cambridge, Mass: MIT Press; 1986:7–57.
22. Antrobus J. Dreaming: cognitive processes during cortical activation and high afferent thresholds. Psych Rev. 1991;98:96–121.
23. Hinton GE, Dayan P, Frey BJ, et al. The "wake-sleep" algorithm for unsupervised neural networks. Science. 1995;268:1158–1161.
24. Antrobus J. Thinking away and ahead. In: Morowitz H, Singer JL, eds. The Mind, the Brain and Complex Adaptive Systems. Reading, Mass: Addison-Wesley; 1995.
25. Antrobus JS: REM and NREM sleep reports: comparison of word frequencies by cognitive classes. Psychophysiology. 1983;20:562–568.
26. Antrobus J, Kondo T, Reinsel R, et al. Summation of REM and diurnal cortical activation. Consciousness Cognition. 1995;4:275–299.
27. LaBerge S. Lucid Dreaming. Los Angeles, Calif: Jeremy Tarcher; 1985.
28. Zimmerman WB. Sleep mentation and auditory awakening thresholds. Psychophysiology. 1970;6:540–549.
29. Hobson JA, Lydic R, Baghdoyan HA. Evolving concepts of sleep cycle generation: from brain centers to neuronal populations. Behav Brain Sci. 1986;9:371–448.
30. Braun AR, Balkin TJ, Wesensten NL, et al. Dissociated pattern of activity in visual cortices and their projections during human rapid eye movement sleep. Science. 1998;279:91–95.
31. Braun AR, Balkin TJ, Wesensten NL, et al. Regional cerebral blood flow throughout the sleep-wake cycle: an $H_2^{15}O$ PET study. Brain. 1997;120:1173–1197.
32. Pompeiano O. Mechanisms of sensorimotor integration during sleep. In: Stellar E, Sprague JM, eds. Progress in Physiological Psychology. New York, NY: Academic Press; 1970:3.
33. Meier B. Speech and thinking in dreams. In: Cavellero C, Foulkes D, eds. Dreaming as Cognition. New York, NY: Harvester Wheatsheaf; 1993:58–76.
34. Hoelscher TJ, Klinger E, Barta SG. Incorporation of concern- and nonconcern-related verbal stimuli into dream content. J Abnorm Psychol. 1981;90:88–91.
35. Maquet P, Peters JM, Aets J, et al. Functional neuroanatomy of human rapid eye-movement in sleep and waking. Nature. 1996;383:163–166.
36. Reinsel R, Antrobus J, Wollman M. Bizarreness in sleep and waking mentation. In: Antrobus J, Bertini M, eds. The Neuropsychology of Dreaming Sleep. Hillsdale, NJ: Erlbaum Associates; 1992:157–186.
37. Hobson JA, Stickgold R, Pace-Schott EF. The neuropsychology of REM sleep dreaming. Neuroreport. 1998;9:R1–R14.
38. Hinton GE, Shallice T. Lesioning an attractor network: investigations of acquired dyslexia. Psychol Rev. 1991;98:74–95.
39. Moffitt A, Kramer M, Hoffman R. The Functions of Dreaming. Albany, NY: State University Press of New York; 1993.
40. Rechtschaffen A, Buchignani C. The visual appearance of dreams. In: Antrobus J, Bertini M, eds. The Neuropsychology of Dreaming Sleep. Hillsdale, NJ: Erlbaum Associates; 1992:143–156.
41. Winson J. The meaning of dreams. Sci Am. 1990;263(5):86–88, 90–92, 94–96.
42. Dement WC. The effect of dream deprivation. Science. 1990;131:1705–1707.
43. Fisher C, Dement WC. Dreaming and psychosis: observations on the dream cycle during the course of an acute paranoid psychosis. Bull Phil Assoc Psychoanal. 1961;11:130–132.
44. Zarcone V, Gulevich G, Pivik T, et al. REM deprivation and schizophrenia. Biol Psychiatry. 1968;1:179–184.
45. Arkin AM, Antrobus J, Ellman S. The Mind in Sleep. New York, NY: Erlbaum Associates; 1978.
46. Lewin I, Singer JL. Psychological effects of REM ("dream") deprivation upon waking mentation. In: Ellman S, Antrobus JS, eds. The Mind in Sleep 2nd ed. New York, NY: Wiley Interscience; 1991:396–412.

39

Dreaming, Imagery, and Perception

Nancy H. Kerr

The metaphors we use to describe mental imagery emphasize its close phenomenological resemblance to perception. Visual imagery, thus, is like "seeing with the mind's eye," or "running a movie in one's head." In perception we record the characteristics of the environment, and in imagery we re-create them. The imagery we experience while dreaming is perhaps even more similar to perceiving, in that the visual, auditory, and other sensory qualities of the dream are hallucinatory in nature and are taken by the dreamer to represent reality. Although dreaming and waking imagery are experienced in virtually all sensory modalities, the predominant sensory experience for most dreamers is visual, and the focus of research on waking imagery has been on visual imagery. Therefore, in considering the relationships among imagery, dreams, and perception, I focus exclusively on visual aspects, with the hope and expectation that research here may inform and stimulate interest in other sensory and representational systems. Throughout the chapter I use the terms *mental imagery* and *visual imagery* to refer to the events that take place in the waking mind in the absence of sensory input, the terms *dream* or *dream imagery* to refer to similar events during sleep, and the term *perception* to refer to the processing of external information.

In the 1960s, in the wake of the dominance of behaviorism in American psychology, the study of mental imagery reemerged as a legitimate topic for research. New and more objective methods were devised for studying it, and mental imagery became a vital topic of interest for the emerging field of cognitive psychology.[1] Coincidentally, the study of dreaming, including dream imagery, was enjoying a revitalization as a result of the 1953 discovery by Aserinsky and Kleitman[2] of the association between rapid eye movement (REM) sleep and dream reporting. The clear phenomenological similarities between imagery experiences during wakefulness and during dreaming invite the supposition that the discoveries and research results from one area would be of eminent interest to researchers in the other. Indeed, the assumption that dream imagery was intimately related to imagery in wakefulness was implicit both in early texts on cognitive psychology[3] and specialty texts on the early research on mental imagery.[4] Cognitive psychologists even adopted the psychophysiological assumptions and methods of the new dream research to study imagery experiences in wakefulness. For example, when research on dreaming appeared to show that the eye movements of REM sleep corresponded to "looking" at images in the dream,[5] researchers were quick to test similar predictions relating eye movements to waking imagery.[6] Unfortunately, when subsequent research failed to uncover any reliable relationship between imagery and eye movements, either in dreaming or waking, the collaborative atmosphere died out and students of waking and dreaming imagery took very different empirical paths in pursuing their related goals. In a recent study of eye movements accompanying waking visual imagery, the researchers acknowledged dream research as a historical source for hypotheses regarding eye movements and imagery, but they dismissed it as an unproductive avenue for empirical study.[7]

There are many reasons for the relative insularity of the study of waking imagery and its neglect of dream phenomena. One of these is the incompatibility of dream data with the computer models of visual imagery that motivate and inform much of the research on waking imagery. Stephen Kosslyn, for example, has formulated one of the most influential and widely researched models of imagery processing based on computer simulations.[8, 9] The model includes a number of components of the imagery processing system, which the computer responds to as separate commands to perform such activities as "retrieving," "rotating," or "zooming in on" an image. The computer program is capable of predicting and reproducing human reaction times in performing standard imagery tasks such as "scanning" or "inspecting" an image of a specific visual stimulus. But the model makes no relevant predictions about dreaming, based as it is on tightly controlled experiments and the constraints of the computer program. It is exactly this incompatibility of dream experiences with computer processes that Neisser[10] cited as one reason why computers will never think exactly like humans. Computers do not dream. And as long as models of waking imagery are based on computer simulation, they exclude the experience of dreaming as well.

But the computer is not wholly, or even mostly, responsible for the bifurcation of research on dreaming and waking imagery. A large measure of the responsibility lies in the vast disparity between the methods favored by students of waking imagery and the methods possible for studying imagery experiences during sleep. Researchers interested in dream imagery are largely dependent on introspection and self-report as determinants of imagery experience. These are exactly the methods eschewed by the new cognitive psychology because of their susceptibility to the charges of subjectivity and unverifiability, which led to their historical rejection. Instead, typical cognitive research paradigms for studying imagery have involved the presentation of stimuli, such as words or pictures, under controlled conditions, and the measurement of verbal or behavioral responses. The work of Allan Paivio,[11, 12] and of Roger Shepard and his associates,[13,14] represent two distinctive and influential approaches to this kind of "input-output" method of studying imagery. A brief consideration of each of their paradigmatic approaches may help to clarify the characteristics of the cognitive approach to imagery research.

In keeping with an early emphasis in cognitive psychology on verbal learning, Paivio's research has focused primarily on the role of mental imagery as a mediator in memory for lists of words and word-pairs. In a typical experiment subjects hear or read the word lists, and subsequently are asked to recall the words and word-pairs. The experimenter systematically varies conditions in the experiment, such as whether the subject is instructed to use imagery or rote rehearsal as a mnemonic strategy, and whether the words refer to concrete, easily imagined items (car, baby), or more abstract ones (theory, justice). The objective dependent variable, the number of words actually recalled, is used to infer whether imagery improves memory. The widely replicated findings that imagery instructions improve recall and that concrete nouns are better remembered than abstract ones have been interpreted as evidence for "dual-coding" visual imagery and verbal processing systems.[11]

Shepard's work, more in line with the emerging "information-processing" approach to cognitive psychology, has relied predominantly on reaction time in a mental rotation task as a gauge of imagery processing. In one typical paradigm, subjects must judge whether two pictures presented at differing rotational angles represent identical figures, or figures that are mirror images of each other. In a similar paradigm, subjects must judge whether a familiar figure, such as the letter *R*, that has been rotated from its upright position, is in its normal or mirror-image form. In both cases, the significant finding is that a linear relationship exists between the degrees of rotation of the judged figure from the comparison or upright figure and the amount of time it takes the subject to make the judgment. Thus, the results provide objective verification of subjects' phenomenological reports that in order to make such judgments, they first must rotate the figure mentally to the appropriate orientation, and then make the comparison. The further the figure must be rotated, the longer it takes to make the judgment. On the basis of these results, Shepard has concluded that mental rotation has an analogue relationship to the actual physical rotation of an object or picture.

These two examples of research approaches to waking imagery illustrate the relative precision with which researchers have been able to manipulate input and measure output in order to infer intervening processing. They also illustrate the impossibility of directly adapting these or similar research methods to the study of dreaming, whose inputs are internal and whose outputs must be mediated by subjective self-report. This is not to say that all cognitive psychologists dismiss dreams as inexplicable or irrelevant to issues of waking imagery. Shepard,[13] for example, frequently cites his own and others' dream imagery as illustrations of the creative powers of imagery. One of his recent theoretical formulations of imagery processes was specifically "motivated . . . by the desire to encompass dreaming, imagining, and thinking."[15(p437)] Unfortunately, the theory has not generated empirically testable hypotheses. The persistent difficulty lies in bridging the gap between theory and research.

The conflict between cognitive psychologists' willingness to extend waking models to dreaming thought and the difficulties of testing those extensions is clearly illustrated in the work of Marcia Johnson. Johnson et al.[16] attempted to test Johnson's model[17] of memory, using memory for dream reports as a measure. They had pairs of subjects who lived together awaken at fixed times each morning and give each other reports either of real dreams or dreams they had made up. Later, subjects were asked to read short excerpts from both their own and partner's reports to judge the source (self or partner) of each excerpt. The somewhat counterintuitive prediction from Johnson's theory was that the subject's own real dreams would be more frequently attributed to the partner than would made-up dreams. The prediction was based on the theoretical assumption that consciously constructed, made-up, dreams are associated with cues from the construction process itself, whereas real dreams are not. They obtained some degree of support for the model's predictions, and concluded that "the model is applicable beyond our previous laboratory studies to more complex, natural memories."[16(p342)] Despite this positive experience with applying the model to dreaming, further research with dreams was not forthcoming. As Johnson later reported, the dream research had been "encouraging, but studying dreams does not allow much in the way of experimental control, so we have attempted to manipulate cognitive operations in the lab."[18(p8)]

Yet, the resistance of dreaming to experimental control does not dictate that this complex, natural source of imagery cannot be studied at all. It is true that the number of studies concerned with dream imagery is a small fraction of those investigating waking imagery. Nevertheless, researchers over the past several decades have produced systematic data on the incidence and nature of dream imagery, and their research questions have often been remarkably similar to those that motivate studies of waking imagery. In the remainder of the chapter I present several research approaches to dreams and dream imagery that argue for the interdependence of dreaming and waking imagery and for the value of including measures of one kind of imagery in the study of the other.

SELECTIVE IMPAIRMENT OF IMAGERY ABILITY AND DREAM EXPERIENCE

One promising approach to understanding the correspondence between waking and dreaming imagery has emerged from investigations of individuals who have lost selective cognitive abilities due to neurological damage. Unfortunately, for many of the same reasons that cognitive psychologists ignored dreaming, this neuropsychological approach to the study of dreaming received little historical attention. Neuropsychologists, like cognitive psychologists, relied on objective test data for primary analysis of deficits in psychological functioning. Reports of deficits in dreaming that accompanied cerebral damage were largely based on patients' spontaneous anecdotal reports, rather than on systematic questioning or data collection. These nonsystematic reports based on case studies have recently been supplemented with a few laboratory-based studies based on REM awakenings, as well as studies that involve more systematic questioning about dreaming of patients whose abilities and characteristics are assessed following cerebral damage.

Farah[19] reported a comprehensive analysis of 37 published cases in which selective loss of visual imagery was reported as a consequence of brain injury. Her primary motivation was to test a model, derived from Kosslyn,[8] for its ability to predict specific kinds of imagery impairment for people with damage to particular parts of the brain. She was able to do this with some degree of success. In addition, in order to show that the imagery deficit was not just a reflection of more generalized cognitive dysfunction or some related deficit, she also analyzed the cases according to other reported impairments. In general, the patients were free of other symptoms. The only cognitive deficit reliably reported for this sample was the concomitant loss or impairment of dreaming. Not all of Farah's case studies explicitly addressed the topic of dreaming, but of the 17 that did, 14 reported some form of dream impairment. Seven reported total loss of dreaming; four, an absence of the visual aspect of dreaming; and three, a severe reduction in dreaming. Farah did not attempt to fit the dream loss cases to her imagery model, and, indeed, the dreaming cases appear to be relatively randomly distributed across her categorical system. The failure of the model to encompass the dream cases, however, should not be taken as refutation of the model or of the potential shared processing mechanisms for waking and dreaming imagery. Unlike the assessment of imagery deficits based on standard waking tests of ability, the basis of determination of dream impairment in the case studies was often casual and incomplete. People's casual observations about their dream experiences in general may be very different from the dream reports they give upon systematic

REM awakenings in a laboratory. And while neuropsychologists may not always be able to sample dreams under controlled conditions, it is clear that more systematic and comprehensive questioning about dream impairment in patients who have suffered neurological damage will allow a better test of its relationship to waking imagery, as well as to injury site.

Complementary to Farah's data on loss of dreaming in imagery-impaired patients are data reported by Greenberg and Farah[20] on the loss of imagery ability in neurological patients who report a loss of dreaming. They examined the case studies of 14 patients for whom loss or alteration of dream recall was a primary symptom following neurological damage. Of the 12 patients for whom information was available on waking imagery ability, all were reported to have an impairment or absence of visual imagery. Localization of damage, especially for those who ceased entirely to recall dreams, was primarily in the left hemisphere, suggesting that dreaming, as well as imaging,[21] may be the product of left hemisphere processes. This is consistent with evidence from sleep laboratory studies that report that commissurotomized subjects,[22] as well as right hemispherectomized patients,[23] are able to report dreams upon awakening from REM sleep. The commissurotomized subjects, who have undergone surgery to relieve epilepsy by severing the neural connections between the hemispheres of the brain, are able to give verbal descriptions only from the isolated left hemisphere. Their verbal reports of dreaming, therefore, like those from patients whose right hemisphere has been removed, are clearly the product of left hemisphere activity.

Doricchi and Violani[24] provided a more extensive survey of cases in which absence or alteration of dreaming was reported following cerebral damage. Although their primary goal was to analyze the distribution of the sites of cerebral damage associated with specific dreaming deficiencies, they did include some analyses of the waking cognitive deficits in their cases. In addition to reviewing a number of cases of cessation of dreaming, these investigators reported nine cases in which patients had experienced the selective loss of the visual component of dreaming. The small number of cases and the variability in sites of damage prevented the authors from any systematic analysis of these patients, although they acknowledged the potentially interesting contribution of such an analysis. On the basis of their literature review, Doricchi and Violani concluded:

> Given the constant concomitance of dream recall and imagery deficits found in the present review it is possible to suggest that the LH [left hemisphere] contribution to the dreaming experience relies at least in part on the same psychological processes that it subserves for waking mental imagery.[24(p120)]

Solms[25] conducted a critical and comprehensive review of the existing literature on changes in patterns of dreaming in patients with cerebral damage, supplemented by data from his own study of such patients. In his literature review, Solms, like Doricchi and Violani, differentiated between patients who reported total cessation of dreaming and those who reported the absence of a visual component to dreaming. Of the 15 patients reported in the literature to have experienced a loss of the visual aspect of dreaming, Solms noted that 91% also were diagnosed with a deficiency in performance on tests of waking visual imagery. On the basis of these cases and the close phenomenological similarities in the two forms of imagery, Solms concluded that the correlated failure of patients to generate visual imagery in wakefulness and to experience visual imagery in dreaming must arise from a common underlying deficit. As further evidence for a linkage between waking deficits and deficits in dream imagery, Solms cited cases in which specific waking deficits, such as the ability to imagine people's faces or form images in color, were accompanied by the same specific deficit in dream imagery.

According to Solms's review, the relationship of waking visual imagery abilities to the total cessation of dreaming is less clear-cut. Of the 47 published cases of patients who experienced a total cessation of dreaming, Solms reported that 20 (43%) patients also showed deficits in waking visual imagery. This number is marginally higher than the 20% of imagery deficits in patients with preserved dreaming, and suggests that there may be multiple causes for the total cessation of dreaming following cerebral trauma.

Solms[25] collected his own set of data to test a number of hypotheses based on the existing literature. Over a 4-year period, he questioned 361 patients about changes in their dream experiences since the onset of their neurological illness, using a series of probes designed to assess the aspects of dreaming in which he was particularly interested. Of these patients, only two reported the absence of visual dream imagery in the continued experience of dreaming. One patient reported a complete cessation of visual dream imagery, which was accompanied by a loss of waking visual imagery ability. The second patient reported a serious disruption in dream imagery, in which he experienced imagery "in parts" or as static, isolated images. This report of disruption to the continuous kinematic aspect of dream imagery is similar to a case described by Kerr and Foulkes[26] based on REM dream reports collected in a sleep laboratory from a patient with damage to the right cerebral cortex. In both cases, the subjects had difficulty performing specific tests of waking visual imagery. The similarity in the reports of dream quality from these two individuals is noteworthy given methodological differences in the data collection. On the basis of his review of the literature and his own investigation, Solms identified at least four variants of the syndrome of nonvisual dreaming: total loss of visual dream imagery, loss of facial dream imagery, loss of color dream imagery, and loss of kinematic dream imagery.

Of his 361 cases, Solms identified 112 who reported total cessation of dreaming following cerebral trauma. Only 3 of these patients also showed serious deficits in waking visual imagery. He attributed this relatively low percentage of visual imagery deficits in his dream cessation cases to the unselected nature of his patients. Patients in previous reports had been selected precisely because of their deficits in imagery or perception. Whereas the loss of waking visual imagery may be a strong predictor of the absence of dream imagery or of dreaming per se, the data Solms presented suggest that the cessation of dreaming due to neurological damage has a modest correlation with waking imagery deficits and is associated with a variety of cognitive disorders.

The implications of these studies for further research are clear. Case studies of individuals with selective loss of cognitive capabilities should include direct analysis of impairments in dreaming as well as in waking thought. Ideally, dream data would be based on systematically elicited, laboratory-monitored dream reports, in which patients were questioned systematically about characteristics of the visual imagery in the dream. Specific models[19] that are employed to assess patterns of imagery loss in wakefulness and their associated neurological sites of damage could then be tested for their predictive power with respect to dreams. Farah's[19] categorical system for analyzing specific kinds of imagery deficits, for example, could be tested for its applicability to dream imagery. Such data would go a long way toward revealing the nature of the shared mechanisms for producing imagery in wakefulness and while dreaming.

INDIVIDUAL DIFFERENCES IN DREAM RECALL

One of the characteristics on which individuals vary widely is the number of dreams they spontaneously recall upon awakening. Some people report recalling many dreams each night, whereas others report recalling a dream rarely, if ever. Most of us fall somewhere between these two extremes, and many nonrecallers are able to report dreams at a normal frequency if they are awakened in the laboratory directly from REM sleep. One theory that dream researchers have suggested to account for these differences in reported dream recall is what has been called the *salience hypothesis*. The premise is that people remember dreams that are especially attention-grabbing because of their vividness, bizarreness, emotionality, or other unusual qualities, and that some people's dreams generally possess more of these qualities than others'. Those people with salient dreams are more likely to remember them. For our purposes, the relevant dimension on which dreams may vary in salience is in the vividness of the visual imagery of the dream experience. If people do differ in the vividness of the visual imagery, an obvious related dimension on which they might also vary is in characteristics of waking imagery. Several researchers have attempted to test this relationship.

Hiscock and Cohen[27] administered a dream frequency questionnaire to a large sample of university students and selected from among them the students at each extreme of the report frequency scale. These students were given three tests of waking imagery. The first was an objective test of performance on a paired-associate (PA) learning task similar to tasks used by Paivio.[28] After an initial test of PA learning as a baseline, half of the infrequent and half of the frequent dream recallers were instructed to use an imagery mnemonic to remember the pairs and the other half were instructed to use verbal rehearsal. The authors reasoned that if frequent dream recallers are also vivid imagers, then they should benefit more from imagery instructions than infrequent recallers whose waking (and dreaming) imagery is less memorable. Although the frequent recallers performed better overall on the PA test, both groups showed an equivalent advantage for imagery instructions over verbal rehearsal instructions on the second testing. Thus, these data did not provide unequivocal support for the salience predictions. The other two measures showed a more direct relationship between waking imagery reports and dream recall. Subjects' scores on both the Betts Questionnaire on the Vividness of Visual Imagery[4] and the Gordon Test of Imagery Controllability[29] differed significantly for frequent and infrequent dream recallers. On the Betts scale, frequent recallers rated their subjective image of a specific item, such as a sunset or a friend's face, as clearer and more vivid than did infrequent recallers. They also reported on the Gordon test a better ability to control and manipulate imagery when asked to visualize such things as an automobile in motion. Although there are clearly reasons to hesitate in interpreting self-report data whose relationship is purely correlational, the findings are at least consistent with a salience hypothesis.

Richardson[30] performed a partial replication of Hiscock and Cohen's study using a sample of 84 subjects without preselection for reported frequency of dream recall. The subjects were administered Hiscock and Cohen's scale for frequency of dream recall as well as Marks' Vividness of Visual Imagery Questionnaire (VVIQ).[31] The VVIQ is similar in format to the Betts scale, and requires subjects to rate the vividness of specific images using a 5-point scale. The results were somewhat complicated because of gender differences in response to the VVIQ with eyes open vs. eyes closed, but in general the findings supported Hiscock and Cohen, with a significant correlation between reported imagery vividness and frequency of dream recall. Although Richardson's results are subject to the same interpretative limitations as Hiscock and Cohen's, they do at least attest to the robustness of the relationship.

Foulkes[32] presented a different kind of evidence linking waking visuospatial skills to dream frequency. However, his data are based on laboratory-collected REM dreams, and thus do not address the spontaneous forgetting of nonsalient dreams. Instead, they are relevant to the question of whether people's abilities to think in visual imagery are related to their abilities to create dream imagery. In his developmental studies of children's dreams, Foulkes included waking tests of a variety of cognitive abilities. Of these, it was tests such as the Block Design subtest of the Wechsler Intelligence Scale for Children (which requires children to construct from blocks a pattern in a visual display) that were the best predictors of frequency of dream report. On the basis of these data, Foulkes suggests that dream reports appear and change developmentally as children acquire the visuospatial cognitive skills necessary for their construction.

On the basis of Foulkes's findings, Butler and Watson[33] proposed that the underlying reason for failure to recall dreams in at least some adults might also reflect poorly developed visuospatial skills. They recruited as subjects 12 men who claimed to dream "rarely or never," and whose failure at dream recall had been verified through a 10-day dream diary. Each subject spent one adaptation night and two experimental nights with standard sleep-stage recordings taken in a sleep laboratory. On experimental nights they were awakened from every REM period and asked for mentation reports. Subjects who reported a dream were asked additional questions regarding its salience, including whether it was visual, and if so, whether the imagery was static or continuous. Subjects were also administered a number of tests of waking cognitive aptitude, including the Block Design subtest from the Wechsler Adult Intelligence Scale and two standard paper and pencil tests of spatial skills. The REM recall rates for these 12 subjects ranged from 0 to 100%, clearly indicating that self-reported infrequent dreamers are not necessarily nonrecallers when dream reports are based on laboratory awakenings. High rates of REM recall among these subjects were correlated significantly with a high proportion of visual and visually continuous dreams, and with high scores on the Block Design and one of the standard tests of visuospatial skill. Again, one must be cautious in interpreting data from a limited number of subjects from a special population. Nevertheless, these data add to the converging evidence indicating a relationship between measures of visual imagery and dream recall.

To date, there has been no attempt to integrate these studies of individual differences in dream recall with models of individual differences based on the same measures of waking imagery. Kosslyn and associates,[34] for example, included the VVIQ as a part of a battery of imagery tests designed to assess patterns of individual differences in imagery abilities that may reflect relative strengths in specific components of imagery processing. Marks[35] reported data based on electroencephalographic (EEG) mapping techniques, which suggest that there are different patterns of brain activation during a mental imagery task for individuals who score high on the VVIQ than for those who score low. It would be interesting to know whether these individual differences are predictive of differences in dream imagery or patterns of brain activity while dreaming as well.

THE VISUAL QUALITIES OF DREAM IMAGERY

In order to test just how similar dream visualization was to perception, Rechtschaffen and Buchignani[36] designed an experiment that allowed a relatively direct comparison of the two experiences. The researchers initially prepared a series of photographs of a single scene that varied on the dimensions of color saturation, brightness, figure clarity, background clarity, and overall hue. They then awakened subjects in a sleep laboratory during REM sleep and asked them to select the photograph that best matched the visual qualities of the imagery of reported dreams. Over 40% of the selections were chosen from photographs whose characteristics were well within the normal range and closely resembled external reality. The most frequent deviation from normal perceptual characteristics was the selection of achromatic pictures for 20% of the dream images, followed by photographs with degraded background detail. Various other deviations from normal perception were reported for other dream reports, but no subject reported highly unusual visual aspects such as double exposure or multiple images. The authors' major conclusion from their research is that visual imagery in dreaming bears a close resemblance to visual perception in wakefulness.

Rechtschaffen and Buchignani's finding that an absence of color in dreams was the most common deviation from normal perception was probably unsurprising. In fact, its relative absence (20%) is low compared to the percentages reported by Kahn and associates.[37] These researchers reviewed a number of studies in which subjects had been asked to estimate the relative frequency with which they dreamed in color. In all of these previous studies the percentages of dreams judged to have been in color were consistently low (14 to 29%). The reviewers contrasted these findings with the results from an experiment of their own in which subjects were awakened from REM sleep in the laboratory and questioned specifically about the visual characteristics of their dreams. Their study produced an average of 83% of dream reports that included color, a number very close to the 80% reported by Rechtschaffen and Buchignani. When subjects are directly aroused from a dream and attention is focused on color, most dreams are reported as in color. It is only when estimates of dream color are based on spontaneous memories for previous dream experiences that the estimates are low. The most parsimonious explanation for these findings is based on the failure to attend to and encode information about color during initial spontaneous dream recall. Thus, this unattended and unrehearsed aspect of the dream is forgotten over time. Indeed, Rechtschaffen and Buchignani considered the 20% incidence of achromatic dreams to be surprisingly high. Perceiving is almost always in color. Why should dreaming be otherwise?

A logical next step to the Rechtschaffen and Buchignani experiment is the extension of the picture comparison procedure to the study of visual imagery experienced during wakefulness. John Antrobus and his associates[38] have taken a first step in this direction. These researchers obtained mentation reports from subjects in a sleep laboratory during REM and non-rapid eye movement (NREM) sleep, as well as during wakefulness. Standard procedures for obtaining content reports were employed in all three conditions, and subjects were asked to select from a series of photographs that varied in brightness and clarity the one that most closely resembled the visual characteristics of imagery in the experience. In an analysis based only on the most vivid imagery reported from each experience, the researchers found NREM imagery to be significantly less bright and clear than REM imagery, with no difference on these dimensions between REM and wakefulness. The REM-NREM finding of differences in imagery qualities replicates previous research based on different methods, but the REM-waking equivalence is somewhat more surprising because it contradicts most anecdotal comparisons of the two.

The picture-comparison method holds strong promise as a means of comparing relatively directly the visual qualities of dreaming and waking imagery. It provides an objective measure against which a recent, explicit experience can be matched, and it allows individual analysis of different characteristics of the experience. It would be interesting to know whether these results extend to the less spontaneous experiences of imagery in wakefulness, such as those studied in typical information-processing paradigms, and to learn more about the relative prevalence of clear, bright imagery in waking vs. dreaming reports. It also would be of interest to include the dimension of color saturation in an assessment of waking imagery to test the generalizability of Rechtschaffen and Buchignani's finding to the waking state.

THE EFFECT OF VISUAL STIMULATION ON DREAM IMAGERY

One question that has driven a large body of research on waking imagery concerns the extent to which concurrent visual stimulation can affect imagery processes. The answer is somewhat complicated. Under some circumstances, for example when subjects are asked to perform concurrent visual perceptual and mental imagery tasks, the two seem to interfere with each other.[39] In other situations, especially when a subject is asked to imagine an object while staring at a screen on which a stimulus appears, the reported image appears to take on the characteristics of the stimulus.[40, 41] Because dreaming takes place with the eyes closed, it may come as a surprise to learn that the question of concurrent visual and imagery processing has also been studied in dreaming.

Of course, even with the subject's eyes closed, it is possible to present bright lights or other stimuli of high contrast to a subject in REM sleep, and to analyze subsequent dream reports for visual content. Such studies have been conducted and there is some evidence that such stimuli may have a minor effect on dream imagery.[42] But in order to test the effects of more specific visual stimuli, such as objects or written words, on dream imagery, Rechtschaffen and Foulkes[43] found it necessary to institute rather unorthodox conditions for dream collection. Subjects in their study slept in a laboratory with their eyes taped open and their pupils chemically dilated. The researchers took precautions to ensure the comfort of their subjects, including a room vaporizer to keep the cornea moist. As surprising as it may seem, physiological recordings indicated that subjects slept normally through all stages of sleep. During an equivalent number of REM and NREM periods, an experimenter entered the subject's room and presented an illuminated object, such as a book or aluminum coffeepot, for a short time in front of the subject's eyes. About 10 sec afterward, the subject was awakened and asked for a dream report. Judges were subsequently asked to match the dream reports to the objects presented and were unable to do so at better than chance levels. Although dream reports contained clear and rich visual imagery, no dream report contained imagery that was an unambiguous example of stimulus incorporation. Thus, at least in the case of dreaming, imagery generation is capable of proceeding independent and to the exclusion of perceptual processing.

It is tempting to interpret these dream data as an extreme example of interference between imagery and perception, in which perception is totally precluded by the vivid imagery of the dream. But two aspects of the dream study suggest that this conclusion is unwarranted. First, mentation reports included all mental activity, thoughts as well as images and dreams. Second, the authors discuss the research as evidence for functional blindness in sleep in general, rather than blindness associated with the presence of visual imagery. The results, however, are clearly inconsistent with reports of stimulus incorporation during waking imagery experiments.[40, 41]

DREAMS OF THE BLIND

For most sighted people, the experience of dreaming is closely associated with the rich visual imagery that accompanies it, and it is difficult to imagine the nature of dreaming in its absence. Thus, they question whether blind people dream or whether blind people's dreams are not in some way impoverished. The response of Elinor Deutsch[44] is typical of a blind person's reaction to these questions.

> The belief held by many people that the blind either do not dream at all or that if they do, their dreams must be very vague and incomplete is . . . entirely erroneous. The majority of people are so accustomed to thinking and forming their mental images almost entirely in terms of vision that they are apt to forget that there are several other sense modalities in terms of which images may be built up. The blind not only dream just as vividly as the sighted but are perhaps less cognizant of the lack of vision when asleep than when awake. The writer, herself blind since birth except for light perception, dreams very frequently and vividly.[44(p288)]

Research interest in the dreams of the blind began very early in psychology's history with an extensive questionnaire study by Joseph Jastrow,[45] whose major findings have been subsequently verified by numerous researchers.[46] The first major finding is that virtually all blind people report experiencing dreams, and that, like Deutsch, they find their dreams to be vivid and self-engaging. One important characteristic on which the dreams of the blind vary, however, is in whether the dream experience includes vision. In general, people born blind, or who became blind before the age of 5, report no visual imagery in their dreams. Those whose blindness occurred at age 7 years or later are likely to continue to experience visual dreaming, often over a lifetime. It is surely no coincidence that the apparent critical age for the incorporation of vision in dreaming coincides with the age identified by Foulkes[32] as the beginning of autonomous dreaming more generally.

Laboratory evidence regarding the organization and characteristics of dreams of the blind provide the strongest kind of evidence for the continuity of the dream experience in blind and sighted people. Kerr et al.[47] studied each of 10 young adults in a sleep laboratory, including two who were totally congenitally blind, two whose congenital blindness permitted perception of contrast and form, two adventitiously blind who lost their vision as teenagers, and four comparison subjects with normal vision. The subjects spent 8 nights in the laboratory and were awakened and asked for mentation reports at sleep onset and during both REM and NREM sleep. Following spontaneous reports of dreaming, the subjects were asked a systematic set of questions about the nature of the experience, including probes for auditory and visual imagery, numbers of people and settings, amount of self-participation, and feelings. The answers to these questions provided the data for comparison across subjects with differing visual status. Blind and sighted subjects were compared on 22 different content categories, and, except for the absence of visual imagery in the congenitally totally blind subjects, the characteristics of the dreams of blind and sighted subjects were indistinguishable from each other. The two subjects with form vision reported a visual aspect to dreaming just as frequently as did sighted subjects, and they described their vision in the dreams as no better or worse than their vision in wakefulness. In contrast, the two adventitiously blind subjects, who each retained some form vision, never reported visual experiences in dreams that matched their impaired perception. Their visual dream experiences, instead, were similar to their experiences in seeing prior to impairment. Thus, visual imagery in dreaming is not a mere reflection of current visual perceptual capabilities, but instead represents an at least partially autonomous cognitive processing system capable of re-creating at night a visual aspect of the world that cannot be directly perceived in wakefulness.

The relatively clear data from research on the dream imagery of blind people should be of special interest to cognitive researchers interested in testing imagery abilities in the blind, whose data are far less clear. A number of researchers have reported similar performance by blind and sighted subjects on tasks such as Shepard's mental rotation,[48, 49] tests of memory for high imagery items[50] or memory for items following imagery instructions,[51] and a variety of other standard imagery performance measures.[52] Other researchers have identified potential limitations in the imagery abilities of blind subjects, especially when the complexity of the material to be imaged is great.[51, 53] Current attempts to resolve these discrepancies have centered on the distinction between "spatial" and "pictorial" components of imagery, which appear to be dissociable processing systems,[54] with imagery limitations in blind people explained by the absence of the visual, but not the spatial, component. If evidence supports this difference as an explanation for waking imagery differences, the very rich dream imagery of the blind is clearly spatial imagery that provides a point of contrast for any "limitations" observed in controlled test situations.

CONCLUSION

Cognitive psychologists have made significant progress over the past several decades in creating and applying experimental methods that reveal the nature and function of imagery in wakefulness. Dream researchers have made parallel progress in developing psychophysiological measures that allow systematic collection of reports of imagery in dreaming. With a few notable exceptions, researchers have chosen to study either waking imagery or dream imagery, with little attention to potential commonalities between the two. The research reported here points to the potential productivity of combining the methodologies to investigate more directly the relationship of waking imagery to dream imagery.

References

1. Holt RR. Imagery: the return of the ostracized. Am Psychol. 1964;19:254–264.
2. Aserinsky E, Kleitman N. Regularly occurring periods of eye motility, and concomitant phenomena during sleep. Science. 1953;118:273–274.
3. Neisser U. Cognitive Psychology. New York, NY: Appleton-Century-Crofts; 1967.
4. Richardson A. Mental Imagery. New York, NY: Springer-Verlag; 1969.
5. Roffwarg HP, Dement WC, Muzio JN, et al. Dream imagery: relationship to rapid eye movements of sleep. Arch Gen Psychiatry. 1962;7:235–258.
6. Antrobus JS, Antrobus JS, Singer JL. Eye movements accompanying daydreaming, visual imagery, and thought suppression. J Abnorm Soc Psychol. 1964;69:244–252.
7. Brandt SA, Stark LW. Spontaneous eye movements during visual imagery reflect the content of the visual scene. J Cogn Neurosci. 1997;9:27–38.
8. Kosslyn SM. Image and Mind. Cambridge, Mass: Harvard University Press; 1980.
9. Kosslyn SM, van Kleek MH, Kirby KN. A neurologically plausible model of individual differences in visual mental imagery. In: Hampson PJ, Marks DF, Richardson JTE, eds. Imagery: Current Developments. New York, NY: Routledge; 1990:31–77.
10. Neisser U. The imitation of man by machine. Science. 1963;139:193–197.
11. Paivio A. Imagery and Verbal Processes. New York, NY: Holt, Rinehart, & Winston; 1971.
12. Paivio A. Mental Representations: A Dual-Coding Approach. New York, NY: Oxford University Press; 1986.
13. Shepard RN. The mental image. Am Psychol. 1978;33:125–137.
14. Shepard RN, Cooper LA. Mental images and their transformations. Cambridge, Mass: MIT Press; 1982.
15. Shepard RN. Ecological constraints on internal representation: resonant kinematics of perceiving, imagining, thinking, and dreaming. Psychol Rev. 1984;91:417–447.
16. Johnson MK, Kahan TL, Raye CL. Dreams and reality monitoring. J Exp Psychol. 1984;113:329–344.
17. Johnson MK. A multiple-entry, modular memory system. In: Bower GH, ed. The Psychology of Learning and Motivation: Advances in Research Theory. Vol 17. New York, NY: Academic Press; 1983:81–116.
18. Johnson MK. Reflection, reality monitoring, and the self. In: Kunzendorf RG, ed. Mental Imagery. New York, NY: Plenum; 1991:3–16.
19. Farah MJ. The neurological basis of mental imagery: a componential analysis. Cognition. 1984;18:245–272.
20. Greenberg MS. Farah MJ. The laterality of dreaming. Brain Cogn. 1986;8:307–321.
21. Farah MJ, Gazzaniga MS, Holtzman JD, et al. A left hemisphere basis for visual mental imagery? Neuropsychologia. 1985;23:115–118.
22. Greenwood P, Wilson DH, Gazzaniga MS. Dream report following comissurotomy. Cortex. 1977;13:311–316.
23. McCormick L, Nielsen T, Ptito M, et al. REM sleep dream mentation in right hemispherectomized patients. Neuropsychologia. 1997;35:695–701.
24. Doricchi F, Violani C. Dream recall in brain-damaged patients: a contribution to the neuropsychology of dreaming through a review of the literature. In: Antrobus JS, Bertini M, eds. The Neuropsychology of Sleep and Dreaming. Hillsdale, NJ: Lawrence Erlbaum Associates; 1992:99–140.
25. Solms M. The Neuropsychology of Dreams. Mahwah, NJ: Lawrence Erlbaum Associates; 1997.
26. Kerr NH, Foulkes D. Right hemispheric mediation of dream visualization: a case study. Cortex. 1981;17:603–610.
27. Hiscock M, Cohen DB. Visual imagery and dream recall. J Res Pers. 1973;7:179–188.
28. Paivio A. A factor-analytic study of word attributes and verbal learning. J Verb Learn Verb Behav. 1968;7:41–49.
29. Gordon R. An investigation into some of the factors that favor the formation of stereotyped images. Br J Psychol. 1949;39:156–167.
30. Richardson A. Dream recall frequency and vividness of visual imagery. J Ment Imagery. 1979;3:65–72.
31. Marks DF. Visual imagery differences in the recall of pictures. Br J Psychol. 1973;64:17–24.
32. Foulkes D. Children's Dreams: Longitudinal Studies. New York, NY: Wiley-Interscience; 1982.
33. Butler S, Watson R. Individual differences in memory for dreams: the role of cognitive skills. Percept Mot Skills. 1985;61:823–828.
34. Kosslyn SM, Brunn J, Cave KR, et al. Individual differences in mental imagery: a computational analysis. Cognition. 1984;18:195–243.
35. Marks DF. On the relationship between imagery, body, and mind. In: Hampson PJ, Marks DF, Richardson JTE, eds. Imagery: Current Developments. New York, NY: Routledge; 1990:1–38.
36. Rechtschaffen A, Buchignani C. The visual appearance of dreams. In: Antrobus JS, Bertini M, eds. The Neuropsychology of Sleep and Dreaming. Hillsdale, NJ: Lawrence Erlbaum Associates; 1992:143–155.
37. Kahn E, Dement W, Fisher C, et al. Incidence of color in immediately recalled dreams. Science. 1962;137:1054–1055.
38. Antrobus J, Hartwig P, Rosa D, et al. Brightness and clarity of REM and NREM imagery: photo response scale. Sleep Res. 1987;16:240.
39. Brooks LR. Spatial and verbal components of the act of recall. Can J Psychol. 1968;22:349–368.
40. Perky CW. An experimental study of imagination. Am J Psychol. 1910;21:442–452.
41. Segal SJ. Processing of the stimulus in imagery and perception. In: Segal SJ, ed. Imagery: Current Cognitive Approaches. New York, NY: Academic Press; 1971:69–100.
42. Dement W, Wolpert E. The relation of eye movements, body

motility, and external stimuli to dream content. J Exp Psychol. 1958;55:543–553.

43. Rechtschaffen A, Foulkes D. Effect of visual stimuli on dream content. Percept Mot Skills. 1965;20:1149–1160.

44. Deutsch ED. The dream imagery of the blind. Psychoanal Rev. 1928;15:288–293.

45. Jastrow J. Fact and Fable in Psychology. New York, NY: Houghton Mifflin; 1900.

46. Kirtley DD. The Psychology of Blindness. Chicago, Ill: Nelson-Hall; 1975.

47. Kerr NH, Foulkes D, Schmidt M. The structure of laboratory dream reports in blind and sighted subjects. J Nerv Ment Dis. 1982;170:247–264.

48. Carpenter PA, Eisenberg P. Mental rotation and the frame of reference in blind and sighted individuals. Percep Psychophys. 1978;23:117–124.

49. Marmor GS, Zaback LA. Mental rotation by the blind: does mental rotation depend on visual imagery? J Exp Psychol Hum Percept Perform. 1976;2:515–521.

50. Craig EM. Role of mental imagery in free recall of deaf, blind, and normal subjects. J Exp Psychol. 1973;97:249–253.

51. Cornoldi C, De Beni R, Roncari S, et al. The effects of imagery instructions on total congenital blind recall. Eur J Cogn Psychol. 1989;1:321–331.

52. Kerr NH. The role of vision in "visual imagery" experiments: evidence from the congenitally blind. J Exp Psychol Gen. 1983;112:265–277.

53. Cornoldi C, Cortesi A, Preti D. Individual differences in the capacity limitations of visuospatial short term memory: research on sighted and totally congenitally blind people. Memory Cogn 1991;19:459–468.

54. Farah MJ, Hammond KJ, Levine DN, et al. Visual and spatial mental imagery: dissociable systems of representation. Cogn Psychol. 1988;20:439–462.

40

Psychophysiology of Dreams

R. T. Pivik

To explore the nature of the relationship between mind and body, scientists have applied physiological probes during various cognitive experiences, and the state of sleep has been most vigorously investigated from this psychophysiological perspective. This focus developed since the 1950s as a result of the availability of technology that allows the continuous monitoring of physiological processes over long periods of time and the discovery of reports of dreaming from a sleep stage characterized by an unexpectedly high degree of physiological activation.[1-7] The early enthusiasm regarding this remarkable correspondence between physiology and mental activity during sleep was evident in the belief of Aserinsky and Kleitman[1] that these physiological measures would allow the determination of "the incidence and duration of periods of dreaming."[1(p274)] These initial observations were seized on by scientists who were influenced by the similarities between hallucinations and dreaming and thought that the capability of identifying moments of dreaming might enable them to understand the physiology of hallucinations and, ultimately, the basis for a fundamental feature of psychosis.

In addition to these considerations, there were other features of sleep physiology and psychology that made the study of mind-body relationships at this time especially appealing. Prominent among these were the wider variations in physiological events and psychological experiences during sleep relative to wakefulness. For example, with few exceptions (notably, 8- to 12-Hz alpha activity), electroencephalographic (EEG) activity typical of wakefulness is desynchronized, low-voltage, mixed-frequency activity, whereas during sleep there are long periods of synchronized activity alternating with episodes of activity similar to that observed during wakefulness, activities peculiar to that state (12- to 14-Hz spindles, 4- to 7-Hz sawtooth waves, K complexes), and marked variation in amplitude (i.e., 10 to 200 μV). Similarly, in contrast to the generally common nature of waking mental activity, cognitive activity during sleep frequently varies from the bizarre to the most mundane. Moreover, attempts to elicit reports of cognitive activity during sleep are often unsuccessful, suggesting that there may be times when mental activity may be absent during sleep, unlike the steady stream of thought that is present during wakefulness.

The impetus to study psychophysiological relationships during sleep was further enhanced by the absence of, or reduction in, potentially confounding variables that are present during wakefulness, such as expectations, stress, environmental distractions, and undetected variations in level of arousal. The confluence of all of these factors—physiological, psychological, and environmental—opened new venues for psychophysiological study and raised the possibility of determining mind-body relationships during sleep that may have been obscured, or perhaps are not even present, during wakefulness.

These considerations highlight the benefits of psychophysiological studies during sleep. Unfortunately, there also are obstacles that complicate both the acquisition and interpretation of data obtained in such studies. It was necessary, for example, to devise methodological procedures and techniques to meet the special demands made for conducting psychophysiological studies in the sleeping human being. On the physiological end, these included the development of methods for maintaining viable recordings continuously for 6 to 8 h while minimizing disturbance to the sleeping subject. Basically, technology and techniques are in common use for the noninvasive overnight recording of a variety of physiological measures, including EEG, eye movement, and autonomic and motor activities.

Although there are a variety of procedures and techniques by which physiological data can be acquired during sleep, there is only one method of accessing psychological experience at this time—through a verbal report provided by the subject. Attempts have been made to obtain these reports from subjects without awakening them, either through posthypnotic suggestions or by attempting to establish meaningful dialog in conjunction with verbalizations that occur spontaneously during sleep, but these attempts have been unsuccessful.[8] Consequently, reports of sleep mentation must be acquired during wakefulness and not directly from the state in which they are thought to be experienced. This introduces a state-dependency confound into these investigations that prompted suggestions that the experiences reported actually occurred during the process of waking up or were confabulations made up by the subject to please the experimenter. Such considerations may account for a small percentage of elicited reports, but on the basis of critical evaluations of the sleep physiological literature, convincing arguments have been produced supporting the belief that these postarousal reports are valid descriptions of cognitive experiences occurring during sleep. Several methods for analyzing the information contained in these reports have been developed, including rating scales,[9] study of the relationship of sleep to waking mentation with the use of free association procedures,[10, 11] or analysis of the reports from a grammatical perspective[10] (see Chapter 37 for a review of these methods).

The discovery of the episodic occurrence during sleep of periods of physiological activation closely associated with reports of dreaming fits comfortably with previous concepts regarding the levels and types of physiological activation required to sustain consciousness. These considerations made it easier to accept the presence of ongoing cognitive experience during a state (sleep) that was previously thought to be not only uniform in nature, but also characterized by unconsciousness. In attempting to map out this new psychophysiological terrain, investigators were challenged with determining physiological correlates that might best identify moments of dreaming. A description of the results of this mapping process is the focus of this chapter.

STATE RELATIONSHIPS

The initial psychophysiological sleep studies triggered by the discovery of the rapid eye movement (REM) sleep–dreaming association were primarily studies of state relationships. Although it was recognized that the REM and nonrapid eye movement (NREM) sleep states were differentially characterized by variations in several physiological measures, the initial studies focused on sustained patterns of EEG activity to index moments of dreaming.[3-7] These early studies predominantly reinforced the initial observations indicating that dreaming essentially was an exclusive attribute of the REM sleep state. Reports of dreaming from NREM periods of sleep were rare (approximately 8% compared with the nearly 80% or higher reported after REM sleep arousals) and were generally discounted as confusional reports generated during the awakening process or as attempts by the subject to produce a report to please the experimenter. At this time, then, it appeared that a unique and unusually high level of mind-body correspondence had been discovered—that is, the mind turned on during REM sleep and turned off at other times during sleep. Despite the prominence and general prevalence of reports substantiating this conclusion, however, there were persistent accumulating reports that seriously challenged the likelihood that the only mentation during sleep occurred during REM sleep. In 1967, Foulkes[12] summarized evidence arguing convincingly for the validity of NREM sleep mentation. Interestingly, contributing to the resistance to accept the possibility of mental activity during sleep other than REM sleep was the

unstated, yet apparently generally accepted, concept of what constituted a *dream*. In the early studies that examined the relationship between REM sleep and dreaming, subjects, on being awakened, were instructed to state "whether or not they had been dreaming," and only reports from subjects who related a "coherent, fairly detailed description of dream content"[5(p341)] were considered to represent dreams. Other reports of having dreamed "without recall of content, or vague, fragmentary impressions of content," were considered negative.[5(p341)] Operational criteria such as these led to reports indicating recall of dreams eight to nine times more often after arousals from REM sleep than after arousals from NREM sleep. The implications and consequences of this restrictive and ill-defined perspective can be appreciated in the following statement.

Initiating a postarousal interview whose opening query requires the subject to decide whether or not a dream has been occurring presupposes an implicitly understood and accepted definition of a dream experience. Although there may well be fundamental features of such experiences during sleep, which together may constitute characteristics of a "standard" dream experience, certainly all of these characteristics may not be present during each dream experience. Furthermore, the psychological experience that we collectively identify as "dreaming" may encompass quite disparate experiences on an individual basis. What one individual may term a bizarre, intense, dreamlike experience may to another seem only moderately bizarre and intense or perhaps even mundane. Nonetheless, the systematic scientific study of material related after arousal from sleep necessitates definitions of dreams. Such definitions have variously characterized the dream as a "verbal report describing an occurrence involving multisensory images and sensations, frequently of a bizarre or unreal nature and involving the narrator himself" (Berger, 1967, p. 16); "the presence of any sensory imagery with development and progression of mental activity" (Kales et al, 1967, p. 556); "any occurrences with visual, auditory, or kinesthetic imagery" (Foulkes, 1962, p. 17)[59]; a "multidimensional conglomerate of an hallucinatory belief in the actual occurrence of an imagined experience which, in turn, tends to be an extended visual, sometimes bizarre, drama" (Antrobus et al, 1978, p. 40); or simply "thinking" (Foulkes, 1978, p. 3).[10] When, instead of attempting to fit elicited reports into a preconceived but vaguely defined mould of the "dream," a more liberal approach was adopted in which more fragmentary, less perceptual reports of "thinking" were accepted as data, a quite different picture of the occurrence of sleep mentation emerged. Using this less restrictive approach, several studies reported recall of material subsequent to NREM sleep periods on more than 50% of the arousals (Foulkes, 1962[59]; Goodenough et al, 1959[81]; Molinari & Foulkes, 1969[135]; Pivik & Foulkes, 1968[66]).[13]*

As evident in some of the above definitions, references to dreams often emphasize the bizarre quality of these experiences. Laboratory dream research has indicated, however, that dreams are not typically bizarre, emotionally loaded experiences, and it has been

---

*For unnumbered references, refer to the original source.

suggested that this popularized, stereotypic view may have originated from biased sampling inherent in spontaneously recalled home dreams.[14, 15]

Although the presence of bizarre aspects in dreams has attracted much scientific attention, other even more common characteristics have been largely ignored. Among such features is a nonreflective quality that is evident in the suspension of judgmental processes during dreams.[16–18] This abandoning of the regulatory functions of self-evaluation characteristic of waking cognitive experiences suggests either limited access to such information during sleep or a discontinuity between specific aspects of waking and sleeping cognitive processes.[19, 20] This passive acceptance of events and images is related to the general lack of awareness during the dream that one is dreaming and contributes to the "single-mindedness" of dreams. This characteristic refers to the tendency for a single train of thoughts and images to be maintained over long periods of time without interruption from other, simultaneously occurring, thoughts and images[17]—a feature that may result from the coupling of increased sensory thresholds with cortical activation during sleep[21] or decoupling of specific cortical and subcortical structures during REM sleep.[20] There are, however, exceptions to this generalization regarding the quality of nonreflectiveness in REM dreams: (1) the sleep-onset REM dream in narcoleptics,[22, 23] (2) the lucid dream,[24] and (3) the nightmare or REM anxiety dream.[25] In each of these conditions, there is a greater appreciation by the dreamer of the sleep mentation, expressed as either a feeling of some control over the mentation (as in the narcoleptic sleep-onset REM dream and in the lucid dream) or an acceptance of dream events as real to the extent that the appropriate cognitive, autonomic, and motor responses are evoked (as in the nightmare). These examples underscore the presence of variations in some of the seemingly fundamental qualitative features of dreaming during REM sleep.

In this regard, it is also important to note that the dream-like features and qualities considered characteristic of REM dreams are present in NREM reports as well, especially reports elicited at sleep onset. Consequently, dreaming is not peculiar to REM sleep. Furthermore, dream-like features may also be found in the mental experiences of normal individuals during relaxed wakefulness.[26–29] The emerging picture suggests that there are conditions under which there may be a high probability for dreaming and that these conditions include reduced environmental sensory input and a loss of voluntary self-control. Although these conditions are relatively maximized during REM sleep, dreaming is not the exclusive property of any state.

If this broader conceptualization of dreaming that removes this cognitive behavior from the confines of REM sleep is accepted, then reductions in the amount of REM sleep may not necessarily translate into reductions in the amount of dreaming. However, for more than a decade after the discovery of REM sleep, there was a virtual identity between the physiological state of REM sleep and the psychological experience of dreaming. This conceptual set was so strong that the initial study that attempted to determine the functional significance of REM sleep and dreaming by preventing the occurrence of this stage of sleep was entitled "the effect of dream deprivation."[30] Indeed, the early experiments in this area were thought to indicate that REM sleep dreaming was essential for psychological normality during wakefulness.[31–33] Since that time, the effects of REM deprivation on cognitive functioning during both sleep and wakefulness have been extensively explored.[34–37] Although the results of this research have raised several interesting questions and pointed to possible psychological correlates of REM sleep deprivation, these data do not support the contention that the prevention of psychological experiences during REM sleep inevitably leads to negative consequences for waking psychological behavior. In fact, for some clinical populations (e.g., specific types of depressed patients), REM sleep deprivation may be associated with improvement in clinical symptoms.[38] The expectation that REM deprivation might have detrimental effects on waking psychological behavior had its roots in the belief that dreaming and waking hallucinatory behavior might share a common substrate.[11, 39, 40] However, if such an interrelationship exists, it remains elusive because studies of the sleep and dreams of mentally ill persons have been unable to demonstrate a consistent increase in adverse effects, either physiological or psychological, during wakefulness as a consequence of REM deprivation (for a review, see Pivik[13]).

While some investigators were grappling with the concepts of dream definition and whether dreaming was an exclusive property of REM sleep, others adopted a quite disparate position. They considered that because the dream report is produced while the subject is awake, and generally at a time of reduced physiological arousal,[41–44] then this report might simply be a consequence of the mind reestablishing contact with the external environment after sleep and not reflect a cognitive experience that occurred during sleep. This position, which attributes all dreaming to processes taking place during the immediate post-arousal period,[45, 46] argues that sleep is a state of unconsciousness and that postarousal reports are constructed from sensory and motor activity, as well as past memories, present during the waking-up process. However, observations that behavioral responses can occur during electroencephalographically defined sleep[47–52] and that subjects can accurately estimate elapsed time during a sleep period[53, 54] or awaken at preselected times without the use of external means[55, 56] argue that sleep is a behaviorally active state in which perception and other forms of information processing occur. The fact that such processes function during sleep is, however, not proof that they are used in the service of dream formation. Still, logical considerations[57] and psychophysiological data (for a review, see Pivik[13]) argue convincingly that reports of cognitive activity obtained after arousals from sleep are indeed descriptions of sleep experiences and not simply experiences generated during the arousal process. It is nevertheless possible that these reports are influenced by activities, both physiological and cognitive, peculiar to this period of awakening and that, as others have suggested,[46] processes at work during the time of awakening require further study.

Although it is clear that mental activity during sleep is not the exclusive property of REM sleep, there are qualitative dimensions along which reports from REM and NREM sleep have been shown to differ. REM reports, for example, are characterized by a greater representation of sensory and motor dimensions, whereas NREM reports show a greater correspondence to the waking life of subjects and are more frequently characterized as thinking than are REM reports.[58-61] In several reports, however, NREM mentation has been characterized as "dreaming" as often as,[62] or more often than,[58, 60, 63-67] "thinking." Although REM and NREM reports can be differentiated when a paired-comparison procedure is used,[63, 68] such between-stage discriminability is not maintained for all REM–NREM stage comparisons. An exception in this regard is mentation associated with arousals made during the transition from wakefulness to sleep, that is, stage 1. Mental activity occurring at this time has been shown to be similar to that from REM sleep along several dimensions, including incidence, report length, hallucinatory quality,[69-72] and perceptual and emotional quality.[73] Dement and Kleitman[4] reported the first study that compared reports from awakenings made at sleep onset with those from subsequent REM periods and observed that subjects' reports were often dream-like, but not as "organized" or "real," as reports from REM periods. Furthermore, because subjects believed they had not been sleeping when the initial reports were elicited, as opposed to being firmly convinced of being asleep before giving the REM reports, the conclusion was drawn that "no dreams were recalled after wakening during the sleep onset stage 1, only hypnogogic reveries."[4(p689)]

The general emphasis on qualitative differences between REM and NREM reports indicated by the preceding review could suggest the existence of state-dependent cognitive processes (i.e., processes specific to REM, NREM, and wakefulness). However, investigations that have controlled for length of report have revealed marked similarities in qualitative features,[74, 75] as well as memory sources of dream imagery,[76] of REM and NREM reports. From these and related data, it has been argued that a single system or process that fluctuates in intensity across states may be responsible for dream generation and that state-dependent processes are not required to account for differences that have been reported.[77-79]

The high positive correlation between reports of mental activity during sleep and low-voltage, mixed-frequency EEG activity characteristic of REM sleep and stage 1 has been generally corroborated by subsequent research. Specifically, recall is greater and reports are more vivid, bizarre, and dream-like after arousals associated with stage 1 EEG patterns[3, 5, 70, 72] than after arousals conducted in association with slower and higher-amplitude EEG activity.[60, 65] This relationship (i.e., between the nature of tonic background EEG activity and the incidence and qualitative aspects of reports from arousals made in association with these patterns) is further substantiated by increases across the night in recall and dream-like features of reports[64, 80-82] that occur in association with a parallel decrease in high-amplitude, slow EEG activity and increase in lower-voltage, fast-frequency activities.

The noted time of night variations in EEG activity points up the necessity to consider such influences on both physiological-state and psychological-experience characteristics that may extend beyond the moment at which these events are sampled. For example, temporal factors (e.g., elapsed time within the sleep stage before arousal) have been shown to influence the incidence and quality of recall in both stage 4[83] and REM sleep.[58, 84, 85] Other factors that may vary during sleep and that may affect the recall of experiences from sleep, if not the experiences themselves, include possible impairment of memory consolidation during sleep[86-91] and the interaction between level of arousal and memory processes.[88, 92, 93] The complexity of interactions among factors influencing recall can be appreciated from the extreme range of individual differences in recall of sleep mentation—extending from subjects who never or rarely recall[80] to those "characterized by relentless epic dreaming that is experienced to occur throughout sleep, leaving [them] fatigued/exhausted during the daytime."[94(p137)]

It is a rather remarkable observation that although the new era of sleep and dream research was initiated by observations in infants,[1] the psychophysiology of sleep in children or adolescents was largely neglected in the wave of investigations that followed. The emphasis placed on the study of dreaming in adults ignored this source of significant information regarding developmental aspects of sleep and how such developmental processes anticipate or contribute to the psychology of sleep in adults. Information is now accumulating regarding the developmental nature of dreaming, and the most extensive studies in this area are by Foulkes.[95] A major conclusion from his normative, longitudinal sleep-laboratory studies on subjects 3 to 15 years old was that "the development of REM dreaming follows a course parallel to the better-documented and well-known stages of waking cognitive maturation."[95(p275)] In these studies, Foulkes[95] observed minimal dream production in the youngest subjects studied (3 to 5 years old), and the content that was reported generally consisted of static imagery in the absence of a developed narrative context. It was not until subjects were within the 7- to 9-year-old range that report frequency increased and more complex content development was present. The longitudinal observations on which these conclusions were based have been replicated in a cross-sectional study using a larger sample of subjects.[96] These data indicate that dreaming is a complex cognitive behavior that requires the maturation of specific analytical skills and refute the general identification during infancy and early childhood of the physiological state of REM sleep as a time when psychological experiences of dreaming must be taking place. These conclusions suggest that before the time these skills required for dream production are developed, REM periods are most likely psychological voids.[95] The correspondence between waking cognitive skills and those reflected in dream production has received support from a study of the formal features of dream content in reading-disabled children that related differences in content to cognitive impairments evident during wakefulness in these children.[97]

To this point, the focus has been on studies emphasizing the importance of tonic background EEG activity as providing an index of the incidence and qualitative aspects of postarousal reports. However, it is clear that at best, this activity provides only a general orientation toward the identification of times when mental activity is present during sleep and does not index precise moments of dreaming. Relationships between sleep mentation and a variety of other physiological measures (e.g., autonomic and motor activities) have also been investigated. In general, measures of the tonic activity of autonomic (e.g., heart rate, respiratory rate, electrodermal activity, and penile erections) and motor (tonic facial muscle activity or stable levels of spinal reflexes) systems have not revealed consistent relationships with either amounts of recall or qualitative features of recalled material (refer to references 13, 98, and 99 for more extensive reviews).

For some measures, the absence of a relationship with mentation is particularly glaring. This is true for the concentrated periods of electrodermal activity occurring during stages 3 and 4[100] and for penile erections or clitoral engorgement, which are normal concomitants of REM sleep.[101–103] It might be expected that these activities would be associated, respectively, with mental activity reflecting high levels of arousal in the case of electrodermal activation or an abundance of manifest sexual references in association with penile tumescence or clitoral engorgement. On the contrary, mental activity recalled from slow-wave sleep is either less dream-like[60] or of a similar dream-like quality[83] relative to reports of NREM mentation from arousals not associated with such electrodermal activation. Similarly, except for those associated with lucid dreaming,[104, 105] reports elicited after arousals from REM sleep contain remarkably little material of an overt sexual nature.[106, 107]

PHASIC INFLUENCES

The general absence of robust psychophysiological relationships between tonic levels of physiological activity and sleep mentation led to a redirection of studies examining the association between cognitive activity and physiological measures during sleep. This reorientation can be summarized as a shift in emphasis from state to event or, in terminology used by Moruzzi[108, 109] to differentiate mechanisms and events underlying sleep states, from tonic to phasic considerations.

A variety of EEG measures that occur intermittently during NREM (K complexes, sleep spindles, and 5- to 6-Hz theta bursts) and REM (theta bursts and 2- to 3-Hz frontal "sawtooth" waves) sleep have been investigated in this regard. In these studies, the presence of phasic EEG events has conferred little or no recall advantage over nonphasic arousals, and with few exceptions (theta bursts and sawtooth waves being associated with greater amounts of primary visual activity [i.e., nonintellectualized visual images] and discontinuity in content, respectively), inconsistent or unremarkable qualitative correlates have been observed (see review in Pivik[110]).

Another type of EEG oscillatory activity has recently drawn the attention of investigators interested in physiological and cognitive processes during sleep. This 20- to 40-Hz high-frequency rhythm has been noted in animals and human beings during both wakefulness and sleep but is present at relatively reduced intensity during NREM sleep.[111–113] It has been speculated that this activity provides a mechanism for integrating multisensory information[114] and that such binding of information may be a neurophysiological correlate of cognition.[115] However, research into the cognitive correlates of this activity is only beginning, and its relationship to sleep cognition remains largely speculative.[116]

The measures most extensively studied within the phasic-tonic framework have been those associated with motor activity (Fig. 40–1). In this regard, an association between discrete muscle activity and specific REM dream content has been reported.[117–119] With respect to motor events, the most conspicuous and extensively studied measure has been eye movements during REM sleep. Such activity has been associated with both increased recall[120, 121] and increased dream-like features (e.g., vividness and emotionality).[122, 123] There is disagreement, however, regarding the extent to which increased eye movement density is associated with increased activity within the dream.[7, 65, 124–127]

Investigators have looked for precise correspondence between eye movements and ongoing mental activity in the context of what has been called the "scanning hypothesis." As suggested by the name, this hypothesis proposes that eye movements generated during REM sleep scan the visual images of the dream in the same way that eye movements during waking scan the environment. Studies examining this hypothesis have produced variable results, ranging from reports of remarkable correspondence between dream activity and associated eye movements to those indicating an absence of such an association (for a review, see Rechtschaffen[99]). Interest in this relationship has continued, with more positive associations between eye movement and dream imagery being observed in lucid dreams[128] and indications from brain imaging studies that the same cortical areas involved in the control of waking eye movements are also active during eye movements in REM sleep.[129] The variability in results noted across studies, which has essentially kept the issue of eye movement–dream content correspondence unresolved, may reflect a range of factors, including limitations in the subject's ability to introspect, the interviewer's knowledge of head–eye movement relationships, interviewing procedures and techniques, and methods of analysis.[13, 130] In fact, Bussel et al.[131] indicated that the ability of subjects to accurately recall

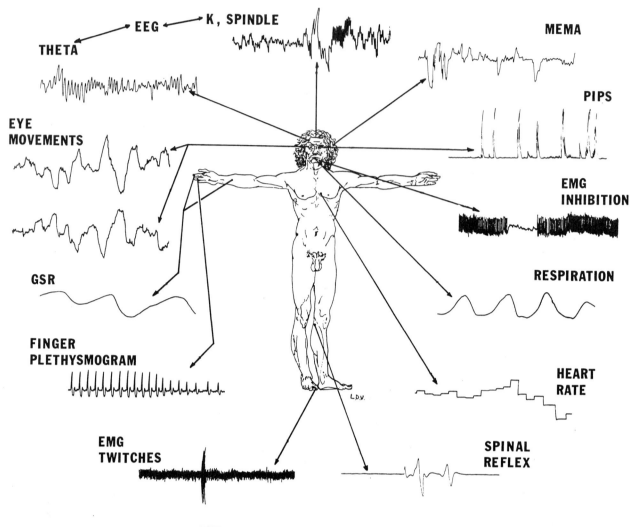

THETA   EEG   K, SPINDLE   MEMA

EYE
MOVEMENTS   PIPS

EMG
INHIBITION

GSR   RESPIRATION

FINGER
PLETHYSMOGRAM   HEART
RATE

EMG
TWITCHES   SPINAL
REFLEX

THE PHASIC PROPORTIONS OF MAN

Figure 40–1. The phasic proportions of man. Various phasically occurring electrophysiological measures that have been investigated in the context of psychophysiological studies of sleep. These variables, with approximate designations of anatomic areas from which they can be recorded, include EEG measures (K complex, spindle, and theta activity); various expressions of muscle activity from auditory (middle ear muscle activity [MEMA]), visual (eye movements, periorbital integrated potentials [PIPS]) and skeletal musculature (facial EMG inhibition, spinal reflexes, and EMG twitches) systems; and autonomic activity (galvanic skin response [GSR], finger plethysmogram, respiration, and heart rate). See the text for a more complete listing and a discussion of phasic variables. (From Pivik RT. Sleep: physiology and psychophysiology. In: Coles MGH, Donchin E, Porges SW, eds. Psychophysiology: Systems, Processes and Applications. New York, NY: Guilford Press; 1986:378–406.)

waking cognitive experiences and related eye movement activity occurring in the few seconds before being interviewed is significantly compromised. The possible bases for discrepant results in both the waking and sleep situations have been previously reviewed, and one conclusion of that review was a call for the appreciation of difficulties intrinsic to establishment of intimate psychophysiological relationships, noting that these difficulties "serve as a reminder that experimental demands need to be carefully considered in the evaluation of negative results."[13(p388)]

It is not uncommon for physiological processes in human beings to be based to some extent on models of these processes in lower animal species and even for fundamental aspects of some cognitive functions, such as information processing, to be studied in the

same way. It is unusual, however, for relatively inaccessible complex cognitive processes in human beings to be based on animal models. It is of interest, therefore, that the model for the study of phasic events in the human being and their relationship to cognitive processes was a physiological event initially described and most extensively studied in the cat. This event, the "ponto-geniculo-occipital (PGO) spike"—an acronym derived from areas of the central nervous system where this activity is most prominent, namely, the pons, the lateral geniculate bodies, and the occipital cortex—has been viewed as a prototypic phasic event because of the widespread anatomic representation[132] and physiological correlates (e.g., eye movements and, most recently, 30- to 40-Hz EEG rhythms[133]) of these events, as well as their distribution during both REM and NREM sleep. However, the correspondence between the occurrence of PGO spike activity in the cat and characteristics of sleep mentation in human beings are, at best, inconsistent.[98] Furthermore, reviews[13, 99, 110] of studies examining differences between reports elicited from arousals in association with tonic or phasic activity during both REM and NREM sleep conclude that these studies have failed to provide evidence of a distinctive differentiation between the content elicited against these markedly different physiological backgrounds. This literature has made it clear that phasic activity is not required for mental activity to be present during sleep, although phasic activity may, perhaps through an arousing effect, enhance the recall of mental activity from both REM and NREM sleep.

Although phasic events could not be used as an index for the presence of mental activity during sleep, it was considered that such activity might be related to specific qualitative features of associated mental activity. The relationship between the presence of phasic activity and qualitative features of associated mentation examined in this context included sensory (primary visual experiences,[134] auditory features[135]) and temporal and cognitive (secondary cognitive elaboration,[136] discontinuity and bizarreness[21, 136, 137]) aspects. However, these studies also were unable to demonstrate a consistent correlation of phasic activity with these qualitative aspects of sleep mentation.

THEORETICAL CONSIDERATIONS AND CONCLUSIONS

The discovery of REM sleep initiated a field of research that has provided unexpected revelations regarding physiological processes and cognitive experience during sleep.[138] At the outset of this new era, psychophysiological studies of sleep were directed toward the possibility of examining and testing the validity of several of the concepts of the most well-known dream theory of the time—that of Freud.[11] As data accumulated, new theories developed that sought to incorporate and integrate the rapidly growing knowledge in this area. For the most part, these theories focused on REM sleep dreaming because of both the strong correlation between these two activities and the perceived differences between REM and NREM sleep in terms of cognitive and physiological characteristics. A listing and brief description of some theories that have been developed will serve to highlight conceptual points of focus that have attracted attention in sleep physiology and psychophysiology. These theories vary in the degree of emphasis placed on cognitive components, ranging from formulations in which dreaming experiences are simply byproducts of other activities that are thought to serve important functions to those in which cognitive features are paramount. Representative of the former grouping in which cognitive activities are incidental to REM sleep physiological activation are theories by Berger,[139] Crick and Mitchison,[140] Hobson and McCarley,[141] and Antrobus.[142, 143] Berger[139] argued that one function of REM sleep was to maintain, via oculomotor activation, visual system activity important for waking binocular coordination. Crick and Mitchison[140] considered REM sleep as a time when the brain rids itself of unwanted memory stores accumulated during waking experience. The activation-synthesis hypothesis[141] of Hobson and McCarley views dreaming as a consequence of the interpretation by the forebrain of the barrage of brainstem activity it receives during REM sleep. As an extension of this hypothesis, Hobson[144] has advanced a more general brain-mind model entitled AIM to account for characteristics of mentation across sleep and waking states. The model is based on three factors, among which the interactions determine the momentary brain state and associated mind state. These factors are activation (A: determined by the level of activity in the reticular activating system), input source (I: referring to the ratio of external relative to internal sensory stimulus strength), and information processing mode (M: operationalized to reflect known variations in aminergic modulation of the cortex). Antrobus[142] also sees the dream as a product of cortical activation and attributes the particular qualitative features of REM sleep mentation to the interpretation of spontaneous activity by the cortex in the absence of external afferent input during a time of high sensory threshold. In this context, he has applied neural network model principles to simulate the characteristics of dreaming.[143] Finally, cognitive theorists such as Foulkes[95] suggest that dreaming depends on abilities to organize experiences in memory and to access and reorganize those experiences independently of external environmental stimulation. This cognitive approach does not rely on specific physiological events to explain dream features and considers dreaming to be a form of thinking.

These theories are, to varying degrees, based on substantive findings; all have heuristic value, but none has been generally accepted. To some extent, the initial fascination of the REM sleep–dreaming association continues to polarize thinking in this area. Foulkes[145] addressed issues related to theories of REM dreaming and noted three problems faced by these theories—problems confronting any state-dependent theory of dreaming. The first general problem underscored the fact that our understanding of REM sleep as a biological process is incomplete and that we may not have sufficient knowledge to explain a cognitive experience as complex as dreaming. The second problem was more philosophical in nature and raised the question of whether psychological experiences can ever be fully explained by even a complete knowledge of the biological correlates of the experience. The third and, in the opinion of Foulkes, "fatal" problem for theories that focus on REM sleep dreams only is that dreaming has been shown not to be restricted to this state but occurs in NREM sleep and even in wakefulness.

It can be expected that the tendency to use particular physiological events or psychological qualities as a foundation for theories of dreaming will continue. However, any theory that attempts to explain the basis for the generation of dreaming and to address issues related to the potential functional significance of this activity must recognize observations indicating the great extent to which dreams consist of mundane experiences (not unlike typical waking thought) and take into account the growing indications of qualitative similarities between REM and NREM experiences. These considerations demand that any viable theory that hopes to explain the generation, process, or function of dreaming cannot be restricted by physiologically defined state boundaries.

Since the discovery of REM sleep, investigations into the psychophysiology of dreaming have undergone shifts in emphasis from state, to event, and, most recently, to a more holistic perspective. Early promises that such studies would yield the secrets of the unconscious mind or perhaps provide a psychophysiological basis for understanding waking hallucinations have not been met. Through these studies, we have, however, learned a great deal about both the biology of sleep and the nature of cognitive activity during sleep. Although it may be disappointing that a reliable, point-for-point correspondence between specific physiological events and specific aspects of cognitive experiences present in postarousal dreaming reports has not been demonstrated, these findings have not discouraged investigators from continuing the assault on mind-body relationships during sleep. Negative results, low correlations, and data trends in this area result, at least in part, from the extreme complexities of the behaviors under study. Even the use of recent technological advances in brain neuroimaging procedures, while offering exciting new insights into physiological processes during sleep,[20, 129, 146] has provided, at best, speculative inferences regarding the neurobiology of dreaming.[147]

The belief of Aserinsky and Kleitman[1] that dreaming was signaled by a specific pattern of physiological events naturally occurring during a time (sleep) when the influence of environmental stimuli and volition are markedly reduced or entirely suspended sparked a fascination for studying these relationships that continues undiminished. Perhaps more than ever before, it is becoming apparent that studies of the characteristics and correlates of dream consciousness prompted by this fascination offer unique insights into our general understanding of cognitive behavior in human beings.[148]

References

1. Aserinsky E, Kleitman N. Regularly occurring periods of eye motility and concomitant phenomena during sleep. Science. 1953;118:273–274.
2. Aserinsky E, Kleitman N. Two types of ocular motility occurring during sleep. J Appl Physiol. 1955;8:1–10.
3. Dement WC. Dream recall and eye movement during sleep in schizophrenics and normals. J Nerv Ment Dis. 1955;122:263–269.
4. Dement WC, Kleitman N. Cyclic variations in EEG during sleep and their relation to eye movements, bodily motility and dreaming. Electroencephalogr Clin Neurophysiol. 1957;9:673–690.
5. Dement WC, Kleitman N. The relation of eye movements during sleep to dream activity: an objective method for the study of dreaming. J Exp Psychol. 1957;53:339–346.
6. Dement WC, Wolpert E. Interrelations in the manifest content of dreams occurring on the same night. J Nerv Ment Dis. 1958;126:568–578.
7. Dement WC, Wolpert E. The relation of eye movements, body motility, and external stimuli to dream content. J Exp Psychol. 1958;55:543–554.
8. Arkin AM. Sleeptalking. In: Ellman SJ, Antrobus JS, eds. The Mind in Sleep. 2nd ed. New York, NY: John Wiley & Sons; 1991;415–436.
9. Winget C, Kramer N. Dimensions of Dreaming. Gainesville, Fla: University Presses of Florida; 1979.
10. Foulkes D. A Grammar of Dreams. New York, NY: Basic Books; 1978.
11. Freud S. The Interpretation of Dreams. New York, NY: Basic Books; 1955 (originally published 1900).
12. Foulkes D. Nonrapid eye movement mentation. Exp Neurol. 1967;19:28–38.
13. Pivik RT. Sleep: physiology and psychophysiology. In: Coles MGH, Donchin E, Porges SW, eds. Psychophysiology: Systems, Processes, and Applications. New York, NY: Guilford Press; 1986:378–406.
14. Foulkes D. Home and laboratory dreams: four empirical studies and a conceptual reevaluation. Sleep. 1979;2:233–251.
15. Weisz R, Foulkes D. Home and laboratory dreams collected under uniform sampling conditions. Psychophysiology. 1970;6:588–596.
16. Kleitman N. The basic rest-activity cycle and physiological correlates of dreaming. Exp Neurol. 1967;19:2–4.
17. Rechtschaffen A. The single-mindedness and isolation of dreams. Sleep. 1978;1:97–109.
18. Meier B. Speech and thinking in dreams. In: Cavallero C, Foulkes D, eds. Dreaming as Cognition. New York, NY: Harvester Wheatsheaf; 1993:58–76.
19. Foulkes D. Children's dreaming. In: Cavallero C, Foulkes D, eds. Dreaming as Cognition. New York, NY: Harvester Wheatsheaf; 1993:114–132.
20. Braun AR, Balkin TJ, Wesensten NJ, et al. Dissociated pattern of activity in visual cortices and their projections during human rapid eye movement sleep. Science. 1998;279:91–95.
21. Reinsel R, Antrobus J, Wollman M. Bizarreness in dreams and waking fantasy. In: Antrobus JS, Bertini M, eds. The Neurophysiology of Sleep and Dreaming. Hillsdale, NJ: Lawrence Erlbaum Associates; 1992:137–183.
22. Ribstein M. Hypnagogic hallucinations. In: Guilleminault C, Dement WC, Passouant P, eds. Narcolepsy. New York, NY: Spectrum; 1976:145–160.
23. Vogel GW. Mentation reported from naps of narcoleptics. In: Guilleminault C, Dement WC, Passouant P, eds. Narcolepsy. New York, NY: Spectrum; 1976:161–168.
24. Tart CT. From spontaneous event to lucidity: a review of attempts to consciously control nocturnal dreaming. In: Wolman M, ed. Handbook of Dreams. New York, NY: Van Nostrand Reinhold; 1979:226–268.
25. Kahn E, Fisher C, Edwards A. Night terrors and anxiety dreams. In: Arkin AM, Antrobus JS, Ellman SJ, eds. The Mind in Sleep. Hillsdale, NJ: Erlbaum; 1978:533–542.
26. Foulkes D, Fleisher S. Mental activity in relaxed wakefulness. J Abnorm Psychol. 1975;84:66–75.
27. Foulkes D, Scott E. An above-zero waking baseline for the incidence of momentarily hallucinatory mentation [abstract]. Sleep Res. 1973;2:108.
28. Galton F. Inquiries Into Human Faculty and Its Development. London, England: JM Dent; 1911 (originally published 1883).
29. Spanos NP, Stam HJ. The elicitation of visual hallucinations via brief instructions in a normal sample. J Nerv Ment Dis. 1979;167:488–494.
30. Dement WC. The effect of dream deprivation. Science. 1960;131:1705–1707.
31. Dement WC, Fisher C. Experimental interference with the sleep cycle. Can Psychiat Assoc J. 1963;8:400–540.
32. Sampson H. Deprivation of dreaming sleep by two methods: 1. Compensatory REM time. Arch Gen Psychiatr. 1965;13:79–86.
33. Sampson H. Psychological effects of deprivation of dreaming sleep. J Nerv Ment Dis. 1966;143:305–317.
34. Ellman SJ, Spielman AJ, et al. REM deprivation: a review. In: Ellman SJ, Antrobus JS, eds. The Mind in Sleep. 2nd ed. New York, NY: John Wiley & Sons; 1991:329–376.
35. Weinstein LN, Schwartz DG, Ellman SJ. Sleep mentation as

affected by REM deprivation: a new look. In: Ellman SJ, Antrobus JS, eds. The Mind in Sleep. 2nd ed. New York, NY: John Wiley & Sons; 1991:377–395.

36. Lewin I, Singer JL. Psychological effects of REM ("DREAM") deprivation upon waking mentation. In: Ellman SJ, Antrobus JS, eds. The Mind in Sleep. 2nd ed. New York, NY: John Wiley & Sons; 1991:396–412.

37. Vogel GW. Review of REM sleep deprivation. Arch Gen Psychiat. 1975;32:749–761.

38. Vogel GW, Thurmond A, Gibbons P, et al. REM sleep reduction effects on depression syndromes. Arch Gen Psychiat. 1975;32:765–777.

39. Jackson H. In: Taylor J, Holmes E, Walshe F, eds. Selected Writings. New York, NY: Basic Books; 1958.

40. Jung CG. The Psychology of Dementia Praecox. New York, NY: Journal of Nervous and Mental Disease Publishing Company; 1944.

41. Broughton RJ. Sleep disorders: disorders of arousal? Science. 1968;159:1070–1078.

42. Felton M, Broughton RJ. Differential effects of arousal from slow wave sleep versus REM sleep [abstract]. Psychophysiology. 1968;5:231.

43. Scott J. Performance after abrupt arousal from sleep: comparison of a simple motor, a visual-perceptual, and a cognitive task. Proceedings of the 77th Annual Convention of the American Psychological Association; 1969:225–226.

44. Tebbs RB. Post-awakening visualization performances as a function of anxiety level, REM or NREM sleep, and time of night (USAF Academy SRI-TR-72-0005, AD-738 630). Colorado Springs, Colo: U.S. Air Force Academy; 1972.

45. Goblot, E. Sur le souvenir des rêves. Rev Philos. 1896;42:288.

46. Hall CS, Raskin R. Do we dream during sleep? Unpublished manuscript, 1980.

47. Brown JN, Cartwright RD. Locating NREM dreaming through instrumental responses. Psychophysiology. 1978;15:35–39.

48. Evans FJ, Gustafson, LA, O'Connell DN, et al. Verbally induced behavioral responses during sleep. J Nerv Ment Dis. 1970;150:171–187.

49. Granda AM, Hammack JT. Operant behavior during sleep. Science. 1961;133:1485–1486.

50. McDonald DG, Schicht WW, Fratier RB, et al. Studies of information processing in sleep. Psychophysiology. 1975;12:624–629.

51. Oswald I, Taylor AM, Treisman AM. Discriminative responses to stimulation during human sleep. Brain. 1960;83:440–453.

52. Williams HC, Morlock HC, Morlock JV. Instrumental behavior during sleep. Psychophysiology. 1966;2:208–216.

53. Carlson VR, Feinberg I, Goodenough DR. Perception of the duration of sleep intervals as a function of EEG sleep stage. Physiol Psychol. 1978;6:497–500.

54. Latash LP, Danilin VP. Subjective estimation of the duration of time periods in night sleep. Nat New Biol. 1972;236:94–95.

55. Moorcroft WH, Kayser KH, Griggs AJ. Subjective and objective confirmation of the ability to self-awaken at a self-predetermined time without using external means. Sleep. 1997;20:40–45.

56. Lavie P, Okensberg A, Zomer J. It's time, you must wake up now. Percept Mot Skills. 1979;49:447–450.

57. Rechtschaffen A. Dream reports and dream experiences. Exp Neurol. 1967;19 (suppl 4):4–15.

58. Foulkes D. Dream reports from different stages of sleep. J Abnorm Soc Psychol. 1962;65:14–25.

59. Foulkes D, Rechtschaffen A. Presleep determinants of dream content: effect of two films. Percept Mot Skills. 1964;19:983–1005.

60. Pivik RT. Mental activity and phasic events during sleep [dissertation]. Stanford, Calif: Stanford University; 1971.

61. Rechtschaffen A, Verdone P, Wheaton J. Reports of mental activity during sleep. Can Psychiatry Assoc J. 1963;8:409–414.

62. Goodenough DR, Lewis HB, Shapiro A, et al. Some correlates of dream reporting following laboratory awakenings. J Nerv Ment Dis. 1965;140:365–373.

63. Bosinelli M, Molinari S, Bagnaresi G, et al. Caratteristiche dell attiva psicofisiologica durante il sonno: un contributo alle tecniche di valutazion. Rivi Sperimentale Freiatria. 1968;92:128–150.

64. Foulkes D. Dream Reports From Different Stages of Sleep [dissertation]. Chicago, Ill: University of Chicago; 1960.

65. Pivik RT, Foulkes D. NREM mentation: relation to personality, orientation time, and time of night. J Consult Clin Psychol. 1968;37:144–151.

66. Rechtschaffen A, Vogel G, Shaikun G. Interrelatedness of mental activity during sleep. Arch Gen Psychiatry. 1963;9:536–547.

67. Zimmerman WB. Psychological and physiological differences between "light" and "deep" sleepers [abstract]. Psychophysiology. 1968;4:387.

68. Monroe LJ, Rechtschaffen A, Foulkes D, et al. Discriminability of REM and NREM reports. J Pers Soc Psychol. 1965;2:456–460.

69. Foulkes D, Spear PS, Symonds J. Individual differences in mental activity at sleep onset. J Abnorm Psychol. 1966;71:280–286.

70. Foulkes D, Vogel G. Mental activity at sleep onset. J Abnorm Psychol. 1965;70:231–243.

71. Vogel GW. Sleep-onset mentation. In: Arkin AM, Antrobus JS, Ellman SJ, eds. The Mind in Sleep. Hillsdale, NJ: Erlbaum; 1978:97–108.

72. Vogel GW, Foulkes D, Trosman H. Ego functions and dreaming during sleep onset. Arch Gen Psychiatry. 1966;14:238–248.

73. Vogel GW, Barrowclough B, Giesler D. Limited discriminability of REM and sleep onset reports and its psychiatric implications. Arch Gen Psychiatry. 1972;26:449–455.

74. Antrobus JS. REM and NREM sleep reports: comparison of word frequencies by cognitive classes. Psychophysiology. 1983;20:562–568.

75. Foulkes D, Schmidt M. Temporal sequence and unit composition in dream reports from different stages of sleep. Sleep. 1983;6:265–280.

76. Cavallero C, Foulkes D, Hollifield M, et al. Memory sources of REM and NREM dreams. Sleep. 1990;13:449–455.

77. Cavallero C, Cicogna P, Natale V, et al. Slow wave sleep dreaming. Sleep. 1992; 15:562–566.

78. Cavallero C, Cicogna P. Memory and dreaming. In: Cavallero C, Foulkes D, eds. Dreaming as Cognition. New York, NY: Harvester Wheatsheaf; 1993:38–57.

79. Foulkes D, Cavallero C. Introduction. In: Cavallero C, Foulkes D, eds. Dreaming as Cognition. New York, NY: Harvester Wheatsheaf; 1993:1–17.

80. Goodenough DR, Shapiro A, Holden M, et al. A comparison of "dreamers" and "nondreamers": eye movements, electroencephalograms and the recall of dreams. J Abnorm Psychol. 1959;59:295–302.

81. Shapiro A, Goodenough DR, Griller RB. Dream recall as a function of method of awakening. Psychosom Med. 1963;25:174–180.

82. Verdone P. Variables Related to the Temporal Reference of Manifest Dream Content. [dissertation]. Chicago, Ill: University of Chicago; 1963.

83. Tracy RL. Tracy LN. Reports of mental activity from sleep stages 2 and 4. Percept Mot Skill. 1974;38:647–648.

84. Kramer M, Roth T, Czaya J. Dream development within a REM period. In: Levin P, Koella WP, eds. Sleep. Basel, Switzerland: Karger; 1975:406–408.

85. Kramer M, Whitman RM, Baldridge B, et al. Dream Psychology and the New Biology of Dreaming: Springfield, Ill: Charles C Thomas; 1969.

86. Goodenough DR. Some recent studies of dream recall. In: Witkin H, Lewis H, eds. Experimental Studies of Dreaming. New York, NY: Random House; 1967:128–147.

87. Goodenough DR. The phenomena of dream recall. In: Abt LE, Riess BF, eds. Progress in Clinical Psychology. Vol 8. New York, NY: Grune & Stratton; 1968:136–153.

88. Goodenough DR. Dream recall: history and current status of the field. In: Arkin AM, Antrobus JS, Ellman SJ, eds. The Mind in Sleep. Hillsdale, NJ: Erlbaum; 1978:113–140.

89. Portnoff G, Baekeland F, Goodenough DR, et al. Retention of verbal materials perceived immediately prior to onset of non-REM sleep. Percept Mot Skills. 1966;22:751–758.

90. Rechtschaffen A. Discussion of experimental dream studies by W. C. Dement. In: Masserman J, ed. Science and Psychoanalysis. Vol. 7: Development and Research. New York, NY: Grune & Stratton; 1964:162–170.

91. Wolpert EA. Two classes of factors affecting dream recall. J Am Psychoanal Assoc. 1972;20:45–58.

92. Akerstedt T, Gillberg M. Effects of sleep deprivation on memory

and sleep latencies in connection with repeated awakenings from sleep. Psychophysiology. 1979;16:49–52.

93. Koulack D, Goodenough DR. Dream recall and dream recall failure: an arousal-retrieval model. Psychol Bull. 1976;83:957–984.

94. Schenck CH, Mahowald MW. A disorder of epic dreaming with daytime fatigue, usually without polysomnographic abnormalities, that predominantly affects women. Sleep Res. 1995;24:137.

95. Foulkes D. Children's Dreams: Longitudinal Studies. New York, NY: John Wiley & Sons, 1982.

96. Foulkes D, Hollifield M, Sullivan B, et al: REM dreaming and cognitive skills at ages 5–8: a cross-sectional study. Int J Behav Dev. 1990;13:447–465.

97. Butler S, Pivik RT. Dreaming in reading disabled children. Dreaming. 1991;1:193–209.

98. Pivik RT. Tonic states and phasic events in relation to sleep mentation. In: Arkin AM, Antrobus JS, Ellman SJ, eds. The Mind in Sleep. Hillsdale, NJ: Erlbaum; 1978:245–271.

99. Rechtschaffen A. The psychophysiology of mental activity during sleep. In: McGuigan FJ, Schoonover RA, eds. The Psychophysiology of Thinking. New York, NY: Academic Press; 1973:153–205.

100. Burch N. Data processing of psychophysiological recordings. In: Proctor LD, Adey WR, eds. Symposium on the Analysis of Central Nervous System and Cardiovascular Data Using Computer Methods. Washington, DC: National Aeronautics and Space Administration; 1965:165–180.

101. Fisher C, Gross J, Zuch J. Cycles of penile erection synchronous with dreaming (REM) sleep. Arch Gen Psychiatry. 1965;12:29–45.

102. Karacan I, Goodenough DR, Shapiro A, et al. Erection cycle during sleep in relation to dream anxiety. Arch Gen Psychiatry. 1966;15:183–189.

103. Cohen HD, Shapiro A. Vaginal blood flow during sleep [abstract]. Psychophysiology. 1970;1:338.

104. LaBerge S, Greenleaf W, Kedzierski B. Physiological responses to dreamed sexual activity during lucid REM sleep. Psychophysiology. 1983;20:454–455.

105. LaBerge S. Lucid Dreaming. Los Angeles, Calif: JP Tarcher; 1985.

106. Fisher C. Dreaming and sexuality. In: Lowenstein R, Newman L, Shur M, et al, eds. Psychoanalysis: A General Psychology. New York, NY: International Universities Press; 1966:537–569.

107. Hall C, Van de Castle RL. The Content Analysis of Dreams. New York, NY: Appleton-Century-Crofts; 1966.

108. Moruzzi G. Active processes in the brain stem during sleep. Harvey Lecture Series. 1963;58:233–297.

109. Moruzzi G. General discussion. In: Aspects Anatomo-Fonctionnels de la Physiologie du Sommeil: Actes du Colloque International sur les Aspects Anatomo-Fontionnels de la Physiologie du Sommeil, Lyon, 1963 (Colloques Internationaux du Centre National de la Recherche Scientifique, No. 127). Paris, France: Centre National de la Recherche Scientifique; 1965:613–650.

110. Pivik RT. Tonic states and phasic events in relation to sleep mentation. In: Ellman SJ, Antrobus JS, eds. The Mind in Sleep. New York, NY: John Wiley & Sons; 1991:214–247.

111. Llinás R, Ribary U. Coherent 40-Hz oscillation characterized dream state in humans. Proc Natl Acad Sci U S A. 1993;90:2078–2081.

112. Franken P, Dijk DJ, Tobler I. et al. High-frequency components of the rat electrocorticogram are modulated by the vigilance states. Neurosci Lett. 1994;167:89–92.

113. Steriade N, Amzica F, Contreras D. Synchronization of fast (30-40 Hz) spontaneous cortical rhythms during brain activation. J Neurosci. 1996;16:392–417.

114. Joliot M, Ribary U, Llinás R. Human oscillatory brain activity near 40 Hz coexists with cognitive temporal binding. Proc Natl Acad Sci U S A. 1994;91:11748–11751.

115. Llinás R, Ribary U, Joliot M, et al. Content and context in temporal thalamocortical binding. In: Buzsaki G, Llinás R, Singer W, et al, eds. Temporal Coding in the Brain. Berlin, Germany: Springer; 1994:251–272.

116. Kahn D, Pace-Schott EF, Hobson JA. Consciousness in waking and dreaming: the roles of neuronal oscillation and neuromodulation in determining similarities and differences. Neuroscience. 1997;78:13–38.

117. Grossman W, Gardner R, Roffwarg H, et al. Limb movement and dream action: are they related? [abstract]. Sleep Res. 1973;2:123.

118. McGuigan FJ, Tanner RG. Covert oral behavior during conversational and visual dreams [abstract]. Psychophysiology. 1970;7:329.

119. Stoyva JM. Finger electromyographic activity during sleep: its relation to dreaming in deaf and normal subjects. J Abnorm Psychol. 1965;70:343–349.

120. Medoff L, Foulkes D. "Microscopic" studies of mentation in stage REM: preliminary report [abstract]. Psychophysiology. 1972;9:114.

121. Pivik RT, Halper C, Dement W. Phasic events and mentation during sleep [abstract]. Psychophysiology. 1969;6:215.

122. Ellman SJ, Antrobus JS, Arkin AM, et al. Sleep mentation in relation to phasic and tonic events—REMP and NREM [abstract]. Sleep Res. 1974;3:115.

123. Hobson JA, Goldfrank F, Snyder F. Respiration and mental activity in sleep. J Psychiatr Res. 1965;3:79–90.

124. Berger RJ, Oswald I. Eye movements during active and passive dreams. Science. 1962;137:601.

125. Firth H, Oswald I. Eye movements and visually active dreams. Psychophysiology. 1975;12:602–605.

126. Hauri P, Van de Castle RL. Psychophysiological parallelism in dreams. Psychosom Med. 1973;35:297–308.

127. Keenan R, Krippner S. Content analysis and visual scanning in dreams. Psychophysiology. 1970;7:302–303.

128. LaBerge S. The postawakening testing technique in the investigation of cognitive asymmetries during sleep. In: Antrobus JS, Bertini M, eds. The Neuropsychology of Sleep and Dreaming. Hillsdale, NJ: Lawrence Erlbaum Associates; 1992:289–303.

129. Hong CC-H, Gillin JC, Dow BM, et al. Localized and lateralized cerebral glucose metabolism associated with eye movements during REM sleep and wakefulness: a positron emission tomography (PET) study. Sleep. 1995;18:570–580.

130. Hong CC-H, Potkin SG, Antrobus JS, et al. REM sleep eye movement counts correlate with visual imagery in dreaming: a pilot study. Psychophysiology. 1997;34:377–381.

131. Bussel J, Dement W, Pivik RT. The eye movement-imagery relationship in REM sleep and waking [abstract]. Sleep Res. 1972;1:100.

132. Brooks DC. Waves associated with eye movement in the awake and sleeping cat. Electroencephal Clin Neurophysiol. 1968;24:532–541.

133. Amzica F, Steriade M. Progressive cortical synchronization of ponto-geniculo-occipital potentials during rapid eye movement sleep. Neuroscience. 1996;72:309–314.

134. Molinari S, Foulkes D. Tonic and phasic events during sleep: psychological correlates and implications. Percept Mot Skills. 1969;29:343–368.

135. Roffwarg HP, Herman J, Lamstein S. The middle ear muscles: predictability of their phasic activity from dream material. Sleep Res. 1975;4:165.

136. Foulkes D, Pope R. Primary visual experience and secondary cognitive elaboration in stage REM: a modest confirmation and an extension. Percept Mot Skills. 1973;37:107–118.

137. Watson RK. Mental correlates of periorbital potentials during REM sleep [dissertation]. Chicago, Ill: University of Chicago; 1972.

138. Aserinsky E. The discovery of REM sleep. J Hist Neurosci. 1996;5:213–227.

139. Berger RJ. Oculomotor control: a possible function of REM sleep. Psychol Rev. 1979;76:144–164.

140. Crick F, Mitchison G. The function of dream sleep. Nature. 1983;304:111–114.

141. Hobson JA, McCarley RW. The brain as a dream state generator: an activation-synthesis hypothesis of the dream process. Am J Psychiatry. 1977;134:1335–1348.

142. Antrobus J. Dreaming: cognitive processes during cortical activation and high afferent thresholds. Psychol Rev. 1991;98:96–121.

143. Antrobus J. Dream theory 1997: toward a computational neurocognitive model. SRS Bull. 1997;3:5–10.

144. Hobson JA. A new model of brain-mind state: Activation level, input source, and mode of processing (AIM). In: Antrobus JS,

Bertini M, eds. The Neuropsychology of Sleep and Dreaming. Hillsdale, NJ: Lawrence Erlbaum: 1992:227–245.

145. Foulkes D. Understanding our dreams. The World and I. 1989;4:296–303.

146. Maquet P, Péters J-M, Aerts J, et al. Functional neuroanatomy of human rapid-eye-movement sleep and dreaming. Nature. 1996;383:163–166.

147. Foulkes D. A contemporary neurobiology of dreaming? SRS Bull. 1997;3:2–4.

148. Foulkes D. Dream research: 1953–1993. Sleep. 1996;19:609–624.

41

Waking Experiences and Dreaming

Joseph De Koninck

HISTORICAL CONSIDERATIONS

Everyone who remembers their dreams will agree that at least some traces of their waking experiences can be found in their content. However, dreams are not simply a replay of preceding waking activity, whether it be mental, emotional, or situational. Instead, their content is often intriguing, leaving the dreamer wondering what they could mean and thus influencing waking thoughts and mood. It is not surprising, therefore, that since the earliest of times human beings have speculated on the origin and the sources of dreams. Their conceptions of what dreams were made of determined the type and extent of attention they were given, and their influence on subsequent waking behavior.

In the most primitive groups, dreams were part of waking reality and therefore could have a major impact on daily life. A dream of adultery could lead to an adultery fine.[1] Similarly, it is interesting to note that in the young child dreams are not separated from waking experiences, which is why a 4-year-old can wake up in bed and refer to a bear that is chasing him and does not understand why his parents do not share his terror. In more evolved ancient societies, dreams were seen as a means by which gods communicated with human beings.[1] Dreams were interpreted to serve as guides for political, social, and everyday decisions. Early books, including the Bible, are filled with examples of the attribution of dreams to divine sources. Temples were constructed specifically to allow individuals to sleep and upon awakening have their dreams interpreted by dream specialists. Greek philosophers, however, attributed dream content to natural sources and were precursors of modern theories of dream formation and significance. For example, Hippocrates proposed that dreams could provide signs of the presence and the source of illnesses. Plato saw dreams as expressions of desires and anger uncontrolled by waking reason. Aristotle devoted an entire book to the topic of dreams, expanding the interest in dreams beyond their natural sources (bodily conditions and internal sensations) and pointing out their influence on subsequent waking thoughts and behavior. He argued that dreams are acts of imagination,[2] and even alluded to the phenomenon of lucid dreaming, that is, the condition wherein dreamers realize they are dreaming and attempt to control the content.

In the Middle Ages, dreams were seen as linked with sins, sex, and demons. They were therefore avoided and had little impact on waking life. The emergence of science in the 19th century brought about several systematic attempts to understand the sources of dreams.[3] But what brought them into the limelight was Freud's theory[4] that dreams were constructed on the basis of repressed childhood conflicts and fantasies, the management of which were at the root of psychological adaptation in adults. For him dreams were important not for their relationship with contemporary life but were instead the "royal road to the unconscious," thereby giving access to repressed conflicts. It is only through psychoanalysis that dreams are meaningful in contemporary psychological adaptation. Freud's immediate followers, however, saw a more direct relationship between dreams and waking daily life. For Adler,[5] dreams reflected the current lifestyle of the dreamer and offered solutions to contemporary problems. Jung[6] believed that waking experience was represented in a compensatory and complementary fashion in dreams, which are creative representations of the "subjective state" of the dreamer.

In all of these conceptions, and when considering the interaction between waking experience and dreams, two main issues must be distinguished: (1) What is the contribution of waking experience to the construction of dreams or how and when does waking experience find its way into dreams? (2) What is the influence of dreaming on subsequent waking activity and experience? Although both issues are ultimately related, and most dream function theories propose answers to both, a better picture of the state of our current knowledge is provided when they are treated separately.

WAKING EXPERIENCE AND THE CONSTRUCTION OF DREAMS

Modern dream research received a tremendous boost from the discovery of rapid eye movement (REM) sleep and its association with a high rate of vivid dream reports.[7] By obtaining a large and systematic sample of the dreaming activity from a single night, it was hoped to determine which waking experiences find their way into dreams, how they are transformed, and when this occurs. However, more than 40 years of laboratory research have revealed that dream construction is very complex and multifactorial. After reporting on the main findings of this research, a review of some factors that seem to mediate the relationship between waking experience and dream content will be presented.

In his classic review, Snyder described the typical dream obtained in the laboratory as "a clear, coherent, and detailed account of a realistic situation involving the dreamer and other people caught up in ordinary activities and preoccupations, and usually talking about them."[8(p148)] From dreams collected over 20 consecutive nights, Kramer and Roth[9] observed that the content exhibited some stability (night-to-night correlations of .46) leaving, however, some 79% of the night-to-night variance unaccounted for. How does this content reflect the preceding waking activity? A host of studies have been carried out in which subjects have been exposed to unusual presleep events. Manipulations of presleep experiences have included social isolation, water deprivation, physical exercise, stressful or unusual films, stressful intellectual activity, and even subliminal stimulation. Other studies have focused on the effects of real-life stress on dream content, such as those associated with serious surgical operations,[10] stressful menstruation,[11] and divorce.[12] The general observations that emerged from these various studies are discussed below.

Incorporation of Waking Events

While traces of the presleep experiences have been observed in dreams, *direct* incorporations have tended to be few. A good example comes from a study of the effects of inverted vision on REM dream content.[13] Subjects wore goggles inverting their visual field for 4 days and REM dreams were collected during the last 2 nights and compared with REM dreams from control conditions. Very few incorporations of inversions of visual fields in dreams were reported and those by only four of the eight participants. The visual inversion experience was instead reflected in dreams by increases in motor and visual difficulties, misfortunes, and dreamer confusion. More effects on dreams have been found following alteration of visual input with tinted goggles,[14] but direct incorporations have tended to be more prominent in the case of real-life stressful experiences.[10] Indeed, the simple fact of placing subjects in a laboratory setting (electrode placement, etc.) has in many studies more prominently influenced the dreams of subjects than artificial manipulations set up by experimenters. Examples of both incorporation and laboratory environment representation are evident in the dream presented next (translated from French).

> I was, that is, I was coming out of here (lab). I had the impression, at least, that I was coming out of here. Then, passing close by the machine on the other side, it was not placed the same way, however, there were

changes. I looked at the machine on the other side . . . then the paper was black. Then there was one of the graphs with lines. I wanted to know what it was. Then I looked at a word but it was upside-down. I am sure because I had to read upside-down. There was a "T", an "R", an "A" and there was also a "C", a "Y" . . . There was also another letter. But I didn't know what it was . . . Let's say that there was not much sense apart from "TRACÉ (most likely the French word referring to EEG tracing.)[13(p19)]

Most incorporations are indeed *indirect* and can take different forms. Examples of how auditory stimulation can be integrated into the dream were provided in an experiment by Berger.[15] He found that a noun, presented while a subject was in REM sleep, could be integrated into REM dreams in three different ways other than by direct incorporation: *assonance* ("Gillian" transformed into "Chile" [Chilean]); *association* (Richard dreams of a shop by the same name); and *representation* (a person with the name appears in the dream).

Certain types of activity, however, do not appear to be incorporated in dreams. Hartmann[16] reported that although reading, writing, and counting are common everyday activities, they are seldom incorporated into dreams.

Time Course of Incorporations

A prevailing observation, which applies to experimentally induced or real-life experiences, is that their incorporation into dreams can be significantly delayed. Michel Jouvet,[17] the renowned sleep neurophysiologist, collected his own home dreams over several years and reported frequently observing a lag of 6 to 9 days before a new environment (e.g., as a result of a trip) would appear in his dreams. Such an observation is consistent with studies of language learning and dreams. English-speaking students undergoing a 6-week French language immersion program maintained a dream diary starting 2 weeks before and continuing until 2 weeks after the course. They slept in the laboratory during four series of nights: one before the course, two during the course, and one after the course. Even though they were required to attend classes conducted entirely in French and were required to speak French all day and evening, it was only after at least 5 days that participants started to incorporate French words into their dreams, and in some subjects it took 1 month before this occurred. Their language learning effort was rather expressed by an increase in verbal communication in dreams.[18] This phenomenon has been further studied by Nielsen and Powell[19] who have labeled it the *dream lag effect*. Marquandt et al.[20] reported that 47% of waking incorporations identified by a group of subjects came from the preceding day, 19% from the preceding week, and the remaining 33% from earlier experiences.

Indeed, there is a relatively sharp decline in references to remote waking experiences in dreams. A study examined temporal references in REM dreams in both young (age 20 to 33 years) and older (age 60 to 77 years) subjects.[21] Interestingly, some elderly subjects reported oneiric elements dating as far back as 50 to 59 years and some younger subjects reported elements dating back about 20 years. When considering only dream temporal references that reportedly had not been accessed by the dreamers' waking conscious awareness since the time of the original experience, descriptive statistics revealed that in the younger subjects, 99% of temporal references fell within the period 10 years ago and 1% within the next 10 years. In elderly subjects, 91.8% of references fell within the most recent decade; 1.9% within the period of 10 to 19 years ago; 1.9%, 20 to 29 years ago; 1.5%, 30 to 39 years ago; 0.6%, 40 to 49 years ago; and 2.3% dated back 50 to 59 years. Contrary to the opinion expressed by many dream researchers, it appears that, although temporal references can date back to a dreamer's remote past, such instances are not common.

Dream Emotionality

It has been commonly observed that the emotional tone of dreams is typically negative. Indeed, normative data suggest that negative emotions and aggressive interactions in dreams are much more frequent than positive emotions and friendly interactions.[22] Most dreams are therefore reported by the dreamers to be unpleasant. This may explain why experimentally induced stress has had little effect on dream emotionality; that is, it may be masked by the already negative tone of the dreams. Again, real-life stress has had more impact on dream emotionality,[10] and extremely stressful life events, such as those experienced by Holocaust survivors and Vietnam War veterans, yield frightful dreams and nightmares which, in many instances, become recurrent dreams.[23, 24]

Waking emotionality as expressed through current concerns has also been considered an important contributor to dream experience. However, research does not support this notion because only 17% of dream narratives can be traced to presleep concerns.[25] When given a description of the daily events or presleep concerns of a dreamer, the layperson is not able to match presleep ideation with nocturnal dreaming,[26] and only in special circumstances have dream specialists been able to match presleep concerns with subsequent dream content.[27]

Continuity vs. Compensation Between Waking and Dreaming

The bulk of the literature supports the notion that the mode of representation of waking activity in dreams is that of continuity, for example, that waking stress induces anxiety in dreams and relaxation induces pleasant dreams. However, instances of compensation have been observed. For example, presleep social isolation has been found to induce dreams filled with social interactions;[28] physical exercise, dreams of rest;[29] and thirst, dreams of drinking.[30]

FACTORS MEDIATING THE REPRESENTATION OF WAKING IN DREAMS

It is clear from the above observations that dreams are not simply a replay of waking activity and concerns but that they draw on these experiences in ways that are complex and little understood. However, a number of mediating factors involved in this process have been identified. The most important of these are discussed below.

Physiology

The psychophysiology of dreams is the subject of Chapter 40 and will not be elaborated on here. However, it must be mentioned that the type of representation of waking experience in dreams varies with sleep physiology and undoubtedly its neurophysiological substrates. Although early studies[7] suggested that dreaming was limited to REM sleep, it has been well demonstrated that dreaming takes place during all sleep stages.[31] Although vivid dreams can be reported from any part of the night and from all sleep stages, there are typically variations in types of mental activity across the sleep cycles, as outlined in Figure 41–1.[35] Sleep-onset mentation is dream-like but tends to be related to the more recent past and is closer to waking fantasy than REM sleep mentation.[32] There is also evidence that dreams reported from nonrapid eye movement (NREM) sleep contain more day residues than dreams from REM sleep. REM dreams, which have been studied much more extensively, show an evolution in content across the night. Verdone[33] observed that as the night progresses, dreams refer to events further in the past of the dreamer's life. This finding was recently replicated in a large group of subjects.[34] It also appears that as the night progresses REM periods become longer and brain activation levels increase, and associated with these changes are dreams with more complex content which do not rely on recent memories but use a broader sample of memory traces. Mental activity during sleep, which is highly emotionally charged, is also related to the time of night and the sleep stage. For example, mental content is rarely recalled from night terrors occurring in slow-wave sleep at the beginning of the night, whereas nightmares are observed in REM periods from the latter part of the night.

Age, Gender, and Social Role

There is clearly an ontogenetic evolution in both the organization and the thematic content of dreams. It has been well documented that children dream more about animals and that these figures are later replaced by human characters. Throughout adulthood, both men's and women's dream narratives refer to family life and work.[36–38] Not surprisingly, themes of death slowly ap-

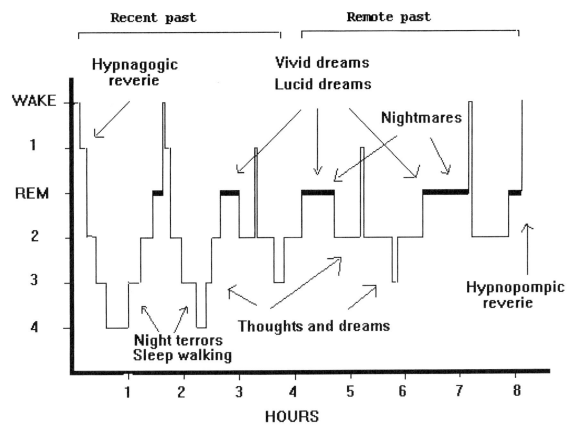

Figure 41-1. General variation in mental activity across the sleep cycles of a night's sleep. This figure depicts the hypnogram of a normal young adult and identifies the various types of mental activity generally obtained when content awakenings are made across the sleep cycles. Vivid dreams can be encountered throughout a night's sleep, but the most vivid and detailed dreams with the longest narrations are most often obtained from REM sleep awakenings. Mental content during the earlier part of the night contains more references to the recent past than that elicited during morning sleep, and mentation from NREM sleep is more likely to contain references to the recent past. (Modified from De Koninck J. Sleep. The common denominator for psychological adaptation. Can Psychol. 1997;38:191–195.)

pear in the dreams of the elderly. On the emotional dimension, dreams become more pleasant with age as their aggressive content is reduced.[36, 38–41]

Gender differences in the content of dreams have been studied extensively. In late adolescence and early adulthood, such differences are particularly noticeable on a number of dream dimensions. Interpersonal and relational issues were found to be more typical of female adolescents' dreams than those of males.[42] Normative data computed by Hall and Van de Castle[22] from college students' dreams indicate that males have, for example, more male characters and more aggression in their dreams than females, who have more friendly interactions[39] and pleasant emotions. The same differences were found a generation later,[43] suggesting a long-lasting impact of biological differences or early socialization, or both. More recent research suggests, however, that social roles enacted in adulthood attenuate some of the gender differences. For instance, compared with homemakers, working mothers were found to have more masculine types of dream imagery, with more aggression and anxiety,[44] and the dreams of women working in traditionally male professions were generally similar to those of men.[36] These findings make sense within the continuity hypothesis, according

to which dreams reflect concerns and preoccupations experienced in the waking state.[45]

Personality and Psychopathology

Modern personality theories assume that personality characteristics shape the content of dreams by making them consistent and continuous with waking experience and personality.[45] For this reason, dream material is used in many forms of psychotherapy. One example of how dreams and personality may be related is the model developed by Rossi[46] which proposed that dreams reflect the state of development of waking personality. He suggested that the passage through various stages of growth in personality development can first be detected in dreams, specifically in the formation of dream scenarios.

However, research attempting to correlate waking personality traits, as measured by personality tests, with dream content has had very limited success.[47] A recent and very interesting conceptualization is the thin-thick boundary personality structure of Hartmann.[48] People with thick boundaries focus on one thing at a time and differentiate clearly between thoughts and feelings, reality and fantasy, and self and others. Thin-boundary people have difficulty focusing on one thing at a time and have a rich fantasy life, sometimes becoming lost in daydreams and unable to distinguish them from reality. Hartmann has found that the latter have a higher dream recall rate and that, in keeping with their waking personality characteristics, their dreams are more vivid, dream-like, nightmare-like, and interactive. More research is needed to determine the importance of this personality dimension in the modulation of dreams.

The relationship between waking personality and dream characteristics has also been studied by examining dream content following changes in waking personality dimensions. Consistent with the continuity model, it has been observed that anxious people have more anxious dreams, that the application of relaxation techniques reducing waking anxiety traits is accompanied by improvements in the pleasantness of dreams,[49] and that systematic desensitization applied to a phobic subject can induce the disappearance of the phobic objects from dreams.[50]

Psychopathological conditions are also reflected in dreams, but not necessarily along with waking personality lines of continuity (for a review of this topic, see Chapter 42). For example, Kramer and Roth[51] reported that schizophrenic patients have brief dreams with little affect, and in an apparently compensatory fashion their dreams have little hallucinatory content. However, Wolman[52] reported that the dreams of some schizophrenic patients, before psychotic reactions emerge in waking, can contain vivid expressions of violence and that the "more patients deteriorate, the less sharp is the line dividing dream from the waking state."[52(p399)] As for depressed patients, they show surprisingly few depressive themes, at least in the manifest content of their dreams. Still, it appears that with improvement in depression, "hostility is decreased while intimacy, heterosexuality, and motility are increased."[51(p379)]

Cognitive Organization

A most interesting conceptualization of dream formation is that of Foulkes[31] who views dreams as "cognitive acts which represent a creative recombination of memory and knowledge."[31(p123)] Before waking experience can be transformed into dreams, it must be integrated cognitively and its expression intertwined with other available memories. Based primarily on his pioneering studies of children's dreams, Foulkes notes that the cognitive organization of dreams follows the cognitive development of the child as described by Piaget. This model extends, however, to dream formation throughout the life span. The study of elderly subjects mentioned above[21] is relevant to this view. In that study, waking autobiographical memory was compared with remoteness of dream content. Large variations between age groups in autobiographical memory were reflected in dreams, thus supporting the notion that dream production mechanisms are somehow related to memory and waking cognitive organization. In the study of the effects of visual inversions, those subjects who incorporated inversions in their dreams generally performed better on tests of adaptation to the visual inversion.[13] It appears that it is only following some cognitive integration of the inversion that it could be reproduced in dreams. Similarly, in the intensive language learning study,[18] those subjects who incorporated French words in their dreams early in the course were those who made the most progress in learning the language. Again, it appears that it is only once the new language is integrated that it can be used in dream production. Along the same lines, Weinstein et al.[53] pointed out that the lack of elaboration in the dreams of schizophrenic patients may be due to their cognitive deficit rather than the psychotic content of their disorder.

According to the cognitive approach, dreams are not dependent on perception but on how the brain thinks during sleep. Dream formation is not attempting to reproduce waking experience as it was perceived, but is using the memory traces available given the arousal state of the system. The higher arousal level during REM sleep would explain how REM dreams can be more elaborated and represent integrations of a wide range of memories from the recent and remote past.

Motivation and Voluntary Control

Spontaneous dream production can be altered by direct or indirect suggestion. Indeed, of all the attempts to influence dream content, by far the most successful has been presleep suggestion.[54] Such suggestions have taken the form of hypnotic, nonhypnotic, and presleep incubation, and all have had some success. For example, with a simple presleep suggestion method subjects have been able to incorporate a phobic object into their dreams and influence their emotional content even in the presence of the phobic object.[55] This presleep suggestion approach has been successful enough to be applied to the treatment of nightmares.[56] Nightmare sufferers are being taught methods of dream control which rest on presleep rehearsal of modified (turned pleasant) nightmare scenarios.

However, the most spectacular way of influencing dream content is lucid dreaming. While it is a natural phenomenon to become aware of dreaming and even staying in a dream state, several authors, following the pioneering work in the 19th century of Hervé de St-Denis,[57] have developed techniques of enhancing this phenomenon.[58] Subjects have been trained to recognize that they are dreaming and to systematically attempt to alter the course of their dreams. They have even been able to signal the onset of lucidity to the experimenter by moving their eyes in a distinctive pattern that can be detected on a polygraph. Such instances of lucidity represent a marked intrusion of waking processes into dreaming and can no longer be considered to represent spontaneous dreaming. The technique can be used effectively for the treatment of nightmares and recurrent dreams.[56]

In brief, while dreams undoubtedly carry traces of waking experience, they have a life of their own. A series of factors, such as memory, sleep physiology, personality, motivation, and cognitive organization, mediate the oneiric expression of waking experience to the point that it is significantly transformed and the dream product constitutes a new cognitive expression.

CONSEQUENCES OF DREAMS ON WAKING EXPERIENCE

It is precisely because dreams are not merely a repetition of waking activity that they can have an impact on subsequent waking activity. Once remembered, they become part of waking thought and can influence the dreamer. The consequences of dreams have been the object of many theories about the functions of dreaming. While the number of these theories is myriad, there is little empirical support for most of them. One reason may be that both researchers and theorists have neglected to take into account the number of variables involved. Figure 41–2 illustrates some of these variables in sequence. Presleep and sleep variables leading to the construction of dreams have been described earlier.

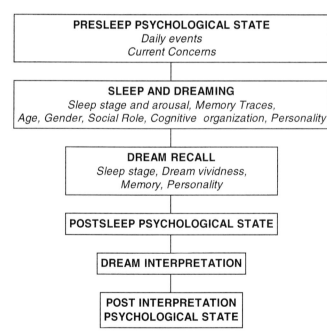

Figure 41–2. Some variables involved in dream formation and possible consequences for waking behavior. Illustrated is the sequence of factors that contribute to the construction of dreams and their potential impact on subsequent waking experience. Dreams appear to be constructed on the basis of a combination of remote past experiences, current concerns, the level of cognitive organization, and the functional level of the sleeping brain. The impact of dreams on subsequent waking experience depends on dream recall, dream mood and content, beliefs about dreams, and dream interpretation. (Modified from De Koninck J. Sources and consequences of dreams: Experimental manipulations and their effects. In: Gachenbac J, Sheikh A, eds. Dream Images: A Call to Mental Arms. Farmingdale, NY: Baywood; 1991:17–30.)

Dream Recall

Once a dream takes place, a most important condition is whether it is recalled, because its influence can depend on whether or not it is remembered. There is some disagreement regarding the factors that determine dream recall.[59] The initial proposition by Freud, that repression was responsible for the forgetting of dreams, has been found to be limited and not sufficient to explain this complex phenomenon. It is recognized, for example, that dreams taking place during REM sleep are more likely to be remembered. Dream characteristics such as vividness and interest favor better recall. Memory factors such as consolidation and interference certainly play a role, and motivation and interest in dreaming are other important factors. Except for the recent conceptualization of personality boundary previously described,[60] personality traits have not been consistently associated with dream recall.

Dream recall sampled by experimental awakenings in the laboratory confirms that mental activity is present throughout sleep. However, in both the laboratory and home environments, what is the influence of dreams that are not recalled or that are briefly remembered and then forgotten? Do they have an impact on waking experience? Little research work has been conducted on this question. According to Freud,[4] dreams that are not remembered are those which fulfill their function as *guardians of sleep*, by preventing the dreamer from waking up and discovering their disguised meaning. Experimentally testing the function of dreams requires treating them as independent variables, manipulating their content, and assessing the effects. However, given the paucity of methods for significantly manipulating dream content without confounding the manipulation with arousal,[61] very little has been achieved.[62]

Recalled Dreams

Once a dream is recalled, the extent of consideration and reflection that it generates and how it is interpreted are crucial determinants of its impact. There have been a number of attempts to examine the effects of remembered dreams, but the methodological approaches are limited and the findings have often been contradictory. Bokert[30] observed that subjects deprived of liquid for 24 h were less thirsty in the morning if they had dreams during which their thirst was slaked. De Koninck and Koulack[63] presented the same stressful film to subjects before sleep and upon awakening in the morning and observed that subjects who incorporated elements of the stressful film in their dreams were more affected by the second presentation of the film. These studies suggest a compensatory effect of dreams and therefore a potential role for dreams in adaptation. Other studies, to the contrary, suggest that incorporation of stressful elements produces tension reduction on a mid- or long-term basis. For example, Cartwright[12] observed that among a group of divorcees, those who had incorporated their ex-spouse in their dreams adapted more easily to the situation than those who did not. Whether their adaptation was somewhat mediated by their dream incorporations or whether the incorporations reflected waking adaptation efforts remains to be established.

Nightmares

If the impact of common dreams on subsequent waking activity is unclear, that of highly charged dreams and nightmares is undeniable. There is even evidence that highly charged dreams can be the source of psychosomatic problems such as migraine headaches.[64] Fortunately, as mentioned above, presleep suggestion and lucid dreaming techniques have been quite successful in alleviating the negative content.[56]

Dreams and the Psychotherapeutic Process

There is, of course, a host of modern psychotherapeutic approaches that use dream interpretation or simply dreams as material for therapeutic processes.[65] In the case of interpretations, therapists and clients look for insights into personality characteristics and motive. In other instances, the dream material is used to derive associations which become part of the therapeutic process. In both cases, it is not the dreams per se that influence waking experience, but what takes place during therapy.

Dreams and Creativity

Perhaps the most intriguing phenomenon associated with dreaming is its creative potential. There have been numerous accounts of discoveries made as a result of dreams containing new associations. Among the best known in this regard were the structure of the benzene ring, the light bulb, and the sewing machine needle. Many writers and artists use their dreams as starting scenarios for their work. In all instances, however, credit must be given to the dreamers who recognized the innovative associations in their dreaming material. Since creative dreams are not frequent, they have eluded systematic study except by those who attempt to provoke creative dream association through lucid dreaming techniques.[66]

Among the attempts to explain the creative potential of dreams, the conception of Klinger[67] deserves attention. He proposed that dreaming is essentially an associative or respondent mental activity. Rather than being limited by operational constraints found in waking thoughts, dreams allow unrestricted sequences of associations between memory traces and cognitive operations. Klinger believes that "Dreams, like play and fantasy, are fractionated, unsystematic approaches that work over the dreamer's real concerns, and in the process sometimes yield solutions by generating new combinations of pre-established schemata,"[67(p83)] and that "Longer respondent sequences following extensive problem-solving effort permit the individual to work over his concerns without the constraints imposed by operant activity and may yield creative solutions."[67(p353)] Hartmann's recent theory on the nature and function of dreaming emphasizes this enhanced connectivity found in the dreaming process. More recent work[68] has suggested that pathways that mediate transmissions between brain structures during REM sleep are different from those during waking and some are simply dissociated. Although such observations cannot be used to explain the peculiarities of dreaming outside of REM sleep, they support the notion of a different nature of cognitive associations that are generated during sleep. It is hoped that future studies will allow us to better understand the underlying brain substrates and tap this unlimited resource.

CONCLUSION

The mind in sleep uses traces of waking experience in highly elusive and selective ways for the construction of dreams. They return to the waking mind original cognitive and emotional creations that are most often ignored, but that can influence psychological adaptation in both positive and negative ways. Dreams remain a fascination for the waking mind and their mysteries are likely to occupy our investigative efforts for many more decades.

Acknowledgments

I thank Monique Lortie-Lussier, Francine Roussy, Jean Grenier, and Mélanie St-Onge for their help in the preparation of this chapter.

References

1. Van de Castle R. The Psychology of Dreaming. New York, NY: General Learning Corp; 1971.
2. Gallop D. Aristotle on Sleep and Dreams. New York, NY: Broadview Press; 1990.
3. Maury A. Le sommeil et les rêves. Paris, France: Didier; 1861.
4. Freud S. The Interpretation of Dreams. New York, NY: Penguin Books; 1991.
5. Adler A. Individual Psychology. London, England: Routledge & Kegan Paul; 1929.
6. Jung CG. Memories, Dreams and Reflections. New York, NY: Vintage; 1961.
7. Aserinsky E, Kleitman N. Regularly occurring periods of eye motility and concomitant phenomena during sleep. Science. 1953;118:273–274.
8. Snyder F. The phenomenology of dreaming. In: Meadow L, Snow L, eds. The Psychodynamic Implications of the Psychophysiological Studies on Dreams. Springfield, Ill: Charles C Thomas; 1970:124–151.
9. Kramer M, Roth T. The stability and variability of dreaming. Sleep. 1979;1:319–325.
10. Breger L, Hunter I, Lane RW. The effects of stress on dreams. Psychol Issues. 1971;7:3.
11. Sirois-Berliss M, De Koninck J. Menstrual stress and dreams: adaptation or interference. Psychiatr J Univ Ottawa. 1982;7:77–86.
12. Cartwright R. Dreams that work: the relation of dream incorporation to adaptation to stressful events. Dreaming. 1991;1:3–9.
13. De Koninck J, Prévost F, Lortie-Lussier M. The effects of inversion of the visual field on REM sleep mentation. J Sleep Res. 1996;5:16–20.
14. Roffwarg H, Herman J, Bowe-Anders C, et al. The effects of

sustained alterations of waking visual input on dream content. In: Arkin AM, Antrobus JS, Ellman SJ. The Mind in Sleep. New York, NY: John Wiley & Sons; 1978.

15. Berger RJ. Experimental modification of dream content by meaningful verbal stimuli. Br J Psychiatry. 1963;109:722–740.

16. Hartmann E. Outline for a theory of the function of dreams. Dreaming. 1996;6:147–170.

17. Jouvet M. Mémoire et "cerveau dédoublé" au cours du rêve à propos de 130 souvenirs de rêve. Annee Praticien. 1979;29:27–32.

18. De Koninck J, Christ G, Hébert G, et al. Language learning efficiency, dreams, and REM sleep. Psychiatr J Univ Ottawa. 1990;15:91–92.

19. Nielsen T, Powell RA. The day-residue and dreams lag effects: a literature review and limited replication of two temporal effects in dream formation. Dreaming. 1992;2:67–78.

20. Marquandt CJG, Bonato RA, Hoffman RF. An empirical investigation into the day-residue and dream lag effects. Dreaming. 1996;6:57–65.

21. Grenier J, St-Onge M, Vachon J, et al. Dreams and autobiographical memory: a study of remote temporal references [abstract]. J Sleep Res. 1998;7:105.

22. Hall C, Van de Castle R. The Content Analysis of Dreams. New York, NY: Appleton-Century-Crofts; 1966.

23. Kramer M, Kinney L. Sleep patterns in trauma victims. Psychiatr J Univ Ottawa. 1988;13:12–16.

24. Lavie P, Kaminer H. Dreams that poison sleep: Dreaming in Holocaust survivors. Dreaming. 1991;1:11–21.

25. Saredi R, Baylor G, Meier B, et al. Current concerns and REM-dreams: a laboratory study of dream incubation. Dreaming. 1997;7:195–208.

26. Roussy F, Camirand C, Foulkes D, et al. Does early-night REM dream content reliably reflect presleep state of mind? Dreaming. 1996;6:121–130.

27. Rados R, Cartwright R. Where do dreams come from? A comparison of presleep and REM sleep thematic content. J Abnorm Psychol. 1982;91:433–436.

28. Wood P. Dreaming and Social Isolation [dissertation]. Chapel Hill, NC: University of North Carolina; 1962.

29. Hauri P. Effects of Evening Activity on Subsequent Sleep and Dreams [dissertation]. Chicago, Ill: University of Chicago; 1967.

30. Bokert E. The effects of thirst and related verbal stimulus on dream reports. Dissertation Abstracts. 1968;28:4753B.

31. Foulkes D. Dreaming: a cognitive-psychological analysis. Hillsdale, NJ: Laurence Erlbaum Associates; 1985.

32. Vogel G. Sleep-onset mentation. In: Ellman SJ, Antrobus JS, eds. The Mind in Sleep. New York, NY: John Wiley & Sons; 1991:125–142.

33. Verdone P. Temporal reference of manifest dream content. Percept Mot Skills. 1965;20:262–271.

34. Roussy F, Raymond I, Gonthier I, et al. Temporal references in manifest dream content: confirmation of increased remoteness as the night progresses. Sleep. 1998; 21(suppl):285.

35. De Koninck J. Sleep, the common denominator for psychological adaptation. Can Psychol. 1997;38:191–195.

36. Lortie-Lussier M, Simond S, Rinfret N, et al. Beyond sex differences: family and occupational roles impact on women's and men's dreams. Sex Roles. 1992;26:79–96.

37. Winget C, Kramer M, Whitman RM. Dreams and demography. Can Psychiatry Assoc J. 1972;17:203–208.

38. Zepelin H. Age differences in dreams, II: distortion and other variables. Int J Aging Hum Dev. 1981;13:37–41.

39. Hall CS, Domhoff GW. Aggression in dreams. Int J Soc Psychiatry. 1963;9:259–267.

40. Foulkes D. Children's Dreams. New York, NY: John Wiley & Sons; 1982.

41. Côté L, Lortie-Lussier M, Roy M, et al. Continuity and change: the dreams of women throughout adulthood. Dreaming. 1996;6:187–199.

42. Winegar RK, Levin R. Sex differences in the object representations in the dreams of adolescents. Sex Roles. 1997;36:503–516.

43. Hall CS, Domhoff GW, Blick KA, et al. The dream of college men and women in 1950 and 1980: a comparison of dream content and sex differences. Sleep. 1982;5:188–194.

44. Lortie-Lussier M, Schwab C, De Koninck J. Working mothers versus homemakers: Do dreams reflect the changing roles of women? Sex Roles. 1985;12:1009–1021.

45. Hall C. The Meaning of Dreams. New York, NY: McGraw-Hill; 1953.

46. Rossi E. Dreams and the Growth of Personality. New York, NY: Pergamon Press; 1972.

47. Domhoff W. Finding Meaning in Dreams. New York, NY: Plenum; 1996.

48. Hartmann E. Boundaries of the Mind: A New Psychology of Personality. New York, NY: BasicBooks; 1991.

49. Busby K, De Koninck J. Short-term effects of strategies for self-regulation on personality dimensions and dream content. Percept Mot Skills. 1978;50:751–765.

50. Koulack D, Lebow MD, Church M. The effects of desensitization on the sleep and dreams of a phobic subject. Can J Behav Sci. 1976;8:418–421.

51. Kramer M, Roth T. Dreams in psychopathology. In: Wolman BB, ed. Handbook of Dreams. New York, NY: Van Nostrand Reinhold; 1979.

52. Wolman B. Dreams and schizophrenia. In: Wolman BB, ed. Handbook of Dreams. New York, NY: Van Nostrand Reinhold; 1979.

53. Weinstein LN, Schwartz DG, Arkin AM. Qualitative aspects of sleep mentation. In: Ellman SJ, Antrobus JS, eds. The Mind in Sleep. New York, NY: John Wiley & Sons; 1991:172–213.

54. Walker PC, Johnson RF. The influence of presleep suggestions on dream content: evidence and methodological problems. Psychol Bull. 1974;81:362–370.

55. De Koninck J, Brunette R. Presleep suggestion related to a phobic object: successful manipulation of reported dream affect. J Gen Psychol. 1991;185:185–200.

56. Halliday G. Direct psychological therapies for nightmares: a review. Clin Psychol Rev. 1987;7:501–523.

57. De St-Denis H. Les rêves et les moyens de les diriger. Paris, France: Tchou; 1964.

58. Gackenbach J, Laberge S. Conscious Mind, Sleeping Brain: Perspectives on Lucid Dreaming. New York, NY: Plenum; 1988:135–154.

59. Goodenough DR. Dream recall: history and current status of the field. In: Ellman SJ, Antrobus JS, eds. The Mind in Sleep. New York, NY: John Wiley & Sons; 1991:125–142.

60. Hartmann E, Elkin R, Garg M. Personality and dreaming: the dreams of people with very thick or very thin boundaries. Dreaming. 1991;1:311–324.

61. De Koninck J. Sources and consequences of dreams: experimental manipulations and their effects. In: Gachenbac J, Sheikh A, eds. Dream Images: A Call to Mental Arms. Farmingdale, NY: Baywood; 1991:17–30.

62. Blagrove M. Dreams as the reflection of our waking concerns and abilities: a critique of the problem-solving paradigm in dream research. Dreaming. 1993;2:205–220.

63. De Koninck JM, Koulack D. Dream content and adaptation to a stressful situation. J Abnorm Psychol. 1975;84:250–260.

64. Levitan H. Dreams which culminate in migraine headache. Psychother Psychosom. 1984;41:161–166.

65. Mahrer AR. Dream Work in Psychotherapy and Self-Change. New York, NY: WW Norton & Co; 1989.

66. Garfield P. Creative dreaming. New York, NY: Simon & Schuster; 1974.

67. Klinger E. The Structure and Function of Fantasy. New York, NY: John Wiley & Sons; 1978.

68. Braun AR, Balkin TJ, Wesensten NJ, et al. Dissociated pattern of activity in visual notices and their projections during human rapid eye movement sleep. Science. 1998;279:91–94.

42

Dreams and Psychopathology

Milton Kramer

There has long been the assumption that there was an intimate relationship between dreams and mental disorders. Epigrammatic statements, that "the madman is a waking dreamer,"[1(p90)] that "dreams [are] a brief madness and madness a long dream,"[2(p90)] that if we "let the dreamer walk about and act like a person awake. . . we [would] have the clinical picture of dementia praecox [schizophrenia]"[3(p86)] and that if "we could find out about dreams, we would find out about insanity,"[4(p45)] reflect the conviction about the close relationship between dreams and profound emotional disturbance. This view enlivened efforts to study dreaming to gain insights into the problems of the mentally ill.

Freud, in the literature review that introduces *The Interpretation of Dreams*,[5] has a section on "The Relations Between Dreams and Mental Diseases." Freud pointed out that when he

> speaks of the relationship of dreams to mental disorders [he] has three things in mind: 1) etiological and clinical connections, as when a dream represents a psychotic state, or introduces it, or is left over from it; 2) modifications to which dream-life is subject in cases of mental disease; and 3) intrinsic connections between dreams and psychosis, analogies pointing to their being essentially akin.[5(p88)]

The published work on dreams and psychopathologic state touches on all three areas of Freud's concern.[6] There are reports of psychotic states appearing to begin with a dream or a series of dreams, and there is certainly a literature which continues to pursue analogies between dreams and psychosis. However, the vast majority of the work that has been done on dreams and psychopathological states devotes itself to the "modifications to which dream life is subject in cases of mental disease" and will be the focus of this report. Freud was of the opinion that as we better understand dreams it will enhance our understanding of psychosis.

There is a potential confusion between a psychopathology of dreams and dreams in a psychopathological state. The former refers to alterations in the dreaming process which may be seen as abnormal. The latter refers to the dreams that are reported by a patient with a mental disorder. A dream that awakens the dreamer in a terrified state, generally with accompanying frightening dream content, a nightmare, would be a psychopathological dream.[7] A dream report from a patient suffering from schizophrenia would be a dream from a person in a psychopathological state. The dream may or may not be unique, either pathognomonically or statistically, to that state. Strangers occurring more frequently in the dreams of schizophrenic than in normal or depressed individuals is a statistical change in dream content in a psychopathological condition.[8]

A psychological examination of the dream is a study of the manifest content of the dream. Jones[9] pointed out that a psychology of dreams must rest on a study of the elements of which it is composed, the manifest dream images. Even Freud pointed out "that in some cases the facade of the dream directly reveals the dream's actual nucleus."[10] However, his almost exclusive focus on the latent dream content and his dismissal of the reported manifest dream retarded the study of dream reports. In 1966 Hall and Van de Castle presented quantitative methods to assess dream content and encouraged a scientific approach to the examination of the dream.

The study of the dream is an undertaking fraught with many difficulties. The dream experience cannot be directly observed and its study is still dependent on the dream report. The dream is experienced during one state, sleep; and reported during another state, wakefulness. The problems of examining verbal reports of inner experiences are compounded by the change in state necessary to obtain the dream report. The study of lucid dreaming[12] opens the possibility of examining the dream experience while it is occurring, but the work so far on lucid dreaming has been more directed at demonstrating its occurrence than utilizing it as a method for studying the dream experience.

The verbal nature of the dream report needs to be expressly addressed. Does the form of the dream obtained in the dream report reflect the dream as experienced or is it a result of the verbal style of the dreamer? An appropriate report of a waking experience becomes a necessary control if the study of the form of the dream is undertaken. For example, is a vague, disjointed report of an experience the same for a subject in describing a waking experience as in describing a dream experience? If it is, then the finding of vagueness or disjointedness cannot be considered a property of the dream experience, but rather an aspect of the dreamer's verbal style.

There are those who see the dream as an ineffable

experience whose essence is destroyed by scientific study, by quantification.[13] This survey is of quantitative reports. Quantification does not have to damage the essence of the dream experience; subtle qualities can be captured.

There are significant methodological issues which influence the content of dream reports. These issues relate to the collection and measurement of the dream report[14] and apply generally to dreams obtained either from nighttime awakenings or from morning reports. (Chapter 37 presents a more detailed discussion of these issues.)

Interest in the dream has been kept alive by the depth psychologists[15] and the man in the street,[16] whereas the scientific study of the dream was significantly stimulated by the discovery of rapid eye movement (REM) sleep.[17, 18] Awakenings from REM sleep permitted a large amount of the dream experience to be recovered relatively close to its time of occurrence. This opened the possibility for manipulative (experimental) studies of dreaming.

Ramsey[19] published in 1953 a review of studies of dreaming. These were all from the pre-REM literature. He cited some 121 articles and books of which 20 at most were of studies of the dreams of six patient groups. The amount of information available from 20 publications would be woefully inadequate to characterize the dreams of psychopathological groups, and appropriately Ramsey concluded that the research was scientifically inadequate. Very few of the studies were so designed and reported that they could be replicated to validate their findings. He found that the dream studies were weak in not (1) adequately describing the population under study, that is their gender, age, intelligence, health, economic status, and education; (2) limiting the group of subjects under study; (3) using control groups; (4) defining more adequately the characteristics of the dreams; (5) treating the data statistically; and (6) controlling for interviewer bias.

The literature dealing with the nature of the relationship between dreaming and mental illness has been reviewed on several occasions[20-24] with the last detailed review published in 1979.[23] The 1979 review focused on 75 reports in 71 articles in six patient groups: schizophrenia, disturbing dreams, depression, alcoholism, chronic brain syndrome, and mental retardation. The scientific adequacy of the publications covered in that review[23] was quite problematical, but a picture of dream content in some psychopathological states began to emerge.

Since that review, only one other review about dream content in psychiatric conditions has appeared.[25] It was of interest in that many of the dream content findings of the previous review[23] were supported and some additional groups were examined. Unfortunately, because only 35 articles covering nine diagnostic groups were cited, the scope of the review was limited. This chapter is an update of the 1979 review[23] and covers some 108 reports from 104 articles. A review of sleep physiology in psychiatric disorders also has been recently published.[26]

DREAM CONTENT IN PSYCHOPATHOLOGIC CONDITIONS

Frosch,[6] in 1976, wrote an evaluative review of "Psychoanalytic Contributions to the Relationship Between Dreams and Psychosis," which provided some partial answers to Freud's questions about the relationship. Frosch concluded

[1] . . . that although there are many apparent similarities between dreams and psychosis, they do differ in some basic respects; certainly insofar as the factors are concerned which play a role in their production [2] . . . that there is no consensus as to whether the manifest dream was of itself a meaningful guide to the presence of psychosis . . . [some] felt it was the latent content that was most telling [while others] seemed to feel that there might be features about the manifest form and content which could be of significance, indicating the presence of a psychosis. It [was] felt by some investigators that the patient's attitude toward the dream, difficulties in differentiating the dream from reality and the persistence of dream-like states invading the waking life may offer clues to the possibly psychotic nature of dreams [and 3] . . . [in regard] to whether there are dreams which presage psychosis, there was some suggestive evidence that this was the case.[6(pp61-62)]

Schizophrenia

The earlier review,[23] based on 30 articles, suggested that schizophrenic patients are less interested in their dreams and that their dreams are more primitive, that is, less complex; more direct; more sexual, anxious, and hostile; and show evidence of their thought disorder in being more bizarre and implausible. Hallucinations and dream content were relatable and the degrees of paranoia awake and in dreaming were similar, contrary to Freud's compensatory view of waking and dreaming in paranoia.[33] Strangers were their most frequent dream character.

The current literature review yielded only six articles on dream content in schizophrenic patients[27-32]—a surprisingly small number. The dreams of schizophrenic patients and their parents have been studied. Male schizophrenic patients in the hospital reported more social alienation and difficulties in adopting a conventional male role, while female schizophrenic patients showed more self-consciousness, envy of the activities of others, and hostility to those who tried to restrict them.[27] A subgroup of female schizophrenic patients reported they were forced to dream.[28] An adult patient, blind since age 3, described visual dreaming while hospitalized for her schizophrenia which was attributed to the regression that accompanied her hospitalization.[29] In the parents of schizophrenic patients, indices of a thought disorder in waking were inversely related to such markers in their dreams.[30]

Psychotherapy of schizophrenic patients showed a

wish fulfillment motive[31] and discussing dreams in a group decreased the insomnia of schizophrenic patients and increased their self-understanding.[32]

There were two reports on the dreams of schizophrenic patients not included in the 1979 review.[23] In a mixed diagnostic population including schizophrenic patients, it was found that increasing anxiety could increase or decrease dream reporting. With increasing anxiety, motion and affect were increased in the dream, whereas a decrease in anxiety in the dream was the first change seen with antipsychotic medication.[33] Dream recall was lower in lobotomized than nonlobotomized patients[34] and both were lower than what has been reported by others in comparable patients.[35]

The few additional articles on dreaming in schizophrenia contributed little to our knowledge of the dreams of these patients. The inattention to dreams in schizophrenia may be part of the shift from the psychological to the biological study of psychiatric disorders, and more particularly to the greater interest in mood disorders than in schizophrenia.[26]

Depression

The 1979 review[23] reported 14 articles related to the dream content of depression. In the current effort, an additional 17 studies, which were published in 15 articles (one article contained three studies),[36–50] were found.

The earlier review[23] provided considerable information about the dream content in depression. The depressed patient was found to dream as frequently as the nondepressed subject, but the dreams were shorter and had a paucity of traumatic or depressive content even after the depression had lifted. Family members were more frequent in their dreams. When hostility was present, it could be directed at or away from the dreamer while in schizophrenia it was directed at the dreamer. The depressed had in their dreams more friendly and fewer aggressive interactions than schizophrenic patients, but more failure and misfortune. With improvement, hostility decreased, while intimacy, motility, and heterosexuality increased.

In examining the dream reports of depressed patients published since 1975, a number of findings corroborate and extend those found in the pre-1975 review,[23] and some additional observations of interest are suggested. It is striking that depressed patients, both in and out of the laboratory, show a decrease in the number of dreams reported,[36, 40] a decrease in recall that correlates with the severity of the depression,[41] and a decrease in the length of the dream report.[38, 39, 42] Shorter laboratory-collected dreams continue even into the remitted state.[43] In a laboratory study in which dreams were collected from men with a major depressive disorder (MDD) no decrease in recall frequency or dream length was noted,[44] whereas in a large series of depressed outpatients treated with an antidepressant medication, a decrease in dream recall frequency was reported in association with improvement in the depression.[40]

How might the apparent contradictions to the observation that dream reporting and dream length decrease in depression be resolved? The continuation of shorter dream reports into the remitted state may reflect that these particular patients were relatively nonverbal compared to control subjects. The male veteran patients with MDD who report no decrease in laboratory dream report frequency or length compared to male controls suggest that there may be a gender difference in verbal reporting, as many of the studies of recall and report length that found decreases include women patients. Verbal reporting may be more emotionally sensitive for women. The observation of decreased report frequency covarying with effective medicinal antidepressant treatment may be the result of the effect of the medication on the recall process.

It was noteworthy that the dreams of unipolar depressed inpatients were described as mundane[45] and the laboratory dreams of hospitalized depressed patients as trivial.[40] Yet, some interesting observations about the content and affects of the dreams of depressed patients have been made. In hospitalized depressed suicide attempters, an increased incidence of death themes was found.[39] Bipolar patients, before their shift to mania, report bizarre dreams with death and injury themes.[36, 45] The shift to mania and happy dreams, it has been suggested, may be a way to avoid painful memories.[46] In a case report[47] some support for increased family role characters in the dreams of depressed patients was found, and in a study of depressed women fewer strangers were reported.[38] However, no increase in family characters was reported until the depression lifted in divorced women,[42] and in another study, no increase in family roles was reported.[40] The association of an increase in family role characters in the dreams of depressed patients is only partially supported by the current data. Beck[51] suggested that an increase in masochism in dreams is a trait characteristic of the depressed patient. This was confirmed in studies of divorced women where it was noted that masochism in their dreams was associated with poor treatment outcome,[48] especially in those women who showed an increase in masochism across the night.[49] An increase in masochism was also noted in remitted depressive patients.[43] In three studies[36, 40, 44] no increase in masochism was found in the dream reports of depressed patients. These latter studies had many, if not all, male patients as subjects.

There has been the interesting suggestion by Hauri[43] that the dreams of the depressed patient are focused on the past, a finding confirmed by Cartwright et al.[42] who pointed out that the past focus diminished with improvement in women suffering from depression. However, Greenberg et al.[37] indicated that in their patients the dreams were both past- and present-focused. Dow et al.[44] showed in comparing post-traumatic stress disorder (PTSD) patients with MDD with those with only MDD that the PTSD patients were the ones with the past focus in their dreams.

In the few studies that have looked at affect in the dreams of depressed patients, not much has been found.[38, 43–45, 49] There is more anxiety in the dreams of stably married women than in depressed divorcees,[50] and there is more anxiety in patients with PTSD than in those with an MDD, but neither have much anxiety.[44] In comparing two depressed patient groups, it was found that the dreams of bipolar patients have more anxiety than those of unipolar patients.[45] Depressed college-age women have less hostility in their dreams than nondepressed subjects[38] and remitted depressive patients have more anger than controls.[43]

The content of the dreams of the depressed patient may have some prognostic implications. Poorly organized dreams without people or the dreamer correlate with a poor treatment response.[37] High masochism scores in dreams of depressed women covary with a decreased likelihood of improvement.[48] In depressed divorcees, an increase in masochism across the night is a poor prognostic sign.[49] Masochism in women may be a marker of the vulnerability to depression,[48] although the data are also open to the interpretation that it is a marker for a greater difficulty in recovering from depression. Depressed divorcees who incorporate the loss in their dreams have more intense dreams and better outcomes.[50]

In summary, in depression there is a decrease in the frequency and length of dream reports. The dreams are commonplace, but have content characteristics of interest. There is an increase in death themes in depressed suicidal patients and in bipolar patients before becoming manic. The presence of an increase in family roles in the dreams of depressed patients may be the case. Masochism in the dreams of depressed patients appears more clearly in women than men and is more likely a trait than a state characteristic. It is evident that a past focus was not universal in depression, nor indeed was it unique to the depressed state. Affects such as anxiety and hostility in depression are not prominent in their dreams.[52] Dream content may have prognostic significance for the response of the depressed patient to treatment.

A most striking implication of these findings about dreaming in depressed patients is that the affective state of the dreamer covaries with the content of the dream and that changes in dreams across the night may contribute to the dreamer's coping capacity, as was proposed in "The Selective Mood Regulatory Function of Dreaming."[53] Changes in dream content across the night alter the affective condition of the dreamer and contribute to the adaptive state of the dreamer the next day.

Post-Traumatic Stress Disorder

A great interest has developed in PTSD since the previous review in 1979.[23] PTSD was only included in the official nomenclature of the American Psychiatric Association in 1980, although it had been described in the psychiatric literature for more than 100 years.[54]

This chapter, rather than dealing with anxiety dreams and nightmares, as was done previously, focuses on dreams in PTSD. Sixty-three studies from 61 articles dating back to 1966 were considered germane to the dreams of patients with this disorder.[44, 55–114]

A general population survey[55] in 1987 described a 1% prevalence of a history of PTSD, a 3.5% prevalence in the civilian population if they have experienced a physical attack or were Vietnam veterans, and a 20% prevalence if they were wounded in Vietnam. Behavioral problems before age 15 years predicted adult exposure to a physical attack or combat wounding. A full PTSD syndrome was common only among veterans. Symptoms of PTSD in the overall population were generally limited to nightmares, trouble sleeping, and jumpiness.

In two studies of civilian populations[56, 57] that were dealing with acute traumas, either the loss of a loved one or the response to a building collapse, disturbed dreaming occurred frequently, but the daytime return of strong feelings[56] and recollections of the event[57] were much more common. The nature of the trauma, civilian or military, and the time since the trauma was experienced affected the frequency and perhaps the nature of the dream experience.

Based on the mentation difference between REM and nonrapid eye movement (NREM) sleep, Ross et al.[58] argued that a sleep disturbance is the hallmark of PTSD. They characterized the dreams of PTSD patients as vivid, affect-laden, disturbing, outside the realm of current waking experience (although representative of an earlier life experience), and easy to recall. They believe that the dream disturbance is relatively specific to the disorder[58] and that PTSD may fundamentally be a disorder of REM sleep mechanisms. However, as the REM nightmare in these subjects occurs early in the night, when there is less REM, and is associated with gross body movements, abnormal NREM sleep mechanisms may be involved as well. Ross et al.[58] speculated that the neural circuitry involved in PTSD may be similar to that in accentuated startle behavior. These authors took exception[59] to Reynold's suggestion,[60] that the dream in PTSD is the same that occurs in traumatized depressive patients, and pointed out that traumatized depressive dreams are not dream-like and do not incorporate the trauma.[42] Ross et al.[58] saw the dream in PTSD as repetitive and more importantly stereotyped.

Kramer[61] proposed that the disturbing dream is more the hallmark of PTSD than the sleep disturbance. Green et al.,[62] in a discussion of diagnostic criteria for PTSD, suggested that the unique aspect of PTSD is indeed the intrusive symptoms, including intrusive images and recurrent dreams and nightmares. They pointed out that not all dreams are direct recapitulations of the trauma. For these authors, intrusive images may be the hallmark of PTSD.

The view of Green et al.[62] is based on the suggestion by Brett and Ostroff[63] who, in a review of theories of PTSD, pointed out that there has been a neglect of post-traumatic imagery, which, they postulate, along with defensive responses to the imagery, is the core of PTSD. They lament a lack of research into the range, content and patterning of the imagery.

Interestingly, Fisher et al.,[64] in an early physiological study of nightmares and night terrors, pointed out that trauma sufferers may have disturbing arousals that can come out of both REM and NREM (stage 4 and stage 2) sleep. This is a view Schlosburg and Benjamin[65] and Kramer, Schoen, and Kinney[66, 67] confirmed. The question remains, does the sleep disturbance in PTSD involve more than REM sleep mechanisms and is the imagery (dreams) reported by PTSD patients (1) stereotyped and (2) REM-bound, as Ross et al.[58] postulated? It is apparent that although the dream report in PTSD is in some cases a re-creation of the traumatic event,[68–72] in many patients this is not the case.[67–69, 73–84] Stereotypy in content is not the hallmark of the dream in PTSD.

There has been repeated observations that the disturbing dream in PTSD tends to occur early rather than late in the night.[67, 70, 78, 85, 86] This timing observation raised questions about the disturbing dream being linked to REM sleep, most of which occurs in the second half of the night. Those studies that have examined the stage of sleep out of which these dreams are reported point out that the disturbing dream is not stage-bound, but may emerge out of REM or NREM sleep.[61, 65–67, 70, 87–89] Interestingly, the disturbing dream is as likely to occur out of REM as out of NREM sleep.[67]

There are several symptoms, such as increased awakenings,[55, 80, 83, 87, 90–92] increased motoric activity,[70, 80, 85, 88, 93] and increased sweating,[89, 94, 95] which are frequent accompaniments of the disturbing dream experience. These symptoms tend to occur early during the night's sleep. In addition, an elevated arousal threshold[96, 97] and increased startle response[98] both occur early in the night. The fundamental alteration in sleep in PTSD may occur in NREM sleep early in the night.

The affective tone of the dream in PTSD has been assumed to be highly disturbing. This view of the terrifying nature of disturbing dreams has not been well supported. Taub et al.[99] pointed out that the experience of the nightmare was less intense than what subjects thought a nightmare was like. Fisher et al.[89] noted that REM nightmares were less intense than night terrors. The affective disturbance in disturbed dreams may be a response to the dream experience rather than intrinsic to the dream itself.[66] Dow et al.[44] found anxiety levels low in the dreams of PTSD patients but higher than in controls. However, Brockway[72] described intense affect in PTSD dreams which diminished with structured group therapy, and Lavie and Kaminer[100] reported an increase in anxiety and hostility in the dreams of poorly adjusted Holocaust survivors.

There has been an effort to describe different types of nightmares that are said to occur in PTSD. A distinction has been made between reenactments of the trauma that are thought to be meaningless and those nightmares that contain other elements and which have meaning associated with them.[68] A contrast was made between dream disturbances associated with extreme terror but without content, related perhaps to the Isakower phenomenon or Lewin's blank dreams and reflecting Piaget's prerepresentational stage, and dream content that goes from pleasant to unpleasant and is related to Piaget's representational stage.[101] These suggest the difference between night terrors and nightmares.[67] Siegel[102] described Holocaust survivors having "miracle dreams" in which a dead relative told them not to give up while in the death camp and which helped sustain them. Siegel[102] also described a traumatic dream in which the dreamer changed from victim to victimizer that covaried with improved waking adaptation. Terr,[81] in describing the post-traumatic nightmares of children, categorized them as dreams that were (1) just of terror, (2) an exact replay of the event, (3) a modified playback of the event, and (4) a disguised nightmare of the event. In a study of disturbed dreamers, it was noted that the content of dreams did not differ between the dream-disturbed and the control group.[66]

Dow et al.[44] suggested that the laboratory collected dreams of PTSD-MDD sufferers were past-focused in contrast to patients with only MDD and controls. Lavie and Kaminer[100] made a similar observation, that in their poorly adjusted Holocaust survivors there was a past focus. In depressed patients, Greenberg et al.[37] noted some patients did and some did not focus on the past in their dreams. Cartwright[50] found that the past focus in the dreams of her depressed divorcing women subjects[42] diminished as the depression lifted, whereas Hauri[43] reported a focus on the past in his remitted depressed patients. A past focus is not unique to any one diagnostic group, does not occur in all patients of that group, and it is not clear, when it does occur, whether it is a state or trait characteristic.

There is an extensive literature[78, 79, 90, 103–108] describing the continuation or reactivation of disturbing dreams 3 to 4 decades after the traumatic event. There is an equally extensive literature linking the current trauma to earlier childhood traumas.[55, 69, 73, 75, 81, 82, 101, 108–111] True et al.[112] pointed out a genetic influence on liability for the reexperiencing symptoms such as disturbing dreams in PTSD. The relationship of the disturbing dream to the life history of the patient remains to be described, although Titchener and Kapp[82] attempted such a formulation in reporting the transformations of the disturbing dream in the survivors of the Buffalo Creek disaster.

Dream recall rates appear to be lowered in PTSD.[66, 67, 83, 88, 100] Patients in a military outpatient clinic reported no difference in nightmare frequency between Vietnam veterans and nonveterans.[113] Dow et al.,[44] in contrast, reported a high rate of recall in a laboratory study of PTSD. Interestingly, when the control groups are better-adjusted former trauma victims, the dream recall rates are even lower[67, 100] than those of active PTSD patients. Military content has been reported higher in the patients' dreams in one study of PTSD,[67] and lower in another.[83] It has been suggested that low dream recall rates in PTSD sufferers are related to efforts to deal with memories of the trauma.[66, 67, 100] What has been particularly striking is that those who have more effectively coped with the trauma have the lowest dream recall rate. Avoidance of dream recall may be an adaptational strategy in PTSD.

The hallmark of PTSD is a disturbance in the psychological aspects of dreaming and possibly of NREM sleep early in the night, but not particularly of REM sleep. Neylan et al.[114] reported that combat experience covaries with dream disturbance to a much greater degree than do difficulties in falling or staying asleep, and that disturbed dreaming occurs only in Vietnam veterans who have PTSD.

An adequate characterization of the phenomenology of the disturbing dream remains to be done. It can be confirmed that the dream is disturbing and that the dream events may be outside the realm of current waking experience. The literature does not support the position that the dream is affect-laden or that the dream is easy to recall. It is not known if the disturbing dream is any more or less vivid then other dreams, although one study found no difference between normals and poorly adjusted and well-adjusted Holocaust survivors[100] in this regard.

Eating Disorders

I found 11 citations to articles or chapters about dreaming associated with eating disorders, providing an initial picture of the dreams of this group of patients. Patients who have eating disorders do not fit the model of alexithymia with its alleged impaired capacity for fantasy and dreaming. They report dreams and are able to use their dreams in treatment.[115, 116] However, it is not clear whether dream recall is normal[117, 118] or decreased[119] in this patient group.

Anorexic patients revealed in their dreams a fear of getting fat, and later in therapy when dreams of being fat appeared they seemed to represent the dreamer as pregnant and vomiting as a delivery.[120] The loss of self in reunion with mother was revealed in the dreams of an anorexic patient in analysis,[121] and death themes were found in the dreams of both anorexic and bulimic patients.[122, 123] The content of the dreams of patients with eating disorders does reflect a preoccupation with food and oral activities.[117–119, 124] Bulimic patients have more hostility in their psychodynamics and in their dreams,[118, 125] whereas anorexic patients have less hostility.[117] Both may have less hostility then normals. Anorexic patients seem more anxious in their dreams[119, 124] than comparison groups.

Alcoholism

In the five articles on dreams of alcoholic patients that were the basis for the pre-1975 review,[23] it was found that these patients have more oral references in their dreams, are more often the object of aggression, and have fewer sexual interactions than nonalcoholic subjects. Interestingly, detoxifying alcoholic patients who dream about drinking maintain sobriety longer.

Five studies dealing with the dreams of alcoholic patients have been published since 1975. It was found that alcoholic patients suffer from nightly nightmares[126, 127] more than controls. In detoxifying alcoholic patients "high cravers" dream more about drinking than "low cravers."[128] In a group of patients detoxifying from drugs of abuse, including alcohol, dreaming about the drug was associated with an increase in the likelihood of a return to drug use.[129] Denizen[130] reported that among Alcoholic Anonymous members who were abstinent, dreaming about drinking was frightening, experienced as a warning, and seemed to reinforce the commitment to abstinence. It is not clear whether dreaming about drinking is a predictor of abstinence or relapse. However, the possibility of dreaming having adaptive significance for these patients is raised by these observations.

Organic Brain Disease

It had been previously reported[23] that there is a decrease in dream reporting associated with increasing age and dementia. In a series of studies[131–133] Sterne and others reported that dreams can be effectively used in psychotherapy with the head-injured who report an increase in threatening dreams, a decrease in sexual dreams, and no change in dream report frequency. No relationship between report frequency and computed tomography–defined brain atrophy was found.[134] Repetitive visual images awake and from sleep awakenings were observed in cases of missile head injury.[135]

Mentally Retarded

In an earlier review of dreams in mentally retarded patients,[23] only four studies were found. Mentally retarded patients dream of home, have simple dreams, and the content of the dreams and Thematic Apperception Test stories are similar. Males who are mentally retarded have more aggressive dreams and dream more about other males, sports, eating, and family members. Females have more color in their dreams and dream more about falling and being chased.

Only two new studies[136, 137] of dreaming in such patients were found in my review that provide limited additional knowledge of the dream life of mentally retarded individuals. One report[136] was of patients in a sheltered workshop, 10% of whose dreams were of deceased loved ones, mostly parents. Most of these dreams were thematically negative. In the second study[137] it was shown that one can use dreams in therapy with these patients.

CONCLUSION

It is apparent that the mysteries of psychosis have not been revealed through the study of dreams. The paucity of studies in some conditions and the relative lack of scientific rigor continue to plague the study of dreaming in psychiatric conditions. However, in some areas, such as depression and PTSD, we do know more about dreaming then we did. The most intriguing insight that emerges from this review is that what one does or does not dream about may be contributing to the waking adaptational process for the dreamer.[49, 53, 67, 10, 128, 129, 138]

Acknowledgments

Without the effective dedicated assistance of Mike Douglas, Valerie Ratchford, and Linda Kittrell, the library staff at Bethesda Oak Hospital, Cincinnati, Ohio, this review could not have been undertaken.

References

1. Kant I, quoted by Freud S. The Interpretation of Dreams. Vols 4 and 5. Standard Edition. London, England: Hogarth Press; 1953:90.
2. Schopenhauer A, quoted by Freud S. The Interpretation of Dreams. Vols 4 and 5. Standard Edition. London, England: Hogarth Press; 1953:90.
3. Jung C. The Psychology of Dementia Praecox. Princeton, NJ: Princeton University Press; 1960:86.
4. Jackson J. In: Taylor J, ed. Selected Writings of John Hughlings Jackson. Vol 2. New York, NY: BasicBooks; 1958:45.
5. Freud S. The Interpretation of Dreams. Vols 4 and 5. Standard Edition. London, England: Hogarth Press; 1953.
6. Frosch J. Psychoanalytic contributions to the relationship between dreams and psychosis—a critical survey. Int J Psychoanal. 1976;5:39–63.
7. Hartmann E. The Nightmare: The Psychology and Biology of Terrifying Dreams. London, England: Harper & Row; 1981.
8. Kramer M, Baldridge B, Whitman R, et al. An exploration of the manifest dream in schizophrenia and depressed patients. Dis Nerv Syst. 1969;30:126–130.
9. Jones R. Dream interpretation and the psychology of dreaming. J Am Psychoanal Assoc. 1965;13:304–319.
10. Freud S. On Dreams. Vol 5. Standard Edition. London, England: Hogarth Press; 1958:667.
11. Hall C, Van de Castle R. The Content Analysis of Dreams. New York, NY: Appleton; 1966.
12. LaBerge S, Rheingold H. Exploring the World of Lucid Dreaming. New York, NY: Ballantine; 1990.
13. Boss M. The Analysis of Dreams. New York, NY: Philosophical Library; 1968.
14. Kramer M, Winget C, Roth T. Problems in the definition of the REM dream. In: Levine E, Koella WP, eds. Sleep 1974: Instinct Neurophysiology, Endocrinology, Episodes, Dreams, Epilepsy and Intracranial Pathology: Proceedings of the Second European Congress of Sleep Research, Rome, Italy, April 8–11, 1974. New York, NY: Karger; 1975:149–161.
15. Kramer M, ed. Dream Psychology and the New Biology of Dreaming. Springfield Ill: Charles C Thomas; 1969.
16. Weiss H. Oneirocritica americana. Bull N Y Public Library. 1969;48:519–541.
17. Aserinsky E, Kleitman N. Regularly occurring periods of eye motility and concomitant phenomena during sleep. Science. 1953;118:273–274.
18. Aserinsky E, Kleitman N. Two types of ocular motility in sleep. J Appl Physiol. 1955;8:1–10.
19. Ramsey G. Studies of dreaming. Psychol Bull. 1953;50:432–455.
20. Kramer M. Manifest dream content in psychopathological states. In: Kramer M, ed. Dream Psychology and the New Biology of Dreaming. Springfield, Ill: Charles C Thomas; 1969:377–396.
21. Kramer M. Manifest dream content in normal and psychopathological states. Arch Gen Psychiatry. 1970;22:149–159.
22. Kramer M, Roth T. Dreams in psychopathologic groups: a critical review. In: Williams R, Karacan I, eds. Sleep Disorders: Diagnosis and Treatment. New York, NY: John Wiley & Sons; 1978:323–349.
23. Kramer M, Roth T. Dreams in psychopathology. In: Wolman B, ed. Handbook of Dreams: Research, Theories and Applications. New York, NY: Van Nostrand Reinhold; 1979:361–387.
24. Kramer M. Dream content in psychiatric conditions: an overview of sleep laboratory studies. In: Perris C, Struwe G, Jansson B, eds. Biological Psychiatry 1981. New York, NY: Elsevier/ North Holland Biomedical Press; 1981:306–309.
25. Mellen R, Duffey T, Craig S. Manifest content in the dreams of clinical populations. J Ment Health Counseling. 1993;15:170–183.
26. Benca R. Sleep in psychiatric disorders. Neurol Clin. 1996;14:739–764.
27. Van de Castle R. Manifest content of schizophrenic dreams. Sleep Res. 1974;3:126.
28. Ohira K, Kato N, Namura I, et al. A psychopathology of schizophrenic dreaming: a feeling of passivity [abstract]. Sleep Res. 1979;8:170.
29. Deutsch H. A case that throws light on the mechanism of regression in schizophrenia. Psychoanal Rev. 1985;72:1–8.
30. Meloy J. Thought organization and primary process in the parents of schizophrenics. Br J Med Psychol. 1984;57:279–281.
31. Ushijima S. On recovery from the post psychotic collapse in schizophrenia. Jpn J Psychiatry Neurol. 1988;42:199–207.
32. Wilmer H. Dream seminar for chronic schizophrenic patients. Psychiatry. 1982;45:351–360.
33. Lesse S. Psychiatric symptoms in relationship to the intensity of anxiety. Psychother Psychosom. 1974;23:94–102.
34. Jus A, Jus K, Villeneuve A, et al. Studies on dream recall in chronic schizophrenic patients after prefrontal lobotomy. Biol Psychiatry. 1973;6:275–293.
35. Solms M. The Neuropsychology of Dreams: A Clinico-Anatomical Study. Mahwah, NJ: Lawrence Erlbaum; 1997.
36. Beauchemin K, Hays P. Prevailing mood, mood changes and dreams in bipolar disorder. J Affect Disord. 1995;35:41–49.
37. Greenberg R, Pearlman C, Blacher R, et al. Depression: variability of intrapsychic and sleep parameters. J Am Acad Psychoanal. 1990;18:233–246.
38. Barrett D, Loeffler M. Comparison of dream content of depressed versus nondepressed dreamers. Psychol Rep. 1992;70:403–406.
39. Firth S, Blouin J, Natarajan C, et al. A comparison of the manifest content in dreams of suicidal, depressed and violent patients. Can J Psychiatry. 1986;31:48–53.
40. Riemann D, Low H, Schredl M, et al. Investigations of morning and laboratory dream recall and content in depressive patients during baseline conditions and under antidepressive treatment with trimipramine. Psychiatr J Univ Ottawa. 1990;15:93–99.
41. Mathew R, Largen J, Claghorn J. Biological symptoms of depression. Psychosom Med. 1979;41:439–443.
42. Cartwright R, Lloyd S, Knight S, et al. Broken dreams: a study of the effects of divorce and depression on dream content. Psychiatry. 1984;47:251–259.
43. Hauri P. Dreams in patients remitted from reactive depression. J Abnorm Psychol. 1976;85:1–10.
44. Dow B, Kelsoe J, Gillen J. Sleep and dreams in Vietnam PTSD and depression. Biol Psychiatry. 1996;39:42–50.
45. Beauchemin K, Hays P. Dreaming away depression: the role of REM sleep and dreaming in affective disorders. J Affect Disord. 1996;41:125–133.
46. Levitan H. The relationship between mania and the memory of pain: a hypothesis. Bull Menninger Clin. 1977;41:145–161.
47. Brenman E. Separation: a clinical problem. Int J Psychoanal. 1982;63:303–310.
48. Cartwright R, Wood E. The contribution of dream masochism to the sex ratio difference in major depression. Psychiatr Res. 1993;46:165–173.
49. Trenholme I, Cartwright R, Greenberg G. Dream dimension differences during a life change. Psychiatr Res. 1984;12:35–45.
50. Cartwright R. Dreams that work: the relation of dream incorporation to adaptation to stressful events. Dreaming. 1991;1:3–9.
51. Beck A. Depression: Clinical, Experimental and Theoretical Aspects. New York, NY: Harper & Row; 1967.
52. Strauch I, Meier B. In Search of Dreams: Results of Experimental Dream Research. Albany, NY: State University of New York Press; 1993:234.
53. Kramer M. The selective mood regulatory function of dreaming: an update and revision. In: Moffitt A, Kramer M, Hoffmann R, eds. The Functions of Dreaming. Albany, NY: State University of New York Press; 1993:139–195.
54. Erichson O. On Concussion of the Spine. New York, NY: Bermingham; 1882; cited by: Modlin H. Is there an assault syndrome? Bull Am Acad Psychiatry Law. 1985;13:139–145.

55. Helzer J, Robins L, McEvoy M. Post traumatic stress disorder in the general population: findings of the epidemiologic catchment area survey. N Engl J Med. 1987;317:1630–1634.

56. Horowitz M, Wilner N, Kaltreider N, et al. Signs and symptoms of post traumatic stress disorder. Arch Gen Psychiatry. 1980;37:85–92.

57. Wilkinson C. Aftermath of a disaster: the collapse of the Hyatt Regency hotel skywalks. Am J Psychiatry. 1983;140:1134–1139.

58. Ross R, Ball W, Sullivan K, et al. Sleep disturbance as the hallmark of post traumatic stress disorder. Am J Psychiatry. 1989;146:697–707.

59. Ross R, Ball W, Sullivan K, et al. Sleep disturbance in post traumatic stress disorder [letter]. Am J Psychiatry. 1990;147:374.

60. Reynold C. Sleep disturbance in post traumatic stress disorder: pathogenetic or epiphenomenal? [editorial]. Am J Psychiatry. 1989;146:695–696.

61. Kramer M. Dream disturbances. Psychiatr Ann. 1979;9:366–376.

62. Green B, Lindy J, Grace M. Post traumatic stress disorder: toward DSM IV. J Nerv Ment Dis. 1985;173:406–411.

63. Brett E, Ostroff R. Imagery and post traumatic stress disorder: an overview. Am J Psychiatry. 1985;142:417–424.

64. Fisher C, Kahn E, Edwards A, et al. A physiological study of nightmares and night terrors. J Nerv Ment Dis. 1973;157:275–298.

65. Schlosberg A, Benjamin M. Sleep patterns in three acute combat fatigue cases. J Clin Psychiatry. 1978;39:546–549.

66. Kramer M, Kinney L. Sleep patterns in trauma victims with disturbed dreaming. Psychiatr J Univ Ottawa. 1988;13:12–16.

67. Kramer M, Schoen L, Kinney L. The dream experience in dream-disturbed Vietnam veterans. In: van der Kolk B, ed. Post Traumatic Stress Disorders: Psychological and Biologic Sequelae. Washington, DC: American Psychiatric Press; 1984:81–95.

68. Schreuder J. Post traumatic re-experiencing in older people: working through or covering up? Am J Psychother. 1996;50:231–242.

69. Kramer M, Schoen L, Kinney L. Nightmares in Vietnam veterans. J Am Acad Psychoanal. 1987;15:67–81.

70. van der Kolk B, Blitz R, Burr W, et al. Nightmares and trauma: a comparison of nightmares after combat with lifelong nightmares in veterans. Am J Psychiatry. 1984;141:187–190.

71. Ross R, Ball W, Dinges D, et al. Rapid eye movement sleep disturbance in post traumatic stress disorder. Biol Psychiatry. 1994;35:195–202.

72. Brockway, S. Group treatment of combat nightmares in post-traumatic stress disorder. J Contemp Psychother. 1987;17:270–284.

73. Lansky M. Nightmares of a hospitalized rape victim. Bull Menninger Clin. 1995;59:4–14.

74. Straker G. Integrating African and Western healing practices in South Africa. Am J Psychother. 1994;48:455–467.

75. Lansky M. The transformation of affect in post traumatic nightmares. Bull Menninger Clin. 1991;55:470–490.

76. Silvan-Adams A, Silvan M. "A dream is the fulfillment of a wish": traumatic dream, repetition compulsion and the pleasure principle. Int J Psychoanal. 1990;71:513–522.

77. Modlin H. Is there an assault syndrome? Bull Am Acad Psychiatry Law 1985;13:139–145.

78. Van Dyke C, Zilberg N, McKinnon J. Post traumatic stress disorder: a thirty year delay in a World War II veteran. Am J Psychiatry. 1985;142:1070–1073.

79. Wells B, Chu C, Johnson R, et al. Buspirone in the treatment of post traumatic stress disorder. Pharmacotherapy. 1991;11:340–343.

80. Melman T, Kulick-Bell R, Ashlock L, et al. Sleep events among veterans with combat-related post traumatic stress disorder. Am J Psychiatry. 1995;152:110–115.

81. Terr L. Children of Chowchilla. In: The Psychoanalytic Study of the Child. Vol 34. New Haven, Conn: Yale University Press; 1979;547–623.

82. Titchener J, Kapp F. Family and character change at Buffalo Creek. Am J Psychiatry. 1976;133:295–299.

83. Dagan Y, Lavie P. Subjective and objective characteristics of sleep and dreaming in war related PTSD patients: lack of relationships [abstract]. Sleep Res. 1991;20A:270.

84. Kellett S, Beail N. The treatment of chronic post-traumatic nightmares using psychodynamic-interpersonal psychotherapy: a single case study. Br J Med Psychol. 1997;70:35–49.

85. Burstein A. Dream disturbance and flashbacks [letter]. J Clin Psychiatry. 1984;45:46.

86. Woodward S, Arsenault E, Bliwise D, et al. The temporal distribution of combat nightmares in vietnam combat veterans [abstract]. Sleep Res. 1991;20:152.

87. Kinzie J, Sack R, Riley C. The polysomnographic effects of clonidine on sleep disorders in post traumatic stress disorder: a pilot study with Cambodian patients. J Nerv Ment Dis. 1994;182:585–587.

88. Hefez A, Metz L, Lavie P. Long-term effects of extreme situational stress on sleep and dreaming. Am J Psychiatry. 1987;144:344–347.

89. Fisher C, Bryne J, Edwards A, et al. A physiological study of nightmares. J Am Psychoanal Assoc. 1970;18:747–782.

90. Mollica R, Wyshak G, Lavelle J. The psychosocial impact of war trauma and torture on Southeast Asian refugees. Am J Psychiatry. 1987;144:1567–1572.

91. Kramer M, Schoen L, Kinney L. Psychological and behavioral features of disturbed dreamers. Psychiatr J Univ Ottawa. 1984;9:102–106.

92. Schoen L, Kramer M, Kinney L. Arousal patterns in non-REM dream disturbed veterans [abstract]. Sleep Res. 1983;12:315.

93. Lavie P, Hertz G. Increased sleep motility and respiration rates in combat neurotic patients. Biol Psychiatry. 1979;14:983–987.

94. Woodward S, Arsenault E, Bliwise D, et al. Physical symptoms accompanying dream reports in combat veterans [abstract]. Sleep Res. 1991;20:153.

95. Wilmer H. The healing nightmare: war dreams of Vietnam veterans. In: Barrett D, ed. Trauma and Dreams. Cambridge, Mass: Harvard University Press; 1996:92.

96. Schoen L, Kramer M, Kinney L. Auditory thresholds in the dream disturbed [abstract]. Sleep Res. 1984;13:102.

97. Dagan Y, Lavie P, Bleich A. Elevated awakening threshold in sleep stage 3–4 in war-related post-traumatic stress disorder. Biol Psychiatry. 1991;30:618–622.

98. Kinney L, Schoen L, Kramer M. Responsivity of night terror patients in sleep [abstract]. Sleep Res. 1983;12:193.

99. Taub J, Kramer M, Arand D, et al. Nightmare dreams and nightmare confabulations. Compr Psychiatry. 1978;19:285–291.

100. Lavie P, Kaminer H. Dreams that poison sleep: dreaming in Holocaust survivors. Dreaming. 1991;1:11–21.

101. Dowling S. Dreams and dreaming in relation to trauma in childhood. Int J Psychoanal. 1983;63:157–166.

102. Siegel L. Holocaust survivors in Hasidic and ultra-Orthodox Jewish populations. J Contemp Psychother. 1980;11:5–31.

103. Watson I. Post traumatic stress disorder in Australian prisoners of the Japanese: a clinical study. Aust N Z J Psychiatry. 1993;27:20–29.

104. Kuch K, Cox B. Symptoms of PTSD in 124 survivors of the Holocaust. Am J Psychiatry. 1992;149:337–340.

105. Goldstein G, Van Kammen W, Shelly C, et al. Survivors of imprisonment in the Pacific theater during World War II. Am J Psychiatry. 1987;144:1210–1213.

106. Defazio V, Rustin S, Diamond A. Symptom development in Vietnam era veterans. Am J Orthopsychiatry. 1975;45:158–163.

107. Archibald H, Long D, Miller C, et al. Gross stress reaction in combat: a 15 year followup. Am J Psychiatry. 1962;119:317–322.

108. Terr L. Chowchilla revisited: the effects of psychic trauma four years after a school-bus kidnapping. Am J Psychiatry. 1983;140:1543–1550.

109. De Saussure J. Dreams and dreaming in relation to trauma in childhood. Int J Psychoanal. 1982;63:167–175.

110. Puk G. Treating traumatic memories: a case report on the eye movement desensitization procedure. J Behav Ther Exp Psychiatry. 1991;22:149–151.

111. Terr L. Life attitudes, dreams and psychic trauma in a group of "normal" children. J Am Acad Child Psychiatry. 1983;22:221–230.

112. True W, Rice J, Eisen S, et al. A twin study of genetic and environmental contributions to liability for post-traumatic stress symptoms. Arch Gen Psychiatry. 1993;50:257–264.

113. Deekin M, Bridenbaugh R. Depression and nightmares among

Vietnam veterans in a military psychiatry outpatient clinic. Mil Med. 1987;152:590–591.

114. Neylan T, Marmar C, Metzler M, et al. Sleep disturbances in the Vietnam generation: findings from a nationally representative sample of male Vietnam veterans. Am J Psychiatry. 1998;155:929–933.

115. Wilson C. Dream interpretation. In: Wilson C, ed. Fear of Being Fat: The Treatment of Anorexia Nervosa and Bulimia. New York, NY: Jason Aronson; 1983:245–254.

116. Wells L. Anorexia nervosa: an illness of young adults. Psychiatr Q. 1980;52:270–282.

117. Hudson J, Bruch H, DeTrinis J, et al. Content analysis of dreams of anorexia nervosa patients [abstract]. Sleep Res. 1978;7:176.

118. Dippel B, Lauer C, Riemann D, et al. Sleep and dreams in eating disorders. Psychother Psychosom. 1987;48:165–169.

119. Frayn D. The incidence and significance of perceptual qualities in the reported dreams of patients with anorexia nervosa. Can J Psychiatry. 1991;36:517–520.

120. Wilson C. The fear of being fat and anorexia nervosa. Int J Psychoanal. 1982–3;9:233–255.

121. Sprince M. Early psychic disturbances in anorexic and bulimic patients as reflected in the psychoanalytic process. J Child Psychother. 1984;10:199–215.

122. Jackson C, Tabin J, Russel J, et al. Themes of death: Helmut Thoma's "anorexia nervosa" (1967): a research note. Int J Eat Disord. 1993;14:433–437.

123. Jackson C, Beumont P, Thornton C, et al. Dreams of death: Von Weizsäcker's dreams in so-called endogenic anorexia: a research note. Int J Eat Disord. 1993;13:329–332.

124. Brink S, Allan J. Dreams of anorexic and bulimic women: a research study. J Anal Psychol. 1992;37:275–297.

125. Levitan H. Implications of certain dreams reported by patients in a bulimic phase of anorexia nervosa. Can J Psychiatry. 1981;26:228–231.

126. Cernovsky Z. MMPI, nightmares in male alcoholics. Percept Mot Skills. 1985;61:841–842.

127. Cernovsky Z. MMPI and nightmare reports in women addicted to alcohol and other drugs. Percept Mot Skills. 1986;62:717–718.

128. Fiss H. Dream content and response to withdrawal from alcohol [abstract]. Sleep Res. 1980;9:152.

129. Christo G, Franey C. Addicts' drug related dreams: their frequency and relationship to six-month outcomes. Subst Use Misuse. 1996;31:1–15.

130. Denizen N. Alcoholic dreams. Alcohol Treat Q. 1988;5:133–139.

131. Stern B, Stern J. On the use of dreams as a means of diagnosis of brain injured patients. Scand J Rehabil Med Suppl. 1985;12:44–46.

132. Stern M, Stern B. Psychotherapy in cases of brain damage: a possible mission. Brain Inj. 1990;4:297–304.

133. Benyakar M, Tadir M, Groswasser Z, et al. Dreams in head-injured patients. Brain Inj. 1988;2:351–356.

134. Nathan R, Rose-Itkoff C, Lord G. Dreams, first memories, and brain atrophy in the elderly. Hillside J Clin Psychiatry. 1981;3:139–148.

135. Askenasy J, Gruskiewicz J, Braun J, et al. Repetitive visual images in severe war head injuries. Resuscitation. 1986;13:191–201.

136. Turner J, Graffam J. Deceased loved ones in the dreams of mentally retarded adults. Am J Ment Retard. 1987;92:282–289.

137. Voelm C, Kossor M, Duran E. Dream work with the mentally retarded. Psychiatr J Univ Ottawa. 1988;13:85–90.

138. Koulack D. To Catch a Dream: Explorations of Dreaming. Albany, NY: State University of New York; 1991.

Abnormal Sleep

Impact, Presentation, and Diagnosis

Michael S. Aldrich

43

Approach to the Patient With Disordered Sleep

Michael S. Aldrich
Michael W. Naylor

Sleep disorders are common in the general population. They can contribute to impaired academic or occupational performance, accidents at work or while driving, disturbances of mood and social adjustment, and decreased marital satisfaction. In addition, sleep disorders may lead to or exacerbate serious medical and psychiatric problems. The clinician should therefore take sleep complaints from a patient seriously and approach the evaluation of such problems in an orderly and systematic fashion.

Patients who complain of disturbed sleep generally describe one or more of three types of problems: insomnia; abnormal movements, behaviors, or sensations during sleep or during nocturnal awakenings; or excessive daytime sleepiness. These sleep complaints are not mutually exclusive, and a given sleep disorder may be associated with more than one type. For example, patients with sleep apnea may complain of insomnia, excessive daytime sleepiness, choking or gasping during the night, or all three.

The foundation for the diagnosis of sleep disorders is the history of the sleep complaint. Ideally, the evaluation includes a history from the patient's bed partner. Many sleep problems are not evident to the patient, and it is often the bed partner who has persuaded the patient to seek evaluation. As with other medical and psychiatric problems, essential information in the diagnosis of sleep disorders is provided by the patient's medical, psychiatric, and family history; a history of the use of medications; an assessment of the psychosocial situation; and the physical, neurological, and mental status examinations.

An assessment is then made on the basis of the clinical evaluation. In many cases, it is possible to make a definitive diagnosis and begin treatment, whereas in others, the diagnosis is presumptive and must be confirmed or excluded by diagnostic studies. If the diagnosis is uncertain, a differential diagnosis is formulated and a plan is developed to determine a definitive diagnosis, if possible. The elements of the evaluation of patients with disordered sleep are reviewed in this chapter, and signs and symptoms that may point to a particular diagnosis are emphasized.

CHIEF COMPLAINT AND HISTORY

Evaluation begins with the chief complaint, which provides a focus for delineating the patient's concerns and eliciting the history. It is often useful to ask why the patient is seeking help at the present time, particularly if the problem has been long-standing. If the chief complaint is from the spouse or bed partner, it is important to determine whether the patient recognizes the problem, is unaware of it, or denies its existence. Many clinicians also obtain a brief patient profile at the beginning of the interview that includes the patient's age, gender, occupational or academic status, marital status, and living arrangements.

There are two kinds of nighttime symptoms: those that occur during sleep, and those that occur during nocturnal awakenings. Symptoms that occur during sleep concern movements or behaviors and often are reported by the spouse or bed partner because the patient may be unaware of the episodes. Examples include twitching or kicking of the legs or arms, chewing movements, sleepwalking, sleeptalking, screams, and violent behavior. Complaints that occur during nocturnal awakenings concern sensations or events and include headaches, wheezing or shortness of breath, palpitations, heartburn, leg cramps, or feelings of paralysis, numbness, or tingling.

Once the chief complaint is delineated, details concerning the sleep problem are sought, including its duration, the circumstances at its onset, the factors that lead to exacerbation or improvement, and any associated symptoms.

The patient's daily schedule is reviewed, including the usual bedtime and estimated time to sleep onset, the number and timing of awakenings, and the time of final awakening. Particularly in children, the bedtime routine, or lack thereof, should be assessed; this information may suggest *limit setting sleep disorder* (see Table 46–1). The method of awakening should be determined: spontaneous, with an alarm, or by a family member. The usual waking schedule should also be determined, including times of work, school, meals, and exercise. It is important to obtain detailed sleep-wake schedules in shiftworkers. A comparison of the patient's weekday and weekend schedules may reveal

significant variations in sleep timing that suggest a *circadian rhythm sleep disorder* (see Chapter 52) or *insufficient sleep syndrome* (see Chapter 5).

Questions assessing the sleep setting may elicit information about factors that cause or aggravate sleep problems. Noise, extreme temperature, uncomfortable sleep surfaces, and frequently changing sleep conditions may all adversely affect sleep continuity and suggest an *environmental sleep disorder*.

For patients with medical or psychiatric diseases, the degree of sleep disturbance usually varies with the severity of the underlying illness. For example, in patients with congestive heart failure, the degree of insomnia may correlate with the severity of orthopnea and paroxysmal nocturnal dyspnea. Similar relationships may occur in patients with sleep disturbance related to depression, asthma, gastroesophageal reflux, and arthritis. In patients with sleep apnea, daytime sleepiness may correlate with seasonal allergies, alcohol use, or other factors that worsen apnea.

Insomnia

Patients with insomnia usually complain that their nocturnal sleep is inadequate in some way. They may describe difficulty falling asleep, frequent awakening, or early morning awakening with inability to return to sleep. The description of insomnia and its course may help determine cause. For example, insomnia that began in early childhood and continues with few remissions may suggest *idiopathic insomnia* (see Chapter 55). The relation of insomnia to stress is also important. If the cause of the stress is clear, such as the recent death of a family member, the diagnosis is likely to be *adjustment sleep disorder* (see Chapter 54). In other patients, however, the nature of the stress may not be immediately apparent. Positive life events, such as a promotion at work or recent marriage, may not be recognized by the patient as stressful.

Specific questions may reveal maladaptive behaviors and thought patterns that contribute to sleep difficulties. Insomniacs may become aroused and anxious when they are preparing for sleep and may worry about their insomnia and its effects on performance at work or at home the following day. Some may sleep better in an unfamiliar sleep setting, which suggests the presence of heightened arousal, frustration, or anxiety in attempting to sleep in the usual environment; these characteristics suggest *psychophysiological insomnia* (see Chapters 56 and 57). Irregular bedtimes, late night exercise, watching television in bed, or going from work directly to bed may interfere with sleep and suggest *inadequate sleep hygiene* (see Chapter 58).

Systematic inquiry into the behaviors and thoughts that accompany nocturnal awakenings is useful and may reveal conscious or unconscious "rewards" for poor sleep. Awakenings followed by inability to return to sleep without eating or drinking alcohol suggest the *nocturnal eating syndrome* (see Chapter 98) or *alcohol-dependent sleep disorder* (see Chapter 99). Patients who report "resting" for up to 8 h at night without sleeping or leaving the bed may have *sleep state misperception*.

Excessive Sleepiness

Patients with daytime sleepiness typically complain of drowsiness that interferes with daytime activities, unavoidable napping, or both. Falling asleep while driving or at other particularly inappropriate or dangerous times is often the impetus that brings the patient to the clinician. Some of these patients complain that they need more sleep at night or that daytime drowsiness occurs regardless of how much sleep is obtained at night.

The situations associated with drowsiness and spontaneous sleep episodes help determine the severity of the problem. Drowsiness and naps either may be limited to sedentary situations in which falling asleep is socially acceptable, such as watching television or reading at home, or may occur at work, while driving, in conversation, sitting on the toilet, or even during sexual intercourse.

Asking patients who complain of sleepiness about other associated symptoms provides essential information. Loud snoring, gasping, snorting, and episodes of apnea suggest the diagnosis of *obstructive sleep apnea-hypopnea syndrome* (see Chapter 74). The relationship of snoring to body position should be determined; snoring may occur in all positions or only in the supine position. A history of episodic muscle weakness with buckling of the knees, laxity of the neck or jaw muscles, or complete loss of muscle tone associated with laughter or other emotions suggests cataplexy and a diagnosis of *narcolepsy* (see Chapter 60). Episodes of partial or total paralysis at the onset or termination of sleep (sleep paralysis) and dream-like auditory, visual, or tactile hallucinations occurring at sleep onset or on awakening (hypnagogic and hypnopompic hallucinations) also suggest narcolepsy. Questions assessing mood are needed to identify patients with *sleep disorder associated with mood disorders* (see Chapter 96).

The sleep-wake schedule may also provide clues to the diagnosis. Short nocturnal sleep time, longer sleep on weekends or days off, and fewer symptoms during vacations when the sleep period is longer suggest the *insufficient sleep syndrome*.

Circadian rhythm sleep disorders should be considered in patients with complaints of nocturnal insomnia and daytime sleepiness. Patients with *delayed sleep phase syndrome* (see Chapter 52) frequently complain of difficulty waking up, morning sleepiness and sluggishness, and difficulty falling asleep at night. Symptoms are worse on days when the patient must awaken by a set time to be at school or work. Patients with *advanced sleep phase syndrome* (see Chapter 52) may complain of evening sleepiness and early morning awakening. The patient's occupation and social schedule may suggest diagnoses of *shift work sleep disorder* (see Chapter 51) or *jet lag syndrome* (see Chapter 50).

Nocturnal Movements, Behaviors, and Sensations

Information from collateral sources is needed for evaluating episodic movements and behaviors during sleep. The bed partner should be asked to describe behaviors and vocalizations during the episodes, to relate episodes to sleep onset and time of night, and to note the degree of the patient's responsiveness during the episode. The patient's ability to recall the events is also significant. Episodes of inconsolable screaming and amnesia during the first third of the night suggest *sleep terrors* (see Chapter 62); episodes of dream-enacting behavior associated with dream recall suggest the rapid eye movement *(REM) sleep behavior disorder* (see Chapter 64).

In patients whose symptoms occur during nocturnal awakenings, the relations to evening activities and medical or psychiatric conditions are often illuminating. Repeated awakenings from sleep with chest discomfort may suggest *sleep-related gastroesophageal reflux, sleep disorder due to peptic ulcer disease* (see Chapter 94), or *nocturnal cardiac ischemia* (see Chapter 86), depending on associated symptoms and underlying diseases. Similarly, complaints of choking during sleep may suggest *obstructive sleep apnea-hypopnea syndrome* when they are accompanied by snoring or *sleep-related gastroesophageal reflux* when they are accompanied by heartburn and a sour taste in the mouth.

MEDICATION USE AND PAST MEDICAL HISTORY

Assessment of medication use is critical because of the wide variety of medications that alter sleep and wakefulness. Some medications, such as theophylline and other bronchodilators, directly affect sleep; others, such as diuretics, have indirect effects. Chronic sedative or hypnotic use raises the possibility of *hypnotic-dependent sleep disorder* (see Table 46–1). Because cold preparations, appetite suppressants, antihistamines, and nonprescription sedatives and stimulants affect sleep, it is important to ask specifically about nonprescription as well as prescription medications.

The history of current or past medical, surgical, and psychiatric illnesses is a source of important information. Seizure disorders, parkinsonism and dementia, arthritic conditions, asthma, ischemic heart disease, migraine or cluster headache, compressive neuropathies, obstructive uropathy, and almost any painful illness can cause significant sleep disturbance. A variety of medical conditions including hypothyroidism, acromegaly, Cushing's syndrome, allergic rhinitis, and some of the mucopolysaccharidoses may contribute to the development of *obstructive sleep apnea syndrome.* Anemia and renal disease may cause or exacerbate *restless legs syndrome* or *periodic limb movement disorder.* In infants and toddlers, milk and other food allergens may cause insomnia. Head trauma may lead to the postconcussion syndrome, often accompanied by disrupted sleep continuity. Information about tonsillectomy, cleft palate repair, nasal trauma or surgery, and other orofacial surgery is essential in patients with suspected obstructive sleep apnea syndrome.

Anxiety disorders, including panic disorder, and mood disorders are psychiatric disturbances that are often accompanied by insomnia, and some patients with depression complain of excessive daytime sleepiness. Exacerbation of schizophrenia and other psychotic disorders are frequently associated with severe sleep disruption.

FAMILY HISTORY

A history of disordered sleep in family members is important information. Specific inquiry should be made about the existence in family members of previously diagnosed sleep disorders or symptoms suggestive of narcolepsy, obstructive sleep apnea, periodic limb movements, enuresis, sleep terrors or sleepwalking, or insomnia. There is a strong genetic contribution to the development of narcolepsy (see Chapter 59), and genetic and familial influences sometimes have a role in the development and expression of obstructive sleep apnea and some of the parasomnias.

SOCIAL HISTORY

Assessment of psychosocial, occupational, and academic functioning as well as of marital satisfaction can yield valuable information about the impact of disordered sleep on the patient's life. When the chief complaint comes from the spouse, the patient may have one of the many sleep disorders whose symptoms may not be noticed by the patient, but the possibility of marital difficulties should also be considered and explored. In patients complaining of excessive sleepiness, potential occupational hazards should be assessed, and special attention should be paid to the assessment of marital, social, and occupational functioning of shift workers. The ability of the work environment to provide support for the patient should be evaluated. For children and adolescents, school performance should be determined.

Alcohol, caffeine, nicotine, and illicit drug use should be determined. Alcohol use or abuse may intensify snoring and obstructive sleep apnea, may be a contributor to insomnia, or may produce long-lasting changes in sleep patterns. Patients who drink heavily on the weekend may complain of sleepiness primarily during the early part of the week. Caffeine use produces significant sleep disturbance in susceptible persons, and nicotine dependency may lead to nocturnal awakenings. Cocaine, amphetamines, barbiturates, and opiates can be associated with major disruption of sleep architecture.

REVIEW OF SYSTEMS

The review of systems may uncover symptoms of medical illnesses that can cause or contribute to sleep disorders. Recent weight gain or increase in collar size increases the likelihood of obstructive sleep apnea syndrome. Particular attention should be paid to the cardiovascular and pulmonary systems because of their relation to breathing and oxygenation during sleep. Angina, orthopnea, paroxysmal nocturnal dyspnea, and wheezing may indicate that sleep disturbance is due to cardiac or pulmonary disease. Heartburn and reflux of gastric contents into the throat when the patient is recumbent may cause nocturnal choking episodes. Leg cramps and neuropathic pain may be accompanied by sleep disruption. Nocturia is a common cause of disturbed sleep, particularly in older men.

PHYSICAL EXAMINATION

Physical examination of the patient with disordered sleep begins with observation. Body habitus often provides clues to potential etiological factors of sleep complaints; thus, obesity with distribution of fat around the neck or midriff suggests the diagnosis of obstructive sleep apnea. Psychomotor slowing, poor hygiene, downcast eyes, blunted affect, or sad facies may suggest major depression and its associated sleep disturbance.

Examination of the head and neck is particularly important in patients with suspected obstructive sleep apnea. Mandibular hypoplasia, craniosynostosis, retrognathia, and other craniofacial abnormalities may indicate the presence of Pierre Robin syndrome, Treacher Collins syndrome, Crouzon's disease, achondroplasia, or other skeletal disorders that are associated with an increased incidence of sleep-related respiratory disturbances. Boggy, edematous nasal mucosa in patients with allergies or deviation of the nasal septum after trauma may compromise nasal patency and predispose the patient to obstructive sleep apnea syndrome. Oropharyngeal findings suggestive of obstructive sleep apnea include an elongated soft palate and uvula; edema and erythema of the peritonsillar pillars, uvula, soft palate, or posterior oropharynx; redundant pharyngeal mucosa; enlarged tongue; and enlarged tonsillar tissue. Examination of the neck may reveal an enlarged thyroid or prominent fatty infiltration suggesting the likelihood of excess retropharyngeal adipose tissue.

Auscultation of the chest may reveal expiratory wheezes in patients with nocturnal asthma attacks. Thoracic abnormalities such as kyphoscoliosis may compromise ventilatory capacity, leading to hypoventilation and nocturnal breathing difficulties. Patients with severe obstructive sleep apnea may have findings consistent with right-sided heart failure including hepatomegaly, ascites, and ankle edema. Cardiac complications of disordered breathing during sleep may be indicated by a cardiac thrust at the left sternal border as a result of right ventricular enlargement or in the left second intercostal space adjacent to the sternum as a result of pulmonary hypertension. Auscultation may reveal a prominent fourth heart sound originating from the enlarged right ventricle and murmurs of pulmonary or tricuspid valve insufficiency.

On abdominal examination, hepatomegaly may suggest that alcohol abuse is contributing to sleep disturbance or, in conjunction with other findings, that congestive heart failure is a factor. Examination of the extremities may reveal joint swelling or deformity, decreased range of motion across affected joints, and thickening of synovial tissue in patients with disordered sleep due to arthritis.

Findings on mental status testing and neurological examination may indicate the presence of a psychiatric or neurological disease that causes or contributes to disturbed sleep. Impairment of short-term memory, judgment, language functions, and abstract reasoning suggests the presence of a dementing illness that may cause insomnia or nocturnal confusion. Assessment of mood may suggest the presence of mania or depression, either of which may be associated with insomnia. Delusional thoughts and agitation may indicate that acute psychosis is the cause of insomnia. Reduced alertness with slurred speech and nystagmus may be signs of hypnotic or sedative abuse. Impaired sensation and reduced or absent tendon reflexes may indicate peripheral neuropathy, sometimes accompanied by nocturnal paresthesias or burning pain.

FORMULATION AND DIAGNOSTIC STUDIES

Once the initial evaluation is complete, the clinician generates a differential diagnosis. The International Classification of Sleep Disorders provides a comprehensive diagnostic approach and is discussed in detail in Chapter 46. On the basis of the relative likelihood of the diagnostic possibilities, appropriate diagnostic studies are ordered (see Chapter 45). Even when the diagnosis is clear, laboratory tests may be required to determine the severity of the condition before the clinician decides on the appropriate treatment.

Additional diagnostic information can be obtained through the use of laboratory or radiological investigations, sleep logs, and sleep laboratory studies. Radiological and laboratory tests may clarify or refine the diagnosis or may indicate its severity. Thyroid function tests or pulmonary function tests may be indicated in some patients with suspected obstructive sleep apnea. If the diagnosis of narcolepsy is under consideration, tissue typing for specific human leukocyte antigens implicated in the genetics of narcolepsy is sometimes helpful. Uremia, anemia, iron deficiency, or other metabolic abnormalities may be present in patients with suspected periodic limb movement disorder or restless legs syndrome. A urine toxicology screen may be diagnostic in cases of insomnia or hypersomnia due to substance abuse.

The sleep log is particularly useful in patients with insomnia or suspected circadian rhythm disturbances. Although a variety of sleep logs exist, a 2-week log in which the patient records bedtime, approximate time of sleep onset, times and durations of awakenings during the sleep period, final awakening time, and nap times during the day is commonly used. The sleep log may provide a new perspective on the sleep problem for both the clinician and the patient; some patients are surprised and relieved to note that their sleep is better than they believed.

Polysomnography can provide confirmatory diagnostic evidence in cases of sleep apnea, narcolepsy, periodic limb movements, nocturnal epilepsy, and sleep terrors and helps determine the severity of these conditions. Its use in the evaluation of insomnia is somewhat controversial but may be beneficial, especially when sleep apnea, periodic limb movements, or sleep state misperception is suspected. The multiple sleep latency test (MSLT), described in Chapter 104, can confirm the presence of excessive sleepiness, quantify its severity, and determine the presence of pathologically early onset of REM sleep; this test is especially useful when it is used the day after polysomnography. Ambulatory sleep-wake recordings, wrist actigraphy, portable monitoring devices that record esophageal acidity, electrocardiogram, or electroencephalogram are useful in selected patients.

CONCLUSIONS

Sleep disorders are prevalent in the general population and are common in patients who consult with physicians and other health care providers. Patients with complaints of sleep disturbance often present a diagnostic challenge to the clinician because of the many possible causes for symptoms and the patients' inability to accurately describe events occurring during sleep. A systematic evaluation generally yields a provisional diagnosis or a set of diagnostic possibilities that can be confirmed or excluded with specific diagnostic tests. With accurate diagnosis and specific interventions, most sleep disorders are treatable.

44

Cardinal Manifestations of Sleep Disorders

Michael S. Aldrich

Sleep disorders are associated with a characteristic set of symptoms and signs. In the evaluation of the patient with a suspected sleep disorder, the physician must know about the manifestations of disordered sleep and must recognize the diagnostic possibilities presented by a particular symptom or sign. This chapter begins with a discussion of sleep as a clinical state in relation to other disturbances of consciousness. The remainder of the chapter is devoted to the cardinal manifestations of sleep disorders, their associated clinical signs and symptoms, and diagnostic considerations.

SLEEP, CONSCIOUSNESS, AND COMA

Sleep is a periodic, natural, and reversible state of altered consciousness. *Consciousness* can be defined as a state of awareness of self and environment that gives meaning or significance to external and internal stimuli. Arousal and cognition, which are required for consciousness, correlate approximately with two major neuroanatomical systems: the arousal system, including the brainstem reticular activating system and the medial diencephalic structures to which it projects; and the cognitive system, including the cerebral cortex, its associated white matter tracts, and subcortical nuclei. The relation between these neuroanatomical systems and sleep and wakefulness is discussed in Chapters 8 and 10.

Loss of either the system responsible for arousal or the system sustaining cognition leads to coma, a state in which awareness of self and environment is lost and there is no meaningful response to external stimuli or inner needs. Patients in coma often have a *sleep-like* appearance, and brief observation of a comatose patient might lead one to the conclusion that the individual is sleeping.

In addition to reversibility, however, sleep and coma have important physiological and metabolic differences. Neurophysiological, neuroanatomical, and neurochemical studies over the past 50 years have demonstrated that sleep, unlike coma, is an active process requiring appropriate interactions of a number of brainstem, diencephalic, and forebrain structures. Sleep can be induced by stimulation of some of the structures that compose the sleep system; lesions of these areas may cause insomnia and disordered sleep-wake regulation. Whereas stupor and coma are associated with depression of cerebral metabolic activity, overall brain metabolism and oxygen use during sleep are altered only slightly.

Two pathological conditions provide evidence that consciousness can be lost while sleep-wake cycles continue. Patients with coma caused by widespread cortical and subcortical damage, due to anoxia, for example, may eventually develop a *persistent vegetative state*. In this state, there is no evidence of awareness or cognition, and cerebral metabolism is markedly reduced;[1, 2] nonetheless, autonomic and vegetative functions are preserved, and sleep-wake cycles are readily identifiable: yawns, chewing, grimacing, and other reflex motor behaviors occur during periods corresponding to physiological wakefulness. In patients with akinetic mutism, a related condition usually caused by large bilateral frontal lobe lesions or diffuse cortical injury, sleep-wake cycles are preserved; during the phase of physiological wakefulness, patients maintain an alert appearance, but they show no evidence of awareness or cognition. In both of these conditions, consciousness has been lost while sleep-wake cycles remain.

Clinical signs associated with sleep onset include eye closure, muscle relaxation, increased regularity of breathing, and brief irregular myoclonic *hypnic jerks* of the distal extremities. During nonrapid eye movement (NREM) sleep, the eyes are deviated upward or are dysconjugate with slow, roving movements, the pupils are small, and the eyelids close smoothly and gradually on release. Muscle tone is reduced but not flaccid, and deep tendon reflexes are present. During rapid eye movement (REM) sleep, breathing is irregular in amplitude and frequency, and brief irregular myoclonic jerks of the face and extremities occur at intervals; these jerks and twitches are much more prominent in infants. If the eyes can be opened without inducing arousal, conjugate rapid eye movements and fluctuations in pupil size can be observed. Muscle tone is flaccid, deep tendon reflexes are markedly reduced or absent, and in males penile erection occurs.

The diagnostic considerations in a patient with a sleep-like appearance include natural or drug-induced sleep, coma, and psychogenic unresponsiveness. In clinical practice, the distinction between sleep and coma is usually readily made because of the reversibility of sleep with stimulation. Problems may sometimes arise in a profoundly sleepy person who is difficult to arouse because of severe sleep deprivation or disruption, or in someone who is in stage 4 sleep and does not arouse easily with stimulation. In such cases, evaluation of pupillary responses, corneal reflexes, oculomotor responses, motor responses, and tendon reflexes, along with behavioral responses to stimulation, helps distinguish sleep and sleepiness from stupor or coma and determine the cause if pathological altered consciousness is present.[3]

Patients with psychogenic unresponsiveness do not usually respond to the types of stimulation that promote wakefulness in sleeping patients, although verbal suggestion is sometimes effective. Examination of the eyes helps diagnose such patients: the dysconjugate gaze; slow, roving eye movements; and gradual eye closure after release of the eyelids that characterize sleep cannot be duplicated in psychogenic states.

The distinction between drug-induced sleep and drug-induced stupor or coma is conceptually, and sometimes clinically, difficult. For example, barbiturates promote sleep in small doses but produce coma in large doses, and there is no clear line separating the alcoholic individual who is "sleeping it off" from one who is in alcoholic stupor. Depressed respirations, lack of arousability, and physiological changes associated with particular drugs are helpful in these clinical situations.

INSOMNIA

Insomnia is the subjective complaint of insufficient or inadequate sleep. It is a subjective complaint not only because it is defined by the patient's experience but also because the required amount of sleep varies from individual to individual. Insomnia is a symptom, like headache, whose medical and psychiatric significance depends on its cause, quality, severity, and chronicity, as well as on other signs and symptoms that may accompany it. There are few, if any, physical signs of insomnia.

The significance of insomnia also depends on its timing—whether it occurs at the beginning, or the end, or in the course of the usual period of sleep. Timing determines the three main types into which insomnia is classified: delayed sleep onset, impaired sleep continuity, and early-morning awakening.

Insomnia is more common among women, older people, and the anxious and depressed. Low socioeconomic status, poor education, chronic medical illness, recent life stresses, and the use of alcohol are also associated with increased incidence of insomnia.

The differential diagnosis of insomnia includes sleep-state misperception and sleep-wake schedule disturbances. Although most patients who complain of poor sleep have objective evidence of disordered sleep when they are assessed polysomnographically, some patients who complain of unrelenting insomnia are found to have normal sleep in the laboratory. This condition, called sleep-state misperception, includes a failure to perceive sleep or sleepiness. Other patients with mild sleep disturbances exaggerate the degree of their sleep disruption.

Patients with sleep-wake schedule disturbances may complain of insomnia. For example, when delayed sleep onset is associated with good sleep continuity and difficulty awakening in the morning, the diagnosis may be a circadian rhythm disturbance, such as eastbound jet lag or delayed sleep phase syndrome. Poor nocturnal sleep and daytime sleepiness may be a consequence of reversal of the sleep-wake schedule, as in nocturnal shift workers who attempt to resume a daytime wake schedule during days off.

The effects of insomnia include sleepiness, fatigue, lack of concentration and alertness, muscle aches, and depression. Compared with normal people, those with insomnia are preoccupied with sleep and sleep habits and describe themselves as tense, anxious, worried, nervous, tired, irritable, and depressed. For many with insomnia, the expectation of poor sleep is a major contributor to continued sleeplessness, and rituals and behaviors whose goal is to induce sleep, either at bedtime or during nocturnal awakenings, may instead exacerbate the insomnia. Although the presence of one or more of these characteristics may help in assessing the patient, none is present in every patient with insomnia.

Symptoms Sometimes Associated With Insomnia

Pain

Pain is a common cause of insomnia, particularly in the elderly. The nocturnal pain and discomfort of arthritis and other rheumatological disorders is a frequent cause of insomnia, and the burning foot pain of diabetic neuropathy and other polyneuropathies is often worse at night. Cluster headaches are precipitated during REM sleep. Chest and epigastric pain during the night may be due to angina, reflux esophagitis, or peptic ulcer disease. Pain from primary tumors and metastatic lesions is also common at night.

Other Nocturnal Symptoms of Medical Illnesses

Besides pain, the symptoms of many medical illnesses and their treatments are associated with insomnia, often because they occur at night or are worse in the supine position. Two of the more common symptoms are nocturia from obstructive uropathy and dyspnea from congestive heart failure and emphysema. Paresthesias from restless legs syndrome or from such nerve compressions as carpal tunnel syndrome are often particularly bothersome at night; immobility from paralysis, ankylosis, or Parkinson's disease is another cause of nocturnal awakenings. Hyperthyroidism and Cushing's disease are among the endocrine disorders occasionally associated with insomnia. Methylxan-thines and beta-adrenergic agonists used in the treatment of asthma and emphysema may disrupt sleep. Finally, the need to awaken to take prescribed medications during the night is an often overlooked cause of disturbed sleep. Medical causes of insomnia are discussed in detail in Section 9.

Anxiety

Many persons with insomnia suffer from anxiety. Anxiety can be manifest at bedtime or during the night as intrusive thoughts, inability to relax, obsessive worrying, and an "overactive" mind while trying to sleep. Emotional or physiological arousal associated with anxiety, and somatic symptoms such as palpitations, increased heart rate, and shortness of breath, may contribute to sleep disturbance. Insomnia associated with anxiety disorders is discussed in Chapter 95.

Depression

Depressive illnesses are almost always associated with sleep disturbance, manifested usually as poor sleep continuity and early-morning awakening, although occasionally as hypersomnia. The sleep patterns and sleep disorders associated with affective disorders are discussed in Chapters 56 and 96.

SLEEPINESS

Sleepiness, which can be viewed as a manifestation of a physiological drive for sleep, has objective and subjective components. Changes in the electroencephalogram (EEG), including mild slowing of the alpha rhythm, and in a variety of performance tasks, particularly those related to vigilance, provide evidence of objective changes related to sleepiness. The sensations, emotions, and thoughts that accompany sleep loss are the subjective components of sleepiness. When sleepiness is chronic and severe, the patient may become less aware of the subjective aspects of sleepiness and so may fall asleep without warning; these episodes are called sleep attacks.

Sleepiness is a normal experience at the end of the day and after prolonged wakefulness, as in the case of a medical intern who has been awake all night. Mild sleepiness is most apparent during passive situations, such as reading, traveling, or watching television. With more severe sleepiness, the patient may have difficulty staying awake during more active situations, such as conversations and meals. Sleepiness is excessive when it occurs at inappropriate or undesirable times, such as at work, while driving, and during social activities. Excessive sleepiness that is not relieved by increased amounts of sleep at night is usually a sign of a sleep disorder.

Chronic or excessive sleepiness is accompanied by lapses of attention and by impaired motor and cognitive abilities, particularly those required by boring tasks. These patients often sleep excessively during the day, may be unable to resist daytime napping, and usually have difficulty attaining full arousal. Chronic sleepiness is diagnosed primarily by history and sleep latency testing; drooping eyelids, repetitive yawning, head-nodding and loss of postural muscle tone, and small pupils may be present on physical examination when sleepiness is severe. Daytime sleepiness is discussed in further detail in Chapter 4.

Sleepiness due to sleep deprivation or to sleep disorders needs to be distinguished from sleepiness associated with clouded consciousness or sedation. Although patients with clouded consciousness due to bihemispheric or brainstem lesions are drowsy, they are usually confused and suffer more inattention and cognitive impairment than is customary with chronic sleepiness.

Clouding of consciousness may progress to stupor or coma. In severe cases of sleep apnea, profound sleepiness and hypoxia- or hypercapnia-induced stupor may coexist. Although ordinarily sleepiness and stupor are easily distinguished, the distinction may be less clear in an intensive care unit, and the possibility that an apparently stuporous patient may be suffering only from severe and chronic sleep loss needs to be considered.

Although chronic sleepiness is usually accompanied by fatigue and a loss of sense of well-being, many patients with complaints of fatigue, listlessness, weakness, loss of energy, and relentless weariness are not sleepy. These patients do not describe the sensation of impending sleep and do not report falling asleep or fighting sleep at inappropriate times; in fact, they more often complain of insomnia. The patient says, "If only I could get some sleep I would feel less tired."

Sleepiness, which can be measured in a number of ways, is commonly assessed clinically by measuring the length of time required to fall asleep when asked to do so, as in the multiple sleep latency test, or when asked to remain awake, as in the Maintenance of Wakefulness Test. Sleepiness may also be assessed by determining the propensity to fall asleep in certain situations. The Epworth Sleepiness Scale (Tables 44–1 and 44–2) is an example.[4] Based on reports from the patient, it correlates with the multiple sleep latency test, although the correlation is not strong.[5] In patients with sleep apnea, this scale is correlated with the respiratory disturbance index, although this correlation also is fairly weak.[6]

Symptoms Sometimes Associated With Sleepiness

Patients with excessive sleepiness may have other symptoms that help determine the cause of the sleepiness. Such symptoms include snoring, apneic episodes, morning headaches, cataplexy, hypnagogic hallucinations, sleep paralysis, automatic behavior, and sleep drunkenness.

SNORING

Snoring is produced by vibration of the soft tissues of the upper airway. It varies in intensity and quality,

Table 44-1. THE EPWORTH SLEEPINESS SCALE

Name: _____
Today's date: _____ Your age (years): _____
Your sex (male = M; female = F): _____

How likely are you to doze off or fall asleep in the following situations, in contrast to feeling just tired? This refers to your usual way of life in recent times. Even if you have not done some of these things recently, try to work out how they would have affected you. Use the following scale to choose the *most appropriate number* for each situation:

0 = would *never* doze
1 = *slight* chance of dozing
2 = *moderate* chance of dozing
3 = *high* chance of dozing

Situation*	Chance of Dozing
Sitting and reading	_____
Watching TV	_____
Sitting, inactive in a public place (e.g., a theater or a meeting)	_____
As a passenger in a car for an hour without a break	_____
Lying down to rest in the afternoon when circumstances permit	_____
Sitting and talking to someone	_____
Sitting quietly after a lunch without alcohol	_____
In a car, while stopped for a few minutes in traffic	_____

Thank you for your cooperation

*The numbers for the eight situations are added together to give a global score between 0 and 24. Table 44-2 shows scores for various conditions.
From Johns MW. A new method for measuring daytime sleepiness: the Epworth Sleepiness Scale. Sleep. 1991;14:540–545.

depending on the time of night, the stage of sleep, the position of the body, the rate of airflow, and the anatomical structure of the individual's nose and throat.[7] Although occasional quiet snoring usually has no pathological significance, loud habitual snoring is a cardinal symptom of obstructive sleep apnea-hypopnea syndrome (OSAHS) and is frequently present years before other symptoms are apparent. Although more than 80% of individuals with OSAHS snore loudly, the absence of snoring does not rule out this diagnosis. For example, patients with neuromuscular disease affecting muscles of the upper airway, chest wall, or diaphragm

may not be able to generate sufficient inspiratory force to cause vibration of soft tissues. Other patients, such as those who have had uvulopalatopharyngoplasty, may not have sufficient floppy airway tissue to vibrate even though airway narrowing is still present.

Snoring of apneic individuals can exceed 80 dB in intensity and may disturb not only the bed partner but family members and even neighbors. Some bed partners sleep so soundly, however, that they are not adequate witnesses to snoring beyond the first hour or two of sleep. A complaint of loud snoring that cannot be verified by objective assessment is sometimes an indication of marital discord.

Snorts, gasps, choking noises, body jerks, and flailing arm movements are often mixed with snoring in patients with obstructive sleep apnea. Loud snoring that has increased in volume or changed in character is particularly suggestive of obstructive sleep apnea. In some patients, as apnea becomes worse and the apneic pauses become longer and more frequent than the snoring, the bed partner may report that snoring has actually improved.

APNEIC EPISODES

Apneic episodes, or *apneas*, are defined as episodes lasting 10 sec or more in which breathing ceases, with or without respiratory effort. Although accurate characterization of apneas can be done only in the sleep laboratory, the bed partner's description may be helpful. For example, if the bed partner reports that apneas are followed by snorts, gasps, and choking noises, the diagnosis is almost always upper airway obstruction. A snore or snort that awakens a patient is usually an indication that an apnea has occurred.

Central apneas often occur at sleep onset or immediately after awakenings. When associated with alternate waxing and waning in the amplitude of respirations, the apneas are part of a respiratory pattern called Cheyne-Stokes respiration and are usually an indication of a metabolic or brain disturbance or heart failure. Apneas after nocturnal seizures may be reported by the bed partner as sleep apnea if the seizure was not observed. In the very obese, shallow breathing may be mistaken for apnea.

Table 44-2. THE GROUPS OF EXPERIMENTAL SUBJECTS, THEIR AGES, AND EPWORTH SLEEPINESS SCALE (ESS) SCORES

Subjects/Diagnoses	Total Number of Subjects (M/F)	Age in Years (mean ±SD)	ESS Scores (mean ±SD)	Range
Normal controls	30 (14/16)	36.4 ±9.9	5.9 ±2.2	2–10
Primary snoring	32 (29/3)	45.7 ±10.7	6.5 ±3.0	0–11
Obstructive sleep apnea syndrome	55 (53/2)	48.4 ±10.7	11.7 ±4.6	4–23
Narcolepsy	13 (8/5)	46.6 ±12.0	17.5 ±3.5	13–23
Idiopathic hypersomnia	14 (8/6)	41.4 ±14.0	17.9 ±3.1	12–24
Insomnia	16 (6/12)	40.3 ±14.6	2.2 ±2.0	0–6
Periodic limb movement disorder	18 (16/2)	52.5 ±10.3	9.2 ±4.0	2–16

From Johns MW. A new method for measuring daytime sleepiness: the Epworth Sleepiness Scale. Sleep. 1991;14:540–545.

MORNING HEADACHES

Morning headache is a nonspecific symptom that can occur in patients with a variety of sleep disorders. Morning headaches are a complaint in about 20% of patients with OSAHS and about 25% of patients with other types of sleep disorders.[8] Hypertension, depression, tension or muscle contraction, migraine, brain tumor, sinus disease, chronic obstructive pulmonary disease, and alcohol consumption can also cause or contribute to morning headaches. For the most part, the quality and location of head pain do not help differentiate sleep disorders from other causes of morning headaches.

A "vascular headache" syndrome with episodes that begin only during sleep may be due to apneic episodes,[7] because treating the episodes may abolish the headaches.

CATAPLEXY

In patients with excessive sleepiness, a history of cataplexy is virtually diagnostic of narcolepsy (see Chapter 60). Cataplexy is a sudden spell of weakness due to a decrease in muscle tone triggered by external or internal stimuli. Its severity ranges from brief sensations of weakness in a few muscles, perceptible only to the patient, to total paralysis of all striated muscles except the muscles of respiration and the sphincters. The most common trigger is laughter; other frequent inciting stimuli include telling or hearing a joke, anger, surprise, joy, fright, intense concentration, and athletic activities. Complete paralysis is uncommon but dramatic; the patient may stagger briefly and then fall to the ground, unable to move yet fully alert.

Physical findings during severe cataplexy include flaccid paralysis, areflexia, reactive pupils, and reduced corneal responses. Occasional twitches similar to those seen in REM sleep may occur. Milder episodes may produce weakness of the knees, twitching of the face, dysarthria, jaw droop, ptosis, blurred or double vision, loss of neck tone, and the need to sit down. Consciousness is preserved initially, although if the episode persists for a minute or more, the patient may enter REM sleep.

Preservation of consciousness at the onset of the attack distinguishes cataplexy from syncope and atonic seizures. The relation of cataplexy to specific inciting factors helps distinguish it from the drop attacks of vertebrobasilar insufficiency; from myasthenia gravis and periodic paralysis, which are also characterized by episodic weakness; and from partial motor seizures, which may be suspected if the cataplectic episodes are associated with facial twitching.

HYPNAGOGIC HALLUCINATIONS

Hypnagogic (onset of sleep) and hypnopompic (end of sleep) hallucinations are auditory, tactile, or visual hallucinations occurring at the interface between waking and sleep. The hallucinations may be pleasant or terrifying. Although "dream-like," they differ from dreams by the lack of full participation of the subject and by the absence of a theme or story. The hallucinations may involve revisualization of scenes from the previous few hours or minutes, often with feelings of weightlessness and loss of balance or support. They last seconds to minutes and often terminate suddenly with a hypnic jerk. Although hypnagogic hallucinations in someone with excessive sleepiness suggest a diagnosis of narcolepsy, they are not diagnostic and can occur in anyone with disturbed sleep or a disrupted sleep schedule.

Their relation to the onset and end of sleep helps distinguish these hallucinations from those associated with migraine and posterior circulation ischemia. Partial seizures arising from the occipital lobes may sometimes be activated by drowsiness; the stereotyped nature of the associated hallucinations helps distinguish them from hypnagogic hallucinations. Patients with evening and nocturnal hallucinations associated with dementia, the "sundown syndrome," or with toxic or psychotic states often believe the hallucinations are real, whereas patients with hypnagogic hallucinations usually know what they are.[9] Peduncular hallucinations, which are associated with some midbrain lesions, are visual and often occur in the evening or at night.[10, 11] Although disordered sleep may accompany them, they are less closely linked than are hypnagogic and hypnopompic hallucinations to sleep onset and offset.

SLEEP PARALYSIS

Sleep paralysis, characterized by flaccid paralysis of skeletal muscles with areflexia, usually occurs at the onset or at the end of sleep, often immediately after an episode of REM sleep. Sleep paralysis differs from cataplexy by its timing and by the absence of a trigger factor. Sleep paralysis usually starts suddenly, lasts a few minutes, and ends either gradually or abruptly; the episode is often terminated by a sound or a touch on the body. During the episode, the patient feels awake or half-awake and unable to move and afterward may describe struggling to move and wake up. When sleep paralysis overlaps with hypnagogic hallucinations, the patient may experience illusions or hallucinations of people in the room or sensations of impending death or suffocation, events so frightening that the patient may maintain a vivid recollection of them for years.

The semiconscious state of sleep paralysis can be distinguished from seizures, syncopal episodes, and periodic paralysis by its association with the beginning and end of sleep, by its termination with noise or touch, and by the immediate return to full consciousness when the episode ends. Although sleep paralysis at the end of a nap or longer sleep period is not uncommon in individuals with disrupted sleep schedules and circadian rhythm disturbances, its occurrence at sleep onset is more suggestive of narcolepsy.

AUTOMATIC BEHAVIOR

Automatic behavior refers to episodes of purposeful but inappropriate behavior occurring in sleepy persons. It is associated with impaired attention and vigilance and with partial or complete amnesia for the events. The episodes may last minutes to hours, during which the subject engages in repetitive, meaningless activity or makes errors resulting from impaired vigilance, such as missing freeway exits, driving through stop signs, or writing nonsense. Sleep-deprived soldiers who fall asleep while marching provide an example of automatic behavior. Narcoleptic patients with automatic behavior may have hallucinations during the episodes.

Polygraph recordings of sleepy subjects engaged in boring tasks show repeated "microsleeps," which are usually NREM sleep in non-narcoleptic subjects but may include features of REM sleep in narcoleptic patients; these microsleeps are probably partly responsible for automatic behavior.

Automatic behavior may be difficult to distinguish from automatisms associated with partial complex seizures, absence status, postictal confusion, transient global amnesia, metabolic or drug-induced confusional states, fugue states, or simply daydreaming. The association with repetitive or boring tasks, the relief with stimulation, and the observation by others of preexisting signs of drowsiness may help differentiate automatic behavior from confusional states. Automatisms associated with partial seizures are often preceded by auras, show greater stereotypy than does automatic behavior, and are usually followed by postictal confusion. Transient global amnesia is usually an isolated event in an elderly patient without an altered level of alertness; the bewilderment that often accompanies transient global amnesia is not part of automatic behavior.

SLEEP DRUNKENNESS

Sleep drunkenness is characterized by an inability to attain full alertness for an extended time after awakening. It usually occurs in the morning and is associated with drowsiness, grogginess, disorientation, incoordination, and automatic behavior, such as repeatedly turning off alarm clocks. The patient may describe very deep sleep at night and may complain of tiredness, poor concentration, job or school difficulties, and morning headaches. Although it occurs most commonly in association with sleep apnea, sleep drunkenness can be seen with idiopathic hypersomnia, after severe sleep deprivation, and occasionally in other disorders that affect the central nervous system arousal system. The usual differential diagnosis is a motivational problem, as in a youth who cannot respond to the alarm clock on school days but has no trouble getting up on holidays.

PARASOMNIAS

Parasomnias are movements and behaviors occurring during sleep. They may be normal or abnormal. The most common normal movements during sleep are hypnic jerks, brief myoclonic jerks occurring at sleep onset. Several types of abnormal movements and behaviors are associated with partial arousals from sleep; these include sleepwalking, sleep-talking, sleep terror, and confusional arousals, conditions that are often associated with difficult arousal and confusion on awakening, with amnesia, and with automatic behavior. Other parasomnias, such as periodic leg movements and head-banging, occur with or without an associated arousal; still others, such as bruxism, are usually not associated with arousal.

SLEEP-TALKING

Sleep-talking is frequent at all ages, more often in females than in males. Although it is most common in stages 1 and 2 of NREM sleep, sleep-talking occurs occasionally in REM sleep. Sleep-talking ranges from coherent sentences to mumbled nonsense, and there is rarely any response to speech by others. Sleep-talking without other associated parasomnias or sleep disturbance is rarely of medical concern.

SLEEPWALKING

Sleepwalking, more common in children than in adults, is most likely to occur during the first third of the night, particularly during the first NREM period (see Chapter 62). The child typically sits up in bed or stands and walks aimlessly with purposeless and clumsy movements. The eyes are open but "glassy" and unseeing. The child may dress or undress, fumble with objects, mumble or moan, and walk to different rooms or even outside the house. The child usually does not respond to voice but often can be led back to bed. Although usually avoiding objects, the child may be injured by falling or by touching hot objects. There is usually no recall or only fragmentary, dream-like recollections of the events. The episodes last 15 sec to 30 min and may be preceded on the EEG by an arousal pattern of synchronous delta activity similar to hypnagogic hypersynchrony.

In most cases, the timing of sleepwalking and the associated behavior make diagnosis straightforward. Occasionally, sleepwalking is a manifestation of a nocturnal complex partial seizure. In such patients, the nocturnal behavior is usually more stereotyped than in primary somnambulism. In the elderly demented patient, nocturnal wandering is more often due to waking disorientation than to sleepwalking.

SLEEP TERRORS AND CONFUSIONAL AROUSALS

Sleep terrors, also called pavor nocturnus or night terrors, are events of NREM sleep, usually occurring during stages 3 and 4. Like sleepwalking, sleep terrors are most common in children. They are characterized by arousal, agitation, and signs of sympathetic over-activity, including large pupils, sweating, tachycardia, tachypnea, and increased blood pressure. The child appears terrified, screams, and is usually inconsolable for several minutes, after which the child relaxes and returns to sleep. Usually there is either amnesia for the events or only a vague memory of monsters, impending death, suffocation, or other terrifying events. Sleep terrors may overlap with sleepwalking, in which walking or running is accompanied by shouting, jumping, and flailing about. Milder episodes, or confusional arousals, may be accompanied only by moaning, muttering, and thrashing (see Chapter 62).

Although sleep terrors can be distinguished from nightmares by the amnesia for the event, the distinction from nocturnal partial complex seizures and REM sleep behavior disorder may be more difficult. Sleep terrors usually occur early in the night and may be precipitated by emotional stress; seizures may occur at any time during the night. The REM sleep behavior disorder, which can also lead to screams and agitated violent behavior, is more common in older persons, can occur at any time of night, and is often associated with vivid dream recall and dream-enacting behaviors.

NIGHTMARES

Nightmares are dreams with vivid and frightening content (see Chapter 66). In contrast to night terrors, nightmares occur during REM sleep, and there is usually immediate awakening and good recall of the dream content. Although anxiety and increased heart rate may follow the nightmare, the extreme autonomic features characteristic of night terrors are rarely present.

REM SLEEP BEHAVIORS

REM sleep behaviors are complex, vigorous, or violent behaviors, sometimes associated with dream-like thoughts and images, that occur during pathological REM sleep. Patients with REM sleep behaviors may complain of sleep disruption, violent behavior with injuries to themself or to the bed partner, or unpleasant and vivid dreams.

Although muscle atonia limits movements in most people during REM sleep to brief twitches, the muscle tone of patients with REM sleep behavior disorders is abnormally preserved during some or all of REM sleep. Patients are usually middle-aged or elderly, and about one third have an associated neurological disease.

REM sleep behaviors may be mistaken for night terrors, nightmares, panic attacks, or seizures. The accompanying dream imagery and mentation, the occurrence in older persons, and the lack of pronounced autonomic activation are features that help differentiate REM sleep behaviors from night terrors. Prominent motor activity is not a feature of nightmares, and nocturnal anxiety and panic attacks are usually not associ-

ated with violent behavior or injuries. Although partial complex seizures are rarely associated with dream enactment, polysomnographic studies may be required to exclude seizures as a cause. REM sleep behavior disorder is discussed in Chapter 64.

HEAD-BANGING

Head-banging, or jactatio capitis nocturna, is characterized by rhythmical forward-and-back head movements, sometimes accompanied by rocking body movements, occurring just before sleep and during stages 1 and 2. The movements are more common in infants and children than in adults and may occur in the prone or supine position. Although the rhythmical movements may resemble seizures and, in rare cases, may be seizures, the occurrence at sleep onset and the duration, as much as 1 h or more, help distinguish head-banging from epilepsy.

PERIODIC MOVEMENTS OF SLEEP

Periodic movements of sleep are rhythmical, repetitive, stereotyped limb muscle contractions, usually affecting the legs, that can be synchronous or asynchronous (see Chapter 65). A typical movement consists of great toe extension, ankle dorsiflexion, and a variable degree of knee and hip flexion or extension. The contractions recur at regular intervals of 10 to 120 sec.

The incidence of periodic movements increases with age and with some neurological and metabolic disorders. These movements may cause insomnia or excessive daytime sleepiness, or they may be asymptomatic and a source of concern and discomfort only to the bed partner. Periodic leg movements frequently accompany sleep apnea, and the main complaint from the bed partner of some patients with sleep apnea may be leg kicks at night.

When periodic movements occur at sleep onset, they must be distinguished from hypnic jerks, which are not periodic, do not predominate in the legs, and persist for only a few minutes after sleep onset. Other movements that may be mistaken for periodic leg movements include dyskinesias, leg cramps, epileptic seizures, and myoclonus due to degenerative neurological disease.

Dyskinesias are choreiform movements and myoclonic jerks that are most common in patients taking excessive amounts of dopamine agonists. They differ from periodic leg movements in that they are often aperiodic, occur in facial as well as in limb muscles, and are present during wakefulness as well as during sleep. Nocturnal leg cramps are painful contractions that produce a visible prolonged muscle tightening as opposed to the brief, painless, repetitive contractions of periodic leg movements. Seizures, particularly partial motor seizures and myoclonic epilepsy, can cause repetitive jerking of the extremities, but the movements seldom occur with a periodicity of greater than 1 sec. Myoclonus associated with degenerative neurological diseases is most prominent during wakefulness and rarely persists into sleep.

References

1. Jennett B, Plum F. The persistent vegetative state: a syndrome in search of a name. Lancet. 1972;1:734–737.
2. Levy DE, Sidtis JJ, Rottenberg DA, et al. Differences in cerebral blood flow and glucose metabolism in vegetative versus locked-in patients. Ann Neurol. 1987;22:673–682.
3. Plum F, Posner JB. The Diagnosis of Stupor and Coma. 3rd ed. Contemporary Neurology Series. Philadelphia, Pa: FA Davis; 1980.
4. Johns MW. A new method for measuring daytime sleepiness: the Epworth Sleepiness Scale. Sleep. 1991;14:540–545.
5. Chervin RD, Aldrich MS, Pickett R, et al. Comparison of the results of the Epworth Sleepiness Scale and the multiple sleep latency test. J Psychosom Res. 1997;42:145–155.
6. Johns MW. Daytime sleepiness, snoring, and obstructive sleep apnea: the Epworth Sleepiness Scale. Chest. 1993;103:30–36.
7. Hoffstein V. Snoring. Chest. 1996;109:201–222.
8. Aldrich MS, Chauncey JB. Are morning headaches part of obstructive sleep apnea syndrome? Arch Intern Med. 1990;150:1265–1267.
9. Buckle P, Kerr P, Kryger M. Nocturnal cluster headache associated with sleep apnea. A case report. Sleep. 1993;16:487–489.
10. Gittinger JW Jr, Miller NR, Keltner JL, et al. Sugarplum fairies, visual hallucinations. Surv Ophthalmol. 1982;27:42–48.
11. McKee AC, Levine DN, Kowall NW, et al. Peduncular hallucinosis associated with isolated infarction of the substantia nigra pars reticulata. Ann Neurol. 1990;27:500–504.

45

Use of Clinical Tools and Tests in Sleep Medicine

Ronald D. Chervin

Many chapters of this textbook describe the clinical and laboratory characteristics of specific sleep disorders. Clinicians use such knowledge, which is essential but not sufficient to identify and assess sleep disorders, in combination with sound clinical reasoning. This chapter reviews a key element of the clinical reasoning process—the value of diagnostic information in evaluations of sleep-related complaints. The material bears on practical decisions clinicians must constantly make: what questions to ask, what parts to examine, what tests to order, what conclusions to draw, and what degree of confidence to invest in those conclusions. The first section of this chapter discusses methodological concepts needed to understand the value of diagnostic information. Subsequent sections provide a review of available data on the value of test results in the evaluation of four common clinical problems: suspected obstructive sleep-disordered breathing, hypersomnolence, insomnia, and parasomnias. The chapter concludes with introductions to more formal clinical decision-making and to cost-effectiveness analysis, methods that are likely to increase in use by physicians and health care managers who must provide optimal care with limited resources. Detailed descriptions of the laboratory procedures mentioned in this chapter are provided in Section 15.

ASSESSMENT OF DIAGNOSTIC VALUE

The value of a diagnostic tool depends on test-specific characteristics but also on the patient sample to be tested. The sensitivity and specificity of a test are largely test-specific characteristics. The sensitivity of a test represents the probability that the test will be positive given that the person has the disorder in question. The specificity of a test represents the probability that the test will be negative given that the person does not have the disorder. Sensitivity and specificity can be determined when another test exists that can be considered a *gold standard*. Tests that are valuable in clinical practice often have high sensitivity and specificity, although for some purposes one can be high and the other low. For example, to screen for a rare but serious disorder, a quick, inexpensive test with high sensitivity but low specificity might be useful to identify patients who require more extensive testing.

The prevalence of the disorder in the tested population also determines the value of the test. The *prevalence* is the proportion of persons who have the disorder or the probability that a randomly selected individual has the disorder. Information on prevalence, sensitivity, and specificity can be used with Bayes' theorem to calculate the positive predictive value (PPV), which is the probability that a patient with a positive test actually has the disorder.[1] Bayes' theorem also allows calculation of the negative predictive value (NPV), which is the probability that a patient with a negative test is truly free of the disorder. The equations can be expressed as:

$$\mathrm{PPV} = \frac{\mathrm{prev^*sens}}{\mathrm{prev^*sens} + (1 - \mathrm{prev})^*(1 - \mathrm{spec})}$$

$$\mathrm{NPV} = \frac{(1 - \mathrm{prev})^*\mathrm{spec}}{(1 - \mathrm{prev})^*\mathrm{spec} + \mathrm{prev}^*(1 - \mathrm{sens})}$$

where prev is prevalence, sens is sensitivity, and spec is specificity. Although prevalence has a strong effect on predictive values, a test with high sensitivity tends to have a high NPV, and a test with high specificity tends to have a high PPV.

After an interview and examination, a clinician may suspect a particular disorder based on many clues besides the knowledge of prevalence. In considering the usefulness of a further test, the pretest probability of disease, rather than the prevalence, and the posttest or posterior probability given a positive or negative test become the relevant values.[2] Tests are valuable to the extent that the posterior probability of disease is significantly lower or higher than the pretest probability.

Other concepts important in the assessment of diagnostic tools include validity and reliability. Valid tests measure what they are intended to measure; reliable tests yield results that are repeatable. The validity of a test can be supported in many different ways: theory; intuition; agreement of experts; comparison with a gold standard, outcome, or other available signs; convergence with expectations based on related findings; or ability to distinguish differences among conditions. The overall reliability of a test is supported by test-retest reliability, interrater reliability, and internal consistency.[3]

EVALUATION FOR OBSTRUCTIVE SLEEP-RELATED BREATHING DISORDERS

History and Questionnaires

The value of interview and questionnaire information has been studied with respect to polysomnographically confirmed diagnoses of obstructive sleep apnea syndrome (OSAS) and, to a much lesser extent, upper airway resistance syndrome (UARS). For primary snoring, no objective measure has been shown to be better than subjective reports.[4]

In the diagnosis of OSAS, overall subjective clinical impressions have inadequate sensitivity and specificity.[5, 6] Combinations of specific symptoms can have sensitivity above 0.90, but the specificity is usually poor (Table 45–1). Although most studies have not reported the PPV and NPV, the sensitivity and specificity results suggest that the NPV of some combinations of symptoms may be good but the PPV is probably poor, especially when the prevalence of OSAS in the tested population is not high.[7] Accordingly, patients without a history suggestive of OSAS usually do not receive further testing for it. Even among patients referred to sleep centers for suspected OSAS, models based on symptoms and demographic features may allow a minority to be classified as apnea free without further tests.[5, 8] However, patients who do have symptoms of OSAS are usually tested.

Although the PPV of symptoms is not high in general, a minority of patients have a clinical picture that is nearly unmistakably diagnostic. The International Classification of Sleep Disorders lists a strongly positive history as adequate to fulfill minimal criteria for a diagnosis of OSAS.[9] In these cases, tests may be useful to define the severity of OSAS but they are not needed to confirm the diagnosis. Perhaps more importantly, in some patients who have multiple, stereotypic symptoms of OSAS, the diagnosis should still be suspected when it is not initially confirmed by oximetry, ambulatory cardiorespiratory sleep studies, or even single-night polysomnography, which are not infallible (see later).

Conclusions about the diagnostic values of specific symptoms are difficult to synthesize from studies with significant methodological differences. The author's clinical impressions are listed in Table 45–2, with reference to adults referred for sleep evaluations. These data are not quantitative or precise, but they provide some indication of the degree to which particular symptoms affect the probability of OSAS. In different populations, clinical values may be quite different. For example, among patients referred specifically for possible OSAS, the symptom of excessive daytime sleepiness (EDS) may[10] or may not[11] be useful in making the diagnosis, and a history of hypertension may be better than a report of snoring as an indication that OSAS is present.[12] In the general population, the symptom with the highest predictive value for OSAS is habitual snoring, although EDS and observed apneas are also useful.[13]

Comparatively less is known about the clinical value of historical symptoms in the diagnosis of UARS. The probability of UARS rather than OSAS may be increased by youth, female gender, and normal body weight.[14, 15] The probability of UARS rather than primary snoring is increased by the presence of EDS or insomnia and may be increased by a history of hypertension, dysmenorrhea, chronic fatigue syndrome, or bruxism.[14, 16, 17] The likelihood of UARS rather than no sleep-related breathing disorder is increased by a history of snoring, but the absence of snoring may not diminish the probability of UARS as much as it does the probability of OSAS.[16]

Physical Examination

Of variables related to body weight, neck circumference and body mass index (BMI; measured in weight [in kg]/height [in m^2]), in this order, correlate best with the presence and severity of OSAS in the general population.[18] Among patients referred for possible OSAS, weight-related variables may also be useful, but their predictive value is not large except in extreme ranges.[5, 6, 8, 10–12, 19–21]

Patients with OSAS who are not obese often have craniofacial abnormalities associated with narrowing of the upper airway.[22] However, much of the literature on craniofacial anomalies concerns the results of cephalometric radiographs or acoustic radiographs rather than bedside findings.[23–25] Reports of oropharyngeal examination findings are often subjective and not quantified. A recently developed quantitative model to aid in the diagnosis of OSAS is based on BMI, neck circumference, and bedside craniofacial measurements that include palatal height, maxillary intermolar distance, mandibular intermolar distance, and overjet.[26] In a series of 300 sleep center patients diagnosed with the use of polysomnography, the model showed a sensitivity of 98% and a specificity of 100% for obstructive sleep apnea. The PPV was 100% and the NPV was 89%, which represent significant improvements in the pretest probabilities of OSAS (85%) and the absence of OSAS (15%), respectively. The predictive value of the model has not yet been reported for other populations of patients, such as those studied specifically for suspected sleep-disordered breathing, those seen in a primary practice setting, or those suspected of having UARS.

Physical findings other than craniofacial features and obesity may also have value in the diagnosis of OSAS, but their values remain poorly defined. As discussed above, a history of hypertension is associated with an increased probability of OSAS, and a high blood pressure measurement also increases the chance that OSAS will be present, especially among persons who are less obese.[27] Nasal obstruction may be an important clue to the presence of OSAS, as may signs of neuropathy or neuromuscular disease.[28, 29]

Nocturnal Polysomnography

A nocturnal, laboratory-based polysomnogram (PSG) is the most commonly used test in the diagnosis

Table 45-1. VALUE OF HISTORICAL OR QUESTIONNAIRE-DERIVED DIAGNOSTIC INFORMATION IN THE DIAGNOSIS OF OBSTRUCTIVE SLEEP APNEA AT SLEEP CENTERS: REPRESENTATIVE STUDIES

Reference	Subjects	Gold Standard	Model	Sensitivity	Specificity	Other Results Provided
Kapuniai et al., 1988[119]	53 sleep center patients	AHI > 10 on PSG	Observed apneas, loud snoring	0.78	0.67	
Crocker et al., 1990[12]	105 sleep center patients	AHI > 15 on PSG	Observed apneas, hypertension, BMI, age	0.92	0.51	
Viner et al., 1991[5]	410 patients referred for suspected sleep apnea	AHI > 10 on PSG	Age, BMI, male sex, snoring	0.94*	0.28*	PPV* = 0.75 with pretest probability of OSA = 0.46
			Subjective impression	0.52	0.70	
Bliwise et al., 1991[120]	1409 patients referred for sleep-related problems	AHI ≥ 10	Usually has . . . Any snoring	Men, 0.97 Women, 0.82	Men, 0.47 Women, 0.79	
			Disruptive snoring	Men, 0.89 Women, 0.71	Men, 0.71 Women, 0.89	
			Nocturnal breath-holding	Men, 0.70 Women, 0.47	Men, 0.88 Women, 0.96	
Haraldsson et al. 1992[121]	42 patients referred for snoring	AI > 10	Habitual snoring, sleep disturbances, sleepiness	0.91	0.74	PPV = 0.56 with pretest probability of OSA = 0.26 NPV = 0.96 with pretest probability of no OSA = 0.74
Hoffstein and Szalai, 1993[6]	594 patients referred for suspected sleep apnea	AHI > 10 on PSG	Age, sex, BMI, observed apneas, pharyngeal examination			Regression model explained 36% of variability in square root-transform of AHI
			Subjective impression	0.60	0.63	
Rauscher et al., 1993[122]	116 patients referred for heavy snoring	AHI > 10	Weight, height, sex, observed apneas, falling asleep while reading	0.94	0.45	
Flemons et al., 1994[11]	180 patients suspected of having sleep apnea	AHI > 10	Habitual snoring, observed gasping/choking, neck circumference, hypertension			PPV* = 0.81 with pretest probability of OSA = 0.45 Model explained 34% of the variation in AHI
Dealberto et al., 1994[10]	129 adults referred for nocturnal PSG	AHI ≥ 10	Loud habitual snoring, observed apneas, sex, age, BMI	0.82	0.68	
Douglass et al., 1994[123]	435 patients with specified sleep disorders and 84 normal control subjects	Followed ICSD[9] criteria and had PSG, but PSG criteria not otherwise specified	Several snoring questions, observed apneas, sweat at night, history of hypertension, nasal obstruction, weight, years of smoking, age, BMI	Men, 0.85 Women, 0.88	Men, 0.76 Women, 0.81	Men: PPV = 0.72, NPV = 0.87 with pretest probability of OSAS = 0.42 Women: PPV = 0.31, NPV = 0.99 with pretest probability of OSAS = 0.09
Deegan and McNicholas, 1996[8]	250 patients referred for suspected sleep-disordered breathing	AHI ≥ 15	Observed apneas Snoring Falls asleep driving Predominant sleep position is supine			PPV = 0.64, NPV = 0.53 PPV = 0.63, NPV = 0.56 PPV = 0.70, NPV = 0.51 PPV = 0.77, NPV = 0.47 With pretest probability of OSA = 0.54 and pretest probability of no OSA = 0.46

*Dependent on cutoff chosen for model results.
AHI, apnea-hypopnea index (number of apneas or hypopneas per hour of sleep); AI, apnea index; BMI, body mass index; NPV, negative predictive value; PPV, positive predictive value; PSG, polysomnography.

Table 45–2. ESTIMATED CLINICAL VALUES OF SPECIFIC SYMPTOMS IN THE DIAGNOSIS OF OSAS, WITH REFERENCE TO PATIENTS REFERRED TO A SLEEP CLINIC

Symptom	Effect on Probability of OSAS	
	Symptom Present	Symptom Absent
Habitual snoring	↑ ↑	↓ ↓ ↓
Loud snoring	↑ ↑ ↑	↓ ↓
Observed apneas	↑ ↑ ↑	↓
Sleepy while driving	↑ ↑	↓
Sleepy while reading	↑	↓ ↓
Morning headaches	↑	↓
Dry mouth on awakening	↑ ↑	↓
Nocturia (>1 episode per night)	↑ ↑	↓
Excessive sweating at night	↑ ↑	↓
Nocturnal reflux	↑ ↑	↓
Sleep maintenance insomnia	↑ ↑	↓ ↓
Nocturnal restlessness	↑	↓ ↓
History of hypertension	↑ ↑	↓
History of stroke	↑ ↑	↓

↑ ↑ ↑, large increase; ↑ ↑, moderate increase; ↑, little or no increase; ↓ ↓ ↓, large decrease; ↓ ↓, moderate decrease; ↓, little or no decrease.
OSAS, obstructive sleep apnea syndrome.

of OSAS, and it is considered a gold standard. In many cases, the PSG also demonstrates the severity of OSAS and can reveal other concurrent sleep disorders. The PSG allows direct monitoring and quantification of the respiratory events and neurophysiological consequences—arousals and awakenings—that are believed to cause daytime symptoms in OSAS. Despite its empirical and intuitive attractiveness, the PSG in isolation is not a perfect test for sleep-related breathing disorders, in large part due to the effects of night-to-night variability, the lack of widely accepted standards for some aspects of polysomnography, and the absence of a high correlation between the severity of abnormal findings and patients' symptoms.

Although a single-night PSG is usually sufficient to diagnose or exclude the diagnosis of OSAS,[30] false-negative test results can occur. Night-to-night biological variability may be particularly high in subjects with low but clinically significant rates of apneas and hypopneas during sleep.[31, 32] In one study, when 11 patients thought likely to have OSAS on clinical grounds were restudied after the initial negative PSGs, 6 were found to have OSAS.[33]

In contrast to widely accepted standards for scoring normal sleep,[34] standards for scoring sleep-related breathing abnormalities are not uniform among laboratories. When research shows what types and severities of sleep-related breathing disorders cause symptoms and complications, clearer standards may emerge. Until that time, however, the clinician must be aware of several variations in practice that make the interpretation of unfamiliar reports more difficult. Most importantly, the definition of an hypopnea varies considerably among laboratories.[35] Many, but not all laboratories, require a duration of at least 10 sec, and

some, but not all, require an associated oxygen desaturation or a variously defined arousal. Although many laboratories require some minimum percentage decrease in airflow signal, most do not measure airflow with a quantitative technique.

The definition of an apnea also varies; some laboratories require complete cessation of airflow, whereas others allow for a small percentage (e.g., 20%) of the original airflow signal. Some laboratories score respiratory arousals not associated with apneas or hypopneas when they detect that sequences of increasing snoring or increasing negative esophageal pressures precede arousals. Most laboratories report a summary measure, called the apnea-hypopnea index (AHI) or the respiratory disturbance index, which represents the sum total of apneas, hypopneas, and—sometimes in the second case—respiratory arousals per hour of sleep. An index of this type is often given the most weight in interpretation of whether the study shows significant sleep-disordered breathing. Other commonly used results—the extent and frequency of oxygen desaturations—are also tallied and reported in differing formats. The result is that interpretation of PSG reports is complicated, requires training and experience, and may not be definitive without clinical information about the patient.

Despite researchers' tendency to use a specified AHI threshold to define OSAS, the clinician cannot succumb to the same temptation. An individual patient with an AHI of 30 is likely to have excessive daytime sleepiness and an increased risk for cardiovascular complications but may not have either. Conversely, a patient with an AHI of 0.3 may still have OSAS (because night-to-night variability exists) or may have another obstructive sleep-related breathing disorder with associated sleepiness and complications.[16, 17] Interpretation of a PSG without knowledge of the patient's clinical presentation can lead to serious underdiagnosis or overdiagnosis. Many clinicians believe that an AHI above 5 suggests OSAS, but a large population-based epidemiological study found that only 22.6% of women and 15.5% of men who met this criterion clearly complained of daytime hypersomnolence.[18] Some patients who meet polysomnographic criteria for OSAS but do not complain of hypersomnolence may have little to gain from treatment.

Future research may refine the ability to monitor aspects of sleep-disordered breathing that affect health and daytime sleepiness. The AHI and minimum oxygen saturation do not correlate well with objectively measured daytime sleepiness,[36] although AHI may correlate better with other complications, such as hypertension.[27] Many patients with UARS have, by definition, excessive daytime sleepiness in the absence of a significant AHI. Additional measures that may prove useful in explaining health-related consequences of sleep-disordered breathing include the frequency of brief electrocortical arousals[37] and esophageal pressure.

In short, the PSG is the single most useful and definitive test in the diagnosis of sleep-related breathing disorders, but the information it provides cannot be reliably interpreted by persons without experience in sleep medicine, summarized on the basis of any single value, or applied to patient care without careful use of additional clinical data. Failure to recognize these limitations, by health care policy makers or clinicians, can deprive a patient of treatment for a dangerous but easily controlled disorder.

Modified Forms of the Polysomnogram

In comparison with the standard PSG, daytime nap studies and split-night studies can reduce the costs of diagnosis. Studies of daytime PSGs have sometimes found a high NPV, if not PPV, for OSAS, but inconsistent results and the lack of further data explain why daytime PSGs are not generally recommended.[7, 38] Split-night studies may save the patient from an extra night in the sleep laboratory, but whether diagnosis and treatment are adequately established in this manner is debated,[38] and the procedure is recommended only for specified patients and circumstances.[39]

Several additional physiological variables can be recorded with a standard PSG, but the additional predictive value they provide has not been well quantified. These additional variables include end-tidal or transcutaneous CO_2 and nasal pressure.[40, 41, 41a, 41b] The monitoring of esophageal pressures greatly facilitates the diagnosis of UARS and is particularly helpful when sleep-disordered breathing is evaluated in patients who lack typical symptoms, signs, or demographics, as do many young, female, or thin individuals.[15, 42] However, criteria for abnormal esophageal pressure recordings, as defined by association with poor outcomes, require further study and refinement.

Portable Recording

The wide range of recordings that can be performed during sleep at a patient's home are designed primarily to test for OSAS, although a portable esophageal catheter has been developed that may offer the potential to diagnose UARS.[43] These portable recordings are less costly than laboratory-based PSGs, and patients usually prefer home studies to laboratory studies. However, the diagnostic value of portable systems is reduced by the inability to make behavioral observations, standardize recording conditions, address technical problems, or make interventions during the night. Cardiorespiratory portable studies may show respiratory events that cannot be assumed to have occurred during sleep and may fail to demonstrate disorders other than OSAS.

Consensus committee reviews of portable monitoring systems have noted that relevant research has focused on many different recording systems, reducing the adequacy of data for any one system.[44] Few studies have compared portable monitors used at home, rather than the laboratory, with laboratory-based PSGs. Several cardiorespiratory recording devices have sensitivities of 95% or more but have lower specificities. Predictive values have rarely been reported. Available evidence on diagnostic value suggests that the use of

portable monitoring should be limited to several specific circumstances[45]: (1) urgent evaluation of patients with severe symptoms when laboratory polysomnography is not readily available, (2) evaluation of patients unable to be studied in a sleep laboratory, and (3) evaluation of response to therapy once the diagnosis has been established and especially if multiple subsequent evaluations will be necessary.

Despite limited validation data for many portable recording devices, those with low costs, high sensitivities, and high specificities have convinced some clinicians that portable studies are cost effective in comparison with PSGs. However, one published model suggested the opposite,[45a] and additional cost-effectiveness analyses should be a priority in coming years because their outcomes are not easy to predict (see later). The need for laboratory-based studies may be obviated by strongly positive portable studies when pretest probability is high, or perhaps by strongly negative portable studies when pretest probability is low.[38] In other situations, the initial performance of portable studies can increase health care dollars spent on the diagnosis of OSAS, on the treatment of patients who do not have OSAS, and on the treatment of medical consequences in patients who have OSAS but escape diagnosis.

Studies of Airway Morphology

Although imaging of the upper airway for research purposes has led to a better understanding of OSAS pathophysiology, such studies are not routinely performed in diagnostic evaluations of patients, in part because findings that predict OSAS or its severity with sufficient accuracy have not been identified. Cephalometric radiography and pharyngoscopy may be useful in the preoperative identification of sites of obstruction and in the selection of appropriate surgical procedures.[46–50] The diagnostic value of cephalometrics may be limited in part because only sagittal-plane dimensions are provided and coronal-plane dimensions may be more pertinent to OSAS.[51] Pharyngoscopy allows three-dimensional anatomic characterization, but whether airway collapse with Mueller's maneuver predicts response to uvulopalatopharyngoplasty is debatable.[52–54] Pharyngoscopy may be particularly valuable if performed during supine sleep.[55]

Computed tomography and magnetic resonance imaging (MRI) studies can show upper airway morphology,[51, 56, 57] and some authors suggest the potential for clinical usefulness,[58] but the value of these techniques in the clinical setting is not well defined. In particular, it is uncertain whether imaging techniques more sophisticated and expensive than cephalometric radiographs and pharyngoscopy provide additional, valuable clinical information.

Ancillary Studies

The complete evaluation of a patient with suspected sleep-disordered breathing frequently includes investigation for common comorbid conditions. For patients with chronic pulmonary diseases, appropriate parts of the evaluation may include awake and asleep arterial blood gas measurements, chest radiographs, pulmonary function tests, and referral to a pulmonologist. A co-morbid neuropathy, myopathy, or brainstem disorder may trigger referral for a neurological evaluation, electromyogram, or brain MRI. Other patients require psychiatric, cardiac, endocrine, renal, or gastrointestinal investigations. Co-morbid conditions should be considered in patients with suspected sleep-disordered breathing, but investigations beyond a complete history and examination are not routinely required unless symptoms or signs of such disorders are present.

EVALUATION OF HYPERSOMNOLENCE

History and Questionnaires

The history provides important clues to the severity of hypersomnolence. Direct inquiry about sleepiness can be supplemented by questions about sleepiness in sedentary situations, such as driving, desk work, reading, or watching TV. The accuracy of these self-assessments has not been extensively studied, but patients may report little of the EDS suggested by family members, clinical signs, or objective tests.[59] In one clinical series, patients' self-assessments of levels of sleepiness showed no significant association with results of the multiple sleep latency test (MSLT).[60]

Questionnaires such as the Epworth Sleepiness Scale (see Chapters 44 and 104) and the Stanford Sleepiness Scale provide a more formal and perhaps reliable measure of EDS.[61–63] The impact of sleepiness on activities of daily living can be assessed with the Functional Outcomes of Sleep Questionnaire.[64] The results of the Epworth scale correlate with subjective assessments of sleepiness and, to a small extent, with MSLT results in some case series but not in one of the largest.[60, 63, 65, 66] Although the Epworth and Stanford scales have some clinical use, such as when monitoring the response to treatment over time, they do not substitute for well-validated objective measures of sleepiness.

Physical Examination

Although the alerting effect of an examination obscures the physical signs of sleepiness in most patients, overt signs of sleepiness—such as the inability to stay awake or to keep eyes open in the examination room—have a high PPV and may obviate the need for additional tests. The examination may also help to distinguish severe sleepiness from stupor due to neurological impairment or drugs. Rarely, ancillary laboratory tests such as an electroencephalogram or drug screen are necessary to help make this distinction.

Nocturnal Polysomnography

Many patients referred to sleep centers for EDS have nocturnal sleep disorders, and polysomnography is of-

ten more notable for the manifestations of such disorders than for signs of EDS. Patients whose EDS is due to insufficient sleep can show shorter sleep latencies, increased sleep efficiency, decreased stage 1 sleep, and increased amounts of rapid eye movement (REM) sleep and deep nonrapid eye movement (NREM) sleep. The polysomnographic variable that best reflects sleepiness, as measured by the mean sleep latency on an MSLT, is nocturnal sleep latency.[36] Polysomnographic measures of sleep pathology, such as the AHI and minimum oxygen saturation, show only low magnitudes of correlation with MSLT results.[36, 67]

Multiple Sleep Latency Test

The mean sleep latency on the MSLT is the most commonly used objective measure in assessment of daytime sleepiness. The MSLT often contributes to diagnosis but is usually not sufficient alone to establish a diagnosis. The mean sleep latency is most useful when it is clearly abnormally low. A patient with a mean sleep latency of 1 min on a properly performed MSLT[68] is unlikely to be exaggerating a complaint of EDS, to have fatigue rather than sleepiness, or to be free of any sleep disorder. The MSLT can help to determine the clinical significance of a sleep disorder or to assess the response to treatment.

Despite clear clinical utility of the MSLT, its interpretation requires knowledge of its limitations. First, the NPV of even a very high mean sleep latency is likely to be less than the PPV of a very low result. When an MSLT is normal, other clinical data also must be considered before a patient is told that he or she does not have EDS. The main reason is that interpretation of the MSLT result is contingent on circumstances being optimally conducive to sleep, and in practice, many factors, such as anxiety, are difficult to control.[69, 70] Another limitation of the MSLT is that results between the extremes are less useful and their interpretation varies among both researchers and clinicians. Formal studies of outcomes associated with different mean sleep latencies are still needed, but until such data are available, clinicians should realize that MSLT results form a continuum without strictly interpretable cutoffs; extreme results, and especially positive ones, contribute more useful information than do middle-range values. Like most other physiological tests, the MSLT is subject to test-retest biological variation, which also must be taken into account when results are interpreted. For example, a patient's mean sleep latency may be 4 min on one day and 7 min on another without any intervening therapy. High test-retest reliability among normal subjects[71] does not necessarily generalize to patients.[72] Interrater reliability can be excellent[73] but adds another source of potential variation in test results.

Finally, interpretation of the mean sleep latency on the MSLT must take into account available data on the validity of the test. The most consistent data in support of the validity of the MSLT were generated in experiments with sleep deprivation, restriction, or fragmentation.[74–77] However, in clinical practice, polysomnographic measures of the severity of sleep disorders may show small[67, 78–80] or insignificant[36, 81, 82] correlation with MSLT results. A clinician should not be surprised if a patient with eight apneic events per hour of sleep has a lower mean sleep latency than a patient who has 50 such events per hour of sleep. Furthermore, despite clear clinical improvement demonstrated by sleep apneics and other patients treated for their sleep disorders, the MSLT does not always reflect the improvement.[16, 81, 83–87]

Evidence that mean sleep latency on the MSLT does not necessarily parallel other measures of sleepiness or reflect patient symptoms may mean that the MSLT does not precisely measure sleepiness. However, the same evidence also can be used to support the importance of the MSLT, which provides unique data that cannot be generated by other methods. Sleepiness may have several aspects, some of which are measured better by the MSLT and some by other means.[88] The investigators who developed the MSLT originally described it as a measure of physiological sleep tendency rather than a direct measure of sleepiness,[89] and the narrower concept may define an important part of the neurophysiological state of sleepiness without capturing the entire concept.

Use of the Multiple Sleep Latency Test in the Diagnosis of Narcolepsy

The MSLT criteria for narcolepsy—two or more sleep-onset REM periods (SOREMPs) and a short mean sleep latency—were once thought to have high sensitivity and specificity, in part because original series suggested that all narcoleptics and no normal control subjects had two or more SOREMPs.[90, 91] Subsequent analyses of two larger groups of patients showed that not 1 of 63 sleepy non-narcoleptic patients met this criterion[92] or that only 1 of 83 non-narcoleptics did so.[93] In the latter study, the PPV of two or more SOREMPs for the diagnosis of narcolepsy was 98%, and the NPV was 89%.

In part because of the changing composition of patients who present for sleep evaluations, later studies did not find the SOREMP criteria to provide such diagnostic accuracy. Two or more SOREMPs were found in 25% of 187 sleep apneics,[94] 17% of 139 normal subjects,[95] and only 83% of 200 narcoleptics who had cataplexy.[96] Among 2083 patients evaluated with MSLTs at one sleep center, the PPV of two or more SOREMPs was 57% and the NPV was 98%.[97] Other MSLT and PSG criteria may have additional uses (Table 45–3), but the data suggest that MSLT results cannot be used alone to diagnose narcolepsy and that the presence of SOREMPs must be interpreted in conjunction with other clinical and polysomnographic findings. In particular, the criterion of two or more SOREMPs cannot be used to diagnose narcolepsy when the patient has untreated OSAS, UARS, or other sleep disorders that can be associated with SOREMPs. When the MSLT does not show two or more SOREMPs, the

Table 45–3. SENSITIVITIES, SPECIFICITIES, AND PREDICTIVE VALUES OF SEVERAL DIFFERENT POLYSOMNOGRAPHIC CRITERIA FOR THE DIAGNOSIS OF NARCOLEPSY AT A SLEEP CENTER

	Sensitivity	Specificity	PPV	NPV
Multiple Sleep Latency Test				
≥2 SOREMPs	0.80	0.93	0.57	0.98
≥2 SOREMPs and MSL <5 min	0.70	0.97	0.70	0.97
≥3 SOREMPs	0.48	0.98	0.77	0.94
≥3 SOREMPs and MSL <5 min	0.46	0.99	0.87	0.94
Nocturnal Polysomnogram				
SOREMP	0.29	0.99	0.68	0.93
SOREMP and sleep latency <10 min	0.27	0.99	0.73	0.92

Republished with permission of the American Sleep Disorders Association, 6301 Bandel Road, Suite 101, Rochester, MN 55901. Figure, M.S. Aldrich, R.D. Chervin, B.A. Malow, *Sleep*, 1997, Vol. 20. Reproduced by permission of the publisher via Copyright Clearance Center, Inc.

MSL, mean sleep latency on multiple sleep latency test; NPV, negative predictive value; PPV, positive predictive value; SOREMPs, sleep-onset rapid eye movement periods.

diagnosis of narcolepsy (in the absence of cataplexy) is less likely but not completely excluded.

Variations of the Multiple Sleep Latency Test and Other Physiological Tests

Results on the Maintenance of Wakefulness Test (MWT) can differ markedly from those of the MSLT,[98] but whether the MWT results are more predictive of adverse effects of sleepiness in daily life remains unknown. The MWT results correlate with measures of sleep apnea severity to about the same extent as MSLT results[99] but may better reflect improvement with treatment.[86] Until more evidence accrues that information from the MWT differs in a clinically meaningful way from that generated with the MSLT, the MSLT will continue to offer the advantages of more published experience, familiarity among clinicians, and relevance to the diagnosis of narcolepsy.

Other MSLT modifications, for which limited validity data exist, include the assignment of a simple performance task during the nap attempts,[69] a formula to combine quantities of sleep stages attained on naps into an overall polygraphic score of sleepiness,[100] calculation of mean wake efficiencies (100 minus percentage of time asleep during nap attempt) as an alternative to mean sleep latencies,[101] and definition of sleep onset not by polysomnography but by a subject's failure to respond to an intermittent light signal.[102] In the clinical setting, none of these modifications have a well-established role in the evaluation of hypersomnolence; neither do a wide range of other physiological tests. Pupillometry, investigated for many years, has not proved to be as useful as was originally hoped.[103, 104] Brainstem auditory evoked potentials may vary with sleepiness but are not a clinically useful measure of sleepiness.[105]

Finally, a variety of performance-based tests are used in research settings to assess variables related to sleepiness, such as the Psychomotor Vigilance Task[106] and the Steer Clear driving simulation test.[107]

EVALUATION OF INSOMNIA

Like EDS, the complaint of inadequate, insufficient, or nonrestorative sleep can have many different causes. Unlike causes of hypersomnia, however, sleep disorders that cause insomnia are most often diagnosed by history alone.[108, 109] In part because the gold standard is not a physiological test, little data are available with which to assess the relative value of individual symptoms. Predictive values for some symptoms are likely to be high because symptoms define the disorders. When a history does not reveal a cause for the insomnia, polysomnography may be useful (see later), but referral to an appropriate specialist for further history taking and evaluation is sometimes necessary. For example, if the sleep clinician cannot thoroughly evaluate a patient for depression, a psychiatrist or psychologist may be better able to establish a diagnosis and treatment regimen that will lead to resolution of the patient's insomnia. Psychometric tests can reveal cognitive differences between insomniacs and normal control subjects,[110] but these tests are not commonly used for diagnostic purposes in the clinical sleep medicine setting.

Sleep logs are an important tool in the evaluation of insomnia,[111] but data on their predictive value have not been published. Logs are not necessary to establish the presence of insomnia but can help to define the severity and to facilitate identification of causes such as inadequate sleep hygiene, delayed sleep phase syndrome, and psychophysiological insomnia.

The physical and mental status examinations may provide clues that the cause of a patient's insomnia is an underlying medical or psychiatric illness such as hyperthyroidism, asthma, benign prostatic hypertrophy, painful lumbar radiculopathy, arthritis, depression, or anxiety. The importance and focus of an examination vary depending on what is learned from the history. In patients with psychiatric causes of insomnia, the mental status examination may reveal valuable diagnostic clues such as pressured speech, thought disorders, depressed affect, or nervousness.

A patient's history and physical examination sometimes suggest that insomnia may be due to central sleep apnea, obstructive sleep apnea, periodic limb movement syndrome, or another physical sleep disorder. In such cases, polysomnography can be an important aid in diagnosis.[109] Clues that a physical cause of insomnia might be present include symptoms of the specific disorders but also some features of the insomnia itself and its response to treatment. For example, insomnia in patients with OSAS often consists of frequent brief awakenings during the night, whereas patients with psychophysiological insomnia rarely report this pattern. If a patient thought to have insomnia due to inadequate sleep hygiene experiences no improvement after successful efforts to correct the behavioral problems, a PSG may shed light on an occult diagnosis. Polysomnography may also be useful in some cases to document the severity of chronic insomnia[112] or to diagnose sleep state misperception. However, the injudicious use of polysomnography can sometimes enhance an insomniac's conviction that symptoms are due to physical rather than behavioral causes or lead to diagnoses that eventually prove irrelevant to the main complaint.

EVALUATION FOR SUSPECTED PARASOMNIAS

Although parasomnias are often diagnosed by history alone,[9] a history taken from a family member may be more contributory than that taken from the patient. Classic descriptions can be diagnostic for disorders such as sleep terrors, rhythmic movement disorder, sleep paralysis, sleep bruxism, and sleep enuresis, but the history in such cases can occasionally be misleading, as in a case of nocturnal behaviors and bed wetting episodes that were shown by polysomnography to occur only when the patient was awake.[113] Furthermore, some common histories for parasomnias lead to a differential diagnosis that frequently requires clarification by polysomnography; for example, the differential diagnosis for a middle-aged adult who presents with behavioral episodes at night may include REM sleep behavior disorder, sleepwalking, and complex partial seizures.

The physical examination of patients evaluated for parasomnias can be useful, but its value is not well quantified. Some signs may suggest sleep apnea as an underlying cause of confusional arousals, sleepwalking, sleep terrors, REM sleep behavior disorder, or nocturnal enuresis. Worn occlusive surfaces of molars can provide key evidence of sleep bruxism. The urogenital examination is important in patients suspected of having impaired sleep-related penile erections, sleep-related painful erections, or sleep enuresis. Endocrine, cardiac, vascular, and neurological examination findings can also show a cause for erectile dysfunction. A neurological examination may suggest a primary cause of sleep enuresis or REM sleep behavior disorder. Similarly, appropriate laboratory findings may be helpful in some cases; for example, a urinalysis may reveal the cause of sleep enuresis.

Few studies have examined the predictive value of polysomnography for parasomnia diagnoses. When the behavior in question occurs during polysomnography, the diagnostic value of the test is likely to be high, especially if appropriate additional recording devices, such as extra EEG leads, extra surface EMG leads, or video monitoring, are used.[114] Unfortunately, polysomnography often fails to document the behavior about which the patient complains—especially in cases of suspected REM sleep behavior disorder, sleepwalking, night terrors, and epilepsy—either because the behavior does not occur on most nights or because the sleep laboratory is not an environment familiar to the patient. Other signs of these parasomnias, besides the behavior in question, are often found on polysomnography, and some signs can have a high PPV. For example, an elevated baseline EMG tone, excessive limb twitching during REM sleep, and normal electroencephalography in a patient whose clinical history is consistent with REM sleep behavior disorder, sleep walking, or epilepsy adds substantially to suspicion of the first diagnosis. The NPP of a completely normal study, however, is less clear. In one series of 122 patients with suspected parasomnias, one or two nights of polysomnography with video monitoring contributed useful diagnostic information in more than 50% of the cases.[114]

BEYOND SENSITIVITY, SPECIFICITY, AND PREDICTIVE VALUE: DECISION AND COST-EFFECTIVENESS ANALYSES

Data on sensitivity, specificity, and pretest probability can be combined with data on the usefulness of different health-related outcomes to construct a decision analysis. A clinical decision analysis typically models a decision between diagnostic or therapeutic alternatives and uses logical rules to integrate information and to obtain the best decision for an individual patient.[2] Decision analysis is particularly useful when, for example, one procedure has a high probability of a small benefit while another procedure has a low probability of a large benefit. Although physicians may attempt a similar mental process, they often do not make optimal use of their beliefs about probabilities and values of outcomes. Decision analysis techniques have not been applied extensively in the sleep medicine literature.

Increasing economic pressures have expanded criteria for the evaluation of diagnostic procedures beyond utility to include cost and cost-effectiveness. Relevant types of economic analyses include (1) studies of the costs of procedures, the costs of treatments, and the costs associated with failure to treat sleep disorders; (2) cost-effectiveness analyses in which different methods to achieve the same end are compared; (3) cost-utility analyses that compare costs per common unit of utility (often quality-adjusted life years); and (4) cost-benefit analyses that compare monetary costs with monetary gains.[115] Such studies, which can focus on health-related outcomes associated with tests and treatments used in sleep medicine, require quantitative information on costs and outcomes.

As an example, the decision of whether to diagnose OSAS with the aid of a PSG, cardiorespiratory home study, or no ancillary test was modeled[45a] based on published figures for the utility of treatment in OSAS,[116] mortality rates when OSAS is untreated,[117] and high sensitivities and specificities reported for one home study device.[118] Polysomnography generated higher utility than the other diagnostic options, even when the pretest probability of OSAS was varied between

0.35 and 0.95. Sensitivity analyses for other key variables in the model suggested that polysomnography was preferable under almost every tested set of circumstances. Moreover, a cost-utility analysis suggested that the magnitude of the advantage of polysomnography over the other options easily justified the added initial expense. This result appeared to reflect the high utility of an OSAS diagnosis and the high costs of treatment of OSAS relative to the costs of an accurate diagnosis: diagnostic mistakes are expensive. These findings highlight the importance of performing decision and cost-utility analyses before conclusions are made about the relative values of tools and tests for the diagnosis of sleep disorders. In addition, the results of such analyses may confirm, for example, that each quality-adjusted life year added by a test for disordered sleep is inexpensive compared with each year added by funded procedures in other fields of medicine.[45a] Health care managers and policymakers will need such data to make decisions about the allocation of increasingly scarce resources.

References

1. Woolson RF. Statistical Methods for the Analysis of Biomedical Data. New York, NY: John Wiley & Sons; 1987.
2. Weinstein MC, Fineberg HV, Elstein AS, et al. Clinical Decision Analysis. Philadelphia, Pa: WB Saunders, 1980.
3. DeVellis RF. Scale Development: Theory and Applications. Newbury Park, Calif: Sage Publications; 1991.
4. Hoffstein V. Snoring. Chest. 1996;109:201–222.
5. Viner S, Szalai JP, Hoffstein V. Are history and physical examination a good screening test for sleep apnea? Ann Intern Med. 1991;115:356–359.
6. Hoffstein V, Szalai JP. Predictive value of clinical features in diagnosing obstructive sleep apnea. Sleep. 1993;16:118–122.
7. Chesson AL, Ferber RA, Fry JM, et al. The indications for polysomnography and related procedures. Sleep. 1997;20:423–487.
8. Deegan PC, McNicholas WT. Predictive value of clinical features for the obstructive sleep apnoea syndrome. Eur Respir J. 1996;9:117–124.
9. American Sleep Disorders Association. International Classification of Sleep Disorders, Revised: Diagnostic and Coding Manual. Rochester, Minn: American Sleep Disorders Association; 1997.
10. Dealberto MJ, Ferber C, Garma L, et al. Factors related to sleep apnea syndrome in sleep clinic patients. Chest. 1994;105:1753–1758.
11. Flemons WW, Whitelaw WA, Brant R, et al. Likelihood ratios for a sleep apnea clinical prediction rule. Am J Respir Crit Care Med. 1994;150:1279–1285.
12. Crocker BD, Olson LG, Saunders NA, et al. Estimation of the probability of disturbed breathing during sleep before a sleep study. Am Rev Respir Dis. 1990;142:14–18.
13. Young T, Hutton R, Finn L, et al. The gender bias in sleep apnea diagnosis: are women missed because they have different symptoms? Arch Intern Med. 1996;156:2445–2451.
14. Guilleminault C, Kim Y, Stoohs R. Upper airway resistance syndrome. Oral Maxillofac Surg Clin North Am. 1995;7:243–256.
15. Guilleminault C, Stoohs R, Kim Y, et al. Upper airway sleep-disordered breathing in women. Ann Intern Med. 1995;122:493–501.
16. Guilleminault C, Stoohs R, Clerk A, et al. A cause of excessive daytime sleepiness: the upper airway resistance syndrome. Chest. 1993;104:781–787.
17. Guilleminault C, Stoohs R, Shiomi T, et al. Upper airway resistance syndrome, nocturnal blood pressure monitoring, and borderline hypertension. Chest. 1996;109:901–908.

18. Young T, Palta M, Dempsey J, et al. The occurrence of sleep-disordered breathing among middle-aged adults. N Engl J Med. 1993;328:1230–1235.

19. Kump K, Whalen C, Tishler PV, et al. Assessment of the validity and utility of a sleep-symptom questionnaire. Am J Respir Crit Care Med. 1994;150:735–741.

20. Stradling JR, Crosby JH. Predictors and prevalence of obstructive sleep apnoea and snoring in 1001 middle aged men. Thorax. 1991;46:85–90.

21. Davies RJ, Ali NJ, Stradling JR. Neck circumference and other clinical features in the diagnosis of the obstructive sleep apnoea syndrome. Thorax. 1992;47:101–105.

22. Ferguson KA, Ono T, Lowe AA, et al. The relationship between obesity and craniofacial structure in obstructive sleep apnea. Chest. 1995;108:375–381.

23. Jamieson A, Guilleminault C, Partinen M, et al. Obstructive sleep apneic patients have craniomandibular abnormalities. Sleep. 1986;9:469–477.

24. Rivlin J, Hoffstein V, Kalbfleisch J, et al. Upper airway morphology in patients with idiopathic obstructive sleep apnea. Am Rev Respir Dis. 1984;129:355–360.

25. Bradley TD, Brown IG, Grossman RF, et al. Pharyngeal size in snorers, nonsnorers, and patients with obstructive sleep apnea. N Engl J Med. 1986;315:1327–1331.

26. Kushida CA, Efron B, Guilleminault C. A predictive morphometric model for the obstructive sleep apnea syndrome. Ann Intern Med. 1997;127:581–587.

27. Young T, Peppard P, Palta M, et al. Population-based study of sleep-disordered breathing as a risk factor for hypertension. Arch Intern Med. 1997;157:1746–1752.

28. Young T, Finn L, Kim H. Nasal obstruction as a risk factor for sleep-disordered breathing: the University of Wisconsin Sleep and Respiratory Research Group. J Allergy Clin Immunol. 1997;99:S757–S762.

29. Labanowski M, Schmidt-Nowara W, Guilleminault C. Sleep and neuromuscular disease: frequency of sleep-disordered breathing in a neuromuscular disease clinic population. Neurology. 1996;47:1173–1180.

30. American Thoracic Society, Medical Section of the American Lung Association. Indications and standards for cardiopulmonary sleep studies. Am Rev Respir Dis. 1989;139:559–568.

31. Wittig RM, Romaker A, Zorick FJ, et al. Night-to-night consistency of apneas during sleep. Am Rev Respir Dis. 1984;129:244–248.

32. Chediak AD, Acevedo-Crespo JC, Seiden DJ, et al. Nightly variability in the indices of sleep-disordered breathing in men being evaluated for impotence with consecutive night polysomnograms. Sleep. 1996;19:589–592.

33. Meyer TJ, Eveloff SE, Kline LR, et al. One negative polysomnogram does not exclude obstructive sleep apnea. Chest. 1993;103:756–760.

34. Rechtschaffen A, Kales A. A Manual of Standardized Terminology, Techniques and Scoring System for Sleep Stages of Human Subjects. Los Angeles, Calif: BIS/BRI, University of California at Los Angeles; 1968.

35. Moser NJ, Phillips BA, Berry DTR, et al. What is hypopnea, anyway? Chest. 1994;105:426–428.

36. Chervin RD, Kraemer HC, Guilleminault C. Correlates of sleep latency on the multiple sleep latency test in a clinical population. Electroencephalogr Clin Neurophysiol. 1995;95:147–153.

37. Philip P, Stoohs R, Guilleminault C. Sleep fragmentation in normals: a model for sleepiness associated with upper airway resistance syndrome. Sleep. 1994;17:242–247.

38. Strohl KP. Timing, number and complexities of sleep studies. Sleep Breathing. 1997;2:45–49.

39. American Sleep Disorders Association Standards of Practice Committee. Practice parameters for the indications for polysomnography and related procedures. Sleep. 1997;20:406–422.

40. American Thoracic Society, Medical Section of the American Lung Association. Standards and indications for cardiopulmonary sleep studies in children. Am J Respir Crit Care Med. 1996;153:866–878.

41. Morielli A, Desjardins D, Brouillette RT. Transcutaneous and end-tidal carbon dioxide pressures should be measured during pediatric polysomnography. Am Rev Respir Dis. 1993;148:1599–1604.

41a. Norman RG, Ahmed MM, Walsleben JA, et al. Detection of respiratory events during NPSG: nasal cannula/pressure sensor versus thermistor. Sleep. 1997;20:1175–1184.

41b. Ballester E, Badia JR, Hernandez L, et al. Nasal prongs in the detection of sleep-related disordered breathing in the sleep apnoea/hypopnoea syndrome. Eur Respir J. 1998;11:880–883.

42. Guilleminault C, Pelayo R, Leger D, et al. Recognition of sleep-disordered breathing in children. Pediatrics. 1996;98:871–882.

43. Tvinnereim M, Mateika S, Cole P, et al. Diagnosis of obstructive sleep apnea using a portable transducer catheter. Am J Respir Crit Care Med. 1995;152:775–779.

44. Ferber R, Millman R, Coppola M, et al. Portable recording in the assessment of obstructive sleep apnea. Sleep. 1994;17:378–392.

45. American Sleep Disorders Association. Practice parameters for the use of portable recording in the assessment of obstructive sleep apnea. Sleep. 1994;17:372–377.

45a. Chervin RD, Murman DL, Malow BA, et al. Cost-utility of three approaches to the diagnosis of sleep apnea: polysomnography, home testing, and empirical therapy. Ann Intern Med. 1999;130:496–505.

46. Riley RW, Powell NB, Guilleminault C. Obstructive sleep apnea syndrome: a review of 306 consecutively treated surgical patients. Otolaryngol Head Neck Surg. 1993;108:117–125.

47. Guilleminault C, Riley R, Powell N. Obstructive sleep apnea and abnormal cephalometric measurements: implications for treatment. Chest. 1984;86:793–794.

48. Sher AE, Schechtman KB, Piccirillo JF. The efficacy of surgical modifications of the upper airway in adults with obstructive sleep apnea syndrome. Sleep. 1996;19:156–177.

49. Woodson BT, Conley SF. Prediction of uvulopalatopharyngoplasty response using cephalometric radiographs. Am J Otolaryngol. 1997;18:179–184.

50. Hans MG, Goldberg J. Cephalometric examination in obstructive sleep apnea. Oral Maxillofac Surg Clin North Am. 1995;7:269–281.

51. Schwab RJ, Gefter WB, Hoffman EA, et al. Dynamic upper airway imaging during awake respiration in normal subjects and patients with sleep disordered breathing. Am Rev Respir Dis. 1993;148:1385–1400.

52. Woodson BT. Examination of the upper airway. Oral Maxillofac Surg Clin North Am. 1995;7:257–267.

53. Sher AE, Thorpy MJ, Shprintzen RJ, et al. Predictive value of Muller maneuver in selection of patients for uvulopalatopharyngoplasty. Laryngoscope. 1985;95:1483–1487.

54. Skatvedt O. Localization of site of obstruction in snorers and patients with obstructive sleep apnea syndrome: a comparison of fiberoptic nasopharyngoscopy and pressure measurements. Acta Otolaryngol (Stockh). 1993;113:206–209.

55. Pringle MB, Croft CB. A grading system for patients with obstructive sleep apnoea: based on sleep nasendoscopy. Clin Otolaryngol. 1993;18:480–484.

56. Schwab RJ, Gupta KB, Gefter WB, et al. Upper airway and soft tissue anatomy in normal subjects and patients with sleep-disordered breathing: significance of the lateral pharyngeal walls. Am J Respir Crit Care Med. 1995;152:1673–1689.

57. Pevernagie DA, Stanson AW, Sheedy PF, et al. Effects of body position on the upper airway of patients with obstructive sleep apnea. Am J Respir Crit Care Med. 1995;152:179–185.

58. Suto Y, Matsuda E, Inoue Y, et al. Sleep apnea syndrome: comparison of MR imaging of the oropharynx with physiologic indexes. Radiology. 1997;201:393–398.

59. Dement WC, Carskadon M, Richardson G. Excessive daytime sleepiness in the sleep apnea syndrome. In: Guilleminault C, Dement WC, eds. Sleep Apnea Syndromes. New York, NY: Alan R. Liss; 1978:23–46.

60. Chervin RD, Aldrich MS, Pickett R, et al. Comparison of the results of the Epworth Sleepiness Scale and the multiple sleep latency test. J Psychosom Res. 1997;42:145–155.

61. Hoddes E, Dement W, Zarcone V. The development and use of the Stanford Sleepiness Scale (SSS). Psychophysiology. 1972;9:150.

62. Herscovitch J, Broughton R. Sensitivity of the Stanford Sleepiness Scale to the effects of cumulative partial sleep deprivation and recovery oversleeping. Sleep. 1981;4:83–92.

63. Johns MW. A new method for measuring daytime sleepiness: the Epworth Sleepiness Scale. Sleep. 1991;14:540–545.

64. Weaver TE, Laizner AM, Evans LK, et al. An instrument to measure functional status outcomes for disorders of excessive sleepiness. Sleep. 1997;20:835–843.

65. Johns MW. Sleepiness in different situations measured by the Epworth Sleepiness Scale. Sleep. 1994;17:703–710.

66. Chervin RD, Aldrich MS. The Epworth Sleepiness Scale may not reflect objective measures of sleepiness or sleep apnea. Neurology. 1999;52:125–131.

67. Chervin RD, Aldrich MS. The relation between MSLT findings and the frequency of apneic events in REM and NREM sleep. Chest. 1998;113:980–984.

68. Carskadon MA, Dement WC, Mitler MM, et al. Guidelines for the multiple sleep latency test (MSLT): a standard measure of sleepiness. Sleep. 1986;9:519–524.

69. Naitoh P, Kelly TL. Modification of the multiple sleep latency test. In: Ogilvie RD, Harsh JR, eds. Sleep Onset: Normal and Abnormal Processes. New York, NY: John Wiley & Sons; 1995:327–338.

70. American Sleep Disorders Association. The clinical use of the multiple sleep latency test. Sleep. 1992;15:268–276.

71. Zwyghuizen-Doorenbos A, Roehrs T, Schaefer M, et al. Test-retest reliability of the MSLT. Sleep. 1988;11:562–565.

72. Roehrs T, Roth T. Multiple sleep latency test: technical aspects and normal values. J Clin Neurophysiol. 1992;9:63–67.

73. Benbadis SR, Qu Y, Perry MC, et al. Interrater reliability of the multiple sleep latency test. Electroencephalogr Clin Neurophysiol. 1995;95:302–304.

74. Carskadon MA, Dement WC. Sleep tendency: an objective measure of sleep loss. Sleep Res. 1977;6:200.

75. Carskadon MA, Dement WC. Effects of total sleep loss on sleep tendency. Percept Mot Skills. 1979;48:495–506.

76. Carskadon MA, Dement WC. Nocturnal determinants of daytime sleepiness. Sleep. 1982;5:S73–S81.

77. Roehrs T, Merlotti L, Petrucelli N, et al. Experimental sleep fragmentation. Sleep. 1994;17:438–443.

78. Guilleminault C, Partinen M, Quera-Salva MA, et al. Determinants of daytime sleepiness in obstructive sleep apnea. Chest. 1988;94:32–37.

79. Roehrs T, Zorick F, Wittig R, et al. Predictors of objective level of daytime sleepiness in patients with sleep-related breathing disorders. Chest. 1989;95:1202–1206.

80. Aldrich MS. Sleep continuity and excessive daytime sleepiness in sleep apnea. Sleep Res. 1990;19:178.

81. Roth T, Hartse M, Zorick F, et al. Multiple naps and the evaluation of daytime sleepiness in patients with upper airway sleep apnea. Sleep. 1980;3:425–439.

82. Cheshire K, Engleman H, Deary I, et al. Factors impairing daytime performance in patients with sleep apnea/hypopnea syndrome. Arch Intern Med. 1992;152:538–541.

83. Lamphere J, Roehrs T, Wittig R, et al. Recovery of alertness after CPAP in apnea. Chest. 1989;96:1364–1367.

84. Engleman HM, Martin SE, Deary IJ, et al. Effect of continuous positive airway pressure treatment on daytime function in sleep apnoea/hypopnoea syndrome. Lancet. 1994;343:572–575.

85. Engleman HM, Cheshire KE, Deary IJ, et al. Daytime sleepiness, cognitive performance and mood after continuous positive airway pressure for the sleep apnoea/hypopnoea syndrome. Thorax. 1993;48:911–914.

86. Sangal RB, Thomas L, Mitler MM. Disorders of excessive sleepiness: treatment improves ability to stay awake but does not reduce sleepiness. Chest. 1992;102:699–703.

87. Phillips BA, Schmitt FA, Berry DT, et al. Treatment of obstructive sleep apnea: a preliminary report comparing nasal CPAP to nasal oxygen in patients with mild OSA. Chest. 1990;98:325–330.

88. Chervin RD, Guilleminault C. Assessment of sleepiness in clinical practice. Nat Med. 1995;1:1252–1253.

89. Carskadon MA, Dement WC. The multiple sleep latency test: what does it measure? Sleep. 1982;5:S67–S72.

90. Mitler MM, Van den Hoed J, Carskadon MA, et al. REM sleep episodes during the multiple sleep latency test in narcoleptic patients. Electroencephalogr Clin Neurophysiol. 1979;46:479–481.

91. Richardson GS, Carskadon MA, Flagg W, et al. Excessive daytime sleepiness in man: multiple sleep latency measurement in narcoleptic and control subjects. Electroencephalogr Clin Neurophysiol. 1978;45:621–627.

92. Mitler MM. The multiple sleep latency test as an evaluation for excessive daytime sleepiness. In: Guilleminault C, ed. Sleeping and Waking Disorders: Indications and Techniques. Menlo Park, Calif: Addison-Wesley; 1982:145–153.

93. Amira SA, Johnson TS, Logowitz NB. Diagnosis of narcolepsy using the multiple sleep latency test: analysis of current laboratory criteria. Sleep. 1985;8:325–331.

94. Biniaurishvili RG, Fry JM, DiPhillipo MA, et al. MSLT REM sleep episodes, excessive daytime sleepiness and sleep structure in obstructive sleep apnea patients [abstract]. Sleep Res. 1994;23:231.

95. Bishop C, Rosenthal L, Helmus T, et al. The frequency of multiple sleep onset REM periods among subjects with no excessive daytime sleepiness. Sleep. 1996;19:727–730.

96. Moscovitch A, Partinen M, Guilleminault C. The positive diagnosis of narcolepsy and narcolepsy's borderland. Neurology. 1993;43:55–60.

97. Aldrich MS, Chervin RD, Malow BA. Value of the multiple sleep latency test (MSLT) for the diagnosis of narcolepsy. Sleep. 1997;20:620–629.

98. Sangal RB, Thomas L, Mitler MM. Maintenance of Wakefulness Test and multiple sleep latency test: measurement of different abilities in patients with sleep disorders. Chest. 1992;101:898–902.

99. Poceta JS, Timms RM, Jeong DU, et al. Maintenance of wakefulness test in obstructive sleep apnea syndrome. Chest. 1992;101:893–897.

100. Roth B, Nevsimalova S, Sonka K, et al. An alternative to the multiple sleep latency test for determining sleepiness in narcolepsy and hypersomnia: polygraphic score of sleepiness. Sleep. 1986;9:243–245.

101. Pollak CP. How should the multiple sleep latency test be analyzed? Sleep. 1997;20:34–39.

102. Bennett LS, Stradling JR, Davies RJ. A behavioral test to assess daytime sleepiness in obstructive sleep apnoea. J Sleep Res. 1997;6:142–145.

103. Yoss RE, Moyer NJ, Hollenhorst RW. Pupil size and spontaneous pupillary waves associated with alertness, drowsiness, and sleep. Neurology. 1970;20:545–554.

104. O'Neill WD, Oroujeh AM, Keegan AP, et al. Neurological pupillary noise in narcolepsy. J Sleep Res. 1996;5:265–271.

105. Sangal RB, Sangal JM. Measurement of P300 and sleep characteristics in patients with hypersomnia: do P300 latencies, P300 amplitudes, and multiple sleep latency and maintenance of wakefulness tests measure different factors? Clin Electroencephalogr. 1997;28:179–184.

106. Kribbs NB, Pack AI, Kline LR, et al. Effects of one night without nasal CPAP treatment on sleep and sleepiness in patients with obstructive sleep apnea. Am Rev Respir Dis. 1993;147:1162–1168.

107. Findley L, Unverzagt M, Guchu R, et al. Vigilance and automobile accidents in patients with sleep apnea or narcolepsy. Chest. 1995;108:619–624.

108. American Sleep Disorders Association. Practice parameters for the use of polysomnography in the evaluation of insomnia. Sleep. 1995;18:55–57.

109. Reite M, Buysse D, Reynolds C, et al. The use of polysomnography in the evaluation of insomnia. Sleep. 1996;18:58–70.

110. Hauri PJ. Cognitive deficits in insomnia patients. Acta Neurol Belg. 1997;97:113–117.

111. Spielman AJ, Nunes J, Glovinsky PB. Insomnia. Neurol Clin. 1996;14:513–543.

112. Costa, Chase M, Sartorius N, et al. Special report from a symposium held by the World Health Organization and the World Federation of Sleep Research Societies: an overview of insomnias and related disorders—recognition, epidemiology, and rational management. Sleep. 1996;19:412–416.

113. Molaie M, Deutsch GK. Psychogenic events presenting as parasomnias. Sleep. 1997;20:402–405.

114. Aldrich MS, Jahnke B. Diagnostic value of video-EEG polysomnography. Neurology. 1991;41:1060–1066.

115. Crawford B. Clinical economics and sleep disorders. Sleep. 1997;20:829–834.

116. Tousignant P, Cosio MG, Levy RD, et al. Quality adjusted life years added by treatment of obstructive sleep apnea. Sleep. 1994;17:52–60.
117. Partinen M, Jamieson A, Guilleminault C. Long-term outcome for obstructive sleep apnea syndrome patients. Chest. 1988;94:1200–1204.
118. Emsellem HA, Corson WA, Rappaport BA, et al. Verification of sleep apnea using a portable sleep apnea screening device. South Med J. 1990;83:748–752.
119. Kapuniai LE, Andrew DJ, Crowell DH, et al. Identifying sleep apnea from self-reports. Sleep. 1988;11:430–436.
120. Bliwise DL, Nekich JC, Dement WC. Relative validity of self-reported snoring as a symptom of sleep apnea in a sleep clinic population. Chest. 1991;99:600–608.
121. Haraldsson PO, Carenfelt C, Knutsson E, et al. Preliminary report: validity of symptom analysis and daytime polysomnography in diagnosis of sleep apnea. Sleep. 1992;15:261–263.
122. Rauscher H, Popp W, Zwick H. Model for investigating snorers with suspected sleep apnoea. Thorax. 1993;48:275–279.
123. Douglass AB, Bornstein R, Nino-Murcia G, et al. The sleep disorders questionnaire, I: creation and multivariate structure of SDQ. Sleep. 1994;17:160–167.

46

Classification of Sleep Disorders

Michael J. Thorpy

The classification of sleep disorders has been of particular interest to physicians since sleep disorders were first recognized. The earliest classification systems were primarily symptom based, and they formed the basis for the modern classifications. In 1990, the widely used International Classification of Sleep Disorders (ICSD) was produced after a 5-year process initiated by the American Sleep Disorders Association (Table 46–1). This classification replaced the Diagnostic Classification of Sleep and Arousal Disorders that was published in 1979.[1] The ICSD development process involved the three major international sleep societies at that time—the European Sleep Research Society, the Japanese Society of Sleep Research, and the Latin American Sleep Society—and resulted in the production of a diagnostic and coding manual, the *International Classification of Sleep Disorders: Diagnostic and Coding Manual.*[2] A revised version of the ICSD with minor revisions to the text was produced in 1997.[3]

The ICSD classification was developed primarily for diagnostic and epidemiological purposes so that sleep disorders can be indexed and morbidity and mortality information could be recorded and retrieved. The classification lists 84 sleep disorders, with each presented in detail and with a descriptive diagnostic text that includes specific diagnostic criteria. The classification manual has led to more accurate diagnoses of sleep symptoms, leading to improved treatment and the stimulation of clinical sleep research.

The main ICSD classification is not a differential diagnostic listing of the sleep disorders; such a listing is presented in the manual to assist the clinician in diagnosing one of three major sleep symptoms: insomnia, excessive sleepiness, or an abnormal event during sleep (Table 46–2).

The ICSD has four major categories: the *dyssomnias,* which are disorders of initiating and maintaining sleep and the disorders of excessive sleepiness; the *parasomnias,* which are disorders that do not primarily cause a complaint of insomnia or excessive sleepiness; *disorders associated with medical or psychiatric disorders;* and the *proposed sleep disorders,* which are disorders for which there is insufficient information to confirm their acceptance as a definitive sleep disorder. This last category was required because of the rapid advance of sleep medicine that resulted in the discovery of several new sleep disorders.

The main categories of the classification, adapted from the *International Classification of Sleep Disorders,*[3] follow:

Dyssomnias

- Intrinsic sleep disorders
- Extrinsic sleep disorders
- Circadian rhythm sleep disorders

Parasomnias

- Arousal disorders
- Sleep-wake transition disorders
- Parasomnias usually associated with rapid eye movement sleep
- Other parasomnias

Medicopsychiatric sleep disorders

- Associated with mental disorders
- Associated with neurological disorders
- Associated with other medical disorders

Proposed sleep disorders

DYSSOMNIAS

The dyssomnias are disorders that produce either insomnia or excessive sleepiness. They are primarily the disorders of the first two sections of the 1979 Diagnostic Classification of Sleep and Arousal Disorders,[1] that is, the disorders of initiating and maintaining sleep (also known as the insomnias) and the disorders of excessive somnolence. The dyssomnias are the major (primary) sleep disorders associated with either disturbed sleep at night or impaired wakefulness.

The dyssomnias contain a heterogeneous group of disorders that have their origin in different systems of the body. For example, a primary disorder of the central nervous system is believed to be the cause of narcolepsy,[10, 11] whereas a physical obstruction in the upper airway may be the sole cause of obstructive sleep apnea syndrome.[17, 18] Some disorders that had been included in the first two sections of the Diagnostic Classification of Sleep and Arousal Disorders are now included in the other sections of the ICSD classification, such as short sleeper[142, 143] and long sleeper.[144, 145]

Table 46-1. THE INTERNATIONAL CLASSIFICATION OF SLEEP DISORDERS

	Recommended ICD-9-CM No.		Recommended ICD-9-CM No.
Dyssomnias		**Other Parasomnias**	
Intrinsic Sleep Disorders		Sleep bruxism[86, 87]	306.8
		Sleep enuresis[88, 89]	780.56-0
Psychophysiological insomnia[4, 5]	307.42-0	Sleep-related abnormal swallowing syndrome[90]	780.56-6
Sleep state misperception[6, 7]	307.49-1	Nocturnal paroxysmal dystonia[91, 92]	780.59-1
Idiopathic insomnia[8, 9]	780.52-7	Sudden unexplained nocturnal death	780.59-3
Narcolepsy[10, 11]	347	syndrome[93, 94]	
Recurrent hypersomnia[12, 13]	780.54-2	Primary snoring[95, 96]	780.53-1
Idiopathic hypersomnia[14, 15]	780.54-7	Infant sleep apnea[97, 98]	770.80
Post-traumatic hypersomnia[16]	780.54-8	Congenital central hypoventilation	770.81
Obstructive sleep apnea syndrome[17, 18]	780.53-0	syndrome[99,100]	
Central sleep apnea syndrome[19, 20]	780.51-0	Sudden infant death syndrome[101, 102]	798.0
Central alveolar hypoventilation syndrome[21, 22]	780.51-1	Benign neonatal sleep myoclonus[103, 104]	780.59-5
Periodic limb movement disorder[23, 24]	780.52-4	Other parasomnia NOS	780.59-9
Restless legs syndrome[25, 26]	780.52-5	**Sleep Disorders Associated With Medical**	
Intrinsic sleep disorder NOS	780.52-9	**or Psychiatric Disorders**	
Extrinsic Sleep Disorders		*Associated With Mental Disorders*	290-319
Inadequate sleep hygiene[27, 28]	307.41-1	Psychoses[105, 106]	292-299
Environmental sleep disorder[29, 30]	780.52-6	Mood disorders[107, 108]	296-301
Altitude insomnia[31,32]	993.2	Anxiety disorders[109, 110]	300
Adjustment sleep disorder[33, 34]	307.41-0	Panic disorder[111, 112]	300
Insufficient sleep syndrome[35, 36]	307.49-4	Alcoholism[113, 114]	303
Limit-setting sleep disorder[37]	307.42-4	*Associated With Neurological Disorders*	320-389
Sleep-onset association disorder[38]	307.42-5	Cerebral degenerative disorders[115]	330-337
Food allergy insomnia[39, 40]	780.52-2	Dementia[116, 117]	331
Nocturnal eating (drinking) syndrome[41, 42]	780.52-8	Parkinsonism[118, 119]	332-333
Hypnotic-dependent sleep disorder[43, 44]	780.52-0	Fatal familial insomnia[120, 121]	337.9
Stimulant-dependent sleep disorder[45, 46]	780.52-1	Sleep-related epilepsy[122, 123]	345
Alcohol-dependent sleep disorder[47]	780.52-3	Electrical status epilepticus of sleep[124, 125]	345.8
Toxin-induced sleep disorder[48]	780.54-6	Sleep-related headaches[126, 127]	346
Extrinsic sleep disorder NOS	780.52-9	*Associated With Other Medical Disorders*	
Circadian Rhythm Sleep Disorders		Sleeping sickness[128, 129]	086
Time-zone change (jet lag) syndrome[49, 50]	307.45-0	Nocturnal cardiac ischemia[130, 131]	411-414
Shift work sleep disorder[51, 52]	307.45-1	Chronic obstructive pulmonary disease[132, 133]	490-494
Irregular sleep-wake pattern[53, 54]	307.45-3	Sleep-related asthma[134, 135]	493
Delayed sleep phase syndrome[55, 56]	780.55-0	Sleep-related gastroesophageal reflux[136, 137]	530.1
Advanced sleep phase syndrome[57, 58]	780.55-1	Peptic ulcer disease[138, 139]	531-534
Non–24-h sleep-wake disorder[59, 60]	780.55-2	Fibrositis syndrome[140, 141]	729.1
Circadian rhythm sleep disorder NOS	780.55-9	**Proposed Sleep Disorders**	
Parasomnias		Short sleeper[142, 143]	307.49-0
Arousal Disorders		Long sleeper[144, 145]	307.49-2
Confusional arousals[61, 62]	307.46-2	Subwakefulness syndrome[146]	307.47-1
Sleepwalking[63, 64]	307.46-0	Fragmentary myoclonus[147]	780.59-7
Sleep terrors[65, 66]	307.46-1	Sleep hyperhidrosis[148, 149]	780.8
Sleep-Wake Transition Disorders		Menstrual-associated sleep disorder[150, 151]	780.54-3
Rhythmic movement disorder[67, 68]	307.3	Pregnancy-associated sleep disorder[152, 153]	780.59-6
Sleep starts[69, 70]	307.47-2	Terrifying hypnagogic hallucinations[154]	307.47-4
Sleeptalking[71, 72]	307.47-3	Sleep-related neurogenic tachypnea[155]	780.53-2
Nocturnal leg cramps[73, 74]	729.82	Sleep-related laryngospasm[156, 157]	780.59-4
Parasomnias Usually Associated With REM Sleep		Sleep choking syndrome[158, 159]	307.42-1
Nightmares[75, 76]	307.47-0		
Sleep paralysis[77, 78]	780.56-2		
Impaired sleep-related penile erections[79, 80]	780.56-3		
Sleep-related painful erections[81, 82]	780.56-4		
REM sleep–related sinus arrest[83]	780.56-8		
REM sleep behavior disorders[84, 85]	780.59-0		

From the American Sleep Disorders Association, Diagnostic Classification Steering Committee; MJ Thorpy, Chairman. International Classification of Sleep Disorders, Revised: Diagnostic and Coding Manual. Rochester, Minn: American Sleep Disorders Association; 1997.
ICD-9-CM, International Classification of Diseases, Ninth Revision, Clinical Modification; NOS, not otherwise specified.

Table 46–2. DIFFERENTIAL DIAGNOSIS OF SLEEP DISORDERS

Insomnia Disorders (Difficulty in Initiating or Maintaining Sleep)

Associated With Behavioral-Psychophysiological Disorders

Adjustment sleep disorder
Psychophysiological insomnia
Inadequate sleep hygiene
Limit-setting sleep disorder
Sleep-onset association disorder
Nocturnal eating (drinking) syndrome
Other

Associated With Psychiatric Disorders

Psychoses
Mood disorders
Anxiety disorders
Panic disorder
Alcoholism
Other

Associated With Environmental Factors

Environmental sleep disorder
Food allergy insomnia
Toxin-induced sleep disorder
Other

Associated With Drug Dependency

Hypnotic-dependent sleep disorder
Stimulant-dependent sleep disorder
Alcohol-dependent sleep disorder
Other

Associated With Sleep-Induced Respiratory Impairment

Obstructive sleep apnea syndrome
Central sleep apnea syndrome
Central alveolar hypoventilation syndrome
Chronic obstructive pulmonary disease
Sleep-related asthma
Altitude insomnia
Other

Associated With Movement Disorders

Sleep starts
Restless legs syndrome
Periodic limb movement disorder
Nocturnal leg cramps
Rhythmic movement disorder
REM sleep behavior disorder
Nocturnal paroxysmal dystonia
Other

Associated With Disorders of the Timing of the Sleep-Wake Pattern

Short sleeper
Time-zone change (jet lag) syndrome
Shift work sleep disorder
Delayed sleep phase syndrome
Advanced sleep phase syndrome
Non–24-h sleep-wake syndrome
Irregular sleep-wake pattern
Other

Associated With Parasomnias (Not Otherwise Classified)

Confusional arousals
Sleep terrors
Nightmares
Sleep hyperhidrosis
Other

Associated With the CNS (Not Otherwise Classified)

Parkinsonism
Dementia
Cerebral degenerative disorders
Sleep-related epilepsy
Fatal familial insomnia
Other

Associated With No Objective Sleep Disturbance

Sleep state misperception
Sleep choking syndrome
Other

Idiopathic Insomnia

Other Causes of Insomnia

Sleep-related gastroesophageal reflux
Fibrositis syndrome
Menstrual-associated sleep disorder
Pregnancy-associated sleep disorder
Terrifying hypnagogic hallucinations
Sleep-related abnormal swallowing syndrome
Sleep-related laryngospasm
Other

Excessive Sleepiness

Associated With Behavioral-Psychophysiological Disorders

Inadequate sleep hygiene
Insufficient sleep syndrome
Limit-setting sleep disorder
Other

Associated With Psychiatric Disorders

Mood disorders
Psychoses
Alcoholism
Other

Associated With Environmental Factors

Environmental sleep disorder
Toxin-induced sleep disorder
Other

Associated With Drug Dependency

Hypnotic-dependent sleep disorder
Stimulant-dependent sleep disorder
Other

Associated With Sleep-Induced Respiratory Impairment

Obstructive sleep apnea syndrome
Central sleep apnea syndrome
Central alveolar hypoventilation syndrome
Sleep-related neurogenic tachypnea
Other

Associated With Movement Disorders

Periodic limb movement disorder
Other

Associated With Disorders of the Timing of the Sleep-Wake Pattern

Long sleeper
Time-zone change (jet lag) syndrome
Shift work sleep disorder
Delayed sleep phase syndrome
Advanced sleep phase syndrome
Non–24-h sleep-wake syndrome
Irregular sleep-wake pattern
Other

Associated With the CNS (Not Otherwise Classified)

Narcolepsy
Idiopathic hypersomnia
Post-traumatic hypersomnia
Recurrent hypersomnia
Subwakefulness syndrome
Fragmentary myoclonus
Parkinsonism
Dementia
Sleeping sickness
Other

Table continued on following page

Table 46–2. DIFFERENTIAL DIAGNOSIS OF SLEEP DISORDERS *Continued*

Other Causes of Excessive Sleepiness

Menstrual-associated sleep disorder
Pregnancy-associated sleep disorder
Other

Other Sleep Disturbances

Associated With Behavioral-Psychophysiological Disorders

Nocturnal eating (drinking) syndrome
Other

Associated With Psychiatric Disorders

Panic disorder
Other

Associated With Sleep-Induced Respiratory Impairment

Primary snoring
Obstructive sleep apnea syndrome
Central sleep apnea syndrome
Central alveolar hypoventilation syndrome
Sleep-related asthma
Chronic obstructive pulmonary disease
Sleep-related neurogenic tachypnea
Other

Associated With Movement Disorders

Sleep starts
Sleepwalking
Sleep terrors
Sleep bruxism
Periodic limb movement disorder

Restless legs syndrome
Rhythmic movement disorder
Sleep paralysis
Nocturnal leg cramps
REM sleep behavior disorder
Nocturnal paroxysmal dystonia
Other

Associated With Parasomnias (Not Otherwise Classified)

Nightmares
Sleeptalking
Sleep enuresis
Sleep-related painful erections
Other

Associated With the CNS (Not Otherwise Classified)

Sleep-related epilepsy
Electrical status epilepticus of sleep
Fragmentary myoclonus
Other

Other Causes of Sleep Disturbance

Sleep-related gastroesophageal reflux
Sleep-related sinus arrest
Sleep-related abnormal swallowing syndrome
Sleep-related laryngospasm
Sleep choking syndrome
Terrifying hypnagogic hallucinations
Other

CNS, central nervous system.

The dyssomnias are divided into three major groups: the intrinsic sleep disorders, the extrinsic sleep disorders, and the circadian rhythm sleep disorders. The divisions are based in part on pathophysiological mechanisms. Because the circadian rhythm sleep disorders share a common chronophysiological basis, they are considered a single group. Both intrinsic and extrinsic factors may be involved in some of the circadian rhythm sleep disorders, so some are subdivided into the two types: intrinsic and extrinsic.

Intrinsic Sleep Disorders

The intrinsic sleep disorders are primary sleep disorders that either originate or develop within the body or arise from causes within the body. This section contains only those disorders that are included in and defined under the group heading of dyssomnias. Some sleep disorders due to processes arising within the body are not listed in the intrinsic section but are listed in the parasomnias, medicopsychiatric, or proposed sleep disorder sections.

The intrinsic sleep disorders include various types of disorders; *psychophysiological insomnia,*[4, 5] *sleep state misperception,*[6, 7] *restless legs syndrome,*[25, 26] and *idiopathic insomnia*[8, 9] are primarily disorders that produce insomnia, whereas *narcolepsy,*[10, 11] *recurrent hypersomnia,*[12, 13] *idiopathic hypersomnia,*[14, 15] and *post-traumatic hypersomnia*[16] are primarily disorders of excessive sleepiness. The next four disorders, *obstructive sleep apnea syndrome,*[17, 18] *central sleep apnea syndrome,*[19, 20] *central*

alveolar hypoventilation syndrome,[21, 22] and *periodic limb movement disorder,*[23, 24] are disorders that can produce a complaint of either insomnia or excessive sleepiness. *Upper airway resistance syndrome* has been recognized as a manifestation of obstructive sleep apnea syndrome and therefore has not been included as a separate diagnosis in the revision of the ICSD.

The term *intrinsic* implies that the primary cause of the disorder is an internal (endogenous) abnormality in physiological or pathological processes within the body. However, it is clear that for some disorders, external factors are important in either precipitating or exacerbating the disorder. The following examples are given to help explain the rationale in organizing the disorders under the group heading of intrinsic.

Post-traumatic hypersomnia[16] is an example of an intrinsic disorder that could not exist without an external event that produced the head injury, but the primary cause of the hypersomnia is of central nervous system origin and is listed in the intrinsic section because the disorder persists after the traumatic event has terminated. Obstructive sleep apnea syndrome can be induced by an external factor, such as alcohol ingestion, but the syndrome would not be possible without the internal factor of upper airway obstruction; in addition, a physiological predisposition to development of the disorder must be present.

Some of the extrinsic sleep disorders have internal factors that are important for the expression of the sleep disturbance, but external factors are essential for continuation of the sleep disturbance, and when they are removed, the sleep disturbance resolves. For example, although the extrinsic adjustment sleep disorder[31, 32] is due to psychologically stressful factors and therefore could be considered internally generated, an external event causes the sleep disturbance, and if it is removed, the sleep disorder resolves. If the sleep disorder continues after removal of the external factor, then an intrinsic sleep disorder may have developed, such as psychophysiological insomnia.[4, 5]

Extrinsic Sleep Disorders

The extrinsic sleep disorders include disorders that originate in or develop from causes outside of the body. External (exogenous) factors are integral in producing these sleep disorders, and removal of the external factors leads to resolution of the sleep disorder. This is not to say that internal factors are not important in the development or maintenance of the sleep disorder, just as external factors can be important in the development or maintenance of an intrinsic sleep disorder. However, the internal factors would not, by themselves, have produced the sleep disorder without the presence of an external factor.

Although there appears to be overlap between some disorders, such as *alcohol-dependent sleep disorder,*[47] *environmental sleep disorder,*[29, 30] and *inadequate sleep hygiene,*[5, 27] the manual text and diagnostic criteria highlight the differences. Some explanation may be helpful.

Inadequate sleep hygiene[27, 28] applies to a sleep disorder that develops out of normal behavioral practices that for another person would not usually cause a sleep disturbance. For example, an irregular bedtime or waketime that might not be important in one person may be instrumental in producing insomnia in another. Although environmental factors can produce a disorder of inadequate sleep hygiene, the diagnosis of an environmental sleep disorder is made only when the environmental factors are particularly abnormal, such as excessive noise or extreme lighting effects that would produce sleep disturbance in most people. Caffeine ingestion in the form of coffee or soda can produce a disorder of inadequate sleep hygiene if the intake is normal and within the limits of common use, whereas stimulant ingestion that is considered excessive or abnormal by normal standards can lead to a diagnosis of a stimulant-dependent sleep disorder.[45, 46] Similarly, sleep that is disrupted by alcohol ingestion that would be considered a socially normal amount can lead to a diagnosis of inadequate sleep hygiene, whereas sleep that is disrupted by alcohol ingestion that is considered by most people to be excessive and taken primarily for sleep purposes can lead to a diagnosis of alcohol-dependent sleep disorder.[45]

Altitude insomnia[31, 32] is sleep disturbance that is due to acute mountain sickness. Insomnia may be the sole manifestation of altitude insomnia, whereas the term *acute mountain sickness* usually applies when other physiological disturbances predominate.

Circadian Rhythm Sleep Disorders

The circadian rhythm sleep disorders comprise the third section of the dyssomnias and are grouped because they share a common underlying chronophysiological basis. The major feature of these disorders is a misalignment between the patient's sleep pattern and the pattern that is desired or regarded as the societal norm. Three circadian rhythm sleep disorders have intrinsic and extrinsic subtypes: *delayed sleep phase syndrome,*[55, 56] *advanced sleep phase syndrome,*[57, 58] and *non–24-h sleep-wake syndrome.*[59, 60]

The underlying problem in the majority of the circadian rhythm sleep disorders is that the patient cannot sleep when sleep is desired, needed, or expected. The wake episodes can occur at undesired times as a result of sleep episodes that occur at inappropriate times; therefore, the patient may complain of insomnia or excessive sleepiness. For several of the circadian rhythm sleep disorders, once sleep is initiated, the major sleep episode is of normal duration with normal rapid eye movement (REM)–nonrapid eye movement (NREM) cycling. Intermittent sleep episodes can occur in some disorders, such as the irregular sleep-wake pattern.[62, 63]

The appropriate timing of sleep within the 24-h day can be disturbed in many other sleep disorders, particularly disorders associated with the complaint of insomnia. Patients with narcolepsy[10, 11] can have a pattern of sleepiness that is identical to that described as due to an irregular sleep-wake pattern.[53, 54] However, because the primary sleep diagnosis is narcolepsy, the patient should not receive a second diagnosis of a circadian rhythm sleep disorder unless the disorder is unrelated to the narcolepsy. For example, a diagnosis of time-zone change (jet lag) syndrome[49, 50] could be stated along with a diagnosis of narcolepsy, if appropriate. Similarly, patients with mood disorders[107, 108] or psychoses[105, 106] can, at times, have a sleep pattern similar to that of delayed sleep phase syndrome.[55, 56]

Some disturbance of sleep timing is a common feature in patients who have a diagnosis of inadequate sleep hygiene.[27, 28] Only if the timing of sleep is the predominant cause of the sleep disturbance and is outside the societal norm would the patient be given a diagnosis of a circadian rhythm sleep disorder. Limit-setting sleep disorder[37] is also associated with an altered time of sleep within the 24-h day. However, the timing of sleep in this disorder is not within the patient's control, nor is it intrinsically induced. If the setting of limits is a function of the caretaker, then the sleep disorder is more appropriately diagnosed within the extrinsic subsection of the dyssomnias, that is, as a limit-setting sleep disorder.[37]

PARASOMNIAS

The parasomnias consist of sleep disorders that are not abnormalities of the processes responsible for sleep and awake states per se but are undesirable physical phenomena that occur predominantly during sleep. The parasomnias are disorders of arousal, partial arousal, and sleep stage transition. Many of the parasomnias are manifestations of central nervous system activation. Autonomic nervous system changes and skeletal muscle activity are the predominant features.

The parasomnias are subdivided into the arousal disorders, the sleep-wake transition disorders, the parasomnias associated with REM sleep, and other parasomnias.

The arousal disorders consist of the classic disorders of arousal: *sleepwalking*,[63, 64] *sleep terrors*,[65, 66] and *confusional arousals*.[61, 62] The sleep-wake transition disorders include disorders that occur in the transition from wakefulness to sleep or from sleep to wakefulness. This group does not include disorders that are clearly associated with REM sleep, such as sleep paralysis.[77, 78] Although some of the sleep-wake transition disorders can occur during sleep or even in wakefulness, such as *rhythmic movement disorder* (jactatio capitis nocturna),[67, 68] the most typical occurrence of these disorders is the transition from wakefulness to sleep. Restless legs syndrome[25, 26] could be considered a sleep-wake transition disorder, but this disorder is not a parasomnia because it is associated primarily with a complaint of insomnia and therefore is listed within the dyssomnias.

The parasomnias usually associated with REM sleep include six disorders that have a close association with the REM sleep stage. Although sleep paralysis[77, 78] generally occurs in the transition from wakefulness to sleep or from sleep to wakefulness, it is listed in this subsection. The association with REM sleep of the other disorders in this group is clear.

The fourth subsection contains parasomnias that are not classified in the previous three sections—the other parasomnias.

Arousal Disorders

The disorders of arousal are disorders associated with impaired arousal from sleep. Their onset in slow-wave sleep is a typical feature. Confusional arousals most commonly occur in children and have features in common with both sleepwalking[63, 64] and sleep terrors.[65, 66] They may be partial manifestations of sleepwalking and sleep terror episodes. Confusional arousals can occur in either disorder or both, or confusional arousals may occur as an isolated sleep disorder.

Sleep-Wake Transition Disorders

The sleep-wake transition disorders are disorders that occur in the transition from wakefulness to sleep, in the transition from sleep to wakefulness, or, more rarely, in sleep stage transitions. All of these disorders can occur commonly in otherwise healthy persons and therefore are regarded as altered physiological processes rather than as pathophysiological changes. Each can occur with an exceptionally high frequency or severity that can lead to discomfort, pain, embarrassment, anxiety, or disturbance of a bedpartner's sleep.

Rhythmic movement disorder[67, 68] is the preferred term for headbanging or jactatio capitis nocturna because several forms of rhythmic activity can occur without predominant headbanging. Although this disorder occurs in sleep stages, it is more commonly associated with drowsiness during sleep onset or in the transition from wakefulness to sleep. Rhythmic movement disorder can also occur during full wakefulness and alertness, particularly in individuals who are mentally retarded. *Sleep starts* (hypnic jerks)[69, 70] are included as a disorder because they rarely cause a sleep-onset insomnia. *Sleeptalking*[71, 72] does not usually have a direct consequence for the patient but can be a source of embarrassment and be disturbing to the sleep of the bedpartner.

Parasomnias Usually Associated With REM Sleep

These parasomnias are typically associated with the REM sleep stage. They are grouped together because some common underlying pathophysiological mechanism related to REM sleep may underlie these disorders.

Nightmares apply to the REM sleep phenomena that are evident by the group heading; therefore, there is little chance of confusing this disorder with that associated with slow-wave sleep—sleep terrors.[65, 66] *REM sleep–related sinus arrest*[83, 85] appears to be relatively rare, and *REM sleep behavior disorder*[84] is more common and sometimes occurs in association with other sleep disorders, such as narcolepsy.

Other Parasomnias

This group of parasomnias includes those that cannot be classified in other sections.

Sleep bruxism[86, 87] and *sleep enuresis*[88, 89] are preferred to the previously used terms, nocturnal bruxism and nocturnal enuresis, because they denote the association with sleep rather than time of day. *Primary snoring*[95, 96] is included because snoring may be associated with the presence of altered cardiovascular status and can be a forerunner to the development of the obstructive sleep apnea syndrome.[17, 18] Primary snoring not only can lead to impaired health but may be a cause of social embarrassment and can disturb the sleep of a bedpartner. Snoring associated with obstructive sleep apnea syndrome is not diagnosed as primary snoring. The disorder *sleep-related abnormal swallowing syndrome*[90] is a rare condition, and there have been few additional reports since the original description. *Nocturnal paroxysmal dystonia* (NPD)[91, 92] is an unusual movement disorder primarily associated with NREM sleep. Although NPD can occur in wakefulness during the major sleep episode, it primarily occurs out of sleep and therefore is classified here rather than as a sleep disorder associated with neurological disease. Some forms of similar motor activity during sleep are due to frontal lobe epilepsy, and these must be distinguished from NPD.

NPD episodes usually last several minutes or longer and do not respond to anticonvulsants.

Sudden unexplained nocturnal death syndrome,[93, 94] which usually occurs in Southeast Asians, has a specific association with sleep and therefore is classified here. *Benign neonatal sleep myoclonus*[103, 104] is a disorder of muscle activity that occurs solely during sleep in infants.

Included in this group are *sudden infant death syndrome*[101, 102] and the *infant sleep-related breathing disorders, infant sleep apnea,*[97, 98] and *congenital central hypoventilation syndrome.*[99, 100] The infant sleep-related breathing disorders can produce dyssomnic features of insomnia or excessive sleepiness. These symptoms are not predominant complaints, however, and usually the disorders are associated with a sudden event noticed to occur during sleep; therefore, they are listed in the parasomnia section.

The inclusion of these infant breathing disorders as sleep disorders requires further explanation. Both the newborn and the young infant sleep a great portion of the day, and the majority of apnea and related respiratory disorders are observed during sleep. Apnea, hypoventilation, and periodic breathing are intrinsic features of infancy that reflect immaturity of the respiratory system rather than pathological processes. Although there is general agreement that apnea associated with prematurity requires diagnosis, surveillance, and treatment, there is far less agreement over the boundaries between pathological and normal manifestations of sleep-related respiratory instabilities in term infants or premature infants who have reached 37 weeks' postconceptional age. The clinical significance of congenital central hypoventilation and obstructive apnea due to a narrow airway is beyond doubt, but there is controversy about the significance of other infant sleep apnea and altered breathing patterns. Some clinicians will be concerned, whereas others will view the same infant as being healthy and the observed phenomenon as a variation of normal. The fear that respiratory instability during sleep may predispose some infants to sudden infant death syndrome[101, 102] confers urgency to clinical management. The majority of cases of sudden infant death syndrome occur when the infant is presumed to be asleep. Even though infant sleep apnea has been implicated as a precursor to sudden infant death syndrome, there is no definitive evidence establishing a direct link; sudden infant death syndrome therefore is discussed separately.

MEDICOPSYCHIATRIC SLEEP DISORDERS

Many medical and psychiatric disorders are associated with disturbances of sleep and wakefulness. The division into medical versus psychiatric is somewhat arbitrary. Psychiatric disorders are common causes of sleep disturbance; this section is divided into three subsections. The first is a listing of the psychiatric disorders that are commonly associated with disturbed sleep or wakefulness; the second indicates the impor-

tance of neurological disorders and their effect on the sleep and wakefulness states; and the third is a listing of disorders that fall into other medical specialty areas but are insufficient in number to warrant a separate subsection.

Only medical disorders commonly seen in the practice of sleep disorder medicine are listed in the medicopsychiatric section. It is recognized that a large number of medical and psychiatric disorders are associated with disturbances of sleep and wakefulness, but an exhaustive list is not provided in the classification.

Sleep Disorders Associated With Mental Disorders

Although most psychiatric disorders can have associated sleep disturbance, the *psychoses,*[105, 106] *mood disorders,*[107, 108] *anxiety disorders,*[109, 110] *panic disorders,*[111, 112] and *alcoholism*[113, 114] are presented here because they are commonly seen in patients presenting with sleep complaints and must be considered in the differential diagnoses. *Panic disorder,*[111, 112] one of the anxiety disorders, can produce a sleep complaint without the occurrence of daytime panic episodes.

Sleep Disorders Associated With Neurological Disorders

Neurological disorders that are commonly associated with sleep disturbance are listed in this section. *Cerebral degenerative disorders,*[115] *dementia,*[116, 117] and *parkinsonism*[118, 119] are commonly recognized neurological disorders associated with sleep disturbance. Epilepsy can be exacerbated by sleep disturbance, and there can be epileptic phenomena that occur predominantly during sleep; therefore, the term *sleep-related epilepsy*[122, 123] is used to denote these forms of epilepsy. Frontal lobe epilepsy can commonly occur out of NREM sleep. Because of its pure association with NREM sleep, *electrical status epilepticus of sleep*[124, 125] is listed separately. Some headache forms, particularly migraine and cluster headaches, can occur predominantly in sleep and are listed under sleep-related headaches.[126, 127]

Sleep Disorders Associated With Other Medical Disorders

A variety of additional medical disorders have features that occur during sleep or cause sleep disturbance. *Sleeping sickness*[128, 129] is included because this disorder is commonly seen in Africa, although it rarely occurs in other continents. Encephalitis lethargica is not included because it is so rare.

Cardiac ischemia during sleep can lead to myocardial infarction or cardiac arrhythmias and may not be symptomatic. *Nocturnal cardiac ischemia*[130, 131] is presented in the classification because of its importance to the health of the population and in the hope of stimulating further research on the causal factors. Myocardial infarction during sleep is not listed because it is rarely seen in the practice of sleep medicine and rarely needs to be included in the differential diagnosis of a patient presenting with sleep complaints.

Chronic obstructive pulmonary disease[132, 133] and sleep-related asthma[134, 135] are sufficiently common in the population to warrant inclusion. Other pulmonary disorders can have sleep-related features but rarely cause sleep disturbances. Many respiratory disorders produce disturbed breathing during sleep that can lead to the development of the central sleep apnea syndrome.[19, 20]

Two gastrointestinal disorders are included in this section: sleep-related gastroesophageal reflux[136, 137] and peptic ulcer disease.[138, 139] The discomfort associated with peptic ulcer disease commonly occurs during the major sleep episode. Although the incidence of peptic ulcer disease appears to be declining in the United States, the incidence in some other countries, notably Japan, is high.

Fibrositis syndrome,[140, 141] also known as fibromyositis syndrome, is included because it is associated with disturbed sleep and an abnormal electroencephalographic pattern during sleep called alpha sleep.

PROPOSED SLEEP DISORDERS

The fourth section of the ICSD, proposed sleep disorders, includes sleep disorders for which insufficient or inadequate information is available to substantiate the unequivocal existence of the disorder. Some of these disorders, such as sleep-related laryngospasm[156, 157] and short sleeper,[142, 143] are controversial as to whether they are disorders in their own right or are at the extreme end of the range of normal physiology.

A short sleeper or long sleeper[144, 145] is a person who has either a shorter or longer sleep episode than is considered normal but has sleep that is not pathological. These patients present with either an inability to sleep or excessive sleepiness; therefore, these disorders are important in the differential diagnoses of these symptoms, and their descriptions are necessary to provide appropriate diagnostic information for clinical purposes.

The subwakefulness syndrome,[146] also known as the subvigilance syndrome, has been described for many years. However, it is unclear whether this is a variant of another disorder of excessive sleepiness, such as idiopathic hypersomnia,[8, 9] or represents a manifestation of a psychological state; therefore, subwakefulness syndrome is presented in the proposed sleep disorders section.

Fragmentary myoclonus,[147] a disorder associated with excessive sleepiness, consists of frequent brief myoclonic jerks that occur at random in many muscle groups. It may be a variant of the normal phasic muscle activity that typically is seen at sleep onset; however, insufficient information is available on this disorder.

Sleep hyperhidrosis,[148, 149] which is also known as night sweats, can be due to a variety of underlying disorders, such as neurological disorders and the obstructive sleep apnea syndrome. An idiopathic form of this disorder occurs but has rarely been described in the literature.

Sleep disturbance characterized by either insomnia or excessive sleepiness can be associated with the menstrual cycle, menopause (menstrual-associated sleep disorder),[150, 151] or pregnancy (pregnancy-associated sleep disorder).[152, 153] Although these sleep disturbances are well recognized to occur commonly, reports of the sleep characteristics of these menstrual states are rare, and the underlying cause of the sleep disturbances is unclear. Whether these sleep disorders are due to a specific and primary effect on sleep mechanisms or another disorder, such as premenstrual stress syndrome or back pain related to pregnancy, is not known.

Terrifying hypnagogic hallucinations[154] are intensely frightening hallucinatory phenomena that occur at sleep onset. Although sometimes associated with other sleep disorders, such as narcolepsy,[10, 11] they can occur in an idiopathic form. Terrifying hypnagogic hallucinations have rarely been described, and their differentiation from unpleasant sleep-onset dreams has not been clearly established.

Sleep-related neurogenic tachypnea,[155] although rarely described as an idiopathic form of tachypnea, can be associated with an underlying neurological disorder.

Sleep-related laryngospasm[156, 157] and the sleep choking syndrome[158, 159] are disorders that occur with a complaint of sleep-related breathing difficulties. Patients with these disorders present because of symptoms similar to those of the obstructive sleep apnea syndrome.[17, 18]

The proposed sleep disorders are described in the anticipation that additional information will be forthcoming in the medical literature to more clearly establish the nature of these disorders.

References

1. Association of Sleep Disorders Centers, Diagnostic Classification of Sleep and Arousal Disorders, prepared by the Sleep Disorders Classification Committee; HP Roffwarg, Chairman. Sleep. 1979;2:1–137.
2. Diagnostic Classification Steering Committee; MJ Thorpy, Chairman. International Classification of Sleep Disorders: Diagnostic and Coding Manual. Rochester, Minn: American Sleep Disorders Association; 1990.
3. American Sleep Disorders Association. International Classification of Sleep Disorders, revised: Diagnostic and Coding Manual. Rochester, Minn: American Sleep Disorders Association; 1997.
4. Hauri PJ, Fischer J. Persistent psychophysiological (learned) insomnia. Sleep. 1986;9:38–53.
5. Reynolds CF, Taska LS, Sewitch DE, et al. Persistent psychophysiologic insomnia: preliminary research diagnostic criteria and EEG sleep data. Am J Psychiatry. 1984;141:804–805.
6. Beutler LE, Thornby JI, Karacan I. Psychological variables in the diagnosis of insomnia. In: Williams RL, Karacan I, eds. Sleep Disorders: Diagnosis and Treatment. New York, NY: John Wiley; 1978:61–100.
7. Carskadon M, Dement W, Mitler M, et al. Self report versus sleep laboratory findings in 122 drug free subjects with the complaint of chronic insomnia. Am J Psychiatry. 1976;133:1382–1388.
8. Hauri PJ, Olmsted E. Childhood onset insomnia. Sleep. 1980;3:59–65.

9. Regestein QR, Reich P. Incapacitating childhood onset insomnia. Comp Psychiatry. 1983;24:244–248.

10. Guilleminault C. Narcolepsy and its differential diagnosis. In: Guilleminault C, ed. Sleep and Its Disorders in Children. New York, NY: Raven Press; 1987:181–194.

11. Mitler MM, Hajdukovic R, Erman M, et al. Narcolepsy. J Clin Neurophysiol. 1990;7:93–118.

12. Reynolds CF, Kupfer DJ, Christianson CL. Multiple sleep latency test findings in Kleine-Levin syndrome. J Nerv Ment Dis. 1984;172:41–44.

13. Takahashi Y. Clinical studies of periodic somnolence: analysis of 28 personal cases. Psychiatr Neurol (Jpn). 1965;10:853–889.

14. Billiard M. Other hypersomnias. In: Thorpy MJ, ed. Handbook of Sleep Disorders. New York, NY: Marcel Dekker; 1990:353–371.

15. Poirier G, Montplaisir J, Lebrun A, et al. HLA antigens in narcolepsy and idiopathic hypersomnolence. Sleep. 1986;9:153–158.

16. Guilleminault C, Faull KM, Miles L, et al. Posttraumatic excessive daytime sleepiness: a review of 20 patients. Neurology. 1980;33:1584–1589.

17. Brouillette RT, Fernbach SK, Hunt CE. Obstructive sleep apnea in infants and children. J Pediatr. 1982;100:31–40.

18. Guilleminault C. Clinical features and evaluation of obstructive sleep apnea. In: Kryger MH, Roth T, Dement WC, eds. Principles and Practice of Sleep Medicine. Philadelphia, Pa: WB Saunders; 1989:552–558.

19. Guilleminault C, Kowall J. Central sleep apnea in adults. In: Thorpy MJ, ed. Handbook of Sleep Disorders. New York, NY: Marcel Dekker; 1990:337–351.

20. Guilleminault C, Quera-Salva MA, Nino-Murcia G, et al. Central sleep apnea and partial obstruction of the airway. Ann Neurol. 1987;21:465–469.

21. Plum F, Leigh RJ. Abnormalities of central mechanisms. In: Hornbein TF, ed. Regulation of Breathing, II. Vol 17: Lung Biology in Health and Disease. New York, NY: Marcel Dekker; 1981:989–1067.

22. Sullivan CE, Issa FG, Berthon-Jones M, et al. Pathophysiology of sleep apnea. In: Saunders NA, Sullivan CE, eds. Sleep and Breathing, Vol 21: Lung Biology in Health and Disease. New York, NY: Marcel Dekker; 1984:299–364.

23. Coleman R. Periodic movements in sleep (nocturnal myoclonus) and restless legs syndrome. In: Guilleminault C, ed. Sleeping and Waking Disorders: Indications and Techniques. Menlo Park, Calif: Addison-Wesley; 1982:265–295.

24. Coccagna G. Restless legs syndrome/periodic leg movements in sleep. In: Thorpy MJ, ed. Handbook of Sleep Disorders. New York, NY: Marcel Dekker; 1990:457–478.

25. Ekbom KA. Restless legs syndrome. Neurology. 1960;10:868–873.

26. Coccagna G. Restless legs syndrome/periodic leg movements in sleep. In: Thorpy MJ, ed. Handbook of Sleep Disorders. New York, NY: Marcel Dekker; 1990:457–478.

27. Bootzin RR, Nicassio PM. Behavioral treatments for insomnia. In: Hersen M, Eisler RM, Miller PM, eds. Progress in Behavior Modification. Vol 6. New York, NY: Academic Press; 1978:1–45.

28. Spielman AJ. Assessment of insomnia. Clin Psychol Rev. 1986;6:11–25.

29. Haskell EH, Palca JW, Walker JM, et al. The effects of high and low ambient temperatures on human sleep stages. Electroencephalogr Clin Neurophysiol. 1981;51:494–501.

30. Thiessen GJ, Lapointe AC. Effect of continuous traffic noise on percentage of deep sleep, waking, and sleep latency. J Acoust Soc Am. 1983;73:225–229.

31. Nicholson AN, Smith PA, Stone BM, et al. Altitude insomnia: studies during an expedition to the Himalayas. Sleep. 1988;11:354–361.

32. Weil JV. Sleep at high altitude. In: Kryger M, Roth T, Dement WC, eds. Principles and Practice of Sleep Medicine. Philadelphia, Pa: WB Saunders; 1989:269–275.

33. Agnew H, Webb W, Williams RL. The first night effect: an EEG study of sleep. Psychophysiology. 1966;7:263–266.

34. Beutler L, Thornby J, Karacan I. Psychological variables in the diagnosis of insomnia. In: Williams RL, Karacan I, eds. Sleep Disorders: Diagnosis and Treatment. New York, NY: John Wiley; 1978:61–100.

35. Carskadon M, Dement W. Effects of total sleep loss on sleep tendency. Percept Motil Skills. 1979;48:495–496.

36. Roehrs T, Zorick F, Sicikelsteel R, et al. Excessive daytime sleepiness associated with insufficient sleep. Sleep. 1983;6:319–325.

37. Ferber R. Sleeplessness in the child. In: Kryger M, Roth T, Dement WC, eds. Principles and Practice of Sleep Medicine. Philadelphia, Pa: WB Saunders; 1989:634.

38. Ferber R. Sleeplessness in the child. In: Kryger M, Roth T, Dement WC, eds. Principles and Practice of Sleep Medicine. Philadelphia, Pa: WB Saunders; 1989:633.

39. Kahn A, Mozin MJ, Casimir G, et al. Insomnia and cow's milk allergy in infants. Pediatrics. 1985;76:880–884.

40. Kahn A, Mozin MJ, Rebuffat E, et al. Difficulty in initiating and maintaining sleep associated with cow's milk allergy in infants. Sleep. 1987;10:116–121.

41. Ferber R. The sleepless child. In: Guilleminault C, ed. Sleep and Its Disorders in Children. New York, NY: Raven Press; 1987:141–163.

42. Stunkard AJ, Grace WJ, Wolfe HG. The night eating syndrome. Am J Med. 1955;7:78–86.

43. Gillin JC, Spinwebber CL, Johnson LC. Rebound insomnia: a critical review. J Clin Psychopharmacol. 1989;9:161–172.

44. Kales A, Soldatos CR, Bixler EO, et al. Rebound insomnia and rebound anxiety: a review. Pharmacology. 1983;26:121–137.

45. Oswald I. Sleep and dependence on amphetamine and other drugs. In: Kales A, ed. Sleep: Physiology and Pathology. Philadelphia, Pa: JB Lippincott; 1969:317–330.

46. Watson R, Hartmann E, Shildkraut J. Amphetamine withdrawal: affective state, sleep patterns and MHPG excretion. Am J Psychiatry. 1972;129:263–269.

47. Pokorny AD. Sleep disturbances, alcohol, and alcoholism: a review. In: Williams RL, Karacan I, eds. Sleep Disorders: Diagnosis and Treatment. New York, NY: John Wiley; 1978:233–260.

48. Friedman PA. Poisoning and its management. In: Braunwald E, Isselbacher KJ, Peterdorf RG, et al, eds. Harrison's Principles of Internal Medicine. 11th ed. New York, NY: McGraw-Hill; 1987.

49. Graeber RC. Sleep and wakefulness in international aircrews. Aviat Space Environ Med. 1986;57(suppl):12.

50. Winget CM, DeRoshio CW, Markley CL, et al. A review of human physiological and performance changes associated with desynchronosis of biological rhythms. Aviat Space Environ Med. 1984;55:1085–1095.

51. Torsvall L, Akerstedt T. Sleepiness on the job: Continuously measured EEG changes in train drivers. Electroencephalogr Clin Neurophysiol. 1987;66:502–511.

52. Walsh JK, Tepas DI, Moss PD. The EEG sleep of night and rotating shift workers. In: Johnson LC, Tepas DI, Colquhoun WP, et al, eds. Biological Rhythms, Sleep and Shift Work. New York, NY: SP Medical and Specific Books; 1981:347–356.

53. Okawa M, Takahashi K, Sasaki H. Disturbance of circadian rhythms in severely brain-damaged patients correlated with CT findings. J Neurol. 1986;233:274–282.

54. Wagner D. Circadian rhythm sleep disorders. In: Thorpy MJ, ed. Handbook of Sleep Disorders. New York, NY: Marcel Dekker; 1990:493–527.

55. Thorpy MJ, Korman E, Spielman AJ, et al. Delayed sleep phase syndrome in adolescents. J Adolesc Health Care. 1988;9:22–27.

56. Weitzman ED, Czeisler CA, Coleman RM, et al. Delayed sleep phase syndrome, a chronobiological disorder with sleep-onset insomnia. Arch Gen Psychiatry. 1981;38:737–746.

57. Kamei R, Hughes L, Miles L, et al. Advanced-sleep phase syndrome studied in a time isolation facility. Chronobiologia. 1979;6:115.

58. Moldofsky H, Musisi S, Phillipson EA. Treatment of advanced sleep phase syndrome by phase advance chronotherapy. Sleep. 1986;9:61–65.

59. Kokkoris CP, Weitzman ED, Pollak CP, et al. Longterm ambulatory monitoring in a subject with a hypernychthemeral sleep-wake cycle disturbance. Sleep. 1980;2:347–354.

60. Weber AL, Cary MS, Conner N, et al. Human non–24-hour sleep-wake cycles in an everyday environment. Sleep. 1980;2:347–354.

61. Ferber R. Sleep disorders in infants and children. In: Riley TL, ed. Clinical Aspects of Sleep and Sleep Disturbance. Boston, Mass: Butterworths; 1985:113–158.

62. Thorpy MJ. Disorders of arousal. In: Thorpy MJ, ed. Handbook of Sleep Disorders. New York, NY: Marcel Dekker; 1990:543.

63. Kales A, Soldatos CR, Bixler EO, et al. Hereditary factors in sleep walking and night terrors. Br J Psychiatry. 1980;137:111–118.

64. Thorpy MJ. Disorders of arousal. In: Thorpy MJ, ed. Handbook of Sleep Disorders. New York, NY: Marcel Dekker; 1990:532.

65. Fisher C, Kahn E, Edwards A, et al. A psychophysiological study of nightmares and night terrors: physiological aspects of the stage 4 night terror. J Nerv Ment Dis. 1973;157:75–98.

66. Thorpy MJ. Disorders of arousal. In: Thorpy MJ, ed. Handbook of Sleep Disorders. New York, NY: Marcel Dekker; 1990:538.

67. Sallustro F, Atwell CW. Body rocking, head banging and head rolling in normal children. J Pediatr. 1978;93:704–708.

68. Thorpy MJ. Rhythmic movement disorder. In: Thorpy MJ, ed. Handbook of Sleep Disorders. New York, NY: Marcel Dekker; 1990:609–629.

69. Broughton R. Pathological fragmentary myoclonus, intensified sleep starts and hypnagogic foot tremor: three unusual sleep-related disorders. In: Koella WP, ed. Sleep 1986. New York, NY: Fischer-Verlag; 1988:240–243.

70. Oswald I. Sudden bodily jerks on falling asleep. Brain. 1959;82:92–93.

71. Aarons L. Evoked sleep talking. Percept Motil Skills. 1970;31:27–40.

72. Arkin AM. Sleep talking: a review. J Nerv Ment Dis. 1966;143:101–122.

73. Jacobsen JH, Rosenberg RS, Huttenlocher PR, et al. Familial nocturnal cramping. Sleep. 1986;9:54–60.

74. Weiner IH, Weiner HL. Nocturnal leg muscle cramps. JAMA. 1980;244:2332–2333.

75. Fisher CJ, Byrne J, Edwards T, et al. A psychophysiological study of nightmares. J Am Psychoanal Assoc. 1970;18:747–782.

76. Hartman E. The nightmare. New York, NY: Basic Books; 1984.

77. Goode GB. Sleep paralysis. Arch Neurol. 1962;6:228–234.

78. Hishikawa Y. Sleep paralysis. In: Guilleminault C, Dement WC, Passouant P, eds. Narcolepsy. New York, NY: Spectrum; 1976:97–124.

79. Fisher C, Schavi RC, Edwards A, et al. Evaluation of nocturnal penile tumescence in the differential diagnosis of sexual impotence: a quantitative study. Arch Gen Psychiatry. 1979;36:431–437.

80. Karacan I, Howell JW. Impaired sleep-related penile tumescence. In: Thorpy MJ, ed. Handbook of Sleep Disorders. New York, NY: Marcel Dekker; 1990:631–640.

81. Karacan I. Painful nocturnal penile erections. JAMA. 1971;215:1831.

82. Matthews BJ, Crutchfield MB. Painful nocturnal penile erections associated with rapid eye movement sleep. Sleep. 1987;10:184–187.

83. Guilleminault C, Pool P, Motta J, et al. Sinus arrest during REM sleep in young adults. N Engl J Med. 1984;311:1006–1010.

84. Schenck CH, Bundlie SR, Ettinger MG, et al. Chronic behavioral disorders of human REM sleep: a new category of parasomnia. Sleep. 1986;9:293–306.

85. Mahowald MW, Schenck CH. REM-sleep behavior disorder. In: Thorpy MJ, ed. Handbook of Sleep Disorders. New York, NY: Marcel Dekker; 1990:567–594.

86. Funch DP, Gale EN. Factors associated with nocturnal bruxism and its treatment. J Behav Med. 1980;3:385–397.

87. Ware JC, Rugh J. Destructive bruxism: sleep stage relationship. Sleep. 1988;11:172–181.

88. Mikkelsen EJ, Rapoport JL. Enuresis: psychopathology, sleep stage, and drug response. Urol Clin North Am. 1980;7:361–377.

89. Brown L. Nocturnal enuresis. In: Thorpy MJ, ed. Handbook of Sleep Disorders. New York, NY: Marcel Dekker; 1990:595–608.

90. Guilleminault C, Eldridge FL, Phillips JR, et al. Two occult causes of insomnia and their therapeutic problems. Arch Gen Psychiatry. 1976;33:1241–1245.

91. Lugaresi E. Nocturnal paroxysmal dystonia. In: Thorpy MJ, ed. Handbook of Sleep Disorders. New York, NY: Marcel Dekker; 1990:551–565.

92. Lugaresi E, Cirignotta F, Montagna P. Nocturnal paroxysmal dystonia. J Neurol Neurosurg Psychiatry. 1986;49:375–380.

93. Baron RC, Thacker SB, Gorelkin L, et al. Sudden death among Southeast Asian refugees. JAMA. 1983;250:2947–2951.

94. Otto CM, Tauxe RV, Cobb LA, et al. Ventricular fibrillation causes sudden death in Southeast Asian immigrants. Ann Intern Med. 1984;100:45–47.

95. Lugaresi E, Cirignotta F, Montagna P. Snoring: Pathogenic, clinical, and therapeutic aspects. In: Kryger M, Roth T, Dement WC, eds. Principles and Practice of Sleep Medicine. Philadelphia, Pa: WB Saunders; 1989:494–500.

96. Waller PC, Bhopal RS. Is snoring a cause of vascular disease? an epidemiological review. Lancet. 1989;1:143–146.

97. Durand M, Cabal L, Gonzalez F, et al. Ventilatory control and carbon dioxide response in preterm infants with idiopathic apnea. Am J Dis Child. 1985;139:717–720.

98. Henderson-Smart DJ. The effect of gestational age on the incidence and duration of recurrent apnea in newborn babies. Aust Paediatr J. 1985;17:273–276.

99. Fleming PJ, Cade D, Bryan MH, et al. Congenital central hypoventilation and sleep state. Pediatrics. 1980;66:425–428.

100. Paton JY, Swaminathan S, Sargent CW, et al. Hypoxic and hypercapneic ventilatory responses in awake children with congenital central hypoventilation syndrome. Am Rev Respir Dis. 1989;140:368–372.

101. Hoppenbrouwers T, Hodgman JE. Sudden infant death syndrome (SIDS): an integration of ontogenetic, pathologic, physiologic and epidemiologic factors. Neuropediatrics. 1982;13:36–51.

102. Merritt TA, Valdes Dapena M. SIDS research update. Pediatr Ann. 1984;13:193–207.

103. Coulter DL, Allen RJ. Benign neonatal sleep myoclonus. Arch Neurol. 1982;39:191–192.

104. Resnick TJ, Moshe SL, Perotta L, et al. Benign neonatal sleep myoclonus: relationship to sleep states. Arch Neurol. 1986;43:266–268.

105. Ganguli R, Reynolds CF, Kupfer DJ. EEG sleep in young, never-medicated, schizophrenic patients: a comparison with delusional and nondelusional depressives and with healthy controls. Arch Gen Psychiatry. 1987;44:36–44.

106. Zarcone VP. Sleep and schizophrenia. In: Williams RL, Karacan I, Moore CA, eds. Sleep Disorders: Diagnosis and Treatment. New York, NY: John Wiley; 1988:165–188.

107. Gillin JC, Duncan W, Pettigrew KD, et al. Successful separation of depressed, normal, and insomniac subjects by EEG sleep data. Arch Gen Psychiatry. 1979;36:85–90.

108. Reynolds CF, Kupfer DJ. Sleep research in affective illness: state of the art circa 1987. Sleep. 1987;10:199–215.

109. Reynolds CF, Shaw DM, Newton TF, et al. EEG sleep in outpatients with generalized anxiety: a preliminary comparison with depressed outpatients. Psychiatry Res. 1983;8:81–89.

110. Rosa RR, Bonnett MM, Kramer M. The relationship of sleep and anxiety in anxious subjects. Biol Psychol. 1983;16:119–126.

111. Hauri PJ, Friedman M, Ravaris CL. Sleep in patients with spontaneous panic attacks. Sleep. 1989;12:323–337.

112. Mellman TA, Unde TW. Electroencephalographic sleep in panic disorder. Arch Gen Psychiatry. 1989;46:178–184.

113. Porkny AD. Sleep disturbances, alcohol and alcoholism: a review. In: Williams RL, Karacan I, eds. Sleep Disorders: Diagnosis and Treatment. New York, NY: John Wiley; 1978:389–402.

114. Wagman A, Allen R. Effects of alcohol ingestion and abstinence on slow wave sleep of alcoholics. In: Gross MM, ed: Alcohol Intoxication and Withdrawal, II. New York, NY: Plenum Press; 1975:453–466.

115. Aldrich M. Sleep and degenerative neurological disorders involving the motor system. In: Thorpy MJ, ed: Handbook of Sleep Disorders. New York, NY: Marcel Dekker; 1990:673–692.

116. Evans LK. Sundown syndrome in institutionalized elderly. J Am Geriatr Soc. 1987;35:101–108.

117. Vitiello MV, Prinz PN. Sleep/wake patterns and sleep disorders in Alzheimer's disease. In: Thorpy MJ, ed. Handbook of Sleep Disorders. New York, NY: Marcel Dekker; 1990:703–718.

118. Mouret J. Difference in sleep in patients with Parkinson's disease. Electroencephalogr Clin Neurophysiol. 1975;38:563–567.

119. Nausieda PA. Sleep in Parkinson's disease. In: Thorpy MJ, ed. Handbook of Sleep Disorders. New York, NY: Marcel Dekker; 1990:719–735.

120. Lugaresi E, Medori R, Montagna P, et al. Fatal familial insomnia and dysautonomia with selective degeneration of thalamic nuclei. N Engl J Med. 1986;315:997–1003.

121. Lugaresi E. Fatal familial insomnia. In: Thorpy MJ, ed. Handbook of Sleep Disorders. New York, NY: Marcel Dekker; 1990:479–489.

122. Degan R, Niedermeyer E, eds: Epilepsy, Sleep and Sleep Deprivation. Amsterdam, Netherlands: Elsevier; 1984.

123. Montplaisir J. Epilepsy and sleep: reciprocal interactions and diagnostic procedures involving sleep. In: Thorpy MJ, ed. Handbook of Sleep Disorders. New York, NY: Marcel Dekker; 1990:643–662.

124. Patry G, Lyagoubi S, Tassinari CA. Subclinical "electrical status epilepticus" induced by sleep in children. Arch Neurol. 1971;24:242–252.

125. Tassinari CA, Bureau M, Dravet C, et al. Epilepsy with continuous spikes and waves during sleep. In: Roger J, Dravet C, Bureau M, et al, eds. Epileptic Syndromes in Infancy, Childhood and Adolescence. London, England: John Libbey Eurotext; 1985:194–204.

126. Dexter JD. Relationship between sleep and headaches. In: Thorpy MJ, ed. Handbook of Sleep Disorders. New York, NY: Marcel Dekker; 1990:663–671.

127. Kayed K, Godtlibsen OB, Sjaastad O. Chronic paroxysmal hemicrania, IV: "REM sleep locked" nocturnal headache attacks. Sleep. 1978;1:91–95.

128. Bert J, Collomb H, Fressy J, et al. Etude electrographique du sommeil nocturne. In: Fischgold H, ed. Le Sommeil de Nuit Normal et Pathologique. Paris, France: Masson; 1965:334–352.

129. Schwartz BA, Escande C. Sleeping sickness: sleep study of a case. Electroencephalogr Clin Neurophysiol. 1970;3:83–87.

130. Muller J, Ludmer PL, Wellick SN, et al. Circadian variation in the frequency of sudden cardiac death. Circulation. 1987;75:131–138.

131. Nowlin JB, Troyer WG Jr, Collins WS, et al. The association of nocturnal angina pectoris with dreaming. Ann Intern Med. 1965;63:1040–1046.

132. Fleetham J, West P, Mezon B, et al. Sleep, arousals and oxygen desaturation in chronic obstructive pulmonary disease: the effect of oxygen therapy. Am Rev Respir Dis. 1982;126:429–433.

133. Flenley C. Chronic obstructive pulmonary disease. In: Kryger M, Roth T, Dement WC, eds. Principles and Practice of Sleep Medicine. Philadelphia, Pa: WB Saunders; 1989:601–610.

134. Douglas NJ. Asthma. In: Kryger M, Roth T, Dement WC, eds. Principles and Practice of Sleep Medicine. Philadelphia, Pa: WB Saunders; 1989:591–600.

135. Montplaisir J, Walsh J, Malo JL. Nocturnal asthma features of attacks, sleep and breathing patterns. Am Rev Respir Dis. 1982;125:18–22.

136. Orr WC. Gastrointestinal disorders. In: Kryger M, Roth T, Dement WC, eds. Principles and Practice of Sleep Medicine. Philadelphia, Pa: WB Saunders; 1989:622–629.

137. Orr WC, Johnson LF, Robinson MG. The effect of sleep on swallowing, esophageal peristalsis, and acid clearance. Gastroenterology. 1984;86:814–819.

138. Segawa K, Nakazawa S, Tsukamoto Y, et al. Peptic ulcer is prevalent among shift workers. Dig Dis Sci. 1987;32:449–453.

139. Stacher G, Presslich B, Starker H. Gastric acid secretion and sleep stages during natural night sleep. Gastroenterology. 1975;68:1455–1499.

140. Moldofsky H, Saskin P, Lue FA. Sleep and symptoms in fibrositis syndrome after a febrile illness. J Rheumatol. 1988;15:1701–1704.

141. Saskin P, Moldofsky H, Lue FA. Sleep and posttraumatic rheumatic pain modulation disorder (fibrositis syndrome). Psychosom Med. 1986;48:319–323.

142. Hartmann E, Baekeland F, Zwilling GR. Psychological differences between short and long sleepers. Arch Gen Psychiatry. 1972;26:463–468.

143. Webb WB. Are short and long sleepers different? Psychol Rep. 1979;44:259–264.

144. Hartmann E, Baekeland F, Zwilling GR. Psychological differences between short and long sleepers. Arch Gen Psychiatry. 1972;26:463–468.

145. Webb WB. Are short and long sleepers different? Psychol Rep. 1979;44:259–264.

146. Roth B. Narcolepsy and Hypersomnia. Basel, Switzerland: Karger; 1980.

147. Broughton R, Tolentino MA, Krelina M. Excessive fragmentary myoclonus in NREM sleep: a report of 38 cases. Electroencephalogr Clin Neurophysiol. 1985;61:123–309.

148. Geschickter EH, Andrews PA, Bullard RW. Nocturnal body temperature regulation in man: a rationale for sweating in sleep. J Appl Physiol. 1966;21:623–630.

149. Lea MJ, Aber RC. Descriptive epidemiology of night sweats upon admission to a university hospital. South Med J. 1985;78:1065–1067.

150. Billiard M, Guilleminault C, Dement WC. A menstruation-linked periodic hypersomnia. Neurology. 1975;25:436–443.

151. Ho A. Sex hormones and the sleep of women. Sleep Res. 1972;1:184.

152. Errante J. Sleep deprivation or postpartum blues? Topics Clin Nurs. 1985;6:9–18.

153. Karacan I, Williams RL, Hursh CJ, et al. Some implications of the sleep pattern of pregnancy for postpartum emotional disturbances. Br J Psychiatry. 1969;115:929–935.

154. Broughton R. Neurology and dreaming. Psychiatr J Univ Ottawa. 1982;7:101–110.

155. Willmer JP, Broughton RJ. Neurogenic sleep related polypnea: a new disorder? Sleep Res. 1989;18:322.

156. Kryger MH, Acres JC, Brownell L. A syndrome of sleep, stridor and panic. Chest. 1981;80:768.

157. Thorpy MJ, Aloe F. Sleep-related laryngospasm. Sleep Res. 1989;18:313.

158. Arnold GE. Disorders of laryngeal function. In: Paparella MM, Shumrick DA, eds. Otolaryngology. Vol 3. Philadelphia, Pa: WB Saunders; 1973:638.

159. Thorpy MJ, Aloe FS. Choking during sleep. Sleep Res. 1989;18:314.

47

Epidemiology of Sleep Disorders

Markku Partinen
Christer Hublin

In the 1980s, the large epidemiological studies on sleep disorders were based on the 1979 sleep disorders classification.[1] In 1990, a new *International Classification of Sleep Disorders* (ICSD) was published. The revised 1997 version of the manual is the most widely used classification system by those working with sleep disorders.[2] Other international classifications include the *International Classification of Diseases, 10th Revision* (ICD-10) published by the World Health Organization and the *Diagnostic and Statistical Manual of Mental Disorders, Fourth Edition* (DSM-IV) published by the American Psychiatric Association.

From the public health viewpoint, the most important sleep problems are insomnia, sleep-related breathing disorders, and excessive daytime sleepiness; these are discussed in detail in this chapter. The prevalence of specific sleep disorders may be found in the corresponding chapters elsewhere in this textbook.

For a general review of epidemiology, the reader is referred to other sources.[3–13] Many clinical epidemiologists, as well as economists, believe in the importance of *evidence-based medicine*. In a critical article, Wright et al.[14] claimed that very little is known about the health effects of sleep apnea, implying that much of the research does not meet the needs of evidence-based medicine.

EARLY STUDIES

The oldest epidemiological studies of sleep length are from the end of the 18th century. Among the most respected studies were those by Clement Dukes from England about the need of sleep by young children. Other well known early studies are by Hertel from Denmark, Bernhard from Germany, and Claparéde from France.[15, 16] According to the reports of that time, 6-year-old children should sleep 10.5 to 13.5 h per night, 15-year-old teenagers should sleep 9 to 10 h per night, and adults should sleep 8 to 8.5 h per night.

In the 1920s through 1930s studies concerned the sleep of schoolchildren, but there were some studies about adults. The average sleep length of adults varied between 7 h 25 min and 8 h 23 min, depending on age.[17, 18] Women slept a little longer than did men, except mentally retarded subjects, for whom the situation was reversed.[19, 20]

Sleep disturbances have been shown to be increased with age. In the study of Laird in 1931,[18] slightly more than 90% of subjects who are 25 years old reported uninterrupted sleep at night, but at the age of 95, 100% reported some wakefulness each night. More than 70% of 509 elderly reported men some difficulty in going to sleep, and more than 40% reported wakefulness during the night. Difficulty going to sleep increased with age. Most men used special techniques to aid them in falling asleep; reading was used by 25%, and relaxation techniques with or without the aid of warm drinks were used by 18%. The author was surprised that 3% used drugs other than alcohol to help them sleep, and 2% used alcohol. This figure should be compared with modern times, when hypnotics are sometimes prescribed too easily.

Many epidemiological studies of sleeping habits have been performed since 1960. In these studies, the average length of sleep varied between 7 and 8 h. In a questionnaire survey, 7.4% of 1278 University of Florida students reported less than 6.5 h of sleep at night, and 13.4% reported more than 8.5 h.[21]

In Scotland, 2446 subjects older than 15 years were questioned. Of subjects in the age group of 65 to 74 years, 18% complained of waking up before 5 AM. This figure decreased 12% after the age of 75 years. Fewer than 10% of men 15 to 64 years old complained of disturbed sleep. In the age group of 65 to 74 years, disturbed sleep was a complaint in 25% of the men and 43% of women.[22]

Many other epidemiological studies have been performed in both the United States and other countries. Bixler et al.[23] determined the prevalence of sleep disorders among 1006 households in the Los Angeles metropolitan area. The prevalence of past or current insomnia was 42.5%, and the prevalence of current insomnia was 32.2%. In the same survey, 7.1% complained of excessive sleep.[23]

INSOMNIA AND USE OF HYPNOTIC AGENTS

Insomnia is the most common sleep-wake–related complaint, and sleeping pills are among the most commonly prescribed drugs in clinical practice at the primary health care level. It is, however, important to remember that insomnia is a symptom, and there can be dozens of causes, many of which require specific therapies. Many of the insomnia diagnoses are quite new as diagnostic entities, and there are few or no studies of their prevalence. Therefore, we concentrate on studies dealing with insomnia in general, its three main manifestations (i.e., trouble falling asleep, trouble staying asleep, and early morning awakening), and the use of hypnotics agents. Subjects range in age from children to adults.

Table 47–1 presents studies on insomnia in general. The heterogeneity of the definitions and methods used is striking, but some clear trends can be seen.

First, insomnia increases with age. About one third of subjects older than 65 years old have more or less continuous insomnia, although at very old age, the levels may be lower. In Australia, 18% of women and 12.6% of men older than 70 years have trouble sleeping nearly every night.[24] In children and adolescents, the prevalence of frequent insomnia is quite variable; in several studies, it is higher than 10%. In middle-aged populations, the frequency of long-standing insomnia seems to be around 10%.

Second, there is a clear gender difference, with insomnia occurring about 1.5 times more often in women than in men; this is especially true in menopausal and postmenopausal women compared with middle-aged men. In a community-based sample of 301 women between 35 and 55 years old, the most common perimenopausal symptoms were dysphoric mood; vasomotor, somatic, and neuromuscular symptoms; and insomnia.[25] More epidemiological studies of insomnia should be focused on postmenopausal women.

Table 47–2 presents another set of studies that provide information on the main manifestations of insomnia. Again, there are considerable differences between the studies both methodologically and in the results, but there are similar trends in general. Trouble falling asleep seems to be the most common manifestation in younger age groups, whereas trouble staying asleep (middle night insomnia or early morning insomnia) is the most frequent form of insomnia in middle-aged and elderly people.

Seasonal differences can occur. Husby and Lingjaerde conducted a questionnaire study in northern Norway.[26] Of the 14,667 respondents from Tromsø, which is situated at about 69 degrees north, 41.7% of the women and 29.9% of the men had occasional insomnia. In their study, complaints of insomnia were more common during the dark period of year than during other times of the year. Insomnia during the midnight-sun period (summer insomnia) decreased with age, whereas the other seasonal types of insomnia increased with age.[26]

The association of psychiatric disorders, especially depression, with insomnia is well known. Primary insomnia and insomnia related to mental disorders are the two most common DSM-IV insomnia diagnoses. The differential diagnosis may be difficult. In a study by Nowell et al.,[27] 216 patients with insomnia were evaluated. Each patient was interviewed by one sleep specialist and one non–sleep specialist. DSM-IV criteria were used. Questions regarding many other contributing factors were included. Of the 216, 99 (46%) were diagnosed as having insomnia related to mental disorders, and 48 (22%) were diagnosed as having primary insomnia. However, a psychiatric disorder was rated as a contributing factor for 77% of patients with a first diagnosis of primary insomnia.[27] In a large U.S. community survey, the prevalence of uncomplicated and complicated insomnia was 4.9% and 3.6%, respectively.[28] Among those with complicated insomnia in the past year, 25% had major depression, 19% abused alcohol, 12% had dysthymia, 9% had panic disorder, 8% abused drugs, 8% had schizophrenia, and 2% had somatization disorder.[28] In a clinical population, 40 young (20 to 40 years old) patients with psychophysiological insomnia were critically evaluated; 48% had some psychiatric disorders according to *Diagnostic and Statistical Manual of Mental Disorders, Revised Third Edition* (DSM-III-R) criteria.[29] In a World Health Organization collaborative study, 25,916 primary health care attenders were evaluated. Sleep problems were present in 27% of the patients. Of the patients with insomnia, 51% had a well-defined ICD-10 mental disorder, mainly depression or anxiety, or abused alcohol, or a combination. Forty percent of insomniacs reported using alcohol and over-the-counter medications to help sleep.[30]

Insomnia is a frequent complaint among many other patient groups. In the study of Dodge et al.,[31] the prevalence of insomnia was 31.8% to 52.4% among adults with respiratory symptoms (e.g., cough, dyspnea, wheeze); among adults without respiratory symptoms, the prevalence was 25.8% to 26.2%.

The prevalence of sleeping problems varies by occupation. In a questionnaire survey of 6268 adults in 40 different occupations, 18.9% of bus drivers complained of having rather or very much difficulty falling asleep. Among male directors and male physicians, the respective percentages were 3.7% and 4.9%. Disturbed nocturnal sleep was complained of the most often by male laborers (28.1% waking up at least three times a night) and female cleaners (26.6%). Disturbed nocturnal sleep was rare among male physicians (1.6%), male directors (7.4%), female head nurses (8.9%), and female social workers (9.4%).[32] Symptoms of work-related stress and burnout also are associated with insomnia. Simple methods, such as the five-item version of the Mental Health Index and some other questions, may be used to effectively screen workers with mental health and sleep problems.[33, 34]

Table 47–3 lists some studies about the use of hypnotic agents. One of the best data about use of hypnotic agents in the United States come from a survey performed in 1979.[35] In a nationally representative probability sample survey of noninstitutionalized adults, 3161 people 18 to 79 years old were surveyed. Insomnia afflicted 35% of all adults during the course of 1 year. Those with serious insomnia tended to be women and older. Many of them had high levels of psychic distress and somatic anxiety, symptoms of depression, and other health problems. During the year before the sur-

Table 47-1. OCCURRENCE OF INSOMNIA IN GENERAL

Reference	N	Study Population (Age Range, y)	Definition	Methods	Occurrence (%)
Saarenpää-Heikkilä et al. (1995)[161]	574	School-age children (7–17)	Sleeplessness	Questionnaire	Often or always: 4 (m), 5 (f) Sometimes: 61 (m), 57 (f)
Tynjälä et al. (1993)[162]	40,202	School-age children (11–16)	Inability to fall asleep twice a week	Questionnaire (in nine countries)	11–12 y: 16.4–33.2 13–14 y: 11.5–25.3 15–16 y: 10.8–26.6
Rimpelä and Rimpelä (1983)[163]	1954	School-age children (12–17)	Difficulties in falling asleep or awakenings during night	Questionnaire	Often or always: 1 (m), 2 (f) Sometimes: 23 (m), 38 (f)
Price et al. (1978)[164]	627	Students (15–18)	Chronic poor sleepers: sleep onset 45 min three times a week or one awakening per night followed by 30 min awake three times a week or three awakenings per night three times a week	Questionnaire	12.6
Kirmil-Gray et al. (1984)[165]	277	Students (13–17)	See Price et al. (1978)[164]	Questionnaire	11
Levy et al. (1986)[166]	379	Students (12–18)	See Price et al. (1978)[164]	Questionnaire	12.5
Lugaresi et al. (1983)[47] Cirignotta et al. (1985)[167]	5713	Population sample (3–94)	Sleeping badly always or almost always	Questionnaire	9.9 (m), 16.8 (f) <20 y: 1.6 20–44 y: 11.9 45–54 y: 20 (m), increase from 20 to 40 (f) >60 y: increase from 20 to 30 (m)
Smirne et al. (1983)[168]	2518	Inpatients (6–92; >90% adults)	Current complaint of insomnia	Questionnaire	12.8
Partinen and Rimpelä (1982)[46]	2016	Population sample (15–64)	Insomnia daily or several times weekly	Telephone interview	7 (m), 9 (f) 15–24 y: 5 25–44 y: 6 45–64 y: 14
Yeo et al. (1996)[169]	2418	Chinese and Malays in Singapore (15–55)	Having insomnia for the past year	Interview at home	15.3%
Hohagen et al. (1991)[170]	1500	Outpatients (18–65)	Severe insomnia including daytime impairment (DSM-III-R)	Questionnaire	19 18–35 y: 11 35–50 y: 21 51–65 y: 27
Ford and Kamerow (1989)[6]	7954	Population sample (18–65+)	Ever a period of 2 weeks or longer with trouble falling asleep, staying asleep, or waking up too early	Direct structured interview using Diagnostic Interview Schedule	7.9 (m), 12.1 (f)
Weissman et al. (1997)[28]	10533	Population sample (18+)	During the past year, ever having a period of 2 weeks or more with trouble falling asleep, staying asleep, or waking	Direct structured interview using Diagnostic Interview Schedule	All types: 11.9 Uncomplicated: 4.9 Complicated: 3.6
Dodge et al. (1995)[31]	1667	Population sample (18–64+)	Current trouble falling asleep, trouble staying asleep, or waking up too early	Questionnaire and interview	18–44 y: 22.8 (m), 30.0 (f) 45–64 y: 31.5 (m), 43.8 (f) >64 y: 36.4 (m), 47.6 (f)
Simon and VonKorff (1997)[171]	373	Primary care patients (18–65)	Nearly every night 2 h to fall asleep; or lying awake 1 h; or waking 2 h early	Interview	10
Husby and Lingjaerde (1990)[26]	14667	Population sample (20–54)	Sleeplessness (yes/no)	Questionnaire	Men: 29.9 Women: 41.0
Hyyppä and Kronholm (1987)[172]	1099	Population sample (29–79)	Sleeplessness	Questionnaire	Often or always: 9.6 (m), 12.8 (f) Sometimes: 57.6 (m), 62.7 (f)
Morgan and Clarke (1997)[173]	1042	Primary care patients (65–80+)	Sleeping problems often or all the time	Questionnaire	65–69 y: 33.2 (m), 44.1 (f) 70–74 y: 39.4 (m), 44.4 (f) 75–79 y: 11.2 (m), 43.8 (f) >80 y: 17.6 (m), 30.8 (f)

f, female; m, male.

Table 47–2. MAIN MANIFESTATIONS OF INSOMNIA

Reference	N	Study Population (Age Range, y)	Methods	Trouble Falling Asleep (%)	Trouble Staying Asleep (%)	Early Morning Awakening (%)
Blader et al. (1997)[174]	987	School-age children (5–12)	Questionnaire	1–2 nights/week: 12.9 ≥3 nights/week: 11.3 ≥4 nights/week: 9.1 (m), 10.0 (f)	1–2 nights/week: 6.0 ≥3 nights/week: 6.5 ≥4 nights/week: 1.5 (m), 3.0 (f)	
Morrison et al. (1992)[175]	943	Cohort (15)	Interview			>4 nights/week: 2.5 (m), 4.4 (f)
Lack (1986)[176]	211	University students (16–50; median, 19)	Questionnaire	Frequently: 13.3	Frequently: 7.6	Frequently: 11.8
Janson et al. (1996)[177]	2394	Population sample (20–45)	Questionnaire	Almost every night: 4.7 ≥3 nights/week: 6.8	Almost every night: 1.4	Almost every night: 1.4 ≥3 nights/week: 5.7
Ohayon (1996)[178]	5622	Population sample (>15)	Telephone interview using the Sleep-Eval expert system		Regularly: 32.8 (m), 45.0 (f)	
Ohayon (1997)[179]	4972	Population sample (>15)	Telephone interview using the Sleep-Eval expert system	Currently: 10.5 (m), 15.3 (f)	Currently: 16.4 (m), 24.8 (f)	Currently: 13.7 (m), 17.8 (f)
Bixler et al. (1979)[23]	1006	Population sample (>18)	Questionnaire	Currently: 14.4 (about two thirds females)	Currently: 22.9 (about two thirds females)	Currently: 13.8 (about two thirds females)
Karacan et al. (1983)[180]	2347	Population sample (18–65+)	Interview	Often or always (no age effect): 6.0 (m), 11.2 (f)	Often or always (significant increase with age): 12.9 (m), 17.4 (f)	Often or always (significant increase with age): 6.2 (m), 8.0 (f)
Kronholm and Hyyppä (1985)[181]	601	Population samples (30–71)	Questionnaire	30–40 y: 4.9% 50–60 y: 10.3% 71 y: 15.3%		30–40 y: 23.9% 50–60 y: 43.3% 71 y: 35.6%
Ganguli et al. (1996)[182]	1050	Population sample (66–97)	Questionnaire	Sometimes or usually: 26.7 (m), 44.1 (f)	Sometimes or usually: 19.2 (m), 35.8 (f)	Sometimes or usually: 13.6 (m), 23.3 (f)
Blazer et al. (1995)[183]	3976	Population sample (≥65; EPESE)	Interview using a questionnaire	Blacks: 14.8 Whites: 16.3	Blacks: 19.9 Whites: 33.8	Blacks: 12.9 Whites: 16.0
Foley et al. (1995)[184]	9282	Population sample (≥65; EPESE)	Interview using a questionnaire	Most of the time: 19.2	Most of the time: 29.7	Most of the time: 18.8
Henderson et al. (1995)[24]	869	Population sample (≥70)	Home interview, use of a computer algorithm	Nearly every night over the previous 2 weeks: 5.1	NA	Nearly every night over the previous 2 weeks: 2.6

EPESE, Established Populations for Epidemiologic Studies in the Elderly; f, female; m, male; NA, not applicable.

Table 47–3. USE OF HYPNOTICS

Reference, Country	N (Age Ranges, y)	Definition of Use	Users (%)
Kirmil-Gray et al. (1984),[165] United States	277 (13–17)	Used medication at least once for disturbed sleep	14.9
Lack (1986),[176] Australia	211 (16–50; median, 19)	At least occasionally	4.7
Janson et al. (1996),[177] Iceland, Sweden, Belgium	2394 (20–45)	At least once weekly	1.3
Ohayon (1996),[178] France	5622 (>15)	Current use	6.8 (m), 12.7 (f)
Simen et al. (1996),[185] Germany	1653 (14–65)	At least once weekly	1
	344 (>65)	At least once weekly	10
Johnson et al. (1998),[186] United States	2181 (18–45)	Use of sleep aids at least some time during the past year	Sleep medication: 18 (36% using for >1 month)
			Alcohol: 13 (15% for >1 month)
			Any substance: 26
Karacan et al. (1983),[180] United States	2347 (18–65+)	Sometimes	3.8 (m), 6.8 (f)
		Often or always	3.3 (m), 4.0 (f)
Partinen et al. (1983),[187] Finland	30,142 (18–69)	For more than 2 months the preceding year	18–29 y: 0.4 (m), 0.3 (f)
			30–39 y: 1.1 (m), 1.0 (f)
			40–49 y: 2.3 (m), 2.3 (f)
			50–59 y: 3.3 (m), 3.9 (f)
			60–69 y: 3.8 (m), 7.5 (f)
Mellinger et al. (1985),[35] United States	3161 (18–79)	Hypnotic use in the past year	2.6
		Hypnotic use regularly for longer than 1 year	0.3 of all adults, 11 of all users of hypnotics (35% of all adults complained of insomnia)
Lopez et al. (1995),[36] Mexico	1000 (18–84)	Use to sleep	5 (50% of men and 14% of women did not report insomnia)
		Frequently	1.4
Hyyppä and Kronholm (1987),[172] Finland	1099 (29–79)	Sometimes	10.7 (m), 15.4 (f)
		Often	1.9 (m), 3.3 (f)
		Almost every evening	1.7 (m), 3.5 (f)
Morgan et al. (1988),[188] Great Britain	1020 (>65)	Sometimes	3
		Often	1
		All the time	12
Asplund (1995),[36a] Sweden	10,216 (pensioners; >65)	Taking hypnotics	<70 y: 7.9 (m), 15.0 (f)
			70–80 y: 14.4 (m), 23.0 (f)
			80+ y: 21.8 (m), 34.9 (f)
Henderson et al. (1995),[24] Australia	Community: 874 Institutions: 59 (≥70)	Taking hypnotics nearly every night over the previous 2 weeks	Community: 14.5 (10.3% among those with no insomnia)
			Institutions: 39.7 (36.5% among those with no insomnia)

f, female; m, male.

vey, 2.6% of adults had used a medically prescribed hypnotic agent; 0.3% of all adults and 11% of all users of hypnotic agents reported using the medication regularly for 1 year or longer. When anxiolytic and antidepressant agents were excluded, 4.3% of adults had used a medically prescribed hypnotic for sleep and 3.1% had used an over-the-counter sleeping pill. It was also found that 85% of serious insomniacs were not treated with either prescribed or over-the-counter medications.[35] The use of hypnotic agents has increased since the 1980s.

In Mexico, 36% of adults have insomnia, and 16% report severe insomnia.[36] Only 10.5% of the insomniacs had been using hypnotic agents, but 3.3% of the insomniacs were using hypnotic agents frequently. Of those 18 to 20 years old, 1.6% had been using hypnotic agents compared with 17% in subjects older than 61 years. Women had significantly more frequent insomnia and took more sleeping pills than men, as in other countries.[36]

In Sweden, 10,216 members of the Swedish Pensioners' Association were surveyed[36a] (see Table 47–3). Hypnotic agents were used by 13.5% of the men and 22.3% of the women. Of the men aged younger than 70 years, 7.9% were receiving such treatment; of those 70 to 80 years old, 14.4% were using hypnotic agents; and of those 80 years old or older, 21.8% were taking hypnotic agents ($P < .0001$). The corresponding frequencies among women were 15.0%, 23.0%, and 34.9%, respectively ($P < .0001$). Hypnotic agents are used by many institutionalized elderly subjects even without insomnia.[24] This is problematic, and it rises an ethical question because the chronic use of hypnotic agents is associated with excessive mortality rates.[37–39] In a Swedish study,[36a] only half of all men and women treated with hypnotic agents in all age groups reported a good night's sleep. Among these subjects, both angina pectoris and cardiac arrhythmia were twice as common as among elderly subjects who experienced poor sleep and were receiving treatment with hypnotic agents. In conclusion, poor health and diseases are overrepresented in elderly persons treated with hypnotic agents.

An excellent way of tracking the use of hypnotic medication of the population is to count unit defined daily doses (DDD) from the sales statistics of pharmacies and hospitals. When one knows the assumed average dose per day for each drug, sales per year, and population of the country, one can calculate DDDs per 1000 inhabitants per day. This method is used in Finnish statistics on medicines. In Finland,[40] for all hypnotic agents, the rate is 38 DDD/1000 inhabitants/day. In 1994, a total of 43.6 million tablets were sold. There are about 5 million inhabitants in Finland. The most commonly used hypnotic agents in Finland is zopiclone (16.3 DDD 1000 inhabitants/day). Other rates were 0.9 DDD/1000 inhabitants/day for triazolam and 14 DDD/1000 inhabitants/day for temazepam. Benzodiazepines are available in all Scandinavian countries; in 1994, the consumption of benzodiazepines (in DDD/1000 inhabitants/day) was 20 in Finland, 24 in Sweden, and 25 in Norway.[40]

DAYTIME SLEEPINESS

Daytime sleepiness is a common complaint (Table 47–4). Snoring is related to daytime sleepiness, as are the use of hypnotic agents, sleep difficulties, irregular sleep-wake schedule, and sleep deprivation. Obstructive sleep apnea syndrome is the most common cause of sleepiness diagnosed in the U.S. or European sleep laboratories. Narcolepsy is less common. In sleep laboratory populations, about 75% of patients with daytime sleepiness have sleep-related breathing disorders (usually obstructive sleep apnea syndrome or upper airway resistance syndrome), 20% have narcolepsy, and 5% have restless legs, periodic movements in sleep, or other disorders that can cause daytime sleepiness.

Definition of Daytime Sleepiness

The feeling of not being alert is common, occurring both as a physiological everday phenomenon and as one symptom of many sleep disorders.[1, 2] In spoken language, this feeling is probably most often called "sleepiness," but the actual meaning varies. By definition, "sleepiness" implies an increased risk of falling asleep,[2] but the complaint of sleepiness is sometimes used to describe physical tiredness, fatigue, and loss of mental alertness without an increase in sleep behavior[1]—conditions often associated with a decreased ability to fall asleep, contrary to true sleepiness.

The results of one of our questionnaire studies[41] exemplify these problems. Among those reporting daytime sleepiness every or almost every day, about one fifth of women and two fifths were habitual snorers,

one fourth had scores suggesting moderate to severe depression, one fourth had insomnia at least every other day, one tenth were regular hypnotic or tranquilizer users, and one tenth reported insufficient sleep. Thus, a "tired" or "sleepy" (in the patient's words) person may have insomnia and not excessive daytime sleepiness (EDS) or hypersomnia. In a multiple sleep latency test study, the patients may have great difficulty falling asleep, contrary to the experience of hypersomniacs and narcoleptics. Sleep researchers know that a proper term for such an insomniac person would probably be "fatigued," but most patients are not researchers, and their descriptions of their symptoms are related to their feelings, emotions, and cultural background. These facts must be taken into consideration when using just one or two items about sleepiness in a questionnaire. However, the issue is even more complex because other studies that use more extensive screening instruments provide similar results.[8, 42]

Occurrence of Daytime Sleepiness

Table 47–4 provides a summary of studies on daytime sleepiness. Depending on the wording, there is about a 100-fold difference in occurrence, ranging from 0.3%[43] to 35.8%,[44] and in the majority of the studies, the range is 5% to 15%. The studies can be grouped according to the type of sleepiness. The prevalence is lowest for hypersomnia-like states (more sleep per 24 hours than normal). Sleep attacks (involuntary sleep episodes during wake) are reported on average in 5% to 10% of subjects up to middle age, and in older persons, the frequency seems to increase to 20% to 30%, without a clear gender difference. Frequent or excessive (subjective) daytime sleepiness occurs in about 10% to 15%, and occurs, more often in school-age children or young adults than in middle-aged adults and more often in females than in males. Results are contradictory regarding occurrences in middle-aged and old adults.[8, 41]

The variability of the results in these studies can be mainly accounted for by differences in the definition of sleepiness and by other methodological aspects, but there probably also are real differences in different populations. Recently, D'Alessandro et al.[45] called attention to the problems of the published studies on EDS; they reviewed seven population-based cross-sectional questionnaire studies[23, 43, 46–50] and concluded that the "prevalence of EDS is an open epidemiological question." They pointed out that the differences in definitions of EDS lead to low comparability of the results, with one additional major problem being how "excessive" should be characterized. There is a need for further studies that use homogeneous definitions and reliable and validated screening instruments in large samples of different general populations.

NARCOLEPSY AND NARCOLEPSY-LIKE SYMPTOMS

The usual prevalence of narcolepsy is about 0.05%, or 50 per 100,000 population.[51–55] However, there is a

Table 47–4. OCCURRENCE OF DAYTIME SLEEPINESS

Reference	N (Gender)	Study Population (Age Range, y)	Definition of Sleepiness (Wording of Questions)	Methods	Occurrence (%)
Hypersomnia-Like States					
Karacan et al. (1976)[43]	1645 (?)	Population sample (18–70)	Too much sleep	Questionnaire	0.3
Bixler et al. (1979)[23]	1006 (m, f)	Population sample (18–80)	Sleeping too much	Questionnaire	7.1 (current, 4.2)
Ford and Kamerow (1989)[6]	7954 (m, f)	Population sample (18–65+)	Ever a period of 2 weeks or longer sleeping too much	Direct structured interview using Diagnostic Interview Schedule	2.8 (m), 3.5 (f)
Sleep Attacks					
Saarenpää-Heikkilä et al. (1995)[161]	574 (m, f)	School-age children (7–17)	Sleeping in lessons often or always	Questionnaire (both subject and parents)	3 (m), 0 (f)
Partinen (1982)[44]	2537 (m)	Army draftees (17–29)	Falling asleep at work	Questionnaire	6.4
Partinen and Rimpelä (1982)[46]	2016 (m, f)	Population sample (15–64)	Involuntary sleep attacks daily or almost daily	Telephone interview	3.4 (m), 2.5 (f)
Billiard et al. (1987)[67]	58,162 (m)	Army draftees (17–22)	Daily sleep episodes	Questionnaire	4.9
Schmidt-Nowara et al. (1991)[49]	1278 (?)	Population sample (?)	Falling asleep often or always	Direct interview using a validated questionnaire	5.7 (inactive in a public place) 13.3 (as passenger in a vehicle) 2.4 (at work)
Klin and Quan (1987)[48]	2187 (?)	Population sample (18–64)	Falling asleep during the day	Questionnaire	12
Johns and Hocking (1997)[42]	331 (m, f)	Australian workers (22–59)	Chance of dozing (ESS >10)	Questionnaire including ESS	10.9 (no gender difference)
Kronholm and Hyyppä (1985)[181]	594 (m, f)	Population sample (30–71)	Irresistible sleep	Questionnaire	12.6 (in 30–40-year-olds) 20.6 (in 50–60-year-olds) 29.1 (in 71-year-olds)
Hyyppä and Kronholm (1987)[172]	1099 (m, f)	Population sample (29–79)	Falling asleep	Questionnaire	7.9 (m), 4.9 (f) (as a passenger often or almost always) 10.9 (m), 7.5 (f) (often or daily in tasks requiring accuracy)
Hays et al. (1996)[189]	3962 (m, f)	Population sample (65–85+)	Most of the time sleepiness, forcing to take a nap	Interview	25.2
Ganguli et al. (1996)[182]	1050 (m, f)	Population sample (66–97)	Ever becoming uncontrollably sleepy so cannot help falling asleep	Interview	18.9 (no gender difference)
Daytime Sleepiness					
Saarenpää-Heikkilä et al. (1995)[161]	574 (m, f)	School-age children (7–17)	Daytime sleepiness always or often	Questionnaire (both subject and parents)	20 (m), 22 (f)
Berg Kelly et al. (1991)[190]	3543 (m, f)	Students (13–18)	Tiredness	Questionnaire	29.3
Partinen (1982)[44]	2537 (m)	Army draftees (17–29)	Excessive daytime sleepiness often or always	Questionnaire	35.8
Partinen and Rimpelä (1982)[46]	2016 (m, f)	Population sample (15–64)	Sleepier than fellow persons	Telephone interview	10 (m), 14 (f)
Lugaresi et al. (1983)[47]	5713 (m, f)	Population sample (3–94)	Sleepiness independent of meal times	Direct interview	8.7
Hyyppä and Kronholm (1987)[172]	1099 (m, f)	Population sample (29–79)	Daytime sleepiness often or always	Questionnaire	17.0 (m), 17.3 (f)
Janson et al. (1996)[177]	2394 (m, f)	Population sample (20–44)	Feeling drowsy in the daytime three times per week	Questionnaire	16.0
Martikainen et al. (1992)[50]	1190 (m, f)	Population sample (36, 41, 46, 50)	Tiredness/sleepiness indicated by (1) more tired than fellow persons, (2) daily compulsory desire to sleep, or (3) feeling tired every day	Questionnaire	6.9 (m), 12.0 (f)

Table 47–4. OCCURRENCE OF DAYTIME SLEEPINESS *Continued*

Reference	N (Gender)	Study Population (Age Range, y)	Definition of Sleepiness (Wording of Questions)	Methods	Occurrence (%)
Hublin et al. (1996)[41]	11,354 (m, f)	Population sample (33–60)	Daytime sleepiness daily or almost daily	Questionnaire	6.7 (m), 11.0 (f)
Ohayon et al. (1997)[8]	4952 (m, f)	Population sample (15–100)	Feeling sleepy during the day on a daily basis at least 1 month greatly (severe sleepiness) or moderately (moderate sleepiness)	Telephone interview using the Sleep-Eval expert system	Severe: 4.4 (m), 6.6 (f) Moderate: 15.2

?, not known, not exactly stated; ESS, Epworth Sleepiness Scale; f, female; m, male.

several 1000-fold difference in the reported frequency rates. The highest figures are from Japan (Table 47–5). Honda et al.[56, 57] interviewed symptomatic Japanese school-aged children selected by questionnaire and found "a suspect of narcolepsy" in 160 per 100,000. A questionnaire study provided an even higher figure of 590 per 100,000 population.[58] The lowest frequency, 0.23 per 100,000 population, is based on seven narcoleptics among 1800 polygraphically examined patients with EDS.[59]

The variable figures are mainly due to differences in methods and in the definition of narcolepsy, but there also may be real differences in frequencies between populations. Generally, studies based solely on questionnaires or using the older and broader narcolepsy entity not requiring cataplexy have provided higher frequency rates. Studies using polygraphical confirmation of narcolepsy or including only cataplectic patients have provided lower frequency rates. However, the 95% confidence intervals for the frequencies overlap or nearly overlap (in size class of 10 per 100,000) in seven of eight evaluable populations. Thus, given the low prevalence rate of the disorder and the relative small numbers of cases in each study, most of the wide variation in the reported frequencies can be attributed to sample variation.

A simple screening method called the Ullanlinna Narcolepsy Scale (UNS) for population studies has been developed and validated.[60] The UNS consists of 11 items assessing cataplexy-like symptoms and the tendency to fall asleep. Using the UNS (excluding more than 99% of the study population), telephone interviews, and polygraphical confirmation of the diagnosis, the prevalence of narcolepsy with clinically significant cataplexy was found to be 26 per 100,000 population in adult Finns.[61]

Although typical cataplexy is practically pathognomonic of narcolepsy, mild forms are difficult to separate from similar physiological phenomena. As mentioned, reports of EDS in the population are common. In the Finnish narcolepsy prevalence study, 29.3% of the population reported (at least once during his or her lifetime) feelings of limb weakness associated with emotions.[61] If this is considered as evidence of cataplexy and combined with the occurrence of daytime

sleep episodes at least 3 days per week, 6.5% of the population would have "fulfilled" the minimal diagnostic criteria for narcolepsy of the ICSD.[2, 61] Therefore, the use of questionnaires only in population studies seems to result in high narcolepsy prevalence rates.

Narcolepsy probably has a multifactorial etiology, and a two-threshold model linking excessive sleepiness without known cause and narcolepsy has been proposed, with the former being a less severe form developed at a lower threshold with fewer predisposing factors.[57, 62] A comparable background has been found for narcolepsy-like symptoms in the population using the UNS and a structural equation model fitting in a large population-based twin sample, suggesting a greater genetic component to the sleepiness subscale of the UNS, whereas environmental components may play more of a role in the development of cataplexy-like symptoms.[63]

SNORING

Snoring is an inspiratory noise caused by vibration of the soft palate and posterior faucial pillars. Snoring corresponds to partial obstruction of the upper airways, and complete obstruction is followed by an apnea. Heavy snoring is practically always present in patients with obstructive sleep apnea syndrome. Some of the prevalence rates of snoring are shown in Table 47–6. Different types of questions account for at least some of the differences in the prevalence rates.

In the first large-scale epidemiological study on snoring,[64] about 24% of San Marino men and 14% of San Marino women were reported to habitually snore (see Table 47–6). In Finland, 9% of adult men and 3.6% of adult women reported snoring always or almost always when asleep.[65]

Snoring was investigated in a survey of respiratory disease among 1222 Hispanic-American adults.[66] The age-adjusted prevalence rate of regular loud snoring was 27.8% in men and 15.3% in women. Among young men in France, habitual snoring was reported by 13.6% of the total sample population.[67] Snoring increases with age up to 60 to 65 years but thereafter decreases.[68–73]

Table 47-5. PREVALENCE STUDIES ON NARCOLEPSY

Reference	Frequency (per 100,000)	95% Confidence Interval*	Base Population (Age Range, y)† Country	Methods‡
Solomon (1945)[51]	20 (190)§	0–48	10,000 (16–34)‖ United States (blacks)	Male population sample
Solomon (1945)[51]	3¶	0.6–5.7	189, 196 (?)‖ United States (whites)	Male population sample
Roth (1962),[52] (1980)[53]	13–20**†† (20-30)§**	NC	? (?) Czechoslovakia	Patient material EEG/polygraphy
Dement et al. (1972)[54]	50‡‡	NC	169 (?)§§ United States	Population sample Newspaper ad‖‖ Telephone interview
Dement et al. (1973)[55]	67¶¶	NC	113 (?)§§ United States	Population sample TV ad‖‖ Telephone interview
Honda (1979),[56] Honda et al. (1983)[57]	160	9–230	12,469 (12–16) Japan	Population sample Questionnaire‖‖ Personal interview
Partinen (1982)[44]	79	6–287	2537 (?)‖ Finland	Male population sample Questionnaire Polygraphy
Franceschi et al. (1982)[193]	40**	0–118	2518 (6–92) Italy	Unselected inpatients Questionnaire‖‖ Polygraphy
Wilner et al. (1988)[59]	0.23**	NC	1800 (30–57) Israel (Jews)	Patient material Polygraphy HLA typing
Martikainen et al. (1992)[50]	168¶	18–604	1190 (36, 41, 46, 50) Finland	Population sample Questionnaire
Tashiro et al. (1992)[58]	590	369–816	4559 (17–59) Japan	Population sample Questionnaire
al Rajeh et al. (1993)[192]	4§	0–13	23,227 (all ages) Saudi-Arabia	Population sample Personal interview Neurological examination
Wing et al. (1994)[193]	1–40§**	NC	342 (?) Hong Kong (Chinese)	Patient material Polygraphy HLA typing
Hublin et al. (1994)[61]	26	0–56	11,354 (33–60) Finland	Population sample Questionnaire‖‖ Telephone interview Polygraphy HLA typing
Ohayon et al. (1996)[194]	40	0–96	4972 (15–100) United Kingdom	Population sample Telephone interview (using the Sleep-Eval expert system)

*95% confidence interval for the frequency of narcolepsy per 100,000 (NC, cannot be computed).
†Number of subjects studied.
‡Also clinical examination in studies 1–3, 9, 11, 14, and 15.
§Reported total narcolepsy frequency (including also noncataplectic cases) or no information on the cataplexy status given.
‖Army recruits.
¶Not reported whether with or without cataplexy.
**Estimated population prevalence based on patient material.
††About 35% of the patients had only one symptom (sleep attacks, cataplexy, or sleep paralysis).
‡‡Estimated from the following data: San Francisco Bay area population (4 million), the newspaper circulation (1.2 million), the number of respondents (196) and interview-confirmed narcolepsy cases (114), the number of persons seeing/not seeing and responding/not responding to a control advertisement.
§§Number of subjects interviewed.
‖‖Used as a screening method.
¶¶Estimated from the following data: number of television homes in Los Angeles area (2,290,200), rating of the number of viewers of the advertisement (56,576), number of respondents (165) and interview-confirmed narcolepsy cases (35), 30% sampling error and errors in making the diagnosis.
HLA, human leucocyte antigen.

Table 47-6. OCCURRENCE OF HABITUAL SNORING

Reference, Population	Methods	Definition/Wording of Habitual Snoring	Gender	N	Age (y)	Prevalence (%)
Lugaresi et al. (1980)[64] San Marino general population	Interview	"Every night" (alternatives: no, sometimes, every night)*	m	2858	3–94	24.1
			f	2855	3–94	13.8
Koskenvuo et al. (1985)[65] Finnish population sample	Postal questionnaire	"Snoring always or almost always"†	m	3847	40–69	9
			f	3864	40–69	3.6
Norton and Dunn (1985)[71] Canadian population sample	Questionnaire filled during a medical visit	Snoring every night (reported by spouses)	m	1411	3rd to 8th decade	13.2
			f	1211		5.6
Billiard et al. (1987)[67] French army draftees	Questionnaire completed under supervision	Snoring habitually	m	58162	17–22	13.6
Gislason et al. (1987)[120] Swedish men	Postal questionnaire	"Loud and disturbing snoring" very often	m	4064	30–69	15.5
Cirignotta et al. (1989)[81] Random sample of Italian men	Postal questionnaire	Snoring always (alternatives: never, rarely, sometimes, often, always)	m	1170	30–69	10.1 all
				890	40–69	11.5
				304	50–59	15.5
Corbo et al. (1989)[70] Italian primary school-age children	Questionnaire filled by parents	Snoring often	Total	1615	6–13	7.3
			m	810	6–13	7.3
			f	815	6–13	7.3
Schmidt-Nowara et al. (1990)[66] Hispanic-American adults	Interview using a questionnaire	"Regular and loud snoring" always (every night	m	482	18 y or older	10.2
			f	724		5.4
Young et al. (1993)[84] State employees in Wisconsin	Postal questionnaire (first stage of the Sleep Cohort study)	Almost every night or every night snoring	m	1670	30–60	35
			f	1843	30–60	28
Ohta et al. (1993)[195] Subjects from four Japanese cities	Questionnaire given during a regular medical checkup	"Habitual snoring"	m, f	3243	Mean, 50 y	12.8–16
Jennum and Sjol (1994)[196] Dannish population sample, part of Dan-MONICA II project	Interview and clinical examinations	Snoring nightly (every night)	m	Total	30–60	19.1
			f	1504	30–60	7.9

*In the San Marino study, there were four alternatives: "no," "I don't know," "yes, sometimes," and "yes, every night."
†In the Finnish studies, five alternatives were used: "I don't know," "never," "sometimes," "often," and "almost always or always."
f, female; m, male.

OBSTRUCTIVE SLEEP APNEA

A Syndrome or a Disease?

Obstructive sleep apnea syndrome (OSAS) is the most common organic disorder causing excessive daytime somnolence in patients seen in sleep disorders clinics. It has recently been suggested that the disorder be called obstructive sleep apnea-hypopnea syndrome (OSAHS).[69] In this chapter, we use the term OSAS instead of OSAHS.

A summary of different prevalence studies is presented later. According to various cross-sectional studies, the lowest rates for the prevalence of OSAS among adult men are 1% to 4%. There is an age relationship, so the prevalence of OSAS among men 40 to 59 years old may be greater than 4% to 8%. OSAS is less common is younger and older age groups.

Is obstructive sleep apnea a syndrome or a disease? Arterial hypertension, for example, is not considered a syndrome, but dementia is a syndrome; the most common causes of dementia are Alzheimer's disease and multiple cerebral infarctions. If the cause of dementia is not known, the proper diagnosis is dementia of unknown origin.

Obstructive sleep apneas are part of the complex of "heavy snorer's disease" as defined by Lugaresi et al[74]; it is interesting to note that the new ASDAs Chicago criteria for sleep-related breathing disorders are close to the original ideas of Lugaresi.

Heavy snoring (i.e., partial upper airway obstruction) even without apneas may influence pulmonary arterial pressure, and it may cause daytime sleepiness and have some health consequences. On the other hand, we know that some heavy snorers have been snoring since childhood until the age of 60 years or older, and they are healthy. The presence of repetitive sleep apneas is a potential determinant of risk in the same way as high blood pressure. It is common medical practice to measure blood pressure. Should recording of breathing during sleep become a common practice? Not for everybody, but perhaps sleep recordings are indicated in some, such as obese patients with newly diagnosed arterial hypertension. We know from epidemiological studies that about 10% to 15% of "occasional or never snorers" may have occasional obstructive sleep apneas.[75] We know from clinical practice that patients with manifest obstructive sleep apnea are almost always heavy snorers but may not be aware of it. Measurement of apneas necessitates a night recording, which may be too costly even with the use of various simple screening methods. The basis of diagnosis is proper history taking (also from cohabiting persons, if possible) and clinical examination.

Patients with kyphoscoliosis and patients with hereditary myopathy may have breathing problems in sleep. The main diagnostic group is "disordered breathing during sleep." The etiological problem arises in many situations. Is a morbidly obese patient, for example, with a body mass index (BMI) of 44 kg/m², a patient with OSAS, the diagnosis may be morbid obesity with obstructive sleep apnea. Morbid obesity is a disease, and it is a risk factor for cardiovascular disease even without sleep apneas. The presence of sleep apneas means a higher risk. Another example is acromegaly with sleep apnea. Such patients do not have essential OSAS but rather symptomatic sleep apnea. The disease (acromegaly) may be treated with pituitary adenomectomy, but the consequence (sleep apnea) often necessitates nasal continuous positive airway pressure or upper airway surgery. This is analogous to a patient with a brain tumor who has symptomatic epilepsy. The primary diagnosis is brain tumor (e.g., glioma), and epilepsy is a symptom caused by the brain tumor.

Sleep apnea should be properly quantified, not only by an apnea index (AI) (or apnea-hypopnea index [AHI]) but also by the length of apnea, degree and number of desaturations, limitation of air flow, cardiac manifestations associated with the breathing events, and so on. An AI of five events per hour of sleep is commonly used as a criterion of OSAS.[76, 77] Recently published criteria have lowered the limit[69]; an overnight monitoring must demonstrate five or more apneas plus hypopnea plus respiratory effort–related arousals per hour of sleep. According to these criteria, a 70-year-old lean man can be diagnosed as having OSAHS, for example, if the following symptoms and findings are present: impaired concentration plus daytime fatigue plus two apneas and five hypopneas per hour of sleep. The criteria must be corrected. The results of an epidemiological study by Bixler et al.[78] supported the need to adjust the diagnostic criteria for age. This study was based on a two-stage general random sample of men 20 to 100 years old. It consisted of a telephone survey (N = 4364) and a sleep laboratory evaluation of a survey subsample (N = 741). The criteria for OSAS were an AHI of at least 10 in sleep laboratory and clinical criteria fulfilled with the presence of daytime symptoms. OSAS was found in 3.3% of the sample, with its maximum prevalence among 45- to 64-year-old men. The prevalence of any type of sleep apnea (central or obstructive) increased with age; however, central apnea appeared to account for this monotonic relationship with age. The severity of sleep apnea, as indicated by both number of events and minimum oxygen saturation, decreased with age when any sleep apnea criteria were used and when control-

ling for BMI. The authors conclude that the prevalence of sleep apnea tends to increase with age but that the clinical meaningfulness of apnea decreases. Based on this study and previous studies, the sleep laboratory criteria used for diagnosis of sleep apnea should be adjusted for age.

It took a long time before the World Health Organization and medical authorities accepted common criteria for arterial hypertension. We hope it takes less time to find commonly accepted criteria for various forms of disordered breathing during sleep. The work of the ICSD[2] and ASDA represent good steps in this direction.[78]

Prevalence

OSAS is characterized by repetitive apneas during sleep. The main symptoms of the disease are loud and irregular snoring, restless sleep, and daytime sleepiness. In Israel, Lavie[79] estimated in a cross-sectional study that the prevalence of the syndrome among male industrial workers is at least 1% (Table 47–7).[80] Peter et al. reported a much higher prevalence of OSAS in a subgroup of industrial workers in Germany, but the method of estimating the prevalence prevents generalization to other industrial workers. Another epidemiological study was conducted in Bologna, Italy.[81] The study population consisted of 3479 men 30 to 69 years old; 2.5% had heavy snorer's disease stage 1 or higher. On the basis of the prevalence of everynight snoring and the results of polysomnography, the authors estimated that the minimal prevalence of sleep apnea in that population was 2.7%, considering an AHI of 10 or more to be pathological. In the age group of 40 to 59 years, the prevalence estimations of OSAS (see Table 47–5) were between 3.4% and 5%.[81] An Australian study by Bearpark et al.[82] found a prevalence rate of 8.5%. These studies gave a good estimate of obstructive sleep apnea but do not indicate how many of their subjects are symptomatic.[80, 82, 83]

The first large epidemiological polysomnographic study was conducted in Madison, Wisconsin. The initial cohort of Young et al.[84] consisted of 602 employed men and women between the ages of 30 and 60 years. These patients underwent overnight polysomnography and were administered a questionnaire. Nine percent of women and 24% of men in this middle-aged group were estimated to have the sleep apnea syndrome, as defined by the combination of an AI exceeding 5 and daytime hypersomnolence. On examination of the subgroup of patients between the ages of 50 and 60, 4% of women and 9.1% of men were found to have an AI exceeding 15.

These figures are somewhat larger than those reported from the Scandinavian countries. Gislason et al.[85] reported a prevalence rate of 1.3% in a Swedish 30- to 69-year-old male population. The prevalence of OSAS among 40- to 50-year-old Finnish men is 0.4% and 1.4%[75] (see Table 47–5). Methodological differences in the study protocol may account for some differences, but other factors may exist.

Table 47–7. OCCURRENCE OF OBSTRUCTIVE SLEEP APNEA AND
OBSTRUCTIVE SLEEP APNEA SYNDROME

Reference, Country	Methods	Subjects N	Age (y)	Criteria	Prevalence %
Lavie (1983),[79] Israel	Questionnaire. PSG recordings and clinical examination for potential patients	1262 (m)	18–67	AI > 10, symptomatic	1.0–5.9
Peter et al (1985),[80] Germany	Questionnaire. PSG recordings and clinical examination for potential patients	354 (m)	25–55	AI > 10, symptomatic	2.3
Telakivi et al (1987),[75] Finland	Questionnaire. PSG recordings and clinical examination for potential patients	1939 (m)	30–69	Snoring, EDS, and RDI > 10	0.4–1.4
Gislason et al. (1988),[85] Sweden	Questionnaire. PSG recordings and clinical examination for potential patients	3201 (m)	30–69	Snoring, EDS, and AHI > 10	0.7–1.9
Cirignotta et al. (1989),[81] Italy	Questionnaire, telephone survey. PSG recordings and clinical examination for potential patients	1170 (m)	30–39 40–59 60–69	AI > 10, symptomatic AI > 10, symptomatic AI > 10, symptomatic	0.2–1.0 3.4–5.0 0.5–1.1
Stradling and Crosby (1991),[198] Great Britain	Ambulatory oximetry recordings at home	893 (m)	35–65	ODI_4 > 20, symptomatic ODI_4 > 10 ODI_4 > 5	0.3 1.0 4.6
Haraldsson et al. (1992),[199] Sweden	Questionnaire. PSG recordings and clinical examination for potential patients	846 (m)	30–69	Positive history and verification of OSAS in PSG	2.8–5.5
Young et al. (1993),[84] Wisconsin	A sample of state employees. PSG recordings and clinical examination for potential patients	352 (m) 250 (f)	30–60 30–60	Hypersomnia and RDI ≥ 5	4.0 (m) 2.0 (f)
Gislason et al. (1993),[200] Iceland	Questionnaire. PSG recordings and clinical examination for potential patients	2016 (f)	40–59	Habitual snoring, EDS and verification of OSAS in PSG	>2.5
Olson et al. (1995),[201] Australia	Questionnaire and home sleep recordings	1233 (m) 969 (f)	35–69	AHI ≥ 15 AHI ≥ 10 AHI ≥ 5	4–18 7–35 14–69
Bearpark et al. (1995),[197] Australia	Ambulatory home sleep recordings (MESAM IV). Estimation of sleep disordered breathing Collection of medical history	294 (m)	40–65	RD ≥ 10 Subjective EDS and RDI ≥ 5	10.0 ≥3.0
Gislason and Benediktsdottir (1995),[109] Iceland	Questionnaire. PSG and examination for suspected patients with habitual snoring or reported apneic episodes	555 children	6 mon to 6 yr	Habitual snoring or apneic episodes, and ODI_4 > 3	>2.9
Esnaola et al. (1995),[87] Spain	Questionnaire, PSG recordings and clinical examination for potential patients	1077 (m)	30–70	AHI ≥ 5 AHI ≥ 10 AHI ≥ 5 and EDS	15.3 13.4 6.5–9.1
Ohayon et al. (1997),[202] Great Britain	Telephone interview (Sleep-EVAL). A sample of the general population. No examinations. No sleep recordings	2078 (m) 2894 (f)	35–64 35–64	NA NA	2.4–4.6 (m) 0.8–2.2 (f)
Kripke et al. (1997),[203] San Diego	Telephone interview. A random sample of 40–64-year-olds living in San Diego. Home interview, home pulse oximeter, and snoring recording	165 (m) 190 (f)	40–64 40–64	ODI_4 > 20 ODI_4 > 20	5.4–13.2 (m) 2.1–8.3 (f)
Bixler et al. (1998),[78] United States	Telephone survey. Random sample of men aged 20–100 y. A sleep laboratory evaluation of a survey subsample	4364 (m) Subsample: 741	20–100	AHI > 10 and clinical criteria fulfilled with daytime symptoms	All: 3.3 45–64 y: 4.7

AHI, Apnea-Hypopnea Index; AI, Apnea Index; EDS, excessive daytime sleepiness; NA, not applicable; ODI_4, Oxygen Desaturation Index (≥4% desaturation); OSAS, obstructive sleep apnea syndrome; PSG, polysomnography; RDI, respiratory disturbance index.

Results from a Spanish study by Duran et al.[86] are in accordance with the figures of Young et al.[84] In the Spanish study, the population consisted of 1077 men 30 to 70 years old. Subjects were interviewed and monitored by MESAM IV (MADAUS electronic sleep apnea monitor). When 885 men were screened, habitual snoring was reported by 49.1% and daytime sleepiness was reported by 22.2%. Based on conventional polysomnography, the prevalence of men having an AHI of more than or equal to 5 was 15.3%, and 9.1% had an AHI of more than or equal to 20. Furthermore, 6.5% of the men met the minimal diagnostic criteria for OSAS with an AHI of more than or equal to 5 plus daytime sleepiness.[87, 88] In an Italian study, 13.7% of the 349 monitored subjects had more than 10 desaturations of at least 4% per hour.[89] A recent study by Bixler et al.[78] showed a mean prevalence rate of 3.3% among men 20 to 100 years old. The peak prevalence, 4.7% (95% confidence interval, 3.1% to 7.1%), was found, supporting other studies, among men 45 to 64 years old. Among the 20- to 44-year-olds and those older than 65 years, the prevalence rate was 1.7%.[78]

Four case-control studies[90–93] have been conducted during the 1980s showing that the prevalence rate of sleep apnea among patients with essential hypertension is 25% or higher. In a case-control study by Worsnop et al.,[94] 38% of the hypertensive subjects and 4% of normotensive had an AHI of higher than 5.

The prevalence rates depend on the base populations. OSAS is most frequent in persons 40 to 65 years old. One can safely estimate that the prevalence rate of OSAS in that age group is around 4% (3% to 8%) in men and 2% in women and that the absolute minimum prevalence of clinically significant OSAS is 1%. Among obese subjects, hypertensives, and some other patient groups, the prevalence rates are significantly higher.

Role of Obesity as a Risk Factor for Snoring and Sleep Apnea

Obesity is an important risk factor for snoring and sleep apnea. Obesity may be measured by the BMI, which is calculated as weight in kilograms divided by square of height in meters.[95] Adults with a BMI of more than 27 kg/m² may be considered obese. Several lines of evidence show that upper body obesity in particular is related to increased risk of cardiovascular disease. The same may be true for heavy snoring and sleep apnea. Using multivariate analysis, Katz et al.[96] reported that neck size is more closely related to severity of sleep apnea than is BMI. Neck size may be easily measured, and it is a useful indicator of upper body obesity.

The frequency of snoring increases with obesity in all published epidemiological reports on snoring. Habitual snoring was found to occur in 7% of men and 2.8% of women with a BMI of less than 27 kg/m² and in 13.9% and 6.1%, respectively, of those above this level.[96] All later studies confirm these findings.

Other Risk Factors for Snoring and Sleep Apnea

Bloom et al.[73] studied risk factors associated with snoring among 2187 subjects representative of a general adult population in Tucson, Arizona. Major independent risk factors for snoring were male gender, age between 40 and 64 years, obesity, and cigarette smoking. Snoring prevalence was slightly increased in subjects who regularly used alcohol or hypnotics. The authors propose that the effect of smoking may be related to the production of upper airway inflammation and edema by cigarette smoke and that smoking cessation may eventually reduce snoring risk.

Alcohol tends to induce obstructive sleep apnea in healthy asymptomatic men[97] and in chronic snorers,[98–101] and it increases the duration and frequency of occlusive episodes in patients with obstructive sleep apnea.[98] This is probably due to the acute centrally depressing effects of alcohol. However, OSAS seems to not be significantly more common among past alcoholics than among nonalcoholics.[102]

An association also exists between hostility and habitual snoring.[103] This could be explained by disturbed sleep of the snorers; disrupted sleep causes daytime sleepiness,[104, 105] which in turn is associated with hostility.[106]

Snoring and Sleep Apnea in Children

Upper airway obstruction with snoring or obstructive sleep apnea is commonly seen in children of all ages.[107] Children may have sleep apnea syndrome similar to that seen in adults.[108] In Italy, 1615 children 6 to 13 years old were categorized according to whether they snored often, occasionally apart from with colds, only with colds, or never. One hundred eighteen children (7.3%) were habitual snorers. Rhinitic children were more than twice as likely to be habitual snorers than were others. There also was a positive correlation between parental smoking and the presence of snoring in children.[70] In Iceland,[109] 3.2% of 555 children 6 months to 6 years old snored often or always at sleep. The estimated minimal prevalence of obstructive sleep apnea in that age group was 3.2%. Adenotonsillar hypertrophy is the most common cause of upper airway obstruction in infants and children.[110]

Sleep Apnea Among Elderly People

The prevalence of everynight snoring seems to decrease after the age of 65 years. However, 19% to 24% of people older than 65 years have more than five apneic events AI of more than 5 per hour of sleep.[111, 112] According to Ancoli-Israel et al.,[113] 62% of elderly people have a respiratory disturbance index (RDI) of more than or equal to 10. Because of its high prevalence in the elderly, sleep apnea has been suggested as one mechanism contributing to sleep-related death. This does not mean that 19% to 24% of elderly persons have sleep apnea syndrome. The clinical significance of the high frequency of sleep apnea among elderly people remains to be seen. In a study, Bixler et al.[77] emphasized the need to adjust the criteria for OSAS in elderly persons.

A cohort of 198 noninstitutionalized elderly individuals (mean age at entry, 66 years) were followed for periods up to 12 years after initial polysomnography.[114] The mortality ratio for sleep apnea, defined as a respiratory disturbance index of more than 10 events per sleep hour, was 2.7 (95% confidence interval, 0.95 to 7.47). These results raise the possibility that "natural" death during sleep in the elderly may be associated with disordered breathing during sleep or with other pathological events during sleep.

Other Patients

Snoring is common among infants and children with Pierre Robin syndrome and among infants with nasal obstruction.[115] Snoring and obstructive sleep apnea are also common in men with acromegaly.[116] Many other syndromes or diseases exist in which upper airways are narrowed; the prevalence of snoring and sleep apnea is increased in all such situations.[117]

Arterial Hypertension

An association between always or almost-always snoring and arterial hypertension has been found in several cross-sectional studies in Italy, Canada, and Scandinavia.[64, 118–120]

In the San Marino study,[64] the relation was particularly significant in the age group of 41 to 60 years; hypertension was present in 15.2% of habitual snorers and in 7.5% of nonsnorers. In the Finnish study, the odds ratio of hypertension between habitual snorers and nonsnorers was 1.94 for men ($P < .0001$).[118] The association remained significant when BMI and age were adjusted. Similar results were found in an Italian case-control study of patients with arterial hypertension and control subjects (R. D'Alessandro et al., unpublished data, 1990). Habitual snoring may be a determinant of risk of arterial hypertension, but occasional snoring is not associated with an increased risk.

The prevalence of snoring, overweight, and systemic hypertension was estimated in a random sample of 4064 Swedish men 30 to 69 years old. Of the responders, 15.5% complained of habitual snoring and 29.6% complained of occasional snoring. There was an age-related increase in the prevalence of snoring up to 60 years. However, habitual snoring was found to be mainly related to BMI ($P < .0001$) and not to age.[120] Altogether, 9.3% of the men reported arterial hypertension, of whom 21.5% were habitual snorers, compared with 14.9% of the nonhypertensives ($P < .01$). The hypertensives also were more often overweight. Logistic multiple regression analyses showed that among subjects 40 to 49 years old, there was an average increase in the predicted prevalence of hypertension from 6.5% among nonsnorers to 10.5% of habitual snorers in the same weight group. For the entire study population, however, the increase was mainly dependent on age and BMI. Thus, the importance of habitual snoring for the prevalence of hypertension varies among age groups.[120] Snoring may influence blood pressure via changes in intrathoracic pressure, obstructive sleep apnea, and nocturnal hypoxemia.

Schmidt-Nowara et al.[66] also found that snorers frequently had hypertension and ischemic heart disease. In contrast to other studies, however, after adjustment for confounding factors, there was no significant effect of snoring per se (odds ratio, 1; 95% confidence interval, 0.7 to 1.5) on hypertension.

Determinants of blood pressure in snorers were studied by Hoffstein et al.[121] Blood pressure was measured, and snoring sound, oxyhemoglobin saturation (SaO$_2$), and thoracoabdominal movements were monitored overnight in 372 snorers.[121] Diastolic blood pressure correlated significantly with BMI, AHI, and mean nocturnal oxygen saturation but not with recorded snoring. However, snoring index correlated with BMI, AHI, and mean nocturnal oxygen saturation.

Polysomnographic recordings have shown that snoring is associated with increased activity of inspiratory muscles and with a marked increase in intrathoracic negative pressure.[122] In heavy snorers, pulmonary artery pressure may increase to pathological levels during sleep. Contrary to what is seen in nonsnorers, systemic arterial pressure also increases slightly and reaches the highest values during rapid eye movement sleep.[64, 123]

The relative influence of BMI and sleep apnea on blood pressure and the prevalence of hypertension was investigated by Carlson et al.[124] in 377 consecutive subjects studied in a sleep laboratory. One hundred twenty-four (33%) had sleep apnea, 153 (41%) were obese, and 93 (25%) had systemic hypertension. Both oxygen desaturations and minimal oxygen saturation were related to BMI ($P < .001$) in patients not taking antihypertensive medication. Systolic and diastolic blood pressures were related to BMI and disease severity. In a multivariate logistic regression analysis, age, BMI, and sleep apnea were all independent predictors of hypertension. The relative risk associated with sleep apnea was 2.1 (cutpoint of 30 desaturations/6 h). Combined obesity and sleep apnea resulted in a 3.9-fold increase in hypertension prevalence.[124] In a German study, 31.1% of the 10.6 hypertensive men and 16.6% of the 391 normotensive men had more than 80 oxygen desaturations below 90% during 8 h of sleep; 44.7% of obese hypertensives and 37.1% of obese normotensives were suspected of having obstructive sleep apnea. Twenty-one hypertensive and 24 normotensive patients were examined by polysomnography. Of the hypertensives, 78.9% had an AI of more than 10 compared with 41.2% of the normotensives. On the whole, patients with arterial hypertension were at a markedly higher risk for obstructive sleep apnea.[125] The results of these two studies are in accordance with earlier case-control studies[90–93] showing that the prevalence of sleep apnea among patients with essential hypertension is 25% or higher. In a recent case-control study by Worsnop et al.,[94] 38% or the hypertensive subjects and 4% of normotensive subjects had an AHI of more than 5. In the latter study, the presence of sleep apnea remained significant after adjustment for BMI, age, sex, and alcohol consumption.[94]

Other reports support these findings. Carlson et al.[126] investigated 377 consecutive subjects studied at a sleep laboratory; 124 (33%) had sleep apnea, 153 (41%) were obese, and 93 (25%) had systemic hypertension. In a multivariate logistic regression analysis, age, BMI, and sleep apnea were all identified as independent predictors of arterial hypertension. The relative risk was 4.3 (40 to 59 years) associated with age, 2.7 (more than 30 kg/m²) associated with obesity, and 2.1 (more than 30 desaturations/6 h in bed) associated with sleep apnea.[124] In another study, 132 randomly selected clinical male patients with arterial hypertension were monitored. Desaturation index of at least 10/h revealed a total prevalence of 27.3%. The prevalence rate increased to 52% in obese patients older than 55 years.[126]

The relationship among arterial hypertension, cardiovascular disease, and OSAS is strongest among middle-aged adults. In elderly persons, the clinical significance of OSAS becomes weaker. In a random sample of 5201 Medicare enrollees 65 years old or older, 33% of the men and 19% of the women reported loud snoring, which was less frequent in those older than 75. Snoring was positively associated with younger age, marital status, and alcohol use in men and with obesity, diabetes, and arthritis in women. Observed apneas were reported by 13% of men and 4% of women. In that elderly population, loud snoring, observed apneas, and daytime sleepiness were not statistically significantly associated with hypertension or prevalent cardiovascular disease.[127]

Obstructive sleep apnea is a common finding among patients with arterial hypertension. According to all of these studies, the prevalence of sleep apnea among patients with essential hypertension is so high (25% or higher) that patients with arterial hypertension should always be queried about their snoring history and possible sleep apnea. Large-scale longitudinal studies are still necessary to determine which patients with arterial hypertension should be monitored for possible sleep apnea. The cost of monitoring and treatment of sleep apnea should be weighed against benefical health effects. A review by Fletcher[128] provides an overview of the relationship between primary hypertension and adult OSAS. The data are taken from the English-language literature through 1993. Logic dictates that clinically symptomatic patients in hypertensive clinics should receive appropriate evaluation for apnea but that broad populations of hypertensive individuals should not be referred for sleep studies.[128]

Snoring, Sleep Apnea, and Heart Disease

An association of habitual snoring with electrocardiographic changes and arrhythmias has been reported.[64, 129] In the study of Schmidt-Nowara et al.,[66] snorers frequently had hypertension and ischemic heart disease. The association with hypertension was not clear, but an effect on myocardial infarction was demonstrable (odds ratio, 1.8; 95% confidence interval, 0.9 to 3.6).

The association of snoring and ischemic heart disease was tested in a population consisting of 3847 men and 3664 women 40 to 69 year old. Reported angina pectoris was associated with habitual snoring among men (risk ratio, 1.9) but not among women (risk ratio, 1.2). Reported myocardial infarction and ischemic heart disease were also associated with habitual snoring. The association was also found after adjustment for arterial hypertension and BMI.[118] These results were confirmed in a prospective follow-up study of 4388 men 40 to 69 year old. The age-adjusted risk ratio of ischemic heart disease between often or always snorers and nonsnorers was 1.91. The 95% confidence interval was 1.18 to 3.09. An additional adjustment for BMI, history of arterial hypertension, smoking, and alcohol use decreased the risk ratio slightly to 1.71 (95% confidence interval, 0.96 to 3.05).[130]

Two hundred successive adult patients entering a medical ward were asked about their sleeping habits and snoring; the mean age of the patients was 57 years.[131] Forty-three patients had entered the hospital because of an acute myocardial infarction, and 157 patients had entered for other reasons. Forty of the 43 patients (93%) with myocardial infarction were often or always snorers. Among the others, there were 111 often or always snorers and 46 occasional or never snorers. The odds ratio of myocardial infarction of patients with often or always snoring compared with never or sometimes snorers was 5.5 (Yates' corrected $\chi^2 = 7.93$; 95% confidence interval for odds ratio, 1.7 to 18). A small case-control study was conducted with 13 patients with myocardial infarction and 13 control subjects. Sleep recordings were performed to assess for possible sleep apneas. Five of the 13 patients with myocardial infarction had more than five apneic events per hour, whereas the corresponding figure among the control patients was 1 of 13. The odds ratio was 7.5.[131]

The occurrence of breathing disorders and hypoxia during sleep was studied in 17 men with coronary artery disease, as demonstrated by coronary angiography, who did not have symptomatic pulmonary disease. Thirteen patients (76%) experienced disordered breathing during sleep; of these, 11 had obstructive apnea, and the other 2 had Cheyne-Stokes respiration. There was an average of 20 episodes of disordered breathing per hour during sleep among the 13 patients, with a mean duration of 24 sec per episode; significant oxygen desaturation occurred in 10 of these 13 patients.[132] There were no episodes of angina pectoris, myocardial infarction, or sudden death. Although cardiac arrhythmias occurred in 12 patients, disordered breathing with hypoxia was not proved to be causative. Therefore, obstructive disordered breathing and nocturnal oxygen desaturation commonly occurred during sleep in patients with coronary artery disease.

In a case-control study with 50 patients with myocardial infarction and 100 control subjects, snoring every night was associated with myocardial infarction. The odds ratio was 2.35 (95% confidence interval, 1.18 to 4.67) when patients were compared with both hospital control and population control subjects. The effect of everynight snoring was independent of smoking, arterial hypertension, diabetes mellitus, and alcohol consumption.[133]

In another case-control study conducted in Australia, 101 male patients with myocardial infarction and 53 male control subjects were investigated.[134] An overnight sleep recording was performed in a sleep laboratory between 6 and 61 days (mean, 24 days) after myocardial infarction, and a significant association of sleep apnea with myocardial infarction was found. The association was independent of age, BMI, arterial hypertension, smoking, and cholesterol level. There was an increase in adjusted risk of myocardial infarction with increasing levels of sleep apnea.[134] Men with an AI of more than 5.3 had 23.3-fold (95% confidence interval, 3.9 to 139.9) the risk of myocardial infarction than did men with an AI of less than 0.4. The mean AI was 6.9 in patients with myocardial infarction versus 1.4 in the control subjects. One possible explanation for an association between sleep apnea and coronary disease is that there are common risk factors, such as male gender, obesity, and smoking. Sleep apnea also is associated with hypertension. However, after adjustment for these factors, the authors still found a highly significant association between sleep apnea and myocardial infarction.[134] As Hung et al.[134] suggest, a possible explanation is that sleep apnea acts together with other known risk factors to accelerate atherosclerosis or to precipitate myocardial ischemia in patients with coronary artery disease. The theory that atherosclerosis may be related to hypoxia has received some experimental support.[135]

Fifty patients 61 ± 6 years old who were diagnosed as having have coronary artery disease by coronary angiography were investigated prospectively. In 25 patients (50%), the AI was more than 10/h sleep. EDS was exhibited by 8 of the 25 patients.[136] The minimum prevalence of OSAS among patients with coronary disease can be estimated as about 16%.

Excessive use of alcohol is associated with increased coronary death.[137] Snoring could be a cofactor. Alcohol tends to induce snoring and obstructive sleep apnea[97, 98] and to increase the duration and frequency of occlusive episodes in patients with obstructive sleep apnea.[98]

Smoking is also associated with coronary disease. Habitual snorers smoke more than do occasional or never snorers.[71, 73] These two factors may be additive, so a habitually snoring smoker is at greater risk for coronary disease than is a habitual snorer who does not smoke.

Snoring and Brain Infarction

The most important factors associated with brain infarction are age, male gender, arterial hypertension, various abnormal cardiac conditions, diabetes mellitus, and cigarette smoking. In addition to these established risk factors, however, there is increasing evidence that suggests a link among habitual, everynight snoring, OSAS, and stroke.

Agnoli et al.[138] studied the relation among the onset of stroke, time of day, and arterial pressure in 200 cases of probable nonembolic infarctions and 56 cases of embolic infarctions. Stroke occurred most commonly during the morning between 6 and 8 AM. In another study, the time of onset of stroke was recorded in 707 patients. Of the 554 cerebral infarctions, 40% occurred between midnight and 6 AM. Onset of cerebral hemorrhage was rare at night.[139] In a study by Tsementzis et al.,[140] cerebral infarction was most common between 10 AM and noon, when the highest blood pressures would be encountered.

An association between cerebral infarction and habitual snoring has been found. In a case-control study of 50 male patients with brain infarction and 100 male control subjects, the risk ratio of brain infarction between habitual or often snorers and occasional or never snorers was 2.8.[141] Between habitual snorers and occasional or never snorers, the risk ratio of stroke was 10.3. The independent contribution of snoring as a risk factor for brain infarction was confirmed in another case-control study of 177 male patients and control subjects matched for age and sex.[142] Again, snoring increased the risk of stroke. After adjustments for several confounding variables, the independent odds ratio relating to snoring and stroke remained at 2.13.[142] Other studies have provided supporting results.[143] In these studies, both men and women have been included. After adjustment for several potential confounders, the odds ratios of snoring "often or almost always" for stroke was 1.7 (95% confidence interval, 1.3 to 2.2).[144] In the study by Smirne et al.,[145] the adjusted (age, gender, obesity, diabetes, dyslipidemia, smoking, use of alcohol, hypertension) odds ratio for "often or always snoring" in relation to ischemic brain infarction was 1.9 (95% confidence interval, 1.2 to 2.9). Neau et al.[146] studied 133 patients 45 to 75 years old and 133 control subjects matched for age and sex. The prevalence of habitual snoring was 23.3% among patients with stroke and 8.3% among their controls. The odds ratio for habitual snoring was 3.4 (95% confidence interval, 1.5 to 7.6). The odds ratio for "often or always snoring" was 1.7 (95% confidence interval 1.03 to 2.93). Even after adjustment for age, sex, arterial hypertension, cardiac arrhythmia, and obesity, the odds ratio of habitual snoring for stroke remained statistically significant (2.9; 95% confidence interval 1.3 to 6.8). The risk of ischemic stroke was especially high among habitually snoring older men with arterial hypertension.[146]

The time of onset of stroke was recorded for an additional 167 consecutive male patients. The median age was 52 years (range, 16 to 60 years). In 70 cases (41.9%), cerebral infarction was noted during sleep or immediately after awakening.[147] Of the 70 infarctions with an onset at night or immediately after awakening, 48 patients had a history of snoring often or always (68.6%). The respective percentage among the other patients was 41.2% (40 of 97). The difference is significant (odds ratio for often or always snoring was 3.1;

95%, Confidence interval, 1.7 to 5.9; $P < .001$). The risk remained elevated when age, arterial hypertension, BMI, smoking, consumption of alcohol, and diabetes mellitus were taken into account.[147]

Physiological rise in blood pressure after awakening in the morning may cause a breakthrough of the autoregulation of the cerebral blood flow. In normal conditions, nothing happens, but under unfavorable conditions, an infarction may follow.

Arterial hypertension is common among patients with sleep apnea. The association of snoring and brain infarction could be in part explained by the high prevalence of habitual snoring and obstructive sleep apnea in patients with arterial hypertension, which is a known risk factor for stroke. However, in epidemiological studies,[148] the effect of habitual snoring remained even after adjustment for arterial hypertension.

Snoring and Sudden Death

An autopsy was performed in 460 consecutive cases of sudden death among 35- to 76-year-old men. The closest cohabiting person to each deceased was interviewed. The mean age was 55.4 years, and the mean BMI was 26.3 kg/m^2. Among the obese snorers (n = 82), apneas had been observed "occasionally," "often," or "habitually" in 49 cases. Death was classified as cardiovascular in 186 cases (40.4%). Cardiovascular cause of death was more common among the habitual and often snorers than among occasional or never snorers. Habitual snorers died more often while sleeping. Habitually snoring was found to be a risk (odds ratio, 4.07; 95% confidence interval, 1.45 to 11.45) for cardiovascular early morning death between 4 and 8 AM.[149]

Warnes and Roberts[150] studied 12 massively obese patients (5 women and 7 men) with a BMI from 41.5 to more than 80 kg/m^2 who had died. Information on the presence or absence of episodes of sleep apnea or hypersomnia was available for 2 women and 4 men. Both women and 2 of the 4 men had a positive history. One of the 2 women and 1 of the 2 men with hypersomnia-sleep apnea had sudden death, and the other 2 patients (1 woman and 1 man) died with right-sided congestive heart failure. There were three other sudden deaths, but unfortunately the authors did not have information about possible sleep apnea in those cases. Only 2 patients had one or more major epicardial coronary arteries narrowed by more than 75%. The authors conclude that these massively obese patients did not have more coronary atherosclerosis than might be expected at their ages.[150] Factors other than atherosclerotic coronary heart disease thus seem to be more important as a cause of premature death in extremely obese subjects. Habitual snoring with partial upper airway obstruction and obstructive sleep apnea syndrome are among the other potential factors.

Snoring and Dementia

The occurrence of snoring was studied in 46 patients with Alzheimer's disease, in 37 patients with multi-infarct dementia, and in a random sample of 124 elderly community residents.[151] The demented patients snored twice as frequently as did the control subjects. No difference in the occurrence of snoring was found between the two types of dementia.[151]

Reynolds et al.[152] found a higher prevalence of sleep apnea among female patients with Alzheimer's disease than among control subjects. Vitiello and Prinz[153] had the same finding when 24 female patients with Alzheimer's disease were compared with 26 control subjects. The mean AHIs among the female control subjects and the patients with Alzheimer's disease were 2 ± 0.4 and 9 ± 3, respectively. There were no significant differences in the amount or severity of apnea activity between 20 male control subjects (AHI-6 ± 1.7) and 20 male patients with Alzheimer's disease (AHI-8 ± 2).[153]

Evolution of Obstructive Sleep Apnea Syndrome

Evolution of OSAS and the effects of treatment are handled in greater detail elsewhere in this textbook. OSAS may be a lethal disease if not treated. There are several studies showing an increased risk of cardiovascular complications and death in patients with at least moderate (AI more than 20) or severe (AI more than 40) OSAS.[154–157] Nasal continuous positive airway pressure is an effective treatment of OSAS. Among obese patients, weight loss is effective as long as the subjects do not gain back the weight. Without a doubt continuous positive airway pressure is an effective and even life-saving treatment of severe continuous positive airway pressure, but well-done prospective epidemiological studies are lacking that concern the long-term effect of continuous positive airway pressure in mild OSAS, in simple snoring, and in upper airway resistance syndrome. Different surgical methods have been developed to treat snoring and OSAS. Uvulopalatopharyngoplasty and different laser techniques have been used to treat snoring and sleep apnea, but there are only a few studies with acceptable epidemiological methodology. More evidence, including randomized controlled trials, is needed. In this perspective, Wright et al.[14] were correct, even though their report lacked many good studies clearly showing that sleep disordered breathing disturbance is associated with cardiovascular disease and that at least severe OSAS must be treated efficiently.

Janson et al.[158] studied the long-term effects of uvulopalatopharyngoplasty in 34 patients with OSAS. Response to treatment was defined as a 50% or greater reduction in AHI and a postoperative AHI of 10 or less. Sixty-four percent were responders at 6 months and 48% were responders at 4 to 8 years after surgery. None of the seven patients with an initial AHI of more than 40 were responders.[158]

OSAS is an important disease. It has also many economical consequences.[159] Much research, however, is needed before sleep researchers can convince others that OSAS and other sleep-related breathing disorders are very important medical problems.

Table 47–8. OCCURRENCE OF PARASOMNIAS

	Childhood		Adulthood	
Diagnosis	Occurrence (%) (Always or Often/ Now and Then)	References	Occurrence (%) (Always or Often/ Now and Then)	References
Sleeptalking	4–14/22–60	161, 204–210	1–5/(3.5-) 20–45	23, 44, 168, 172, 209
Sleep bruxism	4–6/9.5–17	161, 204, 210–213	1–4/5–17	168, 172, 211–214
Sleepwalking	1–3 (–6)/6–29 (–62)	161, 174, 204, 206, 208, 215, 216	0.1–0.6/0.9–3	23, 168, 172, 212, 217
Sleep terrors	3/3.5–15	159a, 161, 174, 206, 210	?	—
Sleep enuresis	1.5–8/6–25	174, 207, 210, 218–224, 228	–/0.07–2.1	168, 172, 217, 225
Nightmares	2–11/15–31	163, 207, 208, 210, 229	3–9 (–47)/5-29 (–69)	23, 160, 172, 217, 226, 227

The lowest and highest frequencies of the original works (references) are given. If the frequency of one study clearly deviates from the others, it is given in parentheses. "Childhood" refers to studies in populations 15 to 20 years old.
–, lower limit not defined or not known; —, not applicable; ?, not known.

PARASOMNIAS

The parasomnias have been identified as a major category of sleep disorders. They represent a group of physiological and behavioral phenomena that occur predominantly during sleep. The parasomnias are disorders of arousal, partial arousal, and sleep stage transition.[2]

Table 47–8 summarizes studies on the occurrence of six parasomnias. The list of publications is not nearly complete because such data seem to be scattered in sources (e.g., among larger health surveys) instead of being identified in literature searches with the use of appropriate key words. Most of the studies are retrospective questionnaire studies that were, performed in variable study populations (patient samples, general population, and so on) and used variable definitions. In other respects, they also are heterogeneous, and the values given must be regarded only as crude ratings. Moreover, as the frequency of parasomnias in children is strongly associated to age, it is difficult (or may even be misleading), for example, to provide occurrence values for enuresis in "childhood."

It is not easy to obtain reliable prevalence rates for parasomnias. One major problem is the definition of different parasomnias and the wording in questionnaires. It seems probable that sleep terror as a medical entity is largely unknown to people, and different types of nocturnal attacks of unpleasant nature (nightmares, panic attacks, and so on) may be reported as "sleep terrors"; there also is a strong correlation between the occurrence of nightmares and the report of sleep terrors.[159a] One additional problem is the obvious risk that the parasomnias occur without being noticed. Unless a cohabiting person reports, the subject may be unaware of the symptoms of sleeptalking or bruxism or of sleepwalking or sleep terror. Recall bias in retrospective questionnaire studies may also be a major factor that affects the results. Salvio et al.[160] found in their study of nightmares in the healthy elderly that the frequency estimates on the basis of sleep logs were more than 10 times higher than retrospective estimates.

References

1. American Sleep Disorders Association. Diagnostic classification of sleep and arousal disorders. Sleep. 1979;2:1–137.
2. American Sleep Disorders Association. International Classification of Sleep Disorder, Revised: Diagnostic and Coding Manual. Rochester, Minn: American Sleep Disorders Association; 1997.
3. MacMahon B, Pugh T. Epidemiology: Principles and Methods. Boston, Mass: Little, Brown; 1970.
4. Feinstein A. Clinical Epidemiology: The Architecture of Clinical Research. Philadelphia, Pa: WB Saunders; 1985.
5. Miettinen O. Theoretical Epidemiology: Principles of Occurrence Research in Medicine. New York, NY: John Wiley; 1985.
6. Ford D, Kamerow D. Epidemiologic study of sleep disturbances and psychiatric disorders: an opportunity for prevention? JAMA. 1989;262:1479–1484.
7. Ohayon MM, Guilleminault C, Paiva T, et al. An international study on sleep disorders in the general population: methodological aspects of the use of the Sleep-EVAL system. Sleep. 1997;20:1086–1092.
8. Ohayon MM, Caulet M, Philip P, et al. How sleep and mental disorders are related to complaints of daytime sleepiness. Arch Intern Med. 1997;157:2645–52.
9. Kraemer HC, Thiemann S. How Many Subjects? Newbury Park, Calif: Sage; 1987.
10. Last J. A Dictionary of Epidemiology. New York, NY: Oxford University Press; 1983.
11. Rothman K. Modern Epidemiology. Boston, Mass: Little, Brown; 1986.
12. Schlesselman JJ. Case-Control Studies. New York, NY: Oxford University Press; 1982.
13. Jenicek M. Méta-Analyse en Médecine. St-Hyacinthe, Québec, Canada: Edisem; 1987.
14. Wright J, Johns R, Watt I, et al. Health effects of obstructive sleep apnoea and the effectiveness of continuous positive airways pressure: a systematic review of the research evidence. Br Med J. 1997;314:851–860.
15. Claparede E. Théorie biologique du sommeil. Arch Psychol. 1905;4:245–349.
16. Dukes C. Sleep in relation to education. J R S Inst. 1905;26:41–44.
17. Camp C. Disturbance of sleep. J Mich Med Soc. 1923;22:133–138.
18. Laird D. The sleep habits of 509 men of distinction. Am Med. 1931;37:271–275.
19. Barry J, Bousfield W. A quantitative determination of euphoria and its relation to sleep. J Abnorm Soc Psychol. 1935;29:385–389.
20. Ladame C. Du sommeil et de quelques-unes de ses modalits chez les aliens. Schweiz Arch Neurol Psychiat. 1923;13:371–390.
21. Webb W. Individual differences in sleep length. Int Psychiatry Clin. 1970;7:44–47.
22. McGhie A, Russell S. The subjective assessment of normal sleep patterns. J Ment Sci. 1962;108:642–654.
23. Bixler EO, Kales A, Soldatos CR, et al. Prevalence of sleep

disorders in the Los Angeles metropolitan area. Am J Psychiatry. 1979;136:1257–1262.

24. Henderson S, Jorm AF, Scott LR, et al. Insomnia in the elderly: its prevalence and correlates in the general population. Med J Aust. 1995;162:22–24.

25. Mitchell ES, Woods NF. Symptom experiences of midlife women: observations from the Seattle Midlife Women's Health Study. Maturitas. 1996;25:1–10.

26. Husby R, Lingjaerde O. Prevalence of reported sleeplessness in northern Norway in relation to sex, age and season. Acta Psychiatr Scand. 1990;81:542–547.

27. Nowell PD, Buysse DJ, Reynolds CF, et al. Clinical factors contributing to the differential diagnosis of primary insomnia and insomnia related to mental disorders. Am J Psychiatry. 1997;154:1412–1416.

28. Weissman MM, Greenwald S, Nino-Murcia G, et al. The morbidity of insomnia uncomplicated by psychiatric disorders. Gen Hosp Psychiatry. 1997;19:245–250.

29. Zucconi M, Ferini-Strambi L, Gambini O, et al. Structured psychiatric interview and ambulatory sleep monitoring in young psychophysiological insomniacs. J Clin Psychiatry. 1996;57:364–370.

30. Costa e Silva JA, Chase M, Sartorius N, et al. Special report from a symposium held by the World Health Organization and the World Federation of Sleep Research Societies: an overview of insomnias and related disorders—recognition, epidemiology, and rational management. Sleep. 1996;19:412–416.

31. Dodge R, Cline MG, Quan SF. The natural history of insomnia and its relationship to respiratory symptoms. Arch Intern Med. 1995;155:1797–1800.

32. Partinen M, Eskelinen L, Tuomi K. Complaints of insomnia in different occupations. Scand J Work Environ Health. 1984;10(6 spec no):467–469.

33. Berwick D, Murphy J, Goldman P, et al. Performance of a five-item mental health screening test. Med Care. 1991;29:169–176.

34. Kuppermann M, Lubeck DP, Mazonson PD, et al. Sleep problems and their correlates in a working population. J Gen Intern Med. 1995;10:10–32.

35. Mellinger GD, Balter MB, Uhlenhuth EH. Insomnia and its treatment: prevalence and correlates. Arch Gen Psychiatry. 1985;42:225–232.

36. Lopez AT, Sanchez EG, Torres FG, et al. Hábitos y trastornos del dormir en residentes del área metropolitana de Monterrey. Salud Mental. 1995;18:14–22.

36a. Asplund R. Sleep and hypnotics among the elderly in relation to body weight and somatic disease. J Intern Med. 1995;238:65–70.

37. Kripke D, Garfinkel L. Excess nocturnal deaths related to sleeping pill and tranquilliser use. Lancet. 1984;1:99.

38. Rumble R, Morgan K. Hypnotics, sleep, and mortality in elderly people. J Am Geriatr Soc. 1992;40:787–791.

39. Kripke DF, Klauber MR, Wingard DL, et al. Mortality hazard associated with prescription hypnotics. Biol Psychiatry. 1998;43:687–693.

40. National Agency for Medicines. Finnish Statistics on Medicines. Helsinki, Finland: National Agency for Medicines; 1995.

41. Hublin C, Kaprio J, Partinen M, et al. Daytime sleepiness in an adult, Finnish population. J Intern Med. 1996;239:417–423.

42. Johns M, Hocking B. Daytime sleepiness and sleep habits of Australian workers. Sleep. 1997;20:844–849.

43. Karacan I, Thornby JI, Anch M, et al. Prevalence of sleep disturbance in a primary urban Florida county. Soc Sci Med. 1976;10:239–244.

44. Partinen M. Sleeping habits and sleep disorders on Finnish men before, during and after military service. Ann Med Milit Fenn. 1982;57(suppl 1):1–96.

45. D'Alessandro R, Rinaldi, R. Cristina E, et al. Prevalence of excessive daytime sleepiness: an open epidemiological problem [letter to the editor]. Sleep. 1995;18:389–391.

46. Partinen M, Rimpelä M. Sleeping habits and sleep disorders in a population of 2,016 Finnish adults. Yearbook of Health Education Research. Helsinki, Finland: National Board of Health; 1982:253–260.

47. Lugaresi E, Cirignotta F, Zucconi M, et al. Good and poor sleepers: an epidemiological survey of the San Marino population. In: Guilleminaolt C, Lugaresi E, eds. Sleep/Wake Disorders: Natural History, Epidemiology, and Long-Term Evolution. New York, NY: Raven Press; 1983:1–12.

48. Klink M, Quan SF. Prevalence of reported sleep disturbances in a general adult population and their relationship to obstructive airway diseases. Chest. 1987;91:540–546.

49. Schmidt-Nowara WW, Wiggins CL, Walch JK. Sleepiness in an adult population: prevalence, validity and correlates. In: Peter JH, Penzel T, von Wichert P, eds. Sleep and Health Risk. New York, NY: Springer-Verlag; 1991:78–83.

50. Martikainen KU, Partinen H, Hasan M, et al. Daytime sleepiness: a risk factor in community life. Acta Neurol Scand. 1992;86:337–341.

51. Solomon P. Narcolepsy in negroes. Dis Nerv Syst. 1945;6:179–183.

52. Roth B. Narkolepsie and Hypersomnie: vom Standpunkt der Physiologie des Schlafes. Berlin, Germany: Volk and Gesundheit; 1962.

53. Roth B. Narcolepsy and Hypersomnia. New York, NY: Karger; 1980:1–301.

54. Dement W, Zarcone V, Varner V, et al. The prevalence of narcolepsy. Sleep Res. 1972;1:148.

55. Dement W, Carskadon M, Ley R. The prevalence of narcolepsy II. Sleep Res. 1973:147.

56. Honda Y. Census of narcolepsy, cataplexy and sleep life among teen-agers in Fujisawa City. Sleep Res. 1979:191.

57. Honda Y, Asaka A, Tanimura M, et al. A genetic study of narcolepsy and excessive daytime sleepiness in 308 families with a narcolepsy or hypersomnia proband. In: Guilleminault C, Lugaresi E, eds. Sleep/Wake Disorders: Natural History, Epidemiology, and Long-Term Evolution. New York, NY: Raven Press; 1983:187–199.

58. Tashiro T, Kanbayashi T, Iijima S, et al. An epidemiological study on prevalence of narcolepsy in Japanese. J Sleep Res. 1992;1(suppl 1):228.

59. Wilner AS, Lavie P, Peled P, et al. Narcolepsy-cataplexy in Israeli Jews is associated exclusively with the HLA DR2 haplotype. Hum Immunol. 1988;21:15–22.

60. Hublin C, Kaprio J, Partinen M, et al. The Ullanlinna Narcolepsy Scale: validation of a measure of symptoms in the narcoleptic syndrome. J Sleep Res. 1994;3:52–59.

61. Hublin C, Kaprio J, Partinen M, et al. The prevalence of narcolepsy: an epidemiological study of the Finnish Twin Cohort. Ann Neurol. 1994;35:709–716.

62. Kessler S. Genetic Factors in Narcolepsy. In: Guilleminault C, Dement WC, Passouant P. Narcolepsy. New York, NY: Spectrum; 1976:285–302.

63. Kaprio J, Hublin C, Partinen M, et al. Narcolepsy-like symptoms among adult twins. J Sleep Res. 1996;5:55–60.

64. Lugaresi E, Cirignotta F, Coggagna G, et al. Some epidemiological data on snoring and cardiocirculatory disturbances. Sleep. 1980;3:221–224.

65. Koskenvuo M, Partinen M, Kaprio J. Snoring and disease. Ann Clin Res. 1985;17:247–251.

66. Schmidt-Nowara WW, Coultas DB, Wiggins C, et al. Snoring in a Hispanic-American population: risk factors and association with hypertension and other morbidity. Arch Intern Med. 1990;150:597–601.

67. Billiard M, Alperovitch A, Perot C, et al. Excessive daytime somnolence in young men: prevalence and contributing factors. Sleep. 1987;10:297–305.

68. Gislason T. Sleep apnea: clinical symptoms, epidemiology and ventilatory aspects. Acta Univ Upps. 1987;78:48.

69. American Academy of Sleep Medicine. Sleep related breathing disorders in adults: recommendations for syndrome definition and measurement techniques in clinical research. Sleep. 1999;22:667–689.

70. Corbo G, Fuciarelli F, Foresi A, et al. Snoring in children: association with respiratory symptoms and passive smoking. Br Med J. 1989;299:1491–1494.

71. Norton PG, Dunn EV. Snoring as a risk factor for disease: an epidemiological survey. Br Med J. 1985;291:630–632.

72. Kauffmann F, Annesi I, Neukirch F, et al. The relation between snoring and smoking, body mass index, age, alcohol consumption and respiratory symptoms. Eur Respir J. 1989;2:599–603.

73. Bloom J, Kaltenborn W, Quan S. Risk factors in a general population for snoring. Importance of cigarette smoking and obesity. Chest. 1988;93:678–683.

74. Lugaresi E, Mondini S, Zucconi M, et al. Staging of heavy snorers' disease: a proposal. Bull Eur Physiopathol Respir. 1983;19:590–594.

75. Telakivi T, Partinen M, Koskenvuo M, et al. Periodic breathing and hypoxia in snorers and controls: validation of snoring history and association with blood pressure and obesity. Acta Neurol Scand. 1987;76:69–75.

76. Berry D, Webb W, Block A. Sleep apnea syndrome: a critical review of the apnea index as diagnostic criterion. Chest. 1984;86:529–531.

77. George C, Kryger M. When is an apnea not an apnea [editorial]. Am Rev Respir Dis. 1985;131:485.

78. Bixler EO, Vgontzas AN, Ten Have T, et al. Effects of age on sleep apnea in men, I: prevalence and severity. Am J Respir Crit Care Med. 1998;157:144–148.

79. Lavie P. Sleep apnea in industrial workers. In: Guilleminault C, Lugaresi E, eds. Sleep/Wake Disorders: Natural History, Epidemiology, and Long-Term Evolution. New York, NY: Raven Press; 1983:127–135.

80. Peter J, Siegrist J, Podszus T, et al. Prevalence of sleep apnea in healthy industrial workers. Klin Wochenschr. 1985;63:807–811.

81. Cirignotta F, D'Alessandro R, Partinen M, et al. Prevalence of every night snoring and obstructive sleep apnoeas among 30-69-year-old men in Bologna, Italy. Acta Neurol Scand. 1989;79:366–372.

82. Bearpark H, Elliott L, Cullen S, et al. Home monitoring demonstrates high prevalence of sleep disordered breathing in men in the Busselton (Western Australia) population. Sleep Res. 1991;20A:411.

83. Partinen M, Telakivi T. Epidemiology of obstructive sleep apnea syndrome. Sleep. 1992;15(suppl 6):S1–S4.

84. Young T, Palta M, Dempsey J, et al. The occurrence of sleep-disordered breathing among middle-aged adults. N Engl J Med. 1993;328:1230–1235.

85. Gislason T, Almqvist M, Eriksson G, et al. Prevalence of sleep apnea syndrome among Swedish men: an epidemiological study. J Clin Epidemiol. 1988;41:571–576.

86. Esnaola S, Duran J, Rubio R, et al. Prevalence of obstructive sleep apnea in the male population of Vittoria-Gasteiz, Spain. Paper presented at: European Seminar on Sleep Disordered Breathing; February 1995.

87. Esnaola S, Duran J, Rubio R, et al. Prevalence of obstructive sleep apnea in the male population of Vittoria-Gasteiz, Spain. Paper presented at: European Seminar on Sleep Disordered Breathing; February 1995; Madrid, Spain.

88. Esnaola S, Duran J, Infante-Rivard C, et al. Diagnostic accuracy of a portable recording device (MESAM IV) in suspected obstructive sleep apnoea. Eur Respir J. 1996;9:2597–2605.

89. Ferini-Strambi L, Zucconi M, Palazzi S, et al. Snoring and nocturnal oxygen desaturations in an Italian middle-aged male population: epidemiologic study with an ambulatory device. Chest. 1994;105:1759–1764.

90. Fletcher E, DeBehnke R, Lavoi M, et al. Undiagnosed sleep apnea in patients with essential hypertension. Ann Intern Med. 1985;103:190–194.

91. Kales A, Bixler E, Cadieux R, et al. Sleep apnoea in a hypertensive population. Lancet. 1984;2:1005–1008.

92. Lavie P, Ben-Yosef R, Rubin A. Prevalence of sleep apnea among patients with essential hypertension. Am Heart J. 1984;108:373–376.

93. Williams A, Houston D, Finberg S, et al. Sleep apnea syndrome and essential hypertension. Am J Cardiol. 1985;55:1019–1022.

94. Worsnop CJ, Naughton MT, Barter CE, et al. The prevalence of obstructive sleep apnea in hypertensives. Am J Respir Crit Care Med. 1998;157:111–115.

95. Khosla T, Lowe F. Indices of obesity derived from body weight and height. Br J Prev Soc Med. 1967;21:122–128.

96. Katz I, Stradling J, Slutsky S, et al. Do patients with obstructive sleep apnea have thick necks? Am Rev Respir Dis. 1990;141:1228–1231.

97. Taasan V, Block A, Boysen P, et al. Alcohol increases sleep apnea and oxygen saturation in asymptomatic men. Am J Med. 1981;71:240–245.

98. Issa F, Sullivan C. Alcohol, snoring and sleep apnea. J Neurol Neurosurg Psychiatry. 1982;45:353–359.

99. Robinson R, White D, Zwillich C. Moderate alcohol ingestion increases upper airway resistance in normal subjects. Am Rev Respir Dis. 1985;132:1238–1241.

100. Mitler M, Dawson A, Henriksen S, et al. Bedtime ethanol increases resistance of upper airways and produces sleep apneas in asymptomatic snorers. Alcoholism. 1988;12:801–805.

101. Scrima L, Hartman P, Hiller F. Effect of three alcohol doses on breathing during sleep in 30-49 year old nonobese snorers and nonsnorers. Alcoholism. 1989;13:420–427.

102. Vitiello M, Prinz P, Personius J, et al. A history of chronic alcohol abuse is not associated with increased nighttime hypoxemia in older males. Sleep Res. 1986;15:178.

103. Koskenvuo M, Kaprio J, Partinen M, et al. Snoring and hostility in men. Sleep Res. 1987;16:371.

104. Roth T, Hartse K, Zorick F, et al. Multiple naps and the evaluation of daytime sleepiness in patients with upper airway sleep apnea. Sleep. 1980;3:425–439.

105. Guilleminault C, Partinen M, Quera-Salva M. Daytime sleepiness in non-narcoleptic subjects: central nervous system hypersomnia and obstructive sleep apneic patients. In: Smirne S, Franceschi M, Forini-Stramb. L, eds. Sleep in Medical and Neuropsychiatric Disorders. Proceedings of the First Milan International Symposium on Sleep, Milan, March 27-28, 1987. Milano, Italy: Masson; 1988:111–121.

106. Sink J, Bliwise D, Dement W. Self-reported excessive daytime somnolence and impaired respiration in sleep. Chest. 1986;90:177–180.

107. Potsic W. Obstructive sleep apnea. Pediatr Clin North Am. 1989;36:1435–1442.

108. Guilleminault C, Tilkian A, Dement WC. The sleep apnea syndromes. Annu Rev Med. 1976;27:465–484.

109. Gislason T, Benediktsdottir B. Snoring, apneic episodes, and nocturnal hypoxemia among children 6 months to 6 years old: an epidemiologic study of lower limit of prevalence. Chest. 1995;107:963–966.

110. Potsic W, Pasquariello P, Baranak C, et al. Relief of upper airway obstruction by adenotonsillectomy. Otolaryngol Head Neck Surg. 1986;94:476–480.

111. Kripke D, Ancoli-Israel S. Epidemiology of sleep apnea among the aged: is sleep apnea a fatal disorder? In: Guilleminault C, Lugaresi E, eds. Sleep/Wake Disorders: Natural History, Epidemiology, and Long-Term Evolution. New York, NY: Raven Press; 1983:137–142.

112. Ancoli-Israel S, Coy T. Are breathing disturbances in elderly equivalent to sleep apnea? Sleep. 1994;17:77–83.

113. Ancoli-Israel S, Kripke DF, Klauber MR, et al. Sleep-disordered breathing in community-dwelling elderly. Sleep. 1991;14:486–495.

114. Bliwise D, Bliwise N, Partinen M, et al. Sleep apnea and mortality in an aged cohort. Am J Public Health. 1988;78:544–547.

115. Cozzi F, Pierro A. Glossoptosis-apnea syndrome in infancy. Pediatrics. 1985;75:836–843.

116. Pekkarinen T, Partinen M, Pelkonen R, et al. Sleep apnoea and daytime sleepiness in acromegaly: relationship to endocrinological factors. Clin Endocrinol. 1987;27:649–654.

117. Kryger M, Roth T, Dement W, eds. Principles and Practice of Sleep Medicine. Philadelphia, Pa: WB Saunders; 1989.

118. Koskenvuo M, Kaprio J, Partinen M, et al. Snoring as a risk factor for hypertension and angina pectoris. Lancet. 1985;1(8434):893–896.

119. Partinen M, Kaprio J, Koskenvuo M, et al. Snoring and hypertension: a cross-sectional study on 12808 Finns aged 24-65 years. Sleep Res. 1983;12:273.

120. Gislason T, Aberg H, Taube A. Snoring and systemic hypertension—an epidemiological study. Acta Med Scand. 1987;222:415–421.

121. Hoffstein V, Rubinstein I, Mateika S, et al. Determinants of blood pressure in snorers. Lancet. 1988;2:992–994.

122. Coccagna G, Cirignotta F, Lugaresi E. Sleep related cardiocirculatory and respiratory changes in normal and pathological conditions. In Smirne S, Franceschi M, Ferini-Strambi L, eds. Sleep in Medical and Neuropsychiatric Disorders: Proceedings of the First Milan International Symposium on Sleep, Milan, March 27-28, 1987. Milano, Italy: Masson; 1988:37–44.

123. Lugaresi E, Cirignotta F, Coccagna G, et al. Clinical significance of snoring. In: Saunders NA, Sulivan CE, eds. Sleep and Breathing. New York, NY: Marcel Dekker; 1984:283–298.

124. Carlson J, Hedner J, Ejnell H, et al. High prevalence of hypertension in sleep apnea patients independent of obesity. Am J Respir Crit Care Med. 1994;150:72–77.

125. Fischer J, Raschke F. Die Pravalenz der Obstruktion der extrathorakalen und intrathorakalen Atemwege bei Patienten mit arterieller Hypertonie. [Prevalence of obstruction of extrathoracic and intrathoracic airways in patients with arterial hypertension]. Pneumologie. 1993(suppl 1);47:151–154.

126. Engel S, Karoff M, Raschke F, et al. Pravalenz des SAS bei Patienten mit primarer arterieller Hypertonie in einer kardiologischen Rehabilitationsklinik. [Prevalence of sleep apnea syndrome with primary arterial hypertension in a cardiologic rehabilitation clinic]. Pneumologie. 1995;49(suppl 1):145–147.

127. Enright PL, Newman AB, Wahl PW, et al. Prevalence and correlates of snoring and observed apneas in 5,201 older adults. Sleep. 1996;19:531–538.

128. Fletcher E. The relationship between systemic hypertension and obstructive sleep apnea: facts and theory. Am J Med. 1995;98:118–128.

129. Shepard JJ. Hypertension, cardiac arrhythmias, myocardial infarction, and stroke in relation to obstructive sleep apnea. Clin Chest Med. 1992;13:437–458.

130. Koskenvuo M, Kaprio J, Telakivi T, et al. Snoring as a risk factor for ischaemic heart disease and stroke in men. Br Med J. 1987;294:16–19.

131. Partinen M, Alihanka J, Lang H, et al. Myocardial infarction in relation to sleep apneas. Sleep Res. 1983;12:272.

132. De Olazabal JR, Miller MJ, Cook WR, et al. Disordered breathing and hypoxia during sleep in coronary artery disease. Chest. 1982;82:548–552.

133. D'Alessandro R, Magelli C, Gamberini G, et al. Snoring every night as a risk factor for myocardial infarction: a case-control study. Br Med J. 1990;300:1557–1558.

134. Hung J, Whitford E, Parsons R, et al. Association of sleep apnoea with myocardial infarction in men. Lancet. 1990;336:261–264.

135. Gainer J. Hypoxia and atherosclerosis: re-evaluation of an old hypothesis. Atherosclerosis. 1987;68:263–266.

136. Andreas S, Schulz R, Werner GS, et al. Prevalence of obstructive sleep apnoea in patients with coronary artery disease. Cor Artery Dis. 1996;7:541–545.

137. Hennekens C, Willet W, Rosner B, et al. Effects of beer, wine, and liquor in coronary deaths. JAMA. 1979;242:1973–1978.

138. Agnoli A, Manfredi M, Mossuto L, et al. Rapport entre les rythmes hemeronyctaux de la tension arterielle et sa pathogenie de l'insuffance vasculaire cerebrale. Rev Neurol. 1975;131:597–606.

139. Marshall J. Diurnal variation in occurrence of strokes. Stroke. 1977;8:230–231.

140. Tsementzis S, Gilla J, Hitchcock E, et al. Diurnal variation of and activity during the onset of stroke. Neurosurgery. 1985;17:901–904.

141. Partinen M, Palomäki H. Snoring and cerebral infarction. Lancet. 1985;2:1325–1326.

142. Palomäki H. Snoring and the risk of ischemic brain infarction. Stroke. 1991;22:1021–1025.

143. Palomäki H, Partinen M, Erkinjuntti T, et al. Snoring, sleep apnea and cerebrovascular disease. Neurology. 1992;6:75–82.

144. Spriggs DA, French JM, Murdy JM, et al. Snoring increases the risk of stroke and adversely affects prognosis. Q J Med. 1992;83:555–562.

145. Smirne S, Palazzi S, Zucconi M, et al. Habitual snoring as a risk factor for acute vascular disease. Eur Respir J 1993;6:1357–1361.

146. Neau J, Meurice J, Paquereau J, et al. Habitual snoring as a risk factor for brain infarction. Acta Neurol Scand. 1995;92:63–68.

147. Palomäki H, Partinen M, Juvela S, et al. Snoring as a risk factor for sleep-related brain infarction. Stroke. 1989;20:1311–1315.

148. Koskenvuo M, Kaprio J, Telakivi T, et al. Snoring as a risk factor for ischaemic heart disease and stroke in men. Br Med J (Clin Res Ed) 1987;294:16–19.

149. Seppälä T, Partinen M, Penttila A, et al. Sudden death and sleeping history among Finnish men. J Intern Med. 1991;229:23–28.

150. Warnes C, Roberts W. The heart in massive (more than 300 pounds or 136 kilograms) obesity: analysis of 12 patients studied at necropsy. Am J Cardiol. 1984;54:1087–1091.

151. Erkinjuntti T, Partinen M, Sulkava R, et al. Snoring and dementia. Age Ageing. 1987;16:305–310.

152. Reynolds C, Kupfer DJ, Taska LS, et al. Sleep apnea in Alzheimer's dementia: correlation with mental deterioration. J Clin Psychiatry. 1985;46:257–261.

153. Vitiello M, Prinz P. Sleep/wake patterns and sleep disorders in Alzheimer's disease. In: Thorpy MJ. Handbook of Sleep Disorders. New York, NY: Marcel Dekker; 1990:703–718.

154. He J, Kryger M, Zorick F, et al. Mortality and apnea index in obstructive sleep apnea. Chest. 1988;94:9–14.

155. Partinen M, Jamieson A, Guilleminault C. Long-term outcome for obstructive sleep apnea syndrome patients: mortality. Chest. 1988;94:1200–1204.

156. Partinen M, Guilleminault C. Daytime sleepiness and vascular morbidity at seven-year follow-up in obstructive sleep apnea patients. Chest. 1990;97:27–32.

157. Lavie P, Herer P, Peled R, et al. Mortality in sleep apnea patients: a multivariate analysis of risk factors. Sleep. 1995;18:149–157.

158. Janson C, Gislason T, Bengtsson H, et al. Long-term follow-up of patients with obstructive sleep apnea treated with uvulopalatopharyngoplasty. Arch Otolaryngol Head Neck Surg. 1997;123:257–262.

159. Ronald J, Delaive K, Roos L, et al. Obstructive sleep apnea patients use more health care resources ten years prior to diagnosis. Sleep Res Online. 1998;1:71–74.

159a. Hublin C, Kaprio J, Partinen M, et al. Limits of self-report in assessing sleep terrors in a population survey. Sleep. 1999;22:89–93.

160. Salvio MA, Wood JM, Schwartz J, et al. Nightmare prevalence in healthy elderly. Psychol Aging. 1992;7:324–325.

161. Saarenpää-Heikkilä OA, Rintahaka PJ, Laippala PJ, et al. Sleep habits and disorders in Finnish schoolchildren. J Sleep Res. 1995;4:173–182.

162. Tynjälä J, Kannas L, Välimaa R. How young Europeans sleep. Health Educ Res. 1993;8.

163. Rimpelä A, Ahlström S. Health Habits Among Finnish Youth. Helsinki, Finland: National Board of Health; 1983:71–83.

164. Price VA, Coates TJ, Thorensen CE, et al. Prevalence and correlates of poor sleep among adolescents. Am J Dis Child. 1978;132:583–586.

165. Kirmil-Gray K, Eagleston J, Gibson E, et al. Sleep disturbance in adolescents: sleep quality, sleep habits, beliefs about sleep, and daytime functioning. J Youth Adolesc. 1984;13:375–384.

166. Levy D, Gray-Donald K, Leech J, et al. Sleep patterns and problems in adolescents. J Adolesc Health. 1986;7:386–389.

167. Cirignotta F, Mondini S, Zucconi M, et al. Insomnia: an epidemiological survey. Clin Neuropharmacol. 1985;8(suppl 1):S49–S54.

168. Smirne S, Franceschi M, Zamproni P, et al. Prevalence of sleep disorders in an unselected inpatient population. In: Guilleminault C, Lugaresi E, eds. Sleep/Wake Disorders: Natural History, Epidemiology and Long-Term Evolution. New York, NY: Raven Press; 1983:61–71.

169. Yeo BK, Perera IS, Kok LP, et al. Insomnia in the community. Singapore Med J. 1996;37:282–284.

170. Hohagen F, Grabhoff U, Ellringmann D, et al. The prevalence of insomnia in different age groups and its treatment modalities in general practice. In: Smirne SFM, Ferini-Strambi L, eds. Sleep and Ageing. Milano, Italy: Masson; 1991:205–215.

171. Simon GE, VonKorff M. Prevalence, burden, and treatment of insomnia in primary care. Am J Psychiatry. 1997;154:1417–1423.

172. Hyyppä M, Kronholm E. How does Finland sleep? Sleeping habits of the Finnish adult population and the rehabilitation of sleep disturbances [in Finnish]. Finland: Publ Soc Ins Inst; 1987;ML:68:1–110.

173. Morgan K, Clarke D. Risk factors for late-life insomnia in a representative general. Br J Gen Pract. 1997;47:166–169.

174. Blader JC, Koplewicz HS, Abikoff H, et al. Sleep problems of elementary school children: a community survey. Arch Pediatr Adolesc Med. 1997;151:473–480.

175. Morrison DN, McGee R, Stanton WR. Sleep problems in adolescence. J Am Acad child Adolesc Psychiatry. 1992;31:94–99.

176. Lack L. Delayed sleep and sleep loss in university students. J Am Col Health. 1986;35:105–110.

177. Janson C, De Backer W, Gislason T, et al. Increased prevalence of sleep disturbances and daytime sleepiness in subjects with bronchial asthma: a population study of young adults in three European countries. Eur Respir J. 1996;9:2132–2138.

178. Ohayon M. Epidemiological study on insomnia in the general population. Sleep. 1996;19(suppl):S7–S15.

179. Ohayon MM, Caulet M, Priest RG, et al. DSM-IV and ICSD-90 insomnia symptoms and sleep dissatisfaction. Br J Psychiatry. 1997;171:382–388.

180. Karacan I, Thornby J, Williams R. Sleep disturbance: a community survey. In: Guilleminault C, Lugaresi E, eds. Sleep/Wake Disorders: Natural History, Epidemiology, and Long-term Evolution. New York, NY: Raven Press; 1983:37–60.

181. Kronholm E, Hyyppä M. Age-related sleep habits and retirement. Ann Clin Res. 1985;17:257–264.

182. Ganguli M, Reynolds CF, Gilby JE. Prevalence and persistence of sleep complaints in a rural older community sample: the MoVIES project. J Am Geriatr Soc. 1996;44:778–784.

183. Blazer DG, Hays JC, Foley DJ. Sleep complaints in older adults: a racial comparison. J Gerontol A Biol Sci Med Sci. 1995;50:M280–M284.

184. Foley DJ, Monjan AA, Brown SL, et al. Sleep complaints among elderly persons: an epidemiologic study of three communities. Sleep. 1995;18:425–432.

185. Simen S, Rodenbeck A, Schlaf G, et al. Sleep complaints and hypnotic use by the elderly—results of a representative survey in West Germany. Wien Med Wochenschr. 1996;146:306–309.

186. Johnson EO, Roehrs T, Roth T, et al. Epidemiology of alcohol and medication as aids to sleep in early adulthood. Sleep. 1998;21:178–186.

187. Partinen M, Kaprio J, Koskenvuo M, et al. Sleeping habits, sleep quality and use of sleeping pills: a population study of 31140 adults in Finland. In: Guilleminault C, Lugaresi E, eds. Sleep/Wake Disorders: Natural History, Epidemiology and Long-Term Evaluation. New York, NY: Raven Press; 1983:29–35.

188. Morgan K, Dalloso H, Ebrahim S, et al. Prevalence, frequency, and duration of hypnotic drug use among the elderly living at home. Br Med J. 1988;296:601–602.

189. Hays JC, Blazer DG, Foley DJ. Risk of napping: excessive daytime sleepiness and mortality in an older community population. J Am Geriatr Soc. 1996;44:693–698.

190. Berg Kelly K, Ehrver M, Erneholm T, et al. Self-reported health status and use of medical care by 3500 adolescents in western Sweden. Acta Pediatr Scand. 1991;80:837–843.

191. Franceschi M, Zamproni P, Crippa D, et al. Excessive daytime sleepiness: a 1-year study in an unselected inpatient population. Sleep. 1982;5:239–247.

192. al Rajeh S, Bademosi O, Ismail H, et al. A community survey of neurological disorders in Saudi Arabia: the Thugbah study. Neuroepidemiology. 1993;12:164–178.

193. Wing YK, Chiu HF, Ho CK, et al. Narcolepsy in Hong Kong Chinese—a preliminary experience. Aust N Z J Med. 1994;24:304–306.

194. Ohayon MM, Priest RG, Caulet M, et al. Hypnagogic and hypnopompic hallucinations: pathological phenomena? Br J Psychiatry. 1996;169:459–467.

195. Ohta Y, Okada T, Kawakami Y, et al. Prevalence of risk factors for sleep apnea in Japan: a preliminary report. Sleep. 1993;16(8 suppl):S6–S7.

196. Jennum P, Sjol A. Self-assessed cognitive function in snorers and sleep apneics. An epidemiological study of 1,504 females and males aged 30-60 years: the Dan-MONICA II Study. Eur Neurol. 1994;34:204–208.

197. Bearpark H, Elliott L, Grunstein R, et al. Snoring and sleep apnea: a population study in Australian men. Am J Respir Crit Care Med. 1995;151:1459–1465.

198. Stradling J, Crosby J. Predictors and prevalence of obstructive sleep apnoea and snoring in 1001 middle age men. Thorax. 1991;46:85–90.

199. Haraldsson PO, Carenfelt C, Tingvall C. Sleep apnea syndrome symptoms and automobile driving in a general population. J Clin Epidemiol. 1992;45:821–825.

200. Gislason T, Benediktsdottir B, Bjornsson J, et al. Snoring, hypertension, and the sleep apnea syndrome: an epidemiologic survey of middle-aged women. Chest. 1993;103:1147–1151.

201. Olson L, King M, Hensley MJ, et al. A community study of snoring and sleep-disordered breathing: prevalence. Am J Respir Crit Care Med. 1995;152:711–716.

202. Ohayon MM, Guilleminault C, Priest RG, et al. Snoring and breathing pauses during sleep: telephone interview survey of a United Kingdom population sample. Br Med J. 1997;314:860–863.

203. Kripke DF, Ancoli-Israel S, Klauber MR, et al. Prevalence of sleep-disordered breathing in ages 40-64 years: a population-based survey. Sleep. 1997;20:65–76.

204. Klackenberg G. Incidence of parasomnias in children in a general population. In: Guilleminault C, ed. Sleep and Its Disorders in Children. New York, NY: Raven Press; 1987:99–114.

205. Reimao RN, Lefevre AB. Prevalence of sleep-talking in childhood. Brain Dev. 1980;2:353–357.

206. Kahn A, An de Merckt C, Rebuffat E, et al. Sleep problems in healthy preadolescents. Pediatrics. 1989;84:542–546.

207. Fisher BE, Wilson AE. Selected sleep disturbances in school children reported by parents: prevalence, interrelationships, behavioral correlates and parenteral attributions. Percept Mot Skills. 1987;64:1147–1157.

208. Rintahaka P, Uusikylä K. Sleeping habits and sleep disorders of Finnish school children. Sleep Res. 1987;208.

209. Hublin C, Kaprio J, Partinen M, et al. Sleeptalking in twins: epidemiology and psychiatric co-morbidity. Behav Genet. 1998;28:289–298.

210. Salzarulo P, Chevalier A. Sleep problems in children and their relationship with early disturbances of the waking-sleeping-rhythms. Sleep. 1983;6:47–51.

211. Reding GR, Rubright WC, Zimmerman SO. Incidence of bruxism. J Dent Res. 1966;45:1198–1204.

212. Hublin C, Kaprio J, Partinen M, et al. Sleep bruxism based on self-report in a nation-wide twin cohort. J Sleep Res. 1998;17:61–67.

213. Lavigne GJ, Montplaisir JY. Restless legs syndrome and sleep bruxism: prevalence and association among Canadians. Sleep. 1994;17:739–743.

214. Glaros AG. Incidence of diurnal and nocturnal bruxism. J Prosthet Dent. 1981;45:545–549.

215. Hublin C, Kaprio J, Partinen M, et al. Prevalence and genetics of sleepwalking—a population-based twin study. Neurology. 1997;4:177–181.

216. Bakwin H. Sleep-walking in twins. Lancet. 1970;2:446–447.

217. Cirignotta F, Zucconi M, Mondini S, et al. Enuresis, sleepwalking and nightmares: an epidemiological survey in the Republic of San Marino. In: Guilleminault C, Lugares; E, eds. Sleep/Wake Disorders: Natural History, Epidemiology, and Long-Term Evolution. New York, NY: Raven Press; 1983:237–241.

218. Devlin JB. Prevalence and risk factors for childhood nocturnal enuresis. Irish Med J. 1991/1992:118–120.

219. Järvelin MR, Vikeväinen-Tervonen L, Moilanen I, et al. Enuresis in seven-year-old children. Acta Paediatr Scand. 1988;77:148–153.

220. Linna SL, Moilanen I, Keistinen H, et al. Prevalence of psychosomatic symptoms in children. Psychother Psychosom. 1991;56:85–87.

221. Hallgren B. Nocturnal enuresis in twins, 1: methods and materials. Acta Psychiatr Scand. 1960;35:73–90.

222. Bakwin H. Enuresis in Twins. Am J Dis Child. 1971;121:222–225.

223. Krantz I, Jylkäs E, Ahlberg BM, et al. On the epidemiology of nocturnal enuresis. Scand J Urol Nephrol Suppl. 1994;163:75–82.

224. Costello EJ, Angold A, Burns BJ, et al. The Great Smoky Mountains study of youth. Arch Gen Psychiatry. 1996;53:1129–1136.

225. Burgio KL, Locher JL, Ives DG, et al. Nocturnal enuresis in community-dwelling older adults. J Am Geriatr Soc. 1996;44:139–143.

226. Wood JMB, Bootzin RR. The prevalence of nightmares and their independence from anxiety. J Abnorm Psychol. 1990;99:64–68.

227. Leung AKC, Robson WLM. Nightmares. J Natl Med Assoc. 1993;85:233–235.

228. Hublin C, Kaprio J, Partinen M, et al. Nocturnal enuresis in a nationwide twin cohort. Sleep. 1998;21:577–583.

229. Hublin C, Kaprio J, Partinen M, et al. Nightmares: familial aggregation and association with psychiatric disorders in a nationwide twin cohort. Am J Med Genet/Neuropsychiatr Genet. 1999;88:329–336.

48

Sleep Medicine, Public Policy, and Public Health

Merrill M. Mitler

William C. Dement

David F. Dinges

Sleep and sleepiness are among the most basic of human behaviors. As amply illustrated throughout this volume, a person's sleep can be disrupted not only by pathological processes but also by the person's lifestyle and by societal demands on the sleep-wake schedule.[1] When sleep disruption occurs, regardless of the reason, the consequences for the individual and, in some circumstances, for society, can be serious. At present, there is only limited recognition of this fundamental fact and of the vast gulf that still exists between gains in the scientific and medical knowledge of sleep and the application of these gains to prevention of personal and public catastrophes.

Sleep specialists constitute an important public policy resource because they have the scientific and medical expertise to affect public policy and reduce unsafe practices associated with sleep and sleepiness. Health professionals have always had a major role in decisions regarding public health issues. One does not have to look far to find cogent examples of behavioral and societal changes that were initiated by and through the health care system that reduced the prevalence of catastrophic outcomes. Physicians advanced the knowledge of linkages between "unseen" microbes and disease, which led to improvements in food preparation and waste disposal. Pulmonologists led the way in reducing cigarette smoking. Emergency department physicians helped implement mandatory seatbelt laws. These and many other public health initiatives have saved millions of lives. Applying what has been learned about the effects of sleepiness on public safety,[2, 3] sleep specialists are contributing to the formulation of public policy on prevention and management of sleepiness on the job and during other safety-sensitive activities such as driving. It can be argued that sleepiness is another "unseen" threat to public health. Just as massive and long-term public educational efforts and government regulations are fundamental components of modern sanitation policy, for example, we must continue to develop similar educational and regulatory approaches to modernize policy concerning sleep.

The purpose of this chapter is to outline key concepts that enable the sleep specialist to approach public policy matters in an informed manner. We also highlight the areas in which the principles of sleep medicine can constructively shape public policy and improve public health.

SLEEP IN MODERN SOCIETY

Sleep, like many other aspects of human activity, has been irrevocably altered by the industrial revolution and its attendant artificial light and cheap energy. Around-the-clock operations are now commonplace, and the time traditionally allocated to sleep has given way to time for more productivity, business, war, and so on. Even today, as societies make the transition from agrarian cultures to industrial powers, some of the more dramatic changes that occur involve sleep. For example, siesta is usually outlawed, and shift work is usually implemented.[4]

The advent of highly technological societies has made poor sleep and substandard levels of wakefulness real (and life-or-death) factors for many human beings. For example, sleepiness-related human errors by people who operate public transportation vehicles, supervise the control of nuclear power stations, and perform 24-h military functions, could cause havoc. Disasters that have occurred on the night shift, such as the event at Three Mile Island nuclear power plant and the grounding of the Exxon Valdez oil tanker, have undermined public trust in these industries.[2]

Technological advances have eliminated many sources of accidents, while sleep deprivation, fatigue, and other human factors have become major causes of failure, error, and accident throughout society. Automation has further potentiated the negative effects of reduced alertness by increasing the amount of monotony involved in many jobs, leaving human beings to stand vigil—an activity that is especially susceptible to sleepiness.[5] At present, human error causes the majority (60 to 90%) of all industrial and transportation accidents.[2]

Unfortunately, with each new wave of technological development, the priority society places on obtaining adequate sleep seems to lessen. Sleep appears to be valued less and less. For example, in 1913, 8- to 12-year-old schoolchildren slept an average of 10.5 h per night[6]; by 1964, the average had dropped to 9.2 h per night.[7] The failure to understand the effect of inadequate sleep on the entire 24-h cycle has created a public health problem. Even modest amounts of daily sleep loss accumulate as a *sleep debt* that is manifest as an increasing tendency to fall asleep[8] and a reduced level of psychomotor performance.[9, 10] Although most people can resist this tendency under normal circumstances, when physical activity is minimal and the circadian reinforcement of sleep is maximal, the likelihood of a lapse in vigilance, a "microsleep," or a longer sleep episode can become high. People who are directly responsible for public health and safety, including, but not limited to, doctors and nurses, work night shifts and long hours, which makes them especially prone to sleepiness-related errors.[11] In work environments where sustained attention is necessary for safety, the probability of an accident rises and falls along with the biological tendency to fall asleep. Thus, catastrophic accidents related to sleepiness and fatigue do not happen at random throughout the day. Rather, they are more likely at times when human beings are most prone to sleep, between midnight and 8 AM and between 1 and 3 PM.[12–14]

THE CHALLENGE

For the most part, the general public does not know the fundamentals of sleep physiology, and people tend to ignore important relationships between sleepiness and accidents. The lay press contains numerous articles about sleep that present topics such as the signs of sleep apnea, the importance of good sleep hygiene for poor sleepers, or the dangers of sleeping pills. These articles seem to be well received by the public, probably because of concern about sleep needs and the negative effects of sleep loss. During the 1990s, the print and broadcasting media presented major stories that raised many of the tough public policy questions with which we continue to grapple, such as how to balance the economic necessities of round-the-clock operations with concerns for the proper rest and safety of workers.

However, unlike these stories, much of the lay press attention to sleep is superficial and narrow. Common features of such articles include a light treatment of "how little sleep we all get because of our hectic modern lifestyles" and feature simplistic self-help ideas and "ask your doctor" suggestions. Superficial articles often underscore the lack of public awareness about the gravity of sleep-related problems. Health care professionals must assume responsibility for the inadequate information about sleep and sleep problems available to the general public. Few people would joke about a drunken colleague at work or about a drunk driver, but many find a sleepy colleague or a sleepy driver more comic than tragic.

The challenge sleep specialists now face is to participate in the development of the comprehensive conceptual paradigms necessary for resolving the economic, social, health, and safety issues associated with people getting proper sleep. Such paradigms are essential if the scientific principles of sleep research are to influence public policy positively. The lessons from other areas of medicine that led to major behavioral changes are instructive. It was not possible to limit communicable diseases without social programs. Automobile crash fatalities and injuries could not be reduced without effective use of seatbelts. Fighting the most common cause of lung cancer required social and political programs to warn consumers about the dangers of smoking and to create smoke-free environments.

Considering the various areas of our modern lives that are especially vulnerable to inappropriate sleepiness, one can see the continued adverse effects of the lack of conceptual paradigms for preventing impairment due to sleepiness. A driver who causes a serious accident will almost always undergo tests for ethanol and perhaps for psychoactive drugs. However, the quality and quantity of the driver's sleep in the previous 24 to 48 h is rarely assessed. This lack of assessment exists despite strong data in prestigious scientific journals that sleep deprivation can be as impairing to driving ability as ethanol intoxication.[15, 16] Although sleep deprivation and ethanol intoxication are both self-imposed conditions of impairment, society views them differently. Being sleep deprived is often considered to be a sign of hard work and worthiness. Being drunk anywhere, but most especially on the job or behind the wheel, is viewed as socially unacceptable.[17]

Teaching people about the dangers of driving when they are impaired by sleepiness will require research on countermeasures such as drowsy-driving detection technologies,[18–21] roadside signs, safe sleeping areas, and tests to assess sleepiness. These concepts are new and quite radical relative to the lax attitude society has held toward sleep. In one study of fatigue and alertness in 80 long-haul truck drivers operating on North American routes with four demanding driving schedules, drivers slept 4.8 h per day. This average appears to be below the level of sleep known to produce increased tendency to fall asleep and to make errors in performance on sedentary tasks that require sustained attention.[10, 22]

Not only will our society need to develop the conceptual paradigm for planning work schedules but also it will need detailed information on the prevalence of sleep-related mishaps and the epidemiological consequences of inadequate sleep. This information is vital for designing paradigmatic approaches and targeting resources where they will do the most good. Presently, much of what we know or suspect about the role of sleep and sleepiness in public and private catastrophes is gleaned inferentially from retrospective studies and time-of-day data. Some prospective efforts to obtain data on sleepiness-related catastrophes are underway, in parallel with attempts to define the biological limits sleep places on the wakefulness of operators in safety-sensitive occupations.[23, 24]

KEY AREAS OF IMPACT

The Role of Sleep in Cardiovascular Mortality and Morbidity

The most likely time for something to go wrong with a patient is in the middle of the night. This central truth of the human condition has been known since biblical times. For example, Solomon's bed was guarded by "sixty valiant men for fear of the night" (Song of Solomon, 3:8). Indeed, disease-related mortality follows the two-peak pattern throughout the 24-h day that has been described for sleep tendency.[25–27] In modern times, the plurality of such deaths is attributed to cardiovascular events, such as heart attack and stroke. The likelihood of suffering a heart attack varies significantly across time of day[28] with a peak between 8 and 10 AM, some 2 h later than the morning peak for mortality.[27] This time shift does not rule out sleep as a contributing factor or condition. There are fundamental properties of sleep physiology that may underlie the shape of the 24-h pattern in disease-related mortality. First, at least part of this time shift may stem from the fact that many people with heart disease get in a habit of sleeping later in the morning. Moreover, aspirin reduces mortality due to myocardial infarct primarily during the morning peak, which suggests that the morning peak may be related to heightened platelet aggregability.[29, 30] Indeed, direct observations of platelet aggregability show diurnal variation with a prominent morning peak.[31] There are sleep-related increases in plasma concentrations of epinephrine and other compounds known to potentiate blood clotting or vasospasm. Such increases may be related to sleep-disordered breathing.[32, 33] Jennum et al.[34] found that morning awake arterial blood pressure and nocturnal arterial blood pressure decreased with nasal continuous positive airway pressure treatment and concluded that these hemodynamic changes were associated with a treatment-related decrease in the number of sleep apnea events, a decrease in sympathetic activity, and an increase in parasympathetic activity. More evidence for the putative role of sleep apnea in the timing of deaths comes from work by Ancoli-Israel and colleagues, who reported that 24% of people over age 65 years had more than 5 apneic events per hour of sleep, and 62% had more than 10 respiratory disturbances per hour of sleep.[35] The high prevalence of sleep apnea coupled with widespread use of bedtime alcohol and sedative hypnotics could have major contributory roles in shaping the 24-h pattern in disease-related mortality.[14, 32, 36, 37]

Transportation

Motor vehicle accidents do not occur randomly throughout the 24-h day but tend to peak during the early morning and midafternoon in accordance with peaks in human sleep tendency.[12, 38–40] Because information relevant to the sleep tendency of drivers is not routinely gathered for automobile accidents,[41] it is dif-ficult to determine precise figures. A study in Great Britain estimated that 27% of drivers who lost consciousness behind the wheel fell asleep, as opposed to fainting, having a seizure, or having a heart attack. However, this 27% accounted for 83% of the fatalities.[42] Other investigators have also observed a high rate of fatality in sleep-related accidents.[14, 43] The increased fatality rate is probably due to the tendency for sleepy drivers to push on rather than stop and sleep, thereby allowing unintended bouts of sleep to occur without warning. Once a driver has fallen asleep, there is little or no attempt to brake or otherwise avoid collision.[14]

Each year in the United States there are approximately 4800 fatal accidents involving trucks and many more nonfatal accidents. The National Transportation Safety Board (NTSB) reported a probable cause of fatigue in 57% of accidents that led to a truck driver's death,[38, 39] although this percentage is disputed by other federal and private entities concerned with trucking safety. The term *fatigue* has been used throughout federal agencies to describe human performance failure attributable to a variety of factors. It is clear from the NTSB's texts that their intended meaning of the term *fatigue* is most congruent with what sleep specialists mean by the term *sleepiness*.[2]

When a truck driver dies in such an accident, between three and four other people are usually also killed.[40] Depending on the involvement of other vehicles and the nature of the cargo, associated damages may be substantial. The mean cost of a crash involving a single large vehicle has been calculated to be $51,000, but when fatalities result, the cost per crash is estimated at $2.7 million.[44] The trucking industry employs approximately 2.5 million drivers, operates 1 million motor carriers, and accounts for 10 billion miles per year of travel on U.S. highways and 5% of the gross domestic product of the United States. Trucks deliver products and materials to every segment of society from local deliveries through transcontinental long hauls. The economic incentives for driving long hours are compelling, and the time-on-task guidelines and regulations promulgated in the 1930s are inadequate in the face of current knowledge of sleep physiology and the forces affecting trucking. Perhaps the understandable fear of harming such a vital industry has prevented the initiation of studies to help reduce accidents due to sleepiness in truck drivers[45]; fortunately, a number of studies have been initiated (Impact of Sleeper Berth Usage on Driver Fatigue [Contract DTFH61-97-C-00068]; Study of the Incidence of Sleep Apnea Among Commercial Truck Drivers [Task A of Contract DTFH61-93-C-00088, TRI Truck and Driver Research]).

Many of the same issues pertaining to the role of sleep in recovery from work and in sleepiness induced by work schedules are fundamental safety issues in other transportation modes. Sleep-related catastrophic accidents on the railroad have also been identified. The NTSB concluded that sleep deprivation with its related impairment was a primary cause in at least four catastrophic railroad accidents between 1987 and 1992.[46]

Maritime transportation typically involves 24-h operations, and sleep deprivation has been the cause of several catastrophes. One of the most dramatic involved the grounding of the supertanker Exxon Valdez on Bligh Reef in Prince William Sound, Alaska, in March 1989. The NTSB determined that a "probable cause of the grounding of the Exxon Valdez was the failure of the third mate to properly maneuver the vessel because of fatigue and excessive workload. . . ."[47(pv)] The grounding of the oil tanker World Prodigy off the coast of Rhode Island is another example of a major maritime accident involving sleep-based fatigue.[48] The NTSB determined that the probable cause was the master's impaired judgment from acute fatigue. The master had been awake for 36 h at the time of the accident.

In each of these transportation areas, little research has been conducted to identify effective measures to counter sleep-based fatigue. Impetus to begin such countermeasure research will be enhanced as more public attention focuses on human error accidents and as top management integrates the real costs of sleepiness-based error accidents into their overall plans for risk management. This has begun in many of these industries, under the aegis of "fatigue management."[49, 50]

Health Care Workers

Many health care workers are on duty for 10- or 12-h shifts, with day and night shifts alternating as frequently as every week. In any work situation, a tired and sleepy worker is less effective and at more risk for an accident. The nature of the risk depends on the nature of the work. When 24-h operations are involved, the likelihood of severe sleep deprivation and other biological rhythm effects is great, and the associated risk for accidents and diminished productivity is consequently much higher.

In 1984, Libby Zion, an 18-year-old college freshman, died in a hospital in New York City. A grand jury found that her death was due to an undiagnosed infection and blamed inadequate supervision of residents and resident fatigue for the failure to institute proper treatment.[51] As a result, New York enacted laws to reduce the total number of hours that residents are permitted to work. Although this is one possible solution to resident fatigue, other approaches, such as providing minimal anchor sleep periods during prolonged work periods that use principles of chronobiology, may be more effective. While the merits of legislated restrictions on work hours for physicians are debated in medical journals and in state legislatures, it is good to remember that, historically, physicians have led in making fundamental changes necessary to accommodate newly understood principles of physiology and medicine. The widespread use of sterile technique in surgery and the modern emphasis on preventive medicine are two good examples.

Hazardous Work

Particularly vulnerable work places include nuclear power plants and 24-h operations involving the production of hazardous or toxic chemicals. The early morning human errors that led to the on-site disaster at Three Mile Island[52] and the environmental disaster at Chernobyl[53, 54] bear all the earmarks of fatigue-related accidents. There have been other summaries of fatigue-related performance failures that resulted in catastrophic outcomes.[55]

Other Sensitive Areas

Sleep specialists encounter patients from all walks of life. It is impossible here to provide an exhaustive list of jobs in which excessive sleepiness constitutes a public health hazard. Some examples include military personnel, firefighters, police officers, emergency utility workers, rescue workers, and Medevac personnel.

Students deserve special mention. Adolescents generally do not sleep enough. They are at risk for a number of serious consequences including daytime sleepiness, poor performance at school, increased incidence of automobile accidents, increased moodiness, and increased use of stimulants and alcohol.[56] Adolescents typically go to bed at an increasingly later bedtime, but their schedules require that they continue to arise early. Some teenagers develop delayed sleep phase syndrome, a pattern that is incompatible with school schedules. Up to 40% of high school and college students are sleep deprived, and laboratory studies[57–59] have documented performance impairment. In addition, tired students are likely to have impaired motivation and unintended sleep episodes.[60, 61]

Because many students beyond the age of 10 y do not get enough sleep, the sleep-deprived individual is the norm. Knowledge of the effects of sleep deprivation in this group has been available since 1980. We must prime parents and educators for constructive changes in the home and the classroom.

Ignoring Sleep Loss: The Challenger Disaster as a Case Study

The sequence of decisions leading up to the Space Shuttle Challenger accident in 1986 is a prime example of human error and poor judgment in a technological society. Sleep deprivation was contributory, if not causal, according to a supplemental report to the investigation.[63] The senior manager's decision to launch was based not on engineering judgments but rather on nonmission-related factors including public image and preset schedules. A Presidential Commission concluded that specific key managers had slept less than 2 h the night before and had been on duty since 1 AM on the day of the launch. The report stated that "time pressure, particularly that caused by launch scrubs and turnarounds, increased the potential for sleep loss and judgment errors" and that working "excessive hours, while admirable, raises serious questions when it jeopardizes job performance, particularly when critical management decisions are at stake."[63(pG5)]

Relieving Sleepiness With Naps: Aviation as a Case Study

Although accidents caused by sleep-based fatigue imperil all modes of transportation, aviation is one mode that has a history of research on the nature of fatigue and on developing countermeasures, primarily through research initiatives at NASA-Ames Research Center. One example of this work serves to illustrate what can be done to reduce sleepiness on the job, but the example also serves to highlight the significant challenges faced by sleep experts in initiating viable sleepiness countermeasures into practice and gaining acceptance by government, industry, labor, and the public.

For transmeridian flight crews, inadequate sleep has been a major source of fatigue.[64, 65] A multidisciplinary research effort was undertaken to evaluate the benefits to long-haul flight crews of preplanned naps while in the air.[66, 67] The results indicated not only that crew members could safely rotate, taking a brief (40-min) nap in flight, but also that the naps enhanced alertness of crews during flight.[68] Interestingly, the brief naps did not eliminate the cumulative sleep debt of crews, but they did appear to provide transient relief from in-flight fatigue, especially on night flights. Clearly, more work of this type is necessary. Its straightforward and cogent approach is based on the time-honored medical concept of reducing a pathogen, *sleepiness*, with an effective countermeasure, *sleep*. However, the example also exposes a problem. Although planned cockpit napping has been adopted by many European and Asian transcontinental air carriers, it has not yet been approved for U.S. carriers by the Federal Aviation Administration, due to political concerns.

DEALING PUBLICLY WITH THE PROBLEMS OF SLEEP

One of the most important reasons for problems in the aforementioned industries is sleep-based fatigue, but as the cockpit napping study serves to illustrate, public action on sleep-based fatigue is lagging. Obviously, the sleep medicine community understands that sleep deprivation will lead to some degree of sleepiness—perhaps to the level of dangerous impairment. Although the public can understand cause and effect relationships, as in "inoculation with a bacillus leads to infection" or "smoking leads to lung disease," society does not extend this level of understanding to "sleep loss leads to accidents." As discussed earlier, society needs a conceptual paradigm for dealing with the causal relationship between sleep loss and human error. Without the necessary concepts, it is difficult to influence public consciousness. In short, our society is in a preparadigmatic crisis. We face problems related to sleepiness, without the paradigm to formulate solutions. Imagine calling in "sleepy" to one's supervisor at work!

Parallels With Driving Under the Influence of Alcohol

The use of alcohol is governed by established policies and laws. These laws exist because alcohol can impair judgment and reflexes on the highway or in other hazardous situations, creating a risk both to the intoxicated person and to innocent people in the vicinity. Enforcement is possible because there is objective, rapid, cheap testing for the presence of alcohol and its concentration in the system: breathalyzer and blood tests.

Sleep loss, depending on the degree, also leads to impairment. In civil cases, if authorities determine that impairment from sleep deprivation has caused an accident, the driver is considered negligent and is liable for civil and criminal penalties. However, the parallel with alcohol ends there because accident investigators have no easy, inexpensive, and reliable measurement of the degree of sleep deprivation. Thus, errors due to falling asleep or impaired performance due to sleep deprivation must always be inferred from the nature of the accident. As the knowledge about sleep-related human error has increased, the involvement of the sleep specialists in litigation has also increased. Because accidents related to sleep are a large public health problem, society will inevitably have to confront issues surrounding the adjudication of sleep-related accidents.[2]

Sleepiness and Alcohol

It is known that sleepiness represents a significant risk to driving safety. Evidence suggests that sleepiness may pose as great a risk to driving safety as does alcohol.[16] Impairment due to alcohol is unquestionably potentiated by sleep deprivation.[15, 16, 69] It is not yet fully appreciated how great a contributory role sleepiness may have in the overall number of transportation accidents involving drug and alcohol use. In a study of fatal-to-the-driver truck accidents, the NTSB found that fatigue plus alcohol or drugs accounted for a large portion of lethal accidents.[38, 39] We may speculate that operating a vehicle while sleepy not only may prompt some people to use stimulants but, more important, may leave individuals unaware of the extent to which they are susceptible to additional performance impairment from alcohol or other depressant drugs.

Liability and Litigation as an Impetus for Change in Public Policy on Sleepiness

As should be obvious from the foregoing discussion, there is a gulf between scientific and medical knowledge about sleep and the application of this knowledge to public policy aimed at preventing personal and public catastrophes. Furthermore, the current lack of understanding that sleep loss causes performance impairments and the paucity of research on countermeasures for sleep-based fatigue retard the formulation of policies for dealing with losses caused by sleep-based fatigue.

Historically, when public policy has been unclear concerning issues surrounding a potentially injurious phenomenon, individuals turn to the courts for adjudication and redress. Precedents stemming from such judicial proceedings often prompt governments to establish policies. Moreover, court precedents can ultimately shape public policy. Because sleep specialists are the only logical source of detailed information concerning sleep physiology, they are often approached by litigators for consultation or to act as expert witnesses. Claims related to sleep physiology arise in all aspects of criminal, workers' compensation, and tort litigation. Knowledgeable and accurate presentations given by experts in sleep medicine will help the public policy process.

U.S. Policy Regarding Sleep

There have been some important achievements in the history of federal policy regarding sleep. All came about through effective communication between federal authorities and individual members or appointed committees representing the community of sleep specialists.

Beginning in the early 1970s, when the Food and Drug Administration developed guidelines for the evaluation of hypnotic efficacy, and moving to the present activities of the National Center for Sleep Disorders Research, our history has been one of activism and success. Here we mention only a few of the important milestones.

In 1979, the Surgeon General's office created Project Sleep to further focus governmental attention on sleep research and sleep disorders.

In 1984, the American Sleep Disorders Association first created an active government affairs committee. The committee's mandate was to provide all three branches of the government with up-to-date information on sleep physiology and current sleep research.

In 1990, the Institute of Medicine prepared a research briefing entitled "Basic Sleep Research." The briefing was prompted, in part, by the Institute of Medicine's recognition that the continuation of basic sleep research in the United States was being threatened by limited training of young researchers, limited research funding, and attacks by animal rights groups on several basic sleep research programs.

In an independent but complementary effort stimulated by the heightened federal interest in the impact of the sleep-wake cycle on society, the Office of Technology Assessment of the U.S. Congress conducted a major review of biological rhythms and their impact in the workplace.[70]

The National Commission for Sleep Disorders Research, in 1993, completed its comprehensive report of its findings.[46] This document called for permanent and concerted government efforts in expanding basic and clinical research on sleep disorders as well as in improving public awareness of the dangers of inappropriate sleepiness.

The National Center for Sleep Disorders Research was subsequently created within the National Institutes of Health. The Center's mandate is to conduct and support research, training, health information dissemination, and other activities with respect to sleep disorders, including biological and circadian rhythm research, basic understanding of sleep, and chronobiology, and to coordinate the activities of the Center with similar activities of other federal agencies. The legislation also mandated development of a National Sleep Disorders Research Plan,[71] which is summarized here:

- Understanding the cellular, molecular, and genetic basis of sleep and its disorders
- Determining the epidemiology of sleep and sleepiness in health and disease
- Identifying the effects of sleep loss on the waking function of the brain, other systems, and behavior
- Elucidating the pathophysiology and optimal management of common sleep disorders
- Developing new technologies to accomplish this task

By any measure, this history indicates that the field of sleep medicine is making itself heard and beginning to influence public policy and public health.

The Role of the Sleep Specialist in Public Policy

When confronted with the sometimes catastrophic consequences of sleepy workers, many people call for onerous penalties for those who deprive workers of sleep. However, such penalties are, in most cases, premature and shortsighted. Devising effective penalties presupposes a general recognition of the problem. The public must view the dangers of fatigue with the same level of concern it now accords to the dangers of, say, *Salmonella*. Without that level of concern, hours of service regulations are as unlikely to be observed now as the principles of modern sanitary practices were observed when typhoid fever was common. Moreover, there needs to be more of a focus on prevention than on punishment.

A relevant lesson comes from Henrik Ibsen's play, *Enemy of the People*. The protagonist, Dr. Stockmann, discovers contamination from a tannery in his town's spring. This is not welcome news because the waters are believed to have health benefits, attracting visitors whose spending is an important source of the town's revenue. Ignoring the contamination and declaring Dr. Stockmann to be an enemy of the people, the town continues to promote commercial aspects of the spring.

Researchers who document the dangers of fatigue in the workplace have begun to feel a certain kinship with Dr. Stockmann. Increasingly, researchers find that our society unwisely requires workers to perform dangerous tasks at times when their physiology would have them sleep. This is an unavoidable effect of shift work, which is compounded by economic forces such as corporate downsizing and just-in-time delivery. Workers now often have longer shifts and less sleep. Yet, at no time before in human history have workers been responsible for the object mass typical of modern trucks, trains, ships, and planes. When present day workers fall asleep on the job, there can be consequences of unprecedented magnitude for the environment and public safety. The news that fatigued workers represent an increasing danger is unwelcome to those who call for our industries to become more productive and efficient. For the moment, the enemy of the people may be identified as the person who decries the dangers posed by sleepy workers—but only for the moment. If sleep specialists bring proper information to bear to the public policy arenas, eventually companies will be unable to treat as "normal costs of doing business" the increasingly large expenses for attorneys and restitution associated with transportation and industrial catastrophes caused by errors of fatigued workers. One possible step in the right direction would be to force litigants in the many lawsuits stemming from fatigue-related industrial and transportation accidents to publish the details of their financial settlements. At present, such settlements are often kept secret by court order. With all such financial settlements made public, a true enemy of the people will be recognized: *worker fatigue in round-the-clock industries*.

SUMMARY

In summary, there is ample precedent for health professionals to assume responsibility, both individually and collectively through their professional organizations, to do whatever they can to improve the health of the public. This includes societal health in its broadest sense: the reduction of risk, the improvement of performance, and the enhancement of quality of life. Indeed, the special expertise of sleep medicine professionals confers a unique and heightened set of obligations to address and the political influence to shape rational public policy. Research indicates that sleep, sleepiness, and inattention related to sleep loss and biological rhythms adversely affect workers. This, in turn, leads to public health problems and underscores the need for wiser public policy concerning sleep and sleep disorders.

It is axiomatic that public policy does not change by itself. It is also axiomatic that public policy can change in a manner that is counterproductive or that poses a threat to the health of the public. There may be economic incentives involved in maintaining or increasing the risks caused by sleep deprivation. It is the responsibility of the professional sleep societies to foster education, understanding, and training of its members in public policy matters and in aspects of the field and the scientific data that have an impact on public policy and public health matters. We also must develop public policy guidelines in areas in which we have expertise, such as through our professional societies' programs for government affairs, so that we may help formulate good public policy and help change poor public policy for the better.

Education and recognition of true risk are necessary first steps toward formulating wise public policy. Just as massive epidemics in crowded cities of the 1800s thrust the notion of disease-carrying microbes into public consciousness, industrial and transportation catastrophes of the 1900s should be forcing worker fatigue into the public consciousness. In the late 1800s, new ways of thinking were required to reduce the risk of microbe-borne disease. This new thinking changed the once common practice of a doctor's dissecting a corpse for anatomy class and then, minutes later, delivering a woman's baby without even washing his hands. Similarly, in the mid-1900s, widespread awareness of the health dangers created by chemical toxins in the environment and the food chain led to changes in the way we think about our personal safety and the way we formulate public policy. Likewise, in the late 1900s, new ways of thinking are required to ensure that people do not make catastrophic mistakes on the job in the 21st century.

References

1. American Sleep Disorders Association. International Classification of Sleep Disorders, Revised: Diagnostic and Coding Manual. Rochester, Minn: American Sleep Disorders Association; 1997.
2. Dinges DF, Graeber RC, Carskadon MA, et al. Attending to inattention. Science. 1989;245:342.
3. Kribbs NB, Getsy J, Dinges DF. Investigation and management of daytime sleepiness in sleep apnea. In: Saunders NA, Sullivan CE, eds. Sleep and Breathing. Vol 2. New York, NY: Marcel Dekker; 1992:575–604.
4. Webb WB, Dinges DF. Cultural perspectives on napping and the siesta. In: Dinges DF, Broughton RJ, eds. Sleep and Alertness: Chronobiological, Behavioral and Medical Aspects of Napping. New York, NY: Raven Press; 1989:247–266.
5. Dinges DF, Broughton RJ. Sleep and Alertness: Chronobiological, Behavioral and Medical Aspects of Napping. New York, NY: Raven Press; 1989.
6. Terman LM, Hocking A. The sleep of school children: its distribution according to age and its relation to physical and mental efficiency. J Educ Psychol. 1913;4:138–147.
7. O'Connor AL. Questionnaire responses about sleep [master's thesis]. Gainesville, Fla: University of Florida; 1964.
8. Rosenthal L, Roehrs TA, Rosen A, et al. Level of sleepiness and total sleep time following various time in bed conditions. Sleep. 1993;16:226–232.
9. Rowland L, Thorne D, Balkin T, et al. The effects of four different sleep-wake cycles on psychomotor vigilance. Sleep Res. 1997;26:627.
10. Dinges DF, Pack F, Williams K, et al. Cumulative sleepiness, mood disturbance, and psychomotor vigilance performance decrements during a week of sleep restricted to 4-5 hours per night. Sleep. 1997;18:267–277.
11. Smith-Coggins R, Rosekind MR, Buccino KR, et al. Rotating shiftwork schedules: can we enhance physician adaptation to night shifts? Acad Emerg Med. 1997;4:951–961.
12. Mitler MM, Carskadon MA, Czeisler CA, et al. Catastrophes, sleep, and public policy: consensus report. Sleep. 1988;11:100–109.
13. Mitler MM, Miller JC. Methods of testing for sleepiness. Behav Med. 1996;21:171–183.
14. Pack AI, Pack AM, Rodgman E, et al. Characteristics of crashes attributed to the driver having fallen asleep. Acc Anal Prev. 1995;27:769–775.
15. Roehrs T, Beare D, Zorick F, et al. Sleepiness and ethanol effects on simulated driving. Alcohol Clin Exp Res. 1994;18:154–158.

16. Dawson D, Reid K. Fatigue, alcohol and performance impairment. Nature. 1997;388:235–235.

17. Dement WC. The perils of drowsy driving. N Engl J Med. 1997;337:783–784.

18. Dinges DF. Technology/scheduling approaches. Proceedings: Managing Fatigue in Transportation: Promoting Safety and Productivity. Washington, DC: National Transportation Safety Board and NASA-Ames Research Center; 1995:53–58.

19. Dinges DF. Validation of psychophysiological monitors. Proceedings: Technical Conference on Enhancing Commercial Motor Vehicle Driver Vigilance. Washington, DC: American Trucking Associations, Federal Highway Administration, National Highway Traffic Administration; 1996:35–41.

20. Dinges DF. The promise and challenges of technologies for monitoring operator vigilance. Proceedings: An International Perspective on Managing Fatigue in Transportation: What We Know and Promising New Directions for Reducing the Risks. Washington, DC: American Trucking Associations; 1997:77–86.

21. Dinges DF, Mallis MM. Managing fatigue by drowsiness detection: can technological promises be realized? In: Hartley L, ed. Managing Fatigue in Transportation: Proceedings of the 3rd Fatigue in Transportation Conference, Fremantle Western Australia, February 1998. Oxford, England: Pergamon; 1998;209–229.

22. Mitler MM, Miller JC, Lipsitz JJ, et al. The sleep of long-haul truck drivers. N Engl J Med. 1997;337:755–761.

23. Dinges DF, Graeber RC, Rosekind MR, et al. Principles and Guidelines for Duty and Rest Scheduling in Commercial Aviation. Washington, DC: NASA Technical Memorandum Report No. 110404, 1996:1–10.

24. Rosekind MR, Neri DF, Dinges DF. From laboratory to flightdeck: promoting operational alertness. Paper presented at: Royal Aeronautical Society's Symposium on Fatigue and Duty Time Limitations—An International Review; September 16, 1997; London, England.

25. von Jenny E. Tageperiodische Einflüsse auf Geburt und Tod. Schweiz Med Wochenschr. 1933;14:15–17.

26. Smolensky M, Halberg F, Sargent F. Chronobiology of the life sequence. In: Ito S, Ogata K, Yoshimura H, eds. Advances in Climatic Physiology. Tokyo, Japan: Igaku Shoin; 1972:281–318.

27. Mitler MM, Hajdukovic RM, Shafor R, et al. When people die. Cause of death versus time of death. Am J Med. 1987;82:266–274.

28. Müller JE, Stone PH, Turi ZG, et al. Circadian variation in the onset of acute myocardial infarction. N Engl J Med. 1985;313:1315–1322.

29. Stampfer MJ, Jakubowski JA, Deykin D, et al. Effect of alternate-day regular and enteric coated aspirin on platelet aggregation, bleeding time and thromboxane A2 levels in bleeding-time blood. Am J Med. 1986;81:400–404.

30. Ridker PM, Manson JE, Buring JE, et al. Circadian variation of acute myocardial infarction and the effect of low-dose aspirin in a randomized trial of physicians. Circulation. 1990;82:897–902.

31. Tofler GH, Brezinski D, Schafer Al, et al. Concurrent morning increase in platelet aggregability and the risk of myocardial infarction and sudden cardiac death. N Engl J Med. 1987;316:1514–1518.

32. Dawson A, Lehr P, Bigby BG, et al. Effect of bedtime ethanol on total inspiratory resistance and respiratory drive in normal nonsnoring men. Alcoholism. 1993;17:256–262.

33. Mitler MM, Dawson A, McNally E. Sleep disorders and coronary disease. In: Zipes DP, Rowlands DJ, eds. Progress in Cardiology. Vol 4/2. Philadelphia, Pa: Lea & Febiger; 1991:99–113.

34. Jennum P, Wildschidtz G, Christensen NJ, et al. Blood pressure, catecholamines and pancreatic polypeptide in obstructive sleep apnea with and without nasal continuous positive airway pressure (nCPAP). Am J Hypertens. 1989;2:847–852.

35. Ancoli-Israel S, Kripke DF, Klauber MR, et al. Sleep-disordered breathing in community-dwelling elderly. Sleep. 1991;14:486–495.

36. Dawson A, Bigby BG, Poceta JS, et al. Effect of bedtime alcohol on inspiratory resistance and respiratory drive in snoring and nonsnoring men. Alcohol Clin Exp Res. 1997;21:183–190.

37. Kripke DF. Chronic hypnotic use: the neglected problem. In: Koella WP, Ruther E, Schulz H, eds. Sleep '84. Stuttgart, Germany: Gustav Fischer Verlag; 1985:338–340.

38. National Transportation Safety Board. Safety Study: Fatigue, Alcohol, Other Drugs, and Medical Factors in Fatal-to-the-Driver Heavy Truck Crashes. Vol 1. Washington, DC: NTSB; 1990:1–181.

39. National Transportation Safety Board. Safety Study: Fatigue, Alcohol, Other Drugs, and Medical Factors in Fatal-to-the-Driver Heavy Truck Crashes. Vol 2. Washington, DC: NTSB; 1990:1–447. Vol NTSB/SS-90/02.

40. US Congress Office of Technology Assessment. Gearing up for Safety: Motor Carrier Safety in a Competitive Environment. Washington, DC: US Government Printing Office; 1988. Publication OTA-SET-382.

41. Pakola SJ, Dinges DF, Pack Al. Review of regulations and guidelines for commercial and non-commercial drivers with sleep apnea and narcolepsy. Sleep. 1995;18:267–277.

42. Parsons M. Fits and other causes of loss of consciousness while driving. QJ M. 1986;58:295–303.

43. Maycock G. Sleepiness and driving: the experience of U.K. drivers. Accid Anal Prev. 1997;29:453–462.

44. US Department of Transportation. The Costs of Highway Crashes. Washington, DC: Federal Highway Administration; 1991.

45. Wylie D, Miller JC, Shultz T, et al. Commercial Driver Fatigue, Loss of Alertness, and Countermeasures. Washington, DC: US Department of Transportation; 1996.

46. National Commission on Sleep Disorders Research. Report of the National Commission on Sleep Disorders Research. Wake Up America: A National Sleep Alert. Washington, DC: US Depart of Health and Human Services; 1993.

47. National Transportation Safety Board. Marine Accident Report—Grounding of the U.S. Tankship EXXON VALDEZ on Bligh Reef, Prince William Sound, Near Valdez, Alaska, March 24, 1989. Washington, DC: National Transportation Safety Board; 1990. NTSB/MAR-90/04.

48. National Transportation Safety Board. Marine Accident Report—Grounding of the Greek Tankship, World Prodigy off the Coast of Rhode Island, June 23, 1989. Washington, DC: National Transportation Safety Board; 1991.

49. Hartley L, ed. Managing Fatigue in Transportation: Proceedings of the 3rd Fatigue in Transportation Conference, Western Australia, February 1998. Oxford, England: Pergamon; 1998.

50. The National Transportation Safety Board, NASA Ames Research Center. Managing fatigue in transportation: promoting safety and productivity. Paper presented at: Managing Fatigue in Transportation: Promoting Safety and Productivity; November 1–2, 1995; Tysons Corner, Va.

51. Asch DA, Parker RM. Sounding board: the Libby Zion case. N Engl J Med. 1988;318:771–775.

52. Moss TH, Sills DL. The Three Mile Island nuclear accident: lessons and implications. Ann N Y Acad Sci. 1981;365:1–341.

53. US Nuclear Regulatory Commission. Report on the Accident at the Chernobyl Nuclear Power Station. Washington, DC: US Government Printing Office; 1987.

54. United States Senate Committee on Energy and Natural Resources. The Chernobyl Accident. Washington, DC: US Government Printing Office; 1986.

55. Lauber JK, Kayten PJ. Sleepiness, circadian dysrhythmia, and fatigue in transportation system accidents. Sleep. 1988;11:503–512.

56. Carskadon MA. Patterns of sleep and sleepiness in adolescents. Pediatrician. 1990;17:5–2.

57. Carskadon MA, Dement WC. Cumulative effects of sleep restriction on daytime sleepiness. Psychophysiology. 1981;18:107–113.

58. Carskadon MA, Mancuso J, Rosekind MR. Impact of part-time employment on adolescent sleep patterns. Sleep Res. 1989;18:114.

59. Wolfson AR, Carskadon MA. Early school start times affect sleep and daytime functioning in adolescents. Sleep Res. 1996;25:177.

60. Strauch I, Meier B. Sleep need in adolescence: a longitudinal approach. Sleep. 1988;11:378–386.

61. Morrison DN, McGee R, Stranton WW. Sleep problems in adolescence. J Am Acad Child Adolesc Psychiatry. 1992;31:94–99.

62. Carskadon MA, Harvey K, Duke P, et al. Pubertal changes in daytime sleepiness. Sleep. 1980;2:453–460.

63. Presidential Commission. Report of the Presidential Commission on the Space Shuttle Challenger Accident. Vol 2, Appendix G. Washington, DC: US Government Printing Office; 1986.

64. Graeber RC, Dement WC, Nicholson AN, et al. International cooperative study of aircrew layover sleep: operational summary. Aviat Space Environ Med. 1986;57:B10–B13.

65. Graeber PC, Lauber JK, Connell LJ, et al. International aircrew sleep and wakefulness after multiple time zone flights: a cooperative study. Aviat Space Environ Med. 1986;57:B3–B9.

66. Rosekind MR, Connell LJ, Dinges DF, et al. Preplanned cockpit rest: EEG sleep and effects on physiological alertness. Sleep Res. 1991;20:129.

67. Dinges DF, Connell LJ, Rosekind MR, et al. Effects of cockpit naps and 24-hour layovers on sleep debt in long-haul transmeridian flight crews. Sleep Res. 1991;20:406.

68. Rosekind MR, Graeber PC, Dinges DF, et al. Crew factors in flight operations, IX: effects of planned cockpit rest on crew performance and alertness in long-haul operations. Moffett Field, Calif: NASA Ames Research Center; 1994.

69. Roehrs TA, Zwyghuizen-Doorenbos A, Zwyghuizen H, et al. Sedating effects of ethanol and time of drinking. Sleep Res. 1989;18:71.

70. US Congress Office of Technology Assessment. Biological Rhythms: Implications for the Worker. Washington, DC: US Government Printing Office; 1991.

71. National Institutes of Health. The National Sleep Disorders Research Plan. Bethesda, Md: National Center for Sleep Disorders Research; 1996.

eight

Disorders of Chronobiology

Fred W. Turek

Introduction: Disorders of Chronobiology

Fred W. Turek

The three other chapters in this section focus on sleep disorders in which the timing of sleep and wake is abnormal relative to either the internal 24-h circadian clock or the normal time for sleep and wake relative to the time when most of the rest of society is asleep and awake. That is, sleep and wake are out of phase with the internal or external environment. It is perhaps worth noting that from an evolutionary perspective, the circadian clock has one major role to play in ensuring the survival of the individual and the species: to regulate the phase of a multitude of circadian rhythms such that specific phase points of these rhythms occur at times relative to each other *(internal synchronization)* or relative to the external environment *(external synchronization)*, in order to optimize the chances that the organism will survive and contribute to the gene pool of future generations. Internal circadian clocks are found in all eukaryotic and at least some prokariotic organisms,[1] indicating that natural selection has placed a high premium from the beginning of life on earth for maintaining proper phase relationships within the internal and between the external environments.

As noted by Monk in Chapter 51, Shift Work, "Working at night must therefore be regarded as an inherently unnatural act." How very true. Indeed, human beings, unlike all other species, are routinely awake when their internal biological clocks are telling them it is time to sleep, and human beings are often trying to sleep when the circadian clock is sending signals throughout the brain and body that it is time to be awake. Human beings are clearly not slaves to their biological clocks and have the ability to cognitively override the temporal signals. Arendt et al. and Monk review the impact of such an override in the two most common situations: during rapid travel across time zones (Chapter 50) (itself an extremely unnatural act never experienced, until recently, by human beings or any other species), and while working at times when diurnal creatures such as ourselves should be asleep (Chapter 51). Of course, fooling mother nature is not easily accomplished and has its price. It can be difficult to perform, either physically or mentally, anywhere near one's capacity at times when the circadian clock is signaling the brain and body it is time to sleep, and trying to sleep at abnormal biological clock times often leads to poor and shortened sleep (Chapter 51). This decrease in the quality and quantity of sleep itself leads to more deficits in alertness and performance during wake times. The combination of sleep loss, being awake at times of diminished capabilities, and the possible abnormal phasing of internal rhythms relative to one another either on an acute or chronic basis can have serious adverse effects on human health, safety, performance, and productivity.[2]

In contrast to the situations of jet lag and shift work, in which human beings voluntarily choose to create temporal disorganization for themselves, there are situations in which such temporal disorganization, either with respect to internal or external time, occurs on an involuntary basis. Some of these phase "disorders" are reviewed by Baker and Zee in Chapter 52 in this section. I put the word *disorders* in quotation marks because these phase disorders are only a problem if the external environment cannot be phase controlled or phase ignored. For example, an individual with delayed sleep phase syndrome may have a major problem if he or she needs to start work early and thus does not obtain sufficient sleep, whereas the same individual may have no problem if his or her job requires him or her to be awake late at night and there are no constraints on when he or she needs to be awake in the morning. Indeed, the same individual may have problems in one society that places a premium on early morning awakening, and he or she may be less of a problem, or no problem at all, if living in a society where the "phase of living" is different.

One final comment. It can be argued that we have only just begun to understand how disorders of chronobiology, or disorders of the circadian clock system, affect sleep. Although most of the discussion about chronobiology disorders has focused on the abnormal timing of sleep and wake, the circadian input to the sleep-wake regulatory mechanisms may include inputs that do much more than control the phase of sleep and wake. There is now considerable evidence to indicate that disrupting the normal sleep-wake cycle has feedback effects on the phase of the circadian clock, and recent data indicate that a mutation in a key genetic component of the circadian clock can influence the duration of sleep in mice.[3] The hypothesis of Edgar et al.[4] that the master circadian clock located in the hypothalamic suprachiasmatic nucleus may produce an "alerting" factor is consistent with the idea that the circadian clock may provide more than just phase information to the sleep-wake system. Finally, it should be noted that throughout many chapters in this book, numerous examples are provided whereby chronobiological disorders may indirectly have adverse effects on sleep. For example, circadian abnormalities in metabolic, respiratory, endocrine, and behavioral rhythms can have severe negative consequences for normal sleep and wake. Thus, at many different levels, improving overall temporal organization may have beneficial effects for improving sleep.

References

1. Turek FW, Van Reeth O. Circadian rhythms. In: Fregly MJ, Blatheis CM, American Physiologica Society. Section 4 Handbook of Physiology. Environmental Physiology. New York NY: Oxford University Press; 1996:1329–1360.
2. Biological Rhythms: Implications for the Worker. Washington, DC: Office of Technology Assessment. US Congress; 1991. Publication OTA-BA-463.
3. Naylor E, Vitaterna MH, Takahashi JT, et al. Sleep in the *Clock* mutant mouse. Sleep. 1998; 21(suppl):9.
4. Edgar DM, Dement WC, Fuller CA. Effect of SCN lesions on sleep in squirrel monkeys: evidence for opponent processes in sleep-wake regulation. J Neurosci. 1993;13:1065–1079.

50

Jet Lag and Sleep Disruption

Josephine Arendt
Barbara Stone
Debra Skene

WHAT IS JET LAG?

The preceding sections of this text book have laid the foundations for understanding the phenomenon of jet lag and for appreciating the various countermeasures that can be taken to minimize this problem. Rapid travel across time zones leads to a mismatch or lack of synchrony between the activity of internal rhythm-generating systems and the local time cues, whether social or environmental.[1, 2] The internal circadian clock adapts slowly to abrupt changes of time cues. It has often been reported that, on average, the clock shifts approximately 1 h per day without countermeasures such that it will take 1 day for each hour of time zone change for adaptation to be complete. This is highly simplistic because the rate of adaptation varies greatly among individuals, with the direction of time zone change (slower toward the east in general) and the rate of shift usually changing in the course of adaptation, being faster in the initial than the final stages. In addition, it is relatively common for travelers to adapt in the "wrong" direction, such as by delaying 16 h instead of advancing 8 h. Reentrainment by "partition," in which some rhythms advance and some delay, has also been reported. In this case, the data must be reevaluated because immediate effects of the environment (*masking*) may have strongly influenced the parameters measured.

Possibly one third of all travelers do not experience jet lag. However, during the state of desynchrony, travelers may experience symptoms such as daytime tiredness, inability to get to sleep at night (after an eastward flight) or early awakening (after a westward flight), disturbed nighttime sleep, impaired daytime alertness and performance, gastrointestinal problems, loss of appetite, inappropriate timing of defecation, and excessive desire to urinate during the night. These symptoms may be just a nuisance for the first few days for a vacationer but may seriously impair the businessperson's ability to function. Aircrew, both civil and military, are of course more exposed than the general population to time zone change; their ability to perform is crucial, and much time has been devoted to developing strategies to combat jet lag in this population.[3, 4]

All of the above symptoms may be ascribed in large part to temporary desynchronization of circadian rhythms. However, the circadian system is also responsible for the organization of the menstrual cycle: air hostesses may have more menstrual problems than the general population.[5] Meals eaten out of phase with the internal clock may give rise to inappropriate pancreatic and metabolic responses, some of which may be long-term risk factors for heart disease.[6] Although to our knowledge there is little evidence that frequent time zone travel affects human life expectancy, there certainly is evidence from other forms of life (e.g., fruit-flies) that life span can be shortened with frequent phase shifting.[7]

CONDITIONS RELATED TO JET LAG

Shift Work

Health problems associated with night shift work are similar to those of jet lag, although travelers adapt with the help of local time cues, whereas shift workers are constantly living at odds with local time cues. Most night shift workers never fully adapt their internal clock to the imposed sleep and work schedule.[8, 9] This is especially true of "fast rotation" schedules, such as 2 to 5 continuous days of night shift interspersed with periods of day shift and rest days. Even permanent night shift workers may not be fully adapted to their schedule. Exceptions to this are many of the night shift workers in isolated situations such as on oil rigs and in the Antarctic.[10, 11] Depending on the schedule, these subjects can fully adapt to a 12-h shift within 4 to 7 days. Such situations are free of the social demands of, for example, family life and entertainment; sleeping quarters are usually quiet and dark; and exposure to natural light is minimized. These observations emphasize the importance of exposure to time cues that may or may not aid adaptation depending on the timing of exposure. For the majority, shift work is a lifetime experience of living out of phase at regular intervals. Many major accidents have been attributed to poor performance during an unadapted night shift. This, coupled with the increased incidence of sleep problems, gastrointestinal disorders, and heart disease,[12] indicates that for economic and health reasons, counter-measures should be developed. Shift work is treated in detail in Chapter 51.

Circadian Sleep-Wake Disorders of Blindness

The light-dark cycle is the major synchronizer of human circadian rhythms. Without this time cue, many blind persons, especially those with no light perception at all, either cannot remain synchronized to the 24-h day-night cycle and "free run" with their own endoge-nous periodicity or take up an abnormal phase position of the internal clock, such that, for example, they consistently have a peak of melatonin production and a trough in core body temperature during the daytime instead of at night.[13–15] The overt consequence often is a strong propensity to nap during the day with poor sleep at night when the clock is out of phase. The tendency to experience these circadian sleep disorders is strongly related to the degree of light perception and to whether a subject with no conscious light perception has no eyes or one or two remaining eyes. However, not all subjects with no light perception (and even those with no eyes) show circadian desynchrony with or without a sleep disorder.[16] In these cases, time cues other than light must be responsible for synchroniza-tion or the endogenous periodicity must be 24 h. Very little is known of other possible circadian-related disor-ders, such as gastrointestinal disturbance and meta-bolic abnormalities, in the blind.

MECHANISMS UNDERLYING STRATEGIC COUNTERMEASURES

General

Circadian rhythms are considered to be internally generated from the central pacemaker, the suprachias-matic nucleus (SCN), in the hypothalamus. Most circa-dian rhythms also have an exogenous component due to direct interaction with the environment (e.g., sup-pression of melatonin secretion by light) or with sleep times (sleep acutely lowers core body temperature) or exercise (which raises core body temperature). Thus, the overt manifestation of a rhythm is the sum of both exogenous and endogenous influences. The exogenous influence is usually known as *masking*.[17] The problems of jet lag are considered to be due to the endogenous component of the rhythm. The direct effects of the environment and of behavior can in principle (but of-ten not in practice) be controlled. To hasten adaptation when this is desirable, it is sensible to exploit both the acute effects of the environment, of behavior, and of drugs, and the strategies designed to hasten adaptation of the internal clock.

Jet lag has never properly been defined, and indeed neither has the cluster of associated problems associ-ated with shift work. In general, many people refer to this "syndrome" as circadian rhythm disorder, and this term will be used here. In our experience, however, the

subjective perception of global "jet lag" is more closely related to sleep disturbance than to any other function. Evidently, sleep disturbance is easier to perceive than, for example, out-of-phase hormones.

Sleep, Alertness, and Performance

Sleep is normally initiated on the rising phase of the melatonin rhythm and on the falling phase of the core body temperature rhythm in the evening (see Chapter 28). Sleep attempted on the rising phase of temperature and falling or baseline melatonin is shorter and associ-ated with more awakenings. This situation is possible with transitions over more than three or four time zones and inevitable over a large number of time zones.

There have been many studies of sleep after trans-meridian flights.[3, 4, 18, 19] In general, the severity of sleep disturbance after a time zone change is dependent on the direction of travel and the number of time zones crossed and is influenced by the timing of the flight itself. After an eastward journey, when sleep is sched-uled in advance of the "home" bedtime, there may be difficulty in falling asleep accompanied by increased wakefulness during the early part of the night, al-though these changes may not be apparent on the first night in the new time zone if the flight involves overnight travel without sleep. Sleep problems may continue for several days after the flight, with reduc-tions in rapid eye movement (REM) sleep and possibly slow-wave sleep, and there may be a compensatory increase in REM sleep several nights later. Sleep distur-bance after a westward flight is usually less persistent, lasting perhaps 2 or 3 days. Sleep is likely to be of good quality in the early part of the night, with in-creased slow-wave activity on the first night due to the long period without sleep. On subsequent nights, when the pressure for slow-wave sleep is less, there may be an increase in REM sleep as bedtime corresponds with early morning in the "home" time zone, when REM sleep predominates and body temperature begins to rise. Awakenings may be evident toward the end of the night at the time corresponding to daytime in the "home" time zone.

The decrements in performance and alertness that arise after transmeridian flights can be attributed at least in part to the reduction in both the quality and quantity of sleep that occurs as a result of the require-ment to sleep at an inappropriate circadian phase. One approach to optimizing performance and alertness is to preserve sleep as much as possible. There are several approaches, such as through the application of sleep-promoting techniques, attention to the circumstances surrounding sleep, the use of hypnotic agents, and the use of chronobiotics, which are drugs that shift the internal clock.[19, 20] Other methods of treatment that may result in improved sleep for aircrew include, for exam-ple, changing duty schedules.

Other Physiological Functions

Compared with sleep, alertness, and performance, far less is known of the precise manifestations of circadian desynchrony with respect to other physiological systems. Any system under control of the circadian pacemaker will be affected by abrupt changes in time cues. Among the functions that merit much closer attention are the cardiovascular, immune, and reproductive systems, all of which are strongly rhythmic.[21] A start has been in the characterization of pancreatic and metabolic responses with respect to the influence of the endogenous clock and exogenous factors such as diet and sleep. Available information suggests that all three factors influence the enteroinsular axis.[22–24]

In principle, however, if it were possible to instantly and reliably shift the circadian clock by any means, all problems due to the endogenous clock would be countered. Thus, a search has been initiated for a treatment that does just this. There is no one solution, although several approaches have met with some success. Two of the major problems in this area are the uncontrollable nature of field studies on jet lag and the fact that so far it has not been possible to simulate time zone change in the laboratory taking into account all the factors that may arise in the field.

COUNTERMEASURES

Sleep Hygiene

It is evident from studies in blind subjects and tolerant shift workers that, at least for some persons, it is quite possible to sleep out of phase without perceived problems. Thus, the initial strategy to alleviate jet lag must be to ensure adequate sleep. Among the techniques or strategies that may be applied to promote sleep are those that aim to ensure that the sleeping environment is optimal: whatever the circadian phase, sleep will be more disturbed if the bedroom environment is noisy and light. If the sleeping environment is not ideal, earplugs and eyeshades can be used to screen unwanted external stimuli. These strategies are frequently used by airline pilots when sleeping in hotels or when they have to obtain rest in the bunk facilities on board the aircraft on long-range flights.[19]

Caffeine and alcohol are known to have detrimental effects on sleep,[25, 26] although alcohol may initially promote sleep onset. It has been suggested that a "jet-lag diet" will speed the adaptation of sleep and other rhythms. With this diet, an evening meal rich in carbohydrates provides a source of tryptophan for serotonin synthesis to assist sleep, and protein-rich meals in the morning will provide tyrosine to enhance catecholamine levels and increase alertness during the day.[27] However, a review of this field of research concludes that there is no evidence to support this idea.[28] The administration of tryptophan has been reported to increase total sleep time on the first night after transmeridian travel westward, although its effects on sleep are considered to be limited.

The use of specifically timed naps before, during, or after flight can in theory and in practice markedly increase alertness.[19, 29] Computer programs are available that enable a prediction of alertness as a function of nap timing.[29] However, napping is frequently not possible either before or during a flight. It often is recommended that the traveler not nap in the destination time zone but instead time meals and sleep to be in synchrony with the new environment. This advice may be hard to follow after a long sleepless flight. Passengers in first, club, and business class will have more opportunity to sleep during the flight because the size and angle of the seats plus the use of foot rests are more conductive to sleep.[19] Sleep during flight should be taken as far as possible during the future nighttime in the destination time zone.

Use of Hypnotic Agents

Another approach to the preservation of sleep involves the use of drugs, and there have been numerous studies on the effects of hypnotic agents.[19, 20, 26] The largest class of hypnotic agents—the benzodiazepines—is known to speed sleep onset, reduce awakenings, and increase total sleep time in normal sleepers and in those with transient or chronic insomnia. In addition, the medications may modify sleep architecture by delaying the appearance of REM sleep, reducing slow-wave sleep, and enhancing sleep spindles. The imidazopyridine zolpidem and the cyclopyrrolone zopiclone have similar effects on the electroencephalogram as the benzodiazepines except that they may increase slow-wave sleep. The overriding factor when considering the potential use of a hypnotic agent is the duration of action of the drug.[19] Clearly, the benefits associated with improved sleep may be masked if use of the hypnotic agent leads to unwanted side effects that diminish alertness after the sleep period. After a transmeridian flight, hypnotics agents with a duration of action of around 3 to 5 h may be useful to sustain sleep during the adaptation phase without having adverse effects on performance. In such situations, the agents are likely to be effective due to their sleep-promoting properties rather than via an effect on shifting circadian rhythms. In addition to their use of hypnotic agents on arrival in a new time zone, passengers may consider the use of medication on the flight to assist in sleep timed to coincide with the nocturnal rest period at the destination. One strategy for business travelers that (anecdotally) appears to be quite successful when traveling from the United Kingdom to the West Coast of the United States is to sleep early on arrival (with the use of a hypnotic agent), conduct meetings on the next morning, and return on the next evening.

Light

Laboratory Studies

The light-dark cycle is the principal time cue for resetting human circadian rhythms. Correctly timed white light of suitable intensity and duration will both phase advance and phase delay circadian rhythms according to a phase response curve.[30, 31] In essence, light of 3000 to 10,000 lux applied soon after the minimum of core body temperature (or the maximum of plasma melatonin) will advance the internal clock; light scheduled soon before the core temperature minimum will phase delay. Phase response curves describing these interactions enable theoretical predictions to be made concerning the timing of light treatment to adapt to phase shift. It is also possible to induce large phase changes of the circadian system with light centered on the core temperature minimum, but this procedure appears to be somewhat unpredictable. It is clearly impractical to expose subjects to light in the middle of the night before departure, although in principle this would be possible during flight through the use of either carefully chosen window seats or artificial means. In addition to its phase-shifting ability, bright light has immediate alerting and temperature-raising properties.[32] It acutely suppresses plasma melatonin production,[33] and this may to some extent be related to the alerting and temperature-raising effects.

Bright light and avoidance of bright light[34] may be useful in helping to facilitate phase shifts of circadian rhythms, although very little research has been conducted in real-life settings. Phase shifts have been produced, however, in laboratory studies that simulate jet lag/shift work situations.[35, 36] A few laboratory studies have measured circadian phase after exposure to bright light (more than 2000 lux) or dim light during the imposed wake time with the use of large (more than or equal to 6 h) abrupt phase shifts of the sleep-wake schedule, either an advance or a delay. The general finding has been that circadian rhythms shifted about 1 h/day in the dim light conditions and as much as 2 to 3 h/day in the bright light conditions. Sleep problems abated as body temperature shifted to align with sleep time. One study suggested that both 3- and 6-h exposures to bright light are equally effective in shifting the temperature rhythm. Thus, extremely long bright light durations throughout the wake period may not be necessary, making the procedure more convenient and feasible. Some laboratory studies have compared different timings of bright light after large abrupt phase advances of the sleep-wake schedule, but there is little consistency in the results. In some cases, there was little difference between the conditions predicted to enhance phase shifting and the conditions predicted to inhibit the phase shift. A full 9 h of moderately bright white light (1200 lux) followed by imposed darkness-sleep applied on a shifting schedule (3 h/day, delay or advance) will reliably advance or delay all circadian rhythms, with no detrimental effects on sleep mood or performance. This "nudging" technique is impractical in many respects but has been used in some specific situations.[37, 38]

Field Studies

The number of field studies of the use of light for jet lag is small, and the results are not very consistent. In general, with the appropriate timing of light exposure, a modest acceleration in the rate of adaptation of circadian rhythms to the new sleep-wake schedule is observed. It is worth noting that except during scheduled light treatments, the subjects in the early field studies were free to engage in activities of their choice, and no attempt was made to limit their exposure to bright light at times when such exposure might hinder reentrainment. Bright light administered under more controlled laboratory conditions after transmeridian flights appeared to speed up reentrainment.[36]

Additional field studies have examined the effects of morning bright light treatment on postflight sleep patterns. For example, exposure to bright white or dim red light for 2 to 3 h on awakening in the morning (centered around 9:30 AM local time) for 3 days after a 6.5- to 10-h advance flight yielded no differences between the groups in any subjective sleep measure. In a second study with objective sleep electroencephalographic recordings after an 8-h advance flight, subjects exposed for 3 days to bright light (3:00 to 6:00 AM local time) showed higher sleep efficiency than those exposed to dim light, with the latter exhibiting prolonged wakefulness during the first half of the night. A recent review by Samel and Wegmann[36] summarized available data. Their conclusion is that there is some evidence that correctly timed bright light may have been effective in accelerating reentrainment.

Many questions remain, including determination of optimum times for light exposure on the first and subsequent treatment days and whether a given, fixed light exposure time is likely to benefit a majority of travelers or whether light treatment should instead be scheduled according to an individual circadian phase marker.[39] A number of computer programs exist that provide the times of exposure and avoidance of bright light for travelers based on the phase response curve for light as a function of direction of flight, number of time zones crossed, and arrival time (see, for example, Houpt et al.[40]).

The avoidance of natural bright light may be the most important consideration. As previously mentioned, shift workers adapt to night shift when shielded from natural light and social time cues.[10, 11] There is good evidence that exposure to natural light when returning home in the early morning after a night shift opposes the delay required to sleep well during the day.[34] When traveling east over more than four or five time zones and arriving in the early morning, subjects will experience light opposed to their adaptation. (Other situations and predicted light avoidance and treatment times are given by Houpt et al.[40])

For aircrew scheduled to return to home base after a brief layover, remaining on home time may be preferable to trying to adjust to local time, eliminating the need for readjustment after the return flight. Indeed, a large proportion of flight personnel report going to bed early after a westward transatlantic flight. In such cases, bright light treatment may be used to maintain entrainment to home time rather than to accelerate reentrainment to new local times.

In addition to effects on alertness, temperature, melatonin levels, and circadian phase shifting, there is a small amount of evidence that bright light can acutely modify some hormonal and metabolic responses after forced phase shift, including attenuation of raised plasma triglyceride levels (Ribeiro, Hampton, Arendt, and Morgan, unpublished observations).

Melatonin

In some respects, melatonin can be considered a "darkness hormone." It is normally produced at night, and the duration of secretion reflects the length of the night. It appears to serve similar functions in all life forms so far studied, acting as a time signal for the organization of daily and annual rhythms.[41] There is little published about the role of melatonin in human reproduction. One study showed there was no effect of long-term melatonin use on the secretion of reproductive hormones in normal men.[41a] In animals that use day length changes to time their seasonal cycles, melatonin indicates the length of the night. For example, a long night of melatonin induces sheep to start breeding in autumn and hamsters (who breed in the summer) to stop breeding. Other seasonal variations such as coat growth are also timed by melatonin. In some species, especially some lower vertebrates and birds, melatonin is essential for the organization of daily (circadian) rhythms. In mammals, it is not essential for circadian organization but appears to reinforce behavior associated with darkness, such as sleep in human beings. It has rapid, transient, mild sleep-inducing effects and lowers alertness and body temperature during the 3 to 4 h after low doses (0.3 to 5 mg); these effects are opposite to the acute effects of bright light. In the same dose range, it can shift the timing of the internal clock to both later and earlier times when the administration is appropriately timed.[41, 42] For light, the appropriate timing can be predicted from a phase response curve (PRC) in subjects whose body clock phase is known. The PRC to melatonin is essentially the reverse of that to light.[43, 44] Melatonin administered about 8 to 13 h before core temperature minimum will phase advance, and melatonin administered about 1 to 4 h after core temperature minimum will phase delay. However, its effects on the circadian system appear to be both more complicated and much weaker than those of light. For example, it is unable to consistently entrain free-running circadian rhythms of core temperature.[44] In subjects synchronized to a normal 24-h environment, the timing of desired phase shifts is relatively simple and can to some extent be judged by habitual sleep times.[42] Optimal timing is not so simple after time zone travel, in shift workers, and in blind subjects. Melatonin is available in the United Kingdom from a licensed manufacturer on prescription; availability varies in other countries. Only licensed preparations have guaranteed content and purity.

Simulated Phase Shifts. At least three studies of melatonin have addressed its possible ability to hasten adaptation to simulated phase shift.[45–47] In environmental isolation, studies using advanced phase shift and suitably timed treatment (5 mg) have shown an increase in the rate of reentrainment of temperature, hormonal, and electrolyte rhythms[45] but with inconsistent effects on sleep. Of particular note was the observation that melatonin was able to specify the direction of reentrainment to advance rather than delay. During a simulated acute 9-h delay of sleep time, the effectiveness of (1) bright light (4 h, 4000 to 7000 lux) for 3 days during the first half of the night shift period, (2) dim red light (50 lux) for the same period, (3) melatonin, and (4) placebo just before and during desired sleep time has been compared. Essentially, only the group receiving bright light showed significant circadian adaptation and improvements in performance, whereas both melatonin and bright light improved sleep.[46]

After a simulated rapid 9-h phase advance, we investigated the ability of melatonin with or without conflicting bright light treatment to hasten adaptation. Melatonin (5 mg fast release) or placebo was taken at 11:00 PM on the first night after the shift and for two additional nights at the same time. Conflicting light (white, 1200 lux) exposure occurred from 8:00 AM through noon during the first 3 days after the shift. Melatonin treatment was (theoretically) timed to be just within a phase advance window, and light treatment was timed to phase delay. Melatonin consistently improved sleep (quality, duration, and night awakenings) compared with placebo even in the presence of inappropriate light, and this appeared to be independent of the direction of phase shift.[47] Daily mean alertness and performance efficiency were higher for all treatments compared with placebo. In a subsequent identical protocol, polysomnographic results indicated that significant differences were found only on the first night after the shift, when total sleep time, sleep efficiency, and stage 1 and stage 2 sleep all increased but slow-wave sleep decreased compared with placebo. There were no effects on REM sleep.[48]

The effects of melatonin were immediately evident before phase adaptation had occurred. They appear to be related to its acute effects on behavior and temperature reinforced by a hastening of phase adaptation. The latter, however, does not appear to play a major role, at least during the first postphase shift days. However, it must be emphasized that simulations of this sort do not fully mimic field conditions. For example, sleep problems last longer in comparable field studies.

Field Studies on Jet Lag. At least nine placebo-controlled field studies[49–58] have reported the use of melatonin to alleviate perceived jet lag (primarily sleep disturbance). Of these, seven were successful in the sense that subjective (and, in one case, objective) measures of sleep and alertness improved compared with placebo. The first study[49, 50] over eight time zones eastward used a time sequence of administration (5 mg melatonin daily) designed to initiate an eastward phase shift before departure by early evening administration (6:00 PM) for 3 days before flight and to reinforce the advance by bedtime (11:00 PM) administration in the new local time zone for 4 days. The results indicated that both subjective jet lag ratings and objective parameters (actigraphic sleep parameters, endogenous melatonin and cortisol) showed more rapid adaptation in the melatonin-treated group (n = 8) than in the placebo group (n = 9). Subjective "jet lag" was significantly correlated with sleep quality. In a larger population (n = 52) of subjects traveling to Australia from the United Kingdom and back, melatonin was timed to phase advance (early evening) for 2 days before departure and 4 days after arrival (at bedtime) eastward and westward for 4 days at local bedtime (a phase delay position after crossing approximately eight time zones). The design was crossover with melatonin outward and placebo on return or vice versa in subjects remaining in Australia for longer than 14 days. Again, a highly significant improvement in subjective jet lag with melatonin was seen,[51] with the caveat, however, that four subjects felt worse on melatonin. With the use of a very similar protocol and dose, subjective measures were improved in 20 subjects, flying from New Zealand to the United Kingdom and back.[52] With no preflight treatment, in a placebo-controlled crossover design after flight over 6, 9, and 11 time zone changes, 5 mg melatonin at bedtime accelerated adaptation of the cortisol rhythm with a consistent, but not significant, improvement of subjective jet lag both eastward and westward in 36 subjects.[53] The effect on cortisol was more significant with a greater number of time zones. Preflight treatment at 10:00 PM and then daily for 3 days after the flight at bedtime (8 mg) led to improved sleep and subjective jet lag in 37 subjects traveling eastward from the United States and Canada to France.[54]

Comperatore et al.[55] used melatonin treatment (10 mg daily) timed just within a theoretical phase advance window and combined with other countermeasures (timed avoidance and exposure to bright light, preflight shift of bedtimes) to adapt to an 8-h advance but with unusual bedtimes (4:00 AM local time) at the destination. The melatonin treatment led to improved sleep duration and cognitive performance compared with the placebo group. Interestingly, given the large dose of 10 mg, mild sleepiness and fatigue were reported only occasionally after ingestion and never after awakening. This dose of melatonin will not be fully cleared from the circulation after an 8-h sleep, and thus such "high" doses, consistent with our experience with 5 mg and that of Waldhauser et al.[55a] with 80 mg, do not appear to lead to hangover effects.

The largest controlled study reported to date involved a total of 320 subjects treated after their flight at bedtime for 4 days after an eastward flight (six to eight time zones). Melatonin (5 mg fast release) was strikingly efficient in improving sleep latency, sleep quality, daytime sleepiness, and fatigue compared with placebo. A lower dose (0.5 mg) of fast-release preparation was less effective, as was a slow-release preparation.[56]

These positive reports are in contrast to the results of two other studies. Petrie et al.[57] used aircrew (n = 52) traveling from Auckland to Los Angeles and returning to Auckland via London. The last leg of the journey was used for the trial. They reported problems with preflight (3 days) melatonin administration but improvement in subjective measures with only postflight treatment. In another large controlled study (249 subjects in four groups) in which 5 or 0.5 mg was taken at bedtime and 0.5 mg was taken on a shifting schedule to phase advance (New York to Oslo), melatonin was completely ineffective at alleviating subjective symptoms of jet lag.[58] It should be noted, however, that all of the previous studies involved subjects either demonstrably or theoretically synchronized to the local environment pretreatment. As with long-haul aircrew, the circadian state of the subjects was unknown before departure, and it is unlikely that 4 days was sufficient for full synchronization to New York time. Because the timing of melatonin is fairly critical, it is possible that the subjects received the treatment at an inappropriate circadian phase before the flight. A method for rapid assessment of circadian phase, suitable for use with minimum training, would be highly desirable.

In both controlled and uncontrolled field studies on the traveling public over the past 10 years,[42, 59] we have observed an overall 50% reduction in subjective assessment of jet lag symptoms (n = 474) using 5 mg fast-release melatonin. For eastward travel, we suggest a single-phase advancing preflight early evening treatment, followed by treatment at bedtime for 4 days after arrival (Table 50–1). For westward travel, we advise

---

Table 50–1. USE OF MELATONIN TO ALLEVIATE JET LAG*

East

When going east, take one capsule (5 mg melatonin, licensed for human experimental use, or placebo) on departure day, if necessary on the flight, between 6 and 7 PM local time. On arrival take a capsule at local bedtime, 10 to 11 PM, for 4 days. If your stopovers are fewer than 4 days, on the evening preceding your next departure, do not take a capsule at bedtime but instead at 6 to 7 PM local time. On arrival, take a capsule daily at the local bedtime 10 to 11 PM for 4 days.

West

When going west, take 1 capsule daily at the local bedtime (11 PM) or later for 4 days after arrival at each stopover and at the destination. If you awake in the very early morning (before 4 AM), you may take another capsule. Be aware that taken as late as this, melatonin may make you sleepy in the morning. Do not take capsules before the flight if going west, except, of course, if your stopover is less than 4 days, when you will be taking them at bedtime on the night before departure.

Please Note

Melatonin can induce sleepiness and lowered alertness. You are advised not to drive or operate heavy or dangerous machinery, or perform equivalent tasks requiring alertness for 4 to 5 hours after taking the medication.

Exclusion Criteria for Anticipation in Study of Arendt and Deacon[42]

You must have permission from your physician to take part. You may not participate in the study if you are a long-haul pilot or air crew or shift worker (this is due to potential difficulties with timing the dose); you or a close blood relative have a psychiatric condition or migraine headaches; you are younger than 18 years old; you know (or suspect) that you are pregnant or intend to become pregnant; you are lactating; you are taking any medication other than minor analgesics or oral contraceptives; and/or you have any disease.

Possible side effects of melatonin treatment are sleepiness (desirable), headache (infrequent), and nausea (very infrequent).

Modified from Arendt J, Deacon S. Treatment of circadian rhythm disorders—melatonin. Chronobiol Int. 1997;14:185–204, by courtesy of Marcel Dekker, Inc.
*Instructions used in field experiments by the authors.
Preflight treatment eastward may not be important, but no comparative data are available.

subjects to take melatonin for 4 days at bedtime (11:00 PM or later: a phase delay time over more than six time zones) in the new time zone. This timing enables the exploitation of both sleep-inducing and phase-shifting effects. The subjective improvement increases with the number of time zones crossed. Short layovers may require specific instructions, and little evidence exists for efficacy in these circumstances.

The majority of published studies have proved treatment to be successful, but there is a need to explore the limitations of the treatment. There is little information on optimal dose or formulation. The pharmacokinetics of fast-release melatonin is extremely variable among individuals, and the question of individual sensitivity has not been addressed. There is no information on long-term safety, although no significant problems have been reported in healthy adults. Successful treatment appears to be associated with the use of subjects synchronized to the local environment before departure. It is a matter for discussion and further experiment whether preflight administration confers any advantages. It is likely to be important given that melatonin can specify the direction of reentrainment,[45] and this must be done before possible exposure to natural bright light or other time cues acting counter to the most rapid direction of reentrainment.

The avoidance of melatonin through the suppression of production by bright light or drugs or, in the future, the use of receptor antagonists is an important consideration. A recent report suggests that the suppression of melatonin with a beta adrenergic antagonist (atenolol) facilitated phase shifts to bright light.[60]

Field Studies on Shift Work. The use of melatonin in adapting to night shift has been reported in two field studies.[61, 62] Both studies used 7-day rotating shift workers, and both studies involved the administration of melatonin at the desired bedtime after the night shift. Early morning melatonin administration, designed to phase delay, significantly improved day sleep duration and quality and night shift alertness. Its effects on various performance tasks were variable. In the other study, melatonin improved the synchrony between endogenous circadian rhythms and daytime sleep.[62] It is a question of considerable importance whether such facilitated adaptation by melatonin is accompanied by consistent changes in work-related performance. However, melatonin clearly shows promise in this area.

Sleep Disorder of Blindness. In a recent epidemiological study in the United Kingdom, 60% of the registered blind subjects who were studied appear to have a sleep disorder as assessed by use of the Pittsburgh Sleep Quality Index, with greater prevalence in individuals with no conscious light perception.[13, 15] Similar statistics have been reported in other studies in the United States, Switzerland, and France. These sleep disturbances vary from delayed sleep phase syndrome to irregular phase position to free-running circadian rhythms in a normal environment. In most blind subjects, poor sleep corresponds to the antiphase of the endogenous melatonin rhythm.[15] Daytime napping is associated with the peak of melatonin production oc-

curring during the day. The situation thus is analogous to jet lag and shift work, in which subjects intermittently must sleep at an inappropriate circadian phase. In blind persons, this is a lifetime problem, and there is an urgent need for an investigation of treatment strategies. For subjects who retain a circadian response to light, bright light treatment is the method of choice. When there is no response to light, techniques using nonphotic time cues (e.g., timed melatonin and exercise) must be explored.

Suitably timed administration of melatonin has provided positive results in stabilizing sleep onset and improving sleep and mood parameters in some, but not all, patients.[63–65] However, data are sparse as to whether, in addition, melatonin can fully synchronize the circadian system to the solar day in blind persons. There appears to be a distinction between the effects of melatonin on behavioral variables (sleep, mood, and performance) and its weak synchronizing activity with respect to strongly endogenous rhythms such as melatonin, core temperature, and cortisol.[66]

Melatonin has been effective when taken at bedtime to treat sleep-wake disorders in multiply disabled children with or without visual loss.[67] These patients have major behavioral problems during the day as well as during the night. Melatonin was found to consolidate sleep to the nighttime and to alleviate daytime problems. Better mood, alertness, and, in some cases, fewer seizures were reported. Many of the patients had tried a number of sedatives without success before becoming stabilized on melatonin. However, there are no data on the circadian status of these subjects, and the mechanism of action has yet to be elucidated.

OTHER STRATEGIES

There is good evidence that timed exercise can shift the human circadian system, although to date primarily delays have been shown.[68] The use of vitamin B12 may sensitize the system to light-induced phase shifts.[69] No field studies have yet shown the effectiveness of these approaches in alleviating jet lag. Preadaptation, by shifting sleep timing, light exposure, and so on, in the desired direction is, of course, a useful, if inconvenient, strategy.

SUMMARY

Although much research involving both animals and human beings demonstrates unequivocally that timed exposure to bright light is an effective means of manipulating the circadian timing system, it appears that more years will be needed to answer the many questions and address the numerous issues necessary to develop effective, reliable, and practical treatment strategies using bright light. Concerns such as optimal intensity, spectral composition, duration and timing of light exposure, individual differences in response to light, and age effects must be addressed if light treatments are to be effective in any setting. Similarly, timed melatonin enhances adaptation to simulated and real night shifts; improves sleep, circadian adaptation, and subjectively perceived jet lag in most field studies; and can stabilize sleep in blind subjects without necessarily entraining all circadian rhythms. Melatonin and light may act in concert to maintain endogenous circadian synchronization. Their combined use should provide optimum phase shifting strategies, although a great deal of further research is needed.

RECOMMENDATIONS FOR TRAVELERS

- Where possible, choose daytime flights to minimize the loss of sleep and fatigue.
- Travel business or first class.
- Avoid large meals out of phase and caffeine and alcohol during the flight, and drink a lot of water.
- Avoid making critical decisions or attending important meetings on the first day after arrival.
- Avoid or seek bright light according to the recommendations of Houpt et al.[40]
- Consider the use of short-acting hypnotic agents during the flight (to sleep during the destination nighttime) and for the first few days after arrival.
- Consider, with the advice of your physician, the use of correctly timed melatonin if a licensed, quality-controlled preparation and use instructions (see Table 50–1) are available. Use the lowest effective dose. Be aware that there are very little short-term and no long-term safety data available.[70]

References

1. Klein KE, Wegmann HM. Significance of circadian rhythms in aerospace operations. Neuilly sur Seine, France: AGARD; 1980; No. 247.
2. Arendt J, Marks V. Physiological changes underlying jet-lag. Br Med J. 1982;284:144–146.
3. Samel A, Wegmann HM, Vejvoda M. Jet lag and sleepiness in aircrew. J Sleep Res. 1995;4:30–36.
4. Nicholson AN, Pascoe PA, Spencer MB, et al. Nocturnal sleep and daytime alertness of aircrew after transmeridian flights. Aviat Space Environ Med. 1986;57(suppl 12):B43–B52.
5. Voge VM. Self-reported menstrual concerns of U.S. Air Force and U.S. Army rated women aircrew. Milit Med. 1996;161:10614–10615.
6. Hampton SM, Morgan LM, Lawrence N, et al. Postprandial hormone and metabolic responses in simulated shift work. J Endocrinol. 1996;151:259–267.
7. Aschoff J, von, Saint Paul U Wever R. Lifetime of flies under influence of time displacement. Naturwissenschaften. 1971;58:574.
8. Akerstedt T. Adjustment of physiological circadian rhythms and the sleep wake cycle to shift work. In: Folkard S, Monk TH, eds. Hours of Work: Temporal Factors in Work Scheduling. New York, NY: John Wiley & Sons; 1985:185–198.
9. Rosa RR, Bonnet MH, Bootzin RR, et al. Intervention factors for promoting adjustment to nightwork and shiftwork. Occup Med. 1990;5:391–415.
10. Ross JK, Arendt J, Horne J, et al. Night-shift work during Antarctic winter: sleep characteristics and adaptation with bright light treatment. Physiol Behav. 1995;57:1169–1174.
11. Barnes R, Arendt J, Forbes M. 6-Sulphatoxymelatonin rhythm in shiftworkers on offshore oil installations during a 2-week 12-h night shift. Neurosci Lett. 1998;241:9–12.
12. Knutsson A. Shift work and coronary heart disease. Scand J Soc. 1989;44:1–36.
13. Lockley SW, Skene DJ, Tabandeh H, et al. Relationship between napping and melatonin in the blind. J Biol Rhythms. 1997;12:16–25.
14. Sack R, Lewy A, Blood M, et al. Circadian rhythm abnormalities in totally blind people: incidence and clinical significance. J Clin Endocrinol Metab. 1992;75:127–134.
15. Lockley SW, Skene DJ, Arendt J, et al. Relationship between melatonin rhythms and visual loss in the blind. J Clin Endocrinol Metab. 1997;82:3763–3770.
16. Czeisler CA, Shanahan TL, Klerman EB, et al. Suppression of melatonin secretion in some blind patients by exposure to bright light. N Engl J Med. 1995;332:6–11.
17. Minors DS, Waterhouse JM. Masking in humans: the problem and some attempts to solve it. Chronobiol Int. 1989;6:29–53.
18. Graeber RC, Sing HC, Cuthbert BN. The impact of transmeridian flight on deploying soldiers. In: Johnson LC, Tepas DI, Colquhoun WP, et al, eds. Biological Rhythms, Sleep and Shiftwork. Lancaster: MTP Press; 1981:513–537.
19. Stone BM, Turner C. Promoting sleep in shiftworkers and international travelers. Chronobiol Int. 1997;14:133–144.
20. Redfern PH. Can pharmacological agents be used effectively in the alleviation of jet-lag? Drugs. 1992;43:146–153.
21. Redfern P, Lemmer B. Physiology and pharmacology of biological rhythms. Berlin-Heidelberg-Handbook of Experimental Pharmacology. Vol 125. New York, NY: Springer-Verlag; 1997.
22. Scheen AJ, Byrne MM, Plat L, et al. Relationships between sleep quality and glucose regulation in normal humans. Am J Physiol. 1996;271:E261–E270.
23. Morgan L, Arendt J, Owens D, et al. Effects of the endogenous clock and sleep time on melatonin, insulin, glucose and lipid metabolism. J Endocrinol. 1998;157:443–451.
24. Van Cauter E, Blackman JD, Roland D, et al. Modulation of glucose regulation and insulin secretion by circadian rhythmicity and sleep. J Clin Invest. 1991;88:934–942.
25. Stone BM. Sleep and low doses of alcohol. Electroencephalogr Clin Neurophysiol. 1980;48:706–709.
26. Walsh JK, Muehlbach MJ, Schweitzer PK. Hypnotics and caffeine as countermeasures for shiftwork-related sleepiness and sleep disturbance. J Sleep Res. 1995;4(suppl 2):80–83.
27. Ehret CF, Scanlon LW. Overcoming Jet Lag. New York, NY: Berkley; 1983.
28. Leathwood P. Circadian rhythms of plasma amino acids, brain neurotransmitters and behaviour. In: Arendt J, Minors DS, Waterhouse JM, eds. Biological Rhythms in Clinical Practice. London, England: Butterworth; 1989:136–159.
29. Akerstedt T, Folkard S. The three process model of alertness and its extension to performance, sleep latency, and sleep length. Chronobiol Int. 1997;14:115–123.
30. Czeisler CA. The effect of light on the human circadian pacemaker. In: Chadwick DJ, Ackrill K, eds. Circadian Clocks and Their Adjustment. Chichester, England: John Wiley & Sons; 1995:254–302, Ciba Foundation Symposium No. 183.
31. Minors DS, Waterhouse JM, Wirz-Justice A. A human phase response curve to light. Neurosci Lett. 1991;133:36–40.
32. Badia P, Myers B, Boecker M, et al. Bright light effects on body temperature, alertness, EEG, and behaviour. Physiol Behav. 1991;50:583.
33. Lewy AJ, Wehr TA, Goodwin FK, et al. Light suppresses melatonin secretion in humans. Science. 1980;210:1267.
34. Koller M, Harma M, Laitinen JT, et al. Different patterns of light exposure in relation to melatonin and cortisol rhythms and sleep of night workers. J Pineal Res. 1994;16:127–135.
35. Czeisler CA, Johnson PJ, Duffy JF, et al. Exposure to bright light and darkness to treat physiologic maladaptation to night-work. N Engl J Med. 1990;322:1253–1259.
36. Samel A, Wegmann HM. Bright light: a countermeasure for jet lag? Chronobiol Int. 1997;14:173–184.
37. Stewart KT, Hayes BC, Eastman CI. Light treatment for NASA shiftworkers. Chronobiol Int. 1995;12:141–151.
38. Deacon S, Arendt J. Adapting to phase-shifts, I: an experimental model for jet lag and shift work. Physiol Behav. 1996;59:665–673.

39. Eastman CI, Boulos Z, Terman M, et al. Light treatment for sleep disorders: consensus report, IV: shift work. J Biol Rhythms. 1995;10:157–166.

40. Houpt TA, Boulos Z, Moore-Ede MC. MidnightSun: software for determining light exposure and phase-shifting schedules during global travel. Physiol Behav. 1996;59:561–568.

41. Arendt J. Melatonin and the Mammalian Pineal Gland. London, England: Chapman Hall; 1995.

41a. Luboshitzky R, Levi M, Shen Orr Z, et al. Long-term melatonin administration does not alter pituitary-gonadal hormone secretion in normal men. Hum Reprod. 2000;15:60–65.

42. Arendt J, Deacon S. Treatment of circadian rhythm disorders—melatonin. Chronobiol Int. 1997;14:185–204.

43. Lewy AJ, Saeeduddin A, Latham-Jackson JM, et al. Melatonin shifts human circadian rhythms according to a phase response curve. Chronobiol Int. 1992;9:380–392.

44. Middleton B, Arendt J, Stone B. Complex effects of melatonin on human circadian rhythms in constant dim light. J Biol Rhythms. 1997;12:467–475.

45. Samel A, Wegman HM, Vejvoda M, et al. Influence of melatonin treatment on human circadian rhythmicity before and after a simulated 9 hour time shift. J Biol Rhythms. 1991;6:235–248.

46. Dawson D, Encel N, Lushington K. Improving adaptation to simulated night-shift: timed exposure to bright light versus daytime melatonin administration. Sleep. 1995;18:11–21.

47. Deacon S, Arendt J. Adapting to phase-shifts, II: effects of melatonin and conflicting light treatment. Physiol Behav. 1995;59:675–682.

48. Stone BM, Turner C, Middleton B, et al. Use of melatonin to adapt to phase shifts: effects on sleep architecture and performance [abstract]. J Sleep Res. 1996;5(suppl 1):221.

49. Arendt J, Aldhous M, Marks V. Alleviation of jet-lag by melatonin: preliminary results of controlled double-blind trial. Br Med J. 1986;292:1170.

50. Arendt J, Aldhous M, Marks M, et al. Some effects of jet-lag and their treatment by melatonin. Ergonomics. 1987;30:1379–1393.

51. Skene DJ, Aldhous M, Arendt J. Melatonin, jet-lag and the sleep-wake cycle. In: Horne J, ed. Sleep '88. Basel, Switzerland: Karger; 1989:39–41.

52. Petrie K, Conaglen JV, Thompson L, et al. Effect of melatonin on jet-lag after long haul flights. Br Med J. 1989;298:705–707.

53. Nickelsen T, Lang A, Bergau L. The effect of 6-, 9- and 11-hour time shifts on circadian rhythms: adaptation of sleep parameters and hormonal patterns following the intake of melatonin or placebo. Adv Pineal Res. 1991;5:303–306.

54. Claustrat B, Brun J, David M, et al. Melatonin and jet-lag: confirmatory result using a simplified protocol. Biol Psychiatry. 1992;32:705–711.

55. Comperatore CA, Lieberman HR, Kirby AW, et al. Melatonin efficiency in aviation missions requiriong rapid deployment and night operations. Aviat Space Env Med. 1996;67:520–524.

55a. Waldhauser F, Saletu B, Trinchard-Lugan I. Sleep laboratory investigations on hypnotic properties of melatonin. Psychopharmacol. 1990;100:222–226.

56. Suhner A, Schlagenhauf P, Johnson R, et al. Comparative study to determine the optimal melatonin dosage form for the alleviation of jet lag. Chronobiol Int. 1998;15:655–666.

57. Petrie K, Dawson, AG, Thompson L, et al. A double blind trial of melatonin as a treatment for jet lag in international cabin crew. Biol Psychiatry. 1993;33:526–530.

58. Spitzer RL, Terman M, Williams JBW, et al. Jet lag: clinical features, validation of a new syndrome-specific scale, and lack of response to melatonin in a randomized double-blind trial. Am J Psychiatry. 1999;156:1392–1396.

59. Arendt J, Skene DJ, Middleton B, et al. Efficacy of melatonin treatment in jet lag, shift work and blindness. J Biol Rhythms. 1997;12:604–618.

60. Deacon S, English J, Tate J et al. Atenolol facilitates light-induced phase shifts in human. Neurosci Lett. 1998;242:53–56.

61. Folkard S, Arendt J, Clark M. Can melatonin improve shift workers' tolerance of the night shift? Some preliminary findings. Chronobiol Int. 1993;10:315–320.

62. Sack RL, Blood ML, Lewy AJ. Melatonin administration promotes circadian adaptation to shift work. Sleep Res. 1994;23:509.

63. Arendt J, Aldhous M, Wright J. Synchronisation of a disturbed sleep-wake cycle in a blind man by melatonin treatment. Lancet. 1988;1:772–773.

64. Aldhous ME, Arendt J. Melatonin rhythms and the sleep wake cycle in blind subjects. J Interdisciplin Cycle Res. 1991;22:84–85.

65. Sack RL, Lewy AJ, Blood ML, et al. Melatonin administration to blind people: phase advances and entrainment. J Biol Rhythms. 1991;6:249–261.

66. Folkard S, Arendt J, Aldhous M, et al. Melatonin stabilises sleep onset time in a blind man without entrainment of cortisol or temperature rhythms. Neurosci Lett. 1990;113:193–198.

67. Jan JE, Espezel H, Appleton RE. The treatment of sleep disorders with melatonin. Dev Med Child Neurol. 1994;36:97–107.

68. Buxton OM, L'Hermite-Baleriaux M, Hirschfeld U, et al. Acute and delayed effects of exercise on human melatonin secretion. J Biol Rhythms. 1997;12:568–574.

69. Honma K, Kohsaka M, Fukuda N, et al. Effects of vitamin B12 on plasma melatonin rhythm in humans: increased light sensitivity phase advances the circadian clock? Experientia. 1992;48:716–720.

70. Arendt J. Safety of melatonin in long term use. J Biol Rhythms. 1997;12:673–682.

51

Shift Work

Timothy H. Monk

Some people cope well with shift work, others poorly. At the extreme, Moore-Ede[1] and others have referred to a shift work maladaptation syndrome in those failing to cope. Several international classifications also refer to a sleep disorder associated with abnormal work hours. The International Classification of Sleep Disorders[2] formally lists shift work sleep disorder as one of the circadian rhythm sleep disorders. The *Diagnostic and Statistical Manual of Mental Disorders*[3] lists shift work type as a subtype of the circadian rhythm sleep disorder (#307.45). Thus, there is increasing acceptance that the difficulties some people experience with shift work should properly be regarded as a disorder worthy of medical diagnosis and treatment.

Although listed within circadian rhythm–related sleep disorders, shift work intolerance is a problem that should not be regarded as *solely* a circadian rhythms ("biological clock") issue, or, indeed, solely a sleep disorders issue, or solely a social and domestic issue. Rather, it is a complex interaction of the three factors, with each factor influencing both of the other factors and the final outcome of shift work tolerance.[4] This chapter discusses shift work research and outlines the beginning of an educational strategy that may improve a patient's ability to cope with shift work.

With about 20% of the U.S. work force now engaged in some form of shift work system,[5] physicians are increasingly confronted with patients whose conditions may be exacerbated by a failure to cope with the repeated changes in schedule that shift work requires. Coping problems stem from factors within the individual (Table 51–1) and from factors relating to work systems (Table 51–2). The long-term health consequences of shift work have been reviewed extensively elsewhere.[6, 7] Results have sometimes been contradictory, but in addition to sleep disorders, gastrointestinal dysfunction and cardiovascular disease have been the major complaints implicated. The aim of this presentation is not to duplicate such reviews but rather to introduce a general conceptual framework within which shift work coping ability may be considered, so that the physician can better understand the various factors that are involved.

Shift work coping ability can be considered to be the product of a mutually interactive triad of factors (Fig. 51–1). Circadian factors stem from the individual's biological clock, which has been shown to be endogenous and self-sustaining under conditions of temporal isolation.[8] Sleep factors are, of course, intimately bound

up with the circadian ones, but have a greater significance for the shift workers themselves and are thus more likely to appear in presenting symptoms.[9] Domestic factors (including social and community aspects) are often neglected in terms of hard research[10] but can be equally important as determinants of shift work coping ability, and certainly influence the behavior of the shift worker in relation to the other two factors.[11] The three factors are discussed in the following sections, with emphasis placed on interactions and interrelationships.

CIRCADIAN FACTORS

One could argue that circadian factors constitute the essential basic determinant of shift work coping ability. Without an endogenous circadian system, sleep could simply be taken "at will," and society would probably be structured in a much less day-oriented fashion. Unfortunately, it is quite clear that, like it or not, *Homo sapiens* is a diurnal species, biologically hard-wired to be active during the day and sleepy at night. Working at night must therefore be regarded as an inherently unnatural act. However, one must avoid the temptation of going too far, of regarding the shift worker's problems as being exclusively circadian in origin and blindly applying "chronohygiene" principles without recognizing all the social and behavioral complexities that are peculiar to the human being. Circadian factors

---

Table 51–1. FACTORS WITHIN AN INDIVIDUAL THAT ARE LIKELY TO CAUSE SHIFT WORK COPING PROBLEMS

Over 50 years of age
Second job for pay ("moonlighting")
Heavy domestic workload
"Morning-type" individuals ("larks")
History of sleep disorders
Psychiatric illness
History of alcohol or drug abuse
History of gastrointestinal complaints
Epilepsy
Diabetes
Heart disease

From Tepas DI, Monk TH. Work schedules. In: Salvendy G, ed: Handbook of Human Factors. New York, NY: John Wiley & Sons; 1987: 819–843. Reprinted by permission of John Wiley & Sons, Ltd.

Table 51–2. FACTORS ASSOCIATED WITH WORK SYSTEMS AND WORK THAT ARE LIKELY TO CAUSE SHIFT WORK COPING PROBLEMS

More than five third shifts in a row without off-time days
More than four 12-h night shifts in a row
First-shift starting times earlier than 7 AM
Rotating hours that change once per week ("weekly rotation")
Less than 48 h off-time after a run of third-shift work
Excessive regular overtime
Backward rotating hours (first to third to second shift)
12-h shifts involving critical monitoring tasks
12-h shifts involving a heavy physical workload
Excessive weekend working
Long commuting times
Split shifts with inappropriate break period lengths
Shifts lacking appropriate shift breaks
12-h shifts with exposure to harmful agents and substances
Overly complicated schedules, which make it difficult to track or plan ahead

From Tepas DI, Monk TH. Work Schedules. In: Salvendy G, ed: Handbook of Human Factors. New York, NY: John Wiley & Sons, 1987: 819–843. Reprinted by permission of John Wiley & Sons, Ltd.

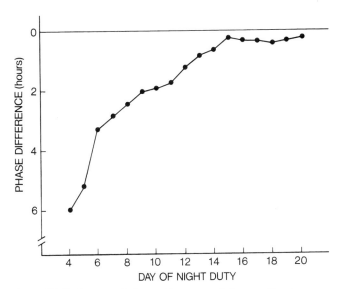

Figure 51–2. Pattern of phase adjustment of the circadian temperature rhythm in two young volunteers working 21 consecutive night shifts. (Data from Monk TH, Knauth P, Folkard S, et al. Memory based performance measures in studies of shift work. Ergonomics. 1978;21:819–826.)

are an important determinant of shift work coping ability, but they are not the only determinant.

The prime negative influence of the circadian system stems from its inability to adjust instantaneously to the changes in routine that shift work schedules require.[12] Figure 51–2 illustrates the process of circadian system realignment (as measured by the temperature rhythm) in two young volunteers who worked 21 consecutive night shifts.[13] As in the jet lag situation (see Chapter 50), the process is a slow one, with more than a week elapsing before complete circadian realignment occurs.

One reason that the circadian realignment of shift workers can take even longer than that associated with jet lag is the difference between the two situations in zeitgeber (time cue giver) influence. In jet lag, both physical (daylight-darkness) and social (e.g., mealtimes

and traffic noise) zeitgebers are *encouraging* the realignment of the circadian system. For the shift worker, however, the physical zeitgebers are resolutely *opposed* to a nocturnal alignment, as are most of the social zeitgebers springing from a day-oriented society. Research has therefore focused on enhancing the zeitgebers that are encouraging a nocturnal circadian orientation. Very bright (greater than 7000 lux) levels of nocturnal workplace illumination coupled with complete darkness for the 8-h-day sleep period at home has been shown, within a week, to phase-shift the circadian systems of young volunteers.[14] However, in a careful series of studies, Eastman and colleagues[15] have shown that bright light–induced phase delays in circadian rhythms may only appear when dark welders' goggles are additionally worn on the commute home from work—a procedure that may be rather unsafe. Further work is therefore needed to evaluate the feasibility of such protocols in actual practice. Another way of enhancing circadian adjustment is by taking melatonin pills—a strategy used by many night workers following the wide exposure given to that hormone in the popular press. While there is some empirical evidence for the effectiveness of melatonin for night workers (albeit those working nine consecutive shifts),[16] there is probably not enough known about the consequences of prolonged melatonin administration for its chronic use in this situation to be advisable. The fact that melatonin is so readily available over the counter in the United States (though not, it should be noted, in most other countries of the world) does not guarantee its safety.

The process of circadian realignment for the night worker can be likened to a salmon leaping up a waterfall; it is difficult to achieve a nocturnal orientation (i.e., reach the top of the waterfall), but easy indeed to fall back down to a diurnal orientation. That asymme-

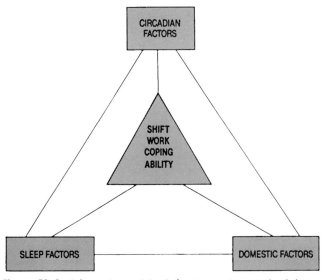

Figure 51–1. Schematic model of the interactive triad of factors influencing shift work coping ability.

try becomes vitally important when social and domestic influences during days off are considered. Thus, although a worker may be a permanent night worker as far as the company is concerned, in reality the individual may be alternating between nocturnal and diurnal orientations, simply because of the social and domestic demands of the individual "weekend" breaks, which require daytime wakefulness. In a reanalysis of field data, I have shown that on the first night after a weekend break, even permanent night workers may have a totally diurnal circadian orientation in their temperature and subjective alertness rhythms.[17]

During the process of circadian realignment, there are three mechanisms by which mood, well-being, and performance efficiency can be adversely affected. First, sleep will be disrupted, and the individual will be in a state of partial sleep deprivation.[18] Second, the new time of wakefulness is likely to tap into the "down phases" of various psychological functions that are normally coincident with sleep in the day-oriented individual.[19] Third, the various individual components of the circadian system will be in a state of disarray, with the normal harmony of appropriate phase relationships destroyed.[20] A good analogy with the biological clock is a symphony orchestra, with a conductor on the rostrum making sure that the various instruments are brought in at the right time. For the night worker, it is as if a second conductor appears on the rostrum, beating at a different time. The rate at which the different instruments switch to the new conductor varies, and until they all do, there is a cacophony, with all harmony lost. In circadian terms, we speak of this cacophony as "desynchronosis" or "internal dissociation." In addition to poor sleep, its symptoms include malaise, gastrointestinal dysfunction, and performance decrements.

Other circadian determinants of shift work coping ability spring from the particular characteristics of the individual's circadian system. Most healthy people have a circadian system that will tend to run slowly (to approximately 24.2 to 25.0 h) in free-running situations in which they are unaware of time cues and are free to choose bedtimes and mealtimes (see Chapter 28). This finding suggests that it might be more congenial to the circadian system to be stretched further (by extending subjective days) than to be shrunk (by contracting them). In the jet lag area, we know this to be the case, with westbound phase adjustment more easily accomplished than eastbound adjustment. In the shift work area, there is only suggestive evidence,[21] but most experts would agree that better circadian realignment results from shift rotation in a "forward" direction (nights, mornings, evenings) than in a "backward" one (evenings, mornings, nights).

Individual differences in circadian system characteristics may also have a role in determining shift work coping ability. One major determinant is habitual sleep need. Those who happen to need 9 h or more of sleep to feel well rested invariably find shift work extremely difficult to cope with.[22] Also, individuals who are "night owls," or "late phasers," in their circadian system often find shift work considerably easier to cope with than do "morning larks," or "early phasers."[22] This finding may be because zeitgeber influences are less potent for late phasers (an advantage for shift workers), or it may be because late phasers have a longer natural free-running period (coping more easily with forward shift rotations), or for the prosaic reason that they can sleep well during the morning (something that night workers often do, because they usually take their recreation after sleep, rather than before it).

Phase differences may also explain why late-middle-aged people often find shift work difficult. A typical case is that of a 50-year-old man who has hitherto been fairly happy with shift work but now finds it increasingly difficult to cope with. In some ways, this is paradoxical, given that he has had many decades of learning shift work coping strategies and that he probably has a quieter house now that his children have grown up and he can afford better housing. The reason for the problem may be that he has become a "morning lark" in circadian phase orientation (most older people are), or that his sleep is becoming more fragile and thus subject to disruption. Campbell[23] has shown that circadian manipulations designed to improve night work tolerance may work much better for young adults than for those in middle age. In addition, Reinberg et al.[24] have shown that older, shift work–intolerant subjects may exhibit circadian rhythms running at periods totally different from the 24-h period of society.

Before the discussion of circadian factors is concluded, the question must be addressed whether circadian realignment is actually desirable, given all the caveats regarding the weekend regression to a diurnal orientation mentioned before. In Europe, many companies are switching to "rapidly rotating" systems in which only one or two shifts are worked at a time, before a different one is worked.[25] Thus, for example, on the "continental" rotation, workers rotate two morning shifts, two evening shifts, and two night shifts, followed by 2 d off. Most European experts favor such systems because they allow the circadian system to retain its diurnal orientation, thus eliminating problems of desynchronosis. Because only one or two night shifts are worked before time off is given, sleep loss and fatigue are minimized. The drawbacks of rapid rotation are the fatigue during the night shifts, which, for some tasks, may render the approach undesirable, and the workers' difficulties in predicting when they will be at work. However, there are undoubtedly many situations in which rapid rotation is worthy of consideration.

SLEEP FACTORS

Sleep is the major preoccupation of most shift workers. In both Europe[26] and the United States,[27] surveys have indicated that night workers get about 5 to 7 h less sleep per week than their day-working counterparts. In his survey of field and laboratory shift work sleep studies, Akerstedt[28] concluded that the shortening in day sleep comes primarily from a reduction in stage 2 and rapid eye movement (REM) sleep, with slow-wave sleep relatively unaffected. Not surprisingly, sleep latency is also reduced, and some studies have found shorter REM latencies to occur.

This sleep loss is sometimes partially recouped on days off but does represent a chronic state of partial sleep deprivation which undoubtedly affects the mood and performance abilities of the shift worker. There are now several well-controlled studies which document the pathological sleepiness levels exhibited by many shift workers, both at work[29] and on the drive home after work.[30] Indeed, one could argue that the latter represents the most dangerous activity that most shift workers ever do, and one which, in aggregate, represents a major public safety concern involving significant loss of life.[31]

Many shift workers assert that if only they could solve their sleep problem, then everything else would be quite tolerable. However, because of the impact of the circadian system on sleep, disrupted sleep may be as much a *symptom* of shift work maladjustment as a *cause* of it. This idea is demonstrated clearly in a study by Walsh et al.,[32] who brought actual shift workers into a sound-attenuated, electrically shielded bedroom for their sleep periods, with the subjects commuting to their work from the laboratory rather than from home. Even in this closely protected environment, there was a highly significant difference in duration between the day sleep of night workers and the night sleep of day workers (306 min vs. 401 min). In addition, there were reliable differences between the polygraphic characteristics of the sleep, with a smaller amount of REM sleep and a greater proportion of slow-wave sleep for the night workers. Thus, even if it were economically feasible, the complete soundproofing and lightproofing of all shift workers' bedrooms would not eradicate the problem of sleep for shift workers.

Circadian factors are not the only ones having an impact on sleep, however. Domestic and social factors (see the next section) are also crucial in determining the shift worker's sleep quality and duration. First, the sleep of the shift worker is not as protected by society's taboos as that of a day worker; for example, no one would think of phoning a day worker at 2 AM, but few would have qualms about phoning a night worker at 2 PM. Similarly, unless the shift worker is in a well-adjusted household, his (and more especially her) sleep is liable to be truncated by the demands of child care, shopping, and household management. In viewing the sleep of shift workers, one must therefore consider both endogenous and exogenous factors that are going to limit sleep time.

Sleep demands may also be as much of an *influence* on the other two factors in the triad as a *product* of their influence. Much domestic disharmony can be attributed to the shift worker's need for sleep at a time when households are usually rather noisy, and impaired mood is a classic symptom of partial sleep loss.[33] Prescribed circadian rhythm coping strategies may not work because the weary shift worker may be asleep when he or she should be experiencing bright light.

Finally, in discussing the sleep of shift workers, one must address the issue of hypnotics. In a study of rotating shift workers, Walsh et al.[34] found that triazolam 0.5 mg could improve the quality and duration of day sleeps. However, the study was also important in demonstrating that the drug had no significant "phase-resetting" effects. Thus, on the third- and fourth-day sleeps in a run of night duty, for which no medication was given, there were no significant differences between those who had been given triazolam on day sleeps 1 and 2 and those who had been given placebo. Moreover when drug and placebo groups were compared in terms of nighttime alertness and performance, no reliable differences emerged, even on the days in which medication was given.[35] One must therefore recognize that hypnotics will probably ameliorate only the *sleep* factor of the triad.

As a general rule, the use of hypnotics is thus inadvisable for shift workers because problems of tolerance and dependence are likely to occur. The only situation in which hypnotics might be appropriate is in rapidly rotating shift systems, in which the occasional day sleep may be improved by hypnotics and no phase resetting is required.

DOMESTIC FACTORS

Human beings are essentially social creatures, and one could argue, as Walker[36] and others[37] have done, that the social and domestic factors are at least as important in shift work as the biological ones. Certainly, if a shift worker's domestic and social life is unsatisfactory, then the individual will not be coping, however well adjusted the sleep and circadian rhythm factors may be. More usually, however, poor domestic adjustment adversely affects the other two factors of the triad. A common example concerns the childcare and household management tasks that can be expected of a female shift worker. Unlike her male colleagues, she is often expected by her spouse to continue to run the household and can thus find herself completely unable to comply with the routine that good sleep hygiene and circadian adjustment might require.

This situation is illustrated by a comparison study[38] between full-time (4 nights per week) and part-time (2 nights per week) female night nurses. Few (36%) of the full-timers had children living with them at home, compared with the part-timers (96%). The study took place over the first 2 nights of a run of duty after some time off. From the sleep records of the two groups shown in Figure 51–3, it is clear that the full-timers were able to make more of a commitment to night work than were the part-timers, in their ability to "sleep in" later in the morning, to take afternoon naps before coming on shift, and to sleep between the two shifts. Indeed, some of the part-timers remained so diurnal in their circadian orientation that they even took brief naps during their "lunch" hour, in the middle of the night shift.

Another aspect of domestic disruption concerns the role of the male shift worker as husband and parent. With regard to the former, there are three major spouse roles that are affected: sexual partner, social compan-

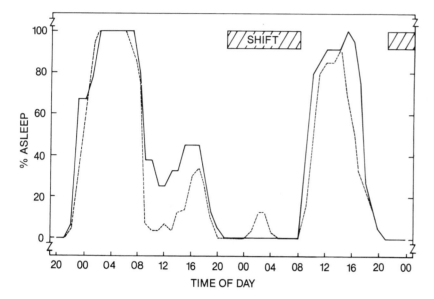

Figure 51–3. Percentage of full-time (*solid line*) and part-time (*dotted line*) night nurses asleep before, during, and after the first of a period of successive night shifts. (Data from Monk TH, Folkard S. Individual differences in shift work adjustment. In: Folkard S, Monk TH, eds. Hours of Work—Temporal Factors in Work Scheduling. New York, NY: John Wiley & Sons; 1985:227–237. Reprinted by permission of John Wiley & Sons, Ltd.)

ion, and protector-caregiver. All three roles are compromised. Perhaps as a consequence, shift work has been shown in a longitudinal follow-up study to increase the risk of divorce by 57%.[39] Although some of the problems are sexual in origin, many spring from the spouse's inability to be there when needed. Feelings of loneliness and insecurity in a wife left alone at home every night, for example, can represent a much more chronic and insoluble problem than that connected with the timing of lovemaking. Similarly, the evening shift, which has minimal impact on the sleep and circadian factors, can have a crushing impact on the role of the shift worker as social companion. With regard to the family role of parent, the evening shift is again the most disruptive. Often during the school week the shift worker may only get to see his or her children when they are asleep in bed. In addition, both spouse and parent roles are heavily disrupted when the shift worker is required to work on weekends.

In addition to disrupted family roles, the shift worker often suffers from social isolation from day-working friends and from religious and community organizations that work under the expectation that evenings or weekends will be free for meetings and activities. One might advance the view that perhaps a shift worker who is denied access to community meetings and social and political associations is as much disadvantaged as a handicapped person who is denied wheelchair access to a museum.

COPING STRATEGIES

As in many fields of endeavor, the task of enumerating all the *problems* connected with shift work is considerably less difficult than that of suggesting the *solutions*, which, in turn, is less difficult than the task of actual *implementation*. The solvency of companies and the livelihood of individuals are at stake, and one must be careful to avoid being too dogmatic or theoretical in one's suggestions for improvement. As this chapter has

sought to demonstrate, the area is a complicated one, with a host of interrelated forces and pressures, many of them impossible to simulate in the laboratory.

Unfortunately, there is no single panacea for shift work and no single "best shift system." What is needed, however, is improved education in the shift work problem for both management and the work force. With regard to the former, management should realize that it has not only a *moral* but also a *financial* obligation to be sensitive to issues of shift work tolerance in the training of its employees and in the selection of shift schedules. Increasing medical, recruiting, and retraining costs dictate that poor employee morale, higher job turnover, and increased accident and absenteeism rates resulting from shift work intolerance can become a financial burden to the company or organization.

Education programs should emphasize the way in which circadian, sleep, and domestic factors can influence shift work coping ability. Workers should be taught good sleep hygiene practice and advised how they can manipulate zeitgebers to their advantage, enhancing those that are working in their favor and attenuating those working against them. In some cases, family counseling may be indicated to discuss solutions to some of the social and domestic problems. The creation of self-help networks can often be of benefit, lessening some of the social and community isolation that many shift workers feel. When educational strategies fail, and the shift schedule cannot be changed, the patient may require a change to a day-working job.

The main task with regard to management education is that of first convincing management that there *is* a problem and that shift work concerns cannot simply be swept under the carpet or dismissed as a problem confined to sick or disgruntled employees who are simply not trying hard enough. Second, management must be informed of the wide range of different shift systems that are available, including the rapidly rotating systems so popular in Europe. Third, management must be taught to recognize the factors (e.g., type of job, nature of work force, average commuting time, male-female ratio, and preponderance of moonlighting) that should influence the selection of the optimal schedule for that work group in that situation. For management, the "carrot" is a happy, healthy, and productive work force; the "stick" is the specter of human error failures, such as that at the Three Mile Island nuclear power plant, and of litigation from a work force that might consider inappropriately selected work schedules to have adversely affected their health or their safety. Such litigation may grow as the applicability of the Americans With Disabilities Act to shift workers is tested in the courts, and as the United States grows increasingly out of step with the fairly restrictive legislation in place elsewhere in the world (e.g., Europe) for the protection of shift workers.[40]

CONCLUSIONS

Although some people cope well with shift work, many others have significant problems that can adversely affect their health and well-being. These problems can become a "shift work sleep disorder," which may be quite debilitating to the patient. Shift work problems can be usefully understood using a multifaceted approach that recognizes the interaction of circadian rhythms, sleep, and social and domestic factors in determining shift work coping ability.

References

1. Moore-Ede MC. Jet lag, shift work, and maladaption. NIPS. 1986;1:156–160.
2. Diagnostic Steering Committee. International Classification of Sleep Disorders: Diagnostic and Coding Manual. Rochester, Minn: American Sleep Disorders Association; 1990.
3. American Psychiatric Association. Diagnostic and Statistical Manual of Mental Disorders. 4th ed. Washington, DC: American Psychiatric Association Press; 1994.
4. Monk TH. Coping with the stress of shift work. Work Stress. 1988;2:169–172.
5. Mellor EF. Shift work and flexitime: how prevalent are they? Monthly Labor Rev. 1986;109:14–21.
6. Rutenfranz J, Colquhoun WP, Knauth P, et al. Biomedical and psychosocial aspects of shift work: a review. Scand J Work Environ Health. 1977;3:165–182.
7. Scott AJ, LaDou J. Shiftwork: Effects on sleep and health with recommendations for medical surveillance and screening. Occup Med. 1990;5:273–299.
8. Moore RY. The suprachiasmatic nucleus and the organization of a circadian system. Trends Neurosci. 1982;5:404–407.
9. Tepas DI, Carvalhais AB. Sleep patterns of shiftworkers. Occup Med. 1990;5:199–208.
10. Akerstedt T, Gillberg M. Night and Shift Work: Biological and Social Aspects. Oxford, England: Pergamon Press; 1990.
11. Tepas DI. Shift worker sleep strategies. J Hum Ergol (Tokyo). 1982;11(suppl):325–326.
12. Aschoff J, Hoffman K, Pohl H, et al. Re-entrainment of circadian rhythms after phase-shifts of the zeitgeber. Chronobiologia. 1975;2:23–78.
13. Monk TH, Knauth P, Folkard S, et al. Memory based performance measures in studies of shiftwork. Ergonomics. 1978;21:819–826.
14. Czeisler CA, Johnson MP, Duffy JF, et al. Exposure to bright light and darkness to treat physiologic maladaptation to night work. N Engl J Med. 1990;322:1253–1259.
15. Eastman CI, Stewart KT, Mahoney MP, et al. Dark goggles and

16. Sack RL, Blood ML, Lewy AJ. Melatonin administration promotes circadian adaptation to night-shift work. Sleep Res. 1994;23:509.
17. Monk TH. Advantages and disadvantages of rapidly rotating shift schedules–a circadian viewpoint. Hum Factors. 1986;28:553–537.
18. Weitzman ED, Kripke DF, Goldmacher D, et al. Acute reversal of the sleep-waking cycle in man. Arch Neurol. 1970;22:483–489.
19. Folkard S, Monk TH. Shiftwork and performance. Hum Factors. 1979;21:483–492.
20. Wever RA. The circadian system of man: results of experiments under temporal isolation. New York, NY: Springer-Verlag; 1979.
21. Czeisler CA, Moore-Ede MC, Coleman RM. Rotating shift work schedules that disrupt sleep are improved by applying circadian principles. Science. 1982;217:460–463.
22. Monk TH, Folkard S. Individual differences in shiftwork adjustment. In: Folkard S, Monk TH, eds. Hours of Work—Temporal Factors in Work Scheduling. New York, NY: John Wiley & Sons; 1985:227–237.
23. Campbell SS. Effects of timed bright-light exposure on shift-work adaptation in middle-aged subjects. Sleep. 1995;18:408–416.
24. Reinberg A, Andlauer P, DePrins J, et al. Desynchronization of the oral temperature circadian rhythm and intolerance to shift work. Nature. 1984;308:272–274.
25. Knauth P, Rutenfranz J, Schulz H, et al. Experimental shift work studies of permanent night, and rapidly rotating, shift systems, II: behaviour of various characteristics of sleep. Int Arch Occup Environ Health. 1980;46:111–125.
26. Knauth P, Landau K, Droge C, et al. Duration of sleep depending on the type of shift work. Int Arch Occup Environ Health. 1980;46:167–177.
27. Tasto DL, Colligan MJ. Health Consequences of Shift Work (Project UR11–4426). Menlo Park, Calif: Stanford Research Institute; 1978.
28. Akerstedt T. Adjustment of physiological circadian rhythms and the sleep-wake cycle to shiftwork. In: Folkard S, Monk TH, eds. Hours of Work—Temporal Factors in Work Scheduling. New York, NY: John Wiley & Sons; 1985:185–197.
29. Akerstedt T, Torsvall L, Gillberg M. Sleepiness and shift work: field studies. Sleep. 1982;5(suppl 2):S95–S106.
30. Richardson GS, Miner JD, Czeisler CA. Impaired driving performance in shiftworkers: the role of the circadian system in a multifactorial model. Alcohol Drugs Driving. 1990;5–6:265–273.
31. Pack AI, Pack AM, Rodgman E, et al. Characteristics of crashes attributed to the driver having fallen asleep. Accident Anal Prev. 1995;27:769–775.
32. Walsh JK, Tepas DI, Moss PD. The EEG sleep of night and rotating shift workers. In: Johnson LC, Tepas DI, Colquhoun WP, et al, eds. The Twenty-Four Hour Workday: Proceedings of a Symposium on Variations in Work-Sleep Schedules. Cincinnati, Ohio: Department of Health and Human Services (NIOSH); 1981:451–465.
33. Horne JA. Why We Sleep: The Functions of Sleep in Humans and Other Mammals. Oxford, England: Oxford University Press; 1988.
34. Walsh JK, Muehlbach MJ, Schweitzer PK. Acute administration of triazolam for the daytime sleep of rotating shift workers. Sleep. 1984;7:223–229.
35. Walsh JK, Schweitzer PK, Anch AM, et al. Sleepiness/alertness on a simulated night shift following sleep at home with triazolam. Sleep. 1991;14:140–146.
36. Walker JM. Social problems of shift work. In: Folkard S, Monk TH, eds. Hours of Work—Temporal Factors in Work Scheduling. New York, NY: John Wiley & Sons; 1985:211–225.
37. Colligan MJ, Rosa RR. Shiftwork effects on social and family life. Occup Med. 1990;5:315–322.
38. Folkard S, Monk TH, Lobban MC. Short and long-term adjustment of circadian rhythms in "permanent" night nurses. Ergonomics. 1978;21:785–799.
39. White L, Keith B. The effect of shift work on the quality and stability of marital relations. J Marriage Fam 1990;52:453–462.
40. US Congress, Office of Technology Assessment. Biological Rhythms: Implications for the Worker (OTA-BA-463). Washington, DC: Government Printing Office; 1991.

52

Circadian Disorders of the Sleep-Wake Cycle

Steven K. Baker

Phyllis C. Zee

The timing and duration of the sleep-wake cycle depend on the synchronization of the endogenous circadian clock with external environmental cycles. The sleep-wake cycle becomes perturbed when these two rhythms become desynchronized (change their phase relation). These dissynchronous states fall into two categories: (1) the terrestrial light-dark (LD) cycle may change relative to circadian timekeeping (shift work sleep disorder and time zone change syndrome), or (2) circadian timekeeping may change relative to the terrestrial LD cycle (delayed sleep phase syndrome, advanced sleep phase syndrome, and non–24-h sleep-wake syndrome). The first circumstance occurs in the presence of a normal circadian timekeeping system and is generally self-limited or resolves with environmental change. The latter circumstance is believed to occur because of a chronic alteration(s) in the circadian pacemaker which results in its inability to achieve a conventional phase relation with the external world. This chapter focuses on the second group of disorders. Because circadian variation in wakefulness and sleep propensity is the most apparent of the many behavioral and physiological outputs of the circadian pacemaker, it is not surprising that the first circadian rhythm disorders to be recognized involved the sleep-wake cycle.[1] Disruptions in the timing of sleep and wakefulness are often associated with sleep deprivation and cause patients to seek medical attention.

Recent advances in the understanding of basic human circadian biology have created new clinical tools for the diagnosis and treatment of several circadian sleep disorders. Increasingly detailed knowledge about how the circadian system responds to photic as well as to nonphotic entraining agents is beginning to offer the opportunity to manipulate circadian rhythms in the clinical setting. Practical therapies that can be used in the "real-life" clinical setting are being defined with increasing clarity.

ENTRAINMENT OF CIRCADIAN RHYTHMS

Animals and human beings removed from the external LD cycle and other time cues (zeitgebers) exhibit a continuing endogenous cycle of sleep and wakefulness in addition to many other physiological and hormonal parameters. The length of this cycle, or free-running period (designated as tau, τ), is probably largely genetically determined, with species and slight individual variation. In the mouse[2] and hamster,[3] genes have been identified which lengthen[2] and shorten,[4] respectively, the free-running period. The mammalian free-running period is generally slightly longer than 24 h in diurnal animals, and slightly shorter than 24 h in nocturnal animals (between 24.5 and 25 h in human beings) and must therefore be synchronized or entrained on a regular basis to the 24-h terrestrial day by external influences.

Entrainment by Light

Light is the major external time cue in mammals, and probably in human beings. The suprachiasmatic nucleus (SCN), in the anterior hypothalamus, is responsible for the generation of circadian rhythmicity in animals.[3, 5] Afferent projections to the SCN from the retina are thought to play the major role in light-induced entrainment of circadian rhythms. The retinohypothalamic tract has been shown to be important for stable entrainment by the LD cycle. Although the prevalent teaching was that in human beings, the effects of light on the circadian system were mediated by the eyes, a recent study suggests that extraocular photic entrainment by other mechanisms may occur.[6]

Although circadian rhythms can be entrained to LD cycles that are not exactly 24 h in duration, entrainment is restricted to cycles with periods that are "close" to 24 h in duration.[7] The range of entrainment can vary from species to species and is dependent on the experimental conditions (e.g., the intensity of the LD cycle, whether the period of the LD cycle is changed gradually or rapidly), but in general animals do not entrain readily to LD cycles that are more than a few hours shorter or longer than the period of the endogenous free-running circadian rhythm. If the period of the LD cycle is too short or too long for entrainment to occur, the circadian rhythm will free-run with a period close to 24 h.

One of the most widely used methods to examine how the LD cycle influences the circadian system has been to expose animals and humans maintained in constant conditions to pulses of light. The effects of the light pulse on a phase reference point of a circadian rhythm (e.g., onset of melatonin, minimum of body temperature) in subsequent cycles is then determined. This approach has demonstrated that light pulses can induce phase advances, phase delays, or have no effect on free-running circadian rhythms. The direction and magnitude of the shifts are strongly dependent on the circadian time at which the light pulse occurs. A phase response curve (PRC) is a plot of the magnitude and direction of the time shift induced by an environmental perturbation as a function of the circadian time at which the perturbation is given. Light pulse PRCs for all organisms share certain characteristics, including the fact that light pulses presented near the onset of the subjective night (the subjective night and subjective day refer to those parts of the circadian cycle that would occur during the dark or light time, respectively, when the organism is exposed to an LD cycle) induce phase delays in the rhythm, whereas light pulses presented in the late subjective night or early subjective day induce phase advances. Czeisler and his colleagues[8, 9] have carried out extensive studies in human beings demonstrating that the LD cycle could entrain human rhythms and that bright light could be used to manipulate human rhythms under a variety of experimental conditions. Bright light (intensities approximating sunlight) is a very strong and reliable entraining agent of human circadian rhythms.[8, 10]

Entrainment by Nonphotic Signals

The role of activity or social cues as synchronizing agents for the human circadian system has been recognized since the early 1970s. Studies by Aschoff et al.[11] showed that scheduled bedtimes, mealtimes, and various social time cues were able to entrain circadian rhythms. More recent studies indicate that sleep and social schedules may phase-shift the circadian clock.[12] In addition, physical exercise during the night can produce a delay shift in human circadian rhythms.[13] These findings raise the possibility that social and physical activity may be useful tools to manipulate circadian rhythms in human beings.[14]

Melatonin

Melatonin, secreted by the pineal gland, has been shown to have an important role in the regulation of circadian rhythms. Melatonin production is regulated by light information to the SCN. It is also likely that melatonin has feedback effects on the SCN. Melatonin receptors are present in the SCN of both rodents[15] and human beings.[16] Recent studies have shown that timed administration of exogenous melatonin can reset the circadian clock in animals[17] and human beings.[18, 19]

CIRCADIAN SLEEP DISORDERS

Delayed Sleep Phase Syndrome

Clinical Manifestations

Delayed sleep phase syndrome (DSPS) is characterized by sleep onset and wake times which are delayed 3 to 6 h relative to conventional sleep-wake times (Fig. 52–1). The typical patient finds it difficult to initiate sleep before 2 to 6 AM and, when free of societal constraints, prefers wake times of 10 AM to 1 PM. Sleep itself is normal.[20, 21] These symptoms are of at least 6 months'—and quite often of many years'—duration. The clinical picture may be that of sleep-onset insomnia. Patients are unable to advance their sleep times despite repeated attempts and may report a history of prolonged sedative-hypnotic drug use, bedtime use of alcohol, behavioral interventions, or psychotherapy.[22] Patients often report feeling most alert in the late evening and score highly as night people on a "morningness-eveningness" scale.[23] Enforced "conventional" wake times may result in chronically insufficient sleep and excessive daytime sleepiness. Sleepiness is greatest in the morning and lessens as the circadian drive for wakefulness peaks in the late afternoon. The syndrome may be associated with daytime irritability and poor school performance in adolescents.[24] In adulthood, the syndrome may be associated with impaired job performance and associated financial difficulty, as well as mari-

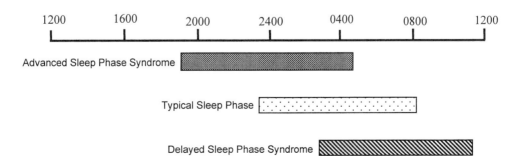

Figure 52–1. Schematic representation of the temporal distribution of sleep and wake in patients with circadian sleep phase disorders. Patients with advanced sleep phase syndrome typically complain of evening sleepiness and either early-morning awakening or sleep disruption. Patients with delayed sleep phase syndrome complain of difficulty initiating sleep usually before 2 AM and have difficulty awakening in the morning.

tal problems.[25] DSPS may be mistaken for depression, in which the sleep-wake cycle may also be delayed (or advanced). Several series, generally from psychiatric clinics, have emphasized an association with depression or other psychopathological disorders.[25, 26]

Prevalence

DSPS has been reported in preadolescence to the 6th decade.[25] It is more common in adolescents and young adults, with a reported prevalence of 7%.[27] In middle-aged adults, the prevalence may be one tenth of that, or 0.7%.[28] In a sleep disorders clinic, 6.7%[21] to 16%[26] of patients seen for a primary complaint of insomnia were believed to have DSPS.

Pathogenesis

It has been pointed out that the tendency for late sleeping is not simply a function of the circadian drive for wakefulness interacting with the sleep homeostat but, analogous to eating or other behaviors mandated by physiology but overlaid by varying individual emotional, social, and medical states, is the product of heterogeneous inputs.[26] Behavioral preference may therefore play a major role in some cases, particularly when enforced risetimes are not required. Delayed exposure to light in the morning may then prevent active advancement of the circadian clock, thus allowing it to drift to a new phase relation with external (sidereal) clock time. Ambient artificial nocturnal light is of insufficient intensity to cause an active phase delay in the human circadian pacemaker. However, the observations that the syndrome persists despite severe social or legal consequences,[29] that it has a high rate of relapse despite initially successful therapy,[22, 30] that other physiological markers of circadian oscillation persist in a delayed pattern despite enforced sleep-wake times,[31] and that the syndrome may in some cases be familial, lend support to the concept of an intrinsic abnormality in the circadian oscillator. Reduced sensitivity of the oscillator to photic entrainment (i.e., a reduction in the amplitude of the advance portion of the PRC to light) has been hypothesized, as has a prolonged τ or free-running period length of the circadian cycle.[22] Alternatively, Pittendrigh and Daan[32] have demonstrated that a strong relationship between the length of τ and the relative areas under the advance portion and delay portion of the PRC exists in many mammals (i.e., the longer τ is, the greater the likelihood that a random light pulse will advance the circadian phase, and the shorter τ is, the more likely a random light pulse will cause a phase delay). τ in nocturnal mammals, whose sleep-wake cycles are "delayed" 180 degrees relative to the solar clock, is short (less than 24 h), while τ in diurnal mammals is generally greater than 24 h. In short-τ mammals, light pulses generally cause phase delays, serving to "push them away" from any light exposure and keep them nocturnal. One might therefore speculate that human DSPS is the result of a shortened, rather than a prolonged τ. The duration and timing of environmental light exposure may play a role

in the expression of the DSPS phenotype. For instance, the prevalence of DSPS may be increased at extreme latitudes.[33]

Mammalian genes that confer altered circadian periodicity to activity have been cloned and characterized[34]; a genetic basis or predisposition to DSPS in human beings probably exists. Familial DSPS has been anecdotally noted.[25] Although these investigators found 11 of 12 patients with DSPS to be HLA DQ1 positive,[25] they were thought to represent different DQ subtypes on the basis of linkage disequilibrium analysis.

Isolated cases of DSPS have been loosely associated with viral infection (Epstein-Barr virus, influenza virus) or birth hypoxia,[25, 35] but no firm causal relationship has ever been made.

Diagnosis

The diagnosis of DSPS is usually made on clinical grounds (see above). A sleep log is usually necessary for confirmation. A morningness-eveningness scale, based on a structured questionnaire to gauge the patient's best time of day, is also useful.[23] Nocturnal polysomnography is sometimes necessary to exclude other sleep-disrupting conditions. When performed during conventional sleep laboratory hours, polysomnography often shows a prolonged sleep-onset latency, as well as a prolonged rapid eye movement (REM) latency, and may sometimes be a clue to the diagnosis in conjunction with an antecedent sleep diary. Actigraphy is also useful in assessing sleep-wake cycles relative to clock time but is generally not widely available clinically (Fig. 52–2A and B). The use of other physiological markers of circadian pacemaker output such as continuous ambulatory recording of body temperature[36] or dim-light melatonin onset (DLMO) may also aid in determining the phase relation of circadian and terrestrial time, although routine clinical availability is also limited (Fig. 52–3). In addition, the rhythm of these markers may be masked by environmental and behavioral influences, thereby confounding their interpretation. In general, the time from sleep onset to body temperature trough is shortened in DSPS.[37] DLMO is probably the most useful marker for circadian pacemaker output.[38] Patients with DSPS are said to have DLMOs which occur after 10 PM.[39] Determining DLMO involves multiple serum measurements in the mid- to late evening and is therefore not practical on a routine basis. Determination of DLMO by measurement of salivary melatonin in patient-collected salivary samples may be clinically feasible in the future.

Therapy

The goal of therapy in DSPS is to resynchronize the circadian clock with the desired 24-h LD cycle. In this sense, Richardson and Malin[1] noted that treatment of DSPS is the same whether it is the result of a primary behavioral or a primary physiological process. Chronotherapy, involving the successive delay of sleep times by 3 h daily over a 5- to 6-day period, until

ACTIGRAPHY

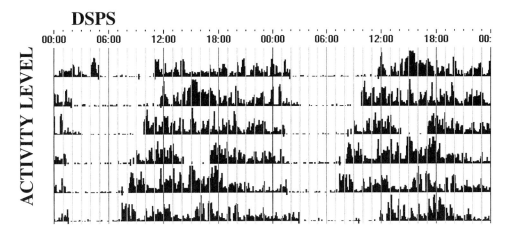

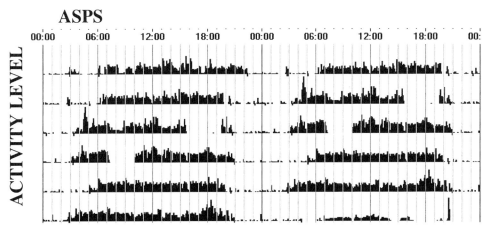

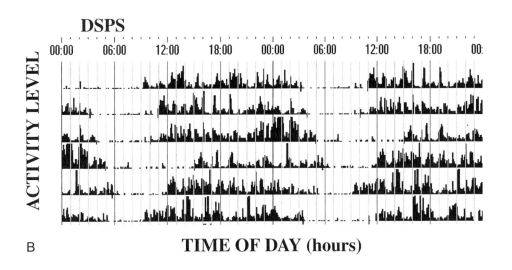

Figure 52–2. *A,* Rest-activity cycle profiles of patients with circadian sleep phase disorders. *Top panel,* Delayed sleep phase syndrome (DSPS) with sleep-onset times of 1:30 AM to 5 AM and wake-up times of 7:30 AM to 12:00 PM. Note that during the last 3 d of the recording, earlier wake times were self-imposed due to work requirements. Despite this, sleep onset continued to be delayed (2 AM). *Lower panel,* Advanced sleep phase syndrome (ASPS), with mean sleep onset between 8:45 PM and mean wake-up time of 4 AM. *B,* Delayed sleep phase syndrome without social constraints. Rest-activity recording of the same patient as in the top panel of *A* without self-imposed wake-up times. Note that sleep onset is more delayed (3 to 6 AM) with corresponding later wake-up times (9 AM to 3 PM).

the desired sleep time is achieved, followed by rigid adherence to a set sleep-wake schedule, was of prolonged success in a small sample of patients in a laboratory setting.[22] In nonlaboratory settings, the potential exists for exposure to daylight levels of illumination to have confounding effects upon the circadian clock, and this approach may be useful only for patients with very prolonged phase delays.[1]

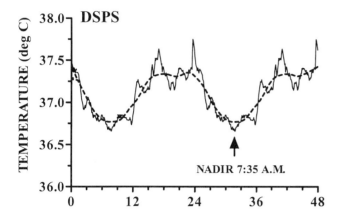

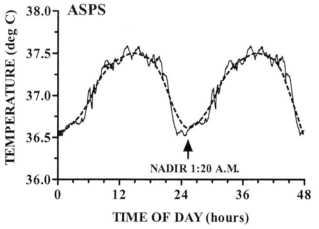

Figure 52–3. Circadian core body temperature profiles of patients with circadian sleep phase disorders. *Top panel,* Delayed sleep phase syndrome (DSPS), with a delayed nadir of the core body temperature of 7:35 AM (normal phase: 4 to 6 AM). *Lower panel,* Advanced sleep phase syndrome (ASPS), with an advanced core body temperature nadir of 1:20 AM.

Because light of daylight intensity likely plays a major role in resetting the human circadian pacemaker,[8, 9, 40] therapy with bright light in the morning—along the advance portion of the human PRC—seems logical and somewhat more convenient than chronotherapy, and was first suggested by Lewy et al.[41, 42] Although a number of case reports of successful application of bright-light therapy in DSPS exist,[43, 44] systematic (i.e., randomized, placebo-controlled, blinded) studies of its effectiveness do not exist. Rosenthal and colleagues[45] found that 2 h of bright-light exposure (2500 lux) in the morning (7 AM to 9 AM), together with light restriction in the evening, successfully phase-advanced (by 1.4 h) circadian rhythms of core body temperature and multiple sleep latencies in 20 patients chosen prospectively after meeting clinical criteria for DSPS.[45] However, a retrospective report from a referral sleep clinic found that only 7 of 20 patients with DSPS treated with bright light alone were able to entrain reliably to a desired sleep schedule.[26] Clinical application of bright-light therapy remains empirical; there are no standard criteria for its use in DSPS. The human PRC to a single 3-h bright-light pulse suggests that a light pulse given slightly before the time of body temperature minimum will result in a maximal phase delay, while a pulse given slightly after the minimum will cause a maximal phase advance (each about 2 h).[40] When light pulses over three successive cycles are used, larger shifts (4 to 7 h) can be produced. Since body temperature minimum is not routinely measured clinically, light therapy is usually timed using sleep logs to estimate the patient's endogenous circadian phase, with a pulse provided (intensity and duration have also not been defined, but 1 to 2 h of 2500 to 10,000 lux is usually used) toward the end of the sleep-wake cycle. Since the portion of the PRC at which the greatest phase advance can be achieved occurs during sleeping hours, light is usually given immediately upon awakening in the morning, which results in a smaller phase advance. The observation that light applied to the popliteal region also can phase-shift the human circadian system[6] may allow light therapy to be used during sleeping hours as well. Because the sleep-wake cycle may not necessarily correlate with circadian phase, particularly in severely delayed individuals, early-morning light could in theory be inadvertently given on the delay portion of the PRC, worsening the problem. Regestein and Pavlova[46] reported a patient who slept later after receiving light exposure at 6 AM.

Administration of exogenous melatonin also shifts the phase of the endogenous circadian clock, although the shifts in human beings occur according to a PRC that is nearly opposite in phase to the PRCs for light exposure: melatonin delays circadian rhythms when administered in the morning and advances them when administered in the afternoon or early evening.[47] Exogenous melatonin given in the afternoon to early evening prior to DLMO will result in a phase advance,[39] acknowledging that DLMO in phase-delayed individuals is later. In a randomized, double-blind, placebo-controlled crossover study of eight patients with DSPS, 5 mg of melatonin administered at 10 PM resulted in a phase advance in all subjects, with a mean advance of sleep-onset time of 82 min and of wake time of 117 min.[35] Upon stopping melatonin, all patients reverted to their previous sleep-wake cycle within 2 to 3 days. The physiological (phase-shifting) dose of melatonin is approximately 0.1 to 0.5 mg, or one-tenth to one-fiftieth of commercially available preparations.[39] Side effects of melatonin at these dose ranges are minimal, although sedative effects occur at higher (80 mg) doses. The combination of morning bright light and early-evening melatonin may be even more efficacious in creating a phase advance, although clinical data are lacking.

Other pharmacotherapies—vitamin B$_{12}$,[48] triazolam,[49] or tricyclic antidepressants or monoamine oxidase inhibitors[25]—do not appear to be effective.

Advanced Sleep Phase Syndrome

Advanced sleep phase syndrome (ASPS) is characterized by habitual and involuntary sleep and wake times that are at least several hours earlier than societal means (see Fig. 52–1). Sleep itself is normal. Individuals often complain of persistent and often irresistible sleepiness in the late afternoon or early evening, often preventing their participation in desired evening activities. Because their circadian drive for wakefulness begins to rise prematurely, they may complain of involuntary early-morning awakening (2 to 5 AM), which occurs even if sleep onset is voluntarily delayed; a diagnosis of depression may be erroneously made. The chronic delay of sleep onset due to professional or social obligations can lead to chronically insufficient sleep and excessive daytime sleepiness, although this occurs less frequently than in DSPS, probably because societal constraints on sleep time are less rigid than on wake time. People may gravitate to professions that are in phase with their endogenous circadian clock, such as farming or anesthesiology.

Epidemiology

The preceding may explain why ASPS is less frequently reported (three case reports exist[50–52]) than DSPS, as it may not be perceived by affected individuals to be pathological. ASPS may have a 1% prevalence in middle-aged adults.[28] Prevalence almost certainly increases with age. Sleep-wake cycles in the elderly are often advanced, characterized by earlier bedtimes and wake times, but whether this is the manifestation of altered circadian pacemaker output or the result of other factors (e.g., sleep is more fragmented in the elderly, which may contribute to daytime sleepiness and earlier bedtimes, social cues change with aging, and so forth) has been questioned. Czeisler and colleagues[53] found that 21 healthy elderly persons (average age, 70 years) without sleep complaints had uniformly earlier sleep and wake times, and uniformly advanced body temperature cycles (measured in constant routine conditions to avoid masking) when compared with younger men. A shortened free-running period length has been shown to occur with aging in mammals and human beings.[9, 54]

Pathogenesis

The cause of ASPS, as with DSPS, is unknown. A shortened free-running period ($\tau = 23.7$ h) has been demonstrated in a 66-year-old woman with advanced sleep and wake times, with intact or even enhanced responsiveness to photic entrainment.[9]

Diagnosis

As in DSPS, diagnosis of ASPS is made on clinical grounds, usually with the use of a sleep log, and actigraphy if available (see Fig. 52–2A). Continuous ambulatory monitoring of body temperature may also gain greater clinical acceptance (see Fig. 52–3). Major affective disorders should be carefully excluded. Polysomnography is sometimes necessary to confirm that sleep is normal and that sleep-disordered breathing, periodic limb movements, or other causes of sleep disruption are not present. Polysomnography should ideally be performed during the patient's normal sleep period; if it is carried out at conventional laboratory hours, a shortened or normal sleep-onset latency and early wake time may be seen. An early REM latency is not seen and may suggest an affective disorder, narcolepsy, or other disorder.[52, 55]

Treatment

A chronotherapeutic approach—advancing bedtime by 3 h every 2 days until the desired bedtime is reached—has been reported,[52] although relapse occurred quickly.[55] Bright-light therapy during the delay portion of the PRC (early evening) is usually tried, although few data on its use in ASPS exist. Bright light from 7 to 9 PM in elderly subjects with sleep maintenance complaints resulted in a phase advance and reduced awakenings.[56]

Melatonin given in the early morning, usually upon awakening, could in theory result in a phase delay, although no data exist on its use in this situation.[39] The sedating effects of melatonin—which can be variable in patients—may limit its usefulness in this regard.

Non–24-Hour Sleep-Wake Syndrome

Non–24-h sleep-wake syndrome (also known as hypernychthemeral syndrome) is believed to be the result of a circadian pacemaker that has no stable phase relation at all to the 24-h LD cycle. Since most people must maintain a regular sleep-wake schedule, the clinical picture is that of periodically recurring problems with sleep initiation, sleep maintenance, and rising, as the circadian cycle of wakefulness and sleep propensity marches through the fixed sleep period time.[57] Without social constraints, sleep onset and wake times are often successively delayed each day (hence the term *hypernychthemeral*), analogous to the free-running state created when all zeitgebers are removed.[58, 59] Because the duration and quality of sleep depend on when it occurs in relation to the circadian cycle,[36] phase "jumps" between two physiologically permissive periods for sustained sleep can be observed.[60–62]

Epidemiology

Non–24-h sleep-wake syndrome is rare and occurs most often in totally blind people.[57, 59, 63–66] In one series, 50% of totally blind subjects had free-running plasma melatonin rhythms[63]; in another, 73% were not entrained to a 24-h sleep-wake rhythm.[67] A number of cases of non–24-h sleep-wake syndrome have been reported in sighted individuals.

Pathogenesis

The cause of non–24-h sleep-wake cycle is not known. Reduced sensitivity to the entraining effects of light is likely the major etiological factor in totally blind individuals, although nonphotic time cues, such as an externally imposed 24-h sleep-wake cycle, also appeared insufficient to entrain the normal free-running period of one totally blind patient.[57] The melatonin rhythm may be damped[68] or nonexistent,[69] or may be normal but delayed.[58, 65] Coexistent mental retardation, which could make it difficult to process social time cues, may contribute to the symptoms in some individuals.[64]

Some totally blind people without conscious perception of light nevertheless exhibit normal suppression of melatonin when exposed to very bright light and do not appear to have sleep difficulties,[67] indicating the existence of a nonvisual photic entrainment system.[6, 67] Sighted individuals may have a reduced sensitivity to the phase-resetting effects of light[58] and may have an increased incidence of psychiatric conditions such as depression or certain personality disorders, which could potentiate the development of the syndrome by changing or removing social time cues.[58]

Non–24-h sleep-wake cycles have developed after chronotherapy for apparent DSPS,[58, 60, 70] prompting the proposal that such therapy could prolong the free-running period to the point where it becomes unentrainable to a 24-h cycle.[70] However, free-running periods that are too short (less than 23 h) or too long (greater than 27 h)[8] for stable entrainment to a 24-h cycle have never been demonstrated in human beings. Because individuals with DSPS tend to receive more light exposure in the delay (late afternoon) portion of their PRC than during the advance portion (early morning), progressive phase delays may sometimes be observed and mistaken for a hypernychthemeral or non–24-h process.[1, 58]

Diagnosis

A sleep log or actigraphy is usually necessary to demonstrate the lack of a relation between the sleep-wake cycle and the 24-h day. Close analysis may reveal two distinct sleep-wake cycle periods, alternation between which can be manifested by phase jumps.[61, 62] Sleep efficiency by actigraphy and polysomnography is usually normal.[58] Overriding behavioral factors predisposing to irregular sleep-wake cycles (substance abuse, dementia, personality or affective disorders) should be considered.

Therapy

Melatonin appears to be emerging as the initial treatment of choice in non–24-h sleep-wake syndrome in blind,[18, 59, 64–66, 71] as well as sighted, patients.[58] Administration is started when the patient's free-running period approaches the normal or desired phase (i.e., sleep-onset times of 10 to 11 PM). Doses sufficient for phase shifting (0.1 to 0.5 mg) are then given at 8 to 9 PM, or near the likely DLMO.[58, 66] Initiating evening dosing when the free-running period is not in the "normal" phase could result in an inappropriate delay or advance of circadian phase, and prolonging the time to entrainment. Bright-light entrainment is an option in sighted patients, or in blind patients who exhibit intact photic suppression of melatonin.[72] Vitamin B[12] has been anecdotally reported to be effective,[48, 73] although the mechanism is unknown. Its role is unclear, particularly as it appears to have no significant clock-resetting activity in patients with DSPS.[74] Benzodiazepines have not been systematically studied; several anecdotal reports of their possible partial effectiveness exist.[48, 73] Entrainment by nonphotic stimuli (e.g., structured social cues) has not been successful.

CONCLUSION

Disorders of the sleep-wake cycle attributed to the disruption of the circadian timing system are characterized by an abnormal temporal distribution of the major sleep period within our 24-h day. Although there is evidence that many of these disorders are the result of alterations in the circadian clock, more studies are needed to confirm this theory. The impact of these disorders is probably larger than estimated, in terms of numbers, misdiagnoses, and health consequences. Most sleep clinics do not yet provide specific diagnostic tools to assess circadian rhythm profiles. Furthermore, many of the proposed therapies, including light, are often considered experimental by the health insurance industry. Application of our expanding knowledge of basic human circadian and sleep physiology to clinical practice remains an important challenge.

References

1. Richardson GS, Malin HV. Circadian rhythm sleep disorders: pathophysiology and treatment. J Clin Neurophysiol. 1996;13:17–31.
2. Vitaterna MH, King DP, Chang AM, et al. Mutagenesis and mapping of a mouse gene, Clock, essential for circadian behavior. Science. 1994;264:719–725.
3. Ralph MR, Foster RG, Davis FC, et al. Transplanted suprachiasmatic nucleus determines circadian period. Science. 1990;247:975–978.
4. Ralph MR, Menaker M. A mutation of the circadian system in golden hamsters. Science. 1988;241:1225–1227.
5. Lehman MN, Silver R, Gladstone WR, et al. Circadian rhythmicity restored by neural transplant. Immunocytochemical characterization of the graft and its integration with the host brain. J Neurosci. 1987;7:1626–1638.
6. Campbell SS, Murphy PJ. Extraocular circadian phototransduction in humans [see comments]. Science. 1998;279:396–399.
7. Pittendrigh CS. Circadian organization and the photoperiodic phenomena. In: Follett BK, Follett DG, eds. Biological Clocks in Seasonal Reproductive Cycles. Bristol, England: John Wright & Sons; 1981.
8. Czeisler CA, Kronauer RE, Allan JS, et al. Bright light induction of strong (type 0) resetting of the human circadian pacemaker. Science. 1989;244:1328–1333.
9. Czeisler CA, Allan JS, Strogatz SH, et al. Bright light resets the human circadian pacemaker independent of the timing of the sleep-wake cycle. Science. 1986;233:667–671.
10. Lewy AJ, Wehr TA, Goodwin FK, et al. Light suppresses melatonin secretion in humans. Science. 1980;210:1267–1269.
11. Aschoff J, Fatranska M, Giedke H, et al. Human circadian rhythms in continuous darkness: entrainment by social cues. Science. 1971;171:213–215.
12. Honma K, Honma S, Nakamura K, et al. Differential effects of bright light and social cues on reentrainment of human circadian rhythms. Am J Physiol. 1995;268(2 pt 2):R528–535.
13. Van Reeth O, Sturis J, Byrne MM, et al. Nocturnal exercise phase delays circadian rhythms of melatonin and thyrotropin secretion in normal men. Am J Physiol. 1994;266(6 pt 1):E964–974.

14. Mouton A, Penev PD, Ruth A, et al. The effects of timed bright light exposure on temperature, mood and performance rhythms in the elderly. Sleep Res. 1996;25:563.

15. Vanecek J, Pavlik A, Illnerova H. Hypothalamic melatonin receptor sites revealed by autoradiography. Brain Res. 1987;435:359–362.

16. Weaver DR, Stehle JH, Stopa EG, et al. Melatonin receptors in human hypothalamus and pituitary: implications for circadian and reproductive responses to melatonin. J Clin Endocrinol Metab. 1993;76:295–301.

17. Redman J, Armstrong S, Ng KT. Free-running activity rhythms in the rat: entrainment by melatonin. Science. 1983;219:1089–1091.

18. Sack RL, Lewy AJ, Blood ML, et al. Melatonin administration to blind people: phase advances and entrainment. J Biol Rhythms. 1991;6:249–261.

19. Lewy AJ, Sack RL, Blood ML, et al. Melatonin marks circadian phase position and resets the endogenous circadian pacemaker in humans. Ciba Found Symp. 1995;183:303–317.

20. Weitzman ED, Czeisler CA, Coleman RM, et al. Delayed sleep phase syndrome: a biological rhythm sleep disorder. Sleep Res. 1979;8:221.

21. Weitzman ED, Czeisler CA, Coleman RM, et al. Delayed sleep phase syndrome. A chronobiological disorder with sleep-onset insomnia. Arch Gen Psychiatry. 1981;38:737–746.

22. Czeisler CA, Richardson GS, Coleman RM, et al. Chronotherapy: resetting the circadian clocks of patients with delayed sleep phase insomnia. Sleep. 1981;4:1–21.

23. Horne JA, Ostberg O. A self-assessment questionnaire to determine morningness-eveningness in human circadian rhythms. Int J Chronobiol. 1976;4:97–110.

24. Thorpy MJ, Korman E, Spielman AJ, et al. Delayed sleep phase syndrome in adolescents. J Adolesc Health. 1988;9:22–27.

25. Alvarez B, Dahlitz MJ, Vignau J, et al. The delayed sleep phase syndrome: clinical and investigative findings in 14 subjects. J Neurol Neurosurg Psychiatry. 1992;55:665–670.

26. Regestein QR, Monk TH. Delayed sleep phase syndrome: a review of its clinical aspects. Am J Psychiatry. 1995;152:602–608.

27. Pelayo R, Thorpy M, Govinski P. Prevalence of delayed sleep phase syndrome among adolescents. Sleep Res. 1988;17:392.

28. Ando K, Kripke DF, Ancoli-Israel S. Estimated prevalence of delayed and advanced sleep phase syndromes. Sleep Res. 1995;24:509.

29. deBeck TW. Delayed sleep phase syndrome—criminal offense in the military? Mil Med. 1990;155:14–15.

30. Ito A, Ando K, Hayakawa T, et al. Long-term course of adult patients with delayed sleep phase syndrome. Jpn J Psychiatry Neurol. 1993;47(3):563–567.

31. Czeisler CA, Richardson GS, Zimmerman JC, et al. Entrainment of human circadian rhythms by light-dark cycles: a reassessment. Photochem Photobiol. 1981;34:239–247.

32. Pittendrigh CS, Daan S. A functional analysis of circadian pacemakers in rodents, II: the variability of phase response curves. J Comp Physiol. 1976;106:253–266.

33. Lingjaerde O, Bratlid T, Hansen T. Insomnia during the "dark period" in northern Norway. An explorative, controlled trial with light treatment. Acta Psychiatr Scand. 1985;71:506–512.

34. King DP, Zhao Y, Sangoram AM, et al. Positional cloning of the mouse circadian clock gene. Cell. 1997;89:641–653.

35. Dahlitz M, Alvarez B, Vignau J, et al. Delayed sleep phase syndrome response to melatonin. Lancet. 1991;337:1121–1124.

36. Czeisler CA, Weitzman ED, Moore-Ede M, et al. Human sleep: its duration and organization depend on its circadian phase. Science. 1980;210:1264–1267.

37. Ozaki N, Iwata T, Itoh A, et al. Body temperature monitoring in subjects with delayed sleep phase syndrome. Neuropsychobiology. 1988;20:174–177.

38. Lewy AJ, Sack RL. The dim light melatonin onset as a marker for circadian phase position. Chronobiol Int. 1989;6:93–102.

39. Lewy AJ, Ahmed S, Sack RL. Phase shifting the human circadian clock using melatonin. Behav Brain Res. 1996;73:131–134.

40. Minors DS, Waterhouse JM, Wirz-Justice A. A human phase-response curve to light. Neurosci Lett. 1991;133:36–40.

41. Lewy AJ, Sack RL, Singer CM. Treating phase typed chronobiologic sleep and mood disorders using appropriately timed bright artificial light. Psychopharmacol Bull. 1985;21:368–372.

42. Lewy AJ, Sack RL, Singer CM. Melatonin, light and chronobiological disorders. Ciba Found Symp. 1985;117:231–252.

43. Akata T, Sekiguchi S, Takahashi M, et al. Successful combined treatment with vitamin B_{12} and bright artificial light of one case with delayed sleep phase syndrome. Jpn J Psychiatry Neurol. 1993;47:439–440.

44. Weyerbrock A, Timmer J, Hohagen F, et al. Effects of light and chronotherapy on human circadian rhythms in delayed sleep phase syndrome: cytokines, cortisol, growth hormone, and the sleep-wake cycle. Biol Psychiatry. 1996;40:794–797.

45. Rosenthal NE, Joseph-Vanderpool JR, Levendosky AA, et al. Phase-shifting effects of bright morning light as treatment for delayed sleep phase syndrome. Sleep. 1990;13:354–361.

46. Regestein QR, Pavlova M. Treatment of delayed sleep phase syndrome. Gen Hosp Psychiatry. 1995;17:335–345.

47. Lewy AJ, Ahmed S, Jackson JM, et al. Melatonin shifts human circadian rhythms according to a phase-response curve. Chronobiol Int. 1992;9:380–392.

48. Okawa M, Mishima K, Nanami T, et al. Vitamin B_{12} treatment for sleep-wake rhythm disorders. Sleep. 1990;13:15–23.

49. Ozaki N, Iwata T, Itoh A, et al. A treatment trial of delayed sleep phase syndrome with triazolam. Jpn J Psychiatry Neurol. 1989;43:51–55.

50. Kamei R, Hughes L, Miles L, et al. Advanced sleep phase syndrome studied in a time isolation facility. Chronobiologia. 1979;6:115.

51. Billiard M, Verge M, Aldaz C, et al. A case of advanced sleep-phase syndrome. Sleep Res. 1993;22:109.

52. Moldofsky H, Musisi S, Phillipson EA. Treatment of a case of advanced sleep phase syndrome by phase advance chronotherapy. Sleep. 1986;9:61–65.

53. Czeisler CA, Dumont M, Duffy JF, et al. Association of sleep-wake habits in older people with changes in output of circadian pacemaker. Lancet. 1992;340:933–936.

54. Weitzman ED, Moline ML, Czeisler CA, et al. Chronobiology of aging: Temperature, sleep-wake rhythms and entrainment. Neurobiol Aging. 1982;3:299–309.

55. Wagner DR. Disorders of the circadian sleep-wake cycle. Neurol Clin. 1996;14:651–670.

56. Campbell SS, Dawson D, Anderson MW. Alleviation of sleep maintenance insomnia with timed exposure to bright light. J Am Geriat Soc. 1993;41:829–836.

57. Klein T, Martens H, Dijk DJ, et al. Circadian sleep regulation in the absence of light perception: chronic non-24-hour circadian rhythm sleep disorder in a blind man with a regular 24-hour sleep-wake schedule. Sleep. 1993;16:333–343.

58. McArthur AJ, Lewy AJ, Sack RL. Non–24-hour sleep-wake syndrome in a sighted man: circadian rhythm studies and efficacy of melatonin treatment. Sleep. 1996;19:544–553.

59. Lapierre O, Dumont M. Melatonin treatment of a non–24-hour sleep-wake cycle in a blind retarded child. Biol Psychiatry. 1995;38:119–122.

60. Kokkoris CP, Weitzman ED, Pollak CP, et al. Long-term ambulatory temperature monitoring in a subject with a hypernychthemeral sleep-wake cycle disturbance. Sleep. 1978;1:177–190.

61. Wollman M, Lavie P. Hypernychthemeral sleep-wake cycle: some hidden regularities. Sleep. 1986;9:324–334.

62. Uchiyama M, Okawa M, Ozaki S, et al. Delayed phase jumps of sleep onset in a patient with non–24-hour sleep-wake syndrome. Sleep. 1996;19:637–640.

63. Sack RL, Lewy AJ, Blood ML, et al. Circadian rhythm abnormalities in totally blind people: incidence and clinical significance. J Clin Endocrinol Metab. 1992;75:127–134.

64. Palm L, Blennow G, Wetterberg L. Correction of non-24-hour sleep/wake cycle by melatonin in a blind retarded boy. Ann Neurol. 1991;29:336–339.

65. Palm L, Blennow G, Wetterberg L. Long-term melatonin treatment in blind children and young adults with circadian sleep-wake disturbances. Dev Med Child Neurol. 1997;39:319–325.

66. Tzischinsky O, Pal I, Epstein R, et al. The importance of timing in melatonin administration in a blind man. J Pineal Res. 1992;12:105–108.

67. Czeisler CA, Shanahan TL, Klerman EB, et al. Suppression of melatonin secretion in some blind patients by exposure to bright light [see comments]. N Engl J Med. 1995;332:6–11.

68. Nakamura K, Hashimoto S, Honma S, et al. A sighted man with non–24-hour sleep-wake syndrome shows damped plasma melatonin rhythm. Psychiatry Clin Neurosci. 1997;51:115–119.

69. Tomoda A, Miike T, Uezono K, et al. A school refusal case with biological rhythm disturbance and melatonin therapy. Brain Dev. 1994;16:71–76.

70. Oren DA, Wehr TA. Hypernychthemeral syndrome after chronotherapy for delayed sleep phase syndrome [letter]. N Engl J Med. 1992;327:1762.

71. Arendt J, Aldhous M, Wright J. Synchronisation of a disturbed sleep-wake cycle in a blind man by melatonin treatment [letter]. Lancet. 1988;1:772–773.

72. Hoban TM, Sack RL, Lewy AJ, et al. Entrainment of a free-running human with bright light? Chronobiol Int. 1989;6:347–353.

73. Kamgar-Parsi B, Wehr TA, Gillin JC. Successful treatment of human non–24-hour sleep-wake syndrome. Sleep. 1983;6:257–264.

74. Okawa M, Takahashi K, Egashira K, et al. Vitamin B_{12} treatment for delayed sleep phase syndrome: a multi-center double-blind study. Psychiatry Clin Neurosci. 1997;51:275–279.

nine

Insomnia

Frank J. Zorick

Evaluation and Management of Insomnia: An Overview

Frank J. Zorick
James K. Walsh

The International Classification of Sleep Disorders[1] defines insomnia as "difficulty in initiating and/or maintaining sleep." Many variations on this definition have been proposed or used in research, and a consensus definition of insomnia has not been reached. A recent working group of the National Center for Sleep Disorders Research stated, "Insomnia is an experience of inadequate or poor quality sleep characterized by one or more of the following: difficulty falling asleep, difficulty maintaining sleep, waking up too early in the morning, nonrefreshing sleep." Insomnia also involves daytime consequences, such as "tiredness, lack of energy, difficulty concentrating, irritability."[2]

The definition of insomnia is not solely a semantic issue or just a conceptual one because the definition used will influence prevalence estimates and associated morbidity rates and calculations of the economic impact of insomnia. In this chapter, _insomnia, difficulty sleeping, sleep problem_, and other similar terms are used interchangeably. Until the threshold of clinically significant sleep disturbance is established and the actual morbidity rate is elucidated, it probably is best to be inclusive in discussions of the prevalence and consequences of insomnia.

EPIDEMIOLOGY

Prevalence

Population prevalence information has largely been obtained through questionnaire and interview surveys inquiring about "difficulty sleeping" without regard to clinical significance or causal factors. Although there is considerable variability in prevalence estimates among studies, this is likely related to the different methodologies used. There is little population-based information on the prevalence of the various diagnostic categories or subtypes of insomnia. Moreover, no study has addressed the issue of clinical significance; that is, when is a report of "difficulty sleeping" pathological, or at what point is medical attention warranted? Nevertheless, insomnia is highly prevalent given the research methods used.

Since the 1980s, a number of investigations have addressed the prevalence of sleep difficulty in the United States. Depending on the exact question and the time frame involved, the prevalence of "difficulty with sleep" ranges from approximately 10 to 50%. Two interview studies inquiring about sleep difficulty "in the past year" in representative national samples of noninstitutionalized adults, 18 to 79 years old, provided estimates of 35% and 34%.[3, 4] Further questioning showed that 17% and 15% indicated that the sleep problem bothered them "a lot." Two surveys of representative samples of the adult U.S. population conducted by the Gallup Organization[5, 6] that asked whether respondents had "ever had difficulty sleeping" reported prevalence rates of 36% and 49%. The same studies found that 9% and 12% reported "regular" or "frequent" sleep difficulty. An earlier study,[7] conducted on a representative national sample, that asked about satisfaction with sleep reported 17% of the sample to be "somewhat or very dissatisfied." The World Health Organization Collaborative Study,[8] which was conducted in 14 countries, found that 15% of general health care attendees had a period of 2 weeks or longer when nearly every night they had "trouble falling asleep or staying asleep."

Ford and Kamerow[9] used a more stringent definition of sleep disturbance to estimate insomnia prevalence in a 6-month time period for those 18 years and older in community samples. Specifically, they required "trouble falling asleep, staying asleep, or waking up too early" that (1) lasted for at least 2 weeks; (2) interfered with their life a lot; and (3) was not always the result of medical illness, medication, or drug/alcohol use; and (4) about which a professional was informed or medications were taken. With this definition, 10.2% of the sample were said to have insomnia and 3% continued to have insomnia at a second interview 1 year later. Another study[10] with rigorous criteria for an insomnia diagnosis examined 1962 consecutive patients in a primary care setting. The insomnia criteria were one or more of the following current symptoms "nearly every night": (1) at least 2 hours to fall asleep, (2) lying awake at least 1 hour, or (3) waking at least 2 hours early. Ten percent of the primary care population reported at least one of these symptoms.

Ohayon,[11] in 1997, published estimates of the various diagnostic subtypes of insomnia based on a representative sample of the French population. A computerized diagnostic tool guided the interviews of 5622 subjects. A total of 12.7% of the sample met the definition of insomnia used in the study (i.e., a sleep complaint lasting 1 month or longer that caused "clinically significant distress or impairment in social, occupational, or other important area of functioning"). Based on the presence or absence of coexisting illnesses, Ohayon estimated the following prevalence rates for subtypes of insomnia: related to a mental disorder, 10.3%; primary, 1.3%; related to a general medical condition, 0.5%; circadian disorder 0.3%; and substance use, 0.2%.

We conclude from these investigations that a reasonable prevalence estimate for chronic insomnia is about 10%. When considering insomnia of any duration or severity, between 30% and 50% of the general population appears to be affected.

Demographics

Both female sex and older age are associated with increased rates of reported sleep difficulty. Virtually all of the investigations cited above indicate that women are about 1.3 times more likely to report insomnia-like sleep problems than are men. Nevertheless, sex differences are small or nonexistent between individuals 20 to 40 years old.

Studies that include samples spanning a wide age range find that the elderly (i.e., older than 65 years) generally have approximately 1.5 times higher prevalence rates of sleep difficulty compared with adults younger than 65 years. Studies specific to older adult populations provide consistent data. A study of a rural community sample of persons 66 to 97 years old found that approximately 50% had at least one insomnia-like complaint "sometimes" or "usually" per year.[12] When restricting the estimate only to those stating they "usually" have one of those complaints, the prevalence fell to less than 20%. Foley et al.[13] examined sleep problems in three community cohorts older than 65 years via the use of interviews. In that study, 42.7% of the sample reported sleep difficulty "most of the time."

Children and adolescents also experience insomnia. In young children, parents are responsible for the identification of a problem. For children 6 months to 2 years old, prevalence rates are roughly 20 to 30%.[14–16] This appears to decrease so that at ages 4 to 8, 10 to 15% have some difficulty with sleep. The prevalence estimates for adolescents are similar to those for adults. Prevalence rates of insomnia in childhood and adolescents do not appear to differ between sexes. Insomnia in children and adolescents is covered in the companion volume to this textbook.[17]

CONSEQUENCES AND CO-MORBIDITY

Relatively little is known about the complications of insomnia or the natural history of insomnia. When co-morbid factors have been identified or postulated, the direction of cause and effect, if any, remains unclear. The natural history of insomnia and the associated complications are likely to differ depending on the chronicity of the problem as well as the diagnostic subtype. Several research areas have been pursued and are summarized here.

Behavioral

Transient insomnia is usually accompanied by reports of daytime sleepiness and performance impairment the next day. This is not surprising because individuals experiencing transient insomnia are usually normal sleepers and the effects of sleep loss on waking function in normal sleepers is well documented (see Chapter 54).

A number of studies have shown that persons reporting more persistent insomnia attribute poor waking function to poor sleep.[3–7] In a nationally representative sample, 27% were negatively affected by poor sleep at least 2 days per week.[7] For those dissatisfied with their sleep, this percentage increased to 70%. A later study[5] found that insomniacs report poor performance at work, memory difficulties, concentration problems, and twice as many fatigue-related automobile accidents as do good sleepers. The latter finding was not replicated in the 1995 study.[6] Nevertheless, there is some additional evidence that accident rates in general[7] and drowsy driving are increased in individuals with poor sleep.[18] A longitudinal study of Navy personnel found that poor sleepers earned fewer promotions, remained at lower pay levels, and received fewer recommendations for reenlistment.[19] Academic performance may also be worse in insomniacs; 21% of poorly sleeping preadolescents had failed at school compared with 11% of good sleepers.[20] Perceived sleep quality was reported to be positively associated with academic performance in medical school.[21]

A small number of laboratory studies of the alertness and performance of chronic insomniacs have found objective deficits in semantic memory, daytime vigilance, and gait and balance[22–25]; however, other investigations have found no differences between insomniacs and noninsomniacs.[26–30] Insomniacs are usually recruited for participation in these laboratory studies, and there is evidence that recruited subjects may not be representative of insomnia patients seeking medical attention.[31] Moreover, the studies generally include insomnia patients or subjects without medical or psychiatric conditions, many of whom would be diagnosed with psychophysiological or primary insomnia. "Hyperarousal" in some subtypes of insomnia may prevent or obscure the deficits that accompany sleep loss.[24, 32] Finally, there are studies of chronic insomnia associated with arthritis[33] and periodic limb movement disorder[34] that show an increase in daytime alertness when sleep is improved with the use of a short-acting hypnotic.

Psychiatric

Information from a variety of sources demonstrates the association between insomnia and psychiatric conditions. The *Diagnostic and Statistical Manual of Mental Disorders, Fourth Edition* (DSM-IV), includes sleep difficulty as a symptom among the diagnostic criteria for several disorders, including major depression, generalized anxiety, and post-traumatic stress.[35] Studies of patients in sleep medicine clinics show that psychiatric illness is common.[36, 37] Samples of unselected psychiatric patients have about a three-fold increase in the frequency of insomnia compared with healthy control subjects and the insomnia severity correlates with the intensity of the psychiatric symptoms.[38] Among samples of outpatients who consulted their general practitioners for insomnia, about 50% presented with psychiatric conditions, and about half of these patients were probably depressed.[39, 40]

Epidemiological research indicates that the prevalence of any psychiatric disorder is two or three times higher in those with insomnia. The risk of depression as a co-morbid state appears to be particularly strong, approximately four times more likely in insomnia patients.[3, 9] Furthermore, a complaint of insomnia may be an early marker for psychiatric disorders such as depression, anxiety conditions, and alcohol abuse.[9] These data raise the possibility that treatment of insomnia may reduce the risk for psychological conditions.

Anxiety has been found to quite common in insomnia patients compared with the general population. Depending on the methods used, about 25 to 40% of insomnia patients are judged to have significant anxiety.[2, 9, 12, 36] Alcohol abuse and other substance abuse is increased in insomniacs relative to good sleepers.[9, 40] The risk for developing new anxiety disorders and alcohol abuse is greater for insomniacs than for noninsomniacs.

Medical

Insomnia has been statistically associated with various medical conditions, including disorders of the cardiovascular, respiratory, gastrointestinal, renal, and musculoskeletal systems (see Section 13). The role of insomnia in the development of various medical conditions has begun to receive attention. For example, in a study of 10,778 men and women 35 to 59 years old, poor sleepers were more than twice as likely as good sleepers to have ischemic heart disease in the next 6 years, and for men, the risk remained significantly higher after controlling for the effects of age, life satisfaction, and neuroticism.[41] Recently, primary insomnia patients have been shown to have impaired immune system function.[42, 43]

Mortality Risk

A small number of epidemiological studies demonstrate increased mortality rates for those who report sleeping less than either 6 or 7 hours per night after controlling for other risk factors.[44, 45] Having "insomnia" often statistically increased the risk of death.[46] One study found that reduced sleep time is a greater mortality risk than smoking, hypertension, and cardiac disease.[46] Sleep disturbance is one of the leading predictors of institutionalization in the elderly, and severe insomnia triples the mortality risk in elderly men.[47] These provocative findings suggest the need for systematic investigation of the link between insomnia, short sleep, and death.

EVALUATION METHODS

Initial Sleep History

The first and most important aspect of the evaluation is the clinical interview and sleep history (Table 53–1). From this initial encounter with the patient, the clinician develops the differential diagnosis and treatment plan. The nature and development of the sleep problem must be elicited. Attention must be paid to daytime symptoms as well as to the complaints about sleep. During this encounter, it will become evident whether the sleep problem is transient or persistent. Furthermore, associated medical and psychiatric disorders or symptoms will be determined. Inquiry about the use of medications, caffeine, alcohol, or recreational drugs is important. The majority of insomnias are secondary to a medical, psychiatric, or behavioral disorder[48]; therefore, the interviewer must inquire carefully and consider thoroughly the possible causes outlined below.

Table 53–1. SLEEP HISTORY IN INSOMNIA PATIENTS

Type of Insomnia

Transient, short term, or acute
Persistent, long term, or chronic
Intermittent

Sleep Pattern

Sleep-onset insomnia
Difficulty maintaining sleep
Early morning awakening
Nonrestorative sleep

Associated Events

Medical illness, medications
Psychosocial stress
Mood changes
Immediate precipitants

Previous Sleep History

Previous sleep quality
Previous episodes of insomnia
Similarity to present problem
Response to treatment

Sleep Hygiene History

Bedtime and arising time
Variations on days off and workdays
Shiftwork or circadian changes
Napping behavior
Exercise, lifestyle
Caffeine, alcohol, substance use

History From Bedpartner

Snoring, irregular breathing
Movements during sleep
Estimates of patient's sleep quality and length
Changes in mood and performance of patient

Medical History

After detailing the nature and development of the sleep complaint, the focus of the interview shifts to the medical history. Sleep is affected by pain and discomfort associated with most medical disorders.[49] Particular attention should be directed to possible rheumatological, pulmonary, cardiac, renal, and neurological disorders. Medication side effects commonly affect sleep symptoms. When the sleep complaint and the course of an illness or a medication regimen are linked historically, a causal relationship is suspected. Often, insomnia will begin coincident with the symptoms of another medical problem or a hospitalization. This will require further investigation to determine causal significance.

Neuropsychiatric History

The most common cause of insomnia is a psychiatric disorder, and a persistent insomnia may predate the development of an affective illness by 1 year or longer.[40, 48] It is important to consider whether a psychiatric disorder is primary in the insomnia complaint. Sleep complaints accompany most, if not all, psychiatric and neurological illnesses, especially anxiety disorders, mood disorders, psychoses, dementia, headache,

convulsive disorders, and movement disorders. Psychoactive drugs whether misused or used therapeutically have great potential for the induction of sleep complaints, particularly insomnia.[50, 51]

Physical Examination

An investigation of the symptoms and confirmation of a medical disorder will occur with examination of the patient. The physician must be able to reasonably explain to the patient whether the insomnia symptom is related to a medical disorder, and this credibly requires a physical examination. In addition, clinical laboratory evaluation or specialty consultation may be required to establish this cause. The physician will look for signs of other sleep disorders such as sleep apnea, which can present as insomnia.[51] For example, the patient's weight, blood pressure, neck size, and appearance of the oropharynx may increase suspicion of sleep disordered breathing (see Chapters 74 and 79).

Mental Status Examination

The sensitivity of the examiner to neuropsychological issues must be high when evaluating an insomnia patient. It is extremely important to include a psychiatric interview with mental status examination as a part of the evaluation of insomnia. Particular attention will be paid to symptoms of anxiety and mood, as well as an assessment of memory, orientation, and cognitive abilities. Subsequently, either dementia or depression may become a significant part of the differential diagnosis. In addition, medications used in treatment of the insomnia have effects on mental status that should be investigated during the evaluation.

The mental status examination describes the present state of psychological functioning of the patient. To accomplish this evaluation requires the establishment of rapport with the patient and cannot be done in a hasty manner. The skillful interviewer not only elicits pertinent information from the patient but also sets the foundation for the physician-patient relationship in later visits. The interaction should avoid technical terms and allow the patient room for self-expression. Observation by the physician of the patient's behavior, activity, attitude, and appearance is an important aspect of the examination.

The examination explores the patient's mood and affect, speech, perception, thought process and content, orientation and cognition, and judgment and insight. The Mini-Mental Status Examination[52] is a brief screening test that assesses orientation, memory, language and intellectual function and is particularly useful in the evaluation of cognitive disorders. *Mood* is defined as sustained and pervasive emotion and is described, for example, as depressed, anxious, joyful, or angry. *Affect* is the patient's present emotional function, which is assessed by the interviewer's observation of the patient's demeanor, facial expression, voice, and nonverbal behaviors. Mood and affect may not be congruent, and this is important to note. Questions such as "How do you feel now?" or "What do you fear the most?" or "How long have you felt this way?" are used to evaluate mood and affect.[53] The sleep physician may consider referral for psychometric evaluation or psychiatric and neurological consultation if the mental status evaluation of the sleep-disordered patient discovers pertinent and significant abnormalities.

Questionnaries and Sleep Diary

Standardized sleep disorder questionnaires are routinely administered to ensure uniform collection of information about the patient's sleep and medical history and associated behavioral and neuropsychological symptoms. The collection of the patient's sleep diary is mandatory when evaluating and treating insomnia.[51, 54] A sleep diary is a record maintained by the patient of sleep-relevant behaviors, such as medications, alcohol use, mood on arising, bedtime and arising times, awakenings, total sleep time, and napping. Patients learn about events and behaviors that are affecting their sleep. This knowledge supports the sleep hygiene education included in the treatment plan of insomnia patients. The sleep diary also is important in monitoring compliance and progress in the treatment.

Psychometric Evaluation

Psychological testing is used as a screening tool or when indicated for more extensive evaluation of neuropsychological symptoms in the patient with insomnia.[55] For screening assessment, mood scales, the Minnesota Multiphasic Personality Inventory, or other self-administered instruments are chosen; these increase the sensitivity of the evaluation concerning associated psychological conditions. More intensive individual testing will, in the indicated patient, increase the diagnostic specificity of the evaluation when psychiatric or neuropsychological diagnoses are suspected.

Physiological Monitoring

There are three types of monitoring of sleep that may contribute to the diagnostic understanding of insomnia. Polysomnography, ambulatory sleep studies, and actigraphy (activity monitoring) have been reported as useful in the evaluation of the sleep-disordered patient. These techniques are used in research protocols of the evaluation and treatment of insomnia[55–59]; however, published clinical standards have not recommended the routine use of physiological recording.[58, 59] Nevertheless, an objective assessment of the patient's sleep should be part of the clinical evaluation in some cases. This decision is based on the preceding evaluation as well as the patient's response to behavioral and pharmacological treatment. If abnormal physiological events in sleep, such as sleep apnea, periodic limb movements, or electroencephalographic abnormalities with arousals are likely etiologic in the insomnia, then polysomnographic monitoring is necessary to confirm this possibility.[51, 55] These abnormalities have medical consequences, in addition to a role in the production of insomnia. The specific role of ambulatory sleep recording in clinical evaluations of insomnia patients is not established.[57] A variety of techniques are used, and the studies may be attended by a technologist. In some cases, the data collected are very similar to that provided by in-laboratory polysomnography; in other cases, the data are difficult to interpret or include limited information. These studies may eventually find a role as screening examinations in the practice of sleep medicine. Standards for actigraphy[59] do not recommend the routine use of actigraphy in a clinical evaluation of disturbed sleep. Actigraphy provides data on multiday activity patterns that can be instructive, particularly for individuals with sleep-wake schedule disorders.[60]

Recent concern about medical costs has influenced the practice standards concerning the use of physiological and objective monitoring in patients with insomnia.[57] On the other hand, although not always diagnostic, monitoring produces a clearer picture of the patient's sleep symptoms by quantifying sleep and related physiology.

CAUSES OF INSOMNIA

The most important concept is that insomnia is a complaint and a symptom and is never the diagnosis. Except for idiopathic (or primary) insomnia and sleep state misperception, this sleep symptom will always be found secondary to a medical, psychiatric, circadian, sleep, behavioral, or environmental disorder. Table 53–2 lists the major differential diagnostic categories of insomnia.[1, 35] The clinician must have a working familiarity with the major causes of insomnia. The primary goal of this section is to acquaint the reader with this conceptual framework so that treatment is rational and planned according to a reasoned diagnosis after a comprehensive evaluation. In addition, the clinician must develop a continuing relationship with the patient. Sometimes, with further interaction and an ongoing evaluation of the patient—in particular, the patient's response to treatment efforts—the diagnostic formulation may change. It is imperative to understand that two or more diagnoses may be relevant and require treatment in the insomnia patient.[50]

In addition to determining the diagnosis as described, it is useful to conceptualize insomnia according to the predisposition and the precipitating and perpetuating factors.[61] Typically, transient, or short-term, insomnia is closely related to a precipitant, which usually makes the cause and treatment plan apparent (see Chapter 54). Typical precipitants are social stress (e.g., divorce, new child, loss, financial difficulty), acute medical stress (e.g., hospitalization, illness, pregnancy, medication side effect), circadian stress (e.g., jet lag, schedule change, shift work), or environmental stress (e.g., new home, travel, noise, bedpartner).

Table 53–2. DIFFERENTIAL DIAGNOSIS
OF INSOMNIA

Psychiatric Disorders (Chapter 56)

Alcoholism, alcohol-dependent sleep disorder
Drug-dependent sleep disorder
Mood disorders
Anxiety disorders
Psychoses

Medical Disorders (Sections 13 and 14)

Respiratory disorders (chronic obstructive pulmonary disease,
  asthma)
Gastroesophageal reflux
Fibromyalgia, other rheumatological diseases

Neurological Disorders (Section 14)

Parkinsonism and other movement disorders
Dementia, degenerative diseases
Cerebrovascular disease
Epilepsy
Headache and other pain syndromes
Fatal familial insomnia

Environmental Disorders (Chapter 54)

Circadian Rhythm Disorders (Section 8)

Time zone change syndrome
Shift work sleep disorder
Delayed or advanced sleep phase syndrome
Irregular sleep pattern

Behavioral Disorders

Psychophysiological insomnia (Chapter 55)
Inadequate sleep hygiene (Chapter 58)
Adjustment sleep disorder

Primary Sleep Disorders

Sleep state misperception (Chapter 55)
Idiopathic insomnia (primary insomnia) (Chapter 55)
Sleep apnea
Restless legs syndrome and periodic limb movements (Chapter 65)
Parasomnias

The development of persistent, or chronic, insomnia is often complex, with a less obvious relationship to a precipitating factor. The precipitant occurred months or years before the evaluation and may no longer be relevant. Predisposition to insomnia is found to be more important in chronic sleep disturbances. Several research findings support predisposition to insomnia that is most often characterized as "hyperarousal."[24, 32, 62] This increased arousal might be physiological, cognitive, or affective; it is likely that these categories overlap. This concept is supported by research findings, such as increased alertness on the multiple sleep latency test, increased heart rate during the sleep period, exaggerated "first-night" effect, increased anxiety on rating scales, and increased rumination during the period of sleep. There is some agreement that predisposition is a useful concept in understanding insomnia, particularly in the psychophysiological (behavioral) and primary insomnias.[63]

Perpetuating factors are quite important in understanding the transformation of an acute, or short-term, sleep problem into a persistent insomnia. Perpetuating factors are patient behaviors and responses that develop during the sleep difficulty and then prolong the short-term sleep disturbance into a long-term disorder

or reinforce predisposition toward insomnia. Most clinicians recognize sleep hygiene behaviors as important perpetuating factors (see Chapter 58). All insomnia treatment programs offer sleep hygiene education as a component of the plan; however, correction of sleep hygiene behaviors as the sole mode of treatment is unlikely to manage the sleep problem.[54] There is more evidence that other perpetuating factors, such as conditioning (learning), internal arousal, and rumination about sleep, play important roles, particularly in psychophysiological insomnia (see Chapters 55 and 57). Other factors such as the inappropriate use of medications and alcohol, secondary changes in circadian rhythm, development of additional medical or psychological symptoms, loss of motivation, and withdrawal from activities are important perpetuating influences.

To summarize, during the assessment of the insomnia patient, the clinician identifies a working medical diagnosis according to the criteria in the International Classification of Sleep Disorders[1] and the cognitive/behavioral framework within which the sleep problem developed.[61, 63] It is important to determine the presence of diagnoses, such as restless legs syndrome, sleep apnea, major depression, or movement disorders, that will require specific medical treatment. Likewise, chronic insomnia requires a behavioral analysis to address the precipitating and perpetuating factors. The psychiatric diagnosis is identified according to the criteria of the DSM-IV[35] after a psychiatric history and mental status examination are conducted. Each evaluative system improves the accuracy of the assessment, and a specific diagnosis (or diagnoses) improves the effectiveness of the treatment plan.

MANAGEMENT AND TREATMENT

The causes of insomnia are many; likewise, the rational treatment plan is varied. The clinician who evaluates and treats insomnia will need to develop understanding and skill in several areas and ideally will function within a multidisciplinary team. The treatment of insomnia can be divided into six areas: cognitive-behavioral, pharmacological, sleep hygiene education, environmental change, medical treatment, and psychiatric treatment. Just as considering the entire differential diagnosis is necessary, it is important to consider potential benefits of each of these therapeutic modalities. In most cases, the treatment plan will use more than one approach. In this section, there are chapters on behavioral therapy (see Chapter 57), and sleep hygiene (see Chapter 58), and pharmacology is covered in Section 5, medical disorders are covered in Section 13, and psychiatric disorders are covered in Section 14.

It is most important that the clinician present a clear treatment plan with definite objectives and engages the patient in that plan. The clinician must present a positive attitude to the patient and explain to the patient the rationale for each step in the treatment program and how progress will be measured. In most cases, it is particularly helpful to the patient to have a specific written treatment plan that can be referred to while at home. Certain general educational material about insomnia and sleep may be useful, but the patient should feel that the treatment plan is geared to his or her particular sleep difficulty. As treatment progresses, referral to this plan and its implementation will focus the patient on the treatment tasks. It is critical for the patient to keep a sleep diary that charts the progress of the therapy. This action directly engages the patient in the treatment process, measures motivation, and provides feedback to the clinician.

Patients come to the sleep medicine specialist with certain expectations concerning the the use of medication. The assessment of the problem and the diagnosis will ordinarily determine the need for and the length of medication treatment. Medication for the symptomatic relief of the insomnia may be indicated early in treatment because this will allow time to initiate the primary interventions. The role of hypnotic medication in the treatment plan must be discussed with the patient before prescription of the medication to elicit patient reactions and to provide realistic expectations.

Suppression of insomnia symptoms in transient or short-term insomnia with a short-acting hypnotic is beneficial because this treatment decreases the likelihood of untoward changes in sleep hygiene behaviors or other factors that could perpetuate the sleep disturbance (see Chapter 54). Typically, when indicated in the symptomatic treatment of transient or short-term insomnia, hypnotic agents are prescribed for 1 to 4 weeks.

For certain chronic insomnia diagnoses, prolonged medication prescription is recommended. For example, patients with the restless legs syndrome, periodic limb movements in sleep, or some parasomnias (e.g., rapid eye movement behavior disorder, nightmares, sleepwalking) may require prolonged prescription of medications to suppress the symptoms. In certain secondary insomnias, medication that alleviates the primary medical, neurological, or psychiatric disorder may be prescribed for prolonged time periods. Anxiety and mood disorders, movement disorders, degenerative neurological disorders, convulsive disorders, pain syndromes, and rheumatological disorders will often require maintenance medication treatment. In all such cases, the use of other treatment modalities, particularly cognitive-behavoral treatment and sleep hygiene education, will be used conjointly with the medical treatment. In secondary sleep disturbances, the symptomatic use of hypnotic medication may play a role in the short term until the primary disorder is under control. Less commonly, symptomatic relief may be prescribed on a long-term basis if unsatisfactory improvement in the sleep symptoms occurs after adequate treatment of the primary disorder.

In psychophysiological insomnia, sleep state misperception, and idiopathic insomnia, the picture is more complex. The primary mode of treatment in psychophysiological insomnia is cognitive and behavioral therapy with sleep hygiene education; medication is not routinely indicated in the behavioral insomnias. Nevertheless, hypnotic agents may aid the treatment process by providing syptomatic relief during the initi-

ation of the behavioral therapy. Sleep state misperception is poorly understood and difficult to classify. This condition may respond, at times, to sleep hygiene education, behavioral approaches, and sedative-hypnotic medication, although most often, it is resistant to treatment. Idiopathic insomnia is a severe, chronic, often lifelong, recalcitrant sleep disturbance. Treatment with all the methods discussed, including medications, may be necessary for management, but this condition may not respond easily or completely to such treatment efforts. Clearly, research leading to the development of a better understanding and more effective treatments for these chronic, difficult-to-manage insomnias is imperative.

Hypnotic–dependent sleep disorder is possible if prolonged pharmacological treatment of insomnia is undertaken. The physician must be aware of this possibility but should not refuse to prescribe symptomatic relief for this reason alone. A criterion for this disorder is not the use of hypnotic agents per se but rather the demonstration of tolerance, increasing doses, ineffectiveness of usual doses, or intense withdrawal symptoms. Withdrawal symptoms are not simply the return of the original symptoms before medication prescription but an increase in the intensity, nature, and number of symptoms. The consideration of substance use/dependence disorder and alcoholism must be included in the sleep medicine evaluation.[35] These conditions would contraindicate the prescription of sedative-hypnotic agents and are an indication for referral to the appropriate specialist. Avoidance of dose escalation beyond the minimal effective dose may reduce the possibility of hypnotic dependence.

To summarize, the clinician must have a clear understanding that insomnia is a symptom and that differential diagnosis, according to published criteria, is required. The context (social, environmental, and medical) within which the sleep complaint developed should be understood. Familiarity with established treatment modes is necessary, as is the ability to implement the developed plan or to refer the patient to another specialist who will carry out the plan. The sleep specialist must explain the treatment to the patient and assess the patient's understanding, motivation, and ability to participate in the plan. The recognition of the lack of understanding or of motivation on the patient's part by the clinician will lead to further inquiry and resolution of these issues before proceding with the insomnia treatment plan.

EXPECTED BENEFITS OF THE EVALUATION AND MANAGEMENT OF INSOMNIA

The most important benefit of the appropriate management of the symptom of insomnia is an accurate diagnosis that leads to rational and effective treatment. The expected resolution of the sleep problem will reduce the effects on daytime function, performance, and mood. With this improvement, the quality of the patient's life will increase.[64, 65] Furthermore, many of the negative aspects associated with insomnia, as outlined in this chapter, are minimized. The co–morbidities, effects on other medical disorders, substance misuse, and psychological symptoms will be lessened. By decreasing the behaviors and practices that perpetuate the sleep disturbance, it is likely that the degree and persistency of the secondary disability and distress will be reduced. Investigation of the patient's sleep symptoms may lead to an appropriate medical evaluation; this may uncover a significant medical disorder that the insomnia heralded. Likewise, careful attention to the insomnia may discover an unrecognized psychiatric, psychosocial, or behavioral disorder. Treatment may not be successful in all cases. Nevertheless, the physician can comfort the patient, provide a realistic analysis, offer understanding, and minimize the untoward effects of the sleep disorder.[54, 65]

CONCLUSIONS

This introductory chapter presents a conceptual overview and a method for the comprehensive evaluation of the patient with insomnia. As this evaluation progresses and the underlying causes become better understood, treatment will be focused in these areas. The remainder of this section on insomnia is divided into five chapters, and each chapter focuses on an issue related to this clinical problem.

References

1. International Classification of Sleep Disorders. Diagnostic and Coding Manual Revised. Diagnostic Classification Steering Committee, Thorpy MJ, Chairman. Rochester, Minn: American Sleep Disorders Association; 1997.
2. National Heart, Lung, and Blood Institute Working Group on Insomnia. Insomnia: assessment and management in primary care. Am Fam Physician. 1999;59:3029–3038.
3. Mellinger GD, Balter MB, Uhlenhuth EH. Insomnia and its treatment: prevalence and correlates. Arch Gen Psychiatry. 1985;42:225–232.
4. Balter MB, Uhlenhuth EH. New epidemiologic findings about insomnia and its treatment. Clin Psychiatry. 1992;53(12 suppl):34–39.
5. Gallup Organization. Sleep in America. Princeton, NJ: The Gallup Organization; 1991.
6. Gallup Organization. Sleep in America: 1995. Princeton, NJ: The Gallup Organization; 1995.
7. Addison RG, Thorpy MJ, Roehrs TA, et al. Sleep/wake complaints in the general population. Sleep Res. 1991;20:112.
8. Ustun TB, Privett M, Lecrubier Y, et al. Form, frequency and burden of sleep problems in general health care: a report from the WHO Collaborative Study on Psychological Problems in General Health Care. Eur Psychiatry. 1996;11(suppl 1):5S–10S.
9. Ford DE, Kamerow DB. Epidemiologic study of sleep disturbances and psychiatric disorders: an opportunity for prevention. JAMA. 1989;262:1479–1484.
10. Simon GE, VonKorff M. Prevalence, burden, and treatment of insomnia in primary care. Am J Psychiatry. 1997;154:1417–1423.
11. Ohayon MM. Prevalence of DSM-IV diagnostic criteria of insomnia: distinguishing insomnia related to mental disorders from sleep disorders. J Psychiatr Res. 1997;31:333–346.
12. Ganguli M, Reynolds CF, Gilby JE. Prevalence and persistence of sleep complaints in a rural older community sample: the MoVIES project. J Am Geriatr Soc. 1996;44:778–784.
13. Foley DJ, Monjan AA, Brown SL, et al. Sleep complaints among elderly persons: an epidemiologic study of three communities. Sleep. 1995;18:425–432.
14. Richman N. A community survey of characteristics of one to two-year-olds with sleep disruptions. J Am Acad Child Psychiatry. 1981;20:281–291.
15. Richman N. Surveys of sleep disorders in children in a general population. In: Guilleminault C, ed. Sleep and Its Disorders in Children. New York, NY: Raven Press; 1987:1125–1237.
16. Lozoff B, Wolf AW, Davis NS. Sleep problems seen in pediatric practice. Pediatrics. 1985;75:477–483.
17. Ferber R, Kryger M. Principle and Practice of Sleep Medicine in the Child. Philadelphia, Pa: WB Saunders; 1995.
18. Schweitzer PK, Engelhardt CL, Hilliker NA, et al. Consequences of reported poor sleep. Sleep Res. 1992;21:260.
19. Johnson LC, Spinweber CL. Quality of sleep and performance in the Navy: a longitudinal study of good and poor sleepers. In: Guilleminault C, Lugaresi E, eds. Sleep-Wake Disorders: Natural History, Epidemiology, and Long-Term Evolution. New York, NY: Raven Press; 1983:13–28.
20. Blum D, Kahn A, Mozin MJ, et al. Relation between chronic insomnia and school failure in preadolescents. Sleep Res. 1990;19:194.
21. Johns MW, Dudley HAF, Masterson JP. The sleep habits, personality and academic performance of medical students. Med Educ. 1976;10:158–162.
22. Sugerman JL, Stern JA, Walsh JK. Daytime alertness in subjective and objective insomnia: some preliminary findings. Biol Psychiatry. 1985;20:741–750.
23. Mendelson WB, Garnett D, Linnoila M. Do insomniacs have impaired daytime functioning? Biol Psychiatry. 1984;19:1261–1263.
24. Bonnet MH, Arand DL. 24-Hour metabolic rate in insomniacs and matched normal sleepers. Sleep. 1995;18:581–588.
25. Hart R, Morin C, Best A. Neuropsychological performance in elderly insomnia patients. Aging Cognition. 1995;2:268–278.
26. Seidel WF, Ball S, Cohen S, et al. Daytime alertness in relation to mood, performance, and nocturnal sleep in chronic insomniacs and noncomplaining sleepers. Sleep. 1984;7:230–238.
27. Church MW, Johnson LC. Mood and performance of poor sleepers during repeated use of flurazepam. Psychopharmacology. 1979;61:309–316.
28. Stone J, Morin CM, Hart RP, et al. Neuropsychological functioning in older insomniacs with or without obstructive sleep apnea. Psychol Aging. 1994;9:231–236.
29. Adam K, Tomeny M, Oswald I. Physiological and psychological differences between good and poor sleepers. J Psychiatric Res. 1986;20:301–316.
30. Broman JE, Lundh LG, Aleman K, et al. Subjective and objective performance in patients with persistent insomnia. Scand J Behav Ther. 1992;21:115–126.
31. Stepanski E, Koshorek G, Zorick F, et al. Characteristics of individuals who do or do not seek treatment for chronic insomnia. Psychosomatics. 1989;30:421–427.
32. Stepanski E, Zorick F, Roehrs T, et al. Daytime alertness in patients with chronic insomnia compared to asymptomatic controls. Sleep. 1988;11:54–60.
33. Walsh JK, Muehlbach MJ, Lauter SA, et al. Effects of triazolam on sleep, daytime sleepiness and morning stiffness in patients with rheumatoid arthritis. J Rheumatol. 1996;23:245–252.
34. Doghramji K, Browman CP, Gaddy JR, et al. Triazolam diminishes daytime sleepiness and sleep fragmentation in patients with periodic leg movements in sleep. J Clin Psychopharmacol. 1991;11:284–290.
35. Diagnostic and Statistical Manual of Mental Disorders. 4th ed. Washington, DC: American Psychiatric Association; 1994.
36. Tan T, Kales JD, Kales A, et al. Biopsychobehavioral correlates of insomnia IV: diagnoses based on DSM-III. Am J Psychiatry. 1984;141:356–362.
37. Buysee D, Reynolds CF 3rd, Hauri PJ, et al. Diagnostic concordance for DSM-IV sleep disorders: a report from the APA/NIMH DSM-IV field trial. Am J Psychiatry. 1994;151:1351–1360.
38. Sweetwood H, Grant I, Kripke DF, et al. Sleep disorder over time: psychiatric correlates among males. Br J Psychiatry. 1980;136:456–462.
39. Charon F, Dramaix M, Mendlewicz J. Epidemiological survey of

insomnia subjects in a sample of 1,761 outpatients. Biol Psychiatry. 1989;21:109.

40. Schramm E, Hohagen F, Kappler C, et al. Mental comorbidity of chronic insomnia in general practice attenders using DSM-III-R. Acta Psychiatr Scand. 1995;91:10–17.

41. Hyyppa MT, Kronholm E. Quality of sleep and chronic illnesses. J Clin Epidemiol. 1989;42:633–638.

42. Irwin M, Fortner M, Clarl C, et al. Reduction of natural killer cell activity in primary insomnia and in major depression. Sleep Res. 1995;24:256.

43. Irwin M, Lacher U, Caldwell C. Depression reduced natural killer cytotoxicity: a longitudinal study of depressed patients and controls. Psychol Med. 1992;22:1045–1050.

44. Kripke D, Simons R, Garfinkel L, et al. Short and long sleep and sleeping pills: Is increased mortality associated? Arch Gen Psychiatry. 1979;36:103–116.

45. Wingard D, Berkman L. Mortality risk associated with sleeping patterns among adults. Sleep. 1983;6:102–107.

46. Kripke D, Ancoli-Israel S, Fell R, et al. Health risk of insomnia. In: Peter JH, Penzel T, Podszus T, et al, eds. Sleep and Health Risk. Heidelberg, Germany: Springer-Verlag; 1991:547–554.

47. Pollack C, Perlick D, Linsner J, et al. Sleep problems in community elderly as predictors of death and nursing home placement. J Community Health. 1990;15:123–135.

48. Nowell PD, Buysse DJ, Reynolds CF III, et al. Clinical factors contributing to the differential diagnosis of primary insomnia and insomnia related to mental disordes. Am J Psychiatry. 1997;154:1412–1416.

49. Mahowald MW, Mahowald ML, Bundlie SR, et al. Sleep fragmentation in rheumatoid arthritis. Arthritis Rheum. 1989;32:974–983.

50. Kupfer DJ, Reynolds CF III. Management of insomnia. N Engl J Med. 1997;336:341–346.

51. Buysse DJ, Reynolds CF III, Kupfer DJ, et al. Clinical diagnoses in 216 insomnia patients using ICSD, DSM IV, and ICD 10 categories. Sleep. 1994;17:630–637.

52. Folstein MF, Folstein S, McHugh PR. Mini-Mental State: a practical method for grading the cognitive state of patients for the clinician. J Psychiatr Res. 1975;12:189–198.

53. Kaplan HI, Sadock BJ. Concise Textbook of Clinical Psychiatry. Baltimore, Md: Williams & Wilkins; 1996.

54. Morin CM, Culbert JP, Schwartz SM. Nonpharmacological interventions for insomnia: a meta-analysis of treatment efficacy. Am J Psychiatry. 1994;151:1172–1180.

55. Zorick FJ, Roth T, Hartse K, et al. Evaluation and diagnosis of persistent insomnia. Am J Psychiatry. 1981;138:769–773.

56. Edinger JD, Fins AI, Goeke JM, et al. The empirical identification of insomnia subtypes: a cluster analytic approach. Sleep. 1996;19:398–411.

57. American Sleep Disorders Standards of Practice Committee. Practice parameters for the indications for polysomnography and related procedures. Sleep. 1997;20:406–422.

58. American Sleep Disorders Standards of Practice Committee. Practice parameters for the use of polysomnography in the evaluation of insomnia. Sleep. 1995;18:55–57.

59. Sadeh A, Hauri PJ, Kripke DF, et al. The role of actigraphy in the evaluation of sleep disorders. Sleep. 1995;18:288–302.

60. Hauri PJ, Wisbey J. Wrist actigraphy in insomnia. Sleep. 1992;15:293–301.

61. Spielman A, Glowinsky P. The natural history of insomnia. In: PJ Hauri, ed. Case Studies in Insomnia. New York, NY: Plenum Press; 1991:1–15.

62. Stepanski E, Glinn M, Zorick F, et al. Heart rate changes in chronic insomnia. Stress Med. 1994;10:261–266.

63. Morin CM. Insomnia: Psychological Assessment and Management. New York, NY: Guilford Press; 1993.

64. Bonnet MH, Arand DL. The consequences of a week of insomnia. Sleep. 1996;19:453–461.

65. Mendelson WB. Long-term follow-up of chronic insomnia. Sleep. 1995;18:698–701.

54

Transient and Short-Term Insomnias

Timothy Roehrs
Frank J. Zorick
Thomas Roth

Transient and short-term insomnias are a heterogeneous group of conditions. The sole unifying feature among these conditions is that they occur in otherwise normal sleepers. Some are related to the environment in which the individual sleeps and others to psychosocial stress. Drugs also can cause transient insomnia, either during the initiation or discontinuation of drug use. Finally, there are transient circadian rhythm disorders, essentially due to abrupt changes in sleep schedule relative to the underlying circadian rhythm of sleepiness and alertness. This chapter describes clinical manifestations and polysomnographic features of transient and short-term insomnias and identifies various treatment issues regarding the different conditions.

EPIDEMIOLOGY

A consensus conference of sleep disorders specialists and psychopharmacologists, convened by the National Institutes of Health (NIH), recognized that the duration of an insomnia complaint has major etiological and treatment implications.[1] Some insomnias are acute conditions, while others are chronic. The consensus conference subdivided insomnia conditions into transient, short-term, and long-term, and defined *transient insomnia* as lasting several days, *short-term* 1 to 3 weeks, and *long-term* more than 3 weeks.[1] This differs somewhat from the International Classification of Sleep Disorders (ICSD) produced by the American Sleep Disorders Association, which distinguishes acute, subacute, and chronic insomnia based on durations of less than 1 month, 1 to 6 months, and greater than 6 months, respectively.[2] The *Diagnostic and Statistical Manual of Mental Disorders, Fourth Edition,* (DSM-IV) of the American Psychiatric Association defines primary insomnia as a condition lasting longer than 1 month and thus excludes shorter-lasting conditions from diagnostic consideration.[2a] Regardless of the differences among systems, all make distinctions, one by exclusion, between transient or short-term conditions and chronic ones. The ICSD and NIH consensus conferees empha-

sized that transient insomnia occurs in persons with a history of normal sleep and with resolution of the precipitating conditions sleep becomes normal once again.

Information regarding the incidence of transient insomnia in the general population is difficult to ascertain as most surveys do not specifically make the transient-chronic distinction. The best information comes from two nationally representative surveys of U.S. adults conducted in 1979 and 1991 (National Sleep Foundation, unpublished data, 1991).[3] In the 1979 survey, about one third (35%) of respondents reported at least some difficulty in the past year falling asleep or staying asleep or both.[3] These 35% described their trouble as "bothering a lot" (17%) or "not that much" (18%). Similar results were found in the 1991 nationally representative survey of sleep complaints conducted by the Gallup Organization in which 36% of respondents reported insomnia and 27% said it was occasional and 9%, chronic (National Sleep Foundation, unpublished data, 1991). The authors of the 1979 survey interpreted the 18% who reported their insomnia as bothering them "not that much" to represent a more transient and short-term insomnia. An additional 14% of the 1979 survey reported having previously experienced sleep troubles, but not during the past year. These 14% also may represent transient insomnias, although the authors did not make such an interpretation. Representative surveys of other nations have yielded slightly lower insomnia prevalences (22 to 25%), although the prevalence of transient insomnia in these surveys is not known because transient vs. chronic distinctions were not made.[4, 5] A survey of the population of Zurich, Switzerland that made transient vs. chronic insomnia distinctions reported that 17% of respondents experienced transient insomnia.[6]

Two demographic characteristics were associated with the insomnia complaints in the 1979 survey. These are findings consistently seen in other more limited surveys and in the 1991 Gallup survey. Women were more likely than men to report sleeping troubles, regardless of severity (National Sleep Foundation, unpublished data, 1991).[3] And the likelihood of insomnia increased with age, although the increases associated with transient insomnia were not as great as those with the more severe insomnia in the 1979 survey.[3] None of the various surveys have carefully assessed the circumstances associated with the transient insomnia complaints (i.e., shift work, jet travel, stress, etc.).

A wide variety of conditions and situations may provoke a transient or short-term insomnia and those that have been documented are discussed later. Regardless of the specific precipitating event or condition, it is felt that there are some common mechanisms. The mechanism common to one subset of conditions is presumed to be central nervous system (CNS) arousal. Thus, any condition or situation that produces CNS arousal, whether a psychological or environmental factor, can potentially disturb sleep. No clear, identifiable, pathophysiological mechanism is associated with these transient insomnias. It is a normal response to stress and an experience most anyone might have. Some have suggested, however, that individuals who have low thresholds for arousal to stress may be more vulnerable than others and experience transient and short-term insomnia more frequently and more severely.[7]

Another subset of transient insomnias occurs due to misalignment of one's sleep-wake schedule with the underlying circadian rhythms. Again, with this subset there is no identifiable pathophysiology; the response is normal and fairly universal. As described earlier, there are individuals who seem less able to tolerate a shifting sleep schedule such as occurs in jet travel across a number of time zones or in the rotating sleep schedule associated with shift work or night work.

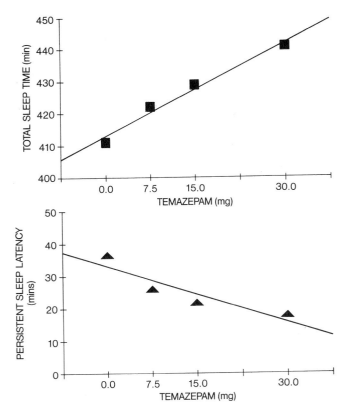

Figure 54–1. Total sleep time and latency to persistent sleep on the first night in the sleep laboratory as a function of temazepam dose. Persistent sleep is defined as 10 min of continuous sleep. (Data plotted are from Roehrs T, Vogel G, Sterling W, et al. Dose effects of temazepam in transient insomnia. Arzneimittelforschung. 1990;40:859–862.)

ENVIRONMENT-RELATED TRANSIENT INSOMNIA

Unfamiliar Sleep Environments

Probably the most universal transient insomnia is the poor sleep experienced in an unfamiliar sleep environment. Early in the modern era of sleep research a "first-night" effect in the sleep laboratory was recognized.[8] Consequently, laboratory studies of sleep have always included an adaptation period of 1 or 2 nights before baseline data are collected. Compared to sleep on subsequent nights, the first night in the laboratory is characterized by increased sleep latency, increased wakefulness during the sleep period, greater amounts of stage 1 (i.e., light) sleep, and typically, an increased latency to rapid eye movement (REM) sleep.[9] In some cases, other aspects of the structure of sleep are altered as well; amounts of REM and delta sleep are reduced. After 1 or 2 nights these alterations in sleep disappear. A recent study comparing first-night effects in home vs. laboratory recordings found comparable disruptions of sleep in chronic insomnia patients and normals on the first night in the laboratory, but at home only insomnia patients showed first-night effects.[10] Thus, for normal people the unfamiliar sleep environment, the laboratory, is specifically sleep disruptive, and for

chronic insomnia patients, sleep recording procedures are further disruptive.

Treatment of a transient insomnia associated with an unfamiliar sleep environment usually would involve reassuring individuals that the experience is natural and endures for 1 or 2 nights. Pharmacotherapy can be considered in cases where sleep disturbance due to an unfamiliar sleep environment is anticipated and optimal sleep for efficient performance the following day is desired. The benzodiazepines are the drugs of choice and the smallest dose of a short-acting compound should be used.[1] One controlled, double-blind study has shown that the transient insomnia experienced on the first night in the sleep laboratory is reversed in a dose-related manner with benzodiazepine hypnotics.[11] Figure 54–1 illustrates the dose effects of temazepam on persistent sleep latency (10 min of uninterrupted sleep) and total sleep time. In fact, the NIH consensus conference cited earlier agreed that transient insomnias were a primary indication for benzodiazepine pharmacotherapy.[1]

Nonconducive Sleep Environments

Noise

Noise seems obvious as a cause of a transient sleep complaint, but identifying noise as the cause of any particular patient's complaint can be difficult. There is a growing literature of basic research on the effects of noise on sleep which can guide the clinical interview and to which clinicians can refer for more complete information.[12, 13] Briefly, the evidence shows that wide variations exist in sensitivity among individuals to sounds during sleep.[14] Furthermore, the meaning or relevance of the sound is also critical.[15] In other words, there is a basis to the commonly held belief that a mother will awaken at the softest whimper of her child, but sleep through a thunderstorm. Consequently, it is important that the clinician not focus solely on the intensity of the noise, but additionally on its informational (i.e., cognitive or emotional) value. Snoring is a perfect example; some bed partners are able to tolerate the most raucous snoring and snorting, whereas others find a soft wheeze extremely offensive and disruptive of their sleep. It also should be recognized that sleep-disruptive noise will not necessarily be remembered when awakening in the morning.[16] As a consequence, a noise-induced sleep disturbance will sometimes result in a complaint of sleepiness or fatigue (the reason is described later) and not insomnia.[17]

Apart from these individual differences in responsiveness to noise during sleep and in the likely clinical presentation, some generalizations can be made. Women are more sensitive to noise than men and sensitivity increases with age.[17, 18] Thus, all these factors must be considered in evaluating the sleep complaint of a patient and the possibility that a noisy sleep environment is the cause.

Studies of the effects of noise on sleep consistently have shown disturbed sleep.[12] The number of body movements, awakenings, and sleep stage shifts are increased. Also, the amount of wakefulness and stage 1 sleep is increased, whereas the amount of delta and REM sleep may be reduced. Sleep stage, time of night, and level of sleepiness are important factors in the disruptive effect of noise. Arousal threshold is higher in stages 3 and 4 than in stages 1 and 2, with REM being intermediate. Controlling for sleep stage, the threshold is higher in the first half of the night than the second half.[19, 20] Sleepiness due to prior sleep deprivation or restriction also heightens arousal threshold, controlling for sleep stage. Differential sleepiness probably accounts for the lowered arousal threshold in the second half of the night, as sleep drive has been partially sated by the first 4 h of sleep. And differential sleepiness may also account for some of the individual differences in the disruptive impact of noise on sleep.[19]

Beyond the usual education and counseling regarding the transitory nature of the insomnia, steps can be taken to protect against recurrence of a problem. Sound attenuation and use of earplugs have been effective; providing "white" noise (e.g., a fan) has been suggested, but its effectiveness is not clear. Again, the use of a short-acting benzodiazepine hypnotic can be considered. Laboratory data clearly indicate that these drugs increase arousal threshold and consequently decrease arousals and wakefulness, resulting in increased sleep time.[21]

Temperature

Temperature is another of those obvious, but clinically difficult factors, important to the quality of sleep. Often, inadequate temperature regulation is attributed by patients to be the cause of a transient sleep complaint. As with noise, there are marked individual differences in sensitivity to temperature variations and in one's optimal sleeping temperature. Transient deviations from optimal temperature clearly do disrupt sleep. Systematic laboratory studies generally show that people sleeping at temperatures above and below thermoneutrality exhibit disturbed sleep. Interestingly, the disturbance usually is not in the facility of falling asleep, but rather in maintaining sleep.[22] The amounts of wakefulness and stage 1 sleep are increased and the amount of REM sleep is decreased. REM sleep seems to be the most sensitive sleep stage to environmental temperature, probably because thermoregulation is suspended during REM sleep. The sleep pattern changes associated with cold and heat are similar, although cold produces more extreme changes in pattern than does heat.[22] There are no data regarding the efficacy of specific treatments for a transient insomnia due to inadequate temperature. However, in most cases temperature adjustment, if that is possible, or the addition of bedclothes, should resolve the transient insomnia.

Sleep Surface

The adequacy of one's sleep surface is the source of a surprising number of insomnia complaints. In a survey of the U.S. public concerning the quality of sleep, conducted by the Gallup Organization, 7% of respondents indicated that their sleeping problems were related to an uncomfortable mattress.[23] However, the few objective studies of sleep surfaces have failed to demonstrate differences in sleep due to sleep surface. In normal individuals, waterbeds had no demonstrable effect on sleep after a 2-week adaptation.[24] Presumably, a change in sleep surface may have a transient effect, but there are no studies of the possible transient effects of sleep surface. The study cited earlier did not present the adaptation data.

Sleep Position

Sleep position also affects the quality of sleep. The usual human sleep posture is horizontal. There are circumstances in which it becomes necessary to sleep with one's back angled from the horizontal (e.g., sleeping in car or airplane seats). Polysomnographic study of the sleep of healthy normals in chairs with back angles of 40, 53, and 72 degrees from the horizontal have shown increased wakefulness during the sleep period and reduced total sleep time compared to sleep in a bed.[25] The extent to which one might adapt to unusual sleep postures is not known. There are individuals who for various health reasons do habitually assume unusual sleep positions, but how the sleep of such persons might be compromised is not known. As with the other nonconducive sleep situations, correction of the situation should resolve the transient insomnia. Again, the use of a short-acting benzodiazepine hypnotic can be considered as prophylactic treatment or as short-term treatment in cases where a nonconducive posture is medically required.

Altitude

Ascent to high altitudes is associated with transient insomnia (see Chapter 18 for a more complete description). Insomnia is one of a complex of symptoms, referred to as acute mountain sickness (AMS), which is experienced initially at high altitude. Sleep at altitudes above 4000 m (13,200 ft) is extremely disturbed, with prolonged sleep latency and increased waking during sleep; overall sleep efficiency is reduced to 70%.[26, 27] Also, the percentage of REM sleep and stage 3–4 sleep are reduced. At lower elevations these disturbances of sleep are not as marked, but relative to sea level they are still evident. In part, the sleep disturbance of altitude is attributed to the disturbed breathing pattern, Cheyne-Stokes respiration, which results from hypoxemia at high altitude. A stress response to the other aspects of AMS, the physiological changes, and the physical illness experienced may also be partially responsible for the sleep disturbance of high altitude. Habituation to these effects is reported clinically to occur within 1 to 2 weeks in high altitude. Pharmacological treatment has taken two approaches: improve the breathing or improve the sleep. At sea level, acetazolamide improved oxygenation and periodic breathing such as Cheyne-Stokes respiration, and at 4000 m, it improved both breathing and sleep.[28] Also, an intermediate-acting benzodiazepine hypnotic, temazepam 10 mg, improved sleep, while having no effect on respiration.[26]

STRESS-RELATED TRANSIENT INSOMNIA

Stress is probably the most frequent cause of a transient or short-term insomnia that is likely to come to the attention of the clinician. In the medical and behavioral literature, *stress* usually is defined as a natural arousal reaction that might have any combination of affective, cognitive, and biological components. To the extent that the arousal reaction is intense enough and persists into the usual sleep period, it may lead to insomnia. The stress can be associated with life events, either positive or negative, or with cognitive expectancies.

Expectancies

The expectancy that sleep will be disturbed will in fact produce disturbed sleep. Individuals on call have been studied on the nights when on call compared with nights when not on call.[29] Sleep is objectively disturbed with more frequent awakenings and lighter sleep when "on call." Another situation in which expectancy of disturbed sleep has in fact produced sleep disturbance is the discontinuation of sleeping pills. A 1992 study found that discontinuation of placebo sleeping pills in both healthy normals and insomnia patients was associated with a reduced sleep efficiency.[30] Each of these situations involving expectancies produces transient insomnias of 1 to 2 nights' duration only. Treatment of each of these expectancy-related insomnias involves education and support. Hypnotics are specifically contraindicated in on call situations because the desired effect of the drug, induction and maintenance of sleep, is directly opposed to the alert, efficient, waking function, which may be required when being called during the middle of the sleep period.

Life Events

Life events may become stressful for an individual and lead to a transient or short-term insomnia. Among laypeople there will be wide variations in awareness and interpretation of the stressful nature of any of the events of everyday life. Consequently, the clinician must evaluate the stressful nature of a particular event or situation for a given patient. The onset of the patient's sleeplessness should be traceable to the particular stressful event or situation to establish that the stress is causing the insomnia. The experience need not necessarily be negative or tragic, such as a loved one's death, other losses, or personal threats; exhilaration associated with positive experiences (i.e., graduation, job promotion, marriage proposal, anticipation of a trip) may also produce insomnia. Or the patient may be ambivalent about the situation and experience that ambivalence as being stressful. With a resolution of the situation or the arousal reaction, sleep usually then becomes normal. Unlike the previously mentioned transient insomnias of 1 to 2 nights, a stress-related insomnia can endure for up to 2 to 3 weeks. It also should be noted that a stress-related transient insomnia can be superimposed on an existing medical or psychiatric condition.

The sleep disturbance of a stress-related insomnia has not been well documented polysomnographically owing to its transitory and unpredictable nature. It is thought to be characterized by any combination of difficulty falling asleep, maintaining sleep, or awakening too early. Correlational studies show a weak relation between questionnaire measures of stress and self-reported sleep symptoms which include nightmares, difficulty falling asleep, awakening during the night, unrefreshing sleep, and restless sleep.[31] Laboratory studies have attempted to create stress-related sleep disturbance by introducing stressors and observing the consequent changes in sleep. They showed that presleep stress delays sleep onset, but no further disturbance of sleep (i.e., increased wakefulness, early awakening, increased stage 1 sleep) has been induced.[32] The failure of laboratory studies to produce extensive sleep disturbances may merely reflect the impotence of the experimental stress manipulation. We noted earlier that stress is a particularly subjective phenomenon. An alternative or additional explanation for the failure to disrupt sleep by various stress manipulations is that not all people may respond to stress with insomnia. One study of presleep stress (2 h of studying) found that poor sleepers slept worse than usual after stress, whereas normal controls were not disturbed by the stress.[33] Earlier (in the Epidemiology section) it was noted that some people may be more prone to transient insomnia than others and these data seem to suggest that.

It has been argued that transient stress-related insomnias may serve as the basis for the development of a chronic psychophysiological insomnia.[34] Evidence regarding such a progression is inconsistent. Some sleep-disordered patients do date the onset of a chronic psychophysiological insomnia to a stressful experience. But correlational data from the general population are not as supportive of such a hypothesis. One retrospective study failed to find a relation between a stress experience and a subsequent chronic insomnia, while another study showed the relation.[31, 35] Regardless, a patient's complaint about a transient insomnia considered to have a stress-related cause should receive therapeutic attention. It should not be dismissed.

Treatment of stress-related insomnias primarily involves reassurance, support, and education. The patient is reassured that the sleep difficulty is a natural response to the stress experience and will resolve in several weeks. The clinician also can educate the patient regarding good sleep hygiene, including consistent bed- and risetimes, avoidance of caffeine and alcohol before bedtime, and avoidance of excessive daytime napping. Alcohol, naps, and extended bedtimes are counterproductive self-help measures often used.[2] The importance of maintaining a standard 7- to 8-h bedtime without supplemental daytime napping, regardless of the daytime fatigue or sleepiness experienced, cannot be overemphasized. Sleeping beyond one's usual risetime or excessive daytime napping after poor nocturnal sleep disrupts circadian rhythms. The disruption of circadian rhythmicity, in turn, reinforces the nocturnal sleep difficulty.

Pharmacotherapy also can be considered in stress-related transient insomnia. When choosing pharmacotherapy, the lowest effective dose of a short-acting benzodiazepine hypnotic should be used. Because a stress-related insomnia may endure beyond 1 to 2 nights, the advisable number of consecutive nights of drug use should be discussed with the patient. Usually, the treatment period should not be more than 3 weeks.[1] The patient should also be apprised of the possibility of experiencing disturbed sleep for 1 to 2 nights when discontinuing the drug.

SLEEP SCHEDULE–RELATED TRANSIENT INSOMNIA

Jet Lag

Jet lag refers to the symptoms experienced after rapid travel across time zones, such as occur in jet aircraft travel. The symptoms include fatigue, malaise, sleepiness during waking hours, and insomnia during sleep periods. It is not jet travel per se, but rather the rapid time zone transition that leads to a misalignment of the sleep schedule with the underlying circadian rhythms that is critical in causing the symptoms. The severity of symptoms depends on the number and rate of time zone transitions (i.e., the extent of the sleep schedule shift) and on the direction of travel (eastward vs. westward).

Extensive research has been conducted on the effects of shifted sleep schedules as occurs in rapid time zone transitions and jet travel. In a westward flight, bedtime is delayed and the result is disturbed sleep in the latter half of the sleep period when, in basal conditions, the individual usually is arising.[36] In the latter half of sleep, there is increased wakefulness and stage 1 sleep. In Figure 54–2A the effect of delaying sleep is illustrated with data from a simulated jet lag study in which the sleep period was shifted by 180 degrees.[37] The minutes of wakefulness were increased compared to baseline during the last 4 h of the shifted sleep period. In contrast, advancing bedtime is required in an eastward flight and consequently increased difficulty falling asleep results. Figure 54–2B illustrates the sleep onset difficulty with data from another jet lag study in which subjects flew from London to Detroit (a 5-h shift) and back.[36] Sleep onset was delayed compared to the baseline after the eastward flight on nights 2 to 5, whereas no delays occurred after the westward flight. Depending on the sleep debt accumulated before or while in flight, one may observe a reduced sleep latency or increased sleep time and sleep efficiency in the first sleep period in the new time zone after the flight. For example, on the first night after the westward flight (see Fig. 54–2B), sleep latency was reduced compared to baseline, probably as a result of lengthening the day to 29 hours. In both schedule shifts (eastward or westward), increased sleepiness and reduced performance during waking periods have been documented. Adaptation to an eastward flight takes longer than that for a westward flight and in extreme shifts can require as long as 7 to 10 days. It is usually suggested that 1 day per time zone crossed is required for adaptation.

Successful treatment of the symptoms of jet lag may include both behavioral techniques and pharmacotherapy. Preparing for a time zone shift while at home by gradually shifting bedtimes in the appropriate direction can be effective. Maintaining the home (basal) sleep-wake schedule in the new time zone can be possible in some circumstances (i.e., small shifts and short stays). There is no evidence to suggest that the various popularized diets have any effect on the symptoms of jet lag.

Jet lag is another of the transient insomnias for which hypnotic pharmacotherapy is an indication.[1] Pharmacological studies have clearly shown that short-acting benzodiazepine agonists restore sleep and daytime alertness in even the most extreme (12 h) sleep schedule shift, although the circadian rhythm of sleepiness-alertness was not shifted.[37] In fact, no studies in human beings have shown that benzodiazepine ago-

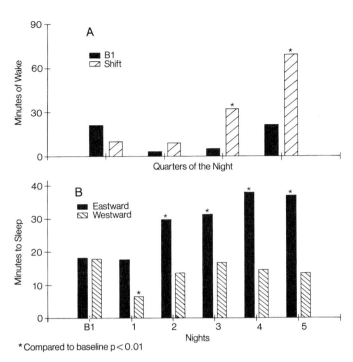

Figure 54–2. *A,* Minutes of wake by quarters (2 h) of the night during a baseline sleep period (12 to 8 AM) and a shifted sleep period (12 to 2 AM) in a simulated jet lag study. *B,* Minutes to sleep on a baseline sleep period and on five sleep periods after an eastward or westward flight requiring a 5-h shift of sleep period in an actual jet lag study. (Data plotted are from Nicholson AN, Pascoe PA, Spencer MB, et al. Sleep after transmeridien flights. Lancet. 1986;2:1206–1208; and Seidel WF, Roth T, Roehrs T, et al. Treatment of a 12-hour shift of sleep schedule with benzodiazepines. Science. 1984;224:1262–1264.)

nists can hasten the adaptation to a new time zone and sleep schedule. The pineal hormone melatonin also has been studied as a treatment for jet lag.[38] Studies have reported improvement in the symptoms of jet lag with melatonin, but the studies have used self-report measures and some have not controlled for the influence of light. Light is known to exert phase-shifting effects and is probably more powerful than melatonin in doing so (see Chapters 28 and 31). Unlike shift work, as discussed later, in jet lag the light-dark cycle is conducive to adaptation. Additionally, both hypnotic and phase-shifting effects of melatonin have been suggested and if melatonin is found to be beneficial, establishing the mechanism may be important to the choice of dose and safety.

Shift Work

The health problems associated with shift work have become a major concern of the Occupational Health and Safety Administration.[39, 40] The symptoms associated with shift work include disturbed and shortened sleep, chronic fatigue, high rates of serious injury and life-threatening job errors, and gastritis and ulcers. For the most part, all of these symptoms can be traced to the disruption of circadian rhythms as a result of eating and sleeping out of phase with one's basal rhythms. These problems appear most frequently in workers on rotating shifts and in permanent night workers who usually shift to conventional sleep-wake schedules on their days off. The insomnia of shift or night work is potentially a chronic problem in that adaptation to the shifted sleep schedule never really occurs as described later. There are clear individual differences in ability to tolerate shift work and many experienced shift workers

become intolerant of shift work in the 5th and 6th decades of life.

The circumstances in a shifting sleep schedule associated with shift work differ from those of jet lag in that environmental time cues (i.e., the light-dark cycle and social patterns) do not shift in phase with the shifted sleep schedule. Consequently, environmental cues remain opposed to the shifted sleep-wake schedule. This difference is important because it is thought that light is the critical circadian rhythm–synchronizing mechanism (circadian rhythm mechanisms are discussed in more detail in Chapters 24 through 31). Whether it is ever possible to fully adapt to a sleep schedule in opposition to environmental cues is not clear. Thus the insomnia associated with the shifting sleep schedule in shift work really may not be transient. However, as yet there is no information on the long-term consequences of shift work. Presumably, shift workers are able to return to conventional sleep schedules without difficulty and with no permanent disruption of circadian rhythmicity and synchronizing mechanisms having occurred. The transient sleep disturbance associated with shift work can be differentiated from the persistent circadian rhythm disorders in which synchronization with conventional sleep-wake schedules and the light-dark cycle is most difficult and may not be possible.

Polysomnographic evaluation of shift workers reveals that they do have shortened and disrupted sleep and also have increased daytime sleepiness. The data show a sleep time of about 5 to 6 h with a reduced sleep efficiency, elevated amounts of stage 1 sleep, and reduced amounts of delta sleep.[41, 42] During waking periods, latency to sleep is reduced (a measure of sleepiness) and the electroencephalogram (EEG) shows increased amounts of alpha and theta activity, which also have been considered signs of sleepiness.[43]

Treatment of an insomnia associated with shift work might include applying chronotherapy techniques and pharmacotherapy. Two chronotherapy principles (delaying sleep periods and slowing shift rotations) have been used successfully to ameliorate the effects of shift work in one field study at a chemical plant.[44] The principle of sleep period delay refers to the direction of the work shift rotation and hence the possible timing of the sleep period: shifting from days, to evenings, to nights (which is the natural tendency of circadian biology—to delay the sleep period). Slowing the rotation implies maintaining each shift for more than 1 week, which is the minimum time necessary for adaptation (given 8-h shifts). Usually, however, it is not within the power of the individual worker to institute such changes. The clinician is left with advising the shift worker to maintain bedtimes and risetimes as consistent as possible and to use naps to supplement the major sleep period. Several controlled laboratory studies have clearly shown that short-acting benzodiazepines improve daytime sleep and consequently improve alertness during the work period.[41, 45] However, the role of pharmacotherapy in insomnia associated with shift work has been controversial because of the potentially chronic nature of the situation. Conservatively, the clinician might advise use of a hypnotic for one or two sleep periods immediately following a sleep schedule shift.

The use of bright light as a rhythm synchronizer in shift and night work is currently being investigated and developed (see Chapter 51) and it may become an important treatment modality. Properly timed exposure to pulses of bright light have been shown to shift circadian phase by as much as 12 h and studies have also assessed constant bright-light exposure during night work.[46–48] The constant light has improved performance and alertness during night work. The necessary intensity of light, duration of exposure, and number of nightly exposures have yet to be determined. Furthermore, the importance of darkness during daytime sleeping and of inappropriate exposure to light during the day in optimizing adaptation to shift and night work is still to be determined.

DRUG-RELATED TRANSIENT INSOMNIA

Drug Discontinuation

A transient insomnia, termed *rebound insomnia*, can be experienced during the discontinuation of short- and intermediate-acting benzodiazepine hypnotics. Several comprehensive reviews of the literature are available.[49, 50] Briefly, rebound insomnia is a 1- to 2-night sleep disturbance relative to that individual's basal sleep and it has been reported in both healthy normals and patients with chronic insomnia. Polysomnographic studies of rebound insomnia have shown an increased latency to sleep onset and wakefulness during the sleep period, producing a reduced total sleep time on the first or second night of a shift from active

drug to placebo.[51] Rebound insomnia appears on discontinuation of all short- and intermediate-acting compounds and can occur even after a single night of drug administration.[52] Rebound does not appear to increase in intensity with increased duration of drug administration, at least in the short term (i.e., 2 weeks). The data indicate that rebound insomnia is associated with drug dose, occurring with high doses beyond which no additional hypnotic efficacy is achieved.[53]

Although rebound insomnia is suggestive of a physiological adaptation of the CNS, it cannot be likened to a withdrawal syndrome and evidence of physiological dependence. It is the experience of a single symptom as opposed to multiple symptoms and is associated with acute drug administration as opposed to chronic drug administration. Also of clinical concern is the extent to which rebound insomnia may lead to behavioral dependence. A study combined human drug self-administration techniques with concurrent evaluation of rebound insomnia to assess the behavioral dependence liability of hypnotics.[54] The study showed the likelihood of self-administering a hypnotic over the 6 nights of evaluation did not increase after rebound insomnia compared to a no-rebound or placebo condition (Fig. 54–3).

Following established principles of pharmacotherapy reduces the likelihood that a given patient may experience rebound insomnia on discontinuing hypnotics. Start with the lowest effective dose and in addition consider the age and health of the patient. Older patients and patients with liver disease achieve higher plasma concentrations of standard hypnotic doses, hence requiring somewhat lower doses. Tapering the dose when discontinuing a short-acting drug has been shown to effectively avoid rebound insomnia[30] (Fig.

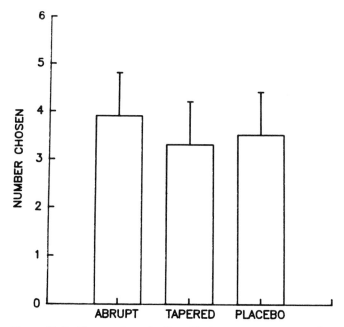

Figure 54–3. The number of pills self-administered over 6 nights after abrupt (6 nights of 0.5 mg triazolam), tapered (3 nights of 0.5 mg, 2 nights of 0.25 mg, and 1 night of 0.125 mg triazolam), or placebo (6 nights of placebo) discontinuation.

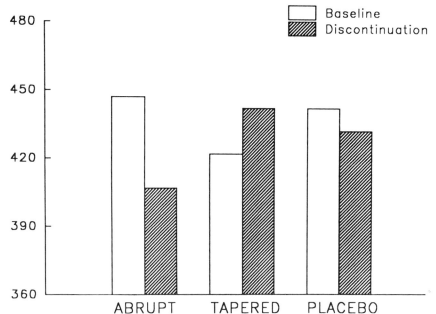

Figure 54–4. Total sleep time (minutes) on the discontinuation night (no pill) after abrupt (6 nights of 0.5 mg triazolam), tapered (3 nights of 0.5 mg, 2 nights of 0.25 mg, and 1 night of 0.125 mg triazolam), or placebo (6 nights of placebo) administration.

54–4). The patient should be assured that rebound insomnia is a 1- to 2-night drug discontinuation effect and not a reflection of his or her natural ability or inability to sleep.

Drug Initiation

Initiation of some pharmacotherapies for various medical conditions may be associated with a transient or short-term insomnia. Some medications have sleep-disruptive side effects, and tolerance may develop to these effects, making the insomnia a transient or short-term problem. However, there is very little systematic clinical or laboratory data addressing this issue. The methylxanthines (i.e., theophylline, caffeine) have stimulatory effects and produce insomnia.[55, 56] The insomnia produced by the methylxanthines is probably transient in that, for example, tolerance to the daytime alerting effects of caffeine has been found to develop rapidly.[57] One would expect a similar rapid development of tolerance to the sleep-disruptive effects of the methylxanthines (i.e., theophylline for respiratory stimulation), although no studies have assessed such tolerance. Beta blockers are disruptive of sleep according to several polysomnographic studies, but the chronic vs. transient nature of that disruption has not been carefully explored.[58] Finally, methylphenidate, a stimulant frequently prescribed for children and young adults with attention-deficit hyperactivity disorder, has a relatively short duration of activity but if administered too close to the sleep period can produce insomnia.[59]

The clinician may avoid such transient drug-related insomnias in several ways. In some cases, an alternative drug that does not cross the blood-brain barrier as readily, but has the same indication, can be chosen. For example, among beta blockers, atenolol does not penetrate the CNS, and objective studies have shown

that it is not disruptive of sleep.[58] Careful attention to the appropriate dose for the given medical condition being treated may sometimes result in the choice of a lower dose and that lower dose leading to reduced CNS penetrance and possible sleep disturbance. The timing of the dosing might also be adjusted such that the drug is less likely to disturb sleep, avoiding afternoon and nighttime dosing, if possible, or giving higher doses in the morning.

References

1. Consensus Conference: Drugs and insomnia. JAMA. 1984; 251:2410–2414.
2. Diagnostic Classification Steering Committee, Thorpy MJ, chairman. International Classification of Sleep Disorders: Diagnostic and Coding Manual. Rochester, Minn: American Sleep Disorders Association; 1990.
2a. American Psychiatric Association: Diagnostic and Statistical Manual of Mental Disorders, Fourth Edition. Washington, DC: American Psychiatric Association; 1994.
3. Mellinger GD, Balter MB, Uhlenhuth EH. Insomnia and its treatment. Arch Gen Psychiatry. 1985;42:225–232.
4. Lugaresi E, Irignotta F, Zucconi M, et al. Good sleepers and poor sleepers: an epidemiological survey of the San Marino population. In: Guilleminault C, Lugaresi C, eds. Sleep/Wake Disorders: Natural History, Epidemiology, and Long-Term Evolution. New York, NY: Raven Press: 1983:1–12.
5. Partinen M, Kaprio J, Koskenvuo M, et al. Sleeping habits, sleep quality, and use of sleeping pills: a population study of 31,149 adults in Finland. In: Guilleminault C, Lugaresi C, eds. Sleep/Wake Disorders: Natural History, Epidemiology, and Long-Term Evolution. New York, NY: Raven Press; 1983:29–36.
6. Angst J, Vollrath M, Koch N, et al. The Zurich study, VII: insomnia: symptoms, classification and prevalence. Eur Arch Psychiatry Clin Neurosci. 1989;238:285–293.
7. Roffwarg H, Erman M: Evaluation and diagnosis of the sleep disorders: implications for psychiatry and other clinical specialties. In: Hales RE, Frances AJ, eds. Psychiatr Update: American Psychiatric Association Annual Review. Vol 4. Washington, DC: American Psychiatric Press; 1985.
8. Agnew H, Webb WB, Williams RI: The first night effect: an EEG study of sleep. Psychophysiology. 1966;2:263–266.

9. Stepanski E, Roehrs T, Saab P, et al. Readaptation to the laboratory in long-term sleep studies. Bull Psychonomic Soc. 1981;17:224–226.
10. Edinger JD, Fins AI, Sullivan RJ, et al. Sleep in the laboratory and sleep at home: comparisons of older insomniacs and normal sleepers. Sleep. 1997;20:1119–1126.
11. Roehrs T, Vogel G, Sterling W, et al. Dose effects of temazepam in transient insomnia. Arzneimittelforschung. 1990;40:859–862.
12. Vallet M, Mouret J. Sleep disturbance due to transportation noise: ear plugs or oral drugs. Experientia. 1984;40:429–437.
13. Lukas JS. Noise and sleep: a literature review and a proposed criteria for assessing effects. J Acoust Soc Am. 1975;58:1232–1242.
14. Rechtschaffen A, Hauri P, Zeitlin M. Auditory awakening thresholds in REM and NREM sleep stages. Percept Mot Skills. 1966;22:927–942.
15. Oswald I, Taylor AM, Treisman M. Discriminative responses to stimulation during human sleep. Brain. 1960;83:440–453.
16. Levine B, Roehrs T, Stepanski E, et al. Fragmenting sleep diminishes its recuperative value. Sleep. 1987;10:590–599.
17. Roth T, Kramer M, Trinder J. The effect of noise during sleep on the sleep patterns of different age groups. Can J Psychiatry. 1972;17:197–201.
18. Lukas JS. Awakening effects of simulated sonic booms and aircraft noise on men and women. J Sound Vibration. 1972;20:457–466.
19. Roehrs T, Merlotti L, Petrucelli N, et al. Experimental sleep fragmentation. Sleep. 1994;17:438–443.
20. Bonnet MH, Johnson LC, Webb W. The reliability of arousal threshold during sleep. Psychophysiology. 1978;15:412–416.
21. Spinweber CL, Johnson LC. Effects of triazolam (0.50 mg) on sleep, performance, memory, and arousal threshold. Psychopharmacology. 1982;76:5–12.
22. Haskell EH, Palca JW, Walker JM, et al. The effects of high and low ambient temperatures on human sleep stages. Electroencephalogr Clin Neurophysiol. 1981;46:29–32.
23. Addison RG, Thorpy MJ, Roth T. A survey of the United States public concerning the quality of sleep. Sleep Res. 1986;16:244.
24. Rosekind M, Phillips R, Rappaport J, et al. Effects of waterbed surface on sleep: a pilot study. Sleep Res. 1976;5:132.
25. Nicholson AN, Stone BM. Influence of back angle on the quality of sleep in seats. Ergonomics. 1987;30:1033–1041.
26. Nicholson AN, Smith PA, Stone BM, et al. Altitude insomnia: studies during an expedition to the Himalayas. Sleep. 1988;11:354–361.
27. Reite M, Jackson D, Cahoon RL, et al. Sleep physiology at high altitude. Electroencephalogr Clin Neurophysiol. 1975;38:463–471.
28. Sutton JR, Houston CS, Mansell AL. Effect of acetazolamide on hypoxemia during sleep at high altitude. N Engl J Med. 1979;301:1329–1331.
29. Torsvall L, Akerstedt T. Disturbed sleep while being on-call: an EEG study of ships' engineers. Sleep. 1988;11:35–38.
30. Roehrs T, Merlotti L, Zorick F, et al. Rebound insomnia in normals and patients with insomnia after abrupt and tapered discontinuation. Psychopharmacology. 1992;108:67–71.
31. Cernovsky ZZ. Life stress measures and reported frequency of sleep disorders. Percept Mot Skills. 1984;58:39–49.
32. Haynes AN, Adams A, Franzen M. The effects of presleep stress on sleep-onset insomnia. J Abnorm Psychol. 1981;90:601–606.
33. Robinson T. Presleep Activity and Sleep Quality of Good and Poor Sleepers [dissertation]. Chicago, Ill: University of Chicago; 1969.
34. Association of Sleep Disorders Centers. Diagnostic classification of sleep and arousal disorders. Sleep. 1979;2:1–137.
35. Healey ES, Kales A, Monroe LJ, et al. Onset of insomnia: role of life-stress events. Psychosom Med. 1981;43:439–451.
36. Nicholson AN, Pascoe PA, Spencer MB, et al. Sleep after transmeridian flights. Lancet. 1986;2:1206–1208.
37. Seidel WF, Roth T, Roehrs T, et al. Treatment of a 12-hour shift of sleep schedule with benzodiazepines. Science. 1984;224:1262–1264.
38. Dawson D, Armstrong SM: Chronobiotics—drugs that shift rhythms. Pharmacol Ther. 1996;69:15–36.
39. Institute of Medicine, National Academy of Sciences. Sleep, biological clocks, and health. In: Health and Behavior. Washington, DC: National Academy Press; 1982.
40. Johnson LC, Tepas DI, Colquhoun WJ, et al, eds. The Twenty-Four Hour Workday. Proceedings of a Symposium on Variations in Work-Sleep Schedules. Washington, DC: US Dept of Health and Human Services; 1981. DHHS publication NIOSH 81-127.
41. Walsh JK, Muehlbach MJ, Schweitzer PK. Acute administration of triazolam for the daytime sleep of rotating shift workers. Sleep. 1984;7:223–229.
42. Anderson H, Chambers MM, Myhre G, et al. Sleep of shiftworkers within the arctic circle. Aviat Space Environ Med. 1984;55:1026–1030.
43. Akerstedt T, Torsvall L, Gillsberg M. Sleepiness and shiftwork: field studies. Sleep. 1982;5:S95–S106.
44. Czeisler CA, Moore-Ede MC, Coleman RM. Rotating shift work schedules that disrupt sleep are improved by applying circadian principles. Science. 1982;217:460–463.
45. Bonnet MH, Mitler M, Gillin JC, et al. Triazolam, sleep satiation, and nocturnal work shift sleepiness and performance. Sleep Res. 1986;15:28.
46. Czeisler CA, Johnson MP, Duffy JF, et al. Exposure to bright light and darkness to treat physiologic maladaptation to night work. N Engl J Med. 1990;322:1253–1259.
47. Campbell SS, Dawson D. Enhancement of nighttime alertness and performance with bright ambient light. Physiol Behav. 1990;48:317–320.
48. Eastman CI. High intensity light for circadian adaptation to a 12-h shift of sleep schedule. Am J Physiol. 1992;263:R428–R436.
49. Gillin JC, Spinweber CL, Johnson LC. Rebound insomnia: a critical review. J Clin Psychopharmacol. 1989;9:161–172.
50. Roehrs T, Vogel G, Roth T. Rebound insomnia: its determinants and significance. Am J Med. 1990;88:39S–42S.
51. Kales A, Scharf M, Kales J. Rebound insomnia: a new clinical syndrome. Science. 1978;201:1039–1040.
52. Merlotti L, Roehrs T, Zorick F, et al. Rebound insomnia: duration of use and individual differences. J Clin Psychopharmacol. 1991;11:368–373.
53. Roehrs TA, Zorick FJ, Wittig RM, et al. Determinants of rebound insomnia. Br J Clin Pharmacol. 1986;22:143–147.
54. Roehrs T, Merlotti L, Zorick F, et al. Rebound insomnia and hypnotic self administration. Psychopharmacology. 1992;107:480–484.
55. Roehrs T, Merlotti L, Halpin D, et al. Effects of theophylline on nocturnal sleep and daytime alertness. Chest. 1995;108:382–387.
56. Rosenthal L, Roehrs T, Zwyghuizen-Doorenbos A, et al. Alerting effects of caffeine after normal and restricted sleep. Neuropsychopharmacology. 1991;4:103–108.
57. Zwyghuizen-Doorenbos A, Roehrs TA, Lipschutz L, et al. Effects of caffeine on alertness. Psychopharmacology. 1990;100:36–39.
58. Kostis JB, Rosen RC, Holzer BC, et al. CNS side effects of centrally-active antihypertensive agents: a prospective, placebo-controlled study of sleep, mood state, and cognitive and sexual function in hypertensive males. Psychopharmacology. 1990;102:163–170.
59. Aoyama T, Sasake T, Kotaki H, et al. Pharmacokinetics and pharmacodynamics of (+)-threo-methylphenidate enantiomer in patients with hypersomnia. Clin Pharmacol Ther. 1994;55:270–276.

55

Primary Insomnia*

Peter J. Hauri

Insomnia may be the basic, root problem in some patients rather than a symptom of some other disease. Specifically, some types of insomnias are not caused by problems such as anxiety, depression, pain, allergy, or restless legs syndrome. For these types of free-standing insomnia, the word *primary* is used in the *Diagnostic and Statistical Manual of Mental Disorders, Fourth Edition* (DSM-IV).[1, 2] This does not imply that such patients are totally free of any medical or psychiatric disorders. It simply means that as far as can be determined, these other disorders are probably not involved in the cause of the insomnia.

The International Classification of Sleep Disorders (ICSD)[3] does not recognize a category of primary insomnia, but discusses three free-standing insomnia subgroups: psychophysiological insomnia, sleep state misperception, and idiopathic insomnia. These three ICSD subgroups empirically make up most of what DSM-IV calls primary insomnia.[4] There is controversy about which classification makes better empirical sense.

It appears that all primary insomniac patients may be hyperaroused. They score high on scales measuring hyperarousal[5] and they are sensation avoiders[6] (suggesting that they may already be overstimulated). They commonly show an increased metabolic rate,[7] increased body temperature, and increased fast activity on the electroencephalogram (EEG)(greater than 20 Hz), both awake and long into sleep.[8, 9] This is in direct opposition to the findings in sleep-deprived normal subjects who show decreased metabolism, decreased body temperature, and increased slow (theta) activity on the EEG. Recent research suggests that insomnia may be much more like caffeine intoxication than like sleep deprivation.[10] When the sleep of normal people is artificially disturbed to resemble that of yoked insomniac patients, the daytime symptoms of the normals were those of sleep deprivation (decreased body temperature, decreased multiple sleep latency test [MSLT] latencies), while the insomniac patients showed the opposite (increased body temperature, increased metabolism, increased MSLT). Indeed, Bonnet and Arand[7] even suggested that insomnia may be the organism's attempt at curing excessive hyperarousal by slowing it down through sleep deprivation!

When comparing subjective estimates of total sleep with sleep assessed by polysomnography, most, but not all, insomniac patients underestimate the amount of time they actually sleep. This may be related to the finding (see earlier) that sufferers from insomnia have more fast EEG frequencies during sleep, which may facilitate cognitive processes and interfere with the normal establishment of mesograde amnesia.[11]

In some insomnia patients, the above-discussed underestimation may be extreme (e.g., "I have not slept for over a week," when the polysomnogram shows 6 h of sleep per night). Such patients are said to suffer from a sleep state misperception syndrome (i.e., they may perceive that they are awake when they are actually asleep). However, on many dimensions, patients with sleep state misperception are very similar to those patients who have "bona fide" insomnia: they seem to have similar difficulties falling asleep when asked to take naps during the day, and they show considerable hyperarousal.[12, 13] They respond to the same treatments (pharmacological, behavioral) as do bona fide insomniac patients. Therefore, some insomnia specialists now question the relevance of sleep parameters assessed by polysomnography when evaluating insomnia.

It will be a matter of clinical judgment and further research to determine whether we are dealing with three separate and distinct subcategories of insomnia, as ICSD[3] implies, or with three general dimensions along which all patients with primary insomnia vary, as DSM-IV maintains.[1] However, the remainder of this chapter is organized according to the ICSD point of view.

PSYCHOPHYSIOLOGICAL INSOMNIA

CASE HISTORY

Mr. R, a 32-year-old laboratory technician, was referred for insomnia after he had twice fallen asleep at the wheel. Mr. R had always been a light sleeper, with sporadic nights of serious insomnia during tense life situations, such as before important examinations. After working as an electronics technician most of his life, he had tried to establish his own manufacturing firm 4 years ago. He had been only lightly insured when soon thereafter an accidental fire destroyed his plant. Bankruptcy ensued, serious depression followed, and Mr. R was treated with psychotherapy and antidepressants. Depression lifted 3 months later, but insomnia remained. A second course of psychotherapy 3 years later ended in his referral to the sleep disorders center because his therapist felt that Mr. R's insomnia was no longer secondary to depression.

Polysomnographic (PSG) recordings on two consecutive nights confirmed serious sleep latency problems: 2 h on the first night and 4.5 h on the second night. Once asleep, Mr. R first slept fitfully for 1 to 3 h, with increased stage 1 sleep and little delta or rapid eye movement (REM) sleep. About 2 h before wake-up time on both nights, he finally fell into a 45-min stage 4 episode, followed by a REM period lasting over 1 h. There was no evidence of respiratory disturbances or periodic leg movements. In the morning, Mr. R rated his night 1 as "better than my average" and his night 2 as "average."

A diagnosis of persistent psychophysiological insomnia was made, and Mr. R's bedtime behavior was examined in detail. Because he typically was worrying about small everyday matters and rehearsing speeches and letters when he could not sleep, he was advised to schedule a 30-min "worry time" immediately after supper each day in which he would write down his worries and possible solutions to them. During that time, he might also write down the letters and speeches that he previously rehearsed at night. At bedtime, he was asked to set the alarm clock and then hide it and read in bed until he fell asleep reading. A few hypnotics were prescribed, to be taken no more than twice per week after particularly poor nights. A late-afternoon increase in exercise was recommended. These measures gradually reduced Mr. R's sleep latency to an average of about 1 h per night. However, Mr. R still felt tense when going to bed. A course of frontalis electromyographic biofeedback and some stress management training were then prescribed, with the result that Mr. R regained his prebankruptcy sleep patterns. He now typically fell asleep in 15 to 20 min. Occasionally, no more than four to six times per month, he would still find that he had to read for 1 to 2 h before feeling sleepy, and on some rare occasions, he then took a short-acting benzodiazepine to help with sleep. He professed satisfaction with this regimen.

Persistent psychophysiological insomnia is often called "learned" insomnia or "behavioral" insomnia. It is diagnosed in patients who complain about insomnia and poor daytime functioning if the sleep pattern of these patients suggests learned sleep-preventing associations. In addition, there is increased somatized tension in such patients (e.g., increased agitation, increased muscle tone, increased vasoconstriction) around the issue of sleep (e.g., thinking about it during the day or trying to sleep). Maladaptive learning can, of course, develop secondary to any chronic insomnia. Psychophysiological insomnia is diagnosed only when these behavioral issues play the *predominant* role in the maintenance of disturbed sleep.

It is natural for all of us to sleep poorly during a period of stress. If stress continues, two maladaptive behaviors may develop. First, being tired and functioning below par after a number of poor nights of sleep, one cannot help but become increasingly concerned about one's sleep. One naturally then tries harder to sleep on subsequent nights. The more one feels sleep-deprived, the harder one tries to sleep; but the harder one tries, the tenser one gets and the less one can actually sleep—thus, a vicious cycle is created. Patients showing this behavior of "trying too hard to sleep" often fall asleep easily when they are distracted (e.g., when they are watching TV, when they are driving, or when they are passively listening to lectures). Second, after a number of frustrating, sleepless nights, one's bedroom or the habits that are leading up to going to bed (e.g., brushing teeth) may become associated with (conditioned to) frustration and arousal. Patients suffering from this maladaptive conditioning often find that they can sleep well anywhere else, but not in their own bedroom.

When the initial stress abates, the bad sleep habits that were naturally acquired during the period of stress will gradually be extinguished in a normal sleeper because they are not reinforced. However, if innate hyperarousal causes occasional poor nights of sleep, then extinction is prevented because any habits that are occasionally reinforced are not extinguished. Said in other words, one can never learn not to worry about sleep if, a few times per month, these worries prove justified. Thus, the insomnia continues for years and decades after the stress has abated and is then labeled *persistent psychophysiological insomnia.*[14]

The sleep disturbance in persistent psychophysiological insomnia may range from mild to severe. It may be difficulty falling asleep or frequent nocturnal awakenings. There is more stage 1 sleep than expected. There may, or may not be, adequate amounts of delta sleep.[15] However, the remaining sleep architecture seems relatively normal. There may be an increase in muscle tension during sleep, as well as an increase in alpha activity (miniarousals). Within the boundaries of a relatively normal personality profile, patients with persistent psychophysiological insomnia tend to be more tense and dissatisfied than are good sleepers. Emotionally, they typically are repressors, denying problems.

About 15% of all insomnia patients seeking help at sleep disorders centers are diagnosed as psychophysiological insomnia.[16] However, a true incidence rate is unknown. It seems likely that many patients with milder forms of this type of insomnia are not seeking help.

Diagnostic Criteria

To be diagnosed with psychophysiological insomnia, patients first have to demonstrate true sleep difficulties that significantly affect their daytime functioning: if sleeping in the laboratory, they show an increased sleep latency, a reduced sleep efficiency, or an increased number and duration of awakenings. A learning component is then demonstrated by interview and history. This typically is done by evaluating the following:

1. Excessive, daily worries about not being able to fall or stay asleep in the absence of excessive

anxiety about other domains of daily living. There are intense efforts to fall asleep that are made each night, accompanied by marked apprehension that these efforts will be unsuccessful.

2. Evidence of trying too hard to sleep, suggested by an inability to fall asleep if desired, but ease of falling asleep when one tries to stay awake but is physically inactive, such as watching TV or reading.

3. Apparently paradoxical improvement in sleep when the patient is away from the usual sleep environment or not carrying out bedtime routines.

4. Evidence of increased somatized tension around the issue of sleep (e.g., increased agitation, increased muscle tension, or increased vasoconstriction).

Obviously, persistent psychophysiological insomnia is diagnosed only if these learning factors seem to play the dominant role in insomnia and if there are no psychiatric or medical diseases that may explain the insomnia. Psychophysiological insomnia is not a catch-all category like "insomnia not otherwise specified." The earlier-described criteria have to be positively satisfied before a patient is classifed as having psychophysiological insomnia.

Differential Diagnosis

The most difficult differential diagnosis is with generalized anxiety disorder. To the extent that the anxiety is pervasive, involving most aspects of waking life, generalized anxiety disorder is the more likely diagnosis. Persistent psychophysiological insomnia becomes more likely if the anxiety focuses exclusively on the patient's inability to sleep. Patients with persistent psychophysiological insomnia typically manage to function as well during the day as their sleep deprivation allows; the pervasive anxiety of the anxiety syndromes interferes with daytime functioning well beyond the fatigue level induced by poor sleep.

Differentiation from affective disorder is difficult in "masked" depression; that is, when the patient does not consciously experience sadness, hopelessness, or helplessness. Attention to the "vegetative signs" of depression may help (especially loss of appetite, energy, or libido, marked diurnal fluctuations, with morning being worst). The association of insomnia with life events that typically might trigger depression (e.g., death of a loved one) helps with diagnosis. Crucial is the diagnostician's sense that chronic depression, although possibly masked, is a primary event rather than a reaction to the frustrations of poor sleep and the resulting fatigue. Also, the psychophysiological insomniac patient typically exhibits a grim, listless, and dour mood, but feelings of sadness, helplessness, and hopelessness are less prominent than they are in depression.

Idiopathic insomnia is differentiated from psychophysiological insomnia by history. To the extent that the insomnia has been chronic and unremitting since early childhood, idiopathic insomnia is more likely, whereas persistent psychophysiological insomnia becomes more probable if there is a clear onset of serious insomnia during a period of stress in adulthood. However, the two conditions shade into each other.

The differentiation of psychophysiological insomnia from sleep state misperception can be made only by objective PSG measures. Again, the two conditions may be on a continuum. Arbitrarily, it is our custom to diagnose psychophysiological insomnia if laboratory sleep latencies are greater than 30 min, if total sleep time in the laboratory is less than 6.5 h, if sleep efficiency is less than 85%, or if patients report that they slept much better in the laboratory than at home. The larger the discrepancy between objective and subjective assessment of sleep, the more sleep state misperception becomes the preferred diagnosis.

A diagnosis of inadequate sleep hygiene is made if such factors directly cause the insomnia, which resolves when sleep hygiene is improved. Psychophysiological insomnia is the preferred diagnosis if learned factors maintain the problem; that is, if patients still sleep poorly even though they now maintain good sleep hygiene.

Treatment

A *multivaried approach* to treatment is indicated, tailored to the individual. For example, if one insomnia patient reports that he gets nervous when he sees the minutes and hours tick by on his bedroom clock, all clocks are removed from the bedroom. However, if another insomnia patient reports that she derives comfort and relaxation when, occasionally, she notices that the bedroom clock has moved much further than she had assumed (thus implying that she must have slept), then the clock remains.

Treatment typically consists of some components from the following three domains: (1) sleep hygiene (see Chapter 58); (2) behavioral treatment (see Chapter 57); and (3) hypnotics (see Chapter 36). Hypnotics are indicated in psychophysiological insomnia for occasional poor nights, to be used no more than once or twice per week. Hypnotics are prescribed to break the vicious cycle of patients' needing sleep so desperately that they seek it too much and thereby become hyperaroused. However, it might be unwise to prescribe hypnotics during the time that behavioral treatment is learned.[17]

Although persons with psychophysiological insomnia rarely become "champion" sleepers after treatment because of their apparently organic predisposition toward poor sleep, most of them can be taught to sleep adequately by using a combination of sleep hygiene, behavioral treatment, and occasional hypnotics.

IDIOPATHIC INSOMNIA

CASE HISTORY

Mrs. I, a 45-year-old professional woman, was self-referred. On interview, she looked tired, grim, and worn-out, and she gave the appearance that she held herself together by sheer willpower. She said that sleep had been her problem "forever." Indeed, her earliest memories were of incidents as a 3-year-old when her parents repeatedly discovered her playing "all night long" while the rest of her family slept.

Grade school was hard. Although not diagnosed at that time, she seems to have had a serious learning disability. She always felt tired and sickly. Nevertheless, she later managed college and law school "by sheer force of will." She also noted during that time that even minor stimulations, such as an interesting evening of conversation, would keep her awake most of the night and that even mild stimulants, such as chocolate or soft drinks with caffeine, did the same.

Over the past 20 years, Mrs. I had undergone many medical evaluations at some of the country's leading medical centers. Nothing was ever found except a general lack of stamina despite her efforts to exercise. Psychological testing showed a generalized feeling of chronic malaise but no noteworthy psychopathological process. Specifically, there were no clear signs of either pathological anxiety or depression. In spite of this, Mrs. I had undergone two intensive courses of psychotherapy during the past 10 years, "to get to the bottom of this," with no success.

In the past, Mrs. I had been tried on most of the available hypnotics, some major tranquilizers, some daytime stimulants, and even some narcotics. Sleep typically improved for a few weeks with each new medication, but Mrs. I habituated to each of them in turn. On a clinical trial of tricyclic antidepressants (up to 200 mg of amitriptyline per day), she had slept much better but had been unable to function because of excessive fatigue during the day, headaches, and ataxia.

Studied in the laboratory for 3 nights, Mrs. I slept fitfully for 2 to 5 h each night, and she was easily aroused, even by faint noises. When disturbed, she was immediately and fully awake. There was excessive stage 1 sleep, almost no delta sleep, and only poorly defined, irregular sleep spindles that occurred rarely, no more than every 3 to 5 min. No respiratory or muscular abnormalities were found, and the alterations between REM and nonrapid eye movement (NREM) sleep seemed normal.

A discussion of sleep hygiene and an intensive course of electromyographic biofeedback improved sleep somewhat, but not markedly so. She was then placed on minute doses of amitriptyline at bedtime, first 10 mg and later 25 mg. This regimen improved her sleep markedly, and she has now been maintained on this medication for 6 years without any apparent decrease in efficacy. To assess her continuous need for amitriptyline, she withdraws from it once a year for 3 weeks during vacation, each time so far with disastrous results. The efficacy of such a small dose of amitriptyline in such patients remains unexplained and deserves further investigation.

Idiopathic insomnia is a lifelong inability to obtain adequate sleep. It may be that these patients are simply hyperaroused on an organic basis.[7] Another explanation, not necessarily different from the hyperaroused hypothesis, might be that this type of insomnia is due to an abnormality in the neurological control of the sleep-wake system. This system is complex. It involves many areas of the reticular activating system (promoting wakefulness), as well as wide-ranging sleep-inducing circuits in the areas of the solitary tract nuclei, the raphe nuclei, and the medial forebrain area, among others. Whether one is awake or asleep depends on the relative dominance of either the arousal system or the sleep system. It seems likely that in such a complex "push-pull" system, not every human being is equally endowed. Some may tend more toward sleep, others toward wakefulness. Idiopathic insomnia may involve the extreme end tending toward arousal, or possibly even a yet-to-be identified neuroanatomical, neurophysiological, or neurochemical weakness in the sleep system, or excessive strength in the arousal system.[18]

Patients who suffer from idiopathic insomnia often have been poor sleepers since birth. Note, however, that most infants or children who sleep poorly should not be classified into this category because the poor sleep in most childhood insomnias can be explained by faulty habit training, by psychological stress, or by other medical or psychological difficulties.

Emotionally, people with idiopathic insomnia are often repressors, denying and minimizing emotional problems. This may be a defense against the common assumption that all persons with insomnia have emotional problems. Although the insomnia seems to be persistent over the entire life span, it can be aggravated by stress. Further, people with idiopathic insomnia often show atypical reactions to medications, such as hypersensitivity (e.g., severe reactions to small amounts of stimulants) or insensitivity (e.g., little sedation from large doses of benzodiazepines).

Diagnostic Criteria

As with all chronic insomnias, there first must be a complaint of disturbed sleep combined with a complaint of decreased functioning during wakefulness. In idiopathic insomnia, the insomnia is long-standing, typically beginning in early childhood without there being any emotional or physical trauma that would explain the early onset. The insomnia complaint is relentless. Sleep improves little or not at all, even in times of good emotional adaptation.

PSG demonstrates severe insomnia, manifested by increased sleep latency, reduced sleep efficiency, and increased number and duration of awakenings. There is often a reversed first-night effect. The only PSG study on idiopathic insomnia[18] also found long periods of REM sleep without actual eye movements. Obviously, idiopathic insomnia is diagnosed only if psychological-behavioral problems have been ruled out and if there are no medical or environmental causes for the sleep disturbance.

Idiopathic insomnia is rarely seen in its pure form.

It seems almost impossible to lead the life of an individual with chronic, serious insomnia without developing other factors that are complicating the picture, such as poor sleep hygiene, learned maladaptive associations, or psychiatric disturbances. Idiopathic insomnia is usually diagnosed only when the history of the insomnia markedly predates the occurrence of these other sleep-disturbing factors.

Differential Diagnosis

The most difficult differential diagnosis is with sleep disturbances during childhood that are caused by psychological or behavioral problems. A chaotic family lifestyle can often lead to poor sleep hygiene in a child, but a toddler with severe idiopathic insomnia may also severely stress a family system and cause, or at least contribute to, a chaotic lifestyle.

There seems to be a continuum from idiopathic insomnia, to psychophysiological insomnia, to insomnia associated with psychiatric difficulties. In idiopathic insomnia, the hyperarousal or neurological predisposition toward poor sleep is so strong that it, in itself, can cause insomnia. In psychophysiological insomnia, an external stress event is necessary to start insomnia in an individual with a lesser predisposition toward poor sleep. At the other extreme, serious psychiatric stress alone apparently can cause insomnia, even in a constitutionally good sleeper.

Short sleepers are differentiated from idiopathic insomniac patients by their daytime functioning. A short sleeper feels and functions well during the day; the idiopathic insomnia patient clearly feels hampered by lack of sleep, showing decreased vigilance and chronic fatigue. However, the MSLT in idiopathic insomnia may often be in the normal range or hyperalert.

Treatment

No consistent treatment approach to childhood-onset insomnia has evolved. Because each case is typically different from any of the others, a highly empirical approach is necessary. Some patients—for example, Mrs. I—have responded to tricyclic antidepressants, either small doses (e.g., amitriptyline 10 mg at bedtime) or larger ones (e.g., trazodone 200 mg). Still others respond to neuroleptic drugs, whereas others respond only to opiates (e.g., hydromorphone 12 mg every other night).[19] In addition to medication, supportive psychological treatment is often necessary, as are behavioral therapy and extremely good sleep hygiene.

SLEEP STATE MISPERCEPTION

CASE HISTORY

Mr. Q, a 25-year-old graduate student, was evaluated for chronic insomnia. Although he claimed that he slept fitfully and for less than 5 h on each of his three consecutive laboratory nights, the PSG showed that he had fallen asleep within 5 min each night and had slept throughout his 8-h sleep time, albeit with somewhat more frequent arousals than is typical for his age (he showed 10 arousals per hour; our norms suggest that five to eight arousals are within normal limits). On the basis of his evaluation, Mr. Q was classified as suffering from sleep state misperception. The sleep laboratory results were explained to the patient, and no treatment was prescribed.

Mr. Q did not believe the laboratory evaluation. He then sought help from a behavioral psychologist who taught him a combination of self-hypnosis, meditation, and relaxation training. Some hypnotics were also prescribed for occasionally poor nights of sleep. This treatment subjectively cured his insomnia; he claimed that he now slept soundly throughout most nights. A repeat evaluation in our sleep laboratory, however, showed no change in any of the PSG-evaluated parameters.

Subjectively, there was a dramatic change in the student's sleep after behavioral treatment. According to the PSG, there was none. Was there a cure? Sleep researchers will disagree on the answer. For the diagnosis of sleep state misperception to be made, there must be a convincing and honest complaint of insomnia by a person who lacks an apparent psychopathological disorder. In addition, sleep duration and quality on the PSG must be normal. This is operationally defined in the ICSD as showing a sleep latency of less than about 20 min, combined with a minimum of 6.5 h of sleep and no increased arousals and awakenings. (Note that the case study above only marginally satisfies these criteria.) Finally, on the MSLT the sleep latency is longer than 10 min. The requirement for a normal MSLT was developed to differentiate patients with sleep state misperception from those with idiopathic hypersomnia who may misinterpret their excessive daytime somnolence as indicating nocturnal insomnia. Defined in the narrow sense of the ICSD,[3] sleep state misperception is a rare insomnia observed in fewer than 5% of those complaining of insomnia.[16] There remain, however, a number of issues.

Most patients underestimate the amount of sleep obtained according to the PSG. Thus, sleep state misperception is a ubiquitous phenomenon, and those so classified may simply be at the extreme of this phenomenon, and not constitute a different nosological entity. Also, the requirement that sleep be entirely normal in this group seems somewhat arbitrary and is not supported by recent research.[12, 15] Finally, there is clearly serious sleep state misperception if a patient claims to have not slept at all in weeks and, on examination in the laboratory, sleeps about 5 h per night; but such a patient does not qualify for this diagnosis according to the criteria of the ICSD.

Our methods of recording sleep may be at fault. For example, Hauri and Wisbey[20] reported that the wrist actigraph often registers wakefulness in such patients (similar to their subjective complaint), whereas the PSG shows them as being asleep. Apparently, patients with sleep state misperception may have frequent wrist movements or similar events that might subjectively suggest to them that they are awake, even though the electroencephalogram shows sleep waves. Thus, it may not be misperception at all. As discussed earlier, the issue is whether sleep as recorded on the PSG is "the essence," or whether other parameters, such as hypermetabolism or fast EEG waves or frequent wrist movements, lie closer to 'the essence' of the sleep experience than the Rechtschaffen and Kales[21] sleep stages.

Diagnostic Criteria

A complaint of persistent insomnia is made while sleep duration and sleep quality are apparently normal. PSG monitoring demonstrates normal sleep latency, a normal number of arousals and awakenings, and normal sleep duration. Also, according to the ICSD criteria, the MSLT shows normal daytime vigilance (greater than 10 min). The context of the sleep complaint indicates no reason to suspect malingering, attention seeking, or any other psychological gain to be derived from the complaints.

Differential Diagnosis

Sleep state misperception can be diagnosed only in the laboratory because one needs to document that sleep is normal. However, because insomnia is a condition that varies dramatically from night to night, even the worst sleepers can occasionally sleep well. Therefore, sleep state misperception is only diagnosed if an individual claims to have slept poorly in the laboratory, even though, on that specific night, the PSG had indicated normal sleep. It is not diagnosed if an insomnia patient happens to sleep well on a given night in the laboratory and then, typically with some embarrassment, reports with surprise the next morning that that particular night had actually been quite good. This latter constellation suggests psychophysiological insomnia (absence of conditioned insomnia response because the sleep laboratory is so different from home).

The criteria for adequate sleep are arbitrary. Cutoff points of 15 to 20 min of sleep latency or 6.5 h of sleep time are suggested by the ICSD. No matter where the exact line is drawn, patients with the diagnosis of sleep state misperception will gradually shade into the category of psychophysiological insomnia. The same may be said for the psychological sphere. Although patients with sleep state misperception are so diagnosed only if they do not carry a DSM-IV psychiatric diagnosis that could explain their complaint, most of them do show some psychological tension and other mild abnormalities.

Treatment

Some patients are relieved when confronted with the fact that they sleep much better than they had feared. Paradoxically, many behavioral treatments,

such as progressive muscle relaxation, biofeedback, stimulus control therapy, or sleep curtailment, are effective in this group. Patients often report that they sleep much better after such treatment, even though a laboratory evaluation cannot document this. An occasional hypnotic is also useful for alleviating the panic that occurs when patients feel that they have slept little for a number of nights. It is interesting that hypnotics are usually perceived as sleep-promoting by these patients, even though they do not improve their sleep according to the Rechtschaffen and Kales criteria.[21]

SUMMARY

Clearly, the final words on primary insomnia have not yet been written and the final diagnostic boundaries have not yet been drawn. Happily, a combination of behavioral therapy, good sleep hygiene, and intelligent use of medication often helps these patients, even though our understanding of them is still poor.

References

1. American Psychiatric Association. Diagnostic and Statistical Manual of Mental Disorders. 4th ed. Washington, DC: American Psychiatric Association Press; 1994.
2. Reynolds CF, Kupfer DJ, Buysse DJ, et al. Subtyping DSM-III-R primary insomnia: a literature review by the DSM-IV work group on sleep disorders. Am J Psychiatry. 1991;148:432–438.
3. Diagnostic Classification Steering Committee, Thorpy MJ, chairman. International Classification of Sleep Disorders: Diagnostic and Coding Manual. Rochester, Minn: American Sleep Disorders Association; 1990.
4. Buysse DJ, Reynold CF, Hauri PJ, et al. Diagnostic concordance for sleep disorders using proposed DSM-IV categories: a report from the APA/NIMH DSM-IV field trial. Am J Psychiatry. 1994; 151:1351–1360.
5. Regestein QR. Specific effects of sedative/hypnotic drugs in the treatment of incapacitating chronic insomnia. Am J Med. 1987;83:909–916.
6. Coursey RD, Buchsbaum M, Frankel BL. Personality measures and evoked responses in chronic insomniacs. J Abnorm Psychol. 1975;84:239–249.
7. Bonnet MH, Arand DL. 24-hour metabolic rate in insomniacs and matched normal sleepers. Sleep. 1995;18:581–588.
8. Freedman RR. EEG power spectra in sleep-onset insomnia. Electroencephalogr Clin Neurophysiol. 1986;63:408–413.
9. Mercia H, Gaillard J. The EEG of sleep onset period in insomnia: a discriminant analysis. Physiol Behav. 1991;52:99–204.
10. Bonnet MH, Arand DL. Caffeine use as a model of acute and chronic insomnia. Sleep. 1992;15:526–536.
11. Perlis ML, Giles DE, Mendelson WB, et al. Psychophysiological insomnia: the behavioral model and a neurocognitive perspective. J Sleep Res. 1997;6:179–188.
12. Bonnet MH, Arand DL. Physiological activation in patients with sleep state misperception. Psychosom Med. 1997;59:533–540.
13. Dorsey CM, Bootzin RR. Subjective and psychophysiologic insomnia: An examination of sleep tendency and personality. Biol Psychiatry 1997;41:209–216.
14. Hauri P, Fisher J. Persistent psychophysiologic (learned) insomnia. Sleep. 1986;9:38–53.
15. Salin PRJ, Roehrs TA, Merlotti LA, et al. Long-term study of the sleep of insomnia patients with sleep state misperception and other insomnia patients. Am J Psychiatry. 1992;149:904–908.
16. Coleman RM. Diagnosis, treatment and follow-up of about 8,000 sleep/wake disorder patients. In: Guilleminault C, Lugaresi E, eds. Sleep/Wake Disorders: Natural History, Epidemiology, and Long-Term Evolution. New York, NY: Raven Press; 1983:87–97.

17. Hauri PJ. Insomnia. Can we mix behavioral therapy with hypnotics when treating insomniacs? Sleep. 1997;20:1111–1118.

18. Hauri P, Olmstead E. Childhood-onset insomnia. Sleep. 1980; 3:59–65.

19. Regestein QR, Reich P. Incapacitating childhood-onset insomnia. Compr Psychiatry. 1983;24:244–248.

20. Hauri P, Wisbey J. Wrist actigraphy in insomnia. Sleep. 1992; 15:293–301.

21. Rechtschaffen A, Kales A, eds. A Manual of Standardized Terminology, Techniques and Scoring System for Sleep Stages of Human Sleep. Los Angeles, Calif: UCLA Brain Information Service/ Brain Research Institute; 1968.

56

Psychiatric Disorders and Insomnia

W. Vaughn McCall
Dianne Reynolds

Insomnia is defined as inadequate or nonrestorative sleep with daytime consequences. The daytime consequences are an essential part of the definition and serve to exclude physiological short sleepers who feel vital and rested during the day. At the other extreme this definition includes patients with severe subjective insomnia who may complain of years of total insomnia and daytime consequences despite polysomnographic (PSG) testing that shows completely normal sleep.[1] This definition of insomnia begins to break down when applied to patients with mania who may sleep little and create numerous problems for themselves and others, yet who still insist that they are alert, vital, and have no daytime consequences from their sleeplessness. Regardless of how insomnia is defined, it is clear that most patients have some type of daytime impairment such as irritability, mild depressed mood, concentration deficits, and subjective fatigue.[2, 3] The presence of a *major* psychiatric disorder, however, is *not* fundamental to the definition of insomnia.

In this chapter we explore the links between insomnia and psychiatric disorders. The sleep disorders associated with specific psychiatric conditions are presented elsewhere in this book.

A complaint of insomnia is common, and as many as one third of Americans report at least one bout of poor sleep in the prior year. Seventeen percent say that they have had severe insomnia in the last year.[4] Psychiatric disorders are also common, with 30% of a community-based sample of Americans endorsing symptoms of a psychiatric disorder in the last year.[5] Chance alone would dictate that two common disorders—insomnia and mental disorders—would overlap. Yet, medicine has long believed that there is a special relationship between insomnia and mental disorders that cannot be explained by chance alone. Hippocrates noted that "insomnolency is connected with sorrow and pains. . . ."[6] In 1922 Klaesi introduced "continuous sleep treatment" as a means of aborting episodes of psychotic excitement.[7] Klaesi believed that pharmacological induction of deep sleep for 10 days with large doses of barbiturates, chloral hydrate, or paraldehyde would break the insomnia-psychosis cycle. Continuous sleep treatment was abandoned as early as 1950 with the advent of phenothiazines.

The scalp electroencephalogram (EEG) was first recorded successfully from human beings in 1929, and sleep EEG investigations of psychiatric disorders soon followed. The sleep EEG has become a powerful *research* tool for understanding psychiatric disease, but PSG testing is not a routine part of clinical management of either psychiatric disorders or insomnia because it has not been shown that outcomes in their management are improved with PSG.[8] Therefore, it remains important to elucidate the relationship between the *clinical* aspects of insomnia and psychiatric disease. Descriptions of the PSG findings in psychiatric disorders are detailed elsewhere in this book; this chapter focuses on the evidence supporting a relationship between insomnia and psychiatric illness. We examine, in turn, the following questions:

1. What are the clinical features of insomnia in different psychiatric disorders, and will these features discriminate among the disorders?
2. Can insomnia be the only symptom of depression?
3. Is insomnia a risk factor for the development of psychiatric disorders?
4. Are primary sleep disorders such as sleep apnea, periodic limb movements, or narcolepsy more common in psychiatric disorders than in the general population?
5. Is the development of a psychiatric disorder a risk factor for the development of chronic insomnia?
6. Does treatment of psychiatric disorders have an impact on the associated insomnia?
7. Does treatment of insomnia with a hypnotic increase the risk of developing a psychiatric disorder?
8. How can sleep loss be both a symptom (insomnia) and a treatment (sleep deprivation) of major depression?

INSOMNIA DURING PSYCHIATRIC DISORDERS

Insomnia is common during the course of psychiatric illness. Insomnia is noted as a diagnostic symptom for mood disorders (i.e., major depression, dysthymia, mania) and anxiety disorders (i.e., generalized anxiety disorder).[9] Still, the presence of insomnia is not *required* to diagnose any of these major psychiatric diagnoses. The number of research articles published on sleep and psychiatric disorders quadrupled from 100 articles annually in the period 1976–1980 to 400 articles annually in 1986–1991.[10] Virtually all of that increase was explained by increases in the number of articles pertaining to the relationship between sleep and depression—comparatively less is known regarding the relationship of sleep and personality disorders, anxiety disorders, schizophrenia, and dementia.

It is estimated that 80% or more of manic-depressive patients have insomnia during an episode of depression.[11] Conversely, 35% of chronic insomniac patients have diagnosable psychiatric disorders.[12] Insomnia is a prominent complaint among depressed outpatients in primary care, and with other somatic symptoms may overshadow complaints of low mood in this setting.[13] Both mood disorder and anxiety disorder patients rate their sleep quality as poorer than nonpsychiatric controls, but it is unclear whether any one disorder is more likely than another to be associated with the perception of poor sleep quality.[14] Classically, early-morning awakening (EMA) is considered specific for a melancholic (i.e., severe) depression. Reynolds et al.[15] compared 14 patients with pseudodementia depression and 28 patients with primary dementia and found higher scores for the EMA item of the Hamilton Rating Scale for Depression (HAMD) in patients with pseudodementia. Similarly, Rodin et al.[16] performed a 3-year longitudinal study of insomnia and depressive symptoms in community-residing elderly people and found that EMA was the insomnia symptom most consistently related to depressed mood. Not all studies, however, have linked EMA to depression. Weissman[17] found that late insomnia was no more specific than initial insomnia in one study of 46 normals and 150 depressed outpatients. Greater severity of middle insomnia, not EMA, separated a comparison of dysthymic mood disorder patients and patients with generalized anxiety.[14] Even if it were true that EMA is more common in groups of depressed insomniac subjects compared with groups of nondepressed insomniac subjects, it would be hazardous to apply this principle to the diagnosis of a single patient. Hohagen et al.[18] examined the stability of the type of sleep complaint (initial, middle, late, initial-middle, initial-late, etc.) over 4 months in 328 insomniac patients identified from a sample of 2512 patients in a general practice. The authors found that 61% of the insomniac patients without EMA at intake were reporting EMA 4 months later if their insomnia had not completely remitted. Similarly, 36% of the insomniac patients who endorsed EMA at intake no longer reported EMA 4 months later if their insomnia had not remitted.[18] The variability of the insomnia pattern was not explained by co-morbid medical or psychiatric disorders or a change in hypnotic use. The authors concluded that clinical subtypes of insomnia are unstable over time, and that single cross-sectional descriptions of insomnia may be misleading.

In contrast, the PSG subtypes of insomnia (i.e., short rapid eye movement [REM] latency in depressive illness) may be stable over time, persisting from the active phase of illness to the remitted phase.[19]

Insomnia may have prognostic significance for depression, independent of its importance in establishing a diagnosis of depression. Fawcett et al[20] examined the rate of completed suicide in 954 patients with major depression. Sixty-eight patients completed suicide in the ensuing 10 years of follow-up. The presence of global insomnia at the time of the diagnosis of depression was one of the few clinical predictors of completed suicide in the first year of follow-up. Global insomnia lost its statistical significance during years 2 to 10 of follow-up. Agargun et al.[21] similarly found that the presence of suicidal thinking during the course of major depression was more common in the patients with insomnia compared with the depressed patients without insomnia. Conversely, the resolution of insomnia during the treatment of a depressed patient is associated with reduced risk of relapse in elderly patients followed through 1 year of continuation therapy for depression.[22]

Insomnia is not a criterion symptom of schizophrenia, but sleep disturbance is common, nonetheless.[23] Patients with schizophrenia may have an insomnia pattern indistinguishable from depressed patients, but day-night reversal is also common, particularly in the paranoid type.[24] The reasons for day-night reversal are unclear, but may be related to heightened perception of threat at nighttime with a corresponding relaxation during the day.[25] Insomnia is also not a criterion symptom for Alzheimer's dementia, but again day-night reversal is common in the advanced stages of the disease.[26, 27] The mechanism for day-night reversal in Alzheimer's disease may be related to degeneration of the suprachiasmatic nucleus and is probably different from the mechanism of day-night reversal in schizophrenia.[28]

Although clinical assessment of the severity and pattern of sleep disturbance may not be sufficiently reliable to discriminate among various psychiatric diagnoses in individual patients, it is sobering to note that the more sophisticated PSG fares no better. Some individual studies have provided evidence for the utility of PSG discriminating among insomnias,[29, 30] but in a meta-analysis Benca et al.[31] concluded that while PSG disturbances were common in psychiatric patients, no single PSG parameter was reliable in discriminating among the diagnoses.

INSOMNIA AS THE SOLE SYMPTOM OF DEPRESSION

The recognition that insomnia is a common symptom of depression opened the door to the concept of monosymptomatic depression—that is, a diagnosis of depression based solely upon the complaint of insomnia. The psychiatric literature has described individuals with alexithymia—literally, patients without words to express their feeling state.[32] These individuals are likely to employ somatic symptoms to communicate psychological distress, and may be particularly common in primary care.[13] The premise of "masked depression" is embedded in these concepts. Patients with masked depression substitute somatic complaints such as insomnia for the traditional core symptoms of depressed mood or loss of pleasure (anhedonia). Among the most common somatic symptoms in masked depression are headache, gastrointestinal distress, pain, and sleep disturbance.[33] Masked depression is a concept that is more popular in Europe than in the United States, judging by the origin of citations on the topic in the last 10 years. Regardless, the *Diagnostic and Statistical Manual of Mental Disorders*[9] makes no allowance for masked depression as either depressed mood or anhedonia must be present to make a diagnosis of major depression. In the absence of sufficient criteria to make a psychiatric diagnosis, we recommend that nonpsychiatric causes of persistent insomnia be considered.

INSOMNIA AS A RISK FACTOR FOR PSYCHIATRIC DISORDERS

Ford et al.[34] examined the importance of insomnia as a risk factor for the development of a new episode of depression. The study included 7954 respondents who were part of the National Institute of Mental Health Epidemiologic Catchment Area study. Respondents underwent a structured interview at two intervals separated by a year for the detection of psychiatric disorders or insomnia, or both. The authors found that respondents with insomnia but no depression at intake were at a 40-fold risk of developing a new episode of major depression and at a 25-fold risk of developing new-onset phobia, obsessive-compulsive disorder, or panic disorder if their insomnia had not remitted at the second interview 1 year later. The authors interpreted the data as suggesting that insomnia may be a modifiable risk factor for preventing new episodes of depression or anxiety disorder, or that the insomnia was simply the "leading edge" of a psychiatric disorder already in development. Similar results, but with smaller relative risks, have been found by Vollrath et al.,[35] Chang et al.,[36] and Dryman and Eaton.[37] Proof that insomnia is a modifiable risk factor for a new-onset psychiatric disorder must wait for a clinical trial that randomizes insomnia patients to treatment vs. no treatment for insomnia and then tracks the respective rates of new episodes of psychiatric disorder.

Wehr et al.[38] make an equally strong case that sleep disturbance is a risk factor for mania. Their case series demonstrate that acute sleep loss from a variety of mechanisms, including work demands, the temporal disruption of travel, or interpersonal stress, may be a direct antecedent of mania. The authors speculated that the insomnia of depression may occasionally be the precipitating factor for mania in patients already at risk of bipolar disorder. The authors suggested that the risk of mania might be reduced if physicians caution bipolar patients to protect their sleep by avoiding intentional sleep deprivation and being conservative in

travel plans requiring crossing multiple time zones, and so forth.

PREVALENCE OF PRIMARY SLEEP DISORDERS IN PSYCHIATRIC POPULATIONS

If sleep disturbance is a risk factor for psychiatric disorders, then we might expect that primary sleep disorders would be overrepresented in psychiatric populations. In general, the evidence has not supported this concern. Obstructive sleep apnea (OSA) and periodic limb movement (PLM) disorder do not appear to be more common in major depression than would be expected in the general population.[39] Conversely, depressed mood and anxiety do not appear to be an intrinsic part of OSA or PLM disorder.[40] It is possible, however, that certain psychotropic medications such as antidepressants may aggravate PLM.[41, 42] Tricyclic antidepressants (TCAs) may have an indirect aggravating effect on OSA by promoting weight gain.[43] OSA may also be a trigger for nocturnal panic attacks.[44] PSG would be helpful in distinguishing OSA from nocturnal panic attacks as both may manifest with nocturnal shortness of breath.

Narcolepsy is usually cataloged with disorders of excessive daytime sleepiness (EDS), but rarely the presentation of narcolepsy may be dominated by complaints of nocturnal sleep disturbance or hallucinations that are subsequently misinterpreted as schizophrenia. Douglass et al.[45, 46] have described such cases and reported that the "schizophrenic" symptoms were reversed with standard analeptic treatment. Although it is premature to recommend PSG or multiple sleep latency test (MSLT) screening for narcolepsy in all patients with a diagnosis of schizophrenia, it seems reasonable to consider testing any patient with presumed schizophrenia and unexplained EDS.

PSYCHIATRIC DISORDER PRECEDING PSYCHOPHYSIOLOGICAL INSOMNIA

Psychophysiological insomnia is defined as resulting from somatized tension and learned sleep-preventing associations.[47] Speilman[48] has suggested that psychophysiological insomnia is usefully conceptionalized as resulting from *predisposing* conditions interacting with *precipitating* circumstances, and maintained by *perpetuating* factors. Psychiatric disorders were identified as the precipitating factor by 10% of 315 patients seeking outpatient treatment for chronic insomnia.[49] A survey of five sleep disorders specialists reported that a prior psychiatric disorder was a contributing factor in 77% of new cases of primary (i.e., psychophysiological) insomnia.[50] Consider the following hypothetical case.

CASE HISTORY

Ms. Jones had always been a good sleeper until she developed an episode of major depression at 40 years of age. She spent many sleepless nights in bed during her depression, racked by suicidal and nihilistic thinking. She came to dread the night and her bedroom. Her symptoms of depression quickly abated with institution of antidepressant therapy, except her insomnia persisted. Antidepressant medications were stopped 6 months later and she remained free of psychiatric symptoms except for her continuing insomnia.

Depression is the precipitating factor in this case example, and the dysphoria associated with the bedroom is the perpetuating factor. There is no information regarding whether the predisposing conditions for depression are the same as or different from the predisposing conditions for insomnia. Behavioral treatment is the preferred treatment for this type of learned insomnia.[51] Most of the early research on behavioral treatment of insomnia was conducted on samples of nonpsychiatrically ill outpatients. Furthermore, it seemed important from a theoretical perspective to treat patients who were living at home because the patient's own bedroom was often the major reinforcing cue for perpetuating the insomnia. This stance appears to have softened, with several reports now advocating the use of behavioral treatment in psychiatrically ill insomniac patients, both in the home[52] and in the hospital.[53] Some behavioral scientists have extended the application of behavioral treatment by suggesting that behavioral treatment of a chronic insomnia associated with a psychiatric disorder may have beneficial effects on nonsleep symptoms of the psychiatric disorder.[54]

EFFECT OF ANTIDEPRESSANT MEDICATIONS ON INSOMNIA

Sleep latency and sleep continuity, as defined by PSG, are generally improved with TCA therapy of the depressed insomnia patient,[55, 56] with some TCAs performing better than others.[57] Trazodone, an older non-TCA antidepressant with sedating properties, also increases subjective total sleep time (TST) or PSG TST in depressed insomniac patients.[58] In contrast, the monoamine oxidase inhibitors (MAOIs) tranylcypromine and phenelzine may induce insomnia.[59, 60] The nocturnal sleep disturbance induced by MAOIs may be so severe as to produce daytime sleepiness.[59, 60]

Several new non-TCA antidepressant medications have been introduced in the United States since 1987 with variable effects on depression-related insomnia. The selective serotonin reuptake inhibitors (SSRIs) have the potential to induce or aggravate insomnia. Multiple investigations have shown that fluoxetine disturbs PSG continuity in depressed adults and children, and this effect may persist for weeks after drug discontinuation.[61-63] Others have reported that paroxetine prolonged sleep latency and produced more wakefulness after sleep onset in nondepressed adult insomniac patients.[64] There is comparatively less information on the

sleep effects of sertraline, but the available information suggests a relatively benign effect on subjective and PSG sleep continuity.[65] Venlafaxine, a serotonin-noradrenaline reuptake inhibitor, may disturb sleep continuity in a manner analogous to the SSRIs.[42]

Nefazodone is an antidepressant with SSRI properties, as well as blockade of 5-hydroxytryptamine (5HT-2A) receptors. Its effect on patient-rated insomnia and PSG-determined sleep disturbance has been compared with fluoxetine in depressed outpatients.[66] Compared with nefazodone, fluoxetine produced less improvement on patient-rated insomnia severity and was associated with PSG-determined deterioration of sleep efficiency (TST/total time in bed). Although the differences between these medications were the primary focus of the investigation, it is equally fascinating that the depressed fluoxetine-treated patients rated their insomnia as improving despite deterioration in their PSG-determined sleep continuity. Discrepancies in patient-rated and PSG-determined sleep are common in psychiatrically ill and nonpsychiatrically ill insomniac patients, thus raising questions regarding whether subjective complaints or objective measures should be the primary determinants of insomnia severity in psychiatric illness.[67, 68]

The evaluation of a continuing complaint of insomnia in a remitted depressed patient is complex. Consideration should be given to antidepressant medication–induced insomnia or a psychophysiological insomnia that was conditioned during the active phase of the depressive illness. If the insomnia is medication-induced, and if lowering the dose or switching to another antidepressant is not a tenable option, then adding trazodone 50 to 100 mg may relieve the insomnia complaint.[69] Other options might include a benzodiazepine hypnotic or behavioral therapy.

HYPNOTIC-INDUCED PSYCHIATRIC DISORDERS

Eighty-five percent of patients with insomnia do not receive treatment.[70] One third of the treated group use an over-the-counter preparation (usually an antihistamine), and two thirds of the treated group receive a prescription medication, usually a benzodiazepine. A small percentage of nondepressed patients with insomnia may receive an antidepressant as a hypnotic with unproven efficacy, but benzodiazepines represent the largest share of prescription treatments for insomnia.[71, 72] Benzodiazepines have other therapeutic actions in addition to their hypnotic action, including antianxiety, muscle relaxant, and anticonvulsant properties.[73] Therefore the subclinical anxiety[2, 3] associated with insomnia may respond to a long-acting benzodiazepine hypnotic (i.e., half-life of the parent compound about 24 h) given at bedtime.

Rarely, benzodiazepine hypnotics may *induce* a major psychiatric disorder. These induced disorders are generally of two types: either an induced depressive disorder, or an induced cognitive disorder. New exposure to benzodiazepine hypnotics was associated with increased risk of depressive symptoms as early as the first week compared with an untreated comparison group, with an overall increased relative risk of 4 in the first month of exposure.[74] Possibly the benzodiazepine was uncovering subclinical depression in these subjects. Benzodiazepine-induced cognitive disorder may include gross disorientation or more subtle isolated memory impairment. Recent initiation of benzodiazepines is associated with a fivefold increased relative risk of cognitive impairment in the elderly compared with nonusers and continuous users of benzodiazepines.[75] Benzodiazepine-induced cognitive dysfunction does not seem to worsen beyond the period of initial administration and remits upon drug discontinuation.[75] The risk of benzodiazepine hypnotic–induced cognitive dysfunction may be related to the pharmacokinetics of the specific medication.[76]

SLEEP LOSS AS BOTH A SYMPTOM AND A TREATMENT OF MAJOR DEPRESSION

Psychiatry is replete with apparent paradoxes. Among them is the riddle of how may sleep loss be both a symptom (insomnia) and a treatment (sleep deprivation) of major depression. Sleep deprivation has been noted to have mood-elevating properties.[77, 78] In the extreme, sleep deprivation can elevate mood to the point of mania, as noted above. More typically, sleep deprivation produces a rapid improvement in the mood of a clinically depressed patient which is observed as early as the first morning after sleep deprivation.[79, 80] The improvement in mood continues usually as long as the sleep deprivation can be maintained, but the patient often relapses with the first recovery sleep.[79, 80]

Mood-elevating sleep deprivation can be effected by (1) total sleep deprivation, (2) selective deprivation of only a portion of the night, usually eliminating the second half of the sleep period, or (3) selective REM sleep deprivation.[78] The finding of an antidepressant effect of selective REM deprivation helped discredit the theory that loss of REM sleep was a potential cause of psychiatric disturbance.[81] All of these approaches are labor-intensive, and although they are useful probes in our understanding of mood disorders, they are impractical for routine clinical use.

The paradox of sleep loss as both a symptom (i.e., insomnia) and a treatment (i.e., sleep deprivation) can be resolved by examining the differences between insomnia and intentional sleep deprivation (Table 56–1). The sleep loss of insomnia typically includes both short (a few seconds) and long (minutes to hours) interruptions of sleep continuity. In contrast, sleep interruption during therapeutic sleep deprivation is usually long (minutes to hours). Despite the reduction in TST, nondepressed insomniac subjects do not have EDS. Instead, they appear to be hyperaroused as measured by the MSLT and whole-body $\dot{V}O_2$.[82, 83] In contrast, systematic sleep deprivation produces EDS and brain hypometabolism in normal volunteers.[84] Systematic sleep deprivation in insomniac patients does result in

Table 56–1. COMPARISON OF INSOMNIA VS. INTENTIONAL SLEEP DEPRIVATION

	Insomnia	Sleep Deprivation
Sleep loss pattern	Erratic, variable	Systematic
Mean sleep latency on MSLT	Normal or elevated	Reduced
Mean waking EEG background	Faster	Slower
Metabolic rate	Higher	Lower
Body temperature	Higher	Lower

EEG, electroencephalogram; MSLT, multiple sleep latency tests.

EDS and hypometabolism similar to that seen in normal volunteers,[83, 85] suggesting that systematic sleep deprivation may offset the metabolic findings seen in nondepressed insomniac subjects. Although the effects of systematic sleep deprivation have not been thoroughly examined in depressed insomniac patients, if the results were similar, it would begin to explain the antidepressant effects of sleep deprivation in this population.

SUMMARY

Insomnia is an integral part of psychiatric disorders. Although insomnia is more common in psychiatric patients compared with nonpsychiatric groups, there is insufficient evidence to confidently differentiate among psychiatric diagnoses based upon the pattern of the insomnia (early, vs. middle, vs. terminal insomnia). Insomnia may precede the development of a major depression, but it is unclear whether this is a modifiable risk factor. It seems more likely that sleep loss is a modifiable risk factor for mania. Primary sleep disorders such as sleep apnea are generally not more prevalent in psychiatric populations compared with nonpsychiatric patient groups. Occasionally, insomnia may persist after the resolution of a major psychiatric disorder, and this may be related to a conditioned arousal response created during the episode of psychiatric illness, or it may be a side effect of psychiatric medications. Treatment of insomnia with benzodiazepines occasionally induces psychiatric disorders. Finally, the observation that sleep loss is both a symptom (insomnia) and a treatment (sleep deprivation) of depression highlights the complexity of the relationship between sleep and psychiatric disorders.

Acknowledgments

Supported in part by NIMH awards MH01090 and MH51552. We thank Dr. Peter Hauri for assistance with Table 56–1.

References

1. McCall WV, Edinger JD. Subjective total insomnia: an example of sleep state misperception. Sleep. 1992;15:71–73.
2. Williams RL, Ware C, Ilaria RL, et al. Disturbed sleep and anxiety.

In: Fann WE, ed. Phenomenology and Treatment of Anxiety. New York, NY: Spectrum Publications; 1979:211–223.

3. Stepanski E, Koshorek G, Zorick F, et al. Characteristics of individuals who do or do not seek treatment for chronic insomnia. Psychosomatics. 1989;30:421–427.

4. Mellinger GD, Mitchell B, Eberhard H, et al. Insomnia and its treatment. Arch Gen Psychiatry. 1985;42:225–232.

5. Kessler RC, McGonagle KA, Zhoa S, et al. Lifetime and 12-month prevalence of DSM-III-R psychiatric disorders in the United States. Arch Gen Psychiatry. 1994;51:8–19.

6. Adams F. The Genuine Works of Hippocrates. Baltimore, Md: Williams & Williams; 1939:48.

7. Kalinowsky L, Hoch P. Somatic Treatments in Psychiatry. New York, NY: Grune & Stratton; 1961:308–309.

8. American Sleep Disorders Association, Standards of Practice Committee. Practice parameters for the use of polysomnography in the evaluation of insomnia: an American Sleep Disorders Association Report. Sleep. 1995;18:55–57.

9. American Psychiatric Association. Diagnostic and Statistical Manual of Mental Disorders. 4th ed. Washington, DC: American Psychiatric Association Press; 1994.

10. Nofzinger EA, Buysse DJ, Reynolds CF, et al. Sleep disorders related to another mental disorder (nonsubstance/primary): a DSM-IV literature review. J Clin Psychiatry. 1993;54:244–255.

11. Goodwin F, Jamieson K. Manic-Depressive Illness. New York, NY: Oxford University Press; 1990:44.

12. Coleman RM, Roffwarg HP, Kennedy SJ, et al. Sleep-wake disorders based on polysomnographic diagnosis: a National Cooperative Study. JAMA. 1982;247:997–1003.

13. Blacker CVR, Clare AW. Depressive disorder in primary care. Br J Psychiatry. 1987;150:737–751.

14. Arriaga F, Paiva T. Clinical and EEG sleep changes in primary dysthymia and generalized anxiety: a comparison with normal controls. Neuropsychobiology. 1990;24:109–114.

15. Reynolds CF, Hoch CC, Kupfer DJ, et al. Bedside differentiation of depressive pseudodementia from dementia. Am J Psychiatry. 1988;145:1099–1103.

16. Rodin J, McAvay G, Timko C. A longitudinal study of depressed mood and sleep disturbances in elderly adults. J Gerontol. 1988;43:45–53.

17. Weissman MM, Prusoff B, Pincus C. Symptom patterns in depressed patients and depressed normals. J Nerv Ment Dis. 1975;160:15–23.

18. Hohagen F, Kappler C, Schramm E, et al. Sleep onset insomnia, sleep maintaining insomnia and insomnia with early morning awakening—Temporal stability of subtypes in a longitudinal study on general practice attenders. Sleep. 1994;17:551–554.

19. Rush AJ, Erman MK, Giles DE, et al. Polysomnographic findings in recently drug-free and clinically remitted depressed patients. Arch Gen Psychiatry. 1986;43:878–884.

20. Fawcett J, Scheftner W, Fogg L, et al. Time related predictors of suicide in major affective disorder. Am J Psychiatry. 1990;147:1189–1194.

21. Agargun MY, Kara H, Solmaz M. Sleep disturbances and suicidal behavior in patients with major depression. J Clin Psychiatry. 1997;58:249–251.

22. Reynolds CF, Frank E, Houck PR, et al. Which elderly patients with remitted depression remain well with continued interpersonal psychotherapy after discontinuation of antidepressant medication? Am J Psychiatry. 1997;154:958–962.

23. Kempenaers C, Kerkhofs M, Linkowski P, et al. Sleep EEG variables in young schizophrenic and depressed patients. Biol Psychiatry. 1988;24:828–833.

24. Benson KL, Zarcone VP. Sleep abnormalities in schizophrenia and other psychotic disorders. In: Oldham JM, Riba MB, eds. Review of Psychiatry. Vol 13. Washington, DC: American Psychiatric Association Press; 1994:677–705.

25. Benca RM. Sleep in psychiatric disorders. Neurol Clin. 1996;14:739–764.

26. Shelton PS, Hocking LB. Zolpidem for dementia-related insomnia and nighttime wandering. Ann Pharmacother. 1997;31:319–321.

27. Prinz PN, Vitiello MV, Raskind MA, et al. Geriatrics: sleep disorders and aging—review article. N Engl J Med. 1990;323:520–526.

28. Colenda CC, Cohen WM, McCall WV, et al. Phototherapy for Alzheimer's disease patients with sleep disturbance: results of a pilot study. Alzheimer Dis Assoc Disord. 1997;11:175–178.

29. Jacobs EA, Reynolds CF, Kupfer DJ, et al. The role of polysomnography in the differential diagnosis of chronic insomnia. Am J Psychiatry. 1988;145:346–349.

30. Gillin JC, Duncan W, Pettigrew KD, et al. Successful separation of depressed, normal, and insomniac subjects by EEG sleep data. Arch Gen Psychiatry. 1979;36:85–90.

31. Benca RM, Obermeyer WH, Thisted RA, et al. Sleep and psychiatric disorders: a meta-analysis. Arch Gen Psychiatry. 1992;49:651–668.

32. Taylor GJ. The alexithymia construct: conceptualization, validation, and relationship with basic dimensions of personality. New Trends Exp Clin Psychiatry. 1994;10:61–73.

33. DeWester JN. Recognizing and treating the patient with somatic-manifestations of depression. J Fam Pract. 1996;43(suppl):S3–515.

34. Ford DE, Kamerow DB. Epidemiologic study of sleep disturbances and psychiatric disorders—an opportunity for prevention? JAMA. 1989;262:1479–1484.

35. Vollrath M, Wicki W, Angst J. The Zurich Study VIII. Insomnia: Association With Depression, Anxiety, Somatic Syndromes, and Course of Insomnia. Eur Arch Psychiatr Neurol Sci. 1989;239:113–124.

36. Chang P, Ford D, Mead L, et al. Insomnia in young men and subsequent depression. Am J Epidemiol. 1997;146:105–114.

37. Dryman A, Eaton WW. Affective symptoms associated with the onset of major depression in the community: findings from the US National Institute of Mental Health Epidemiologic Catchment Area Program. Acta Psychiatr Scand. 1991;84:1–5.

38. Wehr TA, Sack DA, Rosenthal NE. Sleep reduction as a final common pathway in the genesis of mania. Am J Psychiatry. 1987;144:201–204.

39. Reynolds CF, Coble P, Spiker D, et al. Prevalence of sleep apnea and nocturnal myoclonus in major affective disorders: clinical and polysomnographic findings. J Nerv Ment Dis. 1982;170:565–567.

40. Dickel MJ, Mosko SS. Morbidity cut-offs for sleep apnea and periodic leg movements in predicting subjective complaints in seniors. Sleep. 1990;13:155–166.

41. Ware JC, Brown FW, Moorad PJ, et al. Nocturnal myoclonus and tricyclic antidepressants. Sleep Res. 1984;13:72.

42. Salen-Pascual RJ, Gallcia-Polo L, Drucker-Colin R. Sleep changes after four continuous days administration of venlafaxine in normal volunteers. Sleep Res. 1997;26:19.

43. Noyes R, Garvey MJ, Cook BL, et al. Problems with tricyclic antidepressant use in patients with panic disorders or agoraphobia: results of a naturalistic follow-up study. J Clin Psychiatry. 1989;50:163–169.

44. Enns M, Stern M, Kryger M. Successful treatment of comorbid panic disorder and sleep apnea with continuous positive airway pressure. Psychosomatics. 1995;36:585–586.

45. Douglass AB, Hays P, Pazderka F, et al. Florid refractory schizophrenias that turn out to be treatable variants of HLA-associated narcolepsy. J Nerv Ment Dis. 1991;179:12–17.

46. Douglass AB, Shipley JE, Haines RF, et al. Schizophrenia, narcolepsy, and HLA-DR 15, DQ6. Biol Psychiatry. 1993;34:773–780.

47. Diagnostic Steering Committee. International Classification of Sleep Disorders: Diagnostic and Coding Manual. Rochester, Minn: American Sleep Disorders Association; 1990.

48. Spielman AJ. Assessment of insomnia. Clin Psych Rev. 1986;6:11–25.

49. Gagne A, Bastien C, Morin C. Precipitating events of insomnia [abstract]. Sleep Res. 1997;26:281.

50. Nowell PD, Buysse DJ, Reynolds CF, et al. Clinical factors contributing to the differential diagnosis of primary insomnia and insomnia related to mental disorders. Am J Psychiatry. 1997;154:1412–1416.

51. Spielman AJ, Saskin P, Thorpy MJ. Treatment of chronic insomnia by restriction of time in bed. Sleep. 1987;10:45–56.

52. Dashevsky B, Kramer M. Combined behavioral and medicinal treatment of insomnia in psychiatric patients. Sleep Res. 1997;26:200.

53. Morin CM, Kowatch RA, O'Shanick G. Case report: sleep restriction for the inpatient treatment of insomnia. Sleep. 1990;13:183–186.

54. Blais FC, Mimeault V, Morin CM. Treatment of comorbid insomnia and anxiety disorders. Sleep Res. 1997;26:372.

55. Kupfer, DJ. The Sleep EEG in Diagnosis and Treatment of Depression: Basic Mechanisms, Diagnosis and Treatment. New York, NY: Guilford Press; 1986:102–125.

56. Kupfer DJ, Spiker DG, Rossi A, et al. Nortriptyline and EEG sleep in depressed patients. Biol Psychiatry. 1982;17:535–546.

57. Ware, JC, Brown FW, Moorad, PJ, et al. Comparison of trimipramine and imipramine in depressed insomniac patients. Sleep Res. 1984;13:65.

58. Scharf MB, Sachais, BA. Sleep laboratory evaluation of the effects and efficacy of trazodone in depressed insomniac patients. J Clin Psychiatry. 1990;51(suppl):13–17.

59. Joffe RT. Afternoon fatigue and somnolence associated with tranylcypromine treatment. J Clin Psychiatry. 1990;51:192–193.

60. Teicher MH, Cohen BM, Baldessarini RJ, et al. Severe daytime somnolence in patients treated with an MAOI. Am J Psychiatry. 1988;145:1552–1556.

61. Trivedi M, Hoffmann R, et al. Effects of fluoxetine on macro and micro-analytic measures of sleep in patients with major depression [abstract]. Sleep Res. 1997;26:369.

62. Armitage R, Emslie G, Rintelmann J. Effects of fluoxetine on sleep EEG in childhood depression [abstract]. Sleep Res. 1997;26:345.

63. Buysse DJ, Monahan JP, Cherry CR, et al. Persistent effects on sleep EEG following fluoxetine discontinuation. Sleep Res. 1997;26:370.

64. Oswald I, Adam K. Effects of paroxetine on human sleep. Br J Clin Pharmacol. 1986;22:97–99.

65. Cole JO. New directions in antidepressant therapy: a review of sertraline, a unique serotonin reuptake inhibitor. J Clin Psychiatry. 1992;53:333–340.

66. Gillin JC, Rapaport M, Erman MK, et al. A comparison of nefazodone and fluoxetine on mood and on objective, subjective, and clinician-rated measures of sleep in depressed patients: a double-blind, 8-week clinical trial. J Clin Psychiatry. 1997;58:185–192.

67. Weiss BL, McPartland RJ, Kupfer DJ. Once more: the inaccuracy of non-EEG estimations of sleep. Am J Psychiatry. 1973;130:1282–1285.

68. Frankel BL, Coursey RD, Buchbinder R, et al. Recorded and reported sleep in chronic primary insomnia. Arch Gen Psychiatry. 1976;33:615–623.

69. Nierenberg AA, Adler LA, Peselow E, et al. Trazodone for antidepressant-associated insomnia. Am J Psychiatry. 1994;151:1069–1072.

70. Consensus Development Panel, Freedman D, chairman. Drugs and insomnia. JAMA. 1984;251:2410–2414.

71. Wysowski DK, Baum C. Outpatient use of prescription sedative-hypnotic drugs in the United States, 1970 through 1989. Arch Intern Med. 1991;151:1779–1784.

72. Solomon F, White CC, Parron DL, et al. Sleeping pills, insomnia and medical practice. N Engl J Med. 1979;300:803–808.

73. Gilman AG: Goodman and Gilman's The Pharmacological Basis of Therapeutics. 9th ed. Hardman J, Limbird L, eds. New York, NY: McGraw-Hill; 1996:372.

74. Patten SB, Williams JV, Love EJ. Self-reported depressive symptoms following treatment with corticosteroids and sedative-hypnotics. J Psychiatry Med. 1996;26:15–24.

75. Dealberto M-J, McAvay GJ, Seeman T, et al. Psychotropic drug use and cognitive decline among older men and women. Int J Geriatr Psychiatry. 1997;12:567–574.

76. Barbee JG. Memory, benzodiazepines, and anxiety: integration of theoretical and clinical perspectives. J Clin Psychiatry. 1993;54(suppl):86–97.

77. Dessauer M, Goetze U, Tolle R. Periodic sleep deprivation in drug-refractory depression. Neuropsychobiology. 1985;13:111–116.

78. Vogel GW, Vogel F, McAbee RS, et al. Improvement of depression by REM sleep deprivation. Arch Gen Psychiatry. 1980;37:247–253.

79. Wu JC, Bunney WE. The biological basis of an antidepressant response to sleep deprivation and relapse: review and hypothesis. Am J Psychiatry. 1990;147:14–21.

80. Leibenluft E, Wehr TA. Is sleep deprivation useful in the treatment of depression? Am J Psychiatry. 1992;149:159–168.

81. Snyder F. Dynamic aspects of sleep disturbance in relation to mental illness. Biol Psychiatry. 1969;1:119–130.

82. Stepanski E, Zorick F, Roehrs T, et al. Daytime alertness in patients with chronic insomnia compared with asymptomatic control subjects. Sleep. 1988;11:54–60.

83. Bonnet MH, Arand DL. 24-Hour metabolic rate in insomniacs and matched normal sleepers. Sleep. 1995;18:581–588.

84. Bonnet MH, Arand DL. Caffeine use as a model of acute and chronic insomnia. Sleep. 1992;15:526–536.

85. Freedman RR. EEG power spectra in sleep-onset insomnia. Electroencephalogr Clin Neurophysiol. 1986;63:408–413.

57

Behavioral Therapy for Insomnia

Edward J. Stepanski

The current consensus regarding the treatment of chronic insomnia recommends that diagnosis of the cause of the symptom is necessary before an appropriate treatment regimen can be proposed. The insomnia may be secondary to a medical disorder, psychiatric disorder, or sleep disorder, or it may be categorized as "primary." Behavioral treatment programs have been endorsed as most appropriate for patients diagnosed with primary insomnia.[1] The International Classification of Sleep Disorders has four categories for primary insomnia: psychophysiological, inadequate sleep hygiene, idiopathic, and sleep state misperception.[2] In secondary insomnias, although the treatment should be aimed at the underlying medical or psychiatric disorder, behavioral treatment might serve as an adjunctive treatment (Fig. 57–1).

THEORIES OF PRIMARY INSOMNIA

One challenge that confronts insomnia treatment generally and behavioral therapy specifically is understanding the mechanisms underlying primary insomnias. Several theories of insomnia have been proposed to explain causal factors.[3] Physiological arousal, emotional arousal, cognitive arousal, and faulty conditioning are all factors that have been proposed as causes of primary insomnia. The empirical support for regarding each of these theoretical views is equivocal. Heightened physiological arousal in the form of higher core body temperature and increased vasoconstrictions has been reported in poor sleepers before bedtime and during the night.[4] Increased metabolic rate and increased heart rate reactivity have also been shown in insomniacs compared with normal sleepers.[5, 6] Proponents of progressive relaxation procedures believe that physiological hyperarousal at bedtime prevents sleep onset and may lead to fragmented sleep later in the night. It follows that by teaching patients skills that decrease tension, greater control over arousal is achieved, and sleep ability is improved. However, treatment outcome studies using relaxation procedures have shown that basal levels of physiological arousal did not correlate with the level of sleep onset difficulty. In addition, decreases in physiological arousal after relaxation training did not correlate with subsequent changes in sleep onset latency (SOL), even though SOL was significantly reduced.[7–9]

The theory of emotional arousal is based on the consistent finding of abnormal Minnesota Multiphasic Personality Inventory profiles in groups of insomniacs.[10] A common personality style in this population is one that uses repression and denial in response to stress. When these defense mechanisms are used, "internalization" of emotion is expected. Arguing against this position is the lack of correlation between psychometric measures and severity of insomnia.[11] Many individuals with these same personality characteristics have no sleep complaints. It has been argued that the association between personality and sleep can just as easily be interpreted as operating in the opposite causal direction; that is, mood changes may be a response to, rather than a cause of, insomnia.[12]

The role of cognitive arousal in insomnia is supported by the common report in insomniacs of increased rumination with negative content before bedtime. Insomniacs report that cognitive arousal, more than somatic arousal, is to blame for their sleep difficulties.[13] More dysfunctional attitudes and beliefs about sleep have been found in older insomniacs than in asymptomatic sleepers.[14] The group of insomniacs had increased expectations of impairment associated with not sleeping, greater fears of losing control of their sleep, and less belief in their ability to improve their sleep. Theories advocating the primacy of cognitive arousal have not been supported by studies that have manipulated presleep stress.[15, 16] When given cognitive tasks before bedtime, good and poor sleepers slept as well or better than in neutral conditions.

A fourth hypothesis contends that patients have been conditioned to have increased arousal in their sleep environment. This theory is derived from learning research that shows the ability of various stimuli to act as cues in eliciting behavioral responses. Unfortunately, good sleepers have been shown to have the same prevalence of bad sleep habits as do poor sleepers.[17] In addition, some outcome studies have used a "countercontrol" condition (placebo) as a control for stimulus control therapy.[18] Under countercontrol conditions, subjects are given instructions that would be

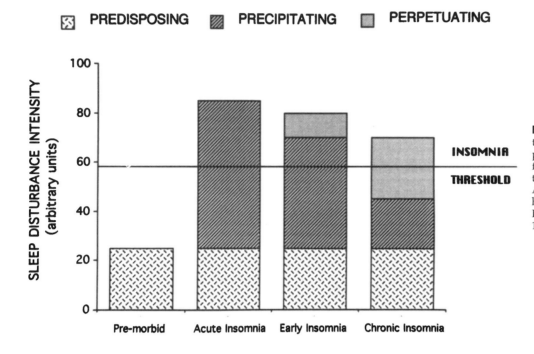

Figure 57–1. Theoretical model of the contribution of predisposing, precipitating, and perpetuating factors in chronic insomnia across time. (Adapted from Spielman AJ, Caruso L, Glovinsky P. A behavioral perspective on insomnia. Psychiatric Clin North Am. 1987; 10:541–553.)

expected to strengthen the conditioned arousal in the bedroom and are opposite those used under stimulus control conditions. Patients must stay in bed when they are unable to sleep and engage in wake activities, and they are also required to spend 30 min each day in bed doing waking activities. Subjects in the countercontrol condition have shown the same improvement in subjective measures of sleep found in the stimulus control condition. Significant improvement in sleep maintenance insomnia has been reported in another study using countercontrol, although no placebo control was available.[19]

Although there are many hypotheses about the causes of insomnia, none of these theories can entirely account for the phenomenon of chronic insomnia. A comprehensive model of acute/chronic insomnia that describes the complex interactions among many contributing factors in the development and maintenance of insomnia has been proposed by Spielman.[20] This model proposes that causes of insomnia can be categorized as predisposing, precipitating, or perpetuating factors (Fig. 57–1). All individuals are hypothesized to have some initial predisposition to disturbed sleep. A tendency toward heightened physiological, emotional, or cognitive arousal would be a predisposing factor in this model. This tendency toward increased arousal is necessary, but not sufficient, for the development of insomnia. Insomnia actually results with exposure to a precipitating factor. An individual with a high predisposition for insomnia may require a minor precipitant (e.g., sleeping in a hotel room) to produce significant insomnia, whereas a person with a low predisposition may require a more significant precipitant (e.g., bereavement) before sleep is adversely affected. A final component in this model is the role of perpetuating factors in maintaining poor sleep. Perpetuating factors are typically poor sleep habits that develop during

episodes of insomnia. Erratic sleep-wake schedules, nocturnal eating, and excessive worry about sleep are examples of perpetuating factors. The use of this theoretical model has obvious application to the clinical task of evaluating and treating patients presenting with complaints of insomnia. By understanding the operative predisposing, precipitating, and perpetuating factors in a specific patient, it should be possible to focus treatment on features relevant to that patient. This is essential for cognitive therapy because not all patients will share the same fears and dysfunctional thoughts regarding the loss of sleep. Behavioral treatments can be categorized according to this model. Most cognitive or behavioral treatments are aimed at ameliorating perpetuating factors, although it could be argued that relaxation treatments operate by modifying the predisposition to arousal. This model also illustrates why behavioral treatment may be helpful, even though the original trigger for the insomnia (e.g., a hospital stay) is no longer active. An understanding of how perpetuating factors maintain poor sleep is critical to the successful treatment of insomnia.

DEVELOPMENT OF BEHAVIORAL PROGRAMS

Relaxation Techniques

The basic tenets of progressive relaxation approaches for insomnia were formulated before 1950, although the majority of controlled studies of these treatments have been conducted since 1970. In the 1920s and 1930s, Dr. Edmund Jacobson published several papers describing techniques that promote muscular relaxation. In 1938, he published a book specifically about insomnia that advocated the use of his new procedure, *progressive relaxation,* as a treatment for this disorder.[21] This treatment teaches patients how to recognize physiological tension and then learn to control this tension. A series of exercises that consist of first tensing and then relaxing each muscle group in a systematic way is taught to the patient. These procedures have since been developed and are described fully elsewhere.[22, 23] Progressive relaxation is initially taught in a 1-h training session; additional sessions to provide feedback and assess proficiency are scheduled as needed. The patient must practice the exercises twice each day, with the second practice session just before bedtime.

Another prominent treatment designed to produce physiological relaxation is electromyographic (EMG) biofeedback. Frontalis muscle tension is measured through an EMG recording, and the patient is given either visual or auditory feedback to indicate the level of tension.[24] Patients are taught relaxation techniques, such as deep breathing, and the immediate feedback helps them discriminate when they are being most successful. In this way, patients are better able to learn how it feels to be relaxed and which behaviors will induce relaxation or increase tension. Biofeedback training sessions are continued until the patient can reliably produce the desired change in the target behavior.

Cognitive arousal, which is experienced as racing thoughts or worrying, has also been hypothesized to produce delayed sleep onset in insomniacs. Therapy for this problem hypothesizes that if patients can learn to control their thoughts, sleep onset can proceed normally. *Meditation* and *guided imagery* are techniques that provide a neutral or pleasant target on which to focus the thought process. Guided imagery consists of having the patient visualize a specific scene that is associated with a calm and relaxed state. As with progressive muscle relaxation, these techniques are first taught during training sessions and then practiced for a 20-min period daily by the patients at home. It may take several weeks of practice before a patient will be able to effectively use the technique for relaxation. These approaches may help by directly inducing relaxation but also act to prevent the patient from engaging in cognitive activity that will cause increased tension (e.g., obsessing about why he or she is not sleeping).

All of these treatments share diffuse relaxation effects in addition to the specific type of relaxation that is intended. For example, practicing meditation decreases physiological arousal in addition to cognitive arousal. This poses a problem in studies trying to isolate a specific mechanism of action for these treatments but affords a bonus in a clinical setting when the cause of arousal may be unknown.

Stimulus Control Therapy

Based not on theory but on his observations of patients, Jacobson also recommended changes in sleep habits that today would be included in sleep hygiene (see Chapter 58) or stimulus control treatment.[21] For example, he states:

> Reading in bed is a bad policy. I warn my patients against it. If they read in order to fall asleep, they have acquired a bad habit, for they accustom themselves to imagining and reflecting in bed in place of relaxing there. Your bed is not the proper place to cultivate an active mind; but if you stimulate yourself with reading matter when you desire to fall asleep, evidently you should not expect the best form of rest to result. It is better practice to do your reading before retiring, and to reserve your bed for relaxation alone.[21(p68)]

An association between the sleep environment and wakefulness can develop. A treatment for this, *stimulus control therapy,* was developed by Bootzin and Nicassio.[25] Stimulus control attempts to break this association by teaching the patient not to engage in "sleep incompatible" behavior in the bedroom and to be in the bedroom only when drowsy or asleep.

The instructions for stimulus control therapy as described by Bootzin and Nicassio[25] are as follows:

1. Lie down intending to go to sleep only when sleepy.
2. Do not use your bed for anything except sleep; that is, do not read, watch television, eat, or worry in bed. Sexual activity is the only exception to this rule. On such occasions, the instructions are to be followed afterward when you intend to go to sleep.
3. If you find yourself unable to fall asleep, get up and go into another room. Stay up as long as you wish and then return to the bedroom to sleep. Although we do not want you to watch the clock, we want you to get out of bed if you do not fall asleep immediately. Remember that the goal is to associate your bed with falling asleep quickly! If you are in bed more than about 10 min without falling asleep and have not gotten up, you are not following this instruction.
4. If you still cannot fall asleep, repeat rule 3. Do this as often as is necessary throughout the night.
5. Set your alarm and get up at the same time every morning regardless of how much sleep you got during the night. This will help your body acquire a consistent sleep rhythm.
6. Do not nap during the day.

Because the patient is only in bed when feeling drowsy or actually sleeping, a positive association between the sleep environment and relaxation is strengthened. Stimulus control therapy may sound easy for both therapist and patient, especially in comparison to relaxation training and sleep restriction therapy (described later); however, as with all behavioral treatment, the patient must be very motivated, and the therapist must provide a coherent explanation of the rationale for these recommendations in addition to ongoing encouragement and monitoring. The practice of simply giving a patient a typed list of the stimulus control instructions is not sufficient.[26]

Sleep Restriction Therapy

Sleep restriction therapy was developed by Spielman et al.[27] and is based on the homeostasis theory of sleep propensity. This treatment seeks to increase homeostatic sleep drive through partial sleep deprivation and thereby improve sleep ability. A strict schedule of bedtimes and arising times is prescribed to try to consolidate sleep and decrease time spent awake during the night. Patients initially reduce their time in bed to the amount of time they are actually sleeping according to their sleep logs but not less than 4.5 h. The arising time is fixed, and the bedtime is manipulated based on the patient's self-reported sleep efficiency. If the sleep efficiency for the prior 5 days is 90% or more, then the patient goes to bed 15 min earlier. If the sleep efficiency is less than 85%, then the bedtime is pushed back later to equal the mean total sleep time of the prior 5 days. This decrease in time in bed is not made for at least 10 days from the beginning of treatment or within 10 days of any other schedule change. Modifications to this original protocol have been suggested.[28] The sleep efficiency needed to make a change in the schedule was lowered by 5% for elderly patients, in keeping with expected reductions in this parameter associated with aging. Further decreases in time in bed after the original reduction are avoided in an effort to improve patient compliance. Finally, a schedule of programmed increases in time in bed has been used, particularly when the patient may have a large subjective component to their insomnia.[29] This programmed increase may be helpful because patients with "subjective" insomnia never report sufficiently high sleep efficiencies to follow the usual criteria for increasing time in bed.

Combined Behavioral Treatment Programs

A recent innovation in the behavioral treatment of insomnia is to combine treatments previously shown to be effective in treatment outcome studies. The rationale for this approach is that the patient is more likely to be exposed to a treatment that works for their specific problem. In addition, a combined treatment model is more like the "real world" in that patients in treatment with a sleep specialist may often receive instruction in more than one behavioral treatment.

Cognitive-Behavioral Therapy

The most widely studied treatment programs are those that combine behavioral treatments and cognitive therapy into a single treatment package.[30, 31] Cognitive-behavioral therapy (CBT) has been used for the treatment of psychological disorders (e.g. anxiety, depression) and was adapted by sleep specialists for use in patients with insomnia. A program of CBT typically consists of 8 to 10 weekly sessions that sequentially provide sleep education, stimulus control techniques, sleep restriction therapy, and cognitive therapy. The cognitive therapy component is aimed at changing un-realistic beliefs and irrational fears regarding sleep or the loss of sleep. An example of an unrealistic belief found commonly in patients with insomnia is the over-estimation of the amount of total sleep time they require to be fully rested. Patients then become anxious if this amount of sleep is not achieved and may become focused on achieving a specific amount of sleep that exceeds their actual physiological sleep need. An example of an irrational fear is that patients may exaggerate the negative consequences of a poor night's sleep. These types of cognitions are hypothesized to escalate the likelihood that patients will experience increased tension and performance anxiety regarding falling asleep, contributing to psychophysiological insomnia. Cognitive therapy is a psychotherapeutic process that targets dysfunctional cognitions regarding sleep. Through cognitive therapy, these beliefs and fears are identified, challenged, and replaced with realistic expectations regarding sleep and daytime function.

A CBT protocol described by Morin[30] consists of eight weekly treatment sessions. Sessions are 60 min long for individual treatment and 90 min long for group treatment. The content of each session is as follows:

Session 1: Overview of treatment program and sleep education
Session 2: Stimulus control and sleep restriction principles introduced
Session 3: Discussion of problems encountered after 1 week of trying the behavioral treatments prescribed in session 2
Session 4: Cognitive therapy introduced
Session 5: Compliance with behavioral therapy assessed, cognitive therapy continued
Session 6: Sleep hygiene education provided, cognitive therapy continued, and compliance with behavioral treatment reevaluated
Session 7: All treatment components reviewed
Session 8: Strategies for avoiding relapse presented

This outline oversimplifies the content of each session but provides a general idea as to the structure of the program. Obviously, there is a strong emphasis on evaluation of compliance and a review of behavioral principles with feedback regarding individual problems with implementation of techniques.

Another treatment program that has been studied combines stimulus control, sleep restriction therapy, and the relaxation response.[32] This program consists of five 30-min sessions spaced every 2 weeks. The context of each session is as follows:

Session 1: Sleep education and sleep hygiene
Session 2: Sleep restriction techniques
Session 3: Modified stimulus control
Session 4: Daytime relaxation response techniques
Session 5: Bedtime relaxation response techniques

Other Behavioral Approaches

Sensory motor rhythm biofeedback seeks to strengthen the patient's ability to produce brain waves in the frequency range of sleep spindles. The elements of this treatment are the same as in EMG biofeedback training as described, except that the feedback is contingent on the electroencephalographic (EEG) frequency.

The use of bright light therapy for circadian causes of insomnia can also be considered a behavioral treatment; this approach is discussed in Chapter 105.

In addition to the specific goals of these approaches, all behavioral treatments share particular nonspecific effects. Of central importance, an increase in self-efficacy is an outcome common to these treatments. Patients learn to rely on their own ability to control sleep. This is in contrast to pharmacological treatment, in which control lies clearly with the medication or prescribing physician. Self-efficacy may be especially relevant for many insomniacs for whom the "lack of control" is a key feature of their sleep complaint.

COMBINED BEHAVIORAL AND PHARMACOLOGICAL TREATMENT

The use of hypnotic medication and behavioral treatment need not be mutually exclusive, and combining these modalities would appear to be a logical approach for certain patients. Unfortunately, data on this topic are sparse. One study compared hypnotic medication alone to medication with stimulus control and relaxation training.[33] Both groups showed equivalent improvement after the 3-week treatment period, but the combined group was significantly better at follow-up 5 weeks after treatment. Hauri[34] compared behavioral treatment alone (sleep hygiene and relaxation) with a combined behavioral and pharmacological treatment. Both groups were improved after treatment, but only the behavioral treatment–alone group maintained this improvement at 10-month follow-up. Morin et al.[35] compared the use of CBT alone, medication alone, combined behavioral/medication treatment, and a drug–placebo condition. Both self-report and polysomnographic measures showed that all three treatments produced significant improvement compared with placebo. Self-report measures collected at 3-, 12-, and 24-month follow-ups found that only the CBT group maintained their improved sleep. In summary, there is agreement among these studies that behavioral treatment will produce long-term improvement and that medication alone will not. Furthermore, outcome for patients using both behavioral treatment and medication appears to be worse than that for behavioral treatment alone. It is possible that patients using medication do not practice the behavioral changes as reliably, or they may attribute their improvement to the medication such that they never internalize a sense of control over insomnia.

BARRIERS TO THE USE OF BEHAVIORAL TREATMENT

Despite recent interest in behavioral approaches, pharmacological treatment is the most commonly used approach for the treatment of insomnia.[36] Given that behavioral treatments have been available for many years, why have they not gained greater acceptance as a viable treatment option to be used at least as often as pharmacological treatment? One possible reason is that behavioral treatment is time intensive for clinicians and patients alike. The practitioner typically must provide up to several hours of instruction, ongoing encouragement and reassurance, and monitoring of patients through sleep logs, often for as long as several months. This level of attention may not be practical for most primary care settings. In addition, most practitioners do not have the expertise to provide this treatment, but they can prescribe hypnotic medication. These treatments are also demanding for the patient who must complete daily monitoring forms, practice techniques daily, make lifestyle changes, and maintain patience, often in the face of considerable fear that the insomnia will not improve. However, patients are increasingly reluctant to rely on "sleeping pills" in the wake of negative press concerning adverse side effects and the danger of addiction. Morin et al.[37] have shown that patients prefer to try behavioral approaches when given the choice between these and pharmacological treatments. They expect behavioral treatment to have fewer side effects and to produce better long-term improvement.

Although the theories described have great intuitive appeal and behavioral therapies have frequently been recommended for insomnia to address these likely underlying causes of the symptom, data from outcome studies are equivocal. Various methods of relaxation training, stimulus control, EMG or sensory motor rhythm biofeedback, autogenic imagery, paradoxical intention, and sleep restriction have all been studied in insomniacs. These studies generally conclude that behavioral treatments have specific effects that lead to significantly improved sleep. There are methodological shortcomings that may explain the inconsistencies among results from different studies.

VALIDITY OF SUBJECTIVE OUTCOME MEASURES

An unusual feature of behavioral treatment outcome research, with respect to sleep disorders research generally, is the reliance on subjective measures of sleep. A large majority of these studies rely exclusively on self-report measures of sleep. There are two issues relevant to the use of subjective ratings as outcome measures. The first issue concerns the suitability of self-report measures based on the operational definition of insomnia. At one extreme, insomnia can be viewed entirely as a subjective experience of inadequate or insufficient sleep, without reference to objectively determined total sleep time or sleep latency. In this view, insomnia has no complications associated with it other than the patient's subjective discomfort. Hence, the goal of therapy is to improve the patient's subjective experience of sleep, and changes in objective total sleep time or sleep latency are not necessary for a successful outcome. At the other extreme, insomnia is seen as the inability to obtain the quality or quantity of sleep to meet the patient's biological requirement. In this view, there are complications (as yet not well defined) associated with the sleep loss. Therapy must both improve the patient's sleep and modify the patient's satisfaction with sleep. To the extent that insomnia is defined by the subjective component, subjective ratings are valid indicators of treatment effectiveness. However, the International Classification of Sleep Disorders nosology also insists that a diagnosis of insomnia is made only when objective abnormalities of sleep are present (sleep state misperception is the only exception). This abnormality is usually defined as a total sleep time of less than 6.5 h.

The second issue concerns the degree to which subjective ratings can be used to infer changes in EEG-defined sleep parameters. It is well documented that insomniacs consistently overestimate SOL and underestimate total sleep time.[38-40] Some authors have claimed that subjective measures are valid measures of polysomnographically defined sleep on the basis of observations that even though subjective measures vary absolutely from EEG measures, the measures covary reliably. Correlation between EEG and self-report measures does not validate the use of self-report ratings as outcome measures. This is illustrated by an abstract[29] in which subjective ratings overestimated SOL by 40 min (50 versus 10 min) and overestimated wake time after sleep onset by almost 2 h (174 versus 64 min). Even if the correlation between these measures is 1.0, sole reliance on the subjective rating would yield misleading results. The decrease in subjective SOL from 50 to 25 min was both statistically and clinically significant; the decrease in polysomnographically defined SOL from 10 to 5 min was neither. This pattern of finding statistically significant improvement with subjective measures of sleep but without significant change in objective measures has occurred in several other studies.[24, 41, 42] This is not to say that subjective measures are irrelevant to improvement in insomnia; it is only to point out that changes in subjective measures do not mean that similar changes have occurred in objectively defined sleep parameters.

An important consideration in the evaluation of the use of subjective ratings is that many reports have found systematic effects of demand characteristics in insomniacs. Most studies using placebo-control groups find significantly improved sleep after treatment in the control group.[43-46] This finding has occurred across studies using various placebo treatments. Relaxation placebos may consist of having the subject "spend 30 min in a quiet place each day relaxing."[47] Borkovec et al.[46] used a "quasidesensitization" procedure that resembled behavioral treatment for anxiety, without promoting actual relaxation. Even a biofeedback placebo has been used in which bogus feedback is given to the subject. In these studies, placebo treatments produced significant change in reported SOL equivalent to that found with "active" treatment after treatment (Table 57–1). This "improvement" on the part of the placebo group presumably is the result of subject expectancy and the need to conform to experimenter demand.

Counterdemand instructions have been used to address the problem of subject expectancy and demand.[43] A counterdemand instruction means that subjects are told not to expect any improvement in the target symptom until after a specific time (e.g., fourth treatment week). The treatment weeks before this time are referred to as the *counterdemand period,* and the specified time is the *positive demand period.* Measurements taken from the counterdemand period are interpreted to reflect effects of treatment because no subject expectancy is yet active. Several studies that have used a placebo control have failed to find differences between active treatment and placebo at the positive demand period but have found differences during counterdemand.[45, 46]

OTHER METHODOLOGICAL PROBLEMS

An additional key issue with this literature concerns subject selection. Often, the subject populations are college students who are self-described poor sleepers. College students are known to have extremely erratic sleep-wake schedules, a high incidence of napping, a high frequency of alcohol use, and other behaviors that negatively affect sleep. The causal factors of disturbed sleep in this group may be different from those found in clinical sample populations, which significantly limits the ability to generalize results obtained with this population. This problem has been remedied in later studies of both clinical populations and groups of older individuals with insomnia.

Some studies have used an unselected clinical group of insomniacs. Perhaps the most vital concern regarding this issue is that in the absence of a more sophisticated nosological system (guidelines for diagnostic categories were not published by the Association of Sleep Disorders Centers until 1979), sleep-onset insomnia was seen as a specific diagnostic entity. This erroneous assumption leads to uninterpretable studies. For example, a common entry criteria for "sleep-onset insomnia" is an average SOL of more than 30 min for at least 6 months. A long SOL in the absence of any other sleep abnormality, such as decreased total sleep time or increased wake time after sleep onset, would be found in phase delay syndrome.[48] Therapies aimed at relaxation would not be expected to substantially change SOL in patients with circadian rhythm disorders. In this respect, the use of a heterogeneous group of insomniacs could be expected to work against obtaining positive treatment results. Furthermore, without objective measures during screening, there is no way to detect the prevalence of subjective insomnia or to definitively rule out another sleep disorder.

REVIEW OF STUDIES USING SUBJECTIVE MEASURES

A list of behavioral treatment outcome studies[7-9, 43-47, 49-56] that rely on subjective measures is presented (see

Table 57-1. SUMMARY OF STUDIES WITH PLACEBO CONTROL CONDITIONS THAT USE ONLY SUBJECTIVE MEASURES

	Sample	Entry Criteria	Placebo Condition	Treatment Studied	Changes in SOL
Borkovec and Fowles (1973)[9]	37 female college students	Long SOL Must discontinue hypnotics	Self-relaxation	PR, HR	All active and placebo treatment better than no treatment; active = placebo
Borkovec et al. (1975)[46]	56 college students	SOL >30 min	Quasi-desensitization	PR, NTR	PR better than NTR and placebo at CTD; PMR, NTR, and placebo better than no treatment at PD
Carr-Kaffashan and Woolfolk (1979)[45]	30 adults	SOL >30 min Duration >6 mo Must discontinue hypnotics	Quasi-desensitization	PR + MED	Active treatment better than placebo at CTD; no difference at PD; no difference in response of moderate vs. severe groups
Espie et al. (1989)[49]	70 adults	SOL >30 min Duration >1 y ASDA diagnostic categories A.1, A.2, or A.9	Imagery relief	PR, SC, PI	Only SC was better than placebo; no difference in TST among groups
Haynes et al. (1977)[50]	12 students, 12 adults	Complaint of insomnia	Subjects told to practice relaxing	EMG, PR	Both active treatments better than placebo; no difference in TST
Lacks et al. (1983)[51]	15 adults, maintenance insomnia	WASO >30 min at least 1 night/week Duration >6 mo Must discontinue hypnotics Rule out medical insomnia	Quasi-desensitization	SC	SOL not studied; no difference between SC and placebo on WASO
Lacks et al. (1983)[44]	64 adults	SOL >30 min at least 1 night/week Duration >6 mo Rule out medical insomnia	Quasi-desensitization	PR, SC, PI	Only SC better than placebo at CTD; all groups same at PD and follow-up
Lick and Heffler (1977)[8]	40 adults	Mean SOL >50 min Hypnotics OK	Mock biofeedback	PR, PR + Tape	"Trend" toward active treatments to be better than placebo ($P < .06$)
Nicassio and Bootzin (1974)[47]	30 adults	SOL >30 min Must discontinue hypnotics	Self-relaxation	AI, PR	Active treatments were compared with placebo and no-treatments and were better; no comparisons to placebo-only were made
Nicassio et al. (1982)[7]	40 adults	Mean SOL >30 min Must discontinue hypnotics Rule out medical insomnia	Mock biofeedback	PR, EMG	Active = placebo; active and placebo better than no treatment
Shealy (1979)[52]	70 college students	Complaint of insomnia	SM; subjects sat in dim light and talked about sleep	PR, PR + SC	PR + SC better than all other conditions; PR = placebo during CTD
Stanton (1989)[53]	45 adults	SOL >30 min Duration >6 mo Must discontinue hypnotics	Quasi-desensitization	HR, SC	HR better than SC and placebo at CTD and PD; SC = placebo at CTD and PD
Steinmark and Borkovec (1974)[43]	48 college students	SOL >30 min Duration >6 mo Must discontinue hypnotics	Quasi-desensitization	PR, PRT	Active treatments better than placebo at CTD; no difference at PD
Turner and Ascher (1979)[54]	50 adults	No medical insomnia Hypnotics OK	Quasi-desensitization	PR, SC, PI	Active treatments together were compared with placebo + no treatments and were better; no comparisons to placebo-only were made
Haynes et al. (1974)[55]	14 college students	Complaint of insomnia	Subjects sat in dim light and talked about sleep	RT	Both active and placebo treatments improved significantly, but active treatment improved significantly more
Edinger et al. (1997)[56]	45 adults with primary insomnia	WASO >60 min	Quasi-desensitization	CBT, PMR	CBT > RT, placebo on WASO

AI, autogenic imagery; CTD, counterdemand; EMG, electromyographic biofeedback; HR, hypnotic relaxation; MED, meditation; NTR, no-tension-release relaxation; PD, positive demand; PI, paradoxical intention; PMR, progressive muscle relaxation; PR, progressive relaxation; PRT, PR + single item desensitization; SC, stimulus control; SM, self-monitoring; SOL, sleep onset latency; Tape, audiotape; TST, total sleep time; WASO, wake time after sleep onset.

Table 57–2. SUMMARY OF OUTCOME STUDIES USING OBJECTIVE MEASURES OF SLEEP

Sample	Entry Criteria	Treatment	Objective Measure	Control Condition	Results
Borkovec et al. (1979)[57] 29 college students (17 subjective, 12 idiopathic insomnia)	SOL >60 min No hypnotics	PR NTR	PSG	NTC	PR < NTR, NTC greater decrease for SOL in idiopathic group No change for subject group Absolute post-treatment values not different
Borkovec and Weerts (1976)[91] 36 college students	SOL >30 min No current hypnotics	PR	PSG	Quasi-desensitization NTC	RT < NTC latency to stage 1 No other differences Subjective; all three groups improved
Coursey et al. (1980)[58] 22 adults	↑ SOL 4 nights/week for >2 y No current hypnotics	EMG AT ES	PSG	ES	5 of 12 subjects receiving BIO or AT met criteria as "responder"
Edinger et al. (1992)[31] 7 older adults (>55 y)	6-mo duration WASO >60 min Daytime symptoms Must discontinue hypnotics	RT CBT	SAD		↓ WASO, ↑ SE with CBT No significant changes with RT
Engle-Friedman et al. (1992)[59] 53 older adults (>47 y)	SOL >45 min, 3 nights/week or >3 awakenings, 3 nights/week or >30 min WASO, 3 nights/week	SH SC RT	PSG	Measurement control	None
Freedman and Papsdorf (1976)[40] 18 young adults	SOL >60 min, 4 nights/week >6-mo duration No current hypnotics	PR EMG	PSG	Placebo relaxation	SOL: PR, EMG < control
Guilleminault et al. (1995)[60] 30 adults (28 clinic patients, 4 recruits from ads)	<6 h TST and >30 min SOL or awake within 2 h of SOL and difficulty returning to sleep No hypnotics for 3 mo	SH SH and exercise SH and bright light	ACT		BL: ↑ TST, ↓ SOL Pre vs post and post vs with SH alone
Hauri (1981)[24] 48 psychophysiological insomniacs	<85% SE or >30 min SOL	Theta SMR Theta/EMG	PSG	NTC	No active treatment group better than control Post-hoc comparisons found that some patients improved
Hauri et al. (1982)[42] 16 psychophysiological insomniacs	Duration ≥2 y <85% SE >30 min SOL Hypnotics OK	SMR	PSG		No differences on objective measures overall ↑ TST and ↓ SOL in subjects receiving appropriate feedback
Jacobs et al. (1993)[32] 12 adults	SOL >60 min for ≥4 nights/week 6-mo duration Daytime symptoms No current hypnotics	Combined behavioral/relaxation program	PSG-H		↓ SOL ↑ SE
Morin et al. (1999)[35] 78 older adults (>55 y)	SOL and/or WASO >30 min for ≥3 nights/week Duration >6 mo Daytime symptoms	CBT pharmacotherapy CBT and pharmacotherapy	PSG	Placebo	All active treatments showed ↓ WASO at post-treatment CBT showed continued improvement at follow-up, pharmacotherapy did not
Morin et al. (1993)[61] 24 older adults (>60 y)	WASO >>30 min for ≥3 nights/week 6-mo duration Daytime symptoms Must discontinue hypnotics	CBT	PSG		↑ SE ↓ WASO ↓ Total wake time

ACT, actigraphy; AT, autogenic training; CBT, cognitive-behavioral therapy; EMG, EMG biofeedback; ES, electrosleep; NTC, no treatment control; NTR, no-tension-release relaxation; PR, progressive relaxation; PSG, polysomnography; PSG-H, PSG performed at home; RT, relaxation training; SAD, sleep assessment device; SC, stimulus control; SE, sleep efficiency; SH, sleep hygiene; SMR, SMR biofeedback; SOL, sleep onset latency; Theta, Theta biofeedback; TST, total sleep time; WASO, wake time after sleep onset.

Table 57–1). Only studies that have a placebo condition are presented. A no-treatment control is inadequate because of the strong expectancy and demand effects that influence self-reports in this population.

Progressive relaxation was used in 12 of these studies, more than any other treatment. Of the studies that directly compared progressive relaxation with placebo (n = 11), five found significant differences (see Table 57–1). This ratio of positive to negative studies (about 1:1) holds up for each type of treatment. The ratio of failure to success does not appear to be related to the type of patient studied or the type of placebo condition used.

REVIEW OF STUDIES USING OBJECTIVE MEASURES

Behavioral treatment outcome studies that used an objective measure of sleep are summarized in Table 57–2. Many of these studies obtained EEG measures of sleep and evaluated relaxation therapy or biofeedback. There are few changes in sleep based on objective measures from studies of relaxation therapy; one exception is a study by Hauri et al.[42] that matched patients with an "appropriate" type of biofeedback treatment based on pretreatment assessment of tension level. In this study, theta feedback was judged as the appropriate treatment for patients with a high level of pretreatment tension, and sensory-motor rhythm feedback was assigned as the appropriate treatment for those with low tension. Significant improvement in sleep parameters was found when patients were compared on the basis of "appropriate" versus "inappropriate" types of biofeedback, even though the overall group did not show systematic improvement.

The results from studies using a treatment package are much more favorable, with consistent improvement demonstrated across all studies. The fact that the greatest improvement was found with the use of treatment packages and with patients matched to treatments may be instructive. It is possible that both of these approaches are successful because they expose patients to the optimal treatment modality. With treatment packages, it is not necessary to predict which treatment is best; all patients are exposed to several treatment modalities.

FUTURE DIRECTIONS

An innovation that may have a significant impact on research in this area is the use of home monitoring. Recent research has found that patients with insomnia had greater variability in their sleep when monitored in the home environment compared with in the laboratory environment.[62] Furthermore, daytime impairment, as measured by multiple sleep latency test, was greater at home than in the laboratory.[63] These findings suggest that the laboratory environment affects patients with insomnia such that studies under laboratory conditions do not accurately reflect their typical sleep or degree of daytime impairment. This laboratory bias may explain why past studies using EEG measures had difficulty showing improved sleep with post-treatment in-laboratory studies, and why at-home studies may better reflect changes in sleep. Also, there is a trend toward increased focus on the daytime consequences of insomnia (e.g., self-reported daytime impairment as an inclusion criteria; see Table 57–2). The inability to consistently demonstrate daytime impairment related to inadequate sleep has been a hindrance to the incorporation of measures of daytime function as outcome measures. The study by Edinger et al.[62] suggests that measures of daytime function obtained outside the laboratory may provide better estimates of insomnia-related impairment.

An obvious goal for research in this area is to understand the mechanisms of treatment so it can be possible to preselect patients who are likely to benefit from behavioral treatment. Earlier work along this line was encouraging (see the discussion of the work of Hauri's et al.[42]), but subsequent attempts have not been successful. In fact, one study found that patients selected for specific treatments based on pretreatment characteristics of their sleep difficulty actually did worse than patients assigned to random treatments.[64] Apparently, a better understanding of patient and treatment dynamics is necessary before patient selection can be possible. One step in this direction is reported in a recent study of the time course of improvement with behavioral treatment.[65] This study reported that Wake time after sleep onset decreased after just one session of CBT, and that total sleep time increased after 4 weeks of treatment. In addition, a subgroup of patients was identified who responded rapidly to treatment, Whereas another subgroup showed much more gradual improvement. The characteristics of these subgroups were analyzed and rapid responders were found to have increased arousal at bedtime, whereas slow responders were likely to have very elevated time in bed. These results are preliminary but serve as an example of the type of research that is needed to allow the preselection of patients for treatment.

References

1. Chesson AL Jr, Anderson WM, Littner M, et al. Practice parameters for the nonpharmacologic treatment of chronic insomnia. An American Academy of Sleep Medicine report. Sleep. 1999;22:1128–1133.
2. American Sleep Disorders Association. The International Classification of Sleep Disorders, Revised: Diagnostic and Coding Manual. Rochester, Minn: American Sleep Disorders Association; 1997.
3. Borkovec T. Insomnia. J Consult Clin Psychol. 1982;50:880–895.
4. Monroe LJ. Psychological and physiological differences between good and poor sleepers. J Abnorm Psychol. 1967;72:255–264.
5. Bonnet M, Arand D. 24-Hour metabolic rate in insomniacs and matched normal sleepers. Sleep. 1995;18:581–588.
6. Stepanski E, Glinn M, Zorick F, et al. Heart rate changes in chronic insomnia. Stress Med. 1994;10:261–266.
7. Nicassio P, Boylan M, McCabe T. Progressive relaxation, EMG biofeedback and biofeedback placebo in the treatment of sleep-onset insomnia. Br J Med Psychol. 1982;55:159–166.
8. Lick J, Heffler D. Relaxation training and attention placebo in the treatment of severe insomnia. J Consult Clin Psychol. 1977;45:153–161.
9. Borkovec TD, Fowles DC. Controlled investigation of the effects of progressive and hypnotic relaxation on insomnia. J Abnorm Psychol. 1973;82:153–158.

10. Kales A, Caldwell A, Preston T, et al. Personality patterns in insomnia. Arch Gen Psychiatry. 1976;33:1128–1134.

11. Stepanski E, Koshorek G, Zorick F, et al. Differences in individuals who do or do not seek treatment for chronic insomnia. Psychosomatics. 1989;30:421–427.

12. Hauri P, Fisher J. Persistent psychopysiologic (learned) insomnia. Sleep. 1986;9:38–53.

13. Lichstein K, Rosenthal T. Insomniacs' perceptions of cognitive versus somatic determinants of sleep disturbance. J Abnorm Psychol. 1980;89:105–107.

14. Morin C, Stone J, Trinkle D, et al. Dysfunctional beliefs and attitudes about sleep among older adults with and without insomnia complaints. Psychol Aging. 1993;8:463–467.

15. Haynes SN, Adams A, Franzen M. The effects of presleep stress on sleep-onset insomnia. J Abnorm Psychol. 1981;90:601–606.

16. Robinson T. Presleep Activity and Sleep Quality of Good and Poor Sleepers [dissertation]. Chicago, Ill: University of Chicago; 1969.

17. Haynes SN, Adams AE, West S, et al. The stimulus control paradigm in sleep-onset insomnia: a multimethod assessment. J Psychosomat Res. 1982;26:333–339.

18. Zwart C, Lisman S. Analysis of stimulus control treatment of sleep-onset insomnia. J Consult Clin Psychol. 1979;47:113–118.

19. Davies R, Lacks P, Storandt M, et al. Countercontrol treatment of sleep-maintenance insomnia in relation to age. Psychol Aging. 1986;1:233–238.

20. Spielman A. Assessment of insomnia. Clin Psychol Rev. 1986;6:11–26.

21. Jacobson E. You Can Sleep Well. New York, NY: McGraw-Hill Book Company; 1938.

22. Bernstein D, Borkovec T. Progressive Relaxation Training. Champaign, Ill: Research Press; 1973.

23. Poppen R. Behavioral Relaxation Training and Assessment. New York, NY: Pergamon Press; 1988.

24. Hauri P. Treating psychophysiologic insomnia with biofeedback. Arch Gen Psychiatry. 1981;38:752–758.

25. Bootzin RR, Nicassio PM. Behavioral treatments for insomnia. In: Hersen M, Eissler R, Miller P, eds. Progress in Behavior Modification. Vol 6. New York, NY: Academic Press; 1978:1–45.

26. Sloan E, Hauri P, Bootzin R, et al. The nuts and bolts of behavioral therapy for insomnia. J Psychosomat Res. 1993;37(suppl 1):19–37.

27. Spielman AJ, Saskin P, Thorpy MJ. Treatment of chronic insomnia by restriction of time in bed. Sleep. 1987;10:45–56.

28. Glovinsky P, Spielman A. Sleep restriction therapy. In: Hauri P, ed. Case Studies in Insomnia. New York, NY: Plenum; 1991:49–63.

29. Rubenstein M, Rothenberg S, Maheswaren S, et al. Modified sleep restriction therapy in middle-aged and elderly chronic insomniacs. Sleep Res. 1990;19:276.

30. Morin C. Insomnia: Psychological Assessment and Management. New York, NY: Guilford Press; 1993.

31. Edinger J, Hoelscher T, Marsh G, et al. A cognitive-behavioral therapy for sleep-maintenance insomnia in older adults. Psychol Aging. 1992;7:282–289.

32. Jacobs G, Benson H, Friedman R. Home-based central nervous system assessment of a multifactor behavioral intervention for chronic sleep-onset insomnia. Behav Ther. 1993;24:159–174.

33. Milby J, Williams V, Hall J, et al. Effectiveness of combined triazolam-behavioral therapy for primary insomnia. Am J Psychiatry. 1993;150:1259–1260.

34. Hauri P. Can we mix behavioral therapy with hypnotics when treating insomniacs? Sleep. 1997;20:1111–1118.

35. Morin C, Colecchi C, Stone J, et al. Behavioral and pharmacological therapies for late-life insomnia. A randomized controlled trial. JAMA. 1999;281:991–999.

36. Mellinger GD, Balter MB, Uhlenhuth EH. Insomnia and its treatment: prevalence and correlates. Arch Gen Psychiatry. 1985;42:225–232.

37. Morin C, Gaulier B, Barry T, et al. Patients' acceptance of psychological and pharmacological therapies for insomnia. Sleep. 1992;15:302–305.

38. Carskadon M, Dement W, Mitler M, et al. Self-reports versus sleep laboratory findings in 122 drug-free subjects with complaints of chronic insomnia. Am J Psychiatry. 1976;133:1382–1388.

39. Rechtschaffen A, Monroe L. Laboratory studies of insomnia. In: Kales A, ed. Sleep: Physiology and Pathology. Philadelphia, Pa: JB Lippincott; 1969.

40. Freedman R, Papsdorf J. Biofeedback and progressive relaxation: treatment of sleep-onset insomnia: a controlled, all-night investigation. Biofeedback Self Regul. 1976;1:253–271.

41. Borkovec T, Weerts T. Effects of progressive relaxation on sleep disturbance: an electroencephalographic evaluation. Psychosom Med. 1976;38:173–180.

42. Hauri P, Percy L, Hellekson C, et al. The treatment of psychophysiologic insomnia with biofeedback: a replication study. Biofeedback Self Regul. 1982;7:223–234.

43. Steinmark S, Borkovec T. Active and placebo treatment effect on moderate insomnia under counterdemand and positive demand instructions. J Abnorm Psychol. 1974;83:157–163.

44. Lacks P, Bertelson A, Gans L, et al. The effectiveness of three behavioral treatments for different degrees of sleep onset insomnia. Behav Ther. 1983;14:593–605.

45. Carr-Kaffashan L, Woolfolk RL. Active and placebo effects in treatment of moderate and severe insomnia. J Consult Clin Psychol. 1979;47:1072–1080.

46. Borkovec T, Kaloupek D, Slama K. The facilitative effect of muscle tension-release in the relaxation treatment of sleep disturbance. Behav Ther. 1975;6:301–309.

47. Nicassio P, Bootzin R. A Comparison of progressive relaxation and autogenic training as treatments for insomnia. J Abnorm Psychol. 1974;83:253–260.

48. Zorick F, Roth T, Hartse K, et al. Evaluation and diagnosis of persistent insomnia. Am J Psychiatry. 1981;138:769–773.

49. Espie C, Lindsay W, Brooks N, et al. A controlled comparative investigation of psychological treatments for chronic sleep-onset insomnia. Behav Res Ther. 1989;27:79–88.

50. Haynes S, Sides H, Lockwood G. Relaxation instructions and frontalis electromyographic feedback intervention with sleep onset insomnia. Behav Ther. 1977;8:644–652.

51. Lacks P, Bertelson A, Sugerman J, et al. The treatment of sleep-maintenance insomnia with stimulus-control techniques. Behav Res Ther. 1983;21:291–295.

52. Shealy RC. The effectiveness of various treatment techniques on different degrees and durations of sleep-onset insomnia. Behav Res Ther. 1979;17:541–546.

53. Stanton H. Hypnotic relaxation and the reduction of sleep onset insomnia. Int J Psychosoat. 1989;36:64–68.

54. Turner RM, Ascher M. Controlled comparison of progressive relaxation, stimulus control, and paradoxical intention therapies for insomnia. J Consult Clin Psychol. 1979;47:500–508.

55. Haynes S, Woodward S, Moran R, et al. Relaxation treatment of insomnia. Behav Ther. 1974;5:555–558.

56. Edinger J, Radtke R, Wohlgemuth W, et al. The efficacy of cognitive-behavioral therapy for sleep-maintenance insomnia [abstract]. Sleep Res. 1997;26:357.

57. Borkovec T, Grayson J, O'Brien G, et al. Relaxation treatment of pseudoinsomnia and idiopathic insomnia: an electroencephalographic evaluation. J Appl Behav Anal. 1979;12:37–54.

58. Coursey R, Frankel B, Gaarder K, et al. A comparison of relaxation techniques with electrosleep therapy for chronic, sleep-onset insomnia: a sleep EEG study. Biofeedback Self Regul. 1980;5:57–73.

59. Engle-Friedman M, Bootzin R, Hazlewood L, et al. An evaluation of behavioral treatments for insomnia in the older adult. J Clin Psychol. 1992;48:77–90.

60. Guilleminault C, Clerk A, Black J, et al. Nondrug treatment trials in psychophysiologic insomnia. Arch Intern Med. 1995;155:838–844.

61. Morin C, Kowatch R, Barry T, et al. Cognitive-behavior therapy for late-life insomnia. J Consult Clin Psychol. 1993;61:137–146.

62. Edinger J, Fins A, Sullivan R, et al. Sleep in the laboratory and sleep at home: comparisons of older insomniacs and normal sleepers. Sleep. 1997;20:1119–1121.

63. Edinger J, Fins A, Sullivan R, et al. Do our methods lead to insomniacs' madness? Daytime testing after laboratory and home-based polysomnographic studies. Sleep. 1997;20:1127–1134.

64. Espie C, Brooks D, Lindsay W. An evaluation of tailored psychological treatment of insomnia. J Behav Ther Exp Psychiatry. 1989;20:143–153.

65. Edinger J. Searching for the dose-response curve in behavioral insomnia therapy [abstract]. Sleep Res. 1997;26:356.

58

Sleep Hygiene

Vincent P. Zarcone, Jr

For decades, beginning with Nathaniel Kleitman's pioneering chapter on sleep hygiene,[1] the budding field of sleep disorders medicine has been concerned with those practices that interfere with normal sleep and contribute to the insomnia complaint. The importance of these sleep hygiene factors has been increasingly emphasized in the last 30 years of development of sleep disorders medicine.

At present, there are two opposing models for all the underlying syndromes that lead to the complaint of insomnia; in both, sleep hygiene is highly emphasized. The International Classification of Sleep Disorders (ICSD) classifies inadequate sleep hygiene (ISH) under the dyssomnias as an extrinsic sleep disorder.[2] It is defined in two ways. The minimal criteria for a tentative diagnosis includes one or more items from the list of maladaptive habits described in this chapter and the complaint of either insomnia or excessive sleepiness. The ICSD suggests that poor sleep hygiene is on the list of syndromes that underlie the insomnia complaint.

The complete diagnostic criteria require the exclusion of psychiatric and medical disorders and the absence of other sleep disorders. Response to a therapeutic trial of sleep hygiene advice is not a criterion. Confusion can result if minimal instead of full criteria are used in research.

The alternative model is to view the insomnia complaint as stemming basically from a genetic predisposition to a physiological disturbance, in either initiation or maintenance of sleep, or both, that is complicated by a number of factors. The second type of model could be referred to as a "disease" model, with poor sleep hygiene as a risk factor. The first is a "complaint"-oriented model in which poor sleep hygiene is a syndrome underlying the complaint. Both models of disturbed nocturnal sleep are multifactorial.

The *Diagnostic and Statistical Manual of Mental Disorders, Fourth Edition* (DSM-IV) diagnosis of primary insomnia "subsumes a number of diagnoses in the ICSD . . . [including] some cases of Inadequate Sleep Hygiene."[3(p557)] In the field trials of the DSM-IV sleep classification primary insomnia was diagnosed in 48 out of 216 patients by sleep specialists. Those same specialists diagnosed 6.2% (with a range of 0 to 16% across centers) of the patients with inadequate sleep hygiene as the primary diagnosis. Of all assigned diagnoses, 34.2% (range: 2 to 64%) were inadequate sleep hygiene in the field trial.[4] Buysse et al.[5] noted in an-

other report that 12 patients diagnosed by ICSD criteria as inadequate sleep hygiene were seen to be suffering from primary insomnia by DSM-IV criteria. It is not clear from the field trial reports that these 12 patients were psychiatrically impaired or that they responded to sleep hygiene advice with a complete resolution of their problem. It is clear that although sleep specialists identified a psychiatric disorder in patients with primary insomnia they also assessed the impact of inadequate sleep hygiene.[6] As well they might, because it is undoubtedly not cost-effective to provide cognitive-behavioral therapy or pharmacological intervention to patients whose primary disability is a result of simple maladaptive learning. These issues of diagnostic and conceptual confusion are further highlighted in the meta-analysis of treatment efficacy of cognitive-behavioral interventions (the most effective being stimulus control and sleep restriction) in 59 studies involving 2102 patients.[7] It can be assumed from the outcomes that a large majority of the patients would have had ICSD diagnoses other than inadequate sleep hygiene because sleep hygiene education was not effective when used alone. No diagnoses are given in the Morin et al. study.[7] At present, there is no longitudinal case series from which the effect of treatment response on final diagnosis can be ascertained. Without such studies it is unlikely that the conundrum created by different diagnostic classification systems, conditioning factors, habits, psychiatric disorders, and physiological predispositions can be unraveled.

Throughout this chapter, an overriding consideration must be the interaction of poor sleep hygiene with many other factors, which leads to disturbed nocturnal sleep. From a practical point of view, sleep hygiene advice, given by itself, probably will be of little benefit to the patient. The advice has to be given with full consideration of the differential diagnosis of the many syndromes that can underlie the complaint of insomnia.

A consensus has developed among those who frequently treat insomnia-complaining patients that a 4- to 6-week trial of sleep hygiene counseling, behavior modification, and the judicious use of hypnotics take place for many but not all patients before nocturnal polysomnography is performed. If the history and physical examination indicate a cause for the complaint, such as narcolepsy, sleep apnea, periodic leg movements, a parasomnia, or a medical condition, then the patient should be referred for further evaluation, including nocturnal polysomnography, to a sleep disorders clinic.

This chapter describes four classes of factors important in sleep hygiene. The first class includes circadian rhythm and the build-up of sleep propensity in the period of consolidated wakefulness; the second factor is age and the changes in sleep physiology that occur with age; the third class includes factors that increase arousal in the sleep setting; and the fourth (a subset of the previous set) category encompasses those common social or recreational drugs that have important effects on sleep, namely, nicotine, caffeine, and ethanol. The model of poor sleep hygiene as a syndrome does not preclude the contribution of sleep hygiene factors to a genetically determined disease. Regardless of the model employed or the complaint of the patient, sleep disorders physicians almost always counsel patients about sleep hygiene.

CIRCADIAN RHYTHM OF SLEEP AND WAKING AND THE EFFECT OF PRIOR WAKEFULNESS

Borbély[8] further elaborated a model suggested by Feinberg[9] for the evolution of sleep in mammalian species. This model includes a circadian oscillator, which determines sleep-wake rhythm, as well as a phylogenetically recently acquired mechanism for increasing the propensity of sleep in proportion to the amount of prior wakefulness. This latter mechanism has survival advantages for mammals because it allows them to coordinate their sleep periods with their status as predator or prey species, that is, their patterns of feeding behavior.

There is considerable variation in the duration of sleep among normal subjects. The variation is unrelated to personality characteristics in the report of Webb and Friel[10] and probably is the normal distribution. The average sleep time for young adults is 7 h, and the standard deviation is 1 h. That means, of course, that there are thousands of people in the United States who need either 5.5 h or less, or 9.5 h or more, of sleep per night. The sleep tendency is biphasic, with another peak of sleepiness approximately 8 h after the termination of the long consolidated sleep period. Napping at any time other than 10 to 15 min during this peak may have deleterious effects on sleep in the next consolidated sleep period of the 24-h day. Naps 10 to 12 h after the major sleep period are particularly likely to disturb subsequent nocturnal sleep.

There has been little systematic study of the normal variation in the timing of sleep in relation to the light-dark cycle. Subjective reports of attributes such as "owl" and "lark" are fairly numerous in the literature.[1] However, reports of systematic studies relating these attributes to the timing of sleep and to seasonal changes, particularly in northern latitudes, have not as yet appeared. The clinical reports of seasonal affective disorder[11] would lead one to believe that there is possibly a normal variation in the timing of sleep among those people who live roughly north of the 35th parallel and that this has some effect on daytime performance and mood. In addition to these circadian and seasonal factors, there are other effects of timing or placement of the sleep period in the 24-h day.

Taub and Berger[12] note that the timing of sleep definitely affects daytime mood and performance independently of duration of sleep. As little a shift as 3 h can result in performance decrements. Patients occasionally report that prolonged sleep to "catch up" can result in daytime grogginess that persists as late as the early evening hours. In addition, the timing of exposure to light is obviously of significance, particularly in northerly or southerly latitudes. Possibly, phase lags can be offset by the administration of a half-hour to 2 h of 2500 lux of bright lights at the appropriate time in the 24-h period, that is, in the early morning (see Chapter 105). Phase advance of the sleep period, that is, falling asleep earlier and arising earlier, may respond to light in the early evening hours to take advantage of the human phase response curve for achieving a more socially acceptable or normative timing of the sleep period.

The behavioral prescription that takes into account all of these "physiological" factors of timing and prior wakefulness is to fix the time out of bed and to follow the awakening by moderate exercise and exposure to light to give an adequate zeitgeber for the timing of the sleep-wake cycle.* Prolonged naps, particularly late in the wake period, should probably be avoided. The length of time in bed should be individualized. In actual practice, this requires an adequately elicited history in which the usual sleep period length and the timing during the period in which the patient did not have symptoms (usually in young adulthood) are determined. A patient who needed 9 h of sleep as a young adult probably cannot spend only 7 h in bed. A careful consideration of the timing of sleep and the avoidance of naps are of obvious importance in any recovery process involved in the treatment of conditioned insomnia or in the treatment of the other syndromes underlying the complaint. It is particularly important to encourage the patient to try at least a 6- to 10-week period in which attention is paid to these important variables of timing of the sleep-wake cycle and the duration of prior wakefulness.

AGE AND SLEEP HYGIENE

Patients over the age of 40 years need to be counseled concerning the normal physiological changes that occur in sleep with aging. Reynolds et al.[13] and Miles and Dement[14] have noted that sleep efficiency and, conversely, the number of wakings and the minutes awake after sleep onset decline and rise precipitously around the age of 45 years. This is true regardless of

---

*Any visitor to Monticello who has knowledge of circadian medicine cannot fail to be impressed by Thomas Jefferson's perspicacity. Every morning of his life there, he rose from his bed as soon as there was enough light to read the clock at the foot of his bed. Perhaps this practice helped him put off his own death until after he had seen the 50th anniversary of the Declaration of Independence.

whether the subject has any degree of sleep apnea or periodic leg movements; the number of wakings in the nocturnal sleep period increases with age, quite dramatically so after the age of 45 years. This phenomenon is an obvious source of interaction with any other conditions that lead to arousal in the sleep setting, such as minor withdrawal syndromes that occur after the nocturnal consumption of alcoholic beverages.

The physiological capacity to initiate sleep at any time of the 24-h day is greatly diminished after the age of 25 years. Although there are no systematic studies on the loss of the capacity to phase-advance sleep or to "make up" for sleep loss on subsequent nights, it probably has some relationship to the loss of the capacity to elaborate slow waves, which mainly occurs in the second decade of life. Patients commonly report irritation with the fact that whereas in the past they could "sleep in" or phase-advance the initiation of their sleep period in relation to the 24-h clock, they no longer can.

AROUSAL IN THE SLEEP SETTING

There are many factors that lead to arousal in the sleep setting. They have been reviewed extensively by Coates and Thoreson,[15] Hauri,[16] and Kirmil-Gray et al.[17] and in an Institute of Medicine report.[18] Most of them are obvious "psychological stressors," for example, deadlines, examinations, job crises, and marital conflict. Some of them, however, are simple habits that are not related to any particular episodic psychological stress.

Of the latter type of stressor, probably the most important is related to the naiveté of some insomnia complainers regarding the rapidity with which they can turn off a sympathetic arousal. The obvious examples are those patients who persist in working on tasks related to their occupations right up to the moment they turn off the lights and attempt to initiate sleep. Other examples are those who retire and continue a review of the previous day's events in an attempt to decide (in a half-awake, half-asleep state) on a plan of action for the next day. Those are obvious habits that need to be discontinued. Other obvious habits have to do with the sleep setting itself. It goes without saying that it should be quiet and dark and that sleep should not be subject to interruption by pets or the need to care for other people. All interfering stimuli should be removed from the bedroom, and the bedroom should be used only for sleep.

Sexual activity is arousing or sedating, depending on the individual. If sexual activity is arousing, then it should occur in some setting other than the one in which the subject desires to sleep—perhaps at a different time of the day other than the hour or so preceding the major sleep period.

Another common arousing stimulus that occurs in patients' bedrooms is an easily visible clock. If the patient is worried about the time remaining in which sleep can be initiated or continued, then looking at a clock will serve only to heighten the arousal state.

The timing and type of meals and the quantity of fluids ingested can be important factors, particularly in those patients complaining of sleep maintenance difficulty.

With respect to psychological stressors, most patients have some vague awareness of the necessity of interposing a period of relaxation between the concerns and psychological stressors of the day and their major or nocturnal sleep period. Any sort of bedtime ritual that breaks the connection between psychological stressors of the preceding day and the sleep period is to be encouraged. Periods of as little as 10 min to as long as an hour need to be evaluated for their benefit in individual patients. Some patients need the assistance of a psychologist to initiate a form of behavioral self-management during this bedtime ritual period. Others can do it on their own; for instance, patients with even severe sympathetic arousal in the sleep setting—such as patients with post-traumatic stress disorder—can benefit from relatively simple techniques of stress management. For instance, taking 10 min to make a list of the psychological stressors that have occurred during the preceding day, along with the plans to deal with each the next day, can be of benefit. The list can be as short as a few words in each category for each psychological stressor and serves to put an end to the activities of the preceding day, particularly if the patient then initiates a period of relaxation after making the list. There are many different techniques employable in the period of relaxation, ranging from meditation to simply reading something that is entertaining and not psychologically stressful, such as Dwight Eisenhower's habit of reading pulp western novels before initiating sleep. The presleep ritual can include behaviors such as assuring oneself that the total sleep environment is safe by locking the doors, making sure that all the fire safety devices are functioning, seeing that the pets are where they belong, and so forth. Nonalcoholic malt drinks or hot baths can be prescribed.

In summary, all four classes of factors can interact in a syndrome of poor sleep hygiene or as risk factors acting with a genetic predisposition to produce a sleep complaint. Poor sleep hygiene can complicate any other syndrome producing the insomnia complaint and must always be considered in any treatment plan. Sleep hygiene instructions are presented in Table 58–1.

EFFECTS OF CAFFEINE, ETHANOL, AND NICOTINE ON SLEEP

Caffeine

There are many studies in the literature, summarized by Curatolo and Robertson[19] in 1983, that indicate that caffeine has deleterious effects on sleep. Caffeine competes for adenosine receptors. Because adenosine is an inhibitory neurotransmitter, there is a net loss of inhibition after caffeine intake.[20] Caffeine produces increases in wakings and decreases in total sleep time during nocturnal sleep. Sensitivity to the effects of caffeine can last as long as 8 to 14 h. There are case reports of patients[21] who are sensitive to as little as the

Table 58–1. SLEEP HYGIENE INSTRUCTIONS

Homeostatic Drive for Sleep

Avoid naps, except for a brief 10- to 15-min nap 8 h after arising; but check with your physician first, because in some sleep disorders naps can be beneficial.

Restrict the sleep period to the average number of hours you have actually slept per night in the preceding week. Quality of sleep is important. Too much time in bed can decrease quality on the subsequent night.

Get regular exercise each day, preferably 40 min each day, of an activity that causes sweating. It is best to finish exercise at least 6 h before bedtime.

Take a hot bath to raise your temperature 2°C for 30 min within 2 h before bedtime. A hot drink may help you relax as well as warm you.

Circadian Factors

Keep a regular time out of bed 7 days a week.

Do not expose yourself to bright light if you have to get up at night.

Get at least one half-hour of sunlight within 30 min of your out-of-bed time. If early-morning awakenings and sleepiness in the evening are problems, then exposure to bright light should be used in the evening and avoided before midmorning.

Drug Effects

Do not smoke to get yourself back to sleep.

Do not smoke after 7 PM, or give up smoking entirely.

Avoid caffeine entirely for a 4-week trial period; limit caffeine use to no more than three cups no later than 10 AM.

Practice light to moderate use of alcoholic beverages. Alcohol can fragment sleep over the second half of the sleep period.

Arousal in Sleep Setting

Keep the clock face turned away, and do not seek out what time it is when you wake up at night.

Avoid strenuous exercise after 6 PM.

Do not eat or drink heavily for 3 h before bedtime. A light bedtime snack may help.

If you have trouble with regurgitation, be especially careful to avoid heavy meals and spices in the evening. Do not retire too hungry or too full. The head of the bed may need to be raised.

Keep your room dark, quiet, well ventilated, and at a comfortable temperature throughout the night. Earplugs and eyeshades are OK.

Practice a bedtime ritual. Reading before lights-out may be helpful if it is not occupationally related.

List problems and one-sentence next steps for the following day. Set aside a worry time. Forgive yourself and others.

Learn simple self-hypnosis to use if you wake up at night. Do not try too hard to sleep; instead, concentrate on the pleasant feeling of relaxation.

Use stress management in the daytime.

Avoid unfamiliar sleep environments.

Be sure that the mattress is not too soft or too firm, and that the pillow is of the right height and firmness.

An occasional sleeping pill is probably all right.

Use the bedroom only for sleep; do not work or do other activities that lead to prolonged arousal.

If possible, make arrangements for caregiving activities (children, others, pets) to be assumed by others.

equivalent of three cups of coffee. The average cup of coffee contains 100 mg of caffeine; a strongly brewed cup of coffee contains 200 mg; tea and cola drinks contain between 50 mg and 75 mg, depending on the type. Caffeinism as a syndrome has to be ruled out in any patient complaining of a nocturnal sleep disturbance. Not infrequently, patients are referred to sleep disorder centers without the referring physician's having obtained a prior history indicating caffeinism. Any person who is consuming 500 mg of caffeine or more per day should be encouraged simply to discontinue the caffeine to see what effect that has on subsequent nocturnal sleep and daytime anxiety associated with the caffeine ingestion. Patients who have other syndromes that cause nocturnal sleep disturbances should be encouraged to discontinue caffeine for at least a 6- to 10-week trial to determine the possible therapeutic benefit of remaining caffeine-free indefinitely.

Ethanol

Ethanol is commonly self-prescribed to initiate sleep; however, in large quantities, it creates sleep maintenance difficulties. This finding is true for socially acceptable doses of ethanol. Of course, the effects of ethanol on sleep in chronic alcoholic individuals are much more profound.[22] The pharmacology of ethanol is too broad a subject for this chapter; however, there is a net sympathetic arousal state that follows the decline in blood alcohol level after even a moderately heavy drinking episode. A "moderately heavy drinking episode" is defined as more than three drinks and fewer than eight. A drink is the equivalent of 1 oz of 100 proof whiskey, 1.5 oz of vodka or gin, 5 oz of wine, 3 oz of port or other fortified wine, and 12 oz of beer. Patients commonly self-prescribe ethanol for sleep latency problems, and they just as commonly report that their subsequent sleep is usually disturbed after ingestion of alcoholic beverages before sleep onset. Awakenings from intense dreaming activity with sweating and headache occur with some frequency. These awakenings are part of the sympathetic arousal that occurs along with catecholamine secretion after even moderate doses of ethanol consumed near bedtime. Ethanol is metabolized at approximately the rate of one drink per hour, so that a patient initiating sleep after a moderate drinking episode should be encouraged to wait at least until the blood alcohol concentration has returned to zero. The sympathetic arousal can persist for as long as 2 or 3 h after the blood alcohol concentration returns to zero, although there are no systematic studies in normal nondrinking subjects or heavy social drinkers of this phenomenon.

Finally, the effects of ethanol on ventilation during sleep have to be considered for any patients who are suspected of having sleep apnea syndromes. It is important in terms of general sleep hygiene to advise middle-aged men and postmenopausal women that ethanol can have important effects on ventilation. Regardless of age or sex, patients who snore heavily would be well advised to limit their ingestion of alcohol or any other sedative-hypnotic and pay attention to the timing of the ingestion and metabolism of the drug in relation to their sleep period.

Nicotine

Laboratory and survey studies indicate that nicotine has much the same effects as caffeine on nocturnal sleep and on subsequent daytime performance and mood.[23, 24] Nicotine has a biphasic effect: at low blood concentrations, mild sedation and relaxation are produced; at higher concentrations, the effect on the same cholinergic mechanism is to produce arousal. These effects can occur in sequence rapidly enough so that smoking during the sleep period results in arousal instead of the desired sedation. Moderate or heavy smokers can actually titrate the effects of ethanol or caffeine with nicotine. That combination of nicotine and caffeine arousal and ethanol sedation can obviously be particularly disturbing to subsequent nocturnal sleep. The patient falls asleep in a net state of mild sedation. When the ethanol is finally metabolized and the nicotine and caffeine blood levels are still effectively high, there is an interaction of the three arousal states. The interaction can profoundly alter sleep maintenance, particularly if the patient is over 45 years old.

References

1. Kleitman N. Sleep and Wakefulness. Chicago, Ill: University of Chicago Press [originally published 1939]. 1963:305–317.
2. American Sleep Disorders Association. The International Classification of Sleep Disorders: Diagnostic and Coding Manual, Revised. Rochester, Minn: American Sleep Disorders Association; 1997.
3. American Psychiatric Association. Diagnostic and Statistical Manual of Mental Disorders. 4th ed. Washington, DC: American Psychiatric Association Press; 1994.
4. Buysse DJ, Reynolds CF III, Hauri PJ, et al. Diagnostic concordance for DSM-IV sleep disorders: a report from the APA/NIMH DSM-IV field trial. Am J Psychiatry. 1994;151:1351–1360.
5. Buysse DJ, Reynolds CF III, Kupfer DJ, et al. Clinical diagnoses in 216 insomnia patients using the International Classification of Sleep Disorders (ICSD), DSM-IV, and ICD-10 categories: a report from the APA/NIMH DSM-IV field trial. Sleep. 1994;17:630–637.
6. Nowell PD, Buysse DJ, Reynolds CF III, et al. Clinical factors contributing to the differential diagnosis of primary insomnia and insomnia related to mental disorders. Am J Psychiatry. 1997;154:1412–1416.
7. Morin CM, Culbert JP, Schwartz SM. Nonpharmacological interventions for insomnia: a meta-analysis of treatment efficacy. Am J Psychiatry. 1994;151:1172–1180.
8. Borbély AA. A two-process model of sleep regulation. Hum Neurobiol. 1982;1:155–204.
9. Feinberg I. Changes in sleep cycle patterns with age. J Psychiatr Res. 1974;10:283–306.
10. Webb WB, Friel J. Sleep stage and personality characteristics of "natural" long and short sleepers. Science. 1971;171:587–588.
11. Lewy AJ, Sack RL, Miller S, et al. Antidepressant and circadian phase shifting effects of light. Science. 1987;235:352–354.
12. Taub JM, Berger RJ. The effects of changing the phase and duration of sleep. J Exp Psychol Hum Percept Perform. 1976;2:30–41.
13. Reynolds CF III, Kupfer DJ, Taska LS, et al. The sleep of healthy seniors: a revisit. Sleep. 1985;8:20–29.
14. Miles LE, Dement WC. Sleep and aging. Sleep. 1980;3:119–220.
15. Coates TJ, Thoresen C. How to Sleep Better. Englewood Cliffs, NJ: Prentice-Hall; 1977.
16. Hauri PJ. The Sleep Disorders: Current Concepts. 2nd ed. Kalamazoo, Mich: Upjohn; 1982.
17. Kirmil-Gray K, Eagleston JR, Thoresen CE, et al. Brief consultation and stress management treatment for drug dependent insomnia: effects on sleep quality, self-efficacy, and daytime stress. J Behav Med. 1985;8:79–99.
18. Institute of Medicine. Sleeping Pills, Insomnias and Medical Practice. Publication no. 10M-79-04. Washington, DC: National Academy of Sciences; 1979.
19. Curatolo PW, Robertson D. The health consequences of caffeine. Ann Intern Med. 1983;98:641–653.
20. Phillis JW, Wu PH. The effect of various centrally active drugs on adenosine uptake by the central nervous system. Comp Biochem Physiol C Pharmacol Toxicol Endocrinol. 1982;72:179–187.
21. Lucas EA, Scheving LE, Halberg F. Circadian rhythmometry before and after relief of delayed sleep onset insomnia following total caffeine withdrawal. In: Takahashi R, Halberg F, eds. Toward Chronopharmacology. London, England: Pergamon Press; 1982:29–42.
22. Zarcone VP. Sleep and alcoholism. In: Weitzman ED, ed. Advances in Sleep Research. New York, NY: Spectrum Publications; 1982. Sleep Disorders: Intersections of Basic and Clinical Research; vol 8.
23. Bale P, White M. The effects of smoking on the health and sleep of sportswomen. Br J Sports Med. 1982;16:149–153.
24. Soldatos CR, Kales JD, Scharf MB, et al. Cigarette smoking associated with sleep difficulty. Science. 1980;207:551–552.

ten

Primary Disorders of Daytime Sleepiness

Christian Guilleminault

Pathophysiology of Narcolepsy

Emmanuel Mignot

In the International Classification of Sleep Disorders, *narcolepsy* is characterized by "excessive sleepiness that typically is associated with cataplexy and other [rapid eye movement] REM sleep phenomena such as sleep paralysis and hypnagogic hallucinations."[1] Disturbed nocturnal sleep is less frequently mentioned but also is central to the narcolepsy syndrome. Many still consider *cataplexy*, which is the sudden occurrence of muscle weakness in association with laughing, joking, or anger, to be a prerequisite for a diagnosis of narcolepsy. A broader definition of narcolepsy includes all patients with daytime sleepiness and abnormal REM sleep, such as sleep-onset REM periods during the multiple sleep latency test (MSLT), sleep paralysis, or hypnagogic hallucinations. The concept of a broad and narrow definition for narcolepsy has been the object of significant controversies over the years.[2, 3] It is important to keep in mind that narcolepsy with cataplexy is more likely to be an etiologically homogeneous disease entity.

Available therapeutic options support the concept of an REM sleep/sleepiness duality in the symptoms of narcolepsy.[4] Excessive daytime sleepiness is typically treated with amphetamine-like stimulants or modafinil. These compounds are effective in reducing daytime sleepiness but have little effect on cataplexy and abnormal REM sleep.[4] Conversely, the most commonly used anticataplectic treatments, antidepressant drugs, alleviate cataplexy and other REM sleep abnormalities but have little effect on daytime sleepiness.[4] Available in-

formation regarding the pathophysiology of narcolepsy is reviewed and discussed; the clinical, diagnostic, and therapeutic aspects of the syndrome are discussed elsewhere in this textbook (see Chapter 60) and are not reviewed here.

PREVALENCE STUDIES IN NARCOLEPSY-CATAPLEXY

Prevalence studies have been performed in several ethnic groups and countries. The best prevalence study was performed in Finland with 11,354 individual twin subjects.[5] All individuals responded to a questionnaire, and subjects with responses suggestive of narcolepsy were contacted by telephone. Clinical interviews and polysomnographic recordings were then conducted if indicated. Three narcoleptic subjects with cataplexy and abnormal MSLT results were identified, leading to a prevalence rate of 0.026%.[5] All three subjects had discordant dizygotic twins. Other, less strictly designed prevalence studies have led to similar prevalence rates (0.02 to 0.067%) in Great Britain, France, the Czech Republic, and the United States (for a review, see Mignot[6]). A study performed in 1945 in black navy recruits also led to a rate of 0.02% in this ethnic group for narcolepsy-cataplexy.[7]

Narcolepsy-cataplexy may be less prevalent in Israel and more prevalent in Japan. Two population-based prevalence studies performed in Japan led to 0.16%

and 0.18% prevalence rates in Japan[8, 9] but in these studies polysomnography was not used to confirm the diagnosis. In Israel, only a few narcoleptic patients were identified when compared to the large population of subjects recruited into sleep clinics.[10] This has led to the suggestion that the prevalence of narcolepsy could be as low as 0.002% in this population.

CANINE NARCOLEPSY, A UNIQUE ANIMAL MODEL OF THE HUMAN CONDITION

Narcolepsy research is greatly facilitated by the existence of a unique animal model, canine narcolepsy. Narcolepsy was first reported in two small breeds of dogs by Knecht et al.[11] and Mitler et al.[12] Early attempts to establish genetic transmission in various breeds were unsuccessful. In 1977, two narcoleptic Doberman pinschers were reported in a single litter.[13] The breeding of these animals led to the demonstration that narcolepsy was transmitted as a single autosomal recessive gene with full penetrance in this breed. A narcoleptic colony of Doberman pinschers was then established and maintained at Stanford University for more than 20 years.

The parallel between human and canine narcolepsy is striking. In MSLT-like procedures, narcoleptic dogs have been shown to have short sleep and REM sleep latencies. The 24-h recording studies show increased sleep fragmentation and proportionally more daytime sleep than in control animals.[4, 14] Finally, as in human narcolepsy, sudden episodes of muscle weakness akin to cataplexy can be observed in association with strong positive emotions, most typically during the presentation of appetitizing food or during play (Fig. 59–1). These episodes usually last a few seconds and preferentially affect the hind legs, neck, or face. Cataplexy may also escalate into complete muscle paralysis with abolition of tendon reflexes. During these episodes, the animal is conscious and most often able to visually track nearby movement. Polysomnographic recording

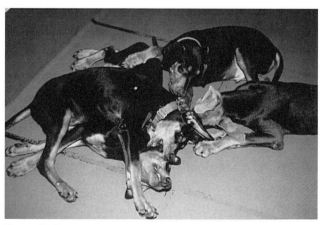

Figure 59–1. Narcoleptic Doberman Pinschers in the middle of a cataplectic attack. Note that the eyes are open. Canine narcolepsy is due to mutations in the hypocretin receptor 2 gene.

indicates a desynchronized, wake-like electroencephalographic pattern at the onset of cataplexy, followed by increased theta activity and genuine REM sleep in long-lasting episodes.[15] A typical picture of a narcoleptic dog in the midst of a cataplectic attack is presented (see Fig. 59–1).

ADRENERGIC UPTAKE INHIBITION MEDIATES THE ANTICATAPLECTIC EFFECTS OF CURRENTLY PRESCRIBED ANTIDEPRESSANT MEDICATIONS

Although cataplexy is difficult to quantify in human beings, this symptom can be easily measured in narcoleptic dogs using a simple behavioral test, the food elicited cataplexy test. In this test, pieces of dog food are lined up on the floor, and the animal is released in the room.[4] A normal dog will complete the test in less than 10 sec, whereas narcoleptic animals, excited by the food, exhibit multiple partial or complete attacks that can be recorded in number and duration. This test has been used to pharmacologically dissect the mode of action of currently prescribed anticataplectic agents.[4] The most commonly prescribed anticataplectic agents are tricyclic antidepressants. These compounds have a complex pharmacological profile that includes monoamine (serotonin, norepinephrine, epinephrine, and dopamine) uptake inhibition and cholinergic, histaminic, and alpha adrenergic blocking effects. Results have shown that inhibition of adrenergic but not dopaminergic or serotoninergic uptake or other properties is critical to the therapeutic efficacy of antidepressant compounds.[16] This observation fits well with available human pharmacological data.[4] Protriptyline, desipramine, and viloxazine, three adrenergic specific uptake blockers with no effect on serotonin transmission, are effective and potent anticataplectic agents (Table 59–1). In contrast, fluoxetine and other selective serotonin uptake inhibitors are active on cataplexy only at relatively high doses, an effect likely to be mediated by the weak adrenergic uptake effects of these compounds and their metabolites.[17] Unfortunately, all available adrenergic uptake blockers are tricyclic antidepressants with significant anticholinergic, antihistaminic, or alpha adrenergic blocking properties.[4, 17] This leaves the clinician with the choice of using either tricyclic antidepressants or high doses of selective serotonin reuptake inhibitors if tricyclic medications are not well tolerated. Novel selective adrenergic uptake inhibitors without anticholinergic effects such as reboxetine are in development in Europe and the United States for the treatment of depression. When available, these compounds may be useful in the management of cataplexy.

The observation that adrenergic uptake blockers are anticataplectic agents correlates well with the potent inhibitory effects of these compounds on REM sleep. It is well established that adrenergic transmission is reduced during REM sleep (see Chapter 9 for a review).

Table 59-1. COMMONLY PRESCRIBED TREATMENTS AND THEIR PHARMACOLOGICAL PROPERTIES

Compound	Pharmacological Properties
Stimulants	
Amphetamine	Increases monoamine release (DA > NE >> 5-HT); blocks monoamine reuptake and monoamine oxidase at high doses; the D-isomer is more specific for dopaminergic transmission and is a better stimulant compound.
Methamphetamine	More lipophilic than amphetamine; increased central penetration; proportionally fewer peripheral side effects
Methylphenidate	Blocks monoamine uptake at lower dose than amphetamine; slightly less effect on monoamine release; short half-life
Pemoline	Dopamine uptake inhibition; low potency; hepatotoxicity
Mazindol	Dopamine and adrenergic uptake blocker; high potency but efficacy limited by peripheral side effects at high doses
Selegiline (L-Deprenyl)	Monoamine oxidase B inhibitor; in vivo conversion into amphetamine
Modafinil	Fewer peripheral side effects; mode of action debated
Anticataplectic Compounds	
Protriptyline	Tricyclic antidepressant; monomoaminergic uptake blocker (NE > 5-HT > DA); anticholinergic effects
Imipramine	Tricyclic antidepressant; monoaminergic uptake blocker (NE = 5-HT > DA); anticholinergic effects; desipramine is an active metabolite.
Desipramine	Tricyclic antidepressant; monoaminergic uptake blocker (NE >> 5-HT > DA); anticholinergic effects
Clomipramine	Tricyclic antidepressant; monoaminergic uptake blocker (5-HT > NE >> DA); anticholinergic effects; desmethylclomipramine (NE >> 5-HT > DA) is an active metabolite; no specificity in vivo
Fluoxetine	Selective serotonin uptake blocker (5-HT >> NE = DA); active metabolite norfluoxetine has more adrenergic effects.
Other	
Gamma hydroxybutyrate	May act via specific, non-GABAergic receptors; reduces dopamine release

DA, dopamine; NE, norepinephrine; 5-HT, 5-hydroxytryptamine (serotonin). For details, see references 93 through 98.

Firing rate in the locus coeruleus has also been shown to decrease during cataplexy in narcoleptic dogs.[18] Adrenergic uptake blockers thus might increase activity in adrenergic projection sites involved in REM sleep regulation. This effect would reverse the effect of decreased locus coeruleus impulse flow normally oc-

curring during natural REM sleep. The fact that serotoninergic uptake blockers, also known to have inhibitory effects on REM sleep, have less or no effect on cataplexy is more surprising. Like adrenergic cells of the locus coeruleus, serotoninergic cells of the raphe nuclei dramatically decrease their activity during REM sleep.[17] This discrepancy could be accounted for by a preferential effect of serotoninergic projections on REM sleep features other than atonia, such as in the control of eye movements. In this model, adrenergic projections may be more important than serotoninergic transmission in the regulation of REM sleep atonia and, thus, cataplexy.[16] The finding that serotonergic cells of the raphe nuclei do not change their activity during cataplexy also substantiates this hypothesis.[19]

INCREASED DOPAMINERGIC TRANSMISSION MEDIATES THE WAKE-PROMOTING EFFECTS OF PRESCRIBED STIMULANT COMPOUNDS

The most commonly prescribed stimulant compounds are amphetamine-like drugs such as dextroamphetamine, methamphetamine, methylphenidate, and pemoline (see Table 59-1). Like tricyclic antidepressant compounds, these drugs are very nonspecific pharmacologically. Their main effect is to globally increase monoaminergic transmission by stimulating monoamine release and blocking monoamine reuptake. Results have demonstrated that the wake-promoting effects of these compounds are secondary to dopamine release stimulation and reuptake inhibition.[20] The mode of action of modafinil is debated, but this compound also selectively inhibits dopamine uptake.[21] Interestingly, compounds selective for dopaminergic transmission have no effect on cataplexy, whereas amphetamine-like compounds with combined dopaminergic and adrenergic effects have some anticataplectic properties at high doses.[16] Adrenergic effects of amphetamine-like stimulants also correlate with the respective effects of these compounds on normal REM sleep.[20] Selective dopaminergic uptake blockers have little effect on REM sleep compared with adrenergic or serotoninergic compounds.[20] The most important effects of dopaminergic uptake blockers are to reduce total sleep time and slow-wave sleep.[20] This preferential effect of dopaminergic uptake blockers on non-REM sleep correlates with electrophysiological data. Unlike adrenergic or serotoninergic neurons, the firing rate of dopaminergic neurons is known to remain relatively constant during REM sleep.[22, 23]

Interestingly, studies in both human beings and narcoleptic dogs have shown that large doses of stimulants are needed to polysomnographically "normalize" narcoleptic subjects. In our narcoleptic Doberman pinscher population, doses of dextroamphetamine equivalent to 60 mg/day were needed to reduce daytime sleep in our narcoleptic population to control levels.[14] In control and narcoleptic animals, however, the dose-response curves for modafinil or amphetamine were parallel. This result suggests that there is no difference in sensitivity to stimulants in narcoleptic animals but that higher doses are needed in narcoleptic animals because of their extreme baseline sleepiness.[14]

CHOLINERGIC SYSTEMS AND THE REGULATION OF CATAPLEXY AND REM SLEEP

Several studies have shown that cholinergic systems are activated during natural REM sleep.[24, 25] REM sleep is facilitated by pharmacological manipulations that increase cholinergic transmission while cholinergic antagonists suppress REM sleep.[24, 25] Finally, REM sleep or REM atonia can also be triggered experimentally in animals by injecting cholinergic agonists into the pontine reticular formation, thus suggesting important REM-triggering systems in the brainstem.[24, 25]

Despite the well-established role of cholinergic transmission in the regulation of REM sleep, cholinergic compounds are not used in the treatment of narcolepsy. Very few studies have investigated the effects of cholinergic compounds in human narcolepsy, and the results have generally been disappointing.[4, 26] In narcoleptic animals, physostigmine, an acetylcholine esterase inhibitor, increases cataplexy, whereas anticholinergic drugs inhibit this symptom.[4] These effects are, however, occurring at high doses in association with numerous peripheral side effects, thus likely explaining the discrepancies between available human and animal data.[4]

Neurochemical and Neuropharmacological Studies in Narcolepsy

The effects of more than 200 compounds with various modes of action have been examined in narcoleptic dogs (for a recent review, see Nishino and Mignot[4]). Because cataplexy is easier to study than sleepiness in dogs, most studies have focused on cataplexy rather than on sleepiness. For cataplexy, the findings were very consistent with pharmacological studies of REM sleep. As is the case for REM sleep, the regulation of cataplexy is modulated positively by cholinergic systems and negatively by monoaminergic tone.[4, 27] Muscarinic M2 or M3 receptors mediate the cholinergic effects, whereas monoaminergic effects are mostly modulated by postsynaptic alpha$_1$ adrenoreceptors.[4]

To determine the neuroanatomical basis for the sleep abnormalities observed in narcolepsy, several complementary approaches have been taken. In both human beings and dogs with narcolepsy, brain neurotransmitter levels and receptors have been measured.[28, 29] In narcoleptic animals, the most consistent abnormalities were observed in the amygdala, where significant increases in dopamine and metabolite levels were reported in two independent studies.[30] This result was interpreted as suggesting decreased dopamine turnover and accumulation of dopamine in presynaptic terminals. Another important finding was the observation of increased muscarinic M2 receptors in the pontine reticular formation,[28, 31] a region in which cholinergic stimulation triggers REM sleep. Less robust abnormalities in norepinephrine and dopamine were also observed in the pontine reticular formation and the preoptic hypothalamus.[30] In human beings, less consistent changes in dopamine receptors and metabolites were reported in the amygdala, brainstem, and caudate.[32–34] Increased D$_2$ binding in the caudate was the most significant finding in two postmortem neurochemical studies[32, 33] and also was observed in narcoleptic dogs.[35] The finding, however, could not be replicated in vivo by several investigators using positron emission tomography imaging studies.[36–38] Finally, in both dogs and human beings, monoamine metabolite levels were measured in the cerebrospinal fluid, with findings generally consistent with abnormal dopaminergic activity.[28, 39] In almost all these studies, serotoninergic transmission was never affected by narcolepsy.[28, 39]

Cholinergic Hypersensitivity Mediates Abnormal REM Sleep in Narcolepsy

The functional significance of these abnormalities has been addressed in experiments in which active pharmacological agents are locally injected or perfused in specific brain areas of freely moving narcoleptic animals. These experiments have shown that widespread hypersensitivity to cholinergic stimulation likely explains abnormal REM sleep tendencies in narcolepsy.[4] As in normal animals, the local injection or perfusion of cholinergic agonists in the pontine reticular formation triggers REM sleep, REM sleep atonia, or both in narcoleptic subjects.[4] In narcoleptic animals, however, much lower doses can trigger muscle atonia, thus suggesting hypersensitivity to cholinergic stimulation. Acetylcholine release was also measured in the pontine reticular formation during cataplexy. As during natural REM sleep, acetylcholine was found to increase during cataplexy in narcoleptic animals but not during emotional stimulation in control animals.[4]

More surprisingly, cholinergic hypersensitivity was also observed in the basal forebrain area,[4, 40] immediately anterior to the preoptic hypothalamus. In this region, cholinergic stimulation also induces cataplexy and abnormal REM sleep in narcoleptic animals.[40] In contrast, extremely high doses of cholinergic agonists were needed to trigger cataplexy-like episodes of muscle paralysis in control dogs. Finally, we also observed that acetylcholine release increases in this brain region not only during cataplexy but also during emotional stimulation in normal animals.[41]

Taken together, these experiments suggest anatomically widespread cholinergic hypersensitivity in narcolepsy. The finding that acetylcholine release is increased in the basal forebrain area during emotional stimulation suggests that this area might be more specifically involved in the induction of cataplexy by emotions.[41]

Site of Action of Monoaminergic Compounds

The site of action of adrenergic compounds on cataplexy is still unknown, but dopaminergic mesolimbic and mesostriatal systems are involved in the regulation of cataplexy and daytime sleepiness. Although the site of action of cholinergic compounds is well established, we have been unable to identify the area in the brain in which adrenergic compounds exert their anticataplectic effects. A possible candidate was the locus coeruleus, but the modulation of its activity with locally administered alpha$_2$ autoreceptor agonists or antagonists did not modify cataplexy.[4] In contrast to this finding, the local administration of dopaminergic autoreceptor agonists into the ventral tegmental area and substantia nigra, two regions that are rich with dopaminergic cell bodies, resulted in very significant changes in both cataplexy and sleepiness.[4, 42] The effect on cataplexy parallels reported effects obtained after the systemic administration of low doses of dopaminergic compounds with preferential effects on dopamine D$_2$/D$_3$ autoreceptors. Dopamine D$_2$/D$_3$ agonists are well known to promote non-REM and REM sleep at low doses, whereas antagonists have opposite and rather stimulating effects.[43–45] It is thus hypothesized that the depression of dopaminergic mesolimbic and nigrostriatal activity with autoreceptor stimulation promotes cataplexy, REM sleep, and daytime sleepiness.

The sleep-modulating effect of dopamine autoreceptor modulation corresponds well with the observation that amphetamine-like dopaminergic stimulants have potent wake-promoting effects. The lack of effects of dopamine-specific amphetamine-like stimulants on cataplexy is, however, surprising because dopaminergic autoreceptor stimulation or blockade modulates both sleepiness and cataplexy.[4, 42, 46] A possible explanation for this discrepancy might be a differential sensitivity of different dopaminergic pathways to uptake inhibition and autoreceptor stimulation. It is also worthwhile to note that mesocorticolimbic systems have been shown to be involved in the control of reward and the expression of pleasurable emotions.[47, 48] Because cataplexy is typically triggered by pleasurable emotions, these pathways could also be involved in the triggering of cataplexy.[42]

GENETIC ALTERATIONS OF THE HYPOCRETIN SYSTEM CAUSE NARCOLEPSY IN ANIMAL MODELS

The positional cloning of the canine narcolepsy gene (canarc-1) was successfully completed in July 1999. In both Dobermans and Labradors with narcolepsy, the disorder is due to exon-skipping mutations in the gene that encodes one of the G-protein–coupled receptors for the neuropeptide hypocretins (Hcrtr2).[49] A report

published soon after this discovery indicated that knockout mice for the natural ligand of this receptor, preprohypocretin, also exhibit sleep abnormalities similar to narcolepsy.[50] Taken together, these two reports implicate hypocretins (also called orexins) and one of their receptors, the hypocretin receptor 2, in the pathophysiology of narcolepsy and in the regulation of REM sleep.[50a]

Hypocretins were first identified by De Lecea et al.[51] using a direct-tag polymerase chain reaction (PCR) subtraction technique aimed at the isolation of hypothalamic specific transcripts. They isolated the preprohypocretin mRNA and showed that the corresponding precursor protein was likely processed into two related peptides, hypocretin-1 and -2. The existence of hypocretins was independently established by Sakurai et al.[52] using biochemical purification and ligand binding to cell lines expressing selected G-coupled orphan receptors. The two orphan receptors were found to bind hypocretin-1, orexin-A (a peptide similar to hypocretin-1), and hypocretin-2 (orexin-B) with different affinity profiles. The first of these receptors, now called hypocretin receptor 1 (Hcrtr1), was shown to selectively bind hypocretin-1, whereas the hypocretin receptor 2 receptor binds both hypocretin-1 and -2 with a similar affinity.[52]

The finding that hypocretin-containing cell bodies were discretely localized to a subregion of the dorsolateral hypothalamus initially suggested a role of this system in the control of feeding.[51, 52] In support of this hypothesis was the observation that centrally administered hypocretin-1 and -2 stimulate appetite in rodents[52] and that preprohypocretin mRNA is upregulated by fasting.[52] Other experiments now suggest a more minor effect of hypocretin in appetite regulation.[53–56] The fact that narcoleptic dogs, which have mutations in the hypocretin receptor 2 locus, do not have significant feeding abnormalities also suggests a more significant role for hypocretins in sleep regulation rather than appetite control.

TOWARD A NEUROANATOMICAL MODEL FOR NARCOLEPSY

How could hypocretin gene defects produce narcolepsy? To date, there is no published study reporting on the sleep-wake effects of hypocretins. The observation that intracerebroventricular administration of hypocretins induces face washing, searching, grooming, and burrowing in rats suggests wake-promoting effects for these peptides,[54] most likely via hypocretin receptor 2 rather than hypocretin receptor 1 stimulation. These two discoveries still remain to be integrated within the existing body of knowledge on sleep regulation and narcolepsy.

As discussed earlier, previous work in canine narcolepsy has demonstrated a role for cholinergic and monoaminergic abnormalities in the pathophysiology of narcolepsy. An anatomically widespread cholinergic hypersensitivity in the pontine reticular formation and in the basal forebrain area might constitute the final

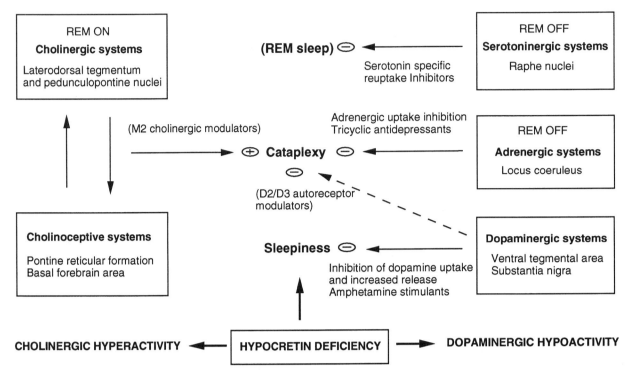

Figure 59–2. Neuropharmacological and neurochemical control of cataplexy and excessive daytime sleepiness. Narcolepsy in animal models is due to genetic alterations in the hypocretin systems. Note that cataplexy, as REM sleep, is regulated by a balance of activity between adrenergic and cholinergic tone. Anticataplectic antidepressant medications are believed to act primarily by increasing adrenergic tone (adrenergic uptake inhibition). Serotoninergic systems are also known to decrease activity during REM sleep, but increasing serotoninergic tone with serotonin uptake blockers reduces REM sleep but not cataplexy in narcoleptic dogs. The most commonly prescribed stimulant compounds promote wakefulness by increasing presynaptically dopaminergic transmission (dopamine uptake inhibition or increased dopamine release). Dopaminergic mechanisms may also be involved in the emotional triggering of cataplexy. (For details, see the text.)

pathway for REM sleep abnormalities in narcolepsy.[4] Other experiments have established an important role for the mesocorticolimbic dopaminergic system in the modulation of cataplexy and daytime sleepiness.[4] Specifically, hypoactive dopaminergic systems may be involved in the regulation of sleepiness (via cortical projections) and in the emotional triggering of cataplexy (via limbic projections).[4] Current neuroanatomical models for the disorder thus suggest a cholinergic/monoaminergic imbalance in narcolepsy (Fig. 59–2).

The finding that hypocretin deficiencies cause narcolepsy in animal models raises the question of how these hypothalamic peptides interact with cholinergic and monoaminergic neuronal groups to generate daytime sleepiness and abnormal REM sleep. Hypocretin neurons project most heavily to the locus coeruleus, and these projections have been shown to be excitatory in nature.[57, 58] As this structure greatly reduces its firing rate during REM sleep, it has been hypothesized that a lowering in hypocretins could decrease locus coeruleus activity, thereby disinhibiting REM sleep and producing narcolepsy.[59] A potential problem with this hypothesis is that the hypocretin receptor subtype present in the locus coeruleus is mostly of type 1 (as opposed to type 2, the subtype mutated in canine narcolepsy).[60] One publication also showed that the firing rate of the locus coeruleus decreases in REM sleep and in cataplexy in narcoleptic dogs.[18] This result suggests that adrenergic cells in the locus coeruleus can still be inhib-

ited during REM sleep and cataplexy via hypocretin receptor 2 independent pathways (possibly receptor 1–mediated).

Little additional information can be gained from our current knowledge of the neuroanatomy of these systems. The neuroanatomical distribution of hypocretin receptor mRNAs was studied in rats by Trivedi et al.[60] Of special interest is the finding that the hypocretin receptor 1 transcript is mostly localized in the ventromedian hypothalamic nucleus, hippocampal formation, dorsal raphe, and locus coeruleus. In contrast, hypocretin receptor 2 mRNA molecules are more abundant in the paraventricular nuclei and in the nucleus accumbens.[60] Hypocretin projections are so diffuse that it is difficult to establish functional significance at this stage. Although the preprohypocretin-positive neurons are discretely localized in the perifornical nucleus and in the dorsal and lateral hypothalamic areas, their projections are widely distributed in the brain.[57, 61] Clearly, these projections could influence monoaminergic and cholinergic systems at many different levels in the central nervous system. As mentioned, hypocretin neurons are known to project to monoaminergic brainstem cell groups, such as the locus coeruleus and the ventral tegmental area, and to cholinoceptive pontine reticular formation and associated cholinergic cell groups.[57] Other major projection sites include the cortex, the basal forebrain area, the nucleus accumbens, and the amygdala.[57] These are consistent with interactions at the level of target projections for hypocretins, mono-amines, and acetylcholine. Experiments aimed at study of the effects of hypocretins on sleep after systemic and central (e.g., intracerebroventricular injection and local perfusion in selected brain areas) administration are now critically needed to establish functional relevance for some of these projections. We expect that the central administration of hypocretins in selected target areas will be wake-promoting and suppress REM sleep via a stimulation of the Hcrtr2 receptor in control, but not in narcoleptic, animals.

Some experiments have suggested that canine narcolepsy is associated with neuronal degeneration in the basal forebrain area and in the amygdala.[62] Functional positron emission tomography imaging studies have shown that these structures are activated during natural REM sleep.[63] Other experiments have established their role in the regulation of emotional behaviors.[64] These results again emphasize the importance of limbic structures in the pathophysiology of narcolepsy, a result that was suggested by previous neuropathological studies in canine narcolepsy.[30]

FAMILIAL ASPECTS OF HUMAN NARCOLEPSY

The familial occurrence of narcolepsy-cataplexy was first reported in 1877 by Westphal.[65] Since then, numerous case reports have appeared in the literature. Narcolepsy had been considered a familial disorder, but studies have shown that earlier reports often were confounded by unrecognized obstructive sleep apnea. One frequently cited publication by Krabbe and Magnussen[66] reports that "narcoleptic" (obese) relatives of a narcoleptic proband would frequently fall asleep while playing cards, falling forward on the table, snoring loudly, and becoming cyanotic during the episodes. In another study, the risk of a first-degree relative to develop narcolepsy-cataplexy has been shown to be only 1 to 2% (for a review, see Mignot[6]). A larger portion of relatives (4 to 5%) may have isolated daytime sleepiness, when other causes of daytime sleepiness have been excluded.[6] These percentages are important to keep in mind because they are helpful in reassuring patients regarding the risk to their children and relatives. A 1 to 2% risk is 10- to 40-fold higher than that in the general population but remains manageable. A 4 to 5% risk for daytime sleepiness is not negligible, but similar values have been reported for excessive daytime sleepiness in the general population independent of narcolepsy.[67-69]

Twin Studies and Environmental Factors in Narcolepsy

The only systematic twin study available was performed by Hublin et al.[5] in white Finns. All three twin individuals identified were dizygotic pairs, so the protocol was not informative to establish concordance in monozygotic twins. Sixteen monozygotic twin reports are available in the literature (for a review, see Mignot[6]). Four to five are discordant for narcolepsy, depending how strictly concordance is determined clinically.[6] Most cases of human narcolepsy therefore require the influence of environmental factors for the pathology to develop.

The nature of the environmental factor involved is still unknown; frequently cited factors are head trauma,[70] sudden change in sleep/wake habits,[71] and various infections.[72, 73] These factors may be involved, but there are no documented studies demonstrating increased frequency compared with control groups.

HUMAN NARCOLEPSY, HLA, AND THE IMMUNE SYSTEM

The observation that narcolepsy is associated with human leukocyte antigen (HLA) *DR2* was first reported in Japan in 1983.[74, 75] It was quickly confirmed in Europe and North America with 90 to 100% of all patients with cataplexy carrying the HLA *DR2* subtype.[76–82] Because many HLA (also called major histocompatibility complex, or MHC)-associated diseases are known to be autoimmune, this discovery led to the hypothesis that narcolepsy may result from an autoimmune insult within the central nervous system. Attempts to verify this possibility have generally been disappointing.[83, 84] Human narcolepsy is not associated with any striking pathological changes in the central nervous system or increased frequency in the occurrence of oligoclonal bands in the cerebrospinal fluid.[83, 84] Similarly, peripheral immunity does not seem to be altered even around disease onset.[83, 84] Lymphocyte $CD4^+/CD8^+$ populations, autoantibody levels, erythrocyte sedimentation rate, and C-reactive protein are within the normal range and were found not to change up to 1 year after disease onset. These studies do not entirely exclude the possibility that an autoimmune mechanism will be discovered in the future. Tissue destruction may be difficult to detect if the pathological process is restricted to a small anatomical area in the central nervous system or is short-lasting around the time of disease onset.

HLA *DQB1*0602* and *DQA1*0102* Are the Actual Narcolepsy Susceptibility Genes

The observation that narcolepsy is HLA-associated but does not seem to be a classic autoimmune disorder led to the hypothesis that HLA *DR2* was only a marker for narcolepsy. To explore this hypothesis, investigators isolated and tested novel markers in the HLA *DR* region and studied neighboring HLA genes (e.g., HLA *DQ*). HLA testing techniques have also changed from serological, antibody-based technology to molecular typing at the DNA level, thus resulting in a further layer of complexity for the clinician. To facilitate the review of this nomenclature, results are summarized in Figure 59–3 and Table 59–2.

At the *DR* level, *DR2* was first split into two sub-

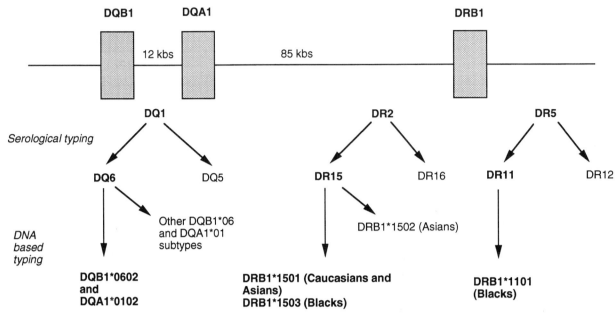

Figure 59–3. HLA *DR* and HLA *DQ* alleles most typically observed in narcolepsy. The HLA *DR* and *DQ* genes are located very close to each other on chromosome 6p21. These genes encode heterodimeric HLA proteins composed of an alpha and a beta chain. In the *DQ* locus, both the *DQ* alpha and *DQ* beta chains have numerous variable residues and are encoded by two polymorphic genes, *DQA1* and *DQB1*, respectively. Polymorphism at the *DR* level is mostly encoded by the *DRB1* gene, so only this locus is depicted in the figure. *DQB1*0602*, a molecular subtype of the serologically defined DQ1 antigen, is the most specific marker for narcolepsy across all ethnic groups. It is always associated with the *DQA1* subtype *DQA1*0102*. In whites and Asians, the associated *DR2* subtype *DRB1*1501* is typically observed with *DQB1*0602* (and *DQA1*0102*) in narcoleptic patients. In blacks, either *DRB1*1503*, a DNA-based subtype of *DR2*, or *DRB1*1101*, a DNA-based subtype of *DR5*, is most frequently observed together with *DQB1*0602*. Other *DRB1* alleles (*DRB1*0301*, *DRB1*0806*, *DRB1*12022*, and *DRB1*1602*) can be observed together with *DQB1*0602* in much rarer cases.

types, *DR15* and *DR16*, with the use of serological typing techniques. *DR15* was then identified in *DR2* narcoleptic subjects. Molecular subtypes of *DR15* were further identified at the *DRB1* level using DNA sequencing or oligotyping. The DR molecule is a heterodimer consisting of a polymorphic *DR* beta chain (encoded by the *DRB* genes) and a monomorphic *DR* alpha chain (encoded by the *DRA* gene), so all the diversity at the level of *DR* can be obtained by molecularly typing the *DRB* genes. *DR15* subtypes recognized at the DNA level were identified as *DRB1*1501* to *DRB1*1508*.[85] In white and Japanese, patients were found to carry the *DRB1*1501* gene, whereas most black narcoleptic patients with the *DR2* antigens were observed to be *DRB1*1503*.[86, 87] A significant number of black patients were also found to be negative for *DR2* and to generally carry the *DR11* subtype *DRB1*1101*.[81, 87]

DQ, another HLA antigen encoded by genes located 85 kb centromeric to *DRB1*, was also studied. Serologically, all patients were initially found to be positive for *DQ1*, a very frequent DQ antigen (see Table 59–2). *DQ1* was then serologically split into *DQ5* and *DQ6*, and all patients found to be positive for *DQ6*. At the molecular level, the *DQA1* and *DQB1* genes encoding the *DQ* molecule are both polymorphic, so typing both the *DQA1* and *DQB1* theoretically is required to identify the biologically active *DQ* antigen. *DQB1* is, however, the most polymorphic of the two genes and usually determines the *DQ* serological specificity. Molecular subtypes of *DQ6* thus are identified at the *DQB1* level

as *DQB1*0601* to *DQB1*0616*. The *DQ6* subtype identified in patients with narcolepsy was found to be *DQB1*0602*.[86, 87]

Studies across ethnic groups have shown that *DQB1*0602* is a better marker for narcolepsy. This is especially important in blacks, in whom many patients are positive for *DQB1*0602* but negative for *DR2*.[81, 86, 87] Subjects were also found to be positive for *DQA1*0102*.[86, 87] Novel DNA markers developed in the HLA *DQ* region have been tested to further map the narcolepsy susceptibility region within the *DQA1*-*DQB1* interval.[86, 87] This segment has been completely sequenced and was shown to contain no new genes.[88] It is also worth noting that in all narcolepsy susceptibility DR-DQ haplotypes identified, both *DQA1*0102* and *DQB1*0602* are present,[87] thus suggesting that the active *DQA1*0102/DQB1*0602* heterodimer is necessary for disease predisposition. A number of other DR-DQ haplotypes in the population carry *DQA1*0102* without *DQB1*0602*, and those do not predispose to narcolepsy.[87] Conversely, although *DQB1*0602* subjects are almost always positive for *DQA1*0102*, rare haplotypes with *DQB1*0602* but without *DQA1*0102* are observed in the control population but not in narcoleptic patients.[87] Both the *DQA1*0102* and *DQB1*0602* alleles thus might be necessary for disease predisposition.[87]

Recent findings in families and in unrelated cases also suggest that most, if not all, of the *DQB1*0602/DQA1*0102* alleles present in the population predispose equally to narcolepsy. One such finding comes

Table 59-2. HLA ALLELE FREQUENCIES IN NARCOLEPTIC AND CONTROL SUBJECTS ACROSS ETHNIC GROUPS

HLA Marker	Frequency in		Notes
	Clearcut Cataplexy	*Control Subjects†*	
HLA *DR2*			
Whites	85–100%	26%	Serological typing (*DR15* and *DR16* are *DR2* subtypes); old
Blacks	65–75%	31%	narcolepsy marker
Japanese	100%	36%	
HLA *DR15*			
Whites	85–100%	23%	Serological or DNA-based typing; most *DR2* antigens are
Blacks	65–75%	29%	*DR15* in controls and patients; almost equivalent to *DR2*
Japanese	100%	35%	
HLA *DRB1*1501*			
Whites	85–100%	22%	DNA-based typing; most *DR15* antigens are *DRB1*1501* in
Blacks	10–20%	7%	whites
Japanese	100%	13%	
HLA *DRB1*1502*			
Japanese (not associated with narcolepsy)	2%	22%	DNA-based typing; Asian antigen; two thirds of the *DR15* antigens are *DRB1*1502* in Japanese; associated with *DQB1*0601*, not *DQB1*0602*
HLA *DRB1*1503*			
Blacks	55–65%	20%	DNA-based typing; African antigen; most *DR15* antigens are *DRB1*1503* in blacks
HLA *DQ1*			
Whites	90–100%	67%	Serological typing (*DQ5* and *DQ6* are *DQ1* subtypes); very
Blacks	>95%	75%	frequent; low specificity; old narcolepsy marker
Japanese	100%	73%	
HLA *DQB1*0602*			
Whites	85–100%	22%	Almost always found with *DRB1*1501* in whites and
Blacks	90–95%	34%	Asians
Japanese	100%	12%	
HLA *DQA1*0102*			
Whites	85–100%	36%	More frequent in controls than *DQB1*0602*; associated with
Blacks	90–95%	48%	many *DQB1*05* and *06* alleles
Japanese	100%	26%	
HLA *DQA1*0102/DQB1*0602*			
Whites	85–100%	22%	Patients with *DQB1*0602* are always *DQA1*0102* positive
Blacks	90–95%	33%	
Japanese	100%	12%	

Narcolepsy values are approximated from references 76 through 82, 86, and 98 through 103.
†Control values are population carrier frequencies compiled from composite panels of 333 U.S. white control subjects[86, 104] (courtesy of S. Hsu), 364 black control subjects[86, 104] (courtesy of M. S. Leffell), and 717 Japanese control subjects.[105]

from multiplex families in whom several patients are positive for *DQB1*0602*. In many cases, *DQB1*0602* has been inherited from different branches of the family (e.g., in one case, from the father, and in another case, from the mother) and thus is not "identical by descent."[6] It also was shown that subjects homozygous for *DQB1*0602* or with the *DQB1*0602/DQB1*0301* are at two to four times increased risk for developing narcolepsy compared with *DQB1*0602* heterozygote subjects.[89, 90] Finally, a study in 509 normal individuals from the Wisconsin Sleep Cohort Study also showed decreased REM sleep latency in normal individuals carrying the HLA subtypes.[91] Overall, the data accumulated to date strongly suggest that the HLA *DQB1* and *DQA1*[91] genes themselves rather than an unknown genetic factor in the region predispose to narcolepsy.

HLA and Narcolepsy in Clinical Practice

The usefulness of HLA typing in clinical practice is limited by several factors. First, the HLA association is very high (more than 90%) only in narcoleptic patients with clear-cut cataplexy[81]; clear-cut cataplexy is defined as episodes of muscle weakness triggered by laughter, joking, or anger. Muscle weakness episodes triggered by anger, stress, other negative emotions, or physical or sexual activity may not be cataplexy if joking or laughing is not mentioned as a triggering factor.[92] In patients without cataplexy or with doubtful cataplexy, HLA *DQB1*0602* frequency is also increased (40% to 60%), but many patients are *DQB1*0602* negative.[81] Second, a large number of control individuals (see Table 59–2) have the HLA *DQB1*0602* marker without having narcolepsy. Finally, a few rare patients with clear-cut cataplexy do not have the HLA *DQB1*0602* marker.[87]

Despite these limitations, HLA typing probably is most useful in atypical cases or in patients with narcolepsy without definite cataplexy. A negative result should lead the clinician to be more cautious in excluding other possible causes of daytime sleepiness such as abnormal breathing during sleep. Practically, it is always more useful to request HLA *DQ* high-resolution typing than *DR2* or *DR15* typing to confirm the diagnosis of narcolepsy. Typical HLA *DR* and *DQ* results are depicted in Table 59–3, together with their interpretation. It is also worthwhile to note that if a patient is homozygous for *DQB1*0602* (subject 2) or heterozygous for *DQB1*0602/DQB1*0301* (subjects 1 and 3), the narcolepsy diagnosis is even more probable. A recent study has shown that 18 to 30% of narcoleptic subjects are *DQB1*0602* homozygous versus 0 to 4% in black and white control subjects.[89] A similar increase in risk was also reported for *DQB1*0602/DQB1*0301* heterozygote.[90] In whites, *DR2* and *DQB1*0602* typing is almost equal, and it probably is unnecessary to retype a patient if he or she has been shown to be *DR2* positive through the use of serological typing techniques (subject 6). Most white subjects with *DR2* are also positive for *DQB1*0602*, but the situation is somewhat different in Asians and blacks (see Table 59–3). It is not necessary to test for *DQA1*0102* because almost all subjects with *DQB1*0602* are also positive for *DQA1*0102* (see Table 59–3). Most HLA typing laboratories do not routinely type for *DQA1*.

HLA *DQB1*0602* Negativity

HLA *DQB1*0602*-negative subjects with typical and severe cataplexy have been reported, but these subjects are exceptionally rare.[87] Interestingly, two partially concordant monozygotic twins reported in the literature were negative for *DQB1*0602*.[6] A number of *DQB1*0602*-negative families have been reported in whom narcolepsy and cataplexy seem to be transmitted as a highly penetrant autosomal dominant trait, with many patients experiencing narcolepsy-cataplexy and other family members having sleepiness and documented REM abnormalities during the MSLT.[6] These results emphasize the fact that HLA typing results should be interpreted in conjunction with a careful family history.

HLA *DQB1*0602*-negative subjects with cataplexy have also been reported in the context of posttraumatic narcolepsy in the United States.[70] This finding requires confirmation in other cultures because the issue could easily be confounded by medicolegal factors in North America.

CAUSE OF HUMAN NARCOLEPSY AND PERSPECTIVES FOR NOVEL TREATMENTS

The cause of human narcolepsy is still unknown, but the identification of the canine gene and the development of a mouse model offer exciting new avenues of research. A recent study has shown that hypocretin levels are undetectable in the cerebrospinal fluid of

Table 59–3. EXAMPLES OF HLA TYPING RESULTS AND THEIR INTERPRETATION

Clinical Case	HLA Typing	Interpretation
35-Year-old white men with clearcut cataplexy	*DRB1*1501, DRB1*1101, DQB1*0602, DQB1*0301*	Compatible with narcolepsy, *DR2* positive, *DQB1*0602* positive
13-Year-old white boy without cataplexy but with sleep-onset REM periods	*DRB1*1501, DRB1*X,† DQB1*0602, DQB1*X*	Compatible with narcolepsy, *DR2* + homozygous, *DQB1*0602* + homozygous
55-Year-old black women with cataplexy	*DRB1*1101, DRB1*X, DQB1*0602, DQB1*0301*	Compatible with narcolepsy, *DR2* negative, *DQB1*0602* positive
32-Year-old Japanese men without cataplexy but with sleep-onset REM periods	*DRB1*1502, DRB1*0405, DQB1*0401, DQB1*06011*	Not typical for narcolepsy, *DR2* positive but *DRB1*1502 DQB1*0602* negative
35-Year-old black men without cataplexy but with sleep-onset REM periods	*DRB1*0302, DRB1*1503, DQB1*0402, DQB1*0602*	Compatible with narcolepsy, *DR2* positive, *DQB1*0602* positive
47-Year-old white women with cataplexy and sleep-onset REM periods	*DR2* positive (insufficient typing resolution)	Compatible with narcolepsy in whites, almost all *DR2* positive are *DQB1*0602* positive
25-Year-old white men with possible cataplexy and two sleep-onset REM periods	*DR1 DR3 DQ1 DQ2* (insufficient typing resolution)	Not typical for narcolepsy, *DQ1* has a low specificity, it is also associated with *DR1, DR6,* and *DR10* but *DQ1* is then not *DQB1*0602*

†X indicates blank or homozygosity. HLA typing results may not always be depicted as shown. HLA *DRB1* results do not need to be requested for clinical purpose if HLA *DQB1*0602* results are provided. *DRB1* typing results are indicated in this table as a reference to older classification. HLA *DRB2, DRB3, DRB4,* or *DRB5* typing results may be reported in addition to HLA *DRB1* typing results but should be ignored. In subject 2, the subject is *DRB1*X* and *DQB1*X*. It is very likely that *DRB1*15-DQB1*0602* is present on both chromosomes, thus indicating homozygosity. A theoretically possible alternative explanation would involve nondetectable *DRB1* and *DQB1* alleles on one of the subject's chromosomes. In subject 3, one of the HLA haplotypes is most probably *DRB1*1101-DQB1*0602* (frequent in blacks), whereas the other haplotypes are *DRB1*1101-DQB1*0301* (frequent in all ethnic groups). HLA typing in parents of subjects 2 and 3 would be required to absolutely establish homozygosity.

most narcoleptic patients.[107] A restricted autoimmune process directed against the hypocretin neurons may thus be the cause of human narcolepsy and explain the HLA association in the human disorder. Alternatively, more complex neuroimmune interactions between hypocretins and HLA system might be involved.[59] Mutations or polymorphisms in hypocretin-related genes might also predispose humans, independently of the HLA association. As mentioned, HLA genetic effects account for only a small portion of the overall genetic risk in first-degree relatives; other predisposing loci are thus likely. Some familial cases of narcolepsy, many of which are not HLA-associated, could be secondary to hypocretin gene mutations of high penetrance.

Experimental results have shown that canine animal heterozygotes for the Hcrtr2 mutation have subclinical abnormalities, such as increased daytime sleepiness. In heterozygous animals, the administration of drugs that increase cholinergic and reduce monoaminergic transmissions has been shown to induce cataplexy at specific developmental times.[27] Hypocretin gene polymorphisms may thus be involved not only in narcolepsy predisposition but also in modulating daytime sleepiness in other sleep disorders.

The identification of hypocretins as key components to the pathophysiology of narcolepsy also opens new therapeutic approaches.[108] The currently prescribed treatments are known to act on the dopaminergic and adrenergic systems and to provide only symptomatic relief. Because most cases of human narcolepsy are unlikely to be due to a complete dysfunction of the hypocretin receptor 2 system, it is possible that the administration of receptor agonists may alleviate it.

References

1. International Classification of Sleep Disorders: Diagnostic and Coding Manual, Revised. Rochester, Minn: American Sleep Disorders; 1997.
2. Guilleminault C, Mignot E, Partinen M. Controversies in the diagnosis of narcolepsy. Sleep. 1994;17:S1–S6.
3. Aldrich M. The clinical spectrum of narcolepsy and idiopathic hypersomnia. Neurology. 1996;46:393–401.
4. Nishino S, Mignot E. Pharmacological aspects of human and canine narcolepsy. Progr Neurobiol. 1997;52:27–78.
5. Hublin C, Kaprio J, Partinene M, et al. The prevalence of narcolepsy: an epidemiological study of the Finnish twin cohort. Ann Neurol. 1994;35:709–716.
6. Mignot E. Genetic and familial aspects of narcolepsy. Neurology. 1998;50(suppl 1):S16–S22.
7. Solomon P. Narcolepsy in Negroes. Dis Nerv Sys. 1945;179–183.
8. Tashiro T, Kambayashi T, Hishikawa Y. An epidemiological study of narcolepsy in Japanese. Proceedings of the 4th International Symposium on Narcolepsy; June 16–17; Tokyo, Japan. 1994:13.
9. Honda Y. Census of narcolepsy, cataplexy and sleep life among teen-agers in Fujisawa city. Sleep Res. 1979;8:191.
10. Lavie P, Peled R. Narcolepsy is a rare disease in Israel. Sleep. 1987;10:608–609.
11. Knecht CD, Oliver JE, Redding R, et al. Narcolepsy in a dog and a cat. J Am Vet Med Assoc. 1973;162:1052–1053.
12. Mitler M, Boysen M, Campbell L, et al. Narcolepsy-cataplexy in a female dog. Exp Neurol. 1974;45:332–340.
13. Baker T, Foutz A, Neyman V, et al. Canine model of narcolepsy: genetic and developmental determinants. Exp Neurol. 1982;75:729–742.
14. Shelton J, Nishino S, Vaught J, et al. Comparative effects of modafinil and amphetamine on daytime sleepiness and cataplexy of narcoleptic dogs. Sleep. 1995;18:817–826.
15. Kushida CA, Baker TL, Dement WC. Electroencephalographic correlates of cataplectic attacks in narcoleptic canines. Electroencephalogr Clin Neurophysiol. 1985;61:61–70.
16. Mignot E, Renaud A, Nishino S, et al. Canine cataplexy is preferentially controlled by adrenergic mechanisms: evidence using monoamine selective uptake inhibitors and release enhancers. Psychopharmacology. 1993;113:76–82.
17. Nishino S, Arrigoni J, Shelton J, et al. Desmethyl metabolites of serotonergic uptake inhibitors are more potent for suppressing canine cataplexy than their parent compounds. Sleep. 1993;16:706–712.
18. Wu MF, Gulyani SA, Yan E, et al. Locus coeruleus neurons: cessation of activity during cataplexy. Neuroscience. 1999; 91:1389–1399.
19. Wu MF, John J, Nguyen FB, et al. Activity of serotonergic cells in the dorsal raphe during cataplexy [Abstract]. Soc Neurosciences. 1999;25:626.
20. Nishino S, Mao J, Sampathkumaran R, et al. Increased dopaminergic transmisson mediates the wake-promoting effects of CNS stimulants. Sleep Res Online. 1998;1:49–61.
21. Mignot E, Nishino S, Guilleminault C, et al. Modafinil binds to the dopamine uptake carrier site with low affinity. Sleep. 1994;17:436–437.
22. Miller JD, Farber J, Gatz P, et al. Activity of mesencephalic dopamine and non-dopamine neurons across stages of sleep and waking in the rat. Brain Res. 1983;273:133–141.
23. Steinfels GF, Heym J, Streckjer RE, et al. Behavioral correlates of dopaminergic activity in freely moving cats. Brain Res. 1983;258:217–228.
24. Gillin J, Salin-Pascual R, Velazquez-Moctezuma J, et al. Cholinergic receptors subtypes and REM sleep in animals and normal controls. In: Cuello A, ed. Progress in Brain Research. New York, NY: Elsevier Science Publishers; 1993:379–387.
25. Hobson JA, Datta S, Calvo JM, et al. Acetylcholine as a brain state modulator: triggering and long-term regulation of REM sleep. In: Cuello AC, ed. Progress in Brain Research: Cholinergic Function and Dysfunction. Amsterdam, Netherlands: Elsevier; 1993.
26. Gillin JC, Horwitz D, Wyatt RJ. Pharmacologic studies of narcolepsy involving serotonin, acetylcholine, and monoamine oxidase. In: Guilleminault C, Dement WC, Passouant P, eds. Narcolepsy: Advances in Sleep Research. Vol 3. New York, NY: Spectrum Publications; 1976:585–603.
27. Mignot E, Nishino S, Hunt-Sharp LE, et al. Heterozygosity at the canarc-1 locus can confer susceptibility for narcolepsy: induction of cataplexy in heterozygous asymptomatic dogs after administration of a combination of drugs acting on monoaminergic and cholinergic systems. J Neurosci. 1993;13:1057–1064.
28. Baker TL, Dement WC. Canine narcolepsy-cataplexy syndrome: evidence for an inherited monoaminergic-cholinergic imbalance. In: McGinty DJ, Drucker-Colin R, Morrison A, et al, eds. Brain Mechanisms of Sleep. New York, NY: Raven Press; 1985:199–233.
29. Aldrich MS. The neurobiology of narcolepsy-cataplexy. Progr Neurobiol. 1993;41:533–541.
30. Miller JD, Faull KF, Bowersox SS, et al. CNS monoamines and their metabolites in canine narcolepsy: a replication study. Brain Res. 1990;509:169–171.
31. Kilduff T, Bowersox SS, Kaitan KI, et al. Muscarinic cholinergic receptors and the canine model of narcolepsy. Sleep. 1986;9:102–107.
32. Kish SJ, Mamelak M, Slimovitch C, et al. Brain neurotransmitter changes in human narcolepsy. Neurology. 1992;42:229–234.
33. Aldrich MS, Hollingsworth Z, Penney JB. Dopamine-receptor autoradiography of human narcoleptic brain. Neurology. 1992;42:410–415.
34. Aldrich MS, Prokopowicz G, Ockert K, et al. Neurochemical studies of human narcolepsy: alpha-adrenergic receptor autoradiography of human narcoleptic brain and brainstem. Sleep. 1994;17:598–608.
35. Bowersox S, Kilduff T, Faul K, et al. Brain dopamine receptor levels elevated in canine narcolepsy. Brain Res. 1987;402:44–48.

36. Khan N, Antonini A, Parkes D, et al. Striatal dopamine D2 receptors in patients with narcolepsy measured with PET and ^{11}C-raclopride. Neurology. 1994;44:2102–2104.

37. Rinne JO, Hublin C, Partinen M, et al. PET study of human narcolepsy: no increase in striatal dopamine D2-receptors. Neurology. 1995;45:1735–1738.

38. MacFarlane JG, List SJ, Moldovsly H, et al. Dopamine D2 receptors quantified in vivo in human narcolepsy. Biol Psychiatry. 1997;41:305–310.

39. Faull KF, Guilleminault C, Berger PS, et al. Cerebrospinal fluid monoamine metabolites in narcolepsy and hypersomnia. Ann Neurol. 1983;13:258–263.

40. Nishino S, Tafti M, Reid M, et al. Muscle atonia is triggered by cholinergic stimulation of the basal forebrain: implication for the pathophysiology of canine narcolepsy. J Neuroscience. 1995;15:4808–4814.

41. Reid M, Nishino S, Tafti M, et al. Neuropharmacological characterization of basal forebrain cholinergic stimulated cataplexy in narcoleptic canines. Exp Neurol. 1998;151:89–104.

42. Reid MS, Tafti M, Nishino S, et al. Local administration of dopaminergic drugs into the ventral tegmental area modulate cataplexy in the narcoleptic canine. Brain Res. 1996;733:83–100.

43. Wauquier A, Clinke GHC, Vand den Broeck WAE, et al. Active and permissive roles of dopamine in sleep-wakefulness regulation. In: Wauquier A, Gaillard JM, Monti JM, Radoulovacki M, eds. Sleep: Neurotransmitters and Neuromodulators. New York, NY: Raven Press; 1985:107–120.

44. Kafi-de-St-Hilaire S, Sovilla JY, Hjorth S, et al. Modifications of sleep parameters in the rat by (+) and (−) 3-PPP. J Neurol Transm. 1985;62:209–217.

45. Monti JM, Jantos H, Fernandez M. Effects of the selective dopamine D-2 receptor agonist quinpirole on sleep and wakefulness in the rat. Eur J Pharmacol. 1989;169:61–66.

46. Nishino S, Arrigoni J, Valtier D, et al. Dopamine D2 mechanisms in canine narcolepsy. J Neurosci. 1991;11:2666–2671.

47. Mirenowicz J, Schultz W. Preferential activation of midbrain dopamine neurons by appetitive rather than aversive stimuli. Nature. 1996;379:449–451.

48. Koob GF, Le Moal M. Drug abuse: hedonic homeostatic dysregulation. 1997;278:52–58.

49. Lin L, Faraco J, Li R, et al. The sleep disorder canine narcolepsy is caused by a mutation in the Hypocretin (Orexin) receptor 2 gene. Cell. 1999;98:365–376.

50. Chemelli RM, Willie JT, Stinton CM, et al. Narcolepsy in orexin knockout mice: molecular genetics of sleep regulation. Cell. 1999;98:437–451.

50a. Siegel JM. Narcolepsy. Sci Am. 2000;282:76–81.

51. De Lecea L, Kilduff TS, Peyron C, et al. The hypocretins: hypothalamus-specific peptides with neuroexcitatory activity. Proc Natl Acad Sci U S A. 1998;95:322–327.

52. Sakurai T, Amemiya A, Ishii M, et al. Orexins and orexin receptors: a family of hypothalamic neuropeptides and G protein–coupled receptors that regulate feeding behavior. Cell. 1998;92:573–585.

53. Edwards CMB, Abusnana S, Sunter D, et al. The effect of the orexins on food intake: comparison with neuropeptide Y, Melanin-concentrating hormone and galanin. J Endocrinol. 1999;160:R7–R12.

54. Ida T, Nakahara K, Katayama T, et al. Effect of lateral cerebroventricular injection of the appetite-stimulating neuropeptide, orexin and neuropeptide Y, on the various behavioral activities of rats. Brain Res. 1999;821:526–529.

55. Lubkin M, Stricker-Krongrad A. Independent feeding and metabolic actions of orexins in mice. Biochem Biophys Res Commun. 1998;253:241–245.

56. Sweet DC, Levine AS, Billington CJ, et al. Feeding response to central orexins. Brain Res. 1999;821:535–538.

57. Peyron C, Tighe DK, van den Pol AN, et al. Neurons containing hypocretin (orexin) project to multiple neuronal systems. J Neurosci. 1998;18:9996–10015.

58. Horwarth T, Peyron C, Diano S, et al. Hypocretin (orexin) activation and synaptic innervation of the locus coeruleus noradrenergic system. J Comp Neurol. 1999;415:145–159.

59. Siegel JM. Narcolepsy: a key role for hypocretins (orexins). Cell. 1999;98:409–412.

60. Trivedi P, Yu H, MacNeil DJ, et al. Distribution of orexin receptor mRNA in the rat brain. FEBS Lett. 1998;438:71–75.

61. Nambu T, Sakurai T, Mizukami K. Distribution of orexin neurons in the adult rat brain. Brain Res. 1999;827:243–260.

62. Siegel JM, Niemhuis R, Gulyani S, et al. Neuronal degeneration in canine narcolepsy. J Neurosci. 1999;19:248–257.

63. Maquet P, Peters J, Aerts J, et al. Functional neuroanatomy of human rapid-eye-movement sleep and dreaming. Nature. 1996;383:163–166.

64. Morris JS, Frith CD, Perrett DI, et al. A differential neural response in the human amygdala to fearful and happy facial expressions. Nature. 1996;383:812–815.

65. Westphal C. Eigenthümliche mit Einschläfen verbundene Anfälle. Arch Psychiatr. 1877;7:631–635.

66. Krabbe E, Magnussen G. On narcolepsy, I: familial narcolepsy. Acta Psychiatr Scand. 1942;17:149.

67. Young T, Palta M, Dempsey J, et al. The occurrence of sleep-disordered breathing among middle-aged adults. N Engl J Med. 1993;328:1230–1235.

68. D'Allessandro R, Rinaldi R, Cristina E, et al. Prevalence of excessive daytime sleepiness: an open epidemiological problem [letter]. Sleep. 1995;18:389–391.

69. Hublin C, Kaprio J, Partinen M, et al. Daytime sleepiness in an adult, Finnish population. J Intern Med. 1996;239:417–423.

70. Lankford DA, Wellman JJ, O'Hara C. Posttraumatic narcolepsy in mild to moderate closed head injury. Sleep. 1994;17:S25–S28.

71. Orellana C, Villemin E, Tafti M, et al. Life events in the year preceding the onset of narcolepsy. Sleep. 1994;17:S50–S53.

72. Roth B. Narcolepsy and Hypersomnia. Basel, Germany: Karger; 1980:310.

73. Mueller-Eckardt G, Meier-Ewert K, Schiefer HG. Is there an infectious origin of narcolepsy? Lancet. 1990;335:424.

74. Honda Y, Asake A, Tanaka Y, et al. Discrimination of narcolepsy by using genetic markers and HLA. Sleep Res. 1983;12:254.

75. Juji T, Satake M, Honda Y, et al. HLA antigens in Japanese patients with narcolepsy: all the patients were DR2 positive. Tissue Antigens. 1984;24:316–319.

76. Mueller-Eckardt G, Meier-Ewert K, Schendel D, et al. HLA and narcolepsy in a German population. Tissue Antigens. 1986;28:163–169.

77. Langdon N, Welsh KI, Van Dam M, et al. Genetic markers in narcolepsy. Lancet. 1984;2:1178–1180.

78. Roth B, Nevsimalova S, Sonka K, et al. A study of occurrence of HLA DR2 in 124 narcoleptics: clinical aspects. Arch Suiss Neurol Psychiatr. 1988;139:41–51.

79. Sachs C, Möller E. The occurrence of HLA-DR2 in clinically established narcolepsy. Acta Neurol Scand. 1987;75:437–439.

80. Billiard M, Seignalet J, Besset A, et al. HLA-DR2 and narcolepsy. Sleep. 1986;9:149–152.

81. Mignot E, Hayduk R, Black J, et al. HLA class II studies in 509 narcoleptic patients. Sleep Res. 1997;26:433.

82. Poirier G, Monplaisir J, Décary F, et al. HLA antigens in narcolepsy and idiopathic central nervous hypersomnolence. Sleep. 1986;9:153–158.

83. Mignot E, Tafti M, Dement W, et al. Narcolepsy and immunity. Adv Neuroimmunol. 1994;5:23–37.

84. Carlander B, Eliaou JF, Billiard M. Autoimmune hypothesis in narcolepsy. Neurophysiol Clin. 1993;23:15–22.

85. Bodmer JG, Marsh SGE, Albert ED, et al. Nomenclature for factors of the HLA system, 1998. Tissue Antigens. 1999;53:407–446.

86. Mignot E, Lin X, Arrigoni J, et al. DQB1*0602 and DQA1*0102 (DQ1) are better markers than DR2 for narcolepsy in Caucasian and black Americans. Sleep. 1994;17:S60–S67.

87. Mignot E, Kimura A, Latterman A, et al. Extensive HLA class II studies in 58 non DRB1*15(DR2) narcoleptic patients with cataplexy. Tissue Antigens. 1997;49:329–341.

88. Ellis M, Hetisimer AH, Ruddy DA, et al. HLA class II haplotype and sequence analysis support a role of DQ in narcolepsy. Immunogenetics. 1997;46:410–417.

89. Pelin Z, Guilleminault C, Rish N, et al. HLA-DQB1*0602 homozygosity increases relative risk for narcolepsy but not disease severity in two ethnic groups. Tissue Antigens. 1998;51:96–100.

90. Mignot E, Lin L, Risch N, et al. Identification of a novel HCA narcolepsy susceptibility subtype, HLA-DQB1*0301. Sleep. 1999;22:S121.

91. Mignot E, Young T, Lin L, et al. Reduction of REM sleep latency associated with HLA-DQB1*0602 in normal adults. Lancet. 1998;351:727.

92. Anic-Labat S, Guilleminault C, Kraemer H, et al. Validation of a cataplexy questionnaire in 983 sleep-disorders patients. Sleep. 1999;22:77–87.

93. Richelson E, Pfenning M. Blockade by antidepressants and related compounds of biogenic amine uptake into rat brain synaptosomes: most antidepressants selectively block norepinephrine uptake. Eur J Pharmacol. 1984;104:277–286.

94. Garattini S, Mennini T. Clinical notes on the specificity of drugs in the study of metabolism and functions of brain monoamines. Int Rev Neurobiol. 1988;29:259–280.

94a. Nomikos GG, Damsma G, Wenkstern D, et al. In vivo characterization of locally applied dopamine uptake inhibitors by striatal microdialysis. Synapse. 1990;6:106–112.

95. Parkes D. Amphetamines and alertness. In: Guilleminault C, Dement WC, Passouant P, eds. Narcolepsy. New York, NY: Spectrum Publication; 1976:643–658.

96. Carlsson A. Drugs acting through dopamine release. Pharmacol Ther. 1975;1:401–403.

97. Heinonen EH, Lammintausta R. A review of the pharmacology of selegiline. Acta Neurol Scand. 1991;84(suppl 136):44–59.

98. Bernasconi R, Mathivet P, Bischoff S, Marescaux C. Gamma-hydroxybutyric acid: an endogenous neuromodulation with abuse potential. Trends Pharmacol Sci. 1999;20:135–141.

99. Neely S, Rosenberg R, Spire J, et al. HLA antigens in narcolepsy. Neurology. 1987;37:1858–1860.

100. Lin L, Kuwata S, Tokunaga K, et al. Analysis of HLA class II genes by single-strand conformation polymorphisms in narcolepsy. In: Tsuji K, Aizawa M, Sasasuki T, eds. HLA 1991: Proceedings of the Eleventh International Histocompatibility Workshop and Conference, New York, NY: Oxford University Press; 1992:333–335.

101. Matsuki K, Honda Y, Juji T. HLA antigens in 206 Japanese patients with narcolepsy and 46 patients with essential hypersomnia. In: Tsuji K, Aizawa M, Sasazuki T, eds. HLA 1991. New York, NY: Oxford University Press; 1989:438–440.

102. Honda Y, Matsuki K. Genetic aspects of narcolepsy. In: Thory M, ed. Handbook of Sleep Disorder. New York, NY: Marcel Dekker; 1990:217–234.

103. Kwon OJ, Peled N, Miller K, et al. HLA class II analysis in Jewish Israeli narcoleptic patients. Hum Immunol. 1995;44:199–202.

104. Fogdell A, Hillert J, Sachs C, et al. The multiple sclerosis- and narcolepsy-associated HLA class II haplotype includes the DRB5*0101 allele. Tissue Antigens. 1995;46:333–336.

105. Fernandez-Vina M, Gao X, Moraes M, et al. Alelles at four HLA class II loci determined by oligonucleotide hybridization and their associations in five ethnic groups. Immunogenetics. 1991;34:299–312.

106. Lin L, Jin L, Kimura A, et al. DQ microsatellite association studies in three ethnic groups. Tissue Antigens. 1997;50:507–520.

107. Nishino S, Ripley B, Overeem S, et al: Hypocretin (orexin) deficiency in human narcolepsy. Lancet. 2000;355:39–40.

108. George CF, Singh SM. Hypocretin (orexin) pathway to sleep. Lancet. 2000;355:6.

60

Narcolepsy

Christian Guilleminault
Angela Anagnos

The word *narcolepsy* was first coined by Gélineau[1] in 1880 to designate a pathological condition characterized by irresistible episodes of sleep of short duration recurring at close intervals. He also wrote that attacks were sometimes accompanied by falls, or "astasias," a condition later referred to as *cataplexy*.[2] In the 1930s, Daniels[3] emphasized the association of daytime sleepiness, cataplexy, sleep paralysis, and hypnagogic hallucinations. Calling these symptoms "the clinical tetrad," Yoss and Daly[4] and Vogel[5] reported a nocturnal sleep-onset rapid eye movement (REM) period in narcoleptic patients, a finding confirmed in the following years.[6–9] In 1975, participants in the First International Symposium on Narcolepsy, which was held in France, defined the syndrome as follows:

> The word "narcolepsy" refers to a syndrome of unknown origin that is characterized by abnormal sleep tendencies, including excessive daytime sleepiness and often disturbed nocturnal sleep and pathological manifestations of REM sleep. The REM sleep abnormalities include sleep onset REM periods and the dissociated REM sleep inhibitory processes, cataplexy and sleep paralysis. Excessive daytime sleepiness, cataplexy, and less often sleep paralysis and hypnagogic hallucinations are the major symptoms of the disease.[1]

The definition strongly emphasizes that the syndrome involves a dysfunction of REM sleep. It ignores, however, the notion that genetic factors are frequently involved in the development of narcolepsy. Moreover, although most cases of narcolepsy are idiopathic, secondary causes of narcolepsy have been described.[10]

EPIDEMIOLOGY AND GENETICS

Narcolepsy is not a rare condition. Its prevalence, about 0.05%,[11, 12] varies among countries because of genetic factors. Males are affected somewhat more often than females. The age at onset varies from childhood to the fifth decade, with a peak in the second decade. Special circumstances, such as an abrupt change in sleep-wake schedule or a severe psychological stress (e.g., death of a relative or divorce), precede the occurrence of the first symptom in half of the cases.

The development of human narcolepsy involves environmental factors acting on a specific genetic background.[13, 14, 14a] More than 85% of all narcoleptics with definite cataplexy share a specific human leukocyte antigen (HLA) allele on chromosome 6, HLA *DQB1*0602*, most often in combination with HLA *DR15*.[15] However, this allele is also present in 12 to 38% of the general population.[16] Some patients with narcolepsy do not have the genetic marker,[17] but the best HLA marker for narcolepsy remains *DQB1*0602* across all ethnic groups.[13] A second gene involved in narcolepsy, the *orexin* (or hypocretin) gene, has been located.[17a–c] It is present in dogs and mice. Mutations have also been noted in narcoleptic animals. This gene is involved in the control of the hypocretin receptor. Hypocretin could not be detected in the cerebrospinal fluid of most people with narcolepsy, suggesting the role of abnormal hypocretin transmission.[17d] These discoveries will most probably change our approach to the diagnosis and treatment of disorders of excessive daytime sleepiness, and particularly narcolepsy. Because this gene is directly involved with the function of a specific receptor, one can foresee the development of agonist and antagonist products that will act at the receptor level. Because of the many pharmacological manipulations that it implies, this discovery will have a major impact on our understandng of many brain functions and sleep controls. A more detailed discussion of the genetic advances in narcolepsy is presented elsewhere (see Chapter 59).

CLINICAL FEATURES

The International Classification of Sleep Disorders diagnostic criteria[18] include the classic tetrad for narcolepsy of excessive daytime sleepiness (EDS), cataplexy, sleep paralysis, and hypnagogic hallucinations. Automatic behaviors and disrupted nighttime sleep also are commonly described. However, not all of these symptoms are present in all patients with narcolepsy.

Sleepiness

Unwanted episodes of sleep recur several times a day—not only under favorable circumstances, such as during monotonous sedentary activity or after a heavy meal but also in situations in which the subject is fully involved in a task. The duration of the episode may vary from a few minutes, if the subject is in an uncomfortable position, to longer than 1 h if the subject is reclining. Narcoleptics characteristically wake up feeling refreshed, and there is a refractory period of 1 to several hours before the next episode occurs.

Apart from sleep episodes, patients may feel abnormally drowsy, resulting in poor performance at work, memory lapses, and even gestural, ambulatory, or speech automatisms.

Cataplexy

Cataplexy is an abrupt and reversible decrease in or loss of muscle tone, most frequently elicited by emotion such as laughter, anger, or surprise, and it may occur in more than two thirds of patients with narcolepsy. It may involve certain muscles or the entire voluntary musculature. Most typically, the jaw sags, the head falls forward, the arms drop to the side, and the knees unlock or buckle.

The severity and extent of cataplectic attacks can vary from a state of absolute powerlessness, which seems to involve the entire voluntary musculature, to a limited involvement of certain muscle groups or to no more than a fleeting sensation of weakness extending more or less throughout the body. Although the extraocular muscles supposedly are not involved, weakness can occur, and the patient may complain of blurred vision. Complete paralysis of extraocular muscles has never been reported, although the palpebral muscle may be affected. Speech may be impaired and respiration may become irregular during an attack. Long breathing pauses have never been recorded, but short pauses similar to those seen during nocturnal REM sleep in normal subjects may occur. In a cataplectic attack, there is a complete loss of muscle tone that can lead to total body collapse and the risk of serious injuries such as skull or other bone fractures. These attacks are not usually dramatic, however, and may go unnoticed by nearby individuals. An attack may consist of only a slight buckling of the knees. Patients may perceive this abrupt and short-lasting weakness and simply stop or stand against a wall. Speech may be broken due to intermittent weakness affecting the arytenoid muscles. As seen during nocturnal REM sleep, the abrupt muscle inhibition is interrupted by sudden bursts of returning muscle tone, which at times even seems enhanced. If the weakness involves only the jaw or speech, the subject may present with wide masticatory movement or an unusual attack of stuttering speech. If it involves the upper limbs, the patient will complain of "clumsiness," reporting activity such as dropping cups or plates or spilling liquids when surprised, laughing, and so on.

The short cataplectic attacks are the most common presentation of cataplexy. Because they do not resemble the "classic" full-blown attack of cataplexy, they are often missed by even skilled physicians without the aid of an electromyographic recording. The duration of each cataplectic attack—whether partial or total—is highly variable, lasting from a few seconds to 30 min.

Attacks can be elicited by emotion, stress, fatigue, or heavy meals. Laughter and anger seem to be the most common triggers, but the attacks can also be induced by a feeling of elation while listening to music, reading a book, or watching a movie. Cataplexy may be induced merely by remembering a happy or funny situation, and it may also occur without clear precipitating acts or emotions.

The physiology of cataplexy has been partially investigated. Cataplexy is associated with an inhibition of the monosynaptic H-reflex and of the multisynaptic tendon reflexes. H-reflex activity is fully suppressed physiologically only during REM sleep, which emphasizes the relationship between the motor inhibitory component of REM sleep and the sudden atonia and areflexia seen during a cataplectic attack. Muscarinic cholinergic regions of the pontine reticular formation and basal forebrain are sites involved in cataplexy via a multisynaptic descending pathway. An increase in postsynaptic D_2 receptors was observed in the amygdala of narcoleptic dogs with impairment of dopamine release, suggesting that an abnormal cholinergic–dominergic interaction could underlie the pathophysiology of narcolepsy.[19]

Sleep Paralysis

This is a terrifying experience that occurs in the narcoleptic on falling asleep or on awakening. Patients find themselves suddenly unable to move the limbs, to speak, or even to breathe deeply. This state is frequently accompanied by hallucinations.

During an episode of sleep paralysis, the patient is unable to move the extremities, to speak, or to open the eyes, although he or she is fully aware of the condition and able to recall it completely later. In many episodes of sleep paralysis, but especially the first occurrence, the patient may be prey to extreme anxiety associated with the fear of dying. This anxiety is often greatly intensified by the terrifying hallucinations that may accompany the sleep paralysis. With more experience with the phenomenon, however, the patient usually learns that episodes are brief and benign, rarely lasting longer than 10 min and always ending spontaneously.

Hallucinations

Sleep onset, either during daytime sleep episodes or at night, may be unpleasant, with vivid auditory or hypnagogic hallucinations. The narcoleptic's hypnagogic hallucinations that accompany sleep paralysis often involve vision. The visual hallucinations usually consist of simple forms (colored circles, parts of objects, and so on) that are constant or changing in size. The image of an animal or a person may present itself abruptly, more often in color. Auditory hallucinations are also common, although other senses are seldom involved. The auditory hallucinations can range from a collection of sounds to an elaborate melody. The patient may also be menaced by threatening sentences or harsh invectives.

Another common and interesting type of hallucination reported at sleep onset involves elementary cenesthopathic feelings (i.e., experiencing picking, rubbing, or light touching), changes in location of body parts (e.g., arm or leg), or feelings of levitation or extracorporeal experiences (e.g., moving the body in space or floating above the bed) that may be quite elaborate. (For example, the patient may report, "I am above my bed and I can also see my body below"; "I am a few feet up and people jump over my body.") The association of sleep paralysis has led researchers to postulate gamma loop involvement in some of these hallucinations. The abrupt motor inhibition that involves the spinal cord motoneurons may lead to a significant decrease in the feedback of information normally used by the central nervous system (CNS) to gauge the position of the body and the relation of the limb segments to each other.

Sleep Disruption

Night sleep is often interrupted by repeated awakenings and sometimes accompanied by terrifying dreams. Ironically, patients may complain of trouble falling asleep and staying asleep at night, although they may fall asleep repeatedly during the daytime.

ONSET OF CLINICAL SYMPTOMS

The first symptoms often develop near the age of puberty; the peak age at which reported symptoms occur is 15 to 25 years, but narcolepsy and other symptoms have been noted as early as 2 years.[20] A second, smaller peak of onset has been noted between 35 and 45 years and near menopause in women.

EDS and irresistible sleep episodes usually occur as the first symptoms, either independently or associated with one or more other symptoms. They are enhanced by high environmental temperature, indoor activity, and idleness. Symptoms may abate with time but never phase out completely. Attacks of cataplexy generally appear in conjunction with abnormal episodes of sleep but may occur as many as 20 years later. They occasionally, but seldom, occur before the abnormal sleep episodes, in which case they are a major source of difficulty in diagnosis. They can vary in frequency from a few episodes during the subject's entire lifetime to one or several episodes per day.

Hypnagogic hallucinations and sleep paralysis do not affect all subjects, are often transitory, and occur commonly in the general population.[21] Disturbed nocturnal sleep seldom occurs in the first stages and generally builds up with age.[22] Narcolepsy leads to a variety of complications, such as driving- or machine-operation–related accidents; difficulties at work leading to disability, forced retirement, or job dismissal; impotence; and depression.[23]

DIAGNOSTIC PROCEDURES: EVALUATION OF SLEEPINESS

The Stanford Sleepiness Scale,[24] a seven-point scale, was developed to quantify the subjective sleepiness of patients, but its reliability in chronically sleepy patients is questionable. The Epworth Sleepiness Scale is also used as an index of sleepiness (see Chapter 104).

Several tests have been designed to objectively evaluate sleepiness. Yoss et al.[25] described the electronic pupillogram as a method of measuring decreased levels of sleepiness. Schmidt and Fortin[23] reviewed the advantages and limitations of the electronic pupillogram in arousal disorders. The size of the pupil is an index of autonomic activity. Berlucchi et al.[26] clearly demonstrated the constriction of the pupil during sleep. A normal, alert individual sitting quietly in total darkness can maintain a stable pupil diameter, usually well above 7 mm, for at least 10 min, without subjective difficulty or pupillary oscillation.[23] The pupillary diameter in excessively sleepy patients is unstable when they are adapting to the dark. There are problems and limitations with this technique. Patients with ocular problems and lesions or autonomic CNS lesions must be identified and excluded. A patient's ability and willingness to cooperate are critical. Excessively sleepy subjects have trouble avoiding lid drooping or closure. Small initial pupil diameters, dark irises, and excessive eye makeup all pose problems. Finally, the data may be difficult to interpret, particularly if recording conditions are not optimal. Although at one time experts did attempt to use pupillography to diagnose narcolepsy, it essentially diagnoses only sleepiness. This test does not distinguish the underlying cause of EDS.

The multiple sleep latency test (MSLT) (see Chapter 104) was designed to measure physiological sleep tendencies in the absence of alerting factors.[27] It consists of five scheduled naps, usually at 10 AM, noon, and 2, 4, and 6 PM, during which the subject is polygraphically monitored in a comfortable, soundproof, dark bedroom, while wearing street clothes. The latency between lights-out time and sleep onset is calculated for each nap. The type of sleep, REM or nonrapid eye movement (NREM) also is noted.[28] After each 20-min monitoring period, patients stay awake until the next scheduled nap. The MSLT records the latency for each nap, the mean sleep latency, and the presence or absence of REM sleep during any of the naps. On the basis of polygraphic recording, REM sleep that occurs within 15 min of sleep onset is considered a sleep-onset REM period.[29]

In normal populations, MSLT scores vary with age, and puberty is a critical landmark. Prepubertal children between the ages of 6 and 11 years appear to be hyper-alert. In postpubertal subjects, mean MSLT scores under 8 min are generally considered to be in the pathological range; those over 10 min are considered to be normal. When the range is between 8 and 10 min, age factors interact, so the test must be interpreted with greater care; mean scores of 8 to 10 min represent a gray area.[30]

An MSLT performed alone has the same drawbacks

as does pupillography—it measures sleepiness regardless of its cause, which may simply be sleep deprivation. The MSLT also ignores repetitive microsleeps that can lead, in borderline cases, to daytime impairment not scored by conventional analysis. To be clinically relevant, the test must be conducted under specific conditions. Subjects must have abstained from medication for a sufficient period (usually 15 days) so that drug interaction is avoided. On the basis of sleep diaries, their sleep-wake schedules are stabilized. On the night preceding the MSLT, the subjects undergo a standard nocturnal polysomnogram. Throughout the total nocturnal sleep period, any sleep-related biological abnormalities responsible for sleep fragmentation and sleep deprivation are recorded.

The nocturnal polysomnogram may indicate the underlying cause of sleepiness; the MSLT indicates the severity of the problem. Once the nocturnal sleep recording has eliminated specific diseases, the MSLT confirms the diagnosis of narcolepsy with the presence of two or more sleep-onset REM periods.

Browman et al.[31] proposed adding to the MSLT a test for the maintenance of wakefulness. This tests the patient's ability to remain awake in a comfortable sitting position in a dark room for five 20-min trials given at 10 AM, noon, and 2, 4, and 6 PM. The test may be helpful in specific pharmacological trials but has proved to be unsatisfactory as a diagnostic procedure.[31] Data from a U.S. multicenter study of more than 500 narcoleptics involved in the investigation of modafinil will be available to help resolve a question concerning the duration of each test; preliminary information suggests that prolonging each test to 30 min probably is better to dissociate pathology from normalcy.

Another procedure that has been used to document sleepiness is a continuous 24- or 36-h polysomnogram that provides information about the number, duration, times, and types of daytime sleep episodes, as well as the disrupted nighttime sleep. In addition, this long polysomnographic recording may identify the dissociated REM sleep inhibitory process characterizing cataplexy with an awake electroencephalogram and electro-oculogram associated with the elimination of chin and muscle twitches typical of REM sleep.

Broughton et al.[32] proposed using auditory-evoked potentials in the evaluation of sleepiness, but this test, which may be helpful in evaluating pharmacological agents, has not been sufficiently discriminative to be used as a diagnostic tool.

POSITIVE DIAGNOSIS OF NARCOLEPSY

There is controversy concerning the criteria needed to confirm narcolepsy in patients with EDS. Clinicians and researchers in Japan have indicated that their U.S. counterparts have given too much credence to polysomnographic criteria and the presence of two or more sleep-onset REM periods at MSLT.[33] In Japan, a positive history of cataplexy associated with EDS is systematically required for the diagnosis of narcolepsy.[33] Undoubtedly, the presence of cataplexy is pathognomonic

of narcolepsy, but it may be difficult to rely on this criterion alone, particularly when cataplexy is partial (i.e., limited to the head and neck or neck and upper arms). Anic-Labat et al.[34] developed a self-administered questionnaire that validated cataplexy in 1000 subjects. Moscovitch et al.,[35] however, caution against the diagnosis of narcolepsy if EDS and two or more sleep-onset REM periods at MSLT are the only positive findings. These authors found that only 84% of the individuals with complaints of EDS and documentation of cataplexy presented with two or more sleep-onset REM periods at MSLT, a replication of findings by Van den Hoed et al.[30] 10 years earlier. They found that all subjects with EDS and cataplexy presented with two or more sleep-onset REM periods at one MSLT if the MSLT was repeated daily for 4 days. Moscovitch et al.[35] recommend that the term *narcolepsy* be used only when EDS and at least a positive history of cataplexy are associated with two or more sleep-onset REM periods. If there is no history of cataplexy, a more descriptive term such as *excessive daytime sleepiness with several sleep-onset REM periods* should be used, even if other symptoms, such as sleep paralysis or hypnagogic hallucinations, exist.

Genetic testing has been used to aid in the clinical diagnosis of narcolepsy. Mignot et al.[36] showed that 40% of subjects with two or more sleep-onset REM periods were positive for *DQB1*0602*. However, narcolepsy was clinically suspected in 60% of these cases; thus, genetic testing alone is not sufficient for the diagnosis of narcolepsy. The requirement of a positive history of cataplexy would eliminate subjects in the developing phase of the syndrome, which can take several years. The use of strict criteria will allow better epidemiological studies. Subjects would be classified as narcoleptic only after the presence of EDS and cataplexy had been reported and abnormal daytime alertness had been confirmed by polysomnographic recording with MSLT. The discovery of the involvement of a second gene in the development of narcolepsy may lead to new diagnostic tests. Hypocretins may one day be measured in the blood of animals and humans. Narcoleptic dogs and mice have mutations that exert an impact directly on the *orexin* (or hypocretin) receptor. This discovery is too recent to have led to new diagnostic approaches. But the facts that a specific known receptor is involved, that some of the brain pathways associated with the receptor have been already studied in mammals, and that pharmacological work has already been performed on the hypocretins suggest strongly as mentioned that new diagnostic avenues will be sought.[17a–d]

PATHOPHYSIOLOGY

Pharmacological Studies

Because few pharmacological data are available for human beings, we review pharmacological studies in canine narcolepsy with cataplexy. This subject is discussed in detail in Chapter 59. In summary, the many pharmacological investigations performed on the dog suggest that an alpha$_{1b}$ receptor is strongly involved in the control of cataplexy.[37] Alpha$_{1b}$ antagonists drastically worsen cataplexy. Stimulation of alpha$_{1b}$ receptors decreases it, as do noradrenergic reuptake blockers and noradrenergic releasing agents. Other receptors, particularly alpha$_2$ receptors, are also involved in cataplexy, as shown by the effect of several alpha$_2$ antagonists, particularly yohimbine, which completely suppresses cataplexy.[38, 39] Central dopamine D$_2$ agonists significantly suppress cataplexy,[40] whereas most D$_2$ agonists aggravate it; this suggests an involvement of "presynaptic dopamine receptors" in the regulation of canine cataplexy. However, experimental data suggest that the effect of D$_2$ compounds on cataplexy is probably mediated by the noradrenergic system.[41, 42]

These investigations indicate that a complex loop involving noradrenergic and cholinergic synapses controls the appearance of canine cataplexy. This loop is similar to that suggested by the pharmacological investigations of REM sleep. The pharmacological investigations of the narcoleptic dog are even more valuable because they provide information useful to the understanding of REM sleep.[43]

Cerebrospinal Fluid Analysis

Studies in human narcoleptics have shown a decrease in dopamine concentration in the cerebrospinal fluid.[44] Studies on narcoleptic dogs performed before and after probenecid administration demonstrated an elevated dopamine turnover with significantly less free homovanillic acid, dihydroxyphenylacetic acid, 3-methoxy-4-hydroxyphenylglycol, and 5-hydroxyindoleacetic acid.[45]

The lower concentration of 5-hydroxyindoleacetic acid in the cerebrospinal fluid of narcoleptic dogs suggests a decreased concentration of the parent amine 5-hydroxytryptamine, a decreased turnover of serotonin in the brain, or both. Similarly, the lower steady-state cerebrospinal fluid concentration of dihydroxyphenylacetic acid and homovanillic acid, as well as the reduced accumulation of dihydroxyphenylacetic acid and homovanillic acid after probenecid, suggests decreased dopamine concentration, decreased turnover, or both. Finally, the lower concentration of 3-methoxy-4-hydroxyphenylglycol after probenecid administration suggests decreased norepinephrine activity.

In most narcolepsy patients, there is an absence of hypocretin in the cerebrospinal fluid.[17d]

Brain Tissue Analysis

Analyses of both human and animal narcoleptic brain tissue suggest dopaminergic dysfunction. In postmortem human autoradiographic studies, striatal dopamine D$_2$ receptor binding was increased in narcolepsy, more so than D$_1$ receptors.[46, 47] However, most in vivo studies with single-photon emission computed tomography[48] and positron emission tomography[49] found no increase in striatal D$_2$ receptor binding in narcolepsy.

Table 60–1. EXAMPLES OF INITIAL TREATMENT PACKAGES (CHILDREN)

Prepubertal Children	Pubertal Children
General Measures	*General Measures*
Contact school to alert teachers	Contact school to alert teachers
Nap at lunch time	Emphasize need for regular
Nap at 4 or 5 PM	nocturnal sleep schedule
	Try to obtain 9 h of nocturnal sleep
	Nap at lunch time and 4 or 5 PM
Medication for Sleepiness	*Medication for Sleepiness*
Methylphenidate 5 mg (2–4 tablets)	Methylphenidate 5 mg (2–6 tablets*) or 20 mg SR in the morning (on empty stomach)
Modafinil 100–200 mg†	Modafinil† 100–400 mg
Medication for Cataplexy‡	*Medication for Cataplexy‡*
Clomipramine 25–50 mg at bedtime	Clomipramine 50 mg at bedtime
Fluoxetine 10–20 mg in the morning	Fluoxetine 10–40 mg in the morning
Venlafaxine (in the morning) 75–150 mg	Venlafaxine (in the morning) 75–150 mg

*Usually 10 mg when waking up on an empty stomach, 5 mg about lunch time, and 5 mg at 3 PM.
†Modafinil is started at 100 mg in the morning for 5 days, and a second dose of 100 mg is then added at lunchtime, if needed. This is usually sufficient in prepubertal children. Pubertal children may require a further increase (after 5 days) to an additional 100 mg in the morning, and if still needed later, another 100 mg at noon.
‡The use of antidepressants for cataplexy is not FDA approved. No medications have specifically received approval by the FDA for use in narcolepsy patients younger than 16 years of age.
SR, sustained-release tablet.

Noradrenergic function has also been found to be abnormal. Two different receptor responses can normally be noted, and two different central alpha$_1$ receptors, so-called high affinity and low affinity, have been identified.[50] The low-affinity central alpha$_1$ noradrenergic receptors are those involved in canine cataplexy.[37, 43]

TREATMENT

In narcolepsy, the goal of all therapeutic approaches is to control the narcoleptic symptoms and to allow the patient to have a full family and professional life. Drug prescriptions must take into account possible side effects, because narcolepsy is a lifelong illness and patients will have to receive medication for years. Tolerance or addiction may occur with some compounds. In addition, hypertension, abnormal liver function, and psychosis are the most commonly reported complications associated with the long-term use of stimulant medications. The treatment of narcolepsy must balance the maintenance of an active life with the avoidance of side effects and tolerance to medications.[51]

Behavioral Approaches

Part of the difficulty in treating patients with narcolepsy involves the patient's frustration over the delay in diagnosis. In 500 narcoleptics surveyed in the United States in the 1980s, the mean time to diagnosis from symptom onset was 15 years. The consequence of this, particularly in a young patient, is the development of reactive depressive symptoms. One of the most important initial treatments is a referral to patient support groups organized by sleep disorders centers, such as the National Sleep Foundation or the Narcolepsy Network. Other support groups exist in most Western European countries and in North America. The American Sleep Disorders Association is an integral resource.

Career counseling is also important because patients and their employers must be educated regarding jobs that patients with narcolepsy should avoid, including shiftwork, on-call schedules, driving and the transportation industry, or any job necessitating continuous attention for long hours without breaks, particularly under monotonous conditions. Some of these difficulties can be overcome if the employer recognizes the importance of short 15- to 20-min naps every 4 h during the daytime.

In addition to scheduled naps, other behavioral approaches include a regular sleep-wake schedule, the avoidance of frequent time zone changes, and overall good sleep hygiene (Tables 60–1 and 60–2).

Pharmacological Treatments

Cataplexy and REM-Related Symptoms

Investigations have shown that muscle atonia is normally associated with REM sleep; REM-associated muscle atonia occurs at inappropriate times during wakefulness in narcoleptic patients and is responsible for cataplexy. Several neurotransmitter systems have been identified as affecting the inhibitory pathways involving the lower motoneurons, particularly muscarinic cholinergic and noradrenergic systems at the alpha$_{1b}$ and D$_2$ receptor levels. The best medications thus are those that target these receptors with the least number of side effects.[52] Tricyclic antidepressants were the first drugs of choice, particularly protriptyline, but the anticholinergic effect led to impotence in more than 40% of male narcoleptics. Most tricyclic antidepressants with significant atropinic side effects are used as a last resource. Similarly, the monoamine oxidase inhibitors are rarely used except for the hybrid selegiline (see below).[53]

Most medications used for cataplexy have a noradrenergic reuptake blocker action. Viloxazine is available in Europe and is very effective in the treatment of cataplexy. The starting dose is 50 to 100 mg in two divided doses with a maximum dose of 200 mg/day.[54]

The most commonly used medications are the serotonin-reuptake blockers that have an active noradrenergic reuptake blocker metabolite; this includes clomipramine and its active metabolite desmethylclomipramine, fluoxetine and its active metabolite norfluoxetine, and zimelidine and its active metabolite norzimelidine.[55, 56] In our experience, we recommend starting with 50 mg clomipramine at bedtime and increasing to a maximum of 200 mg in two divided doses

---

Table 60–2. EXAMPLES OF INITIAL TREATMENT PACKAGES (ADULTS)

General Measures

Avoid shifts in sleep schedule
Avoid heavy meals and alcohol intake
Regular timing of nocturnal sleep: 10:30 PM to 7 AM
Naps: Strategically timed naps, if possible (e.g., 15 min at lunch time, 15 min at 5:30 PM)

Medication for Sleepiness

The effects of stimulant medications vary widely among patients. The dosing and timing of medications should be individualized to optimize performance. Additional doses, as needed, may be suggested for periods of anticipated sleepiness.
Modafinil 100–200 mg (taken when waking up in the morning) or
Methylphenidate 5 mg (3 or 4 tablets) [10 mg when waking up; 5 mg, 30 minutes before lunch; 5 mg near 3 PM; better action is always obtained if the drug is taken on an empty stomach] or 20 mg SR morning (on empty stomach)

If Persistent Difficulties

Methylphenidate (SR): 20 mg in the morning
    5 mg after noon nap
    5 mg at 4 PM or
Modafinil 200 mg in the morning and 100 mg at lunchtime with possible further increase to 200 mg at lunchtime (total daily dosage, 400 mg) or

If No Response

Dextroamphetamine sulfate
(Dexedrine Spansule) (SR): 15 mg on awakening
    5 mg after noon nap
    5 mg at 3:30 or 4 PM
(or 15 mg at awakening and 15 mg after noon nap)

Medication for Cataplexy*

Clomipramine 75–125 mg, or
Viloxazine 150–200 mg, or
Imipramine 75–125 mg, or
Fluoxetine 20–60 mg
Venlafaxine 150–300 mg

---

*Medications may be taken in the evening near bedtime (clomipramine, imipramine); only in the morning (fluoxetine), or in the morning and at lunchtime (viloxazine, venlafaxine). The use of antidepressants for cataplexy is not FDA approved. The only medication specifically approved for use in narcolepsy by the FDA is modafinil.
SR, sustained-release tablet.

---

or with 20 mg fluoxetine in the morning and increasing to 60 to 80 mg/day in two divided doses. The most common dosages are 40 to 60 mg/day of fluoxetine or 100 mg daily of clomipramine.

Common side effects have been well described in previous reports, but there are some side effects that are rarely mentioned that may be more important in narcoleptics.

Appearance of Periodic Limb Movement Syndrome During Sleep. This syndrome is related to the increase in muscle tone induced by these compounds during sleep and may lead to a significant fragmentation of sleep. Levodopa may be useful.[57, 58]

Development of REM Behavior Disorder, Particularly in Older Subjects. Classically, tricyclic antidepressants and serotonin-reuptake blockers "decrease" REM sleep. These drugs eliminate or decrease the muscle atonia of REM sleep and dissociate REM sleep (i.e., electroencephalographic patterns of REM sleep without muscle atonia). Although the absence of muscle atonia limits the ability to score this stage as REM sleep using the international rules,[28] the electroencephalographic pattern and dream state of REM persist. Thus, the individual can "act out" his or her dreams. Although REM behavior disorder is a separate sleep disorder, it may occur in narcoleptics who already have dysfunction of muscle tone control with cataplexy, and this tendency may be enhanced with anticataplectic drugs.

Rebound of Cataplexy and Other REM-Related Symptoms. Abrupt withdrawal of these drugs will induce a significant rebound of cataplexy, sleep paralysis, and hypnagogic hallucinations. Patients should be withdrawn from medications slowly; the recommended withdrawal schedule is one dose every 4 days. Even with such a schedule, cataplexy rebound will be seen. The problem is related to the disappearance of warning signs and the possibility of abrupt, complete falls that may result in bodily injury. Withdrawal experiments performed at Stanford University with the use of clomipramine showed that rebound was noticeable after 72 h and peaked at day 10 after withdrawal, and the normal cataplexy frequency was seen after 15 days. Patients must be warned about this side effect and forbidden from driving during the withdrawal period. When switching medications, our experience has been to add the second drug 16 to 24 h after interruption of the previous medication.[59]

Excessive Daytime Sleepiness

The drugs most widely used to treat EDS (Table 60–3) are the CNS stimulants. Amphetamines were first proposed as a treatment of EDS in narcolepsy by Prinzmetal and Bloomberg in 1935, and the first addiction to amphetamine was reported in 1939.[60] Amphetamines (dextroamphetamines, biamphetamine, metamphetamine), methylphenidate, mazindol, and pemoline are the most commonly used medications for the treatment of EDS.

Methylphenidate and pemoline have been first-line drugs in the treatment of children for many years.[61, 62] The relatively recent reports on the increased risk of liver damage with pemoline, an oxazolidine derivative, have made it a less popular choice in the treatment of children. Pemoline is no longer available in some countries. One of the major problems of these drugs is that in most cases, children are unable to maintain daytime alertness without the appearance of side effects. The clinical effectiveness of these drugs is objectively measured using the MSLT and, more appropriately, maintenance of wakefulness.

Modafinil (200 to 400 mg/day) has been introduced for the treatment of EDS in narcolepsy. The exact mechanism of action of modafinil is unknown, but it requires an intact central alpha$_1$ adrenergic system. Modafinil has little or no effect on dopaminergic activity and has highly selective activity in the CNS relative to amphetamine and methylphenidate.[52, 63] Amphetamines and methylphenidate are classified as stimulant drugs. The activity of modafinil and its mode of action resulted in its being classified as a somnolytic agent.

Drugs that stimulate norepinephrine release and have dopaminergic activity, such as amphetamines and methylphenidate, have had the greatest impact on

Table 60–3. NARCOLEPSY DRUGS CURRENTLY AVAILABLE

	Usual Dosage* (All Drugs Administered Orally)
Treatment of EDS	
Stimulants†	
Dextroamphetamine	5–60 mg/day
Methamphetamine	20–25 mg/day
Methylphenidate	10–60 mg/day
Mazindol	4–8 mg/day (divided dosage)
Modafinil	100–400 mg/day
Adjunct-Effect Drugs (i.e., improve EDS if associated with stimulant)‡	
Protriptyline	2.5–10 mg/day
Viloxazine†	50–200 mg/day
Treatment of Auxiliary Effects	
Antidepressants‡	
With atropinic side effects	
Protriptyline	2.5–20 mg/day
Imipramine	25–200 mg/day
Clomipramine	25–200 mg/day
Desipramine	25–200 mg/day
Without atropinic side effects	
Viloxazine†	50–200 mg/day
Fluoxetine	20–60 mg/day
Experimental Drugs or Drugs Available in Few Countries	
Stimulants	
Codeine (given as stimulant)	
Cataplexy Antagonist and Mild Stimulant	
Gamma hydroxybutyrate	

*Occasionally, depending on clinical response, the dose may be outside the usual dosage range.
†Most stimulants should be administered in divided doses, commonly in the morning and at lunchtime. This is recommended for amphetamines and modafinil. Methylphenidate has a fast elimination rate; the slow-release (SR) formula may be helpful in the morning (e.g., 20 mg SR). If administered by 5-mg increments, the usual timing of methylphenidate administration is every 3 to 4 hours until 1500 hours. Pemoline has been deleted from the list of recommended drugs because of a side effect that may develop years after drug intake.
‡The use of antidepressants for cataplexy is not FDA approved. The only medication specifically approved for use in narcolepsy by the FDA is modafinil.
EDS, excessive daytime somnolence.

sleepiness. The best objective study was reported by Mitler et al.[56, 64] using metamphetamine and evaluating its effect on the MSLT (Fig. 60–1). Compared with dextroamphetamine, metamphetamine accumulates in the CNS and has fewer peripheral side effects. However, our clinical experience does not support this. Our first investigations on narcolepsy and amphetamine treatment occurred in the 1970s.[51] These studies involved narcoleptics who had received amphetamines for at least 5 years, usually longer than 10 years, and who were receiving more than 80 mg/day with a maximum dosage of 300 mg/day. All subjects had periods of EDS on a daily basis, and two thirds of the group had hyperexcitation, nervousness, anxiety, and hypertension. Progressive withdrawal of amphetamines in that population led to lowering of blood pressure in all patients but clear worsening of EDS. After a "drug holiday" of 3 to 4 weeks, patients were prescribed

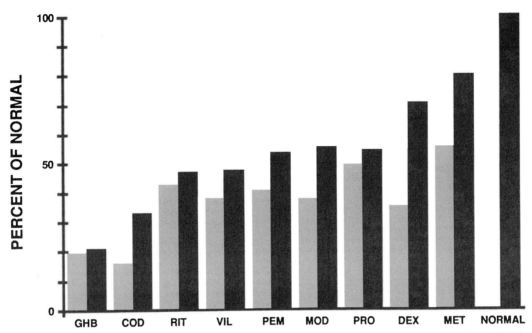

Figure 60–1. Relative efficacy of drugs for treating narcolepsy presented in terms of percentage of normal levels of sleepiness. The lightest shading denotes baseline values. The intermediate shading denotes treatment values. The darkest shading is used only for the normal values. A comparison between drugs in a blind protocol has not been performed. COD, codeine; DEX, dextroamphetamine; GHB, gamma hydroxybutyrate; MET, methylphenidate; MOD, modafinil; PEM, pemoline; PRO, protriptyline; RIT, ritanserin; VIL, viloxazine. (From Mitler MM, Hajdukovic R. Relative efficacy of drugs for the treatment of sleepiness in narcolepsy. Sleep. 1991;14:218–220.)

stimulant medications at a much lower dose. Subjects had a similar improvement in subjective levels of alertness with fewer side effects.

Based on our clinical experience of more than 1000 narcoleptic patients, we use and recommend methylphenidate for the treatment of EDS in children with narcolepsy. Methylphenidate has a short half-life and is available in a slow-release form.[52, 62] In children, there is a problem with noncompliance with medication while at school. The recommended dose is based on weight, and we try to maintain a maximum of 30 mg/ day. The drug is given in the morning (15 mg) and at lunch time (15 mg maximum).

In adults, methylphenidate and amphetamines at dosages of more than 60 mg/day do not significantly improve EDS without the appearance of long-term side effects, including frequent worsening of the nocturnal sleep disruption. The drug is usually administered in three divided doses with a maximum of 20 mg in the morning, 20 mg at lunchtime, and 20 mg at 3 PM—never later. Therefore, short naps are necessary. The combination of pharmacological agents and two short naps provides the best daily response to EDS, with no stimulant drug taken after 3 PM. The slow-release form may provide gradual and delayed response during the daytime. The association between anticataplectic drugs and amphetamine-like medication may enhance the anticataplectic effect of the stimulant medication.[65]

Both the stimulant medications and the anticataplectic drugs are hepatically metabolized, so any liver dysfunction will affect both classes of drug. This promotes the recommendation for regular liver function tests. Mazindol, an imidazolamine, has been helpful in the treatment of EDS in narcolepsy but has not been as

clinically effective as the amphetamines.[66] It has been tried at a dosage of 3 to 8 mg/day, with a mean dose of 5 mg mostly taken in the morning. In declining order, our patients subjectively rate the effectiveness of medications in the treatment of EDS as methylphenidate, pemoline, and then mazindol. None of the currently available stimulants, including the most recent, modafinil, have been tested in parallel with a placebo control in the narcoleptic population.

The two newest compounds are modafinil and γ-hydroxybutyrate (GHB). Modafinil (2-[diphenyl-methyl sulfinyl]acetamide) is a novel stimulant; its mechanism of action is different from amphetamines.[66, 67] Several multicenter studies have been performed in different European and North American countries to evaluate the new compound, with similar results. Most studies used polysomnographic monitoring to evaluate the patients' response to drug. Nocturnal polysomnography was followed by MSLT, maintenance of wakefulness, or both. Subjective sleepiness scales were also used, including the Clinical Global Impression and the Epworth Sleepiness Scale. The results indicate that modafinil had a significant impact on the objective measures of sleepiness; however, the improvement noted on MSLT was never normalized. This suggests that narcolepsy is a complex disorder in which the mechanisms underlying daytime sleepiness are not yet well understood. Cataplexy and the other REM sleep symptoms are not affected by modafinil. The most important benefit of modafinil concerns the few side effects. There are no blood pressure side effects; it is not addictive and therefore has a low potential for abuse. Headache is the most common complaint, and this can be reduced by a slow and progressive increase in dosage.[66] Several studies suggest an initial dose of 400 mg, and headaches were more common than with a progressive 100-mg dose increase every 4 days. Most European studies suggest twice-daily administration, in the morning and at lunchtime. Based on multiple studies (MSLT/maintenance of wakefulness), this mode of drug intake seems to provide better alertness at the end of the day, but compliance with the noon dose was poorer, particularly in the young patients. The most commonly used daily dose in open-label studies has been 300 mg (therapeutic range, 100 to 400 mg/day). Modafinil is administered with anticataplectic medications without problems.

Switching subjects from a stimulant medication to modafinil may lead to the reappearance of narcoleptic symptoms. Patients who have taken a daily dose of amphetamines of 45 mg or more complain of less control over "sleepiness" than with their prior medications. In our clinical population, after 1 month of daily modafinil intake, 20% of the patients previously treated with amphetamines asked to be switched back to their previous drug. This subjective rating of less control over sleepiness with modafinil occurs despite intake at the upper limits of the recommended dose (commonly 400 to 600 mg daily).

Another problem in the switch from amphetamines to modafinil is the appearance of cataplectic attacks and, more rarely, of sleep paralysis in patients previously well controlled with a combination of stimulants and anticataplectic agents, or by amphetamines alone. Amphetamines have a direct impact on the norepinephrine synapse and help to control cataplexy and sleep paralysis. Modafinil causes none of these activities. With the switch to modafinil, patients who had mild REM-related symptoms controlled by the amphetamine intake may thus experience an abrupt recurrence of these symptoms at the time of the switch of medication, and may need an adjunct compound. In patients already taking an anticataplectic drug simultaneously, an increase in the daily intake of this medication may be needed. The combination of modafinil and venlafaxin (100 mg daily) has provided good results in these specific cases. Modafinil produces the best results in stimulant-naïve individuals.

The other new compound is GHB.[68, 69] It is a naturally occurring metabolite of the human nervous system that is found in the highest concentrations in the hypothalamus and basal ganglia. It was shown to induce a normal sequence of non-REM and REM sleep in normal volunteers lasting 2 to 3 h at a dose of 30 mg/kg. The first trials on narcoleptics were performed in the late 1970s.[70, 71] GHB has also been part of a multicenter study in the United States; the study is still under way. The drug is normally taken at bedtime. The dose has varied from 3 to 9 g, with an increase in total nocturnal sleep time and decrease in sleep paralysis, hypnagogic hallucinations, and nightmares. All patients subjectively reported waking up more rested in the morning. Overall, a positive effect on cataplexy is reported. The response is gradual and overall, with a significant decrease in the frequency of cataplectic attacks noted. The impact on daytime sleepiness is not as well documented, and the results of the last large

U.S. multicenter study using objective polysomnographic monitoring are not related to the significant hypnotic effects of the drug. If patients wake up in the middle of the night, they may be confused and disoriented, and they may have episodes of enuresis. A transient worsening of cataplexy during the nocturnal period may occur. Nausea may be reported with a high dosage, as well as sluggishness in the early morning. Overall, patients prefer this drug to the anticataplectic drugs because there are fewer side effects.

SUMMARY

Improvements in the treatment of narcolepsy with the newest compounds provide fewer side effects than occur with the classic stimulants and tricyclic medications. Narcolepsy is a complex syndrome that involves the timing of sleep and wake. Medications with an alerting effect will help but will never completely control the multifaceted problems associated with the syndrome.

Bibliography

Billiard M, ed. Narcolepsy. Sleep. 1994;17(suppl):S1–S115.
Fry JM, ed. Current issues in the diagnosis and management of narcolepsy. Neurology. 1998;50(suppl 1):S1–S48.
Guilleminault C, ed. Narcolepsy. Sleep. 1986;9:99–291.
Guilleminault C, Dement WC, Passouant P, eds. Narcolepsy. New York, NY: Spectrum Publications; 1975.
Honda Y, Juji T, eds. HLA in Narcolepsy. Berlin, Germany: Springer-Verlag; 1988.

References

1. Gélineau J. De la narcolepsie. Gaz Hop (Paris). 1880;53:626–628, 54:635–737.
2. Henneberg R. Über genuine Narkolepsie. Neurol Zbl. 1916;30:282–290.
3. Daniels L. Narcolepsy. Medicine. 1934;13:1–122.
4. Yoss RE, Daly DD. Criteria for the diagnosis of the narcoleptic syndrome. Proc Staff Meet Mayo Clin. 1957;32:320–328.
5. Vogel G. Studies in the psychophysiology of dreams, III: the dream of narcolepsy. Arch Gen Psychiatry. 1960;3:421–425.
6. Rechtschaffen A, Wolpert E, Dement WC, et al. Nocturnal sleep of narcoleptics. Electroencephalogr Clin Neurophysiol. 1963;15:599–609.
7. Takahashi Y, Jimbo M. Polygraphic study of narcoleptic syndrome with special reference to hypnagogic hallucinations and cataplexy. Folia Psychiatr Neurol Jpn. 1963;7(suppl):343–347.
8. Passouant P, Schwab RS, Cadilhac J, et al. Narcolepsie-cataplexie: etude du sommeil de nuit et du sommeil de jour. Rev Neurol (Paris). 1964;3:415–426.
9. Hishikawa Y, Kaneko Z. Electroencephalographic study on narcolepsy. Electroencephalogr Clin Neurophysiol. 1965;18:249–258.
10. Ellis CM, Simmons A, Lemmens G, et al. Proton spectroscopy in the narcoleptic syndrome: is there evidence of a brainstem lesion? Neurology. 1998;50(suppl 1):S23–S26.
11. Dement WC, Zarcone V, Varner V, et al. The prevalence of narcolepsy. Sleep Res. 1972;1:148.
12. Dement WC, Carskadon MA, Ley R. The prevalence of narcolepsy. Sleep Res. 1973;2:147.
13. Mignot E. Genetic and familial aspects of narcolepsy. Neurology. 1998;50(suppl 1):S16–S22.
14. Honda Y, Asaka A, Tanimura M, et al. A genetic study of narcolepsy and excessive daytime sleepiness in 308 families with a

narcolepsy of hypersomnia proband. In: Guilleminault C, Lugaresi E, eds. Sleep/Wake Disorders: Natural History, Epidemiology and Long Term Evolution. New York, NY: Raven Press; 1983:187–199.

14a. Siegel JM. Narcolepsy. Sci Am. 2000;282:76–81.

15. Juji T, Satake M, Honda Y, et al. HLA antigens in Japanese patients with narcolepsy: all the patients were DR2 positive. Tissue Antigens 1984;24:316–319.

16. Guilleminault C, Mignot E, Grumet CA. Familial patterns of narcolepsy. Lancet 1989;2:1376–1379.

17. Guilleminault C, Grumet C. HLA-DR2 and narcolepsy: not all narcoleptic cataplectic patients are DR2. Hum Immunol. 1986;17:1–2.

17a. Ling L, Faraco R, Li R, et al. The sleep disorder canine narcolepsy is caused by a mutation in the hypocretin (orexin) receptor 2 gene. Cell. 1999;98:365–376.

17b. Chemelli RM, Willie JT, Sinton CM, et al. Narcolepsy in orexin knockout mice: molecular genetics of sleep regulation. Cell. 1999;98:437–451.

17c. Peyton C, Tighe DK, van den Pol AN, et al. Neurons containing hypocretin (orexin) project to multiple neuronal systems. J Neurosci. 1998;18:9996–10015.

17d. Nishino S, Ripley B, Overeem S, et al. Hypocretin (orexin) deficiency in human narcolepsy. Lancet. 2000;355:39–40.

18. Diagnostic Classification Steering Committee. The International Classification of Sleep Disorders: Diagnostic and Coding Manual. Rochester, Minn: American Sleep Disorders Association; 1990.

19. Guilleminault C, Heinzer R, Mignot E, et al. Investigations into the neurologic basis of narcolepsy. Neurology. 1998;50(suppl 1):S8–S15.

20. Guilleminault C, Pelayo R. Narcolepsy in prepubertal children. Ann Neurol. 1998;43:135–142.

21. Ohayon MM, Priest RG, Caucet M, et al. Hypnagogic and hypnopompic hallucinations = pathological phenomenon? Br J Psychiatry. 1996;169:459–467.

22. Billiard M, Besset A, Cadilhac J. The clinical and polygraphic development of narcolepsy. In: Guilleminault C, Lugaresi E, eds. Sleep/Wake Disorders: Natural History, Epidemiology, and Long Term Evolution. New York, NY: Raven Press; 1983:187–199.

23. Schmidt HS, Fortin LD. Electronic pupillography in disorders of arousal. In: Guilleminault C, ed. Sleep and Waking Disorders: Indications and Techniques. Menlo Park, Calif: Addison-Wesley; 1981:127–141.

24. Hoddes E, Dement WC, Zarcone V. The development and use of the Stanford Sleepiness Scale (SSS). Psychophysiology. 1972;9:150.

25. Yoss RE, Mayer NJ, Ogle KN. The pupillogram and narcolepsy. Neurology. 1969;19:921–928.

26. Berlucchi G, Moruzzi G, Salva G, et al. Pupil behavior and ocular movements during synchronized and desynchronized sleep. Arch Ital Biol. 1964;102:230.

27. Carskadon MA, Dement WC. The multiple sleep latency test: what does it measure? Sleep. 1982;5:67–72.

28. Rechtschaffen A, Kales AD. A Manual of Standardized Terminology, Techniques and Scoring System for Sleep Stages of Human Subjects. Los Angeles, Calif: UCLA Brain Information Service/Brain Research Institute; 1968.

29. Association of Professional Sleep Societies, APSS Guidelines Committee; Carskadon MA, Chairperson. Guidelines for the multiple sleep latency test (MSLT): a standard measure of sleepiness. Sleep. 1986;9:519–524.

30. Van den Hoed J, Kraemer H, Guilleminault C, et al. Disorders of excessive daytime somnolence: polygraphic and clinical data for 100 patients. Sleep. 1981;4:23–38.

31. Browman CP, Gujavarty KS, Sampson MG, et al. REM sleep episodes during the maintenance of wakefulness tests in patients with sleep apnea syndrome and patients with narcolepsy. Sleep. 1983;6:23–28.

32. Broughton R, Low R, Valley V, et al. Auditory evoked potentials compared to EEG and performance measures of impaired vigilance in narcolepsy-cataplexy. Sleep Res. 1981;10:184.

33. Honda Y, Juji T, eds. HLA in Narcolepsy. Berlin, Germany: Springer-Verlag; 1988.

34. Anic-Labat S, Guilleminault C, Kraemer HC, et al. Validation of a cataplexy questionnaire in 983 sleep-disorders patients. Sleep. 1999;22:77–87.

35. Moscovitch A, Partinen M, Patterson N, et al. Cataplexy in differ-

entiation of excessive daytime somnolence. Sleep Res. 1991;20:301.

36. Mignot E, Jayduk R, Black J, et al. HLA-DQB1*0602 is associated with narcolepsy in 509 narcoleptic patients. Sleep. 1997;20:1012–1020.

37. Mignot E, Guilleminault C, Bowersox S, et al. Effects of alpha-1 adrenoceptor blockade with prazosin in canine narcolepsy. Brain Res. 1988;444:184–188.

38. Fruhstorfer B, Mignot E, Bowersox S, et al. Canine narcolepsy is associated with an elevated number of alpha 2 receptors in the locus coerulus. Brain Res. 1989;500:209–214.

39. Nishino S, Haak L, Shepherd H, et al. Effects of central alpha-2 adrenergic compounds on canine narcolepsy, a disorder of rapid eye movement sleep. J Pharmacol Exp Ther. 1990;253:1145–1152.

40. Nishino S, Arrigoni J, Valtier D, et al. Dopamine D-2 mechanisms in canine narcolepsy. J Neurosci. 1991;11:2666–2671.

41. Langer SZ. Presynaptic regulation of the release of catecholamines. Pharmacol Rev. 1981;32:337–362.

42. Laduron PM. Presynaptic heteroreceptors in regulation of neuronal transmission. Biochem Pharmacol. 1985;34:467–470.

43. Mignot E, Guilleminault C, Dement WC, et al. Genetically determined animal models of narcolepsy, a disorder of REM sleep. In: Driscoll P, ed. Genetically-Defined Animal Models of Neurobehavioral Dysfunction. Cambridge, Mass: Birkhauser; 1992:89–110.

44. Montplaisir J, de Champlain J, Young SN, et al. Narcolepsy and idiopathic hypersomnia: biogenic amines and related compounds in CSF. Neurology. 1982;32:1299–1302.

45. Faull KF, Zeller-DeAmicis LC, Radde L, et al. Biogenic amine concentrations in the brains of normal and narcoleptic canines: current status. Sleep. 1986;9:107–110.

46. Aldrich MS, Hollingsworth Z, Penney JB. Dopamine-receptor autoradiography of human narcoleptic brain. Neurology. 1992;31:503–506.

47. Rinne JP, Hublin C, Partinen M, et al. Striatal dopamine D1 receptors in narcolepsy: a PET study with [¹¹C]NNC756. J Sleep Res. 1996;5:262–264.

48. Hublin C, Launes J, Nikkinen P, et al. Dopamine D2 receptors in human narcolepsy: a SPECT study with ¹²³I-IBZM. Acta Neurol Scand. 1994;90:186–189.

49. Rinne JO, Hublin C, Partinen M, et al. Positron emission tomography study of human narcolepsy: no increase in striatal dopamine D2 receptors. Neurology. 1995;45:1735–1738.

50. Aldrich MS, Prokopowicz G, Ockert K, et al. Neurochemical studies of human narcolepsy: alpha-adrenergic receptor autoradiography of human narcoleptic brain and brainstem. Sleep. 1994;17:598–608.

51. Guilleminault C. Amphetamines and narcolepsy: use of Stanford database. Sleep. 1993;16:199–201.

52. Fry JM. Treatment modalities for narcolepsy. Neurology. 1998;50(suppl 1):S43–S48.

53. Wyatt R, Fram D, Buchbinder R, et al. Treatment of intractable narcolepsy with a monoamine oxidase inhibitor. N Engl J Med. 1971;285:987–999.

54. Guilleminault C, Mancuso J, Quera Salva MA, et al. Viloxazine hydrochloride in narcolepsy: a preliminary report. Sleep. 1986;9:275–279.

55. Langdon N, Bandak S, Shindler J, et al. Fluoxetine in the treatment of cataplexy. Sleep. 1986;9:371–372.

56. Mitler MM, Hajdukovic R. Relative efficacy of drugs for the treatment of sleepiness in narcolepsy. Sleep. 1991;14:218–220.

57. Bedart MA, Montplaisir J, Godbout R. Effect of L-dopa on periodic movements in sleep in narcoleptics. Eur Neurol. 1987;27:35–38.

58. Boivin MA, Montplaisir J, Poirier G. The effect of L-dopa on periodic leg movements and sleep organization in narcolepsy. Clin Neuropharmacol. 1989;12:29–37.

59. Parkes JD. Amphetamines and alertness. In: Guilleminault C, Dement WC, Passouant P, eds. Narcolepsy. New York, NY: Spectrum Publications; 1976:643–657.

60. Prinzmetal M, Bloomberg W. The use of benzedrine for treatment of narcolepsy. JAMA. 1935;105:2051–2054.

61. Yoss RE, Daly DD. Treatment of narcolepsy with Ritalin. Neurology. 1959;9:171–173.

62. Honda Y, Hishikawa Y. Effectiveness of pemoline in narcolepsy. Sleep Res. 1970;8:192.

63. U.S. Modafinil in Narcolepsy Study Group. Randomized trial

of modafinil for the treatment of pathological somnolence in narcolepsy. Ann Neurol. 1998;43:88–97.

64. Mitler M, Erman M, Hajdukovic R. The treatment of excessive somnolence with stimulant drugs. Sleep. 1993;16:203–206.

65. Parkes JD, Dahlitz M. Amphetamine prescription. Sleep. 1993;16:201–203.

66. Parkes JD, Schacter M. Mazindol in the treatment of narcolepsy. Acta Neurol Scand. 1979;60:250–254.

67. Farma L, Galland Y. Treatment of narcoleptics with CRL-40476, an alpha stimulant medication [abstract]. In: Program and Abstracts of the Seventh European Sleep Congress; 1984; Munich, Germany.

68. Scharf MB, Brown D, Woods M, et al. The effects and effectiveness of gamma-hydroxybutyrate in patients with narcolepsy. J Clin Psychol. 1985;46:222–225.

69. Lammers GJ, Arends J, Declerk AC, et al. Gammahydroxybutyrate and narcolepsy: a double-blind placebo-controlled study. Sleep. 1993;16:216–220.

70. Broughton R, Mamelak M. The treatment of narcolepsy-cataplexy with nocturnal gamma hydroxybutyrate. Can J Neurol Sci. 1979;6:1–6.

71. Mamelak M, Scharf MB, Woods M. Treatment of narcolepsy with gamma-hydroxybutyrate: a review of clinical and sleep laboratory findings. Sleep. 1986;9:285–289.

61

Idiopathic Central Nervous System Hypersomnia

Christian Guilleminault
Rafael Pelayo

Idiopathic central nervous system (CNS) hypersomnia is a disorder characterized by chronic sleepiness without cataplexy presumed to be of neurological origin. The daytime sleepiness is not associated with the auxiliary symptoms seen in narcolepsy. Historically, this syndrome has had a number of labels, including essential narcolepsy, independent narcolepsy, nonrapid eye movement (NREM) sleep narcolepsy, functional hypersomnia, and harmonious hypersomnia.[1-6] It is important to clearly differentiate idiopathic hypersomnia from narcolepsy syndrome with its auxiliary symptoms and from daytime sleepiness related to nocturnal sleep disturbances such as sleep apnea or periodic leg movement syndrome.[4] The differential diagnosis of narcolepsy syndrome can be difficult, however, because the two disorders have many similarities, including age of symptom onset, chronicity, and a familial/genetic predisposition. The addition of upper airway resistance syndrome creates a difficult differential diagnosis.[7] Finally, several etiological factors may be responsible for the isolated daytime somnolence seen in idiopathic CNS hypersomnia syndrome, which renders diagnosis and treatment more difficult.

The prevalence of idiopathic CNS hypersomnia is unknown; no study has been performed that allows appropriate determination of the prevalence of the disorder.

CLINICAL FEATURES

Patients complain of long periods of daytime drowsiness that significantly impair their performance. Daytime drowsiness leads to naps that are prolonged, interrupted rarely by short awakenings, and frequently unrefreshing. Nocturnal sleep often is long and undisturbed.[8, 9] In the morning, awakenings are difficult, and sleep "drunkenness" is frequently noted.[10] Patients are hard to awaken; they can be aggressive and verbally and physically abusive during that twilight state if they are awakened, even at their own request. This sleep drunkenness can also be noted when patients are awakened from naps. The unrefreshing quality of napping and the sleep drunkenness associated with

awakenings lead patients to fight sleepiness as long as they can.

During these long periods of drowsiness, patients progressively develop automatic behavior,[11] during which they continue to perform in a semicontrolled way, with short (1- to 4-sec) microsleeps intruding more and more repetitively into the awake state. At times, patients with idiopathic CNS hypersomnia report only these periods of drowsiness and do not report daily long naps. The socioprofessional environment may not be permissive of napping, or subjects may find napping unhelpful, even rendering them less alert than before.

Subjects who do not nap are particularly prone to these periods of drowsiness and automatic behavior. Episodes of automatic behavior are usually signaled by blank stares. Microsleep events can be associated with slow, rolling eye movements on the polysomnographic recording (see later). During these episodes, patients act in an unplanned and often inappropriate way; for example, patients have reported finding themselves miles from their homes while driving or performing inappropriate actions such as sprinkling salt on coffee, putting dirty plates in a clothes dryer and turning on the machine, writing incoherent sentences during classes, having loud and irrelevant bursts of speech, and so on. Amnesia of such occurrences is the rule, although patients are usually aware that they have had one of their "drowsy" episodes when they are later confronted with the results of their automatic behavior.

The age of onset of symptoms varies, but it is frequently between 15 and 30 years, and the condition usually develops progressively over several weeks or months. Once established, symptoms are lifelong, with little change. Worsening has been reported with aging but is poorly documented.

POLYSOMNOGRAPHIC RECORDING FEATURES

Nocturnal recordings must provide an accurate documentation of the night's sleep.[8, 9] The patient should have completed sleep diary forms for at least 1 week before the polysomnographic study. Patients must be set on a regular sleep-wake schedule and must have a minimum of 7 to 7.5 h of nocturnal sleep time. Drugs known to affect sleep, sleep latency, and daytime alertness must be carefully evaluated and should be withdrawn for a minimum of 2 weeks before objective polysomnographic testing. It may be helpful to obtain a urine toxicology sample for drug testing at the time of the polysomnographic evaluation. This initial polysomnographic nocturnal recording may need to be repeated to rule out sleep disordered breathing such as upper airway resistance syndrome.[7]

After the polysomnographic evaluation of nocturnal sleep, a multiple sleep latency test (MSLT) (see Chapter 104) is conducted in a standardized manner the next morning. The combination of the nocturnal polysomnographic monitoring and the MSLT will objectively confirm the clinical diagnosis of CNS hypersomnia. The polysomnographic recording documents the combination of a normal or long nocturnal sleep recording and a short, pathological latency score by MSLT with no sleep-onset rapid eye movement (REM) periods. It is sometimes of interest perform a consecutive second night of polysomnographic monitoring. The first night may be terminated after 7.5 to 8 h of nocturnal sleep to fit the standardized criteria of the MSLT procedure, but it may be of interest to also appreciate ad libitum nocturnal sleep, and this can be done on the second night of monitoring. Patients with CNS hypersomnia, as a rule, have longer and more consolidated nocturnal sleep than do other patients with daytime sleepiness. They have less stage 1 NREM sleep, more total NREM sleep in the second third of the night, more stage 3/4 NREM sleep, less wakefulness in the first and second thirds of the night, and less total wakefulness after sleep onset than do narcoleptic patients. The nocturnal sleep structure and distribution of sleep stages are not strikingly different from those seen in normal subjects.

PATHOPHYSIOLOGY

As the name implies, little is known about the pathophysiology of idiopathic CNS hypersomnia. Research involving cerebrospinal fluid and human leukocyte antigens have shed some, albeit limited, insight into this disorder.

Cerebrospinal Fluid Evaluations

Cerebrospinal fluid analyses have been performed on patients with CNS hypersomnia; no abnormality of cytology or protein content has been shown. Systematic evaluation of the concentrations of the monoamine metabolites[12, 13] homovanillic acid, 3-methoxy-4-hydroxyphenylglycol, 4,3-dihydroxyphenylacetic acid, and 5-hydroxyindoleacetic acid has been performed before and after probenecid ingestion (50 mg/kg orally), and the results have been compared with those in normal control subjects and narcoleptic patients. Samples after probenecid treatment showed significant increases in homovanillic acid and 4,3-dihydroxyphenylacetic acid compared with normal control subjects, but this finding was also noted for narcoleptic patients. The findings of a preliminary study suggest that if the dopamine system seems to be desynchronized from the other amines (on the basis of metabolite data, such as dopamine system malfunction) in narcolepsy, it is the norepinephrine system that seems to be desynchronized in CNS hypersomnia.[14] Despite the preliminary nature of these results, they confirm the differences noted clinically and polysomnographically between CNS hypersomnia and narcolepsy.

Human Leukocyte Antigens in Central Nervous System Hypersomnia

As indicated in Chapter 59, a better understanding of the genetic basis of narcolepsy has come about through the discovery of its link with a class II antigen of the major histocompatibility complex known as DQ6. There also is strong evidence suggesting a genetic predisposition in a small number of patients with CNS hypersomnia. Familial studies of patients with CNS hypersomnia have revealed relatives with a positive history of the same disease. In a human leukocyte antigen (HLA) study that included the DR and DQ loci in those with idiopathic CNS hypersomnia, it was found that, compared with a control population, the frequency of HLA Cw2 was significantly increased.[15] It is interesting that, in contrast to narcoleptics, none of the hypersomanic patients were positive for DR15 or DQ6, but the frequency of HLA DR5 was also increased. However, most cases of the syndrome are isolated and sporadic. It is probable that idiopathic CNS hypersomnia represents a heterogeneous group of patients and that patients with HLA Cw2 may be a specific subgroup.

POSSIBLE SUBGROUPS OF IDIOPATHIC CENTRAL NERVOUS SYSTEM HYPERSOMNIA

On the basis of clinical and genetic features, there appear to be several subgroups of patients with idiopathic CNS hypersomnia.

Subgroup I. This is the smallest group, and it consists of subjects with a positive family history who eventually are shown to have the HLA Cw2 antigen. In this group, in whom two or more affected family members can be identified, associated clinical symptoms suggesting dysfunction of the autonomic nervous system are most commonly seen.[16] The symptoms include headaches, which may be migrainous; mild-to-moderate fainting episodes (syncope); orthostatic hypotension; and, most commonly, peripheral vascular complaints (Raynaud-type phenomena with cold hands and feet).

Subgroup II. This is the group that is best defined.

It consists of individuals who have had a viral infection associated, in some rare and specific cases, with neurological symptoms, such as the Guillain-Barré syndrome. Mononucleosis, hepatitis, and atypical viral pneumonia are the most common primary diseases. Guillain-Barré syndrome is occasionally reported as a primary disease. Idiopathic CNS hypersomnia may occur after infectious mononucleosis or in isolated context. Patients usually complain of tiredness and fatigue related to the initial syndrome. Although other symptoms related to the infectious disease disappear, these patients still require significantly more nocturnal sleep than they did before their illness and feel very tired. To fight the tiredness, they begin to nap.

Patients initially have difficulties in dissociating fatigue related to their viral illness and sleepiness. They generally recognize sleepiness as a complaint when socioeconomic problems arise. Until the problems become pressing, they believe that their symptoms of tiredness will soon disappear. The socioprofessional impairment drives them to consult a clinic soon after the initial viral problem. Guilleminault and Mondini[17] reported that in their study population, consultations for sleepiness occurred 6 to 15 weeks after the onset of the infection.

The only cerebrospinal fluid data available early in the disease process are those obtained on patients with initial Guillain-Barré syndrome in the subgroup; the analysis demonstrated moderate lymphocytosis (30 to 50 cells/mm^3; 30 to 50 × 10^6/L) with the typical mild to moderate protein elevation seen in Guillain-Barré syndrome. A long-term study of the severity of the initial infectious symptoms was unable to identify patients who would develop hypersomnia.[17]

Subgroup III. There is a subgroup of patients with no family or viral history before the onset of the sleep disorder; the daytime somnolence is truly "idiopathic."

POSITIVE DIAGNOSIS

The diagnosis of idiopathic CNS hypersomnia is made by progressive elimination of other causes of excessive daytime sleepiness (EDS). This approach is not satisfactory because no positive testing confirms a specific diagnosis, with the possible exception of the MSLT. The enthusiasm for the term *CNS hypersomnia* has not been enhanced by the growing impression that it covers several causes; however, there undoubtedly is a group of patients with or without clear viral history who present with a disabling syndrome, with a somnolence that responds poorly to stimulant medications. This subgroup is clinically significant. The disabling sleepiness is frequently associated with mild symptoms evoking autonomic nervous system dysfunction: cold hands; cold feet; lightheadedness on standing up, occasionally with drops in systolic blood pressure sufficient to evoke orthostatic hypotension; or dull headache that may be slightly migrainous. Even in the migrainous presentation, the headaches often respond well to stimulant medication.

Polysomnographic monitoring and MSLT are needed to confirm the presence of the syndrome. Classically, no sleep-onset REM periods are seen during a five-nap MSLT. When a large group of narcoleptics and CNS hypersomniacs are compared, the mean sleep latency score is usually higher in the CNS hypersomniac group. Guilleminault et al.[18] reviewed the polysomnographic results of 50 patients with CNS hypersomnia and reported a mean MSLT score of 6.3 ± 3.5 min; only 11% of the population had a score of less than or equal to 3.7 min. Van den Hoed et al.[19] reported a mean MSLT score of 6.5 ± 3.2 min for CNS hypersomniacs versus 3.3 ± 3.3 min for narcoleptics.

DIFFERENTIAL DIAGNOSIS

There are several entities that must be well differentiated from idiopathic CNS hypersomnia.

Narcolepsy is a common differential diagnostic consideration, but it is not the most difficult. The requirement of an association of EDS, a positive history of cataplexy, and the presence of two or more sleep-onset REM periods at up to 4 days of repeated MSLT should allow appropriate differentiation. The narcolepsy syndrome may initially present as isolated EDS, and the positive diagnosis may be in doubt for months or even years. Considering the importance of a proper diagnosis for epidemiological and genetic studies, it is better to classify the disorder as idiopathic hypersomnia until the cataplexy develops. Neither HLA typing nor sleep-onset REM periods are pathognomonic.

The investigations of Van den Hoed et al.[19] and Moscovitch et al.[20] indicate that EDS can occur with one or more sleep-onset REM periods but without cataplexy or other auxiliary symptoms. Of 306 EDS patients without disordered breathing during sleep, Moscovitch et al.[20] found 54 patients who presented with no cataplexy and two or more sleep-onset REM periods and 23 patients with no cataplexy and one sleep-onset REM period. Thus, 25% of the patient groups had no cataplexy and one or more sleep-onset REM periods. Mignot et al.[21] showed that some of these patients can be positive for *DQ6* and may be narcoleptic, but for others this was not true. This large patient group fit the criteria for neither narcolepsy nor idiopathic CNS hypersomnia. At this time, it is recommended that the disorder be classified as *isolated EDS with sleep-onset REM periods.* This patient subgroup is poorly understood. These patients are treated with stimulant medications (methylphenidate, amphetamine, mazindol) at dosages similar to those used for idiopathic CNS hypersomnia. Whether any REM sleep–inhibiting medications would be helpful is unknown. The genetic background and familial histories of these patients also are unknown.

The complaint of sleepiness and the positive MSLT findings may also be similar in patients with significant daytime sleepiness as a sequela of *severe head trauma.*[22] The past medical history, which often includes an initial coma after the head trauma, is enlightening in these cases.

The daytime somnolence seen in association with

communicating hydrocephalus of unknown etiology also does not differ clinically from idiopathic CNS hypersomnia. Imaging of the brain, which confirms the hydrocephalus, distinguishes this syndrome from idiopathic CNS hypersomnia.

A careful history will differentiate patients with idiopathic CNS hypersomnia from those with chronic insufficient nocturnal sleep who have daytime sleepiness. An actigraph recording may be helpful if the history is inconclusive.

Upper Airway Resistance Syndrome

Above all, idiopathic CNS hypersomnia must be distinguished from upper airway resistance syndrome. Clinically, both men and women complain of isolated EDS. Interviews frequently indicate, however, that the patient snores during sleep. In a prospective study performed in a sleep clinic, Guilleminault et al.[7] reported snoring in 100% of the men but an absence of snoring in 25% of the women with the syndrome. However, the subject population of this study was small.[15] Clinical interviews did not provide any additional information.

Examinations of these subjects often reveal a triangular face or a steep mandibular plane, a highly arched palate, a class II malocclusion, and, at times, retroposition of the mandible. All of the patients described have not been obese. Cephalometric radiographs have indicated the presence of a small space behind the base of the tongue (posterior airway space), often near the location of the hyoid bone. The distance between the hyoid bone and the mandibular plane is variable, sometimes small. Several of the nonsnoring women had cervical vertebrae fusions (C3-4, C5-6). These subjects presented repetitive short ("transient") alpha electroencephalographic arousals lasting 3 to 14 sec that regularly interrupted the abnormally high inspiratory efforts. Standard polysomnographic recordings of these subjects evoked the diagnosis on the basis of the presence of these repetitive transient arousals, increases in snoring just before the arousal, and an increase in inspiratory time and a decrease in expiratory time, which were determined with the use of well-calibrated sensors. No significant change in Sa$_{O_2}$ was seen, and the respiratory disturbance index was low (less than 5). Neither obstructive sleep apnea syndrome (Guilleminault et al[23]) nor its subcategory, obstructive sleep apnea-hypopnea syndrome (Gould et al.[24]), was present.

Once the diagnosis has been considered, it must be confirmed. Polysomnographic monitoring with an esophageal balloon or a water-filled esophageal catheter, a face mask, and a pneumotachygraph will demonstrate simultaneous decreases in esophageal pressure with each breath and just before each arousal, one to three breaths before an abrupt decrease in air flow. Clinical investigation may not require the use of a face mask and pneumotachygraph, but measurement of esophageal pressure, an indicator of respiratory effort, is needed. Guilleminault et al.[7] found that tidal volume

could drop a mean of 22% compared with normal breathing in the one to three breaths just preceding transient arousal. Thus, no complete obstruction occurs. A transient decrease in flow precedes and triggers the arousal, but the tidal volume decrease is so transient that pulse oximetry is not significantly affected. The sleep fragmentation occurring with this syndrome is one of the factors leading to the complaint of EDS. The complex diagnostic procedure described can demonstrate the resistance of the upper airway, but it significantly disturbs sleep. It is possible to perform a less complete investigation with only an esophageal balloon or a transducer to measure esophageal pressure, an indirect indicator of upper airway resistance. The diagnosis can be confirmed with the use of nasal continuous positive airway pressure as a therapeutic test. The positive end-expiratory pressure of the nasal continuous positive airway pressure equipment is determined with the use of snoring and esophageal pressure measurements. Guilleminault et al.[7] found that pressures between 4 and 8 cm H$_2$O controlled the repetitive transient arousals in their population. A repeat MSLT during continuous positive airway pressure treatment 1 month later should demonstrate improvement compared with baseline. It is critical that this syndrome be excluded before idiopathic CNS hypersomnia is diagnosed.

Hypersomnia Associated With Mood Disorder

Depression may be associated with a complaint of EDS. The classic depression, monopolar or bipolar, is easy to recognize, and the hypersomnia complaint is not, by far, the predominant symptom. It is more a dysthymia seen after menopause in women and after the fourth decade in men, and it may be associated with a complaint of daytime tiredness, sleepiness, or both. Clinically, patients report a lack of energy, tiredness, fatigue, and sleepiness without really falling asleep. They present symptoms of mood impairment with lack of interest, decreased appetite, and some features of hopelessness but without suicidal ideation. They report cognitive difficulties and a decrease in memory. They spend a large amount of time in bed and acknowledge "resting" more than "sleeping."

Billiard et al.[25] used the term *clinophilia* to indicate the disassociation between "staying in bed for hours during the daytime" in apposition to true excessive sleepiness with repetitive daytime naps. Neuropsychological testing shows moderately elevated scores on the Hamilton Depression Scale or other scales used to evaluate depression. These scales are also commonly mildly elevated with narcolepsy and idiopathic hypersomnia, as in any chronic disorder. In addition, many of these scales include sleep-related symptoms that may be affected by the hypersomnia itself.

Polysomnographic investigation at night may show a decrease in REM sleep latency during the first cycle, but this is variable. The most important finding is a discrepancy between the severity of the reported symptoms and the mild scores obtained on the Epworth Sleepiness Scale, and even more of a discrepancy on the MSLT. If the scores are not necessarily completely normal, they are usually borderline, with mean sleep latency oscillating between 8 and 12 min. Again, this is in contrast to the degree of the complaint.

Chronic Fatigue Syndrome

Chronic fatigue syndrome (see Chapter 87) may be the label given to the patient; often, the clinical presentation is very similar to that seen in patients with dysthymia. Many subjects diagnosed with chronic fatigue syndrome have upper airway resistance syndrome, poor sleep hygiene, mood disorder, and even mild delayed sleep phase syndrome. Patients with chronic fatigue syndrome may complain significantly of their daytime tiredness and sleepiness, but again, there is a very poor correlation between the severity of the complaint and the severity of the neuropsychological test results. The daytime MSLT disassociates EDS from "tiredness," as well; the patients have more tiredness than true sleepiness.

Delayed Sleep Phase Syndrome

Delayed sleep phase syndrome is another consideration (see Chapter 52). Rarely, the daytime symptoms presented by the subject during the morning hours may lead to questions regarding the diagnosis, but an appropriate sleep history, sleep logs covering 15 days, and, if needed, actigraphy performed for 1 week easily indicate a normal total sleep time but abnormal sleep-onset and wake-up times.

TREATMENT

Because the underlying causes of hypersomnia syndrome are unknown, treatment can only be symptomatic. Hypersomnia is a disabling problem that often leads to permanent unemployment and responds poorly to medical treatment.

Behavioral approaches and sleep hygiene techniques must be recommended but have little positive impact alone. They only avoid abrupt worsenings that can temporarily occur with transient sleep deprivation or abrupt time shifts. Daytime naps are long and most commonly nonrefreshing. The list of medications that we have prescribed for patients includes tricyclic antidepressants, monoamine oxidase inhibitors, clonidine, levodopa (isolated or in combination), bromocriptine, amantadine, methysergide, and 5-hydroxytryptophan; none of these drugs have controlled the hypersomnia syndrome well. The only medications that have brought partial, and often intermittent, relief have been the stimulants. Pemoline, which is the mildest, is often inadequate; methylphenidate, mazindol, phenmetrazine hydrochloride, and dextroamphetamine are the most commonly prescribed medications.

A new drug is modafinil.[26] The therapeutic protocols involve maintaining the patient on a daily drug intake sufficiently low to avoid the many side effects, including those involving the liver and cardiovascular system, and yet be helpful. It must be remembered that complete control of daytime sleepiness cannot often be obtained even with significant dosages of stimulant medications; thus, we usually do not prescribe daily therapeutic doses of more than 60 mg of methylphenidate administered in divided dosage, 400 mg of modafinil, or 40 mg of dextroamphetamine. Patients have a lifelong illness, and they will develop tolerance to their medications, so caution must be exercised in prescribing stimulants (Table 61–1).

The mechanism of action of modafinil is not completely understood. It does not seem to have the cardiovascular side effects noted with other stimulants, and it seems to have no addictive properties. The most common side effect is headache, and this negative effect may be eliminated if there is a progressive dose increase over time. The maximum recommended dosage is 400 mg/day. It is recommended to begin with 100 mg in the morning for 1 week and then to increase by 100 mg every 4 to 5 days, while evaluating the effects on symptoms before increasing the dosage. In U.S. trials,[27] the drug was administered once daily in the morning. European data[28, 29] support better coverage during the daytime with a divided intake, in the morning and at lunch time. Once-a-day intake increases compliance, but despite the long half-life of the

---

Table 61–1. TREATMENT APPROACH TO CENTRAL NERVOUS SYSTEM HYPERSOMNIA

Hygiene

One nap daily (noon or late afternoon), no longer than 45 min
Avoid alcohol, heavy meals, sleep deprivation
Avoid shift work
Sleep at least 8.5 h per night

Medication

Initial Treatment

Methylphenidate SR 20 mg morning
Methylphenidate 5 mg tablet 3 PM
If Significant Excessive Daytime Sleepiness
Methylphenidate SR 20 mg morning
Methylphenidate SR 20 mg noon

*Alternative Initial Treatment**

Modafinil may be more effective in stimulant-naive patients
Modafinil 100 mg morning for 1 week to avoid headache
Then increase modafinil as needed by 100 mg every 4 days; maximum dose, 400 mg
Twice-daily dosing (morning and lunch) may provide longer coverage

If Initial Treatment Is Ineffective

Switch to dextroamphetamine (Dexedrine Spansule)
Start with 15-mg dextroamphetamine (SR) morning
May add 15-mg dextroamphetamine (SR) noon
Three 15-mg dextroamphetamine (SR) daily may be prescribed

---

*Patients currently treated with amphetamines will respond less to modafinil than naive patients. Modafinil should, thus, be evaluated in a therapeutic trial before any amphetamine drug is prescribed.
SR, sustained-release.

drug (8 to 14 h), patients may have a lesser effect of the medication at the end of the afternoon to early evening with once-a-day dosing. European data also suggest that modafinil gives a better response in stimulant-naive subjects than in subjects previously treated with stimulants. Modafinil would therefore be a medication to try as a first-line intervention. As with all new medications, not all positive and negative effects of modafinil are probably known.

By 1998, modafinil was available in several countries in Western Europe and was in the late stages of approval in both the United States and Canada. It appears that it can be administered with antidepressants without significant drug interactions, but not all drug interactions are known. Because modafinil is eliminated after metabolism in the liver and by the kidneys, it probably is good clinical practice to check liver function tests once a year in patients ingesting the medication on a chronic basis. This particular recommendation is valid for all stimulants, with pemoline having been more carefully looked at in this regard than any other stimulant.

CONCLUSIONS

Idiopathic CNS hypersomnia is a disabling disease that is understood even less than narcolepsy. A patient's impairment is frequently severe, despite the absence of obvious neurological lesions. At times, the severity of the impairment can place lives in jeopardy (persons with CNS hypersomnia have sustained third-degree burns during automatic behavior episodes or have turned on gas furnaces or stoves without lighting them, leading in one case to a severe explosion). The sleep specialist must be able to convey the seriousness of this chronic disability to the Social Security Administration and other agencies and must objectively and convincingly document the presence of this disorder in view of the long-term prognosis and current absence.

References

1. Berti-Ceroni G, Coccagna G, Gambi D, et al. Considerazioni clinico poligrafiche sulla narcolessia essenziola "a son nolento." Sist Nerv. 1967;19:81–89.
2. Mouret J, Renaud B, Quenin P, et al. Monoamines et regulation de la vigilance: apport et interprétation biochimique des données polygraphiques. In: Girard P, Couteaux R, eds. Les Mediateurs Chimiques. Paris, France: Masson; 1972:139–155.
3. Roth B. Functional hypersomnia. In: Guilleminault C, Dement WC, Passouant P, eds. Narcolepsy: Advances in Sleep Research. Vol 3. New York, NY: Spectrum Publications; 1976:333–350.
4. Roth B. Narcolepsy and Hypersomnia. New York, NY: S. Karger; 1980.
5. Guilleminault C, Faull KF. Sleepiness in non-narcoleptic, non-sleep apneic EDS patients: the idiopathic CNS hypersomnolence. Sleep. 1982;5:S175–S181.
6. Aldrich M. The clinical spectrum of narcolepsy and idiopathic hypersomnia. Neurology. 1996;46:393–401.
7. Guilleminault C, Stoohs R. Clerk A, et al. A cause of excessive daytime sleepiness: the upper airway resistance syndrome. Chest. 1993;104: 781–787.
8. Rechtschaffen A, Roth B. Nocturnal sleep of hypersomniacs. Act Nerv. 1969;11(suppl):229–233.
9. Baker TL, Guilleminault C, Nino-Murcia G, et al. Comparative polysomnographic study of narcolepsy and idiopathic central nervous system hypersomnia. Sleep. 1986;9:232–242.
10. Roth B, Nevsimalova S, Rechtschaffen A. Hypersomnia with "sleep drunkenness." Arch Gen Psychiatry. 1972;26:456–462.
11. Guilleminault C, Phillips R, Dement WC. A syndrome of hypersomnia with automatic behavior. Electroencephalogr Clin Neurophysiol. 1975;38:403–413.
12. Montplaisir J, de Champlain J, Young SN, et al. Narcolepsy and idiopathic hypersomnia: biogenic amines and related compounds. Neurology. 1982;32:1299–1302.
13. Faull KF, Guilleminault C, Berger PA, et al. Cerebrospinal fluid monoamine metabolites in narcolepsy and hypersomnia. Ann Neurol. 1983;13:258–263.
14. Faull KF, Thiemann S, King RJ, et al. Monoamine interactions in narcolepsy and hypersomnia: a preliminary report. Sleep. 1986;9:246–249.
15. Poirier G, Montplaisir J, Decary F, et al. HLA antigens in narcolepsy and idiopathic central nervous system hypersomnolence. Sleep. 1986;9:153–158.
16. Guilleminault C. Disorders of excessive sleepiness. Ann Clin Res. 1985;17:209–219.
17. Guilleminault C, Mondini S. Infectious mononucleosis and excessive daytime sleepiness: a long term follow-up study. Arch Intern Med. 1986;146:1333–1335.
18. Guilleminault C, Partinen M, Quera-Salva MA. Daytime sleepiness in non-narcoleptic subjects: central nervous system hypersomnia and obstructive sleep apneic patients. In: Smirne S, Franceschi M, Ferini-Strambi L, eds. Sleep in Medical and Neuropsychiatric Disorders. Milan, Italy: Masson; 1988:111–124.
19. Van den Hoed J, Kraemer H, Guilleminault C, et al. Disorders of excessive daytime somnolence: polygraphic and clinical data for 100 patients. Sleep. 1981;4:23–38.
20. Moscovitch A, Partinen M, Guilleminault C. The positive diagnosis of narcolepsy and narcolepsy's borderland. Neurology. 1993;43:55–60.
21. Mignot E, Hayduk R, Black J, et al. Extensive HLA class II studies in 58 non-DRB1'15 (DR2) narcoleptic patients with cataplexy. Tissue Antigens. 1997;49:329–341.
22. Guilleminault C, van den Hoed J, Miles L. Post traumatic excessive daytime sleepiness. Neurology 1983;33:1584–1589.
23. Guilleminault C, Tilkian A, Dement WC. The sleep apnea syndromes. Am Rev Med. 1976;27:465–484.
24. Gould GA, Whyte KF, Rhino GB, et al. The sleep hypopnea syndrome. Am Rev Respir Dis. 1990;142:295–300.
25. Billiard M, Cargender B. Troubles primares de l' eueil. Rev Neurol (Paris). 1998;154:111–129.
26. Bastuji H, Jouvet M. Successful treatment of idiopathic hypersomnia and narcolepsy with modafinil. Prog Neuropsychopharmacol Biol Psychiatry. 1988;12:695–706.
27. US Modafinil in Narcolepsy Multicenter Study Group. Randomized trial of modafinil for the treatment of pathological somnolence in narcolepsy. Ann Neurol. 1998;43:88–97.
28. Billiard M, Besset A, Montplaisir J, et al. Modafinil: a double-blind multicentric study. Sleep. 1994;17:S107–S112.
29. Laffont F, Mayer G, Minz M. Modafinil in diurnal sleepiness: a study of 123 patients. Sleep. 1994;17:S113–S115.

eleven

Parasomnias

Mark W. Mahowald

62

NREM Arousal Parasomnias

Roger J. Broughton

Confusional arousals, sleep terrors, and sleep-walking are grouped together in this chapter because they share five fundamental common features. All begin in nonrapid eye movement (NREM) sleep, preferentially in deep slow-wave sleep (SWS) (i.e, in stages 3 and 4), and never or very seldom in rapid eye movement (REM) sleep. Attacks can often be triggered by forced arousals in SWS. Genetic patterns are similar. Episodes combining features of more than one parasomnia may occur. Finally, all three conditions are more common in childhood, when to some degree they may be considered normal, whereas they are less typical in adults.

Although in the early literature these conditions were considered behavioral expressions of dreaming, the ability to trigger attacks by efforts at forced awakening in SWS,[1] regardless of the ongoing state of mental activity, indicated both that they need not express mentation during sleep and that the arousal process itself is abnormal.

This feature also distinguishes these three parasomnias from a large number of others that are associated with arousal as a secondary event rather than as an integral part of their pathogenesis and for which there is no evidence that the arousal process itself is abnormal.

It has therefore been proposed that they be classified as *disorders of arousal*,[2] a concept accepted in the International Classification of Sleep Disorders.[3] Although for many years the NREM arousal disorders appeared to be clinically quite independent from parasomnias occurring during REM sleep, it has long been known that the NREM (usually SWS) arousals inherent in the attacks may, although rarely, appear to be initiated by the onset of REM sleep.[2, 4] In the mid-1990s, an overlap syndrome of patients presenting with both NREM arousal disorders and REM parasomnias, with the latter consisting of either nocturnal wanderings[5] or the REM sleep behavior disorder (RBD),[6] was identified.

Here, these three conditions are discussed in the order of confusional arousals, sleep terrors, and sleepwalking because some behavioral features of confusional arousals are inherent in all three parasomnias and because sleep terrors may occasionally be followed directly by sleepwalking, whereas the reverse order has never been reported.

CONFUSIONAL AROUSALS (NOCTURNAL SLEEP DRUNKENNESS)

Definition

This parasomnia consists of episodes of marked mental confusion during and after arousal from sleep but without the occurrence of any expression of terror or of leaving the bed and walking away. Episodes typically arise from a deep sleep during the first third of the night.

Historical Aspects

Early descriptions of confusional arousals from deep sleep include those in 1840 of Marc,[7] physician to the King of France, who referred to them as *'l'ivresse du sommeil'*, and in 1905 of the German neurologist von Gudden,[8] who referred to them as as *'Schlaftrunkenheit'*; both terms translate literally as "sleep drunkenness." These reports contain excellent documentation of this state in which the brain, for a period of time, is both partially awakened and partially still in the grips of sleep. Direct evidence of this dissociation was provided by the presence of evoked potentials that simultaneously show some features of sleep and others of wakefulness.[2] The term *sleep drunkenness* was later applied by Roth et al.[9] to similar mental slowness and confusion in the morning after the termination of night sleep, a feature that especially characterizes idiopathic hypersomnia (in about 50% of cases). Its original application to behaviors during, rather than after, the sleep period was de-emphasized and often forgotten. Polysomnographic confirmation of the disorder and its usual association with arousals from SWS was first reported in 1965 by Gastaut and Broughton.[1]

Pathophysiology

Even in normal subjects without confusional episodes, experimentally induced arousals in SWS can induce poor memory recall of materials presented after the onset of the arousal[10]; impairment in a variety of performance tasks, including reaction time[11]; and, at times, some degree of mental slowness. These effects in normal subjects are often referred to as *sleep inertia*.[12, 13] Confusional arousals appear to represent simple intensification of this normal process to events that are clinically significant due to their intensity or duration or the nature of the associated behaviors.

Patients with recurrent confusional arousals are typically deep sleepers who are relatively hard to awaken. Although there is evidence that the trait of unusually deep sleep and confusional arousals themselves are both at least in part genetically determined, the molecular basis is unknown. As in the case of sleep terrors and sleepwalking, the probability of an episode of confusional arousal is increased by any factor that deepens sleep or impairs the awakening process, such as young age, recovery from previous sleep deprivation, and the taking of central nervous system (CNS)-depressant substances, including some hypnotic agents and tranquilizers.[14] Triggering factors include any cause of disrupted sleep such as stress, noise, or other arousing stimuli. The probability of episodes of all three parasomnias in fact appears to be enhanced by the simultaneous combination of factors that both deepen and fragment sleep.[15] There are a number of common facilitating and precipitating factors to the three parasomnias; these are summarized in Table 62–1.

Epidemiology

There have been few epidemiological studies that specifically investigated confusional arousals. The episodes occur most commonly in children younger than 5 years and become less frequent with the approach of adolescence.[14] They may also occur in adulthood but are relatively rare. Confusional arousals may be the only parasomnia pattern presented, or they may be associated with sleep terrors or sleepwalking.

Clinical Features

The child or adult awakens only partially, usually from a deep sleep during the first third of the night, and exhibits marked mental confusion with slow mentation, disorientation in time and space, and poor or incomplete responsiveness to external stimuli, includ-

Table 62–1. PREDISPOSING, FACILITATING, AND TRIGGERING FACTORS IN NREM AROUSAL PARASOMNIAS

Predisposing Factors
Genetic factors—family history of same or other NREM aoursal parasomnias

Factors That Deepen Sleep (Increase Slow-Wave Sleep or Increase the Difficulty in Awakening)
Young age
Natural deep sleeper
Recovery from prior sleep deprivation
Onset of CPAP therapy for obstructive sleep apnea
CNS depressant medication (sedatives, hypnotics, alcohol)
Fever
Hypersomniac period (e.g., in Kleine-Levin syndrome)

Factors That Fragment Sleep
Stress
Environmental stimuli
Endogenous stimuli
Pain
Pregnancy
Stimulants
Thyroxine taken in evening
Migraine headache
Tourette's syndrome

CNS, central nervous system; CPAP, continuous positive airway pressure.

Table 62-2. COMPARISON OF THE MOST COMMON FEATURES OF VARIOUS PARASOMNIAS

	Confusional Arousals	Sleep Terrors	Sleepwalking	Nightmares	RDB	Complex PS
Time of night	Early	Early	Early to mid	Late	Late	Any
Sleep stage at start	SWS	SWS	SWS	REM	Dissociated REM	Any
EEG discharges	No	No	No	No	No	Usual
Screams	No	Yes	No	Rare	Rare	Rare
CNS activation	Minimal	Extreme	Minimal	Mild	Mild	Mild
Myoclonus	No	No	No	Rare	Common	Rare
Walking	No	No	Yes	No	Rare	Common
Returns to bed	Stays	Stays	Usual	Stays	Unusual	Unusual
Awakens	Uncommon	Uncommon	Uncommon	Common	Common	Common
Duration	0.5–10 min	1–10 min	2–30 min	3–20 min	1–10 min	5–15 min
Confusion (after)	Usual	Usual	Usual	Very rare	Rare	Usual
Reduced in laboratory	Yes	Yes	Yes	No	No	No
Episodes in wake	No	No	No	No	No	Usual
Age	Child	Child	Child	Adult	Adult	Adult
Genetic transmission	Yes	Yes	Yes	No	No	Rare
Organic CNS lesions	No	No	No	No	Common	Common

CNS, central nervous system; dissociated REM, sleep consisting of REM sleep without atonia; PS, partial epileptic seizures; RBD, REM sleep behavior disorder; SWS, slow-wave sleep (i.e., stages 3 and 4).

ing efforts to provoke full behavioral wakefulness. There may be automatic behaviors such as fingering of bedclothes, picking up an object and speaking into it as though it were a telephone, or other inappropriate activities. Moaning and incomprehensible mumbling or vocalizations may occur. Cognition may be greatly impaired. There are instances of inappropriate or incorrect verbal information having been provided by individuals experiencing a confusional arousal. Confusional arousals may also include aggressive behaviors such as thrashing about in bed or kicking, and can lead to injury to self or others, although this appears to be rarer than in sleep terrors and, especially, sleepwalking. The attacks typically last only 30 sec to 5 min, although longer attacks have been reported. There is retrograde amnesia for the behaviors and for any dream-like or thought-like mentation.[1, 2, 14, 16] The main features of the common parasomnias are compared in Table 62-2.

Differential Diagnosis

Confusional arousals must be distinguished from other conditions that can lead to mental confusion during sleep. The episodes lack the terrified facial expression, piercing cry, and major autonomic features of sleep terrors, as well as the features of leaving the bed and walking about that characterize sleepwalking. RBD[17, 18] is easily distinguished by its typical occurrence in the latter part of the night; the intensity of the motor behaviors, which may include leaping out of bed and myoclonus; the later recall of detailed dreaming; and its association in polysomnograms with patterns of REM sleep without atonia and often with intensified myoclonus or both. Confusional arousals have also been documented to occur with REM sleep awakenings in elderly, demented, and alcoholic patients,[19] who can have further increase in their cognitive difficulties with any state transition; however, the clinical context usually makes the diagnosis easy.

Complex partial epileptic seizures ("psychomotor seizures") of inferomesial temporal or frontal lobe origin[20, 21] may also cause nocturnal confusional episodes, but the latter have a number of distinguishing features. There may be similar partial seizures beginning in daytime wakefulness; interictal or ictal electroencephalographic (EEG) discharges often are present; and epileptic confusional episodes of this type cannot be provoked by forced awakenings.

The movements during confusional arousals may at times raise the possibility of nocturnal paroxysmal dystonia,[22] but in the latter, the onset most often occurs in adulthood, the movements are much more dystonic and at times even ballistic or choreoathetotic, attacks are very stereotyped from episode to episode and often recur across the entire night in all stages of NREM sleep, the confusional element is not predominant, and episodes cannot be triggered by forced arousals.

Diagnostic Evaluation

The minimal clinical features for diagnosis include a complaint by the patient or observer of repeated mental confusion on awakening with the absence of signs of acute fear, walking behaviors, or intense hallucinations. Recurrence during the first part of the night and induction of episodes by forced arousal help confirm the diagnosis.

Polysomnographic recording[1, 14] of an attack helps greatly in the diagnosis. Episodes typically begin with a movement arousal in SWS followed by decreased amplitude of the EEG and the appearance, during the period of mental confusion, of either stage 1 drowsy patterns or a diffuse alpha rhythm that may be slower by 1 to 2 Hz than that of full wakefulness or be poorly reactive to bright light and other arousing stimuli. These brain wave patterns reflect an incomplete awakening that is the basis of the mental confusion experienced by the sleeper. The electrocardiogram does not

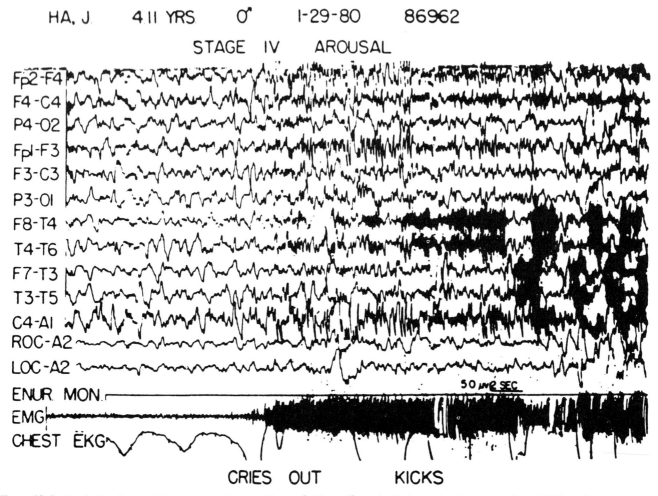

Figure 62–1. Confusional arousal in a young (4 years, 11 months) boy. The episode began in slow-wave sleep (SWS) with an incomplete arousal and consisted of crying out, kicking, and thrashing but no actual scream as in a sleep terror. The EEG shows some reduction in amplitude to a mixed frequency medium voltage pattern but is greatly obscured by muscle artifact. (From Ferber R. Sleep disorders in infants and children. In: Riley TL, ed. Clinical Aspects of Sleep and Sleep Disturbance. Boston, Mass: Butterworths; 1985:113–158.)

show the extreme acceleration characteristic of sleep terrors (Fig. 62–1).

Management

Confusional arousals do not necessarily warrant treatment. Children usually outgrow them. There is no evidence that they harm the patient in any way in their usual benign form. The recurrence, however, of confusional arousals in adults and episodes with repeated self-injury or aggression toward others often require active management. Objects on the bedside table may be removed. Patients may want to minimize any activities involving telephone calls at night or any work demands shortly after awakening. The avoidance of facilitating factors such as periods of sleep deprivation, circadian sleep-wake disturbances, or ingestion of CNS-depressant substances may be all that is needed. The treatment of associated sleep terrors or sleepwalking, if present, may reduce their frequency. During a confusional arousal, there is little point in interfering in any way with its evolution, which is typically quite brief and self-limited and can be allowed to simply "run itself out." Resistance against the spontaneous completion of the episode may in fact provoke aggressive behavior. There are no well-documented drug treatment studies of patients with confusional arousals alone, but patients may respond to the benzodiazepine or tricyclic medication described later for sleep terrors and sleepwalking. It is seldom necessary to prescribe medication other than as short-term therapy, which lasts only a few days or weeks during periods when episodes are more frequent.

SLEEP TERRORS (NIGHT TERRORS, INCUBUS ATTACKS, PAVOR NOCTURNUS, "NREM NIGHTMARES")

Definition

Sleep terrors consist of sitting up during sleep, emitting a piercing cry, and showing behavioral features of acute terror.

Historical Aspects

In children, these parasomnias are often referred to as *pavor nocturnus*, which is the direct Latin translation for "night terror." The term *sleep terrors* is preferable to *night terrors* because episodes may occur during daytime naps as well as during sleep at night. The medieval interpretation was that something, usually the devil, was pressing on the chest of the sleeper, causing feelings of suffocation and terror. This interpretation is the basis of the term *incubus* attack (Latin *in* for "upon," and *cubare* for "to press") sometimes used to designate these attacks in adults. It is also the basis of the synonym "nightmare" in which *mar*, the Teutonic word for "devil," is combined with the usual nocturnal occurrence. Ernst Jones[23] was one of the first to clearly distinguish the sleep terror, which he called the true nightmare, from the terrifying dream. Unfortunately, the term "nightmare" has been used to denote both of these distinctly different parasomnias. Gastaut and Broughton[1] first showed that sleep terrors are not associated with REM sleep and its dream mentation but rather that they begin in deep SWS and are associated with marked tachycardia, tachypnea, and a precipitous decrease in skin resistance. Fisher et al.[16] later confirmed these features and noted that sleep terror severity, when measured as the degree of heart rate increase, is greater after longer durations of prior SWS. This group also introduced the use of benzodiazepine therapy for sleep terrors.[24]

Pathophysiology

Sleep terrors have an important genetic component. They have been described as occurring across three generations of one family.[25] As many as 90% of patients have a family history of sleep terrors or sleepwalking.[26] Although an autosomal dominant pattern of inheritance was first suggested by Hallstrom,[25] others have proposed a two-threshold, multifactorial mode of inheritance.[26] The cause of the remarkable intensity of the arousal remains unexplained. Parkes[27] suggested a lack of endogenous benzodiazepine receptor ligands because benzodiazepine antagonists can induce autonomic disturbances and anxiety episodes that are quite similar to sleep terrors.[28]

Psychopathology is extremely rare in children with sleep terrors, despite the impressive intensity of the attacks. Kales et al.[29] reported it to be much more frequent in adults. These authors found that adults have phobias, depression, or anxiety and often have high scores on the Minnesota Multiphasic Personality Inventory (MMPI) for depression, psychaesthenia, and schizophrenia in association with personality disorders or borderline personality. However, later studies,[30, 31] one involving both sleep terror and sleepwalking patients, have found that the majority of adult patients have essentially normal personality profiles.

Epilepsy is rarely suggested in the mechanism of sleep terrors because ictal fear is an extremely uncommon symptom in complex partial seizures and the EEG at the time never contains discharges. Most patients with sleep terror have daytime EEGs that are entirely normal,[16, 32, 33] although rare cases with minor EEG abnormalities of uncertain clinical significance have been reported.[34] One epileptic patient has been reported who also had sleep terrors and had a typical sleep terror occur with a SWS arousal that evolved into a generalized tonic-clonic grand mal seizure.[35]

During an attack, the polysomnogram shows explosive arousal with marked increases in muscle tone, heart rate, and respiratory rate, plus a rapid decrease in skin resistance. These features suggest a state of cerebral hyperresponsiveness, a concept supported by the tendency for greater heart rate increases in arousal even independent of sleep terror attacks and by daytime exaggerated startle and orienting responses in such patients.[36] Because sleep terror episodes can at times be induced by forced arousals independent of ongoing mental activity, the characteristic subjective features of acute terror, palpitations, and difficulty in breathing all appear to be secondary to the marked tachycardia, tachypnea, and increased muscle tone rather than the inverse.

Epidemiology

The peak prevalence of sleep terrors occurs between 5 and 7 years of age,[37] and the peak frequency of episodes usually occurs soon after the onset of the condition.[38] Recurrent sleep terrors occur in 1 to 6% of prepubertal children.[29, 39, 40] Episodes reduce in frequency with approach of adolescence such that 50% of children no longer have attacks by age 8, and 36% continue to have attacks into adolescence.[38] The prevalence in adults is less than 1%; in most instances, this represents a continuation of episodes since adolescence, although the rare occurrence of onset in adulthood has been reported. The occurrence in boys and girls is about equal.[26, 38]

Clinical Features

Attacks usually arise abruptly from a deep sleep during the first third of the night, although when particularly frequent, they may occur at any time of night. They can also occur during daytime naps. The episodes typically consist of sitting up in bed and producing an intense piercing "primal" scream associated with a facial expression of acute terror. The patient shows marked increases in pulse rate, respiration, widened pupils, and, at times, marked sweating. Subjectively, after becoming fully awake, the person often describes palpitations and difficulty in breathing. Recall of any mental activity is either absent or consists of a single image like a still photograph rather than a series of images typical of a dream.[1, 2, 41] When present, this single image often has features of respiratory oppression such as a pile of rocks on the chest. Although sleep terrors usually have no serious side effects, occasional injuries may occur or violent behavior may be associ-

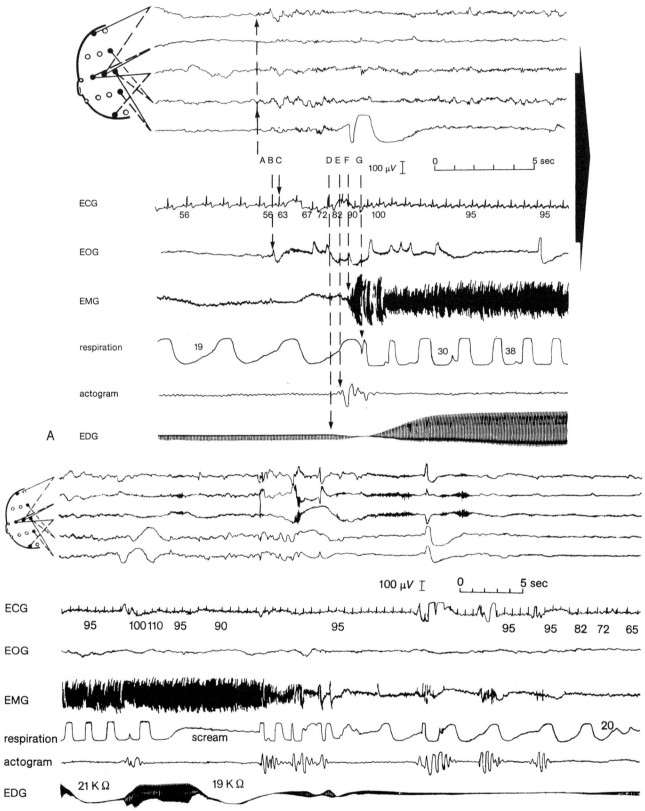

Figure 62–2. Sleep terror in a man. *A,* The episode began in stage 2 sleep and consisted in rapid sequence of some initial EEG synchronization (A), initial eye movement (B), start of tachycardia (C), decreasing skin resistance on the electrodermogram (D), bed movement (E), marked increase in submental muscle tone (F), and start of tachypnea (G), all of which occurred abruptly within 5 sec. *B,* This is followed by extreme tachycardia reaching 110 beats/min, a loud expiratory scream, and continued decreasing skin resistance (sweating) associated with a low-voltage artifacted EEG. Within 40 sec after the start, heart and respiratory rates are at preepisode levels. ECG, electrocardiogram; EDG, electrodermogram; EMG, electromyogram; EOG, electro-oculogram.

ated.[42-44] It seems that adults with heart disease might be at risk during sleep terrors, and it has even been suggested that this parasomnia may be the cause of at least some cases of the so-called unexplained nocturnal death syndrome.[45] Episodes may be triggered by environmental noises, a partner climbing into bed, or other stimuli. After an attack, patients may show difficulty in falling back to sleep. Some develop a form of sleep-onset insomnia for fear of attacks that together with deteriorated sleep quality may produce excessive daytime sleepiness.

The attacks typically last from 30 sec to 5 min—rarely longer. Variations in the typical attack pattern may occur, including partial attacks or direct evolution into sleepwalking, in which case, after the behavior of terror has subsided, the patient leaves the bed and starts to wander about.

Sleep terrors have been described in association with fever,[46] which increases SWS, with the sudden rebound in SWS that occurs when a patient with obstructive sleep apnea is begun on nasal continuous positive airway pressure (CPAP) therapy[47]; with pregnancy,[48] which disrupts sleep; and with NREM sleep arousals during a hypersomniac period in a patient with Kleine-Levin syndrome.[49] Potential facilitating and precipitating factors are summarized in Table 62–1.

Diagnostic Evaluation

The minimal clinical features for a diagnosis of sleep terrors include the occurrence of sudden episodes of terror during sleep, typically during the first third of the night, associated with partial or complete amnesia for events during the episode and the absence of other medical causes of the episode, such as epilepsy.

The polysomnogram during episodes typically shows onset in SWS[1, 2, 16] with rapid activation of the EEG into low-voltage rapid patterns associated with marked tachycardia on the electrocardiographic channel with heart rate often doubling compared with pre-attack levels,[15] tachypnea often interrupted by a slow expiration at the time of the piercing scream, and a precipitous decrease in skin resistance, reflecting the presence of sweating (Fig. 62–2). When attacks recur frequently during a single night of recording, they may also begin in stage 2 sleep. Attack frequency is decreased during laboratory recordings compared with during the normal home sleeping environment.

It is at times possible to precipitate attacks in persons with sleep terrors by simple forced arousal in SWS. Polysomnograms in sleep terror patients on nights without attacks may show frequent direct transitions from SWS to wake[15] (Fig. 62–3), as well as non-event arousals with quite marked increases of heart rate although not to the levels recorded during actual sleep terror episodes.

Differential Diagnosis

REM nightmares[24] are readily distinguished by their usual occurrence during the second half and mainly last third of the night, when REM sleep is most prominent; the recall of detailed dream activity, of which the content becomes threatening to the person before awakening; the rarity of actual screaming as opposed to vocalizations; a lesser degree of palpitations and dyspnea; and the absence of postepisode confusion. Polysomnographic studies confirm their occurrence in REM sleep.

Nocturnal panic attacks may at times clinically resemble sleep terrors, and episodes may arise out of NREM sleep usually stage 2 or 3.[50] Psychopathology

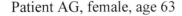

Patient AG, female, age 63

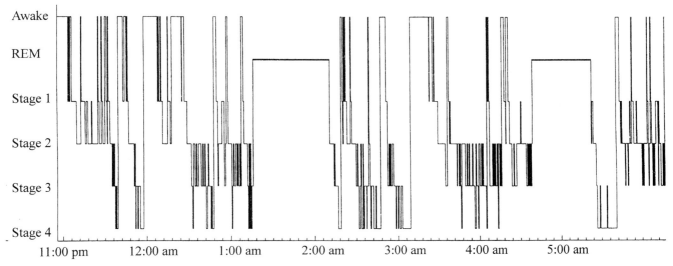

Figure 62–3. Histogram of the sleep of an adult sleep terror patient on a night without episodes. Sleep architecture is characterized by frequent stages shifts during NREM sleep plus high frequency of direct slow-wave sleep (SWS)–to-wake transitions, whereas REM sleep remains unfragmented. SWS-to-wake transitions are rare in normal subjects, with more than two or three a night being exceptional.

is common, and there always are similar episodes in daytime wakefulness, which is not true in patients with sleep terrors.

Confusional arousals seldom are difficult to distinguish because they lack the element of terror and have little autonomic activation.

Complex partial seizures with fear are extremely rare, usually show typical stereotyped automatisms, may be associated with similar episodes beginning in daytime wakefulness, and show a coexistent EEG epileptic discharge. It has been found in patients with epilepsy that attacks of nighttime terror are almost always nonepileptic sleep terror episodes rather than epileptic seizures.[51]

Other conditions may occasionally produce nocturnal fear but typically do so without the acute terror and scream characteristic of sleep terrors; these conditions include obstructive sleep apnea, nocturnal choking syndrome, nocturnal cardiac ischemia, and others, all of which are usually readily distinguished by their typical features.

Management

As in all three NREM arousal disorders, the attacks should be allowed to terminate spontaneously and no effort should be made to interfere. When childhood sleep terrors are rare and cause little family upset, treatment may be unnecessary. Parents should be reassured that the attacks rarely produce harm or injury and that most likely they will be outgrown over a period of several months or a few years.

Facilitating and precipitating causes should be identified and, if possible, avoided; these can include periods of sleep deprivation, ingestion of CNS-depressant substances, and stress.

Diazepam at a dose of 5 to 10 mg before retiring[24, 51] has long been known to be effective for most patients and was introduced because of its known suppression of SWS. Its effectiveness does not parallel that of the degree of SWS reduction, and the mechanism may well relate to reduction in autonomic arousal or reduction in muscle tone increase during the attacks.[52] Unfortunately, the long half-life of diazepam and its metabolites often leads to daytime sedation. Better results have been reported with shorter-acting benzodiazepines such as midazolam,[53] oxazepam, and, especially, clonazepam at the usual evening doses of 10 to 20 mg, 10 to 20 mg, and 0.5 to 2 mg, respectively. Patients unresponsive to benzodiazepines may benefit from treatment with tricyclic antidepressants such as clomipramine, desipramine, or imipramine at the usual doses of 10 to 50 mg before retiring.[54–56] The mechanism of action of tricyclic antidepressants is uncertain but may involve reduced intensity of the onset of REM sleep, which can terminate periods of NREM sleep. In chronic attacks with patients receiving long-term medication, it appears that the episodes themselves are part of the process of fragmented sleep. If the total control of episodes occurs and is sustained for several months, a slow progressive and stepwise withdrawal of medication

may lead to permanent cessation of episodes. In other patients, attacks recur in clusters for several days or weeks, and drug therapy may be necessary only during these periods.

Stress reduction through such techniques as relaxation therapy and autogenic training may be very helpful, as may psychotherapy in adults with psychopathology.[57] Hypnosis has also proved to be useful in individual cases.[58–61]

SLEEPWALKING (SOMNAMBULISM)

Definition

Sleepwalking consists of recurrent episodes in which the subject arises from a deep sleep, typically during the first third of the night, and shows complex behavioral automatisms that include leaving the bed and walking for some distance.

Historical Aspects

Interest in sleepwalking has been reflected in the medical literature for centuries, and the condition was traditionally considered to be acting out a dream. In 1965, Gastaut and Broughton[1] and Jacobson et al.[62] independently confirmed that the condition began in NREM sleep, usually in deep SWS rather than in REM sleep, and that it was associated with little, if any, recall of either dream-like mentation or the behavioral automatisms themselves. It was also noted that forced arousals could precipitate attacks in predisposed individuals.[1, 2, 41]

Pathophysiology

Genetic factors are important in the predisposition to sleepwalking. About 80% of sleepwalkers have an immediate family history of either sleepwalking or sleep terrors,[26] and 10 to 20% have one or more first-degree relatives with sleepwalking.[63–65] There also is an increased occurrence of deep sleepers in the extended family. Sleepwalking has been described in twins, with a higher concordance in monozygotic than in dizygotic pairs.[66] Kales et al.[26] proposed that the mode of inheritance is recessive with incomplete penetrance. Sleeptalking is more frequent in sleepwalkers than in the general population, with an incidence of about 30 versus 5%.[65]

Some have suggested that sleepwalking may be related to CNS "immaturity" expressed in the appearance of high-amplitude slow waves at the start of an episode[41, 62, 67] and in the more frequent than usual persistence of such activity into an older age.[37] However, there has been no compelling evidence for any organic CNS abnormalities in sleepwalkers. Daytime EEGs are usually normal[32, 33] but have occasionally been reported to show minor abnormalities sometimes of epileptiform type; the clinical significance of these remains questionable. No EEG discharges have been reported during typical sleepwalking episodes, and similar behaviors do not occur during daytime wakefulness.

Psychopathology does not appear to be involved in childhood cases,[68] although as in sleep terrors, this may not be true for adults. It has been said that more than 70% of adults with sleepwalking have a coexistent psychiatric diagnosis, usually in the form of a character disorder.[68] Traits that have variously been described in adult-onset cases include impulsivity, antisocial behaviors, and hypomania, and adults may have MMPI scores showing evidence for mania, psychopathic deviation, and schizoid characteristics.[68, 69] Other studies have not confirmed these findings.[6, 30] Moreover, in most instances in which psychopathology is present, it is not usually known whether the personality characteristics predated or followed the onset of sleepwalking.

Deep SWS is important as the matrix from which sleepwalking most commonly takes place. The condition is more common in childhood, when sleep is deeper. The depth of sleep in sleepwalkers is more pronounced than in the population at large,[62] and the occurrence of episodes can be facilitated by a number of factors that increase SWS or the arousal threshold, (i.e, that deepen sleep). These factors include recovery sleep from prior sleep deprivation as in the start of the use of CPAP in patients with sleep apnea,[70] fever,[46] and effects of CNS-depressant medication such as lithium, triazolam, barbiturates, and alcohol.[71-75]

Factors that deepen sleep are usually combined with factors that cause multiple arousals or sleep fragmentation, such as stress, environmental stimuli, pain, and even pregnancy. In sleepwalkers, forced arousals of patients in deep SWS may induce a full-blown episode.[1, 2] Arousals in sleep may also be the role of the heightened incidence of somnambulism in children with migraine[76, 77] or Gilles de la Tourette's syndrome.[78] The potential facilitating and triggering factors are summarized (see Table 62-1).

The fundamental pathophysiology appears to be the inability of the brain to fully awaken from a deep sleep for a period during which complex ambulatory automatisms, including leaving the bed and walking, are elaborated.

Epidemiology

Sleepwalking is common in young children. About 15 to 30% of healthy children have been found to have had at least one episode, and about 3 to 4% of children have frequent episodes.[68, 79, 80] In childhood, the peak age of onset of episodes is at around 5 years of age, with the peak prevalence at about 12 years.[39, 80] Most children outgrow the episodes by age 15. In adults, the prevalence is somewhat greater than that of sleep terrors and is about 1% for chronic sufferers.[68] Adult sleepwalking usually represents a continuation from adolescence, although rarely, adult onset can occur. Sleepwalking is extremely uncommon after the 6th decade, when sleep normally becomes much lighter than earlier. There is no difference in incidence between the genders.[80, 81]

Clinical Features

Sleepwalking episodes usually begin during the first 3 h of sleep as relatively quiescent motor activity in bed in which the subject first sits up, may look about with a relatively blank facial expression, and shows gestural automatic behaviors such as picking at the bedcovers, rearranging the pillows, or other such activities. The person then gets out of bed and may move around the bedroom, go to other rooms, or even, rarely, leave the house. Movements generally are more clumsy and less well executed than those in full wakefulness. Patients may trip over furniture or knock over objects. Often, however, quite complex behaviors[82] may occur, such as attempts at cooking, eating food,[83] playing a musical instrument, or cleaning house. Driving a car during sleepwalking has even been reported.[84] Many movements in the home may in fact appear to be purposeless. There may be verbal utterances, vocalization, or even sleeptalking including full conversations while asleep. There never is, however, the intense scream other than in the rare hybrid attacks that consist of typical sleep terrors evolving into sleepwalking. Self-injuries are not uncommon because sleepwalkers may walk through glass doors, break windows and receive cuts, pound walls and injure their hands, or simply trip and hurt themselves.

During a sleepwalking episode, the subject shows reduced responsiveness to environmental stimuli, including calling of the person's name. Vigorous attempts to awaken subjects often do not lead to full arousal and may induce resistance and even violence. Violence without such resistance to the behaviors appears to be relatively rare. There are a number of episodes of highly aggressive behaviors, including stranglings, stabbings, and even homicidal behaviors, described in sleepwalking. A highly documented instance is the well known case of Ken Parks, a sleepwalker with a strong family history who, after falling asleep at home, arose to drive to the residence of his parents-in-law, strangled his father-in-law into unconsciousness, and lethally stabbed his mother-in-law. The details of history, predisposing factors, precipitating factors, polysomnographic findings, psychiatric and psychological workup, absence of motive or gain, amnesia, and other features best fit a sleepwalking explanation.[85]

Most sleepwalking episodes last less than 15 min, but there are descriptions of episodes with a duration as long a 1 h and, extremely rarely, even longer. At the end of the episode, patients most frequently go back to bed and return quickly to sleep. Children not infrequently crawl into their parents' bed. If awakened during an episode, there typically is a total lack of recall of previous behaviors and of any dream-like or other mentation. In a few instances, there are reported hallucinations.[86] Occasionally, there is partial recall of events, especially those toward the end of the episode. Sleepwalkers who are not awakened and who go back to bed almost never recall the episode the next morning. Sleepwalkers may also show incomplete episodes, which often consist of sitting up and looking about without actually leaving the bed.[1] Patients with sleepwalking show higher incidences than normal of confusional arousals, sleep terrors, and, for children, enuresis nocturna. As previously mentioned, there also is an increased incidence of sleepwalking in patients with migraine-type vascular headache and with Tourette's syndrome.

Diagnostic Evaluation

As in the other NREM arousal parasomnias, diagnosis requires a detailed general medical and sleep history plus a physical examination. Patients in whom seizures are in any way suspected should undergo one or several daytime diagnostic EEGs, and their polysomnograms should include a full-scalp EEG. Although the diagnosis of sleepwalking may often be made by history alone, many patients will benefit from having a polysomnogram performed.

The polysomnogram shows that sleepwalking episodes begin in association with an arousal in stage 3 or 4 of SWS.[1, 2, 41, 62] Although "hypersynchronous" delta waves preceding the arousal have been reported,[41, 62] this finding has not been replicated.[87] The EEG may at times be obscured by muscle artifact. Over several or dozens of seconds, the EEG then decreases in amplitude and increases in frequency, usually with the appearance either of low- to medium-amplitude, mixed-frequency patterns typical of stage 1 or the appearance of a diffuse alpha rhythm 1 to 2 Hz slower than the subject's waking alpha rhythms and unresponsive to eye opening or even intense visual stimulation.[1] Telemetric studies show that these patterns persist throughout the episode[1] (Fig. 62–4). The EEG never shows potentially epileptogenic ("epileptiform") discharges. The electrocardiographic and respiration channels do not contain the extreme tachycardia with tachypnea characteristic of sleep terrors. During the brief

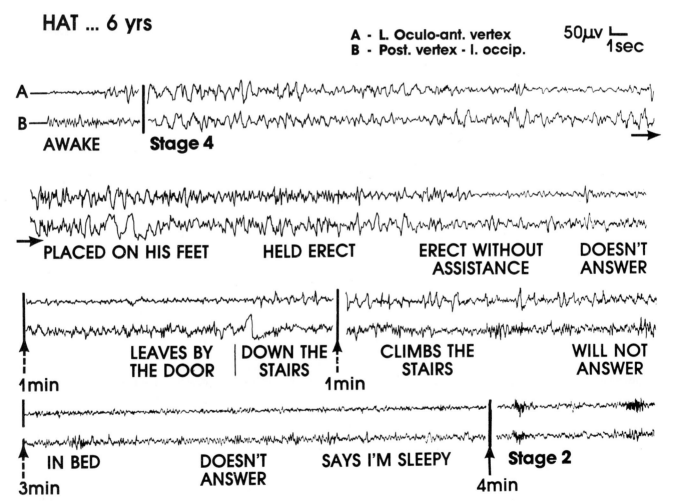

Figure 62–4. Induced sleepwalking recorded by telemetry in a 6-year-old boy. The episode begins during stage 4 sleep when the child was put on his feet. He got out of bed, left the bedroom, and descended three steps outside. He was later led back up the stairs to his bed by the technologist. Three minutes later, on persistent questioning, he mumbled "I'm sleepy" and soon afterward was in stage 2. Several minutes later he was awakened and had no recall of events. The EEG during the entire episode never reached full waking patterns.

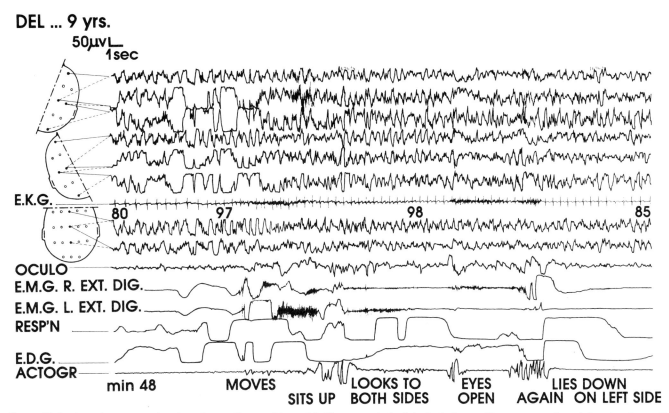

DEL ... 9 yrs.

Figure 62–5. Complex automatism in a sleepwalker, a girl aged 9. She sat up in bed, looked about with eyes opened, and then lay down. To an observer, this behavior appears to represent wakefulness, yet the EEG, as best seen in the unartifacted vertex leads, had significant slow wave activity throughout. After the episode, she was awakened (with some effort) and had no recollection of the episode.

incomplete episodes of sitting and looking about, the EEG may show slow wave activity throughout without apparent lightening of sleep stage[1] (Fig. 62–5). This finding indicates the extraordinary dissociation of behavioral events resembling wakefulness with an EEG of deep sleep.

Independent of the sleepwalking episodes and on nights without attacks, the polysomnogram may show an increased frequency of both slow wave to wake arousals[88] and of brief microarousals with slow waves,[89] both of which appear to represent partial manifestations of the same underlying arousal dysfunction expressed as sleep fragmentation without clinical events but do not represent specific diagnostic features.

There is evidence for a decrease in incidence of sleepwalking episodes in the laboratory, so even those rare patients with almost nightly episodes should have two or more nights reserved in the sleep laboratory. Ambulatory monitoring has also proved to be useful in our laboratories and in those of others[90] in the investigation of the attacks. Videotelemetry[91] is very helpful because it permits the correlation of videotaped behavior and polysomnographic features.

Differential Diagnosis

Usually, the diagnosis of sleepwalking is clear based on history alone. The main features of a number of common parasomnias are summarized in Table 62–2;

however, in some patients there may be confusion with complex partial seizures, "episodic nocturnal wanderings," dissociative disorder, RBD, or even malingering.

Complex partial seizures usually of inferomesial temporal or frontal lobe origin may lead to nocturnal automatisms with walking about. The behaviors are often quite different, however, and most often include highly stereotyped and repeated hand wringing, stomach rubbing, or swallowing. Patients typically do not return to bed. Postictal confusion may be present, and seizures may secondarily generalize into tonic-clonic grand mal attacks. Epileptic seizures may occur in any type of sleep and can be distributed across the night. In some patients, seizures take place only in REM sleep[20] and then are present mainly in the second half of the night and may be associated with vivid dreaming or even nightmares. Similar complex partial seizures may occur in wakefulness. The ictal EEG at night or during daytime attacks usually shows an organized epileptic discharge (although discharges deep in hemispheres or on their mesial surface may not reach scalp electrodes), and between attacks, interictal EEG abnormalities may also be recorded. Patients with attacks and EEG discharges may respond to antiepileptic medication.

Episodic nocturnal wanderings is a term introduced to describe attacks of nocturnal wanderings, often with atypical behavioral features, in which the polysomnogram EEG at the time of the episode does not exhibit an epileptic discharge but daytime EEGs do show potentially epileptogenic discharges; patients with these episodes respond to anticonvulsant medication.[92, 93] The cause of these episodes is not known for certain, but they are presumed to be of epileptic origin.

The nocturnal wanderings of dissociative disorder consist of psychogenic fugue-like states that begin and occur during waking periods at night.[94, 95] Patients have a very high incidence of childhood sexual abuse. Similar daytime psychogenic fugues may be present. Episodes are extremely rare in childhood, when sleepwalking is most common. There is an absence of the usual family history of sleepwalking, sleep terrors, and confusional arousals. Such patients require a detailed psychiatric work-up and treatment.

RBD is usually easily distinguished from sleepwalking by its typically explosive behaviors such as leaping out of bed, often with intense myoclonus; its usual occurrence in the second half of the night, when REM sleep is most common; the detailed recall of dreams; and the typical adult age of the patient. Organic brain pathology may be present. Polysomnography shows REM sleep without atonia both during and outside the episodes.[16, 17]

Nocturnal wanderings beginning in REM sleep have been described in elderly patients with Alzheimer's disease and are readily distinguished by the time of night and the clinical context.[18]

Malingering must also be considered, although it seems unlikely that someone could fabricate an appropriate personal and family history and certainly would not show the typical polysomnographic features on nonevent and event nights.[85]

Confusional awakenings from sleep that are not true sleepwalking episodes may occur in patients taking CNS-depressant substances such as alcohol, sedatives, and hypnotic agents. In such instances, when the patients are awakened, they may have long-lasting mental confusion and some degree of automatic behavior.

Management

Appropriate management requires accurate diagnosis, which in turn necessitates a careful general medical and sleep history, including personal and family history of parasomnias. Essential features are a careful and detailed description of the episodes, the documentation of predisposing and triggering factors, age of onset, and time of night of occurrence. The possibility of an epileptic mechanism should always be raised in patients with an onset of attacks in adulthood, with similar episodes in daytime wakefulness, or, of course, with a known diagnosis of epilepsy. Daytime and nocturnal full-scalp EEGs should be performed in all patients with suspected nocturnal seizures.

In patients in whom predisposing and triggering factors can be determined, every effort should be made to avoid them; these may include self-induced or externally induced periods of sleep deprivation, stresses at school, home, or work, environmental noises, and the taking of alcohol or other CNS-depressant substances (Table 62–1). All efforts should be made to avoid injury

by, for instance, moving dangerous objects from the bedroom, adding special locks to doors or windows, putting heavy drapes in front of windows or glass doors, or other such strategies as are suggested by the details of the patient's typical episodes. During a sleepwalking episode, attempts may be made to gently guide the person back to bed without causing awakening. Many sleepwalkers will, however, ignore such efforts, and strong stimuli may meet resistance or even induce aggression and therefore should be avoided.

In prepubertal sleepwalkers, the condition is often self-limiting, and patients usually outgrow the episodes, probably as sleep lightens. Treatment may then be unnecessary, and parents may usually be reassured that the condition does not reflect serious emotional problems and that the child is not at risk and in time will probably no longer have the attacks. With an onset in adolescence or adulthood, psychiatric aspects may become prominent and, when present, usually require assessment and management. Treatments may then include psychotherapy,[96–98] stress management, or relaxation therapy. Hypnosis,[99, 100] sometimes supplemented by psychotherapy, has proved to be effective and often will long-lasting benefits in a number of patients, especially adults.[61] Success rates of up to 50% have been reported in adult patients with hypnosis alone.[61]

Medication may be helpful. Many patients respond to benzodiazepines, especially triazolam, clonazepam, and diazepam in the usual evening doses. As in the treatment of sleep terrors, these benzodiazepine drugs were introduced because they reduce EEG slow waves; however, there is no correlation between the SWS reduction and the clinical efficacy. Tricyclic drugs such as imipramine, desipramine, and clomipramine in the usual evening doses of 10 to 50 mg may also be effective. A more specific action has been reported for the tricyclic compound amineptine,[101] which is not in North America. Carbamazepine at 100 to 200 mg/day has also been effective in a few patients with sleepwalking. In many patients, sleepwalking episodes occur in clusters for several days or weeks and then disappear for a period of times, only to reappear. In such patients, intermittent drug therapy often is effective, and the complications of long-term drug exposure are avoided. Sometimes, a longer treatment trial, lasting 6 months or more, may be necessary, especially in patients with very frequent episodes or with violent behavior.

The response to drug treatment must be very carefully assessed in these patients. There are a number of potential complications other than usual side effects of medication. There often is a relapse after the discontinuation of medication, especially if withdrawal is rapid. In some patients, benzodiazepines and tricyclic antidepressants may actually precipitate attacks.[72–75] Daytime somnolence may occur, especially with drugs such as diazepam, which have active metabolites with long half-lives. These drugs may also produce nocturnal confusional episodes, especially in the elderly, sometimes with serious falls and fractures. They should therefore either be avoided in this age group or be prescribed with great care and at low doses with careful patient monitoring. As for sleep terrors, it often seems that recurrence of episodes perpetuates the process, leading to further attacks. After patients with initially frequent sleepwalking are totally controlled for 4 to 6 months, it often is possible to reduce medication very progressively over a period of months leading to a lasting cessation of attacks.

References

1. Gastaut H, Broughton RJ. A clinical and polygraphic study of episodic phenomena during sleep. Biol Psychiatry. 1965;7:197–221.
2. Broughton RJ. Sleep disorders: disorders of arousal? Science. 1968;159:1070–1078.
3. Diagnostic Classification Steering Committee. International Classification of Sleep Disorders Diagnostic and Scoring Manual. Rochester, Minn: American Sleep Disorders Association; 1990.
4. Benoit O, Goldenberg-Leygonie F. Is sleepwalking related to REM sleep? Sleep Res. 1977;6:163.
5. Kushida CA, Clerk AA, Kirsch CM, et al. Prolonged confusion with nocturnal wandering arising from NREM and REM sleep: a case report. Sleep. 1995;18:747–764.
6. Schenck CH, Boyd JL, Mahowald MW. A parasomnia overlap disorder involving sleepwalking, sleep terrors and REM sleep behavior disorder in 33 polysomnographically confirmed cases. Sleep. 1997;20:972–981.
7. Marc C. De la Folie. Paris, France: Ballière; 1840.
8. Von Gudden H. Die physiologische und pathologische Schlaftrunkenheit. Arch Psychiatry Nervenkrank. 1905;40:989–1015.
9. Roth B, Nevsimalova S, Sagova V, et al. Neurological, psychological and polygraphic findings in sleep drunkenness. Arch Suisse Neurol Neurochirurg Psychiatr. 1981;129:209–222.
10. Stones M. Memory performance after arousal from different sleep stages. Br J Psychol. 1977;66:177–181.
11. Feltin M, Broughton R. Differential effects of arousal from slow wave versus REM sleep. Psychophysiology. 1968;5:231.
12. Lubin A, Hord DJ, Tracy ML, et al. Effects of exercise, bedrest and napping on performance decrement during 40 hours. Psychophysiology. 1976;13:334–339.
13. Dinges DF. Are you awake? Cognitive performance during the hypnopompic state. In: Bootzin R, Kihlstrom J, Schacter D, eds. Sleep and Cognition. Washington, DC: American Psychological Association; 1990:159–175.
14. Ferber R. Sleep disorders in infants and children. In: Riley TL, eds. Clinical Aspects of Sleep and Sleep Disturbance. Boston, Mass: Butterworths; 1985:113–158.
15. Broughton R. Phasic and dynamic aspects of sleep: a symposium review and synthesis. In: Terzano MG, Halasz P, Declerck AC, ed. Phasic Events and the Dynamic Organization of Sleep. New York, NY: Raven; 1991:85–205.
16. Fisher C, Kahn E, Edwards A, et al. A psychophysiological study of nightmares and night terrors, I: physiological aspects of the stage 4 terror. J Nerv Ment Dis. 1973;157:75–98.
17. Schenck CH, Bundlie SR, Ettinger MG, et al. Chronic behavioral disorders of human REM sleep: a new category of parasomnia. Sleep. 1986;9:293–308.
18. Schenck CH, Bundlie SR, Patterson AL, et al. Rapid eye movement sleep behavior disorder: a treatable parasomnia affecting older adults. JAMA. 1987;257:1986–1989.
19. Hishikawa Y, Sugita Y, Teshima Y, et al. Sleep disorders in alcoholic patients with delerium tremens. In: Karajan I, ed. Psychophysiological Aspects of Sleep. Park Ridge, NJ: Noyes Medical; 1981:109–122.
20. Passouant P. Sleep and epilepsy. In: Koella WP, Levin P, eds. Sleep 1976. Basel, Switzerland: Karger; 1977:37–79.
21. Broughton R. Epilepsy and sleep: a synopsis and prospectus. In: Degen R, Niedermeyer E, eds. Epilepsy, Sleep and Sleep Deprivation. Amsterdam, Netherlands: Elsevier; 1984:317–356.
22. Lugaresi E, Cirignotta F, Montagna P. Nocturnal paroxysmal dystonia. J Neurol Neurosurg Psychiatry. 1986;9:375–380.
23. Jones E. On the Nightmare. Philadelphia, Pa: Hogarth; 1949.
24. Fisher C, Kahn E, Edwards A, et al. A psychophysiological study of nightmares and sleep terrors: the suppression of stage 4 night terrors with diazepam. Arch Gen Psychiatry. 1973;28:252–259.
25. Hallstrom R. Night terror in adults through three generations. Acta Psychiatr Scand. 1972;48:350–352.
26. Kales A, Soldatos CR, Bixler EO, et al. Hereditary factors in sleep walking and night terrors. Br J Psychiatry. 1980;137:111–118.
27. Parks JD. Sleep and Its Disorders. Philadelphia, PA: WB Saunders; 1985:187–241.
28. Dorow R, Howowski R, Paschelke G, et al. Severe anxiety induced by FG-7142, a β-carboline ligand for benzodiazepine receptors. Lancet. 1983;2:98–99.
29. Kales JD, Kales A, Soldatos CR, et al. Night terrors: clinical characteristics and personality patterns. Arch Gen Psychiatry. 1980;37:1413–1417.
30. Hartmann E, Greenwald, D, Brune P. Night terrors–sleepwalking: personality characteristics. Sleep Res. 1982;11:121.
31. Llorente MD, Currier MB, Norman SE, et al. Night terrors in adults: phenomenology and relationship to psychopathology. J Clin Psychiatry. 1992;53:392–394.
32. Christatos C, Dascalov D. Correlations between clinical and electroencephalographic findings in children with night terrors and somnambulism. Acta Neuropsychiatr. 1970;37:61–67.
33. Soldatos CR, Vela-Bueno A, Bixler EO, et al. Sleepwalking and night terrors in adulthood: clinical EEG findings. Clin Electroencephalogr. 1980;11:136–139.
34. Fuster B, Cassells C, Etcheverry M. Epileptic sleep terrors. Neurology. 1954;4:531–540.
35. Passouant P, Billiard M, Paquet J. Terreurs nocturnes et crises épileptiques chez l' enfant. Lyons Méd. 1973;9:547–556.
36. Rogozea R, Florea-Giogoiu V. Responsiveness disturbances in patients with sleep terrors. Neurol Psychiatr (Bucur). 1983;21:83–96.
37. Kurth VE, Gohler I, Knaape H. Untersuchungen über der Pavor Nocturnus bei Kinderen. Psychiatr Neurol Med Psychol (Leipzig). 1965;17:1–7.
38. DiMario FJ, Emery ES. The natural history of night terrors. Clin Pediatr. 1987;26:505–511.
39. Klackenberg G. Incidence of parasomnias in children in a general population. In: Guilleminault C, ed. Sleep and Its Disorders in Children. New York; NY: Raven; 1987:99–115.
40. Beltrammini AV, Hertzig ME. Sleep and bedtime behavior in preschool-aged children. Pediatrics. 1983;71:153–158.
41. Jacobson A, Kales A. Somnambulism: all-night EEG and related studies. In: Kety, SS, Evarts EV, Williams HL, eds. Sleep and Altered States of Consciousness. Baltimore, MD: Williams & Wilkins; 1967:424–455.
42. Rauch PK, Stern TA. Life threatening injuries resulting from sleepwalking and night terrors. Psychosomatics. 1986;27:62–64.
43. Hartmann E. Two case reports: night terrors with sleepwalking, a potentially lethal disorder. J Nerv Ment Dis. 1983;171:503–550.
44. Broughton R, Shimizu T. Dangerous behaviors by night. In: Shapiro C, McCall-Smith A, ed. Forensic Aspects of Sleep. New York; NY: John Wiley & Sons; 1996:65–83.
45. Melles RB, Katz B. Sudden, unexplained nocturnal death syndrome and night terrors. JAMA. 1987;257:2918–2919.
46. Kales JD, Kales A, Soldatos CR, et al. Sleepwalking and night terrors related to febrile illness. Am J Psychiatry. 1979;135:418–424.
47. Pressman M, Meyer TJ, Kendrick-Mohamed J, et al. Night terrors in an adult precipitated by sleep apnea. Sleep. 1995;18:773–775.
48. Synder S. An unusual case of sleep terror in a pregnant patient. Ann J Psychiatry. 1986;143:391.
49. Stirano S, Bilo L, Meo R. An unusual case of Kleine-Levin syndrome associated with sleep terrors. Electroencephalogr Clin Neurophysiol. 1986;64:517–520.
50. Mellman TA, Uhde TW. Electroencephalographic study of nighttime panic attacks. Arch Gen Psychiatry. 1989;46:178–184.
51. Tassinari CA, Mancia D, Della Bernardina B, et al. Pavor nocturnus of nonepileptic nature in epileptic children. Electroencephalogr Clin Neurophysiol. 1972;33:603–607.

52. Broughton R. Pathophysiology of enuresis nocturna, sleep terrors and sleepwalking: current status and the Marseille contribution. In: Broughton R, ed. Henri Gastaut and the Marseille School's Contribution to the Neurosciences. Amsterdam, Netherlands: Elsevier; 1982:401–410.

53. Popiviciu L, Corfariu O. Efficacy and safety of midazolam in the treatment of sleep terrors in children. Br J Clin Pharmacol. 1983;16(suppl):97S–102S.

54. Pesikoff RB, Davis PC. Treatment of pavor nocturnus and somnambulism in children. Am J Psychiatry. 1971;128:778–781.

55. Marshall JR. The treatment of night terrors associated with post-traumatic syndrome. Am J Psychiatry. 1975;132:293–295.

56. Cooper AJ. Treatment of coexistant night-terrors and somnambulism in adults with imipramine and diazepam. J Clin Psychiatry. 1987;48:209–110.

57. Kales JC, Cadieux RJ, Soldatos CR, et al. Psychotherapy with night-terror patients. Am J Psychiatry. 1982;36:399–407.

58. Taboada EL. Night terrors in a child treated with hypnosis. Am J Clin Hypnosis. 1975;17:270–271.

59. Koe GG. Hypnosis treatment of Sleep Terror Disorder: a case report. Am J Clin Hypn. 1989;32:36–40.

60. Kohen DP, Mahowald MW, Rosen GM. Sleep-terror disorder in children: role of self-hypnosis in management. Am J Clin Hypn. 1992;34:233–244.

61. Hurwitz TD, Mahowald MW, Schenck CH, et al. A retrospective outcome study and review of hypnosis as a treatment of adults with sleepwalking and sleep terrors. J Nerv Ment Dis. 1991;179:228–233.

62. Jacobson A, Kales A, Lehmann D, et al. Somnambulism: all-night electroencephalographic studies. Science. 1965;148:975–977.

63. Davies E, Hayes M, Kirman BH. Somnambulism. Lancet. 1970:1:186.

64. Abe K, Shimakawa M. Predisposition to sleep walking. Psychiatr Neurol. 1966;152:306–331.

65. Abe K, Amatomi M, Oda N. Sleepwalking and recurrent sleeptalking in children of childhood sleepwalkers. Am J Psychiatry. 1984;141:800–801.

66. Bakwin H. Sleepwalking in twins. Lancet. 1970;2:446–447.

67. Kales A, Jacobson A, Paulson MJ, et al. Somnambulism: psycho-physiologic correlates, I: all-night EEG studies. Arch Gen Psychiatry. 1966:14:84–94.

68. Kales A, Soldatos C, Caldwell AB, et al. Somnambulism: clinical characteristics and personality patterns. Arch Gen Psychiatry. 1980:37:1406–1410.

69. Sours JA, Frumkin P, Indermill PR. Somnambulism: its clinical significance and dynamic meaning in late adolescence and adulthood. Arch Gen Psychiatry. 1963;9:400–413.

70. Millman RP, Kipp GJ, Carskadon MA. Sleepwalking precipitated by treatment of sleep apnea by nasal CPAP. Chest. 1991;99:750–1.

71. Charney DS, Kales A, Soldatos CR, et al. Somnambulistic-like episodes secondary to combined lithium-neuroleptic treatment. B J Psychiatry. 1979;135:418–424.

72. Glassman JN, Darko D, Gillin JC. Medication-induced somnambulism in a patient with schizoaffective disorder. J Clin Psychiatry. 1986;47:523–524.

73. Huapaya LVM. Somnambulism and bedtime medication. Am J Psychiatry. 1976;133:1207.

74. Huapaya LVM. Seven cases of somnambulism induced by drugs. Am J Psychiatry. 1979;136:985–986.

75. Luchins DJ, Sherwood PM, Gillin JC, et al. Filicide during psychotropic-induced somnambulism: a case report. Am J Psychiatry. 1978;135:1404–1405.

76. Barabas G, Ferrari M, Schemp-Mathews P, et al. Childhood migraine and somnambulism. Neurology. 1983;33:948–949.

77. Giroud M, d'Athis P, Guard O, et al. Migraine et somnambulisme: une enquête portant sur 122 migraineux. Rev Neurol (Paris). 1986;142:42–46.

78. Barabas G, Mathews WS, Ferrari M. Sleepwalking in children with Tourette syndrome. Dev Med Child Neurol. 1984;26:457–460.

79. Fisher BE, Wilson AE. Selected disturbances in school children reported by parents: prevalence interrelationships, behavioral correlates and parental attributions. Percept Mot Skills. 1987;64:1147–1157.

80. Klackenberg G. Somnambulism in childhood: prevalence, course and behavioral correlations. Acta Paediatr Scand. 1982;71:495–499.

81. Cirignotta F, Zucconi M, Mondini S, et al. Enuresis, sleep walking and nightmares: an epidemiological survey in the republic of San Marino. In: Guilleminault C, Lugaresi E, eds. Sleep/Wake Disorders: Natural History, Epidemiology and Long-Term Evolution. New York, NY: Raven; 1983:237–241.

82. Kavey NB, Whyte J, Resor SR, et al. Somnambulism in adults. Neurology. 1990;40:749–752.

83. Whyte J, Kavey NB. Somnambulistic eating: a report of three cases. Int J Eat Disord. 1990;9:577–581.

84. Schenck CH, Mahowald MW. A polysomnographically documented case of adult somnambulism with long-distance automobile driving and frequent nocturnal violence: parasomnia with continuing danger as a non-insane automatism? Sleep. 1995;18:765–772.

85. Broughton R, Billings R, Cartwright R, et al. Homicidal somnambulism: a case report. Sleep. 1994;17:235–264.

86. Kavey NB, Whyte J. Somnambulism associated with hallucinations. Psychosomatics. 1993;34:86–90.

87. Schenck CH, Pareja JA, Patterson AL, et al. Analysis of polysomnographic events surrounding 252 slow-wave sleep arousals in thrity-eight adults with injurious sleepwalking and sleep terrors. J Clin Neurophysiol. 1998;15:159–166.

88. Blatt I, Peled R, Gadoth N, et al. The value of sleep recording in evaluating somnambulism in adults. Electroencephalogr Clin Neurophysiol. 1991;78:407–412.

89. Halasz P, Ujszaszi J, Gadorvo P. Are microarousals preceded by electroencephalographic slow-wave synchronization precursors of confusional awakenings? Sleep. 1985;8:231–238.

90. Guilleminault C, Moscovitch A, Leger D. Forensic sleep medicine: nocturnal wanderings and violence. Sleep. 1995;9:740–748.

91. Mahowald MW, Bundlie SR, Hurwitz TD, et al. Sleep violence–forensic science implications: polygraphic and video documentation. J Forensic Sci. 1990;35:413–432.

92. Pedley TA, Guilleminault C. Episodic nocturnal wanderings responsive to anticonvulsant drug therapy. Ann Neurol. 1977;2:30–35.

93. Maselli RA, Rosenberg RS, Spire J-P. Episodic nocturnal wanderings in non-epileptic young patients. Sleep. 1988;11:156–161.

94. Fleming J. Dissociative episodes presenting as somnambulism. Sleep Res. 1987;16:263.

95. Schenck CH, Milner D, Hurwitz TD, et al. Dissociative disorders presenting as somnambulism: polysomnographic, video and clinical documentation (8 cases). Dissociation. 1989;2:194–204.

96. Reid WH. Treatment of somnambulism in military trainees. Am J Psychiatry. 1975;29:101–105.

97. Gutnik BD, Reid WH. Adult somnambulism: two treatment approaches. Nebr Med J. 1982;67:947–953.

98. Reid WH, Ahmed I, Levie CA. Treatment of sleepwalking: a controlled study. Am J Psychother. 1981;35:27–37.

99. Pai M. Sleepwalking and sleep activities. Br J Psychiatry. 1946;92:756–765.

100. Elsieo TS. The hypnotic treatment of sleepwalking in an adult. Am J Clin Hypnosis. 1975;17:272–276.

101. De Villard R, Dalery J, Mouret J, et al. Le somnambulisme de l'enfant: étude clinique, polygraphique et thérapeutique: à propos de 37 observations. Lyon Med. 1978;240:65–72.

63

Epilepsy and Sleep Disorders

Margaret N. Shouse
Mark W. Mahowald

Sleep, sleep disorders, and epilepsy are frequently associated. It is well known that sleep and sleep deprivation increase the incidence of both parasomnias and seizure activity. Conversely, seizure disorders can affect the wake-sleep cycle.[1-5] Sleep disorders, including parasomnias, may mimic, cause, or even be triggered by epileptic phenomena, and vice versa.

Parasomnias refer to undesirable motor, verbal, or experiential phenomena that occur during sleep.[1, 6] It is these sleep disorders that are most commonly confused with epileptic phenomena. Parasomnias may be conveniently categorized as primary (disorders of sleep states per se) and secondary (disorders of other organ systems that manifest themselves during sleep). The primary sleep parasomnias can be classified according to the sleep state of origin: rapid eye movement (REM) sleep, nonrapid eye movement (NREM) sleep, or miscellaneous (those that occur in either NREM or REM states). The secondary sleep parasomnias can be further classified by the organ system involved.[7]

Epilepsies refer to a host of seizure disorders characterized by uncontrolled, abnormal brain electrical discharges associated with undesirable motor, verbal, or experiential phenomena[8, 9] that often occur during sleep.[2, 3, 9-12] Electroclinical events include *interictal discharges* (IIDs), which are electrographically but not clinically evident, and *ictal events*, which are usually electrographically and clinically evident. There are many ways of classifying seizure disorders.[8] Despite considerable diversity in causes and in specific ictal and interictal discharge characteristics, epileptic seizure manifestations tend to be highly state dependent. NREM sleep is associated with an increased incidence and spread of IIDs; clinical accompaniment is most often associated with localization-related epilepsies originating in the temporal and frontal lobes.[2, 3, 13] REM sleep is a relatively antiepileptic state in that the spread of IID is anatomically localized and clinically evident seizures are usually suppressed.[2, 14-16] Arousal from NREM or REM sleep can also provoke or mimic either seizures or parasomnias.[1, 2, 10, 11, 17-19]

With the advent of neurophysiological monitoring techniques, it has become obvious that state determination is a very complex and dynamic phenomenon that involves multiple neural networks, neurotransmitters, neuropeptides, neurohormones, and a myriad of sleep-promoting substances. Given these complexities, it has become clear that the determination of state may be inexact, with components of two or all three states occurring simultaneously or oscillating rapidly. This concept of state dissociation in animals and human beings has been extensively reviewed.[20, 21]

These mixed or rapidly oscillating states result in fascinating and perplexing clinical phenomena that may easily be confused with epileptic events; conversely, these sleep disorders may be perfectly imitated by epileptic events. Furthermore, other primary sleep disorders may trigger seizures; conversely, seizures may trigger abnormal sleep phenomena. Clinically, there is substantial overlap among epileptic, sleep, and psychiatric phenomena (Table 63–1).

There are five primary determinants of the quality of nighttime sleep and of daytime alertness: (1) homeostatic (duration of prior wakefulness), (2) circadian (biological clock influence), (3) age, (4) drugs, and (5) central nervous system pathology.[22] These factors determine the overall sleep-wake pattern, on which the parasomnias are superimposed. These same factors also play an integral role in epileptic events.

HISTORICAL ASPECTS

In 1965, Gastaut and Broughton[18] reported the clinical and polygraphic characteristics of the sleep-related episodic phenomena in patients. They outlined major symptoms of two major parasomnias: sleepwalking and sleep terrors. Both occur during NREM sleep, usually when the patient emerges from stage 4. Before this study,[18] these parasomnias were associated with seizure disorders. In 1968, Broughton[17] questioned the pathophysiological mechanisms underlying these paroxysmal (sudden) nocturnal events. Although parasomnias and seizure disorders exhibit common features such as abrupt onset, confusion, disorientation, and retrograde amnesia, Broughton proposed that most, if not all, of these episodes could be related to a disorder of arousal rather than to epilepsy.

Table 63–1. OVERLAP BETWEEN SLEEP AND EPILEPTIC PHENOMENA

Symptom	Sleep Disorder	Seizure
Normal sleep phenomena	Sleep starts (hypnic jerks) Nightmares	Seizures manifesting as sleep-onset sensory/motor phenomena or nightmares
Hypersomnia	Sleep deprivation Idiopathic central nervous system	Hypersomnia as a manifestation of having frequent nocturnal seizures resulting in recurrent arousals or hypersomnia as an accompaniment of epilepsy

	Narcolepsy
	    Cataplexy
	    Sleep paralysis
	    Hypnagogic hallucinations
	Automatic behavior
	Recurrent hypersomnia
	    Kleine-Levin syndrome
	    Menstruation related
	Sleep apnea–triggering seizures
		Akinetic
		Fugue states
		    Partial complex seizures
		    Subclinical status
		Poriomania
		Recurrent seizures resulting in prolonged periods of "sleepiness"
		
		Seizures resulting in apnea

Insomnia	Medical Psychiatric Psychological Constitutional	Seizures whose sole manifestation is recurrent arousals

Parasomnias	Disorders of arousal
	    Confusional arousals, sleepwalking, sleep terrors, sleep eating
	REM sleep behavior disorder
	Dreams/nightmares
	Enuresis
	Rhythmic movement disorder
	Periodic limb movement disorder
	Post-traumatic stress disorder
	Cardiopulmonary
	    Cardiac arrhythmias
	    Respiratory dyskinesias
	Gastrointestinal–paroxysmal choking
	Panic disorder
	Psychogenic dissociative disorders
		Mesial frontal, temporal lobe seizures presenting with complex, bizarre behaviors, hypnogenic (nocturnal) paroxysmal dystonia, or autonomic (diencephalic) seizures

Modified from Mahowald MW, Schenck CH. Sleep disorders. In: Engel J Jr, Pedley TA, eds. Epilepsy: A Comprehensive Textbook. Philadelphia, Pa: Lippincott-Raven; 1997:2705–2715.

After Broughton's pioneering work, the concept of an arousal disorder generating parasomnias was accepted, but subsequent studies also suggest that arousal disorders can provoke, represent, or be caused by seizure disorders. Certain predisposing factors in NREM sleep seem to increase IID and ictal epileptic events.[2, 3] The incidence of arousal-related paroxysms, such as sleep spindles, k-complexes, bursts of slow waves, and ponto-geniculo-occipital spikes, is closely associated with the occurrence of generalized or focal epileptiform spikes as well as spike-and-wave and polyspike-and-wave complexes in human and animal epilepsy.[2, 3, 9, 23–29] There also is a statistical relationship between the cyclic alternating pattern of "fluctuating cortical excitability" with both epilepsy and sleep disorders.[27, 28, 30–34]

PATHOPHYSIOLOGY

Many transection, pharmacological, and individual cell recording studies suggest that different neural substrates mediate the circadian sleep-wake cycle, which includes NREM sleep, and the ultradian basic rest activity cycle, which includes REM sleep. The sleep-wake cycle has been localized to antagonistic divisions of the hypothalamus, with sleep-active cells of the preoptic basal forebrain generating NREM sleep.[35–40] REM sleep and its cyclic alternation with waking have been localized to the brainstem reticular formation, particularly cholinergic, noradrenergic, and serotonergic cell populations within the pontine tegmentum.[41–44]

The hypothalamic and brainstem generators of sleep and arousal have diffuse ascending and descending projections[40, 45–48] that give rise to a number of distinguishing physiological characteristics, called *components*. These components can be *tonic* (sustained background activity, such as degree of electroencephalographic [EEG] synchronization and muscle tone) or *phasic* (periodic transients, such as sleep spindles, k-complexes, and muscle twitches). The association of these tonic and phasic events is important to the integrity of sleep states. Dissociation or abnormality of these components likely contributes to a variety of sleep, arousal, and seizure disorders, as well as their interaction.

Direct experimental evidence using dissociative manipulations is best documented with respect to spread of EEG and clinically evident seizures that may coexist with or masquerade as parasomnias.[49] Two state-specific components affecting epilepsy are (1) the degree to which cellular discharge patterns are synchronized and (2) alterations in antigravity muscle tone.[2, 50–53] NREM and drowsiness differ from alert waking and REM sleep in that EEG activity is synchronized and postural muscle tone is diminished. REM sleep differs from NREM in that EEG activity is desynchronized and differs from waking and NREM in that postural muscle tone is absent. REM sleep has sometimes been called "paradoxical sleep"[42] because it is characterized by a "highly active brain in a paralyzed body."[54]

During NREM, virtually every cell in the brain discharges synchronously and may even reach paroxysmal levels similar to those of epileptic states.[55, 56] This occurs to a lesser extent in drowsiness. Lasting oscillations of rhythmic burst-pause firing patterns result in concerted synaptic actions. Synchronous synaptic effects, whether excitatory or inhibitory, are likely to augment the magnitude and propagation of postsynaptic responses, including epileptic discharges. During REM and alert waking, cells discharge asynchronously.[44] The divergent synaptic signals associated with asynchronous discharge patterns are less likely to augment the magnitude or propagation of epileptic EEG discharges.

Skeletal muscle tone also varies by sleep or waking state. Antigravity muscle tone is preserved in NREM and waking,[54, 57] thus permitting seizure-associated and conceivably parasomnia-associated movement. Profound lower motor neuron inhibition occurs in REM,[54, 58] creating virtual paralysis (sparing the diaphragm to permit continued respiration). Disruption of this important component of REM sleep might underlie REM behavior disorder and can influence clinically evident motor seizures.

These different EEG and skeletal motor components can be experimentally dissociated, as depicted in Fig. 63–1.[14] Figure 63–1A shows normal feline REM sleep. Figure 63–1B shows that NREM sleep–like EEG synchrony during REM can be induced by the systemic administration of atropine. Although not shown, atropine also synchronizes the waking EEG. EEG-synchronizing effects are presumably achieved by blocking acetylcholine release from cells in the nucleus basalis of forebrain and pedunculopontine/peribrachial nuclei of brainstem because these are the critical generators of the asynchronous EEG discharges that occur in waking and, to a greater extent, in REM sleep.[40, 59] Figure 63–1C shows the selective loss of postural muscle tone induced by lesioning the pontine generators of REM sleep atonia.[44, 60–64] Neural generators are thought to be cholinoceptive and glutaminergic cells in the brainstem atonia regions,[44, 65] which hyperpolarize lower motoneurons.[58]

Dissociation of these EEG and motor components significantly and differentially influences electrographic and clinical seizure manifestations, as illustrated in Figure 63–2. Figure 63–2A shows the distribution of penicillin-induced spike-wave complexes during intact NREM (left) and REM sleep (right) states. Figure 63–2B shows the effects of atropine administra-

tion. The REM sleep EEG is synchronized, and the spike-wave discharge rate is comparable to that in NREM (compare left with right). Although not shown, atropine similarly synchronizes the waking EEG in conjunction with an increase in spike-wave discharge rate. Unlike waking and NREM sleep, there is no clinical manifestation during REM, presumably because of the skeletal motor paralysis unique to that state. Figure 63–2C shows that a pontine lesion eliminates REM sleep atonia so that a clinically evident myoclonic seizure occurs in REM.

These results are supported by other experimental and clinical findings indicating that substrates of state-specific components rather than integrity of the state per se can be salient determinants of seizure propagation. Agents that synchronize the EEG, such as cholinergic or noradrenergic antagonists, have proconvulsant effects.[66–68] Conversely, agents that desynchronize the EEG discourage epileptic EEG discharge propagation; examples are cholinergic and noradrenergic agonists,[52, 53, 69, 70] as well as β-carbolines such as abecarnil,[71] which act on central benzodiazepine receptors. Finally, pharmacological manipulations that induce atonia, such as carbachol infusion into the brainstem, also block clinical motor accompaniment.[69] Consistent observations have been reported in experimental models of primary generalized epilepsy, such as electroconvulsive shock, penicillin epilepsy, and photosensitive epilepsy,[14, 52, 67] in animal models of localization-related epilepsies, such as limbic system kindling and the cortical alumina cream preparation,[69, 72] as well as in the clinical literature on symptomatic generalized epilepsies, such as the West syndrome.[53] Collectively, the findings confirm that cellular discharge patterns and alterations in tone affect electrographic and clinically evident seizure manifestations in diverse epileptic syndromes, including those that mimic parasomnias.

EPIDEMIOLOGY

There are no definitive epidemiological studies on the coincidence of parasomnias and seizure disorders, although some studies suggest that nocturnal seizures rarely represent parasomnias.[6, 17, 18, 73] Symptoms of parasomnias, such as nightmares, sleep terrors, violent behavior during sleep, sleepwalking, and REM behavior disorder (RBD), resemble seizure disorders, notably partial complex seizures, thus warranting comments on reports of incidence, etiology, and clinical course.

The incidence of epilepsy has been studied most often in industrialized countries, where overall population percentages are similar; available studies conducted in developing countries indicate a higher prevalence than in industrialized countries.[74] The following statistics reflect well-conducted epidemiological studies in the United States.[74] The number of diagnosed patients in the United States is about 2.5 million, with a cumulative lifetime incidence ranging from 1.3 to 3.1% of the population by the age of 80 years. In the United States, epilepsy is the third most common neurological disorder after stroke and Alzheimer's disease. Epilepsies may be classified as generalized (40%),

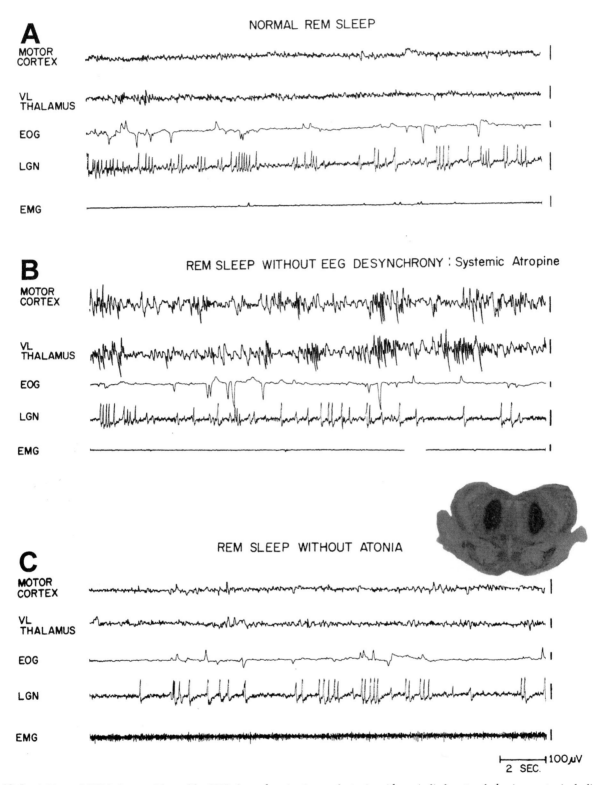

Figure 63–1. *A*, Normal REM sleep, evidenced by EEG desynchronization and atonia with periodic bursts of phasic events, including rapid eye movements and ponto-geniculo-occipital (PGO) spikes. *B*, Systemic atropine selectively abolishes EEG desynchronization. Instead, there is an NREM sleep–like EEG with synchronized background and sleep spindles. However, atonia is intact as are eye movements and PGO spikes. Clustering of PGOs is diminished as customarily reported. *C*, A pontine lesion selectively eliminates atonia. Note presence of tonic EMG activity in the bottom channel of this tracing. (Reprinted from Brain Research, vol 505, Shouse MN, Siegel JM, Wu FM, et al, Mechanisms of seizure suppression during rapid-eye-movement [REM] sleep in cats, 271–282, Copyright 1989, with permission from Elsevier Science.) VL, ventrolateral; EMG, electromyogram; EOG, electro-oculogram; LGN, lateral geniculate nucleus.

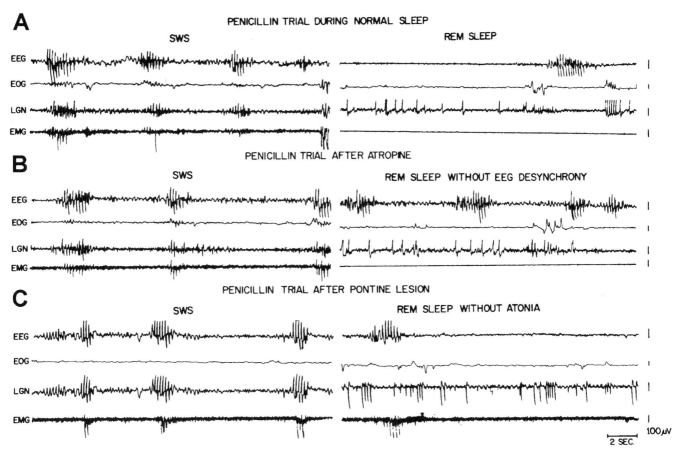

Figure 63–2. Systemic penicillin epilepsy during SWS, the equivalent in human beings of NREM (*left*), and REM (*right*) sleep before (*A*) and after dissociation of REM sleep components (*B* and *C*). Spike-wave paroxysms are visible in the EEG tracing, and myoclonic seizures were associated with EMG discharges in this cat, as long as lower motoneuron activity is present. (Reprinted from Brain Research, vol 505, Shouse MN, Siegel JM, Wu FM, et al, Mechanisms of seizure suppression during rapid-eye-movement [REM] sleep in cats, 271–282, Copyright 1989, with permission from Elsevier Science.) EMG, electromyogram; EOG, electro-oculogram; LGN, lateral geniculate nucleus; SWS, slow-wave sleep.

localization related (57%), or unclassified (3%). Localization-related epilepsies may be further subclassified as partial complex (36%), simple partial (14%), and partial unknown (7%). Localization-related epilepsies, particularly partial complex seizure disorders with tonic-clonic convulsions, are the "prototypic" pure sleep epilepsies, with nearly 60% of the patients exhibiting convulsions only during sleep.[10, 11] Most of these nocturnal seizure disorders are attributed to temporal or frontal lobe foci.[13] Onset can occur at any time, although the average peak age at onset is in adolescence.[10] Electroclinical symptoms tend to persist, and over time ictal and/or IID events are likely to disperse across the sleep-wake cycle.[10, 11, 74]

Reported symptoms suggestive of parasomnias are far more prevalent than epilepsies because many are normal, transient occurrences. The prevalence of sleepwalking ranges from 1 to 15%, that of sleep terrors is unspecified, and that of RBD is estimated at 0.5% of the population.[6, 75] It is becoming clear that sleepwalking in adults is far more commonplace than previously thought, with a prevalence of 3 to 10%.[76, 77] Age at onset of parasomnias such as sleepwalking and sleep terrors is believed to be in childhood, whereas the average age at the onset of RBD is 45 to 55 years. The earlier age at onset of some parasomnias may provide one criterion for differential diagnosis from some nocturnal seizure disorders; however, many parasomnias, like partial complex seizure disorders, do not remit spontaneously.[6, 10, 11, 74] Hereditary factors can be more prevalent in some parasomnias than in partial complex seizure disorders. Still, the most definitive criterion for differential diagnosis is polygraphic evidence of epileptic seizure discharge, and this may be difficult to obtain from surface recordings of patients with deep temporal or frontal lobe foci.[73, 78–84] It is likely that the rarity of nocturnal seizures presenting as other parasomnias is more apparent than real, the correct diagnosis having been overlooked for lack of consideration.

CLINICAL FEATURES

Listed are various areas of overlap and confusion between sleep disorders and seizures, ranging from normal events to hypersomnia, insomnia, and parasomnias (see Table 63–1).

Normal Sleep Phenomena

Sleep Starts. Sleep starts (hypnic jerks) are experienced by many normal individuals during the transition from wake to sleep. The most common is the motor sleep start, a sudden jerk of all or part of the body, occasionally awakening the victim or bedpartner.[85] Variations include the visual (flashes of light, fragmentary visual hallucinations), auditory (loud bangs, snapping noises), and somesthetic (pain, floating, something flowing through the body) sleep starts, occurring without the body jerk.[86-88] Sleep starts represent a normal (although not understood) physiological event and should not be confused with seizures or other neurological conditions. It is likely that the "exploding head syndrome" characterized by a sensation of a loud sound like an explosion or a sensation of "bursting" of the head[89-92] is a variant of a sensory sleep start. Similar phenomena may represent the sole manifestation of a seizure.[93]

Nightmares. Nightmares are frightening dreams that usually awaken the sleeper from REM sleep (see Chapter 66). Unlike disorders of arousal such as sleep terrors (see later), nightmares are not usually associated with prominent motor or vocal behavior, or autonomic excitation, and the arousal results in immediate full wakefulness, with memory for the dream sequence of events that caused the awakening.[94] Seizures may present as recurrent dreams, nightmares, or disorders of arousal such as sleepwalking and sleep terrors. The diagnosis of seizure-related dreams and nightmares may be overlooked if the symptom is misinterpreted as a primary sleep phenomenon.[95-98] Autosomal dominant frontal epilepsy may also present as recurrent "nightmares."[99, 100]

Hypersomnia

Epilepsy. The sole manifestation of nocturnal seizures may be simple arousals, which may or may not be perceived by the patient. If a sufficient number of arousals occur, the resulting sleep fragmentation will present with symptoms of severe excessive daytime

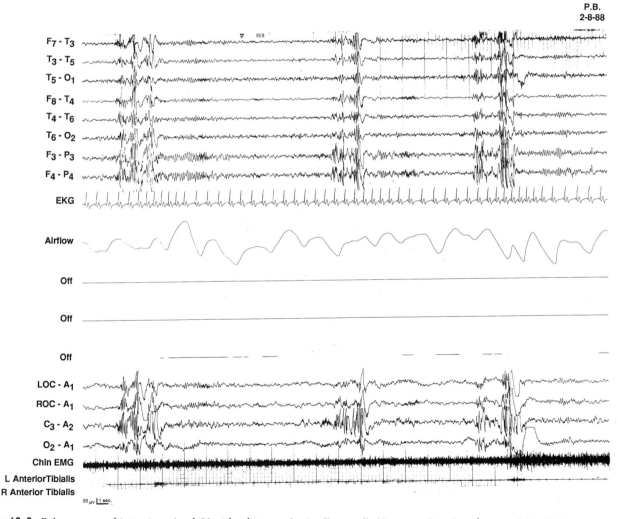

Figure 63–3. Polysomnographic tracing of a child with a history of a "well-controlled" seizure disorder who complained of severe excessive daytime sleepiness. Notice the EEG evidence of arousals, which were the sole manifestation of seizure activity. The seizure-induced arousal index was nearly 100 per hour of sleep, clearly explaining the daytime complaint.

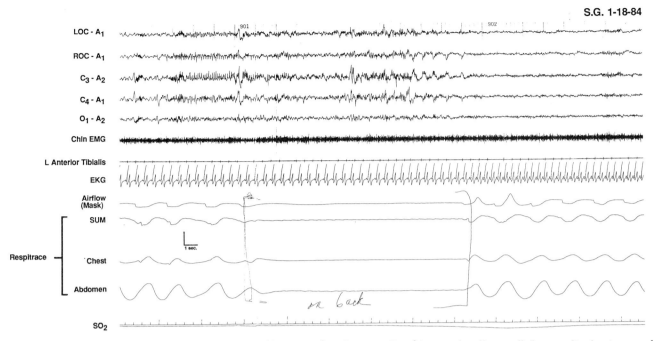

Figure 63–4. Polysomnographic tracing of a 56-year-old man with a long-standing history of well-controlled generalized seizures who developed severe progressive excessive daytime sleepiness. The polysomnogram revealed 22 central apneas per hour as the sole manifestation of seizures. Aggressive medical management was unsuccessful. There was marked improvement in his excessive daytime sleepiness after a right frontal lobectomy. (From Mahowald MW, Schenck CH. Sleep disorders. In: Engel J Jr, Pedley TA, eds. Epilepsy: A Comprehensive Textbook. Philadelphia, Pa: Lippincott-Raven; 1997:2705–2715, with permission.)

sleepiness (Fig. 63–3). These seizure-induced arousals may be associated with very minor motor phenomena.[101]

Some patients with seizures are hypersomnolent during the day, even after the discontinuation of antiepileptic medication. Seizure-free preadolescent children with epilepsy are sleepier than healthy control children. In one study, there was no difference in objective sleepiness in children with epilepsy on or off medication, suggesting that antiepileptic drugs do not necessarily result in daytime sleepiness.[102] Excessive daytime sleepiness in a patient on antiepileptic medications should not summarily be attributed to the medication.[16, 28, 103]

Narcolepsy. Narcolepsy is a genetically determined disorder characterized by excessive daytime sleepiness, cataplexy (the sudden loss of muscle tone triggered by emotionally laden events), sleep paralysis, hypnagogic hallucinations, and automatic behavior during which prolonged, complex activities may be performed without conscious awareness or recall.[104, 105] The "spell-like" nature of some sleep attacks, cataplexy, and sleep paralysis may be mistaken for seizures. Conversely, atonic (epileptic negative myoclonus) or inhibitory seizures may mimic cataplexy,[106–112] and the periods of automatic behavior are often misdiagnosed as partial complex seizures, postictal confusion, or poriomania.[113, 114] The incomplete and waxing and waning nature of cataplexy can imitate tonic-clonic seizure activity.

Periodic Hypersomnia (Kleine-Levin Syndrome). The Kleine-Levin syndrome is a poorly understood condition characterized by recurrent periods of hypersomnia. The often-cited association with adolescent boys and unusual behaviors such as hypersexuality and megaphagia have been overrated.[115] Menstruation-related periodic hypersomnia may represent a variant of the Kleine-Levin syndrome.[116] Similar recurrent episodes of hypersomnia may be caused by "ictal sleep" lasting 13 days at 10- to 60-day intervals.[117, 118]

Sleep-Disordered Breathing. There is an interesting and important relationship between sleep-disordered breathing and seizures. Nocturnal seizures, probably triggered by periods of hypoxemia, may be the presenting symptom in some individuals with obstructive sleep apnea or sleep-related hypoventilation.[119, 120] Furthermore, sleep apnea may exacerbate seizures in patients with epilepsy due to sleep disruption, sleep deprivation, hypoxemia, or decreased cerebral blood flow. Identification and treatment of sleep-disordered breathing in individuals with seizures may improve seizure control.[121–124] Some seizure-like "spells" associated with sleep apnea are actually due to episodes of cerebral anoxia.[125]

Seizures may also cause periods of apnea, often repetitive, and may closely mimic the conditions of obstructive or central sleep apnea.[126–129] Figure 63–4 shows repetitive apneas as the sole manifestation of seizures, and Figure 63–5 shows obstructive sleep apnea inducing electrical seizure activity.

Insomnia

Paroxysmal, otherwise unexplained awakenings may be the sole manifestation of nocturnal seizures and will result in the complaint of insomnia.[130–135] Some

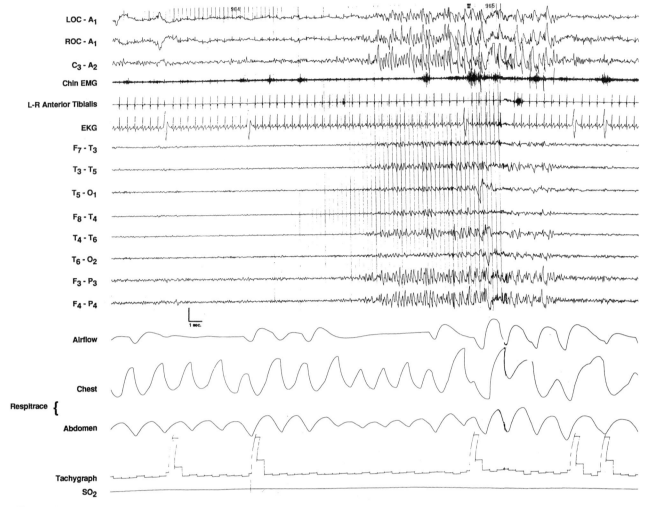

Figure 63–5. Polysomnographic tracing showing electrical seizure activity beginning during an episode of obstructive sleep apnea.

patients with occasional paroxysmal periodic motor attacks during sleep have very frequent (every 20 to 60 sec) subclinical arousals resulting in severe sleep fragmentation.[136] These paroxysmal arousals may be due to deep epileptic foci.[137] The arousal preceding nocturnal seizures may be the initial manifestation of the seizure.[138] Studies in animals support the concept of frequent arousals as the manifestation of a seizures.[29] This may explain the fact that many patients with epilepsy report frequent, otherwise unexplained nocturnal awakenings.[139]

Parasomnias

Disorders of Arousals. Disorders of arousal are the most common and impressive of the NREM sleep parasomnias and may readily be confused with epileptic phenomena (see Chapter 62). These occur on a continuum ranging from confusional arousals to sleepwalking to sleep terrors. The disorders of arousal share common features: a positive family history, suggesting a genetic component; they tend to arise from slow-wave sleep (stages 3 and 4 of NREM sleep), therefore

usually occurring in the first third of the sleep cycle (and rarely during naps); and they are common in childhood and usually decrease in frequency with increasing age.[140–145] They may occur during any stage of NREM sleep, most commonly arising from slow-wave sleep, and may occur late in the sleep period.[146] Contrary to popular opinion, the appearance or persistence of these events into adulthood is usually not associated with significant psychiatric disease.[147–150] A specialized form of disorder of arousal is sleep-related eating.[151–153] A potentially interesting theoretical situation would be eating-induced seizures in such individuals.[154]

Disorders of arousal may difficult to differentiate from nocturnal seizures, and vice versa.[79] Preservation of consciousness during seizures may lead to confusion with disorders of arousal or psychogenic conditions.[155] Crying (dacrystic) or laughing (gelastic) seizures may be misinterpreted as confusional arousals or sleep terrors.[156, 157] Both disorders of arousal and seizures may be related to the menstrual cycle.[158–160]

Arousals of any sort may serve to trigger a disorder of arousal; therefore, any underlying condition resulting in arousal may cause a disorder of arousal, including sleep apnea, gastroesophageal reflux, or seizures, so the clinical event of a sleepwalking or sleep terror episode may in fact represent an epiphenomenon of a completely different underlying sleep disorder.[73] It is common clinical experience to see an improvement in disorders of arousal after the effective treatment of obstructive sleep apnea. Conversely, effective treatment of obstructive sleep apnea with nasal continuous positive airway pressure may result in disorders of arousal, presumably associated with deep NREM sleep rebound.[161, 162] It must be remembered that sleep terrors and seizures may coexist in the same individual.[49]

REM Sleep Behavior Disorder. RBD is a recently described condition in which the anticipated atonia of REM sleep is absent, hypothetically allowing patients to "act out their dreams," often with violent or injurious results (see Chapter 64). RBD is typically a disorder of older men and is frequently misdiagnosed as a nocturnal seizure or psychogenic event. RBD is readily diagnosable with formal sleep studies, which reveal the absence of anticipated somatic muscle atonia of REM sleep. The condition of RBD responds very well to clonazepam.[163] Just as RBD may masquerade as nocturnal seizures, the converse is also true.[164]

Dream/Nightmare Disturbances. As mentioned earlier, dreams (particularly recurrent dreams) or nightmares as the primary manifestation of nocturnal seizures have been well documented.

Enuresis. Enuresis was formerly classified as a "disorder of arousal," implying a relationship with NREM or slow-wave sleep.[17] However, enuresis may occur during either NREM or REM sleep.[165, 166] Enuresis may be the sole manifestation of nocturnal seizures.[73, 167, 168]

Rhythmic Movement Disorder. Rhythmic movement disorder (RMD) refers to a number of behaviors characterized by stereotyped movements (rhythmic oscillation of the head or limbs, head-banging, or body-rocking during sleep) seen most frequently in childhood and, rarely, in adults. RMD may arise from any stage of sleep, may be familial, and is not usually associated with underlying psychiatric or psychological conditions.[169] Rarely, RMD may be the sole manifestation of a seizure.[73]

Periodic Limb Movement Disorder. Periodic limb movement disorder (PLMD) is a polysomnographically determined diagnosis. It is characterized by periodic (every 20 to 30 sec) dorsiflexion of the great toe, foot, or flexion of the entire leg. These movements are not perceived by the patient and may be asymptomatic or be associated with the complaint of either excessive daytime sleepiness or insomnia.[170, 171] When prominent, these movements may be confused with myoclonic seizure activity or may actually represent epileptic phenomena.[172] Propriospinal myoclonus may also be confused with PLMD and present with the complaint of insomnia or sleep-related movements that are bothersome to the bedpartner.[173, 174] PLMD may be particularly dramatic in patients with underlying renal failure.[175, 176]

Post-Traumatic Stress Disorder. Post-traumatic stress disorder is often associated with subjective sleep complaints, including "nightmares" and sleep terror–like experiences.[177] It may be confused with nocturnal panic or seizures manifesting solely as arousals with a fearful effect.

Seizures. The behaviors associated with nocturnal seizures are often bizarre and may masquerade as primary sleep parasomnias, secondary sleep parasomnias, or psychiatric conditions.[178] The following are particularly likely to result in diagnostic dilemmas.

Classified Seizures. These seizures occur frequently during sleep.[8] In many individuals with epilepsy, seizures occur exclusively during sleep, increasing the likelihood of a misdiagnosis of a primary sleep disorder. A conservative estimate is that 10% of patients with epilepsy display seizures exclusively during sleep.[179] One type of seizure that typically occurs predominantly in the sleep period is *'benign childhood epilepsy with centrotemporal spikes'* (also known as benign rolanic epilepsy), which is characterized by unilateral somatosensory onset of paresthesias of the tongue, lips, gums, and cheek with tonic or tonic-clonic movement of the face, lips, tongue, and pharyngeal muscles associated with drooling. The electrical EEG spike discharges are typically activated by sleep[180] (Fig. 63–6).

Unusual Behavioral Seizures. These seizures (usually of frontal lobe origin) may present as bizarre behaviors such as running, loud vocalization, or cursing. The phenomenal behaviors and the tendency to occur during sleep and to cluster in time promote misdiagnosis (usually as a disorder of arousal, RBD, or psychogenic spells).[178, 181–185] Autosomal dominant nocturnal frontal lobe epilepsy may present with predominately or exclusively sleep-related motor behaviors,[186, 187] as may supplementary sensorimotor seizures.[188]

Episodic Nocturnal Wanderings. These respond to anticonvulsants and may be indistinguishable by history from sleepwalking and sleep terrors. The patients ambulate, vocalize, and display violent behavior during sleep. Not all exhibited waking EEG abnormalities. There is growing evidence that many of these cases represent epileptic phenomena and are actually ambulatory automatisms.[75, 80, 189–195]

Nocturnal (Hypnogenic) Paroxysmal Dystonia. Nocturnal paroxysmal dystonia (NPD) is a syndrome characterized by predominantly or exclusively nocturnal episodes of coarse, occasionally violent, movements of the limbs associated with tonic spasms, often occurring multiple times nightly. Vocalization or laughter may occur. EEGs between events are normal; during events, EEGs display movement artifact often without clear evidence of electrical seizure activity.[196, 197] The cyclic alternating pattern of cortical excitability may play a modulatory role in this condition.[34] There is growing and compelling evidence that NPD is a seizure disorder.[81, 198–201] NPD may be unilateral,[83, 196, 202–205] and there can be a familial history.[206] Nocturnal and diurnal paroxysmal dystonia may exist in the same patient, as can reflex and hypnogenic paroxysmal dystonia. There is considerable overlap among the different clinical categories of paroxysmal dyskinesias.[82, 207–209] NPD may be post-traumatic[210] and may coexist with panic disorder.[211]

Carbamazepine is often very effective in eliminating these spells. For exclusively nocturnal spells, late eve-

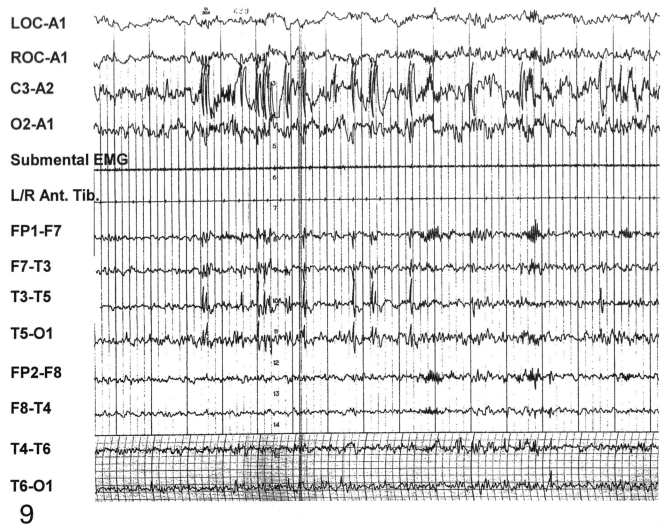

LOC-A1
ROC-A1
C3-A2
O2-A1
Submental EMG
L/R Ant. Tib.
FP1-F7
F7-T3
T3-T5
T5-O1
FP2-F8
F8-T4
T4-T6
T6-O1

9

Figure 63–6. Polysomnographic study showing the prominent state-dependent nature of left-sided centromidtemporal spikes, present almost exclusively during NREM sleep.

ning administration (400 to 600 mg), without daytime doses, may be effective, and better tolerated than regular three times daily dosing. Vigilance level–dependent tonic seizures[212] and familial paroxysmal hypnogenic dystonia[206] likely represent variants of this condition.

Pure Tonic Seizures. These seizures with arousal (or paroxysmal polyspike activity with arousal) have been discussed as seizures presenting as insomnia or hypersomnia due to seizure-induced arousals or sleep fragmentation. An interesting subtype of hypnic tonic postural seizures has been described in 10 children, many with a positive family history.[213] This may be a benign epilepsy syndrome similar to benign childhood epilepsy with centrotemporal spikes,[214] childhood epilepsy with occipital paroxysms,[215, 216] and primary reading epilepsy.[213]

Autonomic/Diencephalic Seizures. These seizures are thought to be rare and could present from sleep with such manifestations as intermittent or paroxysmal apnea,[128, 217] stridor,[218] coughing,[219] laryngospasm,[220, 221] chest pain and arrhythmias,[121, 222–224] paroxysmal flushing, and localized hyperhidrosis.[225, 226] Isolated auto-

nomic symptoms are a well-documented manifestation of seizures and are probably much more common than generally suspected.[205, 227–236] These simple autonomic seizures are easily confused with other primary or secondary sleep parasomnias or are misattributed to disorders of other organ systems.[237]

Electrical Status Epilepticus of Sleep. Electrical status epilepticus of sleep (ESES) may be detected during a polysomnogram performed for other reasons and is characterized by continuous spike-and-wave activity during NREM sleep.[238, 239] ESES is seen in children who may have a history of seizures or neurological dysfunction. The prognosis is variable because ESES can be asymptomatic.[240–242] ESES may share some features with the Landau-Kleffner syndrome.[243, 244]

Cardiopulmonary

Cardiac Arrhythmias. Cardiac arrhythmias may be a manifestation of seizures, masquerading as nocturnal cardiac abnormalities.[222, 223, 245–259] Conversely, primary cardiac events (prolonged QT interval) may present as seizures.[260] Seizures may present as syncope,[261, 262] or vice versa.[263]

Respiratory Dyskinesias. These may occur or persist during the sleep period; examples include (1) segmental myoclonus such as palatal myoclonus[264, 265] or diaphragmatic flutter[266–268] and (2) paroxysmal dystonia.[269] Respiratory dyskinesias may also be the manifestation of neuroleptic-induced dyskinesias, which do not always persist during sleep.[270–273] These dyskinesias should be differentiated from unusual nocturnal seizures that present with primarily or exclusively respiratory symptoms.[126–128]

Gastrointestinal. The sole manifestation of nocturnal seizures may be paroxysmal choking.[274]

Nocturnal Panic Attacks. Nocturnal panic attacks (NPA) may occur in patients with diurnal panic or, rarely, precede the appearance of diurnal panic, or they may be exclusively nocturnal in nature.[275–277] The striking similarity of the symptoms of dream anxiety attack, sleep terror, nocturnal seizures, and nighttime panic urges extreme caution in diagnosis.[278–286] Obstructive sleep apnea can also cause symptoms of NPA.[287] The common association of the affect of "fear" as an accompaniment of nocturnal seizures intensifies their confusion with nocturnal panic.[288–291] It must be remembered that seizures and panic may coexist.[282, 292]

Psychogenic Dissociative States. Complex and potentially injurious behaviors, occasionally confined to the sleep period, may be the manifestation of a psychogenic dissociative state. A history of childhood physical and/or sexual abuse is virtually always present (but may be difficult to elicit). In this condition, unlike other parasomnias or nocturnal seizures, the complex behavior, during EEG monitoring, is seen to arise from clear EEG determined wakefulness.[293] Pseudoseizures may also arise from apparent sleep.[294]

DIAGNOSTIC EVALUATION

As specified, the clinical differentiation between sleep disorders and epileptic events often may be difficult, if not impossible, because primary or secondary sleep phenomena may perfectly mimic epileptic phenomena, and vice versa. Both epileptic and sleep phenomena should be considered in any case of recurrent, stereotyped, and inappropriate unusual sleep-related events.

The decision to further investigate unusual nocturnal events will depend on the clinical situation. The most common condition is the disorder of arousal, which is very common (and normal) in the general population. Simple sleepwalking or sleep terrors can readily be diagnosed clinically. Indications for formal evaluation include behaviors that (1) are potentially injurious or violent, (2) cause disruption for other household members, (3) result in excessive daytime sleepiness, or (4) display unusual clinical features.[295]

Clinical differentiation between sleep disorders and epileptic phenomena may be most difficult, and misdiagnosis in both directions is common, particularly in the absence of a history of diurnal spells. Both waking

and sleep-deprived EEGs may not reveal the diagnosis,[296, 297] necessitating all-night polysomnographic study using a full seizure montage, appropriate paper speed, and continuous video recording.[298] Although exclusively nocturnal seizures may be uncommon, they are routinely misdiagnosed and should never be overlooked as possibly etiologic in any sleep-related behavior that is recurrent, stereotyped, or inappropriate—regardless of the specific nature of that behavior. "Ambulatory" EEG monitoring has led to the misdiagnosis of functional psychiatric disease in a number of our patients subsequently demonstrated to have bona fide nocturnal seizures. Erroneous psychogenic branding is reinforced by the bizarre nature of the spells and by the fact that environmental clues may play a role in the context of psychomotor seizures.[299]

Misdiagnosis is common even after formal and appropriate polysomnographic evaluation. Reasons for misdiagnosis include the following[300]:

1. Obscuration of the scalp EEG by movement artifact
2. Absence of scalp-EEG manifestation of the seizure activity
3. EEG seizure manifestation appearing to be an "arousal" pattern
4. Absence of EEG or clinical postictal period

Extensive polysomnographic monitoring with a full-scalp EEG montage and a paper speed of at least 15 mm/sec is mandatory. Because the clinical events may be infrequent, multiple studies may be necessary to capture an event. Continuous audiovisual monitoring and recording are indicated, and detailed technician observation is invaluable. The difficulties in evaluating unusual sleep-related events emphasize the necessity of extensive, in person laboratory monitoring with interpretation of all data (clinical, EEG, sleep, video, and technologist-provided information) by personnel experienced in both sleep medicine and epileptology.

MANAGEMENT

Effective treatment is available for almost all parasomnias, regardless of cause, and is predicated on an accurate diagnosis. If seizures are responsible for the sleep-wake complaint, treatment is similar to that for other seizure disorders.[301] If a primary sleep disorder (e.g., narcolepsy, sleep apnea, or other parasomnia) is identified, therapy is dictated by the specific diagnosis (see corresponding chapters in this textbook).

CONCLUSIONS

There are various nocturnal paroxysmal events that are not clearly defined with regard to cause. Differential diagnosis of epileptic versus nonepileptic manifestations depends primarily on the use of extracranial recordings, although intracranial EEG recordings are sometimes necessary. Specifically, epileptic seizures originating from mesio-orbito-frontal sites often cannot be recorded extracranially, and attacks of uncertain cause such as sleepwalking, attacks of screaming, and complex automatisms during sleep may be inaccurately diagnosed as parasomnias.[73, 78–80, 302] Some evidence also suggests that short-lasting paroxysmal dystonia attacks represent sleep-related frontal lobe seizures.[81, 83, 84, 302] In other cases, parasomnias coexist with limbic epilepsy without an apparent common cause.[49, 73, 303]

The interface between sleep disorders and epileptic phenomena is vast and compelling because sleep affects seizures and seizures affect sleep. The myriad sleep and epileptic phenomena may perfectly counterfeit one another. A high index of suspicion and a full awareness of the broad spectrum of both sleep and epileptic phenomena are instrumental for an accurate diagnosis. A thorough clinical and laboratory evaluation of unusual phenomena that could be either sleep or seizure related will usually lead to a specific diagnosis, with important and effective therapeutic implications. Continued close collaboration between clinicians and basic science sleep/epilepsy researchers will undoubtedly lead to important advances in the understanding of both sleep and epilepsy, with vital clinical diagnostic and therapeutic implications.

Acknowledgments

We thank our technical and nursing staff as well as Paul R. Farber for computer processing and expertise. This work was supported by the Minnesota Regional Sleep Disorders Center, Hennepin County Medical Center, and the Department of Veterans Affairs.

References

1. Mahowald MW, Schenck CH. Sleep disorders. In: Engel J Jr, Pedley TA, eds. Epilepsy: A Comprehensive Textbook. Philadelphia, Pa: Lippincott-Raven; 1997:2705–2715.
2. Shouse MN, da Silva AM, Sammaritano M. Circadian rhythm, sleep, and epilepsy. J Clin Neurophysiol. 1996;13:32–50.
3. Shouse MN, Martins da Silva A, Sammaritano M. Sleep. In: Engel J Jr, Pedley TA, eds. Epilepsy: A Comprehensive Textbook. Vol 2. Philadelphia, Pa: Lippincott-Raven; 1997:1929–1942.
4. Koridze MG. Effect of petit-mal and generalized seizures on the sleep-wakefulness cycle. Sleep 1978, Fourth European Congress on Sleep Research, Tirgu-Mures. Basel, Switzerland: S. Karger; 1980:713–716.
5. Brazil CW, Walczak TS. Effects of sleep and sleep stage on epileptic and nonepileptic seizures. Epilepsia. 1997;38:56–62.
6. Guilleminault C. Parasomnias. In: Kryger MH, Roth T, Dement WC, eds. Principles and Practice of Sleep Medicine. 2nd ed. Philadelphia, Pa: WB Saunders; 1994:567–601.
7. Mahowald MW, Ettinger MG. Things that go bump in the night—the parasomnias revisited. J Clin Neurophysiol. 1990;7:119–143.
8. Commission Report. Proposal for revised classification of epilepsies and epileptic syndromes. Epilepsia. 1989;30:389–399.
9. Drake ME, Pakalnis A, Phillips BB, et al. Sleep and sleep deprived EEG in partial and generalized epilepsy. Acta Neurol Belg. 1990;90:11–19.
10. Janz D. The grand mal epilepsies and the sleeping-waking cycle. Epilepsia. 1962;3:69–109.
11. Janz D. Epilepsy and the sleeping-waking cycle. In: Vincken PJ, Bruyn GW, eds. Handbook of Clinical Neurology. Vol 15. Amsterdam, Netherlands: North Holland; 1974:457–490.
12. Thomaides TN, Kerezoudi EP, Chaudhuri KR, et al. Study of EEGs following 24-hour sleep deprivation with posttraumatic epilepsy. Eur Neurol. 1992;32:79–82.
13. Hauser WA, Kurland LT. The epidemiology of epilepsy in Rochester, MN. Epilepsia. 1975;16:1–66.
14. Shouse MN, Siegel JM, Wu FM, et al. Mechanisms of seizure suppression during rapid-eye-movement (REM) sleep in cats. Brain Res. 1989;505:271–282.
15. Sammaritano M, Gigli GL, Gotman J. Interictal spiking during wakefulness and sleep and the localization of foci in temporal lobe epilepsy. Neurology. 1991;41:290–297.
16. Malow BA, Kushwaha R, Lin X, et al. Relationship of interictal epileptiform discharges to sleep depth in partial epilepsy. Electroencephalogr Clin Neurophysiol. 1997;102:20–26.
17. Broughton RJ. Sleep disorders: disorders of arousal? Science. 1968;159:1070–1078.
18. Gastaut H, Broughton R. A clinical and polygraphic study of episodic phenomena during sleep. Rec Adv Biol Psychiatry. 1965;7:197–221.
19. Touchon J. Effect of awakening on epileptic activity in primary generalized myoclonic epilepsy. In: Sterman MB, Shouse MN, Passouant P, eds. Sleep and Epilepsy. New York, NY: Academic Press; 1982:239–248.
20. Mahowald MW, Schenck CH. Status dissociatus—a perspective on states of being. Sleep. 1991;14:69–79.
21. Mahowald MW, Schenck CH. Dissociated states of wakefulness and sleep. Neurology. 1992;42:44–52.
22. Roth T, Roehrs TA, Carskadon MA, et al. Daytime sleepiness and alertness. In: Kryger MH, Roth T, Dement WC, eds. Principles and Practice of Sleep Medicine. 2nd ed. Philadelphia, Pa: WB Saunders; 1994:40–49.
23. Halasz P. Generalized epilepsy with spike-wave pattern (GESW) and intermediate states of sleep. In: Sterman MB, Shouse MN, Passouant P, eds. Sleep and Epilepsy. New York, NY: Academic Press; 1982:219–238.
24. Niedermeyer E. Abnormal EEG patterns (epileptic and paroxysmal). In: Niedermeyer E, Lopes da Silva F, eds. Electroencephalography. 2nd ed. Baltimore, Md: Urban and Schwartzenberg; 1987:183–207.
25. Niedermeyer E. Epileptic seizure disorders. In: Niedermeyer E, Lopes da Silva F, eds. Electroencephalography. 2nd ed. Baltimore, Md: Urban and Schwartzenberg; 1987:405–510.
26. Kellaway P, Frost JD Jr, Crawley JW. The relationship between sleep spindles and spike-and-wave bursts in human epilepsy. In: Avoli M, Gloor P, Kostopoulos G, et al, eds. Generalized Epilepsy: Neurobiological Approaches. Boston, Mass: Birkhauser; 1990:36–48.
27. Gigli GL, Calia E, Marciani MG, et al. Sleep microstructure and EEG epileptiform activity in patients with juvenile myoclonic epilepsy. Epilepsia. 1992;33:799–804.
28. Gigli GL, Baldinetti F, Placidi F, et al. Nocturnal sleep and daytime somnolence in untreated temporal lobe epileptics: comparison with normal subjects and changes after carbamazepine administration. J Sleep Res. 1994;3(suppl 1):89.
29. Shouse MN, Langer J, King A, et al: Paroxysmal microarousals in amygdala-kindled kittens: could they be subclinical seizures? Epilepsia. 1995;36:290–300.
30. Terzano MG, Parrino L, Anelli S, et al. Effects of generalized interictal EEG discharges on sleep stability: assessment by means of cyclic alternating pattern. Epilepsia. 1992;33:317–326.
31. Terzano MG, Parrino L, Anelli S, et al. Modulation of generalized spike-and-wave discharges during sleep by cyclic alternating pattern. Epilepsia. 1989;30:772–781.
32. Terzano MG, Parrino L, Garofalo PG, et al. Activation of partial seizures with motor signs during cyclic alternating pattern in human sleep. Epilepsy Res. 1991;10:166–173.
33. Terzano MG, Parrino L, Spaggiari MC. The cyclic alternating pattern sequences in the dynamic organization of sleep. Electroencephalogr Clin Neurophysiol. 1988;69:437–447.
34. Terzano MG, Monge-Strauss M-F, Mikol F, et al. Cyclic alternating pattern as a provocative factor in nocturnal paroxysmal dystonia. Epilepsia. 1997;38:1015–1025.
35. von Economo C. Encephalitis Lethargica: Its Sequellae and Treatment. London, England: Oxford University Press; 1931.
36. Nauta WJH. Hypothalamic regulation of sleep in rats: an experimental study. J Neurophysiol. 1946;9:285–316.
37. Sterman MB, Clemente CD. Forebrain inhibitory mechanisms, II: sleep patterns induced by basal forebrain stimulation in the behaving cat. Exp Neurol. 1962;6:103–117.

38. Sterman MB, Clemente CD. Forebrain inhibitory mechanisms, I: cortical synchronization induced by basal forebrain stimulation. Exp Neurol. 1962;6:91–102.

39. McGinty DJ, Sterman MB. Sleep suppression after basal forebrain lesions in the cat. Science. 1968;160:1253–1255.

40. Jones B. Basic mechanisms of sleep-wake states. In: Kryger MH, Roth R, Dement WC, eds. Principles and Practice of Sleep Medicine. 2nd ed. Philadelphia, Pa: WB Saunders; 1994:145–162.

41. Bremer F. Cerveau isole et physiologie du sommeil. C R Soc Biol (Paris). 1935;118:1235–1242.

42. Jouvet M. Recherches sur les structures nerveuses et les mecanismes responsables des differentes phases due sommeil physiologique. Arch Ital Biol. 1962;100:125–206.

43. Villabalnca J. The electroencephalogram in the chronic cerveau isole cat. Electroencephalogr Clin Neurophysiol. 1965;19:576–586.

44. Siegel J. Brainstem mechanisms generating REM sleep. In: Kryger MH, Roth T, Dement WC, eds. Principles and Practice of Sleep Medicine. 2nd ed. Philadelphia, Pa: WB Saunders; 1994:125–144.

45. McBride RI, Sutin J. Projection of the locus ceruleus and adjacent pontine tegmentum of the cat. J Comp Neurol. 1976;165:265–284.

46. Mugnaini I, Oertel WH. An atlas of the distribution of GABAergic neurons and terminals in the rat CNS as revealed by GAD histochemistry. In: Bjorklund A, Hokfelt T, eds. GABA and Neuropeptides in the CNS, Part I. Amsterdam, Netherlands: Elsevier; 1985:436–608.

47. Jones BE, Beaudet A. Distribution of acetylcholine and catecholamine neurons in the cat brainstem: a choline acetyltransferase and tyrosine hydroxylase immunohistochemical study. J Comp Neurol. 1987;261:15–32.

48. Woolf NJ, Harrison JB, Buckwald JS. Cholinergic neurons of the feline pontomesencephalic tegmentum, II: anatomical projections. Brain Res. 1990;520:55–72.

49. Tassinari CA, Mancia D, Dalla-Bernardina B, et al. Pavor nocturnus of non-epileptic nature in epileptic children. Electroencephalogr Clin Neurophysiol. 1972;33:603–607.

50. Cohen HB, Thomas J, Dement WC. Sleep stages, REM deprivation and electroconvulsive threshold in the cat. Brain Res. 1970;19:317–321.

51. Gloor P. Generalized epilepsy with spike-wave discharge: a reinterpretation of its electroencephalographic and clinical manifestations. Epilepsia. 1979;20:571–588.

52. Rektor I, Bryere P, Valen A, et al. Physostigmine antagonizes benzodiazepine-induced myoclonus in the baboon, Papio papio. Neurosci Lett. 1984;52:91–96.

53. Rektor I, Svejdora M, Silva-Barrat C, et al. Central cholinergic hypofunction in pathophysiology of West's syndrome. In: Wolf P, Dam M, Janz D, et al, eds. Advances in Epileptology. Vol 16. New York, NY: Raven Press; 1987:139–142.

54. Carskadon MA, Dement WC. Normal human sleep: an overview. In: Kryger MH, Roth T, Dement WC, eds. Principles and Practice of Sleep Medicine. 2nd ed. Philadelphia, Pa: WB Saunders; 1994:16–25.

55. Steriade M, McCormick DA, Sejnowski TJ. Thalamocortical oscillations in the sleeping and aroused brain. Science. 1993;262:679–685.

56. Steriade M, Contreras D, Amzica F. Synchronized sleep oscillations and their paroxysmal developments. Trends Neurosci. 1994;17:199–210.

57. Rechtschaffen A, Kales A. A Manual of Standardized Terminology: Techniques and Scoring System for Sleep Stages of Human Subjects. Los Angeles, Calif: UCLA Brain Information Service/Brain Research Institute; 1968.

58. Chase MH, Morales FR. The control of motoneurones during sleep. In: Kryger MH, Roth T, Dement WC, eds. Principles and Practice of Sleep Medicine. 2nd ed. Philadelphia, Pa: WB Saunders; 1994:163–176.

59. Baghdoyan HA, Spotts JL, Snyder SG. Simultaneous pontine and basal forebrain microinjections of carbachol suppress REM sleep. J Neurosci. 1993;13:229–242.

60. Jouvet M, Delorme F. Locus coeruleus et sommeil paradoxal. C R Soc Biol. 1965;159:895–899.

61. Hendricks JC, Morrison AR, Mann GL. Different behaviors during paradoxical sleep without atonia depend upon lesion site. Brain Res. 1982;239:81–105.

62. Henly K, Morrison AR. A re-evaluation of the effects of lesions of the pontine tegmentum and locus coeruleus on phenomena of paradoxical sleep in the cat. Acta Neurobiol Exp. 1974;34:215–232.

63. Sakai K. Executive mechanisms of paradoxical sleep. Arch Ital Biol. 1988;126:239–257.

64. Sakai K, Sastre J-P, Salvert D, et al. Tegmentoreticular projections with special reference to muscular atonia during paradoxical sleep in the cat: an HRP study. Brain Res. 1979;176:233–254.

65. Lai YY, Siegel JM. Medullary regions mediating atonia. J Neurosci. 1988;8:4790–4796.

66. McIntire DC, Saari M, Pappas BA. Potentiation of amygdala kindling in adult or infant rats by injection of 6-hydroxydopamine. Exp Neurol. 1979;63:527–544.

67. Guberman A, Gloor P. Cholinergic drug studies of penicillin epilepsy in the cat. Brain Res. 1982;239:203–222.

68. Applegate CD, Burchfiel JL, Konkol RJ. Kindling antagonism: effects of norepinephrine depletion on kindled seizure suppression after concurrent, alternate stimulation in rats. Exp Neurol. 1986;94:379–390.

69. Velasco M, Velasco F. Brain stem regulation of cortical and motor excitability: effects on experimental and focal motor seizures. In: Sterman MB, Shouse MN, Passouant P, eds. Sleep and Epilepsy. New York, NY: Academic Press; 1982:53–61.

70. Corcoran ME. Characteristics of accelerated kindling after depletion of noradrenaline in adult rats. Neuropharmacology. 1988;27:1081–1084.

71. Coenen AM, Stephens DN, Van Luijtelaar EL. Effects of the beta-carboline abecarnil on epileptic activity, EEG, sleep and behavior of rats. Pharmacol Biochem Behav. 1992;42:401–405.

72. Shouse MN, King A, Langer J, et al. Basic mechanisms underlying seizure-prone and seizure-resistant sleep and awakening states in feline kindled and penicillin epilepsy. In: Wada JA, ed. Kindling 4. New York, NY: Plenum Press; 1990:313–327.

73. Guilleminault C, Silvestri R. Disorders of arousal and epilepsy during sleep. In: Sterman MB, Shouse MN, Passouant PP, eds. Sleep and Epilepsy. New York, NY: Academic Press; 1982:513–531.

74. Hauser WA. Overview: epidemiology, pathology, and genetics. In: Engel J Jr, Pedley TA, eds. Epilepsy: A Comprehensive Textbook. Vol 1. Philadelphia, Pa: Lippincott-Raven; 1997:11–14.

75. Ohayon MM, Caulet M, Priest RG. Violent behavior during sleep. J Clin Psychiatry. 1997;58:369–376.

76. Hublin C, Kaprio J, Partinen M, et al. Prevalence and genetics of sleepwalking: a population-based twin study. Neurology. 1997;48:177–181.

77. Goldin PR, Rosen RC. Epidemiology of nine parasomnias in young adults. Sleep Res. 1997;26:367.

78. Pedley TA, Guilleminault C. Episodic nocturnal wanderings responsive to anticonvulsant drug therapy. Ann Neurol. 1977;2:30–35.

79. Pedley TA. Differential diagnosis of episodic symptoms. Epilepsia. 1983;24(suppl 1):S31–S44.

80. Maselli RA, Rosenberg RS, Spire J-S. Episodic nocturnal wanderings in non-epileptic young patients. Sleep. 1988;11:156–161.

81. Meierkord H, Fish DR, Smith SJM, et al. Is nocturnal paroxysmal dystonia a form of frontal lobe epilepsy? Move Disord. 1992;1:38–42.

82. Montagna P, Cirignotta F, Giovanardi-Rossi P, et al. Dystonic attacks related to sleep and exercise. Eur Neurol. 1992;32:185–189.

83. Lugaresi E, Cirignotta F, Montagna P. Nocturnal paroxysmal dystonia. J Neurol Neurosurg Psychiatry. 1986;49:375–380.

84. Sellal F, Hirsch E, Maquet P, et al. Postures et movements anormaux paroxystiques au cours du sommeil: dystonie paroxystique hypnognique ou epilepsie partielle? Rev Neurol. 1991;147:121–128.

85. Parkes JD. The parasomnias. Lancet. 1986;2:1021–1025.

86. Oswald I. Sudden bodily jerks on falling asleep. Brain. 1959;82:92–103.

87. Dagnino N, Loeb C, Massazza G, et al. Hypnic physiological myoclonus in man: an EEG-EMG study in normals and neurological patients. Eur Neurol. 1969;2:47–58.

88. Lugaresi E, Coccagna G, Cirignotta F. Phenomena occurring during sleep onset in man. In: Popoviciu L, Asgian B, Badiu G, eds. Sleep 1978. Fourth European Congress on Sleep Research, Tirgu-Mures. Basel, Switzerland: S. Karger; 1980:24–27.

89. Declerck AC, Arends JB. An exceptional case of parasomnia: the exploding head syndrome. Sleep-Wake Res Netherlands. 1994;5:41–43.

90. Pearce JMS. Clinical features of the exploding head syndrome. J Neurol Neurosurg Psychiatry. 1989;52:907–910.

91. Sachs C, Svanborg E. The exploding head syndrome: polysomnographic recordings and therapeutic suggestions. Sleep. 1991;14:263–266.

92. Walsleben JA, O'Malley EB, Freeman J, et al. Polysomnographic and topographic mapping of EEG in the exploding head syndrome. Sleep Res. 1993;22:284.

93. Fornazzari L, Farcnik K, Smith I, et al. Violent visual hallucinations and aggression in frontal lobe dysfunction: clinical manifestations of deep orbitofrontal foci. J Neuropsychiatry Clin Neurosci. 1992;4:42–44.

94. Diagnostic Classification Steering Committee. International Classification of Sleep Disorders: Diagnostic and Coding Manual. Rochester, Minn: American Sleep Disorders Association; 1990.

95. Epstein AW, Hill W. Ictal phenomena during REM sleep of a temporal lobe epileptic. Arch Neurol. 1966;15:367–375.

96. Epstein AW. Recurrent dreams: their relationship to temporal lobe seizures. Arch Gen Psychiatry. 1964;10:49–54.

97. Boller F, Wright DG, Cavalieri R, et al. Paroxysmal "nightmares." Neurology. 1975;25:1026–1028.

98. Snyder CH. Epileptic equivalents in children. Pediatrics. 1958;21:308–318.

99. Scheffer IE, Bhatia KP, Lopes-Cendes I, et al. Autosomal dominant nocturnal frontal lobe epilepsy: a distinctive clinical disorder. Brain. 1995;118:61–73.

100. Scheffer IE, Bhatia KP, Lopes-Cendes I, et al. Autosomal dominant frontal epilepsy misdiagnosed as sleep disorder. Lancet. 1994;343:515–517.

101. Zucconi M, Oldani A, Ferini-Strambi L, et al. Nocturnal paroxysmal arousals with motor behaviors during sleep: frontal lobe epilepsy or parasomnia? J Clin Neurophysiol. 1997;14:513–522.

102. Palm L, Anderson H, Elmqvist D, et al. Daytime sleep tendency before and after discontinuation of antiepileptic drugs in preadolescent children with epilepsy. Epilepsia. 1992;33:687–691.

103. Malow BA, Fromes GA, Aldrich MS. Usefulness of polysomnography in epilepsy patients. Neurology. 1997;48:1389–1394.

104. Aldrich MS. Narcolepsy. N Engl J Med. 1990;323:389–394.

105. Nishino S, Mignot E. Pharmacological aspects of human and canine narcolepsy. Prog Neurobiol. 1997;52:27–78.

106. Gambardella A, Reutens DC, Andermann F, et al. Late-onset drop attacks in temporal lobe epilepsy: a reevaluation of the concept of temporal lobe syncope. Neurology. 1994;44:1074–1078.

107. Kanazawa O, Kawai I. Status epilepticus characterized by repetitive asymmetrical atonia: two cases accompanied by partial seizures. Epilepsia. 1990;31:536–543.

108. Guerrini R, Dravet C, Genton P, et al. Epileptic negative myoclonus. Neurology. 1993;43:1078–1083.

109. Lee H, Lerner A. Transient inhibitory seizures mimicking crescendo TIAs. Neurology. 1990;40:165–166.

110. Andermann F, Tenembaum S. Negative motor phenomena in generalized epilepsies: a study of atonic seizures. In: Fahn S, Hallett M, Luders HO, et al. Negative Motor Phenomena. Vol 67. Philadelphia, Pa: Lippincott-Raven; 1995:9–28.

111. So NK. Atonic phenomena and partial seizures. In: Fahn S, Hallett M, Luders HO, et al, eds. Negative Motor Phenomena. Vol 67. Philadelphia, Pa: Lippincott-Raven; 1995:29–39.

112. Noachtar S, Holthausen H, Luders HO. Epileptic negative myoclonus. Neurology. 1997;49:1534–1537.

113. Mayeux R, Alexander MP, Benson DF, et al. Poriomania. Neurology. 1979;29:1616–1619.

114. Fagan KJ, Lee SI. Prolonged confusion following convulsions due to generalized nonconvulsive status epilepticus. Neurology. 1990;40:1689–1694.

115. Smolik P, Roth B. Kleine-Levin syndrome: etiopathogenesis and treatment. Acta Univ Carol Med Monogr. 1988;128:1–94.

116. Billiard M, Guilleminault C, Dement WC. A menstruation-linked periodic hypersomnia. Neurology. 1975;255:436–443.

117. Mothersill IW, Vogt H, Hilfiker P. Epileptic seizures manifesting as sleep, ictal sleep. Sleep Res. 1995;24:410.

118. Wszolek ZK, Groover RV, Klass DW. Seizures presenting as episodic hypersomnolence. Epilepsia. 1995;36:108–110.

119. Kryger MH, Steljes DG, Yee W-C, et al. Central sleep apnoea in congenital muscular dystrophy. J Neurol Neurosurg Psychiatry. 1991;54:710–712.

120. Barthlen GM, Brown LK, Stacy C. Polysomnographic documentation of seizures in a patient with obstructive sleep apnea syndrome. Neurology. 1998;50:309–310.

121. Devinsky O, Eherenberg B, Barthlen GM, et al. Epilepsy and sleep apnea syndrome. Neurology. 1994;44:2060–2064.

122. Vaughn BV, Messenheimer JA, D'Cruz O. The effect of treatment of sleep apnea in patients with epilepsy. Sleep Res. 1994;23:398.

123. Wyler AR, Weymuller EA-J. Epilepsy complicated by sleep apnea. Ann Neurol. 1981;9:403–404.

124. Vaughn BV, D'Cruz OF, Beach J, et al. Improvement of epileptic seizure control with treatment of obstructive sleep apnea. Seizure. 1996;5:73–78.

125. Cirignotta F, Zucconi M, Mondini S, et al. Cerebral anoxic attacks in sleep apnea syndrome. Sleep. 1989;12:400–404.

126. Thach BT. Sleep apnea in infancy and childhood. Med Clin North Am. 1985;69:1289–1315.

127. Wantanabe K, Hara K, Hakamada S, et al. Seizures with apnea in children. Pediatrics. 1982;70:87–90.

128. Walls TJ, Newman PK, Cumming WJK. Recurrent apnoeic attacks as a manifestation of epilepsy. Postgrad Med J. 1981;57:575–576.

129. Monod N, Peirano P, Plouin P, et al. Seizure-induced apnea. Ann NY Acad Sci. 1988;533:411–420.

130. Peled R, Lavie P. Paroxysmal awakenings from sleep associated with excessive daytime somnolence: a form of nocturnal epilepsy. Neurology. 1986;36:95–98.

131. Niedermeyer E, Walker AE. Mesio-frontal epilepsy. Electroencephalogr Clin Neurophysiol. 1971;31:104–105.

132. Benner RP, Atkinson R. Generalized paroxysmal fast activity: electroencephalographic and clinical features. Ann Neurol. 1982;11:386–390.

133. Erba G, Cavazzuti V. Pure tonic seizures with arousal. Sleep Res. 1981;10:164.

134. Erba G, Ferber R. Sleep disruption by subclinical seizure activity as a cause of increased waking seizures and decreased daytime function. Sleep Res. 1983;12:307.

135. Tachibana N, Shinde A, Ikeda A, et al. Supplementary motor area seizure resembling sleep disorder. Sleep. 1996;19:811–816.

136. Sforza E, Montagna P, Rinaldi R, et al. Paroxysmal periodic motor attacks during sleep: clinical and polygraphic features. Electroencephalogr Clin Neurophysiol. 1993;86:161–166.

137. Montagna P, Sforza E, Tinuper F, et al. Paroxysmal arousals during sleep. Neurology. 1990;40:1063–1066.

138. Malow BA, Varma NK. Seizures and arousals from sleep—which comes first? Sleep. 1995;18:783–786.

139. Hoeppner JB, Garron DC, Cartwright RD. Self-reported sleep disorder symptoms in epilepsy. Epilepsia. 1984;25:434–437.

140. Abe K, Amatomi M, Oda N. Sleepwalking and recurrent sleeptalking in children of childhood sleepwalkers. Am J Psychiatry. 1984;141:800–801.

141. Bakwin H. Sleep-walking in twins. Lancet. 1970;2:446–447.

142. Fisher C, Kahn E, Edwards A, et al. A psychophysiological study of nightmares and night terrors, I: physiological aspects of the stage 4 night terror. J Nerv Ment Dis. 1973;157:75–98.

143. Fisher C, Kahn E, Edwards A, et al. A psychophysiological study of nightmares and night terrors, III: mental content and recall of stage 4 night terrors. J Nerv Ment Dis. 1974;158:174–188.

144. Hallstrom T. Night terrors in adults through three generations. Acta Psychiatry Scand. 1972;48:350–352.

145. Kales A, Soldatos C, Bixler EO, et al. Hereditary factors in sleepwalking and night terrors. Br J Psychiatry. 1980;137:111–118.

146. Naylor MW, Aldrich MS. The distribution of confusional arousals across sleep stages and time of night in children and adolescents with sleep terrors. Sleep Res. 1991;20:308.

147. Guilleminault C, Moscovitch A, Leger D. Forensic sleep medicine: nocturnal wandering and violence. Sleep. 1995;18:740–748.

148. Llorente MD, Currier MB, Norman S, et al. Night terrors in adults: phenomenology and relationship to psychopathology. J Clin Psychiatry. 1992;53:392–394.

149. Moldofsky H, Gilbert R, Lue FA, et al. Sleep-related violence. Sleep. 1995;18:731–739.

150. Schenck CH, Hurwitz TD, Bundlie SR, et al. Sleep-related injury in 100 adult patients: a polysomnographic and clinical report. Am J Psychiatry. 1989;146:1166–1173.

151. Schenck CH, Hurwitz TD, Bundlie SR, et al. Sleep-related eating disorders: polysomnographic correlates of a heterogeneous syndrome distinct from daytime eating disorders. Sleep. 1991;14:419–431.

152. Schenck CH, Hurwitz TD, O'Connor KA, et al. Additional categories of sleep-related eating disorders and the current status of treatment. Sleep. 1993;16:457–466.

153. Schenck CH, Mahowald MW. Review of nocturnal sleep-related eating disorders. Int J Eating Disord. 1994;15:343–356.

154. Cirignotta F, Marcacci G, Lugaresi E. Epileptic seizures precipitated by eating. Epilepsia. 1977;18:445–449.

155. Ebner A, Dinner DS, Noachtar S, et al. Automatisms with preserved responsiveness: a lateralizing sign in psychomotor seizures. Neurology. 1995;45:61–64.

156. Armstrong SC, Watters MR, Pearce JW. A case of nocturnal gelastic epilepsy. Neuropsychiatry Neuropsychol Behav Neurol. 1990;3:213–216.

157. Luciano D, Devinsky O, Perrine K. Crying seizures. Neurology. 1993;43:2113–2117.

158. Ichida M, Gomi A, Hiranouchi N, et al. A case of cerebral endometriosis causing catamenial epilepsy. Neurology. 1993;43:2708–2709.

159. Newmark ME, Penry JK. Catamenial epilepsy: a review. Epilepsia. 1980;21:281–300.

160. Schenck CH, Mahowald MW. Two cases of premenstrual sleep terrors and injurious sleepwalking. J Psychosomat Obstet Gynecol 1995;16:79–84.

161. Fietze I, Warmuth R, Witt C, et al. Sleep-related breathing disorder and pavor nocturnus. Sleep Res. 1995;24A:301.

162. Millman RP, Kipp GR, Carskadon MA. Sleepwalking precipitated by treatment of sleep apnea with nasal CPAP. Chest. 1991;99:750–751.

163. Schenck CH, Hurwitz TD, Mahowald MW. REM sleep behavior disorder: a report on a series of 96 consecutive cases and a review of the literature. J Sleep Res. 1993;2:224–231.

164. D'Cruz OF, Vaughn BV. Nocturnal seizures mimic REM behavior disorder. Am J Electroneurodiag Technol. 1997;37:258–264.

165. Gillin JC, Rapoport JL, Mikkelsen EJ, et al. EEG sleep patterns in enuresis: a further analysis and comparison with normal controls. Biol Psychiatry. 1982;17:947–953.

166. Mikkelsen EJ, Rapoport JL, Nee L, et al. Childhood enuresis I: sleep patterns and psychopathology. Arch Gen Psychiatry. 1980;37:1139–1144.

167. Arguner A, Baybas S, Gozukirmizi E, et al. Focal and generalized abnormalities during sleep in cases of enuresis nocturna. In: Popoviciu L, Asgian B, Badiu G, eds. Sleep 1978. Fourth European Congress on Sleep Research, Tirgu-Mures. Basel, Switzerland: Karger; 1980:717–720.

168. Fermaglich JL. Electroencephalographic study of enuretics. Am J Dis Child. 1969;118:473–477.

169. Mahowald MW, Thorpy MJ. Non-arousal parasomnias in the child. In: Ferber R, Kryger MH, eds. Principles and Practice of Sleep Medicine in the Child. Philadelphia, Pa: WB Saunders; 1995:115–123.

170. Montplaisir J, Godbout R, Pelletier G, et al. Restless legs syndrome and periodic limb movements during sleep. In: Kryger MH, Roth T, Dement WC, eds. Principles and Practice of Sleep Medicine, 2nd ed. Philadelphia, Pa; WB Saunders; 1994:589–597.

171. Mendelson WB. Are periodic leg movements associated with clinical sleep disturbance? Sleep. 1996;19:219–223.

172. Lugaresi E, Coccagna G, Mantovani M, et al. The evolution of different types of myoclonus during sleep: a polygraphic study. Eur Neurol. 1970;4:321–331.

173. Plazzi G, Provini F, Ligouri R, et al. Propriospinal myoclonus at the transition from wake to sleep. Sleep Res. 1996;26:438.

174. Montagna P, Provini F, Plazzi G, et al. Propriospinal myoclonus upon relaxation and drowsiness: a cause of severe insomnia. Move Disord. 1997;12:66–72.

175. Kimmel PL. Sleep disorders in chronic renal disease. J Nephrol. 1989;1:59–65.

176. Pressman MR, Benz RL, Peterson DD. High incidence of sleep disorders in end stage renal disease. Sleep Res. 1995;24:417.

177. American Psychiatric Association. Diagnostic and Statistical Manual of Mental Disorders. 4th ed. Washington, DC: American Psychiatric Association; 1994.

178. Stores G, Zaiwalla Z. Misdiagnosis of frontal lobe complex partial seizures in children. Adv Epileptol. 1989;17:288–290.

179. Young GB, Blume WT, Wells GA, et al. Differential aspects of sleep epilepsy. Can J Neurol Sci. 1985;12:317–320.

180. Lerman P. Benign childhood epilepsy with centrotemporal spikes (BECT). In: Engel J Jr, Pedley TA, eds. Epilepsy: A Comprehensive Textbook. Philadelphia, Pa: Lippincott-Raven; 1997:2307–2314.

181. Fusco L, Iani C, Faedda MT, et al. Mesial frontal lobe epilepsy: a clinical entity not sufficiently described. J Epilepsy. 1990;3:123–135.

182. Marsh GG. Neurological syndrome in a patient with episodic howling and violent motor behavior. J Neurol Neurosurg Psychiatry. 1978;41:366–369.

183. Stores G, Zaiwalla Z, Bergel N. Frontal lobe complex partial seizures in children: a form of epilepsy at particular risk of misdiagnosis. Dev Med Child Neurol. 1991;33:998–1009.

184. Sussman NM, Jackel RA, Kaplan LR, et al. Bicycling movements as a manifestation of complex partial seizures of temporal lobe origin. Epilepsia. 1989;30:527–531.

185. Waterman K, Purves SJ, Strauss E, et al. An epileptic syndrome caused by mesial frontal lobe seizure foci. Neurology. 1987;37:577–582.

186. Oldani A, Zucconi M, Ferini-Strambi L, et al. Autosomal dominant nocturnal frontal lobe epilepsy: electroclinical picture. Epilepsia. 1996;37:964–976.

187. Hayman M, Scheffer IE, Chinvarun Y, et al. Autosomal dominant nocturnal frontal lobe epilepsy: demonstration of focal frontal onset and intrafamilial variation. Neurology. 1997;49:969–975.

188. King DW, Smith JR. Supplementary sensorimotor area epilepsy in adults. Adv Neurology. 1996;70:285–291.

189. Montplaisir J, Laveriere M, Saint-Hilaire JM, et al. Sleep and temporal lobe epilepsy: a case study with depth electrodes. Neurology. 1981;31:1352–1356.

190. Drake MEJ. Cursive and cursing epilepsy. Neurology. 1984;34:267.

191. Halbreich U, Assael M. Electroencephalogram with sphenoidal needles in sleepwalkers. Psychiatr Clin. 1979;11:213–218.

192. Spire J-P, Maselli R. Episodic nocturnal wandering: further evidence of an epileptic disorder. Neurology. 1983;33(suppl 2):215.

193. Popoviciu L. Frontier states between sleep incidents and nocturnal epileptic attacks. In: Koella WP, Levin P, eds. Sleep 1976. Third European Congress of Sleep Research, Montpellier, France. Basel, Switzerland: Karger; 1977:65–74.

194. Plazzi G, Tinuper P, Montagna P, et al. Epileptic nocturnal wanderings. Neurology. 1995;45(suppl 4):A332.

195. Goldensohn ES, Gold AP. Prolonged behavioral disturbances as ictal phenomena. Neurology. 1960;10:1–9.

196. Lugaresi E, Cirignotta F. Hypnogenic paroxysmal dystonia: epileptic seizure or a new syndrome? Sleep. 1981;4:129–138.

197. Lugaresi E, Cirignotta F. Nocturnal paroxysmal dystonia. In: Sterman MB, Shouse MN, Passouant P, eds. Sleep and Epilepsy. New York, NY: Academic Press; 1982:507–511.

198. Hirsch E. Abnormal paroxysmal postures and movements during sleep: partial epilepsy or paroxysmal hypnogenic dystonia. In: Horne J, ed. Sleep '90. Tenth European Congress on Sleep Research, Strasbourg, France. Bochum, Germany: Pontenagle Press; 1990:471–473.

199. Hirsch E, Sellal F, Maton B, et al. Nocturnal paroxysmal dystonia: a clinical form of focal epilepsy. Neurophysiol Clin. 1994;24:207–217.

200. Sellal F, Hirsch E. Nocturnal paroxysmal dystonia [letter]. Move Disord. 1993;2:252–253.

201. Tinuper P, Cerullo A, Cirignotta F, et al. Nocturnal paroxysmal

dystonia with short-lasting attacks: three cases with evidence for an epileptic frontal lobe origin of seizures. Epilepsia. 1990;31:549–556.

202. Godbout R, Montplaisir J, Rouleau I. Hypnogenic paroxysmal dystonia: epilepsy or a sleep disorder. A case report. Clin Electroencephalogr. 1985;16:136–142.

203. Lapierre O, Montplaisir J, Remillard G. Therapeutic effect of clobazam in nocturnal paroxysmal dystonia: further support for an epileptic etiology. Sleep Res. 1991;20A:339.

204. Oguni M, Oguni H, Kozasa M, et al. A case with nocturnal paroxysmal unilateral dystonia and interictal right frontal epileptic EEG focus: a lateralized variant of nocturnal paroxysmal dystonia? Brain Dev. 1992;14:412–416.

205. Rosenberg RS, Pasternak JF. Nocturnal paroxysmal dystonia resembling tonic-clonic seizures. Sleep Res. 1990;19:274.

206. Lee BI, Lesser RP, Pippenger CE, et al. Familial paroxysmal hypnogenic dystonia. Neurology. 1985;35:1357–1360.

207. Demirkiran M, Jankovic J. Paroxysmal dyskinesias: clinical features and classification. Ann Neurol. 1995;38:571–579.

208. Lehkuniec E, Micheli F, De-Abelaiz R, et al. Concurrent hypnogenic and reflex paroxysmal dystonia. Move Disord. 1988;3:290–294.

209. Veggiotti P, Zambrino CA, Balottin U, et al. Concurrent nocturnal and diurnal paroxysmal dystonia. Child's Nerv System. 1993;9:458–461.

210. Biary N, Singh B, Bahou Y, et al. Posttraumatic paroxysmal nocturnal hemidystonia. Move Disord. 1994;9:98–99.

211. Stoudemire A, Ninan PT, Wooten V. Hypnogenic paroxysmal dystonia with panic attacks responsive to drug therapy. Psychosomatics. 1987;28:280–281.

212. Rajna P, Kundra O, Halasz P. Vigilance level-dependent tonic seizures—epilepsy or sleep disorder? A case report. Epilepsia. 1983;24:725–733.

213. Vigevano F, Fusco L. Hypnic tonic postural seizures in healthy children provide evidence for a partial epileptic syndrome of frontal lobe origin. Epilepsia. 1993;39:110–119.

214. Holmes GL. Rolandic epilepsy: clinical and electroencephalographic features. In: Degen R, Dreifuss FE, eds. Benign Localized and Generalized Epilepsies of Early Childhood. Amsterdam, Netherland: Elsevier Science Publishers; 1992:29–43.

215. Panayiotopoulos CP. Benign nocturnal childhood occipital epilepsy: a new syndrome with nocturnal seizures, tonic deviation of the eyes, and vomiting. J Child Neurol. 1989;4:43–48.

216. Panayiotopoulos CP. Benign childhood epilepsy with occipital paroxysms. In: Andermann F, Beaumanoir A, Mira L, et al, eds. Occipital Seizures and Epilepsy in Children. London, England: John Libbey; 1993:151–164.

217. Sanmarti FX, Estivial E, Campistol J, et al. Apneic episodes in an infant: exceptional epileptic seizures. Electroencephalogr Clin Neurophysiol. 1985;60:16.

218. Maytal J, Resnick TH. Stridor presenting as the sole manifestation of seizures. Ann Neurol. 1985;18:414–415.

219. Winans HM. Epileptic equivalents, a cause for somatic symptoms. Am J Med. 1949;7:150–152.

220. Ravindran M. Temporal lobe seizure presenting as "laryngospasm." Clin Electroencephalogr. 1981;12:139–140.

221. Amir J, Ashkenazi S, Schonfeld T, et al. Laryngospasm as a single manifestation of epilepsy. Arch Dis Child. 1983;58:151–153.

222. Kiok MC, Terrence CF, Fromm GH, et al. Sinus arrest in epilepsy. Neurology. 1986;36:115–116.

223. Gilchrist JM. Arrhythmogenic seizures: diagnosis by simultaneous EEG/ECG recording. Neurology. 1985;35:1503–1506.

224. Hockman CH, Mauch HP, Hoff EC. ECG changes resulting from cerebral stimulation, II: a spectrum of ventricular arrhythmias of sympathetic origin. Am Heart J. 1966;71:695–700.

225. Metz SA, Halter JB, Porte DJ, et al. Autonomic epilepsy: clonidine blockade of paroxysmal catecholamine release and flushing. Ann Intern Med. 1978;88:189–193.

226. Kuritzky A, Hering R, Goldhammer G, et al. Clonidine treatment in paroxysmal localized hyperhidrosis. Arch Neurol. 1984;41:1210–1211.

227. McLean AJ. Autonomic epilepsy: report of a case with observations at necropsy. Arch Neurol Psychiatry. 1934;32:189–197.

228. Wannamaker BB. Autonomic nervous system and epilepsy. Epilepsia. 1985;26(suppl 1):S31–S39.

229. Connors MH, Sheikholislam BM. Hypothalamic symptomatology and its relationship to diencephalic tumor in childhood. Child's Brain. 1977;3:31–36.

230. Bullard DE. Diencephalic seizures: responsiveness to bromocriptine and morphine. Ann Neurol. 1987;21:609–611.

231. Berger H. Fever: an unusual manifestation of epilepsy. Postgrad Med. 1966;40:479–481.

232. Brogna CG, Lee SI, Dreifuss FE. Pilomotor seizures. Magnetic resonance imaging and electroencephalographic localization of originating focus. Arch Neurol. 1986;43:1085–1086.

233. Cohn DF, Avrahami E, Dalos E. Thermal epilepsy manifest as fever attacks [letter]. Ann Intern Med. 1984;101:569–570.

234. Solomon GE. Diencephalic autonomic epilepsy caused by a neoplasm. J Pediatr. 1973;83:277–280.

235. Mulder DW, Daly D, Bailey AA. Visceral epilepsy. Arch Intern Med. 1954;93:481–493.

236. Van Buren JM. Some autonomic concomitants of ictal automatism: a study of temporal lobe attacks. Brain. 1958;81:505–528.

237. Liporace JD, Sperling MR. Simple autonomic seizures. In: Engel J Jr, Pedley TA, eds. Epilepsy: A Comprehensive Textbook. Philadelphia, Pa: Lippincott-Raven; 1997:549–555.

238. Jayakar PB, Seshia SS. Electrical status epilepticus during slow-wave sleep: a review. J Clin Neurophysiol. 1991;8:299–311.

239. Kobayashi K, Nishibayashi N, Ohtsuka Y, et al. Epilepsy with electrical status epilepticus during slow sleep and secondary bilateral synchrony. Epilepsia. 1994;35:1097–1103.

240. Patry G, Lyagoubi S, Tassinari CA. Subclinical "electrical status epilepticus" induced by sleep in children. Arch Neurol. 1971;24:242–252.

241. Beaumanior A, Grandjean E. Continuous spike and wave discharges during sleep: significance. Electroencephalogr Clin Neurophysiol. 1983;55:18–19.

242. Billard C, Autret A, Laffont F, et al. Electrical status epilepticus during sleep in children: a reappraisal from eight new cases. In: Sterman MB, Shouse MN, Passouant P, eds. Sleep and Epilepsy. New York, NY: Academic Press; 1982:481–494.

243. Maquet P, Hirsch E, Metz-Lutz MN, et al. Regional cerebral glucose metabolism in children with deterioration of one or more cognitive functions and continuous spike-and-wave discharges during sleep. Brain. 1995;118:1497–1520.

244. Genton P, Maton B, Ohihara M, et al. Continuous focal spikes during REM sleep in a case of acquired aphasia (Landau-Kleffner syndrome). Sleep. 1992;15:454–460.

245. Burgerman RS, Sperling M. Cardiac arrhythmias in epilepsy: a study of multiple seizure types. Neurology. 1993;43:A161.

246. Fincham RW, Shivapour ET, Leis AA, et al. Ictal bradycardia with syncope: a case report. Neurology. 1992;42:2222–2223.

247. Frysinger RC, Engel J, Harper RM. Interictal heart rate patterns in partial seizure disorders. Neurology. 1993;43:2136–2169.

248. Iani C, Fusco L, Faedda MT, et al. Cardiac frequency changes during absenses and partial complex seizures. Adv Epileptol. 1989;17:340–342.

249. Keilson MK, Hauser WA, Magrill JP. Electrocardiographic changes during electrographic seizures. Arch Neurol. 1989;46:1169–1170.

250. Lathers CM, Schraeder PL, Weiner FL. Synchronization of cardiac autonomic neural discharge with epileptogenic activity: the lockstep phenomenon. Electroencephalogr Clin Neurophysiol. 1987;67:247–259.

251. Liedholm LJ, Gudjonsson O. Cardiac arrest due to partial epileptic seizures. Neurology. 1992;42:824–829.

252. Mameli P, Mameli O, Tolu E, et al. Neurogenic myocardial arrhythmias in experimental focal epilepsy. Epilepsia. 1988;29:74–82.

253. Oppenheimer SM, Cechetto DF, Hachinski VC. Cerebrogenic cardiac arrhythmias. Cerebral electrocardiographic influences and their role in sudden death. Arch Neurol. 1990;47:513–519.

254. Ossentjuke E, Sterk CJOE, vanLeeuwen WS. Flicker-induced cardiac arrest in a patient with epilepsy. Electroencephalogr Clin Neurophysiol. 1966;20:257–259.

255. Pritchett ELC, McNamara JO, Gallagher JJ. Arrhythmogenic epilepsy: an hypothesis. Am Heart J. 1980;100:683–688.

256. Schott GD, McLeod AA, Jewitt DE. Cardiac arrhythmias that masquerade as epilepsy. Br Med J. 1977;1:1454–1457.

257. Stephenson JBP. Electrocardiographic accompaniments of temporal lobe epileptic seizures. Lancet. 1986;1:1450.

258. Trevathan E, Cascino GD. Partial epilepsy presenting as focal paroxysmal pain. Neurology. 1988;38:329–330.

259. Walsh GO, Masland W, Goldensohn ES. Relationship between paroxysmal atrial tachycardia and paroxysmal cerebral discharges. Bull Los Angeles Neurol Soc. 1972;37:28–35.

260. Pacia SV, Devinsky O, Luciano DJ, et al. The prolonged QT syndrome presenting as epilepsy: a report of two cases and literature review. Neurology. 1994;44:1408–1410.

261. Schraeder PL, Lathers CM, Charles JB. The spectrum of syncope. J Clin Pharmacol. 1994;34:454–459.

262. Reeves AL, Nollet KE, Klass DW, et al. The ictal bradycardia syndrome. Epilepsia. 1996;37:983–987.

263. Bergey GK, Krumholz A, Fleming CP. Complex partial seizure provocation by vasovagal syncope: video-EEG and intracranial electrode documentation. Epilepsia. 1997;38:118–121.

264. Jankovic J, Pardo R. Segmental myoclonus: clinical and pharmacologic study. Arch Neurol. 1986;43:1025–1031.

265. Lapresle J. Palatal myoclonus. Adv Neurol. 1986;43:265–273.

266. Iliceto G, Thompson BL, Day JC, et al. Diaphragmatic flutter, the moving umbilicus syndrome, and "belly dancer's" dyskinesia. Move Disord. 1990;1:15–22.

267. Phillips JR, Eldridge FL. Respiratory myoclonus (Leeuwenhoek's disease). N Engl J Med. 1973;289:1390–1395.

268. Corbett CL. Diaphragmatic flutter. Postgrad Med J. 1977;53:399–402.

269. Sethi KD, Hess DC, Huffnagle VH, et al. Acetazolamide treatment of paroxysmal dystonia in central demyelinating disease. Neurology. 1992;42:919–921.

270. Vertes RP. Brainstem control of the events of REM sleep. Progr Neurobiol. 1984;22:241–288.

271. Kuna ST, Awan R. The irregularly irregular pattern of respiratory dyskinesia. Chest. 1986;90:779–781.

272. Rich MW, Radwany SM. Respiratory dyskinesia: an underrecognized phenomenon. Chest. 1994;105:1826–1832.

273. Wilcox PG, Bassett A, Jones B, et al. Respiratory dysrhythmias in patient with tardive dyskinesias. Chest. 1994;105:203–207.

274. Brown LW, Fry JM. Paroxysmal nocturnal choking: a newly described manifestation of sleep-related epilepsy. Sleep Res. 1988;17:153.

275. Mellman TA, Uhde TW. Patients with frequent sleep panic: clinical findings and response to medication treatment. J Clin Psychiatry. 1990;51:513–516.

276. Rosenfeld DS, Furman Y. Pure sleep panic: two case reports and a review of the literature. Sleep. 1994;17:462–465.

277. Craske MG, Kreuger MT. Prevalence of nocturnal panic in a college population. J Anxiety Disord. 1990;4:125–139.

278. Lesser IM, Poland RE, Holcomb C, et al. Electroencephalographic study of nighttime panic attacks. J Nerv Ment Dis. 1985;173:744–746.

279. Grunhaus L, Birmaher B. The clinical spectrum of panic attacks. J Clin Psychopharmacol. 1985;5:93–99.

280. Hauri P, Friedman M, Ravaris RL, et al. Sleep in agoraphobia with panic attacks. Sleep Res. 1985;14:128.

281. Mellman TA, Uhde TW. Electroencephalographic sleep in panic disorder. Arch Gen Psychiatry. 1989;46:178–184.

282. McNamara ME. Absence seizures associated with panic attacks initially misdiagnosed as temporal lobe epilepsy: the importance of prolonged EEG monitoring in diagnosis. J Psychiatry Neurosci. 1993;18:46–48.

283. Wall M, Tuchman M, Mielke D. Panic attacks and temporal lobe seizures associated with a right temporal lobe arteriovenous malformation: case report. J Clin Psychiatry. 1985;46:143–145.

284. Ghadirian AM, Gauthier S, Bertrand S. Anxiety attacks in a patient with a right temporal lobe meningioma. J Clin Psychiatry. 1986;47:270–271.

285. Drubach DA, Kelly MP. Panic disorder associated with a right paralimbic lesion. Neuropsychiatry Neuropsychol Behav Neurol. 1989;4:282–289.

286. Uhde TW, Stein MB, Post RM. Lack of efficacy of carbamazepine in the treatment of panic disorder. Am J Psychiatry. 1988;145:1104–1109.

287. Edlund MJ, McNamara ME, Millman RP. Sleep apnea and panic attacks. Comprehens Psychiatry. 1991;32:130–132.

288. Daly D. Ictal affect. Am J Psychiatry. 1958;115:97–108.

289. Henriksen GF. Status epilepticus partialis with fear as clinical expression. Epilepsia. 1973;14:39–46.

290. Hermann BP, Melyn M. Effects of carbamazepine on interictal psychopathology in TLE with ictal fear. J Clin Psychiatry. 1984;45:169–171.

291. McLachlan RS, Blume WT. Isolated fear in complex partial status. Ann Neurol. 1980;8:639–641.

292. Spitz MC. Panic disorder in seizure patients: a diagnostic pitfall. Epilepsia. 1991;32:33–38.

293. Schenck CS, Milner DM, Hurwitz TD, et al. Dissociative disorders presenting as somnambulism: polysomnographic, video, and clinical documentation (8 cases). Dissociation. 1989;4:194–204.

294. Thacker K, Devinsky O, Perrine K, et al. Nonepileptic seizures during apparent sleep. Ann Neurol. 1993;33:414–418.

295. Mahowald MW, Rosen GM. Parasomnias in children. Pediatrician. 1990;17:21–31.

296. Passouant P. Historical views on sleep and epilepsy. In: Sterman MB, Shouse MN, Passouant P, eds. Sleep and Epilepsy. New York, NY: Academic Press; 1982:1–6.

297. Billiard M, Echenne B, Besset A, et al. All-night polygraphic recordings in the child with suspected epileptic seizures, in spite of normal routine and post-sleep deprivation EEGs. Electroencephalogr Clin Neurophysiol. 1981;11:450–460.

298. Aldrich MS, Jahnke B. Diagnostic value of video-EEG polysomnography. Neurology. 1991;41:1060–1066.

299. Forster FM, Liske E. Role of environmental clues in temporal lobe epilepsy. Neurology. 1963;13:301–305.

300. Mahowald MW, Schenck CH. Parasomnia purgatory—the epileptic/non-epileptic interface. In: Rowan AJ, Gates JR, eds. Non-Epileptic Seizures. Boston, Mass: Butterworth-Heinemann; 1993:123–139.

301. Dreifuss FE, Porter RJ. Choice of antiepileptic drugs. In: Engel J Jr, Pedley TA, eds. Epilepsy: A Comprehensive Textbook. Philadelphia, Pa: Lippincott-Raven; 1997:1233–1236.

302. Montagna P. Nocturnal paroxysmal dystonia and nocturnal wandering. Neurology. 1992;42(suppl 6):61–67.

303. Geier S, Bancaud J, Talairach J, et al. The seizures of frontal lobe epilepsy: a study of clinical manifestations. Neurology. 1977;27:951–958.

64

REM Sleep Parasomnias

Mark W. Mahowald
Carlos H. Schenck

Parasomnias may be conveniently classified into primary and secondary categories, with the primary consisting of disorders of sleep per se and the secondary consisting of disorders of other organ systems that take advantage of the sleep state to declare themselves (see Chapter 46). The primary parasomnias can be further subcategorized according to the state of sleep during which they occur: rapid eye movement (REM) versus nonrapid eye movement (NREM) (see Chapter 46). Primary parasomnias that occur in both REM and NREM sleep states are in a miscellaneous category.[1–3]

REM SLEEP BEHAVIOR DISORDER

The best-studied REM sleep parasomnia is the REM sleep behavior disorder (RBD). We focus primarily on this recently identified syndrome, the discovery of which was predicted through the use of a corresponding animal model. We also briefly describe other REM sleep parasomnias.

The discovery of REM sleep in 1953 by Aserinsky and Kleitman expanded the states of mammalian being to three: wakefulness, NREM sleep, and REM sleep. Each of these conditions has its own neuroanatomical, neurophysiological, neuropharmacological, and behavioral correlates. The intrusion of components from one state into another may cause severe symptoms in patients.

Numerous physiological phenomena occur during REM sleep,[4–17] and they fall into one of two categories: (1) *tonic* (appearing throughout a REM period) and (2) *phasic* (occurring intermittently during a REM period). Tonic elements include electromyographic (EMG) suppression, low-voltage desynchronized electroencephalography (EEG), high arousal threshold, hippocampal theta rhythm, elevated brain temperature, poikilothermia, olfactory bulb activity, and penile tumescence. Phasic elements include rapid eye movements, middle ear muscle activity, tongue movements, somatic muscle-limb twitches, variability of autonomic activity (cardiac and respiratory), and ponto-geniculo-occipital (PGO) spikes. It is not known whether dreaming occurs tonically or phasically during REM sleep.

Although the synchronizer (pacemaker) for the sleep-wake cycle appears to reside in the suprachiasmatic nucleus of the hypothalamus,[18, 19] the generators or executors of the various REM phenomena, both tonic and phasic, are located in the pons.[8, 20, 21]

The tonic and phasic neurophysiological processes underlying each state can be variously dissociated and recombined across states.[22] For REM sleep, the processes that generally occur in concert may also occur in dissociated form—both experimentally (e.g., REM sleep–deprived animals with PGO spikes occurring in NREM sleep and wakefulness)[23] and in human and animal disease (narcolepsy). In narcolepsy, the best understood dissociated state, the sleep attacks, hypnagogic hallucinations, sleep paralysis, cataplexy, and automatic behavior each represents the intrusion or persistence of one state of being into another (i.e., cataplexy is the inappropriate isolated intrusion of REM sleep atonia [REM atonia] into wakefulness, usually induced by an emotionally laden event).[24, 25] It has recently been shown that the identical medullary cells are responsible for both REM atonia and cataplexy.[26]

Many dissociated conditions involving wakefulness and REM and NREM sleep are theoretically possible and await discovery or better description (i.e., the disorders of arousal—confusional arousals, sleepwalking, sleep terrors). An extreme form, termed *status dissociatus*, is characterized by the complete absence of any conventional sleep-state polygraphic determinants despite the subjective experience of having slept and dreamed has been described.[27] We have recorded striking PSG sleep state admixtures in association with Parkinson's disease, olivopontocerebellar degeneration, narcolepsy, and alcohol withdrawal.

Conventional wakefulness is associated with consciousness and muscle tone; REM sleep is associated with dreaming and muscle atonia. By confining the discussion to wakefulness and REM and by assuming that there must be either consciousness or dreaming and either muscle tone or atonia and recognizing that these states can oscillate rapidly, multiple combinations are possible. The clinical presentation will depend on the baseline state of wakefulness or REM sleep.

Table 64–1 lists the spectrum of the theoretically

Table 64–1. SPECTRUM OF DISSOCIATED AND TRANSITIONAL STATES
INVOLVING WAKEFULNESS AND REM SLEEP

From Wakefulness	Consciousness	Tone	Dream	Atonia	From REM Sleep
Normal waking (ongoing state)	+	+	−	−	Normal waking (normal awakening)
Cataplexy	+	−	−	+	Sleep paralysis
Conscious hallucination	*	+	*	−	Lucid dream with tone
Hypnagogic hallucination (with sleep paralysis)	*	−	*	+	Lucid dream without tone
Conscious delirium (sleep deprivation)	*	†	*	†	Sleep delirium
Automatic behavior (drug withdrawal states)	−	+	+	−	REM sleep behavior disorder (RBD)
Hypnagogic hallucination with intermittent sleep paralysis	−	†	+	†	RBD interruptions
Narcoleptic dream attack with sleep paralysis	−	−	+	+	Normal dream

*Rapidly oscillating shifts in consciousness.
†Rapidly oscillating shifts in muscle tone.
+, present; −, absent.

possible dissociations in wakefulness and REM sleep. Normal wake and dream states are self-explanatory. Cataplexy, sleep paralysis, and hallucinations are common experiences in narcolepsy.[28] Although controversial, a variety of recombinant states may be present in delirium and may explain some of the features of delirium tremens.[29–31] The demonstration of willed movements allowing communication during lucid dreaming in REM sleep established the coexistence of dream and conscious mental activity.[32, 33]

The counterpart of wakeful automatic behavior that arises during REM sleep constitutes the RBD, which is the focus of this chapter.

HISTORICAL ASPECTS

In experiments reported in 1965, bilateral lesions of pontine regions adjacent to the locus ceruleus in cats caused absence of the expected atonia associated with REM sleep, allowing the cats to demonstrate prominent motor behaviors during REM sleep (*oneiric behaviors*).[34] This animal model has been important in further studies demonstrating the similarity between the states of REM and wakefulness[35] and in studies evaluating the state-dependent vulnerability to epileptic activity.[36] In the 1970s, scattered reports of dream-enacting behaviors involving human beings appeared; the polygraphic and behavioral condition was sometimes referred to as "stage 1 REM with tonic electromyogram."[37–40] Recognition of RBD as a distinct clinical disorder followed the report in 1986 of a series of adults with RBD.[41]

PATHOPHYSIOLOGY

The generalized atonia of REM sleep results from active inhibition of motor activity by pontine centers of the peri–locus ceruleus region that exert an excitatory influence on the reticularis magnocellularis nucleus of the medulla via the lateral tegmentoreticular tract. The reticularis magnocellularis nucleus in turn hyperpolarizes spinal motoneuron postsynaptic membranes via the ventrolateral reticulospinal tract.[42, 43] Normally, the atonia of REM sleep is briefly interrupted by excitatory inputs that produce the rapid eye movements and the muscle jerks and twitches characteristic of REM sleep.[44–46]

Most mammals studied (including human beings) exhibit a comparable set of simple REM sleep behaviors during early development,[47–54] which may reflect an adaptive maturational delay in central nervous system inhibitory capacity with heightened endogenous stimulation.[55–57] The rhesus monkey has less vigorous REM sleep movements during infancy compared with its juvenile and adult years,[49] which appears to be an exception to the general rule, but only a small percentage of mammals have been studied during sleep.[58] An in utero study of fetal sheep suggests that there is no wakefulness and that all in utero movements represent phasic REM events.[54] For human beings, a stable pattern of generalized REM atonia with minimal twitching is achieved during early childhood and persists through adulthood (Table 64–2).[59]

Bilateral pontine tegmental lesions in cats will result in a persistent absence of REM atonia associated with prominent motor activity during REM sleep.[6, 15, 34, 43, 60–62] That this represents REM sleep rather than waking activity is supported by the presence of other features typical of REM: loss of thermoregulation, the closed nictitating membrane, miotic pupils (despite signs of autonomic activity), and blunted response to stimuli.[13]

Cats receiving pontine tegmental lesions exhibit a range of REM sleep behaviors that can appear as soon as the second postlesion day. Loss of REM atonia has been shown to be necessary, but not sufficient, to allow the expression of such REM behaviors. The specific site of a pontine lesion determines whether loss of atonia occurs with simple movements or more complex behaviors, suggesting that the pontine tegmentum is responsible for two separate mechanisms of skeletal motor inhibition during REM sleep: the atonia system and a system that suppresses phasic brainstem motor pattern generators.[6] A lesion damaging the atonia mechanism would produce only REM sleep with augmented tone (REM without atonia [RWA]), whereas a lesion affecting both mechanisms (atonia and motor pattern generator suppression) would also release complex behaviors (see Table 64–2), with the stereotypical repertoire being dependent on the precise location of the lesion. Although the classic experimental animal model of RWA involves bilateral peri–locus ceruleus

Table 64–2. MAMMALIAN REM SLEEP BEHAVIORS

Developmental (presumably most mammals)[47–54]
　Orofacial behaviors and limb jerking are present during late prenatal and early postnatal periods. Atonia then becomes more established, and only minimal twitching persists.
Experimental (cats)[6, 15, 34, 43, 60, 61]
　Pontine tegmental lesions release stereotypical behaviors that cluster into four categories:
　　　Unorganized head and limb movements
　　　Orienting, searching behaviors
　　　Attack behaviors
　　　Locomotion
Pathological (animals and human beings)

Animals

Spontaneously occurring RBD has been described in household pets (cats and dogs).[85, 86]

Human Beings

Acute RBD	Etiology
Withdrawal	Alcohol[29–31, 65, 169]
	Meprobamate[37]
	Pentazocine[170]
	Nitrazepam[39]
Intoxication	Biperiden[38]
	Tricyclic antidepressants[66–69, 73]
	Monoamine oxidase inhibitors[70]
	Caffeine[74]

Chronic RBD	
Toxic-metabolic	Tricyclic antidepressants[73]
	Fluoxetine[71]
	Venlafaxine[72]
	Selegiline treatment for Parkinson's disease[105]
	Anticholinergic treatment for Alzheimer's disease[106]
Vascular	Subarachnoid hemorrhage[41]
	Vasculitis (?)[171]
	Ischemic[172]
Tumor	Acoustic neuroma[173]
	Pontine neoplasm[84, 174, 175]
Infectious, postinfectious	Guillain-Barré syndrome[41]
Degenerative	Amyotrophic lateral sclerosis[176]
	Anterior/dorsomedial thalamic syndrome (fatal familial insomnia)[88]
	Dementia (including Alzheimer's disease and diffuse Lewy body disease and corticobasal degeneration)[79, 113, 177–181]
	Demyelinating disorder[182]
	Olivopontocerebellar degeneration[79, 183–187]
	Parkinson's disease[102, 125, 126, 188–190]
	Progressive supranuclear palsy[100, 101, 184, 185]
	Shy-Drager syndrome[186, 191–193]
	Multiple system atrophy[103, 194, 195]
	Normal pressure hydrocephalus[108]
Traumatic	? (See text)
Developmental, congenital, familial	Developmental/congenital/familial[84]
	Narcolepsy[99, 196]
	Tourette's syndrome[109]
	Group A xeroderma pigmentosum[110]
	Mitochondrial encephalomyopathy[107]
Idiopathic[41, 79, 112, 197]	(See text)

RBD, REM sleep behavior disorder.

lesions,[34] it is clear that there are other regions of the central nervous system that can affect muscle tone during REM sleep, including the medulla[63] and possibly even the hypothalamus.[21] Very relevant animal studies have indicated a co-localization of both the locomotor and atonia systems operating during REM

sleep.[64] Given the clear neuroanatomical substrate of an REM behavioral syndrome in cats, "experiments of nature" could be expected, resulting in an analogous disorder in human beings.

RBD in human beings occurs in both an acute and a chronic form. All reported cases of *acute* transient RBD fall in the toxic/metabolic category, with the best studied conditions being the withdrawal states, most commonly involving ethanol.[37] In 1881, Lasegue[65] postulated that dreams and hallucinations may have a common mechanism. Wakeful dreaming has been considered to be a cause of the vivid visual hallucinations associated with delirium tremens.[29–31] Although controversial, dissociated wakeful-REM phenomena may play a major role in delirium tremens. In 1975, Japanese investigators used the phrase *stage 1 REM with tonic EMG* to describe a polygraphic and behavioral condition seen in alcohol and meprobamate withdrawal[37] that appeared to represent RWA. The polygraphic and detailed clinical description of delirium tremens in 1966 by Gross et al.[29] resembles that observed in patients with RBD. Comparable patterns have been described with nitrazepam withdrawal and biperiden intoxication.[38, 39]

Loss of REM atonia induced by medication has been carefully documented in patients receiving tricyclic antidepressants,[66–69] monoamine oxidase inhibitors,[70] fluoxetine,[71] and venlafaxine.[72] One patient, who was receiving clomipramine, experienced motor behavior during sleep that undoubtedly represented loss of REM atonia with dream enactment.[73] Excessive caffeine ingestion has also been implicated.[74] The relation between waking hallucinations and sleeping dreams was extensively reviewed.[75]

The chronic form is most often either idiopathic or associated with neurological disorders. Each basic category of neurological disease (e.g., vascular, neoplastic, toxic/metabolic, infectious, degenerative, traumatic, congenital, and idiopathic, as listed in Table 64–2) could be expected to manifest this disorder. Although RBD has not been reported after infection or trauma, a study of persistent hypersomnolence following Epstein-Barr viral infection (infectious mononucleosis and Guillain-Barré syndrome)[76] and the case of a patient with absent REM sleep as a sequel to a strategically located pontine shrapnel fragment[77] indicate that these categories will eventually be implicated. Rarely, RBD appears to follow significant psychic trauma[78, 79] or to be associated with stress.[80] The phenomenon of stress-related RBD may be explained in part by experience-mediated changes in cortical organization and in synaptic transmission that reflect an impressive plasticity within the central nervous system.[81–83]

The chronic idiopathic category represents patients whose RBD is not associated with psychopathology or detectable neuropathology. A familial association has been documented[84] (Fig. 64–1A and B) and is occasionally suggested historically during clinical evaluations. Interestingly, spontaneously occurring idiopathic RBD has been reported in dogs and cats.[85, 86]

The paucity of nontoxic/metabolic, nonidiopathic, permanent neurological conditions resulting in RBD

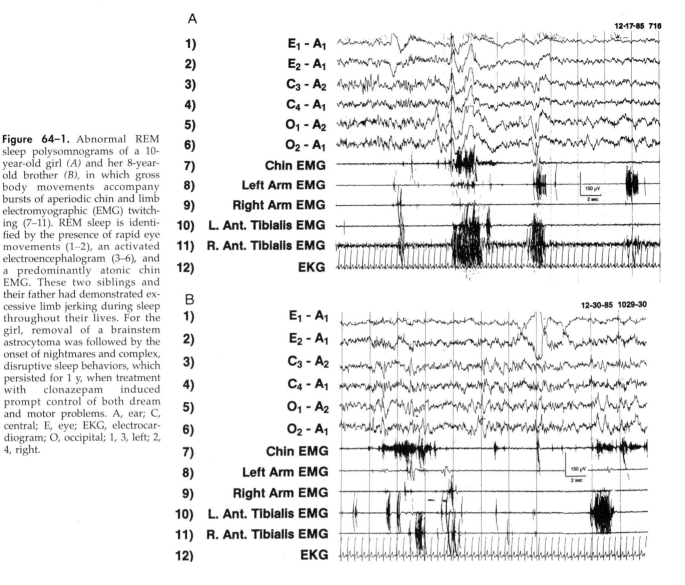

Figure 64–1. Abnormal REM sleep polysomnograms of a 10-year-old girl *(A)* and her 8-year-old brother *(B),* in which gross body movements accompany bursts of aperiodic chin and limb electromyographic (EMG) twitching (7–11). REM sleep is identified by the presence of rapid eye movements (1–2), an activated electroencephalogram (3–6), and a predominantly atonic chin EMG. These two siblings and their father had demonstrated excessive limb jerking during sleep throughout their lives. For the girl, removal of a brainstem astrocytoma was followed by the onset of nightmares and complex, disruptive sleep behaviors, which persisted for 1 y, when treatment with clonazepam induced prompt control of both dream and motor problems. A, ear; C, central; E, eye; EKG, electrocardiogram; O, occipital; 1, 3, left; 2, 4, right.

reflects the fact that structural damage to the intramedullary pontine sleep-generating regions or the more rostral centers infrequently renders the affected individual sufficiently neurologically intact to display RBD.

The pathophysiology of RBD in human beings may be presumed to be similar to that postulated for experimental cats,[6] namely the loss of REM atonia coupled with enhancement of phasic motor drive. However, because approximately 42% (40 of 96) of the patients in our cumulative adult series were considered idiopathic after an extensive neurological evaluation,[87] it appears that identifiable structural neuropathology is not necessary for the genesis of RBD. This view was espoused by a Japanese group: "Excited stage 1 REM" (i.e., RBD) was proposed to result from (1) *functional depression* or destruction of the brainstem structures responsible for atonia and (2) *reduced activity* or destruction of brainstem serotonergic and/or noradrenergic structures responsible for inhibiting phasic activity.[40]

In our group of elderly adults with chronic RBD, we theorize that functional dysregulation associated with

the idiopathic subtype may be triggered by subtle but strategic brain changes that do not primarily affect the brainstem. A compromise in descending inhibition to the brainstem may be sufficient to produce RBD, as strongly suggested in one human case of isolated thalamic degeneration[88] and as theoretically discussed in the context of animal experimentation.[89] It appears that the disinhibition ratio of atonic and phasic mechanisms is crucial to the ongoing manifestation of RBD (Fig. 64–2) and that each mechanism is subject to influences from both within the brainstem and from higher central nervous system centers. This is supported by the results of studies in animals that indicate that multiple neural sites may affect REM atonia.[21, 63] It has been shown that in animals, there is a co-localization of both the locomotor and atonia systems that operate during REM sleep, indicating that RBD may result from an imbalance in REM-related influence on these two systems.[64] In fact, RBD behaviors can emerge despite maintenance of full submental EMG atonia, suggesting hyperactivation of brainstem locomotor centers with-

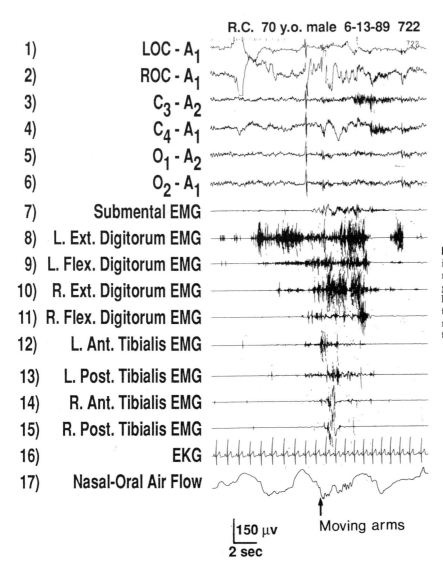

R.C. 70 y.o. male 6-13-89 722

1) LOC - A₁
2) ROC - A₁
3) C₃ - A₂
4) C₄ - A₁
5) O₁ - A₂
6) O₂ - A₁
7) Submental EMG
8) L. Ext. Digitorum EMG
9) L. Flex. Digitorum EMG
10) R. Ext. Digitorum EMG
11) R. Flex. Digitorum EMG
12) L. Ant. Tibialis EMG
13) L. Post. Tibialis EMG
14) R. Ant. Tibialis EMG
15) R. Post. Tibialis EMG
16) EKG
17) Nasal-Oral Air Flow

150 μv
2 sec
Moving arms

Figure 64–2. REM sleep polysomnogram illustrating extensive preservation of submental electromyographic (EMG) atonia (7), despite the emergence of gross arm movements that are noted by the technician and reflected by the prominent twitching in the upper extremity EMGs (8–11). A rapid eye movement (1–2) immediately precedes the onset of complex behaviors.

out compromise of background atonia.[90, 91] Thus, RBD is likely to result from either loss of REM atonia or excessive locomotor drive, or both.

The overwhelming male predominance of RBD raises the intriguing question of hormonal influences, as suggested in male-aggression studies in both animals and human beings.[92, 93] The fact that age-related changes in brain size are more prominent in men may also play a role.[94] The typically late onset of RBD suggests an organic brain factor and may be a manifestation of the reversal or disintegration of ontogeny of state appearance.[53] One highly speculative but tantalizing etiological possibility is that RBD represents a delayed manifestation of REM sleep abnormalities occurring early in development. This explanation invokes the well-documented prolonged effect of pharmacological manipulation on developing neural tissues.[95] In rats, Corner et al.[96] described an RBD-like PSG pattern persisting into adulthood after clomipramine-induced neonatal REM sleep suppression. Another possibility is the presence of neuronal-specific antibodies as described in neurological paraneoplastic syndromes and

the "stiff-man" syndrome.[97] One study failed to identify anti–locus ceruleus–specific antibodies in patients with RBD.[98] As autopsy material becomes available, direct neuropathological examination may provide important correlative information.

RBD and Narcolepsy

There is a higher incidence of RBD in patients with narcolepsy. This association could be expected because both narcolepsy and RBD are disorders characterized by "state boundary control" abnormalities. The tricyclic antidepressants and monoamine oxidase inhibitors that are used to treat cataplexy can trigger or exacerbate RBD in this population.[99]

RBD and Extrapyramidal Disease

RBD may be the first manifestation of Parkinson's disease, progressive supranuclear palsy, or multisystem atrophy and may antedate the appearance of daytime symptoms in these disorders by more than 10 years.[100, 101] In one series, more than one third of men initially diagnosed with idiopathic RBD eventually developed symptoms of Parkinson's disease.[102] Systematic study of patients with such neurological syndromes indicates that RBD and RWA may be far more prevalent than previously suspected. In one large series of patients with multiple system atrophy, 90% were found to have RWA and 69% had clinical RBD.[103] The finding of incidental Lewy body disease in one patient asymptomatic for Parkinson's disease suggests that this condition may explain idiopathic RBD in some older patients.[104] The use of selegiline may trigger RBD in patients with Parkinson's disease and by cholinergic treatment of Alzheimer's disease.[105, 106] Other possible associations include mitochondrial encephalomyopathy, normal pressure hydrocephalus, Tourette's syndrome, and group A xeroderma pigmentosum.[107–110]

EPIDEMIOLOGY

A recent telephone survey of more than 4900 individuals between the ages of 15 and 100 years indicated an overall prevalence of violent behaviors in general during sleep of 2%, one fourth of which were likely due to RBD, giving an overall prevalence rate of RBD of 0.5%.[111]

CLINICAL FEATURES

Cases reported to date indicate strikingly similar clinical features.[41, 79, 112] The presenting complaint is that of vigorous sleep behaviors usually accompanying vivid striking dreams. These behaviors may result in repeated injury, including ecchymoses, lacerations, and fractures. Some of the self-protection measures taken by the patients (e.g., tethering themselves to the bed, using sleeping bags or pillow barricades, or sleeping on a mattress in an empty room) reveal the recurrent and serious nature of these episodes.[112, 113] Chronic RBD is more common in older men and may be preceded by a lengthy prodrome. In some cases, there is a familial predisposition. RBD may be associated with neurological disorders that do not directly involve the brainstem, and in most cases, it is idiopathic. Because effective and safe treatment is available, precise diagnosis is critical.

It should be noted that RBD and other parasomnias may occur in patients in intensive care units. In one series of 20 patients experiencing parasomnias in intensive care units, 17 had RBD (3 developed RBD during admission for neurological disorders, 1 was admitted as a consequence of RBD, and 13 displayed preexisting RBD during the course of hospitalization for other medical conditions).[114] Table 64–3 summarizes our experience with RBD and is the basis for discussing the interlocking facets of this clinical disorder.

Case Histories

The following cases illustrate the idiopathic subtype of RBD and describe the main reason for seeking medical attention. Past history and current neurological and psychiatric evaluations were unremarkable, apart from the findings reported. All four men were known by day to be calm and friendly individuals; their nocturnal behaviors were completely out of (waking) character. Clonazepam was used in each to control problematic behaviors and abnormal dreams. Figure 64–3 illustrates attempted dream enactments during the REM sleep in case 3.

CASE 1

A 77-year-old minister presented with a 20-year history of frequent somniloquy and aggressive behaviors that occurred during "fighting dreams" of defending himself against assaultive children and adults. Although his wife had sustained repeated blows, she remained in bed to protect him from self-harm. Referral was prompted by an injury to his chest from jumping into a table while dreaming. Despite vigorous sleep movements, he generally awakened feeling refreshed; however, fatigue had recently started to interfere with his busy preaching schedule.

His wife recalled a memorable night when "he said he was flying above some trees and there was a phone sitting out there on the table and it was ringing, so he swooped down to answer the phone and, just as he landed, somebody hit him and when he jumped away, he actually bolted out of the bed and was in the hall, just like that."

Medical history was remarkable for coronary artery bypass graft surgery 3 years previously, which was followed by a pronounced depression in consciousness lasting 4 days and a right-sided hemiplegia that gradually resolved. A mild memory deficit ensued, and his preexisting sleep disturbance intensified. Current neurological examination revealed a memory deficit, mild horizontal nystagmus, modest right-sided cogwheel rigidity, and peripheral neuropathy.

CASE 2

A 60-year-old surgeon began to punch and kick his wife and to jump out of bed during nightmares of being attacked "by criminals, terrorists, and monsters who always tried to kill me." Work-related stress was the presumed cause of his sleep disturbance, but the violent behaviors intensified despite retirement 3 years later. He sustained several head lacerations, and his wife once had a severe headache for 2 days after receiving an accidental blow to the ear. The proper diagnosis was established after 11 years. A prodrome of excessive limb and body jerking during sleep had been present for at least 33 years.

Table 64–3. PROMINENT FINDINGS IN 70 CONSECUTIVE PATIENTS WITH POLYGRAPHICALLY DOCUMENTED CHRONIC REM SLEEP BEHAVIOR DISORDER

Categories	Percentage of Patients	Comments
Sex		
Male	90.0 (63/70)	Mean age at onset (N = 70): 52.6 (± SD 16.1) years; range: 9–73
Female	10.0 (7/70)	Mean age at presentation: 59.3 (± 15.4) years; range: 10–77
Prodrome	24.3 (17/70)	Sleeptalking, yelling, limb twitching, and jerking began a mean 22.3 (± 16.8) years before RBD onset; range: 2–48
Chief complaint		
Sleep injury	77.1 (54/70)	Ecchymoses (54); lacerations (24); fractures (5)
Sleep disruption	22.9 (16/70)	
Altered dream process and content	91.4 (64/70)	More vivid, unpleasant, action filled, violent (reported as severe nightmares)
Dream-enacting behaviors	91.4 (64/70)	Talking, laughing, yelling, swearing, gesturing, reaching, grabbing, arm flailing, punching, kicking, sitting, jumping out of bed, crawling, running
Periodic movements of NREM sleep	62.9 (44/70)	Infrequently associated with arousals; involve legs/arms, and occur throughout the entire sleep cycle
Aperiodic movements of NREM sleep	40.0 (28/70)	Infrequently associated with arousals; involve legs/arms, and occur throughout the entire sleep cycle
Elevated percentage of slow-wave (stage 3–4) sleep for age (>58 years)*	84.0 (42/50)	Not associated with prior sleep deprivation; often pronounced: mean percentage for the 42 elevated cases was 25.0 (± 5.8); range: 15–41
Clonazepam treatment efficacy		
Complete	77.2 (44/57)	Rapid control of problem sleep behaviors and altered dreams, sustained for up to 7 years
Partial	12.3 (7/57)	
Total	89.5 (51/57)	
Disorders causally associated with RBD†		

Central nervous system disorders‡	37.5 (24/64)	Degenerative disorders: 11
		  Dementia (5)
		  Parkinsonism (4)
		  Olivopontocerebellar degeneration (1)
		  Shy-Drager syndrome (1)
		Narcolepsy: 7
		Vascular disorders: 3
		  Ischemic cerebrovascular disease (2)
		  Subarachnoid hemorrhage (1)
		Brainstem astrocytoma: 1
		Multiple sclerosis: 1
		Guillain-Barré syndrome: 1

Psychiatric disorders§	9.1 (6/67)	Chronic abstinence states: 3
		  From ethanol abuse (2)
		  From ethanol/amphetamine abuse (1)
		Adjustment disorders: 2
		  (major stressors were divorce and an automobile accident without injury)
		Combined disorder: 1
		  (RBD induced by rapid imipramine withdrawal in a patient with chronic major depression)

Endocrinologic disorder	1.4 (1/70)	64-year-old woman abruptly developed RBD after total parathyroidectomy 10 years previously

Adapted from Schenck CH, Mahowald MW. Polysomnographic, neurologic, psychiatric, and clinical outcome report on 70 consecutive cases with the REM sleep behavior disorder (RBD): sustained clonazepam efficacy in 89.5% of 57 treated patients. Cleve Clin J Med. 1990;57:s10–s24.

*Stage 3–4 percentage elevation was defined as greater than 15% of total sleep time. Twenty patients were excluded from analysis who were younger than 58 years old.

†The timing of onset and clinical course indicated a causal association with RBD.

‡Six patients were excluded from analysis whose neurological disorders had an indeterminate association with RBD.

§Three patients were excluded from analysis whose mood or substance abuse disorders had an indeterminate association with RBD.

RBD, REM sleep behavior disorder.

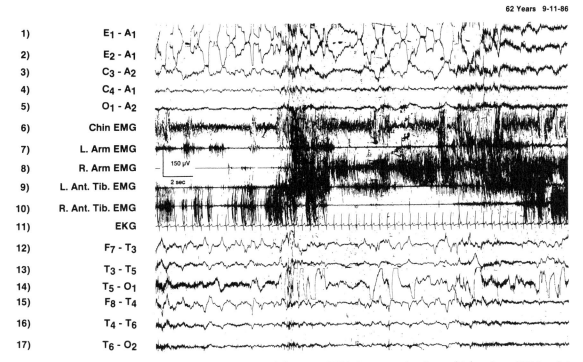

62 Years 9-11-86

Figure 64–3. Polygraphic correlates of nocturnal dream-enacting behaviors. REM sleep contains dense, high-voltage REM activity (1–2) and an activated electroencephalogram (3–5, 12–17). The electrocardiogram (11) has a constant rate of 64 per minute, despite vigorous limb movements, a finding that is consistent with REM sleep and inconsistent with a conventional arousal. Chin EMG tone is augmented with phasic accentuations (6). Arms (7–8) and legs (9–10) show aperiodic bursts of intense EMG twitching, which accompany gross behaviors noted by the technician. This sequence culminates in a spontaneous awakening, when the man reports a dream of running down a hill in Duluth, Minn, and taking shortcuts through backyards, when he suddenly finds himself on a barge that is rocking back and forth. He feels haunted and desperately holds onto anything to prevent falling into the cargo hold, where there are skeletons. He then awakens. F, frontal; O, occipital; T, temporal; 7, 3, 5, 1 left; 8, 4, 6, 2 right.

CASE 3

A 62-year-old industrial plant manager experienced a progressive disorder of "military nightmares" and combative sleep behaviors that had begun 10 years previously, after visiting locations where he had fought in World War II. A psychiatrist diagnosed a post-traumatic stress disorder, but treatment was ineffective because he continued to scream profanities, throw punches, kick, sit up, and jump out of bed while dreaming of being attacked by enemy soldiers. He broke lamps and once kicked a hole in the wall. One dream-incurred head laceration required 10 sutures. He considered his sleep to be sound and had consistent diurnal alertness. He saw four physicians, including two psychiatrists, for this sleep problem before referral to our center. There was a childhood history of sleepwalking.

CASE 4

A 57-year-old retired school principal presented with concern over the possibility of injuring his wife. For 2 years, he had inadvertently punched and kicked her during vivid nightmares of protecting himself and family from aggressive people and snakes. Nocturnal arousals were uncommon, and he felt refreshed most mornings. He developed an adjustment disorder with depressed mood[115] subsequent to a

myocardial infarction 1 year earlier, but treatment with neither desipramine nor trazodone controlled his problematic sleep movements. An MMPI revealed a chronic tendency for somatization. He had two brothers who reported identical sleep and dream disturbances that had persisted since adolescence. One of them tore the headboard off a bed while dreaming of fighting a bear.

Behavioral Features and Their Bases

The history of dream-enacting behavior occurring at least 90 min after sleep onset and as late as the terminal morning awakening strongly suggests an REM sleep disorder, and in our laboratory nearly all such episodes took place within REM sleep. One rare example of an NREM dream enactment (see Fig. 1 in Schenck et al.[41]) was actually a dissociated state in which an RBD process intruded into the transition from stage 3/4 to stage 2 sleep with rapid eye movements, a vivid dream, and behavioral enactment. This case most likely represents a "parasomnia overlap" state (discussed later in Differential Diagnosis).

Idiopathic RBD is a chronic progressive disorder, with increasing complexity, intensity, and frequency of expressed behaviors. Although irregular jerking of the limbs may occur nightly, the major movement episodes appeared intermittently with a minimum frequency of once every 2 weeks to a maximum of four times nightly on 10 consecutive nights. Observed somniloquy runs the spectrum from short and garbled to long winded and clearly articulated. Angry speech with shouting, but also laughter, can emerge. One patient appeared to have a dissociated RBD–lucid dream state in that he could carry on lengthy and coherent conversations with his wife and family while dreaming and incorporate the conversational material into his dreams.

The extended prodrome of prominent limb and body movements during sleep in four patients may reflect a developmental failure to fully establish REM sleep atonia, predisposing them to RBD.

Most patients complained of sleep injury but rarely of sleep disruption. They usually did not awaken due to their violent activity but due to the yelling, often persistent, of their wives. Two conclusions can be drawn. First, chronic RBD is principally a motor disorder and uncommonly also an arousal disorder (in contrast to the periodic leg movements of NREM sleep, a condition with a propensity for symptomatic arousals). Second, the very high arousal threshold constitutes another physiological marker of REM sleep, which is known to have the highest threshold for arousal compared with wakefulness or NREM sleep.[9–11] In addition, the autonomic nervous system generally was not activated during episodes of vigorous REM sleep behaviors, as indicated by Figure 64–3. However, a few patients described episodes of vivid dreaming with behavioral enactment from which they awakened in a terrified state with full subjective autonomic activation.

With rare exception, the violent nocturnal behaviors were completely discordant from the waking personality, supporting the concept that RBD is a state-dependent, neurobehavioral syndrome.

In patients with RBD, arousals from sleep to alertness and orientation is usually rapid and accompanied by complete dream recall (very unlike the confusional arousals observed in the disorders of arousal such as sleepwalking or sleep terrors). After awakening, behavior and social interactions are appropriate, mitigating against an NREM sleep relationship, delirious states, or ictal phenomena but rather further supporting an REM sleep phenomenon. It should be emphasized that the behaviors, although complex and violent, are of briefer duration than those seen in the disorders of arousal. In some individuals, the clinical features contain elements of both RBD and disorders of arousal (see Parasomnia Overlap Syndrome, under Differential Diagnosis). Furthermore, appetitive behaviors (feeding or sexual) have not been seen as a manifestation of RBD in either human beings or the animal model.[6]

REM Behavior Disorder: Both a Dream and a Behavior Disorder

The activation-synthesis model of dream formation (Hobson and McCarley[116, 117]) states that during REM sleep, brainstem generators phasically activate motor, perceptual, affective, cognitive, and amnestic circuits whose information flow is synthesized into dreams by the forebrain and theoretically predicts the dream changes we observed in patients with RBD (see Table 64–3). Intensified activity of these generators or biased activation of particular circuits should induce corresponding changes in dream process and content. We theorize that both these conditions occur to produce RBD. As proposed for pontine-lesioned cats, disinhibition of selective brainstem motor pattern generators accounts for the differential release of stereotypical REM behaviors.[6] This same process may produce both the *behavior* and *dream disorder* of RBD. For example, the generator for violent behaviors may become disinhibited and coactivate both a descending output to the spinal motoneurons and an ascending output to forebrain dream-synthesizing centers, thus producing the simultaneous movement and dreaming. These two outputs from the same generator may be *isomorphic*, so command for dream action (fictive movements) is equivalent to command for actual movements,[118] resulting in "acting out of dreams."

In our series of patients with RBD, all those who acted violently during REM sleep also had violent dreams; in fact, dream recall was most complete after behavioral enactment. The REM sleep behaviors we observed in our patients have never contradicted the reported dream.

Most patients repeatedly experienced a "typical RBD nightmare" that consisted of being attacked by animals or unfamiliar people, few of whom were bizarre in appearance. Characteristically, the dreamer would either fight back in self-defense or attempt to flee. Fear, rather than anger, was the usual accompanying emotion reported. An ironic situation was produced by RBD when a dreaming husband would fight to defend his wife from an aggressor while actually striking her in bed. Her yelling would then awaken him to the unfortunate reality of his violent oneiric activity. In these patients, medication suppressed both the vigorous sleep behaviors and the abnormal dreaming, which adds further support to the activation-synthesis model as described.

One feature of the dream-enacted episodes in this group of patients is that dreams generally are not being played out; rather, distinctly altered, stereotypical, repetitive, and "action-packed" dreams are put on display.

DIAGNOSTIC EVALUATION

Routine medical history-taking should include questions that screen for abnormal sleep movements and altered dreams, especially in older adults; patients of any age with acute or chronic central nervous system disorders, particularly those who have neurological conditions that predispose to RBD, such as Parkinson's disease or multiple system atrophy; or patients receiving psychoactive medications known to trigger RBD. The diagnosis of RBD may be suspected on clinical grounds, but our experience has shown that polysomnographic confirmation is mandatory. The complaint of sleep-related injurious or violent behaviors should be taken very seriously. Reported injuries in our series include lacerations and fractures to the patient, bed partner, or both. RBD has also resulted in subdural hematomas and other serious injuries.[119–121]

Detailed polysomnographic data in these patients have been reported elsewhere.[41, 79, 112] The overall sleep architecture is usually normal, with the expected cycling of NREM and REM sleep. Most of our subjects had excessive slow-wave sleep for age. Although some of the patients were initially thought to have a seizure disorder, accounting for the movements during sleep, neither EEG nor clinical seizure activity has been detected. The conventional scoring parameters of Rechtschaffen and Kales[59] must be modified to allow for the persistence of EMG tone during epochs that are otherwise clearly REM sleep. These periods are similar to the "stage 1 REM with tonic EMG" described by the Japanese,[40] the "stage 1 REM" seen in delirium tremens,[29] and those recorded in the chronic pontine-lesioned cats.[6, 15, 34, 43, 60–62] There is persistence of muscle tone during REM sleep, and it may be strikingly augmented for prolonged periods of time, occasionally lasting much of the REM sleep cycle. The onset of a REM sleep period is often marked by a sudden increase in chin EMG activity or prominent twitching in conjunction with rapid eye movements.

In addition to the intermittent absence of atonia, there are varying amounts of limb twitching (usually far in excess of that observed in normal REM sleep), gross body movements, and complex, often violent, behaviors that correlate with reported dream mentation.

Interestingly, tachycardia may not accompany these impressive movements. A similar lack of autonomic arousal during REM sleep was observed in a study of delirium tremens.[29] This likely represents paresis of the sympathetic nervous system (inactivation of the locus ceruleus) characteristic of REM sleep.[89, 122]

A curious feature of the chin EMG and extremity movements seen during the REM period is the variability of involvement and distribution. The chin EMG may be augmented without body movements or may be atonic despite flailing extremities, as shown in Figure 64–2. The arms and legs often move independently, necessitating monitoring of all limbs. Some patients demonstrated persistent (over the span of several years) lateralization of limb EMG activity or predominant upper or lower extremity movements.

Most patients displayed prominent aperiodic movements of all extremities in every conceivable combination during all stages of NREM sleep. These aperiodic movements are similar but more intense than the fragmentary myoclonus described by Broughton et al.[123, 124] in patients with a wide variety of sleep disorders and occasionally as an incidental observation. Most patients with RBD also showed conventional periodic movements of sleep, usually involving the legs and infrequently associated with arousals. Prolonged periods of aperiodic and periodic movements restricted to the arms were noted occasionally. Figures 64–4A and B

and 64–5 exemplify some of these dissociated wake-REM states.

Prominent changes in sleep patterns likely representing variations of RBD have been described in the drug-induced variety of RWA,[67, 68] narcolepsy,[99] and Parkinson's disease.[125, 126] We have studied individuals with parkinsonism and one each with narcolepsy and advanced olivopontocerebellar degeneration; all had histories highly suggestive of RBD with uninterpretable EEG sleep stages. Their polysomnographic abnormalities consisted of prominent slow and rapid eye movements throughout sleep, associated with an EEG pattern of generalized slowing, which precluded conventional sleep stage scoring. Prominent motor activity during sleep and reported dreams was present; therefore, a spectrum of sleep patterns in RBD appears to exist that range from normal to profoundly abnormal. Consequently, the anticipated RBD polysomnographic pattern may be obscured by additional EEG abnormalities associated with the underlying neurological disorder, necessitating clinical diagnosis. As predicted by the results of experiments in animals, some human beings may be expected to display "asymptomatic RBD," or RWA without behavioral manifestations. In addition to the narcoleptics with RWA who were mentioned, we have seen such cases associated with spinocerebellar degeneration and parkinsonism. As mentioned, commonly prescribed medications such as tricyclic antidepressants, serotonin specific reuptake inhibitors, and venlafaxine may result in RWA or RBD. Figure 64–6 is a dramatic example of venlafaxine-induced RBD in a 9-year-old boy.

Diagnostic Criteria

The minimum diagnostic criteria for RBD that we formulated can be satisfied in either of two ways:

1. History of problematic sleep behavior that is
   * Harmful or potentially harmful or
   * Disruptive of sleep continuity or
   * Annoying to self or bed partner
   and any polysomnographic abnormality listed below
2. No history of problematic sleep behaviors **and** any polysomnographic abnormality listed below **and** any videotaped behavioral abnormality listed below

Polysomnography: At least one of the following during REM sleep:
   * Excessive augmentation of chin EMG tone
   * Excessive chin or limb EMG twitching, or both, regardless of chin EMG tone

Videotaping of behavior: Record at least one of the following during REM sleep:
   * Excessive limb or body jerking, or both
   * Complex movements
   * Vigorous or violent movements

A report of dream changes accompanying the sleep behaviors, such as those listed in Table 64–3, can buttress the history. The determination of what constitutes

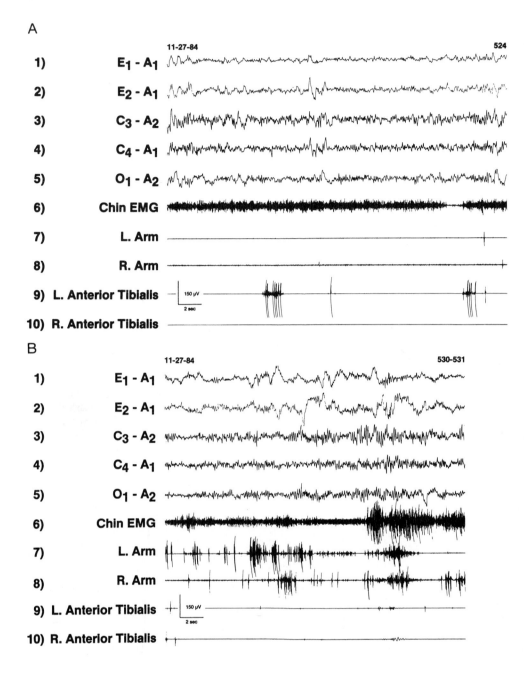

Figure 64–4. Nocturnal polysomnograms that depict contrasting forms of skeletal muscle activity in a 70-year-old man. *A,* Lateralized periodic leg movements appear every 20 to 30 sec throughout a period of stage 2 NREM sleep. *B,* A different pattern emerges 3 min later at the onset of REM sleep, in which both arms have frequent aperiodic movements. Chin atonia does not occur in REM sleep but does appear suddenly in NREM sleep just before a leg movement. This man developed a chronic REM sleep behavioral disorder at the time of subarachnoid hemorrhage 6 years previously. Eye tracings (1–2); electroencephalogram (3–5), REM alpha present in *B;* EMG of chin, arms, and legs (6–10).

excessive EMG augmentation, EMG twitching, or limb jerking requires both meticulous execution of standard recording techniques and an experienced polysomnographer. We recommend that any patient suspected of having RBD undergo a systematic evaluation consisting of the following:

1. A review of sleep-wake complaints (from patient, bed partner, or both)
2. Neurological and psychiatric examinations
3. Sleep laboratory study that includes continuous videotaping of behavior during standard polygrapic monitoring[59] of the electro-oculogram (EOG), EEG, EMG (chin and bilateral extensor digitorum and anterior tibialis muscles), electrocardiogram (ECG), and nasal air flow. We attempt to evaluate each patient during his or her custom-

ary sleeping period for at least 2 consecutive nights. A certified technician makes written observations of ongoing behaviors. The REM density score (REM activity units, 0 to 8 scale/1 min) is determined by use of a standard technique.[127]

4. A multiple sleep latency test[128] administered the day after an overnight sleep study whenever there is a history of associated diurnal fatigue or somnolence

A more extensive neurological evaluation, including multimodal evoked potentials, brain imaging by magnetic resonance imaging (MRI) or computed axial tomography (CAT), or comprehensive neuropsychological testing by methods previously reported,[79] is indicated *only* if there is a suggestion of neurological dysfunction based on history or neurological examination.

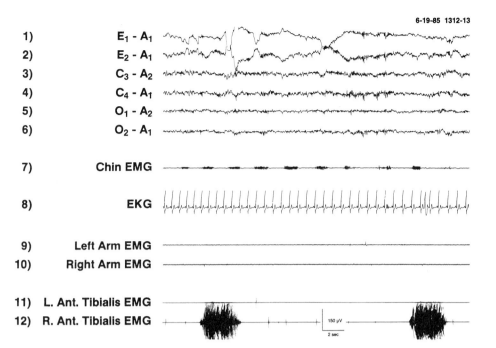

Figure 64–5. Nocturnal polysomnogram of a dissociated state in a 58-year-old man with multiple sclerosis. A pathological process usually confined to NREM sleep—periodic leg movements (12)—has intruded into REM sleep, which has typical rapid eye movements (1–2) and a desynchronized electroencephalogram (3–6). Chin EMG atonia alternates every 3 sec with augmented tone (7).

Differential Diagnosis

RBD can masquerade as many other conditions (Table 64–4). Most conditions in this differential diagnosis represent an initial clinical misdiagnosis in our series, leading to inappropriate and ineffective treatment. The differential diagnosis of these disorders has been extensively reviewed elsewhere.[129] The disorders of arousal, nocturnal seizures, and rhythmic movement disorder are discussed elsewhere in this textbook. It should be remembered that the clinical event (arousal) may not be primary but rather triggered by another, underlying sleep disorder (i.e., apnea leads to arousal, which leads to sleep terror). Nocturnal behaviors induced by obstructive sleep apnea or sleep-related seizures can mimic those of RBD.[130, 131] "Overlap" parasomnias are characterized by a clinical history suggestive of sleepwalking or sleep terrors with polysomnographic features of motor disinhibition during both REM and NREM sleep.[132] It is likely that a recent series of somnambulistic-like behaviors in elderly subjects found to have polysomnographic features of RBD represents this phenomenon.[133] Nocturnal panic disorder is poorly understood and requires more study. It is well established

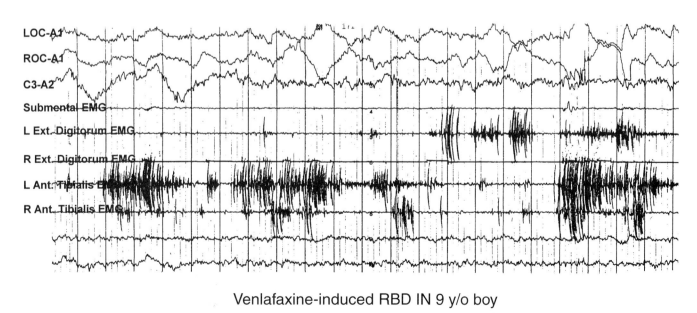

Venlafaxine-induced RBD IN 9 y/o boy

Figure 64–6. Polysomnogram of a 9-year-old boy who developed RBD behaviors coincident with his being placed on 550 mg daily venlafaxine. Note the prominent tonic and phasic muscle activity of the extremities during REM sleep. RBD, REM sleep behavior disorder. (Copyright © MRSDC, Minnesota Regional Sleep Disorders Center.)

Table 64–4. REM SLEEP BEHAVIOR DISORDER: DIFFERENTIAL DIAGNOSIS

Disorders of arousal
    Primary
        Confusional arousals
        Sleepwalking
        Sleep terrors
    Secondary
        Obstructive sleep apnea
        Periodic limb movement disorder
        Gastroesophageal reflux
        Nocturnal seizures
Parasomnia "overlap" syndrome
Nocturnal seizures
Rhythmic movement disorder
Post-traumatic stress disorder
Nocturnal panic disorder
Psychogenic dissociative disorder/conversion hysteria
Malingering

that psychogenic dissociative disorders may arise predominantly or exclusively from the sleep period.[134] Finally, we have seen extremely violent sleep-period behavior thought to represent malingering.[135]

The clinical history alone is insufficient to make the diagnosis, which can be established only with extensive polysomnographic evaluation, including the use of a full seizure montage with a paper speed of at least 15 mm/sec respiratory recording, monitoring of all extremities, continuous audiovisual documentation, and detailed observations made by experienced technicians. The physical and psychological consequences of an erroneous diagnosis are obvious. The impressive response to treatment emphasizes the importance of a definitive diagnosis.[122, 136]

MANAGEMENT

Clonazepam is highly effective in the treatment of RBD. The response to clonazepam is impressive in both degree and duration. It is effective in nearly 90% of cases, with little evidence of tolerance or abuse.[112] The majority of our patients and their bed partners noticed a suppressing effect on problematic sleep behaviors and nightmares within the first week, often beginning on the first night. The initial dose was 0.5 mg at bedtime, with some cases warranting a rapid increase to 1.0 mg. Tolerance has been an infrequent and mild problem despite continuous administration for more than 12 years. A hierarchical benefit often occurred: after an initial period (days or months) of marked suppression of sleep motor activity, moderate amounts of limb twitching re-emerged along with sleep talking and more complex behaviors. Nevertheless, the control of problematic, vigorous behaviors, and the associated nightmares persisted. All instances of drug discontinuation resulted in prompt relapse. Clonazepam may be taken up to 2 h before bedtime by patients complaining of sleep-onset insomnia, prominent limb jerking beginning soon after sleep onset, or excessive morning sedation.

Consideration of the pathophysiological mechanisms of RBD leads directly to an examination of the beneficial effect of clonazepam. This benzodiazepine has been reported to be effective in the control of other motor disorders in various states, such as intention myoclonus,[137] spinal myoclonus,[138] propriospinal myoclonus,[139] rhythmic dystonia[140] and choreiform activity of wakefulness,[141] the motor hyperactivity of bipolar manic states,[142, 143] periodic leg movements of NREM sleep,[144–147] and neuroleptic-induced somnambulism.[148] It is also an anticonvulsant that is prescribed for infantile spasms and myoclonic epilepsy.[149] The specific mechanism of action of clonazepam in RBD is unknown but in part likely reflects its serotonergic property.[150] Disinhibition of REM phasic activity (rapid eye movements and PGO spikes) and hallucinatory behaviors were induced in cats by serotonin-depleting drugs and by selective destruction of serotonergic neurons of the brainstem raphe nuclei (for a review, see Hishikawa et al.[40]). Serotonin administration inhibits motor activity in several animal experimental designs.[151–153] Alcohol-dependent mice in withdrawal—a high-risk state for RBD—had a markedly reduced serotonin metabolism.[154] Many of the neurodegenerative conditions associated with RBD involve monoaminergic systems, including the serotonergic raphe nuclei.[40] Although subtle changes in the polysomnogram after effective clinical treatment with clonazepam have been reported,[155] there are no gross changes in sleep stages or in the absence of atonia.[112] The fact that clonazepam results in striking clinical improvement without discernible effect on the polysomnogram raises the possibility that it acts preferentially on the locomotor systems rather than those affecting REM atonia.

Although tricyclic antidepressants may enhance motor activity during REM sleep, they occasionally are effective in the treatment of RBD.[156] Desipramine, which has been demonstrated to have a serotonergic effect,[157] induced one temporary and one sustained remission of RBD in our patient sample but is less predictably effective than clonazepam. Due to the multiplicity of neural networks involved in REM atonia,[6, 21, 63] it is likely that various medications may be effective in individual cases; likely candidates include dopaminergic and serotonergic compounds. There have been anecdotal unpublished reports of response to L-tryptophan, carbidopa/L-dopa (levodopa), and clonidine. Carbamazepine at 100 mg three times daily was effective in one patient.[158] L-Dopa may be effective, particularly in patients in whom REM sleep behavior disorder is the harbinger of Parkinson's disease.[159] There have been anecdotal reports of response to gabapentin, monoamine oxidase inhibitors, and clonidine.[160] Melatonin has been reportedly effective in one small series.[161] In RBD associated with narcolepsy, the tricyclic antidepressants or monoamine oxidase inhibitors administered for cataplexy may be continued, with clonazepam added.[99] The treatment of Parkinson's disease-associated RBD is the same as for idiopathic RBD.[102] Pallidotomy was effective in one patient.[162]

The other essential therapeutic intervention concerns environmental safety. Clonazepam is not fail-safe:

one patient injured himself during a violent dream 1 year after the initiation of very satisfactory pharmacotherapy. There was no recurrence during the ensuing 5 months, even though the dose was not increased. Potentially dangerous objects should be removed from the bedroom, cushions should be put around the bed, and perhaps the mattress should be placed on the floor and windows protected. We anticipate some cases in which drug intolerance or ineffectiveness will lead to discontinuation, requiring maximal environmental safety.

PERSPECTIVES AND IMPLICATIONS

RBD is an exciting experiment of nature, extending our understanding of state declaration. Its association with narcolepsy and its clinical similarity to "status dissociatus" and the parasomnia overlap syndrome expand the concept of state boundary dyscontrol. The identification of other state declaration errors and their induction by, or response to, specific pharmacological agents promise to unveil much about the neuroanatomy, neurophysiology, neurochemistry, and neuropharmacology of waking and sleep. Such experiments of nature underscore the symbiotic relation between clinical and basic science medicine.

OTHER REM SLEEP PARASOMNIAS

Nightmares. These are thoroughly discussed in Chapter 66.

REM Sleep–Related Sinus Arrest. REM sleep–related sinus arrest[163] was first described by Guilleminault et al. in 1984.[164] It is a cardiac rhythm disorder that affects otherwise healthy young adults of either gender and is characterized by sinus arrest during REM sleep, usually in clusters, with asystoles lasting up to 9 sec. In one case, vocalizations occurred during periods of REM sleep asystole, with a loud scream and a sensation of being "shocked" (but without chest pain or related symptoms) associated with the longest asystole.[165]

Periods of asystole do not occur during NREM sleep and are not associated with sleep apnea. Some patients experience faintness, light-headedness, and blurred vision during abrupt awakenings, and syncope can occur during ambulation after an awakening. In addition, there may be complaints of vague chest pain or tightness or intermittent palpitations during the daytime. However, daytime ECG (including Holter monitoring) is usually completely normal, and angiography, when performed, is unremarkable. The underlying pathophysiology therefore appears to be autonomic dysfunction. The clinical course is unknown. Complications include loss of consciousness and even cardiac arrest due to prolonged asystole. This condition must be considered in case of sudden, unexplained death during sleep. Treatment is usually not indicated, although prophylactic intervention would include a left ventricular–inhibited pacemaker with a low rate limit.

Impaired Sleep-Related Penile Erections. These are discussed Chapter 102.

Sleep-Related Painful Erections. These erections are characterized by penile pain and typically occur during REM sleep.[163] Middle-aged or older men are typically affected; they complain of recurrent awakenings with partial or full erections and pain. The cumulative effects of nightly sleep disruption and sleep loss can result in the additional complaints of insomnia, irritability, anxiety, and daytime somnolence. There usually is a history of normal erections during wakefulness. There is little evidence of underlying psychiatric disease, and pathology of the penis is not usually found. Although the course is not well known, it appears that this condition can become more severe over time. No systematic studies of treatment efficacy have been performed, but clozapine, propranolol, or paroxetine may be effective.[166, 167]

REM Sleep–Related Expiratory Groaning. This has been described but is poorly understood and awaits further definition and therapeutic studies.[168]

Acknowledgments

This work was partly supported by a grant from Hennepin Faculty Associates. We acknowledge our ongoing collaboration with Drs. Scott R. Bundle, Gerald M. Rosen, and Andrea L. Patterson, RPSGT. We are indebted to Traci Oletzke for secretarial support and to our dedicated nurses and technologists.

References

1. Mahowald MW, Ettinger MG. Things that go bump in the night: the parasomnias revisited. J Clin Neurophysiol. 1990;7:119–143.
2. Mahowald MW, Schenck CH. NREM parasomnias. Neurol Clin. 1996;14:675–696.
3. Schenck CH, Mahowald MW. REM parasomnias. Neurol Clin. 1996;14:697–720.
4. Aserinski E, Kleitman N. Regularly occurring periods of eye motility, and concomitant phenomena during sleep. Science. 1953;118:273–274.
5. Steriade M, Hobson JA. Neuronal activity during the sleep-waking cycle. Progr Neurobiol. 1976;6:155–376.
6. Hendricks JC, Morrison AR, Mann GL. Different behaviors during paradoxical sleep without atonia depend upon lesion site. Brain Res. 1982;239:81–105.
7. Gaillard J-M. Biochemical pharmacology of paradoxical sleep. B J Clin Pharmacol. 1983;16:205s–230s.
8. Vertes RP. Brainstem control of the events of REM sleep. Progr Neurobiol. 1984;22:241–288.
9. Huttenlocher PR. Effects of state of arousal on click responses in the mesencephalic reticular formation. Electroencephalogr Clin Neurophysiol. 1960;12:819–827.
10. Williams HL, Tepas DI, Morlock HC. Evoked responses to clicks and electroencephalographic stages of sleep in man. Science. 1962;138:685–686.
11. Hodes R, Suzuki J-I. Comparative thresholds of cortex, vestibular system, and reticular formation in wakefulness, sleep and rapid eye movement periods. Electroencephalogr Clin Neurophysiol. 1965;18:239–248.
12. Pessah MA, Roffwarg HP. Spontaneous middle ear muscle activity in man: a rapid eye movement sleep phenomenon. Science. 1972;178:773–776.
13. Hendricks JC, Bowker RM, Morrison AR. Functional characteristics of cats with pontine lesions during sleep and wakefulness and their usefulness for sleep research. In: Koella WP, Levin P, eds. Sleep 1976. Third European Congress of Sleep Research, Montpellier, France. Basel, Switzerland: Karger; 1977:207–210.

14. Chokroverty S. Phasic tongue movements in human rapid-eye-movement sleep. Neurology. 1980;30:665–668.

15. Jouvet M, Sastre J-P, Sakai K. Toward an etho-ethnology of dreaming. In: Karacan I, ed. Psychophysiological Aspects of Sleep. Park Ridge, NJ: Noyes Medical Publishers; 1981.

16. Morrison A. Paradoxical sleep and alert wakefulness: variations on a theme. In: Chase MH, Weitzman ED, eds. Sleep Disorders: Basic and Clinical Research. New York, NY: S. P. Medical and Scientific Books; 1983.

17. Fisher C, Gross J, Zuch J. Cycle of penile erection synchronous with dreaming (REM) sleep: preliminary report. Arch Gen Psychiatry. 1965;12:29–45.

18. Eastman CI, Mistlberger RE, Rechtschaffen A. Suprachiasmatic nuclei lesions eliminate circadian temperature and sleep rhythms in the rat. Physiol Behavi. 1984;32:357–368.

19. Pickard GE, Turek FW. The suprachiasmatic nuclei: two circadian clocks? Brain Res. 1983;268:201–210.

20. Sakai K. Some anatomical and physiological properties of ponto-mesencephalic tegmental neurons with special reference to the PGO waves and postural atonia during paradoxical sleep in the cat. In: Hobson JA, Brazier MAB, eds. The Reticular Formation Revisited. New York, NY: Raven Press; 1980.

21. Morrison AR. Is the pons the site of rapid eye movement sleep generation in normal individuals? Sleep Res. 1991;20A:57.

22. Steriade M, Ropert N, Kitsikis A, et al. Ascending activating neuronal networks in midbrain core and related rostral systems. In: Hobson JA, Brazier MAB, eds. The Reticular Formation Revisited. New York; NY: Raven Press; 1980:125–167.

23. Dement WC. The biological role of REM sleep (circa 1968). In: Kales A, ed. Sleep Physiology and Pathology. Philadelphia, Pa: JB Lippincott; 1969:245–265.

24. Hishikawa Y, Nan'no H, Tachibana M, et al. The nature of sleep attack and other symptoms of narcolepsy. Electroencephalogr Clin Neurophysiol. 1968;24:1–10.

25. Guilleminault C, Wilson RA, Dement WC. A study on cataplexy. Arch Neurol. 1974;31:255–261.

26. Siegel JM, Nienhuis R, Fahringer HM, et al. Neuronal activity in narcolepsy: identification of cataplexy-related cells in the medial medulla. Science. 1991;252:1315–1318.

27. Mahowald MW, Schenck CH. Status dissociatus: a perspective on states of being. Sleep. 1991;14:69–79.

28. Kales A, Cadieux RJ, Soldatos CR, et al. Narcolepsy-cataplexy, I: clinical and electrophysiologic characteristics. Arch Neurol. 1982;39:164–168.

29. Gross MM, Goodenough D, Tobin M, et al. Sleep disturbances and hallucinations in the acute alcoholic psychoses. J Nerv Ment Dis. 1966;142:493–514.

30. Greenberg R, Pearlman C. Delirium tremens and dreaming. Am J Psychiatry. 1967;124:37–46.

31. Hishikawa Y, Sugita Y, Teshima Y, et al. Sleep disorders in alcoholic patients with delirium tremens and transient withdrawal hallucinations: reevaluation of the REM rebound and intrusion theory. In: Karacan I, ed. Psychophysiological Aspects of Sleep. Park Ridge, NJ: Noyes Medical; 1981:109–122.

32. LaBerge SP, Nagel LE, Dement WC, et al. Lucid dreaming verified by volitional communication during REM sleep. Percept Motor Skills. 1981;52:727–732.

33. Fenwick P, Schatzman M, Worlsey A, et al. Lucid dreaming: correspondence between dreamed and actual events in one subject during REM sleep. Biol Psychiatry. 1984;18:243–252.

34. Jouvet M, Delorme F. Locus coeruleus et sommeil paradoxal. C R Soc Biol. 1965;159:895–899.

35. Morrison AR, Sanford LD, Ball WA, et al. Stimulus-elicited behavior in rapid eye movement sleep without atonia. Behav Neurosci. 1995;109:972–979.

36. Shouse MN, Siegel JM, Wu FM, et al. Mechanisms of seizure suppression during rapid-eye-movement (REM) sleep in cats. Brain Res. 1989;505: 271–282.

37. Tachibana M, Tanaka K, Hishikawa Y, et al. A sleep study of acute psychotic stated due to alcohol and meprobamate addiction. Adv Sleep Res. 1975;2:177–205.

38. Atsumi Y, Kojima T, Matsu'ura M, et al. Polygraphic study of altered consciousness: effect of biperiden on EEG and EOG [in Japanese]. Ann Rep Res Psychotropic Drugs. 1977;9:171–178.

39. Sugano T, Suenaga K, Endo S, et al. Withdrawal delirium in a patient with nitrazepam addiction [in Japanese]. Jpn J EEG EMG. 1980;8:34–35.

40. Hishikawa Y, Sugita Y, Iijima S, et al. Mechanisms producing "stage 1-REM" and similar dissociations of REM sleep and their relation to delirium. Adv Neurol Sci (Tokyo). 1981;25:1129–1147.

41. Schenck CH, Bundlie SR, Ettinger MG, et al. Chronic behavioral disorders of REM sleep: a new category of parasomnia. Sleep. 1986;9:293–308.

42. Sakai K, Sastre J-P, Kanamori N, et al. State-specific neurons in the ponto-medullary reticular formation with special reference to the postural atonia during paradoxical sleep in the cat. In: Pompeiano O, Ajmone Marsan C, eds. Brain Mechanisms and Perceptual Awareness. New York; NY: Raven Press; 1981:405–429.

43. Webster HW, Frideman L, Jones BE. Modification of paradoxical sleep following transections of the reticular formation at the pontomedullary junction. Sleep. 1986;9:1–23.

44. Chase MH. The motor functions of the reticular formation are multifaceted and state-determined. In: Hobson JA, Brazier MAB, eds. The reticular formation revisited. New York, NY: Raven Press; 1980:449–472.

45. Askenasy JJ, Weitzman ED, Yahr MD. Rapid eye movements: expression of a general muscular phasic event of the REM state. Sleep Res. 1983;12:172.

46. Chase MH, Morales FR. Subthreshold excitatory activity and motoneurone discharge during REM periods of active sleep. Science. 1983;221:1195–1198.

47. Emde RN, Koening KL. Neonatal smiling and rapid eye movement states. J Am Acad Child Psychiatry. 1969;8:57–67.

48. Emde RN, Koenig KL. Neonatal smiling, frowning, and rapid eye movement states, II: sleep-cycle study. J Am Acad Child Psychiatry. 1969;8:637–656.

49. Meier GW, Berger RJ. Development of sleep and wakefulness patterns in the infant rhesus monkey. Exp Neurol. 1965;12:257–277.

50. Jouvet-Mournier D, Astic L, Lacote D. Ontogenesis of the states of sleep in rat, cat and guinea pig during the first postnatal month. Dev Psychobiol. 1970;2:216–239.

51. Luce GG. The development of rhythms: youth and age. In: Luce GG, ed. Biological Rhythms in Psychiatry and Medicine. Washington, DC: U.S. Department of Health, Education, and Welfare; 1970. Publication ADM 78-247.

52. Corner MA. Maturation of sleep mechanism in the central nervous system. Exp Brain Res. 1984;(suppl 8):50–66.

53. Corner MA. Ontogeny of brain sleep mechanisms. In: McGinty DJ, Drucker-Colin R, Morrison AR, et al, eds. Brain Mechanisms of Sleep. New York, NY: Raven Press; 1985:175–197.

54. Rigatto H, More M, Cates D. Fetal breathing and behavior measured through a double-wall plexiglas window in sheep. J Appl Physiol. 1986;61:160–164.

55. Roffwarg HP, Muzzio JN, Dement WC. Ontogenetic development of the human sleep-dream cycle. Science. 1966;152:604–619.

56. Corner MA. Spontaneous motor rhythms in early life: phenomenological and neurophysiological aspects. In: Corner MA, Baker RE, van de poll NE, et al, eds. Maturation of the Nervous System. Vol 45. New York, NY: Elsevier; 1978.

57. Denenberg VH, Thoman EB. Evidence for a functional role for active (REM) sleep in infancy. Sleep. 1981;4:185–191.

58. Campbell SS, Tobler I. Animal sleep: a review of sleep duration across phylogeny. Neurosci Biobehav Rev. 1984;8:269–300.

59. Rechtschaffen A, Kales A. A Manual of Standardized Terminology: Techniques and Scoring System for Sleep Stages of Human Subjects. Los Angeles, Calif: UCLA Brain Information Service/ Brain Research Institute; 1968.

60. Henly K, Morrison AR. A re-evaluation of the effects of lesions of the pontine tegmentum and locus coeruleus on phenomena of paradoxical sleep in the cat. Acta Neurobiol Exp. 1974;34:215–232.

61. Trulson ME, Jacobs BL, Morrison AR. Raphe unit activity during REM sleep in normal cats and in pontine lesioned cats displaying REM sleep without atonia. Brain Res. 1981;226:75–91.

62. Friedman L, Jones BE. Study of sleep-wakefulness states by computer graphics and cluster analysis before and after lesions of the pontine tegmentum in the cat. Electroencephalogr Clin Neurophysiol. 1984;57:43–56.

63. Lai YY, Siegel JM. Medullary regions mediating atonia. J Neurosci. 1988;8:4790–4796.

64. Lai YY, Siegel JM. Muscle tone suppression and stepping produced by stimulation of midbrain and rostral pontine reticular formation. J Neurosci. 1990;10:2727–2734.

65. Lasegue C. Le delire alcoolique n'est pas un delire, mais un reve. Arch Gen Med. 1881;88:513–586.

66. Passouant P, Cadilhac J, Ribstein M. Les privations de sommeil avec mouvements oculaires par les anti-depresseurs. Rev Neurol. 1972;127:173–192.

67. Guilleminault C, Raynal D, Takahashi S, et al. Evaluation of short-term and long-term treatment of the narcolepsy syndrome with clomipramine hydrochloride. Acta Neurol Scand. 1976;54:71–87.

68. Besset A. Effect of antidepressants on human sleep. Adv Biosci. 1978;21:141–148.

69. Shimizu T, Ookawa M, Iijuma S, et al. Effect of clomipramine on nocturnal sleep of normal human subjects. Annu Rev Pharmacopsychiatry Res Round. 1985;16:138.

70. Akindele MO, Evans JI, Oswald I. Mono-amine oxidase inhibitors, sleep and mood. Electroencephalogr Clin Neurophysiol. 1970;29:47–56.

71. Schenck CH, Mahowald MW, Kim SW, et al. Prominent eye movements during NREM sleep and REM sleep behavior disorder associated with fluoxetine treatment of depression and obsessive-compulsive disorder. Sleep. 1992;15:226–235.

72. Schutte S, Doghramji K. REM behavior disorder seen with venlafaxine (Effexor). Sleep Res. 1996;25:364.

73. Bental E, Lavie P, Sharf B. Severe hypermotility during sleep in treatment of cataplexy with clomipramine. Israel J Med Sci. 1979;15:607–609.

74. Stolz SE, Aldrich MS. REM sleep behavior disorder associated with caffeine abuse. Sleep Res. 1991;20:341.

75. Mahowald MW, Woods SR, Schenck CH. Sleeping dreams, waking hallucinations, and the central nervous system. Dreaming. 1998;8:89–102.

76. Guilleminault C, Monini S. Mononucleosis and chronic daytime sleepiness:a long-term follow-up study. Arch Intern Med. 1986;146:1333–1335.

77. Lavie P, Pratt H, Sharf B, et al. Localized pontine lesion: nearly total absence of REM sleep. Neurology. 1984;34:118–120.

78. Hefez A, Metz L, Lavie P. Long-term effects of extreme situational stress on sleep and dreaming. Am J Psychiatry. 1987;144:344–347.

79. Schenck CH, Bundlie SR, Patterson AL, et al. REM sleep behavior disorder: a treatable parasomnia affecting older adults. JAMA. 1987;257:1786–1789.

80. Sugita Y, Taniguchi M, Terashima K, et al. A young case of idiopathic REM sleep behavior disorder (RBD) specifically induced by socially stressful conditions. Sleep Res. 1991;20A:394.

81. Cohen LG, Roth BJ, Wassermann EM, et al. Magnetic stimulation of the human cortex, an indicator of reorganization of motor pathways in certain pathological conditions. J Clin Neurophysiol. 1991;8:56–65.

82. Kandel ER. Environmental determinants of brain architecture and of behavior: early experience and learning. In: Kandel ER, Schwartz JH, eds. Principles of Neural Science. New York, NY: Elsevier/North Holland; 1981:620–632.

83. Pons TP, Garraghty PE, Ommaya K, et al. Massive cortical reorganization after sensory deafferentation in adult macaques. Science. 1991;252:1857–1860.

84. Schenck CH, Bundlie SR, Smith SA, et al. REM behavior disorder in a 10 year old girl and aperiodic REM and NREM sleep movements in an 8 year old brother. Sleep Res. 1986;15:162.

85. Hendricks JC, Lager A, O'Brien D, et al. Movement disorders during sleep in cats and dogs. J Am Vet Med Assoc. 1989;194:686–689.

86. Hendricks JC, Morrison AR, Farnbach GL, et al. Disorder of rapid eye movement sleep in a cat. J Am Vet Med Assoc. 1980;178:55–57.

87. Schenck CH, Hurwitz TD, Mahowald MW. REM sleep behavior disorder: a report on a series of 96 consecutive cases and a review of the literature. J Sleep Res. 1993;2:224–231.

88. Lugaresi E, Medori R, Montagna P, et al. Fatal familial insomnia and dysautonomia with selective degeneration of thalamic nuclei. N Engl J Med. 1986;315:997–1003.

89. Morrison AR, Reiner PB. A dissection of paradoxical sleep. In: McGinty DJ, Drucker-Colin R, Morrison A, et al, eds. Brain Mechanisms of Sleep. Vols 97–110. New York, NY: Raven Press; 1985.

90. Schenck CH, Duncan E, Hopwood J, et al. The human REM sleep behavior disorder (RBD): quantitative polygraphic and behavioral analysis of 9 cases. Sleep Res. 1988;17:14.

91. Lapierre O, Montplaisir J. Polysomnographic features of REM sleep behavior disorder: development of a scoring method. Neurology. 1992;42:1371–1374.

92. Moyer KE. Kinds of aggression and their physiological basis. Commun Behav Biol. 1968;2(part A):65–87.

93. Goldstein M. Brain research and violent behavior. Arch Neurol. 1974;30:1–34.

94. Coffey CE, Licke JF, Saxton JA, et al. Sex differences in brain aging: a quantitative magnetic resonance imaging study. Arch Neurol. 1998;55:169–179.

95. Corner MA, Ramakers GJA. Spontaneous firing as an epigenetic factor in brain development-physiological consequences of chronic tetrodotoxin and picrotoxin exposure on cultured rat neocortex neurons. Dev Brain Res. 1992;65:57–64.

96. Corner MA, Mirmiran M, Bour HLMG, et al. Does rapid eye movement sleep play a role in brain development? Progr Brain Res. 1980;53:347–356.

97. Brashear HR, Phillips LH II. Autoantibodies to GABAergic neurons and response to plasmapheresis in stiff-man syndrome. Neurology. 1991;41:1588–1592.

98. Schenck CH, Ullevig CM, Mahowald MW, et al. A controlled study of serum anti-locus ceruleus antibodies in REM sleep behavior disorder. Sleep. 1997;20:349–351.

99. Schenck CH, Mahowald MW. Motor dyscontrol in narcolepsy: rapid-eye-movement (REM) sleep without atonia and REM sleep behavior disorder. Ann Neurol. 1992;32:3–10.

100. Pareja JA, Caminero AB, Masa JF, et al. A first case of progressive supranuclear palsy and pre-clinical REM sleep behavior disorder presenting as inhibition of speech during wakefulness and somniloquy with phasic muscle twitching during REM sleep. Neurologia. 1996;11:304–306.

101. Montplaisir J, Petit D, Decary A, et al. Sleep and quantitative EEG in patients with progressive supranuclear palsy. Neurology. 1997;49:999–1003.

102. Schenck CH, Bundlie SR, Mahowald MW. Delayed emergence of a parkinsonian disorder in 38% of 29 older men initially diagnosed with idiopathic rapid eye movement sleep behavior disorder. Neurology. 1996;46:388–393.

103. Plazzi G, Corsini R, Provini F, et al. REM sleep behavior disorders in multiple system atrophy. Neurology. 1997;48:1094–1097.

104. Uchiyama M, Isse K, Tanaka K, et al. Incidental Lewy body disease in a patient with REM sleep behavior disorder. Neurology. 1995;45:709–712.

105. Louden MB, Morehead MA, Schmidt HS. Activation by selegiline (Eldepryle) of REM sleep behavior disorder in parkinsonism. W V Med J. 1995;91:101.

106. Carlander B, Touchon J, Ondze B, et al. REM sleep behavior disorder induced by cholinergic treatment in Alzheimer's disease. J Sleep Res. 1996;5(suppl 1):28.

107. Nozawa T, Sato Y, Cho T, et al. Polygraphic findings in mitochondrial encephalomyopathy. Sleep Res. 1995;24A:403.

108. Uchiyama M, Tanaka K, Isse K, et al. REM sleep behavior disorder in a case with normal pressure hydrocephalus. Jpn J Psychiatry Neurol. 1991;45:935–936.

109. Trajanovic NN, Shapiro CM, Sandor P. REM sleep behavior disorder in patients with Tourette's syndrome. Sleep Res. 1997;26:524.

110. Kohyama J, Shimohira M, Kondo S, et al. Motor disturbance during REM sleep in group A xeroderma pigmentosum. Acta Neurol Scand. 1995;92:91–95.

111. Ohayon MM, Caulet M, Priest RG. Violent behavior during sleep. J Clin Psychiatry. 1997;58:369–376.

112. Schenck CH, Mahowald MW. Polysomnographic, neurologic, psychiatric, and clinical outcome report on 70 consecutive cases with REM sleep behavior disorder (RBD): sustained clonazepam efficacy in 89.5% of 57 treated patients. Cleve Clin J Med. 1990;57(suppl): s9–s23.

113. Mahowald MW, Bundlie SR, Hurwitz TD, et al. Sleep violence-

forensic science implications: polygraphic and video documentation. J Forens Sci. 1990;35:413–432.

114. Schenck CH, Mahowald MW. Injurious sleep behavior disorders (parasomnias) affecting patients on intensive care units. Intens Care Med. 1991;17:219–224.

115. American Psychiatric Association. Diagnostic and Statistical Manual of Mental Disorders, Third Edition. Washington, DC: American Psychiatric Association; 1987.

116. Hobson JA, McCarley RW. The brain as a dream state generator: an activation-synthesis hypothesis of the dream process. Am J Psychiatry. 1977;134:1335–1348.

117. McCarley RW, Hobson JA. The form of dreams and the biology of sleep. In: Wolman BB, ed. The Handbook of Dreams. New York, NY: Van Nostrand Reinhold; 1979:76–130.

118. McCarley RW. REM dreams, REM sleep and their isomorphisms. In: Chase M, Weitzman ED, eds. Sleep Disorders, Basic and Clinical Research. New York, NY: SP Medical and Scientific Books; 1983:363–393.

119. Dyken ME, Lin-Dyken DC, Seaba P, et al. Violent sleep-related behavior leading to subdural hemorrhage. Arch Neurol. 1995;52:318–321.

120. Gross PT. REM sleep behavior disorder causing bilateral subdural hematomas. Sleep Res. 1992;21:204.

121. Morfis L, Schwartz RS, Cistulli PA. REM sleep behavior disorder: a treatable cause of falls in the elderly. Age Ageing. 1997;26:43–44.

122. Siegel JM. Mechanisms of sleep control. J Clin Neurophysiol. 1990;7:49–65.

123. Broughton R, Tolentino MA. Fragmentary pathological myoclonus in NREM sleep. Electroencephalogr Clin Neurophysiol. 1984;57:303–309.

124. Broughton R, Tolentino MA, Krelina M. Excessive fragmentary myoclonus in NREM sleep: a report of 38 cases. Electroencephalogr Clin Neurophysiol. 1985;61:123–133.

125. Mouret J. Differences in sleep in patients with parkinson's disease. Electroencephalogr Clin Neurophysiol. 1975;38:653–657.

126. Askenasy JJM. Sleep patterns in extrapyramidal disorders. Int J Neurol. 1981;15:62–76.

127. Taska L, Kupfer D. A system for the quantification of phasic ocular activity during REM sleep. Sleep Watchers. 1983;6:15–17.

128. Carskadon MA, Dement WC, Mitler MM, et al. Guidelines for the multiple sleep latency test (MSLT): a standard measure of sleepiness. Sleep. 1986;9:519–524.

129. Mahowald MW, Schenck CH. Parasomnia purgatory: the epileptic/non-epileptic interface. In: Rowan AJ, Gates JR, eds. Non-Epileptic Seizures. Boston, Mass: Butterworth-Heinemann; 1993:123–139.

130. Nalamalapu U, Goldberg R, DePhillipo M, et al. Behaviors simulating REM behavior disorder in patients with severe obstructive sleep apnea. Sleep Res. 1996;25:311.

131. D'Cruz OF, Vaughn BV. Nocturnal seizures mimic REM behavior disorder. Am J END Technol. 1997;37:258–264.

132. Schenck CH, Mahowald MW. A parasomnia overlap disorder involving sleepwalking, sleep terrors and REM sleep behavior disorder: report in 33 polysomnographically confirmed cases. Sleep. 1997;20:972–981.

133. Tachibana N, Sugita Y, Terashima K, et al. Polysomnographic characteristics of healthy elderly subjects with somnambulism-like behaviors. Biol Psychiatry. 1991;30:4–14.

134. Schenck CH, Milner D, Hurwitz TD, et al. Dissociative disorders presenting as somnambulism: polysomnographic, video and clinical documentation (8 cases). Dissociation. 1989;2:194–204.

135. Mahowald MW, Schenck CH, Rosen GR, et al. The role of a sleep disorders center in evaluating sleep violence. Arch Neurol. 1992;49:604–607.

136. Schenck CH, Hurwitz TD, Bundlie SR, et al. Sleep-related injury in 100 adult patients: a polysomnographic and clinical report. Am J Psychiatry. 1989;146:1166–1173.

137. Goldberg MA, Dorman JD. Intention myoclonus: successful treatment with clonazepam. Neurology. 1976;26:24–26.

138. Hoehn MM, Cherington M. Spinal myoclonus. Neurology. 1977;27:942–946.

139. Montagna P, Provini F, Plazzi G, et al. Propriospinal myoclonus upon relaxation and drowsiness: a cause of severe insomnia. Movement Disord. 1997;12:66–72.

140. Sunohara N, Mukoyama M, Mano Y, et al. Action-induced rhythmic dystonia: an autopsy case. Neurology. 1984;34:321–327.

141. Pieris JB, Boralessa H, Lionel NDW. Clonazepam treatment of choreiform activity. Med J Austral. 1976;1:225–227.

142. Chouinard G, Young KN, Annable L. Antimanic effect of clonazepam. Biol Psychiatry. 1983;18:451–466.

143. Feinhar JP, Alvarez WH. Use of clonazepam in two cases of acute mania. J Clin Psychiatry. 1985;46:29–30.

144. Ohstory MA, Vijayan N. Clonazepam treatment of insomnia due to sleep myoclonus. Arch Neurol. 1980;37:119–120.

145. Montplaisir J, Godbout R, Boghen D, et al. Familial restless legs with periodic movements in sleep: electrophysiologic, biochemical and pharmacologic study. Neurology. 1985;35:130–134.

146. Ohanna N, Peled R, Rubin A-H, et al. Periodic leg movements in sleep: effect of clonazepam treatment. Neurology. 1985;35:408–411.

147. Mitler MM, Browman CP, Menn SJ, et al. Nocturnal myoclonus: treatment efficacy of clonazepam and temazepam. Sleep. 1986;9:385–392.

148. Goldbloom D, Chouinard G. Clonazepam in the treatment of neuroleptic-induced somnambulism. Am J Psychiatry. 1984;141:1486.

149. Browne TR. Clonazepam. N Engl J Med. 1978;299:812–818.

150. Chadwick D, Hallet M, Harris R, et al. Clinical, biochemical and physiological features distinguishing myoclonus responsive to 5–hydroxytryptophan, tryptophan with a monoamine oxidase inhibitor and clonazepam. Brain. 1977;100:455–487.

151. Green RA, Gillin JC, Wyatt RJ. The inhibitory effect of intraventricular administration of serotonin on spontaneous motor activity of rats. Psychopharmacology. 1976;51:81–84.

152. Hollister AS, Breese GR, Kuhn CM, et al. An inhibitory role for brain serotonin-containing systems in the locomotor effects of d-amphetamine. J Pharmacol Exp Ther. 1976;198:12–22.

153. Fleisher LN, Simon JR, Aprison MH. A biochemical-behavioral model for studying serotonergic supersensitivity in brain. J Neurochem. 1979;32:1613–1619.

154. Tabakoff B, Hoffman PL. Measures of physical dependence and involvement of serotonin in withdrawal symptomatology. In: Gross MM, ed. Alcohol Intoxication and Withdrawal, IIIa: Biological Aspects of Ethanol. New York, NY: Plenum Press; 1977:547–557.

155. Lapierre O, Casademont A, Montplaisir J, et al. Tonic and phasic features of REM sleep behavior disorder. Sleep Res. 1991;20:276.

156. Matsumoto M, Mutoh F, Naoe H, et al. The effects of imipramine on REM sleep behavior disorder in 3 cases. Sleep Res. 1991;20A:351.

157. Cowen PJ, Gearey DP, Schacter M, et al. Desipramine treatment in normal subjects. Arch Gen Psychiatry. 1986;43:61–67.

158. Bamford C. Carbamazepine in REM sleep behavior disorder. Sleep. 1993;16:33.

159. Tan A, Salgado M, Fahn S. Rapid eye movement sleep behavior disorder preceding Parkinson's disease with therapeutic response to levodopa. Movement Disord. 1996;11:214–216.

160. Mike ME, Kranz AJ. MAOI suppression of RBD refractory to clonazepam and other agents. Sleep Res. 1996;25:63.

161. Kunz D, Bes F, Ziller M. Melatonin in REM sleep behavior disorder. J Sleep Res. 1996;5(suppl 1):114.

162. Rye DB, Dempsay J, Dihenia B, et al. REM-sleep dyscontrol in Parkinson's disease: case report of effects of elective pallidotomy. Sleep Res. 1997;26:591.

163. Diagnostic Classification Steering Committee TM, Chairman. International Classification of Sleep Disorders: Diagnostic and Coding Manual. Rochester, Minn: American Sleep Disorders Association; 1990.

164. Guilleminault C, Pool P, Motta J, et al. Sinus arrest during REM sleep in young adults. N Engl J Med. 1984;311:1106–1110.

165. Rattenborg NC, Lindblom S, Best J, et al. REM sleep-related asystole associated with unusual polysomnographic features: a case history. Sleep Res. 1995;24:324.

166. Steiger A, Benkert O. Examination and treatment of sleep-related painful erections: a case report. Arch Sexual Behav. 1989;18:263–267.

167. Ferini-Strambi L, Zucconi M, Castronovo V, et al. Sleep-related painful erections: clinical and polysomnographic findings. Sleep Res. 1996;25:241.

168. DeRoeck J, Van Hoof E, Cluydts R. Sleep-related expiratory groaning: a case report. Sleep Res. 1983;12:237.
169. Kotorii T, Nakazawa Y, Yokoyama T, et al. The sleep pattern of chronic alcoholics during the alcohol withdrawal period. Folia Psychiatr Neurol Jpn. 1980;34:89–95.
170. Tanaka K, Kameda H, Sugita Y, et al. A case with pentazocine dependence developing delirium upon withdrawal. Psychiatr Neurol Jpn. 1979;81:289–299.
171. Hobson JA. Dreaming sleep attacks and desynchronized sleep enhancement. Arch Gen Psychiatry. 1975;32:1421–1424.
172. Culebras A, Moore JT. Magnetic resonance findings in REM sleep behavior disorder. Neurology. 1989;39:1519–1523.
173. Isono G, Ishii H, Shibata Y, et al. REM sleep with tonic muscle discharge observed in a patient with acoustic neuroma [in Japanese]. Clin Psychiatry. 1979;21:1221–1228.
174. DeBarros-Ferreira M, Chodkiewicz J-P, Lairy GC, et al. Disorganized relations of tonic and phasic events of REM sleep in a case of brain-stem tumor. Electroencephalogr Neurophysiol. 1975;38:203–207.
175. Bianchin MM, Ferreria NP, Fernandes LNT, et al. Dissociated sleep components in a patient with a pontomesencephalic astrocytoma [abstract]. Ann Neurol. 1997;42:470.
176. Minz M, Autret A, Laffont F, et al. A study on sleep in amyotrophic lateral sclerosis. Biomedicine. 1979;30:40–46.
177. Minami R, Harada M. Nocturnal delirium and REM sleep [in Japanese]. Clin Electroencephalogr. 1979;21:315–325.
178. Matsuo R, Iijima S, Sugita Y, et al. Sleep study of aged patients with nocturnal delirium [in Japanese]. Jpn J EEG EMG. 1980;8:38.
179. Turner RS, Chervin RD, Frey KA, et al. Probable diffuse Lewy body disease presenting as REM sleep behavior disorder. Neurology. 1997;49:523–527.
180. Schenck CH, Garcia-Rill E, Skinner RD, et al. A case of REM sleep behavior disorder with autopsy-confirmed Alzheimer's disease: postmortem brain stem histochemical analysis. Biol Psychiatry. 1996;40:422–425.
181. Kimura K, Tachibana N, Aso T, et al. Subclinical REM sleep behavior disorder in a patient with corticobasal degeneration. Sleep. 1997;20:891–894.
182. Schenck CH, Slater GE, Sherman RE, et al. Multiple sclerosis and sleep: survey report and polygraphic detection of REM and NREM motor abnormalities. Sleep Res. 1986;15:163.
183. Shimizu T, Tabushi K, Iijima S, et al. Sleep study in patients with OPCA and related diseases [in Japanese]. Jpn J EEG EMG. 1980;8:38.
184. Shimizu T, Sugita Y, Teshima Y, et al. Sleep study in patients with spinocerebellar degeneration and related diseases. In: Koella WP, ed. Sleep 1980. Basel, Germany: S. Karger; 1981:435–437.
185. Salva MAQ, Guilleminault C. Olivopontocerebellar degeneration, abnormal sleep, and REM sleep without atonia. Neurology. 1986;36:576–577.
186. Sforza E, Zucconi M, Petronelli R, et al. REM sleep behavioral disorders. Eur Neurol. 1988;28:295–300.
187. Tachibana N, Kimura K, Kitajima K, et al. REM sleep without atonia at early stage of sporadic olivopontocerebellar atrophy. J Neurol Sci. 1995;132:28–34.
188. April RS. Observations on parkinsonian tremor in all-night sleep. Neurology. 1966;16:720–724.
189. Stern M, Roffwarg H, Duvoisin R. The parkinsonian tremor in sleep. J Nerv Mental Disord. 1968;147:202–210.
190. Boeve BF, Silber MH, Petersen RC, et al. REM sleep behavior disorder and degenerative dementia with or without parkinsonism: a syndrome predictive of Lewy body disease [abstract]. Neurology. 1997;49:a358–a359.
191. Shimizu T, Sugita Y, Iijima S, et al. Sleep study in Shy-Drager syndrome. Clin Neurol (Jpn). 1981;21:218–227.
192. Shimizu T. A polygraphic study of nocturnal sleep in degenerative diseases: a possible mechanism of nocturnal deliriium in patients with organic brain conditions. Adv Neurol Sci (Tokyo). 1985;29:154–177.
193. Wright BA, Rosen JR, Buysse DJ, et al. Shy-Drager syndrome presenting as a REM behavior disorder. J Geriatr Psychiatry Neurol. 1990;3:110–113.
194. Tison F, Wenning GK, Quinn NP, et al. REM sleep behavior disorder as the presenting symptom of multiple system atrophy. J Neurol Neurosurg Psychiatry. 1995;58:379–380.
195. Tachibana N, Kimura K, Kitajima K, et al. REM sleep motor dysfunction in multiple system atrophy. Sleep Res. 1995;24A:415.
196. Mayer G, Meier-Ewert K. Motor dyscontrol in sleep of narcoleptic patients: a lifelong development? J Sleep Res. 1993;2:143.
197. Ishigooka J, Westendorf F, Oguchi T, et al. Somnambulistic behavior associated with abnormal REM sleep in an elderly woman. Biol Psychiatry. 1985;20:1003–1008.

Restless Legs Syndrome and Periodic Limb Movement Disorder

Jacques Montplaisir

Alain Nicolas

Roger Godbout

Arthur Walters

DESCRIPTION

Restless Legs Syndrome

The restless legs syndrome (RLS) has been described for centuries[1] and was first singled out as a distinct clinical entity by Ekbom in 1945.[2] Patients with RLS usually report dysesthetic sensations when they are at rest. The dysesthesia may be described as "pins and needles," "an internal itch," or "a creeping or crawling sensation." These sensations are generally relieved by agitated motor activity. When symptoms occur, patients move their legs vigorously, flexing, stretching, and crossing them. Only on rare instances is there no dysesthesia immediately preceding the movements of the legs. Symptoms are worse later in the day or at night. Most patients report difficulty falling asleep as both sleepiness and lying down in bed facilitate the occurrence of dysesthesia. On the contrary, several patients fall asleep rapidly but wake up in the middle of the night with paresthesias which force them to rise and walk around to relieve the discomfort. In a recent study of 133 patients, a large majority of RLS patients (84.7%) frequently experienced difficulty falling asleep at night because of RLS and 86% reported that symptoms wake them up frequently during the night.[3] Ninety-four percent reported at least one of these two manifestations. The intensity of sensory and motor symptoms can vary greatly from one patient to another. The severity of RLS can also vary greatly throughout a patient's lifetime. During some periods, motor symptoms may be present several times a day while at other times they may be totally absent, or nearly so.[4] The sudden remissions, lasting for months or even years, are as difficult to explain as the relapses which appear without any apparent reason. In several cases symptoms are present every night and in most patients the severity of symptoms increases with advancing age. Several patients (46.2% of men and 22.2% of women) also report excessive daytime fatigue or somnolence.[3] RLS is sensitive to a variety of influences. For example, symptoms may appear or worsen during pregnancy, especially in patients who have a family history of RLS.[4] Other factors are known to modulate the manifestations of RLS, such as fatigue, a very warm environment, and prolonged exposure to cold.

Several problems may result directly from RLS. The incessant bedtime dysesthesia can cause emotional disturbances in some patients. In severe cases, depression and suicidal thoughts may arise, but RLS should not be confused with the restlessness of anxious patients. RLS may also be responsible for marital difficulties. In several cases of RLS the main complaint comes from the bed partner; in approximately one third of these cases, couples sleep in separate beds because of the discomfort caused by repetitive leg movements.

Periodic Movements During Sleep

The vast majority of patients with RLS have stereotyped repetitive movements once asleep, a condition known as periodic limb movement disorder and also periodic limb movements during sleep (PLMS). However, PLMS also represents a nosological entity distinct from RLS.[5]

Originally called "nocturnal myoclonus," PLMS is best described as rhythmical extensions of the big toe and dorsiflexions of the ankle with occasional flexions of the knee and hip, each movement lasting approximately 0.5 to 5.0 sec with a frequency of about one every 20 to 40 sec (Fig. 65–1). PLMS clusters into episodes, each of which lasts several minutes or even hours. In general, these episodes are more numerous in the first half of the night, but they can also recur

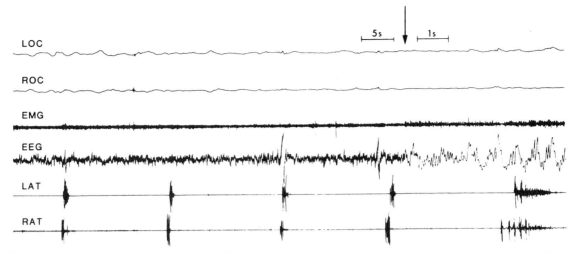

Figure 65–1. Polysomnogram of a patient with restless legs syndrome and periodic leg movements during sleep. Arrow points to a change of chart speed from 3 mm/sec to 15 mm/sec. Left side of the figure shows the periodicity of leg movements, with an inter-event interval of 24.5 sec; right side of the figure illustrates the arousal reaction accompanying leg movements. EEG, left central electroencephalogram; EMG, chin electromyogram; LAT, left anterior tibialis electromyogram; LOC, left electro-oculogram; RAT, right anterior tibialis electromyogram; ROC, right electro-oculogram.

throughout the entire sleep period.[5a] Intense movements may cause arousals[5b] which, if numerous, may lead to nonrestorative sleep. However, mild PLMS can also occur without concomitant nocturnal sleep disruption.

It has been shown that the prevalence of PLMS is correlated with age.[6-12] Whereas PLMS is rare in young people, it is relatively common in the elderly. It is rarely diagnosed in patients under the age of 30 years, is found in 5% of normal subjects aged between 30 and 50 years, in 29% of subjects over 50 years, and in nearly 44% of subjects aged 65 and older.[12]

PLMS co-occurs with a wide range of sleep-wake complaints, including early sleep onset difficulty, nocturnal awakenings, and daytime sleepiness. A multicenter collaborative study involving 18 sleep disorders clinics reported PLMS to be the primary pathological finding in 17% of patients complaining of disorders of initiating and maintaining sleep (insomnia) and in 11% of hypersomniac patients complaining of excessive daytime sleepiness.[13] PLMS also occurs in a wide variety of sleep disorders, including narcolepsy,[14, 15] central,[16] and obstructive[17] sleep apnea syndrome, and rapid eye movement (REM) sleep behavior disorder.[18]

It must be remembered, however, that Bixler et al.[6] found PLMS to be present in 11% of otherwise physically and mentally healthy subjects. Coleman et al.[13] suggested that there is no evidence that PLMS actually causes insomnia.

Similarly, in patients consulting primarily for excessive daytime sleepiness and presenting with an elevated PLMS index, no correlation was found between PLMS index at night, poor sleep efficiency, and daytime somnolence measured by the multiple sleep latency test.[19, 20]

EPIDEMIOLOGY

The prevalence of RLS was first estimated by Ekbom[2] to be 5% of the general population. This estima-

tion was based on the clinical review of 500 patients in his practice. A recent population-based questionnaire survey conducted in 2019 unrelated subjects revealed the presence of leg restlessness at bedtime in 10 to 15% of the responders.[21] A similar prevalence was found among male and female responders. Most cases of RLS in the general population are mild; nevertheless, it is likely that the condition is considerably underdiagnosed.

RLS is thought to be a condition of the middle-age population and in recent studies the mean age of onset was found to be between 27.2 and 41.0 years.[3, 22-24] However, two large surveys[3, 23] found that 38.3% and 45% of RLS patients, respectively, experienced their first symptoms before the age of 20.

CLINICAL EVALUATION

Recently, a consensus emerged from a large international study group on essential criteria for the diagnosis of RLS.[25] This group defined four clinical characteristics of RLS necessary for diagnosis (minimal criteria): (1) a desire to move the limbs usually associated with paresthesias or dysesthesias; (2) motor restlessness, using different motor strategies to relieve the discomfort; (3) symptoms that are worse or exclusively present at rest (i.e., lying, sitting), with at least partial and temporary relief by activity; (4) symptoms that are worse in the evening or during the night (Table 65–1). The group also defined nonessential but common features of RLS as listed in the Table 65–1.

POLYGRAPHIC INVESTIGATION

Polygraphic recording may also be useful in the diagnosis of RLS. In 1988, we developed a test called the Suggested Immobilization Test (SIT) designed to

Table 65–1. DIAGNOSTIC CRITERIA ESTABLISHED BY THE INTERNATIONAL
RESTLESS LEGS SYNDROME STUDY GROUP

Essential Features	Nonessential but Common Features
1. Desire to move the limbs usually associated with paresthesias or dysesthesias 2. Motor restlessness 3. Symptoms are worse or exclusively present at rest with at least partial and temporary relief by activity 4. Symptoms must be worse in the evening or during the night	1. Sleep disturbance and its consequences 2. PLMS 3. Involuntary limb movements while awake and at rest (similar to PLMS and disappearing when patient gets up to walk) 4. Neurological examination: no abnormalities in the primary form, but in the secondary form signs of a peripheral neuropathy or radiculopathy may be present 5. Clinical course: may begin at any age but most severely affected patients are middle to older age; is usually progressive but a static course or remission may occur 6. Family history: sometimes present and suggestive of an autosomal dominant mode of inheritance

PLMS, periodic leg movements during sleep.

quantify periodic leg movements in wakefulness.[26] For the test, patients sit motionless on the bed with legs outstretched and eyes open. Electromyographic (EMG) recording from anterior tibialis muscles indicates that leg movements occur during the SIT. Recently, the sensitivity and the specificity of the SIT was tested in a small number (N = 16) of severe RLS patients and in a group of age-matched normal controls. This method elicited paresthesias and repetitive leg movements in 13 (81%) of the patients with a typical history of RLS.[27] An index of 40 movements per hour was found to discriminate between RLS and controls with a specificity of 81%. However, the SIT has been tested in a small population of severe RLS patients and its sensitivity has never been measured in a large population of RLS patients with various degrees of severity.

The quantification of PLMS is a commonly used sleep laboratory diagnostic procedure for RLS. Diagnostic polysomnography (PSG) always includes central electroencephalography (EEG), electro-oculography (EOG), submental EMG, and bilateral EMG of the anterior tibialis muscles (see Fig. 65–1). Additional EEG and EMG derivations are frequently recorded. The electrographic picture of a single movement can vary from one sustained contraction to a polyclonic burst with a frequency of approximately 5 Hz.[5, 28] Muscular jerks are often associated with polygraphic signs of arousal such as K complexes followed by a train of alpha activity of varying duration, termed *K-alpha complexes*[29, 30] (see Fig. 65–1).

Methods for scoring PLMS were summarized by Coleman.[31] According to standard criteria, PLMS is scored only if it is part of a series of four or more consecutive movements lasting 0.5 to 5.0 sec with an intermovement interval of 4 to 90 sec. A PLMS index (number of PLMS per hour of sleep) greater than 5 for the entire night of sleep is considered pathological. The number of leg movements varies from night to night, especially in individuals with less severe sleep complaints. Recently, a group of 49 patients were recorded for two consecutive nights.[3] On each night, 82% of patients had a PLMS index greater than 5 and 76% met this criterion on both nights. However, with the use of the worse night for each patient, 87.8% were found to

meet the criteria.[3] In a study of 16 RLS patients and 16 normal controls, the sensitivity and the specificity of the PLMS index were tested. When the worst of 2 nights for each patient was used, a PLMS greater than 11 correctly identified RLS patients from normal controls with a sensitivity and a specificity of 81%.[27]

Actigraphy was also used to assess periodic leg movements during waking and during sleep, but this method has never been validated.[32]

ASSOCIATED CONDITIONS

RLS and PLMS have been related to several other medical conditions. Recently, 41 RLS patients underwent electrophysiological evaluation (EMG) and nerve conduction velocities, 15 of which were abnormal (14 had neuropathy of mixed types and one had L5 radiculopathy).[22] Neuropathic RLS may be overrepresented in these patients who were examined at an older age (mean age: 62.7 years). Conversely, RLS was found in only 5.2% of 144 patients presenting with a clinical diagnosis of polyneuropathy.[33] RLS has also been reported in association with lumbosacral radiculopathy,[23] but this association has been less well documented. A controlled study of a large number of RLS patients of different age groups will be needed to assess the association between peripheral neuropathy and RLS.

RLS has also been associated with uremia and 15 to 40% of patients under hemodialysis do actually complain of RLS symptomatology.[4, 34–37] This is dramatic in many patients because hemodialysis requires prolonged periods of immobilization. Several factors may predispose uremic patients to develop RLS, including anemia and peripheral neuropathy. In one case of uremia, symptoms of RLS resolved after kidney transplantation.[38] A high correlation was found for the PLMS index between actigraphic and EMG methods and therefore actigraphic assessment of PLMS may be used for screening purposes. RLS has also been reported in association with iron deficiency anemia.[39, 40] More recently, the iron status was assessed in 18 elderly patients with RLS and 18 matched control subjects. Low serum ferritin levels were found in the RLS patients.[40, 40a, 40b] Ferrous sulfate administered for 2 months to 14 patients resulted in a significant reduction of RLS severity.[40]

In a recent study, 31% of 135 consecutive patients with fibromyalgia had RLS.[41] In another recent study, 21 (30%) of 70 patients with rheumatoid arthritis had RLS.[42] RLS has also been reported to be associated with magnesium deficiency[43] and preliminary data suggest an association of both RLS and PLMS with childhood attention-deficit hyperactivity disorder.[44] PLMS have also been described as the initial clinical manifestations of familial amyloid polyneuropathy.[45]

RLS or PLMS has been reported anecdotally in association with a wide variety of medical conditions.[46–51] However, these associations were found in a limited number of patients. Considering the high prevalence of RLS and PLMS in the general population, these associations should be interpreted with caution. It is also important to know that several medications, including lithium carbonate and tricyclic and other antidepressants, may induce or worsen RLS or PLMS,[52–55] as does withdrawal from a variety of drugs such as anticonvulsants, benzodiazepines, barbiturates, and other hypnotics.[55a]

DIFFERENTIAL DIAGNOSIS

PLMS should be differentiated from other state-dependent motor disorders. Some types of sleep-related "myoclonus" can be observed in normal subjects. The so-called hypnic myoclonus or sleep starts[56, 57] are observed during the transition from wakefulness to sleep. They consist of short massive body movements which involve the extremities of both sides synchronously but which are devoid of periodicity. "Fragmentary myoclonus" occurs as briefer (less than 150 ms) and more diffuse twitch-like jerks, most visible in the hands and face, but free of synchrony and symmetry. Fragmentary myoclonus in the form of phasic REM twitches is normally seen in REM sleep but it may persist throughout all stages of nonrapid eye movement (NREM) sleep in association with several other sleep disorders.[58] Pathological forms of myoclonus are in general suppressed during sleep, but myoclonic epilepsy is specifically activated by awakenings.[59, 60] Propriospinal myoclonus or spinal myoclonus due to other causes, such as structural lesions of the spinal cord, must be distinguished from idiopathic PLMS because these movements may also persist in sleep.[61] However, if there is a spinal cord lesion, signs of spasticity and a sensory level may be present.

Other conditions can also be misdiagnosed as RLS or PLMS. The "painful legs and moving toes" syndrome[62] is characterized by severe pain in one or both feet, sometimes with a sensation of burning, and associated with repetitive, semicontinuous movements of the toes. However, pain is not necessarily worse at night or relieved by activity.

Nocturnal leg cramps[63, 64] are sustained and painful contractions of the leg muscles, mainly the gastrocnemius and the soleus. Nocturnal cramping is a common condition. It is highly prevalent in the elderly[64a] and during pregnancy,[64b] but a recent study of 2527 children[64c] showed an overall incidence of 7.3%. Leg cramps were usually unilateral, ocurred when the children were asleep, and had a mean duration of 1.7 minutes. Several treatments have been used for nocturnal cramps, especially quinine and vitamin E.[64d, 64e] Based on data from cross-over studies, a recent meta-analysis suggested that patients had fewer nocturnal leg cramps in a 4-week period when taking quinine compared to a placebo.[64d] However, given the possible serious side effects of quinine, the benefits and the risks of using quinine should be thoroughly assessed.[64f] Symptomatic treatment, that is, stretching the affected calf muscle by forcible dorsiflexion of the foot, may in many cases be sufficient.

RLS should also be differentiated from akathisia. Neuroleptic-induced akathisia, which is motor restlessness induced by dopamine receptor blocking antipsychotic agents, is not associated with prominent paresthesia, and symptoms are not necessarily worse at night. Inner restlessness rather than leg discomfort is the usual trigger for neuroleptic-induced akathisia. The history of neuroleptic use clarifies the picture. In addition, levodopa (L-dopa) does not suppress akathisia as it does RLS, and in some cases of parkinsonism L-dopa may even trigger akathisia.[65] On the other hand, both RLS and akathisia involve complex alterations in dopamine and iron metabolism.[66, 67] PLMS may occur in neuroleptic-induced akathisia but not in as high a percentage as in RLS.[68, 69]

As mentioned earlier, peripheral neuropathy may be associated with RLS,[33] but peripheral neuropathy in the absence of RLS is not characterized by worsening at rest with relief by activity and worsening at night. Other conditions such as vascular or neurogenic intermittent claudication are frequent causes of leg pain or discomfort, but contrary to RLS they are relieved by rest with the legs outstretched, and worsen during the prolonged upright position or walking.

MEDICAL INVESTIGATION

These observations stress the importance of a careful history-taking and differential diagnosis of RLS and PLMS. Whenever the diagnosis is doubtful, a PSG recording and a thorough neurological examination should be performed. Two consecutive nights of PSG are recommended.[27] As the PLMS index shows night-to-night variability, caution should be taken in drawing conclusions from single-night studies. As a significant number of RLS patients have peripheral neuropathy,[22] a careful clinical examination of sensory and motor functions should be performed. EMG and nerve conduction studies should be done if the examination is suggestive of a peripheral neuropathy or radiculopathy. Given the aforementioned associations with iron, magnesium, and other deficiencies, it is recommended that iron, ferritin, magnesium, and vitamin B_{12} and folate levels be obtained.

TREATMENT

Benzodiazepines

In both double-blind and open-label studies, several benzodiazepines, including clonazepam, nitrazepam, lorazepam, and temazepam, have been used to treat RLS and PLMS. They have been shown to improve the quality of nocturnal sleep,[70–80] even in cases of RLS secondary to uremia. Most PSG studies also showed that benzodiazepines are effective in reducing the number of leg movements per hour of sleep and the number of arousals and awakenings associated with leg jerks. Therefore, at least on a short-term basis, these drugs are useful in improving sleep continuity in RLS and PLMS patients. However, under benzodiazepines, PLMS indices may remain elevated. In addition, benzodiazepines are potent central nervous system (CNS) depressants; they often cause daytime sleepiness and they may induce or aggravate sleep apnea syndrome.

Opioids

The therapeutic action of opioids was mentioned in the original description of RLS by Ekbom.[2] Recently, this effect has been further documented in open and double-blind clinical trials[81–83] where it was found to be reversible by naloxone, an opioid receptor antagonist. Opioids were also found effective in treating PLMS in patients without RLS.[84] The risk of abuse and the danger of addiction theoretically limit the clinical use of opioids in RLS and PLMS, but in our clinical experience the risk of addiction and tolerance is small. The administration of opiates should be limited to patients without a previous history of alcohol or drug abuse. In severe cases, especially in those refractory to benzodiazepines or dopaminergic agents, opiates may be an alternative treatment.

Dopaminergic Agents

Dopaminergic agents are now considered the treatment of choice for RLS. Several open-label and double-blind studies have shown that L-dopa given with a peripheral decarboxylase inhibitor is effective in treating RLS and PLMS.[26, 85–90] A 2-year follow-up study showed long-term beneficial effects of L-dopa in RLS.[89] L-Dopa was also found effective in the treatment of uremic RLS,[91] and in suppressing PLMS in patients with narcolepsy.[92] However, when L-dopa is administered only at bedtime,[86] a rebound of PLMS is often observed in the last part of the night. A controlled study using PSG and a double-blind crossover design also showed that L-dopa administered twice at night produces a significant reduction of RLS occurring at bedtime and of PLMS throughout the night.[26] Morning restlessness was reported in patients chronically treated with L-dopa. Guilleminault et al.[93] found that 35% of RLS patients treated with L-dopa developed morning restlessness; this complaint completely disappeared

within 2 to 6 days after withdrawal from L-dopa. In other studies, treatment-emerging morning restlessness was also found in 8 of 43 patients (18.6%) under L-dopa treatment.[90] An analogous phenomenon is augmentation, where RLS symptoms occur earlier in the afternoon or evening than previously.[94] It is the impression of some clinicians that augmentation may be more of a problem when sustained release preparations are used; this has not been studied rigorously. In rebound, the timing of the reappearance of symptoms is compatible with the timing of withdrawal from medication, whereas in augmentation this is not the case. Augmentation may be due to changes in dopamine receptor sensitivity. In clinical practice, rebound restlessness or augmentation often leads to additional administration of L-dopa during the daytime, reduction of night dosage, or to interruption of treatment.

Other studies have shown that the dopamine D2 receptor agonist bromocriptine was effective in treating RLS and PLMS.[95, 96] However, bromocriptine administration is sometimes associated with frequent and severe side effects quickly leading to cessation of treatment after short-term administration. Recently, pergolide, another D2 receptor agonist, became more and more frequently used in the treatment of RLS.[97–99, 99a] Like bromocriptine, pergolide is an ergoline derivative and has several peripheral side effects, especially nausea and orthostatic hypotension. Nevertheless, pergolide is usually better tolerated than bromocriptine and several patients have been successfully treated for several months with pergolide. It is often necessary to administer domperidone, a peripheral dopamine antagonist, in association with pergolide or bromocriptine, to minimize the side effects of these medications, especially nausea. Over the past year, pramipexole, a full agonist of the D3 receptor, has been used to treat RLS in an open-label fashion.[100] In addition, a crossover placebo-controlled study performed in 10 RLS patients showed a dramatic improvement of RLS symptomatology and a complete suppression of PLMS with pramipexole.[101] Excessive daytime sleepiness has been described as a side effect of pramipexole both in RLS[100, 101] and in Parkinson's disease (PD).[101a] Sudden onset of sleep leading to vehicle accidents was reported in eight PD patients,[101b] including five patients who did not report excessive daytime sleepiness otherwise. None of these patients had a sleep laboratory investigation. Whether pramipexole can trigger sudden onset of sleep without sedation remains to be further documented. This phenomenon was never reported in RLS patients treated with pramipexole.

Ropinirole, another D2-receptor agonist, was also found to improve RLS symptomatology in an open-label clinical trial.[101c]

Other Treatments

Over the years, several other treatments have been proposed for RLS and PLMS, but few of them have been systematically evaluated. In double-blind studies, carbamazepine proved to be effective in reducing nocturnal sleep disruption and RLS symptoms in RLS patients.[102] However, carbamazepine was not found effective in decreasing PLMS or PLMS-associated arousals.[103] In our experience, this medication has limited indications in the treatment of patients with severe PLMS or RLS. Clonidine, an adrenergic agonist, was found in open-label and double-blind studies to have therapeutic effects on RLS but not on PLMS.[104–106] Gabapentin, a new anticonvulsant medication, was also used successfully in the treatment of RLS.[107, 108] Gabapentin may be particularly useful in the painful form of RLS. Most recently, magnesium was found to be successful in treating the symptoms of RLS and PLMS.[109]

Clinical Management of Restless Legs Syndrome

In several patients, RLS occurs sporadically with spontaneous remission lasting weeks or even months.

Therefore, the physician should use pharmacological treatment on an irregular basis or consider a drug holiday when appropriate. Continuous pharmacological treatment should be considered if patients complain of RLS occurring at least 3 nights per week. All treatments are symptomatic and do not influence the course of the illness.[109a] Therefore, the clinician should carefully assess the therapeutic benefit vs. the severity of the side effects. A therapeutic flow chart appears in Table 65–2. Each drug is presented with its commonly used therapeutic dosage, its most frequent side effects, and the appropriate countermeasures. Higher doses may be administered in severe cases.

A questionnaire among sleep experts indicated that dopaminergic agents, then benzodiazepines, followed by opioids, were, in that order of preference, the favored treatments for RLS.[110] Among dopaminergic agents, L-dopa has been used for more than 10 years and its therapeutic effect has been repeatedly confirmed. However, considering the rebound restlessness

Table 65–2. FLOW CHART FOR MANAGEMENT OF RESTLESS LEGS SYNDROME

	Agents	Dosages (mg)	Side Effects	Countermeasures
Step 1	**DA Agonists** Pramipexole Pergolide	0.125–1.0* 0.1–0.5*	Nausea and orthostatic hypotension	Slowly increase dosage *or* use domperidone if available (10–30 mg)
			Insomnia	Use small dose of benzodiazepines in association with DA agonists
			Daytime fatigue and somnolence	Reduce dosage *or* discontinue DA agonists and use levodopa (if severe and persistent)
			Hallucinations	Discontinue DA agonists
			Tolerance	Drug holiday for 2 weeks, then return to lower dosage
Step 2	**DA Precursors** Levodopa with benserazide or carbidopa	Regular or slow release: 100–25, 200–50†	Same as for dopaminergic agonists	See countermeasures for DA agonists above
			Morning rebound or augmentation of RLS in early evening	Use small extra dose of levodopa during daytime *or* reduce dosage *or* combine levodopa with DA agonists or benzodiazepines *or* discontinue levodopa (if severe and persistent)
Step 3	**Benzodiazepines** Clonazepam	0.5–2.0*	Daytime somnolence	Reduce dosage *or* use 1–2 h before bedtime
	Temazepam	15–30*	Tolerance	Drug holiday for 2 weeks, then return to lower dosage
	Nitrazepam	5–10*		
Step 4	**Opiates** Oxycodone	5†	Constipation	Symptomatic treatment
	Propoxyphene Codeine	200* 15–60*	Dependency	Drug holiday *or* withdrawal
Step 5	**Antiepileptic Drugs** Carbamazepine	200–400*	Nephrotoxicity	Monitor blood level regularly and adjust dosage
	Gabapentin	100–400*	Daytime fatigue and somnolence	Reduce dosage

*At bedtime.
†At bedtime; repeated once during the night if needed. Slow release preparation not usually repeated.
DA, dopamine; RLS, restless legs syndrome.

observed with L-dopa therapy, D2 and D3 receptor agonists, and especially pramipexole, are rapidly becoming the first choice of treatment. A recent study showed a persistent effect of pramipexole after daily administration for more than 7.8 months.[110a] The second choice is L-dopa, especially in cases of persistent daytime somnolence induced by dopaminergic agonists. If patients develop insomnia after treatment with dopaminergic agents, a small dose of benzodiazepines may be added. If insomnia persists, if dopaminergic agents are ineffective, or if they generate serious adverse effects, they should be discontinued and replaced by benzodiazepines. Opioids may be used alone or in combination with other therapies. Because of the risk of dependency, opioids should be restricted to severe RLS patients who failed to respond to both dopaminergic agents and benzodiazepines. Other substances, such as carbamazepine, gabapentin, or clonidine, are generally considered less efficacious. However, gabapentin may be useful in painful forms of RLS, particularly if a peripheral neuropathy is present. Iron may be administered for patients with low iron or ferritin levels.

ETIOLOGY AND PHYSIOPATHOLOGY

Genetics

Several studies have reported familial aggregation of RLS and several families have been described where members were affected with RLS over a span of three to five generations.[2, 3, 23, 111-114] The prevalence of RLS patients with at least one first-degree relative affected with RLS was estimated to be around 63%.[3, 22, 23] In these families, 221 of 568 possible first-degree relatives (39%)[3] and 58 of 246 possible first-degree relatives (23.6%)[22] were reported to be afflicted with RLS. In most families, the pedigree suggested an autosomal dominant transmission and men and women were equally afflicted with this condition. Penetrance (the degree to which a gene manifests itself clinically if present) is virtually 100%. In several families, possible anticipation was present, that is, there was a tendency for the symptoms to begin at a younger age in each generation.[114, 114a]

Neural Substrates

There are major controversies with regard to the localization of the neural structures involved in the physiopathology of RLS. There is some evidence of a peripheral origin of RLS. Although muscle biopsy was found normal in most studies, nerve biopsy revealed the presence of axonal atrophy in a large percentage of patients with RLS.[115]

A study by Ondo and Jankovic[22] showed the presence of peripheral neuropathy as assessed by EMG and nerve conduction velocities in 15 out of 41 patients with RLS. The authors suggested that among patients originally diagnosed as having primary RLS, approxi-

mately 35% will turn out to have RLS secondary to peripheral neuropathy. They also found that the percentage of familial cases was much lower in this population (13%) compared with RLS patients without neuropathy (92%). Conversely, only 5.2% of patients with polyneuropathy were found to be affected with RLS.[33]

There is most likely a major contribution of the spinal cord to RLS. RLS or PLMS or both were found during epidural and spinal anesthesia.[116] RLS or PLMS or both were also found in several patients with a spinal cord lesion and even in cases of complete spinal cord transection.[117-120] PLMS was studied by videographic analysis and found to be similar to the Babinski response,[121] which is observed in cortical or spinal cord lesions. However, the Babinski response could also be elicited in 50% of normal subjects following plantar stimulation during NREM sleep.[122] We know that the response to plantar stimulation is normal during wakefulness in patients with RLS and PLMS, but the phenomenon still has to be studied during sleep.

Several electrophysiological studies were performed in patients with RLS. Mixed nerve somatosensory and brainstem auditory evoked responses were found to be normal in patients with RLS and PLMS.[123] Wechsler et al.[124] studied evoked responses after posterior tibialis and median nerve stimulation and found them to be normal. These results led to the conclusion that there is no evidence for a primary afferent sensory disturbance. On the other hand, additional long-latency components of the blink reflex have been reported in patients with PLMS.[125, 126] This observation, although not found in every patient, could indicate that PLMS is operative at the pontine level or more rostrally. It was shown, however, that abnormalities of the habituation of the blink reflex involved the pallidostriatal dopaminergic system.[127] Recently, motor system excitability was measured by means of transcranial magnetic stimulation, and a decrease in intracortical inhibition was found.[127a]

A study using magnetic resonance imaging (MRI) found no anatomical lesion in patients with RLS. However, functional MRI showed that leg-related sensory complaints in RLS were associated with thalamic and cerebellar activation while periodic leg movements in wakefulness were more closely associated with pontine and red nucleus activation. In neither case was any cortical activation found.[128] This result is in agreement with those of backaveraging techniques that found no premovement cortical potentials for PLMS.[5, 129] These data are in support of the involuntary nature of PLMS.

Even if the neurophysiological mechanisms responsible for PLMS are still unknown, the remarkable periodicity of leg movements suggests the presence of an underlying CNS pacemaker.[130] Studies carried out in cats[131, 132] and in human beings[130, 133] during normal sleep, as well as during coma, have reported a 20- to 40-sec periodicity for blood pressure, respiration, intraventricular fluid pressure, pulse frequency, and EEG arousal.[134-139] The periodicity of these functions is comparable to that of PLMS and all these phenomena can be synchronous.[140, 141] These observations and those obtained in patients with spinal cord transection suggest that RLS and PLMS are the behavioral manifestations of a normal CNS (brainstem or spinal) pacemaker that becomes disinhibited under specific circumstances.[142]

Neurotransmitter Dysfunctions

The results obtained with opioids and L-dopa have led to some neuropharmacological hypotheses regarding the pathophysiology of RLS and PLMS. The therapeutic effects of L-dopa and dopamine agonists on RLS and PLMS support the hypothesis that central dopamine may be involved in the physiopathology of these conditions. The fact that the motor restlessness of neuroleptic-induced akathisia can be caused by dopamine receptor–blocking antipsychotic agents is in further support of this hypothesis.[68, 69] Gamma-hydroxybutyrate, a short-acting blocker of dopamine release, was also found to increase RLS and PLMS.[85] High levels of free dopamine and homovanillic acid were also reported in the cerebrospinal fluid of a patient with RLS and PLMS,[85] but normal CSF dopamine metabolite levels were recently found in eight RLS patients.[142a] Brain imagery using single-photo emission computed tomography with D2 receptor ligands shows a decrease in D2 receptor binding sites in the striatum of patients with RLS.[143, 144] A PET study measured nigrostriatal terminal dopamine storage with ^{18}F-Dopa and striatal D2-receptor binding with ^{11}C-raclopride in 13 RLS patients. Both ^{18}F-Dopa and D2-receptor binding were reduced in the caudate and the putamen of RLS patients compared with control subjects.[144a] A recent study[101] showing a complete disappearance of PLMS with pramipexole, a full D3 receptor agonist, raised the possibility of a specific involvement of D3 receptors in the pathophysiology of this condition.

Some observations indicate that RLS and PLMS could be associated with an endogenous opiate system dysfunction.[81–84] It was then postulated that opiate receptors play a major role in the pathophysiology of this condition because the opiate receptor blocker naloxone causes the reappearance of RLS symptoms in opioid-treated patients.[82] However, we know that the effect of L-dopa is not secondary to the action of dopamine on the opioid system as the blockade of opiate receptors by naloxone does not alter the therapeutic effect of L-dopa.[88] On the other hand, a single-case study showed that pretreatment with pimozide, a dopamine receptor antagonist, partially blocks the effect of codeine on RLS.[145]

Several studies have shown interactions between opioid and dopamine systems in many sites, including basal ganglia, brainstem, and spinal cord, but it might be premature to speculate on the respective role of these neurotransmitters in RLS and PLMS. It is hoped that clarification of these interactions may lead to a better understanding of the pathophysiology of RLS and PLMS and to more targeted treatments.

References

1. Willis T. De animae brutorum. London, England: Wells & Scott; 1672.
2. Ekbom KA. Restless legs. Acta Med Scand Suppl. 1945;158:1–123.
3. Montplaisir J, Boucher S, Poirier G, et al. Clinical polysomnographic and genetic characteristics of restless legs syndrome: a study of 133 patients diagnosed with new standard criteria. Mov Disord. 1996;12:61–65.
4. Trenkwalder C, Walters AS, Hening W. Periodic limb movements and restless legs syndrome. Neurol Clin. 1996;14:629–649.
5. Lugaresi E, Cirignotta F, Coccagna G, et al. Nocturnal myoclonus and restless legs syndrome. Adv Neurol. 1986;43:295–307.
5a. Nicolas A, Michaud M, Lavigne G, et al. The influence of sex, age and sleep/wake state on characteristics of periodic leg movements in restless legs syndrome patients. Clin Neurophysiol. 1999;110:1168–1174.
5b. Sforza E, Nicolas A, Lavigne G, et al. EEG and cardiac activation during periodic leg movements in sleep: support for a hierarchy of arousal responses. Neurology. 1999;52:786–791.
6. Bixler EO, Kales A, Vela-Bueno A, et al. Nocturnal myoclonus and nocturnal myoclonic activity in a normal population. Res Commun Chem Pathol Pharmacol. 1982;36:129–140.
7. Ancoli-Israël S, Kripke DF, Mason W, et al. Sleep apnea and periodic movements in sleep in an aging population. J Gerontol. 1985;40:419–425.
8. Crook TH, Kupfer DJ, Hoch CC, et al. Treatment of sleep disorders in the elderly. In: Meltzer HY, ed. Psychopharmacology: The Third Generation of Progress. New York, NY: Raven Press; 1987:1159–1165.
9. Mosko SS, Dickel MJ, Paul T, et al. Sleep apnea and sleep-related periodic leg movements in community resident seniors. J Am Geriatr Soc. 1988;36:502–508.
10. Bliwise DL, Carskadon MA, Dement WC. Nightly variation of periodic movements in sleep in middle aged and elderly individuals. Arch Gerontol Geriatr. 1988;7:273–279.
11. Bannerman C. Sleep disorders in the later years. Postgrad Med J. 1988;84:265–274.
12. Coleman RM, Bliwise DL, Sajben N, et al. Epidemiology of periodic movements during sleep. In: Guilleminault C, Lugaresi E, eds. Sleep/Wake Disorders. Natural History, Epidemiology and Long Term Evolution. New York, NY: Raven Press; 1988:217–229.
13. Coleman RM, Pollak CP, Weitzman ED. Periodic movements in sleep (nocturnal myoclonus): relation to sleep disorders. Ann Neurol. 1980;8:416–421.
14. Wittig R, Zorich F, Piccione P, et al. Narcolepsy and disturbed nocturnal sleep. Clin Electroencephalogr. 1983;14:130–134.
15. Montplaisir J, Godbout R. Nocturnal sleep of narcoleptic patients. Sleep. 1986;9:159–161.
16. Guilleminault C, Crowe C, Quera-Salva MA, et al. Periodic leg movement, sleep fragmentation and central sleep apnea in two cases: reduction with clonazepam. Eur Respir J. 1988;1:762–765.
17. Fry JM, DiPhillipo MA, Pressman MR. Periodic leg movements in sleep following treatment of obstructive sleep apnea with nasal continuous positive airway pressure. Chest. 1989;96:89–91.
18. Mahowald MW, Schenck CH. REM sleep behavior disorder. In: Thorpy MJ, ed. Handbook of Sleep Disorders. New York, NY: Marcel Dekker; 1990:567–593.
19. Nicolas A, Lespérance P, Montplaisir J. Is excessive daytime sleepiness with periodic leg movements during sleep a specific diagnostic category? Eur Neurol. 1988;40:22–26.
20. Mendelson WB. Are periodic leg movements associated with clinical sleep disturbance? Sleep. 1996;19:219–223.
21. Lavigne G, Montplaisir J. Restless legs syndrome and sleep bruxism: prevalence and association among Canadians. Sleep. 1994;17:739–743.
22. Ondo W, Jankovic J. Restless legs syndrome: clinicoetiologic correlates. Neurology. 1996;47:1435–1441.
23. Walters A, Hickey K, Maltzman J, et al. A questionnaire study of 138 patients with restless legs syndrome: the "night-walkers" survey. Neurology. 1996;46:92–95.
24. Bassetti C, Mauerhofer D, Gugger M, et al. Restless legs syndrome: a study of 55 patients. Sleep. 1998;21(suppl):254.
25. The International Restless Legs Syndrome Study Group. Towards a better definition of the restless legs syndrome from the international restless legs syndrome study group. Mov Disord. 1995;10:634–642.

26. Brodeur C, Montplaisir J, Marinier R, et al. Treatment of RLS and PMS with L-dopa: a double-blind controlled study. Neurology. 1988;35:1845–1848.

27. Montplaisir J, Boucher S, Nicolas A, et al. Immobilization tests and periodic leg movements in sleep for the diagnosis of the restless legs syndrome. Mov Disord. 1998;13:324–329.

28. Coccagna G. Restless legs syndrome/periodic movements in sleep. In: Thorpy MJ, ed. Handbook of Sleep Disorders. New York, NY: Marcel Dekker; 1990:457–478.

29. Montplaisir J, Boucher S, Poirier G, et al. Persistence of repetitive EEG arousals in RLS patients treated with L-dopa. Sleep. 1998;19:196–199.

30. MacFarlane JG, Shahal B, Musly C, et al. Periodic k-alpha sleep EEG activity and periodic limb movements during sleep: comparisons of clinical features and sleep parameters. Sleep. 1996;19:200–204.

31. Coleman RM. Periodic movements in sleep (nocturnal myoclonus) and restless legs syndrome. In: Guilleminault C, ed. Sleeping and Waking Disorders: Indications and Techniques. Menlo Park, Calif: Addison-Wesley; 1982:265–295.

32. Kazenwadel J, Pollmächer T, Trenkwalder C, et al. New actigraphic assessment method for periodic leg movements (PLM). Sleep. 1996;18:689–697.

33. Rutkove SB, Matheson JK, Logigian EL. Restless legs syndrome in patients with polyneuropathy. Muscle Nerve. 1996;19:670–672.

34. Callaghan N. Restless legs syndrome in uremic neuropathy. Neurology (Minn). 1966;16:359–361.

35. Sandyk R, Bernick C, Lee SM, et al. L-dopa in uremic patients with the restless legs syndrome. Int J Neurosci. 1987;35:233–235.

36. Roger SD, Harris DCH, Stewart JH. Possible relation between restless legs and anemia in renal dialysis patients. Lancet. 1991;337:1551.

37. Wetter TC, Stiasny K, Kohnen R, et al. Polysomnographic sleep measures in patients with uremic and idiopathic restless legs syndrome. Mov Disord. 1998;13:820–824.

38. Yasuda T, Nishimura A, Katsuki Y, et al. Restless legs syndrome treated successfully by kidney transplantation: a case report. Clin Transplant. 1986;138:138.

39. Matthews WB. Iron deficiency and restless legs. Br Med J. 1976;1:898.

40. O'Keeffe ST, Gavin K, Lavan JN. Iron status and restless legs syndrome in the elderly. Age Ageing. 1994;23:200–203.

40a. Sun ER, Chen CA, Ho G, et al. Iron and the restless legs syndrome. Sleep. 1998;21:381–387.

40b. Early C, Connors JR, Allen RP. RLS patients have abnormally reduced CSF ferritin compared to normal controls. Neurology. 1999;52:A111–A112.

41. Yunus MB, Aldag JC. Restless legs syndrome and leg cramps in fibromyalgia syndrome: a controlled study. Br Med J. 1996;312:1339.

42. Reynolds G, Blake DR, Pall HS, et al. Restless legs syndrome and rheumatoid arthritis. Br Med J. 1986;292:659–660.

43. Popoviciu L, Asgian B, Popoviciu DP, et al. Clinical, EEG, electromyographic and polysomnographic studies in restless legs syndrome caused by magnesium deficiency. Rom J Neurol Psychiatry. 1993;31:55–61.

44. Picchieti DL, Walters AS. Restless legs syndrome and periodic limb movement disorders in children and adolescents. Child Adolesc Psychiatr Clin North Am. 1996;5:729–740.

45. Salvi F, Montagna P, Plasmati R, et al. Restless legs syndrome and nocturnal myoclonus: initial clinical manifestation of familial amyloid polyneuropathy. J Neurol Neurosurg Psychiatry. 1990;53:522–525.

46. Gorman C, Dyck P, Pearson J. Symptoms of restless legs. Arch Intern Med. 1965;115:155–160.

47. Heinze F, Frame B, Fine C. Restless legs and orthostatic hypotension in primary amyloidosis. Arch Neurol. 1967;16:497–500.

48. Spillane JD. Restless legs syndrome in chronic pulmonary disease. Br Med J. 1970;4:796–798.

49. Kotagal S, Chu JY, O'Connor DM. Nocturnal myoclonus—a sleep disturbance in children with leukemia. Ann Neurol. 1984;16:392.

50. Ruiz-Primo E. Is nocturnal myoclonus a common sleep disturbance in children with leukaemia? Dev Med Child Neurol. 1987;29:833.

51. Moldofsky H, Tullis C, Lue FA, et al. Sleep-related myoclonus in rheumatic pain modulation disorder (fibrositis syndrome) and in excessive daytime somnolence. Psychosom Med. 1984;46:145–151.

52. Heiman EM, Christie M. Lithium-aggravated nocturnal myoclonus and restless legs syndrome [letter]. Am J Psychiatry. 1986;143:1191–1192.

53. Ware JC, Brown FW, Moorad PJ, et al. Nocturnal myoclonus and tricyclic antidepressants. Sleep Res. 1984;13:72.

54. Bakshi R. Fluoxetine and restless legs syndrome. J Neurol Sci. 1996;142:151–152.

55. Paik IH, Lee C, Choi BM, et al. Mianserin-induced restless legs syndrome. Br J Psychiatry. 1989;155:415.

55a. American Sleep Disorders Association. The International Classification of Sleep Disorders: Diagnostic and Coding Manual. Rochester, Minn: ASDA; 1990:66.

56. Oswald I. Sudden bodily jerks on falling asleep. Brain. 1985;82:92–103.

57. Dagino N, Loeb C, Massazza G, et al. Hypnic physiological myoclonus in man: an EEG-EMG study in normals and neurological patients. Eur Neurol. 1985;2:47–58.

58. Broughton R, Tolentino MA, Krelina M. Excessive fragmentary myoclonus in NREM sleep: a report of 38 cases. Electroencephalogr Clin Neurophysiol. 1985;61:123–133.

59. Meier-Ewert K, Broughton R. Photomyoclonic response of epileptic subjects during wakefulness, sleep and arousal. Electroencephalogr Clin Neurophysiol. 1967;23:142–151.

60. Touchon J. Effect of awakening on epileptic activity in primary generalized myoclonic epilepsy. In: Sterman MB, Shouse MN, Passouant P, eds. Sleep and Epilepsy. New York, NY: Academic Press; 1982:239–248.

61. Chokroverty S, Walters AS, Zimmerman T, et al. Propriospinal myoclonus: a neurophysiological analysis. Neurology. 1992;42:1591–1595.

62. Spillane JD, Nathan PW, Kelley RE, et al. Painful legs and moving toes. Brain. 1971;94:541–556.

63. Weiner IH, Weiner HL. Nocturnal leg muscle cramps. JAMA. 1980;244:2332–2333.

64. Jacobsen JH, Rosenberg RS, Huttenlocher PR, et al. Familial nocturnal cramping. Sleep. 1986;9:54–60.

64a. Gentili A, Weiner DK, Kuchibhatil M, et al. Factors that disturb sleep in nursing home residents. Aging (Milano). 1997;9:207–213.

64b. Dahle LO, Berg G, Hammar M, et al. The effect of oral magnesium substitution on pregnancy-induced leg cramps. Am J Obstet Gynecol. 1995;173:175–180.

64c. Leung AK, Wong BE, Cho HY. Nocturnal cramps in children: incidence and clinical characteristics. J Natl Med Assoc. 1999;91:329–332.

64d. Man-Son-Hing M, Wells G, Lau A. Quinine for nocturnal leg cramps: a meta-analysis including unpublished data. J Gen Intern Med. 1998;13:600–606.

64e. Connolly PS, Shirley EA, Wasson JH, et al. Treatment of nocturnal leg cramps. A crossover trial of quinine vs vitamin E. Arch Intern Med. 1992;152:1877–1880.

64f. Leclerc KM, Landry FJ. Benign nocturnal leg cramps. Current controversies over use of quinine. Postgrad Med. 1996;99:177–178.

65. Lang AE, Johnson K. Akathisia in idiopathic Parkinson's disease. Neurology. 1987;37:477–481.

66. Brown KW, Glen SE, White TH. Low serum iron status and akathisia. Lancet. 1987;30:1234–1236.

67. O'Loughlin V, Dickie AC, Ebmeier KP. Serum iron and transferrin in acute neuroleptic induced akathisia. J Neurol Neurosurg Psychiatry. 1991;54:363–364.

68. Walters AS, Hening WA, Rubinstein M, et al. A clinical and polysomnographic comparison of neuroleptic-induced akathisia and the idiopathic restless legs syndrome. Sleep. 1991;14:339–345.

69. Lipinski JF, Hudson JI, Cunningham SL, et al. Polysomnographic characteristics of neuroleptic-induced akathisia. Clin Neuropharmacol. 1991;14:413–419.

70. Moldofsky H, Tullis C, Quance G, et al. Nitrazepam for periodic movements in sleep (sleep-related myoclonus). Can J Neurol Sci. 1986;13:52–54.

71. Matthews WB. Treatment of the restless legs syndrome with clonazepam. Br Med J. 1979;281:751.
72. Boghen D. Successful treatment of restless legs with clonazepam. Ann Neurol. 1980;8:341.
73. Oshtory MA, Vijayan N. Clonazepam treatment of insomnia due to sleep myoclonus. Arch Neurol. 1980;37:119–120.
74. Read DJ, Feest TG, Nassim MA. Clonazepam: effective treatment for restless legs syndrome in uraemia. Br Med J. 1981;283:885–886.
75. Boghen D, Lamothe L, Elie R, et al. The treatment of the restless legs syndrome with clonazepam: a prospective controlled study. Can J Neurol Sci. 1986;13:245–247.
76. Ohanna N, Peled R, Rubin AHE, et al. Periodic leg movements in sleep: effect of clonazepam treatment. Neurology. 1985;35:408–411.
77. Mitler MM, Browman CP, Menn SJ, et al. Nocturnal myoclonus: treatment efficacy of clonazepam and temazepam. Sleep. 1986;9:385–392.
78. Bonnet MH, Arand DL. The use of triazolam in older patients with periodic leg movements, fragmented sleep, and daytime sleepiness. J Gerontol. 1990;45:139–144.
79. Horiguchi J, Inami Y, Sasaki A, et al. Periodic leg movements in sleep with restless legs syndrome: effect of clonazepam treatment. Jpn J Psychiatry Neurol. 1992;46:727–732.
80. Peled R, Lavie P. Double-blind evaluation of clonazepam on periodic leg movements in sleep. J Neurol Neurosurg Psychiatry. 1987;50:1679–1681.
81. Trzepacz PT, Violette EJ, Sateia MJ. Response to opioids in three patients with restless legs syndrome. Am J Psychiatry. 1984;141:993–995.
82. Hening WA, Walters A, Kavey N, et al. Dyskinesias while awake and periodic movements in sleep in restless legs syndrome: treatment with opioids. Neurology. 1986;36:1363–1366.
83. Walters AS, Wagner ML, Hening WA, et al. Successful treatment of the idiopathic restless legs syndrome in a randomized double-blind trial of oxycodone versus placebo. Sleep. 1993;16:327–332.
84. Kavey N, Walters AS, Hening W, et al. Opioid treatment of periodic movements in sleep in patients without restless legs. Neuropeptides. 1988;11:181–184.
85. Montplaisir J, Godbout R, Boghen MD, et al. Familial restless legs with periodic movements in sleep: electrophysiological, biochemical, and pharmacological study. Neurology. 1985;35:130–134.
86. Montplaisir J, Godbout R, Poirier G, et al. Restless legs syndrome and periodic movements in sleep: physiopathology and treatment with L-dopa. Clin Neuropharmacol. 1986;9:456–463.
87. Von Scheele C. Levodopa in restless legs. Lancet. 1986;2:426–427.
88. Akpinar S. Restless legs syndrome treatment with dopaminergic drugs. Clin Neuropharmacol. 1987;10:69–79.
89. Von Scheele C, Kempi V. Long-term effect of dopaminergic drugs in restless legs. A 2-year follow-up. Arch Neurol. 1990;47:1223–1224.
90. Becker PM, Jamieson AO, Brown WD. Dopaminergic agents in restless legs syndrome and periodic limb movements of sleep: response and complications of extended treatment in 49 cases. Clin Res. 1993;16:713–716.
91. Trenkwalder C, Stiasny K, Pollmächer T, et al. L-Dopa therapy of uremic and idiopathic restless legs syndrome: a double-blind, crossover trial. Sleep. 1995;18:681–688.
92. Boivin DB, Montplaisir J, Poirier G. The effects of L-dopa on periodic leg movements and sleep organization in narcolepsy. Clin Neuropharmacol. 1989;12:339–345.
93. Guilleminault C, Cetel M, Philip P. Dopaminergic treatment of restless legs and rebound phenomenon. Neurology. 1993;43:445.
94. Allen RP, Earley CJ. Augmentation of the restless legs syndrome with carbidopa/levodopa. Sleep. 1996;19:205–213.
95. Walters AS, Hening WA, Chokroverty S, et al. A double-blind randomized crossover trial of bromocriptine and placebo in restless legs syndrome. Ann Neurol. 1988;24:455–458.
96. Boivin D, Montplaisir J, Lorrain D. Effects of bromocriptine on sleep organization and daytime vigilance in narcolepsy. Sleep Res. 1990;19:55.
97. Silber MH, Shepard JW Jr, Wisbey JA. Pergolide in the management of restless legs syndrome: an extended study. Sleep. 1997;20:878–882.
98. Staedt J, Wabmuth F, Ziemann U, et al. Pergolide: treatment of choice in restless legs syndrome (RLS) and nocturnal myoclonus syndrome (NMS). A double-blind randomized crossover trial of pergolide versus L-dopa. J Neural Transm. 1992;104:461–468.
99. Early CJ, Allen RP. Pergolide and carbidopa/levodopa treatment of the restless legs syndrome and periodic leg movements in sleep in a consecutive series of patients. Sleep. 1997;19:801–810.
99a. Wetter TC, Stiasny K, Winkelmann J, et al. A randomized controlled study of pergolide in patients with restless legs syndrome. Neurology. 1999;52:944–950.
100. Lin SC, Kaplan J, Burger CD, et al. Effect of pramipexole in the treatment of resistant restless legs syndrome. Mayo Clin Proc. 1998;73:497–500.
101. Montplaisir J, Nicolas A, Denesle R, et al. Restless legs syndrome improved by pramipexole: a double-blind randomized trial. Neurology. 1999;52:938–943.
101a. Dalvi A, Ford B. Antiparkinsonian agents. CNS Drugs. 1998;9:291–310.
101b. Frucht S, Rogers JD, Greene PE, et al. Falling asleep at the wheel: motor vehicle mishaps in persons taking pramipexole and ropinirole. Neurology. 1999;52:1908–1919.
101c. Ondo W. Ropinirole for restless legs syndrome. Mov Disord. 1999;14:138–140.
102. Telstad W, Sorensen O, Larsen S, et al. Treatment of the restless legs syndrome with carbamazepine: a double blind study. Br Med J. 1984;89:1–7.
103. Zucconi M, Coccagna G, Petronelli R, et al. Nocturnal myoclonus in restless legs syndrome effect of carbamazepine treatment. Funct Neurol. 1989;4:263–271.
104. Handwerker JV, Palmer RF. Clonidine in the treatment of "restless leg" syndrome. N Engl J Med. 1985;313:1228–1229.
105. Bastani B, Westervelt FB. Effectiveness of clonidine in alleviating the symptoms of "restless legs" [letter]. Am J Kidney Dis. 1987;10:326.
106. Wagner ML, Walters AS, Coleman RG, et al. Randomized, double-blind, placebo-controlled study of clonidine in restless legs syndrome. Sleep. 1996;19:52–58.
107. Mellick GA, Mellick LB. Successful treatment of restless legs syndrome with gabapentin. Sleep Res. 1995;24:290.
108. Adler CH. Treatment of restless legs syndrome with gabapentin. Clin Neuropharmacol. 1997;20:148–151.
109. Hornyak M, Voderholzer U, Hohagen F, et al. Magnesium therapy for periodic leg movements–related insomnia and restless legs syndrome: an open pilot study. Sleep. 1998;21:501–505.
109a. Chesson AL Jr, Wise M, Davila D, et al. Practice parameters for the treatment of restless legs syndrome and periodic limb movement disorder. An American Academy of Sleep Medicine report. Standards of Practice Committee of the American Academy of Sleep Medicine. Sleep. 1999;22:961–968.
110. Hening W, Walters AS, Chockroverty S. Treatment of the restless legs syndrome: current practices of sleep expert. Neurology. 1995;45(suppl 4):A285.
110a. Petit D, Denesle R, Gomez-Mancilla B, et al. A follow-up study of pramipexole in the restless legs syndrome. Sleep Research Online. In press.
111. Boghen D, Peyronnard JM. Myoclonus in familial restless legs syndrome. Arch Neurol. 1976;33:368–370.
112. Godbout R, Montplaisir J, Poirier G. Epidemiological data in restless legs syndrome. Sleep Res. 1987;16:338.
113. Walters AS, Picchietti D, Hening W, et al. Variable expressivity in familial restless legs syndrome. Arch Neurol. 1990;47:1219–1220.
114. Trenkwalder C, Seidel VC, Gasser T, et al. Clinical symptoms and possible anticipation in a large kindred of familial restless legs syndrome. Mov Disord. 1996;11:389–394.
114a. Lazzarini A, Walters AS, Hickey K, et al. Studies of penetrance and anticipation in five autosomal-dominant restless legs syndrome pedigrees. Mov Disord. 1999;14:111–116.
115. Iannaccone S, Zucconi M, Marchettini P, et al. Evidence of peripheral neuropathy in primary restless legs syndrome. Mov Disord. 1995;10:2–9.
116. Watanabe S, Ono A, Naito H. Periodic leg movements during either epidural or spinal anesthesia in an elderly man without sleep-related (nocturnal) myoclonus. Sleep. 1990;13:262–266.
117. Jackson J. Periodic movements of sleep in T10 paraplegic with failure to respond to parlodel. Sleep Res. 1990;19:326.
118. Yokata T, Hirose K, Tanabe H, et al. Sleep-related periodic leg movements (nocturnal myoclonus) due to spinal cord lesions. J Neurol Sci. 1991;104:13–18.
119. Dickell MJ, Renfrow SD, Moore PT, et al. Rapid eye movement

sleep leg movements in patients with spinal cord injury. Sleep. 1994;17:733–738.

120. DeMello MT, Lauro FAA, Silva AC, et al. Incidence of periodic leg movements and the restless legs syndrome during sleep following physical activity in spinal cord injury subjects. Spinal Cord. 1996;34:294–296.

121. Smith RC. Relationship of periodic movements in sleep (nocturnal myoclonus) and the Babinski sign. Sleep. 1985;8:239–243.

122. Fujiki A, Shimizu A, Yamada Y, et al. The Babinski reflex during sleep and wakefulness. Electroencephalogr Clin Neurophysiol. 1971;31:610–613.

123. Mosko SS, Nudleman KL. Somatosensory and brainstem auditory evoked responses in sleep-related periodic leg movements. Sleep. 1986;9:399–404.

124. Wechsler LR, Stakes JW, Shahani BT, et al. Periodic leg movements of sleep (nocturnal myoclonus): an electrophysiological study. Ann Neurol. 1986;19:168–173.

125. Wechsler LR, Stakes J, Shahani BT, et al. Nocturnal myoclonus, restless legs syndrome, and abnormal electrophysiological findings. Ann Neurol. 1987;21:515.

126. Yagnik M, Siao P, Schiff S, et al. Blink reflex in periodic leg movements in sleep. Muscle Nerve. 1989;12:758.

127. Briellman RS, Rosler KM, Hess CW. Blink reflex excitability is abnormal in patients with periodic leg movements in sleep. Mov Disord. 1996;11:710–714.

127a. Tergau F, Wischer S, Paulus W. Motor system excitability in patients with restless legs syndrome. Neurology. 1999;52:1060–1063.

128. Bucher SS, Seelos KC, Oertel WH, et al. Cerebral generators involved in the pathogenesis of the restless legs syndrome. Ann Neurol. 1997;41:639–645.

129. Martinelli P, Coccagna G, Lugaresi E. Nocturnal myoclonus, restless legs syndrome, and abnormal electrophysiological findings. Ann Neurol. 1987;21:515.

130. Lugaresi E, Coccagna G, Mantovani M, et al. Some periodic phenomena arising during drowsiness and sleep in man. Electroencephalogr Clin Neurophysiol. 1972;32:701–705.

131. Oakson G, Steriade M. Slow rhythmic rate fluctuations of cat midbrain reticular neurons in synchronized sleep and waking. Brain Res. 1982;247:277–288.

132. Oakson G, Steriade M. EEG slow-wave amplitudes and their relations to midbrain reticular discharge. Brain Res. 1983;269:386–390.

133. Kjallquist A, Lundberg N, Ponten U. Respiratory and cardiovascular changes during rapid spontaneous variations of ventricular fluid pressure in patients with intracranial hypertension. Acta Neurol Scand. 1964;40:291–317.

134. Coccagna G, Mantovani M, Brignani F, et al. Arterial pressure changes during spontaneous sleep in man. Electroencephalogr Clin Neurophysiol. 1971;31:277–281.

135. Munari C, Calbucci F. Correlations between intracranial pressure and EEG during coma and sleep. Electroencephalogr Clin Neurophysiol. 1981;51:170–176.

136. Scheuler W, Raffelsberger P, Schomatz F, et al. Periodicity of sleep EEG in the second and minutes range—example of application in different alpha activities in sleep. Electroencephalogr Clin Neurophysiol. 1990;76:222–234.

137. Evans BM. Periodic activity in cerebral arousal mechanisms—the relationship to sleep and brain damage. Electroencephalogr Clin Neurophysiol. 1992;83:130–137.

138. Novak P, Lepicovska J, Dostalek C. Periodic amplitude modulation of EEG. Neurosci Lett. 1992;136:213–215.

139. Terzano MG, Mancia D, Salati RM, et al. The CAP as a physiologic component of normal NREM sleep. Sleep. 1985;8:137–145.

140. Terzano MG, Parino L. Clinical applications of cyclic alternating pattern. Physiol Behav. 1993;54:807–813.

141. Montplaisir J, Lapierre O, Lavigne GJ. Le syndrome d'impatiences musculaires: une maladie associée au ralentissement périodique ou apériodique de l'EEG. Neurophysiol Clin. 1994;24:131–140.

142. Trenkwalder C, Bucher SF, Oertel WA. Electrophysiological pattern of involuntary limb movements in the restless legs syndrome. Muscle Nerv. 1996;19:155–162.

142a. Allen RP, Hyland K, Early CJ. Restless legs syndrome (RLS) an L-dopa responsive disorder does not have the CSF abnormalities shown for L-dopa responsive dystonia (DRD). Sleep. 1999;22(suppl 1):s156–s157.

143. Staedt J, Stoppe G, Kögler A, et al. Dopamine D2 receptor alteration in patients with periodic movements in sleep (nocturnal myoclonus). J Neural Transm. 1993;93:71–74.

144. Staedt J, Stoppe G, Kogler A, et al. Single photon emission tomography (SPET) imaging of dopamine D2 receptors in the course of dopamine replacement therapy in patients with nocturnal myoclonus syndrome. J Neural Transm. 1995;99:187–193.

144a. Turjanski N, Lees AJ, Brooks DJ. Striatal dopaminergic function in restless legs syndrome: ^{18}F-dopa and ^{11}C-raclopride PET studies. Neurology. 1999;52:932–937.

145. Montplaisir J, Lorrain D, Godbout, R. Restless legs syndrome and periodic leg movements in sleep: the primary role of dopaminergic mechanism. Eur Neurol. 1991;31:41–43.

66

Dreaming Disorders

Tore A. Nielsen

Antonio Zadra

Because most dreaming disturbances involve a perturbation of emotional expression during sleep, their study may help clarify the role of emotion in dream formation, dream function, and sleep mechanisms. Physiological evidence for emotional activity during rapid eye movement (REM) sleep is substantial. Autonomic system variability increases markedly in conjunction with central phasic activation,[1] as seen especially in measures of cardiac function,[2, 3] respiration,[4] and skin and muscle sympathetic nerve activity.[5, 6] Brain imaging, too, demonstrates increases in metabolic activity in limbic and paralimbic regions during REM sleep (e.g., see references 7, 8), activity similar to that seen during strong emotion in the waking state.[9] These dramatic autonomic fluctuations globally parallel dreamed emotional activity, which is detectable throughout most dreaming when appropriate probes are employed.[10] Most dreamed emotion is negative,[11] primarily fearful,[10] and it may conform to a "surge-like" structure within REM episodes.[12] Isomorphic relationships between physiological and subjective attributes of dreamed emotions have been reported (e.g., see references 13, 14) but are still poorly understood. Nevertheless, many theorists interpret the various peripheral manifestations of phasic ponto-geniculo-occipital (PGO) activity as indicative of dream-related affective activity.[12, 15, 16]

Emotional processes during wakefulness are also implicated in dream disturbances. For the most common disturbances, such as nightmares, dreamed emotion becomes unbearably intense and provokes an awakening; this may lead to further distress which continues to influence waking behavior and mood and may even impair subsequent sleep. Perturbation of dream-related emotion may thus lead to a cycle of sleep disruption and avoidance, insomnia,[17] and psychological distress.[18] This often leads the individual to seek treatment.

However, causal relationships between emotion, dreaming, and other associated symptoms are not well understood. In some instances (e.g., nightmare disorder), emotional disruption may affect primarily sleep-related processes—in which case the dreaming process itself might be considered pathological in some sense.[19] However, the widespread belief in dreaming as an emotionally *adaptive* mechanism also leaves room for the possibility that some dream disturbances are adaptive reactions to more basic pathophysiological factors, rather than signs of a pathological disorder per se. As the pathophysiologies of dream disturbances are still only poorly understood, in this chapter we use the terms *dream disturbance* and *disturbed dreaming* in a neutral sense with respect to this question of etiology.

IDIOPATHIC NIGHTMARES

Historical Aspects

Although the most prevalent form of dream disturbance is the idiopathic nightmare, its cause and psychopathology remain largely unstudied. The *Diagnostic and Statistical Manual of Mental Disorders, Fourth Edition* (DSM-IV)[20] criteria for *nightmare disorder* (Table 66–1) have not changed substantially since the disorder was described as *dream anxiety disorder* in the third, revised (DSM-III-R) and as *dream anxiety attack* in third (DSM-III) editions. This is due, in part, to the fact that little new basic or clinical information about idiopathic nightmares has been published since the initial studies of Fisher et al.[21] and the detailed clinical analyses by Hartmann.[22]

The widely accepted definition of a *nightmare* is a frightening dream that awakens the sleeper, but not all researchers adopt the "awakening" criterion. Some[23] argue that disturbing dreams that awaken merit the designation nightmare, whereas those that do not should be labeled "bad dreams;" whether the person awakens is presumably an indirect measure of the dream's severity. However, the awakening criterion may be an overly conservative estimate of severity. First, among various psychosomatic patients, even the most macabre and threatening dreams do not necessarily produce awakenings.[24, 25] Second, fewer than one fourth of chronic nightmare patients report "always" awakening from their nightmares, and these do not correlate with either nightmare intensity or psychological distress.[17] Third, among subjects with *both* nightmares and bad dreams, approximately 45% of bad dreams have emotional intensities equal to or exceeding those of the average nightmare.[26] Similarly, many researchers define nightmares as disturbing dreams involving *any* unpleasant emotion.[18] This is consistent with many patients' reports that their nightmares involve intensification of unpleasant emotions

Table 66-1. CLINICAL CRITERIA FOR NIGHTMARE DISORDER

DSM-IV Diagnostic Criteria for Nightmare Disorder (307.47)	ICSD-R Diagnostic Criteria for Nightmares (307.47-0)
A. Repeated awakenings from the major sleep period or naps with detailed recall of extended and extremely frightening dreams, usually involving threats to survival, security, or self-esteem. The awakenings generally occur during the second half of the sleep period.	A. The patient has at least one episode of sudden awakening from sleep with intense fear, anxiety, and feeling of impending harm.
B. On awakening from the frightening dreams, the individual rapidly becomes oriented and alert (in contrast to the confusion and disorientation seen in Sleep Terror Disorder and some forms of epilepsy).	B. The patient has immediate recall of frightening dream context
C. The dream experience, or the sleep disturbance resulting from the awakening, causes clinically significant distress or impairment in social, occupational, or other important areas of function.	C. Full alertness occurs immediately upon awakening, with little confusion or disorientation.
D. The nightmares do not occur exclusively during the course of another mental disorder (e.g., a delirium, Posttraumatic Stress Disorder) and are not due to the direct physiological effects of a substance (e.g., a drug of abuse, a medication) or a general medical condition.	D. Associated features include at least one of the following: • Return to sleep after the episode is delayed and not rapid • The episode occurs during the latter half of the habitual sleep period E. Polysomnographic monitoring demonstrates the following: • An abrupt awakening from at least 10 min of REM sleep • Mild tachycardia and tachypnea during the episode • Absence of epileptic activity in association with the disorder F. Other sleep disorders, such as sleep terrors and sleepwalking, can occur.

Data from American Psychiatric Association. Diagnostic and Statistical Manual of Mental Disorders, Fourth Edition. Washington, DC: American Psychiatric Association Press; 1994; and International Classification of Sleep Disorders-Revised: Diagnostic and Coding Manual. Rochester, Minn: American Sleep Disorders Association; 1997.

such as extreme sadness or anger; fear nevertheless remains the most frequently reported emotion.[26]

Prevalence and Frequency

Estimates of nightmare prevalence are complicated by the variety of populations studied and variations in the use of frequency criteria. Lifetime prevalence for a nightmare experience in the general population is unknown but may well approach 100%. If we consider only attack dreams, which are one of the most common nightmare themes, the lifetime prevalence varies from 67%[27] to 90%.[28] Pursuit, a closely related, highly disturbing theme, has a lifetime prevalence of 92% among women and 85% among men.[28] Age is clearly a mediating factor; children, young adult, and adult and elderly groups have nightmares "at least sometimes" with a prevalence of 30 to 90%, 40 to 60% and 60 to 68% respectively.[29]

Nightmares are both more prevalent and more frequent in childhood. In a clinical context,[30] where nightmare problems were defined as lasting for longer than 3 months, their prevalence was 24% for ages 2 to 5, 41% for ages 6 to 10, and 22% for age 11 years. Figures of 5 to 30% (for "often or always") and 30 to 90% (for "at least sometimes") have also been reported for children.[29] Two surveys[31, 32] indicate that 20 to 30% of 5- to 12-year-old children have at least one nightmare in any 6-month period. We found a large gender difference in the recall ("sometimes" or "often") of disturbing dreams at age 13 (boys: 25% vs. girls: 40%) and age 16 (20% vs. 40%) in the same cohort.[33]

Among adults, prevalence nevertheless is high (8 to 25%) when frequencies of "one or more per month" are considered, as in several studies of college and university students.[34-36] Even for higher frequencies—which likely correspond to much of the underdiag-

nosed adult *nightmare disorder* population (e.g., "one or more nightmares per week")—prevalence estimates are consistently elevated, for example, 2 to 6% in college students[34, 35] and about 4% in adults sampled randomly in Iceland, Sweden, Belgium,[37] and Austria.[38] When the question is put as "often or always," young adult prevalence is still 2 to 5%, whereas that of adult and elderly samples is only 1 to 2%.[29] These figures are completely in line with estimates that 4 to 8% of the general population have a "current problem" with nightmares, about 6% have a "past problem,"[39-41] and about 4% of patients spontaneously report a complaint of nightmares to their physicians.[42]

Nightmare prevalence may be elevated in clinical populations, for example, 25% of both chronic male alcoholic patients and female alcohol and drug users report nightmares "every few nights" on the Minnesota Multiphasic Personality Inventory (MMPI).[43, 44] However, other findings of elevated prevalence are difficult to assess because a frequency criterion is not specified, for example, approximately 24% of nonpsychotic patients seen in psychiatric emergency services report nightmares, but with an unknown frequency.[45]

Nightmare frequency is almost always assessed by retrospective self-report, for example, the number of nightmares in the previous week, month, or year. When compared to results from daily home logs, however, *retrospective self-reports underestimate current nightmare frequency by a factor of 2.5 in young adults[36] to a factor of over 10 in the healthy elderly.[46]* In general, a 1-month retrospective estimate is closer to the estimate provided by daily logs than is a 12-month retrospective estimate, and is thus the preferred standard for retrospective assessment. Note, however, that because nightmare prevalence and frequency are both seriously underestimated by such instruments, daily logs are the method of choice.

Pathophysiology

The one available laboratory study of nightmares[21] indicates moderate arousal—in the form of increased heart (HR) and respiration (RR) rates—during some nightmare episodes, but unexpectedly low arousal in most others. Although these early findings constitute the principal empirical basis for diagnostic guidelines such as the DSM-IV, there are serious problems with the work, such as the inclusion of psychiatric and post-traumatic stress disorder (PTSD) patients in the study sample.

We[47, 48] undertook a replication and extension of this early work with a nonpsychiatric sample. Recordings of HR and RR during nine subjects' nightmare and non-nightmare REM sleep episodes confirmed a moderate level of sympathetic arousal during some nightmares. Mean HR for nightmare REM sleep was elevated (by about 6 bpm) only for the 3 mins prior to awakening (Fig. 66–1). Most subjects (78%) showed HR acceleration during nightmare sleep, whereas the same number showed HR *decelerations* during non-nightmare REM sleep. Mean RR was only marginally higher for the last 3 min before awakening.

We also found changes in cortical activity during nightmares.[47] EEG samples from the last 2 min of nightmare sleep, when compared with control samples using a *linked-ear reference montage,* had generally higher absolute and relative alpha (8 to 13 Hz) power, but especially over posterior sites. Using a *scalp-average reference montage,* nightmare sections had higher fast beta (21 to 31 Hz) power over frontotemporal regions. The alpha pattern appears to be an amplification of the "classical posterior alpha" of quiet rest[49] that has been observed for normal REM sleep with an atypical extension from posterior into frontal sites.[50]

Our subjects demonstrated even less sympathetic arousal during nightmares than did those of Fisher et al., likely because they were relatively healthy and untraumatized. The co-occurrence of cortical activation with minimal autonomic change during nightmares may reflect a type of adaptive dissociation between imagery and emotion similar to that attained by behavioral therapies such as systematic desensitization and flooding. Sympathetic inhibition during cortical processing of *potentially* anxiogenic imagery may, in fact, "desomatize" that imagery.[21, 51]

Personality

Although many studies suggest weak to moderate relationships between nightmare frequency and measures of psychopathology,[22, 52, 53] others do not.[18, 36, 54] The seemingly weak relationships between nightmares and psychopathology likely reflect mediating factors, among which two—chronicity and distress—have been given some attention.

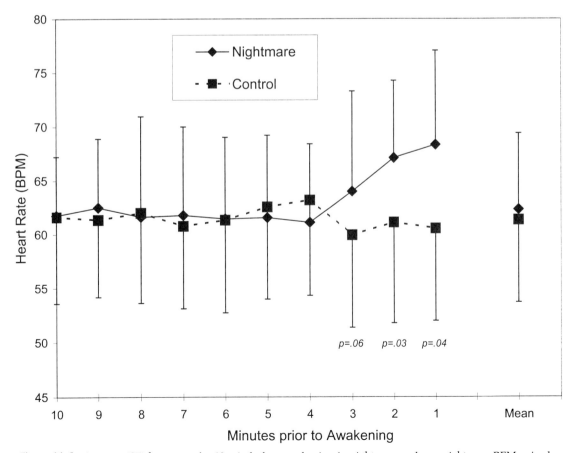

Figure 66–1. Average (SE) heart rate for 10 min before awakening in nightmare and non-nightmare REM episodes.

Nightmare Chronicity. Adults with a lifelong history of frequent nightmares compose a subgroup of idiopathic nightmare sufferers who manifest more psychopathological symptoms than matched controls without nightmares, for example, higher neuroticism and MMPI psychopathology scores.[52, 55] However, Hartmann[22] found that no one measure of psychopathology adequately describes these individuals. He and his colleagues proposed[22, 56] a general "boundary permeability" personality dimension, which at one extreme ("thin boundaries") characterizes lifelong sufferers. "Thin boundary" individuals are more open, sensitive, and vulnerable to intrusions than "thick boundary" subjects, rendering them more sensitive to events not usually viewed as traumatic.[22] Nightmare frequency is positively related to "thin boundary" scores,[57, 58] as well as to hypnotic ability, absorption in fantasy and aesthetic experiences, and creativity.[59]

Nightmare Distress. Nightmare frequency and waking distress over one's nightmares are not equivalent. Nightmare frequency is only moderately related to nightmare distress.[18, 36] Subjects may have only few nightmares (e.g., one per month) yet report high levels of distress, or report many nightmares (e.g., one or more per week) yet low levels of distress. It is the nightmare distress factor that is significantly related to psychopathology, not necessarily the frequency factor.[18]

Effects of Drugs and Alcohol

Numerous classes of drugs trigger nightmares and bizarre dreams, including catecholaminergic agents, beta blockers, some antidepressants, barbiturates, and alcohol. Among catecholaminergic agents, reserpine, thioridazine, and levodopa (L-dopa) are all occasionally associated with vivid dreams and nightmares,[60–63] as are beta blockers such as betaxolol, metropolol, bisoprolol, and propranolol.[64–68] Among the antidepressants, bupropion leads to more vivid dreams and nightmares than do other antidepressants.[69, 70] Bedtime administration of tricyclic and neuroleptic agents leads to a higher recall of frightening dreams than when these are taken in two daily doses,[71, 72] even though normal dream recall remains the same. Neuroleptic and tricyclic drugs appear to render dream affect more dysphoric, rather than to increase dream recall per se. Withdrawal from barbiturates is associated with REM rebound, vivid dreaming, and nightmares.[73, 74] A hypothesis has been advanced that barbiturate suppression of REM sleep, much as with alcohol, causes REM sleep rebound after discontinuation of the drug and consequently longer and more vivid dreams.[75] Several case studies have alerted physicians to the nightmare-inducing effects of specific substances (Table 66–2).

Sleep and dream disturbances follow alcohol withdrawal. Alcoholic patients report more vivid dreams and nightmares following withdrawal than they do during ingestion; although these are more frequent in the week following withdrawal, they are still present in subsequent weeks. The nightmares and insomnia of withdrawal can lead to resumed drinking in an attempt

Table 66–2. DRUGS REPORTED TO INCREASE FREQUENCY OF NIGHTMARES

Drug	Function	Reference
Thiothixene	Neuroleptic	88
Betaxolol	Beta blocker	89
Carbachol	Cholinergic agent	89
Fluoxetine	Antidepressant	90
Naproxen	Nonsteroidal anti-inflammatory agent	92
Verapamil	Antimigraine agent	93
Triazolam	Benzodiazepine hypnotic	238, 239 240
Nitrazepam	Benzodiazepine hypnotic	94
Erythromycin	Antibiotic	95 96

to normalize sleep. In fact, 29 (29%) of a group of 100 alcoholic patients reported further drinking to alleviate nightmares.[76] To illustrate, one 39-year-old man had no difficulty initiating sleep while abstaining, but he was awakened often by nightmares that prevented him from returning to sleep. "The nightmares were of somebody trying to hurt him. He would wake up thrashing and in a sweat and spend the rest of the night pacing and smoking. After he had started drinking . . . he could get no sleep unless he was drunk."[77(p499)] This relationship is also of critical importance because of the danger of alcohol self-medication for PTSD[78, 79] and for other nightmare-producing disorders.

Vivid and macabre dreaming may be central to the delirium tremens (DTs) of acute alcohol withdrawal.[80] Because alcohol suppresses REM sleep, and the percentage of REM sleep (particularly at sleep onset) is extremely elevated in patients with DTs,[77, 81, 82] a theory of DTs hallucinations emphasizing REM rebound and intrusion of dreaming into wakefulness has been proposed.[83] Case studies strongly suggest that hallucinations may seem to continue *uninterrupted* from an ongoing nightmare.[77] DTs sleep appears to be a mixture of REM sleep with "stage 1 REM sleep with tonic EMG [electromyography]," which distinguishes it from the sleep of alcoholic patients without DTs.[84] Some have failed to observe this pattern, however.[85, 86] The similarity of the sleep of patients with DTs to that of REM sleep behavior disorder (RBD) has also been noted.[87]

The neuropharmacological basis of drug-induced or withdrawal-associated disturbed dreaming remains unclear. There may be an imbalance among various neurotransmitter systems such that nightmares are produced by reduced brain norepinephrine and serotonin or increased dopamine and acetylcholine, or a combination of these.[22]

Recurrent Dreaming and Nightmares

Many theories converge on the view that recurrent dreams reflect a lack of progress in resolving daytime emotional preoccupations. Failures in an adaptive function of dreaming may be indicated by a dream series with a repetitive pattern, such as the stating and restating of a problem, yet no depiction of progress. Four points on the "repetition dimension" of dream content[97] may, in fact, reflect different degrees of psychopathological severity. *Repetitive dreams*, such as post-traumatic nightmares, depict—over numerous, highly similar versions—an unresolved experience, for example, a motor vehicle accident or war trauma. *Recurrent dreams* depict conflicts or stressors metaphorically over time, and are also primarily unpleasant in nature.[98, 99] The most frequent recurrent dreams of adults are pseudonightmarish: being endangered (e.g., chased, threatened with injury), being alone and trapped (e.g., in an elevator), facing natural forces (e.g., volcanic eruptions), losing one's teeth. Dreams with less recurrence—*recurrent themes* and *recurrent contents*—both extend over long series and are not so clearly associated with psychopathology. However, they may still have adaptive functions.[97]

Case studies have described changes in repetitive dream elements toward a progressive pattern as a function of successful psychotherapy,[100] as have laboratory studies of women dealing successfully with depressive reactions to divorce.[101, 102] Similarly, subjects with recurrent dreams show less successful adaptation on measures of anxiety, depression, personal adjustment, and life-events stress than those without recurrent dreams.[103, 104] The maintained cessation of recurrent dreaming may also reflect an upturn in well-being.[104]

Treatment

A wide variety of treatments for nightmares have been reported.[23, 105] Although psychotherapy aimed at conflict resolution has traditionally been the treatment of choice,[106, 107] it lacks empirical support. On the other hand, there is much support for diverse cognitive-behavioral interventions that require six or fewer sessions. Systematic desensitization and relaxation techniques, used to countercondition a relaxation response to anxiety-provoking nightmare contents, have been effective in several case studies and in two controlled studies.[54, 108] Imagery rehearsal, which teaches patients to change their remembered nightmares and to rehearse new scenarios, has reduced both nightmare distress and frequency in a recent series of controlled studies.[17, 109, 110] Other treatments with some empirical support are lucid dreaming,[111] eye movement desensitization and reprocessing,[112] and hypnosis.[113]

DISTURBED DREAMING IN OTHER SLEEP DISORDERS

The full extent to which dreaming and various sleep disorders influence one another remains largely unstudied. For several sleep disorders, disturbed dreaming has been identified as a primary symptom (Table 66–3). There are also a number of sleep problems for which disturbed dreaming is a salient factor even though its pathophysiological importance has not been determined. Finally, there are conditions for which dreaming is disturbed, but which nevertheless fall within the normal range of functioning. In all likelihood, whether patients with a particular condition spontaneously disclose that they also suffer from disturbed dreaming will be mitigated by various psychological, sociological, and cultural factors. Many patients

Table 66–3. SLEEP DISORDERS IN WHICH DREAMING IS DISTURBED

Sleep Disorder	Code	Stage	Prevalence	Essential Features
Nightmare disorder	307.47-0 (ICSD)	REM, 2	Children: 5–30%; young adults: 2–5% (see text)	Frightening dreams; awakening
Sleep terrors	307.46-1 (ICSD)	3, 4	Children: 3%; adults: ≤1%	Sudden arousal; piercing scream or cry; autonomic and behavioral manifestations of intense fear
Terrifying hypnagogic hallucinations	307.47-4 (ICSD)	Sleep onset	Rare; narcolepsy: 4–8%	Terrifying dreams similar to those from sleep
Post-traumatic stress disorder nightmares	309.81 (DSM-IV)	REM, 2, 3, 4	Lifetime: 1–14%; at-risk subjects: 3–58%	Persistent reexperiencing of a traumatic event, including recurrent nightmares
Narcolepsy dreams	347 (ICSD)	REM	0.03–0.16%	Excessive sleepiness, cataplexy, sleep paralysis, hypnagogic hallucinations
Sleep paralysis	780.56-2 (ICSD)	Sleep onset or offset	Isolated, normals; 1/lifetime in 40–50%; familial: rare	Paralysis of voluntary muscles; acute anxiety (with or without dreams) is common
REM sleep behavior disorder	780.59-0 (ICSD)	REM	Rare	Intermittent loss of REM sleep; muscle atonia; elaborate motor activity associated with dream (nightmare) mentation
Sleep starts	307.47-2 (ICSD)	Sleep onset	Lifetime: 60–70%; extreme form: rare	Sudden brief jerks associated with sensory flash, hypnagogic dream, or feeling of falling

DSM-IV, *Diagnostic and Statistical Manual of Mental Disorders, Fourth Edition*[20]; ICSD, International Classification of Sleep Disorders.[160]

attribute personal or spiritual significance to dreams or consider them to reflect their "state of sanity" and may therefore hesitate to speak openly about them. Sensitivity to such factors could substantially facilitate research on, and treatment of, dream disturbances.

Post-Traumatic Stress Disorder Nightmares

Recurrent anxiety dreams plague the vast majority of PTSD patients.[114] Disturbed dreaming may, in fact, be the hallmark of delayed PTSD[115, 116]; the content of disturbing dreams (e.g., reliving combat), as well as associated sleep disruptions (e.g., nocturnal awakenings, fear of sleep),[117, 118] may reinforce the illness. A related hypothesis is that disruption of REM sleep control mechanisms—including those governing dreaming—is central to PTSD pathophysiology.[119] Evidence that PTSD produces a variety of changes in REM sleep architecture and in the recall, content, and affective quality of dreaming is consistent with both of these hypotheses. There is evidence of decreased dream recall from REM sleep,[120, 121] as well as increased nightmares or sleep terrors in early REM sleep episodes[122] and in stages 2, 3, and 4 nonrapid eye movement (NREM) sleep.[120, 123, 124] There is also either a decrease[121, 125] or an increase[120, 123] in REM sleep latency, an increase in REM sleep density,[120, 121] a decrease in the number and length of REM sleep periods,[126, 127] and a decrease in total REM sleep time.[120, 128] Any of these associated changes in REM sleep might account for, or be a consequence of, the characteristic dream disturbance in PTSD. The fact that therapeutic interventions directed specifically at nightmares (e.g., imagery rehearsal) can significantly reduce their frequency and associated sleep problems[129] is also consistent with the notion that PTSD is, at root, a disturbance of dreaming or REM sleep, or both.

It is noteworthy that PTSD patients sometimes report nightmares after awakenings from early in the sleep episode,[130] including after awakenings from NREM sleep,[120] which is where sleep terrors are typically found.[131] In fact, PTSD nightmare-associated behaviors, such as autonomic activation, gross body movements, confused arousal, and partial amnesia, greatly resemble those of sleep terrors,[132] suggesting that they may be a phenomenon intermediate between idiopathic nightmares and sleep terrors. A more comprehensive definition of overlapping parasomnic states may be required to fully explain PTSD.[133]

Dream-Interruption Insomnia

Greenberg[134] proposed a subcategory of insomnia, dream-interruption insomnia, on the basis of five patients who reported awakening from sleep "every hour or so" throughout the night. Four of these patients reported a period of intense nightmares just before onset of their insomnia; nightmares then disappeared but subsequently reappeared after treatment with either chlordiazepoxide (Librium) or diazepam (Valium) in three of four cases. This pattern suggested that the awakenings might be a means of defending against anxious dream content, a type of "preemptive strike" against impending nightmares. In the laboratory, Greenberg's patients demonstrated repeated spontaneous awakenings from REM sleep, that is, on an average of 70% of REM episodes, but no consistent reduction in REM sleep time. Treatment reduced the number of REM awakenings almost by half and reduced REM sleep time slightly.

Three cases of dream-interruption insomnia were described by Cartwright[135] and two by Lavie et al.[128] In the latter study, 2 of 11 patients under study for trauma manifested REM-related awakenings; these were also the only two patients who experienced war-related nightmares in the laboratory. Interestingly, most REM interruptions in this study were preceded by increased HR, as is the case for nightmare awakenings.[21] Cartwright[135] reported that psychotherapy focusing on the content of patients' dreams and nightmares is successful in alleviating their insomnia. The notion that insomnia may be due to the expression of conflicts in dreams has been observed by clinicians, even prior to the discovery of REM sleep.[136]

Out of 983 consecutive patients seen at the Sacré-Coeur sleep clinic in Montreal from March 1994 to August 1997, 14 (1.4%) were found to conform to a pattern suggestive of dream-interruption insomnia (mean age: 53.5 ± 15.7 years). Twelve of these patients (85.7%) were male; 2 (14.3%) were female. Of 10 patients who had neither apneas (n = 1; index greater than 5) nor periodic limb movements in sleep (n = 3; index greater than 10), two distinct, but not necessarily independent, patterns of REM interruption were observed (Fig. 66–2). One (panel A) consists of recurrent awakenings early in the REM episode and subsequent curtailment of the episode. This appears as low sleep efficiency, low REM percentage, and high REM efficiency. The second pattern (panel B) is the more common of the two and consists of repeated shorter arousals throughout the REM episode. This appears as moderate to high sleep efficiency, high REM percentage, and very low REM efficiency.

With so few clinical reports of dream-interruption insomnia, its exact prevalence is not known. However, if the problem is, indeed, a variant of nightmare disorder, its prevalence may be substantial, given the high co-morbidity of insomnia with nightmares in the general population. In one sample of 1049 French insomnia patients, 18.3% suffered from nightmares.[137] Many others have confirmed relationships between nightmares and variables associated with insomnia (e.g., sleep-onset latency, night awakenings, restless sleep).[35, 117, 138] Successfully treated nightmare patients also often report improvements in sleep quality.[17, 139]

Whether or how nightmares may trigger dream-interruption insomnia is not known. Although it is clear that nightmares may generate "sleep distress"[18] or a disproportionate fear of the dark,[140] which later may generalize into sleep-onset difficulties, an ability to preempt nightmares would seem to require sustained vigilance or self-monitoring throughout sleep. Another possibility is that inhibitory REM sleep pro-

Hypnogram A

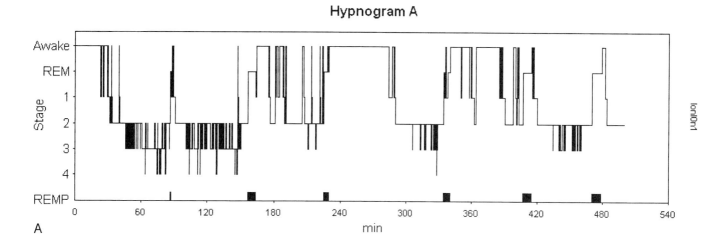

A

Hypnogram B

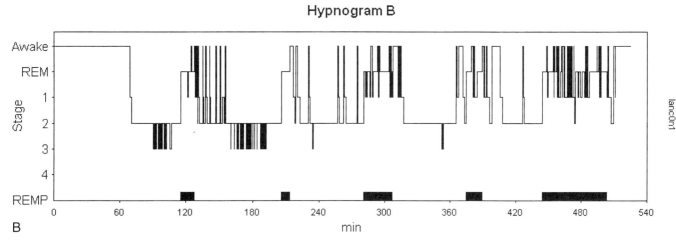

B

Figure 66–2. Hypnograms of two forms of dream-interruption insomnia. *A* illustrates a form consisting of recurrent awakenings early in the REM episode with subsequent curtailment of the episode. This appears polysomnographically as low sleep efficiency, low REM percentage (REMP), and high REM efficiency. *B* illustrates the more common of the two forms: a pattern of repeated brief arousals throughout the REM episode. This appears as moderate to high sleep efficiency, high REMP, and very low REM efficiency.

cesses are unable to completely suppress the "surge-like" nature of anxious dream content[12] or that some particularities of the dream content are more prone to provoke REM sleep microarousals or awakenings. The dream content of some insomniac patients may also be so tightly coupled to activating processes that even minor dream anxieties may trigger an arousal. This idea is supported by the finding that for insomnia patients vivid, frightening, and disrupted dreaming is correlated with shorter REM segments and higher REM densities, whereas for narcolepsy patients it is not.[141] Yet another possibility is that insomnia produces nightmares, particularly insomnia that involves sleep fragmentation and maintenance difficulties. Sleep fragmentation is also known to characterize subjects with frequent snoring—the latter, in turn, is strongly correlated with nightmares.[38, 142, 143] Induced sleep fragmentation also produces sleep paralysis experiences, most of which involve anxiety or terror.[144]

Existential (Grief) Dreams

Employing a method of polythetic (multiattribute) classification, Kuiken and co-workers identified a cate-

gory of experiences referred to as *existential* dreams.[16, 145] They are characterized by distressing emotions (e.g., sadness, despair, guilt), salient bodily feelings (e.g., ineffectuality of action, paralysis), and failures in goal attainment. There is also separation and loss, the appearance of deceased family figures, and an increased sensory vividness that may culminate in an intensely real ending—often with an awakening. This dream type is distinct from the *anxiety* type, identified by the same analytical procedure, which resembles the classic idiopathic nightmare. Existential dreams resemble nightmares in their emotional and sensorial intensity and in their association of vivid apparent reality with arousals from sleep. They differ from them primarily in the specific emotions, bodily feelings, and typical themes that they depict. The clinical importance of existential dreams is their appearance during bereavement, which involves a range of distressing emotions other than fear. Bereavement is also characterized by hallucinations and vivid feelings of the presence of the deceased in both dreaming and waking states.[146, 147] These closely resemble the *presence* dreams of persons with narcolepsy and sleep paralysis (see Narcolepsy).

Existential dreams are common throughout the bereavement period (0 to 5 years after a loss), whereas other dream types are more salient either immediately after (anxiety dreams) or from 3 to 5 years after (transcendent dreams) a loss.[148] The sense of presence of the deceased also remains constant throughout bereavement, whereas hallucinations of the deceased diminish over time.[149] Patients report gaining both personal and spiritual insight from existential dreams, especially 6 to 12 months following their loss.[148]

Epic Dreaming

Long, rambling dream narratives are not unusual in laboratory studies. Nor is the occasional patient complaint of "dreaming all night long" and feeling tired in the morning as a result. In a series of 20 patients, Schenck and Mahowald[150] identified a clinical entity—"epic dreaming"—in which relentless dreaming and daytime fatigue are associated in a chronic fashion.[151] These patients feel that they dream all night and complain of marked daytime fatigue. Their dreams typically involve constant, trivial, or banal physical activity, such as repetitive housework or endless walking through snow or mud, although intense sensations of acceleration or spinning can also occur. Patients describe having a "dream motor running all night long," or "not having the mind shut down during the night."[150] These dreams occur nightly in 90% of affected patients and 4 nights a week in the other 10%.[150] The repetitive quality of epic dreams is reminiscent of some recurrent dream themes and even of some nightmares. Nightmares are, in fact, reported by 70% of these patients, but the epic dreaming pattern is the primary complaint in most cases.[150] Emotional arousal is strangely absent from epic dreams. Nonetheless, the associated sensations of fatigue or exhaustion, as well as the seemingly endless repetitiveness of the dreams, may engender distress and motivate a clinical consultation.

In most cases, polysomnographic evaluation reveals no clinical abnormalities, apart from occasional PLMS (10%) and sleep-disordered breathing (10%); the problem is also more common in women (85%) than in men (15%).[150] The underlying mechanisms of the disorder remain unknown. However, comparative studies of epic dreams with normal dreams, nightmares, and recurrent dreams might shed light on possible pathophysiology, for example, whether the recurrent motor imagery differs from that found in normal dreaming[152] or whether epic dreams are simply long nightmares with an absence of affective intensification.

Changes in dreaming that are possibly related to this disturbance occur in brain-lesioned patients[153] and include increases in both the frequency and the vividness of dream imagery.[154, 155] Either of these changes might render dreaming more memorable and more likely to be perceived as having been continuous through the night. For example, Solms's patient 136, who sustained severe bilateral brain damage following a motor vehicle accident, reported dreaming "far more frequently than before" with the periodic impression of "dreaming all night."[153(p180)] Brain-damaged patients also may report more continuous dreaming, that is, dreaming the same content throughout the night, despite intervening episodes of wakefulness.[153–155] Although brain lesions are not typically suspected in epic-dreaming patients, the neuropsychological evidence points to involvement of the anterior limbic system and suggests that further clues to its cause may be found in associated emotional disturbances (e.g., alexithymia, dysthymia) in these patients. Treatments for epic dreaming (cognitive, hypnosis, relaxation, medications) have proved largely ineffective.[150]

Sleep-Wake Transition Disturbances

Several interrelated dream disturbances occur at the transitions into or out of sleep. These share the attributes of vivid, often intensely real, sensory imagery and disturbing affects such as fear. It may be their close proximity to wakefulness that colors these images with a distinctive reality quality, that is, there may be an interleaving or boundary dissociation of sleep-wake processes at this time. There might be, for example, an intrusion of a reality perception into sleep or of a dreamed object or character into wakefulness (cf. references 156, 157). The nature of the intruding components may well determine the distinctiveness of the transition disturbance, including typical or odd combinations such as a frightening hypnagogic image terminating in a sleep start or incomprehensible sleep-talking accompanying sleep paralysis.

Sleep Starts

Sleep starts, also known as predormital or hypnic myoclonus or hypnagogic or hypnic jerks, are brief phasic contractions of the muscles of the legs, arms, face, or neck that occur at sleep onset. They are often associated with brief, albeit vivid and impactful, dream events. Perhaps the most common of these events is the illusion of suddenly falling that incites a vigorous and startling jerk. Brief sensory flashes also occur; sometimes they may be somatic in nature and somewhat difficult to describe. A subject in Oswald's study, for example, reported "a strange sensation of something passing or flowing through his body, something 'hot' and 'bright.'"[158(p94)] The patients of Sander et al. reported "electric shock-like sensations in the chest" and "focal itchy, sharp, pinprick-like sensations that may occur anywhere."[159(p690)] More complex hypnagogic images may also accompany sleep starts.

Mild starts are a normal—even universal—feature of falling asleep, and a prevalence as high as 60 to 70% has been cited.[160] More extreme starts that can engender difficulties in initiating sleep[161] have been described by Critchley:

> I refer to violent, abrupt sensory and motor phenomena which come on quite unexpectedly, so as to shatter the background of sleeping. The sudden event

of a hallucinatory crash of noise or bang localized within the skull in an explosive fashion is not unfamiliar. Or it may be a sudden blinding flash of light.[162(p105)]

Critchley's claim that these dramatic sensory phenomena are more common in subjects with sensory problems, for example, loud noises among deaf persons, has not been systematically studied.

It is not known whether chronic sleep starts are primarily a disturbance of motor systems, perhaps akin to PLMS, or a disturbance of imagery systems, such that intense images provoke the disruptive reflex activity. Electroencephalographic (EEG) events have been noted to accompany sleep starts,[158] but, more systematic studies of sleep starts and the variety of EEG burst patterns that can accompany drowsiness[163] are needed to clarify this issue.

Terrifying Hypnagogic Hallucinations

Terrifying hypnagogic hallucinations (THHs) are terrifying dreams similar to those from REM sleep; after a sudden awakening at sleep onset there is prompt recall of frightening content.[160] As they arise from sleep-onset REM (SOREM) episodes, they may be aggravated by factors that predispose to this type of sleep, for example, withdrawal from REM-suppressant medication, chronic sleep deprivation, sleep fragmentation, narcolepsy. Other sleep and medical disorders may accompany the condition. Content analyses of THHs are lacking, but clinical and anecdotal reports suggest that the themes of attack and aggression found in REM sleep nightmares are common. THHs are perhaps more anxiety-provoking than most nightmares because of (1) a vivid sense of reality related to their close proximity to wakefulness, and (2) frequently accompanying feelings of paralysis. These features are illustrated in the two following examples.

A Case of Severe THH in a 36-Year-Old Woman With PTSD. At age 19, she was abducted and for more than 3 days, raped, beaten, burned, and subjected to death threats (Russian roulette) by motorcycle gang members. Although she regularly reexperienced these horrors through flashbacks and nightmares, even worse were the THHs with paralysis occurring as she returned to sleep *after* a nightmare. She felt as if she were awake, aroused, and terrified, yet unable to move; time seemed to be extremely drawn out as she experienced "replays" of her torturous experience in slow motion.[164]

THHs in a Healthy 26-Year-Old Practitioner of Esotericism. She reported having had several THHs, but not daytime sleepiness or cataplexy. Her THH included paralysis and vivid tactile, thermal, and auditory images associated with the sense of an assault by an intruder:

> I had just closed my eyes when suddenly I felt the presence of a man behind me. He held me by the hair and pulled it. He had a knife to my throat; I could feel the cold of the blade. He threatened me by saying: "You bitch. If you try to move I will kill you." I tried to scream but was completely unable. I knew it must

be an entity of some kind which would harm me if the dream continued, so I made a huge effort to move my arms and woke up out of the dream.

The suffering during such episodes is exacerbated by the victim's simultaneous sense of wakefulness and inability to move or call for help. Further, the intense anxiety may seriously disrupt sleep. For example, recurrent THHs may disrupt sleep onset sufficiently to produce sleep-onset insomnia.[160] And, as the second example illustrates, the realism of the dream leads readily to attributions about "real" assaults by spiritual entities, especially if the individual lives in a context conducive to such beliefs.[165–167] Prevalence figures for THHs are not available, but an estimate for patients with narcolepsy is 4 to 8%.[29]

Sleep Paralysis

Physiological mechanisms of sleep paralysis (SP) have been studied in some detail,[168, 169] but the relationship of SP to disturbed dreaming remains unclear. SP is a cardinal symptom of narcolepsy and also occurs in healthy persons. Patients seldom present for symptoms of SP alone, although they may when the frequency of their episodes increases, for example, to one per day. The clinical disorder of *sleep paralysis*, either *familial* or *isolated*, occurs at sleep onset or upon awakening from sleep, whereas "normal" feelings of paralysis or ineffectuality are a common feature of dreaming more generally[16] and, especially, of nightmares.[170] According to some,[171] paralysis feelings render hypnagogic hallucinations threatening or terrifying in nature. Frightening SP episodes have also been referred to as *sleep paralysis nightmares*, and their role in the misdiagnosis of hysteria and allegations of abuse described.[172]

Although psychopathology does not seem to be a direct cause of SP,[173] sleep-related life habits are associated with their occurrence in non-narcoleptic populations,[174] for example, poor sleep quality, insufficient sleep, and a proclivity to daytime sleep—all factors that may favor the occurrence of SOREM episodes.[174] In fact, isolated SP episodes have been elicited experimentally (on 72% of trials) by a schedule of sleep interruptions producing SOREM.[144] Of the six SP episodes induced by this method, five occurred during a SOREM episode. The one exception suggests that there may nevertheless be other, subtler factors contributing to SP.

One such factor may be psychopathological, although this likely influences SP indirectly, by its influence on stress and overwork and its subsequent disruptive effects on sleep.[173] Another factor may be rapid resetting of the circadian clock, as is the case with rapid time zone change,[175] or sleeping in the supine position.[173, 176] However, the nature and intensity of imagery generation in both wakefulness and sleep also appears to play a role in the occurrence and frequency of SP. *Imaginativeness*, as indexed by standardized questionnaires, and *vividness of nighttime imagery*, as measured by self-reported frequencies of nightmares and sleep terrors and vividness of dream imagery, are two personality factors found to be *most* predictive of SP occurrence and frequency in a large multivariate study of college students.[173]

SP is typically accompanied by vivid hypnagogic hallucinations. In fact, it is rare to find SP in the absence of other hallucinatory activity. Spanos et al.[173] found that 1.6% (of 387) subjects experienced SP without other attributes. Similarly, of the six experimental SP episodes described, all but one included auditory or visual hallucinations and unpleasant emotions.[144] On the other hand, it is not true that most hypnagogic hallucinations are accompanied by SP. Given this association of SP with hypnagogic hallucinations, it is unclear whether SP is, as some have suggested,[166, 177] a *type of perception*, that is, of ongoing REM sleep muscle atonia. Paralysis sensations—much like dreamed emotions and other sensations—*may be at least partially hallucinatory*. This could account for why SP is often reported to be associated with odd feelings of oppression, pressure on the chest and other body parts, even violent choking and beating. It could also explain how paralysis and felt ineffectuality appear in such a variety in routine dreams and nightmares.[16]

Prevalence Considerations. Multiple SP episodes have a low prevalence, occurring "often or always" in only 0 to 1% of young adults and "at least sometimes" in 7 to 8% of young adults.[29] On the other hand, the International Classification of Sleep Disorders-Revised (ICSD-R)[160] cites the lifetime prevalence of SP at 40 to 50%, which is somewhat higher than other estimates. We found rates of 25 to 36% in surveys of three university psychology student groups (Table 66–4), which are similar to the value of 26% reported for 208 Japanese undergraduates,[178] of 21% for 1798 Canadian undergraduates,[173] and of 34% for 200 sleep-disordered patients.[178a]

Simple methodological differences may explain some of the discrepancies among these estimates. Even a minor change in wording on questionnaires (e.g., replacing "transient paralysis" with "condition") can increase estimates by 5% (from 26 to 31%); use of a culturally identifiable term for SP, such as *kanashibari* in Japan, can increase the estimate by an additional 8% (to 39%).[178] The latter estimate corresponds well with those drawn from other cultures, for example, 37% of 603 Hong Kong undergraduates reporting at least one episode of "ghost oppression," the Chinese equivalent of *kanashibari*.[179] One survey of Newfoundland villagers found as many as 62% admitting to "Old Hag" attacks.[180] Much more work is needed to explain this

large variability and to clarify the role of sociocultural factors in the experiencing and reporting of SP.

Somniloquy With Dream Content

Sleep-talking has been observed in all stages of sleep, but especially in NREM stages 2, 3, and 4.[181] Arkin[181] identified various orders of concordance between sleep speech and later dream reports. For first-order concordances sleep speech exactly matches content in the dream, for example, a subject shouting "No! No!" who dreamed of shouting these words when seeing her baby fall from the bed. For second-order concordances a conceptual or emotional link between sleep speech and the dream is preserved, for example, a nightmare patient dreamed repeatedly of trying to yell "Burglars!" but in reality called out "Mama!" Absence of concordance is also seen: one study of 28 chronic sleep-talkers found it in 16.7% of REM, 32.9% of stage 2, and 38.5% of stage 3/4 sleep episodes.[181] As with SP, it remains unknown why imagery and behavior are dissociated in this manner.

False Awakening

False awakenings are nowhere classified as pathological per se, but they are nevertheless dreaming disturbances that can produce anxious reactions. Two types of false awakening have been distinguished primarily on the basis of the degree of anxious affect associated.[157, 182] Both types typically depict the person as (falsely) waking up from sleep or, in variations, from a dream, and may engender some confusion while dreaming about whether one is actually awake or asleep.

Type 1 awakenings are the more common type and usually depict realistic instances of the person waking up in his or her habitual bed followed by, in many cases, depictions of activities such as dressing, eating breakfast, and setting off for work. Some discrepancy in the imagery may fully awaken the person with the surprising realization that it was "just a dream." The dreams are often repetitive, depicting a succession of awakenings or of setting off for work. The philosopher Bertrand Russell, after having undergone anesthesia, reported seeming to have awakened hundreds of times.[183]

Type 2 false awakenings are less pleasant than type 1 in that the apparent awakenings in bed are accompanied by a "stressed, electrified or tense" atmosphere

Table 66–4. LIFETIME PREVALENCE IN FOUR SAMPLES OF SLEEP PARALYSIS ITEM "BEING HALF AWAKE AND PARALYZED" (TYPICAL DREAMS QUESTIONNAIRE)

	N	Men	Women	Both	Reference
Clinical sample	200	31.6	37.2	34.0	241
University sample 1	132	31.1	37.9	35.6	242
University sample 2	388	18.8	26.7	24.7	Nielsen, Zadra, & Smith (unpublished data, 1998)
University sample 3	107	26.3	30.4	29.0	243
Totals/Averages	**827**	**27.0**	**33.1**	**30.8**	

and feelings of "foreboding or expectancy" that may be "apprehensive or oppressively ominous."[157] There may be hallucinations of ominous or anxiety-provoking sounds, or strange apparitions of persons or monsters.

Both type 1 and type 2 false awakening are frequently associated with experiences of separating from the sleeping body, or *out-of-body experience* (OBE), and of becoming aware of dreaming while dreaming, or *lucid dreaming*.[157] False awakenings are clearly not always about a person's own home and bed, because our research team has elicited them in laboratory subjects.

Pathological and Disturbed Lucid Dreaming

Lucid dreaming is occasionally associated with disturbed or pathological reactions. Typically, lucid dreaming is perceptually vivid—the dreamer often feels awake—with a limited capacity to control the unfolding of some dreamed events. It is often spontaneously triggered within a nightmare and can be used in a therapy context to resolve the distressing contents of recurrent nightmares.[111] However, some have reported diverse negative reactions associated with lucid dreaming, including a type of "burnout" resulting from too frequent intentional use of the mental state, mental confusion, and "quasi-psychotic splits with reality" induced by the overlapping of perceptual and dreamlike mentation, and intense fear associated with the loss of control of the vivid dream contents.[184]

One reported case with polysomnographic evaluation involved a 28-year-old single man with lifelong lucid dreaming who presented to a clinic because 2 years earlier he began to lose control of his lucid dreams.[185] He could no longer escape from dream aggressors, or avoid their beatings and shootings. He experienced uncontrollable sobbing and "being beaten to a pulp."[185] He would awake feeling that he "had been hit by a truck," with severe headaches, muscle pains, and exhaustion. Polysomnographic and psychiatric tests proved normal, with the exception of some MMPI abnormalities. Psychotherapy and hypnotics were ineffective, but the antiepileptic diphenylhydantoin eliminated his symptoms. Adverse reactions to lucid dreaming appear to be rare, but they have not been studied systematically in either normal subjects or at-risk populations.

Narcolepsy

General. During their nocturnal sleep episodes, people with narcolepsy may experience frequent dreams that are intense, vivid, and bizarre.[20, 186] Compared with those suffering from insomnia, patients with narcolepsy report more frightening, recurrent dreams.[141] These may become so vivid and realistic that the patients confuse dreaming with waking reality, incorrectly remember dreams as real events, and develop concerns about losing their sanity.[171, 187] Although such confusions have led to false allegations of sexual abuse,[188] dream-reality confusions can also occur in healthy subjects.[189]

The cause of disturbed dreaming in narcolepsy likely has more to do with the fragmentation of REM sleep[190] than it does with increases in the intensity of REM sleep phasic activity; REM density in persons with narcolepsy is in the normal range.[191, 192] In this respect, disruption of REM sleep mechanisms in narcolepsy resembles that of dream-interruption insomnia (see above).

Patients with narcolepsy are thought to suffer from frightening and macabre hypnagogic hallucinations to a greater extent than are others.[193] These may be as terrifying as REM sleep nightmares.[171] Studies of their content[191, 194] reveal differences from the nocturnal dreams of healthy subjects: they contain less visual and motor imagery, more negative emotions, and more paralysis feelings. Nevertheless, SP and hypnagogic hallucinations occur almost exclusively during SOREM episodes, as opposed to nocturnal REM sleep.[169] A number of characteristic themes have also been described[193, 195] that seem typically nightmarish in nature, for example, human aggressors; threatening insects, snakes, and other animals; and oppressive presences. The majority of hallucinations reported by patients with narcolepsy concern human beings (76%), animals (29.2%), reptiles (22.4%), and monsters or ghosts (21.6%).[195]

Presence Imagery. Dreaming that a presence has entered the premises is closely associated with SP and is thus one of the most frequent hallucination themes reported by persons with either narcolepsy or isolated or familial sleep paralysis.[170, 196, 197] The intruder is often simply sensed as a presence moving about near the bed but without much visual or auditory detail (see reference 193 for examples). More commonly, the presences are associated with intense emotion. They may be perceived as threatening, ransacking the premises, or physically assaulting the patient.

Persons with severe narcolepsy may experience such horrors almost daily. Their hallucinatory vividness may cause severe confusion about the objective reality of events. Thus, if a proper diagnosis is not achieved and the patient not informed about the nature of the hallucinations, there may be a substantial emotional toll. Patients (and sometimes even physicians) may take the hallucinations to be evidence of impending madness, they may seriously misinterpret social events, and they may fail to benefit from treatment because of pressure to conceal their symptoms.

The more frequent occurrence of paralysis, hypnagogic hallucinations, presence imagery, and nightmarish dreaming in persons with narcolepsy is likely due to the fact that the latter tend more easily to shift directly into REM sleep. There is thus greater opportunity for the intercalation of dream contents with waking perceptions. Comparisons between SOREM dreams and regular REM dreams of persons with narcolepsy would be helpful in elucidating the mechanisms of these hallucinatory processes as well as evaluating the relative impact of these disturbed dreams on daytime functioning and distress.

REM Sleep Behavior Disorder

RBD occurs primarily in men over the age of 50 years and is characterized by excessive motor activity and dream-enacting behaviors.[198, 199] (See Chapter 64). These behaviors are often violent and related to ongoing nightmarish dream content. Patients do not appear to enact all of their dreams; just those that involve themes of confrontation, aggression, and violence. A "stereotypic nightmare" of pursuit and threat accompanying RBD episodes has been described.[198] It is visually vivid, with motor hyperactivity in both the dreamed self and other characters.[200] Although nightmares are commonly reported by RBD patients, not all patients recall episodes of overt dream enactment behaviors. Spouses, however, can infer dream content by observing the movements of RBD patients.[200]

The theme of pursuit and assault is the most common typical dream theme reported in our surveys of normal and sleep-disordered individuals (cited earlier); it is possible that the stereotyped disturbed dreaming in RBD is an amplified variation of a normal phenomenon and not a central pathophysiological mechanism of the disorder. Or, it may be that the pervasive threat depicted in RBD dreams reflects either the unique physiological substrate of RBD (sudden muscle tone intrusions into REM sleep) or the menacing psychosociological nature of the disorder (ongoing stress on family integrity). Studies of dream content and sleep-dream relationships are severely lacking.

Clonazepam not only suppresses the abnormal behaviors of REM sleep but also reduces the disturbing dreams associated with them[201, 202]; cessation of the medication is followed by a recurrence of both abnormal behaviors and nightmares.[201]

Sleep Terrors, Somnambulism, and Sleep Violence

Two sleep disorders with similar behavioral and psychophysiological features both implicate disturbed dreaming. Both disorders—sleep terrors and somnambulism—occur in NREM sleep, typically stage 4 sleep early in the night. They have been described as disorders of arousal,[203, 204] or more recently as "partial arousals,"[205] because of the autonomic and motor arousal that propels the patient toward an incomplete wakefulness. Gastaut and Broughton described the "arousal response" as a state of mental confusion and disorientation with automatic behavior, nonresponsiveness to external stimuli, difficulty in being awakened, retrograde amnesia for the episode, and fragmentary or absent recall of dreams. Further, the patient appears to be hallucinating yet displays a waking-like alpha pattern.[206] Despite this appearance of dissociated hallucinating, it was thought that the role of dream content in the arousals was minimal.[203] Later evidence (e.g., see reference 206) suggested that some type of dreaming may accompany most arousals, even though recall for it is impaired. In extreme cases of somnambulism with violence, dream content is often suspected as an immediate cause; indeed, in many cases a macabre nightmare parallels the violent act.

Sleep Terrors

The heart-wrenching screams and terrified facial expressions of a child or adult enduring a sleep terror would prompt a naive observer to conclude that some fearful dream had triggered the reaction. However, the physiological characteristics of terrors are substantially different from those of idiopathic nightmares (Table 66–5) and victims of sleep terrors seldom report that elaborate nightmares are the principal cause of their arousal. Many do report cognitive elements that seem scary enough: glimpses of a monster or strange man, the walls "closing in," and so forth. Over 50% of terror awakenings may produce cognitive activity of some form.[206] This estimate is surprisingly similar to the estimate of recall of mental content after awakenings from NREM sleep more generally.[207] The mental component of terrors may thus stem in part from processes also driving NREM dreaming. Fisher et al.[21] identified two

Table 66–5. DIFFERENTIATION OF NIGHTMARE DISORDER FROM SLEEP TERROR

	Nightmare Disorder	Sleep Terror
Sleep stage	Stage REM (or 2) second half of night	Stages 3 and 4 first half of night
Sleep behaviors	Not typical	Screaming, bolting, etc.
Autonomic activation	None to moderate: increased heart rate, mild or no increase in respiration, eye movement density	Moderate to extreme: tachycardia, rapid breathing, sweating
Awakening	Fully alert, continuing distress	Disorientation, confusion Unresponsive to stimuli
Mentation reports	Detailed, story-like dreams	Absent or fragmentary images, dreams in some cases
Emotions	Primarily fear, anxiety, anger or rage, disgust	Primarily terror, fear, disgust
Return to sleep	Sometimes difficult	Usually easy
Experimental elicitation	Not clearly established	With sudden loud buzzer in some subjects
Complications	Insomnia, sleep avoidance, daytime anxiety, distress	Injury to self or other due to nocturnal behaviors

types of terror-associated dream contents: (1) imagery occurring simultaneously with or just before the arousal, and (2) imagery elaborated subsequent to the awakening and associated with the visible physiological manifestations of anxiety (e.g., fear of suffocating related to sudden respiratory changes).

In many of the reports in Fisher et al., specific hallucinatory contents could be identified that appeared to trigger the terror event.[21] For example, one young man's recurrent, terrified awakenings were regularly associated with images of choking, such as swallowing nails or choking on electrodes. The occurrence of such imagery triggers remains consistent with the disorder of arousal model; the arousal trigger may be cognitive, such as a frightening image, rather than either physiological, such as an apnea,[208] or external, such as a loud buzzer.[206] It is also possible that the relative paucity of dream recall after a terror is due to retrograde amnesia accompanying these awakenings rather than to an absence of content per se. It may be that the extreme autonomic activation of a terror arousal disrupts short-term memory to a great extent. Amnesia has also been suggested to account for lower rates of dream recall from NREM (vs. REM) sleep.[209] Some atypical cases of terror[210] demonstrate little disorientation on arousal and dreams with hallucinatory vividness. However, relatively little data exist on this question.

Somnambulism and Sleep Violence

Somnambulistic actions may be complex, such as dressing or driving a car,[211] and may be performed with substantial dexterity[212]; more often, however, they are mundane, stereotyped, and accompanied by amnesia. It is thus difficult to determine the involvement of cognitive activities in these actions. Although somnambulistic episodes—like nightmares—rarely occur in the laboratory,[208, 213] questionnaires in combination with ambulatory recorders have been useful in eliciting brief imagery reports. Some reports are nightmarish, for example, "someone breaking in," "stones shattering my window," "ceiling falling on bed," "earthquake with bed moving," while others are of more commonplace events, for example, "feed the child," "take the dog out."

In more extreme cases of somnambulistic violence, disturbed dreaming is considered to be a contributing factor.[214] Many case reports[215] suggest that disturbed dreaming can play a considerable role, especially in violent incidents involving complex fight-or-flight reactions. Such reactions do suggest that the patient is reacting to a hallucinated threat. A detailed case study[215] illustrates this point. A 43-year-old man with a benign medical and psychiatric history reported sleep behaviors arising at age 5 and continuing to the present (frequency: five to seven per week). These were often violent excursions from the bed, with complex behaviors suggesting nightmares, for example, stabbing at furniture or the air with knives, swinging and throwing baseball bats, running out of the house. He had suffered numerous lacerations, ecchymoses, and sprained ankles; his wife had suffered bruises, strangulation,

and being hurled into the air, among other insults. At age 25, the patient enacted a dreamed attack by an intruder in his house. He describes how the behaviors seemed to stem from disturbed dreaming:

> . . . he left the house by running through a screen door, entered his automobile and drove 8 kilometers to his parents' home without an accident, and awakened them by pounding on their door.[215(p766)]

While driving, he remembers being aware only of driving to his parents' house to escape an intruder in his house.

He also attempted to strangle his wife while dreaming that he was protecting her. According to his wife:

> He later told me that he was dreaming that someone was trying to strangle me and so he was trying to pry the attacker's hands off me. But actually, his hands were wrapped around my neck, while my hands were around his hands—trying to pry his hands off my neck. It was my screaming that finally woke him up.[215 (p766)]

This patient showed no personality disorder, history of drug abuse, or other pathologic condition that might explain the violence. However, in adult sleepwalkers there is psychopathologic evidence suggestive of difficulties in dealing with aggression.[216] A variety of other clinical features have also been reported,[208] most notably, a DSM-III-R axis II diagnosis of obsessive-compulsive personality disorder in 21% of nonviolent and 50% of violent nocturnal wanderers. Altered sleep has also been noted. Compared with controls, young male somnambulists have more stage 3/4 sleep with hypersynchronous (greater than 10 sec and 150 μV) delta waves, greater stage 3/4 sleep percentage, and more stage 3/4 sleep interruptions.[208, 213] A subgroup also demonstrates theta waves prior to wandering.[208] One seriously violent group revealed less alpha activity and *lower* levels of stage 3/4 sleep compared with nonviolent somnambulists or healthy controls.[217] Although age may explain some discrepant findings for NREM sleep, it remains unknown whether any of these observed sleep characteristics are associated with emotional activity, dream content, or measures of psychopathology in these patients.

DISTURBED DREAMING IN NEUROLOGICAL CONDITIONS

Global Cessation of Dreaming

Changes in the recall of dreams and in their global characteristics as a function of neurological illness have been appreciated ever since Charcot[218, 219] first reported on a patient with complete loss of visual imagery, including loss of visual dreaming. This, and a later case report of complete cessation of dreaming by Wilbrand,[220] stimulated a great deal of interest in dream disturbances under the nosological heading of Charcot-Wilbrand syndrome.[153] In more recent times, interest has been focused on *global cessation of dreaming* (GCD).

Solms's[153] 4-year empirical investigation of dream changes in neurological illness revealed that of the 361 neurological patients seen during this period, 93.4% had undergone a change in some aspect of their dream experience as a function of their condition. Further, 34.9% of the 321 queried about GCD reported that they had ceased dreaming altogether since the onset of their illness. Parietal lobe involvement significantly differentiated patients with and without GCD; 42% of GCD patients had parietal lesions and an additional 7% had lesions in close proximity to parietal lobe ("periparietal"). Parietal involvement in dream recall confirms findings from a previous study on fewer patients.[221] Solms also found that the presence of frontal lobe lesions characterized some patients (8%) with GCD, independent of parietal lobe involvement.[153] This is consistent with the reduced dream recall seen after frontal lobotomy among schizophrenic patients[222] but not with a study[221] finding no such connection. The 43% of GCD cases not linked to either parietal or frontal lesions all had diffuse and nonlocalizable lesions.

Whether there is lateralization of neurological damage in GCD is at present uncertain. Equal distributions of right- and left-sided lesions were found in 45 of 47 cases,[153] whereas the left inferior mesial occipitotemporal cortex has also been implicated.[221] The latter is associated with a syndrome (including right homonymous hemianopia, alexia without agraphia, visual associative agnosia) which is typically explained as a disconnection between right hemisphere visual processes and left hemisphere speech processes. This notion is consistent with the reduced dreaming after corpus callosotomy and in agenesis of the corpus callosum.[223] Our finding of relatively intact dreaming following right hemispherectomy[224] but extremely impoverished recall following left hemispherectomy[225] also clearly supports a left hemisphere lateralization interpretation for GCD. Neuropsychological reviews[226, 227] favor a predominant role for *left* hemisphere processes in dream generation more generally.

Other conditions are known to suppress dream recall, although not to the extent of GCD. In chronic brain syndrome, dream recall from REM sleep deteriorates as the illness progresses from mild (57% recall), to severe (35%), to aged and severe (8%).[228] In Korsakoff's psychosis due to alcoholism, near-normal REM sleep time (29.4%) is seen, but poor dream recall (3%).[229] Patients with permanent amnesia for recent events due to mild encephalitis also have impoverished dreaming; their reports are less frequent than normal (28% vs. 75% of REM awakenings), and simpler, nonsymbolic, repetitious, stereotyped, and lacking in emotions and day residues.[230]

Epilepsy

Disturbances of emotional functioning in the dreams of epilepsy patients are clearly consistent with limbic system participation in the organization of dreaming. Patients with temporal lobe epilepsy who are awakened from REM sleep present more unpleasant emotions in their dreams than do controls[231]; they also have less varied emotions, with a lower frequency but a higher intensity. Although both medicated and nonmedicated patients have higher REM densities than do controls, medicated patients describe their dreams as being more vivid than do the other groups.

The role of the temporal lobe is demonstrated even more specifically by the occurrence of repetitive, painful dream imagery. Case studies[153, 232] indicate that epileptic auras may be incorporated into recurrent nocturnal dreams and that recurrent dream themes may, in turn, appear in the "dreamy state" of a temporal lobe complex partial seizure. REM sleep anomalies, such as rhythmical temporal epileptiform activity, have also been documented.[232] Solms[153] found a 7.9% (out of 114) incidence of recurring nightmares in his neurological sample: five of these presented with definite epilepsy; in two others it was suspected. In six of the seven cases, limbic system involvement could be demonstrated with no evidence of hemispheric predominance.

Dream-Reality Confusions

Intensification and vivification of dreaming to the point of confusion with reality has been described as characteristic of a small (5.3%) subgroup of neurological patients (N = 189)[153] and is illustrated by the following example. A 32-year-old right-handed woman sustained an open skull fracture when a rioter threw a brick through her car window:

> This patient reported that in the first weeks after her injury she experienced frequent and vivid nightmares, which, although bizarre, were very much more realistic than her normal dreams. She had always been a vivid dreamer but she experienced these dreams as being "utterly different." She felt that her dream recall was greatly enhanced, and she stated that she had considerable difficulty convincing herself that the dreams were not real . . . the dreams were always unpleasant . . . one night that there was something wriggling about in her "knickers," so she put her hand down and found (to her extreme horror) a green snake. She then felt something else was there and discovered three smaller snakes. Finally a black snake crawled up into her vagina. She awoke in terror and searched the bed for snakes. . . . On other occasions she would awake from dreams and feel compelled to check all around the house.[153(p192)]

The patient's dreams returned to normal within 2 months of the assault.

There is some evidence consistent with the hypothesis that dream-reality confusions are due to localized anterior limbic lesions. However, there is no one specific pattern of lesions within this region that is selectively associated with the symptom; equal numbers of cases show lesions in the medial prefrontal cortex, anterior cingulate gyrus, basal forebrain nuclei, and anteromedial diencephalic nuclei. The most severe cases also involve medial frontal cortex.

Vivification of dream reality occurs often in a number of other disturbances in which brain damage is not necessarily a contributing factor. For example, dream-reality confusions are well-known in SP and narcolepsy[171] (see above). They also occur in psychotic individuals and were noted as early as 1911 by Ellis to occur in cases of fatal heart disease, hysteria, "some forms of insanity," and "disordered cerebral and nervous conditions."[233(p237)] Indeed, dream-reality confusions can occur in normal persons as a result of dream vivification—what has been referred to as *reality dreaming*.[165] Among the many types of reality dreams are flying dreams, lucid dreams, sexual dreams, urination dreams, and dreams with incorporation of various organic sensations (e.g., pain, hunger).

Prodromal Dreaming and Symptom Incorporation

Many dreams—referred to as *prodromal*—are disturbed by ongoing or anticipated medical conditions (see reference 234 for review). Many direct prodromal expressions of symptoms have been demonstrated in clinical studies. In one study, patients with peripheral or central vestibular diseases reported a selective increase in fearful vestibular imagery (e.g., sensations of flying, rocking, sinking) in their dreams following onset of the illness; home diaries revealed a frequency of 69% of such dreams compared with 20% for control subjects.[235] In a second study,[236] 214 nonacute cardiac patients revealed a strong negative relationship between cardiac ejection fraction and dreamed death references (men) and separation references (women). Garfield[234] also identified a number of dream themes associated with cardiovascular problems; these references were direct (e.g., wounds, pain, or pressure in the arm, heart, chest, or neck), indirect (e.g., clutching or squeezing, references to death, blood, pain), and metaphoric (e.g., explosions). She also proposed that particular illnesses may be associated with certain recurrent themes, for example, gastrointestinal disorders (seeing or eating unpleasant food, dirty water, or feces), pulmonary problems (drowning or moving through polluted water), arthritis (rage or injuring a helpless animal), gynecological or obstetrical problems (difficult birth, pain in the area of the genitals depicted as an attack), dental problems (unusual objects in the mouth), migraine (seeing aura-like patterns, part of the visual field missing). Such themes may often appear in dreams before any overt symptomatology, a phenomenon that has been exploited (and often misunderstood) since the earliest days of medical science.[237]

SUMMARY

Dreaming disturbances implicate perturbation of emotional processes during sleep. They characterize a great variety of sleep disorders and neurological conditions, being at times primary to the etiology and pathophysiology of the disorder (e.g., nightmare disorder),

and at other times secondary associated symptoms (e.g., narcolepsy). Often, REM sleep fragmentation or REM sleep intrusion at the sleep-wake transition is implicated in disturbed dreaming. However, some dreaming disturbances are also frequently seen in NREM sleep disorders such as somnambulism. Most disturbances remain poorly understood because of their intractability to laboratory study and because patients are reluctant to report them in clinical settings. Nevertheless, effective treatments are available for many common disturbances and other treatments are presently under development.

References

1. Parmeggiani PL. The autonomic nervous system in sleep. In: Kryger MH, Roth T, Dement WC, eds. Principles and Practice of Sleep Medicine. 2nd ed. Philadelphia, Pa: WB Saunders; 1994:194–203.
2. Baharav A, Kotagal S, Gibbons V, et al. Fluctuations in autonomic nervous activity during sleep displayed by power spectrum analysis of heart rate variability. Neurology. 1995;45:1183–1187.
3. Verrier RL, Muller JE, Hobson JA. Sleep, dreams, and sudden death: the case for sleep as an autonomic stress test for the heart. Cardiovasc Res. 1996;31:181–211.
4. Orem J. Respiratory neurons and sleep. In: Kryger MH, Roth T, Dement WC, eds. Principles and Practice of Sleep Medicine. 2nd ed. Philadelphia, Pa: WB Saunders; 1994:177–193.
5. Noll G, Elam M, Kunimoto M, et al. Skin sympathetic nerve activity end-effector function during sleep in humans. Acta Physiol Scand. 1994;151:319–329.
6. Takeuchi S, Iwase S, Mano T, et al. Sleep related changes in human muscle and skin sympathetic nerve activities. J Auton Nerv Syst. 1994;47:121–129.
7. Maquet P. Positron emission tomography studies of sleep and sleep disorders. J Neurol. 1997;244(suppl 1):S23–S28.
8. Braun AR, Balkin TJ, Wesensten NJ, et al. Dissociated pattern of activity in visual cortices and their projections during human rapid eye movement sleep. Science. 1997;279:91–95.
9. Paradiso S, Robinson RG, Andreasen NC, et al. Emotional activation of limbic circuitry in elderly normal subjects in a PET study. Am J Psychiatry. 1997;154:384–389.
10. Nielsen TA, Deslauriers D, Baylor GW. Emotions in dream and waking event reports. Dreaming. 1991;1:287–300.
11. Hall C, Van de Castle RI. The Content Analysis of Dreams. New York, NY: Appleton-Century-Crofts; 1966.
12. Kramer M. The selective mood regulatory function of dreaming: an update and revision. In: Moffitt A, Kramer M, Hoffmann R, eds. The Functions of Dreaming. Albany, NY: State University of New York Press; 1993:139–196.
13. Gottschalk LA, Buchsbaum MS, Gillin J, et al. Anxiety levels in dreams: relation to localized cerebral glucose metabolic rate. Brain Res. 538:107–110.
14. Gerne M, Strauch I. Psychophysiological indicators of affect patterns and conversational signals during sleep. In: Koella WP, Ruther E, Schulz H, eds. Sleep '84. Stuttgart, Germany: Fischer; 1985:367–369.
15. Rechtschaffen A. The psychophysiology of mental activity during sleep. In: McGuigan FJ, Schoonoer RA, eds. The Psychophysiology of Thinking: Studies of Covert Processes. New York, NY: Academic Press; 1973:153–205.
16. Kuiken D, Sikora S. The impact of dreams on waking thoughts and feelings. In: Moffitt A, Kramer M, Hoffmann R, eds. The Functions of Dreaming. Albany, NY: State University of New York Press; 1993:419–476.
17. Krakow B, Kellner R, Pathak D, et al. Imagery rehearsal treatment for chronic nightmares. Behav Res Ther. 1995;33:837–843.
18. Belicki K. Nightmare frequency versus nightmare distress: relations to psychopathology and cognitive style. J Abnorm Psychol. 1992;101:592–597.

19. Kramer M. Nightmares (dream disturbances) in posttraumatic stress disorder; implication for a theory of dreaming. In: Bootzin RR, Kihlstrom JF, Schacter DL, eds. Sleep and Cognition. Washington, DC: American Psychological Association; 1992:190–203.

20. American Psychiatric Association. Diagnostic and Statistical Manual of Mental Disorders. 4th ed. Washington, DC: American Psychiatric Association Press; 1994.

21. Fisher C, Byrne J, Edwards A, et al. A psychophysiological study of nightmares. J Am Psychoanal Assoc. 1970;18:747–782.

22. Hartmann E. The Nightmare: The Psychology and the Biology of Terrifying Dreams. New York, NY: BasicBooks; 1984.

23. Halliday G. Direct psychological therapies for nightmares: a review. Clin Psychol Rev. 1987;7:501–523.

24. Levitan HL. The significance of certain catastrophic dreams. Psychother Psychosom. 1976;27:1–7.

25. Van Bork J. An attempt to clarify a dream-mechanism: why do people wake up out of an anxiety dream? Int Rev Psychoanal. 1982;9:273–277.

26. Zadra A, Donderi DC. Variety and intensity of emotions in bad dreams and nightmares. Can Psychol. 1993;34:294.

27. Harris I. Observations concerning typical anxiety dreams. Psychiatry. 1948;11:301–309.

28. Hall CS. The significance of the dream of being attacked. J Pers. 1955;24:168–180.

29. Partinen M. Epidemiology of sleep disorders. In: Kryger MH, Roth T, Dement WC, eds. Principles and Practice of Sleep Medicine. 2nd ed. Philadelphia, Pa: WB Saunders; 1994:437–452.

30. Salzarulo P, Chevalier A. Sleep problems in children and their relationship with early disturbances of the waking-sleeping rhythms. Sleep. 1983;6:47–51.

31. Simonds JF, Parraga H. Prevalence of sleep disorders and sleep behaviors in children and adolescents. J Am Acad Child Adolesc Psychiatry. 1982;21:383–388.

32. Vela-Bueno A, Bixler EO, Dobladez-Blanco B, et al. Prevalence of night terrors and nightmares in elementary school children: a pilot study. Res Commun Psychol Psychiatr Behav. 1985;10:177–188.

33. Nielsen TA, Laberge L, Tremblay R, et al. Prevalence of bad dream recall in 13 and 16 year olds: a longitudinal study. Presented at the 13th Annual Meeting of the Association of Professional Sleep Societies: June 19–24, 1999; Orlando, Fla.

34. Belicki K, Cuddy MA. Nightmares: facts, fictions and future directions. In: Gackenbach J, Sheikh AA, eds. Dream Images: A Call to Mental Arms. Amityville, NY: Baywood; 1991:99–115.

35. Levin R. Sleep and dreaming characteristics of frequent nightmare subjects in a university population. Dreaming. 1994;4:127–137.

36. Wood JM, Bootzin RR. The prevalence of nightmares and their independence from anxiety. J Abnorm Psychol. 1990;99:64–68.

37. Janson C, Gislason T, De Backer W, et al. Prevalence of sleep disturbances among young adults in three European countries. Sleep. 1995;18:589–597.

38. Stepansky R, Holzinger B, Schmeiser-Rieder A, et al. Austrian dream behavior: results of a representative population survey. Dreaming. 1998;8:23–30.

39. Bixler EO, Kales A, Soldatos CR, et al. Prevalence of sleep disorders in the Los Angeles metropolitan area. Am J Psychiatry. 1979;136:1257–1262.

40. Cirignotta F, Zucconi M, Mondini S, et al. Enuresis, sleepwalking, and nightmares: an epidemiological survey in the republic of San Marino. In: Guilleminault C, Lugaresi E, eds. Sleep/Wake Disorder: Natural History, Epidemiology, and Long-Term Evolution. New York, NY: Raven Press; 1983:237–241.

41. Klink M, Quan S. Prevalence of reported sleep disturbances in a general adult population and their relationship to obstructive airways disease. Chest. 1987;91:540–546.

42. Bixler EO, Kales A, Soldatos CR. Sleep disorders encountered in medical practice. Behav Med. 1979;1–6.

43. Cernovsky ZZ. MMPI and nightmares in male alcoholics. Percept Mot Skills. 1985;61:841–842.

44. Cernovsky ZZ. MMPI and nightmare reports in women addicted to alcohol and other drugs. Percept Mot Skills. 1986;62:717–718.

45. Brylowsky A. Nightmares in crisis: clinical applications of lucid dreaming techniques. Psychiatr J Univ Ottawa. 1990;15:79–84.

46. Salvio MA, Wood JM, Schwartz J, et al. Nightmare prevalence in the healthy elderly. Psychol Aging. 1992;7:324–325.

47. Nielsen TA, Zadra A, Germain A. Topography of REM sleep nightmares. Am J Psychiatr. In press.

48. Nielsen TA, Zadra A. Laboratory studies of idiopathic nightmares. In: Abstracts of the Journée académique du département de psychiatrie, Centre Fernand-Séguin, Louis H. Lafontaine Hospital; May 16, 1997; Montreal, Canada.

49. Niedermeyer E. Alpha rhythms as physiological and abnormal phenomena. Int J Psychophysiol. 1997;26:31–49.

50. Cantero JL, Atienza M, Gomez CM, et al: Spectral structure and brain mapping of human alpha activities in different arousal states. Neuropsychobiology 1999;39:110–116.

51. Perlis ML, Nielsen TA. Mood regulation, dreaming and nightmares: evaluation of a desensitization function for REM sleep. Dreaming. 1993;3:243–257.

52. Berquier A, Ashton R. Characteristics of the frequent nightmare sufferer. J Abnorm Psychol. 1992;101:246–250.

53. Levin R, Hurvich MS. Nightmares and annihilation anxiety. Psychoanal Psychol. 1995;12:247–158.

54. Miller WR, DiPilato M. Treatment of nightmares via relaxation and desensitization: a controlled evaluation. J Consult Clin Psychol. 1983;51:870–877.

55. Levin R, Raulin ML. Preliminary evidence for the proposed relationship between frequent nightmares and schizotypal symptomatology. J Pers Dis. 1991;5:8–14.

56. Hartmann E, Elkin R, Garg M. Personality and dreaming: the dreams of people with very thick or very thin boundaries. Dreaming. 1991;1:311–324.

57. Hartmann E. Boundaries of dreams, boundaries of dreamers: thin and thick boundaries as a new personality measure. Psychiatr J Univ Ottawa. 1989;14:557–560.

58. Levin R, Galin J, Zywiak B. Nightmares, boundaries, and creativity. Dreaming. 1991;1:63–74.

59. Belicki K, Belicki D. Predisposition for nightmares: a study of hypnotic ability, vividness of imagery, and absorption. J Clin Psychol. 1986;42:714–718.

60. Hartmann E, Cravens J. The effects of long term administration of psychotropic drugs on human sleep, II: the effects of reserpine. Psychopharmacology. 1973;33:169–184.

61. Kales A, Scharf MB, Bixler EO, et al. Sleep laboratory drug evaluation: thioridazine (Mellaril), a REM enhancing drug. Sleep Res. 1974;3:55–55.

62. Moskovitz C, Moses H, Klawans HL. Levodopa-induced psychosis: a kindling phenomenon. Am J Psychiatry. 1978;135:669–675.

63. Sharf B, Moskovitz C, Lupton MD, et al. Dream phenomena induced by chronic levodopa therapy. J Neural Trans. 1978;43:143–151.

64. Bengtsson C, Lennartsson J, Lindquist O, et al. Sleep disturbances, nightmares and other possible central nervous disturbances in a population sample of women, with special reference to those on antihypertensive drugs. Eur J Clin Pharmacol. 1980;17:173–177.

65. Cove-Smith JR, Kirk CA. CNS-related side-effects with metropolol and atenolol. Eur J Pharmacol. 1985;28:69–72.

66. Davidov ME, Glazer N, Wollam G, et al. Comparison of betaxolol, a new B1-adrenergic antagonist, to propranolol in the treatment of mild to moderate hypertension. Am J Hypertens. 1988;1:206S–210S.

67. Kuriyama S. Bisoprolol-induced nightmares. J Hum Hypertens. 1994;8:731–732.

68. Henningsen NC, Mattiasson I. Long-term clinical experience with atenolol: a new selective beta$_1$-blocker with few side effects from the central nervous system. Acta Med Scand. 1979;205:61–66.

69. Balon R. Bupropion and nightmares. Am J Psychiatry. 1996;153:579–580.

70. Becker RE, Dufresne RL. Perceptual changes with bupropion, a novel antidepressant. Am J Psychiatry. 1982;139:1200–1201.

71. Flemenbaum A. Pavor nocturnus: a complication of single daily tricyclic or neuroleptic dosage. Am J Psychiatry. 1976;133:570–572.

72. Strayhorn JM, Nash JM. Frightening dreams and dosage schedule of tricyclic and neuroleptic drugs. J Nerv Ment Dis. 1978;166:878–880.

73. Kales A, Bixler EO, Tan TL, et al. Chronic hypnotic use: ineffectiveness, drug-withdrawal insomnia, and dependence. JAMA. 1974;227:513–517.

74. Firth H. Sleeping pills and dream content. Br J Psychiatry. 1974;124:547–553.

75. Oswald I, Priest RG. Five weeks to escape the sleeping-pill habit. Br Med J. 1965;2:1093–1095.

76. Hershon HI. Alcohol withdrawal symptoms and drinking behavior. J Stud Alcohol. 1977;38:953–971.

77. Gross MM, Goodenough D, Tobin M, et al. Sleep disturbances and hallucinations in the acute alcoholic psychoses. J Nerv Ment Dis. 1966;142:493–514.

78. Blake DD, Cook JD, Monaco V, et al. Coping patterns in combat-related PTSD: alcohol and drug use. Presented at 24th Annual Association for Advancement of Behavior Therapy Convention, November 1990; San Francisco, Calif.

79. Stewart SH. Alcohol abuse in individuals exposed to trauma—a critical review. Psychol Bull. 1996;120:83–112.

80. Hishikawa Y, Sugita Y, Teshima T, et al. Sleep disorders in alcoholic patients with delirium tremens and transient withdrawal hallucinations—reevaluation of the REM rebound and intrusion theory. In: Karacan I, ed. Psychophysiological Aspects of Sleep. Park Ridge, NJ: Noyes Medical; 1981:109–122.

81. Rowland RH. Sleep onset rapid eye movement periods in neuropsychiatric disorders: implications for the pathophysiology of psychosis. J Nerv Ment Dis. 1997;185:730–738.

82. Johnson LC, Burdick JA, Smith J. Sleep during alcohol intake and withdrawal in the chronic alcoholic. Arch Gen Psychiatry. 1970;22:406–418.

83. Feinberg I. Hallucinations, dreaming and REM sleep. In: Keup W, ed. Origin and Mechanisms of Hallucinations. New York, NY: Plenum; 1970:125–132.

84. Tachibana M, Tanaka K, Hishikawa Y, et al. A sleep study of acute psychotic states due to alcohol and meprobamate addiction. In: Weitzman ED, ed. Advances in Sleep Research. Vol 2. Spectrum; 1975:177–205.

85. Wolin SJ, Mello JK. The effects of alcohol on dreams and hallucinations in alcohol addicts. Ann N Y Acad Sci. 1973;215:266–302.

86. Allen RP, Wagman A, Faillace LA, et al. Electroencephalographic (EEG) sleep recovery following prolonged alcohol intoxication in alcoholics. J Nerv Ment Dis. 1971;153:424–433.

87. Mahowald MW, Schenck CH. REM behavior disorder. In: Kryger MH, Roth T, Dement WC, eds. Principles and Practice of Sleep Medicine. Philadelphia, Pa: WB Saunders; 1994:574–588.

88. Solomon K. Thiothixene and bizarre nightmares: an association? J Clin Psychiatry. 1983;44:77–78.

89. Mort JR. Nightmare cessation following alteration of ophthalmic administration of a cholinergic and a beta-blocking agent. Ann Pharmacother. 1992;26:914–916.

90. Lepkifker W, Dannon PN, Iancu I, et al. Nightmares related to fluoxetine treatment. Clin Neuropharmacol. 1995;18:90–94.

91. Markowitz JC. Fluoxetine and dreaming. J Clin Psychiatry. 1991;52:432–432.

92. Bakht FR, Miller LG. Naproxen-associated nightmares. South Med J. 1991;84:1271–1273.

93. Kumar KL, Hodges M. Disturbing dreams with long-acting verapamil. N Engl J Med. 1988;318:929–930.

94. Girwood RH. Nitrazepam nightmares. Br Med J. 1973;1:353.

95. Black RJ, Dawson TA. Erythromycin and nightmares. Br Med J. 1988;296:1070.

96. Williams NR. Erythromycin: a case of nightmares. Br Med J. 1988;296:214.

97. Domhoff GW. The repetition of dreams and dream elements: a possible clue to a function of dreams. In: Moffitt A, Kramer M, Hoffmann R, eds. The Functions of Dreaming. New York, NY: State University of New York Press; 1993:293–320.

98. Cartwright RD. The nature and function of repetitive dreams: a survey and speculation. Psychiatry. 1979;42:131–137.

99. Zadra AL. Recurrent dreams: their relation to life events. In: Barrett D, ed. Trauma and Dreams. Cambridge, Mass: Harvard University Press; 1996:231–247.

100. Bonime W. The Clinical Use of Dreams. New York, NY: BasicBooks; 1962.

101. Cartwright RD, Lloyd S, Knight S, et al. Broken dreams: a study of the effects of divorce and depression on dream content. Psychiatry. 1984;47:251–259.

102. Cartwright RD. Affect and dream work from an information processing point of view. J Mind Behav. 1986;7:411–427.

103. Zadra AL, O'Brien S, Donderi DC. Dream content, dream recurrence and well-being: a replication with a younger sample. J Imag Cogn Pers. 1998;17:293–311.

104. Brown RJ, Donderi DC. Dream content and self-reported well-being among recurrent dreamers, past-recurrent dreamers, and nonrecurrent dreamers. J Pers Soc Psychol. 1986;50:612–623.

105. Coalson B. Nightmare help: treatment of trauma survivors with PTSD. Psychotherapy. 1995;32:381–388.

106. Freud S. The Interpretation of Dreams. New York, NY: BasicBooks; 1955.

107. Jones E. On the Nightmare. New York, NY: Liveright; 1951.

108. Celluci AJ, Lawrence PS. The efficacy of systematic desensitization in reducing nightmares. J Behav Ther Exp Psychiatry. 1978;9:109–114.

109. Kellner R, Neidhardt J, Krakow B, et al. Changes in chronic nightmares after one session of desensitization or rehearsal instructions. Am J Psychiatry. 1992;149:659–663.

110. Neidhardt EJ, Krakow B, Kellner R, et al. The beneficial effects of one treatment session and recording of nightmares on chronic nightmare sufferers. Sleep. 1992;15:470–473.

111. Zadra AL, Pihl RO. Lucid dreaming as a treatment for recurrent nightmares. Psychother Psychosom. 1997;66:50–55.

112. Marquis J. A report on seventy-eight cases treated by eye movement desensitization. J Behav Ther Exp Psychiatry. 1991;22:187–192.

113. Kingsbury SJ. Brief hypnotic treatment of repetitive nightmares. Am J Clin Hypn. 1993;35:161–169.

114. Van der Kolk BA, Hartmann E, Burr W, et al. A survey of nightmare frequencies in a veterans outpatient clinic. Sleep Res. 1980;9:229–229.

115. Kramer M. Dream disturbances. Psychiatr Ann. 1979;9:50–68.

116. Kramer M, Schoen LW, Kinney L. The dream experience in dream-disturbed Vietnam veterans. In: Van der Kolk BA, ed. PTSD: Psychological and Biological Sequelae. Washington, DC: American Psychiatric Press; 1984:81–95.

117. Krakow B, Tandberg D, Scriggins L, et al. A controlled comparison of self-rated sleep complaints in acute and chronic nightmare sufferers. J Nerv Ment Dis. 1995;183:623–627.

118. Woodward SH, Arsenault EJ, Richardson WB. Trauma-related nightmares are associated with sleep reduction. Sleep Res. 1992;21:134.

119. Ross RJ, Ball WA, Sullivan KA, et al. Sleep disturbance as the hallmark of posttraumatic stress disorder. Am J Psychiatry. 1989;146:697–707.

120. Hefez A, Metz L, Lavie P. Long-term effects of extreme situational stress on sleep and dreaming. Am J Psychiatry. 1987;144:344–347.

121. Greenberg R, Pearlman CA, Gampel D. War neuroses and the adaptive function of REM sleep. Br J Med Psychol. 1972;45:27–33.

122. van der Kolk B, Blitz R, Burr W, et al. Nightmares and trauma: a comparison of nightmares after combat with lifelong nightmares in veterans. Am J Psychiatry. 1984;141:187–190.

123. Kramer M, Kinney L. Sleep patterns in trauma victims with disturbed dreaming. Psychiatr J Univ Ottawa. 1988;13:12–16.

124. Schlosberg A, Benjamin M. Sleep patterns in three acute combat fatigue cases. J Clin Psychiatry. 1978;39:546–549.

125. Reist C, Kauffmann CD, Chicz-Demet A, et al. REM latency, dexamethasone suppression test, and thyroid releasing hormone stimulation test in posttraumatic stress disorder. Neuropsychopharmacol Biol Psychiatry. 1995;19:433–443.

126. Mukilincer M, Glaubman H, Wasserman O, et al. Control-related beliefs and sleep characteristics of posttraumatic stress disorder patients. Psychol Rep. 1989;65:567–576.

127. Kramer M, Kinney L. Is sleep a marker of vulnerability to delayed post traumatic stress disorder? Sleep Res. 1985;14:181.

128. Lavie P, Hefez A, Halperin G, et al. Long-term effects of traumatic war-related events on sleep. Am J Psychiatry. 1979;136:175–178.

129. Krakow B, Tandberg D, Cutchen L, et al. Imagery rehearsal treatment of chronic nightmares in PTSD: a controlled study. Sleep Res. 1997;26:245.

130. Woodward SH, Arsenault EJ, Bilwise DL, et al. The temporal distribution in Vietnam combat veterans. Sleep Res. 1991;20:152.

131. Fisher C, Byrne JV, Edwards A, et al. REM and NREM nightmares. Int Psychiatr Clin. 1970;7:183–187.

132. Blank AS Jr. Clinical detection, diagnosis, and differential diagnosis of post-traumatic stress disorder. Psychiatr Clin North Am. 1994;17:351–383.

133. Schenck CH, Boyd JL, Mahowald MW. A parasomnia overlap disorder involving sleepwalking, sleep terrors, and REM sleep behavior disorder in 33 polysomnographically confirmed cases. Sleep. 1997;20:972–981.

134. Greenberg R. Dream interruption insomnia. J Nerv Ment Dis. 1967;144:18–21.

135. Cartwright R. Dream interruption insomnia. Presented at the Eighth Annual Meeting of the Association of Professional Sleep Societies; June 4–9, 1994; Boston, Mass.

136. Gilman L. Insomnia and Its Relation to Dreams. New York, NY: JB Lippincott; 1958.

137. Ohayon MM, Morselli PL, Guilleminault C. Prevalence of nightmares and their relationship to psychopathology and daytime functioning in insomnia subjects. Sleep. 1997;20:340–348.

138. Cellucci AJ, Lawrence PS. Individual differences in self-reported sleep variable correlations among nightmare sufferers. J Clin Psychol. 1978;34:721–725.

139. Krakow B, Kellner R, Neidhardt J, et al. Imagery rehearsal treatment of chronic nightmares: with a thirty month follow-up. J Behav Ther Exp Psychiatry. 1993;24:325–330.

140. Philip P, Guilleminault C. Adult psychophysiologic insomnia and positive history of childhood insomnia. Sleep. 1996;19:S16–22.

141. Lee JH, Bliwise DL, Lebret-Bories E, et al. Dream-disturbed sleep in insomnia and narcolepsy. J Nerv Ment Dis. 1993;181:320–324.

142. Thoman EB. Snoring, nightmares, and morning headaches in elderly women: a preliminary study. Biol Psychol. 1997;46:275–284.

143. de Groen J, Op den Velde W, Hovens J, et al. Snoring and anxiety dreams. Sleep. 1993;16:35–36.

144. Takeuchi T, Miyasita A, Sasaki Y, et al. Isolated sleep paralysis elicited by sleep interruption. Sleep. 1992;15:217–225.

145. Busink R, Kuiken D. Identifying types of impactful dreams—a replication. Dreaming. 1996;6:97–119.

146. Bowlby J. Attachment and Loss. Vol 1. Attachment. London, England: Hogarth Press; 1969.

147. Parkes CM. Bereavement: Studies of Grief in Adult Life. New York, NY: International Universities Press; 1972.

148. Kuiken D. Euro-North American paths through bereavement. Presented at 12th Annual International Conference of the Association for the Study of Dreams; June 20–24, 1995; New York, NY.

149. Grimby A. Bereavement among elderly people: grief reactions, post-bereavement hallucinations and quality of life. Acta Psychiatr Scand. 1993;87:72–80.

150. Schenck CH, Mahowald MW. A disorder of epic dreaming with daytime fatigue, usually without polysomnographic abnormalities, that predominantly affects women. Sleep Res. 1995;24:137.

151. Zadra AL, Nielsen TA. Epic dreaming: a case report. Sleep Res. 1996;25:148.

152. Porte HS, Hobson JA. Physical motion in dreams—one measure of three theories. J Abnorm Psychol. 1996;105:329–335.

153. Solms M. The Neuropsychology of Dreams. Mahwah, NJ: Lawrence Erlbaum Associates; 1997.

154. Whitty C, Lewin W. Vivid daydreaming: an unusual form of confusion following anterior cingulectomy. Brain. 1957;80:72–76.

155. Lugaresi E, Medori R, Montagna P, et al. Fatal familial insomnia and dysautomania with selective degeneration of thalamic nuclei. N Engl J Med. 1986;315:997–1003.

156. Mahowald MW, Schenck CH. Dissociated states of wakefulness and sleep. Neurology. 1992;42(suppl 6):44–52.

157. Green C, McCreery C. Lucid Dreaming. The Paradox of Consciousness During Sleep. London, England: Routledge; 1994.

158. Oswald I. Sudden bodily jerks on falling asleep. Brain. 1959;82:92–101.

159. Sander HW, Geisse H, Quinto C, et al. Sensory sleep starts. J Neurol Neurosurg Psychiatry. 1998;64:690.

160. International Classification of Sleep Disorders, Revised: Diagnostic and Coding Manual. Rochester, Minn: American Sleep Disorders Association; 1997.

161. Broughton R. Pathological fragmentary myoclonus, intensified "hypnic jerks" and hypnagogic foot tremor: Three unusual sleep-related movement disorders. In: Koella WP, Obal F, Schulz H, et al, eds. Sleep '86. Stuttgart, Germany: Fischer; 1988:240–243.

162. Critchley M. The pre-dormitum. Rev Neurol. 1955;93:101–106.

163. Bartel P, Robinson E, Duim W. Burst patterns occurring during drowsiness in clinical EEGs. Am J Electroncephalogr Technol. 1995;35:283–295.

164. Hudson JI, Manoach DS, Sabo AN, et al. Recurrent nightmares in posttraumatic stress disorder: association with sleep paralysis, hypnopompic hallucinations, and REM sleep. J Nerv Ment Dis. 1991;179:572–573.

165. Nielsen TA. Reality dreams and their effects on spiritual belief: a revision of animism theory. In: Gackenbach J, Sheikh AA, eds. Dream Images: A Call to Mental Arms. Amityville, NY: Baywood; 1991;233–264.

166. Hufford DJ. The Terror That Comes in the Night: An Experience-centered Study of Supernatural Assault Traditions. Philadelphia, Pa: University of Pennsylvania Press; 1982.

167. Fukuda K, Miyasita A, Inugami M, et al. High prevalence of isolated sleep paralysis: kanashibari phenomenon in Japan. Sleep. 1987;10:279–286.

168. Hishikawa Y, Shimizu T. Physiology of REM sleep, cataplexy, and sleep paralysis. Adv Neurol. 1995;67:245–271.

169. Hishikawa Y. Sleep paralysis. In: Guilleminault C, Dement WC, Passouant P, eds. Narcolepsy. New York, NY: Spectrum; 1976;97–123.

170. Liddon SC. Sleep paralysis and hypnagogic hallucinations. Their relationship to the nightmare. Arch Gen Psychiatry. 1967;17:88–96.

171. Broughton RJ. Neurology and dreaming. Psychiatr J Univ Ottawa. 1982;7:101–110.

172. Powell RA, Nielsen TA. Was Anna O.'s black snake hallucination a sleep paralysis nightmare? Dreams, memories, and trauma. Psychiatry. 1998;61:239–248.

173. Spanos NP, McNulty SA, DuBreuil SC, et al. The frequency and correlates of sleep paralysis in a university sample. J Res Pers. 1995;29:285–305.

174. Takeuchi T, Fukuda K, Yamamoto Y, et al. What kind of sleep-related life style affects the occurrence of sleep paralysis in normal individuals? Presented at the 11th annual meeting of the Association of Professional Sleep Societies; June 10–15, 1997; San Francisco, Calif.

175. Snyder S. Isolated sleep paralysis after rapid time zone change ("jet lag") syndrome. Chronobiology. 1983;10:377–379.

176. Fukuda K, Ogilvie R, Takeuchi T. The prevalence of sleep paralysis among Canadian and Japanese college students. Dreaming. 1998;8:59–66.

177. Giaquinto S, Pompeiano O, Somogyi I. Supraspinal inhibitory control of spinal reflexes during natural sleep. Experientia. 1963;19:652–653.

178. Fukuda K. One explanatory basis for the discrepancy of reported prevalences of sleep paralysis among healthy respondents. Percept Mot Skills. 1993;77:803–807.

178a. Nielsen TA, Zadra A, Germain A, Montplaisir J. The 55 typical dreams questionnaire: assessment of 200 sleep patients. Sleep. 1998;21(suppl):286.

179. Wing YK, Lee ST, Chen CN. Sleep paralysis in Chinese: ghost oppression phenomenon in Hong Kong. Sleep. 1994;17:609–613.

180. Ness RC. The Old Hag phenomenon as sleep paralysis: a biocultural interpretation. Cult Med Psychiatry. 1978;2:15–39.

181. Arkin AM. Sleep-Talking: Psychology and Psychophysiology. Hillsdale, NJ: Lawrence Erlbaum Associates; 1981.

182. Green CE. Lucid Dreams. Oxford, England: Institute of Psychophysical Research; 1968.

183. Russell B. Human Knowledge: Its Scope and Limits. London, England: Allen & Unwin; 1948.

184. Gackenbach J, Bosveld J. Control Your Dreams. New York, NY: Harper & Row; 1989.

185. Schenck CH, Mahowald MW. A case of pathologic lucid dreaming presenting to a sleep disorders center. Sleep Res. 1990;19:155.

186. Schredl M. Dream content in narcoleptic patients: preliminary findings. Dreaming. 1998;8:103–107.

187. Zarcone VP, Fuchs HE. Psychiatric disorders and narcolepsy. In:

Guilleminault C, Dement WC, Passouant P, eds. Narcolepsy. New York, NY: Spectrum; 1976:231–255.

188. Hays P. False but sincere accusations of sexual assault made by narcoleptic patients. Med Leg J. 1992;60:1–8.

189. Mazzoni GA, Loftus EF. When dreams become reality. Conscious Cogn. 1996;5:442–462.

190. Montplaisir J, Billiard M, Takahashi S, et al. Twenty-four-hour recording in REM-narcoleptics with special reference to nocturnal sleep disruption. Biol Psychiatry. 1978;13:73–89.

191. Hishikawa Y, Koida H, Yoshino K, et al. Characteristics of REM sleep accompanied by sleep paralysis and hypnagogic hallucinations in narcoleptic patients. Waking Sleep. 1978;2:113–123.

192. Broughton R, Mamelak M. The effects of nocturnal gamma-hydroxybutyrate on sleep/waking patterns in narcolepsy-cataplexy. Can J Neurol Sci. 1980;7:23–31.

193. Ribstein M. Hypnagogic hallucinations. In: Guilleminault C, Dement WC, Passouant P, eds. Narcolepsy. New York, NY: Spectrum; 1976;145–160.

194. Vogel GW. Mentation reported from naps of narcoleptics. In: Guilleminault C, Dement WC, Passouant P, eds. Narcolepsy. New York, NY: Spectrum; 1976;161–168.

195. Honda Y. Clinical features of narcolepsy: Japanese experiences. In: Honda Y, Juji T, eds. HLA in Narcolepsy. New York, NY: Springer Verlag; 1988;24–57.

196. Aldrich MS. Cardinal manifestations of sleep disorders. In: Kryger MH, Roth T, Dement WC, eds. Principles and Practice of Sleep Medicine. 2nd ed. Philadelphia, Pa: WB Saunders; 1994:418–425.

197. Guilleminault C. Narcolepsy syndrome. In: Kryger MH, Roth T, Dement WC, eds. Principles and Practice of Sleep Medicine. Philadelphia, Pa: WB Saunders; 1989:549–561.

198. Mahowald MW, Schenck CH. REM sleep behavior disorder. In: Kryger MH, Roth T, Dement WC, eds. Principles and Practice of Sleep Medicine. 2nd ed. Philadelphia, Pa: WB Saunders; 1994:574–588.

199. Schenck CH, Mahowald MW. REM sleep parasomnias. Neurol Clin. 1996;14:697–720.

200. Schenck CH, Bundlie SR, Ettinger MG, et al. Chronic behavioral disorders of human REM sleep: a new category of parasomnia. Sleep. 1986;9:293–308.

201. Culebras A. Update on disorders of sleep and the sleep-wake cycle. Psychiatr Clin North Am. 1992;15:467–489.

202. Schenck CH, Mahowald MW. Long-term, nightly benzodiazepine treatment of injurious parasomnias and other disorders of disrupted nocturnal sleep in 170 adults. Am J Med. 1996;100:333–337.

203. Gastaut H, Broughton R. A clinical study of episodic phenomena during sleep. In: Wortis S, ed. Recent Advances in Biological Psychiatry. Vol 7. New York, NY: Plenum; 1964.

204. Broughton RJ. Sleep disorders: disorders of arousal? Enuresis, somnambulism, and nightmares occur in confusional states of arousal, not in "dreaming sleep." Science. 1968;159:1070–1078.

205. Mahowald MW, Rosen GM. Parasomnias in children. Pediatrician. 1990;17:21–31.

206. Fisher C, Kahn E, Edwards A, et al. A psychophysiological study of nightmares and night terrors, I: physiological aspects of the stage 4 night terror. J Nerv Ment Dis. 1973;157:75–98.

207. Nielsen TA. Mentation during sleep. The NREM/REM distinction. In: Lydic R, Baghdoyan HA, eds. Handbook of Behavioral State Control. Cellular and Molecular Mechanisms. Boca Raton, Fla: CRC Press; 1998:101–128.

208. Guilleminault C, Moscovitch A, Leger D. Forensic sleep medicine: nocturnal wandering and violence. Sleep. 1995;18:740–748.

209. Antrobus J. REM and NREM sleep reports: comparison of word frequencies by cognitive classes. Psychophysiology. 1983;20:562–568.

210. Lauerma H, Hublin C, Lehtinen I. Chronic and severe nocturnal hallucinosis based on atypical sleep terrors. Nord J Psychiatry. 1994;48:321–324.

211. Fenwick P. Somnambulism and the law: a review. Behav Sci Law. 1987;5:343–358.

212. Kleitman N. Sleep and Wakefulness. Chicago, Ill: University of Chicago Press; 1963.

213. Blatt I, Peled R, Gadoth N, et al. The value of sleep recording in evaluating somnambulism in young adults. Electroencephalogr Clin Neurophysiol. 1991;78:407–412.

214. Broughton RJ, Shimizu T. Sleep-related violence: a medical and forensic challenge. Sleep. 1995;18:727–730.

215. Schenck CH, Mahowald MW. A polysomnographically documented case of adult somnambulism with long-distance automobile driving and frequent nocturnal violence: parasomnia with continuing danger as a noninsane automatism? Sleep. 1995;18:765–772.

216. Kales JD, Kales A, Soldatos CR, et al. Night terrors: clinical characteristics and personality patterns. Arch Gen Psychiatry. 1980;37:1413–1417.

217. Moldofsky H, Gilbert R, Lue FA, et al. Sleep-related violence. Sleep. 1995;18:731–739.

218. Charcot J-M. Un cas de suppression brusque et isolée de la vision mentale des signes et des objets (formes et couleurs) [On a case of sudden isolated suppression of the mental vision of signs and objects (forms and colors)]. Prog Med. 1883;11:568–571.

219. Charcot J-M. Clinical lectures on diseases of the nervous system. In: Savill T, ed, trans. The New Sydenham Society. 3rd ed. London, England: 1889.

220. Wilbrand H. Die Seelenblindheit als Herderscheinung und ihre Beziehung zur Alexie und Agraphie [Mind-blindness as a focal symptom and its relationship to alexia and agraphia]. Wiesbaden, Germany: Bergmann; 1887.

221. Doricchi F, Violani C. Dream recall in brain-damaged patients: a contribution to the neuropsychology of dreaming through a review of the literature. In: Antrobus JS, Bertini M, eds. The Neuropsychology of Sleep and Dreaming. Hillsdale, NJ: Lawrence Erlbaum Associates; 1992:99–129.

222. Jus A, Jus K, Villeneuve A, et al. Studies on dream recall in chronic schizophrenic patients after prefrontal lobotomy. Biol Psychiatry. 1973;6:275–293.

223. Nielsen TA, Montplaisir J, Marcotte R, et al. Sleep, dreaming, and EEG coherence patterns in agenesis of the corpus callosum: comparisons with callosotomy patients. In: Lassonde M, Jeeves MA, eds. Callosal Agenesis: The Natural Split-Brain. New York, NY: Plenum; 1994:109–117.

224. McCormick L, Nielsen TA, Ptito M, et al. REM sleep dream mentation in right hemispherectomized patients. Neuropsychology. 1997;35:695–701.

225. McCormick L, Nielsen T, Ptito M, et al. Case study of REM sleep dream recall after left hemispherectomy. Brain Cogn. 1998;37:M15.

226. Greenberg MS, Farah MJ. The laterality of dreaming. Brain Cogn. 1986;5:307–321.

227. Antrobus JS. Cortical hemisphere asymmetry and sleep mentation. Psychol Rev. 1987;94:359–368.

228. Kramer M, Roth T, Trinder J. Dreams and dementia: a laboratory exploration of dream recall and dream content in chronic brain syndrome patients. Int J Aging Hum Dev. 1975;6:169–178.

229. Greenberg R, Pearlman C, Brooks R, et al. Dreaming and Korsakoff's psychosis. Arch Gen Psychiatry. 1968;18:203–209.

230. Torda C. Dreams of subjects with loss of memory for recent events. Psychophysiology. 1969;6:358–365.

231. Gruen I, Martinez A, Cruzolloa C, et al. Characteristics of the emotional phenomena in the dreams of patients with temporal lobe epilepsy. Salud Ment. 1997;20:8–15.

232. Epstein AW. Effect of certain cerebral hemispheric diseases on dreaming. Biol Psychiatry. 1979;14:77–93.

233. Ellis H. The World of Dreams. Boston, Mass: Houghton Mifflin; 1911.

234. Garfield P. The Healing Power of Dreams. New York, NY: Simon & Schuster; 1991.

235. Doneshka P, Kehaiyov A. Some peculiarities of the dreams of patients with vestibular diseases. Acta Med Croatica. 1978;32:45–50.

236. Smith RC. Do dreams reflect a biological state? J Nerv Ment Dis. 1987;175:201–207.

237. Gallop D. Aristotle on Sleep and Dreams: A Text and Translation with Introduction, Notes and Glossary. Peterborough, Canada: Broadview Press; 1990.

238. Forman JK, Souney PF. Adverse reactions in hospitalized patients receiving triazolam or temazepam. J Geriatr Drug Ther. 1989;3:55–66.

239. Pagel JF Jr. Diagnosis and treatment of insomnia. Am Fam Physician. 1987;35:191–197.

240. Juhl RP, Daughtery VM, Kroboth PD. Incidence of next-day

anterograde amnesia caused by flurazepam hydrochloride and triazolam. Clin Pharmacol. 1984;3:622–625.

241. Nielsen TA, Zadra AL, Germain A, et al. The 55 typical dreams questionnaire: assessment of 200 sleep patients. Sleep. 1998;21(suppl):286.

242. Zadra AL, Nielsen TA. Typical dreams: a comparison of 1958 versus 1996 student samples. Sleep Res. 1997;26:280–280.

243. Zadra AL, Nielsen TA. The 55 typical dreams questionnaire: assessment across 3 student samples. Sleep. 1999; 22(suppl):S175.

67

Bruxism

Gilles J. Lavigne
Christiane Manzini

The International Classification of Sleep Disorders (ICSD)[1] defines *sleep bruxism* (SB) as "a sterotyped movement disorder characterized by grinding or clenching of the teeth during sleep." It is further classified within the parasomnia section because it is considered an undesirable physical phenomenon that includes skeletal muscle activity that is present during sleep. Since SB is probably different in terms of etiology from daytime parafunctional jaw muscle activity,[2, 3] it should be distinguished from teeth clenching, bracing, or gnashing while awake.[4]

SB frequency is reported to be highly variable over time,[3] meaning that it is possible for SB patients to go several nights or even weeks without bruxism grinding episodes. When they do occur, they are typical of either phasic (rhythmical) or tonic (sustained) motor activity in jaw muscles (e.g., masseter and temporalis) with occasional tooth-grinding sounds.[3, 5] This latter element is the major reason people seek consultation: because these sounds are analogous to stone grinding or the cracking of a hardwood floor, they disrupt their bed partner's sleep. The other reasons that people seek help are related to tooth wear (Fig. 67–1); orofacial pain or temporal area headaches; and tooth hypersensitivity to cold air, beverages, and food.

Bruxism without a medical cause is considered the primary or idiopathic form (Table 67–1), whereas SB associated with a medical condition is the secondary form (Table 67–2). If it is noted following drug intake or withdrawal (e.g., neuroleptics that could induce oral tardive dyskinesia and grinding), it is classified as iatrogenic. Several orofacial activities are frequently concomitant: grimacing, chewing automatism, or excessive lip and tongue movements such as thrust or protusion. In this chapter, the term *sleep bruxism* is used for the teeth oromotor grinding–related activities occurring during sleep, as reported by the sleep partner or family, regardless of its primary, secondary, or iatrogenic forms.

HISTORICAL ASPECTS

According to *Dorland's Illustrated Medical Dictionary*,[6] the word *bruxism* comes from the Greek *brychein*, to gnash the teeth. It further defines *bruxism* as the grinding teeth movements that usually occur during sleep, whereas *bruxomania* is the term used for the neurotic habit performed in the daytime. Interestingly, this corresponds to the definition of Marie and Pietkiewicz in 1907,[7] who observed "contagious" grinding in a group of hospitalized patients with cerebellar injury or mental problems. As reviewed by Faulkner,[8] several terms have been used over the years to describe this phenomenon: *occlusal habit neurosis, neuralgia traumatica, bruxomania, teeth gnashing-grinding*, and *parafunction*. It was Frohman, in 1931, who first introduced the term *bruxism*.[8] Today, bruxism is classified as a sleep parasomnia (ICSD[1]), an orofacial parafunction,[4] a craniocervical dyskinesia,[9] a tic, or an automatism.[10] In 1992, the term *brycose* was further suggested for the severe destructive form of bruxism; *brycho-* for movement with teeth contact, and *-ose* for abnormal exaggerated activity.[11]

Over the 20th century, theories regarding the etiology of bruxism swung like a pendulum. The role of peripheral dental occlusion had its moment of glory, and in fact there are still some practitioners convinced of its importance.[12, 13] But the popular trend is toward a global explanation including personality style, one's capacity to adapt to life pressures as induced by his or her psychosocial environment, and brain neurochemi-

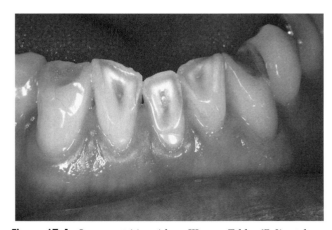

Figure 67–1. Severe attrition (class III; see Table 67–3) at lower anterior tooth level with reduction of crown height (greater than 50%); note the loss of buccal tooth surface and the presence of secondary dentine reaction at the central area (dental canal). This 55-year-old patient had both protrusive-retrusive and lateral jaw displacements while grinding during his sleep as confirmed with audiovideo recordings.

Table 67–1. TYPES OF BRUXISM

Awake Vs. Sleep Time

Awake time—tooth clenching/tapping, jaw bracing without tooth
  contact (grinding is rarely noted during the daytime)
Sleep time—tooth grinding with phasic (rhythmical)/tonic
  (sustained) clenching or mixed (both) jaw muscle contractions

Primary/Idiopathic, Secondary/Iatrogenic Forms

Primary/idiopathic—without known medical or dental causes but
  which could be associated with exacerbating psychosocial
  factors in some patients
Secondary—associated with a medical/psychiatric condition (could
  also be iatrogenic [see Table 67–2])
Iatrogenic—following drug intake/withdrawal

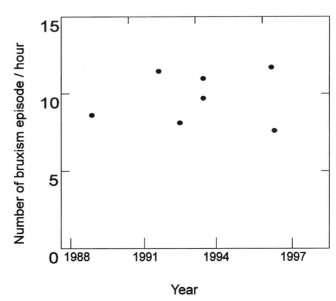

Figure 67–2. Variation, over 8 years (one man between 36 and 44 years of age), of sleep bruxism (SB) frequency (number of episodes per hour of sleep). Although, this patient has had episodes of bruxism every night since childhood, some SB patients may go weeks or months without grinding.

cal and homeostatic sleep-maintaining mechanisms associated with autonomic and motor nervous systems activity.[2, 3, 14–17]

EPIDEMIOLOGY AND RISK FACTORS

Most studies and surveys reporting the prevalence of sleep bruxism (number of positive cases at a given time) are based on subject self-reports regarding clenching during daytime, or both clenching and grinding during sleep. As yet, no longitudinal study using biological recordings has been conducted to estimate

Table 67–2. SECONDARY OR IATROGENIC BRUXISM

Movement Disorders

Oral tardive dyskinesia[60, 130–133]
Oromandibular dystonia (Meige's syndrome)[130, 131, 134, 135]
Parkinson's disease[59, 136, 137]
Tics—simple (grunting) and complex (Tourette's syndrome)[89, 130, 138]

Sleep-Related Disorders

RLS/PLMS (limb myoclonia)[15, 24]
Sleep fragmentary myoclonus: oromandibular-facial-lingual[89, 108, 139]
Apnea/snoring[109]
REM sleep behavior disorders[32, 140]
Epilepsy (not observed yet in our SB sample)[1]

Neurological and Psychiatric-Related Disorders

Cerebellar hemorrhage[141]
Olivopontocerebellar atrophy and Shy-Prager syndrome[32]
Coma[142]
Neurological complication related to Whipple's disease[143]
Mental health problems (e.g., dementia, depression, mental
  retardation)[2, 3, 7, 43, 144]

Drug- or Chemical-Related to Bruxism

Alcohol[2, 145]
Cocaine[146]
Amphetamines[147]
Weight-control drugs such as the amphetamine-derivative
  fenfluramine (Ponderal)[125]
Antidopaminergic: haloperidol (Haldol)[60, 69]
Selective serotonin reuptake inhibitors: fluoxetine (Prozac),
  sertraline (Zoloft)[73, 74]
Calcium inhibitor: flunarizine (Sibelium) in OTD patient[60]

OTD, oral tardive dyskinesia; PLMS, periodic limb movements in sleep; RLS, restless legs syndrome; SB, sleep bruxism.

SB fluctuation (Fig. 67–2) or its persistence in a given individual with respect to age. Moreover, many SB patients are not aware of grinding if they sleep alone or with a "deep sleep" partner. The overall prevalence of daytime clenching "awareness" is reported by approximately 20% of the adult population with more females reporting than males.[18–20] According to parental reports, the incidence of sleep grinding is between 14 and 20% in children younger than 11 years of age. Concomitant oral activities such as biting the nails (onycophagia) is also noted in 9 to 28% of those reporting, and thumb sucking is seen in 21% of children.[21–23] In adults, the prevalence of grinding drops with age: from 13% in those aged 18 to 29 to 3% in those aged 60 years and older, with a mean of 8%. No further gender differences were noted.[24] Caution is necessary in interpreting these numbers, however, because reduced incidence with age can result from an inaccurate estimate due to the high prevalence of denture users in the older population (e.g., greater than 40% in some geographical areas).

Several concomitant risk factors have been linked to SB. Grinding and restless legs syndrome are associated, although only in 10% of the population.[24] Smokers are 1.9 times more at risk of being grinders (significant odds ratio),[25] although it remains to be determined if the variance could be explained by seeing smoking as an oral habit or as a nicotine physiological influence. Another variable related to SB is the concomitant finding of orofacial pain or joint sound or lock at the temporomandibular level; SB patients are three to four times more at risk for pain and jaw limitation.[20, 26] For example, we found that one third of severe SB patients reported moderate pain in the morning, which was associated with a lower frequency of SB episodes per hour of sleep than matched controls.[26, 27] Finally, the prevalence of grinding noted in an institutionalized mentally retarded population is similar to the figure reported in the general population[24, 28]; consequently, mental retardation could not be considered a strong risk factor or as a major factor in the etiological pathophysiology of SB.

PATHOPHYSIOLOGY

A single mechanism or theory cannot explain SB pathophysiology. Rather, this motor activity is more likely the result of biological and psychosocial influences within a given individual. Bruxism probably results from a series of influences that are not obeying a mechanistic model or the logic of an algorithm.

Rhythmical Masticatory Muscle Activity During Sleep in Asymptomatic Sleepers

In the mid- to late 1990s, we recorded masseter electromyographic (EMG) activity in 848 sleep laboratory subjects to assess the specificity of rhythmical masticatory motor activity (RMMA) in the jaw closer muscles. We observed that 58% of our "normal sleepers" (n = 119) exhibited RMMA (three masseter muscle rhythmical contractions in the absence of tooth grinding) during sleep.[16, 29] Gastaut et al.[30] first described the presence of these rhythmical activities in jaw muscles as the "automatismes masticatoires hypniques/diduction-contraction des mâchoires" with grinding if the intensity was elevated. Later, in patients with somnambulism and night terrors, the term *chewing automatism* was used to describe the slow rhythmical masticatory activity.[31] This term was later used in the identification of the orofacial activities noticed with the "REM [rapid eye movement] behavior disorders."[32] Phasic oromotor activity associated with SB is probably an extreme manifestation of an ongoing or natural activity during sleep.

Stress and Psychosocial Influences

As recently as 1949, bruxism was associated with "anxiety and hyperactivity" by several authors, this despite the fact that the Minnesota Multiphasic Personality Inventory (MMPI) and the Cornell Medical Index gave different or confounding outcomes.[33, 34] Recently, the monitoring of 100 patients with bruxism, both during daytime using self-reports of stress and during sleep with portable EMG, revealed a low statistical association (only in eight subjects) between "diurnal perceived stress" and nocturnal change in EMG of the masseter muscle.[35] Interestingly, it was argued that SB subjects, owing to their coping style, are unaware, minimizing, and are more likely to deny the impact of life events on their own stress reactivity.[2, 35] Consequently, the common belief of patients and clinicians that stress triggers SB needs to be reviewed. SB subjects seem to be more task-oriented as a result of their personality and coping style as opposed to being in a pathological stress-related pattern.[2, 35]

Sleep Intrinsic Fluctuations and Reactions

Comparative studies between SB subjects and controls[5, 36–39] have shown that SB patients have a normal sleep organization as assessed by the macrostructure of sleep. They have normal sleep latency and total sleep time, and a normal percentage of the various sleep stages and number of awakenings. They also report a normal amount of time spent awake, as well as sleep efficiency during the night. Thus they do not complain about sleeping poorly.[38] One study reported that some severe bruxers (of an older age than in most published studies) had 20% less REM sleep than would be "expected" from the literature[40]; these data need to be reproduced in a controlled study.

Most SB episodes (60 to 80%) have been scored in sleep stages 1 and 2,[5, 38, 39, 41] although the literature is confusing. It was first reported that SB occurs mainly in REM sleep, but later the authors retracted this statement owing to a methodological error in scoring.[42] Moreover, a high incidence of "destructive" SB, scored from electroencephalographic (EEG) artifacts, was also reported in REM sleep[43] of patients suffering from depression, a condition known to influence REM sleep.

A study in 1998 also supported the lack of correlation between SB and full arousal.[39] Conversely, there are several observations suggesting that SB is associated with microarousals and alterations of sleep microstructure. For example, sleep bruxers showed 30% more body movements than controls,[44] and time-restricted changes in heart rate were seen before and during bruxing episodes.[45–47] As well, 50% of SB episodes are preceded by alpha EEG activity.[41] All of this supports the concept that SB may represent a transient motor and autonomic nervous system manifestation of microarousals.

There is also a growing interest in the existence of periodic changes in several physiological functions that occur at a frequency of approximately one every 20 to 60 sec during sleep; these periodic changes in the EEG are called the cyclic alternating pattern (CAP). There are several findings suggesting that this basic rhythm modulates several other physiological functions, including heart rate, respiration, and motor activity during sleep.[48] Between 60 and 88% of SB episodes have been noted to occur in the active phase A of these CAPs.[39, 49]

Transient EEG activation is also characterized by K complexes and alpha activity in the EEG. In a pilot study of K complexes in SB patients vs. controls completed in 1997, we found, contrary to our expectations, a major decrease in the K complexes of SB patients.[50] In the past, K complexes have been associated with SB,[5, 46] although there has been no controlled study comparing the number, density, or morphology of K complexes in SB with those in normal controls. It remains to be shown if, as suggested for other sleep disorders,[51] these EEG events have, in SB subjects, a protective influence on sleep organization and contribute to the maintenance of sleep continuity.[52, 53]

Oromotor Excitability

Little experimental evidence supports the role of the motor system as a primary factor in the genesis of SB. At best, some very indirect information from animal physiological studies may help us understand how the motor system is comodulated during sleep. First, it was noted that the stimulation of a rabbit's amygdala and the lateral hypothalamus in the limbic area resulted in rhythmical jaw movements[54] and tooth grinding.[55] Furthermore, intracellular recordings of the cat's trigeminal jaw closer and opener motoneurons show that the excitability of these cells is specifically modulated during sleep[56, 57]; from wakefulness to quiet sleep to active sleep (AS or REM), a decline in the tonic jaw EMG level is noted. For human beings, as for animals, it is suggested that fluctuations in the activity of the reticular motor area in relation to sleep modulation could be associated with periodic motor excitation;[56, 58] this, however, remains to be demonstrated.

Catecholamines and Neurochemistry

In 1970, Magee[59] noted that a patient with Parkinson's disease treated with levodopa (L-dopa) for several weeks had exhibited the side effect of grinding his teeth during the day as well as during sleep. This was the initial support for the suggestion that grinding was related to dopaminergic brain-related neurotransmitters,[3, 46] although no evidence came from controlled study. In 1993, this was also reported for some schizophrenic patients treated with neuroleptic drugs as a manifestation of oromandibular tardive dyskinesia.[60] The association of dopamine (DA) and SB from these reports is somewhat weak because it is based on evidence in patients with altered nigrostriatal (basal ganglia) neurochemistry, as well as including those for whom grinding could be a side effect of drug use.

Some evidence gathered during the 1990s further suggests that catecholamines, such as DA and noradrenaline (NA), may have a role in SB pathophysiology. A controlled polysomnographic study done in SB subjects with the catecholamine precursor levodopa (L-dopa) revealed a reduction in SB frequency in comparison to placebo.[61] A similar decrease was noted in two patients receiving bromocriptine, a D2 receptor agonist.[62] Moreover, a more important asymmetrical distribution of DA binding at the nigrostriatal level was noted in SB patients.[63] Regarding the exact significance of this nigrostriatal asymmetry in SB pathophysiology, which remains to be established, we have to consider that a similar DA-striatal asymmetry is also noted in both torticollis and parkinsonian patients.[64–67]

The other catecholamine-related medication reported to reduce SB and tooth grinding is propranolol, a beta-blocker. In an open study, propranolol was reported to reduce polysomnographic SB motor activity in one severe SB subject without medical disorders.[68] This same medication was also associated with a reduction in daytime tooth grinding in two neuroleptic-treated patients presenting with abnormal orofacial movements,[69] but no objective or controlled recordings were done. We do not know, at this time, if the action of propranolol on SB is (1) specific, that is, related to an indirect sedative action or cardiovascular effect by preventing the stress-related responses; or (2) related to the central depression of medullary reticular formation (a brain structure involved in the genesis of rhythmical oromandibular movements[54]) that was reported to inhibit motoneurons, presumably through beta-adrenergic receptors during sleep.[58] Moreover, we have to be cautious in using propranolol since it was reported to have deleterious influences on sleep quality and architecture such as late onset and increased numbers of awakenings and dreams.[70–72]

Also, before interpreting studies using specific pharmacological agents in SB, we have to remember that other neurotransmitters (e.g., 5-hydroxytrytomine [5-HT, serotonin], cholecystokinin, gamma-aminobutyric acid)[16] and drugs (e.g., selective serotonin reuptake inhibitors such as fluoxetine [Prozac][73] or sertraline [Zoloft][74]) are involved in exacerbation of tooth grinding and rhythmical movement modulation,[16, 75] respectively.

Genetics and Familial Predisposition

As yet, no genetic markers have been found for bruxism for the mode of SB transmission. It is, however, interesting to report that between 21 and 50% of SB patients have a direct family member who ground his or her teeth in childhood.[18, 21, 76] Furthermore, studies done with monozygotic and dizygotic twins showed that SB was more frequently observed in monozygotic twins.[77–79] A concomitant finding by a recent Finnish study revealed that childhood SB persisted in a large number of adults (greater than 86.9%).[79] It is therefore possible that genetics play a role in SB. Nevertheless the pattern of inheritance is unknown and the influence of risk factors remains to be assessed.[79]

Possible Role of Local Factors Such as Dental Occlusion

In the 1960s, indirect daytime physiological EMG recordings[80] suggested that tooth occlusal and mechanical interferences were responsible for grinding. Although this concept of "peripheral" causes of SB is still reported to be of interest for some dental clinicians,[12, 13, 81] it is controversial.[14, 82] We have to recall that teeth contacts are not a dominant activity in a 24-h cycle; it has been estimated to occur for approximately 17.5 min/24 h.[83] Moreover, during sleep, oromotor SB-related activity does not always occur with tooth contact; grinding sounds are reported in approximately 30% of the episodes.[5, 36] A conclusion to the debate on the role of dental occlusion in SB is well beyond the scope of this chapter.

Reduced Salivary Flow and Jaw Motor Activity

Another concern is frequently raised. Could RMMA or SB jaw movements reverse the reduced salivary flow which occurs naturally during sleep?[84, 85] To our knowledge, no sleep data directly support this premise, although it is known that chewing movements (similar to those in SB) stimulate salivary flow when people are awake.[86, 87] Moreover, the low salivary flow observed during sleep is probably related to the low swallowing frequency: between 2.1 and 9.1 swallowing movements per hour of sleep are observed, which is much less when compared with the daytime swallowing rate (more than 25 times per hour).[88] It could then be hypothesized that the RMMA could be associated with an increase in salivary flow during sleep to lubricate the oroesophageal tissues. Tooth wear is clinically worse in patients with xerostomia (e.g., Sjögren's syndrome), gastroesophageal reflux, or in bulimic patients who vomit; in some of these cases we noticed a dramatic breakdown of tooth structure. Consequently, specific clinical management has to be planned (see Table 67–8).

CLINICAL FEATURES

Clinicians will be able to diagnose bruxism in their patients using the following clinical features as a guide[1, 3, 4, 38] (Tables 67–3 and 67–4): (1) teeth grinding or tapping sounds noticed by the sleep partner or a family member; (2) complaints of jaw muscle discomfort, fatigue or stiffness, and occasional headaches (e.g., temporalis muscles); (3) the presence of tooth wear (see Fig. 67–1 and Table 67–3); (4) teeth (one or several) sensitive to hot or cold; (5) muscle hypertrophy; (6) temporomandibular joint (TMJ) sound (clicking) or jaw lock (e.g., reduction of opening amplitude); (7) tongue indentation.

Tooth-grinding or tapping sounds have to be objectively distinguished from confounding oral sounds during sleep such as snoring, throat grunting, tongue clicking, or TMJ sounds upon jaw movements.[89] The presence of muscle or TMJ tenderness or pain is usu-

Table 67–3. TOOTH ENAMEL OR CROWN WEAR WITH PRESENCE OF FACETS (SHINY SPOTS)[93]

Class I	Tooth enamel or crown wear with presence of facets (polish-like) or fillings with shiny spots (dry the tooth with air or cotton and use a dental mirror)
Class II	Loss of enamel with dentin exposure and slight reduction of crown height or chipped incisal ridge or cuspids
Class III	Extensive dentin wear (>2 mm²) with lost of crown height (>50%) and flattening of cusps (see Fig. 67–1)

Table 67–4. CLINICAL FEATURES OF BRUXISM

Reported by Patients

During Sleep

Tooth grinding (or tapping)
Sounds noticed by another person

Upon Awakening During Sleep or at Morning

Tooth wear or muscle hypertrophy affecting aesthetics
Jaw muscle discomfort (fatigue or tension) with or without pain
Temporal muscle headache/tenderness
Stiff jaw/reduced mobility/difficulty in biting into food at breakfast
Exacerbation by life pressure/stress
Teeth hypersensitive to cold food (sometimes heat), liquid, air
Frequent tooth restoration failure (e.g., filling, bridge)

Observed by Clinicians

Tooth wear (see Fig. 67–1)/shiny spots on filling
Masseter muscle hypertrophy upon voluntary jaw clenching (less important at temporalis level)
Muscle (masseter, temporalis, pterygoids, sternocleidomastoid) or temporomandibular joint tenderness or pain upon digital palpation
Tongue indendation
Tense personality or hypervigilant patient (subjective appreciation)
Polygraphic observation of jaw muscle activity and of tooth-grinding sounds (audiovideo)

Others

Exacerbation of periodontal disease (controversial issue)
Reduction in salivary flow/xerostomia
Lip/cheek biting
Burning tongue sometimes concomitant with oral habits

ally confirmed by digital palpation. Use of a visual analogue scale (e.g., 0 to 100 mm with no pain and worst pain at both extremes) or a numerical scale (0 to 10) can be used to score the patient's subjective reports. Approximately 1 SB patient in 5 will complain of pain on awakening and occasionally during sleep. The patients with diurnal clenching will mainly report pain toward the end of the afternoon and in the evening.[26, 27]

The presence of tooth wear may represent other problems. Attrition by bruxism is different from attrition resulting from dental work (e.g., crown, bridge, or denture; tooth equilibration with a dental bur) or trauma (e.g., pipe, sports injury, abrasive dust in working milieu, etc.) and from erosion due to chemical (e.g., lemon sucking) or gastroesophageal reflux or vomiting (e.g., bulimia). The wear may also be exacerbated by craniodental morphology, which changes with aging. What is noticed at the time of examination may have no link with the current ongoing muscle activity because bruxism frequency fluctuates over time[3, 36, 90, 91] (see Fig. 67–2). Wear can also be localized to one tooth, a few teeth, or up to a full segment (e.g., lower incisors). The wear pattern can be seen within a normal movement range or with an eccentric jaw position. Finally, although 100% of those with bruxism show tooth wear, so do 40% of those who are asymptomatic.[92] Thus, tooth wear alone cannot be relied upon to make a definite diagnosis. The other factors mentioned above must also be taken into consideration. Tooth sensitivity to temperature stimulations (e.g., cold liquid or air) is also reported following sleep periods with teeth clenching, grinding, or tapping.

Another clinical feature used to recognize SB is the presence of masseter muscle hypertrophy. This is easily seen when the subject is voluntarily clenching the teeth together when a unilateral or bilateral mass will protrude on the side of the face under the zygomatic arch. Upon relaxation, this mass disappears. This needs to be differentiated from the swelling resulting from periodontal abscess or the trauma from wisdom tooth extraction. It should also not be confused with parotid gland tumor or the blockage of Wharton's parotid salivary duct by a calculus, or sustained contraction of the masseter muscle that constricts the salivary flow. This last problem is called the parotid-masseter syndrome.[3]

DIAGNOSTIC EVALUATION

Clinical

The clinical diagnosis of SB is based on the patient's history and orofacial examination. The presence of tooth wear (see Fig. 67–1) could be scored (see Table 67–3) from criteria derived from the literature.[11, 91, 93] To assess tooth wear, dry the tooth with air or cotton and use a dental mirror with a light source. Furthermore, tooth wear can be monitored over time by taking dental arch impressions and visually analyzing wear patterns using casts or models. For research purposes, scanning electron microscopy or computerized laser analysis could be used.[91, 94, 95] Another technique allows the monitoring of wear intensity by using intraoral appliances, for example, the Bruxcore Plate.[96] The validity of this measure for SB frequency assessment is, however, questionable because Bruxcore plate data do not correlate strongly with ongoing SB muscle activity as controlled with ambulatory EMG units[96] and the presence of an oral appliance can influence (increase or decrease) the ongoing EMG activity.[97, 98]

The diagnosis of muscle hypertrophy is made by considering the patient's age and dentofacial morphology, and after ruling out salivary gland swelling caused by infection. The patient is asked to clench the teeth, which induces a protruding mass at the masseter muscle level (rarely the temporalis). Using the fingers, a positive score is given if the contracted muscle volume increases at least twofold. For research purposes, sliding rules or ultrasonography measures can also be done,[99–101] although they are not yet validated for SB diagnostic purposes.

Moreover, we suggest that the following be noted in the patient file: (1) tooth wear location and severity; (2) the presence or absence of masseter muscle hypertrophy; (3) report of sensitive teeth, pain, or tenderness upon digital palpation of muscles and the TMJ; (4) maximum jaw displacement (use the space between both upper and lower central incisors as reference point); and (5) the presence or absence of joint sounds (e.g., TMJ clicking or grating) using finger palpation.

Ambulatory Monitoring

The monitoring of SB motor activity is also possible using other techniques. First, audiovideo home recordings can help to estimate sound frequency and jaw displacement. But without polygraphy it can be very difficult to assess the specificity of oral sounds from snoring, throat grunting, tooth tapping, TMJ clicking, or tooth grinding, or from jaw movements such as swallowing, rumination, typical chewing-like movements, smiling, or orofacial myoclonia, and so forth.[16, 89] Second, ambulatory EMG recordings help to monitor SB at home. The first systems used allowed one-channel masseteric EMG (surface) monitoring during sleep.[97, 102–104] Full ambulatory multichannel (EEG, EMG, electrocardiogram, respiration, movement, etc.) recorders, with a very good-quality EMG signal, are now available (e.g., Embla, Medical Inc., Reykjavik, Iceland; Biosaca, Biosis, Gotheborg, Sweden). Again, although the use of ambulatory recordings allows the monitoring of a patient in his or her own environment, it has some limitations. It is difficult to assess precisely the specificity of EMG activity over the large spectrum of orofacial activities that occurs during sleep such as swallowing, coughing, grunting, sighs, yawning, sleep-talking, smiling, and so forth.[16, 89, 105] Moreover, it should be noted that up to 40% of all orofacial activities scored during sleep (polygraphic and audiovideo recordings) are not specific to SB.[38] Despite these limitations, ambulatory recordings are a valuable complement to sleep laboratory recordings because they allow low-cost monitoring over several nights in the patient's natural environment. The suggested SB scoring algorithm for ambulatory recordings (Table 67–5) needs further validation along with laboratory polysomnography.[104, 106]

Sleep Laboratory

In the sleep laboratory, a highly controlled but less natural milieu, recording the following biological signals frequently completes the diagnosis of SB (see Fig. 67–3): (1) two EEGs (C3A2, 02A1); (2) right and left electro-oculograms (EOGs); (3) EMGs (surface) of both (right and left) jaw masseter and temporalis muscles for SB scoring with chin and suprahyoid muscles to score standard sleep atonia in REM and of the anterior tibialis to rule out periodic leg movements; (4) nasal airflow and microphone recordings for sleep apnea and snoring assessments; (5) audiovideo recordings for specific quantification of jaw and orofacial activities (zoom on face).

These recordings should be done in a temperature-controlled room where light (use black lights for video) and sound are minimal. Before sleep, subjects should swallow, cough, open the jaw vertically and laterally, as well as clench and tap the teeth to help score and assess the EMG signal recognition pattern. All night data are recorded with a computer at a minimum of 128 Hz acquisition speed[38] and analyzed according to the standard Rechtschaffen and Kales criteria.[107] Com-

Table 67–5. CRITERIA SUGGESTED FOR SLEEP BRUXISM DIAGNOSIS USING AMBULATORY AND SLEEP LABORATORY RECORDINGS

Ambulatory[104, 106]

EMG (RMS) level	>10% of maximum (voluntary clench while awake)
EMG periodicity	<5 sec between events
EMG duration	>3 sec
Heart rate change	>5% in beats per minute with an EMG event
Minimum acquisition	16.7-Hz or 0.05-sec frequency for EMG or time resolution

Sleep Laboratory[38]

Mean SB EMG potentials	>20% of the maximum voluntary clench while awake
SB episodes types[5, 38, 43]	
Phasic (rhythmical)	>3 EMG bursts, separated by 2 interburst pauses, in masseter or temporalis muscle lasting >0.25 sec and <2.0 sec
Tonic (sustained)	1 EMG burst lasting >2.0 sec
Mixed	Both phasic and tonic types
Minimum acquisition frequency	128 Hz
Diagnostic cut-off criteria (research)	Sensitivity >72%; specificity >94% Bruxism episodes/h >4 Bruxism bursts/h >25 Minimum episode(s) with grinding 1 per sleep period

EMG, electromyogram; RMS, root mean square of masseter muscle; SB, sleep bruxism.

puter screen segments of 20 or 30 sec can be used. The SB EMG episodes of at least 20% of the maximum voluntary contraction while awake are scored in parallel with audiovideo signals. Three types of SB events are identified (see Table 67–5)—phasic, tonic, or mixed—according to criteria derived from the literature[5, 38, 43] (Fig. 67–3). If bursts of less than 0.25 sec are noticed in temporalis or masseter muscles, they are scored as myoclonic events and separated from bruxism.[89, 108, 108a] We found that 10% of those who were clinically diagnosed with SB had this activity during sleep. Because repetitive myoclonus can be confounded with epileptic spikes, a third night of recording was done with full EEG montage; this did not reveal such neurological disease.

The frequency of SB bursts (single EMG event) are quantified per episode and per hour of sleep, with or without the presence of grinding sounds or leg movement. After training, a strong reliability in scoring the frequencies of events and a moderate capacity to discriminate episode types (i.e., phasic, tonic, or mixed) can be achieved.[38] Again, it is strongly suggested that the audiovideo signal be used in parallel with a polygraphic recording to differentiate SB episodes occurring with snoring, swallowing, major body movement, somniloquy, and so forth.

Other Diagnostic Features

Using the suggested research cut-off criteria to establish a sleep diagnosis of SB (see Table 67–5), bruxism can be correctly predicted in 83.3% of bruxers, as can the asymptomatic status in 81.3% of controls.[38] The clinical use of these research cut-offs needs further validation in a larger population. It is important to note that even if the first night was for habituation, approximately 10% of SB subjects invited to the sleep laboratory did not have a full night of sleep (several awakenings with no habituation to sleep laboratory conditions or refusal to appear on the experimental second night). Following the polygraphic evaluation of severe SB patients, it is important to rule out sleep disorders such as apnea, periodic limb movements in sleep (PLMS), epilepsy, REM behavior disorder, and so on, and other activities (see Tables 67–2 and 67–6).

Sleep architecture variables such as sleep duration, efficiency, number of awakenings, movements, arousal, and sleep stages are not different between SB and asymptomatic controls.[5, 17, 36–39] However, significant sleep-related variables characterizing SB are the following:

- Up to three times more EMG bruxism episodes occur per hour of sleep.[17, 37–39]
- Most SB episodes will usually be scored in light sleep stages (60 to 80% in stages 1 and 2)[5, 17, 37–39, 109] rather than in REM sleep.[40, 43]
- Slightly more SB episodes can be noted when subjects sleep on their back.[109, 110]

No obvious differences were noted in the frequency of periodic leg movements during sleep.[16, 24, 38, 41, 109] At the EEG level, most SB episodes can be observed in relation to the active phase of the CAP[39, 49] and the presence of K complexes is three times less frequent than in asymptomatic matched subjects.[50] Some EEG alpha wave intrusions could also be noted before SB episodes, but the specificity of this observation needs further validation in a controlled study.[40] Finally, as for body movements during sleep, an autonomic response

Table 67–6. DIFFERENTIAL DIAGNOSIS OF SLEEP BRUXISM

EMG/EEG

Natural ongoing rhythmical masticatory muscle activity or chewing automatism

Clenching from muscle spasm with drug intake (e.g., cocaine)

Orofacial/cervical myoclonia, dystonia (Meige's syndrome) or tardive dyskinesia

Abnormal swallowing pattern

Orofacial movements with sighs, somniloquy, smiling, swallowing, coughing, etc.

Epileptic-related activity (be careful with frontal EEG electrode position over temporalis muscle which could give rise to artifact)

Sounds

Tooth grinding with bruxism from a patient with oral tardive dyskinesia, Meige's syndrome, Parkinson's disease, or other neurological condition

Sounds such as snoring, throat grunting, temporomandibular joint sound (click), somniloquy, sigh, etc.*

*EMG and audiovideo recordings help to discriminate.
EEG, electroencephalogram, EMG, electromyogram.

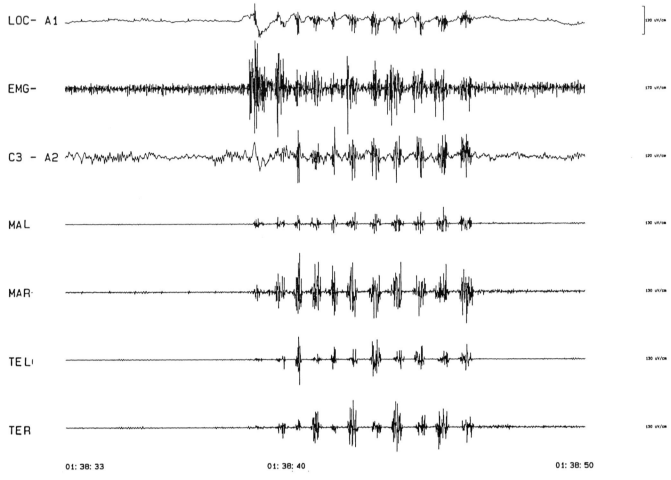

LOC- A1

EMG-

C3 - A2

MA L

MAR·

TE L'

TE R

01: 38: 33   01: 38: 40   01: 38: 50

Figure 67–3. Polygraphic traces of one rhythmical sleep bruxism episode (same subject as in Fig. 67–4). The three upper traces are the left eye (electro-oculogram [EOG] = LOC—A1), submental electromyogram (EMG), and C3A2 electroencephalogram (EEG); all show the rhythmical pattern with movement artifacts in both the EOG and EEG. The left (L) and right (R) masseter (MA) and temporalis (TE) muscle activity is associated with 11 phasic (rhythmical) bursts. In this patient, a co-contraction between closer (MA and TE) and submental opener muscles (EMG) is noted.

is also noted with SB episodes, and acceleration in the heart rate precedes or is concomitant with SB.[5, 17, 41, 45, 106]

MANAGEMENT

As yet, there is no specific cure for bruxism. The clinician's role is to manage these patients with the main goals being the prevention of damage to the orofacial structures and the reduction of sensory complaints. The current types of intervention are oriented toward behavioral, orodental, and pharmacological strategies, but controlled studies that confirm the efficacy of these strategies are lacking. Some of the following recommendations directly address the patient's awareness of the disorder, as well as stress and anxiety management (Table 67–7).

Behavioral strategies should begin with a short and comprehensive explanation of bruxism to the patient, including its definition, causes, and consequences. Next, sleep hygiene instructions are given. The ones we use are derived from Zarcone.[111]

The psychological and behavioral management

strategies for SB have been of major interest for years.[33, 112] No persistent or obvious effects have been obtained with relaxation and tension reduction or exercise strategies,[33, 103, 113] but several patients have reported a sensation of well-being. One study reported a reduction in both EMG activity and grinding frequency following hypnotherapy,[114] but, no control therapy was used. The use of biofeedback, with loud sounds, is also reported to reduce SB EMG activity,[103, 105, 115] but this effect may not last over time without the regular use of the device.

Occlusal appliances, such as a mouth guard or stabilization bite splint, can protect the orofacial structures from damage. The soft mouth guard is usually recommended for use only on a short-term basis because degradation can occur rapidly. The hard occlusal stabilization splint, covering a full dental arch (Fig. 67–4), is particularly useful for patients who are frequent and severe grinders or clenchers.[14] However, not every bruxer finds relief with these orthopedic treatments. Several studies showed a reduction in SB EMG-related levels with short-term use of a splint,[103, 116] an effect that rapidly disappears when patients stop using the

Table 67–7. PALLIATIVE MANAGEMENT
OF SLEEP BRUXISM

Behavioral (With Autocontrol)

Explanation causes/exacerbates SB
Reverse the habit of clenching teeth/bracing jaw during daytime in
  reaction to life pressures
Relaxation, autohypnosis, lifestyle, and sleep hygiene; wind down
  before sleep
Biofeedback
Physical therapy and training (relaxation, breathing)
Psychology (stress/life pressure management
Aversive electrical lip stimulation[148]

Orodental

Mouth guard (soft, short-term)
Bite splint (hard, need follow-up visits)
Dental occlusion (controversy over tooth equilibration and
  orthodontic bite corrections)

**Pharmacological (Short-Term and for
Most Disturbing Conditions)**

Benzodiazepines (e.g., diazepam, clonazepam,* lorazepam*)
Muscle relaxants (e.g., methocarbamol, cyclobenzaprine*)
Serotonin-related: *no effect* for L-tryptophan or amitriptyline but
  exacerbation with fenfluramine, fluoxetine, sertraline[149]
Dopaminergic (e.g., levo-dopa and possibly bromocriptine,*
  pergolide,* or pramipexole,* with domperidone to reduce side
  effects)
Beta blocker (e.g., propranolol*)
Botulinum toxin*

*Of unknown efficacy or may exacerbate sleep disorders (see text).
SB, sleep bruxism.

appliance. Conversely, others found an increase in muscle activity in 20% of hard splint users and in 50% of soft splint users,[97, 98] while others have reported no changes in SB EMG activity.[117, 118] Splints may therefore be considered as "crutches" or "bumpers" which prevent tissue damage or influence oral habits.[119] Clinicians should also be aware that compliance is very low over time; fewer than 20% of patients use the splint after 1 year. Finally, patients should be instructed to keep the hard splint in water to maintain proper hydration, and follow-up is recommended to control appliance stability and oral health.

Tooth equilibration, to reduce occlusal interference, has also been suggested as a treatment for SB.[12, 80] Although the efficacy of such therapy for bruxism is controversial,[4, 14, 16, 82] it is sometimes appropriate following major dental restoration (e.g., crown and bridge work) or orthodontic treatment to restore "oral comfort."

Pharmacological management is indicated on a short-term basis only. Centrally acting drugs in the *benzodiazepine* group and *muscle relaxants* are reported by clinicians to reduce bruxism-related motor activity.[16] To our knowledge, only diazepam and methocarbamol have been tested in an open design.[120, 121] These medications are usually prescribed at bedtime, and patients have to be informed of possible side effects (e.g., not driving in the morning owing to potential drowsiness).

Antidepressants such as the tricyclics have also been recommended for the management of SB.[122] A recent controlled study using ambulatory EMG failed to support the efficacy of a small dose of amitriptyline (25

mg per night) in SB management.[123] But replication with higher doses needs to be done before concluding that amitriptyline is definitively ineffective. The associated xerostomia, as frequently reported in the first few weeks, can be managed (Table 67–8). The use of *selective serotonin reuptake inhibitors* such as fluoxetine and sertraline was reported to induce clenching or grinding.[73, 74] Finally, the use of L-tryptophan (serotonin precursor) in SB management was reported to have no effect[124] and the use of a weight-control medication related to serotonin, fenfluramine (Ponderal), was also noted to exacerbate grinding.[125] Therefore, caution is suggested before using serotonin-related medication in SB management.

The literature on the safe use of *dopamine*-related medications is inconclusive. Patients with chronic antidopaminergic drug exposure (e.g. haloperidol, a dopaminergic antagonist) exhibited iatrogenic grinding similar to that associated with oral tardive dyskinesia,[69] as did L-dopa (a dopaminergic precursor) in a patient already suffering from Parkinson's disease.[59] In SB patients without a medical history, a recent study has

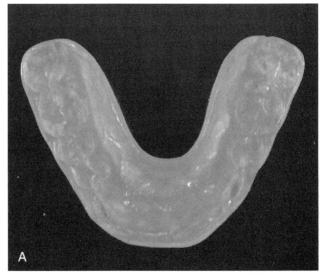

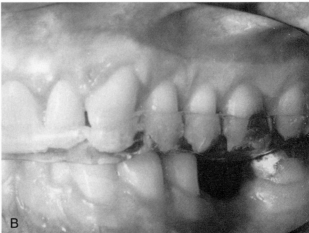

Figure 67–4. *A*, An oral appliance (bite splint) made in hard acrylic to protect the upper teeth from wear associated with grinding. *B*, A similar appliance in the mouth.

Table 67–8. OTHER MODALITIES FOR MANAGEMENT OF SLEEP BRUXISM

For Children and Teenagers

Behavioral managment plus soft mouth guard (replace frequently with growth) can be used with similar behavioral strategies, listed in Table 67–7.

For Hypersensitive Teeth Secondary to Bruxism

0.4% Stannous fluoride gel (e.g., Gel-Kam) as local application, or in mouth guard or splint used concomitantly to reduce clenching

For Dry Mouth (Xerostomia) (Which Could Increase Tooth Wear)

Have a medical evaluation to rule out diabetes, Sjögren's syndrome, etc.
Avoid coffee, tea, colas, etc., in the evening
At bedtime, rinse mouth with water mixed with olive oil to lubricate oral tissues and use a water spray in room.
Upon each night awakening, sip water
Use of a sialagogue, e.g., anetholtrithion (Sialor) or pilocarpine (Salagen), may help, but efficacy is unknown (as yet, no controlled clinical trial related to sleep)

---

shown that acutely administered L-dopa slightly reduced bruxism activity in otherwise healthy SB patients.[61] To avoid waking the patient for the second administration of L-dopa in the middle of the night, a sustained-release drug (e.g., Sinemet CR, levodopa-carbidopa) could be prescribed. So far, not enough studies have been performed on a dopaminergic regimen to consider these in long-term management of SB. It also remains to be demonstrated if, as for PLMS (see Chapter 65), a pharmacological rebound will induce recurrence of SB activity later in the night or during the next day.

Another pharmacological avenue for SB management is the use of a *beta-adrenergic antagonist*, such as propranolol. Two recent case studies reported a reduction of SB in one bruxer without any medical history[68] and in two patients in whom iatrogenic SB was noted secondary to antipsychotic (dopaminergic antagonist) medication.[69] Again, before adrenergic medication becomes a choice for SB management, controlled and double-blind sleep studies are needed to assess efficacy and safety. This is critical because beta-adrenergic antagonists have been reported to disrupt sleep (e.g., increase sleep awakenings) or exacerbate sleep disorders (e.g., REM disorder behavior)[70–72] and have been suggested as a potential risk factor in obstructive sleep apnea.[126]

Botulinum toxin is frequently used in the management of cervicofacial dystonia[127] and it was recently suggested for control of masseter muscle hypertrophy.[128, 129] At this time, no controlled study, with polygraphic recordings, has demonstrated that it has long-term efficacy and safety for SB.

In Table 67–8, further advice is given for the management of SB (1) in children and teenagers; (2) in SB patients of all ages with secondarily hypersensitive teeth; and (3) for the occasional dry mouth and xerostonia brought on by stress and the influence of hormones, age, and drug use (tricyclic antidepressants, benzodiazepine, etc.).

Acknowledgments

The sleep bruxism studies done by the authors were made possible by the support of the Canadian Medical Research Council and the Fonds de recherche en santé du Québec. The following individuals have been involved in these studies: J. Montplaisir (director of the Centre Étude du Sommeil, Hôpital du Sacré-Coeur de Montréal), T. T. T. Dao, A. Gosselin, J. P. Goulet, F. Guitard, F. Lobbezoo, J. P. Lund, M. Major, D. Migraine, P. H. Rompré, S. Rompré, J. P. Soucy, L. TenBokum, and A. Velly-Miguel. Our thanks to Clare Lord for revising the English version of this text and to Francine Bélanger for manuscript preparation.

References

1. Diagnostic Classification Steering Committee, Thorpy MJ, chairman. International Classification of Sleep Disorders: Diagnostic and Coding Manual, Revised. Rochester, Minn: American Sleep Disorders Association; 1997:182–185.
2. Hartman E. Bruxism. In: Kryger MH, Roth T, Dement WC, eds. Principles and Practice of Sleep Medicine. 2nd ed. Philadelphia, Pa: WB Saunders; 1994:598–604.
3. Rugh JD, Harlan J. Nocturnal bruxism and temporomandibular disorders. Adv Neurol. 1988;49:329–341.
4. Okeson JP. Orofacial Pain Guidelines for Assessment, Diagnosis, and Management. Carol Stream, Ill: Quintessence; 1996.
5. Reding GR, Zepelin H, Robinson JE Jr, et al. Nocturnal teeth-grinding: all-night psychophysiologic studies. J Dent Res. 1968;47:786–797.
6. Dorland's Illustrated Medical Dictionary. 28th ed. Philadelphia, Pa: WB Saunders; 1994.
7. Marie, Pietkiewicz Jr. La bruxomanie. Rev Stomatol. 1907;14:107–116.
8. Faulkner KDB. Bruxism: a review of the literature. Part I. Aust Dent J. 1990;35:266–276.
9. Jankovic J. Cranial-cervical dyskinesias: an overview. Adv Neurol 1988;49:1–13.
10. Adams RD, Victor M. Principles of Neurology. New York, NY: McGraw-Hill; 1993.
11. Rozencweig D. Bruxisme et parafonctions: maladies expressives. Coll Natl Occlusodontol (France). 1992;9:95–100.
12. Yustin D, Neff P, Rieger MR, et al. Characterization of 86 bruxing patients and long term study of their management with occlusal devices and other forms of therapy. J Orofac Pain. 1993;7:54–60.
13. Kobayashi Y. Management of bruxism. J Orofac Pain. 1996;10:173.
14. Okeson JP. Management of Temporomandibular Disorders and Occlusion. St Louis, Mo: Mosby–Year Book; 1993.
15. Lavigne GJ, Lobbezoo F, Montplaisir J. The genesis of rhythmic masticatory muscle activity and bruxism during sleep. In: Morimoto T, Matsuya T, Takada T, eds. Brain and Oral Functions. Amsterdam, Netherlands: Elsevier, 1995:249–255.
16. Lavigne GJ, Montplaisir J. Bruxism: epidemiology, diagnosis, pathophysiology, and pharmacology. In: Fricton JR, Dubner RB, eds. Advances in Pain Research and Therapy—Orofacial Pain and Temporomandibular Disorders. New York, NY: Raven Press; 1995:387–404.
17. Sjöholm, T. Sleep Bruxism: Pathophysiology, Diagnosis, and Treatment [doctoral thesis]. Turku, Finland: University of Turkuensis; 1995.
18. Reding GR, Rubright WC, Zimmerman SO. Incidence of bruxism. J Dent Res. 1966;45:1198–1204.
19. Glaros AG. Incidence of diurnal and nocturnal bruxism. J Prosthet Dent. 1981;45:545–549.
20. Goulet JP, Lund JP, Montplaisir J, et al. Daily clenching, nocturnal bruxism, and stress and their association with TMD symptoms. J Orofac Pain. 1993;7:120.
21. Abe K, Shimakawa M. Genetic and developmental aspects of sleeptalking and teeth-grinding. Acta Paedopsychiatry. 1966;33:339–344.
22. Migraine D, Scholte AM, Tremblay R, et al. Bruxism and onychophagy in children: prevalence and relative risk factors. J Dent Res. 1996;75:219.

23. Widmalm SE, Christiansen RL, Gunn SM. Oral parafunctions as temporomandibular disorder risk factors in children. J Craniomandibular Pract. 1995;13:242–246.
24. Lavigne GJ, Montplaisir J. Restless legs syndrome and sleep bruxism: prevalence and association among Canadians. Sleep. 1994;17:739–743.
25. Lavigne GJ, Lobbezoo F, Rompré PH, et al. Cigarette smoking as a risk factor or an exacerbating factor for restless legs syndrome and sleep bruxism. Sleep. 1997;20:290–293.
26. Dao TTT, Lund JP, Lavigne GJ. Comparison of pain and quality of life in bruxers and patients with myofascial pain of the masticatory muscles. J Orofac Pain. 1994;8:350–356.
27. Lavigne GJ, Rompré PH, Montplaisir J, et al. Motor activity in sleep bruxism with concomitant jaw muscle pain. Eur J Oral Sci. 1997;105:92–95.
28. Richmond G, Rugh JD, Dolfi R, et al. Survey of bruxism in an institutionalized mentally retarded population. Am J Ment Retard. 1984;88:418–421.
29. Lavigne GJ, Rompré PH, Poirier G, et al. Rhythmic masticatory muscle activity (RMMA or chewing-automatism) during sleep in normal controls. J Sleep Res. 1998;7:229.
30. Gastaut H, Batini C, Broughton R, et al. Étude électroencéphalographique des phénomènes épisodiques non épileptiques au cours du sommeil. In: Societé electroencé-phalographie et neurophysiologie clinique langue francaise. Le sommeil de nuit normal et pathologique. 2nd ed. Paris, France: Masson & Cie; 1965:217.
31. Halasz P, Ujszaszi J. Chewing automatism in sleep connected with micro-arousals: an indicator of propensity to confusional awakenings? In: Koella WP, Schulz OF, Visser P, eds. Sleep 1986. New York, NY: Fisher; 1988:235–239.
32. Sforza E, Zucconi M, Petronelli R, et al. REM sleep behavioral disorders. Eur Neurol. 1988;28:295–300.
33. Glaros AG, Rao SM. Bruxism: a critical review. Psychol Bull. 1977;84:767–781.
34. Harness DM, Peltier B. Comparison of MMPI scores with self-report of sleep disturbance and bruxism in the facial pain population. J Craniomandibular Pract. 1992;10:70–74.
35. Pierce CJ, Chrisman K, Bennett ME, et al. Stress, anticipatory stress, and psychologic measures related to sleep bruxism. J Orofac Pain. 1995;9:51–56.
36. Dettmar DM, Shaw RM, Tilley AJ. Tooth wear and bruxism: a sleep laboratory investigation. Aust Dent J. 1987;32:421–426.
37. Sjöholm T, Lehtinen I, Helenius H. Masseter muscle activity in diagnosed sleep bruxists compared with non-symptomatic controls. J Sleep Res. 1995;4:48–55.
38. Lavigne GJ, Rompré PH, Montplaisir J. Sleep bruxism: validity of clinical research diagnostic criteria in a controlled polysomnographic study. J Dent Res. 1996;75:546–552.
39. Macaluso GM, Guerra P, Di Giovanni G, et al. Sleep bruxism is a disorder related to the periodic arousals during sleep. J Dent Res. 1998;77:565–573.
40. Boutros NN, Montgomery MT, Nishioka G, et al. The effects of severe bruxism on sleep architecture: a preliminary report. Clin Electroencephalogr. 1993;24:59–62.
41. Bader GG, Kampe T, Tagdae T, et al. Descriptive physiological data on a sleep bruxism population. Sleep. 1997;20:982–990.
42. Reding GR, Zepelin H, Robinson JE Jr, et al. Sleep pattern of bruxism: a revision. Presented at Fourth Association of Professional Sleep Societies Meeting, 1967;4:396.
43. Ware JC, Rugh JD. Destructive bruxism: sleep stage relationship. Sleep. 1988;11:172–181.
44. Sjöholm T, Polo OJ, Alihanka JM. Sleep movements in teethgrinders. J Craniomandibular Disord Fac Oral Pain. 1992;6:184–191.
45. Tani K, Yoshii N, Yoshino I, et al. Electroencephalographic study of parasomnia: sleep-talking, enuresis and bruxism. Physiol Behav. 1966;1:241–243.
46. Satoh T, Harada Y. Electrophysiological study on tooth-grinding during sleep. Electroencephalogr Clin Neurophysiol. 1973;35:267–275.
47. Sjöholm TT, Piha SJ, Lehtinen I, et al. Cardiovascular autonomic control is disturbed in nocturnal teethgrinders. Clin Physiol. 1995;15:349–354.
48. Terzano MG, Parrino L. Clinical applications of cyclic alternating pattern. Physiol Behav. 1993;54:807–813.
49. Zucconi M, Oldani A, Ferini-Strambi L, et al. Arousal fluctuations in non–rapid eye movement parasomnias: the role of cyclic alternating pattern as a measure of sleep instability. J Clin Neurophysiol. 1995;12:147–154.
50. Lavigne GJ, Guitard F, Rompré PH, et al. Low presence of EEG arousal (K-alpha complexes) in sleep bruxism: a controlled study report. Sleep Res. 1997;26:409.
51. Wauquier A, Aloe L, Declerck A. K-complexes: are they signs of arousal or sleep protective? Sleep Res. 1995;4:138–143.
52. Broughton RJ. Phasic and Dynamic Aspects of Sleep: A Symposium Review and Synthesis. New York, NY: Raven Press; 1991.
53. Wauquier A. Aging and changes in phasic events during sleep. Physiol Behav. 1993;54:803–806.
54. Lund JP. Mastication and its control by the brainstem. Crit Rev Oral Biol Med. 1991;2:33–64.
55. Schärer P, Kasahara Y, Kawamura Y. Tooth contact patterns during stimulation of the rabbit brain. Arch Oral Biol. 1967;12:1041–1051.
56. Chase MH, Morales FR. The controls of motoneurons during sleep. In: Kryger MH, Roth T, Dement WC, eds. Principles and Practices of Sleep Medicine. 2nd ed. Philadelphia, Pa: WB Saunders; 1994:163–175.
57. Pedroarena C, Castillo P, Chase MH, et al. Non-reciprocal post-synaptic inhibition of digastric motoneurons. Brain Res. 1990;535:339–342.
58. Gottesmann C. Introduction to the neurophysiological study of sleep: central regulation of skeletal and ocular activities. Arch Ital Biol. 1997;135:279–314.
59. Magee KR. Bruxism related to levodopa therapy. J Am Dent Assoc. 1970;214:147.
60. Micheli F, Pardal MF, Gatto M, et al. Bruxism secondary to chronic antidopaminergic drug exposure. Clin Neuropharmacol. 1993;16:315–323.
61. Lobbezoo F, Lavigne GJ, Tanguay R, et al. The effect of catecholamine precursor L-dopa on sleep bruxism: a controlled clinical trial. Mov Disord. 1997;12:73–78.
62. Lobbezoo F, Soucy JP, Hartman NG, et al. Effects of the D2 receptor agonist bromocriptine on sleep bruxism: report of two single-patient clinical trials. J Dent Res. 1997;76:1610–1614.
63. Lobbezoo F, Soucy JP, Montplaisir J, et al. Striatal D2 receptor binding in sleep bruxism: a controlled study with iodine-123-iodobanzamide and single photon emission computed tomography. J Dent Res. 1996;75:1804–1810.
64. Brücke T, Wenger S, Asenbaum S. Dopamine D2 receptor imaging and measurement with SPECT. Adv Neurol. 1993;60:494–500.
65. Hierholzer J, Cordes M, Sclebosky L, et al. Dopamine D2 receptor imaging with iodine-123-iodobenzamide SPECT in idiopathic rotational torticollis. J Nucl Med. 1994;35:921–927.
66. Knable MB, Jones DW, Coppola R, et al. Lateralized differences in iodine-123-IBZM uptake in the basal ganglia in asymmetric Parkinson's disease. J Nucl Med. 1995;36:1216–1225.
67. Seibyl JP, Marek K, Innis RB. Images in neuroscience. Am J Psychiatry. 1996;153:1131.
68. Sjöholm T, Lehtinen I, Piha SJ. The effect of propranolol on sleep bruxism: hypothetical considerations based on a case study. Clin Auton Res. 1996;6:37–40.
69. Amir I, Hermesh H, Gavish A. Bruxism secondary to antipsychotic drug exposure: a positive response to propranolol. Clin Neuropharmacol. 1997;20:86–89.
70. Nicholson AN, Bradley CM, Pascoe PA. Medications: Effect on sleep and wakefulness. In: Kryger MH, Roth T, Dement WC, eds. Principles and Practice of Sleep Medicine. 2nd ed. Philadelphia, Pa: WB Saunders; 1994:364–372.
71. Danjou P, Puech A, Warot D, et al. Lack of sleep-inducing properties of propranolol (80mg) in chronic insomniacs previously treated by common hypnotic medications. Int Clin Psychopharmacol. 1987;2:135–140.
72. Monti JM. Disturbances of sleep and wakefulness associated with the use of antihypertensive agents. Life Sci. 1987;41:1979–1988.
73. Ellison JA, Stanziani P. SSRI-associated nocturnal bruxism in four patients. J Clin Psychiatry. 1993;54:432–434.
74. Por CH, Watson L, Doucette D, et al. Sertraline-associated bruxism. Can J Clin Pharmacol. 1996;3:123–125.

75. Nakamura Y, Katakura N. Generation of masticatory rhythm in the brainstem. Neurosci Res. 1995;23:1–19.

76. Kuch EV, Till MJ, Messer LB. Bruxing and non-bruxing children: a comparison of their personality traits. Pediatr Dent. 1979;1:182–187.

77. Lindqvist B. Bruxism in twins. Acta Odontol Scand. 1974;32:177–187.

78. Hori A, Hirose G. Twin studies on parasomnias. J Sleep Res. 1995;24:324.

79. Hublin C, Kaprio J, Partinen M, et al. Sleep bruxism based on self-report in a nationwide twin cohort. J Sleep Res. 1998;7:61–67.

80. Ramfjord SP, Mich AA. Bruxism: a clinical and electromyographic study. J Am Dent Assoc. 1961;62:35–58.

81. Leresche L, Truelove EL, Dworkin SF. Temporomandibular disorders: a survey of dentist's knowledge and beliefs. J Am Dent Assoc. 1993;124:90–106.

82. Clark GT, Adler C. A critical evaluation of occlusal therapy: occlusal adjustment procedures. J Am Dent Assoc. 1985;110:743–750.

83. Graf H. Bruxism. Dent Clin North Am. 1969;13:659–665.

84. Schneyer LH, Pigman W, Hanahan L, et al. Rate of flow of human parotid, sublingual, and submaxillary secretions during sleep. J Dent Res. 1956;35:109–114.

85. Gemba H, Teranaka A, Takemura K. Influences of emotion upon parotid secretion in human. Neurosci Lett. 1996;211:159–162.

86. Bradley RM. Salivary secretion. In: Getchell TV, Bartoshuk LM, Doty RL, et al, eds. Smell and Taste in Health and Disease. New York, NY: Raven Press; 1991:127–144.

87. Dodds MWJ, Johnson DA. Influence of mastication on saliva, plaque pH and masseter muscle activity in man. Arch Oral Biol. 1993;38:623–626.

88. Lichter I, Muir RC. The pattern of swallowing during sleep. Electroencephalogr Clin Neurophysiol. 1975;38:427–432.

89. Velly-Miguel AM, Montplaisir J, Rompré PH, et al. Bruxism and other orofacial movements during sleep. J Craniomandibular Dis Fac Oral Pain. 1992;6:71–81.

90. Marbach J, Raphael G, Dohrenwend P, et al. The validity of tooth grinding measures: etiology of pain dysfunction syndrome revisited. J Am Dent Assoc. 1990;120:327–333.

91. Seligman DA, Pullinger AG. The degree to which dental attrition in modern society is a function of age and of canine contact. J Orofac Pain. 1995;9:266–275.

92. Menapace SE, Rinchuse DJ, Zullo T, et al. The dentofacial morphology of bruxers versus non-bruxers. Angle Orthod. 1994;64:43–52.

93. Johansson A, Haraldson T, Omar R, et al. A system for assessing the severity and progression of occlusal wear. J Oral Rehabil. 1993;20:125–131.

94. Teaford MF, Tylenda CA. A new approach to the study of tooth wear. J Dent Res. 1991;70:204–207.

95. Mehl A, Gloger W, Kunzelmann K-H, et al. A new optical 3-D device for the detection of wear. J Dent Res. 1997;76:1799–1807.

96. Pierce CJ, Gale EN. Methodological considerations concerning the use of Bruxcore plates to evaluate nocturnal bruxism. J Dent Res. 1989;68:1110–1114.

97. Clark GT, Beemsterboer PL, Solberg WK, et al. Nocturnal electromyographic evaluation of myofascial pain dysfunction in patients undergoing occlusal splint therapy. J Am Dent Assoc. 1979;99:607–611.

98. Okeson JP. The effects of hard and soft occlusal splints on nocturnal bruxism. J Am Dent Assoc. 1987;114:788–791.

99. Raadsheer MC, Kiliaridis S, Van Eijden MGJ, et al. Masseter muscle thickness in growing individuals and its relation to facial morphology. Arch Oral Biol. 1996;41:323–332.

100. Emshoff R, Bertram S. The ultrasonic value of local muscle hypertrophy in patients with temporomandibular joint disorders. J Prosthet Dent. 1995;73:373–376.

101. Bakke M, Thomsen CE, Vilmann A, et al. Ultrasonographic assessment of the swelling of the human masseter muscle after static and dynamic activity. Arch Oral Biol. 1996;41:133–140.

102. Rugh JD. Electromyographic analysis of bruxism in the natural environment. In: Weinstein P, ed. Advances in Behavioral Research in Dentistry. Seattle, Wash: University of Washington Press; 1978:67–83.

103. Pierce CJ, Gale EN. A comparison of different treatments for nocturnal bruxism. J Dent Res. 1988;67:597–601.

104. Gallo LM, Lavigne GJ, Rompré PH. Reliability of scoring EMG orofacial events: Polysomnography compared ambulatory recordings. J Sleep Res. 1997;6:259–263.

105. Hudzinski LG, Walters PJ. Use of a portable electromyogram integrator and biofeedback unit in the treatment of chronic nocturnal bruxism. J Prosthet Dent. 1987;58:698–701.

106. Ikeda T, Nishigawa K, Kondo K, et al. Criteria for the detection of sleep-associated bruxism in humans. J Orofac Pain. 1996;10:270–282.

107. Rechtschaffen A, Kales A. A Manual of Standardized Terminology, Techniques and Scoring Techniques for Sleep Stages of Human Subjects. Los Angeles, Calif: Brain Research Institute, 1968.

108. Broughton R, Tolentino MA, Krelina M. Excessive fragmentary myoclonus in NREM sleep: a report of 38 cases. Electroencephalogr Clin Neurophysiol. 1985;61:123–133.

108a. Kato T, Montplaisir JY, Blanchet PJ, et al. Idiopathic myoclonus in the oromandibular region during sleep: a possible source of confusion in sleep bruxism diagnosis. Mov Dis. In press.

109. Okeson JP, Phillips BA, Berry DTR, et al. Nocturnal bruxing events in subjects with sleep-disordered breathing and control subjects. J Craniomandibular Dis Fac Oral Pain. 1991;5:258–264.

110. Okeson JP, Phillips BA, Berry DTR, et al. Nocturnal bruxing events in healthy geriatric subjects. J Oral Rehabil. 1990;17:411–418.

111. Zarcone VP. Sleep hygiene. In: Kryger MH, Roth T, Dement WC, eds. Principles and Practice of Sleep Medicine. 3rd ed. Philadelphia, Pa: WB Saunders; 2000.

112. Hathaway KM. Bruxism: definition, measurement, and treatment. In: Fricton JR, Dubner RB, eds. Advances in Pain Research and Therapy—Orofacial Pain and Temporomandibular Disorders. New York, NY: Raven Press; 1995:375–386.

113. Moss RA, Hammer D, Adams HE, et al. A more efficient biofeedback procedure for the treatment of nocturnal bruxism. J Oral Rehabil. 1982;9:125–131.

114. Clarke JH, Reynolds PJ. Suggestive hypnotherapy for nocturnal bruxism: a pilot study. Am J Clin Hypn. 1991;33:248–253.

115. Rugh JD, Johnson RW. Temporal analysis of nocturnal bruxism during EMG feedback. J Periodontol. 1981;52:263–265.

116. Solberg WK, Clark GT, Rugh JD. Nocturnal electromyographic evaluation of bruxism patients undergoing short term splint therapy. J Oral Rehabil. 1975;2:215–223.

117. Holmgren K, Sheikholeslam A, Riise C. Effect of a full-arch maxillary occlusal splint on parafunctional activity during sleep in patient with nocturnal bruxism and signs and symptoms of craniomandibular disorders. J Prosthet Dent. 1993;69:293–297.

118. Macaluso GM, Conversi G, Guerra P, et al. Effect of splint therapy on sleep structure in bruxers. J Dent Res. 1998;77:2305.

119. Dao TTT, Lavigne GJ. Oral splints: the crutches for temporomandibular disorders and bruxism? Crit Rev Oral Biol Med. 1998;9:345–361.

120. Chasins AI. Methocarbamol (Robaxin) as an adjunct in the treatment of bruxism. J Dent Med. 1959;14:166–169.

121. Montgomery MT, Nishioka GJ, Rugh JD, et al. Effect of diazepam on nocturnal masticatory muscle activity. J Dent Res. 1986;65:96.

122. Attanasio R. Nocturnal bruxism and its clinical management. Dent Clin North Am. 1991;35:245–252.

123. Mohamed SE, Christensen LV, Penchas J. A randomized double-blind clinical trial of the effect of amitriptyline on nocturnal masseteric motor activity (sleep bruxism). J Craniomandibular Pract. 1997;15:326–332.

124. Etzel KR, Stockstill JW, Rugh JD, et al. Tryptophan supplementation for nocturnal bruxism: report of negative results. J Craniomandibular Disord Fac Oral Pain. 1991;5:115–119.

125. Lewis SA, Oswald I, Dunleavy PLF. Chronic fenfluramine administration: some cerebral effects. Br Med J. 1971;3:67–70.

126. Longstaff M, Glen R. Do β-blockers pose an unacceptable risk to patients with obstructive sleep apnea (OSA)? Sleep. 1997;20:920.

127. Jankovic J, Brin MF. Therapeutic uses of botulinum toxin. N Engl J Med. 1991;324:1186–1194.

128. Van Zandijcke M, Marchaud MB. Treatment of bruxism with botulinum toxin injections [letter]. J Neurol Neurosurg Psychiatry. 1990;53:530–535.

129. Smyth AG. Botulinum toxin treatment of bilateral masseteric hypertrophy. Br J Oral Maxillofac Surg. 1994;32:29–33.

130. Weiner WJ, Lang AE. Movement Disorders: A Comprehensive Study. New York, NY: Futura; 1989.

131. Jankovic J, Tolosa E. Facial dyskinesias. Adv Neurol. 1988;49:1–13.

132. Bassett A, Remick RA, Blasberg B. Tardive dyskinesia: an unrecognized cause of orofacial pain. Oral Surg Oral Med Oral Pathol. 1986;61:570–572.

133. Klawans HL, Goetz CG, Tanner CM. Common Movement Disorders: A Video Presentation. New York, NY: Raven Press; 1988.

134. Silvestri R, De Domenico P, Di Rosa AE, et al. The effect of nocturnal physiological sleep on various movement disorders. Mov Disord. 1990;5:8–14.

135. Sforza E, Montagna P, Defazio G, et al. Sleep and cranial dystonia. Electroencephalogr Clin Neurophysiol. 1991;79:166–169.

136. Hauser RA, Olanow CW. Orobuccal dyskinesia associated with trihexyphenidyl therapy in a patient with Parkinson's disease. Mov Disord. 1998;8:512–514.

137. Robertson LT, Hammerstad JP. Jaw movement dysfunction related to Parkinson's disease and partially modified by levodopa. J Neurol Neurosurg Psychiatry. 1996;60:41–50.

138. Friedlander AH, Cummings JL. Dental treatment of patients with Gilles de la Tourette's syndrome. Oral Surg Oral Med Oral Pathol. 1992;73:299–303.

139. Aguglia U, Gambardella A, Quattrone A. Sleep-induced masticatory myoclonus: a rare parasomnia associated with insomnia. Sleep. 1998;14:80–82.

140. Tachibana N, Yamanaka K, Kaji R, et al. Sleep bruxism as a manifestation of subclinical rapid eye movement sleep behavior disorder. Sleep. 1994;17:555–558.

141. Pollack IA, Cwik V. Bruxism following cerebellar hemorrhage. Neurology. 1989;39:1262.

142. Pratap-Chand R, Gourie-Devi M. Bruxism: its significance in coma. Clin Neurol Neurosurg. 1985;87:113–117.

143. Tison F, Giendaj-Louvet C, Henry P, et al. Permanent bruxism as a manifestation of the oculo-facial syndrome related to systemic Whipple's disease. Mov Disord. 1992;7:82–85.

144. Stewart JT, Thomas JE, Williams LS. Severe Bruxism in a demented patient. South Med J. 1993;86:476–477.

145. Hartman E. Alcohol and bruxism. N Engl J Med. 1979;301:334.

146. Cardoso FEC, Jankovic J. Cocaine-related movement disorders. Mov Disord. 1993;8:175–178.

147. Ashcroft GW, Eccleston D, Waddell JL. Recognition of amphetamine addicts. Br Med J. 1965;1:57.

148. Nishigawa K, Kondo K, Clark GT. Contingent lip stimulation for sleep associated oral motor dysfunction (bruxism). J Dent Res. 1992;71:151.

149. Gerber PE, Lynd LD. Selective serotonin-reuptake inhibitor–induced movement disorders. Ann Pharmacother. 1998;32:692–698.

68

Violent Parasomnias: Forensic Medicine Issues

Mark W. Mahowald
Carlos H. Schenck

In all of us, even in good men, there is a lawless, wild-beast nature which peers out in sleep.

PLATO, *THE REPUBLIC*

Acts done by a person asleep cannot be criminal, there being no consciousness.[1]

P.J. FITZGERALD

Increasingly, sleep medicine practitioners are asked to render opinions regarding legal issues pertaining to violent or injurious behaviors purported to have arisen from sleep. Such acts, if having arisen from sleep without conscious awareness, would constitute an *automatism*. Automatic behaviors (automatisms) resulting in acts that may result in illegal behaviors have been described in many different medical, neurological, or psychiatric conditions. Medical and psychiatric automatisms arising from wakefulness are reasonably well understood. Advances in sleep medicine have made it apparent that some complex behaviors, occasionally violent or injurious with forensic science implications, are exquisitely state dependent, meaning that they arise exclusively, or predominantly, from the sleep period. Violent behaviors arising from the sleep period are more common than previously thought, being reported by 2% of the adult population.[2] As is discussed later, the medical and legal concepts of automatisms differ greatly.

CASE HISTORY

A 24-year-old single man had a stellar college academic and athletic record, with no history of psychiatric disease or drug or substance abuse. He had no personal or family history of any sleep disorder, and he had absolutely no history of interpersonal violence. In December 1993, after the young man had been living in Japan working as a teacher, he returned to the United States in a very sleep-deprived condition. He estimated that he had slept no more than 15 h during the preceding 4 days. He went to a friend's house where he drank 1½ beers and took one hit of marijuana. His friends noticed his behavior was "peculiar." He and his friends went for a ride (he was a passenger). When they arrived at their destination, he got out of the car and saw a police officer approaching. He told his friends it was "OK," as he knew the officer (which was not true).

He walked over and sat down in the police car. The officer drove him to where his friends were waiting. The officer and the young man each got out of the car and met behind it. The young man viciously attacked the officer, fracturing his jaw and knocking him unconscious. Another officer arrived. The young man was finally subdued by a number of people. According to his friends, his behavior was extremely inappropriate, irrational, and completely out of character for him.

He had no recollection of any of the events—from riding in the car until he "came to" in a hospital. All he remembered from the incident were dream-like images. He stated, "I thought I was in hell." He remembered being held down by a number of arms, but he could not identify bodies or faces. He said that he thought he was in hell because of the burning sensation on his face. In retrospect, he said that this may have been fragmentary imagery of having being held down by the police officer and having been sprayed in the face with Mace. Extensive psychiatric and chemical dependency evaluations performed after the incident were unrevealing.

Based on reports from his friends and the police and on the young man's fragmentary memories, he never denied having committed the violent act. He was charged with a felony. If convicted on the basis of an "insane" automatism, his plan of developing a business in Japan would be destroyed because he could not leave the United States. He wished to have his behavior declared a "noninsane automatism," which would have very different legal consequences. He was convicted, and the case is being appealed.

Modified from Mahowald MW, Schenck CH. Sleep-related violence and forensic medicine issues. In: Chokroverty S, ed. Sleep Disorders Medicine: Basic Science, Technical Considerations, and Clinical Aspects. 2nd ed. Boston, Mass: Butterworth-Heinemann; 1999:729–739.

SLEEP-RELATED VIOLENCE
State-Dependent Violence

The concept that sleep is simply the passive absence of wakefulness is no longer tenable. Not only is sleep an active rather than a passive process, it is now clear that sleep is composed of two completely different states: nonrapid eye movement (NREM) sleep and rapid eye movement (REM) sleep. Therefore, our lives are spent in three entirely different states of being—wakefulness, REM sleep, and NREM sleep. Studies have indicated that bizarre behavioral syndromes can, and do, occur as a result of the incomplete declaration or rapid oscillation of these states.[3, 4] Although the automatic behaviors of some "mixed states" are relatively benign (i.e., shoplifting in narcolepsy),[5] others may be associated with violent or injurious behaviors.

The fact that violent or injurious behaviors may arise in the absence of conscious wakefulness and without conscious awareness raises the crucial question of how such complex behavior can occur. An examination of extensive experimental studies in animals provides preliminary answers. The widely held concept that the brainstem and other more "primitive" neural structures primarily participate in elemental and vegetative rather than behavioral activities is inaccurate. There are overwhelming data documenting that highly complex emotional and motor behaviors can originate from these more primitive structures, without the involvement of higher neural structures such as the cortex.[6–12]

Sleep-Related Disorders Associated With Violence

Violent sleep-related behaviors have been reviewed in the context of automatized behavior in general.[3] There are well-documented cases of (1) somnambulistic homicide, filicide, attempted homicide, and suicide; (2) murders and other crimes with "sleep drunkenness" (confusional arousals); and (3) sleep terrors and sleepwalking (ST/SW) with potential violence or injury. A wide variety of disorders may result in sleep-related violence;[3] conditions are listed in Table 68–1. These conveniently fall into two major categories: neurological and psychiatric.

NEUROLOGICAL CONDITIONS ASSOCIATED WITH VIOLENT BEHAVIORS

Based on extrapolation from animal experimental data to the human condition, it has been shown that structural lesions at multiple levels of the nervous system may result in wakeful violence.[13–16] The results of studies in animals provide insights to violent behaviors in the disorders of arousal, REM behavior disorder (RBD), and sleep-related seizures.

Disorders of Arousal (Confusional Arousals, Sleepwalking/Sleep Terrors)

The disorders of arousal comprise a spectrum ranging from confusional arousals (sleep drunkenness) to

Table 68–1. CONDITIONS ASSOCIATED WITH AUTOMATIC BEHAVIOR

I. Organic neurological disorders
  A. Vascular
    1. Transient global amnesia (including migraine)
  B. Mass lesions
    1. Increased intracranial pressure
    2. Deep midline structural lesions
  C. Toxic/metabolic
    1. Endocrine
    2. Hypoxia/carbon monoxide poisoning
    3. Drugs/alcohol (intoxication/withdrawal)
    4. Thiamine deficiency (Wernicke-Korsakoff syndrome)
  D. Infectious (limbic encephalitis)
  E. Central nervous system trauma
  F. Seizures
  G. Sleep disorders
    1. Disorders of arousal (confusional arousals [sleep drunkenness], sleepwalking, sleep terrors)
    2. REM sleep behavior disorder
    3. Nocturnal seizures
    4. Automatic behavior
      a. Narcolepsy and idiopathic central nervous system hypersomnia
      b. Sleep apnea
      c. Sleep deprivation (including jet lag)
    5. Hypnagogic hallucinations
II. Psychogenic
  A. Dissociative states (may arise exclusively from sleep)
    1. Fugues
    2. Multiple personality disorder
    3. Psychogenic amnesia
  B. Post-traumatic stress disorder
  C. Malingering
  D. Munchausen by proxy

Modified from Mahowald MW, Schenck CH. Sleep-related violence and forensic medicine issues. In: Chokroverty S, ed. Sleep Disorders Medicine: Basic Science, Technical Considerations and Clinical Aspects. 2nd ed. Boston, Mass: Butterworth-Heinemann; 1999.

SW to ST[17, 18] (see Chapter 62). Although there usually is amnesia for the event,[19, 20] vivid dream-like mentation may occasionally be experienced and reported.[21] Contrary to popular opinion, these disorders may actually begin in adulthood and most often are not associated with psychopathology.[21, 22] Population surveys indicate that unlike previously thought, the disorders of arousal are quite prevalent in the adult population, being reported by 3 to 4% of all adults and occurring weekly in 0.4%.[23]

Febrile illness, alcohol, prior sleep deprivation, and emotional stress may serve to trigger disorders of arousal in susceptible individuals.[24–26] Sleep deprivation is well known to result in confusion, disorientation, and hallucinatory phenomena.[27–32] Medications such as sedative/hypnotics, neuroleptics, minor tranquilizers, stimulants, and antihistamines, often in combination with each other or with alcohol, may also play a role.[33–35] Many of the reported medicolegal cases of SW-related violence have involved alcohol consumption in an individual prone to experience spontaneous disorders of arousal.

Confusional arousals, a milder form of SW/ST (sleep drunkenness), occur during the transition between sleep and wakefulness and represent a disturbance of cognition and attention despite the motor behavior of wakefulness, resulting in complex behavior without conscious awareness.[36–38] These may be potentiated by prior sleep deprivation or the ingestion of alcohol or sedative/hypnotics before sleep onset.[39] These episodes of "automatic behavior" occur in the setting of chronic sleep deprivation or other conditions associated with state admixture (shoplifting has been reported during a period of automatic behavior in a narcoleptic.)[5, 40, 41]

Pathophysiology of Disorders of Arousal

The behavioral similarities between documented SW/ST violence in human beings and "sham rage" as seen in the "hypothalamic savage" syndrome are striking.[42] Although it has been assumed that the animals in sham rage preparations are "awake," there is some suggestion that animals in similar preparations are behaviorally awake, yet (partially) physiologically asleep, with apparent "hallucinatory" behavior possibly representing REM sleep dreaming that occurs during wakefulness, dissociated from other REM state markers.[43]

The neural bases of aggression and rage in the cat have been reviewed, indicating that there clearly is an anatomic basis for some forms of violent behavior.[44] The prosencephalic system may serve to control and elaborate rather than initiate behaviors originating from deeper structures.[11] In human beings with confusional arousals (sleep drunkenness), which can result in confusion or aggression, there is clear electroencephalographic evidence of rapid oscillations between wakefulness and sleep.[37, 38] It may be that such behaviors occurring in states other than wakefulness are the expression of motor/affective activity generated by lower structures, unmonitored and unmodified by the cortex.

Other, very important factors beyond the scope of this chapter include (1) the known effect of genetics on violence and (2) the well-demonstrated effects of environmental and social factors on the structure and function of the nervous system.[45] (In one study of 31 individuals awaiting trial or sentencing for murder, none were neurologically or psychiatrically normal.[14]) The plasticity of the nervous system in response to environmental influences is greater than previously thought.[46, 47] Psychobiological and sociocultural factors are undoubtedly operant in both wakeful and sleep-related violence.[48, 49]

The treatment of the disorders of arousal includes both pharmacological (benzodiazepine and tricyclic antidepressant) and behavioral (hypnosis) approaches.[50]

Importantly, there are various associations between obstructive sleep apnea and confusional arousals. Patients with obstructive sleep apnea may experience frequent arousals, which may serve to trigger arousal-induced precipitous motor activity.[51] Therefore, the observed clinical behavior, a confusional arousal, is actually the result of another underlying primary sleep disorder—obstructive sleep apnea. Guilleminault and Silvestri[51(p529)] have made the following observations:

It is well known that adult patients with OSA [obstructive sleep apnea] syndrome present nocturnal wandering during sleep. These patients frequently demonstrate yelling and screaming during sleep, as well as confusion, disorientation, and sleepwalking. . . . The nocturnal hypoxia and the repetitive sleep disruptions secondary to the OSA syndrome readily explain these symptoms.

This is another example of why overnight polysomnographic studies with extensive physiological monitoring are mandatory in the evaluation of problematic motor parasomnias. Disorders of arousal may also be precipitated by adequate or incomplete treatment of sleep apnea with nasal continuous positive airway pressure.[52, 53]

Disorders of Arousal and Human Violence

The commonly held belief that SW and ST are always benign is erroneous: the accompanying behaviors may be violent, resulting in considerable injury to the individual or others or in damage to the environment.[3, 21] To remind us that apparently criminal acts without conscious awareness occurring during sleep drunkenness (formerly termed *somnolentia*) are not a new condition, dramatic cases were described in a classic book on sleep in 1869. The author's conclusion regarding sleep drunkenness was that "it is a natural phenomenon, to which all are liable."[54(p315)]

SW resulting in injury to self or others has been termed *Elpenor's syndrome*, after an incident in Homer's *Odyssey* (Book 10). A youth named Elpenor became intoxicated and fell asleep on the roof of a house. He was suddenly awakened by the noise of others preparing to leave the island of Aeoli, and he ran off the rooftop rather than taking the staircase, sustaining a fatal cervical fracture.

Not only is sleep an active process but also the generators or effectors of many components of both REM and NREM sleep reside in the brainstem and other "lower" centers; it is not surprising that prominent motoric and affective behaviors do occur during sleep. Specific incidents include the following:

- Somnambulistic homicide, attempted homicide, filicide[33, 55–71]
- Murders and other crimes with sleep drunkenness,[25] including sleep apnea[26] and narcolepsy[5]
- Suicide or fear of committing suicide[70, 72–74]
- ST/SW with potential violence or injury;[75–78] these episodes may be drug induced[33, 79, 80]
- Inappropriate sexual behaviors during the sleep state, presumably the results of and admixture of wakefulness and sleep[81–86]

Some dramatic cases have been tried in courts based on the confusional arousal defense. In the *Parks* case in Canada, the defendant drove 23 km, killed his mother-in-law, and attempted to kill his father-in-law. Somnambulism was the legal defense, and he was acquitted.[87] In the *Butler, Pennsylvania* case, a confusional arousal attributed to documented underlying severe obstructive sleep apnea was offered as a criminal defense for a man who fatally shot his wife during his usual sleeping hours. He was found guilty.[88]

REM Sleep Behavior Disorder

RBD represents an experiment of nature that was predicted in 1965 on the basis of animal experiments,[89] and it has since been identified in human beings[40] (see Chapter 64). Normally, during REM sleep, there is active paralysis of all somatic muscles (sparing the diaphragm and eye movement muscles). In RBD, there is the absence of REM sleep atonia, which permits the "acting out" of dreams, often with dramatic and violent or injurious behaviors. The oneiric (dream) behavior demonstrated by cats with bilateral peri–locus ceruleus lesions and by human beings with spontaneously occurring RBD clearly arises from and continues to occur during REM sleep.[40, 89, 90] These oneiric behaviors displayed by patients with RBD are often misdiagnosed as manifestations of a seizure or psychiatric disorder. RBD is usually idiopathic but may be associated with underlying neurological disorders.[40] The overwhelming male predominance (90%) of RBD[91] raises interesting questions of the relation of sexual hormones to aggression and violence.[92, 93] The violent and injurious nature of RBD behaviors has been extensively reviewed previously.[80, 91, 94–96] Treatment with clonazepam is highly effective.[91]

A *parasomnia overlap* syndrome that contains both clinical and polysomnographic features of both disorders of arousal and RBD has been described.[97] Other sleep disorders, such as disorders of arousal, underlying sleep apnea, and nocturnal seizures, may perfectly simulate RBD, again underscoring the necessity for thorough formal polysomnographic evaluation of these patients.[98, 99]

Nocturnal Seizures

The association between seizures and violence has been long debated. It is plain that, on occasion, seizures may result in violent, murderous, or injurious behaviors.[3, 100] Of particular note is the frantic, elaborate, and complex nocturnal motor activity that may result from seizures originating in the orbital, mesial, or prefrontal region.[101–106] *Episodic nocturnal wanderings*, a condition that is clinically indistinguishable from other forms of sleep-related motor activity such as complex SW but responsive to anticonvulsant therapy, has also been described.[107–109] Aggression and violence may be seen preictally, ictally, and postictally. Postictal wanderings may result in confused or violent behaviors.[110, 111] Some postictal violence is induced or perpetuated by the good intentions of bystanders trying to "calm" the patient after a seizure.[112] A fascinating postictal aggression syndrome has been described in which the aggressive behaviors begin hours to days after the confusional postictal period and may last for

hours to several days. Interestingly, as with many other violent states, this is a male phenomenon.[113]

As mentioned, other sleep disorders, such as obstructive sleep apnea or RBD, may masquerade as nocturnal seizures.[99, 114–116] The complex and fascinating relation among epilepsy, sleep, and sleep disorders has been extensively reviewed (see Chapter 63 and reference 117).

Compelling Hypnagogic Hallucinations

Recurrent sexually oriented hypnagogic hallucinations experienced by patients with narcolepsy may be so vivid and convincing to the victim that they may serve as false accusations.[118] The concept of waking hallucinations as the manifestation of wakeful dreaming, often associated with disorders of the central nervous system, has been reviewed previously.[119]

Sleeptalking

Sleeptalking has also been addressed by the legal system: it is interesting to discuss whether utterances made during sleep are admissible in court.[120]

PSYCHIATRIC CONDITIONS

Psychogenic Dissociative States

Waking dissociative states may result in violence.[121] It is now apparent that dissociative disorders may arise exclusively or predominantly from the sleep period.[3, 122] Virtually all patients with nocturnal dissociative disorders who were evaluated at our center were the victims of repeated physical or sexual abuse beginning in childhood.[123]

Post-Traumatic Stress Disorder

Dissociative states and injury related to "nightmare" behaviors have been reported in association with post-traumatic stress disorder.[124, 125] The *limbic psychotic trigger reaction*, in which motiveless unplanned homicidal acts occur, is speculated to represent partial limbic seizures that are kindled by highly individualized and specific trigger stimuli, reviving past repetitive stress.[126] If so, this would be an example of environmentally induced changes in brain function.

Malingering

Although uncommon, *malingering* (the conscious attempt to feign illness—in this case, to obtain documentation of having a disorder of arousal) must also be considered. At our center, we saw a young man who developed progressively violent behaviors that apparently arose from sleep and were directed exclusively at his wife. This behavior included beating her and chasing her with a hammer. After exhaustive neurological, psychiatric, and polysomnographic evaluation, it was determined that this behavior represented malingering. It was suspected that he was attempting to have the sleep center "legitimize" his behaviors should his wife be murdered during one of these episodes.

Munchausen Syndrome by Proxy

In Munchausen syndrome by proxy, a child is reported to have apparently medically serious symptoms that are, in fact, induced by an adult, usually a caregiver and often a parent. The use of surreptitious video monitoring in sleep disorder centers during sleep (with the parent present) has documented the true cause of reported sleep apnea and other unusual nocturnal spells.[127–134]

MEDICOLEGAL EVALUATION

Automatisms and the Law

Actus non facit reum nisi mens sit rea—the deed does not make a man guilty unless his mind is guilty.

PETER FENWICK[86(p125)]

In the United States and the United Kingdom, for a criminal act *(actus rea)* to be criminal, it must be paired with a culpable mental state *(mens rea)*, meaning "knowing intent to commit a crime." The legal definition of automatism is based on this doctrine.

Most of the above-mentioned conditions resulting in violent or injurious behaviors are termed *automatisms*. *Automatism* is difficult to define;[135–137] Fenwick proposed the following definition:

> An automatism is an involuntary piece of behavior over which an individual has no control. The behavior is usually inappropriate to the circumstances, and may be out of character for the individual. It can be complex, coordinated, and apparently purposeful and directed, though lacking in judgment. Afterwards the individual may have no recollection or only partial and confused memory for his actions. In organic automatisms there must be some disturbance of brain function sufficient to give rise to the above features.[86(p125)]

Although the medical concept of automatism is relatively straightforward (complex behavior in the absence of conscious awareness or volitional intent), the judicial concept is quite different. Legally, there are two forms of automatism: *sane* and *insane*. The sane automatism results from an external or extrinsic factor, and the insane automatism results from an internal or endogenous cause. This choice results in two very different consequences for the accused: commitment to a mental hospital for an indefinite period of time if insane or acquittal without any mandated medical consultation or follow-up if sane. For example, a criminal

act resulting from altered behavior due to hypoglycemia induced by the injection of too much insulin would be a sane automatism, whereas the same act due to hypoglycemia caused by an insulinoma would be an insane automatism. By this unscientific paradigm, criminal behavior associated with epilepsy is, by definition, an insane automatism.[135, 138] In the United States, the approach to automatism varies among states.[139]

The current legal system unfortunately must consider a sleep-related violence case strictly in terms of choosing between insane or noninsane automatisms or without any stipulated deterrent concerning a recurrence of SW with criminal charges that was induced by a recurrence of the high-risk behavior. If SW is deemed an insane automatism, then a significant percentage of the general population is "legally insane." Clearly, dialogue between the medical and legal professions regarding this important area would be helpful to both professions and to those arrested during automatisms.[140] For further discussion of this area, consult a book devoted to the various forensic aspects of sleep medicine (see reference 141).

One reasonable approach in dealing with the earlier mentioned automatisms from a legal standpoint would be to add a category of acquittal that allowed for innocence based on a lack of guilt consequent to set diagnoses—specific illnesses that could be categorized by a group of subspecialty clinicians in consultation with the legal profession.[142]

Another suggestion has been a two-stage trial, which would first establish who committed the act and then deal separately with the issue of culpability. The first part would be held before a jury; the second would be held in front of a judge with medical advisors present.[135]

One fortunate, and unexplained, fact is that nocturnal sleep-related violence is hardly ever a reappearing phenomenon.[143] Rarely, recurrence is reported and possibly should be termed a noninsane automatism. Thorough evaluation and effective treatment are mandatory before the patient can be regarded as no longer a menace to society.[144] In some cases, clear precipitating events can be identified and must be avoided to be exonerated from legal culpability. This concept has led to the proposal of two new forensic categories: (1) parasomnia with continuing danger as a noninsane automatism and (2) (intermittent) state-dependent continuing danger.[144–146]

Role of the Sleep Medicine Specialist

With the identification of ever-increasing causes, manifestations, and consequences of sleep-related violence comes an opportunity for sleep medicine experts to educate the general public and practicing clinicians regarding the occurrence and nature of such behaviors and successful treatment. More importantly, the onus is on medical professionals to educate and assist the legal profession in cases of sleep-related violence that result in forensic medicine issues. This often presents difficult ethical problems because most "expert witnesses" are retained by either the defense or the prosecution, leading to the tendency for expert witnesses to become an advocate or a partisan for one side or the other. Historically, this has been fertile ground for the appearance of "junk science" in the courtroom,[147] from Bendectin to triazolam to breast implants. Junk science leads to junk justice and altered standards of care.[148] Much attention has been paid to the existence and prevalence of junk science in the courtroom, with recommendations to minimize its occurrence.

There is some hope that the judicial system is paying more attention to the process of authentic science and may move to accept only valid scientific evidence.[149, 150] In the 1920s, in an attempt to reduce incompetence on the part of expert witnesses, the *Frey* rule was issued, which allowed experts into court only if their testimony was "generally accepted" as valid among other scientists in their field. In 1975, the Federal Rules of Evidence were codified and made no mention of the *Frey* rule, and the standards for expert testimony all but disappeared.[147] In 1993, the *Daubert* decision (after the Bendectin debacle) made it the judge's responsibility to determine the legitimacy of scientific evidence before admitting it.[151] The gatekeeping power (and responsibility) of judges to exclude evidence based on subjective belief or unsupported speculation was further elevated by the U.S. Supreme Court in the *General Electric Co. et al. v Joiner* (No. 96–188) decision.

Forensic Sleep Medicine Experts as Impartial Friends of the Court (amicus curiae)

One infrequently used tactic to improve scientific testimony is to use a court-appointed "impartial expert."[147] When approached to testify, volunteering to serve as a court-appointed expert rather than as one appointed by either the prosecution or defense may encourage this practice. Other proposed measures include the development of a specific section in scientific journals dedicated to expert witness testimony extracted from public documents with request for opinions and consensus statements from appropriate specialists or the development of a library of circulating expert testimony that could be used to discredit irresponsible, professional witnesses.[147] Good science is not determined by the credentials of the expert witness but rather by scientific consensus.[148]

Before accepting any given case, the sleep professional should familiarize himself or herself with this most important issue. A good starting point is a highly informative book, *Galileo's Revenge: Junk Science in the Courtroom.*[147] To address the problem of junk science in the courtroom many professional societies are calling for, and some have developed guidelines for, expert witness qualifications and testimony.[152–154] Similarly, the American Academy of Sleep Medicine and the American Academy of Neurology have adopted their own guidelines, which include the following:[155, 156]

I. Expert witness qualifications
   A. Must have a current, valid, unrestricted license
   B. Must be a diplomate of the American Board of Sleep Medicine

   C. Must be familiar with the clinical practice of sleep medicine and should have been actively involved in clinical practice at the time of the event

II. Guidelines for expert testimony
   A. Must be impartial; the ultimate test for accuracy and impartiality is a willingness to prepare testimony that could be presented unchanged for use by either the plaintiff or the defendant.
   B. Fees should relate to time and effort and not be contingent on the outcome of the claim. Fees should not exceed 20% of the practitioner's annual income.
   C. The practitioner should be willing to submit such testimony for peer review.
   D. To establish consistency, the expert witness should make records from his or her previous expert witness testimony available to the attorneys and expert witnesses of both parties.
   E. The expert witness must not become a partisan or an advocate in the legal proceeding.

Familiarizing oneself with these guidelines may be helpful in a given case because the expert witness from each side should be held to the same standards.[157]

Clinical and Laboratory Evaluation of Sleep-Related Violent Behavior

The history of complex, violent, or potentially injurious motor behavior arising from the sleep period should suggest the possibility of one of the above-mentioned conditions. Our experience with more than 200 cases of sleep-related injury or violence in adults has repeatedly indicated that clinical differentiation, without polysomnographic study, among RBD, disorders of arousal, sleep apnea, and sleep-related psychogenic dissociative states and other psychiatric conditions often is impossible.[158] It is likely that violence arising from the sleep period is more frequent than previously assumed.[159]

As mentioned, the legal implications of automatic behavior have been discussed and debated in both medical and legal literature.[1, 160–164] As with nonsleep automatisms, the identification of a specific underlying organic or psychiatric sleep/violence condition does not establish causality for any given deed. Two questions accompany each case of reportedly sleep-related violence: (1) Is it possible for behavior this complex to have arisen in a mixed state of wakefulness and sleep without conscious awareness or responsibility for the act? (2) Is that what happened at the time of the incident? The answer to the first is often "yes." The second can never be determined with surety because "the thief has fled in the night."

To assist in the determination of the putative role of an underlying sleep disorder in a specific violent act, we have proposed guidelines, modified from Bonkalo (sleepwalking),[25] Walker (epilepsy),[165] and Glasgow (automatism in general)[166] and formulated from our clinical experience:[3]

1. There should be reason (by history or formal sleep laboratory evaluation) to suspect a bona fide sleep disorder. Similar episodes, with benign or morbid outcome, should have occurred previously. (It must be remembered that disorders of arousal may *begin* in adulthood.)
2. The duration of the action is usually brief (i.e., minutes).
3. The behavior is usually abrupt, immediate, impulsive, and senseless—without apparent motivation. Although ostensibly purposeful, it is completely inappropriate to the total situation, out of (waking) character for the individual, and without evidence of premeditation.
4. The victim is someone who merely happened to be present and who may have been the stimulus for the arousal.
5. Immediately after the return of consciousness, there is perplexity or horror, without an attempt to escape, conceal, or cover up the action. There is evidence of lack of awareness on the part of the individual during the event.
6. There usually is some degree of amnesia for the event, but this amnesia need not be complete.
7. In the case of ST/SW or sleep drunkenness, the act may:
   * Occur on awakening (rarely immediately on falling asleep)—usually at least 1 h after sleep onset
   * Occur on attempts to awaken the subject
   * Have been potentiated by alcohol ingestion, sedative/hypnotic administration, or prior sleep deprivation

Most of these conditions are diagnosable, and most are treatable. Clinical evaluation should include a complete review of sleep-wake complaints from both the victim and bedpartner (if available). This should be followed by a thorough general physical, neurological, and psychiatric examination. The diagnosis may only be suspected clinically. Extensive polysomnographic study with an extensive scalp electroencephalographic study at a paper speed of 15 mm/sec, electromyographic monitoring of all four extremities, and continuous audiovisual recording are mandatory for correct diagnosis in atypical cases.[17, 51, 108, 167–172] Establishing the diagnosis of nocturnal seizures may be particularly difficult (see Chapter 63).

The proposition that sleep disorders may be a legitimate defense in cases of violence arising from the sleep period has been met with immense skepticism.[173] To provide credibility, evaluations of such complex cases are best performed in experienced sleep disorders centers with interpretation made by a veteran clinical polysomnographer. Due to the complex nature of many of these disorders, a multidisciplinary approach is highly recommended.[158, 174]

SUMMARY AND FUTURE DIRECTIONS

It is abundantly clear that violence may occur during any one of the three states of being. Violence during REM or NREM sleep may have occurred without conscious awareness and is due to one of a number of completely different disorders. Violent behavior during sleep may result in events that have forensic science implications. The apparent suicide (e.g., leap to death from a second-story window) and assault or murder (e.g., molestation, strangulation, stabbing, shooting) may be the unintentional, nonculpable but catastrophic result of disorders of arousal, sleep-related seizures, RBD, or psychogenic dissociative states. The majority of these conditions are diagnosable and, more important, treatable. The social and legal implications are obvious.

Practitioners in the field of sleep medicine must pursue further productive study and request adequate funding to objectively study the following important questions: What is the true prevalence of these disorders? How are they best and most accurately diagnosed? How can the usually present prodromes be taken seriously? Why is there male predominance in many of the disorders? How can these patients best be treated, or better yet, how can the consequences be prevented? Are "social stressors" truly more prevalent in this population? What is the best way to deal with forensic science issues? What should be done with the offender? What is the likelihood of recurrence? Is such behavior a sane or an insane automatism?[69] How can the potential victim be protected?

More research, both basic science and clinical, is urgently needed to further identify and elaborate on the components of both waking and sleep-related violence, with particular emphasis on neurobiological, neuroplastic, genetic, and socioenvironmental factors.[14–16] The study of violence and aggression will be greatly enhanced by close cooperation among clinicians, basic science researchers, and social scientists.

References

1. Fitzgerald PJ. Voluntary and involuntary acts. In: Guest AG, ed. Oxford Essays in Jurisprudence. Oxford, England: Oxford University Press; 1961:1–28.
2. Ohayon MM, Caulet M, Priest RG. Violent behavior during sleep. J Clin Psychiatry. 1997;58:369–376.
3. Mahowald MW, Bundlie SR, Hurwitz TD, et al. Sleep violence-forensic science implications: polygraphic and video documentation. J Forensic Sci. 1990;35:413–432.
4. Mahowald MW, Schenck CH. Dissociated states of wakefulness and sleep. Neurology. 1992;42:44–52.
5. Zorick FJ, Salis PJ, Roth T, et al. Narcolepsy and automatic behavior: a case report. J Clin Psychiatry. 1979;40:194–197.
6. Grillner S, Dubic R. Control of locomotion in vertebrates: spinal and supraspinal mechanisms. Adv Neurol. 1988;47:425–453.
7. Cohen AH. Evolution of the vertebrate central pattern generator for locomotion. In: Cohen AH, Rossignol S, Grillner S, eds. Neural Control of Rhythmic Movements in Vertebrates. New York, NY: John Wiley & Sons; 1988:129–166.
8. Corner MA. Brainstem control of behavior: ontogenetic aspects. In: Klemm R, Vertes RP, eds. Brainstem Mechanisms of Behavior. New York, NY: John Wiley & Sons; 1990:239–266.
9. Siegel A, Pott CB. Neural substrates of aggression and flight in the cat. Prog Neurobiol. 1988;31:261–283.
10. LeDoux JE. Emotion. In: Montcastle VB, Plum F, Geiger SR, eds. Handbook of Physiology: The Nervous System: Higher Functions of the Brain, Part I. Baltimore, Md: Williams & Wilkins; 1987:419–459.

11. Berntson GG, Micco DJ. Organization of brainstem behavioral systems. Brain Res Bull. 1976;1:471–483.

12. Bandler R. Brain mechanisms of aggression as revealed by electrical and chemical stimulation: suggestion of a central role for the midbrain periaqueductal region. Progr Psychobiol Physiol Psychol. 1988;13:67–154.

13. Weiger WA, Bear DM. An approach to the neurology of aggression. J Psychiatr Res. 1988;22:85–98.

14. Blake PY, Pincus JH, Buckner C. Neurologic abnormalities in murderers. Neurology. 1995;45:1641–1647.

15. Elliott FA. Violence: the neurologic contribution: an overview. Arch Neurol. 1992;49:595–603.

16. Greene AF, Lynch TF, Decker B, et al. A psychological theoretical characterization of interpersonal violence offenders. Aggression Violent Behav. 1997;2:273–284.

17. Mahowald MW, Schenck CH. Parasomnia purgatory: the epileptic/non-epileptic interface. In: Rowan AJ, Gates JR, eds. Non-Epileptic Seizures. Boston, Mass: Butterworth-Heinemann; 1993:123–139.

18. Mahowald MW, Rosen GM. Parasomnias in children. Pediatrician. 1990;17:21–31.

19. Fisher C, Kahn E, Edwards A, et al. A psychophysiological study of nightmares and night terrors, III: mental content and recall of stage 4 night terrors. J Nerv Ment Dis. 1974;158:174–188.

20. American Sleep Disorders Association, Diagnostic Classification Steering Committee. International Classification of Sleep Disorders: Diagnostic and Coding Manual. Rochester, Minn: American Sleep Disorders Association; 1990.

21. Schenck CH, Hurwitz TD, Bundlie SR, et al. Sleep-related injury in 100 adult patients: a polysomnographic and clinical report. Am J Psychiatry. 1989;146:1166–1173.

22. Hartmann E, Greenwald D, Brune P. Night-terrors–sleepwalking. Sleep Res. 1982;11:121.

23. Hublin C, Kaprio J, Partinen M, et al. Prevalence and genetics of sleepwalking: a population-based twin study. Neurology. 1997;48:177–181.

24. Vela Bueno A, Blanco BD, Cajal FV. Episodic sleep disorder triggered by fever: a case presentation. Waking Sleeping. 1980;4:243–251.

25. Bonkalo A. Impulsive acts and confusional states during incomplete arousal from sleep: criminological and forensic implications. Psychiatr Q. 1974;48:400–409.

26. Raschka LB. Sleep and violence. Can J Psychiatry. 1984;29:132–134.

27. Nielsen TA, Dumont M, Montplaisir J. A 20-h recovery sleep after prolonged sleep restriction: some effects of competing in a world record-setting cinemarathon. J Sleep Res. 1995;4:78–85.

28. Williams HL, Morris GO, Lubin A. Illusions, hallucinations and sleep loss. In: West L, ed. Hallucinations. New York, NY: Grune & Stratton, 1962:158–165.

29. Shurley JT. Hallucinations in sensory deprivation and sleep loss. Hallucinations. 1962:87–91.

30. Babkoff H, Sing HC, Thorne DR, et al. Perceptual distortions and hallucinations reported during the course of sleep deprivation. Percep Mot Skills. 1989;68:787–798.

31. Brauchi JT, West LJ. Sleep deprivation. JAMA. 1959;171:1–14.

32. Belenky GL. Unusual visual experiences reported by subjects in the British army study of sustained operations, exercise early call. Milit Med. 1979;144:695–696.

33. Luchins DJ, Sherwood PM, Gillin JC, et al. Filicide during psychotropic-induced somnambulism: a case report. Am J Psychiatry. 1978;135:1404–1405.

34. Huapaya LVM. Seven cases of somnambulism induced by drugs. Am J Psychiatry. 1979;136:985–986.

35. Charney DS, Kales A, Soldatos CR, et al. Somnambulistic-like episodes secondary to combined lithium-neuroleptic treatment. Br J Psychiatry. 1979;135:418–424.

36. Lipowski ZJ. Delirium (acute confusional state). JAMA. 1987;258:1789–1792.

37. Guilleminault C, Phillips R, Dement WC. A syndrome of hypersomnia with automatic behavior. Electroencephalogr Clin Neurophysiol. 1975;38:403–413.

38. Roth B, Nevsimalova S, Sagova V, et al. Neurological, psychological and polygraphic findings in sleep drunkenness. Arch Suisses Neurol Neurochir Psychiatr. 1981;129:209–222.

39. Roth B, Nevsimalova S, Rechtschaffen A. Hypersomnia with "sleep drunkenness." Arch Gen Psych 1972;26:456–462.

40. Mahowald MW, Schenck CH. REM sleep behavior disorder. In: Kryger MH, Dement W, Roth T, eds. Principles and Practice of Sleep Medicine. 2nd ed. Philadelphia, Pa: WB Saunders; 1994:574–588.

41. Parkes JD. Sleep and Its Disorders. Philadelphia, Pa: WB Saunders; 1985.

42. Glusman M. The hypothalamic "savage" syndrome. Assoc Res Nerv Ment Dis. 1974;52:52–92.

43. Kitsikis A, Steriade M. Immediate behavioral effects of kainic acid injections into the midbrain reticular core. Behav Brain Res. 1981;3:361–380.

44. Siegel A, Shaikh MB. The neural bases of aggression and rage in the cat. Aggression Violent Behav. 1997;2:241–271.

45. Valzelli L. Psychobiology of Aggression and Violence. New York, NY: Raven Press; 1981.

46. Pons TP, Garraghty PE, Ommaya K, et al. Massive cortical reorganization after sensory deafferentation in adult Macaques. Science. 1991;252:1857–1860.

47. Edelman GM. Neural Darwinism. New York, NY: Basic Books; 1987.

48. Greene AF, Lynch TF, Decker B, et al. A psychobiological theoretical characterization of interpersonal violence offenders. Aggression Violent Behav. 1997;2:273–284.

49. Golden CJ, Jackson ML, Peterson-Rohne A, et al. Neuropsychological correlates of violence and aggression: a review of the clinical literature. Aggression Violent Behav. 1996;1:3–25.

50. Mahowald MW, Schenck CH. NREM parasomnias. Neurol Clin. 1996;14:675–696.

51. Guilleminault C, Silvestri R. Disorders of arousal and epilepsy during sleep. In: Sterman MB, Shouse MN, Passouant P, eds. Sleep and Epilepsy. New York, NY: Academic Press; 1982:513–531.

52. Millman RP, Kipp GR, Carskadon MA. Sleepwalking precipitated by treatment of sleep apnea with nasal CPAP. Chest. 1991;99:750–751.

53. Pressman MR, Meyer TJ, Kendrick-Mohamed J, et al. Night terrors in an adult precipitated by sleep apnea. Sleep. 1995;18:773–775.

54. Hammond WA. Sleep and Its Derangements. Philadelphia, Pa: JB Lippincott; 1869.

55. Hopwood JS, Snell HK. Amnesia in relation to crime. J Ment Sci. 1933;79:27–41.

56. Tarsh MJ. On serious violence during sleep-walking. Br J Psychiatry. 1986;148:476.

57. Bartholomew AA. On serious violence during sleep-walking. Br J Psychiatry. 1986;148:476–477.

58. Sleepwalking and guilt [editorial]. Br Med J. 1970;2:186.

59. Oswald I, Evans J. On serious violence during sleepwalking. Br J Psychiatry. 1985;147:688–691.

60. Morris N. Somnambulistic homicide: ghosts, spiders, and North Koreans. Res Judicatae. 1951;5:29–33.

61. Fenwick P. Murdering while asleep. Br Med J. 1986;293:574–575.

62. Podolsky E. Somnambulistic homicide. Dis Nerv Syst. 1959;20:534–536.

63. Podolsky E. Somnambulistic homicide. Med Sci Law. 1961;1:260–265.

64. Yellowlees D. Homicide by a somnambulist. J Ment Sci. 1878;24:451–458.

65. Howard C, D'Orban PT. Violence in sleep: medico-legal issues and two case reports. Psychol Med. 1987;17:915–925.

66. Schatzman M. To sleep, perchance to kill. New Scientist. 1986;26:60–62.

67. Lochel M. Sleepwalking in children and adolescents: medical history, child psychiatric and electro-encephalographic aspects. Acta Paedopsychiatr. 1989;52:112–120.

68. Ovuga EBL. Murder during sleepwalking. East Afr Med J. 1992;69:533–534.

69. Brooks AD. Law, Psychiatry, and the Mental Health System. Boston, Mass: Little, Brown; 1974.

70. Bornstein S, Guegen B, Hache E. Syndrome d'Elpenor ou meutre somnambulique? Ann Med-Psychol. 1996;154:195–201.

71. Hamer BA, Payne A. Sleep automatism: clinical study in forensic nursing. Perspect Psychiatr Care. 1993;29:7–11.

72. Kleitman N. Sleep and wakefulness. Chicago, Ill: University of Chicago Press; 1963.

73. Chuaqui C. Suicide and abnormalities of consciousness. Can Psychiatric Assoc J. 1975;20:25–28.

74. Lauerma H. Fear of suicide during sleepwalking. Psychiatry. 1996;59:206–211.

75. Hartmann E. Two case reports: night terrors with sleepwalking: a potentially lethal disorder. J Nerv Ment Dis. 1983;171:503–505.

76. Rauch PK, Stern TA. Life-threatening injuries resulting from sleepwalking and night terrors. Psychosomatics. 1986;27:62–64.

77. Ferber R, Boyle MP. Injury associated with sleepwalking and sleep terrors in children. Sleep Res. 1984;13:141.

78. Chin CN. Sleep walking in adults: two case reports. Med J Malaysia. 1987;42:132–133.

79. Scott AIF. Attempted strangulation during phenothiazine-induced sleep-walking and night terrors. Br J Psychiatry. 1988;153:692–694.

80. Schenck CH, Mahowald MW. Injurious sleep behavior disorders (parasomnias) affecting patients on intensive care units. Intens Care Med. 1991;17:219–224.

81. Wong KE. Masturbation during sleep: a somnambulistic variant? Singapore Med J. 1986;27:542–543.

82. Shapiro CM, Fedoroff JP, Trajanovic NN. Sexual behavior in sleep: a newly described parasomnia. Sleep Res. 1996;25:367.

83. Hurwitz TD, Mahowald MW, Schenck CH, et al. Sleep-related sexual abuse of children. Sleep Res. 1989;18:246.

84. Buchanan A. Sleepwalking and indecent exposure. Med Sci Law. 1991;31:38–40.

85. Rosenfeld DS, Elhajjar AJ. Sleepsex: a variant of sleepwalking. Arch Sex Behav. 1998;27:269–278.

86. Fenwick P. Sleep and sexual offending. Med Sci Law. 1996;36:122–134.

87. Broughton R, Billings R, Cartwright R, et al. Homicidal somnambulism: a case report. Sleep. 1994;17:253–264.

88. Nofzinger EA, Wettstein RM. Homicidal behavior and sleep apnea: a case report and medicolegal discussion. Sleep. 1995;18:776–782.

89. Jouvet M, Delorme F. Locus coeruleus et sommeil paradoxal. CR Soc Biol. 1965;159:895–899.

90. Hendricks JC, Morrison AR, Mann GL. Different behaviors during paradoxical sleep without atonia depend upon lesion site. Brain Res. 1982;239:81–105.

91. Schenck CH, Hurwitz TD, Mahowald MW. REM sleep behavior disorder: a report on a series of 96 consecutive cases and a review of the literature. J Sleep Res. 1993;2:224–231.

92. Goldstein M. Brain research and violent behavior. Arch Neurol. 1974;30:1–34.

93. Moyer KE. Kinds of aggression and their physiological basis. Commun Behav Biol. 1968;2(pt A):65–87.

94. Dyken ME, Lin-Dyken DC, Seaba P, et al. Violent sleep-related behavior leading to subdural hemorrhage. Arch Neurol. 1995;52:318–321.

95. Gross PT. REM sleep behavior disorder causing bilateral subdural hematomas. Sleep Res. 1992;21:204.

96. Morfis L, Schwartz RS, Cistulli PA. REM sleep behavior disorder: a treatable cause of falls in the elderly. Age Ageing. 1997;26:43–44.

97. Schenck CH, Mahowald MW. A parasomnia overlap disorder involving sleepwalking, sleep terrors and REM sleep behavior disorder: report in 33 polysomnographically confirmed cases. Sleep. 1997;20:972–981.

98. Nalamalapu U, Goldberg R, DePhillipo M, et al. Behaviors simulating REM behavior disorder in patients with severe obstructive sleep apnea. Sleep Res. 1996;25:311.

99. D' Cruz OF, Vaughn BV. Nocturnal seizures mimic REM behavior disorder. Am J Electroneurodiag Technol. 1997;37:258–264.

100. Hindler CG. Epilepsy and violence. Br J Psychiatry. 1989;155:246–249.

101. Collins RC, Carnes KM, Price JL. Prefrontal-limbic epilepsy: experimental functional anatomy. J Clin Neurophysiol. 1988;5:105–117.

102. Quesney LF, Krieger C, Leitner C, et al. Frontal lobe epilepsy: clinical and electrographic presentation. In: Porter RL, Mattson RH, Ward AA Jr, et al, eds. Advances in Epileptology: XVth Epilepsy International Symposium. New York, NY: Raven Press; 1984:503–508.

103. Ludwig B, Ajmone Marsan B, Strauss E, et al. Cerebral seizures of probable orbitofrontal origin. Epilepsia. 1987;16:141–158.

104. Waterman K, Purves SJ, Strauss E, et al. An epileptic syndrome caused by mesial frontal lobe seizure foci. Neurology. 1987;37:577–582.

105. Tharp B. Orbital frontal seizures: an unique electroencephalographic and clinical syndrome. Epilepsia. 1972;13:627–642.

106. Williamson PD, Spencer SS. Clinical and EEG features of complex partial seizures of extratemporal origin. Epilepsia. 1986;27(suppl 2):s46.

107. Maselli RA, Rosenberg RS, Spire JP. Episodic nocturnal wanderings in non-epileptic young patients. Sleep. 1988;11:156–161.

108. Pedley TA, Guilleminault C. Episodic nocturnal wanderings responsive to anticonvulsant drug therapy. Ann Neurol. 1977;2:30–35.

109. Plazzi G, Tinuper P, Montagna P, et al. Epileptic nocturnal wanderings. Sleep. 1995;18:749–756.

110. Mayeux R, Alexander MP, Benson DF, et al. Poriomania. Neurology. 1979;29:1616–1619.

111. Borum R, Appelbaum KL. Epilepsy, aggression, and criminal responsibility. Psychiatr Serv. 1996;47:762–763.

112. Fenwick P. The nature and management of aggression in epilepsy. J Neuropsychiatry. 1989;1:418–425.

113. Gerard ME, Spitz MC, Towbin JA, et al. Subacute postictal aggression. Neurology. 1998;50:384–388.

114. Houdart R, Mamo H, Tomkiewicz H. La forme epileptogene du syndrome de Pickwick. Rev Neurol. 1960;103:466–468.

115. Kryger M, Quesney LF, Holder D, et al. The sleep deprivation syndrome of the obese patient. Am J Med. 1974;56:531–539.

116. Guilleminault C. Natural history, cardiac impact and long-term follow-up of sleep apnea syndrome. In: Guilleminault C, Lugaresi E, eds. Sleep/Wake Disorders: Natural History, Epidemiology, and Long-Term Evolution. New York, NY: Raven Press; 1983:107–125.

117. Mahowald MW, Mahowald ML. Sleep disorders. In: Rizzo M, Trandel D, eds. Head Injury and Postconcussive Syndrome. New York, NY: Churchill Livingstone; 1996:285–304.

118. Hays P. False but sincere accusations of sexual assault made by narcoleptic patients. Med Leg Bull. 1992;60:265–271.

119. Mahowald MW, Woods SR, Schenck CH. Sleeping dreams, waking hallucinations, and the central nervous system. Dreaming. 1998;8:89–102.

120. Regina v. Warner. Ontario Rep. Feb 17, 1995:136–157.

121. McCaldon RJ. Automatism. Can Med Assoc J. 1964;91:914–920.

122. Fleming J. Dissociative episodes presenting as somnambulism: a case report. Sleep Res. 1987;16:263.

123. Schenck CH, Milner D, Hurwitz TD, et al. Dissociative disorders presenting as somnambulism: polysomnographic, video and clinical documentation (8 cases). Dissociation. 1989;2:194–204.

124. Coy JD. Letter to editor. J Emerg Med. 1996;14:760–762.

125. Bisson JI. Automatism and post-traumatic stress disorder. Br J Psychiatry. 1993;163:830–832.

126. Pontius AA. Homicide linked to moderate repetitive stresses kindling limbic seizures in 14 cases of limbic psychotic trigger reaction. Aggression Violent Behav. 1997;2:125–141.

127. Rosenberg DA. Web of deceit: a literature review of Munchausen syndrome by proxy. Child Abuse Neglect. 1987;11:547–563.

128. Light MJ, Sheridan MS. Munchausen syndrome by proxy and sleep apnea. Clin Pediatr. 1990;29:162–168.

129. Griffith JC, Slovik LS. Munchausen by proxy and sleep disorders medicine. Sleep. 1989;12:178–183.

130. Byard RW, Beal SM. Munchausen syndrome by proxy: repetitive infantile apnoea and homicide. J Paediatr Child Health. 1993;29:77–79.

131. Samuels MP, McClaughlin W, Jacobson RR, et al. Fourteen cases of imposed upper airway obstruction. Arch Dis Child. 1992;67:162–170.

132. Mydlo JH, Maccia RJ, Kanter JL. Munchausen's syndrome: a medico-legal dilemma. Med Sci Law. 1997;37:198–201.

133. Bryk M, Siegel PT. My mother caused my illness: the story of a survivor of Munchausen by proxy syndrome. Pediatrics. 1997;100:1–7.

134. Shau K, Mouridsen SE. Munchausen syndrome by proxy: a review. Acta Paediatr. 1995;84:977–982.

135. Fenwick P. Automatism, medicine, and the law. Psychol Med Monograph. 1990;17(suppl I):1–27.

136. Jang D, Coles EM. The evolution and definition of the concept of "automatism" in Canadian case law. Med Law. 1995;14:221–238.

137. Fenwick P. Automatism. In: Bluglass R, Bowden P, eds. Principles and Practice of Forensic Psychiatry. Edinburgh, Scotland: Churchill Livingstone; 1990:271–285.

138. Fenwick P. Epilepsy, automatism, and the English law. Med Law. 1997;16:349–358.

139. McCall Smith A, Shapiro CM. Sleep disorders and the criminal law. In: Shapiro C, McCall Smith A, eds. Forensic Aspects of Sleep. Chichester, England: John Wiley & Sons; 1997:29–64.

140. Thomas TN. Sleepwalking disorder and *mens rea*: a review and case report. J Forensic Sci. 1997;42:17–24.

141. Shapiro C, McCall Smith A. Forensic Aspects of Sleep. New York, NY: John Wiley & Sons; 1997:208.

142. Beran RG. Automatisms: the current legal position related to clinical practice and medicolegal interpretation. Clin Exp Neurol. 1992;29:81–91.

143. Guilleminault C, Moscovitch A, Leger D. Forensic sleep medicine: nocturnal wandering and violence. Sleep. 1995;18:740–748.

144. Schenck CH, Mahowald MW. A polysomnographically documented case of adult somnambulism with long-distance automobile driving with frequent nocturnal violence: parasomnia with continuing danger as a noninsane automatism. Sleep. 1995;18:765–772.

145. Schenck CH, Mahowald MW. An analysis of a recent criminal trial involving sexual misconduct with a child, alcohol abuse, and a successful sleepwalking defense: arguments supporting two proposed new forensic categories. Med Sci Law. 1998;38:147–152.

146. Schenck CH, Mahowald MW. Sleepwalking and indecent exposure [letter]. Med Sci Law. 1992;32:86–87.

147. Huber PW. Galileo's Revenge: Junk Science in the Courtroom. New York, NY: Basic Books; 1991.

148. Weintraub MI. Expert witness testimony: a time for self-regulation? Neurology. 1995;45:855–858.

149. Loevinger L. Science as evidence. Jurimetrics J. 1995;153:153–190.

150. Foster KR, Bernstein DE, Huber PW. Phantom Risk: Scientific Inference and the Law. Cambridge, Mass: MIT Press; 1993.

151. *Daubert v Merrell Dow Pharmaceuticals*, 92–102 (9th Cir 1993). [113 S Ct 2768 (1993)].

152. Committee on Medical Liability. Guidelines for expert witness testimony. Pediatrics. 1989;83:312–313.

153. Guidelines for the physician expert witness. American College of Physicians. Ann Intern Med. 1990;113:789.

154. Bone R, Rosenow E. ACCP guidelines for an expert witness. Chest. 1990;98:1006.

155. American Sleep Disorders Association. ASDA guidelines for expert witness qualifications and testimony. APSS Newslett. 1993;8:23.

156. American Academy of Neurology. Qualifications and guidelines for the physician expert witness [newsletter]. Neurology. 1989;39:9A.

157. Mahowald MW, Schenck CH. Complex motor behavior arising during the sleep period: forensic science implications. Sleep. 1995;18:724–727.

158. Mahowald MW, Schenck CH, Rosen GR, et al. The role of a sleep disorders center in evaluating sleep violence. Arch Neurol. 1992;49:604–607.

159. Broughton RJ, Shimizu T. Sleep-related violence: a medical and forensic challenge. Sleep. 1995;18:727–730.

160. Whitlock FA. Criminal Responsibility and Mental Illness. London, England: Butterworths; 1963.

161. Prevezer S. Automatism and involuntary conduct. Criminal Law Rev. 1958:440–452.

162. Prevezer S. Automatism and involuntary conduct. Criminal Law Rev. 1958:361–367.

163. Williams G. Criminal Law. London, England: Stevens & Sons; 1961.

164. Shroder O, Mather NJ. Forensic psychiatry. In: Camps FE, ed. Gradwohl's Legal Medicine. 3rd ed. Chicago, Ill: A. John Wright & Sons; 1976:505.

165. Walker EA. Murder or epilepsy? J Nerv Ment Dis. 1961;133:430–437.

166. Glasgow GL. The anatomy of automatism. N Z Med J. 1965;64:491–495.

167. Soldatos CR, Vela-Bueno A, Bixler EO, et al. Sleepwalking and night terrors in adulthood, clinical and EEG findings. Clin Electroencephalogr. 1980;11:136–139.

168. Halbreich U, Assael M. Electroencephalogram with spheniodal needles in sleepwalkers. Psychiatr Clin. 1978;11:213–218.

169. Popoviciu L, Szabo L, Corfariu O, et al. A study of the relationships of certain pavor nocturnus (PN) attacks with nocturnal epilepsy. In: Popoviciu L, Asgian B, Badiu G, eds. Sleep 1978. Fourth European Congress on Sleep Research. Tirgu-Mures, Romania. Basel, Switzerland: S Karger; 1980:599–605.

170. Dervent A, Karacan I, Ware JC, et al. Somnambulism: a case report. Sleep Res. 1978;7:220.

171. Amir N, Navon P, Silverberg-Shalev R. Interictal electroencephalography in night terrors and somnambulism. Israel J Med Sci. 1985;21:22–26.

172. Broughton R. Childhood sleepwalking, sleep terrors, and enuresis nocturna: their pathophysiology and differentiation from nocturnal epileptic seizures. In: Popoviciu L, Ashian B, Badiu G, eds. Sleep 1978. Fourth European Congress on Sleep Research. Tirgu-Mures, Romania, Basel, Switzerland: S. Karger; 1980:103–122.

173. Guilleminault C, Kushida C, Leger D. Forensic sleep medicine and nocturnal wanderings. Sleep. 1995;18:721–723.

174. Aldrich MS, Jahnke B. Diagnostic value of video-EEG polysomnography. Neurology. 1991;41:1060–1066.

twelve

Sleep Breathing Disorders

Mark H. Sanders

Medications, Sleep, and Breathing

Richard W. Robinson

Clifford W. Zwillich

As the prevalence and clinical importance of sleep-disordered breathing (SDB) have become increasingly apparent, greater interest in the influence of drugs on breathing during sleep has developed. Many medications and certain hormones may profoundly influence breathing, both positively and negatively, during sleep in patients with sleep apnea, pulmonary disorders, and congestive heart failure (CHF). To date, there is no consistently effective pharmacological therapy for the obstructive sleep apnea (OSA) syndrome. This is unfortunate because the presently effective therapeutic modalities require either surgery or the use of cumbersome equipment. The limitations of the various drugs used to treat sleep apnea are discussed in the latter part of this chapter.

DRUGS WITH ADVERSE EFFECTS ON BREATHING DURING SLEEP

Alcohol

Moderate degrees of alcohol intoxication (blood concentrations 100 to 120 mg/dl) decrease hypoxic and hypercapnic ventilatory responses to about 50% of baseline values.[1] The perception of flow-resistive loads is blunted after alcohol ingestion (mean concentration: 133 mg/dl), but ventilatory load compensation is preserved.[2] During wakefulness, irregular breathing patterns with transient apneas can be seen with mild intoxication,[3] but, the effects on overall alveolar ventilation and gas exchange in both normal subjects and nonhypercapnic chronic obstructive pulmonary disease (COPD) patients is negligible.[4, 5] Hypercapnia does not occur even with extreme intoxication until blood concentrations exceed 350 mg/dl.[6]

Although alcohol is only a mild respiratory depressant during wakefulness, it is now widely recognized that it may precipitate or aggravate existing OSA in certain individuals.[7–11] This observation was probably first made anecdotally by the wives of many heavy snorers and patients with sleep apnea.[7]

Asymptomatic persons, particularly men, often have small numbers of apneas during sleep.[12] In many normals, apnea frequency while asleep may increase by a small amount if alcohol is ingested at bedtime.[11] Older people seem to be more vulnerable to this effect of alcohol. However, not all studies in normals have shown increased disordered breathing after bedtime alcohol. Normal women, irrespective of menopausal status, are resistant to development of sleep apnea after modest bedtime alcohol ingestion.[13, 14] Even in men, some studies have shown little or no effect both in normals and in young nonobese snorers.[10, 15] These inconsistent results are probably attributable to differences in the groups of subjects studied. Older, somewhat obese subjects are far more likely to show breathing abnormalities during sleep after alcohol ingestion than are young, healthy people.

In sharp contrast to the mild and inconsistent findings in normals, most people with chronic, habitual snoring or mild OSA typically develop more frequent and more prolonged apneas after alcohol ingestion. Some snorers who have no apneas under baseline conditions develop frank OSA after alcohol use.[9, 16] The tendency for more frequent apneas is seen during the first 1 to 2 h of sleep when blood concentrations are highest.[9, 10]

Maintenance of a patent pharyngeal airway requires that a variety of upper airway muscles generate enough force to overcome the collapsing tendency of the inspiratory negative intrapharyngeal pressure produced by the diaphragm.[17] Several lines of evidence in animals and human beings suggest that alcohol has a depressant influence on the activity of these pharyngeal dilating muscles. Alcohol selectively decreases hypoglossal nerve activity and consequently genioglossal muscle tone at blood concentrations that do not affect phrenic nerve activity.[18, 19] This effect appears less pronounced in women, who are relatively resistant to the development of apneas after alcohol ingestion.[13, 14, 19] In awake normal subjects, pharyngeal inspiratory airflow resistance significantly increases during the first hour after alcohol ingestion[20] (mean blood concentration: 87 mg/dl). Alcohol ingestion in snorers results in collapse of the upper airway when intrapharyngeal pressure is less negative than under control conditions.[21] In addition, higher levels of nasal continuous positive airway pressure (CPAP) are needed to prevent snoring after alcohol ingestion than under control conditions.[16] Interestingly, however, OSA patients using a previously established effective CPAP level do not develop increased apneas.[22] In the presence of externally applied airway occlusion, intoxicated normal males augment inspiratory effort more slowly and require a greater threshold of effort to arouse from sleep[23] (Fig. 69–1). Thus, the development of longer apneas is favored (Fig. 69–2). Because these alcohol effects occur during sleep at a time when the electromyographic (EMG) tone of upper airway muscles is already low,[24] an ideal situation favoring the development of occlusive apneas is present. Heavy snorers and OSA patients who have anatomically narrowed[25] or functionally defective[26] upper airway muscles are most susceptible to alcohol.

Episodes of oxygen desaturation due to hypoventilation occur during sleep in certain patients with severe COPD. One study examining the effects of alcohol on sleep in 20 nonhypercapnic COPD patients[27] found a consistent but small increase in the number and duration of apneas as well as a small increase in the number of premature ventricular contraction. However, the clinical importance of these changes is arguable. Moreover, episodes of hypopnea and oxygen desaturation, which are of greater importance in COPD, did not increase. The reasons for these apparently minor alcohol effects probably include the small amount consumed (mean blood concentration: 40 mg/dl) and the clinically stable condition of the patients, which included a low prealcohol frequency of SDB. A report in

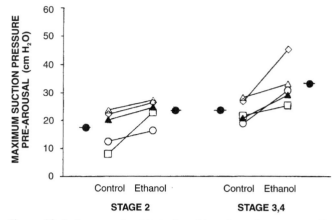

Figure 69–1. In normal subjects breathing through an externally applied resistance, the amount of respiratory effort (negative suction pressure) required to trigger arousal from sleep is increased in both stage 2 and stages 3 and 4 following alcohol consumption. This favors a longer duration of apneas (see Fig. 69–2). (From Berry RB, Bonnet MH, Light RW, 1992, Effect of ethanol on the arousal response to airway occlusion during sleep in normal subjects. American Review of Respiratory Disease, 145:445–452. Official Journal of the American Thoracic Society. © American Lung Association.)

six nonhypercapnic COPD patients noted that bedtime alcohol (mean blood concentration: 129 mg/dl) markedly worsened oxygen saturation, decreased sleep time, and disrupted sleep quality.[28] These effects were especially pronounced during rapid eye movement (REM) sleep as mean Sa_{O_2} fell from 89.6% on placebo night to 81.6% after alcohol ingestion. To our knowledge, the effect of alcohol in hypercapnic COPD patients during sleep has not been examined. However, the above suggest that severe oxygen desaturation may be likely.

Although the short-term effects of alcohol on breathing during sleep have been well studied, the effects of long-term habitual alcohol use are less clear. Several reports suggest that poor sleep quality, as well as apneas and desaturation events, occur with a greater

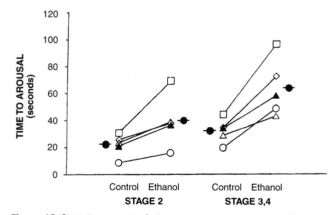

Figure 69–2. Following alcohol, arousal from sleep in both stage 2 and stages 3 and 4 is delayed when normal males breathe through an external resistance. Therefore, apneas are likely to be longer and associated with greater O_2 desaturation. (From Berry RB, Bonnet MH, Light RW, 1992, Effect of ethanol on the arousal response to airway occlusion during sleep in normal subjects. American Review of Respiratory Disease, 145:445–452. Official Journal of the American Thoracic Society. © American Lung Association.)

than expected frequency in abstinent alcoholic subjects, compared with age- and weight-matched controls.[29-31] The clinical relevance of these investigations remains uncertain. Although significantly more SDB was noted in the abstinent alcoholic group, the actual frequency of events and degree of hypoxemia were not impressive. Important unanswered questions are whether SDB is especially severe while the chronic alcoholic individual is actively drinking and whether long-term alcohol use might ultimately irreversibly worsen SDB by permanently altering ventilatory control or upper airway motor function. Two studies by the same investigators[32, 33] suggest that the latter may occur. The authors of these studies proposed that alcohol contributes to the development of hypercapnia in COPD by causing greater sleep hypoxemia, ultimately depressing chemical drives. Another group has observed that edema, a marker of greater hypoxemia, correlates with greater alcohol intake in both COPD and OSA patients. However, there was no correlation in either disease between arterial P_{CO_2} and alcohol consumption.[34, 35] These discrepancies may relate to the inclusion of many females and a lesser overall alcohol consumption in the latter study. Finally, epidemological surveys have suggested that alcohol intake is only weakly or not at all independently associated with snoring or sleep apnea.[36-39] One recent study comparing alcohol intake in OSA patients with age- and weight-matched controls noted no increased alcohol consumption in the patients.[40]

In summary, most normal people will not experience clinically important SDB when they consume alcohol before bedtime. However, certain individuals, particularly obese snorers, may develop frank OSA after bedtime alcohol ingestion. Sleep apnea patients should be strongly advised to avoid alcohol. Patients with COPD who are CO_2 retainers or who have marginal oxygen saturation while awake should also not ingest alcohol near bedtime.

Sedative-Hypnotics

Sedative-hypnotic drugs are widely used in our society; about 20.8 million prescriptions were written in the United States in 1989.[41] Patients with a variety of conditions (alcoholism, COPD, CHF, hypertension) that are clearly associated with SDB often use these agents. Thus, it is important to appreciate how hypnotics affect breathing during sleep.

Benzodiazepines are widely used hypnotic agents. As a class, these drugs are rather mild respiratory depressants. Studies examining the degree to which benzodiazepines affect respiratory chemosensitivity in awake normal subjects have yielded conflicting results.[42] This probably is due to several factors, including interindividual differences in sensitivity to a given drug,[43, 44] route of administration, dosage, and the specific drug studied. From review of multiple reports, a few generalizations may be made. Respiratory depression from oral benzodiazepines is unusual.[45-47] Hypoxic response seems to be more susceptible to depression from these agents than does hypercapnic response.[48-50]

Although the respiratory depressant properties of benzodiazepines appear mild in normal subjects, respiratory depression may be important in certain clinical situations. During acute exacerbations, hypercapnic COPD patients may be highly susceptible to benzodiazepines, and some reports clearly demonstrate worsening hypoventilation and clinical deterioration after administration of recommended dosages of these drugs.[51, 52] Intravenous benzodiazepines, especially diazepam and midazolam, are routinely given during gastrointestinal endoscopy, usually without significant problems.[53] Nevertheless, deaths from respiratory depression and hypoxemia have been reported during endoscopy.[54] About three fourths of midazolam-associated deaths have been respiratory in nature, and over half of these have involved coadministration of an opioid.[55]

Similar to alcohol, neurophysiological data in animals[56] and human beings[57] suggest that benzodiozepines decrease upper airway muscle tone. In a study of healthy adult men intravenous midazolam (0.1 mg/kg) increased supraglottic airway resistance and caused both central and obstructive apneas.[58] In another study the same dose of midazolam produced evidence of airway obstruction in men, whereas in women, even at a dosage of 0.2 mg/kg, upper airway obstruction was infrequently demonstrated.[59] Thus, as with alcohol, women may be relatively resistant to the effects of benzodiazepines on upper airway muscle activity.

The above data suggest that benzodiazepines may promote the development of obstructive apneas in susceptible individuals. A few older reports noted the development of severe upper airway obstruction in OSA patients in whom benzodiazepines were administered as preanesthetics.[7, 60] It is generally advised that hypnotics not be given to individuals with sleep apnea. This recommendation is largely based on reports in the early sleep apnea literature that inconsistently demonstrated an increased apnea frequency in healthy normals[61, 62] or increases in apnea frequency in a few patients with mild SDB.[42, 63] It is probably unwise to draw firm conclusions from these few reports because there is considerable night-to-night variability in apnea frequency in patients with mild SDB, and simple factors such as body position can significantly affect apnea frequency. More recently, several reports have demonstrated that in patients with mild to moderate OSA, hypnotic dosages of benzodiazepines do not produce more frequent apneas or severe oxygen desaturation.[64-69] Despite these data, we recommend avoiding hypnotics in untreated patients with severe OSA, especially those with daytime hypoventilation.

Central sleep apnea syndrome is a heterogeneous disorder with multiple causes. Two reports have demonstrated a decrease in central apneas after benzodiazepine administration.[70, 71] In both studies, the ability of benzodiazepines to reduce arousals, sleep-wake transitions, and sleep fragmentation may have overridden any potential respiratory depressant effects. In the first report, two patients with central apneas associated with frequent arousals due to periodic leg movements experienced a marked reduction in apnea index after

0.5 mg clonazepam. This reduction in apneas was maintained after treatment for 1 week with a 1-mg clonazepam dose at bedtime.[71] The second study involved five men with predominantly central apneas who were otherwise healthy. Compared with placebo, both a 0.125-mg and 0.25-mg dose of triazolam reduced total apnea and central apnea indices by about 50% with no changes in obstructive apnea index.[70] The net effect of triazolam was to increase total sleep time and stage 2 sleep and to decrease arousals and stage transitions. Like the previous investigators, the authors believed that improved sleep quality resulted in fewer central apneas. Because of the small numbers of studies, insufficient data exist to suggest benzodiazepines will help most patients with central sleep apnea. Therefore, the efficacy of any drug treatment must be confirmed with polysomnography, both in the short term and, in the case of benzodiazepines, in the long term, because tolerance to these drugs is well described.

Central apneas associated with oxygen desaturation due to Cheyne-Stokes respiration commonly occur in patients with severe CHF. These patients may complain of poor sleep quality probably due to the frequent arousals that occur during the hyperpneic phase of their periodic breathing. When excessive daytime tiredness occurs it is attributed by patients to poor-quality sleep and they may seek hypnotic medications. Two reports indicate that both short-term[72] and long-term[73] administration of benzodiazepines reduce arousals and improve sleep quality in CHF patients without increasing apneas or the severity of oxygen desaturation. It is not surprising that these weak respiratory depressants do not aggravate this form of SDB because CHF patients with increased chemical drives and lower arterial P_{CO_2} values are most prone to Cheyne-Stokes respiration.[74]

Several studies have reported the effects of various benzodiazepines on SDB in ambulatory, nonhypercapnic COPD patients.[75-79] The evidence suggests that nighttime use of standard doses of these drugs does not produce increased frequency of disordered breathing events or an increased duration or severity of oxygen desaturation after either short-term or long-term[76] administration. Although the baseline (awake) oxygen saturation of most patients was generally normal or only mildly decreased in these studies, several did have some episodes of severe desaturation that did not worsen after benzodiazepine usage. Unfortunately, studies of hypercapnic patients, who are most likely to have severe nocturnal oxygen desaturation, are lacking.

Newer, nonbenzodiazepine hypnotics are becoming increasingly utilized worldwide. These drugs have specific hypnotic activity but lack myorelaxant and respiratory depressant effects. Zolpidem, an imidazopyridine derivative, is widely prescribed worldwide. It does not affect wakeful respiration,[80] and can be safely administered to patients with COPD.[81, 82] When given at twice the usual dosage (20 mg) to 12 sleep apnea patients, it produced an insignificant trend toward more apneas and significantly greater desaturation than did either placebo or flurazepam 30 mg.[64] In a group of nonobese snorers a 10-mg dose resulted in a slight increase in disordered breathing events but no important changes in oxygen saturation.[83] Therefore, this drug should not be considered safer than benzodiazepines to use in patients with sleep apnea syndrome. Zopiclone, a cyclopyrrolone, is used outside of the United States. The limited data suggest it lacks respiratory depressant properties[84] and it produces no detrimental effects in a group of snorers with upper airway resistance syndrome.[85]

The nonbenzodiazepine anxiolytic buspirone does not depress respiration and appears safe for administration to sleep apnea patients.[86] The precipitation of obstructive apneas following chloral hydrate, an infrequently used hypnotic, has been reported in children.[87] The use of barbiturates has dramatically declined and we are aware of no studies examining their effect on breathing during sleep.

In conclusion, sedative hypnotics can probably be safely administered to most patients with mild to moderate sleep apnea, CHF, and nonhypercapnic COPD. It is probably wise to avoid their use in hypercapnic patients with COPD or sleep apnea. If benzodiazepines are required for procedural sedation in patients with known or suspected sleep apnea, careful monitoring should be employed, drug dosages minimized, opiates avoided, and consideration given to postprocedural flumazenil or CPAP or both, until full wakefulness is restored.

Narcotics

Narcotics are powerful respiratory depressants. Administration of a single 10-mg dose of morphine to normal subjects decreases hypoxic and hypercapnic ventilatory response by 60 and 40%, respectively, and causes arterial P_{CO_2} to rise by 2 to 3 mmHg.[88] During the initiation of chronic methadone maintenance in addicts, a 75-mg dose results in hypercapnia and depressed chemical drives of a degree similar to that seen with 10 mg of morphine. With ongoing therapy (longer than 8 months), only hypoxic sensitivity remains depressed; minute ventilation and hypercapnic response no longer fall after the daily dose of methadone.[89] Similarly, compensation for flow-resistive loads is abolished after acute narcotic administration[90] but is restored as tolerance develops during long-term use.[91]

The effects of narcotics on breathing during sleep have not been well evaluated. In one report, no increase in SDB events occurred after either 2- or 4-mg doses of oral hydromorphone in normal subjects,[92] despite a depression of awake minute ventilation and hypoxic response. Unlike with alcohol, no increase in pharyngeal resistance was observed after the two oral narcotic doses. Other investigators have observed that oxycodone did not increase SDB events either in the entire group or in 4 of the 11 patients with sleep apnea.[93] The effects of parenteral narcotics on breathing during sleep in normal subjects or in a large group of sleep apnea patients have not been well examined. However, there is evidence that these drugs may be harmful. Several case reports have documented the occurrence of severe respiratory depression and upper airway obstruction in patients given narcotics in standard doses preoperatively.[94–96] In some instances, polysomnography later revealed severe but previously unrecognized sleep apnea. Data gathered from postoperative respiratory monitoring strongly suggest that narcotic analgesia, compared with regional (local anesthetic) analgesia, is associated with considerably more apneas and greater oxygen desaturation.[97, 98] A synergy in promoting apneas may exist postoperatively in patients given narcotics and general anesthesia, as a dramatic decrease in the frequency of oxygen desaturation episodes occurs when the initial hours of the postoperative period are compared with the last few hours of the monitoring period.[97] At this time, we recommend that narcotics be used with caution in patients known to have sleep apnea. If the need for their use is unavoidable (e.g., postoperatively), the use of nasal CPAP appears to prevent untoward respiratory events.[99] The effect of these drugs in snorers and patients with asymptomatic sleep apnea remains unknown.

Anesthetics

As with other central nervous system depressants, general anesthetics decrease neural input to upper airway muscles to a greater extent than they depress phrenic nerve activity.[100] This is consistent with the common observation that normal subjects will develop upper airway obstruction if, during light general anesthesia, proper positioning of the head and neck is not maintained.[101] These effects are more pronounced in obese patients. In addition, recent data suggest that the upper airway muscles are more sensitive to neuromuscular blocking drugs than either the diaphragm or peripheral muscles.[102] Thus, patients with OSA who have narrow upper airways are particularly vulnerable to airway obstruction following extubation.

Experience with the perioperative management of sleep apnea patients is growing, and guidelines have been published.[103] These patients may have systemic hypertension, cor pulmonale, or cardiac arrhythmias, which thus increases anesthetic risk. On the basis of numerous reports of severe upper airway obstruction, preoperative sedation should never be given on the ward. Because of anatomical features, a difficult intubation should be anticipated. Careful monitoring for respiratory depression and upper airway obstruction is critical in the recovery room, and intensive care unit monitoring should be considered for any sleep apnea patient who has had major surgery or prolonged anesthesia or who is receiving moderate to large doses of narcotics. A European group has reported success following major surgical procedures in OSA patients who were receiving opiates and other sedatives by using CPAP almost continuously for the first 24 to 48 hs following extubation and during all sleep periods thereafter.[99] If possible, regional analgesia is preferable to narcotic usage. Finally, greater than usual oxygen desaturation during apneas may occur after general anesthesia owing to a reduction in functional residual capacity, which depletes oxygen stores, and impairment of hypoxic pulmonary vasoconstriction, which promotes ventilation-perfusion mismatch.

Testosterone

The epidemiology of OSA indicates that there is a higher incidence in men.[104] Asymptomatic men are also more likely to display SDB than are women.[12] Studies in morbidly obese individuals have revealed that sleep apnea is often seen in males but occurs less frequently in women.[105, 106] The information strongly implies that sex hormones influence breathing during sleep.

Sleep apnea may develop in certain individuals during testosterone replacement therapy.[107, 108] Patients with some SDB before replacement are most vulnerable to this testosterone effect. Some patients actually develop many of the classic OSA symptoms and choose to endure the symptoms of androgen deficiency rather than the symptoms of sleep apnea. The mechanism by which testosterone may induce sleep apnea is not understood. In one of the early reports, a female patient was described as developing a "thick tongue" and increased supraglottic airflow resistance while receiving androgen.[107] However, another study did not observe any consistent increase in supraglottic resistance or decreased pharyngeal airway size in subjects receiving testosterone.[109] Similarly, attempts to implicate testosterone-induced changes in chemical ventilatory control[110, 111] have shown conflicting results. The importance of endogenous testosterone in the pathogenesis of sleep apnea is unclear. In adult men with OSA, short-term (1 week) blockade of the testosterone receptor with flutamide[112] and reduction of testosterone levels with progestational agents[113] failed to reduce apneas. In addition, men with established OSA have low testosterone concentrations that rise after successful treatment with CPAP.[114]

Antihypertensives

Systemic arterial hypertension is commonly observed in sleep apnea patients (see Chapters 47 and 73). Moreover, several groups have reported a high prevalence of unsuspected sleep apnea among populations of hypertensive patients.[115, 116] Because therapy for sustained daytime hypertension is generally advisable, consideration of how antihypertensives might influence breathing during sleep is important.

Beta blockers are known to produce nightmares and have disruptive effects on sleep quality in some individuals.[117] One report noted that propranolol seemed to produce or worsen OSA in two patients.[118] However, this was not observed in another study in 10 patients with sleep apnea given propranolol.[119] Recent studies with metoprolol 100 mg daily in hypertensive OSA patients have shown both inconsistent effects on apnea frequency and blood pressure control.[120–122] If a strong indication for beta blockers exists (e.g., coronary artery disease), compliance with CPAP should be ensured as severe bradycardia during apneic events sometimes occurs. Alpha-methyldopa may depress upper airway muscle function (alae nasi electromyogram [EMG]) in both normal subjects and OSA patients,[123] but in one study no detrimental effects on apnea frequency were noted.[124] Clonidine 0.2 mg given to eight OSA patients reduced rapid eye movement (REM) sleep and did not adversely effect the nonrapid eye movement (NREM) apnea index.[125] Current data suggest that angiotension-converting enzyme inhibitors may be the most efficacious class in terms of antihypertensive effect and may even reduce apnea frequency.[120, 122, 126, 127] The limited data for the calcium channel antagonists amlodipine and isradipine suggest no detrimental influences on sleep respiration.[121, 124]

It is reassuring that the prevalence studies to date have not noted any clear association between any specific drug therapy and severe sleep apnea in hypertensive populations.[115, 117] Finally, clinicians treating hypertension should be aware of the very high prevalence of sleep apnea in hypertensive patients refractory to drug therapy.[128, 129]

DRUGS WITH FAVORABLE INFLUENCES

Thyroid Hormone

Alveolar hypoventilation in the absence of severely impaired lung function may occur with hypothyroidism.[130] In some instances, life-threatening hypercapnic respiratory failure is seen with severe myxedema.[131-133] Institution of mechanical ventilation results in prompt improvement in the level of consciousness, and thyroid hormone replacement therapy eventually reverses the respiratory failure. Markedly impaired hypoxic and hypercapnic ventilatory responses are present in patients with hypothyroidism or myxedema,[134] which suggests that attenuation of ventilatory drive may result in their predisposition to respiratory failure. These abnormalities in respiratory drive improve with replacement therapy.

In the early sleep literature, many reports described severe OSA in thyroid-deficient patients.[135, 136] There are several possible mechanisms for OSA with hypothyroidism. These include obesity, macroglossia, impaired upper airway muscle function, deposition of mucopolysaccharides in tissues of the upper airway, and impaired ventilatory control. Among hypothyroid populations snoring is extremely common and OSA is observed frequently.[137, 138] Obesity and increasing age appear to predispose to OSA. Among obese patients, some degree of disordered breathing often persists, even when the euthyroid state is achieved. Conversely, nearly total elimination of sleep apnea is the rule in the nonobese patient once thyroid hormone is adequately replaced. Patients with hypothyroidism and coronary artery disease may have increased nocturnal arrhythmias and angina pectoris with institution of thyroid hormone replacement.[139] This may result from greater apneic oxygen desaturation due to increased oxygen consumption. Temporary use of nasal CPAP has been recommended for such patients. Routine thyroid function testing in all sleep apnea patients is cost-ineffective as fewer than 5% of patients are hypothyroid.[138, 140]

Antidepressants

Protriptyline is a nonsedating tricyclic antidepressant. Observation that this drug seemed to reduce the frequency of sleep apnea episodes in patients with narcolepsy-cataplexy syndrome led to its evaluation in the treatment of OSA.[141] In an uncontrolled study, 11 of 14 patients with OSA displayed decreased apnea frequency and duration when given the drug[142]; however, tolerance to the drug's effect and cardiovascular complications developed. A second uncontrolled study demonstrated that four of nine patients had sustained improvement in daytime symptoms and an associated decrease in apneas.[143] Those with the fewest apneas tended to respond to treatment, whereas patients with more severe OSA did not. Five of the seven patients in this study with more than 50 apneas per hour either failed to respond to protriptyline or could not tolerate the drug's side effects. The major side effects of protriptyline relate to its anticholinergic properties.

A controlled study of the use of protriptyline in five obese men with OSA[144] demonstrated that 2 weeks of therapy produced no changes in body weight, hemoglobin concentration, blood gas values, or hypercapnic ventilatory drive. The major finding was that protriptyline decreased the amount of REM sleep, a known feature of tricyclic antidepressants. This resulted in fewer REM sleep–related apneas per night. Because REM apneas are longer and are associated with greater oxygen desaturation than NREM sleep apneas, indices of nocturnal oxygenation, such as fraction of total sleep time with saturation less than 85%, improved. No changes were found in the total number of apneas, duration of apneas, or arousal frequency, yet symptoms of hypersomnolence improved. Adverse effects on cardiac rhythm were not seen in this study. In fact, bradyarrhythmias tended to improve, perhaps owing to less time spent with severe desaturation or as a result of its anticholinergic effects. Similar effects of protriptyline were seen during 6 months of therapy in three of the above-mentioned five patients. The usual daily dose of protriptyline is between 10 and 30 mg. The larger doses usually needed to achieve the drug's antiapnea action unfortunately result in frequent side effects. The anticholinergic effects, such as dry mouth, constipation, blurred vision, and urinary retention, may be particularly bothersome.

Another report similarly described a decrease in REM sleep with fewer REM apneas during long-term administration of protriptyline to 12 OSA patients.[145] However, there was a change in the pattern of SDB during NREM sleep, in which a decrease in apnea time with an increase in the amount of hypopnea was present. These hypopneas were associated with less severe desaturation and a resultant improvement in nocturnal oxygenation. The authors speculated that protriptyline may in some way affect upper airway muscle tone, a finding of an animal study in which heightened hypoglossal nerve activity after protriptyline administration was seen.[56] As in the previous controlled study, symptoms of hypersomnolence improved, with no decrease in awakenings or apneic arousals. Two double-blind placebo-controlled studies have demonstrated only marginal[146] or no[147] efficacy in sleep apnea patients. In the latter report, patients were preselected on the basis of only mild to moderate OSA. Interestingly, a reduction in REM sleep was not observed in either of these studies.

Nonapneic oxygen desaturation is common in COPD patients, especially those with hypercapnia and borderline oxygen saturation during wakefulness (see Chapter 81). These episodes of desaturation typically occur during REM sleep. Accordingly, the use of a REM sleep-suppressing drug such as protriptyline may be reasonable for treatment of this problem. Two groups found that protriptyline[148, 149] decreased REM sleep and improved nocturnal oxygen saturation, particularly minimal oxygen saturation. Small improvements in wakeful gas exchange were seen in both studies. The decreases in P_{CO_2} were statistically significant in both investigations, and the increase in P_{O_2} was significant in one.[149] The mechanism for improved daytime blood gases is uncertain but is probably not due to increased hypoxic[150] or hypercapnic[144, 150] sensitivity. Similar improvements in nocturnal oxygenation have also been observed in patients with restrictive chest wall disease[151] and muscular dystrophy.[152] Although these observations in patients with mechanical lung dysfunction are interesting, the improvements seen are probably less than would be expected with the use of supplemental oxygen, and the use of protriptyline is greatly limited by its side effects.

In summary, protriptyline affects SDB through two major mechanisms. First, although it has not been universally observed, in most studies the drug has reduced REM sleep. Because REM events are often longer and associated with more severe oxygen desaturation, the net result is improved nocturnal oxygenation. Second, protriptyline probably enhances upper airway motor tone. Unfortunately, the efficacy of protriptyline in the treatment of moderate to severe OSA is not great enough to recommend its routine use. The drug may be useful in patients with mild OSA who have troublesome hypersomnolence and cannot lose weight or use nasal CPAP. Its adjunctive use has also been suggested as a means of lowering nasal CPAP levels in patients requiring uncomfortably high CPAP[153] (greater than 15 cm H_2O). Anticholinergic side effects are a major factor limiting this drug's long-term use.

Experience with antidepressants other than protriptyline is extremely limited. The widely prescribed selective serotonin reuptake inhibitor fluoxetine (Prozac) 20 mg was compared with protriptyline 10 mg in a group of 12 OSA patients.[154] Both drugs significantly reduced REM sleep time and produced modest but significant decreases in NREM apneas and hypopneas. Measures of severity of oxygen desaturation and arousals were not improved by either drug. A response to one drug did not necessarily predict a response to the other. All subjects tolerated fluoxetine, but 3 of 12 could not tolerate protriptyline for the 4-week trial. The efficacy of imipramine,[155] trazodone,[156] and nomifensine[157] has been either marginal or confined to anecdotal reports.

Progestational Agents

In conditions of physiological progesterone elevation, such as the luteal phase of the menstrual cycle and pregnancy, hyperventilation with resultant hypocapnia occurs.[158, 159] Administration of medroxyprogesterone acetate (MPA) to healthy men produces an increase in minute ventilation associated with increased hypoxic and hypercapnic ventilatory responses.[160] The mechanism whereby progestational agents stimulate respiration is not clear. In both normal subjects and COPD patients,[161, 162] hyperventilation persists in the presence of hyperoxia, which implies that chemoreceptors are not crucial to the respiratory stimulant properties of MPA.

It has been shown in both normals and COPD patients that the increment in ventilation and decrement in P_{CO_2} produced by MPA during wakefulness persist during sleep.[163] Improvements in oxygenation are also seen in the COPD patients. However, MPA does not prevent episodes of SDB in COPD patients.[164] With another synthetic progestin, chlormadinone acetate (CMA),[165, 166] the results were generally similar to those observed with MPA. The drug did not benefit those patients with the lowest wakeful P_{O_2} values who had the greatest need for improved nocturnal oxygenation. The improvements in nocturnal oxygenation in COPD patients are too small and occur too inconsistently with progestational agents for their use to be recommended. Clearly, therapy with nocturnal oxygen and even almitrine[167] is likely to improve nocturnal oxygenation to a greater degree.

After menopause, SDB in women occurs with about the same frequency as in asymptomatic men.[168] It has been speculated that this is due to falling endogenous progesterone levels, yet administration of MPA does not significantly affect asymptomatic SDB in postmenopausal women.[169] This was true even when a subgroup of women with the highest frequency of SDB was separately analyzed. The tendency for nasal obstruction to induce apneas during sleep in middle-aged women was not related to menopausal status but rather to body weight, neck circumference, and mandibular-hyoid distance.[170] This is consistent with the observations that severe obesity and upper airway anomalies are especially correlated with sleep apnea in women.[171]

Limited data are available concerning combined estrogen-progesterone replacement therapy. One group has observed that in a group of ovariohysterectomized women, disordered breathing events (apneas and hypopneas) decreased significantly from a mean of 15 to three events per night when sleep after 1 week of placebo was compared with 1 week of combined MPA-conjugated estrogen therapy.[172] The authors speculated that estrogen therapy may increase progesterone receptors, thus enhancing the respiratory stimulant effects of the MPA. Although the elimination of sleep apnea in a postmenopausal woman with combined estradiol and cyclic MPA has been anecdotally described,[173] a recent report has noted no clinically important improvement in SDB in a group of postmenopausal sleep apnea patients with either estrogen or combined hormonal therapy.[174]

Two studies have examined whether breathing during sleep is influenced by physiologically varying progesterone levels in young women. The first compared breathing during sleep in a group of 11 menstruating women during both the follicular (low progesterone) and luteal (high progesterone) phases of the cycle.[175] No changes in any sleep or breathing parameter were observed. The second study compared sleep respiration in women at 36 weeks' gestation with that in the postpartum period (2.5 to 6.0 months after delivery). Mean and minimal oxygen saturation were identical at both times. Apneas and hypopneas, however, were less common during pregnancy. The authors concluded that respiratory stimulation by increased progesterone levels during late pregnancy protects against several potential causes of oxygen desaturation, including a low functional residual capacity, airway closure, and a reduced cardiac output in the supine position.[176] A few case reports have described the development of severe sleep apnea during pregnancy.[177, 178] These patients all appeared to have either mild preexisting sleep apnea or a strong predisposition to it (obesity, retrognathia, hormonal disorders). Thus, it is unclear whether the myriad changes associated with the pregnant state may override the influence of elevated progesterone levels and aggravate or precipitate sleep apnea in the occasional susceptible individual.

The obesity hypoventilation syndrome (OHS) is characterized by severe OSA and daytime hypoventilation (hypercapnia) despite relatively normal pulmonary function. These patients have impaired ventilatory control[179] but are able to normalize their blood gas levels with voluntary hyperventilation.[180] Two studies have clearly shown that administration of progestational agents benefits patients with OHS.[180, 181] The degree of awake hypercapnia decreases, and daytime hypoxemia improves markedly. These improvements are associated with decreases in mean pulmonary artery pressure, lower hematocrit, and fewer signs of right-sided heart failure. In addition, symptoms of hypersomnolence may decrease. Although progestational agents are beneficial in patients with OHS, neither study examined whether these drugs affect the SDB present in such patients. The dose commonly used to obtain an improved level of alveolar ventilation in those with OHS is 20 mg of MPA (Provera) three times per day. This large oral dose is commonly associated with impotence but otherwise is usually well tolerated. The long-term effect of progestational agents in men is presently not known.

The effects of MPA in OSA have been extensively evaluated. Four systematic studies[113, 182–184] have now concluded that MPA does not benefit the majority of

patients with OSA. In all studies, doses of 60 mg or greater per day were used. Only one was performed in a randomized, double-blind manner.[113] Three of the four studies included some patients with daytime hypercapnia. In one of these studies, a minority of patients (four of nine) did have fewer apneas and decreased hypersomnolence.[184] These patients had lower wakeful P_{O_2} values and a tendency toward a higher daytime P_{CO_2}. A later double-blind study,[113] however, did not show any benefit in a hypercapnic (4 of 10) subgroup. CMA has been reported to reduce apnea frequency and improve nocturnal oxygen saturation in a group of nine sleep apnea patients.[185] Close analysis of the data, however, reveals that the reduction in disordered breathing was small and not clinically significant.

In conclusion, the use of progestational agents cannot be recommended for most patients with sleep apnea. We usually reserve the use of MPA for those OHS patients with moderate to severe daytime blood gas derangements or impending cardiorespiratory failure. In this instance, the progestin complements the use of low-flow oxygen and either nasal CPAP or bilevel positive airway pressure (BiPAP). The need for MPA is frequently short-lived; many patients will eventually normalize their blood gas values with definitive therapy for sleep apnea. If patients are intolerant of nasal CPAP and refuse surgical treatment for sleep apnea, MPA may be given on a long-term basis, but its efficacy should be determined with follow-up polysomnography. Finally, progestational agents may improve oxygen saturation during sleep at altitude; however, they are clearly inferior to acetazolamide in this regard.[186]

Almitrine

Almitrine is a respiratory stimulant that is not available for use in many countries. It has been evaluated in Europe mainly in the treatment of COPD but has also been used in syndromes of alveolar hypoventilation[187] and sleep apnea.[188]

Almitrine acts by stimulating peripheral chemoreceptors and accordingly has no effects after bilateral carotid body resection.[189] In COPD, it improves oxygenation by both increasing ventilation and improving ventilation-perfusion matching.[190, 191] The latter action is secondary to increased hypoxic pulmonary vasoconstriction[192] with resultant improved blood flow to better-ventilated lung zones. The present evidence suggests that this drug will improve oxygenation during wakefulness in COPD patients both at rest and with exercise.[193] However, concern has arisen that because of its effects on the pulmonary vasculature, pulmonary artery pressure may increase despite improved oxygenation both at rest and during exercise.[194]

The improvements in oxygenation during wakefulness are sustained during sleep in COPD patients, and episodes of desaturation are both less severe and less frequent with the use of this drug in CO_2-retaining patients.[195] These improvements in nocturnal oxygenation persist with long-term use of the drug.[196] The effects of this drug in treating sleep apnea have been much less encouraging. A study in eight patients found no decrease in the total number of abnormal respiratory events with almitrine use.[188] In studies at altitude, almitrine improves nocturnal oxygen saturation comparably to acetazolamide but increases the amount of periodic breathing owing to enhanced hypoxic sensitivity.[197]

In summary, the use of almitrine in COPD patients during both wakefulness and sleep is controversial. Major concerns relate to its long-term effects on pulmonary artery pressure and a possible association with peripheral neuropathy.[198] There is no basis for the use of almitrine in sleep apnea.

Acetazolamide

Acetazolamide is a carbonic anhydrase inhibitor. By promoting a bicarbonate diuresis, it produces a metabolic acidosis, which stimulates ventilation. One group has found that this drug benefits patients with central sleep apnea,[199] but in a subsequent, smaller study, no benefit was found.[200] This discrepancy may relate to the fact that all patients in the former study were normocapnic while awake, whereas two in the latter study were chronic CO_2 retainers. Such heterogeneity in central sleep apnea patients has been described.

Some patients with predominantly mixed[200] or central[201] apnea have developed purely obstructive apneas of longer duration associated with greater oxygen desaturation after acetazolamide use. This is postulated to be secondary to disproportionate stimulation by the metabolic acidosis of ventilatory muscles relative to the muscles maintaining upper airway patency. Interestingly, however, other studies have demonstrated a moderate but significant decrease in apnea frequency and improved nocturnal oxygen saturation in patients with predominantly obstructive apneas.[147, 202, 203] In one of these reports, the patients had shown no response to protriptyline.[202] In addition, in a recent uncontrolled study of 14 normocapnic central sleep apnea patients, a low dose of acetazolamide (250 mg 1 h before bedtime) reduced central apnea events both on the first night (50% reduction from baseline) and after 1 month of administration[204] (75% reduction from baseline). Obstructive events did not increase and hypersomnolence improved. Decreases in arterial pH were smaller than those observed in previous studies using higher drug doses. Thus, the effects of acetazolamide in a given sleep apnea patient are often unpredictable, and benefits, when present, are often small. The drug may have a role in normocapnic patients with predominantly central apnea. If it is used, follow-up sleep studies should determine drug efficacy.

Acetazolamide is not recommended for use in hypercapnic COPD patients; fewer than half of such patients will increase alveolar ventilation in response to the metabolic acidosis.[205] Therefore, a marked mixed acidosis may ensue.

Acetazolamide probably has its greatest efficacy in treating SDB at high altitude.[186] The usual dose of acetazolamide is 250 mg orally three or four times per day, although a single 250-mg bedtime dose may be equally efficacious. Occasionally, drowsiness and paresthesia may occur. Care must be taken to prevent hypokalemia due to urinary potassium losses.

Nicotine

Nicotine has respiratory stimulant properties. Evidence from animal studies suggests that this drug increases the activity of upper airway muscles to a relatively greater extent than the diaphragm.[206] This provided a rationale for testing the efficacy of this agent in sleep apnea patients. The drug was given in chewing gum form to eight sleep apnea patients. Total apneas were reduced during the first 2 h of sleep, with the reduction being secondary to reduced mixed and obstructive events. The number of central apneas did not change.[207] Unfortunately, its short duration of action and side effects make the use of nicotine gum in sleep apnea somewhat impractical. Data with the nicotine patch in patients with snoring and mild OSA demonstrate poor sleep quality, no reduction in apneas, and frequent side effects.[208]

Theophylline

In addition to being a bronchodilator, theophylline has respiratory stimulant properties.[209] It has been used to treat infants with periodic breathing and central apneas.[210] Although its efficacy as an acute bronchodilator is less than that of inhaled drugs and its potential for toxicity is considerable, the drug enjoys widespread use in treating both asthma and COPD. This occurs despite recommendations by some authorities that use of the drug be markedly curtailed.[211]

Data regarding the effects of theophylline on nocturnal oxygenation in COPD are conflicting.[212, 213] Thus the efficacy of theophylline in improving severely abnormal nocturnal oxygenation in COPD patients remains unestablished. Nocturnal worsening of airflow with bothersome symptoms and frequent awakening is a troublesome problem for many people with asthma. This topic is discussed in Chapter 80. Theophylline is a useful drug for treating nocturnal asthma, particularly in those patients with stable daytime lung function who persist in having nocturnal symptoms despite aggressive anti-inflammatory therapy. The fact that therapeutic drug concentrations can be sustained through the night accounts for the superior efficacy of theophylline, compared with inhaled bronchodilators, which have a short duration of action. A study compared the efficacy of oral sustained-release theophylline with inhaled bitolterol (three puffs every 8 h) in 26 asthmatic patients.[214] The results unequivocally established the superiority of theophylline in terms of improved airway function (morning forced expiratory volume in 1 sec [FEV_1]: 2.47 liters during theophylline vs. 1.79 liters during bitolterol), fewer symptoms, and improved oxygenation. In addition, similar to an aforementioned study in COPD patients,[213] theophylline did not adversely affect any parameter of sleep quality. In many asthmatic patients, it is not necessary to maintain a "therapeutic" theophylline concentration during daytime hours. Conversely, higher concentrations during the night do result in better control of nocturnal asthma. This explains the results of an investigation in which a once-daily theophylline preparation (Uniphyl), given at 7 PM, was more effective than the same total daily dose of a twice-a-day formulation (Theo-Dur) in treating nocturnal asthma.[215] Drug concentrations with once-daily theophylline were more erratic over 24 h but were significantly higher during the nighttime hours. Despite concentrations that were often "subtherapeutic" during the daytime with the once-daily formulation, FEV_1 during the day was similar with both preparations. Thus, nocturnal asthma may be treated in many patients with once-daily dosing of a long-acting preparation given in the evening (7 PM).

The available evidence suggests that theophylline provides either little[216] or no benefit to OSA patients with either short-term[217, 218] or long-term administration.[218] A case report has described a patient with central apnea after surgery for a medullary brain tumor who improved with aminophylline.[219] It has been known for some time that periodic breathing (Cheyne-Stokes respiration) may be stabilized with theophylline[220]; however, the mechanism whereby this effect occurs is not known. Cheyne-Stokes respiration during sleep may be common in many patients with CHF, and it may clinically mimic a typical sleep apnea syndrome. A report in a small group of patients has described a dramatic reduction in Cheyne-Stokes respiration during sleep after theophylline use.[221] The same investigators have reported considerable reductions in both total and central apneic events following 5 days of oral theophylline (mean concentration: 11μg/ml) in 15 CHF patients with periodic breathing. A striking reduction in time spent with an oxygen saturation below 90% from 23% (placebo) to 6% (theophylline) of total sleep time was observed, with no deterioration in sleep quality or increase in cardiac dysrhythmia.[222] Given theophylline's potential for drug interactions and various toxicities in this patient population, it is unlikely that this agent will become widely used.

Pediatricians have become concerned that theophylline may adversely affect behavior, cognitive skills, and school performance in children.[223] The data are conflicting.[224] However, if such effects occur, they are probably not related to theophylline's influences on sleep quality, because a report comparing theophylline and cromolyn in asthmatic children noted no adverse effects of theophylline on sleep quality in the children during theophylline therapy.[225] The effects of the two drugs on pulmonary function were equivalent, but central apneas and episodes of oxygen desaturation during sleep were less frequent in the children during theophylline use.

In summary, theophylline is a useful drug for treatment of nocturnal asthma. Its efficacy in improving clinically significant nocturnal oxygen desaturation in COPD is unproven. Theophylline has no role in treating OSA. It may improve some forms of central sleep apnea syndrome, especially if there is underlying periodic breathing.

MISCELLANEOUS DRUGS

Briefly reviewed here are a variety of other drugs whose influences on breathing during sleep have been examined.

Small quantities of strychnine eliminated apneas in a patient with OSA.[226] This effect was associated with an increase in tensor palatini EMG activity, as well as an increase in genioglossal EMG sensitivity to hypoxia. The authors proposed that strychnine produces blockade of postsynaptic inhibition resulting in more effective pharyngeal dilation, which prevented airway occlusion. Although this fascinating report suggests new avenues of research, this highly toxic drug is unlikely to find important clinical use.

The role of endogenous opiates in regulating respiratory activity has generated much interest. The influence of these substances is generally assessed by determining the consequences of endogenous opiate blockade with naloxone. The available evidence indicates that narcotic antagonists do not produce clinically meaningful benefits to justify their use in OSA patients.[227–229]

The phenothiazine prochlorperazine increases the ventilatory response to hypercapnic hypoxia in both normal subjects and OSA patients[230, 231] studied during wakefulness. This is believed to be due to the dopamine antagonistic properties of phenothiazines. This led to a trial of prochlorperazine in six OSA patients. No clinically significant change in nocturnal apneas occurred.[231] Apnea frequency tended to decrease, but the severity of hypoxemia during apnea worsened. In one case report, bedtime haloperidol 10 mg did not worsen apneas in a patient with severe OSA.[232] In a European study, the phenothiazine hypnotic propiomazine was found not to worsen nocturnal oxygenation in a group of 12 COPD patients.[233] Use of phenothiazine-containing medications may be related to the sudden infant death syndrome.[234] These agents are sometimes used in the pediatric age groups because of their antitussive and antihistaminic properties. A study has found that both central and particularly obstructive apneas increase in infants after promethazine (Phenergan) administration.[235]

In an uncontrolled study, the amino acid L-tryptophan reduced the frequency of obstructive apneas in 15 patients.[236] There was no effect on central apnea. It was speculated that L-tryptophan probably exerts its influence by acting as a serotonin precursor, which recent animal data suggest may be an important stimulator of upper airway motoneuron activity.[237] L-Tryptophan is no longer marketed in the United States owing to the eosinophilia-myalgia syndrome associated with its use.

Nasal obstruction, whether artificially induced or secondary to disease, may produce sleep apnea. Both central and obstructive events may occur. Because most breathing is through the nose during wakefulness and while asleep,[238] when the nose is partially obstructed, greater negative intrapharyngeal pressure is present and suction collapse of the pharynx is favored. This may explain why obstructive events can occur with nasal obstruction. The nose may also contain pressure or flow receptors that regulate respiratory activity.[239–241] The application of negative intrapharyngeal pressure reflexly activates upper airway muscles, an effect blocked by topical anesthesia. Several reports have suggested that topical nasal or orpharyngeal anesthesia may increase SDB.[242–246] In a few central sleep apnea patients, it was found that topical cocaine applied to the upper airway restored a more regular breathing pattern.[247] The authors speculated that this local anesthetic inhibits a reflex initiated by partial pharyngeal collapse that results in central sleep apnea. Finally, in one report a topical nasal decongestant did not reduce apneic frequency in snorers with mild OSA.[248]

Both obstructive and central sleep apnea may occur with acromegaly. Improvements in sleep apnea have been reported with the use of the somatostatin analogue octreotide.[249, 250] Interestingly, the drug's efficacy in reducing apneas does not always correlate with reductions in hormonal concentrations. Apneas in acromegalic patients with severe sleep apnea may persist with biochemical remissions, whereas mild sleep apnea may be eliminated with only partial hormonal responses. Bromocriptine has demonstrated efficacy in reducing apneas in acromegalic but not in other OSA patients.[218, 251] In one series, 4 out of 145 children receiving exogenous growth hormone for diverse reasons developed OSA.[252] In these instances this was related to adenotonsillar hypertrophy and was cured surgically. In a group of children with OSA and enlarged tonsils, a short course of therapy with glucocorticoids did not produce regression in adenotonsillar size or reductions in apneas.[253]

Sabeluzole, an antagonist of glutamate, produced small improvements in SDB without reported side effects in a group of patients with OSA.[259] Interestingly, those with the highest drug concentrations had the greatest response, suggesting that studies with higher drug dosages may be warranted.

Atropine,[255] baclofen,[218] modafinil,[256] flumazenil,[257] and doxapram[258, 259] have failed to demonstrate any consistent benefit when they were given to patients with OSA.

CONCLUSIONS

Information regarding the pharmacology of breathing during sleep is steadily growing. The available evidence suggests that alcohol is detrimental to snorers and patients with OSA and COPD. Its consumption should be avoided within 2 h of bedtime in these groups. The hazards of sedative-hypnotic drugs have probably been overstated. Information regarding opiate effects remains scarce. Effective drug therapy for OSA is not available, but some agents may be efficacious in selected patients with predominantly central apneas.

References

1. Sahn SA, Lakshminarayan S, Pierson DJ, et al. Effect of ethanol on the ventilatory response to oxygen and carbon dioxide in men. Clin Sci Mol Med. 1975;49:33–38.
2. Michiels TM, Light RW, Mahutte CK. Effect of ethanol and naloxone on control of ventilation and load perception. J Appl Physiol. 1983;55:929–934.
3. Johnstone RE, Reier CE. Acute respiratory effects of ethanol in man. Clin Pharmacol Ther. 1973;14:501–508.
4. Sahn SA, Scoggin CH, Chernon B. Moderate alcohol use and chronic obstructive pulmonary disease. Arch Intern Med. 1979;139:429–431.
5. Sovijarvi ARA, Hillbom ME, Poppius H. Effect of ethanol ingestion on blood gases and airway conductance in chronic bronchitis. Bull Eur Physiopathol Respir. 1978;14:409–415.
6. Johnstone RE, Witt RL. Respiratory effects of ethyl alcohol intoxication. JAMA. 1972;222:486.
7. Guilleminault C, Cummiskey J, Dement WC. Sleep apnea syndrome: recent advances. Adv Intern Med. 1980;26:347–372.
8. Guilleminault C, Rosekind M. The arousal threshold: sleep deprivation, sleep fragmentation, and obstructive sleep apnea syndrome. Bull Eur Physiopathol Respir. 1981;17:341–349.
9. Issa FG, Sullivan CE. Alcohol, snoring, and sleep apnea. J Neurol Neurosurg Psychiatry. 1982;45:353–359.
10. Scrima L, Broudy M, Nay K, et al. Increased severity of obstructive sleep apnea after bedtime alcohol ingestion: diagnostic potential and proposed mechanism of actions. Sleep. 1982;5:318–328.
11. Taasan VC, Block AJ, Boysen PG, et al. Alcohol increases sleep apnea and oxygen desaturation in asymptomatic men. Am J Med. 1981;71:240–245.
12. Block AJ, Boysen PG, Wynne JW, et al. Sleep apnea, hypopnea, and oxygen desaturation in normal subjects: a strong male predominance. N Engl J Med. 1979;300:513–517.
13. Block AJ. Alcohol ingestion does not cause sleep-disordered breathing in premenopausal women. Alcoholism. 1984;8:397–398.
14. Block AJ, Hellard DW, Slayton PC. Minimal effect of alcohol ingestion on breathing during the sleep of postmenopausal women. Chest. 1985;88:181–184.
15. Scrima L, Hartman PG, Heller FC. Effect of three alcohol doses on breathing during sleep in 30–49 year old nonobese snorers and nonsnorers. Alcohol Clin Exp Res. 1989;13:420–427.
16. Mitler MM, Dawson A, Henriksen SJ, et al. Bedtime ethanol increases resistance of upper airways and produces sleep apneas in asymptomatic snorers. Alcohol Clin Exp Res. 1988;12:801–805.
17. Remmers JE, deGroot WJ, Sauerland EK, et al. Pathogenesis of upper airway occlusions during sleep. J Appl Physiol. 1978;44:931–938.
18. Bonora M, Shields G, Knuth S, et al. Selective depression by ethanol of upper airway respiratory motor activity in cats. Am Rev Respir Dis. 1984;130:156–161.
19. Krol RC, Knuth SL, Bartlett D. Selective reduction of genioglossal muscle activity by alcohol in normal human subjects. Am Rev Respir Dis. 1984;129:247–250.
20. Robinson RW, White DP, Zwillich CW. Moderate alcohol ingestion increases upper airway resistance in normal subjects. Am Rev Respir Dis. 1985;132:1238–1241.
21. Issa FG, Sullivan CE. Upper airway closing pressures in snorers. J Appl Physiol. 1984;57:528–535.
22. Berry RB, Desa MM, Light RW. Effect of ethanol on the efficacy of nasal continuous positive airway pressure as a treatment for obstructive sleep apnea. Chest. 1991;99:339–343.
23. Berry RB, Bonnet MH, Light RW. Effect of ethanol on the arousal response to airway occlusion during sleep in normal subjects. Am Rev Respir Dis. 1992;145:445–452.
24. Sauerland EK, Harper RM. The human tongue during sleep: electromyographic activity of the genioglossus muscle. Exp Neurol. 1976;51:161–170.
25. Haponik EF, Smith PL, Bohlman ME, et al. Computerized tomography in obstructive sleep apnea. Am Rev Respir Dis. 1983;127:221–226.

26. Issa FG, Sullivan CE. Upper airway closing pressures in obstructive sleep apnea. J Appl Physiol. 1984;57:520–527.

27. Dolly FR, Block AJ. Increased ventricular ectopy and sleep apnea following ethanol ingestion in COPD patients. Chest. 1983;83:469–472.

28. Easton PA, West P, Meatherall RC, et al. The effect of excessive ethanol ingestion on sleep in severe COPD. Sleep. 1987;10:224–233.

29. Tan ETH, Lambie DG, Johnson RH, et al. Sleep apnoea in alcoholic patients after withdrawal. Clin Sci. 1985;69:655–661.

30. Vitiello MV, Prinz PN, Personius JP, et al. A history of chronic alcohol abuse is associated with increased nighttime hypoxemia in older men. Alcohol Clin Exp Res. 1987;11:368–371.

31. LeBon O, Verbanck P, Hoffman G, et al. Sleep in detoxified alcoholics: impairment of most standard sleep parameters and increased risk for sleep apnea, but not for myoclonias—a controlled study. J Stud Alcohol. 1997;58:30–36.

32. Chan CS, Grunstein RR, Bye PTP, et al. Obstructive sleep apnea with severe chronic airflow limitation. Am Rev Respir Dis. 1989;140:1274–1278.

33. Chan CS, Bye PTP, Woolcock AJ, et al. Eucapnea and hypercapnea in patients with chronic airflow limitation. Am Rev Respir Dis. 1990;141:861–865.

34. Jalleh R, Fitzpatrick MF, Mathur R, et al. Do patients with the sleep apnea/hypopnea syndrome drink more alcohol? Sleep. 1992;15:319–321.

35. Jalleh R, Fitzpatrick MF, Jan MA, et al. Alcohol and cor pulmonale in chronic bronchitis and emphysema. Br Med J. 1993;306:374.

36. Enright PL, Newman AB, Wahl PW, et al. Prevalence and correlates of snoring and observed apneas in 5,201 older adults. Sleep. 1996;19:531–538.

37. Jennum P, Sjol A. Snoring, sleep apnoea, and cardiovascular risk factors—the MONICA II study. Int J Epidemiol. 1993;22:439–444.

38. Stradling JR, Crosby JM. Predictors and prevolence of obstructive sleep apnea and snoring in 1001 middle-aged men. Thorax. 1991;46:85–90.

39. Kauffman F, Annesi I, Neukirch F, et al. The relation between snoring and smoking, body mass index, age, alcohol consumption and respiratory symptoms. Eur Respir J. 1989;2:599–603.

40. Olson LG, King MT, Hensley MJ, et al. A community study of snoring and sleep-disordered breating. Am J Respir Crit Care Med. 1995;152:711–716.

41. Wysowski DK, Baum C. Outpatient use of prescription sedative-hypnotic drugs in the United States 1970–1989. Arch Intern Med. 1991;151:1779–1783.

42. Guilleminault C, Cummiskey J, Silvestri R. Benzodiazepines and respiration during sleep. In: Usdin E, Skolnick P, Tallmen JF, et al, eds. Pharmacology of Benzodiazepines. London, England: Macmillan; 1978:229–236.

43. Catchlove RFH, Kafer ER. The effects of diazepam on the ventilatory response to carbon dioxide and on steady-state gas exchange. Anesthesiology. 1971;34:9–13.

44. Catchlove RFH, Kafer ER: The effects of diazepam on respiration in patients with obstructive pulmonary disease. Anesthesiology. 1971;34:14–18.

45. Dobson ME, Yousseff Y, Maddison S, et al. Respiratory effects of lorazepam. Br J Anaesth. 1976;48:611–612.

46. Longbottom RT, Pleuvry BJ. Respiratory and sedative effects of triazolam in volunteers. Br J Anaesth. 1984;56:179–186.

47. Skatrud JB, Begle RL, Busch M. Ventilatory effects of single, high-dose triazolam in awake human subjects. Clin Pharmacol Ther. 1988;44:684–689.

48. Lakshminarayan S, Sahn SA, Hudson L, et al. Effects of diazepam on ventilatory responses. Clin Pharmacol Ther. 1976;20:178–183.

49. Gross JB, Zebrowske ME, Carel WD, et al. Time course of ventilatory depression after thiopental and midazolam in normal subjects and in patients with chronic obstructive pulmonary disease. Anesthesiology. 1983;58:540–544.

50. Alexander CM, Gross JB. Sedative doses of midazolam depress hypoxic ventilatory responses in humans. Anesth Analg. 1988;67:377–382.

51. Clark TJH, Collins JV, Tong D. Respiratory depression caused by nitrazepam in patients with respiratory failure. Lancet. 1971;2:737–738.

52. Model DG, Berry DJ. Effects of chlordiazepoxide in respiratory failure due to chronic bronchitis. Lancet. 1974;2:869–870.

53. Rao S, Sherbaniok RW, Prasad K, et al. Cardiopulmonary effects of diazepam. Clin Pharmacol Ther. 1973;14:182–189.

54. Keeffe EB, O'Connor KW. 1989 ASGE survey of endoscopic sedation and monitoring practices. Gastrointest Endosc. 1990;36:513–522.

55. Bailey PL, Pace NL, Ashburn MA, et al. Frequent hypoxemia and apnea after sedation with midazolam and fentanyl. Anesthesiology. 1990;73:826–830.

56. Bonora M, St. John WM, Bledsoe TA. Differential elevation by protriptyline and depression by diazepam of upper airway respiratory motor activity. Am Rev Respir Dis. 1985;131:41–45.

57. Leiter JC, Knuth SL, Krol RC, et al. The effect of diazepam on genioglossal muscle activity in normal human subjects. Am Rev Respir Dis. 1985;132:216–219.

58. Montravers P, Durevil B, Desmonts JM. Effects of i.v. Midazolam on upper airway resistance. Br J Anaesth. 1992;68:27–31.

59. Masuda A, Haji A, Wakasuji M, et al. Differences in midazolam-induced breating patterns in healthy volunteers. Acta Anaesthesiol. 1995;39:785–790.

60. Simmons FB, Hill MW. Hypersomnia caused by upper airway obstructions: a new syndrome in otolaryngology. Ann Otol Rhinol Laryngol. 1974;83:670–673.

61. Dolly FR, Block AJ. Effect of flurazepam on sleep-disordered breathing and nocturnal oxygen desaturation in asymptomatic subjects. Am J Med. 1982;73:239–243.

62. Carskadon MA, Seidel WF, Greenblait DJ, et al. Daytime carryover of triazolam and flurazepam in elderly insomniacs. Sleep. 1982;5:361–371.

63. Mendelson WB, Garnett D, Gillin JC. Flurazepam induced sleep apnea syndrome in a patient with insomnia and mild sleep-related respiratory changes. J Nerv Ment Dis. 1981;169:261–264.

64. Cirignotta F, Mondini S, Zucconi M, et al. Zolpidem—polysomnographic study of the effect of a new hypnotic drug in sleep apnea syndrome. Pharmacol Biochem Behav. 1988;29:807–809.

65. Cirignotta F, Mondeni S, Gerordi R, et al. Effect of brotizolam on sleep-disordered breating in heavy snorers with obstructive apnea. Curr Ther Res. 1992;51:360–366.

66. Mendelson WB. Safety of short-acting benzodiazepine hypnotics in patients with impaired respiration. Am J Psychiatry. 1991;148:1401.

67. Berry RB, McCasland CR, Light RW. The effect of triazolam on the arousal response to airway occlusion during sleep in normal subjects. Am Rev Respir Dis. 1992;146:1256–60.

68. Hoijer U, Hedner J, Ejnell H, et al. Nitrazepam in patients with sleep apnoea: a double-blind placebo-controlled study. Eur Respir J. 1994;7:2011–2015.

69. Camacho ME, Morin GN. The effect of temazepam on respiration in elderly insomniacs with mild sleep apnea. Sleep. 1995;18:644–645.

70. Bonnet MH, Dexter JR, Arand DL. The effect of triazolam on arousal and respiration in central sleep apnea patients. Sleep. 1990;13:31–41.

71. Guilleminault C, Crowe C, Quera-Salva MA, et al. Periodic leg movement, sleep fragmentation, and central sleep apnoea in two cases: reduction with clonazepam. Eur Respir J. 1988;1:762–765.

72. Biberdorf DJ, Steens R, Millar TW, et al. Benzodiazepines in conjestive heart failure: effects of temazepam on arousability and Cheyne-Stokes respiration. Sleep. 1993;16:529–538.

73. Guilleminault C, Clark A, Labanowski M, et al. Cardiac failure and benzodiazepines. Sleep. 1993;16:524–528.

74. Naughton MT, Benard D, Tam A, et al. Role of hyperventilation in the pathogenesis of central apneas in patients with congestive heart failure. Am Rev Respir Dis. 1993;148:330–338.

75. Block AJ, Dolly FR, Slayton PC. Does flurazepam ingestion affect breathing and oxygenation during sleep in patients with chronic obstructive lung disease? Am Rev Respir Dis. 1984;129:230–233.

76. Cummiskey J, Guilleminault C, Del Rio G, et al. The effects of flurazepam on sleep studies in patients with chronic obstructive pulmonary disease. Chest. 1983;84:143–147.

77. Midgren B, Hansson L, Skeidsvoll H, et al. The effects of nitrazepam and flunitrazepam on oxygen desaturation during sleep

in patients with stable hypoxemic nonhypercapnic COPD. Chest. 1989;95:765–768.

78. Timms RM, Dawson A, Hajdukovic RM, et al. Effect of triazolam on sleep and arterial oxygen saturation in patients with chronic obstructive pulmonary disease. Arch Intern Med. 1988;148:2159–2163.

79. Wedzicha JA, Wallis PJW, Ingram DA, et al. Effect of diazepam on sleep in patients with chronic airflow obstruction. Thorax. 1988;43:729–730.

80. Murciano D, Aubier M, Palacios S, et al. Comparison of zolpidem, triazolam, and flunitrazepam effects on arterial blood gases and control of breathing in patients with severe chronic obstructive pulmonary disease. Chest. 1990;97(suppl):51–52.

81. Steens RD, Poulot Z, Millar TW, et al. Effects of zolpidem and triazolam on sleep and respiration in mild to moderate chronic obstructive pulmonary disease. Sleep. 1993;16:318–326.

82. Girault C, Muir JF, Mihaltan F, et al. Effects of repeated administration of zolpidem on sleep, diurnal and nocturnal respiratory function, vigilance, and physical performance in patients with COPD. Chest. 1996;110:1203–1211.

83. Quera-Salva MA, McCann C, Bondet J. Effects of zolpidem on sleep architecure, night time ventilation, daytime vigilance and performance in heavy snorers. Br J Clin Pharmacol. 1994;37:539–543.

84. Beaupre A, Soucy K, Phillips K, et al. Respiratory center output following zopiclone or diazepam administration in patients with pulmonary disease. Respiration. 1988;54:235–240.

85. Lofaso F, Goldenberg F, Thebault C, et al. Effect of zopiclone on sleep, night-time ventilation, and daytime vigilance in upper airway resistance syndrome. Eur Respir J. 1997; 10:2573–2573.

86. Mendelson WB, Maczaj M, Holt J. Buspirone administration to sleep apnea patients. J Clin Psychopharmacol. 1991;11:71–72.

87. Biban P, Baraldi E, Pettennazzo A, et al. Adverse effect of chloral hydrate in two young children with obstructive sleep apnea. Pediatrics. 1993;92:461–463.

88. Weil JV, McCullough RE, Kline JS, et al. Diminished ventilatory response to hypoxia and hypercapnia after morphine in normal men. N Engl J Med. 1975;292:1103–1106.

89. Santiago TV, Pugliese AC, Edelman NH. Control of breathing during methadone addiction. Am J Med. 1977;62:347–354.

90. Kryger MH, Yacoob O, Dosman J, et al. Effect of meperidine on occlusion pressure responses to hypercapnia and hypoxia with and without external inspiratory resistance. Am Rev Respir Dis. 1976;114:333–340.

91. Santiago TV, Goldblatt K, Winters K, et al. Respiratory consequences of methodone: the response to added resistance to breathing. Am Rev Respir Dis. 1980;122:623–628.

92. Robinson RW, Zwillich CW, Bixler EO, et al. Effects of oral narcotics in sleep disordered breathing in healthy adults. Chest. 1987;91:197–203.

93. Wallers AS, Wagner ML, Hening WA, et al. Successful treatment of the idiopathic restless legs syndrome in a randomized double-blind trial of oxycodone versus placebo. Sleep. 1993;16:327–332.

94. Keamy MF, Cadieux RJ, Kofke WA, et al. The occurrence of obstructive sleep apnea in a recovery room patient. Anesthesiology. 1987;66:232–234.

95. Lamarche Y, Martin R, Reiher J, et al. The sleep apnoea syndrome and epidural morphine. Can Anaesth Soc J. 1986;33:231–233.

96. Samuels SI, Rabinov W. Difficulty reversing drug-induced coma in a patient with sleep apnea. Anesth Analg. 1986;65:1222–1224.

97. Catley DM, Thornton C, Jordan C, et al. Pronounced, episodic oxygen desaturation in the postoperative period: its association with ventilatory pattern and analgesic regimen. Anesthesiology. 1985;63:20–28.

98. Clyburn PA, Rosen M, Vickers MD. Comparison of the respiratory effects of IV infusions of morphine and regional analgesia by extradural block. Br J Anaesth. 1990;64:446–449.

99. Rennotte MT, Baele P, Aubert G, et al. Nasal continuous postive airway pressure in the perioperative management of patients with obstructive sleep apnea submitted to surgery. Chest. 1995;107:367–374.

100. Nishino T, Shirahata M, Toshihide Y, et al. Comparison of changes in the hypoglossal and the phrenic nerve activity in

response to increasing depth of anesthesia in cats. Anesthesiology. 1984;60:19–24.

101. Safar P, Escarraga LA, Chang F. Upper airway obstruction in the unconscious patient. J Appl Physiol. 1959;14:760–764.

102. Isono S, Kochi T, Ide T, et al. Differential effects of vecuronium on diaphragm and geniohyoid muscle in anaesthetized dogs. Br J Anaesth. 1992;68:239–243.

103. Boushra NN. Anaesthetic management of patients with sleep apnoea syndrome. Can J Anaesth. 1996;43:599–616.

104. Guilleminault C, Eldridge FL, Tilkian A, et al. Sleep apnea syndrome due to upper airway obstruction. Arch Intern Med. 1977;137:296–300.

105. Harman E, Wynne JW, Block AJ. Sleep disordered breathing and oxygen desaturation in obese patients. Chest. 1981;79:256–260.

106. Rajola R, Partinen M, Sane T, et al. Obstructive sleep apnea syndrome in morbidly obese patients. J Intern Med. 1991;230:125–129.

107. Johnson MW, Anch AM, Remmers JE. Induction of the obstructive sleep apnea syndrome in a woman by exogenous androgen administration. Am Rev Respir Dis. 1984;129:1023–1025.

108. Sandbloom RE, Matsumato AM, Schoene RB, et al. Obstructive sleep apnea syndrome induced by testosterone administration. N Engl J Med. 1983;308:508–510.

109. Schneider BK, Pickett CK, Zwillich CW, et al. The influence of testosterone on breathing during sleep. J Appl Physiol. 1986;61:618–623.

110. Matsumoto AM, Sandblom RE, Schoene RB, et al. Testosterone replacement in hypogonadal men: effects on sleep apnea, respiratory drives, and sleep. Clin Endocrinol. 1985;22:713–721.

111. White DP, Schneider BK, Santen RJ, et al. Influence of testosterone on ventilation and chemosensitivity in male subjects. J Appl Physiol. 1985;59:1452–1457.

112. Stewart DA, Grunstein RR, Berthon-Jones M, et al. Androgen blockade does not effect sleep-disordered breathing or chemosensitivity in men with obstructive sleep apnea. Am Rev Respir Dis. 1992;146:1389–1393.

113. Cook WR, Benich JJ, Wooten SA. Indices of severity of obstructive sleep apnea syndrome do not change during medroxyprogesterone acetate therapy. Chest. 1989;96:262–266.

114. Grunstein RR. Metabolic aspects of sleep apnea. Sleep. 1996;S218–220.

115. Fletcher EC, DeBehnke RD, Lovoi MS, et al. Undiagnosed sleep apnea in patients with essential hypertension. Ann Intern Med. 1985;103:190–195.

116. Kales A, Cadieux RJ, Shaw LC, et al. Sleep apnea in a hypertensive population. Lancet. 1984;2:1005–1008.

117. Betts TA, Alford C. Beta-blockers and sleep: a controlled trial. Eur J Clin Pharmacol. 1985;28(suppl):65–68.

118. Boudoulas H, Schmidt H, Geleris P, et al. Case reports on deterioration of sleep apnea during therapy with propranolol preliminary studies. Res Commun Chem Pathol Pharmacol. 1983;39:3–10.

119. Fletcher E, Lovoi M, Miller J, et al. Propranolol and sleep apnea [abstract]. Am Rev Respir Dis. 1985;131(suppl):A103.

120. Mayer J, Weichler U, Herres-Mayer B, et al. Influence of metaprolol and cilazapril on blood pressure and sleep apnea activity. J Cardiovasc Pharmacol. 1990;16:952–961.

121. Kantola I, Rauhala E, Erkinjuntti M, et al. Sleep disturbances in hypertension: a double-blind study between isradipine and metoprolol. J Cardiovasc Pharmacol. 1991;18:S41–45.

122. Weichler U, Herres-Mayer B, Mayer J, et al. Influence of antihypertensive drug therapy on sleep pattern and sleep apnea activity. Cardiology. 1991;78:124–130.

123. Lahive K, Weiss JW, Weinberger S. Alpha-methyldopa selectively reduces alae nasi activity. Clin Sci. 1988;74:547–551.

124. Bartel PR, Loock M, Becker P, et al. Short-term antihypertensive medication does not exacerbate sleep-disordered breathing in newly diagnosed hypertensive patients. Am J Hypertens. 1997;10:640–645.

125. Issa FG. Effect of clonidine in obstructive sleep apnea. Am Rev Respir Dis. 1992;145:435–439.

126. Pelttari L, Rauhola E, Kantola I. Effects of antihypertensive medication on hypertension in patients with sleep apnea. Blood Press. 1994;2:S88–91.

127. Grote L, Heitmann J, Kohler U, et al. Effect of angiotensin

converting enzyme inhibition (cilazapril) on blood pressure recording in hypertensive obstructive sleep apneic patients. Blood Press. 1997;6:235–241.

128. Hirshkowitz M, Karacan I, Gurakar A, et al. Hypertension, erectile dysfunction, and occult sleep apnea. Sleep. 1989;12:223–232.

129. Isaksson H, Svanborg E. Obstructive sleep apnea syndrome in male hypertensives, refractory to drug therapy. Nocturnal automatic blood pressure measurements—an aid to diagnosis? Clin Exp Hypertens. 1991;13:1195–1212.

130. Wilson WR, Bedell GN. The pulmonary abnormalities in myxedema. J Clin Invest. 1960;39:42–55.

131. Domm BM, Vassalo CL. Myxedema coma with respiratory failure. Am Rev Respir Dis. 1973;107:842–845.

132. Massumi RA, Winnacker JL. Severe depression of the respiratory center in myxedema. Am J Med. 1964;36:876–882.

133. Nordquist P, Dhuner KG, Stenberg K, et al. Myxedema coma and CO_2 retention. Acta Med Scand. 1960;166:189–194.

134. Zwillich CW, Pierson DJ, Hofeldt FD, et al. Ventilatory control in myxedema and hypothyroidism. N Engl J Med. 1975;292:662–665.

135. Skatrud JB, Iber C, Ewart R, et al. Disordered breathing during sleep in hypothroidism. Am Rev Respir Dis. 1981;124:325–329.

136. Orr WC, Males JL, Imes NK. Myxedema and obstructive sleep apnea. Am J Med. 1981;70:1061–1066.

137. Rajagopal K, Abbrecht PH, Derderian SS, et al. Obstructive sleep apnea in hypothyroidism. Ann Intern Med. 1984;104:491–494.

138. Lin CC, Tsan KW, Chen PJ. The relationship between sleep apnea syndrome and hypothyroidism. Chest. 1992;102:1663–1667.

139. Grunstein RR, Sullivan CE. Sleep apnea and hypothyroidism: mechanisms and management. Am J Med. 1983;85:775–779.

140. Winkelman JW, Goldman H, Piscatelli N, et al. Are thyroid function tests necessary in patients with suspected sleep apnea? Sleep. 1996;19:790–793.

141. Schmidt HS, Clark RW, Hyman PR. Protriptyline: an effective agent in the treatment of the narcolepsy-cataplexy syndrome and hypersomnia. Am J Psychiatry. 1977;134:183–185.

142. Clark RW, Schmidt HS, Schall SF, et al. Sleep apnea: treatment with protriptyline. Neurology. 1979;29:1287–1292.

143. Conway WA, Zorick F, Piccione P, et al. Protriptyline in the treatment of sleep apnoea. Thorax. 1982;37:49–53.

144. Brownell LG, West P, Sweatman P, et al. Protriptyline in obstructive sleep apnea: a double-blind trial. N Engl J Med. 1982;307:1037–1042.

145. Smith PL, Haponik EF, Allen RR, et al. The effect of protriptyline in sleep disordered breathing. Am Rev Respir Dis. 1983;127:8–13.

146. Stepanski EJ, Conway WA, Young DK, et al. A double-blind trial of protriptyline in the treatment of sleep apnea syndrome. Henry Ford Hosp Med J. 1988;36:5–8.

147. Whyte KF, Gould GA, Airlie MAA, et al. Role of protriptyline and acetazolamide in the sleep apnea/hypopnea syndrome. Sleep. 1988;11:463–472.

148. Caroll N, Parker RA, Branthwaite MA. The use of protriptyline for respiratory failure in patients with chronic airflow limitation. Eur Respir J. 1990;3:746–751.

149. Series F, Cormier Y. Effects of protriptyline on diurnal and nocturnal oxygenation in patients with chronic obstructive pulmonary disease. Ann Intern Med. 1990;113:507–511.

150. Simonds AK, Caroll N, Branthwaite MA, et al. Effect of protriptyline on ventilatory responses to hypercapnia and asphyxia in normal subjects. Eur Respir J. 1989;2:758–763.

151. Simonds AK, Parker RA, Branthwaite MA. Effects of protriptyline on sleep-related disturbances of breathing in restrictive chest wall disease. Thorax. 1986;41:586–590.

152. Smith PM, Edwards RH, Calverley PM. Protriptyline treatment of sleep hypoxemia in Duchenne muscular dystrophy. Thorax. 1989;44:1002–1005.

153. Nino-Murcia G, Bliwise D, Keenan S, et al. Treatment of obstructive sleep apnea with CPAP and protriptyline. Chest. 1988;94:1314–1315.

154. Hanzel DA, Proia NG, Hudgel DW. Response of obstructive sleep apnea to fluoxetine and protriptyline. Chest. 1991;100:416–421.

155. Rubin AE, Alroy GG, Peled R, et al. Preliminary clinical experience with imiprimine HCl in the treatment of sleep apnea syndrome. Eur Neurol. 1986;25:81–85.

156. Salazar-Grueso EF, Rosenberg RS, Roos RP. Sleep apnea in olivopontocerebellar degeneration: treatment with trazodone. Ann Neurol. 1988;23:399–401.

157. George CF, West P, Millar T, et al. Trial of a dopaminergic antidepressant in obstructive sleep apnea. Sleep. 1987;10:180–183.

158. England SJ, Farhi LE. Fluctuations in alveolar CO_2 and in base excess during the menstrual cycle. Respir Physiol. 1976;26:157–161.

159. Weinberger SE, Weiss ST, Cohen WR, et al. Pregnancy and the lung. Am Rev Respir Dis. 1980;121:559–581.

160. Zwillich CW, Natalino MR, Sutton FD, et al. Effects of progesterone in chemosensitivity in normal men. J Lab Clin Med. 1978;92:262–269.

161. Skatrud JB, Dempsey JA, Bhansali P, et al. Determinants of chronic carbon dioxide retention and its correction in humans. J Clin Invest. 1980;65:813–821.

162. Skatrud JB, Dempsey JA, Kaiser DG. Ventilatory response to medroxyprogesterone acetate in normal subjects: time course and mechanism. J Appl Physiol. 1978;44:939–944.

163. Skatrud JB, Iber C, Ewart R, et al. Correction of CO_2 retention during sleep in patients with chronic obstructive pulmonary disease. Am Rev Respir Dis. 1981;124:260–268.

164. Dolly FR, Block AJ. Medroxyprogesterone acetate and COPD: effect on breathing and oxygenation in sleeping and awake patients. Chest. 1983;84:394–398.

165. Tatsumi K, Kimura H, Kunitomo F, et al. Effect of chlormadinone acetate on sleep arterial oxygen desaturation in patients with chronic obstructive pulmonary disease. Chest. 1987;91:688–692.

166. Tatsumi K, Kimura H, Kunitomo F, et al. Effect of chlormadinone acetate on ventilatory control in patients with chronic obstructive pulmonary disease. Am Rev Respir Dis. 1986;133:552–557.

167. Daskalopoulou E, Patakas D, Tsara V, et al. Comparison of almitrine bismesylate and medroxyprogesterone acetate on oxygenation during wakefulness and sleep in patients with chronic obstructive lung disease. Thorax. 1990;45:666–669.

168. Block AJ, Wynne JW, Boysen PG. Sleep-disordered breathing and nocturnal oxygen desaturation in post-menopausal women. Am J Med. 1980;69:75–79.

169. Block AJ, Wynne JW, Boysen PG, et al. Menopause, medroxyprogesterone, and breathing during sleep. Am J Med. 1981;70:506–510.

170. Carskadon MA, Bearpark HM, Sharkey KM, et al. Effects of menopause and nasal occlusion on breathing during sleep. Am J Respir Crit Care Med. 1997;155:205–210.

171. Guilleminault C, Quera-Salva, Partmen M. Women and the obstructive sleep apnea syndrome. Chest. 1988;94:983–988.

172. Pickett CK, Regensteiner JG, Woodard WD, et al. Progestin and estrogen reduce sleep-disordered breathing in postmenopausal women. J Appl Physiol. 1989;66:1656–1661.

173. Franklin K, Lundgren R, Rabben T. Sleep apnoea syndrome treated with oestradiol and cyclic medroxyprogesterone. Lancet. 1991;338:251–252.

174. Cistulli PA, Barnes DJ, Grunstein RR, et al. Effect of short-term hormone replacement in the treatment of obstructive sleep apnea in postmenopausal women. Thorax. 1994;49:699–702.

175. Stahl ML, Orr WC, Males JL. Progesterone levels and sleep-related breathing during menstrual cycles of normal women. Sleep. 1985;8:227–230.

176. Brownell LG, West P, Kryger MH. Breathing during sleep in normal pregnant women. Am Rev Respir Dis. 1986;133:38–41.

177. Hostie SJ, Prowse K, Perks WH, et al. Obstructive sleep apnea during pregnancy requiring tracheostomy. Aust N Z J Obstet Gynecol. 1989;29:365–367.

178. Kowall J, Clark G, Nino-Murcia G, et al. Precipitation of obstructive sleep apnea during pregnancy. Obstet Gynecol. 1989;74:453–455.

179. Zwillich CW, Sutton FD, Pierson DJ, et al. Decreased hypoxic ventilatory drive in the obesity-hyperventilation syndrome. Am J Med. 1975;59:343–348.

180. Sutton FD, Zwillich CW, Creagh CE, et al. Progesterone for outpatient treatment of the Pickwickian syndrome. Ann Intern Med. 1975;83:476–479.

181. Lyons HA, Huang CT. Therapeutic use of progesterone in alveolar hypoventilation associated with obesity. Am J Med. 1968;44:881–888.

182. Orr WC, Imes NK, Martin RJ. Progesterone therapy in obese patients with sleep apnea. Arch Intern Med. 1979;139:109–111.

183. Rajagopal KR, Abbrecht PH, Jabbari B. Effects of medroxyprogesterone acetate in obstructive sleep apnea. Chest. 1986;90:815–821.

184. Strohl KP, Hensley MJ, Saunders NA, et al. Progesterone administration and progressive sleep apneas. JAMA. 1981;245:1230–1232.

185. Kimura H, Tatsumi K, Kunitomo F, et al. Progesterone therapy for sleep apnea syndrome evaluated by occlusion pressure responses to exogenous loading. Am Rev Respir Dis. 1989;139:1198–2006.

186. Weil JV. Sleep at high altitude. Clin Chest Med. 1985;6:615–621.

187. Naeije N, Melot C, Naieje R, et al. Ondine's curse: report of a patient treated with almitrine, a new respiratory stimulant. Eur J Respir Dis. 1981;63:342–346.

188. Krieger J, Mangin P, Kurtz D. Effects of a ventilatory stimulant, almitrine bismesylate, in the sleep apnea syndrome. Am Ther Res. 1982;32:697–705.

189. DeBacker W, Bogaert E, Van Maele R, et al. Effect of almitrine bismesylate on arterial blood gases and ventilatory drive in patients with severe chronic airflow obstruction and bilateral carotid body resection. Eur J Respir Dis. 1983;64 (suppl):239–242.

190. Melot C, Naije R. Rothchild J, et al. Improvement in ventilation perfusion matching by almitrine in COPD. Chest. 1983;83:529–523

191. Powles ACP, Tuxen DV, Mahood CB, et al. The effect of intravenously administered almitrine, a peripheral chemoreceptor agonist, on patients with chronic airflow obstruction. Am Respir Dis. 1983;127:284–289.

192. Melot C, Dechamps P, Hallemans R, et al. Enhancement of hypoxic pulmonary vasoconstriction by low dose almitrine bismesylate in normal humans. Am Rev Respir Dis. 1989;139:111–119.

193. Escourrou P, Simonneau G, Ansquer JC, et al. A single orally administered dose of almitrine improves pulmonary gas exchange during exercise in patients with chronic air-flow obstruction. Am Rev Respir Dis. 1986;133:562–567.

194. Macnee W, Connaughton JJ, Rhind GB, et al. A comparison of the effects of almitrine or oxygen breathing on pulmonary artery pressure and right ventricular ejection fraction in hypoxic chronic bronchitis and emphysema. Am Rev Respir Dis. 1986;134:559–565.

195. Connaughton JJ, Douglas NJ, Morgan AD, et al. Almitrine improves oxygenation when both awake and asleep in patients with hypoxia and carbon dioxide retention caused by chronic bronchitis and emphysema. Am Rev Respir Dis. 1985;132:206–210.

196. Gothe B, Cherniack NS, Bachand RT, et al. Long-term effects of almitrine bismesylate on oxygenation during wakefulness and sleep in chronic obstructive pulmonary disease. Am J Med. 1988;84:436–444.

197. Hackett PH, Roach RC, Harrison GL, et al. Respiratory stimulants and sleep periodic breathing at high altitude. Almitrine versus acetazolamide. Am Rev Respir Dis. 1987;135:896–898.

198. Watanabe S, Kanner RE, Cutillo AG, et al. Long-term effect of almitrine bismesylate in patients with hypoxemic chronic obstructive pulmonary disease. Am Rev Respir Dis. 1989;140:1269–1273.

199. White DP, Zwillich CW, Pickett C, et al. Central sleep apnea: improvement with acetazolamide therapy. Arch Intern Med. 1982;142:1816–1819.

200. Sharp JT, Druz WS, D'Souza V, et al. Effect of metabolic acidosis upon sleep apnea. Chest. 1985;87:619–624.

201. Shore ET, Millman RP. Central sleep apnea and acetazolamide therapy. Arch Intern Med. 1983;143:1278.

202. Tojima H, Kunitomo F, Kimura H, et al. Effects of acetazolamide in patients with the sleep apnoea syndrome. Thorax. 1988;43:113–119.

203. Sakumoto T, Nakazawa Y, Hoshizuma Y, et al. Effects of acetozolamide in the sleep apnea syndrome and its therapeutic mechanism. Psychiatry Clin Neurosci. 1995;49:59–64.

204. DeBacker WA, Verbraecken J, Willemen M, et al. Central apnea index decreases after prolonged treatment with acetozolamide. Am J Respir Crit Care Med. 1995;151:87–91.

205. Skatrud JB, Dempsey JA. Relative effectiveness of acetazolamide versus medroxyprogesterone acetate in correction of chronic carbon dioxide retention. Am Rev Respir Dis. 1983;127:405–412.

206. Haxhio MA, Van Lunteren E, Van DeGraff WB, et al. Action of nicotine on the respiratory activity of the diaphragm and genioglossus muscles and the nerves that innervate them. Respir Physiol. 1984;57:153–169.

207. Gothe B, Strohl KP, Levin S, et al. Nicotine. A different approach to the treatment of obstructive sleep apnea. Chest. 1985;89:11–17.

208. Dovila DG, Hurt RD, Offord KP, et al. Acute effects of transdermal nicotine on sleep architecture, snoring, and sleep-disordered breating in nonsmokers. Am J Respir Crit Care Med. 1994;150:469–474.

209. Lakshminarayan S, Sahn SA, Weil JV. Effect of aminophylline on ventilatory responses in normal man. Am Rev Respir Dis. 1978;117:33–38.

210. Kelly DH, Shannon DC. Treatment of apnea and excessive periodic breathing in the full-term infant. Pediatrics. 1981;68:183–186.

211. Lam A, Newhouse MT. Management of asthma and chronic airflow limitation: are methylxanthines obsolete? Chest. 1990;98:44–52.

212. Ebden P, Vatkenen AS. Does aminophylline improve nocturnal hypoxia in patients with chronic airflow obstruction? Eur J Respir Dis. 1987;71:384–387.

213. Berry RB, Desa MM, Branum JP, et al. Effect of theophylline on sleep and sleep-disordered breathing in patients with chronic obstructive pulmonary disease. Am Rev Respir Dis. 1991;143:245–250.

214. Zwillich CW, Neagley SR, Cicutto L, et al. Nocturnal asthma therapy: inhaled bitolterol versus sustained-release theophylline. Am Rev Respir Dis. 1989;139:470–474.

215. Martin RJ, Cicutto LC, Ballard RD, et al. Circadian variations in theophylline concentrations and the treatment of nocturnal asthma. Am Rev Respir Dis. 1989;139:475–478.

216. Mulloy E, McNicholos WT. Theophylline in obstructive sleep apnea: a double-blind evaluation. Chest. 1992;101:753–757.

217. Espinoza H, Antic R, Thornton AT, et al. The effects of aminophylline on sleep and sleep-disordered breathing in patients with obstructive sleep apnea syndrome. Am Rev Respir Dis. 1987;136:80–84.

218. Guilleminault C, Hayes B. Naloxone, theophylline, bromocriptine and obstructive sleep apnea, negative results. Bull Eur Physiopathol Respir. 1981;17:341–349.

219. Raetzo MA, Junod AF, Kryger MH. Effect of aminophylline and relief from hypoxia on central sleep apnoea due to medullary damage. Bull Eur Physiopathol Respir. 1987;23:171–175.

220. Dowell AR, Buckley CE, Cohen R, et al. Cheyne Stokes respiration: a review of manifestations and critique of physiological mechanisms. Arch Intern Med. 1971;127:712.

221. Dowdell WT, Javaheri S, McGinnis W. Cheyne-Stokes respiration presenting as sleep apnea syndrome. Am Rev Respir Dis. 1990;140:871–879.

222. Javaheri S, Parker TJ, Wexler L, et al. Effect of theophylline on sleep-disordered breathing in heart failure. N Engl J Med. 1996;335:562–567.

223. Rachelefsky GS, Wo J, Adelson J, et al. Behavior abnormalities and poor school performance due to oral theophylline use. Pediatrics. 1986;78:1133–1138.

224. Schlleper A, Alcock D, Beaudry P, et al. Effect of therapeutic plasma concentrations of theophylline on behavior, cognitive processing, and affect in children with asthma. J Pediatr. 1991;118:449–455.

225. Avital A, Steljes DG, Pasterkamp H, et al. Sleep quality in children with asthma treated with theophylline or cromolyn sodium. J Pediatr. 1991;119:979–984.

226. Remmers JE, Anch AM, deGroot WJ, et al. Oropharyngeal muscle tone in obstructive sleep apnea before and after strychnine. Sleep. 1980;3:447–453.

227. Orlowski JP, Herrell DW, Moodie DS. Narcotic antagonist therapy of the obesity hypoventilation syndrome. Crit Care Med. 1982;10:604–607.

228. Atkinson RL, Suratt PM, Wilhoit SC, et al. Naloxone improves sleep apnea in obese humans. Int J Obes Relat Metab Disord. 1985;9:233–239.

229. Greenberg HE, Rapoport DM, Rothenberg SA, et al. Endogenous opiates modulate the postapnea ventilatory response in the obstructive sleep apnea syndrome. Am Rev Respir Dis. 1991;143:1282–1287.

230. Olson LG, Hensley MJ, Saunders NA. Augmentation of ventilation response to asphyxia by prochlorperazine in man. J Appl Physiol. 1982;53:637–643.

231. Olson LG, Hensley MJ, Saunders NA. Breathing during sleep: the responses to asphyxia and prochlorperazine in normal subjects and patients with obstructive sleep apnea. Aust N Z J Med. 1983;13:613–620.

232. Sobel SV, Fainman C, Kripke DF. Effect of haloperidol on sleep apnea. Am J Psychiatry. 1985;142:775–776.

233. Midgren B, Hansson L, Ahlmen S, et al. Effects of single dose of propiomazine, a phenothiazine hypnotic, on sleep and oxygenation in patients with stable chronic obstructive pulmonary disease. Respiration. 1990;57:239–242.

234. Kahn A, Blum D. Phenothiazines and sudden infant death syndrome. Pediatrics. 1982;70:75–78.

235. Kahn A, Hasaerts D, Blum D. Phenothiazine-induced sleep apneas in normal infants. Pediatrics. 1985;75:844–847.

236. Schmidt HS. L-Tryptophan in the treatment of impaired respiration in sleep. Bull Eur Physiopathol Respir. 1983;19:625–629.

237. Veasey SC, Panckeri KA, Hoffman EA, et al. The effects of serotonin antagonists in an animal model of sleep disordered breathing. Am J Respir Crit Care Med. 1996;153:776–786.

238. Gleeson K, Zwillich CW, Braier K, et al. Breathing route during sleep. Am Rev Respir Dis. 1986;134:115–120.

239. Mathew OP, Yousef AK, Thach BT. Genioglossus muscle response to upper airway pressure changes: afferent pathways. J Appl Physiol. 1982;52:445–450.

240. Mathew OP, Yousef AK, Thach BT. Influence of upper airway pressure changes in genioglossus muscle respiratory activity. J Appl Physiol. 1982;52:438–444.

241. McBride B, Whitelaw WA. A physiologic stimulus to upper airway receptors in humans. J Appl Physiol. 1981;51:1189–1197.

242. White DP, Cadieux RJ, Lombard RM, et al. The effects of nasal anesthesia on breathing during sleep. Am Rev Respir Dis. 1985;132:972–975.

243. DeWeese EL, Sullivan TY. Effects of upper airway anesthesia on pharyngeal patency during sleep. J Appl Physiol. 1988;64:1346–1353.

244. McNicholas WT, Coffey M, McDonnell T, et al. Upper airway obstruction during sleep in normal subjects after selective topical oropharyngeal anesthesia. Am Rev Respir Dis. 1987;135:1316–1319.

245. Chadwick GA, Crowley P, Fitzgerald MX, et al. Obstructive sleep apnea following topical oropharyngeal anesthesia in loud snorers. Am Rev Respir Dis. 1991;143:810–813.

246. Deegan PC, Mulloy E, McNicholas WT. Topical orophoryngeal anesthesia in patients with obstructive sleep apnea. Am J Respir Crit Care Med. 1995;151:1108–1112.

247. Issa FG, Sullivan CE. Reversal of central sleep apnea using nasal CPAP. Chest. 1986;90:165–171.

248. Brover HM, Block AJ. Effect of nasal spray, positional therapy, and the combination thereof in the asymptomatic snorer. Sleep. 1994;17:516–521.

249. Grunstein RR, Hokk, Sullivan CE. Effect of octreotide, a somatostation analog, on sleep apnea in patients with acromegaly. Ann Intern Med. 1994;121:478–483.

250. Buyse B, Michiels E. Bouillon R, et al. Relief of sleep apnoea after treatment of acromegaly: report of three cases and review of the literature. Eur Respir J. 1997;10:1401–1404.

251. Ziemer DC, Dickson DB. Case report: relief of sleep apnea in acromegaly by bromocriptine. Am J Med Sci. 1988;295:49–51.

252. Gerard JM, Garibaldi L, Myers SE, et al. Sleep apnea in patients receiving growth hormone. Clin Pediatr (Phila). 1997;36:321–326.

253. Al-Ghamdi SA, Manoukian JJ, Morielli A, et al. Do systemic corticosteroids effectively treat obstructive sleep apnea secondary to adenotonsillar hypertrophy? Laryngoscope. 1997;107:1382–1387.

254. Hedner J, Grunstein R, Erikssen B. A double-blind, randomized trial of sabeluzole—a putative glutamate antagonist—in obstructive sleep apnea. Sleep. 1996;19:287–289.

255. Tilkian AG, Guilleminault C, Schroeder JS, et al. Sleep induced apnea syndrome: prevalence of cardiac arrhythmias and their reversal after tracheostomy. Am J Med. 1977;63:348–358.

256. Arnulf I, Homeyer P, Garma L, et al. Modafinil in obstructive sleep apnea–hypopnea syndrome: a pilot study in 6 patients. Respiration. 1997;64:159–161.

257. Schonhofer B, Kohler D. Benzodiozepine receptor antagonist (flumazenil) does not affect sleep-related breathing disorders. Eur Respir J. 1996;9:1816–1820.

258. Houser WC, Schleuter DP. Prolonged doxapram infusion in obesity-hypoventilation syndrome. JAMA. 1978;239:340–341.

259. Suratt PM, Wilhoit SC, Brown ED, et al. Effect of doxapram on obstructive sleep apnea. Bull Eur Physiopathol Respir. 1986;22:127–131.

70

Snoring

Victor Hoffstein

The importance of examining snoring derives from several clinical observations. Although snoring is the most common symptom of sleep apnea, most patients who snore do not have sleep apnea. Nevertheless, many nonapneic snorers present with subjective symptoms similar to those described in patients with sleep apnea, for example, daytime sleepiness, tiredness, difficulty in concentration, headaches, and reduced work performance. In addition, some (but not all) nonapneic snorers have objective physiological findings similar to those of patients with sleep apnea—for example, high blood pressure, cardiac disease, cerebrovascular disease, and endocrine disease or dysfunction such as hypothyroidism, diabetes, or insulin resistance. This raises a possibility that snoring alone, even in the absence of sleep apnea, may be a causative factor in the pathogenesis of the above conditions.

Consequently, we shall review the pathophysiology, clinical features, diagnostic evaluation, and management of snoring. The discussion and recommendations focus only on the evidence obtained from studies examining snoring when it occurs in the absence of sleep apnea. Separating the effect of snoring from apnea is not always simple because both conditions are closely linked, and many investigations dealing with cardiovascular complications and daytime function do not clearly distinguish between apneic and nonapneic snorers.

DEFINITIONS

What is snoring? *The Random House Dictionary of the English Language*[1] defines it as ". . . breathing during sleep with hoarse or harsh sounds as caused by the vibrating of the soft palate." *The New Webster's Dictionary*[2] gives an almost identical definition, with the sole qualifier that the harsh breathing is ". . . through the open mouth and the nose when asleep." Note that both definitions imply something about the pathogenesis, that is, that snoring is produced by the vibrating uvula. The International Classification of Sleep Disorders manual defines *primary snoring* (ICSD 780.53-1) as "loud upper airway breathing sounds in sleep, without episodes of apnea or hypoventilation."[3(p195)] No matter which definition of snoring we adopt, we must remember that it is first and foremost a subjective impression on the part of the listener. This fact has important implications when interpreting the results of studies

investigating various medical aspects of snoring, because the division into snoring and nonsnoring groups may not be entirely accurate. Subjectivity of snoring is a difficult issue that must be taken into account when analyzing, interpreting, and applying the results of many investigations dealing with snoring.

HISTORICAL ASPECTS

Because snoring is such a frequent and invariable accompaniment of human sleep, for many centuries it was probably considered a normal phenomenon. It was only mentioned in literary works, popular books, and in folklore tales as an event that might be a major nuisance to the listener, leading sometimes to rather drastic solutions, including homicide. John Wesley Hardin, a notorious gunfighter from Texas, apparently shot and killed a hotel guest who was asleep and snoring loudly in the adjoining room.[4]

It is difficult to determine when scientific studies on snoring began. George Catlin,[5] the artist who studied the life habits of Native Americans, wrote a book, published in 1872, about breathing during sleep, called *The Breath of Life*. He promoted the idea that daytime health was a consequence of unobstructed nasal breathing at night with the mouth closed; this was common among Native Americans, which in Catlin's opinion accounted for their good general health. He concluded that breathing through the mouth causes snoring, restlessness, and lack of refreshing sleep.

Because Catlin was not a scientist, his views were generally disregarded, and for the next 100 years the topic remained unexplored. This lack of interest is best illustrated by the following fact. The earliest scientific and authoritative book dealing with sleep was *Sleep and Wakefulness*[6] written by Nathaniel Kleitman, and originally published in 1939. This book, which contained 367 pages of text and 4337 references, had only 5 pages devoted to respiration, and just two paragraphs devoted to snoring. Kleitman concluded that snoring is harmless to the sleeper, but can be very annoying to others who may be awake at the time, or have been aroused by the loud noises.[6]

Snorers whose bed partners complained persistently enough about being kept awake by the noise were sometimes referred to an otolaryngologist for surgical cure. There is an extensive otolaryngological literature throughout the 1950s and 1960s dealing with surgical treatment of snoring, including nasal surgery, injection of sclerosing agents into the soft palate, and pharyngeal surgery. Eventually, some otolaryngologists began to realize that in addition to inconveniencing the bed partner, snoring may adversely affect the snorer.[7, 8]

Beginning in the 1970s, concomitant with the recognition of sleep apnea syndrome, snoring assumed a new importance. It was realized that snoring is an almost invariable symptom of obstructive sleep apnea (OSA) and in fact may be a precursor to this disorder. Because the latter condition was found to be associated with daytime tiredness, sleepiness, poor memory, decreased ability to concentrate, and with adverse vascular events such as increased risk of hypertension, strokes, and heart attacks, the question arose as to whether nonapneic snoring had the same health consequences.

The pioneering studies of Lugaresi and colleagues[9] indicated that snoring may be an independent risk factor for hypertension. Lugaresi et al. also noted that even trivial snoring might be the first step in the continuum, which the authors termed *heavy snorer's disease*,[10] eventually leading to full-blown sleep apnea syndrome. Although this orderly progression from normal breathing to snoring and then on to sleep apnea is an attractive and plausible hypothesis, there is no convincing evidence that this is the case. In fact, more than 40% of habitual snorers reported resolution, rather than worsening of their snoring, when asked about it 10 years later.[11]

In addition to the link between snoring and hypertension proposed in 1980 by Lugaresi et al.[9] snoring has been linked to another possible adverse health effect. Guilleminault and colleagues,[12] aside from their seminal work regarding many features of the OSA syndrome, proposed in 1993 that nonapneic snoring may lead to daytime dysfunction by causing sleep fragmentation. They postulated, and demonstrated in several studies, that elevations of upper airway resistance during sleep may lead to arousals and to fragmented sleep. These authors coined the term *upper airway resistance syndrome* (UARS) to describe tired and sleepy patients frequently presenting with snoring whose polysomnography does not confirm sleep apnea.

In the decades that have passed since the publication of Kleitman's book, we have learned that snoring cannot be considered "harmless to the sleeper." At least, it is a potential marker of OSA. At worst, it is a disease characterized by clinical symptoms (daytime dysfunction) and dangerous sequelae, which, if left untreated, may increase the snorer's risk of vascular disease.

PATHOPHYSIOLOGY AND MEASUREMENT OF SNORING

Snoring is a sound produced by the vibrating structures of the upper airway. Direct endoscopic observations of snoring patients during sleep demonstrate that any membranous part of the airway lacking cartilaginous support may vibrate, including the soft palate, uvula, faucial pillars, pharyngeal walls, and the rest of the upper airway, almost to the level of the vocal cords. It is this diffuse, rather than local, involvement of the upper airway that makes successful treatment of snoring so difficult, particularly when techniques directed only to a local modification of the airway segment are employed. Awareness that the entire upper airway may contribute to snoring represents a departure from the previous hypothesis that snoring is a result of a local abnormality within the airway—usually the soft palate and uvula.

Theoretical models[13, 14] indicate that when there exists a specific relationship between flow, airway wall compliance, airway segment geometry (length, width, diameter), and gas density, the airway becomes unstable and begins to vibrate. The sound produced may be perceived as snoring. However, it is too simplistic to think of the pharynx as a structure that becomes hypotonic during sleep and whose walls begin to vibrate. Snoring is a complex acoustical phenomenon that is crucially dependent on the interaction between the various upper airway muscles—tongue, soft palate, and pharynx—which affect the mass and the compliance of airway walls. This interaction is modified by the neural activation of different upper airway muscles, which is exceedingly difficult to model. This was well illustrated by Isono and colleagues,[15] who found in OSA patients that despite achieving inspiratory flow limitation during pharyngeal hypotonia, snoring was not observed. A possible explanation for this is that when the pharyngeal tone is removed, the tongue and the soft palate form a continuous structure (pharyngeal wall), which has a high mass and is not easily set into vibrations. When the pharyngeal tone is restored, the genioglossus becomes active, the tongue moves forward, and the continuity of the pharyngeal wall is disrupted. The consequence of this is reduction in the mass of the pharyngeal wall, which enables it to vibrate with different frequencies than before, thus generating the characteristic snoring sound. This dependence of snoring sound on airway and gas properties is commonly observed in many clinical circumstances. For example, it is well-known that alcohol ingestion, which relaxes the pharyngeal muscles and increases airway wall compliance, thus making the pharynx more "floppy," leads to an increase in snoring. Most recently, Huang et al.[15a] developed a mathematical model of the airway that emphasizes mechanical and neuromuscular interactions in maintenance of airway patency during sleep.

Spectral characteristics of the snoring sound depend on the properties of the segment responsible for the generation of snoring. Because snoring may be generated at several sites along the airway, sometimes at multiple sites simultaneously, it is not surprising that the power spectrum of snoring is wide, encompassing a wide range of frequencies, up to 10,000 Hz. Several investigators studied the spectral characteristics of snoring sounds and pointed out that they depend on route of breathing, stage of sleep, posture, weight, airway wall mass and elasticity, and other factors affecting upper airway properties. Snoring is usually an inspiratory sound, but may also be present during

Table 70–1. PREVALENCE OF SNORING

Authors (y)	Country	N	Men (%)	Women (%)
Lugaresi et al. (1980)[9]	Italy	5713	40	28
Norton et al. (1983)[87]	Canada	279	86	57
Mondini et al. (1983)[88]	Italy	1898	24	14
Koskenvuo et al. (1985)[89]	Finland	7511	9	4
Norton & Dunn (1985)[90]	Canada	2001	71	51
Stradling & Crosby (1990)[18]	United Kingdom	890	10*	
Wiggins et al. (1990)[91]	United States	360	34	18
Bliwise et al. (1991)[92]	United States	1409	40	15
Young et al. (1993)[20]	United States	1255	44	28
Bearpark et al. (1995)[19]	Australia	294	10	
Olson et al. (1995)[93]	Australia	441	52†	
Janson et al. (1995)[22]	Sweden, Iceland, Belgium	2202	5	2–3
Ohayon et al. (1997)[21]	United Kingdom	4972	48	34
Stoohs et al. (1998)[94]	United States	289	6–32‡	
Keenan et al. (1998)[95]	Canada	437	27	

*23% when spouse present.
†Both genders.
‡Age-dependent.

expiration. It occurs in all sleep stages, although it may be more common in stages 2 to 4.

The importance of being able to measure, analyze, and quantify snoring is obvious. First, it is hoped that such measurements can be combined with a realistic model of the airway to determine the site where snoring is generated. Second, these measurements permit study of the relationship between snoring and adverse health outcomes in a more objective fashion. Thirdly, it will become possible to evaluate the effect of treatment objectively.

Several different techniques for measuring and quantifying snoring have been described.[16] Unlike apneas, there is no accepted and uniform way to conduct this measurement. Until such a method is developed, a combination of sound measurements using a calibrated microphone placed in the standard position, and a subjective assessment using currently available questionnaires, should provide a relatively robust and reproducible method of quantifying snoring.

EPIDEMIOLOGY

We know that snoring is common, but estimates of its prevalence vary widely in different populations. Details of several such studies are given in Chapter 47. Table 70–1 shows the marked differences in prevalence found by various investigators.

These differences are probably methodological.[17, 23] Snoring, being a subjective perception, may be reported differently depending on who answers the question (the snorer or the bed partner), and how the question is phrased. For example, Stradling and Crosby[18] found that when the bed partner was present when questions regarding snoring were asked, the prevalence more than doubled—from 10 to 23%. Bearpark et al.[19] found that 15% of self-confessed snorers did not snore at all when studied in the sleep laboratory. Conversely, 15% of those who said they never snore actually snored for at least 50% of the night.

Male predominance, observed in all epidemiological studies, remains unexplained. It may be due to differences in perception of snoring by men and women, or differences in airway collapsibility due to hormonal factors.

The apparent reduction in snoring with age, observed in several studies,[11, 24, 25] is unexpected. It appears to be at odds with the common finding that the prevalence of sleep apnea increases with age. It is possible that the lack of a bed partner, altered perception of snoring, or methodological problems account for this finding. It is noteworthy that when the same cohort of snorers is followed without any interruptions for 10 years, most show increases in apnea-hypopnea index (AHI).[25a]

Finally, does genetics play a role in snoring? Clinical observations suggest that it does. Although there are no familial studies specifically addressing snoring, there are now several studies addressing familial aspects of sleep apnea. The results indicate a strong familial predisposition, raising a possibility that genetic factors may be important in determining the structure and function of the upper airway. Although this evidence is in its early stages, it justifies inquiring about the family history of snoring in all patients who are being assessed for sleep-related breathing disorders.

CLINICAL SIGNIFICANCE OF SNORING

The potential clinical importance of snoring can be illustrated by considering the following questions:

1. Is it a marker of sleep apnea?
2. Is it an independent risk factor for vascular complications, that is, hypertension, cardiovascular, and cerebrovascular disease?
3. Does it cause daytime dysfunction?

These issues, discussed later, remain unresolved.

Snoring as a Marker of Sleep Apnea

The vast majority of patients with sleep apnea snore and have been heavy snorers for many years. Lugaresi et al.[10] recognized this very early when they coined the term *heavy snorer's disease;* this disease has several stages describing the progression from simple snoring to snoring with apneas and daytime dysfunction.

The important issue, however, is not how common snoring is in patients with sleep apnea, but the converse, that is, how common sleep apnea is among snorers. There are no studies specifically addressing the relationship between simple snoring, that is, snoring in completely asymptomatic patients without any daytime dysfunction, and sleep apnea. However, there are many investigations examining the predictive utility of various markers, including snoring, for the diagnosis of sleep apnea.[26-30] Based on the available information, the following generalizations can be made. If snoring is the only symptom, that is, there is no daytime dysfunction, no observed episodes of cessation of breathing at night, and the patient is not obese (body mass index [BMI] less than 27), and is less than 40 years old, the chance of sleep apnea is at most 25%. In obese middle-aged snorers complaining of daytime tiredness or sleepiness, who are observed to stop breathing at night, the chance of sleep apnea approaches 65% (up to 95% reported by some investigators). All studies examining the utility of clinical features for diagnosing sleep apnea agree that snoring alone is not a significant predictor of sleep apnea. However, when snoring is used as one of the variables in a model that includes other features such as gender, age, weight, daytime symptoms, bed partner's observations, and the results of a pharyngeal examination, sleep apnea can be correctly predicted in a high percentage of these patients. Wilson et al.[30a] found that men with a BMI greater than 30 kg/m² and an average snoring sound intensity greater than 38 dB were four times more likely to have a respiratory disturbance index greater than 10. None of the information obtained during the history and physical examination, alone or in various combinations, have sufficient predictive power to replace polysomnography; at best, they can help to prioritize patients for polysomnography in laboratories with long waiting lists.[30]

Snoring and Vascular Disease

The possibility that vascular disease is linked to snoring was raised by Lugaresi et al.[31] in 1975. They demonstrated that episodes of snoring are associated with acute simultaneous elevations of blood pressure. Furthermore, snorers do not exhibit the reduction of blood pressure that is observed in nonsnorers during sleep. These observations raise the possibility that snoring may be an independent risk factor for development of hypertension. There are good physiological reasons to believe that such a relationship might exist. Snoring is usually accompanied by increases in intrathoracic pressure, and may be associated with mild reduction

in oxygen saturation and arousals from sleep—all factors that might lead to increased sympathetic activity during sleep.

To test the hypothesis that snoring is an independent risk factor for hypertension, several groups of investigators embarked on large-scale epidemiological studies, beginning in the early 1970s. They demonstrated a direct and independent link between snoring and hypertension.[31] There is still considerable controversy surrounding this issue.[32] However, the most recent results from the Wisconsin Sleep Cohort lend support to this hypothesis,[33] showing a progressive increase in blood pressure when comparing nonapneic nonsnorers, nonapneic snorers, and apneic snorers. The differences in blood pressure, when adjusted for age, sex, BMI, and use of antihypertensive medications, were small. Not all snorers develop hypertension. Lofaso et al.[34] found that sleep fragmentation was an important factor associated with the higher prevalence of hypertension in snorers. Guilleminault and colleagues[35] successfully treated six nonapneic snorers with nasal continuous positive airway pressure (CPAP) for 1 month and found a clinically significant reduction in blood pressure, from 146/91 to 133/83 mmHg.

The evidence linking snoring and hypertension presented above comes from either cross-sectional epidemiological studies or from small case-controlled studies. It cannot be used to infer (or reject) the existence of a causal relationship between snoring and hypertension.

Most studies examining the association between snoring and vascular disease have concentrated on hypertension, undoubtedly because the outcome variable (blood pressure, or the prevalence of hypertension) is easily measured and can be related to snoring. Other components on the vascular disease spectrum (coronary artery disease, cerebrovascular disease) are more difficult to quantify and relate to snoring. Several studies report a positive association between snoring and cerebral infarction, myocardial infarction, angina pectoris, and other vascular conditions. Nevertheless, there are many uncertainties regarding the classification of subjects into snorers and nonsnorers, the presence of unsuspected sleep apnea, the treatment of confounding factors (e.g., obesity, alcohol, diabetes, hypertension, etc.), which question the validity of a positive association between snoring and these outcomes.[32]

Snoring and Daytime Dysfunction

It is a plausible hypothesis that snoring, a naturally occurring repetitive sound, may, in some snorers, fragment sleep, thus leading to daytime dysfunction.[36-38]

Several investigators in the mid-1980s reported that snorers frequently complain of excessive daytime sleepiness and fatigue and that neuropsychological testing may reveal subtle cognitive deficits. The accepted explanation at the time was the presence of nocturnal hypoxemia in snorers, many of whom turned out to have sleep apnea. However, in 1988 Guilleminault and colleagues[39] were unable to find any correlation between sleepiness, nocturnal oxygenation, and OSA. These authors postulated that abnormalities in sleep architecture are more likely to be significant determinants of daytime sleepiness than respiration. They pointed out that alpha electroencephalographic (EEG) arousals, which frequently occur at the termination of apnea, but may also occur without association with respiratory events, could fragment sleep, thus causing daytime sleepiness.

In 1993 Guilleminault et al.[12] proposed an explanation for why many snorers do not function well during the day. These authors postulated, and demonstrated in several investigations, that these nonapneic patients exhibit a reduction in pharyngeal cross-sectional area during sleep. The reduction in airway area may not reduce the airflow sufficiently to satisfy the criteria for hypopnea, but is enough to increase the resistance of the upper airway. This is associated with increases in inspiratory effort, reduction in tidal volume, and progressively more negative intrathoracic pressure, leading to brief arousals from sleep. The authors termed this constellation of laboratory findings (repetitive arousals and increased upper airway resistance without apneas or hypopneas) and clinical abnormalities (daytime tiredness and sleepiness) *the upper airway resistance syndrome.* Snoring is not a necessary feature of this syndrome because a reduction in upper airway cross-sectional area and increase in upper airway resistance do not automatically imply that the airway walls will vibrate to produce the characteristic snoring sound. The most common use of this term today is to denote nonapneic snorers with daytime symptoms. It is important not to overdiagnose this syndrome by labeling every snorer as having UARS. An analogous situation exists for sleep apnea, which is strictly a laboratory abnormality, vs. sleep apnea syndrome, which is a combination of laboratory abnormality and clinical manifestations. UARS is present only if there are documented elevations in upper airway resistance, sleep fragmentation, and daytime dysfunction (commonly daytime sleepiness and fatigue). The American Academy of Sleep Medicine Task Force[39a] published a report that emphasized the key role of respiratory effort–related arousals, occurring in the absence of apneas and hypopneas, in the pathogenesis of UARS.

Although the original definition of this syndrome requires measurement of upper airway resistance, that is, measurement of pressure and flow, surrogate measures of effort and ventilation may be employed, provided there are no apneas or hypopneas and there are arousals. Such surrogate measures include inductive plethysmography,[39b] strain gauges, oronasal temperature (thermistors or thermocouples), nasal pressures, and the CO_2 concentration in exhaled gas. There is little or no research available to indicate how well these methods compare with the reference standard, that is, esophageal pressure.[39a] Whichever measuring method is selected, it is important to ascertain that it reflects uniquely and accurately the variability of upper airway resistance during sleep. If this is not done, then there is high likelihood of misclassifying hypopneas and thus misdiagnosing UARS as OSA or vice versa. Arousals are usually conventionally diagnosed from the EEG and electromyogram (EMG), although other methods, such as changes in heart rate, ventilation, or other measures of autonomic activity, may become acceptable ways of identifying arousals in the future.

Several observations speak in favor of the association between snoring and daytime dysfunction. First, there is accumulating evidence based on objective measurements of nocturnal respiration that nonapneic snorers are more sleepy during the day and have poorer work performance than nonapneic, nonsnoring controls[39]; the results from the Wisconsin Sleep Cohort Study[40] indicate that even mild sleep-disordered breathing is associated with some neuropsychological impairment. Questionnaire results obtained in over 4000 elderly participants in the Cardiovascular Health Study[41] indicate an association between daytime sleepiness and nocturnal disturbances such as snoring and frequent awakenings. Second, sleep fragmentation caused by brief arousals, some of which may not even satisfy the conventional definition, impairs daytime wakefulness.[42–45] Thirdly, evidence is accumulating that episodes of increased upper airway resistance during sleep, accompanied or not by snoring, may lead to arousals.[45–47]

Ultimately, demonstrating that abolishing snoring in nonapneic patients with daytime dysfunction decreases arousals and improves symptoms confirms the causal relationship between snoring and daytime dysfunction and leads to wider acceptability of the diagnosis of UARS.[47a] There are many unanswered questions regarding the prevalence, diagnosis, and optimal treatment of UARS. One of the important beneficial byproducts of the UARS work is the change in our thinking about snoring. It is no longer considered strictly an acoustical phenomenon, that is, a noise. Instead, our attention is directed toward the underlying pathophysiology of the airway. This is what leads to arousals, sleep fragmentation, and increased sympathetic activity. These events may result in adverse health effects. The awareness of UARS has led to a more careful use of the term "snoring." Patients who snore and have no daytime symptoms are referred to as simple, or primary snorers, whereas patients who snore and have daytime symptoms may have UARS. In this chapter we use the term *nonapneic snoring* to refer collectively to patients with and without UARS.

CLINICAL FEATURES AND DIAGNOSTIC ASSESSMENT

Snoring is a symptom. The purpose of the history and physical examination of a snorer is to determine the likelihood of sleep apnea, decide whether sleep study is necessary, identify the presence of possible risk factors associated with snoring, check if there are anatomical or functional abnormalities whose correction is likely to improve or completely abolish snoring, and to give advice regarding treatment. Which laboratory tests to perform is, to some extent, directed by the findings obtained during the history and physical examination; the major decision in all patients is whether to perform nocturnal polysomnography.

History

As part of the diagnostic assessment, we must ascertain that snoring is indeed present and constitutes a problem. Some bed partners may be particularly sensitive to noise and find it difficult to fall asleep even when exposed to normal breathing sounds. Others may have an ulterior motive for not wanting to sleep with the patient and use snoring simply as an excuse to accomplish this goal. Consequently, we must inquire whether other bed partners, members of the family, or friends who had an occasion to share a room with the patient or observe the patient during sleep also complained about loud and disruptive snoring.

The history is best obtained in the presence of the bed partner. This is important because the snorer is not aware of snoring, and the visit to the physician is usually instigated by the bed partner. If the visit is for a reason other than snoring, and the patient is asked about snoring, it is even more important to have the bed partner present. As we commented earlier, Stradling and Crosby[18] demonstrated that the presence of the bed partner more than doubles the frequency of the affirmative answer when patients are asked about their snoring. In addition, the bed partner helps to determine whether snoring is positional, whether it occurs nightly, and whether it is associated with breathing pauses.

One should then inquire about the risk factors—increase in weight, ingestion of alcohol, allergies, nasal obstruction, use of muscle relaxants, and smoking. If snoring either appeared recently or changed for the worse, it is important to determine whether there was a change in any of the above risk factors. Allergies may contribute to chronic nasal obstruction, thus facilitating snoring.

The interviewer should make an assessment of daytime function and quality of life. Does the snorer wake up feeling refreshed? Is he or she tired or excessively sleepy during the day? Is his or her work performance adequate? Are there any difficulties with memory, ability to concentrate, and the performance of routine tasks? There are several questionnaires, some of them validated, employed in assessing patients with sleep apnea, which are also useful for determining daytime function in snorers. For example, the Epworth Sleepiness Scale,[48] discussed in Chapter 104, is widely used to estimate the effect of sleepiness on daytime function; other questionnaires are used by different investigators.[49, 50] During this part of the interview, particularly if there is evidence of daytime dysfunction, one should ascertain that sleep hygiene is adequate and that there is no sleep restriction that may account for the above symptoms.

Systemic diseases leading to snoring (and usually to sleep apnea) by virtue of interference with upper airway anatomy or function are rare, but should not be overlooked. Examples include hypothyroidism and acromegaly. A routine search for them by biochemical tests of hormone levels is not indicated. There are several uncommon congenital conditions affecting pharyngeal area and collapsibility, such as achondroplasia, dwarfism, fusion of cervical vertebrae (e.g., Klippel-Feil anomaly), and other neck deformities. These are apparent during the physical examination.

Inquiring about any previous surgery or trauma to the upper airways at any site between the nose and the larynx should not be overlooked, because it may affect the local airway area or compliance in such a way as to lead to snoring.

Physical Examination

During the physical examination it is important to document, if applicable, the presence of general or regional obesity (BMI, neck circumference), vascular disease, and local anatomical abnormalities of the upper airway such as nasal polyps and enlarged tonsils or adenoids. It is also useful to make a general note of the pharynx: Is it small and crowded? Is the tongue large? Is the uvula inflamed, bulky, or simply long, hardly lifting off the base of the tongue during phonation? These findings probably do not have therapeutic implications, but they are useful for confirming long-standing snoring and increasing our suspicion of sleep apnea. Detailed examination of the upper airway carried out by an otolaryngologist, including fiberoptic nasendoscopy, should be routine for all habitual snorers seeking medical attention. It is useful for visualizing the anatomical structures, the amount of redundant tissue present, and making a subjective judgment regarding the patient's suitability as a surgical candidate. Simulating snoring or performing Müller's maneuver during endoscopic examination is not useful for determining the site of obstruction and predicting surgical success.

Laboratory Investigations

Laboratory investigations, which usually follow the history and physical examination, are broadly divided into two categories: airway assessment and nocturnal polysomnography. The decision to perform laboratory investigations hinges on whether we are dealing with an asymptomatic or symptomatic snorer. An asymptomatic (also called a simple, or primary) snorer is a patient who presents solely at the instigation of the family or the bed partner because of disruptive snoring. This patient is generally completely healthy and in particular does not have any health problems that are presently thought to be associated with sleep apnea, for example, vascular disease. Generally, such a patient requires no investigations, only treatment of snoring.

There are circumstances, however, when the asymptomatic snorer may require laboratory investigation. For example, if an obvious anatomical anomaly involving the nose or throat is noted, airway assessment directed toward elucidating the nature and the effect of the anomaly may be undertaken. There is no need for nocturnal polysomnography, because it will not alter treatment; even if sleep apnea is demonstrated, surgical correction of the anomaly would still be indicated. However, if surgical treatment is being contemplated in an asymptomatic snorer without an obvious airway abnormality, nocturnal polysomnography should be performed. If sleep apnea is demonstrated, noninvasive approaches may be offered in preference to surgery.

A symptomatic snorer is a patient who, in addition to snoring, has daytime symptoms usually associated with sleep apnea, such as lack of refreshing sleep, daytime tiredness, sleepiness, difficulty concentrating, attention deficit, reduced performance, and so forth. Snorers without the above symptoms but with vascular disease should also be placed in this category. Such patients have a higher likelihood of having either sleep apnea or UARS, and therefore should have full nocturnal polysomnography to establish the appropriate diagnosis and to rule out other reasons for daytime dysfunction, for example, periodic leg movements.

Should detailed airway assessment, whether during wakefulness or during sleep, be carried out in this group of snorers? Provided a full nose and throat examination, which ordinarily includes nasendoscopy, by an ear, nose, and throat specialist is performed, no other assessments during wakefulness are necessary. Only if maxillofacial surgery is contemplated should cephalometric measurements or other radiographic imaging be performed. There is no evidence that simulated snoring, Müller's maneuver, or other airway measurements performed during wakefulness are predictive of sleep apnea or helpful in selecting surgical candidates.

Investigations of the upper airway during sleep consist of direct endoscopic observation of the pharyngeal airway using fiberoptic instruments, and measurements of pressure at multiple sites along the upper airway. These measurements have diagnostic and therapeutic implications. The diagnostic implication is the ability to identify UARS by comparing esophageal pressures measured during quiet breathing without snoring with those obtained during snoring epochs or during epochs preceding the arousals not associated with apneas or hypopneas. The therapeutic implication is the ability to better select candidates for surgery, and thus maximize the chance of success. There are no studies specifically addressing the characteristics of pressure recordings at multiple sites in nonapneic snorers. Therefore, outside of particular research protocols, such measurements cannot be recommended for therapeutic decisions in nonapneic snorers.

TREATMENT

Snoring lies at one end of the spectrum of upper airway dysfunction, which in its most serious form is reflected in OSA. Therefore, it is to be expected that treatment of snoring and sleep apnea overlap. In apneic snorers, whose snoring is a symptom of sleep apnea, treatment of snoring is directed toward treating sleep apnea; if the treatment of sleep apnea is successful, the snoring may be abolished. Various treatments of sleep apnea are discussed in great detail elsewhere in this book. There are some general considerations, unique to snoring, which are relevant to treatment decisions and outcome assessment.

First, should nonapneic snoring be treated at all and by what means? This is a matter of some debate.[51] There are good arguments in favor of treating nonapneic snoring: (1) it is a nuisance to the bed partner and an embarrassment to the snorer; (2) it is the chief complaint responsible for bringing the snorer to medical attention in the first place, and therefore it is inappropriate to disregard it by simply reassuring the snorer and the bed partner that there is no sleep apnea; (3) snoring is aggravated by the same risk factors that are operative in sleep apnea, and therefore dealing with them may prevent the nonapneic snorer from progressing to apnea; and (4) in some patients snoring may cause sleep fragmentation and account for daytime dysfunction. Of the above possibilities, it is the last that suggests that the snorer may have UARS and thus constitutes the strongest indication for treatment. The only situation when one may not treat snoring is when a completely asymptomatic snorer, whose snoring is not disruptive to the bed partner, presents because of a concern that he or she may have sleep apnea. If no apnea is demonstrated, the patient should be reassured and advised about avoidance of risk factors.

Second, what is the best way to assess the outcome of treatment? Superficially, the issue appears to be simple. There is a subjective method, based on responses to specific questions, and an objective method, based on measurement of snoring. However, subjective assessment must take into account that for most patients snoring is a symptom perceived by the bed partner (or other listener), not by the snorer. Consequently, replies to questions about snoring must be given by the bed partner, preferably the one who voiced the initial complaint; this is seldom done and is frequently lost to long-term follow-up because of changes in the lifestyle of the snorer. Objective methods are also problematic, as outlined earlier. There are no standardized measurement techniques and data analysis protocols; most important, there are almost no data to ascertain that the measured sound agrees with the listener's perception of the snoring. Recognizing the above limitations, it is probably more appropriate at this time to assess treatment outcome subjectively using a well-designed questionnaire answered by the person who is qualified to assess differences in snoring before and after intervention.

Surgical Treatment

Most of the studies addressing the surgical treatment of snoring are in the context of sleep apnea, rather than focusing specifically on snoring. Various surgical procedures have been employed. The most common are nasal and pharyngeal surgery. Tongue and jaw surgery (i.e., genioglossal advancement and maxillomandibular osteotomy) are usually performed for apnea rather than for snoring.

Almost all of the studies, with few exceptions, suffer from common limitations:

- Inconsistent endpoint assessment
- Selection bias
- Lack of pre- and postoperative sleep studies
- Differences in surgical techniques
- Failure to take into account the effect of confounding factors
- Short follow-up

These limitations, and their effect on the final outcome of the study, are well described in publications regarding the efficacy of surgical treatments of sleep apnea.[52]

Taking the above limitations into account, review of the surgical literature dealing with snoring allows us to make the following generalizations with respect to the efficacy of different surgical procedures for the treatment of nonapneic snoring.

Nasal Surgery

Nasal obstruction promotes snoring by increasing negative intrathoracic pressure during sleep leading to reduction in the pharyngeal cross-sectional area, pharyngeal collapse, turbulent flow, and vibration of pharyngeal structures. Relief of nasal obstruction, when caused by nasal polyps, significant deviation of the nasal septum, or some other obvious anatomical deformity, may be associated with improvement in snoring in up to 75% of patients.[53] This result is based on subjective, short-term assessment of snoring by the patient, rather than on any objective data.

There is no reliable preoperative test that allows prediction of postoperative success. It is unlikely that nasal surgery alone will cure snoring, but it may improve nasal breathing, thereby making it easier for the patient to tolerate nasal CPAP, although no studies addressing the impact of nasal surgery on CPAP compliance exist. Furthermore, it may be a useful adjunct to other surgical procedures involving the pharynx.

Pharyngeal Surgery

Isolated uvulectomy was discredited as a treatment of snoring in the 1940s. Ikematsu[54] was probably the first to combine uvulectomy with surgery of the palate and pharynx, and report high success rates. His pioneering clinical studies, which were carried out in Japan well before sleep apnea syndrome was described, are of great historical importance, but would not meet the rigorous scientific criteria employed today. Fujita and colleagues[55] modified this procedure and coined the term *uvulopalatopharyngoplasty* (UPPP).

The results of UPPP for treatment of snoring generally indicate a success rate upward of 75%, although the variability among individual studies is high, from less than 50% to 100%.

Friberg and colleagues[56] followed a group of 56 nonapneic, nonobese habitual snorers for 5 years post UPPP. All patients had pre- and postoperative polysomnograms and answered questionnaires regarding their snoring. At the end of 5 years, 49 (87%) patients reported either significant improvement in snoring or complete cure. Other studies[57] reported a similar improvement in snoring, but the dropout rate at the end of 5 years was over 90%. Long-term follow-up is of utmost importance because a seemingly high immediate success rate can drop by 50% within 1 year postoperatively.[58]

Can one predict whether UPPP will be successful in reducing or curing snoring? In patients with sleep apnea a battery of tests during wakefulness and sleep have been done. The former included various imaging techniques of the upper airway (radiography, computed tomography, magnetic resonance imaging), simulated snoring, and Müller's maneuver. The last included pressure measurement along the airway, direct observations using fiberoptic endoscopy, and imaging techniques. None proved to be of good predictive value.

Based on the accumulated experience, the best candidates for pharyngeal surgery are nonapneic snorers who are not obese (BMI less than 27 kg/m²) or who have an obvious anatomical abnormality such as large tonsils. Many snorers have a bulky and inflamed uvula, but this should not be considered as abnormal and serve as an indication for surgery. A bulky uvula is probably a consequence rather than the cause of snoring. Unlike the situation with sleep apnea, there is no meta-analysis of the literature regarding the efficacy of upper airway surgery in the treatment of snoring.

Although many complications of UPPP have been described, such as postoperative bleeding, alterations in speech, regurgitation of food through the nose, even death, these complications are infrequent and overall the procedure is safe. The reason it is not recommended as a first line of treatment is not fear of complications but the availability of noninvasive measures and uncertainty of success.

Laser Surgery

Laser surgery, launched by Kamami[59] in 1990, has been used widely for the treatment of snoring, without a body of rigorous studies demonstrating its efficacy. This undoubtedly accounts for the rather negative recommendation of the American Sleep Disorders Association (ASDA) Standards of Practice Committee issued in 1994, which concluded that LAUP [laser-assisted uvulopalatoplasty] is not recommended for the treatment of sleep-related breathing disorders, including OSA.[60(p747)] This recommendation may be interpreted in its strictest sense as pertaining to snoring when it represents a disorder, as when it is a symptom of sleep apnea or UARS; it may not apply to the asymptomatic nonapneic snorer seeking treatment for social reasons.

LAUP, although similar to conventional UPPP, differs from it in several important respects. First, it is an outpatient, office procedure done under local anesthesia. Second, only partial uvulectomy with resection of adjacent palatal tissue is performed, which is less than the conventional UPPP. Third, it is a sequential procedure performed on average during three office visits.

Although the procedure was originally described as being virtually pain-free, subsequent experience proved that this is not the case; accumulated experience indicates that it is associated with significant postoperative pain, lasting up to several weeks. Very few objective studies documenting the efficacy of this procedure are available, and even fewer studies have attempted any objective assessment of snoring sounds.[61, 62] None of the studies have consistent long-term follow-up data. Based on the limited, short-term (less than 3 years) subjective information, the success rate in improving snoring is 70 to 100%. Measurement of snoring sounds before and after surgery shows that LAUP alters the physical properties of sound (spectral composition and intensity) but not the frequency of snoring (i.e., number of snores per hour of sleep). Similar to the UPPP results, there is a discrepancy between the subjective perception of benefit (which is favorable) and the objective results (much less favorable). For example, a recent retrospective analysis of LAUP carried out by Utley et al.[63] shows 42% success in reducing the respiratory disturbance index to less that 20, but 73% success in reducing snoring. Many of the limitations common to the conventional UPPP literature mentioned above apply here as well (short follow-up time of 4 weeks; few of the original patients available for follow-up, etc.). It appears that even the subjective success rate of surgery falls as the follow-up time increases.

Several studies comparing LAUP with conventional UPPP for snoring failed to find any consistent significant difference between the two procedures.[64, 65] The rate of complications for LAUP is low, similar to UPPP. The main reason for selecting LAUP as opposed to conventional UPPP is avoidance of general anesthesia, rather than a higher success rate or fewer side effects. Although several years have passed since the report of the Standards of Practice Committee of the ASDA,[60] no new data have emerged to justify a less cautious approach than that recommended in 1994.

Other Surgical Procedures

Genioglossal advancement with hyoid myotomy and maxillomandibular osteotomy are procedures used for treatment of OSA. They have not been applied specifically to treat nonapneic snoring.

Diathermy palatoplasty[66] is similar to LAUP as far as tissue removal is concerned, the difference being in the type of cutting tool (diathermy needle rather than laser). The success rate and morbidity in nonapneic snorers are similar to those with LAUP and UPPP.[64]

Radiofrequency tissue volume reduction (somnoplasty) is a new procedure is performed with a local anesthetic in an outpatient setting.[67] It employs radiofrequency energy delivered to the tissues via a long and narrow needle. The tissues are heated and ablated in a relatively localized manner, without damage to adjacent structures. The probe, which delivers energy to the tissues, may be bent and therefore it is theoretically possible to modify the retrolingual area.

The procedure has been described in an experimental laboratory setting[67] and in a group of 22 nonapneic or minimally apneic snorers[68] with an AHI of less than 15. It appears to be a safe procedure, not associated with significant side effects or complications. Follow up at 2 to 3 months revealed a significant reduction in snoring as perceived by the bed partner, and reduction in daytime sleepiness as perceived by the patient. It is too early to properly assess the efficacy of this procedure. Given the paucity of available data, it is in the interest of patients to ensure that the procedure is performed only as part of a clinical study and only by surgeons with the proper technical training.

Nonsurgical Treatment

Weight Loss

Obesity is the most commonly studied risk factor, and the one that has been most consistently shown to be related to snoring and apnea. The relationship is not simply an association, but a causal one. Although not frequently studied specifically for snoring, but usually in the context of sleep apnea, weight loss is definitely beneficial in improving sleep apnea and its most common symptom—snoring. It is not possible to predict the amount of weight loss required to abolish snoring in each individual case, but sometimes even as little as 3 kg is sufficient. The suggested mechanisms include (1) reduction in airway compliance, which may occur with the loss of fatty infiltrates within pharyngeal walls; (2) increase in pharyngeal cross-sectional area; and (3) change in the geometry of the pharynx resulting from the loss of fat from the lateral pharyngeal pads. A review dealing with sleep apnea summarizes the mechanisms, results, and methods (medical and surgical) employed to achieve weight loss.[69]

Avoidance of Alcohol

A common observation, confirmed by several studies, is that alcohol ingestion worsens snoring and apnea. Drinking alcohol before bedtime may convert a nonsnorer into a snorer, a nonapneic snorer into an apneic snorer, and worsen apneas and oxygen desaturation in an apneic snorer.[70] Several mechanisms to explain worsening of snoring, apnea, and oxygen desaturation have been postulated, including increased airway resistance, reduced tone of the upper airway muscles, blunting of the arousal response to resistive load, and reduced functional residual capacity.[71]

The deleterious effect of alcohol on breathing during sleep is directly related to the timing of ingestion before sleep, the amount ingested, and individual's metabolism. The adverse effect is evident for at least 3 h and up to 5 h post ingestion. Snorers who drink alcoholic beverages should be cautioned not to ingest alcohol within 3 to 5 h of going to bed.

Medications

There are no medications that consistently cure or improve snoring in all snorers. There are some medications whose avoidance may improve snoring in some patients. This category usually includes sedatives and muscle relaxants. They can aggravate snoring, frequently without any other significant effects on apneas, hypopneas, or nocturnal oxygen saturation.[72] It is a good general measure, which promotes a healthy lifestyle, to advise snorers to abstain from taking these drugs. However, when they are indicated for treatment of another, coexisting condition (e.g., periodic leg movements) there is no need to avoid prescription of necessary drugs, provided the patient (and physician) is aware of the potential worsening of snoring or the apnea, and adequate follow-up is arranged.

Various medications, most notably protriptyline,[73] nasal lubricants,[74, 75] and nasal decongestants, have been tried to determine if they reduce snoring. The results are inconsistent, studies are few and small, and the side effects of some drugs (e.g., protriptyline, nicotine) are significant enough to prohibit their use for the treatment of snoring.

Nasal decongestants are probably the most common drugs used to reduce snoring in patients with chronic nasal problems. Although most, if not all, studies demonstrate significant reduction in nasal resistance measured during wakefulness, objective evidence of this treatment on reduction in snoring is lacking.[76, 77, 77a] Nocturnal nasal congestion is a common symptom, which occurs regularly or seasonally in up 30% of adults. Patients with rhinitis are twice as likely to be habitual snorers than those without it.[77] It is reasonable to give a trial of nasal decongestants or anti-inflammatory preparations to snorers with rhinitis.

Nasal lubricants, such as phosphocholinamin, may reduce airflow turbulence in the upper airway, alter the pressure-flow relationship, and thus eliminate snoring. However, little data are available[74, 75] to recommend their use for treatment of snoring.

Smoking Cessation

Cigarette smoking has been shown by several investigators to be a risk factor for sleep-disordered breathing, and in particular for snoring. Smoking may lead to inflammation of the pharyngeal airway, causing excessive narrowing and collapsibility of the airway, thus promoting snoring. The link between snoring and smoking has been established on the basis of multivariate regression analysis showing a statistically significant association between smoking and self-confessed snoring. This analysis does not imply a causal relationship but simply an association. There are no studies showing reduction in snoring in patients who quit smoking.

Positional Training

It is a common observation of the bed partners of snorers that snoring is reduced when the snorer lies on his or her side or is semiupright, compared with lying on the back. Investigations in sleep laboratories have confirmed this observation, and indicate that in up to 50% of patients, snoring and apneas are dependent on sleeping position. There are good theoretical arguments to expect that body position might affect snoring. Studies in which the pharyngeal area and stability were measured in normals, nonapneic snorers, and patients with sleep apnea demonstrated reduction in pharyngeal area and stability between the seated and supine position, although no consistent differences between the supine and lateral decubitus position have been demonstrated. The main limitation of these studies is that they were done during wakefulness.

Most investigators agree that there is improvement in OSA in some patients upon assuming the lateral decubitus position, but the effect on snoring is variable; in fact, Braver and Block[76] failed to find any difference in objective measurements of snoring between the supine and lateral positions. Given the benign nature of this treatment, it certainly is worth advising the snorer to avoid sleeping in the supine position. This can be accomplished in several ways: the old-fashioned way involves sewing tennis (or golf) balls along the back of the pajamas, using a special pillow that helps keep the head turned to the side, using a wedge to sleep semiupright, or undergoing behavioral conditioning using various alarms.

Nasal Dilators

A common clinical observation, confirmed by epidemiological studies,[78] is that snoring becomes worse when the nose is obstructed. It is possible to relieve nasal obstruction by mechanical means. The two most popular devices to accomplish this are external and internal nasal dilators. The external dilator is essentially a strip consisting of one or two polyester flat springs with adhesive backing. It is applied to the ridge of the nose and dilates the nares by the recoil forces generated by the springs. The internal dilator is a plastic bar with two end tabs that is inserted into the nares in the region of the nasal valve; it splints the nares by its elastic action.

Both devices produce a significant reduction in nasal resistance. There is much subjective data, based on interviews with snorers, suggesting that these mechanical nasal dilators reduce snoring.[79] However, whenever objective measurements of nocturnal respiration are performed and the results obtained with and without a nasal dilator are compared, either only a trivial reduction in snoring in some patients is found, or no change at all.[80] Given the rather low cost and benign nature of this treatment, there is no harm in recommending it as a therapeutic trial for nonapneic snorers. They will quickly determine for themselves whether it is beneficial.

Oral Appliances

Oral appliances designed to keep the mouth partially closed and the mandible or tongue pushed forward have been available in one form or another since the late 19th century. There are many patents on file, showing sometimes very ingenious designs to accomplish this goal.

At present, all oral appliances may be broadly divided into two categories: tongue-retaining devices[81] and mandibular advancement appliances. There are a few other appliances, such as soft palate lifters and tongue position trainers, but they are almost never used today. Mandibular advancement appliances are either fixed or adjustable. With the fixed type the position of the mandible is locked, whereas with the adjustable appliance the mandible can be moved anteriorly by several millimeters. By far the largest proportion of dental appliances used and manufactured today are the adjustable anterior positioners.

Oral appliances enlarge the pharyngeal area by partially preventing the tongue and perhaps the soft palate from posterior collapse during sleep. They may increase the tone of the genioglossus muscle.

It is difficult to assess the therapeutic effect of oral appliances on snoring from the published data. Most of the studies, in which polysomnography was performed, with and without the appliance, concentrated on sleep apnea. Although patients were asked about their snoring, this was not done consistently in a systematic way; no validated questionnaires were used; follow-up time was either short, not specified, or varied widely among patients within the same study; many different appliances were used; and bed partners were almost never interviewed. Thus the results are highly variable. The reports claim that snoring improves or resolves in 40 to 100% of patients. When polysomnography was employed, it was found that tongue-retaining devices reduced the AHI by approximately 50%. The response rate, defined as the percentage of patients in whom the AHI with the appliance is less than 10, was only 44%; the compliance rate was 38%, with follow-up times varying from a few weeks to several years. The results were better with mandibular advancement appliances; they reduced the AHI by about 60%, the response rate was almost 60%, and the compliance rate was close to 80%. Several recent studies indicate that oral appliances compare favorably with CPAP in terms of reduction in the amount of sleep-disordered breathing, and superior to CPAP in terms of compliance and side effects.[82-84]

The most common complaints voiced by patients who use oral appliances are hypersalivation, sore teeth, sore jaw muscles, and pain in the temporomandibular joints. The last is rare with adjustable appliances. Despite these complaints, patient satisfaction is relatively high, about 80%. The long-term effects of these appliances on teeth alignment, mandibular position, and temporomandibular joints are not known.

In 1995 the task force for the Standards of Practice Committee of the ASDA recommended offering oral appliances to all nonapneic snorers.[85, 86]

Nasal CPAP

This method of treatment is discussed extensively elsewhere. It invariably abolishes snoring, but compliance with CPAP among nonapneic snorers is poor.

SUMMARY

Given the wide choice of different modalities for treatment of snoring discussed above, it is necessary to adopt a systematic approach based on risk factors when recommending treatment for the nonapneic snorer (Fig. 70–1). Frequently, more than one risk factor is present, and that is why the identification of risk factors must be carried out in parallel. Each risk factor can be dealt with as outlined in the algorithm. If the risk factor cannot be modified, or the patient still snores despite appropriate therapy, the pathways converge, and a common approach is followed. There are several common principles, applicable to all patients.

First, lifestyle modification measures should be discussed with particular attention toward removal of the known risk factors (overweight, alcohol, muscle relaxants, smoking). Medical treatment of nasal obstruction, a trial of nasal dilators, and sleep position training should be instituted as appropriate.

Second, patients should be informed about oral appliances. They should be told that the success rate of these appliances is lower than that of CPAP, but the obvious advantage is compactness of the equipment. They should be encouraged to discuss the problem with the dentist who has expertise with oral appliances.

Third, patients should be told about CPAP, that it carries the greatest "guarantee" that snoring will be abolished. Whenever possible, they should be shown the actual equipment, including mask, head straps, and blower. Most sleep disorder centers now have special CPAP clinics where patients can be educated about the equipment, try it on, and select the best-fitting mask. This is of particular importance for nonapneic snorers or those with mild sleep apnea, whose motivation and compliance with CPAP are generally poor.

Last, patients should be informed about surgical approaches. Those with obvious anatomical abnormalities, which are generally a minority of patients, should be offered surgery. Patients should be advised not to expect complete elimination of snoring, informed about comparative success rates with CPAP and oral appliances, and encouraged to consult with the surgeon for discussion of surgical techniques, side effects, recovery time, pain control, and so forth.

After the patient has been informed about the above approaches, he or she will invariably ask for a specific recommendation. The obvious *primum non nocere* approach must prevail—noninvasive treatments must be recommended first, and thus it is the lifestyle modification and oral appliances which should be recommended. Clearly, financial and health insurance considerations may very well influence the course of treatment an individual patient will follow, but these

Risk Factors

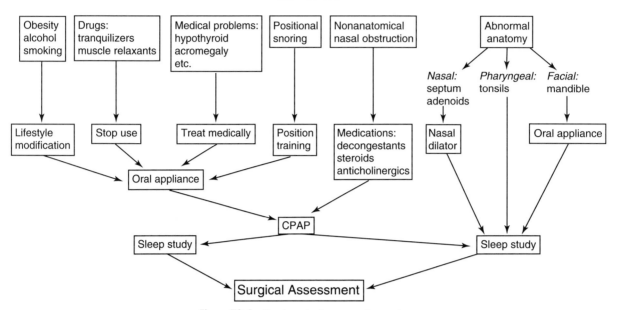

Figure 70–1. Treatment of nonapneic snoring.

considerations should not cloud proper medical advice, which must be based on the available scientific data.

References

1. The Random House Dictionary of the English Language. New York, NY: Random House; 1966.
2. The New Webster's Dictionary and Thesaurus of the English Language. New York, NY: Lexicon Publications; 1991.
3. Diagnostic Classification Steering Committee. International Classification of Sleep Disorders: Diagnostic and Coding Manual. Rochester, Minn: American Sleep Disorders Association; 1990:195.
4. Trachtman P. The Gunfighters. Constable G, ed. New York, NY: Time-Life Books; 1974:176.
5. Catlin G. Breath of Life or Mal-Respiration and Its Effects Upon the Enjoyments and Life of Man. New York, NY: John Wiley & Son; 1872.
6. Kleitman N. Sleep and Wakefulness. Chicago, Ill: University of Chicago Press; 1963:48–52.
7. Robin IG. Snoring. Proc R Soc Med. 1948;41:151–153.
8. Robin IG. Snoring. Proc R Soc Med. 1968;61:575–582.
9. Lugaresi E, Cirignotta F, Piana G. Some epidemiological data on snoring and cardiocirculatory disturbances. Sleep. 1980;3:221–224.
10. Lugaresi E, Mondini S, Zucconi M, et al. Staging of heavy snorers' disease: a proposal. Bull Eur Physiopathol Respir. 1983;19:590–594.
11. Lindberg E, Taube A, Janson C, et al. A 10-year follow up of snoring in men. Chest. 1998;114:1048–1055.
12. Guilleminault C, Stoohs R, Clerk A, et al. A cause of excessive daytime sleepiness: the upper airway resistance syndrome. Chest. 1993;104:781–787.
13. Gavriely N, Jensen O. Theory and measurement of snores. J Appl Physiol. 1993;74:2828–2837.
14. Huang L. Mechanical modeling of palatal snoring. J Acoust Soc Am. 1995;97:3642–3648.
15. Isono S, Feroah TR, Hajduk EA, et al. Interaction of cross-sectional area, driving pressure, and airflow of passive velopharynx. J Appl Physiol. 1997;83:851–859.
15a. Huang L, Williams JE. Neuromechanical interaction in human snoring and upper airway obstruction. J Appl Physiol. 1999;86:1759–1763.
16. Dalmasso F, Prota R. Snoring: analysis, measurement, clinical implications, and applications. Eur Respir J. 1996;9:146–159.
17. Young TB. Some methodological and practical issues of reported snoring validity. Chest. 1991;99:531–532.
18. Stradling JR, Crosby JH. Relation between systemic hypertension and sleep hypoxemia and snoring: analysis in 748 men drawn from general practice. Br Med J. 1990;300:75–78.
19. Bearpark H, Elliott L, Grunstein R, et al. Snoring and sleep apnea: a population study in Australian men. Am J Respir Crit Care Med. 1995;151:1459–1465.
20. Young T, Palta M, Dempsey J, et al. The occurrence of sleep-disordered breathing among middle-aged adults. N Engl J Med. 1993;328:1230–1235.
21. Ohayon MM, Guilleminault C, Priest RG, et al. Snoring and breathing pauses during sleep: telephone interview survey of a United Kingdom population sample. Br Med J. 1997;314:860–863.
22. Janson C, Gislason T, De Backer W, et al. Daytime sleepiness, snoring, and gastro-oesophageal reflux amongst adults in three European countries. J Intern Med. 1995;237:277–285.
23. Gislason T, Janson C, Tomasson K. Epidemiological aspects of snoring and hypertension. J Sleep Res. 1995;4(suppl 1):145–149.
24. Martikainen K, Partinen M, Urponen H, et al. Natural evolution of snoring: a 5-year follow-up study. Acta Neurol Scand. 1994;90:437–442.
25. Honsberg AE, Dodge RR, Cline MG, et al. Incidence and remission of habitual snoring over a 5- to 6-year period. Chest. 1995;108:604–609.
25a. Lindberg E, Elmasry A, Gislason T, et al. Evolution of sleep apnea syndrome in sleepy snorers: a population-based prospective study. Am J Respir Crit Care Med. 1999;159:2024–2027.
26. Crocker BD, Olson LG, Saunders NA, et al. Estimation of the probability of disturbed breathing during sleep before a sleep study. Am Rev Respir Dis. 1990;142:14–18.
27. Flemons WW, Whitelaw WW, Brant R, et al. Likelihood ratios for a sleep apnea clinical prediction rule. Am J Respir Crit Care Med. 1994;150:1279–1285.
28. Kump K, Whalen C, Tishler PV, et al. Assessment of the validity and utility of a sleep-symptom questionnaire. Am J Respir Crit Care Med. 1994;150:735–741.
29. Deegan PC, McNicholas WT. Predictive value of clinical features for the obstructive sleep apnoea syndrome. Eur Respir J. 1996;9:117–124.
30. Pouliot Z, Peters M, Neufield H, et al. Using self-reported questionnaire to prioritize OSA patients for polysomnography. Sleep. 1997;20:232–236.

30a. Wilson K, Stoohs RA, Mulrooney TF, et al. The snoring spectrum: acoustic assessment of snoring sound intensity in 1,139 individuals undergoing polysomnography. Chest. 1999;115:762–770.

31. Lugaresi E, Coccagna G, Farnetti P, et al. Snoring. Electroencephalogr Clin Neurol. 1975;39:59–64.

32. Hoffstein V. Is snoring dangerous to your health? Sleep. 1996;19:506–516.

33. Young T, Finn L, Hla KM, et al. Snoring as a part of dose-response relationship between sleep-disordered breathing and blood pressure. Sleep. 1996;19:S202–S205.

34. Lofaso F, Coste A, Gilain L, et al. Sleep fragmentation as a risk factor for hypertension in middle-aged non-apneic snorers. Chest. 1996;109:896–900.

35. Guilleminault C, Stoohs R, Shiomi T, et al. Upper airway resistance syndrome, nocturnal blood pressure monitoring, and borderline hypertension. Chest. 1996;109:901–908.

36. Bonnet MH. Infrequent periodic sleep disruption: effects on sleep, performance, and mood. Physiol Behav. 1989;45:1049–1055.

37. Martin SE, Engleman HM, Deary IJ, et al. The effect of sleep fragmentation on daytime function. Am J Respir Crit Care Med. 1996;153:1328–1332.

38. Redline S, Strauss ME, Adams N, et al. Neuropsychological function in mild sleep-disordered breathing. Sleep. 1997;20:160–167.

39. Guilleminault C, Partinen M, Quera-Salva MA, et al. Determinants of daytime sleepiness in obstructive sleep apnea. Chest. 1988;94:32–37.

39a. Sleep-related breathing disorders in adults: recommendations for syndrome definition and measurement techniques in clinical research. The Report of an American Academy of Sleep Medicine Task Force. Sleep. 1999;22:667–689.

39b. Loube DI, Andrada T, Howard RS. Accuracy of respiratory inductive plethysmography for the diagnosis of upper airway resistance syndrome. Chest. 1999;115:1333–1337.

40. Kim HC, Young T, Matthews CG, et al. Sleep-disordered breathing and neuropsychological deficits: a population-based study. Am J Respir Crit Care Med. 1997;156:1813–1819.

41. Whitney CW, Enright PL, Newman AB, et al. Correlates of daytime sleepiness in 4578 elderly persons: the cardiovascular health study. Sleep. 1998;21:27–36.

42. Ulfberg J, Carter N, Talbaäck M, et al. Excessive daytime sleepiness at work and subjective work performance in the general population and among heavy snorers and patients with obstructive sleep apnea. Chest. 1996;110:659–663.

43. Collard P, Dury M, Delguste P, et al. Movement arousals and sleep-related disordered breathing in adults. Am J Respir Crit Care Med. 1996;154:454–459.

44. Martin SE, Wraith PK, Deary IJ, et al. The effect of non-visible sleep fragmentation on daytime function. Am J Respir Crit Care Med. 1997;155:1596–1601.

45. Mendelsohn WB. Sleep fragmentation and daytime wakefulness. Am J Respir Crit Care Med. 1997;155:1499–1500.

46. Hoffstein V, Mateika S, Hanly P. Snoring and arousals: a retrospective analysis. Sleep. 1995;10:866–872.

47. Berg S, Nash S, Cole P, et al. Arousals and nocturnal respiration in symptomatic snorers and non-snorers. Sleep. 1997;20:1157–1161.

47a. Exar EN, Collop NA. The upper airway resistance syndrome. Chest. 1999;115:1127–1139.

48. Johns MW. A new method for measuring daytime sleepiness: the Epworth Sleepiness Scale. Sleep. 1991;14:540–545.

49. Kump K, Whalen C, Tishler PV, et al. Assessment of the validity and utility of a sleep-symptom questionnaire. Am J Respir Crit Care Med. 1994;150:735–741.

50. Flemons WW, Reimer MA. Development of a disease-specific health-related quality of life questionnaire for sleep apnea. Am J Respir Crit Care Med. 1998;158:494–503.

51. Strollo PJ, Sanders MH. Significance and treatment of non-apneic snoring. Sleep. 1993;16:403–408.

52. Schechtman KB, Sher A, Piccirillo JF. Methodological and statistical problems in sleep apnea research: the literature on uvulopalatopharyngoplasty. Sleep. 1995;18:659–666.

53. Woodhead CJ, Allen MB. Nasal surgery for snoring. Clin Otolaryngol. 1994;19:41–44.

54. Ikematsu T. Study of snoring, fourth report: therapy. J Jpn Otorhinolaryngol. 1964;64:434–435.

55. Fujita S, Conway W, Zorick F, et al. Surgical correction of anatomic abnormalities in obstructive sleep apnea syndrome: uvulopalatopharyngoplasty. Otolaryngol Head Neck Surg. 1981;89:923–934.

56. Friberg D, Carlsson-Nordlander B, Larsson H, et al. UPPP for habitual snoring: a 5-year follow up with respiratory sleep recordings. Laryngoscope. 1995;105:519–522.

57. Janson C, Hillerdal G, Larsson L, et al. Excessive daytime sleepiness and fatigue in non-apneic snorers: improvement after UPPP. Eur Respir J. 1994;7:845–849.

58. Levin BC, Becker GD. Uvulopalatopharyngoplasty for snoring: long-term results. Laryngoscope. 1994;104:1150–1152.

59. Kamami YV. Laser CO₂ for snoring—preliminary results. Acta Otorhinolaryngol Belg. 1990;44:451–456.

60. Standards of Practice Committee of the ASDA. Practice parameters for the use of laser-assisted uvulopalatoplasty. Sleep. 1994;17:744–748.

61. Walker RP, Gatti WM, Poirier N, et al. Objective assessment of snoring before and after laser-assisted uvulopalatoplasty. Laryngoscope. 1996;106:1372–1377.

62. Ryan CF. Laser assisted uvulopalatoplasty in sleep disordered breathing. Thorax. 1997;52:5–8.

63. Utley DS, Shin EJ, Clerk AA, et al. A cost-effective and rational surgical approach to patients with snoring, upper airway resistance syndrome, or obstructive sleep apnea syndrome. Laryngoscope. 1997;107:726–734.

64. Clarke RW, Yardley MPJ, Davies CM, et al. Palatoplasty for snoring: a randomized controlled trial of three surgical methods. Otolaryngol Head Neck Surg. 1998;119:288–292.

65. Maw J, Marsan J. Uvulopalatopharyngoplasty versus laser-assisted uvulopalatopharyngoplasty in the treatment of snoring. J Otolaryngol. 1997;26:232–235.

66. Yardley MPJ, Clarke RW, Clegg RT. How do we do it: diathermy palatoplasty. J Otolaryngol. 1997;26:284–285.

67. Powell NB, Riley RW, Troell RJ, et al. Radiofrequency volumetric reduction of the tongue: a porcine pilot study for the treatment of obstructive sleep apnea syndrome. Chest. 1997;111:1348–1355.

68. Powell NB, Riley RW, Troell RJ, et al. Radiofrequency volumetric tissue reduction of the palate in subjects with sleep-disordered breathing. Chest. 1998;113:163–174.

69. Strobel RJ, Rosen RC. Obesity and weight loss in obstructive sleep apnea: a critical review. Sleep. 1996;19:104–115.

70. Issa F, Sullivan C. Alcohol, snoring, and sleep apnea. J Neurol Neurosurg Psychiatry. 1982;45:353–359.

71. Dawson A, Bigby BG, Poceta JS, et al. Effect of bedtime alcohol on inspiratory resistance and respiratory drive in snoring and non-snoring men. Alcohol Clin Exp Res. 1997;21:183–190.

72. Schneider H, Grote L, Peter H, et al. The effect of triazolam and flunitrazepam—two benzodiazepines with different half-lives—on breathing during sleep. Chest. 1996;109:909–915.

73. Sériès F, Marc I. Effects of protriptyline on snoring characteristics. Chest. 1993;104:14–18.

74. Hoffstein V, Mateika S, Halko S, et al. Reduction in snoring with phosphocholinamin—a long-acting tissue lubricating agent. Am J Otolaryngol. 1987;8:236–240.

75. Jokic R, Klimaszewski A, Mink J, et al. Surface tension forces in sleep apnea. A randomized double-blind placebo-controlled trial. Am J Respir Crit Care Med. 1998;157:1522–1525.

76. Braver HM, Block AJ. Effect of nasal spray, positional therapy, and combination thereof in the asymptomatic snorer. Sleep. 1994;17:516–521.

77. Braver HM, Block AJ, Perri MG. Treatment for snoring: combined weight loss, sleeping on the side, and nasal spray. Chest. 1995;107:1283–1288.

77a. Lorino AM, Lofaso F, Dahan E, et al: Combined effects of a mechanical nasal dilator and a topical decongestant on nasal airflow resistance. Chest. 1999;115:1514–1518.

78. Young T, Finn L, Kim H, and the University of Wisconsin Sleep and Respiratory Research Group. Nasal obstruction as a risk factor for sleep-disordered breathing. J Allergy Clin Immunol. 1997;99:s757–s762.

79. Löth S, Petruson B. Improved nasal breathing reduces snoring and morning tiredness. Acta Otolaryngol Head Neck Surg. 1996;122:1337–1340.

80. Hoffstein V, Mateika S, Metes A. Effect of nasal dilation on snoring and apneas during different stages of sleep. Sleep. 1993;16:360–365.
81. Cartwright RD, Samelsen CF. The effect of non-surgical treatment for obstructive sleep apnea: the tongue-retaining device. JAMA. 1982;248:705–709.
82. Ferguson KA, Ono T, Lowe A, et al. A randomized crossover study of an oral appliance vs. nasal-continuous positive airway pressure in the treatment of mild-moderate obstructive sleep apnea. Chest. 1996;109:1269–1275.
83. Clark GT, Blumenfeld I, Yaffe N, et al. A crossover study comparing the efficacy of continuous positive airway pressure with anterior mandibular positioning devices on patients with obstructive sleep apnea. Chest. 1996;109:1477–1483.
84. Ferguson KA, Ono T, Lowe AA, et al. A short term controlled trial of an adjustable oral appliance for the treatment of mild to moderate obstructive sleep apnea. Thorax. 1997;52:362–368.
85. Schmidt-Nowara W, Lowe A, Wiegand L, et al. Oral appliances for the treatment of snoring and obstructive sleep apnea: a review. Sleep. 1995;18:501–510.
86. An American Sleep Disorders Association Report. Practice parameters for the treatment of snoring and obstructive sleep apnea with oral appliances. Sleep. 1995;18:511–513.
87. Norton PG, Dunn EV, Haight JSJ. Snoring in adults: some epidemiological aspects. Can Med Assoc J. 1983;128:674–675.
88. Mondini S, Zucconi M, Cirignotta F, et al. Snoring as a risk factor for cardiac and circulatory problems: an epidemiological study. In: Guilleminault C, Lugaresi E, eds. Sleep/Wake Disorders: Natural History, Epidemiology and Long-term Evolution. New York, NY: Raven Press; 1983:99–105.
89. Koskenvuo M, Kaprio J, Partinen M, et al. Snoring as a risk factor for hypertension and angina pectoris. Lancet. 1985;1:893–895.
90. Norton PG, Dunn EV. Snoring as a risk factor for disease: an epidemiological survey. Br Med J. 1985;231:630–632.
91. Wiggins CL, Schmidt-Nowara WW, Coultas DB, et al. Comparison of self- and spouse reports of snoring and other symptoms associated with sleep apnea syndrome. Sleep. 1990;13:245–252.
92. Bliwise DL, Nekich JC, Dement WC. Relative validity of self-reported snoring as a symptom of sleep apnea in a sleep clinic population. Chest. 1991;99:600–608.
93. Olson LG, King MT, Hensley MJ, et al. A community study of snoring and sleep-disordered breathing: prevalence. Am J Respir Crit Care Med. 1995;152:711–714.
94. Stoohs RA, Blum HC, Haselhorst M, et al. Normative data on snoring: a comparison between younger and older adults. Eur Respir J. 1998;11:451–457.
95. Keenan SP, Ferguson KA, Chen-Yeung M, et al. Prevalence of sleep disordered breathing in a population of Canadian grainworkers. Can Respir J. 1998;5:184–190.

71

Central Sleep Apnea

David P. White

Cessation of breathing during sleep can result from obstruction of the upper airway (obstructive apnea), loss of ventilatory effort (central apnea), or a combination of the two. The term *central sleep apnea* is used to describe both the events and the clinical disorder characterized by repeated episodes of apnea during sleep resulting from the temporary loss of ventilatory effort.[1] A central apnea is conventionally defined as a period of at least 10 sec without airflow, during which no ventilatory effort is evident. This condition differs from the obstructive or mixed apnea by the absence of upper airway obstruction and subsequent ventilatory attempts against an occluded airway (Fig. 71–1). Although this chapter is concerned with central sleep apnea, it must be understood that central and obstructive events are rarely seen in isolation. The vast majority of patients with central apneas will also have some obstructive events. This observation suggests that the mechanisms responsible for the different types of apnea must overlap, and research indicates this is likely to be the case.

The muscles of the upper airway (genioglossus and others) behave as respiratory muscles,[2, 3] acting to dilate or stiffen the pharynx on inspiration. If a decrease in or loss of activity occurs in both upper airway muscles and the diaphragm,[4] one of several consequences seems likely. First, the decrement in motor tone of the pharyngeal dilator muscles could produce upper airway occlusion and lead to obstructed ventilatory efforts when diaphragmatic activity resumes (a mixed apnea). On the other hand, if loss of upper airway muscle activity does not lead to obstruction of the pharynx, a pure central apnea will likely be seen. The propensity of the upper airway to collapse may be important in determining whether central or obstructive apneas result when cycling output to respiratory muscles occurs during sleep.

After tracheostomy for obstructive sleep apnea, many patients will develop central apnea, which generally resolves over a period of months.[5, 6] This may also occur when continuous positive airway pressure (CPAP) is initiated to alleviate upper airway obstruction. In addition, it has been observed that the treatment of central apneas with either a respiratory stimulant such as acetazolamide[7] or diaphragmatic pacing[8] can result in obstructive events. Finally, studies report clear narrowing of the pharyngeal airway during purely central apnea. These observations again imply some commonality in the pathophysiology of the various types of apnea, so it is not surprising that central and obstructive apneas are frequently seen in the same individual.

Patients with predominantly central sleep apnea constitute fewer than 10% of apneic individuals in most sleep laboratory populations,[1, 9] with studies suggesting only about 4%.[10, 11] As a result, only a small number of studies with more than a few such patients have been reported, which makes knowledge of this disorder scant. Most of this chapter is dedicated to a discussion of patients with central sleep apnea who breathe normally during the day; however, any patient with hypoventilation during wakefulness will almost certainly have hypoventilation with central apneas at night.

It should be recognized from the beginning that a central pause in respiration can result from a variety of physiological or pathophysiological events. Central apnea does not represent a single entity or result from a single cause; examples include Cheyne-Stokes respi-

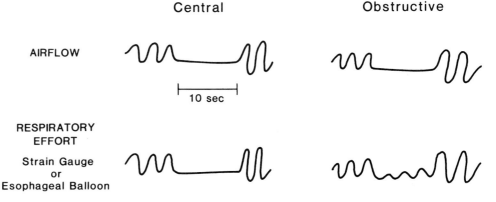

Figure 71–1. The relation between airflow and respiratory effort is demonstrated in both central and obstructive apnea. During a central apnea, there is cessation of airflow for at least 10 sec with no associated ventilatory effort. An obstructive apnea is defined as a similar cessation of airflow but with continued respiratory effort.

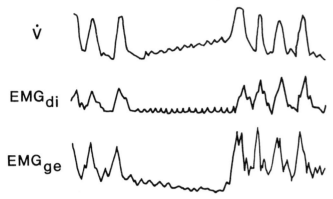

Figure 71-2. During a central apnea, there is complete loss of diaphragmatic (EMG_{di}) and genioglossal (EMG_{ge}) activity, with resumption of activity when breathing begins. $\dot{V}$, flow. (From Onal E, Lopata M, O'Connor T, 1982, Pathogenesis of apnea in hypersomnia–sleep apnea syndrome. American Review of Respiratory Disease, 125:167–174. Official Journal of the American Thoracic Society. © American Lung Association.)

ration, periodic breathing at altitude, and the idiopathic central apnea seen at sea level. Each has a different pathogenesis but is manifested by central apneas during sleep. To understand this disorder, the normal mechanisms controlling ventilation awake and asleep and pathological influences on these mechanisms must be understood. One must also consider all possible causes of central apnea in caring for patients with this disorder.

PATHOPHYSIOLOGY

Because central apneas are defined as pauses in respiration without ventilatory effort, one would expect a complete loss of electromyographic activity of the respiratory muscles during such as apnea, and this has been demonstrated[4] (Fig. 71–2). After the apnea, there is a resumption of normal muscular activity. This finding implies that the neuronal output to the respiratory muscles ceases during central apnea and returns at the end of the ventilatory pause. Central apneas therefore represent a loss of ventilatory drive. Although the cause of central apnea in many cases remains obscure, investigation into the control of breathing during sleep and the association of central apneas with certain disease processes has pointed to a number of possible mechanisms. It should therefore be understood from the beginning that central sleep apnea does not represent a single disease entity but probably is the result of any one of a number of processes that yield instability of respiratory control.

Control of Breathing

Research suggests that ventilation is controlled by a number of processes that have been generally grouped under two headings[12] (see Chapter 16). The first is the automatic or metabolic control system and consists of the chemoreceptors (carotid body for hypoxia and carotid body plus medullary chemoreceptor for hyper-

capnia), vagal intrapulmonary receptors, and numerous brainstem mechanisms that both process the information from these peripheral receptors and control the pattern of breathing. This metabolic system keeps ventilation regular and ensures that the quantity of ventilation occurring at any time is well matched to the metabolic needs of the body. In addition, there is what is called the "behavioral" control system. It seems clear that the activities of normal life, such as talking and eating, as well as excitement, can influence ventilation and are thought of as behavioral or volitional influences. The origin of this neural input to respiration is probably in the forebrain. There also is an apparent ventilatory control process in awake human beings and animals that is referred to as the "wakefulness" stimulus.[12] Although this stimulus is vague, both conceptually and in our understanding of it, it seems that there is increased ventilation associated with the waking state. Although the mechanisms responsible for this effect of wakefulness on ventilation are poorly defined, it has been proposed either to result from the influence of the descending reticular activating system on respiratory pattern generators or to be a product of the tonic input on these ventilatory control areas from nonrespiratory sensory mechanisms such as sight or hearing.[13, 14] The important point, however, is that during wakefulness, ventilation is controlled by both the metabolic and the behavior systems, including possibly this wakefulness stimulus. Ventilation is likely to persist during wakefulness even with the complete absence of metabolic mechanisms.

During sleep, particularly nonrapid eye movement (NREM) sleep, respiration is controlled almost solely by the metabolic control system, with ventilation being tightly linked to afferent input from chemoreceptors and vagal intrapulmonary receptors.[15] This observation was demonstrated in dogs by blocking the input from each of these receptors and monitoring the change in ventilatory pattern (Fig. 71–3). These interventions produced a marked slowing of ventilatory frequency with long apneic periods. Although this has not been carefully demonstrated in human beings, there is evidence suggesting that a similar control system is present in human beings. Oxygen administration, which reduces the hypoxic stimulus to breathing, has been shown to decrease ventilation during sleep and initially prolong apneas in some individuals in whom such events were already present.[16] In addition, hypocapnic alkalosis, which reduces the hypercapnic ventilatory drive, has been shown to produce central apneas in otherwise normal men.[17, 18] This combination of studies indicates the importance of both hypoxic and the hypercapnic influences on breathing during sleep. The implication is that maintenance of neuronal output to the respiratory muscles during sleep may be critically dependent on incoming stimuli, such as those from chemoreceptors.

Considerable investigation has been directed at determining the influence of sleep itself on chemoreceptor activity.[19–22] Although this is still controversial, the majority of the information available suggests the following. First, ventilatory responses to both hypoxia and

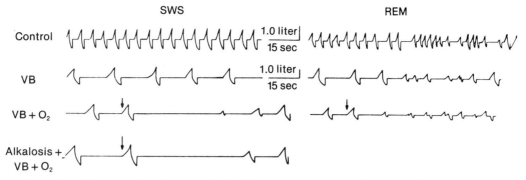

Figure 71–3. Recorder tracing of the same dog showing effects of decreased respiratory afferent stimulation during slow-wave sleep (SWS) and REM sleep. Tracings show inspired and expired volumes. Note change in volume calibration for all records during VB. VB, vagal blockage; Alkalosis + VB + O₂, one breath of 100% oxygen inspired (*at arrow*) during vagal blockage and chronic metabolic alkalosis; VB + O₂, one breath of 100% oxygen inspired (*at arrow*) during vagal blockage. (From Guilleminault C, Dement W, eds. Sleep Apnea Syndromes. New York, NY: Alan R Liss; 1978:58.)

hypercapnia are reduced somewhat during NREM sleep and fall further during rapid eye movement (REM) sleep.[19–22] However, the results of studies indicate that this decrement in ventilatory responses probably is a product of a diminished ability to compensate during sleep for increasing resistive load (rising upper airway resistance) rather than a true loss of chemosensitivity.[23] Therefore, most believe the chemoresponses to be reasonably well maintained during sleep, particularly NREM sleep, and that these chemoreflex mechanisms are probably important in maintaining rhythmic ventilation during sleep.

Pco₂ and Breathing During Sleep

The important role of P_{CO_2} in the maintenance of normal rhythmic ventilation during sleep has been known for years and was outlined by Cherniack.[24, 25] In the normal state, the relationship between increasing P_{CO_2} and ventilation is linear, and it takes only a small rise above the resting P_{CO_2} level to increase ventilation (Fig. 71–4). The hypoxic drive, described by the Pa_{O_2}–ventilation relationship, on the other hand, is a hyperbolic response, with little change in ventilation occurring despite fairly large fluctuations in P_{O_2} around the normal range (see Fig. 71–4). This arrangement yields a stable ventilatory control system for a number of reasons. First, P_{CO_2} probably is the major respiratory

stimulus during sleep, and as stated, the relationship between P_{CO_2} and ventilation is linear. In addition, there are relatively large stores of carbon dioxide in the body such that large increases in ventilation are necessary to produce changes in P_{CO_2}, especially in the central nervous system, where such changes are detected. As a result, a stable, damped feedback system exists. On the other hand, the hypoxic response is neither linear nor damped because oxygen stores in the body (lungs and blood) are small. Changes in P_{O_2} in the normal range, however, have little influence on ventilation, as stated, but any process disturbing this arrangement could make ventilatory control unstable, yielding apnea or cycling breathing. The validity of these observations has been confirmed by a number of investigators.

In his classic studies, Bülow[26] showed that "periodic breathing" during sleep was related to P_{CO_2} in an important way. He observed that apnea or pronounced hypoventilation occurred "only when the preceding P_{CO_2} was relatively low," which suggests that a reduced P_{CO_2} during sleep may decrease the drive to breathe to the point of apnea. Other studies have confirmed the prominent role played by P_{CO_2} in the maintenance of rhythmic breathing during sleep. Skatrud and Dempsey[18, 27] showed that passive, positive-pressure hyperventilation of sleeping subjects yielded apnea by reducing P_{CO_2} only 3 to 6 mmHg below the sleeping value (Fig. 71–5). The actual P_{CO_2} level associ-

Figure 71–4. Schematic representation of normal hypercapnic and hypoxic ventilatory responses. Parentheses enclose normal ranges for P_{CO_2} and P_{O_2}. Little change from the resting P_{CO_2} value is necessary to stimulate ventilation, whereas ventilation is minimally affected by alteration of P_{O_2} in the normal range.

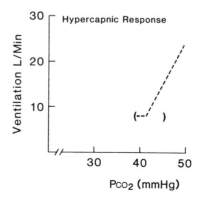

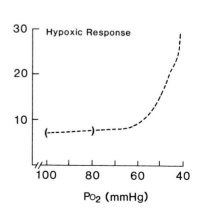

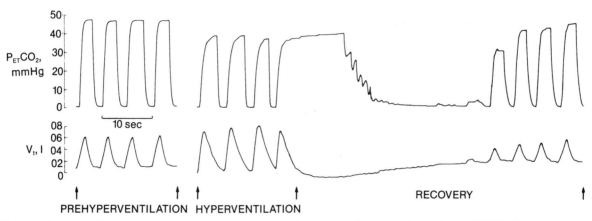

Figure 71–5. Posthyperventilation apnea after 3 min of passive, positive-pressure hyperventilation during NREM sleep. Oxygen saturation was 100% in prehyperventilation, hyperventilation, and recovery periods. Small tidal volume (VT) on first breath after apnea resulted in a poor end-tidal PCO_2 sample that was not representative of the alveolar partial pressure of carbon dioxide during or at the end of the apneic episode. $PETCO_2$, end-tidal PCO_2; VT, tidal volume. (From Skatrud J, Dempsey J. Interaction of sleep state and chemical stimuli in sustaining rhythmic ventilation. J Appl Physiol. 1983;55:813–822.)

ated with apnea often was only 1 to 2 mmHg below the awake value as PCO_2 rose from wakefulness to sleep. Each individual seemed to have an "apnea threshold," a PCO_2 level below which apnea was commonly seen. It seemed, therefore, that the waking PCO_2 level was at or near this apnea threshold, such that waking PCO_2 levels may be inaquate to stimulate ventilation during sleep. It was also demonstrated that the periodic breathing during sleep that is frequently seen with prolonged hypoxia could be abolished by elevating the PCO_2 above the predetermined "apnea threshold." This finding suggests that the hypocapnia induced by hypoxia, not hypoxia itself, is the pivotal element in this periodic breathing. The authors[18] concluded "that effective ventilatory rhythmogenesis in the absence of stimuli associated with wakefulness is critically dependent on chemoreceptor stimulation secondary to PCO_2-[H$^+$]." It should be noted that subsequent studies by this same group now suggest that increased tidal volume (vagal mechanisms) and not low PCO_2 may be the primary mechanism inhibiting respiration after a series of large breaths.[28] However, the concept of hyperventilation ultimately leading to an inhibition of respiration with central apnea (whether secondary to hypocapnia or vagal mechanisms) remains intact and is likely an important one in understanding the pathogenesis of central sleep apnea.

These findings have important implications in the pathogenesis of sleep apnea or periodic breathing seen at altitude, which is discussed in more detail in Chapter 18. It has long been known that human beings acutely exposed to high altitude will have periodic breathing during sleep with central apnea.[29] The previously described studies suggest that this apnea is a product of the hypocapnia induced by hypoxia (hyperventilation) and not of hypoxia itself. Whether hypoxia is a further destabilizing influence on ventilation, as suggested by Cherniack, remains unresolved. It seems that increasing the influence of the hypoxic drive (a hyperbolic, undamped response) might amplify breathing dysrhythmias, but further investigations are necessary to document this.

The previously described series of studies suggest that ventilation is remarkably dependent on the metabolic control system during sleep and that the primary stimulus to respiration during sleep may be arterial PCO_2. Two scenarios are likely to lead to hypoventilation or central apneas during sleep. First, if the PCO_2 drops below a certain level the (*apnea threshold*), breathing is likely to become dysrhythmic. This drop may in part explain the dysrhythmic breathing frequently seen at sleep onset. As an individual changes from wakefulness to stage 1 or 2 sleep, the PCO_2 level that was adequate to stimulate ventilation during wakefulness may be inadequate to do so during sleep, and an apnea occurs. This apnea may arouse the individual, and the process may repeat itself. Once a stable sleep stage is reached, ventilation should become regular under metabolic control. Therefore, any process that leads to frequent sleep-wake transitions over the course of the night (like insomnia) may increase the number of central apneas. In addition, it should be clear that nonrepetitive central apneas in the sleep-wake transition probably are normal events.

Second, with loss of wakefulness, as stated, ventilation becomes completely dependent on metabolic control mechanisms. In individuals with deficient ventilatory control (low or absent hypoxic/hypercapnic responsiveness), respiration during wakefulness may be maintained by behavioral/wakeful stimuli, as described previously. However, during sleep, when these wakeful mechanisms are no longer operative, there is little residual drive to ventilation because metabolic mechanisms are defective. As a result, central apneas frequently ensue.

Based on these comments, the slope of the ventilatory response to hypercapnia (frequently measured during wakefulness) may be an important variable in the development of central apneas during sleep. As stated, in patients with markedly diminished or absent chemosensitivity, some form of sleep-disordered breathing—frequently central apnea—would be expected. If carbon dioxide sensitivity is very low or absent, there would be little stimulus to ventilation during sleep, and central apneas would not be surprising. Patients with disorders such as central alveolar hypoventilation (Ondine's curse)[30] and the obesity-hypoventilation (pickwickian) syndrome would fall into this group.[31, 32] These individuals have virtually no measurable chemosensitivity during wakefulness and tend to hypoventilate during the day. When these patients are asleep, this hypoventilation becomes worse, with further hypoxia and carbon dioxide retention. Apneas, both central and obstructive, are also commonly seen.

Increased hypercapnic sensitivity may also produce problems during sleep. Bradley et al.,[33] in their original report, observed two distinct groups of patients with central apneas. One was similar to the hypoventilating patients described above in that they had hypercapnia during wakefulness and a low hypercapnic ventilatory response (0.6 ± 0.2 L/min/mmHg). In contrast, the other group tended to have low arterial P_{CO_2} levels during wakefulness and a high hypercapnic response (2.9 ± 0.4 L/min/mmHg). In this latter group of patients, it was postulated that the unusually steep hypercapnic response led to respiratory instability with a waxing and waning of ventilation. This is believed to be secondary to intermittent overventilation (yielding hypocapnia) alternating with underventilation (yielding hypercapnia). Such cycling ventilation probably results from the marked increments in ventilation that occur with relatively modest increments in P_{CO_2}.

Bradley et al.[33] subsequently validated these concepts in a number of ways. First, they carefully documented that indeed most apneas in patients with idiopathic central sleep apnea are associated with arousal-induced hyperventilation and subsequent hypocapnia,[34] again emphasizing the importance of P_{CO_2} as a stimulus to breathing during sleep. Second, they noted that patients with central apnea have lower waking and sleeping P_{CO_2} levels associated with higher hypercapnic ventilatory responsiveness compared with normal control subjects.[35] These patients are chronically breathing closer to their P_{CO_2} apnea threshold during sleep. In addition, Grunstein et al.[36] reported a higher incidence of central apnea in patients with acromegaly, noting that the patients with central apnea had quite high ventilatory responsiveness to rising CO_2. Finally, Thalhofer and Dorow[37] confirmed this ventilatory control hypothesis in reporting on three groups of patients with central apnea who were stratified based on their "CO_2 quotient of irritability." Again, there are generally high- and low-drive groups. These observations suggest that abnormalities or even extremes of normality in the metabolic ventilatory control system (hypercapnic response in this case) in either direction (increased or decreased gain) may lead to unstable ventilation during sleep and possibly to central apneas. Ventilatory control abnormalities therefore represent one important cause of central sleep apnea.

Congestive Heart Failure

It has long been known that congestive heart failure is associated with Cheyne-Stokes respiration during wakefulness and sleep. This type of respiration is quite distinct with a crescendo and decrescendo ventilatory pattern with a central apnea or hypopnea at the nadir (Fig. 71–6). It is somewhat different from the previously described central apnea, which has a more abrupt onset and offset. The explanation for this breathing pattern has never been fully understood but probably is a product of respiratory control system instability resulting from a prolonged circulation time and increased ventilatory responsiveness to rising P_{CO_2}.[37a] It has been demonstrated in anesthetized animals that lengthening a normal circulation time can induce Cheyne-Stokes respiration.[38] Such an increased circulation time may produce unstable ventilation due to the delay that occurs between mechanical changes in respiration (hyperpnea or hypopnea) and receptor stimulation resulting from changes in arterial blood gases. If a subject hypoventilates or has an apnea, a substantial period of time will pass before increasing P_{CO_2} or decreasing P_{O_2} is detected at the appropriate receptor. As a result, the apnea or hypopnea is prolonged. When the deoxygenated, hypercapnic blood does reach the receptor, ventilation is stimulated for a disproportionately long period of time because the corrected blood gases are again not presented to the receptor for an extended period of time. Thus, ventilation can wax and wane, with actual apneas occurring at the nadir of this cycle. Whether this is the mechanism of Cheyne-Stokes respiration seen with congestive heart failure is speculative, because a several-fold increase in circulation time is necessary to produce such breathing dysrhythmias in animals.[39] This is probably a greater change than commonly occurs with heart failure. There also is evidence that this prolonged circulation time must be combined with an increased ventilatory responsiveness to rising P_{CO_2} to yield Cheyne-Stokes respiration.[39a] This is likely a similar process to that described in central apnea patients without heart failure. This may, to some extent, explain the variability in its occurrence in patients with heart failure.

It has been demonstrated that patients with Cheyne-Stokes respiration during wakefulness, whether from heart failure or other causes, will continue this respiratory pattern during sleep with frequent apneas.[40] In addition, a number of reports suggest that patients with congestive heart failure without obvious breathing abnormalities during the day may have periodic breathing during sleep.[41–43] One study suggests that 45% of patients with congestive heart failure (left ventricular ejection fraction of less than 40%) have more than 20 central apneas plus hypopneas per hour of sleep.[43] Thus, Cheyne-Stokes respiration during sleep in patients with congestive heart failure is likely to be quite common. These studies also indicate that the hyperpneic phase of this cycling ventilation may lead to frequent arousals and poor sleep quality. In addition, several studies have reported reduced survival rates in individuals with left ventricular failure and Cheyne-Stokes respiration[41, 44, 44a] compared with patients in heart failure who breathed rhythmically. At least two studies specifically associated central apneas during sleep with decreased survival rates in these patients[41, 44a];

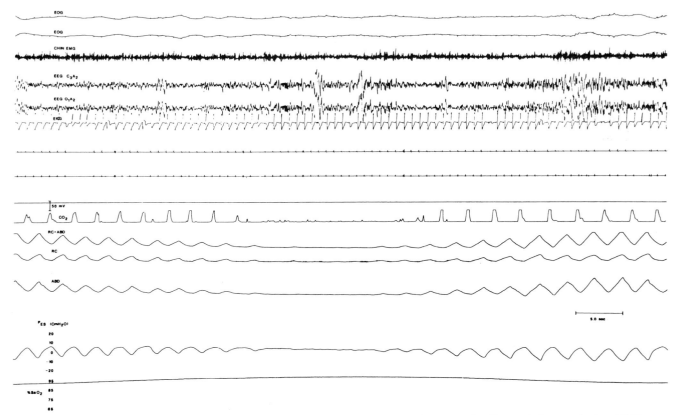

Figure 71–6. Representative tracing in stage 2 NREM sleep showing central apnea at the nadir of a Cheyne-Stokes respiration (CSR) event. Note the gradual decrease and eventual disappearance of esophageal pressure (Pes), abdominal movement (ABD), rib cage movement (RC), and RC + ABD excursions during the central apneic portion of the event, followed by a smooth increase in these tracings. EEG, electroencephalogram; EKG, electrocardiogram; EMG, electromyogram. (From Dowdell WT, Javaheri S, McGinnis W. 1990. Cheyne-Stokes respiration presenting as sleep apnea syndrome. *American Review of Respiratory Disease.* 141:874. Official Journal of the American Thoracic Society. © American Lung Association.)

however, it remains unclear whether this reduced survival rate was a consequence of the breathing dysrhythmia during sleep or of more severe cardiac dysfunction. Whether apneas in patients with congestive heart failure are central or obstructive varies depending on the study; both have been reported. This may be dependent on the characteristics of the individual's upper airway (size, collapsibility), with obstructive events resulting from decreased upper airway muscle tone at the nadir of the respiratory cycle in an individual with a susceptible airway. However, most such events are likely to be central in nature. In conclusion, this series of studies suggest that apneas (often central) are common in patients with congestive heart failure and may be detrimental to sleep quality and possibly the general health of these patients.

It should be noted that Cheyne-Stokes respiration has been reported in patients with neurological disease as well, primarily cerebrovascular disorders[45]; however, the actual ventilatory pattern in these patients has been less well characterized than in patients with congestive heart failure, and the mechanisms remain poorly understood.

Upper Airway

Nasal Obstruction. It is generally acknowledged that the common cold is associated with sleep distur-

bance; the reason for this, however, has remained obscure. It has been demonstrated that nasal obstruction can affect breathing pattern during sleep, with both central and obstructive apneas being reported.[46, 47] A number of investigators have observed sleep-disordered breathing (central and obstructive apneas, as well as hypopneas) in individuals with nasal obstruction, whether occurring naturally, as in allergic rhinitis[48] or deviated nasal septum,[49] or produced artificially.[47] The etiology of these events remains unresolved, although several explanations seem possible. A number of studies suggest that airflow can be detected by receptors in the nose and that these receptor mechanisms may influence respiration.[50] If this is the case, then loss of such input due to obstruction to air flow could alter respiratory pattern. The other possible explanation relates to the simple loss of the nose as a breathing route. Human beings may be more obligate nasal breathers during sleep than was previously appreciated, and the transition to the oral route could prove to be difficult. In addition, the increased negative airway pressures that must be generated to breathe through a partially occluded nasal passage tend to collapse the pharynx during sleep, yielding obstructive apneas.[51] As a result, both central and obstructive events may result from nasal disease, although obstructive events are likely more common.

Upper Airway Receptors (Non-nasal). There also

are early data suggesting that other (non-nasal) pharyngeal airway reflexes may initiate apneas. Davies et al.[52] observed that apneas in infants occurred frequently after the instillation of small boluses of water or warm saline into the oropharynx. They believe this to be a protective reflex. More relevant to adults, Issa and Sullivan[53] reported that pharyngeal airway collapse during sleep may initiate reflexes inhibiting respiration, thus yielding central apneas. In eight patients with predominantly central sleep apnea, they noted that (1) central apneas occurred more frequently when in the supine posture, a position likely to produce pharyngeal collapse during sleep; (2) oropharyngeal anesthesia abolished central apneas in two patients; and (3) high levels of nasal CPAP eliminated all apneas, including central ones. This final observation has been confirmed.[54] Thus, pharyngeal obstruction may yield central apnea, a concept supported by data from studies in animals.[55] This should be kept in mind in evaluating the obese, snoring patient in whom predominantly central apneas are observed in the sleep laboratory. Such patients may respond to therapies aimed at relieving upper airway obstruction.

Neurological Disorders

As stated, ventilation during sleep is highly dependent on the metabolic control system. As a result, any neurological disorder affecting this system could influence the ventilatory pattern while the individual is asleep, possibly leading to central sleep apnea. Various neurological processes have been implicated in the development of central sleep apnea. Patients with autonomic dysfunction,[56, 57] such as the Shy-Drager syndrome, familial dysautonomia, or diabetes mellitus, frequently have apneas that are generally of central origin, although obstructive events are also reported. These patients have also been noted to have erratic breathing during sleep even when central apneas are not obvious.

Because the brainstem is the primary source of both ventilatory pattern generation and the processing of respiratory afferent input from chemoreceptors and intrapulmonary receptors, any disease process affecting this area could influence ventilation during sleep. Damage to the brainstem, particularly the medullary area, may lead to hypoventilation during wakefulness but more commonly affects ventilation during sleep early in the disease. An example is poliomyelitis, a disease well known to damage medullary neurons.[58, 59] In the early stages of the "post-polio syndrome," respiration during wakefulness is normal, although short central apneas or mild hypoventilation may occur during sleep. With progression of this process (which may take decades), ventilation during sleep will become progressively more abnormal, with longer, more frequent apneas, and greater hypoventilation as hypoventilation during wakefulness may become apparent. Finally, some patients may actually require ventilatory support during sleep and wakefulness if the disease progresses that far. Other processes, such as tumor,[60]

infarction,[61] hemorrhage, or encephalitis,[62] can damage the medullary area, leading to breathing dysrhythmias during sleep, with central apneas being a prominent feature.

In addition, if the neural pathways from these medullary respiratory neurons to the motoneurons of the ventilatory muscles are interrupted (without damage to the brainstem itself), the metabolic control of breathing may be affected. This interruption is not an uncommon event after cervical cordotomy,[58, 63] with central apnea being described after this procedure.

Finally, chronic neuromuscular diseases, such as muscular dystrophy or myasthenia gravis,[58] may lead to waking alveolar hypoventilation with further hypoventilation during sleep. This may be associated with central apneas. In fact, as with most post-polio syndrome patients, ventilation during sleep in patients with respiratory muscle disease frequently deteriorates well before waking ventilation is affected. The treatment of these nocturnal apneas and hypoventilation with noninvasive nasal ventilation may delay frank waking respiratory failure.

Summary

The spectrum of disorders associated with central sleep apnea described above is sufficiently wide that definitive statements about the cause of central apnea are frequently difficult to make. It appears that abnormalities of the respiratory control system can produce central apneas. These may be either primary disorders, such as central alveolar hypoventilation, or secondary events, such as those that occur at altitude. Although the mechanisms by which congestive heart failure, nasal obstruction, and dysautonomia produce central apneas are less well defined, the associations are clear. However, many patients with central sleep apnea demonstrate none of these abnormalities, at least within the ability of most physicians to define them. Such patients are currently said to have idiopathic central sleep apnea, which we believe results from increased ventilatory responsiveness to chemical stimuli. As our understanding of this disorder improves, new causes are likely to become evident.

EPIDEMIOLOGY

If abnormal nocturnal breathing is to be understood and recognized, it is important to determine how commonly central apneas occur in normal individuals (see Chapter 17). Sleep-disordered breathing events (apnea and hypopnea, either central or obstructive) are common in normal persons, occur more frequently in men than in women, and increase in men with age and in women after menopause.[64–70] The reported frequency of disordered breathing varies depending on the population studied, the methods used for apnea detection, and the threshold used to define abnormalities. Carskadon and Dement[68] found that 37.5% of all subjects over the age of 62 had apneas or hypopneas, and that most of the time, "when determinations were possible, apneas were primarily of central type." Other studies report an incidence of disordered breathing between 12 and 66%,[65, 66] depending on the population investigated. Lugaresi et al.[69] stated that "central apneas lasting 5-15 sec may appear during light and REM sleep" in normal subjects. The most recent and complete study to date suggests that symptomatic sleep apnea occurs in about 4% of adult men and 2% of women, with most such events being obstructive in origin.[71] Again, apnea type was not always carefully defined, making definitive conclusions difficult.

With the above limitations in mind, a frequency of more than five central apneas per hour of sleep is generally considered abnormal. Although most research-based studies require a greater frequency of events for inclusion, five events per hour remains the current standard. This statement should not indicate that this frequency of central apnea always dictates a need for therapy; it simply represents an upper limit of normal.

In the four studies that specifically considered patients with symptomatic central sleep apnea, no consistent epidemiological trends emerge. Guilleminault et al.,[1] White et al.,[72] and Bradley et al.[33] reported a strong male predominance; Roehrs et al.[9] observed central apneas more commonly in women. No explanation can be offered for this discrepancy. All studies, however, noted this disorder to occur most commonly in middle-aged to elderly individuals, although a few younger patients have been reported. The diagnosis of central sleep apnea should be considered in any patient, regardless of age or gender, whose symptoms suggest its presence.

CLINICAL FEATURES AND CONSEQUENCES

The clinical presentation of patients with central sleep apnea varies dramatically depending on the cause of the apnea (Table 71-1). Patients with alveolar hypoventilation (waking hypercapnia) due to a number of possible causes (see Pathophysiology) make up a substantial percentage of patients with central apnea and generally present with symptoms suggestive of respiratory failure,[33, 73] including cor pulmonale, pe-

ripheral edema, and polycythemia. Restless sleep and daytime sleepiness are also commonly reported[33, 73] in these patients. On the other hand, nonhypoventilating (normocapnic) patients with central apnea have no symptoms of respiratory failure; these patients have a symptom complex that may be similar to that of the patient with obstructive apnea, although differences do exist.[1, 9, 72]

On the basis of several studies[1, 33, 72] and personal experience, it seems that individuals with pure central apnea (nonhypercapnic) less commonly complain of daytime hypersomnolence than do patients with obstructive sleep apnea, although such daytime sleepiness has been commonly described in patients with central apnea.[33] As the proportion of obstructive or mixed events increases in these patients (still with predominantly central apnea), hypersomnolence may become more frequent. The primary complaint of many patients with central apnea tends to be insomnia, restless sleep, or frequent awakenings during the night. Such awakenings may be accompanied by gasping for air or shortness of breath, a rare complaint in the patient with obstructive apnea. Patients with normocapnic central apnea also tend to have a normal body habitus, unlike the characteristically obese patient with obstructive apnea. As a result, patients with central sleep apnea as a group may be clinically distinguishable from those with obstructive apnea, although separation of the two disorders by history alone is often difficult (see Table 71-1).

The frequency and duration of central apneas in the nonhypercapnic group required to produce the clinical symptoms described are difficult to determine from the available literature.[1, 9, 33, 72, 74] The actual number of apneas, either central or obstructive, necessary to yield insomnia, hypersomnolence, or hemodynamic sequelae is unknown. Investigators are still uncertain about which variables should be monitored to predict clinical outcomes in this disorder. Despite this limitation of information, as stated, five central events per hour of sleep are considered the upper limit of normal. Although this number is somewhat arbitrary, we must await new information before a more meaningful figure can be chosen.

As expected, arterial oxygen desaturation occurs with central apneas. How low the saturation falls during a given apnea is likely to be related to the P_{O_2} when ventilation ceased, the duration of the apnea, and the lung volume at which the apnea occurred.[75] Whether ventilatory effort is occurring (obstructive apnea) or not (central apnea) may also have a minor effect on the rate of desaturation.[76] Patients with obstructive apnea generally seem to reach a lower arterial oxygen saturation during an apnea than do individuals with central events; this probably is a product of longer apnea duration, reduced lung volume (lower in patients with obstructive apnea due to obesity), and the presence of ventilatory efforts in the patient with obstructive apnea.

The hemodynamic consequences of central apneas have been poorly investigated. Early studies by Schroeder et al.[77] reported that pulmonary artery pres-

Table 71-1. CLINICAL CHARACTERISTICS OF PATIENTS WITH SLEEP APNEA

Central		Obstructive
Hypercapnic	*Nonhypercapnic*	*Obstructive*
Respiratory failure	Daytime sleepiness	Daytime sleepiness
Cor pulmonale	Insomnia (restless sleep)	Prominent snoring
Polycythemia	Mild and intermittent snoring	Witnessed apneas/ gasping
Daytime sleepiness	Awakenings (± choking, shortness of breath)	Commonly obese
Snoring	Normal body habitus	

sures increased from 26/16 mmHg during wakefulness to 41/26 mmHg during central apneic episodes. A study by Podszus et al.[78] reported virtually no change in pulmonary artery pressure during central apneas or the central component of mixed apneas despite considerable arterial oxygen desaturation; however, it seems highly probable that any elevation in pulmonary pressure associated with central apnea will result from hypoxemia and hypercapnia with the hypoventilating patient with central apnea demonstrating more severe pressure elevations. This concept has been confirmed.[37] There are few data addressing the impact of central apnea on systemic pressures, but Schroeder et al.[77] reported systemic arterial pressures to increase from 155/84 to 188/117 mmHg during central apneas in a small number of patients. In addition, White et al.[79] reported very similar increases in both systemic and pulmonary artery pressures during and after central and obstructive apneas in an anesthetized baboon model. The literature on patients with obstructive apnea suggests that sympathetic activation secondary to arousal is an important component of blood pressure elevation after apnea.[80] This principle likely applies to central events as well.

That dysrhythmic breathing can disrupt normal sleep architecture is well known; however, little information is available that specifically addresses central sleep apnea in this role. White et al.[72] reported an improvement in sleep efficiency and a trend toward more time in deeper (stages 3 and 4) and REM sleep after the treatment of central sleep apnea, which suggests that sleep was disrupted by the apneas. In fact, the six patients reported in that study had a mean of 209 apnea-associated awakenings and arousals during one night before therapy. Roehrs et al.[9] also found a reduction in what is generally considered a normal percentage of stage 3 or 4 sleep and an increase in stage 1 or 2 sleep in a group of patients with about 50% central apneas. The results of these studies suggest that the frequent arousals and awakenings generally associated with the hypercapnia after an apnea can lead to disruption of the normal distribution of sleep stages.

DIAGNOSTIC EVALUATION

The diagnosis of central sleep apnea generally requires a full night's recording of standard polysomnographic variables with a particular focus on respiratory effort. To prove that an apnea is indeed central, it must be documented that there is no respiratory effort throughout the event. This is most effectively and consistently accomplished with an esophageal balloon.[81, 82] Therefore, in the research setting, esophageal pressure should be measured to definitively document apnea type. Recognizing the difficulty in using an esophageal balloon and its infrequent use in clinical practice, other strategies have been used. Most evidence suggests that respiratory inductive plethysmography (RIP), calibrated or uncalibrated, can adequately assess respiratory effort.[81, 82] If there is a complete absence of thoracoabdominal motion (RIP or strain gauges) throughout an apnea, this strongly suggests the event is central in origin. Although recent evidence suggests that chest–abdominal wall motion as a measure of effort may overestimate the frequency of central apnea, rarely will the patient be misclassified with the use of this methodology.[81] A third method of assessing effort would be the use of diaphragmatic electromyelography, although this is frequently difficulty to obtain and therefore cannot always be relied on. Finally, classic teaching has suggested that pulse wave artifacts in the oronasal flow signal indicate a patent airway and, therefore, a central apnea. However, the study by Morrell et al.[83] indicates that this approach cannot be relied on.

Distinguishing central from obstructive hypopneas is extraordinarily difficult and cannot be reliably accomplished with the use of standard monitoring techniques. As a result, central apneas, not hypopneas, must be documented to make a definitive diagnosis of central sleep apnea.

As stated, five central apneas per hour of sleep are considered the upper limit of normal and a greater frequency implies an abnormal state. The number of events per hour that are required to produced symptoms or cardiovascular consequences remains controversial. In a patient with both central and obstructive events, it frequently is difficult to discern the primary abnormality. As a result, no definitive event percentage can be provided that will always indicate a central process. For research purposes, generally 75 to 85% of events must be central for patient inclusion,[33–35] although occasionally a lower percentage has been used.[9] Because obstructive apneas are considerably more common and diagnostic methodologies tend to overestimate the frequency of central apneas,[81, 82] the use of 80% central events as a threshold seems reasonable. This value can be adjusted up or down if the clinical scenario dictates.

To diagnose Cheyne-Stokes respiration, an esophageal balloon again represents the gold standard, but a crescendo-decrescendo pattern of breathing as detected by chest wall–abdominal motion (RIP[84]) is likely to be adequate (see Fig. 71–6). This respiratory pattern commonly has a cycle length of about 60 sec, with 10 min of continuous crescendo-decrescendo breathing often being required to document its existence. In a patient with congestive heart failure (or possible stroke) with this pattern of ventilation (documented using the methods described above), a diagnosis of Cheyne-Stokes respiration can be made comfortably.

TREATMENT

Patients With Alveolar Hypoventilation

Because there are few large series of patients with central sleep apnea, investigation into treatment has been somewhat limited. Two general types of therapeutic approaches have emerged depending on the cause of the central apnea. For the hypercapnic patient with alveolar hypoventilation during wakefulness and worsening hypoventilation during sleep with central apneas, nocturnal ventilation is the most appropriate approach. Initially, such ventilation was accomplished only with tracheostomy with a mechanical respirator, diaphragmatic pacing, or negative-pressure (cuirass) ventilators.[85–87] Newer studies indicate that nocturnal ventilation can be accomplished satisfactorily with a nasal mask and a pressure-cycled ventilator,[88] so the ease of administration of nocturnal ventilation has improved substantially, as has patient acceptance. As stated, most individuals in whom these techniques have been used have some form of central alveolar hypoventilation or respiratory muscle failure with severe nocturnal hypoxia and hypercapnia.

Nonhypercapnic Central Sleep Apnea

For the individual with insomnia, restless sleep, waking hypersomnolence, and mild-to-moderate nocturnal hypoxemia, all secondary to central sleep apnea, a number of therapeutic options are available. First, if any of the previously described conditions known to be associated with central apnea are present (e.g., nasal obstruction, pharyngeal collapse, or congestive heart failure), the abnormality should be treated aggressively and the central apnea reassessed. Second, the results of a review suggest that these central apneas may resolve spontaneously in about 20% of patients.[37] As a result, if the symptoms are not debilitating or other therapies fail, it may be appropriate to follow some patients with central apnea. Third, if the problem persists or if no known predisposing abnormality can be found, several pharmacological approaches can be attempted. Acetazolamide, a carbonic anhydrase inhibitor known to produce a metabolic acidosis and likely a shift in the PCO_2 apnea threshold to a lower value, has been used to treat central sleep apnea.[72] In a series of six patients, acetazolamide (250 mg four times daily) was shown to reduce central apnea substantially in all participants when used over a short period of time (1 to 2 weeks). Long-term use of this medication was assessed in only two individuals and was successful in one and unsuccessful in the other. However, a study[10] of 14 patients with central apnea suggests that acetazolamide may lead to a more sustained improvement in apnea frequency and symptoms (primarily hypersomnolence). Of note, subsequent discontinuation of acetazolamide did not lead to an immediate return of symptoms or events.[11] On the other hand, several studies have reported the development of obstructive apneas after acetazolamide administration in patients previously demonstrated to have central events.[7] The explanation for this remains obscure but may relate to the respiratory stimulating activity of acetazolamide in an individual with a collapsing airway during sleep. When little ventilatory effort is present, the apneas appear central. However, when respiration is stimulated, obstructive events develop. Clearly, follow-up sleep studies are necessary in patients being treated with acetazolamide, particularly if symptoms persist.

Isolated reports of the use of other medications, such as theophylline, naloxone, and medroxyprogesterone acetate, imply that these drugs have little efficacy in the treatment of central apnea.[1] Clomipramine (a tricyclic antidepressant), on the other hand, was found to be successful in several patients in whom it was tried.[1] Theophylline improved apnea in a patient with a damaged brainstem.[89] None of these drugs has been studied systematically, so firm recommendations regarding their use cannot be made.

Nasal CPAP has been shown to be an effective therapy for some patients with central sleep apnea.[53, 54, 90] These patients probably fall into several groups. First, as stated previously, pharyngeal airway collapse or closure during sleep may initiate a reflex inhibition of ventilation in some patients and therefore a central apnea. With nasal CPAP, airway closure is prevented, and such apneas abolished. In obese, snoring patients in whom predominantly central apneas are observed, nasal CPAP may be an effective form of therapy. Second, nasal CPAP has been shown to work well in some patients with congestive heart failure in whom Cheyne-Stokes respiration and central apneas are observed during sleep.[91] Whether CPAF in these patients improves cardiac function, leads to increased oxygen stores in the lung (thus stabilizing ventilation), or improves upper airway patency is controversial at this time; however, it appears to be effective in this heart failure group. Finally, an abstract suggests that CPAP may also be a viable form of therapy in "idiopathic central sleep apnea."[92] The authors observed that CPAP substantially reduced apneas in these patients, which they attributed primarily to a CPAP-induced increase in arterial PCO_2. As a result, PCO_2 was kept above the apnea threshold. Thus, a wide range of patients with central apnea may respond to CPAP, although the final role of this therapeutic modality in central apnea must await further investigation.

A number of studies suggest that oxygen may be a useful method of treating central sleep apnea. Martin et al.[93] observed that central apneas were completely abolished with oxygen administration in two patients during a short-nap study. McNicholas et al.[94] found a considerable reduction in the number of central apneas present in a patient with central alveolar hypoventilation after oxygen therapy was begun. Finally, a study evaluating the effects of low-flow oxygen in nine obese patients with a large component of central apneas reported a considerable reduction in these central events.[95] However, the frequency of obstructive apneas was somewhat increased. Although the mechanism by which oxygen administration reduces central apneas has not yet been established, two explanations seem possible. One relates to the potential destabilizing influence of the hypoxic ventilatory response on respiratory control. As at altitude, with hypoxia an individual will hyperventilate, yielding hypocapnia and alkalosis. As previously stated, hypocapnia may inhibit respiration during sleep. Thus, cycling ventilation may develop with central apneas occurring at the nadir of this periodic breathing. With the administration of oxygen, the hypoxic influence on ventilation may be reduced and breathing regularized. The other possible explanation relates to the fact that hypoxia can be a ventilatory depressant. If respiration is depressed by hypoxia, then central apneas may occur. Oxygen administration in this situation could reduce apneas. Regardless of the mechanism, low-flow oxygen may be an effective treatment for central sleep apnea.

In attempting to treat a patient with predominantly central sleep apnea, one must remember that both central and obstructive apneas are commonly seen in the same individual. In these patients, it is frequently difficult to determine whether the primary cause of the apnea is of central origin, relates to upper airway obstruction, or both. Therefore, in patients who have central apnea with a large component of obstructive events, treatment of the airway obstruction via one of the currently available methods may have beneficial effects on both types of apnea.

Cheyne-Stokes Respiration

The treatment of Cheyne-Stokes respiration requires special comment because it has been the subject of a number of studies. First, as stated, the heart failure (if present) should be treated as aggressively as possible. Optimal medical treatment, however, abolishes the sleep apnea in only a minority of patients who had originally presented with acute left ventricular failure.[95a] Second, should this fail, a number of additional options are available. Nocturnal oxygen administration has been shown to reduce apnea frequency and improve symptoms in several studies of congestive heart failure and Cheyne-Stokes respiration.[96, 97, 97a] Several medications have also demonstrated some efficacy; these include theophylline[98] and possibly hypnotic agents.[99] Finally, as stated, CPAP has been shown to increase cardiac function in these patients when used chronically and may also improve sleep quality. More recently, nasal ventilation has been reported to be helpful in these patients.[100] As a result, a variety of therapeutic options exist for these patients.

SUMMARY

A logical approach to the treatment of central sleep apnea in the symptomatic patient, when one is certain the apneas are of central origin, would be to first rule out treatable causes; these include nasal obstruction, pharyngeal collapse, congestive heart failure, and certainly alveolar hypoventilation. If present, the condition should be corrected. If no such problem is found, the therapeutic approach must be individualized to the patient. First, if the patient is obese and snoring or has heart failure, nasal CPAP may be an appropriate first choice. Second, if the patient is hypoxemic during central apneas or the apneas have a clearly periodic nature, then nocturnally administered oxygen may be most appropriate. Finally, if none of these conditions exists, then acetazolamide (at 250 mg four times daily) should be considered.

One final approach is probably worth consideration.

In the patient with central apneas in whom hypoxemia is not a particular issue but sleep is seriously disrupted, a hypnotic agent might prove useful.[101] If the patient can sleep through the apneas, often deeper stages of sleep (stages 3 and 4) can be attained and apneas diminished. Thus, sleep quality is improved, and the remaining apneas may be of little consequence. However, because hypnotic agents could inhibit ventilation and worsen the problem in some patients, this therapeutic modality must be approached cautiously.

References

1. Guilleminault C, van den Hoed J, Mitler M. Clinical overview of the sleep apnea syndromes. In: Guilleminault C, Dement W, eds. Sleep Apnea Syndromes. New York, NY: Alan R Liss; 1978:1–11.
2. Onal E, Lopata M, O'Connor T. Diaphragmatic and genioglossal EMG responses to isocapnic hypoxia in humans. Am Rev Respir Dis. 1981;124:215–217.
3. Onal E, Lopata M, O'Connor T. Genioglossal and diaphragmatic EMG responses to CO_2 rebreathing in humans. J Appl Physiol. 1981;50:1052–1055.
4. Onal E, Lopata M, O'Connor T. Pathogenesis of apnea in hypersomnia-sleep apnea syndrome. Am Rev Respir Dis. 1982;125:167–174.
5. Fletcher EC. Recurrence of sleep apnea syndrome following tracheostomy: a shift from obstructive to central apnea. Chest. 1989;95:205–209.
6. Guilleminault C, Cummiskey J. Progressive improvement of apnea index and ventilatory response to CO_2 after tracheostomy in obstructive sleep apnea. Am Rev Respir Dis. 1982;126:14–20.
7. Sharp J, Druz W, D'Souza V, et al. Effect of metabolic acidosis upon sleep apnea. Chest. 1985;87:619–624.
8. Hyland R, Hutcheon M, Perl A, et al. Upper airway occlusion induced by diaphragm pacing for primary alveolar hypoventilation: implications for the pathogenesis of obstructive sleep apnea. Am Rev Respir Dis. 1981;124:180–185.
9. Roehrs T, Conway W, Wittig R, et al. Sleep complaints in patients with sleep-related respiratory disturbances. Am Rev Respir Dis. 1985;132:520–523.
10. DeBacker WA, Verbraecken J, Willeman M, et al. Central apnea index decreases after prolonged treatment with acetazolamide. Am J Respir Crit Care Med. 1995;151:87–91.
11. DeBacker WA. Central sleep apnoea, pathogenesis and treatment: an overview and perspective. Eur Respir J. 1995;8:1372–1383.
12. Phillipson EA. Control of breathing during sleep. Am Rev Respir Dis. 1978;118:909–939.
13. Orem J, Lydic R, Norris P. Experimental control of diaphragm and laryngeal abductor muscles by brain stem arousal systems. Respir Physiol. 1979;38:203–221.
14. Sears TA, Newsom-Davis J. The control of respiratory muscles during voluntary breathing. Ann NY Acad Sci. 1968;155:183.
15. Sullivan C, Kozar L, Murphy E, et al. Primary role of respiratory afferents in sustaining breathing rhythm. J Appl Physiol. 1978;45:11–17.
16. Motta J, Guilleminault C. Effects of oxygen administration in sleep-induced apneas. In: Guilleminault C, Dement W, eds. Sleep Apnea Syndromes. New York, NY: Alan R Liss; 1978:137–144.
17. Berssenbrugge A, Dempsey J, Skatrud J. Hypoxic versus hypocapnic effects on periodic breathing during sleep. In: West J, Lahiri S, eds. High Altitude and Man. Bethesda, Md: American Physiological Society; 1984:115–127, Clinical Physiology Series.
18. Skatrud J, Dempsey J. Interaction of sleep state and chemical stimuli in sustaining rhythmic ventilation. J Appl Physiol. 1983;55:813–822.
19. Berthon-Jones M, Sullivan C. Ventilatory and arousal responses to hypoxia in sleeping humans. Am Rev Respir Dis. 1982;125:632–639.

20. Berthon-Jones M, Sullivan C. Ventilatory and arousal responses to hypercapnia in normal sleeping humans. J Appl Physiol. 1984;57:59–67.
21. Douglas N, White D, Pickett C, et al. Hypercapnic ventilatory response in sleeping adults. Am Rev Respir Dis. 1982;126:758–762.
22. Douglas N, White D, Weil J, et al. Hypoxic ventilatory response decreases during sleep in normal man. Am Rev Respir Dis. 1982;125:286–289.
23. White DP. Occlusion pressure and ventilation during sleep in normal humans. J Appl Physiol. 1986;61:1279–1287.
24. Cherniack N. Respiratory dysrhythmias during sleep. N Engl J Med. 1981;305:325–330.
25. Cherniack N. Sleep apnea and its causes. J Clin Invest. 1984;73:1501–1506.
26. Bülow K. Respiration and wakefulness in man. Acta Physiol Scand. 1963;53(suppl 209):1–110.
27. Dempsey JA, Skatrud JB. A sleep induced apneic threshold and its consequences. Am Rev Respir Dis. 1986;133:1163–1170.
28. Chow CM, Xi L, Smith CA, et al. A volume-dependent apnea threshold during NREM sleep in the dog. J Appl Physiol. 1994;76:2315–2325.
29. Weil J, Kryger M, Scoggin C. Sleep and breathing at high altitude. In: Guilleminault C, Dement W, eds. Sleep Apnea Syndromes. New York, NY: Alan R Liss; 1978:119–136.
30. Mellins R, Balfour H, Turino G, et al. Failure of autonomic control of ventilation (Ondine's curse). Medicine. 1970;49:487–504.
31. Tassinari C, Dalla Bernardina B, Cirignotta F, et al. Apnoeic periods and the respiratory related arousal patterns during sleep in the Pickwickian syndrome. Bull Physiopathol Respir. 1972;8:1087–1102.
32. Zwillich C, Sutton F, Pierson D, et al. Decreased hypoxic ventilation drive in the obesity-hypoventilation syndrome. Am J Med. 1975;59:343–348.
33. Bradley TD, McNicholas WT, Rutherford R, et al. Clinical and physiological heterogeneity of the central sleep apnea syndrome. Am Rev Respir Dis. 1986;134:217–221.
34. Xie A, Wong B, Phillipson EA, et al. Interaction of hyperventilation and arousal in the pathogenesis of idiopathic central sleep apnea. Am J Respir Crit Care Med. 1994;150:489–495.
35. Xie A, Rutherford R, Rankin F, et al. Hypocapnia and increased ventilatory responsiveness in patients with idopathic central sleep apnea. Am J Respir Crit Care Med. 1995;152:1950–1955.
36. Grunstein RR, Ho KY, Berthon-Jones M, et al. Central sleep apnea is associated with increased ventilatory responses to carbon dioxide and hypersecretion of growth hormone in patients with acromegaly. Am J Respir Crit Care Med. 1994;150:496–502.
37. Thalhofer S, Dorow P. Central sleep apnea. Respiration. 1997;64:2–9.
37a. Javaheri S. A mechanism of central sleep apnea in patients with heart failure. N Engl J Med. 1999;341:949–954.
38. Lange R, Hecht H. The mechanism of Cheyne-Stokes respiration. J Clin Invest. 1962;41:42–52.
39. Guyton A, Crowell J, Moore J. Basic oscillating mechanism of Cheyne-Stokes breathing. Am J Physiol. 1979;187:185–200.
39a. Wilcox I, McNamara SG, Dodd MJ, et al. Ventilatory control in patients with sleep apnoea and left ventricular dysfunction: comparison of obstructive and central sleep apnoea. Eur Respir J. 1998;11:7–13.
40. Alex CG, Onal E, Lopata M. Upper airway obstruction during sleep in patients with Cheyne-Stokes respiration. Am Rev Respir Dis. 1986;133:42–45.
41. Findley LJ, Zwillich CW, Ancoli-Israel S, et al. Cheyne-Stokes breathing during sleep in patients with left ventricular heart failure. South Med J. 1985;78:11–15.
42. Rees PJ, Clark TSH. Paroxysmal nocturnal dyspnea and periodic respiration. Lancet. 1979;2:1315–1317.
43. Javaheri S, et al. Occult sleep-disordered breathing in stable congestive heart failure. Ann Intern Med. 1995;122:487–492.
44. Hanly P, Zuberi-Khakhar NS. Increased mortality associated with Cheyne-Stokes respiration in patients with congestive heart failure. Am J Respir Crit Care Med. 1996;153:272–276.
44a. Lanfranchi PA, Braghiroli A, Bosimini E, et al. Prognostic value of nocturnal Cheyne-Stokes respiration in chronic heart failure. Circulation. 1999;99:1435–1440.

45. Nachtmann A, Siebler M, Rose G, et al. Cheyne-Stoke respiration in ischemic stroke. Neurology. 1995;45:820–821.
46. Suratt PM, Turner BL, Withoit SC. Effect of intranasal obstruction on breathing during sleep. Chest. 1986;90:324–329.
47. Zwillich C, Pickett C, Hanson F, et al. Disturbed sleep and prolonged apnea during nasal obstruction in normal man. Am Rev Respir Dis. 1981;124:158–160.
48. McNicholas W, Tarlo S, Cole P, et al. Obstructive apneas during sleep in patients with seasonal allergic rhinitis. Am Rev Respir Dis. 1982;126:625–628.
49. Heimer D, Scharf S, Lieberman A, et al. Sleep apnea syndrome treated by repair of deviated nasal septum. Chest. 1983;84:184–185.
50. Ramos J. On the integration of respiratory movements, III: the fifth nerve afferents. Acta Physiol Lat Am. 1960;10:104–113.
51. Wilson S, Thach B, Brouillette R, et al. Upper airway patency in the human infant: influence of airway pressure and posture. J Appl Physiol. 1980;48:500–504.
52. Davies AM, Koenig JC, Thach BT. Upper airway chemoreflex responses to saline and water in preterm infants. J Appl Physiol. 1988;64:1412–1420.
53. Issa F, Sullivan C. Reversal of central sleep apnea using nasal CPAP. Chest. 1986;90:165–171.
54. Hoffstein V, Slutsky AS. Central sleep apnea reversed by continuous positive airway pressure. Am Rev Respir Dis. 1987;135:1210–1212.
55. Mathew OP, Farber JP. Effect of upper airway negative pressure on respiratory timing. Respir Physiol. 1983;54:259–268.
56. Guilleminault C, Briskin J, Greenfield M, et al. The impact of autonomic nervous system dysfunction on breathing during sleep. Sleep. 1981;4:263–278.
57. McNicholas W, Rutherford R, Grossman R, et al. Abnormal respiratory pattern generation during sleep in patients with autonomic dysfunction. Am Rev Respir Dis. 1983;128:429–433.
58. Plum F, Leigh RJ. Abnormalities of central mechanisms. In: Hornbein TF, ed. Regulation of Breathing: Part II. Vol 17. Lung Biology in Health and Disease. New York, NY: Marcel Dekker; 1981:989–1067.
59. Plum F, Swanson AG. Abnormalities in central regulation of respiration in acute and convalescent poliomyelitis. Arch Neurol Psychiatr. 1958;80:267–285.
60. Devereaux M, Keane J, Davis R. Autonomic respiratory failure. Arch Neurol. 1973;29:46–52.
61. Levin B, Margolis G. Acute failure of autonomic respirations secondary to unilateral brainstem infarct. Ann Neurol. 1977;1:583–586.
62. White D, Miller F, Erickson R. Sleep apnea and nocturnal hypoventilation following Western equine encephalitis. Am Rev Respir Dis. 1983;127:132–133.
63. Krieger A, Rosomoff H. Sleep induced apnea: a respiratory and autonomic dysfunction syndrome following bilateral percutaneous cervical cordotomy. J Neurosurg. 1974;39:168–180.
64. Ancoli-Israel S. Epidemiology of sleep disorders. Clin Geriatr Med. 1989;5:347–362.
65. Bixler E, Kales A, Soldatos C, et al. Sleep apneic activity in a normal population. Res Commun Chem Pathol Pharmacol. 1982;36:141–152.
66. Block A, Boysen P, Wayne J, et al. Sleep apnea, hypopnea, and oxygen desaturation in normal subjects. N Engl J Med. 1979;300:513–517.
67. Block A, Wynne J, Boysen P. Sleep-disordered breathing and nocturnal oxygen desaturation in postmenopausal women. Am J Med. 1980;69:75–79.
68. Carskadon M, Dement W. Respiration during sleep in the aged human. J Gerontol. 1981;36:420–425.
69. Lugaresi E, Coccagna G, Cirignotta F, et al. Breathing during sleep in normal and pathological conditions. Adv Exp Med Biol. 1978;99:35–45.
70. Webb P. Periodic breathing during sleep. J Appl Physiol. 1974;37:899–903.
71. Young T, Palla M, Dempsey J, et al. The occurrence of sleep-disordered breathing among middle-aged adults. N Engl J Med. 1993;328:1230–1235.
72. White D, Zwillich C, Pickett C, et al. Central sleep apnea: improvement with acetazolamide therapy. Arch Intern Med. 1982;142:1816–1819.

73. Bradley TD, Phillipson EA. Central sleep apnea. Clin Chest Med. 1992;13:493–505.
74. Guilleminault C, Tilkian A, Dement W. The sleep apnea syndromes. Annu Rev Med. 1976;27:465–484.
75. Findley LJ, Ries AL, Tisi GM, et al. Hypoxemia during apnea in normal subjects: mechanisms and impact of lung volume. J Appl Physiol. 1983;55:1777–1783.
76. Fletcher EC. The rate of fall of arterial oxyhemoglobin saturation on obstructive sleep apnea. Chest. 1989;96:717–722.
77. Schroeder J, Motta J, Guilleminault C. Hemodynamic studies in sleep apnea. In: Guilleminault C, Dement W, eds. Sleep Apnea Syndromes. New York, NY: Alan R Liss; 1978:177–196.
78. Podszus T, Peter JH, Renke A, et al. Pulmonary artery pressure during central sleep apnea. Sleep Res. 1988;17:236.
79. White SG, Fletcher EC, Miller CC. Acute systemic blood pressure elevation in obstructive and nonobstructive breath hold in primates. J Appl Physiol. 1995;79:324–330.
80. Weiss JW, Remsburg S, Garspestad E, et al. Hemodynamic consequences of obstructive sleep apnea. Sleep. 1996;19:388–397.
81. Boudewyns A, Willemen M, Wagemans M, et al. Assessment of respiratory effort by means of strain gauge and esophageal pressure swings: a comparative study. Sleep. 1997;20:168–170.
82. Staats BA, Bonekat HW, Harris CD, et al. Chest wall motion in sleep apnea. Am Rev Respir Dis. 1984;130:59–63.
83. Morrell MJ, Badr S, Harms CA, et al. The assessment of upper airway patency during apnea using cardiogenic oscillations in the airflow signal. Sleep. 1995;18:651–658.
84. Dowdell WT, Javahari S, McGinnis W. Cheyne-Stokes respiration presenting as sleep apnea syndrome. Am Rev Respir Dis. 1990;141:871–879.
85. Coleman M, Boros S, Huseby T, et al. Congenital central hypoventilation syndrome. Am Rev Respir Dis. 1979;119:901–902.
86. Glenn W, Phelps M, Gersten L. Diaphragm pacing in the management of central alveolar hypoventilation. In: Guilleminault C, Dement W, eds. Sleep Apnea Syndromes. New York, NY: Alan R Liss; 1978:333–345.
87. Godfrey C, Man M, Jones R, et al. Primary alveolar hypoventilation managed by negative-pressure ventilators. Chest. 1979;76:219–221.
88. Guilleminault C, Stoohs R, Schnieder H, et al. Central alveolar hypoventilation and sleep: treatment by intermittent positive-pressure ventilation through nasal mask in an adult. Chest. 1989;96:1210–1212.
89. Raetzo MA, Junod AF, Kryger MH. Effect of aminophylline and relief from hypoxia on central sleep apnea due to medullary damage. Bull Eur Physiopathol Respir. 1987;23:171–175.
90. Sullivan CE, Issa FG. Obstructive sleep apnea. Clin Chest Med. 1985;6:633–650.
91. Takasaki Y, Orr D, Popkin J, et al. Effect of nasal continuous positive airway pressure on sleep apnea in congestive heart failure. Am Rev Respir Dis. 1989;140:1578–1584.
92. Rutherford R, Popkin J, Phillipson EA, et al. Effect of CPAP on Cheyne-Stokes respiration and idiopathic central sleep apnea. Am Rev Respir Dis. 1991;143(suppl):A197.
93. Martin R, Sanders M, Gray B, et al. Acute and long-term ventilatory effects of hypoxia in the adult sleep apnea syndrome. Am Rev Respir Dis. 1982;125:175–180.
94. McNicholas W, Carter J, Rutherford R, et al. Beneficial effect of oxygen in primary alveolar hypoventilation with central sleep apnea. Am Rev Respir Dis. 1982;125:773–775.
95. Gold AV, Bleecker ER, Smith PL. A shift from central and mixed sleep apnea to obstructive apnea resulting from low-flow oxygen. Am Rev Respir Dis. 1985;132:220–223.
95a. Tremel F, Pepin J, Veale D, et al. High prevalence and persistence of sleep apnoea in patients referred for acute left ventricular failure and medically treated over 2 months. Eur Heart J. 1999;20:1201–1209.
96. Franklin KA, Eriksson P, Sahlin C, et al. Reversal of central sleep apnea with oxygen. Chest. 1997;111:163–169.
97. Hanly PJ, Millar TW, Steljes DG, et al. The effect of oxygen on respiration and sleep in patients with congestive heart failure. Ann Intern Med. 1989;111:777–782.
97a. Krachman SL, D'Alonzo GE, Berger TJ, et al. Comparison of oxygen therapy with nasal continuous positive airway pressure on Cheyne-Stokes respiration during sleep in congestive heart failure. Chest. 1999;116:1550–1557.
98. Javaheri S, Parker TJ, Wexler L, et al. Effects of theophylline on sleep disordered breathing in stable heart falure: a prospective, double-blind, placebo controlled, crossover study. N Engl J Med. 1996;335:562–567.
99. Biberdorf DJ, Steens R, Millar TW, et al. Benzodiazepines in congestive heart failure: effects of temazepam on arousability and Cheyne-Stokes respiration. Sleep. 1993;16:529–538.
100. Willson GN, Wilcox I, Piper AJ, et al. Treatment of central sleep apnoea in congestive heart failure with nasal ventilation. Thorax. 1998;53(suppl 3):S41–S46.
101. Bonnet MH, Dexter JR, Arand DL. The effect of triazolam on arousal and respiration in central sleep apnea patients. Sleep. 1990;13:31–41.

72

Anatomy and Physiology of Upper Airway Obstruction

Samuel Kuna

John E. Remmers

OBSTRUCTION OF THE PHARYNX DURING SLEEP: THE WHYS AND WHERES

Since the late 1970s, considerable attention has been directed at understanding the pathogenesis of obstructive sleep apnea (OSA). Despite this, we presently possess only fragmentary knowledge of the abnormalities that underlie closure of the upper airway in patients who experience OSA. Nonetheless, three fundamental features are clear:

1. The site of upper airway obstruction lies in the pharynx.
2. The size of the pharyngeal lumen during inspiration depends on the balance between inward, or narrowing, forces resulting from intrapharyngeal suction pressure and outward, or dilating, forces generated principally by pharyngeal muscles.
3. Anatomical abnormalities of the pharynx and its associated structures are commonly present in patients with OSA.

The purpose of this chapter is to review evidence for these generally accepted facts about OSA and to consider new information that relates to the pathogenesis of upper airway obstruction during sleep. This chapter also identifies gaps in our present understanding that appear to be pivotal in developing more effective therapeutic measures. These gaps can be summarized by saying that we know little about specific *whys* and *wheres* of upper airway obstruction during sleep. *Why* is intended to focus attention on the precise causal sequences whereby a particular neural or anatomical abnormality leads to either complete closure or a stable narrowing of the pharynx. *Where* centers on current interest in the relationship between various anatomical or neural disorders and the precise locus of pharyngeal closure or narrowing. What are the regional mechanical characteristics of the different pharyngeal segments, and how do changes in one segment influence behavior in another? These are some of the unanswered or partially answered questions to be addressed.

THE UPPER AIRWAY: GENERAL CONSIDERATIONS

Technically, the upper airway includes the extrathoracic trachea, larynx, pharynx, and nose. The area of greatest interest, in the present context, is the pharyngeal airway, a segment bounded cranially by the nasopharynx and caudally by the glottic chink. Although this segment is of particular interest with regard to OSA, the importance of the nose and nasal resistance cannot be ignored. However, this review focuses on the pharynx because it is the site of upper airway closure or narrowing during sleep. A key feature of the pharynx is that it is not simply an airway; rather, the pharynx is a multipurpose passage—it transmits air, liquid, and solids, and is therefore a common pathway for respiratory, digestive, and phonatory functions.[1, 2] Accordingly, the evolution of the anatomy and neural control of the pharynx has been dictated by the need to serve these multiple ends. For instance, swallowing requires a collapsible tube in which a coordinated neuromuscular action propels oral cavity contents into the esophagus and not into the nose or trachea. Similarly, speaking entails rapid movements of a mobile, collapsible pharyngeal tube controlled by the central nervous system. Finally, the nose and mouth are the sources of large volumes of secretions which must be cleared via the pharynx.

Interspersed and intermingled with these swallowing, secretory, and phonatory functions is airway function: the pharyngeal tube serves as a conduit for airflow connecting the nose with the larynx. Its patency is vital. With the exception of the two ends of the entire respiratory airway tract—that is, the nares and the small intrapulmonary airways—the pharynx is the only collapsible segment of the respiratory tract. This collapsibility of the pharynx probably presented an important evolutionary challenge to mammals. That the pharynx remains open at all times, except during momentary closures associated with swallowing, regurgitation, eructation, and speech, has been well established.[3–6] That the pharynx can be occluded in unconscious individuals is also well recognized.[7] What became apparent in the 1960s is that some people possess an adequate pharyngeal lumen for all respiratory functions while awake but have an obstructed lumen during sleep.[8] We now realize that pharyngeal patency during wakefulness is, in large part, attributable to continual neuromuscular control by the higher nervous system which supervises the action of the pharyngeal muscles and ensures a patent pharynx. The nervous system coordinates the need for a patent airway with the need for swallowing and phonatory functions in such a way that the airway closes only briefly in coordination with respiratory movements of the thoracic pump.

During sleep, apparently, this supervision of the pharyngeal airway by the higher nervous system is, to some extent, altered and, at least in some individuals, this compromises defense of airway patency. When the normal neurological changes that are associated with sleep occur against the background of anatomical abnormalities, severe narrowing or closure of the pharyngeal airway can occur. This occurrence sets the stage for what is referred to as obstructive sleep hypopnea (OSH). OSH connotes a transient reduction in inspiratory flow secondary to elevated upper airway resistance, and OSA constitutes extension of OSH to the limit where upper airway resistance becomes infinite; that is, airflow ceases. Because OSH and OSA appear to represent a continuum, this chapter, for the most part, refers to this spectrum of obstructive processes as obstructive sleep apnea/hypopnea (OSA/H).

FUNCTIONAL PHARYNGEAL ANATOMY

The pharyngeal airway consists of four anatomical subsegments: nasopharynx, velopharynx, oropharynx, and hypopharynx (Fig. 72–1). Structures surrounding

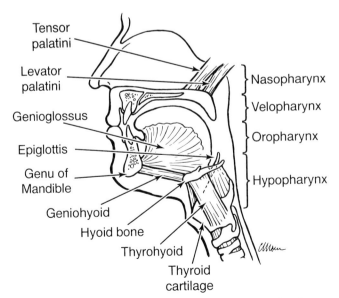

Figure 72–1. Anatomical features of the upper airway. The pharynx consists of four anatomical subsegments: nasopharynx, velopharynx, oropharynx, and hypopharynx.

the pharyngeal airway valve and shape the airway during phonation, and close the airway during deglutition. During inspiration in quiet breathing, pharyngeal structures are pulled inward by subatmospheric intraluminal pressure and in a caudal direction by displacement of the trachea into the thoracic cavity. They return to their resting position during expiration. The size and position of the tongue and soft palate are of particular importance in the maintenance of upper airway patency. Both are highly mobile structures that can occlude the pharyngeal airway. During nasal breathing with the mouth closed, surface adhesive forces help maintain the soft palate in apposition to the base of the tongue and promote contact of the tongue with the mucosa of the fixed-space oral cavity. The base of a tongue that is large relative to the size of the oral cavity may be displaced posteriorly into the pharyngeal air space. Mouth opening can have antagonistic effects on pharyngeal airway patency. Opening the mouth potentially destabilizes the airway by freeing the mucosal attachments of the tongue and soft palate and moving the mandibular point of attachment of the tongue dorsally, allowing the compliant tongue and soft palate to move dorsally and compromise the pharyngeal airway. However, caudal displacement of the mandible may promote velopharyngeal patency by increasing traction on the tonsillar pillars. The anterior and posterior tonsillar pillars form part of the palatal arch and can have a tether-like action on the soft palate. With bite opening, the pillars would pull the soft palate in a caudal and ventral direction.

Contraction of the 20 or more skeletal muscles surrounding the pharyngeal airway dilate the airway as well as stiffen the airway walls.[9, 10] As shown in Figures 72–1 and 72–2, the pharyngeal muscles have complex anatomical relationships.[11] However, for consideration of pharyngeal airway patency during respiration, they can be classified into four groups—that is, the muscles regulating the position of the soft palate, tongue, hyoid apparatus, and posterolateral pharyngeal walls. Contraction of specific muscles within these groups can have antagonistic effects on the pharyngeal airway. For example, contraction of the palatal muscle levator palatini, along with the superior pharyngeal constrictor, closes the velopharyngeal airway, but contraction of other palatal muscles, the palatopharyngeus and glossopharyngeus, opens the velopharynx.[12] Similarly, the extrinsic tongue muscles include tongue protrusors (genioglossus and geniohyoid) and retractors (hyoglossus and styloglossus).

Many pharyngeal muscles, including the medial pterygoid, tensor palatini,[13–15] genioglossus,[16, 17] geniohyoid,[18] and sternohyoid,[19, 20] receive phasic activation during inspiration and tend to promote a patent pharyngeal lumen. Contraction of these muscles promotes ventral movement of the soft palate, mandible, tongue, and hyoid bone, as depicted in Figure 72–3. Although the separate contribution of each of these muscles is not completely clear, their coordinated action is even more difficult to decipher. Nonetheless, a reasonable generalization is that inspiratory motor output to the

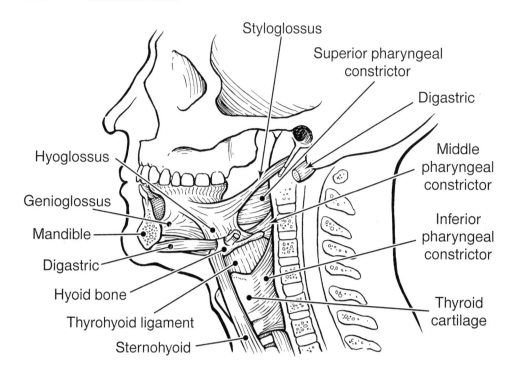

Figure 72–2. Additional anatomical features of the upper airway. Among the many upper airway muscles attaching to the floating hyoid bone are the genioglossus, geniohyoid, hyoglossus, middle pharyngeal constrictor, sternohyoid, and digastric.

muscles of the pharynx and related structures stiffens the pharynx and enlarges its lumen.

Pharyngeal muscles can have different effects when activated in concert than when activated individually. Coactivation of the hyoid muscles is a particularly good example of this phenomenon (see Fig. 72–3).[18] The hyoid bone in human beings does not articulate with any other bony or cartilaginous structure. The position of the relatively compliant ventral pharyngeal wall is, therefore, determined by the numerous muscle attachments to this floating bony structure. Muscles inserting on the hyoid include the geniohyoid and genioglossus. Contraction of these muscles pulls the hyoid in a rostral and ventral direction. Strap muscles originating from the sternum (sternohyoid) and thyroid cartilage (thyrohyoid) also insert on the hyoid and pull it in a caudal direction. With simultaneous contraction of all four muscles, the resultant force vector acting on the hyoid is directed caudally and ven-

trally. This combined effect moves the ventral pharyngeal wall outward and promotes pharyngeal airway patency.

The action of any one pharyngeal muscle depends not only on whether other muscles are simultaneously active but also on precise anatomical arrangements at the time of activation. For instance, the action of pharyngeal dilating muscles in promoting airway patency is significantly compromised when the mouth opens, due to the dorsal movement of its ventral attachments. This decreases the length of the genioglossus and geniohyoid muscles, and hence the force developed by a particular level of efferent neural activity is lessened. Similarly, neck flexion changes the position of the hyoid bone. This alters the anatomical relationships of a variety of muscles acting on the hyoid, shifting the resultant vector of their forces in a more caudal direction.

Other evidence suggests that a particular pharyn-

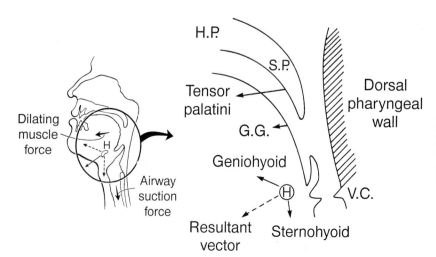

Figure 72–3. A depiction of the action of various muscles on pharyngeal structures. The tensor palatini moves the soft palate (S.P.) ventrally. The genioglossus (G.G.) acts to displace the tongue ventrally. Coactivation of the geniohyoid and sternohyoid act on the hyoid bone (H) to move it ventrally. H.P., hard palate; V.C., vocal cords.

geal muscle may have different mechanical effects on the airway depending on the size of the airway at the time of muscle activation. The superior, middle, and inferior pharyngeal constrictor muscles form the lateral and posterior walls of the pharynx. Activation of the pharyngeal constrictors at relatively high pharyngeal airway volume constricts the airway, but activation at relatively low airway volume dilates the airway.[21] The ability of a given muscle to produce such different mechanical effects may be due to changes in muscle fiber orientation with changes in airway size and shape. In addition, the timing of muscle activation relative to the phase of respiration may play a role in determining the mechanical effects of such activation.[22] The pharyngeal constrictors exhibit phasic activation in expiration under some conditions but become phasically active during inspiration under other conditions.[23–25]

If generally applicable to other pharyngeal muscles, the earlier specific examples may help explain how pharyngeal muscles can play a role in such disparate functions as respiration, deglutition, and phonation. Rather than a separate set of muscles performing one particular function, activation of a given muscle can have diametrically different mechanical effects on the airway depending on what other muscles are simultaneously active, and on precise anatomical arrangements at the time of activation.

Although these concepts appear to be satisfactory in general terms, their application is limited in specific instances. For example, we lack information regarding the mechanical effects of a change in pharyngeal muscle activity on a particular region of the pharyngeal airway. The pharynx is a heterogeneous structure. Fiberoptic observation of the pharyngeal airway in OSA/H patients during sleep indicates that narrowing and closure of the pharynx occur, initially at least, at one specific site.[26] The particular site of obstruction undoubtedly depends on the mechanical factors at that region of the airway. A more useful understanding of the neuromuscular factors controlling airway patency will require knowledge of the regional mechanical effects of pharyngeal muscle activation. Examples of how contraction of individual muscles may enlarge or stiffen particular regions of the pharynx are shown schematically in Figure 72–3. For instance, contraction of the tensor veli palatini is postulated to enhance the stiffness of the most rostral portion of the airway. Similarly, activation of the genioglossus muscle probably increases stiffness in the midregions of the pharynx, whereas, activation of the hyoid muscles could increase the stiffness of the caudal portion of the pharynx and may pull the epiglottis ventrally. These presumed or hypothesized activations, shown schematically in Figure 72–3, lack empirical evidence.

Periodic and Nonperiodic Obstruction of the Pharynx During Sleep

Narrowing of the pharyngeal lumen can produce either periodic or nonperiodic obstruction. The periodic variety is usually associated with periodic pharyngeal occlusion, and the nonperiodic variety frequently constitutes a stable, recurrent hypopneic breath associated with inspiratory flow limitation. A typical polygraphic recording from a patient displaying periodic OSA is shown in Figure 72–4. This tracing shows the well-recognized pattern wherein periods during which airflow is absent are interspersed with somewhat briefer periods during which airflow is present. During the periods of pharyngeal occlusion, oxygen saturation of arterial blood drops progressively and the magnitude of respiratory fluctuations in the esophageal pressure progressively increases. The large burst of submental electromyographic (EMG) activity at the end of the apneic episode is associated with resumption of airflow. That this obstruction lies in the pharynx can be deduced from the transmission of these esophageal pressure fluctuations to the supraglottic space.[16] In nonperiodic airway obstruction, the patient displays a rather stable elevated respiratory resistance associated with sustained arterial oxygen desaturation and repetitive, large inspiratory efforts associated with chin muscle activation.[28–30] An example of such breathing in a symptomatic patient in nonrapid eye movement (NREM) sleep is shown in Figure 72–5. As is the case with periodic occlusion, the location of the obstruction in nonperiodic obstructive hypopnea can be identified as the pharynx by measurement of airflow and supraglottic pressure, which may reveal upper airway resistance exceeding greater than 75 cm H_2O/liter/sec. This tracing also provides insight into a consequence of a collapsible pharyngeal tube—inspiratory flow limitation. Note that despite a progressively larger "driving pressure" (as reflected by abnormally negative esophageal pressure) during an inspiratory effort, airflow remains constant, which indicates increasing resistance during inspiration, presumably resulting from the reduction of the pharyngeal lumen.

THE BALANCE OF PRESSURES CONCEPT

According to the "balance of pressures" concept proposed by Remmers et al.[16] and by Brouillette and Thach,[31] the size of the pharyngeal lumen depends on the balance between outward forces developed by actively contracting muscles and inward forces resulting from subatmospheric intraluminal pressure transmitted into the pharynx from the thoracic cavity during inspiration (Fig. 72–6). In a more general sense, the pharynx is viewed as a collapsible tube and, in the extreme, can be viewed as a Starling resistor. A key step in understanding the behavior of the pharynx in normal and abnormal situations is to separately consider the active forces generated by contracting muscles and the intrinsic mechanical properties of the passive pharynx. Ultimately, the reason the pharynx closes during OSA/H may relate either to abnormal passive mechanics or to disorders of neuromuscular factors, or both. The passive mechanical behavior of the pharynx can be investigated only when neuromuscular influ-

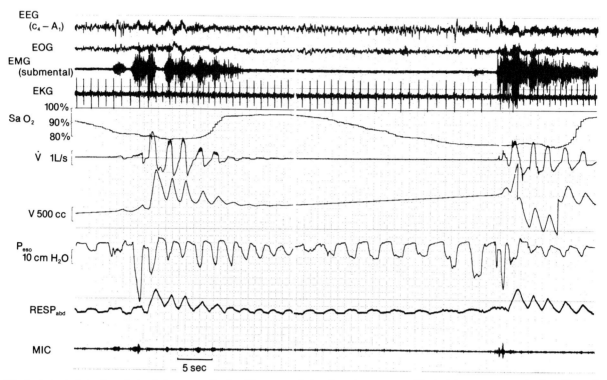

Figure 72–4. A typical tracing derived from a patient with severe obstructive sleep apnea. Bioelectric measurements (top three channels) indicate that the patient is in light sleep between periods of arousals associated with activation of submental electromyogram (EMG). Arterial oxygen saturation (SaO$_2$) decreases periodically and increases after onset of airflow (V̇). Esophageal pressure (P$_{eso}$) and abdominal motion (RESP$_{abd}$) show continuous respiratory efforts. EEG, electroencephalogram; EKG, electrocardiogram; EOG, electro-oculogram; MIC, microphone; V, volume.

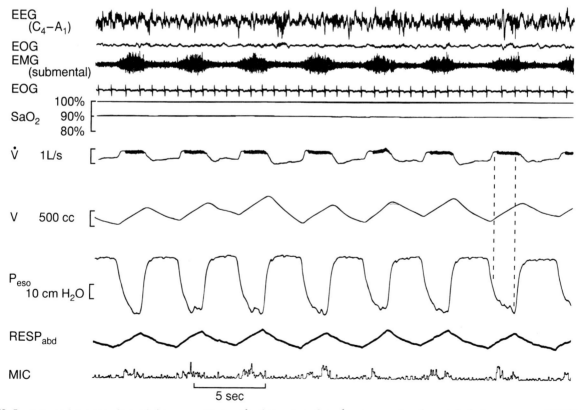

Figure 72–5. A typical tracing derived from a patient with obstructive sleep hypopnea. A submental electromyogram (EMG) indicates rhythmical bursting of pharyngeal inspiratory muscles. SaO$_2$ reveals stable mild hypoxema. Airflow demonstrates flow limitation during inspiration. Despite a progressively larger driving pressure during an inspiratory effort (time between dashed vertical lines), flow remains constant, which indicates increasing resistance during inspiration, presumably resulting from progressive narrowing of the pharyngeal lumen. The thickened tracing at this time results from high-frequency oscillation in airflow caused by snoring. EEG, electroencephalogram; EOG, electro-oculogram; MIC, microphone; P$_{eso}$, esophageal pressure; RESP$_{abd}$, abdominal motion; SaO$_2$, arterial oxygen saturation; V, volume; V̇, airflow.

844

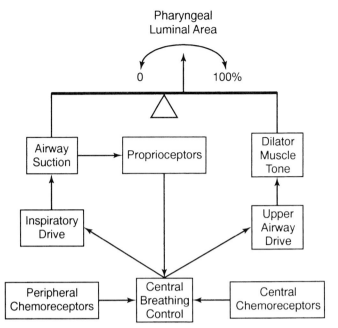

Pharyngeal
Luminal Area

Figure 72–6. Balance of forces that sustain upper airway patency. The two major forces are airway suction pressure and upper airway dilator tone, and these are in turn influenced by other factors.

ences have been suppressed. This can be achieved by inducing complete muscular paralysis under general anesthesia.[32] An alternative approximation to this ideal state is to carry out studies during natural or medicated sleep when a therapeutic level of nasal continuous positive airway pressure (CPAP) is applied because under these circumstances pharyngeal muscles become severely hypotonic.[33–36] In either case, videoendoscopy of the pharynx can be performed and the cross-sectional area can be measured at various levels of nasal airway pressure.

The mechanical features of the passive pharynx can best be described in terms of the relationship between cross-sectional airway area (A) and transmural pressure (P_{tm}). As depicted in Figure 72–7A, transmural

pressure is the difference between intraluminal pressure (P_1) and tissue pressure (P_{ti}): $P_{tm} = P_1 - P_{ti}$. An increase in transmural pressure, caused either by more positive intraluminal pressure or more negative tissue pressure, distends and enlarges the airway area and, conversely, a decrease in transmural pressure, caused either by more negative intraluminal pressure or more positive tissue pressure, narrows the airway.

The overall behavior of the passive pharynx is revealed in a plot of transmural pressure against intraluminal cross-sectional area for each of the four pharyngeal segments, as depicted in Figure 72–7B. Such a plot is referred to as the "tube law" and describes the dependence of cross-sectional area on transmural pressure. The transmural pressure at which area goes to zero is referred to as closing pressure (P_{close}), and the area at which the curve plateaus is referred to as the maximal area. The slope of the line at any point in the relationship ($\Delta A / \Delta P_{tm}$) is referred to as the passive compliance of that particular region of the airway.

STATIC PROPERTIES OF THE PASSIVE PHARYNX

The pressure-area relationship for the velopharynx and oropharynx is shown in Figure 72–8 in anesthetized, paralyzed normal subjects and OSA patients of varying severity.[37] These relationships were measured by viewing the pharyngeal lumen with an endoscope and measuring the cross-sectional area during application of various levels of CPAP to the nasal airway. Of particular importance in interpreting such data is to appreciate that the pressure is transmitted throughout the respiratory system. This means that the pressure-area relationship does not truly describe the tube law for the particular pharyngeal segment. Rather, it describes the intrinsic properties of the pharynx, plus the possible influence of external forces generated by lung volume changes that occur as different airway pressures are applied. Furthermore, luminal pressure does not equal transmural pressure because extramural

Figure 72–7. The concept of transmural pressure (P_{tm}) and a "tube law" of the pharynx are schematized. *A*, P_{tm} is defined as intraluminal pressure (P_1) minus surrounding tissue pressure (P_{ti}). *B*, An increase in P_{tm} results in an increase in the cross-sectional area (A) in accordance with a tube law of the pharynx. The slope of the tube law represents compliance of the pharynx. P_{close}, closing pressure; P_{ti}, tissue pressure.

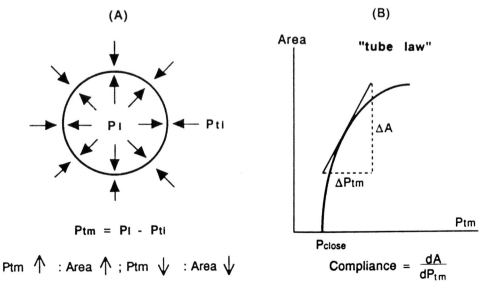

(A)

$$Ptm = Pl - Pti$$

Ptm ↑ : Area ↑ ; Ptm ↓ : Area ↓

(B)

Area   "tube law"

$$Compliance = \frac{dA}{dP_{tm}}$$

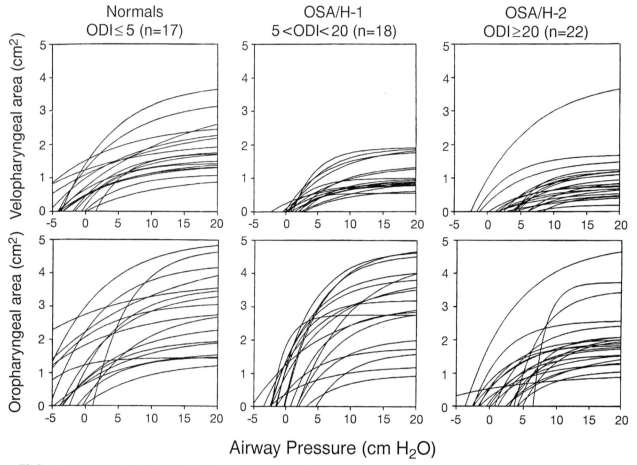

Figure 72–8. Pressure-area relationship at the velopharynx and oropharynx in anesthetized, paralyzed normal subjects and obstructive sleep apnea/hypopnea (OSA/H) patients. Each curve represents the static pressure-area relationship of the passive pharynx of one subject. ODI, oxygen desaturation index (number of oxygen desaturations exceeding 4% from baseline). Group 1 OSA/H patients with an ODI > 5 and < 20. Group 2 OSA/H patients with an ODI ≥ 20. The curves were obtained by fitting measured pressure-area data to an exponential function. Note that velopharyngeal curves of patients with OSA/H lie below and to the right of curves for normal subjects. (From Isono S, Remmers JE, Tanaka A, et al. Anatomy of pharynx in patients with obstructive sleep apnea and in normal subjects. J Appl Physiol. 1997;82:1319–1326.)

pressure, that is, tissue pressure, is not readily measurable and may not be equal to atmospheric pressure. Therefore, the relationship does not describe the pressure-area relationship for the isolated pharynx but, rather, describes the pressure-area relationship for the pharynx plus all surrounding structures.

The pressure-area relationship of the velopharynx and oropharynx approximate an exponential (see Fig. 72–8). As pressure decreases from relatively high to lower levels, the passive compliance of the pharynx, that is, the slope of the curve, continually increases until airway closure occurs. This means that the more narrow the pharyngeal airway becomes, the more susceptible it is to yet further closure. This striking feature is extremely important for the behavior of the pharyngeal airway under a variety of circumstances. Thus, as intraluminal pressure becomes more negative during inspiration, the compliance increases so that a greater reduction in area occurs with further decreases in pressure. This clearly sets the stage for a progressive narrowing of the pharynx under dynamic conditions. As can be seen from the data for normals and OSA/H patients (see Fig. 72–8), closing pressure of the velopha-

rynx, or the pressure at which airway closure occurs, is somewhat higher than that for the oropharynx—reflecting greater collapsibility.

FACTORS INFLUENCING THE STATIC PROPERTIES OF THE PASSIVE PHARYNGEAL AIRWAY

As listed in Table 72–1, a number of mechanical influences impinge on the passive pharyngeal airway to determine whether or not it is fully open, closed, or narrowed. These factors interact with the tube law of the pharynx to determine, at any time, the cross-sectional area of various segments of the pharynx. As indicated in Table 72–1, these factors can be classified as static or dynamic influences.

Static Factors Influencing Behavior of the Passive Pharyngeal Airway

Surface Adhesive Forces

Clinical observation, as well as studies in anesthetized animals, indicates that surface adhesive forces

Table 72–1. MECHANICAL INFLUENCES ON THE PASSIVE PHARYNGEAL AIRWAY

A. Static factors
  1. Surface adhesive forces
  2. Neck and jaw posture
  3. Tracheal tug
  4. Gravity
B. Dynamic factors
  1. Upstream resistance in the nasal airway and pharynx
  2. Bernoulli effect
  3. Dynamic compliance

between opposed luminal surfaces may contribute to airway closure. These same forces may also make restoration of patency more difficult. As the pharyngeal airway narrows, the mucous film lining the surface thickens and further narrows the airway.[38] In addition, a decrease in the size of the pharyngeal lumen means that surface forces exert greater pressure, which would tend to further diminish airway size. Surface adhesive forces may also increase the pressure required to open the closed airway (opening pressure). In support of this concept, the pressure needed to open an already closed airway in patients with OSA/H with positive nasal airway pressure is greater than the closing pressure.[33] Similar findings have been reported in sleeping infants.[39, 40] However, other explanations for these findings need to be considered, such as alterations in pharyngeal geometry after closure that make the closed airway more difficult to open.

Neck and Jaw Posture

A number of studies have indicated that neck flexion tends to close the airway and neck extension acts to open it.[7, 41] This would appear to be particularly true in infants or in obese people. Whether the action is principally on the hypopharynx or on the oropharynx and velopharynx has not been documented, but it seems likely that at least the caudal three segments of the pharynx are narrowed as the neck is flexed.

Jaw posture has also been documented to influence the size of the passive pharyngeal airway. Opening the jaw slightly may actually increase the size of the pharynx by providing more room in the oral cavity for the external portion of the tongue. This may be particularly important if the tongue is large relative to the oral cavity. However, progressive opening of the jaw leads to dorsal movement of the genu of the mandible—that is, the genu moves closer to the dorsal pharyngeal wall because the mandibular condyle of the temporomandibular joint is considerably rostral to the plane of the mandible (Fig. 72–9). This dorsal movement of the genu of the mandible with mouth opening causes the tongue and hyoid apparatus to move dorsally as well, and thereby narrow the pharynx.

Tracheal Tug

Increases in lung volume appear to increase the pharyngeal cross-sectional area and reduce the closing pressure (make it more negative) and compliance of the pharynx.[42–45] This action is probably exerted through axial forces in the trachea—so-called tracheal tug. As lung volume increases, there tends to be a caudal displacement of the intrathoracic trachea which, in turn, exerts caudally directed forces on the pharynx. The development of passive axial tension in the pharyngeal wall tends to open the pharynx when it is at relatively low volumes or small cross-sectional areas.

Gravity

In some situations, gravity can have a major influence on the pressure-area relationship of the passive pharynx. This would appear to be most prominent when there is a coexisting accumulation of submandibular fat.[46] When the mouth is closed, the facial bones and teeth from a rigid container with the only movable portion being the submandibular soft tissues. In other words, the submandibular soft tissues effectively become a diaphragm such that increases in volume of the pharyngeal conduit must be associated with outward movement of the submandibular soft tissues. Conversely, if inward forces are generated in the submandibular soft tissue area, and the mouth is closed, the pharyngeal airway tends to decrease in volume. Consequently, in the supine posture, the action of gravity on submandibular fat tends to narrow the pharyngeal lumen by increasing tissue pressure. Accordingly, for

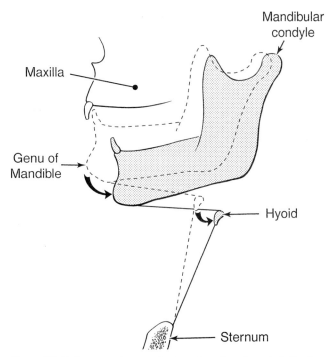

Figure 72–9. Jaw opening results in a dorsal and ventral displacement of the genu of the mandible, as well as the floating hyoid bone, through the many hyomandibular attachments. As a result, the ventral pharyngeal wall structures such as the tongue and epiglottis move inward, decreasing pharyngeal airway size. Neck flexion would have a similar effect on hyoid and ventral pharyngeal position even without a change in the relationship between the mandible and the maxilla.

the same intraluminal pressure, transmural pressure is reduced, and thereby the pharyngeal airway is narrowed.

Dynamic Factors Influencing Behavior of the Passive Pharyngeal Airway

Upstream Resistance Within the Nasal Airway

Airflow is generated through the nose owing to a pressure drop between the nasal inlet and the nasopharynx. This driving pressure for airflow is generated by a reduction in nasopharyngeal pressure owing to active contraction of the diaphragm and other inspiratory pump muscles. Even under normal circumstances the nose has a relatively high resistance and the flow regimen is turbulent. This is, of course, enhanced in situations where the nasal airway is narrowed by mucosal congestion. Accordingly, the increase in nasal resistance that occurs during inspiration is alinear relative to inspiratory airflow such that greater inspiratory airflow leads to disproportionately more negative nasopharyngeal intraluminal pressure. Nasopharyngeal pressure is, effectively, the equivalent of intraluminal pressure for the pharynx if the resistance within the pharynx is relatively low. Accordingly, it can be seen that nasal resistance exerts a direct and striking influence on luminal pressure and, thereby, on transmural pharyngeal pressure. In other words, all other things being equal, increases in nasal resistance will produce corresponding development of greater negative pharyngeal intraluminal pressure and reduced pharyngeal cross-sectional area. The extent to which the lumen narrows depends on regional airway compliance, that is, the relative compliance of each segment.

Upstream Resistance Within the Pharynx

Nasal resistance is that which is most "upstream" in the respiratory system during inspiration. As is the case with nasal resistance, a high resistance existing within the pharynx is associated with a decrease in intraluminal pressure at more caudal (more "downstream") segments during inspiration. In other words, a narrowing at the velopharyngeal level is associated with a further decline in intraluminal pressure during inspiration at sites caudal to the velopharynx, thereby increasing the tendency for closure in the oropharynx and hypopharynx.

Bernoulli Effect

Two types of physical phenomena cause a reduction in intraluminal pressure as gas flows through a tube. These are (1) loss of energy by work done in overcoming flow-resistance aspects of the airway and (2) the Bernoulli effect—that is, the conversion of energy from static to kinetic caused by an increase in the velocity of airflow when the lumen size decreases. The first phenomenon relates to upstream resistance to airflow.

Whenever gas flows through a resistance, potential energy is dissipated in overcoming friction and, consequently, intraluminal pressure decreases. The second phenomenon relates to acceleration of gas as it flows through a narrowed segment of a tube. As mentioned before, this increases kinetic energy of the airstream and hence decreases potential energy—that is, intraluminal pressure. Both phenomena contribute to decreasing pharyngeal intraluminal pressure during inspiration; therefore, both tend to narrow the pharynx during inspiration.

To generate an inspiratory flow through the high-resistance air passage presented by the nose, pharyngeal pressure must fall below pressure at the nares. Because nasal resistance to airflow is highly dependent on flow rate, this pressure drop increases in a highly alinear fashion as flow rate increases. Therefore, nasal resistance greatly contributes to the development of negative intraluminal pressure in the absence of inspiratory flow limitation. However, once inspiratory flow limitation is present, the relatively rigid nasal passage does not contribute to further pressure drop across the collapsible airway segment. By contrast, progressive narrowing of the pharyngeal upstream segment would produce a progressively more negative intraluminal pressure caudal to the site of narrowing, regardless of inspiratory flow limitation, because of increased viscous energy losses in the narrowed region. If the cross-sectional area of the pharyngeal lumen decreases in some regions, the velocity of airflow will be elevated in these regions. This increase in airflow velocity implies an increase in kinetic energy of the airstream and, hence, a decrease in lateral wall pressure. This reduction in lateral wall pressure allows further narrowing of the tube according to the tube law of the pharynx.

Therefore, a reduction in intraluminal pressure is caused by viscous loss of energy upstream of the narrowed segment and an increase in kinetic energy at the stenosis in a most cranial segment. Another source of energy dissipation due to turbulent flow is caused by a rostral, or upstream stenotic, segment reducing luminal pressure in a more caudal, or downstream, segment. This means that the caudal segment of the pharynx tends to narrow during inspiration even though the compliance of the segment is less than that of the cranial segment. Consequently, geometry of the pharynx and intersegmental interdependence are important factors in determining intraluminal pressure distribution along the pharynx.

Dynamic Compliance

During inspiration, the decrease in intraluminal pressure at any point in the pharynx interacts with the dynamic compliance of that segment of the pharynx.[37] If intraluminal pressure at the beginning of inspiration is a value that lies on the steep portion of the pressure-area relationship, the passive pharynx narrows as intraluminal pressure decreases during inspiration. The degree to which pharyngeal cross-sectional area decreases depends on the dynamic compliance of the pharynx.

This mechanical property also influences the likelihood of yet further airway collapse. Specifically, narrowing during inspiration due to a decrease in intraluminal pressure might decrease the area significantly which, in turn, increases the velocity of gas flowing through that segment. This results in further reductions in intraluminal pressure because of the conversion of static to kinetic energy with decreased lateral wall (or distending) pressure. Such a decline in luminal pressure, in turn, tends to further decrease the area and so on. This sequence of events describes dynamic narrowing of the pharynx, which is typically observed under normal conditions if the pharyngeal muscles are relatively hypotonic.

Starling Resistor Model and Critical Pressure

A model of the pharyngeal airway has been advanced and effectively employed that derives from the analogy of the pharyngeal airway to a Starling resistor.[47, 48] In essence, a *Starling resistor* is a term used to describe a highly collapsible tube having infinite compliance at one transmural pressure and low compliance at a higher or lower transmural pressure. The tube is completely closed at one luminal pressure and completely open at a higher luminal pressure. The luminal pressure at which the airway shifts from fully open to fully closed (i.e., the point of infinite compliance) is determined by the extramular pressure and is referred to as the critical pressure (P_{crit}). Although the pressure-area relationship of the passive velopharynx of normals and patients with OSA/H is extremely steep at values of pressure just above closing pressure, the pharynx does not have an infinite compliance at this pressure. Nonetheless, the Starling resistor model and analysis would appear to be an acceptable approximation of the passive pharynx. However, this approach has also been applied in circumstances when the pharyngeal muscles are active and the degree of their activity might vary during the experimental procedures. As discussed later, the activation of pharyngeal dilators can be expected to decrease the compliance of the pharynx, making the Starling resistor a less valid model. Nonetheless, even when used under these circumstances, the approach appears to provide useful information.[49, 50]

The key method in applying the Starling resistor–P_{crit} analysis is to vary upstream (nasopharyngeal) pressure and monitor changes under conditions of inspiratory flow limitation. The extrapolation of a plot of peak flow vs. pharyngeal pressure provides an estimate of P_{crit} Figure 72–10 shows a P_{crit} determination in an OSA/H patient before and following uvulopalatopharyngoplasty. The decrease in P_{crit} from -2.4 cm H_2O before surgery to -8.6 cm H_2O after surgery indicates that the airway is now more resistant to collapse—that is, it takes a greater negative pressure to achieve complete airway closure.

Of particular interest are the results of a study performed under conditions of genioglossal hypotonia initiated by therapeutic levels of nasal CPAP and evaluat-

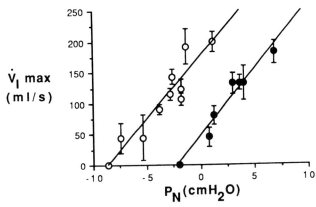

Figure 72–10. Relationship between nose mask pressure (P_N) and maximum inspiratory flow ($\dot{V}_I$ max) in an obstructive sleep apnea/hypopnea (OSA/H) patient before *(closed circles)* and after *(open circles)* uvulopalatopharyngoplasty. Data obtained in an OSA subject on different levels of nasal continuous positive airway pressure during nonrapid eye movement sleep. The x intercept obtained by linear regression of the data is the critical pressure (P_{crit}), the pressure associated with zero flow—that is, airway closure. In this patient, P_{crit} decreased from -2.4 cm H_2O before surgery to -8.6 cm H_2O after surgery. (From Tangel DJ, Mezzanotte WS, White DP. The influence of sleep on tensor palatini EMG and upper airway resistance in normal subjects. J Appl Physiol. 1991;70:2574–2581.)

ing the progressive increase in severity of inspiratory flow limitation and P_{crit} on successive inspiratory efforts when CPAP pressure is reduced.[51] These findings support the concept of progressive airway narrowing of a compromised airway on successive inspiratory efforts.

Factors Modulating Pharyngeal Muscle Activation

Activation of pharyngeal muscles can alter the mechanical characteristics of the passive pharynx detailed earlier. Brainstem motoneurons innervating the pharyngeal muscles receive premotor input from the brainstem respiratory network. Many pharyngeal muscles display spontaneous, phasic activity synchronous with breathing. This is particularly true of the pharyngeal dilator muscles, which enlarge and stiffen the pharynx. The effect of pharyngeal muscle activation on the tube law of the pharynx is shown in Figure 72–11. Under active conditions the pressure-area relationship is shifted upward and to the left. At any given transmural pressure, muscle activation increases area and decreases "effective" compliance. The effect of muscle activation on the tube law is quantitated by the term P_{mus}, the effective pressure exerted by muscle activation that is equivalent to the change in transmural pressure required to yield the equivalent change in area on the passive curve (see Fig. 72–11).

Under certain conditions pharyngeal dilating muscles generally display inspiratory bursting activity together with tonic expiratory activity. Alcohol, sleep deprivation, anesthesia, and sedative-hypnotics suppress respiratory-related pharyngeal muscle activation.[52–59] Additional factors that modulate respiratory-

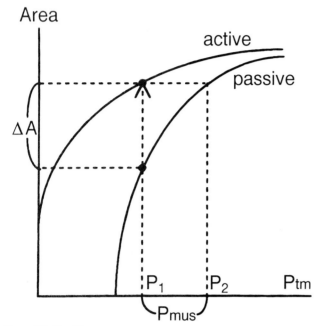

Figure 72-11. The passive curve (i.e., no muscle activation) area can be increased by a rise in transmural pressure (P_{tm}). Such a change occurs with the application of a positive intraluminal pressure, such as with nasal continuous positive airway pressure (CPAP). Contraction of pharyngeal dilators shifts the tube law up and to the left. The muscle contraction increases P_{tm}, and (P_2–P_1) now represents P_{mus} (muscle pressure). A given P_{tm} has identical effects on area change on both the passive and active curves.

related activity of pharyngeal airway motoneurons include proprioceptive feedback, chemical drive, and changes in state (see Fig. 72–6).

Proprioceptive Stimuli

Proprioceptive feedback from thoracic and upper airway receptors can modulate the motor output to pharyngeal muscles. During NREM sleep and general anesthesia in animals, withdrawal of vagally mediated phasic volume feedback by tracheal occlusion during inspiration results in an immediate large augmentation in motor output to many upper airway and chest wall inspiratory pump muscles.[60–62] Neurally mediated upper airway muscle activation also occurs with introduction of subatmospheric pressure into an isolated, sealed upper airway in spontaneously breathing tracheostomized animals.[63–65] Because topical anesthesia of the upper airway inactivates the response, the upper airway receptors mediating this reflex activation are believed to be located superficially in the airway wall.[65, 66] The majority of upper airway respiratory-related afferents appear to be located in the upper trachea and larynx and are carried in the internal branch of the superior laryngeal nerve. Proprioceptive information from the upper airway is also transmitted in the glossopharyngeal and trigeminal nerves.[65, 67] Both intrathoracic and upper airway proprioceptive information may also reduce motor output to the thoracic inspiratory muscles, thereby increasing intraluminal pressure below the site of airway obstruction.[68] The reflex effects

elicited in animals on upper airway and respiratory pump muscles could represent a powerful defense mechanism for the maintenance of upper airway patency during sleep. Ideally, neural reflex activation of pharyngeal muscles by upper airway and thoracic receptors would be initiated by upper airway obstruction and would tend to compensate for airway obstruction by dilating and stiffening the pharynx.

Chemical Stimuli

Respiratory-related pharyngeal muscle activity, which can be absent during quiet breathing, usually appears under hypercapnic or hypoxic conditions.[69–71] It is important to note that these EMG differences are only significant as they relate to their mechanical effects. These electromechanical relationships are largely unexplored, but it appears unlikely that changes in electrical output to upper airway or thoracic pump muscles have a direct, linear relationship to the resulting mechanical changes in the pharyngeal airway.

Recent evidence regarding protrusor and retractor tongue muscles supports the concept that simultaneous activation of "antagonstic" pharyngeal muscles may promote pharyngeal airway patency. Hypercapnia and hypoxia recruit phasic inspiratory activity of not only tongue protrusors but also retractors.[72, 73] Simultaneous activation of these muscles stiffens the pharyngeal airway, making it less susceptible to collapse.

Upper airway and phrenic motoneurons also differ in their response to hypocapnia. Upper airway motoneurons appear to have a higher CO_2 threshold for activation than respiratory pump muscles. With passive hyperventilation in a tracheotomized, vagotomized, anesthetized animal, phasic upper airway motoneuron activity disappears prior to phrenic activity. When the CO_2 level is then allowed to rise, phasic activity first reappears in the phrenic nerve. Thus, cyclical changes in arterial CO_2 around the CO_2 threshold for activation of upper airway motoneuron activity could lead to an imbalance of forces acting on the pharyngeal airway and favor closure.

Changes in State

Perhaps the most convincing evidence demonstrating the overall importance of changes in state on the neuromuscular maintenance of airway patency is that OSA/H is a sleep disorder. That modification of neuromuscular factors by sleep is a normal phenomenon can be inferred from measurements of the supraglottic resistance in normals—that is, resistance from the nares to the region above the glottis. With sleep onset, this resistance rises from the low values (e.g., 1 to 2 cm H_2O/liter/sec) to impressively high values (e.g., 5 to 10 cm H_2O/liter/sec).[74, 75] In heavy snorers, the rise during sleep is even more pronounced, commonly reaching values greater than 50 cm H_2O/liter/sec.[29, 30] Supraglottic airway resistance is abnormally high in OSA/H patients while they are awake and the resistance rises dramatically on going to sleep, reaching infinity with complete airway closure.[13, 74] These obser-

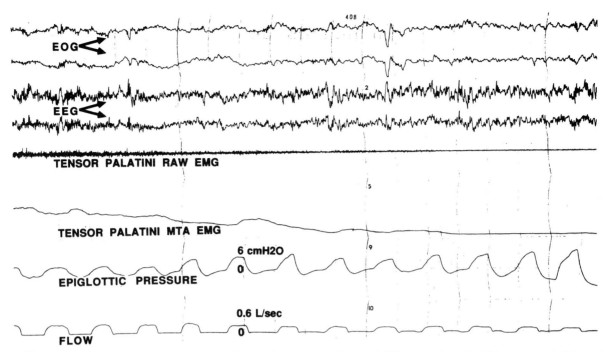

Figure 72-12. Representative airways resistance data during the transition from wakefulness to sleep. A fall in tensor palatini moving time average (MTA) electromyogram (EMG) and associated rise in epiglottic pressure with falling inspiratory flow are shown indicating increased airway resistance. EEG, electroencephalogram; EOG, electro-oculogram. (From Schwartz AR, Schubert N, Rothman W, et al, 1992, Effect of uvulopalatopharyngoplasty on upper airway collapsibility in obstructive sleep apnea, American Review of Respiratory Disease, 145:527–532. Official Journal of the American Thoracic Society. © American Lung Association.)

vations in normal individuals, snorers, and patients with OSA/H indicate that a prompt and reversible change in upper airway caliber occurs with a shift in neural state, and such a behavior is explicable only by a change in neural output to upper airway muscles, which causes a decrease in P_{mus} at one or more sites within the pharyngeal airway. EMG recordings of pharyngeal muscles, such as the genioglossus and tensor palatini, confirm this decrease in pharyngeal muscle activity during the transition from wakefulness to sleep[75, 76] (Fig. 72–12). An even more dramatic reduction in motor output to pharyngeal muscles occurs in a rapid eye movement (REM) sleep, particularly in phasic REM.[77, 78] Although there is striking evidence that sleep compromises the output to pharyngeal dilator muscles, the corresponding effects on inspiratory pump muscles are much less convincing.

Pathogenesis of Pharyngeal Closure

Although there is no doubt that sleep induces a decrease in pharyngeal muscle activity in normal people and in patients with heavy snoring and sleep apnea, the more fundamental question regarding the pathogenesis of OSA/H is whether this decrease in motor output constitutes a key abnormality or whether it occurs against the background of an abnormally narrow passive pharynx, which constitutes the principal pathogenic alteration. Specifically, is the sleep-related decrease in pharyngeal neural activity in patients with OSA/H greater than in normal people? One can hypothesize that a sleep-induced reduction in

pharyngeal muscle activity is the primary abnormality of OSA/H or, alternatively, one can hypothesize that a structural abnormality of the pharynx is the principal pathogenic factor, with the sleep-related decrement in pharyngeal dilator muscle activity playing a permissive role in the development of upper airway closure in OSA/H patients. The former can be referred to as the *neural hypothesis of the pathogenesis of airway occlusion in OSA/H*, and the latter as the *anatomical hypothesis*. Ideally, each hypothesis should be tested critically in a large variety of patients. Pilot studies testing both hypotheses have been reported.

Neural Hypothesis

Does a neural, sleep-related neuromuscular abnormality contribute to OSA/H? There is no evidence at present to indicate the existence of a primary neural abnormality in OSA/H patients, but this may simply reflect our inability to quantify and compare changes from wakefulness to sleep across populations of OSA/H patients and normal subjects. Simple observations lead unequivocally to the conclusion that sleep-induced neuromuscular changes are important in heavy snoring and sleep apnea. This conclusion follows in a straightforward way from the simple observation that neither apnea nor snoring occurs when the patient is awake and that both ensue promptly on sleep onset. Because there is no possibility that anatomical factors can change immediately on going to sleep, one is driven to the conclusion that essential neuromuscular influences dilating the pharyngeal airway are compromised at sleep onset, as shown in Figures 72–12

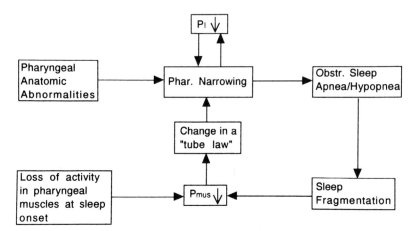

Figure 72–13. A schematic presentation of factors determining pharyngeal narrowing during sleep. P_I, intraluminal pressure; P_{mus}, muscle pressure.

and 72–13. Studies of awake OSA/H patients reveal that the supraglottic resistance is elevated[74] and that the pharyngeal airway lumen is somewhat narrowed.[42, 79, 80] These alterations are apparent despite neural compensations which effectively increase the activity of the genioglossal muscle during wakefulness in patients to a level that is higher than that seen in normals,[81, 82] This indicates that neuromuscular factors during wakefulness play an important compensatory or protective role in increasing P_{mus} of the pharyngeal muscles by shifting the pressure-area relationship of the pharynx, as shown in Figure 72–11. Loss of pharyngeal muscle activity at sleep onset decreases P_{mus} and thereby changes the tube law relationship. This induces pharyngeal narrowing, which becomes more severe as intraluminal pressure falls during inspiration. Whether the level of neuromuscular activation during sleep in OSA/H patients is abnormally reduced as a reflection of a primary abnormality, or reflects a normal sleep-related loss of function, remains a question at issue.

Even if there is no fundamental abnormality of upper airway muscle activation during sleep in OSA/H patients, it is possible that such a reduction may occur secondarily as a result of the disease process. Evidence implicates the nervous system as a secondary contributor in the pathogenesis of OSA/H. These findings reveal a compromise in the response of the genioglossus to increases in the hypercapnic stimulus in normal subjects following sleep deprivation.[57] It can be speculated that the sleep fragmentation associated with OSA/H might produce a similar reduction in P_{mus}, thereby magnifying the effect of sleep on P_{mus}. Such an effect, if operative in patients with OSA/H, can be understood as depicted in Figure 72–13. As described, pharyngeal narrowing caused by anatomical abnormalities interacts with a reduction of P_{mus} caused by sleep onset to initiate sleep apnea and sleep disruption. This, in turn, compromises motor output to pharyngeal muscles, thereby further reducing P_{mus} during sleep. A secondary positive feedback can be postulated whereby the effects of sleep fragmentation further exacerbate the underlying abnormality.

Anatomical Hypothesis

A variety of circumstantial data support the anatomical hypothesis. This principally takes the form of ob-

servations that obstructive sleep apnea is associated with obesity, enlarged tonsils, and facial bony abnormalities.[83–89] Weight loss, tonsillectomy, or correction of the bony abnormalities appears to improve the sleep apnea, indicating that these abnormalities play a role in initiating or perpetuating the disorder. More direct evidence has been supplied by Isono et al.[90] using videoendoscopy in anesthetized, paralyzed patients with sleep-disordered breathing, comparing them with normal individuals (see Fig. 72–8). The patients with sleep-disordered breathing were stratified into two levels depending on their respiratory disturbance index. Both groups of patients with sleep-disordered breathing had a higher closing pressure than did normals. Although the maximum area of the velopharynx was lower in both groups of patients than in the normals, the oropharyngeal area differed significantly from normals only in the more severe sleep-disordered breathing. These results reveal that the anatomy of the velopharynx and oropharynx in patients with sleep-disordered breathing differs from that in age-, weight-, and sex-matched normals. This provides strong support for the anatomical hypothesis, indicating that, independent of neuromuscular factors, structural abnormalities contribute importantly to the pathogenesis of sleep-disordered breathing.

Pharyngeal Muscle Response to Proprioceptive and Chemical Stimuli During Sleep

A key element of the pathogenesis of airway closure in OSA/H is the response of the control system to the airway narrowing or closure during sleep when acting on the background of an underlying anatomical abnormality. As introduced earlier, the system has two methods of responding. One depends on the proprioceptive detection of the negative intrapharyngeal pressure, pharyngeal collapse, or absence of a normal increase in lung volume during inspiration. Such proprioceptively generated afferent messages derived from the lungs or from the pharynx or larynx might initiate compensatory reflexes activating pharyngeal dilator muscles and, perhaps, suppressing the activity of inspiratory pump muscles as described above. However, while operant during wakefulness, these reflexes appear to be suppressed during sleep in normal human beings, and they contribute little to enhance the activity of pharyngeal dilator muscles during sleep in patients with OSA/H.[66, 91–95] In other words, the first line of defense in maintaining a patent pharyngeal airway appears to be lost during sleep. This constitutes a fundamental alteration, one that has profound consequences for the pathogenesis of snoring and OSA/H. However, it is important to note that conflicting, albeit circumstantial, evidence suggests that mechanically induced reflex activation of upper airway muscles may be operant in sleeping human beings. Topical anesthesia of the upper airway, which would reduce proprioceptive afferent feedback, can induce sleep-disordered breathing in normal subjects.[96]

The slower, second line of defense for the control system's response to airway occlusion during sleep is provided by chemical feedback mediated by peripheral and, to some extent, central chemoreceptors. These reflexes appear to be preserved during sleep in normals and, while perhaps somewhat suppressed in patients, nonetheless appear to be operative. After a delay of 6 to 10 sec for circulation of blood to the peripheral chemoreceptors, the central respiratory controller is progressively activated by hypoxia and, to some extent, hypercapnia, present at the peripheral chemoreceptor. This leads to an increase in activation of both pump and pharyngeal airway muscles. If the increase in P_{mus} is less than the decrease in luminal pressure, the airway remains closed. In typical OSA/H, this situation applies during the apneas. Only on arousal with intense activation of the pharyngeal muscles does P_{mus} rise abruptly and exceed the subatmospheric value of luminal pressure.[97]

Interaction of Passive and Active Forces on Pharyngeal Airway Closure During Sleep—A Schematic Model

The overall balance of airway pressure and P_{mus} generated by upper airway muscles for normals and patients with sleep apnea is depicted in Figure 72–14, where a seesaw depicts the balance between luminal pressure and pharyngeal P_{mus} and the angle of equilibrium indicates the pharyngeal luminal area. The position of the fulcrum is determined by the anatomy of the passive pharynx. In awake normals (Fig. 72–14A), equal values of negative luminal pressure and P_{mus} result in a widely dilated pharyngeal area because the anatomy of the pharyngeal airway favors patency— that is, the fulcrum is to the left of center. In contrast, an anatomical abnormality in patients with OSA/H moves the pivot position of the balance to the right of center (Fig. 72–14B). This means that even in the presence of increased upper airway muscle activity and normal intraluminal airway pressure (as may be present during wakefulness), the pharyngeal airway is still smaller than normal. The effect of sleep on these equilibriums under normal conditions and in OSA/H is shown in Fig. 72–14C and 72–14D. In the former case, sleep is associated with a decrease in pharyngeal luminal area because of a sleep-induced decrease in upper

airway muscle activity and a persistence of subatmospheric luminal pressure during inspiration. On the one hand, this means that the airway narrows compared to normal but does not narrow severely. On the other hand, the patient with OSA/H sustains a severe narrowing and closure on entering sleep because sleep-induced loss of upper airway activity occurs against the background of an anatomical impairment and the airway narrows more strikingly.

The Site and Patterns of the Passive Pharynx Narrowing

Using endoscopic methods for evaluating the mechanics of the passive pharynx, Morrison et al.[26] examined a population of OSA/H patients and described the distribution of collapsible segments. According to the extent of narrowing at P_{close}, sites of narrowing were defined as primary site (greater than 75% reduction of the area from the control value) or secondary site (25 to 75% reduction). Three pharyngeal segments—the velopharynx (from the level of the hard palate to the free margin of the soft palate), oropharynx (from the free margin of the soft palate to the tip of the epiglottis), and hypopharynx (from the tip of the epiglottis to the vocal cords)—were examined. In 64 patients with OSA, 47 patients (75%) had more than one site of narrowing in the passive pharynx. Primary velopharyngeal narrowing was observed in 81% of these patients, as shown in Figure 72–15, whereas in half of the patients secondary oropharyngeal and hypopharyngeal narrowing was present.

The soft palate is the most common site of narrowing in the pharynx of OSA/H patients.[12, 26, 98, 99] A stable occlusion in this region is accomplished by a dorsal movement of the tongue due to decreasing oropharyngeal pressure during inspiratory effort. As a result of increasing intraluminal pressure above the P_{close} during expiration, the airway opens and a small amount of expiratory flow is sometimes observed. The collapse at the level of the velopharynx is characterized by movement of both the anterior and lateral walls rather than the more rigid posterior wall. The velopharynx usually shrinks in a sphincter-like fashion, as described by Weitzman et al.[100] The center of the anterior wall, which corresponds to the musculature of the uvula, attaches to the posterior wall first during inspiratory narrowing in some cases. Once the nasopharynx is separated into a double lumen, each lumen determines the maximal level of inspiratory flow in each airway. According to the wave speed theory, when the pharynx is equally divided into two lumina, an approximately 30% reduction of the maximum inspiratory flow is predicted compared with a single lumen, assuming that the total area of the pharynx and the compliance are constant.[101, 102]

A posterior movement of the tongue and uvula causes narrowing of the oropharynx. This agrees with data showing that the onset of occlusion is associated with a decrease in activation of tensor veli palatini and genioglossus muscle activity, both changes allowing a

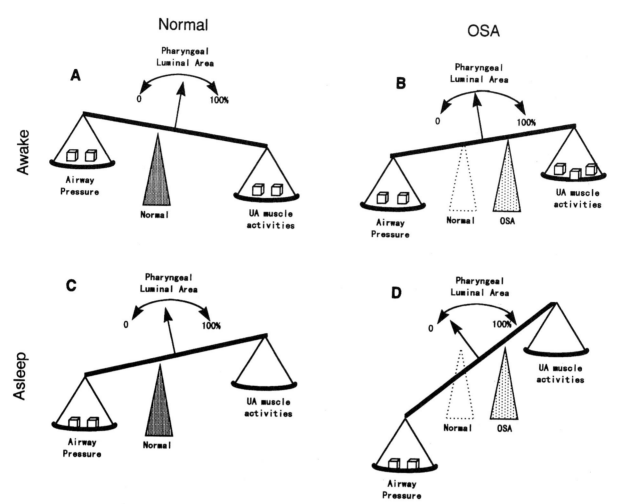

Figure 72–14. Schematic model explaining pharyngeal airway patency, showing upper airway (UA) muscle activities and airway pressure on either side of a fulcrum that represents the intrinsic mechanical properties of the passive pharynx—that is, the anatomy of the pharynx. The fulcrum of sleep apneic subjects *(B and D)* is suggested to be to the right side of normal subjects *(A and C)*. OSA, obstructive sleep apnea. (From Isono S, Remmers JE, Tanaka A, et al. Anatomy of pharynx in patients with obstructive sleep apnea and in normal subjects. J Appl Physiol. 1997;82:1319–1326.)

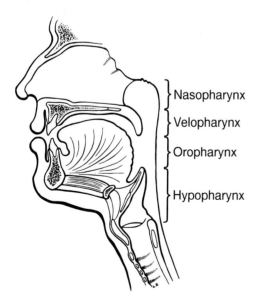

	Primary	Secondary
VP	81%	8%
OP	38%	25%
HP	22%	33%

(64 OSA patients)

Figure 72–15. Observed narrowing of three pharyngeal segments during sleep in 64 obstructive sleep apnea (OSA) patients. Note that a majority of the patients have the primary site at the soft palate and have multiple sites of narrowing. HP, hypopharynx; OP, oropharynx; VP, velopharynx.

posterior movement of anterior soft tissues. Because pressure in the oropharynx decreases during inspiration, occlusion or narrowing of this segment can result from the velopharyngeal occlusion or narrowing, even though compliance of the oropharynx is relatively low. In turn, the tongue can push the soft palate and the epiglottis dorsally, leading to narrowing of the velopharynx and the hypopharynx. Interestingly, pure oropharyngeal occlusion has not been identified yet. Backward movement of the tongue seems to be a key phenomenon for exploration of the interdependence of the pharyngeal segments.

Primary narrowing of the hypopharynx is relatively uncommon in OSA patients, presumably owing to a lesser compliance of this region, compared with that of the other sites. Hypopharyngeal narrowing is usually achieved by posterior movement of the epiglottis, which is subsequently caused by a large negative pressure during inspiration due to upstream stenosis. Once the epiglottis begins to narrow the airway, the airway pressure at the margin of the epiglottis would decrease because of the increased velocity of airflow, and this would promote complete occlusion. Once occlusion has occurred, further inspiratory efforts would tend to maintain rather than release the occlusion. Another observed pattern of epiglottic closure is accomplished by posterior movement of the tongue.

PATHOPHYSIOLOGICAL BASIS FOR TREATMENT OF OBSTRUCTIVE SLEEP APNEA

Current treatments of OSA/H, presented in detail in Chapters 75 through 79 help to illustrate the importance of the above pathophysiological mechanisms underlying OSA/H. In general, most treatments attempt to (1) raise pharyngeal pressure above P_{close}, (2) change the tube law of the passive pharynx, or (3) increase pharyngeal airway muscle activity. Nasal CPAP raises intraluminal pressure above P_{close}. Although nasal CPAP suppresses upper airway muscle activity, it maintains airway patency by establishing a positive transmural pressure along the entire pharyngeal airway, functioning as a pneumatic splint.[35] Oral mandibular advancement devices probably prevent pharyngeal airway closure by shifting the tube law of the passive pharynx upward and to the left—that is, stiffening the airway and decreasing P_{close}. Weight loss and surgical procedures such as uvulopalatopharyngoplasty most probably have similar effects on pharyngeal airway mechanics, as both modalities have been shown to decrease P_{crit}.[49, 50] Other treatments of OSA/H are designed to increase pharyngeal muscle activity. They include avoidance before sleep of alcohol and sedative-hypnotics, known suppressants of pharyngeal muscle activation. Use of pharmacological agents that stimulate upper airway muscle activation[27, 53, 103, 104] have not gained wide acceptance, and implantable hypoglossal nerve stimulators[105] are currently under development. Nonetheless, both modalities illustrate the potential importance of upper airway muscle activa-

tion in the pathogenesis of this disorder. These therapeutic approaches attempt to compensate for the loss of pharyngeal muscle activity during sleep by activating the muscles and shifting the tube law, as shown in Figure 72–11.

OBSTRUCTIVE SLEEP APNEA: A HUMAN DISORDER

We conclude this tour of the *whys* and *wheres* of pharyngeal closure in human beings by posing a quasi-philosophical question: Why does pharyngeal closure occur in sleeping human beings, whereas other mammals appear to exhibit a striking resistance to this? For instance, an extremely obese porcine animal model exhibits hypercapnia and sustained hypoventilation during sleep but does not sustain total pharyngeal airway closure.[106] Only the English bulldog, with its extreme brachiocephalic bony and soft tissue abnormalities, sustains sleep apnea and then only during REM sleep.[107]

Phylogenetic considerations suggest to us that three distinctive features of the pharyngeal anatomy in human beings might underlie our extraordinary propensity to develop OSA/H disorders. First, the hyoid bone is an unarticulated or incomplete structure in the human being. This highly important insertional point for a variety of pharyngeal dilator muscles simply floats in the human being, whereas it is a complete arch anchored against posterior structures of the neck in most mammalian species. Second, human beings exhibit a relatively long pharynx in that there is a substantial distance between the tip of the epiglottis and the free margin of the soft palate—in other words, the oropharyngeal segment is relatively long and the tongue constitutes its ventral wall. Last, human beings, in common with other primates, display a sharp, 90-degree bend in the airflow stream at the level of the nasopharynx such that gas inspired into the nose shifts from a dorsal to a caudal direction.

We hypothesize that all three of these anatomical peculiarities of human beings are probably of recent evolutionary origin and relate strikingly to vocalization and the upright posture. All three combine to provide increased vulnerability of the pharynx to severe narrowing or closure. We speculate that these recent structural changes in the pharynx and the associated acquired vulnerability to pharyngeal narrowing were associated with the development of proprioceptive reflexes and behavioral alterations that ensure a widely patent pharyngeal airway during wakefulness. However, it seems likely that these reflexive and compensatory mechanisms are mediated by higher neural structures and that automatic brainstem mechanisms governing control of breathing do not participate alone in their generation. Overall, therefore, we envision a series of proprioceptively generated reflexes ensuring pharyngeal patency which are mediated at higher levels in the brain and which ultimately have expression at the brainstem respiratory controller. However, much higher nervous system functions are likely not to be preserved during NREM or REM sleep, as this is a time when breathing is controlled principally by automatic brainstem mechanisms alone.

Acknowledgment

The authors wish to express their gratitude to Cheryle Trudel and Ellen Rudisill for their assistance in the preparation of this manuscript.

References

1. Bosma J. Deglutition: pharyngeal stage. Physiol Rev. 1957;37:275–300.
2. Doty R. Neural organization of deglutition. In: Cole CF, ed. Handbook of Physiology. Section 6: Alimentary Canal. Vol 4. Washington, DC: American Physiological Society; 1968:1861–1902.
3. Nishino T, Hiraga K. Coordination of swallowing and respiration in unconscious subjects. J Appl Physiol. 1991;70:988–993.
4. Shelton RL Jr, Bosma JF, Sheets BV. Tongue, hyoid and larynx displacement in swallow and phonation. J Appl Physiol. 1960;15:283–288.
5. Shelton RL Jr, Bosma JF. Maintenance of the pharyngeal airway. J Appl Physiol. 1962;17:209–214.
6. Wilson SL, Thach BT, Brouillette RT, et al. Coordination of breathing and swallowing in human infants. J Appl Physiol. 1981;50:851–858.
7. Safar P, Escarraga LA, Chang F. Upper airway obstruction in the unconscious patient. J Appl Physiol. 1959;14:760–764.
8. Gastaut H, Tassinari CA, Duron B. Polygraphic study of the episodic diurnal and nocturnal (hypnic and respiratory) manifestations of the Pickwickian syndrome. Brain Res. 1986;2:167–186.
9. Fouke JM, Teeter JP, Strohl KP. Pressure-volume behaviour of the upper airway. J Appl Physiol. 1986;61:912–918.
10. Strohl KP, Fouke JM. Dilating forces on the upper airway in anaesthetized dogs. J Appl Physiol. 1985;58:452–458.
11. Van Lunteren E, Strohl KP. Striated muscles of the upper airways. In Mathew OP, Sant'Ambrogio G, eds. Respiratory Function of the Upper Airway. New York, NY: Marcel Dekker; 1988:87–123.
12. Launois SH, Feroah TR, Campbell WN, et al. Site of pharyngeal narrowing predicts outcome of surgery for obstructive sleep apnea. Am Rev Respir Dis. 1993;147:71–94.
13. Anch AM, Remmers JE, Sauerland EK, et al. Oropharyngeal patency during waking and sleep in the Pickwickian syndrome: electromyographic activity of the tensor veli palatini. Electromyogr Clin Neurophysiol. 1981;21:317–330.
14. Hairston LE, Sauerland EK. Electromyography of the human palate: discharge patterns of the levator and tensor veli palatini. Electromyogr Clin Neurophysiol. 1981;21:287–297.
15. Launois SH, Remsburg S, Yang WJ, et al. Relationship between velopharyngeal dimensions and palatal EMG during progressive hypercapnia. J Appl Physiol. 1996;80:478–485.
16. Remmers JE, deGroot WJ, Sauerland EK, et al. Pathogenesis of upper airway occlusion during sleep. J Appl Physiol. 1978;44:931–938.
17. Sauerland EK, Harper RM. The human tongue during sleep: electromyographic activity of the genioglossus muscle. Exp Neurol. 1976;51:160–170.
18. Van de Graaff WB, Gottfried SB, Mitra J, et al. Respiratory function of hyoid muscles and hyoid arch. J Appl Physiol. 1984;57:197–214.
19. Roberts JL, Reed WR, Thach BT. Pharyngeal airway-stabilizing function of sternohyoid and sternothyroid muscles in the rabbit. J Appl Physiol. 1984;57:1790–1795.
20. Rothstein RJ, Narce SL, Borowiecki B De, et al. Respiratory-related activity of upper airway muscles in anesthetized rabbit. J Appl Physiol. 1983;55:1830–1836.
21. Kuna ST, Vanoye CR. Mechanical effects of pharyngeal constrictor activation on pharyngeal airway function. J Appl Physiol. 1999;86:411–417.
22. Hudgel DW, Harasick T. Fluctuation in timing of upper airway and chest wall inspiratory muscle activity in obstructive sleep apnea. J Appl Physiol. 1990;69:443–450.
23. Kuna ST, Smickley JS. Superior pharyngeal constrictor activation in obstructive sleep apnea. Am J Respir Crit Care Med. 1997;156:874–880.
24. Kuna ST, Smickley JS, Vanoye CR. Respiratory-related pharyngeal constrictor muscle activity in normal human adults. Am J Respir Crit Care Med. 1997;155:1991–1999.
25. Kuna ST, Vanoye CR. Respiratory-related pharyngeal constrictor muscle activity in decerebrate cats. J Appl Physiol. 1997;83:1588–1594.
26. Morrison DL, Launois SH, Isono S, et al. Pharyngeal narrowing and closing pressures in patients with obstructive sleep apnea. Am Rev Respir Dis. 1993;148:606–611.
27. Remmers JE, Anch AM, deGroot WJ, et al. Oropharyngeal muscle tone in obstructive sleep apnea before and after strychnine. Sleep. 1980;3:447–453.
28. Lugaresi E, Cocagna G, Cirignotta P. Polygraphic and cineradiographic aspects of obstructive apneas occurring during sleep: physiopathological implication. In: Euler C von, Lagercrantz H, eds. Central Nervous Control Mechanisms in Breathing. Oxford, England: Pergamon Press; 1979:495–501.
29. Skatrud JB, Dempsey JA. Airway resistance and respiratory muscle function in snorers during NREM sleep. J Appl Physiol. 1985;59:328–335.
30. Stoohs R, Guilleminault C. Snoring during NREM sleep: respiratory timing, esophageal pressure and EEG arousal. Respir Physiol. 1991;85:151–167.
31. Brouillette RT, Thach BT. A neuromuscular mechanism maintaining extrathoracic airway patency. J Appl Physiol. 1979;46:772–779.
32. Isono S, Morrison DL, Launois SH, et al. Static mechanics of the velopharynx of patients with obstructive sleep apnea. J Appl Physiol. 1993;75:148–154.
33. Issa FG, Sullivan CE. Upper airway closing pressures in snorers. J Appl Physiol. 1984;57:528–535.
34. Issa FG, Sullivan CE. Upper airway closing pressures in obstructive sleep apnea. J Appl Physiol. 1984;57:520–527.
35. Strohl KP, Redline S. Nasal CPAP therapy, upper airway muscle activation, and obstructive sleep apnea. Am Rev Respir Dis. 1986;134:555–558.
36. Sullivan CE, Issa FG, Berthon-Jones M, et al. Reversal of obstructive sleep apnoea by continuous positive airway pressure applied through the nares. Lancet. 1981;1:862–865.
37. Isono S, Feroah TR, Hajduk EA, et al. Interaction of cross-sectional area, driving pressure, and airflow of passive velopharynx. J Appl Physiol. 1997;83:851–859.
38. Reed WR, Roberts JL, Thach BT. Factors influencing regional patency and configuration of the human infant upper airway. J Appl Physiol. 1985;58:635–644.
39. Menon AP, Schefft GL, Thach BT. Frequency and significance of swallowing during prolonged apnea in infants. Am Rev Respir Dis. 1984;130:969–973.
40. Roberts JL, Reed WR, Mathew OP, et al. Assessment of pharyngeal airway stability in normal and micrognathic infants. J Appl Physiol. 1985;58:190–199.
41. Morikawa S, Safar P, DeCarlo J. Influence of the head-jaw position upon upper airway patency. Anesthesiology. 1981;22:265–270.
42. Hoffstein V, Zamel N, Phillipson EA. Lung volume dependence of pharyngeal cross-sectional area in patients with obstructive sleep apnea. Am Rev Dis. 1984;130:175–178.
43. Rowley JA, Permutt S, Willey S, et al. Effect of tracheal and tongue displacement on upper airway airflow dynamics. J Appl Physiol. 1996;80:2171–2178.
44. Thut DC, Schwartz AR, Roach D, et al. Tracheal and neck position influence upper airway airflow dynamics by altering airway length. J Appl Physiol. 1993;75:2084–2090.
45. Van de Graaff WB. Thoracic influence on upper airway patency. J Appl Physiol. 1988;65:2124–2131.
46. Koenig JS, Thach BT. Effects of mass loading on the upper airway. J Appl Physiol. 1988;64:2294–2299.
47. Smith PL, Wise RA, Gold AR, et al. Upper airway pressure-flow relationships in obstructive sleep apnea. J Appl Physiol. 1988;64:789–795.

48. Schwartz AR, Smith PL, Gold AR, et al. Induction of upper airway occlusion in sleeping normal humans. J Appl Physiol. 1988;64:535–542.

49. Schwartz AR, Schubert N, Rothman W, et al. Effect of uvulopalatopharyngoplasty on upper airway collapsibility in obstructive sleep apnea. Am Rev Respir Dis. 1992;145:527–532.

50. Schwartz AR, Gold AR, Schubert N, et al. Effect of weight loss on upper airway collapsibility in obstructive sleep apnea. Am Rev Respir Dis. 1991;144:494–496.

51. Schwartz AR, O'Donnell CP, Alam D, et al. Passive upper airway properties in obstructive sleep apnea. Am J Respir Crit Care Med. 1996;153:A532.

52. Bonora M, Shields GI, Knuth SL, et al. Selective depression by ethanol of upper airway respiratory motor activity in cats. Am Rev Respir Dis. 1984;130:156–161.

53. Bonora M, St John WM, Bledsoe TA. Differential elevation by protriptyline and depression by diazepam of upper airway respiratory motor activity. Am Rev Respir Dis. 1985;131:41–45.

54. Hershensen M, Brouillette RT, Olsen E, et al. The effect of chloral hydrate on genioglossus and diaphragm and diaphragm activity. Pediatr Res. 1984;18:516–519.

55. Hwang JC, St John WM, Barlett D Jr. Afferent pathways for hypoglossal and phrenic responses to changes in upper airway pressure. Respir Physiol. 1984;55:341–354.

56. Krol RC, Knuth SL, Barlett D Jr. Selective reduction of genioglossal muscle activity by alcohol in normal human subjects. Am Rev Respir Dis. 1984;129:247–250.

57. Leiter JC, Knuth SL, Bartlett D Jr. The effect of sleep deprivation on activity of the genioglossus muscle in man. Am Rev Respir Dis. 1985;132:1242–1245.

58. Leiter JC, Knuth SL, Krol RC, et al. The effect of diazepam on genioglossal muscle activity in normal human subjects. Am Rev Respir Dis. 1985;132:216–219.

59. Nishino T, Shirahata M, Yonczawa T, et al. Comparison of changes in the hypoglossal and the phrenic nerve activity in response to increasing depth of anesthesia in cats. Anesthesiology. 1984;60:19–24.

60. Kuna ST. Inhibition of inspiratory upper airway motoneuron activity by phasic feedback. J Appl Physiol. 1986;60:1373–1379.

61. Van Lunteren E, Strohl KP, Parker DM, et al. Phasic volume-related feedback on upper airway muscle activity. J Appl Physiol. 1984;56:730–736.

62. Van Lunteren E, Van de Graaff WB, Parker DM, et al. Nasal and laryngeal reflex responses to negative upper airway pressure. J Appl Physiol. 1984;56:746–752.

63. Mathew OP. Upper airway negative-pressure effects on respiratory activity of upper airway muscles. J Appl Physiol. 1984;56:500–505.

64. Mathew OP, Abu-Osba YK. Thach BT. Genioglossus muscle responses to upper airway pressure changes: afferent pathways. J Appl Physiol. 1982;52:445–450.

65. Mathew OP, Abu-Osba YK, Thach BT. Influence of upper airway pressure changes on genioglossus muscle respiratory activity. J Appl Physiol. 1982;52:438–444.

66. Horner RL, Innes JA, Holden HB, et al. Afferent pathways for pharyngeal dilator reflex to negative pressure in man: a study using upper airway anesthesia. J Physiol (Lond). 1991;436:31–44.

67. Hwang J, St. John WM, Bartlett D Jr. Respiratory-related hypoglossal nerve activity: influence of anesthetics. J Appl Physiol. 1983;55:785–792.

68. Thach BT, Schefft GL, Pickens DL, et al. Influence of upper airway negative pressure reflex on response to airway occlusion in sleeping infants. J Appl Physiol. 1989;67:749–755.

69. Onal E, Lopata M, O'Connor T. Diaphragmatic and genioglossal electromyogram responses to CO_2 rebreathing in humans. J Appl Physiol. 1981;50:1052–1055.

70. Onal E, Lopata M, O'Connor T. Diaphragmatic and genioglossal electromyogram responses to isocapnic hypoxia in humans. Am Rev Respir Dis. 1981;124:215–217.

71. Weiner D, Mitra J, Salamone J, et al. Effect of chemical stimuli on nerves supplying upper airway muscles. J Appl Physiol. 1982;52:530–536.

72. Fregosi RF, Fuller DD. Respiratory-related control of extrinsic tongue muscle activity. Respir Physiol. 1997;110:295–306.

73. Fuller D, Mateika JH, Fregosi RF. Co-activation of tongue pro-

trudor and retractor muscles during chemotherapy stimulation in the rat. J Physiol. 1998;507:265–276.

74. Anch AM, Remmers JE, Bunce H III. Supraglottic airway resistance in normal subjects and patients with occlusive sleep apnea. J Appl Physiol. 1982;53:1158–1163.

75. Tangel DJ, Mezzanotte WS, White DP. The influence of sleep on tensor palatini EMG and upper airway resistance in normal subjects. J Appl Physiol. 1991;70:2574–2581.

76. Tangel DJ, Mezzanotte WS, Sandberg EJ, et al. The influence of sleep on the activity of tonic postural versus inspiratory phasic muscles in normal men. J Appl Physiol. 1992;73:1053–1066.

77. Pack AI. Changes in respiratory motor activity during rapid eye movement sleep. In: Dempsey JA, Pack AI, eds. Regulation of Breathing. New York, NY: Marcel Dekker; 1995:983–1010.

78. Wiegand L, Zwillich CW, Wiegand D, et al. Changes in upper airway muscle activation and ventilation during phasic REM sleep in normal men. J Appl Physiol. 1991;71:488–497.

79. Haponik EF, Smith PL, Bohlman ME, et al. Computerized tomography in obstructive sleep apnea: correlation of airway size with physiology during sleep and wakefulness. Am Rev Respir Dis. 1983;127:221–226.

80. Suratt PM, Dee P, Atkinson RL, et al. Respiratory function of tomographic features of the pharyngeal airway in obstructive sleep apnea. Am Rev Respir Dis. 1983;127:487–492.

81. Mezzanotte WS, Tangel DJ, White DP. Waking genioglossal EMG in sleep apnea patients versus normal controls (a neuromuscular compensatory mechanism). J Clin Invest. 1992;89:1571–1579.

82. Suratt PM, McTier RF, Wilhoit SC. Upper airway muscle activation is augmented in patients with obstructive sleep apnea compared with that in normal subjects. Am Rev Respir Dis. 1988;137:889–894.

83. Browman CP, Sampson MG, Yolles SF, et al. Obstructive sleep apnea and body weight. Chest. 1984;85:435–436.

84. Guilleminault C, Riley R, Powell N. Obstructive sleep apnea and abnormal cephalometric measurements: implications for treatment. Chest. 1984;86:793–794.

85. Harman EM, Wynne JW, Block AJ. The effect of weight loss on sleep-disordered breathing and oxygen desaturation in morbidly obese men. Chest. 1982;82:291–294.

86. Horner RL, Shea SA, McIvor J, et al. Pharyngeal size and shape during wakefulness and sleep in patients with obstructive sleep apnea. Q J Med. 1989;72:719–735.

87. Leiter JC. Upper airway shape: is it important in the pathogenesis of obstructive sleep apnea? Am J Respir Crit Care Med. 1996;153:894–898.

88. Peiser P, Lavie P, Ovnat A, et al. Sleep apnea syndrome in the morbidly obese as an indication for weight reduction surgery. Ann Surg. 1984;199:112–115.

89. Rivlin J, Hoffstein V, Kalbfleisch J, et al. Upper airway morphology in patients with idiopathic obstructive sleep apnea. Am Rev Respir Dis. 1984;129:355–360.

90. Isono S, Remmers JE, Tanaka A, et al. Anatomy of pharynx in patients with obstructive sleep apnea and in normal subjects. J Appl Physiol. 1997;82:1319–1326.

91. Horner RL, Innes JA, Murphy K, et al. Evidence for reflex upper airway dilator muscle activation by sudden negative airway pressure in man. J Physiol (Lond). 1991;436:15–29.

92. Kuna ST, Smickley JS. Response of genioglossus muscle activity to nasal airway occlusion in normal sleeping adults. J Appl Physiol. 1986;64:347–353.

93. Leiter JC, Daubenspeck JA. Selective reflex activation of the genioglossus in humans. J Appl Physiol. 1990;68:2581–2587.

94. Van de Touw T, O'Neill N, Brancatsiano A, et al. Respiratory-related activity of soft palate muscles: augmentation by negative upper airway pressure. J Appl Physiol. 1994;76:424–431.

95. Wheatley JR, Mezzanotte WS, Tangel DJ, et al. Influence of sleep on genioglossal muscle activation by negative pressure in normal men. Am Rev Respir Dis. 1993;148:597–605.

96. McNicholas WT, Coffrey M, McDonnell T, et al. Abnormal respiration during sleep in normal subjects following selective topical oropharyngeal and nasal anesthesia. Am Rev Respir Dis. 1987;135:1316–1319.

97. Issa FG, Sullivan CE. Arousal and breathing responses to airway occlusion in healthy sleeping adults. J Appl Physiol. 1983;55:1113–1119.

98. Hudgel DW. Variable site of airway narrowing among obstructive sleep apnea patients. J Appl Physiol. 1986;61:1403–1409.

99. Hudgel DW. Palate and hypopharynx—sites of inspiratory narrowing of the upper airway during sleep. Am Rev Respir Dis. 1988;138:1542–1547.

100. Weitzman FD, Pollak CP, Borowiecki B, et al. The hypersomnia-sleep apnea syndrome: site and mechanism of upper airway obstruction. In: Guilleminault C, Dement WD, eds. Sleep Apnea Syndromes. New York, NY: Alan R Liss; 1978:235–248.

101. Pedley TJ, Drozeu JM. Aerodynamic theory: Mechanics of breathing, part 1. In: Macklem PT, Mead J, eds. Handbook of Physiology: Respiration. Vol 3. Bethesda, Md: American Physiological Society; 1986:41–54.

102. Wilson TA, Rodarte JR, Butler JP. Wave-speed and viscous flow limitation: mechanics of breathing, part 1. In: Macklem PT, Mead J, eds. Handbook of Physiology: Respiration. Vol 3. Bethesda, Md: American Physiological Society; 1986:55–61.

103. Brownell LG, West P, Sweatman P, et al. Protriptyline in obstructive sleep apnea: a double blind trial. N Engl J Med. 1982;307:1037–1042.

104. Smith PL, Haponik EF, Allen RR, et al. The effect of protriptyline in sleep disordered breathing. Am Rev Respir Dis. 1983;127:8–13.

105. Schwartz AR, Eisele DW, Hari A, et al. Electrical stimulation of the lingual musculature in obstructive sleep apnea. J Appl Physiol. 1996;81:643–652.

106. Tuck SA, Dort JC, Olson ME, et al. Monitoring respiratory function and sleep in the obese Vietnamese pot-bellied pig. J Appl Physiol. 1999;87:444–451.

107. Hendricks JC, Kovalski RJ, Kline LR. Phasic respiratory muscle patterns and sleep-disordered breathing during rapid eye movement sleep in the English bulldog. Am Rev Respir Dis. 1991;144:1112–1120.

Cardiorespiratory Changes in Sleep-Disordered Breathing

J. Woodrow Weiss

Sandrine H. Launois

Amit Anand

Soon after the first clinical descriptions of obstructive sleep apnea (OSA) appeared in the medical literature, early investigators noted that respiratory events during sleep seemed to have both acute and chronic cardiovascular effects. With the use of invasive hemodynamic monitoring, several early reports documented extreme oscillations in systemic and pulmonary artery pressure and heart rate in association with repetitive episodes of apnea, hypoxemia, and sleep disruption.[1, 2] Then, as the clinical syndrome of sleep apnea was further characterized, additional reports were published noting the frequent association of OSA with decompensated right heart failure and systemic hypertension.[3]

As a consequence of these early reports and subsequent clinical experience, there has been considerable interest in the effects of sleep apnea on the cardiovascular system. In the face of well-established prevalence estimates suggesting that sleep apnea affects millions of otherwise healthy men and women,[4] a contribution of sleep apnea to cardiovascular or cerebrovascular complications has tremendous public health implications. At this time, however, although many studies suggest that OSA contributes to a variety of cardiovascular outcomes, definitive proof for most associations is still lacking. Many published studies are flawed by incomplete definitions, failure to identify and control for important variables of interest, and study designs that do not test the stated hypotheses. In view of the extensive clinical evidence suggesting a causal relation between sleep apnea and cardiovascular dysfunction, convincing confirmatory studies are badly needed. Because of these problems, several well-designed clinical and epidemiological studies have been launched that may prove or disprove a causal association of sleep apnea with cardiovascular disease.

In this chapter, we attempt to summarize the evidence both for and against morbid cardiovascular outcomes of OSA. We begin by describing the acute hemodynamic changes that accompany upper airway obstruction during sleep and contrast normal hemodynamic function during sleep with the changes that occur in patients experiencing obstructive apneas. We then describe the data, which suggest a contribution of OSA to acute cardiovascular complications (myocardial infarction [MI], cerebrovascular events, and cardiac arrhythmias), and close with a discussion of the association of sleep apnea with chronic hemodynamic outcomes (systemic and pulmonary hypertension and left ventricular hypertrophy). Throughout this chapter, we include the results of human studies and relevant animal investigations.

VENTILATORY CONSEQUENCES OF OBSTRUCTIVE SLEEP APNEA

Patients with OSA experience brief episodes of asphyxia during sleep, punctuated by periods of hyperventilation; that is, during the period of obstruction, oxygen saturation falls progressively while carbon dioxide level rises. After arousal and resumption of ventilation, the patient typically takes several recovery breaths. In most patients, these breaths restore normal levels of O_2 and CO_2, but, in some patients, gas exchange never recovers completely between obstructive events.

The severity of the gas exchange derangement measured at apnea termination depends on both the length of the apnea and the oxygen stores in the lung at the onset of the obstruction (Figs. 73–1 and 73–2). Oxygen stores are influenced by lung volume and by intrinsic pulmonary disease. Obesity, which decreases the volume of the lung at end expiration, thus may substantially influence oxygen stores at the onset of an apnea. Obese patients and those with pulmonary disease are likely to experience more severe oxygen desaturations than will patients who are thin and without any pulmonary deficit. In patients without any predisposing factor, apneas of 10 to 20 sec are typically associated with decreases in oxygen saturation of 4% and increases in P_{CO_2} of only 3 to 4 mmHg.

Rapid eye movement (REM) sleep, which is often associated with apnea prolongation and also associated

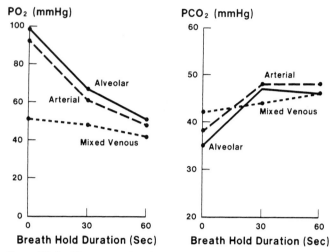

Figure 73–1. Changes in alveolar, arterial, and mixed venous oxygen and carbon dioxide tensions in an anesthetized dog maintained apneic for 60 sec. (From Shepard JW Jr. Gas exchange and hemodynamics during sleep. Med Clin North Am. 1985;69:1243–1264.)

with a decrease in lung volume due to the loss of postural chest wall muscle tone, is another factor that may be associated with more severe oxygen desaturation. In REM sleep, apneas may last up to 60 sec with desaturations below 50% in obese patients or those with severe lung disease. Such decreases in saturation may have marked consequences for the cardiovascular system (see later). Long periods of hypoventilation in REM sleep in such patients may cause PCO_2 to increase above 60 mmHg even if the waking PCO_2 level is near normal.

A final factor that may influence gas exchange during sleep is body position. In the supine posture, obstructions tend to be more complete and desaturations tend to be more severe. Some patients who display minimal desaturations in the lateral position, with SaO_2 remaining at all times greater than 90%, nevertheless display severe desaturations when supine with desaturations below 80%.

When assessing the impact of obstructive apneas on gas exchange, clinicians must remember the curvilinear relation between oxygen saturation and the partial pressure of oxygen in arterial blood (Fig. 73–3). The sigmoid shape of the saturation–partial pressure relation dictates that the same decrease in PO_2 may have markedly different consequences on oxygen saturation depending on the starting PO_2 level; that is, a decrease in PO_2 from 90 to 80 mmHg will decrease oxygen saturation by only 2%, from 97 to 95%. In contrast, a decrease in PO_2 from 50 to 40 mmHg will decrease saturation by almost 10%, from 84 to 75%. Patients who start at a higher PO_2 level are likely to display smaller changes in saturation than those who start at a lower PO_2 level, even when the apnea is the same length. Patients with obesity or underlying lung disease may have normal or near-normal oxygen levels while awake but experience significant decreases with sleep onset. Because of the shape of the oxyhemoglobin dissociation curve, a decrease in saturation with sleep that puts the resting saturation at the steep portion of the curve will amplify the measured gas exchange consequences of the obstructive events.

Although patients with sleep apnea may have profoundly disturbed gas exchange during sleep, the vast majority of patients have normal waking levels of oxygen and carbon dioxide. Sleep apnea alone is likely not sufficient to cause waking hypoventilation. Some patients with sleep disordered breathing do hypoventilate while awake, however, and it seems likely that sleep apnea combined with an abnormal respiratory system (e.g., extreme obesity, chronic obstructive lung disease) may contribute to waking elevations of CO_2 to more than 45 mmHg. The presence of gas exchange abnormalities while awake is significantly associated with right heart failure in patients with sleep apnea (see later).

ACUTE HEMODYNAMIC CONSEQUENCES OF OBSTRUCTIVE SLEEP APNEA

Soon after the clinical entity of sleep apnea was described, investigators began to characterize the acute hemodynamic events that accompany upper airway obstruction during sleep. Numerous recordings have

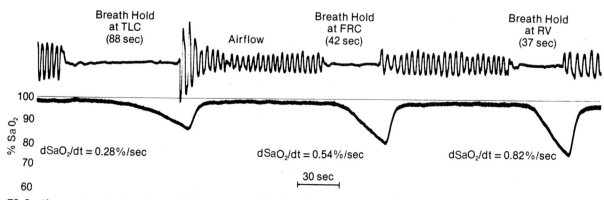

Figure 73–2. Changes in arterial oxyhemoglobin saturation (SaO_2) with maximal breath holds performed by a normal subject in the supine position at total lung capacity (TLC), functional residual capacity (FRC), and residual volume (RV). Note differences in both the extent and the rate of fall of SaO_2. (From Shepard JW Jr. Gas exchange and hemodynamics during sleep. Med Clin North Am. 1985;69:1243–1264.)

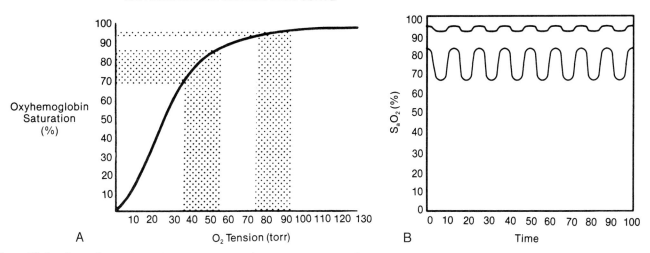

Figure 73–3. The oxyhemoglobin dissociation curve shown in *A* indicates that a 20-mmHg decrease in PaO_2 from a value above 90 mmHg would result in fluctuations in SaO_2 of only several percentage points with periodic breathing *(B)*. In contrast, a 20-mmHg decrease in PaO_2 from an initial value of 55 mmHg would produce an almost identical percentage of reduction in SaO_2. (Modified from Fletcher EC. Sleep, breathing, and oxyhemoglobin saturation in chronic obstructive lung disease. In: Fletcher EC, ed. Abnormalities of Respiration During Sleep. Orlando, Fla: Grune & Stratton; 1986:155–179.)

documented that patients with OSA display oscillations in heart rate, pulmonary and systemic arterial pressure, and cardiac output in association with the apnea-recovery cycle[1, 2, 5, 6] (Fig. 73–4).

These oscillations are made more striking when contrasted with the normal hemodynamic effects of sleep. Considerable data from studies in both animals and human beings indicate that nonrapid eye movement (NREM) sleep is accompanied by a decrease in heart rate and a reduction in systemic arterial pressure.[7–9] Although the magnitude of the decrease is variable, in general, the decrease in both heart rate and pressure is proportional to the depth of sleep.[10] In normal subjects, the decrease in rate and pressure is accompanied by a decrease in muscle sympathetic nerve activity[11]; however, the decrease in sympathetic tone does not imply a decrease in peripheral vascular resistance. In younger normal volunteers, arterial pressure declines during NREM sleep because of a heart rate–mediated decrease in cardiac output, not because of a fall in vascular resistance.[12]

Heart Rate

In patients with OSA, the effects of changes in respiration confound the effects of sleep on heart rate. Initial descriptions of patients with sleep apnea indicated that heart rate typically slows at the end of the obstruction.[13] The oscillations in heart rate were thought to be sufficiently characteristic of sleep apnea that frequency analysis of heart rate during sleep was suggested as a possible diagnostic test for sleep-related obstructions.[14] This heart rate slowing is consistent with the effects of peripheral chemostimulation occurring in the absence of increased ventilation. Hypoxia with increased ventilation is associated with tachycardia, but hypoxia during apnea causes bradycardia.[15] Zwillich et al.[13] were

among the investigators who characterized the heart rate oscillations in patients with sleep apnea who were experiencing upper airway obstructions. These authors compared the heart rate changes in patients with those in normal volunteers performing voluntary breathholds. Tolle et al.[16] quantified the slowing, reporting an 11% decline in heart rate during the apnea compared with during waking.

The nature of the heart rate changes in sleep apnea has been challenged in several studies. For example, Garpestad et al.[17] divided the apnea-recovery cycle into three phases (early apnea, late apnea, and recovery). In this study, heart rate increased progressively from early apnea to late apnea and then increased further after apnea termination; thus, heart rate fluctuated during the apnea-recovery cycle, but the slowest rate occurred at the onset of the apnea, suggesting that chemostimulation did not play an important role. This conflict has yet to be resolved, but some of the discrepancy may relate to differences in measurement techniques and the influence of sleep state. For example, Zwillich et al.[13] compared heart rate at the end of the apnea with the rate during the seconds preceding apnea onset, a period that may include the recovery period of Garpestad et al.[17] In addition, many authors have failed to distinguish REM from NREM sleep. Because desaturations are often more profound during REM and because REM is a state of augmented parasympathetic tone, chemostimulation-mediated bradycardia may be observed more frequently during REM sleep. Substantial sinus pauses may occur, particularly at the end of REM-related apneas.[18]

Arterial Pressure and Cardiac Output

Direct recordings of arterial pressure from patients with OSA show marked surges in pressure typically

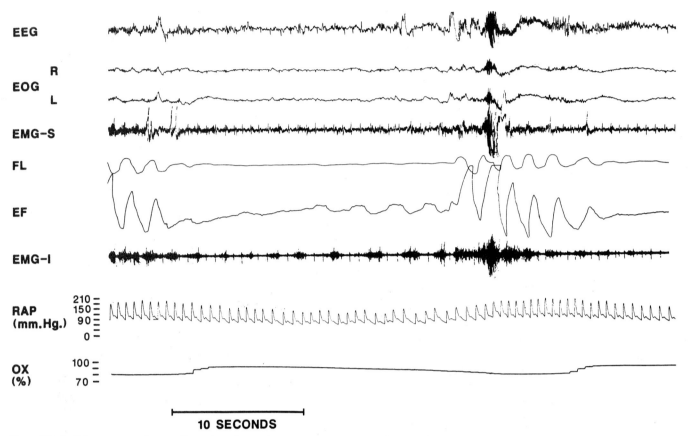

EEG

EOG R
      L

EMG-S

FL

EF

EMG-I

RAP
(mm.Hg.)   210
           150
           90
           0

OX
(%)   100
       70

10 SECONDS

Figure 73–4. Polysomnograph recording of an obstructive event in a patient with sleep apnea. Radial arterial pressure (RAP) recorded from a radial artery catheter shows a marked surge in pressure after termination of the obstructive episode. The peak pressure coincides with nadir of oxygen saturation (OX) measured with an oximetric probe on the ear. EEG, electroencephalograph; EF, respiratory effort measured with a thoracic strain guage; EMG-I, intercostal electromyogram; EMG-S, submental electromyogram; EOG R/L, right and left electro-oculograms; FL, air flow measured by thermistor.

occurring 7 to 10 sec after apnea termination.[5, 6] Arterial pressure is least early in the apnea and increases as the obstruction progresses.[19] The highest pressures of the apnea-recovery cycle occur after the release of upper airway obstruction, coincident with arousal from sleep, resumption of respiration, and the nadir of oxygen saturation. The height of the arterial pressure peak depends, among other factors, on the sleep stage in which the apnea occurs.[20]

The surge in arterial pressure at apnea termination might be due to a sudden increase in cardiac output, an abrupt increase in peripheral vascular resistance, or both. Several studies have examined acute changes in stroke volume associated with obstruction. Garpestad et al.[17] used a nuclear imaging technique to determine left ventricular stroke volume in patients sleeping in a sleep laboratory. These authors reported that stroke volume decreases from early apnea to late apnea, with further reduction at apnea termination. Bonsignore et al.[21] monitored right ventricular stroke volume using an impedance catheter and noted a reduction in stroke volume after the release of upper airway obstruction. Finally, with the use of pulse wave analysis to estimate stroke volume, Escourrou et al.[22] observed that stroke volume falls immediately after apnea termination.

Because heart rate increases as stroke volume de-

creases at end apnea in these studies, the net effect on cardiac output is difficult to predict. In the study by Garpestad et al.,[17] cardiac output fell, but the estimated decrease in stroke volume was less with pulse contour analysis, so Escourrou et al.[22] found that cardiac output increased slightly after the resumption of respiration. Further definition of the cardiac output response depends on the development of monitoring techniques that permit more precise definition of the stroke volume changes.

A decrease or no change in cardiac output at apnea termination would necessitate that vascular resistance increases to account for the surge in arterial pressure. Evidence supporting such an increase comes from the measurement of peripheral sympathetic nerve activity through direct recordings from the peroneal nerve. These recordings indicate that sympathetic activity increases progressively during the apnea, usually falling precipitously after apnea termination.[23] An increase in sympathetic activity might translate into a marked increase in peripheral vascular resistance. Arguing against an increase in vascular resistance as the mechanism for the postapnea pressure increase, however, are reports that atropine blocks the increase in arterial pressure[2] and that suggest heart transplant patients with sleep apnea, who lack the ability to increase heart rate as part of the response to airway occlusion, are unable to increase arterial pressure after termination of the obstruction.[24] These studies suggest that a heart rate–mediated increase in cardiac output is essential to the increase in pressure after obstruction and arousal.

Regardless of the hemodynamic pattern associated with the surge in arterial pressure, it is likely that the hemodynamic events are a consequence of the complex physiological changes that are associated with apnea termination; these include an abrupt increase in lung volume, a sudden change in sleep state, and the nadir of oxygen saturation. Different physiological investigations invoke each of these factors, and the relative contributions of each are as yet uncertain. Ringler et al.[19] studied patients with OSA who were (1) sleeping without intervention and experiencing apneas, (2) sleeping with supplemental oxygen sufficient to ameliorate, but not eliminate, desaturations, and (3) sleeping with the use of nasal continuous positive airway pressure (CPAP) at levels determined to eliminate obstructions while acoustic tones produced brief arousals from sleep. Because supplementary oxygen did not alter the peak arterial pressure after apnea termination, these authors concluded that oxygen desaturation was not necessary to produce the surge in arterial pressure after obstruction. Because acoustic tones sufficient in intensity to disrupt sleep resulted in the same arterial pressure change that occurred after naturally occurring apneas, these authors concluded that arousal from sleep was sufficient to recreate the hemodynamic response to upper airway obstruction during sleep.

Since this study, a number of investigations have examined the conditions leading to the postapnea arterial pressure surge. The picture that emerges is far from clear. Supporting the importance of arousal as a causal factor, Ali et al.[25] reported that nonrespiratory arousals associated with leg movements in a patient with narcolepsy were associated with significant increases in arterial pressure. Similarly, Davies et al.[26] produced tactile arousals in normal individuals during NREM sleep and observed increases in arterial pressure that were proportional to the degree of arousal. Brooks et al.,[27] using a unique animal model of upper airway obstruction during sleep, found that sleep disruption caused by acoustic stimulation raised nocturnal pressure to the same degree as repetitive induced obstructions.

Supporting the importance of chemostimulation as a causal factor is the finding of van den Aardweg and Karemaker,[28] who produced hypoxic breathholds in normal individuals by rebreathing and observed marked elevations of pressure after release of the apnea. Furthermore, Leuenberger et al.[23] recorded sympathetic nervous system activity in patients with sleep apnea during naturally occurring apneas and during apneas in which oxygen supplementation completely abolished desaturations. These authors observed a reduction in the magnitude of the sympathetic response to oxygen supplemented apneas. Morgan et al.[29] measured sympathetic activity during voluntary breathholds in normal volunteers. Although the degree of desaturation was mild in the breathholds unsupplemented with oxygen, oxygen supplementation again reduced the sympathetic responses, causing the authors to suggest that the degree of chemostimulation was augmented by the mild hypercapnia that resulted from the breathhold.

These studies and others suggest that both chemostimulation and sleep disruption likely contribute to the nocturnal oscillations in arterial pressure that occur in patients with sleep apnea. Further definition of the relative importance of these two factors may require more complete characterization of the hemodynamic changes that follow apnea termination. Regardless of the mechanism, these hemodynamic oscillations presumably provide the basis for the cardiovascular events that we review.

ACUTE CARDIOVASCULAR MORBIDITY ASSOCIATED WITH OBSTRUCTIVE SLEEP APNEA

Myocardial Infarction

The extreme nocturnal oscillations in heart rate and arterial pressure observed in patients with OSA make it plausible that sleep apnea contributes to myocardial ischemia. The changes given describe a situation in which peak myocardial oxygen demand (as measured by heart rate and arterial pressure) occurs coincident with the nadir of oxygen desaturation. Current theory indicates that myocardial ischemia also is a consequence of arterial thrombus formation; it may be relevant that physiological evidence suggests increased platelet aggregability in the context of hypoxia further predisposes to myocardial ischemia.[30] Studies of platelet function in patients with sleep apnea and in nonapneic control subjects failed to disclose differences in platelet function while awake, but this study suggested that there might be defective fibrinolysis in patients with apnea.[31] Obviously, these findings must be confirmed.

Despite the physiological plausibility of a relation between sleep apnea to cardiovascular complications and despite numerous clinical anecdotes suggesting a relation between OSA and MI, there is little direct evidence conclusively demonstrating cause-and-effect associations. A number of community-based studies have attempted to relate sleep apnea to myocardial ischemia, but because of the difficulties of identifying individuals with sleep apnea in community-dwelling populations, many of the studies used snoring as a surrogate marker for sleep apnea. In one large cohort reported from Scandinavia, male snorers were found to have an elevated odds ratio for angina pectoris (odds ratio, 2.0; $P < .01$). Such an increased odds ratio might be attributed to other cardiac risk factors associated with sleep apnea, rather than to sleep apnea itself, but this study attempted to correct for many of these potential confounding factors, such as age, body mass index (BMI), and the presence of hypertension.[32] Even after the correction for these variables, snoring conferred an increased risk of angina. Inexplicably, there was no increased risk for angina when women alone were analyzed, suggesting there may be a differential effect of sleep apnea based on gender. Another population-based study was performed in a Mexican American community near Albuquerque, New Mexico.[33] Again, snoring was used as a surrogate for sleep apnea. In this population, snoring conferred an increased odds ratio for MI (1.8), but that ratio was not statistically different than 1. This study also adjusted for standard cardiovascular risk factors. A third community study was reported from Australia.[34] This study was important because home sleep recordings were performed to identify individuals with sleep apnea. After adjustment was made for known risk factors such as age, gender, BMI, smoking, and current alcohol consumption, the odds ratio for coronary disease was 1.4 but the confidence interval included 1.0 (i.e., not statistically significant). Thus, although these studies suggest a small effect of sleep apnea on cardiac ischemia, the magnitude of the effect, if present, is small. Furthermore, these and many other similar cross-sectional prevalence studies are also open to the criticism that the outcome of interest, coronary heart disease, may actually be a risk factor for sleep apnea. This would further confound the results, artificially inflating the risk even after appropriate statistical corrections. Well-designed prospective studies will eliminate this potential source of bias.

In other studies, researchers have attempted to look at the association of sleep apnea with coronary disease through the use of clinical populations. A case-control study examined the occurrence of sleep apnea in women with and without coronary disease.[35] Patients were chosen who had angiographically documented coronary disease. Control subjects without coronary disease were selected from a population registry. Sleep studies were then performed to assess the occurrence of sleep apnea in the two groups. Age, BMI, hypertension, diabetes, and smoking habits were controlled for statistically. In this analysis, sleep apnea (odds ratio, 4.1) conferred approximately the same risk for coronary disease as did hypertension (odds ratio, 3.4). Another case-control study examined the occurrence of apnea in a cohort of patients admitted to the hospital for MI,[36] with a control group chosen from the community. In this study, adjustment also was made for known coronary disease risk factors. The top quartile for apnea index (more than 5.3 apneas/h of sleep) conferred a relative risk for MI of 23.3 compared with the lowest quartile for apnea index. This study can be criticized for the same potential bias cited above, however; MI may increase the risk of sleep apnea, rather than vice versa.

Another way to link sleep apnea to myocardial ischemia is to monitor patients for signs of ischemia during sleep. Koehler et al.[37] took this approach when performing electrocardiographic monitoring for evidence of myocardial ischemia during sleep in 30 patients with and without coronary artery disease.[37] In six subjects (five with coronary artery disease), 85 episodes of nocturnal ischemia were observed. Hanley et al.[38] attempted similar monitoring for silent ischemia in a group of patients with sleep apnea. In this study,

episodes of silent ischemia were common during the night in patients with sleep apnea as measured by ST depression, but interestingly, six of seven patients with ST-T segment abnormalities during sleep had negative exercise studies during the day. Thus, the significance of ST-T segment abnormalities during sleep is uncertain and may occur in the absence of structural coronary artery disease.

Although these studies suggest sleep apnea may contribute to coronary ischemia and MI, the magnitude of this effect remains uncertain. Precise definition of the contribution of sleep apnea to myocardial ischemia awaits further study.

Cerebrovascular Disease

Just as for myocardial ischemia, there are grounds to suspect a contribution of sleep apnea to cerebrovascular disease (see Chapter 90). Cerebral perfusion fluctuates during the apnea-recovery cycle.[39, 40] Furthermore, individual case reports exist suggesting a relation between sleep apnea and cerebrovascular obstruction.[41] Finally, several studies have reported an association of sleep disordered breathing with cerebrovascular occlusion. Although studies exist suggesting an association, compelling evidence is still lacking to determine the magnitude of any increased risk. For example, Dyken et al.[42] considered the prevalence of sleep apnea in a group of patients who had experienced a recent stroke and compared the occurrence in those patients with the prevalence of sleep apnea in a control group without stroke. Sleep apnea was five times as frequent in the group who had an ischemic or a hemorrhagic stroke. In another case-control study of 133 patients after ischemic stroke,[43] even after adjustment for confounding risk factors, habitual snoring conferred an increased risk of stroke (odds ratio, 2.9). These and other studies are biased, however, by the likely contribution of cerebrovascular disease to the development of sleep apnea.

Cardiac Arrhythmias

A number of cardiac arrhythmias have been associated with sleep apnea, both atrial and ventricular. The dramatic changes in arterial pressure, lung volume, and oxygen saturation that occur during the apnea-recovery cycle might be expected to alter left atrial stretch and both atrial and ventricular irritability. Early case series supported an association of sleep apnea with cardiac arrhythmias. For example, one series of 400 patients found cardiac arrhythmias in 48% of patients during overnight recordings, with nonsustained ventricular tachycardia occurring in 8 patients.[44] In addition, 43 of the 400 patients had sinus arrest of 2.5 to 13 sec duration, and 31 had second degree atrioventricular block.

This high prevalence of arrhythmias has not been supported by the results of other series. For example, a smaller series of 23 patients found that only 3 patients had severe bradycardia or heart block, and ventricular arrhythmias decreased from wakefulness to sleep.[45] Flemons et al.[46] reported a series of patients diagnosed at their sleep center who underwent cardiac monitoring. In this study of 173 patients undergoing both polysomnographic and Holter monitoring, sleep apnea was diagnosed in 76 individuals (mean apnea-hypopnea index [AHI], 33 events/h). When individuals diagnosed with sleep apnea were compared with those with AHIs of less than 10 events/h, there was no difference in the frequency of notable atrial or ventricular arrhythmias. In another study, Shepard et al.[47] reported no increase in the frequency of ventricular arrhythmias in 31 male patients with sleep apnea unless oxygen saturation fell below 60% during the obstructions.

Although ventricular arrhythmias seem to be closely related to the degree of desaturation, the cause of bradyarrhythmias in sleep apnea is less certain. Electrophysiological studies in patients with sleep apnea who display prolonged sinus pauses have been reported to be unrevealing,[48] and there is clinical debate as to whether even prolonged episodes of ventricular asystole require electrophysiological intervention because most episodes resolve with effective nasal CPAP therapy.

CHRONIC CARDIOVASCULAR MORBIDITY ASSOCIATED WITH OBSTRUCTIVE SLEEP APNEA

Arterial Hypertension

Early investigators recognized hypertension as a clinical feature of sleep apnea.[3] Until recently, however, the connection between sleep apnea and hypertension was uncertain because of the many confounding factors that are associated with both increased blood pressure and airway obstruction during sleep, such as obesity and alcohol ingestion. There now is a body of physiological and epidemiological evidence that supports a direct contribution of sleep apnea to hypertension.

Some intriguing human studies that suggest a mechanism by which sleep apnea might contribute to hypertension derive from research examining activation of the sympathetic nervous system in patients with sleep apnea. Hedner et al.[49] first noted sympathetic activation in patients experiencing upper airway obstructions and suggested that the sympathetic activation might contribute to increased arterial pressure during the day in the same patients. This connection was strengthened by the demonstration that patients with apnea have augmented sympathetic activity compared with normal volunteers, even while awake[50] (Fig. 73–5). Morgan et al.[51] demonstrated that even a 20-min exposure of nonapneic volunteers to hypoxia combined with mild hypercarbia results in sustained sympathetic activation, suggesting that nocturnal asphyxia, associated with upper airway obstruction, might result in sustained sympathetic activation. Furthermore, Waradekar et al.[52]

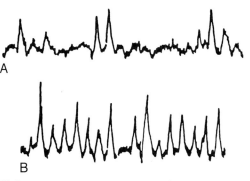

Figure 73–5. Recording of muscle sympathetic nerve activity *(A)* from a normal volunteer and *(B)* from a patient with obstructive sleep apnea before therapy; shown is the high resting sympathetic tone in the patient compared with the normal subject. Recordings are made using microneurography from the peroneal nerve. Subjects were supine, quietly awake. In both subjects, the resting oxygen saturation was more than 96%.

have found that successful treatment with nasal CPAP results in a decline in sympathetic activity. This decline in sympathetic activity is significant because of reports that decreases in arterial pressure occur after CPAP treatment in many patients.[53]

Increased sympathetic activity is not the only possible mechanism by which sleep apnea might contribute to hypertension. Carlson et al.[54] documented that patients with sleep apnea have blunted baroreceptor sensitivity, possibly as a consequence of the repetitive arterial pressure surges that occur during the night. Carlson et al.[55] also found that patients with apnea have faulty endothelium-dependent vasodilation compared with normal control subjects. Finally, patients with sleep apnea have an increased arterial pressure response to transient hypoxic exposure, suggesting that chemoreceptor sensitivity may somehow be altered, possibly further influencing blood pressure.

Two animal models support a connection of sleep apnea to daytime hypertension. Fletcher et al.[56] exposed rats to intermittent hypoxia for 8 h/day and convincingly demonstrated that such intermittent chemostimulation resulted in sustained hypertension in the animals. Another animal model was used to examine the effects on arterial pressure of airway obstructions induced in dogs during sleep.[27] In this model, which mimics the cycle of obstruction and arousal experienced by patients, sleeping occlusions resulted in gradual increases in waking arterial pressure in the animals. Interestingly, sleep disruption induced by acoustic stimuli resulted in nocturnal increases in arterial pressure, similar to those observed with obstructions, but the increase in arterial pressure was not sustained during the nonsleeping hours.

Because of the many risk factors for hypertension that are also associated with sleep apnea, epidemiological investigations that examine the contribution of apnea to elevated arterial pressure have been difficult to perform. A number of early case-control studies that looked at the occurrence of sleep apnea in patients receiving therapy for hypertension failed to account for confounders such as obesity and thus were biased.

Several clinical and population studies have managed to account for many of the more obvious cardiovascular risk factors, however, and many complement the physiological studies. Carlson et al.[57] used multivariate analysis to examine the relative contributions of obesity, age, and sleep apnea to hypertension in a clinic population of patients with apnea. Sleep apnea, defined as more than 30 desaturations in 6 h of sleep, was associated with a relative risk of hypertension of 2.1. The strength of the association of sleep apnea and hypertension is controversial. In an Australian study performed on a community dwelling population screened for sleep apnea with limited home recordings, the odds ratio for hypertension was increased when individuals with OSA were compared with nonsnoring individuals.[34] When the data were adjusted for the possible confounding effects of age, gender, BMI, current alcohol consumption, and smoking, however, the odds ratio fell to a level that was not different from 1.0, suggesting that these other factors accounted for the apparent association of OSA and arterial pressure.

The strongest epidemiological evidence suggesting a causal link between sleep apnea and systemic hypertension was generated by the Wisconsin Sleep Cohort Study.[58] This study examined the prevalence of sleep apnea in a large cohort of state workers in Wisconsin; arterial pressure was monitored with standard cuff inflation as well as 24-h noninvasive monitoring and sleep with overnight polysomnography. Extensive symptom questionnaires are administered with complete assessment of health status. In this population, subjects with an apnea index of more than or equal to five events per hour of sleep had significantly higher blood pressures than did subjects with snoring but without apnea or subjects with neither snoring nor apnea. The effect of sleep disordered breathing on arterial pressure was evident even when the investigators controlled for the effects of weight and gender on the data

Pulmonary Hypertension

Early descriptions of patients with OSA often included clinical features of decompensated right heart failure: edema, hepatomegaly, jugular venous distention, and right ventricular volume overload.[2, 3] Many of these early patients had all of the clinical features of cor pulmonale due to hypoxic lung disease, including erythrocytosis. In view of the repetitive, profound nocturnal desaturations experienced by these patients, it was logical to relate the nocturnal hypoxia to the daytime cardiac decompensation. Subsequently, in an elegant series of studies, Krieger, Weitzenblum, and colleagues[59, 60] showed that approximately 15% of patients with sleep apnea have resting elevations of pulmonary artery pressure. Interestingly, severity of sleep apnea did not correlate with the magnitude of the pulmonary pressure elevation, but waking oxygen level did correlate.

Bradley et al.[61] questioned the relation of sleep apnea and pulmonary hypertension in a review of their patients. These authors suggested that sleep apnea alone is insufficient to produce the clinical syndrome of cor pulmonale and that daytime hypoxia is required for the development of right heart failure in patients with sleep apnea. In this series, all patients with right heart failure had coexisting obstructive lung disease. Other investigators have disputed the requirement for coexisting lung disease, but there are data suggesting that some form of mechanical loading of the respiratory system is necessary, such as obesity or airway disease,[62] sufficient to produce daytime hypoxia.

Some confusion regarding the effect of sleep apnea on the pulmonary circulation has been generated by the distinction between pulmonary hypertension and the clinical syndrome of cor pulmonale. Although the clinical syndrome of cor pulmonale may require daytime hypoxia, there is evidence that sleep apnea alone may cause moderate elevations in pulmonary artery pressures. A study from Australia attempted to clarify this distinction by investigating patients with sleep apnea without coexisting lung disease.[63] With the use of measurement of pulmonary artery pressures noninvasively with an echocardiogram, these authors attempted to assess the effects of nocturnal hypoxia alone on the pulmonary vasculature. In this series, nearly half of the patients with sleep apnea who were studied had pulmonary artery pressures above normal levels. No patients, however, had cor pulmonale, and the height of the pulmonary pressure elevation was generally mild. Thus, it appears that sleep apnea can contribute to pulmonary hypertension but is an unlikely cause of decompensated right heart failure in the absence of coexisting impairment of respiratory function.

Left Ventricular Hypertrophy

Studies suggesting that nocturnal, as well as diurnal, elevations of systemic arterial pressure may increase left ventricular mass have generated interest in the possible role of sleep apnea in left ventricular hypertrophy. Verdecchia et al.[64] studied a population of hypertensive and normotensive individuals with 24-h noninvasive blood pressure recordings. These investigators did not attempt to assess the prevalence of sleep apnea in their study groups. By dividing subjects into those who displayed a normal nocturnal decline of arterial pressure (defined as a decrease of 10% from waking) and those who had no nocturnal decline, these investigators demonstrated that relative increases in arterial pressure at night were an independent risk factor for left ventricular enlargement. Two groups of investigators have attempted to assess the contribution of sleep apnea to left ventricular hypertrophy, hypothesizing that sleep apnea results in repeated elevations in systemic arterial pressure during sleep. These two studies have not resolved the question, however, because they came up with conflicting results—one group identified a contribution of sleep apnea to left ventricular enlargement,[65] and one group found no independent contribution after controlling for appropriate variables.[53] One difficulty in performing such research is identifying suitable control subjects because obesity itself may contribute to left ventricular hypertrophy. Interestingly, the Wisconsin Sleep Cohort Study found a normal decrease in arterial pressure in OSA patients compared with nonapneic individuals using noninvasive ambulatory blood pressure monitors.[58] It thus remains uncertain whether the nocturnal events of sleep apnea further the development of left ventricular hypertrophy independently of daytime elevations of systemic arterial pressure.

SUMMARY

OSA has obvious, at times dramatic, acute hemodynamic consequences. It is attractive to speculate that these acute oscillations in heart rate, arterial pressure, and cardiac output may contribute to acute cardiovascular complications, but the evidence for such a contribution is weak. Many studies are flawed by faulty study design; nevertheless, the physiological events are sufficiently profound that it seems reasonable to caution patients of the potential risk. Evidence for chronic hemodynamic consequences of sleep apnea is more compelling. Physiological and epidemiological data support a contribution of sleep apnea to daytime hypertension, and it seems increasingly evident that sleep apnea may produce mild elevations in pulmonary artery pressure. Patients with sleep apnea and decompensated right heart failure should have additional investigation to identify other causes of pulmonary hypertension. Until there are more data, clinicians should be cautious in justifying therapy of sleep apnea based on the cardiovascular consequences. Nevertheless, patients with severe nocturnal hypoxia likely warrant aggressive treatment, independent of neurocognitive symptoms. Ongoing studies will add substantially to the knowledge of cardiovascular consequences of sleep apnea.

References

1. Coccagna G, Montavani M, Brignani F, et al. Arterial pressure changes during spontaneous sleep in man. Electroencephalogr Clin Neurophysiol. 1971;31:277–281.
2. Tilkian AG, Guilleminault C, Schroeder JS, et al. Hemodynamics in sleep induced apnea. Ann Intern Med. 1976;85:714–719.
3. Guilleminault C, Tilkian A, Dement WC. The sleep apnea syndromes. Annu Rev Med. 1976;27:465–484.
4. Young T, Palta M, Dempsey J, et al. The occurrence of sleep-disordered breathing among middle-aged adults. N Engl J Med. 1993;328:1230–1235.
5. Podzus T, Mayer J, Penzel T, et al. Nocturnal hemodynamics in patients with obstructive sleep apnea. Eur J Respir Dis. 1986;85:714–719.
6. Stoohs R, Guilleminault C. Cardiovascular changes associated with the obstructive sleep apnea syndrome. J Appl Physiol. 1992;72:582–589.
7. Khatri IM, Freis ED. Hemodynamic changes during sleep. J Appl Physiol. 1967;22:867–873.
8. Guazzi M, Zanchetti A. Blood pressure and heart rate during natural sleep of the cat and their regulation by carotid sinus and aortic reflexes. Arch Ital Biol. 1965;103:789–817.
9. Mancia G, Baccelli G, Adams DB, et al. Vasomotor regulation during sleep in the cat. Am J Physiol. 1971;220:1086–1093.
10. Pickering GW, Sleight P, Smyth HS. The relation of arterial pressure to sleep and arousal in man. J Physiol. 1967;191:76P–78P.
11. Somers Vk, Dyken ME, Mark AL, et al. Sympathetic-nerve activity during sleep in normal subjects. N Engl J Med. 1993;328:303–307.
12. Minimasawa K, Tochikubo O, Ishii M. Systemic hemodynamics during sleep in young or middle-aged and elderly patients with essential hypertension. Hypertension. 1994;23:167–173.
13. Zwillich C, Devlin T, White D, et al. Bradycardia during sleep apnea: characteristics and mechanism. J Clin Invest. 1982;69:1286–1292.
14. Guilleminault C, Connolly S, Winkle R, et al. Cyclical variations of the heart rate in sleep apnea syndrome: mechanisms and usefulness of 24h electrocardiography as a screening technique. Lancet. 1984;1:126–131.
15. Daly MD, Hazzeldine JL. The effects of artificially induced hyperventilation on the primary cardiac reflex response to stimulation of the carotid bodies in the dog. J Physiol (Lond). 1963;168:872–879.
16. Tolle FA, Judy WV, Yu P, et al. Reduced stroke volume related to pleural pressure in obstructive sleep apnea. J Appl Physiol. 1983;55:1718–1724.
17. Garpestad E, Katayama H, Parker TA, et al. Stroke volume and cardiac output decrease at termination of obstructive apneas. J Appl Physiol. 1992;73:1743–1748.
18. Imaizumi T. Arrhythmias in sleep apnea. Am Heart J. 1980;100:513–516.
19. Ringler J, Basner RC, Shannon R, et al. Hypoxemia alone does not explain blood pressure elevations after obstructive apneas. J Appl Physiol. 1990;69:2143–2148.
20. Garpestad E, Ringler J, Parker JA, et al. Sleep stage influences the hemodynamic response to obstructive apneas. Am J Respir Crit Care Med. 1995;152:199–203.
21. Bonsignore MR, Marrone O, Romano S, et al. Time course of right ventricular stroke volume and output in obstructive sleep apnea. Am J Respir Crit Care Med. 1994;149:155–159.
22. Escourrou P, Tessier O, Bourgin P. Non-invasive hemodynamics during snoring and sleep apnea. Paper presented at: 3rd International Marburg Symposium on Cardiocirculatory Function During Sleep; 1994; Marburg, Germany.
23. Leuenberger U, Jacob E, Sweer L, et al. Surges of muscle sympathetic nerve activity during obstructive apnea are linked to hypoxemia. J Appl Physiol. 1995;79:581–588.
24. Edwards N, Wilcox I, Keogh A, et al. Hemodynamic responses to obstructive apneas during sleep are attenuated in heart transplant recipients. Am J Respir Crit Care Med. 1997;155:A678.
25. Ali NJ, Davies RJ, Fleetham JA, et al. Periodic movements of the legs during sleep associated with rises in systemic blood pressure. Sleep. 1991;14:163–165.
26. Davies RJ, Belt PJ, Roberts SJ, et al. Arterial blood pressure responses to graded transient arousal from sleep in normal humans. J Appl Physiol. 1993;74:1123–1130.
27. Brooks D, Horner RL, Kozar LF, et al. Obstructive sleep apnea as a cause of systemic hypertension: evidence from a canine model. J Clin Invest. 1997;99:106–119.
28. van den Aardweg JG, Karemaker JM. Repetitive apneas induce periodic hypertension in normal subjects through hypoxia. J Appl Physiol. 1992;72:821–827.
29. Morgan BJ, Denahan T, Ebert TJ. Neurocirculatory consequences of negative intrathoracic pressure vs. asphyxia during voluntary apnea. J Appl Physiol. 1993;74:2969–2975.
30. Kennedy PS, Ware JA, Horak JK, et al. The effect of acute changes in arterial pH and P_{O_2} on platelet aggregation. Microvasc Res. 1981;22:324–330.
31. Rangemark C, Hedner JA, Carlson JT, et al. Platelet function and fibrinolytic activity in hypertensive and normotensive sleep apnea patients. Sleep. 1995;18:188–194.
32. Koskenvuo M, Kaprio J, Partinen M, et al. Snoring as a risk factor for hypertension and angina pectoris. Lancet. 1985;1:893–896.
33. Schmidt-Nowara WW, Coultas DB, Wiggins C, et al. Snoring in a Hispanic-American population: risk factors and association with hypertension and other morbidity. Arch Intern Med. 1990;150:597–601.
34. Olson LG, King MT, Hensley MJ, et al. A community study of snoring and sleep-disordered breathing: health outcomes. Am J Respir Crit Care Med. 1995;152:717–720.

35. Mooe T, Rabben T, Wiklund U, et al. Sleep-disordered breathing in women: occurrence and association with coronary artery disease. Am J Med. 1996;101:251–256.

36. Hung J, Whitford EG, Parsons RW, et al. Association of sleep apnoea with myocardial infarction in men. Lancet. 1990;336:261–264.

37. Koehler U, Dubler H, Glaremin T, et al. Nocturnal myocardial ischemia and cardiac arrhythmia in patients with sleep apnea with and without coronary heart disease. Klin Wochenschr. 1991;69:474–482.

38. Hanley P, Sasson Z, Zuberi N, et al. ST-segment depression during sleep in obstructive sleep apnea. Am J Cardiol. 1993;71:1341–1345.

39. Balfors EM, Franklin KA. Impairment of cerebral perfusion during obstructive sleep apneas. Am J Respir Crit Care Med. 1994;150:1587–1591.

40. Hajak G, Klingelhofer J, Schulz-Varszegi M, et al. Sleep apnea syndrome and cerebral hemodynamics. Chest. 1996;110:670–679.

41. Tikare SK, Chaudhary BA, Bandisode MS. Hypertension and stroke in a young man with obstructive sleep apnea syndrome. Postgrad Med. 1985;78:59–60, 64–66.

42. Dyken ME, Somers VK, Yamada T, et al. Investigating the relationship between stroke and obstructive sleep apnea. Stroke. 1996;27:401–407.

43. Neau JP, Meurice JC, Paquereau J, et al. Habitual snoring as a risk factor for brain infarction. Acta Neurol Scand. 1995;92:63–68.

44. Guilleminault C, Connolly SJ, Winkle RA. Cardiac arrhythmia and conduction disturbances during sleep in 400 patients with sleep apnea syndrome. Am J Cardiol. 1983;52:490–494.

45. Miller WP. Cardiac arrhythmias and conduction disturbances in the sleep apnea syndrome: prevalence and significance. Am J Med. 1982;73:317–321.

46. Flemons WW, Remmers JE, Gillis AM. Sleep apnea and cardiac arrhythmias: is there a relationship? Am Rev Respir Dis. 1993;148:618–621.

47. Shepard JW Jr, Garrison MW, Grither DA, et al. Relationship of ventricular ectopy to oxyhemoglobin desaturation in patients with obstructive sleep apnea. Chest. 1985;88:335–340.

48. Grimm W, Hoffmann J, Menz V, et al. Electrophysiologic evaluation of sinus node function and atrioventricular conduction in patients with prolonged ventricular asystole during obstructive sleep apnea. Am J Cardiol. 1996;77:1310–1314.

49. Hedner J, Ejnell H, Sellgren J, et al. Is high and fluctuating muscle nerve sympathetic activity in the sleep apnoea syndrome of pathogenic importance for the development of hypertension? J Hypertens Suppl. 1998;6:S529–S531.

50. Carlson JT, Hedner J, Elam M, et al. Augmented resting sympathetic activity in awake patients with obstructive sleep apnea. Chest. 1993;103:1763–1768.

51. Morgan BJ, Crabtree DC, Palta M, et al. Combined hypoxia and hypercapnia evokes long-lasting sympathetic activation in humans. J Appl Physiol. 1995;79:205–213.

52. Waradekar NV, Sinoway LI, Zwillich CW, et al. Influence of treatment on muscle sympathetic nerve activity in sleep apnea. Am J Respir Crit Care Med. 1996;153:1333–1338.

53. Davies RJ, Crosby J, Prothero A, et al. Ambulatory blood pressure and left ventricular hypertrophy in subjects with untreated obstructive sleep apnoea and snoring, compared with matched control subjects, and their response to treatment. Clin Sci. 1994;86:417–424.

54. Carlson JT, Hedner JA, Sellgren J, et al. Depressed baroreflex sensitivity in patients with obstructive sleep apnea. Am J Respir Crit Care Med. 1996;154:1490–1496.

55. Carlson JT, Rangemark C, Hedner JA. Attenuated endothelium-dependent vascular relaxation in patients with sleep apnoea. J Hypertens. 1996;14:577–584.

56. Fletcher EC, Lesske J, Behm R, et al. Carotid chemoreceptors, systemic blood pressure, and chronic episodic hypoxia mimicking sleep apnea. J Appl Physiol. 1992;72:1978–1984.

57. Carlson JT, Hedner JA, Ejnell H, et al. High prevalence of hypertension in sleep apnea patients independent of obesity. Am J Respir Crit Care Med. 1994;150:72–77.

58. Hla KM, Young TB, Bidwell T, et al. Sleep apnea and hypertension: a population-based study. Ann Intern Med. 1994;120:382–388.

59. Weitzenblum E, Krieger J, Apprill M, et al. Daytime pulmonary hypertension in patients with obstructive sleep apnea syndrome. Am Rev Respir Dis. 1988;138:345–349.

60. Chaouat A, Weitzenblum E, Krieger J, et al. Pulmonary hemodynamics in the obstructive sleep apnea syndrome: results in 220 consecutive patients. Chest. 1996;109:380–386.

61. Bradley TD, Rutherford R, Lue F, et al. Role of diffuse airway obstruction in the hypercapnia of obstructive sleep apnea. Am Rev Respir Dis. 1986;134:920–924.

62. Leech JA, Onal E, Baer P, et al. Determinants of hypercapnia in occlusive sleep apnea syndrome. Chest. 1987;92:807–813.

63. Sajkov D, Cowie RJ, Thornton AT, et al. Pulmonary hypertension and hypoxemia in obstructive sleep apnea syndrome. Am J Respir Crit Care Med. 1994;149:416–422.

64. Verdecchia P, Schillaci G, Guerrieri M, et al. Circadian blood pressure changes and left ventricular hypertrophy in essential hypertension. Circulation. 1990;81:528–536.

65. Hedner J, Ejnell H, Caidahl K. Left ventricular hypertrophy independent of hypertension in patients with obstructive sleep apnoea. J Hypertens. 1990;8:941–946.

Clinical Features and Evaluation of Obstructive Sleep Apnea-Hypopnea Syndrome

Ali G. Bassiri

Christian Guilleminault

DEFINITIONS

Obstructive sleep apnea (OSA) is characterized by episodes of complete or partial pharyngeal obstruction during sleep. When these apneas and hypopneas are combined with symptoms such as daytime somnolence, the term *obstructive sleep apnea-hypopnea syndrome* (OSAHS) is applied.[1] The term *obstructive sleep apnea syndrome* is also widely used.

Apnea is defined as the cessation of air flow for a minimum of 10 sec. Apneas are usually associated with sleep fragmentation (electroencephalographic arousal) and a 2 to 4% drop in oxygen saturation.[1,2] Although the definition of hypopnea has not been standardized, many centers use a definition of hypopnea that includes a 30 to 50% reduction in airflow for a minimum of 10 sec.[1,2] The lack of consensus regarding the precise definition of *hypopnea* arises from not knowing which aspects of sleep disturbances lead to daytime symptoms and other pathological manifestations—is it the number or duration of the respiratory effort–related arousals (RERAs), or the quality or depth of inter-arousal sleep? In our center, a 50% reduction in airflow must be terminated by an arousal or followed by a minimum 2% reduction in oxygen saturation to be scored as a hypopnea.

OSAHS is defined as daytime sleepiness and an apnea-hypopnea index (AHI) of at least five apneas plus hypopneas per hour of sleep. Thus, OSAHS is defined using two dimensions: sleepiness and the number of obstructive breathing events per hour.[1] See Chapter 79 and Table 79–1 for definitions of OSAHS severity.

The upper airway resistance syndrome (UARS) is a sleep breathing disorder in which there is increased breathing effort during periods of increased upper airway resistance but in the absence of hypopnea or apneas. These patients also present with daytime sleepiness.

EPIDEMIOLOGY

Sleep apnea was first discovered during the polysomnographic monitoring of severely obese patients with the pickwickian syndrome.[3] Subsequent research confirmed that OSAHS can also be seen in obese patients without daytime hypoventilation (hypercapnia) as well as in nonobese patients. Epidemiological studies estimate that 2 to 5% of the population meet the minimal diagnostic criteria,[4–7] and two community-based studies have found that about 2% of women and 4% of men between 30 and 60 years old are affected by OSAHS.[8,9]

MORTALITY

Most studies of OSAHS and mortality rates have been based on sleep clinic study populations and often have been limited by retrospective design, absence of control groups, and the potential for referral bias. Furthermore, the increased prevalence of obesity and hypertension in sleep clinics is likely to affect conclusions related to mortality rates in OSAHS.[10]

The possibility of increased mortality rates in OSAHS was initially raised by studies showing that aggressive treatment with tracheostomy is associated with a lower mortality rate.[11–13] Subsequent studies seem to indicate that mortality rates may be different depending on the age of the patient, being higher in middle-aged men and elderly women.[14–18] Further large-scale prospective trials are needed before definitive conclusions can be made.

PATHOPHYSIOLOGY

OSA is characterized by narrowing at one or more sites along the upper airway. These locations may be at the retropalatal region (area between the soft palate and the posterior pharyngeal wall, including the uvula and the tonsils), the retroglossal region (area between the base of the tongue and the posterior pharyngeal wall), or, less commonly, the hypopharyngeal region (area between the tip of the epiglottis and the laryngeal vestibule).[19–21] Snoring is thought to result from the vibration of soft tissues within the upper airway and usually is the earliest symptom. Obesity may exacerbate the narrowing in part due to the increased adiposity of the neck.[22]

The patency of the upper airway is maintained by muscles, such as the genioglossus, that are phasic inspiratory muscles. This mechanism may be blunted during sleep. In patients with a preexisting narrow upper airway, the pharynx may collapse, resulting in apneas and hypopneas.[23, 24] The resulting apneas and hypopneas may in turn cause pressure fluctuations, which in time lead to pharyngeal muscle damage and hypertrophy, further compromising the airway.[25] The result is a vicious cycle of worsening OSAHS.

In the presence of hypopneas and apneas, there is an increased effort of breathing (as reflected by increasingly negative pleural pressures), and this is believed to lead to subsequent arousals and, hence, fragmented sleep. It is important to note that increased breathing effort may occur during periods of increased upper airway resistance but in the absence of hypopnea or apneas, as is seen in UARS.[26–28] In UARS, the increased airway resistance itself leads to a progressive increase in respiratory effort and subsequent arousal and sleep fragmentation.[26–28] Fragmented sleep and the pathophysiological changes associated with disrupted breathing are thought to account for the symptoms and complications of OSAHS.

CLINICAL SYMPTOMS

The most common symptoms or observations made by a bedpartner are snoring, excessive daytime sleepiness, nocturnal snorting and gasping, and witnessed apneas (Table 74–1).[29, 30] Nocturnal symptoms tend to be more specific for OSAHS than are daytime symptoms; daytime symptoms are usually a result of abnormal sleep regardless of the cause.

Table 74–1. SYMPTOMS OF OBSTRUCTIVE SLEEP APNEA-HYPOPNEA SYNDROME

Nighttime	Daytime
Snoring	Sleepiness
Witnessed apnea	Fatigue
Choking	Morning headaches
Dyspnea	Poor concentration
Restlessness	Decreased libido or impotence
Nocturia	Decreased attention
Diaphoresis	Depression
Reflux	Decreased dexterity
Drooling	Personality changes

Nocturnal Symptoms

Although the absence of reported snoring does not definitely exclude a diagnosis of OSAHS or UARS, virtually all patients snore. Snoring can be extremely loud. A characteristic pattern is that of loud snoring or brief gasps that alternate with episodes of silence typically lasting 20 to 30 sec.[29, 30] Snoring often precedes the complaint of daytime sleepiness,[30] and the intensity increases with weight gain and bedtime alcohol intake. Snoring is not uncommonly a factor in marital discord; in one study, 46% of the patients slept in separate bedrooms from their partners.[30] Interestingly, pregnancy is associated with an increase in snoring due to the upward displacement of the diaphragm and nasopharyngeal edema. Although up to 30% of pregnant women snore, overt OSAHS is uncommon.[31–33]

Apneic episodes are reported by about 75% of bedpartners.[34] The cessation of breathing can cause considerable anxiety, and many bedpartners shake the patient for the fear that breathing may not resume.[29] Respiratory movements can usually be observed during these periods of obstructive apneas, especially in milder cases. In more severe cases, it is not unusual to have an initial period during which there are no observable chest wall movements. Such episodes correspond to *mixed apneas*, which have an initial central component. Apneic episodes are usually terminated by gasps, chokes, snorts, vocalizations, or brief awakenings. Bedpartners will report a sudden cessation of snoring followed by a loud snort and a resumption of snoring. Although some patients awaken with a sensation of having stopped breathing, most are unaware of the apneas or the events leading to their termination. Others, particularly the elderly, remain aware of the frequent awakenings and can actually present with a complaint of insomnia and unrefreshing sleep.[29]

About half the patients with OSAHS report restlessness (tossing and turning) and diaphoresis, usually in the neck and upper chest area.[29, 30, 35] These symptoms are probably related to increased breathing efforts during periods of upper airway obstruction. Bedpartners readily attest to excessive body movements because these can at times be violent. Patients without bedpartners usually notice disheveled bedsheets in the morning.

A sensation of choking or dyspnea that interrupts sleep is reported in 18 to 31% of patients.[29, 30, 35, 36] During episodes of upper airway obstruction, respiratory efforts tend to decrease intrathoracic pressure (Müller maneuver) and lead to an increase in venous return from the extremities. This increase in venous return has been documented to increase the pulmonary capillary wedge pressure[37] and may contribute to the sensation of dyspnea. Because nocturnal dyspnea also may occur in congestive heart failure, it is important to inquire about other typical symptoms to distinguish heart failure from OSAHS.[38] It is not unusual for the two disorders to coexist. In our experience, dyspnea (or choking sensation) from OSAHS usually resolves quickly on awakening.

Esophageal reflux is another frequently observed

symptom among patients with OSAHS. Reflux results from increased gastric pressures during periods of upper airway obstruction and a subsequent increase in breathing effort and abdominal pressure.[29] Patients report awakening with heartburn, and in one case, reflux led to laryngospasm.[39]

Nocturia is a relatively common symptom.[30] In our experience, 28% of patients report four to seven nightly trips to the bathroom. Rarely, an adult patient may complain of enuresis. Increased intraabdominal pressure, confusion associated with arousals, and increased secretion of atrial natriuretic peptide[40] have been postulated to contribute to the cause of nocturia.

About 74% of patients report dry mouth and the need to drink water either in the morning or during the night.[29, 30] Drooling occurs in 36%.[30] These symptoms are most likely the result of mouth breathing, commonly seen in patients with OSAHS.

Daytime Symptoms

Daytime fatigue or sleepiness is the most common complaint of patients with OSAHS.[29, 30, 35, 36] Sleepiness may be subtle, such as midafternoon drowsiness during a group meeting or occasional naps; severe, such as falling asleep while eating or talking; or catastrophic, such as falling asleep while driving. In general, it is not normal to feel sleepy after a meal or while watching television. Such drowsiness usually indicates some degree of sleep deprivation, and OSAHS may be the underlying factor.

It is essential to inquire about sleepiness during the operation of motor vehicles, not only because of the increased risk of accidents[41, 42] but also because the safety of innocent bystanders is involved. The symptoms may be subtle. Some drivers recall an occasional honk from the car behind alerting them to the changing of the traffic light. Others routinely roll down the windows or drink coffee to stay awake. These reports indicate abnormal sleepiness and should never be dismissed. Patients may have difficulty distinguishing sleepiness from fatigue; some of our patients evaluated for chronic fatigue syndrome were eventually diagnosed with OSAHS.

Patients may report clumsiness in tasks requiring dexterity, concentration, attention, memory, or judgment. Such difficulties may be so severe that job performance or even the ability to maintain employment is affected. Such intellectual impairment can be detected on neuropsychological testing.[43] Treatment with nasal continuous positive airway pressure, however, has been shown to improve some of the symptoms, such as depression and fatigue.[44]

Personality changes, such as aggressiveness, irritability, anxiety, or depression, may be observed. As a consequence, family and social life can suffer considerably. Friends and family members may become less inclined to include patients in everyday events and decision making. This alienation may in turn lead to depression in the patient.

In our experience, a third of the patients also report decreased libido or impotence. In fact, patients with primary complaints related to erection and ejaculation seen at the Stanford Sleep Disorders Clinic are more likely to have an underlying diagnosis of OSAHS than any other organic cause.

Morning or nocturnal headaches are reported in about half of patients[30] and often are described as dull and generalized.[29] They usually last 1 to 2 h and may prompt the ingestion of analgesics.[29] A study from a headache clinic found OSAHS to be the main cause of nocturnal or morning headaches.[45] None of these patients had been investigated for OSAHS. Other sleep disorders, such as periodic limb movements, also caused headaches; hence, patients with morning headaches should be asked about sleep habits and symptoms.

Not all symptoms will be observed in any one individual. There also is a notable lack of specificity for many of these symptoms, with significant overlap with other disorders such as depression or hypothyroidism. Careful inquiry about other symptoms can differentiate OSAHS from these disorders.

CLINICAL EXAMINATION

As with any other patient, a complete physical examination is required to assess a patient suspected of having OSAHS. Special attention, however, must be given to the evaluation of body habitus and the upper airway.

Obesity and Neck Circumference

Measurement of height, weight, and the calculation of body mass index ([BMI] weight in kg/height in m^2), as well as the measurement of neck circumference, should be obtained in every patient. Katz et al.[46] found that the mean neck circumference (measured at the superior border of the cricothyroid membrane, with the patient in the upright position) was 43.7 ± 4.5 cm (mean ± SD) in patients with OSAHS and 39.6 ± 4.5 cm in patients without OSAHS ($P = .0001$). Another study found a correlation between neck circumference and the severity of OSAHS.[47] In their morphometric model of OSAHS, Kushida et al.[48] found the cut-off level of 40 cm as having a sensitivity of 61% and a specificity of 93% for OSAHS, regardless of the sex of the patient.

Upper Airway

The purpose of the upper airway examination is to identify structures or abnormalities that potentially narrow the airway and increase its resistance during sleep. The patient should preferably be examined in the seated and supine positions because the latter may provide a relatively better reflection of the anatomy during sleep and frequently aggravates snoring and OSAHS.

The presence of retrognathia and dental overbite should be identified. The craniofacial dysmorphism that leads to OSAHS can involve a delayed growth of the mandible, narrowing the caliber of the upper airway and producing retrognathia.[49] Dental malocclusion and dislocation of the temporomandibular joint during mouth opening may also contribute to an airway predisposed to collapse.

The tongue should be examined for the presence of macroglossia. The uvula and soft palate are assessed for size, length, and height. Edema or erythema of the uvula may indicate repetitive vibration trauma from snoring. A low-lying soft palate and uvula are commonly seen in patients with OSAHS, and the retropalatal area can be a site of occlusion in these patients. Tonsillar hypertrophy and the size of the tonsillar pillars (occasionally referred to as "redundant tissue") should be noted.

A visual estimate of the space between the back of the tongue and the posterior pharyngeal wall should be made because the retroglossal area commonly is a site of airway obstruction during sleep. Accurate visualization of this area, however, may require endoscopy.

Finally, one should inspect the nose for septal deviation, evidence of trauma, or any other abnormality that may lead to nasal obstruction. Although the nasal obstruction alone is rarely the sole cause of OSAHS, it may nevertheless contribute to increased airway resistance.

Kushida et al.[48] described four measurements that characterize the narrow airway: palatal height, maxillary intermolar distance, mandibular intermolar distance, and overjet. Routine visual estimate of these parameters in patients with and without OSAHS will quickly familiarize the examiner with the typical appearance of the narrow upper airway (Table 74–2).

PREDICTIVE VALUE OF CLINICAL EXAMINATION

Hoffstein and Szalai[34] studied 594 patients referred to their sleep laboratory and found that clinical impression alone is not sufficient to identify patients with OSAHS. Subjective impression had a sensitivity of 60% and a specificity of 63%. The positive predictive value for snoring was 49%; bedpartner's observation of apnea, 56%; and nocturnal choking, 44%. Physical examination of the pharynx revealed that 54% of the patients had an abnormal pharynx (bulky or long uvula that failed to elevate from the base of the tongue during phonation, large tonsils, or small and narrow pharyngeal orifice). In contrast, 35% of the patients without OSAHS had an abnormal pharynx. The authors concluded that history and physical examination (including blood pressure and BMI) can predict OSAHS in only about 50% of the patients. Definitive diagnosis requires a sleep study.

LABORATORY EVALUATION

Although hypothyroidism is associated with OSAHS, the role of the routine measurement of thyroid function in patients with OSAHS is not entirely clear.[50, 50a] Winkelman et al.[51] discovered hypothyroidism in 3 of 103 patients (2.9%) with OSAHS versus 1 of 135 control subjects (0.7%). The difference was not significant, and the authors concluded that routine thyroid function test measurements are not indicated in the absence of signs or symptoms of hypothyroidism, unless the patients are in a high-risk group (women older than 60 years). Similarly, there is little to be gained with the routine measurement of lung function in the absence of lung disease.

RISK FACTORS

Certain risk factors can strengthen a clinical suspicion of OSAHS. The strongest risk factors for OSAHS are obesity and age of more than 65 years.[52–61]

Obesity, defined as a BMI of more than 28 kg/m², is present in 60 to 90% of patients with OSAHS. Central obesity measurements such as the hip-to-waist ratio or neck circumference exhibit a better correlation with OSAHS than does BMI, especially in subjects with a BMI of less than 28 kg/m². In one morphometric model, a BMI of at least 25 kg/m² had a sensitivity of 93% and a specificity of 74% for OSAHS.[48]

Male gender has also been shown to be a risk factor. In studies of community-dwelling individuals, the male-to-female ratio for OSAHS is 2 to 3:1, whereas in clinic-based studies, the male-to-female ratio for OSAHS is 10 to 90:1.[52] The risk in females increases with obesity and postmenopausal status.[62–65]

A positive family history increases the risk of OSAHS by twofold to fourfold.[66–68] Studies by Redline et al.[66] and Guilleminault et al.[68] revealed that relatives of OSAHS patients had a 21 to 84% chance of having OSAHS compared with 10 to 12% of the control subjects.

Several studies have shown that OSAHS is exacerbated by alcohol ingestion, especially around bedtime.[69–71] Alcohol ingestion reduces the activity of the genioglossus muscle, which is involved in maintaining

Table 74–2. CLINICAL FEATURES ASSOCIATED WITH OBSTRUCTIVE SLEEP APNEA-HYPOPNEA SYNDROME

Obesity (BMI >28 kg/m²)
Neck circumference >40 cm
Enlarged nasal turbinates
Deviated nasal septum
Narrow mandible
Narrow maxilla
Dental overjet and retrognathia
Cross-bite and dental malocclusion (class 2)
High and narrow hard palate
Elongated and low-lying uvula
Prominent tonsillar pillars
Enlarged tonsils and adenoids
Macroglossia

BMI, body mass index.

the patency of the upper airway. Decreased genioglossal activity can predispose to upper airway collapse and apneas.

Additional potential risk factors include race (with African Americans, Mexican Americans, and Pacific Islanders having a higher risk of OSAHS[72–75]) and disorders such as Marfan's disease, Down's syndrome, and the Pierre-Robin syndrome.[52, 76]

Isolated studies have implicated tobacco use[77] and low vital capacity as independent risk factors of OSAHS.[73, 78]

OSAHS may be aggravated by certain factors such as sedatives, sleep deprivation, and supine posture.[1, 79–81] Respiratory allergies and nasal congestion may also aggravate snoring and OSAHS.[82] All of these factors should be identified during the initial clinical evaluation.

OBSTRUCTIVE SLEEP APNEA-HYPOPNEA SYNDROME AND OTHER MEDICAL DISEASES

Hypertension

It has been suggested that hypertension represents a clinical marker for the presence of OSA. More than 40% of patients with OSAHS are reported to have daytime hypertension, whereas about 30% of middle-aged men with primary hypertension are thought to have occult sleep apnea.[83–88] Although some have questioned the evidence,[89] most researchers believe the relationship between the AHI or respiratory disturbance index (RDI) and blood pressure is well established even when the effects of obesity are accounted for.[90–94] Young et al.[94] studied 1060 men and women 30 to 60 years old who completed an overnight polysomnogram and observed a dose-response relation between RDI and blood pressure, independent of known confounding factors. Furthermore, in many patients, the treatment of OSAHS reduces daytime systemic blood pressure.[95] It therefore is prudent to inquire about symptoms of OSAHS in patients with hypertension.

Pulmonary Disorders

Pulmonary Hypertension

In patients with pulmonary hypertension, it is prudent to eliminate all causes of hypoxemia, including nocturnal hypoxemia. Whether OSAHS causes pulmonary hypertension remains controversial. Most studies have concluded that sleep apnea alone is unlikely to lead to pulmonary hypertension.[96–101] Daytime hypoxia, most commonly due to an underlying lung disease, is usually necessary. A recent study by Sajkov et al.,[101] however, found mild pulmonary hypertension in some patients without lung disease, although the degree of hypertension did not correlate with the severity of apnea. It appears, then, that sleep apnea may cause mild pulmonary hypertension but is not sufficient to

lead to right heart failure.[102] Given these findings, the decision to perform polysomnography in patients with pulmonary hypertension and cor pulmonale should be based on the presence of other characteristic symptoms of OSAHS.

Asthma and COPD

Asthmatic patients have a diurnal variation in airway function, with the lowest air flow at 4 AM. If concomitant OSAHS is present, adequate treatment may improve the control of asthma via unknown mechanisms.[103] Patients with nocturnal or refractory asthma should be questioned about the presence of snoring and witnessed apneas. If clinical suspicion is present, a polysomnogram should be performed. Chronic obstructive pulmonary disease and its relationship with sleep are discussed in Chapter 81.

Cardiac Disorders

Ischemic Heart Disease

Although there are conflicting studies, there is evidence favoring an association between OSAHS and ischemic heart disease, and it may well be that the relation is causal.[104–111] It certainly is worthwhile to inquire about OSAHS in patients whose cardiac symptoms are nocturnal or difficult to control. Nocturnal hypoxemia and autonomic nervous system activity during apnea may well predispose susceptible patients to ischemia. Cardiovascular consequences of OSAHS are discussed in Chapter 73.

Arrhythmia

In one of the only controlled studies, Hoffstein and Mateika[112] prospectively studied 458 patients suspected of having OSAHS. They found a 58% prevalence of arrhythmia in patients with OSAHS (AHI more than 10) versus 42% in nonapneic control subjects during sleep ($P < .0001$), including both supraventricular and ventricular arrhythmias. The patients with arrhythmias had more severe apnea and nocturnal hypoxemia. Another study showed a reduction in the number of premature ventricular contractions after tracheostomy.[113]

The most common arrhythmia seen during apneic episodes is bradycardia during the apneic phase followed by tachycardia at the termination of the obstruction.[29] Other arrhythmias recorded during apneic events include sinus arrest, sinus bradycardia, second-degree heart block, atrial tachycardia, paroxysmal atrial fibrillation, atrial flutter, premature ventricular contractions, and unsustained ventricular tachycardia.[114]

Although further studies are needed for definitive conclusions, it seems that OSAHS patients are more prone to cardiac arrhythmias. When confronted with patients with rhythm abnormalities that occur predominantly during sleep, assessment for the signs and symptoms of OSAHS is prudent. The treatment of concomitant OSAHS may decrease the propensity to arrhythmias.

Neurological Disorders

Cerebrovascular Disease (see Chapter 90)

A study of 400 stroke victims with age- and gender-matched control subjects revealed an odds ratio of 3.2 for stroke in patients with snoring.[115] Another case-control study found an odds ratio of 8.0 for snoring along with observed apneas, sleepiness, and obesity.[116] Dyken et al.[117] prospectively performed polysomnography in 24 patients who had a recent stroke and 27 control subjects. OSA was found in 77% of stroke patients and 23% of control subjects ($P < .02$); it is difficult to state whether OSAHS led to stroke, or vice versa. Strokes that compromise the function of the hypoglossal nerve would affect the function of the genioglossal muscle and can potentially predispose to OSA. Such patients may not tolerate treatment for OSAHS. Furthermore, it is not clear whether treatment of OSAHS alters the prognosis. At this point the routine investigation of stroke patients for OSAHS cannot be recommended (see Chapter 90).

Parkinson's Disease

It is well known that patients with Parkinson's disease are predisposed to OSAHS, particularly those with autonomic abnormalities.[29] Abnormal upper airway and chest wall muscle activities are thought to be the cause. Patients with parkinsonism who complain of disturbed sleep and daytime somnolence should first have their medications optimized. The improved upper airway muscle motility may help reduce the propensity to OSAHS. If symptoms persist, polysomnography is warranted. The latter study may also uncover periodic limb movements, which occur with a higher frequency in patients with Parkinson's disease.

OSAHS has been reported in disorders such as postpoliomyelitis,[118] muscular dystrophy,[119] and syringobulbomyelia.[120] In fact, any myopathy or neuropathy that affects the function of the genioglossus muscle or causes dysphagia can predispose to OSAHS.

Endocrinological Disorders

Hypothyroidism

Although routine testing for hypothyroidism is probably not indicated in the evaluation of the patient with possible OSAHS, the clinician should recognize that this disorder predisposes to OSAHS. Postulated mechanisms include macroglossia, upper airway myopathy, and abnormalities in ventilatory control. Furthermore, restoration of the euthyroid state may reduce the frequency of apnea and hypopneas.[121, 122] Therefore, patients with hypothyroidism should be questioned regarding snoring and daytime somnolence. If OSAHS is diagnosed, the treatment of OSAHS and hormone replacement should be initiated simultaneously, especially in patients with ischemic heart disease. After hypothyroidism has been corrected, a repeat sleep study can determine whether continued OSAHS treatment remains indicated.

Acromegaly

Acromegaly predisposes to OSAHS.[123] Macroglossia and increased soft tissues of the upper airway are thought to be the mechanisms that decrease the caliber of the upper airway. The treatment of OSAHS can reduce symptoms of daytime fatigue but obviously is not a substitute for correction of the underlying cause.

Hematological Disorders

Sickle Cell Disease

Hypoxia is well known to exacerbate sickle cell crisis, and treatment for OSAHS has been reported to resolve the painful vaso-occlusive crisis characteristic of this disease.[124] The RDI, however, has not been found to correlate with the severity of sickle cell anemia.[125] Nevertheless, one should inquire about the symptoms of OSAHS in patients with sickle cell disease. The treatment of OSAHS may significantly improve the frequency of the painful crisis.

Finally, infectious mononucleosis, leukemia, lymphoma, or malignancies that promote an increased mass of the pharyngeal lymphoid tissues can all predispose the patient to OSAHS. OSAHS may resolve after successful treatment of the underlying disease. In selected cases, the appropriate treatment of OSAHS may improve the patient's quality of life.

OBSTRUCTIVE SLEEP APNEA-HYPOPNEA SYNDROME AND OTHER SLEEP DISORDERS

In a general population survey in England, OSAHS was found to occur in 10.3% of persons with night terrors and 3.8% of persons with somnambulism, once psychiatric disorders were eliminated.[126] In our experience, treatment of the underlying OSAHS can frequently reduce the severity of night terrors and somnambulism.

One should remember that OSAHS precipitates a form of sleep deprivation; as such, OSAHS can aggravate any disorder that in turn is exacerbated by sleep deprivation such as narcolepsy. Finally, it is not uncommon to simultaneously diagnose both OSAHS and disorders such as periodic limb movements. In such cases, it may be difficult to distinguish the degree to which each disease contributes to the patient's symptoms. Because of all of these facts, we prefer to treat OSAHS first before attempting to correct any other concomitantly present sleep disorder.

LABORATORY ASSESSMENT FOR SLEEP APNEA

Polysomnography

The indications for polysomnography were published in 1997 by the American Sleep Disorders Association Standards of Practice Committee.[127] Measurement techniques and syndrome definitions were published in 1999.[1] Full-night polysomnography is routinely indicated for most patients suspected of having a sleep-related breathing disorder. Esophageal manometry is used at some centers to more accurately gauge respiratory effort. Split-night studies are occasionally used in which the first half of the night is used for diagnosis and the second half is used for continuous positive airway pressure titration. Although further studies are needed, Strollo et al.[128] have shown comparable results to full-night polysomnography. The main problem with split-night studies is that the architecture of sleep is not constant throughout the night. Specifically, stage 3 and 4 sleep predominate in the first half of the night, whereas rapid eye movement sleep (when apneas are more likely to appear) predominates in the second half. As such, split-night studies may in theory underestimate the severity of OSAHS.

A cardiorespiratory sleep study involving the measurements of air flow, respiratory effort, oxygen saturation, and heart rate may be an acceptable alternative, provided that negative results are followed by a full-night polysomnography. The advantage of this system is its portability and the ability to monitor the patient's sleep at home. A review of seven studies on portable ambulatory monitoring systems reported sensitivities of 78 to 100% and specificities of 67 to 100%.[129] One problem with such devices is the inability to detect hypopneas and apneas associated with arousals only. Newer, more sophisticated equipment is available that allows the recording of electroencephalography; such systems may help increase the accuracy of these ambulatory units.

The distinction between obstructive apnea (airflow cessation with continued respiratory effort) and central apnea (airflow and respiratory effort cessation) is not thought to influence therapy except in rare cases when apneas are exclusively central.[127] Patients typically have both types of apneas, and the AHI (also called the RDI) does not distinguish between central and obstructive apneas.

An RDI of at least 5 along with daytime sleepiness defines OSAHS,[1] although several laboratories use an RDI of at least 10.[127] The severity of OSAHS should be based not only on the RDI but also on the degree of daytime sleepiness and other polysomnographic features, such as degree of sleep fragmentation, oxygen desaturation, and presence of cardiac arrhythmias. By definition, the UARS is associated with an RDI of less than 5. The hallmark of UARS is progressive increase in respiratory effort (as measured by esophageal manometry) in the absence of an obvious reduction in airflow and maintenance of SaO_2 above 90% terminating with an arousal and a return of effort to baseline.[26, 27] UARS may be present in the absence of snoring.

Overnight pulse oximetry is occasionally used as a screening test to identify patients who may benefit from OSAHS evaluation, but this test is not a substitute for polysomnography.[127] The pitfalls of nocturnal oximetry include the failure to detect apneas and hypopneas associated with arousals but without significant oxygen desaturation, the failure to detect UARS, and the potential for displacement of the oximeter. Furthermore, not all oxygen desaturations are due to apneas. In otherwise healthy individuals, oxygen saturation can drop as low as 90 ± 3%.[130] In patients with chronic obstructive pulmonary disease, hypoventilation is commonly observed during the rapid eye movement stage of sleep and may lead to oxygen desaturation independent of any apneas.[131-134] Similarly, obese patients may have oxygen desaturation due to a decrease in functional residual capacity or hypoventilation, independent of apneas.[135, 136] It therefore is important to follow-up any abnormal pulse oximetry study with a formal sleep evaluation.

MULTIPLE SLEEP LATENCY TEST AND THE MAINTENANCE OF WAKEFULNESS TEST

Occasionally, it becomes important to quantify daytime somnolence (see Chapter 104). There are two tests available in clinical practice: the multiple sleep latency test (MSLT) and the Maintenance of Wakefulness Test (MWT). The MSLT is more commonly used; it measures the ability of an individual to fall asleep. The MWT is administered under similar conditions, but it tests the ability of an individual to stay awake.

The MSLT consists of a series of five nap opportunities spaced at 2-h intervals during which the individual tries to fall asleep.[137, 138] Each trial is terminated after either 20 min of wakefulness, 15 min of sleep (clinical protocol), or three 30-sec epochs of sleep (research protocol). Time to sleep onset is measured and averaged over all naps; this value is called the sleep latency. Sleep latency of less than 5 min is considered severe sleepiness, more than 5 min to 10 min is considered moderate sleepiness, and more than 10 min is considered normal. The MSLT can be used to quantify the severity of daytime sleepiness and to assess response to therapy. Its use in narcolepsy is described in Chapter 104.

The MWT consists of a series of four to five trials spaced 2 h apart during which the individual tries to remain awake under conditions of minimal stimulation.[139, 140] Each trial is terminated either at sleep onset (defined as the occurrence of one epoch of any stage of sleep) or if sleep onset is not achieved by 20 min. Again, the sleep latency is measured. A multicenter study of 64 normal subjects defined impairment in wake tendency as a mean sleep latency of less than 11 min.[140] The MWT may be a more useful test than the MSLT in assessing the ability of an individual such as a pilot or truck driver to stay awake, but normative data are lacking for many age groups.

SUMMARY

A full assessment of the symptoms and signs, followed by an overnight sleep recording, is necessary for the diagnosis of OSAHS. As more physicians become familiar with the clinical presentation of OSAHS, the number of patients diagnosed with this disorder will increase. This should lead to appropriate treatment and a decrease in the morbidity and mortality rates associated with this disorder.

References

1. American Academy of Sleep Medicine. Sleep related breathing disorders in adults: recommendations for syndrome definition and measurement techniques in clinical research. Sleep. 1999;22:667–689.
2. Butkov N. Atlas of Clinical Polysomnography. Vol II. Ashland, Ore: Synapse Media Inc; 1996;184–189.
3. Gastaut H, Tassinari CA, Duron B. Polygraphic study of the episodic diurnal and nocturnal (hypnic and respiratory) manifestations of the Pickwick syndrome. Brain Res. 1965;2:167–186.
4. Bresnitz EA, Goldberg R, Kosinski RM. Epidemiology of obstructive sleep apnea. Epidemiol Rev. 1994;16:210–227.
5. Redline S, Young T. Epidemiology and natural history of obstructive sleep apnea. Ear Nose Throat J. 1993;72:20–26.
6. Olson LG, King MT, Hensley MJ, et al. A community study of snoring and sleep-disordered breathing: prevalence. Am J Respir Crit Care Med. 1995;152:711–716.
7. Kripke DF, Ancoli-Israel S, Klauber MR, et al. Prevalence of sleep-disordered breathing in ages 40–64 years: a population-based survey. Sleep. 1997;20:65–76.
8. Young T, Palta M, Dempsey J, et al. The occurrence of sleep-disordered breathing among middle-aged adults. N Engl J Med. 1993;328:1230–1235.
9. Ohayon MM, Guilleminault C, Priest RG, et al. Snoring and breathing pauses during sleep: telephone interview survey of a United Kingdom population sample. Br Med J. 1997;314:860–863.
10. Lavie P, Herer P, Peled R, et al. Mortality in sleep apnea patients: multivariate analysis of risk factors. Sleep. 1995;18:149–157.
11. Partinen M, Jamieson A, Guilleminault C. Long-term outcome for obstructive sleep apnea syndrome patients: mortality. Chest. 1988;94:1200–1204.
12. Partinen M, Guilleminault C. Daytime sleepiness and vascular morbidity at seven-year follow-up in obstructive sleep apnea patients. Chest. 1990;97:27–32.
13. Thorpy MJ, Ledereich PS, Glovinsky PB, et al. Five and ten years survival of patients with obstructive sleep apnea: the Montefiore long-term follow-up study [abstract]. Sleep Res. 1987;17:264.
14. He J, Kryger MH, Zorick FJ, et al. Mortality and apnea index in obstructive sleep apnea: experience in 385 male patients. Chest. 1988;94:9–14.
15. Lavie P, Herer P, Peled R, et al. Mortality in sleep apnea patients: a multivariate analysis of risk factors. Sleep. 1995;18:149–157.
16. Ancoli-Israel S, Klauber MR, Kripke DF, et al. Sleep apnea in female patients in a nursing home. Chest. 1989;96:1054–1058.
17. Bliwise DL, Bliwise NG, Partinen M, et al. Sleep apnea and mortality in an aged cohort. Am J Public Health. 1988;78:544–547.
18. Ancoli-Israel S, Kripke DF, Klauber MR, et al. Morbidity, mortality and sleep-disordered breathing in community dwelling elderly. Sleep. 1996;19:277–282.
19. Hudgel DW. Mechanisms of obstructive sleep apnea. Chest. 1992;101:541–549.
20. Bonsignore MR, Marrone O, Insalaco G, et al. The cardiovascular effects of obstructive sleep apnea: analysis of pathogenic mechanisms. Eur Respir J. 1994;7:786–805.
21. Shepard JW Jr, Thawley SE. Localization of upper airway collapse during sleep in patients with obstructive sleep apnea. Am Rev Respir Dis. 1990;141:1350–1355.
22. Horner RL, Mohiaddin RH, Lowell DG, et al. Sites and sizes of fat deposits around the pharynx in obese patients with obstructive sleep apnoea and weight matched controls. Eur Respir J. 1989;2:613–622.
23. Guilleminault C, Mondini S. The complexity of obstructive sleep apnea syndrome: need for multi-diagnostic approaches before considering treatment. Bull Eur Physiopathol Respir. 1983;19:595–599.
24. Mezzanotte WS, Tangel DJ, White DJ. Waking genioglossal electromyogram in sleep apnea patients versus normal controls: a neuromuscular compensatory mechanism. J Clin Invest. 1992;89:1571–1579.
25. Petrof BJ, Hendricks JC, Pack AI. Does upper airway muscle injury trigger a vicious cycle in obstructive sleep apnea? A hypothesis. Sleep. 1996;19:465–471.
26. Guilleminault C, Stoohs R. The upper airway resistance syndrome. Sleep Res. 1991;20:250.
27. Guilleminault C, Stoohs R, Clerk A, et al. A cause of excessive daytime sleepiness: the upper airway resistance syndrome. Chest. 1993;104:781–787.
28. Guilleminault C, Stoohs R, Kim Y-D, et al. Upper airway sleep-disordered breathing in women. Ann Intern Med. 1995;122:493–501.
29. American Sleep Disorders Association. The International Classification of Sleep Disorders, Revised: Diagnostic and Coding Manual. Rochester, Minn: American Sleep Disorders Association; 1997:52–58.
30. Kales A, Cadieux RJ, Bixler EO, et al. Severe obstructive sleep apnea, I: onset, clinical course, and characteristics. J Chron Dis. 1985;38:419–425.
31. Feinsilver SH, Hertz G. Respiration during sleep in pregnancy. Clin Chest Med. 1992;13:637–644.
32. Charbonneau M, Falcone T, Cosio MG, et al. Obstructive sleep apnea during pregnancy. Am Rev Respir Dis. 1991;144:461–463.
33. Loube DI, Poceta JS, Morales MC, et al. Self-reported snoring during pregnancy: association with fetal outcome. Chest. 1996;109:885–889.
34. Hoffstein V, Szalai JP. Predictive value of clinical features in diagnosing obstructive sleep apnea. Sleep. 1993;16:118–122.
35. Maislin G, Pack AI, Kribbs NB, et al. A survey screen for prediction of apnea. Sleep. 1995;18:158–166.
36. Coverdale SGM, Read DJC, Woolcock AJ, et al. The importance of suspecting sleep apnea as a common cause of excessive daytime sleepiness: further experience from the diagnosis and management of 19 patients. Aust N Z J Med. 1980;10:284–288.
37. Buda AJ, Schroeder JS, Guilleminault C. Abnormalities of pulmonary artery wedge pressure in sleep-induced apnea. Int J Cardiol. 1981;1:67–74.
38. Yamashiro Y, Kryger MH. Review: sleep in heart failure. Sleep. 1993;16:513–523.
39. Guilleminault C, Miles L. Differential diagnosis of obstructive apnea syndrome: the abnormal esophageal reflux and laryngospasm during sleep [abstract]. Sleep Res. 1980;16:410.
40. Krieger J, Laks L, Wilcox I, et al. Atrial natriuretic peptide release during sleep in patients with obstructive sleep apnoea before and during treatment with nasal continuous positive airway pressure. Clin Sci. 1989;77:407–411.
41. George CF, Nickerson PW, Hanly PJ, et al. Sleep apnoea patients have more automobile accidents. Lancet. 1987;2:447.
42. Findley LJ, Unverzadt M, Suratt P. Automobile accidents in patients with obstructive sleep apnea. Am Rev Respir Dis. 1988;138:337–340.
43. Greenberg GD, Watson RK, Deptula D. Neuropsychological dysfunction in sleep apnea. Sleep. 1987;10:254.
44. Derderian SS, Bridenbaugh RH, Rajagopal KR. Neuropsychologic symptoms in obstructive sleep apnea improve after treatment with nasal continuous positive airway pressure. Chest. 1988;94:1023–1027.
45. Paiva T, Farinha A, Martins A, et al. Chronic headaches and sleep disorders. Arch Intern Med. 1977;157:1701–1705.
46. Katz I, Stradling J, Slutsky AS, et al. Do patients with obstructive sleep apnea have thick necks? Am Rev Respir Dis. 1990;141:1228–1231.
47. Davies RJO, Stradling JR. The relationship between neck circumference, radiographic pharyngeal anatomy, and the obstructive sleep apnoea syndrome. Eur Respir J. 1990;3:509–514.
48. Kushida CA, Efron B, Guilleminault C. A predictive morphometric model for the obstructive sleep apnea syndrome. Ann Intern Med. 1997;127:581–587.

49. Jamieson A, Guilleminault C, Partinen M, et al. Obstructive sleep apnea patients have craniomandibular abnormalities. Sleep. 1986;9:469–477.
50. Rajagopal KR, Abbrecht PH, Derderian SS. Obstructive sleep apnea in hypothyroidism. Ann Intern Med. 1984;101:471–474.
50a. Skjodt NM, Atkar R, Easton PA. Screening for hypothyroidism in sleep apnea. Am J Respir Crit Care Med. 1999;160:732–735.
51. Winkelman JW, Goldman H, Piscatelli N, et al. Are thyroid function tests necessary in patients with suspected sleep apnea? Sleep. 1996;19:790–793.
52. Strohl KP, Redline S. Recognition of obstructive sleep apnea. Am J Respir Crit Care Med. 1996;154:279–289.
53. Levinson PD, McGarvey ST, Carlisle CC, et al. Adiposity and cardiovascular risk factors in men with obstructive sleep apnea. Chest. 1993;103:1336–1342.
54. Rajala RM, Partinen M, Sane T, et al. Obstructive sleep apnea in morbidly obese patients. J Intern Med. 1991;230:125–129.
55. Phillips B, Cook Y, Schmitt F, et al. Sleep apnea: prevalence of risk factors in the general population. South Med J. 1989;82:1090–1092.
56. Bloom JW, Kaltenborn WT, Quan SF. Risk factors in the general population for snoring: importance of cigarette smoking and obesity. Chest. 1988;93:678–683.
57. Dealberto M-J, Ferber C, Garma L, et al. Factors related to sleep apnea syndrome in sleep clinic patients. Chest. 1994;105:1753–1758.
58. Grunstein R, Wilcox I, Yang T, et al. Snoring and sleep apnoea in men: association with central obesity and hypertension. Int J Obes. 1993;17:533–540.
59. Katz I, Stradling J, Slutsky A, et al. Do patients with obstructive sleep apnea have thick necks? Am Rev Respir Med. 1990;141:1228–1231.
60. Davies RJO, Stradling J. The relationship between neck circumference, radiographic pharyngeal anatomy, and obstructive sleep apnea syndrome. Eur Respir J. 1990;3:509–514.
61. National Commission on Sleep Disorders Research. Wake Up America: A National Sleep Alert. Vol 1. Washington, DC: National Commission on Sleep Disorders Research; 1993.
62. Wilhoit SC, Suratt PM. Obstructive sleep apnea in premenopausal women: a comparison with men and with post-menopausal women. Chest. 1987;91:654–658.
63. Leech JA, Onal E, Dulberg C, et al. A comparison of men and women with occlusive sleep apnea syndrome. Chest. 1988;94:983–988.
64. Guilleminault C, Quera-Salva A, Partinen M, et al. Women and the obstructive sleep apnea syndrome. Chest. 1988;93:104–109.
65. Richmond RM, Elliot LM, Burns CM, et al. The prevalence of obstructive sleep apnoea in an obese female population. Int J Obes. 1994;18:173–177.
66. Redline S, Tishler PV, Williamson J, et al. The familial aggregates of sleep apnea. Am J Respir Crit Care Med. 1995;151:682–687.
67. Pillar G, Lavie P. Assessment of the role of inheritance in sleep apnea syndrome. Am J Respir Crit Care Med. 1995;151:688–691.
68. Guilleminault C, Partinen M, Hollman K, et al. Familial aggregates in obstructive sleep apnea syndrome. Chest. 1995;107:1545–1551.
69. Taasan VC, Block AJ, Boysen PG, et al. Alcohol increases sleep apnea and oxygen desaturation in asymptomatic men. Am J Med. 1981;71:240–245.
70. Krol RC, Knuth SL, Bartlett D Jr. Selective reduction of genioglossal muscle activity by alcohol in normal human subjects. Am Rev Respir Dis. 1984;129:247–250.
71. Scrima L, Broudy M, Nay KN, et al. Increased severity of obstructive sleep apnea after bedtime alcohol ingestion: diagnostic potential and proposed mechanism of action. Sleep. 1982;5:318–328.
72. Kripke DF, Ancoli-Israel S, Klauber MR, et al. U.S. population estimate for disordered sleep breathing: high rates in minorities. Sleep Res. 1995;24:268.
73. Redline S, Hans M, Pracharktam N, et al. Differences in the age distribution and risk factors for sleep-disordered breathing in blacks and whites. Am J Respir Crit Care Med. 1994;149:577.
74. Schmid-Nowara WW, Coultas D, Wiggins C, et al. Snoring in a Hispanic-American population: risk factors and association with hypertension and other morbidity. Arch Intern Med. 1990;150:597–601.
75. Grunstein RR, Lawrence S, Spies JM, et al. Snoring in paradise: the Western Samoa Sleep Survey. Eur Respir J. 1989;2(S5):4015.
76. Cistulli P, Sullivan CE. Sleep apnea in Marfan's syndrome. Am Rev Respir Dis. 1993;147:645–648.
77. Wetter D, Young T, Bidwall T, et al. Smoking as a risk factor for sleep disordered breathing. Arch Intern Med. 1994;154:2219–2224.
78. Bliwise DL, Bliwise NG, Partinen M, et al. Sleep apnea and mortality in an aged cohort. Am J Public Health. 1988;78:544–547.
79. Roth T, Roehrs T, Zorick F, et al. Pharmacological effects of sedative-hypnotics, narcotic analgesics, and alcohol during sleep. Med Clin North Am. 1985;69:1281–1288.
80. Mendelson WB, Garnett D, Gillin JC. Flurazepam-induced sleep apnea syndrome in a patient with insomnia and mild sleep-related respiratory changes. J Nerv Ment Dis. 1981;169:261–264.
81. Dolly FR, Block AJ. Effects of flurazepam on sleep-disordered breathing and nocturnal oxygen desaturation in asymptomatic subjects. Am J Med. 1982;73:239–243.
82. Lavie P, Fischel N, Zomer J, et al. The effects of partial and complete mechanical occlusion of the nasal passages on sleep structure and breathing in sleep. Acta Otolaryngol (Stockh). 1983;95:161–166.
83. Fletcher EC. The relationship between systemic hypertension and obstructive sleep apnea: facts and theory. Am J Med. 1995;98:118–128.
84. Stradling JR. Sleep apnea and systemic hypertension. Thorax. 1989;44:984–989.
85. Hoffstein V. Blood pressure, snoring, obesity, and nocturnal hypoxemia. Lancet. 1994;344:643–645.
86. Hoffstein MD, Chan CK, Slutsky AS. Sleep apnea and systemic hypertension: a causal association review. Am J Med. 1991;91:190–196.
87. Working Group on OSA and Hypertension. Obstructive sleep apnea and blood pressure: what is the relationship? Blood Press. 1993;2:166–182.
88. Waller PC, Bhopal RS. Is snoring a cause of vascular disease? Lancet. 1989;1:143–146.
89. Stradling J, Davies RJO. Sleep apnea and hypertension: what a mess! Sleep. 1997;20:789–793.
90. Hla KM, Young TB, Bidwell T, et al. Sleep apnea and hypertension: a population-based study. Ann Intern Med. 1994;120:382–388.
91. Carlson JT, Hedner JA, Ejnell H, et al. High prevalence of hypertension in sleep apnea patients independent of obesity. Am J Respir Crit Care Med. 1994;150:72–77.
92. Kiselak J, Clark M, Pera V, et al. The association between hypertension and sleep apnea in obese patients. Chest. 1993;104:775–780.
93. Silverberg DS, Oksenberg A. Essential hypertension and abnormal upper airway resistance during sleep. Sleep. 1997;20:794–806.
94. Young T, Peppard P, Palta M, et al. Population-based study of sleep-disordered breathing as a risk factor for hypertension. Arch Intern Med. 1997;157:1746–1752.
95. Mayer J, Becker H, Brandenberg U, et al. Blood pressure and sleep apnea: results of long term nasal continuous positive airway pressure therapy. Cardiology. 1991;79:84–92.
96. Bradley TD, Rutherford R, Grossman RF, et al. Role of daytime hypoxemia in the pathogenesis of right heart failure in the obstructive sleep apnea syndrome. Am Rev Respir Dis. 1985;131:835–839.
97. Weitzenblum E, Krieger J, Apprill M, et al. Daytime pulmonary hypertension in patients with obstructive sleep apnea syndrome. Am Rev Respir Dis. 1988;138:345–349.
98. Apprill M, Weitzenblum E, Krieger J, et al. Frequency and mechanism of daytime pulmonary hypertension in patients with obstructive sleep apnoea syndrome. Cor Vasa. 1991;33:42–49.
99. Podzus T, Bauer W, Mayer J, et al. Sleep apnea and pulmonary hypertension. Klin Wochenschr. 1986;64:131–134.
100. Laks L. Pulmonary arterial pressure in sleep apnea. Sleep. 1993;16:S41–S43.
101. Sajkov D, Cowie RJ, Thornton AT, et al. Pulmonary hypertension and hypoxemia in obstructive sleep apnea syndrome. Am J Respir Crit Care Med. 1994;149:416–422.

102. Weiss WJ, Remsburg S, Garpestad E, et al. Hemodynamic consequences of obstructive sleep apnea. Sleep. 1996;19:388–397.
103. Chan CS, Woolcock AJ, Sullivan CE. Nocturnal asthma: role of snoring and obstructive sleep apnea. Am Rev Respir Dis. 1988;137:1502–1504.
104. Koskenvuo M, Kaprio J, Partinen M. Snoring as a risk factor for hypertension and angina pectoris. Lancet. 1985;1:893–896.
105. Norton PG, Dunn EV. Snoring as a risk factor for disease: an epidemiological survey. Br Med J. 1985;291:630–632.
106. Koskenvuo M, Kaprio J, Telakivi T. Snoring as a risk factor for ischemic heart disease and stroke in men. Br Med J. 1987;294:16–19.
107. Waller PC, Bhopal RS. Is snoring a cause of vascular disease? An epidemiological review. Lancet. l989;1:143–146.
108. Hung J, Whitford EG, Parsons RW, et al. Association of sleep apnoea with myocardial infarction in men. Lancet. 1990;336:261–264.
109. Saito T, Yoshikawa T, Sakamoto Y, et al. Sleep apnea in patients with acute myocardial infarction. Crit Care Med. 1991;19:938–941.
110. Koehler U, Schafer H. Is obstructive sleep apnea (OSA) a risk factor for myocardial infarction and cardiac arrhythmias in patients with coronary heart disease (CHD)? Sleep. 1996;19:283–286.
111. Hillman DR. Sleep apnea and myocardial infarction. Sleep. 1993; 16:S23–S24.
112. Hoffstein V, Mateika S. Cardiac arrhythmias, snoring, and sleep apnea. Chest. 1994;106:466–471.
113. Guilleminault C, Simmons FB, Motta J, et al. Obstructive sleep apnea and tracheostomy: long term follow-up experience. Arch Intern Med. 1981;141:985–988.
114. Guilleminault C, Connolly S, Winkle R. Cardiac arrhythmia during sleep in 400 patients with obstructive sleep apnea. Am J Cardiol. 1983;52:490–494.
115. Spriggs D, French JM, Murdy JM. Historical risk factors for stroke: a case control study. Age Ageing. 1990;19:280–287.
116. Palomaki H. Snoring and the risk of brain infarction. Stroke. 1991;22:1021–1025.
117. Dyken ME, Somers VK, Yamada T, et al. Investigating the relationship between stroke and obstructive sleep apnea. Stroke. 1996;27:401–407.
118. Hill K, Robbins AW, Messing R, et al. Sleep apnea syndrome after poliomyelitis. Am Rev Respir Dis. 1983;127:129.
119. Skatrud J, Iber C, McHugh W, et al. Determinants of hypoventilation during wakefulness and sleep in diaphragmatic paralysis. Am Rev Respir Dis. 1980;121:587.
120. Haponik EF, Givens D, Angelo J. Syringobulbia-myelia with obstructive sleep apnea. Neurology. 1983;33:1046.
121. Rajagopal KR, Abbrecht PH, Derderian SS, et al. Obstructive sleep apnea in hypothyroidism. Ann Intern Med. 1984;101:491–494.
122. Grunestein RR, Sullivan CE. Sleep apnea and hypothyroidism: Mechanisms and management. Am J Med. 1988;85:775–779.
123. Perks WH, Horrocks PM, Cooper RA, et al. Sleep apnoea in acromegaly. Br Med J. 1980;280:894.
124. Sidman JD, Fry TL. Exacerbation of sickle cell disease by obstructive sleep apnea. Arch Otolaryngol Head Neck Surg. 1988;114:916–917.
125. Brooks LJ, Koziol SM, Chiarucci KM, et al. Does sleep-disordered breathing contribute to the clinical severity of sickle cell anemia? J Pediatr Hematol Oncol. 1996;18:135–139.
126. Ohayon M, Guilleminault C, Priest RC. Night terrors, sleepwalking, and confusional arousals in the general population: their frequency and relationship to other sleep and mental disorders. J Clin Psych. 1999;60:268–276.
127. Polysomnography Task Force, American Sleep Disorders Association Standards of Practice Committee. Practice parameters for the indications for polysomnography and related procedures. Sleep. 1997;20:406–422.
128. Strollo PJ Jr, Sanders MH, Constantino JP, et al. Split-night studies for the diagnosis and treatment of sleep-disordered breathing. Sleep. 1996;19:S255–S259.
129. Ferber R, Millman R, Coppola M, et al. Portable recording in the assessment of obstructive sleep apnea. ASDA standards of practice. Sleep. 1994;17:378–392.
130. Gries RE, Brooks LJ. Normal oxyhemoglobin saturation during sleep. Chest. 1996;110:1489–1492.
131. Skatrud JB, Dempsey JA, Iber C, et al. Correction of CO_2 retention during sleep in patients with chronic obstructive pulmonary diseases. Am Rev Respir Dis. 1981;124:260–268.
132. Hudgel DW, Martin RJ, Capehart M, et al. Contribution of hypoventilation to sleep oxygen desaturation in chronic obstructive pulmonary disease. J Appl Physiol. 1983;55:669–677.
133. George CF, West P, Kryger MH. Oxygenation and breathing pattern during phasic and tonic REM in patients with chronic obstructive pulmonary disease. Sleep. 1987;10:234–243.
134. Fletcher EC, Gray BA, Levin DC. Non-apneic mechanisms of arterial oxygen desaturation during rapid-eye movement sleep. J Appl Physiol. 1983;54:632–639.
135. Tucker DH, Sieker HO. The effects of change in body position on lung volumes and intrapulmonary gas mixing in patients with obesity, heart failure, and emphysema. J Clin Invest. 1960;39:787–791.
136. Kryger MH. Restrictive lung diseases. In: Kryger MH, Roth T, Dement WC, eds. Principles and Practice of Sleep Medicine. Philadelphia, Pa: WB Saunders; 1994:769–775.
137. Carskadon MA, Dement WC, Mitler MM, et al. Guidelines for the multiple sleep latency test (MSLT): a standard measure of sleepiness. Sleep. 1986;9:519–524.
138. Richardson G, Carskadon M, Flagg W, et al. Excessive daytime sleepiness in man: multiple sleep latency measurements in narcoleptics and control subjects. Electroencephalogr Clin Neurophysiol. 1978;45:621–627.
139. Mitler MM, Gujavarty KS, Browman CP. Maintenance of wakefulness test: a polysomnographic technique for evaluating treatment efficacy in patients with excessive somnolence. Electroencephalogr Clin Neurophysiol. 1982;53:658–661.
140. Doghramji K, Mitler MM, Sangal B, et al. A normative study of the maintenance of wakefulness test (MWT). Electroencephalogr Clin Neurophysiol. 1997;103:554–562.

Medical Therapy for Obstructive Sleep Apnea-Hypopnea Syndrome

Mark H. Sanders

A great deal has been learned about the obstructive sleep apnea-hypopnea syndrome (OSAHS) since sleep-related obstructive apneas were polysomnographically demonstrated by Gastaut et al.[1] in the mid-1960s. Investigators and clinicians now have a greater understanding of the nature of upper airway dysfunction during sleep and recognize that it is a common disorder with a significant adverse impact on the quality of life and longevity.[2-11] It also appears likely that increased upper airway resistance without reduced airflow, or hypopnea,[12] even in the absence of apnea or oxyhemoglobin desaturation, may precipitate sleep fragmentation. This has been termed the *upper airway resistance syndrome* (UARS).[13] In this chapter, OSAHS refers to the clinical spectrum of sleep-disordered breathing, from apnea, to hypopnea, to UARS.[13a] Obstructed breathing *events* (which include apnea, hypopnea, and respiratory effort-related arousals) are referred to as *OSA/H*.

Given the potential, and indeed likely pathophysiological heterogeneity across patients with OSAHS, and the general inability to reliably identify the operative mechanisms in specific patients, a number of therapeutic approaches have been developed that are directed toward one or more of the possible pathophysiological processes. The only universally successful therapies for sleep-related upper airway dysfunction are those that specifically bypass or reverse the obstruction, independent of the responsible mechanism and anatomical site. In this regard, tracheotomy was the first intervention to unequivocally provide a patent airway to OSAHS patients during sleep. However, as a result of the medical and psychosocial morbidity associated with this procedure,[14-16] less invasive treatment options became necessary. Positive airway pressure is a noninvasive treatment that almost always maintains upper airway patency during sleep, regardless of the level of obstruction above the epiglottis. In this chapter, a variety of nonsurgical therapeutic strategies for the care of OSAHS patients are discussed. Positive airway pressure therapy, the current nonsurgical therapeutic mainstay, is discussed in Chapter 76, and oral appliance therapy in Chapter 78. These modalities provide substantial therapeutic benefit and have undergone significant development since publication of the previous edition of this book.

The following discussion primarily addresses practical issues associated with treatment strategies, grouped by category, that is, pharmacological agents, mechanical devices, and so forth. The physiological bases for these interventions, as well as positive pressure therapy and treatment with oral appliances, are addressed in other chapters. In addition, although this chapter is generally organized in order of increasing therapeutic aggressiveness, it does not necessarily represent a treatment algorithm. The approach to treatment should be tailored to the requirements of the individual patient to arrive at the optimal result with the greatest possible expediency.

A relatively small percentage of patients have nonobstructive or central sleep-disordered breathing. A detailed discussion of central sleep apnea, including current therapeutic concepts, is provided in Chapter 71.

WHEN TO TREAT OBSTRUCTIVE SLEEP APNEA/HYPOPNEA

Patients with symptoms or signs attributable to OSAHS, such as excessive daytime sleepiness or fatigue, episodic choking or gasping resulting in awakening from sleep, morning headaches, nocturnal dysrhythmias or arrhythmias, and so on, should be treated. In addition, early data indicate that the presence of 20 or more apneas per hour of sleep may predict early mortality,[10] and consideration should be given to initiating therapy on this basis alone. Some studies suggest that milder degrees of OSAHS contribute to neurocognitive dysfunction and the presence of systemic arterial hypertension,[17-19] and perhaps the cardiovascular status of the patient should also be incorporated into the decision analysis of when and how aggressively treatment should be applied. It is clear that further studies are needed to define and validate the decision-making process. In the following discussion, it is assumed that the decision to treat the patient has been made on the basis of available clinical and objectively derived physiological data collected during sleep.

COEXISTENT CONDITIONS THAT PREDISPOSE TO, PRECIPITATE, OR WORSEN UPPER AIRWAY DYSFUNCTION DURING SLEEP

Regardless of the severity of a patient's OSAHS, one should identify and address any coexistent medical or lifestyle issues that may promote upper airway dysfunction during sleep. Although eliminating these conditions may not obviate the need for further intervention, it may simplify any additional therapy that may be necessary.

Obesity

Obesity is prevalent among patients with OSAHS[20–22] and constitutes a risk factor for this disorder.[23] The evidence suggests that obesity compromises upper airway function by altering pharyngeal size or geometry. Previous studies have demonstrated a direct relationship between lung volume and pharyngeal cross-sectional area in OSAHS patients and snorers.[24–26] Although this is consistent with the possibility that the association between obesity and upper airway dysfunction during sleep is mediated by its effect on lung volume, these data were collected from awake patients. Other investigators have found no relationship between the severity of OSAHS and functional residual capacity.[27] In addition, increasing end-expiratory lung volume by applying continuous negative extrathoracic pressure has not consistently alleviated OSAHS.[28, 29] It is therefore unlikely that improvement in OSAHS following weight reduction is due to increased lung volume.

The adverse effect of obesity on upper airway function may be mediated through a direct mechanical influence on upper airway geometry. Studies in animals have indicated that upper airway resistance is influenced by mass loading of the anterior neck, which may simulate the clinical scenario of excessive adipose tissue deposits in this area.[30] Further support for a significant pathophysiological role of cervical obesity is provided by the observation that changes in pressure surrounding the neck are transmitted to the airway lumen and that cyclical pressure fluctuations in the pharyngeal fat pad coincide with intrapharyngeal pressure fluctuations.[31, 32] These data also support the relevance of the observation that OSAHS patients have "thick" necks[33] and that increased neck circumference is a predictive factor for OSAHS.[34–36] Furthermore, velopharyngeal collapsibility increases with increasing neck circumference, at least in awake OSAHS patients.[37]

The presence of intrapharyngeal fat deposition may also be of pathophysiological significance. Several groups of investigators have observed increased intrapharyngeal adipose tissue or increased lateral fat pad size on magnetic resonance imaging of OSAHS patients.[38, 41] The significance of a space-occupying intrapharyngeal mass for pharyngeal function has been demonstrated in an animal model with increased upper airway resistance, which is related to the magnitude of inflation of a balloon catheter in the region of the upper airway lateral fat pad.[32, 42]

Whatever the mechanism mediating the relationship between obesity and OSAHS, it has been well documented that either medical or surgical weight reduction often has a substantial ameliorative impact on this disorder.[27, 43–49] Although weight reduction may have a beneficial impact on upper airway function during sleep, it is likely that the degree of improvement is not linearly related to the amount of weight that is lost. Browman et al.[44] performed sequential polysomnograms on a patient during a dietary weight reduction program. Although there was a reduction in sleep apnea index as body weight decreased, the relationship was plotted on a semilogarithmic scale (Fig. 75–1), indicating that the absolute relationship between the variables is curvilinear. This parallels the impression of many clinicians that a critical reduction in body weight must be achieved before there is a significant reduction in OSA/H. The magnitude of this weight reduction probably varies across patients and even a relatively modest weight loss may provide a significant benefit for some patients.[45]

Although it is clear that there remains a population of nonobese OSAHS patients and that there are some patients who do not obtain benefit from weight reduction,[27, 45] obese patients should always be encouraged to lose weight. A multidisciplinary team approach to weight reduction, encompassing lifestyle and dietary modification and pharmacological and surgical options, may optimize clinical results. Not only does this have a beneficial impact on overall health, it also has a high likelihood of reducing the severity of upper airway dysfunction during sleep. If not eliminating the need for further therapy, weight reduction may minimize the required degree of aggressiveness. Conceivably, the "nonresponders" reflect those who have not lost sufficient weight or have coexistent craniofacial abnormalities.

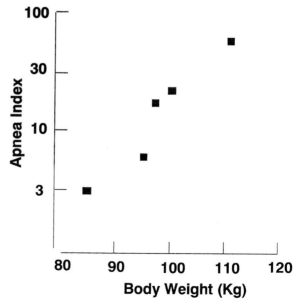

Figure 75–1. Change in apnea frequency during sleep as body weight changes in a single patient. (From Browman CP, Sampson MG, Yolles SF, et al. Obstructive sleep apnea and body weight. Chest. 1984;85:435–436.)

Tobacco Use

Tobacco use is known to have a detrimental effect on sleep. Cigarette smokers have more difficulty initiating and maintaining sleep, as well as having increased daytime sleepiness.[50] Although there are a variety of possible explanations for this, including the impact of nicotine withdrawal, it is conceivable that one mechanism is through an association between smoking and sleep-disordered breathing. Smokers have a four- to five-fold greater risk than those who never smoke of having at least moderate sleep-disordered breathing.[51] Heavy smokers are at greatest risk. Cigarette smoking may contribute to upper airway dysfunction during sleep by eliciting mucosal edema and increased upper airway resistance. It is obvious that tobacco use should be discouraged on the basis of its adverse, multisystem effects.

In light of this discussion, the observation that nicotine administered as gum reduces apnea frequency over the first several hours of sleep[52] is of conceptual if not practical interest. The short duration of action of this mode of delivery precludes effective therapeutic application of nicotine gum for OSAHS. Unfortunately, additional studies subsequently demonstrated that there was no clinically significant reduction in the frequency of disordered breathing after application of transdermal nicotine patches, which have an extended duration of delivery. Apnea duration and snoring intensity were reduced, although the magnitude of the latter was insufficient to be therapeutically useful. Adverse effects were observed in conjunction with the transdermal patch, including reduced total sleep time, sleep efficiency, and rapid eye movement (REM) sleep. Other side effects, including gastrointestinal complaints, lightheadedness, and tremor, were also reported.

Sleep Deprivation

We live in a sleep-deprived society.[53] In addition to the adverse impact of sleep deprivation on performance, several lines of evidence suggest that absolute deprivation, as well as repetitive sleep disruption, may also predispose to or worsen existing OSA/H. Sleep deprivation is associated with blunted hypoxic and hypercapnic ventilatory chemoresponsiveness, at least during wakefulness,[54, 55] and may prolong apneas and hypopneas with consequently greater oxyhemoglobin desaturation, by depressing the arousal response.[56, 57] In addition, Sériès et al.[29] noted that upper airway collapsibility increased after sleep fragmentation but not following short-term sleep deprivation.

In general, patients should be encouraged to maintain good sleep hygiene, although this advice is often unheeded because of social and financial pressures. It may be useful to remind them that to do otherwise may have an adverse impact on their sleep-disordered breathing and contribute to a vicious cycle in which insufficient or fragmented sleep promotes OSA/H, which in turn promotes poor-quality sleep.

Modification of Body Position During Sleep

A bed partner's prompting constitutes one of the oldest interventions for snoring and OSA/H, attesting to the recognition that upper airway dysfunction may be particularly notable during sleep in the supine position. In many patients, the frequency of sleep-disordered breathing events is substantially greater during sleep in the supine position than in the lateral recumbent position.[58-62] Sleeping in the supine position may increase the probability of upper airway occlusion owing to the effect of gravity on the tongue, which tends to relapse posteriorly and come into apposition with the posterior pharyngeal wall. If, indeed, as previously suggested, the mass of soft tissue in the anterior cervical region enhances the propensity for upper airway dysfunction,[30, 33] it is reasonable to speculate that this factor interacts with body position to compromise upper airway patency during sleep.

The presence of body position dependency is inversely related to the degree of obesity,[58] with a greater likelihood that more obese patients will have OSA/H regardless of position. On the other hand, it should not be assumed that a patient with normal body weight has position-dependent OSA/H[58] and the presence or absence of obesity is not an invariable predictor of supine position–dependent sleep-disordered breathing. Furthermore, it has been suggested that there is no effect of body position specifically during REM sleep[62] and that position-related alterations in overall apnea frequency are due to the impact during nonrapid eye movement (NREM) sleep. Similarly, body position has no effect on the duration of apnea. This suggests that the arousal mechanism is influenced by sleep stage, but not by body position.

Sleeping with the head and trunk elevated at a 30- to 60-degree angle to the horizontal, ameliorates OSA/H.[63, 64] Upper airway closing pressure (the magnitude of negative pressure, which, when applied to the airway, results in occlusion) is more negative (indicating greater stability) in the 30-degree head-elevated position than in the supine and lateral recumbent positions during NREM sleep.[64] Opening pressure (the magnitude of nasal continuous positive airway pressure, or CPAP, that eliminates apnea, hypopneas, and oxyhemoglobin desaturation) is less in the head-elevated position than in the supine position but not significantly different from the lateral recumbent position. These data suggest that 30-degree head elevation may be more effective in stabilizing the upper airway than sleeping in the lateral recumbent position, but that head elevation may not reduce the required magnitude of CPAP relative to lateral recumbency.

The data are sufficiently suggestive that body position influences upper airway patency during sleep in some patients to warrant specific questioning of the patient and bed partner with regard to this issue. In addition, one should objectively evaluate sleep and breathing in this context. If there is sufficient amelioration of OSA/H, as well as maintenance of acceptable oxygenation and sleep continuity in the lateral recumbent position during REM and NREM sleep, therapeutic management of body position during sleep may be considered. The "sleep ball," or similar technique to facilitate maintenance of the lateral recumbent position during sleep, may be employed. This technique entails sewing a pocket into the back of the patient's sleeping garment and placing an object, such as one or more tennis or golf balls, within the pocket. Alternatively, the objects may be placed in a sock, which is safety-pinned to the back of the sleeping garment. Over time, the patient may become trained to sleep in this position, without the need for a physical reminder. The clinician must also recognize the practical issues involved with prescribing a head-elevated position because this may require a wedge on which the patient sleeps (cumbersome with regard to sharing a bed) or a specialized and potentially costly bed. These issues notwithstanding, head-elevated body-position modification may be useful for some OSAHS patients.

In addition to affecting OSA/H frequency, body position may influence central apnea. We have seen several patients with supine body position–dependent mixed and central apneas. Issa and Sullivan[65] also remarked on the presence of supine position–dependent central apnea in patients with predominantly obstructive apnea. It has been postulated that occlusion of the upper airway in the supine position is an important element in the pathogenesis of these central apneas. Sanders et al.[66] suggested that upper airway obstruction during exhalation could result in prolonged, low-level expiratory airflow, which is generally below the threshold for detection by the usual recording techniques, thereby simulating true central apnea. Similarly, several more recent studies, employing videoendoscopy, have reinforced the presence of upper airway occlusion during otherwise central apneas.[67, 68] On the other hand, Issa and Sullivan[65] postulated that supine position–dependent (gravity-related) apposition of the pharyngeal walls precipitates central apnea via reflex inhibition of ventilation. In any case, the tendency for amelioration of these central apneas by nasal CPAP,[65, 66, 69] or in some cases by maintaining the lateral recumbent body position, supports a pathophysiological role of upper airway obstruction in these events.

In summary, manipulation of body position to promote sleeping in the lateral recumbent posture or with a 30- to 60-degree head elevation may lead to clinically significant amelioration of OSA/H in some patients. It is therefore important to analyze each patient's historical and polysomnographic data with this in mind. The potential impact of variation in body position should be considered when critically evaluating published reports describing the effects of other therapeutic interventions for OSAHS. In addition, the effect of variations in head, neck, and shoulder position on upper airway patency during sleep remains to be fully investigated.

PHARMACOLOGICAL AGENTS THAT ADVERSELY AFFECT UPPER AIRWAY FUNCTION DURING SLEEP

Alcohol

Bed partners and housemates were probably the first to recognize the association between alcohol consumption and upper airway dysfunction during sleep. A detailed discussion of the physiological effect of alcohol on the upper airway is provided in Chapter 69. It is clear, however, that alcohol evokes obstructive apnea in individuals who otherwise only snore, and increases apnea frequency in patients with preexisting OSA/H.[56, 70–73] There are limited and conflicting data regarding the contribution of alcohol to the development of upper airway dysfunction in individuals who otherwise do not snore or have apnea during sleep.[71, 72] In addition to increasing the frequency of sleep-disordered breathing events, alcohol consumption increases the duration of these events.[74, 75]

Alcohol may also have a particularly adverse impact on daytime alertness in OSAHS patients. The hypnotic effect of this agent is enhanced in the presence of underlying sleepiness. Similarly, alcohol consumption superimposed on sleepiness, as in sleep deprivation, is associated with worse driving simulator test performance compared with sleep deprivation and placebo.[76] Thus, it would be expected that alcohol would have a notably greater detrimental impact on daytime alertness in OSAHS patients who have increased basal sleepiness.

The key message is that patients with OSAHS, treated or untreated, would be best served by abstinence from alcohol. Although this is good advice, not all patients will follow it. If a patient is unwilling to completely abstain, he or she should be told to limit alcohol intake and not to consume alcohol for a time prior to bedtime that is sufficient to permit the blood alcohol level to fall to a negligible level. Furthermore, although there is inconsistency in the literature regarding the impact of alcohol on the requisite magnitude of the positive pressure prescription,[77–79] patients who are unlikely to modify their alcohol consumption should have a therapeutic trial under their usual lifestyle conditions. Thus, therapy needs to be proved successful despite the presence of exogenous as well as endogenous influences on the pathophysiological processes. These include not only alcohol consumption but other factors, including body position during sleep (some patients may only be able to sleep in the supine position) and the need for treatment with pharmacological agents that may adversely effect upper airway stability during sleep (e.g., benzodiazepines).

While alcohol represents a pharmacological agent with a potentially adverse impact on the upper airway, there are other, often-prescribed drugs with similar destabilizing effects on the upper airway during sleep.

Benzodiazepines

A detailed overview of the physiological effects of benzodiazepines on sleep and breathing is provided in Chapter 69. Although the effect of every benzodiazepine on breathing during sleep has not been evaluated, flurazepam has been the subject of several investigations. Although this agent may worsen OSA/H in some patients who otherwise have minimal sleep-disordered breathing,[80–82] reports addressing the impact on breathing during sleep in otherwise healthy have provided inconsistent results.[82, 83]

There have been a limited number of studies examining the impact of benzodiazepines other than flurazepam and diazepam. In a group of patients with mild insomnia and sleep apnea (respiratory disturbance index or RDI: 8.8 ± 5.3, mean $\pm$ SE), 15 to 30 mg of temazepam did not significantly increase the RDI or alter the degree of oxyhemoglobin desaturation, compared with placebo.[84] On the other hand, although no significant increase in the group average RDI was observed following 0.25 mg of triazolam to a group of patients with mild chronic obstructive pulmonary disease, the investigators were careful to note that individual patients met their criteria for worsened sleep-disordered breathing after administration of this agent.[85]

Thus, owing to the small populations evaluated in published investigations, as well as the conflicting results of these studies, the safety of benzodiazepine administration to OSAHS patients remains uncertain and the issue remains debatable.[86] Although in usual hypnotic doses, benzodiazepines may not present a substantial risk for provoking OSA/H in otherwise normal patients, in view of the inconclusive data regarding the margin of safety, it is wise to avoid this class of agents in patients who have been diagnosed with OSAHS and those with risk factors for this disorder.

Narcotics and Anesthetics

Although there has not been a systematic assessment of the effect of intravenous narcotics on breathing during sleep, there have been anecdotal reports of clinically significant upper airway obstruction developing after administration of these agents.[87–89] At least when delivered intravenously, narcotics have properties that heighten concern regarding their safety in the setting of OSA/H. These are discussed in detail in Chapter 69. In contrast to the impact of intravenously administered narcotics, normal subjects failed to demonstrate a change in breathing during sleep after *oral* administration of hydromorphone hydrochloride, in 2- and 4-mg doses.[90] It may not be valid, however, to extrapolate these results to the administration of higher doses of narcotics or give narcotics to patients who have, or are at risk of, upper airway dysfunction during sleep. Because of these concerns it is judicious to withhold, or at least minimize, narcotics given to patients with OSAHS or those with risk factors for this disorder. There may, of course, be instances where good medical practice requires analgesia, as in the postoperative or periprocedural (e.g., bronchoscopy or colonoscopy) setting. Under these circumstances, if non-narcotic or non-ventilatory depressant agents cannot provide adequate pain control, and if the risk is deemed clinically acceptable, minimal doses of narcotics may be administered and the patient carefully monitored, with immediate availability of an experienced airway management team to emergently reestablish upper airway patency

if the need arises. Patients who are already on nasal CPAP for OSAHS should use this therapy in the postoperative or periprocedural period, although they may have increased pressure requirements in the presence of narcotics and following general anesthesia. The latter can also promote upper airway instability by selectively reducing innervation to the upper airway dilator muscles.[91] If patients have not previously required aggressive intervention for OSAHS, nasal CPAP therapy at appropriate levels, empirically determined if necessary, should be considered until there is no longer a need for drugs with the potential to destabilize the upper airway. A review of anesthesia management in patients with OSAHS was provided by Boushra.[89]

Barbiturates

There has been no systematic assessment of the impact of barbiturates on upper airway function during sleep. However, like alcohol, this class of agents selectively reduces the neural output via the hypoglossal nerve, reduces the tone of the upper airway dilator muscles, and predisposes to upper airway occlusion during sleep.[92, 93] Thus, to avoid barbiturates in patients who are predisposed to, or are known to have, sleep-disordered breathing.

Testosterone

A few patients have been reported to experience exacerbation of OSA/H after the administration of testosterone.[94–96] Plausibility of an association between OSA/H and androgen administration is supported by the recognition of a greater prevalence of OSAHS in males than in premenopausal females.[97–99] In addition, there may be an increase in upper airway resistance during wakefulness and worsening of OSA/H during testosterone therapy.[94, 96, 100] On the other hand, no difference in OSA/H was observed in dialysis patients during and without androgen administration,[101] and androgen blockade with flutamide has been shown to have no impact on sleep-disordered breathing in men.[102]

Thus, while the magnitude of the risk of precipitating or exacerbating sleep-disordered breathing with testosterone administration is uncertain and probably variable among individuals, it is reasonable to specifically monitor these patients clinically for signs and symptoms consistent with abnormal breathing during sleep. If there are any developments in this regard, objective evaluation is warranted.

HYPOTHYROIDISM

The physiological relationship between thyroid function and sleep-disordered breathing is addressed in Chapters 69 and 93. Although the magnitude of the clinical association between hypothyroidism and OSAHS is not clear, there are considerable data in support of the former reflecting a risk factor for the latter.[103–106] On the other hand, Winkelman et al.[107] reported a similar prevalence of chemical hypothyroidism in OSAHS patients and individuals without OSAHS. These authors concluded that screening for thyroid dysfunction is not indicated in OSAHS patients unless there are corroborating signs and symptoms.

The utility of objectively screening OSAHS patients for hypothyroidism is an important question because all other things being equal, OSAHS patients may benefit substantially from thyroid replacement with a reduction of the apnea frequency.[105] On the other hand, efforts to contain the cost of medical care dictate circumspection when ordering diagnostic studies. At present, however, on the basis of the data suggesting that thyroid replacement improves upper airway function during sleep, patients with OSAHS should be evaluated for hypothyroidism with a thyroid-stimulating hormone (TSH) assay. In addition, hypothyroid patients (and their bed partners) should be specifically interviewed and examined to detect factors that raise the probability that OSAHS is present.

Although OSA/H may be reduced after initiation of thyroid replacement therapy, the degree of improvement may be insufficient to obviate the need for additional treatment.[105, 108] It is therefore important to repeat objective assessment of breathing during sleep after restoration of the euthyroid state. Grunstein and Sullivan[108] made the important observation that thyroid replacement in patients with untreated OSAHS may precipitate cardiac complications attributable to ischemia in the setting of augmented metabolism in the presence of persistent nocturnal hypoxemia. For this reason, as well as for the benefit of more rapid relief of OSAHS, the authors suggested treatment with nasal CPAP during thyroid replacement. Conceivably, this recommendation could be broadened to include successful oral appliance therapy. This strategy appears useful until an objective reassessment can be performed when the patient is clinically and chemically euthyroid and further management decisions can be made based on the additional data.

MECHANICAL DEVICES AND TECHNIQUES FOR MAINTENANCE OF UPPER AIRWAY PATENCY DURING SLEEP (EXCLUSIVE OF POSITIVE AIRWAY PRESSURE AND ORAL APPLIANCES)

Nasopharyngeal Airway

Although the concept of nasopharyngeal intubation to maintain upper airway patency during sleep was addressed in the literature as long ago as the 1970s,[109] there have been relatively few reports describing its use.[110, 111]

At best, nasopharyngeal intubation has limited therapeutic utility. A substantial proportion of patients do not tolerate this intervention and of those who do,

only about two thirds may have a clinically significant improvement in sleep-disordered breathing as defined by a reduction in disordered breathing event frequency of 65%, or an apnea index of less than 5 and an apnea-hypopnea index (AHI) of less than 10.[111] Some of these patients continued to experience notable oxyhemoglobin desaturation and there was no major improvement in sleep quality and architecture. Thus, the limited available data suggest that there is substantial patient intolerance of this form of therapy and many of the apparent "responders" still have a noteworthy degree of sleep-disordered breathing, as well as persistently abnormal sleep quality and architecture. In selected patients, however, especially those in whom other, usually more successful, noninvasive therapies have failed, a trial of this modality may be considered. Alternating nostrils in which the nasopharyngeal airway is placed, in conjunction with adequate lubrication (avoiding substances that may cause lipoid pneumonia), may improve acceptance.

Electrical Stimulation of the Upper Airway

Phasic activity of the upper airway dilators during inspiration is generally increased during wakefulness in OSAHS patients compared with control subjects.[112–114] This is consistent with ongoing physiological compensation for compromised upper airway patency. This compensatory augmentation may be diminished during sleep and consequently, upper airway dilator muscle tone becomes insufficient to overcome those factors promoting airway occlusion. It is therefore reasonable to speculate that external augmentation of upper airway dilator muscle activity will enhance luminal patency during periods when these occlusive forces are operative and natural compensatory mechanisms are reduced.

Attempts to stimulate the upper airway dilator muscles using transcutaneous submental or transhyoidal electrodes, as well as intraoral electrodes, have met with either disappointing results or concern regarding the possible impact of unintentional patient arousal.[115–117] In contrast, promising results have been obtained using direct intramuscular genioglossal or hypoglossal stimulation. Unilateral electrical stimulation of those branches of the hypoglossal nerve supplying the genioglossus muscle reduces (i.e., makes more negative) the upper airway critical closing pressure (P_{crit}) or increases maximal inspiratory airflow in feline and canine models.[118, 119] Schwartz et al.[120] applied direct electrical stimulation to the genioglossus muscle in several OSAHS patients. The electrical stimulus was triggered by the development of negative intrapharyngeal or esophageal pressure, consistent with the onset of inspiration. In a small number of patients, this reduced the number of inspiratory flow-limited breaths by about 50% and also the AHI (Fig. 75–2). Electrical stimulation did not appear to induce arousal because there was no change in the electroencephalogram immediately following the stimulus train compared with the period immediately prior to application of the stimulus, nor

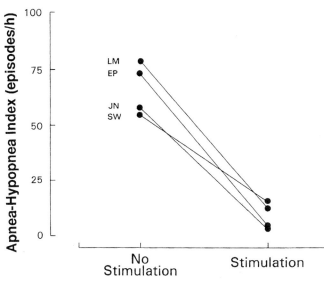

Figure 75–2. Impact of direct electrical stimulation of the genioglossus muscle in four patients with obstructive sleep apnea/hypopnea. (From Schwartz AR, Eisele DW, Hari A, et al. Electrical stimulation of the lingual musculature in obstructive sleep apnea. J Appl Physiol. 1996;81:643–652.)

was there a difference in the heart rate across the periods before, during, or after stimulation. In a small group of OSAHS patients with inspiratory airflow limitation, unilateral hypoglossal nerve stimulation employing electrodes applied directly either to the main hypoglossal nerve trunk or specifically to those branches innervating the genioglossus muscle increased maximal inspiratory airflow.[121] The impact on apnea and hypopnea events was not specifically reported, although in one patient discontinuation of stimulation for one breath resulted in airway obstruction (Fig. 75–3). Although no arousals were observed during stimulation, notable bradycardia, which was attributed to vagal nerve stimulation, developed in one participant in whom the stimulus was applied to the hypoglossal nerve trunk.

The results of hypoglossal nerve stimulation are encouraging but require confirmation in larger studies. The data suggesting that stimulation does not precipitate arousal is of particular importance, but whether this remains the case in patients after the initial treatment period and reduction of sleep pressure requires confirmation. Additionally, the limited available data suggest that electrical stimulation improves, but may not eliminate, OSA/H. If the impact of this intervention is incomplete, it may be related to the unilateral stimulation technique (one would be reluctant to implant bilateral electrodes owing to concern regarding potential bilateral nerve trauma), the importance of other, unstimulated upper airway muscles, or factors related to upper airway lateral wall instability. Finally, a durable and reliable system is needed.[118] These issues notwithstanding, electrical stimulation techniques are exciting new prospects for the treatment of OSAHS patients.

Nasal Dilators

Elevated nasal resistance may promote upper airway closure during sleep.[122, 123] Although the therapeutic benefit is controversial, about 10% of patients with snoring and apnea have been reported to improve following administration of mucosal vasoconstrictors.[124] Kerr et al.[124a] showed that when nasal resistance was reduced by 73% in OSAHS patients with nasal obstruction, by using nasal vestibular stents and topical vasoconstrictors, there was no signifcant effect on sleep architecture oxygenation or apnea index. A variety of devices have become available, which mechanically dilate the anterior nasal valve to reduce nasal airway resistance and putatively decrease the propensity toward OSA/H.

Hoijer et al.[125] assessed the impact of an external nasal dilator in 10 snorers, 7 of whom had an apnea index in excess of 5. The average apnea index fell from 18 to 6.4 and the minimum oxyhemoglobin saturation also improved while asleep with the nasal dilator, although saturation remained severely reduced in those patients with more severe baseline desaturation. Although snoring intensity was reduced, there was no subjective effect of the nasal dilator on arousal frequency or daytime sleepiness after 10 nights of use. Neither the hypopnea index, nor objectively measured arousal frequency, was reported in this study and it is therefore possible that neither the AHI nor the arousal index was favorably affected by the nasal dilator. It is

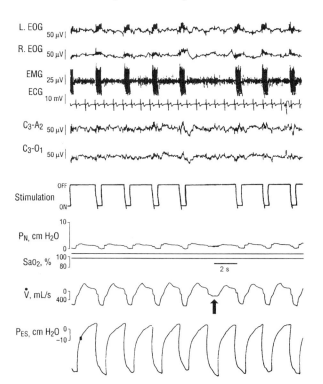

Figure 75–3. The effect of repetitive hypoglossal nerve stimulation in a patient with obstructive sleep apnea/hypopnea. The arrow indicates one breath during which stimulation was not provided; note the reduction in airflow and the increased esophageal pressure swing, which is consistent with upper airway obstruction. ECG, electrocardiogram; EMG, electromyogram; EOG, electro-oculogram. (From Eisele DW, Smith PL, Alam DS, et al. Direct hypoglossal nerve stimulation in obstructive sleep apnea. Arch Otolaryngol Head Neck Surg. 1997;123:57–61. Copyright 1997, American Medical Association.)

also noteworthy that only 4 patients expressed a desire to continue to use the nasal dilator. In contrast, Hoffstein et al.[126] concluded that dilation of the anterior nasal valve using an external dilator has no impact on sleep-disordered breathing, nadir of desaturation, and mean oxyhemoglobin saturation, although a reduction in snoring intensity was noted. However, as the authors indicated, it is possible that their results may have been biased by the absence of a randomized treatment order.

Employing an intranasally applied dilator, Scharf et al.[127] reported that a significant proportion of 20 participants had improved subjective sleepiness scores, morning concentration, and subjective quality of sleep, reduced sleepiness on awakening and number of awakenings. However, using a numerical scale, there was no difference in subjective sleep depth, refreshing quality of sleep, morning sleepiness, sleep quality, number of awakenings, and other subjective parameters. A significant number of bed partners reported decreased snoring loudness but no change in snoring regularity. Unfortunately, there was no objective assessment of sleep and breathing, either at study entry or with the nasal dilator. In another study, cyclic alternating pattern (CAPs) sequences in nonapneic snorers were reduced during use of an intranasally applied dilator, suggesting improved sleep continuity.[128]

Bahammam et al.[128a] performed a double-blind randomized controlled study of 15 UARS patients using external nasal dilators. They found that treatment reduced stage 1 sleep and had a small positive effect on oxygen desaturation time but no additional effects on sleep architecture or sleep-disordered breathing.

The literature suggests that these devices may offer some benefit for a few selected patients, but are of no proven value for most OSAHS patients.

PHARMACOLOGICAL THERAPY

Protriptyline

In the late 1970s, protriptyline, a nonsedating tricyclic antidepressant, was reported to reduce apnea episodes and increase daytime alertness in patients with narcolepsy-cataplexy.[129] Conceptually, protriptyline may reduce OSA/H by reducing the duration of REM sleep[130] and by increasing the tone of the upper airway dilator muscles[131] with increased hypoglossal and recurrent laryngeal nerve activity. Protriptyline may alter the distribution of obstructive apneas and hypopneas with a decreased frequency of the former and increased frequency of the latter.[132] The clinical significance of converting obstructive apneas to hypopneas is not clear because both may result in arousals, autonomic nervous system activation, and potentially deleterious cardiovascular impact. Although protriptyline administration may result in a statistically significant reduction in sleep-disordered breathing in study populations,

breathing and oxygenation during sleep generally remain abnormal.[133]

It is of interest, however, that despite a persistently elevated arousal frequency, the study participants receiving protriptyline reported subjective improvement in daytime sleepiness.[130] This has led to speculation that this agent has specific "alerting" properties over and above any effect on breathing. This has clinical relevance in that changes in symptoms after initiation of protriptyline therapy cannot be used as a reflection of physiological changes in breathing during sleep and objective assessment is required to evaluate the therapeutic impact.

Protriptyline has a number of side effects, primarily related to its anticholinergic properties, that further limit its use.[130, 134] Side effects include dry mouth, urinary hesitancy, constipation, confusion, and ataxia, and some patients were forced to discontinue this medication because of side effects. However, no worsening of significant cardiac dysrhythmias were observed at the dosages employed (up to 30 mg/d). The potential for dysrhythmias associated with protriptyline should, however, be recognized. Careful assessment of patients for whom use of this agent is planned or provided is needed.

In summary, owing to its lack of clinically significant therapeutic impact, in conjunction with troublesome side effects, protriptyline is not generally considered to be a standard intervention in the treatment of OSAHS.

Oxygen

In addition to sleep fragmentation, many of the clinically and physiologically evident consequences of OSAHS are attributable to nocturnal hypoxemia. Thus, prevention of hypoxemia is a worthwhile therapeutic goal in OSAHS patients. Several studies, however, reported that administration of supplemental oxygen to OSAHS patients may significantly increase apnea duration with associated hypercapnia and respiratory acidosis.[135–137] However, although there was an initial prolongation of apnea duration in a group of eucapnic OSAHS patients, Martin et al.[137] observed a significantly reduced apnea frequency with no change in the mean apnea duration after 30 min of oxygen administration compared with a period of room air breathing. This resulted in decreased apnea time and maintenance of satisfactory oxyhemoglobin saturation over the study period (Fig. 75–4). Additionally, the bradycardia that accompanied apnea was eliminated by supplemental oxygen administration. Gold et al.[138] subsequently reported that supplemental oxygen administration was associated with a statistically, but probably not clinically significant, reduction in apnea frequency, particularly during NREM sleep, as well as improved oxyhemoglobin saturation. Apnea duration increased slightly by an average of 4 to 7 sec across the study group. There was no improvement in subjective or objective measures of daytime sleepiness during the period of nocturnal oxygen supplementation.

The above considerations notwithstanding, the evi-

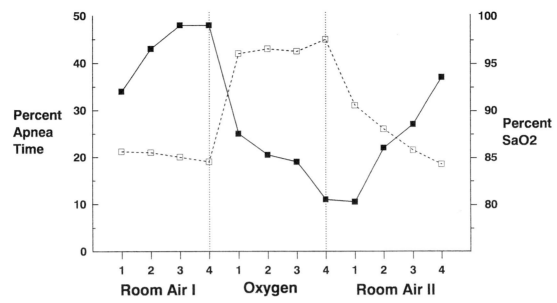

Figure 75–4. Mean percent apnea time for eight patients *(closed squares, solid line)* and the average nadir of oxyhemoglobin saturation per apnea *(open squares, dashed line)* for each 7.5-min interval during the three study periods (Room Air I, Oxygen, Room Air II). (Adapted from Martin RJ, Sanders MH, Gray BA, et al. Acute and long-term ventilatory effects of hypoxia in the adult sleep apnea syndrome. Am Rev Respir Dis. 1982;125:175–180.)

dence suggests that providing supplemental oxygen during sleep is not effective in reducing the frequency of apnea and increasing daytime alertness to stand alone as therapy for most patients. On the other hand, there may be a subpopulation of patients who are asymptomatic with regard to the consequences of sleep fragmentation (i.e., hypersomnolence) or have a minimal frequency of OSA/H events, but who experience unacceptable oxyhemoglobin desaturation during sleep. In these patients, increasing nocturnal oxyhemoglobin saturation may be the major, if not the only, therapeutic goal. The degree and duration of oxyhemoglobin desaturation that is ultimately harmful remains to be determined.[139] However, patients with coronary artery or cerebrovascular disease and only a marginally elevated frequency of abnormal breathing events during sleep, but with unacceptable oxyhemoglobin desaturation during those events, might benefit from supplemental oxygen.[140, 141] Outcome studies are clearly needed to determine at what level of desaturation there is a cost-benefit justification for providing oxygen therapy. Because of the possibility of severe prolongation of apnea, at least during the first several minutes of oxygen administration, initial trials of oxygen therapy should be monitored. Monitoring is also necessary to determine the flow of supplemental oxygen required for maintenance of acceptable oxyhemoglobin saturation.

In addition to providing sole therapy in selected patients with OSAHS, oxygen may be a useful adjunct to positive airway pressure (CPAP or bilevel positive airway pressure).[142] OSAHS patients who are sufficiently hypoxemic or borderline hypoxemic during wakefulness to warrant supplemental oxygen therapy will usually meet the criteria for this therapy during sleep, even if positive airway pressure treatment maintains upper airway patency.[143] Thus, the addition of supplemental oxygen to the positive airway pressure system may be necessary in some patients. One should be careful, however, to determine if persistent desaturation on CPAP is related to hypoventilation resulting from the high mechanical impedance to expiration or the increased dead space–tidal volume ratio that may be associated with this modality.[144] In these circumstances bilevel positive airway pressure may permit sufficient reduction of expiratory pressure to avoid significant hypoventilation and desaturation and obviate the need for supplemental oxygen.

Transtracheal Oxygen Delivery

Several studies have described the impact of transtracheal oxygen administration to OSAHS patients.[145–147] Although suggestive of a favorable impact, the data are too limited to provide substantive insight into the clinical utility of this mode of oxygen delivery, or to determine if it provides meaningful benefit over less invasive methods. If the transtracheal route is effective and superior to nasal cannulas in reducing OSA/H, it could be the result of stimulation of flow or temperature-sensitive receptors in the upper airway. Large, well-designed studies are necessary to evaluate the role of this intervention. The frequency and severity of complications resulting from transtracheal oxygen therapy in a predominantly obese patient population has not been elucidated. Availability of this information is essential before this therapeutic modality can be accepted. At present, transtracheal oxygen should be considered investigational in the treatment of OSAHS patients.

Agents With an Uncertain or Limited Therapeutic Role

Stimulants

There are a number of reasons why an OSAHS patient who is thought to be on adequate treatment to reverse upper airway dysfunction and maintain acceptable oxyhemoglobin saturation, as well as sleep continuity, may still complain of disturbing diurnal sleepiness or lack of alertness. Indeed, mean sleep latency improves during CPAP therapy, but in many cases does not return to clearly normal values.[148] Under these circumstances, the clinician must consider the possibility of noncompliance with the treatment regimen (e.g., CPAP, oral appliances, body position modification), an inadequate prescription (e.g., CPAP level or mandibular advancement), changing external factors (e.g., weight gain, medications, sleep hygiene, shift work, other medical or psychiatric disorders), or a nonpulmonary sleep-wake disorder, to name a few. However, even after these issues have been addressed, some patients remain unacceptably and perhaps dangerously sleepy or inattentive. Stimulants may provide symptomatic benefit for these patients.

Historically, amphetamines have been the class of agents employed as stimulants. Unfortunately, this group of drugs has considerable potential for harmful cardiovascular consequences, as well as adverse psychiatric and sleep effects. Modafinil is thought to be a central alpha$_1$ agonist with possible dopaminergic properties.[149] Limited studies have suggested that modafinil increases daytime alertness and vigilance and memory performance without significant side effects in patients with or without OSAHS.[149, 150] There was no change in the AHI or the nadir of oxyhemoglobin saturation on modafinil in OSAHS patients. Much more work is necessary before modafinil or any stimulant drug can be recommended for OSAHS patients. The safety, efficacy, and indications must be clearly elucidated. Although potentially useful, application of stimulants even if "safe," should be considered only in patients with impaired alertness despite known reversal of physiologically significant consequences of OSAHS. Prescription of stimulants without a diagnostic evaluation risks masking important persistent and significant sleep-related pathological condition that may negatively affect the quality and duration of the patient's life, independent of the issue of daytime sleepiness.[10, 17, 140, 141, 151–159]

Serotonin Agonists

Several studies have suggested that serotonin may mediate both upper airway dilator muscle and diaphragm activity.[133, 160] It has been further postulated that the reduction in upper airway dilator muscle tone, particularly during REM sleep, is due to withdrawal of serotonin-related excitatory input to the hypoglossal motor neurons.[161] If these postulates are true, it could have substantial implications for the treatment of patients with OSAHS.

Buspirone is an anxiolytic agent, whose mechanism of action is believed to be at least partly mediated through serotonin receptors in the central nervous system.[162, 163] Several animal studies have suggested that administration of buspirone augments ventilation during wakefulness and sleep and enhances ventilatory responsiveness to carbon dioxide.[162, 163] In addition, the apneic threshold for CO_2 is reduced by an average of 3.7 mmHg.

The above data suggest that as a class of agents, serotonin agonists may have a therapeutic role in OSAHS. Although, theoretically, buspirone has characteristics that may provide therapeutic benefit in OSAHS there are insufficient data on which to base judgments regarding its safety or efficacy. Other serotonin agonists have been evaluated to limited degrees. Following administration of fluoxetine 20 mg/d, one study found a statistically significant reduction in the apnea-hypopnea frequency, from 57 ±9 to 34 ±6 (mean ± SE), although there was wide intersubject variability and there was no significant impact on arousal frequency.[133] Fluoxetine increased sleep latency, independent of its effect on sleep-disordered breathing, and reduced the percentage of REM sleep. Although these results are disappointing, knowledge regarding the relationship between the serotoninergic system, sleep, and breathing is continuing to evolve. There is reason to be hopeful that further knowledge of the relevant receptors will result in more effective interventions.

A discussion of OSAHS therapy employing serotonin-related agents would be incomplete without cautionary mention of L-tryptophan. Several studies were published in the 1980s on the impact of L-tryptophan in the treatment of OSAHS.[164, 165] The evidence for consistent, clinically significant amelioration of OSA/H was at best arguable. It was subsequently observed that L-tryptophan has an unacceptable safety profile and should not be used owing to its association with development of the eosinophilia-myalgia syndrome.[166, 167]

Agents With No Therapeutic Indications for Obstructive Sleep Apnea/Hypopnea

A variety of agents have been administered to OSAHS patients and found to be ineffective or harmful.

Progesterone augments hypercapnic ventilatory chemosensitivity and resting ventilation in some normals and some patients with chronic obstructive pulmonary disease.[168–170] In addition, a hormonal influence in the pathogenesis of OSAHS is suggested by the results of epidemiological studies, which show a greater prevalence of OSAHS in men and postmenopausal women compared with premenopausal women.[97] This has provided the basis for trials of progestational agents in patients with OSAHS. Several early studies of small groups of patients concluded that medroxyprogesterone acetate (MPA) might be beneficial in selected patients.[171–173] However, subsequent placebo-controlled investigations demonstrated that although MPA aug-

Table 75–1. PHARMACOLOGICAL AGENTS WITH NO THERAPEUTIC INDICATION FOR OBSTRUCTIVE SLEEP APNEA-HYPOPNEA SYNDROME

Agent	Action	References
Progestational agents	Hormone; ventilatory stimulant	97, 168–178
Acetazolamide	Carbonic anhydrase inhibitor	179, 180
Theophylline	3'5'-Phosphodiesterase inhibitor; adenosine antagonist	181–184
L-Tryptophan	Serotonin precursor	164–167
Naloxone	Opiate antagonist	185
Bromocriptine	Dopamine receptor agonist	185
Baclofen	Analogue of gamma-aminobutyric acid (GABA)	186
Almitrine	Piperazine derivative; stimulates peripheral chemoreceptors	187
Chlorimipramine	Tricyclic antidepressant	188
Prochlorperazine	Phenothiazine	189

ments awake hypercapnic ventilatory responsiveness, there is no reduction in disordered-breathing time or disordered-breathing event frequency or duration.[174, 175] Studies investigating another progestational agent, chlormadinone acetate (CMA), found similar ventilation-augmenting properties and similarly disappointing therapeutic efficacy for OSAHS.[176–178]

The literature, therefore, suggests that progestational agents, at least MPA and CMA, have little effectiveness in the treatment of eucapnic OSAHS patients. Too little data are available that address the impact of progestational agents specifically in hypercapnic OSAHS patients to speculate on their clinical utility in this patient population.

Other agents with no current therapeutic indication for OSAHS are summarized in Table 75–1.

CONCLUSIONS

Unfortunately, it cannot be claimed that great advances have been made in the medical treatment of OSAHS, exclusive of positive pressure and oral appliance therapy, since the last edition of this book. Our current understanding of the pathogenesis and pathophysiology of sleep-disordered breathing remains incomplete, but our knowledge base is expanding into the neuronal and molecular biological aspects of the elements that control upper airway function and breathing during sleep. It is anticipated that once a paradigm of the normal mechanisms has been developed, information regarding the pathogenesis of OSAHS will be forthcoming. With this knowledge, specifically targeted pharmacological intervention will not be long in coming. In the meantime, clinicians can take satisfaction that virtually all patients can be effectively treated by at least one of the available modalities. Although positive airway pressure remains the most definitive and consistently successful treatment for OSAHS, consideration of "medical" factors is often rewarding. This is particularly true with respect to the

various elements that represent predisposing factors toward upper airway dysfunction during sleep, because reversal of these conditions may eliminate the need for more aggressive intervention.

Acknowledgments

Supported in part by NHLBI training grant #5T32HL07563-07.

References

1. Gastaut H, Tassinari CA, Duron B. Etude polygraphique des manifestations épisodique (hyponique et respiratoires), diurnes et nocturne, du syndrome de Pickwick. Rev Neurol (Paris). 1965;112:568–579.
2. Carskadon MA, Dement WC. Respiration during sleep in the aged human. J Gerontol. 1981;36:420–423.
3. Lavie P. Incidence of sleep apnea in a presumably healthy working population: a significant relationship with excessive daytime sleepiness. Sleep. 1983;6:312–318.
4. Bixler EO, Kales A, Cadieux RJ, et al. Sleep apneic activity in older healthy subjects. J Appl Physiol. 1985;58:1597–1601.
5. Gislason T, Almqvist MEG, Taube A, et al. Prevalence of sleep apnea syndrome among Swedish men—an epidemiological study. J Clin Epidemiol. 1988;41:571–576.
6. Berry DTR, Webb WB, Block AJ. Sleep apnea syndrome: a critical review of the apnea index as a diagnostic criterion. Chest. 1984;86:529–531.
7. Berry DTR, Webb WB, Block AJ, et al. Sleep-disordered breathing and its concomitants in a subclinical population. Sleep. 1986;9:478–483.
8. Ancoli-Israel S, Klauber M, Kripke DF, et al. Sleep apnea in female patients in a nursing home. Increased risk of mortality. Chest. 1989;96:1054–1058.
9. Partinen M, Jamieson A, Guilleminault C. Long-term outcome for obstructive sleep apnea syndrome patients: mortality. Chest. 1988;94:1200–1204.
10. He J, Kryger MH, Zorick FJ, et al. Mortality and apnea index in obstructive sleep apnea: experience in 385 male patients. Chest. 1988;94:9–14.
11. Partinen M, Guilleminault C. Daytime sleepiness and vascular morbidity at seven-year follow-up in obstructive sleep apnea patients. Chest. 1990;97:27–32.
12. Redline S, Sanders M. Hypopnea, a floating metric: implications for prevalence, morbidity estimates and case finding. Sleep. 1997;20:1209–1217.
13. Guilleminault C, Stoohs R. Upper airway resistance syndrome. Am Rev Respir Dis. 1991;143:A589.
13a. Sleep-related breathing disorders in adults: recommendations for syndrome definition and measurement techniques in clinical research. The Report of an American Academy of Sleep Medicine Task Force. Sleep. 1999;22:667–689.
14. Lugaresi E, Coccagna G, Mantovani M, et al. Effects of tracheostomy in two cases of hypersomnia with periodic breathing. J Neurol Neurosurg Psychiatry. 1973;36:15–26.
15. Kenan PD. Complications associated with tracheostomy: prevention and treatment. Otolaryngol Clin North Am. 1979;12:807–816.
16. Conway WA, Victor LD, Magilligan DJ Jr, et al. Adverse effects of tracheostomy for sleep apnea. JAMA. 1981;246:347–350.
17. Hla KM, Young TB, Bidwell T, et al. Sleep apnea and hypertension. Ann Intern Med. 1994;120:382–388.
18. Young T, Palta M, Dempsey J, et al. The occurrence of sleep-disordered breathing among middle-aged adults. N Engl J Med. 1993;328:1230–1235.
19. Young T, Finn L, Hla KM, et al. Snoring as part of a dose-response relationship between sleep-disordered breathing and blood pressure. Sleep. 1996;19(suppl 10):s202–s205.
20. Guilleminault C, Tilkian A, Dement WC. The sleep apnea syndromes. Annu Rev Med. 1976;27:465–484.
21. Guilleminault C, Eldridge FL, Tilkian A, et al. Sleep apnea syndrome due to upper airway obstruction: a review of 25 cases. Arch Intern Med. 1977;137:296–300.

22. Wittels EH. Obesity and hormonal factors in sleep and sleep apnea. Med Clin North Am. 1985;69:1265–1280.

23. Lloyd J. Saturday conference: sleep apnea syndrome. South Med J. 1983;76:1417–1420.

24. Hoffstein V, Zamel N, Phillipson EA. Lung volume dependence of pharyngeal cross-sectional area in patients with obstructive sleep apnea. Am Rev Respir Dis. 1984;130:175–178.

25. Bradley TD, Brown IG, Grossman R, et al. Pharyngeal size in snorers, non-snorers, and patients with obstructive sleep apnea. N Engl J Med. 1986;315:1327–1331.

26. Rivlin J, Hoffstein V, Kalbfleisch J, et al. Upper airway morphology in patients with idiopathic obstructive sleep apnea. Am Rev Respir Dis. 1984;129:355–360.

27. Suratt PM, McTier RF, Findley LJ, et al. Changes in breathing and the pharynx after weight loss in obstructive sleep apnea. Chest. 1987;92:631–637.

28. Abbey NC, Cooper KR, Kwentus JA. Benefit of nasal CPAP in obstructive sleep apnea is due to positive pharyngeal pressure. Sleep. 1989;12:420–422.

29. Sériès F, Cormier Y, La Forge J, et al. Mechanisms of the effectiveness of continuous positive airway pressure in obstructive sleep apnea. Sleep. 1992;15(6):s47–s49.

30. Koenig JS, Thach BT. Effects of mass loading on the upper airway. J Appl Physiol. 1988;64:2294–2299.

31. Wolin AD, Strohl KP, Acree BN, et al. Responses to negative pressure surrounding the neck in anesthetized animals. J Appl Physiol. 1990;68:154–160.

32. Winter WC, Gampper T, Gay SB, et al. Lateral pharyngeal fat pad pressure during breathing. Sleep. 1996;19:s178–s179.

33. Katz I, Stradling J, Slutsky AS, et al. Do patients with obstructive sleep apnea have thick necks? Am Rev Respir Dis. 1990;141:1228–1231.

34. Davies RJO, Stradling JR. The relationship between neck circumference, radiographic pharyngeal anatomy, and obstructive sleep apnoea syndrome. Eur Respir J. 1990;3:509–514.

35. Hoffstein V, Mateika S. Differences in abdominal and neck circumferences in patients with and without obstructive sleep apnoea. Eur Respir J. 1992;5:377–381.

36. Hoffstein V, Mateika S. Predicting nasal continuous positive airway pressure. Am J Respir Crit Care Med. 1994;150:486–488.

37. Ryan CF, Love LL. Mechanical properties of the velopharynx in obese patients with obstructive sleep apnea. Am J Respir Crit Care Med. 1996;154:806–812.

38. Horner RL, Mohiaddin RH, Lowell DG, et al. Sites and sizes of fat deposits around the pharynx in obese patients with obstructive sleep apnoea and weight matched controls. Eur Respir J. 1989;2:613–622.

39. Shelton KE, Woodson H, Gay S, et al. Pharyngeal fat in obstructive sleep apnea. Am Rev Respir Dis. 1993;148:462–466.

40. Schwab RJ, Gupta KB, Hoffman EA, et al. Differences in upper airway soft tissue anatomy in normal subjects and patients with sleep-disordered breathing. Am Rev Respir Dis. 1993;147:A947.

41. Schwab RJ. Diagnostic imaging in the diagnostic evaluation of the upper airway. In: Rose BD, ed. UpToDate. Vol version 5.3. Wellesley, Mass; UpToDate;1999.

42. Winter WC, Goumpper T, Gay SB, et al. Enlargement of the lateral pharyngeal fat pad space in pigs increases upper airway resistance. J Appl Physiol. 1995;79:726–731.

43. Harman EM, Wynne JW, Block AJ. The effect of weight loss on sleep-disordered breathing and oxygen desaturation in morbidly obese men. Chest. 1982;82:291–294.

44. Browman CP, Sampson MG, Yolles SF, et al. Obstructive sleep apnea and body weight. Chest. 1984;85:435–436.

45. Smith PL, Gold AR, Meyers DA, et al. Weight loss in mildly to moderately obese patients with obstructive sleep apnea. Ann Intern Med. 1983;103:850–855.

46. Peiser J, Lavie P, Ovnat A, et al. Sleep apnea syndrome in the morbidly obese as an indication for weight reduction surgery. Ann Surg. 1984;199:112–115.

47. Schwartz AR, Gold AR, Schubert N, et al. Effect of weight loss on upper airway collapsibility in obstructive sleep apnea. Am Rev Respir Dis. 1991;144:494–498.

48. Charuzi I, Lavie P, Peiser J, et al. Bariatric surgery in morbidly obese sleep-apnea patients: short- and long-term follow-up. Am J Clin Nutr. 1992;55:594s–596s.

49. Sugarman HJ, Fairman RP, Sood RK, et al. Long-term effects on gastric surgery for treating respiratory insufficiency of obesity. Am J Clin Nutr. 1992;55:597s–601s.

50. Phillips B, Danner F. Cigarette smoking and sleep disturbance. Arch Intern Med. 1995;155:734–737.

51. Wetter DW, Young TB, Bidwell TR, et al. Smoking as a risk factor for sleep-disordered breathing. Arch Intern Med. 1994;154:2219–2224.

52. Gothe B, Strohl KP, Cherniack NS. Nicotine: a different approach to treatment of obstructive sleep apnea. Chest. 1985;87:11–17.

53. Bonnet MH, Arand DL. We are chronically sleep deprived. Sleep. 1995;18:908–911.

54. Schiffman PL, Trontell MC, Mazar MF, et al. Sleep deprivation decreases ventilatory response to CO_2 but not load compensation. Chest. 1983;84:695–698.

55. White DP, Douglas NJ, Pickett CK, et al. Sleep deprivation and the control of ventilation. Am Rev Respir Dis. 1983;128:984–986.

56. Guilleminault C, Rosekind M. The arousal threshold: sleep deprivation, sleep fragmentation, and obstructive sleep apnea syndrome. Bull Eur Pathophysiol Respir. 1981;17:341–349.

57. Bowes G, Woolf GM, Sullivan CE, et al. Effect of sleep fragmentation on ventilatory and arousal responses of sleeping dogs to respiratory stimuli. Am Rev Respir Dis. 1980;122:899–908.

58. Cartwright RD. Effect of sleep position on sleep apnea severity. Sleep. 1984;7:110–114.

59. Cartwright RD, Lloyd S, Lilie J, et al. Sleep position training as treatment for sleep apnea syndrome: a preliminary study. Sleep. 1985;8:87–94.

60. Chaudhary BA, Chaudhary TK, Kolbeck RC, et al. Therapeutic effect of posture in sleep apnea. South Med J. 1986;79:1061–1063.

61. Phillips BA, Okeson J, Paesani D, et al. Effect of sleep position on sleep apnea and parafunctional activity. Chest. 1986;90:424–429.

62. George CF, Millar TW, Kryger MH. Sleep apnea and body position during sleep. Sleep. 1988;11:90–99.

63. McEvoy RD, Sharp DJ, Thornton AT. The effects of posture on obstructive sleep apnea. Am Rev Respir Dis. 1986;133:662–666.

64. Neill AM, Angus SM, Sajkov D, et al. Effects of sleep posture on upper airway stability in patients with obstructive sleep apnea. Am J Respir Crit Care Med. 1997;155:199–204.

65. Issa FG, Sullivan CE. Reversal of central sleep apnea using nasal CPAP. Chest. 1986;90:165–171.

66. Sanders MH, Rogers RM, Pennock BE. Prolonged expiratory phase in sleep apnea: a unifying hypothesis. Am Rev Respir Dis. 1985;131:401–408.

67. Badr MS, Toiber F, Skatrud JB, et al. Pharyngeal narrowing/occlusion during central sleep apnea. J Appl Physiol. 1995;78:1806–1815.

68. Morrell MJ, Badr MS, Harms CA, et al. The assessment of upper airway patency during apnea using cardiogenic oscillations in the airflow signal. Sleep. 1995;18:651–658.

69. Sanders MH. Nasal CPAP effect on patterns of sleep apnea. Chest. 1984;86:839–844.

70. Issa FG, Sullivan CE. Alcohol, snoring and sleep apnea. J Neurol Neurosurg Psychiatry. 1982;45:353–359.

71. Scrima L, Broudy M, Nay KN, et al. Increased severity of obstructive sleep apnea after bedtime alcohol ingestion: diagnostic potential and proposed mechanism of action. Sleep. 1982;5:318–328.

72. Taasan VC, Block AJ, Boysen PG, et al. Alcohol increases sleep apnea and oxygen desaturation in asymptomatic men. Am J Med. 1981;71:240–245.

73. Remmers JE. Obstructive sleep apnea: a common disorder exacerbated by alcohol. Am Rev Respir Dis. 1984;130:153–155.

74. Gleeson K, Zwillich CW, White DP. The influence of increasing ventilatory effort on arousal from sleep. Am Rev Respir Dis. 1990;142:295–300.

75. Berry RB, Bonnet MH, Light RW. Effect of ethanol on the arousal response to airway occlusion during sleep in normal subjects. Am Rev Respir Dis. 1992;145:445–452.

76. Roehrs T, Beare D, Zorick F, et al. Sleepiness and ethanol effects on simulated driving. Alcohol Clin Exp Res. 1994;18:154–158.

77. Berry RT, Desa MM, Light RW. Effect of ethanol on the efficacy of nasal continuous positive airway pressure as a treatment of obstructive sleep apnea. Chest. 1991;99:339–343.

78. Mitler MM, Dawson A, Henriksen SJ, et al. Bedtime ethanol increases resistance of upper airways and produces sleep apneas in asymptomatic snorers. Alcohol Clin Exp Res. 1988;12:801–805.
79. Teschler H, Berthon-Jones M, Wessendorf T, et al. Influence of moderate alcohol consumption on obstructive sleep apnoea with and without AutoSet nasal CPAP therapy. Eur Respir J. 1996;9:2371–2377.
80. Dolly FR, Block AJ. Effect of flurazepam on sleep-disordered breathing and nocturnal desaturation in asymptomatic subjects. Am J Med. 1982;73:239–243.
81. Mendelson WB, Garnett D, Gillin JC. Flurazepam-induced sleep apnea syndrome in a patient with insomnia and mild sleep-related respiratory changes. J Nerv Ment Dis. 1981;160:261–264.
82. Guilleminault C, Silvestri R, Mondini S, et al. Aging and sleep apnea: action of benzodiazepine, acetazolamide, alcohol and sleep deprivation in a healthy elderly group. J Gerontol. 1984;39:655–661.
83. Guilleminault C, Cummiskey J, Silvestri R. Benzodiazepines and respiration during sleep. In: Usdin E, Skolnick P, Tallman JF, et al, eds. Pharmacology of Benzodiazepines. London, England: Macmillan; 1982:229–236.
84. Camacho ME, Morin CM. The effect of temazepam on respiration in elderly insomniacs with mild sleep apnea. Sleep. 1995;18:644–645.
85. Steens RD, Pouliot Z, Millar TW, et al. Effects of zolpidem and triazolam on sleep and respiration in mild to moderate chronic obstructive pulmonary disease. Sleep. 1993;16:318–326.
86. Hanly P, Powles P. Hypnotics should never be used in patients with sleep apnea. J Psychosom Res. 1993;37(suppl 1):59–65.
87. Rafferty TD, Ruskis A, Sasaki C, et al. Perioperative considerations in the management of tracheostomy for the obstructive sleep apnea patient. Br J Anaesth. 1980;52:619–621.
88. Cately DM, Thornton C, Jordan C, et al. Pronounced episodic oxygen desaturation in the postoperative period: its association with ventilatory pattern and analgesic regimen. Anesthesiology. 1985;63:20–28.
89. Boushra NN. Anesthetic management of patients with sleep apnea syndrome. Can J Anaesth. 1996;43:599–616.
90. Robinson RW, Zwillich CW, Bixler EO, et al. Effects of oral narcotics on sleep-disordered breathing in healthy adults. Chest. 1987;91:197–203.
91. Nishino T, Shirahata M, Yonezawa T, et al. Comparison of changes in the hypoglossal and phrenic nerve activity in response to increasing depth of anesthesia in cats. Anesthesiology. 1984;60:19–24.
92. Brouillette RT, Thach BT. A neuromuscular mechanism maintaining extrathoracic airway patency. J Appl Physiol. 1979;46:772–779.
93. Drummond GB. Influence of thiopentone on upper airway muscles. Br J Anaesth. 1989;63:212–221.
94. Johnson MW, Anch AM, Remmers JE. Induction of the sleep apnea syndrome in a woman by exogenous androgen administration. Am Rev Respir Dis. 1984;129:1023–1025.
95. Sandblom RE, Matsumoto RB, Schoene RB, et al. Obstructive sleep apnea syndrome induced by testosterone administration. N Engl J Med. 1983;308:508–510.
96. Schneider BK, Pickett CK, Zwillich CW, et al. Influence of testosterone on breathing during sleep. J Appl Physiol. 1986;61:618–623.
97. Block AJ, Wynne JW, Boysen PG. Sleep-disordered breathing and nocturnal oxygen desaturation in post-menopausal women. Am J Med. 1980;69:75–79.
98. Block AJ, Boysen PG, Wynne JW, et al. Sleep apnea, hypopnea and oxygen desaturation in normal subjects: a strong male predominance. N Engl J Med. 1979;300:513–517.
99. Block AJ, Wynne JW, Boysen PG, et al. Menopause, medroxyprogesterone and breathing during sleep. Am J Med. 1981;70:506–510.
100. Cistulli PA, Grunstein RR, Sullivan CE. Effect of testosterone administration on upper airway collapsibility during sleep. Am J Respir Crit Care Med. 1994;149:530–532.
101. Millman RP, Kimmel PL, Shore ET, et al. Sleep apnea in hemodialysis patients: the lack of testosterone effect on its pathogenesis. Am Rev Respir Dis. 1984;129:A252.
102. Stewart DA, Grunstein RR, Berthon-Jones M, et al. Androgen blockade does not affect sleep-disordered breathing or chemosensitivity in men with obstructive sleep apnea. Am Rev Respir Dis. 1992;146:1389–1393.
103. Skatrud J, Iber C, Ewart R, et al. Disordered breathing during sleep in hypothyroidism. Am Rev Respir Dis. 1981;124:325–329.
104. Orr WC, Males JL, Imes NK. Myxedema and obstructive sleep apnea. Am J Med. 1981;70:1061–1066.
105. Rajagopal KR, Abbrecht PH, Derderian SS, et al. Obstructive sleep apnea in hypothyroidism. Ann Intern Med. 1984;101:491–494.
106. Pelttari L, Rauhala E, Polo O, et al. Upper airway obstruction in hypothyroidism. J Intern Med. 1995;236:177–181.
107. Winkelman JW, Goldman H, Piscatelli N, et al. Are thyroid function tests necessary in patients with suspected sleep apnea? Sleep. 1996;19:790–793.
108. Grunstein RR, Sullivan CE. Sleep apnea and hypothyroidism: mechanisms and management. Am J Med. 1988;85:775–779.
109. Kravath RE, Pollack CP, Borowiecki B. Hypoventilation during sleep in children who have lymphoid airway obstruction treated by nasopharyngeal tube and tonsillectomy and adenoidectomy. Pediatrics. 1977;59:865–871.
110. Afzelius L-E, Elmqvist D, Hougaard K, et al. Sleep apnea syndrome—an alternative treatment to tracheostomy. Laryngoscope. 1981;91:285–291.
111. Nahmias JS, Karetzky MS. Treatment of the obstructive sleep apnea syndrome using a nasopharyngeal tube. Chest. 1988;94:1142–1147.
112. Mezzanotte WS, Tangel DJ, White DP. Influence of sleep onset on upper airway muscle activity in apnea patients versus normal controls. Am J Respir Crit Care Med. 1996;153:1880–1887.
113. Mezzanotte WS, Tangel DJ, White DP. Waking genioglossal EMG in sleep apnea patients versus normal controls (a neuromuscular compensatory mechanism). J Clin Invest. 1992;89:1571–1579.
114. Suratt PM, McTier RF, Wilhoit SC. Upper airway muscle activation is augmented in patients with obstructive sleep apnea compared with that in normal subjects. Am Rev Respir Dis. 1988;137:889–894.
115. Miki H, Hida W, Chonan T, et al. Effects of electrical stimulation during sleep on upper airway patency in patients with obstructive sleep apnea. Am Rev Respir Dis. 1989;140:1285–1289.
116. Edmonds LC, Daniels BK, Stanson AW, et al. The effects of transcutaneous electrical stimulation during wakefulness and sleep in patients with obstructive sleep apnea. Am Rev Respir Dis. 1992;146:1030–1036.
117. Guilleminault C, Powell N, Bowman B, et al. The effect of electrical stimulation on obstructive sleep apnea. Chest. 1995;107:67–73.
118. Goding GS, Eisele DW, Testrman R, et al. Relief of upper airway obstruction with hypoglossal nerve stimulation in the canine. Laryngoscope. 1998;108:162–169.
119. Schwartz AR, Thut DC, Russ B, et al. Effect of electrical stimulation of the hypoglossal nerve on airflow mechanics in the isolated upper airway. Am Rev Respir Dis. 1993;147:1144–1150.
120. Schwartz AR, Eisele DW, Hari A, et al. Electrical stimulation of the lingual musculature in obstructive sleep apnea. J Appl Physiol. 1996;81:643–652.
121. Eisele DW, Smith PL, Alam DS, et al. Direct hypoglossal nerve stimulation in obstructive sleep apnea. Arch Otolaryngol Head Neck Surg. 1997;123:57–61.
122. Suratt PM, Turner BL, Wilhoit SC. Effect of intranasal obstruction on breathing during sleep. Chest. 1986;90:324–329.
123. Lavie P, Fischel N, Zomer J, et al. The effects of partial and complete mechanical occlusion of the nasal passages on sleep architecture and breathing during sleep. Acta Otolaryngol. 1983;95:161–166.
124. Fairbanks DNF, Fairbanks DW. Obstructive sleep apnea: therapeutic alternatives. Am J Otolaryngol. 1992;13:265–270.
124a. Kerr P, Millar T, Buckle P, et al. The importance of nasal resistance in obstructive sleep apnea syndrome. J Otolaryngol. 1992;21:189–195.
125. Hoijer U, Ejnell H, Hedner J, et al. The effects of nasal dilation on snoring and obstructive sleep apnea. Arch Otolaryngol Head Neck Surg. 1992;118:281–284.

126. Hoffstein V, Mateika S, Metes A. Effect of nasal dilation on snoring and apneas during different stages of sleep. Sleep. 1993;16:360–365.

127. Scharf MB, Brannen DE, McDonnold M. A subjective evaluation of a nasal dilator on sleep and snoring. Ear Nose Throat J. 1994;73:395–401.

128. Scharf MB, McDonnold MD, Zaretsky NT, et al. Cyclic alternating pattern sequences in non-apneic snorers with and without nasal dilation. Ear Nose Throat J. 1996;75:617–619.

128a. Bahammam AS, Tate R, Manfreda J, et al. Upper airway resistance syndrome: effect of nasal dilation, sleep stage, and sleep position. Sleep. 1999;22:592–598.

129. Schmidt HS, Clark RW, Hyman PR. Protriptyline: an effective agent in the treatment of the narcolepsy-cataplexy syndrome and hypersomnia. Am J Psychiatry. 1977;134:183–185.

130. Brownell LG, West P, Sweatman P, et al. Protriptyline in obstructive sleep apnea. A double blind trial. N Engl J Med. 1982;307:1037–1042.

131. Bonora M, St John WM, Bledsoe TA. Differential elevation by protriptyline and depression by diazepam of upper airway respiratory muscle activity. Am Rev Respir Dis. 1985;131:41–45.

132. Smith PL, Haponik EF, Allen RP, et al. The effects of protriptyline in sleep-disordered breathing. Am Rev Respir Dis. 1983;127:8–13.

133. Hanzel DA, Proia NG, Hudgel DW. Response of obstructive sleep apnea to fluoxetine and protriptyline. Chest. 1991;100:416–421.

134. Conway WA, Zorick F, Piccione P, et al. Protriptyline in the treatment of sleep apnoea. Thorax. 1982;37:49–53.

135. Motta J, Guilleminault C. Effects of oxygen administration in sleep-induced apneas. In: Guilleminault C, Dement WC, eds. Sleep Apnea Syndromes. New York, NY: Alan R Liss; 1978:137–145.

136. Kimoff RJ, Cheong TH, Olha AE, et al. Mechanisms of apnea termination in obstructive sleep apnea. Role of chemoreceptor and mechanoreceptor stimuli. Am J Respir Crit Care Med. 1994;149:707–714.

137. Martin RJ, Sanders MH, Gray BA, et al. Acute and long-term ventilatory effects of hyperoxia in the adult sleep apnea syndrome. Am Rev Respir Dis. 1982;125:175–180.

138. Gold AR, Schwartz AR, Bleecker ER, et al. The effect of chronic nocturnal oxygen administration upon sleep apnea. Am Rev Respir Dis. 1986;134:925–929.

139. Sanders MH, Rogers RM. Sleep apnea: when does better become benefit? Chest. 1985;88:320–321.

140. Hanly P, Sasson Z, Zuberi N, et al. ST-segment depression during sleep in obstructive sleep apnea. Am J Cardiol. 1993;71:1341–1345.

141. Franklin KA, Nilsson JB, Sahlin C, et al. Sleep apnoea and nocturnal angina. Lancet. 1995;345:1085–1087.

142. Sanders MH, Kern N. Obstructive sleep apnea treated by independently adjusted inspiratory and expiratory positive airway pressures via nasal mask. Physiologic and clinical implications. Chest. 1990;98:317–324.

143. Piper AJ, Sullivan CE. Effects of short-term NIPPV in the treatment of patients with severe obstructive sleep apnea and hypercapnia. Chest. 1994;105:434–440.

144. Martin T, Sanders M, Atwood C. Correlation between changes in $PaCO_2$ and CPAP in obstructive sleep apnea (OSA) patients. Am Rev Respir Dis. 1993;147:A681.

145. Chauncey JB, Aldrich MS. Preliminary findings in the treatment of obstructive sleep apnea with transtracheal oxygen. Sleep. 1990;13:167–174.

146. Elmer JC, Farney RJ, Walker JM, et al. The comparison of transtracheal oxygen with other therapies for obstructive sleep apnea. Am Rev Respir Dis. 1988;137:311A.

147. Farney RJ, Walker JM, Elmer JC, et al. Transtracheal oxygen, nasal CPAP and nasal oxygen in five patients with obstructive sleep apnea. Chest. 1992;101:1228–1235.

148. Engleman HM, Martin SE, Deary IJ, et al. Effect of continuous positive airway pressure treatment on daytime function in sleep apnoea/hypopnoea syndrome. Lancet. 1994;343:572–575.

149. Lyons TJ, French J. Modafinil: the unique properties of a new stimulant. Aviat Space Environ Med. 1991;62:432–435.

150. Arnulf I, Homeyer P, Garma L, et al. Modafinil in obstructive sleep apnea-hypopnea syndrome: a pilot study in 6 patients. Respiration. 1997;64:159–161.

151. Bradley TD, Rutherford R, Grossman RF, et al. Role of daytime hypoxemia in the pathogenesis of right heart failure in the obstructive sleep apnea syndrome. Am Rev Respir Dis. 1985;131:835–839.

152. Buda AJ, Schroeder JS, Guilleminault C. Abnormalities of pulmonary artery wedge pressures in sleep-induced apnea. Int J Cardiol. 1981;1:67–74.

153. Findley LJ, Barth JT, Powers DC, et al. Cognitive impairment in patients with obstructive sleep apnea and associated hypoxemia. Chest. 1986;90:686–690.

154. Fletcher EC, Lesske J, Qian W, et al. Repetitive, episodic hypoxia causes diurnal elevation of blood pressure in rats. Hypertension. 1992;19:555–561.

155. Fletcher EC. The relationship between systemic hypertension and obstructive sleep apnea: facts and theory. Am J Med. 1995;98:118–128.

156. Guilleminault C, Connolly S, Winkle RA. Cardiac arrhythmia and conduction disturbances during sleep in 400 patients with sleep apnea syndrome. Am J Cardiol. 1983;52:490–494.

157. Somers VK, Mark AL, Abboud FM. Potentiation of sympathetic nerve response to hypoxia in borderline hypertensive subjects. Hypertension. 1988;11:608–612.

158. Somers VK, Mrk AL, Abboud FM. Sympathetic activation by hypoxia and hypercapnia—implications for sleep apnea. Clin Exp Hypertens. 1988;A10(suppl 1):413–422.

159. Zwillich C, Devlin T, White D, et al. Bradycardia during sleep apnea. Characteristics and mechanism. J Clin Invest. 1982;69:1286–1292.

160. Richmonds C, Hudgel DW. Hypoglossal and phrenic motoneuron responses to serotoninergic active agents in rats. Respir Physiol. 1996;106:153–160.

161. Veasy SC, Panckeri KA, Hofman EA, et al. The effects of serotonin antagonists in an animal model of sleep-disordered breathing. Am Rev Respir Crit Care Med. 1996;153:776–786.

162. Mendelson WB, Martin JV, Rapoport DM. Effects of buspirone on sleep and respiration. Am Rev Respir Dis. 1990;141:1527–1530.

163. Garner SJ, Eldridge FL, Wagner PG, et al. Buspirone, an anxiolytic drug that stimulates respiration. Am Rev Respir Dis. 1989;139:946–950.

164. Schmidt HS. L-Tryptophan in the treatment of impaired respiration during sleep. Bull Eur Physiopathol Respir. 1983;19:625–629.

165. Schmidt HS. Combined L-Tryptophan and protriptyline in the treatment of obstructive sleep apnea. Sleep Res. 1985;14:209.

166. Strumpf IJ, Drucker RD, Anders KH, et al. Acute eosinophilic pulmonary disease associated with the ingestion of L-Tryptophan-containing products. Chest. 1991;99:8–13.

167. Hertzman PA, Blevins WL, Mayer J, et al. Association of the eosinophilia-myalgia syndrome with the ingestion of tryptophan. N Engl J Med. 1990;322:869–873.

168. Zwillich CW, Natalino MR, Sutton FD, et al. Effects of progesterone on chemosensitivity in normal men. J Lab Clin Med. 1978;92:262–269.

169. Skatrud JB, Dempsey JA, Kaiser DG. Ventilatory response to medroxyprogesterone acetate in normal subjects: time course and mechanisms. J Appl Physiol. 1978;44:939–944.

170. Skatrud JB, Dempsey JA, Bhansali P, et al. Determinants of carbon dioxide retention and its correction in humans. J Clin Invest. 1980;65:813–821.

171. Orr WC, Imes NK, Martin RJ. Progesterone therapy in obese patients with sleep apnea. Arch Intern Med. 1979;139:109–111.

172. Hensley MJ, Saunders NA, Strohl KP. Medroxyprogesterone treatment of obstructive sleep apnea. Sleep. 1980;3:441–446.

173. Strohl KP, Hensley MJ, Saunders NA, et al. Progesterone administration and progressive sleep apneas. JAMA. 1981;245:1230–1232.

174. Rajagopal KR, Abbrecht PH, Jabbari B. Effects of medroxyprogesterone acetate in obstructive sleep apnea. Chest. 1986;90:815–821.

175. Cook WR, Benich JJ, Wooten SA. Indices of severity of obstructive sleep apnea syndrome do not change during medroxyprogesterone acetate therapy. Chest. 1989;96:262–266.

176. Kimura H, Hayashi F, Yoshida A, et al. Augmentation of CO_2 drives by chlormadinone acetate, a synthetic progesterone. J Appl Physiol. 1984;56:1627–1632.

177. Tatsumi K, Kimura H, Kunitomo F, et al. Effect of chlormadinone acetate on sleep arterial oxygen desaturation in patients with chronic obstructive pulmonary disease. Chest. 1987;91:688–692.

178. Kimura H, Tatsumi K, Kunitomo F, et al. Progesterone therapy for sleep apnea syndrome evaluated by occlusion pressure responses to exogenous loading. Am Rev Respir Dis. 1989;139:1198–1206.

179. Whyte KF, Gould GA, Airlie AA, et al. Role of protriptyline and acetazolamide in the sleep apnea/hypopnea syndrome. Sleep. 1988;11:463–472.

180. Sharp JT, Druz WS, D'Souza V, et al. Effect of metabolic acidosis upon sleep apnea. Chest. 1985;87:619–624.

181. Dowell AR, Heyman A, Sieker HO, et al. Effect of aminophylline on respiratory-center sensitivity and in pulmonary emphysema. N Engl J Med. 1963;273:1447–1453.

182. Lakshminarayan S, Sahn SA, Weil JV. Effect of theophylline on ventilatory responses in normal man. Am Rev Respir Dis. 1978;117:33–38.

183. Marias OAS, McMichael J. Theophylline ethylenediamine in Cheyne-Stokes breathing. Lancet. 1937;2:437–440.

184. Espinoza H, Antic R, Thornton AT, et al. The effects of aminophylline on sleep and sleep-disordered breathing with obstructive sleep apnea syndrome. Am Rev Respir Dis. 1987;136:80–84.

185. Guilleminault C, Hayes B. Naloxone, theophylline, bromocriptine, and obstructive sleep apnea. Bull Eur Physiopathol Respir. 1983;19:632–634.

186. Guilleminault C, Flagg WH, Coburn SC, et al. Baclofen trial in myotonic dystrophy patients. Acta Neurol Scand. 1978;57:232–238.

187. Krieger J, Mangin P, Kurtz D. Effects of almitrine in the treatment of sleep apnea syndromes. Bull Eur Physiopathol Respir. 1983;19:630.

188. Krieger J, Mangin P, Kurtz D. Sleep apnea syndrome: effects of chlorimipramine in subjects with stable body weight. Rev Electroencephalogr Neurophysiol Clin. 1979;9:250–257.

189. Olson LG, Hensley MJ, Saunders NA. Breathing during sleep: the responses to asphyxia and prochlorperazine in normal subjects and patients with obstructive sleep apnoea. Aust N Z J Med. 1983;13:613–620.

76

Continuous Positive Airway Pressure for Sleep Breathing Disorders

Ronald Grunstein
Colin Sullivan

HISTORICAL DEVELOPMENT

Nasally applied continuous positive airway pressure (CPAP) is now the established treatment for obstructive sleep apnea-hypopnea syndrome (OSAHS) and for some forms of central apnea. Studies have provided information on different aspects of usage and compliance, as well as efficacy, of CPAP therapy. In this chapter, these data are reviewed with emphasis on the practical use of CPAP therapy in clinical practice. The successful use of nasal masks to deliver CPAP to the upper airway has, in turn, led to the use of nasal masks with various ventilatory modes, including pressure support and volume-cycled ventilation. This has revolutionized the management of chronic respiratory failure and is discussed extensively in Chapter 83.

The historical development of CPAP has followed four phases. Nasal CPAP therapy for sleep apnea was first described by our group in Sydney in 1981,[1] but it was not until about 1985 that it began to be recognized as a realistic form of long-term therapy in other centers.[2] In part, this delay arose out of the difficulty in attaching masks using a Silastic glue, as well as some conceptual difficulties with the design of a CPAP breathing circuit for home use.[3] Although patients needed to use an adhesive to attach the mask, the prompt relief of sleepiness led to an increasing number of users. By 1985, over one hundred patients were using this therapy on a regular basis.[4] The second phase came with technical improvements in design and when the development of nasal CPAP moved out of university hospital–based research groups and into the commercial arena. In 1986, we commenced using molded Silastic masks worn using head straps and within a few years there were at least six companies producing commercial versions of the device.

Since the publication of the last edition of this book, two subsequent phases of CPAP development have occurred. The evidence base of CPAP has improved both in quantity and quality, driven by both the demands of government funding authorities and health maintenance organizations (HMOs) and the availability of industry sponsorship with the increasing commercial success of companies selling CPAP equipment.[5] Nevertheless, clinical trials of CPAP raise difficult issues of study design with problems with placebos and "sham" CPAP. It is often too simplistic to try and perform the same type of trials required for pharmaceutical registration with a mechanical device such as CPAP. More recently, we have entered the phase of automatically titrating CPAP devices ("intelligent CPAP") which has major implications for the delivery of healthcare to patients with sleep apnea and the traditional sleep laboratory–patient relationship.[6]

Nasal CPAP also has taken a long time to gain credibility, as there has been an erroneous belief that a cure for sleep apnea was available by surgery, or, more recently, with oral appliances. The long-term success of CPAP therapy places an onus on advocates of surgical or dental therapies for sleep apnea to demonstrate long-term efficacy in controlled studies. Importantly, some forms of surgical treatment may reduce subsequent success rates for CPAP compliance. Thus, nasal CPAP remains the gold standard for treatment of moderate to severe OSAHS, and consensus groups have published indications for its use.[6a] The absence of any viable pharmacological therapy for sleep apnea[7] suggests that this will remain the situation for the foreseeable future.

NASAL CONTINUOUS POSITIVE AIRWAY PRESSURE: MODE OF ACTION

The original experiments with CPAP followed from the concept that closure of the oropharynx was the result of an imbalance in the forces that normally keep the upper airway open (see Chapter 72). The most concise early formulation of this model was presented by Remmers and colleagues in 1978.[8] In the first description of CPAP use for treatment of OSAHS by Sullivan et al. in 1981,[1] it was suggested that nasal

CPAP acts as a pneumatic splint to prevent collapse of the pharyngeal airway, that is, elevating the pressure in the oropharyngeal airway and reversing the transmural pressure gradient across the pharyngeal airway (Fig. 76–1). This notion has been subsequently confirmed by a number of studies which either demonstrate the "pneumatic splint" by endoscopic or other imaging or show that CPAP does *not* increase upper airway muscle activity by reflex mechanisms.[9] Detailed magnetic resonance imaging (MRI) has confirmed the pneumatic splinting effect of CPAP and its ability to reduce upper airway edema secondary to chronic vibration and occlusion of the airway.[10]

The manner in which the pressure is administered is crucial to achieving adequate pressures in the oropharynx; the static pressure and the pressure during inspiratory efforts must be considered. The apparatus providing the pressure at the nasal airway must have the "capacitance" to maintain any given pressure during inspiration (Fig. 76–2).

CPAP and Central Apnea

Regardless of the mechanism, nasal CPAP has been documented to be effective in eliminating both mixed and obstructive apneas.[11] Some central apneas, particularly those observed in patients with predominantly obstructive events, are also eliminated by nasal CPAP[11] (Fig. 76–3). Clearly, some central apneas are associated with increased upper airway resistance and it could be argued that it is better to consider apnea classification as being CPAP responsive or CPAP nonresponsive. CPAP is also effective in central apneas associated with cardiac failure (see later).

PRACTICAL ASPECTS OF TREATMENT

Currently, most patients commence CPAP under supervision, usually in a hospital-based sleep laboratory.

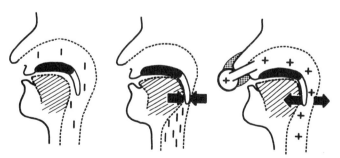

Figure 76–1. Mechanism of upper airway occlusion and its prevention by nasal continuous positive airway pressure (CPAP). When the patient is awake *(left)*, muscle tone prevents collapse of the upper airway during inspiration; during sleep, the tongue and soft palate are sucked against the posterior oropharyngeal wall *(middle)*. CPAP with low pressure provides a pneumatic splint and keeps the upper airway open *(right)*. (Adapted from Sullivan CE, Issa FG, Bethon-Jones M, et al. Reversal of obstructive sleep apnea by continuous positive airway pressure applied through the nares. Lancet. 1981;1:862–865.)

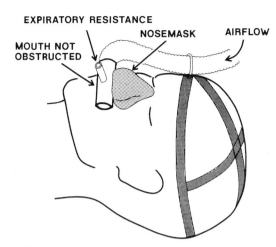

Figure 76–2. Diagram of method of applying continuous positive airway pressure by nose mask. (From Sullivan CE, Issa FG, Berthon-Jones M, et al. Home treatment of obstructive sleep apnea with continuous positive airway pressure applied through a nosemask. Bull Eur Physiopathol Respir. 1984;20:49–54.)

Economic pressures within health systems are challenging this approach and moving in the direction of less intensive staffing or even home commencement of CPAP. As part of this economic rationalization, health authorities are expecting some evidence base for clinical practice with CPAP titration.

Initially, more severe cases of sleep apnea were considered for CPAP, often patients with some degree of hypoventilation. Early reports of potential side effects of inadequate CPAP pressure in patients with impaired arousability to chemical stimuli[12] emphasized the importance of close hospital-based supervision. Our understanding of the potential risks, improved technology, and other positive pressure options (see later) have reduced concerns. However, irrespective of the location or method of CPAP titration, there is a clear demand for proper patient assessment (i.e., does the patient have awake respiratory failure or marked hypoxemia in sleep?), which, in turn, requires specific physician training and experience. CPAP titration is not appropriate for a primary or family practice setting or one where there is no trained medical supervision of the process.

Similarly, trained technologists are required to provide patient education, technical aspects of titration, and follow-up. Although discussed later, it is important to emphasize that the dominant determinants of CPAP usage are patient understanding of the therapy and close professional support irrespective of the mask type, CPAP manufacturer, or mode of delivery. This type of education and support cannot be provided by untrained staff.

The First Night

Sleeping with a nose mask and feeling the pressure sensation of CPAP, although not necessarily uncomfortable, are certainly novel experiences for the patient. Physician explanation, video programs, and mask "ac-

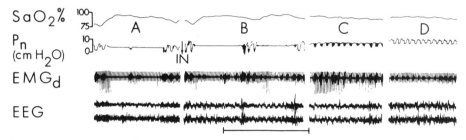

Figure 76–3. Polygraphic records demonstrating prevention of central sleep apnea by continuous positive airway pressure (CPAP) applied through the nose. SaO_2, arterial oxyhemoglobin saturation (scale 100 to 75%); P_n, nasal pressure (scale 0 to 15 cm H_2O); EMG_d, diaphragm electromyogram; EEG, electroencephalogram; time scale is in seconds. Patient is in the supine position. *A,* Note the presence of central apnea at a nasal CPAP of 2 cm H_2O. *B,* Elevation of nasal CPAP to 6.6 cm H_2O changes the apnea from a central to a mixed type. Further increase of nasal CPAP to 10 cm H_2O (not shown) leads to a change in the apnea pattern from a mixed to an obstructive apnea. *C,* Loud, continuous snoring occurs when the nasal CPAP is elevated to 11.5 cm H_2O. *D,* Finally, at a nasal CPAP of 14.5 cm H_2O, the patient breathes with an open airway. (Adapted from Issa FG, Sullivan CE. Reversal of central sleep apnea using nasal CPAP. Chest. 1986;90:165–171.)

climation" sessions prior to commencing CPAP are routine in many centers. Although the benefits of these techniques have not been fully scientifically evaluated, it is obvious that patient education about CPAP will be beneficial in reducing anxiety and improving acceptance. Current evidence provides support for the benefit of more intensive patient education in CPAP usage.[13]

On the first night of treatment, it is important to ensure that the CPAP level finally determined is sufficient not only to prevent apnea and oxyhemoglobin desaturation but also to prevent respiratory-related arousals in all sleep stages and in all postures of sleep (Fig. 76–4). *Thus, simple apnea prevention is not the endpoint of CPAP titration.* It is important to ensure that

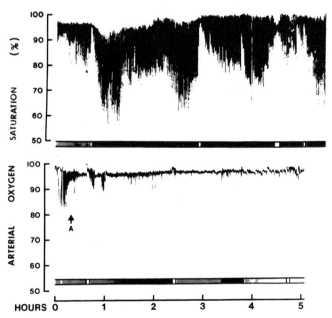

Figure 76–4. All-night recordings of arterial hemoglobin saturation in one of the earliest patients to use home continuous positive airway pressure (CPAP). *Upper panel,* control night; *lower panel,* CPAP trial night; hatched bar, NREM sleep; closed bar, REM sleep; open bar, awake. A CPAP of 7 cm H_2O was applied at arrow A and continued for the rest of the night. (Adapted from Sullivan CE, Issa FG, Berthon-Jones M, et al. Reversal of obstructive sleep apnea by continuous positive airway pressure applied through the nares. Lancet. 1981;1:862–865.)

the airflow-CPAP pressure tracing is normal and not "chopped off" to avoid residual partial airway obstruction[5] (Fig. 76–5). It is important to correct this flow limitation as it may indicate residual upper airway obstruction, potentially causing arousal.[14] Since the first development of CPAP, we have used pressure transducers to measure airflow rather than thermistors. Studies have emphasized the importance of proper flow measurement in CPAP titration using pressure-flow transducers rather than thermistors or other more indirect airflow measures.[15] Other workers have also used respiratory effort (esophageal pressure monitoring)[16] or upper airway impedance to determine the optimal CPAP level.[17] From our clinical experience, the practical applicability of esophageal pressure monitoring in determining the correct CPAP level is questionable. Another endpoint that theoretically could help determine the optimal CPAP level is whether the pressure prevents respiratory-related arousals. Although acute (one-night) studies suggest that flow limitation correction may be the preferred method of CPAP titration, long-term data are sparse. In one study, it appears that CPAP compliance is improved in patients where correction of flow limitation is used as a CPAP titration endpoint, despite there being no difference in measured sleepiness.[18]

When the correct CPAP level is reached and the airway is open, sleep should no longer be fragmented by repetitive arousals. In fact there is often "rebound" slow-wave and rapid eye movement (REM) sleep[19] (Fig. 76–6). This rebound phase of recovery from severe sleep fragmentation lasts about a week; the duration and intensity of these rebound sleep episodes decrease quickly after the first night of treatment.[19] However, the improvement in sleep architecture is usually immediate and can be used as a sign of an effective CPAP level. Continued frequent arousals may indicate that a critical level of upper airway resistance persists, especially if associated with flow limitation. Continued snoring is another sign of inadequate CPAP pressure. There are other data demonstrating that hysteresis exists in CPAP normalizing upper airway resistance—that is, to eliminate inspiratory flow limitation, higher pressures are required during upward titration of CPAP compared with downward titration from

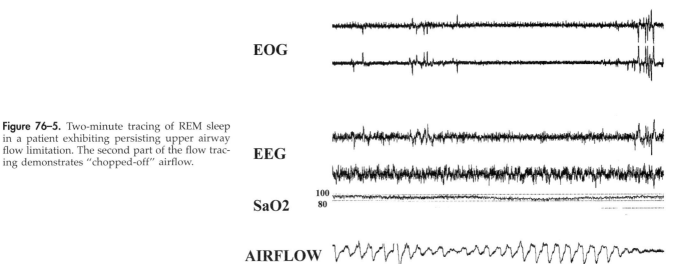

Figure 76–5. Two-minute tracing of REM sleep in a patient exhibiting persisting upper airway flow limitation. The second part of the flow tracing demonstrates "chopped-off" airflow.

higher pressures.[20] Considering the length of time CPAP has been used in patients with sleep apnea, there are surprisingly little published data on the variability in CPAP pressure with posture or sleep stage. Some evidence exists for higher pressure requirements with the supine posture.[21] Although intuitive from upper airway physiology studies,[22] it is not entirely clear whether higher CPAP levels are required in REM sleep.

It would appear that a CPAP level accurately set on one night is effective on subsequent nights.[23] Early work and clinical experience suggested this was the case, but the use of autotitrating CPAP (auto-CPAP) technology in the home has provided the research methodology to test this.[24] When caring for patients who respond immediately to CPAP but who report continued daytime sleepiness on home treatment, it may be appropriate to empirically increase CPAP pressure, assuming that the laboratory study underestimated the pressure requirement. There is also a range of factors which may have an impact on CPAP pressure in the home. Weight gain may lead to a need for a

higher CPAP setting.[25] Heavy alcohol consumption may affect CPAP pressure, presumably owing to the effect of alcohol in depressing upper airway neuromuscular tone.[26] However, moderate alcohol consumption does not affect CPAP pressure.[27] Nasal congestion or a different posture in the home may also lead to different pressure requirements. This issue of varying CPAP requirements has led to interest in developing "intelligent" CPAP systems that vary the pressure according to the presence of upper airway flow limitation (see later). It is also important to recognize that even patients with obvious sleep apnea, apparently responsive to CPAP, may have other causes of sleepiness.

Treatment of Decompensated Patients With Cardiorespiratory Failure

Patients with carbon dioxide retention, heart failure, extreme nocturnal hypoxemia (i.e., SaO_2 50% or less), or severe ischemic heart disease require close supervision

Figure 76–6. Recordings demonstrating the rapid onset of REM sleep soon after obstructive apnea was prevented by nasal continuous positive airway pressure (CPAP). P, nasal airway pressure. Note that the onset of each episode of obstructive apnea *(left side)* is accompanied by fadeout of electromyogram (EMG). Apneas were prevented when nasal CPAP was increased *(arrow A)*. Note the fadeout of postural EMG activity *(arrow B)* preceding the changes in electroencephalogram (EEG) and electro-oculogram (EOG) characteristic of REM sleep *(arrow C)*. (From Sullivan CE, Issa FG, Berthon-Jones M, et al. Pathophysiology of sleep apnea. In: Saunders NA, Sullivan CE, eds. Sleep and Breathing. New York, NY: Marcel Dekker; 1984:299–364.)

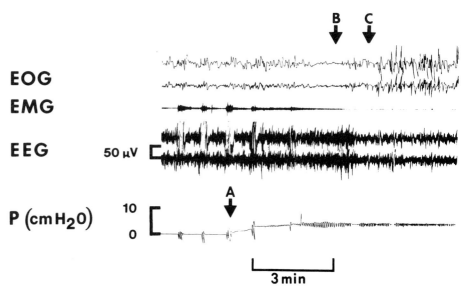

when commencing CPAP. In many of these patients, the nurse or technician will need to provide close attention for most of the first night; often such patients sleep well episodically but awaken confused and pull off the mask repeatedly throughout the night. After the first few nights, these patients typically settle down and sleep with the CPAP unit without the need for intensive nursing. These are the patients in whom hypoxic encephalopathy and CO_2 narcosis combine with excessive daytime sleepiness to produce a difficult management problem. This type of patient often becomes agitated and disoriented during the night, almost certainly because of the severe blood gas disturbance. The previous choice of therapy for these patients was intubation or urgent tracheostomy. Intubation may still be the appropriate option; however, in trained hands, nasally applied CPAP or noninvasive ventilation (see Chapter 83) will readily control the breathing disturbance during sleep. Many of these patients have both upper airway obstruction and hypoventilation and nasal CPAP may not be adequate to normalize gas exchange.[28] Increasingly, the clinical approach in these patients is to employ bilevel positive airway pressure therapy. Auto-CPAP approaches are inappropriate in such patients.

Can CPAP Be Commenced on the Same Night Sleep Apnea Is Diagnosed? The Split-Night Study

It has been suggested that CPAP can be initiated on the same night the diagnosis is established.[29] This would imply set laboratory policies on CPAP initiation and CPAP pre-education in all patients. The success of this procedure with abbreviated diagnostic and subsequent CPAP pressure determination is variable, with some patients requiring retitration. Early data[29] indicated that after such a "split-night" study, a majority of patients still required a subsequent change in CPAP pressure, mask, or a switch to bilevel positive airway pressure.[29] More recent work from the same group has been more positive about split-night studies.[30] Yama-Shiro and Kryger[31] identified a subset of patients for whom a split-night study provided insufficient time for CPAP titration to achieve a satisfactory prescription. Patients with milder degrees of sleep-disordered breathing (SDB) (apnea-hypopnea index [AHI] less than 20) in whom the titration is initiated later in the night (because prolonged monitoring was required to establish a diagnosis) were more likely to have unsuccessful split-night titrations. Other workers have suggested that CPAP can be titrated during the day.[32] In this study, both daytime and nocturnal CPAP titration studies yielded sufficient amounts of REM and nonrapid eye movement (NREM) sleep to help determine CPAP settings. The diurnal and nocturnal CPAP titrations resulted in comparable therapeutic pressures, resolution of SDB, and 1-week compliance.

Although such split-night or day studies may appear attractive from a short-term economic point of view, incorrect treatment prescription may result in CPAP failure and more frequent outpatient visits with CPAP problems. The need for further sleep studies may negate short-term financial advantages. Also, economic analyses from the United States may be inappropriate for other health systems with lower costs. The long-term utility of split-night studies is unproven as yet. Clearly, the usefulness of split-night studies would be enhanced by ensuring that patients are adequately educated about CPAP and adequate time is allowed for titration. It is possible but speculative at this stage, depending on outcome studies, whether a combination of split-night titration and subsequent home autotitration may be an adequate strategy.

Can CPAP Be Commenced at Home?

There may be theoretical economic advantages of starting CPAP at home and avoiding a formal polysomnographic CPAP titration, but outcome studies showing true cost utility are not available. In one hospital-based study, CPAP titration using laboratory-measured respiratory variables produced only similar CPAP levels, as did full polysomnography.[33] Other workers have claimed that CPAP compliance is decreased in patients assessed only with respiratory monitoring.[34] Home CPAP titrations were first reported in the United States[35] where patients were given progressively increasing nightly CPAP settings at home with CPAP pressure and oxygen saturation monitoring. These records were then assessed each day to determine the "success" or "failure" of CPAP. Respiratory therapists attended at home and provided training at the beginning of treatment. Technicians spent 1 to 2 h with the patient. Patients were begun on 5 cm or 7 cm of nasal CPAP. Bed partners were present in 10 of 11 cases and the patient was expected to report a reduction in snoring to minimal or absent levels, as well as an improvement in daytime hypersomnolence. A maximum CPAP pressure of 10 cm was set. The authors reported that the cost of this procedure was $600 compared to $1200 to $1800 for a full sleep study. It is important to recognize that, in this study, incremental increases in CPAP were given on successive nights, not on the same night. This retrospective study was the first formal report of both complete diagnostic and CPAP treatment outside a sleep laboratory. The sleep architecture and arousal frequency in patients were unknown in this study. Alternative home treatment approaches have employed a technologist staying overnight and setting the pressure, using some form of respiratory monitoring, with subjective responses equivalent to in-hospital CPAP commencement.[36] However, any cost savings with this approach are minimized owing to the costs of supervision.

White and Gibb[37] recently compared laboratory CPAP with polysomnography with home CPAP titrated by modem from a central laboratory. Six weeks later, no difference could be found in CPAP efficacy or compliance.[37] Other workers have found reasonable utility with unattended in-hospital CPAP titration in patients with mild to moderate disease rather than severe OSAHS.[38] Other studies have suggested that equations can be determined which would allow an empirical CPAP level to be set, potentially preventing the need for any investigation of CPAP efficacy.[39] Again, long-term outcome data are lacking. Moreover, it is important in all home CPAP titration studies to include patients from diverse backgrounds and education levels to properly assess whether such a therapeutic strategy works in all groups. The clinician should be cognizant of the fact that only after careful selection criteria are fulfilled should a patient be a candidate for home titration. Such criteria should include adequate support in the home, good cognitive function, and patient communication skills.

PROBLEMS AND SIDE EFFECTS

Side effects reported by the patient are usually, but not exclusively, related to pressure or airflow or the mask-nose interface (Table 76–1). Side effects are important for CPAP usage; patients who complain of side effects use CPAP less frequently than those without side effects.[40] However, dangerous complications of nasal CPAP therapy are extremely rare and represent isolated case reports in the literature, including pulmonary barotrauma, pneumocephalus, increased intraocular pressure, tympanic membrane rupture, and subcutaneous emphysema after facial trauma.[41–44] It is clear that caution should be used when implementing CPAP therapy postneuro- or facial surgery. Irritating side effects such as aerophagy and musculoskeletal chest discomfort (presumably related to increased lung volumes) have also been reported.[44]

Nasal Congestion

Nasal congestion is a common side effect of CPAP therapy.[45] Although most patients experience initial self-limiting nasal congestion, at least 10% complain of persistent nasal stuffiness to some degree after 6

months of therapy.[45] There appear to be many reasons for nasal symptoms. CPAP may provoke pressure-sensitive mucosal receptors, leading to vasodilation and mucus production. In some patients, it may unmask allergic rhinitis by restoring the nasal route of breathing after years of "mouth breathing." In others, fixed nasal obstruction with polyps or a deviated septum may produce symptoms. Mouth leaks also cause increased nasal resistance.[46]

Treatment of nasal congestion will depend on the exact cause. Mouth leak may be minimized by ensuring that the correct CPAP pressure is used avoiding arousals. Sometimes, it may be necessary to use chin straps. These are often uncomfortable and acclimation to this device is often necessary. Heated, rather than cold, pass-over humidification is necessary to treat nasal congestion.[46, 46a] Nasal congestion can be treated with antihistamines, topical steroids, or topical saline sprays, and humidification of the circuit will improve nasal dryness. Intranasal ipratropium bromide can be helpful in abating CPAP-induced rhinorrhea.

Patients with persistent symptoms of nasal congestion or those with obvious nasal obstruction should have nasopharyngoscopy performed and may require corrective surgery for an obstructive lesion such as polyps, marked mucosal thickening, or deviated septum. However, in our experience, such nasal obstruction needs to be quite marked to be significant. Most patients with chronic nasal congestion affecting their ability to tolerate CPAP benefit from attempts to reduce mouth leak with chin straps or by adding a humidification system to their CPAP circuit. There are no available objective data on the effect of nasal decongestants or humidification on compliance rates.

Oronasal masks have been tried for some years to treat mouth leak. This has been given added impetus by the need for these masks for patients with hypoventilation disorders on bilevel devices. Currently, there is no evidence that face mask CPAP improves compliance in patients with mask leak.[47]

The Interface

Initially, masks were custom-made but in the mid-1980s new forms of plastic self-sealing masks became more convenient to use. Mask technology has improved greatly, but it is reasonable to say that mask comfort remains a pivotal influence on CPAP acceptance and compliance. Poorly fitting masks will cause air leakage and a drop in pressure leading to persistent sleep apnea and sleep fragmentation. The leak is usually the source of considerable discomfort; if it is directed toward the eye, it may cause conjunctivitis.[48] A common problem with a poorly fitting mask is the development of bruising or even ulceration of the bridge of the nose; this is usually the result of applying too much tension on the headband by pulling the top of the mask too tightly onto the bridge of the nose. This is an area where there is little subcutaneous tissue to cushion the mask, and it is therefore vulnerable to pressure injury.

Table 76–1. SIDE EFFECTS OF NASAL CONTINUOUS POSITIVE AIRWAY PRESSURE

Problem	Side Effect
Nasal	Rhinorrhea
	Nasal congestion, oronasal dryness
	Epistaxis
Mask	Skin abrasion/rash
	Conjunctivitis from air leak
Flow-related	Chest discomfort
	Aerophagy
	Sinus discomfort
	Claustrophobia
	Difficulty exhaling
	Pneumothorax (very rare)
	Pneumoencephaly (very rare)
Noise	
Partner intolerance	
Inconvenience	

Anecdotally, the newer generation of mask types is associated with fewer mask-fit problems. Nevertheless, certain patients become claustrophobic when using nasal CPAP. Changing the interface prescription from a nasal mask to less confining nasal prongs may correct that problem. If a proper seal at the nares is achieved, there appears to be no significant difference between nasal prongs and mask in the pressure prescription. However, nasal prongs may cause irritation in the nares and are infrequently tolerated in the long term. Newer interfaces are constantly being developed to address mask problems. However, it is reasonable to say for some patients, particularly younger patients with mild disease, that aesthetic problems with CPAP, regardless of interface, preclude this treatment modality.

An infrequent but difficult problem is the patient who has no upper front teeth. The upper teeth provide the rigid structure against which the lower part of the mask can be pulled. If there is no dentition, the mask simply rolls around the top gums into the mouth, with loss of an adequate seal. The problem may be rectified by providing a denture[49] or possibly, in the future, an oronasal mask (see below).

The Pressure Level and Airflow

Although frequently mentioned as a problem, there is no convincing evidence that the CPAP level impairs compliance (see Autotitrating CPAP below). Some patients may complain of increased resistance to expiration or the sensation of too much pressure in the nose. For these patients, a CPAP unit with a ramp feature may be worth considering. The ramp allows the pressure to increase to the optimal CPAP pressure gradually over a set time interval (usually 5 to 30 min). No published data indicate that a ramp feature improves acceptance or compliance with CPAP, however. A case of "ramp abuse" has been reported where continuous patient application of the ramp function led to undertreatment of sleep apnea.[50] If that approach is not effective, a bilevel positive airway pressure system, in which inspiratory positive airway pressure and expiratory positive airway pressure can be adjusted independently, may be used, as this approach lowers mean airway pressure and resistance to expiration. Again, it is not clear whether these approaches will improve compliance. Limited data indicated that use of bilevel devices do not affect CPAP usage greatly.[51]

Patients occasionally find the air generated by the CPAP unit too warm or too cold. If moving the machine from the floor to a bedside table, heating the bedroom, or placing tubing under the blankets does not correct the problem, incorporating a heated humidifier into the circuit may help. Bed partners may also experience cold air on their bodies from the expiratory port of the device.

Another complaint, also usually from the bed partner, is that the CPAP machine generates too much noise. Removing the machine from the bedside or placing it in a closet may remedy the problem. Extra tubing may be needed and it is important to recheck pressures if nonstandard tubing is used. Noise or a changing level of noise may be a problem in some auto-CPAP devices due to the nature of their motors. It is also important to consider the altitude of the patients' home. One report has found varying pressure performances at varying altitudes among CPAP machines, although most modern machines are altitude-compensated.[52]

Comparison With Other Treatments

One of the great advantages of nasal CPAP is that it is immediately and demonstrably effective in relieving OSAHS.[53] The other advantage is that it can be offered on a "trial" basis and withdrawn if not tolerated, in contrast to surgical options. This is particularly important in milder cases of OSAHS, or where the contribution of OSAHS to the patient's symptomatology is unclear. Few studies have attempted to compare CPAP with other treatments for OSAHS using formal protocols. The conclusion of most of these studies is that CPAP is the appropriate therapy for moderate to severe sleep apnea.[53–56]

COMPLIANCE

General Issues

Compliance is a complicated term which has come into medical use in general when referring to a patient administered pharmacological therapy. Strictly speaking, the word evolved in the context of clinical drug trials and implied one of the following: (1) adherence of patients to following medical advice and prescriptions; (2) adherence of investigators to following a protocol and related administrative responsibilities; and (3) adherence of sponsors to regulatory and other legal responsibilities.[57] In terms of mechanical therapies, compliance may be interpreted in different ways (see below). In general, more accurate methods of true compliance are possible with devices such as CPAP.

It is important to recognize that at least 40 to 50% of patients do not use medications as prescribed.[58] In general, compliance is not associated with age, sex, educational or economic status, or personality or characteristics of a disease, including diagnosis or severity or frequency of symptoms.[59] Others have reported that physicians cannot predict which of their patients will be compliant.[60] Therefore, it appears that compliance is not easily associated with any factor that might be used in everyday practice to make predictions about patients' behavior. Recently, Rand and colleagues[61] found that, despite efforts to enhance compliance, over 70% of patients with chronic obstructive lung disease in a clinical trial did not comply with their prescribed drug treatment. Moreover, 15% of the patients deliberately "dump" their medications in order to appear to be following the physician's orders. It is reasonable to assume that more than half of patients on long-term medication use their therapy differently from their physician's prescription.

There are several factors associated with improved compliance.[59] These include simplicity of the regimen, family support, the patient's perception that his or her disease is serious, belief that the proposed therapy will be effective, patient understanding of the rationale of treatment, provision of accurate details of the treatment planned, and a close patient-clinician relationship, including close clinician supervision of therapy. Interestingly, a review of six drug trials for various illnesses has showed that in five of them the compliant patients did significantly better irrespective of whether they were on an active drug or placebo! Strategies for improvement of compliance include patient education, prescriber education, and simplifying treatment regimens.[58–60]

Compliance and CPAP

How do these general issues in compliance affect CPAP? In assessing the long-term results of CPAP, different words have been used, including "acceptance," "tolerance," "adherence," "usage," "compliance," and "efficacy," in descriptions of the patient-CPAP interaction. To a large extent these terms describe different measures. "Acceptance" and "tolerance" are subjective terms used in early studies, whereas more recent studies measure CPAP "usage" or "compliance" utilizing time meters or more sophisticated devices that measure both run-time and pressure delivery. True "efficacy" studies have yet to be performed, as they would need to measure total sleep time over a set period and compare this with CPAP usage and the actual number of respiratory events not prevented by CPAP. Nevertheless, when one looks at all the CPAP usage data currently available, compliance with CPAP devices compares favorably with medication use. We have previously suggested various terms used in relation to CPAP usage[5] which are listed in Table 76–2. The criteria

set for the terms may vary; for example, good compliance for one group may be 6 h of CPAP, 6 nights per week, whereas for others such criteria may be too strict.

Several specific factors affect CPAP compliance studies, including machine cost, the technical advances in masks, and prescriber motivation. In some countries machines are provided free of cost, whereas in others, the cost may vary between U.S. $1000 and $3000. This may lead to variable acceptance and prescription of the therapy. In addition, there have been rapid changes in CPAP technology. Current machines are quieter, with better masks, and with a ramp facility to slowly increase the pressure over the first period of sleep. Many CPAP usage studies have used superseded equipment, and compliance data need to be continually updated to verify whether these technical changes do actually influence CPAP use or are purely cosmetic marketing ploys. This situation is analogous to clinical trials of new medications within the same drug class, for example, comparative studies of beta blockers.

Unlike the study of Rand and colleagues,[61] it appears that CPAP "dumping" is not a major factor. If a CPAP mask is taken off the face, then there is detectable drop in pressure. If patients were simply switching on their machine and leaving the mask on the floor, then there would be a major discrepancy between "machine-on" time and "mask-on-face" time. This is not the case, as simultaneous studies of CPAP use and pressure delivery at the mask revealed a high correlation between usage and compliance.[62]

"Dosage" studies are not available for CPAP. Do patients have to use CPAP every night to receive beneficial therapeutic effects? Mean CPAP use of less than 4 h per night produces a demonstrable reduction in sleepiness.[63] Another study showed that one night off CPAP in compliant CPAP users led to a recurrence in daytime sleepiness.[64] A number of "biological" markers of CPAP usage may exist in all or certain patient subgroups.[65] However, these studies have not simultaneously measured the biological endpoint and objectively measured CPAP usage. At this stage all criteria set for CPAP usage or nonusage or compliance or noncompliance[62, 63] are essentially arbitrary. However, it is clear that even partial-night CPAP use can lead to measurable clinical improvement. It has been suggested that at least some sleep apnea patients use CPAP for only part of the night because they derive a satisfactory degree of symptomatic benefit from that limited application.[66] That observation would be in keeping with previous observations that sleep restriction of greater than 4 h will increase sleep propensity greatly, and that 4 h of adequate sleep may be the minimum requirement for acceptable daytime performance.[67] Newer-generation CPAP devices that allow monitoring of more precise patterns of use (i.e., time at pressure on individual nights) undoubtedly will give us insight into the minimal duration of CPAP use that is "acceptable" to decrease daytime sleepiness and, possibly, to modify the vascular consequences of sleep apnea.

Partial-night CPAP can also lead to improvement in underlying sleep apnea severity, even on the same

Table 76–2. SUGGESTED TERMINOLOGY DESCRIBING PATIENT INTERACTION WITH CONTINUOUS POSITIVE AIRWAY PRESSURE

Term	Definition
Acceptance	The proportion of patients who meet selection criteria for CPAP treatment *and* actually proceed to have their CPAP pressure level determined
Prescription	The proportion of patients who accept CPAP *and* commence home treatment
Adherence	The proportion of patients prescribed CPAP who *report* that they are continuing to use CPAP
Tolerance	The proportion of patients who *report* that they are able to use CPAP without side effects; often can be used interchangably with "adherence"
Usage	The proportion of patients with CPAP machines switched on more than an arbitrary period of time
Compliance	The proportion of patients *using* CPAP machines *and delivering* a preset level (i.e., the mask is likely to be on the patient's face)

night when CPAP is not used.[66] Hers et al.[66] reported that, when CPAP was discontinued after 4 h, there was a persistent beneficial effect on oxyhemoglobin saturation and sleep continuity during the remainder of the night. They hypothesized that the persistent improvement was attributable to improved sleep continuity achieved during the initial portion of the night while on CPAP, improving upper airway stability during the latter portion of the night after the CPAP was removed.

Studies of CPAP Usage

Early data from our center suggested that there was a high level of long-term acceptance of CPAP.[4] However, these patients had more severe forms of apnea, were highly motivated by staff, and their subjective reports could not be corroborated by objective data. These early patients had to use a Silastic sealant to glue a fiberglass mask onto their face. Interestingly, as the glue was provided by the sleep laboratory, glue usage provided a primitive form of objective measurement and it was clear at this early stage of CPAP development that "usage" was very variable.

In the paragraphs below, using the terminology suggested in Table 76–2, available data on how patients interact with CPAP are discussed under separate headings.

How Many Patients Will Accept CPAP?

Little accurate data are available on this point as most studies only discuss patient data from the night of CPAP pressure determination or later. There are little published data that address this issue. In one study, 70% of patients offered a CPAP trial night accepted.[68] Others have reported that 76% of patients offered a trial of CPAP took their machines home.[69]

How Many Patients Will Agree to Prescription of Home CPAP?

The percentage of patients who refuse CPAP after an in-hospital trial is variable. Two studies have reported prescription rates in excess of 80%,[70, 71] while other authors observed only a 58% prescription rate after an in-hospital trial.[72] There are many potential sources of prescription rate variability, including machine cost, which has a major impact in Australia; whether more than one night of in-hospital CPAP trial is possible; and the original selection criteria for CPAP. For example, we often first try certain patients with severe forms of sleep apnea on CPAP simply on economic grounds, knowing that it is likely to be less effective and poorly tolerated compared with more expensive forms of therapy such as nasal ventilation. In Australia, it has been estimated that CPAP purchase rates nationally are over 50%, based on a calculation comparing new CPAP machine sales provided by manufacturers with national insurance data on multiple sleep study frequency.[73] In other words, over 50% of patients completing a sleep laboratory trial end up purchasing a CPAP machine or having one purchased for them by the health system.

How Many Patients Will Continue to Use CPAP Long-Term?

When compliance is assessed by subjective means, a 65 to 90% compliance rate with positive airway pressure therapy has been reported.[5] The patient's perception of improvement and not the severity of sleep apnea generally predicts compliance with CPAP.[5, 44] Covert monitoring of CPAP has demonstrated that compliance with nasal CPAP was substantially less than in previous studies where compliance was reported on the basis of subjective patient data.[62] That study indicated that nasal CPAP was used 46% of the time, equal to or greater than 4 h for 70% of the observed nights, and compliance at 1 month predicted compliance at 3 months. Other studies have confirmed this degree of usage, their data indicating that (1) patients subjectively overestimate CPAP use and (2) long-term compliance may be less than desirable when use is monitored objectively.

Weaver et al.[74] observed in 32 patients on CPAP that approximately half the subjects were consistent users of CPAP at 9 weeks (average of 6.2 h per night), while the other half had a wide range of daily use, averaging 3.45 h per night on the nights CPAP was used. The percentage of days skipped was significantly correlated with decreased nightly duration and the two groups differed significantly in the nightly duration of CPAP use by the fourth day of treatment.

What Baseline Indicators Influence CPAP Usage?

Data from the general compliance literature suggest that it is hard for physicians to predict good compliers at the time of initiation of therapy. This may be the case for medications, but it may be a different situation for a mechanical treatment such as CPAP. In addition, CPAP provides immediate reinforcement of its efficacy in many patients with relief of daytime sleepiness. Therefore it is possible that the severity of symptoms has some role in maintaining usage of CPAP. Several studies have confirmed this hypothesis—that is, that patients with good objective usage or reported adherence are sleepier at baseline[62, 70, 75]—although other studies have not found this relationship.[64] Although multiple sleep latency test (MSLT)–measured daytime sleepiness improves following CPAP,[63] baseline MSLT scores do not appear to predict CPAP compliance.[62, 76] It is controversial whether the amount of improvement in MSLT scores will predict compliance in contrast to MSLT results at baseline.[62, 76] It is possible that in sleep apnea the MWT (Maintenance of Wakefulness Test) may be a better predictor of CPAP use, but this is untested. Recent work by Bennett et al.[77] indicated that sleep fragmentation measured by a electroencephalographic (EEG) neural network analysis or movement events on video recordings are reasonably correlated with CPAP compliance.[77] Other factors that may be related to reduced usage include previous palatal surgery,[70] absence of hypoxemia,[75] and fewer years of education.[62] Surprisingly, in two larger series, the CPAP pressure level was not higher in those having difficulties using CPAP.[70, 78] These two studies found no obvious predictors of usage.[70, 78]

Does Physician or Technologist Motivation or Support Improve Usage?

It would seem obvious that the more positive the reinforcement given to patients, the more likely the patient will use CPAP as prescribed. This has been questioned by one study[79] which showed no advantage of regular telephone advice, although the crossover nature of this study's design has been described as flawed.[80] Discrepant results on patient education have been reported by Kribbs and co-workers.[62, 64] They showed that a protocol[64] urging subjects to be as compliant as possible was more successful than lesser degrees of intervention.[62] Clearly these authors recognize that patient support and motivation will have a great influence on compliance. More recent work has provided more evidence that compliance can be improved by early intervention and education.[13] In a preliminary report, intensive CPAP support led to improved CPAP compliance at 1 month.[81]

Impact of Bilevel Positive Airway Pressure on Obstructive Sleep Apnea Management

Sanders and Kern[82] first reported the potential benefits and efficacy of reducing the expiratory positive airway pressure (EPAP) level relative to inspiratory pressure (IPAP) in the management of OSAHS. Previous work had shown that there are differences in the magnitudes of the forces destabilizing the upper airway during inspiration and expiration.[83, 84] A device that permitted independent adjustment of EPAP and IPAP demonstrated that obstructive SDB can be eliminated at lower levels of EPAP compared with conventional nasal CPAP therapy.[82] The authors speculated that such a device may reduce the adverse effects associated with nasal CPAP therapy and improve long-term therapeutic compliance. There are no convincing data that bilevel positive airway pressure is more effective than CPAP in patients with OSAHS and normal awake respiratory function. One report has observed that there is no difference in hours of device use in patients with OSAHS randomized to either bilevel positive airway pressure or CPAP.[51] However, in the same study, a higher proportion of patients "adhered" (see Table 76–2) to bilevel positive airway pressure compared with CPAP.[51] More data are needed before widespread use of the more costly bilevel positive airway pressure devices can be advocated in patients with OSAHS.

Management of CPAP Failure

What constitutes CPAP failure? This is a subjective issue and practice will vary from center to center in the absence of hard data addressing the diverse health consequences of varying degrees of sleep apnea. Kribbs et al.[62] defined CPAP failure as the "use of CPAP for less than 4 hours per night on 70% of the nights and/or lack of symptomatic improvement." The specific figure of 4 h was based on minimal criteria for adequate sleep from the general sleep literature on average sleep duration and the figure of 70% of nights was an arbitrary figure based on the authors' expert clinical opinion.[62] Based on the *objective* part of this definition,[19] 54% of 35 patients were CPAP failures. Others would argue that even 3 h of CPAP will produce measurable improvement in health outcomes.[80]

Clearly, it is important to identify the cause of CPAP failure. Some of the commonest side effects and potential solutions have been mentioned. Claustrophobia is frequently a major cause of complete CPAP failure. Ear, nose, and throat assessment may be appropriate in looking for any structural reasons to explain CPAP failure. Our practice is to run through a checklist including looking for the possibility of secondary gain. Some patients with OSAHS, because of the nature of their illness, are receiving, or are potential recipients of, some form of social welfare. A subset of these patients may not have the incentive to improve their fitness for work by use of the CPAP device to increase alertness.

It is important also to consider if an incorrect diagnosis has been made. It is rare in the setting of comprehensive nocturnal respiratory monitoring or full polysomnography to make a false-positive diagnosis of SDB. However, it is more common to attribute patient symptoms to the degree of SDB when there may be other coexisting disorders (recognized or unrecognized). An example of this may include patients with mild sleep apnea and narcolepsy or idiopathic hypersomnolence where CPAP may be totally ineffective in abolishing sleepiness to any extent. Others have claimed that obesity *per se* can cause sleep disturbance and sleepiness and that it is possible that sleep apnea may not be contributory to symptoms in all patients with obesity and sleep apnea.[85]

Provided the physician recognizes the potential causes of symptoms, a CPAP trial may be warranted and then CPAP failure may be a diagnostic endpoint. In some patients with SDB, CPAP may be inadequate to manage the respiratory disorder. For example, patients with obesity-hypoventilation syndrome may require nasal ventilation initially or, in some cases, over a long term. In other patients, low-flow oxygen needs to be administered in conjunction with CPAP.

Sometimes, we admit patients who have CPAP failure to hospital for a period of intensive inpatient training. The success of such treatment has not been investigated objectively. However, after exhausting all the relevant causes of CPAP failure, and if the patient with sleep apnea is completely intolerant of all varieties of nasal CPAP therapy (including bilevel positive airway pressure or nasal ventilation) despite intensive inpatient training, the following issues need to be considered:

1. What is the potential risk of leaving the patient untreated?
2. How much does the patient want to be treated, knowing the medical answer to question 1?
3. If the patient and physician agree on trying a different treatment, what should it be? This would usually occur in patients where

   • Coexisting sleepiness is seriously impairing daytime function.
   • Coexisting disease may be exacerbated by sleep apnea with risk to the patient (this risk may at times be a potential risk due to lack of hard data in the medical literature).
   • There is evidence of severe hypoxemia or awake cardiorespiratory failure even without sleepiness.

HEALTH OUTCOMES AND NASAL CONTINUOUS POSITIVE AIRWAY PRESSURE

One of the most notable features of sleep apnea research over the past 3 years has been the increasing controversy over health outcomes in sleep apnea.[80, 86, 87] In the early years of CPAP clinical research, dramatic improvements in small, highly selected groups were observed and reported as justification for continuing to investigate and treat patients. However, sleep apnea and CPAP therapy have entered clinical practice at the same time that public health authorities are increasingly seeking outcome data from randomized controlled studies as a way of allocating healthcare resources. Two systematic reviews of sleep apnea and its treatment, one from the United Kingdom[86] and one from Australasia,[86, 88] have aroused controversy over some of their conclusions. Both studies pointed out the lack of robust outcome data from randomized controlled trials in sleep apnea, but differed in their opinion on the efficacy of CPAP. Essentially, the Australasian study[88] accepted the overwhelming number of "before-and-after" studies supporting CPAP efficacy, whereas the U.K. report[86] questioned the use of such evidence at all. This is particularly controversial as there is a wealth of data in these before-and-after studies, including studies showing improvement in sleep quality,[19] daytime sleepiness,[44] endocrine function,[65] driving simulator performance,[89] and quality of life.[90]

One of the basic problems in outcomes research with nasal CPAP is the lack of an appropriate placebo. Unlike drug studies, placebo or sham CPAP has limitations. A lower than therapeutic CPAP level may be uncomfortable, partly therapeutic, or even dangerous.[80] In the past few years, a number of randomized controlled studies of CPAP efficacy have been performed.[91–94] These studies have looked at outcomes related to sleepiness and general psychosocial performance. Significant improvements were identified, particularly in MSLT results. These results would seem to justify ongoing prescription of nasal CPAP in patients reporting sleepiness. Obviously, larger trials are required, looking at a wider range of outcomes, particularly those outcomes "understood" by clinical epidemiologists involved in healthcare budgets. Evidence of a positive impact of CPAP on productivity, quality of life, motor vehicle accidents, and cardiovascular outcomes will be needed to compete with other medical conditions seeking limited health resources.

Retrospective and preliminary data indicate that CPAP reduces hospital admissions and health costs.[95, 96] As mentioned above, several groups have performed randomized controlled trials using conservative therapy, oral placebo, or even sham CPAP as the control arm.[97] All studies have indicated positive neurobehavioral outcomes. At this stage, a similar level of evidence is lacking for cardiovascular outcomes.

SPECIAL USES OF NASAL CONTINUOUS POSITIVE AIRWAY PRESSURE

Diagnostic Dilemmas

Occasionally, patients present with severe daytime sleepiness with polysomnographic evidence of surprisingly mild sleep apnea. Others may present with a combination of sleep disorders, such as sleep apnea and periodic movements in sleep, in which the dominant cause of daytime sleepiness is uncertain and treatment with agents such as clonazepam may cloud the issue. In these patients, a short trial of CPAP is extremely useful to the clinician for determining the role of sleep apnea in producing daytime sleepiness. One report has suggested that CPAP may improve periodic movements in patients who also have sleep apnea.[98] A CPAP trial can be used in patients with mild sleep apnea who are also on antihypertensive or psychiatric medications. In this group of patients, daytime sleepiness may well be related to medication.

Endocrine Disorders

Sleep apnea is common in both hypothyroidism and acromegaly (see Chapter 93). In hypothyroidism, only some patients have their sleep apnea cured by restoration of the euthyroid state. Nasal CPAP is an ideal interim treatment for sleep apnea until it can be determined whether thyroxine has cured or significantly improved the condition. CPAP is also effective in the cardiovascular complications experienced by some patients beginning thyroxine therapy. In acromegaly, CPAP is particularly useful in managing sleep apnea in patients when the effect of surgery or other therapeutic modalities (such as a somatostatin analogue) is being evaluated. Patients with this disorder often have difficulties in obtaining a satisfactory mask fit and may need special customized masks. Their excessive sweating will often lead to the hardening of some plastic masks.

CPAP and Upper Airway Surgery

Some patients undergoing upper airway surgery for sleep apnea are temporarily tracheostomized for prevention of perioperative complications. These patients can avoid tracheostomy if nasal CPAP is commenced before surgery; in our experience, it can be used in the perioperative period, provided the patient has used this form of therapy previously. Certainly, in a patient with sleep apnea who awakens from anesthesia from upper airway surgery or even other procedures, CPAP can prevent any upper airway obstruction in the recovery room.[99] It has been reported that previous upper airway surgery may impair subsequent compliance with CPAP, possibly due to increased mouth leak.[100] In those patients who could not use nasal CPAP after surgery, evaluation with an oronasal mask might be helpful.

Sleep Apnea and Chronic Lung Disease

On the spectrum of SDB, there are many patients with a combination of OSAHS and chronic airflow limitation. These patients may exhibit both repetitive apneas and characteristic REM-related hypoventilation.[28] Depending on the degree of lung function abnormality, CPAP therapy may need to be supplemented with low-flow oxygen, usually at a rate of 2 liters/min. Mezzanotte et al.[101] have shown improved waking respiratory muscle function after CPAP in patients with a combination of OSAHS and chronic airflow limitation. However, current clinical practice suggests that bilevel positive pressure devices are now more appropriate in such patients, at least in the short term (see Chapter 81). CPAP may be beneficial in cystic fibrosis patients with mild degrees of SDB. An additional effect may be improved clearance of secretions during sleep.[102]

Cardiac Failure

Sleep apnea is common in patients with cardiac failure.[103, 104] A number of studies have reported the presence of central sleep apnea in patients with ventricular dysfunction. It has been suggested that central apnea may be an adverse prognostic factor in such patients.[105] OSAHS, as a common disorder, is frequently found in patients with cardiac failure of various causes, such as coronary artery disease, hypertension, and idiopathic cardiomyopathy. It has been suggested that OSAHS may cause or exacerbate ventricular dysfunction by a number of mechanisms. These include increasing left ventricular afterload through the combined effects of elevations in systemic blood pressure and the generation of exaggerated negative intrathoracic pressure, and by activating the sympathetic nervous system through the influence of hypoxia and arousals from sleep.[106]

Use of nasal CPAP in OSAHS in cardiac failure patients is associated with an improvement in left ven-

tricular function (LVF). Nasal CPAP improved LVF (measured by ejection fraction) in eight obese men with idiopathic cardiomyopathy.[107] Cessation of CPAP resulted in a decrease in LVF. Recently, Tkacova et al.[108] reported increased blood pressure and left ventricular transmural pressure in a group of pharmacologically treated cardiac failure patients. CPAP reversed these changes markedly, including reducing left ventricular afterload in these patients.

In contrast to OSAHS, central sleep apnea is usually considered to be the result of cardiac failure.[106] A number of studies, including some with a randomized controlled design, have demonstrated improvement in various endpoints with CPAP treatment in patients with cardiac failure and central apnea. These endpoints include reduced mitral regurgitant fraction,[109] atrial natriuretic factor secretion,[109] inspiratory muscle strength,[110] reduced left ventricular afterload,[106] increasing P_{CO_2} toward normal, and norepinephrine concentrations.[106] The effect on mortality is unknown.

There have been some studies that question the use of nasal CPAP in patients with cardiac failure.[111, 112] There are ongoing large-scale studies examining the role of CPAP in such patients, but based on current evidence it would appear reasonable practice to treat sleep apnea aggressively in patients with cardiac failure and symptoms of sleep apnea.

AUTOTITRATING CONTINUOUS POSITIVE AIRWAY PRESSURE

Development and Rationale

Since the early days of CPAP development, individuals have conceptualized a device that could simultaneously detect upper airway obstruction and apply the necessary increase in CPAP to prevent the obstruction. Similarly, if the airway was not obstructed the device would lower the pressure until imminent obstruction was detected and the pressure would be increased again to prevent obstruction. In this way there would be a stepwise increase or decrease in pressure across the night with the overall aim of preventing airway obstruction. It was speculated that such a device could deliver a lower average CPAP pressure across the night and in turn possibly improve compliance. Moreover, if pressure requirements vary with changes in upper airway resistance (nasal obstruction, alcohol or sedative use), then an auto-CPAP machine would, in theory, adjust to these changes, unlike a fixed-pressure machine. Naturally, the utility of such a device would require a very robust detection algorithm quantifying a logical measure of airflow obstruction. Without such an algorithm, short periods of apnea may occur, leading to arousals and defeating the purpose of such a device. An overnight tracing from one such device is shown in Figure 76–7.

Such a device could also be used to determine the CPAP level in the home over several nights without the need for a full laboratory diagnosis. In this mode, it would also assist patients previously established on

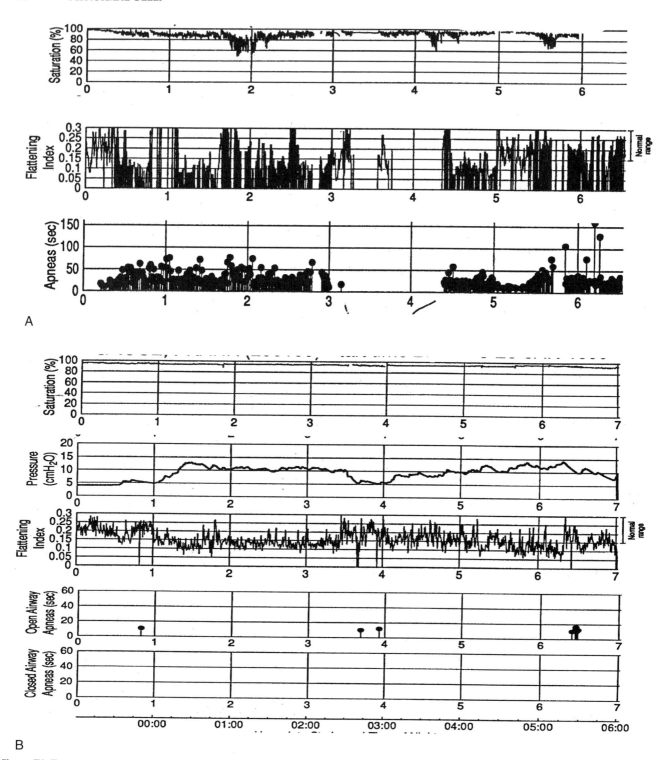

Figure 76–7. Auto-titrating continuous positive airway pressure (auto-CPAP) tracing of a patient with severe obstructive sleep apnea before *(A)* and on nasal CPAP treatment *(B)*. In *B*, CPAP level varies automatically to prevent flow limitation (denoted by an arbitrary index based on flattening of the shape of the inspiratory flow curve) and apneas.

home CPAP who encountered problems with their therapy. Economic benefits could accrue if auto-CPAP reduced technician time, eliminated in-hospital polysomnography for CPAP titration, or reduced clinic visits of patients with CPAP compliance problems.

Potential problems with auto-CPAP include overcompensation for mask or mouth leaks with a possibil-

ity of unnecessarily high pressures (Fig. 76–8). This, in turn, could lead to a worsening air leak. Other potential problems include undertreatment due to slow responses to airway obstruction or even the presence of central apnea or hypoventilation (Fig. 76–9), which may not be detected if flow limitation is the only endpoint used by the device's diagnostic algorithm.

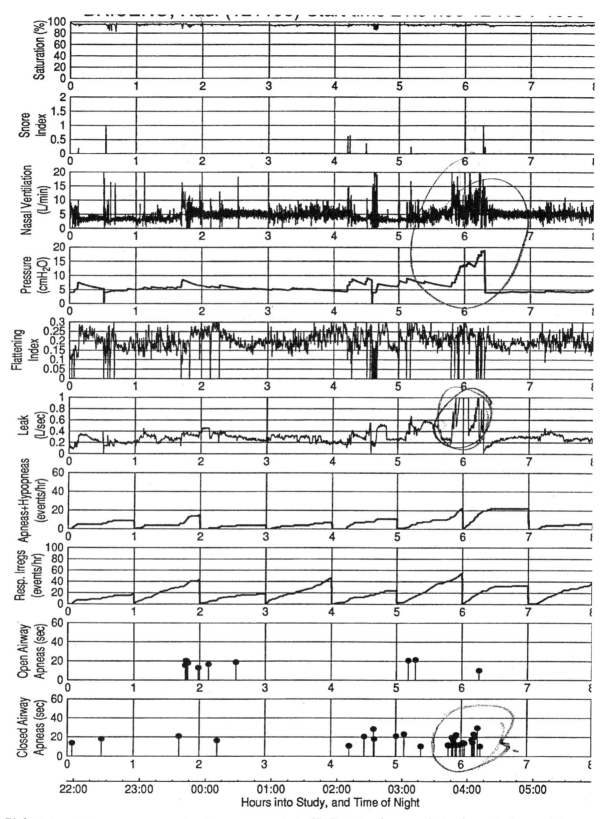

Figure 76–8. Auto-titrating continuous positive airway pressure (auto-CPAP) tracing from one device demonstrating persisting apneas with constant increase in pressure in the presence of a mask leak (roughly circled areas). The pressure rises over a 22-min period from 6 cm to nearly 20 cm, eventually resulting in the patient attempting to pull the mask off and a drop in pressure.

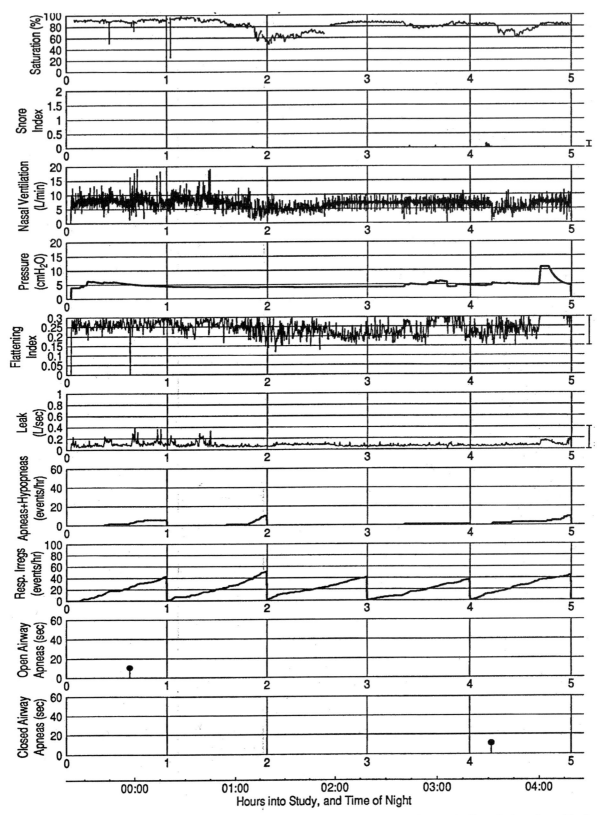

Figure 76–9. Patient with long-standing sleep apnea and obesity. Evidence of marked reduction in SaO$_2$ during sleep. No increase in continuous positive airway pressure (CPAP) with auto-CPAP presumably due to nondetection of any upper airway obstruction, flow limitation, or snoring.

The first published report of such a self-titrating CPAP device was in 1993.[113] Subsequently, a number of such devices utilizing different algorithms were described.[38, 114-117] Some of these devices have a diagnostic mode of operation which will not be discussed here. Also, the algorithms for operation of these devices are usually proprietary information, and cannot be easily compared. There are no significant studies comparing different types of autotitrating devices. However, the literature describing the efficacy of auto-CPAP machines is expanding rapidly and is summarized in the following paragraphs.

Do Auto-CPAP Devices Determine CPAP Levels Accurately?

There are reasonable data supporting the utility of auto-CPAP devices in determining optimal CPAP in selected patients in the sleep laboratory. Our initial data showed reasonable efficacy of the device in eliminating upper airway obstruction.[117] Maximal pressures were similar and the median pressure delivered across the night was lower than in separate manual CPAP titrations of the same patient.[117] However, there are important methodological issues which must be considered, particularly before drawing inferences regarding the success of auto-CPAP in the home. We discuss these below. In the final analysis, data from unattended home studies with auto-CPAP are not available as yet.

As mentioned above, there are differences between auto-CPAP devices, particularly related to their method of detecting upper airway obstruction. These differences would make it important *not* to extrapolate findings from one auto-CPAP device to another.

When comparing technician- and auto-CPAP–determined pressures, it is important that the technician and machine are trying to obtain the same titration outcomes. For example, in one study, workers demonstrated similar efficacy of auto-CPAP in determining pressures equivalent to manual CPAP titration for subsequent fixed-pressure use.[118] These authors also reported a lower respiratory disturbance index on an auto-CPAP device. However, in this study, although the auto-CPAP detected flow limitation, the manual titration was reported as using only elimination of apneas and hypopneas as an endpoint. This would be a potential explanation for the lower respiratory disturbance index with auto-CPAP. Eliminating snoring is not the same as eliminating flattening of the airflow tracing and related arousals.[119] Also, it may be inappropriate to depend on a flow signal provided by the auto-CPAP device itself and for research and comparative purposes independent verification should be obtained. Finally, data obtained in the sleep laboratory with technician supervision cannot be extrapolated to home, unattended CPAP titration where correction of a leak or mask adjustment is not possible. For example, when comparing auto-CPAP with manual pressure determination, one group of investigators excluded periods of mask leak or "high sudden unusual increases in pressure" from their analysis of auto-CPAP titration.[120] Other work has shown mask leaks to be a significant problem in auto-CPAP, as well as manual titration.

Sharma et al.[115] using a different type of auto-CPAP device, found failure to increase pressure and failure to maintain minimum pressure in 7 out of 20 patients. Stradling et al.[121] investigated whether use of an auto-CPAP device in the sleep laboratory influenced subsequent acceptance of CPAP. Acceptance of CPAP was slightly higher in the auto-CPAP group, but unfortunately the study was not double-blinded, which limits the conclusions.

Do Auto-CPAP Devices Improve Compliance and Usage?

Two studies have suggested that home use of an auto-CPAP device leads to increased CPAP usage. Meurice et al.[122] reported 1.4 h more nightly use with an auto-CPAP device allowed to vary +2 or −4 cm around a previously laboratory-determined effective pressure. Konermann et al.[123] reported 0.8 h more usage with another type of device. In neither of these studies were the investigators blinded, which is necessary in this type of comparative study. In another study, where the investigators were apparently blinded, no difference in usage was observed.[124]

Do Auto-CPAP Devices Have Cost Benefits? Home Auto-CPAP—Current Status

Cost-benefit analyses of methods of CPAP treatment are difficult to perform. Assessments of costs will vary according to the type of health system and the location of patients. Benefit assessment must be standardized and reproducible to allow extrapolation to clinical practice. One report suggests that use of auto-CPAP in determining the CPAP level will produce cost savings with reduced laboratory investigation time,[125] but larger and better-designed studies are needed.

Another potential benefit would accrue if home use of auto-CPAP produced better health outcomes. At this stage, there is no evidence that this is the case. Commercial auto-CPAP units are substantially more expensive than fixed-pressure devices. Wide acceptance of home auto-CPAP will require extensive outcome studies to justify the extra cost.

Part of the rationale for auto-CPAP was the hypothesis that a substantially reduced CPAP level would be better tolerated by patients and increase the number of patients able to continue home use. However, in most auto-CPAP studies, the median pressure level is 70 to 80% of the peak autoset or manually determined pressure.[126] Clearly, for most patients, positional and sleep stage differences do not produce large CPAP variance across the night. Moreover, there is no evidence that lower CPAP pressures are associated with better compliance. Similarly, there is evidence that moderate alcohol consumption does not affect the CPAP pressure requirement.[70, 78, 90] Auto-CPAP does not appear to easily correct the flow limitation caused by acute nasal congestion.[127] In addition, concern has been raised over inadequate correction of sleep apnea using one auto-CPAP system[128] or cases where central apneas appear after adequate correction of obstructive events.[129] Given the current costs of auto-CPAP devices, there is no rationale, at this stage, for their use as a home device replacing cheaper fixed-pressure CPAP. Even if the CPAP level required to treat sleep apnea decreases over time in compliant patients, such changes in pressure are usually small. It is not clear what the advantage of lowering pressure would be in patients who are, presumably, successfully established on therapy.

CONCLUSION

Nasal CPAP is the standard form of treatment for patients with moderate to severe symptomatic OSAHS or forms of central sleep apnea that respond to CPAP. Correction of flow limitation appears to be the most practical and effective endpoint for pressure titration. Severe side effects are rare, but nasal and mask problems may limit compliance. Compliance varies from 40 to 80% depending on the study and is probably influenced by how much education and support are provided to the patient. Randomized controlled studies are now offering an evidence-based rationale for CPAP treatment in addition to the plethora of "before-and-after" studies performed in the 1980s. Auto-CPAP is a major technological step forward in CPAP development, but its widespread applicability will depend on studies showing cost benefit, improved compliance, and better health outcomes for these devices.

Acknowledgments

Supported by grants from the National Health and Medical Research Council, and the New South Wales Department of Health, Australia.

References

1. Sullivan CE, Issa FG, Berthon-Jones M, et al. Reversal of obstructive sleep apnea by continuous positive airway pressure applied through the nares. Lancet. 1981;1:862–865.
2. Lombard RM Jr, Zwillich CW. Medical therapy of obstructive sleep apnea. Med Clin North Am. 1985;69:1317–1335.
3. Bradley TD, Phillipson EA. The treatment of sleep apnea—separating the wheat from the chaff. Am Rev Respir Dis. 1983;128:583–586.
4. Grunstein RR, Dodd MJ, Costas L, et al. Home nasal CPAP for sleep apnea—acceptance of home therapy and its usefulness. Aust N Z J Med. 1986;16:635.
5. Grunstein RR. Sleep-related breathing disorders, 5: nasal continuous positive airway pressure treatment for obstructive sleep apnoea. Thorax. 1995;50:1106–1113.
6. Levy P, Pepin JL. Auto-CPAP: an effective and low-cost procedure in the management of OSAHSS? Eur Respir J. 1998;12:753–755.
6a. Loube DI, Gay PC, Strohl KP, et al. Indications for positive airway pressure treatment of adult obstructive sleep apnea patients: a consensus statement. Chest. 1999;115:863–866.
7. Grunstein RR, Hedner JA, Grote L. Therapy of sleep apnea. Drugs 1999. In press.
8. Remmers JE, De Groot WJ, Sauerland EK, et al. Pathogenesis of upper airway occlusion during sleep. J Appl Physiol. 1978;44:931–938.
9. Strohl KP, Redline S. Nasal CPAP therapy, upper air-way muscle activation and obstructive sleep apnea. Am Rev Respir Dis. 1986;134:555–558.
10. Schwab RJ, Pack AI, Gupta KB, et al. Upper airway and soft tissue structural changes induced by CPAP in normal subjects. Am J Respir Crit Care Med. 1996;154(4 pt 1):1106–1116.
11. Issa FG, Sullivan CE. Reversal of central sleep apnea using nasal CPAP. Chest. 1986;90:165–171.
12. Krieger J, Weitzenblum E, Monassier JP. Dangerous hypoxemia during continuous positive airways pressure treatment of obstructive apnea. Lancet. 1983;2:1429–1430.
13. Chervin RD, Theut S, Bassetti C, et al. Compliance with nasal CPAP can be improved by simple interventions. Sleep. 1997;20:284–289.
14. Montserrat JM, Ballester E, Olivi H, et al. Time-course of stepwise CPAP titration. Behavior of respiratory and neurological variables. Am J Respir Crit Care Med. 1995;152:1854–1859.
15. Hosselet JJ, Norman RG, Ayappa I, et al. Detection of flow limitation with a nasal cannula/pressure transducer system. Am J Respir Crit Care Med. 1998;157:1461–1467.
16. Sforza E, Krieger J, Bacon W, et al. Determinants of effective continuous positive airway pressure in obstructive sleep apnea. Role of respiratory effort. Am J Respir Crit Care Med. 1995;151:1852–1856.
17. Lorino AM, Lofaso F, Duizabo D, et al. Respiratory resistive impedance as an index of airway obstruction during nasal continuous positive airway pressure titration. Am J Respir Crit Care Med. 1998;158:1465–1470.
18. Meurice JC, Paquereau J, Denjean A, et al. Influence of correction of flow limitation on continuous positive airway pressure efficiency in sleep apnoea/hypopnoea syndrome. Eur Respir J. 1998;11:1121–1127.
19. Issa FG, Sullivan CE. The immediate effects of nasal continuous positive airway pressure treatment on sleep pattern in patients with obstructive sleep apnea syndrome. Electroencephalogr Clin Neurophysiol. 1986;63:10–17.
20. Condos R, Norman RG, Krishnasamy I, et al. Flow limitation as a noninvasive assessment of residual upper-airway resistance during continuous positive airway pressure therapy of obstructive sleep apnea. Am J Respir Crit Care Med. 1994;150:475–480.
21. Pevernagie DA, Shepard JW Jr. Relations between sleep stage, posture and effective nasal CPAP levels in OSAHS. Sleep. 1992;15:162–167.
22. Issa FG, Sullivan CE. Upper airway closing pressures in snorers. J Appl Physiol. 1984;57:528–535.
23. Jokic R, Klimaszewski A, Sridhar G, et al. Continuous positive airway pressure requirement during the first month of treatment in patients with severe obstructive sleep apnea. Chest. 1998;114:1061–1069.
24. Willson G, Grunstein RR, Doyle J, et al. Domiciliary use of autoset nasal continuous positive airway pressure (nCPAP): feasibility, efficacy and night to night variability. Sleep Res. 1996;25:210.
25. Miljeteigh H, Hoffstein V. Continuous positive airway pressure for treatment of obstructive sleep apnea. Am Rev Respir Dis. 1993;147:1526–1530.
26. Issa FG, Sullivan CE. Alcohol, snoring and sleep apnea. J Neurol Neurosurg Psychiatry. 1982;45:353–359.
27. Berry RB, Desa MM, Light RW. Effect of ethanol on the efficacy of nasal continuous positive airway pressure as a treatment for obstructive sleep apnea. Chest. 1991;99:339–343.
28. Becker HF, Piper AJ, Flynn WE, et al. Breathing during sleep in patients with nocturnal desaturation. Am J Respir Crit Care Med. 1999;159:112–118.
29. Sanders MH, Kern NB, Costantino JP, et al. Adequacy of prescribing positive airway pressure therapy by mask for sleep apnea on the basis of a partial-night trial. Am Rev Respir Dis. 1993;147:1169–1174.
30. Strollo PJ Jr, Sanders MH, Costantino JP, et al. Split-night studies for the diagnosis and treatment of sleep-disordered breathing. Sleep. 1996;19(suppl 10):S255–259.
31. Yamashiro Y, Kryger MH. CPAP titration for sleep apnea using a split-night protocol. Chest. 1995;107:62–66.
32. Rosenthal L, Nykamp K, Guido P, et al. Daytime CPAP titration: a viable alternative for patients with severe obstructive sleep apnea. Chest. 1998;114:1056–1060.
33. Montserrat JM, Alarcon A, Lloberes P, et al. Adequacy of prescribing nasal continuous positive airway pressure therapy for

the sleep apnoea/hypopnoea syndrome on the basis of night time respiratory recording variables. Thorax. 1995;50:969–971.

34. Krieger J, Sforza E, Petiau C, et al. Simplified diagnostic procedure for obstructive sleep apnoea syndrome: lower subsequent compliance with CPAP. Eur Respir J. 1998;12:776–779.

35. Coppola MP, Lawee M. Measurement of obstructive sleep apnea syndrome in the home—the role of portable sleep apnea recording. Chest. 1993;104:19–25.

36. Waldhorn RE, Wood K. Attended home titration of nasal continuous positive airway pressure therapy for obstructive sleep apnea. Chest. 1993;104:1707–1710.

37. White DP, Gibb TJ. Evaluation of the Healthdyne NightWatch system to titrate CPAP in the home. Sleep. 1998;21:198–204.

38. Juhasz J, Schillen J, Urbigkeit A, et al. Unattended continuous positive airway pressure titration. Clinical relevance and cardio-respiratory hazards of the method. Am J Respir Crit Care Med. 1996;154:359–365.

39. Hoffstein V, Mateika S. Predicting nasal continuous positive airway pressure. Am J Respir Crit Care Med. 1994;150:486–488.

40. Engleman HM, Asgari-Jirhandeh N, McLeod AL, et al. Self-reported use of CPAP and benefits of CPAP therapy: a patient survey. Chest. 1996;109:1470–1476.

41. Strumpf DA, Harrop P, Dobbin J, et al. Massive epistaxis from nasal CPAP therapy. Chest. 1989;95:1141.

42. Jarjour NN; Wilson P. Pneumocephalus associated with nasal continuous positive airway pressure in a patient with sleep apnea syndrome. Chest. 1989;96:1425–1426.

43. Kramer NR, Fine MD, McRae RG, et al. Unusual complication of nasal CPAP: subcutaneous emphysema following facial trauma. Sleep. 1997;20:895–897.

44. Strollo PJ Jr, Sanders MH, Atwood CW. Positive pressure therapy. Clin Chest Med. 1998;19:55–68.

45. Pepin JL, Leger P, Veale D, et al. Side effects of nasal continuous positive airway pressure in sleep apnea syndrome. Study of 193 patients in two French sleep centers. Chest. 1995;107:375–381.

46. Richards GN, Cistulli PA, Ungar RG, et al. Mouth leak with nasal continuous positive airway pressure increases nasal airway resistance. Am J Respir Crit Care Med. 1996;154:182–186.

46a. Martins de Araújo MT, Vieira SB, Vasquez EC, et al. Heated humidification or face mask to prevent upper airway dryness during continuous positive airway pressure therapy. Chest. 2000;117:142–147.

47. Mortimore IL, Whittle AT, Douglas NJ. Comparison of nose and face mask CPAP therapy for sleep apnoea. Thorax. 1998;53:290–292.

48. Stauffer JL, Fayter NA, McClure BJ. Conjunctivitis from nasal CPAP apparatus. Chest. 1984;86:802.

49. Bucca C, Carossa S, Pivetti S, et al. Edentulism and worsening of obstructive sleep apnoea. Lancet. 1999;353:121–122.

50. Pressman MR, Peterson DD, Meyer TJ, et al. Ramp abuse. A novel form of patient noncompliance to administration of nasal continuous positive airway pressure for treatment of obstructive sleep apnea. Am J Respir Crit Care Med. 1995;151:1632–1634.

51. Reeves-Hoche MK, Hudgel DW, Meck R, et al. Continuous versus bilevel positive airway pressure for obstructive sleep apnea. Am J Respir Crit Care Med. 1995;151:443–449.

52. Fromm RE Jr, Varon J, Lechin AE, et al. CPAP machine performance and altitude. Chest. 1995;108:1577–1580.

53. Lojander J, Maasilta P, Partinen M, et al. Nasal-CPAP, surgery, and conservative management for treatment of obstructive sleep apnea syndrome. A randomized study. Chest. 1996;110:114–119.

54. Rodenstein D, Collard P, Aubert G. OSAHS treatment UPPP vs N-CPAP. Chest. 1995;107:584–585.

55. Ferguson KA, Ono T, Lowe AA, et al. A randomized crossover study of an oral appliance vs nasal-continuous positive airway pressure in the treatment of mild-moderate obstructive sleep apnea. Chest. 1996;109:1269–1275.

56. Anand VK, Ferguson PW, Schoen LS. Obstructive sleep apnea: a comparison of continuous positive airway pressure and surgical treatment. Otolaryngol Head Neck Surg. 1991;105:382–390.

57. Spilker B. Guide to Clinical Trials. New York, NY: Raven Press; 1991.

58. Ley P. Communicating With Patients: Improving Communication, Satisfaction and Compliance. New York, NY: Chapman & Hall; 1988:61–63.

59. Haynes RB, Taylor DW, Sackett DL. Compliance in Health. Baltimore, Md: John Hopkins University Press; 1979.

60. Mushlania AI, Apple FA. Diagnosing potential non-compliance: physician's ability in a behavioural dimension of medical care. Arch Intern Med. 1977;137:318–321.

61. Rand CS, Wise RA, Nides N, et al. Medication adherence in a clinical trial. Am Rev Respir Dis. 1992;146:1559–1564.

62. Kribbs NB, Pack AI, Kline LR, et al. Objective measurement of patterns of nasal CPAP use by patients with obstructive sleep apnea. Am Rev Respir Dis. 1993;147:887–895.

63. Engleman HM, Martin SE, Deary IJ, et al. Effect of continuous positive airway pressure treatment on daytime function in sleep apnoea/hypopnoea syndrome. Lancet. 1994;343:572–575.

64. Kribbs NB, Pack AI, Kline LR, et al. Effects of one night without nasal CPAP treatment on sleep and sleepiness in patients with obstructive sleep apnea. Am Rev Respir Dis. 1993;147:1162–1168.

65. Grunstein RR, Handelsman DJ, Lawrence S, et al. Neuroendocrine dysfunction in sleep apnea: reversal by nasal continuous positive airways pressure. J Clin Endocrinol Metab. 1989;68:352–358.

66. Hers V, Liistro G, Dury M, et al. Residual effect of nCPAP applied for part of the night in patients with obstructive sleep apnoea. Eur Respir J. 1997;10:973–976.

67. Dinges DF, Pack F, Williams K, et al. Cumulative sleepiness, mood disturbance, and psychomotor vigilance performance decrements during a week of sleep restricted to 4–5 hours per night. Sleep. 1997;20:267–277.

68. Rauscher H, Popp W, Wanke T, et al. Acceptance of CPAP therapy for sleep apnea. Chest. 1991;100:1019–1023.

69. Pieters T, Collard P, Aubert G, et al. Acceptance and long-term compliance with nCPAP in patients with obstructive sleep apnoea syndrome. Eur Respir J. 1996;9:939–944.

70. Waldhorn RE, Herrick TW, Nguyen MC, et al. Long-term compliance with nasal continuous positive airway pressure therapy of obstructive sleep apnea. Chest. 1990;97:33–38.

71. Meurice JC, Dore P, Paquereau J, et al. Predictive factors of long term compliance with nasal continuous positive airway pressure treatment in sleep apnea syndrome. Chest. 1994;105:429–433.

72. Rauscher H, Formanek D, Popp W, et al. Nasal CPAP and weight loss in hypertensive patients with obstructive sleep apnea. Thorax. 1993;48:529–533.

73. Grunstein R. Investigation and treatment of sleep apnea in Australia 1991–95. Am J Respir Crit Care Med. 1997;155:A133.

74. Weaver TE, Kribbs NB, Pack AI, et al. Night-to-night variability in CPAP use over the first three months of treatment. Sleep. 1997;20:278–283.

75. Rolfe I, Olson LG, Saunders NA. Long-term acceptance of continuous positive airway pressure in obstructive sleep apnea. Am Rev Respir Dis. 1991;144:1130–1133.

76. Engleman HM, Martin SE, Douglas NJ. Compliance with CPAP therapy in patients with sleep apnea/hypopnea syndrome. Thorax. 1994;49:263–266.

77. Bennett LS, Langford BA, Stradling JR, et al. Sleep fragmentation indices as predictors of daytime sleepiness and nCPAP response in obstructive sleep apnea. Am J Respir Crit Care Med. 1998;158:778–786.

78. Hoffstein V, Viner S, Mateika S, et al. Treatment of obstructive sleep apnea with nasal continuous positive airway pressure. Patient compliance, perception of benefits, and side effects. Am Rev Respir Dis. 1992;145:841–845.

79. Fletcher E, Luckett RA. The effect of positive reinforcement on hourly compliance in continuous positive airway pressure users with obstructive sleep apnea. Am Rev Respir Dis. 1991;143:936–941.

80. Douglas NJ. Systematic review of the efficacy of nasal CPAP. Thorax. 1998;53:414–415.

81. Hoy CJ, Vennelle M, Douglas NJ. Can CPAP use be improved? Am J Respir Crit Care Med. 1997;155:A304.

82. Sanders MH, Kern N. Obstructive sleep apnea treated by independently adjusted inspiratory and expiratory positive airway pressures via nasal mask: physiological and clinical implications. Chest. 1990;98:317–324.

83. Mahadevia AK, Onal E, Lopata M. Effects of expiratory positive airway pressure on sleep-induced respiratory abnormalities in patients with hypersomnia-sleep apnea syndrome. Am Rev Respir Dis. 1983;128:708–711.

84. Sanders MH, Moore SE. Inspiratory and expiratory partitioning

of airway resistance during sleep in patients with sleep apnea. Am Rev Respir Dis. 1983;127:554–558.

85. Vgontzas AN, Bixler EO, Tan TL, et al. Obesity without sleep apnea is associated with daytime sleepiness. Arch Intern Med. 1998;158:1333–1337.

86. Wright J, Johns R, Watt I, et al. Health effects of obstructive sleep apnoea and the effectiveness of continuous positive airways pressure: a systematic review of the research evidence. Br Med J. 1997;22;314:851–860.

87. Fricker J. Measuring the best way to get a good night's sleep. Lancet. 1997;350:122.

88. Australian Health Technology Advisory Committee (Draft Report). The Effectiveness and Cost Effectiveness of Nasal Continuous Positive Airway Pressure in the Treatment of Obstructive Sleep Apnea in Adults. Canberra, Australia: Australian Government Publishing Services; 1996.

89. Findley LJ, Fabrizio MJ, Knight H, et al. Driving simulator performance in patients with sleep apnea. Am Rev Respir Dis. 1989;140:529–530.

90. Meslier N, Lebrun T, Grillier-Lanoir V, et al. French survey of 3,225 patients treated with CPAP for obstructive sleep apnoea: benefits, tolerance, compliance and quality of life. Eur Respir J. 1998;12:185–192.

91. Engleman HM, Martin SE, Kingshott RN, et al. Randomised placebo controlled trial of daytime function after continuous positive airway pressure (CPAP) therapy for the sleep apnoea/hypopnoea syndrome. Thorax. 1998;53:341–345.

92. Redline S, Adams N, Strauss ME, et al. Improvement of mild sleep-disordered breathing with CPAP compared with conservative therapy. Am J Respir Crit Care Med. 1998;157(3 pt 1):858–865.

93. Ballester E, Badia JR, Hernandez L, et al. Evidence of the effectiveness of continuous positive airway pressure in the treatment of sleep apnea/hypopnea syndrome. Am J Respir Crit Care Med. 1999;159:495–501.

94. Engleman HM, Kingshott RN, Wraith PK, et al. Randomized placebo-controlled crossover trial of continuous positive airway pressure for mild sleep apnea/hypopnea syndrome. Am J Respir Crit Care Med. 1999;159:461–467.

95. Kryger MH, Roos L, Delaive K, et al. Utilization of health care services in patients with severe obstructive sleep apnea. Sleep. 1996;19(suppl 9):S111–116.

96. Peker Y, Hedner J, Johansson A, et al. Reduced hospitalization with cardiovascular and pulmonary disease in obstructive sleep apnea patients on nasal CPAP treatment. Sleep. 1997;20:645–653.

97. Jenkinson C, Davies RJO, Mullins R, et al. Comparison of therapeutic and subtherapeutic nasal continuous positive airway pressure for obstructive sleep apnea: a randomized prospective parallel trial. Lancet. 1999;353:2100–2105.

98. Yamashiro Y, Kryger MH. Acute effect of nasal CPAP on periodic limb movements associated with breathing disorders during sleep. Sleep. 1994;17:172–175.

99. Rennotte MT, Baele P, Aubert G, et al. Nasal continuous positive airway pressure in the perioperative management of patients with obstructive sleep apnea submitted to surgery. Chest. 1995;107:367–374.

100. Mortimore IL, Bradley PA, Murray JA, et al. Uvulopalatopharyngoplasty may compromise nasal CPAP therapy in sleep apnea syndrome. Am J Respir Crit Care Med. 1996;154(6 pt 1):1759–1762.

101. Mezzanotte WS, Tangel DJ, Fox AM, et al. Nocturnal nasal continuous positive airway pressure in patients with chronic obstructive pulmonary disease. Influence on waking respiratory muscle function. Chest. 1994;106:1100–1108.

102. Regnis JA, Piper AJ, Henke KG, et al. Benefits of nocturnal nasal CPAP in patients with cystic fibrosis. Chest. 1994;106:1717–1724.

103. Hanly PJ, Millar TW, Steljes DG, et al. Respiration and abnormal sleep in patients with congestive heart failure. Chest. 1989;96:480–488.

104. Javaheri S, Parker TJ, Liming JD, et al. Sleep apnea in 81 ambulatory male patients with stable heart failure. Types and their prevalences, consequences, and presentations. Circulation. 1998;97:2154–2159.

105. Hanly PJ, Zuberi-Khokhar NS. Increased mortality associated with Cheyne-Stokes respiration in patients with congestive heart failure. Am J Respir Crit Care Med. 1996;153:272–276.

106. Naughton MT, Bradley TD. Sleep apnea in congestive heart failure. Clin Chest Med. 1998;19:99–113.

107. Malone S, Liu PP, Holloway R, et al. Obstructive sleep apnoea in patients with dilated cardiomyopathy: effects of continuous positive airway pressure. Lancet. 1991;338:1480–1484.

108. Tkacova R, Rankin F, Fitzgerald FS, et al. Effects of continuous positive airway pressure on obstructive sleep apnea and left ventricular afterload in patients with heart failure. Circulation. 1998;98(1):2269–2275.

109. Tkacova R, Liu PP, Naughton MT, et al. Effect of continuous positive airway pressure on mitral regurgitant fraction and atria natriuretic peptide in patients with heart failure. J Am Coll Cardiol. 1997;30:739–745.

110. Granton JT, Naughton MT, Benard DC, et al. CPAP improves inspiratory muscle strength in patients with heart failure and central sleep apnea. Am J Respir Crit Care Med. 1996;153:277–282.

111. Davies RJ, Harrington KJ, Ormerod OJ, et al. Nasal continuous positive airway pressure in chronic heart failure with sleep-disordered breathing. Am Rev Respir Dis. 1993;147:630–634.

112. Liston R, Deegan PC, McCreery C, et al. Haemodynamic effects of nasal continuous positive airway pressure in severe congestive heart failure. Eur Respir J. 1995;8:430–435.

113. Berthon-Jones M. Feasibility of a self-setting CPAP machine. Sleep. 1993;16:S120–121.

114. Behbehani K, Yen FC, Burk JR, et al. Automatic control of airway pressure for treatment of obstructive sleep apnea. Trans EEE Biomed Eng. 1995;42:1007–1016.

115. Sharma S, Wali S, Pouliot Z, et al. Treatment of obstructive sleep apnea with a self-titrating continuous positive airway pressure (CPAP) system. Sleep. 1996;19:497–501.

116. Séries F, Marc I. Efficacy of automatic continuous positive airway pressure therapy that uses an estimated required pressure in the treatment of the obstructive sleep apnea syndrome. Ann Intern Med. 1997;127:588–595.

117. Berthon-Jones M, Lawrence S, Sullivan CE, et al. Nasal continuous positive airway pressure treatment: current realities and future. Sleep. 1996;19(suppl 9):S131–135.

118. Teschler H, Berthon-Jones M, Thompson AB, et al. Automated continuous positive airway pressure titration for obstructive sleep apnea syndrome. Am J Respir Crit Care Med. 1996;154(3 pt 1):734–740.

119. Clark SA, Wilson CR, Satoh M, et al. Assessment of inspiratory flow limitation invasively and noninvasively during sleep. Am J Respir Crit Care Med. 1996;154:1755–1758.

120. Lloberes P, Ballester E, Montserrat JM, et al. Comparison of manual and automatic CPAP titration in patients with sleep apnea/hypopnea syndrome. Am J Respir Crit Care Med. 1998;158:713–722.

121. Stradling JR, Barbour C, Pitson DJ, et al. Automatic nasal continuous positive airway pressure titration in the laboratory: patient outcomes. Thorax. 1997;52:72–75.

122. Meurice JC, Marc I, Séries F. Efficacy of auto-CPAP in the treatment of obstructive sleep apnea/hypopnea syndrome. Am J Respir Crit Care Med. 1996;153:794–798.

123. Konermann M, Sanner BM, Vyleta M, et al. Use of conventional and self-adjusting nasal continuous positive airway pressure for treatment of severe obstructive sleep apnea syndrome: a comparative study. Chest. 1998;113:714–718.

124. Teschler H, Berthon-Jones M. Intelligent CPAP systems: clinical experience. Thorax. 1998;53:S49–S54.

125. Berkani M, Lofaso F, Chouaid C, et al. CPAP titration by an auto-CPAP device based on snoring detection: a clinical trial and economic considerations. Eur Respir J. 1998;12:759–763.

126. Grunstein RR, Willson GN, Lawrence S, et al. Automatically adjusting nasal CPAP—one year experience in a sleep laboratory. Sleep Res. 1996;25:211.

127. Lafond C, Séries F. Influence of nasal obstruction on auto-CPAP behaviour in the treatment of obstructive sleep apnea/hypopnea syndrome. Thorax. 1998;53:780–783.

128. Hoster M, Schlenker E, Ruhle KH. Computer-assisted nCPAP settings in comparison with conventional methods. Pneumologie. 1997;51(suppl 3):754–757.

129. Boudewyns A, Van de Heyning P, De Backer W. Appearance of central apnoea in a patient treated by auto-CPAP for obstructive sleep apnoea. Respir Med. 1998;92:891–893.

77

Surgical Therapy for Obstructive Sleep Apnea-Hypopnea Syndrome

Robert W. Riley

Nelson B. Powell

Kasey K. Li

Christian Guilleminault

Obstructive sleep apnea-hypopnea syndrome (OSAHS) can be the cause of disabling sleepiness that impairs the patient's well-being and, at times, may be life-threatening. In this chapter, we use the more commonly utilized term, *obstructive sleep apnea syndrome* (OSAS) to describe these patients. The first treatment used to control this syndrome was surgical and dates back to the initial studies that focused on pickwickian subjects. Kuhlo[1] is credited with performing the first tracheostomy with the intention of bypassing upper airway obstruction that occurred during the sleep of morbidly obese patients. Since its initial treatment, selective surgical approaches have been developed to address specific regions of anatomical obstruction in patients with OSAS. The currently accepted surgical methods and future modalities are subsequently reviewed.

It is now well known that the contributing causes that lead to OSAS are multifactorial, but generally they all entail a negative influence on the delicate balance necessary for airway maintenance during sleep. Ideally, medical and surgical approaches strive to intervene at identified levels of obstruction. Medical approaches, including continuous positive airway pressure (CPAP) bilevel positive airway pressure, weight loss, body position during sleep, and avoidance of alcohol and sedating medications,[2, 3] are most commonly employed and are discussed in detail elsewhere in this section. Patients who are unable or unwilling to comply with medical management may be surgical candidates.

SURGERY FOR OBESITY

Because obesity is a major risk factor for the development of OSAS, surgical approaches for OSAS directed at forced weight loss have been advocated. Both the vertical banded gastroplasty and the gastric bypass are currently used to produce malabsorption and restrict gastric volume for weight control[4] and thus improve OSAS. However, these operations have associated mortality (0.3 to 1.6%) and significant perioperative complications including wound infection, deep venous thrombosis, pulmonary embolism, and subphrenic abscess, as well as delayed complications such as micronutrient deficiencies (up to 70%) with potential hematologic and neurologic consequences, persistent vomiting, and maladaptive eating behavior (20 to 30%).[5–10] Furthermore, poor long-term outcome with significant weight gain to and above the preoperative weight level have been reported.[11, 12] Even in series with successful results, the average postoperative weight plateaus to 30 to 70% above ideal weight.[6, 13–16] Although OSAS has been shown to improve in a majority of patients after significant weight loss, many patients continue to have significant apnea,[17–19] and one report has demonstrated recurrence of sleep apnea despite maintenance of weight loss several years after bariatric surgery.[20] Therefore, bariatric surgery should only be considered in patients with body mass index (BMI, kg/m^2) greater than 40, or greater than 35 in combination with other co-morbidity including life-threatening cardiopulmonary problems, severe diabetes mellitus, sleep apnea, obesity-related pulmonary hypertension, and degenerative joint disease.[4]

SURGERY INVOLVING THE UPPER AIRWAY

Surgical management of OSAS is currently directed to site-specific anatomic regions involved in OSAS (Table 77–1). Physicians referring an OSAS patient for

Table 77–1. SURGICAL PROCEDURES FOR TREATMENT OF OBSTRUCTIVE SLEEP APNEA SYNDROME AT DESIGNATED LEVELS

Bypass All Upper Airway Obstructions

Tracheotomy

Selectively Eliminate One or Several Specific Abnormalities in the Upper Airway

Nasal reconstruction
Uvulopalatopharyngoplasty
Mandibular osteotomy with genioglossus advancement
Hyoid myotomy with suspension
Maxillomandibular advancement osteotomy
Base of tongue resection

surgery should investigate each individual patient's associated problems thoroughly for a full understanding of the associated variables. For instance, some OSAS patients have a specific anatomic upper airway abnormality; hence, treatment such as weight loss alone often does not resolve their symptoms. Further clinical investigation in this patient group may reveal an abnormality of this type that will be particularly amenable to correction with a specific surgical procedure. In fact, we (M. Partinen, MD, and C. Guilleminault, MD, unpublished data, 1993) have learned, as an extension of the study by Jamieson et al., that obese patients may have only minor cranial mandibular abnormalities, whereas thin patients may have considerable facial derangements.[21] Findings such as these should help the clinician to develop specific treatment plan.

During the comprehensive evaluation of the patient with OSAS, it may become evident that a surgical alternative may be preferable to medical management, particularly in younger or middle-aged adults, who may thereby be spared years of nightly attachment to a CPAP machine. Presurgical evaluations therefore, are mandatory to detect any anatomic abnormalities that may be present and evaluate their significance in the context of the level of severity of the patient's OSAS. This investigation requires not only the classic nocturnal polysomnographic recording but also a thorough evaluation of how these individual factors affect OSAS (Table 77–2). Several of these factors will vary, depending on the age of the subject, weight, nocturnal

Table 77–2. PARAMETERS MONITORED AND EVALUATED IN OBSTRUCTIVE SLEEP APNEA SYNDROME

Oxygen desaturations
  Frequency and levels of SaO_2 drops
  The nadir and total events and time desaturated below
  90%-80%-70%, and so on
Carbon dioxide retention
Cardiac arrhythmias
Hemodynamic changes
  During sleep and awake
Negative intrathoracic pressures sleep architecture
Degree of fatigue and sleepiness

alcohol intake, co-morbid lung disease, and possibly most important, anatomy of the individual patient.

IDENTIFICATION OF SITE OF ANATOMIC REGIONS PRODUCING OBSTRUCTION DURING SLEEP

Although the etiology of OSAS is not well understood, the areas producing anatomic obstruction are well defined.[22–30] OSAS can thus be ideally viewed as a surgically responsive problem due to the presence of regional areas of "disproportionate anatomy" (nose, palate, base of tongue, pharyngeal wall). The availability of methods to identify such regions are essential for directing decision-making with respect to surgical treatment. A systematic approach to this evaluation will allow for the use of a surgical protocol that results in improved clinical outcomes.

General Clinical Evaluation

The patient's weight, overall body habitus, and skeletal facial pattern should be documented. A detailed examination centers around attention to the three major anatomic regions of the potential obstruction: nose, palate (*oropharynx*), and base of tongue (*hypopharynx*). A nasal examination should be done at rest and during deep inspiration allowing assessment during dynamic breathing to evaluate whether there is adequate alar support and nasal valve function. Nasal septal deflection, turbinate enlargement, webs, polyps, or masses are potentially important in the patient with OSAS. The oral cavity should be examined by assessing the state of dental health and the character of oral mucous membranes. Examination of the pharynx should include documentation of the length of the soft palate, the character of the soft tissues, and the presence or absence of tonsils.

The facial skeletal portion of the examination can be done by evaluating the overall position of the upper and lower jaw as well as their relationship. The overall size of the tongue should always be evaluated relative to the space available; that is, a tongue of normal size may look considerably larger in a patient with mandibular deficiency (*retrognathia*). Fujita[31, 32] (Table 77–3) proposed a classification to define and categorize areas of obstruction. A laryngeal examination is essential on all patients because there may be laryngeal dysfunction secondary to webs, cysts, tumors, or vocal cord paralysis.[33] The character of the epiglottis can be important, especially if it is omega-shaped (*folded*).[34]

Table 77–3. CLASSIFICATION OF OBSTRUCTIVE REGIONS BY FUJITA

Type I	Palate (normal base of tongue)
Type II	Palate and base of tongue
Type III	Base of tongue (normal palate)

The presence of "floppy" redundant supraglottic mucosa and tissue also should not be overlooked because it is yet another potentially specific variable in the obstructive process. In many patients with OSAS, it is found that examination of the posterior pharyngeal wall and larynx is virtually impossible because of a brisk gag reflex, a large tongue, and the over abundance of soft tissue. In such cases, evaluation should be done during fiberoptic nasopharyngolaryngoscopy. Lateral cephalometric radiographs assist in the overall evaluation of the soft tissue and bony configuration. Other upper airway imaging methods that can be used are magnetic resonance imaging (MRI), volumetric computed tomographic (CT) scans, cine studies, and acoustic reflections.[35] Many of these methods are more investigational than routine. The usual methods are described in the following sections.

Fiberoptic Nasopharyngolaryngoscopy

A flexible fiberoptic scope can be used to evaluate the nasal airway, pharynx, and larynx. Maneuvers such as Müller's have been evaluated by Sher et al.[36] and Katsantonis et al.[37] in an attempt to identify areas of potential obstruction and thus more accurately predict the likelihood of success of surgical procedures directed at the pharyngeal level. During the fiberoptic evaluation, it is important to rule out any abnormal pathological change at each region. Photographs or videotapes are useful primarily because they can be reviewed in the course of therapy and compared with postoperative studies.

Radiographic Evaluation

Cephalometric radiographs and CT, which may include three-dimensional (3-D) scans, have been used to evaluate patients with OSAS.[38-43] 3-D CT is usually reserved as an investigational tool. The cephalometric radiograph has been the simplest and most practical upper airway imaging technique. It is a lateral radiographic view of the head detailing the bone and soft tissue landmarks (Fig. 77–1). Data from these films help preoperative and postoperative evaluation of the airway space. Although there are limitations to this technique, this film does provide information about the skeletal anatomic structure and reliable data on the posterior airway space, hyoid position, and soft palate.

We originally used cephalometric radiographs to evaluate uvulopalatopharyngoplasty (UPPP) failure in 1984[23] and over the years reported on the correlation of these two-dimensional (2-D) studies with 3-D volumetric CT scans.[38, 39] This correlation gave us confidence in evaluating the posterior airway space with this method, and it has been a reliable and relatively inexpensive tool. The limitations of the cephalometric head film are obvious in that the patient is evaluated while awake and seated, and it is not a dynamic study obtained during sleep. It should be cautioned that overuse of this technique by itself to determine the exact

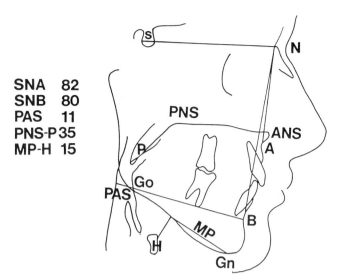

Figure 77–1. Cephalometric analysis used for evaluation of patients with obstructive sleep apnea syndrome. SNA 82° (SD ± 2), maxilla to cranial base; SNB 80° (SD ± 2), mandible to cranial base; PAS 11 mm (SD ± 1), posterior airway space; PNS-P 37 mm (SD ± 3), length of soft palate; MP-H 15.4 mm (SD ± 3), distance of hyoid from inferior mandible. MP-H, mandibular plane—hyoid; PNS-P, posterior nasal spine—point B; SNA, Sella-Nasion—point A; SNB, Sella-Nasion—point B. (From Riley RW, Powell NB, Guilleminault C. Obstructive sleep apnea syndrome: a surgical protocol for dynamic upper airway reconstruction. J Oral Maxillofac Surg. 1993;51:742–747.

surgical intervention is not recommended. In summary, a thorough clinical head and neck evaluation combined with fiberoptic nasopharyngolaryngoscopy and radiographic imaging should assist the physician in better isolating and directing management at the region or regions of obstruction in OSAS.[38-40]

SURGICAL TREATMENT PHILOSOPHY

Objective tests (polysomnogram [PSG], multiple sleep latency test [MSLT]), history, and clinical examination establish the severity of the syndrome. The clinician must decide if the criteria for therapy are met and with this knowledge develop a treatment plan. Because the potential exists for upper airway narrowing at multiple sites in a given OSAS patient, it may be necessary for surgical intervention to address more than one anatomic level with the objective of total upper airway reconstruction (UAR) (Table 77–4).

Although we consider OSAS a surgical problem, medical management is usually included in the formu-

Table 77–4. SURGICAL TREATMENT PHILOSOPHIES

Treatment to cure
Logically directed management
Full disclosure of options and risks
Stage surgical management
Follow-up of all treatment

lation of any treatment philosophy. Medical management primarily uses the modalities of positive airway pressure (CPAP or bilevel positive airway pressure)[41–44] and weight loss.[45–48] Positive airway pressure is currently the most frequently used treatment. This is due, in part, to the fact that it is successful, at least initially, and can give almost instant relief to most patients. At Stanford University, approximately 85% of those patients seen with OSAS are treated medically. This still leaves a significant number of patients (15%) who initially reject medical management in favor of surgical therapy. These individuals are usually younger or active older patients. We also see a large group who have failed nasal CPAP therapy for one reason or another.[49–52]

The primary goal of surgical treatment is to eliminate sleep-disordered breathing. For reporting purposes, we define a *surgical responder* as a patient with a *normal sleep study*, which is defined as normalization of respiratory events and relief from hypoxemia and fragmented sleep. Previous reporting methods have defined responders as those who were 50% improved; however, this can no longer be considered valid. Tracheostomy has, in the past, been the gold standard to assess surgical outcomes; however, tracheostomy has been replaced by CPAP. We have instituted a revised surgical goal to define *cure* that will compare and compete directly with the results of CPAP or bilevel positive airway pressure. To meet and better attain this goal, we adopted a surgical protocol that combines the evaluation, the indications for treatment, the treatment philosophies, and a two-phase approach to surgical intervention. A surgical plan is selected by meticulously identifying the possible region or regions of upper airway obstruction and applying the specific surgical indications to the area involved. Staging of the surgical approach is selected after assessing the results of our various examinations coupled with the reported experience of others. Our two-phase surgical protocol has individual stages in each phase and was adopted to meet the previous described goals (Fig. 77–2). Tra-

cheostomy is not included in our protocol. Nasal CPAP has all but eliminated the need for tracheostomy. The only potential candidates for tracheostomy are those patients with severe, life-threatening sleep apnea (i.e., respiratory disturbance index [RDI] greater than 60, SaO_2 less than 60%) who are intolerant of nasal CPAP.

Because there are potentially three levels of obstruction (i.e., nose, palate, base of tongue), one must be willing to treat each individually for sufficient upper airway stabilization. We suggest nasal reconstruction for any patient who has notable obstruction of the nasal airway (e.g., deviated septum, collapsed ala, or enlarged turbinates).[53]

UPPP is an operative procedure for the removal of redundant tissue at the oropharyngeal level (Type I Fujita),[54–56] and if this regional obstruction is not recognized, it can effect the overall results. Base of tongue (hypopharyngeal) obstruction is managed currently by three techniques: (1) limited mandibular osteotomy with genioglossus advancement and hyoid myotomy-suspension (GAHM), (2) maxillomandibular surgical procedure for advancement of the maxilla and mandible (MMO),[57–69] and (3) base of tongue surgery (e.g., midline glossectomy via surgical or laser excision).[70–72] Midline glossectomy[70–72] and transpalatal advancement pharyngoplasty[73, 74] are occasionally performed for the management of tongue base and palatal obstruction, respectively. However, these procedures have not gained wide acceptance as compared to the procedures described next due to the potential complications as well as the lack of consistent results.[70–74]

THE TWO-PHASE SURGICAL APPROACH TO THERAPY

We have established a two-phase approach to direct treatment of suspected regions of obstruction during sleep. Phase I surgical intervention includes nasal reconstruction, UPPP, and limited mandibular osteotomy

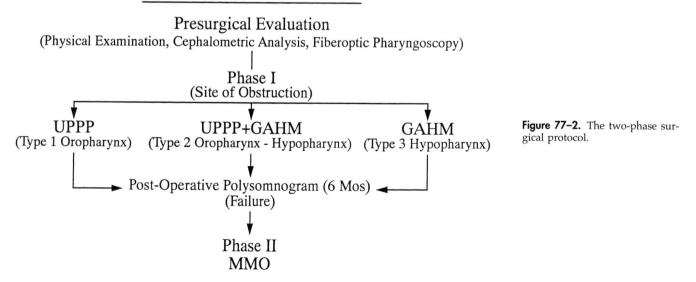

SURGICAL PROTOCOL

Presurgical Evaluation
(Physical Examination, Cephalometric Analysis, Fiberoptic Pharyngoscopy)

Phase I
(Site of Obstruction)

UPPP
(Type 1 Oropharynx)

UPPP+GAHM
(Type 2 Oropharynx - Hypopharynx)

GAHM
(Type 3 Hypopharynx)

Post-Operative Polysomnogram (6 Mos)
(Failure)

Phase II
MMO

Figure 77–2. The two-phase surgical protocol.

with genioglossus advancement. Should the patient need one or all three, each would be completed before moving on to phase II. Each patient who has undergone phase I surgery is allowed a period of healing followed by a PSG assessment to determine the outcome. It is important to reevaluate between phases. Individuals with persistent OSAS following phase I surgery become candidates for phase II (MMO). The published data has shown that control of OSAS occurs in approximately 60% of patients following phase I and greater than 90% following phase II.[57, 64–66] It is important to review all possible surgical plans with the patient and the family well in advance of surgery and to clearly point out the rationale for this approach. Combining phase I and phase II as one surgical procedure should be vigorously discouraged because of significant increased morbidity, including immediate postoperative airway obstruction and death.

Our concern for postoperative airway compromise from surgery has prompted us to further establish a CPAP surgical protocol.[75] Any patient who can tolerate CPAP and has an RDI greater than or equal to 40 and oxygen desaturation of 80% or less is placed on CPAP 2 weeks before surgery. The patient is maintained on CPAP immediately after extubation and remains on CPAP until 2 weeks before the postoperative PSG (4 to 6 months). Patients with severe sleep apnea (RDI greater than 60, SaO$_2$ less than 70%) who are intolerant of nasal CPAP should be considered as candidates for temporary tracheostomy.

As always, there are exceptions to this treatment protocol; in many instances, local resources, experience, and expertise dictate the type of surgical therapy a patient may receive. This is due to the fact that some of the procedures require surgeons with multiple disciplinary training, and such surgeons may not be available in the patient's community. In such cases, individual surgical treatment must be left to the choice of the surgeon and the patient.

Surgical Procedures

Tracheostomy

Tracheostomy was described as the first surgical treatment for OSAS. The success was due to the fact that it bypassed the upper airway. In most centers, it is now a limited procedure. This is due to poor acceptance by the patient and the fact that CPAP can compete with the results of tracheostomy. There are occasions, however, when tracheostomy may be safer for the patient such as in the presence of morbid obesity or when there is a need to ensure adequate airway in the interim period of multistep procedures. The indications of tracheostomy are listed in Table 77–5.

Nasal Reconstruction (Phase I)

It is important that nasal airway be clear for normal respiration both asleep and awake. Olson[53] has reported the effects of nasal obstruction in OSA. Nasal

Table 77–5. INDICATIONS FOR TRACHEOTOMY

Morbid obesity
Severe facial skeletal deformity (mandibular deficiency) with excessive daytime somnolence
Hypoxemia (SaO$_2$ ≤ 70%)
Significant cardiac arrhythmias

obstruction may also interfere with the optimal use of nasal CPAP. Nasal obstruction during sleep may cause the patient to open the mouth and autorotate the mandible back, thus allowing the base of tongue to drift to the pharynx and further add to the obstruction.

Three anatomical areas of the nose that require examination in detail are the alar cartilage and nasal valve region, the septum, and the turbinates. Indications for nasal procedures are listed in Table 77–6. The procedures to correct nasal valve narrowing and alar collapse, septal deformities, and turbinate hypertrophy have been well described in the head and neck literature and can be appropriately modified for use in OSA. Proper staging of the nasal reconstruction during this sequential intervention of the airway should be planned carefully. Nasal procedures are usually performed at the end of phase I reconstruction. This is particularly important if the patient requires nasal CPAP for airway protection. Nasal reconstruction is a highly successful operation, and improvement can be expected in a majority of the patients.

Pharyngeal Reconstruction (Phase I): Uvulopalatopharyngoplasty

UPPP was proposed by Ikematsu[76] in 1964 for the treatment of habitual snoring. Fujita and colleagues[54–56] subsequently adopted this technique for the treatment of OSAS as well as snoring. The rationale for UPPP has been established by studies showing obstruction during sleep at the oropharyneal region. Consequently, this procedure was originally thought to be an alternative to tracheostomy in OSAS. Unfortunately, however, because of disappointing and variable results, it became clear that the oropharyneal region was only one of the potential regions of obstruction. Techniques such as fiberoptics, electromyography (EMG), fluoroscopy, CT, and MRI were used to confirm and better define the obstructive process. Indications for UPPP are listed in Table 77–7.

UPPP is an excellent method to manage obstruction isolated to the oropharyngeal region. The surgical procedure is easily done under general anesthesia and includes the removal of a portion of the soft palate,

Table 77–6. INDICATIONS FOR NASAL RECONSTRUCTION

Nasal valve collapse
Septal deviations
Turbinate hypertrophy refractory to medical management

Table 77–7. OBSTRUCTION AT THE PHARYNGEAL LEVEL (FUJITA TYPE I AND TYPE III): INDICATIONS FOR UVULOPALATOPHARYNGOPLASTY

Long soft palate
Redundant lateral pharyngeal wall
Excess tonsillar tissues

uvula, and any residual tonsillar tissue that may be present.[77–79] The procedure was discussed frequently during the 1990s; therefore, a detailed technique is not presented. For review of the general technique of UPPP, see Figure 77–3. Unfortunately, UPPP is most uncomfortable for the patient, and this creates the incorrect image to both the patient and the referring medical colleague that this surgery is extensive. The procedure is relatively simple, and proper patient education helps resolve this aspect of the stigma associated with this procedure.

At present, there are reports that this site of intervention provides approximately a 20 to 50% reduction in respiratory events.[80–86] In a meta-analysis, Sher et al.[87] reported a 39% success rate of UPPP for correcting OSAS. UPPP has seldom been credited with curing moderate or severe OSAS. Although there is often an improvement in sleep-disordered breathing following UPPP, the degree of improvement is frequently insufficient to define surgical success. The temptation to improve the results by taking additional tissue should be resisted because the potential complications dramatically increase. As noted earlier, the incomplete response to UPPP is almost always due to the fact that other regions of obstruction exist. We suggest that UPPP is probably overused as an isolated procedure by those who have failed to identify other existing obstructive sites.

Alternate Procedure for Pharyngeal Reconstruction

Uvulopalatal Flap

We developed and reported the uvulopalatal flap (UPF) as a modification of the UPPP.[88] The goal was to reduce the risk of nasopharyngeal incompetence and nasal stenosis. The technique is demonstrated in Figure 77–4. The method involves initially grasping the uvula with toothed forceps and reflecting it toward the hard-soft palate junction. The opening to the nasal pharynx is examined and assessment of the amount of mucosa to be removed is made. The mucosa is excised as diagrammed and a portion of the uvula is excised. The flap is repositioned and closed with 3-0 Vicryl sutures. Redundant lateral wall tissue is then excised as needed.

Eighty patients were examined in a prospective and consecutive manner. The study variables included age, gender, BMI, palatal length, RDI, lowest oxygen desaturation during sleep, and subjective snoring scale. There was no statistically significant difference between the UPPP group and the UPF group. There were no significant complications in the UPF group. Using a visual analogue scale to assess pain, there was significantly less pain in the UPF group compared with the UPPP group.

Laser-Assisted Uvulopalatoplasty

Laser-assisted uvulopalatoplasty (LAUP), an office-based surgical procedure, was introduced by Kamami[89] in 1990 as a new approach to the treatment of snoring. This technique progressively shortens and tightens the uvula and palate through a series of carbon dioxide laser incisions and vaporizations. Most of the uvula is amputated and the soft palate is incised by vertical trenches up to the muscular sling, 1 to 2 cm lateral to the uvula. Additionally, mucosal or tonsillar pillar tissue is vaporized as needed (Fig. 77–5). There are several studies evaluating the efficacy of LAUP for OSAS, but most are flawed by method discrepancies or statistical inadequacies such as ill-defined criteria for response for lack of adequate follow-up. Kamami indicated that 40% of patients were cured, with no definition of cure except for 50% improvement in RDI. His responders' RDI decreased from 41.5 to 16.9, and the entire group had an average RDI improvement from 41.3 to 20.3. Walker et al.[90] achieved a 48% success rate; however, 21% had worsening of their disease, 15%

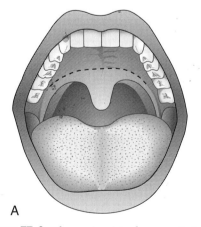
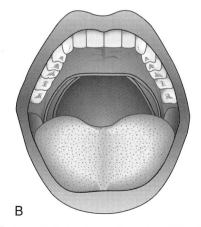
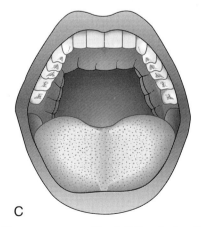

A   B   C

Figure 77–3. The uvulopalatopharyngoplasty technique. *A,* Redundant soft palate and tonsillar pillar mucosa are outlined. *B,* Tonsils, tonsillar pillar mucosa, and posterior soft palate have been excised. The extent of soft palate excision is determined by placing traction on the uvula and noting the position of the mucosal crease. *C,* Mucosal flaps of the lateral pharyngeal wall and nasal palatal muscle are advanced to the anterior pillar and oral mucosa of the soft palate. The wound is closed with 3-0 Vicryl braided suture. (From Troell RJ, Strom CG. Surgical therapy for snoring. Fed Pract. 1997;14:29–52.)

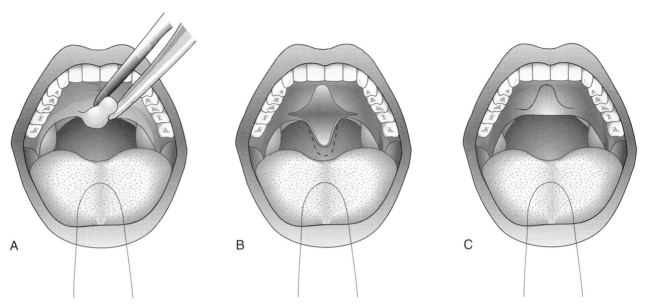

Figure 77–4. The reversible uvulopalatal flap technique. *A,* Local anesthetic injected, uvula reflected to identify mucosal crease of muscular sling. *B,* Knife or pinpoint cautery removes mucosa on proposed flap site. *C,* Wound is closed with a half-buried suture of 3-0 Vicryl braided suture at tip of the uvula and simple interrupted sutures along the mucosal closure. (From Troell RJ, Strom CG. Surgical therapy for snoring. Fed Pract. 1997;14:29–52.)

had no significant change, and 36% had a postoperative RDI greater than 20. The mean RDI of the responders decreased from 24.5 to 3.4, while nonresponders remained unchanged, 39.5 to 39.2. Surgical success (responders) was defined as a postoperative RDI of 10 or less. There is concern regarding the safety of performing upper airway surgery on an ambulatory basis, especially with respect to the early postoperative period secondary to surgical trauma and edema. Terris et al.,[91] in patients with a mean postoperative RDI of 11.3, revealed a doubling of the RDI, a fourfold increase in the apnea index (AI), stable oxygen saturation, and a decrease in the cross-sectional area of as much as 48%

at 72 h. They concluded that patients with mild OSAS (RDI less than 20, SaO_2 greater than 85%) may be offered LAUP, but those with moderate to severe OSAS should be counseled on other more prudent surgical options such as UPPP, UPF, or hypopharyngeal reconstructive techniques.

Mandibular Osteotomy With Genioglossus Advancement (Phase I)

The mandible, tongue, and hyoid complex is a determinant in the pathophysiology of OSAS at the hypopharyngeal level.[92–95] The rationale for surgical inter-

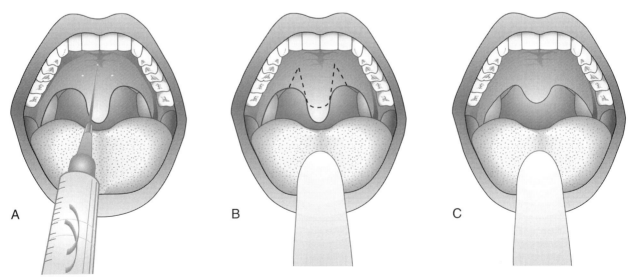

Figure 77–5. The laser-assisted uvulopalatoplasty technique. *A,* Local anesthetic injected. *B,* The CO_2 laser is used to excise vertical trenches of the soft palate on either aspect of the uvula up to the muscular sling; 30 to 90% of the uvula is amputated or vaporized. *C,* The postoperative result necessitates 4 to 5 weeks for complete healing and scarring to produce traction forces to improve the airway patency. (From Troell RJ, Strom CG. Surgical therapy for snoring. Fed Pract. 1997;14:29–52.)

ventions at the tongue base (hypopharynx) is to minimize the posterior displacement of this structure during sleep. Surgical intervention at this level attempts to enlarge the posterior airway space and thus alleviate obstruction at this level.

This limited surgical procedure is used in phase I of our protocol as conservative treatment for obstruction at the hypopharyngeal level. It is considered a maxillo-facial technique because an osteotomy is performed to advance the tongue at the genial tubercle attachment. The surgery is limited in that the jaw and teeth do not move; only the genial tubercle and genioglossus-hyoid complex are advanced. The limiting factor in this forward movement is the thickness of the anterior portion of the mandible. This advancement places tension on the tongue musculature and thereby limits the posterior displacement during sleep. It must be appreciated that in this limited procedure, no additional room for the tongue is anatomically created. This is contrasted with a total mandibular advancement (phase II), which not only places further tension on the genioglossus but also creates more physical space for the tongue. The hyoid myotomy and suspension is not a maxillofacial procedure and is described separately. Table 77–8 outlines the specific indications for the limited osteotomy genioglossus advancement procedure. It is important to obtain selected baseline information before surgery to assist the surgeon in planning the selected bone and soft tissue manipulation. A radiographic analysis should include a lateral cephalometric head film and a panoramic dental radiograph. The cephalogram documents skeletal deformities and soft tissue airway narrowing. It further assists in assessing anatomic and airway changes following surgery. The dental film depicts the course of the inferior alveolar nerve canal and mental foramen. It further shows the anatomy of the anterior teeth and potential pathologic processes (e.g., periodontal disease, cyst).

Surgery may be performed under general anesthesia or intravenous (IV) sedation technique. The surgical technique has been previously described in detail. The technique depicted (Fig. 77–6) is a modification of previous descriptions. The current technique creates less surgical trauma by advancing only the genioglossus muscle with the genial tubercle instead of a major portion of the mandibular symphysis as in the earlier procedure. It is recommended because there is reduced

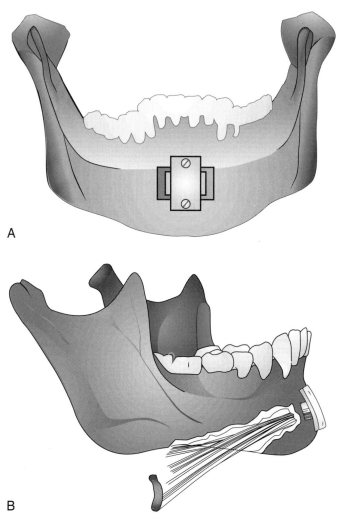

A

B

Figure 77–6. The limited mandibular osteotomy with genioglossus advancement procedure. A rectangular window of symphyseal bone consisting of the geniotubercle is advanced anteriorly, rotated to allow bony overlap, and immobilized with a titanium screw. *A,* Anterior view. *B,* Lateral view. (From Troell RJ, Powell NB, Riley RW. Hypopharyngeal airway surgery for obstructive sleep apnea syndrome. Semin Respir Crit Care Med. 1998;19:175–183.)

postoperative morbidity while similar results are achieved.

The surgical approach is intraoral and sublabial. The cut is made just below the mucogingival junction, and a subperiosteal flap is developed to expose the anterior mandible and mental nerves. The genial tubercle and genioglossus muscle can be identified with the aid of the lateral cephalometric head film and by finger palpation in the floor of the mouth. It is recommended that the superior horizontal bone cut be approximately 5 mm below the root apices and the inferior horizontal bone cut be approximately 10 mm above the inferior border. The lateral and vertical bone cuts should not be extended beyond the canine teeth. It is recommended to initially outline the rectangular osteotomy and then complete all four osteotomies. It is important to maintain parallel walls. Before completing the osteotomy, a titanium screw is placed in the outer cortex to control and manipulate the fragment. The genioglossus

---

Table 77–8. SPECIFIC INDICATIONS FOR SURGICAL INTERVENTION WITH MANDIBULAR OSTEOTOMY WITH GENIOGLOSSUS ADVANCEMENT

A respiratory disease index of 20 or greater, excessive daytime somnolence with respiratory disease index of less than 20, or both

Oxygen saturation below an SaO_2 of 90%

A body mass index < 33

Patients with severe obstructive sleep apnea syndrome who are being prepared for maxillomandibular osteotomy in a step sequence in our phased protocol

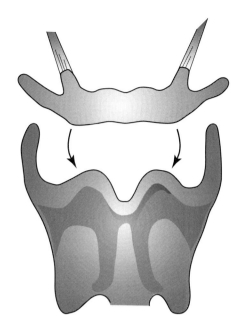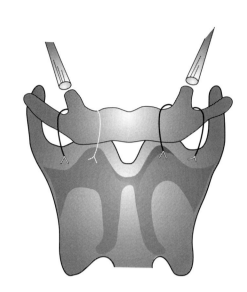

Figure 77–7. The modified hyoid myotomy and suspension procedure. The hyoid bone is isolated, the inferior body dissected clean, the majority of the suprahyoid musculature remains intact. The hyoid is advanced over the thyroid lamina and immobilized with sutures placed through the superior aspect of the thyroid cartilage. (From Troell RJ, Powell NB, Riley RW. Hypopharyngeal airway surgery for obstructive sleep apnea syndrome. Semin Respir Crit Care Med. 1998;19:175–183.)

fragment is advanced and partially rotated as depicted. The outer cortex and marrow are removed. The inner cortex is rigidly fixed with a 2.0-mm titanium screw. It is important to emphasize that this current osteotomy does not violate the inferior border of the mandible. Violation of the inferior border significantly increases the risk of pathologic mandibular fracture.

Hyoid Myotomy-Suspension (Phase I)

The rationale for including the hyoid procedure in the treatment of base of tongue obstruction is the fact that, anatomically, the hyoid complex is an integral part of the hypopharynx, both statically and dynamically. Movement laterally forward improves the posterior airway space. Lateral radiographs taken of patients on CPAP at their preset therapeutic pressure levels (cm H_2O) show an improved opening at the valecular level that is also seen after a hyoid procedure. Numerous reports have supported the concept that surgical intervention at the hyoid complex level improves the hypopharyngeal airway. Kaya[96] is credited with the first report, followed by Patton et al.[97, 98] A hyoid myotomy with suspension has been performed as part of phase I treatment but is not always included at the same time as genioglossus advancement. This is due to the fact that in our population of severe OSAS patients (RDI greater than 60, SaO_2 less than 60%, BMI greater than 33) we have generally combined the genioglossus advancement with UPPP. The added insult to the infrahyoid region was thought to be inappropriate in many patients of this group. We have also found, when evaluating patients following UPPP and genioglossus advancement, that the posterior airway space is improved and the patient symptomatically better, thus a hyoid procedure may not be necessary. For these reasons we have elected to use hyoid myotomy and suspension only in some patients, and as a separate surgical step. However, we often perform genioglossus advancement and hyoid myotomy simultaneously when a UPPP has been done previously. The original description of the hyoid suspension technique involves suspending the hyoid to the anterior mandible with fascia lata. The technique has subsequently been modified and currently involves suspension of the hyoid to the superior thyroid cartilage as shown in Figure 77–7.[99]

The surgical approach is through a horizontal skin incision above the hyoid bone. The dissection is carried inferiorly along the suprahyoid musculature to the body of the hyoid. The body of the hyoid is isolated, which involves removing the infrahyoid muscles from the body of the hyoid. The suprahyoid muscles are left intact. If the hyoid lacks mobility, the stylohyoid ligament is amputated from the lesser cornu. The hyoid is suspended anteriorly to the superior thyroid cartilage with four engaged permanent sutures. It is recommended that a surgical drain be placed for 1 to 2 days to prevent seroma or hematoma formation. It is important not to extend beyond the lesser cornu because of the risk to the superior laryngeal nerve.

Maxillomandibular Advancement Osteotomy (Phase II Surgery)

Mandibular movement forward helps clear hypopharyngeal obstruction. Our group and others have previously noted this finding.[100–103] In fact, it has been previously reported that mandibular setback for the correction of mandibular prognathism has produced OSAS.[104] Indications for the use of maxillomandibular advancement (phase II) are outlined in Table 77–9.

The rationale for this surgical treatment is specifically to treat refractory hypopharyngeal (base of tongue) obstruction. Patients enter phase II surgical management usually after they have undergone preparatory steps of phase I and have failed to respond fully. Although some authors have advocated maxillomandibular advancement as the first intervention, it is usu-

Table 77–9. MAXILLOMANDIBULAR
ADVANCEMENT

Severe obstructive sleep apnea syndrome
Morbid obesity, body mass index > 33
Satisfactory desire and health to undergo and recover from surgery
Failure of other froms of treatment both medically and surgically

ally recommended for patients with significant craniofacial disorders (e.g., maxillomandibular deficiency) in whom advancement of the midface and mandible will improve dental occlusion and facial esthetics in conjunction to the treatment of OSAS.

The practice of maxillomandibular advancement as the primary treatment modality is generally not advocated due to the acceptable cure rate with the less invasive phase I surgery in a significant number of patients.

In the two-phase protocol, patients entering phase II surgical management already have the nasal airway and soft palate sufficiently treated and, most commonly, have already undergone base of tongue surgery with the mandibular osteotomy with genioglossus advancement. Failure of phase I usually involves persistent obstruction of the hypopharyngeal (base of tongue) level. The maxillomandibular advancement procedure creates further tension and physical room for the tongue thus expanding the posterior airway space. Achieving such clearance necessitates a major advancement of the maxilla and mandible.

In summary, the goals of phase II are to clear the posterior airway space at the hypopharyngeal level by moving the maxillary and mandibular complex forward. It is important to achieve maximal advancement while maintaining a stable osteotomy, an acceptable dental occlusion, and a balanced aesthetic appearance. It is also important to plan the movements to minimize relapse or excessive stress at the temporomandibular joint complex. This surgical procedure is often conducted in coordination with an orthodontist who understands the goals of this surgical treatment. Orthodontic intervention improves the chances of a satisfactory dental occlusion following surgery. It is sometimes necessary for economic reasons to use arch bars in a fashion similar to that used for mandibular fractures. Arch bars takes the place of orthodontic brackets and are adapted to the teeth with stainless steel wires. This form of treatment has an increased risk of a postoperative malocclusion but, on the whole, has been satisfactory. The maxillomandibular advancement procedure has been used for many years to correct skeletal facial deformities for malocclusion in children and young adults. It is well described in the maxillofacial surgical literature.[105] Suffice it to say that the standard methods are used except for some modifications. The modifications include maximal advancement of the mandible by at least 10 mm. The maxillary and mandibular osteotomy sites are stabilized with rigid interosseus fixation that requires a minimum of four titanium plates in the maxilla and bicortical screw and plate fixation of the mandible. It is also recommended to use skeletal fixation wires on the nasal

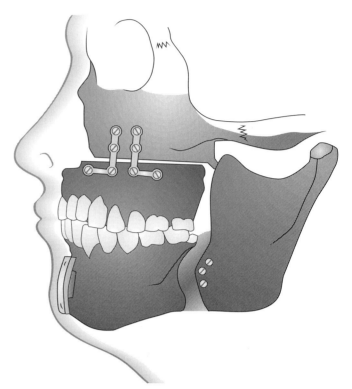

Figure 77–8. The maxillomandibular advancement osteotomy procedure (lateral view). Lefort I maxillary osteotomy with rigid plate fixation and a bilateral sagittal split mandibular osteotomy with bicortical screw fixation. The advancement is at least 10 mm. A previous genioglossus advancement is shown. (From Troell RJ, Powell NB, Riley RW. Hypopharyngeal airway surgery for obstructive sleep apnea syndrome. Semin Respir Crit Care Med. 1998;19:175–183.)

aperture of the maxilla and the inferior border of the mandible. Intermaxillary fixation is usually maintained for 7 to 10 days. The patient's occlusion usually does not change and, therefore, the maxilla and mandible usually move an equal distance. If a patient has a class II malocclusion *(mandibular deficiency)*, it is possible to achieve a class I *(normal)* occlusion and this is considered after orthodontic evaluation (Fig. 77–8).

SURGICAL PROTOCOL CLINICAL OUTCOMES

The results of our surgical protocol are shown in Table 77–10.[66] In all, 239 patients entered phase I treat-

Table 77–10. SURGICAL PROTOCOL RESULTS

Surgery Groups		Patient Success/ Total Patients	Success Rate (%)
Phase I	GAHM + UPPP	133/223	60
	GAHM	4/6	66
	UPPP	8/10	80
	Total	**145/239**	**61**
Phase II	MMO	24/24	100

GAHM, genioglossus advancement and hyoid myotomy; MMO, maxillomandibular advancement osteotomy; UPPP, uvulopalatopharyngoplasty.

Table 77-11. PHASE I SURGICAL PROTOCOL

OSAS Severity		Patient Success/ Total Patients	Success Rate (%)
Mild	(RDI <20) (LSAT >85)	20/26	77
Moderate	(RDI 20–40) (LSAT >80)	45/58	78
Moderate-Severe	(RDI 40–60) (LSAT >70)	36/51	71
Severe	(RDI >60) (LSAT <70)	44/104	42

LSAT, low oxyhemoglobin desaturation; OSAS, obstructive sleep apnea syndrome; RDI, respiratory disturbance index.

Table 77-13. SURGICAL OUTCOMES PHASE II: MAXILLOMANDIBULAR ADVANCEMENT OSTEOTOMY

Surgery Groups	No. of Patients Success/Total	Success Rate (%)
Failed phase I	83/36	97
Skeletal deformity (without UPPP)	10/11	91
Failed UPPP*	73/78	94
Total	**166/175**	**95**

*Outside referral—severe obstructive sleep apnea syndrome.
UPPP, uvulopalatopharyngoplasty.

ment, with most requiring genioglossus advancement and hyoid suspension plus UPPP. Treatment was successful for 61% of the patients (i.e., postoperative RDI less than 20 *and* minimum of 50% reduction in RDI with only a few brief falls below 90%). The results were based on the 6-month postoperative PSG and included analysis of changes in sleep architecture and sleep disorders breathing. The mean pretreatment RDI in the success group was 48.3. The preoperative nasal CPAP and postoperative mean RDI were 7.2 and 9.5, respectively (*P* = NS). The mean follow-up duration was 9 months. Most of the patients who underwent unsuccessful phase I therapy had severe OSAS (mean RDI, 61.9) and morbid obesity (mean BMI, 32.3).

Patients treated with phase I surgery were further evaluated by comparing the measurements of surgical success with those of OSAS severity (Table 77–11). Patients with mild to moderately severe OSAS had the highest frequency of success (approximately 70%). Surgical success declined to 42% with patients who had severe OSAS.

Of the original 239 patients, 94 failed phase I surgery. Of the 94 patients, 24 elected to have phase II surgical treatment. Most of the patients who declined phase II surgery were older, with a mean age of 51.8 y. The mean age of patients entering phase II treatment was 43.5 y. All the patients who elected phase II surgery had a successful outcome (Table 77–12). The mean RDI improved from 75.1 to 9.6, and mean low oxyhemoglobin desaturation (LSAT) level improved from

64.0% to 86.7%. The nasal CPAP mean RDI and mean SaO$_2$ nadir were 8.2 and 87.5%, respectively (*P* = NS).

Between 1988 and 1995, 175 patients completed phase II reconstruction. Of these 175 patients, 166 have had a successful outcome (i.e., postoperative RDI less than 20 *and* minimum of 50% reduction in RDI with only a few brief falls below 90%) (Table 77–13). The mean pretreatment RDI was 72.3. The mean postoperative RDI and nasal CPAP RDI were 7.5 and 8.2, respectively (*P* = NS). The mean low oxyhemoglobin saturation following surgery improved dramatically and was not statistically significant from the nasal CPAP results.

To date, we have reviewed 55 patients for long-term follow-up of phase II surgery. Of the 55, 33 patients have had long-term follow-up PSG. There have been 18 patients who have refused long-term PSG; however, interviews dealing with the subjective symptoms of OSAS have been reviewed. Four patients have been lost to follow-up. The long-term PSG data are shown on Table 77–14. Thirty patients have shown continued surgical success long term. Three patients showed initial success, only to relapse to OSAS. The preoperative RDI was 69.6, and the postoperative and long-term RDI was 8.9 and 7.7, respectively. The 6-month and long-term oxyhemoglobin desaturation shows similar improvement over the preoperative value. The mean follow-up was 39 months, with a range of 12 to 110 months. Of the 18 patients who were subjectively reviewed by the author, 16 patients had continued good subjective correction. There was no progressive snoring, absence of apnea, and no excessive daytime sleepi-

Table 77-12. SURGERY AND CPAP TREATMENT OUTCOMES

	Phase I (145 Patients)			Phase II (24 Patients)		
	Pretreatment	CPAP	Postsurgery	Pretreatment	CPAP	Postsurgery
RDI	47.3 (SD 25.8)	7.2 (SD 4.9)	9.5 (SD 9.5)	75.1 (SD 26.7)	8.2 (SD 2.9)	9.6 (SD 2.9)
LSAT	72.3 (SD 12.9)	86.4 (SD 11.0)	86.6 (SD 4.5)	64.0 (SD 15.9)	87.5 (SD 6.9)	86.7 (SD 7.0)
TST	360 (SD 72)	363 (SD 67)	379 (SD 63)	379 (SD 58)	376 (SD 69)	388 (SD 56)
% St 3-4	4.4 (SD 5.6)	11.1 (SD 10.8)	8.5 (SD 7.7)	2.7 (SD 4.3)	11.0 (SD 13.3)	8.2 (SD 6.7)
% REM	11.9 (SD 5.8)	18.3 (SD 7.0)	17.7 (SD 5.6)	8.1 (SD 3.1)	21.2 (SD 8.4)	21.5 (SD 6.1)
BMI	29.2 (SD 5.2)		28.8 (SD 4.9)	31.4 (SD 6.5)		30.9 (SD 6.0)

BMI, body mass index; CPAP, continuous positive airway pressure; LSAT, low oxyhemoglobin desaturation; RDI, respiratory disturbance index; St, stage; TST, total test time.

Table 77–14. LONG-TERM POLYSOMNOGRAPHIC RESULTS (N = 30)

	RDI	LSAT	Months
Preoperative	69.6 ± 27.9	68.5 ± 14.3	
Postoperative	8.9 ± 5.5	85.4 ± 4.6	6
Postoperative (long-term)	7.7 ± 5.3	86.4 ± 3.7	39 ± 24*

*Range: 12 to 110 months.
LSAT, low oxyhemoglobin desaturation; RDI, respiratory disturbance index.

ness. One patient had a subjective failure with recurrence of snoring and daytime fatigue. One patient had subjective recurrence of his OSAS and his primary care physician referred him for a PSG, which showed recurrence of his OSAS. In general, recurrence of disease was associated with significant weight gain.

RISK MANAGEMENT AND COMPLICATIONS

Life-threatening complications have been associated with sleep apnea surgery. Fairbanks,[106] on the basis of a national survey, reported 16 fatalities and 7 near fatalities from UPPP in the early postoperative period. Respiratory obstruction, secondary to pharmacological sedation and surgical edema, were the most frequently sited causes. Several authors have cautioned against the use of narcotics in OSAS patients undergoing surgery.[107–110]

In 1988, we prospectively reviewed 10 severe OSAS patients undergoing surgical treatment.[75] The patients were maintained on nasal CPAP while in hospital following surgery. Patients were on supplemental O_2 while awake and placed on CPAP while sleeping. The patients were monitored in the intensive care unit (ICU) for the 1st day and then for an additional day in the surgical ward. In spite of a mean pretreatment RDI of 87 and a mean LSAT of 51.5%, the mean postoperative LSAT during the hospital stay was 93%. We concluded that nasal CPAP protected postoperative OSAS patients from airway obstruction and hypoxemia.

Based on this review, a risk management surgical protocol was developed in 1988 for OSAS patients.

1. Patients with an RDI greater than 40 and LSAT less than 80 begin on nasal CPAP at least 2 weeks before surgery and continue nasal CPAP postoperatively until a PSG (in 6 months) is performed to document outcome. All patients, however, are encouraged to attempt nasal CPAP before surgery.
2. Anesthesia is induced and patients are intubated with the surgeons present, and an awake fiberoptic intubation is performed if there are any concerns from the surgeon or anesthesiologist about the airway.
3. All patients are extubated when awake in the operating room immediately following surgery.
4. All patients undergoing multiple procedures

(UPPP, maxillofacial surgery) or a single procedure in which the patient has significant co-existing medical problems (hypertension, coronary artery disease) are monitored in the ICU for the 1st day following surgery and then in the surgical ward. Oximetry is monitored throughout the hospital stay.
5. Patients with nasal CPAP must use the machine during all periods of sleep following surgery. All other patients are maintained on humidified oxygen (35%) via face tent.
6. Analgesia consists of IV morphine sulfate or meperidine HCl in the ICU. IV narcotics are administered by a nurse in graduated doses (e.g., morphine sulfate 1 to 5 mg every 1 to 3 h as required) while monitoring respiratory rate. All nurses caring for OSAS patients have been educated regarding the mechanisms of sleep apnea and the use of narcotics. Patient-controlled analgesia is not recommended. Intramuscular meperidine HCl and oxycodone elixir are used in the surgical ward. Oral hydrocodone is used following discharge.
7. Requirements for discharge are adequate oral intake of fluids, satisfactory pain control, stable or resolving surgical edema, and the use of nasal CPAP.

The outcomes review of the risks management protocol was performed on 182 consecutively treated OSAS patients undergoing 210 surgical procedures in 1995.[111] Data examined were the patient's age, gender, weight (BMI), facial skeletal development, coexisting medical problems, complications with anesthetic induction and extubation, postoperative vital signs, medication requirements for all postoperative days, ICU days, and total hospital stay.

The review concluded that patients undergoing surgical reconstruction of the airway for OSAS have coexisting medical problems that can complicate therapy, and clearly cardiovascular disease (CV) is the most significant. Of the study group, 40% (72 patients) gave a positive history of CV disease. This included hypertension in 31% (56 patients), arrhythmia in 5.5% (10 patients), and coronary artery disease in 3.3% (6 patients). All patients received an electrocardiogram (ECG) before surgery, and 41% (75 patients) were interpreted as abnormal (axis deviations, S-T segment changes, T-wave abnormalities), which could require further evaluation. This did not include the 16 patients with either arrhythmia or previous myocardial infarction. A significant portion of OSAS patients had difficulty with induction and intubation for general anesthesia (18.6%). Men with neck circumference greater than 46 cm and associated skeletal deformities (mandibular deficiency [SNB, Sella-Nasion-Point B, less than 75 degrees] and low hyoid [MP-H greater than 30 cm]) should be carefully evaluated and considered for fiberoptic intubation. Extubating the patients when they are awake in the operating room was also best for airway protection. The majority of the patients required both intraoperative (58%) and postoperative (70%) antihypertensives during their hospital stay. Individuals with no postoperative history of hypertension also had a significant incidence of requiring IV antihypertensive medications following surgery (63%). Aggressive treatment of hypertension may be attributed to the fact that no immediate postoperative bleeding occurred in any patient. In spite of the concern others have expressed about the use of parenteral and oral narcotics in OSAS surgery, this review has shown that IV MS is safe when administered in a monitored setting. Nasal CPAP protects the airway and reduces the risk of potentially life-threatening hypoxemia (mean LSAT day 1 of 94.8% and LSAT day 2 of 95.5%). The mean hospital stay for phase I was 2.1 days and for phase II was 2.2 days. The risk of UPPP include postoperative bleeding (less than 1%), infection (2%), transient nasal reflux (less than 12%), partial lateral palatal stenosis (less than 1%), and altered speech (0%). The complications associated with the genioglossus advancement and hyoid suspension include infection (less than 2%), need for root canal therapy (less than 1%), permanent anesthesia (less than 6%), seroma (less than 2%), mandibular fracture (0%), aspiration (0%), and death (0%). Maxillomandibular advancement osteotomy had similar complications as previously stated. There were no significant episodes of bleeding or infection. There has been an 80% resolution of anesthesia to the cheek and chin area (between 6 and 12 months). There has been skeletal relapse with 15% of the patients developing a malocclusion; however, this has been a minor skeletal relapse (less than 20%) and has not affected OSAS symptoms. No deaths have occurred.

NEW TECHNOLOGY: RADIOFREQUENCY VOLUMETRIC TISSUE REDUCTION

Radiofrequency (RF) applications have been investigated previously for both medical and surgical use.

Biophysics of radiofrequency energy (Rfe) are unique. Rfe is delivered in a unipolar or bipolar fashion from an electrode. An RF energy provides alternating current to an electrode to generate low heat energy (40° to 90°C) sufficient to denature tissue protein. An RF needle may be placed percutaneously so that only the tissue adjacent to the unprotected portion of the needle will undergo ablation. A precise targeting of tissues requiring treatment is possible with RF. The physical properties of RF concerning heat dispersement are favorable for controlling lesion size. RF energy dispersement is proportional to $1/radius^4$. This rapid drop off of energy from the source is useful in the treatment of lesions that contain, or are near, vital structures. Lesion size can further be controlled by the diameter and the length of the needle electrode, as well as treatment duration and total energy in joules (watts $\times$ seconds). The biophysics of Rfe lends itself to the potential treatment of disproportionate anatomy in OSAS.

A prospective investigation was undertaken in an animal model to assess the feasibility of RF volumetric tongue reduction.[112] A porcine animal model was selected to evaluate histologic and volumetric changes in tongue tissue. The Rfe was delivered by a custom-fabricated needle electrode and an RF generator to the tongue tissue. Microultrasonic crystals were used to measure 3-D changes (*volumetric reduction*). The lesion size correlated well with increasing Rfe delivery. Histologic assessment, performed serially over time (1 hour through 3 weeks), showed a well-circumscribed lesion with normal healing progression and no peripheral damage to nerves. Volumetric analysis determined a mild initial edematous response that promptly tapered at 24 h (Fig. 77–9). At 10 days after RF, a 26.3% volumetric reduction was documented at the treatment site. The results of this animal investigation led to an assessment of RF volumetric tissue reduction of the palate and its affect on snoring. With investigational review board approval, a prospective randomized study using

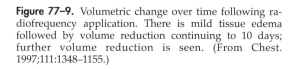

Figure 77–9. Volumetric change over time following radiofrequency application. There is mild tissue edema followed by volume reduction continuing to 10 days; further volume reduction is seen. (From Chest. 1997;111:1348–1155.)

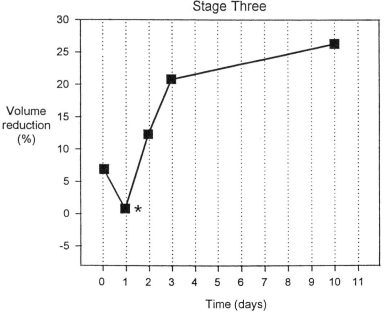

25 volunteers was undertaken.[113] Patients underwent midline soft palate volumetric reduction under local anesthesia. Pain, speech, swallowing, edema, snoring, sleep variables, and quality of life issues were assessed. All patients were snorers seeking treatment and met the pretreatment PSG criteria of an RDI of less than 15. Pretreatment snoring was reduced in the study group by an overall mean of 77%. Each treatment session showed additional palatal shrinkage and associated reduction in snoring. The mean number of treatment sessions was 6.6. Epworth Sleepiness Scale scores improved by 39%. Speech and swallowing were not affected. Pain was minimal and of short duration. Over-the-counter medications (acetaminophen) was the first choice for pain relief. Adverse effects were negligible and there were no infections. We concluded that RF volumetric reduction is a viable treatment for airway narrowing in OSAS. Ongoing clinical trials are currently investigating the safety and efficacy of this technology for the treatment of base of tongue obstruction in OSAS.

CONCLUSION

The management of OSAHS requires a multidisciplinary treatment approach. A systematic evaluation followed by a rational step-wise surgical protocol in carefully selected patients can achieve a reliable long-term cure. New surgical techniques and evolving technology may potentially offer less invasive treatment modalities with broader patient acceptance and improved therapeutic results.[114]

Radiofrequency volumetric tissue reduction has also been assessed for the treatment of turbinate hypertrophy.[115, 116] This approach may be useful in those patients in whom nasal obstruction caused by turbinate hypertrophy leads to a sleep-breathing disorder.

References

1. Kuhlo W, Doll E, Franck MD. Erfolgreiche Behandlung eines Pickwick Syndroms durch eine Dauertrachekanuele. Dtsch Med Wochenschr. 1969;94:1286–1290.
2. Kribbs NB, Pack AI, Kline LR, et al. The effects of one night without nasal CPAP treatment on sleep and sleepiness in patients with obstructive sleep apnea. Am Rev Respir Dis. 1993;147:1162–1168.
3. Kribbs NB, Pack AI, Kline LR, et al. Objective measurement of patterns of nasal CPAP used by patient with obstructive sleep apnea. Am Rev Respir Dis. 1993;147:887–895.
4. NIH Consensus Development Panel. National Institutes of Health Consensus Development Conference Statement. Gastrointestinal surgery for severe obesity. Ann Intern Med. 1991;115:956–961.
5. Yale CE. Gastric surgery for morbid obesity. Complications and long-term weight control. Arch Surg. 1989;124:941–946.
6. Mason EE, Maher JW, Scott DH, et al. Ten years of vertical banded gastroplasty for severe obesity. Probl Gen Surg. 1992;9:280–289.
7. Halverson JD. Metabolic risk of obesity surgery and long-term follow up. Am J Clin Nutr. 1992;55:602S–605S.
8. Amaral JF, Thompson WR, Caldwell MD, et al. Prospective hematologic evaluation of gastric exclusion surgery for morbid obesity. Ann Surg. 1985;201:186–193.
9. Halverson JD. Micronutrient deficiencies after gastric bypass for morbid obesity. Am Surg. 1986;52:594–598.
10. Griffen WO, Young VL, Stevenson CC. A prospective comparison of gastric and jejunoileal bypass procedures for morbid obesity. Ann Surg. 1977;186:501–509.
11. Ramsey-Stewart G. Vertical banded gastroplasty for morbid obesity: weight loss at short and long-term follow up. Aust N Z J Surg. 1995;65:4–7.
12. Wolfel R, Gunther K, Rumenapf G, et al. Weight reduction after gastric bypass and horizontal gastroplasty for morbid obesity. Eur J Surg. 1994;160:219–225.
13. Benotti PN, Hollingsworth J, Mascioli EA, et al. Gastric restrictive operations for morbid obesity. Am J Surg. 1989;157:150–155.
14. MacDonald KG, Pories WJ. Roux gastric bypass or vertical banded gastroplasty. Probl Gen Surg. 1992;9:321–331.
15. MacLean LD, Rhode B, Forse RA. Late results of vertical banded gastroplasty for morbid obesity. Surgery. 1990;107:20–27.
16. Yale CE, Weiler SJ. Weight control after vertical banded gastroplasty for morbid obesity. Am J Surg. 1991;162:13–18.
17. Smith PL, Gold AR, Meyers DA, et al. Weight loss in mildly to moderately obese patients with obstructive sleep apnea. Ann Intern Med. 1985;103:850–855.
18. Charuzi I, Lavie P, Jochanan P, et al. Bariatric surgery in morbidly obese sleep-apnea patients: short- and long-term follow-up. Am J Clin Nutr. 1992;55:594S–596S.
19. Rajala R, Partinent M, Sane T, et al. Obstructive sleep apnoea syndrome in morbidly obese patients. J Intern Med. 1991;230:125–129.
20. Pillar G, Peled R, Lavie P. Recurrence of sleep apnea without concomitant weight increase 7.5 years after weight reduction surgery. Chest. 1994;106:1702–1704.
21. Jamieson A, Guilleminault C, Partinen M, et al. Obstructive sleep apneic patients have craniomandibular abnormalities. Sleep. 1986;9:469–477.
22. Shepard J, Gefter W, Guilleminault C, et al. Evaluation of the upper airway in patients with obstructive sleep apnea. Sleep. 1991;14:361–371.
23. Riley R, Guilleminault C, Powell NB, et al. Palatopharyngoplasty failure, cephalometric roentgenograms, and obstructive sleep apnea. Otolaryngol Head Neck Surg. 1985;93:240–244.
24. Lavie P, Fischel N, Zomer J, et al. The effects of partial and complete mechanical occlusion of the nasal passages on sleep structure and breathing in sleep. Acta Otolaryngol. 1983;95:161–166.
25. Olsen K, Kern E, Westbrook P. Sleep and breathing disturbance secondary to nasal obstruction. Otolaryngol Head Neck Surg. 1981;89:804–810.
26. Zwillich CW, Pickett C, Hanson FN, et al. Disturbed sleep and prolonged apnea during nasal obstruction in normal men. Am Rev Respir Dis. 1981;124:158–160.
27. Rojewski TE, Schuller DE, Clark RW, et al. Videoendoscopic determination of the mechanism of obstruction in obstructive sleep apnea. Otolaryngol Head Neck Surg. 1984;92:127–131.
28. Rivlin J, Hoffstein V, Kalbfleisch J, et al. Upper airway morphology in patients with idiopathic obstructive sleep apnea. Am Rev Respir Dis. 1984;129:355–360.
29. Remmers JE, DeGrott WJ, Sauerland EK, et al. Pathogenesis of upper airway occlusion during sleep. J Appl Physiol. 1978;44:931–938.
30. Crumley R, Stein M, Gamsu G, et al. Determination of obstructive site in obstructive sleep apnea. Laryngoscope. 1987;97:301–308.
31. Fujita S. Pharyngeal surgery for obstructive sleep apnea and snoring. In: Fairbanks D, Fujita S, Ikematsu T, et al. Snoring and Obstructive Sleep Apnea. New York, NY: Raven Press; 1987:101–128.
32. Fujita S, Conway WA, Sickleested JM, et al. Evaluation of the effectiveness of uvulopalatopharyngoplasty. Laryngoscope. 1985;95:70–74.
33. Anonsen C. Laryngeal obstruction and obstructive sleep apnea syndrome. Laryngoscope. 1990;100:775–778.
34. Kletzker GR, Bastian RW. Acquired airway obstruction from histologically normal, abnormally mobile supraglottic soft tissues. Laryngoscope. 1990;100:375–379.
35. Adair NE, Matthew BL, Haponik EF. Techniques to assist selec-

tion of appropriate therapy for patients with obstructive sleep apnea. Otolaryngol Head Neck Surg. 1991;2:81–86.

36. Sher AE, Thorpy MJ, Shrintzen RJ, et al. Predictive value of Muller maneuver in selection of patient for uvulopalatopharyngoplasty. Laryngoscope. 1985;95:1483–1487.

37. Katsantonis GP, Mass CS, Walsh JK. The predictive efficacy of the Muller maneuver in uvulopalatopharyngoplasty. Laryngoscope. 1989;99:677–680.

38. Riley R, Guilleminault C, Herran J, et al. Cephalometric analyses and flow volume loops in obstructive sleep apnea patients. Sleep. 1983;6:304–307.

39. Riley R, Powell N, Guilleminault C. Current surgical concepts for treating obstructive sleep apnea syndrome. J Oral Maxillofac Surg. 1987;43:149–157.

40. Riley R, Powell N, Guilleminault C. Cephalometric roentgenograms and computerized tomographic scans in obstructive sleep apnea. Sleep. 1986;9:514–515.

41. Rapoport DM, Sorkin B, Garay SM, et al. Reversal of the "Pickwickian syndrome" by long-term use of nocturnal nasal-airway pressure. N Engl J Med. 1982;307:931–933.

42. Sanders MH, Moore SE, Eveslage J. CPAP via nasal mask: a treatment for occlusive sleep apnea. Chest. 1983;83:144–145.

43. Sullivan CE, Berthon-Jones M, Issa FG, et al. Reversal of obstructive sleep apnoea by continuous positive airway pressure applied through the nares. Lancet. 1981;1:862–865.

44. Sanders MH, Kern N. Obstructive sleep apnea treated by independently adjusted inspiratory and expiratory positive airway pressure via nasal mask: physiologic and clinical implications. Chest. 1990;93:317–324.

45. Jamieson A. Obesity and sleep disordered breathing. Soc Behav Med. 1988;10:107–112.

46. Browman C, Sampson M, Yolles S, et al. Obstructive sleep apnea and body weight. Chest. 1984;85:435–436.

47. Guilleminault C. Weight loss in sleep apnea. Chest. 1989;96:703–704.

48. Rubinstein I, Colapinto N, Rotstein L, et al. Improvement in upper airway function after weight loss in patients with obstructive sleep apnea. Am Rev Respir Dis. 1988;138:1192–1195.

49. Nino-Murcia G, Crowe C, Bliwise D, et al. Nasal CPAP: follow-up of compliance and adverse effects. Sleep Res. 1987;16:398.

50. Nino-Murcia G, Crowe C, Bliwise D, et al. Nasal CPAP: follow-up of compliance and adverse effects. West J Med. 1989;150:165–169.

51. Sanders MH, Gruendl CA, Rogers RM. Patient compliance with nasal CPAP therapy for sleep apnea. Chest. 1986;90:330–333.

52. Waldhorn RE, Herrick TW, Nguyen MC, et al. Long-term compliance with nasal continuous positive airway pressure therapy of obstructive sleep apnea. Chest. 1990;97:33–38.

53. Olsen K. The role of nasal surgery in the treatment of obstructive sleep apnea. Otolaryngol Head Neck Surg. 1991;2:63–68.

54. Fujita S, Conway W, Zorick F, et al. Surgical correction of anatomic abnormalities in obstructive sleep apnea syndrome: uvulopalatopharyngoplasty. Otolaryngol Head Neck Surg. 1981;89:923–934.

55. Simmons FB, Guilleminault C, Silvestri R. Snoring, and some obstructive sleep apnea can be cured by oropharyngeal surgery. Arch Otolaryngol. 1983;109:503–507.

56. Hernandez SF. Palatopharyngoplasty for obstructive sleep apnea syndrome. Am J Otolaryngol. 1982;3:229–236.

57. Riley R, Powell N, Guilleminault C. Maxillofacial surgery and obstructive sleep apnea: a review of 80 patients. Otolaryngol Head Neck Surg. 1989;101:353–361.

58. Powell N, Guilleminault C, Riley R, et al. Mandibular advancement and obstructive sleep apnea syndrome. Bull Eur Physiopathol Respir. 1983;19:607–610.

59. Powell N, Riley R, Guilleminault C. Maxillofacial surgery for obstructive sleep apnea. In: Partinen M, Guilleminault C, eds. Obstructive Sleep Apnea Syndrome: Clinical Research and Treatment. New York, NY: Raven Press; 1989:153–182.

60. Riley R, Guilleminault C, Powell N, et al. Mandibular osteotomy and hyoid bone advancement for obstructive sleep apnea: a case report. Sleep. 1984;7:79–82.

61. Riley R, Powell N, Guilleminault C, et al. Maxillary, mandibular, and hyoid advancement: an alternative to tracheostomy in obstructive sleep apnea syndrome. Otolaryngol Head Neck Surg. 1986;94:584–588.

62. Riley R, Powell N, Guilleminault C. Inferior sagittal osteotomy of the mandible with hyoid myotomy-suspension: a new procedure for obstructive sleep apnea. Otolaryngol Head Neck Surg. 1986;94:589–593.

63. Riley RW, Powell NB, Guilleminault C. Inferior mandibular osteotomy and hyoid myotomy suspension for obstructive sleep apnea: a review of 55 patients. J Oral Maxillofac Surg. 1989;47:159–164.

64. Riley RW, Powell NB, Guilleminault C. Maxillary, mandibular, and hyoid advancement for treatment of obstructive sleep apnea: a review of 40 patients. J Oral Maxillofac Surg. 1990;48:20–26.

65. Riley RW, Powell NB. Maxillofacial surgery and obstructive sleep apnea syndrome. Otolaryngol Clin North Am. 1990;23:809–826.

66. Riley RW, Powell NB, Guilleminault C. Obstructive sleep apnea syndrome: a review of 306 consecutively treated surgical patients. Otolaryngol Head Neck Surg. 1993;108:117–125.

67. Waite PD, Wooten V, Lachner J, et al. Maxillomandibular advancement surgery in 23 patients with obstructive sleep apnea syndrome. J Oral Maxillofac Surg. 1989;47:1256–1261.

68. Hochban W, Brandenburg U, Hermann PJ. Surgical treatment of obstructive sleep apnea by maxillomandibular advancement. Sleep. 1994;17:624–629.

69. Hochban W, Conradt R, Brandenburg U, et al. Surgical maxillofacial treatment of obstructive sleep apnea. Plast Reconstr Surg. 1997;99:619–626.

70. Fujita S, Woodson T, Clark J, et al. Laser midline glossectomy as a treatment for obstructive sleep apnea. Laryngoscope. 1991;101:805–809.

71. Woodson BT, Fujita S. Clinical experience with lingualoplasty as part of the treatment of severe obstructive sleep apnea. Otolaryngol Head Neck Surg. 1992;107:40–48.

72. Mickelson SA, Rosenthal L. Midline glossectomy and epiglottidectomy for obstructive sleep apnea syndrome. Laryngoscope. 1997;107:614–619.

73. Woodson BT, Toohill RJ. Transpalatal advancement pharyngoplasty for obstructive sleep apnea. Laryngoscope. 1993;103:269–276.

74. Woodson BT. Retropalatal airway characteristics in uvulopalatopharyngoplasty compared with transpalatal advancement pharyngoplasty. Laryngoscope. 1997;107:735–740.

75. Powell N, Riley R, Guilleminault C. Obstructive sleep apnea, continuous positive airway pressure, and surgery. Otolaryngol Head Neck Surg. 1988;99:362–369.

76. Ikematsu T. Study of snoring, fourth report: therapy (in Japanese). Jpn Otorhinolaryngol. 1964;64:434–435.

77. Katsantonis G. Uvulopalatopharyngoplasty for obstructive sleep apnea and snoring. Otolaryngol Head Neck Surg. 1991;2:100–103.

78. Fairbanks D. Operative techniques of uvulopalatopharyngoplasty. Otolaryngol Head Nedk Surg. 1991;2:104–106.

79. Ikematsu T, Fujita S, Simmons FB, et al. Uvulopalatopharyngoplasty: variations. In: Fairbanks D, Fujita S, Ikematsu T, et al, eds. Snoring and Obstructive Sleep Apnea. New York, NY: Raven Press; 1987:129–170.

80. Sher A. Obstructive sleep apnea and the otoloaryngologist—1991. AAO-HNS Bull. Sept 1991:12–14.

81. Katsantonis GP, Walsh JK. Somnofluoroscopy: its role in the selection of candidates for uvulopalatopharyngoplasty. Otolaryngol Head Neck Surg. 1986;94:56–60.

82. Simmons FB, Guilleminault C, Laughton M. The palatopharyngoplasty operation for snoring and sleep apnea: an interim report. Otolargynol Head Neck Surg. 1984;92:375.

83. Fujita S. UPPP for sleep apnea and snoring. Ear Nose Throat J. 1984;64:74.

84. Gislason T, Lindholm CE, Alimqvist M, et al. Uvulopalatopharyngoplasty in the sleep apnea syndrome. Arch Otolaryngol Head Neck Surg. 1988;114:45–51.

85. Dickson RI, Blokmanis A. Treatment of obstructive sleep apnea by uvulopalatopharyngoplasty. Laryngoscope. 1987;97:1054–1059.

86. Conway W, Fujita S, Zorick F, et al. Uvulopalatopharyngoplasty: a onc-year followup. Chest. 1985;88:385–387.

87. Sher AE, Schechtman KB, Piccirillo JF. The efficacy of surgical

modifications of the upper airway in adults with obstructive sleep apnea syndrome. Sleep. 1996;19:156–177.

88. Powell NB, Riley RW, Guilleminault C, et al. A reversible uvulopalatal flap for snoring and obstructive sleep. Sleep. 1996;19:593–599.

89. Kamami YV. Laser CO_2 for snoring-preliminary results. Acta Otorhinolaryngol Belg. 1990;44:451–456.

90. Walker RP, Grigg-Damberger MM, Gopalsami C, et al. Laser-assisted uvulopalatoplasty for snoring and obstructive sleep apnea: results in 170 patients. Laryngoscope. 1995;105:938–943.

91. Terris DJ, Clerk AA, Norbash AM, et al. Characterization of postoperative edema following laser-assisted uvulopalatoplasty using MRI and polysomnography: implication for the outpatient treatment of obstructive sleep apnea syndrome. Laryngoscope. 1996;106:124–128.

92. Lowe A, Gionhaku N, Takeuchi K, et al. Three dimensional reconstructions of the tongue and airway in adult subjects with obstructive sleep apnea. Am J Orthod. 1986;90:364–374.

93. Lowe A. The tongue and airway. Otolaryngol Clin North Am. 1990;23:677–698.

94. Rivlin J, Hoffstein V, Kalbfleisch J, et al. Upper airway morphology in patients with idiopathic obstructive sleep apnea. Am Rev Respir Dis. 1984;129:355–360.

95. Rojewski TE, Schuller DE, Clark RW, et al. Synchronous video recording of the pharyngeal airway and polysomnograph in patients with obstructive sleep apnea. Laryngoscope. 1982;92:246–250.

96. Kaya N. Sectioning the hyoid bone as a therapeutic approach for obstructive sleep apnea. Sleep. 1984;7:77–78.

97. Patton TJ, Thawley SE, Water RC, et al. Expansion hyoid-plasty: a potential surgical procedure designed for selected patients with obstructive sleep apnea syndrome. Experimental canine results. Laryngoscope. 1983;93:1387–1396.

98. Patton TJ, Ogura JH, Thawley SE. Expansion hyoidplasty. Otolaryngol Head Neck Surg. 1984;92:509–519.

99. Riley RW, Powell NB, Guilleminault C. Obstructive sleep apnea and the hyoid: a revised surgical procedure. Otolaryngol Head Neck Surg. 1994;111:717–721.

100. Bear SE, Priest JH. Sleep apnea syndrome: correction with surgical advancement of the mandible. J Oral Surg. 1980;38:543–549.

101. Kuo PC, West RA, Bloomquist DS, et al. The effect of mandibular osteotomy in three patients with hypersomnia and sleep apnea. Oral Surg Oral Med Oral Pathol. 1979;48:385–392.

102. Wittig R, Wolford G, Conway W, et al. Mandibular advancement as a treatment of sleep apnea syndrome. In: Abstracts and Proceedings of the Fourth Congress of Sleep Research; Bologna, Italy; 1983:360.

103. Powell NB, Guilleminault C, Riley RW, et al. Mandibular advancement and obstructive sleep apnea syndrome. Bull Eur Physiopathol Respir. 1983;19:607–610.

104. Riley RW, Powell NB, Guilleminault C, et al. Obstructive sleep apnea syndrome following surgery for mandibular prognathism. J Oral Maxillofac Surg. 1987;45:450–452.

105. Bell W, Proffit W, White R. Surgical Correction of Dental Facial Deformities. Philadelphia, Pa: WB Saunders; 1980.

106. Fairbanks D. Uvulopalatopharyngoplasty complications and avoidance strategies. Otolaryngol Head Neck Surg. 1990;102:239–245.

107. Esclamado RM, Glenn MG, McCulloch TM, et al. Perioperative complications and risk factors in the surgical treatment of obstructive sleep apnea syndrome. Laryngoscope. 1989;99:1125–1129.

108. Gabrielczyk MR. Acute airway obstruction after uvulopalatopharyngoplasty for obstructive sleep apnea syndrome. Anesthesiology. 1988;69:941–943.

109. Kravath RE, Pollak CP, Borowiecki B, et al. Obstructive sleep apnea and death associated with surgical correction of velopharyngeal incompetence. J Pediatr. 1980;96:645–648.

110. Polo O, Brissaud L, Fraga J, et al. Partial upper airway obstruction in sleep after uvulopalatopharyngoplasty. Arch Otolaryngol Head Neck Surg. 1989;115:1350–1354.

111. Riley RW, Powell NB, Guilleminault C, et al. Obstructive sleep apnea surgery: risk management and complications. Otolaryngol Head Neck Surg. 1997;117:648–562.

112. Powell NB, Riley RW, Troell RJ, et al. Radiofrequency volumetric reduction of the tongue: a porcine pilot study for the treatment of obstructive sleep apnea syndrome. Chest. 1997;111:1348–1355.

113. Powell NB, Riley RW, Troell RJ, et al. Radiofrequency volumetric tissue reduction of the palate in subjects with sleep-disordered breathing. Chest. 1998;113:1163–1174.

114. Powell NB, Riley RW, Guilleminault C. Radiofrequency tongue base reduction in sleep-disordered breathing: a pilot study. Otolaryngol Head Neck Surgery. 1999;120:656–664.

115. Li KK, Powell NB, Riley RW, et al. Radiofrequency volumetric tissue reduction for treatment of turbinate hypertrophy: a pilot study. Otolaryngol Head Neck Surg. 1998;119:569–573.

116. Smith TL, Correa AJ, Kuo T, et al. Radiofrequency tissue ablation of the inferior turbinates using a thermocouple feedback electrode. Laryngoscope. 1999;109:1760–1765.

Oral Appliances for Sleep Breathing Disorders

Alan A. Lowe

Oral appliances for the treatment of snoring and of obstructive sleep apnea (OSA) fall into two main categories: those which hold the tongue forward and those which reposition the mandible (and the attached tongue) forward during sleep. Before treating either snoring or OSA with any oral appliance, a complete assessment by a knowledgeable physician or sleep disorder specialist is mandatory. If treatment with an oral appliance is indicated, the physician provides a dentist who has skill and experience in oral appliance therapy with a written referral or prescription and a copy of the diagnostic report. Because of the obvious life-threatening implications of a number of sleep disorders, it is imperative that oral appliance therapy commence only after a complete medical assessment.

The American Sleep Disorders Association (ASDA) reviewed the available literature in 1995 and recommended that oral appliances be used in patients with primary snoring or mild OSA and in patients with moderate to severe OSA who are intolerant of or refuse treatment with nasal continuous positive airway pressure (nCPAP).[1, 2] For some patients, combination therapy with other treatments such as weight loss, surgery, and nCPAP may be indicated and this must be coordinated by the attending sleep physician.

The purpose of this chapter is to provide an overview of the seven most frequently used oral appliances and guidelines for their use. A titration sequence for one representative adjustable oral appliance is outlined because this clinical procedure is often not well understood by many sleep physicians.

Current evidence suggests that the pathogenesis of OSA involves a combination of reduced upper airway size and altered upper airway muscle activity. Features and size of the upper airway have been characterized by cephalometry,[3] computed tomography (CT),[4, 5] and magnetic resonance imaging (MRI).[6] A high apnea index (AI) was seen in association with a large tongue and soft palate volume, a retrognathic mandible, an anteroposterior discrepancy between the maxilla and mandible, an open bite tendency between the incisors, and obesity.[6] Cephalograms may be useful to estimate the volume of the tongue, nasopharynx, and soft palate, but not the oropharynx or hypopharynx.[7] Tongue posture appears to have a substantial effect on upper airway morphology.[8] The tongue cross-sectional area increases and the oropharyngeal cross-sectional area decreases when OSA patients change their body position from upright to supine.[6] Oral appliances are believed to have a direct effect on mandibular posture, and consequently affect airway size.

Three-dimensional (3-D) analyses have increased our understanding of the mechanisms of different forms of treatment, including oral appliances[9, 10] and nCPAP,[6] and have helped predict the response to upper airway surgery.[11] Tongue and soft palate volumes increase as the body mass index increases,[5] which confirms the potential importance of weight loss as an effective treatment for the control of OSA. In response to nCPAP, an increase in pharyngeal volume and a decrease in tongue volume due to the resolution of upper airway edema have been identified.[6] Distinct OSA subgroups may provide some insight into the contribution of obesity to OSA,[12] and skeletal subtypes are of considerable importance[13] when selecting the oral appliance. Although the control of tongue posture is extremely complex,[14, 15] an abnormality in genioglossus (GG) timing in OSA subjects has been demonstrated.[16] The duration of the inspiratory GG activity and the total GG activity cycle are shorter in patients with OSA. Oral appliance therapy relates directly to the pathophysiology of OSA and this chapter reviews these interactions in light of current knowledge for each of the seven most frequently used appliances.

CLINICAL PROTOCOL FOR ORAL APPLIANCE THERAPY

A therapy sequence is suggested by the Sleep Disorders Dental Society for the management of oral appliances in patients who are being treated for snoring or OSA.

1. Medical assessment by the attending physician or sleep specialist. Prior to referral to a dentist, the physician should check that the patient has sufficient teeth (at least eight in each of the upper and lower jaws) and that they have no limitations in forward jaw movement (greater than 5 mm) or jaw opening (greater than 25 mm). Full upper and lower dentures may preclude the use of a mandibular

repositioner, but some of these patients may have a good treatment response with a tongue-retaining device (TRD). Partial dentures that replace four or fewer teeth do not preclude oral appliance use. Evidence of a past history of a temporomandibular joint abnormality or chronic joint pain may, depending on its severity, preclude the use of oral appliances in some patients. Severe occlusal wear (more than 20% of the clinical crown) may indicate severe bruxism and complicate oral appliance therapy. The size of the mandible is not a reliable predictor of treatment success. Oral appliances do not appear to work as well in the morbidly obese patient, although exceptions have been documented.

2. Overnight polysomnogram as required by the physician or sleep specialist.
3. Written referral or prescription and diagnostic report sent to the dentist or dental specialist.
4. Oral examination.
   a. Medical and dental histories.
   b. Soft tissue and intraoral assessment.
   c. Periodontal evaluation.
   d. Temporomandibular joint and occlusal examination.
   e. Intraoral habit assessment.
   f. Examination of teeth and restorations.
   g. Initial dental radiographs if not taken in the preceding 6 months.
      i. Panoramic or full-mouth survey.
      ii. Cephalometric radiograph (optional).
   h. Diagnostic plaster models as appropriate for the specific oral appliance.
5. Appliance determination.
   a. Consideration of mandibular repositioner vs. tongue retainer and whether a boil-and-bite type or a custom-made appliance is indicated.
   b. Design, fabrication, fitting, instructions, and training.
   c. Subjective symptom evaluation.
6. Refer patient back to attending physician for assessment or repeat overnight sleep study.
7. Possible modification, redesign, or remake of the appliance as required based on subjective resolution of symptoms, patient compliance, and follow-up sleep study.
8. Recall dental appointments at least every 6 months for the first 2 years to monitor subjective effectiveness, fit, comfort, and temporomandibular joint and dental status.

OVERVIEW OF ORAL APPLIANCES

Table 78–1 lists the oral appliances that have received 510k market clearance from the Food and Drug Administration (FDA) for the treatment of snoring or OSA. Dentists are aware of this classification system

Table 78–1. ORAL APPLIANCES FOR THE TREATMENT OF SNORING AND OF OBSTRUCTIVE SLEEP APNEA

Device	Manufacturer	Snoring	OSA
Adjustable PM Positioner	Jonathan A. Parker, DDS	√	√
Adjustable Soft Palate Lifter	Ortho Publications Inc.	√	X
Adjustable TheraSnore	Distar, Inc.	√	X
Dental Anti-Snoring Device	Ortho Publications Inc.	√	X
DESRA	D.S.R.A. Inc.	√	X
Elastic Mandibular Advancement, Titration (EMA-T)	Frantz Design, Inc.	√	√
Elastic Mandibular Advancement (EMA)	Frantz Design, Inc.	√	√
Elastomeric Sleep Appliance	Village Park Orthodontics	√	√
Equalizer Airway Device	Sleep Renewal Inc.	√	√
Herbst	Orthodontics, State University of New York at Buffalo	√	√
Klearway	Great Lakes Orthodontics, Ltd.	√	√
NAPA	Great Lakes Orthodontics, Ltd.	√	√
OSAP	Snorefree, Inc.	√	√
PM Positioner	Jonathan A. Parker, DDS	√	√
Silencer	Silent Knights Ventures, Inc.	√	√
SILENTNITE	Glidewell Laboratories	√	X
Sleep-In Bone Screw System	Influence Inc.	√	√
SNOAR Open Airway Appliance	Kent J. Toone, DDS	√	√
Snore-Cure	Ortho-Tain, Inc.	√	X
Snore-Ezzer	Snore-Ezzer	√	X
Snorefree	Scott Feldman, DDS, Norman Shapiro, DDS	√	X
Snore Guard	Snore Guard	√	X
Snoremaster Snore Remedy	The Snoremaster Co.	√	X
Snore-No-More	Great Lakes Orthodontics, Ltd.	√	X
Snore Peace	Snore Peace Group	√	X
Snore Tec	Marketing Technologies, Inc.	√	X
Snor-X Mouth Guard	Snor-X, Inc.	√	X
Snoring Control Device	Kenneth Hilsen, DDS	√	X
TAP Anti-Snoring Device	Nellcor Puritan Bennett, Inc.	√	X
TheraSnore	Distar, Inc.	√	X
Thornton Oral Appliance	W. Keith Thornton, DDS	√	√
Tongue-Retaining Device (TRD)	Advanced Medical Equipment	√	X

√, has received market clearance from the Food and Drug Administration; X, has not received market clearance from the Food and Drug Administration; OSA, obstructive sleep apnea.

and select appliances accordingly. The FDA has granted 510k market clearance for snoring for 32 different oral appliances. Only 14 oral appliances have received market clearance for both snoring and OSA. We review below seven widely used appliances as examples of this treatment approach.

Since a previous overview of oral appliance design, when only 13 appliances were commercially available,[17] and since publication of the ASDA position papers,[1, 2] two significant advances in this field have occurred. Adjustable appliances which allow titration of the mandibular position over time and the use of materials and designs that significantly improve intraoral retention are major improvements. Of the more than 55 oral appliances currently on the market (not all have received FDA market clearance), only seven are fully adjustable, and only three have undergone controlled or randomized clinical trial. Dentists realized early on that determining the correct jaw position was the most difficult step in using oral appliances successfully. Considerable variations in the initial comfort range of the anteroposterior movement of the mandible, and differences in the speed and amount of forward jaw position that any given patient could tolerate were found. Single jaw position or nonadjustable appliances often need to be remade if the initial jaw position proves to be inadequate. Gradual titration forward of the mandible without the necessity of making a new appliance each time became the objective, and adjustable appliances were invented and marketed.

A subgroup of patients, particularly those who suffer from sleep bruxism,[18] often experiences considerable jaw discomfort in the morning after wearing a rigid hard acrylic single jaw position oral appliance. A need to develop oral appliances that could allow for lateral jaw movement, as well as some degree of vertical jaw opening, was identified. At the same time, major advances in dental materials significantly improved the flexibility and strength of thermosensitive acrylic resin materials. Appliances made of temperature-sensitive material that the patient could heat in hot water before insertion and that would cool and harden somewhat intraorally were found to have considerable more retention than traditionally designed cold cure acrylic appliances. The combination of adjustability, lateral and vertical jaw movement, increased retention, and better-defined titration protocols have significantly improved the effectiveness of oral appliances since they were last reviewed.

Each of the oral appliances has a primary effect on either the tongue or the tongue and mandible together. Several appliances move the mandible anteriorly—for example, the Herbst, Klearway, mandibular repositioner, PM Positioner, Snore Guard, and TheraSnore. The tongue is affected by all the appliances either by direct forward movement of the muscle itself or by changes secondary to an altered mandibular rest position. The TRD is the most commonly used oral appliance that has a direct effect on tongue posture.

Herbst

Variations of the Herbst appliance (Fig. 78–1) have been used effectively in orthodontics for many years.[19–21] Herbst is a registered trademark of Dentaurum, Inc., Newton, Pa. This removable appliance is available from most orthodontic laboratories and is highly effective in advancing the mandible.[22] The plunger mechanism holds the mandible forward in both the open and closed positions[23] and allows for easy adjustments of forward mandibular positions. The Herbst appliance offers the advantages of permitting forward jaw opening and some limited side-to-side jaw movements compared with the other more rigid mandibular repositioning appliances.[24] Clark et al.[25] suggested the use of bilateral interarch elastics to keep the jaw closed during sleep and the incorporation of interproximal ball clasps to increase retention. In 15 subjects who underwent sleep studies before and after appliance insertion, oxygen desaturation levels improved markedly and the respiratory disturbance index (RDI) decreased from a mean of 48.4 to 12.4 four months after the insertion of a Herbst appliance.[25] A 39% decrease in stage 1 sleep together with increases in stages 2, 3, and 4, and a 50% increase in rapid eye movement (REM) sleep were seen. Some 73% of the subjects were able to utilize the Herbst appliance successfully at the 18-month follow-up and no increase in facial pain or jaw dysfunction was seen.

The left-hand side of Figure 78–2 provides a superimposition of supine before-and-after cephalometric tracings of a subject fitted with a Herbst appliance in our laboratory. The RDI decreased from 44.3 to 24.6 and significant increases in the cross-sectional areas of the oropharynx (from 386.4 to 739.5 mm^2) and the hypopharynx (from 73.7 to 267.6 mm^2) were seen. Although great care must be exercised when one uses two-dimensional cephalometric films[26] to evaluate 3-D airway size,[7] it appears that a forward mandibular position is effective in reducing the severity of the OSA and that the airway tube is significantly altered.

Klearway

The Klearway (see Fig. 78–1) differs in several ways from other appliances currently available on the market. It works by keeping the teeth together and holding the lower jaw and tongue forward during sleep to open the airway. The klearway possesses retention characteristics designed to keep the appliance in the mouth during all the various complex jaw movements that can occur during sleep. Klearway provides full occlusal coverage of both arches and is designed not to encroach on tongue space. Furthermore, it facilitates the very slow and gradual movement of the mandible by permitting the patient to adjust the appliance according to his or her own comfort level with the guidance of the attending dentist. This fully adjustable oral appliance is much more comfortable to wear than a single jaw position appliance which often may require time-consuming and expensive remakes to place the mandible in the ideal forward position required to adequately open the airway. Fabricated of thermoactive acrylic, Klearway becomes pliable for easy insertion and conforms securely to the dentition for an excellent fit while

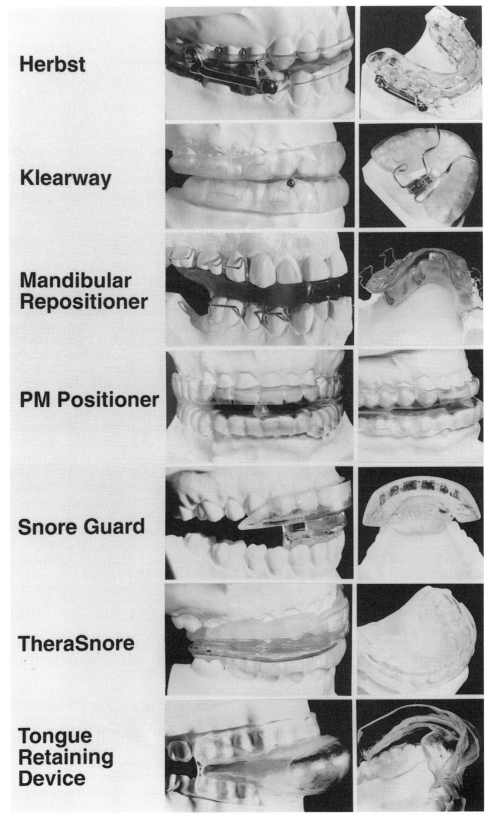

Herbst

Klearway

Mandibular Repositioner

PM Positioner

Snore Guard

TheraSnore

Tongue Retaining Device

Figure 78–1. Lateral and superior and inferior views of seven oral appliances used for the treatment of snoring or obstructive sleep apnea.

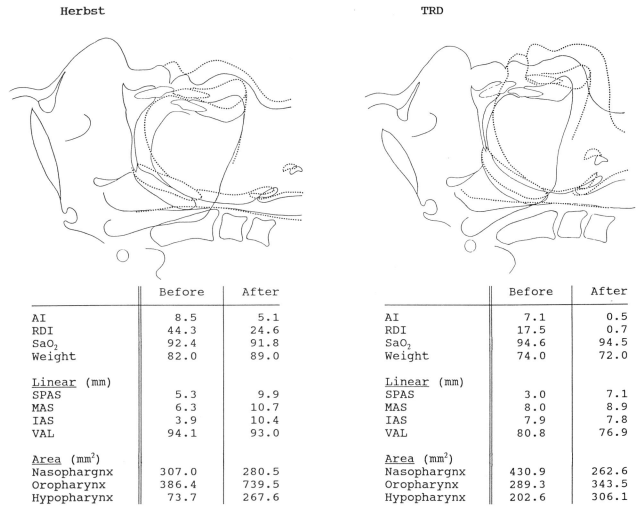

Herbst

	Before	After
AI	8.5	5.1
RDI	44.3	24.6
SaO$_2$	92.4	91.8
Weight	82.0	89.0
Linear (mm)		
SPAS	5.3	9.9
MAS	6.3	10.7
IAS	3.9	10.4
VAL	94.1	93.0
Area (mm^2)		
Nasophargnx	307.0	280.5
Oropharynx	386.4	739.5
Hypopharynx	73.7	267.6

TRD

	Before	After
AI	7.1	0.5
RDI	17.5	0.7
SaO$_2$	94.6	94.5
Weight	74.0	72.0
Linear (mm)		
SPAS	3.0	7.1
MAS	8.0	8.9
IAS	7.9	7.8
VAL	80.8	76.9
Area (mm^2)		
Nasophargnx	430.9	262.6
Oropharynx	289.3	343.5
Hypopharynx	202.6	306.1

Figure 78–2. Cephalometric superimpositions of supine before *(solid line)*-and-after *(broken line)* appliance insertion tracings. A Herbst appliance was used on the left and a tongue-retaining device (TRD) on the right. AI, apnea index; IAS, inferior airway space; MAS, middle airway space; RDI, respiratory disturbance index; SPAS, superior posterior airway space; VAL, vertical airway length.

significantly decreasing soft tissue and tooth discomfort. A total of 44 forward positions are available in increments of 0.25 mm which covers a full 11-mm range of anteroposterior movement. Such small increments help avoid rapid forward jaw movements, which can cause significant patient discomfort.

The Klearway allows the patient to feel less restricted and thus less claustrophobic—a sensation experienced by a small number of patients during the first few nights of wear. Once warmed under hot water and inserted, the acrylic resin hardens as it cools to body temperature and firmly affixes itself to both arches. Lateral and vertical jaw movement is permitted, which enables the patient to yawn, swallow, and drink water without dislodging the appliance. Patients with bruxism are also very comfortable with this appliance because it does not prevent jaw movements during sleep.

In a comparison of 38 patients from three sites,[27] the RDI was reduced to less than 15 per hour in 80% of a group of moderate OSA patients and in 61% of a group of severe OSA patients. Fiberoptic videoendoscopy documented that the airway size was significantly in-

creased at the level of the velopharynx.[27] In another preliminary study, covert compliance data measured with a newly developed miniaturized temperature-sensitive monitor embedded in the appliance indicated that it was worn for a mean of 6.8 h per night.[28, 29]

Patients with mild temporomandibular joint discomfort or bruxism can usually wear the Klearway with ease because comfort of the temporomandibular joint and the dentition over the long term are criteria employed to establish the therapeutic jaw position. Totally edentulous patients may not be suited for treatment with mandibular repositioners because they usually do not have enough intraoral retention to keep the appliance in the mouth during sleep. Patients with edentulous maxillary arches and adequate teeth in the lower arch may respond favorably to Klearway therapy. If the patient wears the appliance every night and is comfortable for 1 month, instruct the patient to activate the appliance by turning the screw on the top of the appliance two times per week until the next appointment. Each turn or activation in the direction of the arrow will move the lower jaw forward gradually in 0.25-mm increments, which has a direct effect on the

3-D size of the airway. The Klearway appliance has been shown to be particularly effective in increasing the size of the velopharynx.[27] Have the patient insert the tip of the key into the hole on the side of the expansion screw at the base of the arrow. Turn or push the key toward the direction of the arrow imprinted in the metal expansion screw which shows the correct movement to advance the lower jaw. Once the key is completely turned from one side to the other, remove it and a new hole will appear for the next turn. If the key is removed before a new hole appears after the completed turn, the patient may be unable to fully place the key in the new hole. Always remove the key after turning. Turning the key opposite to the direction of the arrow will close the expansion screw and retract the mandible. If significant jaw or joint discomfort occurs, advise the patient to stop turning the screw until the next visit.

Some patients stop snoring and feel more rested shortly after the Klearway is inserted and no further advancement of the mandible is required. Others may require 2 or 3 months of slow and gradual forward repositioning before a significant treatment effect is noted. When the patient or bed partner reports a cessation of snoring and a resolution of symptoms, further advancement of the mandible may not be required and the appliance is considered titrated. The expansion screw should be tied off with stainless steel ligature wire or filled in with cold cure acrylic to prevent any further movement of the screw. The patient should be referred back to his or her physician or sleep specialist for assessment at this time.

If the oral appliance has been shown to be effective and the patient is comfortable, 6-month recall appointments should be scheduled by the patient's attending dentist. At each appointment, check the status of the occlusion and verify that the appliance has not been distorted. Minor cracks in the appliance can be repaired at chairside with cold cure acrylic. Expansion screws may self-close over time and therefore should always be permanently stabilized for long-term Klearway wear. The overall management of the patient's particular sleep disorder remains the responsibility of the attending physician. In conclusion, the Klearway adjustable mandibular advancement appliance, made from thermoelastic acrylic resin, has a direct effect on airway size, is consistently well worn throughout the night, and significantly improves the sleep quality of OSA patients.

Mandibular Repositioner

In 1934, Pierre Robin[30] described glossoptosis (tongue obstruction) due to mandibular hypotrophy together with the design of a functional appliance cast in one piece to move the mandible forward. Since then, many variations[31] in mandibular repositioning appliances (see Fig. 78–1) have been used to effect growth, change the airway size, and alter the dentition. Meier-Ewert et al.[32] were the first to describe a rigid mandibular repositioning appliance to move the man-

dible 3 to 5 mm forward, which was effective in reducing OSA. In a group of seven subjects, the mean AI was reduced from 38.0 to 12.1.[33] Using the same appliance in a sample of 44 subjects, an AI reduction from 50.4 to 23.1 was achieved.[34] Reports based on single case studies[35–37] also documented the use of similar appliances. Ichioka et al.[37] found that mandibular advancements of 5 to 7 mm reduced the mean AI from 32.2 to 9.9 in a sample of 14 subjects. Bonham et al.[38] evaluated a group of 12 patients who were fitted with a mandibular repositioning appliance to the most comfortable protrusive position. The mean AI was reduced from 53.8 to 36.0 after insertion of the mandibular repositioning appliance. None of the patients complained about temporomandibular joint discomfort during the treatment.

The Esmarch prosthesis advances the mandible forward 3 to 5 mm and was found to reduce the mean AI from 65.0 to 31.0 in 30 subjects[39] and the mean RDI from 43.3 to 18.2 in 67 subjects.[40] Other reports have confirmed the efficacy of mandibular repositioners. Menn et al.[41] found that 16 (70%) of 23 patients were good responders and Cohen[42] reported a 60% success rate in a group of patients with RDIs greater than 20. Loube et al.[43] have suggested the use of mandibular repositioners for the treatment of upper airway resistance syndrome. A mandibular repositioning appliance for edentulous patients has also been described.[44] Clark[45] recently reviewed the use of mandibular repositioners and found them to be effective for the treatment of snoring and mild to moderate OSA. A small group of patients discontinued wear because of temporomandibular joint or jaw muscle discomfort and a limited number revealed occlusal changes. Lowe and Schmidt-Nowara[46] reviewed the evidence of effectiveness, especially in light of the addition of titratable appliances, and concluded that in all large case studies, patients with higher RDIs had a lower proportion of treatment success compared with patients with less severe OSA.

Lowe et al.[9] reported on the effects of a mandibular repositioning appliance for the treatment of OSA in a subject whose RDI was reduced from 57.3 to 2.3. Figure 78–3 provides before-and-after appliance insertion 3D reconstructions of CT scans from lateral, superior, and posterior views. The lateral view after appliance insertion on the right reveals a rotated mandible and a more superiorly placed tongue. The 3D spatial interactions from the superior view indicate an anteroposterior elongation of the total airway after insertion of the appliance. In addition, the dorsal aspect of the tongue is narrower and more superior. The posterior view reveals an overall larger airway, which was quantified as a net 27.6% increase in volume from 12.3 to 15.7 cc.[7] This significant increase in airway size, especially in the oropharynx, could decrease the potential for tissue collapse during negative inspiratory pressure and thus have a direct effect on the resolution of the OSA.

PM Positioner

The PM Positioner (see Fig. 78–1) and the Adjustable PM Positioner have received FDA market clearance for

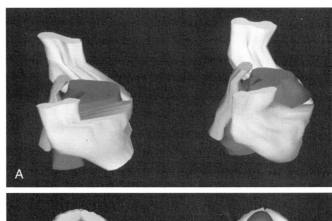

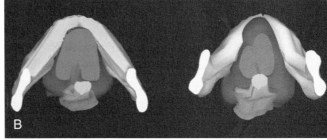

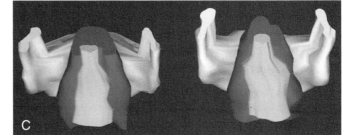

LATERAL

SUPERIOR

POSTERIOR

BEFORE   AFTER

Figure 78–3. *A–C,* Before-and-after appliance insertion three-dimensional reconstructions from lateral, superior, and posterior views. The mandible is shown in white, the tongue in dark gray, and the oropharynx in light gray.

the treatment of snoring and OSA. Formed from a thermoplastic material, the PM Positioner is softened in warm water before insertion into the mouth. The Adjustable PM Positioner can be used to advance the mandible by using a wire instrument to turn the screws located on both sides of the appliance. Initial bite registrations are taken at 65 to 75% of maximum protrusion and the incisors are separated by approximately 5 mm in the treatment position. Parker et al.,[47] based on a study of 15 OSA patients, reported a mean decrease in RDI from 25.8 to 7.3, a mean increase in the lowest oxygen saturation from 78.2 to 83.8%, and an increase in the percentage of REM sleep from 14 to 18.8% with the PM Positioner.

Snore Guard

The Snore Guard (see Fig. 78–1) is a boil-and-bite appliance that is easy to fit and adjust directly on the patient and appears to be well tolerated. The mandible is positioned 3 mm behind maximum protrusion with a 7 mm opening. The appliance covers the anterior teeth only and is lined with a soft polyvinyl for patient comfort. The Snore Guard has received FDA market clearance only for the treatment of snoring. Schmidt-

Nowara et al.[48] found that after 7 months of use in 68 patients, 51 (75%) of the patients were using the appliance regularly. Snoring was decreased in all but one patient and eliminated in 29. In 20 OSA patients, polysomnography revealed a mean RDI decrease from 47.4 to 19.7. In addition, oxygenation and sleep disturbance were improved.

Ferguson et al.[49] compared the efficacy, side effects, patient compliance, and preference between 4 months of Snore Guard and nCPAP therapies in a randomized, prospective, crossover study in patients with mild to moderate OSA. The RDI was lower with nCPAP than with the oral appliances. Forty-eight percent of the patients who used the Snore Guard experienced a reduction of RDI to less than 10 per hour and relief of symptoms, 24% were compliance failures, and 28% were treatment failures. Four people refused to use nCPAP after using the Snore Guard. Some 62% of the patients who used nCPAP were overall treatment successes, 38% were compliance failures, and there were no treatment failures. Side effects were more common and the patients were less satisfied with nCPAP. Seven patients were treatment successes with both treatments; six of these patients preferred Snore Guard and one preferred nCPAP as a long-term treatment. The Snore Guard is an effective treatment in some patients with mild to moderate OSA and is associated with fewer side effects and greater patient satisfaction than nCPAP. The advantages of the Snore Guard are its relatively low cost and reduced clinical time required by the dentist. However, it is nonadjustable, it may apply excessive pressure to the lower anterior teeth in some patients, and retention problems may develop over time.

TheraSnore

The adjustable TheraSnore (see Fig. 78–1) is the only adjustable boil-and-bite appliance available on the market and has received FDA market approval only for the treatment of snoring. The appliance consists of upper and lower trays that snap together by means of four locking mechanisms. The trays are made of a thermoplastic material surrounded by a harder polycarbonate frame. The TheraSnore can be adjusted forward or backward in 1.5-mm increments. The upper tray is designed to fit over the maxilla and the lower tray prevents the tongue and jaw from dropping backward during sleep. The appliance is fitted to the patient's centric arc, or the mandible can be advanced by using the position indicators on the appliance. In 13 patients with OSA, Schmidt-Nowara et al.[50] documented with MRI an increase in the retropalatal and retroglossal spaces with a Snore Guard or TheraSnore in place. Using the same sample of patients, Schwab et al.[51] found that the increase in cross-sectional area was related to a reduction in the thickness of the lateral pharyngeal walls. Miyazaki et al.[52] evaluated the TheraSnore in 11 OSA patients and found that 40% of the patients had more than a 10% increase in their lowest oxygen saturation level and 70% demonstrated more than a 5% increase. The average RDI decreased from 49.5 to 32.0, and 60% of the patients reported an improvement in subjective symptoms.

Tongue-Retaining Device

The TRD is a custom-made appliance (see Fig. 78–1) with an anterior bulb, which, by means of negative pressure, holds the tongue forward during sleep.[53] For those patients with blocked nasal passages, a modified TRD with lateral airway tubes to permit mouth breathing is also available. The FDA has granted market clearance for the TRD for the treatment of snoring. The TRD appliance is particularly useful in patients who have a large tongue. It is an effective alternative to a mandibular repositioner in patients with a compromised dentition or who are edentulous.

The TRD is the only appliance that has been studied in various body positions and in conjunction with other forms of therapy. Cartwright[54] evaluated 14 subjects and found a mean AI reduction from 54.4 to 22.7 after insertion of the TRD. In addition, improved sleep and significantly fewer and shorter apneic events were seen. The sleep architecture showed a change toward a more normal pattern with less light sleep and more

delta-wave and more REM sleep immediately after treatment began. The results were comparable with the rate reported for patients who had been treated either by tracheotomy or uvulopalatopharyngoplasty. In a group of 16 male patients,[54] those with a substantial worsening of the AI while in the supine sleep position were more responsive to the TRD than those who were equally affected in both the lateral and supine positions. The AI in untreated subjects was twice as high while supine as it was in the lateral position.[55] When obesity, age, and the position ratio were used in a discriminant function analysis, these three variables predicted TRD success (as defined by an AI of less than 6 or a 50% reduction in AI) correctly for 13 (81%) of the patients. In a sample of 30 male patients,[56] 20 (66%) tried on the TRD alone or in conjunction with other treatments were improved at the 1-year point. Samelson[57] found that the TRD was effective in 80% of subjects who had used it for 3 years or more. In another TRD report,[58] a group of 12 subjects were treated with the TRD alone or in conjunction with some behavioral therapy such as sleep position training[59] or weight loss. A mean RDI reduction from 37.0 to 17.3 was observed in this first group. In another group of more severe apneic patients, the TRD was used in conjunction with a submucous resection of the septum or a uvulopalatopharyngoplasty. The TRD appears useful either alone or in conjunction with other treatments in patients with a wide range of apnea severity provided that the apnea is more severe in the supine position and the patient's weight is not greater than 50% above the ideal body weight.

In another study,[60] a sample of 60 adult males with RDI values greater than 12.5 who had two or more times the apnea rate during supine sleep in comparison with their lateral sleep rate were assigned to four treatment groups: TRD only, posture alarm, TRD plus posture alarm,[61] and health habits instruction. Some 73% of the TRD group and 80% of the TRD plus posture alarm group were improved. The 15 subjects treated with the TRD alone had a reduction in mean RDI from 27.4 to 11.4. Patency of the nasal airway and an initially low side index were the two factors significantly related to successful control of OSA with the TRD. For the 15 subjects in the TRD plus posture alarm group, lower initial obesity and higher weight loss during treatment were the factors associated with best success. A mean RDI reduction from 30.7 to 7.9 was seen for the latter group.

The effects of the TRD on baseline tongue muscle activity have been studied. Ono et al.[62] found that the TRD has different effects on the awake GG muscle activity in control subjects and OSA patients. In awake OSA patients, the TRD reduces GG muscle activity and corrects the delayed timing of the muscle before an apneic period during sleep.[63] The TRD may counteract fatigue in the tongue muscles and fluctuations in the activity of the GG muscle. In addition, the TRD may provide a pneumatic splint to enlarge the upper airway similar to that seen with nCPAP.

The right-hand side of Figure 78–2 provides a superimposition of supine before-and-after cephalometric tracings of a subject fitted with a TRD in our laboratory.

The mandible and tongue are both positioned forward. A significant reduction in RDI from 17.5 to 0.7 is noted. The cross-sectional area of the oropharynx is increased from 289.3 to 343.5 mm² and the hypopharynx is increased from 202.6 to 306.1 mm².

CONTRAINDICATIONS

Several contraindications to the use of oral appliances have been suggested, but not all are applicable to any one appliance. Obviously, they should only be used for the treatment of obstructive, not central, sleep apnea as quantified by overnight polysomnograms. If oral appliances simply rotate the mandible down and back and a predisposing constriction of the hypopharynx exists, the OSA may worsen.

Oral appliances are not well tolerated by patients with arthritis, crepitus, or other significant temporomandibular joint symptoms. However, mild joint problems may be lessened by the forward jaw position. Sufficient healthy teeth to anchor the oral appliance are required for most appliances. Allergic rhinitis and nasal obstructions may also be contraindications in selected patients. Finally, oral appliances can only be used in cooperative patients who are motivated to wear the appliance during sleep on a regular and consistent basis.

CONSIDERATIONS FOR FUTURE STUDY

Several questions require further study. How can one easily identify the obstruction site in a cost-effective way? Which patients are ideally suited for an oral appliance? Which appliance will be most effective in the individual patient? What is the long-term patient compliance with these appliances? Are there any long-term deleterious effects on the temporomandibular joint or dentition? A long-term prospective study of the frequency and amount of occlusal changes is definitely required. Numerous simple solutions exist for the correction of minor tooth position changes and long-term monitoring of these patients is definitely required.

SUMMARY

Oral appliances are effective to varying degrees and appear to work as a result of an increase in airway space, the provision of a stable anterior position of the mandible, advancement of the tongue or soft palate, and possibly by a change in GG muscle activity. Oral appliance therapy for snoring or OSA is simple, reversible, quiet, and cost-effective, and may be indicated in patients who are unable to tolerate nCPAP or who are poor surgical risks. The appliances should be used during sleep for life, must be comfortable for the patient, and ideally should have full occlusal coverage to prevent vertical changes to the dentition over time.

The selection of patients suitable for oral appliance therapy must be made by the attending physician. The dentist then selects the oral appliance. Documentation of the obstruction site is very useful if such an assessment is available. Although traditional cephalometry can predict with some accuracy the volume of the tongue, soft palate, and nasopharynx, it is not a reliable indicator of oropharynx or hypopharynx size.[7] If a small oropharynx is documented on the basis of CT or MRI evaluations, any appliance that could enlarge the airway by either advancing the tongue alone or advancing the mandible and the tongue together could be useful. If a disproportionately large tongue is seen or if the patient is edentulous or dentally compromised, a TRD could be effective. The TRD is even more effective if it is used in conjunction with behavioral modifications. Mandibular repositioners all are effective in changing the 3D size of the airway tube.[62, 63] Oral appliances have an effect on the tongue muscle either by advancing the mandible, holding the tongue forward, or altering the vertical dimension and thus affecting baseline tongue activity.[10, 11]

Patients demand alternatives to surgery and nCPAP and the usefulness of oral appliances for the effective treatment of snoring and OSA is no longer in question. Three comparisons of oral appliances and nCPAP have been completed,[49, 64, 65] and a strong patient preference for, as well as efficacy of, oral appliances has been demonstrated. In addition, oral appliances have been found to be effective in patients who have not been treated successfully with uvulopalatopharyngoplasty.[66] If the initial assessment is coordinated by the attending physician and good communication is established with the dentist involved, a significant number of subjects with snoring or mild to moderate OSA can be treated effectively with oral appliances.

Acknowledgments

Research undertaken by me and discussed in this chapter was supported by grants from the Medical Research Council of Canada, the British Columbia Lung Association, and the National Centres of Excellence, Inspiraplex. The Klearway was invented by me at the University of British Columbia. International patents have been obtained by the university and specific licensees are assigned the rights to manufacture and distribute the appliance worldwide.

References

1. Schmidt-Nowara W, Lowe A, Wiegand L, et al. Oral appliances for the treatment of snoring and obstructive sleep apnea: a review. Sleep. 1995;18:501–510.
2. American Sleep Disorders Association Standards of Practice Committee. Practice parameters for the treatment of snoring and obstructive sleep apnea with oral appliances. Sleep. 1995;18:511–513.
3. Lowe A, Santamaria J, Fleetham J, et al. Facial morphology and obstructive sleep apnea. Am J Orthod Dentofacial Orthop. 1986;90:484–491.
4. Lowe A, Gionhaku N, Takeuchi K, et al. Three-dimensional CT reconstructions of tongue and airway in adult subjects with obstructive sleep apnea. Am J Orthod Dentofacial Orthop. 1986;90:364–374.
5. Lowe A, Fleetham J, Adachi S, et al. Cephalometric and CT predictors of apnea index severity. Am J Orthod Dentofacial Orthop. 1995;107:589–595.

6. Ryan C, Lowe A, Li D, et al. Magnetic resonance imaging of the upper airway in obstructive sleep apnea before and after chronic nCPAP therapy. Am J Respir Crit Care Med. 1991;144:939–944.

7. Lowe A, Fleetham J. Two- and three-dimensional analysis of tongue, airway and soft palate size. In: Norton ML, ed. Atlas of the Difficult Airway. St Louis, Mo: Mosby–Year Book; 1991:74–82.

8. Pae E, Lowe AA, Sasaki K, et al. A cephalometric and electromyographic study of upper airway structures in the upright and supine position. Am J Orthod Dentofacial Orthop. 1994;106:52–59.

9. Lowe A, Fleetham J, Ryan F, et al. Effects of a mandibular repositioning appliance used in the treatment of obstructive sleep apnea on tongue muscle activity. In: Suratt PM, Remmers JE, eds. Sleep and Respiration. New York, NY: Wiley-Liss; 1990:395–405.

10. Smith SD. A three-dimensional airway assessment for the treatment of snoring and/or sleep apnea with jaw repositioning intraoral appliances: a case study. J Craniomandibular Pract. 1996;14:332–343.

11. Ryan C, Lowe A, Li D, et al. Three dimensional upper airway computed tomography in OSA: a prospective study in patients treated by uvulopalstopharyngoplasty. Am J Respir Crit Care Med. 1991;144:428–432.

12. Tsuchiya M, Lowe A, Pae E, et al. Obstructive sleep apnea subtypes by cluster analysis. Am J Orthod Dentofacial Orthop. 1992;101:533–542.

13. Lowe AA, Ono T, Ferguson KA, et al. Cephalometric comparisons of craniofacial and upper airway structure by skeletal subtype and gender in patients with obstructive sleep apnea. Am J Orthod Dentofacial Orthop. 1996;110:653–664.

14. Lowe A. Neural control of tongue posture. In: Taylor A, ed. Neurophysiology of the Jaws and Teeth. London, England: Macmillan; 1990:322–368.

15. Lowe A. The tongue and airway. Otolaryngol Clin North Am. 1990;23:677–698.

16. Adachi S, Lowe A, Ryan C, et al. Genioglossus muscle activity and inspiratory timing in obstructive sleep apnea. Am J Orthod Dentofacial Orthop. 1993;104:138–145.

17. Lowe AA. Dental appliances for the treatment of snoring and obstructive sleep apnea. In: Kryger M, Roth T, Dement W, eds. Principles and Practice of Sleep Medicine. 2nd ed. Philadelphia, Pa: WB Saunders; 1994:722–735.

18. Sjöholm T, Piha S, Mantyvaara J, et al. Spectral analysis of circulation in teethgrinders: correlation with masseter activity during sleep. J Dent Res. In press.

19. Herbst E. Dreissigjährige Erfahrungen mit dem Retentionsscharnier. Zahnartzl Rundschau. 1934;42:1515–1524, 1563–1568, 1611–1616.

20. Pancherz H. The Herbst appliance—its biologic effects and clinical use. Am J Orthod. 1985;87:1–20.

21. McNamara J, Howe R. Clinical management of the acrylic splint appliance. Am J Orthodont Dentofacial Orthop. 1988;82:142–149.

22. Clark G. OSA and dental appliances: the use of dental appliances to treat common sleep disorders has proved to be effective. Calif Dent Assoc J. 1988;16:26–33.

23. Rider E. Removable Herbst appliance for treatment of obstructive sleep apnea. J Clin Orthod. 1988;22:256–257.

24. Clark G, Nakano M. Dental appliances for the treatment of obstructive sleep apnea. J Am Dent Assoc. 1989;118:611–619.

25. Clark GT, Arand D, Chung E, et al. Effect of anterior mandibular positioning on obstructive sleep apnea. Am J Respir Crit Care Med. 1993;147:624–629.

26. Hoffstein V, Weiser W, Haney R. Roentgenographic dimensions of the upper airway in snoring patients with and without obstructive sleep apnea. Chest. 1991;100:81–85.

27. Lowe AA, Sjöholm TT, Ryan F, et al. Treatment, airway and compliance effects of a titratable oral appliance. Sleep. In press.

28. Lowe AA, Sjöholm TT, Low W, et al. Validity testing of a small intraoral compliance monitor. J Dent Res. 1997;76:238.

29. Lowe AA, Sjöholm TT, Low W, et al. Intraoral compliance monitoring of Klearway appliance wear. Paper presented at: Inspiraplex Annual Meeting; April 1997, Montreal, Canada.

30. Robin P. Glossoptosis due to atresia and hypotrophy of the mandible. Am J Dis Child. 1934;48:541–547.

31. Boraz R, Martin H, Michel J. Sleep apnea syndrome: report of case. J Dent Child. 1979;46:50–52.

32. Meier-Ewert K, Schafer H, Kloss W. Treatment of sleep apnea by a mandibular protracting device. In: Proceedings of the Seventh European Congress on Sleep Research; Munich, Germany: 1984:217.

33. Kloss W, Meier-Ewert K, Schafer H. Zur Therapie des obstruktiven Schlaf-apnoe-syndroms. Fortschr Neurol Psychiatrie. 1986;54:267–271.

34. Meier-Ewert K, Brosig B. Treatment of sleep apnea by prosthetic mandibular advancement. In: Peter JH, Podszus T, von Wichert P, eds. Sleep Related Disorders and Internal Diseases. New York, NY: Springer-Verlag; 1987:341–345.

35. Soll B, George P. Treatment of OSA with a nocturnal airway-patency appliance. N Engl J Med 1985;313:386.

36. Bernstein A, Reidy R. The effects of mandibular repositioning on obstructive sleep apnea. J Craniomandibular Pract. 1988;6:179–181.

37. Ichioka M, Tojo N, Yoshizawa M, et al. A dental device for the treatment of obstructive sleep apnea: a preliminary study. Otol Head Neck Surg. 1991;104:555–558.

38. Bonham P, Currier G, Orr W, et al. The effect of a modified functional appliance on obstructive sleep apnea. Am J Orthod Dentofacial Orthop. 1988;94:384–392.

39. Mayer G. Efficacy evaluation of Esmarch prosthesis and cephalometric analysis. Sleep Res. 1990;19:251.

40. Miyazaki S, Meier-Ewert K. Cephalometric indications for successful prosthetic treatment of sleep apnea [abstract]. Sleep Res. 1990;19:260.

41. Menn SJ, Loube DI, Morgan TD, et al. The mandibular repositioning device: role in the treatment of obstructive sleep apnea. Sleep. 1996;19:794–800.

42. Cohen R. Obstructive sleep apnea: oral appliance therapy and severity of condition. Oral Surg Oral Med Oral Pathol. 1998;85:388–392.

43. Loube DI, Andrada T, Shanmagum N, et al. Successful treatment of upper airway resistance syndrome with an oral appliance. Sleep Breathing. 1997/98;2:98–101.

44. Meyer J, Knudson R. Fabrication of a prosthesis to prevent sleep apnea in edentulous patients. J Prosthet Dent. 1990;63:448–451.

45. Clark GT. Mandibular advancement devices and sleep disordered breathing. Sleep Med Rev. 1998;2:163–174.

46. Lowe AA, Schmidt-Nowara WW. Oral appliance therapy for snoring and apnea. In: Pack A, Lenfant C, eds. Pathogenesis, Diagnosis and Treatment of Sleep Apnea. New York, NY: Marcel Dekker. In press.

47. Parker JA, Kathawalla S, Ravenscraft S, et al. A prospective study evaluating the effectiveness of a mandibular repositioning appliance (PM Positioner) for the treatment of moderate obstructive sleep apnea [abstract]. Sleep. 1999;22:S230.

48. Schmidt-Nowara W, Meade T, Hays M. Treatment of snoring and obstructive sleep apnea with a dental orthosis. Chest. 1991;99:1378–1385.

49. Ferguson KA, Ono T, Lowe AA, et al. A randomized crossover study of an oral appliance vs nasal–continuous positive airway pressure in the treatment of mild–moderate obstructive sleep apnea. Chest. 1996;109:1269–1275.

50. Schmidt-Nowara WW, Williamson MS, Olivera DL, et al. The effect of a dental appliance for snoring on upper airway anatomy. Am J Respir Crit Care Med. 1993;147:682A.

51. Schwab RJ, Gupta KB, Duong D, et al. Upper airway soft tissue structural changes with dental appliances in apneics. Am J Respir Crit Care Med. 1996;153:A719.

52. Miyazaki S, Itasaka Y, Tada H, et al. Efficacy of TheraSnore in the treatment of sleep apnea. Jpn J Clin Otorhinolaryngol. 1997;94:32–37.

53. Samelson C. The role of tongue retaining device in treatment of snoring and obstructive sleep apnea. CDS Review. October 1988;44–47.

54. Cartwright R. Predicting response to the tongue retaining device for sleep apnea syndrome. Arch Otolaryngol. 1985;111:385–358.

55. Cartwright R. Effect of sleep position on sleep apnea severity. Sleep. 1984;7:110–114.

56. Cartwright R, Samelson C, Lilie J, et al. Testing the tongue retaining device for control of sleep apnea [abstract]. Sleep Res. 1986;15:111.

57. Samelson C. A survey of the effectiveness of the tongue retaining device for the control of snoring and/or obstructive sleep apnea [abstract]. Sleep Res. 1989;18:299.

58. Cartwright R, Stefoski D, Caldarelli D, et al. Toward a treatment logic for sleep apnea: the place of the tongue retaining device. Behav Res Ther. 1988;26:121–126.

59. Cartwright R, Lloyd S, Lilie J, et al. Sleep position training as treatment for sleep apnea syndrome: a preliminary study. Sleep. 1985;8:87–94.

60. Cartwright R, Ristanovic R, Diaz F, et al. A comparative study of treatments for positional sleep apnea. Sleep. 1991;14:546–552.

61. Cartwright R, Diaz F, Ristanovic R. Comparing two treatments for positional sleep apnea: TRD and posture alarm [abstract]. Sleep Res. 1990;18:202.

62. Ono T, Lowe AA, Ferguson KA, et al. The effect of the tongue retaining device on awake genioglossus muscle activity in patients with obstructive sleep apnea. Am J Orthod Dentofacial Orthop. 1996;110:28–35.

63. Ono T, Lowe AA, Ferguson KA, et al. A tongue retaining device and sleep-state genioglossus muscle activity in patients with OSA. Angle Orthod. 1996;66:273–280.

64. Ferguson KA, Ono T, Lowe AA, et al. A short term controlled trial of an adjustable oral appliance for the treatment of mild–moderate obstructive sleep apnea. Thorax. 1997;52:362–368.

65. Clark GT, Blumenfeld I, Yoffe N, et al. A crossover study comparing the efficacy of continuous positive airway pressure with anterior mandibular positioning devices on patients with obstructive sleep apnea. Chest. 1996;109:1477–1483.

66. Millman RP, Rosenberg CL, Carlisle CC, et al. The efficacy of oral appliances in the treatment of persistent sleep apnea after uvulopalatopharyngoplasty. Chest. 1998;113:992–996.

Management of Obstructive Sleep Apnea-Hypopnea Syndrome: Overview

Meir H. Kryger

The purpose of this chapter is to outline a practical, useful approach to the overall management of patients with obstructive sleep apnea syndrome (OSAS). The reader is directed to Chapters 75 through 78 for a more detailed review of the most commonly used therapeutic modalities. Until about 20 years ago the only treatment was tracheostomy. There have been broad advances in the evolution of rational treatment modalities. What follows is a consensus of current thoughts on the management of adult patients with OSAS. The reader must recognize that authorities are not unanimous and that controversies about evaluation and therapy[1-6] do exist in this rapidly changing field. In many instances, diagnostic and therapeutic choices are limited by the local medical environment.[7]

DEFINITIONS

OSAS is not a disease but rather a final common pathway of many diseases. This pathway has typical clinical and physiological features. The spectrum of sleep breathing disorders ranges from nonapneic snoring, to asymptomatic apneas, to more severe apneas causing physiological and clinical abnormalities. When possible, the definitions used in this chapter reflect those accepted by most of the expert groups involved in sleep medicine.[7a] In most cases, OSAS is caused by a disorder associated with upper airway obstruction. Wherever possible, the site and the cause of the obstruction should be determined so that the most rational and efficacious treatment can be instituted. In most cases obesity is the cause of OSAS; in about 20% of cases another specific medical diagnosis will be found to be the cause.[8]

OSAS (also called obstructive sleep apnea-hypopnea syndrome [OSAHS]) is defined by a combination of symptoms and laboratory findings.[7a] The symptoms may be excessive daytime sleepiness not better explained by other factors and two or more of the following not better explained by other factors: choking or gasping during sleep, recurrent awakenings from sleep, unrefreshing sleep, daytime fatigue, and impaired concentration. The overnight sleep study should demonstrate a respiratory disturbance index (RDI) of five or more obstructed breathing events per hour. These events include any combination of obstructive apnea/hypopneas or respiratory effort–related arousals (RERAs). The severity of sleep apnea can be defined by two dimensions obtained by history and laboratory evaluation (Table 79–1).[7a] A patient can be mild in one dimension but severe in the other, and the overall severity of the syndrome should reflect the most severely affected dimension.

THE INITIAL HISTORY

In the majority of cases, patients with sleep apnea present with excessive daytime sleepiness (EDS), neuropsychiatric symptoms, or cardiorespiratory features. Males and females have similar presenting features.[9] The practitioner must learn to elicit these findings. Unfortunately, sleep apnea is often missed even though patients have had symptoms for years.[10, 11]

Table 79–1. DIMENSIONS AND SEVERITY OF OBSTRUCTIVE SLEEP APNEA SYNDROME

Dimension	Mild	Moderate	Severe
Sleepiness or unintended sleep episodes	During activities requiring *little* attention (e.g., watching television)	During activities requiring *some* attention (e.g., business meeting)	During activities requiring *active* attention (e.g., driving a car)
Sleep-related obstructive breathing events per hour	5–15	15–30	>30

The Presenting Complaint

Excessive Daytime Sleepiness

EDS is by far the most common presenting complaint.[12] The more severe the apnea, the more sleepiness disrupts activities of daily living.[13] Patients fall asleep and stay asleep in inappropriate settings and at inappropriate times. Such patients may frequently sleep in excess of 12 h each day.[14] Early in the disorder the sleepiness may be present during low stimulation (e.g., watching television) and in more severe cases may be present during active states (e.g., driving a car). These patients have an increased automobile accident rate.[15–17] Patients may fall asleep during the day, even while driving, without realizing they had done so.[18] The practitioner can usually elicit from the patient a history of almost always falling asleep while a passenger in a car or while at the theater, movie, ballet, and so forth. As a result, many patients with sleep apnea have stopped going to such events. The patient and family eventually consider falling asleep while driving or after dinner "normal." Some patients with objectively confirmed sleepiness may deny the symptom (Fig. 79–1). Almost all patients have had embarrassing episodes of falling asleep. We have encountered patients who fell asleep (and snored loudly) *during* their wedding ceremony, at funerals, and during job interviews. These embarrassments frequently cause marital strife. In some cases, the patient does not feel that there is any problem, even though the EDS is severe. Some patients may even deny that EDS is present, even though they are obviously sleepy clinically and EDS is documented by objective tests.[12] Even patients with mild sleep apnea have a measurable deficit in vigilance.[19] The physician should attempt to obtain the following information for considering the various causes of EDS.[20]

1. Does the patient make loud "snoring" noises or stop breathing while asleep? The snoring is not steady or continuous but cyclical; periods of loud snoring or snorting alternate with quieter intervals. This information is best elicited by talking to the spouse or roommate.
2. Does the patient feel refreshed after a nap? Most patients with sleep apnea are still sleepy or foggy after awakening. Most patients with narcolepsy-cataplexy feel refreshed immediately on awakening. We have not encountered sleep apnea patients with cataplexy or sleep paralysis.
3. Does the patient have hypnagogic hallucinations? Although these are characteristic of narcolepsy, we have also had several patients with sleep apnea who had this feature.
4. Does the patient sleep an adequate amount at night, and is the patient less sleepy on nonworking days when sleeping in? This information is needed for determining whether the patient has chronically deficient sleep.
5. Does alcohol, even in moderate amounts, cause an inappropriate hangover or headaches?[21, 22] As reviewed in Chapter 69, alcohol worsens the apneic episodes.

Cardiorespiratory Features

A surprisingly large number of patients are referred because their spouses are concerned that patients stop breathing during sleep.[23] Other spouses focus on the loud respiratory noises that terminate the apneas. The snoring may cause sleeplessness in the spouse and result in deterioration of personal relationships.[24] The noises have a disturbing quality about them; loud gasps, snorts, and loud snores often alternate with silent periods. The disturbing nature of the noises has often been present for decades. Amazingly, some patients seek medical assistance only when symptoms such as breathlessness during wakefulness or peripheral edema appear—even though sleepiness may have been present for years. Peripheral edema should be a clue that the patient may have daytime hypoxemia or lung disease.[25] Patients with nocturnal angina pectoris may be found to have obstructive apnea.[26] Some patients may be referred for the finding of asymptomatic bradyarrhythmia.[27]

Neuropsychiatric Symptoms

Nocturnal headaches, often coming on in early morning, are probably caused by hypercapnia-induced cerebral vasodilation during sleep, similar to what occurs in patients who have chronic obstructive pulmonary disease with hypercapnia. It has been shown that precapillary arteriolar dilation occurs, and that blood flow decreases during long apneas, but it is unclear whether it is hypoxemia, hypercapnia, acidemia, or a combination of these factors that is important.[28, 29]

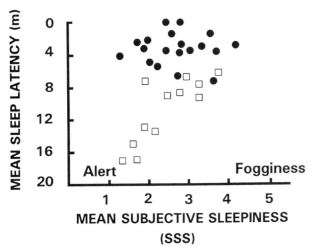

Figure 79–1. The relationship between objective sleepiness (sleep latency) and subjective sleepiness (SSS) in normal individuals (*squares*) and sleep apnea patients (*circles*). Note that there was a correlation among normal individuals but not among apnea patients. (Adapted from Dement WC, Carskadon MA, Richardson GW. Excessive daytime sleepiness in the sleep apnea syndrome. In: Guilleminault C, Dement WC, eds. Sleep Apnea Syndrome. New York, NY: Alan R Liss, 1978:23–46.)

Other neuropsychiatric symptoms include poor memory, deteriorating intellectual function manifested as poor work or school performance, and altered states of consciousness manifested as "automatic" behavior or morning drunkenness or frank psychosis.[30–32] Some patients will appear to be depressed. Patients with even mild apnea may have a poor quality of life with problems in social and family relationships and behavioral impairment.[33, 34]

Other Features

Some patients with sleep apnea will present to their physicians with one of the less common features of apnea (e.g., impotence) or will be suspected of having sleep apnea during the evaluation of another disorder (e.g., hypothyroidism or acromegaly). The review of systems, described next, should explore these features. Rarely, patients will first come for medical attention while being treated for an unrelated medical problem. For example, some patients will be evaluated for "unexplained" polycythemia.[35] Patients may become apneic after receiving medications (sedative-hypnotics or opiate analgesics) or may become "difficult to wean" from mechanical ventilation after surgery.[36, 37] Patients developing renal failure (with its increased ventilatory effort secondary to acidemia, which may collapse the upper airway) may also develop obstructive apnea.[38, 39] In patients with renal failure being treated with peritoneal dialysis, another factor playing a role is the volume of dialysate; the greater the volume of dialysate, the more severe the hypoxemia.[40] OSAS may result in nocturia.[40a] Some apnea patients present with proteinuria or a nephrotic syndrome, the pathophysiological mechanism of which is not yet understood.[41–43] OSAS patients may also have seizures during sleep,[44, 45] or may be found to have a patent foramen ovale.[46]

Pertinent Review of Systems

The review of systems should focus on features supporting the presence of apnea, features suggesting the cause of the apnea, and features that will indicate other diagnostic possibilities.

Table 79–2 lists the features elicited from the patient that are consistent with obstructive apnea. The features suggesting the cause of the apnea include relationship to weight; nasal obstruction (seasonal[47] or chronic[48, 49]); characteristics of hypothyroidism (cold intolerance, weight gain, hair loss, voice change, previous treatment for thyroid disease) or acromegaly[50, 51] (reduced visual fields, coarse facial features, enlarged jaw, enlarging glove and shoe size); or other medical conditions that can cause apnea (e.g., retrognathia in rheumatoid arthritis).

Cardiovascular diseases are so often seen in OSA, that the practitioner should consider this disorder in patients with arterial hypertension,[52, 53] coronary heart disease,[54] transient ischemic attack, and stroke.[55] Sleep apnea is also a risk for coronary artery disease in women.[56]

Table 79-2. CLINICAL PRESENTATION IN OBSTRUCTIVE SLEEP APNEA SYNDROME

Common Reasons for Referral

Excessive daytime sleepiness
Loud snoring or apnea observed by bed partner
Obesity

Less Common Reasons for Referral

Nocturnal headaches
Enuresis
Gastroesophageal reflux
Impotence
"Seizures" at night
Postanesthetic respiratory failure
Psychiatric disorders
    Altered states of consciousness
    Depression
    Psychosis
Abnormal findings during medical assessment
    Polycythemia
    Respiratory failure during wakefulness
    Proteinuria or nephrotic syndrome
Sleepiness associated with other conditions
    Anatomical upper airway obstruction
    Hypothyroidism
    Acromegaly
    Renal failure
    Achondroplastic dwarfism
    Arterial hypertension
    Neuromuscular disorders

Drugs may induce or worsen existing sleep apnea: growth hormone,[57] alcohol (frequently),[22] beta blockers (rarely),[58, 59] testosterone (rarely),[60] and flurazepam (rarely).[61] The *family history* often reveals other family members with similar problems.[62–64] The *medical history* should note remote thyroid disease, poliomyelitis, encephalitis, and head trauma. The last three are more often factors with central sleep apnea.

PHYSICAL EXAMINATION

The almost caricature-like presentation of the obese, plethoric man with large jowls and thick neck,[65] asleep and snoring in the waiting room, is common. Indeed, neck circumference correlates with apnea index[66] and arterial hypertension.[67] Visceral fat accumulation is more common in OSAS,[68] and fat accumulation anterolateral to the upper airway is more common even in relatively nonobese OSAS patients.[69] These same factors play a role in female OSAS patients.[70] There may be racial differences in apnea presentation: young blacks seem to be at increased risk for more severe apnea, and on average the diagnosis is made 10 years before diagnosis in whites.[71]

One should note any obvious skeletal or soft tissue abnormalities, including retrognathia or micrognathia, enlarged tonsils,[72] achondroplasia,[73] the Arnold-Chiari malformation,[74] acromegaly,[50, 51] cleft palate,[75] chest wall deformity, Marfan's syndrome,[76] goiter,[77] or the stigmata of Cushing's disease,[78] muscular dystrophy, or remote poliomyelitis.[79] All these conditions have been associated with sleep apnea.

The following findings are often made: conjunctival injection (particularly in the morning), periorbital and eyelid edema, peripheral edema, and systemic hypertension. The patient may also have the floppy eyelid syndrome, which may be bilateral or unilateral,[80] with the upper lid being lax and easily everted with ptosis, lower lid ectropion, and rarely corneal complications.

One *must* carefully examine the upper airway in an attempt to locate a possible cause of upper airway obstruction. If necessary, evaluation by an ear, nose, and throat (ENT) specialist should be undertaken. The following structures must be examined directly or indirectly: nose (to exclude nasal obstruction caused by a deviated septum or by inflammatory or allergic polyps); mouth (to exclude facial or jaw deformity or an overjet or enlarged tongue); base of tongue (to exclude posterior bulging or large epiglottis); larynx (to exclude tumors or paralyzed vocal cords); and throat (to exclude enlarged tonsils and adenoids; large, beefy soft palate and uvula; and tumors).

Massive obesity may make it difficult to elicit subtle physical findings suggesting venous hypertension or pulmonary hypertension, because the internal jugular vein will be under centimeters of fat tissue. Peripheral edema is common in these patients and may reflect severe venostasis either caused by venous obstruction secondary to the massive obesity or related to pulmonary hypertension and cor pulmonale. The presence of respiratory failure and cor pulmonale may be a clue that there is also chronic obstructive lung disease—the overlap syndrome.[81]

It must be stressed, however, that in many patients the physical examination appears to be entirely normal. Thus, a normal physical examination cannot exclude sleep apnea.

CONFIRMING THE DIAGNOSIS

Polysomnography

If OSAS is suspected clinically,[82] polysomnography must be done, if possible.[83, 84] There is some debate about the extent of monitoring required for diagnosis; most investigators suggest that all neurophysiological variables, as well as respiratory variables, be recorded,[85, 86] whereas others believe that more limited monitoring (oximetry and breathing patterns) is adequate.[87] Some even suggest the use of self-adjusting automatic continuous positive airway pressure (CPAP) systems to both document the apnea and determine CPAP levels.[88] What is clear is that clinical evaluation alone is neither adequately sensitive nor accurate.[87, 89, 90] Some patients who snore heavily and continuously may have periodic hypopnea instead of apnea, and they may have a syndrome indistinguishable from total occlusion of the airway. This has been called the sleep hypopnea syndrome.[91]

Polysomnography is done to (1) confirm the diagnosis, (2) ascertain the severity of the physiological disturbances during sleep, which will then act as a guide to further therapy, and (3) evaluate the response to nasal CPAP. Monitoring should include all sleep stages, in particular, rapid eye movement (REM) sleep. Patients may require more CPAP during REM than during the other sleep stages.[92, 93]

Some patients with the upper airway resistance syndrome (UARS) who do not develop frank apneas may have subtle polysomnographic changes or may require the measurement of pleural pressure to document their physiological abnormalities.[94] For example, these patients may have a sequence of breaths with increasing respiratory effort that cause arousals, called RERAs.[7a] Even though there may be lack of frank apneas, the patients may have PSG abnormalities similar to those of OSAS patients.[94a] It has been suggested that examination of the breathing pattern may help document UARS: prior to arousal there may be evidence of flow limitation (plateauing of flow) and arousal may be associated with increased tidal volume and variation in respiratory cycle time.[95]

"Screening" by either Holter monitoring or measuring oxygen saturation alone during sleep is *not* adequate for excluding sleep apnea with certainty. For example, in one study, only 66% of patients could be diagnosed with use of oximetry alone by an experienced physician.[87] Other studies have suggested that nocturnal oximetry is also not cost-effective.[96] Home oximetry alone has significant limitations.[97] Although such screening may be useful in severe OSA, it is likely that detailed polysomnography is needed in milder forms of apnea, particularly in thin people without baseline hypoxemia.[98] Computerized screening systems (see Chapter 101) and their validity and place in clinical assessment are a matter of intense current investigation.[97–99]

Ideally, polysomnography should include an entire night to indicate the patient's usual sleep and a second night to evaluate the response to CPAP therapy, if indicated. Some centers combine the non-CPAP and CPAP titration studies into a single night. This appears to be adequate in 60 to 80% of patients.[100, 101] In the remainder the CPAP level may be incorrect. Unless there is a mechanism to quickly restudy these patients, we and others[102] believe it is prudent to have at least an entire night on CPAP therapy. In our experience, mask problems and mouth leaks may not become apparent in abbreviated testing. In addition, counseling and teaching is much more likely to be effective if the patient has had a good night's sleep. Some laboratories suggest using automated CPAP machines to determine the ideal CPAP level, rather than a technician.[103–105] Some centers suggest the use of remote monitoring and CPAP titration.[106] These issues are discussed in more detail in Chapter 101.

In many patients with a clear-cut history confirmed by others, it will not be necessary to document sleepiness. Some laboratories use the Epworth Sleepiness Scale as an index of the sleep propensity.[107–109] The score of this test has been correlated with the respiratory disturbance index. It must always be remembered that there may be wide differences between a patient's subjective evaluation of sleepiness and objective testing.[8, 110] The multiple sleep latency test (MSLT; see

Chapter 104) is the most widely used test. A variant of this test, the Maintenance of Wakefulness Test (MWT) is used in addition in some centers.[111] In this test, patients are asked to remain awake in a sleep-inducing environment and then are monitored for sleep onset. The authors of this report believe that although the MSLT primarily measures sleepiness, the MWT measures alertness, and that in some patients there may be a discrepancy between the two.[112] Some patients with low MSLT scores are able to stay awake when instructed; paradoxically, some patients with low MWT scores were unable to fall asleep during the MSLT.

Other Evaluations

If the presence of obstructive apnea is confirmed, then an anatomical obstruction may be present. Thus, tests to evaluate the location of the obstruction may be indicated. It is best that such tests be done and interpreted by institutions used to dealing with sleep apnea patients. Cephalometrics,[113] computed tomography, magnetic resonance imaging, upper airway tomography, endoscopy,[114, 115] and fluoroscopy[116–118] have all been used to evaluate the geometry of the upper airway. The utility of such tests in the overall management of the typical apnea patient has not been established. It must be emphasized that all these tests are used to determine the site of obstruction, not to diagnose the presence of OSAS. One must be aware of the limitations of all these tests; some of these evaluations may be position sensitive in that obstruction may be present in one posture but not the other. A test that requires obtaining data over many breaths—for example, magnetic resonance imaging—may not indicate the true geometry of the upper airway, which is most abnormal during inspiration. Collaboration with an ENT specialist may be valuable. In some cities, evaluation by experienced orthodontists may also add useful information to the investigation of these patients.

Routine evaluations that may help in the overall management of the patients are hematocrit, which is sometimes elevated in these patients; arterial blood gas analysis to determine whether the patient has respiratory failure; pulmonary function tests, when lung or chest wall or neuromuscular disease is suspected; thyroid function assessments (thyroid-stimulating hormone level) when signs or symptoms of hypothyroidism are present[119, 119a]; and imaging of the skull and growth hormone determination if acromegaly is suspected. OSAS patients also may have a high prevalence of glaucoma.[119b]

During the initial interaction with the patient, the physician can decide on the urgency of evaluation and whether the patient must be hospitalized. In general, if the patient has features of ventilatory failure, peripheral edema, hematocrit in excess of 50%, an elevated arterial P_{CO_2}, severe neural impairment with continuous uncontrollable sleepiness, or obtundation, we believe the patient should be hospitalized, and the condition should be diagnosed and treated quickly. Polysomnography in the critically ill will help direct therapy and may avoid endotracheal intubation.[120]

If the Polysomnogram Is "Negative"

A negative polysomnogram most often will rule out OSAS. If, however, the patient has a history strongly suggestive of obstructive apnea (snoring, observed apnea, EDS) and the polysomnogram is negative, more information may be required. It must always be remembered that the first polysomnogram may be negative, and the test may have to be repeated.[121–123] Also, if the patient routinely uses alcohol or sedatives but did not use them before testing, then the test may be negative. One must also bear in mind that CPAP use in the days prior to evaluation may also lead to a negative study.[124] The physician should ascertain that other conditions resulting in EDS, such as periodic limb movements in sleep, have been excluded by monitoring of the anterior tibialis electromyogram.

The recording may show subtle changes. In some patients, there are many arousals or chains of K complexes that are correlated with a change in the breathing pattern (usually an increase of tidal volume without a preceding apnea).[7a, 94a, 125] This finding suggests that in these patients arousal occurs immediately on occlusion without the development of overt apnea. These events, which do not meet the criteria for apnea or hypopnea, are classified as RERAs. This variant of obstructive apnea has been called the upper airway resistance syndrome (UARS) by the Stanford University group.[94, 126] Measurement of esophageal pressure in such patients may confirm that the arousals are in response to respiratory effort. I believe these patients should be treated and sent home with a 2-week trial of CPAP. The pressure required to reduce arousals should be used.

In the absence of a diagnosis, the MSLT may be required to rule out narcolepsy and to confirm hypersomnolence.

INDICATIONS FOR TREATMENT

Guidelines for the use of nasal CPAP have been published.[127] The apnea (or apnea-hypopnea) index, the number of episodes per hour of sleep, is the most widely used measure of sleep-breathing abnormalities. RERAs may be included in quantifying abnormal breathing events to yield the RDI.[7a] Although an apnea index of 5 is frequently suggested as the upper limit of normal, the actual apnea index or the severity of sleep fragmentation that would require treatment is not clear. Relying on a single measure as an indication for treatment is probably an oversimplification: prognosis may be affected by age, the presence and severity of oxygen desaturation, the severity of sleep fragmentation, and the presence of hypertension.[128] It has been shown that an apnea index exceeding 20 results in a higher mortality (Fig. 79–2) than does an index less than 20 in untreated patients.[129] Thus, all patients with an apnea index of more than 20 should be treated. Some have recommended that an apnea-hypopnea index or an RDI of 30 or more be required for treatment of symptomatic patients.[6, 127] It has been reported that an apnea index in excess of 5 is associated with an increased risk

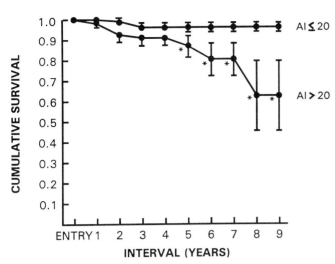

Figure 79–2. Effect of apnea index (AI) on mortality. Probability of cumulative survival for patients with an AI equal to or less than 20 (*top line*, 142 patients) or exceeding 20 (*bottom line*, 104 patients). All these patients were males and were untreated. (From He J, Kryger MH, Zorick FJ, et al. Mortality and apnea index in obstructive sleep apnea. Chest. 1988;94:9–14.)

for myocardial infarction that is greater than the risk imposed by hypertension or obesity.[130] It seems prudent to treat those patients with an apnea-hypopnea index of 5 to 20 if they are symptomatic with sleepiness and if they have an additional risk factor (high cholesterol level, high blood pressure, cigarette smoking). We currently treat those patients with an apnea index less than 20 if daytime sleepiness can be confirmed. Some patients with UARS may require treatment even if the apnea index is normal or snoring is absent.[126]

THERAPY

In the majority of patients, nasal CPAP is the cornerstone of treatment.[6, 127, 130a] Before this treatment is discussed, general measures and options when an anatomical abnormality is found are first reviewed. Less commonly used and evolving treatments have been reviewed elsewhere.[131, 131a] If it is ascertained that the patient does not require urgent treatment (see later), the following general measures are instituted.

General Measures

Dietary control of weight is extremely important and, in our experience, may be successful.[132–134] We have had enough patients who had abolition of their sleep apnea after sometimes even modest weight loss that we embark on this course with all our obese patients. This approach requires a dedicated dietary service. The long-term results of the treatment of obesity with use of current methods are not encouraging, however.[135] Weight reduction programs that focus on behavioral techniques may show a significant response at 6 months (with a concomitant reduction in apnea index), but frequently the weight has returned to pretreatment

levels at 2 years.[136] In one series only 4% of patients had a "cure" of apnea related to weight loss.[137] In some disorders such as Prader-Willi syndrome, in which obesity, sleepiness, and sleep-disordered breathing coexist, normalizing weight may improve the sleep-disordered breathing but the sleepiness may remain,[138] suggesting that the hypersomnia may be primary in these patients. There is much to be learned about how to manage weight in sleep apnea.

Abstinence from alcohol before bedtime is an important part of therapy.[22] It has been reported that if the patient is receiving CPAP therapy, moderate alcohol use at bedtime may be acceptable.[139] We do not encourage any alcohol use because the patients may forget to put on the CPAP mask, or the mask may come off, which would put the patient at risk because moderate alcohol intake interferes with the arousal response to airway occlusion, even in normal subjects.[140] In general, patients should not receive any hypnotics or sedatives.

Treating the commonly found high blood pressure with drugs alone is frequently unsuccessful in apnea patients.[59] If a patient has arterial hypertension and is being treated with beta blockers or alpha-methyldopa, other alternatives to treatment of the hypertension (e.g., captopril or enalapril) should be considered. We have had patients whose apnea worsened with beta blockade treatment.

It has been reported, in short-term studies involving small numbers of patients, that alertness in OSAS can be improved by modafinil.[141] In the absence of more data this drug cannot be recommended.

Recommendations about driving are reviewed elsewhere.[15] The practitioner must be familiar with the driving regulations and the legal implications for the local state or jurisdiction. One study employing 24-h monitoring showed that sleep occurred during driving in one third of the patients on the day they were monitored[18]! It is important that the patient at risk be told not to operate a motor vehicle until treated. If required by law, the automobile driving license authorities should be notified by the family physician. Treatment is expected to reduce the accident rate.[16]

Matching Treatment to the Patient

After the general measures have been instituted and the patient is not at risk, one may consider the different choices for long-term therapy. (See Chapters 75 to 78.)

If Apnea Is Caused by a Specific Condition

If a specific disease has caused sleep apnea, then if possible, the disease should be treated. Although these are uncommon causes of apnea, the diseases that should be treated include acromegaly,[51] sarcoidosis,[142] carcinoid syndrome,[143] hypothyroidism,[119] goiter (with or without hypothyroidism),[77] and lymphoma.[144]

If a Specific Upper Airway Abnormality Is Found

Nasal Obstruction. Because nasal obstruction is a risk factor for sleep-disordered breathing,[145] if it is present, it is important to distinguish obstruction caused by anatomical abnormalities, such as a deviated nasal septum, from a narrowed nasal airway secondary to inflammation, as in chronic rhinitis.[47-49] If the nasal obstruction is secondary to an anatomical defect, one should refer the patient to an ENT surgeon to determine whether surgical therapy is indicated.[49] We have seen patients with sleep apnea due to nasal obstruction who had an excellent response when the nasal airway was corrected surgically. On the other hand, we have seen apnea patients with nasal obstruction treated surgically who *did not* respond to nasal surgery. Thus, in some cases, the nasal obstruction does not cause the apnea. Patients should not be painted an overoptimistic picture about how their apnea will respond to surgery. If the problem appears to be chronic rhinitis, one should determine whether the rhinitis is allergic or vasomotor in origin or whether it is associated with chronic sinusitis. If it is thought, on clinical grounds, that the rhinitis is allergic, then a trial with an inhaled nasal steroid, such as fluticasone, is indicated for 1 month. One may also add an oral decongestant, recognizing that many have sedation as a side effect. Thus, one of the nonsedating antihistamines or pseudoephedrine should be used. Radiofrequency volume reduction of the turbinates may be helpful in selected patients.[145a]

Enlarged Tonsils or Adenoids. If these are present, they should be removed in a patient with OSAS.[72] Again, we have had some excellent results with surgery in adult patients with sleep apnea who had markedly enlarged tonsils and adenoids.

Face Skeletal Abnormality. If an insufficient upper airway is thought to be caused by micrognathia, retrognathia, or another skeletal abnormality, the patient should be evaluated by an expert—an ENT surgeon, a dental surgeon, or an orthodontist.[146-150] In some cases, the patient may have to be seen by several such specialists because therapy may involve a change in the bite and thus may require prolonged orthodontic treatment. Patients with mild to moderate obstructive apnea with an overjet can be treated by an oral appliance, which is inserted into the mouth at bedtime[151-153] (see also Chapter 78). Such patients may require assessment after initiation of treatment as there may be improvement in snoring but continuation of apnea.[154]

If No Specific Upper Airway Obstruction Is Found

Nasal CPAP (see Chapter 76). This treatment can be used in the majority of patients with OSAS and is currently the treatment of choice.[130a, 155, 156] The circuits that are commercially available are well designed and relatively quiet, and the masks are comfortable and tight-fitting. Addition of humidification may improve compliance, and heated humidification may offer some advantages over cold humidification.[156a, 156b] The major reasons for lack of success with nasal CPAP are nasal complications and intolerance of the noise of the system by the patient or family. Some patients develop a panic reaction or "claustrophobia" when they are on the nasal CPAP circuit. We have had some patients

who have had such a severe panic reaction with nasal CPAP therapy that even though they were hypersomnolent, they required, temporarily, a benzodiazepine at bedtime to stay on the nasal CPAP! This is not a course that is recommended, except under unusual circumstances.

The level of CPAP should be determined objectively while the patient is sleeping, with data being obtained in all sleep stages. The patient should generally use the same model of machine that was shown to be effective because different machines with the same pressure settings may have different characteristics.[157] In the majority of patients, the amount of pressure required is between 6 and 12 cm H_2O. We have had some thin patients with, for example, retrognathia who required much less pressure (4 to 5 cm H_2O), and some obese patients with sleep apnea will require 15 to 20 cm H_2O. These extremes are unusual, however. Some patients who are uncomfortable with CPAP may benefit from the use of systems that increase the pressure slowly (Ramp devices) as they fall asleep, or the use of self-adjusting units, which result in the use of lower overall mean pressure during the night. The latter systems may result in improved sleep quality and compliance.[158] Others will accept bilevel positive airway pressure systems that allow a reduction of the expiratory pressure. On the average, the expiratory pressure will be about 5 cmH_2O less than the inspiratory pressure.[159] Several self-titrating CPAP systems are currently available.[103] The place of these systems in therapy is not clear at present.

Patients should use CPAP or bilevel positive airway pressure all night every night because even 1 night without treatment reverses almost all the gains in daytime alertness.[160] In addition CPAP should be used during daytime naps because patients may have apneic episodes anytime they fall asleep.[18] Many devices can be powered by a 12-V direct current power supply, which is useful for truckers.

Some patients with severe hypoventilation will benefit from bilevel positive airway pressure used as an intermittent positive-pressure device.[161] In such cases, the expiratory pressure used is the pressure required to abolish the obstructions, while the inspiratory pressure is increased until there is elimination of the episodes of hypoxemia. Occasionally, oxygen will have to be added to the system.

Uvulopalatopharyngoplasty (see Chapter 77). This and other surgical procedures for sleep apnea should be attempted only in centers with experienced ENT surgeons, anesthesiologists, and recovery room staff familiar with the management of such patients.[162, 163] The results published to date on uvulopalatopharyngoplasty (UPPP), whether using traditional techniques or laser-assisted, in sleep apnea are variable.[164-169] In most series about 40 to 50% of patients may have the number of apneic episodes reduced by about half. Thus we cannot recommend this as sole therapy in patients with severe sleep apnea. As yet, no single test has emerged that can predict with more than 90% certainty that UPPP will be successful.[166, 170] The centers with the best data are those whose evaluations include dynamic endoscopic assessment of the upper airway with Valsalva's and Müller's maneuvers.[166] The immediate complications of this type of surgery are the possibility of obstruction of the upper airway in the postoperative period, bleeding, and severe sore throat, which may last for several weeks. More long-term complications may include nasal regurgitation and difficulty in pronouncing certain sounds. One must remember, however, that after UPPP, snoring decreases, because some of the vibrating tissues that cause the snoring noises have been removed, but the patient may still have severe but silent obstructive apnea! The role of radiofrequency volumetric tissue reduction for sleep apnea, is not currently known, although there may be advantages in using this treatment for asymptomatic snorers.[171]

In terms of definitive long-term therapy, there are advantages to both nasal CPAP and UPPP. Nasal CPAP is fairly noninvasive, but it is likely the patients must use the device for as long as they live. Although the present failure rate from UPPP is greater than that with nasal CPAP, when it is effective UPPP can "cure" the problem, so the patient does not require long-term pharmacological or airway therapy.

Drug Therapy. A trial of drug therapy is indicated in a small number of patients who satisfy specific criteria. Because apnea is so well treated by nasal CPAP, drug therapy is used only if CPAP is ineffective or not available.

Patients with sleep apnea and the obesity-hypoventilation syndrome (with hypoventilation while awake as demonstrated by a $PaCO_2$ greater than 48 mmHg with a forced expiratory volume in 1 sec greater than 1 liter) may deserve a trial of medroxyprogesterone acetate (60 mg/d).[172] Before CPAP or bilevel pressure was available, we had excellent results in several patients who met these criteria. This therapy does not work in the more common obese patients with sleep apnea who do not have hypoventilation while awake.[173–175] If medroxyprogesterone acetate is used long-term, its efficacy should be monitored closely. Some laboratories use medroxyprogesterone acetate to complement the use of nasal CPAP or bilevel positive airway pressure in obesity-hypoventilation syndrome in patients with severe blood gas abnormalities or impending cardiorespiratory failure. In such patients, medroxyprogesterone acetate is used only until the hypoventilation has resolved.

If a patient has obesity and mild to moderate obstructive apnea without hypercapnia, and CPAP is not an option, we may initiate a trial of protriptyline.[176–178] We use a dose of 10 mg twice daily and may adjust it upward or downward, depending on clinical response or side effects. About half of the patients receiving protriptyline develop severe anticholinergic side effects (dry mouth, impotence, constipation, and urinary hesitancy).[177] In some patients with hypnagogic hallucinations or morning drunkenness, these unpleasant symptoms may disappear with therapy. Surprisingly, there is subjective improvement in symptoms similar to that obtained with CPAP, even though CPAP treatment results in dramatically improved polysomnographic changes, whereas protriptyline improves the polysomnogram little.[179] In the postmenopausal woman with

obstructive apnea, estrogens alone may improve the apnea, and the combination of estrogen and cyclic progestins may improve the apnea even further.[180]

Surgery for Weight Loss. Although some centers have reported improvement after such surgery,[181] until they have been evaluated in larger series, such operations cannot be widely recommended for obese sleep apnea patients.

Follow-up

One expects that successful treatment of apnea will improve symptoms in the patient,[130a, 182, 183, 183a] as well as the quality of life for both the patient and his or her family.[2, 24] Compliance with treatment can be improved by interventions and support, such as weekly phone calls, and education about sleep apnea.[183a, 184] Intervention and follow-up seem most effective when done at the start of treatment,[184] as the pattern of CPAP usage may be established quite early, perhaps within the first week.[185] Compliance may be highest in those who are sleepiest with the highest apnea-hypopnea index.[185a]

After 1 night of CPAP use, there is some improvement in daytime sleepiness,[186] but the patient will still be sleepier than normal. Although the number of arousals may decrease with short-term CPAP, sleep architecture may remain abnormal.[186a] After 3 nights of nasal CPAP, the amount of time spent sleeping each 24 h decreases from about 12 to 8 h.[14] After 2 weeks, there is further improvement to the point at which the MSLT may be in the normal range. Thus, recovery of alertness requires at least several nights. Patients first starting CPAP therapy may complain of excessive dreaming or nightmares. This occurs because CPAP results in a REM rebound, and the extent of the rebound correlates best with the degree of oxygen desaturation before therapy.[187] Nasal CPAP treatment is associated with improvement in mood,[188] psychological function,[189] and daytime performance as indicated by a reduction in automobile accident rates.[190] Some cognitive function, such as short-term memory, may still be abnormal after treatment, suggesting that irreversible nervous system damage may have occurred.[32, 191]

Whatever therapy is employed, one must ensure that the patient is compliant and that the treatment is having its desired effect. If the patient is obviously much improved clinically, with abolition of EDS and resolution of polycythemia or right-sided heart failure, it is unlikely that a sleep study will add useful data. The abolition of snoring after UPPP does *not* necessarily mean that silent OSAS is not present. In the patient who has had UPPP, because there may be edema of the upper airway for some time after surgery, there may be temporary worsening of the apnea. It is recommended that polysomnography be performed within a few days of surgery; if results are normal, a late postoperative test is not necessary.[192] If the early test result is abnormal, it might be best to evaluate the patient again when another steady state has been reached, which would be several months after surgery. Thereafter, additional evaluation should be done as directed by the patient's clinical status.

When Therapy Fails

Serious complications of CPAP (pneumocephalus[193] and meningitis[194]) appear to be very rare. Recurrent episodes of acute sinusitis, or communications between the nasal airway and the cerebrospinal fluid (as may occur with trauma to the skull), are probably a contraindication to the use of nasal CPAP, and other therapies should be evaluated.

Most (60 to 80%) patients prescribed CPAP use the equipment and perceive the treatment to be effective.[195] Compliance with CPAP is higher in patients whose main complaint was daytime sleepiness, those with more years of education, and those with a high posttreatment energy level.[196] Compliance is not affected by whether the machine is supplied essentially cost-free.[195] If a patient or the family does not notice improvement in symptoms, there are more likely to be adverse comments about the equipment.[195]

If the patient with documented sleep apnea still has EDS on CPAP, the patient will require reevaluation. First one must ascertain that the patient is compliant with the treatment and then that the CPAP level that is prescribed is being delivered by the system. A mechanical problem with the CPAP system (e.g., deterioration of the mask) must be looked for. Then one might retest the patient to confirm the CPAP pressure. Finally, one may be left with a patient who has another sleep disorder causing EDS. Our laboratory has encountered many patients with sleep apnea who also had narcolepsy or periodic limb movements. We have also had patients with all three disorders. If these disorders are thought to contribute to EDS, they should be treated.

If the patient was prescribed nasal CPAP and this could not be tolerated, the patient should be reassessed before surgical therapy is contemplated. One must make sure that the failure of the nasal CPAP was not related to nasal obstruction, because UPPP will not improve matters if nasal obstruction was an important cause of the OSAS. Heated humidification may be helpful in improving compliance.[156a, 156b] If the patient had difficulty in tolerating the pressure and could not fall asleep on CPAP, then a device that allows the independent application of inspiratory and expiratory pressure (bilevel positive airway pressure) or a Ramp device may be tried first before UPPP is considered. In some patients with difficulty in tolerating CPAP, modification of sleeping position (elevation) may substantially reduce the therapeutic CPAP level.[197]

If the primary treatment was UPPP and if this did not resolve the sleep apnea, the patient may still benefit from nasal CPAP. However, about half the patients with previous UPPP were noncompliant on CPAP in one report.[196] Even these patients who have failed both UPPP and CPAP treatment may benefit from the use of an oral appliance.[198] Preliminary studies are now evaluating the efficacy of radiofrequency tongue volume reduction.[198a]

If nasal CPAP, oral appliances, UPPP, and drug therapy all have failed, maxillofacial surgery may be an option. Such surgery is not routinely performed for sleep apnea in many centers, and the cost may be high because of the complexity of the procedure and the associated orthodontic therapy.[149] When all other approaches have been exhausted, the patient can still be treated with a tracheostomy. Before resorting to tracheostomy, the use of transtracheal air should be considered.[149a] Although tracheostomy is invasive, it is a highly effective form of therapy, and with the use of a fenestrated tube, the patient can be restored to virtually a normal life. Long-term follow-up of such patients indicates that the serious complication rate is low and patient acceptance is high.[199] It is my impression that far fewer than 5% of patients at present will require tracheostomy treatment. Patients who have been treated with tracheostomy may have episodes of central apnea for several months after insertion of the tracheostomy. If the patient continues to be symptomatic and a repeated sleep study shows that the patient is having episodes of hypoventilation or prolonged central apneas, the patient may at that point be a candidate for mechanical ventilation used overnight. An extremely small number of patients will require such aggressive treatment.

MANAGEMENT OF OBSTRUCTIVE SLEEP APNEA IN THE CRITICALLY ILL PATIENT

If a patient has any features suggestive of risk of death (respiratory failure or obtundation), we believe that such patients should be hospitalized and monitored in an intensive care unit. Such patients, particularly those who have severe carbon dioxide retention, may require emergent treatment; it is paramount that a diagnostic sleep study be done as soon as possible.[120] In our experience, treating such patients with oxygen if they are hypoxic may cause severe carbon dioxide retention. If the patient is found to have OSAS, the appropriate urgent therapy is nasal CPAP or bilevel positive airway pressure. This treatment improves daytime blood gas levels in those initially hypoxic and hypercapnic.[200] If the patient has hypoventilation without episodes of apnea or obstructive hypopnea, administration of medroxyprogesterone acetate 60 mg/d, with monitoring until there is a response, may be indicated; in our experience, such patients may also respond to nasal CPAP or bilevel positive airway pressure. Monitoring in an intensive care setting is important until the patient has shown clinical improvement. If the patient has severe hypercapnia, one must initially resist the temptation to intubate the patient and place the patient on a mechanical ventilator. It is when patients with hypercapnia are difficult to arouse or are obtunded that we recommend they be mechanically ventilated. We cannot emphasize enough that these patients must have their mental status and their physiological parameters, oxygen saturation, and carbon dioxide levels monitored continuously. In the patient with hypercapnia who is treated with nasal CPAP, mechanical ventilation, or medroxyprogesterone, the reduction in P_{CO_2} may be rapid and may cause a serious alkalosis, which may require treatment.

It is known that polycythemia results in a marked reduction in cerebral blood flow.[201–203] Phlebotomy to reduce elevated hematocrit is indicated when the hematocrit is well in excess of 55% and especially if the patient has neurological complaints.[203] The major sequela of an elevated hematocrit and its concomitant hyperviscosity is a "fogginess," which may be difficult to ascertain in a sleepy patient. Lowering of the hematocrit to less than 55% may result in improved alertness[204] ("lifting of the fog"), but the patient may still have severe sleepiness.

OTHER MEDICAL AND SURGICAL PROBLEMS IN THE PATIENT WITH SLEEP APNEA

Sleep apnea patients may, in addition to their apnea, have other medical and surgical conditions. At times, these conditions (chronic bronchitis, bronchial asthma, heart disease) may worsen breathing during sleep, and they must be treated as aggressively as in any other patient with those disorders. Some apnea patients may have severe gastroesophageal reflux, which will improve with CPAP treatment.[205]

Patients with OSAS and coronary heart disease are especially at risk.[10] They may develop myocardial ischemic episodes when hypoxic; most of the episodes occur during REM sleep and may be resistant to coronary vasodilator treatment (nitrates). Sleep may be disrupted by both the myocardial ischemia–caused pain and apnea-related arousals. Indeed OSAS should be suspected in any patient with nocturnal angina pectoris. Treatment with CPAP may reduce not only the nighttime ischemic episodes but also those during the daytime.[26]

I have also observed that in some patients with OSAS, paroxysmal atrial arrhythmias may begin almost exclusively during sleep; often impressive polyuria may accompany the episodes. Digoxin, in my experience, may increase the number of such episodes.[206] Some patients with idiopathic dilated cardiomyopathy may have severe obstructive apnea, and treatment of the apnea may result in improvement in left ventricular performance.[207]

When a patient known to have sleep apnea is treated surgically, the patient is particularly at risk because of the effect of anesthesia both on the control of respiration and on the tone of the upper airway musculature. There is surprisingly little in the medical literature about anesthesia in the sleep apnea patient.[208–211] Caution and close monitoring, especially in the postoperative period, are mandatory.

In general, sleep apnea patients should not receive sedatives or opiate analgesics unless their airway is under control. The standard premedications often used in surgery are not appropriate for these patients. If the patient is scheduled to have an inhalational anesthetic by mask and will not have tracheal intubation (as might occur with a minor surgical procedure such as cystoscopy), then the use of a nasopharyngeal tube may be all that the patient requires for stability of the airway to be maintained. The tube should not be withdrawn after the procedure until the patient is awake and alert or is on a CPAP system. In the recovery room, such patients should be monitored with oximetry to ensure adequate oxygenation.

Some sleep apnea patients, after receiving any anesthetic agent, may take an extremely long time to "wake up." Patient-controlled analgesia using morphine is generally contraindicated in such patients unless they are being monitored and there are strict limits on the amount of opiate being administered.[36]

When a patient has a major surgical procedure that requires tracheal intubation, there are several additional important issues. Because of the vulnerability of the airway, awake intubation using, if possible, a fiberoptic laryngoscope without muscle relaxants is recommended. Also, the patient's upper airway may be at risk immediately after extubation. Such patients will require either CPAP or bilevel positive airway pressure. It is my experience that a patient receiving opiate analgesics will require higher CPAP pressures. In addition, some patients with obstructive apnea who receive opiates may develop severe central apneas and will require either nasal ventilation or nasal bilevel positive airway pressure. It is impractical to do polysomnography in the recovery room or the intensive care unit, but observing the patient and examining the oximetry trace may help determine whether such a patient is receiving adequate pressure in this setting.

After major surgery, such as coronary artery bypass surgery, the patient may sleep on and off for several days, depending on the degree of pain and the amount of analgesia. Such patients may require ventilatory assistance whenever they are asleep and, for the first 1 or 2 days, may require a nasal airway. The patient's nose should be examined frequently for areas of pressure or necrosis if the mask is worn for prolonged periods of time. As prophylaxis, the patient should have more than one mask of slightly different sizes so that there are different pressure points. Patients who have had a sternotomy or thoracotomy may complain of severe chest wall pain the morning after they have been on CPAP. This might be related to the stretching of the incision by the increased intrathoracic pressure. We have found that temporarily switching to bilevel positive airway pressure for several weeks up to 3 months reduces the morning chest pain. After operations involving the chest or the upper abdominal wall, the patient may develop atelectasis, and oxygen may have to be entrained into the CPAP or bilevel positive airway pressure system. High oxygen flow rates of 5 to 10 liters/min or more may have to be added to maintain oxygenation due to the varying flow rates required to maintain pressure, leaks in the system, and the nature of the valves.

OSAS patients who have had heart transplants may be at particular risk of developing serious cardiac arrhythmias because the denervated allograft may not be able to respond to hypoxia.[212]

References*

1. Wright J, Johns R, Watt I, Melville A, et al. Health effects of obstructive sleep apnoea and the effectiveness of continuous

*Bibliography of articles on sleep and breathing available at: http://www.sleep.umanitoba.ca/resprefs.htm. Accessed January 4, 2000.

positive airways pressure: a systematic review of the research evidence. Br Med J. 1997;314:851–860.

2. Stradling JR, Davies RJ. The unacceptable face of evidence-based medicine [editorial]. J Eval Clin Pract. 1997;3:99–103.

3. Stradling J. Sleep apnoea and the misuse of evidence-based medicine [see comments]. Lancet. 1997;349:201–202.

4. Douglas NJ. Systematic review of the efficacy of nasal CPAP. Thorax. 1998;53:414–415.

5. Gibson GJ. Public health aspects of obstructive sleep apnea. Thorax. 1998;53:408–409.

6. Australian Health Technology Advisory Committee. The Effectiveness and Cost Effectiveness of Nasal Continuous Airway Pressure in the Treatment of Obstructive Sleep Apnea in Adults. Canberra, Australia: Government Public Services; 1996.

7. Gitanjali R. Establishing a sleep polysomnography laboratory in India—problems and pitfalls. Sleep. 1998;21:331–332.

7a. American Academy of Sleep Medicine. Sleep-related breathing disorders in adults: recommendations for syndrome definition and measurement techniques in clinical research. Sleep. 1999;22:667–689.

8. Langevin B, Sukkar F, Léger P, et al. Sleep apnea syndromes of a specific etiology: review and incidence from a sleep laboratory. Sleep. 1992;15(suppl):S25–S32.

9. Young T, Hutton R, Finn L, et al. The gender bias in sleep apnea diagnosis. Are women missed because they have different symptoms? Arch Intern Med. 1996;156:2445–2451.

10. Ball EM, Simon RD Jr, Tall AA, et al. Diagnosis and treatment of sleep apnea within the community. The Walla Walla Project. Arch Intern Med. 1997;157:419–424.

11. Kryger MH, Roos L, Delaive K, et al. Utilization of health care services in patients with severe obstructive sleep apnea. Sleep. 1996;19(9 suppl):S111–S116.

12. Dement WC, Carskadon MA, Richardson G. Excessive daytime sleepiness in the sleep apnea syndrome. In: Dement WC, Guilleminault CG, eds. Sleep Apnea Syndrome. New York, NY: Alan R Liss; 1978.

13. Rosenthal L, Bishop C, Guido P, et al. The sleep/wake habits of patients diagnosed as having obstructive sleep apnea. Chest. 1997;111:1494–1499.

14. Cassel W, Vogel M, Moog R, et al. 24 hours spontaneous sleep, multiple sleep latencies, reaction time and subjective sleepiness in patients with obstructive sleep apnea. Sleep Res. 1991;20A:527.

15. Pakola SJ, Dinges DF, Pack AI. Review of regulations and guidelines for commercial and noncommercial drivers with sleep apnea and narcolepsy. Sleep. 1995;18:787–796.

16. Cassel W, Ploch T, Becker C, et al. Risk of traffic accidents in patients with sleep-disordered breathing: reduction with nasal CPAP. Eur Respir J. 1996;9:2606–2611.

17. Teran-Santos J, Jimenez-Gomez A, Cordero-Guevara J. The association between sleep apnea and the risk of traffic accidents. Cooperative Group Burgos-Santander. N Engl J Med. 1999;340:847–851.

18. Noda A, Ito R, Okada T, et al. Twenty-four-hour ambulatory oxygen desaturation and electrocardiographic recording in obstructive sleep apnea syndrome. Clin Cardiol. 1998;21:506–510.

19. Redline S, Strauss ME, Adams N, et al. Neuropsychological function in mild sleep-disordered breathing. Sleep. 1997;20:160–167.

20. Guilleminault CG, Dement WC. Two hundred thirty-five cases of excessive daytime sleepiness: diagnosis and tentative classification. J Neurol Sci. 1997;31:13–27.

21. Krol RC, Knuth SL, Bartlett D. Selective reduction of genioglossus muscle activity by alcohol in normal human subjects. Am Rev Respir Dis. 1984;129:247–250.

22. Issa FG, Sullivan CE. Alcohol, snoring and sleep apnea. J Neurol Neurosurg Psychiatry. 1982;45:353–359.

23. Kryger MH, Mezon BJ, Acres JC, et al. Diagnosis of sleep breathing disorders in a general hospital. Experience and recommendations. Arch Intern Med. 1982;142:956–958.

24. Kiely JL, McNicholas WT. Bed partners' assessment of nasal continuous positive airway pressure therapy in obstructive sleep apnea. Chest. 1997;111:1261–1265.

25. Whyte KF, Douglas NJ. Peripheral edema in the sleep apnea/hypopnea syndrome. Sleep. 1991;14:354–356.

26. Franklin KA, Nilsson JB, Sahlin C, et al. Sleep apnoea and nocturnal angina. Lancet. 1995;345:1085–1087.

27. Stegman SS, Burroughs JM, Henthorn RW. Asymptomatic bradyarrhythmias as a marker for sleep apnea: appropriate recognition and treatment may reduce the need for pacemaker therapy. Pacing Clin Electrophysiol. 1996;19:899–904.

28. Poceta SJ, Rieke K, Mitler M, et al. Transcranial Doppler ultrasound during obstructive sleep apnea. Sleep Res. 1991;20A:374.

29. Netzer N, Werner P, Jochums I, et al. Blood flow of the middle cerebral artery with sleep-disordered breathing: correlation with obstructive hypopneas. Stroke. 1998;29:87–93.

30. Guilleminault C, Billiard M, Montplaisir J, et al. Altered states of consciousness in disorders of daytime sleepiness. J Neurosci. 1975;26:377–393.

31. Beretinni WH. Paranoid psychosis and sleep apnea syndrome. Am J Psychiatry. 1980;137:493–494.

32. Montplaisir J, Bédard A, Richer F, et al. Neurobehavioral manifestations in obstructive sleep apnea syndrome before and after treatment with CPAP. Sleep. 1992;15(suppl):S17–S19.

33. Isaac L, Gall R, Kryger M. Quality of life in patients with mild sleep apnea. Sleep. 1993;16(suppl):S59–S61.

34. Jenkinson C, Stradling J, Petersen S. Comparison of three measures of quality of life outcome in the evaluation of continuous positive airways pressure therapy for sleep apnoea. J Sleep Res. 1997;6:199–204.

35. Carlson J, Hedner J, Fagerberg B, et al. Secondary polycythemia associated with nocturnal apnea: no relation to plasma erythropoietin. Sleep Res. 1991;20A:412.

36. VanDercar DH, Martinez AP, De Lisser EA. Sleep apnea syndromes: a potential contraindication for patient-controlled analgesia. Anesthesiology. 1991;74:623–624.

37. Vidhani K, Langham BT. Obstructive sleep apnoea syndrome: Is this an overlooked cause of desaturation in the immediate postoperative period? Br J Anaesth. 1997;78:442–443.

38. Auckley DH, Schmidt-Nowara W, Brown LK. Reversal of sleep apnea hypopnea syndrome in end-stage renal disease after kidney transplantation. Am J Kidney Dis. 1999;34:739–744.

39. Pressman MR, Benz RL, Schleifer CR, et al. Sleep disordered breathing in ESRD: acute beneficial effects of treatment with nasal continuous positive airway pressure. Kidney Int. 1993;43:1134–1139.

40. Mendelson W, Wadhwa NK, Seliger M, et al. Effects of peritoneal dialysis on sleep disordered respiration in patients with end stage renal disease. Sleep Res. 1991;20A:436.

40a. Weiss JP, Blaivas JG. Nocturia. J Urol. 2000;163:5–12.

41. Wesson DE, Kurtzman J, Frommer JP. Massive obesity and nephrotic proteinuria with a normal renal biopsy. Nephron. 1985;40:235–237.

42. Sklar AH, Bashir A, Chaudhary RH. Reversible proteinuria in obstructive sleep apnea syndrome. Arch Intern Med. 1988;148:87–89.

43. Sklar AH, Bashir A, Chaudhary RH. Nocturnal urinary protein excretion rates in patients with sleep apnea. Nephron. 1989;51:35–38.

44. Kryger MH, Quesney LF, Holder D, et al. The sleep deprivation syndrome of the obese patient. Am J Med. 1974;56:531–539.

45. Barthlen GM, Brown LK, Stacy C. Polysomnographic documentation of seizures in a patient with obstructive sleep apnea syndrome. Neurology. 1998;50:309–310.

46. Shanoudy H, Soliman A, Raggi P, et al. Prevalence of patent foramen ovale and its contribution to hypoxemia in patients with obstructive sleep apnea. Chest. 1998;113:91–96.

47. McNicholas WT, Tarlo S, Cole P, et al. Obstructive apneas during sleep in patients with seasonal allergic rhinitis. Am Rev Respir Dis. 1982;126:625.

48. Olson KD, Kern EB, Westbrook PR. Sleep and breathing disturbance secondary to nasal obstruction. Otolaryngol Head Neck Surg. 1981;89:804.

49. Lavie P, Zomer J, Eliaschar I, et al. Excessive daytime sleepiness and insomnia. Association with deviated nasal septum and nocturnal breathing disorders. Arch Otolaryngol. 1982;108:373.

50. Mezon BJ, West P, Maclean JP, et al. Sleep apnea in acromegaly. Am J Med. 1980;69:615–618.

51. Buyse B, Michiels E, Bouillon R, et al. Relief of sleep apnea after treatment of acromegaly: report of three cases and review of the literature. Eur Respir J. 1997;10:1401–1404.

52. Stoohs RA, Gingold J, Cohrs S, et al. Sleep-disordered breathing and systemic hypertension in the older male. J Am Geriatr Soc. 1996;44:1295–1300.

53. Worsnop CJ, Naughton MT, Barter CE, et al. The prevalence of obstructive sleep apnea in hypertensives. Am J Respir Crit Care Med. 1998;157:111–115.

54. Schafer H, Ewig S, Hasper E, et al. Sleep apnea as a risk marker in coronary heart disease. Z Kardiol. 1996;85:768–775.

55. Bassetti C, Aldrich MS, Chervin RD, et al. Sleep apnea in patients with transient ischemic attack and stroke: a prospective study of 59 patients. Neurology. 1996;47:1167–1173.

56. Mooe T, Rabben T, Wiklund U, et al. Sleep-disordered breathing in women: occurrence and association with coronary artery disease. Am J Med. 1996;101:251–156.

57. Gerard JM, Garibaldi L, Myers SE, et al. Sleep apnea in patients receiving growth hormone. Clin Pediatr (Phila). 1997;36:321–326.

58. Rauhala E, Kantola I, Polo O, et al. Poor effect of antihypertensive medication in obstructive sleep apnea patients. Sleep Res. 1991;20A:446.

59. Boudoulas H, Schmidt H, Geleris P, et al. Case reports on deterioration of sleep apnea during therapy with propranolol—preliminary studies. Res Commun Chem Pathol Pharmacol. 1983;39:3–10.

60. Sandblom RE, Matsumoto AM, Schoene RB, et al. Obstructive sleep apnea syndrome induced by testosterone administration. N Engl J Med. 1983;308:508–510.

61. Mendelson WB, Garnett D, Gillin JC. Flurazepam-induced sleep apnea syndrome in a patient with insomnia and mild sleep related respiratory changes. J Nerv Ment Dis. 1981;169:261–264.

62. Strohl KP, Saunders NA, Feldman T, et al. Obstructive sleep apnea in family members. N Engl J Med. 1978;299:969.

63. Redline S, Tosteson T, Tishler PV, et al. Studies in the genetics of sleep apnea: familial aggregation of symptoms associated with sleep-related breathing disturbances. Am Rev Respir Dis. 1992;145:440–444.

64. Redline S, Leitner J, Arnold J, et al. Ventilatory-control abnormalities in familial sleep apnea. Am J Respir Crit Care Med. 1997;156:155–160.

65. Katz I, Stradling J, Slutsky AS, et al. Do patients with obstructive sleep apnea have thick necks? Am Rev Respir Dis. 1990;141:1228–1231.

66. Flemons WW, Remmers JE, Whitelaw WA, et al. The clinical prediction of obstructive sleep apnea. Am Rev Respir Dis. 1992;145(pt 2):A722.

67. Marabini A, Chan-Yeung M, Fleetham JA, et al. Smoking and obesity indicators as predictors of snoring and sleep-apnea. Relation with diastolic blood pressure. Am Rev Respir Dis. 1992;145(pt 2):A867.

68. Shinohara E, Kihara S, Yamashita S, et al. Visceral fat accumulation as an important risk factor for obstructive sleep apnoea syndrome in obese patients. J Intern Med. 1997;241:11–18.

69. Mortimore IL, Marshall I, Wraith PK, et al. Neck and total body fat deposition in nonobese and obese patients with sleep apnea compared with that in control subjects. Am J Respir Crit Care Med. 1998;157:280–283.

70. Carskadon MA, Bearpark HM, Sharkey KM, et al. Effects of menopause and nasal occlusion on breathing during sleep. Am J Respir Crit Care Med. 1997;155:205–210.

71. Redline S, Tishler PV, Hans MG, et al. Racial differences in sleep-disorderd breathing in African-Americans and Caucasians. Am J Respir Crit Care Med. 1997;155:186–192.

72. Mangat D, Orr WC, Smith RO. Sleep apnea, hypersomnolence, and upper airway obstruction secondary to adenotonsillar enlargement. Arch Otolaryngol. 1977;103:383.

73. Mogayzel PJ Jr, Carroll JL, Loughlin GM, et al. Sleep-disordered breathing in children with achondroplasia. J Pediatr. 1998;132:667–671.

74. Abourg F, Dougui M, Knani J, et al. Sleep apnea syndromes and Arnold-Chiari malformation. Rev Mal Respir. 1990;7:159–161.

75. Abramson DL, Marrinan EM, Mulliken JB. Robin sequence: obstructive sleep apnea following pharyngeal flap. Cleft Palate Craniofac J. 1997;34:256–260.

76. Cistulli P, Sullivan C. Sleep apnea in Marfan's syndrome. Sleep Res. 1991;20A:413.

77. Deegan PC, McNamara VM, Morgan WE. Goitre: a cause of obstructive sleep apnoea in euthyroid patients. Eur Respir J. 1997;10:500–502.

78. Shipley JE, Schteingart DE, Tandon R, et al. Sleep architecture and sleep apnea in patients with Cushing's disease. Sleep. 1992;15:514–518.

79. Steljes D, Kryger MH, Kirk BW, et al. Sleep in postpolio syndrome. Chest. 1990;98:133–140.

80. McNab AA. Floppy eyelid syndrome and obstructive sleep apnea. Ophthal Plast Reconstr Surg. 1997;13:98–114.

81. Wietzenblum E, Krieger J, Oswald M, et al. Chronic obstructive pulmonary disease and sleep apnea syndrome. Sleep. 1992;15(suppl):S33–S35.

82. Pouliot Z, Peters M, Neufeld H, et al. Using self-reported questionnaire data to prioritize OSA patients for polysomnography. Sleep. 1997;20:232–236.

83. American Sleep Disorders Association Standards of Practice Committee. Practice parameters for the indications for polysomnography and related procedures: an American Sleep Disorders Association report. Sleep. 1997;20:406–422.

84. Chesson AL Jr, Ferber RA, Fry J, et al. The indications for polysomnography and related procedures: an American Sleep Disorders Association review. Sleep. 1997;20:423–487.

85. Phillipson EA, Remmers JE, eds: Indications and standards for cardiopulmonary sleep studies. Am Rev Respir Dis. 1989;139:559–568.

86. McAvoy RD. Guidelines for Respiratory Sleep Studies. Sydney, Australia: Thoracic Society of Australia and New Zealand; 1988.

87. Douglas NJ, Thomas S, Jan MA. Clinical value of polysomnography. Lancet. 1992;339:347–350.

88. Gugger M. Comparison of ResMed AutoSet (version 3.03) with polysomnography in the diagnosis of the sleep apnoea/hypopnoea syndrome. Eur Respir J. 1997;10:587–591.

89. Haponik EF, Smith PL, Meyers DA, et al. Evaluation of sleep-disordered breathing. Is polysomnography necessary? Am J Med. 1984;77:671.

90. Hoffstein V, Szalai JP. Predictive value of clinical features in diagnosing sleep apnea. Sleep. 1993;16:118–122.

91. Gould GA, Whyte KF, Rhind GB, et al. The sleep hypopnea syndrome. Am Rev Respir Dis. 1988;137:895–898.

92. Issa FG, Sullivan CE. Upper airway closing pressures in obstructive sleep apnea. J Appl Physiol. 1984;57:520–527.

93. Sullivan CE, Issa FG. Obstructive sleep apnea. Clin Chest Med. 1985;6:633.

94. Guilleminault C, Stoohs R, Clerk A, et al. A cause of daytime sleepiness: the upper airway resistance syndrome. Chest. 1993;104:781–787.

94a. Loube DI, Andrada TF. Comparison of respiratory polysomnographic parameters in matched cohorts of upper airway resistance and obstructive sleep apnea syndrome patients. Chest. 1999;115:1519–1524.

95. Bloch KE, Li Y, Sackner MA, et al. Breathing pattern during sleep disruptive snoring. Eur Respir J. 1997;10:576–586.

96. Epstein LJ, Dorlac GR. Cost-effectiveness analysis of nocturnal oximetry as a method of screening for sleep apnea-hypopnea syndrome. Chest. 1998;113:97–103.

97. Anderson B, Keenan SP, Wiggs B, et al. 2%, 3% or 4% arterial oxygen desaturations as a screening test for suspected obstructive sleep apnea? Am Rev Respir Dis. 1992;145(pt 2):A723.

98. Collard PH, Aubert G, Rodenstein DO. Value of nocturnal pulse oximetry as a screening tool for sleep apnea-hypopnea syndrome. Am Rev Respir Dis. 1992;145(pt 2):A724.

99. White DP, Gibb TJ. Evaluation of a computerized polysomnographic system. Sleep. 1998;21:188–196.

100. Iber C, O'Brien C, Schluter J, et al. Single night studies in obstructive sleep apnea. Sleep. 1991;14:383–385.

101. Strollo PJ Jr, Sanders MH, Costantino JP, et al. Split-night studies for the diagnosis and treatment of sleep-disordered breathing. Sleep. 1996;19(suppl):S255–S259.

102. Jamieson A. Split-night studies: a new standard? Forcing the examination of outcome. Sleep. 1991;14:381–382.

103. Stradling JR, Barbour C, Pitson DJ, et al. Automatic nasal continuous positive airway pressure titration in the laboratory: patient outcomes. Thorax. 1997;52:72–75.

104. Teschler H, Berthon-Jones M, Thompson AB, et al. Automated

continuous positive airway pressure titration for obstructive sleep apnea syndrome. Am J Respir Crit Care Med. 1996;154:734–740.

105. Lloberes P, Ballester E, Montserrat JM, et al. Comparison of manual and automatic CPAP titration in patients with sleep apnea/hypopnea syndrome. Am J Respir Crit Care Med. 1996;154(6, pt 1):1755–1758.

106. White DP, Gibb TJ. Evaluation of Healthdyne NightWatch system to titrate CPAP in the home. Sleep. 1998;21:198–204.

107. Johns MW. A new method for measuring sleepiness: the Epworth Sleepiness Scale. Sleep. 1991;14:540–545.

108. Johns MW. Daytime sleepiness, snoring, and obstructive sleep apnea: the Epworth Sleepiness Scale. Chest. 1993;103:30–36.

109. Johns MW. Reliability and factor analysis of the Epworth Sleepiness Scale. Sleep. 1992;15:376–381.

110. Mendelson WB. Sleepiness and hypertension in obstructive sleep apnea. Chest. 1992;101:903–909.

111. Poceta JS, Timms RM, Jeong D, et al. Maintenance of wakefulness test in obstructive sleep apnea syndrome. Chest. 1992;101:893–897.

112. Sangal RB, Thomas L, Michigan T, et al. Maintenance of wakefulness test and multiple sleep latency test: measurement of different abilities in patients with sleep disorders. Chest. 1992;101:898–902.

113. Kushida CA, Elfron B, Guilleminault C. A predictive morphometric model for the obstructive sleep apnea syndrome. Ann Intern Med. 1997;127:581–587.

114. Suratt PM, Dee P, Atkinson RL, et al. Fluoroscopic and computed tomographic features of the pharyngeal airway in obstructive sleep apnea. Am Rev Respir Dis. 1983;127:487–492.

115. Haponik EF, Bleecker ER, Allen RP, et al. Abnormal inspiratory flow volume curves in patients with sleep apnea disordered breathing. Am Rev Respir Dis. 1981;124:571–574.

116. Guilleminault C, Hill MW, Simmons FB, et al. Obstructive sleep apnea: electromyographic and fiberoptic studies. Exp Neurol. 1978;62:48–67.

117. Rojewski TE, Schuller DE, Clark RW, et al. Synchronous video recording of the pharyngeal airway and polysomnograph in patients with obstructive sleep apnea. Laryngoscope. 1983;92:246–250.

118. Smith TH, Baska RE, Francisco CB, et al. Sleep apnea syndrome: diagnosis of upper airway obstruction by fluoroscopy. J Pediatr. 1978;93:891–892.

119. Winkelman JW, Goldman H, Piscatelli N, et al. Are thyroid function tests necessary in patients with suspected sleep apnea? Sleep. 1996;19:790–793.

119a. Skjodt NM, Atkar R, Easton PA. Screening for hypothyroidism in sleep apnea. Am J Respir Crit Care Med. 1999;160:732–735.

119b. Mojon DS, Hess CW, Goldblum D, et al. High prevalence of glaucoma in patients with sleep apnea syndrome. Ophthalmology. 1999;106:1009–1012.

120. Buckle PM, Pouliot Z, Millar T, et al. Polysomnography in acutely ill intensive care unit patients. Chest. 1992;102:288–291.

121. Dean RJ, Chaudhary BA. Negative polysomnogram in patients with obstructive sleep apnea syndrome. Chest. 1992;101:105–108.

122. Meyer TJ, Eveloff J, Kline LR, et al. One negative polysomnography does not exclude OSA. Am Rev Respir Dis. 1992;145(pt 2):A724.

123. Meyer TJ, Eveloff SE, Kline LR, et al. One negative polysomnogram does not exclude obstructive sleep apnea. Chest. 1993;103:756–760.

124. Baetz M, Jokic R, Fitzpatrick MF. Sleep apnea blown away by CPAP. Chest. 1998;113:258.

125. Guilleminault C, Stoohs R, Duncan S. Snoring, I: daytime sleepiness in regular heavy snorers. Chest. 1991;99:40–48.

126. Guilleminault C, Stoohs R, Clerk A, et al. From obstructive sleep apnea syndrome to upper airway resistance syndrome: consistency of daytime symptoms. Sleep. 1992;15(suppl):S13–S16.

127. Loube DI, Gay PC, Strohl KP, et al. Indications for positive airway pressure treatment of adult obstructive sleep apnea patients: a consensus statement. Chest. 1999;115:863–866.

128. Noda A, Okada T, Yasuma F, et al. Prognosis of the middle-aged and aged patients with obstructive sleep apnea. Psychiatry Clin Neurosci. 1998;52:79–85.

129. He J, Kryger MH, Zorick FJ, et al. Mortality and apnea index in obstructive sleep apnea: experience in 385 male patients. Chest. 1988;94:9–14.

130. Hung J, Whitford EG, Parsons RW, et al. Association of sleep apnoea with myocardial infarction in men. Lancet. 1990;336:261–264.

130a. Jenkinson C, Davies RJO, Mullins R, et al. Comparison of therapeutic and subtherapeutic nasal continuous positive airway pressure for obstructive sleep apnoea: a randomized prospective parallel trial. Lancet. 1999;353:2100–2105.

131. Aubert G. Alternative therapeutic approaches in sleep apnea syndromes. Sleep. 1992;15(suppl):S69–S72.

131a. Loube DI. Technologic advances in the treatment of obstructive sleep apnea syndrome. Chest. 1999;116:1426–1433.

132. Browman CP, Sampson MG, Yolles SF, et al. Obstructive sleep apnea and body weight. Chest. 1984;85:435–438.

133. Smith PL, Gold AR, Meyers DA, et al. Weight loss in mildly to moderately obese patients with obstructive sleep apnea. Ann Intern Med. 1985;103:850–855.

134. Wittels EH, Thompson S. Obstructive sleep apnea and obesity. Otolaryngol Clin North Am. 1990;23:751–760.

135. Bray GA. Barriers to the treatment of obesity. Ann Intern Med. 1991;115:152–153.

136. Kajaste S, Telakivi T, Pihl S, et al. Effects of a weight reduction program on sleep apnea: a two-year follow-up. Sleep Res. 1991;20A:332.

137. Noseda A, Kempenaers C, Hoffmann G, et al. Sleep apnea and nocturnal ventilatory assistance (nCPAP): 5-year experience in the conventional system. Rev Med Brux. 1997;18:64–69.

138. Harris JC, Allen RP. Is excessive daytime sleepiness characteristic of Prader-Willi syndrome? The effects of weight change. Arch Pediatr Adolesc Med. 1996;150:1288–1293.

139. Berry RB, Desa MM, Light RW. Effect of ethanol on the efficacy of nasal continuous positive airway pressure as a treatment for obstructive sleep apnea. Chest. 1991;99:339–343.

140. Berry RB, Bonnet M, Light RW. Effect of ethanol on the arousal response to airway occlusion during sleep in normal subjects. Am Rev Respir Dis. 1992;145:445–452.

141. Arnulf I, Homeyer P, Garma L, et al. Modafinil in obstructive sleep apnea–hypopnea syndrome: a pilot study in 6 patients. Respiration. 1997;64:159–161.

142. Turner GA, Lower EE, Corser BC, et al. Sleep apnea in sarcoidosis. Sarcoidosis Vasc Diffuse Lung Dis. 1997;14:61–64.

143. Milkiewicz P, Olliff S, Johnson AP, et al. Obstructive sleep apnoea syndrome (OSAS) as a complication of carcinoid syndrome treated successfully by hepatic artery embolization. Eur J Gastroenterol Hepatol. 1997;9:217–220.

144. Espinosa G, Alarcon A, Morello A, et al. Obstructive apnea syndrome during sleep secondary to a pharyngeal lymphoma. Improvement with continuous pressure treatment of the upper airway. Arch Bronconeumol. 1996;32:547–549.

145. Young T, Finn L, Kim H. Nasal obstruction as a risk factor for sleep-disordered breathing. The University of Wisconsin Sleep and Respiratory Research Group. J Allergy Clin Immunol. 1997;99:S757–762.

145a. Li KK, Powell NB, Riley RW, et al. Radiofrequency volumetric tissue reduction for treatment of turbinate hypertrophy: a pilot study. Otolaryngol Head Neck Surg. 1998;119:569–573.

146. Lowe A, Fleetham J, Ryan F, et al. Effects of a mandibular repositioning appliance used in the treatment of obstructive sleep apnea on tongue muscle activity. Prog Clin Biol Res. 1990;345:395–404.

147. Loew AA, Santamaria JD, Fleetham JA, et al. Facial morphology and obstructive sleep apnea. Am J Orthod Dentofacial Orthop. 1986;90:484–490.

148. Riley RW, Powell NB, Guilleminault C. Maxillofacial surgery and obstructive sleep apnea: a review of 80 patients. Otolaryngol Head Neck Surg. 1989;101:353–361.

149. Riley RW, Powell NB, Guilleminault C. Maxillofacial surgery and nasal CPAP: a comparison of treatment for obstructive sleep apnea syndrome. Chest. 1990;98:1421–1425.

149a. Series F, Forge JL, Lampron N, et al. Transtracheal air in the treatment of obstructive sleep apnoea hypopnoea syndrome. Thorax. 2000;55:86–87.

150. Conradt R, Hochban W, Brandenburg U, et al. Long-term fol-

low-up after surgical treatment of obstructive sleep apnoea by maxillomandibular advancement. Eur Respir J. 1997;10:123–128.

151. American Sleep Disorders Association. Practice parameters for the treatment of snoring and obstructive sleep apnea with oral appliances. Sleep. 1995;18:511–513.

152. Schmidt-Nowara W, Lowe A, Wiegand L, et al. Oral appliances for the treatment of snoring and obstructive sleep apnea: a review. Sleep. 1995;18:501–510.

153. Ferguson KA, Ono T, Lowe AA, et al. A short-term controlled trial of an adjustable oral appliance for the treatment of mild to moderate obstructive sleep apnoea. Thorax. 1997;52:362–368.

154. Marklund M, Franklin KA, Sahlin C, et al. The effect of a mandibular advancement device on apneas and sleep in patients with obstructive sleep apnea. Chest. 1998;113:707–713.

155. Sullivan CE, Issa FG, Berthon-Jones M, et al. Reversal of obstructive sleep apnoea by continuous positive airway pressure applied through the nares. Lancet. 1981;1:862–865.

156. Sullivan CE, Issa FG, Berthon-Jones M, et al. Home treatment of obstructive sleep apnea with continuous positive airway pressure applied through a nose mask. Bull Eur Physiopathol Respir. 1984;20:49–54.

156a. Massie CA, Hart RW, Peralez K, et al. Effects of humidification on nasal symptoms and compliance in sleep apnea patients using continuous positive airway pressure (CPAP). Sleep. 1999;22:S228.

156b. Kline LR, Carlson P, NCPAP. Acceptance and compliance is altered by humidification. Sleep. 1999;22:S230.

157. Demirozu MC, Chediak AD, Nay KN, et al. A comparison of nine nasal continuous positive pressure machines in maintaining mask pressure during simulated inspiration. Sleep. 1991;14:259–262.

158. Konermann M, Sanner BM, Vyleta M, et al. Use of conventional and self-adjusting nasal continuous positive airway pressure for treatment of severe sleep apnea syndrome. Chest. 1998;113:714–718.

159. Sanders MH, Kern N. Obstructive sleep apnea treated by independently adjusted inspiratory and expiratory positive airway pressures via nasal mask. Chest. 1990;98:317–324.

160. Kribbs NB, Pack AI, Kline LR, et al. Effects of one night without nasal CPAP treatment on sleep and sleepiness in patients with obstructive sleep apnea. Am Rev Respir Dis. 1993;147:1162–1168.

161. Waldhorn RE. Nocturnal nasal intermittent positive pressure ventilation with bi-level positive pressure (BiPap) in respiratory failure. Chest. 1992;101:516–521.

162. Sher AE, Schechtman KB, Piccirillo JF. The efficacy of surgical modifications of the upper airway in adults with obstructive sleep apnea syndrome. Sleep. 1996;19:156–177.

163. American Sleep Disorders Association. Practice parameters for the treatment of obstructive sleep apnea in adults: the efficacy of surgical modifications of the upper airway. Sleep. 1996;19:152–155.

164. Fujita S, Conway W, Zorick F, et al. Surgical correction of anatomic abnormalities in obstructive sleep apnea syndrome: Uvulopalatopharyngoplasty. Otolaryngol Head Neck Surg. 1981;89:923–934.

165. Cotton RT. Uvulopalatopharyngoplasty. Arch Otolaryngol. 1983;109:502.

166. Sher AE, Thorpy MJ, Spielman AJ, et al. Predictive value of Müller maneuver in selection of patients for uvulopalatopharyngoplasty. Laryngoscope. 1985;95:1483–1487.

167. Zorick F, Roehrs T, Conway W, et al. Effects of uvulopalatopharyngoplasty on the daytime sleepiness associated with sleep apnea syndrome. Bull Eur Physiopathol Respir. 1983;19:600–603.

168. Fairbanks DNF, Fujita S, eds. Snoring and Obstructive Sleep Apnea. New York, NY: Raven Press; 1994.

169. Langin T, Pepin JL, Pendelbury S, et al. Upper airway changes in snorers and mild sleep apnea sufferers after uvulopalatopharyngoplasty (UPPP). Chest. 1998;113:1595–1603.

170. Shepard JW Jr, Olsen KD. Uvulopalatopharyngoplasty for treatment of obstructive sleep apnea. Mayo Clin Proc. 1990;65:1260–1267.

171. Powell NB, Riley RW, Troell RJ, et al. Radiofrequency volumetric tissue reduction of the palate in subjects with sleep-disordered breathing. Chest. 1998;113:1163–1174.

172. Sutton JD Jr, Zwillich CW, Creagh EE, et al. Progesterone for the outpatient treatment of Pickwickian syndrome. Ann Intern Med. 1975;83:476–479.

173. Orr WC, Imes NK, Martin RJ. Progesterone therapy in obese patients with sleep apnea. Arch Intern Med. 1979;139:109–111.

174. Strohl KP, Hensley MJ, Saunders NA, et al. Progesterone administration and progressive sleep apneas. JAMA. 1980;245:1230–1232.

175. Rajagopal KR, Abbrecht PH, Jabbari B. Effects of medroxyprogesterone acetate in obstructive sleep apnea. Chest. 1986;90:815–821.

176. Brownell LG, West P, Sweatman P, et al. Protriptyline in obstructive sleep apnea. N Engl J Med. 1982;307:1037–1042.

177. Brownell LG, Perez-Padilla R, West P, et al. The role of protriptyline in obstructive sleep apnea. Bull Eur Physiopathol Respir. 1983;19:621–624.

178. Smith PL, Haponik EF, Allen RP, et al. The effects of protriptyline in sleep-disordered breathing. Am Rev Respir Dis. 1983;127:8–13.

179. Popkin J, Rutherford R, Lue F, et al. A one-year randomized trial of nasal CPAP versus protriptyline in the management of obstructive sleep apnea. Sleep Res. 1988;17:237.

180. Franklin K, Lundgren R, Rabben T. Sleep apnoea syndrome treated with oestradiol and cyclic medroxyprogesterone. Lancet. 1991;338:251–252.

181. Sugerman HG, Fairman RP, Baron PL, et al. Gastric surgery for respiratory insufficiency of obesity. Chest. 1986;89:81–86.

182. Engleman HM, Martin SE, Deary IJ, et al. Effect of CPAP therapy on daytime function in patients with mild sleep apnoea/hypopnoea syndrome. Thorax. 1997;51:114–119.

183. Engleman HM, Martin SE, Kingshott RN, et al. Randomised placebo controlled trial of daytime function after continuous positive airway pressure (CPAP) therapy for the sleep apneoea/hypopnoea syndrome. Thorax. 1998;53:341–345.

183a. Hoy CJ, Vennelle M, Kingshott RN, et al. Can intensive support improve continuous positive airway pressure use in patients with the sleep apnea/hypopnea syndrome? Am J Respir Crit Care Med. 1999;159:1096–1100.

184. Chervin RD, Theut S, Bassetti C, et al. Compliance with nasal CPAP can be improved by simple interventions. Sleep. 1997;20:284–289.

185. Weaver TE, Kribbs NB, Pack AI, et al. Night-to-night variability in CPAP use over the first three months of treatment. Sleep. 1997;20:278–283.

185a. McArdle N, Devereux G, Heidarnejad H, et al. Long-term use of CPAP therapy for sleep apnea-hypopnea syndrome. Am J Respir Crit Care Med. 1999;159:1108–1114.

186. Lamphere J, Roehrs T, Wittig R, et al. Recovery of alertness after CPAP in apnea. Chest. 1989;96:1364–1367.

186a. Loredo JS, Ancoli Israel S, Dimsdale JE. Effect of continuous positive airway pressure vs placebo continuous positive airway pressure on sleep quality in obstructive sleep apnea. Chest. 1999;116:1545–1549

187. Aldrich M, Eiser A, Lee M, et al. Effects of continuous positive airway pressure on phasic events of REM sleep in patients with obstructive sleep apnea. Sleep. 1989;12:413–419.

188. Engleman HM, Cheshire KE, Deary IJ, et al. Daytime sleepiness and cognitive performance and mood after continuous positive airway pressure for the sleep apnea/hypopnea syndrome. Thorax. 1993;48:911–914.

189. Charbonneau M, Tousignant P, Lamping DL, et al. The effects of nasal continuous positive airway pressure (nCPAP) on sleepiness and psychological functioning in obstructive sleep apnea (OSA). Am Rev Respir Dis. 1992;145(pt 2):A168.

190. Surrat PM, Findley LJ. Effect of nasal CPAP on auto simulator performance and on self-reported auto accidents in patients with sleep apnea. Am Rev Respir Dis. 1992;145(pt 2):A169.

191. Naegele B, Pepin JL, Levy P, et al. Cognitive executive dysfunction in patients with obstructive sleep apnea syndrome (OSAS) after treatment. Sleep. 1998;21:392–397.

192. Sanders MH, Costantino JP, Johnson JT. Polysomnography early after uvulopalatopharyngoplasty as a predictor of late postoperative results. Chest. 1990;97:913–919.

193. Jarjour NN, Wilson P. Pneumocephalus associated with nasal continuous airway pressure in a patient with sleep apnea syndrome. Chest. 1989;96:1425–1426.

194. Bamford CR, Quan SF. Bacterial meningitis—a possible complication of nasal continuous positive airway pressure in obstructive sleep apnea syndrome and a mucocele. Sleep. 1993;16:31–32.

195. Hoffstein V, Viner S, Mateika S, et al. Treatment of obstructive sleep apnea with nasal continuous positive airway pressure. Am Rev Respir Dis. 1992;145:841–845.

196. Kribbs, NB, Pack AI, Kline LR, et al. Objective measurement of patterns of nasal CPAP use by patients with obstructive sleep apnea. Am Rev Respir Dis. 1993;147:887–895.

197. Neill AM, Angus SM, Sajkov D, et al. Effects of sleep posture on upper airway stability in patients with obstructive sleep apnea. Am J Respir Crit Care Med. 1997;155:199–204.

198. Millman RP, Rosenberg CL, Carlisle CC, et al. The efficacy of oral appliances in the treatment of persistent sleep apnea after uvulopalatopharyngoplasty. Chest. 1998;113:992–996.

198a. Powell NB, Riley RW, Guilleminault C. Radiofrequency tongue base reduction in sleep-disordered breathing: a pilot study. Otolaryngol Head Neck Surg. 1999;120:656–664.

199. Staats BA, Offord KP, Richardson JW, et al. Long-term followup of obstructive sleep apnea patients treated with tracheostomy. Sleep Res. 1988;17:262.

200. Krieger J, Weitzenblum E, Kessler R, et al. Effects of treatment with nasal CPAP on arterial blood gases and pulmonary artery pressure in patients with sleep apnea syndrome. Am Rev Respir Dis. 1992;145(pt 2):A442.

201. Humphrey PRD, Marshall J, Russell RWR, et al. Cerebral blood-flow and viscosity in relative polycythemia. Lancet. 1979;2:873–876.

202. Thomas DJ, Marshall J, Russell RWR, et al. Effect of hematocrit on cerebral blood-flow in man. Lancet. 1977;2:941–943.

203. Thomas DJ, Marshall J, Russell RWR, et al. Cerebral blood-flow in polycythemia. Lancet. 1977;2:161–164.

204. Willison JR, DuBoulay GH, Paul EA, et al. Effect of high hematocrit on alertness. Lancet. 1980;1:846–848.

205. Kerr P, Shoenut JP, Millar T, et al. Nasal CPAP reduces gastroesophageal reflux in obstructive sleep apnea syndrome. Chest. 1992;101:1539–1544.

206. Coumel P, Attuel P, Lavallee JP, et al. Syndrome d'arythmie auriculaire d'origine vagale. Arch Mal Coeur. 1978;71:645.

207. Malone S, Liu PP, Holloway R, et al. Obstructive sleep apnea in patients with dilated cardiomyopathy: effects of continuous positive airway pressure on left ventricular ejection fraction. Lancet. 1991;338:1480–1483.

208. Wang M, Tu P, Chen T, et al. Anesthetic implications and complications of uvulopalatopharyngoplasty in the sleep apnea syndrome. Ma Tsui Hsueh Tsa Chi. 1989;27:191–196.

209. Chung F, Crago RR. Sleep apnoea syndrome and anesthesia. Can Anaesth Soc J. 1991;29:439–445.

210. Craddock M, Lees DE. Anesthesia for obstructive sleep apnea patients: risks, precautions, and management. In: Fairbanks DNF, ed. Snoring and Obstructive Sleep Apnea. 2nd ed. New York, NY: Raven Press, 1994:211–217.

211. Rafferty TD, Ruskis A, Sasaki C, et al. Perioperative considerations in the management of tracheostomy for obstructive sleep apnea patients. Br J Anaesth. 1980;52:619–622.

212. Madden BP, Shenoy V, Dalrymple-Hay M, et al. Absence of bradycardic response to apnea and hypoxia in heart transplant recipients with obstructive sleep apnea. J Heart Lung Transplant. 1997;16:394–397.

80

Asthma

Neil J. Douglas

Asthma, a disease characterized by widespread bronchoconstriction, occurs in about 5% of the population. The bronchoconstriction is almost totally reversible with therapy. Besides spasm of bronchial smooth muscle, other causes of the airflow obstruction are viscous bronchial secretions and inflammation and swelling of the mucosa and submucosa. The airways of asthmatic patients are hyperresponsive; bronchoconstriction may follow exposure to allergens (pollen, animal dander) or nonallergenic stimuli (viral infections, cold, fumes, etc.). In many patients, asthma is worse at night or in the early morning, when the patient coughs or wheezes. These symptoms reflect overnight bronchoconstriction, which occurs in over two thirds of asthmatic patients.[1, 2] Although the cause of such nocturnal bronchospasm remains uncertain, its management has become easier in the past decade.

The observation that many asthmatic patients wheeze at night is not new. In 1698, Dr. (later Sir) John Floyer, himself asthmatic, wrote:

> I have observed the fit always to happen after sleep in the night. . . . At first waking, about one or two of the clock in the night, the fit of asthma more evidently begins, the breath is very slow . . . the diaphragm seems stiff and tied. . . . It is not without much difficulty moved downwards.[3]

Despite the clarity of this description, 2½ centuries passed before nocturnal asthma received much further attention.

The forced expiratory volume in 1 sec (FEV_1) and peak flow rates fall overnight in patients with asthma,[4-6] the fall being over 50% in some patients. Patients with such overnight bronchoconstriction have been called "morning dippers"[7] (Fig. 80–1). In asthmatic patients recovering from recent exacerbations, about one third have bronchoconstriction during the night; another third have bronchoconstriction before sleep and continue to have it overnight.[1] Thus, two thirds of these patients have their lowest flow rates between 10 PM and 8 AM. The mean amplitude of variation of peak flow rates was 29% of the highest recorded value in this study.[1] A population-based study found that 85% of asthmatic patients complained about being woken from time to time by their asthma. Thus, significant nocturnal bronchoconstriction is common in asthma.

CIRCADIAN RHYTHM OF AIRWAY CALIBER

Most normal people also have circadian changes in airway caliber with mild nocturnal bronchoconstriction.[5, 9, 10] Although circadian changes in flow rate are synchronous in asthmatic patients and normal subjects, asthmatic patients have a far greater variation in their peak flow rates.[5, 9] The largest series comparing circadian changes in peak flow in healthy subjects and unstable asthmatic patients[9] shows that the changes in flow rate are synchronous in asthmatic and normal subjects, whereas the amplitude of peak flow rate changes is far greater in asthmatic patients (50%) than in normal subjects (8%). Thus, nocturnal bronchoconstriction in asthma appears to be an exaggeration of the normal circadian changes in airway caliber. Asthmatic patients are hyperreactive to constrictor stimuli; thus, nocturnal bronchoconstriction in asthmatic patients is probably an expression of hyperresponsiveness to the factors that produce mild nocturnal bronchoconstriction in normal subjects.

Synchronization of Circadian Rhythm

As with some other circadian rhythms, the major synchronizing factor is sleep. Overnight sleep deprivation reduces, but does not abolish, nocturnal airway

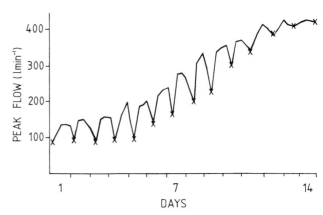

Figure 80–1. Peak flow rate over a 2-week period in a 62-year-old nonallergic asthmatic woman. The flow rate on waking is indicated with a cross. There is marked "morning dipping." (From Douglas NJ. Asthma at night. Clin Chest Med. 1985;6:663–674.)

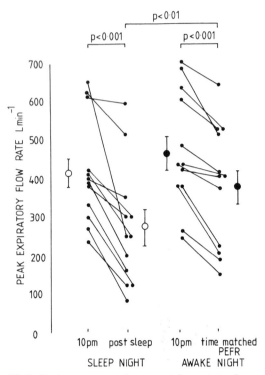

Figure 80–2. Peak expiratory flow at night and in the morning on both the asleep and the awake nights. All patients developed bronchoconstriction on both nights, but although the 10 PM peak flow rates were not significantly different, morning peak flow was higher after the awake night. (From Catterall JR, Rhind GB, Stewart IC, et al. Effect of sleep deprivation on overnight bronchoconstriction in nocturnal asthma. Thorax. 1986;41:676–680.)

narrowing[11, 12] (Fig. 80–2). In asthmatic shift workers, sleep time determines the timing of "nocturnal" airway narrowing,[13, 14] with rapid inversion of airway caliber changes with inversion of sleep pattern. That some overnight airway narrowing persists even if patients are kept awake all night could be due to a lag between altered sleep times and readjustment of circadian rhythms.[15]

MECHANISMS AND CAUSES OF NOCTURNAL AIRWAY NARROWING

Factors that have been suggested but seem unlikely primary causes of nocturnal airway narrowing include the sleeping posture,[4] interruption of bronchodilator or other treatment,[8] and allergens in bedding.[4]

Posture is not a major factor because patients who lie in bed throughout the 24 h continue to exhibit overnight bronchoconstriction,[4] and lying down does not produce sustained bronchoconstriction.[16] The treatment interval is not critical; regular spacing of treatment throughout the 24 h does not abolish nocturnal bronchospasm,[8] and nocturnal wheeze is a presenting complaint of many untreated asthmatic patients.

Allergens

It is unlikely that allergens in bedding are prime causes of nocturnal asthma, because avoidance of such allergens[6, 17] does not abolish nocturnal airway narrowing. In addition, overnight bronchoconstriction occurs in both allergic and nonallergic asthmatic patients[1, 2] and in normal people.[5, 9, 10] Allergic factors can, however, produce nocturnal wheeze; experimental allergen inhalation can cause bronchoconstriction on subsequent nights[18] (Fig. 80–3), and scrupulous exclusion of allergens can reduce circadian changes in peak flow rates and the frequency and severity of asthmatic attacks.[6, 17, 19]

These findings suggest that allergic reactions—and particularly, perhaps, late or delayed allergic reactions—are important in the development of nocturnal wheeze in some patients. There is a close relationship between the extent of nocturnal airway narrowing and the degree of airway twitchiness or bronchial reactivity.[20] It seems likely that such allergen exposure increases bronchial reactivity in predisposed patients and thus may result in nocturnal bronchoconstriction.

Airway Cooling

Cold, dry air causes bronchoconstriction in asthmatic patients.[21] It has been suggested that nocturnal asthma might be caused either by breathing cooler air at night or by bronchial wall cooling as a result of the overnight decrease in body core temperature. It seems unlikely that inspired air temperature and humidity are important because overnight bronchoconstriction persists in normal subjects when temperature and humidity are kept constant throughout the 24-h day.[10] Nevertheless, it has been reported that breathing warm, humid air (36 to 37°C, 100% saturation) overnight, compared with breathing room air (23°C, 17 to 24% saturation) overnight, abolished nocturnal bron-

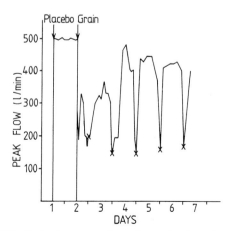

Figure 80–3. Peak flow rates throughout the day after bronchial challenge with placebo and then after challenge with grain dust, which initiates nocturnal bronchoconstriction. The crosses indicate morning flow rates. (Redrawn from Davies RJ, Green M, Schofield NM. Recurrent nocturnal asthma after exposure to grain dust. Am Rev Respir Dis. 1976;114:1011–1019.)

choconstriction in six of seven asthmatic patients.[22] It is not clear how well the patients slept when breathing the warm, humid air. If it kept them awake, this could explain the lack of bronchoconstriction.

Gastroesophageal Reflux

There seems to be a high incidence of gastroesophageal reflux (GER) in people with asthma, especially in those with nocturnal wheeze.[22a, 23] The GER may be clinically "silent."[22a] Although esophageal acid infusion in the early morning can produce alterations in respiratory timing, which suggests bronchoconstriction,[24] there is no convincing evidence that spontaneous GER causes either nocturnal bronchoconstriction[25, 26] or clinically significant bronchoconstriction at other times.[27] A histamine type 2 (H_2) receptor blocker in patients with symptomatic GER and nocturnal wheeze showed a small, but significant, improvement in nocturnal asthma symptoms but no change in morning peak flow rate.[28] Similarly, gastric acid suppression with omeprazole improved nocturnal but not daytime asthma symptoms.[22a]

Mucociliary Clearance

Mucociliary clearance is impaired during sleep,[29] and the accumulation of mucus in the airways could contribute to nocturnal airway narrowing. However, this accumulation seems unlikely to be a major factor in nocturnal wheeze, because bronchodilators are rapidly effective.

Bronchial Hyperreactivity

Bronchial responsiveness to inhaled histamine and allergens increases throughout the night.[30, 31] However, the airways are narrower at this time, and thus the increased response could reflect greater initial bronchomotor tone at night rather than any change in mucosal permeability or receptor or neuromuscular function. A skin prick test for allergens and histamine shows marked circadian variation; maximal effects are in the late evening, and a minimum is reached by early morning.[32] Thus, there may be circadian variations in reactivity, although the changes in sensitivity to skin tests are about 8 h ahead of the circadian changes in airway reactivity.

Endogenous Opioids

Because naloxone does not significantly alter overnight bronchoconstriction,[33] changes in endogenous opioids are unlikely to be important.

Is Nocturnal Wheeze Related to Sleep Stage?

Several groups have recorded electroencephalograms (EEGs) in sleeping asthmatic patients and noted

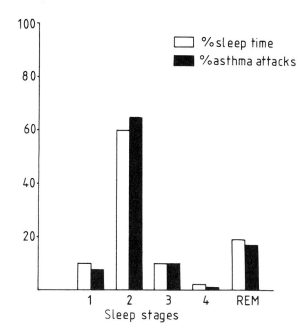

Figure 80–4. Comparison of percentage of night spent in each sleep stage with percentage of asthmatic awakenings from that stage. The asthmatic attack frequency was proportional to the frequency of each sleep stage. (Redrawn from Kales A, Beall GN, Bajor GF, et al. Sleep studies in asthmatic adults: relationship of attacks to sleep stage and time of night. J Allergy. 1968;41:164–173.)

the stage when patients awoke with attacks of asthma. Although an early study suggested that the patients awoke more frequently from rapid eye movement (REM) sleep than would be expected by chance,[34] this has not been confirmed.[35–37] The largest of these studies found that asthmatic attacks were randomly distributed throughout the stages of sleep in proportion to the amount of time spent in each sleep stage[35] (Fig. 80–4). Studies[36, 37] suggesting that slow-wave sleep may protect against asthmatic attacks are based on too few data to allow such a firm conclusion about a sleep state that takes up a relatively small proportion of sleep time. In addition, arousal from sleep in response to increased resistance is decreased in slow-wave sleep.[38] All these studies must be interpreted with caution, because the "asthmatic episodes" were usually loosely defined.[34–36]

When asthmatic patients were deliberately awakened from either REM sleep or nonrapid eye movement (NREM) sleep during 2 nights in a sleep laboratory and asked to perform forced expiratory maneuvers immediately on waking,[39] analysis of the FEV_1 obtained at time-matched awakenings in each subject showed that the FEV_1 was lower when the patients were awakened from REM sleep than from NREM sleep. However, the difference between REM sleep and NREM sleep averaged only 200 ml, whereas the overnight fall in FEV_1 was about 800 ml.

Esophageal pressure measurements suggest that pulmonary resistance does not differ between sleep stages[11] or may be slightly higher during slow-wave sleep.[40] Although these studies were based on small numbers of subjects who slept poorly, and one study measured total respiratory and not just pulmonary resistance,[40] it appears likely that there is little difference in the degree of airway narrowing between sleep stages.

Breathing Patterns During Sleep

Expiratory time would be expected to lengthen during bronchospasm, and this was initially thought to be increased in REM sleep in asthmatic patients.[41] Subsequent studies[42] have shown that there is no overall change in mean expiratory time between sleep stages but that expiratory time becomes markedly more variable in REM sleep, in keeping with the general irregularity in frequency and depth of breathing in that stage.[43, 44]

Like normal subjects,[44] asthmatic patients decrease their ventilation from wakefulness to the different sleep stages,[42] ventilation being lower during NREM sleep than during wakefulness, with the lowest levels tending to occur in REM sleep.[45] Paradoxical movement of the rib cage during REM sleep in adolescent asthmatic patients (aged 15 years, SD 1 year) has been reported.[45] This movement was not found in older asthmatic patients studied in our laboratory.[42] Because such paradoxical chest movement during REM sleep is common in early life,[46] it seems likely that the paradox reflects the compliance of youthful chest walls rather than any abnormality specific to asthma.

Whether there is any other abnormality of breathing pattern during sleep in asthmatic patients is unclear. We found a small, but significant, increase in irregular breathing in asthmatic patients due almost entirely to more apneas in asthmatic patients,[41] but others have found no such changes.[45, 47] The increased number of apneas in our study may have been the result of the

study's having been performed in the early summer, when the patients may have had mild rhinitis. This factor was unfortunately not noted at the time; it has only since become clear that nasal obstruction could cause apneas.[48, 49] In addition, the asthmatic patients in our study slept poorly, with more intervening wakefulness and drowsiness, which would predispose to apneas. The apneas were few and brief and were not associated with undue hypoxemia; thus, their clinical significance is dubious.

Lung volume falls during sleep, and this could contribute to increasing resistance to airflow because airway caliber will drop as lung volume decreases. However, it appears that this is not a major cause of sleep-related airway narrowing, although it may contribute.[50]

Reports suggest that some nocturnal asthmatic patients who snore or have obstructive sleep apnea may develop worsening of their asthma, perhaps as a reflex response to their upper airway vibration. Nasal continuous positive airway pressure therapy may be extremely helpful in such cases[51, 52] (Fig. 80–5).

Causes of Nocturnal Asthma: Conclusions

Nocturnal asthma is largely a sleep-synchronized circadian rhythm in airway caliber. How this results in airway narrowing is discussed below.

MECHANISMS AND EFFECTOR SYSTEMS FOR NOCTURNAL AIRWAY NARROWING
Autonomic Function

Bronchial muscle receives efferent innervation from the parasympathetic system via the vagus nerve, but

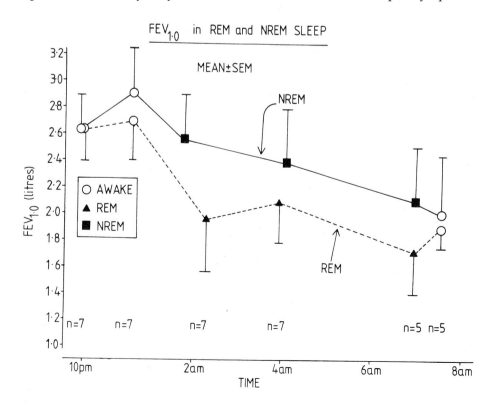

Figure 80–5. FEV_1 in seven asthmatic patients who were studied on 2 nights with time-matched, as far as possible, awakenings from REM sleep on 1 night and from NREM sleep on the other. FEV_1 was significantly lower after awakening from REM sleep. (Data from Shapiro C, Catterall JR, Montgomery I, et al. Do asthmatics suffer bronchoconstriction during rapid eye movement sleep? Br Med J. 1986;292:1161–1164.)

there is no evidence of direct sympathetic innervation to the muscle in human beings, although there are sympathetic nerves to the airway and some probably terminate on the vagal ganglia in the bronchial wall. Circulating (or inhaled) catechols probably cause bronchodilation by acting directly on bronchial smooth muscle. There is also a third component of the autonomic nervous system, which passes in the vagus nerve and produces bronchodilation, possibly using vasoactive intestinal peptide as a transmitter.[53]

Parasympathetic Nervous System

Parasympathetic tone tends to be increased at night.[54] Heart rate changes in parallel with alterations in peak flow rate in some asthmatic patients suggest that vagal activity might be important.[7] Cholinergic blockade with either inhaled ipratropium[55] or intravenous atropine[56] suggests that an increase in airway parasympathetic tone contributes significantly to the development of nocturnal asthma. However, increased vagal tone does not account for all the nocturnal airway narrowing.[55, 56]

Sympathetic Nervous System

There have been no studies of intrinsic sympathetic tone in nocturnal asthma. The bronchodilator response to infused epinephrine is unchanged at night[57]; thus, circadian changes in beta-adrenergic receptor sensitivity cannot explain nocturnal asthma.

Nonadrenergic, Noncholinergic Nervous System

The activity of the nonadrenergic, noncholinergic bronchodilating system has been shown to be impaired in the early morning.[58] This may contribute to the development of overnight bronchoconstriction.

Circadian Variation of Hormones

Cortisol. Nocturnal breathlessness in asthmatic patients is most marked when the urinary excretion of 17-hydroxycorticosteroid is at its nadir.[59] Peak flow rates parallel changes in the levels of circulating steroids.[1] This relationship is not causal; overnight falls in peak flow rate remain unchanged if plasma levels of 11-hydroxycorticosteroids are kept constant by infusion of hydrocortisone. In addition, therapy with large doses of steroids does not abolish morning dipping.[4] Thus, it seems unlikely that circadian changes in circulating cortisol levels are important in the pathogenesis of nocturnal bronchoconstriction.

Catecholamines and Other Mediators. Circulating cathecholamine levels show diurnal changes, with a nocturnal nadir.[60] Urinary catecholamine excretion falls to a minimum coincidental with the lowest peak flow rates in some patients.[61] However, catechol infusion does not abolish nocturnal airway narrowing.[62]

Airway Inflammation. It has been suggested that plasma histamine rises as airway caliber narrows at night.[57] However, this conclusion probably rested on imperfect methods and has not been confirmed.[63] Some,[64, 65] but not all,[66] studies have shown increased inflammatory cells in bronchoalveolar lavage fluid obtained at 4 AM from patients with nocturnal asthma. Increased inflammation has also been reported in the alveolar tissue of patients with nocturnal asthma at 4 AM, but the significance of this is unknown.[67] Leukotrienes are increased at night in patients with nocturnal asthma.[67a]

Causes of Nocturnal Bronchoconstriction: Conclusions

Airway narrowing at night is a normal physiological phenomenon, more obvious in asthmatic patients because their airways are already narrower by day. The major cause is a sleep-synchronized circadian rhythm probably effected largely by changes in the autonomic tone to the airways, with increased parasympathetic bronchoconstrictor tone and decreased nonadrenergic, noncholinergic bronchodilator function in the early morning.

CONSEQUENCES OF NOCTURNAL BRONCHOCONSTRICTION

Nocturnal wheezing causes inconvenience and disturbed sleep and probably also hypoxemia and death.

Sleep Disturbance

The major complaint of patients with nocturnal wheeze is that their sleep is interrupted and that they sometimes feel tired in the daytime. This sleep disruption has been confirmed by EEG studies,[35–37, 41, 68] which show a decreased sleep efficiency[37] with increased intervening wakefulness and drowsiness[37, 41] and, in one study, a decrease in total sleep time,[35] compared with age-matched normal subjects. This sleep disruption probably results in the impairment in daytime cognitive function in patients with nocturnal asthma in comparison with age- and education-matched normal subjects.[68] There was no evidence that this impairment in cognitive function was due to drug therapy.[68] Indeed, treatment of nocturnal asthma has been reported to improve cognitive function, but this improvement could have been due to increased familiarity with the tests.[69] Nevertheless, the potential damage to daytime cognitive function, work, and school performance caused by nocturnal sleep disruption underlines the importance of intensifying therapy in patients with nocturnal asthma.

Patients with acute, severe asthma often have several worsening nights with little or no sleep during their attacks. Sleep deprivation for as little as 24 h can reduce ventilatory drive by as much as one third,[70] and such a blunting of drive may be a factor, along with fatigue and continuing bronchospasm, in the subsequent development of hypoxemia and hypercapnia in some of these patients.

Hypoxemia

Patients with nocturnal asthma can undoubtedly become hypoxemic during the night,[37, 41, 71] but the hypoxemia is rarely severe; in stable asthmatic patients studied at sea level, the lowest saturation is normally in the range of 85 to 95%.[41, 42] However, there have been no comparable studies in unstable patients with nocturnal asthma, and it seems likely that these patients may become more hypoxemic, and hypoxemia is a normal accompaniment of spontaneous or induced[72] bronchoconstriction by day. Indeed, in one report,[37] there were two episodes of desaturation that lasted for 5 min before the patients woke with nocturnal wheeze. On the other hand, another study of six attacks of nocturnal wheeze found none to be associated with significant hypoxemia.[73]

In stable asthmatic adults, we found no correlation between the extent of hypoxemia and the degree of overnight bronchoconstriction[41]; indeed, the extent of nocturnal hypoxemia appears to be predictable from the level of oxygenation during wakefulness, which suggests that preexisting rather than nocturnal events determine the extent of hypoxemia during sleep. However, in asthmatic children, it was found that nocturnal desaturation correlated with the percentage fall in FEV_1 overnight and that bronchodilators reduced nocturnal desaturation.[71] It is possible that the altitude (1600 m) at which this study was performed exaggerated the desaturation, which makes such a relationship more obvious than it is at sea level.

Nocturnal Asthmatic Attacks

Asthmatic patients present with attacks more frequently by night than by day, both to their family physician and to the emergency department.[74] This timing is inconvenient to all concerned.

Deaths

Fortunately, deaths from asthma are now uncommon. There has been controversy over whether there is a nocturnal excess of deaths from asthma.[47, 75, 76] Although two studies showed no increase in deaths at night,[47, 76] combining the four largest published series[47, 75–76, 77] revealed that 93 of the 219 deaths occurred between midnight and 8 AM, which indicates a significant ($P < .01$ by χ^2) excess of nocturnal deaths. With subdivision according to the place, there was an excess nocturnal rate for the 146 deaths that occurred at home

($P < .05$). The same trend was seen for the 73 deaths occurring in hospital; this was not significant ($0.15 > P > 0.10$). The death rate is, of course, higher at night than by day in the general population,[78] but this averages only a 5% increase between midnight and 8 AM, in contrast to the 28% increase observed in these asthmatic patients.

Excess nocturnal mortality could be due to many factors, including the inability of hypoxia,[79, 80] hypercapnia,[81, 82] or increased airflow resistance[38, 83] to awaken sleeping subjects rapidly, with resultant delays in taking treatment, reticence to summon family or medical help at night, and delay in the arrival of medical assistance. Eight of 10 ventilatory arrests in asthmatic patients in hospital occurred in the early morning,[84] which suggests that the unavailability of medical assistance is not a major factor. One of the most important causes of nocturnal death seems to be the occurrence of nocturnal bronchospasm. The two asthmatic patients who died at night during a prospective study were both morning dippers,[85] which suggests that nocturnal bronchoconstriction can be life-threatening. Thus, the morning dip pattern of asthma should be sought and recognized as potentially dangerous when it is marked in unstable asthmatic patients.

TREATMENT

Nocturnal bronchoconstriction is a sign of inadequate control of asthma, and the new development of nocturnal wheeze in a patient must be regarded as a dangerous sign requiring monitoring and urgent treatment. Nocturnal wheeze often responds to increasing conventional daytime maintenance treatment with either prophylactic agents or bronchodilators.[13, 86–88a] Only when optimal daytime control does not abolish nocturnal symptoms should additional treatment be directed at nocturnal wheeze.

Inhalation of bronchodilators immediately before sleep, repeated whenever the patient is awakened by wheeze, is the initial treatment of choice; side effects are few. However, conventional inhaled beta$_2$ agonists last only around 4 h, and most people sleep for longer than that. Inhaled ipratropium may last slightly longer,[55, 89] but this increased duration has proved disappointing in clinical practice.

For those for whom these treatments are insufficient, long-acting bronchodilators—either inhaled or oral—should be used. Salmeterol is a beta$_2$ agonist that lasts over 12 h after inhalation. We have shown that salmeterol improves symptoms, overnight peak flow rates, and sleep quality in nocturnal asthma[90] (Figs. 80–6, 80–7, and 80–8). Formoterol, another long-acting inhaled agent, has been shown to improve overnight lung function.[91]

In terms of oral bronchodilators, there appears to be little to choose, from the bronchodilation point of view, between oral theophyllines[37, 92–94] and oral beta$_2$ agonists.[94, 95] Both can markedly reduce nocturnal symptoms, and the choice will largely be determined by whether the patient develops side effects. These

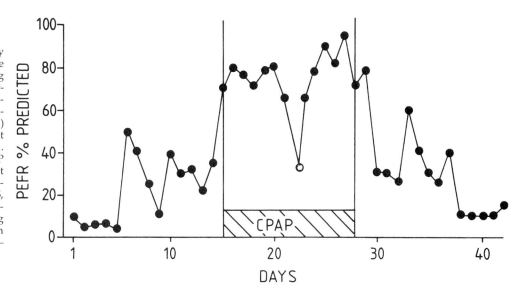

Figure 80–6. Peak expiratory flow rate (PEFR), as percentage predicted, at 3 AM in a snoring asthmatic patient measured during a control period, during a period of nocturnal continuous positive airway pressure (CPAP) therapy, and during a subsequent period after CPAP withdrawal. The open circle during the CPAP period represents a single night when the CPAP period was withdrawn. (Redrawn from Chan CS, Woolcock AJ, Sullivan CE. Nocturnal asthma: role of snoring and obstructive sleep apnea. Am Rev Respir Dis. 1988;137:1502–1504.)

agents can often be taken effectively once a day immediately before going to bed, thus reducing daytime side effects.[92] Theophylline absorption tends to be lower at night than in the morning.[96] This finding is not due to diurnal variations in theophylline absorption or disposition[97] but probably results from differences between nocturnal and morning gastric content, physical activity, and posture. However, it is important to be aware of this difference, because larger dosages can be given at night. It has been reported that oral theophyllines disturb sleep, as judged by the EEG in patients with

nocturnal asthma, despite improving nocturnal symptoms and overnight changes in flow rates.[98] However, there was no evidence of sleep disturbance in a medium-term study of normal subjects placed on theophylline.[99] Oral beta$_2$ agonists produce similar improvements in respiratory function and symptoms and certainly do not impair sleep in patients with nocturnal asthma.[100]

There have been relatively few studies comparing long-acting inhaled beta$_2$ agonists with other agents in the management of nocturnal asthma.[101, 101a] One study showed no major difference in efficacy between salmeterol and oral theophylline, although there were marginal benefits in favor of salmeterol in terms of frequency of arousals from sleep and improved quality of life.[101] Another study showed that salmeterol compared with theophylline resulted in less deterioration in

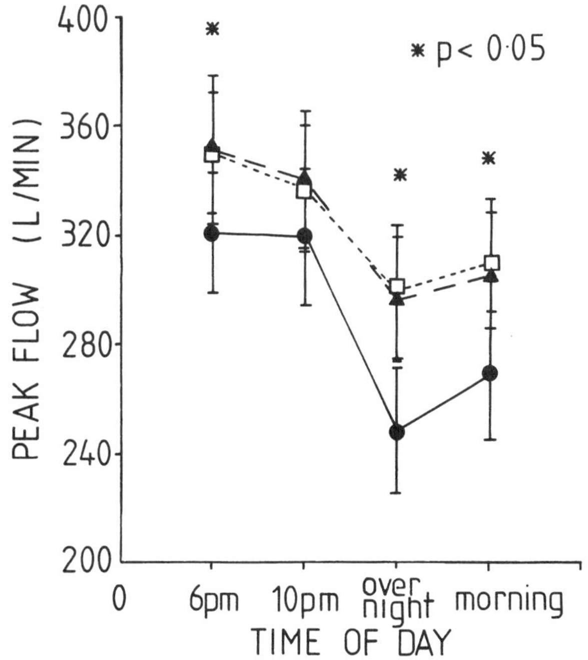

Figure 80–7. Mean (SE) peak expiratory flow rate in 18 asthmatic patients receiving placebo (●) or salmeterol 50 μg (□) or 100 μg (▲) twice daily. (Redrawn from Fitzpatrick MF, Mackay TM, Driver H, et al. Salmeterol in nocturnal asthma: a double blind, placebo controlled trial of a long acting inhaled β₂ agonist. Br Med J. 1990;301:1365–1368.)

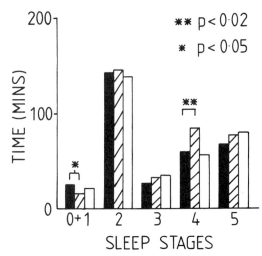

Figure 80–8. Mean (SE) time spent in each sleep stage by 18 asthmatic patients receiving placebo (*solid bar*) or salmeterol 50 μg (*hatched bar*) or 100 μg (*open bar*) twice daily. (Redrawn from Fitzpatrick MF, Mackay T, Driver H, et al. Salmeterol in nocturnal asthma: a double blind, placebo controlled trial of a long acting inhaled β₂ agonist. Br Med J. 1990;301:1365–1368.)

nighttime lung function and improvement in subjective sleep quality.[101a] Salmeterol was superior to oral slow release terbutaline in terms of the number of nights free of awakenings, morning peak flow rates, and assessment of clinical efficacy.[102] Salmeterol 50 μg twice daily was similar in efficacy to fluticasone 250 μg twice daily in improving nocturnal asthma.[103] It seems likely that inhaled long-acting bronchodilators will gradually take over from oral long-acting bronchodilators because side effects seem to be fewer.

Patients who do not respond to these measures will require oral steroid therapy. A small minority will need further immunosuppression such as methotrexate, which has been shown to improve symptoms and FEV_1.[104]

In the small minority of asthmatic patients whose nocturnal airway narrowing relates to their snoring or obstructive apneas, continuous positive airway pressure therapy should be tried.[51, 52]

CONCLUSIONS

Although there have been advances in our understanding of both pathophysiology and therapeutics, overnight wheeze remains a problem for many patients with the common condition of asthma.[105] Overnight wheeze is caused by a circadian rhythm in airway caliber which is at least partially controlled by neural factors. Development of long-acting inhaled bronchodilators has simplified the management of these symptoms.

References

1. Connolly CK. Diurnal rhythms in airway obstruction. Br J Dis Chest. 1979;73:357–366.
2. Turner-Warwick M. The definition and recognition of nocturnal asthma. R Soc Med Int Congr Symp Ser. 1984;73:3–5.
3. Floyer J. A Treatise of the Asthma. London, England: Wilkin; 1698.
4. Clark TJH, Hetzel MR. Diurnal variation of asthma. Br J Dis Chest. 1977;71:87–92.
5. Lewinsohn HC, Capel LH, Smart J. Changes in forced expiratory volume throughout the day. Br Med J. 1960;1:462–464.
6. Reinberg A, Gervais P. Circadian rhythms in respiratory functions, with special reference to human chronophysiology and chronopharmacology. Bull Physiopathol Respir. 1972;8:663–675.
7. Turner-Warwick M. On observing patterns of airflow obstruction in chronic asthma. Br J Dis Chest. 1977;71:73–86.
8. Fitzpatrick MF, Martin K, Fossey E, et al. Snoring, asthma and sleep disturbance in Britain: a community based survey. Eur Respir J. 1993;6:531–535.
9. Hetzel MR, Clark TJH. Comparison of normal and asthmatic circadian rhythms in peak expiratory flow rate. Thorax. 1980;35:732–738.
10. Kerr HD. Diurnal variation of respiratory function independent of air quality. Arch Environ Health. 1973;26:144–153.
11. Ballard RD, Saathoff MC, Patel DK, et al. Effect of sleep on nocturnal bronchoconstriction and ventilatory patterns in asthmatics. J Appl Physiol. 1989;67:243–249.
12. Catterall JR, Rhind GB, Stewart IC, et al. Effect of sleep deprivation on overnight bronchoconstriction in nocturnal asthma. Thorax. 1986;41:676–680.
13. Connolly CK. The effect of bronchodilators on diurnal rhythms in airway obstruction. Br J Dis Chest. 1981;75:197–203.
14. Hetzel MR, Clark TJH. Does sleep cause nocturnal asthma? Thorax. 1979;34:749–754.
15. Perkoff GT, Eik-Nes K, Nugent CA, et al. Studies of the diurnal variation of plasma 17-hydroxycorticosteroids in man. J Clin Endocrinol. 1959;19:432–433.
16. Whyte KF, Douglas NJ. Posture and nocturnal asthma. Thorax. 1989;44:579–581.
17. Scherr MS, Peck LW. The effects of high efficiency air filtration system on night time asthma attacks. W V Med J. 1977;73:144–148.
18. Davies RJ, Green M, Schofield NM. Recurrent nocturnal asthma after exposure to grain dust. Am Rev Respir Dis. 1976;114:1011–1019.
19. Platts-Mills TAE, Mitchell EB, Nock P, et al. Reduction of bronchial hyper-reactivity during prolonged allergen avoidance. Lancet. 1982;2:675–677.
20. Ryan G, Latimer KM, Dolovich J, et al. Bronchial responsiveness to histamine: Relationship to diurnal variation of peak flow rate, improvement after bronchodilator, and airway calibre. Thorax. 1982;37:423–429.
21. Deal EC, McFadden ER, Ingram RH, et al. Role of respiratory heat exchange in production of exercise-induced asthma. J Appl Physiol. 1979;46:467–475.
22. Chen WY, Chai H. Airway cooling and nocturnal asthma. Chest. 1982;81:675–680.
22a. Kiljander TO, Salomaa ER, Hietanen EK, et al. Gastroesophageal reflux in asthmatics: a double-blind, placebo-controlled crossover study with omeprazole. Chest. 1999;116:1257–1264.
23. Martin ME, Grunstein MM, Larsen GL. The relationship of gastroesophageal reflux to nocturnal wheezing in children with asthma. Ann Allergy. 1982;49:318–322.
24. Davis RS, Larsen GL, Grunstein MM. Respiratory response to intraesophageal acid infusion in asthmatic children during sleep. J Allergy Clin Immunol. 1983;72:393–398.
25. Hughes DM, Spier S, Riulin J, et al. Gastroesophageal reflux during sleep in asthmatic patients. J Pediatr. 1983;102:666–672.
26. Nagel RA, Brown P, Perks WH, et al. Ambulatory pH monitoring of gastro-oesophageal reflux in "morning dipper" asthmatics. Br Med J. 1988;297:1371–1373.
27. Perpina M, Pellicer C, Marco V, et al. The significance of the reflex bronchoconstriction provoked by gastroesophageal reflux in bronchial asthma. Eur J Respir Dis. 1985;66:91–97.
28. Goodall RJR, Earis JE, Cooper DN, et al. Relationship between asthma and gastro-oesophageal reflux. Thorax. 1981;36:116–121.
29. Bateman JRM, Pavia D, Clarke SW. The retention of lung secretions during the night in normal subjects. Clin Sci. 1978;55:523–527.
30. De Vries K, Goei JT, Booy-Noord H, et al. Changes during 24 hours in the lung function and histamine hyperreactivity of the bronchial tree in asthmatic and bronchitic patients. Int Arch Allergy. 1962;20:93–101.
31. Gervais P, Reinberg A, Gervais C, et al. Twenty-four hour rhythm in the bronchial hyperactivity to house dust mite in asthmatics. J Allergy Clin Immunol. 1972;59:207–213.
32. Smolensky MH, Reinberg A, Queng JT. The chronobiology and chronopharmacology of allergy. Ann Allergy. 1981;47:234–251.
33. Al-Damluji S, Thompson PJ, Citron KM, et al. Effect of naloxone on circadian rhythm in lung function. Thorax. 1983;38:914–918.
34. Ravenscroft K, Hartmann EL. The temporal correlation of nocturnal asthmatic attacks and the D-state. Psychophysiology. 1968;4:396–397.
35. Kales A, Beall GN, Bajor GF, et al. Sleep studies in asthmatic adults: relationship of attacks to sleep stage and time of night. J Allergy. 1968;41:164–173.
36. Kales A, Kales JD, Sly RM, et al. Sleep patterns of asthmatic children: all-night electroencephalographic studies. J Allergy. 1970;46:300–308.
37. Montplaisir J, Walsh J, Malo JL. Nocturnal asthma features of attacks, sleep and breathing patterns. Am Rev Respir Dis. 1982;125:18–22.
38. Gugger M, Molloy J, Gould GA, et al. Ventilatory and arousal responses to added inspiratory resistance during sleep. Am Rev Respir Dis. 1989;140:1301–1307.
39. Shapiro C, Catterall JR, Montgomery I, et al. Do asthmatics suffer bronchoconstriction during rapid eye movement sleep? Br Med J. 1986;292:1161–1164.

40. Bellia V, Cuttitta G, Insalaco G, et al. Relationship of nocturnal bronchoconstriction to sleep stages. Am Rev Respir Dis. 1989;140:363–367.

41. Catterall JR, Douglas NJ, Calverley PM, et al. Irregular breathing and hypoxaemia during sleep in chronic stable asthma. Lancet. 1982;1:301–304.

42. Morgan AD, Rhind GB, Connaughton JJ, et al. Breathing and oxygenation during sleep in patients with nocturnal asthma. Thorax. 1987;42:600–603.

43. Aserinsky E. Periodic respiratory pattern occurring in conjunction with eye movements during sleep. Science. 1965;150:763–766.

44. Douglas NJ, White DP, Pickett CK, et al. Respiration during sleep in normal man. Thorax. 1982;37:840–844.

45. Tabachnik E, Muller NL, Levison H, et al. Chest wall mechanics and patterns of breathing during sleep in asthmatic adolescents. Am Rev Respir Dis. 1981;124:269–273.

46. Knill R, Andrews W, Bryan AC, et al. Respiratory load compensation in infants. J Appl Physiol. 1976;40:357–361.

47. MacDonald JB, Seaton A, Williams DA. Asthma deaths in Cardiff 1963–74: 90 deaths outside hospital. Br Med J. 1976;1:1493–1495.

48. McNicholas WT, Tarlo S, Cole P, et al. Obstructive apneas during sleep in patients with seasonal allergic rhinitis. Am Rev Respir Dis. 1982;126:625–628.

49. Zwillich CW, Pickett C, Hanson FN, et al. Disturbed sleep and prolonged apnea during nasal obstruction in normal men. Am Rev Respir Dis. 1981;124:158–160.

50. Ballard RD, Irvin CG, Martin RJ, et al. Influence of sleep on lung volume in asthmatic patients and normal subjects. J Appl Physiol. 1990;68:2034–2041.

51. Chan CS, Woolcock AJ, Sullivan CE. Nocturnal asthma: role of snoring and obstructive sleep apnea. Am Rev Respir Dis. 1988;137:1502–1504.

52. Guilleminault C, Quera-Salva MA, Powell N, et al. Nocturnal asthma: snoring, small pharynx and nasal CPAP. Eur Respir J. 1988;1:902–907.

53. Matsuzaki Y, Hamasaki Y, Said SI. Vasoactive intestinal peptide: a possible transmitter of nonadrenergic relaxation of guinea pig airways. Science. 1980;210:1252–1253.

54. Baust W, Bohnert B. The regulation of heart rate during sleep. Exp Brain Res. 1969;7:169–180.

55. Catterall JR, Rhind GB, Whyte KF, et al. Is nocturnal asthma caused by changes in airway cholinergic activity? Thorax. 1988;43:720–724.

56. Morrison JF, Pearson SB, Dean HG. Parasympathetic nervous system in nocturnal asthma. Br Med J. 1988;296:1427–1429.

57. Barnes P, Fitzgerald G, Brown M, et al. Nocturnal asthma and changes in circulating epinephrine, histamine and cortisol. N Engl J Med. 1980;303:263–267.

58. Mackay TW, Fitzpatrick MF, Douglas NJ. Non-adrenergic, non-cholinergic nervous system and overnight airway calibre in asthmatic and normal subjects. Lancet. 1991;338:1289–1292.

59. Reinberg A, Ghata J, Sidi E. Nocturnal asthma attacks: their relationship to the circadian adrenal cycle. J Allergy. 1963;34:323–330.

60. Reinberg A, Halberg F, Ghata J, et al. Rhythme circadien de diverse fonction physiologiques de l'homme adulte sain, actif et au repos. J Physiol Paris. 1969;61(suppl 2):383.

61. Soutar CA, Carruthers M, Pickering CAC. Nocturnal asthma and urinary adrenaline and noradrenaline excretion. Thorax. 1977;32:677–683.

62. Morrison JFJ, Teale C, Pearson SB, et al. Adrenaline and nocturnal asthma. Br Med J. 1990;301:473–476.

63. Fitzpatrick MF, Mackay T, Walters C, et al. Circulating histamine and eosinophil cationic protein levels in nocturnal asthma. Clin Sci. 1992;83:227–232.

64. Martin RJ, Cicutto LC, Smith HR, et al. Airways inflammation in nocturnal asthma. Am Rev Respir Dis. 1991;143:351–357.

65. Mackay TW, Wallace WAH, Howie SEM, et al. Role of inflammation in nocturnal asthma. Thorax. 1994;49:257–262.

66. Jarjour NN, Busse WW, Calhoun WJ. Enhanced production of oxygen radicals in nocturnal asthma. Am Rev Respir Dis. 1992;146:905–911.

67. Kraft M, Djukanovic R, Wilson S, et al. Alveolar tissue inflammation in asthma. Am J Respir Crit Care Med. 1996;154:1505–1510.

67a. Kraft M. Corticosteroids and leukotrienes: chronobiology and chronotherapy. Chronobiol Int. 1999;16:683–693.

68. Fitzpatrick MF, Engleman H, Whyte KF, et al. Morbidity in nocturnal asthma: sleep quality and daytime cognitive performance. Thorax. 1991;46:569–573.

69. Weersink EJ, van Zomeren EH, Koeter GH, et al. Treatment of nocturnal airway obstruction improves daytime cognitive performance in asthmatics. Am J Respir Crit Care Med. 1997;156:1144–1150.

70. White DP, Douglas NJ, Pickett CK, et al. Sleep deprivation and the control of ventilation. Am Rev Respir Dis. 1983;128:984–986.

71. Smith TH, Hudgel DW. Arterial oxygen desaturation during sleep in children with asthma and its relation to airway obstruction and ventilatory drive. Pediatrics. 1980;66:746–751.

72. Stewart IC, Parker A, Catterall JR, et al. Effect of bronchial challenge on breathing patterns and arterial oxygenation in stable asthma. Chest. 1989;95:65–71.

73. Issa FG, Sullivan CE. Respiratory muscle activity in thoracoabdominal movement during acute episodes of asthma during sleep. Am Rev Respir Dis. 1985;132:999–1004.

74. Horn CR, Clark TJH, Cochrane GM. Is there a circadian variation in respiratory morbidity? Br J Dis Chest. 1987;81:248–251.

75. Cochrane GM, Clark TJH. A survey of asthma mortality in patients between ages 35 and 64 in the Greater London hospitals in 1971. Thorax. 1975;30:300–305.

76. MacDonald JB, MacDonald ET, Seaton A, et al. Asthma deaths in Cardiff 1963–74: 53 deaths in hospital. Br Med J. 1976;2:721–723.

77. British Thoracic Association. Death from asthma in two regions of England. Br Med J. 1982;285:1251–1255.

78. Smolensky M, Halberg F, Sargent F. Chronobiology of the life sequence. In: Itoh S, Ogata K, Yoshimura H, eds. Advances in Climatic Physiology. Berlin, Germany: Springer-Verlag; 1972:281–318.

79. Berthon-Jones M, Sullivan CE. Ventilatory and arousal responses to hypoxia in sleeping humans. Am Rev Respir Dis. 1982;125:632–639.

80. Douglas NJ, White DP, Weil JV, et al. Hypoxic ventilatory response decreases during sleep in normal men. Am Rev Respir Dis. 1982;125:286–289.

81. Berthon-Jones M, Sullivan CE. Ventilation and arousal responses to hypercapnia in normal sleeping adults. J Appl Physiol. 1984;57:59–67.

82. Douglas NJ, White DP, Weil JV, et al. Hypercapnic ventilatory response in sleeping adults. Am Rev Respir Dis. 1982;126:758–762.

83. Iber C, Berssenbrugge A, Skatrud JB, et al. Ventilatory adaptations to resistive loading during wakefulness in non-REM sleep. J Appl Physiol. 1982;52:607–614.

84. Hetzel MR, Clark TJH, Branthwaite MA. Asthma: analysis of sudden deaths and ventilatory arrests in hospital. Br Med J. 1977;1:808–811.

85. Bateman JRM, Clarke SW. Sudden death in asthma. Thorax. 1979;34:40–44.

86. Carpentiere G, Merino S, Castello F. Effect of inhaled fenoterol on the circadian rhythm of expiratory flow in allergic bronchial asthma. Chest. 1983;83:211–214.

87. Horn CR, Clark TJH, Cochrane GM. Inhaled therapy reduces morning dips in asthma. Lancet. 1984;1:1143–1145.

88. Neagley SR, White DP, Zwillich CW. Breathing during sleep in stable asthmatic subjects. Influence of inhaled bronchodilators. Chest. 1986;90:334–337.

88a. Canadian Asthma Consensus Group. Canadian Asthma Consensus Report. CMAJ 1999;161(11 suppl):S1–S62.

89. Douglas NJ, Sudlow MF, Flenley DC. The effect of an inhaled atropine-like agent on normal airway function. J Appl Physiol. 1979;46:256–262.

90. Fitzpatrick MF, Mackay T, Driver H, et al. Salmeterol in nocturnal asthma: a double blind, placebo controlled trial of a long acting inhaled b_2 agonist. Br Med J. 1990;301:1365–1368.

91. Maesen FPV, Smeets JJ, Gubbelmans HLL, et al. Formoterol in the treatment of nocturnal asthma. Chest. 1990;98:866–870.

92. Barnes PJ, Greening AP, Neville L, et al. Single-dose slow-

release aminophylline at night prevents nocturnal asthma. Lancet. 1982;1:299–301.

93. Davies PDO, Fennerty AG, Benfield GFA, et al. Twice daily slow-release theophylline versus placebo for "morning dipping" in asthma. Br J Clin Pharmacol. 1984;17:335–340.

94. Fairfax AJ, McNabb WR, Davies HJ, et al. Slow-release oral salbutamol and aminophylline in nocturnal asthma: relation of overnight changes in lung function and plasma drug levels. Thorax. 1980;35:526–530.

95. Milledge JS, Morris J. A comparison of slow-release salbutamol with slow-release aminophylline in nocturnal asthma. J Int Med Res. 1979;7:106–110.

96. Scott PH, Tabachnik E, MacLeod S, et al. Sustained-release theophylline for childhood asthma: evidence for circadian variation of theophylline pharmacokinetics. J Pediatr. 1981;99:476–479.

97. Taylor DR, Duffin D, Kinney CD, et al. Investigation of diurnal changes in the disposition of theophylline. Br J Clin Pharmacol. 1983;16:413–416.

98. Rhind GB, Connaughton JJ, McFie J, et al. Sustained release choline theophyllinate in nocturnal asthma. Br Med J. 1985;291:1605–1607.

99. Fitzpatrick MF, Engleman HM, Boellert F, et al. Effect of therapeutic theophylline levels on the sleep quality and daytime cognitive performance of normal subjects. Am Rev Respir Dis. 1992;145:1355–1358.

100. Stewart IC, Rhind GB, Power JT, et al. Effects of sustained release terbutaline on symptoms and sleep quality in patients with nocturnal asthma. Thorax. 1987;42:797–800.

101. Selby C, Engleman HM, Fitzpatrick MF, et al. Inhaled salmeterol or oral theophylline in nocturnal asthma? Am J Respir Crit Care Med. 1997;155:104–108.

101a. Wiegand L, Mende CN, Zaidel G, et al. Salmeterol versus theophylline: sleep and efficacy outcomes in patients with nocturnal asthma. Chest. 1999;115:1525–1532.

102. Brambilla C, Chastang C, George D, et al. Salmeterol compared with slow release terbutaline in nocturnal asthma. A multicentre randomised double blind double dummy sequential clinical trial. Allergy. 1994;49:421–426.

103. Weersink EJ, Douma RR, Postma DS, et al. Fluticasone propionate, salmeterol xinafoate, and their combination in the treatment of nocturnal asthma. Am J Respir Crit Care Med. 1997;155:1241–1246.

104. Mullarkey MF, Lammert JK, Blumenstein BA. Long term methotrexate treatment in corticosteroid dependent asthma. Ann Intern Med. 1990;112:577–581.

105. D'Ambrosio CM, Mohsenin V. Sleep in asthma. Clin Chest Med. 1998;19:127–137.

81

Chronic Obstructive Pulmonary Disease

Neil J. Douglas

In the late 1950s, Robin and colleagues[1, 2] reported that "alveolar" carbon dioxide tension rose by 10 mmHg during sleep in seven patients with emphysema and chronic hypercapnia and that four exhibited Cheyne-Stokes respiration during sleep. Subsequent studies that involved the use of an early oximeter demonstrated that arterial oxygen saturation fell in patients with chronic obstructive pulmonary disease (COPD) during sleep; the authors noted that the lowest oxygen saturations during sleep occurred in those who had the lowest oxygen saturations during wakefulness.[3] These findings were subsequently confirmed on the basis of arterial blood gas tension measurements,[4] and later studies that combined electroenceph-

alographic sleep staging with arterial blood gas tension measurements demonstrated that the most severe hypoxemia and hypercapnia occurred during rapid eye movement (REM) sleep.[5–7]

The development of accurate oximeters allowed the continuous measurement of arterial oxygen saturation during sleep in patients with COPD. Douglas et al.[8] reported that the majority of hypoxemic episodes occurred during REM sleep (Fig. 81–1) and that during these episodes, arterial oxygen tension dropped to as low as 26 mmHg. These observations have been widely confirmed[9–13] in studies that indicate hypoxemia is most marked during REM sleep, particularly during periods within REM sleep, when eye movements are

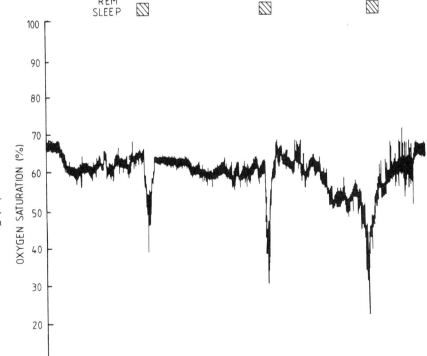

Figure 81–1. Overnight oxygen saturation in a patient with chronic obstructive pulmonary disease. Shaded areas represent REM sleep during which marked oxygen desaturation occurs.

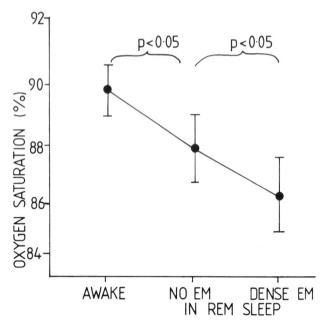

Figure 81–2. Oxygen saturation in 18 patients with chronic obstructive pulmonary disease during wakefulness and REM sleep; REM sleep is subdivided into periods when there are no eye movements (EM) or periods when there are frequent eye movements (dense EM). (Redrawn from George CF, West P, Kryger MH. Oxygenation and breathing pattern during phasic and tonic REM in patients with chronic obstructive pulmonary disease. Sleep. 1987;10:234–243.)

frequent[11–14] (Fig. 81–2). Patients become more hypoxemic during sleep than during exercise,[15] and because patients with COPD spend much more time sleeping than exercising, sleep is a more significant cause of hypoxemic load for these patients. Arterial carbon dioxide tension rises during these hypoxemic episodes, although the additional elevation in carbon dioxide tension usually is relatively small.[5, 6, 8, 15, 16]

MECHANISMS OF HYPOXEMIA DURING SLEEP IN CHRONIC OBSTRUCTIVE PULMONARY DISEASE

Many factors have been proposed as causes of hypoxemia during sleep in COPD, including hypoventilation, a decrease in functional residual capacity, and ventilation-perfusion mismatching.

Hypoventilation

Minute ventilation decreases during all sleep stages compared with wakefulness in normal subjects[17] and in patients with COPD.[13] The reduction in ventilation from wakefulness to nonrapid eye movement (NREM) sleep is small, but during REM sleep, there is intermittent marked hypoventilation.[17, 18] This hypoventilation in normal subjects is most severe during periods of frequent eye movements,[19, 20] when tidal volume falls substantially.

The typical REM sleep–related desaturation in COPD is accompanied by hypoventilation and not by apneas[11, 13, 14, 21] (Fig. 81–3). Although ventilation had not been accurately measured in sleeping patients with COPD, their breathing pattern during REM sleep is similar to that in normal subjects.[12] It has been estimated that alveolar ventilation in normal subjects is about 40% lower during bursts of eye movements in REM sleep than during wakefulness.[16, 18] Because patients with COPD have raised physiological dead spaces, the rapid shallow breathing during bursts of eye movements in REM sleep would be expected to produce an even greater decrease in alveolar ventilation than occurs in normal subjects. This contributes significantly to their REM sleep–related hypoxemia, and it has been suggested that such hypoventilation would be adequate to account for all the hypoxemia observed in REM sleep in patients with COPD.[22]

Many factors contribute to hypoventilation during sleep. In NREM sleep, ventilation falls in normal subjects despite an increase in respiratory effort as measured on the basis of occlusion pressure.[23, 24] It is likely that this hypoventilation in NREM sleep is in part due to the increase in upper airway resistance that occurs during NREM sleep.[25, 26] Furthermore, the ventilatory response to added respiratory resistance is impaired during NREM sleep,[24, 27] which allows hypoventilation to occur. There also may be loss of the "wakefulness drive to breathing," which contributes to hypoventilation during NREM sleep[28] and an effect from the fall in basal metabolic rate during sleep.[29]

The marked intermittent hypoventilation during REM sleep seems unlikely to be due to further increases in upper airway resistance because overall airway resistance is no greater in REM sleep than in NREM sleep, at least in normal subjects.[26] Furthermore, although few measurements have been made, it appears that the ventilatory response to inspiratory resistance is similar in NREM and REM sleep.[24, 27] During REM sleep, there is altered brainstem function with phasic activity of respiratory neurons in animals.[30] It seems that such central diminution in respiratory output may be a major factor in producing REM sleep–related hypoventilation. During REM sleep, there is hypotonia of postural muscles, including the intercostal muscles,[31] so that the rib cage contributes less to ventilation.[20, 32] This further decreases ventilation during REM sleep in hyperinflated patients with COPD in whom the flattened diaphragm pulls in the flaccid lower chest wall, with resultant highly inefficient ventilation. This may explain why patients with COPD become relatively more hypoxemic during sleep than do patients with pulmonary fibrosis.[33] In addition, the "postural" hypotonia of REM sleep involves not only the intercostal muscles but also the accessory muscles of respiration,[34] which may be important in maintaining adequate ventilation in patients with COPD.

The hypoventilation of REM sleep is accompanied by a marked diminution of both the hypoxic[28, 35] and hypercapnic[36, 37] ventilatory responses. The normal defense mechanisms of the body to the resulting hypoxemia and hypercapnia are diminished.

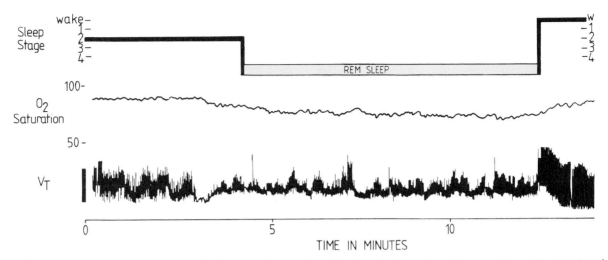

Figure 81–3. Tidal volume V_T, O_2 saturation, and sleep stage in a patient with chronic obstructive pulmonary disease illustrated in the drop in O_2 saturation and irregular hyperventilation during REM sleep. (Redrawn from Fletcher EC, Gray BA, Levin DC. Non-apneic mechanisms of arterial oxygen desaturation during rapid-eye movement sleep. J Appl Physiol. 1983;54:632–639.)

Decrease in Functional Residual Capacity

Functional residual capacity decreases during REM sleep in normal subjects.[26] Earlier reports that included the use of inductive plethysmography, which may not be accurate during sleep,[38] suggested that functional residual capacity also fell during REM sleep in patients with COPD.[13] However, body plethysmographic studies indicate that functional residual capacity does not change during sleep in patients with COPD, although these data were gathered in only five patients.[39]

Ventilation-Perfusion Mismatching

It is inevitable that additional ventilation-perfusion mismatching occurs in patients with COPD during the marked hypoventilation of REM sleep. This is supported by evidence that cardiac output is maintained during these episodes of hypoventilation, which indicates changes in global ventilation-perfusion matching.[21, 22] Unfortunately, technology does not allow assessment of the importance of ventilation-perfusion matching relative to the other mechanisms involved. Techniques for quantifying ventilation-perfusion mismatch are reliant on a steady state of both ventilation and metabolism; certainly, the former does not occur during REM sleep when ventilation is extremely variable.[22] This negates many of the arguments previously advanced for the importance of ventilation-perfusion mismatching. For example, it has been suggested that the greater decrease in alveolar P_{O_2} compared with the rise in arterial P_{CO_2} indicates the importance of ventilation-perfusion changes[5, 6] during REM sleep in patients with COPD. However, because the body stores of carbon dioxide are much larger than those of oxygen,[22] the transient episodes of hypoventilation that occur during REM sleep produce much greater decreases in P_{O_2} than rises in P_{CO_2}, which is exactly what has been observed.[22]

Chronic Obstructive Pulmonary Disease Combined With Obstructive Sleep Apnea-Hypopnea Syndrome

Both COPD and obstructive sleep apnea-hypopnea syndrome (OSAHS) are common.[40–42] These two conditions can coexist in some patients, although the prevalence of sleep apnea-hypopnea syndrome (SAHS) in patients with COPD who attend respiratory clinics seems to be no greater than the prevalence of SAHS in the normal population. In a small minority of patients with COPD, perhaps about 2%, nocturnal hypoxemia results from obstructive apneas or hypopneas in addition to REM sleep–related hypoventilation. Viewed in a different way, one study suggested that 10% of patients with SAHS may have some degree of coexisting COPD.[43] In patients with both conditions, the pattern of nocturnal desaturation is different; frequent desaturation results in a broad band saturation trace rather than the relatively clearly defined "spike" desaturation typically found in REM sleep (see Fig. 81–1). Hypercapnic patients with COPD may have narrower upper airways when awake, predisposing them to SAHS.[44]

Summary

Hypoventilation is the major cause of hypoxemia during REM sleep in patients with COPD. There may be additional contributions from ventilation-perfusion mismatching and a decrease in functional residual capacity. In a small minority of patients with COPD, there may also be coexisting OSAHS.

CONSEQUENCES OF SLEEP HYPOXEMIA

Hypoxemia during sleep in patients with COPD has significant cardiovascular and neurophysiological effects, may have hematological consequences, and may contribute to the incidence of nocturnal death.

Cardiac Dysrhythmias

Patients with COPD have more ventricular ectopic beats during sleep,[45] although in most patients there is no direct relation between ventricular ectopic frequency and oxygen saturation.[46] In a minority of the most hypoxic patients, a significant relation could be found between ventricular ectopic frequency and nocturnal oxygen saturation.[46] Flick and Block[45] found a nonsignificant tendency for nocturnal oxygen therapy to reduce ectopic frequency; there is no evidence that such ectopic beats are of clinical importance.

Hemodynamics

Pulmonary arterial pressure rises as oxygen saturation falls during REM sleep.[7, 8, 47] Coccagna and Lugaresi[7] observed in 12 patients with COPD that mean pulmonary arterial pressure rose from 37 to 55 mmHg during REM sleep as the average arterial oxygen tension fell from 56 to 43 mmHg. Boysen et al.[47] observed an inverse correlation between oxygenation and mean pulmonary arterial pressure, and although individual values varied widely, on average a 1% fall in oxygen saturation led to a 1-mmHg rise in mean pulmonary arterial pressure. During these REM hypoxemic episodes, cardiac output increases little, if at all.[21, 22]

The clinical significance of these transient episodes of pulmonary arterial pressure elevation is unknown; however, in rats, intermittent hypoxemia induced by breathing 12% oxygen for as little as 2 h each day for 4 weeks significantly elevated right ventricular mass, even when individual episodes of hypoxia were as short as 30 min[48] (Fig. 81–4). It thus seems possible that the intermittent REM sleep hypoxemia in patients with COPD has similar effects on the human myocardium. Indeed, REM sleep hypoxemia in COPD may have effects on the myocardium similar to those of maximal exercise when an assessment is made in terms of either myocardial oxygen consumption[49] or left ventricular ejection.[50]

Polycythemia

Intermittent hypoxemia in rats results in an elevation of red cell mass[42] (see Fig. 81–4); the nocturnal desaturation in patients with COPD might also stimulate erythropoiesis. Morning erythropoietin levels have been found to be raised in some patients with COPD.[51, 52]

A study compared red cell masses and pulmonary hemodynamics of 36 patients with COPD who desaturated at night to at least 85% with more than 5 min spent below 90% saturation with those of 30 patients who did not so desaturate.[53] Those with nocturnal de-

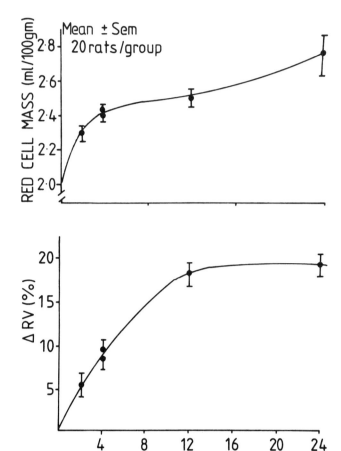

Figure 81–4. Red cell mass and change in right ventricular mass in rats made hypoxic for the number of hours per day indicated for 4 weeks. The two datasets at the 4-h time point represent groups of rats made hypoxic for 4 h on one occasion per day and rats made hypoxic for 30 min on eight occasions per day. ΔRV, change in right ventricular mass. (Redrawn from Moore-Gillon JC, Cameron IR. Right ventricular hypertrophy and polycythemia in rats after intermittent exposure to hypoxia. Clin Sci. 1985;69:595–599.)

saturation had significantly higher daytime pulmonary arterial pressures and red cell masses than did the nondesaturators. Although these differences could have resulted from the nocturnal events, the nocturnal desaturators also had significantly poorer daytime oxygenation levels, which could account for the hemodynamic and hematological differences.

Nocturnal erythropoietin rises only in patients with COPD whose oxygen saturations fall below 60% at night.[54] This suggests that the relatively minor degree of nocturnal desaturation reported by Fletcher et al.[55] may be of little hematological consequence.

Sleep Quality

Both subjective[55] and objective[56–58] assessments indicate that patients with COPD sleep poorly compared with healthy subjects. Although arousals and sleep fragmentation are common during episodes of desaturation,[57, 58a] the extent of sleep disruption is at least as great in relatively normoxic patients with COPD.[58] Despite these reports of poor sleep, there is no objective evidence of daytime sleepiness as assessed by the multiple sleep latency test in patients with COPD.[59]

Death During Sleep in Chronic Obstructive Pulmonary Disease

Death has been reported to occur at night more often in patients with COPD than in age-matched control patients, and death at night was especially common in patients with COPD who had hypoxemia and carbon dioxide retention.[60] In hypoxemic patients with COPD, nocturnal death is more common in those breathing air than in those receiving nocturnal oxygen therapy[61]; however, care must be taken not to equate death at night with death during sleep.

Consequences of Chronic Obstructive Pulmonary Disease Combined With Obstructive Sleep Apnea-Hypopnea Syndrome

Patients with both COPD and OSAHS are more likely to develop pulmonary hypertension,[62] right-sided heart failure,[63, 64] and carbon dioxide retention[65] than are patients with SAHS alone. Indeed, these complications develop earlier in patients with COPD and OSAHS than in patients with COPD alone. Certainly, many patients with COPD and OSAHS and these complications have relatively good lung function. This seems likely to be due to their having two causes for nocturnal hypoxemia, resulting in more severe nocturnal hypoxemia than would have occurred if they had only one such condition.

Prediction of Nocturnal Oxygenation

In 1962, Trask and Cree[3] reported that the patients with COPD who were most hypoxic during sleep were those who were the most hypoxic when awake. Subsequently, oxygenation during wakefulness in patients with COPD has been demonstrated to be related to both the mean and lowest levels of oxygenation during sleep[12, 66, 67, 67a] and to the extent of desaturation during sleep.[10] Because the hypoxemic complications of pulmonary hypertension and polycythemia relate to the patient's absolute arterial oxygenation rather than to the change in saturation, I believe that the more important relation is that between absolute levels of nocturnal oxygenation and measurements that can be taken during wakefulness. Several different equations relating these variables have been derived, and although each is statistically significant,[12, 66, 67] their clinical significance is limited because the scatter around the regression lines is wide,[67] especially for the more

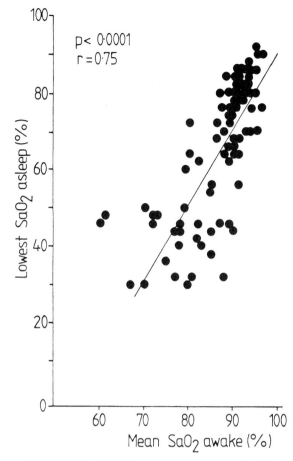

Figure 81–5. Relationship between mean oxygen saturation (Sa_{O_2}) awake and lowest oxygen saturation during sleep in 97 patients with COPD. (Redrawn from Connaughton JJ, Catterall JR, Elton RA, et al. Do sleep studies contribute to the management of patients with severe chronic obstructive pulmonary disease? Am Rev Respir Dis. 1988;138:341–345.)

severely hypoxemic patients (Fig. 81–5). Regression relations show that the extent of nocturnal hypoxemia relates not only to daytime oxygenation but also to daytime arterial carbon dioxide tension[66, 67] and to the duration of REM sleep.[67]

These relations are derived from the consideration of patients with a wide range of arterial oxygen tension when awake. Considerable attention has been paid to the concept of "nocturnal desaturators" among patients whose awake arterial oxygen tension is above 60 mmHg.[68] Of 152 such patients with COPD, Fletcher et al.[68] found that 41 were able to desaturate (defining desaturation arbitrarily as having an oxygen saturation below 90% for at least 5 min with a trough saturation of 85% or lower). These nocturnal desaturators could not be predicted in terms of respiratory function or history; however, mean arterial oxygen tension when awake was significantly lower (70 versus 76 mmHg) and arterial carbon dioxide tension was higher (41 versus 38 mmHg) compared with patients who did not desaturate during sleep. This group of patients would be expected to desaturate more readily than the remainder on the basis of the regression relations.[12, 66, 67]

The clinical significance of such nocturnal desaturation is unproved (see earlier).

CLINICAL VALUE OF SLEEP STUDIES IN CHRONIC OBSTRUCTIVE PULMONARY DISEASE

Studies of breathing and oxygenation during sleep in patients with COPD could be of clinical relevance by (1) detecting unsuspected cases of SAHS, (2) detecting which patients had clinically important excess nocturnal hypoxemia, (3) guiding which patients might benefit from nocturnal oxygen therapy, and (4) determining the optimal inspired oxygen concentration for nocturnal oxygen therapy. The last two roles are discussed in the section on Treatment of Nocturnal Hypoxemia in Chronic Obstructive Pulmonary Disease.

There is no evidence that the prevalence of SAHS is increased in patients with COPD,[12] although large population studies are lacking. When SAHS and COPD coexist, the typical symptoms of SAHS[69, 70] are present, and it appears that sleep studies do not yield unsuspected cases of SAHS.[12, 67] Thus, all patients with COPD should be questioned about the occurrence of symptoms of SAHS; if major symptoms are elicited, polysomnography should be performed.

Oxygenation during sleep can be predicted on the basis of awake arterial blood gas tensions[12, 66, 67] or ventilatory responses during wakefulness.[10] All of these predictions leave considerable unexplained residual variance, but it is unclear whether this is of clinical significance. Measurement of the extent of nocturnal hypoxemia in such patients has been held to be a useful guide for treatment.[71] To clarify the clinical importance of this variability among patients in the extent of nocturnal hypoxemia, Connaughton et al.[67] studied the relation between nocturnal oxygen saturation and survival in 97 patients with severe COPD followed up

for a median of 70 months. Both the mean nocturnal oxygen saturation and the lowest nocturnal oxygen saturation were significantly related to survival; the lower the nocturnal oxygenation, the worse the prognosis. However, neither nocturnal measure significantly improved the prediction of survival that could be obtained from the easier and cheaper measurements of vital capacity or oxygen saturation when awake.[67]

These data[67] were also analyzed to determine the significance of the scatter around the regression relation between measurements of oxygen saturation and $PaCO_2$ when awake and oxygen saturation during sleep. The patients were divided into those who had excess nocturnal hypoxemia, defined as those whose oxygen saturation during sleep was lower than that predicted on the basis of their awake oxygen saturation and arterial PCO_2, and those who became less hypoxemic than predicted at night. There was no difference in survival rates at a median of 70 months between those with excess nocturnal hypoxemia and those who became less hypoxemic at night than might be predicted based on the awake oxygenation and $PaCO_2$ (Fig. 81–6). Thus, measurement of nocturnal oxygenation does not yield useful prognostic information in addition to that obtained during wakefulness. A recent study found no significant relation between the magnitude of nocturnal hypoxemia and the extent of daytime pulmonary hypertension,[72] again suggesting that the contribution of the additional hypoxemia during sleep to overall daytime pulmonary arterial pressure is relatively small.

There seems to be no clinical advantage, therefore, in performing routine polysomnography in patients with COPD, although undoubtedly there are many research areas requiring clarification by this technique. The only situation for which I believe clinical polysomnography is indicated in patients with COPD is when SAHS is suspected due to either symptoms or the development of hypoxemic complications, cor pulmonale, and polycythemia in patients whose daytime arterial oxygen tension is greater than 60 mmHg.

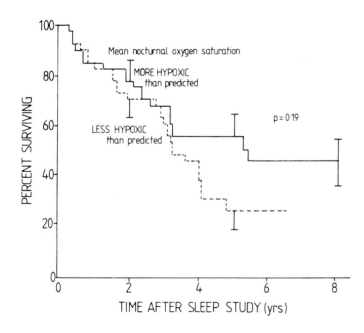

Figure 81–6. Survival curves for patients who are more hypoxic than predicted from their awake oxygen saturation and carbon dioxide level compared with those who are less hypoxic than predicted. There was no significant difference in the survival curves in the two groups. (Redrawn from Connaughton JJ, Catterall JR, Elton RA, et al. Do sleep studies contribute to the management of patients with severe chronic obstructive pulmonary disease? Am Rev Respir Dis. 1988;138:341–345.)

TREATMENT OF NOCTURNAL HYPOXEMIA IN CHRONIC OBSTRUCTIVE PULMONARY DISEASE

Oxygen Therapy

Not surprisingly, nocturnal oxygen therapy improves oxygenation during sleep in patients with COPD.[8, 10, 73] Some nocturnal desaturation still occurs, particularly during REM sleep, although the hypoxemia experienced will not be so profound. A few patients will report morning headaches due to carbon dioxide retention as a result of nocturnal oxygen therapy. This may be a particular problem in patients with coexisting SAHS,[73] and I regard it as an indication for polysomnography.

The patients who become most severely hypoxemic at night are those with daytime hypoxemia.[67] Long-term domiciliary oxygen therapy remains the only treatment shown by controlled clinical trials to prolong life in such patients.[74, 75] Because the period of oxygen administration almost always includes the night, it is possible that some of the benefit of oxygen therapy is due to diminishing of the rise in pulmonary arterial pressure during REM sleep.[76]

In both the Nocturnal Oxygen Therapy Trial[75] and Medical Research Council Study,[76] the inspired oxygen concentration used was selected entirely on the basis of daytime arterial oxygen tension. There is no information that indicates the level of nocturnal oxygenation required to optimize survival, so there is at present no proven role for studies of breathing and oxygenation during sleep in patients who are being started on nocturnal oxygen therapy. Despite that, some have suggested the studies should be performed to ensure that an arbitrary oxygen saturation is achieved throughout the night. This situation might have to be reviewed as further evidence accumulates. Two studies in patients with daytime arterial tensions of greater than 60 mmHg but with nocturnal desaturation reported that nocturnal oxygen therapy did not improve patient survival rates.[77, 78] The only patients in whom I suggest that polysomnography be performed in relation to oxygen therapy in COPD are those who develop morning headaches with oxygen therapy because this may indicate coexisting SAHS.

Some[56, 73] but not all[57, 79] find that the correction of nocturnal hypoxemia improves sleep quality in patients with COPD. This divergence of opinion may have resulted from the patients having differing severities of daytime hypoxemia; also, some studies[57, 73] have not randomized the order of oxygen- and air-breathing nights and have not incorporated a familiarization night. It seems likely that severely hypoxemic patients with COPD sleep better while receiving nocturnal oxygen therapy, although a carefully designed randomized study of a large number of patients is needed to clarify this.

Almitrine

The use of almitrine can raise arterial oxygen tension in patients with COPD. In a randomized double-blind study, 50 mg almitrine twice daily for 2 weeks improved oxygenation during sleep in patients with COPD but did not alter sleep quality.[80] This effect is maintained for at least 1 year.[81]

It was hoped that the combination of almitrine and nocturnal oxygen therapy might produce greater improvements in oxygenation and right-sided heart pressures than those obtained with the use of either agent alone, but this hope has not been fulfilled. If anything, there was a tendency for pulmonary arterial pressure to be higher with the combination of almitrine and oxygen than with the use of oxygen alone.[82]

The role for almitrine in patients with COPD is not yet clear, and further work on this interesting agent is required. Neither the dosage to be used[83] nor the importance of the peripheral neuropathy that can be associated with its use has been defined.

Protriptyline

In an uncontrolled trial, Séries et al.[84] found that 20 mg protriptyline daily improved nocturnal oxygenation in 11 patients with COPD, with the improvement appearing to result from the suppression of REM sleep. However, all patients experienced mouth dryness, and 6 of the 11 patients also reported dysuria. The results of a nonrandomized, nonblinded trial[85] suggested that protriptyline may improve daytime arterial oxygen and carbon dioxide tensions in patients with COPD, but again, side effects were common, causing cessation of therapy within 10 weeks in 4 of 14 patients. The acceptability of long-term protriptyline and its effect on survival remain to be assessed.

Medroxyprogesterone Acetate

Skatrud and Dempsey[86] reported that medroxyprogesterone acetate improved arterial oxygen tension and reduced arterial carbon dioxide tension during both wakefulness and NREM sleep in 5 of 17 hypercapnic patients with COPD. However, in a double-blind, placebo-controlled trial, Dolly and Block[87] found no significant change in the lowest oxygen saturation during sleep in 19 patients with COPD who were taking medroxyprogesterone acetate. In addition, medroxyprogesterone acetate may cause troublesome side effects, including impotence in many patients. The clinical role of the drug appears to be limited.

Acetazolamide

In five patients with hypercapnic COPD, acetazolamide improved both arterial oxygen tension when awake and nocturnal oxygenation but did not alter arterial carbon dioxide tension during sleep in two of the five patients.[86] However, the side effects of paresthesia, nephrolithiasis, and acidosis may limit the acceptability of acetazolamide.

Theophylline

The use of oral theophyllines may improve overnight oxygen saturation and transcutaneous carbon dioxide levels.[88, 89] and morning peak flow rates[90] but may[89] or may not[88, 90, 91] improve sleep quality. In a study of 11 patients with COPD,[92] intravenous theophylline infusion did not improve overnight oxygenation.

Beta Agonists and Anticholinergic Bronchodilators

The use of oral sustained-release salbutamol had no effect on sleep, oxygenation, or morning FEV_1 in 14 patients with moderately severe COPD.[93] In a placebo-controlled, randomized, double-blind trial involving 36 patients, ipratropium bromide improved oxygenation and sleep quality.[93a]

Negative-Pressure Ventilation

Negative-pressure ventilation can reduce arterial carbon dioxide tension and increase respiratory muscle strength in COPD.[94, 95] It may also suck closed the upper airways, resulting in apneas and impaired sleep,[96] which raises significant doubts about the value of this technique in many patients with COPD.

Continuous Positive Airway Pressure

Nocturnal continuous positive airway pressure has been reported to improve inspiratory muscle strength and 12-min walking distances in eight patients with COPD[97] without altering nocturnal oxygenation or sleep quality. These data require confirmation.

Intermittent Positive-Pressure Ventilation by Nasal Mask

Nocturnal intermittent positive-pressure ventilation (NIPPV) via a nasal mask was developed for use in patients with chest wall or neuromuscular disorders.[98–101] Some patients with COPD find this technique to be acceptable, and it has a theoretical advantage over long-term oxygen therapy of reducing, rather than raising, arterial carbon dioxide tension. In patients who can tolerate NIPPV, improvements in arterial blood gas tensions and sleep may be achieved,[100, 102] but nocturnal oxygenation is improved more with nocturnal oxygen therapy than with NIPPV alone.[103] Simultaneous nasal NIPPV and nocturnal oxygen therapy produced greater improvements in daytime arterial oxygen and carbon dioxide tensions and overnight arterial carbon

dioxide tension, sleep quality, and quality of life than did oxygen therapy alone in a randomized control trial of 14 patients with COPD.[104] A more-detailed review of NIPPV is given in Chapter 83.

Inspiratory Muscle Training

Inspiratory muscle training may improve nocturnal oxygenation in some patients with COPD.[105]

Hypnotics Agents

Many patients with COPD receive hypnotic agents when they complain of sleep disturbance. Hypnotic agents should not be used in hypercapnic patients because ventilatory responses may be further inhibited and acute or chronic respiratory failure may be precipitated. In normocapnic patients with COPD, benzodiazepines have been found to increase sleep duration in some[106–108] but not all[109] studies, but the frequency and severity of nocturnal hypoxemia may increase.[106] Thus, even in normocapnic patients, hypnotic agents should be used only with great care.

Alcohol

Alcohol consumption before sleep may worsen nocturnal hypoxemia[110] and increase ventricular ectopic frequency[111] in patients with COPD. Evidence suggests that heavy alcohol consumption by patients with COPD may lead to hypercapnic respiratory failure,[44] to right-sided heart failure,[112] and to an increase in hypopneas and desaturation during sleep.[44] These data require further analysis; in particular, the interrelation between excess alcohol consumption and body weight requires further clarification. The combined results of the four studies[44, 110–112] suggest that alcohol consumption should be discouraged in such patients, and this may in particular apply to alcohol ingestion in the evening.

Treatment of Chronic Obstructive Pulmonary Disease Combined With Obstructive Sleep Apnea-Hypopnea Syndrome

There are remarkably few data indicating how to treat patients who have both COPD and OSAHS. A nonrandomized study found that patients with both conditions improved their daytime arterial blood gas tensions (Fig. 81–7) and pulmonary arterial pressures when they were adequately treated for SAHS but not when they received domiciliary oxygen therapy in the absence of adequate therapy for OSAHS.[113] It is important to recognize coexisting OSAHS in such patients and to treat it appropriately, usually with continuous positive airway pressure therapy. In some who are markedly hypoxemic at both day and night, despite continuous positive airway pressure, supplemental oxygen may have to be added to the continuous positive

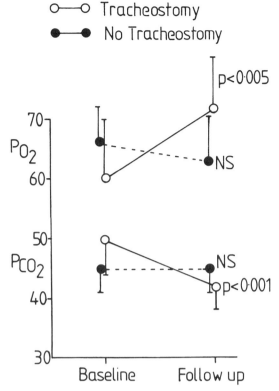

Figure 81–7. Arterial oxygen (P_{O_2}) and carbon dioxide (P_{CO_2}) tensions (in mmHg) in patients with both COPD and sleep apnea at baseline and subsequent follow-up; open circles indicate those who were treated with tracheostomy, and closed circles indicate those who were treated by other techniques, which largely consisted of long-term oxygen therapy. The *P* values indicate significant improvements in arterial blood gas tensions in the patients treated with tracheostomy. (Redrawn from Fletcher EC, Schaaf JW, Miller J, et al. Long-term cardiopulmonary sequelae in patients with sleep apnea and chronic lung disease. Am Rev Respir Dis. 1987;135:525–533.)

airway pressure line. In such patients, NIPPV administered via a nasal mask may be a viable alternative.

Conclusions

Patients with COPD become hypoxemic during sleep, particularly during episodes of dense eye movements in REM sleep. The measurement of nocturnal hypoxemia and breathing pattern in individual patients does not provide prognostic information that significantly adds to the more simple measurements of oxygenation and lung function during wakefulness. In a small minority of patients with COPD, SAHS coexists, and any patient with COPD and a history suggestive of SAHS should undergo full polysomnography. Those found to have SAHS should be aggressively treated. Domiciliary oxygen therapy is the treatment of choice for patients with COPD who are hypoxemic at day and night, but the roles of respiratory stimulants and of IPPV via a nasal mask may grow.

References

1. Robin ED, Whaley RD, Crump CH, et al. The nature of the respiratory acidosis of sleep and of the respiratory alkalosis of hepatic comas [abstract]. J Clin Invest. 1957;36:924.
2. Robin ED. Some interrrelations between sleep and disease. Arch Intern Med. 1958;102:669–675.
3. Trask CH, Cree EM. Oximeter studies on patients with chronic obstructive emphysema, awake and during sleep. N Engl J Med. 1962;266:639–642.
4. Pierce AK, Jarrett CE, Werkle G, et al. Respiratory function during sleep in patients with chronic obstructive lung disease. J Clin Invest. 1966;45:631–636.
5. Koo KW, Sax DS, Snider GL. Arterial blood gases and pH during sleep in chronic obstructive pulmonary disease. Am J Med. 1975;58:663–670.
6. Leitch AG, Clancy LJ, Leggett RJE, et al. Arterial blood gas tensions, hydrogen ion, and electroencephalogram during sleep in patients with chronic ventilatory failure. Thorax. 1976;31:730–735.
7. Coccagna G, Lugaresi E. Arterial blood gases and pulmonary and systemic arterial pressure during sleep in chronic obstructive pulmonary disease. Sleep. 1978;1:117–124.
8. Douglas NJ, Calverley PMA, Leggett RJE, et al. Transient hypoxemia during sleep in chronic bronchitis and emphysema. Lancet. 1979;1:1–4.
9. Wynne JW, Block AJ, Hemenway J, et al. Disordered breathing and oxygen desaturation during sleep in patients with chronic obstructive lung disease (COLD). Am J Med. 1979;66:573–579.
10. Fleetham JA, Mezon B, West P, et al. Chemical control of ventilation and sleep arterial oxygen desaturation in patients with COPD. Am Rev Respir Dis. 1980;122:583–589.
11. Skatrud JB, Dempsey JA, Iber C, et al. Correction of CO_2 retention during sleep in patients with chronic obstructive pulmonary diseases. Am Rev Respir Dis. 1981;124:260–268.
12. Catterall JR, Douglas NJ, Calverley PMA, et al. Transient hypoxemia during sleep in chronic obstructive pulmonary disease is not a sleep apnea syndrome. Am Rev Respir Dis. 1983;128:24–29.
13. Hudgel DW, Martin RJ, Capehart M, et al. Contribution of hypoventilation to sleep oxygen desaturation in chronic obstructive pulmonary disease. J Appl Physiol. 1983;55:669–677.
14. George CF, West P, Kryger MH. Oxygenation and breathing pattern during phasic and tonic REM in patients with chronic obstructive pulmonary disease. Sleep. 1987;10:234–243.
15. Mulloy E, McNicholas WT. Theophylline improves gas exchange during rest, exercise and sleep in severe chronic obstructive pulmonary disease. Am Rev Respir Dis. 1993;148:1030–1036.
16. Midgren B, Hansson L. Changes in transcutaneous P_{CO_2} with sleep in normal subjects and in patients with chronic respiratory diseases. Eur J Respir Dis. 1987;71:384–387.
17. Douglas NJ, White DP, Pickett CK, et al. Respiration during sleep in normal man. Thorax. 1982;37:840–844.
18. Aserinsky E. Periodic respiratory pattern occurring in conjunction with eye movements during sleep. Science. 1965;150:763–766.
19. Gould GA, Gugger M, Molloy J, et al. Breathing pattern and eye movement density during REM sleep in man. Am Rev Respir Dis. 1988;138:874–877.
20. Millman RP, Knight H, Kline LR, et al. Changes in compartmental ventilation in association with eye movements during REM sleep. J Appl Physiol. 1988;65:1196–1202.
21. Fletcher EC, Gray BA, Levin DC. Non-apneic mechanisms of arterial oxygen desaturation during rapid-eye movement sleep. J Appl Physiol. 1983;54:632–639.
22. Catterall JR, Calverley PMA, MacNee W, et al. Mechanism of transient nocturnal hypoxemia in hypoxic chronic bronchitis and emphysema. J Appl Physiol. 1985;59:1698–1703.
23. White DP. Occlusion pressure and ventilation during sleep in normal humans. J Appl Physiol. 1986;61:1279–1287.
24. Gugger M, Molloy J, Gould GA, et al. Ventilatory and arousal responses to added inspiratory resistance during sleep. Am Rev Respir Dis. 1989;140:1301–1307.
25. Lopes JM, Tabachnik E, Muller NL, et al. Total airway resistance and respiratory muscle activity during sleep. J Appl Physiol. 1983;54:773–777.
26. Hudgel DW, Martin RJ, Johnson B, et al. Mechanics of the respiratory system and breathing pattern during sleep in normal humans. J Appl Physiol. 1984;56:133–137.

27. Wiegand L, Zwillich CW, White DP. Sleep and the ventilatory response to resistive loading in normal men. J Appl Physiol. 1988;64:1186–1195.
28. Douglas NJ, White DP, Weil JV, et al. Hypoxic ventilatory response decreases during sleep in normal men. Am Rev Respir Dis. 1982;125:286–289.
29. White DP, Weil JV, Zwillich CK. Metabolic rate and breathing during sleep. J Appl Physiol. 1985;59:384–391.
30. Orem J. Medullary respiratory neuron activity: relationship to tonic and phasic REM sleep. J Appl Physiol. 1980;48:54–65.
31. Tabachnik E, Muller NL, Bryan AC, et al. Changes in ventilation and chest wall mechanics during sleep in normal adolescents. J Appl Physiol. 1981;51:557–564.
32. White JES, Drinnan MJ, Smithson AJ, et al. Respiratory muscle activity during rapid eye movement (REM) sleep in patients with chronic obstructive pulmonary disease. Thorax. 1995;50:376–382.
33. Midgren B. Oxygen desaturation during sleep as a function of the underlying respiratory disease. Am Rev Respir Dis. 1990;141:43–46.
34. Johnson MW, Remmers JE. Accessory muscle activity during sleep in chronic obstructive pulmonary disease. J Appl Physiol. 1984;57:1011–1017.
35. Berthon-Jones M, Sullivan CE. Ventilatory and arousal responses to hypoxia in sleeping humans. Am Rev Respir Dis. 1982;125:632–639.
36. Douglas NJ, White DP, Weil JV, et al. Hypercapnic ventilatory response in sleeping adults. Am Rev Respir Dis. 1982;126:758–762.
37. Berthon-Jones M, Sullivan CE. Ventilation and arousal responses to hypercapnia in normal sleeping adults. J Appl Physiol. 1984;57:59–67.
38. Whyte KF, Gugger M, Gould GA, et al. Accuracy of the respiratory inductive plethysmograph in measuring tidal volume during sleep. J Appl Physiol. 1991;71:1866–1871.
39. Ballard RD, Clover CW, Suh BY. Influence of sleep on respiratory function in emphysema. Am J Respir Crit Care Med. 1995;151:945–951.
40. Franceschi M, Zamproni P, Crippa D, et al. Excessive daytime sleepiness: a 1-year study in an unselected in-patient population. Sleep. 1982;5:239–247.
41. Lavie P. Incidence of sleep apnea in a presumably healthy, working population: a significant relationship with excessive daytime sleepiness. Sleep. 1983;6:312–318.
42. Stradling JR, Crosby JH. Predictors and prevalence of obstructive sleep apnoea and snoring in 1001 middle aged men. Thorax. 1991;46:85–90.
43. Chaouat A, Weitzenblum E, Krieger J, et al. Association of chronic-obstructive pulmonary disease and sleep apnoea syndrome. Am J Respir Crit Care Med. 1995;151:82–86.
44. Chan CS, Bye PTP, Woolcock AJ, et al. Eucapnia and hypercapnia in patients with chronic airflow limitation: the role of the upper airway. Am Rev Respir Dis. 1990;141:861–865.
45. Flick MR, Block AJ. Nocturnal versus diurnal cardiac arrhythmias in patients with chronic obstructive pulmonary disease. Chest. 1979;75:8–11.
46. Shepard JW, Garrison MW, Grither DA, et al. Relationship of ventricular ectopy to nocturnal oxygen desaturation in patients with chronic obstructive pulmonary disease. Am J Med. 1985;78:28–34.
47. Boysen PG, Block AJ, Wynne JW, et al. Nocturnal pulmonary hypertension in patients with chronic obstructive pulmonary disease. Chest. 1979;76:536–542.
48. Moore-Gillon JC, Cameron IR. Right ventricular hypertrophy and polycythemia in rats after intermittent exposure to hypoxia. Clin Sci. 1985;69:595–599.
49. Shepard JW, Schweitzer PK, Keller CA, et al. Myocardial stress: exercise versus sleep in patients with COPD. Chest. 1984;86:366–374.
50. Levy PA, Guilleminault C, Fagret D, et al. Changes in left ventricular ejection fraction during REM sleep and exercise in chronic obstructive pulmonary disease and sleep apnoea syndrome. Eur Respir J. 1991;4:347–352.
51. Miller ME, Garcia JF, Cohen RA, et al. Diurnal levels of immunoreactive erythropoietin in normal subjects and subjects with chronic lung disease. Br J Haematol. 1981;49:189–200.
52. Wedzicha JA, Cotes PM, Empey DW. Serum immunoreactive erythropoietin and hypoxic lung disease with and without polycythemia. Clin Sci. 1985;69:413–422.
53. Fletcher EC, Luckett RA, Miller T, et al. Pulmonary vascular hemodynamics in chronic lung disease patients with and without oxyhemoglobin desaturation during sleep. Chest. 1989;95:757–764.
54. Fitzpatrick MF, McMahon G, Whyte KF, et al. Does oxygen desaturation during sleep cause release of erythropoietin in patients with COPD? Clin Sci. 1993;84:319–324.
55. Cormick W, Olsen LG, Hensley MJ, et al. Nocturnal hypoxemia and quality of sleep in patients with chronic obstructive lung disease. Thorax. 1986;41:846–854.
56. Calverley PMA, Brezinova V, Douglas NJ, et al. The effect of oxygenation on sleep quality in chronic bronchitis and emphysema. Am Rev Respir Dis. 1982;126:206–210.
57. Fleetham J, West P, Mezon B, et al. Sleep, arousals and oxygen desaturation in chronic obstructive pulmonary disease. Am Rev Respir Dis. 1982;126:429–433.
58. Brezinova V, Catterall JR, Douglas NJ, et al. Night sleep of patients with chronic ventilatory failure and age-matched controls: number and duration of ECG episodes of intervening wakefulness and drowsiness. Sleep. 1982;5:123–130.
58a. Sandek K, Andersson T, Bratel T, et al. Sleep quality, carbon dioxide responsiveness and hypoxaemic patterns in nocturnal hypoxaemia due to chronic obstructive pulmonary disease (COPD) without daytime hypoxaemia. Respir Med. 1999;93:79–87.
59. Orr WC, Shamma-Othman Z, Levin D, et al. Persistent hypoxemia and excessive daytime sleepiness in chronic obstructive pulmonary disease. Chest. 1990;97:583–585.
60. McNicholas WT, Fitzgerald MX. Nocturnal deaths in patients with chronic bronchitis and emphysema. Br Med J. 1984;289:878.
61. Douglas NJ. Breathing during sleep in patients with respiratory disease. In: Guilleminault C, Partinen M, eds. Obstructive Sleep Apnea Syndrome. New York, NY: Raven Press; 1990:37–48.
62. Weitzenblum E, Krieger J, Apprill M, et al. Daytime pulmonary hypertension in patients with obstructive sleep apnea syndrome. Am Rev Respir Dis. 1988;138:345–349.
63. Bradley TD, Rutherford R, Grossman RF, et al. Role of daytime hypoxemia in the pathogenesis of right heart failure in the obstructive sleep apnea syndrome. Am Rev Respir Dis. 1985;131:835–839.
64. Whyte KF, Douglas NJ. Peripheral edema in the sleep apnea/hypopnea syndrome. Sleep. 1991;14:354–356.
65. Bradley TD, Rutherford R, Lue F, et al. Role of diffuse airway obstruction in the hypercapnia of obstructive sleep apnea. Am Rev Respir Dis. 1986;134:920–924.
66. McKeon JL, Muree-Allan K, Saunders NA. Prediction of oxygenation during sleep in patients with chronic obstructive lung disease. Thorax. 1988;43:312–317.
67. Connaughton JJ, Catterall JR, Elton RA, et al. Do sleep studies contribute to the management of patients with severe chronic obstructive pulmonary disease? Am Rev Respir Dis. 1988;138:341–345.
67a. Little SA, Elkholy MM, Chalmers GW, et al. Predictors of nocturnal oxygen desaturation in patients with COPD. Respir Med. 1999;93:202–207.
68. Fletcher EC, Miller J, Devine GW, et al. Nocturnal oxyhemoglobin desaturation in COPD patients with arterial oxygen tensions above 60 mmHg. Chest. 1987;92:604–608.
69. Guilleminault C, van den Hoed J, Mitler MM. Clinical overview of the sleep apnea syndromes. In: Guilleminault C, Dement WC, eds. Sleep Apnea Syndromes. New York, NY: Alan R Liss; 1978:1–12.
70. Whyte KF, Allen MB, Jeffrey AA, et al. Clinical features of the sleep apnoea/hypopnoea syndrome. Q J Med. 1989;72:659–666.
71. Phillipson EA, Remmers JE, Chairmen. Indications and standards for cardiopulmonary sleep studies. Am Rev Respir Dis. 1989;139:559–568.
72. Chaouat A, Weitzenblum E, Kessler R, et al. Sleep-related O_2 desaturation and daytime pulmonary haemodynamics in COPD patients with mild hypoxaemia. Eur Respir J. 1997;10:1730–1735.
73. Goldstein RS, Ramcharan V, Bowes G, et al. Effect of supplemental nocturnal oxygen on gas exchange in patients with severe obstructive lung disease. N Engl J Med. 1984;310:425–429.

74. Nocturnal Oxygen Therapy Trial Group. Continuous or nocturnal oxygen therapy in hypoxemic chronic obstructive lung disease: a clinical trial. Ann Intern Med. 1980;93:391–398.

75. Medical Research Council Working Party Report. Long-term domiciliary oxygen therapy in chronic hypoxic cor pulmonale complicating chronic bronchitis and emphysema. Lancet. 1981;1:681–686.

76. Fletcher EC, Levin DC. Cardiopulmonary hemodynamics during sleep in subjects with chronic obstructive pulmonary disease: the effect of short- and long-term oxygen. Chest. 1984;85:6–14.

77. Fletcher EC, Donner CF, Midgren B, et al. Survival in COPD patients with the daytime PaO₂ > 60 mmHg, with or without nocturnal oxygen desaturation. Chest. 1992;101:649–655.

78. Fletcher EC, Luckett RA, Goodnight-White S, et al. A double-blind trial of nocturnal supplemental oxygen for sleep desaturation in patients with chronic obstructive pulmonary disease and daytime PaO₂ above 60 mmHg. Am Rev Respir Dis. 1992;145:1070–1076.

79. McKeon JL, Murree-Allen K, Saunders NA. Supplemental oxygen and quality of sleep in patients with chronic obstructive lung disease. Thorax. 1989;44:184–188.

80. Connaughton JJ, Douglas NJ, Morgan AD, et al. Almitrine improves oxygenation when both awake and asleep in patients with hypoxia and carbon dioxide retention caused by chronic bronchitis and emphysema. Am Rev Respir Dis. 1985;132:206–210.

81. Gothe B, Cherniack NS, Bachand RT, et al. Long-term effects of almitrine bismesylate on oxygenation during wakefulness and sleep in chronic obstructive pulmonary disease. Am J Med. 1988;84:436–443.

82. Ruhle KH, Kempf P, Mossinger B, et al. Einfluss von almitrin, einem chemorezeptoren Stimulator, auf die nachtliche Hyperkapnie und dem pulmonarteriellen druck unter O₂ Atmung bei chronisch obstruktiver Lungenerkrankung. Prax Clin Pneumol. 1988;42:411–414.

83. Howard P. Hypoxia, almitrine and peripheral neuropathy. Thorax. 1989;44:247–250.

84. Séries F, Cormier Y, La Forge J. Changes in day and in night time oxygenation with protriptyline in patients with chronic obstructive lung disease. Thorax. 1989;44:275–279.

85. Séries F, Cormier Y. Effects of protriptyline on diurnal and nocturnal oxygenation in patients with chronic obstructive pulmonary disease. Ann Intern Med. 1990;113:507–511.

86. Skatrud JB, Dempsey JA. Relative effectiveness of acetazolamide versus medroxyprogesterone acetate in correction of carbon dioxide retention. Am Rev Respir Dis. 1983;127:405–412.

87. Dolly FR, Block AJ. Medroxyprogesterone acetate in COPD: effect on breathing and oxygenation in sleeping and awake patients. Chest. 1983;84:394–398.

88. Berry RB, Desa MM, Branum JP, et al. Effect of theophylline on sleep and sleep-disordered breathing in patients with chronic obstructive pulmonary disease. Am Rev Respir Dis. 1991;143:245–250.

89. Mulloy E, McNicholas WT. Theophylline improves gas exchange during rest, exercise and sleep in severe chronic obstructive pulmonary disease. Am Rev Respir Dis. 1993;148:1030–1036.

90. Man GCW, Chapman KR, Habib AS, et al. Sleep quality and nocturnal respiratory function with once-daily theophylline (Uniphyl) and inhaled salbutamol in patients with COPD. Chest. 1996;110:648–653.

91. Martin RJ, Pak J. Overnight theophylline concentrations and effects on sleep and lung function in chronic obstructive pulmonary disease. Am Rev Respir Dis. 1992;145:540–544.

92. Ebden P, Vathenen AS. Does aminophylline improve nocturnal hypoxia in patients with chronic airflow obstruction? Eur J Respir Dis. 1987;71:384–387.

93. Veale D, Cooper BG, Griffiths CJ, et al. The effect of controlled-release salbutamol on sleep and nocturnal oxygenation in patients with asthma and chronic obstructive pulmonary disease. Respir Med. 1994;88:121–124.

93a. Martin RJ, Bartelson BL, Smith P, et al. Effect of ipratropium bromide treatment on oxygen saturation and sleep quality in COPD. Chest. 1999;115:1338–1345.

94. Brown NMT, Marino WD. Effective daily intermittent rest of respiratory muscles in patients with severe chronic airflow limitation. Chest. 1984;85:59S–60S.

95. Crop AJ, Di Marco AF. Effects of intermittent negative pressure ventilation on respiratory muscle function in patients with severe chronic obstructive pulmonary disease. Am Rev Respir Dis. 1987;135:1056–1061.

96. Levy RD, Bradley TD, Newman SL, et al. Negative pressure ventilation: effects on ventilation during sleep in normal subjects. Chest. 1989;95:95–99.

97. Mezzanotte WS, Tangel DJ, Fox AM, et al. Nocturnal nasal continuous positive airway pressure in patients with chronic obstructive pulmonary disease: influence on waking respiratory muscle function. Chest. 1994;106:1100–1108.

98. Ellis ER, Bye PTP, Bruderer JW, et al. Treatment of respiratory failure during sleep in patients with neuro-muscular disease. Am Rev Respir Dis. 1987;135:148–152.

99. Kerby GR, Mayer LS, Pringleton SK. Nocturnal positive pressure ventilation via nasal mask. Am Rev Respir Dis. 1987;135:738–740.

100. Carroll N, Branthwaite MA. Control of nocturnal hypoventilation by nasal intermittent positive pressure ventilation. Thorax. 1988;43:349–353.

101. Clinical indications for noninvasive positive pressure ventilation in chronic respiratory failure due to restrictive lung disease, COPD, and nocturnal hypoventilation—a consensus conference report. Chest. 1999;116:521–534.

102. Elliot MW, Simmonds AK, Carroll MP, et al. Domiciliary nocturnal nasal intermittent positive pressure ventilation in hypercapnic respiratory failure due to chronic obstructive lung disease: effect on sleep and quality of life. Thorax. 1992;47:342–348.

103. Lin CC. Comparison between nocturnal nasal positive pressure ventilation combined with oxygen therapy and oxygen monotherapy in patients with severe COPD. Am J Respir Crit Care Med. 1996;154:353–358.

104. Meecham Jones DJ, Paul EA, Jones PW, et al. Nasal pressure support ventilation plus oxygen compared with oxygen therapy alone in hypercapnic COPD. Am J Respir Crit Care Med. 1995;152:538–544.

105. Heijdra YF, Dekhuijzen PNR, van Herwaarden CLA. Nocturnal saturation improves by target-flow inspiratory muscle training in patients with COPD. Am J Respir Crit Care Med. 1996;153:260–265.

106. Block AJ, Dolly FR, Slayton PC. Does flurazepam ingestion affect breathing and oxygenation during sleep in patients with chronic obstructive lung disease? Am Rev Respir Dis. 1984;129:230–233.

107. Wedzicha JA, Wallis PJW, Ingram DA, et al. Effect of diazepam on sleep in patients with chronic airflow obstruction. Thorax. 1988;43:729–730.

108. Midgren B, Hansson L, Skeidsvoll H, et al. The effects of nitrazepam and flunitrazepam on oxygen desaturation during sleep in stable hypoxemic nonhypercapnic COPD. Chest. 1989;95:765–768.

109. Cummiskey J, Guilleminault C, Rio GD, et al. The effects of flurazepam on sleep studies in patients with chronic obstructive pulmonary disease. Chest. 1983;84:143–147.

110. Easton PA, West P, Meatherall RC, et al. The effect of excessive ethanol ingestion on sleep in severe chronic obstructive pulmonary disease. Sleep. 1987;10:224–233.

111. Dolly FR, Block AJ. Increased ventricular ectopy and sleep apnea following ethanol ingestion in COPD patients. Chest. 1983;83:469–472.

112. Jalleh R, Fitzpatrick MF, Jan MA, et al. Alcohol and cor pulmonale in chronic bronchitis and emphysema. Br Med J. 1993;306:374.

113. Fletcher EC, Schaaf JW, Miller J, et al. Long-term cardiopulmonary sequelae in patients with sleep apnea and chronic lung disease. Am Rev Respir Dis. 1987;135:525–533.

82

Restrictive Lung Disorders

Meir H. Kryger

Lung volume is determined by the balance of two forces—the elasticity of the lung, which tends to reduce lung volume, and the normal outward recoil of the thoracic cage, which tends to increase lung volume. Restriction of lung expansion may thus be due to disorders of the lungs (intrapulmonary restriction) or to disorders of structures surrounding the lungs (extrapulmonary restriction).[1] The physiological consequences of these two types of lung restriction are different, resulting in varying effects on respiratory control. In general, patients with intrapulmonary restriction have stimulation of pulmonary vagal receptors with resultant hyperventilation. Patients with extrapulmonary restriction may develop blunting of chemical drives to breathe and hypoventilation. On the basis of differences during the awake state, one would expect these two groups to behave differently during sleep. Lung restriction is most commonly seen in four conditions: obesity, pregnancy, kyphoscoliosis, and interstitial lung disease. Patients with neuromuscular diseases may also have a restriction of lung expansion. These patients are reviewed in Chapter 91.

OBESITY

Obesity, the excessive accumulation of fat and the resulting generalized increase in body mass, is associated with increased morbidity from arterial hypertension, diabetes mellitus, and degenerative joint disease. Fat has also been implicated in the development of cardiomyopathy.[2] Obese patients also have compromised respiratory function while awake and upright.[3] Their ventilatory function may become worse when they assume the supine position and worsen even more when they sleep.[4]

Awake Respiration in Obesity

Obese people have increased metabolic demands, which are reflected by an increased oxygen uptake ($\dot{V}O_2$) and higher carbon dioxide production ($\dot{V}CO_2$).[5] Thus, to maintain normal PaO_2 and $PaCO_2$, they must maintain a high level of alveolar ventilation. The work of breathing is increased in obesity owing mainly to the extreme stiffness (reduced compliance) of the thoracic cage, which results from the accumulation of adipose tissue in and around the ribs, abdomen, and diaphragm.[6] The energy expended in ventilation in obese people is substantially greater than that actually required to overcome the stiffness of the chest wall. Thus, it appears that the respiratory muscles are inefficient, consuming excess energy.[7]

The volume of the lungs when the respiratory muscles are relaxed (the functional residual capacity [FRC]) is determined by the natural tendency of the lungs to assume a smaller volume (like an inflated balloon) and by the tendency of the chest wall to spring out. At the relaxation volume, these two forces are equal and opposite in direction. With obesity, the tendency of the chest wall to spring out is reduced—hence, the lower relaxation volume.[8]

During expiration, when a certain lung volume is reached, airways at the lung bases begin to close. This airway closure, and the volume at which it occurs, is called closing volume. Perfusion may continue to lung units having closed airways, which results in mismatching of ventilation and perfusion ($\dot{V}/\dot{Q}$) and causes hypoxemia. In obesity, because of the low relaxation volume, ventilation may occur at volumes lower than the closing volume, which explains the hypoxemia common in obese persons.[4]

Obesity and the Supine Position

In the supine position, the weight of the diaphragm and the abdomen is applied to the lungs. In addition, the chest wall in obesity is stiffer in the supine than in the upright position.[9] Thus, FRC is lower in the supine position, which exacerbates the hypoxemia caused, in part, by ventilation occurring at lung volumes below the closing volume. When asleep there is a further increase in the work of breathing related to upper airway obstruction.[10]

Breathing During Sleep

Abnormalities in breathing pattern in normal persons increase with age and weight.[11] Obese patients with and without the obesity-hypoventilation syndrome (OHS) (see below), may demonstrate the following breathing abnormalities in sleep.

No Demonstrable Change in Breathing Pattern With Heavy Snoring. Some patients may have severe snoring but without hypoxemia. When such patients have increased respiratory effort–related arousals (RERAs) during sleep, and excessive daytime sleepiness, their symptoms fit the criteria for upper airway resistance syndrome.[12]

Hypoxemia With No Demonstrable Change in Breathing Pattern. This phenomenon is most likely related to the low lung volumes in the supine position. Some obese patients may have an SaO_2 in the range of 90 to 94% during nonrapid eye movement (NREM) sleep, with further reductions during rapid eye movement (REM) sleep. Some patients may demonstrate long periods of hypoventilation. The lack of overt apneas in these patients may reflect normal drives to breathe and an absence of upper airway obstruction. In contrast to the cyclic hypoxemia described next, some OHS patients will demonstrate severe continuous hypoxemia with no abnormalities in the pattern of breathing. The cause of the hypoxemia is hypoventilation, and I have seen several such patients whose sleep $PaCO_2$ is in excess of 100 mmHg.

Periodic Hypoxemia Without Apneas. Swings in SaO_2 may be present without overt apneas. In some cases, these may be related to periodic changes in ventilation or to incomplete upper airway occlusion—the sleep hypopnea syndrome. Such patients may have the same sequelae as do those with apnea, including multiple arousals, cyclic hypoxemia, sleepiness, and right-sided heart failure.[13] Such patients may represent a transition between normality and the sleep apnea syndrome.

Sleep Apnea and Hypoventilation. Although many obese patients develop the sleep apnea syndrome, some do not.[14] Weight itself is not sufficient to cause sleep apnea. About 40% of men and 3% of women with a body mass index (BMI) exceeding 45 may be expected to have sleep apnea severe enough to warrant treatment.[15] It is likely that the distribution of fat with an associated anatomical upper airway obstruction is a key element in the genesis of sleep apnea. Increased compliance of the walls of the upper airway may also be present, making it more collapsible.[16, 17] Obese sleepy patients fall into two distinct groups: those having hypoventilation while awake and asleep, who as a group have reduced chemical drives to breathe; and those without hypoventilation while awake. The former group of patients have OHS, also popularized as the "pickwickian syndrome" (see below). They have more severe polycythemia, pulmonary hypertension, and cor pulmonale than do obese patients without awake hypoventilation. In my experience, hypoventilation in the awake state is present in about 10% of sleepy, obese patients.[18–20] About half of sleep apnea patients with a BMI exceeding 40 would be expected to have awake hypoventilation.[21] It is not clear whether sleep respiration in patients who have OHS with sleep apnea is different from that in obese patients who have sleep apnea without hypoventilation during wakefulness. Diagnostic criteria for sleep hypoventilation syndromes have been published.[21a] The patient has one or more features of chronic hypoventilation (cor pulmonale, pulmonary hypertension, daytime sleepiness, erythrocytosis, awake hypercapnea) and an overnight sleep study that documents an increase in PCO_2 of more than 10 mmHg, or oxygen desaturation not explained by apnea or hypopnea. Occasionally, OHS patients may have only continuous hypoventilation during sleep without apneas. Obstructive sleep apnea-hypopnea syndrome (OSAHS) is discussed in greater detail in Chapters 73 to 79.

Obesity-Hypoventilation Syndrome: Pickwickian Syndrome

Some obese patients hypoventilate not only during sleep but also while awake and thus have an elevated $PaCO_2$. These patients usually have polycythemia,[18] as well as pulmonary hypertension.[20] Respiratory mechanics and weight do not adequately explain why a few obese patients develop hypoventilation during waking, whereas the majority do not. Indeed hypoventilation may occur with only mildly impaired ventilatory function.[18] Control of respiration plays a role. If the limiting factor is simply the stiffness of the respiratory system, these patients should demonstrate increased muscle work, compared with obese patients without hypoventilation during waking.[22] They do not. The chemical drives to breathe—both hypoxic and hypercapnic—have been found to be reduced in OHS.[23–25] These responses may normalize with weight loss[26] but in some cases may be inherited. That reduced drive plays a role in many of the features of OHS is shown by the sometimes dramatic improvement when these patients are treated with progestational agents.[27] Pulse therapy using medroxyprogesterone acetate has been suggested as helpful in postmenopausal women with OHS.[27a] Progesterone increases chemical drives to breathe without altering lung mechanics.

PREGNANCY

Respiration

In several ways, pregnant women have the impairment of lung function seen in the morbidly obese. These alterations in respiratory function can theoretically lead to reduced maternal oxygenation during sleep. The risk factors potentially worsening gas exchange are low FRC and the supine position.[28, 29] The changes in lung function are greatest with highest fundal position, which usually occurs at 36 weeks of gestation in primigravidas. Residual volume and FRC are both reduced maximally at this time.[30] Airway closure can occur above FRC at the end of pregnancy,[31] with resultant increased perfusion of low $\dot{V}/\dot{Q}$ regions in the lung, just as in the obese. There is also exacerbation of these factors in the supine position, which further worsens gas exchange.[32] Modest hypoxemia may occur in awake, supine pregnant women despite the increase in tidal volume[28] and resulting hyperventilation that accompany pregnancy.[32] There is evidence that the oxyhemoglobin dissociation curve is shifted to the right in pregnancy.[33] Thus, at a given level of PaO_2, SaO_2 would be lower. Reduction in FRC during pregnancy decreases lung oxygen stores. Any apnea or hypoventilation during sleep can thus exhaust the reduced oxygen stores more rapidly, similar to what has been observed with apnea during succinylcholine paralysis in pregnancy.[34] An additional factor that may induce apneas in sleep is respiratory alkalosis, similar to the situation found with acute exposure to high altitude (see Chapter 18).

In spite of the many factors that may potentially cause sleep hypoxemia in pregnancy, physiologically significant maternal arterial oxygen desaturation has not been documented in normal, sleeping pregnant women.[35, 36] Surprisingly, even in multiple pregnancy (up to quadruplets) SaO_2 was always maintained above 90%.[37] In fact, there is a significant reduction in apnea and hypopnea frequency and duration. One important difference between pregnancy and obesity is the high progesterone level in the pregnant woman. Production of progesterone, a hormone with respiratory stimulant properties,[38] is greatly increased in pregnancy. This greater level of progesterone is thought to be responsible for increasing alveolar ventilation.[39, 40] Progesterone levels at 36 weeks of gestation are approximately 10 times greater than peak menstrual cycle levels (150 vs. 15 mg/ml).[41] Progesterone increases alveolar ventilation by increasing tidal volume, not breathing frequency.[42, 43] Thus, physiological mechanisms in the normal pregnant woman protect the fetus from potential hypoxemia. Sleep hypoxemia might occur in pregnant women with concurrent respiratory disease or obesity when high progesterone levels may not provide sufficient protection. In addition, with uteroplacental insufficiency, even small reductions in maternal oxygenation might compromise fetal oxygen delivery.

Sleep Quality and Architecture

Sleep is disrupted in most pregnant women,[44] with increased complaints of restless sleep, low back pain, and leg cramps.[36] Low back pain occurs in more than half of all pregnancies. In about a third of the patients, the pain increases during the night and disturbs sleep.[45] Many pregnant women change their normal sleeping position to a left tilt[46] which minimizes the aortocaval compression syndrome. Sleep efficiency is reduced because time in bed increases while sleep time does not change, and there is increased wake time after sleep onset; sleep latency is normal.[36] There is an increased amount of stage 1 sleep and a reduction in REM sleep. There is also an increase in the number of awakenings during pregnancy.[36] Periodic movements in sleep or the development of restless legs syndrome is common during pregnancy.[47] I am unaware of studies of women who complain of restless sleep and shortness of breath. Preliminary data suggest that women with preeclampsia have reduced sleep quality with major postural shifts, increased amounts of wakefulness, and periodic movements in sleep.[48] Preexisting sleep disorders, such as sleepwalking and narcolepsy, can be expected to continue into pregnancy.[49]

I do not recommend pharmacological treatment of the disorders causing restlessness and insomnia in pregnancy. If symptoms persist in the postdelivery period and drug therapy is being considered, the clinician and patient should be aware of potential side effects in the mother which interfere with her ability to care for the baby, and that the medication may be present in breast milk.

Upper Airway Obstruction and Obstructive Sleep Apnea-Hypopnea Syndrome in Pregnancy

Some women snore only when they are pregnant.[50] In a large study involving 502 women, at the end of pregnancy, 23% of the women snored nightly; 4% of them snored before becoming pregnant.[51] Hypertension developed in 14% of the snorers versus 6% of the nonsnorers. Several other abnormalities were more common in the snorers: preeclampsia (10% of snorers, 4% of nonsnorers); fetal growth retardation (7.1% of snorers, 2.6% of nonsnorers); and an Apgar score of less than 7 (more common in infants born to snorers). Some pregnant women develop nocturnal nasal congestion.[52] In some women, the snoring during pregnancy may be a marker of the development of OSAHS,[53] which may rarely result in pulmonary hypertension.[53a] Pregnant women with sleep apnea that began either before[54, 55] or after[53] pregnancy occurred may be putting the fetus at great risk, although this has not been documented.[56] Grossly obese primiparas with a snoring history and subjective nocturnal arousals all had infants with asymmetrical intrauterine growth retardation.[57] Sleep studies were not done on this group of women.

A trial of external nasal dilation may be warranted in snorers without apnea.[52] In pregnant OSAHS patients, because of the potential danger to both mother and fetus, treatment should be instituted as early as possible with continuous positive airway pressure (CPAP).[53, 53a, 56] Tracheostomy has been performed on pregnant women[54] for sleep apnea, but it must be remembered that in such patients it may be difficult to intubate the trachea because of obesity or mandibular abnormalities. I have encountered apnea patients in the immediate postpartum period who were not able to awaken to their newborn baby's cries and thus had to be treated emergently. Pregnant women with hypoventilation syndromes may require nocturnal nasal intermittent positive-pressure ventilation to reverse nocturnal hypoxemia and pulmonary hypertension.[58]

Pregnancies in obese women with or without apnea may be further complicated by gestational diabetes[43]; cesarean section may need to be performed. Again, the physician should be prepared to encounter perioperative problems in airway management and hypoxemia, particularly when opiate analgesics are used.[18]

KYPHOSCOLIOSIS

Kyphoscoliosis, which affects the thoracic spine and causes thoracic cage deformity, is usually idiopathic in origin but may be a result of many diseases, including paralytic poliomyelitis, neurofibromatosis, Pott's disease, ankylosing spondylitis, and Marfan's syndrome.

Depending on the cause and degree of spinal curvature, it can produce respiratory failure at ages ranging from adolescence to late adulthood.[59] Scoliosis by itself is insufficient to cause respiratory failure. About 100 degrees of curvature is present in kyphoscoliosis patients with respiratory failure; in most of the studies reporting sleep in kyphoscoliosis, the spinal deformity has been in this range.[60–62]

Although, in some cases, hypoventilation during wakefulness is chronic, in most it appears to be precipitated episodically by infections and less frequently by pulmonary emboli or ingestion of respiratory depressant agents, such as hypnotics or opiates. Patients with chronic hypoventilation will have the sequelae of chronic hypoxemia, polycythemia, pulmonary hypertension, and cor pulmonale. Between episodes of acute respiratory failure, these patients have the rapid, shallow breathing pattern of a marked restrictive defect. This breathing pattern increases the ventilation of dead space; because the chest wall is so stiff, attempts to increase tidal volume result in steep increases in the work of breathing. The deformity also causes abnormal distribution of inspired air, with consequent atelectasis and $\dot{V}/\dot{Q}$ mismatching. The small tidal volumes probably promote airway closure and thus perpetuate the atelectasis. Another factor that may play a role is the low FRC. Patients with a low FRC have low oxygen stores in the lungs. If such a patient becomes apneic, oxygen uptake from the lungs into the pulmonary circulation will continue and cause a precipitous fall in alveolar P_{O_2}.

Control of ventilation in kyphoscoliosis may be abnormal for two reasons. First, if the kyphoscoliosis was caused by poliomyelitis, the defect in respiratory drive may be secondary to involvement of the respiratory control system in the medulla or may be due to weakness of the respiratory muscles. Second, the blunting of drive may be acquired and may be related to the enormous mechanical load, as may occur with obesity. Respiratory failure may first occur in patients with post-poliomyelitic kyphoscoliosis 20 to 30 years after their acute infection and recovery.

The ventilatory response to hypercapnia may be markedly reduced.[59, 63] This blunting of hypercapnic drive may be due to mechanical impairment alone. However, when hypercapnia is present, peak ventilation remains well below the patient's maximal minute ventilation, which suggests a primary defect in ventilatory drive. Hypoxic ventilatory drive may also be blunted in some patients. Interestingly, when made hypoxic and hypercapnic in the laboratory, the patients may not have the sensation of dyspnea. Traditionally, chemical drives to breathe are quantified by measuring ventilation as Sa_{O_2} is lowered or as Pa_{CO_2} is raised. In the presence of lung disease, the pressure generated by the respiratory muscles (measured 0.1 sec after the onset of inspiration [$P_{0.1}$]) is thought to be more reliable than ventilation as a measure of ventilatory drive. Chemical drives to breathe are difficult to interpret in this population because the thoracic distortion may interfere with both the ventilatory and the $P_{0.1}$ responses to chemical stimuli.

Quality of Sleep

Patients may complain of excessive daytime sleepiness and disrupted nocturnal sleep.[60] Some patients have severe nocturnal or morning headaches. The headaches are probably caused by severe carbon dioxide retention during sleep. Both hypercapnia and hypoxia are known to increase cerebral blood flow by vasodilation, which is the likely mechanism by which these headaches occur.[64] Sleep studies show that sleep in these patients is "lighter," with an increase in stage 1 and a reduction in stage 2 sleep.[61]

Breathing Patterns

Patients may have a Cheyne-Stokes respiration pattern (i.e., a periodic breathing pattern with or without apneas), severe central apneas or hypoventilation (primarily during REM sleep),[61] and obstructive apneas.[60] Apnea duration is substantially greater in REM sleep than in NREM sleep. In one case, a patient spent 77% of REM time apneic.[61] In fact, the longest apneas I have ever encountered have been in patients with kyphoscoliosis. The cause of the REM apneas is unclear but may be linked to REM sleep–related loss of tone in the primary and accessory muscles of respiration.

The hypoventilation of sleep results in elevation of Pa_{CO_2}, there being a positive correlation between awake Pa_{CO_2} and the nocturnal rise in Pa_{CO_2}[65, 66]; that is, hypercapnic patients have the greatest increases in P_{CO_2} during sleep.

Oxygenation

The Sa_{O_2} was much lower in REM sleep than in NREM sleep, and the lowest Sa_{O_2} of the night was less than 60% in most of the reported cases.[60–62, 67] Patients with cor pulmonale had the most severe drops in Sa_{O_2}.[61]

What are the factors that seemed related to the oxygen desaturation? In one report, elevated hematocrit, hypoxemia during the awake state, and cor pulmonale were present in two of the five patients with severe oxygen desaturation.[61] It is interesting that the degree of impairment of lung function did not seem to correlate with desaturation during sleep. The patients with the lowest vital capacity and forced expiratory volume in 1 sec (FEV_1) were not those with the most sleep desaturation.

The gender of the patients may play a role. All the patients in one report were men,[60] and in the other, the only two patients who desaturated severely were men; the two women who had the most impaired lung function desaturated little during sleep.[61] However, I have encountered several women with kyphoscoliosis secondary to poliomyelitis who had severe breathing abnormalities during sleep.

Spillover Daytime Sequelae

In one report, four patients with severe kyphoscoliosis and a previous history of poliomyelitis had hypercapnic respiratory failure during waking that seemed related to abnormalities in sleep.[68] When these patients were mechanically ventilated at night, the daytime hypoventilation resolved. This finding suggested that one of two mechanisms may be involved in producing spillover hypoventilation. One is respiratory muscle fatigue. These patients must generate high pleural pressures to maintain tidal volume in the presence of altered mechanics. The respiratory muscles, which may be abnormal in the first place, may fatigue during the night.[69] The other possible mechanism causing hypoxemia is a progressive loss of lung volume during sleep. It is believed that low tidal volume breathing with no or few sighs promotes airway closure and microatelectasis.

Therapeutic Implications

Patients with kyphoscoliosis, respiratory failure, and cor pulmonale have a poor prognosis. Little has been published about the treatment of sleep problems in kyphoscoliosis.

Tracheostomy alone, which has been used in the past in an attempt to reduce anatomical dead space, is probably not indicated unless severe obstructive apnea is documented. The use of tracheostomy does not result in consistent improvement in respiratory failure.[68, 70]

The uncontrolled administration of CPAP in kyphoscoliosis patients without obstructive apnea may have detrimental effects. Because of the extreme stiffness of the chest wall, increasing FRC may result in the patient's having to generate great pressure to breathe in. Patients with kyphoscoliosis have developed acute respiratory failure with the institution of CPAP.

Intermittent positive-pressure ventilation has been shown to improve, temporarily, lung mechanics and gas exchange and reduce the work of breathing in awake patients with kyphoscoliosis.[59, 68, 70, 71] The improvement, however, is maintained only for up to 3 h,[70] and high inspiratory pressures are required.[68] In one patient, intermittent positive-pressure ventilation was applied for 10 min each waking hour for a consistent effect on blood gases to be obtained.[59]

Tracheostomy and chronic nighttime ventilation with high inflation pressures had a dramatic effect in four patients, resulting in a change in $PaCO_2$ during wakefulness from 59.8 to 38.3 mmHg, in PaO_2 from 37.5 to 67.8 mmHg, and in hemoglobin concentration from 18.1 to 14.7 g/dl.[68] This form of therapy has been useful for long-term support and suggests strongly that the respiratory failure during wakefulness may be a spillover from sleep abnormalities.

Nasal ventilation using either a traditional ventilator or a bilevel positive airway pressure device can also be expected to be effective (see Chapter 83).[72–75a] Encouraging results have been reported over 3 months with use of bilevel positive airway pressure, with reduction in nocturnal carbon dioxide retention and improvement in daytime somnolence and the sensation of dyspnea.[73] In the latter report, if patients did not have coexisting obstructive apnea, the inspiratory pressure used was the highest that was tolerated by the patient while the expiratory pressure was 2 to 4 cm H_2O. If the patients had obstructive apnea, the expiratory pressure value was the previously determined effective CPAP level while the inspiratory pressure level was increased until there was the elimination of oxygen desaturations. When bilevel positive airway pressure is stopped once patients have had clinical improvement, within a week they have a return of daytime sleepiness, morning headaches, dyspnea, and a loss of energy.[74]

I have had patients with post-poliomyelitic kyphoscoliosis who had been sleeping on rocking beds for decades. Several developed progressive nocturnal respiratory failure and required other modalities of ventilation. Determining the most appropriate ventilatory modality may involve trial and error. These patients can be ventilated noninvasively by use of a negative pressure (Emerson) ventilator.[76] Intermittent positive-pressure ventilation or CPAP, both administered by a nasal mask, may also be effective.[72] These modalities should be evaluated in a setting in which their effects can be monitored. When ventilation is not possible with these "noninvasive" modalities, a tracheostomy may become necessary.

Medications in the Nonventilated Patient

Although breathing oxygen-enriched gas mixtures is known to increase waking values of $PaCO_2$ in kyphoscoliosis patients already hypercapnic, it is not known whether the benefit of increased PaO_2 offsets the rise in $PaCO_2$.[59] I have seen several hypercapnic kyphoscoliotic patients who became comatose with oxygen administration. Thus, the sensorium and $PaCO_2$ should be monitored closely until the patient is stable. It has been shown that while oxygen will increase SaO_2 during sleep in these patients, dyspnea, morning headache, and sleepiness are not systematically improved in contrast to improvement in patients with these symptoms documented with ventilatory support.[75]

Because the most severe oxygen desaturations occur in REM sleep, suppression of REM sleep may theoretically be of benefit. Protriptyline (see Chapter 69), a nonsedating tricyclic antidepressant, has been evaluated in eight patients with chest wall restriction.[62] A dose of 10 to 20 mg at bedtime reduced REM sleep by about 50%. Oxygenation was significantly improved while the patients were asleep and awake. Hypercapnia was also improved during sleep. Anticholinergic side effects were not a severe problem in this report; however, seven of the eight patients were women, who are less likely than are men to develop urinary hesitancy.

I have evaluated medroxyprogesterone acetate and acetazolamide in a single kyphoscoliosis patient with REM sleep–related central apneas and cor pulmonale. Acetazolamide alone did not reduce apnea frequency but reduced mean apnea duration from about 39 to 21 sec and increased mean SaO_2 in REM sleep from 71.3 to 76.5% ($P < .05$). Unfortunately, this medication did not resolve the cor pulmonale. Medroxyprogesterone acetate alone in this same patient had no effect on apnea duration or frequency or on sleep SaO_2 and did not resolve the cor pulmonale. The combination of acetazolamide and medroxyprogesterone acetate improved the cor pulmonale.

INTERSTITIAL LUNG DISEASE

The accumulation of abnormal cells, tissues, or fluid in the interstitial space of the lung alters the mechanical properties of the lung, making it substantially stiffer and increasing its recoil, which reduces lung volume. Although interstitial lung disease can be caused by over a hundred diseases, the disorders most commonly responsible are idiopathic pulmonary fibrosis (also called interstitial pneumonitis or cryptogenic fibrosing alveolitis), sarcoidosis, occupational dust exposures, malignancy, and reaction to drugs.[1] Patients with interstitial lung disorders have a rapid, shallow breathing pattern thought to be related to lung vagal stimulation by the pathological process in the lungs. The resultant level of ventilation is usually excessive for the level of carbon dioxide production, which causes hypocapnia to occur.[77] These patients have very disrupted sleep, with more arousals, sleep-stage changes, and sleep fragmentation than normal subjects monitored with similar instrumentation have.[78, 79] The multiple arousals could be related to coughing or to chemical stimuli. Patients with SaO_2 less than 90% had more disrupted sleep than did those with SaO_2 above 90%. Sleep stages were also redistributed, with a marked increase in stage 1 and a reduction in REM sleep.

In studies of SaO_2 during sleep, three patterns of oxygen desaturations have been reported.[77] In the first, and most common, oxygen desaturation occurred primarily during REM sleep and seemed to be related to episodic hypoventilation. The lower the baseline SaO_2, the greater the fall in SaO_2 from awake to REM sleep.[80] In the second pattern, there were sustained falls in SaO_2 during both REM sleep and NREM sleep. The third group of patients consisted of those who snored, some of whom had the classic obstructive sleep apnea syndrome. Although a low incidence of apnea and hypopnea was found in the authors' series, it was found that patients with interstitial lung disease with SaO_2 less than 90% had drops in SaO_2 when they snored.[79] Profound hypoxemic episodes tend to be brief and rare, and the maximal fall in SaO_2 is similar to that seen during maximal exercise.[81] Because the hypoxemic episodes may be brief, the mean sleep SaO_2 may fall only slightly from awake values.[81]

Low oxygen saturation of the night is related to awake PaO_2, age, and lung compliance. Low SaO_2 could be reasonably predicted from awake PaO_2 and age by the following equation[82]:

$$\text{Predicted low } SaO_2 = 75 + 0.23(PaO_2) - 0.2(\text{age})$$

Breathing frequency tends to remain high but may decrease during sleep. Transcutaneous PCO_2 may stay the same as at awake levels,[83] or it may increase by levels similar to those seen in normal subjects.[66] Hypoventilation does not seem to occur.[66, 80] Thus, although many reflexes are inhibited by the sleep state, those that maintain the rapid breathing pattern remain during sleep. Apnea frequency is low in these patients, perhaps reflecting a high drive to breathe. Control of breathing does appear to be important in maintaining ventilation in interstitial fibrosis; patients with lower hypercapnic ventilatory responses have greater falls in SaO_2 during sleep.[80] Obstructive sleep apnea has been described in patients with disorders that may cause interstitial lung diseases, including rheumatoid arthritis[84] and sarcoidosis.[85]

Therapeutic Implications

In view of the high drive to breathe and the low incidence of apnea, it is unlikely that nocturnal oxygen therapy would cause either significant apneas or hypoventilation. In the absence of any literature dealing with indications for nocturnal oxygen therapy in this group, it seems prudent to start with the criteria of the Nocturnal Oxygen Therapy Trial Group.[86] One would use supplemental oxygen if awake PaO_2 is less than 55 mmHg or if it is less than 60 mmHg in the presence of hypoxemic complications (polycythemia or peripheral edema). However, because many of these patients desaturate rapidly with minimal exercise, criteria for home oxygen therapy should be more liberal, and many centers use exercise oximetry as a guide in determining the need for home oxygen. Some patients may need oxygen therapy only with exercise. Respiratory stimulants probably do not have a role in interstitial lung disease because respiratory drive is usually already high.

References

1. Warren CPW. Lung restriction. In: Kryger M, ed. Introduction to Respiratory Medicine. New York, NY: Churchill Livingstone; 1990:45–73.
2. Alpert MA, Hashimi MW. Obesity and the heart. Am J Med Sci. 1993;306:117–123.
3. Luce JM. Respiratory complications of obesity. Chest. 1980;78:4.
4. Mark P, Varon J. The obese patient in the ICU. Chest. 1998;113:492–498.
5. Dempsey JA, Reddan W, Balke B, et al. Work capacity determinants and physiologic cost of weight-supported breathing in obesity. J Appl Physiol. 1966;21:1815–1820.
6. Naimark A, Cherniack RM. Compliance of the respiratory system and its components in health and obesity. J Appl Physiol. 1960;15:377–382.
7. Fritts HW, Filler J, Fishman AP, et al. The efficiency of ventilation during voluntary hyperpnea: studies in normal subjects and in dyspneic patients with either chronic pulmonary emphysema or obesity. J Clin Invest. 1959;38:1339–1348.
8. Bedell GN, Wilson WR, Seebohm PM. Pulmonary function in obese persons. J Clin Invest. 1958;37:1049–1061.
9. Sharp JT, Henry JP, Sweany SK, et al. Effects of mass loading the respiratory system in man. J Appl Physiol. 1964;19:959–966.
10. Pankow W, Hijjeh N, Schuttler F, et al. Effect of noninvasive ventilation on work of breathing in obesity. Med Klin. 1997;92(suppl 1):54–60.

11. Block AJ, Boysen PG, Wynne JW, et al. The sleep hypopnea and oxygen desaturation in normal subjects. N Engl J Med. 1979;300:513–517.

12. Exar EN, Collop NA. The upper airway resistance syndrome. Chest. 1999;115:1127–1139.

13. Gould G, Whyte KF, Rhind GB, et al. The sleep hypopnea syndrome. Am Rev Respir Dis. 1988;137:895–898.

14. Harman E, Wynne JW, Block AJ, et al. Sleep disordered breathing and desaturation in obesity bypass patients [abstract]. Am Rev Respir Dis. 1979;119:125.

15. Vgontzas AN, Tan TL, Bixler EO, et al. Sleep apnea and sleep disruption in obese patients. Arch Intern Med. 1994;154:1705–1711.

16. Hoffstein V, Brown I, Zamel N, et al. Changes in pharyngeal size with recumbency and the application of continuous positive airway pressure in patients with obstructive sleep apnea. Am Rev Respir Dis. 1986;133:A147.

17. Schwartz AR, Smith PL, Gould AR, et al. Induction of obstructive sleep apnea in normal individuals. Am Rev Respir Dis. 1986;133:A307.

18. Brzecka A, Zukowska H, Werynska B. Chronic alveolar hypoventilation in obstructive sieep apnea syndrome. Pol Merkuriusz Lek. 1996;1:8–10.

19. Kessler R, Chaouat A, Weitzenblum E, et al. Pulmonary hypertension in the obstructive sleep apnea syndrome: prevalence, causes and therapeutic consequences. Eur Respir J. 1996;9:787–794.

20. Ahmed Q, Chung-Park M, Tomashefski JF Jr. Cardiopulmonary pathology in patients with sleep apnea/obesity hypoventilation syndrome. Hum Pathol. 1997;28:264–269.

21. Laaban JP, Orvoen-Frija E, Cassuto D, et al. Mechanisms of diurnal hypercapnia in sleep apnea syndromes associated with morbid obesity. Presse Med. 1996;25:12–16.

21a. American Academy of Sleep Medicine. Sleep-related breathing disorders in adults: recommendations for syndrome definition and measurement techniques in clinical research. Sleep. 1999;22:667–689.

22. Lourenco RV. Diaphragm activity in obesity. J Clin Invest. 1969;48:1609–1614.

23. Gilbert R, Sipple JH, Auchincloss JH. Respiratory control and work of breathing in obese subjects. J Appl Physiol. 1961;16:21–26.

24. Pedersen J, Torp-Pedersen E. Ventilatory insufficiency in extreme obesity. Acta Med Scand. 1960;167:343–351.

25. Zwillich CW, Sutton FO, Pierson DJ, et al. Decreased hypoxic ventilatory drive in the obesity-hypoventilation syndrome. Am J Med. 1975;59:343–347.

26. Burwell CS, Robin ED, Whaley RD, et al. Extreme obesity associated with alveolar hypoventilation—a pickwickian syndrome. Am J Med. 1956;21:811–818.

27. Lyons HH, Huang CT. Therapeutic use of progesterone in alveolar hypoventilation associated with obesity. Am J Med. 1968;44:881–888.

27a. Saaresranta T, Polo-Kantola P, Irjala K, et al. Respiratory insufficiency in postmenopausal women: sustained improvement with short-term medroxyprogesterone acetate. Chest. 1999;115:1581–1587.

28. Thompson KJ, Cohen ME. Vital capacity observations in normal pregnant women. Surg Gynecol Obstet. 1938;66:591.

29. Prowse CM, Gaensler EA. Respiratory and acid base changes during pregnancy. Anesthesiology. 1965;26:381.

30. Cugell DW, Frank NR, Gaensler EA, et al. Pulmonary function in pregnancy, I: serial observations in normal women. Am Rev Tuberc. 1953;67:568–597.

31. Holdcroft A, Bevan DR, O'Sullivan JC, et al. Airway closure and pregnancy. Anaesthesia. 1979;32:517–523.

32. Awe RJ, Nicorta MB, Newson TD, et al. Arterial oxygen and alveolar-arterial gradients in term pregnancy. Obstet Gynecol. 1979;53:182–186.

33. Kambam JR, Handte RE, Brown WR, et al. Effect of pregnancy on oxygen dissociation [abstract]. Anesthesiology. 1983;59:A39.

34. Archer GW, Marx GF. Arterial oxygen tension during apnea in parturient women. Br J Anaesth. 1974;46:358–360.

35. Brownell LG, West P, Kryger MH. Breathing during sleep in normal pregnant women. Am Rev Respir Dis. 1986;133:38–41.

36. Hertz G, Fast A, Feinsilver SH, et al. Sleep in normal late pregnancy. Sleep. 1992;15:246–251.

37. Nikkola E, Ekblad UU, Ekholm EM, et al. Sleep in multiple pregnancy: breathing patterns, oxygenation and periodic leg movements. Am J Obstet Gynecol. 1996;174:1622–1625.

38. Lyons HA. Centrally acting hormone and respiration. Pharmacol Ther. 1976;2:743–751.

39. Jaffe RB, Josimovich JB. Endocrine physiology of pregnancy. In: Danford DN, ed. Obstetrics and Gynecology. Hagerstown, Md: Harper & Row; 1977:286–298.

40. Yannone ME, McCurdy JR, Coldfien A. Plasma progesterone levels in normal pregnancy, labour and the puerperium. Am J Obstet Gynecol. 1968;101:1058–1061.

41. Mishell DR, Davajan V. Reproductive Endocrinology, Infertility and Contraception. Philadelphia, Pa: FA Davis; 1979:123–124.

42. Kryger MH, McCullough RE, Collins D, et al. Treatment of excessive polycythemia of high altitude with respiratory stimulant drugs. Am Rev Respir Dis. 1978;117:445–464.

43. Pernoll ML, Metcalfe J, Kovach PA, et al. Ventilation during rest and exercise in pregnancy and post partum. Respir Physiol. 1975;25:295.

44. Suzuki S, Dennerstein L, Greenwood KM, et al. Sleeping patterns during pregnancy in Japanese women. J Psychosom Obstet Gynaecol. 1994;15:19–26.

45. Fast A, Shapiro D, Ducommun EJ, et al. Low-back pain in pregnancy. Spine. 1987;12:368–371.

46. Mills GH, Chaffe AG. Sleeping positions adopted by pregnant women of more than 30 weeks gestation. Anaesthesia. 1994;49:249–250.

47. McParland P, Pearce JM. Restless legs syndrome in pregnancy. Case reports. Clin Exp Obstet Gynecol. 1990;17:5–6.

48. Ekholm E, Polo O, Rauhala ER, et al. Sleep quality in preeclampsia. Am J Obstet Gynecol. 1992;167:1262–1266.

49. Berlin RM. Sleepwalking disorder during pregnancy: a case report. Sleep. 1988;11:298–300.

50. Littner MR. Snoring in pregnancy. Disease or not? Chest. 1996;109:859–861.

51. Franklin KA, Holmgren PÅ, Jönsson F, et al. Snoring, pregnancy-induced hypertension, and growth retardation of the fetus. Chest. 2000;117:137–141.

52. Turnbull GL, Rundell OH, Rayburn WF, et al. Managing pregnancy-related nocturnal nasal congestion. The external nasal dilator. J Reprod Med. 1996;41:897–902.

53. Kowall J, Clark G, Nino-Murcia G, et al. Precipitation of obstructive sleep apnea during pregnancy. Obstet Gynecol. 1989;74(pt 2):453–455.

53a. Lewis DF, Chesson AL, Edwards MS, et al. Obstructive sleep apnea during pregnancy resulting in pulmonary hypertension. South Med J. 1998;91:761–762.

54. Hastie SJ, Prowse K, Perks WH, et al. Obstructive sleep apnoea during pregnancy requiring tracheostomy. Aust N Z J Obstet Gynaecol. 1989;29(pt 2):365–367.

55. Conti M, Izzo V, Muggiasca ML, et al. Sleep apnoea syndrome in pregnancy: a case report. Eur J Anaesthesiol. 1988;5:151–154.

56. Charbonneau M, Falcone T, Cosio MG, et al. Obstructive sleep apnea during pregnancy. Therapy and implications for fetal health. Am Rev Respir Dis. 1991;144:461–463.

57. Schoefeld A, Ovadia Y, Neri A, et al. Obstructive sleep apnea (OSA)—implications in maternal-fetal medicine. A hypothesis. Med Hypotheses. 1989;30:51–54.

58. Pieters T, Amy JJ, Burrini D, et al. Normal pregnancy in primary alveolar hypoventilation treated with nocturnal nasal intermittent positive pressure ventilation. Eur Respir J. 1995;8:1424–1427.

59. Bergofsky EH, Turinto GM, Fishman AP. Cardiorespiratory failure in kyphoscoliosis. Medicine (Baltimore). 1959;38:263.

60. Guilleminault C, Kurland G, Winkle R, et al. Severe kyphoscoliosis, breathing, and sleep. The "Quasimodo" syndrome during sleep. Chest. 1981;79:6.

61. Mezon BL, West P, Israels J, et al. Sleep breathing abnormalities in kyphoscoliosis. Am Rev Respir Dis. 1980;122:617.

62. Simonds AK, Parker RA, Branthwaite MA. Effects of protriptyline on sleep related disturbances of breathing in restrictive chest wall disease. Thorax. 1986;41:586–590.

63. Kafer ER. Respiratory function in paralytic scoliosis. Am Rev Respir Dis. 1974;110:450.

64. Kryger M. Pathophysiology of Respiration. New York, NY: John Wiley & Sons; 1981:218.

65. Sawicka EH, Branthwaite MA. Respiration during sleep in kyphoscoliosis. Thorax. 1987;42:801–808.

66. Midgren B, Hansson L. Changes in transcutaneous P_{CO_2} with sleep in normal subjects and in patients with chronic respiratory diseases. Eur J Respir Dis. 1987;71:388–394.

67. Midgren B. Oxygen desaturation during sleep as a function of the underlying respiratory disease. Am Rev Respir Dis. 1990;141:43–46.

68. Hoeppner VH, Cockcroft DW, Dosman JA, et al. Night-time ventilation improves respiratory failure in secondary kyphoscoliosis. Am Rev Respir Dis. 1984;129:240.

69. Levine S, Henson D, Levy S. Respiratory muscle rest therapy. Clin Chest Med. 1988;9:297–309.

70. Bruderman I, Stein M. Physiologic evaluation and treatment of kyphoscoliotic patients. Ann Intern Med. 1961;55:94.

71. Sinha R, Bergofsky EH. Prolonged alteration of lung mechanics in kyphoscoliosis by positive pressure hyperinflation. Am Rev Respir Dis. 1972;106:47.

72. Ellis ER, Grunstein RR, Chan S, et al. Noninvasive ventilatory support during sleep improves respiratory failure in kyphoscoliosis. Chest. 1988;94:811–815.

73. Waldhorn RE. Nocturnal nasal intermittent positive pressure ventilation with bi-level positive pressure (BiPap) in respiratory failure. Chest. 1992;101:516–521.

74. Hill NS, Eveloff SE, Carlisle CC, et al. Efficacy of nocturnal nasal ventilation in patients with restrictive thoracic disease. Am Rev Respir Dis. 1992;145:365–371.

75. Masa JF. Noninvasive positive pressure ventilation and not oxygen may prevent overt ventilatory failure in patients with chest wall disease. Chest. 1997;112:207–213.

75a. Clinical indications for noninvasive positive pressure ventilation in chronic respiratory failure due to restrictive lung disease, COPD, and nocturnal hypoventilation—a consensus conference report. Chest. 1999;116:521–534.

76. Pfister M, Keller R. Periodic nocturnal ventilation using an Emerson chest respirator as an alternative to permanent tracheostomy with positive pressure ventilation in patients with idiopathic scoliosis and severe global respiratory insufficiency. Schweiz Med Wochenschr. 1988;118:1371–1374.

77. Lourenco RV, Turino GM, Davidson LA, et al. The regulation of ventilation in diffuse pulmonary fibrosis. Am J Med. 1965;38:199–216.

78. Bye PT, Issa F, Berthon-Jones M, et al. Studies of oxygenation during sleep in patients with interstitial lung disease. Am Rev Respir Dis. 1984;129:27–32.

79. Perez-Padilla R, West P, Lertzman M, et al. Breathing during sleep in patients with interstitial lung disease. Am Rev Respir Dis. 1985;132:224–229.

80. Tatsumi K, Kimuar H, Kunitomo F, et al. Arterial oxygen desaturation during sleep in interstitial pulmonary disease. Correlation with chemical control of breathing during wakefulness. Chest. 1989;95:962–967.

81. Midgren B, Hansson L, Eriksson L, et al. Oxygen desaturation during sleep and exercise in patients with interstitial lung disease. Thorax. 1987;42:353–356.

82. Rajagopal KR, Derderian SS, Culpepper WJ, et al. Sleep and nocturnal oxygenation in patients with restrictive pulmonary disease. Sleep Res. 1991;20A:445.

83. Shea SA, Winning AJ, McKenzie E, et al. Does the abnormal pattern of breathing in patients with interstitial lung disease persist in deep, non-rapid eye movement sleep? Am Rev Respir Dis. 1989;139:653–658.

84. Offers E, Herbort C, Dumke K, et al. Complicated course of rheumatoid arthritis with pulmonary involvement, myocardial fibrosis and sleep apnea syndrome. Pneumologie. 1996;50:906–911.

85. Turner GA, Lower EE, Corser BC, et al. Sleep apnea in sarcoidosis. Sarcoidosis Vasc Diffuse Lung Dis. 1997;14:61–64.

86. Nocturnal Oxygen Therapy Trial Group. Continuous or nocturnal oxygen therapy in hypoxemic chronic obstructive lung disease. Ann Intern Med. 1980;93:391–398.

83

Noninvasive Ventilation for Sleep Breathing Disorders

Dominique Robert

Patrick Leger

Patients requiring long-term mechanical ventilatory assistance (LTMV) were initially those who had sequelae of poliomyelitis or Duchenne's muscular dystrophy (DMD). Either noninvasive ventilation (negative pressure body ventilators, positive pressure via mouthpiece, or both) or invasive ventilation (via tracheotomy) was used.[1–10] Early experience with LTMV revealed that patients with essentially no ventilatory function could be maintained on continuous support, whereas individuals who retained partial ventilatory function could do well by receiving intermittent ventilatory assistance (e.g., during sleep).[7, 11, 12] It was recognized that continuous positive airway pressure and intermittent positive pressure ventilation could be comfortably delivered, noninvasively, through a nasal mask.[13–20] In light of its successful application, the use of noninvasive positive pressure ventilation (NPPV) for LTMV increased substantially, both in patients with restrictive disorders due to neuromuscular or chest wall disorders and, to a somewhat lesser degree, to patients with lung parenchymal disorders such as chronic obstructive pulmonary disease (COPD). Nocturnal NPPV has also been proposed in a few instances of central obstructive sleep apnea syndrome. This chapter focuses on the treatment of patients who require NPPV during sleep to achieve physiological and clinical improvement while asleep as well as during wakefulness. In addition, we contrast treatments with NPPV and negative pressure modalities.

HISTORICAL PERSPECTIVE

Long-term ventilatory support began during the poliomyelitis epidemics of the 1950s. At that time, the only available method of providing noninvasive ventilatory assistance was via negative pressure such as use of the the "iron lung." The clinical outcome remained dismal, however, until workers in Copenhagen started performing tracheotomy, through which intermittent positive pressure ventilation was provided by manual inflation.[21, 22] To replace manual inflation, Lassen successfully used an experimental positive pressure ventilator.[22, 23] Subsequently, ventilatory support through the use of positive pressure via tracheostomy became widely used throughout Europe, and the mortality rates in succeeding epidemics were markedly reduced. Many patients with poliomyelitis survived the acute phase but, due to permanent neuromuscular damage, did not regain the adequate ability to breathe spontaneously. As a result, they received chronic ventilatory support either with positive pressure (predominantly in Europe) or with negative pressure (predominantly in North America).

Experience with long-term ventilated poliomyelitis survivors in the 1960s proved that it was possible for these patients to live a long and active life with assisted ventilation.[10, 12] Positive pressure via a tracheostomy or negative pressure ventilation was frequently used into the 1980s to provide LTMV support to patients with other diseases such as DMD, thoracic deformities, or lung and chest wall structural abnormalities associated with tuberculosis and thoracoplasty, as well as a few individuals with COPD.[8, 9, 12, 24–27] During this same period of time, there was a large and unique experience with NPPV with the use of a lip seal mouthpiece during sleep and a mouthpiece during wakefulness in poliomyelitis survivors and DMD patients with good clinical results.[10]

The therapeutic results associated with LTMV assistance were very good in patients with restrictive disorders. In addition, it was noted that many patients were greatly improved with the use of only nocturnal ventilation, which reversed daytime chronic hypoventilation and alleviated the clinical signs of cor pulmonale.[7, 11, 12, 28] This in turn decreased the need for hospitalization due to acute failure and prolonged patient survival for many years. Surprisingly, the application of either positive or negative long-term ventilation in patients with these disorders did not become popular, probably because of the invasive nature of tracheostomy and the practical difficulties associated with the use of negative pressure ventilation, even with the relatively simpler poncho or cuirass devices.

In the 1980s, the introduction of nasal continuous positive airway pressure (CPAP) using commercially made nasal masks to treat sleep apnea[13] facilitated the emergence of noninvasive NPPV, particularly during sleep, as a feasible therapeutic option. This practice spread to many centers throughout the world. Subsequently, successful LTMV with the use of NPPV was reported at a number of centers.[14–18, 20, 29–33] Two additional reasons favored a more expanded application of NPPV in the 1990s: (1) a small portable machine was capable of independently adjusting inspiratory and expiratory pressure; these bilevel machines did not present a clear advantage compared with CPAP and probably were used in a minority of patients with sleep apnea but appeared to be a simple and less expensive ventilator by which to provide NPPV[34]; and (2) the successful use of NPPV to treat acute ventilatory failure in patients with underlying chronic respiratory insufficiency promoted the concept in the medical community that because NPPV is efficient in acute failure, it can also be useful in the treatment of chronic ventilatory failure.[35–37]

INDICATIONS FOR THE USE OF NOCTURNAL NONINVASIVE POSITIVE PRESSURE VENTILATION

Diseases That Might Be Treated With Noninvasive Positive Pressure Ventilation

Consensus recommendations concerning the clinical indications for noninvasive ventilation have been published.[37a] The principal diseases that may benefit from NPPV therapy are shown in Table 83–1. All of the diseases may be sufficiently severe to cause alveolar hypoventilation that impairs the quality of life or is life threatening. As they pertain to the initiation of noctur-

---

Table 83–1. DISEASES THAT CAN BENEFIT FROM NONINVASIVE POSITIVE PRESSURE VENTILATION

Restrictive Disorders (VC $\downarrow\downarrow$, FEV$_1$ $\downarrow\downarrow$; FEV$_1$/FVC$\rightarrow$; RV $\downarrow$; TLC $\downarrow$)

Chest Wall

No worsening	Kyphoscoliosis
Slow worsening	Sequelae of tuberculosis

Neuromuscular

Slow worsening (>15 y)	Spinal muscular atrophy, acid maltase deficit
Intermediate worsening (5–15 y)	Duchenne's muscular dystrophy, myotonic myopathy
Rapid worsening (0–5 y)	Amyotrophic lateral sclerosis

Obstructive Diseases (VC $\downarrow$ or $\rightarrow$; FEV$_1$ $\downarrow\downarrow$; FEV$_1$/FVC $\downarrow\downarrow$; RV $\uparrow\uparrow$; TLC $\uparrow\uparrow$)

COPD

Bronchiectasis

Normal Lungs (with abnormal central ventilatory control; PFTs normal)

Idiopathic Hypoventilation

Obesity Hypoventilation Syndrome

Symbols indicate actual value compared with theoretical value: $\downarrow\downarrow$ or $\uparrow\uparrow$, important decrease or increase; $\downarrow$, moderate decrease; $\rightarrow$, normal; COPD, chronic obstructive pulmonary disease; FEV$_1$, forced expiratory volume in 1 sec; PFT, pulmonary function of testing; RV, residual volume; TLC, total lung capacity; VC, vital capacity.

Table 83–2. CLINICAL FEATURES OF HYPOVENTILATION

Shortness of breath during activities of daily living in the absence of paralysis
Orthopnea in disorders of diaphragmatic dysfunction
Poor sleep quality: insomnia, nightmares, frequent arousals
Nocturnal or early morning headaches
Daytime fatigue and sleepiness, loss of energy
Decrease in intellectual performance
Loss of appetite
Loss of weight
Appearance of recurrent complications: respiratory infections
Cor pulmonale

---

nal NPPV therapy, the primary considerations include (1) the relative contribution of chest wall, neuromuscular, and pulmonary parenchymal disorders; (2) the natural evolution of the disease process to anticipate the future need for evolution from NPPV exclusively during sleep, to diurnal ventilatory assistance; and (3) the associated comorbidity that may dominate the prognosis.

Clinical Severity

The presence of clinical or physiological markers of hypoventilation reflects one way to define disease severity as it relates to the consideration of nocturnal NPPV. Clinical symptoms indicating the consequences of hypoventilation (Table 83–2) must be carefully evaluated. Hypoventilation is defined by increased arterial carbon dioxide tension (PaCO_2) and high serum bicarbonate levels with associated reduction in arterial oxygen tension (PaO_2). There are no validated values above which NPPV is definitely indicated, but many clinicians consider treatment for patients with an awake PaCO_2 level of more than 50 to 55 mmHg and a PaO_2 level of less than 65 mmHg. The degrees of severity are schematically presented in Table 83–3, all representing different states in which NPPV may be considered. Clinical symptoms and daytime hypoventilation are associated with the most important level of severity. Chronic daytime hypoventilation is an important indicator of a very low respiratory reserve and should be considered an unstable state prone to life threatening acute failure that may be triggered by minimal additional factors. Sleep-related hypoventilation is invariably present in patients with diurnal hypoventilation, and there is no need to prove it with polysomnography except to rule out apnea. An FEV$_1$ less than 40%, a PaCO_2 greater than 45 mmHg, and a base excess equal to or greater than 4 mmol/L may be helpful in predicting hypoventilation during sleep.[37b] In patients with mild or moderate severity (see Table 83–3), limited cardiopulmonary sleep studies are required for the recognition of nocturnal hypoventilation that may occur throughout all sleep stages but in some cases exclusively during rapid eye movement (REM) sleep. The recognition of nocturnal hypoventilation requires measurements of SpO_2 (oxygen saturation level measured by pulse oximeter) and tcPCO_2 (transcutaneous PCO_2) or capnography as part of a full polysomnogram (PSG),

Table 83–3. DEGREES OF SEVERITY BASED ON CLINICAL SIGNS AND PHYSIOLOGICAL MEASUREMENTS

Clinical Signs*	Diurnal Hypoventilation†	Nocturnal Hypoventilation‡	Severity
Yes	Yes	Yes	Severe
Yes	No	Yes	Moderate
No	No	Yes	Mild
No	No	No	No

*Symptoms of chronic ventilatory failure (see Table 83–2).
†PaO_2 less than 65 mmHg and $PaCO_2$ of more than 50–55 mmHg.
‡Proved at least with overnight SpO_2, possibly associated with CO_2 recording (transcutaneous or capnography).

which will facilitate assessment of the unique or combined mechanisms of hypoventilation (nonobstructive hypoventilation, central or obstructive apnea-hypopnea) and the impact on sleep that may result in daytime symptoms (e.g., arousals leading to hypersomnolence). Nevertheless, due to the complexity and cost of full PSG or because PSG may not be available, fewer physiological parameters may be recorded. At least in the absence of clinically suspected sleep apnea, SpO_2 may be recorded alone because desaturations occur simultaneously with increase in $PaCO_2$. Although there are no consensus statements addressing the duration and degree of hypoventilation, it seems reasonable, although unproved, that hypoventilation must be present throughout sleep (nonrapid eye movement [NREM] plus REM) to have severe clinical consequences. In these patients, management requires expertise in sleep medicine and experience with NPPV.

Pulmonary function tests help define and quantify the ventilatory-respiratory disease but are poorly correlated with chronic hypoventilation in individual cases.

Indications for Nocturnal Noninvasive Positive Pressure Ventilation

Indications for NPPV must balance several points: (1) the disease process and its natural rate of progression, (2) the severity at the time of decision, and (3) the

patient's willingness to undertake this therapy, which is a mandatory requirement.

In clinical practice, NPPV is initiated either electively or in the context of acute ventilatory failure. In the latter circumstance, the long-term necessity for NPPV should be reevaluated in follow-up of the patient after the acute episode because as the clinical condition stabilizes, the indications for NPPV may change. Indications are listed in Table 83–4. NPPV is indicated in patients with restrictive diseases (chest wall and neuromuscular) in the presence of symptoms attributable to either diurnal or nocturnal hypoventilation.[38–40] The required duration of NPPV depends on the natural progression of the ventilatory impairment inherent to the underlying disease process. With increasing ventilator dependency, the daily duration of NPPV may be progressively extended from sleep time alone to throughout the 24-h period[32, 41] or a tracheostomy could be performed.[12, 42] Conversely, in COPD, NPPV could be indicated as an option only in patients with symptoms of hypoventilation or hypoventilation contributing to hypoxemia, provided that long-term oxygen therapy has already been optimally adjusted.

There are limited data regarding the use of NPPV as prophylaxis against acute ventilatory failure or to increase survival rates in patients who do not have chronic ventilatory failure. However, although frequently criticized on methodological grounds, one study reported that there was no benefit of such use in patients with muscular dystrophy.[43]

Table 83–4. INDICATIONS FOR NONINVASIVE POSITIVE PRESSURE VENTILATION BASED ON DISEASE PROCESS AND SEVERITY

Disease	Clinical Sign* Plus Diurnal Hypoventilation†	Clinical Sign Plus Nocturnal Hypoventilation‡	Only Nocturnal Hypoventilation	Neither Clinical Signs nor Hypoventilation	Maintainance on Nocturnal NPPV (y)
Scoliosis	Yes	Yes	Perhaps	No	>10–20
Tuberculosis	Yes	Yes	No	No	10
Neuromuscular slow	Yes	Yes	No	No	10–15
Neuromuscular intermediate	Yes	Yes	No	No	5
Neuromuscular severe	Yes	Yes	No	No	0–5
COPD	Perhaps	No	No	No	1–5
Bronchiectasis	Yes	Perhaps	No	No	1–5
Obesity hypoventilation	Yes	Yes	Perhaps	No	>10–20

*Symptoms of chronic ventilatory failure (see Table 83–2).
†PaO_2 less than 65 mmHg and $PaCO_2$ of more than 50–55 mmHg.
‡Documented at least with overnight SpO_2, possibly associated with CO_2 recording (transcutaneous or capnography).
COPD, chronic obstructive pulmonary disease; NPPV, noninvasive positive pressure ventilation.

Patients Who Require Continuous Assistance With Noninvasive Positive Pressure Ventilation

With time, many patients, particularly those with progressive neuromuscular disease, require ventilatory assistance during wakefulness as well as during sleep. At this point, the clinician must reconsider the suitability of NPPV. It is evident that an interface such as a nasal mask, which functions well during sleep, would be generally inappropriate during wakefulness. Thus, when both diurnal and nocturnal NPPV ventilation are required, the interface may vary with the period of use (e.g., nasal NPPV at night and NPPV via mouthpiece during the day). Such an application has been reported by different teams in the treatment of stable patients with neuromuscular disease, such as those with sequelae of poliomyelitis, high-level spinal cord injury, or DMD.[9, 41, 44, 45] Nevertheless, some clinicians have expressed a preference for tracheostomy when 24-h or nearly 24-h ventilatory assistance is required, often because tracheostomy ensures the airway and facilitates secretion removal.[12, 38, 46, 47] The continuation of NPPV assumes that the medical team, patient, family, and caregivers have a good understanding of secretion removal techniques; however, this represents an important clinical issue that may remain problematic under the best of circumstances during the provision of NPPV. There is no clear answer as to whether, and beyond what duration, a ventilator patient is better or more safely ventilated by tracheostomy or NPPV. In our experience, patients with DMD who have been using NPPV for 16 to 20 h/day and subsequently converted to ventilatory assistance via tracheostomy demonstrate weight gain and psychological improvement. This may be related to the fact that during the daytime, ventilatory assistance is consistently delivered via the tracheostomy, thereby releasing the patient of the obligation to repeatedly access the mouthpiece for a few assisted breaths and then leave it. This debate will probably continue; in the end, the decision to convert to tracheostomy will be highly dependent on the philosophy and capabilities of the clinical team as well as those of the patient and his or her family and environment. It is essential that a discussion of such issues be started early in the patient's course, well before the imperative arises, and that an expert team in the field of LTMV be involved.

Contraindications

The only major contraindications to nasal intermittent positive pressure ventilation (NIPPV) occur in patients with upper airway dysfunction who are prone to swallowing difficulties and aspiration (particularly frequent in amyotrophic lateral sclerosis) or neurological disorders that render a patient insufficiently cooperative.

Positive Versus Negative Pressure to Deliver Noninvasive Ventilation

As reported, negative pressure ventilation with the use of either an iron lung, poncho, or cuirass was successfully and predominantly used for LTMV until the mid-1980s.[3, 6, 7, 9, 11, 27, 41, 48–51] Currently, negative pressure is applied in a limited number of cases and essentially in those with neuromuscular diseases. In the last decade, the reported application of negative pressure ventilatory assistance was limited to short-term or physiological studies[52–63] and to one long-term study of patients with chest wall diseases.[63] There is little interest in LTMV using negative pressure. Explanations for this lack of enthusiasm include the relatively lower efficacy in providing ventilatory support compared with NPPV in patients with altered pulmonary/chest wall mechanics and in those who have comorbid sleep apnea. In addition, negative pressure ventilation may precipitate sleep apnea.[32, 64–70] From a patient-use perspective, negative pressure modalities are cumbersome and relatively impractical. In this regard, the literature suggests that particularly in patients with nonneuromuscular diseases, long-term compliance with negative pressure ventilation is poor due to discomfort.[58, 59, 62]

TECHNICAL CONSIDERATIONS

Methods of Noninvasive Positive Pressure Ventilation

Interfaces

Choices of interface include nasal masks, mouthpieces, face masks, and various combinations.[71] Table 83–5 lists the advantages, disadvantages, and indications for each interface. Properly fitting a patient with an interface that is both comfortable and relatively airtight is the first step in enhancing the success of NPPV from both patient compliance and clinical efficiency perspectives.

Nasal Interface. There are many nasal interfaces available. If manufacturers' instructions related to the selection of an appropriate size are closely followed and the tools offered for this purpose are used, commercial nasal masks should be the first choice. Recognizing that it is impossible to fit all patients with the same style mask, the clinician should provide the patient with several models and sizes from which to choose.

Difficulties in finding a commercial mask that fits comfortably and is without leaks can be addressed by using a custom-fit mask. Custom nasal masks are used extensively in Europe but rarely in North America.[71, 72] Special consideration is necessary with custom-molded nasal masks to prevent compression of the nares, which would increase airway resistance and adversely influence the quality of ventilation. When using volume-preset ventilation, custom nasal interfaces limit leaks and dead space and therefore seem to be more appropriate than commercial masks.[73]

Table 83–5. ADVANTAGES, DISADVANTAGES, AND INDICATIONS OF INTERFACES

Interface	Advantages	Disadvantages	Indication
Nasal mask	Physiological Natural humidification Can speak and expectorate	Damage nasal bridge Mouth leaks	First interface to use
Commercially made	Large choice Easy to size		First choice
Custom made	Large contact area with face, limiting skin damage	Time consuming Risk of nares compression	Second choice More indicated for volume- than for pressure-preset ventilation
Mouth piece: lip seal industrial or customized	Better control of leaks	Cannot expectorate or talk Aerophagia Initial hypersalivation Dental pain Orthodontic problem Nasal leaks No physiological humidification	Nasal obstruction Massive oral air leaks Intermittent daytime ventilation
Oronasal mask: industrial or customized	Control of oral air leaks	Less choice available for long-term use Difficult to size Claustrophobia Dead space Facial skin necrosis	Nocturnal use Massive air leaks

Oral Interface. Nocturnal lip seal ventilation was the first interface to be used for noninvasive ventilation in postpoliomyelitis patients.[10] In patients with major mouth leaks and nasal obstruction, a mouthpiece is an alternative to nasal ventilation for nocturnal ventilation.[74] Commercial and custom-made intraoral mouthpieces are available. The application of oral interfaces is associated with some specific challenges. It is sometimes necessary to occlude the nares (e.g., with cotton pledgets) to limit nasal leaks during sleep. In addition, aerophagia is more frequently reported with mouth ventilation. It is important to counsel the patient and caregiver that the patient should avoid eating shortly before using a mouthpiece or oronasal (see discussion below) interface and should report nausea or vomiting. In fact, if gastroesophageal reflux or vomiting occurs, there are risks for aspiration because the mouth is more or less occluded with the mouthpiece.

Oronasal Interface. When mouth leaks are significant and prevent adequate ventilatory support, a full face or oronasal mask may be indicated. Oronasal mask ventilation is used extensively during acute respiratory failure,[35, 36] and some clinicians estimate that as many as 30 to 40% of their patients who receive chronic ventilatory assistance use this type of interface.[75, 76] As with nasal masks, proper sizing minimizes leaks and increases tolerance. However, an acceptable fit with a mask may be difficult to achieve in some patients. Oronasal masks can add significant dead space, and ventilator settings must be adjusted accordingly. A custom oronasal mask can be an alternative for the patient in a stable state when noninvasive ventilation can be expected for a long time.[74] A combination of interfaces for the same patient should also be considered for the ventilator-dependent patient who requires assistance both night and day.

When using oronasal interfaces, there are specific safety issues that must be considered. Because the oral airway is not free for breathing in the event of mechanical failure of the ventilatory assist device, the oronasal interface or the circuit should incorporate a safety valve to permit entrainment of fresh air. As with the use of a mouthpiece interface during sleep and discussed previously, there is concern about the risks of aspiration, and similar precautions should be taken.

Ventilator and Settings

Ventilators Used for Noninvasive Positive Pressure Ventilation

The two basic principles for delivering intermittent positive pressure ventilation are related to the use of different types of ventilators: volume preset and pressure preset. *Volume-preset ventilators* used in the home environment involve either a bellows system or a piston in a cylinder and are characterized by low electric consumption and low noise. *Pressure-preset ventilators* usually use blower systems with valving to develop pressure and are characterized by consistently higher electric consumption and level of noise. Blower systems may deliver flow during expiration, allowing the maintenance of positive end-expiratory airway pressure (PEEP) or expiratory positive airway pressure (EPAP). Some home volume-preset ventilators can also deliver PEEP. The advantage of volume-preset ventilation is that the delivered inspiratory volume is held constant while inspiratory pressure varies when respiratory system compliance or resistance changes. The disadvantage is the absence of volume compensation in the presence of air leaks that frequently occur at the junction between skin and mask or through the mouth when using a nasal interface during sleep. Conversely, an advantage of pressure-preset devices is that leaks will be compensated by increased flow to maintain the pressure. A disadvantage of these devices is that the delivered tidal volume will vary when respiratory system compliance or resistance changes, potentially resulting in overventilation or underventilation.

Each of the above two fundamental modes of ventilatory assistance may be set to deliver inspiration at a fixed (control) or variable (assist) frequency. The assist mode may be set with or without a minimal frequency; the patient is allowed to trigger the ventilator to deliver inspiratory assistance. Depending on the specific device, triggering may be sensed by either pressure or flow changes in the circuit, which correspond to a spontaneous effort to breathe. Although flow triggering has been shown to be slightly superior to pressure triggering with respect to reduction in the work of breathing,[77, 78] clinically significant superiority has yet to be demonstrated.

Variations in pressure-preset ventilation have been developed. Ventilator inspiration may be discontinued when airflow approximates zero, indicating that the tidal volume has been completely delivered (pressure support) or a preset inspiratory duration has been reached (pressure control). In NPPV, the former is principally used with the idea that synchronization between patient need and effort would be optimal. In the pressure-preset ventilators, blowers limit PEEP at a preset level.

Choice of Ventilator

The decision for selecting volume- or pressure-preset ventilatory assistance should be made on the basis of several issues: capacity to control nocturnal hypoventilation, ability to control mouth leaks, ability to detect patient demand, patient comfort, and the need for accessory equipment (e.g., alarms, internal batteries). There are few studies that compare volume- and pressure-preset ventilators; in short-term studies,[79, 80] there were no major differences in the correction of hypoventilation in restrictive and COPD patients. Nevertheless, Schönhofer et al.[81] showed that of 28 patients who were adequately ventilated with the volume-preset mode and who then were consecutively ventilated with the pressure-preset mode, significant worsening occurred after 4 weeks in 10 patients. They were converted again to volume-preset ventilators, and after 4 months, all had improved.

Intrinsic PEEP and the consequent requirement for increased inspiratory effort to trigger the ventilator occur frequently in patients with COPD. It therefore is logical to begin ventilation in patients with a ventilator able to confidently establish PEEP (pressure support). It is also important to note that numerous pressure-preset ventilators do not incorporate an expiratory valve but have single tubing with a calibrated leak. In this case, continuous PEEP or EPAP must be maintained to avoid or, more frequently, minimize CO_2 rebreathing.[82, 83] Upper airway instability during sleep (e.g., sleep apnea–hypopnea or upper airway resistance syndrome) represents another indication to begin ventilation with pressure support ventilation and PEEP or EPAP.

When issues of internal and external battery power and ability to have the ventilator mounted on the wheelchair are important considerations, the tendency is to begin NPPV with volume-preset ventilation, particularly for patients with neuromuscular diseases.

These are general guidelines for beginning NPPV. The most important rule of thumb is to consider the main characteristics of different modes (Table 83–6) and for the clinician to remain flexible by trying alternative approaches if problems occur.

Initiation of Noninvasive Positive Pressure Ventilation

The goals of NPPV include provision of patient comfort, synchrony with the ventilator, improvement in sleep, and improvement in arterial blood gases on and off ventilation. It is good general practice to first select and adjust the ventilator settings while the patient is awake, ensuring physiological adequacy and patient comfort for at least 1 or 2 h. Next, the clinician should assess the impact during and after nocturnal use. Sub-

Table 83–6. RESPECTIVE INDICATIONS FOR VOLUME- AND PRESSURE-PRESET VENTILATORS FOR HOME MECHANICAL VENTILATION

	Volume Preset	Pressure Preset
Advantages	Tidal volume always delivered Internal batteries	Comfort Responsive to patient demand PEEP Leak compensation Tidal volume variable
Disadvantages	Decrease of tidal volume in presence of leaks No leaks compensation Poor response to patient demand Desynchronization	Decrease in V_t when resistance increases Failure to maintain pressure and to cycle with massive leaks Variability of FIO_2
First choice	Neuromuscular patients Need for battery	COPD Chest wall or tuberculosis
Second choice	Failure of pressure preset	Failure of volume preset

COPD, chronic obstructive pulmonary disease; PEEP, positive end-expiratory airway pressure.

sequent modification of the settings should be made as necessary according to the results.

If one begins with pressure-preset ventilation, suggested initial settings are a pressure support mode at an inspiratory pressure support of 10 cm H_2O. Some or all criteria, such as a decrease in spontaneous respiratory rate, patient comfort, an increase in inspiratory tidal volume (V_t) to approximately 10 ml/kg, and a decrease in $Paco_2$ on the arterial blood gases, will indicate the effectiveness of ventilatory assistance. If necessary, the pressure level may be progressively increased to achieve evidence of improvement. Pressure support of higher than 20 cm H_2O is rarely necessary and frequently is not well tolerated. With the single circuit ventilators (a single tube connecting the patient's interface with the device), the ventilator setting range does not allow PEEP or EPAP of less than 2 to 4 cm H_2O due to concerns regarding CO_2 rebreathing, although under experimental conditions, higher PEEP or EPAP may be necessary to eliminate rebreathing.[83] Clinical implications of this rebreathing risk are unknown, and increasing PEEP above the minimal obligatory level for that reason is not usually recommended. Indeed, under clinical circumstances, without patient symptoms, it may be difficult to detect the presence of rebreathing. The addition of PEEP should conceptually improve patient triggering when intrinsic PEEP exists in patients with COPD,[84, 85] but there is no long-term study proving its clinical usefulness. In addition, as PEEP increases, so does the risk for air leakage. Practically speaking, PEEP above 4 to 6 cm H_2O is difficult to maintain on a long-term basis.

Initial suggested settings for volume-preset ventilation are to adjust the frequency of delivered breaths close to the spontaneous breathing frequency of the patient, a ratio of inspiratory time to total breathing cycle time (T_i/T_{tot}) between 0.33 and 0.5, and a tidal volume of around 10 ml/kg. A back-up frequency in both volume- and pressure-preset ventilation is determined according to the patient's respiratory drive, sensitivity of the triggering, the potential for hyperinflation, and comfort (while awake). If the patient is unable to effectively trigger the ventilator, the back-up frequency should be set close to the spontaneous frequency of the patient during sleep. Pressure support ventilation without a back-up frequency or low frequency can be used and could limit hyperinflation in patients with COPD.[86]

Supplemental O_2 should be added into the ventilator circuit when starting NPPV in patients requiring oxygen while awake.

After establishing the initial ventilator settings during wakefulness, the next step is to apply nocturnal NPPV and to judge adequacy. When possible, nocturnal recordings should be performed to document the adequacy of ventilation. Ideally, expiratory V_t, airway pressure (P_{aw}), SpO_2, $TcCO_2$ or capnography, thorax and abdomen diameters, and sleep staging will permit assessment. When resources are not available to perform these detailed recordings, it is recommended that the clinician records what is possible and, at the least, evaluate SpO_2. In addition to obtaining objective infor-

mation while the patient is asleep, clinical data about tolerance and comfort should be obtained as well as arterial blood gases during spontaneous breathing. Reduction in $Paco_2$ after several nights confirms the efficacy of NPPV. When no nighttime recordings are available, evidence of a good tolerance and a decrease in $Paco_2$ may be sufficient documentation that the settings are adequate. If the results are not satisfactory, alterations must be made to the settings, and their effects must be rechecked. In most cases, a few days are necessary to succeed.

Follow-Up

Clinical follow-up, including an assessment of symptoms of hypoventilation and daytime arterial blood gases, should be conducted one or two times per year. When possible, night recordings identical to those used for initiating NPPV are useful. At any time, when there are indications of unsatisfactory results, suboptimal NPPV must be suspected and evaluation undertaken, including recording during sleep on NPPV with use of as comprehensive assessment as possible. A change in ventilator modality or settings may be indicated. Increasing the total duration of NPPV use per day may be necessary, particularly when the underlying disease has progressed.

When Should Patients Use Noninvasive Positive Pressure Ventilation?

Nasal ventilation is mainly used at night for physiological and practical reasons but should be encouraged during daytime naps. Schönhofer et al.[81] recently observed that in the short term, awake ventilatory support provided results that were very similar to those for 8 consecutive hours during the night.

MANAGEMENT OF COMPLICATIONS

Air Leaks During Noninvasive Positive Pressure Ventilation

Leaks are present to some degree in all patients who use NPPV during sleep. The major adverse effects are reduction in the efficiency of ventilation and sleep fragmentation.[87, 88] The mechanism responsible for leaks may be related to decreased muscle tone of the oral pharynx during sleep, to a very resistant chest wall, or to glottic occlusion in response to hypocapnia,[89] making leakage the path of least resistance. A variety of measures have been suggested to address problematic mouth leaks, including the prevention of neck flexion, ventilating in a semirecumbent position, discouraging the mouth from opening and preventing the fall of the mandible by use of a chin strap or a cervical collar, decreasing the peak inspiratory pressure, using PEEP or EPAP as necessary to prevent or treat upper airway obstruction, preventing hyperventilation and hypocapnia, and, if using a volume-preset ventilator, attempting pressure ventilation with leak compensation. Changes from nasal to mouth or oronasal ventilation could also be considered.

Nasal Dryness, Congestion, and Rhinitis

Humidification is not usually necessary in noninvasive ventilation, but for some patients, nasal and mouth dryness (usually related to leaks) can be a source of discomfort. A pass-over, or heated, humidifier can be used in this situation or for patients with high sputum production (e.g., bronchiectasis, cystic fibrosis). Heat/moisture exchangers are not well adapted for continuous-flow systems because of low efficiency due to high inspiratory flow or because they create additional resistance in the ventilator circuit.

Aerophagia

Aerophagia is frequently reported by patients, but it is rarely intolerable and not always only related to NPPV.[90] Aerophagia is usually dependent on the level of inspiratory pressure and is more commonly seen when using volume or mouthpiece ventilation. The incidence decreases considerably if the peak inspiratory pressure is kept below 25 cm H_2O pressure. If aerophagia occurs, patient discomfort is the main problem. To address this problem, efforts should be made to reduce the inspiratory pressure by increasing the inspiratory time (when using a volume-limited ventilator) or reducing the V_t. When using a pressure ventilator, reducing the inspiratory pressure may alleviate aerophagia. When adopting these strategies, however, care should be taken to ensure that these measures do not have an unacceptable impact on patient comfort or adequacy of ventilatory assistance.

OUTCOMES WITH NOCTURNAL NONINVASIVE POSITIVE PRESSURE VENTILATION

In this section, we present (1) the effect of NPPV when used at night; (2) the effects on daytime respiratory function during spontaneous breathing; (3) the effect on hospitalization days, which is closely related to health improvement; and (4) the continuation of NPPV, which is closely related to survival.

Effects of Noninvasive Positive Pressure Ventilation During Ventilatory Assistance

During ventilatory assistance, gas exchange is improved as shown by overnight records of SpO_2 and $TcPCO_2$.[39, 76, 81, 88, 91–95] Nevertheless, significant episodes of transient hypoventilation may persist and appear to be related to mouth leaks.[87, 88]

Theoretically, respiratory muscles are rested during NPPV. Although this has been shown to be partially true during wakefulness,[96] this has not been assessed during sleep. Sleep duration usually improves during NIPPV, as shown by an increased total sleep time from 265 ± 63 to 298 ± 82 min.[91, 94, 97–101] Among five series studying COPD, three have shown improvement and two have shown worsening. The two series reporting outcome in restrictive patients have shown improvement. Sleep efficiency in eight studies were similar, from 70 ± 9 to $73 \pm 11\%$[39, 91, 92, 94, 97, 98, 100] in COPD and restrictive patients. No significant changes were reported in the percentage of NREM and REM sleep. When measured, the number of arousals did not change[39, 88, 99, 100]; thus, NPPV improves nocturnal hypoventilation, but the improvement in sleep quality is inconsistent.

Effects on Daytime Respiratory Function During Spontaneous Breathing

The following data relate to patients who are able to spontaneously breathe at least 8 h during the day and who use nocturnal NPPV. A comparison of arterial blood gases, maximal inspiratory pressure, and vital capacity during wakefulness before and after NPPV is summarized in Tables 83–7 and 83–8. As opposed to improvements seen in patients with restrictive disorders,[86] it appears that there is little or no improvement with NPPV in patients with COPD. Three studies assessed[91, 101, 102] the impact of NPPV in COPD; only one demonstrated some improvement.[102]

Three main hypotheses have been proposed to explain the improvements noted in patients with restrictive disorders, including improved respiratory muscle strength, resetting of the chemoreceptors, and decrease in the ventilatory load. First, it has been suggested that ventilatory assistance rests the respiratory muscles, thus reversing fatigue; however, the change in the ventilatory pattern observed in some patients using noc-

Table 83–7. RESPONSE TO NONINVASIVE MECHANICAL VENTILATION: DAYTIME ARTERIAL BLOOD GASES DURING SPONTANEOUS BREATHING

| | | Arterial Blood Gases (mmHg) | | | |
| | | Pao_2 | | $Paco_2$ | |
Disease	Patients/ Studies	Base	Change	Base	Change
COPD*	221/13‡	55 ± 14	5 ± 5	54 ± 7	-4 ± 4
KS, TB*	483/14§	53 ± 9	12 ± 5	55 ± 5	-14 ± 10
NM†	138/12‖	64 ± 7	15 ± 6	57 ± 3	-11 ± 5

*NPPV.
†NPPV and negative pressure ventilation.
‡Data from references 30, 38, 40, 76, 91–93, 98, 100, 102, and 111–113.
§Data from references 18, 20, 30, 38, 39, 81, 87, 97, 105, 107, 111, and 114–116.
‖Data from references 7, 15, 16, 40, 54, 57, 67, 88, 94, and 117–119.
COPD, chronic obstructive pulmonary disease; KS, kyphoscoliosis; NM, neuromuscular diseases; NPPV, noninvasive positive pressure ventilation; TB, tuberculosis.

Table 83–8. VITAL CAPACITY AND MAXIMUM INSPIRATORY PRESSURE RESPONSES
TO NONINVASIVE POSITIVE PRESSURE VENTILATION

Disease	Vital Capacity (ml)			Maximal Inspiratory Pressure (cm H$_2$O)		
	Patients/Studies	Base	Change	Patients/Studies	Base	Change
COPD	35/3*	1980 ± 228	+57 ± 143	52/4‡	−48 ± 2	−1 ± 11
KS, TB	178/5†	1097 ± 219	+110 ± 98	112/10§	−39 ± 6	−14 ± 10

*Data from references 91, 93, and 113.
†Data from references 20, 87, 107, 115, and 116.
‡Data from references 91, 98, 102, and 112.
§Data from references 20, 39, 81, 91, 97, 98, 102, 107, 112, and 116.
COPD, chronic obstructive pulmonary disease; KS, kyphoscoliosis; TB, tuberculosis.

turnal NPPV, as characterized by lower frequency and higher V$_t$, means that muscles could develop more force per breath.[81] Second, a hypothesis suggests that in response to chronic hypercapnia, the respiratory centers change their set-point, which perpetuates the hypoventilation rather than trying to generate nonsustainable ventilatory muscle effort. This nonvolitional interaction between muscles and the respiratory centers could reflect "central wisdom."[33, 103–105] Third, a hypothesis suggests that an improvement in respiratory mechanics, present during spontaneous breathing, reduces the ventilatory load and increases the efficiency of the muscles. One study has shown transitory improvement of dynamic compliance in kyphoscoliosis after hyperinflation[106]; however, the generally modest improvement in vital capacity often associated with increased maximal inspiratory pressure does not favor the hypothesis of changes in respiratory mechanics.

Even if the mechanisms that explain the efficacy of nocturnal assisted ventilation are unknown, it is evident that improvement is more or less related to the normalization, or at least the improvement, of hypoventilation.[61, 93] The minimum mandatory duration of assistance is unknown.[107]

In general, it is likely that in addition to reducing the burden of breathing during use in patients with chest wall or neuromuscular diseases, NPPV has a favorable impact on ventilatory mechanics or muscle function during spontaneous breathing, even in cases of intrinsic neuromuscular abnormality. Conversely, in patients with COPD, ventilatory assistance has no apparent favorable influence on the parenchymal abnormality, and thus little or no benefit is conferred by unloading of the ventilatory muscles.

Effects on Hospitalization

The home care system in France allows precise tabulation of the days that patients spend in the hospital. A comparison between the year before and the first and second years after beginning nocturnal NPPV reveals a significant reduction in the number of days of hospitalization: 34 versus 6 days during the first year and 5 days during the second for scoliosis; 31 versus 10 and 9 days for the sequelae of tuberculosis; and 18 versus 7 and 2 days for patients with DMD. By contrast, the number of hospital days for patients with COPD decreased significantly only during the first year on NIPPV: 49 versus 17 and 25 days.[38] For patients with bronchiectasis, there was no statistical change in the number of hospital days after the initiation of NIPPV.[38, 108]

Withdrawal From Therapy, Continuation, and Survival According to Different Causes

There are few studies reporting results concerning withdrawal (defined as stopping NPPV for reasons other than death, tracheostomy, or lung transplantation), continuation, and survival with NPPV of patients with different diseases. Moreover, interpretation of existing studies is confounded by the absence of control groups and no correlation with the age of the patients. Table 83–9 reviews the results of several series with a 5-year follow-up.[33, 40, 76, 95, 104, 105, 109, 110] Patient adherence with NPPV is very good for tuberculosis, poliomyelitis, DMD, and bronchiectasis (99 to 100%), not as good for kyphoscoliosis (93 to 99%), and worse for patients with COPD (85 to 92%). Overall, 5 years' continuation is more than 70% for chest wall disorders and poliomyelitis and less than 70% for DMD, COPD, and bronchiectasis. Differences in continuation between different series in tuberculosis, DMD, and COPD are probably related to different medical practices.[38] On the other hand, differences in continuation in bronchiectasis are related to survival and probably to age. A comparison of NPPV with tracheostomy in terms of either continuation or survival reveals the same range.[12] Finally, except for a study by Sivasothy et al.,[76] the results in patients with COPD are approximately the same as those obtained with long-term O$_2$ therapy. The relatively high NPPV continuation reported by Sivasothy et al. at 5 years, compared with other studies,[40, 109] is probably related to patient selection. The majority of patients (18 of 26) did not receive long-term O$_2$ before starting NPPV, whereas the number was only 6 of 50 in the study of Leger et al.,[109] indicating that the levels of severity were certainly different. In summary, it appears that NPPV compliance is good in patients with neuromuscular and chest wall disorders but probably substantially less satisfactory in COPD. Furthermore,

Table 83–9. LONG-TERM EVOLUTION OF PATIENTS ON NONINVASIVE POSITIVE PRESSURE VENTILATION ACCORDING TO CAUSE

Disease, Author	No. of Patients/ Age (y)	NPPV Continuation (%) at 5 Years	NPPV Withdrawal*	Tracheostomy	Death
Scoliosis					
Simonds and Elliott[40]	47/49	79	1 (2%)	NA tech†	7 (9%)
Leger et al.[109]	105/57	73	7 (7%)	5 (5%)	15 (14%)
Tuberculosis					
Simonds and Elliott[40]	20/61	94	0	NA tech	1 (5%)
Leger et al.[109]	80/64	68	1 (1%)	11 (14%)	17 (21%)
Poliomyelitis					
Simonds and Elliott[40]	30/51	100	0	NA tech	0
Duchenne's muscular dystrophy					
Leger et al.[109]	16/21	47	0	7 (44%)	2 (13%)
Simonds et al.[110]	23/20	73	0	NA tech	5 (22%)
COPD					
Simonds and Elliott[40]	33/57	43	5 (15%)	NA tech	6 (19%)
Leger et al.[109]	50/63	31	4 (8%)*	12 (24%)	15 (30%)
Sivasothy et al.[76]	26/66	68	0		6 (23%)
Bronchiectasis					
Simonds and Elliott[40]	13/41	<20	0	NA tech	7 (54%)
Leger et al.[109]	25/55	62	0	2 (8%)	6 (24%)
Benhamou et al.[95]	14/64	29	0	NA tech	10 (71%)

*Lung transplantations are not included in the patients who were withdrawn.
†Nonavailable technique.
COPD, chronic obstructive pulmonary disease; NPPV, noninvasive positive pressure ventilation.

survival does not depend on tracheostomy as a salvage therapy, except perhaps in patients with DMD.

SUMMARY

Chronic ventilatory support with the use of NPPV improves and stabilizes the clinical course of many patients with chronic ventilatory failure. The results appear to be better in patients with restrictive disorders than in those with COPD. Among patients with neuromuscular disorders, results are better in slowly progressive cases. In patients with restrictive disorders, the benefit of NPPV is reflected by the improvements in survival rates, blood gas composition, and clinical stability. Due to its relative simplicity and its noninvasive nature, NPPV permits LTMV to be an acceptable option to patients who would not otherwise have been treated if tracheostomy were the only alternative. In this way, nocturnal NPPV represents progress.

References

1. Bertoye A, Garin JP, Vincent P, et al. Le retour á domicile des insuffisants respiratoires chroniques appareillés. Lyon Med. 1965;38:389–410.
2. Bertrand A, Milane J. Domiciliary assisted respiration in the Languedoc-Roussillon region. MMW Munch Med Wochenschr. 1977;119:1647–1652.
3. Wiers PWJ, Le Coultre R, Dallinga OT, et al. Cuirass respirator treatment of chronic respiratory failure in scoliotic patients. Thorax. 1977;32:221–228.
4. Bolot JF, Robert D, Chemorin B, et al. Assisted ventilation at home by tracheotomy in subjects with chronic respiratory insufficiency. Minerva Med. 1977;68:409–414.
5. Robert D, Chemorin B, Gerard M, et al. Results of home assisted ventilation of non-paralytic and tracheostomized chronic respiratory insufficient patients. Rev Fr Mal Respir. 1979;7:408–412.
6. Alexander MA, Johnson EW, Petty J, et al. Mechanical ventilation of patients with late stage Duchenne muscular dystrophy: management in the home. Arch Phys Med Rehabil. 1979;60:289–292.
7. Curran FJ. Night ventilation by body respirators for patients in chronic respiratory failure due to late stage Duchenne muscular dystrophy. Arch Phys Med Rehabil. 1981;62:270–274.
8. Bach J, Alba A, Pilkington LA, et al. Long-term rehabilitation in advanced stage of childhood onset, rapidly progressive muscular dystrophy. Arch Phys Med Rehabil. 1981;62:328–331.
9. Splaingard ML, Frates RC Jr, Harrison GM, et al. Home positive-pressure ventilation: twenty years' experience. Chest. 1983;84:376–382.
10. Bach JR, Alba AS, Bohatiuk G, et al. Mouth intermittent positive pressure ventilation in the management of postpolio respiratory insufficiency. Chest. 1987;91:859–864.
11. Garay SM, Turino GM, Goldring RM. Sustained reversal of chronic hypercapnia in patients with alveolar hypoventilation syndromes: long-term maintenance with noninvasive nocturnal mechanical ventilation. Am J Med. 1981;70:269–274.
12. Robert D, Gerard M, Leger P, et al. Permanent mechanical ventilation at home via a tracheotomy in chronic respiratory insufficiency. Rev Fr Mal Respir. 1983;11:923–936.
13. Sullivan CE, Issa FG, Berthon-Jones M, et al. Reversal of obstructive sleep apnea by continuous positive airway pressure applied through the nares. Lancet. 1981;1:862–865.
14. Bach JR, Alba A, Mosher R, et al. Intermittent positive pressure ventilation via nasal access in the management of respiratory insufficiency. Chest. 1987;92:168–170.
15. Kerby GR, Mayer LS, Pingleton SK. Nocturnal positive pressure ventilation via nasal mask. Am Rev Respir Dis. 1987;135:738–740.
16. Ellis ER, Bye PTP, Bruderer JW, et al. Treatment of respiratory failure during sleep in patients with neuromuscular disease: positive-pressure ventilation through a nose mask. Am Rev Respir Dis. 1987;135:148–152.
17. Carroll N, Branthwaite MA. Intermittent positive pressure ventilation by nasal mask: technique and applications. Intens Care Med. 1988;14:115–117.
18. Leger P, Jennequin J, Gerard M, et al. Nocturnal mechanical ventilation in intermittent positive pressure at home by nasal

route in chronic restrictive respiratory insufficiency: an effective substitute for tracheotomy [letter]. Presse Med. 1988;17:874.

19. Segall D. Noninvasive nasal mask-assisted ventilation of Duchenne muscular dystrophy. Chest. 1988;93:1298–1300.

20. Ellis ER, Grunstein RR, Chan S, et al. Noninvasive ventilatory support during sleep improves respiratory failure in kyphoscoliosis. Chest. 1988;94:811–815.

21. Wackers GL. Modern anesthesiological principles for bulbar polio: manual IPPR in the 1952 polio-epidemic in Copenhagen. Acta Anaesthesiol Scand. 1994;38:420–431.

22. Severinghaus JW, Astrup P, Murray JF. Blood gas analysis and critical care medicine. Am J Respir Crit Care Med. 1998;157:114–122.

23. Engström CG. Treatment of severe cases of respiratory paralysis by the Engström universal respirator. Br Med J. 1954;18:666–669.

24. Fischer DA, Prentice WS. Feasibility of home care for certain respiratory-dependent restrictive or obstructive lung disease patients. Chest. 1982;82:739–743.

25. Braun NMT, Marino WD. Effects of daily intermittent rest of respiratory muscles in patients with severe chronic airflow limitation. Chest. 1984;85 (suppl):59s.

26. Fulkerton WJ, Wilkins JK, Esbenshade AM, et al. Life threatening hypoventilation in kyphoscoliosis: successful treatment with a molded body brace-ventilator. Am Rev Respir Dis. 1984;129:185–187.

27. Splaingard ML, Frates RC, Jefferson LS, et al. Home negative pressure ventilation: report of 20 years of experience in patients with neuromuscular disease. Arch Phys Med Rehabil. 1985;66:239–242.

28. Hoeppner VH, Cockcroft DW, Dosman JA, et al. Nighttime ventilation improves respiratory failure in secondary kyphoscoliosis. Am Rev Respir Dis. 1984;129:240–243.

29. Ellis ER, McCauley B, Mellis C, et al. Treatment of alveolar hypoventilation in a six-year-old girl with intermittent positive pressure ventilation through a nose mask. Am Rev Respir Dis. 1987;136:188–191.

30. Carroll N, Branthwaite M. Control of nocturnal hypoventilation by nasal intermittent positive ventilation. Thorax. 1988;43:349–353.

31. Leger P, Jennequin J, Gerard M, et al. Home positive pressure ventilation via nasal mask for patients with neuromuscular weakness or restrictive lung or chest-wall disease. Respir Care. 1989;34:73–77.

32. Bach J, Alba AS. Management of chronic alveolar hypoventilation by nasal ventilation. Chest. 1990;97:52–57.

33. Elliott MW, Mulvey DA, Moxham J, et al. A. Domiciliary nocturnal nasal intermittent positive pressure ventilation in COPD: mechanisms underlying changes in arterial blood gas tensions. Eur Respir J. 1991;4:1044–1052.

34. Strumpf DA, Carlisle CC, Millman RP, et al. An evaluation of the Respironics BiPAP Bi-Level CPAP device for delivery of assisted ventilation. Respir Care. 1990;35:415–422.

35. Brochard L, Isabey D, Piquet J, et al. Reversal of acute exacerbations of chronic obstructive lung disease by inspiratory assistance with a face mask. N Engl J Med. 1990;323:1523–1530.

36. Meduri GU, Conoscenti CC, Menashe P, et al. Noninvasive face mask ventilation in patients with acute respiratory failure. Chest. 1989;95:865–870.

37. Bott J, Carroll MP, Conway JH, et al. Randomised controlled trial of nasal ventilation in acute ventilatory failure due to chronic obstructive airways disease. Lancet. 1993;341:1555–1557.

37a. Clinical indications for noninvasive positive pressure ventilation in chronic respiratory failure due to restrictive lung disease, COPD, and nocturnal hypoventilation—a consensus conference report. Chest. 1999;116:521–534.

37b. Hukins CA, Hillman DR. Daytime predictors of sleep hypoventilation in Duchenne muscular dystrophy. Am J Respir Crit Care Med. 2000;161:166–170.

38. Leger P, Bedicam JM, Cornette A, et al. Nasal intermittent positive pressure ventilation: long-term follow-up in patients with severe chronic respiratory insufficiency. Chest. 1994;105:100–105.

39. Masa JF, Celli BR, Riesco JA, et al. Noninvasive positive pressure ventilation and not oxygen may prevent overt ventilatory failure in patients with chest wall diseases. Chest. 1997;112:207–213.

40. Simonds AK, Elliott MW. Outcome of domiciliary nasal intermittent positive pressure ventilation in restrictive and obstructive disorders. Thorax. 1995;50:604–609.

41. Curran FJ, Colbert AP. Ventilator management in Duchenne muscular dystrophy and postpoliomyelitis syndrome: twelve years' experience. Arch Phys Med Rehabil. 1989;70:180–185.

42. Strumpf DA, Millman RP, Hill NS. The management of chronic hypoventilation. Chest. 1990;98:474–480.

43. Raphael JC, Chevret S, Chastang C, et al. Randomised trial of preventive nasal ventilation in Duchenne muscular dystrophy: French Multicentre Cooperative Group on Home Mechanical Ventilation Assistance in Duchenne de Boulogne Muscular Dystrophy. Lancet. 1994;343:1600–1604.

44. Bach J. Noninvasive options for ventilatory support of the traumatic high level quadriplegic patient. Chest. 1990;98:613–619.

45. Bach JR, Alba AS, Saporito LR. Intermittent positive pressure ventilation via the mouth as an alternative to tracheostomy for 257 ventilator users. Chest. 1993;103:174–182.

46. Robert D, Willig TN, Paulus J, et al. Long-term nasal ventilation in neuromuscular disorders: report of a consensus conference. Eur Respir J. 1993;6:599–606.

47. Raphael JC, Chevret S, Auriant I, et al. Long-term ventilation at home in adults with neurological diseases. Rev Mal Respir. 1998;15:495–505.

48. Drinker P, McKhann CF. The use of a new apparatus for the prolonged administration of artificial respiration. JAMA. 1929:1658–1660.

49. Collier CR, Offeldt JE. Ventilatory efficiency of the cuirass respirator in totally paralyzed chronic poliomyelitis patients. J Appl Physiol. 1954;6:532–538.

50. O'Leary J, King R, Leblanc M, et al. Cuirass ventilation in childhood neuromuscular disease. J Pediatr. 1979;94:419–421.

51. Dunkin LJ. Home ventilatory assistance. Anaesthesia. 1983;38:644–649.

52. Driver AG, Blackburn BB, Marcuard SP, et al. Bilateral diaphragm paralysis treated with cuirass ventilation. Chest. 1987;92:683–685.

53. Goldstein RS, Molotiu N, Skrastins R, et al. Reversal of sleep-induced hypoventilation and chronic respiratory failure by nocturnal negative pressure ventilation in patients with restrictive ventilatory impairment. Am Rev Respir Dis. 1987;135:1049–1055.

54. Goldstein RS, Molotiu N, Skrastins R, et al. Assisting ventilation in respiratory failure by negative pressure ventilation and by rocking bed. Chest. 1987;92:470–474.

55. Cropp A, Dimarco F. Effects of intermittent negative pressure ventilation on respiratory muscle function in patients with severe chronic obstructive pulmonary disease. Am Rev Respir Dis. 1987;135:1056–1061.

56. Gutièrrez M, Berozia T, Contreras G, et al. Weekly cuirass ventilation improves blood gases and inspiratory muscle strength in patients with chronic air-flow limitation and hypercarbia. Am Rev Respir Dis. 1988;138:617–623.

57. Kinnear W, Hockley S, Harvey J, et al. The effects of one year of nocturnal cuirass-assisted ventilation in chest wall disease. Eur Respir J. 1988;1:204–208.

58. Zibrack JD, Hill NS, Federman EC, et al. Evaluation of intermittent long-term negative-pressure ventilation in patients with severe chronic obstructive pulmonary disease. Am Rev Respir Dis. 1988;138:1515–1518.

59. Celli B, Criner G, Bermudez M, et al. Controlled trial of external negative pressure ventilation in patients with severe chronic airflow obstruction. Am Rev Respir Dis. 1989;140:1251–1256.

60. Ambrosino N, Montagna T, Nava S, et al. Short term effect of intermittent negative pressure ventilation in COPD patients with respiratory failure. Eur Respir J. 1990;3:502–508.

61. Levine S, Levy SF, Henson DJ. Effect of negative pressure ventilation on ventilatory muscle endurance in patients with severe chronic obstructive pulmonary disease. Am Rev Respir Dis. 1992;146:722–729.

62. Shapiro SH, Ernst P, Gray-Donald K, et al. Effect of negative pressure ventilation in severe chronic obstructive pulmonary disease. Lancet. 1992;340:1425–1429.

63. Jackson M, Kinnear W, King M, et al. The effects of five years of nocturnal cuirass-assisted ventilation in chest wall disease. Eur Respir J. 1993;6:630–635.

64. Kinnear WJ, Shneerson JM. Assisted ventilation at home: is it worth considering? Br J Dis Chest. 1985;79:313–351.

65. Levy RD, Bradley TD, Newman SL, et al. Negative pressure ventilation: effects on ventilation during sleep in normal subjects. Chest. 1989;95:95–99.

66. Belman MJ, Soo Hoo GW, Kuei JH, et al. Efficacy of positive vs negative pressure ventilation in unloading the respiratory muscles. Chest. 1990;98:850–856.

67. Heckmatt JZ, Loh L, Dubowitz V. Night-time nasal ventilation in neuromuscular disease. Lancet. 1990;335:579–582.

68. Bach JR, Penek J. Obstructive sleep apnea complicating negative-pressure ventilatory support in patients with chronic paralytic/restrictive ventilatory dysfunction. Chest. 1991;99:1386–1393.

69. Levy RD, Cosio MG, Gibbons L, et al. Induction of sleep apnea with negative pressure ventilation in patients with chronic obstructive lung disease. Thorax. 1992;47:612–615.

70. Hill NS, Redline S, Carskadon MA, et al. Sleep-disordered breathing in patients with Duchenne muscular dystrophy using negative pressure ventilators. Chest. 1992;102:1656–1662.

71. Bach JR, Sortor SM, Saporito LR. Interfaces for non-invasive intermittent positive pressure ventilatory support in North America. Eur Respir Rev. 1993;3:254–259.

72. Cornette A, Mougel D. Ventilatory assistance via the nasal route: masks and fitting. Eur Respir Rev. 1993;3:250–253.

73. Tsuboi T, Ohi M, Kita H, et al. The efficacy of a custom-fabricated mask on gas exchange during nasal intermittent positive pressure ventilation. Eur Respir J. 1999;13:152–156.

74. Bach JR, McDermott IG. Strapless oral-nasal interface for positive pressure ventilation. Arch Phys Med Rehabil. 1990;71:910–913.

75. Criner GJ, Travaline JM, Brennan KJ, et al. Efficacy of a new full face mask for noninvasive positive pressure ventilation. Chest. 1994;106:1109–1115.

76. Sivasothy P, Smith IE, Shneerson JM. Mask intermittent positive pressure ventilation in chronic hypercapnic respiratory failure due to chronic obstructive pulmonary disease. Eur Respir J. 1998;11:34–40.

77. Kackmareck RM, Hess D. Equipment required for home mechanical ventilation. In: Tobin MJ, ed. Principles and Practice of Mechanical Ventilation. New York, NY: McGraw-Hill; 1994:111–154.

78. Nava S, Ambrosino N, Bruschi C, et al. Physiological effects of flow and pressure triggering during non-invasive mechanical ventilation in patients with chronic obstructive pulmonary disease. Thorax. 1997;52:249–254.

79. Meecham Jones DJ, Wedzichia JA. Comparison of pressure and volume preset nasal ventilator systems in stable chronic respiratory failure. Eur Respir J. 1993;6:1060–1064.

80. Elliott MW. A comparison of different modes of noninvasive ventilatory support: effects on ventilation and inspiratory muscle effort. Anaesthesia. 1994;49:279–283.

81. Schönhofer B, Sonneborn M, Haidl P, et al. Comparison of two different modes for noninvasive mechanical ventilation in chronic respiratory failure: volume versus pressure controlled device. Eur Respir J. 1997;10:184–191.

82. Ferguson GT, Gilmartin M. CO_2 rebreathing during BiPAP ventilatory assistance. Am J Respir Crit Care Med. 1995;151:1126–1135.

83. Lofaso F, Brochard L, Touchard D, et al. Evaluation of carbon dioxide rebreathing during pressure support ventilation with airway management system (BiPAP) devices. Chest. 1995;108:772–778.

84. Nava S, Ambrosino N, Rubini F, et al. Effect of nasal pressure support ventilation and external PEEP on diaphragmatic activity in patients with severe stable COPD. Chest. 1993;103:143–150.

85. Appendini L, Patessio A, Zanaboni S, et al. Physiologic effects of positive end expiratory pressure and mask pressure support during exacerbation of chronic obstructive pulmonary disease. Am J Respir Crit Care Med. 1994;149:1069–1076.

86. Restrick LJ, Fox NC, Braid G, et al. Comparison of nasal pressure support ventilation with nasal intermittent positive pressure ventilation in patients with nocturnal hypoventilation. Eur Respir J. 1993;6:364–370.

87. Bach JR, Robert D, Leger P, et al. Sleep fragmentation in kyphoscoliotic individuals with alveolar hypoventilation treated by NIPPV. Chest. 1995;107:1552–1558.

88. Meyer TJ, Pressman MR, Benditt J, et al. Air leaking through the mouth during nocturnal nasal ventilation: effect on sleep quality. Sleep. 1997;20:561–569.

89. Delguste P, Aubert-Tulkens G, Rodenstein DO. Upper airway obstruction during nasal intermittent positive pressure hyperventilation in sleep. Lancet. 1991;338:1295–1297.

90. Hill NS. Complications of NPPV. Respir Care. 1997;42:432–442.

91. Strumpf DA, Millman RP, Carlisle CC, et al. Nocturnal positive-pressure ventilation via nasal mask in patients with severe chronic obstructive pulmonary disease. Am Rev Respir Dis. 1991;144:1234–1239.

92. Elliott MW, Simonds AK, Carroll MP, et al. Domiciliary nocturnal nasal intermittent positive pressure ventilation in hypercapnic respiratory failure due to chronic obstructive lung disease: effects on sleep and quality of life. Thorax. 1992;47:342–348.

93. Meecham Jones DJ, Paul EA, Jones PW, et al. Nasal pressure support ventilation plus oxygen compared with oxygen therapy alone in hypercapnic COPD. Am J Respir Crit Care Med. 1995;152:538–544.

94. Barbé F, Quera-Salva MA, de Lattre J, et al. Long-term effects of nasal intermittent positive-pressure ventilation on pulmonary function and sleep architecture in patients with neuromuscular diseases. Chest. 1996;110:1179–1183.

95. Benhamou D, Muir JF, Raspaud C, et al. Long-term efficiency of home nasal mask ventilation in patients with diffuse bronchiectasis and severe chronic respiratory failure. Chest. 1997;112:1259–1266.

96. Carrey Z, Gottfried SB, Levy RD. Ventilatory muscle support in respiratory failure with nasal positive pressure ventilation. Chest. 1990;97:150–158.

97. Goldstein RS, De Rosie JA, Avendano MA, et al. Influence of noninvasive positive pressure ventilation on inspiratory muscles. Chest. 1991;99:408–415.

98. Lin CC. Comparison between nocturnal nasal positive pressure ventilation combined with oxygen therapy and oxygen monotherapy in patients with severe COPD. Am J Respir Crit Care Med. 1996;154:353–358.

99. Gozal D. Nocturnal ventilatory support in patients with cystic fibrosis: comparison with supplemental oxygen. Eur Respir J. 1997;10:1999–2003.

100. Krachman SL, Quaranta AJ, Berger TJ, et al. Effects of noninvasive positive pressure ventilation on gas exchange and sleep in COPD patients. Chest. 1997;112:623–628.

101. Jones SE, Packham S, Hebden M, et al. Domiciliary nocturnal intermittent positive pressure ventilation in patients with respiratory failure due to severe COPD: long-term follow up and effect on survival. Thorax. 1998;53:495–498.

102. Renston JP, DiMarco AF, Supinski GS. Respiratory muscle rest using nasal BiPAP ventilation in patients with stable severe COPD. Chest. 1994;105:1053–1060.

103. Berthon-Jones M, Sullivan CE. Time course of change in ventilatory response to CO_2 with long term CPAP therapy for obstructive sleep apnea. Am Rev Respir Dis. 1987;135:144–147.

104. Fernandez E, Weinert P, Meltzer E, et al. Sustained improvement in gas exchange after negative pressure ventilation for 8 hours per day on 2 successive days in chronic airflow limitation. Am Rev Respir Dis. 1991;144:390–394.

105. Hill NS, Eveloff SE, Carlisle C, et al. Efficacy of nocturnal nasal ventilation in patients with restrictive thoracic disease. Am Rev Respir Dis. 1992;145:365–371.

106. Bergowsky EH. Respiratory failure in disorders of the thoracic cage. Am Rev Respir Dis. 1979;119:643–669.

107. Schönhofer B, Geibel M, Sonneborn M, et al. Daytime mechanical ventilation in chronic respiratory insufficiency. Eur Respir J. 1997;10:2840–2846.

108. Gacouin A, Desrues B, Lena H, et al. Long-term nasal intermittent positive pressure ventilation (NIPPV) in sixteen consecutive patients with bronchiectasis: a retrospective study. Eur Respir J. 1996;9:1246–1250.

109. Leger P, Petitjean T, Langevin B, et al. Long term effects of nocturnal nasal positive pressure ventilation at home. In: Robert D, Make B, Leger P, et al, eds. Home Mechanical Ventilation. Paris, France: Arnette-Blackwell; 1995:217–232.

110. Simonds AK, Muntoni F, Heather S, et al. Impact of nasal ventilation on survival in hypercapnic Duchenne muscular dystrophy. Thorax. 1998;53:949–952.

111. Laier-Groeneveld G, Hûttemenn U, Criée CP. Nasal inspiratory positive pressure ventilation. Eur Respir Rev. 1992;2:389–397.

112. Clini E, Vitacca M, Foglio K, et al. Long-term home care programmes may reduce hospital admissions in COPD with chronic hypercapnia. Eur Respir J. 1996;9:1605–1610.

113. Perrin C, El Far Y, Vandenbos F, et al. Domiciliary nasal intermittent positive pressure ventilation in severe COPD: effects on lung function and quality of life. Eur Respir J. 1997;10:2835–2839.

114. Waldhorn RE. Nocturnal nasal intermittent positive pressure ventilation with bilevel positive airway pressure (BiPAP) in respiratory failure. Chest. 1992;101:516–521.

115. Leger P, Robert D, Langevin B, et al. Indications of home mechanical ventilation in patients with chest wall deformities due to idiopathic kyphoscoliosis or sequelae of tuberculosis. Eur Respir Rev. 1992;2:362–368.

116. Jackson M, Smith I, King M, et al. Long term non-invasive domiciliary assisted ventilation for respiratory failure following thoracoplasty. Thorax. 1994;49:915–919.

117. Piper AJ, Sullivan CE. Effects of long term nocturnal nasal ventilation on spontaneous breathing during sleep in neuromuscular and chest wall disorders. Eur Respir J. 1996;9:1515–1522.

118. Vianello A, Bevilacqua M, Salvador V, et al. Long-term nasal intermittent positive pressure ventilation in advanced Duchenne's muscular dystrophy. Chest. 1994;105:445–448.

119. Sawicka EH, Loh L, Branthwaite MA. Domiciliary ventilatory support: an analysis of outcome. Thorax. 1988;43:31–35.

thirteen

Medical and Neurological Disorders

Christian Guilleminault

Sleep-Related Cardiac Risk

Richard L. Verrier
Murray A. Mittleman

In healthy people, sleep is generally salutary and restorative. Ironically, during sleep in patients with respiratory or heart disease, the brain can precipitate breathing disorders, myocardial ischemia, arrhythmias, and even death. Our recent observation that 20% of myocardial infarctions (MIs) and 15% of sudden deaths occur during the period from midnight to 6 AM projects to an estimated 250,000 nocturnal MIs and 38,000 nocturnal sudden deaths annually in the U.S. population.[1] The latter figure is equivalent to 91% of the number of fatalities due to automobile accidents and is 20% more than the number of deaths due to HIV infection. Thus, sleep is not a protected state. Furthermore, the nonuniform distribution of deaths and MIs during nighttime is consonant with provocation by pathophysiological triggers. Precise characterization of the precipitating factors for nocturnal cardiac events is, however, incomplete. While death during sleep can be presumed to be painless, in many cases it is premature, as it occurs in infants and adolescents and in adults with ischemic heart disease, for whom the median age is 59 years. High-risk populations for nocturnal cardiorespiratory events include a number of sizable patient groups (Table 84–1).

The two main factors implicated in nocturnal cardiac events are sleep state–dependent surges in autonomic activity and depression of respiratory control mechanisms, which affect a vulnerable cardiac substrate. The brain, in subserving its needs for periodic reexcitation during rapid eye movement (REM) sleep and dreaming, imposes significant demands on the heart by inducing bursts in sympathetic nerve activity, which reaches levels higher than during wakefulness. In susceptible individuals, such neural activity may compromise coronary artery blood flow, as metabolic demand outstrips supply, and may trigger sympathetically mediated life-threatening arrhythmias. Impairment of ventilation during sleep by obstructive sleep apnea can generate reductions in arterial oxygen saturation. Obstructive sleep apnea afflicts 5 to 10 million Americans, or 2 to 4% of the population,[2] and has been strongly implicated, when severe, in the etiology of hypertension, ischemia, arrhythmias, MI, and sudden death in people with coexisting ischemic heart disease. Atrial fibrillation may be triggered by autonomic or respiratory disturbances during sleep in certain patient populations. An additional challenge is presented by nonrapid eye movement (NREM) sleep, when hypotension may lead to malperfusion of the heart and brain as a result of a lowered blood pressure gradient through stenosed vessels. These conditions may be confounded by medications that cross the blood-brain barrier, altering sleep structure and provoking nightmares with severe cardiac autonomic discharge. Finally, an insidious component of the problem of nocturnal risk results from the fact that many people are unaware of their

Table 84-1. PATIENT GROUPS AT POTENTIALLY INCREASED RISK FOR NOCTURNAL CARDIAC EVENTS

Indication (U.S. Patients/Year)	Possible Mechanism
Angina, myocardial infarction, arrhythmias, ischemia, or cardiac arrest at night	The nocturnal pattern suggests a sleep state–dependent autonomic trigger or respiratory distress; 20% of myocardial infarctions (~250,000 cases/year) and 15% of sudden deaths (~38,000) occur between midnight and 6 A.M.[1]
Unstable angina, non-Q-wave infarction, Prinzmetal's angina	Nondemand ischemia and angina and non-Q-wave infarction peak between midnight and 6 A.M.[16, 40, 59, 67, 73, 74, 95]
Acute myocardial infarction (1.5 million)	Disturbances in sleep, respiration, and autonomic balance may be factors in nocturnal arrhythmogenesis.[34–36, 59, 62, 82–88]
Spousal or family report of highly irregular breathing, excessive snoring, or apnea in patients with coronary disease (5–10 million patients with apnea)	Patients with hypertension or coronary artery disease should be screened for the presence of sleep apnea, which conduces to hypertension,[102, 104, 105, 107, 109, 110] ischemia,[146] arrhythmia,[145–147] and atrial fibrillation[207] and is a risk factor for lethal daytime cardiac events,[152–154] including myocardial infarction.[150]
Heart failure (4.6 million)	20% of sudden deaths in heart failure patients occur between midnight and 6 A.M.[130]
Long Q–T syndrome	The profound cycle-length changes associated with sleep may trigger pause-dependent torsades de pointes in these patients.[161]
Near-miss or siblings of sudden infant death syndrome victims	Crib death commonly occurs during sleep with characteristic cardiorespiratory symptoms.[164, 175–179]
Asians with warning signs of sudden unexplained nocturnal death (SUNDS)	SUNDS is a sleep-related phenomenon in which night terrors may play a role.[196, 198]
Atrial fibrillation (2.5 million)	29% of episodes occur between midnight and 6 A.M.[202, 203] Respiratory and autonomic mechanisms are suspected.
Patients on cardiac medications (13.5 million patients with cardiovascular disease)	Beta blockers and calcium channel blockers that cross the blood-brain barrier may increase nighttime risk, as poor sleep and violent dreams may be triggered.[92, 208, 209] Medications that increase the Q–T interval may conduce to pause-dependent torsade de pointes during the profound cycle-length changes of sleep. Because arterial blood pressure is decreased during nonrapid eye movement sleep, additional lowering by antihypertensive agents may induce a risk of ischemia and infarction due to lowered coronary perfusion.[4, 58, 59, 61, 79, 97]

respiratory or cardiac distress at night and take no corrective action. Thus, sleep presents unique autonomic, hemodynamic, and respiratory challenges to the diseased myocardium that cannot be monitored by daytime diagnostic tests.

Filling gaps in medical knowledge of sleep-related cardiac events would be expected to affect nocturnal therapy, as attention has been drawn to the potential of medications to disrupt sleep or to be rendered ineffective or deleterious by sleep state–dependent autonomic or hemodynamic profiles. There is also growing appreciation of the fact that the importance of monitoring nocturnal arrhythmias extends beyond identifying sleep state–dependent triggers of cardiac events, as nighttime ischemia, arrhythmias, autonomic activity, and respiratory disturbances carry predictive value for daytime events (Table 84–2).

In this chapter we discuss the pathophysiological mechanisms responsible for sleep-related cardiac morbidity and mortality.

AUTONOMIC ACTIVITY AND CIRCULATORY FUNCTION DURING SLEEP

The generalized decrease in mean heart rate and arterial blood pressure at the onset of sleep and throughout NREM sleep, which occupies 80% of sleep time, has prompted the assumption that sleep is a period of relative autonomic inactivity. NREM sleep, the initial stage, is characterized by marked stability of autonomic regulation with a high degree of parasympathetic neural tone[3, 4] and prominent respiratory sinus arrhythmia.[5] Baroreceptor gain is high and contributes to the stability of arterial blood pressure and to overall cardiovascular homeostasis.[6–9] Muscle sympathetic nerve activity is stable, falls with the transition from awake to NREM sleep, and decreases progressively with depth of sleep,[3, 10, 11] reaching half the awake value during stage 4.[3] Short-lasting increases in muscle sympathetic nerve activity, heart rate, and arterial blood pressure accompany the appearance of high-amplitude K complexes during stage 2.[3, 10, 11] Heart rate accelerations may even precede the electroencephalographic (EEG) arousals of stage 2 and REM.[12] During transitions from NREM to REM sleep, bursts of vagus nerve activity may result in pauses in heart rhythm and frank asystole.[13, 14] Transitions between REM and NREM sleep elicit posture shifts that are associated with varying degrees of autonomic activation and attendant changes in heart rate and arterial blood pressure.[15, 16] These shifts in body position increase in frequency as people age and sleep becomes fragmented.

Autonomic nervous system activity is dramatically altered when REM sleep is initiated (Fig. 84–1). REM sleep is marked by profound muscle sympathetic nerve activation, in terms of both frequency and amplitude,[3, 10, 11] which attain levels significantly higher than in

Table 84-2. PREDICTIVE VALUE OF NOCTURNAL CARDIORESPIRATORY STATUS

Because parasympathetic nerve activity is elevated during sleep in normal individuals, lack of circadian pattern of HRV and BRS may be readily monitored for increased risk of cardiac events.[28, 30, 32–36, 141, 142, 211a, 211b]

Nondemand nocturnal ischemic episodes may disclose a critical underlying coronary lesion, coronary vasospasm, or transient coronary artery stenosis.[59]

In elderly subjects, nighttime multifocal ventricular ectopic activity predicts increased mortality from cardiac causes independently of clinically evident cardiac diseases.[47]

Elevated nighttime heart rate (>90 bpm) following myocardial infarction is a predictor of fatal events.[28]

Q–T interval dispersion during sleep is an indicator of increased risk of sudden death in heart failure patients[132] and discriminates patients with cardiac disease from normals.[46]

Sleep apnea conduces to hypertension,[102, 104, 105, 107, 109, 110] ischemia,[146] arrhythmia,[145–147] and atrial fibrillation,[207] and is a risk factor for lethal daytime cardiac events,[152–154] including myocardial infarction.[150]

Cheyne-Stokes respiration accelerates deterioration in cardiac function in heart failure patients[123, 125]; the apnea/hypopnea index predicts poor prognoses in these patients.[125a]

Hypertensive patients with <10% nocturnal decline in blood pressure are at increased risk of cerebrovascular insult,[112, 113] frequent or complex ventricular arrhythmias,[114] and increased organ damage,[112, 115, 116] including cardiac hypertrophy.[117, 118]

Nocturnal hypertension is a marker of left ventricular filling impairment.[121]

Autonomic dysfunction is evident with sleep monitoring for heart rate variability, but not daytime autonomic testing, in patients with multiple sclerosis,[212] systemic sclerosis,[213] muscular dystrophy,[214] dementia of the Alzheimer's type,[215] and Parkinson's disease.[215]

It should be emphasized that direct measurement of cardiac sympathetic nerve activity or of vagus nerve activity has never been achieved in any species. Autonomic activity during sleep has been monitored by measuring peroneal muscle sympathetic nerve activity[3, 10, 11] and plasma catecholamine concentrations.[25] A decrease in average levels of epinephrine but not norepinephrine mirrors the generalized sleep-induced decline in heart rate and arterial blood pressure. Plasma cortisol is depressed during sleep; increased levels are initiated at 5 AM.[26]

In the absence of readily achieved, direct measures of cardiac-bound nerve activity, heart rate variability (HRV), an analytical technique that employs mathematical transformations of heart rate, has emerged as a widely accepted method for measuring cardiac sympathetic vs. parasympathetic neural dominance.[27] Decreased HRV, indicating a decline in parasympathetic nerve activity, is an established indicator of risk for sudden cardiac death following MI.[27, 28] Power spectral analyses of HRV reveal a generalized increase in vagus nerve activity and a decrease in cardiac sympathetic nerve activity across the sleep period,[28–30] probably reflecting the dominance of total sleep time by NREM sleep. High frequency (HF) HRV is a general indicator of cardiac parasympathetic tone and includes the effects of respiration. The low- to high-frequency ratio (LF/HF) is widely accepted as an approximation of cardiac-bound sympathetic nerve activity, as validated by studies involving beta-adrenergic receptor blockers.[27] HRV studies employing 5-min intervals provide results consistent with muscle nerve recording, indicating increased HF and decreased LF (or parasympathetic nerve dominance) in NREM sleep, but decreased HF and increased LF (or predominant sympathetic

wakefulness.[3] Sympathetic nerve activity is concentrated in short, irregular periods which are most striking when accompanied by intense eye movements.[3] These bursts trigger intermittent increases in heart rate and arterial blood pressure to levels similar to those in wakefulness with increased variability.[3, 6, 7, 10–12] Significant surges and pauses in heart rate during REM sleep have been described in several species,[13, 14, 17–20] including human beings.[10–12] Cardiac efferent vagal tone and baroreceptor regulation are generally suppressed during REM sleep, and breathing patterns may become highly irregular and may lead, in susceptible individuals, to oxygen desaturation.[5] Thus, while subserving the neurochemical functions of the brain, REM sleep can disrupt cardiorespiratory homeostasis. The brain's increased excitability during REM sleep can also trigger major surges in sympathetic nerve activity to the skeletal muscular beds, accompanied by muscular twitching,[3, 19] which interrupts the generalized skeletal atonia of REM.[21] The peripheral autonomic status characterized by muscle sympathetic nerve recording is compatible with reduced neuronal activity in the brainstem and other regions of the brain[22] and reduced cerebral blood flow[23] during NREM sleep and, during REM sleep, with increased brain activity in several discrete regions to levels above waking values.[23, 24]

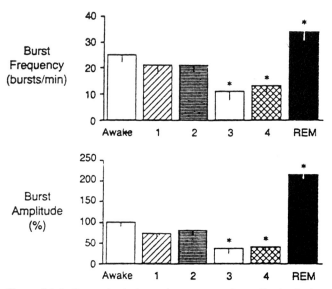

Figure 84-1. Sympathetic burst frequency and amplitude during wakefulness, NREM sleep (eight subjects), and REM sleep (six subjects). Sympathetic activity was significantly lower during stages 3 and 4 (*$P < .001$). During REM sleep, sympathetic activity increased significantly ($P < .001$). Values are means ± SEM. (From Somers VK, Dyken ME, Mark AL, et al. Sympathetic nerve activity during sleep in normal subjects. N Engl J Med. 1993;328:303–307. Copyright © 1993 Massachusetts Medical Society. All rights reserved.)

nerve activity) in REM sleep and during wakefulness.[12] In normal people, the increase in HRV measures of cardiac sympathetic nerve activity at onset of REM sleep is initiated prior to[12, 31] the transition from NREM sleep as classically defined from the polysomnographic record.

The typical circadian pattern of decreased nocturnal cardiac sympathetic nerve activity as described by heart rate and HRV studies is altered in patients with coronary artery disease[32, 33] or MI,[28, 30, 34–36] suggesting either increased nocturnal cardiac sympathetic nerve activity or decreased parasympathetic nerve activity in comparison to normals. The HF component has been observed[33] to decrease ~10 min before onset of ischemia. In unmedicated patients with a recent MI, the LF/HF ratio was significantly increased during both REM and NREM sleep, in contrast to normals, in whom this ratio during REM sleep is similar to awake levels and higher than during NREM sleep.[35, 36] The conclusions were reached that MI decreases the capacity of the vagus nerve to be activated during sleep, resulting in unbridled cardiac sympathetic nerve activity,[35] and that loss of rise in the HF component is characteristic of post-MI patients with residual ischemia.[36]

REM sleep dreams, which may be vivid, bizarre, emotionally intense, and illogical, commonly generate the emotions of anger and fear. As these emotions have been linked in wakefulness to the onset of MI and sudden death,[37] it is reasonable to hypothesize that when these affective states are evoked during dreaming, they may trigger lethal events. This possibility is illustrated by a case report of recurrence of ventricular fibrillation in a 39-year-old man with normal coronary arteries and coronary function while sleeping. A subsequent sleep study determined that ventricular premature beats were substantially increased during REM and that dreams at the same hour that fibrillation had occurred were emotionally charged.[38]

These sleep state–dependent profiles of autonomic activity have significant potential to affect coronary function and cardiac electrical stability in patients with ischemic heart disease.

PATIENTS AT RISK FOR NOCTURNAL SUDDEN DEATH AND MYOCARDIAL INFARCTION

Nocturnal Cardiac Events and Arrhythmias

The circadian pattern of cardiac events demonstrates a general nocturnal trough in incidence of MI and sudden death, ischemic events, and arrhythmias in patients with ischemic heart disease.[1, 4, 39–42] This decrement is coordinate with lessened metabolic demands during NREM sleep, which occupies ~80% of sleep time. But surges in cardiac sympathetic nerve activity have been implicated in nocturnal arrhythmias[43, 44] and ischemia. The specific mechanisms of REM-induced cardiac events include direct effects on electrophysiological status or indirect consequences of heart rate

and arterial blood pressure accelerations, which may disrupt plaques and lead to intra-arterial platelet aggregates, releasing proarrhythmic constituents such as thromboxane A_2. In some cases, arrhythmia frequency may be enhanced during NREM sleep, when latent foci are exposed by the generalized reduction in heart rate,[45] or when hypotension exacerbates impaired coronary perfusion. The increase in Q–T interval dispersion during sleep in survivors of sudden cardiac death[46] may provide clues regarding arrhythmia generation because of changes in repolarization of the heartbeat. The impact of sleep states on arrhythmogenesis is more complex when there are respiratory abnormalities or changes in cardiac mechanical function due to infarction or disease. The value of nocturnal monitoring for cardiac arrhythmias, as indicators of generalized electrical instability, was demonstrated in unselected elderly patients, as nighttime multifocal ventricular ectopic activity predicted increased cardiac mortality.[47]

Nocturnal Ischemia and Angina

Accurate assessment and treatment of nocturnal angina has been a subject of concern for over 2 centuries. Heberden in 1768 described angina which "will often oblige [the patients] to rise up out of their bed every night for many months altogether."[48] John Hunter, the well-known 18th-century surgeon, reported chest pains that "seized him in his sleep so as to awaken him."[49] As early as 1923, MacWilliam[50] postulated that the mechanisms of nocturnal ventricular fibrillation and angina were stimulation of sympathetic nerves and increased arterial blood pressure. He described "reflex excitations, dreams, nightmares, etc., sometimes accompanied by extensive rises of arterial blood pressure (hitherto not recognized), increased heart action, changes in respiration, and various reflex effects" and noted "the suddenness of development of the functional disturbances in arterial blood pressure, heart action, etc., in the dreaming state . . . ." He documented greater stress on the circulatory system during dreaming than during wakefulness with arterial blood pressures reaching 200 mmHg. In the middle of this century, the renowned cardiologists Paul Dudley White[48] and Samuel Levine[51] remarked on the frequency of MI and angina in sleep and suggested an association with dreams.

Ischemic activity is an important marker of prognosis in cardiac patients, and characteristics of both REM and NREM sleep may conduce to nocturnal ischemia and angina. The dramatic descriptions cited above can be referred largely to demand-related episodes attributable to the increased sympathetic nerve activity, metabolic demands, and heart rate surges of REM sleep. The few studies in cardiac patients that have employed sleep staging have concluded that in the absence of significant depression of left ventricular function, nocturnal ischemic events occur primarily during REM sleep.[52–54] In stable coronary artery disease patients, ischemia is largely attributable to bouts of sympathetically mediated surges in heart rate and resultant metabolic demands in flow-limited, stenotic coronary arteries.[4, 16, 33, 34, 39–42, 53–58] Nowlin and co-workers[53] attributed nocturnal angina to heightened blood pressure after performing detailed, multisession polysomnographic analysis of four patients with advanced coronary artery disease and nocturnal angina pectoris and established that attacks of nocturnal angina occurred predominantly during REM sleep (32 of 39 recordings) and were associated with heart rate acceleration. Dream content, in patients who could describe it, included awareness of chest pain and involved strenuous physical activity or emotions of fear, anger, or frustration.

That nocturnal ischemia is generated by mechanisms in addition to sympathetic nerve activity and unsatisfied metabolic demands is indicated by the finding that nighttime ischemic events remain, although less frequent, in patients receiving beta-blockade therapy, the primary therapy that effectively reduces the overall incidence and suppresses the morning peak in cardiac events by containing sympathetic nerve activity and demand-related ischemia.[42, 55, 59, 60] In fact, ischemic events in patients with severe coronary disease or acute coronary syndromes who received beta-blockade therapy exhibit a significant nocturnal peak.[42, 59] Possible mechanisms of non–demand-related ischemia include decreased coronary perfusion pressure due to the nighttime trough in heart rate[42, 61] and arterial blood pressure, especially during NREM sleep,[4, 62] and increased coronary vasomotor tone.[55, 61] These factors acting in concert decrease the metabolic threshold for induction of nocturnal ischemia, which has a nadir between 1 AM and 3 AM.[16, 56, 61, 63] During these hours in patients with stable coronary disease, Benhorin and colleagues[61] observed that ischemia can be provoked at heart rates of 83 bpm, in contrast to 96 bpm during midday and that its incidence was not affected by beta blockade. Patel et al.[59] noted that nocturnal ischemia is attended by heart rate elevations of 6 bpm or less in patients with unstable angina receiving beta-adrenergic blocking agents. Figueras et al.[63] found in patients with angina at rest and coronary stenosis greater than 70% that the incidence of resting angina was highest at night and concluded that nocturnal decline in ischemic threshold facilitated development of transmural ischemia. Mancia[4] hypothesized that the hypotension of NREM sleep is a major contributor to nocturnal ischemia, because it "reduces the volume and velocity of blood flow, favoring the development of thrombi and embolic and ischemic phenomena before and after arousal." It has also been postulated that ischemia provoked by transient thrombus formation[64, 65] is attributable to the nocturnal nadir in endogenous fibrinolytic activity,[64, 66–68] the peak in plasminogen activator inhibitor,[65, 66] increasing blood viscosity or hypercoagulability at night,[66, 69] and increased free-radical generation.[70]

Nondemand nocturnal ischemia is prevalent in patients with more severe coronary disease,[16, 42, 71, 72] acute coronary syndromes,[59, 73] and Prinzmetal's angina.[16, 40, 67, 74] This distribution of patient populations suggests that endothelial dysfunction plays an important role in nocturnal ischemia. Indeed, it has been concluded that

nondemand nocturnal ischemic episodes disclose a critical underlying coronary lesion, coronary vasospasm, or transient coronary artery stenosis.[59] Stern and Tzivoni[72] reported nondemand nocturnal ischemia in 97 patients with fixed abnormal ST-T segment changes during the day. The ST-T segment depression became more pronounced during sleep, with T-wave inversion, in 23 patients (24%); in these patients, ischemia lasted for 1 to 3 h, was not associated with tachycardia or other markers of REM sleep, and was silent in 21 of 23 (91%) patients. Selwyn and associates[71] documented 26% of ischemic episodes in patients with frequent angina between 10 PM and 6 AM, with a significant peak between 4 AM and 6 PM. Langer et al.[73] determined that there was no significant rise in metabolic activity during 10 min before onset of ischemia in sleeping patients with unstable angina. Andrews et al.[42] observed in patients with more advanced stable coronary disease that non–demand-related ischemic episodes cluster between midnight and 6 AM. Patel and colleagues[59] documented a nocturnal peak in ischemic events in their study of patients with the acute coronary syndromes of unstable angina and non–Q-wave MI who were receiving optimal medical therapy aimed at containing demand-related ischemia (Fig. 84–2). This single nocturnal peak in ischemic episodes between midnight and 6 AM involved 36% of all ischemic episodes. Episodes of unstable angina also clustered at night, with 38% occurring during these 6 h.

Patients with Prinzmetal's variant angina experience no nighttime decrease in the incidence of nocturnal ischemia.[40, 42, 74] The incidence of these episodes doubles during the second half of the sleep period, when REM is more frequent[40] and ischemia is both demand-related[54, 75] and non–demand-related.[16, 40, 74] In these individuals, REM sleep is associated with coronary vasospasm, leading to nocturnal ischemia and angina.[54] Otsuka and colleagues[75] observed in eight patients with Prinzmetal's angina that the episodes of nocturnal angina occurred exclusively during REM sleep and were accompanied by ventricular premature beats and ventricular tachycardia. Masuda et al.[67] discovered that the nocturnal peak in ischemic activity in patients with variant angina coincided with a nadir in fibrinolytic activity.

Impaired breathing and oxygen desaturation are not prerequisites of nocturnal ischemic episodes in patients with coronary disease. Investigators have demonstrated that ischemia need not be concomitant with decreased oxygen saturation[76, 77] and recorded episodes of ischemia[76] or oxygen desaturation[78] were not accompanied by apnea.

Thus, treatment of nocturnal ischemia and angina requires attention to several distinct mechanisms that may occur in a single patient. Demand-related ischemic episodes can be effectively contained by beta-adrenergic blockade,[58, 59] but antihypertensive treatment does not reduce[79] the nocturnal incidence of non–demand-related ischemia. The use of vasodilators to treat nondemand episodes due to endothelial dysfunction is the subject of current discussion.[58] The incidence of nocturnal ischemic activity in patients with unstable angina and

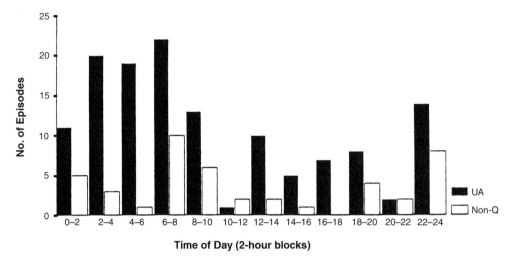

Figure 84–2. The circadian variation of ischemic activity based on 2-h time blocks for the study population. There is a single peak of ischemic activity at night between 10 PM and 8 AM and no morning peak in ischemia activity is apparent. More than 64% of episodes occurred during this time period ($P < .001$ compared with daytime). The circadian distribution of episodes of unstable angina (UA) and non-Q-wave myocardial infarction (Non-Q) is similar to the overall pattern of ischemic activity. (From Patel DJ, Knight CJ, Holdright DR, et al. Pathophysiology of transient myocardial ischemia in acute coronary syndromes. Characterization by continuous ST-segment monitoring. Circulation. 1997;95[5]:1185–1192.)

non–Q-wave infarction who were receiving optimal medical therapy suggests that current approaches to management do not adequately address the factors involved.[59] The lack of sleep staging and arterial blood pressure monitoring in coronary patients with nocturnal ischemia leaves unidentified any contribution by autonomic and hemodynamic activity dictated by sleep states. Such monitoring would also disclose the prevalence of the established proischemic influences of nocturnal arousal and rising from bed.[32, 80, 81]

Post–Myocardial Infarction Patients

During the first weeks following MI, many pathophysiological disturbances act in concert. Sleep is significantly disturbed,[62, 82] and nocturnal oxygen desaturation, especially in patients with impaired left ventricular function, may be generalized or episodic and directly provoke tachycardia, ventricular premature beats, and ST segment changes[82–86] (Fig. 84–3). Both the duration and number of nighttime ischemic events is increased, consonant with increased cardiac sympathetic nerve activity[34, 59, 87, 88] or decreased parasympathetic nerve activity[35] (Fig. 84–4), particularly in patients with residual ischemia.[36] Nocturnal levels of norepinephrine are increased and nocturnal secretion of melatonin, an endogenous hormone that suppresses sympathetic nerve activity, is impaired.[89] These symptoms become normal over time so that within the first 6 months, ventricular tachycardia during sleep is relatively rare and is characteristic of patients whose heart rates in sleep had averaged greater than 80 bpm at the time of the crisis.[84] If the nighttime heart rate remains high, averaging over 90 bpm, the risk of fatal events is increased,[28] further underscoring the importance of enhanced sympathetic nerve activity during sleep.

The most detailed study to date of sleep in post-MI patients was performed in 1978 by Broughton and Baron[62] who reported on the sleep and cardiovascular condition of 12 patients, aged 33 to 70 years, following severe MI, first during their stay in the intensive care unit and then in the hospital ward. They noted a "marked disturbance of nocturnal sleep patterns . . . characterized by high amounts of wakefulness, stage 1, and number of awakenings, and REM density and low amounts of REM sleep, shorter REM periods with prolonged REM latencies. Sleep efficiency was substantially reduced."[62] All of these sleep quality parameters improved in parallel with time after MI until on day 9 the only remaining abnormal feature was high content of NREM sleep stages 3 and 4. REM density peaked on postinfarction nights 3 and 4 and NREM sleep on night 4. On subsequent hospital visits after discharge, the patients described terrifying dreams, suggesting that REM suppression was followed by REM rebound more than 2 weeks following the crisis. Importantly, Broughton and Baron observed that NREM sleep provoked nocturnal angina and awakening. They postulated that the hypotension associated with NREM sleep resulted in a diminution in perfusion pressure of the major coronary and collateral vessels supplying the mechanically compromised myocardium. The decreased heart rates typical of NREM, however, were not observed, and heart rates were higher in NREM sleep than in wakefulness on half the nights recorded, indicating enhanced cardiac sympathetic nerve activity even in NREM. In half of the cases, the electrocardiogram (EKG) amplitude decreased during anginal attacks. T-wave alternans, a marker of vulnerability to lethal arrhythmias,[90, 91] appeared in the EKG of one postinfarction patient during angina in NREM sleep.

There are few published reports of the effects of experimental induction of MI on sleep. Snisarenko[92] found significant elevations in heart rate in both the acute (4 to 10 d) and subacute (3 to 12 months) periods

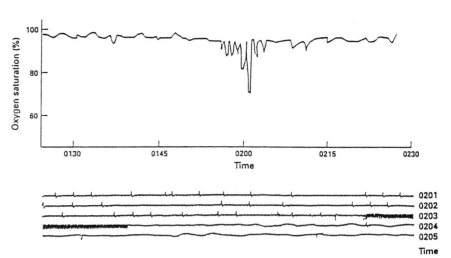

Figure 84–3. Importance of monitoring nocturnal oxygen saturation in postinfarction patients. Simultaneously occurring nonsustained ventricular tachycardia and hypoxemia measured by pulse oximetry in a patient on the third night after infarction. The patient died on the following day of cardiogenic shock. (From Galatius-Jensen S, Hansen J, Rasmussen V, et al. Nocturnal hypoxemia after myocardial infarction: association with nocturnal myocardial ischaemia and arrhythmias. Br Heart J. 1994;72:23–30.)

following MI in a feline model. In the acute period these were accompanied by increased wakefulness, decreased HRV, and severely disordered sleep. In the intervening weeks, sleep quality recovered fully until, in the subacute period, beta blockade with propranolol led to renewed, pronounced disturbances in sleep structure, with increased wakefulness, reduction in REM sleep, and prolongation of stages 1 and 2 of NREM sleep. The author attributed these results to reflex activation of adrenergic, noradrenergic, and dopaminergic nerves in several brain structures following coronary artery ligation. Skinner and colleagues[93] documented ventricular ectopic activity but not ventricular fibrillation during NREM sleep in pigs following MI. This pattern may be attributable to slowing of the heart rate and increased vagus nerve activity during NREM

sleep, which can inhibit the normal overdrive suppression of ventricular rhythms by sinoatrial node pacemaker activity and result in firing of latent ventricular pacemakers and triggered activity.

Nocturnal Myocardial Infarction

The dynamic perturbations in autonomic nervous system activity both independent of and in conjunction with disturbances in breathing, particularly apnea, are likely to constitute important triggers of MI at night. REM-induced surges in sympathetic nerve activity have the potential to provoke tachycardia and hypertension, alterations that carry the potential for inducing MI secondary to coronary artery plaque rupture as well as inappropriate decreases in the myocardial oxygen supply–demand relationship or alpha-adrenergically mediated coronary vasoconstriction. Alternatively, in a starkly opposite manner, the hypotension of slow-wave sleep may lead to malperfusion of the myocardium due to reduced coronary perfusion pressure through stenotic vessel segments. In the early phase of MI, when there is impaired myocardial contractility, the attendant reductions in systemic pressure may precipitate ischemic attacks. Thus, several investigators[59, 94–97] have attributed nocturnal MI and ischemia to the relative hypotension of NREM sleep, which "reduces the volume and velocity of blood flow, favoring the development of thrombi and embolic and ischemic phenomena before and after arousal."[4] Mancia[4] therefore advocated avoiding drugs that enhance the hypotension of NREM sleep and prescribing antihypertensive medications only for daytime therapy. He echoed the argument of Floras,[79] who observed that antihypertensive treatment did not reduce the incidence of nocturnal MI and ischemia. Further evidence of the risk of hypotension-induced infarction has been provided by Kleitman et al.,[95] who reported that the incidence of subendocardial MI clustered at 2 AM to 4 AM, simultaneous with the nadir in arterial blood pressure. Tsuda et al.[97] also documented a peak in MI in the early morning when arterial blood pressure was lowest in patients on anti-

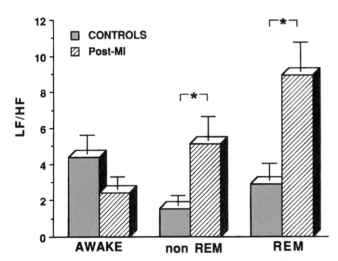

Figure 84–4. Bar graphs indicating mean ± SEM of the low- to high-frequency ratio (LF/HF) from spectral analysis of the heart rate during the awake state *(left)*, during nonrapid eye movement (non REM) sleep *(middle)*, and during rapid eye movement (REM) sleep *(right)* in normal subjects and in postmyocardial infarction (post-MI) patients ($*P < .01$ when comparing control subjects vs. post-MI patients). (From Vanoli E, Adamson PB, Ba-Lin, et al. Heart rate variability during specific sleep stages: a comparison of healthy subjects with patients after myocardial infarction. Circulation. 1995;91[7]:1918–1922.)

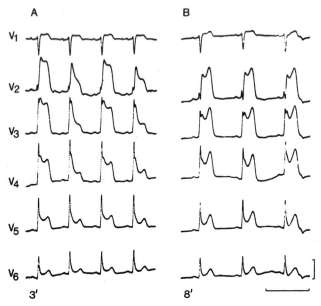

Figure 84–5. *A,* Alternation in precordial leads V$_2$ to V$_5$ 3 min after onset of nocturnal angina during transmural myocardial infarction. *B,* 8 min after beginning of pain, alternation has disappeared. (From Cinca J, Jansa MJ, Moréna H, et al. Mechanism and time course of the early electrical changes during acute coronary artery occlusion. An attempt to correlate the early ECG changes in man to the cellular electrophysiology in the pig. Chest. 1980;77:499–505.)

hypertensive medications. Other factors known to contribute to MI are operative during sleep, including increased ventricular diastolic pressures and volumes due to the fluid shifts resulting from assuming a supine posture, unfavorable alterations in the balance of fibrinolytic and thrombotic factors,[64–70] and chronic or episodic oxygen desaturation.[62, 82–86] It is unknown which of these factors contributed in the case report of onset of nocturnal angina and transmural MI[98] in which T-wave alternans, a new marker of risk for lethal tachyarrhythmias,[90, 91] was recorded during sleep (Fig. 84–5). Alternans, evident in the precordial leads, disappeared as the ischemia and pain were resolved.

Specific patient groups experience an increased incidence of nighttime MIs. The hourly rate of non-Q-wave infarction has been observed not to decline at night.[59, 95] In diabetic patients,[99] the hourly daytime and nighttime incidences of MI are roughly equivalent. In a Japanese population, Hayashi et al.[100] observed a 4- to 6-AM primary peak in sudden cardiac death due to MI. The subgroup analysis of Hjalmarson et al.[101] of nearly 4800 patients concluded that certain patients were more likely to have nighttime than daytime onset of non-Q-wave infarction if they had previously had an MI. These patients were more often older than 70 years of age, female, diabetic, with either previous MI or congestive heart failure, and on beta-blocker therapy at the time of the event.

Hypertension

Sleep apnea is an established risk factor for systemic hypertension independent of the influences of age and obesity.[102–105] A causal relationship is supported by the dose-dependent, linear relationship of sleep-disordered breathing to elevated arterial blood pressure[105] and by experimental evidence that intermittent airway occlusion increased daytime arterial blood pressure by more than 15 mmHg within 3 months.[106] The putative mechanisms are reflex activation of the sympathetic nerves due to nocturnal hypoxia[106–109] and impaired baroreceptor sensitivity.[110] This possibility is underscored by the finding of an enhanced chemoreceptor reflex in borderline hypertensive subjects, which results in exaggerated increases in sympathetic nerve activity during hypoxia.[107] The findings linking apnea and hypertension provide an important opportunity for diagnosis and treatment of hypertension in this subset of patients. Increased risk of hypertension due to snoring in the absence of apnea has not been demonstrated.[111]

Hypertensive patients whose nighttime arterial blood pressure declines less than 10% from day to night (called "nondippers") are at increased risk of cerebrovascular insult,[112, 113] frequent or complex ventricular arrhythmias,[114] and increased organ damage,[112, 115, 116] including cardiac hypertrophy.[117, 118] Large-population studies have documented a nocturnal peak in sudden cardiac death among hypertensive women[119] (Fig. 84–6). Pickering and James[120] argued that the pathological basis for this increased risk is the challenge of a higher average 24-h arterial blood pressure. An alternative explanation may be that a high average nocturnal diastolic arterial blood pressure is a powerful marker of left ventricular filling impairment, itself a strong indicator of cardiovascular risk.[121] Faulty baroreceptor activation may account for the fact that arterial blood pressure during sleep remains significantly elevated in these hypertensive patients, who typically show evidence of central hypersympathetic nerve activity with

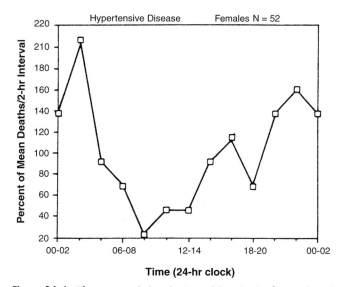

Figure 84–6. The temporal distribution of female deaths attributed to hypertensive disease peaked at 1 AM. The temporal concentration was statistically significant ($P < .01$). (Reprinted from *American Journal of Medicine*, vol. 82, Mitler MM, Hajdukovic RM, Shafor R, et al. When people die. Cause of death versus time of death, 266–274, Copyright 1987, with permission from Excerpta Medica Inc.)

an increased number of microarousals, reduced length and depth of NREM sleep, and a shortened REM latency.

Heart Failure

Sleep in heart failure patients is highly fragmented; arousals and state changes may occur at a rate of up to 50 per hour.[122, 123] More than half of heart failure patients suffer from sleep-related breathing disorders,[123a] and the common appearance of Cheyne-Stokes respiration can impair cardiac function and increase mortality.[123–125] The apnea-hypopnea index has been determined to be a powerful independent predictor of poor prognoses in clinically stable congestive heart failure patients.[125a] Decreased oxygen saturation[126] and elevated sympathetic nerve activity[127] are typical and attributable to disordered breathing. Continuous positive airway pressure (CPAP) may improve sleep, exercise tolerance, cognitive function,[128] and left ventricular ejection fraction.[129] Moser and colleagues[130] registered their surprise that the 20% incidence of nocturnal sudden cardiac death was not higher in view of the high incidence of sleep abnormalities and oxygen desaturation in these patients. Elevated sympathetic neural tone in heart failure patients is associated with increased mortality.[131] The contribution of increased autonomic activity is further underscored by the recent determination that Q–T interval dispersion, a marker of heterogeneity of repolarization that is increased during sleep in survivors of sudden cardiac death,[46] is an indicator of arrhythmic events in patients with heart failure.[132, 133] An affective component is suggested by Smith's[134] conclusion that the severity of cardiac dysfunction in patients with heart failure is reflected in an increasing number of dream references to death and separation, introducing significant negative states such as depression and loss of will to survive.

Elderly Patients

Aging presents additional challenges in terms of disturbed sleep, which, when it occurs, may be associated with depression, poor health, daytime angina, a limited activity level,[135] and cardiac arrhythmias.[136] Initiating a moderately intense exercise program significantly improves sleep quality in formerly sedentary older people.[137] Nocturnal ischemia is not uncommon in older patients with vascular disease who experience regular episodes of oxygen desaturation and increased heart rate.[138] Conflicting evidence has been presented of increased risk for nighttime MI and sudden cardiac death in the elderly.[96, 101, 139, 140] An impairment in baroreceptor sensitivity,[141] a measure of the capacity for reflex vagus nerve activation,[8] and increased LF power of heart rate variability[142] are evident at night in susceptible elderly patients. Given this autonomic background, it is not surprising that nighttime multifocal activity in elderly patients is a predictor of cardiac mortality.[47]

The severe stress of living near the epicenter of a major earthquake has recently been reported as a trigger of nocturnal cardiac death, especially in the elderly.[113] Individuals more than 60 years old with coronary heart disease were affected for several months following the Hanshin-Awaji 1995 earthquake, and the incidence of events was positively associated with earthquake damage. The nocturnal cardiovascular death rate (between 11 PM and 5 AM) was increased by 80% over the previous year.

Respiratory Challenges: Apnea, Chronic Obstructive Lung Disease, and Snoring

Sleep apnea due to airway obstruction is estimated to affect 2 to 4% of adults,[2] or 5 to 10 million Americans. Such derangements in respiratory function can play a subtle and insidious role in disrupting myocardial perfusion, even in people without cardiac disease.[143, 144] Respiratory challenges during sleep evolve from the necessity of maintaining control over two fundamentally different types of musculature: somatic, which is responsible for oxygen exchange, and autonomic, which involves the heart and vasculature and is responsible for blood transport.[5] Malperfusion of the myocardium may result from loss of regulation of either or both systems in patients with ischemic heart disease.

A large body of evidence indicates that apneic episodes and oxygen desaturation are highly conducive to nocturnal ischemia, bradyarrhythmias, and tachyarrhythmias in patients with coronary artery disease[145–147] and are a risk factor for development of hypertension (see earlier). A great majority (more than 80%) of episodes of nocturnal ischemia are precipitated during REM sleep, when apneic activity is high and hypoxemia is cumulative.[146] Elevated plasma adenosine levels, a marker of myocardial ischemia, are associated with hypoxemia in patients with severe apnea.[148] Apnea that produces severe, chronic oxygen desaturation (to less than 65%) is highly conducive to ventricular ectopy and tachycardias. The postulated mechanism of arrhythmogenesis during apnea is the accompanying surges in arterial blood pressure and sympathetic nerve activity.[3, 107, 109, 149] Patients with sleep apnea experience high levels of sympathetic nerve activity, even during wakefulness.[109] In these patients, nerve activity and blood pressure were increased above wakefulness, especially during stage 2 and REM sleep. Sympathetic activity peaked at 246 to 299% of baseline during the final 10 sec of apneic events during REM and stage 2 sleep, respectively. CPAP treatment attenuated the elevations in blood pressure and sympathetic nerve activity. However, apnea does not provoke arrhythmia in patients without serious cardiac or respiratory comorbidity[147] and is not a prerequisite of oxygen desaturation[78] or ischemic events[76] in patients with cardiac disease. The facts that MI and sudden cardiac death may be unheralded by prodromes and that the presence of cardiovascular disease is frequently underdiagnosed provide a rationale for investigating whether apnea may be provoking nocturnal arrhythmias in individual patients.

Sleep apnea has been strongly implicated in the occurrence of MI. Cardiac patients in the highest quartile of apnea severity maintain a risk for MI of 23.3 times that of patients in the lowest quartile ($P <$ .001).[150] The postulated mechanisms include reduced myocardial oxygen supply due to bradycardia, asystole, and impaired respiration; the analyses were controlled for hypertension. Further possible mechanisms are apnea-induced increases in whole-blood viscosity, plasma fibrinogen concentration, and platelet activation, which may be independent risk factors for cardiovascular events.[151, 151a]

When apneas exceed a frequency of 20 per hour, the risk of death is greatly increased, particularly in patients less than 50 years of age.[152] Death following a prolonged apnea has been witnessed.[153] Half of the deaths in apnea patients occur between midnight and 8 AM.[154] Apneas also predispose patients to lethal daytime events, and 71% of the total deaths are due to cardiovascular causes.[154] Thus, death in apnea patients is predominantly of cardiovascular origin and is not confined to the sleeping period.

Patients with chronic obstructive lung disease are also at increased nighttime cardiac risk. Nocturnal oxygen desaturation may be of sufficient magnitude to be arrhythmogenic. This condition may elicit ST segment and T-wave changes, prolong the Q–T interval, and increase ventricular premature beats at night compared to daytime.[155]

Increased sleep-related risk of cardiac events has been attributed to snoring in several large population studies, adjusted for age, obesity, and hypertension. A direct causal link has not been demonstrated, as many investigations were not adjusted for the possibility that sleep apnea, which is not uncommon in habitual snorers, is at the root of the apparent excess risk.[156] Thus, because heavy snoring is a conspicuous phenomenon commonly associated with apnea, a known risk factor for MI, cardiac death, hypertension, ischemia, and arrhythmias, the possible presence of apnea should be investigated when heavy snoring is reported. The established contribution of smoking[157] and excessive alcohol consumption to both snoring and apnea suggests additional confounding mechanisms as well as therapeutic options.

Nocturnal Asystole and Q–T Interval Prolongation

In individuals who are physically fit, such as athletes[158] and female heavy laborers,[159] pauses in nighttime heart rate and even heart block are well documented and are attributed to enhanced vagal tone. Although heightened vagal tone is generally cardioprotective, sleep-induced surges in vagal activity[13, 14] may trigger bradycardias and asystoles in otherwise healthy individuals. Guilleminault and colleagues[160] observed striking periods of sinus arrest of 9 sec or less during REM sleep in young adults who were apparently nor-

mal with respect to cardiac function. It was concluded that the nocturnal asystoles were the result of exaggerated, if not abnormally elevated, vagal tone, as muscarinic receptor blockers significantly reduced the duration of the nocturnal asystoles but did not prevent them.

In patients with cardiac disease, especially those on class III antiarrhythmic drugs, nocturnal asystolic events can set the stage for arrhythmias, as abrupt changes in cycle length are conducive to early and late afterdepolarizations and to the lethal arrhythmia, torsade de pointes. In patients with damaged endothelium, surges in vagus nerve activity could result in vasoconstriction due to impaired release of endothelium-derived relaxing factor. Nocturnal heart rate pauses may be particularly arrhythmogenic in a subset of patients with the long Q–T syndrome who have mutations on SCN5A, the sodium channel gene.[161] The asystoles occur almost exclusively at rest or during sleep, when the Q–T interval is further prolonged.[162]

Sudden Infant Death Syndrome

Sudden infant death syndrome (SIDS), the leading cause of mortality in infants between 1 week and 1 year of age, accounts for one third of all deaths during the first year of life and occurs during sleep.[163] The definition of the syndrome is a "diagnosis of exclusion," that is, it includes all causes "which remain unexplained after a thorough case investigation, including performance of a complete autopsy, examination of the death scene, and review of the clinical history."[163] Thus, SIDS may be attributable to a variety of etiologies which challenge the developing cardiorespiratory system.[164] Among environmental influences, the increased risk of SIDS during the winter season is well documented[165, 166] and is not related to bronchiolitis.[167] Conflicting evidence has been provided regarding the relative increase in risk attributable to prone sleeping.[168–172]

A genetic susceptibility that may interact with environmental factors has been implicated by a 5.8-fold increase in recurrence of SIDS within families.[173] Tishler and colleagues[174] reported a significant incidence of deficits in ventilatory responses to hypoxia in families with apnea. Failure to respond to cardiorespiratory challenges during sleep may result from a binding deficit in the arcuate nucleus of SIDS infants,[175] as muscarinic cholinergic activity in this structure at the ventricular medullary surface is postulated to be involved in cardiorespiratory control.

The fatal event in SIDS victims is characterized by hypotension and bradycardia[176] and appears to be attributable to a deficit in the normal reflex coordination of heart rate, arterial blood pressure, and respiration during sleep.[175, 177] Heart rates in infants who later died of SIDS are generally higher and exhibit a reduced range, suggesting altered autonomic control.[177, 178] Autonomic instability has also been documented in NREM sleep in infants with aborted SIDS events.[177, 179] Recent evidence from a 19-year study of more than

33,000 infants determined that significant prolongation of the Q–T interval, the period of repolarization in the cardiac cycle, is strongly associated with SIDS.[180] These data suggest that SIDS may be attributed to a developmental abnormality in cardiac sympathetic innervation that can increase the risk of ventricular arrhythmia. T-wave alternans, an EKG indicator of heightened vulnerability to sudden cardiac death,[90, 91] has been reported in a chest lead on the first day of life in an infant who became a SIDS victim.[181]

Passive cigarette smoking is a very significant modifiable risk factor in SIDS. Reduction of 61% in the number of SIDS deaths has been projected if smoking were eliminated from infants' environments.[169–172, 182] A dose-dependent effect has been demonstrated.[170] Maternal smoking during pregnancy is also implicated.[182–184] Established SIDS risk factors of preterm birth and low birth weight increased risk more than 15-fold among smokers[184] but not at all among nonsmokers. Illegal drug use increases risk of SIDS by more than four-fold.[182] The mechanisms may include impairment in chemoreceptor responsiveness due to decreased sensitivity to carbon dioxide in infants of substance-abusing mothers.[185] Nicotine may operate through a combination of effects to account for the increase in SIDS due to passive smoking. It is known to increase sleep apnea[157] and to affect chemoreceptor activation of respiration adversely,[186, 187] dulling the response to hypoxia.[188] Nicotine and its metabolites have been found at autopsy in the pericardial fluid of SIDS infants.[189, 190] Epicardial nicotine is associated with hypopnea[191] and affects the sinoatrial node and epicardial neural fibers to induce hypotension and bradycardia,[192, 193] the documented symptomatology of the final event in SIDS infants.[176]

Sudden Unexplained Nocturnal Death Syndrome

The most striking association between sudden death and sleep has been reported in young, apparently healthy Southeast Asian men (see Chapter 85). These deaths are named *lai-tai* ("sleep death") in Laos, *pokkuri* ("sudden and unexpected death") in Japan, *bangungut* ("to rise and moan in sleep") in the Philippines, and "sudden unexplained nocturnal death (SUNDS)" in the United States, where the phenomenon occurs among immigrants. Autopsies have established that cardiovascular disease is absent, but, in some instances, that conduction pathways are developmentally abnormal.[194, 195] Companions have reported that the immediate symptoms are onset of agonal respirations during sleep,[196, 197] along with vocalization, violent motor activity, nonarousability, rapid irregular deep breathing, perspiration, heart rate surges, and severe autonomic discharge. Several victims revived by vigorous massage reported sensations of airway obstruction, chest discomfort or pressure, and numb and weak limbs. When these symptoms recurred within weeks to months, they culminated in death.[198] Three victims who had been resuscitated from ventricular fibrillation then experienced recurring fibrillation in hospital during sleep accompanied by similar moaning vocalizations.[196] In these three patients, there was no evidence of atherosclerosis or structural abnormalities and no sleep apnea, but creatine kinase levels were markedly elevated and potassium was depressed. The Brugada syndrome is typically nocturnal and, like SUNDS, strikes males almost exclusively. The electrocardiographic "Brugada sign," involving right bundle branch block with ST segment elevation in the right precordial leads[199] and arrhythmogenic right ventricular cardiomyopathy,[200] suggests a common etiology.

Atrial Fibrillation

Atrial fibrillation is a prevalent arrhythmia with serious consequences in terms of increased morbidity and mortality and is more frequently triggered at night than during any other 8-h period.[201–203] Current estimates are that 2.5 million patients experience this arrhythmia, which is associated with a doubling of overall mortality and of mortality due to cardiovascular disease.[204, 205] Approximately 40% of symptomatic episodes of atrial fibrillation have their onset between midnight and 8 AM,[202] with a peak incidence at midnight[203] (Fig. 84–7). The nocturnal pattern is nonuniform, suggesting triggering by physiological processes. Atrial fibrillation is provoked by periods of intense vagus nerve activity[206] associated with sleep states or as part of the postprandial vagomimetic response. In animals, administration of acetylcholine or intense stimulation of the vagus nerve can cause heterogeneity of atrial repolarization and atrial fibrillation.[206] Enhanced adrenergic activity may interact in a complex manner with changes in vagal tone to affect atrial refractoriness and dispersion of repolarization and to

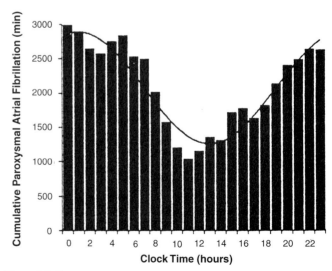

Figure 84–7. Hourly total duration of paroxysmal atrial fibrillation accumulated in the total of 150 patients. A single-harmonic fit is represented by the curved line. A prominent circadian rhythm is present, with a peak at midnight and a nadir at 11 AM. (From Yamashita T, Murakawa Y, Sezaki K, et al. Circadian variation of paroxysmal atrial fibrillation. Circulation. 1997;96[5]:1537–1541.)

alter intra-atrial conduction to increase propensity to atrial fibrillation.[205, 206] Risk of atrial fibrillation is increased by 2.8-fold if breathing during sleep is disordered,[207] which can provoke nocturnal hypoxemia, sympathetic nerve activity, and hemodynamic stress. However, few records exist of concurrent monitoring of sleep and nocturnal onset of atrial fibrillation.

Sleep-Disrupting Effects of Medications

Several important medications that are widely prescribed for cardiac patients, including antihypertensive agents, beta blockers that cross the blood-brain barrier, and calcium channel blockers, have the potential to disrupt sleep[92, 208, 209] (Fig. 84–8). In particular, the lipophilic beta blockers (pindolol, propranolol, and metoprolol) disrupt sleep, increasing the total number of awakenings and total wakefulness compared with placebo and with the nonlipophilic atenolol.[208] Penetration of the blood-brain barrier occurs with prolonged therapy, when these distinctions may become less apparent.[210] In addition, pindolol, which has intrinsic sympathomimetic activity, increases REM latency and, as a result, decreases REM sleep time.[208] Sleep disruption may provoke daytime fatigue and lethargy, symptoms widely reported by patients taking beta blockers and which may prompt discontinuation of the medication or noncompliance. It has been postulated that the mechanism of sleep disruption by beta-adrenergic blocking agents is their well-known tendency to deplete endogenous melatonin,[211] a key sleep-regulating hormone that moderates sympathetic nerve activity. An additional important side effect of these beta blockers[208] and of calcium channel blockers[209] is their potential to provoke nightmares. Sleep disturbance has also been documented in conjunction with the widely employed antiarrhythmic agent amiodarone.[209a, 209b] Finally, pharmacological agents (e.g., barbiturates) and ventilation treatments (e.g., CPAP) have the capability to induce REM deprivation and to create the conditions for subsequent rebound phenomena with arrhythmogenic potential.

The therapeutic regimen may require adjustment to allow for the circadian variation in circulatory and autonomic nervous system activity. Mancia[4] has suggested that pharmacological therapy, which exacerbates the hypotensive effect of NREM sleep, may introduce the potential risk of thrombosis and embolism in patients with stenotic lesions in the heart or brain. Floras[79] determined that the nocturnal incidence of MI was not diminished in patients treated with antihypertensive agents and suggested that the agents induced nocturnal hypotension. Tsuda et al.[97] identified a peak in MI coincident with the nadir in blood pressure in patients on antihypertensive medication. Thus, special attention should be given to the hemodynamic effects of antihypertensive drugs and vasodilators[4, 58, 59, 61, 79, 97] to avoid precipitating cardiac events by inducing profound hypotension.

CONCLUSIONS

Sleep exerts a major impact on the health of the cardiac patient. In a sense, the diseased heart and lungs are unwitting victims of the needs of the sleeping brain, which commands dramatic alterations in autonomic and respiratory activity. A sizable population experiences cardiac events during sleep, with identifiable high-risk groups (see Table 84–1). Sleep also presents unusual opportunities to monitor the cardiac patient, as there is growing appreciation of the fact that nighttime heart rate, blood pressure, ischemia, arrhythmias, and respiratory disturbances carry predictive value for daytime events (see Table 84–2). Daytime tests cannot

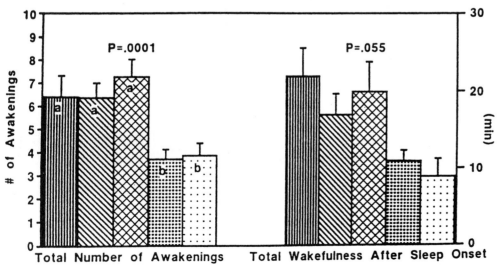

SLEEP CONTINUITY

Figure 84–8. Polysomnographic measures of sleep continuity in 30 healthy male subjects during 1 night following 1 week of treatment with beta blockers or placebo. Lipophilic beta blockers pindolol (PIND), propranolol (PROP), and metoprolol (METOP) significantly disturbed sleep, as indicated by the number of awakenings, which was significantly reduced with nonlipophilic atenolol (ATEN). (From Kostis JB, Rosen RC. Central nervous system effects of beta-adrenergic-blocking drugs: the role of ancillary properties. Circulation. 1987;75[1]:204–212.)

substitute for nighttime monitoring of the cardiac patient, as treadmill exercise testing and daytime ambulatory monitoring cannot replicate the autonomic, hemodynamic, or respiratory changes that uniquely accompany sleep. Improved identification of the precise triggers of nocturnal cardiac events may be anticipated when technologies are integrated for monitoring sleep state, respiration, and cardiovascular variables.

Acknowledgments

Supported by grant HL50078 from the National Heart, Lung, and Blood Institute and ES 08129 from the National Institutes of Environmental Health, National Institutes of Health, Bethesda, Md. The authors thank Sandra Verrier for her editorial contributions.

References

1. Lavery CE, Mittleman MA, Cohen MC, et al. Nonuniform nighttime distribution of acute cardiac events: a possible effect of sleep states. Circulation. 1997;5:3321–3327.
2. Young T, Palta M, Dempsey J, et al. The occurrence of sleep-disordered breathing among middle-aged adults. N Engl J Med. 1993;328:1230–1235.
3. Somers VK, Dyken ME, Mark AL, et al. Sympathetic nerve activity during sleep in normal subjects. N Engl J Med. 1993;328:303–307.
4. Mancia G. Autonomic modulation of the cardiovascular system during sleep. N Engl J Med. 1993;328:347–349.
5. Harper RM, Frysinger RC, Zhang J, et al. Cardiac and respiratory interactions maintaining homeostasis during sleep. In: Lydic R, Biebuyck JF, eds. Clinical Physiology of Sleep. Bethesda Md: American Physiological Society; 1988.
6. Coccagna G, Mantovani M, Brignani F, et al. Laboratory note. Arterial pressure changes during spontaneous sleep in man. Electroencephalogr Clin Neurophysiol. 1971;31:277–281.
7. Snyder F, Hobson JA, Morrison DF, et al. Changes in respiration, heart rate, and systolic blood pressure in human sleep. J Appl Physiol. 1964;19:417–422.
8. Smyth HS, Sleight P, Pickering GW. Reflex regulation of arterial pressure during sleep in man. A quantitative method of assessing baroreflex sensitivity. Circ Res. 1969;24:109–121.
9. Conway J, Boon N, Jones JV, et al. Involvement of the baroreceptor reflexes in the changes in blood pressure with sleep and mental arousal. Hypertension. 1983;5:746–748.
10. Hornyak M, Cejnar M, Elam M, et al. Sympathetic muscle nerve activity during sleep in man. Brain. 1991;114:1281–1295.
11. Okada H, Iwase S, Mano T, et al. Changes in muscle sympathetic nerve activity during sleep in humans. Neurology. 1991; 41:1961–1966.
12. Bonnet MH, Arand DL. Heart rate variability: sleep stage, time of night, and arousal influences. Electroencephalogr Clin Neurophysiol. 1997;102:390–396.
13. Dickerson LW, Huang AH, Nearing BD, et al. Primary coronary vasodilation associated with pauses in heart rhythm during sleep. Am J Physiol. 1993;264:R186–196.
14. Verrier RL, Lau RT, Wallooppillai U, et al. Primary vagally mediated decelerations in heart rate during tonic rapid eye movement sleep in cats. Am J Physiol. 1998;43:R1136–1141.
15. Hobson JA, Spagna T, Malenka R. Ethology of sleep studied with time-lapse photography: postural immobility and sleep-cycle phase in humans. Science. 1979;201:1251–1253.
16. Quyyumi AA, Efthimiou J, Quyyumi A, et al. Nocturnal angina: precipitating factors in patients with coronary artery disease and those with variant angina. Br Heart J. 1986;56:346–352.
17. Kirby DA, Verrier RL. Differential effects of sleep stage on coronary hemodynamic function. Am J Physiol. 1989; 256:H1378–1383.
18. Kirby DA, Verrier RL. Differential effects of sleep stage on coronary hemodynamic function during stenosis. Physiol Behav. 1989;45:1–4.
19. Dickerson LW, Huang AH, Thurnher MM, et al. Relationship between coronary hemodynamic changes and the phasic events of rapid eye movement sleep. Sleep. 1993;16:550–557.
20. Rowe K, Moreno R, Lau RT, et al. Heart rate surges during REM sleep are associated with theta rhythm and PGO activity in the cat. Am J Physiol. 1999;277:R843–R849.
21. Khatri IM, Freis ED. Hemodynamic changes during sleep. J Appl Physiol. 1967;22:867–873.
22. Siegel JM. Mechanisms of sleep control. J Clin Neurophysiol. 1990;7:49–65.
23. Townsend RE, Prinz PN, Obrist WD. Human cerebral blood flow during sleep and waking. J Appl Physiol. 1973;35:620–625.
24. Maquet P, Peters J, Aerts J, et al. Functional neuroanatomy of human rapid-eye-movement sleep and dreaming. Nature. 1996; 383:163–166.
25. Dodt C, Breckling U, Derad I, et al. Plasma epinephrine and norepinephrine concentrations of healthy humans associated with nighttime sleep and morning arousal. Hypertension. 1997; 30(1 pt 1):71–76.
26. Weitzman ED, Fukushima D, Nogeire C, et al. Twenty-four hour pattern of the episodic secretion of cortisol in normal subjects. J Clin Endocrinol Metab. 1971;33:14–22.
27. Task Force of the European Society of Cardiology and the North American Society of Pacing and Electrophysiology. Heart rate variability: standards of measurement, physiological interpretation and clinical use. Circulation. 1996;93:1043–1065.
28. Touboul P, Andre-Fouet X, Leizorovica A, et al. Risk stratification after myocardial infarction. A reappraisal in the era of thrombolysis. The Groupe d'étude du pronostic de l'infarctus du myocarde (GREPI). Eur Heart J. 1997;18:99–107.
29. Baharav A, Kotagal S, Gibbons V, et al. Fluctuations in autonomic nervous activity during sleep displayed by power spectrum analysis of heart rate variability. Neurology. 1995;45:1183–1187.
30. Klingenheben T, Rapp U, Hohnloser SH. Circadian variation of heart rate variability in post-infarction patients with and without life-threatening ventricular tachyarrhythmias. J Cardiovasc Electrophysiol. 1995;6:357–364.
31. Otzenberger H, Simon C, Gronfier C, et al. Temporal relationship between dynamic heart rate variability and electroencephalographic activity during sleep in man. Neurosci Lett. 1997; 229:173–176.
32. Huikuri HV, Niemela MJ, Ojala S, et al. Circadian rhythms of frequency domain measures of heart rate variability in healthy subjects and patients with coronary artery disease. Effects of arousal and upright posture. Circulation. 1994;90:121–126.
33. Vardas PE, Kochiadakis GE, Manios EG, et al. Spectral analysis of heart rate variability before and during episodes of nocturnal ischaemia in patients with extensive coronary artery disease. Eur Heart J. 1996;17:388–393.
34. Marchant B, Stevenson R, Vaishnav S, et al. Influence of the autonomic nervous system on circadian patterns of myocardial ischaemia: comparison of stable angina with the early postinfarction period. Br Heart J. 1994;71:329–333.
35. Vanoli E, Adamson PB, Ba-Lin, et al. Heart rate variability during specific sleep stages: a comparison of healthy subjects with patients after myocardial infarction. Circulation. 1995; 91:1918–1922.
36. Cerati D, Nador F, Maestri R, et al. Influence of residual ischaemia on heart rate variability after myocardial infarction. Eur Heart J. 1997;18:78–83.
37. Verrier RL, Mittleman MA. Life-threatening cardiovascular consequences of anger in patients with coronary heart disease. Cardiol Clin. 1996;14:289–307.
38. Lown B, Temte JV, Reich P, et al. Basis for recurring ventricular fibrillation in the absence of coronary heart disease and its management. N Engl J Med. 1976;294:623–629.
39. Beamer AD, Lee TH, Cook EF, et al. Diagnostic implications for myocardial ischemia of the circadian variation of the onset of chest pain. Am J Cardiol. 1987;60:988–1002.
40. Nademanee K, Intrachot V, Josephson MA, et al. Circadian variation in occurrence of transient overt and silent myocardial ischemia in chronic stable angina and comparison with Prinzmetal angina in men. Am J Cardiol. 1987;60:494–498.
41. Behar S, Reicher-Reiss H, Goldbourt U, et al. Circadian variation in pain onset in unstable angina pectoris. Am J Cardiol. 1991; 67:91–93.

42. Andrews TC, Fenton T, Toyosaki N, et al for the Angina and Silent Ischemia Study Group (ASIS). Subsets of ambulatory myocardial ischemia based on heart rate activity: circadian distribution and response to anti-ischemic medication. Circulation. 1993;98:92–100.

43. Smith R, Johnson L, Rothfeld D, et al. Sleep and cardiac arrhythmias. Arch Intern Med. 1972;130:751–753.

44. Rosenblatt G, Hartman E, Zwilling GR. Cardiac irritability during sleep and dreaming. J Psychosom. 1973;17:129–134.

45. Otsuka K, Yanaga T, Ichimaru Y, et al. Sleep and night-type arrhythmias. Jpn Heart J. 1982;23:479–486.

46. Molnar J, Rosenthal JE, Weiss JS, et al. QT interval dispersion in healthy subjects and survivors of sudden cardiac death: circadian variation in a 24-hour assessment. Am J Cardiol. 1997;79:1190–1193.

47. Raiha IJ, Piha SJ, Seppanen A, et al. Predictive value of continuous ambulatory electrocardiographic monitoring in elderly people. Br Med J. 1994;309:1263–1267.

48. White PD. Heart Disease. 3rd ed. New York, NY: Macmillan; 1944:87.

49. Home E. Life of John Hunter, In: Major RH, ed. Classic Descriptions of Disease. 4th ed. Springfield, Ill: Charles C Thomas; 1955:423.

50. MacWilliam JA. Blood pressure and heart action in sleep and dreams: their relation to haemorrhages, angina, and sudden death. Br Med J. 1923;22:1196–2000.

51. Levine S. Clinical Heart Disease. Philadelphia, Pa: WB Saunders; 1951:816.

52. Kales A, Kales JD. Evaluation, diagnosis, and treatment of clinical conditions related to sleep. JAMA. 1970;213:2229–2232.

53. Nowlin JB, Troyer WG Jr, Collins WS, et al. The association of nocturnal angina pectoris with dreaming. Ann Intern Med. 1965;63:1040–1046.

54. King MJ, Zir LM, Kaltman AJ, et al. Variant angina associated with angiographically demonstrated coronary artery spasm and REM sleep. Am J Med Sci. 1973;265:419–422.

55. Mulcahy D, Cunningham D, Crean P, et al. Circadian variation of total ischaemic burden and its alteration with anti-anginal agents. Lancet. 1988;1:755–759.

56. Quyyumi AA, Wright CA, Mockus LJ, et al. Mechanisms of nocturnal angina pectoris: Importance of increased myocardial oxygen demand in patients with severe coronary artery disease. Lancet. 1984;1:1207–1209.

57. Deedwania PC, Nelson JR. Pathophysiology of silent myocardial ischemia during daily life: hemodynamic evaluation by simultaneous electrocardiographic and blood pressure monitoring. Circulation. 1990;92:1296–1304.

58. Deedwania PC. Increased demand versus reduced supply and the circadian variations in ambulatory myocardial ischemia. Therapeutic implications [editorial]. Circulation. 1993;98:328–331.

59. Patel DJ, Knight CJ, Holdright DR, et al. Pathophysiology of transient myocardial ischemia in acute coronary syndromes. Characterization by continuous ST-segment monitoring. Circulation. 1997;95:1185–1192.

60. Peckova M, Fahrenbruch CE, Cobb LA, et al. Circadian variations in the occurrence of cardiac arrests. Initial and repeat episodes. Circulation. 1998;98:31–39.

61. Benhorin J, Banai S, Moriel M, et al. Circadian variations in ischemic threshold and their relation to the occurrence of ischemic episodes. Circulation. 1993;97:808–814.

62. Broughton R, Baron R. Sleep patterns in the intensive care unit and on the ward after acute myocardial infarction. Electroencephalogr Clin Neurophysiol. 1978;45:348–360.

63. Figueras J, Cinca J, Balda F, et al. Resting angina with fixed coronary artery stenosis: Nocturnal decline in ischemic threshold. Circulation 1986;74:1248–1254.

64. Andreotti F, Davies GJ, Hackett DR, et al. Major circadian fluctuations in fibrinolytic factors and possible relevance to time of onset of myocardial infarction, sudden cardiac death, and stroke. Am J Cardiol. 1988;62:635–637.

65. Bridges AB, McLaren M, Scott NA, et al. Circadian variation of tissue plasminogen activator and its inhibitor, von Willebrand factor antigen, and prostacyclin stimulating factor in men with ischemic heart disease. Br Heart J. 1993;69:121–124.

66. Tofler GH, Stone PH, Maclure M, et al. Analysis of possible triggers of acute myocardial infarction (the MILIS study). Am J Cardiol. 1990;66:22–27.

67. Masuda T, Ogawa H, Miyao Y, et al. Circadian variation in fibrinolytic activity in patients with variant angina. Br Heart J. 1994;71:156–161.

68. Kurnik PB. Circadian variation in the efficacy of tissue-type plasminogen activator. Circulation. 1995;91:1341–1346.

69. Talan MI, Engel BT. Morning increase in whole blood viscosity: a consequence of a hemostatic nocturnal haemodynamic pattern. Acta Physiol Scand. 1993;147:179–183.

70. Bridges AB, Scott NA, McNeill GP, et al. Circadian variation in white blood cell aggregation and free radical indices in men with ischaemic heart disease. Eur Heart J. 1992;13:1632–1636.

71. Selwyn AP, Fox K, Eves M, et al. Myocardial ischaemia in patients with frequent angina pectoris. Br Med J. 1978;2:1594–1596.

72. Stern S, Tzivoni D. Dynamic changes in the ST-T segment during sleep in ischemic heart disease. Am J Cardiol. 1973;32:17–20.

73. Langer AL, Freeman MR, Armstrong PW. ST-segment shift in unstable angina: pathophysiology and association with coronary anatomy and hospital outcome. J Am Coll Cardiol. 1989;13:1495–1502.

74. Araki H, Koiwaya Y, Nakagaki O, et al. Diurnal distribution of ST-segment elevation and related arrhythmias in patients with variant angina: a study by ambulatory ECG monitoring. Circulation. 1983;67:995–1000.

75. Otsuka K, Yanaga T, Watanabe H. Variant angina and REM sleep [letter]. Am Heart J. 1988;115:1343–1346.

76. Keyl C, Lemberger P, Rodig G, et al. Hypoxaemia and myocardial ischaemia on the night before coronary bypass surgery. Br J Anaesth. 1994;73:157–161.

77. Smith HL, Sapsford DJ, Delaney ME, et al. The effect on the heart of hypoxemia in patients with severe coronary artery disease. Anaesthesia. 1996;51:211–218.

78. Pollock JS, Kenny GN. Effect of lorazepam on oxygen saturation before cardiac surgery. Br J Anaesth. 1993;70:219–220.

79. Floras JS. Antihypertensive treatment, myocardial infarction, and nocturnal myocardial ischaemia. Lancet. 1988;2:994–996.

80. Barry J, Campbell S, Yeung AC, et al. Waking and rising at night as a trigger of myocardial ischemia. Am J Cardiol. 1991;67:1067–1072.

81. Parker JD, Testa MA, Jimenez AH, et al. Morning increase in ambulatory ischemia in patients with stable coronary artery disease. Importance of physical activity and increased cardiac demand. Circulation. 1994;99:604–614.

82. Galatius-Jensen S, Hansen J, Rasmussen V, et al. Nocturnal hypoxemia after myocardial infarction: association with nocturnal myocardial ischaemia and arrhythmias. Br Heart J. 1994;72:23–30.

83. Spudge DD, Seires SF, Maron BJ, et al. Prevalence of arrhythmias during 24-hour Holter electrocardiographic monitoring and exercise testing in patients with obstructive and nonobstructive hypertrophic cardiomyopathy. Circulation. 1979;59:866–875.

84. Møller M, Lyager Nielsen B, Fabricius J. Paroxysmal VT during repeated 24-hr ambulatory electrographic monitoring of post-MI patients. Br Heart J. 1980;43:447–453.

85. Davies SW, John LM, Wedzicha JA, et al. Overnight studies in severe chronic left heart failure: arrhythmias and oxygen desaturation. Br Heart J. 1991;65:77–83.

86. Cripps T, Rocker G, Stradling J. Nocturnal hypoxia and arrhythmias in patients with impaired left ventricular function. Br Heart J. 1992;68:382–386.

87. Mickley H, Pless P, Nielsen JR, et al. Circadian variation of transient myocardial ischemia in the early out-of-hospital period after first acute myocardial infarction. Am J Cardiol. 1991;67:927–932.

88. Casolo GC, Stroder P, Signorini C, et al. Heart rate variability during the acute phase of myocardial infarction. Circulation. 1992;95:2073–2079.

89. Brugger P, Marktl W, Herold M. Impaired nocturnal secretion of melatonin in coronary heart disease. Lancet. 1995;345:1408.

90. Nearing BD, Huang AH, Verrier RL. Dynamic tracking of car-

diac vulnerability by complex demodulation of the T-wave. Science. 1991;252:437–440.

91. Rosenbaum DS, Jackson LE, Smith JM, et al. Electrical alternans and vulnerability to ventricular arrhythmia. N Engl J Med. 1994; 330:235–241.

92. Snisarenko AA. Cardiac rhythm in cats during physiological sleep in experimental myocardial infarction and beta-adrenergic receptor blockade. Cor Vasa. 1986;38:306–314.

93. Skinner JE, Mohr DN, Kellaway P. Sleep-stage regulation of ventricular arrhythmias in the unanesthetized pig. Circ Res. 1975;37:342–349.

94. Gibson RS, Boden WE, Theroux P, et al. Diltiazem and reinfarction in patients with non–Q-wave myocardial infarction. Results of a double-blind, randomized, multicenter trial. N Engl J Med. 1986;315:423–429.

95. Kleitman NS, Schechtman KB, Young PM, et al, and the Diltiazem Reinfarction Study Investigators. Lack of diurnal variation in the onset of non-Q-wave infarction. 1990;91:548–555.

96. Hansen O, Johannsson BW, Gullberg B. Circadian distribution of onset of acute myocardial infarction in subgroups from analysis of 10,791 patients treated in a single center. Am J Cardiol. 1992;69:1003–1008.

97. Tsuda M, Hayashi H, Kanematsu K, et al. Comparison between diurnal distribution of onset of infarction in patients with acute myocardial infarction and circadian variation of blood pressure in patients with coronary artery disease. Clin Cardiol. 1993; 16:543–547.

98. Cinca J, Janse MJ, Moréna H, et al. Mechanism and time course of the early electrical changes during acute coronary artery occlusion. An attempt to correlate the early ECG changes in man to the cellular electrophysiology in the pig. Chest. 1980; 77:499–505.

99. Fava S, Azzopardi J, Muscat HA, et al. Absence of circadian variation in the onset of acute myocardial infarction in diabetic subjects. Br Heart J. 1995;74:370–372.

100. Hayashi S, Toyoshima H, Tanabe N, et al. Daily peaks in the incidence of sudden cardiac death and fatal stroke in Niigata Prefecture. Jpn Circ J. 1996;60:193–200.

101. Hjalmarson A, Gilpin EA, Nicod P, et al. Differing circadian patterns of symptom onset in subgroups of patients with acute myocardial infarction. Circulation. 1989;90:267–275.

102. Williams AJ, Houston D, Finberg S, et al. Sleep apnea syndrome and essential hypertension. Am J Cardiol. 1985;55:1019–1022.

103. Carlson JT, Hedner JA, Ejnell H, et al. High prevalence of hypertension in sleep apnea patients independent of obesity. Am J Respir Crit Care Med. 1994;150:72–77.

104. Hla KM, Young TB, Bidwell T, et al. Sleep apnea and hypertension. A population-based study. Ann Intern Med. 1994;120:382–388.

105. Young T, Peppard P, Palta M, et al. Population-based study of sleep-disordered breathing as a risk factor for hypertension. Arch Intern Med. 1997;157:1746–1762.

106. Brooks D, Horner RL, Kozar LF, et al. Obstructive sleep apnea as a cause of systemic hypertension. Evidence from a canine model. J Clin Invest. 1997;99:106–109.

107. Somers VK, Mark AL, Abboud FM. Potentiation of sympathetic nerve responses to hypoxia in borderline hypertensive subjects. Hypertension. 1988;11:608–612.

108. Van den Aardweg JG, Karemaker JM. Repetitive apneas induce periodic hypertension in normal subjects through hypoxia. J Appl Physiol. 1992;72:821–827.

109. Somers VK, Dyken ME, Clary MP, et al. Sympathetic neural mechanisms in obstructive sleep apnea. J Clin Invest. 1995; 1897–1904.

110. Carlson JT, Hedner JA, Sellgren J, et al. Depressed baroreflex sensitivity in patients with obstructive sleep apnea. Am J Respir Crit Care Med. 1996;154:1490–1496.

111. Hoffstein V. Blood pressure, snoring, obesity, and nocturnal hypoxaemia. Lancet. 1994;344:643–645.

112. Verdecchia P, Schillaci G, Gatteschi C, et al. Blunted nocturnal fall in blood pressure in hypertensive women with future cardiovascular morbid events. Circulation. 1993;98:986–992.

113. Kario K, Matsuo T, Kobayashi H, et al. Nocturnal fall of blood pressure and silent cerebrovascular damage in elderly hypertensive patients. Advanced silent cerebrovascular damage in extreme dippers. Hypertension. 1997;27:130–135.

114. Schillaci G, Verdecchia P, Borgioni C, et al. Association between persistent pressure overload and ventricular arrhythmias in essential hypertension. Hypertension. 1996;28:284–289.

115. Parati G, Pomidossi G, Albini F, et al. Relationship of 24-hour blood pressure mean and variability to severity of target organ damage in hypertension. J Hypertens. 1987;5:93–98.

116. Fagher B, Valind S, Thulin T. End-organ damage in treated severe hypertension: close relation to nocturnal blood pressure. J Hum Hypertens. 1995;9:605–610.

117. Verdecchia P, Schillaci G, Guerrieri M, et al. Circadian blood pressure changes and left ventricular hypertrophy in essential hypertension. Circulation. 1990;91:523–536.

118. Muiesan ML, Rizzoni D, Zulli R, et al. Regression of cardiac hypertrophy and night-time blood pressure reduction. J Hypertens. 1993;11(suppl 5):S5300–S5301.

119. Mitler MM, Hajdukovic RM, Shafor R, et al. When people die. Cause of death versus time of death. Am J Med. 1987; 82:266–274.

120. Pickering TG, James GD. Determinants and consequences of the diurnal rhythm of blood pressure. Am J Hypertens. 1993; 6:166S–169S.

121. Galderisi M, Petrocelli A, Alfieri A, et al. Impact of ambulatory blood pressure on left ventricular diastolic dysfunction in uncomplicated arterial systemic hypertension. Am J Cardiol. 1996; 77:597–601.

122. Yamashiro Y, Kryger MH. Sleep in heart failure. Sleep. 1993; 16:513–523.

123. Bradley TD, Floras JS. Pathophysiologic and therapeutic implications of sleep apnea in congestive heart failure. J Card Failure. 1996;2:223–240.

123a. Javaheri S, Parker TJ, Liming JD, et al. Sleep apnea in 81 ambulatory male patients with stable heart failure: types and their prevalences, consequences, and presentations. Circulation. 1998;97:2154–2159.

124. Blackshear JL, Kaplan J, Thompson RC, et al. Nocturnal dyspnea and atrial fibrillation predict Cheyne-Stokes respirations in patients with congestive heart failure. Arch Intern Med. 1995; 155:1297–1302.

125. Hanly PJ, Zuberi-Khokhar NS. Increased mortality associated with Cheyne-Stokes respiration in patients with congestive heart failure. Am J Respir Crit Care Med. 1996;153:272–276.

125a. Lanfranchi PA, Braghiroli A, Bosimini E, et al. Prognostic value of nocturnal Cheyne-Stokes respiration in chronic heart failure. Circulation 1999;99:1435–1440.

126. Munger MA, Stanek EJ, Nara AR, et al. Arterial oxygen saturation in chronic congestive heart failure. Am J Cardiol. 1994; 73:180–185.

127. Naughton MT, Benard DC, Liu PP, et al. Effects of nasal CPAP on sympathetic activity in patients with heart failure and central sleep apnea. Am J Respir Crit Care Med. 1995;152:473–479.

128. Andreas S, Clemens C, Sandholzer H, et al. Improvement of exercise capacity with treatment of Cheyne-Stokes respiration in patients with congestive heart failure. J Am Coll Cardiol. 1996;27:1486–1490.

129. Granton JT, Naughton MT, Benard DC, et al. CPAP improves inspiratory muscle strength in patients with heart failure and central sleep apnea. Am J Respir Crit Care Med. 1996;153:277–282.

130. Moser DK, Stevenson WG, Woo MA, et al. Timing of sudden death in patients with heart failure. J Am Coll Cardiol. 1994; 24:963–967.

131. Woo MA, Stevenson WG, Moser DK, et al. Patterns of beat-to-beat heart rate variability in advanced heart failure. Am Heart J. 1992;123:704–710.

132. Barr CS, Naas A, Freeman M, et al. QT dispersion and sudden unexpected death in chronic heart failure. Lancet. 1994;343:327–329.

133. Tomaselli GF, Beuckelmann DJ, Calkins HG, et al. Sudden cardiac death in heart failure: the role of abnormal repolarization. Circulation. 1994;90:2534–2539.

134. Smith RC. Do dreams reflect a biological state? J Nerv Ment Dis. 1987;175:201–207.

135. Newman AB, Enright PL, Manolio TA, et al. Sleep disturbance, psychosocial correlates, and cardiovascular disease in 5201 older adults: the Cardiovascular Health Study. J Am Geriatr Soc. 1997;45:1–7.

136. Asplund R. Sleep and cardiac disease amongst elderly people. J Intern Med. 1994;236:65–71.
137. King AC, Oman RF, Brassington GS, et al. Moderate-intensity exercise and self-rated quality of sleep in older adults. A randomized controlled trial. JAMA. 1997;277:32–37.
138. Goldman MD, Reeder MK, Muir AD, et al. Repetitive nocturnal arterial oxygen desaturation and silent myocardial ischemia in patients presenting for vascular surgery. J Am Geriatr Soc. 1993; 41:703–709.
139. Thompson DR, Pohl JE, Sutton TW. Circadian variation in the frequency of onset of chest pain in elderly patients with acute myocardial infarction. Age Ageing. 1992;21:99–102.
140. Aronow WS, Ahn C. Circadian variation of primary cardiac arrest or sudden cardiac death in patients aged 62 to 100 years (mean 82). Am J Cardiol. 1993;71:1455–1456.
141. Parati G, Frattola A, Di Rienzo M, et al. Effects of aging on 24-h dynamic baroreceptor control of heart rate in ambulant subjects. Am J Physiol. 1995;268:H1606–1612.
142. Yamasaki Y, Kodama M, Matsuhisa M, et al. Diurnal heart rate variability in healthy subjects: effects of aging and sex difference. Am J Physiol. 1996;271:H303–310.
143. Hanly P, Sasson Z, Zuberi N, et al. ST-segment depression during sleep in obstructive sleep apnea. Am J Cardiol. 1993; 71:1341–1345.
144. Franklin KA, Nilsson JB, Sahlin C, et al. Sleep apnoea and nocturnal angina. Lancet. 1995;345:1085–1087.
145. Guilleminault C, Connolly SJ, Winkle RA. Cardiac arrhythmia and conduction disturbances during sleep in 400 patients with sleep apnea syndrome. Am J Cardiol. 1983;52:490–494.
146. Koehler U, Dübler H, Glaremin T, et al. Nocturnal myocardial ischemia and cardiac arrhythmias in patients with sleep apnea with and without coronary heart disease. Klin Wochenschr. 1991;69:474–482.
147. Flemons WW, Remmers JE, Gillis AM. Sleep apnea and cardiac arrhythmias. Is there a relationship? Am Rev Respir Dis. 1993; 148:618–621.
148. Findley LF, Boykin M, Fallon T, et al. Plasma adenosine and hypoxemia in patients with sleep apnea. J Appl Physiol. 1988; 64:556–561.
149. Leroy M, Van Surell C, Pilliere R, et al. Short-term variability of blood pressure during sleep in snorers with or without apnea. Hypertension. 1996;28:937–943.
150. Hung J, Whitford EG, Parsons RW, et al. Association of sleep apnoea with myocardial infarction in men. Lancet. 1990; 336:261–264.
151. Chin K, Ohi M, Kita H, et al. Effects of NCPAP therapy on fibrinogen levels in obstructive sleep apnea syndrome. Am J Respir Crit Care Med. 1996;153:1972–1976.
151a. Eisensehr I, Ehrenberg BL, Noachtar S, et al. Platelet activation, epinephrine, and blood pressure in obstructive sleep apnea syndrome. Neurology. 1998;51:188–195.
152. He J, Kryger MH, Zorick FJ, et al. Mortality and apnea index in obstructive sleep apnea. Experience in 385 male patients. Chest. 1988;94:9–14.
153. Partinen M, Jamieson A, Guilleminault C. Long-term outcome for obstructive sleep-apnea syndrome patients: mortality. Chest. 1988;94:1200–1204.
154. Thorpy MJ, Ledereich PS, Burack B. Death in patients with obstructive sleep apnea. Sleep Res. 1990;19:301.
155. Holford FD, Mithoefer JC. Cardiac arrhythmias in hospitalized patients with chronic obstructive pulmonary disease. Am Rev Respir Dis. 1973;108:879–885.
156. Waller PC, Bhopal RS. Is snoring a cause of vascular disease? Lancet. 1989;1:143–146.
157. Jarvik ME. Beneficial effects of nicotine. Br J Addict. 1991; 86:571–575.
158. Bjornstad H, Storstein L, Meen HD, et al. Ambulatory electrocardiographic findings in top athletes, athletic students and control subjects. Cardiology. 1994;94:42–50.
159. Bortkiewicz A, Palczynski C, Makowiec-Dabrowska T, et al. Cardiac arrhythmia in women performing heavy physical work. Int J Occup Med Environ Health. 1995;9:23–31.
160. Guilleminault CP, Pool P, Motta J, et al. Sinus arrest during REM sleep in young adults. N Engl J Med. 1984;311:1006–1010.
161. Schwartz PJ, Priori SG, Locati EH, et al. Long QT syndrome patients with mutations of the SCN5A and HERG genes have differential responses to Na+ channel blockade and to increases in heart rate. Implications for gene-specific therapy. Circulation. 1995;92:3381–3386.
162. Molnar J, Zhang F, Weiss J, et al. Diurnal pattern of QTC interval: how long is prolonged? Possible relation to circadian triggers of cardiovascular events. J Am Coll Cardiol. 1996; 27:76–83.
163. Sudden infant death syndrome—United States, 1983–1994. MMWR. 1996;45:859–863.
164. Schwartz PJ, Southall DP, Valdes-Dapena M, eds. The sudden infant death syndrome: cardiac and respiratory mechanisms and interventions. Ann N Y Acad Sci. 1988:533.
165. Haglund B, Cnattingius S, Otterblad-Olausson P. Sudden infant death syndrome in Sweden, 1983–1990: Season at death, age at death, and maternal smoking. Am J Epidemiol. 1995;142:619–624.
166. Douglas AS, Allan TM, Helms PJ. Seasonality and the sudden infant death syndrome during 1987–9 and 1991–3 in Australia and Britain. Br Med J. 1996;312:1381–1383.
167. Gupta R, Helms PJ, Jolliffe IT, et al. Seasonal variation in sudden infant death syndrome and bronchiolitis—a common mechanism? Am J Respir Crit Care Med. 1996;154:431–435.
168. Dwyer T, Ponsonby AL, Blizzard L, et al. The contribution of changes in the prevalence of prone sleeping position to the decline in sudden infant death syndrome in Tasmania. JAMA. 1995;273:783–789.
169. Klonoff-Cohen HS, Edelstein SL. A case-control study of routine and death scene sleep position and sudden infant death syndrome in Southern California. JAMA. 1995;273:790–794.
170. Klonoff-Cohen HS, Edelstein SL, Lefkowitz ES, et al. The effect of passive smoking and tobacco exposure through breast milk on sudden infant death syndrome. JAMA. 1995;273:795–798.
171. Fleming PJ, Blair PS, Bacon C, et al. Environment of infants during sleep and risk of the sudden infant death syndrome: results of 1993–1995 case-control study for confidential inquiry into stillbirths and deaths in infancy. Confidential Enquiry into Stillbirths and Deaths Regional Coordinators and Researchers. Br Med J. 1996;313:191–195.
172. Brooke H, Gibson A, Tappin D, et al. Case-control study of sudden infant death syndrome in Scotland, 1992–5. Br Med J. 1997;314:1516–1520.
173. Oyen N, Skjaerven R, Irgens LM. Population-based recurrence risk of sudden infant death syndrome compared with other infant and fetal deaths. Am J Epidemiol. 1996;144:300–305.
174. Tishler PV, Redline S, Ferrette V, et al. The association of sudden unexpected infant death with obstructive sleep apnea. Am J Respir Crit Care Med. 1996;153:1857–1863.
175. Kinney HC, Filiano JJ, Sleeper LA, et al. Decreased muscarinic receptor binding in the arcuate nucleus in sudden infant death syndrome. Science. 1995;269:1446–1450.
176. Meny RF, Carroll JL, Carbone MT, et al. Cardiorespiratory recordings from infants dying suddenly and unexpectedly at home. Pediatrics. 1994;93:43–49.
177. Harper RM, Bandler R. Finding the failure mechanism in sudden infant death syndrome [news]. Nature Med. 1998;4:157–158.
178. Schechtman VL, Harper RK, Harper RM. Aberrant temporal patterning of slow-wave sleep in siblings of SIDS victims. Electroencephalogr Clin Neurophysiol. 1995;94:95–102.
179. Pincus SM, Cummins TR, Haddad GG. Heart rate control in normal and aborted-SIDS infants. Am J Physiol. 1993;264:R638–646.
180. Schwartz PJ, Stramba-Badiale M, Segantini A, et al. Prolongation of the QT interval and the sudden infant death syndrome. N Engl J Med. 1998;338:1709–1714.
181. Smith TA, Mason JM, Bell JS, et al. Sleep apnea and QT interval prolongation—a particularly lethal combination. Am Heart J. 1979;97:505–507.
182. Blair PS, Fleming PJ, Bensley D, et al. Smoking and the sudden infant death syndrome: results from 1993–5 case-control study for confidential inquiry into stillbirths and deaths in infancy. Confidential Enquiry into Stillbirths and Deaths Regional Coordinators and Researchers. Br Med J. 1996;313:195–198.
183. MacDorman MF, Cnattingius S, Hoffman HJ, et al. Sudden infant death syndrome and smoking in the United States and Sweden. Am J Epidemiol. 1997;146:249–257.

184. Schellscheidt J, Oyen N, Jorch G. Interactions between maternal smoking and other prenatal risk factors for sudden infant death syndrome (SIDS). Acta Paediatr. 1997;96:857–863.

185. Wingkun JG, Knisely JS, Schnoll SH, et al. Decreased carbon dioxide sensitivity in infants of substance-abusing mothers. Pediatrics. 1995;95:864–867.

186. Holgert H, Hokfelt T, Hertzberg T, et al. Functional and developmental studies of the peripheral arterial chemoreceptors in rat: effects of nicotine and possible relation to sudden infant death syndrome. Proc Natl Acad Sci U S A. 1995;92:7575–7579.

187. Slotkin TA, Lappi SE, McCook EC, et al. Loss of neonatal hypoxia tolerance after prenatal nicotine exposure: implications for sudden infant death syndrome. Brain Res Bull. 1995;38:69–75.

188. Cutz E, Ma TK, Perrin DG, et al. Peripheral chemoreceptors in congenital central hypoventilation syndrome. Am J Respir Crit Care Med. 1997;155:358–363.

189. Milerad J, Majs J, Gidlund E. Nicotine and cotinine levels in pericardial fluid in victims of SIDS. Acta Pediatr 1994;93:59–62.

190. Rajs J, Rasten-Almqvist P, Falck G, et al. Sudden infant death syndrome: postmortem findings of nicotine and cotinine in pericardial fluid of infants in relation to morphological changes and position at death. Pediatr Pathol Lab Med. 1997;17:83–97.

191. Evans RG, Ludbrook J, Michalicek J. Use of nicotine, bradykinin and veratridine to elicit cardiovascular chemoreflexes in unanesthetized rabbits. Clin Exp Pharmacol Physiol. 1991;18:245–254.

192. Staszewska-Barczak J. Prostanoids and cardiac reflexes of sympathetic and vagal origin. Am J Cardiol. 1983;52:36A–45A.

193. Barber MJ, Mueller TM, Davies BG, et al. Phenol topically applied to canine left ventricular epicardium interrupts sympathetic but not vagal afferents. Circ Res. 1984;55:532–544.

194. Kirschner RH, Eckner FA, Baron RC. The cardiac pathology of sudden, unexplained nocturnal death in Southeast Asian refugees. JAMA. 1986;256:2700–2705.

195. Goh KT, Chao TC, Heng BH, et al. Epidemiology of sudden unexpected death syndrome among Thai migrant workers in Singapore. Int J Epidemiol. 1993;22:88–95.

196. Otto CM, Tauxe RV, Cobb LA, et al. Ventricular fibrillation causes sudden death in Southeast Asian immigrants. Ann Intern Med. 1984;101:45–47.

197. Pollanen MS, Chiasson DA, Cairns J, et al. Sudden unexplained death in Asian immigrants: recognition of a syndrome in metropolitan Toronto. Can Med Assoc J. 1996;155:537–540.

198. Munger RG. Sudden death in sleep of Laotian-Hmong refugees in Thailand: a case-control study. Am J Public Health. 1987;77:1187–1190.

199. Viskin S, Belhassen B. Polymorphic ventricular tachyarrhythmias in the absence of organic heart disease: classification, differential diagnosis, and implications for therapy. Prog Cardiovasc Dis. 1998;41:17–34.

200. Tada H, Aihara N, Ohe T, et al. Arrhythmogenic right ventricular cardiomyopathy underlies syndrome of right bundle branch block, ST-segment elevation, and sudden death. Am J Cardiol. 1998;91:519–522.

201. Gabathuler J, Adamec R. Triggering of paroxysmal auricular fibrillation. Study using continuous electrocardiographic recording (Holter system) [in French]. Arch Mal Coeur Vaiss. 1985;78:1255–1262.

202. Rostagno C, Taddei T, Paladini B, et al. The onset of symptomatic atrial fibrillation and paroxysmal supraventricular tachycardia is characterized by different circadian rhythms. Am J Cardiol. 1993;71:453–455.

203. Yamashita T, Murakawa Y, Sezaki K, et al. Circadian variation of paroxysmal atrial fibrillation. Circulation. 1997;96:1537–1541.

204. Kannel WB, Abbott RD, Savage DD, et al. Epidemiologic features of chronic atrial fibrillation: the Framingham study. N Engl J Med. 1982;306:1018–1022.

205. Josephson ME. Atrial flutter and fibrillation. In: Josephson ME, ed. Clinical Cardiac Electrophysiology Techniques and Interpretations. Philadelphia, Pa: Lea & Febiger; 1992:275–310.

206. Allessie M. Reentrant mechanisms underlying atrial fibrillation. In: Zipes DP, Jalife J, eds. Cardiac Electrophysiology: From Cell to Bedside. Philadelphia, Pa: WB Saunders; 1995.

207. Mooe T, Gullsby S, Rabben T, et al. Sleep-disordered breathing: a novel predictor of atrial fibrillation after coronary bypass surgery. Coron Artery Dis. 1996;7:475–478.

208. Kostis JB, Rosen RC. Central nervous system effects of beta-adrenergic blocking drugs: the role of ancillary properties. Circulation. 1987;75:204–212.

209. Kumar KL, Hodges M. Disturbing dreams with long-acting verapamil [letter]. N Engl J Med. 1988;318:929–930.

209a. Bucknall CA, Keeton BR, Curry PV, et al. Intravenous and oral amiodarone for arrhythmias in children. Br Heart J. 1986;56:278–284.

209b. Landolina M, Peccoz PB, Piscitelli G, et al. Side effects during therapy with low dosage amiodarone. G Ital Cardiol. 1984;14:723–726.

210. Walle PO, Westergren G, Dimenas E, et al. Effects of 100 mg of controlled-release metoprolol and 100 mg of atenolol on blood pressure, central nervous system-related symptoms, and general well being. J Clin Pharmacol. 1994;34:742–747.

211. Garrick NA, Tamarkin L, Taylor PL, et al. Light and propranolol suppress the nocturnal elevation of serotonin in the cerebrospinal fluid of rhesus monkeys. Science. 1983;221:474–476.

211a. LaRovere MT, Bigger JT Jr, Marcus FI, et al. Baroreflex sensitivity and heart-rate variability in prediction of total cardiac mortality after myocardial infarction. ATRAMI (Autonomic Tone and Reflexes After Myocardial Infarction) Investigators. Lancet. 351:478–484, 1998.

211b. Chakko S, Mulingtapang RF, Huikuri HV, et al. Alterations in heart rate variability and its circadian rhythm in hypertensive patients with left ventricular hypertrophy free of coronary artery disease. Am Heart J. 1993;126:1364–1372.

212. Ferini-Strambi L, Rovaris M, Oldani A, et al. Cardiac autonomic function during sleep and wakefulness in multiple sclerosis. J Neurol. 1995;242:639–643.

213. Ferri C, Emdin M, Giuggioli D, et al. Autonomic dysfunction in systemic sclerosis: time and frequency domain 24 hour heart rate variability analysis. Br J Rheumatol. 1997;36:669–676.

214. Yotsukura M, Sasaki K, Kachi E, et al. Circadian rhythm and variability of heart rate in Duchenne-type progressive muscular dystrophy. Am J Cardiol. 1995;76:947–951.

215. Ferini-Strambi L, Smirne S. Cardiac autonomic function during sleep in several neuropsychiatric disorders. Neurology. 1997;244:S29–S36.

85

Cardiac Arrhythmias

Anne M. Gillis

Changes in the balance of parasympathetic tone and sympathetic tone associated with different sleep states may contribute to differences in the frequency of arrhythmias observed between sleep states and between sleep and wakefulness.[1, 2] Some investigators have suggested that the profound changes in autonomic tone that occur during sleep states, particularly during rapid eye movement (REM) sleep, or during the transitions between sleep states in patients with underlying structural heart disease, may increase their risk for life-threatening ventricular arrhythmias.[2-4] Other investigators have suggested that cardiac arrhythmias during sleep may be an important cause of death in patients with obstructive sleep apnea (OSA)[5, 6] as well as in infants experiencing the sudden infant death syndrome (SIDS).[7-9] The focus of this chapter is on the mechanisms that contribute to the genesis or suppression of cardiac arrhythmias during sleep as well as on the clinical relevance of various arrhythmias that may be observed during sleep.

MECHANISMS OF ARRHYTHMOGENESIS

Spontaneous depolarizations normally arise in the sinus node and are conducted by way of the specialized conduction system to the endocardial Purkinje network and myocardium. Sinus impulses are normally conducted through specialized atrial conduction tracts to the atrioventricular (AV) node. Impulses then travel along the bundle of His, which bifurcates into a right and left bundle, to the Purkinje network on the endocardium. Both the sinus node and the AV node are richly innervated and hence both heart rate and conduction through the AV node are modulated by changes in autonomic tone.[10]

Arrhythmias may arise owing to abnormalities of impulse formation or impulse propagation (Table 85–1). Abnormalities of impulse formation include abnormal automaticity and triggered automaticity. Reentry involves abnormalities of impulse propagation.

Sympathetic activation may initiate arrhythmias by direct effects on cardiac electrophysiology or indirectly by effects on heart rate, blood pressure, and coronary blood flow.[1, 7, 11, 12] Increased circulating catecholamines or release of norepinephrine at nerve terminals activates alpha- and beta-adrenergic receptors, which increase intracellular cyclic adenosine monophosphate and calcium.[12] Under certain conditions, these effects may result in the development of delayed afterdepolarizations and trigger arrhythmias[13] or increase spatial heterogeneity of the electrophysiological effects, resulting in increased dispersion of repolarization and increased risk for arrhythmogenesis.[14] In normal animals, stimulation of sympathetic fibers shortens the ventricular effective refractory period and lowers the ventricular fibrillation (VF) threshold.[7, 11, 12, 15] In the setting of myocardial ischemia, sympathetic stimulation induces VF.[7, 15, 16] These effects are attenuated by beta-adrenoceptor blocking agents or stellate ganglionectomy.[2, 7, 11, 12] The antiarrhythmic effect of beta-adrenergic receptor blockers may be in part due to central adrenergic receptor blockade.[2, 17]

Table 85–1. MECHANISMS OF CARDIAC ARRHYTHMIAS

Mechanism	Description
Abnormal automaticity	Spontaneous depolarization occurs in partially depolarized cells. May be mechanism of some atrial tachycardias and accelerated junctional rhythms.
Triggered automaticity	Impulse formation occurs as a result of oscillations of the membrane potential termed *afterdepolarizations*. Afterdepolarizations are classified as early when they interrupt or delay normal repolarization. Early afterdepolarizations are believed to be the mechanism of torsades de pointes ventricular tachycardia. Delayed afterdepolarizations follow complete repolarization of the action potential. Catecholamines increase the amplitude of afterdepolarizations. Delayed afterdepolarizations are believed to be the mechanism of some digitalis-induced tachycardias.
Reentry	Requires a circuit, unidirectional block, and sufficiently slow conduction such that the transit time around the circuit exceeds the longest effective refractory period of participating cells. The autonomic nervous system may modulate reentry by modulating the effective refractory period in the circuit. This is the mechanism of atrial flutter and supraventricular tachycardia in the Wolff-Parkinson-White syndrome. This is believed to be the mechanism of most sustained ventricular tachycardias following a myocardial infarction.

Parasympathetic activation may inhibit the genesis of arrhythmias by direct effects on cardiac electrophysiology or indirectly by effects on heart rate or inhibition of excitatory sympathetic reflexes.[2, 7, 11, 12] Vagus nerve stimulation slows the heart rate, prolongs the ventricular effective refractory period, and increases the VF threshold in normal and ischemic myocardium.[2, 7, 11, 12, 16, 18] The effects of vagal stimuli on cardiac electrophysiology are dependent on the level of cardiac sympathetic tone and are most marked under conditions of increased sympathetic activity.[11, 16] These effects are likely mediated through muscarinic receptors because they are blocked by atropine. Thus, the balance of sympathetic-parasympathetic tone significantly modulates cardiac arrhythmias.

AUTONOMIC INFLUENCES ON ELECTROPHYSIOLOGICAL PARAMETERS DURING SLEEP

Sleep is characterized by a dominance of parasympathetic tone and a decrease in sympathetic activity.[19–21] The decrease in heart rate observed during sleep is secondary to increased parasympathetic activity, although a reduction in sympathetic tone also appears to be important because a further reduction in heart rate is observed during sleep in vagotomized cats.[19] The tonic and phasic heart rate changes are completely eliminated only by combined vagotomy and bilateral stellectomy. The reduction in heart rate observed during REM sleep is due primarily to predominance of parasympathetic tone, whereas the striking increase in heart rate that heralds the burst of REM is mainly caused by a phasic inhibition of parasympathetic activity.[19, 21] The bradycardia following a REM burst is due to a phasic reduction in sympathetic activity, as well as an increase in parasympathetic activity.

In normal human subjects, the decrease in heart rate and blood pressure observed in nonrapid eye movement (NREM) sleep is associated with a reduction in peripheral sympathetic nerve activity as measured by direct microneurographic recordings, whereas increases in heart rate and blood pressure are observed during REM sleep and correlate with marked increases in sympathetic activity compared to wakefulness[22] (Fig. 85–1). Although these studies were conducted in normal subjects, it can be hypothesized that REM sleep is a period of potential cardiovascular risk, particularly in patients with coronary or cerebrovascular disease.[5, 23]

Power spectral analysis of the heart rate has been performed by a number of investigators to assess the control of heart rate during sleep in normal volunteers and in patients with ischemic heart disease.[21, 24–30] Decreases in the low- to high-power frequency ratio during NREM sleep are consistent with the dominance of parasympathetic tone during NREM sleep, and increases in this ratio during REM sleep are consistent with the dominance of sympathetic tone. Reduced heart rate variability associated with ischemic heart disease may be a marker of risk of sudden cardiac death.[31] An increase in the low- to high-power fre-

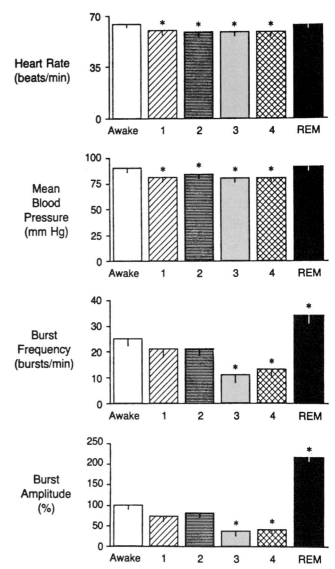

Figure 85–1. Heart rate, mean blood pressure, sympathetic burst frequency, and burst amplitude during wakefulness and NREM sleep (eight subjects) and REM sleep (six subjects). Heart rate and blood pressure were significantly lower during all phases of NREM sleep compared to wakefulness or REM sleep (*$P < .001$). Sympathetic activity was lower during stages 3 and 4, whereas during REM sleep sympathetic activity increased significantly (*$P < .001$). Values are mean ± SEM. (From Somers VK, Dyken ME, Mark AL, et al. Sympathetic-nerve activity during sleep in normal subjects. N Engl J Med. 1993;328:303–307. Copyright © 1993 Massachusetts Medical Society. All rights reserved.)

quency ratio has been reported during NREM sleep compared with wakefulness, and a further increase has been observed during REM sleep in patients following a myocardial infarction[28] (Fig. 85–2). A loss of the circadian variation of heart period variability has been reported in patients with heart disease, particularly those at risk of ventricular tachycardia.[30] Thus, myocardial infarction or other forms of heart disease may reduce or eliminate vagal dominance during sleep. This may alter the risk for cardiac arrhythmias and predispose to increased risk at night.[31, 32]

The ventricular effective refractory period has also

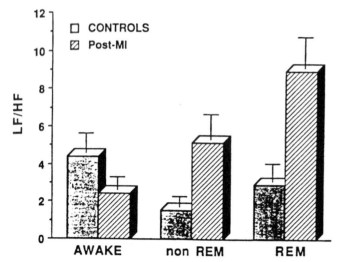

Figure 85–2. Bar graph indicating mean ± SEM of the low- to high-frequency ratio (LF/HF) from spectral analysis of the heart rate during the awake state *(left)*, nonREM sleep *(middle)*, and REM sleep *(right)* in normal subjects and in postmyocardial infarction (Post-MI) patients. (*P < .01 comparing normal subjects to post-MI patients). (From Vanoli E, Adamson PB, Ba-Lin, et al. Heart rate variability during specific sleep stages. A comparison of healthy subjects with patients after myocardial infarction. Circulation. 1995;91[7]:1918.)

been observed to be prolonged during both REM and slow-wave sleep in chronically instrumented cats.[7] The prolongation of the ventricular effective refractory period is similar in REM and NREM sleep. This prolongation is abolished following administration of muscarinic blocking agents but not prevented by bilateral stellectomy, suggesting that these changes are mediated by variation in cardiac vagal tone. However, in human beings, the prolongation of the ventricular effective refractory period observed during sleep is abolished by beta-adrenergic receptor blockers, suggesting that withdrawal of sympathetic tone or modulation of sympathetic tone by vagal innervation determines these effects[33] (Fig. 85–3). Shorter refractory periods promote reentry by reducing the wavelength or the total mass of tissue required for maintenance of the reentrant circuit. Thus, the longer refractory periods observed during sleep likely account for the lower incidence of arrhythmias and sudden death reported during sleep.

In human beings, circadian variations of a number of cardiac electrophysiological variables have been observed.[33–36] Prolongation of the atrial effective refractory period, the AV nodal effective refractory period, the right ventricular effective refractory period, and the QT interval of the surface electrocardiogram (EKG) were observed during the evening and early morning in 12 patients undergoing serial bedside electrophysiological testing.[34] In association with the prolongation of refractoriness in atrial, AV nodal, ventricular, and accessory pathway tissue, a decrease in the inducibility of reciprocating tachycardia has also been observed in patients with the Wolff-Parkinson-White syndrome.[36]

The QT interval, a surface EKG measure of ventricular repolarization, is prolonged during sleep, and this prolongation is independent of changes in heart rate.[37] We have previously reported that QT interval prolongation during sleep is predominantly due to inactivity and presumed withdrawal of sympathetic tone.[38] Consistent with this conclusion, other investigators correlating QT interval changes with power spectral analysis concluded that enhanced sympathetic activity during the day was a major determinant of the diurnal variation in the QT interval.[39] We have not observed differences in QT interval prolongation comparing REM and NREM sleep.[38] The expected circadian variation of the QT interval, with shortening on arousal, is blunted in heart transplant recipients and is absent in patients with diabetic autonomic neuropathy.[40] The slight decrease in the QT interval observed in the morning in patients with denervated hearts is probably secondary to increased concentrations of circulating catecholamines associated with assumption of the upright posture. The circadian variation of the QT interval corrected for heart rate is also blunted by beta-adrenergic receptor blockers and amiodarone.[41] The greatest variability between hourly minimal and maximal QT interval corrected for heart rate has been observed within the first hour after awakening.[42] Because increased dispersion of repolarization is a risk factor for sudden cardiac death, this time might be a particularly vulnerable period for arrhythmogenesis.[43–45]

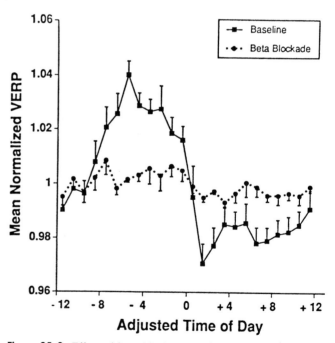

Figure 85–3. Effect of beta blockade on the circadian variation in ventricular effective refractory periods (VERP). Mean hourly VERPs at baseline and during beta blockade adjusted according to the hour of waking (waking hour = 0 h) measured at a pacing cycle length of 400 ms (150 bpm). VERPs for each subject were normalized to the subject's 24-h mean value to correct for intersubject variability in the absolute measures of VERP. The circadian variation of VERP and the marked shortening of VERP around the hour of awakening are abolished by beta blockade. Data are paired. (From Kong TQ Jr, Goldberger JJ, Parker M, et al. Circadian variation in human ventricular refractoriness. Circulation. 1995;92[6]:1507.)

In summary, increased parasympathetic activity during sleep significantly influences cardiac electrophysiology, causing marked slowing of the heart rate, slowing of conduction in AV nodal tissue, and prolongation of cardiac refractory periods. Such effects would be expected to suppress arrhythmogenesis. The beneficial effects of sleep on cardiac electrical stability are supported by the low incidence of sudden cardiac death during sleep[46] and the decreased probability of inducing supraventricular tachycardia in patients with the Wolff-Parkinson-White syndrome.[36]

HEART RATE AND RHYTHM DURING SLEEP IN NORMAL SUBJECTS

The most frequently observed changes in the heart rhythm observed during sleep are sinus bradycardia and sinus arrhythmia. The diurnal variation of heart rate has been studied in healthy populations of varying ages.[47–50] The mean heart rates and minimal heart rates recorded during wakefulness and sleep in young adults between 22 and 28 years of age are shown in Table 85–2.[47, 48] Males have slower heart rates during sleep than females, and this difference persists in older subjects, although the magnitude of the difference in heart rates between day and night decreases with age.[49, 50] The higher heart rates observed during sleep in the elderly suggests less dominance of parasympathetic tone during sleep compared with younger subjects. Sinus pauses have been documented predominantly at night in 30% of healthy subjects ranging in age from 40 to 79 years.[50] However, sinus pauses greater than 2-sec duration are rare in subjects with a normal EKG. In contrast, marked sinus bradycardia and sinus pauses are frequently observed during sleep in highly trained athletes.[51, 52] These differences are presumed to be secondary to increased vagal tone in athletes.

Sleep state does significantly modulate some atrial arrhythmias. We have observed abnormal periods of sinus arrest up to 9 sec in duration during REM sleep in young adults without structural heart disease[53] (Fig. 85–4). We hypothesized that this arrhythmia was due to enhanced vagal activity during REM sleep. This theory is supported in part by the partial response to atropine documented in these subjects. The incidence of such profound asystole during REM sleep is suspected to be low. It must be emphasized that the isolated finding of sinus arrest during sleep in the absence of symptoms does not warrant therapeutic intervention.

Sinus arrest and AV block have also been observed predominantly during REM sleep in some experimental animals.[54] The majority of episodes follow REM bursts, and the incidence of episodes increases with increasing duration of REM sleep. These bradyarrhythmias tend to disappear following vagotomy. Other investigators have also observed pauses 1 to 8 sec in duration during transitions from slow-wave sleep to sleep characterized by desynchronized electroencephalographic (EEG) rhythms in chronically instrumented dogs.[55]

ATRIOVENTRICULAR BLOCK DURING SLEEP

First-degree and Wenckebach AV block frequently occur in normal subjects during sleep[49–52, 56–58] and are believed to be secondary to the effects of increased parasympathetic activity on AV node conduction during sleep. There does not appear to be a consistent relationship between sleep stage and these conduction disturbances. Viitasalo et al.[59] reported that short-term heart rate accelerations preceded the majority of episodes of second-degree AV block that developed during sleep in healthy men, leading these investigators to hypothesize that rapid autonomic changes during sleep rather than centrally mediated cortical arousals initiated these events. A circadian variation of heart rate response in patients with chronic atrial fibrillation (AF) has been reported with slowest ventricular rates observed in the nocturnal hours and the most rapid ventricular rates observed during the daytime.[60] These

Table 85–2. HEART RATES AND SINUS PAUSES IN 50 NORMAL YOUNG MEN AND WOMEN

	Men		Women	
	Mean ± SD	Range	Mean ± SD	Range
Wake period				
Average heart rate (bpm)	80 ± 7.0	67–90	90 ± 11	65–120
Minimum heart rate (bpm)	53 ± 6.0	37–65	56 ± 7.0	40–70
Longest sinus pause (sec)	1.36 ± 0.16	1.00–1.68	1.23 ± 0.15	0.88–1.64
Sleep period				
Average heart rate (bpm)	56 ± 6.0	45–70	66 ± 9.0	47–84
Minimum heart rate (bpm)	43 ± 5.0	33–55	48 ± 6.0	37–59
Longest sinus pause (sec)	1.62 ± 0.20	1.20–2.06	1.47 ± 0.20	1.08–1.92

Data from Brodsky M, Wu D, Denes P, et al. Arrhythmias documented by 24-hour continuous electrocardiographic monitoring in 50 male medical students without apparent heart disease. Am J Cardiol. 1977;39:390–395; and Sobotka PA, Mayer JH, Bauernfeind RA, et al. Arrhythmias documented by 24-hour continuous ambulatory electrocardiographic monitoring in young women without apparent heart disease. Am Heart J. 1981;101:753–759.

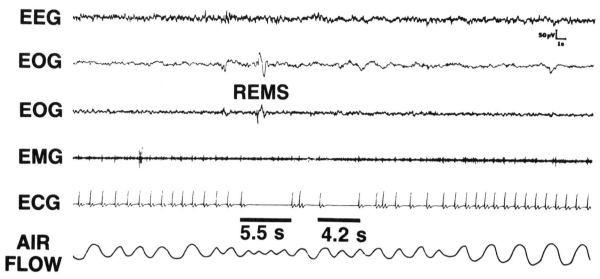

EEG

EOG

REMS

EOG

EMG

ECG

AIR FLOW

5.5 s   4.2 s

Figure 85–4. Polygraphic recording during REM sleep (REMS). Sinus arrest occurs in this patient in association with a burst of REM. ECG, electrocardiogram; EEG, electroencephalogram; EMG, electromyogram; EOG, electro-oculogram. (From Guilleminault C, Pool P, Motta J, et al. Sinus arrest during REM sleep in young adults. N Engl J Med. 1984;311:1006–1010. Copyright © 1984 Massachusetts Medical Society. All rights reserved.)

variations in heart rate response likely reflect modulation of AV node refractoriness by the autonomic nervous system (ANS).

SUPRAVENTRICULAR TACHYCARDIAS DURING SLEEP

A circadian variation of the onset of sustained supraventricular tachycardia has been described with the time of peak incidence occurring at 4 PM and the time of lowest incidence occurring at 4 AM.[61] Other investigators have reported a bimodal distribution of the time of onset of supraventricular tachycardia, with peaks occurring in the morning (6 AM to 12 PM) and evening (6 PM to 12 AM).[62] This bimodal time of onset was most characteristic for AF, whereas other supraventricular tachyarrhythmias tended not to have a distinct evening peak. Kupari et al.[62] also observed an absence of the morning peak in onset of supraventricular tachycardia in patients taking beta-adrenoceptor blocking agents. Fluctuations in autonomic tone contributing to the circadian variation of atrial and AV node refractory periods may explain the variation in the timing of onset of supraventricular tachycardia.[34–36, 63] The mechanism of the evening peak in the incidence of some supraventricular tachyarrhythmias is not known. Certainly factors such as shift work and evening recreational activities must be considered. Another possible explanation is that the mechanism of initiation of supraventricular tachycardia in the evening is different (i.e., vagally induced). This phenomenon has been described for AF and flutter, which have been observed to begin during sleep or at rest in some people.[64, 65]

ATRIAL FIBRILLATION DURING SLEEP

Vagal stimulation may cause significant bradycardia, which may predispose to some arrhythmias, for example, vagally mediated AF that has been described to occur during sleep.[64, 65] The mechanism of this arrhythmia is believed to be bradycardia-dependent increased dispersion of atrial repolarization, which predisposes to intra-atrial reentry.[14] Cardiac pacing at rates above those that trigger AF has been reported to be antiarrhythmic in some patients.[65, 66] A circadian periodicity of the onset of AF has been described with some investigators reporting peaks in the morning and early evening[62] and others reporting increases after lunch and at midnight. Yamashita et al.[67] also observed a circadian variation in the maintenance and termination of AF episodes with episodes tending to be shorter in duration if they were initiated in the morning (Fig. 85–5). Although this pattern appears surprising, it is possible that increased vagal tone at night facilitates the maintenance of AF.

VENTRICULAR ARRHYTHMIAS DURING SLEEP

The influence of sleep on ventricular arrhythmias and sudden cardiac death has attracted considerable attention. A number of investigators have studied the relationship between sleep and ventricular arrhythmias, but the results have been inconsistent. Some investigators have observed a decrease in ventricular arrhythmias during sleep,[68–71] whereas others have reported no change in ventricular arrhythmia frequency during sleep.[71–74] Rosenberg et al.[75] identified a small group of patients who had more ventricular premature depolarizations (VPDs) at night than during the daytime. A number of factors may explain these apparent inconsistencies. These include heterogeneous populations; small numbers of experimental subjects; the effects of medications, including beta-adrenoceptor blocking agents; and the use of ambulatory vs. sedentary patients in different studies.

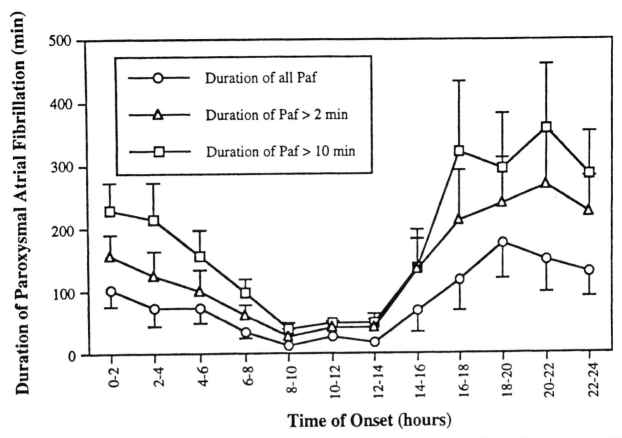

Figure 85–5. Differences in the duration of paroxysmal atrial fibrillation (Paf) depending on the time of onset. Data are mean ± SEM. ○, duration of all episodes; △, duration of episodes lasting longer than 2 min; □, duration of episodes lasting longer than 10 min. (From Yamashita T, Murakawa Y, Sezaki K, et al. Circadian variation of paroxysmal atrial fibrillation. Circulation. 1997;96[5]:1537–1541.)

The circadian variation of VPDs is generally characterized by an abrupt increase in VPD frequency, which peaks between 6 and 11 AM.[69, 71] The mechanism of this morning increase in arrhythmias is not well understood. However, neurohumoral mechanisms associated with assumption of the upright posture may be involved.[76] A circadian variation in VPDs is not present in all subjects with frequent VPDs. The observation that beta-adrenoceptor blocking agents eliminate the morning increase in VPD frequency and sudden cardiac death further supports the hypothesis that altered sympathetic tone throughout the day contributes to the circadian variation of ventricular arrhythmias.[71, 77–81] We have observed a suppression of the expected circadian variation of ventricular arrhythmias in patients with severe left ventricular dysfunction[71] (Fig. 85–6). Persistent increased sympathetic tone, loss of vagal activity, hypoxia, or increased circulating catecholamines during the night secondary to congestive heart failure may be important factors contributing to the loss of this circadian rhythm in these patients. Changes in autonomic tone during sleep that are characterized by changes in heart rate variability have been observed in some patients with ischemic heart disease.[28–30]

Ventricular tachycardia (VT) and VF are the most common causes of sudden cardiac death. A circadian variation of sudden cardiac death,[46, 81–88] VT, and VF[78, 89–94] with a peak in the morning following arousal have also been described. The circadian variation of sudden cardiac death is shown in Figure 85–7.[46] The greatest risk of sudden cardiac death is observed in the first 3 h after awakening. Increased circulating catecholamine concentrations associated with arousal may contribute to the morning increase in sudden cardiac death. A circadian variation in defibrillation thresholds has also been reported with a morning peak (15.1 ±1.2 J) compared with the afternoon (13.1 ± 0.9 J, $P < .05$). These differences correlate with higher failures of the first shock delivered by an implantable cardioverter defibrillator to successfully terminate an arrhythmia when it occurs in the morning. Interestingly, the circadian variation of sudden cardiac death is blunted in patients in hospital, and this change may reflect alterations in day-night or sleep-wake cycles[46] (Fig. 85–8).

Patients with severely compromised left ventricular function have been reported to demonstrate a more uniform distribution of ventricular tachyarrhythmias, which likely reflects the sympathovagal imbalance in this subgroup.[91] Beta-adrenergic receptor blocking therapy eliminates the circadian variation of sudden cardiac death and sustained VT, supporting the hypothesis that the morning surge in sudden death is related to increased sympathetic tone associated with arousal and increased activity.[81, 88, 95–97] Other investigators have reported that antiarrhythmic therapy eliminates the circadian pattern of ventricular tachyarrhythmia recur-

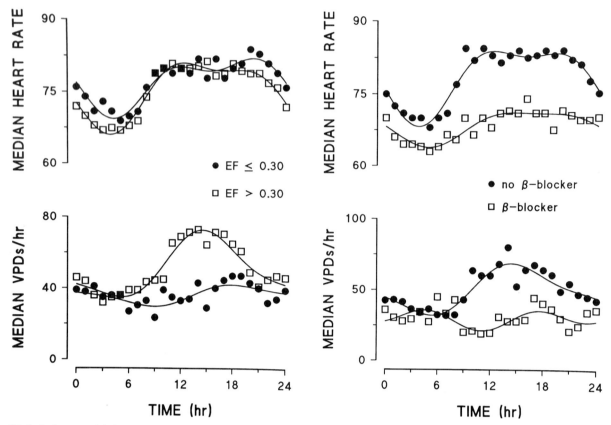

Figure 85–6. Influence of left ventricular dysfunction on circadian variation of heart rate and ventricular premature contractions (VPDs, ventricular premature depolarizations) in patients with left ventricular dysfunction following myocardial infarction. *Top left,* Hourly median heart rate for patients according to left ventricular ejection fraction (EF): EF ≤ 0.30 (black circles) and > 0.30 but ≤ 0.45 (open squares). *Lower left,* Hourly median VPD frequency for patients according to EF. Curves are fitted to a two-harmonic cosinor function. The circadian variation of VPD frequency is eliminated in patients with EF ≤ 0.30. *Right panels,* Effect of beta blockers on circadian variation of heart rate and VPDs. *Top right,* Beta blockers blunt the circadian variation of the heart rate. □, patients on beta blockers; •, patients not on beta blockers. *Lower right,* Circadian variation of VPDs is absent in patients receiving beta blocker therapy. Curves are fits of data to a two-harmonic cosinor function. (Reprinted from Gillis AM, Peters RW, Mitchell LB, et al. Effects of left ventricular dysfunction on the circadian variation of ventricular premature complexes in healed myocardial infarction. American Journal of Cardiology, vol 69, 1009–1014, Copyright 1992, with permission from Excerpta Medica Inc.)

rence.[90] Because the majority of patients studied were receiving amiodarone therapy, this effect may reflect the beta-adrenergic receptor blocking activity of amiodarone.

The electrophysiological substrate for sudden cardiac death does not seem to manifest a substantial diurnal variation. McClelland et al.[98] did not observe a significant difference in the VT induction rate between morning or afternoon electrophysiological studies, which led the investigators to conclude that a circadian variation in electrical instability could not explain the morning peak in ventricular tachyarrhythmias. These investigators did not perform studies during the night; it is possible that a nocturnal trough in tachycardia induction would have been observed, as has been reported for supraventricular tachycardias.[36] Although the electrical substrate for VT or VF may not vary throughout the day, frequent ventricular premature beats, which may trigger VT or VF, and platelet aggregability, which may trigger acute ischemia, manifest similar circadian patterns as those reported for sudden death.

Asystole and pulseless bradycardia may also cause sudden cardiac death. These latter arrhythmias tend to be more evenly distributed during the daytime, but a decrease in event frequency was still observed at nighttime.[86]

SLEEP STATE AND VENTRICULAR ARRHYTHMIAS

A number of investigators have attempted to determine whether sleep state independently influences ventricular arrhythmia frequency. In general, there is no consistent relationship between sleep state and VPD frequency. Some patients have more VPDs during the wake-sleep transition period compared with sleep transition periods (e.g., NREM–REM),[73] whereas others experience an increase in VPD frequency during REM.[70, 74] Lown et al.[100] reported a patient with recurrent VF during REM sleep in the absence of documented structural heart disease. Thus, the surge in sympathetic tone associated with REM sleep may in some instances provoke life-threatening arrhythmias.

The relationship between VPD frequency and heart rate is likely an important determinant of the diurnal

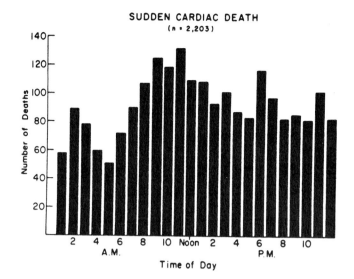

SUDDEN CARDIAC DEATH
(n = 2,203)

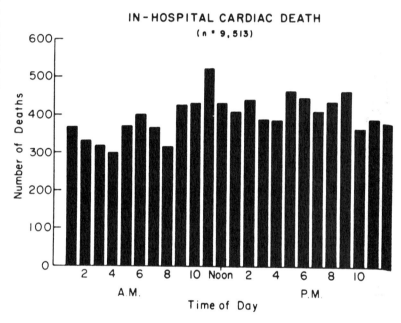

IN-HOSPITAL CARDIAC DEATH
(n = 9,513)

Figure 85–7. *Top,* Time of day of out of hospital to sudden cardiac death (<1 h from onset of symptoms to death) for 2203 persons dying in Massachusetts in 1983. A significant circadian rhythm is present ($P < .001$) with a morning peak between 7 and 11 AM and a secondary peak between 5 and 6 PM. *Bottom,* The time of day of in-hospital cardiac death for 9513 persons dying in Massachusetts in 1983. For these hospitalized patients the time of cardiac death is almost randomly distributed over the 24-h period, although there was a trend toward fewer deaths from midnight to 6 AM. (From Muller JE, Ludmer PL, Willich SN, et al. Circadian variation in the frequency of sudden cardiac death. Circulation. 1987;75[1]:131–138.)

variability of VPD frequency.[72, 101] Many of these subjects manifested an increase in VPD frequency with increasing heart rate. Flat curves, that is, no relationship between heart rate and VPD frequency or a decrease in VPD frequency with increasing heart rate, are less frequently observed. Although heart rate appears to be the major determinant of VPD variability in many patients, sleep state–dependent effects may also exist.

Although significant effects of sleep state on ventricular arrhythmia frequency have not been consistently observed in human beings, important effects of sleep state on ventricular arrhythmia frequency have been observed in pigs during acute ischemia.[102] The highest incidence of ventricular arrhythmias was observed during NREM sleep compared with the awake state and with REM sleep. Furthermore, the VF latency during transient coronary artery occlusion was shortest during NREM sleep compared with REM sleep and

the awake state. These observations are somewhat surprising because one might have predicted a higher incidence of arrhythmias during the awake state when resting sympathetic tone is predicted to be higher. However, the mechanisms of arrhythmogenesis during acute ischemia are complex and differ considerably from the mechanisms of arrhythmias that develop late following a myocardial infarction. The balance of parasympathetic-sympathetic tone may differ considerably between sleep states, and this factor may explain differences in arrhythmogenesis observed between REM and NREM sleep.[19, 21] Furthermore, the size and depth of a myocardial infarction (transmural vs. subendocardial) may be important because sympathetic fibers are located on the epicardium, whereas parasympathetic fibers are found in the endocardium.[1] These factors may account for the diverse effects of sleep on cardiac arrhythmias noted in human beings.

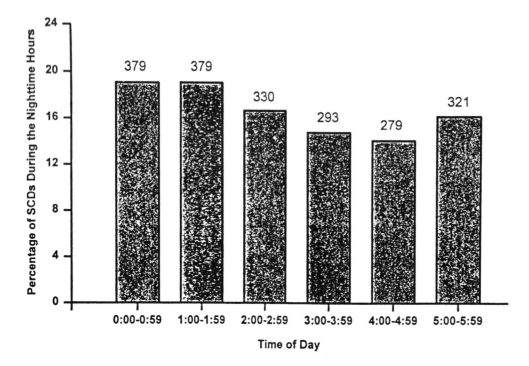

Figure 85–8. The hourly incidence of sudden cardiac death (SCD) onset from 12 studies involving 1981 patients with onset between midnight and 5:59 AM. The number above each bar indicates the number of sudden cardiac deaths observed each hour. (From Lavery CE, Mittleman MA, Cohen MC, et al. Nonuniform nighttime distribution of acute cardiac events. A possible effect of sleep states. Circulation. 1997; 96[10]:3321–3327.)

There are certain subsets of patients in whom ventricular arrhythmias are more common during sleep than wakefulness. Patients with nocturnal hypoxemia either secondary to cardiac or pulmonary disease may experience a nighttime increase in ventricular arrhythmias.[103–107] In these patients, the nocturnal increase in VPD frequency is associated with significant oxygen desaturation (SaO_2 less than 80%). Neurological abnormalities are more common in patients with an increase in VPDs during sleep compared with matched controls, suggesting that neurological or neurohumoral factors also play an important role in the mechanism of ventricular arrhythmia exacerbation by sleep.[75] In some patients, increased VPD frequency during sleep is related to the development of bradycardia. The mechanism in these cases may be enhanced automaticity or triggered automaticity arising from altered repolarization.[1, 13, 14]

As already indicated, some investigators have suggested that arousals during sleep may be associated with electrical instability.[7, 70, 73] An example of this is a case report of a 14-year-old girl who experienced repeated episodes of life-threatening ventricular tachyarrhythmias when awakened from sleep by loud auditory stimuli such as an alarm clock or music.[108] The mechanism of arrhythmogenesis appeared to be increased sympathetic activity because the episodes could be prevented by beta-adrenoceptor blocking agents. Observations such as this, coupled with reports that VPD frequency may be increased during wake-sleep transition periods,[70, 73] suggest that arousal from sleep may be a factor in the sudden cardiac death that occurs during sleep.

Nocturnal episodes of sudden cardiac death and VT exhibit nonuniform distributions[4] (see Fig. 85–8). This observation is consistent with the hypothesis that sleep state–dependent fluctuations in the ANS may trigger cardiovascular events that could precipitate arrhythmias. For instance, increased sympathetic tone during phasic REM sleep may decrease coronary artery flow in stenotic vessels, precipitating acute ischemia followed by the development of arrhythmias and sudden death.[2–4, 109]

ARRHYTHMIAS DURING OBSTRUCTIVE SLEEP APNEA

Significant bradycardia has been observed during episodes of OSA, and the degree of bradycardia correlates with the duration of apnea.[110, 111] Administration of oxygen and atropine eliminates the bradycardia, although in some cases the duration of apnea lengthens.[110] A characteristic pattern of a progressive bradycardia followed by abrupt tachycardia on resumption of breathing has been observed during apneic episodes in patients with OSA and an intact nervous system.[111] This cyclical variation of the heart rate is not observed in patients with autonomic dysfunction or in heart transplant recipients. Cyclical variation of the heart rate is a specific (95%) but not very sensitive (48%) indicator of OSA.[112]

Cardiac arrhythmias have frequently been observed during sleep in patients with OSA. Marked sinus bradycardia and sinus arrest are the arrhythmias most commonly observed.[113, 114] Guilleminault et al.[115] observed sinus arrest in 10% and second-degree AV block in 5% of 400 patients with OSA. Severe OSA, morbid obesity, REM sleep, and the severity of desaturation during apneas are independent predictors of heart block developing during apnea.[116] Oxygen reduces apnea-induced bradycardia despite an overall lengthening of the apneic period.[110] Continuous positive airway pressure (CPAP) therapy also eliminates the nocturnal episodes of sinus arrest and heart block in patients with OSA.[117] The episodes of sinus arrest and heart block occurring during OSA are likely vagally mediated because they are eliminated by atropine and electrophysiological abnormalities were not detected in patients with OSA and periods of asystole.[118] Permanent cardiac pacemakers are generally not indicated for the management of sinus arrest or heart block in patients with OSA unless the arrhythmia persists despite adequate treatment.

In patients with OSA, the prevalence of VT has been reported to range from 3 to 13% and VPDs to range from 20 to 67%.[113–115] The prevalence of ventricular arrhythmias is probably related to the severity of OSA and the severity of oxygen desaturation.[104] Guilleminault and co-workers have demonstrated that arrhythmias, including ventricular arrhythmias, resolve following tracheostomy.[114, 115]

Cardiac arrhythmias, including marked sinus bradycardia, AV block, and ventricular arrhythmias, have been documented in healthy subjects, and the incidence of these arrhythmias increases with age.[47–50] We have prospectively evaluated the prevalence of cardiac arrhythmias in 196 patients undergoing polysomnographic study and EKG monitoring for the evaluation of suspected OSA.[119] The prevalence of significant cardiac arrhythmias was low in patients with and without OSA and did not differ between the two groups (Table 85–3). The higher frequency of arrhythmias reported by previous investigators likely reflects patient populations with more severe disease.[104, 113–115, 120–122] This is consistent with the observations of Hoffstein and Mateika[107] who saw a significant increase in the prevalence of cardiac arrhythmias in patients with severe OSA. Thus, although some patients with severe OSA have arrhythmias that clearly are associated with severe apnea and oxygen desaturation, the majority of arrhythmias observed in this population are likely unrelated to the OSA syndrome.

The mechanism of ventricular arrhythmias associated with severe OSA is likely enhanced automaticity or triggered activity. Patients with OSA have evidence of autonomic dysfunction manifested by increased sympathetic tone and blunted baroreceptor function, which might increase their risk for sudden cardiac death.[123]

Death in patients with OSA is predominantly due to cardiac causes and half of deaths occur between midnight and 8 AM.[124] However, the mechanism of these deaths remains uncertain.

CONGESTIVE HEART FAILURE

Sleep in patients with severe congestive heart failure is highly fragmented, with frequent arousals and sleep changes.[125] The distribution of sleep is abnormal with an increased density of stage 1 and reduction in the density of deeper sleep stages. Respiration is also abnormal with frequent episodes of Cheyne-Stokes respirations, which may be characterized by profound hypoxia in the setting of prolonged apneas.[126, 127] Although one might predict that these pathophysiological changes would predispose to arrhythmia development, there is little information to support this. Moser et al.[128] did not observe a high incidence of arrhythmic deaths at night in patients with severe congestive heart failure.

SUDDEN INFANT DEATH SYNDROME

Sleep-induced arrhythmias may be a factor in the sudden infant death syndrome (SIDS).[7–9] It has been hypothesized that changes in ANS activity during sleep could precipitate an arrhythmia resulting in sudden death. Some potential abnormalities of autonomic

Table 85–3. PREVALENCE OF ARRHYTHMIAS IN PATIENTS WITH AND WITHOUT SLEEP APNEA

Study	Patients (N)	Sinus Arrest (%)	Second-Degree AV Block (%)	VPBs >10/h (%)	VPBs >30/h (%)	Complex VPBs (%)	VT (%)
Flemons et al.[119]							
No sleep apnea	97	1.0	4.1	8.2	6.2	4.1	2.1
(95% CI)		(0.2–5.6)	(1.6–10.1)	(4.2–15.4)	(2.9–12.8)	(1.6–10.1)	(0.5–7.2)
Sleep apnea	76	5.3	1.3	6.6	2.6	1.3	0
(95% CI)		(2.2–12.6)	(0.4–6.9)	(2.9–14.4)	(0.8–8.9)	(0.4–6.9)	(0–4.5)
Shepard et al.[104]	31	10	6	NR	0	55	3
Bolm-Audorff et al.[120]	30	NR	10	30	15*	45	15
Boudoulas et al.[121]							
No apnea	59	0	NR	NR	3†	0	0
Sleep apnea	61	3	NR	NR	7†	13	5
Guilleminault et al.[115]	400	11	8	NR	20†	NR	3
Miller[122]	23	9	4	NR	9	9	0
Tilkian et al.[113]	25	36	16	NR	NR	NR	8
	15	33	13	NR	NR	66	13

Modified from Flemons WW, Remers JE, Gillis AM, 1993, Sleep apnea and cardiac arrhythmias. Is there a relationship? *American Review of Respiratory Disease*, vol 148, 618–621. Official Journal of the American Thoracic Society. © American Lung Association.
*Greater than 100/h.
†Greater than 120/h.
AV, atrioventricular; CI, confidence interval; NR, not reported; VPBs, ventricular premature beats; VT, ventricular tachycardia.

Table 85–4. SUMMARY OF POTENTIAL NEUROCARDIAC MECHANISMS IN SUDDEN INFANT DEATH SYNDROME

Autonomic Derangement	Cardiac Mechanism	Comments
Excess vagal activity due to sleep-induced apnea	Asystole	This could occur in association with apnea and hypoxia.[7] It is unclear whether the infant heart could be permanently arrested by sustained hypervagotonia.
	Asystole degenerating to ventricular fibrillation	Prolonged asystole could precipitate ventricular fibrillation
Sleep-induced surges in sympathetic activity	Ventricular fibrillation	In the absence of functional abnormalities it is unlikely that the increases in sympathetic activity observed during sleep are of a sufficient magnitude to trigger ventricular fibrillation. Arousal from sleep could be a factor.[70, 108]
Developmental imbalance in sympathetic innervation to the heart	Ventricular fibrillation	Experimental studies in puppies suggest that inhomogeneity of sympathetic innervation occurs during development, a pattern that has been shown to be arrhythmogenic.[129] The prolongation of QT intervals that has been observed in infants is also suggestive of sympathetic nervous system imbalance.[9, 130]

Modified from Verrier RL, Kirby DA. Sleep and cardiac arrhythmias. Ann N Y Acad Sci. 1988;533:238–251.

function that might initiate a cardiac arrhythmia and SIDS have been reviewed by Verrier and Kirby[7] and are shown in Table 85–4. Although increased vagal tone is thought to have antiarrhythmic properties (increased thresholds for VT and VF), it is possible that the excess vagal tone that might occur during episodes of apnea could lead to profound bradycardia and asystole. Guilleminault[8] has observed significant bradycardia or sinus arrest in 38 of 594 infants studied following an episode of near-miss SIDS. In the vast majority of these subjects, the arrhythmias observed during sleep were secondary to apnea and hypoventilation. Another possible mechanism of sudden cardiac death in SIDS victims is VF secondary to increased sympathetic nervous system activity during REM sleep. Against this hypothesis is the absence of any documented abnormalities of the myocardium or conduction system in victims of SIDS.[7, 9] In addition, ventricular arrhythmias have been infrequently observed in infants following an episode of near-miss SIDS.[4]

A third possible mechanism of SIDS is a developmental imbalance of the ANS, which could lead to inhomogeneity of depolarization and repolarization within the myocardium.[7, 9] Kralios and Millar[129] studied the functional development of cardiac sympathetic nerves in puppies between 1 and 6 weeks of age. These investigators observed a regression of functional maturation of all nerves except for the ventrolateral branch of the left stellate ganglion in the third week of life. If regional sympathetic imbalance with left sympathetic predominance does develop at some point during maturation, this might provide the substrate for the development of VF.[9] Such a change might explain the prolongation of the QT interval that occurs in normal infants between 2 and 4 months of age.[130] Although ventricular tachyarrhythmia associated with prolongation of the QT interval has been proposed as a potential mechanism of SIDS, significant prolongation of the QT interval has not been documented in 100 infants studied following near-miss SIDS.[8] However, in support of the developmental imbalance hypothesis are the observations by several investigators of decreased heart rate variability during NREM sleep in near-miss SIDS victims and in the siblings of SIDS victims.[131, 132] A similar decrease in heart rate variability has been observed in patients who are at high risk of sudden cardiac death following a myocardial infarction.[31, 32]

Thus, changes in autonomic tone that occur during sleep could precipitate life-threatening cardiac arrhythmias in infants through several mechanisms. However, their role in SIDS remains unknown.

SUDDEN UNEXPLAINED NOCTURNAL DEATH

The syndrome of sudden unexplained nocturnal death (SUND) in Southeast Asian immigrants has also attracted considerable attention.[133–142] VF has been documented in some of the victims, but the mechanism of this electrical instability and its possible relationship to sleep state is not completely understood.[136, 138] SUND in young adult males has several clinical similarities to SIDS: there is no known preexisting disorder, otherwise healthy young adults are affected, and the autopsy reveals no cause. SUND has been reported in the Philippines (*bangungut*, moaning and dying during sleep), in Japan (*pokkuri*, sudden unexplained death at night), in Thailand (*lai-tai*, died during sleep), and in Laos (*non-latia*), as well as in other Southeast Asian countries and in some of the islands of the Pacific. Immigrants from these endemic areas are also at high risk. The victims are healthy, young adult males who either die in their sleep or appear to moan or temporarily arouse from sleep and then die suddenly. Abnormal agonal respirations have been reported by witnesses. Sometimes, patients are awakened from an event by vigorous stimulation, only to die later.[135] Thiamine deficiency[137] and hypokalemia[139] have both been hypothesized as important pathogenetic factors. These factors, however, do not explain the overwhelming number of males with this disorder. The hypokalemia hypothesis is based on the finding that within endemic areas, such as Thailand, there may be isolated regions where there are clustering of SUND cases in the same regions where there are disorders associated with hypokalemia: hypokalemic periodic paralysis and endemic distal renal tubular acidosis. In some cases, the serum potassium concentration was found to be low in subjects whose deaths were consistent with SUND and who had relatives with distal renal tubular acidosis.[139, 140] Investigators have reported patients who were admitted late at night or in the early morning with sudden onset of muscle weakness, cardiac arrhythmias, and very low potassium concentrations.[139] The authors contended that this group of patients survived because of rapid treatment, but if they had died, the disorder would have been consistent with SUND. In Thailand, not only is there clustering of SUND, hypokalemic periodic paralysis, and endemic distal renal tubular acidosis in the same regions but also those same regions are often associated with poor dietary potassium intake and consequent lower serum potassium levels in the general population. Whether poor diet plays a role in people who die of SUND in other parts of the world is unknown. The QT interval has been reported to be prolonged in 100 Laotian refugees at risk for SUND who had a history of poor thiamine status and seizure-like episodes during sleep.[143] QT interval prolongation, particularly in the setting of hypokalemia, would predispose individuals to torsades de pointes VT, which can precipitate VF.[44]

Nademannee et al.[138] studied 27 Thai men who survived a cardiac arrest due to ventricular fibrillation at night or who had symptoms similar to the clinical presentation of SUND. These investigators observed a right bundle branch block and precordial injury pattern in 59% of patients, which correlated with spontaneous VF as well as the induction of VF, abnormalities of the signal-averaged EKG, and increased risk of death (Fig. 85–9). These investigators have observed dynamic changes in the EKG and have speculated that sympathetic stimulation may correct these abnormalities. These electrophysiological abnormalities are consistent with the Brugada syndrome.[144, 145] The genetic basis of these electrophysiological abnormalities has been identified as mutations of the sodium channel.

Based on the observations of Nadamanee et al.,[138] the 12-lead EKG and a signal-averaged EKG may be useful tools for identifying patients at high risk for SUND. Survivors of near-miss sudden cardiac death and such high-risk patients should likely be treated with an implantable cardioverter defibrillator.

THERAPEUTIC IMPLICATIONS

Most cardiac arrhythmias that are observed during sleep are benign. The presence of structural heart disease should be ruled out in such patients by careful history, physical examination, and review of a 12-lead EKG. The management of more serious arrhythmias such as complete heart block, supraventricular tachy-

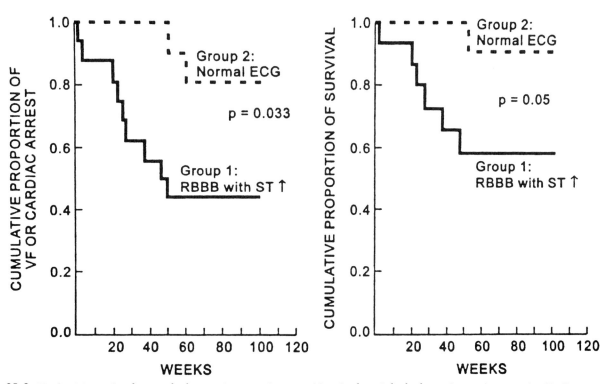

Figure 85–9. Kaplan-Meier plot showing high mortality rate due to sudden death and the high incidence of ventricular fibrillation (VF) and cardiac arrest occurring in patients with suspected sudden unexplained nocturnal death syndrome (SUNDS) who had right bundle branch block (RBBB) and a precordial injury pattern in electrocardiogram (ECG) leads V_1 through V_3 (Group 1) compared with patients without these clinical markers (Group 2). (From Nadamanee K, Veerakul G, Nimmannit S, et al. Arrhythmogenic marker for the sudden unexplained death syndrome in Thai men. Circulation. 1997;96[8]:2595–2600.)

cardia, and VT should be directed toward identifying reversible causes (e.g., severe hypoxemia secondary to poorly controlled heart failure or OSA). The decision to institute treatment must be individualized and will be determined by the risk of cardiovascular morbidity or mortality. Persistent bradycardia with heart rates less than 40 bpm lasting for hours in asymptomatic individuals does not require intervention. If patients are on an antiarrhythmic therapy that might contribute to nocturnal bradycardia, the need for drug therapy and the dose of the drug should be reevaluated. If nocturnal atrial fibrillation is heralded by bradycardia or sinus pauses, then drugs contributing to this trigger should be reevaluated (e.g., digoxin, beta blockers, or calcium channel blockers). If such drugs are required long-term, then pacing may be a therapeutic option. It is tempting to speculate that modulation of either parasympathetic or sympathetic tone might be beneficial in some cases, but current data are limited and largely anecdotal.

Acknowledgments

Supported by the Medical Research Council of Canada, PG-11888 and the Heart and Stroke Foundation of Alberta. Dr. Gillis is a Senior Scholar of the Alberta Heritage Foundation for Medical Research.

References

1. Zipes DP. Autonomic modulation of cardiac arrhythmias. In: Zipes DP, Jalife J, eds. Cardiac Electrophysiology: From Cell to Bedside. 2nd ed. Philadelphia, Pa: WB Saunders; 1995:441–454.
2. Verrier RL, Muller JE, Hobson JA. Sleep, dreams and sudden death: the case for sleep as an autonomic stress test for the heart. Cardiovasc Res. 1996;31:118–211.
3. Verrier RL, Dickerson LW. Autonomic nervous system and coronary blood flow changes related to emotional activation and sleep. Circulation. 1991;83(4 suppl):II81–II83.
4. Lavery CF, Mittleman MA, Cohen MC, et al. Nonuniform nighttime distribution of acute cardiac events. A possible effect of sleep states. Circulation. 1997;96:3321–3327.
5. He J, Kryger MH, Zorick FJ, et al. Mortality and apnea index in obstructive sleep apnea: experience in 385 male patients. Chest. 1988;94:9–14.
6. Partinen M, Jamieson A, Guilleminault C. Long-term outcome for obstructive sleep apnea syndrome patients. Chest. 1988;94:1200–1204.
7. Verrier RL, Kirby DA. Sleep and cardiac arrhythmias. Ann N Y Acad Sci. 1988;533:238–251.
8. Guilleminault C. SIDS, near-miss SIDS and cardiac arrhythmia. Ann N Y Acad Sci. 1988;533:358–367.
9. Schwartz PJ. The quest for the mechanisms of the sudden infant death syndrome: doubts and progress. Circulation. 1987;75:677–683.
10. James TN. The sinus node as a servo mechanism. Circ Res. 1973;32:302.
11. Schwartz PJ, Priori SG. Sympathetic nervous system and cardiac arrhythmias. In: Zipes DP, Jalife J, eds. Cardiac Electrophysiology: From Cell to Bedside. Philadelphia, Pa: WB Saunders; 1990:330–342.
12. Podrid PJ, Fuchs T, Candinas R. Role of the sympathetic nervous system in the genesis of ventricular arrhythmia. Circulation. 1990;82(suppl 1):103–113.
13. Wit AL, Rosen MR. After depolarizations and triggered activity. In: Fozzard HA, Haber ES, Jennings RB, eds. The Heart and Cardiovascular System. New York, NY: Raven Press; 1986;1449–1490.
14. Han J, Millet D, Chizzonitti B, et al. Temporal dispersion of

15. Verrier RL, Thompson PL, Lown B. Ventricular vulnerability during sympathetic stimulation: role of heart rate and blood pressure. Cardiovasc Res. 1974;8:602–610.
16. Lown B, Verrier RL. Neural activity and ventricular fibrillation. N Engl J Med. 1976;294:1165–1170.
17. Carpeggiani C, Landisman C, Montaron M-F, et al. Cryoblockade in limbic brain (amygdala) prevents or delays ventricular fibrillation after coronary artery occlusion in psychologically stressed pigs. Circ Res. 1992;70:600.
18. Kent KM, Smith ER, Redwood DR, et al. Beneficial electrophysiologic effects of nitroglycerine during acute myocardial infarction. Am J Cardiol. 1974;33:513–516.
19. Baust W, Bohnert B. The regulation of heart rate during sleep. Exp Brain Res. 1969;7:169–180.
20. Mancia G, Zanchetti A. Cardiovascular regulation during sleep. In: Orem J, ed. Physiology in Sleep. New York, NY: Academic Press; 1980:1–55.
21. Zemaityte D, Varoneckas G, Sokolov E. Heart rhythm during sleep in ischemic heart disease. Psychophysiology. 1984;21:290–298.
22. Somers VK, Dyken ME, Mark AL, et al. Sympathetic nerve activity during sleep in normal subjects. N Engl J Med. 1993;328:303–307.
23. Mancia G. Autonomic modulation of the cardiovascular system during sleep. N Engl J Med. 1993;328:347–349.
24. Furlan R, Guzzetti S, Crivellar W, et al. Continuous 24-hour assessment of neural regulation of systemic arterial pressure and RR variabilities in ambulant subjects. Circulation. 1990;81:537–547.
25. Huikuri HV, Kessler KM, Terracall E, et al. Reproducibility and circadian rhythm of heart rate variability in healthy subjects. Am J Cardiol. 1990;65:391–393.
26. Huikuri HV, Niemela MJ, Ojala S, et al. Circadian rhythms of frequency domain measures of heart rate variability in healthy subjects and patients with coronary artery disease. Effects of arousal and upright posture. Circulation. 1994;90:121–126.
27. Raetz SL, Richard CA, Garfinkel A, et al. Dynamic characteristics of cardiac R-R intervals during sleep and waking states. Sleep. 1992;14:526.
28. Vanoli E, Adamson PB, Ba-Lin, et al. Heart rate variability during specific sleep stages: a comparison of healthy subjects with patients after myocardial infarction. Circulation. 1995;91:1918–1922.
29. Panina G, Khot UN, Nunziata E, et al. Assessment of autonomic tone over a 24-hour period in patients with congestive heart failure: relation between mean heart rate and measures of heart rate variability. Am Heart J. 1995;129:748–753.
30. Klingenheben T, Rapp U, Hohnloser SH. Circadian variation of heart rate variability in post infarction patients with and without life-threatening ventricular tachyarrhythmias. J Cardiovasc Electrophysiol. 1995;6:357–364.
31. Kleiger RE, Miller JP, Bigger JT Jr, et al. Decreased heart rate variability and its association with increased mortality after acute myocardial infarction. Am J Cardiol. 1987;59:256–262.
32. LaRovere MT, Specchia G, Mortara A, et al. Baroreflex sensitivity, clinical correlates and cardiovascular mortality among patients with a first myocardial infarction: a prospective study. Circulation. 1988;78:816–824.
33. Kong TQ, Goldberger JJ, Parker M, et al. Circadian variation in human ventricular refractoriness. Circulation. 1995;92:1507–1516.
34. Cinca J, Moya A, Figueras J, et al. Circadian variations in the electrical properties of the human heart assessed by sequential bedside electrophysiologic testing. Am Heart J. 1986;112:315–321.
35. Cinca J, Moya A, Bardaji A, et al. Circadian variations of electrical properties of the heart. Ann N Y Acad Sci. 1989;604:222–233.
36. Cinca J, Moya A, Bardaji A, et al. Daily variability of electrically induced reciprocating tachycardia in patients with atrioventricular accessory pathways. Am Heart J. 1987;114:327–333.
37. Browne KF, Prystowsky E, Heger JJ, et al. Prolongation of the Q-T interval in man during sleep. Am J Cardiol. 1983;52:55–59.
38. Gillis AM, MacLean KE, Guilleminault C. The QT interval dur-

ing wake and sleep in patients with ventricular arrhythmias. Sleep. 1988;11:333–339.

39. Murakawa Y, Inoue H, Nozaki A, et al. Role of sympathovagal interactions in diurnal variation of QT interval. Am J Cardiol. 1992;69:339–343.

40. Bexton RS, Vallin HO, Camm AJ. Diurnal variation of the QT interval: influence of the autonomic nervous system. Br Heart J. 1986;55:253–258.

41. Sarma JSM, Singh BN. Circadian rhythmicity of heart rate and myocardial repolarization: implications for the prevention of ventricular fibrillation. In: Singh BN, Wellens HJJ, Hiraoka M, eds. Electropharmacological Control of Cardiac Arrhythmias. To Delay Conduction or to Prolong Refractoriness? Mount Kisco, NY: Futura; 1994:441–455.

42. Molnar J, Zhang F, Weiss J, et al. Diurnal pattern of the QTc interval: how long is prolonged? Possible relation to circadian triggers of cardiovascular events. J Am Coll Cardiol. 1996;27:76–83.

43. Day CP, McComb JM, Campbell RWF. QT dispersion: an indication of arrhythmia risk in patients with long QT intervals. Br Heart J. 1990;63:342–344.

44. Hii TJY, Wyse DG, Gillis AM, et al. Precordial QT interval dispersion as a marker of torsade de pointes: disparate effects of class Ia antiarrhythmic drugs and amiodarone. Circulation. 1992;86:1376–1382.

45. Priori SG, Napolitano C, Diehl L, et al. Dispersion of the QT interval. A marker to therapeutic efficacy in the idiopathic long QT syndrome. Circulation. 1994;89:1681–1689.

46. Muller JE, Ludmer PL, Willich SN, et al. Circadian variation in the frequency of sudden cardiac death. Circulation. 1987;75:131–138.

47. Brodsky M, Wu D, Denes P, et al. Arrhythmias documented by 24-hour continuous electrocardiographic monitoring in 50 male medical students without apparent heart disease. Am J Cardiol. 1977;39:390–395.

48. Sobotka PA, Mayer JH, Bauernfeind RA, et al. Arrhythmias documented by 24-hour continuous ambulatory electrocardiographic monitoring in young women without apparent heart disease. Am Heart J. 1981;101:753–759.

49. Bjerregaard P. Mean 24 hour heart rate, minimal heart rate and pauses in healthy subjects 40–79 years of age. Eur Heart J. 1983;4:44–51.

50. Kantelip J-P, Sage E, Duchene-Marullaz P. Findings on ambulatory electrocardiographic monitoring in subjects older than 80 years. Am J Cardiol. 1986;57:398–401.

51. Vitasalo MT, Kala R, Eisalo A. Ambulatory electrocardiographic recording in endurance athletes. Br Heart J. 1982;47:213–220.

52. Ector H, Bourgois J, Verlinden M, et al. Bradycardia, ventricular pauses, syncope, and sports. Lancet. 1984;2:591–594.

53. Guilleminault C, Pool P, Motta J, et al. Sinus arrest during REM sleep in young adults. N Engl J Med. 1984;311:1006–1010.

54. Otsuka K, Kawakami T, Saito H, et al. REM sleep and bradyarrhythmia episodes in rats. J Electrocardiol. 1989;22:235–240.

55. Dickerson LW, Huang AH, Nearing BD, et al. Primary coronary vasodilation associated with pauses in heart rhythm during sleep. Am J Physiol. 1993;264:R186–R196.

56. Nagashima M, Matsushima M, Ogawa A, et al. Cardiac arrhythmias in healthy children revealed by 24-hour ambulatory ECG monitoring. Pediatr Cardiol. 1987;8:103–108.

57. Nevins DB. First- and second-degree A-V heart block with rapid eye movement sleep. Ann Intern Med. 1972;76:981–983.

58. Otsuka K, Ichimaru Y, Yanaga T. Studies of arrhythmias by 24-hour polygraphic recordings: relationship between atrioventricular block and sleep states. Am Heart J. 1983;105:934–940.

59. Viitasalo M, Halonen L, Partinen M, et al. Sleep and cardiac rhythm in healthy men. Ann Med. 1991;23:135–139.

60. Raeder EA. Circadian fluctuations in ventricular response to atrial fibrillation. Am J Cardiol. 1990;66:1013–1016.

61. Irwin JM, McCarthy EA, Wilkinson WE, et al. Circadian occurrence of symptomatic paroxysmal supraventricular tachycardia in untreated patients. Circulation. 1988;77:298–300.

62. Kupari M, Koskinen P, Leinonen H. Double-peaking circadian variation in the occurrence of sustained supraventricular tachyarrhythmias. Am Heart J. 1990;120:1364–1369.

63. Waxman MB, Wald RW, Cameron D. Interactions between the autonomic nervous system and tachycardias in man. Cardiol Clin. 1983;1:143–185.

64. Coumel P, Ledercq JF, Attuel P, et al. Autonomic influences in the genesis of atrial arrhythmias: atrial flutter and fibrillation of vagal origin. In: Narula SO, ed. Cardiac Arrhythmias: Electrophysiology, Diagnosis and Management. Baltimore, Md: Williams & Wilkins; 1979:243–255.

65. Coumel P, Friocourt P, Mugica J, et al. Long-term prevention of vagal atrial arrhythmias by atrial pacing at 90/minute: experience with 6 cases. Pacing Clin Electrophysiol. 1983;6:552–560.

66. Attuel P, Pellerin D, Mugica J, et al. DDD pacing: an effective treatment modality for recurrent atrial arrhythmias. Pacing Clin Electrophysiol. 1988;11:1647–1654.

67. Yamashita T, Murakawa Y, Sezaki K, et al. Circadian variation of paroxysmal atrial fibrillation. Circulation. 1997;96:1537.

68. Lown B, Tykocinski M, Garfein A, et al. Sleep and ventricular premature beats. Circulation. 1973;48:691–701.

69. Raeder EA, Hohnloser SH, Graboys TB, et al. Spontaneous variability and circadian distribution of ectopic activity in patients with malignant ventricular arrhythmia. J Am Coll Cardiol. 1988;12:656–661.

70. Pickering TG, Johnston J, Honour AJ. Comparison of the effects of sleep, exercise and autonomic drugs on ventricular extrasystoles, using ambulatory monitoring of electrocardiogram and electroencephalogram. Am J Med. 1978;65:575–583.

71. Gillis AM, Peters RW, Mitchell LB, et al. Effects of left ventricular dysfunction on the circadian variation of ventricular premature complexes. Am J Cardiol. 1992;69:1009–1014.

72. Gillis AM, Guilleminault C, Partinen M, et al. The diurnal variability of ventricular premature depolarizations: influence of heart rate, sleep and wakefulness. Sleep. 1989;12:391–399.

73. Smith R, Johnson L, Rothfeld D, et al. Sleep and cardiac arrhythmias. Arch Intern Med. 1972;130:751–753.

74. Rosenblatt G, Hartmann E, Zwilling GR. Cardiac irritability during sleep and dreaming. J Psychosom Res. 1973;17:129–134.

75. Rosenberg MJ, Uretz E, Denes P. Sleep and ventricular arrhythmias. Am Heart J. 1983;106:703–709.

76. Muller JE, Tofler GH, Stone PH. Circadian variation and triggers of onset of acute cardiovascular disease. Circulation. 1989;79:733–743.

77. Lucente M, Rebuzzi AG, Lanza GA, et al. Circadian variation of ventricular tachycardia in acute myocardial infarction. Am J Cardiol. 1988;622:670–674.

78. Twidale N, Taylor S, Heddle WF, et al. Morning increase in the time of onset of sustained ventricular tachycardia. Am J Cardiol. 1989;64:1204–1206.

79. Aronow WS, Ahn C, Mercando AD, et al. Effects of propranolol on circadian variation of ventricular arrhythmias in elderly patients with heart disease and complex ventricular arrhythmias. Am J Cardiol. 1995;75:514–516.

80. Behrens S, Ehlers C, Bruggemann T, et al. Modification of the circadian pattern of ventricular tachyarrhythmias by beta-blocker therapy. Clin Cardiol. 1997;20:253–257.

81. Aronow WS, Ahn C, Mercando AD, et al. Circadian variation of sudden cardiac death or fatal myocardial infarction is abolished by propranolol in patients with heart disease and complex ventricular arrhythmias. Am J Cardiol. 1994;74:819–821.

82. Willich SN, Goldberg RJ, Maclure M, et al. Increased onset of sudden cardiac death in the first three hours after awakening. Am J Cardiol. 1992;70:65–68.

83. Aronow WS, Ahn C. Circadian variation of primary cardiac arrest or sudden cardiac death in patients aged 62 to 100 years (mean 82). Am J Cardiol. 1993;71:1455–1456.

84. Buff DD, Fleisher JM, Roca JA, et al. Circadian distribution of in-hospital cardiopulmonary arrests on the general medical ward. Arch Intern Med. 1992;152:1282–1288.

85. Levine RL, Pepe PE, Fromm RE, et al. Prospective evidence of a circadian rhythm for out-of-hospital cardiac arrests. JAMA. 1992;267:2935–2937.

86. Arntz H-R, Willich SN, Oeff M, et al. Circadian variation of sudden death reflects age-related variability in ventricular fibrillation. Circulation. 1993;88:2284–2289.

87. Behrens S, Ney G, Fisher SG, et al. Effects of amiodarone on the circadian pattern of sudden cardiac death (Department of Veterans Affairs Congestive Heart Failure–Survival Trial of Antiarrhythmic Therapy). Am J Cardiol. 1997;80:45–48.

88. Peters RW, Muller JE, Goldstein S, et al. Propranolol and the morning increase in the frequency of sudden cardiac death (BHAT study). Am J Cardiol. 1989;63:1518–1520.

89. Lampert R, Rosenfeld L, Batsford E, et al. Circadian variation of sustained ventricular tachycardia in patients with coronary artery disease and implantable cardioverter-defibrillators. Circulation. 1994;90:241–247.

90. Wood MA, Simpson PM, London WB, et al. Circadian pattern of ventricular tachyarrhythmias in patients with implantable cardioverter-defibrillators. J Am Coll Cardiol. 1995;25:901–907.

91. Toffer GH, Gebara OCE, Mittleman MA, et al. Morning peak in ventricular tachyarrhythmias detected by time of implantable cardioverter/defibrillator therapy. Circulation. 1995;92:1203–1208.

92. Mallavarapu C, Pancholy S, Schwartzman D, et al. Circadian variation of ventricular arrhythmia recurrences after cardioverter-defibrillator implantation in patients with healed myocardial infarcts. Am J Cardiol. 1995;75:1140–1144.

93. Behrens S, Galecka M, Bruggemann T, et al. Circadian variation of sustained ventricular tachyarrhythmias terminated by appropriate shocks in patients with an implantable cardioverter defibrillator. Am Heart J. 1995;130:79–84.

94. d'Avila A, Wellens F, Andries E, et al. At what time are implantable defibrillator shocks delivered? Evidence for individual circadian variance in sudden cardiac death. Eur Heart J. 1995;16:1231–1233.

95. Lichstein E, Morganroth J, Harris TR, et al. (for the BHAT Study Group). Effect of propranolol on ventricular arrhythmia: the Beta-Blocker Heart Attack Trial experience. Circulation. 1983;67(suppl 1):I5–I10.

96. Willich SN, Linderer T, Wegscheider K, et al. Increased morning incidence of myocardial infarction in the ISAM study: absence with prior beta-adrenergic blockade. Circulation. 1989;80:853–858.

97. Behrens S, Ehlers C, Bruggemann T, et al. Modification of the circadian pattern of ventricular tachyarrhythmias. Clin Cardiol. 1997;20:253.

98. McClelland J, Halperin B, Cutter J, et al. Circadian variation in ventricular electrical instability associated with coronary artery disease. Am J Cardiol. 1990;65:1351–1357.

99. Venditti FJ, John RM, Hull M, et al. Circadian variation in defibrillation energy requirements. Circulation. 1996;94:1607–1612.

100. Lown B, Temte JV, Reich P, et al. Basis for recurring ventricular fibrillation in the absence of coronary heart disease and its management. N Engl J Med. 1976;294:623–629.

101. Winkle RA. The relationship between ventricular ectopic beat frequency and heart rate. Circulation. 1982;66:439–446.

102. Skinner JE, Mohr DN, Kellaway P. Sleep-stage regulation of ventricular arrhythmias in the unanesthetized pig. Circ Res. 1975;37:342–349.

103. Flick MR, Block AJ. Nocturnal vs diurnal cardiac arrhythmias in patients with chronic obstructive pulmonary disease. Chest. 1979;75:8–11.

104. Shepard JW Jr, Garrison MW, Grither DA, et al. Relationship of ventricular ectopy to nocturnal oxygen desaturation in patients with chronic obstructive pulmonary disease. Am J Med. 1985;78:28–34.

105. Findley LJ, Blackburn MR, Goldberger AL, et al. Apneas and oscillation of cardiac ectopy in Cheyne-Stokes breathing during sleep. Am Rev Respir Dis. 1984;130:937–939.

106. Galatius-Jensen S, Hansen J, Rasmussen V, et al. Nocturnal hypoxia after myocardial infarction: association with nocturnal myocardial ischaemia and arrhythmias. Br Heart J. 1994;72:23–30.

107. Hoffstein V, Mateika S. Cardiac arrhythmias, snoring, and sleep apnea. Chest. 1994;106:466–471.

108. Wellens HJJ, Vermeulen A, Durrer D. Ventricular fibrillation occurring on arousal from sleep by auditory stimuli. Circulation. 1972;46:661–665.

109. Kirby DA, Verrier RL. Differential effects of sleep stage on coronary hemodynamic function. Physiol Behav. 1989;45:1017–1020.

110. Zwillich C, Devlin T, White D, et al. Bradycardia during sleep apnea: characteristics and mechanism. J Clin Invest. 1982;69:1286–1292.

111. Guilleminault C, Connolly S, Winkle R, et al. Cyclical variation of the heart rate in sleep apnoea syndrome: mechanisms and usefulness of 24 h electrocardiography as a screening technique. Lancet. 1984;1:126–131.

112. Flemons WW, McDonald M, Kim D, et al. The sensitivity, specificity and likelihood ratios of cyclical variation for the diagnosis of sleep apnea. Am Rev Respir Dis. 1993;147:811.

113. Tilkian AG, Guilleminault C, Schroeder JS, et al. Sleep-induced apnea syndrome: prevalence of cardiac arrhythmias and their reversal after tracheostomy. Am J Med. 1977;63:348–358.

114. Guilleminault C, Simmons FB, Motta J, et al. Obstructive sleep apnea syndrome and tracheostomy: long-term follow-up experience. Arch Intern Med. 1981;141:985–988.

115. Guilleminault C, Connolly SJ, Winkle RA. Cardiac arrhythmia and conduction disturbances during sleep in 400 patients with sleep apnea syndrome. Am J Cardiol. 1983;52:490–494.

116. Peter JH, Koehler U, Groto L, et al. Manifestations and consequences of obstructive sleep apnea. Eur Respir J. 1995;8:1572–1583.

117. Becker H, Brandenburg U, Peter JH, et al. Reversal of sinus arrest and atrioventricular conduction block in patients with sleep apnea during nasal continuous positive air way pressure. Am J Respir Crit Care Med. 1995;151:215–218.

118. Grimm W, Hoffman J, Menz V, et al. Electrophysiologic evaluation of sinus node function and atrioventricular conduction in patients with prolonged ventricular asystole during obstructive sleep apnea. Am J Cardiol. 1996;77:1310–1314.

119. Flemons WW, Remmers JE, Gillis AM. Sleep apnea and cardiac arrhythmias: is there a relationship? Am Rev Respir Dis. 1993;148:618–621.

120. Bolm-Audorff U, Kohler U, Becker E, et al. Nächtliche Herzrhythmus-störungen bei Schlafapnoe-syndrome. Dtsch Med Wochenschr. 1984;109:853–856.

121. Boudoulas H, Schmidt HS, Clark RW, et al. Anthropometric characteristics, cardiac abnormalities and adrenergic activity in patients with primary disorders of sleep. J Med. 1983;14:223–239.

122. Miller WP. Cardiac arrhythmias and conduction disturbances in sleep apnea syndrome. Am J Med. 1982;73:317–321.

123. Cortelli P, Parchi P, Storza E, et al. Cardiovascular autonomic dysfunction in normotensive awake subjects with obstructive sleep apnea syndrome. Clin Autonom Res. 1994;4:57–62.

124. Thorpy MJ, Ledereich PS, Burack B, et al. Death in patients with obstructive sleep apnea. Sleep Res. 1990;19:301.

125. Yamashiro Y, Kryger MH. Sleep in heart failure. Sleep. 1993;16:513–523.

126. Javaheri S, Parker TJ, Wesler L, et al. Occult sleep-disorders breathing in stable congestive heart failure. Ann Intern Med. 1995;122:487–492.

127. Davies SW, John LM, Wedzicha JA, et al. Overnight studies in severe chronic left heart failure: arrhythmias and oxygen desaturation. Br Heart J. 1991;65:77–83.

128. Moser DK, Stevenson WG, Woo MA, et al. Timing of sudden death in patients with heart failure. J Am Coll Cardiol. 1994;24:963–967.

129. Kralios FA, Millar CK. Functional development of cardiac sympathetic nerves in newborn dogs: evidence for asymmetrical development. Cardiovasc Res. 1978;12:547–554.

130. Schwartz PJ, Montemerlo M, Facchini M, et al. The QT interval throughout the first 6 months of life: a prospective study. Circulation. 1982;66:496–501.

131. Leistner HL, Haddad GG, Epstein RA, et al. Heart rate and heart rate variability during sleep in aborted sudden infant death syndrome. J Pediatr. 1980;97:51–55.

132. Kluge KA, Harper RM, Schechtman VL, et al. Spectral analysis assessment of respiratory sinus arrhythmia in normal infants and infants who subsequently died of sudden infant death syndrome. Pediatr Res. 1988;24:677–682.

133. Baron RC, Thacker SB, Gorelkin L, et al. Sudden death among Southeast Asian refugees. JAMA. 1983;250:2947–2951.

134. Otto CM, Tauxe RV, Cobb LA, et al. Ventricular fibrillation causes sudden cardiac death in Southeast Asian immigrants. Ann Intern Med. 1984;100:45–47.

135. Munger RG. Sudden death in sleep of Laotian-Hmong refugees in Thailand: a case-control study. Am J Public Health. 1987;77:1187–1190.

136. Munger RG, Weniger BG, Warintrawat S, et al. Sudden death in sleep of South-East Asian refugees. Lancet. 1986;2:1093–1094.

137. Munger RG, Booton EA. Thiamine and sudden death in sleep of Southeast Asian refugees. Lancet. 1990;1:1154–1155.

138. Nademanee K, Veerakul G, Nimmannit S, et al. Arrhythmogenic marker for the sudden unexplained death syndrome in Thai men. Circulation. 1997;96:2595–2600.

139. Nimmannit S, Malasit P, Chaovakul V, et al. Pathogenesis of sudden unexplained nocturnal death (*lai tai*) and endemic distal renal tubular acidosis. Lancet. 1991;1:930–932.

140. Nimmannit S, Malasit P, Chaovakul V, et al. Potassium and sudden unexplained nocturnal death. Lancet. 1990;1:116–117.

141. Pressman MR, Marinchak RA, Kowey PR, et al. Polysomnographic and electrocardiographic findings in a sudden unexplained nocturnal death syndrome (SUNDS) survivor. Sleep Res. 1993;22:313.

142. Munger RG, Prineas RJ, Crow RS, et al. Prolonged QT interval and risk of sudden death in South-East Asian men. Lancet. 1991;338:280–281.

143. Munger RG, Prineas RJ, Crow RS, et al. Prolonged QT interval and risk of sudden death in South-East Asian men. Lancet. 1991;338:280–281.

144. Alings M, Wilde A. "Brugada" syndrome. Clinical data and suggested pathophysiologic mechanism. Circulation. 1999;99:666–673.

145. Gussak I, Antzelevitch C, Bjerregaard P, et al. The Brugada syndrome: clinical electrophysiologic and genetic aspects. J Am Coll Cardiol. 1999;33:5–15.

86

Hypertension, Ischemic Heart Disease, and Stroke

Charles F. P. George

Diseases of the cardiovascular system account for considerable rates of morbidity and mortality in North Americans and can account for up to 50% of medical admissions to hospital. Although there have been major advances in the understanding of risk factors, prevention, and treatment of coronary artery disease, our knowledge is still incomplete and morbidity rates are still very high.

Since the 1970s, the field of sleep medicine has grown tremendously, and our understanding of the interaction of sleep and other medical conditions has made great gains. With respect to cardiovascular disease, recognition of the importance of the sleep-wake cycle and other circadian rhythm interaction has led to major improvements in the understanding of the mechanisms of transient myocardial ischemia, myocardial infarction, sudden cardiac death, and stroke. This in turn has provided the rationale for new therapeutic interventions and stimulated much further research in this important area. Other chapters deal with central nervous system regulation of cardiac function (Chapter 13), sleep-related cardiac risk (Chapter 84), arrhythmias (Chapter 85), and cerebrovascular disease (Chapter 90); in this chapter, the sleep-related aspects of hypertension, ischemic heart disease, and cerebrovascular accidents are discussed.

HISTORICAL ASPECTS

The ability to synchronize physiological functions with the environment is well recognized and occurs in many biological functions, including hormone secretion and autonomic nervous system function, as well as the sleep-wake cycle. Although variations in onset of acute myocardial infarction with time of day were noted in the 1970s,[1] interest in circadian aspects of cardiovascular function remained low until the observation by Muller et al.[2] in 1985 that acute myocardial infarction has a higher incidence during the morning hours. Since then, interest in the circadian variation in cardiovascular physiology has increased exponentially. The demonstration of 24-h and other periodical changes in the physiology of the cardiovascular system dates back at least to the 19th century.[3] The first research to reveal periodicity in onset of symptoms of myocardial infarction was that of Master,[4] although he did not focus on this. In 1976, Smolensky et al.[5] commented on the data of Master, but the comment probably did not reach the cardiology field at large. As pointed out by Muller et al.,[2] reports from 1966 through 1976[6–11] contained similar data on periodicity of symptoms of myocardial infarction but again went relatively unnoticed. Even the World Health Organization report of the Myocardial Infarction Community Registers did not stimulate major clinical research in circadian physiology.[12] Since the work of Muller et al. in 1985, however, there has been much more interest in the subject.

EPIDEMIOLOGY

Hypertension

Diurnal variation is well described in both normal persons and patients with hypertension, with significant falls in blood pressure occurring at night during sleep.[13–15] During normal nonrapid eye movement (NREM) sleep, systolic blood pressure is 5 to 14% lower than that during quiet wakefulness.[16, 17] Blood pressure is higher during rapid eye movement (REM) sleep than during NREM sleep but does not reach awake levels. Individuals with this 24-h blood pressure profile have been labeled "dippers." This dipper pattern has been observed in most patients with essential hypertension. It is not clear whether these individuals experience a reduction in the nocturnal decline in blood pressure or failure in appropriate blood pressure rise during the daytime. The flattened 24-h blood pressure pattern in "nondippers" occurs in a minority of patients with essential hypertension and patients with secondary forms of hypertension and in patients with renal insufficiency.[18] The clinical significance of nondipper status is not entirely clear,[19] and although an understanding of circadian differences in blood pressure has been enhanced by 24-h ambulatory blood pressure monitoring, the limited reproducibility of circadian variation in blood pressure dippers and nondippers calls into question the usefulness of such a designation.[20] Ambulatory blood pressure recordings are more strongly associated with hypertensive end-organ damage than with isolated blood pressure readings, but it is the awake period that is most responsible for end-organ damage, and after controlling for age, the lack of normal nocturnal fall in blood pressure is not associated with an increase in left ventricular mass or in arterial disease. Age-related changes in carotid artery wall thickness and plaque among nondippers may reflect a contribution of altered baroreceptor function to the lack of normal nocturnal and supine blood pressure decreases.

Myocardial Infarction

The Multicentre Investigation of Limitation of Infarct Size (MILIS),[2] which was designed to evaluate the role of propranolol or hyaluronidase therapy in limiting infarct size in acute myocardial infarction, provided additional information on the time of onset of chest pain. Serial determination of plasma creatine kinase–MB activity, obtained for the assessment of infarct size, also permitted objective assessment of time of onset of myocardial infarction. In 703 patients, there was marked circadian periodicity in the onset of pain with a peak incidence between 6 AM and noon, and there was excellent correlation between symptom-based and enzyme-deduced times of onset of myocardial infarction. A smaller secondary peak in onset of myocardial infarction was observed between 7 and 8 PM. This pattern is illustrated in Figure 86–1, *top*.[21]

The Intravenous Streptokinase in Acute Myocardial Infarction (ISAM) study, which included 1741 patients, also demonstrated that the incidence of acute myocardial infarction markedly increased between 6 AM and noon, with a peak incidence from 8 to 9 AM and a minimum incidence between midnight and 1 AM.[22] The Physicians Health Study, a randomized, double-blind placebo-controlled trial of alternate-day aspirin intake (325 mg), examined the effect of aspirin on the incidence of myocardial infarction among 22,071 U.S. male physicians without a previous history of myocardial infarction. This large study also demonstrated the early morning peak in myocardial infarction.[23]

Depending on type of patients studied, other circadian patterns of infarction have been reported, although small populations may account for the differences.[24–27] An analysis of more than 7500 patients in the Thrombolysis in Myocardial Ischemia (TIMI) III study demonstrated similar circadian patterns of ischemia for unstable angina and non–Q wave (subendocardial) infarction.[28] Not all diabetics, however, exhibit a circadian rhythm in the onset of myocardial infarction, possibly due to differences in autonomic tone.[9]

In addition to circadian variation in the incidence of myocardial infarction, a *circaseptan* (day of the week) or *circannual* (every 12 months) pattern, or both, may also be seen. For example, Monday is associated with increased risk,[30] as are the winter months (January through March).[31] Differences in incidence between working versus retired patients may reflect differences in mechanisms or risk factors for myocardial infarction.

There is a wealth of information supporting the circadian variation in the onset of acute myocardial infarction. The mechanisms involved in this circadian

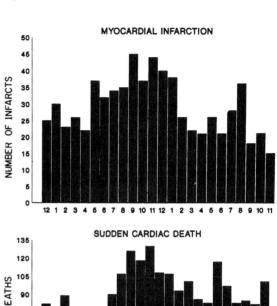
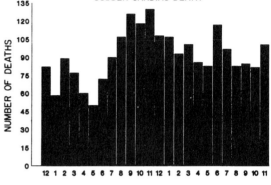
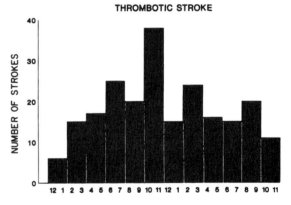
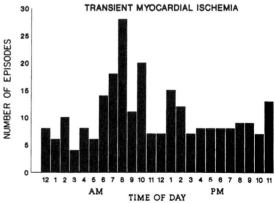

Figure 86–1. Bar graphs of time of day of onset of myocardial infarction, sudden cardiac death, stroke, and transient myocardial ischemia in four different patient groups. Number of events (*y*-axis) shown across 24 h (*x*-axis). Each disorder exhibits a prominent increase of onset in the period from 6 AM to noon. (From Muller JG, Tofler GH, Stone PH. Circadian variation and triggers of onset of acute cardiovascular disease. Circulation. 1989;79:733–743.)

variation in ischemia and therapeutic implications are addressed.

Transient Myocardial Ischemia

Although the relation between specific sleep stages and myocardial ischemia is not yet clear, the relation of the entire sleep period (as part of the rest-activity cycle) to transient ischemia is fairly well characterized and understood. Clinical studies have demonstrated circadian variations in ischemic episodes during daily routine activities, with the peak incidence of ST-segment depression occurring in the morning hours between 6 AM and noon[31, 32] (see Fig. 86–1, *bottom*). This early morning increase is further accentuated when the time of awakening and body position are taken into account.[33–35] This circadian variation in silent myocardial ischemia may continue even after infarction.[36] Soon after infarction (4 to 8 weeks), transient myocardial ischemia may become more frequent as the time after discharge from hospital increases, possibly related to increased activity and increased myocardial oxygen demand.[37]

Although not all study patients have been similar, there clearly is a circadian pattern in patients with typical angina with ischemic attacks clustered between 6 AM and noon. In patients who have had a myocardial infarction, the time from the infarction seems to have an effect on the strength of the circadian rhythm with differences between morning and evening peaks in transient ischemia. Other factors must also be responsible in this particular patient group.

Variant (Atypical) Angina

Originally defined by Prinzmetal et al.,[38] variant angina is characterized by angina at rest in association with transient ST-segment elevation (2 mm or greater), both of which can be reversed with the use of nitroglycerin. These episodes (and those of patients with typical angina) are most often silent but can be detected with Holter monitoring. In contrast to silent ischemia and myocardial infarction, these episodes occur most frequently during the nocturnal hours.

Holter monitoring in large numbers of patients[39] with variant angina demonstrates circadian variation in ST elevation, with the peak between 5 and 6 AM. Provoked attacks of coronary artery spasm, whether by exercise[40] or pharmacological stimulation (e.g., ergonovine[41]), also are subject to the same circadian pattern. Exercise in the morning results in more attacks of angina, and less ergonovine is needed in the morning to induce an attack. Figure 86–2 illustrates differences in the time of onset of variant angina compared with other patients with rest angina in the absence of ST-segment elevation.[42] Differences in these circadian patterns imply different mechanisms of ischemia.

Nocturnal angina may be a manifestation of sleep apnea in a patient with coronary artery disease.[42a] Treatment of the apnea may improve both nighttime and daytime ischemia.

Sudden Cardiac Death

Because of the relation between acute myocardial infarction and sudden death and with recognition of the circadian variation in onset of acute myocardial infarction, it is not surprising that sudden cardiac death would conform to similar circadian variability. Two large studies from Boston have addressed this area. From the time of out-of-hospital death (based on death certificates), a circadian rhythm was obvious, with a primary peak between 10 and 11 AM and a secondary peak from 5 to 6 PM[43] (see Fig. 86–1). Analysis of The

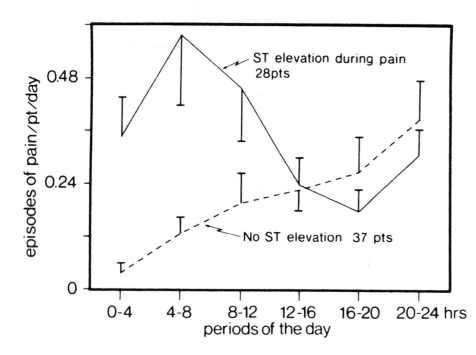

Figure 86–2. Episodes of angina throughout the day in patients with ST-segment elevation during pain (*solid line*) and without ST-segment elevation (*dashed line*). The peak incidence is from 4 to 8 AM in variant angina patients (with ST-segment elevation) and between 8 PM and midnight in other patients with rest angina (without ST-segment elevation). Although coronary spasm is the cause of variant angina, the different circadian patterns in other patients with rest angina imply a different mechanism for their attacks. (From Bogaty P, Waters DD. Circadian patterns in coronary disease: the mournfulness of morning. Can J Cardiol. 1988;4:5–11.)

Framingham Heart Study population for time of sudden cardiac death again demonstrated a circadian rhythm with a peak incidence between 7 and 9 AM.[44] Other studies of time of death support these conclusions.[45–47] A summary of 49 separate studies involving more than 400,000 deaths[45] notes a peak at 6 AM peak for all deaths. A subgroup of patients with death due to cardiovascular causes had a circadian rhythm peak at 10 AM. The effects of sleep on cardiac arrhythmias, including sudden cardiac death, are further discussed in Chapters 84 and 85.

Cerebrovascular Accidents (Strokes)

A circadian rhythm exists in the onset of stroke. Although earlier studies[48–52] have suggested that this pattern applied primarily for ischemic stroke (see Fig. 86–1), data indicate that such a pattern applies to all types of stroke. A meta-analysis of 31 published studies on stroke (consisting of 11,816 patients) found an early morning (6 AM and noon) peak incidence in ischemic, hemorrhagic, or all strokes combined with the increase being predominantly within the first hour after awakening.[53] This circadian variation is also apparent for transient ischemic attacks. The relation of cerebral event to time of awakening is again noted and is examined in Pathophysiology.

Of interest is that in addition to a circadian rhythm in stroke, there is a clear circannual rhythm (every 12 months) in stroke. The maximum occurrence in winter months (January through March) is well documented.[50] Although the mechanisms are not clear, it has been suggested that cold temperatures may alter the fibrinolytic system, decrease levels of antithrombin III, and cause an increase in blood viscosity. There also is some evidence that stroke is more common in snorers (see Chapters 47 and 90). In addition, changes in autonomic nervous system activity during sleep in ischemic stroke may influence the development of cardiac arrhythmias in the poststroke period[54]—the influence of sleep on arrhythmias is discussed in Chapter 85.

PATHOPHYSIOLOGY

Hypertension

Although changes in cardiac output or peripheral resistance may account for blood pressure differences between NREM and REM sleep, the mechanism or mechanisms for diurnal variation in blood pressure are uncertain. With age, there is increased blood pressure variability, particularly in women, but this appears to be confined to wakefulness rather than sleep.[55] There is debate regarding the contribution of changes in physical activity,[14] as opposed to cyclic alteration in the sympathetic nervous system, the renin-angiotensin-aldosterone system, cortisol secretion, and atrial natriuretic peptide secretion.[56–59] Shift workers have rapid reversal of their circadian blood pressure profile that coincides with changes in wakefulness, sleep, and work. Changes in these hormones follow an endogenous circadian rhythm that is independent of posture and physical activity. Studies comparing quadriplegic patients with immobilized but neurologically intact patients demonstrate a markedly diminished diurnal blood pressure variation in the quadriplegic patients. Although nighttime blood pressure is similar in both groups, the expected daytime rise in systolic and diastolic blood pressures is absent in quadriplegic patients. This suggests that the increase in blood pressure during waking hours in neurologically intact subjects is a consequence of diurnal variation in sympathetic activity (which is absent in quadriplegic patients with sympathetic decentralization), which is independent of changes in physical activity. Sympathetic antagonists such as metoprolol will not abolish this circadian rhythm, although beta blockers are effective in treating hypertension.[60, 61]

In patients with congestive heart failure, there appears to be a blunting of the circadian pattern of blood pressure that is positively correlated with the degree of left ventricular dysfunction.[62] This may be due to increased sympathetic activity or altered neurohumoral mechanisms associated with the heart failure. Figure 86–3 illustrates the expected circadian variation of heart rate and blood pressure in normal subjects and the absence of this rhythm in patients with significant heart failure.

In patients with essential hypertension, the magnitude of circadian blood pressure change may be related to the degree of left ventricular hypertrophy. This effect may be restricted to women, although there is considerable controversy. The mechanism responsible for this blunting of the expected nocturnal fall in systolic and diastolic pressures is not clear.

The recognition of hypertension and its circadian variation is important because it allows not only for accurate diagnosis but also for better assessment of therapy.[62a, 62b] It is well established that 24-h recordings of blood pressure can predict the presence of hypertensive heart disease and vascular disease and are superior to casual blood pressure measurements.[63, 63a]

MECHANISMS OF ISCHEMIA AND RELATION TO CIRCADIAN DISTRIBUTION OF CARDIOVASCULAR EVENTS

There are multiple factors that singly or in combination promote the development of transient ischemia (myocardial or cerebral). In the setting of an appropriate (vulnerable) atherosclerotic plaque, these factors may induce plaque rupture, propagate thrombosis, and produce myocardial infarction or sudden cardiac death.

In patients with coronary artery disease, myocardial ischemia (symptomatically expressed as angina) typically develops in the setting of exertion. With exercise, increased myocardial oxygen is needed to meet the demands of exercise but cannot be delivered in the setting of reduced coronary blood flow. With exercise,

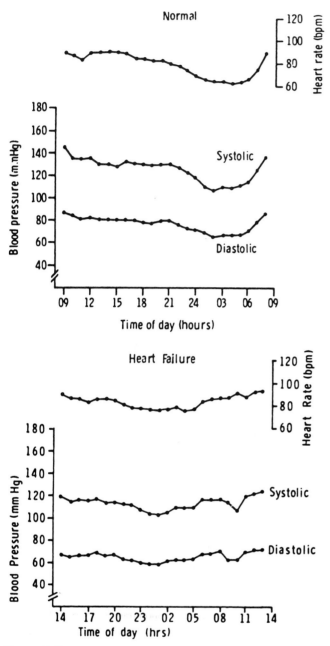

Figure 86–3. Hourly mean values of intra-arterial blood pressure and heart rate in 22 normal subjects and 22 patients with heart failure. Note reduced circadian amplitude in patients with heart failure. (From Caruana MP, Lahiri A, Cashman PMM, et al. Effects of chronic congestive heart failure secondary to coronary artery disease on the circadian rhythm of blood pressure and heart rate. Am J Cardiol. 1988;62:755–759.)

there is a significant increase in heart rate and blood pressure, both of which are factors in increasing myocardial oxygen demand. However, transient ischemia with little or no preceding increase in heart rate or blood pressure must be explained on the basis of reduced oxygen delivery (reduced coronary blood flow, coronary vasoconstriction). In many cases, both mechanisms may apply because there may be more than one trigger for ischemia.

Physical activity and mental stress are two factors

that play key roles in precipitating angina associated with myocardial ischemia.[64, 65] The majority of ischemic episodes are preceded by a possible triggering event, ranging from usual activity to stressful physical or mental activity, with the greater likelihood of ischemia occurring during activities perceived to be most physically or mentally stimulating.[66, 67] In fact, patients may frequently exhibit greater increases in peak systolic arterial pressure during mental stress than during exercise. Personally relevant mental stress appears to be the most potent type of mental stress in terms of both frequency and magnitude of ischemia. Most mental stress–induced ischemic episodes are silent and occur at heart rates significantly lower than those noted during exercise. Both systolic and diastolic blood pressures increase during mental stress–induced ischemia, suggesting that increased myocardial oxygen demands play a role in the pathophysiology of mental stress–induced transient ischemia. Mental arithmetic tasks have also been shown to result in paradoxical restriction of irregular or stenotic coronary artery segments[68, 69]; in contrast, vessel diameter increases in normal arteries when arithmetic tasks are performed. Thus, although myocardial oxygen demands rise after mental stress, as indicated by increases in systolic blood pressure, ischemia is also due to a primary decrease in coronary blood flow.

The mechanism by which an activity triggers ischemia has been the subject of considerable controversy, primarily over the relative contribution of decreases in myocardial oxygen supply versus increases in myocardial oxygen demand. The view that transient ischemia is due to decreases in coronary artery flow is supported by observations in vitro and in animal studies that atherosclerotic arteries show exaggerated vascular sensitivity to norepinephrine, histamine, and serotonin. A paradoxical vasoconstrictor response to acetylcholine has also been demonstrated in patients.[70–72]

In ambulatory patients with proved coronary artery disease, episodes of transient myocardial ischemia are frequent and most often silent during assessment of heart rate changes by Holter monitoring or the use of simultaneous electrocardiographic and blood pressure measurements.[73] Such events are often preceded by increases in heart rate and blood pressure, suggesting that increased myocardial oxygen demands play a significant role in silent ischemia. However, changes in coronary artery tone and blood flow can also play roles. Other possible triggers of myocardial ischemia or coronary thrombosis include cigarette smoking and assumption of the upright posture. Cigarette smoking causes a decrease in myocardial blood flow (as measured by decreased rubidium-82 uptake).

The effect of sleep stage on the development of myocardial ischemia seems to be quite clear in the canine model, although the relation in human beings is still unclear. In dogs with normal coronary arteries, small but significant reductions in heart rate and left circumflex coronary blood flow and an increase in coronary vascular resistance were seen in slow-wave sleep.[74, 75] During REM sleep, there were pronounced, phasic increases in heart rate (35%) and coronary blood flow (35%) lasting 15 to 20 sec.[74] In dogs with coronary artery stenosis (60%), however, the phasic REM increases in heart rate resulted in a 38% decrease in coronary blood flow and a 56% increase in coronary vascular resistance.[75] These surges are eliminated by bilateral stellectomy, indicating that they were mediated by the sympathetic nervous system. Thus, changes in autonomic tone may be important in the genesis of nocturnal ischemia. However, the increase in heart rate itself may be a compounding factor because diastolic perfusion time is reduced at higher heart rate. There is a very high correlation ($r = .96$) between changes in heart rate and coronary blood flow.

In humans, the relation between sleep stage and nocturnal angina is not as clear.[76–79] A meta-analysis of 12 studies clearly demonstrates a nonuniform nighttime distribution of acute cardiac events. This is consistent with the hypothesis that sleep state–dependent fluctuations in autonomic nervous system activity trigger major cardiovascular events[79]; however, mechanisms of nocturnal angina are still not completely understood. Patients with nocturnal angina may have sleep apnea. Treatment of the apnea may ameliorate the angina.[42a] The specific abnormality in apnea (e.g., hypoxemia, increased sympathetic tone) that is responsible is not known.

Morning increases in several physiological factors may predispose to myocardial ischemia and cardiovascular events. For example, the increase in blood pressure on awakening with an attendant heart rate increase may cause plaque rupture. Coronary arterial tone is increased, and this could further reduce flow through a previously fixed, stenotic vessel. Increase in blood viscosity and increased platelet aggregation on assuming the upright posture (Fig. 86–4), as well as reduction in circulating tissue-type plasminogen activator activity, may promote a state of relative hypercoagulability. Such a thrombotic tendency may increase the likelihood that a new thrombus may propagate over small plaque fissures and lead to occlusion.[80]

Changes in thrombotic tendency in themselves are likely insufficient to precipitate coronary ischemia, and the effect may be different in unstable patients. Changes in fibrinopeptide A (FPA; a specific product of fibrinogen cleavage by thrombin and a useful index of fibrin formation in vivo) are a result of, rather than the cause of, variant angina.[81] In this type of patient, the nocturnal increase in FPA, in conjunction with nocturnal ischemia, can be suppressed with heparin (an inhibitor of thrombin activation), whereas angina attacks and their circadian variation continue. Plasma FPA levels, and thus thrombin formation, are increased in patients with variant angina as a consequence of coronary spasm. Coronary spasm probably causes injury to the coronary endothelium and may trigger the coagulation cascade. Whether this leads to coronary obstruction resulting in stable angina or acute myocardial infarction likely depends on the degree of activation of the fibrinolytic system.

Although there is coincidence of 24-h periodicity of disease onset and physiological processes, the degree to which disease periodicity results from a true endoge-

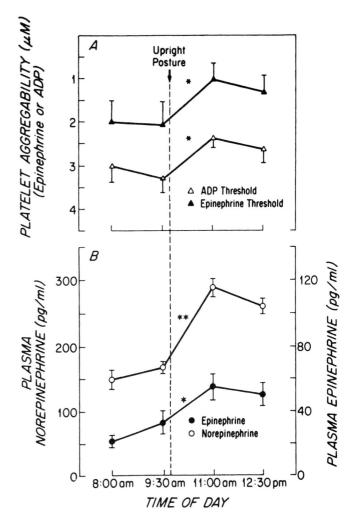

Figure 86–4. *A,* Plot of minimum concentration of adenosine diphosphate (ADP) and epinephrine required to produce biphasic aggregation on day of experimental activity. Scale of y-axis is inverted so that increasing aggregability is represented by upward sloping line. Subjects were awakened and lights were turned on after the 8 AM sample. After the 9:30 AM sample, subjects first assumed upright posture. After the 11 AM sample, subjects showed and walked up and down three flights of stairs (mean ± standard error of the mean [SEM] of 16 subjects). *B,* Plasma concentrations of epinephrine and norepinephrine on day of experimental activity (mean ± SEM of 13 subjects). Duncan's post hoc test of consecutive samples (two-way analysis of variance): *P < .05; **P < .01. (From Brezinski DA, Tofler GH, Muller JE, et al. Morning increase in platelet aggregability: association with the upright posture. Circulation. 1988;78:35–40.)

nous circadian rhythm or from the daily rest-activity cycle is only partially characterized. For example, cortisol secretion has an endogenous circadian rhythm independent of daily activities, whereas circadian rhythm of platelet aggregability is dependent on body position. Heart rate, blood pressure, plasma norepinephrine levels, and plasma renin activity exhibit an underlying endogenous circadian variation that is amplified by awakening (assuming the upright posture and exercise).[80] Indeed, the rest-activity cycle may be the major determinant of disease onset because adjustment for time of awakening shows that the onset of infarction and increases in transient ischemia follow awakening.

The changes in plasma norepinephrine and epinephrine concentrations associated with assumption of the upright posture and increased platelet aggregability are shown (see Fig. 86–4). Thus, rising at night is often associated with episodes of myocardial ischemia, and like the morning events on rising, it is an important trigger of ischemia in patients with coronary artery disease. With understanding of the effect of rising on vascular tone, platelet aggregability,[82] and so on, it might come as no surprise that cerebrovascular accidents are concentrated on awakening. Coexisting abnormalities in cerebrovascular autoregulation may compound the postural change in blood pressure and further contribute to cerebral ischemia.

Effect of Treatment on Circadian Variation in Hypertension and Transient Ischemia

The identification of circadian rhythm in transient ischemia and the recognition of the physiological processes that promote it have led to the hope of more rational therapy and improved quality of life. A review of previous works suggests that although standard therapies (e.g., beta blockers, calcium channel blockers, aspirin) reduce symptoms, some of their beneficial effects may be related to effects on circadian rhythms in transient ischemia. Moreover, in attempt to match the treatment of hypertension with circadian blood pressure rhythm, new drug formulations are being designed to provide optimal drug concentrations during the early morning hours while still maintaining antihypertensive activity throughout the day.

Beta Blockers

Since the early 1980s, beta blockers (e.g., atenolol, metoprolol, propranolol) have been part of post–myocardial infarction care. Analysis of data from several studies involving beta-blocker trials reveals similar findings. Beta blockers reduce the incidence of sudden death, and they reduce the early morning circadian peak in sudden death or myocardial infarction.[83] Analysis of the MILIS[2] database revealed that patients who were receiving beta blockers at the time of myocardial infarction did not have a morning peak in the incidence of myocardial infarction. This also was seen in the ISAM study, in which patients receiving beta blockers did not have an increased morning incidence of myocardial infarction.[19] The Beta-Blocker Heart Attack Trial (BHAT) was a randomized, double-blind placebo-controlled study of propranolol in the prevention of death and complications after acute myocardial infarction. In this study, propranolol had its major effect in the early morning hours.[84]

Beta blockers also reduce the morning incidence in transient myocardial ischemia, and this reduction will probably apply to all beta blockers without intrinsic sympathomimetic activity (e.g., pindolol) when administered to have a 24-h effect.[83–87] Because of their varying durations of action, the dosing schedule will vary among agents.

There are at least three possible mechanisms by which beta blockers reduce angina and alter the circadian variation in myocardial ischemia; these include effects on blood pressure and heart rate, cardiac arrhythmias, and platelet/clotting mechanisms. Beta blockers reduce heart rate and blood pressure. Although circadian variation in blood pressure is maintained with the use of beta blockers, the reduction in peak systolic values decreases the intravascular forces that can lead to plaque rupture and development of ischemia.

Results from the BHAT study revealed a decrease in complex ventricular ectopy and, in particular, a reduction in the increase that occurs with awakening. Whether this is a secondary reduction in ischemia (and secondary arrhythmia) or a direct myocardial and arrhythmia threshold effect is uncertain. The effect of beta blockers may be in the central nervous system in regions related to stress. Finally, beta blockers may have weak antiplatelet effects, although this is still somewhat controversial.[88, 89]

Calcium Channel Blockers

Calcium channel antagonists are effective agents for reducing transient myocardial ischemia. Verapamil, which is effective in lowering heart rate and blood pressure, reduces both symptomatic and asymptomatic myocardial ischemia. The effects of verapamil on circadian variation of ischemia are unknown. However, newer preparations of verapamil, which take into account circadian changes in blood pressure, can have significant benefits in the treatment of hypertension. A controlled-onset, extended-release preparation of verapamil, dosed at bedtime, is highly effective in reducing blood pressure and heart rate in the early morning hours while maintaining activity for 24 h. Furthermore, it is not associated with excessive hypotension in the middle of the sleep period, when blood pressure is typically lowest in patients with essential hypertension.[90]

Diltiazem also reduces silent and symptomatic ischemia but does not seem to completely abolish the morning increase in episodes. Nifedipine does not lower heart rate and when used as monotherapy is incomplete in altering myocardial ischemia. Some studies have reported no influence on ischemic circadian variability,[35] but this may have been due to dosage and frequency of administration. Although a reduction in circadian distribution of ischemia can be shown using nifedipine (mean dose, 80 mg/day) in four divided doses,[91] this form of therapy (four times a day) has been linked to orthostatic hypotension and possibly ischemic changes, so it is no longer recommended.

Angiotensin-Converting Enzyme Inhibitors

Angiotensin-converting enzyme inhibitors (ACEIs) are effective and very important drugs in the treatment of hypertension and congestive heart failure. There is little question that these medications decrease cardiac morbidity rates and are extremely cost-effective thera-

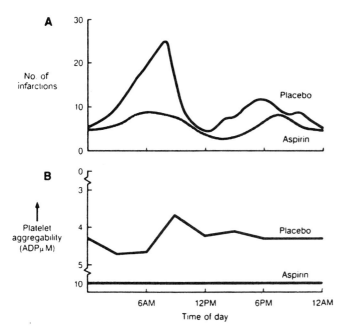

Figure 86–5. Number of infarctions *(A)* and platelet aggregability *(B)* in relation to time of day for patients taking either aspirin or placebo. Aspirin abolishes the morning peak in myocardial infarction. (From Ridker PM, Manson JE, Buring JE, et al. Circadian variation of acute myocardial infarction and the effect of low dose aspirin in a randomized trial of physicians. Circulation. 1990;82:897–902.)

pies. ACEIs do not appear to influence the circadian rhythm in blood pressure or cause excessive hypotension during sleep in contrast to some calcium channel drugs and therefore may be safer medications in patients with preexisting vascular disease.[92, 93] There are no data on the effects of ACEIs on sleep and sleep structure.

Aspirin

Increased platelet aggregation in the morning and on assuming the upright posture may contribute to the observed circadian variation in onset of acute myocardial infarction. The Physicians Health Study[23] revealed that aspirin was associated with a mean reduction in infarction of 44.8% over the entire 24-h period, with a 59.3% reduction during morning waking hours compared with a 34.1% reduction during the remaining hours of the day. The placebo group showed a bimodal circadian variation in the onset of myocardial infarction, whereas the aspirin group did not, primarily due to an absent morning peak. The reduction in death with the use of aspirin is due in large part to elimination by aspirin of the morning effects on platelet aggregability[94] (Fig. 86–5).

Although the mechanisms for transient ischemia are likely similar for cardiac and cerebral events, little work has been done to assess the effect of treatment on circadian distribution of cerebral ischemia.

SUMMARY

The circadian variation of cardiovascular events, including myocardial infarction, sudden cardiac death,

transient myocardial ischemia, and thrombotic stroke, that is characterized by a morning peak and night time nadir has been well documented. The effects are significantly attenuated by beta blockers and aspirin, suggesting that increased sympathetic tone and increased platelet aggregability are important factors that contribute to the diurnal variation of these cardiovascular events.

References

1. Pell S, D'Alonzo CA. Acute myocardial infarction in a large industrial population: report of a 6 year study of 1356 cases. JAMA. 1979;185:831–838.
2. Muller JE, Stone PH, Turi ZG, et al. Circadian variation in the frequency of onset of acute myocardial infarction. N Engl J Med. 1985;313:1315–1322.
3. Guillaume AC. Etudes sur le mechanisme neuropsychique de l'hypertension arterielle: physiologie et physiopathologie des reactions tensionelles à l'emotion. Biol Med (Paris). 1959;48:252–320.
4. Master AM. The role of effort and occupation (including physicians) in coronary occlusion. JAMA. 1960;174:942–948.
5. Smolensky MH, Tatar SE, Bergman SA, et al. Circadian rhythmic aspects of human cardiovascular function: a review by chronobiologic statistical methods. Chronobiologia. 1976;3:337–371.
6. Bok KD, Kreuzenbeck W. Spontaneous blood-pressure variations in hypertension: the effect of antihypertensive therapy and correlations with the incidence of complications. In: Gross F, ed. Antihypertensive Therapy: Principles and Practice: An International Symposium. New York, NY: Springer-Verlag; 1966:224–241.
7. Johansson BW. Myocardial infarction in Malmo, 1960–1968. Acta Med Scand. 1972;191:505–515.
8. Myers A, Dewar HA. Circumstances attending 100 sudden deaths from coronary artery disease with coroner's necropsies. Br Heart J. 1975;37:1133–1143.
9. Pedoe HT, Clayton D, Morris JN, et al. Coronary heart-attacks in East London. Lancet. 1975;2:833–838.
10. Churina SK, Ganelina IE, Volpert EI. On the distribution of the incidence of acute myocardial infarction within a 24 hour period [in Russian]. Kardiologia. 1975;15:115–118.
11. Gyarfas I, Cxukas A, Horvath-Gaudi I. Analysis of the diurnal periodicity of acute myocardial infarction attacks. Sante Publique (Bucur). 1976;19:77–84.
12. Myocardial Infarction Community Registers. Results of a WHO international collaborative study coordinated by the regional office for Europe. In: Public Health in Europe, No. 5. Copenhagen, Denmark: Regional Office for Europe (World Health Organization); 1976:1–232.
13. Miller-Craig MW, Bishop CN, Raftery EG. Circadian variation of blood pressure. Lancet. 1978;1:795–797.
14. Pickering TG. The influence of daily activity on ambulatory blood pressure. Am Heart J. 1988;116:1141–1145.
15. Richards AM, Nicholls MG, Espiner EA, et al. Diurnal patterns of blood pressure, heart rate and vasoactive hormones in normal man. Clin Exp Hypertens. 1986;A8:153–166.
16. Khatri IM, Freis ED. Hemodynamic changes during sleep. J Appl Physiol. 1967;23:964–970.
17. Coccagna G, Montovani M, Brignani F, et al. Arterial pressure changes during spontaneous sleep in man. Electroencephalogr Clin Neurophysiol. 1971;31:277–281.
18. Mansoor GA, White WB. Ambulatory blood pressure and cardiovascular risk stratification. J Vasc Med Biol. 1994;5:61–68.
19. Roman MJ, Pickering TG, Schwartz JE, et al. Is the absence of a normal nocturnal fall in blood pressure (nondipping) associated with cardiovascular target organ damage? J Hypertens. 1997;15:969–978.
20. Mochizuki Y, Okutami M, Donfeng Y, et al. Limited reproducibility of circadian variation in blood pressure dippers and nondippers. Am J Hypertens. 1998;11:403–409.
21. Muller JG, Tofler GH, Stone PH. Circadian variation and triggers

of onset of acute cardiovascular disease. Circulation. 1989;79:733–743.

22. Willich SN, Pohjola-Sintonen S, Bhatia SJS, et al. Suppression of silent ischemia by metoprolol without alteration of morning increase of platelet aggregability in patients with stable coronary artery disease. Circulation. 1989;79:557–565.

23. Ridker PM, Manson JE, Buring JE, et al. Circadian variation of acute myocardial infarction and the effect of low dose aspirin in a randomized trial of physicians. Circulation. 1990;82:897–902.

24. Hjalmarson A, Gilpen EA, Nicod P, et al. Differing circadian patterns of symptom onset in subgroups of patients with acute myocardial infarction. Circulation. 1989;80:267–275.

25. Kleinman NS, Schechtman KB, Young PM, et al. Lack of diurnal variation in the onset of non-Q wave infarction. Circulation. 1990;81:548–555.

26. Thompson DR, Blandford RL, Sutton TW, et al. Time of onset of chest pain in acute myocardial infarction. Int J Cardiol. 1985;7:139–146.

27. Thompson DR, Sutton TW, Jowett NI, et al. Circadian variation in the frequency of onset of chest pain in acute myocardial infarction. Br Heart J. 1991;65:177–178.

28. Cannon CP, McCabe CH, Stone PH, et al. Circadian variation in the onset of unstable angina and non-Q-wave acute myocardial infarction (the TIMI III Registry and TIMI IIIB). Am J Cardiol. 1997;79:253–258.

29. Fava S, Azzopardi J, Muscat HA, et al. Absence of circadian variation in the onset of acute myocardial infarction in diabetic subjects. Br Heart J. 1995;74:370–372.

30. Willich SN, Lowel H, Lewis M, et al. Weekly variation of acute myocardial infarction: increased Monday risk in the working population. Circulation. 1994;90:87–93.

31. Spielberg C, Falkenhahn D, Willich SN, et al. Circadian, day-of-week, and seasonal variability in myocardial infarction: comparison between working and retired patients. Am Heart J. 1996;132:579–585.

32. Rocco MB, Barry J, Campbell S, et al. Circadian variation of transient myocardial ischemia in patients with coronary artery disease. Circulation. 1987;75:395–400.

33. Quyyumi AA, Mockus L, Wright C, et al. Pathology of ambulatory ST segment changes in patients with varying severity of coronary artery disease. Br Heart J. 1985;53:186–193.

34. Shea MJ, Deanfield JE, Wilson R, et al. Transient ischemia in angina pectoris: frequent silent events with everyday activities. Am J Cardiol. 1985;56:34E–38E.

35. Mulcahy D, Keegan J, Cunningham D, et al. Circadian variation of total ischemic burden and its alterations with anti-anginal agents. Lancet. 1988;2:755–759.

36. Currie P, Saltissi S. Transient myocardial ischemia after acute myocardial infarction. Br Heart J. 1990;65:299–303.

37. Mickley H, Pless T, Nielsen JR, et al. Circadian variation of transient myocardial ischemia in the early out of hospital period after first acute myocardial infarction. Am J Cardiol. 1991;67:927–932.

38. Prinzmetal M, Kennamer R, Merliss R, et al. Angina pectoris, I: a variant form of angina pectoris. Am J Med. 1959;27:375–388.

39. Araki H, Koiwaya Y, Nakagaki D, et al. Diurnal distribution of ST segment elevation and related arrhythmias in patients with variant angina: a study by ambulatory ECG monitoring. Circulation. 1983;67:995–1000.

40. Yasue H, Omote S, Takizawa A, et al. Circadian variation of exercise capacity in patients with Prinzmetal's variant angina: role of exercise induced coronary arterial spasm. Circulation. 1979;59:938–948.

41. Waters DD, Miller DD, Bouchard A, et al. Circadian variation and variant angina. Am J Cardiol. 1984;54:61–64.

42. Bogarty P, Waters DD. Circadian patterns in coronary disease: the mournfulness of morning. Can J Cardiol. 1988;4:5–11.

42a. Franklin KA, Nilsson JB, Sahlin C, et al. Sleep apnea and nocturnal angina. Lancet. 1995;345:1085–1087.

43. Muller JE, Ludmer PL, Willich SN, et al. Circadian variation in the frequency of sudden cardiac death. Circulation. 1987;75:131–138.

44. Willich SN, Levy D, Rocco MB, et al. Circadian variation in the incidence of sudden cardiac death in The Framingham Heart Study population. Am J Cardiol. 1987;60:801–806.

45. Smolensky M, Hulberg F, Sargent F. Chronobiology of the life sequence. In: Itoh S, Ogata K, Yoshimur A, eds. Advances in Climatic Physiology. New York, NY: Springer-Verlag; 1972:281–318.

46. Mitler MM, Hajdukovic RM, Shafer R, et al. When people die: cause of death vs. time of death. Am J Med. 1987;82:266–274.

47. Peckova M, Fahrenbruch CE, Cobb LA, et al. Circadian variations in the occurrence of cardiac arrests: initial and repeat episodes. Circulation. 1998;98:31–39.

48. Marler JR, Price TR, Clark GL, et al. Morning increase in onset of ischemic stroke. Stroke. 1989;20:473–476.

49. Argentino C, Toni D, Rasura M, et al. Circadian variation in the frequency of ischemic stroke. Stroke. 1990;21:387–389.

50. Pasqualetti P, Natali G, Casale R, et al. Epidemiological chrono-risk of stroke. Acta Neurol Scand. 1990;81:71–74.

51. Gallerani M, Manfredini R, Ricci L, et al. Chronobiological aspects of acute cerebrovascular diseases. Acta Neurol Scand. 1993;87:482–487.

52. Marsh EE, Biller J, Adams HP, et al. Circadian variation in onset of acute ischemic stroke. Arch Neurol. 1990;47:1178–1180.

53. Elliott WJ. Circadian variation in the riming of stroke onset: a meta-analysis. Stroke. 1998;29:992–996.

54. Giubilei F, Strano S, Lino S, et al. Autonomic nervous activity during sleep in middle cerebral artery infarction. Cerebrovasc Dis. 1998;8:118–123.

55. Jaquet F, Goldstein IB, Shapiro D. Effects of age and gender on ambulatory blood pressure and heart rate. J Hum Hypertens. 1998;12:253–257.

56. Thurton MB, Deegan T. Circadian variations of plasma catecholamines, cortisol and immunoreactive insulin concentrates in supine subjects. Clin Chem Acta. 1974;55:389–350.

56a. Munakata M, Imai Y, Abe K, et al. Involvement of the hypothalamo-pituitary-adrenal axis in the control of circadian blood pressure rhythm. J Hypertens. 1988;6(suppl 4):544–546.

57. Colantonio D, Pasqualetti P, Casale R, et al. Is atrial natriuretic peptide important in the circadian rhythm of blood pressure? Am J Cardiol. 1988;63:1166.

58. Portaluppi F, Montanari L, Bagni B, et al. Circadian rhythms of atrial natriuretic peptides, blood pressure, and heart rate in normal subjects. Cardiology. 1989;76:428–432.

59. Krum H, Louis WJ, Brown DJ, et al. Diurnal blood pressure variation in quadriplegic chronic spinal cord injury patients. Clin Sci. 1991;80:271–276.

60. Krum H, Howes LG, Rowe PR, et al. Steady state [³H]noradrenaline kinetics in quadriplegic chronic spinal cord injury. J Autonom Pharmacol. 1990;10:221–226.

61. Caruana MP, Lahiri A, Cashman PMM, et al. Effects of chronic congestive heart failure secondary to coronary artery disease on the circadian rhythm of blood pressure and heart rate. Am J Cardiol. 1988;62:755–759.

62. Verdecchia P, Schillaci B, Borgioni C, et al. Gender, day-night blood pressure changes and left ventricular mass in essential hypertension: dippers and peakers. Am J Hypertens. 1995;8:193–196.

62a. Imai Y, Ohkubo T, Tsuji I, et al. Clinical significance of nocturnal blood pressure monitoring. Clin Exp Hypertens. 1999;21:717–727.

62b. Imai Y. Prognostic significance of ambulatory blood pressure. Blood Press Monit. 1999;4:249–256.

63. White WB, Schullman P, McCabe EJ, et al. Average daily blood pressure, not office blood pressure, determines cardiac function in patients with hypertension. JAMA. 1989;261:873–877.

63a. Mallion JM, Baguet JP, Siche JP, et al. Clinical value of ambulatory blood pressure monitoring. J Hypertens. 1999;17:585–595.

64. Barry J, Selwin AP, Nabel EG, et al. Frequency of ST segment depression produced by mental stress in stable angina pectoris from coronary artery disease. Am J Cardiol. 1988;61:989–993.

65. Mittleman MA, Maclure M, Tofler GH, et al. Triggering of acute myocardial infarction by heavy exertion: protection against triggering by regular exertion. N Engl J Med. 1993;329:1677–1683.

66. Freeman LJ, Nickson PGF, Sallabank P, et al. Psychological stress and silent myocardial ischemia. Am Heart J. 1987;114:477–482.

67. Rozanski A, Bairey CN, Crantz DS, et al. Mental stress and the induction of silent myocardial ischemia in patients with coronary artery disease. N Engl J Med. 1988;318:1005–1012.

68. Rebecca G, Wagner R, Zebede T, et al. Pathogenic mechanisms

causing transient myocardial ischemia with mental arousal in patients with coronary artery disease [abstract]. Clin Res. 1986;34:338A.

69. Deanfield JE, Shea M, Kensett M, et al. Silent myocardial ischemia due to mental stress. Lancet. 1984;2:1001–1005.

70. Ginsburg R, Bristow MR, Davis K, et al. Quantitative pharmacologic responses of normal and atherosclerotic isolated human epicardial coronary arteries. Circulation. 1984;69:430–440.

71. Ganz P, Alexander RW. New insights into the cellular mechanisms of vasospasm. Am J Cardiol. 1985;56:11E–15E.

72. Ludmer PL, Selwyn AP, Shook TL, et al. Paradoxical vasoconstriction induced by acetylcholine in atherosclerotic coronary arteries. N Engl J Med. 1986;315:1046–1061.

73. Deedwania PC, Nelson JR. Pathophysiology of silent myocardial ischemia during daily life: hemodynamic evaluation by simultaneous electrocardiographic and blood pressure monitoring. Circulation. 1990;82:1296–1304.

74. Kirby DA, Verrier RL. Differential effects of sleep stage on coronary hemodynamic function. Am J Physiol. 1989;256:H1378–H1383.

75. Kirby DA, Verrier RL. Differential effects of sleep stage on coronary hemodynamic function during stenosis. Physiol Behav. 1985;45:1017–1020.

76. Murao S, Harumi K, Katayama S, et al. All night polysomnographic studies of natural angina. Jpn Heart J. 1972;13:295–305.

77. Nowlin JB, Troyer WE, Collins WS, et al. The association of nocturnal or angina pectoris with dreaming. Ann Intern Med. 1965;63:1040–1046.

78. Karacan I, Williams RL, Taylor WJ. Sleep characteristics of patients with angina pectoris. Psychosomatics. 1969;10:280–284.

79. Lavery CE, Mittleman MA, Cohen MC, et al. Nonuniform nighttime distribution of acute cardiac events: a possible effect of sleep states. Circulation. 1997;96:3321–3327.

80. Brezinski DA, Tofler GH, Muller JE, et al. Morning increase in platelet aggregability: association with the upright posture. Circulation. 1988;78:35–40.

81. Ogawa N, Yasue H, Oshima S, et al. Circadian variation of plasma fibrinopeptide A level in patients with variant angina. Circulation. 1989;80:1617–1626.

82. Barry J, Campbell S, Yeung AC, et al. Waking and rising at night is a trigger of myocardial ischemia. Am J Cardiol. 1991;67:1067–1072.

83. Willich SN, Linderer T, Wegscheider K, et al. Increased morning incidence of myocardial infarction in the ISAM study: absence with prior beta-adrenergic blockade. Circulation. 1989;80:853–858.

84. Peters RW, Muller JE, Goldstein S, et al. Propranolol and the morning increase in the frequency of sudden cardiac deaths (BHAT study). Am J Cardiol. 1989;63:1518–1520.

85. Imperi GA, Lambert CR, Roy K, et al. Effects of titrated beta blockade (metoprolol) on silent myocardial ischemia in ambulatory patients with coronary artery disease. Am J Cardiol. 1987;60:519–524.

86. Cohn PF, Lawson WE. Effects of long acting propranolol on A.M. and P.M. peaks in silent myocardial ischemia. Am J Cardiol. 1989;63:872–873.

87. Lambert CR, Coy K, Imperi G, et al. Influences of beta-adrenergic blockade defined by time series analysis on circadian variation of heart rate and ambulatory myocardial ischemia. Am J Cardiol. 1989;64:835–839.

88. Green D, Rossi EC, Haring O. The Beta-Blocker Heart Attack Trial: studies of platelets and factor VIII. Thromb Res. 1982;28:261–267.

89. Vilen L, Jutti J, Swedbert K, et al. ADP induced platelet aggregation and metroprolol treatment of myocardial infarction patients. Acta Med Scand. 1985;217:15–20.

90. White WB, Anders RJ, MacIntyre JM, et al, and the Verapamil Study Group. Nocturnal dosing of a novel delivery system of verapamil for systemic hypertension. Am J Cardiol. 1995;76:375–380.

91. Nesto RW, Phillips RT, Kett KG, et al. Effect of nifedipine on total ischemia activity and circadian distribution of myocardial ischemic episodes in angina pectoris. Am J Cardiol. 1991;67:128–132.

92. Takabatake T, Ohta H, Yamamoto Y, et al. Effect of atenolol or enalapril on diurnal changes of blood pressure in Japanese mild to moderate hypertensives: a double blind, randomised, crossover trial. J Hum Hypertens. 1991;5:199–204.

93. Azuma T, Matsubara T, Nagai Y, et al. Effects of antihypertensives on circadian blood pressure in hypertensive patients with previous brain infarction. J Hum Hypertens. 1997;11:637–640.

94. McCall NT, Tofler GH, Schafer AI, et al. The effect of enteric coated aspirin on the morning increase in platelet activity. Am Heart J. 1991;121:1382–1388.

87

Chronic Fatigue Syndrome and Fibromyalgia

Ralph Pascualy
Dedra Buchwald

OVERVIEW

This chapter reviews current evidence of the relationships between sleep disturbance and fibromyalgia (FM) and chronic fatigue syndrome (CFS). We discuss strategies directed toward sleep improvement as an essential treatment tool.

Rheumatologists are now well aware of the co-morbidity of sleep disturbance with the fatigue, depression, and pain of rheumatic disease.[1-5] The majority of patients with a rheumatic disease complain of chronic fatigue.[1, 2] However, clinical study of sleep disturbance in rheumatic disease is a relatively recent endeavor. Moldofsky's studies[6] of the alpha electroencephalographic (EEG) anomaly found in nonrapid eye movement (NREM) sleep in FM and other rheumatic diseases focused clinicians on the importance of evaluating and treating patients not only for their rheumatic disease and its associated pain but also for sleep disturbance.

There is a great deal of controversy surrounding symptoms of chronic pain and fatigue and their relationship to sleep abnormalities. Some respected authorities have questioned whether CFS and FM even exist, and it has been suggested that these may be fad diagnoses.[7-9] There is a controversy in the literature about whether abnormal sleep causes the daytime symptoms, or whether the disorders cause the abnormal sleep. There is further controversy about whether the sleep abnormalities in these patients are diagnostic. In the background of these controversies, one issue is inescapable: patients labeled with these disorders and with complaints of fatigue and pain will be referred to sleep specialists. Because of the controversies, the reader should be advised that the approach outlined in this chapter may not be one that is universally accepted.

In clinical practice, many patients who have been diagnosed as having FM or CFS do not meet research criteria for these conditions. Often they also have coexisting multiple psychiatric, medical, and psychosocial problems. The healthcare industry that has grown around patients with these and other syndromes can result in self-diagnosis or in patients' identification with FM or CFS as a simple explanation for their complex difficulties. Many experienced physicians acknowledge that some well-characterized patients have puzzling and severe medical syndromes consistent with the classic descriptions of these conditions apparently free of confounding factors. Unfortunately, the overzealous labeling of patients with complex psychiatric, psychosocial, and medical factors as having CFS has led to widespread disbelief and skepticism among physicians that many patients labeled with these syndromal diagnoses do not have real pathological conditions that can be treated. These views or biases about the reality of the syndromes in general, or their applicability to specific patients, can become an obstacle to careful clinical assessment of their sleep disorder and the delivery of effective treatment.

CHRONIC FATIGUE SYNDROME

Chronic fatigue syndrome is defined as a disorder characterized by generalized incapacitating fatigue of at least 6 months' duration that is medically unexplained and is associated with impaired physical and mental functioning[10, 11] and complaints of poor-quality sleep.[12, 13] Fatigue is a common symptom in the community[1-4] and a frequent complaint in clinical practice, being reported by at least 20% of patients seeking medical care.[5, 14-17] Typically, the fatigue is transient, self-limiting, and explained by prevailing circumstances. However, a minority of patients experience persistent and disabling fatigue. In some cases, such fatigue may result from medical diseases such as anemia or hypothyroidism. However, in other individuals, chronic fatigue cannot be readily explained by organic illness and may represent CFS.

CFS is an illness characterized by profound disabling fatigue lasting at least 6 months accompanied by symptoms of sleep disturbance, musculoskeletal pain, and neurocognitive impairment.[18] As its name implies, CFS is a symptom-based diagnosis without distinguishing physical examination or routine laboratory findings. Although infectious, immunological, autonomic nervous system, neuroendocrine, sleep disorder, and psychiatric mechanisms have been investigated, a unifying etiology for CFS has yet to emerge. Regardless of the pathogenesis, those with CFS have substantially impaired functional status similar to other chronic diseases, resulting in significant personal and economic morbidity.[19-21] Treatment for CFS is generally supportive and symptom-based. However, there does appear to be a role for antidepressant pharmacotherapy, physiotherapy, and cognitive behavioral therapy in some patients with CFS. Advances in care for CFS require comprehensive investigation into its pathophysiology, including sleep.

CFS has been reported worldwide and case definitions have been developed by the Centers for Disease Control and Prevention (CDC), and British and Australian researchers.[13, 22, 23] Although diagnostic criteria only recently have been formulated, CFS is unlikely to be a new entity. Several clinical syndromes, both sporadic and epidemic, have been described previously that, in retrospect, appear to share key clinical features. These include neurasthenia, benign myalgic encephalitis, and "chronic Epstein-Barr virus (EBV) infection." In 1987, a group of epidemiologists, researchers, and clinicians convened by the CDC developed a consensus statement on the salient clinical characteristics of the syndrome.[23a] Chronic EBV infection was renamed CFS, thus removing the implication that EBV is the etiologic agent and emphasizing the syndrome's most striking feature. This original CDC case definition consisted of 2 major and 14 minor (11 symptom and 3 physical examination) criteria. A case of CFS was required to have at least 6 months of unexplained debilitating fatigue and eight minor criteria. In 1994, the CDC directed the formulation of a new international case definition which incorporated major components of the original criteria.[11] This new case definition eliminated the physical examination criteria, reduced the number of required symptoms, and clarified exclusionary conditions. Like that of FM, the CFS case definition now includes patients with most nonpsychotic psychiatric disorders.[22] However, in contrast to the guidelines for diagnosing FM, the CFS criteria are not empirically based and have never been subjected to rigorous scrutiny.

FIBROMYALGIA

Fibromyalgia, a common form of nonarticular rheumatism, is another illness associated with fatigue. Although its hallmark is diffuse muscle pain and stiffness, patients almost invariably report sleep disturbances, severe fatigue, and often a constellation of other symptoms virtually identical to CFS.[24-26] Like CFS, FM is of unknown etiology and affects primarily women.[24-26] Routine laboratory tests also are generally normal; the physical examination, however, is remarkable for painful tender points.[25] A small body of work suggests there is extensive overlap between these conditions, and some investigators believe they may represent the same condition.[26-29]

Only recently have formal, widely accepted criteria for FM been developed. In the past, a variety of definitions were in use, some of which required fewer tender points or the presence of other signs and symptoms such as skin roll tenderness, irritable bowel syndrome, swelling, paresthesias, or disturbed sleep. In 1990, the American College of Rheumatology (ACR) endorsed a case definition for FM based on the presence of widespread musculoskeletal pain and tender points of a specified number and location. More specifically, a diagnosis of FM required the presence of 11 of 18 (9 bilateral) tender points. Nonmusculoskeletal features were not incorporated into the case definition because they were not found to improve its operating characteristics. Although current ACR diagnostic criteria, as outlined by Wolfe et al.,[30] do not list sleep disorders, early diagnostic criteria for FM included abnormal sleep characteristics (e.g., nonrestorative sleep, alpha intrusion into the EEG of NREM sleep).[31, 32] Histological, metabolic, muscle strength, and tenderness studies all point to pain generated by central nervous system (CNS) mechanisms.[33] It is surprising that despite their remarkably different diagnostic criteria, CFS and FM have many similarities.

The almost universal presence of disordered sleep in FM patients and the widely observed improvement in pain symptoms with improved sleep emphasize the importance of access to sleep specialists experienced in treating these conditions.

ROLE OF PAIN, PSYCHIATRIC DISORDERS, AND OTHER ILLNESS-ASSOCIATED FACTORS IN DISTURBANCE OF SLEEP

Pain

The relationship between pain and disturbed sleep is complex, and appears to be bidirectional: pain during the day makes sleep more difficult; disturbances in sleep exacerbate pain.[34] Pain has been reported to be the most disruptive factor in the lives of patients with rheumatic disease,[17-20] and is perhaps the most commonly suggested cause of sleep disturbance in these patients. Other somatic factors that have been suggested include stiffness,[21] muscular discomfort,[35] and cognitive arousal.[36] Several prospective studies have examined the characteristics and correlates of daily changes in chronic musculoskeletal pain intensity.[27, 37-41] A recent study of attention to pain found it to be a function of the individual's sleep quality.[34]

The ability of pain to disrupt sleep has been objectively demonstrated; conversely, it has been suggested that disturbed sleep may exacerbate pain.[42-44]

Numerous investigators have sought to clarify the complex dynamics of the relationship between pain and sleep. Two prospective, within-person studies showed that the variability in the intensity of chronic musculoskeletal pain[40] and the quality of sleep in healthy volunteers[45] are predictive of the changes in emotional well-being that occur from day to day. Totterdell and colleagues[45] found that a given night's sleep quality was more likely to predict the following day's mood and minor physical symptoms than were a given day's mood and symptoms able to predict the following night's sleep quality. Another study found that a morning-after sleep diary by 46 chronic pain patients correlated with their retrospective ratings of pain severity.[46]

Interesting evidence of long-term chronological sequencing of sleep disturbance and chronic pain intensity emerged from a study of patients with rheumatoid arthritis (RA). Nicassio and Wallston[47] showed that baseline pain levels could predict sleep disturbance that would occur 2 years in the future. However, the reverse was not true: baseline sleep disturbance did not predict long-term changes in pain.

Attention to pain and its relationship to pain intensity and poor sleep quality in patients with FM has been studied by Affleck et al.[34] In one 30-d study, 50 women with FM were asked to recall their ratings of subjective sleep quality, pain intensity, and attention to pain using a palmtop computer. Poor sleepers reported significantly more pain than did women with higher quality of sleep. Their studies also supported other reports that a night of poor sleep tended to be followed by a significantly more painful day, and vice versa. Affleck's group has also found that individuals who are in greater pain pay more attention to it; and within-person analyses confirmed that they do so especially on more painful days. When individuals are compared, attention to pain is not related to sleep: poorer sleepers are not more likely to pay attention to their pain. However, within the individual, attention to pain is linked with changes in sleep regardless of changes that occur in pain intensity.

The role of psychological factors in the sleep-pain picture needs further study. It is not known whether attention to pain is associated with negative or intrusive thoughts and emotions or other psychological correlates.[46] It is possible that the mechanisms regulating somatic attention may be impaired by poor sleep, resulting in amplified attention to nociceptive stimuli. In particular, dysphoric mood can result from poor sleep, and is known to heighten attention to pain and other somatic symptoms.[34, 39] Brooks and McFarlane[15] found that anxiety and depression were common in patients with RA, with a prevalence between 20 and 80%. These rates are similar to those found in other chronic diseases.[16] Another hypothesis is that poor sleep impairs cognitive coping strategies that would aid in distraction from pain,[47] so that attention to pain is greater following a poor night's sleep.

Recent research reflects the increasing interest in the complex interaction between psychological and somatic processes in FM.[48] The sleep disturbance associated with FM has been interpreted as a vigilant arousal state during sleep.

The psychobiological interpretation of the perpetuation of FM symptoms suggests that heightened somatic attention acts to maintain altered thresholds for nociceptive stimulation.[49, 50] Although the underlying mechanisms remain poorly understood, this explanation is generally consistent with the view of FM as a disorder of pain modulation associated with altered neurosensory processing of painful stimuli and amplification of

pain sensations.[51, 52] CFS patients do not report more attention to their pain that do those with RA.[52] And there is evidence from both laboratory and field studies that somatic attention increases pain, whereas distraction reduces it.[53, 54]

These studies support the hypothesis that nonrestorative sleep may exacerbate pain complaints in patients with FM. Furthermore, the relation between sleep and attention to pain is bidirectional: the greater the attention to pain during the day, the poorer the sleep the following night; and the more disturbed the night's sleep, the more attention to pain the following day.

Neuropsychiatric Factors

A detailed review of neuropsychiatric factors is beyond the scope of this chapter. The most striking and clinically relevant problem is the difficulty in assessing the presence and severity of coexisting major and chronic depression. The classic vegetative symptoms required for these diagnoses may be present but are experienced and reported by the patient as caused solely by pain or sleep disturbance. Similarly the loss of social function and interest in pleasurable activities used to identify anhedonia (depression-associated pervasive loss of pleasure) may be experienced and reported as a "physical incapacity" accompanied by a denial of depressed mood, rather than as an understandable reaction to the physical symptoms.

The empirical use of antidepressants is often necessary but their failure does not rule out a significant affective component in the face of multiple striking vegetative symptoms. Conversely, a substantial improvement with a thorough and expert course of antidepressant therapy in the face of significant ongoing disability experienced as secondary to pain or fatigue needs to be carefully diagnosed rather than assuming that it represents a partially treated depression.

Neuropsychiatric factors in the relationship between sleep and pain are being explored, including the degree to which coexisting psychiatric disorders and developmental trauma are important features. Psychiatric disorders of particular importance include the somatiform and affective disorders. Developmental trauma, including physical and sexual abuse, also appear to be associated factors that affect pain focus and its regulation by sleep. It will be necessary to unravel the unavoidable confounder, that sleep disturbance is a common feature of affective disorders and that symptoms of depression are a common outcome of chronic pain, disturbed sleep, and developmental trauma.

Cognition

Cognitive deficits and associated performance decrements affect coping capabilities and thus have important implications for the treatment of these disorders. Similarities in the cognitive impairment found in patients with FM and CFS suggest a functional similarity between FM and CFS. Smith et al.[55] investigated memory, attention, and motor skills in 57 patients with

CFS and 19 controls. They found that CFS patients reported more depression, anxiety, physical symptoms, and cognitive difficulties and had psychomotor impairments, difficulty maintaining attention, and slower performance on semantic memory and logical reasoning tasks. Sandman et al.,[56] Altay et al.,[57] and Scheffers et al.[58] reported similar discordances. Further research should determine whether these cognitive impairments may be secondary to clinical depression.[59–61] For example, performance deficits like those in FM and CFS patients also occur in co-morbid disorders that also have disordered sleep (i.e., temporomandibular joint disorder).[61, 62] Thus, the performance deficits reported in depression may result from disordered sleep, fatigue, and somatic malaise, rather than from the cognitive components of depression. Nonrestorative sleep may thus leave affected individuals with cognitive deficits and little energy to apply cognitive and behavioral coping strategies that could help them distract themselves from their pain[63, 69] or fully cooperate with medical therapy.

POTENTIAL MECHANISMS IN FIBROMYALGIA

Neurohormones

Growth hormone (GH) is secreted primarily during stage 4 sleep. Approximately one third of FM patients show low levels of insulin-like growth factor I (somatomedin C), an indicator of GH production.[65] Administration of GH has been shown to improve sleep in patients with FM, compared with controls receiving a placebo.[66]

Elevated cerebrospinal fluid (CSF) levels of substance P have been found in patients with FM.[67] Substance P is a neuroactive peptide that is widely distributed throughout the nervous system, and some researchers suspect that it may contribute to arousals; however, its role in sleep regulation requires further investigation.[68]

Several studies have noted a decrease in CSF and blood serum levels of serotonin in FM patients.[69, 70] Low CNS levels of serotonin may be partially responsible for decreases in delta sleep and may predispose these patients to experience alpha intrusion. Sallanon et al.[71] reported that 5-hydroxytryptamine (5-HT, a serotonin precursor) is released by axons in the basal hypothalamus during waking. The authors postulated that 5-HT might induce sleep-promoting factors that are secondarily responsible for slow-wave and rapid eye movement (REM) sleep.[71] As further evidence implicating serotonin, low doses of tricyclic antidepressants (e.g., amitriptyline), which affect CNS serotonin metabolism, are able to reduce alpha intrusion and improve sleep quality in patients with FM.[23, 72] Plasma melatonin levels were found to be increased in women with FM but normal in women with CFS.[72a] The significance of these findings is unclear, but the data suggest that there is no rationale for the use of medications in these patients.

Neurotransmitters

Several nuclei in the thalamus are attracting interest for their potential role in the regulation of sleep and the pathogenesis of abnormal sleep. Neuroimaging studies indicate that regional cerebral blood flow (rCBF) to the thalamus and caudate nucleus is decreased in FM patients compared with normal controls.[29] These brain structures are involved in encoding and inhibiting pain transmission, and studies in the cat have shown that ablation of the thalamus leads to severe, persistent insomnia.[73–75] Clinical evidence also has linked lesions in the dorsal medial nucleus of the thalamus with a loss of GH secretion during delta sleep.[76] Thus, abnormal thalamic rCBF may play a role in both the GH secretion abnormalities and the disordered sleep of patients with FM.

POLYSOMNOGRAPHIC STUDIES

Chronic Fatigue Syndrome

Subjective reports of unrefreshing sleep and debilitating, chronic fatigue are characteristic of CFS.[77, 78] One hypothesis suggests that the daytime fatigue and other symptoms of CFS may result from a sleep disorder.[79, 80]

A number of studies have appeared to confirm this hypothesis. Polysomnography has revealed objective abnormalities in the sleep of many of the subjects studied, including significantly decreased sleep efficiency and REM sleep and intrusion of alpha rhythm in NREM sleep.[13, 81–84] A pilot study of the sleep of carefully selected CFS patients (excluding major depression)[10] found that patients with CFS felt less refreshed by their sleep and slept less efficiently than healthy controls. However, a follow-up study,[85] excluding major depression and primary sleep disorders from the sample population, replicated the findings of the pilot study but found that major sleep abnormalities occur in only a minority of carefully screened CFS patients.

This conclusion differs from previous reports of studies that used a less restrictive definition of CFS.[85] Increased alpha activity did not appear to be characteristic of the sleep of CFS patients. Unlike major depression, in which clear EEG changes are seen in most patients (reduced REM latency, reduced slow-wave sleep, and poor sleep continuity), and in FM, in which alpha intrusion in NREM sleep may be a marker, CFS does not at present seem to have an objective "sleep fingerprint."

Fibromyalgia

FM patients commonly describe their sleep as being light, restless, easily disturbed by noise, and unrefreshing.[86] Insomnia and early wakening are also frequent FM complaints, along with the consciousness of dreaming or thinking during sleep. FM patients also report awakening with stiffness, aching, and fatigue, even after 6 to 8 h of sleep. When they do, rarely, awaken feeling rested, they have less discomfort or fatigue during the following day.[87, 88]

For some 30 years, a number of investigators have been monitoring sleep in patients with FM to attempt to tease out the role of disruptive sleep and altered sleep architecture in the symptoms of this disorder.

Alpha-delta sleep (alpha rhythm appearing during delta, or stage 4, sleep) was first reported by Hauri and Hawkins in 1973 in nine psychiatric patients with somatic malaise and fatigue.[88a] Moldofsky et al.[42] later identified alpha-delta sleep in FM patients, and implicated sleep in the pathophysiology of FM. In addition to alpha intrusion, polysomnography clearly shows that, compared with controls, FM patients have less slow-wave sleep (corrected for age), less REM sleep, and less total sleep time. They also have a greater number of arousals and awakenings, and more long awakenings (greater than 10 mins).[22] These are all non-specific findings of disturbed sleep.

Alpha intrusion is an abnormal sleep EEG rhythm characterized by alpha wave activity (8 to 13 Hz) that is superimposed on the EEG of sleep.[89] Normally, the alpha rhythm is associated with relaxed wakefulness (with eyes closed). Its anomalous appearance in the sleep EEG is accompanied by indications of vigilance during sleep, and with the subjective experience of unrefreshing sleep.[25] Since Moldofsky's observations, much of the research on alpha intrusion has involved FM patients, although alpha intrusion can also occur in patients with RA and CFS.[90, 91] One important concept is that there may be a difference between tonically appearing alpha activity during NREM sleep (the alpha-delta phenomenon, appearing throughout NREM sleep), and the phasically occurring alpha frequency activity induced by external stimulation (the alpha intrusion phenomenon, appearing intermittently during NREM sleep). These may be different phenomena, and these facts must be taken into account in subsequent studies of alpha-delta sleep.[92]

To explore the relationship between pain, arousal, and alpha intrusion, Moldofsky et al.[42] measured musculoskeletal tenderness in 10 drug-free patients with FM using a 20-lb dolorimeter and found an increase in dolorimeter scores in all subjects, and alpha rhythm intrusion in seven subjects. In another study of normal controls, alpha-delta sleep coincided with auditory stimuli during stage 4 sleep deprivation. Perlis et al.[93] found similar results looking at alpha sleep, the perception of sleep, information processing, muscle tenderness, and arousability in 20 FM patients. Alpha sleep correlated with the subject's perception of shallow sleep and with increased arousals in response to external stimuli.[93] Thus, alpha sleep looks, both subjectively and objectively, like shallow sleep. To underscore the complicated nature of any relationship between external stimulus–generated intrusion of alpha activity into NREM sleep, a recent study found that delta wave sleep interruptions caused no significant lowering of the pain threshold.[94]

Pharmacological evidence from Moldofsky's group further implicates alpha intrusion in the symptomatology of FM. Administration of chlorpromazine and L-tryptophan (which increase delta sleep) in patients with FM demonstrated that the alpha-delta frequency is related to pain, energy, and mood: the more alpha activity occurring during sleep, the greater the increase in overnight pain.[26] These results strongly suggest that alpha intrusion is a nonspecific indicator for unrefreshing sleep.[26]

Spectral analysis of EEG and of alpha and delta power supports this hypothesis.[28, 95, 96] Branco et al.[28] prospectively studied the alpha-delta ratio across sleep cycles and calculated alpha and delta power in 14 normal controls and 10 patients with FM. Nine of 10 patients and none of the controls exhibited alpha-delta sleep. The anomaly increased exponentially during the night.[28] Spectral analysis of EEG by Drewes et al.[97] showed that patients with FM displaced more power in the higher-frequency bands (alpha) and less in the lower-frequency bands throughout NREM sleep and in all sleep cycles. The subjects were 12 women with FM and 14 control women.

Drewes's group has extensively analyzed data on alpha-delta sleep in FM. Using cluster analysis to obtain additional information from the sleep EEG, they showed a characteristic EEG pattern in patients with FM, compared with matched controls, which was independent of the stage of sleep. Drewes et al. consistently found that these FM patients had decreased delta power and increased power in the alpha frequency bands.[97] They have also produced evidence that deep pain can alter sleep architecture, increasing alpha activity. They observed how painful stimuli affected the sleep EEG of 10 normal subjects. During slow-wave sleep they induced muscle pain (6% hypertonic saline), joint pain (computer-controlled pneumatic stimulation of the second proximal interphalangeal joint), and cutaneous pain (green-blue argon laser light applied to the skin).[44] An arousal effect occurred during muscle and joint (but not cutaneous) stimulation, with a decrease in delta (0.5 to 3.5 Hz) and an increase in alpha (8 to 10 Hz) activity.[44] This work has not been replicated.

Delta, or stage 4, sleep is the stage that is most significantly disturbed by alpha rhythm in patients with rheumatoid disease. The fragmentation of normal sleep architecture by frequent arousals may be as important, or more so, than the decrease in the amount of delta sleep.[98, 99] Molony et al.,[99] for example, reported that patients with FM had three times more micro-arousals per hour (brief sleep interruptions lasting 5 to 19 sec) than control subjects. These results provide further evidence of poor sleep quality with frequent interruptions in the sleep of FM patients. Although it is tempting to associate these "arousals" with the complaint of nonrestorative sleep and FM, if such were the case, then patients with obstructive sleep apnea, with literally hundreds of arousals nightly, would be expected to have symptoms of FM. In fact, the incidence of FM in patients with obstructive sleep apnea is no higher than in the general population.[100]

Critique of Studies

Although objective studies of CFS demonstrate the importance of sleep disorders as a differential diagnosis for CFS, many studies of sleep in CFS have, unfortunately, been flawed: subjects have been self-selected[82, 83]; primary sleep disorders (obstructive sleep apnea, periodic limb movement in sleep, narcolepsy) have not been excluded[81–84]; depression[84] and anxiety disorders, both of which are common among both CFS and sleep disorders patients,[101] have not been excluded. Thus the data do not clarify the role of sleep disorders in the etiology of CFS or determine whether there is a characteristic CFS sleep disturbance.

While alpha intrusion is found in many FM patients, and can be induced during sleep in normal controls using deep pain stimuli, not all investigators agree on the significance of the alpha EEG finding. It can also be found in normal subjects, and is not a constant feature of well-diagnosed FM patients.[79, 102, 103] Alpha intrusion has been observed to occur not only in delta sleep but in all stages of NREM sleep. Thus alpha intrusion appears to be a nonspecific finding that correlates with the subjective feeling of nonrestorative sleep. It may suggest a state of increased arousability leading to fragmented sleep and thus to complaints of nonrestorative sleep.[104]

The amount of alpha intrusion correlates with objective measurements of pain. Conversely, a decrease in the amount of alpha rhythm results in a decrease in pain measurements. These data support the widely reported improvement in pain symptoms that reliably follows the improvement of sleep in FM patients. One clinically striking argument against sleep disturbance causing the development of FM or chronic musculoskeletal pain is the lack of correlation between the often severely disordered sleep of patients with severe sleep apnea of many years' duration and the development of the CFS and FM syndromes. The hundreds of nightly arousals and awakenings experienced by these patients far exceed the experimentally induced arousals that have been reported to cause myalgia in the above-referenced studies.

DIAGNOSIS, TREATMENT, AND REFERRAL ISSUES

Patients with CFS, FM, and other pain syndromes may have faced substantial skepticism and neglect from physicians and others prior to establishing a supportive treatment relationship with a practitioner sympathetic to their condition. If the physician is unfamiliar with the clinical features of these disorders or communicates his or her own disbelief, the process of care may have a poor outcome even if a competent sleep assessment is carried out. Failure to understand the patients' explanatory models of their syndrome and the role sleep plays in their difficulties can lead to noncompliance or therapeutic failure.

Careful assessment of the patient's explanatory model and expectations with nonjudgmental acceptance is essential. In some instances where a physician has a strong negative bias toward these syndromes, referral to a more neutral colleague may be in the patient's best interest.

Diagnosis

The goals for assessing sleep disorders in CFS, FM, and related disorders of pain and fatigue are as follows:

- Accurately diagnose sleep disorders that can have specific treatment separate from the underlying rheumatological symptoms. Diagnostic polysomnography is often required, but care needs to be taken to avoid (1) pursuing nonspecific symptoms such as fatigue in the absence of specific sleep symptoms: for example, excessive daytime sleepiness, chronic snoring, and so on; (2) writing off the patient's sleep-related symptoms as secondary to other pathologic conditions without a careful assessment.
- Identify the role of pain and other rheumatological symptoms that perpetuate disordered sleep in order to improve the management of the underlying condition. This is in contrast to treating disordered sleep directly, that is, better pain management to improve sleep rather than sedative-hypnotics to improve sleep and, secondarily, hoping to relieve pain.
- Identify maladaptive sleep behaviors that contribute and perpetuate disordered sleep patterns.
- Assess the patient's explanatory model regarding the role of sleep in the illness and provide accurate information to support effective interventions and realistic goals: for example, an FM patient with severe dyssomnia and untreated depression, who feels strongly that if she could obtain more "deep sleep" her symptoms and occupational disability would be cured.
- Because somatiform, anxiety, and affective disorders have a striking prevalence in patients with these syndromes, a formal psychiatric assessment should be considered and integrated into the findings and treatment of any sleep disorder. The clinician should expect this task to be challenging, because the psychiatric symptoms may be difficult to separate from symptoms associated with the underlying condition, and the patient may experience his or her symptoms as being nonpsychiatric in nature.

Treatment

The goals for treating sleep disorders in patients with these disease conditions are as follows:

- Prevent progression of a dyssomnia from a transient or episodic problem to a chronic sleep disturbance.
- Improve the pain and disability associated with the underlying illness.
- Modify effective sleep therapies in light of the patient's underlying illness and explanatory model.
- Manage expectations of global improvement and focus on specific limited changes in target symptoms.

- Eliminate inaccurate and unproductive patient focus on improved sleep as a panacea.

Many therapeutic options that may interact with some or all of these factors are available. There are two types of intervention: nonpharmacological and pharmacological therapy.

Nonpharmacological

Nonpharmacological interventions include patient education and maintenance of good sleep hygiene, and behavioral and psychological therapies. Multiple etiologic factors are usually present and each must be recognized and addressed. Traditional good sleep hygiene rules need to be modified as follows to be effective in this patient population:

1. Sleep only when sleepy, and only as much as is needed to feel refreshed. Patients with FM and CFS may report the ability to sleep for excessive periods of time without any improvement in function, daytime alertness, or decreased symptomatology. Whenever the ability to sleep exceeds the patient's maximal restorative sleep time, attempts should be made to curtail sleep behaviors. Many patients will find standard sleep-restriction techniques intolerable as they feel an overwhelming need to rest in bed even if they are not sleeping. Understanding these needs will lead to a compromise that will allow therapeutic goals to be achieved.
2. Maintain a regular wake-up time. Variability in function, fatigue, and pain symptoms may result in great variability in wake-up time. In FM, CFS, and more severe rheumatological conditions, realistic intervention often requires the assistance of another individual. Classic reliance on alarm clocks and other self-administered techniques has a high failure rate.
3. Exercise daily, but not within 3 to 6 hs of sleep time. Exercise is an essential part of rehabilitation in these disorders, if only to prevent a vicious circle of deconditioning, decreased activity, and increasing fatigue with diminished function. The limitations of many of these patients, particularly when beginning any type of salutary physical activity program, preclude the type of vigorous aerobic activity that would affect core body temperature and the reported effects on sleep onset. Unless exercise is demonstrated by diaries to have a negative effect on sleep, obtaining exercise at any time of day should take precedence.
4. Eliminate excesses of noise and room temperature. Do not use caffeine, alcohol, and nicotine in the evening. Avoid going to bed on a full stomach.
5. Use sleep medication only occasionally if the insomnia is intolerable. This recommendation does not apply readily to most patients in these diagnostic categories. Many FM and CFS patients will indeed require sleep-promoting medications during illness flare-ups or as chronic treatments.
6. During times when sleeping is difficult, use the bedroom for sleep and sex only. More severely disabled patients may "live" in their bedrooms. Concerted efforts can be made to arrange other resting places as a way to improve function and morale and to diminish excessive sleeping.

Basic patient education about sleep hygiene is helpful both alone and in concert with other interventions. Formal behavioral and psychological interventions include cognitive therapy, stimulus control, biofeedback, relaxation, sleep restriction, psychotherapy, and multidisciplinary group programs.[105] A survey of the effectiveness of nonpharmacological treatment, a meta-analysis of 17 studies,[106] found that in patients who received active treatment, improvement ranged from 26 to 59%, while mean improvement in placebo patients was 30%.

Patient support groups, while useful, may provide patients with incorrect or poorly understood information that has a serious impact on the assessment process.

Pharmacological

There are no specific sleep-related pharmacological interventions for these disorders, so sleep specialists must rely on a very accurate clinical assessment to guide symptomatic therapy. Nevertheless, certain clinical observations can be of benefit, particularly in complex patients with CFS or FMS who often have been treated by several physicians.

1. The clinician should not expect that successful treatment of disordered sleep will explain or cure the patient's fatigue and impairments in function. These often are multifactorial. Limited but significant improvements can be achieved within a background of more severe unremitting complaints. Patient satisfaction with limited improvement can be very high and can allow increased cooperation with other therapies.
2. These patients may complain of extreme sensitivity to low doses of medications, so dosing should be adjusted accordingly. Although this sensitivity feature has not been statistically proved, it is widely reported by experienced clinicians.
3. Widespread anecdotal clinical experience suggests that low-dose tricyclic antidepressants such as amitriptyline may be of particular benefit in diminishing pain and improving sleep fragmentation.
4. Sedative-hypnotics may be useful as long-term adjuvants, as long as they are used on an intermittent basis, a clear and significant improvement on sleep is documented, and the dose is not increased beyond the initial therapeutic dose.
5. Affective disorders should be considered and treated even in the absence of a complaint of depressed mood if other criteria for an affective disorder are present. The medication history of not responding to antidepressants should be checked carefully to be sure that therapeutic levels were used.

6. When sleep is disturbed and significant pain complaints are present during the night, every effort should be made to be sure that optimal therapy of the underlying disorder has been achieved. Collaboration with the appropriate specialists should be pursued prior to attempting to induce sleep.

7. Some patients with CFS may have neurally mediated hypotension that may respond to treatment.[107, 108] Randomized studies are in progress.[109] The effect of treatment on sleep is unknown.

Indications for Referral to a Sleep Center

The indications for polysomnography have been reviewed recently and certainly apply to this patient population. Clear symptoms of a specific sleep disorder should trigger further assessment rather than an assumption that the fatigue is predominantly explained by the main diagnosis. The presence of nonrestorative sleep and disturbed sleep patterns is ubiquitous in this population, so additional factors need to be considered to make an appropriate referral.

1. The presence of significant excessive daytime sleepiness distinct from complaints of fatigue should suggest the need for sleep medicine consultation. A careful history that distinguishes wakefulness problems from fatigue (lack of energy) may be time-consuming and difficult to obtain.

2. Sleep questionnaires that focus on specific sleep-related disorders such as restless legs syndrome, sleep-related breathing disorders, and narcolepsy can provide valuable information and set specific criteria for referral.

3. Sleep consultation, even in the absence of a specific sleep disorder, can be cost-effective if patient education and guidance are provided in identifying and correcting maladaptive responses to disturbed sleep. Written recommendations specific to the patient's condition and habits can be very useful to the referring physician as he or she attempts to manage the patient's care over time and as sleep complaints wax and wane in importance to the patient.

References

1. Goldenberg DL. Fatigue in rheumatic disease. Bull Rheum Dis. 1995;44:103.
2. McCarty DJ. Clinical picture of rheumatoid arthritis. In: McCarty DJ, Koopman WJ, eds. Arthritis and Allied Conditions, Philadelphia, Pa: Lea & Febiger; 1993:788.
3. Crosby LJ. Factors which contribute to fatigue associated with rheumatoid arthritis. J Adv Nurs. 1991;16:974–981.
4. Tack BB. Self-reported fatigue in rheumatoid arthritis: a pilot study. Arthritis Care Res. 1990;3:154–157.
5. Schur P. Clinical features of SLE. In: Kelley W, Harris E, Ruddy S, et al, eds. Textbook of Rheumatology. Philadelphia, Pa: WB Saunders Co; 1993:1018.
6. Moldofsky H. Sleep and fibrositis syndrome. Rheum Dis Clin North Am. 1989;15:91–103.
7. Bohr TW. Fibromyalgia syndrome and myofascial pain syndrome. Do they exist? Neurol Clin. 1995;13:365–384.
8. Bohr T. Problems with myofascial pain syndrome and fibromyalgia syndrome. Neurology. 1996;46:593–597.
9. Cohen ML. Fibromyalgia syndrome, a problem of tautology. Lancet. 1993;342:906–909.
10. Sharpe M, Archard LC, Banatvala JE, et al. A report—chronic fatigue syndrome: guidelines for research. J R Soc Med. 1991;84:118–121.
11. Fukuda K, Straus SE, Hickie I, et al. Chronic fatigue syndrome: a comprehensive approach to its definition and management. Ann Intern Med. 1994;121:953–959.
12. Sharpe M, Hawton KE, Seagroatt V, et al. Patients who present with fatigue: a follow up of referrals to an infectious diseases clinic. Br Med J. 1992;305:147–152.
13. Schaefer KM. Sleep disturbances and fatigue in women with fibromyalgia and chronic fatigue syndrome. J Obstet Gynecol Neonatal Nurs. 1995;24:229–233.
14. Bates D, Schmitt W, Buchwald D. Prevalence of fatigue and chronic syndrome in a primary care practice. Arch Intern Med. 1993;153:2759–2765.
15. Brooks PM, McFarlane AC. Psychological aspects of arthritis. New Stand Arthritis Care. 1996;1:9–11.
16. Hawley DJ, Wolfe F. Anxiety and depression in patients with rheumatoid arthritis: a prospective study of 400 patients. J Rheumatol. 1988;15:932–941.
17. Bayley TRL, Haslock I. Night medication in rheumatoid arthritis. Gen Pract. 1976;26:591–594.
18. Wojtulewski JA, Walter J. Treatment of sleep disturbance in arthritis with chlormezanone. Curr Med Res Opin. 1983;8:456–460.
19. Hart FD, Taylor RT, Huskisson EC. Pain at night. Lancet. 1970;1:881–884.
20. Leigh TJ, Bird HA, Hindmarch I, et al. A comparison of sleep in rheumatic and non-rheumatic patients. Clin Exp Rheumatol. 1987;5:363–365.
21. Condie R. Chlormezanone in the treatment of insomnia due to rheumatic stiffness. Curr Med Res Opin. 1979;6:217–220.
22. Shapiro CM, Devins GM, Hussain MRG. Sleep problems in patients with medical illness. Br Med J. 1993;306:1532–1535.
23. Watson R, Liebmann KO, Jenson J. Alpha-delta sleep: EEG characteristics, incidence, treatment, psychological correlates in personality. Sleep Res. 1985;14:226.
23a. Holmes GP, Kaplan JE, Gantz NM, et al. Chronic fatigue syndrome: a working case definition. Ann Intern Med. 1988;108:387–389.
24. Pilowsky I, Crettenden I, Townley M. Sleep disturbance in pain clinic patients. Pain. 1985;23:27–33.
25. Anch AM, Lue FA, MacLean AW, et al. Sleep physiology and psychological aspects of fibrositis (fibromyalgia) syndrome. Can J Exp Psychol. 1991;45:179–184.
26. Moldofsky H, Lue FA. The relationship of alpha delta EEG frequencies to pain and mood in "fibrositis" patients with chlorpromazine and L-tryptophan. Electroencephalogr Clin Neurophysiol. 1980;50:71–80.
27. Linton S, Gotestam K. Relations between pain, anxiety, mood, and muscle tension in chronic pain patients: a correlational study. Psychother Psychosom 1985;43:90–95.
28. Branco J, Atalaia A, Paiva T. Sleep cycles and alpha-delta sleep in fibromyalgia syndrome. J Rheumatol. 1994;21:1113–1117.
29. Affleck G, Tennen H, Urrows S, et al. Individual differences in the day-to-day experiences of chronic pain: a prospective daily study of rheumatoid arthritis patients. Health Psychol. 1991;19:419–426.
30. Wolfe F, Smythe HA, Yunus MB, et al. The American College of Rheumatology 1990 Criteria for the Classification of Fibromyalgia: report of multi-center criteria committee. Arthritis Rheum. 1990;33:160–172.
31. Smythe HA, Moldofsky H. Two contributions to understanding "fibrositis" syndrome. Bull Rheum Dis. 1977;28:928–931.
32. Yunus M, Masi AT, Calabro JJ, et al. Primary fibromyalgia (fibrositis): clinical study of 50 patients with matched normal controls. Semin Arthritis Rheum. 1990;33:160–172.
33. Simms RW. Fibromyalgia: muscle; chronic pain syndrome. Am J Med Sci. 1998;315:346–350.
34. Affleck G, Urrows S, Tennen H, et al. Sequential daily relations

of sleep, pain intensity, and attention to pain among women with fibromyalgia. Pain. 1996;68:363–368.

35. Cohen L. A controlled study of Trancopal in sleep disturbances due to rheumatic disease. J Intern Med Res. 1978;6:111–114.

36. Lichstein KL, Rosenthal TL. Insomniacs' perception of cognitive versus somatic determinates of sleep distribution. J Abnorm Psychol. 1980;89:105–107.

37. Moldofsky H, Chester W. Pain and mood patterns in patients with rheumatoid arthritis: a prospective study. Psychosom Med. 1970;32:309–318.

38. Persson L, Sjoberg L. Mood and somatic symptoms. J Psychosom Res. 1987;31:499–511.

39. Geisser M, Gaskin M, Robinson M, et al. The relationship of depression and somatic focus to experimental and clinical pain in chronic pain patients. Psychol Health. 1993;8:405–415.

40. Affleck G, Tennen H, Urrows S, et al. Neuroticism and the pain-mood relation in rheumatoid arthritis: insights from a prospective daily study. J Consult Clin Psychol. 1992;60:119–126.

41. Affleck G, Tennen H, Urrows S, et al. Person and contextual features of stress reactivity: individual differences in relations of undesirable daily events with mood disturbance and chronic pain intensity. J Pers Soc Psychol. 1994;66:329–340.

42. Moldofsky H, Scarsbrick P, England R, et al. Musculoskeletal symptoms and non-REM sleep disturbance in patients with "fibrositis syndrome" and healthy subjects. Psychosom Med. 1975;37:341–351.

43. Moldofsky H, Scarsbrick P. Induction of neurasthenic musculoskeletal pain syndrome by selective sleep stage deprivation. Psychom Med. 1976;38:35–44.

44. Drewes AM, Nielsen KD, Arendt-Nielsen L, et al. The effect of cutaneous and deep pain on the electroencephalogram during sleep: an experimental study. Sleep. 1997;20:632–640.

45. Totterdell P, Reynolds S, Parkinson B, et al. Associations of sleep with everyday mood, minor symptoms, and social interaction experience. Sleep. 1991;17:446–475.

46. Haythornthwaite J, Hegel M, Kerns R. Development of a sleep diary for chronic pain patients. J Pain Symptom Manage. 1991;6:65–72.

47. Nicassio P, Wallston K. Longitudinal relationships among pain, sleep problems, and depression in rheumatoid arthritis. J Abnorm Psychol. 1992;101:514–520.

48. Wolfe F, Smythe H, Yunus M, et al. The American College of Rheumatology 1990 criteria for the classification of fibromyalgia. Arthritis Rheum. 1990;33:160–172.

49. Geisser M, Gaskin M, Robinson M, et al. The relationship of depression and somatic focus to experimental and clinical pain in chronic pain patients. Psychol Health. 1993;8:405–415.

50. Alexander R, Alexander M, Bradley L, et al. Negative affectivity in association with pain perception in patients with fibromyalgia: support for sensory decision theory model. Arthritis Rheum. 1995;38(suppl):s270.

51. Rice J. "Fibrositis" syndrome. Med Clin North Am. 1986;70:455–468.

52. Gaston-Johansson F, Gustafsson M, Felldin R, et al. A comparative study of feelings, attitudes, and behaviors of patients with fibromyalgia and rheumatoid arthritis. Soc Sci Med. 1990;31:941–947.

53. Worthington P. The effects of imagery content, choice of imagery content, and self-verbalization on the self control of pain. Cogn Ther Res. 1978;2:225–240.

54. Beers T, Karoly P. Cognitive strategies, expectancy, and coping style in the control of pain. J Consult Clin Psychol. 1979;47:179–180.

55. Smith AP, Behan PO, Bell W, et al. Behavioural problems associated with the chronic fatigue syndrome. Br J Psychol. 193;84:411–423.

56. Sandman CA, Barron JL, Nackoul K, et al. Memory deficits associated with chronic fatigue immune dysfunction syndrome. Biol Psychiatry. 1993;33:618–623.

57. Altay HT, Toner B, Brooker H, et al. The neuropsychological dimensions of postinfectious neuromyasthenia (chronic fatigue syndrome): a preliminary report. Int J Psychiatry Med. 1990;20:141–149.

58. Scheffers MK, Johnson RJ, Grafman J, et al. Attention and short-term memory in chronic fatigue syndrome patients: an event-related potential analysis. Neurology. 1992;42:1667–1675.

59. Sletvold H, Stiles TC, Landro NI. Information processing in primary fibromyalgia, major depression, and healthy controls. J Rheumatol. 1995;22:137–142.

60. Joyce E, Blumenthal S, Wessely S. Memory, attention, and executive function in chronic fatigue syndrome. J Neurol Neurosurg Psychiatry. 1996;60:495–503.

61. Marshall PS, Forster M, Callies A, et al. Cognitive slowing and working memory difficulties in chronic fatigue syndrome. Psychosom Med. 1997;59:58–66.

62. Romanelli GG, Tenenbaum GO. Characteristics and response to treatment of post-traumatic temporomandibular disorder: a retrospective study. Clin J Pain. 1992;8:6–17.

63. Karoly P, Ruehlman L. Goal cognition and its clinical implications: development and preliminary validation of four motivational assessment instruments. Assessment. 1995;2:113–129.

64. Lawson K, Reesor K, Keefe F, et al. Dimensions of pain-related cognitive coping: cross-validation of the factor structure of the coping strategy questionnaire. Pain. 1990;43:194–204.

65. Bennett RM, Clark SR, Campbell SM, et al. Low levels of somatomedia C in patients with the fibromyalgia syndrome: a possible link between sleep and muscle pain. Arthritis Rheum. 1992;35:1113–1116.

66. Bennett RM, Clark SR, Burchkhardt CS, et al. A double-blind placebo controlled study of growth hormone therapy in fibromyalgia [abstract]. J Musculoskeletal Pain. 1995;3:110.

67. Vaeroy H, Helle R, Forre O, et al. Elevated CSF levels of substance P and high incidence of Raynaud phenomenon in patients with fibromyalgia: new features for diagnosis. Pain. 1988;32:21–26.

68. Cooper JR, Bloom FE, Roth RH. The Biochemical Basis of Neuropharmacology. New York, NY: Oxford University Press; 1986:362–366.

69. Russell IJ, Michalek JE, Vipario GA, et al. Platelet H-imipramine uptake receptor density and serum serotonin levels in patients with fibromyalgia/fibrositis syndrome. J Rheumatol. 1992; 19:104–109.

70. Vaeroy H, Helle R, Forre O, et al. Cerebrospinal fluid levels of β-endorphin in patients with fibromyalgia (fibrositis syndrome). J Rheumatol. 1988;15:1894–1896.

71. Sallanon M, Buda C, Janin M, et al. Implications of serotonin in sleep mechanisms: induction, facilitation? In: Wauquier A, Monte JM, Gaillard JM, et al, eds. Sleep: Neurotransmitters and Neuromodulators. New York, NY: Raven Press; 1985:136.

72. Carette S, McCain GA, Bell DA, et al. Evaluation of amitriptyline in primary fibrositis. Arthritis Rheum. 1986;29:655–659.

72a. Korszun A, Sackett-Lundeen L, Papadopoulos E, et al. Melatonin levels in women with fibromyalgia and chronic fatigue syndrome. J Rheumatol. 1999;26:2675–2680.

73. Villablanca J. Role of the thalamus in sleep control: sleep-wakefulness studies in chronic diencephalic and athalamic cats. In: Petre-Quadens O, Schlag JD, eds. Basic Sleep Mechanisms. New York, NY: Academic Press; 1974:51.

74. Jurko MF, Andy OJ, Webster CL. Disorderal sleep patterns following thalamotomy. Clin Electroencephalogr. 1971;2:213–217.

75. Lugaresi E. The thalamus and insomnia. Neurology. 1992; 42(suppl 6);28–33.

76. Culebras A, Miller M. Dissociated patterns of nocturnal prolactin, cortisol and growth hormone secretion after stroke. Neurology. 1984;34:361–366.

77. Moldofsky H. Scarisbrick P, Englan R, et al. Musculoskeletal symptoms and non-REM sleep disturbance in patients with "fibrositis syndrome" and healthy subjects. Psychosom Med. 1975;37:341–351.

78. Anch A, Lue F, MacLean A, et al. Sleep physiology and psychological aspects of the fibrositis (fibromyalgia) syndrome. Can J Psychol. 1991;45:179–184.

79. Shaver JFL, Lentz M, Landis CA, et al. Sleep, psychological distress, and stress arousal in women with fibromyalgia. Res Nurs Health. 1998;20:247–257.

80. Huller RF, Moser RJ. Chronic fatigue: psyche or sleep? Arch Intern Med. 1990;150:1116–1117.

81. Whelton C, Saskin P, Salit H, et al. Post-viral fatigue syndrome and sleep. Sleep Res. 1988;17:307.

82. Krupp LB, Jandorf L, Coyle PK, et al. Sleep disturbance in chronic fatigue syndrome. J Psychosom Res. 1993;37:325–331.

83. Buchwald DS, Pascualy R, Bombardier C, et al. Sleep disorders in patients with chronic fatigue. Clin Infect Dis 1994;18(suppl 1):568–572.

84. Whelton CL, Salit I, Moldofsky H. Sleep, Epstein-Barr virus infection, musculoskeletal pain, and depressive symptoms in chronic fatigue syndrome. J Rheumatol. 1992;19:939–943.

85. Schramm E, Hohagen F, Grasshoff U, et al. Test-retest reliability and validity of the structured interview for sleep disorders according to the DSM-III-R. Am J Psychiatry. 1993;150:867–872.

86. Campbell SM, Clark S, Tindall EA, et al. Clinical characteristics of fibrositis, I: a "blinded" controlled study of symptoms and tender points. Arthritis Rheum. 1983;26:817–825.

87. Wolfe F, Cathey MA. Prevalence of primary and secondary fibrositis. J Rheumatol. 1983;10:965–968.

88. Hyyppa MT, Kronholm E. Nocturnal motor activity in fibromyalgia patients with poor sleep quality. J Psychosom Res. 1995;39:85–91.

88a. Hauri P, Hawkins DR. Alpha-delta sleep. Electroencephalogr Clin Neurophysiol. 1973;34:233–237.

89. McNamara ME. Alpha sleep: a mini review and update. Clin Electroencephalogr 1993;24:192–193.

90. Moldofsky H, Saskin P, Lue FA. Sleep and symptoms in fibrositis syndrome after a febrile illness. J Rheumatol. 1988;15:1701–1704.

91. Moldofsky H, Lue FA, Smythe H. Alpha EEG sleep and morning symptoms of rheumatoid arthritis. J Rheumatol. 1983;10:373–379.

92. Pivik RT, Harman K. A reconceptualization of EEG alpha activity as an index of arousal during sleep: all activity is not equal. J Sleep Res. 1995;4:131–137.

93. Perlis ML, Giles DE, Bootzin RR, et al. Alpha sleep and information processing, perception of sleep, pain, and arousability in fibromyalgia. Int J Neurosci. 1997;89:265–280.

94. Battafarano DF, Danning CL, Ward JA, et al. The effects of delta wave sleep interruption on pain thresholds and fibromyalgia-like symptoms in healthy subjects: correlations with insulin-like growth factor I. J Rheumatol. 1998;25:1180–1186.

95. Drewes AM, Nielsen KD, Taagholt SJ, et al. Sleep intensity in fibromyalgia: focus on the microstructure of the sleep process. Br J Rheumatol. 1995;34:629–635.

96. Smythe HA. Studies of sleep in fibromyalgia: techniques, clinical significance, and future directions. Br J Rheumatol. 1995;34:897–900.

97. Drewes AM, Gade J, Nielsen KD, et al. Clustering of sleep electroencephalographic patterns in patients with the fibromyalgia syndrome. Br J Rheumatol. 1995;34:1151–1156.

98. Jennum P, Drewes AM, Andreasen A, et al. Sleep and other symptoms in primary fibromyalgia and in healthy controls. J Rheumatol. 1993;20:1756–1759.

99. Molony RR, MacPeek DM, Schiffman PL, et al. Sleep, sleep apnea, and the fibromyalgia syndrome. J Rheumatol. 1986;13:797–800.

100. Donald F, Esdaile JM, Kimoff JR, et al. Musculoskeletal complaints and fibromyalgia in patients attending a respiratory disease clinic. J Rheumatol. 1996;23:1612–1616.

101. Reynolds CF, Kupfer DJ. Sleep research in affective illness: state of the art circa 1987. Sleep. 1987;19:119–215.

102. Schueler W, Stinhoff D, Kubrick S. The alpha-sleep pattern. Neuropsychobiology. 1983;10:183–189.

103. Horns JA, Shackell BS. Alpha-like EEG activity in non-REM sleep and fibromyalgia (fibrositis) syndrome. Electroencephalogr Clin Neurophysiol. 1991;79:271–276.

104. Schueler W, Stinshoff D, Kubicki S. The alpha sleep pattern: different from other sleep patterns and effects of hypnotics. Neuropsychobiology. 1983;10:183–189.

105. Bennett RM. Multidisciplinary group programs to treat fibromyalgia patients. Rheum Dis Clin North Am. 1996;22:351–367.

106. Lacks P, Morin CM. Recent advances in the assessment and treatment of insomnia. J Consult Clin Psychol. 1992;60:586–594.

107. LaManca JJ, Peckerman A, Walker J, et al. Cardiovascular response during head-up tilt in chronic fatigue syndrome. Clin Physiol. 1999;19:111–120.

108. Wilke WS, Fouad-Tarazi FM, Cash JM, et al. The connection between chronic fatigue syndrome and neurally mediated hypotension. Cleve Clin J Med. 1998;65:261–266.

109. Rowe RC, Calkins H. Neurally mediated hypotension and chronic fatigue syndrome. Am J Med. 1998;105(3A):15S–21S.

88

Parkinsonism

Michael S. Aldrich

Parkinson's disease and related movement disorders are common neurological diseases, particularly in older persons. Although the daytime phenomena of Parkinson's disease have been well recognized since the early 1800s,[1] the frequent nocturnal symptoms, which occur in as many as 75% of patients,[2] and the associated sleep abnormalities were not systematically studied until the 1960s. Its characteristic pathological features have been known since the early 20th century, but its cause is still uncertain.

Parkinson's disease is an idiopathic disorder characterized clinically by resting tremor, rigidity, bradykinesia, and loss of postural reflexes and pathologically by distinctive degenerative changes. When fully developed, the clinical picture is unmistakable. The patient maintains a stiff, flexed posture with few adjustments of position. Movements are slow, the face is expressionless with infrequent blinking, and the voice is soft and monotonous. The gait is slow and shuffling with small steps, and the loss of postural reflexes, along with the flexed posture, may lead to a *festinating gait* as the patient attempts to keep up with his or her center of gravity. A coarse *resting tremor* of the hands is present when the hands are immobile, but the tremor diminishes or disappears with motion or with complete relaxation, as in stage 1 sleep.

Idiopathic Parkinson's disease progresses slowly but inexorably. Walking becomes increasingly difficult and finally impossible. Speech becomes inaudible, and normal swallowing may virtually cease, making eating impossible and requiring the placement of a feeding tube. Death generally occurs 10 to 25 years after the onset of the disease due to inanition or the complications of an immobile, bedridden state.

Similar clinical features occur with secondary parkinsonism, caused by drugs, toxins, infections, and brain lesions. Currently, the most common causes of secondary parkinsonism are medications that block dopamine receptors, such as the phenothiazines and butyrophenones. Other causes include manganese intoxication, carbon monoxide poisoning, viral encephalitis, bilateral basal ganglia infarctions, frontal meningiomas, and hypoparathyroidism with basal ganglia calcification. Methylphenyltetrahydropyridine, a toxin chemically related to heroin, causes parkinsonism by producing a selective degeneration of the substantia nigra.[3, 4]

Parkinsonian features are included among other neurological signs and symptoms in several other progressive degenerative neurological disorders. A distinctive feature of *progressive supranuclear palsy* (Steele-Richardson-Olszewski syndrome) is the progressive inability to move the eyes voluntarily, although reflex eye movements are preserved. Pronounced rigidity of the neck and face is common, and the disorder is not responsive to dopaminergic medications. *Multiple system atrophy* refers to a group of disorders that cause degeneration of the basal ganglia, substantia nigra, cerebellum, and other brain regions. At least four clinical entities fall within this spectrum: Shy-Drager syndrome, olivopontocerebellar degeneration, striatonigral degeneration, and parkinsonism-amyotrophy. The manifestations of these disorders include varying combinations of ataxia, eye movement abnormalities, autonomic failure, motoneuron degeneration, dementia, and parkinsonism. Although the major emphasis in this chapter is on Parkinson's disease, much of the discussion applies to secondary parkinsonism and to the other degenerative disorders associated with parkinsonism.

A variety of psychological and physiological processes can lead to disruption of the normal rhythm of the sleep-wake cycle in patients with parkinsonism. First, when the brain is subject to a degenerative process such as parkinsonism, which affects the neurophysiological and neurochemical systems responsible for sleep organization, sleep disruption is likely to occur. Second, the behavioral, respiratory, and motor system phenomena accompanying the disease may produce nocturnal symptoms. Third, the medications used in its treatment may induce new symptoms, such as nightmares or nocturnal movements. All of these effects on sleep have implications for treatment planning.

HISTORICAL ASPECTS

The clinical features of Parkinson's disease were described by James Parkinson in 1817 in *Essay on the Shaking Palsy*. In addition to his description of daytime symptoms, Parkinson noted that "sleep becomes much disturbed" and that the terminal stage of the disease is associated with "constant sleepiness, with slight delirium, and other marks of extreme exhaustion."[1(p17)] Charcot, in the 19th century, described the impact of severe rigidity and bradykinesia on sleep:

This need of change of position is principally exhibited at night in bed. . . . Half an hour, a quarter of an hour, has scarcely elapsed until they require to be turned again, and if . . . not . . . gratified they give vent to moans, which . . . testify to the intense uneasiness they experience."[5(p147)]

The epidemic of encephalitis lethargica in the early 20th century, the major cause of secondary parkinsonism at that time, focused increased attention on the disorder, but despite the writings of Parkinson and Charcot, the sleep problems accompanying parkinsonism received relatively little attention until the 1950s and 1960s, when the first polysomnographic recordings of parkinsonian patients were performed.

PATHOPHYSIOLOGY

Neuronal depletion and gliosis of pigmented areas of the brainstem are the most striking pathological features of Parkinson's disease.[6] The loss of dopaminergic input from the substantia nigra leads to a marked reduction in dopamine content of the basal ganglia. The occurrence of parkinsonism in intravenous users of methylphenyltetrahydropyridine, a narcotic derivative that is selectively neurotoxic to neurons in the zona compacta of the substantia nigra,[4, 7] indicates the importance of these dopamine-containing neurons in the pathogenesis of Parkinson's disease.

Although loss of dopaminergic neurons of the substantia nigra is responsible for most of the daytime clinical features of Parkinson's disease, other brain abnormalities may account for some of the sleep-wake abnormalities described later in this chapter. Serotonergic neurons originating in the dorsal raphe nuclei are reduced in number, as are noradrenergic neurons originating in the region of the locus coeruleus.[8] Cholinergic neurons of the pedunculopontine nucleus, implicated in the control of REM sleep, are also reduced in number.[9] Because the noradrenergic, serotonergic, and cholinergic systems have all been implicated in the control and regulation of sleep, abnormalities in these systems may account for some of the sleep disturbance in patients with parkinsonism.

Abnormalities of the mesocorticolimbic dopamine system, as well as the mesostriatal system, are apparent in Parkinson's disease and may contribute to sleep-wake disturbances.[10] Dopamine neurons with cell bodies in the ventral tegmental area of the brainstem project to the cerebral cortex, where the predominant dopamine receptor is the D_1 type.[11] The administration of dopamine D_1 receptor agonists produces electroencephalographic (EEG) desynchronization and behavioral arousal,[12] whereas the administration of antagonists produces sedation,[13] consistent with an arousal function for the ventral tegmental projection neurons. High doses of dopamine D_2 receptor agonists, such as apomorphine, reduce total sleep time[14]; however, very low doses induce sleep and increase the amount of slow-wave sleep. Low doses of apomorphine also induce sleep when injected into the ventral tegmental area, an effect that is blocked by dopamine receptor autoantagonists, suggesting that dopamine D_2 autoreceptors play a role

in the mediation of sleep through autoinhibition of the firing rate of ventral tegmental dopaminergic neurons.[15, 16] The arousing effects of higher doses of D_2 agonists may be due to effects at postsynaptic receptors.

Dopamine also appears to be involved in the regulation of rapid eye movement (REM) sleep through effects mediated by D_1 and D_2 receptors. Dopamine D_1 receptor antagonists increase the amount and duration of REM sleep, whereas D_1 agonists suppress REM sleep.[17, 18] REM sleep is also suppressed by high doses of D_2 agonists.[14] The site of action for the effects of these agents on REM sleep is unknown.

Drugs that enhance activity of dopamine systems, including levodopa (L-dopa), the biochemical precursor of dopamine and norepinephrine, and such dopamine agonists as bromocriptine and pergolide, are frequently used in the treatment of Parkinson's disease and can have significant effects on sleep. In normal persons, L-dopa reduces the amount of REM sleep,[19] an effect that may be due to increased activity of dopamine, norepinephrine, or both. L-Dopa also reduces the serotonin, tryptophan, and tyrosine contents of the brain.[20–22] Consequently, the effects of L-dopa on sleep may be due in part to effects on serotonergic neurons. Dopamine agonists that act directly on dopamine D_2 receptors, such as apomorphine and bromocriptine, have little effect on noradrenergic or serotonergic neurons but still alter sleep-wake patterns, presumably through effects on mesocortical dopamine pathways.

Several other aspects of Parkinson's disease also contribute to sleep disturbance (Table 88–1).

EPIDEMIOLOGY

Parkinson's disease is primarily a disease of the elderly: the prevalence increases with age from about

Table 88–1. CONTRIBUTORS TO SLEEP DISRUPTION IN PARKINSON'S DISEASE

Cause	Consequence
Neurochemical changes affecting cholinergic and monoaminergic systems	Impaired sleep-wake control, reduced REM sleep
Bradykinesia and rigidity	Reduction in the number of normal body shifts during sleep, leading to discomfort and awakenings; impaired ability to use the bathroom at night
Periodic leg movements, tremor, and medication-induced myoclonus	Arousals
REM sleep behavior disorder	Disrupted REM sleep
Abnormal motor activity affecting respiratory and upper airway muscles	Sleep-disordered breathing
Medication effects	Increased time awake at night, reduced REM sleep
Depression and anxiety	Difficulty falling asleep, early morning awakening
Dementia	Nocturnal confusional episodes

0.9% among persons 65 to 69 years old to 5% among persons 80 to 84 years old.[23] Although substantial numbers of middle-aged persons have Parkinson's disease, few have an onset before the age of 30. About 60% of cases occur in men. Sleep problems are common: in one series of consecutive patients with Parkinson's disease, 67% had difficulty initiating sleep and 88% had difficulty maintaining sleep.[24]

CLINICAL FEATURES

Difficulty falling asleep and difficulty remaining asleep are the most common sleep-related complaints. Nocturnal vocalizations and spontaneous daytime dozing are also common,[24] and inability to turn over in bed and to get out of bed to use the bathroom are two especially bothersome complaints.

Sleep disturbance tends to increase with disease progression, and daytime drowsiness becomes increasingly common. Older patients with on-off phenomena and those with hallucinations are particularly likely to have severe sleep disruption.[25, 26] Depression and dementia, which commonly accompany late-stage Parkinson's disease, are usually associated with increased severity of sleep disturbance, including nocturnal vocalizations and hallucinations, and sometimes the REM sleep behavior disorder.[27]

The abnormal sleep features associated with Parkinson's disease include disturbed sleep-wake organization and sleep stage patterns, abnormal motor activity, and disturbed breathing.

Sleep-Wake Organization

Although sleep disturbance tends to increase with age, in people with Parkinson's disease, the severity of sleep disruption is greater than that in healthy individuals of comparable age. The most consistent abnormality is sleep fragmentation. Polysomnographic studies have demonstrated increased sleep latency and frequent awakenings, with as much as 30 to 40% of the night spent awake.[28, 29] The sleep latency and the number of awakenings tend to increase in proportion to the severity of waking parkinsonian symptoms.[30] Increased amounts of stage 1 sleep and reduced amounts of stage 3 and 4 sleep and REM sleep are also common, and the duration of REM periods may be reduced, although in milder cases sleep architecture may be normal or nearly so.[28] Patients with rigidity appear to have less REM sleep than those with normal tone during sleep.[31] REM sleep and total sleep time are often markedly reduced in patients with nocturnal hallucinations.[26]

EEG features of sleep may change; for example, the number of sleep spindles during slow-wave sleep is reduced,[29, 30] and EEG alpha activity may be prominent during REM sleep.[31]

Sleep disturbances also occur in related degenerative disorders. For example, progressive supranuclear palsy is associated with insomnia, poorly formed or absent spindles, increased amounts of slow wave activity during REM sleep, and decreased amounts of REM sleep; these abnormalities tend to worsen with disease progression.[32] Patients with Shy-Drager syndrome may have increased sleep latency and increased numbers of awakenings, along with reductions in REM sleep and stage 3 and 4 sleep.[33]

Motor Activity During Sleep

Although parkinsonian motor symptoms are most prominent during wakefulness, they are not completely abolished during sleep. Both tremor and altered muscle tone occur to varying degrees in the different stages of sleep.

The tremor of parkinsonism is enhanced by maintenance of posture and reduced by movement and relaxation. Although Parkinson noted the occurrence of tremor during sleep, the fact that the tremor usually disappears at the onset of sleep has led some observers to believe that tremor does not occur in sleep at all. In fact, tremor does disappear with the onset of stage 1 sleep, in some cases before alpha EEG activity is entirely gone.[34, 35] Furthermore, tremor is rarely present during stage 3 and 4 sleep and is not associated with spindles or K complexes.

Tremor may appear, however, in stages 1 and 2 and with awakenings, arousals, and body movements.[36] Tremor may also appear for a few seconds during sleep stage changes, during bursts of rapid eye movements, and shortly before or after an REM period. Tremor amplitude varies considerably during sleep and is usually less than 50% of the waking amplitude.[35] Tremor often improves or disappears during the first 1 to 2 h after awakening, suggesting that in some patients sleep may have a beneficial effect on it.

In contrast to the quiescence of sleep in normal persons, increased muscle tone and abnormal simple and complex movements are common during the sleep of patients with parkinsonism.[37] Patterns of simple motor activity during sleep include repeated blinking at the onset of sleep, rapid eye movements during non-rapid eye movement (NREM) sleep, blepharospasm at the onset of REM sleep, and prolonged tonic contractions of limb extensor or flexor muscles during NREM sleep (Fig. 88–1).[31] During REM sleep, prolonged elevations of muscle tone may occur as well as more complex movements, vocalizations, and fully developed REM sleep behavior disorder. Furthermore, the REM sleep behavior disorder may appear years before the onset of daytime symptoms of Parkinson's disease or other related degenerative disorders.[38–42]

Periodic leg movements occur in up to one third of patients with parkinsonism and even more commonly in the elderly. Fragmentary irregular myoclonic twitches and jerks of the extremities may also occur, mainly during light NREM sleep. Repetitive muscle contractions followed by tremor may occur, particularly in limbs with waking manifestations of the disease, resulting in extension of the great toe, finger, or foot.

Spontaneous circadian variations in the severity of

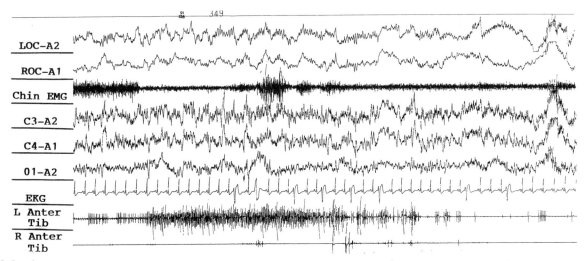

Figure 88–1. This 42-sec interval of NREM sleep was recorded from a 72-year-old man with Parkinson's disease. The tracing shows a 15- to 20-sec muscle contraction in the left leg. Isolated muscle potentials occurred before and after the muscle contraction and also were apparent in the right leg. The EEG electrodes (A1, A2, C3, C4, O1, O2) are named according to the International 10–20 system. Chin EMG, submental surface electromyogram; EKG, electrocardiogram; L Anter Tib and R Anter Tib, surface electrodes over the left and right anterior tibialis muscles, respectively; LOC, left outer canthus electro-oculogram; ROC, right outer canthus electro-oculogram. (From SLEEP MEDICINE: SLEEP AND ITS DISORDERS by Michael S. Aldrich, copyright © 1999 by Oxford University Press, Inc. Used by permission of Oxford University Press, Inc.)

motor symptoms are frequent in idiopathic Parkinson's disease. In one third to one half of patients, symptoms are mildest in the morning on arising, a phenomenon sometimes referred to as *sleep benefit*.[43–45] In other patients, bradykinesia is severe in the morning and eases in the afternoon and evening. Early morning foot dystonia may occur just before waking or soon thereafter.

Some patients with familial early-onset Parkinson's disease show marked diurnal variations in rigidity and dystonia, with little rigidity soon after arising but progressively increasing rigidity, tremor, and dysarthria as the day goes on. These symptoms are improved with naps.[46] Similar diurnal fluctuations have been observed in patients with hereditary progressive dystonia and in patients with a combination of idiopathic dystonia and parkinsonism; in these patients, the dystonic movements may improve after brief rest periods as well as after nighttime sleep.[47, 48]

Respiratory Disorders of Sleep in Parkinsonism

Waking pulmonary function is frequently disturbed in a pattern that suggests that these patients may be at risk for obstructive, sleep-related respiratory disturbances. Waking obstructive ventilatory deficits are common in moderate-to-severe Parkinson's disease and apparently are caused by a combination of upper airway obstruction, probably due at least in part to abnormal tone in upper airway muscles, and respiratory muscle incoordination with decreased effective muscle strength.[49] Although these deficits correlate to some extent with the severity of rigidity and tremor, they do not improve to any great extent with administration of L-dopa. In some patients, upper airway endoscopy has shown intermittent airway closure due to dyskinetic movements of glottic and supraglottic

structures caused by either the disease itself or dopaminergic medications.[50] Swallowing disturbances are common and are further evidence of pharyngeal dysfunction.[51]

Although nocturnal respiration is normal in some patients with parkinsonism, other patients show disorganized patterns of respiration with central apneas, obstructive apneas, or episodes of hypoventilation.[52, 53] The severity of these respiratory abnormalities tends to be greater in patients with autonomic disturbance.[53]

Sleep-related respiratory disturbances and associated excessive daytime sleepiness are regularly present in patients with Shy-Drager syndrome, a multisystem disorder with impaired autonomic function as a prominent feature. In some of these patients, daytime respiratory abnormalities include reduced ventilatory responses to hypercapnia and hypoxia.[54, 55] Polysomnographic studies have demonstrated obstructive sleep apnea as well as other abnormal breathing patterns, including central sleep apnea, variable-amplitude respirations, and arrhythmic respirations.[55–58] Abnormal vocal cord function, leading to stridor and laryngeal stenosis or obstruction, appears to be a major contributor to abnormal breathing during sleep.[59]

Both hemodynamic and respiratory abnormalities may occur during sleep in patients with Shy-Drager syndrome, including increased systemic arterial pressure during REM and slow-wave sleep and sudden phasic swings of blood pressure.[33] The autonomic failure of Shy-Drager syndrome can lead to reductions in systemic blood pressure during obstructive apneas.[56]

DIAGNOSTIC EVALUATION

A number of factors may contribute to sleep disturbance in parkinsonism, including neurochemical changes, medications, motor activity during sleep,

sleep-wake schedule abnormalities or circadian rhythm disturbances, and respiratory disorders (see Table 88–1). To determine which factors are most important, clinical history, examination, and polysomnographic evaluation are used.

Sleep disturbance is rarely the presenting complaint in a patient with previously undiagnosed parkinsonism. More commonly, the diagnosis has been established, and the patient complains of insomnia, daytime sleepiness, or both. The history of the sleep complaint should include all the features the physician would obtain from any patient with a sleep complaint. It is necessary to determine whether the onset of the disease preceded or followed the onset of the sleep problem. A careful description from the bedpartner is essential to determine the presence and frequency of movements during sleep (and their timing), arousals and awakenings, and periods of daytime sleepiness. A history of diurnal variation in tremor and rigidity may be apparent independent of the effects of medications.

The medication schedule is significant. If dopaminergic medications are not prescribed in the evening, nocturnal rigidity may contribute to the sleep disturbance; on the other hand, excessive evening doses of dopamine agonists may induce sleep-onset insomnia. Anticholinergic medications may contribute to existing autonomic dysfunction, with consequent effects on the amount of REM sleep and on respiratory activity during sleep. The timing of daytime sleepiness may be helpful in determining whether dopaminergic or anticholinergic medications are aggravating or improving the sleepiness.

Patients with parkinsonian disorders appear to be particularly susceptible to schedule disturbances, and if daytime sleepiness and nighttime insomnia are unrelated to the medication schedule, such problems as sleep phase delay or advance and sleep-wake cycle inversion may be present.

On physical examination, the patient shows the usual signs of parkinsonism. The patient with a sleep disturbance may show signs of autonomic dysfunction, such as orthostatic hypotension, lack of change in the heart rate with the Valsalva maneuver, and the absence of sweat in the axillas, which may be due to anticholinergic medications as well as to parkinsonism. An irregular waking respiration pattern is suggestive of Shy-Drager syndrome. Signs suggestive of a multisystem disorder may be present, such as cognitive or eye movement abnormalities or cerebellar or pyramidal tract dysfunction.

Some patients with parkinsonism and sleep disturbance require a polysomnogram for diagnosis of the cause of the sleep disorder, particularly when daytime sleepiness is present. Simultaneous closed-circuit television monitoring and surface electromyelographic monitoring of all four extremities or of flexors and extensors in one extremity often are helpful if nocturnal myoclonic movements or the REM sleep behavior disorder is contributing to the sleep disturbance. If daytime sleepiness is a prominent complaint, a multiple sleep latency test will help to determine its severity and its circadian variation. It is usually best to record the patient while he or she is on the usual medication schedule, but if medications appear to be a major factor in the sleep disturbance, definite diagnosis may require two or more nights of recording under different treatment regimens.

TREATMENT

The treatment of sleep disturbances in patients with parkinsonism is rarely straightforward because treatment of the disease may affect the sleep disorder. Sleep fragmentation, nocturnal movements and vocalizations, abnormal muscle tone during sleep, and sleep-wake schedule disturbances can all be caused by parkinsonism or by its treatment with dopamine agonists. The biphasic actions of dopaminergic medications must be kept in mind: low doses of these medications may promote sleep,[60] whereas high evening doses that increase sleep latency and disrupt sleep in the first half of the night may improve sleep continuity in the second half of the night. In patients with advanced disease, on-off phenomena (freeze attacks) and profound akinesia may cause severe sleep disruption and REM sleep deprivation.[61] Finally, when managing the sleep disturbance of parkinsonism, the physician must balance the effects on sleep of changes in medication dosage with the effects of such changes on daytime parkinsonian symptoms.

The first step in the treatment of insomnia in Parkinson's disease is to assess psychosocial and behavioral factors that may be contributing to sleep disturbance. Improvements in sleep hygiene and such simple measures as placing a portable commode at the bedside may lead to substantial improvements. Concurrent psychiatric disorders should be addressed. In advanced stages of the disease, the patient's spouse should be encouraged to sleep in a different bed or room; inadequate rest for the spouse or other caregiver may make the patient's sleep disturbance intolerable and lead to institutionalization.

The next step is to consider adjustment of the timing of medication administration. For the patient with a principal complaint of insomnia who does not have nocturnal hallucinations or vocalizations, it is often useful to add a small dose of dopaminergic medication at bedtime, such as 100 mg of L-dopa combined with 25 mg of carbidopa (Sinemet 25/100) with a second similar dose at 2 or 3 AM if the patient awakens. Low doses of dopamine agonists or of L-dopa combined with carbidopa (Sinemet) tend to improve sleep continuity.[61, 62] A bedtime dose of a controlled-release formulation containing 200 mg of L-dopa and 50 mg of carbidopa appears to be particularly useful. Trials of several different agents in varying doses are usually warranted if sleep is not improved. The variability of response to dopaminergic medications probably reflects differences in the cause of sleep disturbance and the severity of the disease, differences in individual sensitivity to medication, and the effects of concurrent medications. Factors that may contribute to improved sleep during treatment with dopamine agonists include decreased rigidity and bradykinesia with consequent improvement in nocturnal mobility, reduced numbers of periodic limb movements, and normalization of sleep muscle activity.[62, 63] Early morning bradykinesia often is also improved.

Unfortunately, when used during the day or in the evening, dopaminergic medications may induce entirely new sleep problems. Vivid dreams, nightmares, and night terrors occur in up to 30% of patients with parkinsonism who are taking L-dopa,[64] especially those with dementia, and may necessitate a reduction in the afternoon or evening doses. Nocturnal vocalizations and behaviors due to REM sleep behavior disorder usually respond to clonazepam, as they do in patients with idiopathic REM sleep behavior disorder. Bedtime doses of levodopa may provide some benefit as well.[39] For the demented patient with Parkinson's disease, nocturnal confusion and hallucinations often are so disruptive that only minimal doses of dopaminergic agonists can be used and the management of sleep disturbance and daytime symptoms becomes exceedingly difficult. In such cases, small doses of clozapine at bedtime are sometimes helpful.

Other patients develop fragmentary nocturnal myoclonus and periodic leg movements during NREM sleep after taking L-dopa for extended periods. These complications may be due to medication-induced dysregulation of serotonin activity.[65, 66] Insomnia due to dyskinetic nocturnal movements may respond to reduced doses of dopamine agonists or to benzodiazepines such as clonazepam, temazepam, or triazolam.

If insomnia is unresponsive to these measures, the judicious use of short-acting benzodiazepines for a few days or weeks may help to normalize the sleep-wake schedule. Although in theory, improved nighttime sleep may lead to reductions in morning tremor and rigidity, in practice, these changes may be hard to assess. Tricyclic antidepressants with sedating properties, such as amitriptyline, are frequently helpful for sleep-onset insomnia. The anticholinergic effects of tricyclic antidepressants may have therapeutic benefits for daytime parkinsonian symptoms as well, but they can induce nocturnal delirium in patients with cognitive impairment.

The treatment of sleep-related respiratory disturbances in parkinsonism is similar to the treatment of such problems in other patients. In patients with obstructive apneas and hypopneas, nasal continuous positive airway pressure offers the best chance of success and can be used effectively by most patients with parkinsonism until the advanced stages of the disease are reached. Upper airway surgery may help some patients with redundant palatal or pharyngeal tissue, but the abnormal motor activity of the upper airway remains present after surgery. For patients with multiple system atrophy and severe vocal cord dysfunction, tracheostomy often is necessary.

References

1. Parkinson J. Essay on the Shaking Palsy. London, England: Sherwood, Neely, and Jones; 1817:17.

2. Nausieda PA, Glantz R, Weber S, et al. Psychiatric complications of levodopa therapy of Parkinson's disease. In: Hassler RG, Christ JF, eds. Advances in Neurology. Vol 40. New York, NY: Raven Press; 1984:271–277.

3. Langston JW, Ballard PA, Tetrud JW, et al. Chronic parkinsonism in humans due to a product of meperidine-analog synthesis. Science. 1983;219:979–980.

4. Langston JW, Forno LS, Rebert CS, et al. Selective nigral toxicity after systemic administration of 1-methyl-4-phenyl-1,2,5,6-tetrahydropyridine (MPTP) in the squirrel monkey. Brain Res. 1984;292:390–394.

5. Charcot JM. Lectures on the Diseases of the Nervous System [trans. by G. Sigerson]. London, England: The New Sydenham Society; Lecture V, 1877:147.

6. Forno LS. Neuropathology of Parkinson's disease. J Neuropathol Exp Neurol. 1996;55:259–272.

7. Burns RS, Chiueh CC, Markey SP, et al. A primate model of parkinsonism: selective destruction of dopaminergic neurons in the pars compacta of the substantia nigra by N-methyl-4-phenyl-1,2,3,6-tetrahydropyridine. Proc Natl Acad Sci U S A. 1983;80:4546–4550.

8. Jellinger K. Pathology of parkinsonism. In: Fahn S, Marsden CD, Jenner P, et al, eds. Recent Developments in Parkinson's Disease. New York, NY: Raven Press; 1986:33–66.

9. Zweig RM, Jankel WR, Hedreen JC, et al. The pedunculopontine nucleus in Parkinson's disease. Ann Neurol. 1989;26:41–46.

10. Javoy-Agid F, Agid Y. Is the mesocortical dopaminergic system involved in Parkinson's disease? Neurology (NY). 1980;30:1326–1330.

11. De Keyser J, Ebinger G, Vauquelin G. Evidence for a widespread dopaminergic innervation of the human cerebral neocortex. Neurosci Lett. 1989;104:281–285.

12. Ongini E, Caporali MG, Massotti M. Stimulation of dopamine D-1 receptors by SKF 38393 induces EEG desynchronisation and behavioral arousal. Life Sci. 1985;37:2327–2333.

13. Bo P, Ongini E, Giorgetti A, et al. Synchronization of the EEG and sedation induced by neuroleptics depend upon blockade of both D_1 and D_2 dopamine receptors. Neuropharmacology. 1988;27:799.

14. Cianchetti C. Dopamine agonists and sleep in man. In: Wauquier A, Gaillard JM, Monti JM, et al, eds. Sleep: Neurotransmitters and Neuromodulators. New York, NY: Raven Press; 1985:121–134.

15. Bagetta G, De Sarro G, Priolo E, et al. Ventral tegmental area: site through which dopamine D_2-receptor agonists evoke behavioural and electrocortical sleep in rats. Br J Pharmacol. 1988;95:860–866.

16. Svensson K, Alfoldi P, Hajos M, et al. Dopamine autoreceptor antagonists: effects of sleep-wake activity in the rat. Pharmacol Biochem Behav. 1987;26:123–129.

17. Trampus M, Ferri N, Monopoli A, et al. The dopamine D_1 receptor is involved in the regulation of REM sleep in the rat. Eur J Pharmacol. 1991;194:189–194.

18. Trampus M, Ongini E. The D_1 dopamine receptor antagonist SCH 23390 enhances REM sleep in the rat. Neuropharmacology. 1990;10:889–893.

19. Gillin JC, Post RM, Wyatt RJ, et al. REM inhibitory effect of L-dopa infusion during human sleep. Electroencephalogr Clin Neurophysiol. 1973;35:181–186.

20. Everett GM, Borcherding JW. L-Dopa: effect on concentrations of dopamine, norepinephrine, and serotonin in brains of mice. Science. 1970;168:849–850.

21. Karobath M, Diaz J-L, Huttunen MO. The effect of L-dopa on the concentrations of tryptophan, tyrosine and serotonin in rat brain. Eur J Pharmacol. 1971;14:393–399.

22. Fahn S, Snider S, Prasad ALN, et al. Normalization of brain serotonin by L-tryptophan in levodopa-treated rats. Neurology (NY). 1975;25:861–865.

23. de Rijk MC, Tzourio C, Breteler MM, et al. Prevalence of parkinsonism and Parkinson's disease in Europe: the Europarkinson Collaborative Study: European Community Concerted Action on the Epidemiology of Parkinson's disease. J Neurol Neurosurg Psychiatry. 1997;62:10–15.

24. Factor SA, McAlarney T, Sanchez-Ramon JR, et al. Sleep disorders and sleep effect in Parkinson's disease. Mov Disord. 1990;4:280–285.

25. Menza MA, Rosen RC. Sleep in Parkinson's disease: the role of depression and anxiety. Psychosomatics. 1995;36:262–266.
26. Comella CL, Tanner CM, Ristanovic RK. Polysomnographic sleep measures in Parkinson's disease patients with treatment-induced hallucinations. Ann Neurol. 1993;34:710–714.
27. Smith MC, Ellgring H, Oertel WH. Sleep disturbances in Parkinson's disease patients and spouses. J Am Geriatr Soc. 1997;45:194–199.
28. Kales A, Ansel RD, Markham CH, et al. Sleep in patients with Parkinson's disease and normal subjects prior to and following levodopa administration. Clin Pharmacol Ther. 1971;12:397–406.
29. Bergonzi P, Chiurulla C, Gambi D, et al. L-Dopa plus dopa-decarboxylase inhibitor: sleep organization in Parkinson's syndrome before and after treatment. Acta Neurol Belg. 1975;75:5–10.
30. Friedman A. Sleep pattern in Parkinson's disease. Acta Med Pol. 1980;21:193–199.
31. Mouret J. Differences in sleep in patients with Parkinson's disease. Electroencephalogr Clin Neurophysiol. 1975;38:653–657.
32. Aldrich MS, Foster NL, White RF, et al. Sleep abnormalities in progressive supranuclear palsy. Ann Neurol. 1989;25:577–581.
33. Martinelli P, Coccagna G, Rizzuto N, et al. Changes in systemic arterial pressure during sleep in Shy-Drager syndrome. Sleep. 1981;4:139–146.
34. April RS. Observations on parkinsonian tremor in all-night sleep. Neurology (NY). 1966;16:720–724.
35. Stern M, Roffwarg H, Duvoisin R. The parkinsonian tremor in sleep. J Nerv Ment Dis. 1968;147:202–210.
36. Fish DR, Sawyers D, Allen PJ, et al. The effect of sleep on the dyskinetic movements of Parkinson's disease, Gilles de la Tourette syndrome, Huntington's disease, and torsion dystonia. Arch Neurol. 1991;48:210–214.
37. van Hilten B, Hoff JI, Middelkoop HA, et al. Sleep disruption in Parkinson's disease: assessment by continuous activity monitoring. Arch Neurol. 1994;51:922–928.
38. Schenck CH, Bundlie SR, Mahowald MW. Delayed emergence of a parkinsonian disorder in 38% of 29 older men initially diagnosed with idiopathic rapid eye movement sleep behaviour disorder. Neurology. 1996;46:388–393.
39. Tan A, Salgado M, Fahn S. Rapid eye movement sleep behavior disorder preceding Parkinson's disease with therapeutic response to levodopa. Mov Disord. 1996;11:214–216.
40. Uchiyama M, Isse K, Tanaka K, et al. Incidental Lewy body disease in a patient with REM sleep behavior disorder. Neurology. 1995;45:709–712.
41. Turner RS, Chervin RD, Frey KA, et al. Probable diffuse Lewy body disease presenting as REM sleep behavior disorder. Neurology. 1997;49:523–527.
42. Plazzi G, Corsini R, Provini F, et al. REM sleep behavior disorders in multiple system atrophy. Neurology. 1997;48:1094–1097.
43. Currie LJ, Bennett JP Jr, Harrison MB, et al. Clinical correlates of sleep benefit in Parkinson's disease. Neurology. 1997;48:1115–1117.
44. Merello M, Hughes A, Colosimo C, et al. Sleep benefit in Parkinson's disease. Mov Disord. 1997;12:506–508.
45. Marsden CD, Parkes J, Quinn N. Fluctuations of disability in Parkinson's disease: clinical aspects. In: Marsden CD, Fahn S, eds. Movement Disorders. London, England: Butterworth Scientific; 1981:96–122.
46. Yamamura Y, Sobue I, Ando K, et al. Paralysis agitans of early onset with marked diurnal fluctuation of symptoms. Neurology (NY). 1973;23:239–244.
47. Sunohara N, Mano Y, Ando K, et al. Idiopathic dystonia-parkinsonism with marked diurnal fluctuation of symptoms. Ann Neurol. 1985;17:39–45.
48. Segawa M, Hosaka A, Miyagawa F, et al. Hereditary progressive dystonia with marked diurnal fluctuation. Adv Neurol. 1976;14:215–233.
49. Hovestadt A, Bogaard JM, Meerwaldt JD, et al. Pulmonary function in Parkinson's disease. J Neurol Neurosurg Psychiatry. 1989;52:329–333.
50. Vincken WG, Gauthier SG, Dollfuss RE, et al. Involvement of upper-airway muscles in extrapyramidal disorders: a cause of airflow limitation. N Engl J Med. 1984;311:438–442.
51. Bushmann M, Dobmeyer SM, Leeker L, et al. Swallowing abnormalities and their response to treatment in Parkinson's disease. Neurology. 1989;39:1309–1314.
52. Hardie RJ, Efthimiou J, Stern GM. Respiration and sleep in Parkinson's disease. J Neurol Neurosurg Psychiatry. 1986;49:1326.
53. Apps MCP, Sheaff PC, Ingram DA, et al. Respiration and sleep in Parkinson's disease. J Neurol Neurosurg Psychiatry. 1985;48:1240–1245.
54. Chokroverty S, Sharp JT, Barron KD. Periodic respiration in erect posture in Shy-Drager syndrome. J Neurol Neurosurg Psychiatry. 1978;41:980–986.
55. McNicholas WT, Rutherford R, Grossman R, et al. Abnormal respiratory pattern generation during sleep in patients with autonomic dysfunction. Am Rev Respir Dis. 1983;128:429–433.
56. Guilleminault C, Tilkian A, Lehrman K, et al. Sleep apnoea syndrome: states of sleep and autonomic dysfunction. J Neurol Neurosurg Psychiatry. 1977;40:718–725.
57. Guilleminault C, Briskin JG, Greenfield MS, et al. The impact of autonomic nervous system dysfunction on breathing during sleep. Sleep. 1981;4:263–268.
58. Kenyon GS, Apps MCP, Traub M. Stridor and obstructive sleep apnea in Shy-Drager syndrome treated by laryngofissure and cord lateralization. Laryngoscope. 1984;94:1106–1108.
59. Isozaki E, Naito A, Horiguchi S, et al. Early diagnosis and stage classification of vocal cord abductor paralysis in patients with multiple system atrophy. J Neurol Neurosurg Psychiatry. 1996;60:399–402.
60. Leeman AL, ONeill CJ, Nicholson PW, et al. Parkinson's disease in the elderly: response to and optimal spacing of night time dosing with levodopa. Br J Clin Pharmacol. 1987;24:637–643.
61. Askenasy JJM, Yahr MD. Suppression of REM rebound by pergolide. J Neural Transm. 1984;59:151–159.
62. Askenasy JJM, Yahr MD. Reversal of sleep disturbance in Parkinson's disease by antiparkinsonian therapy: a preliminary study. Neurology (NY). 1985;35:527–532.
63. Lang AE, Quinn N, Brincat S, et al. Pergolide in late-stage Parkinson disease. Ann Neurol. 1982;12:243–247.
64. Scharf B, Moskovitz C, Lupton MD, et al. Dream phenomena induced by chronic levodopa therapy. J Neural Transm. 1978;43:143–151.
65. Klawans HL, Goetz C, Bergen D. Levodopa-induced myoclonus. Arch Neurol. 1975;32:331–334.
66. Vardi J, Glaubman H, Rabey J, et al. EEG sleep patterns in Parkinsonian patients treated with bromocryptine and L-dopa: a comparative study. J Neural Transm. 1979;45:307–316.

89

Dementia

Donald L. Bliwise

Dementing illnesses encompass a wide variety of nonreversible conditions, including Alzheimer's disease (AD), Parkinson's disease (PD), progressive supranuclear palsy, Huntington's disease, Creutzfeld-Jakob disease, fatal familial insomnia, and multi-infarct (vascularized) dementia. This chapter reviews current knowledge of dementing illness with emphasis on sleep-wake patterns in AD with occasional reference to vascular dementia/stroke and PD. See Chapters 88 and 90 for more detailed discussions of these latter conditions.

The largest proportion (as high as 70%) of demented patients suffer from primary degenerative dementia (AD). Most of the studies examining sleep in dementia probably include mostly cases of AD, but diagnostic imprecision often makes it difficult to know precisely which type of dementia patients have been studied. AD is typically diagnosed by exclusion of other reversible dementias (e.g., dementia due to folate deficiency, hypothyroidism, or metabolic or toxic conditions). Very few studies involving sleep have gone beyond such an exclusionary diagnosis to acquire neuropathological verification of AD or have related sleep patterns to specific brain lesions. The National Institute of Neurological and Communication Disorders and Stroke guidelines[1] suggest use of a three-level system to indicate diagnostic uncertainty in the diagnosis of AD, classifying patients as having definite, probable, or possible disease. With rare exception,[2, 3] nearly all sleep studies use patients in the last two categories. Unfortunately, in some cases in which the patients were only crudely screened, the weaker diagnosis of possible AD was more likely.

ELECTROENCEPHALOGRAPHIC WAVEFORMS IN DEMENTIA

The electroencephalographic (EEG) waveforms in dementia differ from normal. Automated stage scoring recognition programs are of little utility in attempting to determine electrophysiological state in such patients. The waking EEG of demented patients typically shows abundant, diffuse slow-wave activity encompassing both delta (0 to 3 Hz) and theta (3 to 7 Hz) frequencies[4, 5]; focal slowing occurs less frequently unless a localized stroke has occurred or a lesion exists.[6, 7] Some studies have shown correlations between diffuse EEG slowing

in AD and pathology-verified amyloid plaques and neurofibrillary tangles.[8] In addition, both the incidence and frequency of dominant occipital (alpha) activity decrease in dementia,[9, 10] even in very mild, early-stage AD.[11]

The slowing of EEG activity in dementia may make discriminations between sleep and wakefulness, as well as among various sleep stages, difficult. Systematic behavioral observations may be helpful in validation of electrophysiological state.[12] Diffuse waking slow-wave activity is demonstrated in Figure 89–1 in a polysomnogram in a demented patient. Typically, such activity is mistaken for sweat or other artifact. During nonrapid eye movement (NREM) sleep, the "carryover" of such abnormal delta activity makes it difficult to discriminate normal (0.5 to 2.0 Hz) delta wave activity occurring during sleep. Figure 89–2 shows exaggerated slow-wave activity during NREM sleep in a dementia patient. Discrimination between normal and abnormal delta waves during sleep may be aided by careful examination of the frequency component of the EEG, which is often slower than the minimum cut-off value (0.5 Hz) used by Rechtschaffen and Kales to define normal delta waves. Because of these interpretive difficulties, some have favored scoring of NREM sleep in such patients as "indeterminate,"[13] and a 1998 reliability study of scoring sleep in such patients suggests that higher interrater NREM scoring reliability was achieved when NREM stages were collapsed in this way.[14] Slow-wave activity may persist into rapid eye movement (REM) sleep as well. Figure 89–3 demonstrates slow-wave activity during an epoch of REM sleep.

These difficulties have led many researchers to attempt computerized waveform analysis for research purposes. Spectral analysis of the waking EEGs of demented patients generally shows the greatest differences from elderly controls in delta or theta power relative to alpha measures.[15–18] Topographically, both right[19] and left[15, 20] temporal areas have been suggested as most likely to be abnormal. A major limitation in nearly all of these studies is their cross-sectional design. Longitudinal studies are required to adequately tease apart issues of severity, stage of disease, and length of dementing illness. In one of the few such studies, Coben et al.[16] reported that increased theta power showed the earliest alterations in the progression of AD over time. This was followed by decreased alpha power, and then finally, increased delta power.

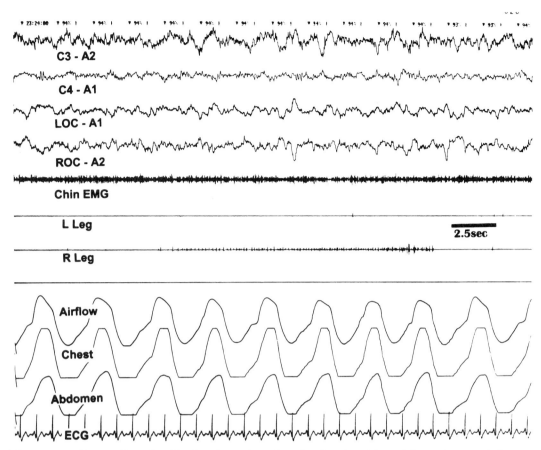

Figure 89–1. Polysomnographic recording of waking in a dementia patient showing slow delta activity on the central electroencephalographic (EEG) channel. ECG, electrocardiogram; EMG, electromyogram.

Some investigators have questioned whether such techniques provide any incremental information regarding diagnosis. Waking theta activity (higher percentage and lower frequency) provided high specificity but only marginal sensitivity in identifying patients with mild AD[21-23] but more recent work suggests the value of REM EEG as a marker for such slowing. Theta and delta (2 to 8 Hz) spectral power at occipital placements within artifact-free epochs of tonic REM sleep provided high specificity and sensitivity in early-stage mild AD.[24-26] Hassainia et al.[27] reported greater effects in frontal and temporal regions, and Petit et al.[28] also suggested that asymmetry was more conspicuous during REM in AD patients. These results, suggesting that REM EEG is a particularly sensitive marker of AD, might reflect deterioration of critical cholinergic structures (e.g., nucleus basalis of Meynert) also responsible for EEG desynchronization, though a pharmacological intervention with a cholinesterase inhibitor[29] showed no significant effects on sleep in AD. More recent data suggest better discrimination between AD patients and controls with these measures than with single-photon emission computed tomography (SPECT).[30]

SLEEP ARCHITECTURE

The subpopulation of demented patients studied in the sleep laboratory is almost certainly biased by selec-

tion factors. Many demented patients are known to "sundown" (see later), and the most profoundly demented patients simply cannot tolerate the laboratory procedures, although there are a few studies in which grossly demented patients have been studied.[31]

More sleep disruption in demented patients relative to aged controls has been shown in a number of studies, as well as in a meta-analysis.[32] Typically reported findings include lower sleep efficiency, higher stage 1 percentage, and greater frequency of arousals and awakenings.[33-35] Evidence that measures such as sleep efficiency and number of awakenings closely parallel the level of severity of dementia is impressive,[31, 35, 36] although use of such information to classify patients vs. controls was powerful only for moderate (as opposed to mild) levels of dementia.[36] Decreases in stages 3 and 4 sleep have also been noted in dementia,[31, 34, 35] although two research groups failed to find such differences.[12, 13] Meta-analysis[32] also suggested no differences between demented patients and controls, but gross overrepresentation of the patient pools generating those findings may have played a role. Some studies have reported elevated stages 3 and 4 sleep in dementia, but this probably represented the effect of including pathological delta activity as stages 3 and 4 sleep (see Fig. 89–2). Decreases in spindling activity have also been noted in dementia.[31]

Abnormalities in REM sleep are of particular interest in AD because the integrity of cholinergic systems may

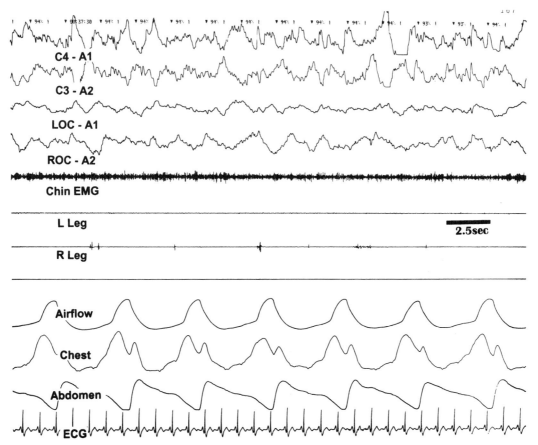

Figure 89–2. Polysomnographic recording of NREM sleep in a dementia patient showing excessively slow (less than 0.5 Hz) delta wave activity; because of difficulty discriminating normal sleep-related delta activity from such pathological delta activity, scoring of "indeterminate" NREM sleep in dementia patients is preferred. ECG, electrocardiogram; EMG, electromyogram.

be related to both REM sleep and AD. Although REM sleep is probably dependent on multiple neurotransmitter systems, the role of acetylcholine and its precursors in the induction of REM sleep has been shown in both human and animal studies. In addition, AD is known to be characterized by reduced levels of choline acetyltransferase. These findings suggest that measurements related to REM sleep should be attenuated in AD. We have previously mentioned the extent to which EEG desynchronization in REM sleep (spectral power of theta and delta frequency bands relative to higher frequencies) may reflect cholinergic integrity of basal forebrain mechanisms. REM sleep as a function of total sleep time has been suggested to be decreased in dementia in some[31, 35] but not all[34, 36] studies. Severity may play a role in the discrepancies; in one study, group differences in REM time were present only when comparing patients with moderate and severe AD with controls.[37] Positive relationships between higher psychometric test performance and higher REM sleep amounts have been reported.[37, 38] An animal model for such decreased REM sleep in dementia has been proposed by Stone et al.[39]

Lengthened REM latency in dementia relative to controls is an inconsistent finding,[35] with some studies finding no apparent differences,[3, 13] and others even suggesting a trend for shorter REM latency.[33] If REM latency is lengthened in dementia, this may have diagnostic usefulness because REM latency is typically shortened in affective disorders (see Chapter 96), and the differential diagnosis between dementia and depression is a common problem in geriatrics. Disagreement over definitions of REM latency (e.g., whether wake time after sleep onset is included and how sleep onset is defined) may play a role in determining how sensitive and specific an indicator for dementia and depression this measure may be.[34] Other measures of REM, such as REM density[40] or low-frequency power spectra in REM EEG[41] may yet yield higher classification accuracy.

Several studies have employed total or REM sleep deprivation as probes to differentiate depressive syndromes and dementia in old age.[42–45] These studies suggested that both elderly depressed *and* demented patients rebound from total sleep deprivation with increased sleep efficiency on recovery sleep, although the depressed patients continue to show somewhat lower sleep efficiencies after sleep deprivation.[44] REM latencies increased in both groups following sleep deprivation, whereas REM latency decreased in aged controls. REM sleep deprivation produced little evidence of REM rebound in depressed people, but a modest increase in REM activity in AD.[43] Given the common mixed clinical presentation of depression and dementia

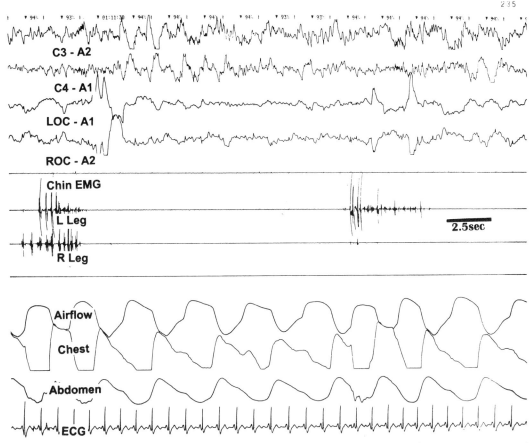

Figure 89–3. Polysomnographic recording of rapid eye movement (REM) sleep in a dementia patient showing continuation of abnormal delta and slow theta activity on both central and occipital electroencephalographic (EEG) channels. ECG, electrocardiogram; EMG, electromyogram.

in late life, the question arises as to whether sleep following sleep deprivation can differentiate these syndromes. Using total sleep deprivation, Buysse et al.[42] reported that elderly depressed patients with cognitive symptoms showed more robust REM rebound effects than did demented patients with depressive symptoms, although the reasons why the former group should show greater REM rebound effects than a purely depressed group subjected specifically to REM deprivation[43] are unclear.

SLEEP APNEA

Sleep apnea has been associated with impaired reaction time, memory, and executive function[46–51] (for reviews, see references 52, 53). This raises the possibility that more severe forms of global mental impairment, such as dementia, might be associated with sleep apnea. The high prevalence of both sleep apnea (see Chapter 3) and dementia in the older population also lends some credence to this hypothesis.

Of all neurotransmitters affected by hypoxia, the metabolism of acetylcholine (the transmitter system markedly affected in AD) is most closely related to oxidative metabolic pathways.[54] Studies demonstrating hypoxic effects on acetylcholine in animals rely on

sustained continuous hypoxic exposure,[54, 55] not the intermittent changes in oxygenation characteristic of sleep apnea. If such a mechanism was common in dementia, one would expect to see relatively severe sleep apnea in AD patients on a routine basis. Although some studies show that AD patients may, statistically, have more sleep apnea than elderly controls,[56, 57] these results are not uniform.[58, 59] Moreover, even among the former studies, the magnitude of the group differences are hardly overwhelming. Although the memory impairments and subtle effects of psychomotor slowing in sleep apnea patients are undeniably real, these effects are vastly different from the substantial decrements in intellectual abilities that occur in AD.

Sleep apnea may be associated with certain cases of dementia related to cerebrovascular disease, sometimes called multi-infarct dementia or vascular dementia. Patients with strokes often show high levels of sleep-disordered breathing,[60–62] although the interpretation of this finding is equivocal because sleep apnea may have occurred subsequent to stroke rather than preceding it. Patients with vascular dementia appeared to have higher rates of sleep-disordered breathing relative to patients with AD.[63, 64] Epidemiological evidence has linked snoring and stroke[65–67] and many studies suggest that cerebrovasomotor regulation may be affected by apnea[68, 69] (see Chapters 47, 70, 90). Some studies have shown that sleep apnea in stroke patients was associated with lower rates of survival and poorer functional capacity.[61] Treatment with nasal continuous positive airway pressure (CPAP) was shown to improve vasomotor reactivity of the right middle cerebral artery to hypercapnia in middle-aged sleep apnea patients.[69]

Should the older dementia patient with sleep apnea be treated with CPAP? It may well be that if the dementia is due to Alzheimer's-type degeneration, treatment of sleep apnea may do little to impede the course of the dementia. If the patient with sleep apnea and AD is somnolent and incurs a decreased quality of life because of that hypersomnolence, however, treatment of sleep apnea may be beneficial and positively affect the patient's remaining years. Depending on the level of incapacity and extent of confusion, application of CPAP may be more or less difficult. Experience dictates that a concerned and involved caregiver (spouse, adult child, nursing home personnel) may make the critical difference in the success of instituting such treatments. Before the sleep medicine specialist initiates sleep apnea treatment in a patient with presumed AD, ethical considerations should be weighed carefully. The inevitable decline of the patient and the duress on the family must be considered. The slow insidious "death of the mind" experienced by these patients and observed by their caregivers may predispose those caregivers to grasp at a false hope for a miracle cure. Although a few anecdotal case reports suggest that dementia patients with sleep apnea may show dramatic improvements,[70, 71] reversible dementias are not common. Clarfield[72] estimated that only about 3% of all dementia cases from *any* cause are potentially reversible. The sleep medicine specialist should be clear at the outset with members of the family about what is reasonable and unreasonable to expect from instituting treatment for sleep apnea in such patients.

NOCTURNAL AGITATION AND SUNDOWNING

Definitions and Prevalence

Many demented patients "sundown" during the evening hours or during the night, and sleep medicine specialists are often asked to offer diagnostic and/or treatment recommendations regarding such cases. Nocturnal agitation may be the single most common cause of institutionalization in demented geriatric patients.[73, 74] Families may be able to tolerate mental confusion, the memory loss, and to some extent the incontinence of a demented family member. When the caregivers' sleep is disrupted night after night by an agitated, demented patient, this may well be what leads the caregiver to resort to institutionalization. In fact, actigraphic studies of caregivers of demented patients have shown that bedtime and arising times of demented patients coincide with peaks of caregiver activity.[75]

Sundowning is often considered to represent nocturnal delirium. However, *delirium*, defined as a psychiatric syndrome characterized by a transient disorganization of a wide range of cognitive functions due to widespread derangement of cerebral metabolism,[76] is a psychiatric diagnosis, not a description of behavior. Nocturnal exacerbation of delirium has been recognized since the time of Hippocrates,[76] and the *Diagnostic and Statistical Manual of Mental Disorders, Fourth Edition* (DSM-IV)[77] notes strong associations with aberrations in the sleep-wake cycle. Delirium, which can occur at any age, is seen in a wide variety of toxic, metabolic, infectious, nutritional, and substance-induced states, may frequently, but not invariably, accompany dementia.[78] For example, acute dystonic reactions in psychiatric patients receiving neuroleptic medication tended to peak in the time interval between 4 and 8 PM.[79]

One can operationally define *sundowning* without regard to etiology as temporally specific agitation occurring in the evening or nighttime hours,[80, 81] although there is little consensus on how the descriptor is used. The term is employed frequently in clinical geriatrics,[82] and one study even attempted systematic treatment for "sundown syndrome" without even bothering to define it.[83] In the first apparent attempt to investigate sundowning,[84] patients were brought into a dark room for about an hour during the day. The patients were reported to become delirious shortly after this. This study was poorly controlled and has never been replicated.

Because few studies use rigorous definitions for sundowning, figures are scarce about its prevalence. As many as 50% of geriatric patients may be delirious on admission to a general medical unit or develop delirium during an acute care hospital stay,[85, 86] although other studies place these figures somewhat lower, at about 20%.[87, 88] One assumes that most of these patients experienced sleep disturbance as part of their delirium. These high prevalence figures may reflect the broad time referent used in some of these studies. By contrast, when examining a shorter time frame, much lower prevalences were found.[89, 90]

In nursing home populations, the prevalence of sundowning has been variously estimated as 25%,[91] 12.4%,[92] and 14%.[93] Estimates from in-home caregivers range from 28%[94] to 24%.[95] Other studies of well-characterized patients with AD have noted clinically significant sleep disturbance in about 40% of the patients studied[96] and sleep disturbance associated with the APOE 3/4 genotype relative to the APOE 4/4 and 3/3 subtypes,[97] although it was unclear if this sleep disturbance was accompanied by sufficient agitation and confusion to warrant the label of sundowning. In many of these studies, the time sampling frame was also unspecified, thus leaving open the possibility that sundowning may have occurred at some point in the course of the dementia rather than concurrently with evaluation.

Several studies have reported agitation to be most likely in the early evening hours. This has been documented using videomonitoring of wandering,[98] hour-by-hour caregiver logs,[99] actigraphy,[100] and in-person real-time behavioral observations.[80, 101, 102] For further review of this literature, see reference 81.

A different perspective on temporal specificity of agitation has been offered by Exum et al.,[103] who viewed agitation from the standpoint of treatment rather than behavior description. As needed, psychoactive medication served as a proxy for disruptive behavior, and the authors presented data suggesting that milieu-derived factors, such as the patient-to-staff ratio and shift change, related to such medication use. The authors' interpretation of their results portrayed sundowning as a factitious construct, embedded in the social context of harried nurses and aides caring for often difficult patients. Though an intriguing notion, combined data across patients and types of dosages of medications make it difficult to reach conclusions about patients' behavior from these types of data.

Associated Factors and Etiology

Observation of sleep in institutionalized patients indicates that the severity of dementia is correlated with the extent of sleep disruption at night.[104] However, factors associated with the behavioral syndrome of sundowning are unclear. Evans[92] noted that nursing home patients who experienced sundowning were more likely to be demented, have recent room transfers, be incontinent, and have fewer medical diagnoses than those who did not experience sundowning. Other variables that might be expected to relate to sundowning (e.g., visual or auditory impairment; use of psychotropic, cardiovascular, or analgesic medications; morning-afternoon differences in blood pressure and temperature), however, did not differentiate the groups. In one study,[94] it was noted that caregiver-reported sundowning in noninstitutionalized patients with AD was related to a faster rate of decline in selected mental abilities, but not to general level of function. Although not explicitly examining nocturnal delirium, a 1996 prospective study examining the development of delirium over 9 days in a geriatric population reported that the onset of delirium was associated with malnutrition (serum albumin less than 30 g/liter), use of physical restraints, insertion of a bladder catheter, addition of four or more medications, and any iatrogenic events (infections, pulmonary embolism, falls, fecal impaction).[105]

Cohen-Mansfield et al.[106–110] suggested that agitated, aggressive behaviors were more related to physical pain and relatively recent surgery, whereas nonaggressive agitated behaviors were related to cognitive impairment and impairment in activities of daily living. Previous psychiatric history appeared unrelated to agitation, although past stressful events (e.g., financial problems, Holocaust experiences, death of spouse) were related to nonaggressive physical behavior.[109] Nursing home residents with higher levels of cognitive functioning were more verbally agitated.[107]

Several different sleep-specific or chronobiologically based causes can be postulated as underlying sundowning. Agitation during the nocturnal hours and arising from sleep might be suggestive of REM dyscontrol mechanisms or sleep interruption as an underlying cause. Agitation arising in the early evening hours not preceded by sleep might be more suggestive of the influence of chronobiological mechanisms.

REM Dyscontrol

The first suggestion that nocturnal confusion was related to REM sleep mechanisms was the early study of Feinberg et al.[33] In their study of sleep in DSM-II–defined chronic brain syndrome patients, the authors found that 3 of 15 patients awakened out of REM sleep in "states of delirium with fixed ideas . . . of an everyday nature rather than bizarre."[33(p133)] Although in the mid-1980s, idiopathic REM behavior disorder (RBD) patients were described as nondemented[111] (see Chapter 64), the spectrum of REM dyscontrol syndromes has now broadened considerably to include dementing disorders.[112] For example, a substantial number of idiopathic RBD patients have been shown to develop later PD.[113] Additionally known connections between basal ganglia outputs (globus pallidus and substantia nigra), known to deteriorate in PD, and brainstem centers known to modulate REM sleep atonia,[114] have substantial functional impact upon state-dependent motor control in a variety of neurodegenerative conditions.[115] Given these neuroanatomical considerations, it is of interest that primary caregivers of PD patients reported patients to have greater nocturnal agitation (but not more total agitation) relative to caregivers of AD patients.[116]

It is important to stress that certain elements of neurodegenerative disease may be common to both AD and PD. Lewy bodies, a neuropathological finding that is often a hallmark of PD, may also be found in AD, and RBD with autopsy-confirmed Lewy bodies has been described.[117–119] Aberrant motor control during REM sleep may thus occur across a variety of dementias including both PD *and* AD. For example, a clinicopathological study reported that AD patients with Lewy body findings on neuropathological examination were far more likely to have clinical histories involving hallucinations than AD patients without such results,[120] though no description was offered regarding whether the hallucinations were nocturnal.

Forced Awakening From Sleep

Demented patients who are awakened frequently during sleep are the most agitated.[92] Nocturnal bed checks by staff are related to many types of aggressive behavior during the daytime hours in nursing home patients.[110] Episodes of interrupted sleep were more likely to be associated with agitated behavior if the awakenings occurred during the postsunset period.[80]

It is ironic that in the United States, adequate nursing home care often includes policies that *ensure* multiple nightly awakenings of nursing home residents by staff. Owing largely to the standards of care set by the Agency for Health Care Policy and Research within the Department of Health and Human Services, mandatory checks of bedding and bedclothes for dampness are considered components of adequate nursing home care to prevent bedsores caused by moisture. Even from the standpoint of geriatricians concerned with incontinence, such awakenings may be unnecessary. Schnelle et al.[121] have noted that many incontinent nursing home residents awakened for position changes during the night have considerable spontaneous mobility during their sleep which would obviate the need for such awakenings. Environmental noise within nursing homes is also considered a major disruptive influence on sleep. Nearly 30% of all actigraphically assessed awakenings could be traced to inadvertent environmental noise, from sources such as intercoms, staff vocalizations, cleaning equipment, and linen carts.[122] The resident in a nursing home is exposed on average to 32 noise events per night in excess of 60 dB.[123]

Chronobiological Influences

Given the relative temporal specificity of agitation for the late-afternoon/early-evening time period, the possibility exists that the circadian timing system may prompt or otherwise facilitate such behaviors. Although no studies have yet linked physiological measures of diurnal variability to such sundowning, the time of day when agitation is most likely in demented patients may correspond to the maximum of the body temperature cycle and the wake-maintenance zone described in a number of studies of human circadian rhythms. The wake-maintenance zone represents a period of maximal circadian alertness and occurs about 8 h before the body temperature minimum, typically several hours before bedtime.[124] In a demented patient with compromised mental faculties, the wake-maintenance zone may represent a period of heightened vulnerability for agitation. Alternatively, demented patients may show so-called day-night reversal, in which sleep is displaced primarily to the daytime hours and wakefulness occurs nocturnally. In such cases, a patient's nocturnal behavior may be similar to behavior occurring during the daytime but it becomes far more disruptive to caregivers at night. Some have even suggested that sundowning in a nursing home, at least as reflected in as needed medication usage, may indeed be more a function of staffing and shift changes than of real temporal alterations in patients' behavior.[103]

Speculation that elements of the circadian timing system may be involved in sundowning arises partly from the observation that the suprachiasmatic nucleus, (SCN), the center that controls circadian rhythms in mammals (see Chapter 28), undergoes substantial deterioration in AD.[125] The deterioration of the hypothalamus in AD has been shown to be specific for the SCN and not include the adjacent supraoptic or paraventricular nuclei.[126] Although limited to the extent that severely agitated dementia patients cannot undergo polysomnographic or other physiological measurements, available data are at least suggestive that circadian rhythms may be altered in demented patients. The relative proportion of daytime sleep (as a percentage of 24-h sleep) was higher in severely demented, institutionalized patients (14%) than in noninstitutionalized

moderately (5%) or mildly (2%) demented patients.[31, 35] Other studies of institutionalized and noninstitutionalized AD patients have reported or implied reduced amplitude in rhythms of actigraphically monitored rest and activity,[75, 127–129] behaviorally observed sleep and wakefulness,[102] heart rate,[130] blood pressure,[131] and melatonin,[132, 133] but a few studies report no differences from controls in body temperature rhythms in amplitude[134–137] and phase.[135, 136] Data on phase relationships appear to conflict. One study of body temperature[137] and several actigraphic studies have reported apparent phase delays in AD patients,[137–139] but another 1997 study did not.[75] Gillin et al.[140] reported phase advances in body temperature in male AD patients, but phase delays in female AD patients relative to controls. Additionally, several other studies have shown that caregivers report earlier bedtimes and wake-up times in AD patients relative to healthy elderly persons, suggesting a phase advance.[141, 142] Cortisol rhythms have variously been reported to be no different in AD relative to controls[143] or possibly present higher amplitudes (higher nocturnal values) relative to controls.[144] Finally, Okawa et al.[145] reported "disorganized" and apparently desynchronized temperature rhythms in demented nursing home patients relative to nondemented nursing home patients (Fig. 89–4). Some of the patients with disorganized temperature rhythms also demonstrated nocturnal behavior disruption.

Data on rhythms in dementias other than AD are quite rare but are important in suggesting how chronobiology may be affected by dementing disease. Cerebrovascular white matter disease (subcortical vascular dementia) might be expected to disrupt major outputs from the SCN such as the thalamus, internal capsule, and selected midbrain regions,[146] and three separate studies have reported comparisons between measures of rhythms in AD and subcortical vascular dementia. All reported patients with vascular dementia having greater disruption of sleep-wake or body temperature rhythms.[147–149] In at least one of these studies, computed tomography (CT) imaging suggested that cases with a greater likelihood of white matter lucencies (highest proportion in internal or outer capsule, thalamus, and periventricular region) were related to greater 24-h sleep-wake disruption.[147] Few studies are available of rhythms in PD, a neurodegenerative disease characterized primarily by dopaminergic neuronal loss within the striatum and substantia nigra, which may only minimally affect hypothalamic structures.[150] The temperature rhythms for a small number of these patients have been reported to be similar to those in age-matched controls[151] and melatonin rhythms in de novo unmedicated patients did not differ from controls.[152] Furthermore, PD patients as a group did not appear sleepy on the multiple sleep latency test (MSLT), even when medications were taken into account.[153] These data are compatible with the notion that key features of time-keeping mechanisms, including both the SCN and its outputs, may be more or less disrupted in patients with specific kinds of dementing illness. The data are consistent with older case reports, which suggested that lesions of the third ventricle and

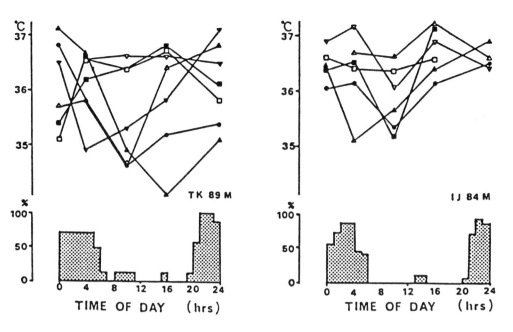

Figure 89–4. Examples of "disorganized" body temperature curves in two highly demented nursing home patients. Curves show 7 days of oral temperature data, based on intermittent sampling every 3 h. Bottom graphs indicate observed sleep episodes. Note wide day-to-day variation in peaks and troughs of the temperature cycle, suggesting dysfunction in the circadian timing system. (From Okawa M, Mishima K, Hishikawa Y, et al. Circadian rhythm disorders in sleep-waking and body temperature in elderly patients with dementia and their treatment. Sleep. 1991;14:478–485.)

the hypothalamic region were associated with aberrations of the sleep-wake and/or body temperature cycle.[154–157]

Treatments

Treatments for sundowning and nocturnal agitation represent one of the most vexing problems for the sleep disorders specialist. Ascertainment of probable cause should inform treatment to whatever extent possible (Table 89–1). First, it is well worth emphasizing that medical causes of nocturnal agitation, including, but not limited to, polypharmacy, bladder catheterization, low serum albumin indicative of malnutrition, fecal impactions, and infections, should be addressed.[105]

The institutional environment provides its own unique set of challenges for the treatment of nocturnal agitation. One early study reported that physicians' use of antipsychotics in nursing homes was directly related to case load in the facility[158]; newer studies suggest that sedative-hypnotic use was associated with higher hospital costs and longer hospital stays in the acute care setting, even after controlling for levels of disease.[159] Following adoption of the 1987 Omnibus Budget Reconciliation Act guidelines for nursing home care, most nursing homes within the United States now dispense far fewer psychotropic medications than in years before the passing of these guidelines.[160] Much of the danger attributable to the use of such medications arose from studies suggesting associations between injurious falls and the use of psychotropic drugs.[161] Just as in the noninstitutionalized, nondemented aged population (see Chapter 3), psychotropic medication use in the institutionalized geriatric population is not necessarily associated with a resolution of sleep problems; several studies in institutionalized patients have now shown that sleep problems persist.[162–164] Reducing medication should always at least be considered before instituting a new medication regimen.

The standard of care requiring elderly residents of nursing homes to be awakened for bedclothing changes to prevent bedsores hastened by urinary incontinence is poorly considered from the standpoint of sleep and wakefulness. Obviously, the exigencies of

Table 89–1. CLINICAL MANAGEMENT OF SUNDOWNING

Presumed Etiology	Potential Treatments
Medical causes (e.g., fecal impaction, infection, polypharmacy, malnutrition)	Alleviate primary medical problem
Environmental nocturnal interruptions	Assess spontaneous mobility in bed and potential for pressure sores; weigh necessity of bed checks; reduce staff noise
Rapid eye movement dyscontrol	Attempt clonazepam but in severe dementia consider selective dopamine antagonists (e.g., clozapine, risperidone) (see Table 89–2)
Dysfunction of chronobiological or homeostatic sleep-wake regulation	*Nonpharmacological:* enhance daytime illumination; restrict daytime napping; institute mild physical activity to extent possible
	Pharmacological: attempt zolpidem, zaleplon, customary benzodiazepine hypnotics, but which may be ineffective; antipsychotics are usually required; newer antipsychotics (see Table 89–2) are usually preferred to traditional antipsychotics (thioridazine, haloperidol)
	Melatonin: use judiciously in patients with possible cardiac and/or cerebrovasular disease (see text)

any particular patient requiring this type of preventive intervention would have to be determined on a case-by-case basis, but if sleep disturbance and nocturnal agitation result from such nocturnal interruption, such a policy might require reconsideration.[121, 165] Similarly, the disruptive influences of the nursing home environment itself cannot be overstated. Poorly informed staff with little understanding of the rudiments of sleep hygiene (e.g., light, noise) can seriously undermine the suitability of the nighttime environment for sleep.[122] In some cases, other aspects of nursing home policy (e.g., waxing floors) may be at issue.

Treatment of REM dyscontrol has been highlighted elsewhere in this book (see Chapter 64). Whereas clonazepam may be the preferred medication for nondemented outpatients with RBD,[111] site-specific dopamine antagonists, such as risperidone or clozapine (Clozaril), may also be considered in dementia patients. Beneficial effects of such medications in parkinsonian patients experiencing dopamimetic psychosis have been documented.[166–168] Given the heterogeneity of neuropathological findings across dementia syndromes (e.g., Lewy bodies are a neuropathological finding in AD as well as PD; also, see earlier), there is no reason to believe that use of such medications might not also be indicated for AD patients or other neurodegenerative conditions showing REM-specific agitation. Other medications having potentially selective dopaminergic antagonist properties include olanzapine[169] and quetiapine (Table 89–2). Although little published data exist regarding the use of these medications in dementia, some use might be indicated. Caution is suggested, however, with regard to olanzapine, since two groups have reported adverse effects with this medication in PD.[170–171]

The vast majority of cases of disturbed sleep in dementia are likely to reflect dysfunction of the chronobiological or homeostatic regulation of sleep secondary to the changes within the central nervous system. Pharmacologically, a diverse array of medications have been tried to promote sleep and reduce agitation in dementia (see review in reference 172). Although many studies did not specifically target nocturnal agitation as an outcome,[172] medications for which anecdotal success has been reported in the treatment of agitation include carbamazepine,[173] valproate,[174] antidepressants such as trazodone,[175] lithium carbonate,[176] L-deprenyl,[177] pindolol,[178] and propranolol.[179] Benzodiazepines such as triazolam have not been shown to be successful in helping AD patients to sleep.[180] Few clinical studies with site-specific benzodiazepine agonists (zolpidem, zaleplon) in frankly demented patients have been reported, although in one report,[181] which included approximately 60 demented patients, a relatively high dose of zolpidem (20 mg) was shown to improve patients' sleep based on nursing ratings. Biochemically, site-specific benzodiazepine agonists might be expected to be good medications for sleep in AD patients because postmortem studies showed a preferential binding for the gamma-aminobutyric acid (GABA$_A$) receptor complex in frontal cortex of AD patients relative to other benzodiazepines.[182] Adverse reactions at modest dosages (10 mg) have been reported in younger patients, however, suggesting cautious use in cognitively impaired elderly.[183]

Traditionally, older antipsychotics such as haloperidol 0.5 to 1.0 mg and thioridazine[184] 10 to 25 mg have been shown to improve sleep and reduce nocturnal agitation in demented patients. Haloperidol and thioridazine both have undesirable long-term sequelae. The former may exacerbate extrapyramidal symptoms or lead to tardive dyskinesia, whereas the latter may lead to orthostatic hypotension. Because of these untoward effects, most clinicians treating agitated patients prefer the newer antipsychotics such as clozapine, risperidone, olanzapine, and quetiapine, which in general, may have a slightly more favorable side effect profile (see Table 89–2). Of particular concern with clozapine is the possibility of agranulocytosis, which necessitates frequent white blood cell counts.

Melatonin (see Chapter 31) represents another possible treatment of the nocturnal sleep disturbance and agitation of the demented patient. Several studies have suggested utility of melatonin 2 mg as a hypnotic for elderly subjects with disturbed sleep.[185, 186] The clinical relevance of these data for dementia, however, remains uncertain because the studies relied on actigraphic measurements as their primary outcome and they did not specify the type or extent, if any, of dementia cases in their populations. In 1998, Hughes et al.[187] published a double-blind, placebo-controlled, crossover polysomnographic study of melatonin in *nondemented* geriatric

Table 89–2. NEW GENERATION ANTIPSYCHOTICS POTENTIALLY USEFUL FOR TREATMENT OF SUNDOWNING

	Clozapine*	Olanzapine	Quetiapine	Risperidone
Typical initial bedtime dose	12.5–75 mg	2.5–5 mg	25–100 mg	1–4 mg
Sedation	+++	+++	++	+
Extrapyramidal symptoms	+	+	+	+
Anticholinergic effects	+++	+++	—	—
Orthostatic hypotension	++	++	++	+
Primary sites of action	Dopamine D$_4$ receptor antagonist	Multiple receptor antagonist (5HT$_2$, D$_{1-4}$, M$_{1-5}$, H$_1$)	Multiple receptor antagonist (5HT$_{1/2}$, D$_{1/2}$, alpha$_{1/2}$ adrenoceptors, H$_1$)	Dopamine D$_2$ receptor, 5-HT$_2$ antagonist

*Requires monitoring for agranulocytosis.
—, negligible; +, mild; ++, moderate; +++, marked; 5-HT, 5-hydroxytryptamine (serotonin); D, dopaminergic; H, histamine; M, muscarinic.

patients that showed melatonin to have sleep-promoting and body temperature–lowering effects but to have minimal effects on sleep maintenance and sleep continuity. Perhaps more relevant are preliminary data from Singer et al.[188–190] who presented preliminary actigraphic data from ongoing double-blind, crossover, placebo-controlled clinical trials examining the effects of melatonin 0.5 mg and 10 mg in a well-characterized severely demented AD population. Results have been mixed to date with only the higher dose offering any possibility of an effect. Given the controversy over whether melatonin truly has hypnotic properties, the extent to which these may be independent of its ability to induce phase shifts, and its potential role as a vasoconstrictor,[191] the use of melatonin in demented patients is unproved with potentially adverse effects in elderly patients with cardiac or cerebrovascular disease.

Nonpharmacological management of sundowning can include enhanced daytime light exposure, restriction of daytime napping, and institution of structured social and physical activity. The net effects of age-dependent visual impairment such as macular degeneration, possible optic nerve neuropathy (often associated with AD),[192] and low daytime light exposures (often below 300 lux)[80, 193] are to reduce illumination as a relevant zeitgeber in the demented patient. Several studies suggest beneficial effects of light therapy,[145, 194–198] although differences in timing and duration of light exposure varied across studies. Whether enhanced illumination in these studies improved sleep and behavior by enhancing rhythmicity or merely by keeping patients awake remains unclear. Curtailment of daytime napping may in itself be useful. Demented nursing home patients who were awake during the day were more likely to be asleep at night; those asleep during the day were more likely to be awake at night.[102] Low-voltage, low-current transcranial electrical stimulation at increasing frequencies of 14 to 80 Hz administered during the daytime was shown to improve nocturnal sleep, presumably by at least partially enhancing daytime alertness.[199] Physical activity was tested as an intervention to improve sleep in nursing home patients with only minimal success, but the physical activity was very slight and probably not aerobic.[200] Okawa et al.[145] have reported success with an omnibus treatment package of mild activity, exposure to light, and presumed sleep restriction, but no alteration in temperature rhythm was seen subsequent to alteration in sleep. Finally, as a last resort, some nursing facilities have instituted a regularly scheduled nocturnal activities hour (e.g., 2 to 4 AM) to minimize disruption of staff and other residents. Obviously, sleep disturbance at the very end of life may be exceedingly difficult to treat and may require creative environmental manipulations in addition to pharmacological management.

References

1. McKhann G, Drachman D, Folstein M, et al. Clinical diagnosis of Alzheimer's disease: report of the NINCDS-ADRDA work group under the auspices of Department Health and Human Services Task Force on Alzheimer's disease. Neurology. 1984;34:939–944.
2. Prinz PN, Vitiello MV, Bokan J, et al. Sleep in Alzheimer's dementia. In: Von Hahn E, Emser W, Kurtz D, et al, eds. Sleep, Aging, and Related Disorders. Basel, Switzerland: Karger; 1987:128–142. Interdisciplinary Topics in Gerontology; vol 22.
3. Blois R, Pawlak C, Rossi JM, et al. Sleep EEG findings in Alzheimer and Pick's dementia. In: Smirne S, Franceschi M, Ferini-Strambi L, eds. Sleep and Aging. Milan, Italy: Masson; 1991:65–70.
4. Mundy-Castle AC, Hurst LA, Beerstecher DM, et al. The electroencephalogram in the senile psychoses. Electroencephalogr Clin Neurophysiol. 1954;6:245–252.
5. Obrist WD, Henry CE. Electroencephalographic findings in aged psychiatric patients. J Nerv Ment Dis. 1958;126:254–267.
6. Gloor P, Ball G, Schaul N. Brain lesions that produce delta waves in the EEG. Neurology. 1977;27:326–333.
7. Soininen H, Partanen VJ, Helkala E-L, et al. EEG findings in senile dementia and normal aging. Acta Neurol Scand. 1982;65:59–70.
8. Muller HF, Schwartz G. Electroencephalograms and autopsy findings in geropsychiatry. J Gerontol. 1978;33:504–513.
9. Otomo E: Electroencephalography in old age: dominant alpha pattern. Electroencephalogr Clin Neurophysiol. 1966;21:489–491.
10. Busse EW, Wang HS. The electroencephalographic changes in late life: a longitudinal study. J Clin Exp Gerontol. 1979;1:145–158.
11. Prinz PN, Vitiello MV. Dominant occipital (alpha) rhythm frequency in early stage Alzheimer's disease and depression. Electroencephalogr Clin Neurophysiol. 1989;73:427–432.
12. Allen SR, Seiler WO, Stahelin HB, et al. Seventy-two-hour polygraphic and behavior recordings of wakefulness and sleep in a hospital geriatric unit: comparison between demented and nondemented patients. Sleep. 1987;10:143–159.
13. Reynolds CF III, Kupfer DJ, Taska LS, et al. EEG sleep in elderly depressed, demented, and healthy subjects. Biol Psychiatry. 1985;20:431–442.
14. Williams ML, Irbe D, Ansari FP, et al. Stage scoring reliability for nocturnal polysomnography in patients with Parkinson's disease. Sleep. 1998;21:171.
15. Breslau J, Starr A, Sicotte N, et al. Topographic EEG changes with normal aging and SDAT. Electroencephalogr Clin Neurophysiol. 1989;72:281–289.
16. Coben LA, Danziger W, Storandt M. A longitudinal EEG study of mild senile dementia of Alzheimer type: changes at 1 year and at 2.5 years. Electroencephalogr Clin Neurophysiol. 1985;61:101–112.
17. Penttila M, Partanen JV, Soininen H, et al. Quantitative analysis of occipital EEG in different stages of Alzheimer's disease. Electroencephalogr Clin Neurophysiol. 1985;60:1–6.
18. Coben LA, Danziger WL, Berg L. Frequency analysis of the resting awake EEG in mild senile dementia of the Alzheimer type. Electroencephalogr Clin Neurophysiol. 1983;55:372–380.
19. Duffy FH, Albert MS, McAnulty G. Brain electrical activity in patients with presenile and senile dementia of the Alzheimer type. Ann Neurol. 1984;16:439–448.
20. Rice DM, Buchsbaum MS, Starr A, et al. Abnormal EEG slow wave activity in left temporal areas in senile dementia of the Alzheimer type. J Gerontol. 1990;45:M145–M151.
21. Brenner RP, Reynolds CF, Ulrich RF. Diagnostic efficacy of computerized spectral versus visual EEG analysis in elderly normal, demented, and depressed subjects. Electroencephalogr Clin Neurophysiol. 1988;69:110–117.
22. Coben LA, Chi D, Snyder AZ, et al. Replication of a study of frequency analysis of the resting awake EEG in mild probable Alzheimer's disease. Electroencephalogr Clin Neurophysiol. 1990;75:148–154.
23. Brenner RP, Ulrich RF, Spiker DG, et al. Computerized EEG spectral analysis in elderly normal, demented, and depressed subjects. Electroencephalogr Clin Neurophysiol. 1986;64:483–492.
24. Larsen LH, Prinz PN. EKG artifacts suppression from the EEG. Electroencephalogr Clin Neurophysiol. 1991;79:241–244.
25. Larsen LH, Prinz PN, Moe KE. Quantitative analysis of the

EEG during REM sleep: methodology. Electroencephalogr Clin Neurophysiol. 1992;83:24–35.

26. Prinz PN, Larsen LH, Moe KE, et al. EEG markers of early Alzheimer's disease in computer selected tonic REM sleep. Electroencephalogr Clin Neurophysiol. 1992;83:36–43.

27. Hassainia F, Petit D, Nielsen T, et al. Quantitative EEG and statistical mapping of wakefulness and REM sleep in the evaluation of mild to moderate Alzheimer's disease. Eur Neurol. 1997;37:219–224.

28. Petit D, Montplaisir J, Lorrain D, et al. Spectral analysis of the rapid eye movement sleep electroencephalogram in right and left temporal regions: a biological marker of Alzheimer's disease. Ann Neurol. 1992;32:172–176.

29. Petit D, Montplaisir J, Lorrain D, et al. THA does not affect sleep or EEG spectral power in Alzheimer's disease. Biol Psychiatry. 1993;33:753–754.

30. Montplaisir J, Petit D, McNamara D, et al. Comparisons between SPECT and quantitative EEG measures of cortical impairment in mild to moderate Alzheimer's disease. Eur Neurol. 1996;36:197–200.

31. Prinz PN, Peskind ER, Vitaliano PP, et al. Changes in the sleep and waking EEGs of nondemented and demented elderly subjects. J Am Geriatr Soc. 1992;30:86–93.

32. Benca RM, Obermeyer WH, Thisted RA, et al. Sleep and psychiatric disorders: a meta-analysis. Arch Gen Psychiatry. 1992;49:651–668.

33. Feinberg I, Koresko RL, Heller N. EEG sleep patterns as a function of normal and pathological aging in man. J Psychiatr Res. 1967;5:107–144.

34. Bliwise DL, Tinklenberg J, Yesavage JA, et al. REM latency in Alzheimer's disease. Biol Psychiatry. 1989;25:320–328.

35. Prinz PN, Vitaliano PP, Vitiello MV, et al. Sleep, EEG, and mental function changes in senile dementia of the Alzheimer type. Neurobiol Aging. 1982;3:361–370.

36. Vitiello MV, Prinz PN, Williams DE, et al. Sleep disturbances in patients with mild-stage Alzheimer's disease. J Gerontol. 1990;45:M131–M138.

37. Vitiello M, Bokan J, Kukull W, et al. Rapid eye movement sleep measures of Alzheimer type dementia patients and optimally healthy aged individuals. Biol Psychiatry. 1984;19:721–734.

38. Benson K, Cohen M, Zarcone VP Jr. REM sleep time and digit span impairment in alcoholics. J Stud Alcohol. 1978;39:1488–1498.

39. Stone WS, Altman HJ, Berman RF, et al. Association of sleep parameters and memory in intact old rats and young rats with lesions in the nucleus basalis magnocellularis. Behav Neurosci. 1989;103:755–764.

40. Bahro M, Riemann D, Stadtmuller G, et al. REM sleep parameters in the discrimination of probable Alzheimer's disease from old-age depression. Biol Psychiatry. 1993;34:482–486.

41. Moe KE, Larsen LH, Prinz PN, et al. Major unipolar depression and mild Alzheimer's disease: differentiation by quantitative tonic REM EEG. Electroencephalogr Clinical Neurophysiol. 1993;86:238–246.

42. Buysse DJ, Reynolds CF, Kupfer DJ, et al. Electroencephalographic sleep in depressive pseudodementia. Arch Gen Psychiatry. 1988;45:568–575.

43. Reynolds CF, Buysse DJ, Kupfer DJ, et al. Rapid eye movement sleep deprivation as a probe in elderly subjects. Arch Gen Psychiatry. 1990;47:1128–1136.

44. Reynolds CF, Kupfer DJ, Hoch CC, et al. Sleep deprivation as a probe in the elderly. Arch Gen Psychiatry. 1987;44:982–990.

45. Hoch CC, Buysse DJ, Reynolds CF. Sleep and depression in late life. Clin Geriatr Med. 1989;5:259–274.

46. Berry DTR, Webb WB, Block AJ, et al. Nocturnal hypoxia and neuropsychological variables. J Clin Exp Neuropsychol. 1986;8:229–238.

47. Telakivi T, Kajaste S, Partinen M, et al. Cognitive function in middle-aged snorers and controls: role of excessive daytime somnolence and sleep-related hypoxic events. Sleep. 1988;11:454–462.

48. Greenberg GD, Watson RK, Deptula D. Neuropsychological dysfunction in sleep apnea. Sleep. 1987;10:254–262.

49. Yesavage JA, Bliwise D, Guilleminault C, et al. Preliminary communication: intellectual deficit and sleep-related respiratory disturbance in the elderly. Sleep. 1985;8:30–33.

50. Cheshire K, Engleman H, Deary I, et al. Factors impairing daytime performance in patients with sleep apnea/hypopnea syndrome. Arch Intern Med. 1992;152:538–541.

51. Naegele B, Thouvard V, Pepin JL, et al. Deficits of cognitive executive functions in patients with sleep apnea syndrome. Sleep. 1995;18:43–52.

52. Bliwise DL. Neuropsychological function and sleep. Clin Geriatr Med. 1989;5:381–394.

53. Bliwise DL. Is sleep apnea a cause of reversible dementia in old age? J Am Geriatr Soc. 1996;44:1407–1409.

54. Gibson GE, Pulsinelli W, Blass JP, et al. Brain dysfunction in mild to moderate hypoxia. Am J Med. 1981;70:1247–1254.

55. Shimada M. Alteration of acetylcholine synthesis in mouse brain cortex in mild hypoxic hypoxia. J Neural Transm. 1981;50:233–245.

56. Hoch CC, Reynolds CF, Nebes RD, et al. Clinical significance of sleep-disordered breathing in Alzheimer's disease: preliminary data. J Am Geriatr Soc. 1989;37:138–144.

57. Hoch CC, Reynolds CF III, Kupfer DJ, et al. Sleep disordered breathing in normal and pathologic aging. J Clin Psychiatry. 1986;47:499–503.

58. Smallwood RG, Vitiello MV, Giblin EC, et al. Sleep apnea: relationship to age, sex, and Alzheimer dementia. Sleep. 1983;6:16–22.

59. Bliwise DL, Yesavage JA, Tinklenberg J, et al. Sleep apnea in Alzheimer's disease. Neurobiol Aging. 1989;10:343–346.

60. Bassetti C, Aldrich MS, Chervin RD, et al. Sleep apnea in patients with transient ischemic attack and stroke. Neurology. 1996;47:1167–1173.

61. Good DC, Henkle JQ, Gelber D, et al. Sleep-disordered breathing and poor functional outcome after stroke. Stroke. 1996;27:252–259.

62. Mohsenin V, Valor R. Sleep apnea in patients with hemispheric stroke. Arch Phys Med Rehabil. 1995;76:71–76.

63. Erkinjuntti T, Partinen M, Sulkava R, et al. Sleep apnea in multi-infarct dementia and Alzheimer's disease. Sleep. 1987;10:419–425.

64. Manni R, Marchioni E, Romani A, et al. Sleep apnea in vascular and primary degenerative dementia. In: Koella WP, Obal F, Schulz H, et al, eds. Sleep 86. New York, NY: Fischer; 1988;427–429.

65. Koskenvou M, Kaprio J, Telakivi T, et al. Snoring as risk factor for ischaemic heart disease and stroke in men. Br Med J. 1987;294:16–19.

66. Partinen M, Palomaki H. Snoring and cerebral infarction. Lancet. 1985;2:1325–1326.

67. Palomaki H. Snoring and the risk of ischemic brain infarction. Stroke. 1991;22:1021–1025.

68. Balfors EM, Franklin KA. Impairment of cerebral perfusion during obstructive sleep apnea. Am J Respir Crit Care Med. 1994;150:1587–1591.

69. Diomedi M, Placidi F, Cupini LM, et al. Cerebral hemodynamic changes in sleep apnea syndrome and effect of continuous positive airway pressure treatment. Neurology. 1998;51:1051–1056.

70. Legall D, Hubert P, Truelle JL, et al. Le syndrome d' apnée du sommeil: une cause curable de déterioration mentale. Presse Med. 1986;15:260–261.

71. Scheltens PH, Visscher F, Keimpema ARJV, et al. Sleep apnea syndrome presenting with cognitive impairment. Neurology. 1991;41:155–156.

72. Clarfield AM. The reversible dementias: do they reverse? Ann Intern Med. 1988;109:476–486.

73. Sanford JRA. Tolerance of debility in elderly dependents by supporters at home: Its significance for hospital practice. Br Med J. 1975;3:471–473.

74. Pollak CP, Perlick D, Linsner JP, et al. Sleep problems in the community elderly as predictors of death and nursing home placement. J Commun Health. 1990;15:123–135.

75. Pollak CP, Stokes PE. Circadian rest-activity rhythms in demented and nondemented older community residents and their caregivers. J Am Geriatr Soc. 1997;45:446–452.

76. Lipowski ZJ. Delirium: Acute Brain Failure in Man. Springfield, Ill: Charles C Thomas; 1980.

77. American Psychiatric Association. Diagnostic and Statistical

Manual of Mental Disorders, Fourth Edition. Washington, DC: American Psychiatric Association Press; 1994.

78. Lipowski ZJ. Delirium in the elderly patient. N Engl J Med. 1989;320:578–582.

79. Mazurek MF, Rosebush PI. Circadian pattern of acute, neuroleptic-induced dystonic reactions. Am J Psychiatry. 1996;153:708–710.

80. Bliwise DL, Carroll JS, Lee KA, et al. Sleep and sundowning in nursing home patients with dementia. Psychiatry Res. 1993;48:277–292.

81. Bliwise DL. What is sundowning? J Am Geriatr Soc. 1994;42:1009–1011.

82. Kane RL, Ouslander JG, Abrass IB. Essentials of Clinical Geriatrics. New York, NY: McGraw-Hill; 1984.

83. Ginsburg R, Weintraub M. Caffeine in the "sundown syndrome": report of negative results. J Gerontol. 1976;31:419–420.

84. Cameron DE. Studies in senile nocturnal delirium. Psychiatr Q. 1941;15:47–53.

85. Warshaw GA, Moore JT, Friedman W, et al. Functional disability in the hospitalized elderly. JAMA. 1982;248:847–850.

86. Gillick MR, Serrell NA, Gillick LS. Adverse consequences of hospitalization in the elderly. Soc Sci Med. 1982;16:1033–1038.

87. Johnson J. Delirium in the elderly: incidence, diagnosis, management, and functional status in general medical patients. Gerontologist. 1987;27:243A.

88. Hogue C, Gottlieb G, Evans L. Delirium: elderly orthopedic surgical patients. Gerontologist. 1986;26:186A.

89. O'Dell C, Aronow WS, Cameron D. Delirium in the nursing home. Gerontologist. 1986;26:26A.

90. Liston EH. Delirium in the aged. Psychiatr Clin North Am. 1982;5:49–66.

91. Cohen-Mansfield J, Watson V, Meade W, et al. Does sundowning occur in residents of an Alzheimer unit? Int J Geriatr Psychiatry. 1989;4:293–298.

92. Evans LK. Sundown syndrome in institutionalized elderly. J Am Geriatr Soc. 1987;35:101–108.

93. Cohen-Mansfield J, Marx MS, Rosenthal AS. A description of agitation in a nursing home. J Gerontol. 1988;32:M77–M84.

94. Bliwise DL, Yesavage JA, Tinklenberg JR. Sundowning and rate of decline in mental function in Alzheimer's disease. Dementia. 1992;3:335–341.

95. Little JT, Satlin A, Sunderland T, et al. Sundown syndrome in severely demented patients with probable Alzheimer's disease. J Geriatr Psychiatry Neurol. 1995;8:103–106.

96. Reisberg B, Borenstein J, Salob SP, et al. Behavioral symptoms in Alzheimer's disease: phenomenology and treatment. J Clin Psychiatry. 1987;48:9–15.

97. Cacabelos R, Rodriguez B, Carrera C, et al. APOE-related frequency of cognitive and noncognitive symptoms in dementia. Methods Find Exp Clin Pharmacol. 1996;18:693–706.

98. Martino-Saltzman D, Blasch BB, Morris RD, et al. Travel behavior of nursing home residents perceived as wanderers and nonwanderers. Gerontologist. 1991;31:666–672.

99. O'Leary P, Haley W, Paul P. Behavioral assessment in Alzheimer's disease: use of a 24-hr log. Psychol Aging. 1993;8:139–143.

100. Jacobs D, Ancoli-Israel S, Parker L, et al. Twenty-four-hour sleep/wake patterns in a nursing home population. Psychol Aging. 1989;4:352–356.

101. Burgio L, Scilley K, Hardin JM, et al. Studying disruptive vocalization and contextual factors in the nursing home using computer-assisted real-time observation. J Gerontol B Psychol Sci Soc Sci. 1994;49:230–239.

102. Bliwise DL, Bevier WC, Bliwise NG, et al. Systematic 24-hr behavioral observations of sleep and wakefulness in skilled-care nursing facility. Psychol Aging. 1990;5:16–24.

103. Exum ME, Phelps BJ, Nabers KE, et al. Sundown syndrome: is it reflected in the use of PRN medications for nursing home residents? Gerontologist. 1993;33:756–761.

104. Bliwise DL, Hughes M, McMahon PM, et al. Observed sleep/wakefulness and severity of dementia in an Alzheimer's disease special care unit. J Gerontol Med Sci. 1995;50:M303–M306.

105. Inouye SK, Charpentier PA. Precipitating factors for delirium in hospitalized elderly persons: predictive model and interrelationship with baseline vulnerability. JAMA. 1996;275:852–857.

106. Cohen-Mansfield J, Billig N, Lipson S, et al. Medical correlates of agitation in nursing home residents. Gerontology. 1990;36:150–158.

107. Cohen-Mansfield J, Marx MS, Rosenthal AS. Dementia and agitation in nursing home residents: how are they related? Psychol Aging. 1990;5:3–8.

108. Cohen-Mansfield J, Marx MS, Rosenthal AS. A description of agitation in a nursing home. J Gerontol. 1988;32:M77–M84.

109. Cohen-Mansfield J, Marx MS. Do past experiences predict agitation in nursing home residents? Int J Aging Hum Dev. 1989;28:285–294.

110. Cohen-Mansfield J. The relationship between sleep disturbances and agitation in a nursing home. Int J Aging Health. 1990;2:42–57.

111. Schenck CH, Bundlie SR, Ettinger MG, et al. Chronic behavioral disorders of human REM sleep: a new category of parasomnia. Sleep. 1986;9:293–308.

112. Mahowald MW, Schenck CH. Status dissociatus—a perspective on states of being. Sleep. 1991;14:69–79.

113. Schenck CH, Bundlie SR, Mahowald MW. Delayed emergence of a Parkinsonian disorder in 38% of 29 older men initially diagnosed with idiopathic rapid eye movement sleep behavior disorder. Neurology. 1996;46:388–393.

114. Rye DB. Contributions of the pedunculopontine region to normal and altered REM sleep. Sleep. 1997;20:757–788.

115. Rye DB, Bliwise DL. Movement disorders specific to sleep and the nocturnal manifestations of waking movement disorders. In: Watts RL, Koller WC, eds. Movement Disorders: Neurologic Principles and Practice. New York, NY: McGraw-Hill; 1997:687–713.

116. Bliwise DL, Watts R, Watts N, et al. Disruptive nocturnal behavior in Parkinson's disease and Alzheimer's disease. J Geriatr Psychiatry Neurol. 1995;8:107–110.

117. Uchiyama M, Isse K, Tanaka K, et al. Incidental Lewy body disease in a patient with REM sleep behavior disorder. Neurology. 1995;45:709–712.

118. Schenck C, Mahowald M, Silber M, et al. Lewy body variant of Alzheimer's disease (AD) identified by post-mortem ubiquitin staining in a previously reported case of AD associated with REM sleep behavior disorder. Biol Psychiatry. 1997;42:527–528.

119. Boeve BF, Silber MH, Ferman TJ, et al. REM sleep behavior disorder and degenerative dementia. Neurology. 1998;51:363–370.

120. Ala TA, Yang K-H, Sung JH, et al. Hallucinations and signs of parkinsonism help distinguish patients with dementia and cortical Lewy bodies from patients with Alzheimer's disease at presentation: a clinicopathological study. J Neurol Neurosurg Psychiatry. 1997;62:16–21.

121. Schnelle JF, Ouslander JG, Simmons SF, et al. Nighttime sleep and bed mobility among incontinent nursing home residents. J Am Geriatr Soc. 1993;41:903–909.

122. Schnelle JF, Cruise PA, Alessi CA, et al. Sleep hygiene in physically dependent nursing home residents: behavioral and environmental intervention implications. Sleep. 1998;21:515–523.

123. Schnelle JF, Ouslander JG, Simmons SF, et al. The nighttime environment, incontinence care, and sleep disruption in nursing homes. J Am Geriatr Soc. 1993;41:910–914.

124. Strogatz SH, Kronauer RE, Czeisler CA. Circadian pacemaker interferes with sleep onset at specific times each day: role in insomnia. Am J Physiol. 1987;253:R172–R178.

125. Swaab DF, Fliers E, Partiman TS. The suprachiasmatic nucleus of the human brain in relation to sex, age, and senile dementia. Brain Res. 1985;342:37–44.

126. Goudsmit E, Hofman MA, Fliers E, et al. The supraoptic and paraventricular nuclei of the human hypothalamus in relation to sex, age, and Alzheimer's disease. Neurobiol Aging. 1990;11:529–536.

127. Witting W, Kwa IH, Eikelenboom P, et al. Alterations in the circadian rest-activity rhythm in aging and Alzheimer's disease. Biol Psychiatry. 1990;27:563–572.

128. Satlin A, Teicher MH, Lieberman HR, et al. Circadian locomotion activity rhythms in Alzheimer's disease. Neuropsychopharmacology. 1991;5(suppl 2):115–126.

129. Hopkins RW, Rindlisbacher P. Fragmentation of activity periods in Alzheimer's disease. Int J Geriatr Psychiatry. 1992;7:805–812.

130. Reynolds V, Marriott FHC, Waterhouse J, et al. Heart rate varia-

tion, age, and behavior in subjects with senile dementia of Alzheimer type. Chronobiol Int. 1995;12:37–45.

131. Otsuka A, Mikami H, Katahira K, et al. Absence of nocturnal fall in blood pressure in elderly persons with Alzheimer type dementia. J Am Geriatr Soc. 1990;38:973–978.

132. Uchida K, Okamoto N, Ohara K, et al. Daily rhythm of serum melatonin in patients with dementia of the degenerate type. Brain Res. 1996;717:154–159.

133. Dori D, Casale G, Solerte SB, et al. Chrononeuroendocrinological aspects of physiological aging and senile dementia. Chronobiologia. 1994;21:121–126.

134. Touitou Y, Reinberg A, Bogdan A, et al. Age-related changes in both circadian and seasonal rhythms of rectal temperature with special reference to senile dementia of Alzheimer type. Gerontology. 1986;32:110–118.

135. Prinz PN, Christie C, Smallwood R, et al. Circadian temperature variation in healthy aged and in Alzheimer's disease. J Gerontol. 1984;39:30–35.

136. Prinz PN, Moe KE, Vitiello MV, et al. Entrained body temperature rhythms are similar in mild Alzheimer's disease, geriatric onset depression, and normal aging. J Geriatr Psychiatry Neurol. 1992;5:65–71.

137. Satlin A, Volicer L, Stopa EG, et al. Circadian locomotor activity and core-body temperature rhythms in Alzheimer's disease. Neurobiol Aging. 1995;16:765–771.

138. Satlin A, Teicher MH, Liebermann HR, et al. Circadian locomotor activity rhythms in Alzheimer's disease. Neuropsychopharmacology. 1991;5:115–126.

139. Ancoli-Israel S, Klauber MR, Jones DW, et al. Variations in circadian rhythms of activity, sleep, and light exposure related to dementia in nursing-home patients. Sleep. 1997;20:18–23.

140. Gillin JC, Kripke DF, Campbell SS. Ambulatory measures of activity, light, and temperature in elderly normal controls of patients with Alzheimer's disease. Bull Clin Neurosci. 1989;54:144–148.

141. Bliwise DL, Tinklenberg JR, Yesavage JA. Timing of sleep and wakefulness in Alzheimer's disease. Biol Psychiatry. 1992;31:1163–1165.

142. Ancoli-Israel S, Klauber MR, Gillin JC, et al. Sleep in non-institutionalized Alzheimer's disease patients. Aging Clin Exp Res. 1994;6:451–458.

143. Christie JE, Whalley LJ, Dick H, et al. Plasma cortisol concentrations in the functional psychoses and Alzheimer type dementia: a neuroendocrine day approach in drug-free patients. J Steroid Biochem. 1983;19:247–250.

144. Davis KL, Davis BM, Greenwald BS, et al. Cortisol and Alzheimer's disease, I: basal studies. Am J Psychiatry. 1986;143:300–305.

145. Okawa M, Mishima K, Hishikawa Y, et al. Circadian rhythm disorders in sleep-waking and body temperature in elderly patients with dementia and their treatment. Sleep. 1991;14:478–485.

146. Meijer JH, Rietveld WJ. Neurophysiology of the suprachiasmatic circadian pacemaker in rodents. Physiol Rev. 1989;69:671–707.

147. Meguro K, Ueda M, Kobayashi I, et al. Sleep disturbance in elderly patients with cognitive impairment, decreased daily activity and periventricular white matter lesions. Sleep. 1995;18:109–114.

148. Mishima K, Okawa M, Satoh K, et al. Different manifestations of circadian rhythms in senile dementia of Alzheimer's type and multi-infarct dementia. Neurobiol Aging. 1997;18:105–109.

149. Aharon-Peretz J, Masiah A, Pillar T, et al. Sleep-wake cycles in multi-infarct dementia and dementia of the Alzheimer type. Neurology. 1991;41:1616–1619.

150. Matzuk MM, Saper CB. Preservation of hypothalamic dopaminergic neurons in Parkinson's disease. Ann Neurol. 1985;18:552–555.

151. Dowling GA. A comparative study of sleep and temperature rhythm in older women with and without Parkinson's disease [abstract]. Sleep Res. 1996;25:409.

152. Fertl E, Auff E, Doppelbauer A, et al. Circadian secretion pattern of melatonin in de novo parkinsonian patients: evidence for phase-shifting properties of L-dopa. J Neural Transm Park Dis Dement Sect. 1993;5:227–234.

153. Dihenia BH, Rye DB, Bliwise DL. Daytime alertness in Parkinson's disease. Sleep Res. 1997;26:550.

154. Cohen RA, Albers HE. Disruption of human circadian and cognitive regulation following a discrete hypothalamic lesion: a case study. Neurology. 1991;41:726–729.

155. Torch WC, Hirano A, Solomon S. Anterograde transneuronal degeneration in the limbic system: clinical anatomic correlation. Neurology. 1977;27:1157–1163.

156. Schwartz WJ, Busis NA, Hedley-Whyte ET. A discrete lesion of ventral hypothalamus and optic chiasm that disturbed the daily temperature rhythm. J Neurol. 1986;233:1–4.

157. Davison C, Demuth EL. Disturbances in sleep mechanism: a clinicopathologic study. Arch Neurol Psychiatry. 1946;55:111–125.

158. Ray WA, Federspeil CF, Schaffner W. A study of antipsychotic drug use in nursing homes: epidemiologic evidence suggesting misuse. Am J Public Health. 1980;70:485–491.

159. Yuen EJ, Zisselman MH, Louis DZ, et al. Sedative-hypnotic use by the elderly: Effects on hospital length of stay and costs. J Ment Health Administration. 1997;24:90–97.

160. Shorr RI, Fought RL, Ray WA. Changes in antipsychotic drug use in nursing homes during implementation of the OBRA-87 regulations. JAMA. 1994;271:358–362.

161. Ray WA, Griffin MR, Schaffner W, et al. Psychotropic drug use and risk of hip fracture. N Engl J Med. 1987;316:363–369.

162. Seppala M, Rajala T, Sourander L. Subjective evaluation of sleep and the use of hypnotics in nursing homes. Aging Clin Exp Res. 1993;5:199–205.

163. Gilbert A, Innes JM, Owen N, et al. Trial of an intervention to reduce chronic benzodiazepine use among residents of aged-care accommodation. Aust N Z J Med. 1993;23:343–347.

164. Monane M, Glynn RJ, Avorn J. The impact of sedative-hypnotic use on sleep symptoms in elderly nursing home residents. Clin Pharmacol Ther. 1996;59:83–92.

165. Cruise PA, Schnelle JF, Alessi CA, et al. The nighttime environment and incontinence care practices in nursing homes. J Am Geriatr Soc. 1998;46:181–186.

166. Factor SA, Brown D, Molho ES, et al. Clozapine: a 2-year open trial in Parkinson's disease patients with psychosis. Neurology. 1994;44:544–546.

167. Lew MF, Waters CH. Clozapine treatment of Parkinsonism with psychosis. J Am Geriatr Soc. 1993;41:669–671.

168. Rabey JM, Treves TA, Neufeld MY, et al. Low-dose clozapine in the treatment of levodopa-induced mental disturbances in Parkinson's disease. Neurology. 1995;45:432–434.

169. Wolters EC, Jansen EN, Tuynman-Qua HG, et al. Olanzapine in the treatment of dopaminomimetic psychosis in patients with Parkinson's disease. Neurology. 1996;47:1085–1087.

170. Jimenez-Jimenez FJ, Tallon-Barranco A, Orti-Pareja M, et al. Olanzapine can worsen parkinsonism. Neurology. 1998;50:1183–1184.

171. Friedman J. Olanzapine in the treatment of dopaminomimetic psychosis in patients with Parkinson's disease. Neurology. 1998;50:1195–1196.

172. McGaffigan S, Bliwise DL. The treatment of sundowning: a selective review of pharmacological and nonpharmacological studies. Drugs Aging. 1997;10:10–17.

173. Tariot PN, Erb R, Leibovici A, et al. Carbamazepine treatment of agitation in nursing home patients with dementia: a preliminary study. J Am Geriatr Soc. 1994;42:1160–1166.

174. Sival RC, Haffmans PMJ, van Gent PP, et al. The effects of sodium valproate on disturbed behavior in dementia. J Am Geriatr Soc. 1994;42:906–909.

175. Houlihan DJ, Mulsant BH, Sweet RA, et al. A naturalistic study of trazodone in treatment of behavioral complications of dementia. Am J Geriatr Psychiatry. 1994;2:78–85.

176. Williams KH, Goldstein G. Cognitive and affective responses to lithium in patients with organic syndrome. Am J Psychiatry. 1979;136:800–803.

177. Schneider LS, Pollock VE, Zemansky MF, et al. A pilot study of low-dose l-deprenyl in Alzheimer's disease. J Geriatr Psychiatry Neurol. 1991;4:143–148.

178. Greendyke RM, Kanter DR. Therapeutic effects of pindolol on behavior disturbances associated with organic brain disease: a double-blind study. J Clin Psychiatry. 1986;47:423–426.

179. Weiler PG, Goodman TA. The use of propranolol in Alzheimer's disease patients with disruptive behavior. Curr Ther Res. 1987;42:364–374.

180. McCarten JR, Kovera C, Maddox MK, et al. Triazolam in Alzheimer's disease: pilot study on sleep and memory effects. Pharmacol Biochem Behav. 1995;52:447–452.

181. Shaw SH, Curson H, Coquelin JP. A double-blind, comparative study of zolpidem and placebo in the treatment of insomnia in elderly psychiatric in-patients. J Int Med Res. 1992;20:150–161.

182. Lloyd GK, Lowenthal A, Javoy-Agid F, et al. GABA$_A$ receptor complex function in frontal cortex membranes from control and neurological patients. Eur J Pharmacol. 1991;197:33–39.

183. Ansseau M, Pitchot W, Hansenne M, et al. Psychotic reactions to zolpidem. Lancet. 1992;339:809.

184. Stotsky B. Multicenter study comparing thioridazine with diazepam and placebo in elderly, nonpsychotic patients with emotional and behavioral disorders. Clin Ther. 1984;6:546–549.

185. Haimov I, Lavie P, Laudon M, et al. Melatonin replacement therapy in elderly insomniacs. Sleep. 1995;18:598–603.

186. Garfinkel D, Laudon M, Nof D, et al. Improvement of sleep quality in elderly people by controlled-release melatonin. Lancet. 1995;346:541–544.

187. Hughes RJ, Sack RL, Lewy AJ. The role of melatonin and circadian phase in age-related sleep-maintenance insomnia: assessment in a clinical trial of melatonin replacement. Sleep. 1998;21:52–68.

188. Singer C, McArthur A, Hughes R, et al. High dose melatonin administration and sleep in the elderly [abstract]. Sleep Res. 1995;24A:151.

189. Singer CM, Moffit MT, Colling ED, et al. Low dose melatonin administration and nocturnal activity levels in patients with Alzheimer's disease [abstract]. Sleep Res. 1997;26:752.

190. Singer C, Colling E, Moffit M, et al. Melatonin and sleep in patients with Alzheimer's disease. Sleep. 1998;21(suppl):248.

191. Krause DN, Barrios VE, Duckles SP. Melatonin receptors mediate potentiation of contractile responses to adrenergic nerve stimulation in rat caudal artery. Eur J Pharmacol. 1995;276:207–213.

192. Hinton DR, Sadun AA, Blanks JC, et al. Optic-nerve degeneration in Alzheimer's disease. N Engl J Med. 1986;315:485–487.

193. Ancoli-Israel S, Jones DW, Hanger MA, et al. Sleep in the nursing home. In: Kuna ST, Scroft PM, Remmers JE, eds. Sleep and Respiration in Aging Adults. New York, NY: Elsevier; 1991:77–84.

194. Meltzer-Brody S, Mouton A, Ge YR, et al. Effects of scheduled bright light exposure on subjective measurements of vigor in residents of an assisted living facility. Sleep Res. 1994;23:504.

195. Satlin A, Volicer L, Ross V, et al. Bright light treatment of behavioral and sleep disturbances in patients with Alzheimer's disease. Am J Psychiatry. 1992;149:1028–1032.

196. Castor D, Woods D, Pigott K, et al. Effect of sunlight on sleep patterns of the elderly. J Am Acad Physician Assist. 1991;4:321–326.

197. Lovell BB, Ancoli-Israel S, Gevirtz R. Effect of bright light treatment on agitated behavior in institutionalized elderly subjects. Psychiatry Res. 1995;57:7–12.

198. Mishima K, Okawa M, Hishikawa Y, et al. Morning bright light therapy for sleep and behavior disorders in elderly patients with dementia. Acta Psychiatr Scand. 1994;89:1–7.

199. Hozumi S, Hori H, Okawa M, et al. Favorable effect of transcranial electrostimulation on behavior disorders in elderly patients with dementia: a double-blind study. Int J Neurosci. 1996;88:1–10.

200. Alessi CA, Schnelle JF, MacRae PG, et al. Does physical activity improve sleep in impaired nursing home residents? J Am Geriatr Soc. 1995;43:1098–1102.

90

Cerebrovascular Diseases

Claudio Bassetti
Ronald Chervin

Cerebrovascular disease and sleep disorders are among the most common neurological problems and would occur together commonly by chance alone. In addition, however, each condition may cause the other and each may arise from similar predisposing factors. Clinicians who treat patients with stroke or sleep disorders should be aware of the likely co-morbidity and clinical implications.

As emphasized in this chapter, most of the research on stroke and sleep disorders has focused on obstructive sleep apnea (OSA) in patients with ischemic stroke or on changes in sleep architecture after stroke. The chapter starts with a brief introduction to cerebrovascular disease and then reviews some of the earliest reports on altered sleep and breathing following stroke. Circadian aspects of stroke are then discussed. The next section focuses on evidence that sleep-disordered breathing might cause stroke and, conversely, that stroke can lead to several types of sleep-disordered breathing. The chapter concludes with some discussion of sleep-related symptoms and changes in sleep architecture that can occur after stroke.

Defined as a focal neurological deficit of acute onset and vascular origin, stroke has an incidence rate of 1.7 to 17.9 per 1000 per year and is the most common neurological disease to warrant hospitalization.[1] Transient ischemic attacks (TIAs), in which neurological deficits resolve within 24 h, account for about 20% of acute cerebrovascular deficits and intracerebral hemorrhage for about 15%. The remaining 65% are ischemic strokes. Some of the well-recognized causes and risk factors for ischemic and hemorrhagic stroke are shown in Table 90–1. Treatment of acute stroke includes anticoagulants or agents that inhibit platelet aggregation.[2] Fibrinolytic agents can be effective in the first 3 h after ischemic stroke.[3] Other treatments under evaluation include neuroprotective agents and endovascular stenting or balloon dilation of stenotic vessels. Surgery may be considered in noncomatose patients with accessible (e.g., cerebellar) hemorrhages. Primary prevention of stroke includes treatment of hypertension and hypercholesterolemia, anticoagulation for atrial fibrillation, and endarterectomy in some patients with significant (70% or greater) carotid stenosis.[4, 5] After an ischemic stroke, prevention of further events often involves aspirin (alternatively clopidogrel), which reduces the relative risk of stroke recurrence by about 23%.[6] Anticoagulation and endarterectomy are the treatment of choice in some situations.[7, 8] Beyond these traditional considerations in stroke, the remainder of this chapter discusses growing evidence that sleep disorders and especially OSA are important to the etiology, morbidity, and treatment of stroke.

HISTORICAL REMARKS

Changes in sleep and breathing were reported in stroke patients as early as the beginning of the 19th century. In 1818 John Cheyne first described periodic breathing in a patient with cardiac disease and "apoplexy."[9] Hughlines Jackson later recognized that Cheyne-Stokes respiration frequently accompanies bilateral hemispheric stroke (quoted in reference 10). Hiccup in the course of medullary stroke was first reported by Vieusseux in 1810 (quoted in reference 11). Symptoms of obstructive sleep apnea were first recognized in a patient with intracerebral hemorrhage by Broadbent in 1877.[12] Charles Beevor described the loss of voluntary respiratory control in a patient with pseudobulbar palsy (quoted in reference 13). Although central apnea in the course of progressive paralysis was described by Weir Mitchell in 1890,[14] failure of automatic respiration during sleep (later called "Ondine's curse") after brainstem stroke was first reported by Ratto in 1955.[15] Hypersomnia following stroke was mentioned by MacNish in 1830,[16] but it was only at the beginning of this century that thalamic and mesencephalic stroke, in particular, were implicated.[17, 18] In 1883 Charcot[19] first reported that a patient lost dream recall after a presumed parieto-occipital stroke. Lhermitte[20] coined the term peduncular hallucinosis in 1922 to describe vivid, colorful, and dream-like hallucinations following midbrain stroke. Asymmetry of the electroencephalogram (EEG) during sleep, with reduction of spindling over the affected hemisphere, was first observed in stroke patients by Cress and Gibbs in 1948.[21] During subsequent decades, other authors described abnormalities of nonrapid eye movement (NREM) and rapid eye movement (REM) sleep in patients who had brainstem stroke.[22, 23]

Table 90–1. SOME CAUSES OR RISK FACTORS FOR STROKE

Ischemic Stroke and Transient Ischemic Attack

Large artery disease (macroangiopathy with artery-to-artery embolic occlusion)
Small artery disease (microangiopathy)
Cardioembolism
Arterial dissection
Migraine
Vasculitis
Coagulopathy
Hypertension
Cigarette smoking
Hypercholesterolemia
Diabetes mellitus
Alcohol or drug abuse
Male sex
Age
Race (blacks > whites)
Positive family history
Treatment with estrogens
Increased blood levels of fibrinogen and homocysteine
Elevated hematocrit
Atrial fibrillation
Carotid stenosis
Ischemic heart disease

Hemorrhagic Stroke

Acute hypertension
Chronic hypertension
Cerebral amyloid angiopathy
Anticoagulation and thrombolysis
Coagulopathies
Vascular malformations
Cerebral venous thrombosis
Intracranial tumors
Trauma

CIRCADIAN RHYTHMS AND STROKE

Ischemic stroke, like myocardial infarction and sudden death, occurs most frequently in the morning hours, particularly after awakening, between 6 AM and noon (Fig. 90–1). A meta-analysis of 31 publications reporting the circadian timing of 11,816 strokes found a 49% increase in stroke of all types (ischemic stroke, hemorrhagic stroke, TIA) between 6 and 12 AM.[26] A recent study found a higher frequency of strokes on awakening in thrombotic (29%) and lacunar (28%) stroke than in embolic stroke (19%).[27] There was no difference in circadian rhythm between first and recurrent stroke. Possible explanations for this pattern have focused on circadian or postural changes in platelet aggregation, thrombolysis, blood pressure, heart rate, and catecholamine levels that occur after awakening and resumption of physical and mental activities.[28] The highest incidence in the early hours of the morning can be overestimated because of patients who awaken with stroke. Treatment with aspirin does not modify the circadian pattern of stroke onset.[29, 31]

Whereas intracerebral and subarachnoid hemorrhages rarely occur at night,[25] 20 to 40% of ischemic strokes present at night. This suggests that sleep may represent a vulnerable phase for a subset of patients

with cerebrovascular disease.[25] Although preliminary studies have not found any significant difference in time of stroke onset between patients with and without sleep apnea,[30, 31] cardiovascular changes produced by apneas do appear to precipitate cerebrovascular events in some instances.[32, 33]

Acute brain infarction—particularly when the right hemisphere and the insula are affected—can disturb normal circadian variation in autonomic functions (e.g., heart rate) and contribute to increased poststroke cardiovascular morbidity.[34–36] Acute stroke also may alter other circadian functions such as sleep-related secretion of growth hormone.[37]

Actigraphy in a few patients with acute stroke and multi-infarct dementia has demonstrated sleep-wake cycles to be disrupted, shortened, lengthened, or shifted.[38, 39] In patients who awaken from coma caused by large hemispheric or brainstem strokes, a polyphasic sleep-wake rhythm often precedes the reappearance of a monophasic rhythm.[40] Alteration of circadian variation in core temperature was documented in a patient with a focal (neoplastic) lesion of the ventral hypothalamus,[41] but never following acute stroke. However, hyperthermia—which may, in some cases, imply diencephalic dysfunction—correlates with stroke severity and represents a bad prognostic sign after acute stroke.[42]

SLEEP-DISORDERED BREATHING AND STROKE

Snoring and Sleep Apnea as Vascular Risk Factors

Snoring that is present always or almost always (habitual snoring) occurs in 44% of middle-aged men and 28% of middle-aged women,[43] and represents a risk factor for stroke.[44] The odds ratios for stroke and snoring reportedly range from 2.1 to 3.3.[45] Stroke that occurs during sleep may be associated with habitual snoring and poor outcome.[46, 47] Some epidemiological reports of associations between snoring and stroke may not have controlled for potential confounding factors.[48] However, at least one large study that compared well-adjusted and unadjusted odds ratios for snoring and stroke showed similar, robust associations either way.[49]

Whether snoring causes or contributes to stroke remains a subject of debate.[49–51] Habitual snoring is strongly associated with obstructive sleep apnea-hypopnea syndrome (OSAHS), and most epidemiological studies of snoring have not separated out the effect of OSAHS.

Several findings have suggested plausible physiological mechanisms by which obstructive sleep-disordered breathing could cause stroke. Chronically, OSAHS of different degrees of severity, upper airway resistance syndrome, and isolated snoring are all associated with hypertension,[52–54] which in turn is an important risk factor for stroke. Furthermore, OSAHS may cause myocardial infarction and arrhythmias, either of which could also act as an intermediate variable in an effect of OSAHS on risk for stroke.[55] Neurohum-

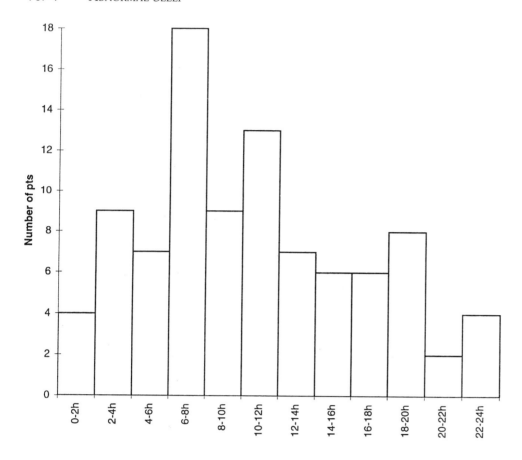

Figure 90–1. Estimated onset time of symptoms in 93 consecutive patients with acute ischemic stroke.

eral consequences of OSAHS may contribute to diabetes, increased platelet aggregation, decreased fibrinolysis, and increased atherogenesis.[56] Finally, high mortality of patients with OSAHS—largely a result of vascular disease[57, 58]—is reduced with treatment, perhaps because of beneficial changes in cardiac function,[58, 59] blood pressure,[60] and coagulation.[61, 62]

Individual apneas and hypopneas during sleep may be accompanied by decreased cardiac output, cardiac

arrhythmias, systemic hypotension or hypertension, vasodilation due to hypoxia and hypercapnia, and increased intracranial pressure.[63–65] The type, duration, and timing of respiratory events may affect hemodynamic consequences. Obstructive apneas of long duration and those that occur during REM sleep may be particularly detrimental.[32, 66–69] Large fluctuations in cerebral blood velocities (or flow) occur in association with apneic events and arousals (Fig. 90–2). Cheyne-

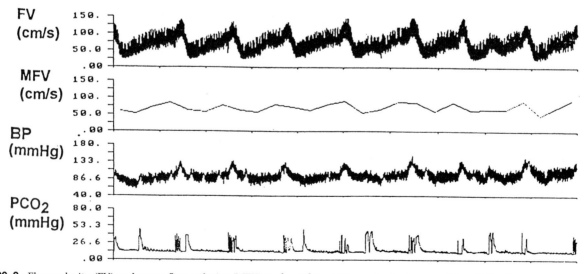

Figure 90–2. Flow velocity (FV) and mean flow velocity (MFV) in the right middle cerebral artery, peripheral blood pressure (BP), and end-expiratory P_{CO_2} in a patient with obstructive sleep apnea. Intervals with low end-expiratory P_{CO_2} show apneic episodes. (From Hajak G, Klingelhöfer J, Schulz-Varszegi M, et al. Sleep apnea syndrome and cerebral hemodynamics. Chest. 1996;110[3]:670–679.)

Stokes respiration (CSR) may precipitate brain ischemia.[69–71] A direct link between OSAHS and nocturnal cerebrovascular ischemic events has been demonstrated for retinal infarcts of embolic origin[72] and in single patients with TIA or minor stroke.[33, 73] A role of OSAHS in vascular dementia remains speculative.[74]

Neurological deficits left by stroke can also cause sleep-disordered breathing (see below), so the high prevalence of OSAHS in stroke patients cannot be completely explained by stroke predilection in patients with OSAHS. However, patients with TIA have no residual deficit yet suffer from OSAHS just as frequently as do patients with ischemic stroke.[30, 75] This finding suggests that OSAHS is more often a risk factor for stroke than a consequence of it.

In comparison to OSAHS, much less is known about the relation between other sleep disorders and stroke. However, any disorder that causes frequent arousals is likely to cause transient increases in blood pressure,[76] may thereby lead to hypertension, and could, in theory, increase the risk for stroke. Some evidence suggests that periodic limb movement disorder is associated with hypertension.[77, 78] Patients who obtained more than 8 h of sleep per night and had daytime sleepiness—most but not all of whom may have had OSAHS—were found to have an increased risk for stroke and coronary disease.[79] In another large epidemiological study an association between insomnia and hypertension was found, although persons treated for hypertension reported insomnia less frequently.[80]

Sleep-Disordered Breathing After Transient Ischemic Attacks and Stroke

Breathing disturbances affect more than 50% of patients who have had a stroke and are more common during sleep than during wakefulness.[75, 81–83] Supratentorial stroke is often associated with CSR and infratentorial stroke with OSA, central hyperventilation, central apnea, apneustic breathing, and ataxic breathing. Identification of specific types of breathing disorders after stroke has limited value for neuroanatomical localizing (see below).[75, 81, 82] In a single patient, different breathing disturbances may be observed in different sleep stages.[75, 84] For example, CSR may predominate in light sleep and OSA in REM sleep (Fig. 90–3).

As a consequence of brain vulnerability to hypoxia and cardiovascular instability, sleep-disordered breathing may impede recovery of ischemic but not yet irreversibly damaged brain tissue. Furthermore, sleep-disordered breathing may predispose to serious complications, such as aspiration or respiratory arrest, and contribute to short-term morbidity and mortality of stroke patients.[85, 86]

Obstructive Sleep Apnea

Studies of patients with acute stroke have found that 69 to 95% have OSA, as defined by an apnea-hypopnea index (AHI, or number of apneas and hypopneas per hour of sleep) greater than 10.[87–89] Despite methodological differences in selection of patients and assessment of breathing during sleep, all studies found moderate to severe obstructive sleep apnea (AHI greater than 20 to 30) in 30 to 50% of patients.

Although patients at risk for cerebrovascular disease frequently have OSA before they experience a stroke, some develop the sleep disorder as a consequence of stroke. Infarction of the medulla can impair breathing directly, and strokes in other areas can affect breathing indirectly, for example, when pain or pulmonary complications result.[90] In a prospective study of 128 patients with acute stroke or TIA, independent predictors of AHI included both premorbid health factors such as age, body mass index, and diabetes, as well as stroke outcome measures such as clinical severity.[30] Late observations suggest that recovery from stroke may be accompanied by improvement of sleep-disordered breathing.[95]

The frequency of OSA in stroke or TIA patients rivals or exceeds that frequency among patients tested at sleep centers specifically for suspected sleep-disordered breathing.[91, 92] This high frequency, in combination with epidemiological and physiological evidence that OSA may cause stroke, suggests that clinicians should investigate the possibility of sleep-disordered breathing in patients who have had a TIA or ischemic stroke. What such an investigation should comprise has not been extensively studied. However, in a series of 36 patients with recent strokes or TIAs, sleepiness and other common symptoms of OSA had only a 64% sensitivity and 67% specificity for OSA as defined by AHI equal to or greater than 10.[89] These findings support the use of objective sleep studies to supplement information provided by the patient. Such studies could potentially include oximetry and cardiorespiratory monitoring, but these are preferable to laboratory polysomnography in only a minority of patients suspected to have sleep apnea.[93] The so-called intelligent continuous positive airway pressure (CPAP) machines[94, 95] may provide an alternative to laboratory studies in the future.

The optimal timing of sleep studies after stroke or TIA is unknown. Although studies within days of a stroke might be less representative of the baseline condition attained several weeks to months after the ischemic event, treatment of OSA soon after stroke could potentially minimize further damage to injured neural tissue and improve outcome. The presence of OSA in stroke patients is associated with poor outcome,[87, 88] but whether OSA worsens outcome is not known. In addition, effectiveness of CPAP in patients with stroke may be limited by reduced compliance[95] and deserves further study.

Cheyne-Stokes Respiration

CSR is a type of periodic breathing in which central apneas and hypopneas are separated by crescendo-decrescendo respiratory patterns. The CSR can be observed in newborns, at high altitude in healthy adults, and particularly in older people.[96] The CSR has been well described in bihemispheric stroke, heart failure,

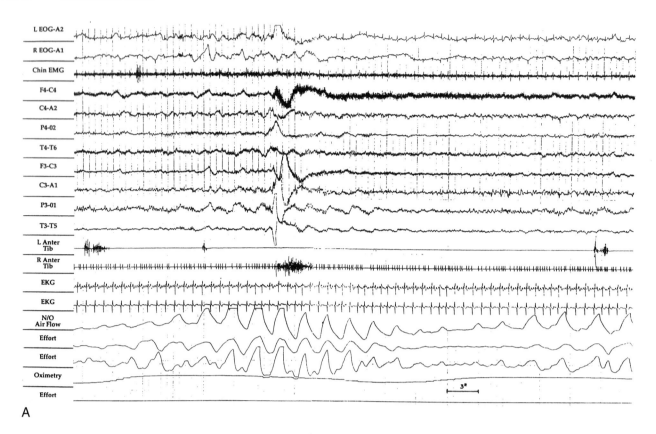

A

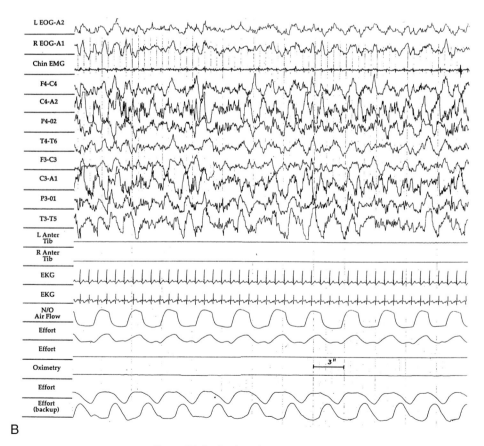

B

Figure 90–3. *See legend on opposite page*

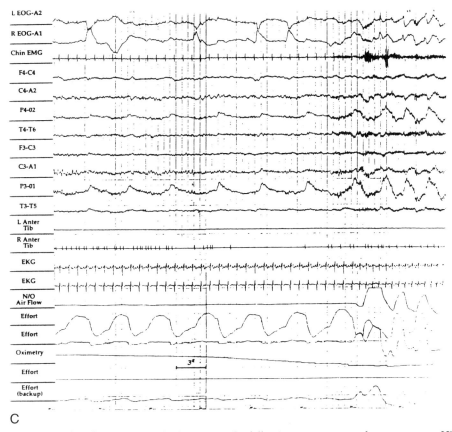

C

Figure 90–3. A 65-year-old man with right middle cerebral artery stroke following aortocoronary bypass surgery. History revealed habitual snoring but no hypersomnia. Clinical examination showed severe neurological deficits (Scandinavian Stroke Score of 20/58[186]) but no signs of heart failure. *A*, Polysomnogram (PSG) recorded 48 d after stroke onset documented severe sleep apnea with Cheyne-Stokes–like respiration predominantly in light NREM sleep; *B*, essentially normal breathing in deep NREM sleep; and *C*, obstructive events mainly in rapid eye movement (REM) sleep. The apnea-hypopnea index (AHI) was 104. Sleep-disordered breathing improved (AHI = 2) in a second PSG when continuous positive airway pressure reached 8 cm H_2O. EKG, electrocardiogram; EMG, electromyogram; EOG, electro-oculogram. (From Bassetti C, Aldrich MS, Quint D. Sleep-disordered breathing in patients with acute supra- and infratentorial stroke. Stroke. 1997;28[9]:1765–1772.)

somnolence, and brain edema with increased intracranial pressure.[10, 97, 98] Recent studies have shown, however, that CSR is also frequent in awake patients without cardiac disease who have had a unilateral hemispheric or infratentorial stroke.[75, 99, 100] Furthermore, CSR and OSA can occur in the same patient and either may exacerbate the other[75, 83, 99] (see Fig. 90–3). Whether CSR without OSA should be treated in acute stroke remains unknown: treatment may protect the patient from several potentially detrimental consequences of CSR, including hypoxemia, recurrent arousals, and reduction of cerebral perfusion.[70] The CSR may improve with oxygen or theophylline[99, 101] or with CPAP when OSA is also present.[75]

Other Breathing Disturbances

In comparison to CSR and OSA, other breathing abnormalities following *hemispheric strokes* have not been as well studied. Such abnormalities can include selective impairment of behavioral or volitional respiratory control with preservation of metabolic control mechanisms. After cerebral stroke, voluntary chest movements are reduced on the paralyzed side.[102]

Strokes in the frontal cortex, basal ganglia, or capsula interna may cause *respiratory apraxia*, with impairment of voluntary modulation of breathing amplitude and frequency, leaving patients unable to take a deep breath or hold the breath.[102, 103]

Several abnormal patterns of breathing, though uncommon, can occur after *brainstem stroke*, especially during sleep or with decreased levels of consciousness. Sustained respiratory rates above 25 to 30/min in the absence of hypoxemia (*neurogenic hyperventilation*) were originally described in six comatose patients with ventrotegmental pontine strokes,[104] but were subsequently attributed to stimulation of lung and chest wall afferent reflexes due to pulmonary congestion.[105, 106] Neurogenic hyperventilation after stroke usually indicates a poor prognosis.[83, 85] Inspiratory breath-holding (*apneustic breathing*), originally described in two patients with bilateral ventrotegmental mediocaudal (infratrigeminal) pontine stroke,[107] is rare and usually secondary to basilar artery occlusion.[106] Erratic variations in breathing frequency and amplitude (ataxic or *Biot's breathing*), and failure of automatic breathing (central sleep apnea or *Ondine's curse*), usually imply a lateral medullary stroke, often bilateral.[108–110] Damage to the medullary reticular formation and nucleus ambiguus may be sufficient to cause a loss of automatic breathing, while a lesion that also includes the nucleus tractus solitarius is necessary to cause failure of both automatic and voluntary respiration.[110] Volitional breathing can be impaired by brainstem strokes involving corticobulbar and corticospinal pathways at pontine and medullary levels.[102, 103] *Hiccup* is not uncommon after brainstem and particularly medullary stroke,[111, 112] occasionally occurs in supratentorial strokes, and may become chronic in some cases.[113] *Yawning* can accompany hypersomnia in patients with thalamic lesions, for example,[39] and may occur as a release phenomenon after extensive corticospinal lesions (e.g., locked-in syndrome[114]).

Spinal cord stroke can impair both automatic and voluntary breathing control.[102, 115] The topography and extent of the lesion can determine respiratory effects. Anterior spinal artery strokes can affect reticulospinal pathways, located anteriorly in the lateral columns of the first three cervical segments, which are crucial for automatic breathing.[115, 116] In contrast, posterior spinal artery strokes can damage corticospinal pathways in the dorsolateral spinal cord and impair voluntary control of breathing. Strokes that extend up to the C1 level usually cause severe respiratory insufficiency and necessitate ventilatory support.

Control of central apneas and ataxic breathing usually requires assisted ventilation. Hiccup can be treated with neuroleptics or baclofen.[117]

SLEEP CHANGES AFTER STROKE

Relatively little is known about changes in sleep and related physiological processes after stroke. Future research in this area could potentially provide insight into the role of sleep in restorative and healing processes, host defenses, and memory consolidation.[118–120] In addition, changes in sleep architecture after strokes that involve identified brain structures may improve understanding of the neuroanatomy and neurophysiology that underlie normal sleep.[121–124]

Clinical Sleep Disturbances

Hypersomnia

Hypersomnia, defined as a reduced latency to sleep, increased sleep, or excessive daytime sleepiness, can be caused by a stroke that results in deficient arousal ("passive hypersomnia"), increased production of sleep ("active hypersomnia"), or both in some cases.[39] Insomnia (see below), sleep deprivation, drugs, endocrine changes, and systemic complications secondary to acute stroke (e.g., fever, infections) may contribute to hypersomnia. Hypersomnia is frequently associated with decreased motor activation (akinetic mutism) and depressed mood. In patients with strokes that affect the reticular formation or the paramedian thalamus, periods of hypersomnia may alternate with periods of insomnia, suggesting that normally the role of these brain areas extends beyond maintenance of arousal to regulation of the sleep-wake cycle. Façon and co-

workers[125] described, for example, a 78-year-old patient with a tegmental mesencephalic infarct in whom severe, persistent hypersomnia was accompanied by an inversion of the sleep-wake cycle with nocturnal agitation.

Hypersomnia can occur after bilateral and sometimes unilateral strokes in the paramedian thalamus and mesencephalon, especially when affected structures include the dorsomedial nucleus, intralaminar nuclei, centromedian nucleus, and the most cephalic portions of the ascending reticular activating system.[125–128] Such strokes may cause initial coma or, conversely, manic delirium, hyperalertness, and insomnia before hypersomnia evolves.[129] Other areas in which stroke can occasionally produce hypersomnia include the caudate, striatum, tegmental pons, median regions of the medulla, and cerebral hemispheres, the last when a large lesion occurs, on the left more than on the right, and anteriorly more than posteriorly.[130–134]

Patients with bilateral paramedian thalamic infarcts may develop pseudohypersomnia that consists of increased behavioral rather than true sleep.[135, 136] They may appear to sleep as much as 20 h/d. Such patients yawn, stretch, close their eyes, assume a sleeping posture, complain of a constant urge to sleep, and doze when left alone.[135, 136] However, some are able to control this behavior when stimulated or given explicit, active tasks to perform. The "presleep" behavior, as it has been described, may be compulsive in that removal of the patient from bed can result in repeated attempts to lie down and adopt a sleeping posture. However, during what appear to be daytime sleep periods, relatively quick responses to questions or requests suggest wakefulness. Polysomnography demonstrates during most of the time an absence of NREM and REM sleep except during the nocturnal phase of the circadian cycle (see below). Two other findings in patients with paramedian thalamic strokes can include an upgaze palsy and a Korsakoff-like amnesia with confabulation; with hypersomnia, these features constitute the so-called diencephalic triad. Additional somatic symptoms and signs are gait instability, skew deviation, Horner's syndrome, and hypogeusia-hyposmia. Other vegetative symptoms of thalamic strokes include hyperphagia, sexual disinhibition, and mood changes. Extension to the mesencephalon is suggested by the presence of downgaze palsy, third nerve palsy, motor deficits, and unusual sleep postures. Hypersomnia can persist for months to years and may eventually evolve into "thalamic dementia," which is characterized by a state of apathy, psychomotor slowing, attentional deficits, and depressed mood.[39] In a series of 12 patients, Bassetti et al.[39] reported the persistence of disabling hypersomnia for more than 8 months in three patients with bilateral thalamic stroke and in two patients with unilateral thalamic stroke that extended to the subthalamus. Treatment of thalamic hypersomnia is rarely effective, although some benefit may be provided by levodopa, bromocriptine, methylphenidate, modafinil, or mazindol.[39, 135, 137]

Hypersomnia with hyperphagia (Kleine-Levin–like syndrome) was reported after multiple cerebral strokes.[138] In another patient, narcolepsy with a classic tetrad of symptoms developed after cardiac arrest and pontine stroke despite the absence of the HLA-DR2 haplotype.[139]

Insomnia

Mild to moderate insomnia is a frequent, usually nonspecific, and multifactorial complication of acute stroke that may predispose to delirium or other mental status changes and may slow functional recovery. Recurrent arousals, sleep discontinuity, and sleep deprivation can result from preexisting disorders (e.g., congestive heart failure, chronic pulmonary disease); sleep-disordered breathing; medications; infections and fever; inactivity; environmental disturbances (e.g., noise, medical controls and tests, light); and emotional stress. Insomnia directly related to brain damage (agrypnia) is less common but occurs, occasionally in association with inversion of the sleep-wake cycle and depressive symptoms,[140] in patients with thalamic,[141] thalamomesencephalic,[20] and large tegmento-basal pontine stroke.[23, 142] Van Bogaert[141] reported a patient with thalamohypothalamic stroke who experienced almost complete insomnia during more than 2 months. One patient with locked-in syndrome due to bilateral basal pontine stroke with some extension to the pontine tegmentum experienced nearly complete, polysomnographically documented insomnia for 6 months.[142]

Treatment of insomnia in acute stroke includes placement of patients in private rooms at night; protection from nocturnal light, noise, and unnecessary arousals; increased mobilization with exposure to light during the day; and, when unavoidable, temporary use of hypnotics that are relatively free of cognitive side effects, such as zolpidem.[143]

Parasomnias

The REM sleep behavior disorder, in which patients are thought to "act out" dreams, occurs with loss of physiological REM atonia. Although in most cases the cause of REM sleep behavior disorder is either an unknown or neurodegenerative process, lacunar stroke in the tegmentum of the pons has also been implicated.[144] Clonazepam 0.5 to 2.0 mg at bedtime is the treatment of first choice in REM sleep behavior disorder.

A reduction in physiological NREM sleep myoclonus was described in the hemiplegic limbs of a few stroke patients.[145] Periodic leg movements in sleep can increase[146] or decrease after unilateral hemispheric stroke and may persist after spinal stroke.[147]

Hallucinations and Altered Dreaming

Patients with strokes in the pontomesencephalic or mesencephalic tegmentum and in the paramedian thalamus may experience peduncular hallucinosis of Lhermitte, characterized by complex, often colorful, dreamlike visual hallucinations, particularly in the evening and at sleep onset.[20, 148–150] Peduncular hallucinosis may represent a release of REM sleep mentation.[151] It can be associated with insomnia,[20] but fortunately resolves spontaneously in most cases. The Charles Bonnet syn-

drome generally involves less complex visual hallucinations that also occur in the setting of diminished arousal. These hallucinations, "release phenomena" after stroke that involves visual loss, may be limited to a hemianopic field.[152–155] Cessation or reduction of dreaming occurs in the Charcot-Wilbrand syndrome and is occasionally limited to alteration of the visual component of the dream (as in the original patient described by Charcot). This syndrome can occur in patients with parieto-occipital, occipital, or deep frontal strokes and the lesions are often bilateral.[156, 157] Patients frequently, but not invariably, show deficient revisualization (referred to as visual irreminiscence), topographical amnesia, and prosopagnosia.[19, 158] Conversely, REM sleep characteristics may be normal.[156] Focal (temporal) seizures secondary to stroke can lead to the syndrome of dream-reality confusion or to recurrent nightmares, which may be more frequent in right-sided lesions and can be controlled with antiepileptics.[157, 159] Hallucinations as well as increased frequency or vividness of dreaming may occur following stroke, particularly after thalamic, parietal, and occipital stroke.[160, 168]

Sleep Architecture Changes

Abnormalities in sleep architecture are common after acute stroke but result only in part from acute brain damage (see Insomnia). Changes in sleep architecture depend upon (1) patient and health characteristics present before the stroke (e.g., age, respiratory disturbances); (2) topography and extent of the lesion; (3) associated complications of stroke (e.g., fever, infections, breathing disturbances); (4) drug treatment; and (5) time after stroke onset. Even patients without brain damage who are admitted to an intensive care unit after acute myocardial infarction can have a decreased total sleep time, sleep efficiency, REM sleep, and slow-wave sleep.[162] Some changes in sleep architecture are more specifically related to brain damage (see below): examples are persistent alteration of spindling and slow-wave sleep in supratentorial stroke, and persistent REM sleep abnormalities in infratentorial stroke. In patients with brain damage, however, changes in sleep behavior and sleep EEG do not always correlate. In patients with diffuse cortical, thalamic, or pontine stroke, for example, sleep-wake physiological cyclicity in eyelid tone, respiration, temperature, and motor activity may occur despite prominent EEG abnormalities.[39, 40] In patients with thalamic and mesencephalic stroke, daytime sleep-like behavior may be accompanied by a variety of EEG patterns, including diffuse low voltage alpha-beta activity, NREM stage 1 sleep, diffuse slow-wave activity, and REM sleep.[39, 40, 136]

Supratentorial Stroke

Reductions in NREM sleep, total sleep time, and sleep efficiency can follow acute supratentorial stroke. Decreased spindles, K complexes, and slow-wave sleep may predict poor outcome when found after large hemispheric strokes.[21, 163–166] Reduction of spindling can be ipsilateral[167] or bilateral[164, 165, 168] to unilateral stroke (Fig. 90–4). Rarely, spindling and slow-wave sleep in-

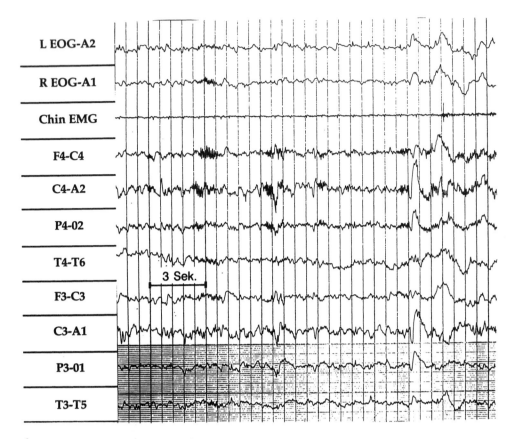

A

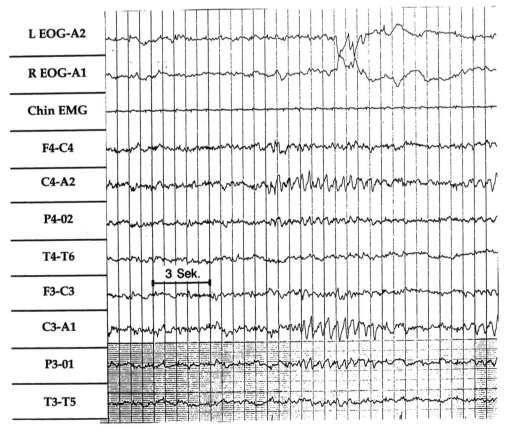

B

Figure 90–4. A 58-year-old man with a moderately severe left middle cerebral artery stroke (Scandinavian Stroke Score of 33/58[186]). Polysomnography recorded 9 d after stroke onset showed mild obstructive sleep apnea (apnea-hypopnea index = 16). *A*, In NREM sleep, spindling decreased ipsilaterally, with three spindles per hour recorded at C3 and 172 per hour at C4. *B*, In REM sleep sawtooth waves were symmetrical. EMG, electromyogram; EOG, electro-oculogram.

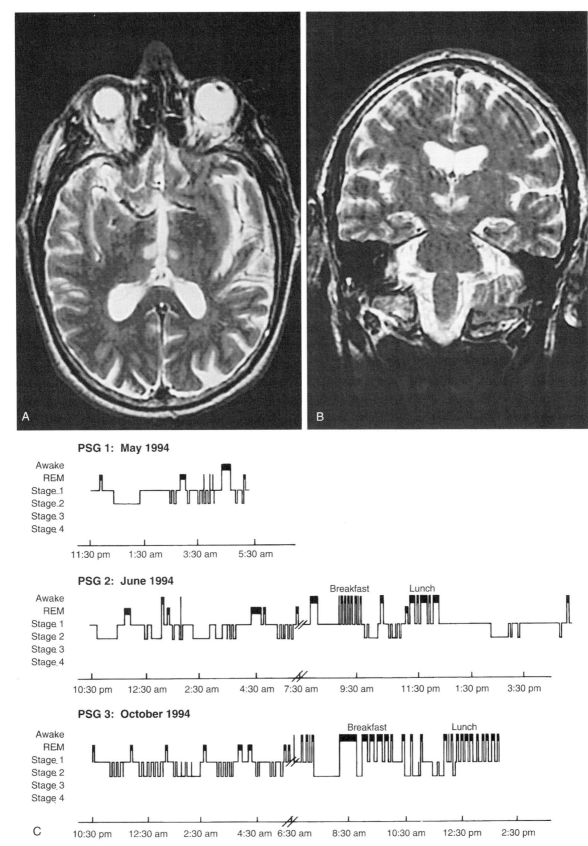

Figure 90–5. *A* and *B*, 60-year-old man with severe hypersomnia after bilateral paramedian thalamic ischemic stroke. He initially appeared to sleep more than 19 h/d. Other findings included an upgaze palsy and amnesia. *C*, Prolonged polysomnographic recording (PSG) 1 and 9 weeks after stroke documented (1) disruption of nocturnal NREM sleep with decreased spindling (automatic sleep spindle counts of 34/h on PSG 1 and 116/h on PSG 2), (2) absent slow-wave sleep, and (3) less severe disruption of REM sleep. The patient was awake during only 30% of daytime hours, remaining for the most part "suspended" in a drowsy state (NREM stage 1 sleep). At 6 months moderate hypersomnia persisted (sleep behavior over 12 h/d). Prolonged PSG showed some recovery of nocturnal spindling (162/h) and improved REM sleep but continued absence of slow-wave sleep. During daytime there was an improvement in wakefulness (54% of time). (From Bassetti C, Mathis J, Gugger M, et al. Hypersomnia following paramedian thalamic stroke. Ann Neurol. 1996;39[4]:471–480.)

crease in the acute stage of large middle cerebral artery stroke.[37, 168, 169] In some such cases, the increase in scored slow-wave sleep may reflect a generalized increase in delta activity during both sleep and wakefulness.[170] Changes in sleep spindle and slow-wave activity usually, but not always, coincide.[39]

Transient reductions in REM sleep can occur in the first days after supratentorial stroke,[164, 165, 168] and changes in REM sleep may persist after large hemispheric strokes with poor outcome.[169] Sawtooth waves can be decreased bilaterally in large hemispheric strokes, especially those that involve the right side.[168, 171]

Changes in sleep architecture after hemispheric stroke probably do not have high localizing value.[165] Some reports suggest, however, that right-sided strokes can preferentially decrease REM sleep and REM density,[172, 173] and that left-sided strokes can selectively reduce NREM stage 4 sleep.[172] Cortical blindness has been associated with a reduction of rapid eye movements.[174] Spindling and, to a lesser degree, slow-wave activity and K complexes appear to be particularly reduced in paramedian thalamic strokes.[39, 136, 137] In severe hypersomnia following paramedian thalamic strokes, prolonged polygraphic recordings can demonstrate an almost continuous state of light NREM stage 1 sleep (Fig. 90–5), perhaps reflecting inability to make the transition from wakefulness to sleep or to produce full wakefulness.[136] In these patients, REM sleep can occur at night and during the day despite the absence of slow-wave sleep.[39]

Like the EEG of wakefulness,[175] the sleep EEG probably undergoes a reorganization after acute damage, but data on this subject are scarce. Hachinski et al.[168] reported that during clinical recovery from a large left hemispheric stroke, one patient had progressive deterioration of the sleep EEG on the right side. In patients with paramedian thalamic stroke, recovery from hypersomnia may occur despite the persistence of significant NREM sleep changes.[89, 136, 137, 176]

Infratentorial Stroke

Bilateral, paramedian infarcts in the pontine tegmentum or large bilateral infarcts in the ventrotegmental pons can lead to reduction in NREM and, especially, REM sleep.[133, 177–179] Normal sleep EEG features such as sleep spindles, K complexes, and vertex waves may be completely lost.[177, 180] Patients usually present clinically with crossed or bilateral sensorimotor deficits, oculomotor disturbances, and, at least initially, disturbances of consciousness. In rare instances, the only focal finding in a patient with severe sleep EEG changes may be a horizontal gaze palsy.[181] Patients with abnormal sleep architecture may complain of insomnia, but isolated REM sleep loss can persist for years without cognitive or behavioral consequences.[182]

Bilateral infarction near, but not in, the pontine tegmentum, or infarction of this area only on one side, usually does not alter sleep architecture. Reported examples have included patients with bilateral pontomedullary junction infarcts, bilateral ventral pontine infarcts with locked-in syndrome, and unilateral pon-

tine tegmental infarcts.[180, 183] However, exceptions have also been described: a patient with a hematoma in the left pontine tegmentum had an ipsilateral abnormal EEG during REM sleep (despite normal rapid eye movements and muscle atonia),[184] and a second patient with a hematoma in the right pontine tegmentum had increased NREM stages 1 and 2 sleep and increased total sleep time in the setting of clinical hypersomnia.[133]

Occasionally, NREM or REM sleep may be altered selectively. Strokes that affect the pontomesencephalic junction tegmentum and the raphe nucleus can lead to a moderate to marked decrease in total sleep time with reduction in NREM sleep but no major changes in REM sleep.[23] Infarctions of the paramedian thalamus and of the lower pons have been associated with absence of slow-wave sleep but preservation of REM sleep and appearance of REM at sleep onset.[39, 179] In contrast, infarction in the lower pons can cause an almost completely selective decrease in REM sleep.[180] Increased REM sleep has been noted in one patient who had an infarct in the mesencephalic tegmentum and in another with an infarct in the pontomedullary junction.[185]

CONCLUSIONS

Sleep disorders and especially sleep-disordered breathing are common in patients who have ischemic stroke. Each condition is a potential cause of the other. Detection and treatment of sleep-disordered breathing may be an effective strategy in efforts to prevent initial stroke or stroke recurrence.

Survivors of stroke can develop hypersomnia, insomnia, or other sleep disturbances that may hamper mental and physical recovery from acute brain damage. In the future, a better understanding of how sleep architecture changes after strokes that affect specific brain regions may provide crucial insight into the neurophysiology of sleep.

References

1. Bonita R. Epidemiology of stroke. Lancet. 1992;339:342–344.
2. International Stroke Trial Collaborative Group. The International Stroke Trial (IST): a randomized trial of aspirin, subcutaneous heparin, both, or neither among 19435 patients with acute ischaemic stroke. Lancet. 1997;349:1569–1581.
3. The National Institute of Neurological Disorders and Stroke rt-PA Stroke Study Group. Tissue plasminogen activator for acute ischemic stroke. N Engl J Med. 1995;333:1581–1587.
4. Executive Committee for the Asymptomatic Carotid Atherosclerosis Study (ACAS). Endarterectomy for asymptomatic carotid artery stenosis. JAMA. 1995;273:1421–1428.
5. Barnett HJM, Eliasziw M, Meldrum HE. Drugs and surgery in the prevention of ischemic stroke. N Engl J Med. 1995;332:238–248.
6. Antiplatelet Trialist's Cooperation. Collaborative overview of randomized trials of antiplatelet therapy, I: prevention of death, myocardial infarction, and stroke by prolonged antiplatelet therapy in various categories of patients. Br Med J. 1994;308:81–106.
7. North American Symptomatic Carotid Endarterectomy Trial Collaborators (NASCET). Beneficial effect of carotid endarterectomy in symptomatic patients with high-grade carotid stenosis. N Engl J Med. 1991;325:444–453.

8. European Carotid Surgery Trialists' Collaborative Group. MRC European Carotid Surgery Trial: interim results for symptomatic patients with severe (70–99%) or with mild (0–29%) carotid stenosis. Lancet. 1991;337:1235–1243.

9. Cheyne J. A case of apoplexy in which the fleshy part of the heart was converted into fat. Dublin Hosp Rep. 1818;2:216–218.

10. Brown HW, Plum F. The neurologic basis of Cheyne-Stokes respiration. Am J Med. 1961;30:849–869.

11. Romano J, Merritt HH. The singular affection of Gaspard Vieusseux. Bull Hist Med. 1941;9:72–79.

12. Broadbent WH. On Cheyne-Stokes respiration in cerebral hemorrhage. Lancet. 1877;1:307–309.

13. Oppenheim H. Lehrbuch der Nervenkrankheiten. Berlin, Germany: S. Karger; 1913.

14. Mitchell SW. Some disorders of sleep. Am J Med Sci. 1890;100:109–127.

15. Goldblatt D. Ondine's curse. Semin Neurol. 1995;15:218–223.

16. Lavie P. The touch of Morpheus: pre-20th century accounts of sleepy patients. Neurology. 1991;41:1841–1844.

17. Freund SC. Zur Klinik und Anatomie der vertikalen Blicklähmung. Neurol Zentralbl. 1913;32:1215–1229.

18. Claude H, Loyez M. Ramollissement du noyau rouge. Rev Neurol. 1912;23:40–51.

19. Charcot M. Un cas de suppression brusque et isolée de la vision mentale des signes et des objects (formes et couleurs). Prog Med. 1883;2:568–571.

20. Lhermitte MJ. Syndrome de la calotte du pédoncule cérébral. Les troubles psycho-sensoriels dans les lésions mésocéphaliques. Rev Neurol. 1922;29:1359–1365.

21. Cress CH, Gibbs EL. Electroencephalographic asymmetry during sleep. Dis Nerv Syst. 1948;9:327–329.

22. Chase TN, Moretti L, Prensky AL. Clinical and electroencephalographic manifestations of vascular lesions of the pons. Neurology. 1968;18:357–368.

23. Freemon FR, Salinas-Garcia RF, Ward JW. Sleep patterns in a patient with brainstem infarction involving the raphae nucleus. Electroencephalogr Clin Neurophysiol. 1974;36:657–660.

24. Muller JE, Stone PH, Turi ZG, et al. Circadian variation in the frequency of onset of acute myocardial infarction. N Engl J Med. 1985;313:1315–1322.

25. Wroe SJ, Sandercock P, Bamford J, et al. Diurnal variation in incidence of stroke: Oxfordshire community stroke project. Br Med J. 1992;304:155–157.

26. Elliott WJ. Circadian variation in the timing of stroke onset. A meta-analysis. Stroke. 1998;29:992–996.

27. Lago A, Geffner D, Tembl J, et al. Circadian variation in acute ischemic stroke. A hospital-based study. Stroke. 1998;29:1873–1875.

28. Krantz DS, Kop WJ, Gabbay FH, et al. Circadian variation of ambulatory myocardial infarction. Triggering by daily activities and evidence for an endogenous circadian component. Circulation. 1996;93:1364–1371.

29. Marsh EE, Biller J, Adams HP, et al. Circadian variation in onset of acute ischemic stroke. Arch Neurol. 1990;47:1178–1180.

30. Bassetti C, Aldrich MS. Sleep apnea in acute cerebrovascular diseases: final report on 128 patients. Sleep. 1999;22:217–223.

31. Bassetti C, Aldrich MS. Nighttime versus daytime TIA and ischemic stroke: a prospective study of 110 patients. J Neurol Neurosurg Psychiatry. 1999;67:463–467.

32. Bassetti C, Jung HH, Hess CW. Near cardiac death following REM sleep: polysomnographic case report. J Sleep Res. 1997;6:57–58.

33. Rivest J, Reiher J. Transient ischemic attacks triggered by symptomatic sleep apneas [abstract]. Stroke. 1987;18:293.

34. Sander D, Klingelhöfer J. Changes of circadian blood pressure patterns and cardiovascular parameters indicate lateralization of sympathetic activation following hemispheric brain infarction. J Neurol. 1995;242:313–318.

35. Korpelainen JT, Sotaniemi KA, Huikuri HV, et al. Circadian rhythm of heart rate variability is reversibly abolished in ischemic stroke. Stroke. 1997;28:2150–2154.

36. Yoon BW, Morillo CA, Cechetto DF, et al. Cerebral hemispheric lateralization in cardiac autonomic control. Arch Neurol. 1997;54:741–744.

37. Culebras A, Miller M. Absence of sleep-related elevation of growth hormon level in patients with stroke. Arch Neurol. 1983;40:283–286.

38. Aharon-Peretz J, Masiah A, Pillar T, et al. Sleep-wake cycles in multi-infarct dementia and dementia of the Alzheimer type. Neurology. 1991;41:1616–1619.

39. Bassetti C, Mathis J, Gugger M, et al. Hypersomnia following thalamic stroke. Ann Neurol. 1996;39:471–480.

40. Passouant P, Cadilhac J, Baldy-Moulinier M. Physiopathologie des hypersomnies. Rev Neurol. 1967;116:585–629.

41. Schwartz WJ, Busis NA, Hedley-Whyte ET. A discrete lesion of ventral hypothalamus and optic chiasm that disturbed the daily temperature rhythm. J Neurol. 1986;233:1–4.

42. Reith J, Jorgensen HS, Pedersen PM, et al. Body temperature in acute stroke: relations to stroke severity, infarct size, mortality, and outcome. Lancet. 1996;347:422–425.

43. Young T, Palta M, Dempsey J, et al. The occurrence of sleep-disordered breathing among middle-aged adults. N Engl J Med. 1993;328:1230–1235.

44. Koskenvuo M, Kaprio J, Telakivi T. Snoring as a risk factor for ischaemic heart disease and stroke in men. Br Med J. 1987;294:16–19.

45. Partinen M. Ischaemic stroke, snoring and ostructive sleep apnea. J Sleep Res. 1995;4:156–159.

46. Palomäki H, Partinen M, Juvela S, et al. Snoring as a risk factor for sleep-related brain infarction. Stroke. 1989;20:1311–1315.

47. Spriggs DA, French JM, Murdy JM, et al. Snoring increases the risk of stroke and adversely affects prognosis. Q J Med. 1992;303:555–562.

48. Wright J, Johns R, Watt I, et al. Health effects of obstructive sleep apnoea and the effectiveness of continuous positive airways pressure: a systematic review of the research evidence. Br Med J. 1997;314:851–860.

49. Waller PC, Bhopal RS. Is snoring a cause of vascular disease. Lancet. 1989;2:143–146.

50. Hoffstein V. Is snoring dangerous to your health? Sleep. 1996;19:506–516.

51. Bassetti C. Habitual snoring, sleep apnoea, and stroke prevention. J Neurol Neurosurg Psychiatry. 1997;62:303.

52. Silverberg DS, Oksenberg A. Essential hypertension and abnormal upper airway resistance during sleep. Sleep. 1997;20:794–806.

53. Brooks D, Horner RL, Kozar L-F, et al. Obstructive sleep apnea as a cause of systemic hypertension. J Clin Invest. 1997;99:106–109.

54. Young T, Peppard P, Palta M, et al. Population-based study of sleep-disordered breathing as a risk factor for hypertension. Arch Intern Med. 1997;157:1746–1752.

55. Barnett HJM, Eliasziw M, Meldrum HE. Drugs and surgery in the prevention of ischemic stroke. N Engl J Med. 1995;332:238–248.

56. Dean RT, Wilcox I. Possible atherogenic effects of hypoxia during obstructive sleep apnea. Sleep. 1993;16:S15–S22.

57. He J, Kryger MH, Zorick FJ, et al. Mortality and apnea index in obstructive sleep apnea. Experience in 385 male patients. Chest. 1988;94:9–14.

58. Malone S, Liu PP, Holloway R, et al. Obstructive sleep apnea in patients with dilated cardiomyopathy: effects of continuous positive airway pressure. Lancet. 1991;338:1480–1484.

59. Wilcox I, Grunstein RR, Hedner JA, et al. Effect of nasal continuous positive airway pressure during sleep on 24-hour blood pressure in obstructive sleep apnea. Sleep. 1993;16:539–544.

60. Fletcher EC. Can the treatment of sleep apnea syndrome prevent the cardiovascular consequences? Sleep. 1996;19:S67–S70.

61. Bokinsky G, Miller M, Ault K, et al. Spontaneous platelet activation and aggregation during obstructive sleep apnea and its response to therapy with nasal continuous positive airway pressure. Chest. 1995;108:625–630.

62. Chin T, Ohi M, Kita H, et al. Effects of NCPAP therapy on fibrinogen levels in obstructive sleep apnea syndrome. Am J Respir Crit Care Med. 1996;153:1972–1976.

63. Jennum P, Börgesen SE. Intracranial pressure and obstructive sleep apnea. Chest. 1989;95:279–283.

64. Fischer AQ, Chaudhary BA, Taormina MA, et al. Intracranial hemodynamics in sleep apnea. Chest. 1992;102:1402–1406.

65. Bonsignore MR, Marrone E, Insalaco G, et al. The cardiovascular

effects of obstructive sleep apnoeas: analysis of pathogenetic mechanisms. Eur Respir J. 1994;7:786–805.

66. Garpestad E, Ringler J, Parker JA, et al. Sleep stage influences the hemodynamic response to obstructive apneas. Am J Respir Crit Care Med. 1995;152:199–203.

67. Somers VK, Dyken ME, Mark AL, et al. Parasympathetic hyperresponsiveness and bradyarrhythmias during apnea in hypertension. Clin Auton Res. 1992;2:171–176.

68. Somers VK, Abboud FM. Chemoreflexes—responses, interactions and implications for sleep apnea. Sleep. 1993;16:S30–S34.

69. Netzer N, Werner P, Jochums I, et al. Blood flow of the middle cerebral artery with sleep-disordered breathing. Stroke. 1998;29:87–93.

70. Wardlaw JM. Cheyne-Stokes respiration in patients with acute ischaemic stroke: observations on middle cerebral artery blood velocity changes using transcranial Doppler ultrasound. Cerebrovasc Dis. 1993;3:377–380.

71. Hajak G, Klingelhöfer J, Schulz-Varszegi M, et al. Sleep apnea syndrome and cerebral hemodynamics. Chest. 1996;110:670–679.

72. Bruno A, Biller J, Adams JP, et al. Retinal infarction during sleep and wakefulness. Stroke. 1990;21:1494–1496.

73. Pressman MR, Schetman WR, Figueroa WG, et al. Transient ischemic attacks and minor stroke during sleep. Stroke. 1995;26:2361–2365.

74. Erkinjuntti T, Partinen M, Sulkawa R, et al. Sleep apnea in multiinfarct dementia and Alzheimer's disease. Sleep. 1987;10:419–425.

75. Bassetti C, Aldrich MS, Quint D. Sleep-disordered breathing in patients with acute supra- and infratentorial stroke. Stroke. 1997;28:1765–1772.

76. Horner RL. Autonomic consequences of arousal from sleep: mechanisms and implications. Sleep. 1996;19:S193–S195.

77. Ali NJ, Davies RJ, Fleetham JA, et al. Periodic movements of the legs during sleep associated with rises in systemic blood pressure. Sleep. 1991;14:163–165.

78. Espinar-Sierra J, Vela-Bueno A, Luque-Otero M. Periodic leg movements in sleep in essential hypertension. Psychiatry Clin Neurosci. 1997;51:103–107.

79. Qreshi AI, Giles WH, Croft JB, et al. Habitual sleep patterns and risk for stroke and coronary disease: a 10-year follow-up from NHANES I. Neurology. 1997;48:904–910.

80. Gislason T, Almqvist M. Somatic diseases and sleep complaints. An epidemiological study of 3201 Swedish men. Acta Med Scand. 1987;221:475–481.

81. Lee MC, Klassen AC, Resch JA. Respiratory pattern disturbances in ischemic cerebral vascular disease. Stroke. 1974;5:612–616.

82. Lee MC, Klassen AC, Heaney LM, et al. Respiratory rate and pattern disturbances in acute brainstem infarction. Stroke. 1976;7:382–385.

83. North JB, Jennett S. Abnormal breathing patterns associated with acute brain damage. Arch Neurol. 1974;31:338–344.

84. Power WR, Mosko SS, Sassin JF. Sleep-stage dependent Cheyne-Stokes respiration after cerebral infarct: a case study. Neurology. 1982;32:763–766.

85. Rout MW, Lane DJ, Wollner L. Prognosis in acute cerebrovascular accidents in relation to respiratory pattern and blood gas tensions. Br Med J. 1971;3:7–9.

86. Norrving B, Cronquist S. Lateral medullary infarction. Prognosis in an unselected series. Neurology. 1991;41:244–248.

87. Good DC, Henkle JQ, Gelber D, et al. Sleep-disordered breathing and poor functional outcome after stroke. Stroke. 1996;27:252–259.

88. Dyken ME, Somers VK, Yamada T, et al. Investigating the relationship between stroke and obstructive sleep apnea. Stroke. 1996;27:401–407.

89. Bassetti C, Aldrich M, Chervin R, et al. Sleep apnea in the acute phase of TIA and stroke. Neurology. 1996;47:1167–1173.

90. Dempsey JA, Smith CA, Harms CA, et al. Sleep-induced breathing instability. Sleep. 1996;19:236–247.

91. Deegan PC, McNicholas WT. Predictive value of clinical features for the obstructive sleep apnoea syndrome. Eur Respir J. 1996;9:117–124.

92. Viner S, Szalai JP, Hoffstein V. Are history and physical examination a good screening test for sleep apnea. Ann Intern Med. 1991;115:356–359.

93. American Sleep Disorders Association. Practice parameters for the use of portable recording in the assessment of obstructive sleep apnea. Sleep. 1994;17:372–377.

94. Gugger M, Mathis J, Bassetti C. Accuracy of an intelligent CPAP machine with in-built diagnostic abilities in detecting apneas: a comparison with polysomnography. Thorax. 1995;50:1199–1201.

95. Milanova M, Pfäffli B, Gugger M, Bassetti C. Sleep apnea in acute stroke: diagnosis, treatment and follow-up in 100 patients. Sleep Research Online. 1999;2(suppl 1):405.

96. Cherniack NS. Respiratory dysrhythmias during sleep. N Engl J Med. 1981;305:325–330.

97. Heyman A, Birchfield RI, Sieker HO. Effects of bilateral cerebral infarction on respiratory center sensitivity. Neurology. 1958;8:694–700.

98. Ropper AH, Shafran B. Brain edema after stroke. Clinical syndrome and intracranial pressure. Arch Neurol. 1984;41:26–29.

99. Nachtmann A, Siebler M, Rose G, et al. Cheyne-Stokes respiration in ischemic stroke. Neurology. 1995;45:820–821.

100. Hudgel DW, Devadatta P, Quadri M, et al. Mechanism of sleep-induced periodic breathing in convalescing stroke patients and healthy elderly subjects. Chest. 1993;104:1503–1510.

101. Javaheri S, Paker TJ, Wexler L, et al. Effect of theophylline on sleep-disordered breathing in heart failure. N Engl J Med. 1996;335:562–567.

102. Plum F. Neurological integration of behavioral and metabolic control of breathing. In: Porter R, ed. Ciba Foundation Breuer Centenary Symposium: Breathing. London, England: J & A Churchill; 1970:159–181.

103. Munschauer FE, Mador J, Ahuja A, et al. Selective paralysis of voluntary but not limbically influenced automatic respiration. Arch Neurol. 1991;48:1190–1192.

104. Plum F. Mechanisms of "central" hyperventilation. Ann Neurol. 1982;11:636–637.

105. Siderowf LJ, Balcer LJ, Kenyon LC, et al. Central neurogenic hyperventilation in an awake patient with pontine glioma. Neurology. 1996;46:1160–1162.

106. Plum F, Posner JB. The Diagnosis of Stupor and Coma. 3rd ed. Philadelphia, Pa: FA Davis; 1980.

107. Plum F, Alvord EC. Apneustic breathing in man. Arch Neurol. 1964;10:101–112.

108. Levin BE, Margolis G. Acute failure of automatic respirations secondary to unilateral brainstem infarct. Ann Neurol. 1977;1:583–586.

109. Hunziker A, Frick P, Regli F, et al. Zentralbedingte chronische alveoläre Hypoventilation bei Malazien in der Medulla oblongata. Beitrag zum Wallenberg-Syndrom. Dtsch Med Wochenschr. 1964;89:676–680.

110. Bogousslavsky J, Khurana R, Deruaz JP, et al. Respiratory failure and unilateral caudal brainstem infarction. Ann Neurol. 1990;28:668–673.

111. Milandre L, Lucchini P, Khalil R. Les infarctus latérobulbaires. Distribution, étiologies et pronostic de 40 cas identifiés par IRM. Rev Neurol. 1995;151:714–721.

112. Currier RD, Giles CL, deJong RN. Some aspects on Wallenberg's lateral medullary syndrome. Neurology. 1961;11:778–791.

113. Al Deeb SM, Sharif H, Al Moutaery K, et al. Intractable hiccup induced by brainstem lesion. J Neurol Sci. 1991;103:144–150.

114. Bauer G, Gerstenbrand F, Hengl W. Involuntary motor phenomena in the locked-in syndrome. J Neurol. 1980;223:191–198.

115. Howard RS, Thorpe J, Barker R, et al. Respiratory insufficiency due to high anterior cervical cord infarction. J Neurol Neurosurg Psychiatry. 1998;64:358–361.

116. Newsom-Davis J. Autonomous breathing. Arch Neurol. 1974;30:480–483.

117. Burke AM, White AB, Brill N. Baclofen for intractable hiccup. N Engl J Med. 1988;319:1354.

118. Benca RM, Quintans J. Sleep and host defenses: a review. Sleep. 1997;20:1027–1037.

119. Zepelin H: Mammalian sleep. In: Kryger MH, Roth T, Dement WC, eds. Principles and Practice of Sleep Medicine. Philadelphia, Pa: WB Saunders; 1994:69–80.

120. Steriade M, Amzica F. Coalescence of sleep rhythms and their chronology in corticothalamic networks. Sleep Res [serial online]. 1998;1:1–10.

121. Werth E, Achermann P, Borbély A. Fronto-occipital EEG power gradients in human sleep. J Sleep Res. 1997;6:102–112.

122. Werth E, Achermann P, Dijk DA, et al. Spindles frequency activity in the sleep EEG: individual differences and topographic distribution. Electroencephalogr Clin Neurophysiol. 1997;102:535–542.

123. Braun AR, Balkin TJ, Wesensten NJ, et al. Regional cerebral blood flow throughout the sleep-wake cycle. An H2l5O study. Brain. 1997;120:1173–1197.

124. Maquet P, Péters JM, Aerts J, et al. Functional neuroanatomy of human rapid-eye-movement sleep and dreaming. Nature. 1996;383:163–166.

125. Façon E, Steriade M, Wertheim N. Hypersomnie prolongée engendrée par des lésions bilatérale du système activateur médial. Le syndrome thrombotique de la bifurcation du tronc basilaire. Rev Neurol. 1958;98:117–133.

126. Castaigne P, Buge A, Escourolle R, et al. Ramollissement pédonculaire médian tegmento-thalamique avec ophtalmoplégie et hypersomnie. Etude anatomo-clinique. Rev Neurol. 1962; 106:357–361.

127. Castaigne P, Lhermitte F, Buge A, et al. Paramedian thalamic and midbrain infarcts: clinical and neuropathological study. Ann Neurol. 1981;10:127–148.

128. Bassetti C, Bogousslavsky J. Impaired consciousness and sleep. In: Caplan L, Bogousslavsky J, eds. Stroke Syndromes. Cambridge, England: Cambridge University Press; 1995:108–117.

129. Walther H. Ueber einen Dämmerzustand mit triebhafter Erregung nach Thalamusschädigung [dissertation]. Bern, Switzerland: University of Bern; 1945.

130. Niedermeyer E, Coyle PK, Preziosi TS. Hypersomnia with sudden sleep attacks ("symptomatic narcolepsy") on the basis of vertebrobasilar artery insufficiency. A case report. Waking Sleeping. 1979;3:361–364.

131. Caplan LR, Schmahmann JD, Kase CS, et al. Caudate infarcts. Arch Neurol. 1990;47:133–143.

132. Albert ML, Silverberg R, Reches A, et al. Cerebral dominance for consciousness. Arch Neurol. 1976;33:453–454.

133. Arpa J, Rodriguez-Albarino R, Izal E, et al. Hypersomnia after tegmental potnine hematoma: case report. Neurologia. 1995;10:140–144.

134. Bassetti C, Bogousslavsky J, Mattle H, et al. Medial medullary infarction: Report of seven patients and review of the literature. Neurology. 1997;48:882–890.

135. Catsman-Berrevoets CE, Harskamp F. Compulsive pre-sleep behaviour and apathy due to bilateral thalamic stroke. Neurology. 1988;38:647–649.

136. Guilleminault C, Quera-Salva MA, Goldberg MP. Pseudo-hypersomnia and pre-sleep behaviour with bilateral paramedian thalamic lesions. Brain. 1993;116:1549–1563.

137. Bastuji H, Nighoghossian N, Salord F, et al. Mesodiencephalic infarct with hypersomnia: sleep recording in two cases. J Sleep Res. 1994;3:16.

138. Drake ME. Kleine-Levine syndrome after multiple cerebral infarctions. Psychosomatics. 1987;28:329–330.

139. Rivera VM, Meyer JS, Hata T, et al. Narcolepsy following cerebral hypoxic ischemia. Ann Neurol. 1986;19:505–508.

140. Stern RA, Bachmann DL. Depressive symptoms following stroke. Am J Psychiatry. 1991;148:351–356.

141. Van Bogaert M. Syndrome de la calotte protubérantielle avec myoclonie localisée et troubles du sommeil. Rev Neurol (Paris). 1926;45:977–988.

142. Girard P, Gerrest F, Tommasi M, et al. Ramollissement géant du pied de la protubérance. Lyon Med. 1962;14:877–892.

143. Krachmann SL, D'Alonzo GE, Criner GJ. Sleep in the intensive care unit. Chest. 1995;107:1713–1720.

144. Culebras A, Moore JT. Magnetic resonance findings in rem sleep behavior disorder. Neurology. 1989;39:1519–1523.

145. Dagnino N, Loeb C, Massazza G, et al. Hypnic physiological myoclonias in man: an EEG-EMG study in normals and neurological patients. Eur Neurol. 1969;2:47–58.

146. Dyken ME, Rodnitzky RL. Periodic, aperiodic, and rhythmic motor disorders of sleep. Neurology. 1992;42(suppl 6):68–74.

147. Yokota T, Hirose K, Tanabe H, et al. Sleep-related periodic leg movements (nocturnal myoclonus) due to spinal cord lesion. J Neurol Sci. 1991;104:13–18.

148. Van Bogaert 1. L'hallucinose pédonculaire. Rev Neurol. 1927;43:608–617.

149. Feinberg WF, Rapcsack SZ. Peduncular hallucinosis following paramedian thalamic infarction. Neurology. 1989;39:1535–1536.

150. Geller TJ, Bellur SN. Peduncular hallucinosis: magnetic resonance imaging confirmation of mesencephalic infarction during life. Ann Neurol. 1987;21:602–604.

151. Mahowald MK, Schenck CH. Dissociated states of wakefulness and sleep. Neurology. 1992;42(suppl 6):44–52.

152. Teunisse RJ, Cruysberg JR, Hoefnagels WH, et al. Visual hallucinations in psychologically normal people: Charles Bonnet's syndrome. Lancet. 1996;347:794–797.

153. Martin R, Bogousslavsky J, Regli F. Striatocapsular infarction and "release" visual hallucinations. Cerebrovasc Dis. 1992; 2:111–113.

154. Vaphiades MS, Celesia GG, Brigell MG. Positive spontaneous visual phenomena limited to the hemianopic field in lesions of central visual pathways. Neurology. 1996;47:408–417.

155. Lepore FE. Spontaneous visual phenomena with visual loss: 104 patients with lesions of retinal and neural afferent pathways. Neurology. 1990;40:444–447.

156. Bischof M, Gutbrod C, Bassetti C. Peduncular hallucinosis and cessation of dreaming after bilateral posterior cerebral artery stroke. J Sleep Res. 1998;7:24.

157. Solms M. The Neuropsychology of Dreams. Mahwah, NJ: Lawrence Erlbaum Associates; 1997.

158. Murri L, Massetani R, Siciliano G, et al. Dream recall after sleep interruption in brain-injured patients. Sleep. 1985;8:356–362.

159. Boller F, Wright D, Cavalieri R, et al. Paroxysmal "nightmares." Neurology. 1975;25:1026.

160. Grünstein AM. Die Erforschung der Träme als eine Methode der topischen Diagnostik bei Grosshirnerkrankungen. Zeitschr Gesamte Neurol Psychiatrie 1924;93:416–420.

161. Gloning K, Sternbach I. Ueber das Träumen bei zerebralen Herdläsionen. Wien Zeitschr Nerv. 1953;6:302–329.

162. Broughton R, Baron R. Sleep patterns in the intensive care unit and on the ward after acute myocardial infarction. Electroencephalogr Clin Neurophysiol. 1978;45:348–360.

163. Karacan I, Hirschkowitz M, Tamura K, et al. Prognostic indicators of sleep EEG patterns in cerebrovascular disease. Part II. Relationship of clinical outcome to microsleep parameters. Sleep Res. 1979;8:231.

164. Hachinski V, Mamelak M, Norris JW. Prognostic Value of Sleep Morphology in Cerebral Infarction. Amsterdam, Netherlands: Excerpta Medica; 1978.

165. Bassetti C, Aldrich M, Quint D. Sleep abnormalities following supratentorial stroke. Neurology. 1997;48:A278.

166. Sumra RS, Pathak SN, Singh N, et al. Polygraphic sleep studies in cerebrovascular accidents. Neurol India. 1972;20:1–7.

167. Greenberg R. Cerebral cortex lesions: the dream process and sleep spindles. Cortex. 1966;2:357–366.

168. Hachinski V, Mamelak M, Norris JW. Clinical recovery and sleep architecture degradation. Can J Neurol Sci. 1990;17:332–335.

169. Giubilei F, Iannilli M, Vitale A, et al. Sleep patterns in acute ischemic stroke. Acta Neurol Scand. 1992;86:567–571.

170. Yokohama E, Nagata K, Hirata Y, et al. Correlation of EEG activities between slow-wave sleep and wakefulness in patients with supratentorial stroke. Brain Topogr. 1996;8:269–273.

171. Bassetti C, Aldrich MS, Quint D. Sleep abnormalities in hemispheric stroke. Sleep Res. 1997;26:320.

172. Körner E, Flooh E, Reinhart B, et al. Sleep alterations in ischemic stroke. Eur Neurol. 1986;25:104–110.

173. Ribeiro Pinto L, Baptistas Silva A, Tufik S. Rapid eye movements density in patients with stroke [abstract]. Sleep Res. 1994;076.

174. Appenzeller O, Fischer AP. Disturbances of rapid eye movements during sleep in patients with lesions of the nervous system. Electroencephalogr Clin Neurophysiol. 1968;25:29–35.

175. Hirose G, Saeki M, Kosoegawa H, et al. Delta waves in the EEGs of patients with intracerebral hemorrhage. Arch Neurol. 1981;38:170–175.

176. Mathis J, Bassetti C, Gugger M, et al. Pattern of recovery of hypersomnia and polysomnographic changes in patients with unilateral and bilateral paramedian thalamic stroke. Sleep Res. 1996;5:136.

177. Autret A, Laffont F, De Toffol B, et al. A syndrome of REM and

non-REM sleep reduction and lateral gaze paresis after medial tegmental pontine stroke. Arch Neurol. 1988;45:1236–1242.

178. Cummings JL, Greenberg R. Sleep patterns in the "locked-in" syndrome. Electroencephalogr Clin Neurophysiol. 1977;43:270–271.

179. Tamura K, Karacan I, Williams RL, et al. Disturbances of the sleep-waking cycle in patients with vascular brain stem lesions. Clin Electroencephalogr. 1983;14:35–46.

180. Markand ON, Dyken ML. Sleep abnormalities in patients with brainstem lesions. Neurology. 1976;26:769–776.

181. Valldeoriola F, Santamaria J, Graus F, et al. Absence of REM sleep, altered NREM sleep and supranuclear horizontal gaze palsy caused by a lesion of the pontine tegmentum. Sleep. 1993;16:184–188.

182. Obrador S, Reinoso-Suarez F, Carbonell J, et al. Comatose state maintained during eight years following a vascular ponto-mes-

encephalic lesion. Electroencephalogr Clin Neurophysiol. 1975;38:21–26.

183. Bassetti C, Mathis J, Hess CW. Multimodal electrophysiological studies including motor evoked potentials in patients with locked-in syndrome: report of six patients. J Neurol Neurosurg Psychiatry. 1994;57:1403–1406.

184. Kushida CA, Rye DB, Nummy D. Cortical asymmetry of REM sleep EEG following unilateral pontine hemorrhage. Neurology. 1991;41:598–601.

185. Popoviciu L, Asgian B, Corfarici D, et al. Anatomoclinical and polygraphic features in cerebrovascular diseases with disturbances of vigilance. In: Tirgu-Mures L, Popoviciu L, Asgia B, et al, eds. Sleep 1978: Fourth European Congress on Sleep Research. New York, NY: Karger; 1980:165–169.

186. Scandinavian Stroke Study Group. Multicenter trial of hemodilution in ischemic stroke: background and study protocol. Stroke. 1985;16:885–890.

91

Neuromuscular Disorders

Charles F. P. George

Disease of nerve, neuromuscular junction, or muscle can lead to muscle weakness and to general fatigue. This tiredness can affect the patient's sense of well-being and may influence the perception of how well he or she has slept. When the neuromuscular process affects muscles of respiration, inadequate ventilation may progress to respiratory failure and death. There have been many reports of sleep and breathing in these patients, and we are beginning to understand the mechanisms for nocturnal changes in breathing and oxygenation and how these contribute to the morbidity and progression of clinical disease.

PATHOPHYSIOLOGY

The diaphragm is the major muscle of respiration during wakefulness and sleep. During nonrapid eye movement (NREM) sleep, there is an overall reduction in ventilation related to sleep state and in response to increased impedance of the respiratory system. However, rib cage activity is maintained, albeit reduced, as is diaphragmatic activity. The importance of the diaphragm is particularly evident during rapid eye movement (REM) sleep. During REM sleep, there is postsynaptic inhibition of somatic motoneurons, which causes further reduction or even complete loss of tone in rib cage and other accessory muscles of respiration, but which leaves the diaphragm relatively unaffected. Thus, any process affecting the diaphragm, whether a myopathy or a process involving its innervation, might be expected to cause significant changes in breathing and oxygenation during sleep.

In patients with bilateral diaphragmatic paralysis, marked oxygen desaturations can occur in REM sleep.[1-3] The REM sleep–related inhibition of intercostal and accessory muscles leads to profound hypoventilation in this sleep stage because patients with diaphragmatic paralysis are totally dependent on intercostal and accessory muscles for breathing. As noted previously, this suppression of accessory respiratory muscle tone is a normal concomitant of REM sleep and is seen in normal subjects and patients with lung diseases.[4-6] Depending on the type of neuromuscular disorder, breathing abnormalities during sleep may be present as central apneas, obstructive apneas, or periods of prolonged hypoventilation.

Specific Disorders

Degenerative Diseases

Sleep disturbances such as insomnia, hypersomnia, circadian rhythm disturbances, parasomnia, and sleep-disordered breathing have been recorded in degenerative neurological disorders. In amyotrophic lateral sclerosis (ALS), although ALS has not been shown to affect the sleep-regulating areas of the brain, it is likely that indirect effects of the disease cause the sleep disruption. Periodic limb movements associated with arousals and sleep-disordered breathing contributed to the sleep disruption in some ALS patients. However, some patients without any respiratory disturbance or periodic limb movements still have sleep fragmentation, independent of age. This suggests other factors contributing to disturbed sleep such as anxiety, depression, pain, choking, excessive secretions, fasciculations and cramps, and the inability to get comfortable or turn oneself freely in bed. Orthopnea, a frequent complaint in ALS, may also contribute to sleep disruption.[7, 8]

Various sleep and breathing abnormalities have been described in poliomyelitis. Abnormalities in central regulation of breathing in acute and convalescent poliomyelitis were described in 1958 by Plum and Swanson.[9] Subsequently, central, mixed, and obstructive events have been noted.[10] Sleep and breathing abnormalities are seen not only in patients who are on respiratory assistance (rocking beds) during sleep but also before ventilatory assistance is initiated.[11] Sleep abnormalities include decreased sleep efficiency, increased arousal frequency, and varying degrees of apnea and hypopnea. After treatment of these sleep and breathing abnormalities, many symptoms frequently attributed to the "post-polio syndrome" improve. Thus, although not all symptoms may be explained, daytime symptoms may be explained by poor sleep quality and abnormal respiration during sleep. Inherited metabolic diseases such as subacute necrotizing encephalomyelopathy (Leigh's disease) typically present in childhood and may be associated with respiratory disturbance. Rarely, this disease may present in adulthood with automatic respiratory failure during sleep.[12]

In general, diseases of peripheral nerves are not characterized by abnormalities of respiration. Hereditary motor and sensory neuropathy (Charcot-Marie-Tooth disease) is characterized by chronic degeneration of peripheral nerves and roots, resulting in distal muscle atrophy, beginning in the feet and legs and later involving the hands. However, the association of this disease with diaphragmatic dysfunction has recently been reported, making these patients susceptible to sleep-disordered breathing.[13]

Disease of Neuromuscular Junction

Myasthenia gravis is a disorder of the neuromuscular junction characterized by weakness and fatigability of skeletal muscles. As a result of diaphragmatic weakness, sleep breathing abnormalities can occur. Younger patients with shorter duration of illness are least likely to experience any sleep-related hypoventilation or oxygen desaturation,[14] while older patients with moderately increased body mass index, abnormal total lung capacity, and abnormal daytime blood gases are most likely to develop hypopneas or apneas, particularly during REM sleep.[15]

Disorders of Muscle

From all published series on any neuromuscular disorders, more data exist for myotonic dystrophy (MD) than any other single condition. This autosomal dominant form of muscular dystrophy is distinguished by its unique topography, associated myotonia, and occurrence of dystrophic changes in nonmuscular tissues.

In myotonic dystrophy, there is consistent involvement of facial, masseter, levator palpebrae, sternocleidomastoid, forearm, hand, and pretibial muscles; MD is, in a sense, a distal myopathy. However, pharyngeal and laryngeal muscles may be involved as well as respiratory muscles, particularly the diaphragm. Involvement of these respiratory muscles may predispose to breathing and oxygenation changes during sleep. There has been ample evidence for the occurrence of documented periods of alveolar hypoventilation, predominantly in REM sleep,[16–18] obstructive apneas,[19] and central apneas.[20] However, the development of sleep-breathing abnormalities in MD is not simply due to muscle weakness. When sleep and breathing in MD patients are compared with nonmyotonic respiratory muscle weakness patients and with control subjects, periods of hypoventilation and apneas (central and obstructive) occurred in MD and at higher frequencies than in nonmyotonic patients with the same degree of muscle weakness (measured by maximal inspiratory and expiratory pressures).[21] This finding adds further evidence that respiratory muscle weakness alone does not account for abnormal breathing in MD.

The observation of decreased ventilatory response to hypoxic and hypercapnic stimuli[17, 22–25] and extreme sensitivity to sedative drugs has suggested a central origin of the breathing impairments. Whereas response of ventilation to increased carbon dioxide is a standard technique for assessing control of respiration, in MD the respiratory muscles must transduce the chemical stimulus. When these muscles are abnormal, as in MD, it becomes difficult to interpret a reduced ventilatory response. That is, chemoreceptor activity and efferent activity to muscles may be intact, but weak or inefficient respiratory muscles may not permit a normal ventilatory response to a hypoxic stimulus. Measuring mouth pressure developed at the beginning of a transiently occluded breath (occlusion pressure, $P_{0.1}$) can also be used as a measure of respiratory center output.[26]

In MD, $P_{0.1}$ may be as high as or higher than that of control subjects at rest and during stimulated breathing, although overall ventilation is lower.[23, 27] The finding of high transdiaphragmatic pressure (P_{di}), despite overall lower ventilation, suggests that increased impedance of the respiratory system accounts for incomplete transformation into ventilation of normal or increased respiratory center output. Magnetic stimulation of the cortex, in conjunction with phrenic nerve recordings, will test the corticospinal tract to phrenic motor neuron pathways and is a reliable method for diagnosing and monitoring patients with impaired central respiratory drive.[28] Using transcortical and cervical magnetic stimulation demonstrates that more than 20% of myotonic patients have impaired central respiratory drive.[29] The recent finding of neuronal loss in the dorsal central, ventral central, and subtrigeminal medullary nuclei in MD patients with alveolar hypoventilation[30] and the severe neuronal loss and gliosis in the tegmentum of the brainstem[31] also support a central abnormality.

Thus, there may be central or peripheral abnormalities contributing to disordered breathing in MD: central drive may be decreased (as reflected in sensitivity to sedation or decreased ventilatory response to chemical stimuli) or increased (as reflected in $P_{0.1}$). When drive ($P_{0.1}$) is increased and there is no muscle weakness (normal or increased P_{di}), reduced ventilatory response is due to incomplete transformation of the stimulus, probably because of increased impedance of the respiratory system. The addition of muscle weakness (i.e., reduced P_{di}) may further contribute to reduced ventilatory response.[22]

Other muscular dystrophy patients may develop similar breathing abnormalities during sleep although not all do so and the data are few. With progression of their illness, patients with Duchenne muscular dystrophy develop progressive inspiratory muscle weakness and rib cage deformities associated with kyphoscoliosis and thus develop extraparenchymal restrictive lung disease. (Chapter 82 deals with sleep in restrictive lung disease, where it will be pointed out that patients with restrictive lung disease are at risk for oxygen desaturation during sleep.) While some Duchenne patients may develop hypoventilation in all stages with significant desaturation during REM sleep,[32] others have only infrequent apneas or hypopneas during REM sleep but little oxygen desaturation and near-normal sleep architecture.[33]

Such differences may reflect varying degrees of muscle weakness, as well as differences in residual lung function. Despite severe restrictive disease and marked scoliosis,[32] preservation of end-expiratory lung volumes (functional residual capacity), with attendant higher oxygen stores and little change in volumes between sitting and supine position, helped defend against sleep-related hypoventilation and significant desaturation. As a consequence of hypoventilation or apnea during sleep, myotonic dystrophy patients may develop frequent oxygen desaturation and arousal, leading to sleep fragmentation and excessive daytime sleepiness.[19] Indeed, this association of cyanosis and hypersomnolence in myotonic dystrophy has been known for many years.[34]

However, disturbances of sleep architecture and daytime symptoms may not be related to sleep-disordered breathing in these types of patients. There may be excessive daytime sleepiness but minimal sleep-disordered breathing and sleep disruption insufficient to account for the degree of sleepiness, which suggests a central cause for the somnolence.[35] Waking cognitive impairment cannot be attributed to the effect of nocturnal sleep apnea or sleep disruption but probably represents a direct effect of central nervous system lesions. Thus, although sleepiness appears to be secondary to sleep apnea in some patients, in others there may be a central basis.

Sleep may be disturbed in the absence of sleep-disordered breathing in Duchenne muscular dystrophy[36]: many arousals from sleep (not related to breathing pattern changes), more than double the normal sleep-stage changes and awakenings, and marked reduction in the amount of REM sleep. In these patients, frequent arousals and reduced REM sleep may, in some way, be related to quadriplegia and the resultant inability to reposition oneself or to accompanying joint contractures, Abnormalities in sleep and breathing have been reported in isolated series of patients with various other neuromuscular disorders, such as congenital myopathies (nemaline or congenital fiber-type disproportion myopathy[37–39]) or metabolic myopathies (mitochondrial myopathy [Kearns-Sayre] syndrome,[40–42] acid maltase deficiency).[43–45] In all of these cases, there are various alterations in control of breathing and varied breathing pattern changes, including hypoventilation, obstruction, and central apnea. Severe central sleep apnea and marked oxygen desaturation, particularly during REM sleep, resulting in hypoxia-induced nocturnal seizures, as well as pulmonary hypertension, excessive daytime sleepiness, heart failure, and morning headaches, may be seen in congenital muscular dystrophy,[46] while obstructive sleep apnea has also been described in Thomsen's disease (myotonia congenita).[47]

CLINICAL FEATURES

Patients with neuromuscular weakness may present with no symptoms of disturbed sleep or abnormal breathing or may have severe respiratory failure with excessive daytime sleepiness. Disturbed sleep, early-morning headaches, daytime fatigue, and hypersomnolence are common symptoms. Depending on the degree of sleep fragmentation, complaints of insomnia may predominate. Orthopnea may be a frequent symptom if the diaphragm is involved or when muscle weakness is severe. Even patients who have very mild muscle weakness may have unrecognized significant abnormalities in breathing during sleep.

DIAGNOSTIC EVALUATION

All patients with neuromuscular disease should be questioned carefully about sleep duration and sleep quality. Nonrestorative sleep or daytime sleepiness may be the early signs of disturbed sleep due to respiratory insufficiency. Tiredness and fatigue are commonly used by patients to indicate sleepiness, and physicians should not automatically assume that these are due solely to the neuromuscular disease. Other symptoms to consider are frequency of napping, rest periods during the day, and symptoms which could be explained on the basis of sleepiness such as decreased memory, decreased attention span, decreased performance, or an increase in errors at work. However, none of these symptoms are sufficiently sensitive or specific. There is some evidence to suggest that patients with even mild symptoms may have significant sleep-breathing abnormalities. These can be detected by careful recordings of sleep and breathing using overnight polysomnography or properly validated ambulatory recording devices.[48] Whether detecting these early will have any impact in the long run is uncertain.

Pulmonary function tests and arterial blood gases may be helpful in predicting sleep hypoventilation in Duchenne's muscular dystrophy. An FEV_1 less than 40% predicted, a $PaCO_2$ greater than 45 mm Hg, and a base excess of 4 or more mmol/L may indicate that there is a risk of sleep hypoventilation, and it has been suggested that when these abnormalities are present, polysomnography be done.[48a] These criteria may be useful in other neuromuscular disorders as well (see Chapter 83).

EPIDEMIOLOGY

Although reports of abnormal sleep and breathing in neuromuscular diseases have been increasing, and while several studies dealing with the treatment of respiratory insufficiency contain fairly large numbers of patients,[49–52] there are almost no studies which examine the prevalence of sleep-disordered breathing in neuromuscular disease patients. One study from New Mexico[48] attempted to gather information from its entire clinic population of over 300 patients. (This clinic provides free care, including neurological, orthopedic, and physical therapy services, and such access assures that virtually all patients with neuromuscular disease from the state will be referred.) Although complete data are available on only 60 patients (20% of the clinic population), they demonstrate that sleep and breathing abnormalities are or may be present in more than 40% of patients being routinely followed at a neuromuscular diseases clinic.[48] Such a high prevalence should not be surprising given the vulnerability of such patients to sleep-related reductions in muscle tone and overall ventilation. What is more surprising is that many physicians would not have thought to inquire about abnor-

Table 91–1. EXAMPLES OF NEUROMUSCULAR
DISORDERS CAUSING SLEEP
BREATHING DISORDERS

Disorder	References
Diseases of Muscle	
Muscular Dystrophies	
Myotonic dystrophy	16–21, 27, 34
Duchenne muscular dystrophy	32, 33
Thomsen's disease (myotonia congenita)	46, 47
Congenital Myopathies	
Nemaline myopathy	38
Congenital fiber-type disproportion	37
Diseases of Nerve	
Degenerative	
Amyotrophic lateral sclerosis	7, 8
Poliomyelitis	9–11
Leigh's disease	12
Peripheral Neuropathy	
Charcot-Marie-Tooth disease	13
Disease of Neuromuscular Function	
Myasthenia gravis	14, 15
Metabolic Myopathies	
Mitochondrial myopathy (Kearns-Sayre syndrome)	39–41
Acid maltase deficiency	42, 43

malities of sleep. Table 91–1 summarizes neuromuscular disorders causing sleep-breathing abnormalities.

TREATMENT OF SLEEP ABNORMALITIES IN NEUROMUSCULAR DISEASE

Various therapies may be considered to improve nocturnal hypoventilation or offset the attendant oxygen desaturation. Supplemental oxygen has been used to obviate the REM sleep–related oxygen desaturation in patients with Duchenne muscular dystrophy. However, little improvement in sleep ensues.[53] Because most of the hypoventilation occurs during REM sleep, pharmacological manipulation of REM sleep by use of tricyclic antidepressants is a theoretical option and has been attempted using protriptyline. In a small study of patients with Duchenne muscular dystrophy, marked improvement in the nocturnal oxygen saturation profile[54] was seen. These results are similar to protriptyline's effectiveness in patients with restrictive lung disease[55]; however, anticholinergic side effects certainly limit the widespread use of such therapy.

Inspiratory muscle training has demonstrated improved waking respiratory failure in one patient with acid maltase deficiency.[44] This patient had abnormal sleep architecture that was unchanged by the muscle training, but there was major improvement in the nocturnal oxygen profile. Muscle weakness can obviously lead to nocturnal hypoventilation and worsening of oxygenation. Repeated nocturnal asphyxia may lead to increased muscle weakness, which begets further oxygen desaturation, and reversal of the hypoxemia

may arrest the muscle weakness. Such a case was reported by Olsen et al.[56] In this instance, nocturnal ventilation ablated nocturnal hypoxemia in a patient with acid maltase deficiency, and muscle weakness did not progress over an 8-year period.

Since the days of the poliomyelitis epidemics, mechanical ventilation has been a mainstay in supporting ventilation in patients with poliomyelitis. Rocking beds, negative pressure tank ventilator, and positive-pressure ventilation via tracheostomy have usually been the long-term options. Indeed, many patients are still successfully managed with this form of therapy.[49–51] However, all of these options are cumbersome, severely limit the mobility of patients, and, in the case of tracheostomy, may have unwanted complications. Over the years, other forms of assisted ventilation have been developed, including phrenic nerve pacing, cuirass ventilation, nasal continuous positive airway pressure (CPAP), and nasal intermittent positive-pressure ventilation. In contrast to CPAP (in which airway pressures are constant), the bilevel positive airway pressure (BiPAP) system allows different positive pressures on inspiration and expiration. By adjusting the inspiratory pressures higher than the expiratory pressures, the BiPAP system emulates a conventional positive-pressure ventilatory device and may be used as a means of enhancing ventilation. This is an effective treatment for a number of neuromuscular diseases[52] and in the early stages may be as effective as a conventional ventilator. If, however, this is insufficient, nasal intermittent positive-pressure ventilation with a small ventilator can be used. This last form is rapidly becoming the preferred means of assisting ventilation because of its relative simplicity and because it obviates the need for tracheostomy and its attendant problems. Nasal ventilation has been used predominantly nocturnally for post-poliomyelitis patients and in other neuromuscular disorders[57–65] and has even been used almost continuously in patients with severe post-poliomyelitis respiratory insufficiency.[61] In almost every case, not only is the nocturnal ventilation normalized, but daytime respiratory failure and excessive sleepiness are improved as well. In the report by Steljes et al.,[11] use of nasal intermittent positive-pressure ventilation allowed one patient to return to work; another patient who had been constrained by having to rely on a rocking bed for nocturnal ventilatory support could travel for the first time in years.

The Decision to Assist Nocturnal Ventilation

When patients present with disrupted sleep, snoring, excessive daytime sleepiness, and unexplained development of peripheral edema or polycythemia, sleep studies will characterize the breathing disorder, and the decision to assist ventilation is an easy one. For those with obstructive sleep apnea, nasal CPAP or BiPAP will be the preferred treatment; patients with predominantly hypoventilation or central apnea and oxygen desaturation should be managed with BiPAP or full nasal ventilation (if tolerated). For a detailed review of noninvasive ventilation, see Chapter 83. However a change in SaO$_2$ alone is insufficient for deciding whether the patient needs ventilatory assistance. Patients may not be "allowing" themselves to fall asleep, and thus the main abnormality is abnormal sleep structure. In these individuals, the endpoint for successful nasal ventilation is not improvement in SaO$_2$ but rather improvement in sleep structure.

Only recently is there beginning to emerge a consensus[66] on the management of severe progressive neuromuscular disorders, in which respiratory failure plays only a part and in which other systems are severely affected (e.g., ALS). Issues such as quality of life must be taken into account. Without specific guidance from the published literature, each patient must be assessed in detail, with the clinician always bearing in mind that nocturnal (and later, 24-h) ventilation will treat only one (albeit important) aspect of the disorder.

CONCLUSIONS

Patients with neuromuscular disease have variable degrees of extrapulmonary lung restriction, muscle weakness, and reduction in drives to breathe. Available evidence suggests that sleep is disrupted either because of severe nocturnal breathing abnormalities and oxygen desaturation or possibly because of factors still unknown. While the range of nocturnal respiratory abnormality is great, there does not appear to be a good correlation with the degree of muscle impairment and development of sleep abnormalities. Indeed, in some patients, there may be severe sleep-breathing abnormalities, even though the respiratory muscles are still able to generate more than adequate pressure. Treatment of nocturnal breathing abnormalities markedly improves both daytime symptoms and function and can be achieved by a variety of ventilatory assist devices. Nasal CPAP and, in some cases, nasal positive-pressure ventilation are rapidly becoming the preferred routes of ventilatory support in these groups of patients. With further improvements in this mode of therapy, it is likely to become the standard in years to come. Prompt recognition and treatment of sleep-disordered breathing is of significant benefit to the patient's well-being, will reduce morbidity, and is likely to improve survival.

References

1. Newsom-Davis J, Goldman M, Loh L, et al. Diaphragm function and alveolar hypoventilation. Q J Med. 1975;45:87–100.
2. Kreitzer SM, Feldman NT, Saunders NA, et al. Bilateral diaphragmatic paralysis with hypercapnic respiratory failure. Am J Med. 1978;65:89–95.
3. Skatrud J, Iber C, McHugh W, et al. Determinants of hypoventilation during wakefulness and sleep in diaphragmatic paralysis. Am Rev Respir Dis. 1980;121:587–593.
4. Muller NL, Francis DW, Gurwitz D, et al. Mechanisms of hemoglobin desaturation during REM sleep in normal subjects and in patients with cystic fibrosis. Am Rev Respir Dis. 1980;121:463–469.
5. Johnson MW, Remmers JE. Accessory muscle activity during sleep in chronic obstructive pulmonary disease. J Appl Physiol. 1984;57:1011–1017.
6. Millman BP, Knight H, Kline LR, et al. Changes in compartmental ventilation in association with eye movements during REM sleep. J Appl Physiol. 1988;65:1196–1202.
7. Ferguson KA, Strong MJ, Ahmad D, et al. Sleep-disordered breathing in amyotrophic lateral sclerosis. Chest. 1996;110:664–669.
8. David WS, Bundlie SR, Mahdavi Z. Polysomnographic studies in amyotrophic lateral sclerosis. J Neurol Sci. 1997;152(suppl 1):S29–S35.
9. Plum F, Swanson AG. Abnormalities in central regulation of respiration in acute and convalescent poliomyelitis. Arch Neurol Psychiatry. 1958;80:267–285.
10. Guilleminault C, Motta J. Sleep apnea syndrome as a long-term sequelae of poliomyelitis. In: Guilleminault C, Dement WC, eds: Sleep Apnea Syndrome. New York, NY: Alan R Liss; 1978:309–315.
11. Steljes DG, Kryger MH, Kirk BW, et al. Sleep in postpolio syndrome. Chest. 1990;98:133–140.
12. Cummiskey J, Guilleminault C, Davis R, et al. Automatic respiratory failure: sleep studies and Leigh's disease. Neurology. 1987;37:1876–1878.
13. Chan CK, Mohsenin V, Loke J, et al. Diaphragmatic dysfunction in siblings with hereditary motor and sensory neuropathy (Charcot-Marie-Tooth disease). Chest. 1987;91:567–570.
14. Manni R, Piccolo G, Sartori I, et al. Breathing during sleep in myasthenia gravis. Ital J Neurol Sci. 1995;16:589–594.
15. Quera-Salva MA, Guilleminault C, Chevret S, et al. Breathing disorders during sleep in myasthenia gravis. Ann Neurol. 1992;31:8692.
16. Kilburn KH, Eagan JT, Sieker HO, et al. Cardiopulmonary insufficiency in myotonic and progressive muscular dystrophy. N Engl J Med. 1954;261:1089–1096.
17. Coccagna G, Mantovani M, Parchi C, et al. Alveolar hypoventilation and hypersomnia in myotonic dystrophy. J Neurol Neurosurg Psychiatry. 1975;38:977–984.
18. Coccagna G, Martinelli P, Lugaresi E. Sleep and alveolar hypoventilation in myotonic dystrophy. Acta Neurol Belg. 1982;82:185–194.
19. Guilleminault C, Cummiskey J, Motta J, et al. Respiratory and hypodynamics study during wakefulness and sleep in myotonic dystrophy. Sleep. 1978;1:19–31.
20. Cirignotta F, Mondini S, Zucconi M, et al. Sleep related breathing impairments in myotonic dystrophy. J Neurol. 1987;235:80–85.
21. Gilmartin JJ, Cooper BG, Griffiths CJ, et al. Breathing during sleep in patients with myotonic dystrophy and non-myotonic respiratory muscle weakness. Q J Med. 1991;78:21–31.
22. Serisier DE, Mastaglia FL, Gibson GJ. Respiratory muscle function and ventilatory control, I: in patients with motor neurone disease, II: in patients with myotonic dystrophy. Q J Med. 1982;51:205–226.
23. Begin R, Bureau MA, Lupien L, et al. Pathogenesis of respiratory insufficiency in myotonic dystrophy. Am Rev Respir Dis. 1982;125:312–318.
24. Carroll JE, Zwillich LW, Weil JV. Ventilatory response in myotonic dystrophy. Neurology. 1977;27:1125–1128.
25. Gillam PMS, Heaf PJD, Kaufman L, et al. Respiration in dystrophic myotonia. Thorax. 1964;19:112–120.
26. Whitelaw WA, Derenne JP, Milic-Emili J. Occlusion pressure as a measure of the respiratory centre output in conscious man. Respir Physiol. 1975;23:181–199.
27. Begin P, Mathieu J, Almirall J, et al. Relationship between chronic hypercapnia and inspiratory-muscle weakness in myotonic dystrophy. Am J Respir Crit Care Med. 1997;156:133–139.
28. Zifko UA, Hahn AF, Remtulla H, et al. Central and peripheral respiratory electrophysiological studies in myotonic dystrophy. Brain. 1996;119:1911–1922.
29. Zifko U, Remtulla H, Power K, et al. Transcortical and cervical magnetic stimulation with recording of the diaphragm. Muscle Nerve. 1996;19:614–620.
30. Ono SF, Kanda F, Takahashi K, et al. Neuronal loss in the medullary reticular formation in myotonic dystrophy: a clinicopathological study. Neurology. 1996;46:A171.
31. Ono S, Kurisaki H, Sakuma A, et al. Myotonic dystrophy with alveolar hypoventilation and hypersomnia: a clinicopathological study. J Neurol Sci. 1995;128:225–231.

32. Smith PEM, Edwards BHT, Calverley PMA. Ventilations and breathing pattern during sleep in Duchenne muscular dystrophy. Chest. 1989;96:1346–1351.

33. Manni R, Ottolini A, Cerveri I, et al. Breathing patterns and HbSₐO₂ changes during nocturnal sleep in patients with Duchenne muscular dystrophy. J Neurol. 1989;236:391–394.

34. Adie WJ, Greenfield JG. Dystrophica myotonia. Brain. 1923;46:73–127.

35. Broughton R, Stuss D, Kates M, et al. Neuropsychological deficits and sleep in myotonic dystrophy. Can J Neurol Sci. 1990;17:410–415.

36. Redding GJ, Okamoto GA, Guthrie RD, et al. Sleep patterns in non-ambulatory boys with Duchenne muscular dystrophy. Arch Phys Med Rehabil. 1985;66:818–821.

37. Riley DJ, Santiago RV, Daniele RP, et al. Blunted respiratory drive in congenital myopathy. Am J Med. 1977;63:459–466.

38. Maayan C, Springer C, Armen Y, et al. Nemaline myopathy as a cause of sleep hypoventilation. Pediatrics. 1986;77:390–395.

39. Wilson DO, Sanders MH, Dauber JH. Abnormal ventilatory chemosensitivity and congenital myopathy. Arch Intern Med. 1987;147:1773–1777.

40. Carroll JE, Zwillich C, Weil JV, et al. Depressed ventilatory response in oculocraniosomatic neuromuscular disease. Neurology. 1976;26:140–146.

41. Weng TR, Schultz GE, Chang HC, et al. Pulmonary function and ventilatory response to chemical stimuli in familial myopathy. Chest. 1985;88:488–495.

42. Kotagal S, Archer CR, Walsh JK, et al. Hypersomnia, bithalamic lesions, and altered sleep architecture in Kearns-Sayre syndrome. Neurology. 1985;35:574–577.

43. Bellamy D, Newsom-Davis JM, Mickey BP, et al. A case of primary alveolar hypoventilation associated with mild proximal myopathy. Am Rev Respir Dis. 1975;112:867–873.

44. Martin RJ, Sufit RI, Ringel SP, et al. Respiratory improvement by muscle training in adult-onset acid maltase deficiency. Muscle Nerve. 1983;6:201–203.

45. Margolis ML, Howlett P, Goldberg R, et al. Obstructive sleep apnea syndrome in acid maltase deficiency Chest. 1994;105:947–949.

46. Kryger MH, Steljes DG, Yee WC, et al. Central sleep apnea in congenital muscular dysrophy. J Neurol Neurosurg Psychiatry. 1991;54:710–712.

47. Striano S, Meo R, Bilo L, et al. Sleep apnea syndrome in Thomsen's disease. A case report. Electroencephalogr Clin Neurophysiol. 1983;56:323–325.

48. Labanowski M, Schmidt-Nowara W, Guilleminault C. Sleep and neuromuscular disease: frequency of sleep-disordered breathing in a neuromuscular disease clinic population. Neurology. 1996;47:1173–1180.

48a. Hukins CA, Hillman DR. Daytime predictors of sleep hypoventilation in Duchenne muscular dystrophy. Am J Respir Crit Care Med. 2000;161:166–170.

49. Howard RS, Wiles CM, Hirsch NP, et al. Respiratory involvement in primary muscle disorders: assessment and management. Q J Med. 1993;86:175–189.

50. Chalmers RM, Howard RS, Wiles CM, et al. Use of the rocking bed in the treatment of neurogenic respiratory insufficiency. Q J Med. 1994;87:423–429.

51. Iber C, Davies SF, Mahowald MW Nocturnal rocking bed therapy: improvement in sleep fragmentation in patients with respiratory muscle weakness. Sleep. 1989;12:405–412.

52. Guilleminault C, Philip P, Robinson A. Sleep and neuromuscular disease: bilevel positive airway pressure by nasal mask as a treatment for sleep disordered breathing in patients with neuromuscular disease J. Neurol Neurosurg Psychiatry. 1998;65:225–232.

53. Smith PEM, Edwards RHT, Calverley PMA. Oxygen treatment of sleep hypoxemia in Duchenne muscular dystrophy. Thorax. 1989;44:997–1001.

54. Smith PEM, Edwards RHT, Calverley PMA. Protriptyline treatment of sleep hypoxemia in Duchenne muscular dystrophy. Thorax. 1989;44:1002–1105.

55. Simons AK, Parker RA, Branthwaite MA. Effects of protriptyline on sleep related disturbance of breathing in restrictive chest wall disease. Thorax. 1986;41:586–590.

56. Olsen LG, Hensley MJ, Saunders NA, et al. Sleep breathing and lung disease. In: Saunders NA, Sullivan CE, eds. Sleep and Breathing. New York, NY: Marcel Dekker; 1984;517–558.

57. Kerby GR, Mayer LS, Pingleton SK. Nocturnal positive pressure ventilation via nasal mask. Am Rev Respir Dis. 1987;135:738–740.

58. Segall D. Noninvasive nasal mask-assisted ventilation in respiratory failure of Duchenne muscular dystrophy. Chest. 1988;93:1298–1300.

59. Ellis ER, Grunstein RR, Chan S, et al. Noninvasive ventilatory support during sleep improves respiratory failure in kyphoscoliosis. Chest. 1988;94:811–815.

60. Rodenstein DO, Stanescu, DC, Delguste P, et al. Adaptation to intermittent positive pressure ventilation applied through the nose during day and night. Eur Respir J. 1989;2:473–478.

61. Bach JR, Alba AS, Shin D. Management alternatives for postpolio respiratory insufficiency: assisted ventilation by nasal or oral-nasal interface. Am J Phys Med Rehabil. 1989;68:264–271.

62. Heckmatt JZ, Loh L, Dubowitz V. Night-time nasal ventilation in neuromuscular disease. Lancet. 1990;335:579–581.

63. Barbe F, Quera-Salva MA, deLattre J, et al. Long-term effects of nasal intermittent positive pressure ventilation on pulmonary function and sleep architecture in patients with neuromuscular diseases. Chest. 1996;110:1179–1183.

64. Bonekat HW. Noninvasive ventilation in neuromuscular disease. Crit Care Clin. 1998;14:775–797.

65. Guilleminault C, Philip P, Robinson A. Sleep and neuromuscular disease: bilevel positive airway pressure by nasal mask as a treatment for sleep disordered breathing in patients with neuromuscular disease. J Neurol Neurosurg Psychiatry. 1998;65:225–232.

66. Clinical indications for noninvasive positive pressure ventilation in chronic respiratory failure due to restrictive lung disease, COPD, and nocturnal hypoventilation—a consensus conference report. Chest. 1999;116:521–534.

92

Sleep and Infectious Disease

Suzan E. Jaffe

Although for centuries it has been postulated that rest and sleep facilitate the recuperative process, scientific data supporting this hypothesis are limited. Infectious processes—mild or severe, acute or chronic, organ specific or generalized—are typically associated with fever and fatigue. Unlike fever, which is easily and objectively assessed, the sensation or complaint of "fatigue or sleepiness" is much more subjective and individual. Extensive research from animal models demonstrates that bacterial, viral, and fungal infections induce complex changes in sleep, but clinical data on human sleep during infectious disease are scarce and highly anecdotal. This is puzzling because the complaint of fatigue or daytime tiredness is second only to pain as the most commonly heard symptom by physicians throughout the Western World. Persons with any type of acute infectious process are rarely advised to undergo sleep evaluation and testing, despite complaints of sleep disturbance. More often, clinicians examine patients who present with sleep disturbances of a more persistent or chronic nature.

This chapter provides a review of the limited information available concerning the clinical and polysomnographic (PSG) features, including management recommendations, of central nervous system (CNS) infections and other non-CNS infective illnesses. HIV infection has risen at epidemic proportions. Sleep complaints are commonly associated with HIV infection and have precipitated interest in the study of sleep in this population. Due to the gravity of HIV infection, especially when it involves the nervous system, a detailed discussion of sleep research findings in this area is provided at the end of the chapter.

PATHOPHYSIOLOGY

Sixty-eight years ago, von Economo[1] reported viral-induced CNS lesions as evidence that the hypothalamus was involved in sleep regulation. It was not until the 1980s that sleep was actually recorded during the course of infection and that sleep pattern alterations were observed in human subjects.

Research studies in both animals and human beings have demonstrated that modulators of the immune response appear to be critical in the regulation of sleep stages, particularly slow-wave sleep (SWS; sleep stages 3 and 4).[2-6] The investigators concluded that immune system regulators in the brain, referred to as *cytokines*, are the key elements in the humoral regulation of the sleep response to infection and in the physiological regulation of sleep.

A variety of peptides and lipids with immunomodulating effects have been identified and shown to promote sleep in studies in animals; these include factor S, muramyl peptides (bacterial cell wall products [MPs]), interleukin-1 (IL-1), alpha-interferon, tumor necrosis factor, vasoactive intestinal peptide, prostaglandin D_2, and delta sleep–inducing peptide. Shoham et al.[7] found that MPs induced the synthesis and release of the immunologically active, inflammatory mediator IL-1 in the host. Chedid[8] suggested that MPs and IL-1 are immunopeptides and regulate T-cell activity. MPs are pyrogenic and have the capacity to enhance sleep. Even when the febrile response is blocked by antipyretic agents, an increased amount of SWS persists. This effect is thought to be mediated by IL-1.[3] In studies in animals, warming of the hypothalamus facilitates SWS production.[9] In human beings, the most effective technique of producing an increase in SWS is by increasing core body temperature.[10, 11] Mechanisms for such results include an increase in cerebral restitution or a build-up of some substance within the brain that promotes the production of SWS.[12]

Investigations in animals have explored the molecular mechanisms responsible for the propensity to sleep during infection primarily by challenging rabbits with either viral, fungal, bacterial, or protozoan pathogens. Rabbits show changes in sleep patterns, characterized by increases in SWS, followed by an inhibition of SWS. The extent of the observed effects is dependent on the specific microbe, the dose of the infectious substance, and the route of administration.[13-16] Rapid eye movement (REM), on the other hand, is observed to be inhibited during fungal and bacterial infections in animal models.[17]

In a clinical study, researchers documented preliminary findings suggesting that even the common cold (rhinovirus type 23) is associated with sleep disruption and possible reduced attentiveness. The symptomatic subjects demonstrated declining minutes of consolidated sleep (non–stage 1) on PSG compared with the control (asymptomatic) subjects. In addition, sleep efficiency significantly dropped in the symptomatic group of subjects. Despite a lack of change on multiple sleep latency test, mean reaction time on an auditory vigilance task was slowed in the symptomatic group, whereas it remained unchanged in the control subjects.

There also was a decline in the Profile of Mood States inventory for "vigor" in the symptomatic group, suggesting a possible decrease in daytime alertness.[18] With the exception of this preliminary work and data presented on HIV-infected people later in this chapter, PSG data on this population are virtually nonexistent.

In summary, (1) the increased need for sleep and the increased sleep disruption (i.e., increased wakefulness during sleep) that occur at different times during the course of an infectious process result from dynamic changes in specific cytokines during the host's response to infectious confrontations,[2-4, 13] (2) changes in sleep induced by infection seem to be of recuperative value of the host,[3, 7, 14] and (3) sleep deprivation is associated with changes in immune function.[10, 12, 15]

CENTRAL NERVOUS SYSTEM INFECTIONS AND CLINICAL FEATURES

Encephalitis

Encephalitis refers to a number of different infections of the CNS that cause tissue inflammation. Sleep disturbances are among the most common neurological symptoms in patients with acute or chronic encephalitis.[19] Such infections can be bacterial or viral in origin; examples include Guillain-Barré syndrome, herpes, measles, poliomyelitis, mumps, Reye's syndrome, influenza, aseptic meningitis, rabies, and mononucleosis. These infections are associated with a myriad of symptoms, but one of the most common is disordered sleep, either excessive daytime sleepiness (EDS) or insomnia. Unfortunately, due to the paucity of clinical research in this area, it is impossible to say for certain what actual mechanisms are responsible for such sleep disruption.

Polysomnographic Features. In a study by Guilleminault and Mondini,[20] 12 patients between the ages of 14 and 26 years were thought to have been infected with the Epstein-Barr virus. Ten had diagnosed infectious mononucleosis, and two had Guillain-Barré syndrome. Patients were evaluated 4.5 to 7 months after the onset of clinical symptoms. All subjects reported daytime sleepiness that was corroborated by PSG. Sleep studies consistently demonstrated prolonged nocturnal sleep times. When questioned at a 2-year follow-up evaluation, although no subject had other neurological sequelae, all reported disabling daytime drowsiness and napped regularly. These patients also reported long nocturnal sleep times. The authors concluded that encephalitis, perhaps involving the hypothalamus, caused this chronic disruption of sleep-wake patterns.[20]

Sleeping Sickness (African Trypanosomiasis)

This disease received its name because victims experienced severe sleepiness. This infection is rarely seen outside of Africa and is caused by a parasitic (protozoan) infection with *Trypanosoma*, which is transmitted by the tsetse fly. During the acute phase, patients are often febrile and manifest tender lymphadenopathy and severe headache. A ring-shaped erythema develops with painful subcutaneous swelling of the hands, feet, and periorbital tissues. The signs and symptoms reappear over months to years. Neuropathological examination of the brain reveals a diffuse inflammatory process involving the rostral midbrain, hypothalamus, and basal forebrain. The exact prevalence is unknown, but it is very common in endemic regions of tropical Africa.

African sleeping sickness is distinguished by the progressive involvement of the CNS, terminating with infection wherein there are extensive inflammatory changes with lymphoplasmocytic infiltration.[21] In the early stages of this disease, when the parasite penetrates the brain, causing acute inflammation, there is a concurrent meningoencephalitis with associated severe lethargy. During this phase of the illness, characteristically a vacant facial expression is observed, as are ptosis and sometimes a droopy lower lip. Spontaneous speech is often minimal, and patients become sedentary and listless. A myriad of associated symptoms may occur depending on the extent of nervous system involvement. Tremor of the hands and tongue, or choreiform movements, are sometimes observed. Frequently, patients have seizures, and there may be loss of sphincter control. Ophthalmoplegia is often present.[22, 23]

Meningitis, which can occur quite early in the course of infection, results in a collapse of the choroid plexus and movement of the parasite into certain localized brain areas, and encephalitis ensues. The encephalitis involves a chronic, rampant inflammation with perivascular infiltrations of B cells, plasma cells, inactivated T cells, and macrophages. Vasogenic edema occurs as the blood-brain barrier is damaged. Alterations (elevations) in the cytokine/mediator network are documented that may play a role in the observed hypersomnia.[24] These patients are often described as sleepy by day and restless by night. Such symptoms can last for months to several years before reaching the terminal stages.[21-23] If untreated, this disorder usually results in death. Death most often is due to status epilepticus, coma, hyperpyrexia, or secondary infection.

Polysomnographic Features. Even during waking electroencephalography (EEG), the PSG recording is usually characterized by alpha and theta rhythms of low amplitude, interrupted by bursts of high-amplitude delta waves. In the early stages of the disease, there is loss of all the transient properties of stage 1 and 2 nonrapid eye movement (NREM) sleep, including sleep spindles, K complexes, and vertex sharp waves. Eventually, all stages of NREM sleep become unrecognizable, and the EEG becomes homogeneous, with either diffuse high-amplitude slow waves or diffuse theta and lower-amplitude delta activity. Patients present with a disorganization of the circadian alternation of sleeping and waking during the early phase of this illness. The overall sleep cycle is distorted as well; stages 1 and 4 are often missing. These individuals often have very fragmented nocturnal sleep with resultant sleep-maintenance insomnia and severe daytime lethargy.[25] In the advanced state, the majority of patients demonstrate recurrent 3- to 7-sec duration epochs of lower-amplitude waves in the beta and alpha frequencies or, occasionally, theta activity, associated with brief episodes of tachycardia, alterations in breathing patterns, and increased muscle tone. Such events are thought to represent "microarousals."[24] Epileptiform discharges may be recorded during such episodes. Stage REM sleep persists, although it may partially intrude other sleep stages and also occur with sudden awakening. In fact, relatively normal REM sleep patterns are preserved until death.

In one case, reported by Buguet et al.,[26] a 24-hour PSG recording was performed on a patient with sleeping sickness who presented with an atypical neurological syndrome. *Trypanosoma gambiense* was found in a lymph gland puncture and the cerebrospinal fluid, and a serological immunofluorescence test was positive. REM sleep and wakefulness presented normal PSG characteristics. The patient had eight sleep periods during the 24-h recording; these sleep periods occurred during the daytime and at night, constituting the typical diurnal sleepiness and nocturnal fitfulness of sleeping sickness. On all occasions, REM latency was short, and two sleep-onset REM periods were observed. Wakefulness and REM sleep had a circadian rhythmicity, whereas NREM sleep, total sleep time, and deep sleep had an ultradian periodicity.[26] In most cases of African sleeping sickness, daytime drowsiness and listlessness eventually progress to stupor, and the EEG shows increasing slow waves accompanied by spike-and-wave complexes. The patient ultimately dies in a coma.

Fatal Familial Insomnia and Other Prion Diseases

A *prion* is a protein that can replicate itself and cause disease. Unlike a bacterial or viral agent that needs DNA or RNA to reproduce, prions can multiply and invade healthy cells, even though they do not carry genetic properties. They "pirate" the genetic material from the cells they invade, thus gaining the ability to reproduce. There are various types of prion diseases, including Gerstman-Straussler-Scheinker syndrome (GSS), fatal familial insomnia (FFI), Kuru disease, and Creutzfeldt-Jakob disease (CJD). Abnormal prion protein is deposited as amyloid structure in the brain of the patients with these diseases. Mutation of the prion protein gene exists in some of these diseases.[27] Sleep data on such individuals, however, are sparse.

Fatal Familial Insomnia

FFI was first described in 1986, and it remains a very rare autosomal dominant prion disease that leads to death within 7 to 32 months. With an age of onset of 35 to 60 years, the pathology of FFI has been shown to consist of a buildup of prion particles in the brains of affected individuals.[28] The most common symptom is progressive insomnia that quickly develops into a virtual total lack of sleep. As the insomnia worsens and the amount of sleep deteriorates, autonomic and somatomotor manifestations occur, accompanied by cognitive changes and stuporous episodes. Stuporous periods are often associated with semipurposeful automatic gestures mimicking dream content.[29] Vegetative symptoms can occur in correlation with the insomnia, such as hyperhidrosis, tachycardia, tachydyspnea, arterial hypertension, fever, salivation, constipation, urinary difficulties, and impotence.[30] Neurological somatomotor symptomatology is progressive and often present after a few months, including dysarthria, deep hyperreflexia, dystonic posturing, ataxia, and spontaneous and evoked myoclonus. Eventually, the stupor becomes persistent, and individuals die while in a comatose state.[31] In the terminal stages, extreme body wasting and adrenal insufficiency are reported. Bronchopulmonary infections are common.[32]

Pathophysiology. The specific location of the lesions causing this disease underscores the role of the thalamus in the regulation of the sleep-wake cycle. Pathological findings at autopsy have revealed severe atrophy, neuronal loss, and reactive gliosis of the anterior and dorsomedial nuclei of the thalamus. Other thalamic nuclei (centromedian, pulvinar, reticular, and others) were less profoundly affected. In the deep layers of the cerebral cortex, moderate gliosis was evident, specifically in the frontal and temporal areas. Unlike other prion diseases, spongiosis is not observed. The prion protein PrPsc is detected in the brain, and there is a pathogenic mutation at codon 178 of the gene encoding this protein, coupled with methionine at codon 129.[33–35]

Polysomnographic Features. The prominent background rhythm of the EEG in FFI is an alpha rhythm. In the few recordings available, the alpha rhythm was observed to become progressively slower and more diffuse. Characteristic features of SWS are absent throughout the course of illness. In later stages of the disease, recordings have shown periodic spike complexes at intervals of 1 to 2 sec, despite normal visual, acoustic, and somatosensory-evoked potentials. A diminished or absent sympathetic skin response has also been observed. In follow-up recordings, these patients have demonstrated virtually only a few minutes of physiological sleep, if any. Benzodiazepines and barbituates, when administered, were observed to activate the characteristic electrical patterns of pharmacologically induced sleep.

In one study, a 53-year-old patient underwent a 52-day recording (by wrist actigraphy) and detailed PSG. During the course of illness, periods of abrupt unconsciousness and dream-like states were observed. Repeated PSGs showed slow background EEG activity (7 to 8 Hz) and the complete absence of any sleep pattern. During the days before the patient's death, the EEG demonstrated progressively slower EEG background with periodic sharp waves, a complete disappearance of any 24-h rest-activity rhythm, and the loss of circadian rhythms. Weight loss, endocrine and autonomic changes, and the complete loss of SWS (preceding death) were similar to that clinically observed in sleep-deprived rats.[36]

Autonomic and Endocrine Function in Fatal Familial Insomnia. Parasympathetic tests have been found to be normal, yet studies of cardiovascular function have demonstrated heightened baseline and increased evoked sympathetic activities. Frequently elevated heart rates, respiratory rates, body temperature, and systemic arterial pressure have been recorded with diminished circadian oscillations.

Elevations in serum and urinary catecholamine and cortisol levels have also been documented. Reduced circadian fluctuations were observed in levels of growth hormone, prolactin, follicle-stimulating hormone, luteinizing hormone, corticotropin, and cortisol. Melatonin secretion did not display the usual increase during darkness.

Neuropsychological and Neuroradiological Findings. On repeated neuropsychological tests, patients exhibit mainly frontal lobe disturbances, such as problems with attention and memory. Such testing is impeded by the patients' decreasing vigilance, as their levels of alertness wane. Cognitive function appears preserved until impaired consciousness makes testing futile.

Computed tomography scans and magnetic resonance imaging of the brain have been reported as normal. In three cases, positron emission tomography scans demonstrated glucose hypometabolism in the thalamus and putamen.[30–32, 35]

Kuru Disease

Kuru disease is a transmissible, rapidly progressive, and neurologically fatal disease found in the Fore tribe of New Guinea. The disease affects mostly adult women and children of either gender. The cause is probably a slow-acting virus transmitted via cannibalism. Although sleep-wake disturbances are reported, PSG data have not been recorded.

Creutzfeldt-Jakob Disease

CJD is classified as either sporadic or familial. It is a prion-related subacute encephalopathy that manifests extensive neuronal degeneration and spongiform pathological changes, especially in the neocortex. It is a fatal disease that casts an unyielding fog across the brain. Classic CJD presents as a rapidly progressive dementia with myoclonus, and it is usually associated with the presence of pseudoperiodic sharp-wave complexes on EEG. EEG patterns are dramatically altered during both sleep and wakefulness. During the initial phase of disease, the normal sleep architecture (alternating NREM-REM periods) is maintained, but this sleep organization is lost as disease becomes more profound.

In one serial PSG study, a series of eight 24-h PSG recordings were performed during the last 3 months of the life of a 68-year-old woman. The PSG findings included (1) sustained sequences of slow sharp waves or diphasic slow waves recurring at 0.5- to 1.5-sec intervals, (2) discontinuous pseudoperiodic discharges, and (3) NREM sleep–like pattern, with dominant 0.5- to 4-Hz activities.[37]

Clinically, CJD is associated with a rapid mental and physical decline to akinetic mutism and death, often occurring within 3 to 4 months. Cerebellar ataxia, extrapyramidal features, cortical blindness, and pyramidal signs are also commonly observed.[38]

Gerstmann-Straussler-Scheinker Disease

The most common mutation carrying GSS is associated with the proline-to-leucine point mutation of codon 102 of the prion protein gene. GSS is a very rare disease, typically characterized by ataxia and progressive dementia. PSG data have not been recorded for persons infected with this disease, even though sleep disturbances have been described.

SLEEP IN HIV INFECTION

Ever since HIV was identified as the causal agent for AIDS, complaints of fatigue and sleep disturbance have been reported throughout the literature. These sleep-related symptoms have been recognized as key clinical features of HIV-infected persons.[39, 40] It has been well documented that during the clinical latency phase of HIV infection, the CNS may be infected and begin to manifest subtle dysfunction.[41] Soon after infection with HIV, the level of virus in the body becomes high and most patients feel like they have the flu (e.g., fever, swollen lymph nodes, and sleep disturbances). Neurobehavioral and pathological data indicate that the CNS becomes infected with HIV soon after the virus enters the body. In HIV infection, the effects of cytokines on the sleep center may be present regardless of whether the HIV has actually infiltrated the brain.

Pathophysiology of Sleep Disturbances Associated With HIV Infection

Studies have documented an increase in specific peptides in the blood of HIV-infected persons.[42] It has been suggested that the somnogenic immune peptide tumor necrosis factor and IL-1β may be influential in the sleep changes and fatigue experienced by HIV-infected individuals. It is postulated that the altered somnogenic cytokines are involved in the excessive desire to sleep that is associated with infections, especially in patients with active infection. It seems plausible that this mechanism could contribute to the observed sleep disturbances in the HIV-infected population.

Investigations in Animals

The mobilization of specific and nonspecific immunological pathways has repeatedly shown disruption of the regulation mechanisms of sleep and wakefulness. Darko described sleep disturbances in cats infected with the feline immunodeficiency virus. These changes are reportedly similar to those of human beings infected with HIV. Increases in the total number of minutes spent in SWS, a shift of SWS to the latter sleep periods, increased arousals, and increased time awake during the sleep periods were observed.[42]

Clinical Features of HIV Infection

The first investigation of sleep in HIV-infected persons was performed in a small cohort of homosexual men in 1986. These early studies demonstrated prominent changes in sleep architecture and persistent sleep complaints in asymptomatic and symptomatic HIV-infected men. The sleep architecture differed between the HIV-infected men and HIV-negative control subjects, specifically in that the HIV-infected subjects demonstrated increased wakefulness and an increase in the total number of minutes of SWS. SWS and REM sleep were also observed to be more evenly dispersed throughout the night than normally expected. In particular, SWS was prevalent during the second half of recorded sleep.[43] The high incidence of sleep disturbances in HIV-infected men and observed changes in the NREM-REM cycle could not be accounted for on the basis of anxiety or depression.[44-46] These preliminary studies have since been corroborated by others.[47-49] One such study reported that fatigue and sleep disturbances contributed significantly to morbidity and disability in HIV-infected men, especially those in the later stages of disease. The most striking finding of this study demonstrated that HIV-infected patients had a significant interference in their driving ability due to sleepiness compared with control subjects.[50]

In a retrospective analysis of data collected since 1986, 111 polysomnograms were completed on 51 HIV-infected men at different stages of disease progression. Of these, 12 had died, 28 were lost to follow-up, and 11 remained in contact with the investigators. Repeat PSG was performed on two subjects. Subjective data on the entire group were collected through both written questionnaires and telephone interviews. Immunological parameters (CD4$^+$ absolute cell count) were also obtained. Eight subjects were taking antiretroviral and/or antibacterial agents, and four were hospitalized for HIV-related illnesses within the past year. This study demonstrated that as early as 3 years after HIV infection occurs, there is a significant difference in the following sleep parameters: (1) total SWS is increased in long-term survivors, (2) sleep is more efficient in the long-term survivors, with fewer arousals, (3) long-term survivors demonstrate a longer total sleep time, and (4) sleep complaints were significantly less frequent in the survivors, even as far back as baseline testing.[53] Figure 92–1 shows representative histograms depicting sleep architecture as the disease progresses compared with a normal HIV-seronegative subject.[52]

Repeated studies concluded that daytime fatigue and poor sleep quality may be an early indication of a declining immune system. As time passes, a declining immune system (as measured by decreasing CD4$^+$ counts and opportunistic infections) is associated with an increase in sleep complaints and daytime fatigue (Table 92–1). Perhaps the insomnia and fatigue experienced by HIV-infected persons are influenced by fluctuations in levels of specific cytokines. The persistent finding of increased SWS in long-term survivors may be related to an increase in somnogenic cytokines, demonstrating an enhanced ability to fight the HIV infection. The decrease in SWS as disease progresses may reflect an immune system that is failing. Similar disturbances of sleep may occur in HIV-infected children.[52a]

In summary, clinical studies on HIV-infected persons at different stages of disease progression have shown the following:

1. Early HIV infection is associated with an increase in total SWS.
2. The progressive deterioration of immunological function, secondary to advancing disease (as measured by CD4$^+$ counts and the incidence of opportunistic infections), is associated with a progressive decline in the quantitative amount of SWS across the night.
3. Reports of mild daytime fatigue and difficulty

Table 92-1. SLEEP COMPLAINTS AND POLYSOMNOGRAPHIC FINDINGS IN HIV INFECTION

Stage of Infection	Subjective Complaints	Polysomnographic Findings
Early infection; asymptomatic (CD4$^+$ > 400)	Difficulty initiating and maintaining sleep (mild) Daytime fatigue (mild and intermittent)	Increased total SWS SWS during terminal sleep cycles Alteration of NREM-REM cycles Frequent alpha-NREM anomaly
Some clinical symptoms (CD4$^+$ > 200)	Increased difficulty maintaining sleep Daytime fatigue (moderate) Trouble concentrating Mild memory disturbances	Decrease in total SWS Decrease in sleep efficiency Increased arousals Increasingly disorganized NREM-REM cycles
Terminal stages (CD4$^+$ < 200)	Very poor sleep quality Increased fatigue and periods of lethargy Severe difficulty maintaining sleep	Diminished or absent SWS Very poor sleep efficiency Complete absence of recognizable NREM-REM cycles Spontaneous arousals from all sleep stages

SWS, slow-wave sleep.

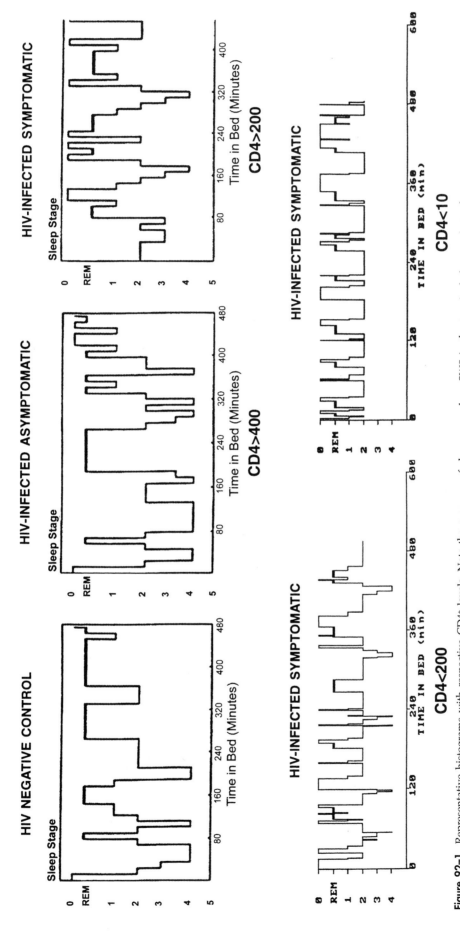

Figure 92–1. Representative histograms with respective CD4+ levels. Note the presence of slow-wave sleep SWS in the terminal sleep cycle in the asymptomatic subject as well as the increased amount of total SWS. As CD4+ levels fall and HIV disease progresses, observe decreasing SWS and alterations in sleep architecture. Observe the increased arousals in subjects with CD4+ levels below 400. The last histogram shows a striking absence of SWS as CD4+ level falls below 10. (Data from Jaffe Norman SE, Chediak AD. Long term follow up of sleep and immune function in 11 HIV-infected men. Sleep Res. 1996;25:433; Norman SE. Sleep disturbances associated with HIV infection. In: Smirne S, Franceschi M, Ferini-Strambi L, et al, eds. Sleep, Hormones and Immunological System. Milano, Italy: Masson SpA; 1992:45–57; Norman SE, Chediak AD, Freeman C, et al. Sleep disturbances in men with asymptomatic HIV infection. Sleep. 1992; 15:150–155; and Rothenberg S, Zozula R, Funesti J, et al. Sleep habits in asymptomatic HIV-seropositive individuals. Sleep Res. 1990;19:342.)

initiating sleep occur in the majority of HIV-infected individuals before an obvious decline in clinical status.

4. Repeated analyses reveal that CD4$^+$ levels inversely correlate with the frequency of sleep-onset problems in subjects complaining of current sleep disturbances.[53–55]

5. The cyclic pattern of sleep is destroyed in patients with end-stage AIDS, and the ability to organize the cortical neuronal system to a protective sleep state appears lost, perhaps due to neural microstructure destruction.[56]

6. Frequent sleep complaints (specifically, severe difficulty maintaining sleep and daytime fatigue) are common during the terminal stages of the disease.

7. Findings from a retrospective analysis support and strengthen preliminary reports that PSG aberrations and subjective sleep complaints occur early in the course of HIV infection, well before any clinical manifestations of HIV-related disease (Table 92–2).

NON–CENTRAL NERVOUS SYSTEM INFECTIONS AND CLINICAL FEATURES

Non-CNS infections that exhibit fatigue/tiredness often or usually include classic infectious mononucleosis, Lyme disease, tuberculosis, cat-scratch disease, interstitial cystitis, sinusitis, hepatitis B and C, influenza, cyclospora, human brucellosis, and cytomegalovirus mononucleosis. In hepatitis, cyclospora, mononucleosis (classic), influenza, and Lyme disease, the sleepiness typically persists after treatment is completed.

Classic Infectious Mononucleosis

Caused by a double-stranded DNA virus of the herpesvirus group called Epstein-Barr virus, infectious mononucleosis is an acute and generally benign disease. Clinically, it is most often observed in teenagers (typically at age 15 to 25 years) and presents with fever, sore throat, and swollen lymph glands. Sometimes, a rash is noted on the trunk and extremities at the onset of the illness, as well as splenomegaly. During the prodromal period of classic infectious mononucleosis, which lasts 7 to 14 days, an individual experiences fatigue, generalized malaise, headache, and myalgias. In some cases, individuals develop chronic tiredness despite the absence of neurological complications. Such patients crave longer nocturnal sleep periods and despite longer sleep periods complain of persistent daytime fatigue. Although naps may help relieve daytime symptoms during the early phases of recovery, in the chronic stages, the tiredness persists, and naps, despite their length (lasting 1 to 2 h), are nonrefreshing.

Epstein-Barr virus infection in adults can be severe, with debilitating fever, malaise, and fatigue (pharyngitis, cervical adenopathy, and splenomegaly are minimal). The symptom of excessive sleepiness has not been found to be associated with snoring, sleep apnea, or other primary sleep disorders. Classic infectious mononucleosis is also associated with night sweats and a restless nighttime sleep.[57]

The limited number of multiple sleep latency tests performed on these patients have corroborated these subjective complaints with mean sleep latency scores ranging from 1 to 8 min.[58] Chronic fatigue syndrome is not discussed in this section; this lifelong debilitating disorder is discussed in Chapter 87.

Other Non–Central Nervous System Infections

Cyclospora is a disease caused by a human parasite, and it often first presents with symptoms of profound fatigue. Other symptoms are gastrointestinal, including watery diarrhea, abdominal pain, nausea and vomiting, and anorexia and weight loss. The symptom of fatigue or anorexia may persist for weeks after the gastrointestinal symptoms have subsided.[59]

Human brucellosis is a disease of animals that is transmissible to human beings (zoonosis). It has continued to be a problem in countries in which brucellosis in domestic animals is not controlled.[60] Subclinical to chronic disease states exist with an incubation period lasting weeks to months. There are very few early physical findings; subsequently, persons are often considered to have "psychosomatic" complaints.[61] As the disease progresses, patients have multiple nonspecific complaints, with lethargy and fatigue being markedly pronounced along with body aches, fever, night sweats, anorexia, and depression.

Lyme disease is a systemic, tick-borne spirochetal disease characterized by skin lesions, accompanied by wide range of clinical characteristics, including fatigue, headache, stiff neck, chills, arthralgia, abdominal pain, and nausea and vomiting.[61] Because these individuals often present with such nonspecific complaints of "fatigue" or "tiredness," testing for Lyme disease is commonly performed.[62]

The most frequent finding in *cytomegalovirus mononucleosis* is fever, usually accompanied by profound fatigue and malaise.[63]

Table 92–2. SUBJECTIVE SLEEP DISTURBANCES AND CD4$^+$ DATA

Sleep-Wake Parameter	No. of Subjects (% of Total)
Increase in awakenings	7 (64)
Daytime sleepiness and/or naps	7 (64)
Insomnia	5 (45)
Sedatives and/or tranquilizers	3 (27)
CD4$^+$ < 200	3 (27)

$n = 11$.
Follow-up at mean of 81.3 months.[51]
Data from retrospective analysis by S. E. Jaffe, December 1997, unpublished.

MANAGEMENT

Stimulants and Excessive Daytime Sleepiness

The only medications that may help symptoms of acute or persistent fatigue and EDS probably are stimulants. There is, unfortunately, no controlled follow-up of such cases. Amphetamines in general have been shown to elevate mood, increase effort, prevent fatigue, increase vigilance, stimulate respiration, and cause electrical and behavioral arousal from natural or drug-induced sleep. The specific mechanism of action by which stimulants enhance wakefulness is not known. These effects are thought to be caused by both brainstem reticular activating system and cortical stimulation.[64] It has been documented by PSG that stimulants, such as the amphetamines and methylphenidate, decrease sleepiness, increase sleep latency, increase REM sleep latency, and reduce the proportion of REM sleep. Nocturnal sleep disturbance also is commonly observed.

Anecdotally, it is reported that methylphenidate is useful in the treatment of drowsiness associated with chronic hepatic disease, specifically hepatitis B. In severe cases of infectious mononucleosis, the sleepiness has been reported to respond poorly to stimulant drugs, resulting in persistent disability.[58] In a study of the efficacy of modafinil in the treatment of diurnal sleepiness, a group of 123 subjects were administered the test drug. Even though the majority of subjects were diagnosed with narcolepsy, 23 carried the diagnosis of "hypersomnia; 6 with disrupted nocturnal sleep"—the causes of these diagnoses were not delineated. Overall, 80% of the subjects reported a "good or excellent" response to their daytime symptoms of EDS.[65] This suggests that a trial of modafinil might be effective when symptoms of fatigue persist after the patient has fully recovered from the infection process.

Treatment recommendations for sleep disturbances in infections are primarily geared toward symptomatic relief. First and foremost, the cause of the infection must be determined and treated aggressively, if treatable. Unfortunately, as described here, many of these infections are serious and few, if any, treatment interventions have been examined systematically in controlled studies.

In general, if the infected person survives, the sleep disturbances should abate spontaneously as the patient recovers from the acute illness. In more chronic conditions, such as HIV infection, hepatitis, and chronic Epstein-Barr virus infection, the sleep disturbances can wax and wane, typically becoming worse if the patient's physical condition declines. In fatal diseases, such as FFI, CJD, Kuru disease, and GSS, it is unlikely that any specific treatment will improve sleep. Traditional sedative-hypnotics, such as benzodiazepines and barbiturates, have been shown to be ineffective in treating FFI. Atropine, hydroxytryptophan, and carbidopa have been shown to markedly worsen the symptoms of FFI.

Persons with HIV infection who have used sedative, antidepressant, or antianxiolytic medications have reported mild to moderate improvement in their sleep, in both initiating sleep and maintaining sleep. When HIV-infected patients have been treated aggressively for depressive syndromes, an improvement in their cognitive functioning has been reported.[66] Unfortunately, these study subjects were not screened for sleep disturbances, and hence the effects of stimulants specifically related to changes in sleep were not reported. Zidovudine (AZT) therapy in the treatment of AIDS has also been thought to aggravate insomnia in many individuals.

It has been well documented that sleep hygiene improves sleep quality and decreases daytime symptoms of fatigue in otherwise healthy individuals. Because sleep is recognized as a restorative process, it is reasonable to suggest that improved sleep quality, or even increased sleep time, may help, even if only symptomatically, those with certain infectious diseases. Improved sleep may increase opportunities for recovery, especially in those immunocompromised by HIV or other infectious agents. Behavioral interventions and good sleep hygiene techniques should therefore be discussed with appropriate patients. It is unlikely these techniques would worsen sleep, but to date there is no conclusive evidence to support that such treatment will actually improve sleep quality or survival.

In general, for complaints of insomnia, the intermittent use of prescription hypnotics, antidepressants, or tranquilizers may be necessary, but the chronic use of such medications should be discouraged in most infections. These drugs are known to alter normal sleep architecture, decreasing the amount of REM sleep and possibly affecting SWS as well. The chronic use of sedating drugs, including antihistamines and alcohol, may also produce nocturnal respiratory depression and worsening sleep apnea (when present), further fragmenting sleep, as well, resulting in an increase in morning lethargy and overall daytime sluggishness. Such symptomatology could mask changes in a patient's mental status and decrease motor performance. There is no doubt that sleep should be carefully monitored during serious infection; the close monitoring of sleep during treatment clinical trials may assist in determining therapeutic success.

SUMMARY

Sleep disorders caused by infections involving the CNS are often life-threatening conditions, whereas non-CNS infections tend to be less critical. If sleep is affected as the result of the infectious process, it is often marked by poor sleep maintenance and daytime fatigue (mild to severe). Such sleep disturbances, if persistent, may seriously affect an individual's ability to remain employed, to take care of normal day-to-day obligations, to perform activities of daily living, and so on. In chronic nervous system infections, such as HIV infection, or in non-CNS infections, such as chronic Epstein-Barr infection, the sleep disturbances may last for years. Although preliminary research has suggested that improved sleep during early HIV infection may increase longevity, this research needs further validation. Because patients with infectious diseases are so rarely evaluated by sleep specialists, an understanding of these processes is still limited. Future research is indicated to determine what, if any, interventions will be beneficial and which may be detrimental to these individuals.

References

1. von Economo C. Sleep as a problem of localization. J Nerv Ment Dis. 1930;71:249–259.
2. Krueger JM, Obal F, Johanssen L, et al. Endogenous slow wave sleep substances: a review. In: Wacquier A, Dugovic C, Radulovacki M, eds. Slow Wave Sleep: Physical, Pathophysiological and Functional Aspects. New York, NY: Raven Press; 1989:75–89.
3. Moldofsky H, Lue FA, Eisen J, et al. The relationship of interleukin-1 and immune functions to sleep in humans. Psychosom Med. 1986;48:309–318.
4. Krueger JM, Kubillus S, Shoham S, et al. Enhancement of slow-wave sleep by endotoxin and lipid A. Am J Physiol. 1986:R591–R597.
5. Dinarello CA, Krueger JM. Introduction of interleukin-1 by synthetic and naturally occurring muramyl peptides. FASEB J. 1986;45:2545–2548.
6. Shoham S, Davenne D, Krueger JM. Muramyl dipeptide, amphetamine and physostigmine: effects on sleep of rabbits. Physiol Behav. 1987;41:179–185.
7. Shoham S, Ahokas RA, Blatteis CM, et al. Effects of muramyl dipeptide on sleep, body temperature and plasma copper after intracerebral ventricular administration. Brain Res. 1987;419:223–228.
8. Chedid L. Synthetic muramyl peptides: their origin, present status and future prospects. FASEB J. 1986;45:2531–2533.
9. Berger R, Palca JW, Walker JM, et al. Relations between body temperatures, metabolic rate and slow wave sleep in men. Sleep Res. 1986;15:42.
10. Shapiro CM, Bortz R, Mitchell D. Slow wave sleep: a recovery period after exercise. Science. 1981;214:1253–1254.
11. Horne JA. Functional aspects of human slow wave sleep (HSWS). In: Wacquier A, Dugovic C, Radulovacki M, eds: Slow Wave Sleep: Physical, Pathophysiological and Functional Aspects. New York, NY: Raven Press; 1989:109–111.
12. Walter J, Davenne D, Shoham S, et al. Brain temperature changes coupled to sleep states persist during interleukin-1 enhanced sleep. Am J Physiol. 1986;250:R96–R103.
13. Krueger JM, Takahashi S, Kapas L, et al. Cytokines in sleep regulation. Adv Neuroimmunol. 1995;5:171–188.
14. Krueger JM, Toth LA. Cytokines as regulators of sleep. Ann N Y Acad Sci. 1994;739: 299–310.
15. Krueger JM. Somnogenic activity of immune response modifiers. TIPS. 1990;11:122–126.
16. Krueger JM, Kubillus S, Shoham S, Davenne D. Enhancement of slow wave sleep by endotoxin and lipid A. Am J Physiol. 1996;R591–R597.
17. Krueger JM, Obal F Jr. Sleep factors. In: Saunders NA, Sullivan CE, eds. Sleep and Breathing. 2nd ed. New York, NY: Marcel Dekker; 1994:79–112.
18. Benham H, Roehrs T, Koshorek G, Fortier J, et al. Effects of rhinovirus type 23 on sleep and daytime function [abstract]. Sleep. 1998;21(suppl):176.
19. Booss J, Esiri MM. Viral encephalitis: pathology, diagnosis and management. Boston, Mass: Blackwell Scientific; 1986.
20. Guilleminault C, Mondini S. Mononucleosis and chronic daytime sleepiness. Arch Intern Med. 1986;146:1333–1335.
21. Philip KA, Dascombe MJ, Fraser PA, et al. Blood brain barrier damage in experimental African trypanosomiasis. Ann Trop Med Parasitol. 1994;88:606–616.
22. Mulligan HW, ed. The African Trypanosomiasis. London, England: Allen & Irvin; 1970.
23. Schwartz BA, Escande C. Sleeping sickness: sleep study of a case. Electroencephalogr Clin Neurophysiol. 1970;3:83–87.
24. Pentreath VW, Baugh PJ, Lavin DR. Sleeping sickness and the central nervous system. Onderstepoort J Vet Res. 1994;61:369–377.
25. Jones B. Sleeping sickness. In: Carskadon MA, ed. Encyclopedia of Sleep and Dreaming. New York, NY: MacMillan; 1993:504.
26. Buguet A, Gati R, Sevre JP, et al. 24 hour polysomnographic evaluation in a patient with sleeping sickness. Electroencephalogr Clin Neurophysiol. 1989;72:471–478.
27. Udaka F, Fujisawa M, Kameyama M. Creutzfeldt-Jakob disease (CJD) and Gerstmann-Straussler-Scheinker syndrome. Nippon Rinsho. 1997;55:972–977.
28. Lugaresi E, Medori R, Montagna P, et al. Fatal familial insomnia and dysautonomia with selective degeneration of thalamic nuclei. N Engl J Med. 1986;315:997–1003.
29. Seilhean D, Duyckaerts C, Hauw JJ. Fatal familial insomnia and prion diseases. Rev Neurol. 1995;151:225–230.
30. Lugaresi E, Baruzzi A, Cacciari E, et al. Lack of vegetative and endocrine circadian rhythms in fatal familial thalamic degeneration. Clin Endocrinol. 1987;26:573–580.
31. Cortelli P, Parchi P, Contin M, et al. Cardiovascular dysautonomia in fatal familial insomnia. Clin Autonom Res. 1991;1:15–21.
32. Medori R, Gambetti PL, Montagna P, et al. Familial progressive insomnia, impairment of the autonomic functions, degeneration of the thalamic nuclei: a new disease? [abstract]. Neurology (NY). 1985;1(suppl 35):145.
33. McLean CA, Storey E, Gardner RJ, et al. The D178N "fatal familial insomnia" mutation associated with diverse clinicopathologic phenotypes in an Australian kindred. Neurology. 1997;49:552–558.
34. Medori R, Tritscher J, LeBlanc AA, et al. Fatal familial insomnia, a prion disease with a mutation at codon 178 of the prion protein gene. N Engl J Med. 1992;326:444–449.
35. Lugaresi E. Thalamus and sleep. Neurology. 1992;42(suppl 6):28–33.
36. Plazzi G, Schutz Y, Cortelli P, et al. Motor overactivity and loss of motor circadian rhythm in fatal familial insomnia: an actigraphic study. Sleep. 1997;20:739–742.
37. Terzano MG, Parrino L, Pietrini V, et al. Precocious loss of physiological sleep in a case of Creutzfeldt Jakob disease: a serial polygraphic study. Sleep. 1995;18:849–858.
38. Roos RP. Prion diseases. In: Baker HF, Ridley RM, eds. Methods on Molecular Medicine. Totowa, NJ: Humana Press; 1996:317.
39. Wilson IB, Cleary PD. Clinical predictors of functioning in persons with acquired immunodeficiency syndrome. Med Care. 1996;34:610–623.
40. Walker K, McGown A, Jantos M, et al. Fatigue, depression, and quality of life in HIV-positive men. J Psychosoc Nurs Ment Health Serv. 1997;35:32–40.
41. Resnick L, Berger JR, Shapshak P, et al. Early penetration of the blood brain barrier by HIV. Neurology. 1988;38:9–14.
42. Darko DF, Mitler MM, Propero-Garcia O, et al. Sleep and lentivirus infection: parallel observations obtained from human and animal studies. SRS Bull. 1996;2:43–51.
43. Norman SE, Resnick L, Cohn MA, et al. Sleep disturbances in HIV-seropositive patients. Letter. JAMA. 1988;26:922.
44. Norman SE, Chediak AD, Kiel M, et al. Sleep disturbances in HIV infected homosexual men. AIDS. 1996;4:775–781.
45. Perkins DO, Leserman J, Stern RA, et al. Somatic symptoms and HIV infection: relationship to depressive symptoms and indicators of HIV disease. Am J Psychiatry. 1995;152:1776–1781.
46. Brown S, Atkinson H, Malone J, et al. Relating subjective sleep complaints, immune status and psychological state in HIV. Paper presented at: VI International Conference on AIDS, June 1990, San Diego.
47. O'Dell MW, Meighen M, Riggs RV. Correlates of fatigue in HIV infection prior to AIDS: a pilot study. Disabil Rehabil. 1996; 18:249–254.
48. Cohen FL, Ferrans CE, Vizgirda V, et al. Sleep in men and women infected with human immunodeficiency virus (HIV) infection. Holist Nurs Pract. 1996; 10:33–43.
49. Fukunishi I, Hayashi M, Matsumoto T, et al. Liaison psychiatry and HIV infection, I: avoidance coping responses associated with depressive symptoms accompanying somatic complaints. Psychiatry Clin Neurosci. 1997;51:1–4.
50. Darko DF, McCutchan JA, Kripke DF, et al. Fatigue, sleep distur-

bances, disability and indices of progression of HIV infection. Am J Psychiatry. 1992;149:514–520.

51. Jaffe Norman SE, Chediak AD. Long term follow up of sleep and immune function in 11 HIV-infected men. Sleep Res. 1996;25:433.

52. Norman SE. Sleep disturbances associated with HIV infection. In: Smirne S, Franceschi M, Ferini-Strambi L, et al, eds. Sleep, Hormones and Immunological System. Milano, Italy: Masson SpA; 1992:45–57.

52a. Franck LS, Johnson LM, Lee K, et al. Sleep disturbances in children with human immunodeficiency virus infection. Pediatrics. 1999;104:e62.

53. Norman SE, Chediak AD, Freeman C, et al. Sleep disturbances in men with asymptomatic HIV infection. Sleep. 1992;15:150–155.

54. Rothenberg S, Zozula R, Funesti J, et al. Sleep habits in asymptomatic HIV-seropositive individuals. Sleep Res. 1990;19:342.

55. Darko D, McCutchan J, Kripke D, et al. Fatigue, sleep disturbances, disability and indices of progression of HIV infection. Am J Psychiatry. 1992;149:514–520.

56. St. Kubicki H, Henkes H, Terstegge K, et al. AIDS related sleep disturbances: a preliminary report. In: St. Kubicki H, Henkes H, Bienzle H, et al, eds. HIV and Nervous System. Stuttgart, Germany: Gustav Fischer; 1988:97–105.

57. Magnussen CR, Chessin LN, Dolin R. Infectious mononucleosis and mono-like syndromes. In: Reese RE, Betts RF, eds. A Practical Approach to Infectious Diseases. 3rd ed. Boston, Mass: Little, Brown & Co; 1991:499–503.

58. Guilleminault C. Mononucleosis. In: Carskadon MA, ed. Encyclopedia of Sleep and Dreaming. New York, NY: MacMillan; 1993:381.

59. Taylor AP, Davis LJ, Soave R. Cyclospora. In: Remington JS, Swarts MN, eds. Current Clinical Topics in Infectious Diseases. Boston, Mass: Blackwell Science; 1997:256–268.

60. Young EJ. Human brucellosis. In: Kass EH, Platt R, eds. Current Therapy in Infectious Disease–2. Toronto, Ontario, Canada: BCDecker; 1986:369–371.

61. Markowitz LE, Steere AC. Lyme disease. In: Kass EH, Platt R, eds. Current Therapy in Infectious Disease–2. Toronto, Ontario, Canada: BCDecker; 1986:373–375.

62. Lightfoot RW Jr, Luft BJ, Rahn DW, et al. Empiric parental antibiotic treatment of patients with fibromyalgia and fatigue and a positive serologic result for Lyme disease: a cost effective analysis. Ann Intern Med. 1993;119:503–509.

63. Cheeseman SH. Cytomegalovirus infections. In: Gorbach SL, Bartlett JG, Blacklow NR, eds. Infectious Diseases. 2nd ed. Philadelphia, Pa: WB Saunders; 1998:1655–1662.

64. Parkes D. Introduction to the mechanism of action of different treatments of narcolepsy. Sleep. 1994;17:S93–S96.

65. Laffont F, Mayer G, Minz M. Modafinil in diurnal sleepiness: a study of 123 patients. Sleep. 1994;17:S113–S115.

66. Masand PS, Tesar GE. Use of stimulants in the medically ill. Psychiatric Clin North Am. 1996;19:515–547.

93

Endocrine Disorders

Ronald Grunstein

There are many diverse associations between human endocrine function and sleep. Importantly, neuroendocrine and metabolic physiology is often influenced by behavioral states of sleep and wakefulness (see Chapter 20). Extensive research in this area has flourished due to the development of better assays of endocrine function, paralleling the growth of human sleep research stimulated by the availability of polysomnography. Endocrine rhythms have often been labeled either sleep-related (when the predominant change in fluctuation is nocturnal) or circadian (when the rhythm appears to be regulated by an internal clock rather than periodic changes in the external environment). The predominant influences are intrinsic circadian rhythmicity and sleep, which interact to varying degrees to produce the characteristic 24-h rhythm of each hormone. Conversely, aberrations of normal endocrine function may influence sleep or alter state-affected parameters such as breathing or the electroencephalogram (EEG). This chapter concentrates on these changes, limiting discussion to particular endocrine disorders in adults and children.

ACROMEGALY AND OTHER GROWTH HORMONE DISORDERS

Acromegaly is a condition of growth hormone (GH) excess in adults characterized by the insidious development of coarsening of facial features, bony proliferation, and soft tissue swelling.[1] It is usually secondary to a GH-producing pituitary adenoma, which may be either a micro- or macroadenoma. Rarely, the GH excess commences prior to puberty and closure of the epiphyses and then the condition is termed *gigantism*. It occurs with equal frequency in both sexes with a prevalence of 50 to 70 cases per million. The clinical features may be due to the local effects of an expanding pituitary mass in addition to the effects of excess GH secretion which include disordered somatic cell growth and insulin resistance. The mortality of untreated or partially treated acromegaly is about double the expected rate in healthy subjects matched for age.[2] Acromegaly was first described as a clinical entity by Marie in 1876. Ten years later, Roxburgh and Collis[3] described daytime sleepiness and Chappell and Booth[4] observed upper airway obstruction as features of acromegaly, but the association between sleep apnea and acromegaly was only described 90 years later.[5]

Prevalence of Sleep Apnea in Acromegaly

Sleep-disordered breathing is extremely common in acromegaly. We have previously estimated that 60% of our unselected patients with acromegaly have sleep apnea[6] (Fig. 93–1). Almost all of our patients were noted to have heavy snoring. In a Finnish study, using the static-charged bed respiratory screening device, 10 of 11 patients had sleep apnea (91%) compared with 29.4% of the general population.[7] In the only other large study of sleep apnea prevalence, Rosenow and co-workers[8] studied 54 patients with treated acromegaly from a larger sample of 100 patients. They excluded patients with previously known sleep apnea. Despite these exclusion criteria, 21 (39%) of these remaining 54 patients had sleep apnea. Treatment of acromegaly may also have reduced prevalence as well as the limited monitoring techniques used in the study. Sleep apnea was associated with increasing age and tended to be more common in males and in females over 50 years old. Obesity does not appear to be a predisposing factor to sleep apnea in acromegaly.[6–8] Increases in body mass index in acromegaly may be due to increased muscle mass rather than the increased body fat typically seen in obesity.[1]

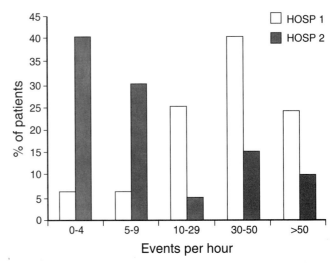

Figure 93–1. Prevalence of sleep apnea in acromegaly in two cohorts in Sydney, Australia. In hospital 1, which has a sleep laboratory, almost all patients with acromegaly have sleep apnea. In hospital 2, a regional endocrine center without sleep investigation facilities, 60% of patients have sleep apnea (defined by respiratory disturbance index > 5).

Etiology of Central and Obstructive Sleep Apnea in Acromegaly

The first reports of sleep apnea in acromegaly suggested that macroglossia was an important etiological factor in producing sleep apnea by narrowing the hypopharynx and collapsing backward in sleep.[9] However, endoscopy during apneic periods[10] revealed no posterior movement of the tongue, suggesting that macroglossia was not the primary factor in upper airway obstruction. In this report, primary pharyngeal collapse into the laryngeal vestibule was observed. Attempted treatment with a nasopharyngeal airway past the tongue did not prevent apnea. Pelttari et al.[7] observed no dynamic narrowing behind the tongue on nasopharyngoscopy. One study suggested that craniofacial changes explained why some people with acromegaly had obstructive sleep apnea (OSA) while others did not.[10a]

We have observed a high rate of central apnea in patients with acromegaly[6] (34% of the total group of patients with sleep apnea). Others,[11] using full sleep studies, reported that two of their three patients with sleep apnea and acromegaly had predominantly or exclusively central apnea. A waxing-and-waning central apnea pattern of breathing on static charge–sensitive bed studies has also been reported as more common in acromegaly as opposed to typical upper airway obstruction.[7]

The high prevalence of central apnea in acromegaly suggests that abnormalities of central respiratory control are involved. This has been supported by our finding that patients with central sleep apnea had significantly lower awake arterial carbon dioxide levels than those with obstructive apnea[6,12] and increased ventilatory responsiveness was observed in the central group[12] (Fig. 93–2). Central apnea occurs in association

with a wide range of disorders and many potential mechanisms have been described, including disordered central respiratory control.[12] The precise cause in acromegaly is unclear, but there are a number of hypotheses, including alterations in central somatostatin pathways disinhibiting respiratory control.[12] Other mechanisms include an effect of GH on central respiratory control, either directly or by altering metabolic rate, inducing central apnea. This is supported by the correlation between GH hypersecretion and the prevalence of central apnea.[6, 12] Interestingly, apparent central apneas have been observed in beagles exposed to medroxyprogesterone, which in turn causes GH increases and an acromegaly-like condition.[12]

Disease Activity in Acromegaly and Sleep Apnea

In view of the morbidity and mortality of acromegaly, it is important to define active and inactive (cured) disease. High circulating insulin-like growth factor 1 (IGF-1) and GH levels reflect increased GH production and therefore disease activity. Studies describing "cure" following pituitary surgery often use inadequate criteria of disease inactivity.[1] True cure involves observing a physiological 24-h GH secretion, normal IGF-1 levels, and normal GH responses to glucose. Even in patients with acromegaly and normal IGF-1 and GH profiles, GH secretory patterns are still different from normals.

Most studies have observed persisting sleep apnea despite treatment of acromegaly by pituitary surgery. We have found no correlation between disease activity and sleep apnea severity.[6] There were no significant differences in mean GH and IGF-1 levels in patients with and without sleep apnea. In this study, 23 patients had detailed 24-h GH secretory profiles and 16 had sleep apnea (2 predominantly central and 14 predominantly obstructive). In this subgroup with more extensive GH measurements, no significant differences in mean GH and GH pulsatility were found between patients with and without sleep apnea. In contrast, Rosenow et al.[8] have reported lower GH levels in patients with milder sleep apnea. Studies using octreotide, a somatostatin analogue, have shown powerful GH reduction with a parallel decrease in apnea severity.[12] However, even in this study, there was no relationship between the decrease in apnea and the decrease in GH levels.[12]

At present, it is not known what proportion of patients with both sleep apnea and acromegaly will have complete resolution of their sleep apnea after cure of acromegaly. This will require careful prospective studies accurately monitoring true cure of acromegaly. However, it is clear that sleep apnea does occur in cured acromegaly. The combination of inactive acromegaly and sleep apnea may occur for a number of reasons. Firstly, sleep apnea is a common disorder and may be coincident to acromegaly in patients with other risk factors for sleep apnea. Secondly, it may take a long time following normalization of GH secretion for the effects of acromegaly to resolve or there may be

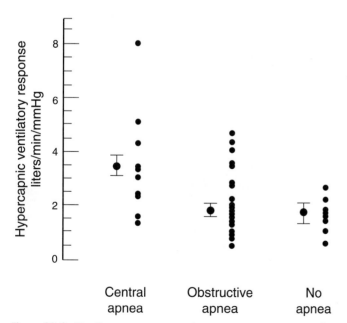

Figure 93–2. Ventilatory responses to hypercapnia in patients with acromegaly. Patients with predominantly central sleep apnea have increased ventilatory responses.

permanent effects on upper airway function or sleep-breathing regulation.

Although there appears to be no relationship between disease activity and severity of sleep apnea, patients with central sleep apnea have much higher IGF-1 and fasting GH levels compared with patients with obstructive apnea.[6, 12]

Morbidity and Mortality of Acromegaly and Sleep Apnea

The adverse health risks of both acromegaly and sleep apnea are well established. Both disorders are associated with an increased risk of hypertension.[1] In acromegaly, the blood pressure level is sometimes reduced by successful transsphenoidal surgery. One postulated mechanism for hypertension in acromegaly is sodium and water retention secondary to GH overproduction.[1]

We have found strong links between hypertension and sleep apnea in our patients with acromegaly, suggesting that sleep apnea may be another important mechanism causing hypertension.[6] Over 50% of our patients with both acromegaly and sleep apnea had hypertension. All patients who did not have sleep apnea were normotensive. Patients who were hypertensive had significantly higher respiratory disturbance indices and a greater degree of sleep hypoxemia than those who were normotensive. Mean 24-h GH and IGF-1 levels and the degree of obesity were not significantly different in those with hypertension compared with those without hypertension. Using multiple regression, both the respiratory disturbance index and age were found to be independent predictors of hypertension.[6]

Somnolence has long been recognized as part of the clinical spectrum of acromegaly. Although sleep apnea is the most likely cause, a direct effect of increased GH in promoting sleep and sleepiness has been suggested.[13] Alternatively, sleepiness in the absence of sleep apnea may be due to the effects of radiotherapy.[14] Wright et al.[2] reviewed the causes of death in patients with acromegaly at four London hospitals and found an excess of deaths due to cardiovascular and respiratory causes. They commented, "The excess of deaths due to respiratory disease was an unexpected finding for which there was no obvious explanation." This finding was inexplicable as there is no apparent excess of chronic lung disease in acromegaly. Lung function is usually normal or supernormal. With our new understanding of the high prevalence of sleep apnea in acromegaly, it is likely that this is the mechanism of the deaths attributed at that time to respiratory disease. Another potential link is sleep apnea and upper airway obstruction complicating anesthesia in these patients. One recent Swedish report of deaths in acromegaly found five postoperative deaths out of 62 total consecutive deaths in patients with acromegaly.[15]

Does Acromegaly Cause Nonrespiratory Sleep Disorders?

Early descriptions of sleepiness in patients with acromegaly suggested a link with narcolepsy.[16] However, subsequent data have clearly shown this not to be the case. Rather, the dominant sleep disorder caused by acromegaly is sleep apnea.

However, it has also been suggested that GH excess is associated with daytime sleepiness and reduced rapid eye movement (REM) sleep.[13] This study reported only subjective sleepiness and, again, limited airflow measurement did not allow full exclusion of upper airway obstruction. Pituitary adenectomy led to an increase in REM sleep, possibly related to suppression of GH secretion. Other possible causes of sleepiness in patients with acromegaly include cerebral irradiation[14] or even misdiagnosing the neuromuscular fatigue due to acromegalic myopathy as sleepiness.

Growth Hormone Deficiency

Adults with sleep apnea appear to have relative GH deficiency which is reversible by nasal continuous positive airway pressure (CPAP)[17, 18] (Fig. 93–3). This deficiency in untreated patients is likely related to abnormal sleep structure (see Chapter 20). In individuals with primary GH deficiency, a reduction in power in delta sleep has been observed.[19] There are little data on GH-inducing sleep apnea in hypopituitary patients. We have observed one case of a child with Turner's syndrome developing sleep apnea after GH administration (unpublished observation) and others have reported[20] four children developing sleep apnea (two obstructive, two mixed) after GH administration.

SEX HORMONE DISORDERS

Male Hormonal Disorders

Several case reports in the early 1980s described development of sleep apnea following testosterone therapy.[21–23] Others[24] reported the development of sleep apnea in a 54-year-old woman with renal failure following androgen administration. The sleep apnea re-

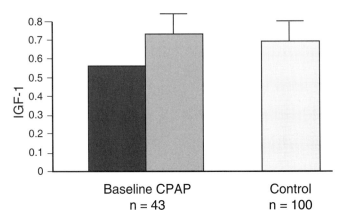

Figure 93–3. Insulin-like growth factor 1 (IGF-1) levels in sleep apnea in 43 men before (*black bar*) and 3 months after nasal continuous positive airway pressure (CPAP) therapy (*gray bar*). IGF-1 levels increase to similar levels observed in a control group of 100 hospital volunteers (mean age 40 years).

solved on withdrawal of the medication and recurred when the drug was reintroduced. These researchers also observed an increase in supraglottic resistance following androgen administration.[24] More recently, sleep apnea associated with an endogenous benign testosterone-producing ovarian tumor has been described.[25] The OSA resolved after tumor removal. These cases certainly suggest that testosterone may be important in the regulation of breathing during sleep and in the pathogenesis of sleep apnea. Testosterone also was reported to exacerbate sleep apnea in a 13-year-old boy, associated with an increase in upper airway collapsibility during sleep.[26]

Two studies have systematically examined the sleep-breathing effects of exogenous testosterone on hypogonadal patients. Matsumoto et al.[27] studied five patients and observed development of sleep apnea in one patient and worsening of preexisting sleep apnea in another. There was no effect in the other three patients. Schneider and co-workers[28] investigated 11 hypogonadal men before and after testosterone replacement. There was a significant increase in apneas in the group as a whole, but clinically significant increases occurred in only three patients. The two studies show that testosterone-induced or -exacerbated sleep apnea is not a consistent finding in hypogonadal patients. The clinical message from these studies is that patients commencing on androgen replacement should be questioned closely for sleep apnea symptomatology and monitored during the course of their therapy to check if such symptoms develop. The possibility of more extensive use of testosterone therapy in eugonadal men for contraception or for "andropause" will likely bring testosterone-induced apnea into clinical practice.

Testosterone also influences sleep architecture. In a study of pharmacologically induced hypogonadism,[29] with and without gonadal steroid replacement, hypogonadal males had reduced 24-h prolactin levels and percentage of stage 4 sleep in the hypogonadal state compared with testosterone replacement. Melatonin secretion is increased in male patients with gonadotropin-releasing hormone (Gn-RH) deficiency and in low-testosterone hypergonadotropic hypogonadal patients.[30] However there are no data on the prevalence of sleep disturbance in these patients.

Low testosterone levels have been reported in men with sleep apnea.[17, 31] In the largest study,[17] hormone level suppression by sleep apnea was independent of age, degree of obesity, and presence of awake hypoxemia and hypercapnia. Testosterone levels increase with treatment of sleep apnea using nasal CPAP or even successful uvulopalatopharyngoplasty.[17, 31] These androgen abnormalities in sleep apnea (decreased sex hormone–binding globulin [SHBG] and free and total testosterone) are qualitatively as well as quantitatively distinct from those reported in aging (increased SHBG, decreased free and total testosterone) and obesity (decreased SHBG and total testosterone, normal free testosterone). Importantly, despite the fall in plasma free and total testosterone levels, there was no increase in basal plasma gonadotropin (luteinizing hormone [LH], follicle-stimulating hormone) levels. These findings, together with the retention of pituitary sensitivity to exogenous Gn-RH in sleep apnea,[32] point to a hypothalamic abnormality as the cause of the fall in testosterone levels. This explanation would be similar to the postulated level of the dysfunction of the GH-IGF-1 axis in sleep apnea. The lack of change in plasma LH levels does not imply that LH secretion is entirely normal in men with sleep apnea because LH is secreted in an intermittent fashion.[33] It is certainly possible that pulsatile LH secretion is abnormal in sleep apnea but no published data are available.

The potential causes of this hypothalamic abnormality are essentially similar to those involved in reduced GH secretion. Testosterone levels are significantly reduced by sleep deprivation and fragmentation.[34] Therefore, sleep fragmentation in sleep apnea may lead to disruption of sleep-entrained rhythms in LH and testosterone. Hypoxemia in sleep apnea may be involved, as, unlike GH, there are several reports of low sex steroid levels in chronic airflow limitation in studies with small patient numbers.[35] In other larger studies,[16] the apparent effects of awake hypoxemia and impaired lung function were entirely accounted for by sleep hypoxemia. It is possible that the sexual dysfunction reported in sleep apnea may be mediated by the sex hormone changes seen in sleep-disordered breathing. The low testosterone levels may also interact with low IGF-1 levels and impair anabolism. Androgens may exacerbate sleep apnea and it is possible that the fall in androgen levels may be part of an adaptive homeostatic mechanism to reduce sleep-disordered breathing. However, androgen-lowering therapy with the nonsteroidal androgen antagonist flutamide did not alter sleep-disordered breathing or awake ventilatory drive.[36]

Female Sex Hormones and Sleep

Many women in the premenopausal time of their life have disturbed sleep; the transition into menopause is associated with worsening sleep in women who do not use hormone replacement.[37] Estrogen replacement therapy in postmenopausal women subjectively improves sleep quality and sleep initiation, decreases nocturnal restlessness and awakenings, and reduces daytime tiredness.[38] Large studies of the direct long-term effects of female sex hormones on sleep architecture are not available. However, in a study of short-term estrogen replacement in premenopausal women, improved sleep efficiency, fewer wakenings, and increased REM sleep were observed in the treated group.[39]

The low prevalence of sleep apnea in premenopausal women compared with women after the menopause and the increase in prevalence of sleep-disordered breathing among postmenopausal women have led to studies examining the therapeutic role of progestational hormones in sleep apnea.[40] The level of awake genioglossus electromyogram (EMG_{gg}) is higher in the luteal phase, followed by the follicular phase, and lowest in postmenopausal women.[41] Importantly, EMG_{gg}

increases after hormone therapy. Progesterone levels fall after menopause and progestogens have been shown to stimulate ventilation during the luteal phase of the menstrual cycle, in pregnancy, in normal male subjects, and in conditions of alveolar hypoventilation.[40]

In general, the therapeutic results for progestogens have been disappointing. Recent reports, including a double-blind study at high doses,[40] have revealed no improvement in indices of sleep apnea severity. Block et al.[42] were unable to demonstrate a protective effect of progesterone upon postmenopausal women with sleep apnea syndrome. The apparent "protection" of premenopausal status against sleep apnea has provoked some interest in hormone replacement as a therapy for sleep apnea in women. Pickett and co-workers[43] used combined therapy with both progestogen and an estrogen in women who had a surgical menopause. They demonstrated improvement, but the pretreatment apnea severity was very mild. Estrogen alone or in combination with progesterone on sleep-disordered breathing had no effect on sleep apnea in 15 postmenopausal women with moderate OSA despite a doubling of serum estrogen.[44] It is still possible that longer-term or higher-dose treatment may provide more positive results.

It is important to recognize that menopause is associated with increased central obesity. Whether this is a specific menopausal effect or simply reflects aging is unclear.[45] However, this increasing central obesity may explain the association between menopause and sleep apnea prevalence. Some female hormonal disorders are associated with obesity and in this way possibly linked to sleep apnea. Obesity occurs in approximately 50% of hyperandrogenic anovulatory women, some of whom also have non–insulin-dependent diabetes mellitus (NIDDM). One example of this is the polycystic ovary syndrome.[46]

Prolactinoma

Short-term administration of prolactin (PRL) and even long-term hyperprolactinemia in animals increases REM sleep.[47] In one study,[48] sleep in drug-free patients with prolactinoma (mean PRL levels: 1450 ± 1810 ng/ml; range between 146 and 5106 ng/ml) was compared with that of matched controls. The patients had secondary hypogonadism but no other endocrine abnormalities. They spent more time in slow-wave sleep (SWS) than the controls. REM sleep variables did not differ between the groups. It appears that chronic excessive enhancement of PRL levels exerts different influences on the sleep EEG in humans compared with the enhanced REM sleep produced by hyperprolactinemia in rats. These findings are in accordance with reports of good sleep quality in patients with prolactinoma.

THYROID

Hypothyroidism and Sleep Apnea

Apneic breathing in myxedema was noted by Massumi and Winnacker[49] and the presence of sleep apnea

was later confirmed by others.[50] Though myxedema coma is now rare, in retrospect many cases were probably due to severe sleepiness and obtundation secondary to severe sleep apnea, coupled with the hypercapnic respiratory failure of sleep apnea. Several mechanisms have been suggested to explain the association between sleep apnea and hypothyroidism. These include reduced upper airway patency due to myxedematous infiltration of tissues, impaired function of upper airway muscles, and reduced central drive to upper airway muscles.[51]

Several studies have questioned the strength of the association between sleep apnea and hypothyroidism. Lin et al.[52] studied 20 hypothyroid patients. All reported snoring but only two patients had moderate to severe OSA and three had mild OSA. Pelttari and co-workers[53] compared 26 patients with hypothyroidism with 188 euthyroid controls. Fifty percent of the hypothyroid patients and 29.3% of the control subjects had at least some episodes of partial or complete upper airway obstruction. Severe obstruction with episodes of repetitive apnea was present in 7.7% of the patients and in 1.5% of the controls. However, this association was largely explained by coexisting obesity and male sex. It has also been claimed that routine thyroid function testing in sleep apnea is not cost-effective[54] except in certain high-risk groups such as elderly women. Several large studies have been completed with conflicting conclusions on the strength of the association between sleep apnea and hypothyroidism and whether all OSA patients should be screened for this disorder.[54a–54c] It is likely that the prevalence of the association in sleep apnea cohorts is too low and further case-control studies in larger cohorts of sleep apnea patients are needed. In contrast, there are no large prospectively collected data on hypothyroid patients. It has been asserted that the prevalence of sleep apnea in this group is high.[55]

The effect of adequate thyroid hormone replacement on sleep apnea in hypothyroidism has been variable. Orr et al.[56] described three obese patients with myxedema and sleep apnea and reported cure of sleep apnea when they became euthyroid. Other case reports[51] describe similar cures. Rajagopal et al.[55] noted a significant reduction in apnea index for both obese and nonobese patients. The mean apnea index fell from 99.5 to less than 20 in the six obese patients without weight change, and in all patients there was an associated decrease in apnea duration. The three nonobese patients reduced their apnea indices to less than 5 after achieving euthyroid status. In contrast, in another study of 10 patients,[51] only two of them had a complete resolution of their sleep apnea when they became euthyroid. Five patients had moderate improvement in their sleep apnea though they continued to require nasal CPAP, whereas three patients had worsening in their apnea frequency.

The failure of sleep apnea to resolve after thyroxine treatment supports the view of a chance rather than causal association. An alternative explanation may be that hypothyroidism induces long-term changes in upper airway mechanics[57] or breathing control that do not resolve immediately after a euthyroid state is achieved.

However, in two sleep apnea case-control studies, past hypothyroidism did not appear to be a risk factor for sleep apnea.[54, 54a]

A number of studies have suggested a link between sleep apnea and cardiovascular complications in the initial stages of thyroid hormone replacement therapy. It is well recognized that rapid restoration of the euthyroid state in hypothyroid patients may entail significant cardiovascular morbidity and mortality.[51] This is particularly so in the elderly or those with preexisting cardiovascular disease. We observed one male patient with extremely long apneas lasting over 2 min, yet oxyhemoglobin desaturation only fell to 64%.[51] Undoubtedly, his low metabolic rate and oxygen consumption (reduced to 50% of normal) contributed to his ability to maintain such saturation despite long apneas. After commencing thyroxine treatment, there may be a more rapid increase in basal metabolic rate and oxygen consumption than clearance of abnormal myxedematous mucoprotein from the upper airway and normalization of depressed ventilatory responses. Long apneas may then be associated with a lower oxyhemoglobin saturation as the oxygen consumption rate increases, therefore posing a potential risk of dangerous hypoxemia for a patient with compromised coronary blood supply. We have also observed two female patients who had cardiac complications after commencing thyroxine prior to a sleep study and to the use of nasal CPAP therapy. One had a myocardial infarction with residual nocturnal angina after her thyroxine dosage was increased. Her nocturnal angina resolved after nasal CPAP was commenced. Another had nocturnal ventricular arrhythmias and unstable angina noted after thyroxine was commenced. Both complications resolved with CPAP therapy. We are also aware of an elderly obtunded patient with myxedema and with witnessed long apneas who died in her sleep 24 h after commencing a minimal dose of 25 μg of thyroxine. No sleep study had been performed and no CPAP treatment had been initiated. Abouganem et al.[58] reported extreme bradycardia and hypotension complicating sleep apnea in a patient with myxedema successfully managed with nasal CPAP prior to commencing thyroxine. Orr et al.[56] described a myxedematous patient with OSA and cardiac arrhythmias who had a tracheostomy performed resolving both the OSA and the arrhythmias. It would seem appropriate to institute thyroid hormone replacement cautiously in patients with hypothyroidism, sleep apnea, and probable cardiovascular disease.

Sleep Quality in Hypothyroidism

Sleepiness has long been observed as a symptom in hypothyroidism. Although sleep apnea may be one cause, a primary central effect on sleep is also possible in some patients. Marked reduction in SWS has been seen in patients with hypothyroidism which is reversible with treatment.[59] In congenital hypothyroidism, increased movement in sleep and reduced REM sleep have been noted.[60]

Hyperthyroidism and Sleep

A number of studies have shown an association between hyperthyroidism and sleep disturbance. This is not surprising in view of theoretical links between increased metabolic rates and insomnia.[61] Hyperthyroid patients complain of insomnia and have consequent impairment in mood.[62] However, these changes are not obvious in asymptomatic hyperthyroidism detected on random testing.[63] In addition, definitive controlled studies of sleep in hyperthyroid patients are lacking.

DISORDERED CORTICOSTEROID SECRETION AND SLEEP

Patients with corticosteroid excess secondary to Cushing's disease are characterized by truncal obesity, hypertension, and depression. In the only published data, about one third of patients appear to have sleep apnea.[64] Patients with Cushing's disease who do not have sleep apnea exhibit poorer sleep continuity, shortened REM latency, and increased first REM period density compared with normal subjects.[65] Other workers have suggested that, apart from insufficient inhibition of hypothalamic-pituitary-adrenal secretory activity during early sleep, patients with Cushing's disease have reduced SWS.[66] Interestingly, reduced SWS occurs in Addisons disease,[67] suggesting that normal cortisol secretion is needed for maintenance of SWS.

DIABETES AND OBESITY

Diabetes and Central Obesity

No specific sleep architecture abnormalities are associated with diabetes. Even hypoglycemic episodes during sleep are not apparently associated with EEG evidence of arousal.[68] Periodic movements in sleep may be more common in diabetes (see Chapter 65), and sleep may be disrupted in those with painful neuropathy.[69] Sleep apnea is common in diabetes and even more common in diabetic patients with autonomic neuropathy.[70] The fundamental link between diabetes and sleep apnea is through a co-association with obesity.[71]

Central obesity is often a more crucial determinant of morbidity and mortality than total adiposity.[72] Centrally obese individuals have increased risk of cardiovascular and cerebrovascular disease, diabetes, hypertension, hyperlipidemia, hyperuricemia, and insulin resistance relative to peripherally obese individuals. Central obesity is the commonest metabolic abnormality in sleep apnea. In sleep apnea, the predominant pattern of obesity is central.[73] The health risks of obesity and sleep apnea are similar and data are complicated by mutually confounding variables.[73] Attempts at separating the two disorders have suggested that both are additive in the pathogenesis of obesity-related morbidity.

Central obesity is a powerful epidemiological predictor of sleep apnea,[73, 74] and weight reduction may lead to marked improvement in sleep apnea severity. However, there are certainly less data addressing the reverse possibility—that sleep apnea may promote the development of obesity.[18] Unfortunately, no long-term longitudinal studies examining the developmental relationship between upper airway obstruction and obesity exist. It is tempting to think that chronic intermittent hypoxia and sleep fragmentation over years in sleep apnea can lead to changes in central control of energy regulation, appetite control, feeding, and metabolism, which would promote weight gain and thus worsen sleep apnea further. Moreover, if this is the case, could this vicious circle be broken by successful CPAP therapy? Or are there clear interindividual differences in underlying hypothalamic function leading to divergent responses in energy balance in patients with sleep apnea?

During sleep, energy expenditure (EE) typically fails, relative to the awake basal state.[61] In severe sleep apnea, sleep EE appears to increase during apneic sleep and fails with CPAP therapy[75] (Fig. 93–4). This would seem to be paradoxical—such EE changes would favor weight loss prior to CPAP and weight gain after CPAP. However, the 24-h EE may be different in untreated sleep apnea with reduced spontaneous physical activity (fidgeting, routine physical activities) due to fatigue and sleepiness producing a net decrease in EE, despite increased EE in sleep due to respiratory effort and sleep fragmentation. Other intriguing data suggest that patients with sleep apnea may have altered serotonergic sensitivity in the hypothalamus. Hudgel and coworkers[76] observed that the cortisol response to L-5-hydroxytryptophan (L-5HTP), a serotonin precursor, was elevated relative to control nonapneic subjects and was not readily explained by changes in weight. Subsequent data have shown that treatment with nasal CPAP reverses the elevated cortisol response to serotoninergic stimulation.[77] These investigators have speculated that the exaggerated cortisol responses in sleep apnea indicate supersensitivity of postsynaptic serotoninergic receptors in the hypothalamus caused by a serotoninergic "deficient" state induced by sleep apnea. Certainly, short periods of sleep deprivation in human beings and animals produce evidence of increased serotonin turnover[78]; whether chronic sleep fragmentation and hypoxemia in sleep apnea produce serotonin depletion in the hypothalamus and other regions is entirely speculative.

Interestingly, there are parallel findings of a serotonin-deficient state in central obesity.[79] Bjorntorp[79] has described a cluster of disorders associated with central obesity, including abnormalities of the hypothalamic-pituitary-end organ axis (low GH and testosterone, high cortisol), a "defeat" reaction to stress with psychosocial disability, and carbohydrate craving promoted by a low serotoninergic state. Specific serotoninergic agonists have been used as treatments in central obesity. The observed low testosterone and GH in sleep apnea also occur in central obesity. In central obesity, recombinant GH appears to reduce central body fat.[80] Perhaps, restoration of GH secretion during sleep with nasal CPAP in sleep apnea may have similar effects. A recent report suggests that nasal CPAP will reduce visceral fat deposits even without change in body mass index in patients with sleep apnea.[81]

Another area of common ground is insulin sensitivity. Central obesity is associated with hyperinsulinemia and insulin resistance.[72, 79] Certainly, some data also point to increased insulin levels in sleep apnea independent of weight and central obesity.[29] Nasal CPAP also improves insulin sensitivity in NIDDM.[70] However, in community cohorts, any relationship between

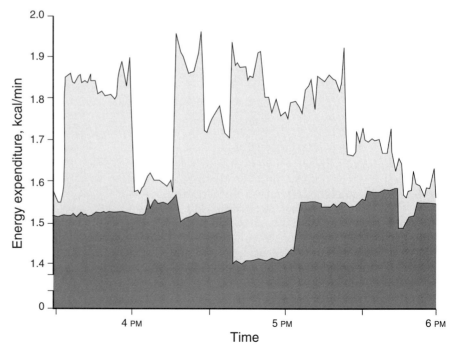

Figure 93–4. Sleep energy expenditure (SEE) curve for a subject (age 26, body mass index 40 kg/m²) with severe obstructive sleep apnea before treatment with nasal continuous positive airway pressure (CPAP) *(top curve)* and reduction in SEE with CPAP therapy *(bottom curve)*. (Adapted from Stenlöf K, Grunstein RR, Hedner J, et al. Energy expenditure in obstructive sleep apnea: effects of treatment with continuous positive airway pressure. Am J Physiol. 1996; 271:E1036–1043.)

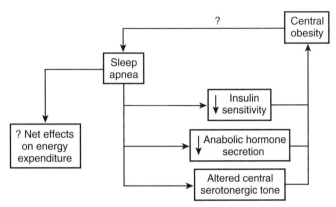

Figure 93–5. Factors involved in the relationship between central obesity and sleep apnea. Sleep apnea is linked with reduced insulin sensitivity and secretion of anabolic hormones which would favor development of central obesity. The observed changes in serotonergic "tone" in sleep apnea would also theoretically promote the obese state. Although continuous positive airway pressure treatment of sleep apnea will reduce energy expenditure, the net effects of sleep apnea on energy expenditure are unknown.

sleep apnea and insulin resistance appears to be mediated by obesity.[83]

In summary, diabetes and central obesity, in particular, are closely linked to sleep-breathing disorders. A schema of the association between sleep apnea and central obesity is outlined in Figure 93–5.

Can Obesity Cause Nonrespiratory Sleep Disturbances?

Some genetic forms of obesity are associated with somnolence. One important example is the Prader-Willi syndrome (PWS).[84–86] A number of groups have suggested that although sleep apnea is common in PWS, a primary hypersomnolence disorder may be associated with this condition.[84–86] This is possible, though residual degrees of sleep apnea persisted in most of these sleepy PWS patients after weight loss.[84–86] Moreover, none of these studies used pressure flow measuring techniques to fully quantify the degree of residual upper airway obstruction, nor reported on CPAP effects on sleepiness in these patients.

Recently, Vgontzas and co-workers[87] have argued that daytime sleepiness is a frequent complaint of obese patients even among those who do not have sleep apnea. They investigated 73 obese patients without sleep apnea who were consecutively referred for treatment of their obesity, and 45 controls matched for age. Obese patients compared with controls were sleepier on objective testing during the day and their nighttime sleep was more disturbed. Although intriguing, it would be important to confirm these findings using rigorous measurement of upper airway resistance and arousals. If proved, it may indicate that somnogeneic cytokines, such as tumor necrosis factor-alpha and interleukins, produced by central fat masses[88, 89] can cause daytime sleepiness, which is distinct from arousals and sleep fragmentation produced by upper airway obstruction.

References

1. Melmed S. Acromegaly. N Engl J Med. 1990;322:966–977.
2. Wright AD, Hill DM, Lowy C, et al. Mortality in acromegaly. Q J Med. 1970;39:1–16.
3. Roxburgh F, Collis AJ. Notes on a case of acromegaly. Br Med J. 1886;2:63–65.
4. Chappell WF, Booth JA. A case of acromegaly with laryngeal symptoms and pharyngeal symptoms. J Laryngol Otol. 1886;1:142–150.
5. Laroche C, Festal G, Poenaru S, et al. Une observation de respiration périodique chez une acromégalie. Ann Med Intern. 1976; 127:381–385.
6. Grunstein RR, Ho KY, Sullivan CE. Acromegaly and sleep apnea. Ann Intern Med. 1991;115:527–532.
7. Pelttari L, Polo O, Rauhala E, et al. Nocturnal breathing abnormalities in acromegaly after adenomectomy. Clin Endocrinol (Oxf). 1995;43:175–182.
8. Rosenow F, Reuter S, Deuss U, et al. Sleep apnoea in treated acromegaly: relative frequency and predisposing factors. Clin Endocrinol (Oxf). 1996;45:563–569.
9. Mezon BJ, West P, MacLean JP, et al. Sleep apnea in acromegaly. Am J Med. 1980;69:615–618.
10. Cadieux RJ, Kales A, Santen RJ, et al. Endoscopic findings in sleep apnea associated with acromegaly. J Clin Endocrinol Metab. 1982;55:18–22.
10a. Hochban W, Ehlenz K, Conradt R, et al. Obstructive sleep apnea in acromegaly: the role of craniofacial changes. Eur Respir J. 1999;14:196–202.
11. Perks WH, Horrocks PM, Cooper RA, et al. Sleep apnea in acromegaly. Br Med J. 1980;280:894.
12. Grunstein RR, Ho KY, Berthon-Jones M, et al. Central sleep apnea is associated with increased ventilatory response to carbon dioxide and hypersecretion of growth hormone in patients with acromegaly. Am J Respir Crit Care Med. 1994;150:496–502.
13. Astrom C, Christensen L, Gjerris F, et al. Sleep in acromegaly before and after treatment with adenomectomy. Neuroendocrinology. 1991;53:328–331.
14. Faithfull S. Patients' experiences following cranial radiotherapy: a study of the somnolence syndrome. J Adv Nurs. 1991;16:939–946.
15. Bengtsson BA, Eden S, Ernst I, et al. Epidemiology and long term survival in acromegaly. Acta Med Scand. 1988;223:327–335.
16. Barnes AJ, Pallis C, Joplin GF. Acromegaly and narcolepsy. Lancet. 1979;2:332–333.
17. Grunstein RR, Handelsman DJ, Lawrence S, et al. Neuroendocrine dysfunction in sleep apnea: reversal by nasal continuous positive airway pressure. J Clin Endocrinol Metab. 1989;68:352–358.
18. Grunstein RR. Metabolic aspects of sleep apnea. Sleep. 1996; 19(suppl):S218–220.
19. Astrom C, Jochumsen PL. Decrease in delta sleep in growth hormone deficiency assessed by a new power spectrum analysis. Sleep. 1989;12:508–515.
20. Gerard JM, Garibaldi L, Myers SE, et al. Sleep apnea in patients receiving growth hormone. Clin Pediatr (Phila). 1997;36:321–326.
21. Sandblom RE, Matsumoto AM, Schoene RB, et al. Obstructive sleep apnea induced by testosterone administration. N Engl J Med. 1983;308:506–510.
22. Strumpf IJ, Reynolds SF, Vash P, et al. A possible relationship between testosterone, central control of ventilation, and the Pickwickian syndrome [abstract]. Am Rev Respir Dis. 1978;117:A183.
23. Harman E, Wynne JW, Block AJ. The effect of weight loss on sleep disordered breathing and oxygen desaturation in morbidly obese men. Chest. 1982;82:291–293.
24. Johnson MW, Arch AM, Remmers JE. Induction of the obstructive sleep apnea syndrome in a woman by exogenous androgen administration. Am Rev Respir Dis. 1984;129:1023.
25. Dexter DD, Dovre EJ. Obstructive sleep apnea due to endogenous testosterone production in a woman. Mayo Clin Proc. 1998;73:246–248.
26. Cistulli PA, Grunstein RR, Sullivan CE. Effect of testosterone administration on upper airway collapsibility during sleep. Am J Respir Crit Care Med. 1994;149:530–532.
27. Matsumoto AM, Sandblom RE, Schoene RB, et al. Testosterone

replacement in hypogonadal males: effects on obstructive sleep apnea, respiratory drives and sleep. Clin Endocrinol (Oxf). 1985;22:713–717.

28. Schneider BK, Pickett CK, Zwillich CW, et al. Influence of testosterone on breathing during sleep. J Appl Physiol. 1986;61:618–624.

29. Leibenluft E, Schmidt PJ, Turner EH, et al. Effects of leuprolide-induced hypogonadism and testosterone replacement on sleep, melatonin, and prolactin secretion in men. J Clin Endocrinol Metab. 1997;82:3203–3207.

30. Luboshitzky R, Wagner O, Lavi S, et al. Abnormal melatonin secretion in male patients with hypogonadism. J Mol Neurosci. 1996;7:91–98.

31. Santamaria JD, Prior JC, Fleetham JA. Reversible reproductive dysfunction in men with obstructive sleep apnea. Clin Endocrinol (Oxf). 1988;28:461–470.

32. Stewart DA, Grunstein RR, Sullivan CE, et al. Neuroendocrine changes in sleep apnea are not related to a pituitary defect. Sleep Res. 1989;18:308.

33. Pincus SM, Mulligan T, Iranmanesh A, et al. Older males secrete luteinizing hormone and testosterone more irregularly, and jointly more asynchronously, than younger males. Proc Natl Acad Sci U S A. 1996;93:14100–14105.

34. Akerstedt T, Palmblad J, de la Torre B, et al. Adrenocortical and gonadal steroids during sleep deprivation. Sleep. 1980;3:23–30.

35. d'A Semple P, Beastall GH, Brown TM, et al. Sex hormone suppression and sexual impotence in hypoxic pulmonary fibrosis. Thorax. 1984;39:46.

36. Stewart DA, Grunstein RR, Berthon-Jones M, et al. Androgen blockade does not affect sleep-disordered breathing or chemosensitivity in men with obstructive sleep apnea. Am Rev Respir Dis. 1992;146:1389–1393.

37. Owens JF, Matthews KA. Sleep disturbance in healthy middle-aged women. Maturitas. 1998;30:41–50.

38. Polo-Kantola P, Erkkola R, Helenius H, et al. When does estrogen replacement therapy improve sleep quality? Am J Obstet Gynecol. 1998;178:1002–1009.

39. Thomson J, Oswald I. Effect of oestrogen on the sleep, mood, and anxiety of menopausal women. Br Med J. 1977;2:1317–1319.

40. Cook WR, Benich JJ, Wooten SA. Indices of severity of obstructive sleep apnea syndrome do not change during medroxyprogesterone acetate therapy. Chest. 1989;96:262–266.

41. Popovic RM, White DP. Upper airway muscle activity in normal women: influence of hormonal status. J Appl Physiol. 1998;84:1055–1062.

42. Block AJ, Wynne JW, Boysen PG, et al. Menopause, medroxyprogesterone and breathing during sleep. Am J Med. 1980;70:506–510.

43. Pickett CK, Regensteiner JG, Woodard WD, et al. Progestogen and estrogen reduce sleep-disordered breathing in post-menopausal women. J Appl Physiol. 1989;66:1656–1661.

44. Cistulli PA, Barnes DJ, Grunstein RR, et al. Effect of short-term hormone replacement in the treatment of obstructive sleep apnoea in postmenopausal women. Thorax. 1994;49:699–702.

45. Colombel A, Charbonnel B. Weight gain and cardiovascular risk factors in the post-menopausal woman. Hum Reprod. 1997;12(suppl 1):134–145.

46. Goudas VT, Dumesic DA. Polycystic ovary syndrome. Endocrinol Metab Clin North Am. 1997;26:893–912.

47. Obal F Jr, Kacsoh B, Bredow S, et al. Sleep in rats rendered chronically hyperprolactinemic with anterior pituitary grafts. Brain Res. 1997;25;755:130–136.

48. Frieboes RM, Murck H, Stalla GK, et al. Enhanced slow wave sleep in patients with prolactinoma. J Clin Endocrinol Metab. 1998;83:2706–2710.

49. Massumi RA, Winnacker JL. Severe depression of the respiratory center in myxedema. Am J Med. 1964;36:876–882.

50. Duron B, Quinchard J, Fullana N. Nouvelles recherches sur le mécanisme des apnées du syndrome de pickwick. Bull Physiopathol Respir. 1972;8:1277–1288.

51. Grunstein RR, Sullivan CE. Hypothyroidism and sleep apnea. Mechanisms and management. Am J Med. 1988;85:775–779.

52. Lin CC, Tsan KW, Chen PJ. The relationship between sleep apnea syndrome and hypothyroidism. Chest. 1992;102:1663–1667.

53. Pelttari L, Rauhala E, Polo O, et al. Upper airway obstruction in hypothyroidism. J Intern Med. 1994;236:177–181.

54. Winkelman JW, Goldman H, Piscatelli N, et al. Are thyroid function tests necessary in patients with suspected sleep apnea? Sleep. 1996;19:790–793.

54a. Kapur VK, Koepsell TD, deMaube J, et al. Association of hypothyroidism and obstructive sleep apnea. Am J Respir Crit Care Med. 1998;158:1379–1383.

54b. Sjokdt NM, Aktar R, Easton PA. Screening for hypothyroidism in sleep apnea. Am J Respir Crit Care Med. 1999;160:732–735.

54c. Mickelson SA, Lian T, Rosenthal L. Thyroid testing and thyroid replacement in patients with sleep disordered breathing. Ear Nose Throat J. 1999;78:768–771.

55. Rajagopal KR, Abbrecht PH, Derderian SS, et al. Obstructive sleep apnea in hypothyroidism. Ann Intern Med. 1984;101:471–474.

56. Orr WC, Males JL, Imes NK. Myxedema and obstructive sleep apnea. Am J Med. 1981;70:1061–1066.

57. Petrof BJ, Kelly AM, Rubinstein NA, et al. Effect of hypothyroidism on myosin heavy chain expression in rat pharyngeal dilator muscles. J Appl Physiol. 1992;73:179–187.

58. Abouganem D, Taylor AL, Donna E, et al. Extreme bradycardia during sleep apnea caused by myxedema. Arch Intern Med. 1987;147:1497–1499.

59. Ruiz-Primo E, Jurado JL, Solis H, et al. Polysomnographic effects of thyroid hormones in primary myxedema. Electroencephalogr Clin Neurophysiol. 1982;53:559–564.

60. Hayashi M, Araki S, Kohyama J, et al. Sleep development in children with congenital and acquired hypothyroidism. Brain Dev. 1997;19:43–49.

61. Bonnet MH, Berry RB, Arand DL. Metabolism during normal, fragmented and recovery sleep. J Appl Physiol. 1991;71:1112–1118.

62. Huang YR, Wang GH. Study on quality of sleep and mental health in patients with hyperthyroidism. Chung Hua Hu Li Tsa Chih. 1997;32:435–439.

63. Schlote B, Schaaf L, Schmidt R, et al. Mental and physical state in subclinical hyperthyroidism: investigations in a normal working population. Biol Psychiatry. 1992;32:48–56.

64. Shipley JE, Schteingart DE, Tandon R, et al. Sleep architecture and sleep apnea in patients with Cushing's disease. Sleep. 1992;15:514–518.

65. Shipley JE, Schteingart DE, Tandon R, et al. EEG sleep in Cushing's disease and Cushing's syndrome: comparison with patients with major depressive disorder. Biol Psychiatry. 1992;32:146–155.

66. Born J, Fehm HL. Hypothalamus-pituitary-adrenal activity during human sleep: a coordinating role for the limbic hippocampal system. Exp Clin Endocrinol Diabetes. 1998;106:153–163.

67. Gillin JC, Jacobs LS, Snyder F, et al. Effects of decreased adrenal corticosteroids: changes in sleep in normal subjects and patients with adrenal cortical insufficiency. Electroencephalogr Clin Neurophysiol. 1974;36:283–289.

68. Porter PA, Byrne G, Stick S, et al. Nocturnal hypoglycaemia and sleep disturbances in young teenagers with insulin dependent diabetes mellitus. Arch Dis Child. 1996;75:120–123.

69. Backonja M, Beydoun A, Edwards KR, et al. Gabapentin for the symptomatic treatment of painful neuropathy in patients with diabetes mellitus: a randomized controlled trial. JAMA. 1998;280:1831–1836.

70. Brooks B, Cistulli PA, Borkman M, et al. Effect of nasal continuous positive airway pressure treatment on insulin sensitivity in patients with type II diabetes and obstructive sleep apnea. J Clin Endocrinol Metab. 1994; 79:1681–1685.

71. Ficker JH, Dertinger SH, Siegfried W, et al. Obstructive sleep apnoea and diabetes mellitus: the role of cardiovascular autonomic neuropathy. Eur Respir J. 1998;11:14–19.

72. Bjorntorp P. Obesity. Lancet. 1997;350:423–426.

73. Grunstein RR, Wilcox I, Yang TS, et al. Snoring and sleep apnoea in men: association with central obesity and hypertension. Int J Obesity. 1993;17:533–540.

74. Grunstein RR, Stenlöf K, Hedner J, et al. Impact of self reported sleep apnea symptoms on psycho-social performance in the Swedish Obese Subjects (SOS) Study. Sleep. 1995;18:635–643.

75. Stenlöf K, Grunstein RR, Hedner J, et al. Energy expenditure in obstructive sleep apnea: effects of treatment with continuous positive airway pressure. Am J Physiol. 1996;271:E1036–1043.

76. Hudgel DW, Gordon EA, Meltzer HY. Abnormal serotonergic

stimulation of cortisol production in obstructive sleep apnea. Am J Respir Crit Care Med. 1995;152:186–192.

77. Hudgel DW, Gordon EA. Serotonin-induced cortisol release in CPAP-treated obstructive sleep apnea patients. Chest. 1997;111:632–638.

78. Heiser P, Dickhaus B, Opper C, et al. Platelet serotonin and interleukin-1 beta after sleep deprivation and recovery sleep in humans. J Neural Transm. 1997;104:1049–1058.

79. Bjorntorp P. Neuroendocrine abnormalities in human obesity. Metabolism. 1995;44(suppl 2):38–41.

80. Johannsson G, Marin P, Lonn L, et al. Growth hormone treatment of abdominally obese men reduces abdominal fat mass, improves glucose and lipoprotein metabolism, and reduces diastolic blood pressure. J Clin Endocrinol Metab. 1997;82:727–734.

81. Chin K, Shimizu K, Nakamura T, et al. Changes in intra-abdominal visceral fat and serum leptin levels in patients with obstructive sleep apnea following nasal continuous positive airway pressure. Circulation. 1999;100:706–712.

82. Grunstein RR, Stenlof K, Hedner J, et al. Impact of obstructive sleep apnea and sleepiness on metabolic and cardiovascular risk factors in the Swedish Obese Subjects (SOS) Study. Int J Obesity. 1995:151:410–418.

83. Stoohs RA, Facchini F, Guilleminault C. Insulin resistance and sleep-disordered breathing in healthy humans. Am J Respir Crit Care Med. 1996;154:170–174.

84. Harris JC, Allen RP. Is excessive daytime sleepiness characteristic of Prader-Willi syndrome? The effects of weight change. Arch Pediatr Adolesc Med. 1996;150:1288–1293.

85. Vgontzas AN, Kales A, Seip J, et al. Relationship of sleep abnormalities to patient genotypes in Prader-Willi syndrome. Am J Med Genet. 1996;67:478–482.

86. Vgontzas AN, Bixler EO, Kales A, et al. Daytime sleepiness and REM abnormalities in Prader-Willi syndrome: evidence of generalized hypoarousal. Int J Neurosci. 1996;87:127–139

87. Vgontzas AN, Bixler EO, Tan TL, et al. Obesity without sleep apnea is associated with daytime sleepiness. Arch Intern Med. 1998;158:1333–1337.

88. Katsuki A, Sumida Y, Murashima S, et al. Serum levels of tumor necrosis factor-alpha are increased in obese patients with noninsulin-dependent diabetes mellitus. J Clin Endocrinol Metab. 1998;83:859–862.

89. Vgontzas AN, Papanicolaou DA, Bixler EO, et al. Elevation of plasma cytokines in disorders of excessive daytime sleepiness: role of sleep disturbance and obesity. J Clin Endocrinol Metab. 1997;82:1313–1316.

94

Gastrointestinal Disorders

William C. Orr

NOCTURNAL GASTROINTESTINAL SYMPTOMS

The manifestation of gastrointestinal symptoms during sleep is quite familiar to the practicing gastroenterologist. Perhaps the most obvious and common example is the occurrence of epigastric pain characteristically awakening the patient from sleep in the early morning hours. This pattern of awakening from sleep is quite predictable by the patient and can help significantly in establishing an empirical diagnosis of duodenal ulcer disease. Patients may also have awakenings from sleep with symptoms that ostensibly are not related to gastrointestinal disorders. For example, individuals may complain of sleep disruption secondary to awakening from sleep with chest pain, heartburn, or regurgitation into the throat. Asthmatics may awaken from sleep by the exacerbation of bronchial asthma that can be secondary to gastroesophageal reflux (GER). Numerous studies are accumulating to suggest that respiratory complications secondary to gastroesophageal reflux are common, and these symptoms are noted primarily secondary to sleep-related GER.[1]

Other symptoms encountered by the practicing gastroenterologist that may occur during the day but whose occurrence during sleep adds a disconcerting dimension to the symptom include nocturnal diarrhea, fecal incontinence, chest pain, or the respiratory disorders noted above. Although a denial of symptoms thought to be related to gastrointestinal problems such as GER does not necessarily preclude the occurrence of the sleep-related abnormalities, a positive symptom history would enhance the probability of the existence of a nocturnal gastrointestinal disorder.

NOCTURNAL ACID SECRETION IN DUODENAL ULCER DISEASE

Patients with duodenal ulcer disease maintain a circadian pattern of gastric acid secretion, and studies have shown that the levels of secretion are enhanced.[2] This study shows that the peak of basal acid secretion occurs at approximately midnight, with minimal acid secretion occurring during the day in the absence of food ingestion. In addition, as reviewed in Chapter 21, there does not appear to be any relation between the stages of sleep and gastric acid secretion. However, the study by Orr et al.[3] demonstrated a failure to inhibit acid during the first 2 h of sleep in patients with duodenal ulcer disease. Multicenter trials with bedtime administration of histamine (H$_2$) receptor antagonists have documented the efficacy of healing duodenal ulcers through nocturnal acid suppression.[4, 5] These studies uniformly documented that duodenal ulcer–healing rates were at least as good with a once-a-day, bedtime dose of these potent acid-suppressing compounds as with the more conventional multiple daily dosing regimens. Howden et al.[6] reviewed the published data on nocturnal dosing of H$_2$ receptor antagonists in more than 12,000 patients with duodenal ulcer disease. They concluded that nocturnal dosing showed a clear advantage over multiple daily doses. These data strongly support the notion that nocturnal acid suppression alone is sufficient to heal a duodenal ulcer.

Other studies in patients with refractory duodenal ulcer suggest that nocturnal acid suppression is not only sufficient but also necessary for duodenal ulcer healing. In a study by Gledhill et al.,[7] it was demonstrated that a reduction in nocturnal acid secretion through parietal cell vagotomy produced an enhanced healing rate in patients who were unresponsive to conventional cimetidine treatment. In a similar study by Galmiche et al.,[8] 20 patients with duodenal ulcer who were resistant to conventional cimetidine treatment received 150 mg ranitidine twice daily for 6 weeks. They demonstrated that in 8 patients, the ulcer was healed, whereas in 12 patients, the ulcer remained unhealed. Patients whose ulcer healed had a substantial suppression of nocturnal acid secretion, whereas patients whose ulcer again failed to heal maintained a nocturnal peak in gastric acid secretion. A subsequent study found that in persons who have had a parietal cell vagotomy, nocturnal acid secretion was significantly greater in those who experienced ulcer recurrence than in those who did not.[9] Further support for the important role of nocturnal acid secretion in the pathogenesis of duodenal ulcer disease comes from data showing that the maintenance of a modest degree of nocturnal acid suppression will effectively prevent the recurrence of duodenal ulcer disease.[10, 11] These studies compared the use of 150 mg ranitidine at bedtime with 400 mg cimetidine at bedtime and found ranitidine to be superior in the prevention of ulcer recurrence. This finding is most likely due to the increased potency of ranitidine and its enhanced effectiveness in producing nocturnal acid suppression. A study actually documenting effective nocturnal acid suppression by 150 mg ranitidine at bedtime was reported by Santana et al.,[12] who concluded that "it may be relevant to the pathogenesis of duodenal ulceration that the short-lived decrease in nocturnal acidity observed in this study is sufficient to prevent relapse of ulceration in most patients."

Therapeutic Considerations

The data reviewed concerning ulcer healing and the prevention of ulcer relapse strongly suggest that suppression of nocturnal gastric acid secretion is an important element in ulcer pathogenesis and healing. This observation does not imply that the numerous other factors (such as *Helicobacter pylori*) that have been implicated in the pathogenesis of duodenal ulcer disease are not equally important; it simply strongly affirms that nocturnal acid secretion appears to be an important element in ulcer formation. Even though the pathogenesis of duodenal ulcer disease is complex, these data appear to make it clear that ulcer healing will not occur, or will be severely retarded, without effective nocturnal acid suppression.

GASTROESOPHAGEAL REFLUX DURING SLEEP

GER, particularly with its familiar symptom of heartburn, is recognized as a common phenomenon. Most normal people will experience occasional bouts of heartburn. About 7% of the normal population experiences heartburn nearly every day.[13] Most patients who present to a physician with a complaint of heartburn can be readily treated with simple alterations in lifestyle, such as the avoidance of certain provocative foods and the use of antacid therapy. The familiarity of this symptom and its rapid response in most instances to relatively simple therapeutic measures belie the severity and potential complications of this disease process. As will be reviewed, the complications of GER appear to be the result of recurrent episodes of sleep-related GER.

Attention has been focused on the importance of different patterns of GER associated with waking and sleeping.[14] These patterns were documented in studies involving 24-h monitoring of the distal esophageal pH. GER is identified when the pH falls below 4 for a period of more than 30 sec, and the reflux episode is arbitrarily terminated when the pH reaches 4 or 5. In this landmark study, Johnson and DeMeester[14] described two different patterns of reflux. Reflux in the upright position occurs most often postprandially and usually consists of two or three reflux episodes that are rapidly cleared (2 to 3 min). Reflux in the supine position is usually associated with sleep and with more prolonged clearance time.

These studies documented highly significant increases in acid–mucosa contact time in patients with esophagitis, and these differences were most impressive when the supine position or sleep interval was considered; that is, there was a greater difference between patients and control subjects in the supine position as opposed to in the upright position. These investigators have also asserted that even though acid–mucosa contact time may be equivalent in the upright and supine positions, the prolonged acid clearance times associated with sleep appeared to result in greater damage to the esophageal mucosa.[15] In another study, the same investigators attempted to correlate the relation between the patterns of GER, as determined by 24-h esophageal pH monitoring, and the endoscopic evaluation of the esophageal mucosa.[16] They identified patients as primarily *upright* (waking) *refluxers,* *supine* (sleep) *refluxers,* and those whose reflux was evident throughout the 24-h day, whom they termed *combined refluxers.* The severity of endoscopic change according to three grades of esophagitis was determined. Grade 1 esophagitis was defined simply as distal erythema and friability; grade 2 esophagitis was when mucosal erosions are noted; and grade 3 esophagitis involved more severe ulcerations and strictures. Their data indicated that an increasing incidence of nocturnal acid exposure was associated with more severe esophageal mucosal damage. An additional study compared the results of 24-h esophageal pH monitoring in patients who had either normal findings on endoscopy or erosive esophagitis.[17] The results of this study showed that total acid exposure time and the number of reflux episodes requiring longer than 5 min to clear were found to most reliably discriminate these two groups of patients. Furthermore, these authors found that 50% of the patients with reflux symptoms had normal 24-h pH monitoring and that 29% of the patients with erosive esophagitis also had normal pH studies. It is of interest that the most effective variable in distinguishing the two groups of patients was the number of episodes requiring longer than 5 min to clear (to pH 4). An extension of these findings comes from a study by Orr et al.[18] in which 24-hour pH monitoring was accomplished in a group of symptomatic patients with heartburn and normal endoscopic results and a group of patients with severe complications of GER, including erosive esophagitis, stricture, and Barrett's esophagus. The results showed that the best discriminator among the two groups was the number of episodes of prolonged acid clearance (longer than 5 min) in the supine position. These episodes appear to be more likely to occur during sleep, and this finding certainly confirms the notion that prolonged acid clearance is an important determinant in the development of esophagitis. Other investigators have not been as enthusiastic in their support of nocturnal GER as an important factor in the pathogenesis of reflux esophagitis. De Caestecker et al.[19] found that postprandial acid exposure was the best predictor of the severity of esophagitis, and their results led them to conclude that nocturnal reflux was substantially less important in the production of esophagitis.

ESOPHAGEAL ACID CLEARANCE DURING SLEEP

As previously noted, acid clearance during sleep seems to be an important contributing factor in the development of reflux esophagitis. The process of acid clearance has been well studied by Helm et al.,[20] who described a two-factor theory of acid clearance. They proposed that acid clearance takes place in two phases: an initial phase, termed *volume clearance*, and a second phase, termed *acid neutralization*. Their data indicate that the vast majority of the volume of refluxed material is cleared from the esophagus quite rapidly by the first two or three swallows. There remains a coating of acid on the esophageal mucosa, which keeps the esophageal pH well below 4. Subsequent swallows serve to deliver saliva to the distal esophagus, and with its potent buffering capacity, the distal esophageal pH is returned to its normal level (5.5 to 6.5). A subsequent study confirmed these findings in that acid clearance was found to be independent of the swallowing rate but significantly altered by an anticholinergic drug that inhibits salivation.[21]

Both swallowing frequency and salivation have been shown to be markedly depressed during sleep; as a result, one would hypothesize a prolongation of acid clearance during sleep.[22, 23] Lichter and Muir[22] have shown that swallowing occurs sporadically during sleep, and there are long periods (longer than 30 min) without swallowing. Overall, the rate of swallowing during sleep is approximately six swallows per hour, and the swallows usually occur in association with a movement arousal. The highest frequency of these events is in stages 1 and 2 and rapid eye movement (REM) sleep.[22] Similarly, a study by Orr et al.[24] showed a 50% reduction in swallows, which was required for the clearance of infused acid during sleep. Studies have focused specifically on the issue of the parameters of esophageal acid clearance during sleep. A model that incorporates the clearance of infused acid (15.0/ml 0.1 N HCl) during sleep was used in these studies. As opposed to simply analyzing spontaneous GER, this allowed the infusion of acid into the distal esophagus during specific periods of documented sleep (REM versus nonrapid eye movement [NREM]), and it allowed the precise timing of infusions such that the amount of sleep before each infusion could be relatively well controlled. This model also permitted a precise comparison of acid clearance during waking and during sleep under well-controlled conditions.

The initial study in this series involved a comparison of acid clearance during sleep in normal volunteers and patients with mild-to-moderate esophagitis.[24] The results revealed that sleep infusions in both groups were associated with a statistically significant prolongation of acid clearance time. In minutes, the absolute clearance time was nearly doubled in both groups. However, there was no significant difference between the clearance times in the patients and in the control subjects. The latter finding is believed to be a somewhat academic point because, as noted previously, normal persons rarely have reflux during sleep, whereas it is somewhat more common in patients with esophagitis. In addition, it was clear from the polysomnographic observations that clearance was invariably associated with an arousal from sleep, and if this did not occur, there was a marked prolongation in acid clear-

ance time. To more precisely evaluate this notion, clearance intervals that were associated with greater or less than 50% of waking during the clearance interval were compared. The clearance trials that involved more than 50% of waking had significantly faster clearance times. These data led to the conclusion that both arousal responses and waking are important elements in the response to an acidic distal esophagus.

To more carefully evaluate the motor functioning of the esophagus during sleep and the associated arousals from sleep, a subsequent study was performed using a specially designed esophageal probe (Konigsberg Instruments, Inc., Los Angeles, California) to monitor not only distal esophageal pH but also esophageal peristalsis.[25] This study also confirmed the importance of arousal responses in the efficient clearance of acid from the distal esophagus. The test was performed on normal volunteers who had a negative acid perfusion test; that is, they did not show any sensitivity to acid dripped in the distal esophagus and could not distinguish acid from water in the esophagus. However, the determination of arousal responses to these two different substances infused during sleep revealed that the acid infusions produced a significantly greater number of arousal responses. In addition, an exponential relation was described between the percentage of waking during the acid clearance interval and the acid clearance time; that is, the greater the amount of waking during the acid clearance interval, the faster the clearance time. Again, this finding substantiates those from the previous study of patients with esophagitis. This study did not document any difference between peristaltic parameters during sleep and during waking.

To more definitively test the hypothesis that complications of GER are associated with prolonged acid clearance, a group of 13 patients with Barrett's esophagus was studied.[26] Barrett's esophagus is a condition believed to be related to chronic, severe GER, which results in the replacement of normal esophageal squamous epithelium with gastric columnar epithelium. The results of this study proved to be quite surprising in that the patients with Barrett's esophagus were shown to have significantly faster acid clearance during sleep and waking compared with the control subjects. These data were, however, quite compatible with previous results in documenting the importance of arousal responses in the clearance process. The patients with Barrett's esophagus showed both a higher frequency of arousal responses and a shorter latency to the first swallow than did the control subjects.

Further illustrating the importance of these parameters in differentiating the patients with Barrett's esophagus from the control subjects is the fact that they could not be distinguished on the basis of any parameters associated with esophageal motor functioning, such as the amplitude of the peristaltic contraction or the esophageal transit time. It is especially notable in this study that there were a remarkable number of episodes of spontaneous GER in the group with Barrett's esophagus compared with the control subjects. These data led to the conclusion that the severe esophagitis in the patients with Barrett's esophagus is acquired through repeated episodes of spontaneous GER during sleep, which are associated with a prolongation of the acid clearance time (even though this was demonstrated to be faster than in normal control subjects, the acid clearance still is substantially longer than that occurring during waking).

Therapeutic Considerations

The results of previously cited studies suggest that the pattern of GER during waking and sleep is important in that sleep-related reflux produces a prolongation of acid clearance.[17, 18] Additional documentation of the importance of this pattern of the prolongation of acid clearance comes from studies that have shown that the back-diffusion of hydrogen ions in the esophagus is directly related to the duration of acid–mucosa contact time.[27] Further evidence for the importance of nocturnal GER comes from a clinical study that documented individuals with symptoms of nocturnal heartburn, as well as dysphagia and chest pain, were much more likely to have demonstrable esophageal disease.[28]

These results, as well as those described in the cited studies, tend to substantiate the time-honored clinical approach to persistent reflux, which is the suggestion that the patient sleep with the head of the bed elevated. This clinical axiom has survived for decades with little in the way of objective documentation that it actually is an efficacious approach to GER. Johnson and DeMeester[29] specifically tested this clinical axiom. Using intraesophageal pH monitoring during sleep, they demonstrated that sleeping with the head of the bed elevated produced a 67% improvement in the acid clearance time; however, the frequency of reflux episodes remained unchanged.[29] The use of a cholinergic drug (bethanechol) that produces an elevation in lower esophageal sphincter pressure and increases esophageal peristaltic efficiency resulted in a decrease in both reflux frequency (30%) and acid clearance time (53%). The authors concluded that nocturnal reflux was most responsive to these therapeutic modalities.

The use of H_2 receptor antagonists to suppress gastric acid secretion has been shown to be effective in the relief of heartburn.[30, 31] One study using 24-h ambulatory esophageal pH assessments in patients with symptomatic heartburn and documented GER demonstrated that increasing doses (40 mg at bedtime, 20 mg twice daily, and 40 mg twice daily) of an H_2 receptor antagonist (famotidine) produced increasing reductions in daytime and total acid–mucosa contact.[32] The three dosing regimens were equally effective in reducing nocturnal acid contact time. Thus, in contrast to duodenal ulcer disease, it does not appear that only bedtime dosing is adequate to treat GER. However, these data suggest that GER can be adequately controlled through effective gastric acid suppression. An interesting finding was reported by Kerr et al.,[33] who showed that the administration of nasal continuous positive airway pressure to patients who are being treated for obstructive sleep apnea had the additional therapeutic benefit of reducing GER and consequent esophageal acid contact time. Similar improvement was reported in pa-

tients with GER without apnea.[34] Also of interest with regard to sleep apnea syndrome is a study by Graf et al.[35] that determined that patients with sleep apnea have a high incidence of GER. The authors further determined that there is no relation between severity of sleep apnea and GER, nor is there any relation between apneic events and reflux events.

Of considerable interest is the fact that studies have documented that commonly consumed sedating drugs such as benzodiazepines and alcohol have been shown to prolong acid clearance during sleep.[36, 37] A study by Vitale et al.[36] showed that alcohol consumption approximately 3 h before sleep resulted in marked prolongation of the clearance of spontaneous episodes of GER. In another investigation of the effect of the administration of commonly used hypnotic drugs, a decrease was shown in the arousal latency and a prolongation was shown in the acid clearance time with triazolam.[37]

To summarize, these studies on acid clearance during sleep lend increasing support to the idea that sleep is a time of considerable risk for patients with reflux esophagitis and that intact afferent arousal mechanisms are important in allowing normal acid clearance from the distal esophagus. Furthermore, commonly ingested sedating compounds such as hypnotic drugs and alcohol appear to result in a prolongation of acid clearance time, which might make otherwise benign GER a more clinically significant event.

PULMONARY COMPLICATIONS OF NOCTURNAL GASTROESOPHAGEAL REFLUX

Nocturnal wheezing in persons with asthma and chronic nocturnal cough are pulmonary symptoms that have been linked to the occurrence of GER.[1, 37a, 37b] The GER may be clinically "silent," and treatment of the GER may reduce nocturnal asthma symptoms.[37b] In fact, a much greater incidence of nocturnal symptoms was identified in asthmatics who were subsequently found to have GER.[38] In the same study, symptoms such as night cough, nocturnal wheezing, shortness of breath, and other upper gastrointestinal complaints, especially when positionally induced, were significantly more common in asthmatics with GER than in those without reflux. David et al.[39] documented the fact that 47% of patients with chronic bronchitis have GER, and they noted that the most striking abnormality in these patients was a significant impairment of acid clearance. Results of the studies reviewed strongly suggest that prolonged acid clearance is most likely to occur during sleep. Furthermore, Sontag et al.[40] documented that an abnormal degree of GER is substantially more common in a group of unselected asthmatics than in control subjects. Cuttitta et al.[1] concluded that GER duration may determine the severity of nocturnal bronchoconstriction in asthmatics with GER. A study by Orr et al.[41] provided data with regard to esophageal function in another group of patients with lung dysfunction (i.e., chronic obstructive pulmonary disease). In this study, patients with chronic obstructive pulmonary disease failed to show any reflex bronchial constriction to esophageal acid infusion, and their nocturnal and diurnal acid exposure times were completely normal on 24-h pH monitoring. Thus, with regard to the relation between pulmonary functioning and reflux during sleep, it appears that there is something unique to the asthmatic patient.

Only rarely does a patient develop acute or chronic inflammatory lung disease as the direct consequence of GER. Orringer[42] commented in an editorial concerning respiratory systems in patients with GER: "Far more commonly than is generally appreciated, however, gastroesophageal reflux triggers a variety of respiratory symptoms in the absence of actual aspiration of gastric contents into the tracheal bronchial tree." He points out that because GER-related symptoms generally occur in the supine position during sleep and are generally resolved by assuming the upright position, symptoms such as shortness of breath may be confused with paroxysmal nocturnal dyspnea. Although it is clear that there are pulmonary symptoms that suggest nocturnal GER in their pathogenesis, daytime symptoms suggesting GER are not as consistently obvious. In a study of patients with esophageal pH and symptoms indicative of pulmonary aspiration, only approximately half of the patients had a significant symptom of heartburn.[43] The common symptoms associated with GER are not necessarily reliable indicators of the physiological presence of GER, particularly in patients with chronic pulmonary symptomatology.

Of considerable interest is the fact that there are a number of parameters of GER that are believed to be related to the likelihood of pulmonary aspiration and subsequent damage to the lung parenchyma; two of these are volume refluxed and pH of the refluxant. Questions concerning esophageal responsiveness to these critical stimuli during sleep were addressed subsequent to a previous study from our laboratory that suggested arousals to esophageal acid stimulation were enhanced during sleep.[25] It was shown that in normal asymptomatic volunteers with a negative acid perfusion test (no distinction between acid and water infused into the esophagus), acid provoked a marked increase in arousal responses during sleep. This suggested that esophageal responsivity was altered during sleep and that the enhanced arousal responses and shortened latency to swallowing were endogenous mechanisms designed to protect the tracheal bronchial tree from the aspiration of esophageal contents. Another parameter of importance may be the degree of proximal acid migration with the esophagus. Tuchman et al.[44] have shown in cats that tracheal stimulation with minute amounts of acid produces a markedly greater bronchoconstrictive response than occurs with much larger volumes placed in the distal esophagus. In addition, in infants, Kahn et al.[45] demonstrated that proximal esophageal acid contact acts as a strong arousal stimulus.

These study results are compatible with the notion that responses to a noxious and potentially dangerous stimulus such as acid are altered or amplified under circumstances of increased risk, (i.e., decreased level of consciousness such as the sleeping state). This hypothesis was tested by investigating the effect of parameters that would produce increased risk of pulmonary aspiration. As noted, two of these parameters are volume and pH. An increasing volume of reflux into the esophagus would be considered a greater risk for pulmonary aspiration, and it would be hypothesized that larger volumes would produce more prompt and vigorous responses. To test this hypothesis, three different volumes of 0.1 N HCl were infused into the distal esophagus during waking and sleep.[46] The data revealed that acid clearance was more rapid for the higher volumes; during waking, the latency to the first swallow was not noted to be significantly different, but subsequent to acid infusion during sleep, the latency clearly progressively decreased with increasing volume. Similarly, the latency to the arousal from sleep was significantly reduced with increasing volume.

In a follow-up study, as a further test of the hypothesis of differential esophageal acid sensitivity during sleep, the effect of different pH levels infused with constant volume was studied.[47] It has been well established, for example, that aspiration of fluid into the lungs at a relatively high pH (above 3.0) does not produce any significant damage to the lungs.[48] However, considerable damage and, in some instances, death can occur with the aspiration of more acidic gastric contents. In a study by Orr and Johnson,[47] acid (0.1 N HCl) was infused into the esophagus at a constant volume (15 ml) and pH 1.2, 3.0, and 5.0. These data also indicated that esophageal acid sensitivity is enhanced during sleep compared with during the waking state. Arousal latency, for example, was shown to be significantly decreased with an infusion of the lowest pH compared with the highest pH, and the latency to the first swallow was significantly decreased with pH 1.2 compared with 5.0. No differences were noted with infusions in the waking state. Data from these two experiments are quite consistent with the notion that the esophagus responds differentially during sleep to stimuli that would be considered to produce an increased risk of esophageal injury or pulmonary aspiration.

Published observations that acid in the distal esophagus can induce a reflex bronchoconstriction, presumably leading to pulmonary symptoms, have markedly changed the views on the medical significance of the relation between GER and pulmonary symptoms. If the latter occur only in the presence of true aspiration of gastric contents, obviously the significance of this complication diminishes substantially because it is well known that this is a relatively rare phenomenon. Mansfield and Stein[49] documented that acid alone in the distal esophagus produced an increase in pulmonary resistance when reflux symptoms occurred during the acid infusion. These studies were performed in 15 asthmatic patients, all of whom had a positive acid perfusion test (i.e., reproduction of typical substernal pyrosis with acid infusion into the esophagus). In a subsequent, more well-controlled study,[50] the same investigators noted that the increased pulmonary resistance and decreased air flow occurred only in patients with a positive acid perfusion test. In both of these studies, symptoms were relieved with antacid ingestion, further substantiating the notion that the pulmonary changes were reflexly induced by the presence of acid in the distal esophagus.

Obviously, GER can occur during waking or sleep; therefore, symptom induction by this mechanism would be expected to occur both during the daytime and at night. However, Spaulding et al.[50] noted that decreased air flow was apparent when the patients began to experience reflux symptoms. In our experience, symptom provocation in most people with esophagitis may take 5 min or longer with the acid perfusion test, so one might extrapolate from this that the esophagus must be perfused for a period of several minutes before symptoms will occur. From the results of previous studies, it is suspected that this would most commonly occur with nocturnal GER.

A clinical study by Goodall et al.[51] documented significant resolution of nocturnal symptoms only in those asthmatics treated with an H₂ receptor antagonist (cimetidine). There also was significant improvement in reflux symptoms in 14 of the 18 patients studied. In a clinical study by Harper et al.,[52] respiratory symptoms in a group of asthmatics with predominant nocturnal wheezing showed significant abatement with treatment for GER with 150 mg of ranitidine twice daily. The authors specifically commented in their discussion that GER should be considered in the pathogenesis of asthma symptoms, particularly in persons with nocturnal wheezing. These data lend additional support to the notion that the adequate treatment of reflux symptoms can substantially improve asthmatic symptoms. Although the presence of the clinical symptoms of GER in patients with pulmonary disease is notable, as emphasized previously, the presence of GER as a contributing factor to the pulmonary disease cannot be ruled out on the basis of an absence of symptoms of GER. This was again emphasized in a study by Berquist et al.[53] in which they documented the presence of "silent" physiological reflux in a group of asthmatic patients who were asymptomatic with regard to reflux symptoms.

In an excellent review, Murphy and Johnson[54] pointed out that the relationship among small airway disease, GER, and symptoms can be difficult to document historically because small airway resistance due to bronchial asthma can intensify at night and not be causally related. It seems clear, however, that regardless of the mechanism, empiric therapy can determine this relation by resolving pulmonary symptoms through a reduction in nocturnal GER.

The physiological and clinical data noted earlier suggest a relation between asthmatic symptoms, particularly nocturnal wheezing, and a reflex bronchoconstriction caused by GER. Despite the numerous studies noted, controversy remains, and any parsimonious explanation of these phenomena must account for some significant negative data. For example, in an excellent study by Tan et al.,[55] patients with nocturnal wheezing were studied at night with the use of respiratory and polysomnographic monitoring. These data showed no relation between spontaneous GER and pulmonary resistance measures, nor was there any relation with the exogenous infusion of acid. Similarly, in another study in patients with chronic obstructive pulmonary disease and varying degrees of reversible lung disease, acidification of the distal esophagus did not produce any notable change in respiratory resistance or conductance. Furthermore, these patients did not exhibit any alterations in daytime or nocturnal GER as noted with 24-h pH monitoring.

Further documentation of the relation between nocturnal pulmonary symptoms and nocturnal aspiration of gastric contents comes from a study by Chernow et al.[56] They used a scintiscanning technique that involved the instillation of a radionuclide into the stomach before sleep and a lung scan the next morning to identify any radioactivity. Their study documented positive scans in three of six patients suspected of having nocturnal pulmonary aspiration. In the patients with positive scans, they also documented the presence of prolonged episodes of reflux during sleep. It is of interest that a similar study documented a positive lung scan in 45% of normal persons who had a radionuclide placed in the posterior pharynx during sleep.[57] These data suggest that subtle pulmonary aspiration occurs in normal persons during sleep, and a somewhat more sensitive approach to this diagnosis would include placing the radionuclide directly into the stomach, as was done by Chernow et al.[56] It is particularly interesting that Huxley et al.[57] found that depressed consciousness markedly enhanced the rate of positive lung scans and that of the normal persons who were studied, those who reported multiple awakenings (arousals) during sleep uniformly had negative scans. These data suggest that arousals from sleep, as emphasized earlier, are important elements in response to acid in the upper airway.

Similar techniques used by Chernow et al.[56] have been applied to asthmatic patients with nocturnal wheezing. These investigators did not find evidence of pulmonary aspiration in this population of patients and proposed that the technique itself may lack adequate sensitivity or that pulmonary aspiration is relatively uncommon in asthmatic persons with nocturnal symptoms. Although the actual aspiration of gastric contents into the lungs may be uncommon,[58] there are numerous studies suggesting that the aspiration of gastric contents is not necessary to produce symptoms. The study by Tuchman et al.[44] noted previously suggested that a reflex gradient exists from the distal esophagus to the posterior pharyngeal airway and results in increasing intensity of reflex bronchoconstriction when acid is introduced in these areas. Although there have been some studies suggesting that proximal esophageal acid exposure can produce symptoms such as chronic cough, there are no definitive studies related to the occurrence of these symptoms and their relation to polysomnographically monitored sleep and esophageal acid exposure.

COMPLICATIONS OF NOCTURNAL GASTROESOPHAGEAL REFLUX IN CHILDREN

The complications of nocturnal GER in infants and children are similar to those noted in adults (i.e., pulmonary aspiration and the exacerbation of bronchial asthma) but, in addition, sleep apnea appears to be another documented consequence of nocturnal GER.[59] Clinical symptoms suggestive of nocturnal GER include persistent wheezing, cough, radiographic evidence of pneumonitis or pneumonia, and apnea. The documentation of abnormal GER in children is somewhat more difficult because reflux and regurgitation are considerably more common in this age group than in adults.

Jolley et al.[60] studied 24 asymptomatic children between the ages of 12 and 14 years with symptoms and complications of GER. The symptomatic children were clearly separated from the control subjects in terms of overall scores of GER. They point out, however, that although both groups of patients experienced reflux in the upright and supine positions, reflux was rarely noted in control subjects sleeping in the supine position longer than 2 h postprandially. They suggest that studies of distal esophageal pH during sleep would be particularly useful in children suspected of having complications related to clinically significant GER. In another study that included 24-h distal esophageal pH monitoring, Jolley et al.[61] found that episodes of GER lasting longer than 5 min during sleep significantly distinguished a group of infants and children with associated respiratory symptoms and complications.

A great deal of interest, and some controversy, has centered on the relation among GER, apnea, and sudden infant death. Much of the interest in this area stemmed from an observation by Herbst et al.,[62] who documented a case of sudden infant death that clearly appeared to be secondary to recurrent GER. In a subsequent study, this same group described apnea associated with reflux in a group of infants with respiratory distress.[60] Of particular interest in this study is the fact that the investigators were able to induce apnea with the instillation of acid into the esophagus. This induction of apnea could not be done with the instillation of water or formula. Although clinically there appears to be little doubt that there are occasional instances when apnea (either central or obstructive) is noted to be secondary to episodes of GER, most of the well-controlled studies in this area do not appear to substantiate a consistent relation between these two phenomena.[63–65] Of interest, however, is a report by Spitzer et al.[66] that describes a consistent relation between waking GER and obstructive apnea. Jolley et al.[67] suggested a relation between the occurrence of sudden infant death syndrome and the pattern of sleep-related GER. More specifically, the mean acid clearance time was a parameter consistently noted to be abnormally prolonged in this group. Jolley et al.[61, 67] used sleep monitoring to determine the relation between GER and pulmonary symptoms in infants. They also used these studies to determine the need for fundoplication in infants Their studies have shown excellent results in reducing both GER and pulmonary symptoms. These infants were essentially refractory to standard medical therapy but have shown excellent responses to fundoplication for reduction in GER.

INTESTINAL MOTILITY

Due to the technological and practical difficulties in monitoring intestinal activity, particularly in patients, relatively little has been done in terms of acquiring data on intestinal motility during sleeping and waking in patient populations of interest. However, some data have been gradually appearing in the medical literature. One study that used 24-h ambulatory monitoring of small intestinal motility in patients with irritable bowel syndrome was accomplished by Kellow et al.[68] Although nocturnal motor patterns did not differentiate the patient group from the control subjects, it was noted that there was a marked prolongation in phase II of the migrating motor complex (MMC; see Chapter 21 for definition) in the waking state in patients with irritable bowel syndrome (IBS). The notable lack of motility activity during sleep led these investigators to suggest that the changes in motor functioning noted were primarily the result of reactions to various "stressful" events occurring in the waking state. However, in a subsequent study, this group of investigators noted a marked increase in REM sleep in patients with IBS.[69] These data were interpreted as lending additional support to their speculation that this syndrome has a central nervous system pathogenesis.

In another study that examined the MMC in the patient with cyclic unipolar depression, Talley et al.[70] noted that during the depressed phase, there was a reduction in the number of MMCs and an increase in the mean interval between MMCs compared with the euthymic phase. They did not, however, document any relation between sleep stages and MMC activity in this patient. The authors noted that these results constitute "the first documentation of an association between psychiatric disease per se and motor functions of the upper intestine."

In another study that examined the effects of alcohol on the MMC, Charles et al.[71] showed that alcohol reduces phase II of the MMC during sleep (although the authors did not polysomnographically monitor sleep). The authors noted that the actual contractions during phase II were enhanced, and they interpreted this to suggest that these findings were more related to the central effects of alcohol than to the local effects. They pointed out that much of the alcohol would be metabolized by the time the actual effects on the amplitude were noted.

The observation by Kumar et al.[69] that REM sleep was enhanced in patients with IBS has prompted a number of investigations into sleep and functional bowel disorders to include IBS and functional dyspepsia. Using subjective reports of sleep quality, Goldsmith and Levin[72] documented that the exacerbation of IBS symptoms and poor sleep show a strong correlation. The obvious problems of a subjective study without physiological measurement of sleep are noted by Wingate,[73] one of the authors of the original study on IBS and sleep. Wingate points out that the occurrence of waking symptomatology may unduly influence the perception of the previous night's sleep, and without polysomnographic documentation of sleep, this influence cannot be discounted.

The original study by Kumar et al.[69] documenting the enhancement of REM sleep in patients with IBS reported on only six individuals who had a single night of sleep subsequent to small bowel intubation for monitoring of intestinal motility. With a small number of subjects and no attempt to adapt individuals to the laboratory setting (even though a control group was used), there is a high probability that these results were spurious. Orr et al.[74] attempted to replicate this study while at the same time noninvasively monitoring a gastrointestinal measure so that more natural sleep could be obtained. Nine patients with IBS and nine control subjects were studied with full polysomnographic monitoring and gastric electrical activity monitored by the surface electrogastrogram. In this study, a statistically significant increase in REM sleep was documented in the patients with IBS, but the absolute level of REM sleep was not nearly in the range reported by Kumar et al.[69] In addition, specific electrogastrographic changes were found to be associated with sleep in normal subjects that were not noted in patients with IBS. Normal volunteers showed a significant decrease in the spectral amplitude of the EGG three-cycle-per-minute rhythm during NREM sleep compared with during waking. Of interest is the fact that during REM sleep, the amplitude was significantly increased to levels approaching those in the waking state. The patients with IBS failed to significantly modulate the amplitude of the dominant frequency of the gastric electrical rhythm during any of these states of consciousness. The lack of modulation of the dominant frequency of the electrogastrographic amplitude during sleep in patients with IBS raises the possibility that other autonomic abnormalities may be unmasked by further study of physiological functioning during sleep.

In a study in patients with nonulcer dyspepsia (characterized by epigastric postprandial bloating, nausea, or early satiety), two thirds of 65 patients with nonulcer dyspepsia complained of general sleep disturbances suggestive of nonrestorative sleep (i.e., numerous wakenings after sleep onset, morning awakenings without feeling rested).[75] These were significantly more common than noted in control subjects, and 65% of those complaining of sleep disturbance attributed their sleep problem to their abdominal symptoms. Ten patients were also studied for a 24-h period with intestinal manometric monitoring, and a change in the rhythmicity of the MMC was found in the functional dyspeptic patients characterized by a significant decrease in the number of MMCs during the nocturnal recording interval.

Collectively, these results from various sleep investigations in patients with functional bowel disorders suggest not only that there are sleep disturbances noted in this patient population but also that the sleep disturbances may contribute to altered gastrointestinal functioning. Certainly, these studies confirm the notion that there are central nervous system alterations in patients with functional bowel disorders and that these alterations are perhaps uniquely identified during sleep.

Future studies on sleep in patients with functional bowel disorders will undoubtedly provide additional understanding of the pathophysiology of the brain-gut axis and its alterations during sleep.

Bassotti et al.[76] monitored colonic motility for 24 h in normal volunteers and in patients with chronic constipation. Although they documented a decrease in the number and duration of mass movements in the patients with chronic constipation, as well as a circadian pattern of decrease in mass movements during the night, no significant difference was noted between patients and control subjects with regard to the circadian pattern itself. In a similar study, Ferrara et al.[77] monitored the motor activity of the distal colon, rectum, and anal canal over a 24-h interval in patients with slow-transit constipation. These patients were compared with 10 healthy control subjects. The patients with slow-transit constipation were noted to have impaired responses to feeding as well as on awakening from sleep in the morning.

Another interesting observation concerning alterations in anorectal functioning during sleep concerns a study by Orkin et al.[78] in which the authors monitored rectal motor activity during sleep in patients who have undergone ileal-anal anastomosis. They noted that decreases in anal resting pressure coupled with marked minute-to-minute variations in pressure during sleep occurred in control subjects and in patients and, when particularly profound, led to nocturnal fecal incontinence in some patients.

CONCLUSIONS

It appears that there is an important relation between sleep and the development of various acid peptic diseases, such as duodenal ulcer disease and GER disease. The pathogenesis and treatment of these disorders relate in large measure to the control of acid secretion during sleep. The suppression of nocturnal acid secretion appears to be an essential element in the healing of duodenal ulcers, and the occurrence of nocturnal GER is an unquestionably important aspect of the development of serious complications of this disorder. Continuous monitoring of the distal esophageal pH to document nocturnal GER is emerging as an important and useful diagnostic tool. The respiratory complications of GER also appear to be associated with sleep-related GER. In addition, prolonged monitoring of small and large bowel motility appears to be a promising tool in further understanding the pathogenesis of various gastrointestinal diseases and how these diseases may be altered by sleeping and waking. An awareness of these sleep-related phenomena is becoming an important element in the practice of state-of-the-art gastroenterology, and future research will undoubtedly further substantiate the important role of sleep in the pathogenesis of gastrointestinal disease.

References

1. Cuttitta G, Cibella F, Visconti A, et al. Spontaneous gastroesophageal reflux and airway patency during the night in adult asthmatics. Am J Respir Crit Care Med. 2000;161:177–181.

2. Feldman M, Richardson CT. Total 24-hour gastric acid secretion in patients with duodenal ulcer: comparison with normal subjects and effects of cimetidine and parietal cell vagotomy. Gastroenterology. 1986;90:540–544.

3. Orr WC, Hall WH, Stahl ML, et al. Sleep patterns and gastric acid secretion in duodenal ulcer disease. Arch Intern Med. 1976; 136:655–660.

4. Kildebo S, Aronsen O, Bernersen B, et al. Cimetidine, 800 mg at night, in the treatment of duodenal ulcers. Scand J Gastroenterol. 1985;20:1147–1150.

5. Colin-Jones DG, Ireland A, Gear P, et al. Reducing overnight secretion of acid to heal duodenal ulcers: comparison of standard divided dose of ranitidine with a single dose administered at night. Am J Med. 1984;77:116–122.

6. Howden CW, Jones DB, Hunt RH. Nocturnal doses of H_2 receptor antagonists for duodenal ulcer. Lancet. 1985;1:647–648.

7. Gledhill T, Buck M, Paul A, et al. Comparison of the effects of proximal gastric vagotomy, cimetidine, and placebo on nocturnal intragastric acidity and acid secretion in patients with cimetidine resistant duodenal ulcer. Br J Surg. 1983;70:704–706.

8. Galmiche JP, Tranvouez JL, Denis P, et al. L'enregistrement nocturne du pH gastrique permet-il de prévoir la réponse thérapeutique des ulc; geres duodenaux sév; ageres traites par la ranitidine? Gastroenterol Clin Biol. 1985;9:583–589.

9. Gotthard R, Strom M, Sjodahl R, et al. 24-h study of gastric acidity and bile acid concentration after parietal cell vagotomy. Scand J Gastroenterol. 1986;21:503–508.

10. Gough KR, Bardhan KD, Crowe JP, et al. Ranitidine and cimetidine in prevention of duodenal ulcer relapse. Lancet. 1984;2:659–662.

11. Silvis SE. Final report on the United States multicenter trial comparing ranitidine to cimetidine as maintenance therapy following healing of duodenal ulcer. J Clin Gastroenterol. 1985; 7:482–487.

12. Santana IA, Sharma BK, Pounder RE, et al. 24-Hour intragastric acidity during maintenance treatment with ranitidine. Br Med J. 1984;289:1420.

13. Nebel OT, Fornes MF, Castell DO. Symptomatic gastroesophageal reflux: incidence and precipitating factors. Am J Dig Dis. 1976;21:953–956.

14. Johnson LF, DeMeester TR. Twenty-four hour pH monitoring of the distal esophagus. Am J Gastroenterol. 1974;62:325–332.

15. DeMeester TR, Johnson LF, Guy JJ, et al. Patterns of gastroesophageal reflux in health and disease. Ann Surg. 1976;184:459–470.

16. Johnson LF, DeMeester TR, Haggitt RC. Esophageal epithelial response to gastroesophageal reflux, a quantitative study. Am J Dig Dis. 1978;23:498–509.

17. Schlesinger PK, Honahue PE, Schmid B, et al. Limitations of 24-hour intraesophageal pH monitoring in the hospital setting. Gastroenterology. 1985;89:797–804.

18. Orr WC, Allen ML, Robinson M. The pattern of nocturnal and diurnal esophageal acid exposure in the pathogenesis of erosive mucosal damage. Am J Gastro. 1994;89:509–512.

19. De Caestecker, Blackwell JH, Brown J, et al. When is acid reflux most damaging to the esophagus? [abstract]. Gastroenterology. 1985;88:1360.

20. Helm JF, Dodds WJ, Hogan WJ, et al. Acid neutralizing capacity of human saliva. Gastroenterology. 1982;83:69–74.

21. Allen ML, Orr WC, Woodruff DM, et al. The effects of swallowing frequency and transdermal scopolamine on esophageal acid clearance. Am J Gastroenterol. 1985;80:669–672.

22. Lichter J, Muir RC. The pattern of swallowing during sleep. Electroencephalogr Clin Neurophysiol. 1975;38:427–432.

23. Schneyer LH, Pigman W, Hanahan L, et al. Rate of flow of human parotid, sublingual, and submaxillary secretions during sleep. J Dent Res. 1956;35:109–114.

24. Orr WC, Robinson MG, Johnson LF. Acid clearing during sleep in the pathogenesis of reflux esophagitis. Dig Dis Sci. 1981;26:423.

25. Orr WC, Johnson LF, Robinson MG. The effect of sleep on swallowing, esophageal peristalsis, and acid clearance. Gastroenterology. 1984;86:814–819.

26. Orr WC, Lackey C, Robinson MG, et al. Acid clearance and reflux during sleep in Barrett's esophagus. Gastroenterology. 1983;84:1265.

27. Johnson LF, Harmon JW. Experimental esophagitis in a rabbit

model: clinical relevance. J Clin Gastroenterol. 1986;8 (suppl 1):26–44.

28. Anderson LIB, Madsen PV, Dalgaard P, et al. Validity of clinical symptoms in benign esophageal disease, assessed by questionnaire. Acta Med Scand. 1987;221:171–177.

29. Johnson LF, DeMeester TR. Evaluation of the head of the bed, bethanechol, and antacid foam tablets on gastroesophageal reflux. Dig Dis Sci. 1981;26:673–680.

30. Behar J, Brand DL, Brown FC, et al. Cimetidine in the treatment of symptomatic gastroesophageal reflux: a double-blind controlled trial. Gastroenterology. 1978;74:441–448.

31. Sontag S, Glaxo, GERD Research Group. Ranitidine therapy for gastroesophageal reflux disease. Results of a large double-blind trial. Arch Intern Med. 1987;147:1485–1491.

32. Orr WC, Robinson MG, Humphries T. Dose response effect of famotidine on patterns of gastroesophageal reflux. Aliment Pharmacol Ther. 1988;2:229–235.

33. Kerr P, Shoenut P, Millar T, et al. Nasal CPAP reduces gastroesophageal reflux in obstructive sleep apnea syndrome. Chest. 1992;101:1539–1544.

34. Kerr P, Shoenut JP, Steens RD, et al. Nasal CPAP: a new treatment for nocturnal gastroesophageal reflux. J Clin Gastroenterol. 1993;17:276–280.

35. Graf KI, Karaus M, Heinemann S, et al. Gastroesophageal reflux in patients with sleep apnea syndrome. Zeitschrift Gastroenterol 1995;33:689–693.

36. Vitale GC, Cheadle WG, Patel B, et al. The effect of alcohol on nocturnal gastroesophageal reflux. JAMA. 1987;258:2077–2079.

37. Orr WC, Robinson MG, Rundell OH. The effect of hypnotic drugs on acid clearance during sleep. Gastroenterology. 1985; 88:1526.

37a. Field SK. Gastroesophageal reflux and asthma: are they related? J Asthma. 1999;36:631–644.

37b. Kiljander TO, Salomaa ER, Hietanen EK, et al. Gastroesophageal reflux in asthmatics: a double-blind, placebo-controlled crossover study with omeprazole. Chest. 1999;116:1257–1264.

38. Perrin-Foyalle M, Bell A, Kofman J, et al. Asthma and gastroesophageal reflux: results of a survey of over 250 cases. Poumon Coeur. 1980;36:225–230.

39. David P, Denis P, Nouvet G, et al. Lung function and gastroesophageal reflux during chronic bronchitis. Bull Eur Physiopathol Respir. 1982;18:81–86.

40. Sontag SJ, O'Connell S, Khandelwal S, et al. Most asthmatics have gastroesophageal reflux with or without bronchodilator therapy. Gastroenterology. 1990;99:613–620.

41. Orr WC, Shamma-Othman Z, Allen M, et al. Esophageal function and gastroesophageal reflux during sleep and waking in patients with chronic obstructive pulmonary disease. Chest. 1992; 101:1521–1525.

42. Orringer MB. Respiratory symptoms and esophageal reflux. Chest. 1979;76:618–619.

43. Pelligrini CA, DeMeester TR, Johnson LF, et al. Gastroesophageal reflux and pulmonary aspiration: incidence, functional abnormality, and results of surgical therapy. Surgery. 1979;86:110–119.

44. Tuchman DN, Boyle JT, Pack AI, et al. Comparison of airway responses following tracheal or esophageal acidification in the cat. Gastroenterology. 1984;87:872–881.

45. Kahn A, Rebuffate E, Sottiaux M, et al. Arousals induced by proximal esophageal reflux in infants. Sleep. 1991;14:39–42.

46. Orr WC, Robinson MG, Johnson LF. The effect of esophageal acid volume on arousals from sleep and acid clearance. Chest. 1991;99:351–355.

47. Orr WC, Johnson LF. Responses to different levels of esophageal acidification during waking and sleep. Dig Dis Sci. 1998;43:241–245.

48. Terry PB, Fuller SD. Pulmonary consequences of aspiration. Dysphagia. 1989;3:179–183.

49. Mansfield LE, Stein MR. Gastroesophageal reflux and asthma: a possible reflex mechanism. Ann Allergy. 1978;41:224–226.

50. Spaulding HS, Mansfield LE, Stein MR, et al. Further investigation of the association between gastroesophageal reflux and bronchoconstriction. J Allergy Clin Immunol. 1982;69:516–521.

51. Goodall RJR, Earis JE, Cooper DN, et al. Relationship between asthma and gastro-oesophageal reflux. Thorax. 1981;36:116–121.

52. Harper PC, Bergner A, Kaye MD. Antireflux treatment for

asthma: improvement in patients with associated gastroesophageal reflux. Arch Intern Med. 1987;147:56–60.

53. Berquist WE, Rachelefsky GS, Rawshan N, et al. Quantitative gastroesophageal reflux and pulmonary function in asthmatic children and normal adults receiving placebo, theophylline, and metaproterenol sulfate therapy. J Allergy Clin Immunol. 1984;73:253–258.

54. Murphy JR, Johnson LF. Sleep and the respiratory complications of gastroesophageal reflux. Pract Gastroenterol. 1993;17:16–29.

55. Tan WC, Martin RJ, Pandey R, et al. Effects of spontaneous and simulated gastroesophageal reflux on sleeping asthmatics. Am Rev Respir Dis. 1990;141:1394–1399.

56. Chernow B, Johnson LF, Janowitz WR, et al. Pulmonary aspiration as a consequence of gastroesophageal reflux: a diagnostic approach. Dig Dis Sci. 1979;24:839–844.

57. Huxley EJ, Viroslav J, Gray WR, et al. Pharyngeal aspiration in normal adults with depressed consciousness. Am J Med. 1978;64:564–568.

58. Ghaed N, Stein MR. Assessment of a technique for scintigraphic monitoring of pulmonary aspiration of gastric contents in asthmatics with gastroesophageal reflux. Ann Allergy. 1979;42:306–308.

59. Herbst JJ, Minton SD, Book LS. Gastroesophageal reflux causing respiratory distress and apnea in newborn infants. J Pediatr. 1979;95:763.

60. Jolley SG, Johnson DG, Herbst JJ, et al. An assessment of gastroesophageal reflux in children by extended pH monitoring of the distal esophagus. Surgery. 1978;84:16–24.

61. Jolley SG, Herbst JJ, Johnson DG, et al. Esophageal pH monitoring during sleep identifies children with respiratory symptoms from gastroesophageal reflux. Gastroenterology. 1981;80:1501–1506.

62. Herbst JJ, Book LS, Bray PF. Gastroesophageal reflux in the "near miss" sudden infant death syndrome. J Pediatr. 1978;92:73.

63. Ariagno RL, Guilleminault C, Baldwin R, et al. Movement and gastroesophageal reflux in awake term infants with "near miss" SIDS, unrelated to apnea. J Pediatr. 1982;100:894.

64. Jeffrey HE, Reid I, Rohilly P, et al. Gastroesophageal reflux in "near miss" sudden infant death infants in active but not quiet sleep. Sleep. 1980;3:393.

65. Walsh JK, Farrell MK, Keenan WJ, et al. Gastroesophageal reflux in infants: relation to apnea. J Pediatr. 1981;99:197.

66. Spitzer AR, Boyle JT, Tuchman DN, et al. Awake apnea associated with gastroesophageal reflux: a specific clinical syndrome. J Pediatr. 1984;104:200–204.

67. Jolley SG, Halpern LM, Tunell WP, et al. The risk of sudden death from gastroesophageal reflux. J Pediatr Surg. 1991;26:691–696.

68. Kellow JE, Gill RG, Wingate DL. Prolonged ambulant recordings of small bowel motility demonstrate abnormalities in the irritable bowel syndrome. Gastroenterology. 1990;98:1208–1218.

69. Kumar D, Thompson PD, Wingate DL, et al. Abnormal REM sleep in the irritable bowel syndrome. Gastroenterology. 1992;103:12–17.

70. Talley NJ, Camilleri M, Orkin BA, et al. Effect of cyclical unipolar depression on upper gastrointestinal motility and sleep. Gastroenterology. 1989;97:775–777.

71. Charles F, Evans DF, Castillo FD, et al. Daytime indigestion of alcohol alters nighttime jejunal motility in man. Dig Dis Sci. 1994;39:51–58.

72. Goldsmith G, Levin JS. Effect of sleep quality on symptoms of irritable bowel syndrome. Dig Dis Sci. 1993;38:1809–1814.

73. Wingate D. An association between poor sleep quality and the severity of IBS symptoms [letter]. Dig Dis Sci. 1994;39:2350–2351.

74. Orr WC, Crowell MD, Lin B, et al. Sleep and gastric function in irritable bowel syndrome: derailing the brain-gut axis. Gut. 1997;41:390–393.

75. David D, Mertz H, Fefer L, et al. Sleep and duodenal motor activity in patients with severe non-ulcer dyspepsia. Gut. 1994;35:916–925.

76. Bassotti G, Gaburri M, Imbimbo BP, et al. Alimentary tract and pancreas: colonic mass movements in idiopathic chronic constipation. Gut. 1988;29:1173–1179.

77. Ferrara A, Pemberton JH, Hanson RB. Motor responses of the sigmoid, rectum and anal canal in health and in patients with slow transit constipation (STC). Gastroenterology. 1991;100:A441.

78. Orkin BA, Soper NJ, Kelly KA, et al. Influence of sleep on anal sphincter pressure in health and after ileal pouch-anal anastomosis. Dis Colon Rectum. 1992;35:137–144.

fourteen

Psychiatric Disorders

J. Christian Gillin

Anxiety Disorders

Thomas W. Uhde

"Are you worried or anxious about something?" This probably is the most commonly asked question of individuals complaining of insomnia. Underlying this question is the almost universal belief that anxiety causes insomnia. Despite this widespread assumption, few studies have investigated the sleep of patients with anxiety disorders. The lack of empirically based information is striking given the high lifetime prevalence (about 8%) of anxiety disorders in U.S. citizens. This chapter provides a review of the diagnostic criteria, sleep features, and treatment of sleep-related problems in patients with panic disorder, generalized anxiety disorder, social phobia, post-traumatic stress disorder, simple phobias, and obsessive-compulsive disorders.

PANIC DISORDER

Phenomenology and Demography

The characteristic feature of panic disorder is recurrent, unexpected *panic attacks* (Table 95–1), which are acute episodes of severe anxiety associated with a wide array of somatic symptoms, such as chest pain, heart palpitations, tachycardia, psychosensory disturbances (i.e., changes in sound or light intensity, alterations in the perception of time, floating or turning sensations, depersonalization or derealization), gastrointestinal discomfort, and lightheadedness. Classic panic attacks reach peak severity within 10 min and are short lived (i.e., seconds to minutes).

Not all people who have panic attacks have a *panic disorder*. A few individuals may experience infrequent panic attacks for years without conspicuous changes in their health. More often, however, panic attacks are complicated by anticipatory anxiety (i.e., apprehension about future attacks), and many patients worry about possible underlying medical disorders (e.g., heart disease). Such concerns, if lasting for 1 month or longer after the panic attack or attacks, justify the designation of panic disorder.

Patients also may become frightened of places or situations in which unexpected panic attacks have occurred. The actual avoidance of places (e.g., bridges, tunnels, airplanes) or situations (e.g., driving, shopping, traveling) in which unexpected panic attacks, limited-symptom attacks, or panic-like symptoms have occurred in the past is referred to as *agoraphobia* (Table 95–2).

The natural course of panic disorder is characterized by the following sequential events: (1) unexpected (also referred to as *spontaneous* or *uncued*) panic attacks and (2) apprehension about future panic attacks (i.e., *anticipatory* or *generalized anxiety*). Many patients with panic disorder also develop two additional complications: (1) secondary fears (i.e., *phobia*) and (2) increasing constriction of lifestyle due to the avoidance of these secondary fears (i.e., agoraphobia).[1] Patients may proceed rapidly along this pathological continuum or remain at any particular stage without acquiring further complications; therefore, individuals may report varying admixtures (i.e., frequency and/or severity) of sleep or wake panic attacks, anticipatory or generalized anxiety, band

Table 95–1. DSM-IV CRITERIA FOR PANIC ATTACK

A discrete period of intense fear or discomfort, in which four (or more) of the following symptoms developed abruptly and reached a peak within 10 min:
Palpitations, pounding heart, or accelerated heart rate
Sweating
Trembling or shaking
Sensations of shortness of breath or smothering
Feeling of choking
Chest pain or discomfort
Nausea or abdominal distress
Feeling dizzy, unsteady, lightheaded, or faint
Derealization (feelings of unreality) or depersonalization (being detached from oneself)
Fear of losing control or going crazy
Fear of dying
Paresthesias (numbness or tingling sensations)
Chills or hot flashes

Reprinted with permission from the *Diagnostic and Statistical Manual of Mental Disorders, Fourth Edition.* Copyright 1994 American Psychiatric Association.
DSM-IV, *Diagnostic and Statistical Manual of Mental Disorders, Fourth Edition.*

Table 95–3. DSM-IV CRITERIA FOR PANIC DISORDER WITHOUT AGORAPHOBIA

A. Both 1 and 2:
  1. Recurrent unexpected panic attacks
  2. At least one of the attacks has been followed by 1 month (or more) of one (or more) of the following:
     a. Persistent concern about having additional attacks
     b. Worry about the implications of the attack or its consequences (e.g., losing control, having a heart attack, "going crazy")
     c. A significant change in behavior related to the attacks
B. The absence of agoraphobia
C. The panic attacks are not due to the direct physiological effects of a substance (e.g., a drug of abuse, a medication) or a general medical condition (e.g., hyperthyroidism)
D. The panic attacks are not better accounted for by another mental disorder such as *Social phobia* (e.g., occurring on exposure to feared social situations), *Specific phobia* (e.g., on exposure to a specific phobic situation), *Obsessive-compulsive disorder* (e.g., on exposure to dirt in someone with an obsession about contamination), *Post-traumatic stress disorder* (e.g., in response to stimuli associated with severe stressor), or *Separation anxiety* (e.g., in response to being away from home or close relatives).

Reprinted with permission from the *Diagnostic and Statistical Manual of Mental Disorders, Fourth Edition.* Copyright 1994 American Psychiatric Association.
DSM-IV, *Diagnostic and Statistical Manual of Mental Disorders, Fourth Edition.*

agoraphobia. Depending on the absence or presence of agoraphobia, respectively, patients are given a diagnosis of panic disorder *without* or *with* agoraphobia (Tables 95–3 and 95–4).

Panic disorder affects approximately two to three times as many women as men. The average age at onset of panic attacks is 22 years, although even prepubescent children have experienced full-blown panic attacks and agoraphobia. Agoraphobia without a history

of panic attacks is also recognized in the *Diagnostic and Statistical Manual of Mental Disorders, Fourth Edition* (DSM-IV) nomenclature but is an extremely rare (or nonexistent) condition.

The DSM-IV makes no mention of sleep panic attacks, so no official diagnostic pathways are provided for the differential diagnosis of patients who present with sleep panic attacks. It is unclear what DSM-IV diagnosis a patient with only sleep panic attacks should receive, although the 1991 National Institutes of Health Consensus Development Conference acknowledged that panic disorder is a condition in which panic attacks may "also occur during sleep."[2]

Most patients report that a greater proportion of their panic attacks occur during wake versus sleeping states. There is, however, an important subgroup of patients with panic disorder who experience a majority of their panic attacks during sleep.

In this chapter, the terms *nocturnal panic* and *sleep panic* are synonymous and refer to the same phenomenon.

Table 95–2. CRITERIA FOR AGORAPHOBIA*

A. Anxiety about being in places or situations from which escape might be difficult (or embarrassing) or in which help may not be available in the event of having an unexpected or situationally predisposed panic attack or panic-like symptoms. Agoraphobic fears typically involve characteristic clusters of situations that include being outside the home alone, being in a crowd or standing in a line, being on a bridge, and traveling in a bus, train, or automobile.
  Note: Consider the diagnosis of *Specific phobia* if the avoidance is limited to one or only a few specific situations or *Social phobia* if the avoidance is limited to social situations.
B. The situations are avoided (e.g., travel is restricted) or else are endured with marked distress or with anxiety about having a panic attack or panic-like symptoms or require the presence of a companion.
C. The anxiety or phobic avoidance is not better accounted for by another mental disorder, such as *Social phobia* (e.g., avoidance limited to social situations because of fear of embarrassment), *Specific phobia* (e.g., avoidance limited to a single situation, like elevators), *Obsessive-compulsive disorder* (e.g., avoidance of dirt in someone with an obsession about contamination), *Post-traumatic stress disorder* (e.g., avoidance of stimuli associated with a severe stressor), or *Separation anxiety disorder* (e.g., avoidance of leaving home or relatives).

*Agoraphobia is not a DSM-IV codable disorder. Code the specific disorder in which the agoraphobia occurs (e.g., *Panic disorder with agoraphobia* or *Agoraphobia without history of panic disorder*).
DSM-IV, *Diagnostic and Statistical Manual of Mental Disorders, Fourth Edition.*

Table 95–4. DSM-IV CRITERIA FOR PANIC DISORDER WITH AGORAPHOBIA

A. Meets the criteria for *Panic disorder*
B. Meets the criteria for *Agoraphobia*

Reprinted with permission from the *Diagnostic and Statistical Manual of Mental Disorders, Fourth Edition.* Copyright 1994 American Psychiatric Association.
DSM-IV, *Diagnostic and Statistical Manual of Mental Disorders, Fourth Edition.*

CASE HISTORY 1: SLEEP PANIC

Ms. B. is a 30-year-old woman with a 17-year history of panic disorder. Her first lifetime episode of panic attacks awakened her from sleep at the age of 13. Both this initial and subsequent sleep panic attacks were characterized by abrupt arousals from sleep without dream recall. She denied somnambulism. Her sleep panic attacks were associated with a sense of impending doom, heart palpitations, shortness of breath, and lightheadedness that lasted for several minutes.

The patient experienced her first daytime panic attack at the age of 15, approximately 2 years after her first sleep panic attack. Her daytime awake panic attacks, which were similar in quality to her sleep panic attacks, often were unpredictable or triggered by exercise. It was not unusual for Ms. B. to have many episodes of daytime awake or sleep panic attacks within 24 h. Despite her frequent daytime wake and sleep panic attacks, she reported minimal degrees of avoidance behavior.

During the month before her admission to the National Institute of Mental Health, Ms. B. had had 35 sleep panic attacks and 30 wake panic attacks. Treatment consisted of imipramine and alprazolam. She had a total response (i.e., complete blockade of wake and sleep panic attacks) on this drug combination, although she relapsed when these drugs were discontinued during a later pregnancy.

CASE HISTORY 2: SLEEP PANIC AND SLEEP AVOIDANCE

Ms. C. is a 26-year-old single woman with a 10-year history of panic disorder with agoraphobia. Her first daytime panic attack developed at home while reading a newspaper. The occurrence of several additional panic attacks within the next several weeks led to an extensive medical and neurological workup. No evidence of neurological or cardiovascular disease was identified. Her daytime wake panic attacks featured heart palpitations, tachycardia, sweating, hand tremors, hot flashes, chest tightness, psychosensory disturbances, and shortness of breath. The patient was treated for several years with insight-oriented psychotherapy that improved her ability to deal with stressful family issues but had no effect on the frequency or severity of her daytime wake panic attacks. Ms. C. gradually developed multiple fears typical of agoraphobia (i.e., fear of elevators, grocery shopping, bridges, crowded places, and public transportation) and became unable to travel beyond a 1-mile radius of her home. These avoidance behaviors increasingly dominated her life, leading to complete disability in terms of work and social function.

Several years after the onset of daytime wake panic attack, Ms. C. developed sleep panic attacks. The patient had a history of nightmares but stated that her sleep panic attacks were quite different in quality from her nightmares. She denied any dream content associated with her sleep panic attacks. Ms. C. described awakening from sleep with a pounding chest, sweating, numbness in her hands, and a choking sensation. She also had a fear that she might die of suffocation. Ms. C. quickly became frightened of sleeping ("I didn't want to die in my sleep") and developed a progressive pattern of bizarre sleep behaviors (e.g., sleeping in a sitting position, sleeping in a chair, sleeping without bedspreads, lowering or raising the temperature in the room, and asking a friend or family member to sleep in a nearby room). These behaviors were intentionally promulgated by the patient in an attempt to obtain rest without "sleeping to the point of panic." A consequence of her sleep phobia, however, was the development of chronic intermittent sleep deprivation and an apparent increase in the frequency and severity of both sleep and wake panic attacks.

Sleep Complaints and Electroencephalography

Subjective Complaints. Insomnia; restless, broken, or "fitful" sleep; and nocturnal (i.e., during sleep) panic attacks are common complaints in patients with panic disorder.[2–7] Sixty-five percent of patients with panic disorder have a history of nocturnal panic attacks, and 30 to 45% report repeated episodes throughout their lifetimes.

Unquestionably, the most disturbing and disabling sleep problem in panic disorder is nocturnal panic (i.e., sleep panic attacks). Nocturnal panic attacks are characterized by an abrupt arousal from sleep and, on awakening, a sense of impending doom, fear, palpitations, shortness of breath, chest discomfort, feelings of unreality, and hot or cold flashes. Sleep panic symptoms are similar in quality, severity, and duration to wake panic attacks, although dyspnea may be more common in nocturnal than in wake panic attacks. Not surprisingly, patients with panic disorder with nocturnal panic attacks report higher rates of insomnia, especially nonrestorative sleep and frequent awakenings, than do those without.[3, 7, 8]

Perhaps the most serious downstream complication of nocturnal panic attacks is chronic intermittent sleep deprivation.[9] As presented in Case 2 and Figure 95–1, patients with nocturnal panic attacks develop secondary anticipatory anxiety and avoidance behaviors in a manner identical to the development of agoraphobia in patients with wake panic attacks. Specifically in response to nocturnal panic attacks, many patients develop a conditioned fear and avoidance of sleep. The resultant sleep deprivation causes a worsening of anxiety.[10] In fact, clinical experience suggests that the subgroup of patients with nocturnal wake panic attacks is especially vulnerable to sleep deprivation–induced increases in both wake and nocturnal panic attacks. We reported that patients with panic disorder, particularly those with nocturnal attacks, are particularly vulnerable to the anxiogenic effects of relaxation.[11] This information, combined with the knowledge that sleep deprivation itself produces sedation and a "drive" toward relaxation, led to the proposal that "relative increases in P_{CO_2} may form a common mechanism for the pan-

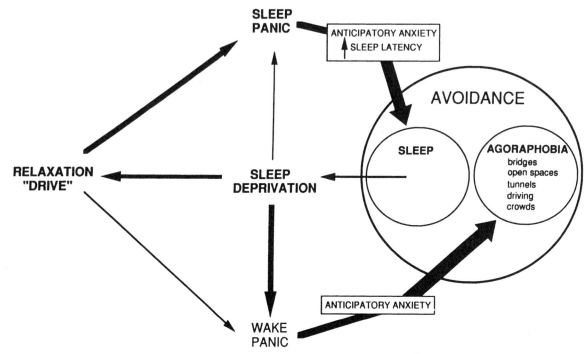

Figure 95–1. Classic panic disorder: Individuals who experience "spontaneous" panic attacks while awake often become fearful about having future panic attacks (i.e., "anticipatory anxiety"). The context associated with the spontaneous panic attacks may be viewed as causative in nature and, as a result, individuals may then develop secondary fears and may avoid situations (e.g., crowds) and/or places (e.g., bridges, tunnels, and crowds) associated with the original panic attacks. Sleep panic attacks: Individuals with sleep panic attacks develop a pattern of fear and avoidance similar to the course of illness found in patients with classic panic disorder. The occurrence of sleep panic attacks may produce a secondary fear of sleeping (i.e., conditioned fear of sleep) followed by a pattern of chronic-intermittent sleep deprivation. Emerging evidence suggests that sleep deprivation may trigger or exacerbate the frequency and severity of "wake" and "sleep" panic attacks.

icogenic effects of CO_2 inhalation, sleep-induced panic attacks, and relaxation-induced panic attacks"[9, 11] (see Fig. 95–1). Within this context, it is interesting that Stein et al.[12] reported that patients with panic disorder have an increased rate of microapneas (5 to 10 sec) during sleep compared with a healthy control group. These converging lines of evidence suggest a possible role for abnormal respiratory or brain CO_2 "receptor" dysfunction in panic disorder.

Patients with sleep panic attacks are often embarrassed about their fear of sleep, especially adult men, and may invent excuses for their poor sleep habits (e.g., "I have too much work to go to bed"). In truth, they have developed a conditioned fear of sleep and sleeping. Patients will pursue a number of strategies to obtain "rest without sleeping," such as sitting up in bed; reclining in a chair; turning on the radio, television, or bright lights; or changing the temperature of the bedroom to uncomfortably low or high degrees. If not thwarted by the shame of having a "silly fear of sleep," they may even request that a friend or spouse watch them sleep or be immediately available in case of a nocturnal panic attack.

Patients with panic disorder can accurately differentiate between sleep panic attacks (nonrapid eye movement [NREM] events without cognitions or vivid imagery[3, 6, 13]) and dream anxiety attacks (rapid eye movement [REM] events associated with elaborate dream content), although both panic attacks and night-

mares may be associated with autonomic activation (i.e., increased respiratory or heart rate, or both).

Knowledge regarding the sleep electroencephalographic (EEG) correlates of sleep panic attacks is insufficient to draw undisputed conclusions. Nevertheless, converging lines of evidence suggest that sleep panic attacks can be distinguished from night terrors, nightmares, sleep apnea, or the flashback nightmares of post-traumatic stress disorder.

Sleep panic attacks are NREM-related events, usually emerging from late stage 2 or early stage 3 sleep.[6, 13] Most nocturnal panic attacks occur within 3 h of sleep onset. Sleep panic attacks are short lived, lasting approximately 2 to 8 min. Nocturnal panic attacks are not associated with dreams, cognition, or imagery. When EEG-verified nightmares do take place in people with a history of coexisting panic attacks and nightmares, subjects consistently discriminate between their REM-related nightmares and stage 2 or 3 nocturnal panic attacks (see Case 2).

Bell et al.[14] speculated about a possible connection between sleep paralysis and sleep-related panic attacks. It is well known that sleep paralysis can be a frightening experience. The authors, however, found that 9 of 25 subjects (35%) with isolated sleep paralysis also reported a history of wake panic attacks unrelated to the experience of paralysis; 4 of these individuals (16%) with isolated sleep paralysis met full diagnostic DSM-III criteria of panic disorder. Controlled studies have not reported an unusually high rate of sleep paralysis among patients with panic disorder. Nevertheless, it is possible that patients with sleep paralysis have an increased rate of panic disorder but that panic disorder itself is not associated with an increased risk of sleep paralysis. The true association, if any, between sleep panic attacks and sleep paralysis must be determined in future studies.

What about traditional objective measures of EEG sleep recording? Cumulative evidence indicates that REM indices (i.e., REM latency, REM density, REM percent, number and progression of REM periods, REM interruptions) are essentially normal in patients with panic disorder.[6, 13, 15–17] The percentages of stage 1, stage 2, and delta sleep have consistently been found to be normal in patients with panic disorder compared with normal control subjects.

The original National Institute of Mental Health study[17] and two subsequent studies[6, 11] reported an increase in movement time among patients with panic disorder. At first, we thought that panic disorder might be a syndrome characterized by an increase in arousal throughout the sleep-wake cycle. In an attempt to confirm this hypothesis, we investigated a second group of patients with panic disorder[13] and found a nonsignificant increase in movement time (14.5 ± 7.6 min) in a group of 13 patients with panic disorder compared with 7 normal control subjects (11.3 ± 8.2 min). Although these findings were not significant, the results were in the direction of increased movement time in the patients with panic disorder. Of interest, we also found that the six patients with sleep panic attacks had the lowest levels of movement time (10.2 ± 7.6 min), whereas the patients without sleep panic attacks had the highest levels of movement time (16.0 ± 12.2 min; P = NS). We subsequently reexamined the one patient who had a sleep panic attack in the 1984 study[17] and found that this individual had the lowest amount of movement time of the nine patients investigated. Based on these observations, combined with independent lines of evidence suggesting a role for relaxation-induced panic attacks, the author postulates that *increased* movement during sleep may actually confer a degree of compensatory protection against, rather than provoke or represent a pathological correlate of, sleep panic attacks.

Given the high prevalence of subjective complaints of insomnia in patients with panic disorder, one might expect to uncover marked disturbances in initiation and maintenance of sleep. Patients with panic disorder, as a group, have EEG documented evidence of difficulty falling asleep and reduced sleep efficiency. However, the severity of these problems, as documented by polysomnography, is less impressive than might be anticipated given the degree of subjective distress. The mean sleep latency and sleep efficiency in patients with panic disorder across four studies (with available data) were only 32.0 ± 10.9 and 84.5 ± 4.4 min, respectively, compared with the values of 19.1 ± 11.4 and 89.4 ± 5.9 min in the normal control subjects. Emerging data suggest that patients with sleep panic attacks may have the greatest problems with maintaining sleep, although

this is highly variable and not uniformly observed across case reports or controlled studies.

Taken together, the observations of several research teams indicate that complaints of insomnia and sleep panic attacks are reported by a majority of patients with panic disorder. The sleep EEG generally corroborates complaints of restless broken sleep, although as a group, the sleep architecture of patients with panic disorder is surprisingly "normal." Sleep panic attacks (when evaluated in patients with pure panic disorder under controlled conditions) appear to be linked in most cases with late stage 2 or early stage 3 sleep. Case reports of panic disorder,[14, 18–20] often involving patients with atypical panic disorder or medical imposters of panic disorder, provide less consistent evidence for a specific linkage between sleep panic and stage 2 or 3 sleep. In part, this lack of consistency among the case reports of "real world" clinical medicine probably reflects the fact that many different sleep or medical conditions may be associated, at one time or another, with frightening arousals from sleep or complex sleep behaviors.[21–24] These issues should be taken into consideration when interpreting or conducting research designed to improve understanding of sleep panic attacks. Although complaints of insomnia or sleep panic attacks probably oscillate with the changing course of panic disorder, it is unknown whether insomnia, sleep panic attacks, or both can arise as independent problems during otherwise quiescent periods of illness.

Treatment

The aim of drug treatment is to block panic attacks (wake and nocturnal panic attacks) and to eliminate secondary fears and avoidance behaviors (e.g., sleep phobias). The removal of exogenous (e.g., caffeine) factors or the correction of maladaptive behaviors (e.g., sleep deprivation) that often exacerbate panic disorder should also be an integral part of the treatment program. The ultimate goal is a return of the patient to a totally normal lifestyle.

Historically, tricyclic antidepressants (i.e., imipramine), monoamine oxidase inhibitors (MAOIs) (i.e., phenelzine), and high-potency benzodiazepines (i.e., alprazolam, clonazepam) have been the main drugs used to block daytime wake panic attacks. Selective serotonin reuptake inhibitors (SSRIs) (e.g., fluoxetine) have been found to be effective in the treatment of panic disorder. Clinicians, however, should be vigilant about fluoxetine-related insomnia. Clinical practice further suggests that many older antidepressant medications (e.g., desipramine, nortriptyline, amitriptyline, doxepin) are probably effective in the treatment of classic panic disorder (i.e., patients with typical daytime wake panic attacks).

Not all antidepressant compounds, however, are useful in the treatment of panic disorder. Bupropion, trazodone, and protriptyline tend to be ineffective or low in potency or poorly tolerated by most patients with panic disorder. Even drugs effective in the treatment of some other anxiety conditions may prove to be ineffective in the treatment of panic disorder (e.g., propranolol, buspirone). Cognitive-behavioral techniques are also valuable in the treatment of avoidance behaviors and panic attacks. There is little information regarding the treatment of patients with panic disorder who have nocturnal panic attacks; whether patients *with* sleep panic attacks respond to the same or different medications as do patients *without* sleep panic attacks remains a question for future research. In an open clinical trial of patients with panic disorder who have frequent sleep panic attacks (i.e., patients who had more frequent sleep panic attacks than daytime wake panic attacks),[25] tricyclic antidepressants (i.e., imipramine) were found to be effective. The prevalence and treatment of patients with sleep panic attacks without histories of daytime wake panic attacks are unknown. Until treatment strategies with data-based proved efficacy are developed,[26] it is recommended that patients with sleep panic attacks accompanied by sleep deprivation be treated with an antipanic agent and be instructed on normal sleep hygiene (see Chapter 58).

GENERALIZED ANXIETY DISORDER

Phenomenology and Demography

The earmark of generalized anxiety disorder is *chronic* anxiety (Table 95–5). Individuals with generalized anxiety disorder are recognized by friends as being "nervous," "tense," "uptight," and "always worrying."

It is difficult to determine the exact prevalence of generalized anxiety disorder. Some experts argue that it is a rare disorder and that many patients given the diagnosis of generalized anxiety disorder actually have low-grade panic disorder, whereas other lines of evidence suggest 1-month prevalence rates in the range of 2.5 to 4.6%. In clinical practice, an equal proportion of men and women meet the criteria for generalized anxiety disorder. The mean age of illness onset is approximately 21 years, with a range of 16 to 26 years.

Emerging data suggest that genetic factors might play a less salient role in generalized anxiety disorder than in panic disorder. Nevertheless, there is a higher rate of generalized anxiety disorder in first-degree relatives of probands with generalized anxiety disorder than in first-degree relatives of normal control subjects.

CASE HISTORY 3: TYPICAL PRESENTATION

Mr. D. is a 43-year-old married engineer with a 15-year history of chronic tension and generalized anxiety. His anxiety symptoms began shortly after the death of his father. Additional signs or symptoms of his generalized anxiety disorder included chronic tension, constant worrying about either his job performance or marriage, bouts of fatigue (viewed by the patient as a consequence of chronic stress), shortness of breath, motor agitation (usually lower extremities), sweating, and hot flashes. Mr. D.'s concerns were almost always unrealistic; for example, he had received many outstanding evaluations regarding his work performance and was highly regarded within the industry. Nevertheless, he harbored a fear that he was inept and would be fired.

Major life events triggered a marked exacerbation in the severity of the above symptoms. During periods of stress, Mr. D. also predictably developed "globus hystericus," urinary frequency, and a wide array of abdominal complaints. He also sought the advice of several different physicians.

At the height of his distress, Mr. D. had significant sleep disturbance (particularly early and middle insomnia) lasting for weeks or months. He denied suicidal ideation, melancholia, sleep panic attacks, nightmares, somnambulism, loud snoring, sleep paralysis, obsessions, compulsions, or social anxiety.

Treatment consisted of cognitive behavioral therapy plus alprazolam pharmacotherapy. This treatment approach resulted in an immediate and sustained improvement in his sleep complaints, although complete control of his generalized anxiety and associated gastrointestinal problems required 12 months of intensive cognitive behavioral therapy.

Sleep Complaints and Electroencephalography

Disturbances in sleep can be quite severe and prolonged (Case 3). From 50 to 70% of patients with generalized anxiety disorder report trouble sleeping,[27–29] with 30% reporting moderate-to-severe symptoms. Patients with generalized anxiety disorder will often, but not always, report that they cannot "stop worrying," "relax," or "stop thinking about problems" at bedtime.

Two research teams have investigated the polysomnography of patients with mixed anxiety disorders, including cohorts of patients with generalized anxiety disorder. Akiskal et al.[30] reported that anxious patients have problems initiating and maintaining sleep. Sitaram et al.[31] reported that a mixed group of patients with generalized anxiety disorder and panic disorder had increased time awake compared with normal control subjects. Although it is difficult to extrapolate findings from these mixed groups of anxious patients to those with *pure* generalized anxiety disorder, the aforementioned findings parallel observations made by Reynolds et al.[32] who found increased sleep latencies, increased time awake, and reduced delta wave sleep in patients with generalized anxiety disorder compared with depressed outpatients.

In summary, patients with generalized anxiety disorder report poor quality of sleep characterized by initial or middle insomnia and restless broken sleep. Polysomnographic studies in patients with admixtures of anxious symptoms largely confirm this subjective perception as indicated by problems initiating and maintaining sleep.

Treatment

Historically, benzodiazepines have been the mainstay in the management of generalized anxiety disorder. Although benzodiazepines (e.g., alprazolam, clonazepam) continue to have a major role in the

Table 95–5. DSM-IV CRITERIA FOR GENERALIZED ANXIETY DISORDER

A. Excessive anxiety and worry (apprehensive expectation) occur more days than not for at least 6 months, about a number of events or activities (such as work or school performance).
B. The person finds it difficult to control the worry.
C. The anxiety and worry are associated with three (or more) of the following six symptoms (with at least some symptoms present for more days than not for the past 6 months). **Note:** Only one item is required in children.
   1. Restlessness or feeling keyed up or on edge
   2. Being easily fatigued
   3. Difficulty concentrating or mind going blank
   4. Irritability
   5. Muscle tension
   6. Sleep disturbance (difficulty falling or staying asleep, or restless unsatisfying sleep)
D. The focus of the anxiety and worry is not confined to features of an axis 1 disorder—the anxiety or worry is not about having a panic attack (as in *Panic disorder*), being embarrassed in public (as in *Social phobia*), being contaminated (as in Obsessive-compulsive disorder), gaining weight (as in *Anorexia nervosa*), having multiple physical complaints (as in *Somatization disorder*), or having multiple illness (as in *Hypochondriasis*)—and the anxiety and worry do not occur exclusively during *Post-traumatic stress disorder*.
E. The anxiety, worry, or physical symptoms cause clinically significant distress or impairment in social, occupational, or other important areas of functioning.
F. The disturbance is not due to the direct physiological effects of a substance (e.g., a drug of abuse, a medication) or a general medical condition (e.g., hyperthyroidism) and does not occur exclusively during a mood disorder, psychotic disorder, or pervasive development disorder.

Reprinted with permission from the *Diagnostic and Statistical Manual of Mental Disorders, Fourth Edition*. Copyright 1994 American Psychiatric Association.
DSM-IV, *Diagnostic and Statistical Manual of Mental Disorders, Fourth Edition*.

treatment of generalized anxiety disorder, several lines of evidence indicate that SSRIs may also be valuable in the treatment of generalized anxiety disorder. Although tricyclic antidepressants are seldom prescribed as a first-line drug, imipramine was found to be effective in a controlled study.

Clinical experience suggests that improvement in insomnia parallels the overall benefits associated with benzodiazepine treatment; however, the relation of insomnia to treatment outcome requires double-blind, placebo-controlled studies.

SOCIAL PHOBIA

Phenomenology and Demography

The patient with social phobia is fearful of scrutiny; situations that elicit anxiety may be circumscribed (e.g., writing, speaking, or eating in public) or generalized (e.g., most social interactions).[33] Underlying the social phobia is a fear of doing or saying something that would be embarrassing or humiliating. The patient with social phobia may worry about an upcoming social event or formal gathering for weeks in advance. In the workplace, social phobic patients may appear "shy," "quiet," and "passive" or, in contrast, outgoing and highly competent. Outside the structured environment of work, however, the latter individual with social phobia will become profoundly uncomfortable and might totally avoid any situation in which casual exchanges are the norm (e.g., dinner meetings) (Table 95–6).

Many patients with social phobia report that they always have been "shy"; blushing often is a special problem for the social phobic patient. Other symptoms

Table 95–6. DSM-IV CRITERIA FOR SOCIAL PHOBIA

A. A marked and persistent fear of one or more social or performance situations in which the person is exposed to unfamiliar people or to possible scrutiny by others. The individual fears that he or she will act in a way (or show anxiety symptoms) that will be humiliating or embarrassing. **Note:** In children, there must be evidence of the capacity for age-appropriate social relationships with familiar people and the anxiety must occur in peer settings, not just in interactions with adults.
B. Exposure to the feared social situation almost invariably provokes anxiety, which may take the form of a situationally bound or situationally predisposed panic attack. **Note:** In children, the anxiety may be expressed by crying, tantrums, freezing, or shrinking from social situations with unfamiliar people.
C. The person recognizes that the fear is excessive or unreasonable. **Note:** In children, this feature may be absent.
D. The feared social or performance situations are avoided or are endured with intense anxiety or distress.
E. The avoidance, anxious anticipation, or distress in the feared social or performance situation(s) interferes significantly with the person's normal routine, occupational (academic) functioning, or social activities or relationships or there is marked distress about having the phobia.
F. In individuals younger than 18 years, the duration is at least 6 months.
G. The fear or avoidance is not due to the direct physiological effects of a substance (e.g., a drug of abuse, a medication) or a general medical condition and is not better accounted for by another mental disorder (e.g., *Panic disorder with* or *without agoraphobia, Separation anxiety disorder, Body dysmorphic disorder, Pervasive developmental disorder,* or *Schizoid personality disorder*).
H. If a general medical condition or another mental disorder is present, the fear in Criterion A is unrelated to it, e.g., the fear is not of Stuttering, trembling in Parkinson's disease, or exhibiting abnormal eating behavior in Anorexia Nervosa or Bulimia Nervosa.
Specify whether *Generalized:* if the fears include most social situations (also consider the additional diagnosis of *Avoidant personality disorder*).

Reprinted with permission from the *Diagnostic and Statistical Manual of Mental Disorders, Fourth Edition*. Copyright 1994 American Psychiatric Association.
DSM-IV, *Diagnostic and Statistical Manual of Mental Disorders, Fourth Edition*.

especially dreaded, and perhaps occurring more frequently, in social phobic patients are sweating, tremors, and stuttering. Any overt sign of discomfort (tremors in voice, motor tics) that might be visualized by another person is distressing to the social phobic patient. One of these symptoms ("I sweat too much"; "I have the shakes") might be the chief and exclusive complaint of the social phobic patient when seeking treatment from his or her family physician. A careful history, however, will uncover a wider array of complaints typical of the patient with social phobia.

Social phobia affects about as many men as women. The onset is often in early childhood, and painful memories of being embarrassed at school when asked to make an oral presentation are not uncommon. Social phobia is often associated with panic disorder. Alcohol and drug abuse are associated risk factors in this disorder, particularly in men.

CASE HISTORY 4: TYPICAL PRESENTATION

Mr. E. is a 20-year-old college student who recently dropped out of school because of his "inability to attend classes." The patient described himself as having always been "quiet, maybe even shy," although he had been able to initiate and maintain companionship with a small circle of friends during high school. Mr. E. was an excellent student throughout high school and had enjoyed participating in a small number of structured extracurricular activities (e.g., yearbook staff). Mr. E. was a physically attractive young man, and although he enjoyed organized school functions related to sporting events, he found unstructured social occasions to be "less interesting" to him. He had become friendly with one or two girls during high school, but did not develop any sustained relations of a romantic nature. In fact, his relative lack of heterosexual experience was gradually becoming an area of worry ("I wasn't very comfortable or particularly good in those types of situations"). Informal social situations (e.g., meeting in the hallway or after-school activities) were particularly stressful but did not result in marked avoidance behaviors or dysphoria. Mr. E. graduated near the top of his class and, at that time, was viewed as someone with a promising future.

Mr. E. attended a small college with an excellent academic reputation. His academic performance was above average during the first semester. However, a number of events and situations contributed to his dropping out of school during the second semester. Several courses involved classroom participation (i.e., speaking in public). Although he understood the facts, the idea of speaking in public was accompanied by extreme nervousness and a fear of making a "fool" of himself. He began to worry in advance about whether the professor would call on him the next day. Sometimes he would fret about this at night, but he denied any problems with sleep; in fact, sleep provided a sense of relief from his distress, and he found himself going to bed slightly earlier than usual.

His classroom behavior underwent a transformation. He arrived at the classroom "not too early, not too late" and picked a seat in an attempt to remain inconspicuous. How-

ever, he recalled that his attempt to maintain an unobtrusive presence once resulted in an instructor asking him to "join the class" up front. This was a particularly traumatic event that resulted in an increased fear of attending not only this class but also other classes. He had a number of unpleasant symptoms while sitting in class (or just thinking about going to classes), such as sweating, hot flashes, hand tremors, skipped heartbeats, and abdominal discomfort. Eventually, Mr. E. became unable to attend classes.

Sleep Complaints and Electroencephalography

Subjective complaints of insomnia are common in patients with social phobia if the clinician elicits specific information regarding sleep habits. It is fairly rare, however, for a patient with social phobia to present with sleep disturbances as his or her chief or major complaint. It is possible that individuals with pervasive social anxiety or generalized type of social phobia are more prone to have sleep problems than are patients with the more circumscribed forms of the disorder (e.g., public speaking).[33, 34] Polysomnography is in large part normal, with sleep latency and sleep efficiency being similar in patients with social phobia and in normal control subjects.[34, 35] REM latency, REM distribution, REM progression, and REM density are normal in social phobia. Because of the increased movement time reported in patients with panic disorder, Brown et al.[35] evaluated movement times in social phobic and normal control (N) subjects. The movement times were almost identical (social phobic, 9.5 ± 6.1 min; normal control, 10.2 ± 5.3 min; $P = NS$).

In summary, information suggests that most social phobic patients have normal total sleep time and normal sleep efficiency. These EEG findings are fully consistent with self-reports of normal quality and quantity of sleep in patients with social phobia. Secondary sleep problems may develop in patients who attempt to self-medicate with alcohol. At first, alcohol consumption may be beneficial in both reducing social anxiety and promoting a subjective sense of "deep" sleep. As alcohol misuse increases, particularly if consumed in increasing quantities at late-night social functions, some patients will experience disrupted sleep and nightmares during the second half of the night. These sleep complaints are unrelated to the social phobia per se and appear to be directly related to the amount and pattern of alcohol consumption.

Treatment

Social phobia can be effectively treated with not only cognitive-behavioral treatments but also drug therapies. Four classes of medications are effective in the treatment of social phobia: high-potency benzodiazepines (i.e., alprazolam, clonazepam), MAOI antidepressants (i.e., phenelzine, tranylcypromine), SSRIs (i.e., fluoxetine, paroxetine), and in selective cases, beta blockers (i.e., atenolol, propranolol). Clinical experience suggests that patients with specific social phobias (e.g., public speaking) may respond to beta-blockers, whereas the more generalized, pervasive forms of social phobia may require MAOI antidepressants (i.e., phenelzine) to achieve an optimal response. Core symptoms of social phobia can be effectively treated with both cognitive-behavioral and drug therapies. A combination of psychosocial and drug therapies may be necessary to achieve an optimal response. In rare circumstances, a social phobic patient may have problems with the scrutiny associated with sexual performance or sleeping with a partner; such fears may have a negative impact on sleeping habits. Once these issues are identified and appropriately treated, there is an immediate return to the patient's preexisting normal sleep habits.

OBSESSIVE-COMPULSIVE DISORDER

Phenomenology and Demography

The key signs and symptoms of this disorder are obsession or compulsions. Obsessions are thoughts or ideas recognized by the patient as being irrational. Patients will invariably depict their thoughts, ideas, or images in one of the following ways: "senseless," "foolish," "nonsensical," "absurd," "pointless," "stupid," "ridiculous," "preposterous," "ludicrous," "asinine," "idiotic," "outrageous," "embarrassing," "disgraceful," or "crazy." Despite the apparent belief that the thoughts or images are irrational, the patient cannot rid himself or herself of the obsessions. Obsessions can also take the form of impulses. In fact, impulses often are the most disturbing or frightening type of obsession (e.g., the impulse to kill someone you love or the fear that one has already injured another person, such as unwittingly hit someone while driving an automobile).

Compulsions are repetitive but deliberate behaviors performed by the patient in response to a particular obsession (Table 95–7). The compulsions are performed in a predictable fashion according to specific rules in an attempt to lessen, neutralize, or ward off distressing obsessions. Typical compulsions, however, cannot reasonably be expected to rid the person of the dreaded event (e.g., "catching AIDS"), or the otherwise normal behavior (e.g., washing one's hands) is exaggerated in degree (e.g., washing one's hands 100 times in a precise and stereotyped manner). There is an inner drive to perform the act, although the individual usually resists the compulsion. Like obsessions, almost all individuals recognize the illogical nature of their compulsions and, as a result, actively resist the urge to act. Examples of classic compulsions include hand-washing and checking.

Obsessive-compulsive disorder is not an uncommon disorder, with a lifetime prevalence of approximately 2.5%. The disorder is about equally distributed among men and women. The age of onset is adolescence or early adulthood, and the disorder often fluctuates in intensity throughout life.

CASE HISTORY 5: TYPICAL PRESENTATION

Mr. G. was a 23-year-old man who worked as an aide to an elected government official. His chief complaint was the repetitive thought that he might suddenly hit or kill someone. He had no history of aggression or arrests for antisocial behavior and was regarded as a scholar and gentleman by his friends.

He viewed his thoughts of "acting in an impulsive manner" as "irrational" and "impossible...not anything I would do." Nevertheless, he could not get the thought out of his mind. He also developed the "stupid" notion that if he read or saw a picture of violence in the newspaper, he might somehow do the same thing. He again viewed this idea as "irrational" but had developed a series of repetitive behaviors that would prevent him from acting on these impulses. If he inadvertently glanced at a story involving violence, he had a specific series of actions to reverse its impact. Thus, he would start reading the paper again and turn the pages of the newspaper in a specific manner without looking at the story.

Mr. G. gradually adopted a similar approach to reading the newspaper each day; that is, he would read the same sections of the newspaper in the same precise manner. If he had an "irrational idea" (e.g., shooting someone) while reading an article, he felt compelled to reread the article many times until he was absolutely sure that he had had the correct philosophical attitude that would prevent his acting on the obsession. This was often quite difficult, sometimes requiring his reading the story over and over again. Sometimes, he would be unsure about his success in this regard and return, later in the day, to reread the story. He viewed both his obsessions and compulsion as "idiotic" but disabling. He denied sleep problems during his adulthood.

At the age of 13, he had suffered through a period during which he had the repetitive "stupid" thought that he might kill his grandfather by giving him germs. Before visiting his grandfather he would wash his hands over and over—first turning on the faucet with his right hand and then using the soap in a particular way, and so on. If he made a mistake in the routine, he would start over until he was able to wash his hands in the appropriate manner.

During this stressful period, he recalls having difficulty sleeping and worrying that he had given his grandfather deadly germs. He would sometimes awaken in a "start" and go check to see whether his grandfather was still alive. He would then return to bed, worry, and recheck his grandfather many times during the night. The day after a night of repetitive checking was often associated with daytime fatigue and poor performance in school.

Sleep Complaints and Electroencephalography

Many patients with obsessive-compulsive disorder have little or no problems with sleep. When a disrup-

Table 95–7. DSM-IV CRITERIA FOR OBSESSIVE-COMPULSIVE DISORDER

A. Either obsessions or compulsions:

Obsessions

1. Recurrent and persistent thoughts, impulses, or images that are experienced, at some time during the disturbance, as intrusive and inappropriate and that cause marked anxiety or distress.
2. The thoughts, impulses, or images are not simply excessive worries about real-life problems.
3. The person attempts to ignore or suppress such thoughts, impulses, or images or to neutralize them with some other thought or action.
4. The person recognizes that the obsessional thoughts, impulses, or images are a product of his or her own mind (not imposed from without as in thought insertion).

Compulsions

1. Repetitive behaviors (e.g., hand washing, ordering, checking) or mental acts (e.g., praying, counting, repeating words silently) that the person feels driven to perform in response to an obsession, or according to rules that must be applied rigidly.
2. The behaviors or mental acts are aimed at preventing or reducing distress or preventing some dreaded event or situation; however, these behaviors or mental acts either are not connected in a realistic way with what they are designed to neutralize or prevent or are clearly excessive.

B. At some point during the course of the disorder, the person has recognized that the obsessions or compulsions are excessive or unreasonable. **Note:** This does not apply to children.

C. The obsessions or compulsions cause marked distress, are time consuming (take more than 1 h a day), or significantly interfere with the person's normal routine, occupational (or academic) functioning, or usual social activities or relationships.

D. If another axis 1 disorder is present, the content of the obsessions or compulsions is not restricted to it (e.g., preoccupation with food in the presence of an eating disorder, hair pulling in the presence of trichotillomania, concern with appearance in the presence of body dysmorphic disorder, preoccupation with drugs in the presence of a substance use disorder, preoccupation with having a serious illness in the presence of hypochondriasis, preoccupation with sexual urges in the presence of a paraphilia, or guilty ruminations in the presence of major depressive disorder).

E. The disturbance is not due to the direct physiological effects of a substance (e.g., a drug of abuse, a medication) or a general medical condition.

Reprinted with permission from the *Diagnostic and Statistical Manual of Mental Disorders, Fourth Edition.* Copyright 1994 American Psychiatric Association.

DSM-IV, *Diagnostic and Statistical Manual of Mental Disorders, Fourth Edition.*

tion in sleep does occur, it is usually linked in obvious ways to the underlying psychiatric condition. For example, delayed sleep onset or multiple awakenings may take place as a consequence of the person's need to check that doors are locked, that alarms are appropriately engaged, and that gas stoves have been turned off. Such sleep problems were evident in Mr. G., who, as a result of repeatedly checking his grandfather at night, experienced a significant disruption in his normal sleep-wake cycle. Analogous to Mr. G.'s fear of contaminating his grandfather with germs, Insel et al.[36] noted that patients with cleaning rituals are particularly stressed by standard research procedures (e.g., attaching leads) and may have marked difficulty sleeping in the laboratory.

Insel et al.[36] conducted a sleep EEG study in *adult* patients with obsessive-compulsive disorder. This research team investigated the sleep of 14 patients with obsessive-compulsive disorder, 9 of whom complained of previous sleep problems. In general, polysomnography confirmed the patients' aforementioned sleep complaints. Moreover, several (but not all) findings in adults in the study of Insel et al.[36] corresponded with the EEG findings in adolescents with obsessive-compulsive disorder.[37] Both adult and adolescent patients with obsessive-compulsive disorder tend to have poor quality of sleep as indicated by significantly decreased total sleep and increased awake movement time and by nonsignificant increases and decreases, respectively, in sleep latency and sleep efficiency. In contrast to the findings in adolescents, the adults with obsessive-compulsive disorder did not have significant differences in total or percent time in stage 4 or delta sleep.

Both studies, however, found a significant decrease in the total time in stage 2 (adolescents also had a significant decrease in the percent of stage 2 time that was not evident in the adults).

Of interest, REM latency also was significantly reduced in the adult patients with obsessive-compulsive disorder (48.4 ± 8.8 versus 80.8 ± 5.5 min, $P < .05$); moreover, the obsessive-compulsive patients with and without concurrent symptoms of depression both had shortened REM latencies compared with their respective normal control group, whereas there was no difference in REM latency between the two subgroups (depressed versus nondepressed) of patients with obsessive-compulsive disorder. These observations suggest that REM latency may be decreased in patients with obsessive-compulsive disorder, independent of the coexisting presence of depressive symptomatology.

Insel et al.[36] also found a significant decrease in REM efficiency on the second night of sleep recording that was not present on the first adaptation night. Other REM indices (i.e., REM density, number of REM periods, and total REM time), however, were not significantly different between the patients with obsessive compulsive disorder and normal control subjects.

Because the reduced REM latency found in the patients with obsessive-compulsive disorder has been most often associated with major depression (see Chapter 96), the National Institute of Mental Health team compared their findings in patients with obsessive-compulsive disorder with a comparison group of 14 age-matched patients with major depression.[36] There were few significant differences between the obsessive-compulsive and depressed patients; specifically, the two groups did not differ on REM latency (48.4 ± 8.8 versus 47.3 ± 5.1 min, P = NS), REM density (1.68 ± 0.12 versus 1.69 ± 0.14 min, P = NS), REM efficiency (83.7 ± 7.9 versus 88.5 ± 11.9 min, P = NS), number of REM periods (3.8 ± 0.2 versus 3.9 ± 0.3 min, P = NS), or total REM time (75.7 ± 3.9 versus 85.2 ± 7.2 min), although there was a trend for the obsessive-compulsive patients to have a lower REM density than the depressed patients. In fact, the only significant between-group difference was that obsessive-compulsive patients had greater amounts of stage 1 and stage 3 sleep than the depressed patients.

Overall, the subjective and objective findings in two small studies (a total of 9 adolescents and 14 adults with obsessive-compulsive disorder) suggest that patients with this disabling anxiety disorder often may experience poor-quality sleep, that is, sleep is broken, restless, shortened, and, in adults, associated with less delta sleep. Whether these disturbances are exclusively limited to and are a direct consequence of intrusive thoughts, ruminations, worry, and associated compulsions that represent the core symptoms of obsessive-compulsive disorder has yet to be determined in a decisive manner.

Treatment

Treatment is targeted toward the removal of obsessions or compulsions. Although obsessive-compulsive disorder tends to be one of the more severe anxiety disorders, both pharmacotherapy and psychosocial treatments appear to be effective in the treatment of this condition; most effective are drugs that produce changes in the serotonergic neurotransmitter system (e.g., clomipramine, fluoxetine, fluvoxamine). Not all drugs with serotonergic action have beneficial effects in the treatment of obsessive-compulsive disorder (e.g., zimelidine and trazodone).

Specialized cognitive behavioral treatments are also useful in treating obsessive-compulsive disorder, particularly in terms of the compulsive rituals associated with this condition. Despite promising results with these psychosocial treatments, many patients with more severe illness do not achieve a satisfactory response. A small number of patients with severe, disabling, and treatment-refractory obsessive-compulsive disorder may respond to psychosurgery (i.e., cingulotomy and capsulotomy). Because of the complex and often disabling nature of this disorder, treatment frequently requires a combination of drug therapies and newly developed behavioral techniques.

Patients with obsessive-compulsive disorder rarely present with insomnia as their primary concern. Nevertheless, sleep disturbances probably are fairly common in obsessive-compulsive disorder. A careful history will often uncover a pattern of sleep disruption in obsessive-compulsive patients, perhaps particularly in those with checking or washing rituals. Although complaints often focus on difficulty falling or maintaining sleep, it has yet to be determined whether these problems are connected to the obsessive-compulsive disorder itself or to the comorbid symptoms of depression that are inevitably found in most patients with obsessive-compulsive disorder. Clinical experience suggests that sleep improves with the successful treatment of the core symptoms of obsessive-compulsive disorder. In the patient with insomnia, the selection of a drug to treat obsessions, compulsions, or both should be considered in relation to the sedating versus activating properties of the serotonergic class of agents. Clomipramine is more sedating, whereas fluoxetine and fluvoxamine tend to induce or worsen insomnia. In the obsessive-compulsive patient with insomnia, fluoxetine should be started at very low doses and titrated to therapeutic levels as tolerated. Clinical experience suggests that trazodone, at low doses (i.e., 50 to 100 mg), might be useful in counteracting the insomnia associated with fluoxetine pharmacotherapy.

POST-TRAUMATIC STRESS DISORDER

Phenomenology

This disorder is characterized by the reliving or reexperiencing of a previous traumatic event. The trauma is one that is beyond the scope of normal life events and would be experienced by almost anyone as profoundly disturbing. After the trauma, the individual develops a constellation of symptoms such as intrusive recollections of the event, crying, anxiety or fear (particularly when exposed to stimuli associated with the original trauma), hypervigilance, and hyperstartle.

It is very common for patients with post-traumatic stress disorder to complain of sleep disturbances (Table 95–8). Patients may have problems initiating sleep or have nightmares about the trauma; they can repeatedly relive the event in their sleep. These nightmares may reoccur for weeks or months. If the original trauma occurred during sleep (e.g., a fire), the individual may develop particular problems with sleep (i.e., a conditioned fear of sleep). Some patients with post-traumatic disorder may have dissociative episodes, with or without aggressive behavior.

An avoidance of stimuli that remind the individual of the original trauma may develop; conversely, the individual may suddenly find himself or herself reexperiencing the trauma only to later discover that an unrecognized stimulus associated with the original trauma actually triggered the response. Major depression is commonly associated with post-traumatic stress disorder.

It is not unusual for an individual who has survived a major trauma to experience guilt regarding his or her survival. Alcohol and drug abuse, anxiety disorders, and major depression appear to be increased in patients with post-traumatic stress disorder. Certain personality traits (e.g., neuroticism), prior life experiences (e.g., separation), and family history of anxiety may be risk factors for post-traumatic stress disorder.

Table 95–8. DSM-IV CRITERIA FOR POST-TRAUMATIC STRESS DISORDERS

A. The person has been exposed to a traumatic event in which both of the following were present.
1. The person experienced, witnessed, or was confronted with an event or events that involved actual or threatened death or serious injury, or a threat to the physical integrity of self or others.
2. The person's response involved intense fear, helplessness, or horror. **Note:** In children, this may be expressed instead by disorganized or agitated behavior.
B. The traumatic event is persistently reexperienced in one (or more) of the following ways:
1. Recurrent and intrusive distressing recollections of the event, including images, thoughts, perceptions. **Note:** In young children, repetitive play may occur in which themes or aspects of the trauma are expressed.
2. Recurrent distressing dreams of the event. **Note:** In children, there may be frightening dreams without recognizable content.
3. Acting or feeling as if the traumatic event were recurring (includes a sense of reliving the experience, illusions, hallucinations, and dissociative flashback episodes, including those that occur on awakening or when intoxicated).
4. Intense psychological distress at exposure to internal or external cues that symbolize or resemble an aspect of the traumatic event.
5. Physiological reactivity on exposure to internal or external cues that symbolize or resemble an aspect of the traumatic event.
C. Persistent avoidance of stimuli associated with the trauma and numbing of general responsiveness (not present before the trauma), as indicated by three (or more) of the following:
1. Efforts to avoid thoughts, feelings, or conversations associated with the trauma
2. Efforts to avoid activities, places, or people that arouse recollections of the trauma
3. Inability to recall an important aspect of the trauma
4. Markedly diminished interest or participation in significant activities
5. Feeling of detachment or estrangement from others
6. Restricted range of affect (e.g., unable to have loving feelings)
7. Sense of foreshortened future (e.g., does not expect to have a career, marriage, children, or a normal life span)
D. Persistent symptoms of increased arousal (not present before the trauma), as indicated by two (or more) of the following:
1. Difficulty falling or staying asleep
2. Irritability or outbursts of anger
3. Difficulty concentrating
4. Hypervigilance
5. Exaggerated startle response
E. Duration of the disturbance (symptoms in criteria B, C, and D) is longer than 1 month.
F. The disturbance causes clinically significant distress or impairment in social, occupational, or other important areas of functioning.
Specify if
Acute: Duration of symptoms is less than 3 months
Chronic: Duration of symptoms is 3 months or longer
Specify if
With delayed onset: Onset of symptoms is at least 6 months after the stressor.

Reprinted with permission from the *Diagnostic and Statistical Manual of Mental Disorders, Fourth Edition.* Copyright 1994 American Psychiatric Association.
DSM-IV, *Diagnostic and Statistical Manual of Mental Disorders, Fourth Edition.*

CASE HISTORY 6: TYPICAL PRESENTATION

Ms. H. is a 25-year-old college student who reported problems with anxiety and nightmares. She had no previous problems with nightmares until 2 days ago, after having been kept hostage and repeatedly raped for approximately 10 h. She had been raped at knifepoint, although between the aggressive acts the rapist had attempted to carry on casual conversation. She believed that she would not survive the night.

The rapist escaped in the morning, after she had been tied to her bed. She attended classes the next day and did not report the assault to authorities until the second day.

On the second night, she had a nightmare about the rape. Subsequently, she found it almost impossible to fall asleep, and when she did, her sleep was restless; she would often awaken from a nightmares about the rape. She denied sleepwalking. Ms. H. had crying jags and was easily startled when approached by unfamiliar men. She repeatedly thought about the rape, reliving the night in a step-by-step fashion, and feeling that she was responsible for the assault. Despite her best efforts to forget about the rape, Ms. H. had intrusive thoughts about the event that resulted in increased dysfunction (e.g., thinking about the rape while eating dinner with friends or during examinations). Ms. H. found herself socially withdrawing. She also became increasingly irritable about minor inconveniences and angry with her closest friends.

All of the above symptoms persisted for about 6 months. After this interval of time, her nightmares began to decrease in frequency, although she continued to have bouts of irritability, crying jags, and a heightened startle response when approached by men.

Sleep Complaints and Electroencephalography

Sleep disturbances are commonly reported in patients with post-traumatic stress disorder; moreover, insomnia, anxiety arousals, or nightmares during sleep may represent the primary complaint of some patients.[38] From 59 to 68% of patients with post-traumatic stress disorder or individuals exposed to major stressors report frequent "nightmares."[38–42] These rates of anxiety arousals in patients with post-traumatic stress disorder appear to be higher than those found in students or the general population.[42–44] Therefore, the increased rate of "nightmares" appears to be a true phenomenon, rather than an artifact of retrospective bias or recall.

The content and associated emotions (e.g., fear, terror, anger) of the "nightmares" are similar to or identical to those experienced during the original trauma. The patient with post-traumatic stress disorder is conceptualized as "reliving" the original trauma; identical "nightmares," therefore, are often repeated night after night. The cognition and images associated with the anxiety arousals are analogous to "bad" memories.

Several lines of evidence suggest that the anxiety arousals in patients with post-traumatic stress disorder are REM-related nightmares,[43] although anxious awakenings may also occur during NREM stages of sleep.[46, 47] Many of the anxiety arousals from sleep in patients with post-traumatic stress disorder, however, are similar in quality to true nightmares (i.e., there are cognition and/or vivid images, strong emotions, and full recall of the "dream"). Like sleep panic attacks and night terrors, many anxiety arousals in patients with post-traumatic stress disorder occur early in the sleep cycle. REM sleep behavior disorder has also been reported in patients with post-traumatic stress disorder[23] (see Chapter 64).

Patients with post-traumatic stress disorder or individuals undergoing major stressors have been found to have both shortened and normal-to-prolonged REM latencies.[48-53] Based on these limited observations, it appears that anxiety arousals in post-traumatic stress disorder may emerge from both REM and NREM stages of sleep. Although there is no consistent pattern of altered REM parameters (i.e., REM latency, REM density, REM progression, or percent REM sleep) across studies, it is nevertheless impressive how often *some* type of REM-related abnormality is reported in patients with post-traumatic stress disorder.

Treatment

Patients with this anxiety disorder not only have the core symptoms of the syndrome (e.g., intrusive thoughts, flashbacks, etc.) but also frequently report depression, anxiety, alcohol or drug abuse, insomnia, "nightmares," or other parasomnias. Patients with post-traumatic stress disorder also have a high rate of personality disorders. The treatment of post-traumatic stress disorder, therefore, requires not only therapy for intrusive thoughts, memories, flashbacks, or nightmares but also the management of a number of related complications (e.g., drug abuse) or comorbid axis I (e.g., major depression) or axis II (e.g., antisocial) conditions. Good care often demands the use of combined treatments (e.g., pharmacological and psychosocial) to control multiple target symptoms.

Converging data indicate that a wide range of medications might be effective in the treatment of *individual patients* with post-traumatic stress disorder. The large number of different classes of medications (i.e., lithium, clonidine, carbamazepine, fluoxetine, clonazepam, MAOIs, tricyclic antidepressants, buspirone) reported to be effective in case reports, open treatment trials, or controlled trials underscores the heterogeneous symptomatic nature of post-traumatic stress disorder and its high rate of comorbidity with other medical or psychiatric conditions. It is possible that different patients respond to different psychotropic agents *because* they actually have different pharmacologically responsive comorbid conditions (e.g., major depression or panic disorder). It remains unclear whether any class of medication is effective in reducing the frequency or intensity of core symptoms of post-traumatic stress

disorder. At the present time, the key term in relation to pharmacotherapy of post-traumatic stress disorder is *individualized treatment*.

Many psychotherapies are also used in the direct or adjunctive treatment of post-traumatic stress disorder. It is beyond the scope of this chapter to review in detail the psychosocial treatments reported to be useful in the management of post-traumatic stress disorder. Like the pharmacotherapies, the role of psychosocial interventions in the treatment of patients with post-traumatic stress disorder appears promising but must be developed and administered on a case-by-case basis.

Several authors have implied or explicitly noted that improvement in sleep disturbances, including nightmares, insomnia, or both, usually coincides with the overall benefits of successful drug therapy.[54-60]

The degree of improvement or unimprovement in sleep, respectively, appears to be associated with an equally impressive or unimpressive amelioration in the other core symptoms of the disorder. Whether a single drug or drug combination can be identified or developed that specifically blocks post-traumatic-related nightmares or NREM anxiety arousals requires additional research.

SPECIFIC PHOBIA

Phenomenology and Demography

The main characteristic of specific phobia is the fear of a circumscribed situation or object. Exposure to the feared situation or object invokes severe anxiety; avoidance of the feared stimulus is common but not inevitable. Specific phobia often begins in childhood; the greatest proportion of persons with specific phobia is children. The phobia must be evident for a minimum of 6 months before a child or adolescent younger than 18 years meets DSM-IV criteria for this disorder. Classic examples of simple phobia include insects (e.g., spiders), animals (e.g., dogs), situations (e.g., elevators, airplanes, tunnels, bridges), blood or body injury, or natural events (e.g., storms). Specific phobia is often viewed by laypersons as a minor problem in daily living, yet it can be seriously disabling. Simple phobia occurs about equally in men and women. As a group, specific phobia may have different causes. Blood/illness/injury phobias, for example, have high familial transmission rates, whereas other specific phobia has little or no familial aggregation (Table 95–9).

CASE HISTORY 7: FEAR-RELATED INSOMNIA

J. is a 9-year-old boy who had refused to remain in his room after bedtime. Typically, he would return to his parents' bedroom after being in his room for 1 to 2 h. His typical complaint was, "I can't sleep; I don't know why, I just can't sleep." J. would easily fall asleep if he was allowed to remain in his parents' bedroom. In contrast, if he were taken back to his own room or encouraged to go back to his room, he often would return later in an apparent state of anxiety.

J. had normal developmental milestones, was popular among his peers, and was a good student. He denied any problems either at school or at home. The parents denied marital discord.

Perplexed by this problem, the parents attempted a number of interventions: (1) allowing J. to remain in the parents' room (to be carried to his own bedroom after sleep onset), (2) comforting J. in his own room until falling asleep, and (3) strong encouragement.

After a period of offering this type of reassurance and support, J. related the following information: he was frightened of an illusion of a human face on a fixture in the bathroom that was within direct visual contact of his bed. When the bathroom door was left open to provide light, this "face kept looking at me." If J. closed the door, his room became "black and scary." J. was a rather mature boy and felt silly about his fears.

When J. was assured that his fears were normal for a person his age, his room was equipped with a night light, and he was given permission to close the bathroom door, his fear of sleeping in his own room totally resolved.

Sleep Complaints

Disturbances in sleep are not a typical trait of specific phobia. When sleep disturbances are present, they are tightly linked to the phobic stimulus. As illustrated in the vignette (Case 7), J. developed sleep complications only as a consequence of a normal childhood fear.

Treatment

There is little role for pharmacotherapy in the treatment of specific phobia. The benefit of behavioral and cognitive therapies is well documented; they produce sustained elimination of most specific phobia. Some simple phobia (e.g., blood drawing) may require specialized techniques (e.g., biofeedback techniques). Sleep disturbances associated with specific phobia are rare, and when present, they respond in parallel with the effective treatment of the main phobia. Normal fears (e.g., fear of the dark in children) that may result in disruption of sleep patterns almost always respond to education (i.e., age-appropriate examination of the risk) and emotional support.

SUMMARY

The anxiety disorders are often, but not always, associated with disturbances in initiating and maintaining sleep.[61] Different anxiety disorders appear to be associated with different types and severities of sleep disturbances. Patients with social and specific phobia appear to have largely normal sleep unless the phobic stimulus is somehow linked with the bedroom or sleeping environment. Many patients with obsessive-

compulsive disorder have poor-quality sleep as documented by increased sleep latency, decreased total sleep time, and increased movement time. There is great variation in the severity of sleep disturbances associated with obsessive-compulsive disorder; some patients report no problems whatsoever, and other patients relate significant distress with initiating and maintaining sleep. The early report of Insel et al.[36] of shortened REM latency in obsessive-compulsive disorder, a seminal finding at the time, could not be replicated by two independent research teams.[62, 63] The polysomnographic correlates of subjective sleep complaints in obsessive-compulsive disorder remain unclear. It is likely, however, that the major sleep disturbances associated with obsessive-compulsive disorder are idiosyncratic consequences of the primary anxiety disorder (e.g., decreased sleep latency and impaired sleep efficiency due to compulsive checking at bedtime) or possibly comorbid conditions (e.g., major depression).

Patients with generalized anxiety disorder, like other

Table 95–9. DSM-IV CRITERIA FOR SPECIFIC PHOBIA

A. Marked and persistent fear that is excessive or unreasonable, cued by the presence or anticipation of a specific object or situation (e.g., flying, heights, animals, receiving an injection, seeing blood).
B. Exposure to the phobic stimulus almost invariably provokes an immediate anxiety response, which may take the form of a situationally predisposed panic attack. **Note:** In children, the anxiety may be expressed by crying, tantrums, freezing, or clinging.
C. The person recognizes that the fear is excessive or unreasonable. **Note:** In children, this feature may be absent.
D. The phobic situation(s) are avoided or are endured with intense anxiety.
E. The avoidance, anxious anticipation, or distress in the feared situation(s) interferes significantly with the person's normal routine, occupational (or academic) functioning, or social activities or relationships or there is marked distress about having the phobia.
F. In individuals younger than 18 years, the duration is at least 6 months.
G. The anxiety, panic attacks, or phobic avoidance associated with the specific object or situation are not better accounted for by another mental disorder such as *Obsessive-compulsive disorder* (e.g., fear of dirt in someone with an obsession about contamination), *Post-traumatic stress disorder* (e.g., avoidance of stimuli associated with a severe stressor), *Separation anxiety disorder* (e.g., avoidance of school), *Social phobia* (e.g., avoidance of social situations because of fear of embarrassment), *Panic disorder with agoraphobia*, or *Agoraphobia without history of panic disorder.*
Specify type
Animal type
Natural environment type (e.g., heights, storms, water)
Blood-injection-injury type
Situational type (e.g., airplanes, elevators, enclosed places)
Other type (e.g., phobic avoidance of situations that may lead to choking, vomiting, or contracting an illness; in children, avoidance of loud sounds or costumed characters)

Reprinted with permission from the *Diagnostic and Statistical Manual of Mental Disorders, Fourth Edition.* Copyright 1994 American Psychiatric Association.
DSM-IV, *Diagnostic and Statistical Manual of Mental Disorders, Fourth Edition.*

Table 95–10. DIFFERENTIATION OF SLEEP AROUSALS

	Sleep Panic Attacks	Nightmares	Night Terrors	Post-traumatic Nightmares	Sleep Apnea
Demographics	Adults M>F	Children and adults F>M	Children M>F	Children and adults	Adult M>F
Clinical features	Abrupt arousal to full	Variable arousal	Confused, nonreactive behavior consciousness	Variable/ dissociative	Incomplete arousal
	No dream recall	Vivid imagery/ elaborate content	Retrograde amnesia	Reliving trauma	Patient unaware (snoring)
	Moderate autonomic activation	Mild or variable autonomic activation	Extreme autonomic activation	Extreme autonomic activation	
EEG correlates	NREM (early delta)	REM	NREM (sustained delta)	REM/NREM	All stages
Associated features	Similar wake attacks Agoraphobia	Stressful life events	Somnambulism	Post-traumatic	Obesity, hypertension, somnolence

F, female; M, male.

individuals complaining of chronic stress, tension, or free-floating anxiety, may have significant reductions in total sleep time and sleep efficiency. Clinical experience suggests these disturbances, when present, are tightly linked to distressful cognitions and pathological worry about stressors of daily living. Improvement in insomnia closely parallels the successful amelioration of core anxiety symptoms.

Panic disorder and post-traumatic stress disorder, unlike the other primary anxiety disorders, are often associated with recurrent frightening arousals from sleep. These events are designated *sleep-panic* or *nocturnal-panic* attacks in patients with panic disorder and *anxiety* or *threatening dreams* in post-traumatic stress disorder. As illustrated in Table 95–10, sleep or nocturnal panic attacks and post-traumatic stress disorder–related anxiety dreams can be differentiated from each other and additional parasomnias according to a number of clinical and polysomnographic parameters. The major polysomnographic distinction between sleep panic attacks and post-traumatic stress disorder–related anxiety dreams is that sleep panic attacks occur in late stage 2 or early stage 3 sleep, whereas anxiety dreams tend to be associated with REM stage sleep.

Although nocturnal panic attacks in patients with panic disorder are NREM events, the best evidence (albeit inconsistent and complex) suggests a key role for REM stage sleep in the pathophysiology of anxiety dreams. Several but not all[64, 65] investigators have found *some* REM architectural change in post-traumatic stress disorder. Frightening awakenings, both with and without dream content, take place during or immediately after REM stage sleep[66–69]; other REM or REM-related abnormalities include increased REM density, decreased REM latency (less often), greater proportion of REM epochs, periodic limb movements, and prolonged twitch bursts.[65–70] Ross et al.[67] suggested that the types of muscle activation seen in patients with post-traumatic stress disorder is also observed in patients with REM behavior disorder (see Chapter 64). If so, this provides a possible theoretical model for conceptualizing the temporal coexistence of dream anxiety and motor agitation seen in some patients with post-trau-

matic stress disorder. Sleep panic attacks, especially as reported by patients with otherwise classic panic disorder, are not associated with dream content, visual images, auditory or tactile sensations, cognitions, or thrashing movements during sleep.

Unlike sleep panic attacks, both classic nightmares (nontraumatic) and post-traumatic stress disorder–related anxiety dreams are characterized by vivid images, cognitions, and strong emotions. Posttraumatic stress disorder–related anxiety dreams are so real in quality that some patients experience sleep-related dissociative episodes and report "reliving" past traumatic events in their sleep.

There are some similarities between nocturnal panic attacks and nightmares and anxiety dreams (Table 95–10). Increased autonomic arousal may be associated with all three phenomena, and both sleep panic attacks and anxiety dreams in post-traumatic stress disorder tend to occur early in the sleep cycle. Patients with panic disorder and post-traumatic stress disorder may develop secondary fears of sleep; such conditioned fear responses and avoidance behaviors, however, are quite rare in the other anxiety disorders. On the other hand, we have seen patients with isolated sleep paralysis develop profound fear of sleep and sleeping. The putative association between both nocturnal panic attacks and isolated sleep paralysis with sleep avoidance behaviors is noteworthy given the reported increased incidence of isolated sleep paralysis in blacks with panic disorder.[14, 71]

The role of sleep deprivation in the cause, maintenance, or exacerbation of sleep panic attacks, anxiety dreams, or sleep paralysis is poorly understood and requires investigation. Increasing evidence indicates that the anxiety disorders can be distinguished from major depression on the basis of differential responses to sleep deprivation. Patients with major depression experience marked but transient symptomatic improvement after sleep deprivation. In contrast, patients with anxiety disorders report either significant worsening (e.g., panic disorder)[9, 10] or no change (e.g., social phobia and generalized anxiety disorder)[72] in symptoms after sleep deprivation.

Effective treatment of the core symptoms of most anxiety disorders will almost always result in a corresponding improvement in associated sleep disturbances. Patients with a mixed anxiety (e.g., panic disorder) and sleep disorder (e.g., sleep apnea) may prove refractory to traditional interventions. If sleep disturbances persist after the successful treatment of the primary anxiety disorder, the clinician should reevaluate the patient for other possible medical or sleep disorders.

References

1. Uhde TW, Boulenger J-P, Roy-Byrne PP, et al. Longitudinal course of panic disorder: clinical and biological considerations. Prog Neuropsychopharmacol Biol Psychiatry. 1985;9:39–51.
2. National Institutes of Health Consensus Development Conference. Panic: Consensus Statement. Bethesda, Md: National Institutes of Health; 1991.
3. Sheehan DV, Ballenger J, Jacobsen G. Treatment of endogenous anxiety with phobic, hysterical and hypochondriacal symptoms. Arch Gen Psychiatry. 1980;37:51–59.
4. Mellman TA, Uhde TW. Sleep panic attacks: new clinical findings and theoretical implications. Am J Psychiatry. 1989;146:1204–1207.
5. Taylor CB, Sheikh J, Agras WS, et al. Self report of panic attacks: agreement with heart rate changes. Am J Psychiatry. 1986;143:478–482.
6. Uhde TW. Treating panic and anxiety. Psychiatr Ann. 1986;16:536–541.
7. Hauri PJ, Friedman M, Ravaris CL. Sleep in patients with spontaneous panic attacks. Sleep. 1989;12:323–337.
8. Krystal JH, Kosten TR, Southwick S, et al. Neurobiological aspects of PTSD: review of clinical and preclinical studies. Behav Ther. 1989;20:177–198.
9. Craske MG, Barlow DH. Nocturnal panic. J Nerv Ment Dis. 1989;177:160–167.
10. Uhde TW. The anxiety disorders. In: Kryger MH, Roth T, Dement WC, eds. Principles and Practice of Sleep Medicine. Philadelphia, Pa: WB Saunders; 1994:871–898.
11. Roy-Byrne PP, Uhde TW, Post RM. Effects of one night's sleep deprivation on mood and behavior in patients with panic disorder: comparison with depressed patients and normal controls. Arch Gen Psychiatry. 1986;43:895–899.
12. Uhde TW, Mellman TA. Commentary on "Relaxation-induced panic (RIP): when resting isn't peaceful." Integr Psychiatry. 1987;5:101–104. Reprinted with publisher's erratum, 1988;6:147–149.
13. Stein MB, Millar TW, Larsen DK, et al. Irregular breathing during sleep in patients with panic disorder. Am J Psychiatry. 1995;152:1168–1173.
14. Mellman TA, Uhde TW. Electroencephalographic sleep in panic disorder: a focus on sleep-related panic attacks. Arch Gen Psychiatry. 1989;46:178–184.
15. Bell CC, Shakoor B, Thompson B, et al. Prevalence of isolated sleep paralysis in black subjects. J Natl Med Assoc. 1984;76:501–508.
16. Dube S, Jones DA, Bell J, et al. Interface of panic and depression: clinical and sleep EEG correlates. Psychiatry Res. 1986;19:119–133.
17. Mellman TA, Uhde TW. Sleep in panic and generalized anxiety disorders. In: Ballenger JC, ed. Neurobiology of Panic Disorder. Frontiers in Clinical Neuroscience. Vol 8. New York, NY: Alan R Liss; 1990:365–376.
18. Uhde TW, Roy-Byrne PP, Gillin JC, et al. The sleep of patients with panic disorder: a preliminary report. Psychiatry Res. 1984;12:251–259.
19. Gastaut H, Dongier M, Broughton R, et al. Electroencephalographic and clinical study of diurnal and nocturnal anxiety attacks. Electroencephalogr Clin Neurophysiol. 1964;17:475.
20. Herman R. Nocturnal panic in a depressed patient: pathophysiological implications. Biol Psychiatry. 1988;24:432–436.
21. Lesser IM, Poland RE, Holcomb C, et al. Electroencephalographic study of nighttime panic attacks. J Nerv Ment Dis. 1985;173:744–746.
22. Kales JD, Kales A, Soldatos CR et al. Night terrors: clinical characteristics and personality patterns. Arch Gen Psychiatry. 1980;37:1413–1417.
23. Mahowald MW, Bundlie SR, Hurwitz TD, et al. Sleep violence—forensic science implications: polygraphic and video documentation. J Forensic Sci. 1990;35:413–432.
24. Mahowald MW, Schenck CH. REM sleep behavior disorder. In: Kryger MH, Roth T, Dement WC, eds. Principles and Practice of Sleep Medicine. Philadelphia, Pa: WB Saunders; 1989:389–401.
25. Schenck CH, Milner DM, Hurwitz TD, et al. A polysomnographic and clinical report on sleep-related injury in 100 adult patients. Am J Psychiatry. 1989;146:1166–1173.
26. Mellman TA, Uhde TW. Patients with frequent sleep panic: clinical findings and response to medication treatment. J Clin Psychiatry. 1990;51:513–516.
27. Uhde TW, Tancer ME, Gurguis GNM. Chemical models of anxiety: evidence for diagnostic and neurotransmitter specificity. Int Rev J Psychiatry. 1990;2:367–384.
28. Anderson DJ, Noyes R, Crowe RR. A comparison of panic disorder and generalized anxiety disorder. Am J Psychiatry. 1984;141:572–575.
29. Hoehn-Saric R, McLeod DR. Generalized anxiety disorder in adulthood. In: Hersen M, Last CG, eds. Handbook of Child and Adult Psychopathology: A Longitudinal Perspective. New York, NY: Pergamon Press; 1990:247–260.
30. Akiskal HS, Lemmi H, Dickens H, et al. Chronic depression, part 2: sleep EEG differentiation of primary dysthymic disorders from anxious depression. J Affect Dis. 1984;6:287–295.
31. Sitaram N, Dube S, Jones D, et al. Acetylcholine and alpha-adrenergic sensitivity in the separation of depression and anxiety. Psychopathology. 1984;17:24–39.
32. Reynolds CF, Shaw PH, Newton TF, et al. EEG sleep in outpatients with generalized anxiety: a preliminary comparison with depressed outpatients. Psychiatry Res. 1983;8:81–89.
33. Uhde TW, Tancer ME, Black B, et al. Phenomenology and neurobiology of social phobia: comparison with panic disorder. J Clin Psychiatry. 1991;52(suppl):31–40.
34. Stein MB, Kroft CD, Walker JR. Sleep impairment in patients with social phobia. Psychiatry Res. 1993;49:251–256.
35. Brown TM, Black B, Uhde TW. The sleep architecture of social phobia. Biol Psychiatry. 1994;15:420–421.
36. Insel TR, Gillin JC, Moore A, et al. The sleep of patients with obsessive-compulsive disorder. Arch Gen Psychiatry. 1982;39:1372–1377.
37. Rapoport J, Elkins R, Langer DH, et al. Childhood obsessive-compulsive disorder. Am J Psychiatry. 1981;138:1545–1554.
38. Mellman TA, Davis GC. Combat-related flashbacks in posttraumatic stress disorder: phenomenology and similarity to panic attacks. J Clin Psychiatry. 1985;46:379–382.
39. Archibald HC, Long DM, Miller C, et al. Gross stress reaction in combat: a 15-year follow-up. Am J Psychiatry. 1962;119:317–322.
40. DeFazio VJ, Rustin S, Diamond A. Symptom development in Vietnam era veterans. Am J Orthopsychiatry. 1975;45:158–163.
41. Horowitz MJ, Wilner N, Kaltreider N, et al. Signs and symptoms of posttraumatic stress disorder. Arch Gen Psychiatry. 1980;37:85–92.
42. van der Kolk BA, Hartmann E, Burr A, et al. A survey of nightmare frequencies in a veterans outpatient clinic. Sleep Res. 1980;9:229.
43. Ross RJ, Ball WA, Sullivan KA, et al. Sleep disturbance as the hallmark of posttraumatic stress disorder. Am J Psychiatry. 1989;146:697–707.
44. Belicky D, Belicky K. Nightmares in a university population. Sleep Res. 1982;11:116.
45. Feldman MJ, Hersen M. Attitudes toward death in nightmare subjects. J Abnormal Psychol. 1967;72:421–425.
46. Schlosberg A, Benjamin M. Sleep patterns in three acute combat fatigue cases. J Clin Psychiatry. 1978;39:546–549.
47. van der Kolk B, Blitz R, Burr W, et al. Nightmares and trauma: a comparison of nightmares after combat with lifelong nightmares in veterans. Am J Psychiatry. 1984;141:187–190.
48. Cartwright RD. Rapid eye movement sleep characteristics during

and after mood-disturbing events. Arch Gen Psychiatry. 1983;40:197–201.

49. Greenberg R, Pearlman CA, Gampel D. War neuroses and the adaptive function of REM sleep. Br J Med Psychol. 1972;45:27–33.

50. Kauffman CD, Reist C, Djenderedjian A, et al. Biological markers of affective disorders and posttraumatic stress disorder: a pilot study with desipramine. J Clin Psychiatry. 1987;48:366–367.

51. Kramer M, Kinney L. Sleep patterns in trauma victims with disturbed dreaming. Psychiatr J Univ Ottawa. 1988;13:12–16.

52. Lavie P, Hefez A, Halperin G, et al. Long-term effects of trumatic war-related events on sleep. Am J Psychiatr. 1979;136:175–178.

53. van Kammen W, Christiansen C, van Kammen D, et al. Sleep and the POW experience. Sleep Res. 1987;16:291.

54. Lipper S, Davidson JRT, Grady TA, et al. Preliminary study of carbamazepine in post traumatic stress disorder. Psychosomatics. 1986;27:849–854.

55. Kolb LC, Burris BC, Griffiths S. Propranolol and clonidine in the treatment of post traumatic disorders of war. In: van der Kolk BA, ed. Post Traumatic Stress Disorder: Psychological and Biological Sequelae. Washington, DC: American Psychiatric Press; 1984:97–107.

56. Lowenstein RJ, Hornstein N, Farber B. Open trial of clonazepam in the treatment of post traumatic stress symptoms in multiple personality disorder. Dissociation. 1988;1:3–12.

57. Johnson R, Nasdahl C, Ayubi MA, et al. Buspirone in the treatment of posttraumatic stress disorder. Pharmacotherapy. 1991;11:340–343.

58. Wells BG, Chu C-C, Johnson R, et al. Buspirone in the treatment of posttraumatic stress disorder. Pharmacotherapy. 1991;11:340–343.

59. Kinzie JD, Leung P. Clonidine in Cambodian patients with post-traumatic stress disorder. J Nerv Ment Dis. 1989;177:546–550.

60. Hogben GL, Cornfield RB. Treatment of traumatic war neurosis with phenelzinel. Arch Gen Psychiatry. 1981;38:440–445.

61. Benca RM, Obermeyer WH, Thisted RA, et al. Sleep and psychiatric disorders: a meta-analysis. Arch Gen Psychiatry. 1992;49:651–668.

62. Robinson D, Walsleben J, Pollack S, et al. Nocturnal polysomnography in obsessive-compulsive disorder. Psychiatry Res. 1998;80:257–263.

63. Hohagen F, Lis S, Krieger S, et al. Sleep EEG of patients with obsessive-compulsive disorder. Eur Arch Psychiatry Clin Neurosci. 1994;243:273–278.

64. Hurwitz TD, Mahowald MW, Kuskowski M, et al. Polysomnographic sleep is not clinically impaired in Vietnam combat veterans with chronic posttraumatic stress disorder. Biol Psychiatry. 1998;44:1066–1073.

65. Woodward SH, Friedman MJ, Bliwise DL. Sleep and depression in combat-related PTSD inpatients. Biol Psychiatry. 1996;39:182–192.

66. Ross RJ, Ball WA, Dinges DF, et al. Rapid eye movement sleep disturbance in posttraumatic stress disorder. Biol Psychiatry. 1994;35:195–202.

67. Ross RJ, Ball WA, Dinges DF, et al. Motor dysfunction during sleep in posttraumatic stress disorder. Sleep. 1994;17:723–732.

68. Mellman TA, Kulick-Bell R, Ashlock LE, et al. Sleep events among veterans with combat-related posttraumatic stress disorder. Am J Psychiatry. 1995;152:110–115.

69. Mellman TA, Nolan B, Hebding J, et al. A polysomnographic comparison of veterans with combat-related PTSD, depressed men, and non-ill controls. Sleep. 1997;20:46–51.

70. Dow BM, Kelsoe JR Jr, Gillin JC. Sleep and dreams in Vietnam PTSD and depression. Biol Psychiatry. 1996;39:42–50.

71. Paradis CM, Friedman S, Hatch M. Isolated sleep paralysis in African Americans with panic disorder. Cult Divers Ment Health. 1997;3:69–76.

72. Labbate LA, Johnson MR, Lydiard RB, et al. Sleep deprivation in social phobia and generalized anxiety disorder. Biol Psychiatry. 1998;43:840–842.

96

Mood Disorders

Ruth M. Benca

Disturbed sleep is characteristic of patients with mood disorders, and changes in sleep patterns are among the diagnostic criteria for these illnesses. In epidemiological surveys of the general adult population, 14 to 20% of subjects with significant complaints of insomnia showed evidence of major depression, whereas rates of depression were less than 1% in those without sleep complaints.[1, 2] An assessment of the lifetime prevalence of sleep disturbance and psychiatric disorders in young adults also found greatly increased rates of major depression in patients with sleep complaints (31.1% for those with insomnia, 25.3% for those with hypersomnia, and 54.3% for those with both insomnia and hypersomnia) in comparison with those with no sleep complaints (2.7%).[3]

The association between insomnia and depression may be even greater in clinical samples. A study of patients presenting to general medical clinics found that the symptoms of sleep disturbance and fatigue had the greatest positive predictive values (61% and 69%, respectively) for significant depressive symptoms.[4] Studies of diagnostic patterns in sleep disorders centers have found that the most common primary diagnosis in patients presenting with a complaint of insomnia is a psychiatric illness, particularly depression. In a multicenter study of patients evaluated by clinical interview and polysomnography, a diagnosis of insomnia related to psychiatric disorders was made in 35% of cases, and half of those had mood disorders.[5] In a more recent study, the International Classification of Sleep Disorders (ICSD) diagnosis of sleep disorder associated with mood disorder was diagnosed in over half of insomnia and medical and psychiatric patients evaluated by clinical interview in sleep disorders centers.[6]

There may also be an increased association between primary sleep disorders and psychiatric disorders. For example, patients with sleep apnea or narcolepsy appear to have elevated levels of anxiety, depression, and substance abuse.[7–12]

It has historically been assumed that mood disorders cause changes in sleep patterns. Possible explanations for sleep disturbance include the increased anxiety and arousal experienced by most patients, abnormalities in circadian rhythms, and the fact that neurobiological systems involved in mood and behavior may also mediate sleep.

Sleep changes, however, may affect mood disorders as well, and some epidemiological data support this contention. Subjects who reported insomnia at both initial interview and at 1-year follow-up interview were more likely to have developed a new major depression (odds ratio: 39.8) than were subjects whose insomnia had resolved by the second interview (odds ratio: 1.6).[2] In a subsequent study using a similar two-wave longitudinal design, Breslau et al.[3] found that a history of sleep disturbance in the baseline interview was associated with an increased risk for new onset of major depression, anxiety disorders, substance abuse disorders, and nicotine dependence. The association appeared to be strongest between sleep disturbance and major depression, even when depression was defined on criterion symptoms other than sleep disturbance.

A long-term prospective study found that men who reported insomnia or difficulty sleeping under stress while in medical school showed significantly increased relative risks (2.0 and 1.8, respectively) for development of major depression during a median follow-up period of 34 years.[13] These data suggest that insomnia is predictive of depression and may contribute to the development of mood disorders.

CLASSIFICATION AND PATHOPHYSIOLOGY

Mood disorders are subclassified into bipolar disorders and depressive disorders.[14] Bipolar disorder is diagnosed in patients who have experienced at least one manic episode; most patients have had depressive episodes as well. Manic episodes are described in Table 96–1 and are characterized by elevated or irritable mood. Other symptoms may include decreased sleep (usually perceived as decreased need for sleep), grandiosity, rapid thought and speech, psychomotor agitation, distractibility, or hedonistic indulgences such as shopping sprees, drinking, or sexual activity. During a hypomanic episode, the mood disturbance and some of the associated symptoms are present but not as severe as in a full manic episode. Individuals with cyclothymia have alternating episodes of hypomania and depressed mood.

Depressive disorders include major depressive disorder, diagnosed in people who have experienced one or more major depressive episodes. Diagnostic criteria for major depression are listed in Table 96–2. At least five symptoms must be present for the same 2-week

Table 96–1. CRITERIA FOR MANIC EPISODE

A. A distinct period of abnormality and persistently elevated, expansive, or irritable mood, lasting at least 1 week (or any duration if hospitalization is necessary).

B. During the period of mood disturbance, three (or more) of the following symptoms have persisted (four if the mood is only irritable) and have been present to a significant degree:
   1. Inflated self-esteem or grandiosity
   2. Decreased need for sleep (e.g., feels rested after only 3 h of sleep)
   3. More talkative than usual or pressure to keep talking
   4. Flight of ideas or subjective experience that thoughts are racing
   5. Distractibility (i.e., attention too easily drawn to unimportant or irrelevant external stimuli)
   6. Increase in goal-directed activity (either socially, at work or school, or sexually) or psychomotor agitation
   7. Excessive involvement in pleasurable activities that have a high potential for painful consequences (e.g., engaging in unrestrained buying sprees, sexual indiscretion, or foolish business investments)

C. The symptoms do not meet criteria for a mixed episode.

D. The mood disturbance is sufficiently severe to cause marked impairment in occupational functioning or in usual social activities or relationships with others, or to necessitate hospitalization to prevent harm to self or others, or there are psychotic features.

E. The symptoms are not due to the direct physiological effects of a substance (e.g., a drug of abuse, a medication, or other treatment) or a general medical condition (e.g., hyperthyroidism).

Note: Manic-like episodes that are clearly caused by somatic antidepressant treatment (e.g., medication, electroconvulsive therapy, light therapy) should not count toward a diagnosis of bipolar I disorder.

Modified with permission from the *Diagnostic and Statistical Manual of Mental Disorders, Fourth Edition.* Copyright 1994 American Psychiatric Association.

tween acute episodes. As the overall duration of illness increases, individual episodes may occur more frequently and last longer.

Over the years, various subclassifications of depressive disorders have been developed. The earliest distinctions were based upon presumed differences in the causes of endogenous depression, which occurred in the absence of environmental or neurotic or characterological factors, and reactive depression, which represented responses to external stressors. However, in many cases of depression, both biological and environmental factors are involved, making the classification of a particular episode as endogenous vs. reactive (or nonendogenous) difficult. Another system defined de-

Table 96–2. CRITERIA FOR MAJOR DEPRESSIVE EPISODE

A. Five (or more) of the following symptoms have been present during the same 2-week period and represent a change from previous functioning; at least one of the symptoms is either (1) depressed mood or (2) loss of interest or pleasure.
Note: Do not include symptoms that are clearly due to a general medical condition, or mood-incongruent delusions or hallucinations.
   1. Depressed mood most of the day, nearly every day, as indicated by either subjective report (e.g., feels sad or empty) or observation made by others (e.g., appears tearful)
   Note: In children and adolescents, can be irritable mood.
   2. Markedly diminished interest or pleasure in all, or almost all, activities most of the day, nearly every day (as indicated by either subjective account or observation made by others)
   3. Significant weight loss when not dieting or weight gain (e.g., a change of more than 5% of body weight in a month), or decrease or increase in appetite nearly every day
   Note: In children, consider failure to make expected weight gains.
   4. Insomnia or hypersomnia nearly every day
   5. Psychomotor agitation or retardation nearly every day (observable by others, not merely subjective feelings of restlessness or being slowed down)
   6. Fatigue or loss of energy nearly every day
   7. Feelings of worthlessness or excessive or inappropriate guilt (which may be delusional) nearly every day (not merely self-reproach or guilt about being sick)
   8. Diminished ability to think or concentrate, or indecisiveness, nearly every day (either by subjective account or as observed by others)
   9. Recurrent thoughts of death (not just fear of dying), recurrent suicidal ideation without a specific plan, or a suicide attempt or a specific plan for committing suicide

B. The symptoms do not meet criteria for a mixed episode.

C. The symptoms cause clinically significant distress or impairment in social, occupational, or other important areas of functioning.

D. The symptoms are not due to the direct physiological effects of a substance (e.g., a drug of abuse, a medication) or a general medical condition (e.g., hypothyroidism).

E. The symptoms are not better accounted for by bereavement, that is, after the loss of a loved one, the symptoms persist for longer than 2 months or are characterized by marked functional impairment, morbid preoccupational with worthlessness, suicidal ideation, psychotic symptoms, or psychomotor retardation.

Modified with permission from the *Diagnostic and Statistical Manual of Mental Disorders, Fourth Edition.* Copyright 1994 American Psychiatric Association.

period, and at least one symptom must be either depressed mood or loss of interest or pleasure. Other symptoms of major depressive episodes include insomnia or hypersomnia, weight gain or loss, increased or decreased psychomotor activity, decreased energy, poor concentration, feelings of worthlessness or guilt, or suicidal thoughts. Suicidal ideation is common in more severe depression, and up to 15% of patients ultimately commit suicide. Individuals who are chronically depressed for at least 2 years but do not meet the full criteria for major depression during that period are classified as dysthymic.

Mood disorders tend to appear in the 3rd decade of life, but first occurrences of major depression, in particular, can appear at any point in the life span. Major depression is a common disorder and is reported to have a lifetime prevalence of 5 to 12% in men and 10 to 25% in women.[15] Bipolar disorder, on the other hand, affects only about 1% of the population and shows no gender predilection. Both illnesses occur with increased frequency in first-degree relatives of affected individuals.

Most episodes of depression or mania last fewer than 6 months, and patients tend to recover fully be-

pression as primary or secondary. Primary depression referred to any case that was not preceded by another psychiatric disorder, whereas secondary depression occurred following, or in conjunction with, another psychiatric illness. Depressed patients also have been classified as psychotic (delusional) or nonpsychotic (nondelusional), depending on the presence or absence of psychotic symptoms. One purpose of these classifications has been to determine if subgroups with similar clinical features showed evidence of common pathophysiological mechanisms. Currently, major depressive episodes may be categorized with one of several specifiers. Melancholic features include either loss of pleasure in all, or almost all, activities or a lack of improvement in mood in response to normally pleasurable stimuli. Patients with melancholic features also may complain of early-morning awakening and diurnal variation in mood, with depression worse in the morning. Depressed patients with atypical features, in contrast, show significant mood reactivity to positive events. They characteristically show significant weight gain and hypersomnia during periods of depression. Patients with catatonic features have psychomotor disturbances, which may range from excessive, purposeless motor activity, to catalepsy, stupor, or mutism. Overall, no specific biological marker has been identified, although certain subgroups tend to show evidence of more significant biological disturbances, such as sleep abnormalities. In both bipolar and major depressive disorders, sleep disturbances are more severe during acute episodes of illness but may persist during periods of partial or complete remission.

Although the pathophysiological mechanisms of mood disorders have not yet been identified precisely, it is hypothesized that abnormalities in central nervous system monoaminergic systems are responsible. It has been suggested that relative deficiencies in noradrenergic, serotonergic, or dopaminergic neurotransmission may lead to depression.[16, 17] Antidepressant treatments, including tricyclic antidepressants, monamine oxidase inhibitors, electroconvulsive therapy, and the newer antidepressants, all increase monoaminergic neurotransmission. They also may precipitate mania in susceptible individuals, which supports the theory that mania may be related to increased monaminergic activity.

Studies using a variety of structural and functional brain imaging techniques have suggested that mood disorders are associated with abnormalities in specific brain regions which are known to be involved in emotional regulation (reviewed in references 18, 19, 20). Abnormalities in prefrontal cortex have been documented most consistently in patients with major depression and bipolar disorder; they include decreased volume and reduced blood flow and metabolism. Decrements in area, blood flow, and metabolism in the basal ganglia have also been found in most studies of depressive patients. The evidence for structural or functional abnormalities in temporal lobe, limbic regions, and the thalamus is more equivocal at present. Many of the brain regions implicated in depression also appear to be involved in the regulation of sleep

and wakefulness (see Chapter 10), which suggests that dysfunction in particular brain regions may lead to both mood and sleep abnormalities.[21]

SUBJECTIVE SLEEP COMPLAINTS AND POLYSOMNOGRAPHIC FINDINGS

Clinical Features of Sleep

Most patients with major depression complain of insomnia. Specific features may include difficulty falling asleep, frequent nocturnal awakenings, early-morning awakening, nonrestorative sleep, decreased total sleep, and disturbing dreams. In addition, some patients with insomnia report increased daytime fatigue, and they may attempt to compensate with daytime napping.[22] Episodes of recurrent depression are often preceded by several weeks of subjectively reported increases in sleep disturbance.[23]

Most patients with bipolar disorder also report insomnia while depressed, but a significant percentage of patients with bipolar depression develop symptoms of hypersomnia, with extended nocturnal sleep periods, difficulty awakening, and excessive daytime sleepiness.[24] Similarly, patients with seasonal affective disorder (Table 96–3), a major depressive disorder occurring during the winter months, also show hypersomnia.[25] During manic periods, however, patients usually report significantly reduced amounts of total sleep, often with a subjective sense of a decreased need for sleep. In many cases, switches into manic episodes are preceded by periods of sleeplessness.

Polysomnographic Findings

Major depression has been studied polysomnographically more than any other psychiatric disorder,

---

Table 96–3. CRITERIA FOR SEASONAL PATTERN SPECIFIER

A. There has been a regular temporal relationship between the onset of major depressive episodes in bipolar I or bipolar II disorder or major depressive disorder, recurrent, and a particular time of the year (e.g., regular appearance of the major depressive episode in the fall or winter).
  Note: Do not include cases in which there is an obvious effect of seasonal-related psychosocial stressors (e.g., regularly being unemployed every winter).

B. Full remissions (or a change from depression to mania or hypomania) also occur at a characteristic time of the year (e.g., depression disappears in the spring).

C. In the last 2 years, two major depressive episodes have occurred that demonstrate the temporal seasonal relationships defined in criteria A and B, and no nonseasonal major depressive episodes have occurred during the same period.

D. Seasonal major depressive episodes (as described above) substantially outnumber the nonseasonal major depressive episodes that may have occurred over the individual's lifetime.

Modified with permission from the *Diagnostic and Statistical Manual of Mental Disorders, Fourth Edition.* Copyright 1994 American Psychiatric Association.

and the majority of patients have shown objective sleep disturbances. Sleep abnormalities in depression have been grouped into three general categories[26]:

1. *Sleep continuity disturbances.* The earliest polysomnographic sleep studies in depressed patients showed prolonged sleep latency, increased wakefulness during sleep, and early-morning awakening, which resulted in sleep fragmentation and decreased sleep efficiency.[27–30] Other studies comparing groups of depressed patients with age-matched normal controls have subsequently confirmed these findings of disturbed sleep continuity.[32–38]

2. *Slow-wave sleep (SWS) deficits.* Another early finding was that patients with depression had decreased amounts of SWS.[28, 39] SWS decrements were not merely a result of sleep continuity disturbances because they did not correlate significantly with total sleep loss or sleep fragmentation.[40–43] The evidence to date supports the finding of SWS reductions in patients with mood disorders[44]; significant loss of SWS has been reported in a number of studies.[32, 33, 35, 45] However, not all groups of depressed patients have shown SWS abnormalities in comparison with controls.[36, 46–49]

   Computer analyses have shown that SWS loss is most significant during the first nonrapid eye movement (NREM) period, and that depressive patients appeared to have reduced delta wave power and delta wave counts across the night.[45, 46, 50, 51] Abnormalities in SWS distribution have also been observed, with a decrease in slow-wave activity in the first NREM period relative to the second NREM period.[50]

3. *Rapid eye movement (REM) sleep abnormalities.* A number of changes in REM parameters have been reported, with the earliest finding that REM latency (period of time from sleep onset to REM sleep onset) was significantly reduced in depression.[40, 52–54] Over the years, reduced REM latency has proved to be one of the most robust and specific features of sleep in depressed patients.[32, 33, 35, 38, 44, 47, 48, 55–60] Other reported abnormalities in the REM sleep of patients with depression include prolonged duration of the first REM period,[32, 45, 61] and increased rate of rapid eye movements (increased REM density) during REM sleep.[35, 38, 59, 62] Increased percentage of REM sleep has also been observed.[32, 38, 58] Common sleep complaints and polysomnographic abnormalities are listed in Table 96–4.

Although these polysomnographic features listed earlier have been documented most extensively in patients with major depression, studies of manic subjects have reported similar findings.[36, 63] In contrast, dysthymic subjects tended to show sleep patterns comparable to normal controls.[55, 64] Hypersomnic patients with bipolar depression did not show reduced REM latency consistently, and although they complained of daytime

Table 96–4. SLEEP ABNORMALITIES IN DEPRESSION

Subjective Complaints	Polysomnographic Findings
Insomnia, including	Sleep continuity disturbances
Difficulty falling asleep	Prolonged sleep latency
Increased awakening at night	Increased wake time during sleep
Early morning awakening	Increased early-morning wake time
Decreased amounts of sleep	Decreased total sleep time
Less "deep" sleep	Slow-wave sleep (SWS) deficits
	Decreased SWS amount
	Decreased SWS percentage of total sleep
Disturbing dreams	REM sleep abnormalities
	Reduced REM latency
	Prolongation of the 1st REM period
	Increased REM activity (total number of eye movements during the night)
	Increased REM density (REM activity/total REM time)
	Increased REM percentage of total sleep

sleepiness, their sleep latency, as measured on the multiple sleep latency test (MSLT), was relatively normal.[65]

Further analyses have been performed to determine whether subtypes of mood disorders could be distinguished by polysomnographic testing. Several studies have explored the differences between endogenous vs. nonendogenous and primary vs. secondary depressions. Some investigators have reported reduced REM latency in endogenous and primary depression in comparison with nonendogenous and secondary groups, respectively,[56, 61, 62, 66–68] whereas other investigators were unable to distinguish subtypes.[34, 69–71] Overall, analyses of sleep patterns in patient groups by diagnostic subtypes have not been particularly fruitful either for diagnostic purposes or as a means to identify biologically similar subgroups.

Other attempts have been made to correlate sleep abnormalities with specific symptoms, duration, or global severity of illness. Significant sleep disturbances were not seen in depressed patients who did not meet criteria for major depression and in individuals with depressed mood but not a mood disorder[72]; this finding suggested that a depressed mood alone does not produce the polysomnographic abnormalities of depression. Giles et al.[73] have shown that the symptoms of terminal insomnia, decreased appetite, anhedonia, and unreactive mood were more strongly associated with reduced REM latency in patients with endogenous depression. A 1997 multivariate analysis of sleep variables and depressive symptoms found that a constellation of 15 depressive symptoms, including depressed mood, weight loss, decreased libido, disturbed sleep, anxiety, and self-blame, were correlated with nine sleep variables, particularly decreased delta activity, increased stage 1 sleep percentage, and increased REM activity.[74] These findings have been interpreted as suggesting that the relationship between sleep abnormalities and depression is based on associations between a number of core depressive symptoms and predominantly NREM sleep abnormalities.

Some studies showed that severely ill patients, particularly those with psychotic features, had more significant sleep disturbances.[40, 68, 75–78] In other studies, however, clinical ratings of depression did not correlate significantly with sleep abnormalities.[32, 79, 80] Furthermore, a number of studies failed to find correlations between overall duration of illness, or number of episodes of illness and severity of sleep disturbances.[81–83] Giles et al.[84] reported similar REM latency reductions in patients suffering recurrent vs. first episodes of depression, which was interpreted as showing that depression did not cause reduced REM latency because repeated episodes of illness did not have additive effects on REM latency measures. A more recent study found that patients with multiple episodes of depression had significantly increased phasic REM sleep and poorer sleep efficiency in comparison with patients experiencing their first depressive episode.[85] Thus, additive effects of illness may affect some, but not all, sleep parameters associated with depression.

There is evidence to suggest that the duration of the depressive episode may also correlate with the degree of observed sleep abnormalities. In studies of middle-aged patients, REM sleep abnormalities were more pronounced during the early phase of a recurrent episode in comparison with a more chronic phase of a previous episode.[83, 86] A more recent study of elderly subjects found that both REM and NREM sleep abnormalities were more severe in patients during the early phase of a depressive episode in comparison with patients who had been depressed for longer periods of time.[87] These findings suggest that more significant REM sleep abnormalities may be associated with an earlier phase of the depressive episode or recurrence.

The presence of sleep disturbance does not necessarily indicate that a patient is acutely ill at the time of study. Several studies have reported sleep abnormalities in patients in remission as well as during episodes of illness. Some sleep abnormalities may be more severe in acute vs. remitted phases, including increased REM density and reduced sleep efficiency.[88–91] However, reduced REM sleep latency and decreased SWS can persist for prolonged periods of time in otherwise asymptomatic individuals.[70, 82, 91–94] Thus, sleep disturbances—particularly reduced REM sleep latency and SWS abnormalities—may be trait markers for some patients with mood disorders rather than simply indications of an acute state of illness. The persistence of sleep abnormalities in the absence of clinical illness has been interpreted in two ways: (1) sleep disturbance may indicate a biological susceptibility to depression and predate the illness, or (2) sleep changes may be caused by depression and persist much longer than other affective symptoms.[26]

The hypothesis of reduced REM latency as a trait rather than a state marker is further supported by data from family studies. First-degree relatives with major depression tend to show concordance in REM latency measures.[84] Furthermore, first-degree relatives of probands with major depression and short REM latency are themselves more likely to show reduced REM latency and SWS deficits, even without a personal history of a mood disorder.[82, 95] Another study compared nonpsychiatrically ill subjects who had at least one first-degree relative with a mood disorder (high-risk probands) with healthy subjects without any family history of psychiatric illness (normal probands). Although their affected first-degree relatives were not characterized polysomnographically, the high-risk probands showed increased phasic REM sleep and reduced SWS in comparison with the normal probands.[96] These data suggest familial transmission of polysomnographic features of sleep associated with depression. Ongoing longitudinal studies will determine whether the sleep abnormalities confer increased risk for development of mood disorders.

Age strongly affects the relationship between sleep patterns and mood disorders. A 1990 analysis of age and gender effects in depressive people showed that REM latency, SWS amount, and sleep efficiency declined with age, and that SWS amounts were greater in females than males.[97] Younger groups with depression were generally indistinguishable from controls in most sleep parameters.[44] Although some studies have reported sleep differences—particularly reduced REM latency—in younger depressed patients,[57, 58, 60, 98] others have not found significant sleep abnormalities in depressed children and adolescents.[99–103] The interaction of depression and age on sleep parameters has led some investigators to suggest that depression may accelerate the effects of aging on sleep.[104–107] This is probably not the case because some sleep parameters that change with age do not show increased effects of depression. For example, elderly patients with depression do not tend to have significant reductions in SWS compared with controls; the absence of a difference may result from both groups having very little SWS by that time.[44] The duration of the first REM period, sleep latency, and other sleep-continuity measures also do not show evidence of depression-age interactions.[44] In summary, although adult groups of patients are more easily distinguished from controls, the effects of age on sleep in depression cannot yet be explained easily. As discussed earlier, depressed mood per se is not the initial determinant of the sleep disorder of people with depression. Perhaps the depressed mood in young and old patients results from different pathogenic processes, and it is only the depressive process in older people that is associated with anomalies of sleep.

Sensitivity and Specificity

The potential diagnostic utility of polysomnography in mood disorders is dependent on the specificity and sensitivity of the sleep abnormalities. Although most patients with mood disorders show significant sleep abnormalities on electroencephalography (EEG) testing in comparison with normal controls, so do other psychiatric patients.[44]

Most studies have assessed sensitivity and specificity of either REM latency alone or combinations of sleep parameters for distinguishing mood disorder patients from normal controls. Short REM latency alone has shown sensitivities of up to 70% and even higher degrees of specificity in identifying depressed patients.[84, 108] However, one of the problems in attempting to define cut-off values for REM latency has been the lack of a standardized definition of REM latency. Different definitions (yielding different calculated values of REM latency) show varying degrees of sensitivity and specificity for depression.[109, 110] REM density (number of eye movements divided by REM time) has been shown to distinguish people with depression from controls,[111, 112] but it is also a parameter without a uniformly accepted definition.

Discriminative analyses using multiple sleep parameters have been relatively successful in separating depressed patients from controls and insomniacs[33] or from those with anxiety disorders.[110] Sleep variables distinguished elderly depressive patients from demented patients as well. In comparison to patients with dementia, patients with depression showed shorter REM latency, increased REM percentage of total sleep, and more early-morning awakening[113]; patients with dementia produced fewer sleep spindles and K complexes in NREM sleep.

A detailed comparison of sleep variables in patients with mood disorders, other patient groups, and normal controls was performed using meta-analysis,[44] a statistical technique for combining data from different studies. Data from 177 polysomnographic studies of patients with psychiatric disorders, dementia, and narcolepsy (for comparison) were included. Significant sleep disturbances were identified in all patient groups in comparison with age-matched controls, although mood disorders groups showed the greatest number of abnormalities. Although patients with mood disorders showed significant sleep continuity disturbances and decreased amounts of SWS compared with controls, groups of patients with mood disorders were generally not distinguishable from other illness categories in these parameters. For REM sleep parameters, other groups with psychiatric illnesses had abnormalities similar to those with mood disorders. In particular, groups of patients with schizophrenia, borderline personality, and eating disorders showed reduced REM latency in analyses of controlled studies or all available (including uncontrolled) studies. Thus, the meta-analysis suggested that REM latency was not useful in distinguishing patients with mood disorders from all other patient groups; mean REM latency values were not always significantly different from mood disorders for several other disorders, including borderline personality and narcolepsy. However, REM latency reductions in comparison with normal controls were more robust in mood disorders groups than in groups with other psychiatric disorders, and thus were relatively specific.

The fact that REM latency reductions can be found in patients with psychiatric disorders other than primary major depression has led to speculation that the presence of short REM latency may signify the presence of a concomitant depressive illness. Alternatively, it may indicate common biological factors in different disorders. Short REM latency has been reported occasionally in panic disorder,[112, 114] post-traumatic stress disorder,[115, 116] eating disorders,[117, 118] alcoholism,[119] schizophrenia, and schizoaffective disorder.[120–123] Each of these disorders can be accompanied by depression, but decreased REM latency could not be accounted for by coexisting depression in all studies.[123] However, short REM latency has been demonstrated more consistently in borderline personality disorder, which is characterized by instability of affect and a high rate of depression.[124–129] Clearly, reduced REM latency may be seen in patients with secondary depression, but it is not yet known whether reduced REM latency is a specific indicator of past or current depression.

Correlation of Sleep Findings With Other Markers

Attempts have been made to correlate changes in sleep parameters with other biological abnormalities in depression. Many patients with depression show dysregulation of their hypothalamic-pituitary-adrenal axis, characterized by excessive cortisol secretion. They also show a lack of cortisol suppression in response to challenge with dexamethasone.[130, 131] One question that has been addressed is whether people with depression who fail to reduce cortisol secretion in response to the dexamethasone suppression test (DST) are the same people who exhibit short REM latency. Although the two groups (DST nonsuppressors and those with short REM latency) are not identical, the two parameters tend to be correlated.[49, 132–135] In addition to showing an abnormal response to dexamethasone, people with depression tend to secrete excessive daily amounts of cortisol, and cortisol hypersecretors tend to have reduced REM latency.[136] Cortisol may also show an abnormal pattern of secretion; an earlier cortisol nadir and an earlier rise were observed in some[137–139] but not all groups with depression.[140]

Correlations between circadian rhythms of body temperature and REM sleep patterns also have been studied. Depressed individuals had elevated nocturnal temperature means[141, 142] and decreased amplitudes of the temperature rhythm.[143, 144] In some studies, a possible phase advance of the temperature curve has been described, including earlier appearances of maximal and minimal body temperatures.[143, 145, 146] A more recent study of unipolar depressed outpatients during periods of illness and remission failed to document differences in nocturnal or circadian body temperatures in comparison with healthy controls; however, sleep parameters were not reported for these subjects.[147] Short REM latency has been significantly correlated with both flatter amplitudes of temperature rhythm[148] and higher mean nocturnal temperatures.[141]

DIAGNOSIS AND TREATMENT OF SLEEP DISTURBANCE IN PATIENTS WITH MOOD DISORDERS

The diagnosis of a mood disorder is often complicated by the failure of the patient to recognize the nature of the illness. Patients with mood disorders may present to primary care physicians or sleep clinics with complaints of insomnia alone. People with depression often try to deny the presence of an emotional disturbance and attribute their symptoms of fatigue, poor concentration, and loss of interest to sleep loss. The strong association between mood disorders and insomnia has been suggested in recent surveys of the general population, which have demonstrated that depression is prevalent in individuals with significant sleep disturbance.[1, 2] Recognition of major depression is important for determining appropriate treatment and must include careful assessment of possible suicide risk, given the high rate of suicide in this patient group. Obviously, patients with suicidal ideation should not be given potentially lethal amounts of hypnotics or antidepressants.

Although this chapter focuses on primary mood disorders, it should be emphasized that depression is a common feature of many other illnesses that are also associated with sleep disruption. Depressive symptoms are common in people with chronic medical illnesses, as well as those suffering from other psychiatric disorders, including alcoholism or substance abuse, anxiety disorders, schizophrenia, eating disorders, somatoform disorders, and personality disorders. Even though objective sleep abnormalities characteristic of depression are not routinely found in populations with secondary depression, these patients commonly complain of poor sleep. In addition to appropriate diagnostic and therapeutic interventions for the primary medical and psychiatric illnesses, adjunctive antidepressant treatment may be helpful to many of these patients.

Mood disorders and the accompanying sleep disturbances may be treated with medication, psychotherapy, or a combination of both. Patients meeting criteria for major depression with moderate-to-severe symptoms usually are treated with medication (Table 96–5). Slightly over one half of all depressed patients improve regardless of the choice of drug. Individuals with the melancholic type of depression, including diurnal variation in mood, loss of interest or pleasure, lack of mood reactivity to environmental stimuli, early-morning awakening, and weight loss, have a significantly greater response rate to somatic therapies. The tricyclic antidepressants and most of the newer agents are roughly equivalent in terms of overall clinical efficacy, although individual patients may respond preferentially to particular drugs. The initial choice of antidepressant is therefore often made on the basis of a side effect profile of the drug; patients with agitated depression and severe insomnia might be started on a more sedating antidepressant, for example. Pharmacological treatments for mood disorders all have significant effects on sleep, including both the tendency to normalize sleep patterns by treating the underlying illness, as well as direct effects on sleep.

Serotonin selective reuptake inhibitors (SSRIs) are currently the most widely prescribed class of drugs for depression in the United States. Along with some of the other newer agents (e.g., bupropion, mirtazapine, nefazodone, and venlafaxine) they have become first-line agents because of their safety and improved side effect profiles in comparison to the older tricyclics and monoamine oxidase inhibitors (MAOIs). SSRIs, bupropion, and venlafaxine can cause significant sleep disruption and worsen insomnia in some patients, however.[149–153] In contrast, nefazodone, trazodone, and mirtazapine are sedating and may improve sleep initiation and maintenance.

Although the use of tricyclic antidepressants has diminished because of the associated side effects and greater toxicity, these drugs may be effective in patients who fail to improve with SSRIs or other, newer antidepressants. Most tricyclics are quite sedating and may be helpful to patients with insomnia. In fact, low doses of tricyclics such as amitriptyline have commonly been prescribed for insomnia, although there are no controlled studies on the use of tricyclics as hypnotics in the absence of significant depression.

Patients who fail to improve with other agents, and those with atypical features (hypersomnia, increased appetite) or a significant component of anxiety, may respond to MAOIs. The drawback to using these agents is the danger of hypertensive crisis if used in combination with sympathomimetic drugs or with foods containing tyramine. Severely depressed patients, including those with psychotic features or strong suicidal intent, may require a course of electroconvulsive therapy (ECT). Antipsychotics are also used in combination with antidepressants in delusional or psychotic patients. Commonly used antidepressants, their dose ranges, and their side effects are listed in Table 96–5.

Many antidepressant medications have REM-suppressant effects, which has led to the theory that some antidepressants work by causing selective REM sleep deprivation.[154] MAOIs are the most potent suppressors of REM sleep, and they may virtually eliminate REM sleep for prolonged periods of treatment.[155–157] Tricyclics, SSRIs, and venlafaxine also reduce REM amounts and prolong REM latency.[151, 153, 157a–157d] ECT has also been reported to prolong REM sleep latency but has little effect on REM sleep amount.[159] Not surprisingly, abrupt cessation of REM sleep–suppressing antidepressants is associated with REM sleep rebound, with accompanying symptoms of bizarre, intense, or frightening dreams and sleep fragmentation.[160]

Some of the newer antidepressants, however, do not suppress REM sleep, suggesting that REM sleep suppression is not necessary for clinical efficacy. Trazodone and nefazodone are relatively sedating drugs with no consistent effects on REM sleep patterns. Bupropion, a more activating agent, has been reported to cause increases in REM sleep.[161]

Antidepressants may also show a variety of other effects on sleep. Some patients complain of "hangover" effects from the more anticholinergic agents. Fluoxetine has been associated with frequent eye movements in NREM sleep, which may persist for prolonged periods following cessation of treatment; the clinical significance of this effect is unknown.[162] Tricyclic antidepressants and SSRIs have been implicated in precipitating or exacerbating restless legs or periodic leg movements, and thus may exacerbate symptoms of insomnia

Table 96–5. TREATMENT OF MAJOR DEPRESSION

Medication	Usual Therapeutic Dosage Range (mg)	Pharmacological Mechanism	Side Effects	Effects on Sleep
Heterocyclic antidepressants Amitriptyline (Elavil) Imipramine (Tofranil) Doxepin (Sinequan) Nortriptyline (Pamelor) Clomipramine (Anafranil) Desipramine (Norpramin) Protriptyline (Vivactil)	75–150 75–200 75–150 75–150 100–250 100–200 15–60	Inhibit serotonin and norepinephrine reuptake Anticholinergic Antihistaminergic	*Anticholinergic* effects (drugs listed in decreasing order of severity): blurred vision, dry mouth, urinary retention, orthostatic hypotension, flushing, tachycardia, confusion, others Other side effects include: liver toxicity, lowering of seizure threshold, sweating Weight gain	Sedation (drugs listed in decreasing order); clomipramine, desipramine, and protriptyline may be nonsedating or even activating) REM sleep suppression Increased stage 2 sleep
Monoamine oxidase inhibitors Phenelzine (Nardil) Tranylcypromine (Parnate)	45–90 10–30	Inhibit monoamine oxidase, increasing norepinephrine, serotonin, and dopamine	Hypertensive crisis in combination with tyramine-containing foods or sympathomimetics Anticholinergic effects Dizziness, agitation, liver toxicity Weight gain	Insomnia Potent REM sleep suppression
Serotonin selective reuptake inhibitors (SSRIs) Fluoxetine (Prozac) Paroxetine (Paxil) Sertraline (Zoloft)	20–60 20–60 50–200	Inhibit serotonin transporter	Gastrointestinal disturbances Sexual dysfunction Anxiety, agitation	Insomnia REM sleep suppression Increased eye movements in NREM sleep
Trazodone (Desyrel) Nefazodone (Serzone)	150–600 300–600	Inhibits serotonin reuptake Serotonin-2 receptor antagonist	Few anticholinergic effects Priapism Nausea, dizziness, dry mouth	Significant sedation REM sleep suppression Increased slow-wave sleep Sedation
Bupropion (Wellbutrin)	225–450	Inhibits norepinephrine and dopamine reuptake	Gastrointestinal upset Lowering of seizure threshold	Insomnia Increased REM sleep
Venlafaxine (Effexor)	150–375	Inhibits serotonin, norepinephrine, and dopamine reuptake	Anxiety Anorexia	Insomnia
Mirtazapine (Remeron)	15–45	Alpha$_2$-adrenoceptor antagonist Serotonin-2 receptor antagonist	Increased appetite, weight gain Dizziness	Sedation

by this mechanism in some patients.[163–165] REM behavior disorder also has been reported following administration of various antidepressants.[162, 166]

Patients with bipolar disorders generally require the use of mood stabilizers (Table 96–6). Lithium carbonate is the treatment of choice for most manic patients, although neuroleptics may also be required during the acute phase of a manic episode. The anticonvulsants carbamazepine and valproate sodium also have been found to be effective treatments for patients with bipolar disorders who cannot be controlled with lithium, and may be used alone or in combination with lithium. The efficacy of both lithium and the anticonvulsants is dependent on achieving adequate plasma drug levels. Mood-stabilizing agents have more potent antimanic than antidepressant effects, and depressed patients with bipolar disorders may require antidepressant medication in addition.

Lithium carbonate may prolong REM latency and suppress REM sleep time.[167] In manic patients, it has been shown to increase SWS amounts as well. Lithium and the mood-stabilizing anticonvulsants can lead to increased daytime sleepiness, particularly at higher plasma levels. Lithium has also been reported to induce restless legs syndrome.[168]

In treating patients with mood disorders and prominent sleep disturbances, it is important to focus on the psychiatric illness rather than the sleep complaint alone; as the acute illness resolves, so may the sleep problem. In mild to moderate cases of depression or hypomania, insomnia can be an important target symptom and a gauge of treatment efficacy. The degree of sleep disturbance is not always linked with the clinical course of a mood disturbance, however. For example, fluoxetine was found to be equally effective in ameliorating depression in comparison to nefazodone, but significantly more disruptive of sleep.[169, 170]

Nevertheless, the choice of a specific drug regimen should be influenced by the patient's sleep complaint. Patients with agitated depression or mania and total insomnia may initially require a benzodiazepine or a sedating neuroleptic medication if psychosis is present.

It may be particularly important to treat insomnia in mania, because sleep loss might be a trigger for manic episodes in some patients. For depressed patients with insomnia, more highly sedating antidepressants can be administered in a single dose at bedtime. Although the mood stabilizers (lithium carbonate, carbamazepine, or valproate sodium) need to be given in divided doses throughout the day to maintain adequate plasma levels, they also tend to be sedating, and a larger proportion of medication may be given at bedtime. If antipsychotic medications are indicated, they should also be given at bedtime to obtain maximal benefit from their sleep-inducing effects.

When treating sleep disorders associated with depression, it is usually necessary to administer antidepressant medications in full therapeutic dosages. Low doses of antidepressants are commonly prescribed for a variety of sleep disorders, including insomnia and sleep apnea and some parasomnias, but they may not be effective for treatment of the insomnia that accompanies a major depression. An adequate clinical trial of an antidepressant usually requires a minimum of 3 weeks at a therapeutic dose (see Table 96–5).

Insomnia occurring in patients treated with activating antidepressants (e.g., SSRIs or bupropion), or which persists in spite of treatment with other antidepressants or mood stabilizers, may require additional pharmacotherapy. Trazodone has been shown to be effective as a hypnotic in patients with chronic insomnia with and without depression,[171, 172] and is frequently combined with other antidepressants to improve sleep.[173] Hypnotics such as zolpidem and triazolam can usually be safely combined with antidepressants, although care should be taken when combining drugs that are metabolized by the cytochrome P-450 system, such as the SSRIs, nefazodone, benzodiazepines (alprazolam, clonazepam, diazepam, and triazolam), and zolpidem.

Patients with mood disorders and chronic sleep disturbances tend to develop a superimposed component of psychophysiological insomnia and can probably benefit from behavioral therapies as well. Relaxation or stimulus-control techniques may be helpful in some

Table 96–6. TREATMENT OF MANIA

Medication	Usual Dosage Range	Side Effects	Effects on Sleep
Lithium carbonate	600–1800 mg/d—plasma level (0.7–1.5 mEq/l)	Increased white blood cell count Polyuria, polydipsia Diabetes insipidus Decreased thyroid function Weight gain Gastrointestinal upset Tremor	Sedation Increased total sleep May increase slow-wave sleep, decrease REM sleep
Carbamazepine	800–1200 mg/d—plasma level (4–12 μg/ml)	Bone marrow suppression (rare) Liver toxicity Rashes	Sedation
Valproate sodium	30–60 mg/kg/d—plasma level (50–100 μg/ml)	Gastrointestinal upset Liver toxicity Tremor Weight gain Rashes	Mild sedation No significant effects on sleep

cases. Patients with significant insomnia should be instructed in the basic aspects of sleep hygiene (see Chapter 58). The use of stimulants such as caffeine and nicotine should be discouraged. Likewise, alcohol must be avoided for its negative effects on both sleep and affective illnesses. For patients with significant hypersomnia, sleep restriction (i.e., limiting the number of hours in bed) may be indicated.

For patients with winter depression and hypersomnia, bright-light therapy has been shown to be effective, either alone or in combination with antidepressant medication. Light therapy and its use in treating depression is reviewed in detail in Chapter 105. Patients with severe hypersomnia may also benefit from stimulant medications.

Finally, for patients with mood disorders and significant insomnia or hypersomnia that does not respond to appropriate pharmacotherapy of the underlying illness, it is important to consider the possibility of a concomitant primary sleep disorder. Patients with narcolepsy or sleep apnea have been reported to have higher rates of depression[9, 174]; both sleep disorders are associated with nocturnal sleep disruption, daytime fatigue, and hypersomnia, or impaired daytime concentration, all of which may be confused with the "vegetative" symptoms of depression.

Treatment of Mood Disorders With Sleep Deprivation

A variety of sleep manipulations have been shown to have antidepressant effects, although they have not come into widespread clinical use. They include selective deprivation of REM sleep, partial and total sleep deprivation, and, possibly, phase advance of the sleep period relative to clock time.[175–177] A single night of sleep deprivation was shown to have antidepressant effects with response rates of 50% or greater in a number of studies.[178–180] Antidepressant effects peaked by the afternoon following a night of total sleep loss[177]; it has been suggested that the mood switch process occurs in the early-morning hours.[181] Patients with endogenous depression and a more pronounced diurnal pattern of illness had better responses to sleep deprivation.[179, 182, 183] A study of depressed adolescents suggested that more severely ill patients may benefit more from sleep deprivation than mildly depressed subjects, who showed no significant effects of sleep deprivation on mood[184]; remitted patients and healthy controls reported worsening of mood following sleep deprivation, consistent with other reports.[185] The major drawback to total sleep deprivation as a therapy for depression, however, has been the immediate reversibility of the antidepressant effects by recovery sleep, including short naps.[180, 186, 187]

The mood-elevating effects of sleep deprivation were most dramatically demonstrated by reports that sleep deprivation triggered manic episodes in some patients with bipolar depression.[188, 189] Furthermore, manic episodes are often immediately preceded by periods of sleeplessness, suggesting that decreased sleep may contribute to mania.[190–193]

Chronic REM sleep deprivation also improved depressive symptomatology.[194] However, unlike total sleep deprivation, the antidepressant effects took several weeks to appear and were not immediately reversed following recovery sleep.

Antidepressant effects have been produced by partial sleep deprivation, particularly during the latter half of the night, which proportionately reduced REM more than NREM sleep.[195, 196] Like total sleep deprivation, partial deprivation was immediately effective and had comparable response rates.[197] It has been suggested that sleep during the early-morning hours is more "depressogenic,"[198] and that the antidepressant effect of sleep deprivation accrues from avoiding sleep during this period. Antidepressant effects of total sleep deprivation may be prolonged if sleep is phase-advanced during the period immediately following a night of sleep deprivation.[199, 200] Sleep-phase advance may also potentiate the effects of antidepressant medications.[201] Intermittent partial sleep deprivation on one or more nights per week may also be useful as a prophylactic or adjunctive treatment for depression.[202, 203]

Although the mechanism for the antidepressant effects of sleep deprivation is not known, functional neuroimaging studies suggest the effects may be mediated by effects on limbic structures. Increased rates of glucose metabolism[204] and blood flow[205–207] in amygdala and cingulate have been reported in depressed subjects who respond to sleep deprivation. Normalization of activity in these limbic structures was associated with a decrease in depression.[204]

CLINICAL APPLICATION OF SLEEP STUDIES

Sleep studies may be increasingly useful in psychiatry, both for diagnosis and treatment evaluation. Although a specific psychiatric diagnosis cannot be made solely on the basis of polysomnographic data, sleep studies can sometimes answer specific questions. For example, reduced REM latency may suggest a concomitant diagnosis of depression in patients with significant anxiety complaints or dementia. Although in most patients with mood disorders sleep complaints are usually related to the underlying psychiatric illness, in some cases a sleep study may help in diagnosis of an occult primary sleep disorder. Both sleep apnea and periodic leg movements can disrupt nocturnal sleep and lead to fatigue and poor concentration during the day, which are also symptoms of depression. In depressed patients whose sleep complaints continue in spite of aggressive treatment and resolution of depressed mood, a sleep study should be considered for further evaluation. In some cases, medications also may be responsible for precipitating or exacerbating sleep disorders (i.e., tricyclic antidepressants and periodic leg movements, benzodiazepines and sleep apnea).

The potential prognostic utility of sleep studies in

mood disorders has not yet been fully realized. It is possible that specific sleep abnormalities may be predictive of treatment response. Several studies have suggested that patients with reduced REM sleep latency may be more likely to respond to antidepressant medications than those with nonreduced REM sleep latency.[208, 209] A multicenter study comparing response to fluoxetine vs. placebo, however, found no difference in response rates in patients with short vs. normal REM sleep latencies.[210] In one study of depressed inpatients, the response to amitriptyline was related to a more severe initial depression rating and less baseline stage 4 sleep.[211] However, another study found no correlations between sleep variables and response to cognitive therapy.[212]

Alternatively, medication-induced changes in sleep patterns may be correlated with antidepressant effects. For patients with depression and reduced REM latencies, it has been shown that the REM-suppressing effects of an antidepressant medication predicted clinical efficacy.[157b] The amount of REM sleep suppression during the first night of treatment with tricyclic antidepressants correlated with eventual antidepressant response in several studies.[34, 75, 157b, 214] Prolongation of REM latency alone was less consistent in predicting treatment response. Furthermore, the efficacy of REM sleep deprivation in treating depression was correlated positively with both greater suppression of REM sleep early in the treatment, as well as increased REM rebound during recovery sleep.[215] Increased amounts of REM sleep rebound following abrupt discontinuation of amitriptyline were also indicative of clinical response to the drug[157c]; in this case, the amount of rebound may have reflected the amount of prior deprivation. Studies of treatment-resistant depression may clarify whether sleep studies can play a role in evaluating potential treatment efficacy more quickly than the standard 3- to 6-week clinical trial.

Furthermore, sleep variables may be helpful in identifying individuals susceptible to developing affective illnesses or relapses. Kupfer et al.[216] have shown that a decreased delta sleep ratio (average delta wave counts in the first vs. second NREM periods) correlated with an increased risk of relapse. Healthy adolescents with increased phasic REM sleep and a trend for shorter REM sleep latency were more likely to develop new-onset depression than subjects with normal sleep patterns.[217] Short REM latency also appeared to be correlated with earlier recurrence of illness.[218, 219] If reduced REM latency or other sleep abnormalities indicate a susceptibility to depression, it might be useful to consider whether patients with subjective sleep complaints and short REM latency should be treated prophylactically with antidepressants.

Finally, in interpreting sleep studies in clinical settings, it is important to bear in mind that reduced REM latency can be present in a variety of conditions other than mood disorders. As mentioned previously, short REM latency has been reported in some groups of patients with schizophrenia, borderline personality, eating disorders, and alcoholism. Early appearance of REM sleep, of course, is also characteristic of narco-

Table 96–7. CLINICAL CONDITIONS IN WHICH REDUCED REM SLEEP LATENCY HAS BEEN REPORTED

Psychiatric disorders
  Mood disorders
  Borderline personality disorder
  Eating disorders
  Anxiety disorders
  Alcoholism
  Schizophrenia
Narcolepsy
Following cessation of treatment with REM sleep–suppressing
    drugs
  Benzodiazepines
  Antidepressants
During alcohol withdrawal
During recovery sleep following sleep deprivation

lepsy. Short REM latency and REM sleep rebound commonly occur in patients who have been withdrawn recently from antidepressant medications, benzodiazepines, or alcohol. Following sleep deprivation, REM latency reductions may occur during recovery sleep, although usually not during the first night. Common causes of reduced REM latency are listed in Table 96–7.

THEORETICAL ISSUES

Both the objective measures of sleep disturbance in depression and the "sleep therapies" of depression emphasize the close association between sleep and depression and suggest that an understanding of the physiology of sleep may contribute to a better understanding of the pathophysiology of depression. A number of models have been proposed to account for the known relationships between sleep and depression.

The REM Pressure Hypothesis

Related to the observation that REM sleep deprivation has antidepressant effects, Vogel and co-workers have postulated that depression may be caused by excessive amounts of REM sleep and the resulting decrease in REM pressure.[194, 220] According to this view, the sleep deprivation therapies work by suppressing REM sleep and thus increasing REM pressure. In addition, most antidepressant medications suppress REM sleep for prolonged periods of time, a point that Vogel and co-workers have used to support their hypothesis.[194, 215, 220] Further evidence for a relationship between increased REM pressure and antidepressant response is suggested by the positive correlations between clinical response and either REM suppression early in the course of treatment with tricyclics[75, 157b, 214, 221] or REM rebound following cessation of REM sleep deprivation or tricyclic administration.[157b, 215] The fact that a number of effective medications (e.g., bupropion, nefazodone, and trazodone) do not reduce REM sleep, however, suggests that REM sleep suppression is not necessary for an antidepressant response.

The Cholinergic-Aminergic Imbalance Hypothesis

Considerable evidence suggests that REM sleep is promoted by cholinergic activation within the medial pontine reticular formation and inhibited by aminergic (serotonergic and noradrenergic) activation.[222–224] Thus, either enhanced cholinergic neurotransmission or diminished aminergic neurotransmission could account for the short REM latency and elevated REM density and, possibly, reduced total sleep time and sleep efficiency of depression.[225–228a] Increased cholinergic activation may also suppress SWS; recent animal studies have demonstrated that pontine reticular formation neurons inhibit delta wave production by thalamocortical neurons.[229] Furthermore, these same changes might account for the hypothalamic-pituitary-adrenal axis activation of depression.[230, 231] This interpretation of the sleep and neuroendocrine abnormalities of depression would also be consistent with the cholinergic-aminergic imbalance hypothesis of affective disorders originally proposed by Janowsky et al.[232] Cholinergic, muscarinic receptor supersensitivity has been proposed to play an important role in the pathophysiology of depression, particularly the sleep changes.[228] Normal volunteers treated with scopolamine, a muscarinic antagonist, for 3 days and studied during a period of withdrawal showed many of the sleep changes typical of depression, including short REM latency, elevated REM density, and shortened sleep.[228, 233] Consistent with the cholinergic supersensitivity hypothesis, depressed patients, compared with control subjects, show faster REM sleep induction with the muscarinic agonists arecoline[59, 234–238] and RS-86[239] and more frequent awakening with infusions of physostigmine (an anticholinesterase).[240] Increased sensitivity to cholinergic REM sleep induction, like short REM latency, may also be a marker of depression, because concordance in twin and family studies has been demonstrated.[241, 242]

The Phase-Advance Hypothesis

The phase-advance hypothesis suggests that the circadian oscillator controlling REM sleep, temperature, and cortisol is phase-advanced in depressed patients.[145, 243–245] That is, when a depressed patient retires at midnight, the NREM-REM cycles are similar to the NREM-REM cycles of a normal person beginning at about 6 AM. Wehr and Wirz-Justice[198] proposed the internal phase coincidence model to explain REM sleep abnormalities in depression. They hypothesized that REM sleep is phase-advanced relative to the sleep-wake cycle in depressives, and that depression results from awakening at sensitive circadian phases. Several studies in normal subjects have confirmed that an acute phase delay in bedtime results in REM sleep changes similar to those seen in depression.[246, 247] In some ways, the concepts are similar to the independent suggestion of Vogel et al.,[215] that the sleep of depressed patients mimics the extended sleep of normal subjects.

The phase-advance hypothesis would account for the short REM latency and, possibly, the increased length and duration of the first REM period. However, it is not clear that short REM latency at night invariably means phase advance of the REM circadian system. For example, Kupfer et al.[248] reported that REM latency during daytime naps was correlated with REM latency at night. Schulz and Tetzlaff[249] also reported that REM latency was short in depressed patients after awakenings at night. Thus, the available data suggest that REM latency is short whenever sleep occurs in depressed patients. Furthermore, other studies have suggested that REM sleep does not appear to be phase-advanced when measured relative to "clock" time (i.e., REM sleep appeared to occur at the same time of night, but earlier relative to sleep onset).[250] As described earlier, the data on circadian temperature rhythms do not show a consistent phase advance in depressed patients, but suggest instead that, if anything, the nocturnal temperature of depressed patients is elevated.[143] Although several studies suggest a phase advance of the cortisol rhythm in depression, the effect is relatively small. Partially as a result of their study of the circadian temperature rhythm, Schulz and Lund[148] have hypothesized that circadian rhythms are "flat" (i.e., have reduced amplitude) in depression. Finally, although phase advance of bedtime has been shown to have antidepressant effects and has been proposed to support the phase-advance hypothesis,[244, 251] not all studies have been able to confirm the antidepressant effects of phase advance.[252]

The Two-Process Model of Sleep Regulation: The Process S Deficiency Hypothesis of Depression

Borbély[253] proposed that sleep is regulated by the interaction of two processes: a homeostatic, sleep-inducing process (process S), which rises exponentially during wakefulness and declines exponentially during sleep; and a circadian process (process C), which reflects an internal clock that governs circadian propensity for sleep (see Chapter 29). He suggested that process S is deficient in patients with depression.[254] Process S is considered to be an inhibitor of REM sleep; therefore, the less delta sleep (which reflects process S), the shorter the REM latency, the longer the first REM period, and the higher the REM density. Because process S is inferred from the time course of delta activity (or, more technically, EEG power density in the low-frequency range) across the night, this hypothesis reflects the reduction of stage 4 sleep in depression. The hypothesis also was suggested by the antidepressant effect of total and partial sleep deprivation, because process S increases with sleep deprivation. When compared with normal control subjects, depressed patients show a reduction of both the integrated EEG power density and the average delta count (delta waves per minute).[45, 255] Although the mechanism for the loss of stage 4 sleep is unknown, it is of interest that Lindstrom et al.[256] reported that the cerebrospinal fluid levels of delta sleep–inducing peptide were low in people with depression and schizophrenia.

CONCLUSIONS

All of these hypotheses offer theoretical interpretations of the known sleep disturbances of depression, but none of them account for all the known "facts" about sleep and depression. The REM pressure hypothesis does not account for decreased sleep continuity or SWS reductions, and the cholinergic-aminergic hypothesis does not explain the antidepressant effects of sleep deprivation. The phase-advance hypothesis does not offer a ready, experimentally verified explanation for hypothalamic-pituitary-adrenal activation or response to sleep deprivation. The process S deficiency hypothesis does not explain the mechanism of the antidepressant drugs or the therapeutic effects of selective REM deprivation. No experimental study, based on the premises of the cholinergic-aminergic hypothesis, the phase-advance hypothesis, or the process S deficiency hypothesis, has produced depression in normal volunteers or euthymic depressed patients, although a number of pharmacological challenge studies have shown effects on sleep similar to depression compatible with the cholinergic-aminergic hypothesis. Indeed, actually testing the premises and underlying assumptions of these hypotheses may prove to be difficult. Finally, none of the hypotheses have addressed the lack of specificity of sleep disturbances, that is, the fact that short REM latency and other abnormalities have been found in patients lacking major depressive disorders.

However, despite the lack of an ideal theory, there is considerable evidence to suggest that sleep is biologically linked to mood disorders. Perhaps the most basic question is whether a causal link exists between sleep and depression, regardless of the specific mechanism involved. For example, does depression cause sleep abnormalities? This is probably not the case, because many people with depression, particularly younger patients, fail to exhibit short REM latency, reduced SWS, or sleep disruption. Also, depression-like sleep patterns are seen during remission and in first-degree relatives without depression. Alternatively, does the abnormal sleep pattern specifically lead to an increased susceptibility to depression, as suggested by some of the longitudinal and family studies? This is also unlikely, because narcolepsy patients with short REM latency are not invariably depressed, and inducing "depressive" sleep patterns in normals with cholinergic agents does not cause depression. A third possibility is that separate biological processes can lead to the clinical syndrome of depression or the characteristic sleep abnormalities. Whether the psychiatric illness, the sleep disturbance, or both are expressed may depend on other biological factors. Continued study of sleep in mood disorders—and the psychiatric disorders in general—will elucidate neuropharmacological and genetic mechanisms involved in sleep regulation and psychiatric illnesses. An understanding of the sleep abnormalities and sleep disorders commonly found in patients with mood disorders can lead to more effective clinical management of this large patient population.

References

1. Mellinger GD, Balter MB, Uhlenhuth EH. Insomnia and its treatment. Prevalence and correlates. Arch Gen Psychiatry. 1985;42:225–232.
2. Ford DE, Kamerow DB Epidemiologic study of sleep disturbance and psychiatric disorders: an opportunity for prevention? JAMA. 1989;262:1479–1484.
3. Breslau N, Roth T, Rosenthal L, et al. Sleep disturbance and psychiatric disorders: a longitudinal epidemiological study of young adults. Biol Psychiatry. 1996;39:411–418.
4. Gerber PD, Barrett JE, Barrett JA, et al. The relationship of presenting physical complaints to depressive symptoms in primary care. J Gen Intern Med. 1992;7:170–173.
5. Coleman RM, Roffwarg HP, Kennedy SJ, et al. Sleep-wake disorders based on a polysomnographic diagnosis. A national cooperative study. JAMA. 1982;247:997–1003.
6. Buysse DJ, Reynolds CF III, Kupfer DJ, et al. Clinical diagnoses in 216 insomnia patients using the International Classification of Sleep Disorders (ICSD), DSM-IV and ICD-10 categories: a report from the APA/NIMH DSM-IV Field Trial. Sleep. 1994;17:630–637.
7. Beutler LE, Ware JC, Karacan I, et al. Differentiating psychological characteristics of patients with sleep apnea and narcolepsy. Sleep. 1981;4:39–47.
8. Guilleminault C, Dement WC. Sleep apnea syndromes and related sleep disorders. In: Williams RL, Karacan I, eds. Sleep Disorders: Diagnosis and Treatment. New York, NY: John Wiley & Sons; 1978:9–28.
9. Guilleminault C, van den Hoed J, Mitler MM. Clinical overview of the sleep apnea syndromes. In: Guilleminault C, Dement WC, eds. Sleep Apnea Syndromes. New York, NY: Alan R Liss; 1978:1–12.
10. Kales A, Soldatos CR, Bixler EO, et al. Narcolepsy-cataplexy, II: psychosocial consequences and associated psychopathology. Arch Neurol. 1982;39:169–171.
11. Reynolds CF III, Taska LS, Sewitch DE, et al. Persistent psychophysiologic insomnia: preliminary research diagnostic criteria and EEG sleep data. Am J Psychiatry. 1984;141:804–805.
12. Reynolds CF III, Kupfer DJ, McEachran AB, et al. Depressive psychopathology in male sleep apneics. J Clin Psychiatry. 1984;45:287–290.
13. Chang PP, Ford DE, Mead LA, et al. Insomnia in young men and subsequent depression. The Johns Hopkins Precursors Study. Am J Epidemiol. 1997;146:105–114.
14. Diagnostic and Statistical Manual of Mental Disorders, Fourth Edition. Washington, DC: American Psychiatric Association; 1994.
15. Boyd JH, Weissman MM. Epidemiology of affective disorders. A reexamination and future directions [review]. Arch Gen Psychiatry. 1981;38:1039–1046.
16. Bunney WE, Davis JM. Norepinephrine in depressive reactions. Arch Gen Psychiatry. 1965;13:483–494.
17. Schildkraut JJ. The catecholamine hypothesis of affective disorders: a review of supporting evidence. Am J Psychiatry. 1965;122:509–522.
18. Soares JC, Mann JJ. The functional neuroanatomy of mood disorders. J Psychiatr Res. 1997;31:393–432.
19. Soares JC, Mann JJ. The anatomy of mood disorders—review of structural neuroimaging studies. Biol Psychiatry. 1997;41:86–106.
20. Drevets WC. Functional neuroimaging studies of depression: the anatomy of melancholia. Annu Rev Med. 1998;49:341–361.
21. Rye DB. Contributions of the pedunculopontine region to normal and altered REM sleep. Sleep. 1997;20:757–788.
22. Claghorn JL, Mathew RJ, Weinman ML, et al. Daytime sleepiness in depression. J Clin Psychiatry. 1981;42:342–343.
23. Perlis ML, Giles DE, Buysse DJ, et al. Self-reported sleep disturbance as a prodromal symptom in recurrent depression. J Affect Disord. 1997;42:209–212.

24. Detre TP, Himmelhoch JM, Swartzburg M, et al. Hypersomnia and manic-depressive disease. Am J Psychiatry. 1972;128:1303–1305.

25. Rosenthal NE, Sack DA, Gillin JC, et al. Seasonal affective disorder. A description of the syndrome and preliminary findings with light therapy. Arch Gen Psychiatry. 1984;41:72–80.

26. Reynolds CF III, Kupfer DJ. Sleep research in affective illness: state of the art circa 1987. Sleep. 1987;10:199–215.

27. Oswald I, Berger RJ, Jaramillo RA, et al. Melancholia and barbiturates: a controlled EEG, body and eye movement study of sleep. Br J Psychiatry. 1963;109:66–78.

28. Diaz-Guerrero R, Gottlieb JS, Knott JR. The sleep of patients with manic-depressive psychosis, depressive type: an electroencephalographic study. Psychosom Med. 1946:399–404.

29. Gresham SC, Agnew HW Jr, Williams RL. The sleep of depressed patients: an EEG and eye movement study. Arch Gen Psychiatry. 1965;13:503–507.

30. Zung W, Wilson W, Dodson W. Effect of depressive disorders on sleep EEG responses. Arch Gen Psychiatry. 1964;10:429–445.

31. Leranth C, MacLusky NJ, Shanabrough M, et al. Catecholaminergic innervation of luteinizing hormone–releasing hormone and glutamic acid decarboxylase immunopositive neurons in the rat medial preoptic area. An electron-microscopic double immunostaining and degeneration study. Neuroendocrinology. 1988;48:591–602.

32. Berger M, Doerr P, Lund RD, et al. Neuroendocrinological and neurophysiological studies in major depressive disorders: are there biologial markers for the endogenous subtype? Biol Psychiatry. 1982;17:1217–1242.

33. Gillin JC, Duncan WC, Pettigrew KD, et al. Successful separation of depressed, normal, and insomniac subjects by EEG sleep data. Arch Gen Psychiatry. 1979;36:85–90.

34. Goetz RR, Puig-Antich J, Ryan ND, et al. Electroencephalographic sleep of adolescents with major depression and normal controls. Arch Gen Psychiatry. 1987;44:61–68.

35. Kupfer DJ, Ulrich RF, Coble PA, et al. Electroencephalographic sleep of younger depressives. Arch Gen Psychiatry. 1985;42:806–810.

36. Linkowski P, Kerkhofs M, Rielaert C, et al. Sleep during mania in manic-depressive males. Eur Arch Psychiatry Neurol Sci. 1986;235:339–341.

37. Mendelson WB, Sack DA, James SP, et al. Frequency analysis of the sleep EEG in depression. Psychiatry Res. 1987;21:89–94.

38. Waller DA, Hardy BW, Pole R, et al. Sleep EEG in bulimic, depressed, and normal subjects. Biol Psychiatry. 1989;25:661–664.

39. Hawkins DR, Mendels J. Sleep disturbance in depressive syndromes. Am J Psychiatry. 1966;123:682–690.

40. Kupfer DJ, Foster FG. Interval between onset of sleep and rapid-eye-movement sleep as an indicator of depression. Lancet. 1972;2:684–686.

41. Kupfer DJ, Foster FG, Detre TP. Sleep continuity changes in depression. Dis Nerv Syst. 1973;34:192–195.

42. Kupfer DJ, Reynolds CF III, Grochocinski VJ, et al. Aspects of short REM latency in affective states: a revisit. Psychiatry Res. 1986;17:49–59.

43. Kupfer DJ, Grochocinski VJ, McEachran AB. Relationship of awakening and delta sleep in depression. Psychiatry Res. 1986;19:297–304.

44. Benca RM, Obermeyer WH, Thisted RA, et al. Sleep and psychiatric disorders: a meta-analysis. Arch Gen Psychiatry. 1992;49:651–668.

45. Borbély AA, Tobler I, Loepfe M, et al. All-night spectral analysis of the sleep EEG in untreated depressives and normal controls. Psychiatry Res. 1984;12:27–33.

46. Kupfer DJ, Frank E, Ehlers CL. EEG sleep in young depressives: first and second night effects. Biol Psychiatry. 1989;25:87–97.

47. Kupfer DJ, Reynolds CF III, Ehlers CL. Comparison of EEG sleep measures among depressive subtypes and controls in older individuals. Psychiatry Res. 1989;27:13–21.

48. Quitkin FM, Rabkin JG, Stewart JW, et al. Sleep of atypical depressives. J Affect Disord. 1985;8:61–67.

49. Thase ME, Himmelhoch JM, Mallinger AG, et al. Sleep EEG and DST findings in anergic bipolar depression. Am J Psychiatry. 1989;146:329–333.

50. Kupfer DJ, Reynolds CF III, Ulrich RF, et al. Comparison of automated REM and slow-wave sleep analysis in young and middle-aged depressed subjects. Biol Psychiatry. 1986;21:189–200.

51. Reynolds CF III, Kupfer DJ, Taska LS, et al. Slow wave sleep in elderly depressed, demented and healthy subjects. Sleep. 1985;8:155–159.

52. Hartmann E, Verdone P, Snyder F. Longitudinal studies of sleep and dreaming patterns in psychiatric patients. J Nerv Ment Dis. 1966;142:117–126.

53. Mendels J, Hawkins DR. Sleep and depression: a controlled EEG study. Arch Gen Psychiatry. 1967;16:344–354.

54. Snyder F. Dynamic aspects of sleep disturbance in relation to mental illness. Biol Psychiatry. 1969;1:119–130.

55. Akiskal HS, Lemmi H, Dickson H, et al. Chronic depressions. Part 2. Sleep EEG differentiation of primary dysthymic disorders from anxious depressions. J Affect Disord. 1984;6:287–295.

56. Akiskal HS, Lemmi H, Yerevanian B, et al. The utility of the REM latency test in psychiatric diagnosis: a study of 81 depressed outpatients. Psychiatry Res. 1982;7:101–110.

57. Emslie GJ, Roffwarg HP, Rush AJ, et al. Sleep EEG findings in depressed children and adolescents. Am J Psychiatry. 1987;144:668–670.

58. Emslie GJ, Rush AJ, Weinberg WA, et al. Children with major depression show reduced rapid eye movement latencies. Arch Gen Psychiatry. 1990;47:119–124.

59. Jones DA, Kelwala S, Bell J, et al. Cholinergic REM sleep induction response correlation with endogenous major depressive subtype. Psychiatry Res. 1985;14:99–110.

60. Lahmeyer HW, Poznanski EO, Bellur SN. EEG sleep in depressed adolescents. Am J Psychiatry. 1983;140:1150–1153.

61. Feinberg M, Gillin JC, Carroll BJ, et al. EEG studies of sleep in the diagnosis of depression. Biol Psychiatry. 1982;17:305–316.

62. Foster FG, Kupfer DJ, Coble PA, et al. Rapid eye movement sleep density. An objective indicator in severe medial-depressive syndromes. Arch Gen Psychiatry. 1976;33:1119–1123.

63. Hudson JI, Lipinski JF, Frankenburg FR, et al. Electroencephalographic sleep in mania. Arch Gen Psychiatry. 1988;45:267–273.

64. Arriaga F, Rosado P, Paiva T. The sleep of dysthymic patients: a comparison with normal controls. Biol Psychiatry. 1990;27:649–656.

65. Nofzinger EA, Thase ME, Reynolds CF III, et al. Hypersomnia in bipolar depression: a comparison with narcolepsy using the multiple sleep latency test. Am J Psychiatry. 1991;148:1177–1181.

66. Coble PA, Foster FG, Kupfer DJ. Electroencephalographic sleep diagnosis of primary depression. Arch Gen Psychiatry. 1976;33:1124–1127.

67. Kerkhofs M, Kempenaers C, Linkowski P, et al. Multivariate study of sleep EEG in depression. Acta Psychiatr Scand. 1988;77:463–468.

68. Kupfer DJ, Frank E. The relation of EEG sleep to vital depression. J Affect Disord. 1984;7:249–263.

69. Giles DE, Schlesser MA, Rush AJ, et al. Polysomnographic findings and dexamethasone nonsuppression in unipolar depression: a replication and extension. Biol Psychiatry. 1987;22:872–882.

70. Puig-Antich J, Goetz RR, Hanlon C, et al. Sleep architecture and REM sleep measures in prepubertal major depressives. Arch Gen Psychiatry. 1983;40:187–192.

71. Thase ME, Kupfer DJ, Spiker DG. Electroencephalographic sleep in secondary depression: a revisit. Biol Psychiatry. 1984;19:805–814.

72. Cohen DB. Dysphoric affect and REM sleep. J Abnorm Psychol. 1979;88:73–77.

73. Giles DE, Roffwarg HP, Schlesser MA, et al. Which endogenous depressive symptoms relate to REM latency reduction? Biol Psychiatry. 1986;21:473–482.

74. Perlis M, Giles D, Buysse D, et al. Which depressive symptoms are related to which sleep electroencephalographic variables? Biol Psychiatry. 1997;42:904–913.

75. Kupfer DJ, Foster FG, Reich L, et al. EEG sleep changes as predictors in depression. Am J Psychiatry. 1976;133:622–626.

76. Reynolds CF III, Newton TF, Shaw DH, et al. Electroencephalographic sleep findings in depressed outpatients. Psychiatry Res. 1982;6:65–75.

77. Spiker DG, Coble PA, Cofsky J, et al. EEG sleep and severity of depression. Biol Psychiatry. 1978;13:485–488.

78. Zarcone VP, Benson KL. Increased REM eye movement density in self-rated depression. Psychiatry Res. 1983;8:65–71.

79. Feinberg M, Carroll BJ, Greden JF, et al. Sleep EEG, depression rating scales, and diagnosis. Biol Psychiatry. 1982;17:1453–1458.

80. Kumar A, Shipley JE, Eiser AS, et al. Clinical correlates of sleep onset REM periods in depression. Biol Psychiatry. 1987;22:1473–1477.

81. Buysse DJ, Reynolds CF III, Houck PR, et al. Age of illness onset and sleep EEG variables in elderly depressives. Biol Psychiatry. 1988;24:355–359.

82. Giles DE, Etzel BA, Reynolds CF III, et al. Stability of polysomnographic parameters in unipolar depression: a cross-sectional report. Biol Psychiatry. 1989;25:807–810.

83. Kupfer DJ, Frank E, Grochocinski VJ, et al. Electroencephalographic sleep profiles in recurrent depression. Arch Gen Psychiatry. 1988;45:678–681.

84. Giles DE, Roffwarg HP, Rush AJ. A cross sectional study of the effects of depression on REM latency. Biol Psychiatry. 1990;28:697–704.

85. Thase ME, Kupfer DJ, Buysse DJ, et al. Electroencephalographic sleep profiles in single-episode and recurrent unipolar forms of major depression, I: comparison during acute depressive states. Biol Psychiatry. 1995;38:506–515.

86. Kupfer DJ, Ehlers CL, Frank E, et al. EEG sleep profiles and recurrent depression. Biol Psychiatry. 1991;30:641–655.

87. Dew MA, Reynolds CF III, Buysse DJ, et al. Electroencephalographic sleep profiles during depression. Effects of episode duration and other clinical and psychosocial factors in older adults. Arch Gen Psychiatry. 1996;53:148–156.

88. Kerkhofs M, Hoffmann G, De Martelaere V, et al. Sleep EEG recordings in depressive disorders. J Affect Disord. 1985;9:47–53.

89. Knowles JB, Cairns J, MacLean AW, et al. The sleep of remitted bipolar depressives: comparison with sex and age-matched controls. Can J Psychiatry. 1986;31:295–298.

90. Schulz H, Lund RD, Cording C, et al. Bimodal distribution of REM sleep latencies in depression. Biol Psychiatry. 1979;14:595–600.

91. Thase ME, Fasiczka AL, Berman SR, et al. Electroencephalographic sleep profiles before and after cognitive behavior therapy of depression. Arch Gen Psychiatry. 1998;55:138–144.

92. Hauri PJ, Chernik D, Hawkins DR, et al. Sleep of depressed patients in remission. Arch Gen Psychiatry. 1974;31:386–391.

93. Rush AJ, Erman MK, Giles DE, et al. Polysomnographic findings in recently drug-free and clinically remitted depressed patients. Arch Gen Psychiatry. 1986;43:878–884.

94. Lee JH, Reynolds CF III, Hoch CC, et al. Electroencephalographic sleep in recently remitted, elderly depressed patients in double-blind placebo-maintenance therapy. Neuropsychopharmacology. 1993;8:143–150.

95. Giles DE, Kupfer DJ, Rush AJ, et al. Controlled comparison of electrophysiological sleep in families of probands with unipolar depression. Am J Psychiatry. 1998;155:192–199.

96. Lauer CJ, Schreiber W, Holsboer F, et al. In quest of identifying vulnerability markers for psychiatric disorders by all-night polysomnography. Arch Gen Psychiatry. 1995;52:145–153.

97. Reynolds CF III, Kupfer DJ, Thase ME, et al. Sleep, gender and depression: an analysis of gender effects on the electroencephalographic sleep of 302 depressed outpatients. Biol Psychiatry. 1990;28:673–684.

98. Emslie GJ, Rush AJ, Weinberg WA, et al. Sleep EEG features of adolescents with major depression. Biol Psychiatry. 1994;36:573–581.

99. Appelboom-Fondu J, Kerkhofs M, Mendlewicz J. Depression in adolescents and young adults—polysomnographic and neuroendocrine aspects. J Affect Disord. 1988;14:35–40.

100. Dahl RE, Puig-Antich J, Ryan ND, et al. EEG sleep in adolescents with major depression: the role of suicidality and inpatient status. J Affect Disord. 1990;19:63–75.

101. Khan AU, Todd S. Polysomnographic findings in adolescents with major depression. Psychiatry Res. 1990;33:313–320.

102. Puig-Antich J, Goetz RR, Hanlon C, et al. Sleep architecture and REM sleep measures in prepubertal children with major depression: a controlled study. Arch Gen Psychiatry. 1982;39:932–939.

103. Young W, Knowles JB, MacLean AW, et al. The sleep of childhood depressives: comparison with age-matched controls. Biol Psychiatry. 1982;17:1163–1168.

104. Gillin JC, Duncan WC, Murphy DL, et al. Age-related changes in sleep in depressed and normal subjects. Psychiatry Res. 1981;4:73–78.

105. Knowles JB, MacLean AW. Age-related changes in sleep in depressed and healthy subjects. Neuropsychopharmacology. 1990;3:251–259.

106. Lauer CJ, Riemann D, Wiegand M, et al. From early to late adulthood: changes in EEG sleep of depressed patients and healthy volunteers. Biol Psychiatry. 1991;29:979–993.

107. Ulrich RF, Shaw DH, Kupfer DJ. Effects of aging on EEG sleep in depression. Sleep. 1980;3:31–40.

108. Somoza E, Mossman D. Optimizing REM latency as a diagnostic test for depression using receiver operating characteristic anaysis and information theory. Biol Psychiatry. 1989;27:990–1006.

109. Knowles JB, MacLean AW, Cairns J. Definitions of REM latency: some comparisons with particular reference to depression. Biol Psychiatry. 1982;17:993–1002.

110. Reynolds CF III, Shaw DH, Newton TF, et al. EEG sleep in outpatients with generalized anxiety: a preliminary comparison with depressed outpatients. Psychiatry Res. 1983;8:81–89.

111. King D, Akiskal HS, Lemmi H, et al. REM density in the differential diagnosis of psychiatric from medical-neurologic disorders: a replication. Psychiatry Res. 1981;5:267–276.

112. Lauer CJ, Garcia D, Pollmacher T, et al. All-night EEG sleep in anxiety disorders and major depression. In: Horne J, ed. Sleep '90. Bochum, Germany: Pontenagel Press; 1991.

113. Reynolds CF III, Kupfer DJ, Houck PR, et al. Reliable discrimination of elderly depressed and demented patients by electroencephalographic sleep data. Arch Gen Psychiatry. 1988;45:258–264.

114. Uhde TW, Roy-Byrne P, Gillin JC, et al. The sleep of patients with panic disorder: a preliminary report. Psychiatry Res. 1985;12:251–259.

115. Greenberg R, Pearlman CA, Gampel D. War neuroses and the adaptive function of REM sleep. Br J Med Psychol. 1972;45:27–33.

116. Kauffman CD, Reist C, Djenderedjian A, et al. Biological markers of affective disorders and posttraumatic stress disorder: a pilot study with desipramine. J Clin Psychiatry. 1987;48:366–367.

117. Katz JL, Kuperberg A, Pollack CP, et al. Is there a relationship between eating disorder and affective disorder? New evidence from sleep recordings. Am J Psychiatry. 1984;141:753–759.

118. Neil JF, Merikangas JR, Foster FG, et al. Waking and all-night sleep EEG's in anorexia nervosa. Clin Electroencephalogr. 1980;11:9–15.

119. Gillin JC, Smith TL, Irwin M, et al. Short REM latency in primary alcoholic patients with secondary depression. Am J Psychiatry. 1990;147:106–109.

120. Hiatt JF, Floyd TC, Katz PH, et al. Further evidence of abnormal non-rapid-eye-movement sleep in schizophrenia. Arch Gen Psychiatry. 1985;42:797–802.

121. Kupfer DJ, Broudy D, Spiker DG, et al. EEG sleep and affective psychosis: schizoaffective disorders. Psychiatry Res. 1979;1:173–178.

122. Reich L, Weiss BL, Coble PA, et al. Sleep disturbance in schizophrenia. Arch Gen Psychiatry. 1975;32:51–55.

123. Zarcone VP, Benson KL, Berger PA. Abnormal rapid eye movement latencies in schizophrenia. Arch Gen Psychiatry. 1987;44:45–48.

124. Akiskal HS, Yerevanian BI, Davis GC, et al. The nosologic status of borderline personality: clinical and polysomnographic study. Am J Psychiatry. 1985;142:192–198.

125. Akiskal HS. Subaffective disorders: dysthymic, cyclothymic and bipolar II disorders in the "borderline" realm. Psychiatr Clin North Am. 1981;4:25–46.

126. Bell J, Lycaki H, Jones DA, et al. Effect of preexisting borderline personality disorder on clinical and EEG sleep correlates of depression. Psychiatry Res. 1983;9:115–123.

127. Lahmeyer HW, Val E, Gaviria M, et al. EEG sleep, lithium transport, dexamethasone suppression, and monoamine oxidase

activity in borderline personality disorder. Psychiatry Res. 1988;25:19–30.

128. McNamara ME, Reynolds CF III, Soloff PH, et al. EEG sleep evaluation of depression in borderline patients. Am J Psychiatry. 1984;141:182–186.

129. Reynolds CF III, Soloff PH, Kupfer DJ, et al. Depression in borderline patients: a prospective EEG sleep study. Psychiatry Res. 1985;14:1–15.

130. Asnis GM, Halbreich U, Ryan ND, et al. The relationship of the dexamethasone suppression test (1 mg and 2 mg) to basal plasma cortisol levels in endogenous depression. Psychoneuroendocrinology. 1987;12:295–301.

131. Carroll BJ, Feinberg M, Greden JF, et al. A specific laboratory test for the diagnosis of melancholia. Standardization, validation, and clinical utility. Arch Gen Psychiatry. 1981;38:15–22.

132. Ansseau M, Scheyvaerts M, Doumont A, et al. Concurrent use of REM latency, dexamethasone suppression, clonidine and apomorphine tests as biological markers of endogenous depression: a pilot study. Psychiatry Res. 1985;12:261–272.

133. Kerkhofs M, Missa J-N, Mendlewicz J. Sleep electroencephalographic measures in primary major depressive disorder: distinction between DST suppressor and nonsuppressor patients. Biol Psychiatry. 1986;21:225–228.

134. Mendlewicz J, Kerkhofs M, Hoffmann G, et al. Dexamethasone suppression test and REM sleep in patients with major depressive disorder. Br J Psychiatry. 1984;145:383–388.

135. Rush AJ, Giles DE, Roffwarg HP, et al. Sleep EEG and dexamethasone suppression test findings in outpatients with unipolar major depressive disorders. Biol Psychiatry. 1982;17:327–341.

136. Asnis GM, Halbreich U, Sachar EJ, et al. Plasma cortisol secretion and REM period latency in adult endogenous depression. Am J Psychiatry. 1983;140:750–753.

137. Halbreich U, Asnis GM, Shindledecker R, et al. Cortisol secretion in endogenous depression, I: basal plasma levels. Arch Gen Psychiatry. 1985;42:904–908.

138. Jarrett DB, Coble PA, Kupfer DJ. Reduced cortisol latency in depressive illness. Arch Gen Psychiatry. 1983;40:506–511.

139. Linkowski P, Mendlewicz J, Leclercq R, et al. The 24-hour profile of adrenocorticotropin and cortisol in major depressive illness. J Clin Endocrinol Metab. 1985;61:429–436.

140. Sachar EJ, Hellman L, Roffwarg HP, et al. Disrupted 24-hour pattern of cortisol secretion in psychotic depression. Arch Gen Psychiatry. 1973;28:19–24.

141. Avery DH, Wilschiodtz G, Smallwood RG, et al. REM latency and core temperature relationships in primary depression. Acta Psychiatr Scand. 1986;74:269–280.

142. Lund RD, Kammerloher A, Dirlich G. Body temperature in endogenously depressed patients during depression and remission. In: Wehr TA, Goodwin FK, eds. Circadian Rhythms in Psychiatry. Pacific Grove, Calif: Boxwood Press; 1983:77–88.

143. Avery DH, Wildschiodtz G, Rafaelsen O. REM latency and temperature in affective disorder before and after treatment. Biol Psychiatry. 1982;17:463–470.

144. Tsujimoto T, Yamada N, Shimoda K, et al. Circadian rhythms in depression, part II: circadian rhythms in inpatients with various mental disorders. J Affect Disord. 1990;18:199–210.

145. Wehr TA, Gillin JC, Goodwin FK. Sleep and circadian rhythms in depression. In: Chase M, ed. Sleep Disorders: Basic and Clinical Research. New York, NY: Spectrum; 1983:195–225.

146. Wehr TA, Muscettola G, Goodwin FK. Urinary 3-methoxy-4-hydroxyphenylglycol circadian rhythm: early timing (phase advance) in manic-depressives compared with normal subjects. Arch Gen Psychiatry. 1980;37:257–263.

147. Monk TH, Buysse DJ, Frank E, et al. Nocturnal and circadian body temperatures of depressed outpatients during symptomatic and recovered states [published erratum appears in Psychiatry Res. 1994;54:309]. Psychiatry Res. 1994;51:297–311.

148. Schulz H, Lund R. Sleep onset REM episodes are associated with circadian parameters of body temperature. A study in depressed patients and normal controls. Biol Psychiatry. 1983;18:1411–1426.

149. Armitage R, Yonkers K, Cole D, et al. A multicenter, double-blind comparison of the effects of nefazodone and fluoxetine on sleep architecture and quality of sleep in depressed outpatients. J Clin Psychopharmacol. 1997;17:161–168.

150. Armitage R, Emslie G, Rintelmann J. The effect of fluoxetine on sleep EEG in childhood depression: a preliminary report. Neuropsychopharmacology. 1997;17:241–245.

151. Staner L, Kerkhofs M, Detroux D, et al. Acute, subchronic and withdrawal sleep EEG changes during treatment with paroxetine and amitriptyline: a double-blind randomized trial in major depression. Sleep. 1995;18:470–477.

152. Hendrickse WA, Roffwarg HP, Grannemann BD, et al. The effects of fluoxetine on the polysomnogram of depressed outpatients: a pilot study. Neuropsychopharmacology. 1994;10:85–91.

153. Luthringer R, Toussaint M, Schaltenbrand N, et al. A double-blind, placebo-controlled evaluation of the effects of orally administered venlafaxine on sleep in inpatients with major depression. Psychopharmacol Bull. 1996;32:637–646.

154. Vogel GW, Buffenstein A, Minter K, et al. Drug effects on REM sleep and on endogenous depression. Neurosci Biobehav Rev. 1990;14:49–63.

155. Bowers M, Kupfer DJ. Central monoamine oxidase inhibition and REM sleep. Brain Res. 1971;35:561–564.

156. Wyatt RJ, Fram DH, Buchbinder R, et al. Treatment of intractable narcolepsy with a monoamine oxidase inhibitor. N Engl J Med. 1971;285:987–991.

157. Wyatt RJ, Fram DH, Kupfer DJ, et al. Total prolonged drug-induced REM sleep suppression in anxious-depressed patients. Arch Gen Psychiatry. 1971;24:145–155.

157a. Kupfer DJ, Spiker DG, Rossi A, et al. Nortriptyline and EEG sleep in depressed patients. Biol Psychiatry. 1982;17:535–546.

157b. Gillin JC, Wyatt RJ, Fram DH, et al. The relationship between changes in REM sleep and clinical improvement in depressed patients treated with amitriptyline. Psychopharmacology. 1978;59:267–272.

157c. Kupfer DJ, Perel JM, Pollock BG, et al. Fluroxamine vs desipramine: comparative polysomnographic effects. Biol Psychiatry. 1991;29:23–40.

157d. Roth T, Zorick F, Wittig R, et al. The effects of doxepin HCl on sleep and depression. J Clin Psychiatry. 1982;43:366–368.

158. Parrott AC, Hindmarch I. The Leeds Sleep Evaluation Questionnaire in psychopharmacological investigations—a review [review]. Psychopharmacology. 1980;71:173–179.

159. Grunhaus L, Tiongco D, Pande A, et al. Monitoring of antidepressant response to ECT with polysomnographic recordings and dexamethasone suppression test. Psychiatry Res. 1988;24:177–185.

160. Hartmann E, Cravens J. The effects of long term administration of psychotropic drugs on human sleep, III: the effects of amitriptyline. Psychopharmacologia. 1973;33:185–202.

161. Nofzinger EA, Reynolds CF III, Thase ME, et al. REM sleep enhancement by bupropion in depressed men. Am J Psychiatry. 1995;152:274–276.

162. Schenck CH, Mahowald MW, Kim SW, et al. Prominent eye movements during NREM sleep and REM sleep behavior disorder associated with fluoxetine treatment of depression and obsessive-compulsive disorder. Sleep. 1992;15:226–235.

163. Ware JC, Brown FW, Moorad PJ, et al. Nocturnal myoclonus and tricyclic antidepressants. Sleep Res. 1984;13:72.

164. Salin-Pascual RJ, Galicia-Polo L, Drucker-Colin R. Sleep changes after 4 consecutive days of venlafaxine administration in normal volunteers. J Clin Psychiatry. 1997;58:348–350.

165. Bakshi R. Fluoxetine and restless legs syndrome. J Neurol Sci. 1996;142:151–152.

166. Schenck CH, Mahowald MW. Motor dyscontrol in narcolepsy: rapid-eye-movement (REM) sleep without atonia and REM sleep behavior disorder. Ann Neurol. 1992;32(1):3–10.

167. Kupfer DJ, Reynolds CF III, Weiss BL, et al. Lithium carbonate and sleep in affective disorders: further considerations. Arch Gen Psychiatry. 1974;30:79–84.

168. Terao T, Terao M, Yoshimura R, et al. Restless legs syndrome induced by lithium. Biol Psychiatry. 1991;30:1167–1170.

169. Gillin JC, Rapaport M, Erman MK, et al. A comparison of nefazodone and fluoxetine on mood and on objective, subjective, and clinician-rated measures of sleep in depressed patients: a double-blind, 8-week clinical trial [published erratum appears in J Clin psychiatry. 1997;58:275]. J Clin Psychiatry. 1997;58:185–192.

170. Rush AJ, Armitage R, Gillin JC, et al. Comparative effects of

nefazodone and fluoxetine on sleep in outpatients with major depressive disorder. Biol Psychiatry. 1998;44:3–14.

171. Parrino L, Spaggiari MC, Boselli M, et al. Clinical and polysomnographic effects of trazodone CR in chronic insomnia associated with dysthymia. Psychopharmacology. 1994;116:389–395.

172. Scharf MB, Sachais BA. Sleep laboratory evaluation of the effects and efficacy of trazodone in depressed insomniac patients. J Clin Psychiatry. 1990;51(suppl):13–17.

173. Nierenberg AA, Aadler LA, Peselow E, et al. Trazodone for antidepressant-associated insomnia. Am J Psychiatry. 1994; 151:1069–1072.

174. Roth B, Nevsimalova S. Depression in narcolepsy and hypersommia. Schweiz Arch Neurol Psychiatr. 1975;116:291–300.

175. Gillin JC. The sleep therapies of depression. Prog Neuropsychopharmacol Biol Psychiatry. 1983;7:351–364.

176. Leibenluft E, Wehr TA. Is sleep deprivation useful in the treatment of depression? Am J Psychiatry. 1992;149:159–168.

177. Wu JC, Bunney WE. The biological basis of an antidepressant response to sleep deprivation and relapse: review and hypothesis. Am J Psychiatry. 1990;147:14–21.

178. Post RM, Kotin J, Goodwin FK. Effects of sleep deprivation on mood and central amine metabolism in depressed patients. Arch Gen Psychiatry. 1976;33:627–632.

179. Pflug B, Tolle R. Disturbance of the 24-hour rhythm in endogenous depression and the treatment of endogeneous depression by sleep deprivation. Int Pharmacopsychiatry. 1971;6:187–196.

180. Van den Burg W, Van den Hoofdakker RH. Total sleep deprivation on endogenous depression. Arch Gen Pschiatry. 1975;32:1121–1125.

181. Bouhuys AL. Towards a model of mood responses to sleep deprivation in depressed patients. Biol Psychiatry. 1991;29:600–612.

182. Fahndrich E. Effects of sleep deprivation on depressed patients of different nosological groups. Psychiatry Res. 1981;5:277–285.

183. Riemann D, Wiegand M, Berger M. Are there predictors for sleep deprivation response in depressed patients? Biol Psychiatry. 1990;29:707–710.

184. Naylor MW, King CA, Lindsay KA, et al. Sleep deprivation in depressed adolescents and psychiatric controls. J Am Acad Child Adolesc Psychiatry. 1993;32:753–759.

185. Pilcher JJ, Huffcutt AI. Effects of sleep deprivation on performance: a meta-analysis. Sleep. 1996;194:318–326.

186. Knowles JB, Southmayd SE, Delva N, et al. Five variations of sleep deprivation in a depressed woman. Br J Psychiatry. 1979;135:403–410.

187. Wiegand M, Berger M, Zulley J, et al. The influence of daytime naps on the therapeutic effect of sleep deprivation. Biol Psychiatry. 1987;22:386–389.

188. Wehr TA. Sleep-loss as a possible mediator of diverse causes of mania. Br J Psychiatry. 1991;159:576–578.

189. Wehr TA, Goodwin FK, Wirz-Justice A, et al. 48-hour sleep-wake cycles in manic-depressive illness: naturalistic observations and sleep deprivation experiments. Arch Gen Psychiatry. 1982;39:559–565.

190. Knowles J, Waldron J, Cairns J. Sleep proceding the onset of a manic episode. Biol Psychiatry. 1979;14:671–675.

191. Sitaram N, Gillin JC, Bunney WE Jr. The switch process in manic-depressive illness: circadian variation in time of switch and sleep and manic ratings before and after switch. Acta Psychiatr Scand. 1978;58:267–278.

192. Wehr TA, Sack DA, Rosenthal NE. Sleep reduction as a final common pathway in the genesis of mania. Am J Psychiatry. 1987;144:201–204.

193. Leibenluft E, Albert PS, Rosenthal NE, et al. Relationship between sleep and mood in patients with rapid-cycling bipolar disorder. Psychiatry Res. 1996;63:161–168.

194. Vogel GW, Thurmond A, Gibbons P, et al. REM sleep reduction effects on depression syndromes. Arch Gen Psychiatry. 1975;32:765–777.

195. Sack DA, Dancan W, Rosenthal NE, et al. The timing and duration of sleep in partial sleep deprivation therapy of depression. Acta Psychiatr Scand. 1988;77:219–224.

196. Schilgen B, Tolle R. Partial sleep deprivation as therapy for depression. Arch Gen Psychiatry. 1980;37:267–271.

197. Szuba MP, Baxter LRJ, Fairbanks LA, et al. Effects of partial sleep deprivation on the diurnal viration of mood and motor activity in major depression. Biol Psychiatry. 1991;30:817–829.

198. Wehr TA, Wirz-Justice A. Internal coincidence model for sleep deprivation and depression. In: Koella WP, ed. Sleep 1980. Basel, Switzerland: Karger, 1981:26–33.

199. Vollmann J, Berger M. Sleep deprivation with consecutive sleep-phase advance therapy in patients with major depression: a pilot study. Biol Psychiatry. 1993;33:54–57.

200. Berger M, Vollmann J, Hohagen F, et al. Sleep deprivation combined with consecutive sleep phase advance as a fast-acting therapy in depression: an open pilot trial in medicated and unmedicated patients. Am J Psychiatry. 1997;154:870–872.

201. Sack DA, Nurnberger J, Rosenthal NE, et al. Potentiation of antidepressant medications by phase advance of the sleep-wake cycle. Am J Psychiatry. 1985;142:606–608.

202. Christodoulou GN, Malliaras DE, Lykouras EP, et al. Possible prophylactic effect of sleep deprivation. Am J Psychiatry. 1978;135:375–376.

203. Papadimitriou GN, Christodoulou GN, Katsouyanni K, et al. Therapy and prevention of affective illness by total sleep deprivation. J Affect Disord. 1993;27:107–116.

204. Wu JC, Gillin JC, Buchsbaum MS, et al. Effect of sleep deprivation on brain metabolism of depressed patients. Am J Psychiatry. 1992;149:538–543.

205. Ebert D, Feistel H, Barocka A. Effects of sleep deprivation on the limbic system and the frontal lobes in affective disorders: a study with Tc-99m-HMPAO SPECT. Psychiatry Res. 1991;40:247–251.

206. Ebert D, Kaschka WP, Loew T, et al. Cortisol and beta-endorphin responses to sleep deprivation in major depression—the hyperarousal theories of sleep deprivation. Neuropsychobiology. 1994;29:64–68.

207. Ebert D, Feistel H, Kaschka W, et al. Single photon emission computerized tomography assessment of cerebral dopamine D2 receptor blockade in depression before and after sleep deprivation—preliminary results. Biol Psychiatry. 1994;35:880–885.

208. Rush AJ, Giles DE, Jarrett RB, et al. Reduced REM latency predicts response to tricyclic medication in depressed outpatients. Biol Psychiatry. 1989;26:61–72.

209. Svendsen K, Christensen PG. Duration of REM sleep latency as predictor of effect of antidepressant therapy: a preliminary report. Acta Psychiatr Scand. 1981;64:238–243.

210. Heiligenstein JH, Faries DE, Rush AJ, et al. Latency to rapid eye movement sleep as a predictor of treatment response to fluoxetine and placebo in nonpsychotic depressed outpatients. Psychiatry Res. 1994;52:327–339.

211. Mendlewicz J, Kempenaers C, de Maertelaer V. Sleep EEG and amitryptiline treatment in depressed inpatients. Biol Psychiatry. 1991;30:691–702.

212. Jarrett RB, Rush AJ, Khatami M, et al. Does the pretreatment polysomnogram predict response to cognitive therapy in depressed outpatients? A preliminary report. Psychiatry Res. 1990;33:285–299.

213. Gillin JC, Wyatt RJ, Frame DH, et al. The relationship between changes in REM sleep and clinical improvement in depressed patients treated with amitriptyline. Psychopharmacology. 1978;59:267–272.

214. Kupfer DJ, Spiker DG, Coble PA, et al. Sleep and treatment prediction in endogenous depression. Am J Psychiatry. 1981;138:429–434.

215. Vogel GW, Vogel F, McAbee RS, et al. Improvement of depression by REM sleep deprivation. New findings and a theory. Arch Gen Psychiatry. 1980;37:247–253.

216. Kupfer DJ, Frank E, McEachran AB, et al. Delta sleep ratio. A biological correlate of early recurrence in unipolar affective disorder. Arch Gen Psychiatry. 1990;47:1100–1105.

217. Rao U, Dahl RE, Ryan ND, et al. The relationship between longitudinal clinical course and sleep and cortisol changes in adolescent depression. Biol Psychiatry. 1996;40:474–484.

218. Giles DE, Jarrett RB, Roffwarg HP, et al. Reduced rapid eye movement latency: a predictor of recurrence in depression. Neuropharmacology. 1987;1:33–39.

219. Reynolds CF III, Perel JM, Frank E, et al. Open-trial maintenance nortriptyline in geriatric depression: survival analysis and pre-

liminary data on the use of REM latency as a predictor of recurrence. Psychopharmacol Bull. 1989;25:129–132.

220. Vogel GW. A review of REM sleep deprivation. Arch Gen Psychiatry. 1975;32:749–761.

221. Hochli D, Riemann D, Zulley J, et al. Initial REM sleep suppression by clomipramine: a prognostic tool for treatment response in patients with a major depressive disorder. Biol Psychiatry. 1986;21:1217–1220.

222. Karczmar AG, Longo VG, De Carolis AS. A pharmacological model of paradoxical sleep: the role of cholinergic and monamine systems. Physiol Behav. 1970;5:175–182.

223. McGinty DJ. Sleep mechanisms: biology and control of REM sleep. Int Rev Neurobiol. 1982;23:391–436.

224. Shiromani PJ, Gillin JC, Henriksen SJ. Acetylcholine and the regulation of REM sleep: basic mechanisms and clinical implications for affective illness and narcolepsy. Annu Rev Pharmacol Toxicol. 1987;27:137–156.

225. Sitaram N, Gillin JC, Bunney WEJ. Cholinergic and catecholaminergic receptor sensitivity in affective illness: strategy and theory. In: Post RM, Ballenger JC, eds. Neurobiology of Mood Disorders. Baltimore, Md: Williams & Wilkins; 1984:629–651.

226. McCarley RW, Massaquoi SG. A limit cycle mathematical model of the REM sleep oscillator system. Am J Physiol. 1986;251(6 pt 2):R1011–1029.

227. McCarley RW. REM sleep and depression: common neurobiological control mechanisms. Am J Psychiatry. 1982;139:565–570.

228. Gillin JC, Sitaram N, Duncan WC. Muscarinic supersensitivity: a possible model for the sleep disturbance of primary depression. Psychiatry Res. 1979;1:17–22.

228a. McCarley RW, Greene RW, Massaquoi SG. Sleep abnormalities in depression: a cellular neurobiological perspective. Arch Gen Psychiatry. 1993.

229. Steriade M, Curro Dossi RC, Nunez A. Network modulation of a slow intrinsic oscillation of cat thalamocortical neurons implicated in sleep delta waves: cortically induced synchronization and brainstem cholinergic suppression. J Neurosci. 1991;11:3200–3217.

230. Risch SC, Janowsky DS, Mott MA, et al. Central and peripheral cholinesterase inhibition: effects on anterior pituitary and sympathomimetic function. Psychoneuroendocrinology. 1986;11:221–230.

231. Berger M, Doerr P, von Zerssen D. Physostigmine infleunce on DST results. Am J Psychiatry. 1982;141:469–470.

232. Janowsky DS, Davis JM, El-Yousef MK, et al. A cholinergic-adrenergic hypothesis of mania and depression. Lancet. 1972;2:632–635.

233. Sagales T, Erill S, Domino EF. Effects of repeated doses of scopolamine on the electroencephalographic stages of sleep in normal volunteers. Clin Pharmacol Ther. 1975;18:727–732.

234. Dube S, Kumar N, Ettedgui E, et al. Cholinergic REM induction response: separation of anxiety and depression. Biol Psychiatry. 1985;20:408–414.

235. Gillin JC, Sutton L, Ruiz C, et al. The cholinergic rapid eye movement induction test with arecoline in depression. Arch Gen Psychiatry. 1991;48:264–270.

236. Sitaram N, Gillin JC. Development and use of pharmacological probes of the CNS in man: evidence of colinergic abnormality in primary affective illness. Biol Psychiatry. 1980;15:925–955.

237. Sitaram N, Nurnberger JI Jr. Gershon ES, et al. Cholinergic regulation of mood and REM sleep: potential model and marker of vulnerability to affective disorder. Am J Psychiatry. 1982;139:571–576.

238. Dahl RE, Ryan ND, Perel J, et al. Cholinergic REM induction test with arecoline in depressed children. Psychiatry Res. 1994;51:269–282.

239. Berger M, Hochli D, Zulley J, et al. Cholinomimetic drug RS 86, REM sleep, and depression. Lancet. 1985;8447:1385–1386.

240. Berger M, Lund RD, Bronisch T, et al. REM latency in neurotic and endogenous depression and cholinergic REM induction test. Psychiatry Res. 1983;10:113–123.

241. Nurnberger JJ, Sitaram N, Gershon ES, et al. A twin study of cholinergic REM induction. Biol Psychiatry. 1983;18:1161–1165.

242. Sitaram N, Dube S, Keshavan M, et al. The association of supersensitive cholinergic REM-induction and affective illness within pedigrees. J Psychiatr Res. 1987;21:487–497.

243. Papousek M. Chronobiological aspects of cyclothymia [in German]. Fortschr Neurol Psychiatr. 1975;43:381–440.

244. Kripke DF, Mullaney DJ, Atkinson M, et al. Circadian rhythm disorders in manic-depressives. Biol Psychiatry. 1978;13:335–351.

245. Wehr TA, Wirz-Justice A, Goodwin FK, et al. Phase advance of the circadian sleep-wake cycle as an antidepressant. Science. 1979;206:710–713.

246. Surridge-David M, MacLean A, Coulter ME, et al. Mood change following an acute delay of sleep [published erratum appears in Psychiatry Res. 1988;24:121]. Psychiatry Res. 1987;22:149–158.

247. David MM, MacLean AW, Knowles JB, et al. Rapid eye movement latency and mood following a delay of bedtime in healthy subjects: do the effects mimic changes in depressive illness? Acta Psychiatr Scand. 1991;84:33–39.

248. Kupfer DJ, Gillin JC, Coble PA, et al. REM sleep, naps, and depression. Psychiaty Res. 1981;5:195–203.

249. Schulz H, Tetzlaff W. Distribution of REM latencies after sleep interruption in depressive patients and control subjects. Biol Psychiatry. 1982;17:1367–1376.

250. Buysse DJ, Jarrett DB, Miewald JM, et al. Minute-by-minute analysis of REM sleep timing in major depression. Biol Psychiatry. 1990;28:911–925.

251. Riemann D, Hohagen F, Konig A, et al. Advanced vs. normal sleep timing: effects on depressed mood after response to sleep deprivation in patients with a major depressive disorder. J Affect Disord. 1996;37:121–128.

252. Elsenga S, Van den Hoofdakker RH. Clinical effects of several sleep-wake manipulations on endogenous depression. Sleep Res. 1983;12:326.

253. Borbély AA. A two process model of sleep regulation. Hum Neurobiol. 1982;1:195–204.

254. Borbély AA, Wirz-Justice A. Sleep, sleep deprivation and depression: a hypothesis derived from a model of sleep regulation. Hum Neurobiol. 1982;1:205–210.

255. Kupfer DJ, Ulrich RF, Coble PA, et al. Application of automated REM and slow wave sleep analysis, II: testing the assumption of the two-process model of sleep regulation in normal and depressed subjects. Psychiatry Res. 1984;13:335–343.

256. Lindstrom LH, Ekman R, Walleus H, et al. Delta-sleep inducing peptide in cerebrospinal fluid from schizophrenics, depressives and healthy volunteers. Prog Neuropsychopharmacol Biol Psychiatry. 1985;9:83–90.

97

Schizophrenia

Kathleen L. Benson

Vincent P. Zarcone, Jr.

Most clinicians who can make the comparisons agree that schizophrenia is the most devastating psychiatric illness. Perhaps it is the most devastating of all illnesses. Since the pioneering descriptive studies of Bleuler,[1] the course of the illness has changed little. Roughly one fourth of patients recover complete social and occupational function. One fifth are severely incapacitated for the rest of their lives and essentially require hospitalization. The remainder require numerous outpatient interventions and rehospitalizations for the rest of their life.

Standard antipsychotic treatment shortens hospitalization at the time of psychotic episodes, but it does not alter the recovery process or the outcomes given above, although the newer or novel antipsychotic drugs may lower the number of rehospitalizations. Also, the benefits of antipsychotics do not accrue without cost. Traditional antipsychotics such as haloperidol and thiothixene are associated with movement disorders such as tardive dyskinesia and with death from the neuroleptic malignant syndrome; the newer antipsychotics such as clozapine involve other risks such as agranulocytosis.

The human suffering is immense. Schizophrenia has a high suicide rate; most suicides occur early and thus the disease causes "a greater loss of total years of expected life"[2(p631)] than any other psychiatric disorder. In the mid-1980s, schizophrenia cost the United States between $10 and $20 billion per year.[2, 3]

HISTORICAL ASPECTS

Abnormalities of REM Sleep

Dreaming has many similarities to psychosis. As Jackson[4] and Wundt[5] noted, we all become temporarily insane every night of our lives. Dreaming sleep is a state in which hallucinations, perceptual distortions, bizarre thinking, and temporary delusions are intimately mixed with more normal thought and perceptual processes. This similarity led to the speculation that schizophrenia is an intrusion of the dream state into wakefulness. The hope engendered by the early discovery of the association between dreaming and rapid eye movement (REM) sleep was that schizophrenia might represent an intrusion of the REM sleep state into wakefulness, or at least that REM sleep was somehow abnormal in schizophrenia.

REM Sleep Time

Early polygraphic studies of sleep were aimed at testing the above hypothesis. The first was Dement's[6] groundbreaking study in 1955, which showed that schizophrenic patients do not have an abnormal temporal distribution of rapid eye movements during nocturnal sleep. Rechtschaffen et al.[7] looked for indices of REM sleep occurring during the waking state of schizophrenic patients. They reported an absence of two or more electrophysiological signs of REM sleep occurring simultaneously in the waking state in five schizophrenic patients. Thus, the first polygraphic studies of sleep in schizophrenic patients found no evidence of gross abnormalities of nocturnal REM sleep or of an intrusion of REM sleep into wakefulness. However, they did not rule out the possibility of more subtle REM sleep abnormalities in schizophrenia. Such possibilities were pursued for several years.

Koresko et al.[8] found that there was essentially little difference in REM time in seven hallucinating patients compared with four nonhallucinating patients. This study did not support the hypothesis that hallucinations in schizophrenia were a spillover of REM sleep into wakefulness, as the REM sleep intrusion hypothesis implied more abnormalities of REM sleep in hallucinating patients than in nonhallucinating patients. Also, in a longitudinal study of acutely disturbed schizophrenic patients, REM sleep did not appear to be abnormally shortened in the waxing phase of the psychosis.[9] In general, however, the early studies demonstrated that nocturnal REM sleep time and percentage of total sleep time were not abnormal in schizophrenia.

There is, however, some evidence that in schizophrenia the REM rebound following REM sleep deprivation might be abnormal. Studies reported by Zarcone et al.,[10] Gillin et al.,[11] and Jus et al.[12] showed a REM rebound failure in acutely symptomatic schizophrenic patients. Contradictory evidence was reported in two studies that found normal REM rebound in schizophrenic patients. Thus, the majority of studies indicated that REM rebound following REM sleep deprivation by awakenings is abnormally reduced or absent in acute schizophrenia; however, the mechanism of this abnormality and its relation to the symptoms of schizophrenia remain unknown.

REM Sleep Phasic Events

Historically, the finding of REM rebound failure in acutely symptomatic schizophrenic patients led to the REM phasic event intrusion hypothesis. According to this hypothesis, REM rebound is impaired in acute schizophrenia because REM phasic events, seen as the driving force of REM sleep, leak from REM sleep into nonrapid eye movement (NREM) sleep and into wakefulness. Such leakage would be associated with a decrease in REM phasic events during REM sleep and, indirectly, a reduction of REM sleep duration. The occurrence of phasic REM events in wakefulness was speculated to cause the thought disorders or attention deficits of schizophrenia. An animal model of the REM phasic intrusion hypothesis was developed by Dement et al.[13] Cats depleted of serotonin by chronic administration of parachlorophenylalanine (PCPA) showed a release of ponto-geniculo-occipital (PGO) spikes from REM sleep into NREM sleep and wakefulness. The PGO spikes are phasic events during REM sleep that appear to drive REM sleep. In the animal model, the PGO spikes during wakefulness were associated with "hallucination-like" behavior, that is, orienting responses with no stimuli in the environment. If a PCPA-treated cat were REM-deprived, it showed a REM rebound failure and a continuation of the redistribution of PGO spikes into the waking state. Chlorpromazine reversed the rebound failure and decreased the hallucination-like orienting responses.

Somewhat more recently, an attempt was made to test the REM phasic event intrusion hypothesis in schizophrenic patients. Given that there is no direct way to record PGO spike-like activity from surface electrodes in human subjects, possible indirect indicators of PGO activity were utilized. These included surface recordings of phasic integrated potentials (PIPs) of the ocular muscles and middle ear muscle activity (MEMA). However, a comprehensive study of PIPs and MEMAs failed to show any significant abnormality in their NREM-REM distribution in schizophrenic patients in comparison with schizoaffective and depressive patients and nonpsychiatric controls.[14]

Phasic REM activity has also been studied in schizophrenia. Because the number of eye movements (EMs) in REM sleep is, in part, dependent on the availability of background stage REM time, measures of EM density have been employed to guard against this confounding effect. EM density is typically computed as the ratio of EM frequency to stage REM minutes. Gulevich et al.[15] noted a trend toward increased EM density in schizophrenic patients relative to nonpsychiatric controls. In contrast, Feinberg et al.[16] found no difference in EM density between schizophrenic patients and controls; however, within the schizophrenic patients, EM density was higher in the hallucinating than the nonhallucinating patients. A recent study confirmed and extended the observations of Feinberg et al. using computerized measures of EM detection. Benson and Zarcone[17] found no difference in EM density between schizophrenic patients, nonpsychiatric controls, and patients with major depressive disorder. Within the schizophrenic group, EM density was positively correlated with ratings of hallucinatory behavior from the Brief Psychiatric Rating Scale (BPRS).

REM Latency

While the studies reported above have revealed few abnormalities of REM time or REM sleep EM density in schizophrenia, many studies of nocturnal sleep in schizophrenia have observed that the latency to the onset of the first REM period is less than normal. Since 1965, 12 studies[15, 16, 18–27] have compared the REM latency of unmedicated schizophrenic patients with that of nonpsychiatric controls. Seven[15, 18–21, 24, 25] of the 12 studies found significant between-group differences with the schizophrenic patients demonstrating short REM latencies. Even among those studies finding no between-group differences, a bimodal distribution of REM latency values in schizophrenic patients has been observed; this bimodality demonstrates that there are subgroups of schizophrenic patients with sleep-onset REM periods.[16, 23, 26, 28]

Abnormalities of NREM Sleep

Slow-Wave Sleep

While short REM latencies in schizophrenia have been documented by several investigators, there is some lack of agreement about the mechanism underlying the shortening of the latency to the first REM period. In 1969, Feinberg et al.[29] suggested that a slow-wave or delta sleep deficit in the first NREM period (i.e., that interval of time between sleep onset and the first REM period) could be responsible for the passive advance or early onset of the first REM period. Alternatively, short REM latencies could represent an active, or primary alteration of REM sleep mechanisms.

We turn now to a discussion of slow-wave sleep because slow-wave sleep deficits are one of the most reliably reported abnormalities found in schizophrenia. In visually scored polysomnography, slow-wave sleep is reported as the summation of sleep stages 3 and 4, with stage 4 sleep having the greater incidence of underlying slow-wave activity. In the Feinberg et al. 1969 study,[29] stage 3 measures did not differentiate schizophrenic patients from controls; only stage 4 sleep was significantly reduced in the schizophrenic patients relative to the controls. This identical observation was made by Caldwell and Domino[30] in their study of 25 chronic schizophrenic patients medication-free for a minimum of 2 years. In addition to this basic observation, they reported an absence of stage 4 sleep in 10 (40%) of the 25 schizophrenic patients. In the intervening decades, some[21, 31] but not all[23–26] studies have observed stage 4 or slow-wave sleep deficits in schizophrenic patients relative to nonpsychiatric controls.

These inconsistencies may in part be attributed to the inherent insensitivity of visual scoring to underlying differences in delta band or slow waveform (0 to 3 Hz) incidence and amplitude. Those studies[20, 22, 27] utilizing digital or computer processing of electroencephalographic (EEG) waveforms during sleep have substantiated the degradation of slow-wave incidence and amplitude in schizophrenic patients relative to nonpsychiatric controls.

Sleep Efficiency

The sleep of schizophrenic patients is characterized by poor sleep efficiency.[21–27, 32] Often this takes the form of long sleep-onset latencies and reduced total sleep. Sleep continuity is also impaired by long periods of waking after sleep onset. Probably the most consistently reported abnormality noted in empirical studies of sleep patterns in schizophrenia is a marked increase in sleep-onset latency. Typically, sleep-onset latency in healthy controls ranges from 10 to 20 min; in contrast, sleep latency in schizophrenic patients exceeds 30 min, and is often in the 50- to 100-min range. Van Kammen et al.[33] have reported that severe insomnia is one of the prodromal symptoms associated with psychotic decompensation; according to van Kammen et al.,[33] this severe insomnia may actually precede the occurrence of ratable symptoms of relapse.

Clinical Correlates

Having reviewed the characteristic alterations found in the sleep of schizophrenic patients, the issue of how these alterations relate to clinical presentation remains. Over the past 3 decades, several sleep centers have addressed this issue. Global severity is typically, though not always, measured by the BPRS.[34] Global severity has been associated with increased wake time, reduced REM time, reduced slow-wave sleep, and short REM latencies.[23, 24, 35] Psychosis or psychotic symptoms are a component of global severity. Depending on the clinical instrument, a psychosis assessment may include ratings of unusual thought content, conceptual disorganization, delusions, and hallucinatory behavior. Aggregated, these psychotic symptoms are often referred to as "positive" symptoms of schizophrenia. Positive or psychotic symptoms have been associated with increased REM sleep EM density,[16, 17] short REM latencies[24, 26] (sleep-onset REM periods in particular[36]), reduced sleep efficiency,[37] and prolonged sleep latencies.[38] "Negative" symptoms refer to another component of global severity and include symptoms of affective flattening, alogia, avolition, anhedonia, and attentional impairment. Negative symptoms have been linked to slow wave sleep deficits[22, 39–41] and short REM latencies.[24, 28] While REM latency in schizophrenia is unrelated to severity of depression[24] or family history of affective illness,[26] greater REM sleep time and REM sleep EM activity in schizophrenia have been associated with suicidality.[42, 43] Finally, longitudinal outcome studies have observed that poor clinical and psychosocial outcome is associated with both short REM latency[28, 44] and slow-wave sleep deficits.[45]

Broadly viewed, these studies failed to produce a consistent picture. This lack of consistency may reflect the variety of rating scales and instruments used to assess clinical symptoms, different quantifications of sleep parameters, effects of sample size, medication status, patient characteristics such as chronicity, subtype (e.g., paranoid), and gender, and finally the nearly exclusive use of a cross-sectional design. These studies point to the need for longitudinal assessments documenting how changes in clinical state affect sleep parameters.

PATHOPHYSIOLOGY

The pathophysiology of the sleep abnormalities found in schizophrenic patients is unknown. There are, however, theoretical models that have been advanced, as well as several demonstrated neurobiological correlates of these abnormalities.

Neuroanatomical Abnormalities

One such theoretical model was advanced by Irwin Feinberg[46] in 1983. According to this model, an error may occur in the programmed decrease in synaptic density during the adolescence of some schizophrenic patients, resulting in decreased capability for synchronous delta band or slow-wave EEG activity; this decreased capability would reveal itself as a slow-wave sleep deficit. This theory implies a permanent brain structural defect and is consistent with Luby and Caldwell's[47] report of no homeostatic recovery of slow-wave sleep in schizophrenic patients following 85 h of total sleep deprivation.

Brain anatomical defects in schizophrenia have frequently been observed in imaging studies,[48] as well as in postmortem analyses.[49] Pfefferbaum et al.[48] demonstrated that the ventricular system is larger in schizophrenic patients than in nonpsychiatric controls; in a related study, ventricular enlargement in schizophrenia was associated with reduced cortical gray matter.[50] Van Kammen et al.[39] have reported a significant negative correlation between the amount of stage 4 sleep in schizophrenic patients and the lateral ventricular-to-brain ratio (VBR) using computed tomography (CT) imaging. In a replication, Benson et al.[51] reported that all measures of slow-wave sleep were inversely related to ventricular system volume in schizophrenia even after ventricular volume was corrected for normal variation in age and head size. Because ventricular system volume in schizophrenic patients has been associated with reduced cerebral gray matter, both studies provide indirect and modest support for Feinberg's theory that changes in synaptic density may underlie slow-wave sleep deficits in schizophrenia. Feinberg et al.[52] have also described an association between the delta waveform amplitude of slow-wave sleep and the cerebral metabolic rate. Using phosphorus 31-magnetic resonance spectroscopy, Keshavan et al.[40] have shown that decreased brain anabolic processes are associated with slow-wave sleep deficits in psychotic disorders, primarily schizophrenia, and have suggested that this association may be explained by developmental abnormalities in cortical synaptic pruning, as suggested by Feinberg.

Brain anatomical features have also been related to abnormalities of sleep efficiency, another robust characteristic of the sleep disturbance found in schizophrenia. The van Kammen et al. study[39] reported a negative correlation between total sleep time and the size of the third ventricle. The third ventricle-to-brain ratio was studied by Keshavan et al.[53] and found to be inversely correlated with sleep maintenance. Finally, Lauer et al.[26] reported that the VBR as imaged by CT is positively associated with measures of awakening in drug-naive schizophrenic patients. In summary, these studies suggest that the sleep disturbances in schizophrenia may have underlying brain neuroanatomical concomitants contributing to a more trait-like rather than state-like presentation of these abnormalities.

Neurotransmitter Systems and Psychopharmacology

Serotonin

For decades, research studies have noted that serotonin (5-hydroxytryptamine, 5-HT) plays a key role in sleep regulation. The association of stage 4 sleep deficits in schizophrenia with a serotonin defect was reported by Benson et al.[54] who demonstrated that cerebrospinal fluid (CSF) levels of the 5-HT metabolite, 5-hydroxyindole acetic acid (5-HIAA), are positively correlated with stage 4 and slow-wave sleep time in unmedicated schizophrenic patients. In a separate study, Benson et al.[55] also demonstrated that the serotonin defect underlying stage 4 sleep deficits in some schizophrenic patients appears to be resistant to ritanserin, an experimental agent with strong 5-HT-2 antagonism. In this study, visually scored stage 4 sleep was virtually absent at baseline; furthermore, there was no increase in stage 4 sleep after the administration of ritanserin 10 mg, a drug and dose shown to produce a 100% increase in slow-wave sleep time in normals.[56] Although ritanserin did not increase stage 4 sleep in these patients, it did increase the incidence and amplitude of underlying slow or delta band waveforms. It also promoted sleep continuity; the amount of waking after sleep onset, the number of awakenings after sleep onset, and the amount of stage 1 sleep were significantly reduced. These effects were related to plasma levels of ritanserin.

The newer or novel antipsychotics like clozapine and risperidone are also noted for their serotonin antagonism. However, in a longitudinal study[57] of clozapine's effects on sleep in schizophrenic patients, screened to exclude those with clozapine-induced fever, clozapine significantly decreased slow-wave sleep;

it did, however, increase total sleep time, sleep efficiency and NREM stage 2 sleep. With respect to sleepiness or sedation, serotonergic antagonism should not be viewed to the exclusion of other neurotransmitter involvement. For example, clozapine is associated with significantly more sleepiness than risperidone, but clozapine's binding profile to the 5-HT-2 receptor is markedly less than that of risperidone; possibly, the sedative effect of clozapine may be associated with its greater histaminergic blockade.

Norepinephrine

As reported earlier in this chapter, van Kammen et al.[33] have demonstrated that severe insomnia is one of the prodromal symptoms associated with psychotic decompensation and that this severe insomnia may actually precede the occurrence of ratable symptoms of relapse. Van Kammen and colleagues also observed that increased CSF levels of norepinephrine and its metabolite, 3-methoxy-4-hydroxyphenylglycol (MHPG), are associated with this relapse-related insomnia.

The Cholinergic-Dopaminergic Hypothesis of Schizophrenia

Given the prominent role assigned to dopaminergic dysfunction in the pathophysiology of schizophrenia, there is surprisingly little information on the relationship of sleep abnormalities in schizophrenia to dopaminergic abnormalities. As reported above, CSF levels of the serotonin metabolite 5-HIAA are correlated with slow-wave sleep in schizophrenia. Benson et al.[54] also observed a similar, but weaker, association with CSF homovanillic acid (HVA), the metabolite of dopamine. This association may derive from the fact that HVA and 5-HIAA are often highly intercorrelated in CSF analyses. The role of dopamine per se in sleep abnormalities in schizophrenia certainly warrants explicit attention; however, such studies may likely be confounded by long-term exposure to the dopamine antagonist properties of antipsychotics. Thaker et al.[35] observed that patients with longer antipsychotic exposure as well as tardive dyskinesia have more abnormalities of REM time and REM latency during medication-free sleep recordings than do schizophrenic patients with a briefer history of antipsychotic exposure without tardive dyskinesia.

Studies elucidating the role of cholinergic mechanisms in the development of sleep abnormalities in schizophrenia are few and are, in large part, confined to extrapolations from studies of patients with affective illness. Most studies have looked at the effect of cholinergic agents on REM latency. Arecoline, a muscarinic receptor agonist, reduces REM latency, whereas scopolamine, a muscarinic antagonist, prolongs REM latency.[58] The finding that arecoline tends to reduce REM latency led to the development of the Cholinergic REM Induction Test (CRIT).[59] In this test, arecoline is infused approximately 25 min after the first REM period; the dependent measure is the elapsed time from the infusion to the start of the second REM period. Compared with a placebo infusion, arecoline shortens this interval. The CRIT has been used primarily in the study of affective illness. Typically, the postinfusion latency to the second REM period is shorter in depressive patients than in healthy controls, prompting the speculation that REM sleep abnormalities in depression reflect cholinergic supersensitivity. Given the fact that both schizophrenic and mood disorder patients exhibit short REM latencies, abnormalities in the cholinergic regulation of REM sleep initiation may be present in schizophrenic patients as well. Riemann et al.[60] have demonstrated that schizophrenic patients respond similarly to depressive patients using the CRIT, suggesting that short REM latencies in schizophrenic patients may also reflect some cholinergic supersensitivity. Consistent with this hypothesis of a hyperexcitable cholinergic system is the recent observation of Garcia-Rill et al.[61] noting an above-normal number of mesopontine cholinergic neurons in schizophrenia.

Independent of sleep abnormalities, a link between cholinergic hyperactivity and schizophrenia has been proposed as part of a comprehensive model of cholinergic-dopaminergic interaction in schizophrenia. Tandon and Greden[62] suggest that cholinergic hyperactivity is related to the development of negative symptoms in schizophrenia. According to their model, cholinergic activity increases as a protective mechanism when faced with elevated dopaminergic activity and psychotic exacerbation. Negative symptoms accompany this cholinergic hyperactivity. With effective treatment, dopamine activity might normalize, but some residual cholinergic hyperactivity would persist; the presence of negative symptoms would reflect this residual cholinergic hyperactivity.

EPIDEMIOLOGY

Schizophrenia affects between 0.4 and 2.7% of the population; the mean lifetime prevalence is 1.0% worldwide. Schizophrenia is equally common in both sexes. While the age of onset is usually in the second decade of life, the disorder seems to begin earlier in males than in females. The course is variable; most schizophrenic patients recover to levels where they can function occupationally and socially. The course is modified considerably by the use of antipsychotic agents and hospitalization, which is usually brief, on the order of 4 to 6 weeks. There is much residual dysphoria and depressed mood, particularly early in the course of the illness.

As indicated earlier, there is considerable impairment, high suicidality, and strong familial patterns. Family studies indicate that schizophrenia is, at least in part, genetically determined, although there are high rates of discordance in monozygotic twin, which indicates that the environment has considerable influence.

CLINICAL FEATURES

The Diagnosis of Schizophrenia

Currently, the criteria for the diagnosis of schizophrenia are based on the work of three prominent clinicians: Bleuler, Kraepelin, and Schneider; they are most recently defined in the *Diagnostic and Statistical Manual of Mental Disorders, Fourth Edition* (DSM-IV)[63] and are summarized below.

A. Characteristic symptoms include two or more of the following, each present for a significant portion of time during a 1-month period: (1) delusions; (2) hallucinations; (3) disorganized speech, for example, frequent derailment or incoherence; (4) grossly disorganized or catatonic behavior; and (5) negative symptoms such as affective flattening, alogia, or avolition. Note that only one criterion A symptom is required if delusions are bizarre or hallucinations consist of a voice keeping up a running commentary on the person's behavior or thoughts, or two or more voices conversing with each other.

B. Marked deterioration in function in areas such as work, interpersonal relations, or self-care.

C. Continuous signs of disturbance persist for at least 6 months.

D. Schizoaffective disorder and mood disorder with psychotic features have been ruled out.

E. Drugs of abuse or medications or general medical conditions have been excluded.

F. If there is a history of a developmental disorder, such as autistic disorder, the additional diagnosis of schizophrenia is made only if prominent delusions or hallucinations are also present for at least 1 month.

Subjective Complaints

As Bleuler pointed out over 90 years ago, "In schizophrenia, sleep is habitually disturbed."[1(p168)] Since Bleuler, there have been many similar descriptions. For example, Mark Vonnegutt stated in *Eden Express* that at the onset of his first schizophrenic episode, "I realized that this meant I could never sleep again,"[64(p12)] and R. D. Laing in *The Divided Self* observed that the patient before the first episode is "persecuted by his own insight and lucidity" and so lacks "the assurance" required for sleep.[65(p119)]

Sleep disturbance, particularly at the onset of the first psychotic symptoms, and with each subsequent relapse, can be marked. The sleep of schizophrenic patients who are in a state of psychotic agitation is characterized by prolonged periods of total sleeplessness. In times of less severe psychotic agitation, sleep, when it comes, may be characterized by a marked insomnia—long sleep-onset latencies, reduced total sleep time, and sleep fragmented by bouts of waking. There is a fairly frequent reversal of sleep and wake so that the patient sleeps in the daylight hours, preferring to do so because it relieves him or her of some of the responsibility and anxiety of interacting with other people. Schizophrenic patients can also experience profoundly disturbing, terrifying hypnagogic hallucinations. Many also suffer from nightmares. Although there are no systematic studies, anecdotal clinical reports indicate that alcohol and substance abuse can both disturb sleep and cause the patient to relapse.

DIAGNOSTIC EVALUATION

Because there is no consensus that sleep abnormalities can reliably differentiate among psychiatric disorders, the sleep disorders specialist is not likely to be asked to apply polysomnography to assist in the differentiation of schizophrenia from other psychiatric disorders. For example, the most compelling sleep disturbance associated with schizophrenia is a profound insomnia associated with periods of psychotic agitation. Across psychiatric categories, schizophrenic patients, as a group, tend to have longer sleep-onset latencies than depressive patients or patients with borderline personality disorder; however, their sleep latencies do not differ on a group basis from patients with schizoaffective disorder,[21] psychotic depression,[22] or mania.[25] Outside of the major psychiatric disorders, prolonged sleep-onset latencies are also associated with psychophysiological insomnia and delayed sleep phase syndrome. Among schizophrenic patients, there is a broad range of sleep-onset latencies; consequently, even this variable cannot be used definitively as a diagnostic indicator.

While short REM latencies, including sleep-onset REM periods, are often observed in schizophrenias, similar REM latency values have also been noted in schizoaffective disorder,[21] major depression,[21, 25] delusional depression,[22] and mania.[25] Like REM latency, stage 4 sleep deficits lack diagnostic specificity and are found in other psychiatric disorders such as major depressive disorder,[66] borderline personality disorder,[67] and post-traumatic stress disorder.[68] Finally, all-night measures of REM sleep EM activity do not reliably differentiate schizophrenic patients from patients with major depressive disorder,[17] delusional depression,[22] or mania.[25]

Douglass et al.[69] have suggested that the sleep clinic may be of considerable use in differentiating schizophrenia from narcolepsy, which can present with a strong hallucinatory component. This may be particularly important due to the fact that a mistake in diagnosis can result in very high risk-benefit ratios for the patients. Sleep studies may also assist in the differential diagnosis of other sleep disorders associated with excessive daytime somnolence in schizophrenic patients for whom oversedation with antipsychotics may be suspected. It is obvious that schizophrenic patients who are sleepy have to be approached in the same manner as any other patient referred to the sleep disorders specialist. Given the higher prevalence of co-morbidity of sleep disorders seen in schizophrenic patients, causes of excessive daytime somnolence in schizophrenic patients other than antipsychotic sedation have to be strongly entertained.

Our experience with insomnia complainers indicates that it is extremely rare for an undiagnosed schizophrenic patient to be referred to a sleep clinic because of an insomnia complaint. However, it is not rare for depressed patients or patients with borderline personality disturbance to be referred. The sleep disorders physician should be aware of the possibility that mood disorder and personality disturbance may not be diagnosed by the referring physician.

Co-Morbidity

Subjectively experienced sleep disturbance is common in schizophrenic patients; this disturbance more often takes the form of early or middle insomnia.[70] While this sleep disturbance may only reflect their psychiatric illness, schizophrenic patients can also suffer from a variety of other sleep disorders. Some of the most common include inadequate sleep hygiene, environmental sleep disorders, sleep disorders associated with the abuse of or withdrawal from alcohol and illicit drugs, and irregular sleep-wake patterns. Wirz-Justice et al.[71] recently described a schizophrenic patient with a near-arrhythmic circadian rest-activity cycle which was improved by clozapine.

The incidence of intrinsic dyssomnias is also high in psychiatric populations. In our experience,[72] 25 to 30% of male schizophrenic patients are co-morbid for clinically significant sleep-disordered breathing or periodic limb movement (PLM)·disorder or both; 15% of schizophrenic patients screened in our clinic had sleep-disordered breathing, 11% had PLM disorder, and 2% had both. Both of these disorders have a profound impact on sleep fragmentation and daytime somnolence. More recently, Ancoli-Isreal et al.[73] have observed even greater impairment. Forty-eight percent of the schizophrenics in their study had a respiratory disturbance index (RDI) of 10 or greater; 14% had a movement index of 5 or more limb movements per hour of sleep. In this study, schizophrenic patients with an RDI of 10 or more reported significantly more symptoms of daytime sleepiness that those patients with an RDI of less than 10. Depending on the level of symptomatology, many schizophrenic patients with sleep-disordered breathing can be effectively treated with nasal continuous positive airway pressure or bilateral positive airway pressure and demonstrate relatively the same degree of compliance as nonschizophrenic patients.

MANAGEMENT

The standard treatment of schizophrenia is with hospitalization at the time of the onset of the first episode and at subsequent relapses so that antipsychotic medicine can be administered and psychosocial intervention can be planned and initiated. The standard, rapid administration of antipsychotic medications usually produces sedation. For example, haloperidol 5 to 10 mg intramuscularly every 2 h is commonly administered until the patient is sedated or less psychotic. The side effects of antipsychotics are in three major groups. Group A includes the drugs which produce prominent extrapyramidal side effects and includes haloperidol, fluphenazine, trifluperazine, and butaperazine. Group B comprises the antipsychotics that produce hypotension, anticholinergic effects, and moderate or marked sedation. It includes chlorpromazine and thioridazine. Group C is a mixture of groups A and B which include thiothixene and perphenazine. The standard practice is to give group B drugs to younger, more agitated patients who are in good medical health and free of cardiovascular disease, and to reserve the group A drugs with the extrapyramidal side effects for the elderly, hypertensive, or patients with cardiovascular disease.

The chronic administration of traditional antipsychotics do alter sleep architecture. In general, studies[74-77] have shown that these agents uniformly produce some sedation such as an increase in total sleep, reduced sleep latency, and reduced waking after sleep onset. Of the newer or novel antipsychotics, clozapine is the most sedating. Risperidone, olanzapine, and sertindole are less sedating and are similar to traditional antipsychotics in their sedation profiles.[78] Polysomnographic studies[57, 79] of schizophrenic patients treated with clozapine show clozapine to have strong consolidating effects on sleep similar to the effects of classic antipsychotics such as haloperidol; these effects include increased total sleep, decreased sleep latency, decreased waking after sleep onset, and increased sleep efficiency. In addition, clozapine causes more consolidation of NREM sleep, that is, increasing stage 2 and decreasing stage 1, relative to classic antipsychotics.

One of the oldest clinical maxims in the treatment of schizophrenia is to give the entire dose of antipsychotic at bedtime. Both typical and atypical antipsychotics have long half-lives and reach steady-state plasma concentrations and can be given once a day. This dosing schedule takes advantage of the sedative properties of the medication. If the patient is able to sleep through the night, the stress level for the caregivers can be greatly diminished. Judicious intermittent use of benzodiazepine tranquilizers and hypnotics may be important, particularly in the first 3 to 4 weeks after discharge, because many patients have persistent high levels of anxiety even after the acute psychosis has remitted. Because many patients now have addiction problems, close supervision of benzodiazepines by family or other caregivers is important. The ordinary guidelines for the use of hypnotics should be followed and sleep-related breathing disorders should be ruled out. Additionally, patients with schizoaffective disorder and those with impulse control problems are often treated with mood stabilizers such as valproate. This usually has a continuing beneficial effect on sleep.

The new generation of atypical antipsychotics seems to have effects on negative symptoms. Thus the patient may become more active with consequently increased consolidation of daytime alertness and the homeostatic drive for sleep. Patients should be encouraged to "go with the medicine" and avoid naps and social withdrawal. Within the next few years, the use of atypical antipsychotics may change the practice of greatly decreasing or discontinuing traditional antipsychotic medication because of their associated risk of extrapyramidal side effects, especially tardive dyskinesia. Often this practice results in relapse. Sleep complaints are frequently prodromal signs of relapse, as described by van Kammen et al.[33] and noted earlier in this chapter. Hopefully, the use of atypical antipsychotics for relapse prevention will preclude this clinical dilemma.

Another prominent side effect of the atypical antipsychotics is akathisia, that is, intense restlessness and pacing. It can lead to significant sleep disruption and relapse; thus it is very important to treat it with anticholinergics or propranolol. The latter has a favorable effect on sleep but does have to be given in divided doses. Amantadine is also helpful and can be used if the patient is asthmatic and cannot take propranolol. Akathisia can be differentiated from restless legs syndrome by history, but it is important to remember that both restless legs syndrome and sleep-related periodic limb movements can occur in the same patient. The incidence of akathisia is much lower with the atypical antipsychotics. It is not yet known what effect these newer medications have on restless legs or periodic limb movements, particularly those which might arise after treatment with typical antipsychotics.

These interventions include counseling of family members, occupational rehabilitation, and a complete evaluation of the physical health of the patient. This physical evaluation might lead to consultation with a sleep disorders clinician. Both inpatient and outpatient psychiatrists are increasingly aware of the high prevalence and treatment options for schizophrenic patients co-morbid for sleep disorders such as sleep-disordered breathing and periodic limb movements. The schizophrenic patient is also a good candidate for sleep hygiene counseling. Many patients, in order to isolate themselves socially and avoid painful interactions with other people, develop many bad habits in relation to sleep initiation and sleep maintenance, including sleep reversals and polyphasic sleep patterns sometimes complicated by heavy self-prescribed administration of alcohol or other psychoactive drugs. There are no systematic studies of the application of sleep hygiene to inpatient groups of schizophrenic patients. However, there is every reason to believe that patients would respond to sleep hygiene counseling and to relaxation training to help sleep initiation, sleep maintenance, and stress management. Most schizophrenic patients are seen ideally in long-term follow-up in day hospitals and outpatient clinics. The opportunity exists to work with a patient on sleep hygiene to improve his or her overall level of function. It is important to note that the immediate application of sleep disorders medicine interventions and sleep hygiene advice will undoubtedly benefit schizophrenic patients as they do any other medical or psychiatric patients. Education of the medical community, patients, and their families is already feasible and should be done immediately.

References

1. Bleuler E. Dementia Praecox. New York, NY: International University Press; 1950:168–169.

2. Kaplan HI, Saddock BJ. Comprehensive Textbook of Psychiatry, 4th ed. Baltimore, Md: Williams & Wilkins; 1985.

3. Nicholi AM, ed. The New Harvard Guide to Psychiatry. Cambridge, Mass: Harvard University Press; 1988:259–295.

4. Jackson JH. In: Taylor J, Holmes G, Walshe FMR, eds. Selected Writings of John Hughlings Jackson. Vol 2. New York, NY: BasicBooks; 1958:412.

5. Wundt W. Outlines of Psychology. East St Clair Shores, Mich: Scholarly Publication; 1897.

6. Dement W. Dream recall and eye movements during sleep in schizophrenics and normals. J Nerv Ment Dis. 1955;122:263–269.

7. Rechtschaffen A, Schulsinger F, Mednick S. Schizophrenia and physiological indices of dreaming. Arch Gen Psychiatry. 1964;10:89–93.

8. Koresko R, Snyder F, Feinberg I. "Dream time" in hallucinating and non-hallucinating schizophrenic patients. Nature. 1963; 199:1118–1119.

9. Kupfer DJ, Wyatt RJ, Scott J, et al. Sleep disturbance in acute schizophrenic patients. Am J Psychiatry. 1970;126:1213–1223.

10. Zarcone VP, Azumi K, Dement W, et al. REM phase deprivation and schizophrenia: II. Arch Gen Psychiatry. 1975;32:1431–1436.

11. Gillin JC, Buchsbaum MS, Jacobs LS, et al. Partial sleep deprivation, schizophrenia and field articulation. Arch Gen Psychiatry. 1974;30:653–662.

12. Jus K, Gagnon-Binette M, Desjardins D, et al. Effets de la déprivation du sommeil rapide pendant la première et la seconde partie de la nuit chez les schizophrènes chroniques. La Vie Med Can Fr. 1977;6:1234–1242.

13. Dement W, Zarcone V, Ferguson J, et al. Some parallel findings in schizophrenic patients and serotonin-depleted cats. In: Sankar D, ed. Schizophrenia: Current Concepts and Research. Hicksville, NY: PJD Publications; 1969:775–811.

14. Benson KL, Zarcone VP. Testing the REM sleep phasic event intrusion hypothesis of schizophrenia. Psychiatry Res. 1985;15:163–173.

15. Gulevich GD, Dement WC, Zarcone VP. All-night sleep recordings of chronic schizophrenics in remission. Comp Psychiatry. 1967;8:141–149.

16. Feinberg I, Koresko RL, Gottlieb F. Further observations on electrophysiological sleep patterns in schizophrenia. Comp Psychiatry. 1965;6:21–24.

17. Benson KL, Zarcone VP. REM sleep eye movement activity in schizophrenia and depression. Arch Gen Psychiatry. 1993;50:474–482.

18. Jus K, Bouchard M, Jus AK, et al. Sleep EEG studies in untreated long-term schizophrenic patients. Arch Gen Psychiatry. 1973;29:386–390.

19. Stern M, Fram D, Wyatt R, et al. All night sleep studies of acute schizophrenics. Arch Gen Psychiatry. 1969;20:470–477.

20. Hiatt JF, Floyd TC, Katz PH, et al. Further evidence of abnormal NREM sleep in schizophrenia. Arch Gen Psychiatry. 1985;42:797–802.

21. Zarcone VP, Benson KL, Berger PA. Abnormal rapid eye movement latencies in schizophrenia. Arch Gen Psychiatry. 1987;44:45–48.

22. Ganguli R, Reynolds CF, Kupfer DJ. EEG sleep in young, never medicated, schizophrenic patients: a comparison with delusional and nondelusional depressives and with healthy controls. Arch Gen Psychiatry. 1987;44:36–45.

23. Kempenaers C, Kerkhofs M, Linkowski P, et al. Sleep EEG variables in young schizophrenic and depressive patients. Biol Psychiatry. 1988;24:833–838.

24. Tandon R, Shipley JE, Taylor S, et al. Electroencephalographic sleep abnormalities in schizophrenia. Arch Gen Psychiatry. 1992;49:185–194.

25. Hudson JI, Lipinski JF, Keck PE, et al. Polysomnographic characteristics of schizophrenia in comparison with mania and depression. Biol Psychiatry. 1993;34:191–193.

26. Lauer CJ, Schreiber W, Pollmächer T, et al. Sleep in schizophrenia: a polysomnographic study on drug-naïve patients. Neuropsychopharmacology. 1997;16:51–60.

27. Keshavan MS, Reynolds CF, Miewald JM, et al. Delta sleep deficits in schizophrenia. Arch Gen Psychiatry. 1998;55:443–448.

28. Taylor SF, Tandon R, Shipley JE, et al. Sleep onset REM periods in schizophrenic patients. Biol Psychiatry. 1991;30:205–209.

29. Feinberg I, Braum N, Koresko RL, et al. Stage 4 sleep in schizophrenia. Arch Gen Psychiatry. 1969;21:262–266.

30. Caldwell DF, Domino EF. Electroencephalographic and eye movement patterns during sleep in chronic schizophrenic patients. Electroencephalogr Clin Neurophysiol. 1967;22:414–420.

31. Traub AC. Sleep stage deficits in chronic schizophrenia. Psychol Rep. 1972;31:815–820.

32. Martin J, Jones DW, Caliguiri MP, et al. 24-hour sleep patterns in older schizophrenia patients. J Schiz Res. In press.

33. Van Kammen DP, van Kammen WB, Peters JL, et al. CSF MHPG, sleep and psychosis in schizophrenia. Clin Neuropharmacol. 1986;9(suppl 4):575–577.

34. Overall JE, Gorham DR. The brief psychiatric rating scale. Psychol Rep. 1962;10:799–812.

35. Thaker GK, Wagman AMI, Tamminga CA. Sleep polygraphy in schizophrenia: Methodological issues. Biol Psychiatry. 1990; 28:240–246.

36. Howland RH. Sleep-onset rapid eye movement periods in neuropsychiatric disorders: implications for the pathophysiology of psychosis. J Nerv Ment Dis. 1997;185:730–738.

37. Neylan TC, van Kammen DP, Kelley ME, et al. Sleep in schizophrenic patients on and off haloperidol therapy. Arch Gen Psychiatry. 1992;49:643–649.

38. Zarcone VP, Benson KL. BPRS symptom factors and sleep variables in schizophrenia. Psychiatry Res. 1997;66:111–120.

39. Van Kammen DP, van Kammen WM, Peters J, et al. Decreased slow-wave sleep and enlarged lateral ventricles in schizophrenia. Neuropsychopharmacology. 1988;1:265–271.

40. Keshavan MS, Pettegrew JW, Reynolds CF, et al. Biological correlates of slow wave sleep deficits in functional psychoses: ^{31}P-magnetic resonance spectroscopy. Psychiatry Res. 1995;57:91–100.

41. Keshavan MS, Miewald J, Haas G, et al. Slow-wave sleep and symptomatology in schizophrenia and related psychotic disorders. J Psychiatr Res. 1995;29:303–314.

42. Keshavan MS, Reynolds CF, Montrose D, et al. Sleep and suicidality in psychotic patients. Acta Psychiatr Scand. 1994;89:122–125.

43. Lewis CF, Tandon R, Shipley JE, et al. Biological predictors of suicidality in schizophrenia. Acta Psychiatr Scand. 1996;94:416–420.

44. Goldman M, Tandon R, DeQuardo JR, et al. Biological predictors of 1-year outcome in schizophrenia in males and females. Schizophr Res. 1996;21:65–73.

45. Keshavan MS, Reynolds CF III, Miewald J, et al. Slow-wave sleep deficits and outcome in schizophrenia and schizoaffective disorder. Acta Psychiatr Scand. 1995;91:289–292.

46. Feinberg I. Schizophrenia: caused by a fault in programmed synaptic elimination during adolescence? J Psychiatr Res. 1983;17:319–334.

47. Luby ED, Caldwell DF. Sleep deprivation and EEG slow wave activity in chronic schizophrenia. Arch Gen Psychiatry. 1967;17:361–364.

48. Pfefferbaum A, Zipursky RB, Lim KO, et al. Computed tomographic evidence for generalized sulcal and ventricular enlargement in schizophrenia. Arch Gen Psychiatry. 1988;45:633–640.

49. Bogerts B, Meetz E, Schonfeldt-Bausch R. Basal ganglia and limbic system pathology in schizophrenia. Arch Gen Psychiatry. 1985;42:784–791.

50. Zipursky RB, Lim KO, Sullivan EV, et al. Widespread cerebral gray matter volume deficits in schizophrenia. Arch Gen Psychiatry. 1992;49:195–205.

51. Benson KL, Sullivan EV, Lim KO, et al. Slow wave sleep and CT measures of brain morphology in schizophrenia. Psychiatry Res. 1996;60:125–134.

52. Feinberg I, Thode HC, Chugani HT, et al. Gamma distribution model describes maturational curves for delta wave amplitude, cortical metabolic rate and synaptic density. J Theor Biol. 1990;142:149–161.

53. Keshavan MS, Reynolds CF, Ganguli R, et al. Electroencephalographic sleep and cerebral morphology in functional psychosis: a preliminary study with computed tomography. Psychiatry Res. 1991;39:293–301.

54. Benson KL, Faull KF, Zarcone VP. Evidence for the role of serotonin in the regulation of slow wave sleep in schizophrenia. Sleep. 1991;14:133–139.

55. Benson KL, Csernansky JG, Zarcone VP. The effect of ritanserin

on slow wave sleep deficits and sleep continuity in schizophrenia. Sleep Res. 1991;20:170.

56. Idzikowski C, Mills F, Glennard R. 5-hydroxytryptamine-2 antagonist increases human slow wave sleep. Brain Res. 1986;378:164–168.

57. Hinze-Selch D, Mullington J, Orth A, et al. Effects of clozapine on sleep: a longitudinal study. Biol Psychiatry. 1997;42:260–266.

58. Gillin JC, Sitaram N, Mendelson WB. Acetylcholine, sleep, and depression. Hum Neurobiol. 1982;1:211–219.

59. Gillin JC, Sitaram N, Nurnberger JI, et al. The cholinergic REM induction test. Psychopharmacol Bull. 1983;19:668–670.

60. Riemann D, Hohagen F, Krieger S, et al. Cholinergic REM induction test: muscarinic supersensitivity underlies polysomnographic findings in both depression and schizophrenia. J Psychiatr Res. 1994;28:195–210.

61. Garcia-Rill E, Biedermann JA, Chambers T, et al. Mesopontine neurons in schizophrenia. Neuroscience. 1995;66:321–335.

62. Tandon R, Greden JF. Cholinergic hyperactivity and negative schizophrenia symptoms. Arch Gen Psychiatry. 1989;46:745–753.

63. American Psychiatric Association. Diagnostic and Statistical Manual of Mental Disorders. 4th ed. Washington, DC: American Psychiatric Association Press; 1994:273–290.

64. Vonnegutt M. Eden Express. New York, NY: Praeger Publications; 1975:12.

65. Laing RD. The Divided Self. Baltimore, Md: Penguin Books; 1960:119.

66. Kupfer DJ, Ulrich RF, Coble PA, et al. Application of automated REM and slow wave sleep analysis, II: testing the assumptions of the two-process model of sleep regulation in normal and depressed subjects. Psychiatry Res. 1985;13:335–343.

67. Benson KL, King A, Gordon D, et al. Sleep patterns in borderline personality disorder. J Affect Disord. 1990;18:267–273.

68. Kraemer M, Kinney L. Sleep patterns in trauma victims with disturbed dreaming. Psychiatr J Univ Ottawa. 1988;13:12–16.

69. Douglass AB, Hays P, Pazderka F, et al. Florid refractory schizophrenias that turn out to be treatable variants of HLA-associated narcolepsy. J Nerv Ment Dis. 1991;179:12–18.

70. Haffmans PM, Hoencamp E, Knegtering HJ, et al. Sleep disturbance in schizophrenia. Br J Psychiatry. 1994;165:697–698.

71. Wirz-Justice A, Cajochen C, Nussbaaum P. A schizophrenic patient with an arrhythmic circadian rest-activity cycle. Psychiatry Res. 1997;73:83–90.

72. Benson KL, Zarcone VP. Sleep abnormalities in schizophrenia and other psychotic disorders. In: Oldham JM, Riba MB, eds. Review of Psychiatry. Vol 13. Washington, DC: American Psychiatric Press; 1994:677–705.

73. Ancoli-Israel S, Martin J, Jones DW, et al. Sleep disordered breathing and periodic limb movements in sleep in older patients with schizophrenia. Biol Psychiatry. 1999;45:1426–1432.

74. Nofzinger EA, van Kammen DP, Gilbertson MW, et al. Electroencephalographic sleep in clinically stable schizophrenic patients: two-weeks versus six-weeks neuroleptic free. Biol Psychiatry. 1993;33:829–835.

75. Adam K, Allen S, Carruthers-Jones I, et al. Mesoridazine and human sleep. Br J Clin Pharmacol. 1976;3:157–163.

76. Hartmann E, Cravens J. The effects of long term administration of psychotrophic drugs on human sleep, IV: the effects of chlorpromazine. Psychopharmacology (Berl). 1973;33:203–218.

77. Brannen JO, Jewett RE. Effects of selected phenothiazines on REM sleep in schizophrenics. Arch Gen Psychiatry. 1969;21:284–290.

78. Casey DE. Side effect profiles of new antipsychotic agents. J Clin Psychiatry. 1996;57(suppl 11):40–52.

79. Wetter TC, Lauer CJ, Gillich G, et al. The electroencephalographic sleep pattern in schizophrenic patients treated with clozapine or classical antipsychotic drugs. J Psychiatr Res. 1996;30:411–419.

98

Eating Disorders

Ruth M. Benca
Regina C. Casper

Anorexia nervosa and bulimia nervosa are classified as eating disorders and both are characterized by abnormalities in eating behavior as a result of fear of losing control and becoming overweight (Table 98–1). The pursuit of thinness in anorexia nervosa invariably leads to pathological weight loss and malnutrition, whereas in bulimia nervosa bouts of binge eating often followed by vomiting result in sometimes unpredictable metabolic and endocrine changes with large weight fluctuations within the normal range of body weight. Following eating binges, patients with bulimia attempt to prevent weight gain by vomiting, using diuretics or laxatives, restricting food intake, or exercising excessively. Hormone and metabolic disturbances are regularly associated with anorexia nervosa; their presence and severity are largely functions of the weight loss and nutritional deficiencies.[1]

Anorexia nervosa and bulimia nervosa occur almost exclusively in women, with female-to-male ratios of 20:1 for anorexia nervosa and 4:1 for bulimia nervosa. Anorexia nervosa typically occurs in early or middle adolescence, whereas bulimia nervosa has its onset in mid- to late adolescence or early adulthood. Bulimia nervosa is 5 to 10 times more common than anorexia nervosa.

Eating disorders are unusual in patients older than 40 years of age, and then they usually reflect a chronic condition. The current mortality rate for anorexia nervosa is about 5%, from either the disease itself or suicide. Suicidal ideation may occur at an increased rate in bulimia nervosa as well; the overall mortality rate is unknown, but it is lower than in anorexia nervosa and most often the result of metabolic or physiological disturbances secondary to vomiting.

There is an increased incidence of major depression in patients with bulimia nervosa, which has led to speculation that the two categories may be related biologically.[2] Although like patients with major depressive disorder,[3] those with anorexia and bulimia may show abnormally elevated cortisol secretion both at baseline[4, 5] and following administration of dexamethasone,[6–9] profound underweight has been shown to account for these changes in anorexia nervosa, and intermittent caloric restriction contributes to these changes in bulimia nervosa.[10, 11] A further biological link between eating disorders and depressive disorders is suggested by the fact that antidepressant drugs have been shown to be effective in the treatment of bulimia nervosa.[12, 13] In addition, patients with bipolar depression may present with hyperphagia, often accompanied by hypersomnia (see Chapter 96). All patients with significant eating abnormalities and sleep disturbance should, therefore, be evaluated for mood disorders.

SLEEP COMPLAINTS

Patients with anorexia nervosa rarely if ever complain of insomnia. Quite to the contrary, people with

---

Table 98–1. CRITERIA FOR EATING DISORDERS

Anorexia Nervosa

A. Refusal to maintain body weight at or above a minimally normal weight for age and height (e.g., weight loss leading to maintenance of body weight less than 85% of that expected; or failure to make expected weight gain during period of growth, leading to body weight less than 85% of that expected).

B. Intense fear of gaining weight or becoming fat, even though underweight.

C. Disturbance in the way in which one's body weight or shape is experienced, undue influence of body weight or shape on self-evaluation, or denial of the seriousness of the current low body weight.

D. In postmenarcheal females, amenorrhea, i.e., the absence of at least three consecutive menstrual cycles. (A woman is considered to have amenorrhea if her periods occur only following hormone, e.g., estrogen, administration.)

Bulimia Nervosa

A. Recurrent episodes of binge eating. An episode of binge eating is characterized by both of the following:
   1. Eating, in a discrete period of time (e.g., within any 2-h period), an amount of food that is definitely larger than most people would eat during a similar period of time and under similar circumstances.
   2. A sense of lack of control over eating during the episode (e.g., a feeling that one cannot stop eating or control what or how much one is eating)

B. Recurrent inappropriate compensatory behavior in order to prevent weight gain, such as self-induced vomiting; misuse of laxatives, diuretics, enemas, or other medications; fasting; or excessive exercise.

C. The binge eating and inappropriate compensatory behaviors both occur, on average, at least twice a week for 3 months.

D. Self-evaluation is unduly influenced by body shape and weight.

E. The disturbance does not occur exclusively during episodes of anorexia nervosa.

Modified with permission from the *Diagnostic and Statistical Manual of Mental Disorders, Fourth Edition.* Copyright 1994 American Psychiatric Association.

anorexia nervosa tend to use the time gained by their reduced need for sleep for activities and exercise. Insomnia and decreased amounts of sleep are common, as long as weight is subnormal.[14] People with bulimia nervosa frequently binge into or throughout the night and tend to fall asleep after midnight, often sleeping through the morning hours. Increased amounts of sleep may occur following eating binges.

Bulimia nervosa patients anecdotally report sleepwalking and binge eating, occasionally even shopping for food during the night after having fallen asleep with partial recollection of the episode. Sometimes the only evidence of the behavior is the presence of store receipts or partially eaten food the next morning. Guirguis[15] reported a case of a 32-year-old woman who went on uncontrollable nightly eating binges in a dream-like state. Gupta[16] found 11 (34%) of 32 bulimia nervosa patients to have experienced sleep-related eating; this behavior was reported to be similar to that in other parasomnias in that patients often did not awaken completely while eating nor did they have recall of the behavior the next morning. A majority of the subjects reported sleepwalking as children; episodes of sleep-talking and recurrent bruxism were reported less frequently. Parasomnias have not been described in restricting anorexia nervosa. Clinical experience and published reports suggest that parasomnias deserve to be investigated more systematically in bulimia nervosa or in conditions associated with binge eating (see Sleep-Related Eating Disorders later).

POLYSOMNOGRAPHIC FINDINGS

Polysomnographic studies have been performed on patients with eating disorders to define the sleep disturbances and to determine whether eating disorders and major depression share biological markers, such as sleep electroencephalogram (EEG) alterations. As discussed in Chapter 96, sleep in depression is characterized by sleep continuity disruption, decreased slow-wave sleep (SWS) amounts, and rapid eye movement (REM) abnormalities consistent with increased REM sleep drive. A number of studies have been performed on patients with anorexia nervosa, bulimia nervosa, and mixed eating disorders. In general, patients with bulimia nervosa are not easily distinguishable from age-matched controls.[17–21] Anorexia nervosa patients have been found to have significant decrements in sleep efficiency, total sleep time, or SWS amounts, singly or in combination.[18–23] Reduced REM latency, the sleep abnormality most specific for depression, was reported in several studies.[22, 24, 25] Paradoxically, REM density was reduced in comparison with controls in two studies.[4, 22]

The failure to demonstrate consistent sleep abnormalities in patients with eating disorders does not necessarily imply that they do not share common features with those having depression. In four studies,[17, 23, 25, 26] age-matched groups with major depression were included, and these groups with depression generally failed to show robust differences in comparison with controls. Only one depressed group exhibited reduced REM latency,[25] three groups had disturbed sleep continuity,[17, 23, 25] and two groups showed increased REM density,[25, 26] but no other sleep abnormality was reported. Eating disorders groups were not significantly different from the groups with depression, except for a decrease in REM density[17, 26] or increase in nocturnal awakenings.[23]

Because some with eating disorders showed reduced REM sleep latency, investigators have questioned whether short REM latency in a patient with an eating disorder might signify the presence of concurrent depressive symptoms or a concomitant affective disorder. Indeed, Katz et al.[24] found a significant negative correlation between Hamilton depression ratings and REM latency in patients with eating disorders. A study by Walsh et al.[21] failed to find a similar association between Hamilton scores and REM latency; however, they did find that subgroups of patients with eating disorders who also qualified for a diagnosis of major depression tended to have shorter REM latency than those without major depression. On the other hand, two studies have failed to document reduced REM latency in eating disorders patients with depressive illness,[20, 26] although one study reported increased REM density in patients with depressive disorders and eating disorders.[20]

Although sleep studies have not reliably distinguished eating disorders groups from either controls or groups of depressed patients, this does not necessarily mean that sleep is unaffected in patients with eating disorders. The major problem with most recent studies on sleep in eating disorders has been the failure to consider those factors that specifically affect sleep patterns in these patients, including age, gender, weight loss, and nutritional status.

Age

One explanation for the failure to find many significant abnormalities in either eating disorders or depressive groups is that the groups studied may have been too young to exhibit the full spectrum of sleep abnormalities; in all cases mean group ages were between 20 and 30 years old. As discussed in Chapter 96, age has profound effects on sleep in depression. Younger patient groups often fail to show the characteristic sleep abnormalities. The lack of studies of patient groups with mean ages over 30 years makes it difficult to determine whether patients with eating disorders have sleep abnormalities in common with those with depression and difficult to define the effects of age on sleep in eating disorders. On the other hand, the early age at onset, especially for anorexia nervosa, suggests that if patients beyond the age of 30 years are being studied, either they have been chronically ill for many years and thus would represent selective treatment-resistant cases, or, if their symptoms have developed in their late 20s, they would be considered atypical cases. Thus, it may not be possible to explore the effects of age on sleep in eating disorders patients, nor may the potential "depressive" effects of eating disorders on sleep become fully expressed, if most treatment-responsive patients have long had remission by the age at which sleep abnormalities become most pronounced.

Gender

The effects of gender on sleep in eating disorders are impossible to determine, because too few patients studied were male. A previous study of the effects of gender on sleep in depression has shown that SWS amounts declined less significantly with age in females than in males, although other parameters did not appear to be affected.[27]

Weight Loss

In addition to the possible effects of depression on sleep in eating disorders, the degree of weight loss may strongly influence sleep patterns. Some of the first data on the effects of starvation on sleep were obtained from animal studies. Food deprivation caused severe insomnia and significantly increased activity in rats.[28, 29] Early clinical studies suggested that weight loss was responsible for insomnia during acute starvation and strongly associated with insomnia in populations with psychiatric illness, whereas hypersomnia was more commonly found during periods of significant weight gain.[14, 30] Several studies have been performed to assess the effects of weight gain on sleep in anorexia nervosa. During periods of severely reduced weight, patients with anorexia reported of insomnia and reduced amounts of total sleep; following treatment and significant weight gain, patients reported increased amounts of sleep and decreased wakefulness during sleep hours.[14] Similar results were obtained in polygraphic studies of patients with anorexia, with significant increases in total sleep, SWS, and REM sleep amounts following weight gain.[31, 32] In other studies, Levy et al. found significant positive correlations between percentage of ideal body weight (IBW) and SWS amount in one study,[19] and between percentage of IBW and total sleep time and sleep efficiency in another.[20] Others have failed to confirm significant relationships between percentage of IBW and sleep parameters in eating disorders patients.[18, 26] Possible explanations for these discrepancies include the independent effects of drug treatment and psychotherapy in some of the earlier studies, and differences in correlations performed within individual patients over time vs. cross-sectional studies of patients.

Nutritional Status

The eating habits of patients with anorexia nervosa vary so markedly that the only common denominator is profoundly reduced caloric intake, generally between 400 to 800 kcal/d. However, the composition of the food differs widely, from consumption of only apricot juice for weeks or months, to lettuce and rice cakes or boiled eggs and tea. On the other hand, for patients with bulimia nervosa the amount of calories consumed during one binge can fluctuate from a few hundred to several thousand, depending upon binge frequency, and can amount to a maximum of 10,000 to 30,000 kcal/d. Some patients with bulimia prefer high fat foods such as ice cream or chocolate cake, whereas others may binge on meat or bread. Similarly, vomiting may occur immediately following a binge or at variable intervals thereafter, resulting in considerable differences in absorption. Thus, in order to determine whether nutritional factors influence sleep, it is necessary to obtain detailed dietary records or to stabilize the patient's condition on a controlled diet under supervision.

Virtually none of the recent studies of sleep in eating disorders reported the eating behavior, body weight changes, or caloric intake during the week preceding sleep studies; any of these factors may influence sleep patterns. Acute fasting in humans, rats, and birds has been shown to increase SWS amounts.[33–37] With prolonged starvation resulting in increased protein catabolism, wake time increased, and both SWS and REM sleep amounts were significantly reduced.[34, 36]

Conversely, ingestion of food may lead to sleepiness. Animal studies have shown that fat-containing food in the gastrointestinal tract causes drowsiness.[38]

A number of studies have assessed the effects of eating on sleepiness in normal human subjects. A high calorie, high carbohydrate noontime meal led to a prolonged duration of postprandial sleep in a group of healthy men.[39] Orr et al.[40] found that solid but not liquid meals led to decreased sleep latencies, but could not detect a difference in the soporific effects of high fat vs. high carbohydrate meals. Similarly, both high fat–low carbohydrate and low fat–high carbohydrate meals increased sleepiness and reduced sleep latency in a study by Wells and colleagues.[41] A previous study by Wells and Read found subjective sleepiness increased by both types of meals, but more so by high fat content.[42] It is not clear whether increased sleep following feeding is caused by specific food substances, endogenous peptides released in response to food, or the increased metabolic rate following eating. The sleep-promoting effects of the gastrointestinal peptide cholecystokinin (CCK), released in response to food intake, have been assessed in several studies. Direct administration of CCK to rats has been shown to have sleep-inducing effects in some studies,[43–45] and CCK caused drowsiness in humans.[46] Others studies, however, have failed to confirm hypnotic effects of CCK.[47–49] Normal subjects who had ingested high fat–low carbohydrate meals had higher plasma CCK levels and greater subjective sleepiness than those who had eaten low fat–high carbohydrate meals.[50] Geracioti and Liddle[51] found subnormal CCK levels postprandially in 14 women with bulimia nervosa, although fasting CCK plasma levels were similar in comparison with normal subjects. Bombesin, another gut-associated peptide released in response to feeding, has also shown sleep-promoting effects in rats.[52–54] Finally, the amino acid L-tryptophan, a precursor of serotonin, may have sleep-inducing effects, and bedtime snacks have been reported to have variable effects on sleep.[30] Typically, patients with anorexia nervosa maintain low fat, low carbohydrate, and low protein diets and thus are unlikely to benefit from any direct sleep-inducing effects from their food.

Sensitivity and Specificity of REM Latency

The polysomnographic findings from studies of patients with eating disorders were compared with those of groups of patients with affective disorders and normal controls of comparable ages using meta-analysis,[55] a statistical technique for combining data from different studies. Depending on whether eating disorders groups were compared with their own controls or with a larger pool of age-matched controls, they showed tendencies toward decreased total sleep and sleep efficiency and reduced REM latency. In comparison with those with affective disorders, they seemed to show less significant disruption of sleep continuity, and REM latency was indistinguishable (in controlled studies) or prolonged (for all studies combined). Of interest was the fact that although REM latency was not reduced in the studies of eating disorders patients compared with their own matched controls in the meta-analysis, REM latency appeared to be significantly reduced when compared with a larger pool of control data in the same age group. This discrepancy could be explained by the somewhat shorter-than-average REM latencies reported for control groups in the few studies of eating disorders. Because of the lack of robust findings in eating disorders patients in the age groups tested, it is generally not possible to use sleep markers to distinguish them reliably from normals or from those with depression. Thus, the issue as to whether REM latency is reduced in eating disorders, or whether short REM latency in patients with eating disorders represents a component of major depressive illness, has yet to be resolved.

CORRELATION OF SLEEP FINDINGS WITH OTHER MARKERS

The cholinergic REM induction test has been performed to assess the possibility of abnormal cholinergic regulation of REM sleep in eating disorders. People with depressive disorder tend to show abnormally rapid appearance of REM sleep in response to cholinomimetic agents (see Chapter 96). In tests of the responses of anorexia nervosa patients to the cholinergic REM sleep induction test (RIT), Sitaram et al.[56] found that a majority of patients with both anorexia nervosa and major depression showed more rapid REM sleep induction in response to arecoline. However, in later studies by Lauer et al.,[18, 26] no differences in anorexia nervosa patients were demonstrated in comparison with controls. Although an age-matched group with depression showed more rapid REM sleep onset following the RIT,[26] normal RIT responses were observed in patients with anorexia nervosa, including those with concomitant major depression.

A single study of cortisol responses and sleep in nondepressed bulimic patients found that although the group showed elevated baseline and post–dexamethasone suppression test (DST) cortisol levels, REM latency values were not reduced on average.[4] Furthermore, no significant correlation was found between reduced REM latency and DST nonsuppression.

TREATMENT

The treatment of an eating disorder is based upon a comprehensive assessment of the patient and the family. Treatment interventions vary and depend on the patient's age, premorbid functioning, duration of illness, severity of weight loss, the presence of coexisting psychiatric disorders or, in bulimia nervosa, the frequency of the binge eating–purging episodes.

Anorexia Nervosa

Hospitalization in specialty treatment programs is generally required for patients who have lost in excess of 25% of IBW or who have a body mass index (BMI = kg/m^2) of less than 15, as well as for patients who refuse to drink fluids, or patients who have been unsuccessful in gaining weight in supervised outpatient treatment. No medications currently exist to treat the resistance to weight gain or the anxiety and guilt associated with eating and the fear of becoming overweight in anorexia nervosa; food is the only effective antidote. Depending upon the co-morbid diagnosis, antidepressant or antianxiety drugs may be indicated. Sleeping medications are generally contraindicated because patients' sleep disturbances promptly improve with balanced nutrition sufficient for weight gain. Persistent sleep problems may indicate a depressive illness or unresolved emotional conflicts. The patient's reasons for her strong investment in the weight loss process need to be explored in psychotherapy. Similarly, the family's dysfunctional expectations and interaction pattern require attention through family treatment. Patients with restricting anorexia have been shown to share particular personality characteristics, including greater-than-normal tendencies toward perfectionism, self-control, inhibition, and conscientiousness, whereas those with bulimic anorexia nervosa tend to be more expressive and dramatic.[57] Treatment needs to take these personality differences into account. Treatment therefore occurs at several levels simultaneously: a supervised, clearly spelled-out nutritional regimen; regular body weight measurements to ensure age- and height-adequate weight gain; treatment of dysfunctional personality characteristics to bring about changes in attitude, beliefs, and self-concept; treatment of psychiatric symptoms through individual, family, and peer group therapy; and occasionally pharmacotherapy. The goal is to help the patient relinquish her excessive reliance on body weight for improving her self-esteem and to use food again as nourishment so that she can gain control over herself and her life and proceed in growth and development through age-appropriate ways.

Bulimia Nervosa

Bulimia nervosa is largely treated on an outpatient basis, unless the bulimic behavior significantly disrupts work and psychosocial functioning or results in life-threatening medical symptoms or suicidality. Cognitive-behavioral methods and nutritional education are used first to assist the patient in organizing and controlling her eating behavior. In addition, antidepressant drugs, especially monoamine oxidase inhibitors (such as phenelzine)[57a] and selective serotonin reuptake inhibitors (such as fluoxetine),[57b] have been shown to reduce the urge to eat. Because in bulimia nervosa emotional distress or uncontrollable feelings trigger eating binges, individual, family, and group psychotherapy are generally necessary to explore dysfunctional interpersonal relationships or to treat a coexisting psychiatric disorder. Maturational issues germane to adolescence or young adulthood—such as lack of a sense of identity, a poor self-concept, and struggle with self-definition or separation-autonomy issues—are usually in the foreground. Thus, in bulimia nervosa, character and family issues need to be addressed so that eating can again serve a nutritional function instead of controlling emotions.

Sleep abnormalities usually resolve with return to more normal weight and eating behaviors. Persistent sleep disturbance may indicate the need for further assessment of possible psychiatric or medical causes of insomnia, including primary sleep disorders. Patients with bulimia nervosa have increased rates of alcoholism and substance abuse disorders, as well as depression, all of which can significantly affect sleep.[58, 59]

SLEEP-RELATED EATING DISORDERS

Episodes of uncontrolled sleep-related eating have been described in association with a variety of other primary sleep and psychiatric disorders, including sleepwalking, periodic limb movements, narcolepsy, obstructive sleep apnea, triazolam abuse, nicotine or alcohol abstinence, mood disorders, and anxiety disorders.[60–63a] Sleepwalking and bulimia nervosa are the most common primary diagnoses in these patients,[64] who tend to be female and overweight. The disorder usually begins in adulthood and is characterized by eating episodes which occur after sleep onset. Patients will often ingest large amounts of high calorie foods on a nightly basis, which leads to weight gain. Sometimes patients will consume foods that they would normally not eat while awake. They usually have little or no memory of the episode the next day, and they are frequently sloppy or careless during the binges, which

can result in injuries (e.g., burns or cuts incurred while preparing food). In contrast to bulimia nervosa, patients with nocturnal eating syndrome never purge, although they may restrict intake or exercise during the day.

Sleep-related eating differs from nocturnal eating syndrome, which was originally described as a combination of insomnia and nocturnal binge eating with morning anorexia.[65] Patients with nocturnal eating syndrome also have recurrent awakenings from sleep associated with inability to get back to sleep without eating.[66] Patients are fully awake during these episodes and able to remember them the next day. As in the case of the sleep-related eating disorders described above, these patients appear to have increased rates of other primary psychiatric and sleep disorders, although the presence of primary sleep disorders or eating disorders are exclusionary criteria for the diagnosis.[62, 67] The patients are also frequently overweight and female, with onset of the disorder in adulthood.

It is likely that these categories of nocturnal eating syndrome and sleep-related eating disorder overlap, and both are clearly heterogeneous. In the various published series of patients with these disorders, careful clinical evaluation has suggested that somnambulism, periodic movements in sleep, and eating disorders are relatively common in this population.[63, 64] Because the disorders do not clearly fit the diagnostic criteria for primary eating disorders, it has been argued that they should be considered as a separate diagnostic entity from other sleep or eating disorders. Polygraphic studies have suggested that 50 to 70% of patients with sleep-related eating disorders show evidence of SWS parasomnias.[61, 63] In addition, cases of sleep apnea, periodic movements in sleep, and narcolepsy were also documented in these reports. No consistent abnormalities in overall sleep architecture have otherwise been described.

Successful treatment of these disorders has been reported with clonazepam, dopaminergic agents, or opiates, individually or severally, for patients with sleepwalking or periodic limb movement disorders. Antidepressants such as fluoxetine or trazodone may also be helpful to some patients, particularly those with underlying mood disorders. Disappointingly, behavioral treatments have been largely unsuccessful in treating sleep-related eating disorders.

CONCLUSION

The eating disorders, anorexia nervosa and bulimia nervosa, are most prevalent during adolescence and young adulthood, respectively—an age range in which sleep tends to be least disturbed by psychiatric illness. Nevertheless, sleep disturbances are not uncommon in patients with anorexia nervosa or bulimia nervosa, and sleep abnormalities have been documented. Virtually all polysomnographic studies in eating disorders performed from the mid-1980s to the late 1990s focused on the question of whether sleep changes indicate the presence of a coexisting affective illness.[68, 69] This question is difficult to answer, at best, in part because young patients, even if they are depressed, lack significant sleep abnormalities. Sleep-related eating disorders were increasingly recognized throughout the 1990s, and further work will be required to define these syndromes more clearly, as well as develop effective treatments for them.

However, the study of sleep and eating disorders may yield important clues about the effects of various physiological parameters on human sleep. Patients with anorexia nervosa can provide an opportunity to learn about the effects of chronic starvation, extreme weight loss, or undernutrition on sleep. In addition, the impact of hypercaloric intake on sleep in previously starving subjects, as well as the disturbed sleep patterns and sleep-related behaviors of bulimia nervosa patients, requires further study.

References

1. Casper RC, Kirschner B, Sandstead HH, et al. An evaluation of trace metals, vitamins, and taste function in anorexia nervosa. Am J Clin Nutr. 1980;33:1801–1808.
2. Levy AB, Dixon KN, Stern SL. How are depression and bulimia related? Am J Psychiatry. 1989;146:162–169.
3. Carroll BJ, Feinberg M, Greden JF, et al. A specific laboratory test for the diagnosis of melancholia. Standardization, validation, and clinical utility. Arch Gen Psychiatry. 1981;38:15–22.
4. Byrne B, Nino-Murcia G, Gaddy JR, et al. Sleep patterns and dexamethasone suppression in nondepressed bulimics. Biol Psychiatry. 1990;27:454–456.
5. Casper RC, Pandy GN, Jaspan JB, et al. Hormone and metabolite plasma levels after oral glucose in bulimia and healthy controls. Biol Psychiatry. 1988;24:663–674.
6. Gwirtsman HE, Roy-Byrne P, Yager J, et al. Neuroendocrine abnormalities in bulimia. Am J Psychiatry. 1983;140:559–563.
7. Hudson JI, Pope HG Jr, Jonas JM, et al. Hypothalamic-pituitary-adrenal-axis hyperactivity in bulimia. Psychiatry Res. 1983;8:111–117.
8. Levy AB, Dixon KN. DST in bulimia without endogenous depression. Biol Psychiatry. 1987;22:783–786.
9. Walsh BT, Katz JL, Levin J, et al. Adrenal activity in anorexia nervosa. Psychosom Med. 1978;40:499–506.
10. Casper RC, Chatterton RT Jr, Davis JM. Alterations in serum cortisol and its binding characteristics in anorexia nervosa. J Clin Endocrinol Metab. 1979;49:406–411.
11. Fichter MM, Pirke KM, Holsboer F. Weight loss causes neuroendocrine disturbances: experimental study in healthy starving subjects. Psychiatry Res. 1986;17:61–72.
12. Walsh BT, Stewart JW, Roose SP, et al. A double-blind trial of phenelzine in bulimia. J Psychiatr Res. 1985;19:485–489.
13. Pope HG Jr, Hudson JI, Jonas JM, et al. Bulimia treated with imipramine: a placebo-controlled, double-blind study. Am J Psychiatry. 1983;140:554–558.
14. Crisp AH, Stonehill E, eds. Sleep, Nutrition and Mood. London, England: John Wiley & Sons; 1971.
15. Guirguis WR. Sleepwalking as a symptom of bulimia. Br Med J. 1986;293:587–588.
16. Gupta MA. Sleep-related eating in bulimia nervosa—an underreported parasomnia disorder. Sleep Res. 1991;20:182.
17. Hudson JI, Pope HG Jr, Jonas JM, et al. Sleep EEG in bulimia. Biol Psychiatry. 1987;22:820–828.
18. Lauer CJ, Zulley J, Krieg J, et al. M. EEG sleep and the cholinergic REM induction test in anorexic and bulimic patients. Psychiatry Res. 1988;26:171–181.
19. Levy AB, Dixon KN, Schmidt H. REM and delta sleep in anorexia nervosa and bulimia. Psychiatry Res. 1987;20:189–197.
20. Levy AB, Dixon KN, Schmidt H. Sleep architecture in anorexia nervosa and bulimia. Biol Psychiatry. 1988;23:99–101.
21. Walsh BT, Goetz RR, Roose SP, et al. EEG-monitored sleep in anorexia nervosa and bulimia. Biol Psychiatry. 1985;20:947–956.
22. Neil JF, Merikangas JR, Foster FG, et al. Waking and all-night sleep EEG's in anorexia nervosa. Clin Electroencephalogr. 1980;11:9–15.
23. Delvenne V, Kerkhofs M, Appelboom Fondu J, et al. Sleep polygraphic variables in anorexia nervosa and depression: a comparative study in adolescents. J Affect Disord. 1992;25:167–172.
24. Katz JL, Kuperberg A, Pollack CP, et al. Is there a relationship between eating disorder and affective disorder? New evidence from sleep recordings. Am J Psychiatry. 1984;141:753–759.
25. Waller DA, Hardy BW, Pole R, et al. Sleep EEG in bulimic, depressed, and normal subjects. Biol Psychiatry. 1989;25:661–664.
26. Lauer CJ, Krieg J-C, Riemann D, et al. A polysomnographic study in young psychiatric inpatients: major depression, anorexia nervosa, bulimia nervosa. J Affect Disord. 1990;18:235–245.
27. Reynolds CF III, Kupfer DJ, Thase ME, et al. Sleep, gender and depression: an analysis of gender effects on the electroencephalographic sleep of 302 depressed outpatients. Biol Psychiatry. 1990;28:673–684.
28. Jacobs BL, McGinty DJ. Effects of food deprivation on sleep and wakefulness in the rat. Exp Neurol. 1971;30:212–222.
29. Treichler FR, Hall JF. The relationship between deprivation, weight loss and several measures of activity. J Compr Physiol Psychol. 1962;55:348–349.
30. Evans FJ. Sleep, eating, and weight disorders. In: Richard K, ed. Eating and Weight Disorders. New York, NY: Springer; 1983:147–178.
31. Crisp AH, Stonehill E, Fenton GW. The relationship between sleep, nutrition and mood: a study of patients with anorexia nervosa. Postgrad Med J. 1971;47:207–213.
32. Lacey JH, Crisp AH, Kalucy RS, et al. Weight gain and the sleeping electroencephalogram: study of 10 patients with anorexia nervosa. Br Med J. 1975;6:556–558.
33. MacFadyen UM, Oswald I, Lewis SA. Starvation and human slow-wave sleep. J Appl Physiol. 1973;35:391–394.
34. Dewasmes G, Cohen-Adad F, Koubi H, et al. Sleep changes in long-term fasting geese in relation to lipid and protein metabolism. Am J Physiol. 1984;247(4 pt 2):R663–671.
35. Dewasmes G, Buchet C, Geloen A, et al. Sleep changes in emperor penguins during fasting. Am J Physiol. 1989;256:R476–R480.
36. Dewasmes G, Duchamp C, Minaire Y. Sleep changes in fasting rats. Physiol Behav. 1989;46:179–184.
37. Karacan I, Rosenbloom AL, Londono JH, et al. The effect of acute fasting on sleep and the sleep-growth hormone response. Psychosomatics. 1973;14:33–37.
38. Fara JW, Rubinstein EH, Sonnenschein RR. Visceral and behavioral responses to intraduodenal fat. Science. 1969;166:110–111.
39. Zammit GK, Kolevzon A, Fauci M, et al. Postprandial sleep in healthy men. Sleep. 1995;18:229–231.
40. Orr WC, Shadid G, Harnish MJ, et al. Meal composition and its effect on postprandial sleepiness. Physiol Behav. 1997;62:709–712.
41. Wells AS, Read NW, Idzikowski C, et al. Effects of meals on objective and subjective measures of daytime sleepiness. J Appl Physiol. 1998;84:507–515.
42. Wells AS, Read NW. Influences of fat, energy, and time of day on mood and performance. Physiol Behav. 1996;59:1069–1076.
43. Antin J, Gibbs J, Holt J, et al. Cholecystokinin elicits the complete behavioral sequence of satiety in rats. J Comp Physiol Psychol. 1975;89:784–790.
44. Kapas L, Obal FJ, Alföldi P, et al. Effects of nocturnal intraperitoneal administration of cholecystokinin in rats: simultaneous increase in sleep, increase in EEG slow-wave activity, reduction of motor activity, suppression of eating, and decrease in brain temperature. Brain Res. 1988;438:155–164.
45. Mansbach RS, Lorenz DN. Cholecystokinin (CCK-8) elicits prandial sleep in rats. Physiol Behav. 1983;30:179–183.
46. Stacher G, Bauer H, Steinringer H. Cholecystokinin decreases appetite and activation evoked by stimuli arising from the preparation of a meal in man. Physiol Behav. 1979;23:325–331.
47. Rojas-Ramirez JA, Crawley JN, Mendelson WB. Electroencephalographic analysis of the sleep-inducing actions of cholecystokinin. Neuropeptides. 1982;3:129–138.
48. Riou F, Cespuglio R, Jouvet M. Endogenous peptides and sleep in

the rat, I: peptides decreasing paradoxical sleep. Neuropeptides. 1982;2:243–254.

49. De Saint Hilaire-Kafi Z, Depoortere H, Nicolaidis S. Does cholecystokinin induce physiological satiety and sleep? Brain Res. 1989;488:304–310.

50. Wells AS, Read NW, Uvnas-Moberg K, et al. Influences of fat and carbohydrate on postprandial sleepiness, mood, and hormones. Physiol Behav. 1997;61:679–686.

51. Geracioti TD Jr, Liddle RA. Impaired cholecystokinin secretion in bulimia nervosa. N Engl J Med. 1988;319:683–688.

52. Gibbs J, Fauser DJ, Rowe EA, et al. Bombesin suppresses feeding in rats. Nature. 1979;282:208–210.

53. Gibbs J, Smith GP. Satiety: the roles of peptides from the stomach and the intestine. Fed Proc. 1986;45:1391–1395.

54. De Saint Hilaire-Kafi Z, Gibbs J, Nicolaidis S. Satiety and sleep: the effects of bombesin. Brain Res. 1989;478:152–155.

55. Benca RM, Obermeyer WH, Thisted RA, et al. Sleep and psychiatric disorders: a meta-analysis. Arch Gen Psychiatry. 1992; 49:651–668.

56. Sitaram N, Gillin JC, Bunney WEJ. Cholinergic and catecholaminergic receptor sensitivity in affective illness: strategy and theory. In: Post RM, Ballenger JC, eds. Neurobiology of Mood Disorders. Baltimore, Md: Williams & Wilkins; 1984:629–651.

57. Casper RC, Hedeker D, McClough JF. Personality dimensions in eating disorders and their relevance for subtyping. J Am Acad Child Adolesc Psychiatry. 1992;31:830–840.

57a. Walsh BT, Wilson GT, Loeb KL, et al. Medication and psychotherapy in the treatment of bulimia nervosa. Am J Psychiatry. 1997;154:523–531.

57b. Fluoxetine Bulimia Nervosa Collaborative Study Group. Fluoxetine in the treatment of bulimia nervosa. A multicenter, placebo-controlled, double-blind trial. Arch Gen Psychiatry. 1992;49:139–147.

58. Hatsukami D, Eckert E, Mitchell JE, et al. Affective disorder and substance abuse in women with bulimia. Psychol Med. 1984;14:701–704.

59. Lacey JH, Moureli E. Bulimic alcoholics: some features of a clinical sub-group. Br J Addict. 1986;81:389–393.

60. Schenck CH, Hurwitz TD, O'Connor KA, et al. Additional categories of sleep-related eating disorders and the current status of treatment. Sleep. 1993;16:457–466.

61. Schenck CH, Hurwitz TD, Bundlie SR, et al. Sleep-related eating disorders: polysomnographic correlates of a heterogeneous syndrome distinct from daytime eating disorders. Sleep. 1991;14:419–431.

62. Manni R, Ratti MT, Tartara A. Nocturnal eating: prevalence and features in 120 insomniac referrals. Sleep. 1997;20:734–738.

63. Winkelman JW. Clinical and polysomnographic features of sleep-related eating disorder. J Clin Psychiatry. 1998;59:14–19.

63a. Winkelman JW, Herzog DB, Fara M. The prevalence of sleep-related eating disorder in the psychiatric and non-psychiatric populations. Psychol Med. 1999;29:1461–1466.

64. Schenck CH, Mahowald MW. Review of nocturnal sleep-related eating disorders. Int J Eat Disord. 1994;15:343–356.

65. Stunkard AJ, Grace WJ, Wolff HG. The night-eating syndrome: a pattern of food intake among certain obese patients. Am J Med. 1955;19:78–86.

66. Diagnostic Classification Steering Committee. The International Classification of Sleep Disorders: Diagnostic and Coding Manual. Rochester, Minn: American Sleep Disorders Association; 1990.

67. Spaggiari MC, Granella F, Parrino L, et al. Nocturnal eating syndrome in adults. Sleep. 1994;17:339–344.

68. Strober M, Katz JL. Do eating disorders and affective disorders share a common etiology? A dissenting opinion. Int J Eat Disord. 1987;6:171–180.

69. Casper RC. The dilemma of homonymous symptoms for evaluating comorbidity between affective disorders and eating disorders. In: Maser JD, Cloninger CR, eds. Comorbidity of Mood and Anxiety Disorders. Washington, DC: American Psychiatric Press, 1990:253–269.

99

Medication and Substance Abuse

J. Christian Gillin
Sean P. A. Drummond

Psychoactive substances are widely used in all cultures. Many of these substances are used according to social or medical norms. These include alcohol, sedatives, hypnotics, anxiolytics, caffeine, tobacco, stimulants (such as prescription amphetamines for narcolepsy), and opioids (for medical analgesia). But psychoactive substances can also be abused or misused. In the United States, 18% of the population experiences a substance abuse disorder during their lifetime. About 20% of the patients in general medical facilities and about 35% of patients in general psychiatric units present with substance abuse disorders.

Nearly all psychoactive substances affect the sleep-wake cycle, for better or worse. For this reason, sleep disorders clinicians should routinely assess substance use and abuse in their patients, including prescription and over-the-counter drugs, recreational drugs, tobacco and caffeine, health foods, steroids or body-building aids, and botanical and natural substances (such as melatonin, valerian, or Saint John's Wort). In this chapter, we focus primarily on substances of abuse and dependence.

The terms used to describe psychoactive substances are often misleading, controversial, or arbitrary. The words *addiction* and *drug abuse*, for example, have been used extensively to condemn any drug with withdrawal symptoms. These drugs include methadone, amphetamine, sleeping pills, and anxiolytics. On the other hand, considerable scientific and clinical experience supports their value in the treatment of medical illnesses. For example, benzodiazepines are valuable in the long-term clinical management of generalized anxiety disorder or chronic insomnia; amphetamines can be useful to treat attention deficit disorder or narcolepsy; methadone is used in the management of heroin abuse. For these reasons, the word *addiction* is used less and less in the scientific literature. Table 99–1 defines some of the terms used to describe effects of psychoactive substances.

Substance-related disorders are divided into two groups according to the *Diagnostic and Statistical Manual of Mental Disorders, Fourth Edition* (DSM-IV)[1]: (1) substance use disorders (substance dependence, substance abuse); and (2) substance-induced disorders (including substance intoxication, substance withdrawal, and substance-induced sleep disorder). The nature of the disorder is usually a function of the dose and duration of substance use, the pharmacological characteristics of the substance, and idiosyncratic nature of the user.

Substance abuse is defined as recurrent and significant adverse consequences related to repeated use of the substance (Table 99–2). These problems include failure to meet obligations, hazardous behaviors, legal problems, and other persistent problems.

Substance dependence is associated with repeated self-administered use of the substance despite significant substance-related problems (Table 99–3). It is usually characterized by drug craving, significant time spent

---

Table 99–1. COMMONLY USED TERMS RELATED TO DRUGS OF ABUSE AND DEPENDENCE

Intoxication: A reversible substance-specific syndrome of maladaptive behavior or psychological changes associated with the recent exposure of a drug acting on the central nervous system. Significant changes may include belligerence, mood lability, cognitive impairment, and poor judgment (e.g., hallucinations associated with lysergic acid diethylamide [LSD] or drunkenness with alcohol).

Tolerance: Following repeated exposure to a drug, a given dose of the drug produces a reduced effect or, conversely, higher doses are needed to induce the effects previously induced by the initial dose (e.g., increased doses of morphine may be needed to control severe pain over a period of time).

Cross-Tolerance and Cross-Dependence: The ability of one drug to suppress manifestations of dependence produced by another drug and to maintain the physical dependence (e.g., between alcohol and barbiturates or benzodiazepines).

Withdrawal: New physical and psychological manifestations following abrupt cessation of a dependence-producing drug (e.g., development of panic disorder during withdrawal from a benzodiazepine hypnotic in a patient without a history of panic disorder).

Relapse: The recurrence of the original condition from which the patient suffered on discontinuing an effective medical treatment (e.g., reemergence of mania after cessation of a mood stabilizer).

Rebound: The exaggerated expression of the original condition sometimes experienced by patients during immediate cessation of an effective treatment (e.g., emergence of insomnia that is worse than it was before treatment when discontinuing a short-acting benzodiazepine hypnotic).

Table 99-2. DSM-IV CRITERIA FOR SUBSTANCE ABUSE

A. A maladaptive pattern of substance use, leading to clinically significant impairment or distress, as manifested by one (or more) of the following, occurring within a 12-month period:
  (1) Recurrent substance use resulting in a failure to fulfill major role obligations at work, school, or home (e.g., repeated absences or poor work performance related to substance use; substance-related absences, suspensions, or expulsions from school; neglect of children or household)
  (2) Recurrent substance use in situations in which it is physically hazardous (e.g., driving an automobile or operating a machine when impaired by the substance use)
  (3) Recurrent substance-related legal problems (e.g., arrests for substance-related disorderly conduct)
  (4) Continued substance use despite having persistent or recurrent social or interpersonal problems caused or exacerbated by the effects of the substance (e.g., arguments with spouse about consequences of intoxication, physical fights)
B. The symptoms have never met the criteria for Substance Dependence for this class of substance.

Reprinted with permission from the *Diagnostic and Statistical Manual of Mental Disorders, Fourth Edition.* Copyright 1994 American Psychiatric Association.
DSM-IV, *Diagnostic and Statistical Manual of Mental Disorders, Fourth Edition.*

---

in substance procurement, compulsive substance use, pharmacological tolerance, and withdrawal symptoms upon discontinuation. As implied earlier, substance dependence should not be equated with withdrawal symptoms, which are not necessarily associated with drug-seeking behavior. Because tolerance and withdrawal are often associated with increased risk of immediate medical problems and relapse, the diagnosis of the substance dependence should include the specifier *with physiological dependence* or *without physiological dependence.* Furthermore, four remission specifiers can be applied if none of the criteria for substance dependence or abuse have been present for at least 1 month: *early full remission* (less than 12 months), *early partial remission* (one or more criteria for dependence or abuse have been met but not the full criteria), *sustained full remission* (none of the criteria have been met for 12 months or longer), and *sustained partial remission* (one or more criteria have been met but not full criteria for dependence or abuse for 12 months or longer). The remission specifiers are important not only because relapse is most likely during the 1st year of abstinence but also because many physiological and psychological signs and symptoms persist for long periods of time. For example, sleep disturbances can persist for months to years despite continued sobriety from alcohol.

The clinical states associated with different classes of substances are shown in Table 99-4. According to the DSM-IV criteria, substance-induced mental disorders include substance-induced delirium, dementia, persisting amnesia disorder, psychotic disorder, mood disorder, anxiety disorder, and sexual dysfunction. Of particular importance to sleep researchers and clinicians, sleep disorders are commonly associated with alcohol, stimulants (amphetamine, cocaine, methylphenidate), opioids, and sedative-hypnotics during both intoxication and withdrawal. In addition, caffeine can produce

insomnia during intoxication, whereas nicotine is associated with insomnia typically during withdrawal. It should be noted that most of these substances produce a variety of mental, psychological, and physiological disorders, including delirium, psychosis, mood disorder, anxiety disorder, or sexual dysfunction.

The DSM-IV diagnostic criteria for substance-induced sleep disorders are presented in Table 99-5. The diagnosis requires that the sleep disorder be sufficiently severe to warrant special attention and cause significant distress or impairment. Specific subtypes include alcohol, amphetamines, caffeine, and opioids. The disorder can manifest as insomnia, hypersomnia, parasomnia, or mixed type.

GENERAL CONSIDERATIONS IN THE CLINICAL MANAGEMENT OF SUBSTANCE USE IN CLINICAL SLEEP DISORDERS

During the evaluation of patients who use psychoactive substances, the clinician should remember that their use, abuse, and misuse are multifaceted and mul-

Table 99-3. DSM-IV CRITERIA FOR SUBSTANCE DEPENDENCE

A maladaptive pattern of substance use, leading to clinically significant impairment or distress, as manifested by three (or more) of the following, occurring at any time in the same 12-month period:
(1) Tolerance, as defined by either of the following:
  (a) A need for markedly increased amounts of the substance to achieve intoxication or desired effect
  (b) Markedly diminished effect with continued use of the same amount of the substance
(2) Withdrawal, as manifested by either of the following:
  (a) The characteristic withdrawal syndrome for the substance (refer to criteria A and B of the criteria sets for withdrawal from the specific substances)
  (b) The same (or a closely related) substance is taken to relieve or avoid withdrawal symptoms
(3) The substance is often taken in larger amounts or over a longer period than was intended
(4) There is a persistent desire of unsuccessful efforts to cut down or control substance use
(5) A great deal of time is spent in activities necessary to obtain the substance (e.g., visiting multiple doctors or driving long distances), use the substance (e.g., chain-smoking), or recover from its effects
(6) Important social, occupational, or recreational activities are given up or reduced because of substance use
(7) The substance use is continued despite knowledge of having a persistent or recurrent physical or psychological problem that is likely to have been caused or exacerbated by the substance (e.g., current cocaine use despite recognition of cocaine-induced depression or continued drinking recognition that an ulcer was made worse by alcohol consumption)
Specify if:
With physiological dependence: Evidence of tolerance or withdrawal (i.e., either Item 1 or 2 is present)
Without physiological dependence: No evidence of tolerance or withdrawal (i.e., neither Item 1 nor Item 2 is present)
Course specifiers (see text for definitions):
  Early Full Remission
  Early Partial Remission
  Sustained Full Remission
  Sustained Partial Remission
  On Agonist Therapy
  In a Controlled Environment

Reprinted with permission from the *Diagnostic and Statistical Manual of Mental Disorders, Fourth Edition.* Copyright 1994 American Psychiatric Association.
DSM-IV, *Diagnostic and Statistical Manual of Mental Disorders, Fourth Edition.*

Table 99–4. CLINICAL STATES ASSOCIATED WITH DIFFERENT CLASSES OF SUBSTANCES

	Delirium	Psychotic Disorder	Mood Disorder	Anxiety	Sexual Dysfunction	Sleep Disorder
Alcohol	I/W	I/W	I/W	I/W	I	I/W
Stimulants	I	I	I/W	I/W	I	I/W
Caffeine				I		I
Cannabis	I	I		I		
Hallucinogens	I	I	I	I		
Inhalants	I	I	I	I		
Nicotine						W
Opioids	I	I			I	I/W
Phencyclidine	I	I	I	I		
Sedatives/hypnotic	I	I/W	I/W	W	I	I/W

Reprinted with permission from the *Diagnostic and Statistical Manual of Mental Disorders, Fourth Edition.* Copyright 1994 American Psychiatric Association.
I, intoxication; W, withdrawal.

tidetermined in clinical practice.[2-5] The following general guidelines may be helpful.

Denial

Most substance abusing patients deny to themselves and others the amount, duration, and negative consequences of substance use. Clinicians must be proactive in determining whether and to what extent the patient uses these substances. Various laboratory tests are available to detect use of substances, including relatively simple, inexpensive measures that can be used routinely in the sleep laboratory, such as breathalyzers for measuring alcohol and carbon monoxide (which is associated with smoking). Urine toxicology screens may detect recent use, depending on the length of time the compound is found in the urine (Table 99–6). In order to ensure reliability of toxicology screening, a chain of accountability must be established from the collection of urine or blood to the final laboratory procedure. Following permission from the patient, it is helpful to review the situation with the patient's family or friends, not only to help with diagnosis but also to engage them in long-term clinical management. Issues of confidentiality are important in establishing a trust-

Table 99–5. DSM-IV DIAGNOSTIC CRITERIA FOR SUBSTANCE-INDUCED SLEEP DISORDER

A. A prominent disturbance in sleep that is sufficiently severe to warrant independent clinical attention.
B. There is evidence from the history, physical examination, or laboratory findings of either (1) or (2):
 (1) The symptoms in criterion A developed during, or within a month of, substance intoxication or withdrawal
 (2) Medication use is etiologically related to the sleep disturbance
C. The disturbance is not better accounted for by a Sleep Disorder that is not substance induced. Evidence that the symptoms are better accounted for by a Sleep Disorder that is not substance induced might include the following: the symptoms precede the onset of the substance abuse (or medication use), the symptoms persist for a substance period of time (e.g., a month) after cessation of acute withdrawal or severe intoxication, or are substantially in excess of what would be expected given the type or amount of substance used or the duration of use; or there is other evidence that suggests the existence of an independent non-substance-induced Sleep Disorder (e.g., history of recurrent non-substance-related episodes).
D. The disturbance does not occur exclusively during the course of a delirium.
E. The sleep disturbance causes clinically significant distress or impairment in social, occupational, or other important areas of functioning.
Specific Subtype: Alcohol, Amphetamine, Caffeine, Cocaine, Opioids, Sedative, Hypnotic, Anxiolytics, or Other.
Specify type:
Insomnia type: If the predominant sleep disturbance is insomnia.
Hypersomnia type: If the predominant sleep disturbance is Hypersomnia.
Parasomnia type: If the predominant sleep disturbance is Parasomnia.
Mixed type: If more than one sleep disturbance is present and none predominates.
Specify if:
With onset during intoxication
With onset during withdrawal

Reprinted with permission from the *Diagnostic and Statistical Manual of Mental Disorders, Fourth Edition.* Copyright 1994 American Psychiatric Association.
DSM-IV, *Diagnostic and Statistical Manual of Mental Disorders, Fourth Edition.*

Table 99–6. APPROXIMATE DURATION OF DETECTABILITY OF DRUGS IN URINE

Drugs	Retention Time
Amphetamine and Methamphetamine	48 h
Barbiturates	
Short-acting (secobarbital, pentobarbital)	24 h
Medium-acting (amobarbital, butabarbital)	48–72 h
Long-acting (phenobarbital)	2–3 wk
Benzodiazepines (at Therapeutic Doses)	3 d
Cannabinoids	
Occasional user	3 d
Daily user	10 d
Heavy daily user	3–4 wk
Cocaine	6–8 d
Cocaine metabolites	2–4 d
Ethyl Alcohol	7–12 h
Methaqualone	7 d
Narcotics	
Codeine	48 h
Heroin (as morphine)	36–72 h
Hydrocodone	24 h
Hydromorphone	48 h
Methadone	3 d
Morphine	48–72 h
Oxycodone	24 h
Propoxyphene	6–48 h

ing doctor-patient relationship and to protecting the patient's reputation.

Multiple Substance Use

Psychoactive substances are rarely used alone, even in the social setting. Smoking and alcohol or "uppers" (e.g., amphetamines, cocaine) and "downers" (e.g., barbiturates, benzodiazepines, alcohol) are often used together or sequentially.

Co-Morbidity and Dual Diagnosis

Misuse of psychoactive substances is often associated with other psychiatric or medical disorders. For example, about 30% of patients with major depression and about 60% of patients with bipolar disorder met rigorous diagnostic criteria for substance abuse. Likewise, many patients with substance abuse meet diagnostic criteria for psychiatric disorders, serious medical disorders or complications, or sleep disorders. Long-term goals must be set to manage all symptomatic disorders.

Long-Term Goals

The clinical management of patients with substance abuse or dependence disorders usually has as its goals (1) achieving a substance-free lifestyle, (2) maximizing multiple facets of life-functioning, and (3) preventing relapse.

Pharmacodynamic Properties of Drugs of Abuse

The direct effects of abused drugs are usually opposite to the effects displayed during withdrawal. For example, following nightly use of sedative hypnotics or alcohol, the withdrawal syndrome is usually characterized by physiological and psychological activation, ranging from insomnia to seizures. Likewise, following use of stimulants such as amphetamine or cocaine, the withdrawal syndrome is usually typified by sedation, lethargy, and dysphoria. Drugs with common mechanisms of action usually have similar direct effects, similar withdrawal syndromes, and cross-tolerance. The mechanisms involved in the acute and chronic effects, as well as the withdrawal syndromes, of drugs of abuse are complicated and not fully understood.[6] Nevertheless, as a simplification, alcohol, benzodiazepines, and barbiturates all appear to enhance neurotransmission of gamma-aminobutyric acid (GABA), an inhibitory neurotransmitter in the central nervous system (CNS). This concept may help explain the similarities of their effects.

Pharmacokinetic Properties of Drugs of Abuse

The time of day a drug of abuse is taken, its duration of action, and the dosage largely determine how sleep and wakefulness will be affected, not only during initial effects but during withdrawal. For example, short-acting sedatives, such as alcohol, short half-life benzodiazepines, and, possibly, nicotine promote sleep when administered at bedtime but, unlike long-acting sedatives, may result in early morning awakening as the subject enters withdrawal at the end of the night. Many people, and not just drug abusers, take all three before going to bed. As will be described later, the addition of coffee taken after dinner may potentiate the stimulating withdrawal effects of alcohol, nicotine, or a short-acting sedative taken before lights out, again increasing early morning awakening.

Other drug interactions may also be clinically important. Some drugs, for example, have additive or synergistic effects on the CNS, such as the combination of benzodiazepines, alcohol, and opioids. Some drugs affect absorption. For example, antacids reduce plasma concentrations of benzodiazepines. Drugs may speed or slow the metabolism of other drugs, especially by affecting the cytochrome P-450 system, a collection of at least 30 hepatic isoenzymes responsible for the oxidative metabolism of many endogenous and exogenous compounds.[4] For example, benzodiazepine plasma concentrations can be increased by valproic acid, selective serotonin reuptake inhibitors (such as fluoxetine), erythromycin, nefazodone, and cimetidine, all of which inhibit hepatic P-450 enzymes, which metabolize benzodiazepines. In contrast, carbamazepine lowers benzodiazepine concentrations by inducing P-450 enzymes. Other drugs of abuse that are metabolized by the P-450 system include the opioids codeine, oxycodone, pentazocine, and methadone. Whether or not these drug interactions are clinically significant in substance abuse and dependence is not clearly established, but further experience may demonstrate their usefulness.

Long half-life substances have the potential for other types of problems. For example, a long-acting sedative administered before bedtime may promote sleep at night, but "hangover" effects occur the next morning. With nightly use, long half-life sedatives and their active metabolites gradually accumulate in the body, especially in the elderly. This suggests that the effects, good and bad, not only increase with repeated administration but also last longer the longer the drug has been administered. In general, steady-state levels of the substance are reached in about four to five half-lives when the substance is taken on a regular basis; likewise, it takes about four to five half-lives to rid the body of the substance once intake is stopped. Some tolerance to the effects of most drugs may ameliorate the accumulation of the drug. Withdrawal symptoms generally appear faster and with more intensity with short-acting drugs compared with long-acting drugs. For example, "rebound insomnia" is typical with triazolam but not flurazepam.

Table 99–7. ORGANIZATIONS PROVIDING ADDITIONAL INFORMATION ON THE TREATMENT OF SUBSTANCE ABUSE

Organization	Telephone Number*	Internet Address*
National Institute on Alcohol Abuse and Alcoholism	301-443-3860	www.niaaa.nih.gov
National Cancer Institute	800-4-CANCER	www.nci.nih.gov
American Lung Association	800-586-4872	www.lungusa.org
National Institute on Drug Abuse	888-644-6432	www.nida.nih.gov
National Clearinghouse for Alcohol and Drug Information	800-729-6686	www.health.org
Self-help 12-step groups	Call the regional offices	
Alcoholics Anonymous		www.alcoholicsanonymous.org
Cocaine Anonymous		www.ca.org
Narcotics Anonymous		www.wsoinc.org

*Telephone numbers in the United States and Internet addresses were valid at time of publication.

In general, the elderly not only metabolize drugs more slowly than the young but also may be more affected at a lower blood concentration. Although the popular stereotype of the drug abuse is a young person, it should not be forgotten than the elderly often abuse alcohol, sedative hypnotics, and other substances.

Additional Information

Information about the treatment of specific substances of abuse, including written material, can be obtained by both physicians and consumers from the various organizations listed in Table 99–7.

SLEEP AND SPECIFIC SUBSTANCES

Alcohol and Alcoholism

In the United States, of those who drink alcohol, about 10% of men and 3 to 5% of women develop serious alcohol-related life problems.[7, 8] Between 20 and 50% of men and 6 and 10% of women in general medical-psychiatric settings suffer from alcoholism. Nevertheless, only 20 to 50% of alcoholic patients are recognized and diagnosed in clinical practice. Most alcoholic people do not identify themselves as such. In addition to medical and psychiatric history and physical examination, the CAGE Questionnaire has been shown to increase the identification of alcohol abusers[9] (Table 99–8). A positive answer to two or more questions indicates that the patient is at risk. Laboratory tests also may help identify alcohol abusers. These tests measure blood and breath alcohol concentrations, liver enzymes (such as gamma-glutamyl transferase, aspar-

tate aminotransferase), alanine aminotransferase, high-density lipoprotein phospholipids, apolipoproteins and angiotensin I and angiotensin II, and mean corpuscular volume. Because genetic factors appear to predispose people to certain types of alcoholism, patients should be asked specifically about alcohol use and abuse in the family.

Effects of Alcohol on Sleep in Nonalcoholics

Alcohol may be mildly stimulating in some people,[10] but more commonly it has a transient sedative effect, especially in sleepy or anxious individuals. It is probably the most frequently used sleeping aid in the general population. In a survey of 18- to 45-year-olds in the general population, 13% reported using alcohol in the previous year to sleep. Of this 13%, 15%, or about 2% of the general population, had used it regularly for 1 month or more; an additional 5% of the population used both alcohol and a hypnotic in order to sleep.[11]

When given to normal controls shortly before bedtime, alcohol tends to shorten sleep latency and to increase nonrapid eye movement (NREM) sleep and to reduce rapid eye movement (REM) sleep in the first hours following ingestion at night.[12, 13] Alcohol, however, is metabolized relatively rapidly: about one glass of wine or 1/2 pint of beer per hour. Therefore, after four to five drinks in the hours before bedtime, alcohol concentrations in blood approach zero about halfway through the night.[14] As a consequence, the individual is likely to be in withdrawal and to experience shallow, disrupted sleep, increased REM sleep, dream recall or nightmares, and sympathetic arousal including tachycardia and sweating in the last half of the night. Sleep may also be interrupted by gastric irritation, headache, a full bladder, and a "rebound wakefulness." Although alcohol increases sleep at the beginning of the night, it decreases sleep at the end of the night. It also increases the risk of falls during the night. The effects of alcohol may be more pronounced in the elderly compared with younger individuals because a given dose produces higher concentrations in blood and brain in the former. With nightly use of alcohol, some tolerance develops to the sedative and REM-suppressing effects of alcohol.

Little is known about the effects of alcohol in babies, but some studies suggest that alcohol (or marijuana) in mother's milk helps their infants to go to sleep easily

---

Table 99–8. THE CAGE QUESTIONNAIRE FOR DETECTION OF HEAVY ALCOHOL USE

Have you ever felt you should Cut down on your drinking?
Have you felt Annoyed by people criticizing your drinking?
Have you ever felt Guilty about your drinking?
Do you require an "Eye-opener" in the morning to steady yourself or to get rid of a hangover?

but to sleep less well overall than those babies who did not ingest alcohol.[15] Furthermore, Scher et al[16] reported that infants whose mothers drank one drink per day during the first trimester of pregnancy showed more sleep disruptions than infants born to nondrinking women. The full significance of these observations is unknown.

The adverse effects of alcohol may continue after blood alcohol concentrations are zero. For example, moderate drinking in the late afternoon—the so-called "happy hour"—may disrupt sleep during the last half of the night, long after alcohol has disappeared from the blood.[17] Likewise, when alcohol is administered in the morning, its sedative and detrimental effects continue on the multiple sleep latency test (MSLT) and a divided attention task and in simulated driving in the afternoon after the point when breath ethanol is undetectable.[18]

Interestingly, the sedative effects of alcohol in normal subjects may reflect an "unmasking" of prior sleep loss.[19] Sleepiness potentiates the sedative effects of alcohol. For example, the risk of an automobile accident is probably greater following consumption of alcohol by a sleep-deprived individual compared with a rested driver.

It should be noted that no systematic scientific data exists, to our knowledge, about the effects of alcohol taken at low doses at bedtime on sleep in nonalcohol, chronic insomniacs who regularly use alcohol to promote sleep at night. We do not know if tolerance has developed to the side effects or the soporific benefits of alcohol. In other words, we have little information on whether a "nightcap" is helpful or harmful in individuals who imbibe every night.

Sleep-Related Disturbances in Alcoholics

Alcoholic patients commonly report insomnia, hypersomnia, circadian rhythm disturbances, and parasomnias.[20, 21] As alcohol dependence develops, patients often report difficulty sleeping without a drink.[22] Objective measures bear out the subjective complaints, finding long sleep latencies; poor sleep efficiencies; and decreased total sleep, slow-wave sleep (SWS), and REM sleep.[23-25] Peripheral neuropathies may occur during these periods if the subject lies for long periods without moving in a position that exerts pressure on nerves.

The normal circadian patterns of sleep and wakefulness may become disrupted in alcoholics. Some patients develop *polyphasic sleep-wake cycles*, for example during a binge, characterized by short periods of sleep induced by drinking, followed by short periods of wakefulness.

Finally, alcohol consumption at both the social and pathological levels may lead to diurnal hypersomnolence. Hypersomnia may result from (1) the direct hypnotic effects of alcohol following daytime consumption, especially in sleep-deprived individuals; (2) the accumulative effects of alcohol and sleep deprivation may sometimes be followed by periods of hypersomnia or near coma; (3) other primary sleep disorders such as apnea and periodic limb movements during sleep

(PLMs); or (4) "terminal sleep," which can occur during withdrawal after delirium tremens and is a prolonged, deep sleep. Terminal sleep may be associated with a loss of delta and REM sleep, as well as with behavioral disturbances such as pavor nocturnus.[26]

Alcohol and Formal Sleep Disorders

As mentioned already, the DSM-IV defines a substance-induced sleep disorder, alcohol subtype, which occurs in association with either intoxication or withdrawal, and which manifests itself as insomnia, hypersomnia, parasomnia, or mixed type (see Table 99–5). In contrast, the International Classification of Sleep Disorders (ICSD)[27] defines an alcohol-dependent sleep disorder in insomniac individuals without a diagnosis of alcoholism who have used alcohol as a bedtime sleep aid for over 30 days (Table 99–9).

Alcohol Sleep-Related Breathing and Periodic Limb Movements

Alcohol increases the likelihood of snoring, greater inspiratory resistance, and apneic events in nonalcoholic individuals without a history of obstructive sleep apnea-hypopnea syndrome (OSAHS) or snoring.[28] It apparently does this by potentiating upper airway atonia and inspiratory resistance,[29-31] although some

---

Table 99–9. INTERNATIONAL CLASSIFICATION OF SLEEP DISORDERS DIAGNOSTIC CRITERIA: ALCOHOL-DEPENDENT SLEEP DISORDER (780.52-3)

A. A complaint of insomnia.
B. The complaint is temporally associated with more than one attempt to withdraw from bedtime alcohol ingestion.
C. The alcohol must have been taken daily as a bedtime sleep aid for at least 30 days.
D. Polysomnographic monitoring during alcohol ingestion demonstrates:
  1. Frequent awakenings, particularly during REM sleep in the latter half of the night, when the alcohol blood level declines
  2. Increased slow wave sleep percentage
  3. Upon withdrawal of alcohol, more marked sleep disruption, with an increased number and duration of awakenings
E. No evidence of a medical or psychiatric disorder producing the insomnia. This disorder must be distinguished from alcoholism.
F. Does not meet the criteria for other sleep disorders producing a primary complaint of insomnia.
Minimal Criteria: A plus B plus E.
Severity Criteria:
Mild: Mild insomnia as defined above. Few if any symptoms in excess of those required to make the diagnosis.
Moderate: Moderate insomnia as defined above. Additional non-sleep-related symptoms of alcohol use may be present, causing mild to moderate psychosocial impairment.
Severe: Severe insomnia as defined above. Alcohol use produces non-sleep-related symptoms that markedly interfere with occupational or social functioning.
Duration Criteria:
Acute: Duration less than 3 months.
Subacute: Duration longer than 3 months but less than 12 months.
Chronic: Duration 12 months or longer.

From Diagnostic Classification Steering Committee. The International Classification of Sleep Disorders: Diagnostic and Coding Manual. Rochester, Minn: American Sleep Disorders Association; 1990.

studies report minimal effects of moderate alcohol on breathing or saturation in patients with mild to severe apnea.[32] Nevertheless, sleep-disordered breathing (i.e., apneas, hypopneas, and desaturations) increase in an age-dependent manner in abstinent alcoholic patients,[33] particularly over the age of 60 years.[34] The risk of PLMs was increased threefold with alcohol consumption in a general sleep disorders clinic sample,[35] but PLMs were not increased in another study of abstinent alcoholic patients.[33]

The effects of alcohol on both sleep-related breathing and PLMs may increase daytime sleepiness and fatigue. The risk of a fatigue-related automobile accident is increased fivefold in obstructive sleep apnea (OSA) patients who consume alcohol at the rate of two drinks or more per day compared with patients who drink little or not at all.[36] In addition, the combination of alcohol, OSA, and snoring increase the risk of heart attacks, stroke, and sudden death.

Sleep During Recovery and Abstinence in Alcoholics

Abnormal sleep patterns persist for months to years during abstinence. At about the 2nd or 3rd week of abstinence, alcoholic patients show prolonged sleep latency; reduced total sleep time, especially NREM sleep and SWS; and increased *REM density* (a measure of ocular activity during REM sleep).[37, 38] Patients with a history of secondary depression have shorter REM latency and greater REM percentage than patients without depression.[38]

Even after 1 to 2 years of abstinence, sleep tends to be shortened, shallow, and fragmented. REM percentage is often elevated.[33, 39–41] Figure 99–1 shows the slow recovery of total sleep time and lack of recovery in REM sleep in male veteran primary alcoholic patients over the course of 14 months of abstinence. Only a few abstinent, recovering alcoholic patients have been studied for 1 year or more, and they continued to show low levels of SWS and other subjective and objective sleep abnormalities.[39, 41, 42]

Sleep Measures May Predict Relapse in Recovering Alcoholics

Does poor sleep contribute to relapse during subacute and long-term abstinence? Many patients rationalize drinking because they say it helps them sleep, at least at the beginning of the night during the first days of renewed drinking. In an inpatient experimental ward, recovered alcoholic patients were given the opportunity to drink alcoholic beverages; those with subjective sleep complaints were more likely to drink than those without sleep problems.[43] Resumption of drinking appears to increase SWS and decrease wakefulness during the night, which may reinforce the impression that alcohol reduces complaints of sleep and daytime fatigue. Unfortunately, as drinking continues, both objective and subjective sleep patterns generally worsen.

Increasing evidence suggests that either objective or subjective sleep measures during the acute and sub-

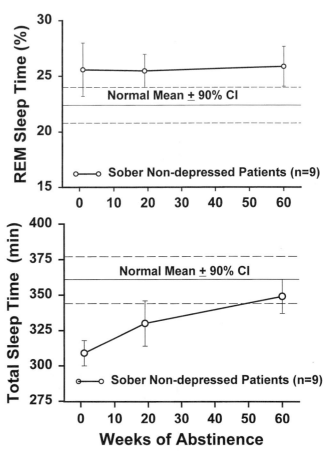

Figure 99–1. Polygraphic sleep recordings for REM percentage and total sleep time in nine male, sober, recovering, primary nondepressed, alcoholic patients for more than 1 year. Note that both measures differ from age-matched normal controls for most of the recovery period. Values for the patients are mean ± SEM, for normal controls mean ± 90% confidence interval.

acute abstinent recovery periods predict abstinence or relapse within 2 to 12 months. In the 1970s, Allen and Wagman[44–46] suggested that low levels of SWS at baseline were associated with poor sobriety at 2 months after discharge from an inpatient alcohol sleep research unit. More recently, elevated REM sleep measures (short REM latency, increased REM percentage and REM density) at about 2 weeks of abstinence predicted relapse at 3 months after discharge in primary alcoholic patients with and without secondary depression.[47–49] Although age, duration and severity of alcoholism, marital status, employment, hepatic enzymes, cognitive performance, and depression ratings did not discriminate abstainers from relapsers, polygraphic sleep measures correctly classified about 75 to 80% of alcoholic patients. In the whole group of patients (both nondepressed and depressed alcoholics), elevated REM density during the first 1 to 2 weeks of abstinence was the best predictor of relapse at 3 months after discharge from the 1 month inpatient alcohol treatment program. In contrast, at about 5 months of abstinence, the REM sleep measures no longer predicted relapse or abstinence at about 1 year; nevertheless, long objective sleep latency and poor sleep efficiency (e.g., insomnia) at that time was associated with relapse by the end of the 1st year.[42] In a longitudinal study of alcoholic patients who were initially evaluated at an average of 32 days of sobriety, patients who relapsed at an average of 5 months differed from those who remained sober on both subjective and objective sleep measures. After controlling for a variety of measures, polygraphic sleep latency was the best predictor of relapse.[41] Different sleep measures may reflect different phases of the protracted physical withdrawal syndrome associated with recovery from alcoholism.

Treatment of Alcoholism and Alcohol-Induced Sleep Disorders

Successful treatment of sleep disorders in alcoholic patients should be conducted as part of an overall treatment plan. Clinical sleep disorder specialists are well positioned to diagnose alcohol abuse and dependence because sleep disturbances are common in these disorders. We and many other clinicians have been consulted by patients complaining of insomnia or daytime fatigue and sleepiness who were ultimately found to have alcohol-related problems. Furthermore, the chronic insomnia and other sleep problems of the long-term abstinent, recovering alcoholic patient poses therapeutic challenges to the field of sleep disorder medicine. Treatment needs of the alcoholic patient vary with the severity and phase of the alcohol problems and may involve inpatient and outpatient treatment; medical, psychiatric, family, and social therapy; and pharmacological treatment.

The overall treatment of alcoholism and its withdrawal is too broad a topic to be covered in detail here. Physicians are advised to consult substance abuse treatment texts for specifics.[4, 7, 8, 50, 51] Abrupt termination of chronic ethanol ingestion may precipitate an acute alcohol withdrawal syndrome, beginning sometimes within a few hours of the last drink and lasting more or less 1 week. Following long periods of heavy drinking, abrupt reduction of drinking triggers autonomic hyperactivity (tachycardia, hypertension, diaphoresis, tremor, fever, respiratory alkalosis); gastrointestinal (GI) manifestations (anorexia, nausea, vomiting); psychological manifestations (agitation, anxiety, restlessness, hallucinations); and neurological signs (seizures). Importantly, sleep disturbance is common, including sleep onset insomnia with significant loss of total sleep time and SWS, and increased REM sleep, fragmented sleep, and wakefulness.

During acute alcohol withdrawal and detoxification, patients are frequently admitted to an inpatient setting or specialized detoxification center and treated with a benzodiazepine taper to reduce the autonomic hyperactivity, psychological manifestations, and sleep disturbances, and to prevent seizures, which typically occur about 7 to 48 h after the last drink. In the case of chronic alcoholism, typical detoxification with benzodiazepines include chlordiazepoxide (25 to 50 mg orally), diazepam (10 to 20 mg orally), or lorazepam (2 to 4

mg orally), repeated every 1 to 2 h until the patient is mildly sedated.[8, 51] Delirium tremens comprise a constellation of severe withdrawal symptoms, including hyperpyrexia (104°F or 40°C), electrolyte and fluid disturbances, disorientation, hallucinations, and tremor. Beta blockers can also be used to treat withdrawal symptoms, but their efficacy in treating delirium and seizures is not well established. Patients may suffer from nutritional, vitamin, and electrolyte deficiencies, such as thiamine, folate, magnesium, potassium, and vitamins A, D, or K. For alcoholics who are withdrawing abruptly, expert medical consultation and evaluation are needed promptly to ameliorate the acute withdrawal syndromes, to treat acute medical problems, and to prevent or treat serious medical consequences of alcoholism, such as Wernicke-Korsakoff syndrome, alcoholic dementia, cerebellar degeneration, hepatitis, cirrhosis, and pancreatitis.

During the first weeks of abstinence, a sizeable proportion of primary alcoholic patients meet diagnostic criteria for major depressive disorder. Fortunately, depression in many patients spontaneously improves with the nonspecific treatment in an inpatient alcohol recovery unit.[52]

Following the withdrawal period, it is necessary to take the long-term view in the prevention of relapse, much like the lifetime management of diabetes, hypertension, or bipolar disorder. Long-term treatment may use psychological and psychosocial treatments; referral to self-help groups, residential care, spiritual centers, and religious activities; and pharmacological therapies. Psychological interventions include cognitive behavioral therapy, interpersonal therapy, family counseling, occupational therapy, and motivational enhancement therapy. The most prevalent self-help group is Alcoholics Anonymous,[50, 53] although others such as Rational Recovery also exist in a more limited fashion. Pharmacological interventions include disulfiram (Antabuse) and calcium carbimide (Temposil or Abstem), which is not available in the United States. Naltrexone hydrochloride (ReVia), an antagonist of endogenous endorphin receptors, has been approved by the Food and Drug Administration for the prevention of relapse in alcoholic patients as an adjunct to good psychosocial treatments; it appears to reduce the subjective pleasure normally induced by drinking alcohol.[54–56] A promising experimental drug for treatment of alcoholism, acamprosate, is a direct $GABA_A$ agonist.

Many clinicians and alcoholic patients believe that successful alleviation of insomnia and other sleep complaints will enhance these long-term goals in the subacute and chronic abstinent phases. Unfortunately, the treatment of alcohol-related sleep problems has not been well studied. Few well developed guidelines have been accepted by the clinical community, in general, but the following clinical issues should be considered.

1. Maximize the general health and nutrition of the recovering alcoholic patient, including clinical management of sleep apnea and PLMs. Patients with PLMs should be treated with the dopamine-related medications rather than benzodiazepines or opioids.

2. Seek to improve the overall quality of sleep in patients, through both sleep hygiene instructions (see Chapter 58) and circadian regulation of the sleep-wake cycle. Bright-light therapy improved objective and subjective measures of sleep during the first 4 days of abstinence in one study.[57] Another study suggested that light therapy had antidepressant benefits in abstinent alcoholics with winter depression.[58] The connection reported between insomnia and relapse suggests that patients should be screened for sleep initiation and maintenance problems and those problems should be specifically targeted.

3. Should sedatives be administered to abstinent alcoholics with insomnia? Except for management of acute symptoms of withdrawal, benzodiazepines or other sleeping pills are generally not recommended in managing abstinent alcoholics.[3] They are cross-tolerant with alcohol and can be abused or misused themselves. Sedating antidepressants might be helpful for the abstinent, insomniac alcoholic patient, but this treatment has not been studied well enough to evaluate the benefits and problems. They may be misused if the patients resume drinking. Serotonin-specific reuptake inhibitors (SSRIs) have been largely unsuccessful in the prevention of relapse in alcoholic patients, perhaps because of SSRIs' detrimental effects on sleep continuity. Again, cognitive-behavioral approaches such as sleep hygiene instructions and stimulus-control should be included in any treatment plan, regardless of the use of pharmacotherapy. Further information on alcohol can be found in Table 99–7 and through

the National Institute of Alcohol and Alcoholism, the National Clearinghouse for Alcohol and Drug Information, and Alcoholics Anonymous.

Anxiolytics and Sedative Hypnotics

Sedative hypnotics have been popular since antiquity, especially for the induction of sleep. Older drugs include alcohol, bromide, chloral hydrate, paraldehyde, and barbiturates. About a century ago, chloral hydrate was a widely abused addictive substance. For reasons poorly understood, it passed out of fashion as an abused drug even before the introduction of the newer sedative hypnotics. Barbiturates were abused for many decades, but less so now because their use has declined dramatically since the introduction of the benzodiazepines.

At present, the major anxiolytics and sedative-hypnotic drugs include the benzodiazepines and miscellaneous drugs (zolpidem, chloral hydrate, and zaleplon) (Table 99–10). Other similar drugs, which are infrequently used in clinical practice for the management of insomnia or anxiety, include barbiturates, methyprylon, meprobamate, and others. These drugs probably increase the effects of GABA, an inhibitory neurotransmitter in the brain. When the GABA receptor is stimulated, the chloride channel on neuronal membranes is opened, which allows negatively charged chloride ions to cross the cell membrane, thereby hyperpolarizing the cell. Benzodiazepines exert their agonist effects on the $GABA_A$ receptor chloride ion channel. The opposite effect is achieved by benzodiazepine *inverse agonists*, such as the experimental agent beta carboline, which

Table 99–10. SUMMARY OF BENZODIAZEPINES AND HYPNOTIC AGENTS

Drug	Plasma Peak (h)	Half-Life (h)	Active Metabolites	Half-Life (h)	Dose Equivalent	Duration
Alprazolam	1–2	12–15	Alpha-hydroxy-alprazolam	6	0.5	Short
Chlordiazepoxide	1–4	7–28	Desmethylchlor-diazepam	5–30	12.5	Long
			Demoxepam	14–95		
			Desmethyldiazepam	25–100		
			Oxazepam	3–24		
Clonazepam	1–2	18–56	None		0.25	Long
Clorazepate	1–2		Desmethyldiazepam	25–100	7.5	Long
			Oxazepam	3–24		
Diazepam	½–2	20–50	Desmethyldiazepam	25–100	5	Long
			Oxazepam	3–24		
Estazolam	2	10–24	None	—	1	Short
Flurazepam			n-Desalkylflurazepam	32–100	15	Long
Lorazepam	1–3 ⅓ IM	10–24	None	—	1	Short
Midazolam		1–6	1-Hydroxy-methyl-midazolam	—	1–3	Short
Oxazepam	1–4	3–24	None	—	15	Short
Prazepam	4–6		Desmethyldiazepam	25–100	10	Long
			Oxazepam	3–24		
Quazepam	1–3	39	2-Oxoquazepam	75	7.5	Long
			n-Desalkyl-2-oxoquazepam			
Temazepam	2½	7–14	None	—	15	Short
Triazolam	1–1½	2–5	None	—	0.25	Short
Zaleplon	1	1	None	—	10	Short
Zolpidem	1–2	2–5	None	—	10	Short

close the ion channel; they are anxiolytic and lower the seizure threshold. Finally, receptor *antagonists*, such as flumazenil, are essentially neutral ligands, neither increasing nor decreasing the effects of GABA. Flumazenil, however, can displace either agonists or inverse agonists. For this reason, it can be used to reverse sedation produced by a benzodiazepine overdose. The sedative hypnotics differ from one another to some degree in the exact mechanisms of action, but this common enhancement of GABA neurotransmission is probably responsible for the tendency for cross-tolerance between these drugs and alcohol.

Both clinical experience and laboratory studies in animals indicate that abuse and dependence can occur with the sedative hypnotics. In self-administration paradigms in laboratory animals, for example, benzodiazepines and zolpidem are positively reinforcing, although to a lesser extent than stimulants (amphetamine and cocaine) and barbiturates. Benzodiazepines with a rapid onset of action (lorazepam, diazepam, and alprazolam) are more likely to be self-administered than those with a longer onset of action (oxazepam, halazepam, or chlordiazepoxide). In a similar fashion, in the barbiturate family, the short-acting pentobarbital and secobarbital appear to have more euphoria and abuse potential than phenobarbital, which has a longer onset of action. Buspirone does not appear to induce self-administration in animals or people.

In general usage, benzodiazepines are not usually strongly reinforcing or pleasurable for most individuals. Abusers of sedative hypnotics usually prefer pentobarbital to diazepam. Sedative-hypnotic abuse occurs predominately in the context of polysubstance abuse, particularly to reduce the adverse effects of stimulants, to self-medicate withdrawal from heroin or alcohol, or to produce intoxication when no other drugs are available. Other individuals at high risk for sedative-hypnotic abuse include those with a history of sedative hypnotic abuse, sedative-hypnotic dependence, or alcoholism, or those who are current substance abusers, who are seeking pharmacological therapy for anxiety or depression. Current alcohol use should always be carefully evaluated before prescribing a sedative hypnotic to anyone, even if there is no known suggestion of substance abuse. Alcohol use increases the risk of cross-tolerance and withdrawal symptoms in benzodiazepine users, probably because both potentiate brain GABA neurotransmission. A strong family history of substance abuse should also be considered a risk factor because genetic factors play a role in the etiology of these disorders.

Many patients with mood disorders, anxiety and panic disorder, or severe insomnia take benzodiazepines daily for long periods. Nevertheless, the risk of serious physical or behavioral dependency appears to be low. Epidemiological surveys estimate that about 2.6% of the adult population in the United States has used a hypnotic agent within the past year. About three quarters of hypnotic users take them for fewer than 2 weeks. Of the hypnotic users, about 10 to 11% (0.3% of the total sample) have taken the hypnotic more or less nightly for a year. Only about 35% of the insomniacs have actually taken sleeping pills. The reality is that many individuals with insomnia and other disorders are not using medications or other therapies that might be of benefit. The use of sleeping pills in the United States appears to be about average compared with other industrialized nations around the world.

Concerns have been raised for decades about the benefits and risks of long-term treatment with benzodiazepines at more or less conventional doses. Nevertheless, little empirical data exists about the benefits and risks associated with long-term treatment of insomnia. If patients were randomly assigned in a double-blind fashion to hypnotic therapy or placebo for long periods of time (9 to 12 months), which group would fare better over time? We do not have the answer to that simple question at this time. We do know, however, from relatively short-term sleep laboratory studies (2 to 4 weeks) that the placebo group usually improves over time compared with the pretreatment baseline and that some pharmacological tolerance develops to benzodiazepines. The benefits of the active drug compared with the placebo *(the effect size)* are usually statistically significant but weak. Insomnia, even chronic insomnia, probably has a fluctuating course and is influenced by nonpharmacological factors, for example, the attention of the experimenters, the expectation of help, and the sleep hygiene schedules associated with sleep laboratory studies. A major study would be required to do justice to the question of long-term benefits and hazards of current chronic hypnotic usage.

Long-term therapy with benzodiazepines and zolpidem raises concerns about the risk of tolerance and physical dependence. Some pharmacological tolerance is expected, suggesting that the doses may increase somewhat with nightly or daily use. Furthermore, some withdrawal symptoms are common when benzodiazepines or zolpidem is stopped suddenly, for example withdrawal insomnia, suggesting physical dependence. Physical withdrawal symptoms are usually greater following long-term use of short-acting (e.g., triazolam, alprazolam) as compared with long-acting (diazepam, flurazepam, temazepam) benzodiazepines.[59, 60] In general, however, the withdrawal syndrome associated with benzodiazepines and zolpidem is generally milder than those associated with barbiturates and other nonbenzodiazepine sedative hypnotics. With few exceptions, serious, acute withdrawal problems are rare after long-term treatment (6 to 12 months) at the recommended doses. The incidence of drug-seeking behavior or escalating doses with benzodiazepine therapy is low.[61]

In evaluating the risks and benefits of sedative-hypnotic therapy in a patient, it is helpful to distinguish *drug-seeking behavior* from *therapy-seeking behavior*. The former involves drug use in a nontherapeutic context, at the expense of other activities, in excessive nontherapeutic amounts, with discriminable subjective effects, and on a chronic basis leading to tolerance and physical dependence. In contrast, with therapy seeking behavior the drug is taken for its therapeutic efficacy and is self-administered at a therapeutic dose for an appropriate period under medical supervision. Nevertheless, clinicians and patients should be wary and cautious about long-term use of sedative hypnotics.

In evaluating the clinical changes associated with discontinuation of drug therapy, it is useful to distinguish three groups of symptoms: (1) reemergence of the original symptoms for which the medication was ordered; (2) transient exacerbation of typical original symptoms, such as rebound insomnia for 1 to 2 nights after abrupt withdrawal from a short-acting benzodiazepine, such as triazolam, in insomniac patients; and (3) emergence of new symptoms. The first two usually occur with conventional therapy for short periods; rebound insomnia, for example, has been reported after only 1 or 2 nights of therapy. The third type, the emergence of new symptoms, usually occurs after prolonged, high-dose treatment, for example, starting 1 to 2 days after stopping a short-acting benzodiazepine or starting 3 to 8 days after stopping a long-acting benzodiazepine. Symptoms include anxiety, insomnia, nightmares, seizures, psychosis, hyperpyrexia, and even death. In addition, however, some clinicians have noted a protracted, low-dose withdrawal syndrome that emerges about 1 to 7 days after the discontinuation of a benzodiazepine or the reduction of the drug dose to a lower therapeutic dose.[62] Symptoms include anxiety, agitation, insomnia, nightmares, tachycardia, palpitations, anorexia, muscle spasms, increased sensitivity to light and sounds, and paresthesias. The protracted syndrome can last for months and can be severe and disabling. Risk factors for the low-dose benzodiazepine withdrawal syndrome may include a family or personal history of alcoholism, daily consumption of alcohol or other sedatives, and use of short-acting, high milligram potency benzodiazepines. These protracted syndromes and their treatment are discussed in other texts.[63–65]

The ICSD defines a hypnotic-dependent sleep disorder, which is associated with withdrawal symptoms worse than the original complaint in individuals who used a hypnotic at night for at least 3 weeks (Table 99–11).

Treatment of Withdrawal From Sedative Hypnotics

If withdrawal from long-term use of sedative hypnotics is desired, it should be done slowly and carefully. Patients should be cautioned of the potential withdrawal and rebound effects, especially insomnia and anxiety. Reemergence of the symptoms originally medicated may be a major risk factor for resumption of use. In fact, reemergence of some symptoms (e.g., panic attacks) may actually warrant resumption of use, although insomnia does not usually fall into that category.

The protocols for detoxification depend on the type of use by the patient.[4, 51, 62, 66]

Therapeutic Doses. If a patient has been taking therapeutic doses for a long time without escalating the prescribed dose, tapering can usually be done with the same medication, although switching from a short half-

Table 99–11. INTERNATIONAL CLASSIFICATION OF SLEEP DISORDERS DIAGNOSTIC CRITERIA: HYPNOTIC-DEPENDENT SLEEP DISORDER (780.52-0)

A. A complaint of insomnia or excessive sleepiness.
B. Nearly daily use of a hypnotic agent for at least 3 weeks.
C. Hypnotic withdrawal is associated with exacerbation of the primary complaint, which is often judged to be worse than the original sleep problem.
D. Daytime symptoms during drug withdrawal of nausea, muscle tension, aches, restlessness, and nervousness.
E. Polysomnographic monitoring demonstrates:
  1. Normal sleep architecture while on medication; or
  2. An increased sleep latency, reduced total sleep time and sleep, efficiency with reduced stages 3, 4, and REM sleep, and an increased stage 1 and 2 sleep, during withdrawal of medication.
F. Other medical or psychiatric disorders cannot account for the primary symptom, e.g., mood disorders.
G. Other sleep disorders can be present, but do not account for the primary symptom.

Minimal Criteria: A plus B plus C.
Severity Criteria:
Mild: Mild insomnia or mild excessive sleepiness as defined above.
Moderate: Moderate insomnia or moderate excessive sleepiness as defined above. Withdrawal is marked by a rebound in the subjective complaint, which is often worse than that prior to hypnotic use.
Severe: Severe insomnia or severe excessive sleepiness as defined above. Other features of central nervous system drug ingestion or withdrawal may be seen, such as performance deficits, severe anxiety, and incoordination or ataxia.
Duration Criteria:
Acute: Duration 3 months or less.
Subacute: Duration longer than 3 months but less than 1 year
Chronic: Duration 1 year or longer.

From Diagnostic Classification Steering Committee. The International Classification of Sleep Disorders: Diagnostic and Coding Manual. Rochester, Minn: American Sleep Disorders Association; 1990.

life drug to a long half-life drug may reduce some withdrawal symptoms. Initial tapering (e.g., to 50% of the original dosage) is often easier than later transitions from 50 to 25% of the original dose and then through the last transition from 25% of the original dose to zero. In addition, psychological treatments for the emergent symptoms may reduce the continued need for the sedative hypnotics. Tapering alprazolam may be particularly difficult when low doses are reached (1 mg or less to zero dose); it may help to reduce the rate of dose reduction to 0.125 to 0.25 mg per week. Alternatively, the patient can be gradually switched from the short half-life alprazolam to the long half-life clonazepam over the course of a week, and then slowly tapered off. Diazepam does not appear to be as useful as clonazepam in covering withdrawal from alprazolam. Some clinicians have also recommended a taper with carbamazepine (approximately 200 mg twice a day, adjusted to a serum level of 4 to 10 μg/ml), starting once the patient has been tapered to the lowest dose tolerated.

High Dose Sedative-Hypnotic Use. Unlike most opioid and stimulant abusers, many sedative-hypnotic abusers do not belong to the drug-seeking culture. Instead, some escalate beyond therapeutic doses in a misguided attempt to treat anxiety or insomnia. Patients abusing high doses of sedative hypnotics for long periods of time are at great risk for medical complications during withdrawal, including delirium, psychosis, seizures, and, rarely, death. Withdrawal may require hospitalization in these patients, particularly in individuals with a history of seizures, medical problems, poor psychosocial supports, and difficulties during past attempts to withdraw. Patients are usually switched to a long half-life benzodiazepine, such as chlordiazepoxide or clonazepam, which is cut by 30% of the original dose after 2 days, and then cut further each day by 5%. Sometimes, withdrawal from high doses must be conducted gradually in the outpatient setting (i.e., 5% reduction of the original dose per week). Even with these slow, gradual tapers, patients often experience anxiety, insomnia, lethargy, and dysphoria. Some, but not all, addiction clinicians recommend pretreatment with carbamazepine 200 to 800 mg per day, which may reduce withdrawal symptoms during the taper.

Sedative-Hypnotic Abuse in the Context of Polysubstance Abuse. For patients who are abusing different sedative-hypnotics concomitantly (benzodiazepines, alcohol, barbiturates), it is recommended to switch first to a single, long half-life benzodiazepine and discontinue alcohol or the barbiturates. Once the patient is stabilized, withdrawal from the benzodiazepine can begin. For patients who have been using both sedative hypnotics and opiates, withdrawal from the former is more serious than from the latter. Therefore, patients may be switched off the opiate onto methadone, if they are not already on it, and then withdrawn from the sedative hypnotic with a long half-life.

It is often difficult to judge how much sedative hypnotics and which ones the patient is taking (Table 99–12). Therefore, the physician may have difficulty establishing the initial dose to be used in withdrawal. The pentobarbital challenge test[4, 51] has been used to determine sedative tolerance and to estimate crossover treatment dose in patients who are estimated to have taken a daily dose of 400 to 1200 mg pentobarbital (equivalent to 40 to 120 mg diazepam). When the patient is no longer intoxicated, he or she is given an oral dose of pentobarbital, 200 mg. One hour later, the patient is examined for evidence of intoxication, such as nystagmus, slurred speech, ataxia, or sedation. If the patient has nystagmus on lateral gaze, or is otherwise

intoxicated after taking pentobarbital 200 mg, he or she has probably been taking less than the equivalent of 800 mg per day. These patients can be stabilized on pentobarbital 100 to 200 mg every 6 h. If the patient falls asleep, it is unlikely that he or she has tolerance to the drugs; these patients do not need further detoxification. If 200 mg has no effect, it is likely that the patient was taking a minimal daily dose of 800 mg or its equivalent. These patients should be given 100 mg pentobarbital every 2 h until symptoms develop or a maximum dose of 500 mg pentobarbital has been reached. The total dose needed to produce intoxication is the patient's 6-h pentobarbital equivalent; the total daily dose can be determined by multiplying the 6-h dose by 4. After 2 days of treatment with pentobarbital, substitute 30 mg of phenobarbital for each 100 mg pentobarbital and give it in three divided doses for 2 days. The dose of phenobarbital should then be given for 2 more days and then reduced by 30 mg per day.

Withdrawal from sedative hypnotics may also be facilitated by administration of propranolol (10 to 40 mg three times a day), a beta-adrenergic blocker, or by clonidine (0.1 mg twice a day to 0.2 mg three times a day), an alpha$_2$ agonist. These two drugs may ameliorate anxiety and autonomic side effects, but they do not affect the risk of seizures.

Nonpharmacological therapy may be helpful in reducing the anxiety, sleep problems, dysphoria, and fatigue that usually accompany long-term withdrawal from sedative hypnotics. These include group support, relaxation therapy, meditation, cognitive behavioral therapy, hypnosis, family and marital therapy, sleep hygiene, daytime exercise, and so forth. Further information can be found in Table 99–7, from the National Institute of Drug Abuse, and from the National Clearinghouse for Alcohol and Drug Information.

Caffeine

Caffeine and other methylxanthines are stimulants found not only in coffee but also in tea; cola; chocolate; cocoa; and over-the-counter (OTC) analgesics, cold remedies, and stimulants.[67] A normal cup of brewed coffee contains about 100 to 150 mg of caffeine and a cup of instant coffee about 85 to 100 mg of caffeine; tea contains about 60 to 75 mg per cup; cola contains about 40 to 75 mg per 12 oz drink; cocoa holds about 50 mg per cup; OTC cold preparations have about 15 to 60 mg per tablet; and OTC stimulants contain about 100 to 200 mg.

Individuals differ in their response to caffeine, with some people becoming over-stimulated with as little as 250 mg.[68, 69] Others are less affected, especially chronic users who appear to develop some tolerance to the stimulating effect of caffeine. Caffeine intoxication is characterized by restlessness, nervousness, excitement, insomnia, flushed face, GI disturbances, and other symptoms. Ingesting 500 mg of caffeine has the same altering effects as about 5 mg of amphetamine. For most people, doses of caffeine above 1 g may produce insomnia, dyspnea, delirium, and arrhythmias. Doses

Table 99–12. DOSE CONVERSIONS FOR SEDATIVE-HYPNOTIC DRUGS

Benzodiazepines	Dose (mg)	Barbiturates	Dose (mg)
Alprazolam	1	Amobarbital	100
Chlordiazepoxide	25	Butabarbital	100
Clonazepam	2	Butalbital	100
Clorazepate	15	Pentobarbital	100
Diazepam	10	Phenobarbital	30
Flurazepam	15	Secobarbital	100
Halazepam	40		
Lorazepam	2		
Oxazepam	10		
Prazepam	10		
Temazepam	15		

above 5 g can be fatal. Although the half-life of caffeine is about 3 to 7 h, the effects may last as long as 8 to 14 h. Therefore, caffeine may have significant effects on sleep at night even if it is consumed in the late afternoon or early evening. Six cups or more of coffee throughout the day are likely to cause insomnia at night, even if not taken shortly before bedtime. Under the circumstances, a vicious cycle can easily develop: although a few cups of coffee may reduce daytime sleepiness, this amount is sufficient to disrupt sleep at night and, therefore, exacerbate or perpetuate the daytime sleepiness. The effects of caffeine are prolonged in children and pregnant women, who may become toxic at relatively low doses, as well as the elderly and patients with hypothyroidism. In addition, caffeine may trigger panic attacks in some patients with panic disorder.

Caffeine has been used to produce experimental models of insomnia.[69] Many people, however, develop tolerance, and apparently sleep well, by subjective report. Caffeine has an important role in combating daytime fatigue and sleepiness in normal people.[70-74] From the perspective of sleep-wake regulation, caffeine appears to promote wakefulness by blocking adenosine receptors in the brain. Adenosine may be an endogenous sleep-promoting substance.[75]

The combination of alcohol and caffeine can produce insomnia synergistically several hours later.[76] The two drugs are frequently consumed together, for example, at dinner. The two substances initially have opposing effects when taken together: alcohol is sedative and counteracts the stimulating effects of caffeine. The half-life of alcohol, however, is shorter than that of caffeine. Four to 6 h after consumption, blood levels of alcohol have fallen to near zero. Therefore, the subject goes into the arousing, withdrawal effects of alcohol at the same time that the blood levels of caffeine remain relatively high. Similar synergistic effects in coffee drinkers at bedtime may also occur in individuals who take a short-acting sleeping pill at bedtime and, perhaps, in cigarette smokers who go into withdrawal from nicotine at the end of the night.

Many patients and their doctors fail to recognize that caffeine may contribute to complaints of anxiety, insomnia, or other disorders. For patients with such symptoms who consume three or more cups of coffee per day (about 400 to 500 mg caffeine), gradual tapering off all caffeine may be helpful. Abrupt withdrawal, however, should be avoided because irritability, dysphoria, fatigue, sleepiness, headache, and flu-like symptoms may ensue about 18 to 24 h after the last dose.[77] These withdrawal symptoms suggest that heavy users of caffeine may develop dependence and may self-administer it to avoid the uncomfortable symptoms. Sleep-related difficulties associated with caffeine can be classified under the DSM-IV criteria for a substance-induced sleep disorder, caffeine subtype. In addition, DSM-IV defines research criteria for caffeine withdrawal, which include marked fatigue or drowsiness after abrupt cessation of high amounts of caffeine daily.

Nicotine

Nicotine is addicting.[78-80] This concept was long rejected and has only recently been officially recognized by the federal government and by most biomedical investigators. Consistent with this characterization, most smokers report that they would like to quit, that they have tried unsuccessfully to quit, that they recognized that smoking is hazardous to their health, and that they often smoke to avoid the withdrawal symptoms that appear 1 to 2 h after the last smoke. Furthermore, controlled, double-blind studies show that smokers do not like and do not select tobacco without nicotine when compared with tobacco with nicotine. In addition to smoking, nicotine may be administered in chewing tobacco, snuff, and nicotine gum and patches. Tolerance to the effects of nicotine are both gained and lost quickly. The DSM-IV diagnostic criteria for nicotine withdrawal are shown in Table 99–13.

About 20% of the adult population in the United States currently smokes cigarettes, 4% smoke pipes or cigars, and 3% use smokeless tobacco.[1] It is estimated that 20 to 50% of smokers meet diagnostic criteria for nicotine dependence. Nicotine dependence is about two to three times higher in patients with other psychiatric disorders than in the general population. About half of people who smoke experience nicotine withdrawal.

The plasma half-life of nicotine is about 2 h. Therefore, for the average smoker who smokes throughout the day, plasma concentrations of nicotine increase over the course of the day and fall throughout the night, although they remain detectable in the morning. A rough but simple measure of nicotine dependence is to ask how long the smoker can go in the morning before the first cigarette: 30 minutes or less suggests that the smoker is strongly dependent on nicotine.[80] The dose-response pharmacological effects of nicotine are complex, with ganglionic stimulation at low doses and ganglionic blockade at high doses.

Table 99–13. DSM-IV DIAGNOSTIC CRITERIA FOR 292.0 NICOTINE WITHDRAWAL

A. Daily Use of Nicotine for at least several weeks.
B. Abrupt cessation of nicotine use or reduction in the amount of nicotine used, followed within 24 hours by four (or more) of the following signs:
  (1) dysphoria or depressed mood
  (2) insomnia
  (3) irritability, frustration, or anger
  (4) anxiety
  (5) difficulty concentrating
  (6) restlessness
  (7) decreased heart rate
  (8) increased appetite or weight gain
C. The symptoms of Criterion B cause clinically significant distress or impairment in social, occupational, or other important areas of functioning.
D. The symptoms are not due to a general medical condition and are not better accounted for by another mental disorder

Reprinted with permission from the *Diagnostic and Statistical Manual of Mental Disorders, Fourth Edition.* Copyright 1994 American Psychiatric Association.
DSM-IV, *Diagnostic and Statistical Manual of Mental Disorders, Fourth Edition.*

The Effects of Nicotine on Sleep

The direct effects of nicotine on sleep in nonsmokers are not well characterized.[81, 82] Some evidence suggests that it has sedating effects at low doses and alerting effects at high doses. Both PSG and questionnaire studies report increased sleep latency as well as increased arousals and difficulty staying asleep at night in active smokers vs. nonsmokers.[81] Interestingly, nicotine may have novel effects in nonsmoking depressed patients compared with normal controls, in that it increased rather than decreased REM sleep,[83, 85] Some studies suggest that smoking is a risk factor for sleep-disordered breathing.[84] During acute withdrawal from nicotine, sleep tends to worsen in smokers, with increased arousals at night followed by sleepiness on the MSLT the next day.[86, 87] Furthermore, the nicotine patch, which is used as replacement therapy on smoking cessation, has been reported to have mixed results with regard to sleep complaints[88, 89] and does not provide clinically significant improvements in sleep-disordered breathing, although it may ameliorate other symptoms such as poor mood.

Cigarette smoking accelerates the metabolism of many drugs, including diazepam, lorazepam, oxazepam, imipramine, and caffeine. Perhaps for these pharmacodynamic and pharmacokinetic reasons, cigarette smokers report less sedation than nonsmokers with diazepam, chlordiazepoxide, and chlorpromazine.

General Considerations in the Treatment of Smoking

Smokers vary considerably in their need for help in quitting. Many quit on their own, but in general, quitting is more difficult for people dependent on nicotine compared with cocaine. Depressed patients have greater difficulty quitting than nondepressed smokers. The Fagerstrom Tolerance Questionnaire is a clinically validated short questionnaire that measures tolerance and dependence to nicotine in smokers.[80] Sleep disorder clinicians are in a good position to motivate smokers to quit. Over 80% of smokers who are trying to quit report inadequate sleep, anxiety, and irritability.[90] Many specialized clinical treatment programs, both commercial and noncommercial, are now available to help smokers quit. In addition, clinically proven pharmacological aids include the nicotine transdermal patch, nicotine polacrilex gum, clonidine, and bupropion. Further information on smoking can be found in Table 99–7 and from the National Cancer Institute, the American Lung Association, and the National Institute on Drug Abuse.

Stimulants

Stimulants such as amphetamine, methylphenidate, fenfluramine, and pemoline may have important therapeutic effects, especially in narcolepsy[90] and attention deficit disorder and, occasionally, in patients with obesity or depression, negative symptom schizophrenia, or other apathetic states. When taken in moderation for short periods of time, these stimulants counteract excessive daytime sleepiness and sleep loss and improve mood, performance, and endurance. Unfortunately, these drugs can be abused.[4, 51, 91, 92] Pemoline apparently has less abuse potential, perhaps because it has a slower, more prolonged onset of action and less euphoric effects compared with the other drugs. Other stimulants are often used as anorectics, including phendimetrazine, diethylpropion, mazindol, phentermine, and phenylpropanolamine.

Cocaine is a product of the coca plant.[92, 93] The freebase or "crack" is prepared by a simple extraction from the salt, cocaine hydrochloride. Coca leaf has long been used by different cultures, including the Indians of the Andes, by chewing with alkaline materials. This method produces a mild high, with an onset of 5 to 10 min and lasting about an hour. More commonly, it is taken by cocaine abusers by intranasal "snorting," intravenous (IV) administration, or smoking freebase. Smoking freebase cocaine acts in seconds and results in an intense high lasting several minutes. Smoking produces the most medical and psychiatric symptoms. The combined use of cocaine and ethyl alcohol results in a metabolic product by the liver, cocaethylene, which has intense and long-lasting cocaine-like effects.

The amphetamines, such as methamphetamine ("speed"), are also taken IV, by snorting, or by smoking ("ice"). Smoking gives an intensive and relatively long-lasting high. Other stimulants that may be abused include phenmetrazine, methylenedioxyamphetamine, and 3,4-methylenedioxymethamphetamine ("ecstasy"); the latter two drugs also possess lysergic acid diethylamide–like hallucinogenic properties. In addition, propylhexedrine, which is an active ingredient of Benzedrex nasal decongestant inhalants, can be prepared as "stovetop speed" for IV use by heating with hydrochloric acid.

Cocaine, amphetamine, methylphenidate, and many of the other stimulants apparently enhance neurotransmission of norepinephrine, dopamine, and serotonin, primarily by reuptake blockade or increased release of the neurotransmitter.[6]

The diagnosis of stimulant abuse may require both clinical suspicion and laboratory confirmation. Patients may present with intoxication; symptoms of withdrawal including hypersomnia and dysphoria, overdose, psychosocial correlates of stimulant abuse (job loss, marital difficulties, legal and financial problems); or medical, psychiatric, or sleep-wake disorders. Signs and symptoms of acute stimulant intoxication include sweating, tachycardia, elevated blood pressure, dilated pupils (mydriasis), hyperactivity, confusion, and disorientation. With repeated use, tolerance develops quickly and dosage escalation is common. Other common symptoms include hypervigilance, paranoid ideation and delusions, full-blown psychosis, parasitosis, sterotypy, bruxism, violent behavior, and disrupted sleep-wake patterns. Stimulant abusers are at risk for serious medical complications, including cardiovascular collapse, arrhythmias, myocardial infarction, seizures, strokes, infections and HIV conversion, hyperthermia, pulmonary problems, and obstetrical complications. Patients may present with nasal bleeding and nasal septal perforation from snorting, headaches, fatigue, insomnia, anxiety, depression, and chronic hoarseness. Toxicology screens on urine or serum may confirm the diagnostic suspicion, including radioimmunoassay, enzyme immunoassay, or gas chromatography-mass spectrometry for parent compounds or metabolites, such as the long half-life benzoylmethylecgonine for cocaine.

Acute withdrawal is not usually life-threatening in stimulant abusers but usually produces craving, sleep disturbances, hyperphagia, fatigue and lassitude, and depression (including suicidal risk), lasting for days to months.

Modafinil is a promising new stimulant for the treatment of narcolepsy and sleepiness.[94] It appears to have a unique mode of action compared with other stimulants.[95–97] At this time, it appears to be much safer, less likely to be abused, and to have fewer side effects than other stimulants, but time will tell.

Sleep in Stimulant Use and Withdrawal

Relatively few studies have investigated sleep patterns during stimulant use or after withdrawal from stimulant dependence, and only a subset of these have used PSG data to assess sleep. Amphetamine, methylphenidate, pemoline, and cocaine prolong sleep latency and REM latency and reduce total sleep time and REM time, presumably by stimulating dopaminergic arousal systems or, in the case of fenfluramine, releasing serotonin.[98–100] Tolerance may develop with long-term administration, not only in addicted patients but also in patients with legitimate medical reasons for taking amphetamines or methylphenidate, such as narcolepsy or attention-deficit disorder.[101] During bouts or runs of stimulant abuse, individuals may go for days without sleep, followed by periods of hypersomnia. With chronic use of stimulants at low to moderate doses, tolerance may develop to the sleep, anorectic, autonomic, and euphoric effects of stimulants, although activation of mood and behavior may persist. Stimulant abusers also use sedatives or alcohol in order to promote sleep and reduce anxiety.

The main subjective complaint on withdrawal is difficulty falling asleep, with one study reporting subjectively long sleep latencies for an entire 28-d study period.[102] The objective sleep data contains some inconsistencies, due perhaps to the specific drugs abused by the subjects (e.g., diet pills vs. methamphetamine), the quantity and frequency of use, and the age of the subjects studied. For example, although some studies reported greatly increased amounts of total sleep time compared to control or normative data during the first few days of withdrawal,[105, 106] one other reported no differences.[104] The sleep abnormalities related to stimulant withdrawal include lowered sleep efficiency, increased nocturnal wake time, increased amounts of stage 1 sleep and REM sleep, and shortened REM latency.[106] Sleep does not improve much during the first 2 weeks of abstinence, with the possible exception of a decrease in nocturnal wake time, stage 1 sleep, and

REM density.[106] These measures were still abnormal compared with normative data in both studies, however. Lisuride, a drug with dopaminergic properties, significantly prolonged REM latency and reduced REM time in stimulant abusers during withdrawal.[107]

Some stimulant abusers may develop depressed mood during acute and subacute withdrawal.

Stimulants and Sleep Disorders

In the ICSD, a stimulant-dependent sleep disorder is "characterized by reduction of sleepiness or suppression of sleep by central stimulants, and resultant alterations in wakefulness following drug abstinence"[27(p107)] (Table 99–14). This schema includes not only illicit stimulants but also caffeine, theophylline, and thyroid hormones. In the VA San Diego Healthcare System's Sleep Disorders Clinic, several stimulant-dependent patients have been diagnosed with sleep apnea who reported initially using stimulants as a self-medication for daytime hypersomnolence. Clinicians should screen

---

Table 99–14. INTERNATIONAL CLASSIFICATION OF SLEEP DISORDERS DIAGNOSTIC CRITERIA: STIMULANT-DEPENDENT SLEEP DISORDER (780.52-1)

A. A complaint of insomnia or excessive sleepiness.
B. The complaint is temporally associated with the use or withdrawal of a stimulant medication.
C. The use of stimulant medication leads to disruption of the habitual sleep period, or more than one attempt to withdraw from the stimulant leads to the development of symptoms of excessive sleepiness.
D. Polysomnographic monitoring demonstrates:
   1. Sleep disruption with reduced sleep efficiency and an increased number and duration of awakenings; and, upon withdrawal of the stimulant,
   2. An MSLT that demonstrates a mean sleep latency of less than 10 minutes.
E. Other medical or psychiatric disorders producing insomnia or excessive sleepiness may coexist.
F. Does not meet the criteria for other sleep disorders producing a primary complaint of insomnia or excessive sleepiness.
Note: If the clinical features are indicative, a diagnosis of psychoactive substance dependence or abuse should be additionally stated and coded on axis C, e.g., amphetamine abuse, and use the following code numbers: amphetamine or similarly acting sympathomimetic abuse, 305.70; amphetamine or similarly acting sympathomimetic dependence, 304.40.
Minimal Criteria: A plus B plus C.
Severity Criteria:
Mild: Mild insomnia or mild excessive sleepiness as defined above. Few if any symptoms in excess of those required to make the diagnosis.
Moderate: Moderate insomnia or moderate excessive sleepiness as defined above. Additional non–sleep-related symptoms of stimulant use may be present, causing mild to moderate impairment.
Severe: Severe insomnia or severe excessive sleepiness as defined above. Stimulant use produces non–sleep-related symptoms that markedly interfere with occupational or social functioning.
Duration Criteria:
Acute: Duration 3 weeks or less.
Subacute: Duration longer than 3 weeks but less than 6 months.
Chronic: Duration 6 months or longer

From Diagnostic Classification Steering Committee. The International Classification of Sleep Disorders: Diagnostic and Coding Manual. Rochester, Minn: American Sleep Disorders Association; 1990.

patients who use excessive stimulants (such as caffeine) for sleep disorders, such as apnea, PLMs, or narcolepsy.

Before prescribing stimulants, sleep disorder specialists must objectively document the diagnosis and reasons for treatment. This concern reinforces the importance of establishing a diagnosis of narcolepsy by objective means. Objective diagnosis not only protects the physician against charges of malpractice, misdiagnosis, and "script writing" but also ultimately helps the narcoleptic patient obtain legitimate prescriptions in localities where family physicians and pharmacies are reluctant to supply stimulants. Likewise, patients who are prescribed stimulants need careful monitoring and education to ensure proper use. The first reported case of an amphetamine-induced psychosis occurred in a narcoleptic patient.

Treatment of Stimulant Abuse

Acute intoxication with amphetamine, cocaine, or other stimulants can be serious and life-threatening. In the case of severe intoxication, the patients should be treated in an emergency department or hospital in order to provide close observation and intensive medical and psychiatric management. The psychotic symptoms and violence may be treated with haloperidol, a dopamine receptor antagonist which seems to be safer and more effective than phenothiazines. Diazepam is also useful, as are physical restraints. Ammonium chloride (500 mg orally every 4 h) may promote renal excretion of amphetamine if renal and hepatic function are normal.

The signs and symptoms of chronic stimulant use vary from person to person and depend on patterns of use and dosage. Low dose users may experience elevation of mood and activation while developing tolerance to the anorectic, autonomic nervous system, and sleep effects. Symptoms may emerge only during withdrawal or if the dosage is increased. About half of subjects who abuse stimulants for 3 months or more develop psychotic symptoms, especially paranoid ideation. Continued exposure to stimulants appears to sensitize or "kindle" the CNS so that even small doses elicit psychosis despite prolonged abstinence.

Withdrawal symptoms are common and important, not only following stimulant abuse but also after therapeutic use, as in narcolepsy or hyperactivity. As mentioned earlier, hypersomnia and a rebound of REM sleep are to be expected almost immediately. Dysphoria or even severe depression, with suicidal ideation, often develop about 48 to 72 h after the last dose and can persist for months. Animal studies suggest that brain concentrations of serotonin, dopamine, and norepinephrine remain reduced for months after administration of amphetamine compounds for 6 months or more. No well-established pharmacological treatments for stimulant abuse are currently available, although some investigators have suggested that administration of antidepressants may reduce dysphoria and the risk of relapse.

The treatment of stimulant dependence has traditionally been psychological and psychosocial, as physi-ological stimulant dependence and withdrawal was not formally recognized until the DSM-IV was published in 1994. Cognitive-behavioral, supportive, and psychodynamic therapies have each been used with some success. Comorbid depression is a risk factor for relapse and must therefore also be addressed in the treatment of stimulant dependence. Further information can be found in Table 99–7 and through the National Institute on Drug Abuse, the National Clearinghouse for Alcohol and Drug Information, Narcotics Anonymous, and Cocaine Anonymous.

Opioids

When morphine was isolated from opium in 1803, it was named *morphine* after the Greek god responsible for dreams, Morpheus. Ironically, modern research has shown that short-term administration of morphine, heroin, and other opiates to normal volunteers or abstinent addicts reduces REM sleep rather than increasing it, and also reduces total sleep time, sleep efficiency, and SWS.[108]

The term *opiate* was originally derived from opium, which was obtained from the poppy plant, *Papaver somniferum*. The word *opioid* initially referred to synthetic drugs not derived from opium.[109–111] Today, the term *opioid* generally refers to natural, semisynthetic, and synthetic substances with opiate-like activity, including meperidone, methadone, and hyromorphone. They are agonists at any of several endogenous opiate-like receptors, which are present in the brain, the gut, and elsewhere in the body. More than a dozen endogenous opioid peptides have been identified, falling into three different families: endorphins, enkephalins, and dynorphins. In addition, many different types of receptors have been characterized, including mu, kappa, delta, and sigma receptors. Because of the complexity of these systems, it has been difficult to identify the normal physiological roles of the endogenous opioid peptides and receptors. The effects of opioid drugs depend on the complex net agonist and antagonist action at a variety of receptor sites and depend on the dose.

Naloxone and naltrexone are relatively pure opioid receptor antagonists, that is, they bind to the receptor but do not activate it. In contrast, nalorphine and buprenorphine are mixed partial agonists. They share properties associated with both methadone and naltrexone. When present in sufficiently high concentrations, naloxone and naltrexone compete for the binding sites of the opioid receptor and block the opioid effects of the agonists. Naloxone, for example, blocks the euphoria, respiratory depression, and pupillary constriction produced by morphine and other opioid agonists. Naloxone or naltrexone have been used to reverse opioid overdose and respiratory depression in newborns, to diagnose opioid physical dependence, and to prevent readdiction in detoxified individuals. Individuals who are dependent on opioids are exquisitely sensitive to opioid antagonists. In contrast, nondependent individuals usually show no change when administered antagonists at the normally used clinical doses. Naloxone, however, inhibits REM sleep in normal subjects at large doses compared with those used to reverse the effects of exogenously administered opioids.[112]

The most commonly abused opioids include morphine, heroin, hydromorphine, and oxycodone (components of Percodan and Percocet). Heroin is metabolized in the body to morphine. The half-life of most narcotics is typically fairly short: 4 to 7 h for codeine, morphine, hydromorphine, methadone, and propoxyphene; 3 to 5 h for oxycodone and pentazocine; and 2 to 4 h for meperidine. Nevertheless, the frequency with which these drugs are used by established substance abusers varies considerably: about every 2 to 3 h with meperidine, dilaudid, and codeine; about every 4 to 6 h with heroin and morphine, and about every 8 to 12 h with methadone.[113] Methadone is rarely abused. Because of its relatively long half-life, it has been used to treat chronic opioid addicts. It generally lacks the euphoric effects of heroin, morphine, or commonly abused narcotics.

Opioids induce analgesis, sedation, apathy, poor concentration, mood changes, nausea, and vomiting. Rapid IV administration of an opioid causes a warm skin flushing and a "rush" that lasts about 45 sec, associated with pleasure, relaxation, and satisfaction. Opioids also initially reduce secretion of gonadotropin-releasing hormone and corticotopin-releasing hormone. Constipation and pupillary constriction (miosis) are common. At high doses or overdose, respiratory depression is a danger, leading to death in some cases. Opioids are also absorbed subcutaneously and intramuscularly from the gut, nasal mucosa (as in snorting), and the lung (as in smoking opium). With repeated administration, tolerance to the pleasurable and neuroendocrine effects develops and dose escalation begins.

As mentioned earlier, the opioids tend to reduce total sleep time and REM sleep when first administered to a nontolerant pain-free subject. (In patients with pain, however, narcotics may increase sleep). Opioids have also been used to treat restless legs syndrome with and without PLMs.[114] With chronic administration, tolerance develops to most of these effects. For example, the REM suppressing effects to morphine are lost within a week,[109] although the arousing effects may persist. Although early studies reported that methadone does not induce insomnia, a more recent study reported that chronic administration of methadone leads to disrupted sleep architecture and increased arousals.[115]

The mechanism by which morphine inhibits REM sleep may involve inhibition of acetylcholine in the pontine reticular formation[116] and direct agonist effects at specific mu receptors.[117]

Opioid abusers usually seek medical attention because of overdose, withdrawal, or medical complications such as HIV infection, hepatitis, or endocarditis. They rarely seek help during active intoxication, which is characterized by euphoria, tranquility, and drowsiness. Pupils are generally constricted. Overdose, however, is potentially lethal as a result of respiratory depression. if patients do not reveal their use of opioids, the clinician's level of suspicion may be raised by needle puncture marks; "tracks" or scars along veins; hand edema secondary to thrombosed veins in the arm; thrombophlebitis; abscesses or ulcers; ulceration of the nasal septum from "snorting" heroin or cocaine; cigarette burns or scars occurring while falling asleep; piloerection, which is a sign of opioid withdrawal; jaundice; and monilial infections or "thrush" of the mouth, which is a sign of AIDS. As a consequence of the addiction, patients often have endocarditis, cardiac arrhythmias, multiple infarcts of the lungs, pulmonary fibrosis, pulmonary edema, tuberculosis, pneumonia, hepatitis, seizures, osteomyelitis, chronic constipation or diarrhea, and pancreatitis. A urine toxicology screen should be ordered.

The intensity of withdrawal symptoms from opioids depends on the dose and duration of use, rate of removal of the drug from opiate receptors in the brain and elsewhere, and extent of continuous use. Generally, the shorter the half-life of the drug, the greater the intensity of the withdrawal symptoms will be. For short-acting drugs such as heroin and morphine, the early symptoms may occur between 8 and 12 h after the last dose, whereas peak symptoms occur between 48 and 72 h. Onset of symptoms during withdrawal from meperidine may begin within 3 h and peak at 8 to 12 h. In contrast, for long-acting drugs such as methadone or l-acetyl-α-methadol, onset of symptoms may be delayed for 1 to 3 d and peak symptoms for 3 to 5 d. Peak symptoms of withdrawal occur after about 8 to 12 h of abstinence with meperidine, 48 to 72 h with heroin, and about 72 to 96 h with methadone. The majority of symptoms are over after about 5 to 10 d during withdrawal from heroin and after about 14 to 21 d for methadone. In addition, protracted withdrawal symptoms, including somatic concerns, poor self-image, and disturbed sleep, may last for weeks following acute withdrawal from opioid drugs.

The signs and symptoms of opiate withdrawal vary with early, middle, and late phases of abstinence. During the early phase, yawning, lacrimation, rhinorrhea, and sweating are common. The middle phase is characterized by restless sleep, dilated pupils, anorexia, irritability, and gooseflesh. Finally, the late phase may be associated with increased severity of earlier symptoms, tachycardia, nausea, vomiting, diarrhea, abdominal cramps, depression, weakness, and pain. Death rarely, if ever, occurs with opioid withdrawal.

Detoxification from opioids often involves the use of methadone.[4, 51, 109–111] The goal is to reduce distressing symptoms associated with withdrawal. This is achieved by treating objective clinical signs rather than subjective symptoms, which may be difficult to assess in an opioid-dependent individual with a history of drug-seeking. Four sets of objective signs are monitored:

1. An increase of 10 heartbeats per minute or a heart rate of 90 in the absence of prior tachycardia
2. An increase in systolic blood pressure greater than 10 mm Hg or a blood pressure greater than 160/95 in the absence of known hypertension
3. Dilated pupils
4. Sweating, gooseflesh, rhinorrhea, or lacrimation.

When two or more of these four criteria are met, administer methadone 5 to 10 mg by mouth every 4 h. Methadone should be administered every 4 h as needed, not usually exceeding 40 mg over the first 24 h. The next day, the total dose is usually administered in two divided doses. Thereafter, the dose is tapered by 5 mg per day until the patient is totally withdrawn. Patients are also sometimes withdrawn with clonidine, which is not likely to be abused and which is not a controlled substance. Clonidine can be used in addition to methadone or alone. Following a test dose of 0.025 to 0.05 mg, it is usually prescribed in a dose of 0.15 to 0.3 mg per day in three divided doses. It can cause hypotension and is withheld if blood pressure falls below 90/60 mm Hg. Patients are usually stabilized for 4 days for short-acting opioids such as meperidine and heroin and for 2 weeks for methadone. After that time, the drug is tapered over 4 to 6 d. Other withdrawal protocols are discussed elsewhere.[4, 51, 110, 111]

Although these treatments may suppress the autonomic signs of withdrawal and improve EEG sleep measures, they may not affect symptoms such as restlessness, lethargy, insomnia, and craving. For example, at least one study has reported that patients undergoing methadone detoxification reported problems with initiating and maintaining sleep, inadequate total sleep time, and poor sleep quality compared with controls.[118] However, the same study also reported that treatment with naltrexone (an opioid antagonist) decreased sleep latency and increased total sleep time compared with control subjects. Treatment with clonidine is often complicated by hypotension, insomnia, fatigue, and sedation during the day. Clonidine is also contraindicated in patients with cardiac, renal, or metabolic disorders.

Insomnia is one of the most troublesome symptoms of withdrawal, particularly because it weakens the patient's resolve to remain drug-free. Flurazepam is reported to be well liked and tolerated by patients during withdrawal, but many of these patients have abused benzodiazepines in the past and it should be used cautiously, if at all.[111] Sedating antidepressants, such as amitriptyline, doxepine, trazodone, and diphenhydramine have also been used.

Long-term prevention of relapse in opioid abusers involves pharmacological agents, such as methadone or bupromorphine, deconditioning and cognitive-behavioral therapy, individual and group therapy, and therapeutic communities. Further information may be found in Table 99–7 and from the National Institute of Drug Abuse, the National Clearinghouse for Alcohol and Drug Information, and Narcotics Anonymous.

Acknowledgments

Supported by grants from the Department of Veterans Affairs, NIMH 30914-22, NIH RO1 RR00827, and F31 MH11452.

References

1. American Psychiatric Association. Diagnostic and Statistical Manual of Mental Disorders. 4th ed. Washington DC: American Psychiatric Association; 1994.

2. Galanter M, Kleber HD, eds. The American Psychiatric Textbook of Substance Abuse Treatment. Washington, DC: American Psychiatric Association; 1994.

3. Schuckit MA. Drug and Alcohol Abuse: A Clinical Guide to Diagnosis and Treatment. 3rd ed. New York, NY: Plenum; 1988.

4. Goldberg RJ. Practical Guide to the Care of the Psychiatric Patient. 2nd ed. St. Louis, Mo: CV Mosby; 1998.

5. Ciraulo DA, Shader RI, eds. Clinical Manual of Chemical Dependence. Washington, DC: American Psychiatric Press; 1991.

6. Koob G, Le Moal M. Drug abuse: hedonic homeostatic dysregulation. Science. 1997;278:52–58.

7. Gallant D. Alcohol. In: Galanter M, Kleber HD, eds. Textbook of Substance Abuse Treatment. 1st ed. Washington, DC: American Psychiatric Press; 1994:67–89.

8. Ciraulo DA, Renner JA. Alcoholism. In: Ciraulo DA, Shader RI, eds. Clinical Manual of Chemical Dependence. 1st ed. Washington, DC: American Psychiatric Press; 1991:1–93.

9. Perdrix A, Decrey H, Pécoud A, et al. Detection of alcoholism in general practice: applicability of the CAGE test by the general practitioner. Schweiz Med Wochenschr. 1995;125:1772–1778.

10. Papineau KL, Roehrs TA, Petrucelli N, et al. Electrophysiological assessment (the multiple sleep latency test) of the biphasic effects of ethanol in humans. Alcohol Clin Exp Res. 1998;22:231–235.

11. Johnson EA, Roehrs T, Roth T, et al. Epidemiology of alcohol and medication as aids to sleep in early adulthood. Sleep. 1998;21:178–186.

12. Yules RB, Lippman ME, Freedman DX. Alcohol administration prior to sleep: the effect of EEG sleep stages. Arch Gen Psychiatry. 1967;16:94–97.

13. Lobo LL, Tufik S. Effects of alcohol on sleep parameters of sleep-deprived healthy volunteers. Sleep. 1997;20:52–59.

14. Madsen BW, Rossi L. Sleep and Michael-Menten elimination of ethanol. Clin Pharmacol Ther. 1980;27:114–119.

15. Mennella JA, Gerrish CJ. Effects of exposure to alcohol in mother's milk on infant sleep. Pediatrics. 1998;101:E2.

16. Scher MS, Richardson GA, Coble PA, et al. The effects of prenatal alcohol and marijuana exposure: disturbances in neonatal sleep cycling and arousal. Pediatr Res. 1988;24:101–105.

17. Landolt HP, Roth C, Dijk DJ, et al. Late-afternoon ethanol intake affects nocturnal sleep and the sleep EEG in middle-aged men. J Clin Psychopharmacol. 1996;16:428–436.

18. Roehrs T, Beare D, Zorick F, et al. Sleepiness and ethanol effects on simulated driving. Alcohol Clin Exp Res. 1994;18:154–158.

19. Zwyghuizen-Doorenbos A, Roehrs T, Timms V. Individual differences in the sedating effects of alcohol. Alcohol Clin Exp Res. 1990;14:400–404.

20. Gross MM, Hastey JM. Sleep disturbances in alcoholism. In: Tarter RE, Sugerman A, eds. Alcoholism: Interdisciplinary Approaches to an Enduring Problem. Reading, Mass: Addison-Wesley; 1976:257–309.

21. Zarcone V. Alcoholism and sleep. In: Passonant P, Oswald I, eds. Pharmacology of the State of Alertness. Oxford, England: Pergamon Press; 1979:9–38.

22. Mello NK, Mendelson JH. Behavioral studies of sleep patterns in alcoholics during intoxication and withdrawal. J Pharmacol Exp Ther. 1970;175:94–112.

23. Allen RP, Wagman A, Faillace LA, et al. Electroencephalographic (EEG) sleep recovery following prolonged alcohol intoxication in alcoholics. J Nerv Ment Dis. 1971;153:424–433.

24. Adamson J, Burdick JA. Sleep of dry alcoholics. Arch Gen Psychiatry. 1973;28:146–149.

25. Benca RM, Obermeyer WH, Thisted RA, et al. Sleep and psychiatric disorders: a meta-analysis. Arch Gen Psychiatry. 1992;49:651–668.

26. Kotorii T, Nakazawa Y, Yokoyama T. Terminal sleep following delirium tremens in chronic alcoholics—polysomnographic and behavioral study. Drug Alcohol Depend. 1982;10:125–134.

27. Diagnostic Classification Steering Committee. The International Classification of Sleep Disorders: Diagnostic and Coding Manual, Revised. Rochester, Minn: American Sleep Disorders Association; 1997.

28. Dawson A, Lehr P, Bigby BG, et al. Effect of bedtime ethanol on total inspiratory resistance and respiratory drive in normal nonsnoring men. Alcohol Clin Exp Res. 1993;17:256–262.

29. Krol RC, Knuth SL, Bartlett D Jr. Selective reduction of genioglossal muscle activity by alcohol in normal human subjects. Am Rev Respir Dis. 1984;129:247–250.

30. Stradling JR, Crosby JH. Predictors and prevalence of obstructive sleep apnoea and snoring in 1001 middle aged men. Thorax. 1991;46:85–90.

31. Dawson A, Bigby BG, Poceta JS, et al. Effect of bedtime alcohol on inspiratory resistance and respiratory drive in snoring and nonsnoring men. Alcohol Clin Res. 1997;21:183–190.

32. Teschler H, Berthon-Jones M, Wessendorf T, et al. Influence of moderate alcohol consumption on obstructive sleep apnoea with and without AutoSet nasal CPAP therapy. Eur Respir J. 1996;9:2371–2377.

33. Le Bon O, Verbanck P, Hoffmann G, et al. Sleep in detoxified alcoholics: impairment of most standard sleep parameters and increased risk for sleep apnea, but not for myclonias—a controlled study. J Stud Alcohol. 1997;58:30–36.

34. Aldrich MS, Shipley JE, Tandon R, et al. Sleep disordered breathing in alcoholics: association with age. Alcohol Clin Exp Res. 1993;17:1179–1183.

35. Aldrich MS, Shipley JE. Alcohol use and periodic limb movements of sleep. Alcohol Clin Exp Res. 1993;17:192–196.

36. Aldrich MS, Chervin RD. Alcohol use, obstructive sleep apnea, and sleep-related motor vehicle accidents [abstract]. Sleep Res. 1997;26:308.

37. Gillin JC, Smith TL, Irwin M, et al. EEG sleep studies in "pure" primary alcoholism during subacute withdrawal: relationships to normal controls, age, and other clinical variables. Biol Psychiatry. 1990;27:447–488.

38. Gillin JC, Smith TL, Irwin M, et al. Short REM latency in primary alcoholics with secondary depression. Am J Psychiatry. 1990;147:106–109.

39. Williams HL, Rundell OH. Altered sleep physiology in chronic alcoholics: reversal with abstinence. Alcohol Clin Exp Res. 1981;2:318–325.

40. Ehlers CL, Phillips E, Parry BL. Electrophysiological findings during the menstrual cycle in women with and without late luteal phase dysphoric disorder: relationship to risk for alcoholism? Biol Psychiatry. 1996;39:720–732.

41. Brower KJ, Aldrich MS, Hall JM. Polysomnographic and subjective sleep predictors of alcoholic relapse. Alcohol Clin Exp Res. 1998;22:1864–1871.

42. Drummond SPA, Gillin JC, Smith TL, et al. The sleep of abstinent pure primary alcoholic patients: natural course and relationship to relapse. Alcohol Clin Exp Res. 1998;22:1796–1802.

43. Skoloda TE, Alterman AI, Gottheil E. Sleep quality reported by drinking and nondrinking alcoholics. In: Gottheil EL, ed. Addiction Research and Treatment: Converging Trends. New York, NY: Pergamon Press; 1979:102–112.

44. Allen RP, Wagman AM. Do sleep patterns relate to the desire for alcohol? Adv Exp Med Biol. 1975;59:495–508.

45. Allen RP, Wagman AM, Funderburk FR, et al. Slow wave sleep: a predictor of individual differences in response to drinking? Biol Psychiatry. 1980;15:345–348.

46. Wagman AM, Allen RP, Funderburk FR, et al. EEG measures of functional tolerance to alcohol. Biol Psychiatry. 1978;13:719–778.

47. Clark CP, Gillin JC, Golshan S, et al. Increased REM sleep density at admission predicts relapse by three months in primary alcoholics with a lifetime diagnosis of secondary depression. Biol Psychiatry. 1998;43:601–607.

48. Gillin JC, Smith TL, Irwin M, et al. Increased pressure for rapid eye movement sleep at time of hospital admission predicts relapse in nondepressed patients with primary alcoholism at 3-month follow-up. Arch Gen Psychiatry. 1994;51:189–197.

49. Clark CP, Gillin JC, Golshan S, et al. Polysomnography and depressive symptoms in primary alcoholics with and without a lifetime diagnosis of secondary depression and in patients with primary major depression. J Affect Disord. 1999;52:177–185.

50. Bean-Bayog M. Alcoholics Anonymous. In: Ciraulo DA, Shader RI, eds. Clinical Manual of Chemical Dependence. 1st ed. Washington, DC: American Psychiatric Press; 1991:359–375.

51. Weiss RD, Greenfield SF, Mirin SM. Intoxication and withdrawal syndromes. In: Hyman SE, Tesar GE, eds. Manual of Psychiatric Emergencies. 3rd ed. Boston, Mass: Little Brown; 1994:279–293.

52. Brown SA, Inaba RK, Gillin JC, et al. Alcoholism and affective disorder: clinical course of depressive symptoms. Am J Psychiatry. 1995;152:45–52.

53. Emrick CD. Alcoholics Anonymous and other 12-step groups. In: Galanter M, Kleber HD, eds. Textbook of Substance Abuse Treatment. 1st ed. Washington, DC: American Psychiatric Press; 1994:351–358.

54. O'Malley SS, Jaffe AJ, Chang G, et al. Naltrexone and coping skills therapy for alcohol dependence: a controlled study. Arch Gen Psychiatry. 1992;49:881–887.

55. Volpicelli JR, Alterman AI, Hayashida M, et al. Naltrexone in the treatment of alcohol dependence. Arch Gen Psychiatry. 1992;49:876–880.

56. Volpicelli JR, Alterman AI, O'Brien CP. Naltrexone and alcohol dependence: some methodological issues [reply]. Arch Gen Psychiatry. 1994;51:335–336.

57. Schmitz M, Frey R, Pichler P, et al. Sleep quality during alcohol withdrawal with bright light therapy. Prog Neuropsychopharmacol Biol Psychiatry. 1997;21:965–977.

58. Avery DH, Bolte MA, Ries R. Dawn simulation treatment of abstinent alcoholics with winter depression. J Clin Psychiatry. 1998;59:36–42.

59. Gillin JC, Spinweber CL, Johnson LC. Rebound insomnia: a critical review. J Clin Psychopharmacol. 1989;9:161–172.

60. Hallfors DD, Saxe L. The dependence potential of short half-life benzodiazepines: a meta-analysis. Am J Public Health. 1993;83:1300–1304.

61. Grad RM. Benzodiazepines for insomnia in community-dwelling elderly: a review of benefit and risk. J Fam Pract. 1995;41:473–481.

62. Smith DE, Wesson DR. Benzodiazepines and other sedative hypnotics. In: Galanter M, Kleber HD, eds. The American Psychiatric Press Textbook of Substance Abuse Treatment. Washington, DC: American Psychiatric Press; 1994:179–190.

63. Salzman C. Benzodiazepine Dependence, Toxicity and Abuse: A Task Force Report of the American Psychiatric Association. Washington, DC: American Psychiatric Association; 1990.

64. Brenner PM, Wolf B, Rechlin T, et al. Benzodiazepine dependence: detoxification under standardized conditions. Drug Alcohol Depend. 1991;29:195–204.

65. Ciraulo DA, Sands BF, Shader RI, et al. Anxiolytics. In: Ciraulo DA, Shader RI, eds. Clinical Manual of Chemical Dependence. Washington, DC: American Psychiatric Press; 1991:135–174.

66. Kunkel EJ, Rodgers C, DeMaria PA Jr, et al. Use of high dose benzodiazepines in alcohol and sedative withdrawal delirium. Gen Hosp Psychiatry. 1997;19:286–293.

67. Greden JF. Caffeinism and caffeine withdrawal. In: Lowinson JH, Ruiz P, eds. Substance Abuse: Clinical Problems and Perspectives. Baltimore, Md: Williams & Wilkins; 1981:274–286.

68. James JE. Acute and chronic effects of caffeine on performance, mood, headache, and sleep. Neuropsychobiology. 1998;38:32–41.

69. Bonnet MH, Arand DL. Caffeine use as a model of acute and chronic insomnia. Sleep. 1992;15:526–536.

70. Johnson LC, Freeman CR, Spinweber CL, et al. Subjective and objective measures of sleepiness: effect of benzodiazepine and caffeine on their relationship. Psychophysiology. 1991;28:65–71.

71. Kelly TL, Mitler MM, Bonnet MH. Sleep latency measures of caffeine effects during sleep deprivation. Electroencephalogr Clin Neurophysiol. 1997;102:397–400.

72. Rosenthal L, Roehrs T, Zwyghuizen-Doorenbos A, et al. Alerting effects of caffeine after normal and restricted sleep. Neuropsychopharmacology. 1991;4:103–108.

73. Penetar D, McCann U, Thorne D, et al. Caffeine reversal of sleep deprivation effects on alertness and mood. Psychopharmacology (Berl). 1993;112:359–365.

74. Zwyghuizen-Doorenbos A, Roehrs T, Lipschutz L, et al. Effects of caffeine on alertness. Psychopharmacology. 1990;100:36–39.

75. Portas CM, Thakkar M, Rainnie DG, et al. Role of adenosine in behavioral state modulation: a microdialysis study in the freely moving cat. Neuroscience. 1997;79:225–235.

76. Stradling JR. Recreational drugs and sleep. Br Med J. 1993;306:573–575.

77. Hughes JR, Higgins ST, Bickel WK, et al. Caffeine self administration, withdrawal, and adverse effects among coffee drinkers. Arch Gen Psychiatry. 1991;48:611–617.

78. Jones RT. Tobacco. In: Ciraulo DA, Shader RI, eds. Clinical

Manual of Chemical Dependence. Washington, DC: American Psychiatric Press; 1991:321–344.

79. Ockene JK, Kristeller JL. Tobacco. In: Galanter M, Kleber HD, eds. Textbook of Substance Abuse Treatment. 1st ed. Washington, DC: American Psychiatric Press; 1994:157–177.

80. Fagerstrom KO. Measuring degree of physical dependence to tobacco smoking with reference to individualization of treatment. Addict Behav. 1978;3:235–241.

81. Davila DG, Hurt RD, Offord KP, et al. Acute effects of transdermal nicotine on sleep architecture, snoring, and sleep-disordered breathing in nonsmokers. Am J Respir Crit Care Med. 1994;150:469–474.

82. Gillin JC, Lardon M, Ruiz C, et al. Dose-dependent effects of transdermal nicotine on early morning awakening and rapid eye movement sleep time in nonsmoking normal volunteers. Clin Psychopharmacol. 1994;14:264–267.

83. Salin-Pascual RJ, De La Fuente JR, Galicia-Polo L, et al. Effects of transdermal nicotine on mood and sleep in nonsmoking major depressed patients. Psychopharmacology. 1995;121:476–479.

84. Wetter DW, Young TB, Bidwell TR, et al. Smoking as a risk factor for sleep-disordered breathing. Arch Intern Med. 1994;154:2219–2224.

85. Salin-Pascual RJ, Drucker-Colin R. A novel effect of nicotine on mood and sleep in major depression. Neuroreport. 1998;9:57–60.

86. Prosise GL, Bonnet MH, Berry RB, et al. Effects of abstinence from smoking on sleep and daytime sleepiness. Chest. 1994;105:1136–1141.

87. Wolter TD, Hauri PJ, Schroeder WJ, et al. Effects of 24-hour nicotine replacement on sleep and daytime activity during smoking cessation. Prev Med. 1996;25:601–610.

88. Hughes JR, Higgins ST, Bickel WK. Nicotine withdrawal versus other drug withdrawal syndromes: similarities and dissimilarities. Addiction. 1994;89:1461–1470.

89. Hughes JR, Hatsukami D. Signs and symptoms of tobacco withdrawal. Arch Gen Psychiatry. 1986;43:289–294.

90. Mittler MM. Evaluation of treatment with stimulants in narcolepsy. N Engl J Med. 1995;17:103–106.

91. Gawin FH, Khalsa ME, Ellinwood E Jr. Stimulants. In: Galanter M, Kleber HD, eds. Textbook of Substance Abuse Treatment. 1st ed. Washington, DC: American Psychiatric Press; 1994:111–139.

92. Goff DC, Ciraulo DA. Cocaine. In: Ciraulo DA, Shader RI, eds. Clinical Manual of Chemical Dependence. Washington, DC: American Psychiatric Press; 1991:233–259.

93. Withers NW, Pulvirenti L, Koob GF, et al. Cocaine abuse and dependence. J Clin Psychopharmacol. 1995;15:63–78.

94. Boivin DB, Montplaisir J, Petit D, et al. Effects of modafinil on symptomatology of human narcolepsy. Clin Neuropharmacol. 1993;16:46–53.

95. Lin JS, Roussel B, Akaoka H, et al. Role of catecholamines in the modafinil and amphetamine induced wakefulness, a comparative pharmacological study in the cat. Brain Res. 1992;591:319–326.

96. Touret M, Sallanon-Moulin M, Jouvet M. Awakening properties of modafinil without paradoxical sleep rebound: comparative study with amphetamine in the rat. Neurosci Lett. 1995;189:43–46.

97. Engber TM, Dennis SA, Jones BE, et al. Brain regional substrates for the actions of the novel wake-promoting agent modafinil in the rat: comparison with amphetamine. Neuroscience. 1998;87:905–911.

98. Post RM, Gillin JC, Goodwin FK, et al. The effect of orally administered cocaine on sleep of depressed patients. Psychopharmacology. 1974;37:59–66.

99. Gillin JC, van Kammen D, Bunney WE Jr. Pimozide attenuates effects of d-amphetamine in EEG sleep patterns in psychiatric patients. Life Sci. 1978;22:1805–1810.

100. Lewis SA. Comparative effects of some amphetamine derivatives on human sleep. In: Costa E, Garattini S, eds. Amphetamines and Related Compounds. New York, NY: Raven Press; 1970:873–888.

101. Feinberg I, Hibi S, Cavness C, et al. Sleep amphetamine effects in MBDS and normal subjects. Arch Gen Psychiatry. 1974;31:723–731.

102. Weddington WW, Brown BS, Haertzen CA, et al. Changes in mood, craving, and sleep during short term abstinence reported by male cocaine addicts. Arch Gen Psychiatry. 1990;47:861–868.

103. Watson R, Bakos L, Compton P, et al. Cocaine use and withdrawal: the effect on sleep and mood. Am J Drug Alcohol Abuse. 1992;18:21–28.

104. Gossop MR, Bradley BP, Brewis RK. Amphetamine withdrawal and sleep disturbance. Drug Alcohol Depend. 1982:10:177–183.

105. Thompson PM, Gillin JC, Golshan S, et al. Polygraphic sleep measures differentiate alcoholics and stimulant abusers during short-term abstinence. Biol Psychiatry. 1995;38:831–836.

106. Watson R, Hartmann E, Schildkraut JJ. Amphetamine withdrawal: affective state sleep patterns, and MHPG excretion. Am J Psychiatry. 1972;129:39–45.

107. Gillin JC, Pulvirenti L, Withers N, et al. The effects of lisuride on mood and sleep during acute withdrawal in stimulant abusers: a preliminary report. Biol Psychiatry. 1994;35:843–849.

108. Kay D, Pickworth W, Neider G. Morphine-like insomnia in nondependent human addicts. Br J Clin Pharmacol. 1981;11:159–169.

109. Staedt J, Wassmuth F, Stoppe G, et al. Effects of chronic treatment with methadone and naltrexone on sleep in addicts. Eur Arch Psychiatry Clin Neurosci. 1996;246:305–309.

110. Kleber HD. Opioids: detoxification. In: Galanter M, Kleber HD, eds. Textbook of Substance Abuse Treatment. 1st ed. Washington, DC: American Psychiatric Press; 1994:191–208.

111. Jaffe JH, Epstein S, Ciraulo DA. Opioids. In: Ciraulo DA, Shader RI, eds. Clinical Manual of Chemical Dependence. Washington, DC: American Psychiatric Press; 1991:95–134.

112. Sitaram N, Gillin JC. The effect of naloxone on normal human sleep. Brain Res. 1982;244:387–392.

113. Senay EC. Opioids: methadone maintenance. In: Galanter M, ed. Textbook of Substance Abuse Treatment. 1st ed. Washington, DC: American Psychiatric Press; 1994:209–221.

114. Montplaisir J, Lapierre O, Warnes H, et al. The treatment of the restless leg syndrome with or without periodic leg movements in sleep. Sleep. 1992;15:391–395.

115. Kay D. Human sleep and EEG through a cycle of methadone dependence. Electroencephalogr Clin Neurophysiol. 1975;38:35–43.

116. Lydic R, Keifer JC, Baghdoyan HA, et al. Microdialysis of the pontine reticular formation reveals inhibition of acetylcholine release by morphine. Anesthesiology. 1993;79:1003–1012.

117. Cronin A, Keifer JC, Baghdoyan HA, et al. Opioid inhibition of rapid eye movement sleep by a specific mu receptor agonist. Br J Anaesth. 1995;74:188–192.

118. Oyefeso A, Sedgwick P, Ghodse H. Subjective sleep-wake parameters in treatment-seeking opiate addicts. Drug Alcohol Depend. 1997;48:9–16.

fifteen

Methodology

Max Hirshkowitz

Monitoring and Staging Human Sleep

Mary A. Carskadon
Allan Rechtschaffen

The goal of this chapter is to summarize the procedures for monitoring and evaluating sleep in the laboratory setting. This material will not substitute for the standard manual; rather, one hopes it will be complementary. After recommended techniques and procedures are summarized, a few problematic areas are discussed briefly.

Although it is possible to monitor continuously and concurrently the activity of dozens of systems during sleep, one need measure just three systems to assess sleep according to standard criteria.[1] This standard system of sleep recording and staging criteria is firmly rooted in the U.S. sleep research tradition, and although certain of its criteria have been challenged in recent years, it is the only system established by a consensus of experts.

Among the earliest descriptions of electroencephalographic (EEG) activity during sleep were those from the laboratory of Loomis et al.[2] These authors described five stages of sleep but failed to distinguish rapid eye movement (REM) sleep. Not until the landmark work of Kleitman's group at the University of Chicago was REM sleep described,[3] a description made possible by the addition of electro-oculography (EOG) to the recording paradigm. The first comprehensive description of the nocturnal pattern of nonrapid eye movement (NREM) and REM sleep in human beings[4] remains the foundation of modern human sleep research and represents one of the most outstanding scientific

achievements of the 20th century. The standard sleep staging system[1] modified the EEG and EOG categorizations of Dement and Kleitman[4] primarily by adding electromyography (EMG). The addition of EMG to the criteria was based on the research of Berger[5] in human beings and Jouvet[6] in cats, which linked muscle atonia with REM sleep. The EMG provided a more stable marker for REM sleep than the intermittent bursts of rapid eye movements.

PROCEDURES FOR MONITORING SLEEP

The EEG is the core measurement of polysomnography. The four stages of NREM sleep are distinguished from each other principally along this dimension.

Electroencephalogram

Application. The reliable recording of EEG begins with accurate measurement of the skull according to the international 10–20 system of electrode placement.[7] A skilled technologist can make the requisite measurements in 10 min. The "eyeball" or "rule-of-thumb" placement of EEG electrodes is not recommended because of the marked variability of electrode locations

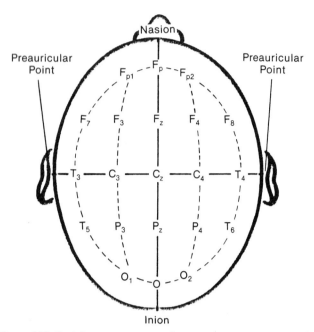

Figure 100–1. Schematic diagram showing measurements for the 10–20 electrode placement system. Measurements are made at 10 and 20% of the distances from inion to nasion, from left to right preauricular points, and around the circumference of the head. Intersecting points denote electrode placements. The most common placements for recording the electroencephalogram (EEG) during sleep are C3 (left central), C4 (right central), O1 (left occipital), and O2 (right occipital). (Redrawn from Harner PF, Sannit T. A Review of the International Ten-Twenty System of Electrode Placement. Quincy, Mass: Grass Instrument Company; 1974.)

such practices engender, regardless of the technologist's skills.

Figure 100–1 illustrates the 10–20 placement system, by which a grid is placed over the skull and points of intersection denote electrode placement locations. The name of the system derives from measurements made at intervals of 10 or 20% of the total distance between landmarks. The four landmarks of the system are the nasion, inion (external occipital protuberance), and left and right preauricular points. Thus, the measurements are specific to each individual.

After measurements are made, the hair is separated and the scalp is cleaned in preparation for electrode application. In the past, technologists have used coarse-grained compounds to abrade the scalp, enabling better signal conduction. This practice has recently been discouraged in response to the increased risk of infection from bloodborne viruses.[8] Thorough cleansing and removal of dead skin layers by brisk rubbing with gauze are generally sufficient to ensure adequate conduction when the electrode is applied over a good conducting medium. The EEG electrodes for overnight sleep studies are generally attached to the scalp using small patches of gauze soaked in collodion and dried with compressed air. The conducting medium may be added through a small hole in the electrode cup, or if it is placed in the cup before application, an airtight seal will prevent evaporation for at least 24 to 36 h.

Derivations. The standard manual[1] recommends referential recording of one EEG lead, either C3 or C4,

referenced to an indifferent auricularly placed electrode on the contralateral mastoid or ear lobe: hence C3/A2 or C4/A1. The recommended sleep staging criteria, therefore, are intended to be used with this single, central EEG lead. The recommendations of the original committee acknowledged that use of a single EEG channel was largely an economic issue for most laboratories, which at that time were limited to eight-channel recording systems on which two subjects were generally recorded simultaneously. Nevertheless, this economically dictated approach has proved to be a remarkably robust system.

Sleep stage scoring does not require measurement of focal EEG activity or regional comparisons, as might be performed in an EEG laboratory. Rather, all of the EEG waveforms used to distinguish sleep stages are well visualized at C3 or C4, particularly when signal amplitudes are optimized, with the relatively large interelectrode distance afforded by a contralateral reference. Thus, vertex sharp waves and K complexes, which are maximal over the vertex, are clearly evident at C3 and C4; high-voltage slow waves characteristic of deep NREM sleep are seen maximally in frontal regions yet show clearly on central derivations; alpha rhythm, by contrast, is maximal over the occipital poles but can be characterized centrally in most human beings.[9, 10]

Therefore, only C3/A2 or C4/A1 is used in the standard assessment of sleep stages. Many laboratories, however, routinely record an occipital EEG (usually O1/A2 or O2/A1) as an adjunct to the central EEG, particularly for assessing sleep onset or arousals during sleep. Certain laboratories also routinely record from frontal placements. When the latter procedure is used for sleep staging, however, there is a tendency to observe a somewhat greater quantity of the deep NREM sleep stages (stages 3 and 4); therefore, such use should be documented in any published reports.

Electro-Oculogram

There are two primary reasons to record eye movement activity during sleep. The most obvious is to record the cardinal sign of REM sleep—the phasic bursts of rapid eye movements—which is an essential sleep stage scoring criterion. In addition, the onset of sleep in most human beings is heralded or accompanied by slow, rolling eye movements, which also occur with transitions to stage 1 during the night. Although these slow eye movements (SEMs) are not essential to sleep staging, they often provide very useful information.

The EOG recordings are based on the small electropotential difference from the front to the back of the eye. The cornea is positive with respect to the retina. Thus, the eyeball exists in the head as a potential field within a volume conductor. Because of this essentially constant potential difference, movement of the eyes can be measured from electrodes placed beside the eyes. An electrode nearest the cornea will register a positive potential; an electrode nearest the retina will register a negative potential. As the eye moves, the positions of the cornea and retina change relative to the fixed position of the electrode, and a potential change will register as a pen deflection at the polysomnograph.

Application. Standard EOG placements include the right outer canthus (ROC) and the left outer canthus (LOC). According to the standard manual,[1] the EOG electrodes should be offset from horizontal, one slightly above and one slightly below the horizontal plane. In this manner, the electrodes can detect horizontal and vertical eye movements. The EOG electrodes are usually applied with tape to a skin surface that has been thoroughly cleansed. An airtight seal over the electrode will protect the conductivity of the electrode jelly for approximately 24 h. The collodion electrode application technique is greatly discouraged for EOG leads because of the risk of splashing collodion into the eyes.

Derivations. The standard manual[1] recommends continuous referential recording of two EOG leads: one outer canthus placement referred to the auricular reference on the opposite side and the other to the same auricular reference (e.g., ROC/A1 and LOC/A1). Certain laboratories[11] routinely use a contralateral reference for each outer canthus placement (ROC/A1 and LOC/A2). In the latter case, the contralateral references maximize the signal amplitude for both EOGs and equalize the amplitudes of pen deflections for conjugate eye movements. Either technique provides the capability to distinguish eye movements from electrode artifact. For example, in a montage recording ROC/A1 on one channel and LOC/A2 on another, conjugate eye movements will register as out-of-phase pen deflections; EEG activity reflected in the EOG channels (e.g., K complexes) will be seen as in-phase deflections; and electrode artifacts will register in phase or in only one channel.

When a major goal of an experiment is to determine more precisely the direction of eye movements, the EOG may be simultaneously recorded from horizontal and vertical placements. Thus, in addition to placements on the outer canthi, electrodes would be placed supraorbitally and infraorbitally. For exact determination of eye position, direct current (DC) recordings are recommended.

Electromyogram

In a standard polysomnographic recording, the EMG from muscles beneath the chin is used as a criterion for staging REM sleep.[1] The EMG recordings from other muscle groups are sometimes used to assess certain sleep disorders. For example, the anterior tibialis EMG is important to evaluate patients who have periodic movements in sleep. The intercostal EMG may be used to monitor respiratory effort. Most EMG recordings during sleep require taping electrodes to the skin over the muscle group of interest.

Application. Three electrodes are placed beneath the chin, overlying the mentalis/submentalis muscles. These placements, rather than others, are recom-

mended for the sake of convenience. The chin is very accessible, and the electrode wires can be drawn together with the others to form a bundle or "pony tail" at the back of the head. As in preparation for the EEG and EOG leads, the skin is thoroughly cleansed of oils and dead skin cells before applying the electrodes, which are generally secured with tape. Particularly in the case of a patient with a beard, the EMG electrodes may be affixed using a collodion-soaked gauze pad in the manner of the EEG leads.

Derivations. The EMG is recorded bipolarly. Any combination of the three placements can be used; the pair selected should produce the record of highest quality. The primary reason for using three electrodes (even though only two are recorded at any given time) is to ensure that there is always a back-up electrode in case of failure of one placement. Availability of a back-up is important, especially if electrodes remain in place during the daytime when subjects are eating and talking. To monitor bruxism, one EMG may be offset to a location over the masseter muscle.

General Considerations for Recording Sleep

A minimal four-channel montage for recording sleep is shown in Table 100–1. If channels are limited, it is possible to use a single EOG channel, although this practice is discouraged. If more channels can be devoted to the sleep portion of the recording, an occipital EEG will be the most helpful addition. When limited to four sleep channels, some laboratories begin a night's recording with a central and an occipital EEG, a single EOG, and an EMG. After sleep onset, the occipital EEG is replaced with the second EOG.[11] Depending on the purpose of the recording, other selected parameters will be added to the montage to record respiration, heart rate, blood pressure, esophageal pH, penile circumference, or any of the many other available systems. To correlate other events with sleep stages, it is most convenient to output all signals to a single device. When more than one recording device is used, it is helpful if they are linked to a single time-code generator.

Most sleep laboratories use a standard chart paper speed of 10 or 15 mm/sec. Slower speeds are discouraged because clear visualization of alpha rhythm and

Table 100–1. MONTAGE FOR MONITORING SLEEP STATES

Parameter	Derivation	Back-Up or Option
EEG	C3/A2	C4/A1
EOG	ROC/A1	ROC/A1
	and	and
	LOC/A1	LOC/A2
EMG	Mentalis/submentalis	
If additional channels are available, add the following:		
EEG	O1/A2	O2/A1
EOG	Infraorbital/supraorbital	

sleep spindles becomes extremely difficult. Faster paper speeds are unusual because of the generally prohibitive expense of the recording chart paper. A sensitivity that gives a pen deflection of 7.5 or 10.0 mm for a 50-μV signal is recommended for the EEG and EOG channels. The chin EMG amplification is often adjusted after the recording has begun so that an acceptable EMG recording is obtained. A known calibration of the central EEG leads is *essential* because of the amplitude criterion for scoring NREM stage 3 and 4 sleep. A calibration of 50 μV/cm is common. Greater amplification of the EEG may result in pen blocking during slow-wave sleep (stages 3 and 4), especially in younger subjects. Lower amplification may result in difficulty observing small-amplitude sleep spindles.

Electroencephalographic filtering should allow suitable visualization of a fairly wide range of signals, from slow waves (2 cps or less) to sleep spindles (12 to 14 cps). A high-frequency filter setting in the range of 30 to 35 cps will generally pass through the essential waveforms, while minimizing high-frequency (e.g., EMG) interference. A time constant of 0.3 sec or slower (corresponding to a half-amplitude low-frequency filter setting of about 0.3 cps) is recommended to ensure adequate coverage of slow wave activity.

The same settings are recommended for EOG channels. This filtering will pass both the rapid eye movements essential to scoring REM sleep and the SEMs characteristic of sleep onset and transitional stage 1 sleep. A faster time constant has been used in certain laboratories to reduce the "contamination" of EOG by EEG signals. In slow-wave (stages 3 and 4) sleep, however, the EEG activity seen in the EOG channels (with a slow time constant) tends to have fewer overriding fast components than the central leads and may therefore be helpful in distinguishing the slow EEG components. Thus, the slower time constant for EOGs may be doubly helpful.

The EMG is generally recorded with a much higher setting on both high- and low-pass filters. A low-pass setting of 70 or 75 cps is common (with notch filtering of alternating current [AC] interference, e.g., 60 Hz). High-pass filtering at 10 cps (time constant = 0.015 sec) is useful to prevent slow signals from interfering with the EMG tracing. The standard manual recommends a time constant for EMG of 0.1 sec or faster.[1] The absolute amplitude of EMG activity is not relevant to polysomnography; the emphasis, rather, is on relative changes in EMG amplitude. Thus, the EMG level is adjusted at the start of the record to provide an amplitude permitting such comparisons. An amplification of 20 μV/cm at the start of the recording will usually approximate a reasonable EMG level.

A number of special cases may require modification of the sensitivity, filter, and time constant settings just described. In certain patients (especially older individuals), the amplitude of the EEG using the standard gain may be so small that the record is extremely difficult to evaluate. The gain may be increased so that a 50-μV pulse gives a pen deflection of 15 mm. By contrast, the amplitude of the EEG in some young children is so great that the pen sweep is not large

enough to register the signal. In this instance, the sensitivity of EEG channels (and EOG channels) may be reduced so that a 50-μV pulse causes a pen deflection of 5 mm.

The EEG and EOG channels may also pick up a very low-frequency artifact related to sweat. If extreme, "sweat artifact" can make the record virtually unscorable. When a correction cannot be made by re-referencing or by lowering the room temperature, the low-frequency cutoff may be set at 1.0 cps (time constant = 0.1 sec). This step is recommended only in extreme cases in adults; in children, sweat artifact usually does not need to be extreme to justify changing the low-frequency filter because children have such pervasive slow wave activity in stages 3 and 4 sleep. One should never use the 5-cps low-frequency cutoff setting for the EEG because the slow frequencies of stage 3 and 4 sleep would be lost entirely.

A sleep tracing requires constant vigilance during the night, and a key concern is that the technologist stays awake and alert. The recording must be observed frequently to check for paper jams, ink clogs, recording artifacts, changes in pen alignment, and so forth. This requirement for technologist vigilance makes the process of laboratory sleep recording a labor-intensive procedure; however, it also eliminates the necessity of retesting because of lost data, which may occur when out-of-laboratory procedures are used.

PROCEDURES FOR STAGING SLEEP

General Considerations

The standard sleep staging manual[1] provides detailed guidelines and criteria for staging normal human sleep. The following material does not supersede the manual but is intended to be supplementary.

Several general concepts, referring primarily to the EEG, are helpful when one approaches sleep stage scoring. It should first be noted that the sleep research community has adopted the EEG convention of "negative up," which simply means that a signal of negative polarity is shown as an upward pen deflection. Second, a number of the standard guidelines refer to the frequency of the EEG waves. Frequency is measured as cycles (each cycle is the complete series of potential changes before the series repeats) per second. A few common EEG frequency bands are as follows:

1. Alpha rhythm: 8 to 13 cps
2. Beta rhythm: more than 13 cps
3. Delta rhythm: less than 4 cps
4. Theta rhythm: 4 to 7 cps

The amplitude measures used in sleep staging are taken from trough to peak (or peak to trough) of the wave, rather than from baseline or zero crossing to peak or trough.

When a sleep recording is scored, it is customary to divide the chart into convenient segments and to assign a sleep stage value to each segment or epoch. The most common epoch length is 30 or 20 sec, which

Table 100–2. PARTIAL LISTING OF EVENTS THAT MAY BE CODED WITHIN OR ACROSS EPOCHS

Body movement	Penile tumescence
Movement arousal	T_{up}
Transient arousal	T_{max}
Microsleep episodes	T_{down}
K-alpha complex	Heart rate irregularities
Esophageal pH abnormalities	Asystole
Respiratory abnormalities	Premature ventricular
Apnea	contraction (PVC)
Obstructive	Premature atrial contraction
Central	(PAC)
Mixed	Tachycardia
Hypopnea (usually ≥10 sec)	Bradycardia
Obstructive	Oxygen saturation
Central	Below 90%
Mixed	Below 80%
Paradoxical respiration	REM phasic events
Cheyne-Stokes respiration	Twitches
Periodic breathing	Rapid eye movements
Periodic movements	Middle ear muscle activity
With arousal	Periorbital integrated
Without arousal	potentials

corresponds to a single page of chart paper 300 mm wide recorded with a chart speed of 10 or 15 mm/ sec. A 1-min scoring epoch has also been used (see particularly Williams et al.[12]), although such a long epoch may overlook stage changes of relatively short duration.[13] A scoring epoch shorter than 20 sec is considered too tedious by most groups, although epochs as short as 3 sec have been used for specific research purposes.

Each epoch is assigned a score that most appropriately characterizes the predominant pattern occurring during that interval. Thus, the purpose of epoch staging is to determine the single descriptive factor that most fully characterizes the epoch. Any number of additional codes may be used to denote activities or events occurring within (or across) an epoch. Thus, for example, the standard manual describes "movement arousals," which are short-lived events occurring within an epoch but not descriptive of the majority of the epoch. With the increasing application of polysomnography to clinical assessments, the variety of possible events to be evaluated has grown markedly. Table 100–2 gives a partial listing of events that are coded by various laboratories. To date, these events have usually been defined within each laboratory because standard consensus descriptions are generally lacking. Laboratories typically select those events that are of local experimental or clinical relevance. Event coding is an extremely valuable adjunct to sleep staging but is not a substitute for sleep staging.

Sleep Staging in Normal Adult Human Beings

The following material summarizes the criteria described in the standard manual[1] for staging normal human sleep. Although these criteria apply most specifically to adults, they have also been used to characterize sleep in children and adolescents.[14, 15] A separate set of criteria, however, is generally deemed necessary in newborns[16] and older infants.[17] The standard sleep staging criteria in adults, according to the three electrographic parameters, are outlined in Table 100–3 and described below.

Relaxed Wakefulness. The majority of human beings show an EEG of rhythmic alpha activity (in the range of 8 to 13 cps) when relaxed with the eyes closed (Fig. 100–2). This activity is maximal occipitally but also often occurs centrally. This rhythmic EEG pattern attenuates with attention, as well as when the eyes are open (Fig. 100–3), at which time the waking EEG pattern is best characterized as one of relatively low voltage and mixed frequency. In an excessively sleepy individual, rhythmic alpha activity may be present when the eyes are open and may attenuate with eye closure; in this case, alpha attenuation is related to the intrusion of stage 1 sleep.

When a person is awake, control of eye movements is voluntary. The waking EOG tracing generally consists of rapid eye movements and eye blinks when the eyes are open and few or no eye movements with the eyes closed. Involuntary slow, rolling eye movements (with eyes closed) often characterize the EOG in the seconds to minutes preceding the EEG change to stage 1 sleep.

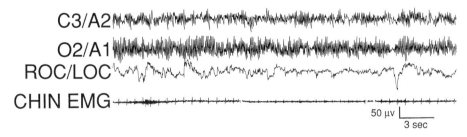

Figure 100–2. Rhythmic EEG alpha activity is clearly evident in the C3/A2 and O2/A1 tracings of this young adult male volunteer who is awake with his eyes closed. Figures 100–2 to 100–7 and 100–9 to 100–13 are all taken from an overnight recording of a 19-year-old normal male volunteer. All leads were recorded on a Grass Instruments Company Model 78 polygraph. The central and occipital EEGs and the electro-oculograms (EOGs) used a low-frequency cutoff of 0.3 cps, a high-frequency cutoff of 30 cps, and sensitivity of 50 μV/cm. The electromyogram (EMG) was recorded with a low-frequency cutoff of 10 cps, high-frequency cutoff of 60 cps, and sensitivity of 20 μV/cm. Paper speed was 10 mm/sec. In Figures 100–2 to 100–5, the EOG is monitored with a single lead (ROC/LOC). In Figures 100–9 to 100–13, the occipital tracing has been dropped, and the EOG is recorded from two leads, ROC/A1 and LOC/A2. (See text for comments on the latter procedure.)

Table 100–3. OUTLINE OF SLEEP SCORING CRITERIA ACCORDING TO STANDARD MANUAL

Stage/State	EEG	EOG	EMG
Relaxed Wakefulness	**Eyes closed:** rhythmic alpha (8–13 cps); prominent in occipital; attenuates with attention **Eyes open:** relatively low voltage, mixed frequency	Voluntary control; REMs or none; blinks; SEMs when drowsy	Tonic activity, relatively high; voluntary movement
NREM			
Stage 1	Relatively low voltage, mixed frequency May be theta (3–7 cps) activity with greater amplitude Vertex sharp waves Synchronous high-voltage theta bursts in children	SEMs	Tonic activity, may be slight decrease from waking
Stage 2	**Background:** relatively low voltage, mixed frequency **Sleep spindles:** waxing, waning, 12–14 cps (≥0.5 sec) **K complex:** negative sharp wave followed immediately by slower positive component (≥0.5 sec); spindles may ride on Ks; Ks maximal in vertex; spontaneous or in response to sound	Occasionally SEMs near sleep onset	Tonic activity, low level
Stage 3	≥20 ≤50% high amplitude (>75 μV), slow frequency (≤2 cps); maximal in frontal	None, picks up EEG	Tonic activity, low level
Stage 4	>50% high amplitude, slow frequency	None, picks up EEG	Tonic activity, low level
REM	Relatively low voltage, mixed frequency Sawtooth waves Theta activity; slow alpha	Phasic REMs	Tonic suppression; phasic twitches
Movement Time	Obscured	Obscured	Very high activity
*Anomalous Sleep**	Similar to REM	Phasic REMs	Tonic activity; phasic twitches

*Described in reference 44.
Modified from Rechtschaffen A, Kales A, eds. A Manual of Standardized Terminology: Techniques and Scoring System for Sleep Stages of Human Subjects. Los Angeles, Calif: UCLA Brain Information Service/Brain Research Institute; 1968.

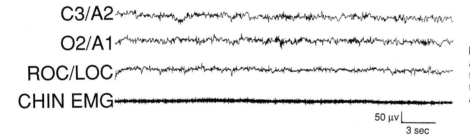

Figure 100–3. Attenuation of waking EEG alpha activity with eyes open is illustrated in this tracing. Note the characteristic "relatively low-voltage, mixed-frequency" EEG activity.

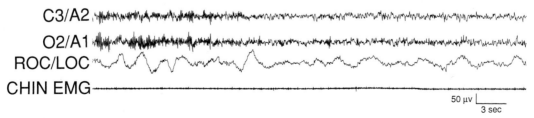

Figure 100–4. A transition from wakefulness to stage 1 sleep is illustrated in this figure, which clearly shows the attenuation of alpha that marks the onset of stage 1 sleep. As described in Figure 100–3 for an EEG of wakefulness with the eyes open, the EEG pattern of stage 1 sleep is described as one of "relatively low voltage, mixed frequency." Note, too, the presence of slow eye movements in the EOG tracing.

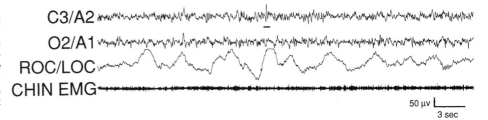

Figure 100–5. Vertex sharp waves are a common feature of the onset of stage 1 sleep. Few were seen in this volunteer, however, although one *(underlined)* is illustrated in this figure. Note that the vertex sharp wave is visible in the C3/A2 lead, but not in the O2/A1 lead, emphasizing localization to the vertex region.

The EMG shows tonic activity of a relatively high level. Voluntary movements produce phasic increases of EMG amplitude. In very relaxed individuals, waking EMG tonus may be indistinguishable from NREM sleep.

NREM Sleep. The four NREM sleep stages are distinguished, as mentioned previously, principally by changes in EEG pattern. The EOG and EMG patterns contribute little to NREM sleep staging, except in the case of transitional stage 1 NREM sleep, in which both may be useful. Therefore, the discussion below will focus on EEG.

Stage 1. The transition from wakefulness to stage 1 sleep (Fig. 100–4) is most clearly visualized on the EEG when the waking pattern has well-defined rhythmic alpha activity. It is for this reason that an occipital derivation is frequently added to the sleep recording montage, because waking alpha is most prominent in this cortical region. The EEG pattern of stage 1 is described as relatively low-voltage, mixed-frequency activity. Especially during stage 1 sleep occurring at the beginning of the night, vertex sharp waves (Fig. 100–5) are common. In addition, the EEG activity with the highest relative amplitude during stage 1 sleep is generally in the theta (3 to 7 cps) range. Bursts of relatively high-voltage, very synchronous theta activity are common during the onset of stage 1 sleep in children and young adolescents (Fig. 100–6).

The SEMs commonly precede the EEG transition to stage 1 sleep from wakefulness. Although the onset of SEMs usually leads the EEG transition by only 1 or 2 min, the lead time may occasionally—particularly in daytime recordings—be as long as 15 min.[18] Slow eye movements are very useful to distinguish stage 1 sleep transitions occurring during stage 2 NREM sleep or REM sleep.

Muscle tone is maintained during all NREM sleep stages and registers as low-amplitude EMG activity. There generally is no discrete change in EMG amplitude in the wake-to-sleep transition, although a gradual diminution of the EMG signal amplitude may occur within moments of the transition. During NREM sleep, the EMG is most helpful for distinguishing movement arousals, which are useful in certain stage change decisions. In addition, a rise in EMG activity often will be the only discrete indicator of a transition to stage 1 sleep within a REM sleep episode (see Fig. 100–12).

Stage 2. The background EEG of stage 2 NREM sleep is a pattern of relatively low-voltage, mixed-frequency activity. Stage 2 is distinguished from stage 1 on the basis of two specific EEG patterns that occur sporadically on this mixed-frequency background: the sleep spindle and K complex (Fig. 100–7). Because these stage 2 defining EEG patterns occur episodically, the standard staging criteria[1] provide for a default to stage 1 sleep if neither a sleep spindle nor a K complex occurs within a 3-min span when the EEG is of relatively low voltage and mixed frequency (the "3-min" rule).

In their most pure presentation, sleep spindles, have a waxing and waning spindle shape (Fig. 100–8), composed of waves in the range of 12 to 14 cps, with a duration of about 0.5 to 1.5 sec.[19] Sleep spindles are a common feature of mammalian sleep, and when recorded using identical techniques, they are indistinguishable, for example, between human beings and cats.[20] Sleep spindle activity occurs during stage 2 sleep, with a frequency of about three to eight spindles per minute in normal adults[21] or insomniac adults,[22] and spindle rate appears to be a fairly stable individual characteristic.[21] "Incipient sleep spindles" may appear near the stage 1 to stage 2 transition early during sleep; however, "the presence of a spindle should not be defined unless it is of at least 0.5 sec duration, i.e., one should be able to count 6 or 7 distinct waves within the half-second period."[1]

From an ontogenetic perspective, sleep spindles in the human being usually develop before age 3 months.[23, 24] In mentally retarded infants, sleep spindles are slower to develop and occur less frequently than

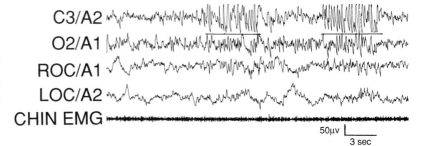

Figure 100–6. Very high-voltage, highly synchronous theta activity *(underlined)* is common during sleep onset stage 1 in children and young adolescents. This phenomenon is illustrated here in a tracing from a 14-year-old male volunteer. (Recording parameters are as described in the legend for Figure 100–2, with the exception that EEGs were recorded with a low-frequency cutoff of 1.0 cps.)

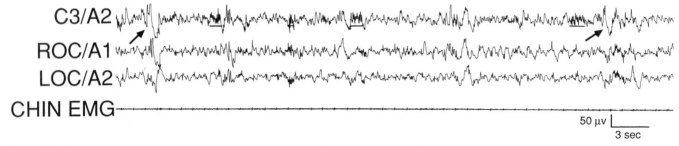

Figure 100–7. A stage 2 sleep pattern is illustrated in this figure. The arrows indicate K complexes, and sleep spindles are underlined. Note that K complexes are seen in the EOG tracings but are distinct from eye movements because the EOG tracings are in phase with one another. The last K complex in this figure illustrates the coincidence of a sleep spindle and a K complex, seen as relative low-voltage activity of spindle frequency (12 to 14 cps) on the trailing portion of the K complex.

in normal infants.[25] In old persons, sleep spindles tend to lose their classic morphology and have a slightly slower frequency, lower amplitude, and shorter duration[26, 27] than in the young adult. Benzodiazepine hypnotics tend to increase the density of sleep spindles in stage 2 sleep.[22, 28]

Sleep spindles* are absent in stage 1 NREM but may occur in REM sleep, particularly in subjects or patients whose sleep has been restricted or fragmented. If a single sleep spindle occurs in the middle of a REM sleep episode, it is not considered to be indicative of a stage change. If, however, two sleep spindles bracket half a scoring epoch or longer with no REMs intervening, the interval between spindles is considered a stage 2 sleep interruption of the REM episode.

The K complex (see Fig. 100–7) is another sleep-specific EEG waveform that is characteristic of stage 2 sleep. This paroxysmal wave complex consists of a "well-delineated negative sharp wave which is immediately followed by a positive component. The total duration of the complex should exceed 0.5 sec."[1] The standard manual provides no amplitude criterion for K complexes. There usually is very little difficulty in discerning K complexes in stage 2 sleep. The following definition used by electroencephalographers for the term *complex* is very helpful when a K complex distinction is in doubt, as may occur in stage 3 and 4 sleep, when it is sometimes difficult to differentiate K complexes from high-voltage slow wave activity. A complex is a "group of two or more waves, clearly distinguished from background activity and occurring with

_____
*The term *K complex* may be substituted for *sleep spindle* throughout this paragraph.

a well-recognized form or recurring with consistent form."[29] A key part of this definition is that the complex is distinct from the ongoing background activity, which makes the K complex in stage 2 very clear, whereas the same morphology embedded within a series of high-voltage, slow wave activity during stage 3 or 4 would probably not stand out from the background.

K complexes are maximal over the vertex. It is very common for spindle activity (12 to 14 cps) to ride over the K complex. In young adults, the typical density of K complexes in stage 2 is about 1 to 3 per minute,[21, 30, 31] although there is considerable individual variability. K complexes occur spontaneously during stage 2 sleep and are also evoked in response to auditory stimuli.

At the beginning of the night, SEMs may infrequently and only very briefly persist after the appearance of sleep spindles and K complexes. Because the EOG channels also register EEG activity, K complexes can reflect on these channels (see Fig. 100–7). They are generally easily distinguished from rapid eye movements because the pens on the two channels deflect in phase and because the central EEG amplitude of a K complex is usually much greater than any EEG activity related to eye movements. The EMG during stage 2 sleep is tonically active, generally at a low amplitude relative to wakefulness.

Stages 3 and 4. The EEG of stage 3 and 4 sleep is defined by the presence of high-voltage slow wave activity (Figs. 100–9 and 100–10). In stage 3 sleep, "at least 20 per cent but not more than 50 per cent of the epoch consists of waves of 2 cps or slower which have amplitudes greater than 75 μV from peak to peak (the difference between the most negative and positive points of the wave)."[1] In stage 4 sleep, such waves predominate (more than 50% of the epoch). Sleep spindles can occur during stages 3 and 4, as can K complexes; however, they are only infrequently distinct from the background EEG activity, particularly in stage 4 sleep. Eye movements do not occur during stage 3 and 4 sleep, although the EOG will register the high-voltage slow wave activity. The EMG during stages 3 and 4 is tonically active, although the tracing may occasionally achieve very low levels, nearly indistinguishable from that of REM sleep.

REM Sleep. Staging REM sleep requires the coinci-

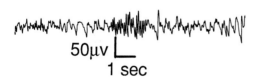

Figure 100–8. A sleep spindle from stage 2 sleep in a normal 16-year-old adolescent girl is illustrated in this figure. The activity is grossly spindle shaped, with waxing and waning amplitude. Elderly volunteers and many patients with sleep disorders no longer have spindles with this morphology. The "spindles" tend to be shorter and of lower amplitude in such individuals.

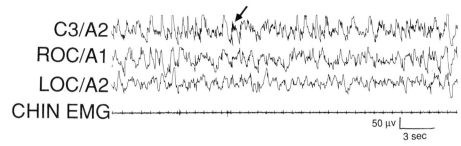

Figure 100–9. Stage 3 sleep is scored when the EEG pattern consists of high-voltage (≥75 µV), slow (≤2 cps) activity in 20% or more, but less than 50%, of a scoring epoch, as illustrated in this figure. Sleep spindles may occur in stage 3 sleep; the arrow indicates a spindle in this example of stage 3 sleep. Note that the EOG tracings pick up the high-voltage, slow wave activity, which can be seen in the ROC and LOC leads as in-phase deflections.

dence of specific activities in all three electrographic measures: "activated" or "desynchronized" EEG, bursts of rapid eye movements, and suppression of EMG activity (Fig. 100–11). The REM sleep EEG pattern is characterized as one of "relatively low voltage, mixed frequency."[1] An EEG pattern called sawtooth waves—because of their notched morphology—is fairly common during REM sleep,[32] particularly in proximity to eye movements, but is by no means a universal phenomenon. Thus, the presence of sawtooth activity is not required for staging REM sleep, although it may be very useful in equivocal instances. Sawtooth waves achieve the highest amplitude at the vertex[33] and, like much other REM sleep EEG activity, have a frequency in the theta range. Activity in the alpha range (usually 1 to 2 cps slower than waking alpha activity) may also be seen in the REM sleep EEG.[34]

Ponto-geniculo-occipital (PGO) spikes are a definitive feature of feline REM sleep,[35] and rhythmic hippocampal theta activity is a prominent REM feature in many primates, cats, dogs, and rodents.[36] In cats, PGO spikes occur singly in the transition to REM sleep and in bursts during REM sleep, usually leading other REM sleep phasic events. The scalp EEG routinely recorded in human beings is not clearly related to these characteristic REM sleep patterns of other species. Hodes and Dement,[37] however, suggested that K complexes in human beings may be an analog of the pre-REM PGO spikes because both pre-REM events are similarly associated with EMG and reflex suppression. Depth EEG recordings in human beings have also suggested the presence of PGO spikes in REM sleep.[38]

The EOG reveals bursts of rapid eye movements

at intervals during REM sleep (see Fig. 100–11). The acronym REM originated with these eye movements, of course, although the term is now used to denote the full constellation of physiological events constituting this state. The density of rapid eye movement bursts within REM sleep varies with time of night; thus, earlier REM episodes contain fewer rapid eye movements than do later REM episodes.[39] The episodic nature of this sign of REM sleep often requires the sleep record scorer to scan the chart in advance of the epoch currently under scrutiny. The criteria of the standard manual[1] provide contingencies for such contextual decisions, as will be described below.

For an epoch to be considered REM sleep, in addition to the activated EEG and REM bursts, an EMG recorded in the manner described previously must obtain its lowest value. A universal feature of REM sleep in the intact organism is the tonic suppression of skeletal muscle tone and reflexes via a circuit that involves pontine activation of medullary inhibitory centers and culminates in postsynaptic hyperpolarization of brainstem and spinal motoneurons.[40] Superimposed on this background of tonic motor inhibition can be seen occasional twitches of distal muscles. In household pets, for example, paws, face, and whiskers show twitches in REM sleep. In human polysomnographic recordings, twitches appear as very short-lived EMG elevations, usually in proximity to eye movement bursts (see Fig. 100–11). Prolonged EMG elevation (15 sec or longer) in REM sleep, even in the absence of an EEG change, requires a stage shift (Fig. 100–12). Brief EMG elevations associated with an alteration in EEG or EOG activity (i.e., movement arousal) may signal a stage

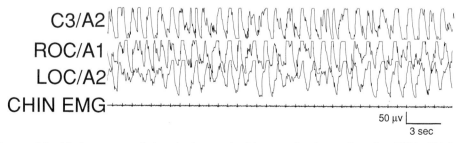

Figure 100–10. As illustrated in this figure, stage 4 sleep is characterized by a predominance (less than 50%) of high-voltage slow waves in the EEG. In this sample tracing, the slow wave EEG amplitude is so great that the pen-swing limitation of the recorder is exceeded and pen "blocking" distorts the wave shapes.

change, depending on the relative size of this movement and duration of the EEG and EOG alterations.

Both REM sleep and NREM stage 2 sleep require the presence of episodic events: bursts of rapid eye movements in REM sleep and spindles or K complexes in stage 2. In both, the background EEG is similar, that is, relatively low voltage, mixed frequency. Scoring transitions from stage 2 to REM sleep (Fig. 100–13) and from REM level to stage 2, as well as stage 2 interruptions of REM sleep (Fig. 100–14), is therefore sometimes problematic. Two fundamental guidelines in the standard manual[1]—listed below—enable one to deal with virtually every contingency.

1. Any section of record contiguous with stage REM sleep in which the EEG shows relatively low voltage and mixed frequency is scored stage REM sleep regardless of whether rapid eye movements are present, providing EMG is at the stage REM level and there are no intervening movement arousals.
2. An interval of relatively low-voltage, mixed-frequency EEG record between two sleep spindles or K complexes is considered stage 2 regardless of EMG level, if there are no rapid eye movements or movement arousals during this interval and if the interval is less than 3 min long.

The manual provides a variety of specific examples that apply these guidelines, and the reader is urged to review them.

Movement Time. Gross postural readjustments are fairly common during sleep, often occurring in the vicinity of REM episodes.[4] When such movements arise from sleep, immediately precede sleep, and obscure the EEG activity (and usually the EOG as well) for at least one half the scoring epoch, that epoch is designated "movement time." If this pattern is preceded or followed by wakefulness, it is scored as an awake pattern.

Considerations for Staging Sleep in Pathologies

The standard manual was developed to provide guidelines for staging sleep in normal adult human beings, and its recommendations are suitable for many pathologies as well. Nevertheless, full characterization of sleep in a number of sleep-related pathologies at times requires one to depart from the standard procedures. The following material briefly reviews certain issues that may arise in specific disorders and suggests alternatives for addressing these issues.

Narcolepsy. The sleep of patients with narcolepsy is characterized by sleep onset REM episodes (the occurrence of rapid eye movements within 15 min of sleep onset), mixtures of stage 2 and REM sleep, and numerous arousals relative to normal persons.[41] Each of these phenomena can be characterized using the guidelines of the standard manual. Particular care is often required, however, and one may wish to use additional procedures, such as adding a vertical EOG, to assist in identifying a brief, early REM episode. An early REM episode may not last sufficiently long to characterize a full epoch (e.g., longer than 15 sec) as REM sleep; its occurrence may nonetheless be diagnostically relevant and must be noted.

The most problematic area with narcolepsy generally involves patients who are medicated with tricyclic antidepressants. Tricyclics are commonly noted to have an REM-suppressant effect[42]; however, a REM-like state—characterized by an elevated EMG in the presence of an activated EEG and phasic rapid eye movements—occurs with a periodicity similar to that of REM sleep.[43] One might characterize this as an "anomalous" state, as shown in Table 100–3. Thus, epochs of anomalous sleep may be accounted for outside the standard criteria and staged as neither REM nor NREM sleep.[44]

Sleep Apnea Syndromes. Patients with sleep apnea syndromes experience a great increase in the frequency of arousals from sleep and in the number of body movements. Both types of activity have an impact on sleep staging. For example, a patient may be clearly asleep and apneic for 10 sec, and movement associated with the termination of the apnea may obscure the remainder of the epoch (Fig. 100–15). Another common occurrence in patients with sleep apnea syndromes is the appearance of K complexes almost exclusively at the termination of apneas. If scored exclusively using the standard guidelines, sleep might never be found in such patients or might appear as only stage 1 and movement time. The following suggestions (modified from Flagg and Coburn[45]) for scoring sleep in such patients attempt to account for these pathological events.

1. Follow standard guidelines for entry into stage 1 from wakefulness and stage 2 from stage 1. (Coding "microsleep" episodes [less than half the epoch with stage 1 EEG] at the onset of sleep may be useful.)
2. Once stage 2 sleep is scored, continue stage 2 through any arousal that does not result in a transition to wakefulness (more than half the epoch with waking EEG). (Coding "transient arousals" [see below] may be useful.)
3. In REM sleep, ignore EMG elevations that are clearly associated with snoring.
4. In adults, stages 3 and 4 may be combined. (Some investigators[45] recommend combining stages 2, 3, and 4 in patients with sleep apnea. Such crude categorization may obscure clinically relevant information and is not recommended, particularly for children.)

Alpha-Delta Sleep. An EEG pattern of alpha intrusion into NREM sleep was first noted in patients with psychiatric disorders.[46] The pattern was described as "a mixture of 5–20 per cent delta waves (more than 75 μV, 0.5–2 cps) combined with relatively large amplitude, alpha-like rhythms (7–10 cps). These alpha rhythms are usually 1–2 cps slower than waking alpha." A similar pattern has been related to a complaint of "nonrestorative" sleep in patients with musculoskeletal pain or fibrositis.[47] This EEG pattern might legitimately be scored as NREM stage 1 or 2, but the

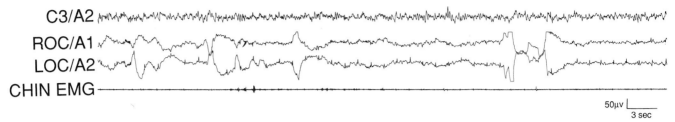

Figure 100–11. REM sleep is scored when the EEG pattern is one of relatively low voltage, mixed frequency; the EMG is tonically suppressed; and the EOG shows rapid eye movements. Each of these REM sleep components is present in this figure. The early and late portions of the figure, in which eye movement bursts occur along with EMG twitches in the earlier portion, might be characterized as "phasic" REM sleep, whereas the intervening segment containing no eye movements might be called "tonic" REM sleep. Note that eye movements appear as out-of-phase deflections in the ROC and LOC tracings.

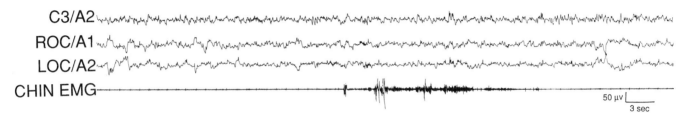

Figure 100–12. This figure shows an example of stage 1 sleep interrupting an REM episode. The interruption is seen as a tonic increase in EMG activity lasting longer than 50% of the scoring epoch. This change is scored even if the EEG pattern shows no discernible difference and even if no slow eye movements occur.

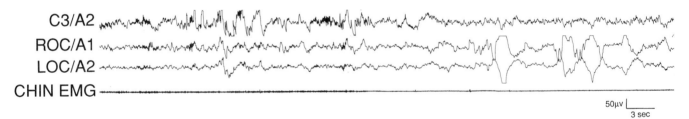

Figure 100–13. This figure illustrates a transition from stage 2 NREM sleep to REM sleep, in which the three markers of REM sleep occur in fairly close proximity. EMG suppression leads the EEG desynchronization by a few seconds, and bursts of rapid eye movements occur several seconds later. It is not uncommon for several minutes to elapse during such a transition.

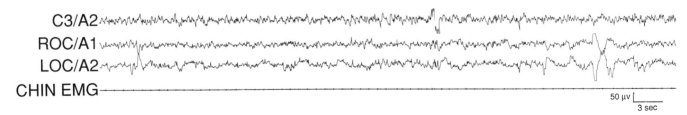

Figure 100–14. In this figure, an isolated K complex occurs in the midst of an REM episode. The episode is staged as REM sleep despite the K complex (refer to Rule 1). Had a second K complex or sleep spindle occurred, spanning more than 50% of the scoring epoch, the interval would be staged as stage 2 sleep, even if the background EEG resembled the REM pattern and the EMG were at the REM sleep level.

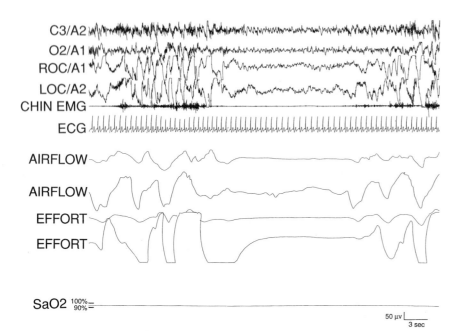

Figure 100–15. Sleep onset is aborted by a large movement associated with the termination of an episode of sleep apnea. Note that the "scorable" portion of this epoch contains only about 12 sec of stage 1 sleep, which is insufficient to characterize the entire 30-sec epoch. For this type of occurrence, the coding of a microsleep event might be useful, along with the coding of an apneic event.

clinical implications of this type of "sleep" require that it be noted and remarked on. Thus, one might define a separate sleep "stage" or use an "event" code to make this pattern accessible for separate analysis.

Transient Arousals. Many sleep disorders involve frequent, brief arousals that do not alter sleep stage scoring but that may be clinically relevant. Such arousals are a common feature of normal aging as well. Clinical implications of these brief arousals have been shown in several types of study. For example, brief arousals induced experimentally into the sleep of normal volunteers resulted in daytime sleepiness, even though the total amount of sleep was unchanged.[48] In addition, spontaneously occurring transient arousals in elderly subjects have been correlated with waking alertness level.[49] This type of arousal occurs frequently in patients with sleep apnea syndromes, periodic movements in sleep, and other sleep disorders. Therefore, cataloguing such events may be relevant in several clinical and nonclinical populations. The following definition has been proposed for transient arousals[49]: "any clearly visible EEG arousal (usually alpha rhythm) lasting two seconds or longer, but not associated with any stage or state change in the epoch scoring. These brief arousals are sometimes, but not always, associated with a body movement or respiration event." To this definition we add the recommendation that transient arousals in REM sleep be coded only when EEG alpha activity is associated with another sign of arousal (e.g., increased heart rate, EMG elevation, or respiration irregularity) because alpha activity is a fairly common feature of REM sleep.[34] A task force of the American Sleep Disorders Association (ASDA) has defined a set of scoring rules and has provided examples for coding EEG arousals during sleep.[50]

The ASDA coding system has initiated a renewed interest in sleep-related arousals, an aspect of sleep staging that has beleaguered sleep researchers and clinicians for decades. For example, a 1999 task force of the American Academy of Sleep Medicine focused on the role of repiratory-effort related arousal events in helping define the severity of the obstructive sleep apnea-hypopnea syndrome[50a] (see Chapters 79 and 101). Furthermore, as more investigators examine sleep in newly described sleep disorders and other medical disorders, this interest in sleep fragmentation strengthens. For example, the description of upper airway resistance syndrome (UARS)[51] rekindled interest in EEG arousals because the respiratory signs of UARS are less obvious than those in frank obstructive sleep apnea syndrome (OSAS) and only subtle indicators may be available.[52] In addition, the ASDA arousal staging system and related research have stimulated an examination or reexamination of arousals in other disorders such as allergic rhinitis,[53, 54] juvenile rheumatoid arthritis,[55] and Parkinson's disease.[56]

Others have begun to examine variations of the ASDA arousal scoring schema, and still others suggest that non-EEG markers may be important and even more reliable signs of arousal than the EEG. Pitson and Stradling,[57] for example, note that transient changes in blood pressure may signify arousals more reliably than cortical EEG, although Lofaso et al.[58] indicate that autonomic changes are highly correlated with the extent of EEG arousals. Less well studied is the possibility that certain sleep fragmenting phenomena are associated with subcortical events not visible in the cortical EEG signal. One suspects that such may be the case in sleep studies of children who manifest few cortical arousals even with prominent OSAS.

Automatic Sleep Stagers

Although many groups in the United States continue to analyze sleep data using human hand scoring of polysomnographic or digitally acquired tracings, several systems for automatically staging sleep have been proposed, and a number are commercially available.[59-66] Certain of these systems are based on the standard guidelines, although several approaches that confront the sleep staging issues more from the perspective of available technologies have also been used. Thus, instead of adapting digital computer technology to human eyeball scoring criteria, they use such techniques as frequency spectra analysis or multidimensional scaling,[59] adaptive segmentation and fuzzy subset theory,[60] or expert systems approaches.[61] No single automated stager has yet emerged as the ideal alternative to hand scoring, and space does not permit a review of available systems. The following questions are offered as a basis for evaluating automatic sleep staging systems (see Chapter 110):

1. Has the system been validated against another known assessment technique?
2. Is the system valid for the types of studies for which it will be used—for example, sleep only, sleep and breathing, sleep and movements, and so forth?
3. Is the system valid for the types of patients in whom it will be used—for example, sleep apneics versus narcoleptics, medicated versus non-medicated patients, and so on?
4. Is the system valid for the age groups in whom it will be used—children versus adults versus the elderly?
5. Is the system compatible with available laboratory hardware?
6. Does the system require excessive operator input (e.g., knob turning, "tweaking," fine tuning) that takes time equivalent to hand scoring?
7. Does the system provide output verification? That is, can the raw data be reviewed?
8. If the system does not automatically assess relevant events, can hand-scored events be accurately correlated to the stager's output?
9. Is the system sufficiently flexible to support future forseeable applications? Such applications might include changes in patient population, recording equipment, research orientation, and so forth.
10. Is the system supported by accessible consultants?

SUMMARIZING SLEEP STAGE DATA

After the sleep data are scored, they must be summarized into a comprehensible form. No consensus format has been achieved, and certain areas of controversy exist; however, a number of conventions are fairly common and include the following types of analysis. (Alternate calculation paradigms are sometimes used and have been noted where appropriate.) Figure 100–16 shows the output of one type of sleep data summary sheet.

Stages

A summary of the night will invariably include the time spent in each of the sleep stages, as well as time awake and movement time. This type of summary is relatively straightforward and noncontroversial. Calculation of percentage distributions is not quite as clear cut, as various groups may calculate sleep stage percentages based on total recording time (dark time), total sleep time (total NREM stages 1 to 4 plus REM), or sleep period time (time from sleep onset to sleep offset, including intervening arousals). The example in Figure 100–16 begs the question by using all three alternatives.

Latencies

The topic of latencies is associated with a certain amount of controversy, particularly because the type of patient may affect the appropriateness of specific definitions. Thus, although sleep latency, defined as elapsed time from lights out until the first of three consecutive epochs of stage 1 or the first of any other stage, may be appropriate for normal, noncomplaining individuals or for hypersomnolent patients, it may not be appropriate for patients with sleep onset insomnia. One alternative to the above definition requires stage 2 sleep (spindle or K complex) to define sleep onset.[65] To account for instances in which a patient may have 2 or 3 min of sleep followed by a lengthy awakening, definitions that require, for example, 5 consecutive min of sleep have been suggested by others.[66] The issue of the definition of sleep onset is nontrivial because latencies to stage 4 or REM sleep are generally calculated from sleep onset. Certain analysis programs have the capability to provide several calculations of sleep onset, whereas others provide the flexibility to redefine the criterion for individual cases. In the absence of a comprehensive database, it is not possible to make a sweeping generalization. A "safe" alternative for most clinical studies is probably to choose the conservative "5-min" rule or even a 10-min rule, although a briefer requirement might be more appropriate for patients with sleep apnea syndromes, in whom frequent awakenings may preclude such a "sleep onset" entirely.

Once a definition of sleep onset is established, determining stage 3 or 4 or REM latency is fairly straightforward: elapsed time from the (start of) defined sleep onset to the first epoch of stage 3 (or 4) or REM sleep. Certain groups may apply a "three-epoch" rule to this definition, that is, three consecutive epochs of the target stage are required. One point of dispute regarding REM latency calculation concerns whether or not to include any waking intervals that may occur between sleep onset and REM onset.[67] No firm recommendation can be made; however, it is still generally assumed that waking is included in the calculation, unless otherwise noted. Such considerations are crucial when data are compared across groups, which is particularly relevant when one uses norms from another laboratory.

T.A.

Subject's name:	T.A.
Subject's gender:	M
Subject's age:	14.0000 years
Subject's date of birth:	1/11/73
Subject's Tanner stage:	
Recording date:	1/11/87
Name of study:	T/A
Group:	
Recording condition:	PRETREATMENT
Recording technician:	CARSKADON
Scoring technician:	MANCUSO
Data entry technician:	MANCUSO

Minimum epoch length:	0.4800 minutes (Epoch 478 of Page 11)
Maximum epoch length:	0.5294 minutes (Epoch 965 of Page 10)
Average epoch length:	0.4975 minutes

	Epochs	Minutes	%TDT	%SPT	%TST
TDT	1179	586.50	-	-	-
SPT	1067	530.95	90.53	-	-
TST	1031	513.00	87.47	96.62	-
WASO	38	18.93	3.23	3.56	3.69
WAFA	82	41.00	6.99	7.72	7.99
TS1	93	46.09	7.86	8.68	8.98
TS2	546	272.43	46.45	51.31	53.11
TS3	92	45.62	7.78	8.59	8.89
TS4	167	82.91	14.14	15.61	16.16
TNREM	898	447.05	76.22	84.20	87.14
TREM	115	56.98	9.71	10.73	11.11
TSW	259	128.53	21.91	24.21	25.05
TWT	148	73.50	12.53	13.84	14.33
TMT	18	8.97	1.53	1.69	1.75

Rem Summary:

	REM1	REM2	REM3	REM4	TOTAL	MEAN
TT	3.93	8.95	21.80	27.20	61.89	15.47
REMT	2.95	8.95	21.80	23.27	56.98	14.24
S1	0.00	0.00	0.00	2.95	2.95	0.74
S2	0.98	0.00	0.00	0.00	0.98	0.25
WT	0.00	0.00	0.00	0.98	0.98	0.25
MT	0.00	0.00	0.00	0.00	0.00	0.00
SEG	2	1	1	3	7	1.75
Cycles	192.77	111.64	104.66	111.89	520.95	130.24

End of last REM from end of night: 51.00

Analysis by fraction (1/3):

	1	2	3
Wake	0.00	6.98	12.20
SW	91.94	13.18	23.41
REM	0.00	11.90	45.08

T/A, PRETREATMENT

Milestones:

Lights out:	22:14:00 (Epoch 27 of Page 1)
Sleep onset:	22:28:33 (Epoch 57 of Page 1)
Last sleep epoch:	7:19:00 (Epoch 602 of Page 13)
End of night:	8:00:30 (Epoch 685 of Page 13)

	REM	NREM	WAKE
Body movement (1)	1	43	1
Transient arousal (2)	0	4	0
Slow eye movement (4)	0	4	4
Microsleep (5)	0	0	5
Central Apnea/Hypopnea (7)	2	6	0
Obstructive Apnea/Hypopnea (A)	0	83	0
Mixed Apnea/Hypopnea (B)	0	1	0
SaO2<90% (C)	0	21	0
SaO2<80% (D)	0	0	0

Latencies (minutes):

Lights out to S1	13.58
Lights out to S2	14.55
Lights out to S3	23.50
Lights out to S4	26.00
Lights out to sleep onset	13.58
LO to 10 minutes continuous sleep	14.55
Sleep onset to slow wave	8.95
Sleep onset to REM	188.83

Figure 100–16. A sleep stage summary sheet is illustrated here. This sample represents only one of many possible summary formats. The data are taken from a night of sleep recorded in a 14-year-old boy with enlarged tonsils and adenoids who had moderately disordered breathing during sleep. The 25-min combining rule was used to define REM periods. The following definitions were used to derive specific items presented in this summary: TDT, total dark time (elapsed time from lights out to end of night); SPT, sleep period time (elapsed time from sleep onset to last epoch of sleep); TST, total sleep time; WASO, wake time after sleep onset; WAFA, wake time after final awakening; TS1 to TS4, total amount of stage 1, 2, 3, and 4 sleep; TNREM, total stages 1 + 2 + 3 + 4 sleep; TREM, total amount of REM sleep; TSW, total amount of stages 3 + 4 sleep; TWT, total amount of wakefulness; TMT, total amount of movement time. Definitions in the REM summary are as follows: TT, total time of the REM episode; REMT, amount of REM sleep; S1, S2, WT, and MT, as defined above; SEG, number of REM sleep segments within the REM period; cycles, elapsed time from sleep onset to end of first REM period, from end of first to end of second REM period, and so on. All other items are self-explanatory.

Cycles

A description of the NREM-REM cycle is a common feature of the night's sleep summary. Unfortunately, the defining characteristics for such a description are not standardized, and therefore, a number of idiosyncratic approaches have been used. One common way of defining cycles is as the elapsed time from the end of each REM episode to the end of the next REM episode, whereas another uses the time from the start of one REM episode to the start of the next. The consequences of choosing one alternative over the other

have not been clearly established. Another difficulty for defining REM cycles arises from the fact that REM sleep episodes are noncontinuous—that is, as described above, REM sleep may be interrupted by stages 1 or 2, wakefulness, or movement time. Thus, one must choose a "combining rule" for defining REM episodes, which in turn defines the cycle. In the past, combining rules of 0, 5, 10, 15, and 25 min have been used.[68] (Thus, a new REM cycle is begun when the NREM interval exceeds the time designated by the combining rule.) When data are evaluated using a number of alternatives, a 15- to 25-min rule is generally recom-

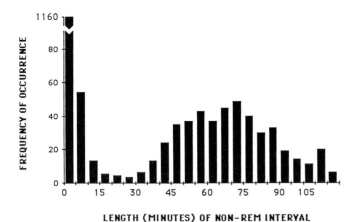

Figure 100–17. A frequency histogram illustrating the distribution of NREM (wakefulness, NREM sleep, and/or movement time) intervals of various duration during REM sleep episodes. Data are combined from the second laboratory night recorded in 82 adolescents, 18 young adults, and 26 elderly adults. Virtually no intervals of 15 to 30 min were recorded in these volunteers, suggesting that a combining rule in the range of 15 to 30 min will reflect the cyclic organization of REM sleep. (A 25-min combining rule was used in the sleep stage summary sheet in Figure 100–16.)

mended.[68] Dement[69] originally recommended a 25-min combining rule based on the frequency distribution of NREM intervals separating epochs of REM sleep. We replicated this finding, as illustrated in Figure 100–17, confirming Dement's results in adolescent, adult, and elderly volunteers. These data suggest that a combining rule of 15 to 30 min will provide the best description of REM sleep in human beings.

Partitioning the Night

For many years, it has been a common practice to examine at least waking, slow-wave (stages 3 + 4) sleep, and REM sleep by thirds of the night. This practice, at least for REM sleep, seems to have originated in early studies of insomnia and sleeping pills.[70] Its usefulness derives primarily from normative studies in young adults, in which one sees a predominance of stage 3 and 4 NREM sleep in the first third of sleep and a predominance of REM sleep toward the last third of sleep. In insomniacs, preferential distribution of waking to a third of the night may provide insight regarding the type of sleep problem.[71] Although these specific comparisons are not always useful or appropriate, the "thirds of night" analysis remains a valuable thumbnail description of a night's sleep. Other variations of this partitioning technique may use halves or quarters of the night or even hour-by-hour assessment (Fig. 100–18).

Events

Events coded during sleep (see Table 100–2) are frequently tabulated according to whether they occurred in NREM or REM sleep. Finer distinctions are rarely made. When the event spans more than one epoch (e.g., respiratory disturbance), it is recommended that it be catalogued according to the stage in which it began.

Figure 100–18. The sleep data summary may partition the night in one of several ways, depending on the purpose of the study or the questions being asked. The example in this figure, based on the night summarized in Figure 100–16, illustrates partitioning by thirds, quarters, and halves of the night and hour-by-hour across the night.

Analysis by fraction (1/3):

	1	2	3
Wake	0.00	6.98	12.20
SW	91.94	13.18	23.41
REM	0.00	11.90	45.08

Analysis by fraction (1/4):

	1	2	3	4
Wake	0.00	1.00	8.45	9.72
SW	79.29	12.65	19.48	17.11
REM	0.00	2.95	20.09	33.93

Analysis by fraction (1/2):

	1	2
Wake	1.00	18.18
SW	91.94	36.59
REM	2.95	54.03

Analysis by interval (60 minutes):

	1	2	3	4	5	6	7	8	9
Wake	0.00	0.00	0.00	0.00	5.50	1.48	3.47	0.00	17.53
SW	43.82	22.67	25.45	0.00	0.00	17.50	1.98	13.19	3.91
REM	0.00	0.00	0.00	2.95	4.55	4.41	21.80	0.00	23.27

Sleep Histogram

Another way to examine events is in correlation with the ongoing pattern of nocturnal sleep, as visualized using histogram plotting techniques. Figure 100–19 shows an example of such a plot. Sleep stages and transitions are illustrated in the upper portion of the plot and show the unfolding of sleep versus time. This type of graphic display has been used from the earliest modern sleep studies.[4] Events are usually plotted below the histogram, aligned temporally with their occurrence. This plotting technique provides a sometimes very helpful visual representation of the data, and many software packages that provide data reduction of sleep stages and events also have such plotting capabilities.

WHY STAGE SLEEP?

A number of investigators and clinicians coming to the field of sleep from other disciplines question the necessity for evaluating sleep stages, particularly in clinical conditions. Thus, for example, a pulmonary specialist may question sleep staging in a patient with apnea for whom the key issues to the specialist may be length of apnea, degree of desaturation, cardiac arrhythmias, and so forth. A urologist's focus may be penile circumference, which does not require distinctions of sleep staging. Thus, an argument can be and has been made for focusing on the pathological event rather than sleep per se. A few counterarguments are offered below.

Regulatory Physiology Differs From Waking to NREM to REM Sleep

As increasing numbers of systems are evaluated during naturally occurring wakefulness and sleep, it has become quite clear that many regulatory mechanisms are affected by state.[72] For example, the ventilatory responses to oxygen and carbon dioxide (see Chapter 16) are somewhat damped in NREM sleep and may be absent in REM sleep.[73, 74] Another dramatic example concerns thermoregulation. Thermoregulatory responses are only slightly altered in NREM sleep and virtually totally lacking in REM sleep.[75] Such marked state-dependent alterations in regulatory physiology must be taken into account to assess fully the implications of observed sleep-related pathologies.

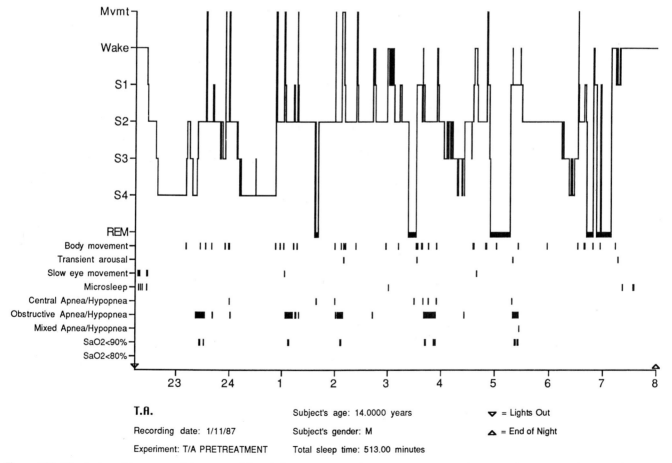

Figure 100–19. A sleep histogram of the same night of sleep summarized in Figure 100–16 is shown in this figure. The sleep histogram provides a graphic display of the night using an analog plot of sleep-wake stages across time *(upper portion).* Arrayed beneath this plot are event markers, which are temporally aligned.

Pathological Events Disturb Sleep

Patients with sleep apnea syndromes, for example, have markedly disrupted sleep. In children, the disruption may preferentially reduce stage 3 and 4 sleep,[76] and sleep apnea may be associated with growth problems[77]; in adults, sleep apnea is more likely to occur during, and be disruptive of, REM sleep.[78] The possible clinical relevance of such a sleep disturbance in a child is obvious but cannot be appreciated if sleep states are not evaluated. Documentation of recovery sleep following treatment may also provide insights into therapeutic efficacy that may be unrelated to the pathological events (apneas) per se.

Arousals consequent to sleep pathologies are also clinically relevant and require assessment to fully characterize the pathology. Thus, as mentioned previously, arousals are clearly related to daytime sleepiness.[48, 49] In the case of sleep apnea syndromes, a given treatment may improve the apnea–as documented by maintenance of SaO_2 at more than 85%, reduction in cardiac arrhythmias, and conversion of apneas to hypopneas– yet the patient may still suffer arousals from sleep sufficient to impair waking function or to be associated with a vulnerability to unintentional sleep episodes. Hence, it is relevant to evaluate sleep and arousals, as well as the respiratory function in such patients. Arousals may be a relevant issue in the case of periodic movements during sleep, as well. One study has documented clinical improvement of patients in whom periodic movements during sleep were treated with benzodiazepine hypnotics, although the number of movements was unchanged from pretreatment.[79] The number of associated arousals and the amount of transitional stage 1 sleep were reduced, however, a factor that would have been overlooked had sleep staging not been performed.

Sleep State May Affect Pathology

It has been known for many years that penile tumescence occurs in association with REM sleep in normal males of virtually all ages.[80] This phenomenon has been capitalized on to assess erectile dysfunction by recording REM sleep–related nocturnal penile tumescence (NPT).[81] Various clinicians, however, have attempted to perform studies of NPT in patients outside the sleep laboratory using such techniques as the "postage stamp method."[82] Other methodological considerations aside[83] (because the argument obtains even if appropriate NPT techniques are used without monitoring sleep stage), one cannot achieve a valid test of NPT if sleep is not assessed. This is true simply because an "abnormal" NPT can result if REM sleep is abnormal, disrupted, or absent. Sleep disorders themselves may have an impact on NPT as well.[84] Therefore, without evaluating sleep, it is not possible to determine whether tumescence did not occur because erectile function was impaired or sleep was disturbed.

Another example again concerns sleep apnea syndromes. As mentioned previously, sleep apneas in a percentage of adult patients may occur preferentially in REM sleep.[78] It has been suggested that diagnostic assessment of sleep apneas can be performed by monitoring respiration during a daytime nap.[85] In this case, in particular, sleep monitoring is essential because REM sleep may not occur during a daytime nap (depending on the time of the nap[86]), and therefore, the severity of sleep apnea may be very greatly underestimated. Without documentation of sleep state, such important clinical judgments (including optimal continuous positive airway pressure) may not be possible.[86a]

An Abnormal Sleep Architecture May Be a Marker of Pathology

Patients with narcolepsy often enter sleep through REM sleep, rather than experiencing the normal transition from waking to NREM sleep.[41, 87] Because the symptom presentation of narcolepsy is variable,[88] it is relevant to document the sleep onset transition in patients with complaints of hypersomnolence. Relatively short REM onset latencies are also thought to be a marker of endogenous depression.[89]

In summary, laboratory monitoring and staging of sleep remain important components in the assessment of patients with sleep disorders. The techniques derive directly from the earliest studies following the discovery of REM sleep in the 1950s, and some might criticize that the procedures have not kept pace with technological advances. Because automated, ambulant systems that are inexpensive, validated, and reliable are marketed, it is likely that polysomnography will advance accordingly.

The Newborn Infant

Because of rapid changes in the nervous system after birth, the well-defined *stages* seen in the adult are not present, and special criteria are used to define *states*. The standard scoring manual for neonates[16] defines sleep states using behaviors, respiration, eye movements, the EEG, and muscle tone. The following states were defined: active-REM sleep, quiet sleep, and indeterminate sleep. Criteria for defining these states with examples of sleep recordings in neonates are found in the standard scoring manual for neonates.[16]

Acknowledgments

We thank Lisa Donovan for typing the manuscript, Joan Mancuso for assembling the figures, and Sharon Keenan, REEGT, RPSGT, for her comments on the technical accuracy of the manuscript.

References

1. Rechtschaffen A, Kales A, eds. A Manual of Standardized Terminology: Techniques and Scoring System for Sleep Stages of Human Subjects. Los Angeles, Calif: UCLA Brain Information Service/Brain Research Institute; 1968.
2. Loomis AL, Harvey EN, Hobart GA. Electrical potentials of the human brain. J Exp Psychol. 1936;19:249–279.

3. Aserinsky E, Kleitman N. Regularly occurring periods of eye motility, and concomitant phenomena, during sleep. Science. 1953;118:273–274.

4. Dement WC, Kleitman N. Cyclic variations in EEG during sleep and their relation to eye movements, body motility, and dreaming. Electroencephalogr Clin Neurophysiol. 1957;9:673–690.

5. Berger RJ. Tonus of extrinsic laryngeal muscles during sleep and dreaming. Science. 1961;134:840.

6. Jouvet M, Michel M. Correlations electromyographiques du sommeil chez le chat décortique et mesencephalique chronique. CR Soc Biol (Paris). 1959;153:422–425.

7. Jasper HH (Committee Chairman). The ten twenty electrode system of the International Federation. Electroencephalogr Clin Neurophysiol. 1958;10:371–375.

8. Grass ER. A Second AIDS Alert. Quincy, Mass: Grass Instrument Company Bulletin; September 1–2, 1985.

9. Blake H, Gerard RW, Kleitman N. Factors influencing brain potentials during sleep. J Neurophysiol. 1939;2:48–60.

10. Brazier MAB. The electrical fields at the surface of the head during sleep. Electroencephalogr Clin Neurophysiol. 1949;1:195–204.

11. Carskadon MA. Basics for polygraphic monitoring of sleep. In: Guilleminault C, ed. Sleeping and Waking Disorders: Indications and Techniques. Menlo Park, Calif: Addison-Wesley: 1982:1–16.

12. Williams RL, Karacan I, Hursch CJ. EEG of Human Sleep: Clinical Applications. New York, NY: John Wiley & Sons; 1974.

13. Carskadon MA. The second decade. In: Guilleminault C, ed: Sleeping and Waking Disorders: Indications and Techniques. Menlo Park, Calif: Addison-Wesley; 1982:99–125.

14. Coble PA, Kupfer DJ, Taska LS, et al. EEG sleep of normal healthy children, part I: findings using standard measurement methods. Sleep. 1984;7:289–303.

15. Carskadon MA, Orav EJ, Dement WC. Evolution of sleep and daytime sleepiness in adolescents. In: Guilleminault C, Lugaresi E, eds. Sleep/Wake Disorders: Natural History, Epidemiology, and Long-Term Evolution. New York, NY: Raven Press; 1983:201–216.

16. Anders T, Emde R, Parmelee A, eds. A Manual of Standardized Terminology: Techniques and Criteria for Scoring of States of Sleep and Wakefulness in Newborn Infants. Los Angeles, Calif: UCLA Brain Information Service/Brain Research Institute; 1971.

17. Guilleminault C, Souquet M. Sleep states and related pathology. In: Korobkin R, Guilleminault C, eds. Advances in Perinatal Neurology. New York, NY: Spectrum; 1979:225–247.

18. Carskadon MA. Determinants of daytime sleepiness: adolescent development, extended and restricted nocturnal sleep [dissertation]. Stanford, Calif: Stanford University; 1979.

19. DiPerri R, Meduri M, DiRosa AE, et al. Sleep spindles in healthy people, I: quantitative, automatic analysis in young-adult subjects. Boll Soc Ital Biol Sper. 1977;53:983–989.

20. Dement WC. The nature and function of sleep. In: Reynolds D, Sjoberg A, eds. Neuroelectric Research: Electroneuroprosthesis, Electroanesthesia, and Nonconvulsive Electrotherapy. Springfield, Ill: Charles C Thomas; 1970:171–204.

21. Gaillard J-M, Blois R. Spindle density in sleep of normal subjects. Sleep. 1981;4:385–391.

22. Johnson LC, Spinweber CL, Seidel WF, et al. Sleep spindle and delta changes during chronic use of a short-acting and a long-acting benzodiazepine hypnotic. Electroencephalogr Clin Neurophysiol. 1983;55:662–667.

23. Crowell DH, Kapuniai LE, Boychuk RB, et al. Daytime sleep stage organization in three-month-old infants. Electroencephalogr Clin Neurophysiol. 1982;53:36–47.

24. Ellingson RJ. Development of sleep spindle bursts during the first year of life. Sleep. 1982;5:39–46.

25. Shibagaki M, Kiyono S, Watanabe K. Spindle evolution in normal and mentally retarded children: a review. Sleep. 1982;5:47–57.

26. Prinz PN, Raskind M. Aging and sleep disorders. In: Williams R, Karacan I, eds. Sleep Disorders: Diagnosis and Treatment. New York, NY: John Wiley & Sons; 1978:303–321.

27. Principe JC, Smith JR. Sleep spindle characteristics as a function of age. Sleep. 1982;5:73–84.

28. Hirschkowitz M, Thornby JI, Karacan I. Sleep spindles: pharmacologic effects in humans. Sleep. 1982;5:85–94.

29. Van Leeuwen S (chairman). Proposal for an EEG terminology by the Terminology Committee of the International Federation for Electroencephalography and Clinical Neurophysiology. Electroencephalogr Clin Neurophysiol. 1966;20:293–304.

30. Johnson LC, Karpan WE. Autonomic correlates of the spontaneous K complex. Psychophysiology. 1968;4:444–452.

31. Halász P, Pál I, Rajna P. K complex formation of the EEG in sleep: a survey and new examinations. Acta Physiol Acad Sci Hung 1985;65:3–35.

32. Berger RJ, Olley P, Oswald I. The EEG, eye movements and dreams of the blind. Q J Exp Psychol. 1962;14:182–186.

33. Yasoshima A, Hayashi H, Iijima S, et al. Potential distribution of vertex sharp wave and saw-toothed wave on the scalp. Electroencephalogr Clin Neurophysiol. 1984;58:73–76.

34. Johnson LC, Nute C, Austin MT, et al. Spectral analysis of the EEG during waking and sleeping. Electroencephalogr Clin Neurophysiol. 1967;23:80.

35. Jouvet M. Neurophysiology of the states of sleep. Physiol Rev. 1967;47:117–177.

36. Freemon FR. Sleep Research: A Critical Review. Springfield, Ill: Charles C Thomas; 1972.

37. Hodes R, Dement WC. Depression of electrically induced reflexes ("H-reflexes") in man during low voltage EEG "sleep." Electroencephalogr Clin Neurophysiol. 1964;17:617–629.

38. Salzarulo P, Lairy GC, Bancaud J, et al. Direct depth recording of the striate cortex during REM sleep in man: are there PGO potentials? Electroencephalogr Clin Neurophysiol. 1975;38:192–202.

39. Aserinsky E. The maximal capacity for sleep: rapid eye movement density as an index of sleep satiety. Biol Psychiatry. 1969;1:147–159.

40. Chase MH. Synaptic mechanisms and circuitry involved in motoneuron control during sleep. Int Rev Neurobiol. 1983;24:213–258.

41. Montplaisir J, Billiard M, Takahashi S, et al. Twenty-four-hour recording in REM-narcoleptics with special reference to nocturnal sleep disruption. Biol Psychiatry 1978;13:73–89.

42. Passouant P, Cadilhac J, Ribstein M. Les privations de sommeil avec mouvements oculaires par les antidépresseurs. Rev Neurol. 1972;127:173–192.

43. Passouant P, Cadilhac J, Billiard M, et al. La suppression du sommeil paradoxal par la clomipramine. Thérapie. 1973;28:379–392.

44. Raynal DM. Polygraphic aspects of narcolepsy. In: Guilleminault C, ed. Narcolepsy. New York, NY: Spectrum, 1976:669–684.

45. Flagg WH, Coburn SC. Appendix 2: polygraphic aspects of sleep apnea. In: Guilleminault C, Dement WC, eds. Sleep Apnea Syndromes. New York, NY: Alan R Liss, 1978:357–363.

46. Hauri P, Hawkins DR. Alpha-delta sleep. Electroencephalogr Clin Neurophysiol. 1973;34:233–237.

47. Moldofsky H, Scarisbrick P, England R, et al. Musculoskeletal symptoms and nonREM sleep disturbance in patients with "fibrositis syndrome" and healthy subjects. Psychosom Med. 1975;37:341–351.

48. Stepanski E, Salava W, Lamphere J, et al. Experimental sleep fragmentation and sleepiness in normal subjects: a preliminary report. Sleep Res. 1984;13:193.

49. Carskadon MA, Brown ED, Dement WC. Sleep fragmentation in the elderly: relationship to daytime sleep tendency. Neurobiol Aging. 1982;3:321–327.

50. Guilleminault C. EEG arousals: scoring rules and examples. Sleep. 1992;15:173–184.

50a. American Academy of Sleep Medicine. Sleep related breathing disorders in adults: recommendations for syndrome definition and measurement techniques in clinical research. Sleep. 1999;22:667–689.

51. Exar EN, Collop NA. The upper airway resistance syndrome. Chest. 1999;115:1127–1139.

52. Hosselet JJ, Norman RG, Ayappa I, et al. Detection of flow limitation with a nasal cannula/pressure transducer system. Am J Respir Crit Care Med. 1998;157:1461–1467.

53. Lavie P, Gertner R, Zomer J, et al. Breathing disorders in sleep associated with "microarousals" in patients with allergic rhinitis. Acta Otolaryngol. 1981;92:529–533.

54. Craig TJ, Teets S, Lehman EB, et al. Nasal congestion secondary to allergic rhinitis as a cause of sleep disturbance and daytime fatigue and the response to topical nasal corticosteroids. J Allergy Clin Immunol. 1998;101:633–637.

55. Zamir G, Press J, Tal A, et al. Sleep fragmentation in children with juvenile rheumatoid arthritis. J Rheumatol. 1998;25:1191–1197.
56. Stocchi F, Barbato L, Nordera G, et al. Sleep disorders in Parkinson's disease. J Neurol. 1998;245:S15–S18.
57. Pitson DJ, Stradling JR. Autonomic markers of arousal during sleep in patients undergoing investigation for obstructive sleep apnoea, their relationship to EEG arousals, respiratory events and subjective sleepiness. J Sleep Res. 1998;7:53–59.
58. Lofaso F, Goldenberg F, Dortho MP, et al. Arterial blood pressure response to transient arousals from NREM sleep in nonapneic snorers with sleep fragmentation. Chest. 1998;113:985–991.
59. Burger D, Cantani P, West J. Multidimensional analysis of sleep electrophysiological signals. Biol Cybern. 1977;26:131–139.
60. Gath I, Bar-on E. Computerized method for scoring of polygraphic sleep recordings. Comput Prog Biomed. 1980;11:217–223.
61. Ray SR, Lee WD, Morgan CD, et al. Computer sleep stage scoring—an expert system approach. Int J Biomed Comput. 1986;19:43–61.
62. Gaillard J-M, Tissot R. Principles of automatic analysis of sleep records with a hybrid system. Comput Biomed Res. 1973;6:1–13.
63. Smith JR, Karacan I, Lang M. Automated analysis of human sleep EEG. Waking Sleep. 1978;2:75–82.
64. Martens WLJ, Declerck AC, Kums DJThm, et al. Considerations on a computerized analysis of long-term polygraphic recordings. In: Stefan H, Burr W, eds. EEG Monitoring. Stuttgart, Germany: Gustav Fischer; 1982:265–274.
65. Agnew HW, Webb WB. Measurement of sleep onset by EEG criteria. Am J EEG Technol. 1972;12:127–134.
66. Webb WB. Recording methods and visual scoring criteria of sleep records: comments and recommendations. Percept Mot Skills. 1986;62:664–666.
67. Kupfer DJ, Targ E, Stack J. Electroencephalographic sleep in unipolar depressive subtypes: support for a biological and familial classification. J Nerv Ment Dis. 1982;170:494–498.
68. Webb WB, Dreblow LM. The REM cycle, combining rules and age. Sleep. 1982;5:372–377.
69. Dement WC. Physiology of Dreaming [dissertation]. Chicago, Ill: University of Chicago; 1958.
70. Kales A, Allen C, Scharf M, et al. Hypnotic drugs and their effectiveness: all-night EEG studies of insomniac subjects. Arch Gen Psychiatry. 1970;23:226–232.
71. Kales A, Bixler EO, Vela-Bueno A, et al. Biopsychobehavioral correlates of insomnia, III: polygraphic findings of sleep difficulty and their relationship to psychopathology. Int J Neurosci. 1984;23:43–56.
72. Orem J, Barnes CD, eds. Physiology in Sleep. New York, NY: Academic Press; 1980.
73. Phillipson EA, Sullivan CE, Read DJ, et al. Ventilatory and waking responses to hypoxia in sleeping dogs. J Appl Physiol. 1978;44:512–520.
74. Phillipson EA, Kozar LF, Rebuck AS, et al. Ventilatory and waking responses to CO$_2$ in sleeping dogs. Am Rev Respir Dis. 1977;115:251–259.
75. Parmeggiani PL. Temperature regulation during sleep: a study in homeostasis. In: Orem J, Barnes CD, eds. Physiology in Sleep. New York, NY: Academic Press; 1980:98–145.
76. Guilleminault C, Eldridge FL, Simmons FB, et al. Sleep apnea in eight children. Pediatrics. 1976;58:23–31.
77. Brouillette RT, Fernbach SK, Hunt CE. Obstructive sleep apnea in infants and children. J Pediatr. 1982;100:31–40.
78. Sackner MA, Lauda J, Forrest T, et al. Periodic sleep apnea: chronic sleep deprivation related to intermittent upper airway obstruction and central nervous system disturbance. Chest. 1975;67:164–171.
79. Mitler MM, Browman CP, Menn SJ, et al. Nocturnal myoclonus: treatment efficacy of clonazepam and temazepam. Sleep. 1986;9:385–392.
80. Karacan I. The developmental aspect and the effect of certain clinical conditions upon penile erection during sleep. Excerpta Med. 1966;150:2356–2359.
81. Karacan I. The clinical value of nocturnal erection in the prognosis and diagnosis of impotence. Hum Sex. 1970;4:27–34.
82. Barry JM, Blank B, Bioleau M. Nocturnal penile tumescence monitoring with stamps. Urology. 1980;15:171–172.
83. Karacan I, Aslan C, Williams RL. Reliability of stamp ring as indicator of penile rigidity in the diagnosis of impotence. Sleep Res. 1982;11:202.
84. Pressman MR, DiPhillips MA, Kendrick JI, et al. Problems in the interpretation of nocturnal penile tumescence studies: disruption of sleep by occult sleep disorders. J Urol. 1986;136:595–598.
85. Goode GB, Slyter HM. Daytime polysomnogram diagnosis of sleep apnea. Trans Am Neurol Assoc. 1980;105:367–370.
86. Karacan I, Finley W, Williams R, et al. Changes in stage 1-REM and stage 4 sleep during naps. Biol Psychiatry. 1970;2:261–265.
86a. Oksenberg A, Silverberg DS, Arons E, et al. The sleep supine position has a major effect on optimal nasal continuous positive airway pressure: relationship with rapid eye movements and non-rapid eye movements sleep, body mass index, respiratory disturbance index, and age. Chest. 1999;116:1000–1006.
87. Vogel G. Studies in the psychophysiology of dreams, III: the dreams of narcolepsy. Arch Gen Psychiatry. 1960;3:421–428.
88. Zarcone V. Narcolepsy: a review of the syndrome. N Engl J Med. 1973;288:1156–1166.
89. Kupfer DJ. A psychobiologic marker for primary depressive disease. Biol Psychiatry. 1976;11:159–174.
90. Harner PF, Sannit T. A Review of the International Ten-Twenty System of Electrode Placement. Quincy, Mass: Grass Instrument Company; 1974.

101

Monitoring Respiratory and Cardiac Function

Meir H. Kryger

The documentation of a sleep breathing disorder requires objective measurements. The focus of this chapter is to review methodologies of monitoring the breathing pattern and detecting abnormalities. The transducers used to monitor the sequelae of abnormal respiration (abnormal gas exchange) and the instruments used for the acquisition of data (polysomnographs and computers) also are be reviewed. Also provided are the procedures followed in most laboratories. There is some disagreement about what methodology is appropriate, and expert committees have made recommendations about what measurements are optimal.[1, 2, 2a] Local medical resources may vary, and the clinician may be forced to make management decisions with less-than-adequate diagnostic information, possibly putting the patient at risk.

DEFINITIONS

Many terms have been used for abnormal breathing during sleep, including apnea, hypopnea, sleep disordered breathing, sleep-related breathing disorder, and periodic breathing. Adjectives that have been used to classify these events include obstructive, central, and mixed. Surprisingly, until recently there were no widely accepted "official" consensus definitions of these terms or how to document them.[2a, 3, 4] What follows is the author's interpretation of what most experts mean by the use of the terms.

Apnea is the complete cessation of breathing for more than 10 sec in adults and 3 sec in infants.

Hypopnea refers to a reduction in, but not cessation of, ventilation.

Respiratory effort-related arousal (RERA) events refers to obstructed events that do not meet the criteria for apnea or hypopnea but that nevertheless cause an arousal from sleep.[2a]

Sleep disordered breathing, or *sleep-related breathing disorder*, refers to any respiratory abnormality that would include apnea, hypopnea, and RERA events.

Periodic breathing refers to a regularly repeating pattern in which normal or increased ventilation alternates with decreased or absent ventilation. Cheyne-Stokes respiration, which is found in heart failure and at high altitude, is an example of periodic breathing.

Obstructive is the adjective used to classify the events as being caused by obstruction of the upper airway.

Central is the adjective used to classify the events as being due to decreased output to the muscles of inspiration from the respiratory control system in the central nervous system.

Mixed refers to events that have features of both obstructive and central in the same event. In scoring, many laboratories consider a mixed event to be obstructive.

Individual authors have included *oxygen desaturation* as an additional factor used to define sleep-disordered breathing and hypopnea.

The most widely used frequency measure is the number of *events per hour* of sleep. Most laboratories report the *apnea index* or the *apnea-hypopnea index*. The *respiratory disturbance index* includes apneas, hypopneas, and RERAs.

Severity of sleep breathing disorders can be defined using two dimensions: a clinical one (e.g., sleepiness, see Table 79–1); and a laboratory one, which is done by determining the number of sleep related breathing events (apneas, hypopneas, and RERAs) per hour of sleep: mild, 5 to 15; moderate, 15 to 30; severe, more than 30.

There is no consensus on how to best report the frequency of the physiological changes in the upper airway resistance syndrome. A reasonable measure seems to be the number of *arousals per hour* related to obstructive breathing events (e.g., RERAs).

MONITORING BREATHING PATTERNS AND EFFORT

Rib Cage and Abdominal Motion

During normal breathing, contraction of the major muscle of inspiration, the diaphragm, causes both expansion of the rib cage and downward movement of the diaphragm. These movements cause the pressure around and in the lung to become negative relative to atmosphere. This ambient air–lung pressure gradient results in air flow into the lung. Thus, a change in lung volume is the sum of the volume changes of the structures surrounding the lungs, the rib cage, and the abdomen.[5] Other respiratory muscles (intercostal, sternocleidomastoid, and so on) also play a role in stabilizing the thoracic cage.

Some erroneously interpret the abdominal and rib cage motion changes to imply separate activity of abdominal and thoracic respiratory muscles; this is not the case. Virtually all the changes in abdominal and rib cage volumes (including paradoxical motion) can be explained by changes in the respiratory muscles directly inserting onto the thoracic cage, as described later.

Normally, the enlargement of the thorax and the outward movement of the abdominal wall occur together, that is, they are *in phase*. For a given change in lung volume, one can thus quantify a change in rib cage volume and abdominal volume. For a given breath, the relative contributions of the rib cage and abdominal compartments also can be determined. If it is assumed that the abdominal and rib cage fractional contributions are constant, then changes in lung volume can be measured by calibrating transducers sensitive to rib cage and abdominal displacement. The relative rib cage and abdominal contributions may change with posture and with the changes in muscle tone occurring in sleep; thus, the devices (mentioned later) can be calibrated, but their calibration may change markedly during the night.

Causes of Abdominal–Rib Cage Paradox

Paradoxical motion of the rib cage and abdomen occurs with loss of tone of the diaphragm, with loss of tone of the other respiratory muscles, or with complete or partial upper airway obstruction.

Loss of Tone of the Diaphragm. When the diaphragm ceases contraction and becomes flaccid, it merely transmits and reacts to pressure changes around it, instead of generating pressure changes. In this situation, when the other respiratory muscles contract, the rib cage is enlarged, and pleural pressure becomes negative, sucking the diaphragm into the chest. This condition results in an increase in rib cage volume and a reduction in abdominal volume.

Loss of Tone of the Accessory Respiratory Muscles. When the accessory muscles lose tone, the rib cage, particularly the upper part of the rib cage, becomes unstable. When the diaphragm then contracts, the negative intrathoracic pressure causes the unstable part of the thorax to be sucked in during inspiration.

Partial Upper Airway Obstruction. With partial upper airway obstruction, the diaphragm must generate very strong negative pressures for inspiration to occur. As the diaphragm contracts, it both pushes out the abdomen and creates great negative intrathoracic pressure. This highly negative intrathoracic pressure may overcome the mechanisms maintaining chest wall stability (accessory muscle tone and rigidity of the cage) and cause the least stable portions of the rib cage to move inward with inspiration. This inward movement of the rib cage is a problem mainly in the very young, who have a pliable rib cage.

Complete Upper Airway Obstruction (Obstructive Apnea). With complete upper airway obstruction, there obviously is no movement of air into the lungs. Because the volume change is zero, the volume change of the abdomen (caused by diaphragmatic contraction) is equal and opposite in direction to the volume change of the rib cage. This volume change is a pathognomonic finding in obstructive sleep apnea.

METHODS TO DETECT CHANGES IN LUNG VOLUME

Strain Gauges

A strain gauge consists of a sealed elastic tube filled with an electrical conductor, usually mercury, through which an electric current is passed.[6] When length is constant, current and resistance are constant. Stretching the strain gauge changes the length and cross-sectional area of the fixed-volume conductor, resulting in proportional increases in resistance. Current varies inversely to the length of the gauge, thereby becoming an index of gauge length.

These gauges, which thus are sensitive to length, can be used to qualitatively detect breathing abnormalities. They may also be used, when calibrated, to quantitatively measure dynamic volume changes.[7] To quantify actual volume changes, the transducers must be calibrated against an independent volume-measuring system. The number and length of the gauges may vary, depending on the application. When it is not critical to measure exact volumes (as in many clinical applications), a short strain gauge placed on the chest or abdominal wall may yield an adequate signal. When more exact volume measurements are required, two or more circumferential gauges may be used. One could then use multiple linear regression techniques to obtain calibration factors for each transducer.[7] In practice, two gauges—one for the rib cage and one for the abdomen—can produce adequate precision for measuring changes in lung volume. The rib cage gauge is placed at the level of the axilla, and the abdominal gauge is placed just superior to the iliac crest. Once the gauges are calibrated, the sum of the rib cage and abdominal excursions will describe volume changes.

Differentiation of apnea type (central or obstructive) is not possible based on the summed rib cage and abdominal volume signals alone. Paradoxical rib cage and abdominal movement, which is common during an obstructive apnea, results in zero summed net volume change because the abdominal and rib cage volumes change in equal and opposite directions. Similarly, central apnea (a cessation of all respiratory effort) is characterized by zero summed net volume change.

To determine whether respiratory effort is present, an additional recording of either a rib cage or an abdominal transducer or of pleural pressure is required. If the gauge is being used solely as a relative index of respiratory movements, a single uncalibrated abdominal transducer will suffice.

The optimal working range of a mercury-filled strain gauge is narrow. An understretched gauge may not produce a measurable change in resistance with change in its length. An overstretched gauge produces a high level of resistance. Both of these conditions preclude the gauge from correctly detecting changes in length. It is suggested that an unstretched gauge, if placed circumferentially, be at least 20% smaller than the circumference of the torso. Over time, there is deterioration in the function of the gauge due to the constant current through the conductor.

Piezoelectric transducers are also being used to monitor respiratory motion. These sensors are sensitive to changes in length; however, they are not usually calibrated in typical sleep laboratory applications.

Inductance Plethysmography

Changes in the cross-sectional area of the rib cage and abdominal compartments can be measured electronically by determining changes in inductance. Inductance is a property of electrical conductors characterized by the opposition to a change of current flow in the conductor.

Transducers are placed around the rib cage and abdomen, the physiological equivalent of conductors. Each transducer consists of an insulated wire, sewn into the shape of a horizontally oriented sinusoid onto an elasticized band. Changes in lung volumes alter the cross-sectional areas of the rib cage and abdomen, with a proportional change in the diameter of each transducer; this change directly affects the self-inductance of the transducer.[8] Considerations concerning transducer placement, volume calibration, and apnea identification are identical to those applied to strain gauges.

Additional factors must be considered in using these devices: there is sensitivity to artifact during changes in body position because the elasticized band may migrate from its original site, and the size of the band makes it deformable. All of these factors may adversely affect the accuracy and stability of the original volume calibration. As mentioned previously, the relative contributions of rib cage and abdomen may change with sleep and changes in posture, thereby causing the initial calibration to become less accurate.

Calibrated inductance plethysmography has been suggested as a method to infer the changes of upper airway resistance syndrome.[9] The following have been described: snoring may lead to rib cage/abdominal asynchrony with increased thoracic breathing and increased breathing cycle time taken up by inspiration; before arousal, one may detect evidence of flow limitation; and arousals may lead to increased variation of respiratory cycle time and increased tidal volume.

Impedance Pneumography

Impedance defines the combined effects of two previously discussed properties of an electrical conductor: *resistance* and *inductance*. In physical terms, when impedance pneumography is used, the conductor is the thorax. Impedance is measured by applying a small current across the thorax using a pair of electrodes placed at the site of maximal thoracic excursion. Changes in transthoracic impedance are related to variations in the amount of conductive materials (liquids, including interstitial fluid, blood, and lymph, and tissue) and nonconductive material (air) between the electrodes. The conductive and nonconductive materials obviously affect the total impedance differently. Increased air in the lung increases impedance, and increased fluid in the thorax decreases impedance. A recording of both the volume of air exchanged and the total impedance changes may allow the differentiation of air-related and fluid-related changes in impedance.[10] If total impedance is recorded in a single channel, both air volume–related and fluid-related changes are measured. Changes in impedance in obstructive apnea are complex. During apnea, lung volume decreases, whereas the negative intrathoracic pressure likely temporarily pools blood in the pulmonary circulation. For these reasons, a precise measurement of respiratory volume and pattern may not be possible. Another potential problem with impedance pneumography is electrical interference caused by other measuring devices.

Other Methods Used to Measure Volume

The static charge–sensitive bed technology has been evaluated in sleep disorders.[11] The transducer is part of a thin mattress that responds to the slightest movement (even as a result of the heartbeat) from the person sleeping on it. The amplitude of the respiratory signal varies with body position but otherwise is stable; thus, the device has not been calibrated to volume.

Other techniques have been used to measure volume changes, including magnetometers, body plethysmography, canopy with neck seal, barometric method, and pneumotachography, but they are not commonly used in a clinical setting.[12–16]

METHODS TO DETECT CHANGES IN RESPIRATORY EFFORT

Pleural Pressure

Esophageal pressure measurements are used in some centers as an index of inspiratory effort. In our experience, esophageal balloons are unacceptable by many patients for all-night studies. Newer, thin, catheter-tip piezoelectric transducers may be better tolerated. In patients with apneas only of the central type, it may be necessary to document the lack of respiratory efforts with esophageal pressure measurements.

The measurement of esophageal pressure during inspiration may also be very helpful in the diagnosis of the upper airway resistance syndrome. The classic findings include pleural pressure that becomes progressively more negative until an arousal (sometimes associated with an audible snort) occurs (Fig. 101–1). After arousal, the pleural pressure swings temporarily decrease, to be followed by the next cycle of increased swings and arousal. At times, arousal may not be associated with visible electroencephalographic changes but may be inferred from automatic nervous system changes documented by a change in heart rate.[4, 17] The presence of frequent (more than 10 per hour) cycles of negative pleural pressure swings and arousals (visible on electroencephalogram or inferred from other measures) in the sleepy patient without significant apnea is presumptive evidence of upper airway resistance syndrome (see Fig. 101–1).

Respiratory Muscle Electromyography

Several centers use electrodes on the chest wall in an attempt to measure respiratory muscle electromyog-

raphy (Fig. 101–2) as an indirect measure of effort (C. Ware, personal communication). Electrode pairs are placed in an intercostal space on the right anterior chest until an optimal signal is attained; this may require trial and error. We are unaware of any standardized technique to obtain this measurement, which nevertheless seems to be promising.

METHODS USED TO DETECT AIR FLOW

Apnea is defined as cessation of air flow. As mentioned later, occasionally, unidirectional occlusion occurs, in which there is no air flow in inspiration but tiny puffs in expiration. The air flow can be evaluated either by measuring it directly using a pneumotachograph or by detecting chemical or physical differences between expired air and ambient air.

Pneumotachography

Several types of pneumotachographs based on different physical principles are in use: differential pres-

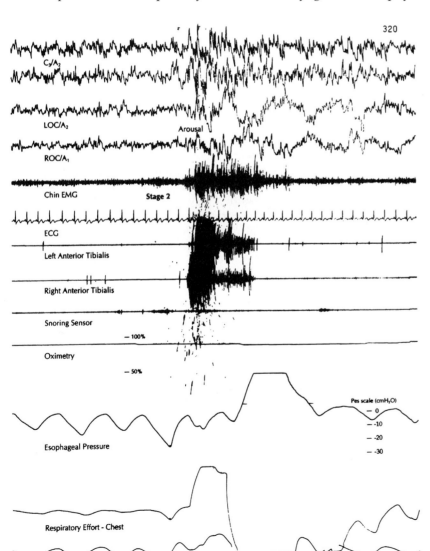

Figure 101–1. Esophageal pressure in the upper airway resistance syndrome. The esophageal pressure swing was greatest just before the arousal. (From Butkov N. Atlas of Clinical Polysomnography. Ashland, Ore: Synapse Media; 1996:224.)

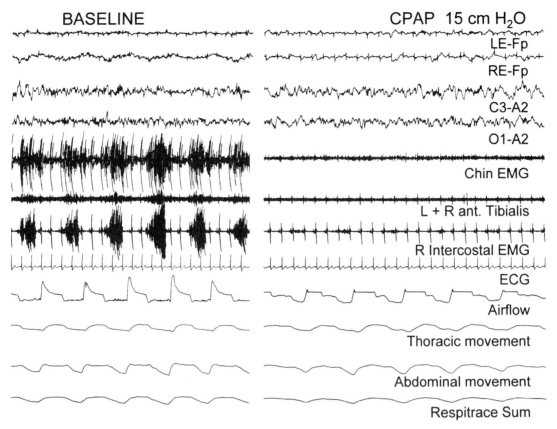

BASELINE   **CPAP 15 cm H$_2$O**

LE-Fp

RE-Fp

C3-A2

O1-A2

Chin EMG

L + R ant. Tibialis

R Intercostal EMG

ECG

Airflow

Thoracic movement

Abdominal movement

Respitrace Sum

Figure 101–2. Surface respiratory (R intercostal) muscle EMG in sleep apnea. *Left,* The respiratory EMG is dramatically increased. *Right,* This signal is reduced on nasal CPAP. (Courtesy of Dr. Catesby Ware.)

sure air flow transducers, ultrasonic flowmeters, and hot wire anemometers. This discussion focuses on the differential pressure flow transducer, which is the most widely used transducer.

Air flow is directed through a cylinder. Before exiting the cylinder, air passes through a small resistive field, usually small parallel tubes or a grill that promotes laminar flow. The pressure drop across this resistive field is measured by a differential manometer. When flow is laminar, there is a linear relation between the pressure differences and flow. The pressure-flow relation is altered by changes in gas density, viscosity, and temperature. Heating is required to prevent condensation on the resistive element, so calibration should be done when the pneumotachograph is heated. Correction factors can be used to minimize the error introduced by alterations in these physical factors. The flow signal may be integrated electronically or digitally to obtain volume.

In sleep research applications, the pneumotachograph is usually connected to a face mask. Although this pneumotachograph and face mask combination is the most accurate means of assessing the volume of air flow, it is a relatively large, uncomfortable device, making it often unsuitable for many clinical respiratory studies during sleep. In awake patients, invasive devices alter breathing pattern; tidal volume increases, and breathing frequency is either decreased or unchanged. Some of the newer bilevel positive airway pressure and continuous positive airway pressure

(CPAP) machines have pneumotachographs built in; so therefore, these devices can be used to monitor airflow and ventilation. Cardiogenic oscillations, which are markers of central apnea, can be detected with these systems.[17a]

Nasal Airway Pressure

During inspiration, airway pressure is negative relative to atmosphere, and during expiration, airway pressure is positive relative to atmosphere. Some investigators have suggested that measurement of these pressure changes in the nasal airway may be used to estimate air flow.[18, 19] It has been shown that such a pressure signal resembles that obtained with a pneumotachograph.[18] This measurement appears to be much more sensitive in the detection of the type of flow limitation seen in the upper airway resistance syndrome than the thermistor[19] (Fig. 101–3). Air flow limitation is inferred when a plateau is present on the pressure trace during inspiration. It has been shown that such a system tracks changes in upper airway resistance and flow limitation in patients.[20] Such a system requires careful attention to signal conditioning. The optimal signal is obtained by using a DC amplifier; if an AC amplifier is used, then a long time constant filter should be used. A short time constant filter may result in artifacts[19] (Fig. 101–4). The role of this relatively new methodology is not entirely clear because

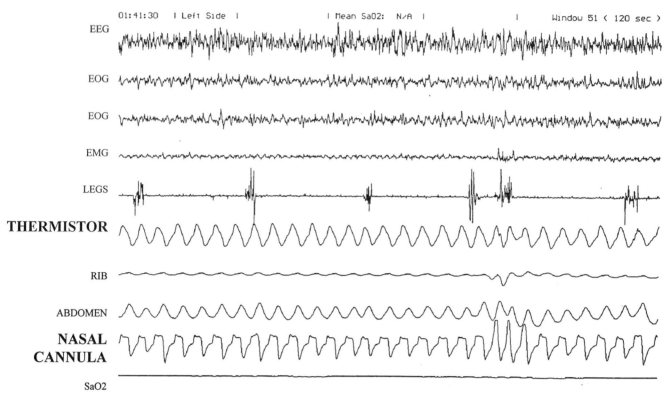

Figure 101–3. A 120-sec section from a nocturnal polysomnogram (NPSG) in a subject undergoing simultaneous recording with a conventional thermistor and with a nasal cannula used for recording pressure . In this subject, there is nothing in the thermistor tracing to suggest a respiratory event, with only a suggestion of a movement indicated in the rib and abdominal inductance plethysmographic tracings. However, in the nasal cannula tracing, the end of a hypopnea and the beginning of another are easily detected. Notice the plateaus (chopped off tops) of the pressure traces during hypopnea. (Courtesy of Dr. David Rappaport.)

some patients may not breathe via the nose. It does, however, seem more sensitive than the thermistor.

Thermistor

During inspiration, air is rapidly heated so that air in the lungs reaches core body temperature. There is a large temperature difference between air coming from the respiratory system (body temperature) and air going into the respiratory system. Simply measuring temperature in front of the nose and mouth can be used to detect expiration.

A thermistor is a thermally sensitive resistor that is supplied with a constant but low current. The use of a low current reduces the tendency of the thermistor to heat itself. Thermistors are designed to maximize the sensing area while minimizing the size and mass of the sensor. This design results in the thermistor being more sensitive to changes in air flow. Small temperature changes should produce large resistance changes. Care must be taken to ensure that the operating temperature of the thermistor is below body temperature; otherwise, expiratory air flow may not always be detected. An unheated thermistor cannot accurately differentiate prolonged inspiratory activity from a respiratory pause. A thermistor ceases being an air flow sensor if it touches the skin because it will remain at body temperature.

Thermistors are placed in the path of air flow from the nose and mouth. Expired air flow heats the sensor, increasing its resistance, and inspiratory air flow cools the sensor to ambient temperature, resulting in a relative decrease in the resistance, which can then be recorded.

Expired Carbon Dioxide Sensing

Air leaving the lungs has a much higher concentration of CO_2 than ambient air. There is always a large CO_2 difference between air coming from the respiratory system and air going into the respiratory system. Thus, simply measuring CO_2 in front of the nose and mouth can detect expiration. An infrared analyzer is frequently used to measure the concentration of CO_2.

The CO_2 pressure offers several advantages over measuring nasal pressure or using thermistors. First, in some patients, the end of breath concentration may yield an end-tidal P_{CO_2}. Because the catheters sampling CO_2 may also entrain some room air, the CO_2 measured is likely to be lower than the end-tidal P_{CO_2}; thus, an elevated P_{CO_2} should be accepted as real, indicating that true P_{CO_2} is even higher. Thus, this is the only noninvasive measurement sampling the airstream that can potentially confirm hypoventilation. Second, the shape of the expired curve may offer useful information. When a patient originally demonstrates an ex-

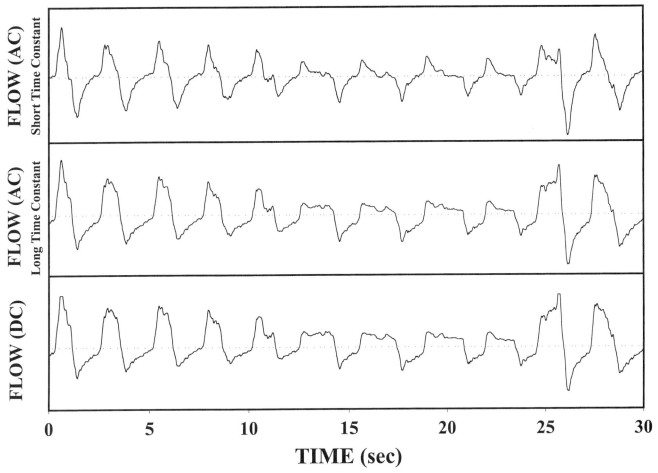

Figure 101–4. A flow limitation event recorded from the nasal cannula measuring pressure simultaneously amplified by three different amplifiers. The bottom signal is from a DC amplifier with no filtering. The top two signals are from AC amplifiers with low-frequency filters with time constants of 1.6 *(top)* and 5.3 *(middle)*. The short time constant filter *(top)* causes the flow signal to decay to baseline rapidly during a period of relatively constant flow (flow limitation plateau). The longer time constant filter *(middle)* provides reasonably good reproduction of these constant flows.

pired CO_2 curve with a clearcut plateau, the loss of the plateau or the curve becoming smaller or dome shaped indicates a change in breathing pattern, usually a reduction in expiratory volume. Third, during central apnea, the CO_2 tracing may show cardiogenic oscillations. These oscillations are the result of small volume displacements caused by the beating heart. These oscillations are synchronized to the heartbeat, and they prove that the upper airway is wide open (Fig. 101–5). The catheter system should be of low volume and the analyzer set on its fastest response to detect these oscillations.

Infants and children with upper airway obstruction may develop severe hypoventilation during sleep without frank apnea; this can be detected by measuring expired CO_2, but it cannot be detected with a thermistor.[21]

Problems and Artifacts in Detecting Apnea

Because a thermistor and devices monitoring expired gases cannot reliably differentiate among a pro-

longed inspiration, central apnea, or obstructive apnea, they are almost always used in conjunction with a device sensitive to lung volume or respiratory effort.

Extreme care must be taken when classification of respiratory activity is based on the relation between detection of air flow and respiratory effort. In some cases, patients may have complete occlusion on inspiration but small puffs on expiration, which can be detected by thermistor or CO_2 analyzer. Such patients are erroneously categorized as having *hypopneas* or even normal, unobstructed breathing. An example of this phenomenon is seen in Figure 101–6. Air flow is recorded simultaneously from a CO_2 analyzer and a pneumotachograph. During the obstructive apnea, periods of expiratory air flow occur (recorded by the pneumotachograph and CO_2 analyzer) in the absence of inspiratory flow (obvious in the pneumotachograph recording, and unclear in the CO_2 recording). Without the information from the pneumotachograph, one would interpret the recording from the CO_2 analyzer as evidence of uninterrupted inspiratory and expiratory air flow.

As mentioned previously, an additional useful find-

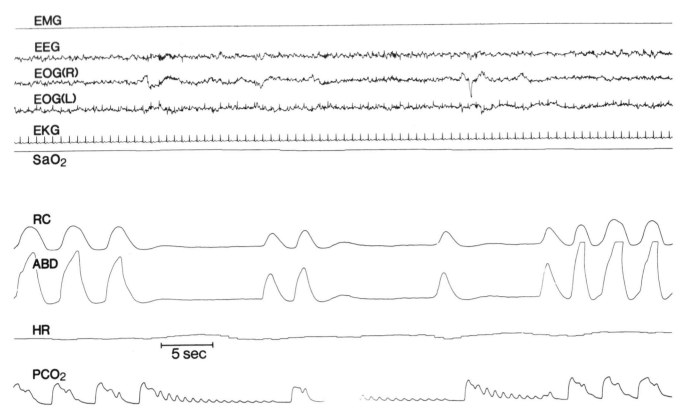

Figure 101–5. Cardiogenic oscillations in CO_2 are seen in the bottom channel in this example of central apnea. The presence of these oscillations, synchronous with the heartbeat, proves that the upper airway is patent.

ing when recording expired CO_2 is the occurrence of cardiogenic oscillations. When the typical CO_2 changes of expiration are absent, one cannot differentiate among a prolonged inspiration, obstructive apnea, or central apnea. In this setting, the presence of prolonged cardiogenic oscillations only is proof that the upper airway is patent and that central apnea is present.

CONTINUOUS POSITIVE AIRWAY PRESSURE AS A DIAGNOSTIC TOOL

Response to nasal CPAP in the laboratory (normalizing gas exchange, sleep structure, and heart rate) is

evidence supporting the diagnosis of sleep disordered breathing. Some CPAP systems have built-in diagnostic capabilities.[22] Occasionally, in some difficult cases, the only way to determine the presence and significance of sleep disordered breathing is a therapeutic trial of nasal CPAP; a positive response (improvement in sleepiness) can be used to support, for example, the diagnosis of sleep disordered breathing. At this time, we believe there is insufficient published data to support the widespread use of nasal CPAP as a diagnostic tool for the routine patient suspected of having OSAS. In selected patients (e.g., patients suspected of having UARS, but with inconclusive PSGs), such an approach may be helpful.

ERROR IN DETECTING APNEA

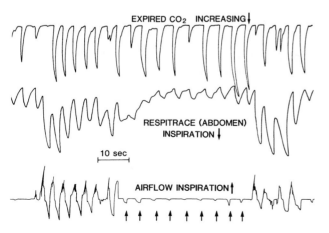

Figure 101–6. An example of the limitations of noninvasive air flow detection. *Top,* Air flow is detected with the CO_2 analyzer. *Middle,* Respiratory inductance plethysmograph (RIP). *Bottom,* Air flow measured with a pneumotachograph. With each apnea-related expiratory deflection documented by the pneumotachograph *(arrows, bottom),* there is a sustained shift in the baseline of the RIP. This suggests an incremental decrease in functional residual capacity resulting from absent inspirations with continued small expiratory puffs. If only the top two tracings were available, this pattern would have been mistakenly called hypoventilation or hypopnea, when it is clearly total occlusion on inspiration. (From West P, Kryger MH. Sleep and respiration: terminology and methodology. Clin Chest Med. 1985;6:706.)

MONITORING BLOOD GAS CHANGES

It is highly invasive to measure the oxygen content of the blood directly from an indwelling arterial catheter during sleep. Intermittent sampling also fails to detect the incidence and severity of hypoxemia, which is now known to be highly variable in sleep. A report that reviewed in detail all the devices being used for the noninvasive assessment of blood gases is recommended.[23]

Pulse Oximetry

Noninvasive technologies allow the continuous monitoring of oxygen saturation of arterial blood (SaO_2).[24-28] Pulse oximeters use spectrophotoelectrical principles to determine SaO_2 from a two-wavelength light transmitter and receiver placed on either side of a pulsating arterial vascular bed. Digit, ear, and nasal sites are recommended by the manufacturers. The amplitude of light detected by the receiver is dependent on the magnitude of the change in arterial pulse, the wavelengths transmitted through the arterial vascular bed, and the SaO_2 of the arterial hemoglobin. These devices are said to be sensitive only to tissues that pulsate; thus, venous blood, connective tissue, skin pigment, and bone theoretically do not interfere with the measurement of SaO_2. A minimal pulse amplitude must be detected by the devices to prevent erroneous measurements. Dyshemoglobinemias, however, may cause problems. The correct alignment of the light transmitter and receiver is critical to the proper operation of pulse oximeters. If the sensor is applied to a digit, that digit must be immobilized. Significant bending of the digit may restrict the ability of the devices to detect pulsatile flow, the absence of which precludes SaO_2 determinations. Although all pulse oximeters are based on similar technology,[26] they have very different response characteristics, which depend on sensor location and manufacturer.[27] Indeed, the same model by the same manufacturer may have different software versions, which may result in differing performance.[29, 30] The difference in the response characteristics and dependence on sensor locations cannot be overemphasized (Fig. 101–7). Some oximeters may entirely miss episodes of hypoxemia easily detectable by other oximeters and thus may lead to an incorrect diagnosis and treatment (Fig. 101–8). The sensors are very lightweight and thus can be used in neonates.

In reflectance pulse oximetry, the light transmitter and receiver are on the same surface. The light, which is transmitted into the vascular bed, is scattered, absorbed, and reflected, and thus only a small proportion of the light returns to the receiver. Reflectance devices deal with weaker pulse signals and therefore are more sensitive to changes in blood pressure and motion artifacts.

It is beyond the scope of this chapter to review the specific manufacturers and all their models.[29, 31] There are, however, a few generalizations that seem appropriate.

Sensor Locations. In our experience, for most adults, the ear is the preferred location. In the presence of poor perfusion, we apply a trace amount of a vasodilator (nonylic acid vanillylamide and nicotinic acid, Finalgon ointment [Boehringer Ingelheim]). This is a powerful cutaneous vasodilator, and the technician must be careful to avoid contact of this ointment with

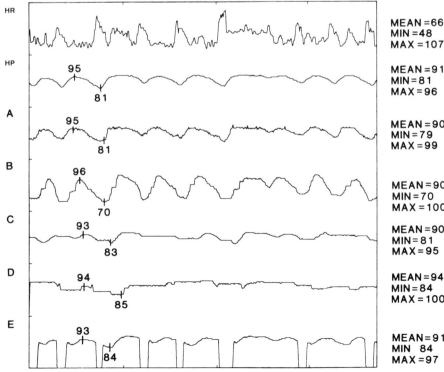

Figure 101–7. Heart rate (HR) and SaO_2 during 5 min in a patient with sleep apnea. HP, Hewlett Packard oximeter; A to E, five different pulse oximeters. The scales for the six oximeters are identical. The numbers on the tracings represent the instantaneous SaO_2 measured during the peak and through of an apneic episode. The numbers to the right of the figure are the mean, standard deviation, and minimum and maximum values for HR and SaO_2 for the six oximeters. Note that C and D do not track SaO_2 and that E has numerous artifacts.

HR   MEAN=66±11 MIN=48 MAX=107

HP   95 81   MEAN=91.5±3.5 MIN=81 MAX=96

A   95 81   MEAN=90.5±4.5 MIN=79 MAX=99

B   96 70   MEAN=90.5±5.75 MIN=70 MAX=100

C   93 83   MEAN=90±3.25 MIN=81 MAX=95

D   94 85   MEAN=94.5±3.5 MIN=84 MAX=100

E   93 84   MEAN=91.5±3.25 MIN 84 MAX=97

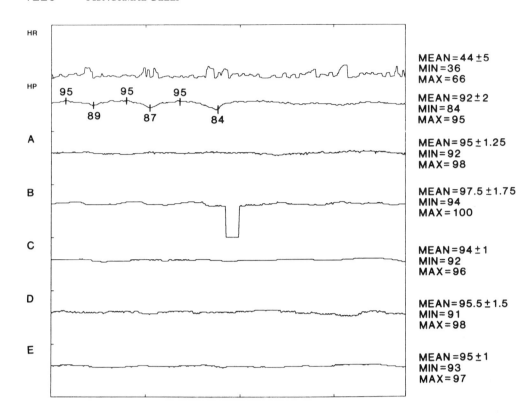

HR

MEAN=44±5
MIN=36
MAX=66

HP   95   95   95
           89   87   84

MEAN=92±2
MIN=84
MAX=95

A

MEAN=95±1.25
MIN=92
MAX=98

B

MEAN=97.5±1.75
MIN=94
MAX=100

C

MEAN=94±1
MIN=92
MAX=96

D

MEAN=95.5±1.5
MIN=91
MAX=98

E

MEAN=95±1
MIN=93
MAX=97

Figure 101–8. Heart rate and SaO_2 during 5 min in a patient with sleep apnea and bradycardia. Tracings are taken from six oximeters, as described in Figure 101–7. In this example, three apneic episodes are missed entirely by all the pulse oximeters. This patient's problem would have been missed entirely by pulse oximetry screening.

eyes. We have used this ointment (which is not available in all countries) for more than 10 years without any problems. When the ear site is not usable, reflectance pulse oximeter sensors on the forehead or another well-perfused surface may be used.

Instrument Filters. Most pulse oximeters filter the SaO_2 signal. For some devices, the filter algorithms use the heart rate; thus, the degree of filtering becomes inversely related to rate, and at very low heart rates the signal is heavily filtered.[27] The greater the filtering, the less likely is the detection of brief, mild hypoxemic episodes.[32] We recommend that the least filtering (i.e., the fastest response) be used.

Potential Problems. Because pulse oximeters use two wavelengths of light in the process of estimating SaO_2, they are unable to distinguish three or more hemoglobin species. In the presence of carboxyhemoglobin, the SaO_2 will be overestimated in heavy smokers, whose carboxyhemoglobin level may reach 10 to 20%.[33] In the presence of a rising methemoglobin concentration, SaO_2 measured by oximetry will plateau toward 85%, regardless of whether the true SaO_2 is much higher or lower.[34] Because light is transmitted through tissue, pigment in the skin may degrade oximeter performance, with the device indicating a "probe off" or "perfusion low" message.[35] Although probe connectors from one manufacturer may perfectly fit into the unit of another, the wiring may be incompatible, and severe burns may result.[36] Pressure-related injuries to the digits have also been reported.[37]

Transmittance Oximetry

This technique (with the use of Hewlett-Packard model 47201A) uses the absorption of transmitted light to calculate the SaO_2. Fiberoptic bundles in a cable transmit and detect eight wavelengths of light. Transmittance characteristics of each light wavelength have been correlated with independently measured SaO_2. The device is unaffected by skin color and sensor movement, although ambient light and poor perfusion may interfere with proper SaO_2 measurement. At low SaO_2 values, this device may give falsely low readings, and a correction equation is required for SaO_2 values below 65%.[24] Recalibration is recommended at 4-h intervals. The sensor mount distributed by the manufacturer is not serviceable when using the instrument during sleep. Alternatively, the patient's head may be wrapped with padded gauze, with the sensor attached to the ear and secured to the gauze. An additional layer of gauze is used to anchor the sensor. The Hewlett-Packard oximeter has excellent electronic response characteristics. The disadvantages of this oximeter are the weight and heat generation of the sensor. It is no longer being manufactured.

Intravascular oximetry using fiberoptic sensors in systemic arteries or the pulmonary artery is too highly invasive for routine clinical use.

Measurement of Transcutaneous Oxygen and Carbon Dioxide

The estimation of PaO_2 from the surface of the skin is dependent on the oxygen flux through the skin, local oxygen consumption, and the diffusion barrier of the skin.[38] This measurement technique is most commonly used in neonates, whose skin is thin.

Accurate measurement of transcutaneous PO_2 ($tcPO_2$)

requires maximal dilation of the local vasculature in the upper dermis, which is achieved by heating it to 43°C. Heating, however, shifts the oxyhemoglobin dissociation curve to the right, increases the resistance of the skin stratum corneum to oxygen permeation, increases the metabolic rate of the dermal tissue, and increases the rate of cutaneous blood flow. The shift in the oxyhemoglobin dissociation curve and the increase in metabolic rate effectively cancel each other out, leaving permeability and flow as the dependent factors in correlating $tcPO_2$ and PaO_2. An important advantage of heating is that the amount of blood present is maximal and $tcPO_2$ will thereby be unaffected by small changes in blood supply to the tissue.

The $tcPO_2$ may be misinterpreted when the state of blood flow is unknown. When flow and PaO_2 are adequate, $tcPO_2$ reflects PaO_2. Under conditions of compromised flow and adequate PaO_2, $tcPO_2$ will change with flow. If SaO_2 and flow are compromised, $tcPO_2$ tracks oxygen delivery.

The accuracy of transcutaneous measurement also depends on correct sensor application. To convert $tcPO_2$ measurements to PaO_2 values precisely, a calibration curve for each subject is required; this is a prohibitive step. In practice, the $tcPO_2$ measurements are thus used to track, in relative terms, the status of arterial oxygen content. The responsiveness of the device is not adequate to rapidly track the blood gas changes of short apneas (less than 30 sec) because oxygen diffuses slowly across the skin. The conditions that govern the transcutaneous measurement of PCO_2 are similar to those described for PaO_2. Transcutaneous blood gas determinations are of greatest value in neonates. A review concluded that in adults there was little clinical use for the measurement of $tcPO_2$; the authors were only modestly enthusiastic about transcutaneous PCO_2.[23] The use of transcutaneous PCO_2 is highly recommended to assess hypoventilation in children who may present without frank apnea but with continuous hypoventilation.[21]

METHODS USED TO MEASURE PULSE PRESSURE WAVES AND SYSTEMIC ARTERIAL BLOOD PRESSURE

Most laboratories do not include the continuous measurement of blood pressure (BP) in routine clinical evaluations. The techniques mentioned below are currently practiced primarily in a research setting.

Many pulse oximeters now include an output that tracks the pulse pressure, an index of the magnitude of the pulsation occurring at the site of the oximetry sensor. Pulse transit time (PTT) is the time taken for the pulse pressure wave to travel from the heart (R-wave on EKG), to the periphery. When pleural pressure is negative, there is a drop in blood pressure and thus a lengthening of pulse transit time; the progressive increase in pleural pressure during obstructive apnea is associated with a progressive rise in the amplitude

of PTT oscillations; during central apnea, this does not occur. Thus, it has been suggested that the measurement of PTT may be a noninvasive estimate of inspiratory effort, which could be used to differentiate obstructive from central apnea.[39, 40]

Automatic self-inflating arm cuff sphygmomanometers are likely to be too "invasive" to be used routinely in the sleep laboratory because the patient may arouse when the cuff inflates. A continuous measurement of BP can be obtained using a device consisting of a minature cuff that fits on the finger. The first generation of the device (Finapres, Datex-Ohmeda Inc.) was validated in the anesthesia setting[41, 42] and has been used in a sleep laboratory setting.[43] The current generation of this device (Portapres Model-2, TNO-TPD Biomedical Instrumentation, The Netherlands) can be used for prolonged periods because the measurements are obtained alternately from adjacent fingers, minimizing the risk of injury to the digits. In addition, there is automatic hydrostatic correction if the arm is moved. Measurements are sensitive to movement artifacts caused by flexion of the fingers, perhaps explaining the increased variability of the measurements. In general, this technique is acceptable for continuous measurement of mean BP.[43a, 43b]

METHODS OF DATA COLLECTION

Polysomnography

Is polysomnography (PSG) required in the evaluation of patients suspected of having a respiratory sleep disorder? Yes, in almost all cases.[44] A single, brief clinical observation alone is an ineffective screening or diagnostic procedure for detecting the presence or severity of sleep apnea.[45] Thus, recording while the patient sleeps is required. In most cases, all-night PSG is recommended. Although some laboratories perform nap studies in the afternoon, there are problems with this approach, with the diagnostic yield being only about 75% at best.[46] First, rapid eye movement sleep is usually not attained, and this is the period of greatest interest. Second, if a study is nondiagnostic, a night study is usually required for definitive diagnosis. Most laboratories have abandoned the study of afternoon naps for determining the diagnosis of sleep apnea because, in so many cases, a night study is eventually required and the nap study was "wasted." Some laboratories combine diagnostic and CPAP titration studies (split-night testing) during the same night. This approach has been reported to be acceptable for about 80% of patients.[47] Because some problems,[48] such as mask fit and mouth leaks, may not be apparent after a CPAP device is worn for a short time and because of potential scheduling problems and extra costs associated with travel, we believe it is prudent to record an entire night on CPAP in patients who live far away from the laboratory. Whether a 20% inadequate outcome of split-night testing is offset by a potential monetary saving is a matter of debate because these patients may require retesting and will be inadequately treated until on the proper level of CPAP.

What variables are recorded is a matter of controversy, and four levels of recording montages have been defined (see Table 110–3). Most investigators recommend the recording of oximetry, effort to breathe, air flow, electrocardiography, and neurophysiological variables (including electroencephalography [EEG], electro-oculography [EOG], submental electromyography [EMG], and anterior tibialis EMG)[44, 49]; others believe that monitoring oximetry (alone or with videorecording),[50] thoracoabdominal movement, and the anterior tibialis EMG may be sufficient.[51] Surprisingly, nocturnal oximetry alone is not cost effective because of poor diagnostic accuracy.[2]

Most laboratories use a multichannel paper recorder to collect cardiorespiratory and neurophysiological data. Most of the instruments used to monitor respiration have an analog output in the range of 0 to 5 V DC and require signal conditioning. Because respiratory variables change relatively slowly compared with neurophysiological waveforms, filtering of these signals within reason (down to the range of 3 to 15 Hz) results in little loss of accuracy or frequency response. There may be phase shifts between measurements, which in some cases may be the result of physiology (i.e., circulation time determines the maximal response of oximeters) or of the instruments themselves. For example, some oximeters filter the signals internally. The recording speed required to stage sleep (10 to 15 mm/sec) is adequate to have a good representation of all the respiratory waveforms. This paper speed is adequate to detect the presence of most cardiac arrhythmias but may not be fast enough to analyze the type of arrhythmia in detail. In our laboratory, if we are concerned about analyzing types of cardiac arrhythmias in detail, we use a portable tape-recording system and analyze the data on screen or on paper at the standard 25 mm/sec used in ECG.

Screening Systems

Systems that monitor a subset of the channels recorded during PSG are being used by some laboratories in the investigation of sleep-related respiratory disorders.[52] Apart from a reduction in the stress and discomfort to the patient, there are potential savings of both time and money. Ambulatory monitoring used as a diagnostic screening tool is not a substitute for a detailed evaluation of patients; in fact, even detailed laboratory PSG may have false-negative results.[37, 53, 54] In our experience, screening with oximetry alone may result in false-negative results (i.e., few O_2 desaturations are detected in some patients with apnea). One study reported that oximetry alone interpreted by a very experienced physician could be used to diagnose apnea in only 66% of patients.[51] Another study found that screening oximetry was not cost effective because of poor diagnostic accuracy.[2] Home oximetry alone has significant limitations[55]; although this may be useful in severe obstructive sleep apnea, it is likely that a detailed PSG is necessary in milder forms of sleep disordered breathing, particularly in thin persons without baseline hypoxemia.[56] There are several reasons for this: the slow time constant of the oximeter (see Figs. 101–7 and 101–8); the patient with a very high awake PaO_2 level may have trivial SaO_2 level drops with apneas because the PaO_2 is on the flat portion of the oxyhemoglobin dissociation curve; and it is unknown whether the patient slept during the test. Also, such a screening test cannot aid in the diagnosis of patients with daytime sleepiness who have narcolepsy or periodic leg movements. Thus, many patients with a "negative" screening test result still require PSG; because of poor diagnostic accuracy, oximetry alone is not cost effective.[2]

The addition of a measure of ventilation to oximetry improves diagnostic accuracy somewhat; however, in one study, even when both oximetry and the static charge-sensitive bed were used, the recording was not conclusive in 34% of the population.[11] Some newer screening systems also analyze snoring signals as well as SaO_2.[57]

We do not recommend screening in a patient strongly suspected of having apnea. If the test shows positive results, the patient almost always requires a detailed study before definitive therapy is recommended. If the test shows negative results, the patient is usually restudied in detail to ensure the result was not a false-negative or to look for other sleep pathologies.

Ambulatory monitoring methods are problematic because some systems, limited by mass storage technology, cannot easily record all the sleep data digitally in high resolution (see Chapter 110). Such systems are also prone to record artifacts. Screening systems and their validity and place in clinical assessment are a matter of intense investigation and debate.[55]

Electrocardiography. Twenty-four-hour ECG is sometimes used as a screening tool. Patients may exhibit cyclic bradycardia (even asystole) and tachycardia.[58] Dangerous-looking premature ventricular contractions also may be present.[58] One of the problems with the use of ECG monitoring as a screening test is that not all patients, and in particular those with autonomic neuropathy (e.g., Shy-Drager syndrome), exhibit these changes. In one report, 27% of patients with an apnea index of more than 20 did not have this response.[11]

Portable Data Acquisition Systems. Miniaturized sensors, preamplifiers, and amplifiers exist for EEG, ECG, oxygen saturation, respiration, body temperature, and body movement testing. Computer programs in some commercially available systems control the collection and storage of the physiological data.[52] Obstructive and central apneas, hypopneas, hypoxemia, and rib cage and abdominal paradoxes are recognized and encoded. To save on mass storage, data compression techniques are used to facilitate extended monitoring in some systems. Tidal volume, heart rate, and SaO_2 can be recorded for each breath during an all-night sleep study. These data can then be transferred to a computer for detailed analysis, report generation, and archival storage.

Computer Data Acquisition and Analysis (see Chapter 110). Computerized systems have been used in research laboratories and in clinical laboratories to evaluate respiration during sleep.[59] Some laboratories are even evaluating the use of computerized systems for unattended CPAP titration[60] or for titration in the home setting with remote monitoring.[61] Computer systems that allow paperless data acquisition are constantly being introduced for both laboratory and home use[61, 62]; at least 32 systems were marketed by 17 manufacturers by 1992.[63]

Because of the reduction in price and increased capability for mass storage, systems are available to collect all the data for all electrodes and transducers at appropriate sample rates. Such systems allow for very high resolution analysis of the data and thus require large mass storage memory devices. Some of the systems in which the technician scores the record from the screen are problematic because the resolution of the display may not be adequate to show discrete waveforms with a frequency exceeding 10 to 12 Hz. Other computerized systems process the signals during collection using waveform analytic techniques with or without artificial intelligence algorithms to stage sleep. Such systems are expensive, and most have not been validated for all the pathologies likely to be seen in a laboratory. High-tech devices also require a high level of support, which may not be available in some parts of the world.[64] It thus is difficult to recommend computerized systems as the sole data collection method for widespread routine clinical use. Some believe that available computerized systems can replace paper recordings.[62]

As hardware and software improve, as the cost of mass storage decreases, as technical support becomes more widely available throughout the world, and when validated, such systems will become a useful addition to the clinical sleep laboratory.

STANDARDS

A detailed review[65] of indications and practice parameters[66] for polysomnography were published in 1997. These guidelines are official documents of the American Sleep Disorders Association (now called the American Academy of Sleep Medicine) and are recommended to all readers. Similarly, the reader is directed to the recommendations for syndrome definitions and measurement techniques formulated by the same association.[2a]

Although once very few facilities were able to evaluate patients with sleep breathing disorders, with the use of widely available technology and recording systems, the type of disorder, its severity, and CPAP titration can be achieved for patients in many communities.

References

1. Stradling JR, Davies RJ, Pitson DJ. New approaches to monitoring sleep-related breathing disorders. Sleep. 1996;19(suppl):S77–S84.

2. Epstein LJ, Dorlac GR. Cost-effectiveness analysis of nocturnal oximetry as a method of screening for sleep apnea-hypopnea syndrome. Chest. 1998;113:97–103.

2a. American Academy of Sleep Medicine. Sleep related breathing disorders in adults: recommendations for syndrome definition and measurement techniques in clinical research. Sleep. 1999;22:667–689.

3. George CF, Kryger MH. When is an apnea not an apnea? Am Rev Respir Dis. 1985;131:485–486.

4. Douglas NJ, Martin SE. Arousals and the sleep apnea/hypopnea syndrome. Sleep. 1996;19(suppl):S196–S197.

5. Konno K, Mead J. Measurement of the separate volume changes of ribcage and abdomen during breathing. J Appl Physiol. 1967;22:407–422.

6. Shapiro A, Cohen HD. The use of mercury capillary length gauges for the measurement of the volume of thoracic and diaphragmatic components of human respiration: a theoretical analysis and a practical method. Trans N Y Acad Sci Ser II. 1965;27:634–649.

7. Loveridge B, Perez-Padilla R, West P, et al. Comparison of the stability of the respiratory inductance plethysmograph versus mercury strain gauges in measuring ventilation. Am Rev Respir Dis. 1984;129:A82.

8. Chadha TS, Watson H, Birch S, et al. Validation of respiratory inductive plethysmography using different calibration procedures. Am Rev Respir Dis. 1982;125:644–649.

9. Bloch KE, Li Y, Sackner MA, et al. Breathing pattern during sleep disruptive snoring. Eur Respir J. 1997;10:576–586.

10. Victorin L, Olsson T. Transthoracic impedance: a tool for the evaluation of air and fluid changes in the lung. In: Stetson JB, Swyer PR, eds. Neonatal Intensive Care. St. Louis, Mo: Warren H. Green; 1976.

11. Svanborg E, Larsson H, Carlsson-Nordlander B, et al. A limited diagnostic investigation for obstructive sleep apnea syndrome. Chest. 1990;98:1341–1345.

12. Dawson A. Pneumotachography. In: Clausen JL, Ziment I, eds. Pulmonary Function Testing: Guidelines and Controversies. New York, NY: Academic Press; 1982.

13. Dubois A, Botelho SY, Bedell GN, et al. A new method for measuring airway resistance in man using a body plethysmograph: values in normal subjects and in patients with respiratory disease. J Clin Invest. 1956;35:327.

14. Epstein RA, Epstein MAF, Haddad GG, et al. Practical implementation of the barometric method for measurement of tidal volume. J Appl Physiol. 1980;49:1107–1115.

15. Sharp JT, Druz WS, D'Souza V, et al. Use of the respiratory magnetometer in diagnosis and classification of sleep apnea. Chest. 1980;3:350–353.

16. Sorkin B, Rapoport DM, Falk DB, et al. Canopy ventilation monitor for quantitative measurement of ventilation during sleep. J Appl Physiol. 1980;48:724–730.

17. Martin SE, Wraith PK, Deary IJ, et al. The effect of nonvisible sleep fragmentation on daytime function. Am J Respir Crit Care Med. 1997;155:1596–1601.

17a. Ayappa I, Norman RG, Rapoport DM. Cardiogenic oscillations on the airflow signal during continuous positive airway pressure as a marker of central apnea. Chest. 1999;116:660–666.

18. Montserrat JM, Farre R, Ballester E, et al. Evaluation of nasal prongs for estimating nasal flow. Am J Respir Crit Care Med. 1997;155:211–215.

19. Norman RG, Ahmed MM, Walsleben JA, et al. Detection of respiratory events during NPSG: nasal cannula/pressure sensor versus thermistor. Sleep. 1997;20:1175–1184.

20. Hosselet J-J, Norman RG, Ayappa I, et al. Detection of flow limitation with a nasal cannula/pressure transducer system. Am J Respir Crit Care Med. 1998; 157(pt1):1461–1467.

21. Morielli A, Desjardins D, Brouillette RT. To assess hypoventilation during pediatric polysomnography both transcutaneous and end-tidal CO_2 should be measured. Am Rev Respir Dis. 1992;145:A180.

22. Gugger M. Comparison of ResMed AutoSet (version 3.03) with polysomnography in the diagnosis of the sleep apnoea/hypopnoea syndrome. Eur Respir J. 1997;10:587–591.

23. Clark JS, Votteri B, Ariagno RL, et al. Noninvasive assessment of blood gases. Am Rev Respir Dis. 1992;145:220–232.

24. Douglas NJ, Brash HM, Wraith PK, et al. Accuracy, sensitivity to carboxyhemoglobin, and speed of response of the Hewlett-Packard 47201A Ear Oximeter. Am Rev Respir Dis. 1979;119:311–313.
25. Rebuck AS, Chapman KR, D'Urzo A. The accuracy and response characteristics of a simplified ear oximeter. Chest. 1983;83:860–864.
26. Taylor MB, Whitwam MB. The accuracy of pulse oximeters: a comparative clinical evaluation of five pulse oximeters. Anaesthesia. 1988;43:229–232.
27. West P, George CF, Kryger MH. Dynamic in-vivo response characteristics of three oximeters: Hewlett-Packard 47201A, Biox III, and Nellcor N-100. Sleep. 1987;10:263–271.
28. Yelderman M, New W. Evaluation of pulse oximetry. Anesthesiology. 1983;59:349–352.
29. Hannhart B, Haberer JP, Saulnir C, et al. Accuracy and precision of 14 pulse oximeters. Eur Respir J. 1991;4:115–119.
30. Hannhart B, Michalski H, Delorme N, et al. Reliability of six pulse oximeters in chronic obstructive pulmonary disease. Chest. 1991;99:842–846.
31. Severinhaus JW, Naifeh KH, Koh SO. Errors in 14 pulse oximeters during profound hypoxia. J Clin Monit. 1989;5:72–81.
32. Farré R, Montserrat JM, Ballester E, et al. Importance of the pulse oximeter averaging time when measuring oxygen desaturation in sleep apnea. Sleep. 1998;21:386–390.
33. Barker SJ, Tremper KK, Hufstedler S. The effects of carbon monoxide inhalation on pulse oximetry and transcutaneous PO_2. Anesthesiology. 1987;66:677–679.
34. Tremper KK, Barker SJ. Pulse oximetry. Anesthesiology. 1989;70:98–106.
35. Ries AL, Prewitt LM, Johnson JJ. Skin color and ear oximetry. Chest. 1989;96:287–290.
36. Murphy KG, Secunda JA, Rockoff MA. Severe burns from a pulse oximeter. Anesthesiology. 1990;73:350–352.
37. Meyer TJ, Eveloff J, Kline LR, et al. One negative polysomonography does not exclude OSA. Am Rev Respir Dis. 1992;145:A724.
38. Lubbers DW. Theoretical basis of the transcutaneous blood gas measurements. Crit Care Med. 1981;9:721–733.
39. Pitson DJ, Stradling JR. Value of beat-to-beat blood pressure changes, detected by pulse transit time, in the management of the obstructive sleep apnoea syndrome. Eur Respir J. 1998;12:685–692.
40. Argod J, Pepin JL, Levy P. Differentiating obstructive and central sleep respiratory events through pulse transit time. Am J Respir Crit Care Med. 1998;158:1778–1783.
41. Kurki T, Smith NT, Nead N, et al. Noninvasive continuous blood pressure measurement from the finger: optimal measurement conditions and factors affecting reliability. J Clin Monit. 1987;3:6–13.
42. Van Egmond J, Hasenbos M, Crul JF. Invasive vs non-invasive measurement of arterial pressure. Br J Anaesthiol. 1985;57:433–443.
43. Mateika JH, Slutsky AS, Hoffstein V. The effect of snoring on mean arterial blood pressure during non-REM sleep. Am Rev Respir Dis. 1992;145:141–152.
43a. Omboni S, Parati G, Castiglioni P, et al. Estimation of blood pressure variability from 24-hour ambulatory finger blood pressure. Hypertension. 1998;32:52–68.
43b. Voogel AJ, van Montfrans GA. Reproducibility of twenty-four-hour finger arterial blood pressure, variability and systemic hemodynamics. J Hypertens. 1997;15:1761–1765.
44. Phillipson EA, Remmers JE (Chairs). American Thoracic Society Consensus Conference on Indications and Standards for Cardio-pulmonary Sleep Studies. Am Rev Respir Dis. 1989;139:559–568.
45. Haponick EF, Smith PL, Meyers DA, et al. Evaluation of sleep-disordered breathing: is polysomnography necessary? Am J Med. 1984;77:671–677.
46. Arias A, Antonio M, Dandamudi N, et al. Diagnostic yield of daytime nap polysomnography. Am Rev Respir Dis. 1992;145:A724.
47. Iber C, O'Brien C, Schluter J, et al. Single night studies in obstructive sleep apnea. Sleep. 1991;14:383–385.
48. Jamieson A. Split-night studies: a new standard? Forcing the examination of outcome. Sleep. 1991;14:381–382. Editorial.
49. McAvoy RD. Guidelines for Respiratory Sleep Studies. Sydney, Australia: Thoracic Society of Australia and New Zealand; 1988.
50. British Thoracic Society. Facilities for the diagnosis and treatment of abnormal breathing during sleep including nocturnal ventilation. BTS News. 1990;5:7–10.
51. Douglas NJ, Thomas JMA. Clinical value of polysomnography. Lancet. 1992;339:347–350.
52. Emsellem HA. Verification of sleep apnea using a portable sleep apnea screening device. South Med J. 1990;83:748–752.
53. Dean RJ, Chaudhary BA. Negative polysomnogram in patients with obstructive sleep apnea syndrome. Chest. 1992;101:105–108.
54. Meyer TJ, Eveloff SE, Kline LR, et al. One negative polysomnogram does not exclude obstructive sleep apnea. Chest. 1993;103:756–760.
55. Keenan SP, Anderson B, Wiggs B, et al. The predictive accuracy of screening techniques in patients with suspected obstructive sleep apnea. Am Rev Respir Dis. 1992;145:A723.
56. Collard PH, Aubert G, Rodenstein DO. Value of nocturnal pulse oximetry as a screening tool for sleep apnea-hypopnea syndrome. Am Rev Respir Dis. 1992;145:A724.
57. Issa F, Morrison D, Hajduk E, et al. Digital monitoring of sleep apnea using SaO_2 and snoring signals. Am Rev Respir Dis. 1992;145:A722.
58. Guilleminault C, Connolly S, Winkle R, et al. Cyclical variation of the heart rate in sleep apnea syndrome: mechanisms and usefulness of 24 h electrocardiography as a screening technique. Lancet. 1984; 1:126–131.
59. West P, Kryger MH. Continuous monitoring of respiratory variables during sleep by microcomputer. Methods Inf Med. 1983;22:198–203.
60. Guilleminault C, Stoohs R, Miles L, et al. Unattended CPAP titration: toward a smart machine. Am Rev Respir Dis. 1992;145:A725.
61. White DP, Gibb TJ. Evaluation of Healthdyne NightWatch system to titrate CPAP in the home. Sleep. 1998;21:198–204.
62. White DP, Gibb TJ. Evaluation of a computerized polysomnographic system. Sleep. 1998;21:188–196.
63. Zimmerman JT, Torch WC, Reichert JA. A comparison of sleep-data-acquisition and analysis systems and computerized-paperless polysomnography. J Polysomnogr Technol. June 1992:30–44.
64. Gitanjali R. Establishing a sleep polysomnography laboratory in India: problems and pitfalls. Sleep. 1998;21:331–332.
65. Chesson AL Jr, Ferber RA, Fry J, et al. The indications for polysomnography and related procedures: an American Sleep Disorders Association Review. Sleep. 1997;20:423–487.
66. American Sleep Disorders Association Standards of Practice Committee. Practice parameters for the indications for polysomnography and related procedures: an American Sleep Disorders Association Report. Sleep. 1997;20:406–422.

102

Assessment of Sleep-Related Erections

J. Catesby Ware
Max Hirshkowitz

Penile erections normally occur in two situations: during sexual arousal and during rapid eye movement (REM) sleep. After German physiologists published the first scientific report on periodic sleep-related erections (SREs) in 1944,[1] Fisher et al.[2] and Karacan[3] determined that these erections occurred in association with REM sleep. (The physiology of SREs is reviewed in detail in Chapter 23.) SREs begin at age 3 to 6 months[4, 5] and occur in healthy male human beings of all ages, as well as in other mammals. In the flaccid penis, blood drawn from the corpora cavernosa has a PO_2 similar to that of venous blood (25 to 43 mmHg).[6] Regular penile vasodilation during sleep probably provides the oxygenation, nutrition, and waste removal necessary to maintain erectile capability, thus adding a new meaning to the adage "Use it or lose it."

In addition, SREs (also referred to as nocturnal penile tumescence [NPT]) are diagnostically useful in the evaluation of impotence. Men with abnormal SREs are likely to have impairment in physiological systems underlying normal erectile functioning; thus, SREs are sensitive to organic factors that impair erectile functioning. Patients with abnormal SREs typically have abnormalities in vascular, neurological, or hormonal systems necessary for normal sexual functioning; however, sleep appears to insulate SREs from psychological factors. For example, viewing a video before sleep, regardless of whether its content is neutral, dysphoric, or sexually explicit, does not affect subsequent erections.[7] Nevertheless, the isolation of these sleep erections from psychiatric illnesses is not complete. Depression, a problem associated with altered sleep,[8] may result in an abnormal SRE pattern.[9] Furthermore, even after the treatment of depression, patients have greater SRE variability than normal subjects.[9] Depression or any disorder that alters the basic sleep pattern, particularly REM sleep, may alter the SRE pattern.

PROCEDURES

This chapter focuses on the procedures for the assessment of impotence, particularly on SRE monitoring. We describe in detail the traditional recording technique for measuring SREs that involves the use of penile plethysmography with strain gauges and polysomnography. SRE data obtained in a vacuum is of limited usefulness, so the diagnostic assessment of a patient complaining of impotence requires several steps. The process includes a history and physical examination, an explanation of the procedures to the patient, calibration and the placement of correct-size strain gauges, measurement of penile rigidity and observation of the penis in its most erect state, and the determination of sleep stages, particularly REM sleep.

History and Physical Examination

In addition to the normal information usually obtained during the history, specific questions concerning the patient's sexual ability are helpful, such as: What is the maximum erection currently obtainable? What is the minimum percentage of a full erection necessary to achieve penetration? Is there pain during erection? Is there penile curvature? Is there any change in sensitivity or numbness? Is there any change in level of sexual desire? Can the patient ejaculate? Can he ejaculate with a soft penis? Does he have a regular sexual partner? How does the partner respond? What are the patient's expectations for sexual performance? What is his sexual experience? When was the last successful intercourse? Is the problem partner specific? Is there any difference in erection with different sexual practices?

During the physical examination, careful palpation of the penis for Peyronie's plaques is important. If there are other indications of hormonal abnormalities, an assay for testosterone and prolactin can be particularly helpful.

Assessment of Co-Morbidity Factors

Cardiovascular, endocrine, genitourinary, neurological, and psychiatric conditions commonly exist in patients with impotence. Disorders accompanying altered SREs include diabetes mellitus,[10–13] hypogonadism,[14] chronic obstructive pulmonary disease,[15] alcoholism,[16, 17] spinal lesions,[18] end-stage renal disease,[19] and hypertension.[20] Although the SRE pattern continues to some degree, the changes are often profound. For example, compared with potent subjects, SREs in patients with diabetes have smaller maximum circumference increases (often less than 10 mm) and greater variability in the circumference of each episode. Detumescence may be prolonged; penile rigidity is low (often less than 500 g); SREs occur less frequently and have a shorter duration.

Hypogonadism is of particular interest. Decreased testosterone traditionally was thought to primarily reduce sexual drive. However, recent data indicate that testosterone affects SREs. Reduction in testosterone with gonadotropin-releasing hormone agonist lowers SREs in normal subjects without affecting REM sleep.[21] In addition, the withdrawal of androgen replacement therapy in hypogonadal men results in diminished SREs without changing the sleep patterns.[14] Thus, endocrine functions, not just psychosexual factors, influence erectile arousal mechanisms.

Medications

Several classes of drugs adversely affect erectile function in men. Some medications reduce SREs by altering penile physiology; other pharmacological agents suppress erections as a result of REM sleep disruption. Consequently, it is essential to acquire a thorough drug history. Antihypertensives and other medications that affect autonomic nervous system functioning have the potential to interfere with sexual function. Other medications associated with erectile failure include antidepressants, antiandrogens, and antipsychotics. In addition, cimetidine, disulfiram, atropine, digoxin, and cancer chemotherapy agents may cause iatrogenic impotence. Conversely, trazodone increases the duration of SREs in young normal males.[22] Three antidepressants do not reduce REM sleep: nefazodone,[23] bupropion,[24] and trimipramine.[25] These medications also appear less likely to impair sexual functioning than other antidepressants.

Polysomnography

Recording

Traditional SRE evaluation requires a full polysomnographic study. In addition to the transducers used to assess sleep and respiratory problems, a technician places strain gauges around the base of the penis (base gauge) and behind the glans at the coronal sulcus (sometimes called tip gauge). Strain gauges are loops of mercury-filled Silastic tubing with a small wire inserted in each end that are sealed and tied together[26] so that a small electrical current can pass through the mercury. Penile expansion produces elongation and thinning of the gauge, so increased resistance reflects a circumference increase. The circumference changes indicate the underlying dynamics of penile erections. The process involves initial vasodilatation and filling of the corpora cavernosa, maintenance of the tumescence, and detumescence. Table 102–1 summarizes SRE recording procedures and interpretations.

The measurement of only penile circumference changes is inadequate. Proper assessment requires the measurement of rigidity because normal penile circumference increases can occur without rigidification. Some patients may have a 2-cm circumference increase with little increase in rigidity. Conversely, although less common, some patients have normal rigidity even with little circumference increase (i.e., a maximum circumference increase [MCI] of less than 10 mm). It is crucial to measure rigidity during the maximal circumference of a representative SRE.

For a clinical diagnosis, the few awakenings made to measure rigidity have little consequence on the overall sleep pattern, but for some research studies, these awakenings may be unacceptable. On the first night in the laboratory for normal subjects, the technician has only 6 min per episode (on average) to decide whether the patient has reached an MCI and to measure rigidity.[27] In patients with pathology, this window of opportunity is usually shorter; therefore, well before it is time to measure rigidity, the technician must prepare the force gauge, videotape, and camera.

Although the first episode of tumescence may be unstable, it often indicates the minimum circumference increase and duration of subsequent episodes. The technician typically skips measuring rigidity during the first erection and takes a measurement during the second erection episode if the tip circumference reaches at least the circumference achieved during the first erection and stabilizes. Later, if the patient has tumescence with greater circumference than that accompanying the best (highest) rigidity value, the technician takes additional measurements.

No device provides a continuous measure of the resistance of the penis to buckling; consequently, accuracy depends on the technician's skill at judging when to measure penile rigidity using a force gauge. To measure penile rigidity, we awaken the patient and remind him of the procedure. (The patient is given an explanation of the rigidity measurement procedure during the office intake, during the tour of the facilities after the office intake, and during the wiring in the evening before bed.) To quickly measure rigidity, the technician pulls down the covers and the patient's pajamas, stabilizes the patient's penis at the base between the index finger and thumb, and applies the force gauge to the tip of the penis, parallel to the longitudinal axis. The technician increases the force gradually until either the penile shaft buckles or the meter reaches 1000 g. The technician then photographs the penis and instructs the patient to inspect and estimate the percentage of a full erection. This patient estimate can sometimes be informative. The entire procedure takes less than 30 sec. Generally, this is not sufficient time for detumescence to occur. A normal healthy male is usually able to achieve an axial rigidity of 750 to 1200 g. Rigidities of 500 to 749 g are potentially functional. Rigidities of less than 500 g are abnor-

Table 102-1. TECHNICAL PROCEDURES AND POSSIBLE PROBLEMS

Procedure	Description or Purpose	Potential Problems
Gauge calibration	Gauges and amplifiers are calibrated on standard-size cylinders.	Gauge size does not match calibration cylinder.
Gauge sizing and placement	Gauges should be approximately 0.5 cm less than flaccid penile circumference. Place one around penile base and one behind the glans at the coronal sulcus.	Gauges that are not perpendicular to the axis of penis will roll as they stretch. An unsecured tip gauge on an uncircumsized patient may slide over the end of the penis. Too small a gauge loses linearity. Too large a gauge loses sensitivity.
Beginning the recording	The recording should indicate a circumference close to that of calibration cylinder.	A circumference reading greater than baseline may indicate incorrect placement, a gauge that is too small, a broken gauge, or a penile erection.
Artifact detection	Technician must be able to recognize and eliminate artifact during study.	Common problems include a broken gauge, a tip gauge off the penis, or too little slack to gauge to allow for penile erection.
Rigidity measurement	Measure rigidity at maximum circumference.	Measuring not at maximum results in lower rigidity values and can result in a false-positive study.
Visual observation and photography	Observe and photograph the erection when measuring rigidity. This can document anatomical abnormalities and help resolve any discrepancies between rigidity reading and technician estimates of fullness of erection.	If the rigidity readings are less than normal, to ensure measurements are made at appropriate times, repeat the procedure during the night.
Postcalibration	This documents normal functioning of gauges and helps validate abnormal circumference changes during study.	If handled improperly, gauges may break during their removal in the morning.
Multinight recording	Testing usually requires two studies to determine rigidity and ability to maintain erections.	Poor sleep or a sleep disorder (e.g., sleep apnea) may necessitate additional recording nights.
Comparison with norms	This is necessary to account for age-related changes.	There may be disturbed sleep or abnormal sleep architecture.

mally diminished and rarely are adequate to achieve penetration.

The patient estimate during rigidity measurement reveals a subgroup of patients with normal SREs who estimate their erections as far below normal and insufficient for intercourse. These patients may indicate that they have little or no erection notwithstanding the presence of a physiologically normal erection. Possibly, these patients also obtain full erections during sexual activity but have a distorted perception of their degree of erection. It is likely that individuals with *penis state misperception* require different treatment than patients with psychogenic impotence arising from performance anxiety. This perceptual discrepancy is a possible variant of the body dysmorphic disorder described in the *Diagnostic and Statistical Manual of Mental Disorders, Fourth Edition.*[28]

Visual Observation

The process of awakening the patient to measure rigidity allows detection of abnormalities that may not be obvious in the flaccid penis, such as a marked curve or bend in the penis caused by Peyronie's disease.

Consider the example of a 35-year-old, physically healthy man diagnosed with schizoid personality disorder and psychogenic impotence. He presented with a 2-year history of an inability to obtain an erection sufficient for penetration. His tumescence pattern and rigidity were normal; however, he had a 75-degree upward bend in his penis. Examination of his penis during the office visit failed to detect a small plaque on the dorsal surface of his penis, and therefore the diagnosis of Peyronie's disease was missed. In addition, either the patient had failed to mention the bend during several interviews or he was not aware of it.

In some cases, photographic documentation of a normal SRE helps to persuade the patient of his ability to achieve a full erection. Photographing the erection is also helpful when considering surgical correction of Peyronie's disease. Documentation of the erect state, before and after surgery, can be desirable. Finally, a photograph of the erection at the time of rigidity measurement provides independent evidence for cross-validating buckling (rigidity) values.

Number of Nights

An SRE evaluation usually requires two nights of polysomnography, although for some patients, a single night is sufficient to make a diagnosis. One study night usually suffices when a completely normal SRE pattern occurs. It is worth noting that many patients have reduced REM sleep during the first night sleeping in the laboratory.[29] Because REM sleep is a key ingredient for evaluating SREs, a second night is often required. Although the patient may obtain a full erection during the first night, shortened REM sleep episodes will prevent accurate determination of his ability to maintain these erections. On the second night, the patient sleeps undisturbed to determine the duration of his erections. Short-duration SREs may accompany a complaint of inability to maintain erections. An extreme example occurs in some spinal cord–injured patients who obtain brief rigid erections (reflex erections) without the ability to sustain them.[18]

On the second night, if MCI exceeds that occurring during the first-night rigidity measurement and the maximal rigidity on the first night was less than 750 g, the patient must return for a third night to collect additional rigidity measurements. During the second night, if a full erection occurs near the patient's scheduled arising time, measuring rigidity may obviate the need for a third recording session.

Scoring and Summarizing Data

SRE Measures. Parameters needed for diagnosis include SRE frequency, magnitude, and duration. In addition, indices of sleep continuity, integrity, and architecture complete the necessary quantitative picture of SREs. Four points—T_{up}, T_{max}, T_{down}, and T_{zero}— characterize an episode of penile tumescence; these are defined in Table 102–2 and illustrated in Figure 102–1.

Sleep Measures. Sleep, especially REM sleep, provides the essential physiological milieu for SREs. Polysomnography during sleep erection assessment provides a number of benefits. Polysomnography prevents a false-positive test—that is, an abnormal erection pattern due to abnormal sleep. If the duration of REM sleep is short, the erectile duration may be short as a result of sleep disturbance rather than erectile pathophysiology. This often occurs during first-night evaluations conducted in a noisy hospital environment. It may also occur when a patient's medication suppresses REM sleep (e.g., medications with anticholinergic properties and many antidepressants). A false-positive test increases the likelihood of misdiagnosis, resulting in invasive treatment for the patient's impotence.

Sleep Disorders. Because older men are particularly susceptible to sleep disturbances[30] and more likely to complain of impotence, assessment of sleep is an important part of the SRE evaluation. Sleep apnea is exceedingly common in men with erectile dysfunction.[31, 32] In a group of 1025 patients complaining of impotence, more than 25% had significant obstructive sleep apnea (apnea frequency of 10 or greater per hour of sleep).[33] Periodic limb movements in sleep also occur at a remarkably high rate in men with erectile dysfunction. Of 768 consecutively evaluated impotent men,

Table 102–2. SLEEP-RELATED ERECTION SCORING, TABULATION, AND SUMMARY PARAMETERS

Parameter	Description
Maximum circumference increase (MCI)	The overall MCI above the flaccid state (baseline) that occurs during the recording period. The MCI also is determined for each tumescence episode.
T_{up} (tumescence up)	The beginning of tumescence. This is the point where there has been more than a 2-mm circumference increase above the baseline for 2 min. The term T_{up} also refers to the time between the points T_{up} and T_{max}.
T_{max} (tumescence maximum)	The point where penile circumference reaches 75% of the MCI for the entire night. T_{max} also refers to the time between the points T_{max} and T_{down}. If the MCI for a particular episode does not reach 75%, T_{max} for that episode begins and ends at the maximal point for that episode and T_{down} begins in the next minute.
T_{down} (tumescence down)	Begins where the circumference falls below the 75% T_{max} criterion and continues to T_{zero}. The term T_{down} also identifies the time between the points T_{down} and T_{zero}.
T_{zero} (tumescence zero)	The point where penile circumference reaches 2 mm or less above the baseline.
Tumescence episodes (TE)	Number of SREs during the sleep period. This closely parallels the number of REM periods. Episodes that overlap REM sleep by at least 1 min (REM-related episodes) may be tabulated separately.
Total tumescence time (TTT)	Minutes during the recording in which penile circumference is more than 2 mm above the baseline. This is usually 125 ± 50 min.
Percentage total tumescence time (%TTT)	Percentage of the sleep period (interval from sleep onset to final awakening) during which there was a more than 2-mm increase in penile circumference above baseline.
Fluctuations (FLUC)	Transient decreases in circumference during T_{max}. The circumference drops below 75% of the MCI and may approach, but does not reach, baseline. Fluctuations may accompany anxiety-laden dreams and may occur to a greater degree in patients with vascular outflow problems. Because fluctuations allow for increased blood flow through the penis, they may be physiologically important during an erection.
TTT-to-REM sleep ratio (TTT/REM)	Ratio of total tumescence time to REM sleep time facilitates comparisons between records with different durations of REM sleep.
T_{max}-to-REM sleep ratio (T_{max}/REM)	Ratio of the total duration of maximal tumescence (minutes between the points T_{max} and T_{down}) to REM sleep duration. This measures the erectile system's ability to maintain tumescence in the presence of an appropriate stimulus (i.e., REM sleep).
T_{up}–REM sleep onset differential (T_{up}–REM_{on})	Time between T_{up} and the beginning of REM sleep. In healthy subjects, T_{up} may precede an episode of REM sleep. In this situation, T_{up}–REM_{on} is a positive number. It is a negative number when tumescence onset follows the onset of REM.
REM sleep–T_{zero} offset differential (REM_{off}–T_{zero})	Time between the end of REM sleep and the end of tumescence. If tumescence ends before the end of REM sleep, the measure is a negative number. When tumescence ends after REM sleep, it is a positive number. In healthy subjects and patients free from vascular impotence, it may measure sympathetic activity because alpha-adrenergic receptor blocking will dramatically prolong REM_{off}–T_{zero}.

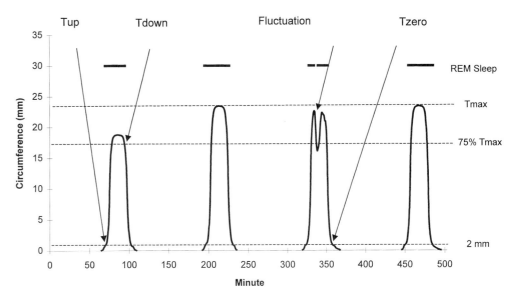

Figure 102–1. Normal sleep-related erection pattern illustrating T_{up}, T_{down}, T_{max}, a fluctuation, and T_{zero}. Note that the illustrated points actually occur on each of the four erections. The duration of T_{max} is measured from when circumference reaches more than 75% of the maximum circumference increase (T_{max}) to when it drops below the 75% line. REM sleep is indicated by the dark bars above the erections. Circumference is given in millimeters.

54% had 15 or more leg movements per hour of sleep.[34] These disorders may suppress REM sleep, increase penile strain gauge artifact due to increased movement, or directly contribute to impotence.

Sleep apnea may result in cardiovascular problems.[35] In addition, hypoxia insults associated with apnea events and obesity-related hypoventilation may lower testosterone levels. The treatment of obstructive sleep apnea appears to increase testosterone levels and reverse a decrease in sexual function in some men.[36] Also, excessive daytime sleepiness, a prominent symptom of sleep apnea, can overwhelm the libido and result in falling asleep in bed rather than sexual activity.

Interpreting SRE Results

Several questions are helpful to interpret the results.
Does the Patient Have Sustained REM Sleep Episodes? During wakefulness, sexual stimulation initiates penile erections. During sleep, REM sleep provides an analog to sexual stimulation. Interpretation of a polysomnographic SRE recording must be within the context of REM sleep. The amount of REM sleep required for a valid study depends on both the patient's complaint and the pattern of penile erections. Some patients complain of difficulty maintaining penile erections, and polysomnography reveals full but brief erections. Fragmented and short REM sleep episodes make it impossible to determine whether the short-duration erections reflect abnormal penile physiology or the REM sleep interruption. In others, brief REM sleep interruptions or short-duration REM periods do not substantially alter episodes of penile erections. Under these circumstances, the REM sleep fragmentation is irrelevant.

When the patient complains of an inability to obtain a full erection, REM sleep duration must be sufficient to obtain a stable maximum circumference for measuring rigidity. Although approximately 100 min of REM sleep occur during a normal night, this duration may not be necessary. One sustained 20-min REM episode may be sufficient to determine whether the patient can obtain and maintain a normal erection. If a patient is taking medication, however, one normal erection at the end of the sleep period may not indicate that the patient can function normally during the day. It is possible that the medication suppresses erectile capability during wakefulness and the early part of the night. As the night progresses, blood levels may decline during sleep and allow a normal erection to occur toward the end of the night.

Does the Erection Progress Normally to the Maximum Circumference Increase? In normal REM SREs, T_{up} is steep and steady. The development of an erection from onset to T_{max} takes approximately 10 min.

Does the Erection Continue Throughout the REM Episode? Once reached, the maximal erectile phase should remain throughout most of the REM episode. Small oscillations (several millimeters) are common; however, an inability to sustain tumescence for more than 1 or 2 min during a normal REM sleep episode is unusual. Such a pattern suggests venous leakage or some other penile pathophysiology. Detumescence typically starts just before the end of REM sleep and continues for 10 to 20 min (time from T_{down} to T_{zero}). The time from the end of REM sleep to T_{zero} ($REM_{off}-T_{zero}$) is typically 5 to 10 min.

Does Detumescence Proceed Quickly After the End of REM Sleep? *Detumescence* is a physiologically active phase with increased sympathetic activity and vasoconstriction. Even to maintain the flaccid penis, some degree of sympathetic tone is necessary. The inability to proceed through detumescence rapidly *(fuzzy detumescence)* suggests an alteration in autonomic functioning. Block of the sympathetic nervous system pharmacologically with, for example, trazodone, may result in tumescence continuing long after the end of REM sleep.[22]

Does Penile Buckling Force Indicate Functional Erectile Capacity? Evidence suggests that 500 g is the minimal force required to achieve penetration under circumstances conducive to intercourse.[37] These data derive from direct measures during vaginal insertion, confidence ratings made by normal subjects, and success–failure judgments made by patients. The presence of an erection with at least 750 g rigidity suggests adequate capacity for achieving penetration. There are several exceptions. A patient complaining of difficulty maintaining an erection after achieving full tumescence may have completely rigid but short-lived tumescence episodes during sleep. Other instances in which rigidity values must be complemented by other measures are in assessment of men with spinal injuries, the pelvic steal syndrome,[38] and Peyronie's disease.

Are Penile Pulsations Present? The resolution of the recording must be sufficient to detect penile pulsations. Pulsations are transient circumference increases that last approximately 1 sec. Pulsations result from contractions of the bulbocavernosus and ichiocavernosus muscles. They normally occur during T_{up} and the first part of T_{max} at a frequency of several per minute. They occur less frequently in patients with organic problems.[39] The absence of pulsations may indicate either gauge artifact (i.e., no true tumescence) or a problem of neurological origin.

How Do SREs Compare With Age-Matched Normative Data? Sleep-related erections change with age in normal subjects.[27] These changes occur not only as a result of changes in sleep pattern but also apparently as a result of erectile capability. Table 102–3 illustrates statistically reliable but modest changes with age. Importantly, these data indicate that sleep erections persist throughout life in healthy subjects. A comparison of the number and duration of erections in patients with age-matched normative values is helpful when interpreting nocturnal penile tumescence.

Does the Patient Have an Agenda? Concurrent polysomnography during SRE testing safeguards against undetected intentional manipulation of data. Some patients strongly prefer one treatment over another. To fake an "organic pattern," a patient assessed without polysomnography need only remove the strain gauge or stay awake. A diagnosis of organic impotence may increase the chance of obtaining a penile prosthesis, help obtain a more favorable judgment from a jury in an accident compensation case, or affect the ruling in a sexual assault trial.

Table 102–3. APPROXIMATE RANGE FOR SELECTED SRE PARAMETERS AT DIFFERENT AGES

Age (y)	Total Tumescence (min)	REM-Related Tumescence* (%)	No. of Episodes
20–29	100–200	20–30	2–5
30–49	65–165	19–29	2–5
40–49	60–160	14–24	2–4
50–59	60–160	13–23	2–4
60–69	40–140	12–22	1–3

In the presence of normal REM sleep, patient values less than the lower range suggest an abnormal SRE pattern.
Data derived from Ware JC, Hirshkowitz M. Characteristics of penile erections during sleep. J Clin Neurophysiol. 1992;9:78–87.
*(TTT/REM) × 100.
SRE, sleep-related erection.

SUMMARY

The measurement of SREs provides an objective assessment of erectile capability but must be combined with a clinical assessment. Performed correctly, a diagnostic evaluation of SREs consists of the following measures.

1. *Measurement of sleep pattern* is performed to prevent false-positive tests, to ease artifact detection, and to detect subject manipulation of data. An additional benefit is that the information obtained from sleep studies may be helpful in determining the presence of depression or sleep-related pathology.
2. *Measurement of penile circumference patterns* is performed to determine the number, magnitude, and duration of erections. An ability to obtain and maintain an erection within REM sleep suggests an intact erectile physiology.
3. *Measurement of penile rigidity* is performed to determine erectile quality. The maximal circumference is not a guaranteed indicator of rigidity; thus, interpretation of the study requires rigidity measurements during MCIs.
4. *Visual inspection of the penis during an erection* is performed to determine penile anatomic problems that may not be obvious when the penis is flaccid. During an awakening when tumescence is present, asking the patient to estimate the degree of his erection allows identification of a penis state misperception.

Accurate diagnostic methods become more essential as knowledge of the mechanisms controlling penile erections increases and as treatment techniques become more refined. When treatment options were limited to penile prosthesis, psychotherapy, or sex therapy, impotence was classified as either organic or psychogenic. The degree of physical impairment and precise cause often made little difference. With improved surgical techniques and advancements in pharmacotherapy, detailed information concerning erectile function is more important to help match the treatment with the cause. Sleep erection monitoring provides a wealth of information to facilitate therapeutic decisions. Polysomnographic assessment of SREs still represents the most unbiased, objective, noninvasive tool for differentially diagnosing erectile dysfunction in men.

References

1. Ohlmeyer P, Brilmayer H, Hullstrung H. Periodische vorgange in schaf pflug. Arch Ges Physiol. 1944;248:559–560.
2. Fisher C, Gross J, Zuch J. Cycle of penile erection synchronous with dreaming (REM) sleep: preliminary report. Arch Gen Psychiatry. 1965;12:29–45.
3. Karacan I. The effect of exciting presleep events on dream reporting and penile erections during sleep [dissertation]. Brooklyn, NY: Department of Psychiatry, Downstate Medical Center Library, New York University; 1965.
4. Karacan I. The developmental aspect and the effect of certain clinical conditions upon penile erection during sleep. Proceedings of the IV World Congress of Psychiatry, Madrid, September 1966. Excerp Med Int Congr Series. 1996;150:2356 2359.

5. Korner A. REM organization in neonates. Arch Gen Psychiatry. 1968;19:330–340.

6. Kim N, Vardi Y, Padma-Nathan H, et al. Oxygen tension regulates the nitric oxide pathway: physiological role in penile erection. J Clin Invest. 1993;91:437–422.

7. Ware, JC, Hirshkowitz, M, Thornby J, et al. Sleep-related erections: effects of presleep sexual arousal. J Psychosomat Res. 1997; 42:547–553.

8. Benca RM, Obermeyer WH, Thisted RA, et al. Sleep and psychiatric disorders: a meta-analysis. Arch Gen Psychiatry. 1992; 49:651–668.

9. Nofzinger EA, Thase ME, Reynolds CF, et al. Sexual function in depressed men: assessment by self-report, behavioral, and nocturnal penile tumescence measures before and after treatment with cognitive behavior therapy. Arch Gen Psychiatry. 1993; 50:24–30.

10. Hirshkowitz M, Karacan I, Rando KC, et al. Diabetes, erectile dysfunction, and sleep-related erections. Sleep. 1990;13:53–68.

11. Karacan I, Salis PJ, Ware JC, et al. Nocturnal penile tumescence and diagnosis in diabetic impotence. Am J Psychiatry. 1978; 135:191–197.

12. Schiavi RC, Stimmel BB, Mandeli J, et al. Diabetes mellitus and male sexual function: a controlled study. Diabetologia. 1993; 36:745–751.

13. Zuckerman M, Neeb M, Ficher M, et al. Nocturnal penile tumescence and penile responses in the waking state in diabetic and nondiabetic sexual dysfunctionals. Arch Sex Behav. 1985;14:109–129.

14. Cunningham GR, Hirshkowitz M, Korenman SG, et al. Testosterone replacement therapy and sleep-related erections in hypogonadal men. J Clin Endocrinol Metab. 1990;70:792–797.

15. Fletcher EC, Martin RJ. Sexual dysfunction and erectile impotence in chronic obstructive pulmonary disease. Chest. 1982; 81:413–421.

16. Karacan I, Moore CA. Sexual dysfunction in alcoholic men. In: Wheatley D, ed. Psychopharmacology and Sexual Disorders. British Association for Psychopharmacology Monograph. Oxford, England: Oxford University; 1983:113–122.

17. Snyder S, Karacan I. Effects of chronic alcoholism on nocturnal penile tumescence. Psychosomat Med. 1981;43:423–429.

18. Halstead LS, Dimitrijevic M, Karacan I, et al. Impotence in spinal cord injury: neurophysiological assessment of diminished tumescence and its relation to supraspinal influences. Curr Concepts Rehab Med. 1984;1:8–14.

19. Karacan I, Dervent A, Cunningham G, et al. Assessment of nocturnal penile tumescence as an objective method for evaluating sexual functioning in ESRD patients. Dialysis Transplant. 1978;7:872–876, 890.

20. Karacan I, Salis PJ, Hirshkowitz M, et al. Erectile dysfunction in hypertensive men: sleep-related erections, penile blood flow, and musculovascular events. J Urol. 1989;142:56–61.

21. Hirshkowitz M, Moore CA, O'Connor S, et al. Androgen and sleep-related erections. J Psychosomat Res. 1997;42:541–546.

22. Saenz de Tejada I, Ware JC, Blanco R, et al. Pathophysiology of prolonged penile erection associated with trazodone use. J Urol. 1991;145:60–64.

23. Ware JC, Rose, FV, McBrayer R. The acute effects of nefazodone, trazodone and buspirone on sleep and sleep-related penile tumescence in normal subjects. Sleep. 1994;6:544–550.

24. Nofzinger EA, Reynolds CF 3rd, Thase ME, et al. REM sleep enhancement by bupropion in depressed men. Am J Psychiatry. 1995;152:274–276.

25. Ware JC, Brown FW, Moorad PJ, et al. Effects on sleep: a double-blind study comparing trimipramine to imipramine in depressed insomniac patients. Sleep. 1989;12:537–549.

26. Karacan I. A simple and inexpensive transducer for quantitative measurements of penile erection during sleep. Behav Res Methods Instrum. 1969;1:251–252.

27. Ware JC, Hirshkowitz M. Characteristics of penile erections during sleep. J Clin Neurophysiol. 1992;9:78–87.

28. American Psychiatric Association. Diagnostic and Statistical Manual of Mental Disorders. 4th ed. Washington, DC: American Psychiatric Association; 1994:466–468.

29. Agnew HW, Webb WB, Williams RL. The first night effect: an EEG study of sleep. Psychophysiology. 1966;2:263–266.

30. Miles LE, Dement WC. Sleep and aging. Sleep. 1980;3:119–220.

31. Schmidt HS, Wise HA. Significance of impaired penile tumescence and associated polysomnographic abnormalities in the impotent patient. J Urol. 1981;126:348–352.

32. Pressman MR, DiPhillipo MA, Kendrick JI, et al. Problems in the interpretation of nocturnal penile tumescence studies: disruption of sleep by occult sleep disorders. J Urol. 1986;136:595–598.

33. Hirshkowitz M, Karacan I, Arcasoy MO, et al. Prevalence of sleep apnea in men with erectile dysfunction. Urology. 1990; 36:232–234.

34. Hirshkowitz M, Karacan I, Arcasoy MO, et al. The prevalence of periodic limb movements during sleep in men with erectile dysfunction. Biol Psychiatry. 1989;26:541–544.

35. Weiss JW, Remsburg S, Garpestad E, et al. Hemodynamic consequences of obstructive sleep apnea. Sleep. 1996;19:388–397.

36. Santamaria JD, Prior JC, Fleetham JA. Reversible reproductive dysfunction in men with obstructive sleep apnoea. Clin Endocrinol (Oxf). 1988;28:461–470.

37. Karacan I, Moore CA, Sahmay S. Measurement of pressure necessary for vaginal penetration [abstract]. Sleep Res. 1985;14:269.

38. Michal V, Kramar R, Pospichal J. External iliac "steal syndrome." J Cardiovasc Surg. 1978;19:355–357.

39. Allen RP, Smolev JK. Bulbo-ischio-cavernosus muscle activity in determining etiology for organic impotence. In: Virag R, Virag H, eds. Proceedings of the First World Meeting on Impotence. Paris, France: CERI; 1984:95–99.

103

Assessment Techniques for Insomnia

Arthur J. Spielman

Chien-Ming Yang

Paul B. Glovinsky

This chapter discusses the various methods by which clinicians evaluate the complaint of insomnia. Although insomnia is an extremely common complaint, it can still be a difficult problem to evaluate, let alone to treat, because insomnia is symptomatic of a wide variety of disorders, has a number of different manifestations, and often follows a variable course. One of the main challenges facing the clinician is to avoid attempting to treat "last night's sleep problem" and to instead address the major factors underlying the symptom. The methods discussed here have evolved to address this challenge. Although few investigators will apply this list exhaustively, a working knowledge of methods drawn from the array discussed here will prove to be very helpful when confronted with the inconstancy and persistence of insomnia.

Certain methods of assessment are beyond the scope of this chapter. We are omitting specialized techniques that have been developed to assess sleep disturbance in children, and we are foregoing discussion of the assessments that have been devised to further research protocols, even though some of these techniques have been proposed as potentially useful in the clinical setting. Our aim is to address the needs of the clinician by providing descriptions of assessment techniques that have proved to be useful in clinical practice rather than to list more esoteric research methodologies. Finally, we do not cover the various methods of assessing daytime sleepiness, which is a major complaint of only a subgroup of insomniac patients (see Chapter 104).

MODELS OF THE PATHOGENESIS OF INSOMNIA

The assessment of any disorder is typically directed toward identifying the factors producing and maintaining the condition, as well as toward gauging the individual's preexisting vulnerability to the disorder. Although this model may be applied to the evaluation and treatment of the insomnia disorders, the fit is not always comfortable. Despite careful inquiry, the cause and pathogenesis of a substantial proportion of the insomnia disorders often remain unsettled. Nevertheless, the characteristics and consequences associated with a particular case of insomnia usually can be well delineated. Furthermore, the factors maintaining the disturbance can usually be isolated. Effective treatments for insomnia target these features. The clinician often is working on multiple levels, addressing current maladaptations while building a case for pathogenesis that may direct longer-term treatment interventions. This broader inquiry requires the consideration of all potential causes. With this in mind, we briefly review the major theoretical models that describe the purported mechanisms responsible for the insomnia disorders.

Psychiatric and Psychological Conditions

Insomniacs, clinicians, and normally good sleepers have long recognized the close connection between psychological distress and poor sleep. Correlative research has shown that excessive anxiety, depression, and severe psychopathology are associated with sleep disturbance.[1-5] A series of studies has replicated and refined the personality patterns that are associated with insomnia, and a theory has been generated that it is the internalization of conflicts that produces physiological arousal in vulnerable individuals.[6,7] The sense of helplessness that is so often part and parcel of the insomnia disorders is another contribution to insomnia that must be appreciated and addressed by the clinician.[8-10]

Organic factors associated with psychiatric conditions or acute states that promote wakefulness or impair sleep have also been identified; these factors include the lack of cortisol suppression, enhanced cholinergic mechanisms, and reduced slow-wave sleep[11-13] (see Section 14).

Learned Insomnia and the Vicious Circle

The repeated experience of poor sleep night after night promotes an association between sleeplessness and both presleep activities and the sleep setting.[14] Once these connections are established, the bedtime rituals and bedroom environment become cues for poor sleep. This is how the worry about sleeplessness becomes a self-fulfilling prophecy. Studies in animals that have shown classic conditioning of sleep and wakefulness support this learning model of insomnia.[15, 16]

Physiological Arousal

The global reduction in metabolism and a broad range of physiological processes is a hallmark of the transition to sleep. It is not surprising that heightened physiological arousal, indexed by such changes as increased body temperature, heart rate, and muscle tension, is incompatible with sleep.[17-19] Patients may be unaware of their hyperarousal, however, posing a problem for the diagnostician. Furthermore, systematic work has not yielded a practical, valid, and objective method of assessing level of arousal. This domain remains a challenge for the clinical evaluation.

Inadequate Sleep Hygiene

Practices and activities of everyday living have long been known to be capable of promoting or preventing sleep.[20] These practices of good or poor sleep hygiene have been the subject of more systematic focus.[21-23] Paradoxically, some of the very same behaviors that the insomniac engages in to improve sleep or daytime functioning, such as napping, daytime coffee, and evening alcohol, will also contribute to poor sleep.

Cognitive Factors: Arousal and Beliefs

The buzz of the overactive mind can interfere with falling asleep as well as interrupt and awaken the sleeper.[24-27] Sometimes, insomnia can be readily attributed to the worries and cares of life. In other cases, the would-be sleeper is baffled to learn that benign planning and reflections of the day can also cause sleeplessness. Of course, because substantial mental processing occurs subconsciously, the irritating thought may not be available for scrutiny. Alternatively, sleep may be disrupted by cognitive style rather than by mental content. Jumping from one thought to another without a sense of order or completion is not at all conducive to sleep.

The poor sleeper begins to anticipate the consequences of poor sleep, such as cloudy consciousness, fatigue, and irritability during the next day. A dread of the struggles of both night and day produces worry and arousal that are self-defeating. The anticipatory anxiety that results from past poor sleep has become the cause of future sleep disturbance. This vicious circle serves to perpetuate an insomnia, regardless of its original trigger.

Beliefs and self-attribution may act like self-fulfilling prophecies. The insomniac who assumes that mild sleep loss leads to an impaired immune system, disease, and death has raised the stakes on falling asleep. Faced with these dire consequences, going to sleep becomes a daunting task. Similarly, labeling oneself an insomniac may be a depressing thought that is damaging to the self. The label becomes worrisome and interferes with sleep.

Primary Sleep Disorders

The technological advances of polysomnography have illuminated the physiological processes that take place under the cover of dark. Monitoring of breathing and limb movements during sleep has revealed that some individuals with insomnia complaints have arousals induced by sleep-disordered breathing; in others, brief awakenings are triggered by periodically occurring movements.[28, 29]

Sleep Disorders Secondary to Medical Conditions

Trouble sleeping can also be the result of the pain, discomfort, and the pathophysiology associated with medical conditions (see Section 13). Although trouble sleeping is often transient and confined to the time during which the patient is symptomatic, this is not always the case. The patient may be taking medications that interfere with sleep, and a learned insomnia may develop due to the repeated association of sleeplessness and bedroom cues. The patient may start to spend too much time in bed to "rest and get healthy," leading to a weakening of the circadian sleep-wake cycle. Alternately, the patient may have begun using hypnotic medication on a regular basis and have difficulty stopping because of anticipatory anxiety and the physiological effects of discontinuation of the drug. Regardless of the specific route, troubled sleep initiated by medical illness can readily lead to chronic insomnia.

Circadian Rhythm Disorders

The explication of the mechanisms responsible for the nearly 24-h rhythmic regulation of biological and behavioral processes has enhanced understanding of normal and abnormal sleep.[30, 31] The periodic occurrence of sleep-wake cycles has been shown to be controlled by the timing, duration, and intensity of time cues. The ability of the most salient time cue, *bright light*, to shift the time of sleep onset and offset has suggested that aberrant clock mechanisms or poorly timed cue delivery may be implicated in some insomnia disorders.

Predisposing, Precipitating, and Perpetuating Factors

A simple conceptual model provides organization by dividing the multiple determinants of insomnia just

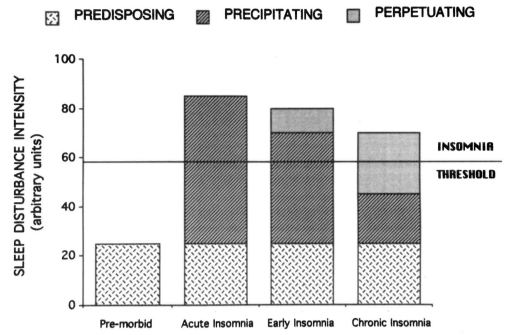

Figure 103-1. Schematic of the development of an unspecified type of chronic insomnia and the changing factors that play a role over the course of the disorder. (Adapted from Spielman AJ, Caruso L, Glovinsky PB. A behavioral perspective on insomnia. In: Erman M, ed. Psychiatr Clin North Am. 1987;10:541–553.)

reviewed into predisposing, precipitating, and perpetuating factors (Fig. 103–1).[23, 32] Clinical evaluation of all three components enables treatment planning to comprehensively address both the current conditions producing and sustaining the insomnia and the individual's vulnerability to future bouts of sleep disturbance.

SURVEY OF THE ASSESSMENT METHODS OF SLEEP DISORDERS CENTERS

To obtain a sense of evaluation procedures for insomnia, we conducted a quasirandom telephone survey of 40 sleep disorders centers, which represents more than 10% of the centers certified by the American Sleep Disorders Association. We learned that a majority of centers used structured rating scales and questionnaires as adjuncts in the evaluation of patients complaining of insomnia. More than two thirds of the centers send questionnaires to the patient before the initial visit. Although virtually all centers use sleep logs, only about one third of patients fill out a sleep log before the sleep consultation. About three fourths of centers formally evaluate some of their patients for depression, whereas fewer than half evaluate their patients for anxiety. Although only a handful of centers use a separate instrument to assess beliefs and attitudes about sleep, this domain is often measured in sleep questionnaires. Two thirds of patients fill out a sleep and medical history questionnaire, and a similar number are evaluated by the clinician with the use of a semistructured interview. Half of the insomniacs have an evaluation by a psychologist or psychiatrist. After the initial consultation, a fourth of patients undergo nocturnal polysomnography. In the four centers that use actigraphy, only about 10% of patients receive this type of evaluation.

Unfortunately, most of the sleep logs, sleep history questionnaires, and semistructured interviews are custom made, unpublished, and unique to each center. Because of the absence of commonly accepted standard instruments, the lists that follow include published and unpublished methods even though they are not in common use. We refer to an instrument as *published* when the reference includes either a blank questionnaire or all the items, responses, and scoring necessary for use. Scales referred to as *available on request* can be purchased or obtained from the authors. The material in the tables is listed by date, except for Table 103–4 (assessment of specific causes), which groups according to categories.

The following methods are arranged by the order in which clinicians typically proceed.

METHODS

Questionnaires, Diaries, and Logs

One of the best methods for obtaining a more balanced, comprehensive overview of a complaint of persistent insomnia is to have the patient fill out retrospective questionnaires, inventories of current status, and prospective sleep diaries or logs. The following is an overview of the major varieties of retrospective instruments available to the clinician.

Retrospective Instruments

A main benefit of adopting a guided retrospective approach to the assessment of insomnia is that it aids in forming an accurate picture of the sleep disturbance.

Providing prompts to recognition memory as opposed to relying solely on recall, the patient is helped to gain a broader perspective on the problem. There is less need to focus only on those aspects that, in the judgment of the patient, would justify clinical attention.

Sleep and Medical History Questionnaires. Most useful if filled out by the patient before the first visit, sleep and medical history questionnaires can broach potentially sensitive topics for the patient's consideration in privacy, while also giving notice that the inquiry will necessarily be a broad one if the patient's complaint is to be adequately addressed. They also have the benefit of introducing the "long view" and of moving the patient from the role of hapless victim of the vagaries of sleep into that of a coinvestigator.[22, 24] When the patient commits his or her experience to paper, there is the opportunity for reflection and revision common to all writing processes, which fosters a more considered and reliable assessment.

These methods do generate problems. The most obvious is that they often take a fair amount of the clinician's time to review. One such example is the venerable Cornell Medical Index.[33] This long form constains 195 items and is comprehensive with a standard format. In addition to a review of the patient's past medical history and current symptoms, with or without a questionnaire, it is essential to carefully consider the effects of all medications over the course of the insomnia disorder. This is partly accomplished with the sleep diary (see below), which asks the patient to list medication use. However, because the patient starts filling out the diary after the evaluation has begun, there is no examination of the effect of drugs at earlier stages, during the development of the insomnia. The clinical interview is the best way to weave together the features of medication use (e.g., type, amount, time of administration, frequency, side effects, withdrawal effects on discontinuation, and degree of drug toler-ance) with other treatments and coping strategies and the effect of these approaches on the sleep disturbance.

There are two types of sleep history questionnaires. One assesses the adequacy and quality of sleep, and the other, more comprehensive type, also includes a survey of potential etiological factors (Tables 103–1 and 103–2). In our survey of sleep disorders centers, we found that the overwhelming majority of clinicians use a sleep history questionnaire that is of their own design. In the past, little psychometric work has been conducted to design a valid and reliable survey for insomnia.

There also are more subtle problems associated with the use of questionnaires. They can create a false sense on the part of both patient and clinician that the inquiry has been comprehensive. There is a danger that in the interests of expediency, the clinician may choose "not to cover the same ground" as the questionnaire. Alternately, due to the patient's positive response bias, the clinician may be obliged to follow-up more intensively than would be otherwise necessary merely to rule out various diagnostic possibilities, and the interview will be prolonged. In other cases, patients simply are not capable of providing a faithful account by these means. However, even when a well-designed questionnaire is completed by an accurate historian, there is ample opportunity for confusion. For these reasons, leaving the history taking to the form is tantamount to leaving out the history altogether. Rather than being misused in this way, questionnaires are properly used to structure the ensuing inquiry and to serve as an outline and guarantee that attention will be paid to all relevant areas as well as to the particular "flags" that are raised by the patient's responses.

Psychopathology and Personality Questionnaires. Although insomnia can result from a wide array of medical, environmental, and chronobiological conditions, the high prevalence of psychopathology in pa-

Table 103–1. SLEEP QUALITY QUESTIONNAIRES

Scale Name (Source)	No. of Items	Format	Scale Description
Published			
Post-sleep inventory[51] (page 989)	30	13-point bipolar scales	All assess the quality and adequacy of sleep. None survey etiological factors.
Leeds Sleep Evaluation Questionnaire[52] (pages 178–179)	10	Visual-analogue scales Assesses medication effects	
The St. Mary's Hospital Sleep Questionnaire[53] (pages 96–97)	14	Yes/no Frequency and severity ratings Fill in the blanks	
Pittsburgh Sleep Quality Index[54] (pages 209–213)	24	Severity and frequency ratings Mainly symptom checklists A global score composed of a number of categories	
Sleep Impairment Index[55] (pages 199–200)	15	Severity ratings Mainly symptom checklists	
Available on Request			
Sleep Questionnaire[56]	59	Mainly frequency ratings	
Insomnia Symptom Questionnaire[57]	13	Visual-analogue scales	

Table 103–2. SLEEP HISTORY QUESTIONNAIRES

Scale Name (Source)	No. of Items	Format	Scale Description
Published			
Sleep Questionnaire and Assessment of Wakefulness[58] (pages 384–413)	863	Yes/no Symptom checklist Frequency and severity ratings Fill in the blanks Not specific to insomnia	All assess the quality and adequacy of sleep and survey etiological factors.
Sleep History Questionnaire[59] (pages 63–65)	48	Yes/no Fill in the blanks Links between particular questions and semistructured interview for follow-up	
Sleep History Analysis[60] (page 24)	20	Yes/no Fill in the blanks	
Available on Request			
Sleep Disorders Questionnaire[61]	176	Derived from Sleep Quality and Assessment of Wakefulness Frequency and severity ratings Not specific to insomnia	
Brock Sleep and Insomnia Questionnaire[62]	103	Yes/no Severity and frequency ratings Fill in the blanks Separate sections on five diagnostic entities and a drug inventory	

tients with insomnia makes careful attention to this domain particularly important. Specific disorders, such as depression, anxiety disorder, chaotic personality organizations, and psychotic disorders, may play a direct role in the genesis of an insomnia. Even when overt psychopathology is not present, certain types of personality configuration may predispose toward insomnia. For example, an individual who is prone to internalize conflict often experiences hyperarousal as a result. Detail-oriented perfectionists may not allow themselves a respite from the day's challenges; instead, these problems are brought into bed for further reflection. Persons with ruminative personalities may become caught in a cycle of misgivings or strategizing rather than settling into sleep.

Screening for psychopathology and personality typing are readily accomplished through the use of assessment instruments (Table 103–3). A large number of tests have been developed that permit valid inferences to be drawn about a patient's psychological makeup. Some cast a wide net and are useful in characterizing a broad range of pathology; others have a more specific focus. In all cases, the use of psychological assessments does not relieve the clinician of the responsibility of evaluating the patient's mental status. Often, clinical judgment is confirmed and treatment can proceed with greater assurance, whereas at other times, discrepancies between these forms of assessment may lead to fruitful new avenues of inquiry.

The Minnesota Multiphasic Personality Inventory (MMPI) is a widely used instrument that yields a personality profile and alerts the clinician to the possible existence of a wide range of psychopathology.[34] Extensive research has demonstrated that specific MMPI patterns are associated with insomnia.[6, 7] If such personal-

ity configurations or psychopathologies are found, the clinician may bring specific remedies to bear on the sleep disturbance—for example, cognitive therapy or pharmacotherapy for depression may in turn relieve the symptom of early morning awakening. Instruction in self-hypnosis may allow those who are prone to somaticizing a way to redirect their attention from physical discomfort, thereby alleviating a sleep-onset insomnia.

The MMPI has several drawbacks. Its comprehensive nature requires a lengthy administration. Although this is typically done before the initial visit, it can cause consternation in patients who feel they are being diverted back toward the general practice of psychology just when they thought they had reached a specialist who would focus on the complaint at hand. Depending on the type of scoring used, the turnaround time for results from the MMPI also can be long. Finally, the MMPI may be susceptible to some bias in the sleep disorders setting because questions regarding sleep disturbance contribute to the scoring of some clinical scales (such as the Depression scale) and these items may receive more pronounced endorsement in the sleep clinic than they might otherwise have garnered.

Two instruments—the Beck Depression Inventory[35] and the Spielberger State-Trait Anxiety Scale[36]—deserve mention because they are in widespread use in sleep disorders centers, are relatively easy to administer and interpret, and target the most common types of psychopathology associated with insomnia—depression and anxiety. Because they offer a quick assessment of the intensity of depression or anxiety, these scales allow for rapid intervention in patients who may be at risk for serious psychological distress. When choosing a scale, it

Table 103–3. ASSESSMENT OF PSYCHOPATHOLOGY AND PERSONALITY

Scale Name (Source)	No. of Items	Format	Scale Description
Published			
Hamilton Rating Scale of Depression[63] (pages 61–62)	21	Clinician rating of severity based on patient interview	Semistructured interview for depression Clinician needed for administration
Beck Depression Inventory[64] (pages 561–571)	21	Four levels of severity description	Assesses depressive state with a cognitive emphasis
Self Rating Depression Scale[65] (page 65)	20	Four-point frequency ratings	Depression survey
Beck Anxiety Inventory[66] (page 895)	21	Four-point severity ratings	Anxiety survey
Available on Request			
Symptom Checklist Revised[67]	90	Five-point frequency ratings	Psychiatric symptoms and descriptions Norms for different samples Nine primary symptom dimensions and three global indices Narrative interpretation may be obtained
Profile of Mood Scales[68]	65	Five-point severity ratings	Adjectives that describe mood states Norms published
State-Trait Anxiety Inventory[69]	40	Four-point severity ratings	Separate scales measure current and long-standing anxiety
Minnesota Multiphasic Personality Inventory—2[70]	567	True/false	Nine clinical subscales measure enduring personality and psychopathology Response bias correction Skilled interpretation necessary or narrative summary needs to be obtained

is important to become familiar with the content of the items that yield the scaled score because different instruments may focus on different aspects of a disorder. For example, one depression scale may emphasize the biological features of the disturbance, whereas another may focus on cognitive abnormalities. There is no single appropriate scale, but the clinician should be aware of the particular slant of the selected instrument. As with all questionnaires, these inventories are susceptible to response bias on the part of the individual patient. Some people tend to deny or minimize, others aim to give the clinician what he or she is thought to expect, others are careless in responding, and still others harbor some motivation to exaggerate their symptoms. The more comprehensive inventories such as the MMPI build in monitoring of various types of response bias, whereas shorter scales necessarily place greater, unchecked emphasis on relatively few endorsements.

Inventories of Cognitive and Somatic Arousal. Cognitive style will often determine whether an individual is predisposed toward developing insomnia. Although all people must deal with some degree of stress in their lives, there is a great deal of variation in how this is accomplished. Some lucky souls can literally "sleep on it" when confronted with a problem, but many persons dwell on issues, obsessing over them until too aroused to fall asleep. When the particular problem to be overcome is lack of sleep, the consequences can be especially pernicious. Several authors have described a "vicious cycle" in which concern over the possibility of not sleeping will lead to hyperarousal as evening approaches, reaching such a peak that by bedtime, sleep truly is an impossibility. Past experiences of insomnia reinforce the belief that sleep will

once more prove elusive, setting the stage for another evening of anxiety and failure to sleep.[3, 24, 37]

Many patients insist with bewilderment that there is nothing particularly upsetting that they are dealing with in their lives, yet their minds continue to race at night. Initially, their thoughts range over all sorts of seemingly trivial issues, eventually gravitating to the fact that sleep is not occurring. It may in fact be that the contents of one's thoughts do not necessarily lead directly to arousal; rather, the problem may lie with the thought process itself: half-completed thoughts, racing, and the repetition of themes may represent operating characteristics of a mind that is temporarily incapable of sleep.

One reason why hyperarousal so effectively forestalls sleep is that once triggered, it takes a long time for baseline conditions of arousal to be reestablished. It has been noted that the response to a perceived threat is rapid, which makes sense from an evolutionary perspective, whereas the "fall time" to a level of calm that would be conducive to sleeping is prolonged.[38] This view leads to several practical consequences in terms of treating insomnia. It is important to prevent runaway hyperarousal if at all possible, because at that point, the battle for timely sleep is lost. The nature of the thoughts and activities taking place in the hours before attempting to fall asleep gain in importance. An interim goal of establishing 15 or so min of relative calm is a reasonable aim rather than having the patient "try" to fall asleep.

Several inventories are available that help the clinician gauge the extent to which cognitively induced and somatic hyperarousal may be expected to interfere with sleep (Table 103–4). These scales have the benefit of

Table 103-4. ASSESSMENT OF SPECIFIC CAUSES

Scale Name (Source)	No. of Items	Format	Scale Description
Published			
Morningness-Eveningness[71] (pages 100–103)	19	Four-point severity ratings Time of day items	Feeling and functioning best rhythm
Sleep Behavior Self Rating Scale[72] (pages 414–415)	20	Frequency ratings	Activities, practices, and circumstances of the day that affect sleep
Sleep Hygiene Awareness and Practice Scale[59] (pages 75–76)	32 +	Frequency and effect on sleep ratings	Activities, practices, and circumstances of the day that affect sleep
Sleep Hygiene Questionnaire[60] (page 38)	10	Yes/no	Activities, practices, and circumstances of the day that affect sleep
Pre-Sleep Arousal Scale[73] (page 266)	16	Five-point severity ratings	Assesses cognitive and somatic arousal at bedtime
Arousability Predisposition Scale[74] (page 420)	12	Frequency ratings	Assesses cognitive and somatic arousal
Sleep Disturbance Questionnaire[75] (page 153)	12	Five-point severity ratings	Assesses sleep hygiene and cognitive and somatic arousal
Beliefs and Attitudes About Sleep Scale[55] (pages 201–204)	30	Visual-analogue scale	Surveys dysfunctional sleep-related cognitions

targeting a factor that often perpetuates an insomniac condition regardless of whether other factors originally precipitated it. They can help to interrupt the vicious cycle of insomnia by preventing the patient from catastrophizing the consequences of poor sleep and to instead adopt a more detached, dispassionate attitude toward the disturbance. This in itself is often very beneficial to therapy. The clinician should be aware, however, of the potential for confrontation and harm to the therapeutic alliance that can occur by implying that a patient's beliefs are "faulty" and "unrealistic" and that the patient is engaging in "catastrophizing."

It is also important to try to assess the degree of physiological activation that is fueling the fire of arousal. Muscle tension, psychomotor agitation, and heart pounding are reported by some insomniacs, and the role of treatments based on de-arousal suggests that an assessment of this domain is relevant to a comprehensive evaluation of sleep disturbance.

Assessment of Sleep Hygiene and Feeling Best Rhythm. As noted above, it often is the quality of the hours spent before sleep is attempted that determines whether sleep will come easily. This argument applies to the entire day, not just the evening hours. The amount of physical activity, bedrest, and light exposure obtained during the day will affect one's propensity for sleep, the timing of that sleep, and its quality. Overconsumption of caffeine, exposure to dreadful television news stories in the evening, extended periods of reading in bed, and other aspects of poor sleep hygiene will ultimately prove counterproductive, whereas regular bedtimes and an evening "buffer period" in which to wind down from the day's events will over time be beneficial. Several authors have developed scales that assess these factors (see Table 103–4).

The timing of the propensity for sleep and activity differs among individuals, and tendencies toward greater activity in either the morning or evening hours may be constitutional. This disposition toward being either a "morning lark" or a "night owl" is assessed by a number of circadian-typing scales; the best known is a questionnaire developed by Horne and Ostberg[39] (see Table 103–4).

Prospective Sleep Diaries (Sleep Logs)

Retrospective instruments such as those described above have the advantage of being able to quickly summarize events occurring over a long period of time, but along with this comes the distortion inevitably introduced when collapsing and distilling descriptions. Memories are often incomplete or selective. In the case of insomnia, there is a natural tendency to focus on the worst experiences and perhaps to amplify their importance. These pitfalls can be countered through the use of a prospective sleep diary or sleep log (Table 103–5). Sleep logs have an intuitive appeal, are user friendly, and allow for repeated, accurate sampling of target behaviors, whether lying in bed awake or consuming coffee, in a prospective manner that increases the reliability of the measure. Filling out a sleep log directs the patient's attention to aspects of behavior that might otherwise be overlooked and in some versions presents the information in a graphical format that allows the clinician to quickly survey large amounts of data. Patterns are easily discerned from the visual cues of these graph-type logs. On the other hand, more precise information is obtained from fill-in-the-grid or question-type formats. Filling out a 2-week sleep log before the initial evaluation also provides a baseline against which treatment response may be measured.

Sleep logs have potential drawbacks as well. Some obsessive patients will feel compelled to provide such accurate and complete information that the very act of logging clock times of various events will interfere with sleep. Even in less extreme cases, the act of logging information on a night-by-night basis will often work against the therapeutic goal of instilling a "longer view" in the patient toward the sleep disturbance.

Table 103–5. SLEEP DIARIES

Scale Name (Source)	No. of Items	Format	Scale Description
Published			
Daily Sleep Diary[59] (page 71)	10	Severity ratings Fill in the blanks	All diaries assess sleep pattern and quality as well as presleep activities and practices.
Sleep Log and Day Log[60] (pages 72–73)	11	Fill in the blanks Severity ratings Grid for daily activities	
Sleep Diary[55] (page 210)	10	Five-point severity ratings Fill in the blanks	
Pittsburgh Sleep Diary[76] (pages 113–114)	24	Five-point frequency ratings Visual-analogue scales Fill in the blanks	
Sleep Log[77] (page 140)	9	Graphical depiction of sleep over time Five-point severity ratings Fill in the blanks	
Available on Request			
Sleep Log[78]	12	Graphical depiction of sleep over time Fill in the blanks	

The Initial Consultation

Questionnaires and prospective logs certainly have their role in the assessment of insomnia, but it is in the face-to-face setting of the consultation that the clinician's skills and knowledge will find full expression. Questionnaires do not ask follow-up questions. They cannot achieve the degree of nuance often necessary to decide, for example, whether episodes of awakening with gasping and palpitations likely represent a nocturnal anxiety attack or an apneic disturbance. They cannot probe for further examples or establish the context in which an event of interest occurs. It is up to the clinician, too, to recognize internal inconsistencies in a patient's history and to encourage the patient to be more exacting in his or her recollections to establish a more accurate reconstruction. Finally, within the course of the interaction itself, there may arise facets of the history that were not apparent even to the patient and that would likely be wholly overlooked on a questionnaire.

A standard history-taking format will usually serve well to elicit the essential features of an insomnia; however, an empirical study has shown that the non–sleep specialist clinician asks few questions of the insomnia patient.[40] The skilled clinician will try to start close to the patient's experience, allowing the patient the opportunity to present the gist of the presenting problem with sufficient idiosyncratic detail to ensure both parties that the patient's experience is not being fit too neatly and quickly into a preformed diagnostic category. As these details emerge, the clinician is generating hypotheses regarding the genesis of the insomnia and the factors that are maintaining it. These hypotheses are then tested via further questioning. For example, if it appears that a sleep-onset difficulty relates to concerns about performance at work, the clinician might ask about patterns in the severity of the disturbance and find that it is exacerbated on Sunday night, whereas the patient has experienced some asymptomatic periods during vacations.

After a working formulation has been established and a preliminary differential diagnosis is settled on, the clinician will generally systematically survey the various domains that might have a bearing on the problem, such as the past medical history, family history, current psychosocial context, and so on. Even when the clinician is fairly certain of the cause of an insomnia and confident of an appropriate course of treatment, it still is important to piece together a comprehensive picture of the background conditions out of which the disturbance evolved. There may be other ancillary or independent problems that also require attention.

The consultation interview is critical for establishing the trust and working alliance that will be necessary to carry the patient successfully through the treatment phase, especially when that treatment may involve changes in habits or lifestyle that are difficult to implement. The clinician must demonstrate caring, openness, and an ability to listen and understand—while bearing in mind that the patient is by definition in distress and likely to focus more on the extreme than on the typical experience to garner aid.

Several semistructured interviews have been developed that help guide inquiry into a complaint of insomnia (Table 103–6). They have the advantage of cueing the clinician to cover relevant domains, and both include a survey of sleep hygiene practices. As with the use of any interview guide, the skilled clinician will be alert to instances where departures from the guide must be made to fully follow up on the patient's experience.

Testing and Referrals

Most clinicians working in the field of sleep disorders will, in virtually every case, accumulate information

Table 103–6. SEMISTRUCTURED SLEEP INTERVIEWS

Scale Name (Source)	No. of Items	Format	Scale Description
Published			
Structured Sleep History Interview[59] (pages 66–69)	53 +	Open-ended questions	All interviews survey a wide range of symptoms and etiological factors.
Insomnia Interview Schedule[55] (pages 195–198)	77	Open-ended questions Yes/no Severity ratings Fill in the blanks	
CCNY Insomnia Interview[79] (pages 421–426)	41 +	Open-ended questions Symptom checklists Severity ratings Rating of the degree to which factors co-vary with sleep disturbance Diagnostic entities linked to particular questions	

from the broad categories covered above—retrospective questionnaires, prospective logs, and interviews. Referrals for testing or evaluation by another specialist will generally be made more judiciously, based on the information gathered during the evaluation process. Sometimes, the history will be sufficiently strong to warrant polysomnographic testing to confirm or rule out physiological disturbance during sleep, such as sleep apnea or periodic limb movement disorder, before any treatments are applied. Similarly, further clinical evaluation may be indicated if the history is suggestive of psychiatric disturbance or specific disorders, such as hyperthyroidism or cardiac arrhythmia, that may be accompanied by insomnia. In other cases, testing or referral to a specialist will take place after a poor response to initial treatment is documented, to widen the base of potentially helpful information.

The Nocturnal Polysomnogram

The nocturnal polysomnogram (NPSG) is the standard objective measure of sleep (see Chapter 100). Over the past 30 years, a large body of research and clinical experience has accumulated regarding both normal sleep parameters and variants seen in disordered sleep. Evaluation with polysomnography allows the clinician to objectively compare the patient's sleep characteristics with normative data and with data gathered within various clinical populations to clarify the diagnosis. The NPSG is also helpful in uncovering covert disorders, such as periodic limb movement disorder, that might otherwise escape detection, especially if there is no bedpartner available to observe sleep. In addition to characterizing sleep, polysomnography affords the clinician several indices of arousal that may prove especially helpful in characterizing and addressing cases of insomnia; these include such measures as the percentage of nonrapid eye movement (NREM) stage 1 transitional sleep, the number of transient arousals, the number of stage changes across the record, and the intrusion of alpha wave activity into deeper sleep. Finally, polysomnography allows a comparison to be made between objective parameters such as total sleep time or the number of awakenings exceeding a specified duration with the patient's subjective estimate of these same parameters. Sometimes, a large discrepancy between objective parameters and their corresponding subjective estimates represents the core of the presenting problem.[41, 42]

The NPSG does have drawbacks, such as its expense, reflecting both its labor-intensive character and the investment in costly technology required. One consequence of the costliness is that only one or two nights of data are typically obtained, resulting in a very limited sample of sleep. Given the increased night-to-night variability of sleep in insomnia, this may result in a biased estimate. In addition, the effect of sleeping in a sleep laboratory can result in an inaccurate representation of the patient's sleep, either exaggerating sleep difficulties—the classic "first night effect"[43]—or, paradoxically, resulting in better sleep than that typically obtained at home—the "reverse first night effect."[44] This latter effect can occur when associations have been established between the insomniac's bedroom environment and the experience of sleeping poorly that make continued insomnia more likely. These maladaptive cues are missing from the sleep laboratory, so sleep is improved there. Because of these drawbacks associated with the NPSG, it is not indicated as a first-line diagnostic tool in the assessment of insomnia according to American Sleep Disorders Association guidelines.[45]

Actigraphy

Actigraphy is a relatively low-cost method of estimating sleep parameters, such as total sleep time and the timing and duration of prolonged awakenings[15, 46–48a] (see Chapter 109). An actigraph is a device that records gross motor movements. Not much bigger than a wristwatch, it is attached to a limb and can be worn day or night without interfering with normal sleep or daily functioning. It can record motor activity (or in the case of presumed sleep, the lack thereof) across many days and nights with the use of various sampling rates. The collected data are usually downloaded to a computer for analysis. The cost-effectiveness of actigraphy allows for multiple nights of sampling, avoiding the sampling error associated with the NPSG. However, it can overestimate the amount of sleep obtained in insomniacs, who do not move much during the night even when awake. Furthermore, the various actigraphs available commercially have not been standardized. They have different sensitivities with regard to the detection of movement and differing algorithms for converting raw data points into estimates of sleep and wakefulness.

Laboratory Urinalysis and Blood Work

Analyses of urine and blood samples routinely conducted by commercial laboratories at the behest of physicians in general medical practice may also prove helpful in the assessment of selected patients complaining of insomnia. Levels of thyroid-stimulating hormone and follicle-stimulating hormone and blood count profiles will be of help in evaluating whether hyperthyroidism, menopause, or infection is playing a role in the sleep disturbance. A survey of the methods used to assess the numerous medical conditions associated with insomnia is beyond the scope of this chapter (see Section 13). We comment on the assessment of the conditions of restless legs syndrome and periodic limb movement disorder (PLMD). Although the pathophysiology of these conditions is still under investigation, a subset of patients may have anemia, which can be assessed by obtaining ferritin levels.[49] Obtaining a set of blood panels on every insomnia patient is not recommended because of the low yield; however, when there is sufficient reason to suspect an underlying medical cause of insomnia and testing proves negative, this will allow behavioral interventions to be applied with more confidence and persistence.

Commonplace Technologies

Ubiquitous devices such as telephone answering machines or digital watches can be helpful in the assessment of insomnia. For example, patients complaining that they "get no sleep at all, or at best, just 1 or 2 hours" can be instructed to call on an hourly basis into a telephone answering machine equipped with a time stamp when they are unable to sleep. This provides an objective record of at least intermittent wakefulness across the night and may be useful in cases of sleep state misperception. Digital watches that have an hourly chime function can be used to cue the patient to rate alertness or mood. Audio or video tape recordings can be useful as screening tools in those cases where sleep-maintenance difficulties are suspected as being secondary to a physiological disturbance such as sleep apnea.

Trial Treatment as Assessment

There are cases in which after a thorough history has yielded a probable cause underlying a patient's complaint of insomnia, the most expeditious means of verifying that supposition is through the application of a trial treatment. Of course, reasoning that a diagnostic impression is correct because improvement follows treatment is not necessarily the case; just because a cold improves after a few days of drinking chamomile tea does not mean that chamomile deficiency caused the cold in the first place. Similarly, good sleep hygiene practices are helpful for all sleepers, not just those whose sleep difficulties stem specifically from poor sleep hygiene. However, if poor sleep hygiene is suspected as a causative factor, instruction in better practices can efficiently treat those who are correctly targeted while not doing harm to those whose insomnia arises from other causes.

Another condition that deserves mention in this regard is sleep-maintenance insomnia due to suspected PLMD during sleep.[50] Very often, this condition responds to treatment with dopamine agonists or opioid drugs. These drugs are not of general benefit in other types of sleep-maintenance insomnia; therefore, if a case of suspected PLMD shows a positive response to these drugs, this can usually be taken as indirect evidence that PLMD was the underlying culprit. Note that a positive response to one of the sedative-hypnotic medications, which can also be helpful in treating cases of insomnia due to PLMD, would not yield information regarding the presence of PLMD. This class of drug would be expected to benefit many different types of insomnia whether due to PLMD or not.

SUMMARY

There are very few medical or psychological disorders that are associated with as diverse an array of diagnostic procedures as those summarized here in connection with the assessment of insomnia. This heterogeneity mirrors the multiple facets of the complaint, ranging through physical discomfort, psychological distress, cognitive deficiencies, behavioral impairment, and social disruption. Full evaluation of the complaint requires a multidimensional approach because those aspects of the sleep disorder that are most salient or distressing to the patient—and the facets where it might prove most amenable or recalcitrant to treatment—will vary among individuals. The clinician who is prepared to meet a complaint of insomnia on its own terms, drawing across the range of diagnostic methods described in this chapter, will come to a more complete understanding of the problem and be better able to formulate effective recommendations for its treatment.

References

1. Kumar A, Vaidya AK. Anxiety as a personality dimension of short and long sleepers. J Clin Psychol. 1984;40:197–198.

2. Mellinger GD, Balter MB, Uhlenhuth EH. Insomnia and its treatment: prevalence and correlates. Arch Gen Psychiatry. 1985;42:225–232.

3. Reynolds CF, Kupfer DJ. Sleep research in affective illness: state of the art. Sleep. 1987;10:199–215.

4. Sweetwood HL, Kripke DF, Grant I, et al. Sleep disorder and psychobiological symptomatology. Psychosom Med. 1976;38:373–378.

5. Vollrath M, Wicki W, Angst J. The Zurich Study, VIII: insomnia: association with depression, anxiety, somatic syndromes, and course of insomnia. Eur Arch Psychiatry Neurol Sci. 1989;239:113–124.

6. Kales A, Caldwell AB, Preston TA, et al. Personality patterns in insomnia. Arch Gen Psychiatry. 1976;33:1128–1134.

7. Kales A, Kales JD. Evaluation and Treatment of Insomnia. New York, NY: Oxford University Press; 1984.

8. Espie CA, Lindsay WR. Paradoxical intention in the treatment of chronic insomnia: six case studies illustrating variability in therapeutic response. Behav Res Ther. 1985;23:703–709.

9. Killen JD, Coates TJ. The complaint of insomnia: what is it and how do we treat? Clin Behav Ther Rev. 1979;1:1–15.

10. Lacks P. Behavioural Treatment for Persistent Insomnia. New York, NY: Pergamon Press; 1987.

11. Carroll BJ, Feinberg M, Greden JF, et al. A specific laboratory test for the diagnosis of melancholia: standardization, validation and clinical utility. Arch Gen Psychiatry. 1981;38:15–22.

12. Czeisler CA, Moore-Ede MC, Regestein QR, et al. Episodic 24-hour cortisol secretory patterns in patients awaiting elective cardiac surgery. J Clin Endocrinol Metab. 1976;42:273–283.

13. Sitaram N, Gillin JC. Development and use of pharmacological probes of the CNS in man: evidence of cholinergic abnormality in primary affective illness. Biol Psychiatry. 1980;15:925–955.

14. Bootzin RR, Rider SP. Behavioral techniques and biofeedback for insomnia. In: Pressman MR, Orr WC, eds. Understanding Sleep: The Evaluation and Treatment of Sleep Disorders. Washington, DC: American Psychological Association; 1997:315–338.

15. Sterman MD, Clemente CD, Wyricka W. Forebrain inhibitory mechanisms: conditioning of basal forebrain induced EEG synchronization and sleep. Exp Neurol. 1963;7:404–417.

16. Sterman MB, Szymusiask R, McGinty D. Quantitative analysis of basal forebrain stimulation effects: sleep induction, sleep conditioning, and state distribution. Paper presented at: 5th International Congress of Sleep Research; July 1987; Copenhagen, Denmark.

17. Bonnet MH, Arand DI. 24-Hour metabolic rate in insomniacs and matched normal sleepers. Sleep. 1995;19:581–588.

18. Freedman R, Sattler HI. Physiological and psychological factors in sleep-onset insomnia. Abnorm Psychol. 1982;91:380–389.

19. Johns MW, Gay MP, Masterton JP, et al. Relationship between sleep habits, adrenocortical activity and personality. Psychosomat Med. 1971;3:499–508.

20. Kleitman N. Sleep and Wakefulness. Chicago, Ill: University of Chicago Press; 1939.

21. Hauri P. The Sleep Disorders. 2nd ed. Kalamazoo, Mich: Upjohn; 1982.

22. Hauri PJ. Consulting about insomnia: a method and some preliminary data. Sleep. 1993;16:344–350.

23. Spielman AJ. Assessment of insomnia. Clin Psychol Rev. 1986;6:11–26.

24. Espie CA. The Psychological Treatment of Insomnia. New York, NY: Wiley; 1991.

25. Hauri P, Linde S. No More Sleepless Nights. New York, NY: John Wiley & Sons; 1990.

26. Monroe LJ. Psychological and physiological differences between good and poor sleepers. J Abnorm Psychol. 1967;72:255–264.

27. Torsvall L, Akerstedt T. Disturbed sleep while being on-call: an EEG study of ship's engineers. Sleep. 1988;11:35–38.

28. Guilleminault C, Eldridge F, Dement WC. Insomnia, narcolepsy, and sleep apneas. Bull Physiopathol Respir. 1972;8:1127–1138.

29. Symonds CP: Nocturnal myoclonus J Neurol Neurosurg Psychiatry. 1953;16:166–171.

30. Moore-Ede MC, Czeisler CA, Richardson GS. Circadian timekeeping in health and disease, I: basic properties of circadian pacemakers. N Engl J Med. 1983;309:469–476.

31. Moore-Ede MC, Czeisler CA, Richardson GS. Circadian timekeeping in health and disease, II: clinical implications of circadian rhythmicity. N Engl J Med. 1983;309:530–536.

32. Spielman AJ, Caruso L, Glovinsky PB. A behavioral perspective on insomnia. Psychiatr Clin North Am. 1987;10:541–553.

33. Brodman K, Erdmann AJ Jr, Lorge I, et al. The Cornell Medical Index: an adjunct to medical interview. JAMA. 1949;140:530–534.

34. Butcher JN, Dahlstrom WG, Graham JR, et al. MMPI-2: Minnesota Multiphasic Personality Inventory–2: Manual for Administration and Scoring. Minneapolis, Minn: University of Minnesota Press; 1989.

35. Beck AT, Ward CH, Mendelson M, et al. An inventory for measuring depression. Arch Gen Psychiatry. 1961;4:561–571.

36. Spielberger CD, Gorsuch RL, Lushene R, et al. The State-Trait Anxiety Inventory for Adults. Palo Alto, Calif: Mind Garden; 1983.

37. Morin CM. Insomnia: Psychological Assessment and Management. New York, NY: The Guilford Press; 1993.

38. Hauri PJ. Personal communication, 1985.

39. Horne JA, Ostberg O. A self-assessment questionnaire to determine morningness-eveningness in human circadian rhythms. Int J Chronobiol. 1976;4:97–110.

40. Everitt DE, Avoran J. Clinical decision-making in the evaluation and treatment of insomnia. Am J Med. 1990;89:357–362.

41. Frankel BL, Coursey RD, Buchbinder R, et al. Recorded and reported sleep in chronic primary insomnia. Arch Gen Psychiatry. 1976;33:615–623.

42. McCall WV, Edinger JD. Subjective total insomnia: an example of sleep state misperception. Sleep. 1992;15:71–73.

43. Agnew HW Jr, Webb WB, William RI. The first night effect: an EEG study of sleep. Psychophysiology. 1966;2:263–266.

44. Hauri PJ, Olmstead EM. Reverse first night effect in insomnia. Sleep. 1989;12:97–105.

45. Standards of Practice Committee of the American Sleep Disorders Association. Practice parameters for the use of polysomnography in the evaluation of insomnia. Sleep. 1995;18:55–57.

46. Hauri PJ, Wisbey J. Wrist actigraphy in insomnia. Sleep. 1992;15:293–301.

47. Jean-Louis G, von Gizycki H, Zizi F, et al. Determination of sleep and wakefulness with the actigraph data analysis software (ADAS). Sleep. 1996;19:739–743.

48. Sadeh A, Hauri PJ, Kripke D, et al. The role of actigraphy in the evaluation of sleep disorders. Sleep. 1995;18:288–302.

48a. Standards of Practice Committee of the American Sleep Disorders Association. Practice parameters for the use of actigraphy in the clinical assessment of sleep disorders. Sleep. 1995;18:285–287.

49. Early C, Sun E, Chen C, et al. Iron relation to periodic leg movements and sleep disturbance in patients with the restless legs syndrome. Sleep. 1998;21(suppl):142.

50. American Sleep Disorders Association. International Classification of Sleep Disorders, Revised: Diagnostic and Coding Manual. Rochester, Minn: American Sleep Disorders Association; 1997.

51. Webb WB, Bonnet M, Blume G. A post-sleep inventory. Percept Motor Skills. 1976;43:987–993.

52. Parrott AC, Hindmarch I. The Leeds Sleep Evaluation Questionnaire in psychopharmacological investigations—a review. Psychopharmacology. 1980;71:173–179.

53. Ellis BW, Johns MW, Lancaster R, et al. The St. Mary's Hospital Sleep Questionnaire: a study of reliability. Sleep. 1981;4:93–97.

54. Buysse DJ, Reynolds CF III, Monk TH, et al. The Pittsburgh Sleep Quality Index: a new instrument for psychiatric practice and research. Psychiatry Res. 1989;28:193–213.

55. Morin CM. Insomnia: Psychological Assessment and Management. New York, NY: The Guilford Press; 1993.

56. Domino G, Blair G, Bridges A. Subjective assessment of sleep by sleep questionnaire. Percept Motor Skills. 1985;59:163–170.

57. Spielman AJ, Saskin P, Thorpy MJ. Treatment of chronic insomnia by restriction of time in bed. Sleep. 1987;10:45–56.

58. Miles I. Sleep Questionnaire and assessment of wakefulness (SQAW). In: Guilleminault C, ed. Sleeping and Waking Disorders: Indications and Techniques. Menlo Park, Calif: Addison Wesley; 1982:384–413.

59. Lacks P. Behavioral Treatment for Persistent Insomnia. New York, NY: Pergamon Press; 1987.

60. Hauri P, Linde S. No More Sleepless Nights. New York, NY: Wiley; 1990.

61. Douglass AB, Bornstein RF, Nino-Murcia G, et al. The Sleep Disorders Questionnaire, I: creation and multivariate structure of SDQ. Sleep. 1994;17:160–167.

62. Cote KA, Ogilvie RD. The Brock Sleep and Insomnia Questionnaire: phase I. Sleep Res. 1992;22:356.

63. Hamilton M. A rating scale for depression. J Neurol Neurosurg Psychiatry. 1960;23:56–62.

64. Beck AT, Ward CH, Mendelson M, et al. An inventory for measuring depression. Arch Gen Psychiatry. 1961;4:561–571.

65. Zung WWK. A self-rating depression scale. Arch Gen Psychiatry. 1965;12:63–70.

66. Beck AT, Epstein N, Brown G, et al. An inventory for measuring clinical anxiety. J Consult Clin Psychol. 1988;56:893–897.

67. Derogatis LR. SCL-90-R: Administration, Scoring, and Procedures Manual. Baltimore, Md: Clinical Psychometrics Research; 1977.

68. McNair DM, Lorr M, Droppleman LF. EDITS manual for the Profile of Mood States. San Diego, Calif: Educational and Industrial Testing Service; 1981.

69. Spielberger CD, Gorsuch RL, Lushene R, et al. The State-Trait Anxiety Inventory for Adults. Palo Alto, Calif: Mind Garden; 1983.

70. Butcher JN, Dahlstrom WG, Graham JR, et al. MMPI-2: Minnesota Multiphasic Personality Inventory, 2. Manual for Administration and Scoring. Minneapolis, Minn: University of Minnesota Press; 1989.

71. Horne JA, Ostberg O. A self-assessment questionnaire to determine morningness-eveningness in human circadian rhythms. Int J Chronobiol. 1976;4:97–110.

72. Kazarian SS, Howe MG, Csapo KG. Development of the Sleep Behavior Self-Rating Scale. Behav Ther. 1979;10:412–417.

73. Nicassio PM, Mendlowitz DR, Fussell JJ, et al. The phenomenology of the pre-sleep state: the development of the pre-sleep arousal scale. Behav Res Ther. 1985;23:263–271.

74. Coren S. Prediction of insomnia from arousability predisposition scores: scale development and cross-validation. Behav Res Ther. 1988;26:415–420.

75. Espie CA, Brooks DN, Lindsay WR. An evaluation of tailored psychological treatment of insomnia. J Behav Ther Exp Psychiatry. 1989;20:143–153.

76. Monk TH, Reynolds CF III, Kupfer DJ, et al. The Pittsburgh Sleep Diary. J Sleep Res. 1994;3:111–120.

77. Spielman AJ, Glovinsky PB. The diagnostic interview and differential diagnosis for complaints of insomnia. In: Pressman MR, Orr WC, eds. Understanding Sleep: The Evaluation and Treatment of Sleep Disorders. Washington, DC: American Psychological Association; 1997:125–160.

78. Metrodesign Associates/Charles Pollak, MD, 90 Clinton Street, Homer, NY 13077; 1989.

79. Spielman AJ, Anderson MW. The clinical interview and treatment planning as a guide to understanding the nature of insomnia: the CCNY insomnia interview. In: Chokroverty S, ed. Sleep Disorders Medicine: Basic Science, Technical Considerations, and Clinical Aspects. 2nd ed. Boston, Mass: Butterworth-Heinemann; 1998:385–426.

104

Evaluating Sleepiness

Merrill M. Mitler
Mary A. Carskadon
Max Hirshkowitz

Excessive sleepiness during work activities is a serious, potentially life-threatening condition that affects not only sleepy individuals but also their families, co-workers, and society in general. The current conceptualization of sleep regulation involves two processes: one process is circadian, and the other is homeostatic. The effect of these processes on self-reported, biological, and behavioral measures of sleepiness is a topic of continuing research. With the growth and increasing interest in sleep disorders, tools are needed not only for conducting research but also for clinically assessing patients for sleepiness. It is helpful to remember that all tools have optimal uses and limitations. Although one may use a hammer to fasten screws, a screwdriver works better. Thus, one should consider the assessment goal when choosing a technique, consider the advantages and limitations, and carefully follow specific evaluation protocols.

The focus of this chapter is clinical assessment; therefore, special attention is directed to three specific measurement issues. The first issue relates to individual differences in measurements of within-subjects comparisons versus between-subjects comparisons. For example, if the increase in sleepiness can be precisely measured in a before-and-after experimental design, the initial value for one person will exceed the final value for another. Consequently, this superb metric for indexing relative sleepiness is unable to establish whether the patient in your office is excessively sleepy.

The second issue concerns self-report. In a clinical situation, a rational, self-aware, objective, scrupulously honest individual who is a good historian and has no agenda other than obtaining treatment for affliction still presents a few problems involving impairment of self-assessment due to chronic sleepiness itself. Of course, this best case scenario is relatively uncommon. With increasing frequency, sleep specialists are being asked to make assessments for regulatory and judicial purposes, so parameters of testing have become more crucial.

The third issue is that clinical testing of sleepiness usually involves testing during the daytime. A large number of studies and normative data exist for physiologically based metrics of daytime sleepiness. If it is clinically necessary to assess sleepiness during the night, such as in shift workers, the choices of validated tools are generally limited to performance tests. Although physiologically based metrics can readily be used to detect nighttime drops in alertness in normal and sleep-deprived volunteers, the guidelines as to what degree of sleepiness is *pathological* during the night have not been established; it is *normal* to be very sleepy at 4:00 AM.

One traditional conceptualization for characterizing sleepiness involved three factors: physiological sleepiness, manifest sleepiness, and introspective sleepiness.[1] This model provides a useful organizational device for understanding sleepiness measurement, but different measurements may index quite different (although related) phenomena. Physiological sleepiness can be thought of as the underlying biological drive to sleep; consequently, the primary index is the speed with which an individuals falls asleep. Manifest sleepiness can be considered from three perspectives: behavioral signs of sleepiness, inability to volitionally remain awake, and performance deficit on psychomotor or cognitive tasks. The common thread is the transformational effect of underlying sleepiness on outward behavior and abilities. Finally, introspective sleepiness concerns an individual's self-assessment of an internal state. Although the manifest and introspective measures may stem from the same underlying drive state, individual differences factor in and modify the measurable phenomena. It is not merely illogical to attempt to use these measures interchangeably; it misses the importance of the differences between them.

PHYSIOLOGICAL SLEEPINESS

Multiple Sleep Latency Test

If sleepiness is considered a motivational drive state, the rapidity with which an individual falls asleep can be used to evaluate the intensity of the drive. As such, sleep deprivation decreases latency to sleep on subsequent sleep opportunities. Awake-dependent drive for sleep builds across the normal waking day, is opposed by a circadian-dependent drive for alertness in the evening, and then rapidly rises to maximal levels as sleep deprivation and circadian factors combine in the nighttime hours.[2] During the normal nighttime hours, the physiological drive to sleep quickly reaches maximum levels, and sleep onset becomes almost immediate when sleep opportunities are provided. Physiological sleepiness is standardly indexed using the multiple sleep latency test (MSLT). An MSLT is a series of nap opportunities (four to six) presented at 2-h intervals beginning approximately 2 h after initial (morning) awakening (for details, see Carskadon et al.[3]). Individuals undergoing an MSLT are instructed to *allow themselves to fall asleep* or *to not to resist falling asleep*. Subjects are tested under standardized conditions in their street clothes and are not permitted to remain in bed between nap test sessions. Similarly, subjects should not engage in vigorous pretest activity because it will alter test outcome.[4] Standardization of testing conditions is necessary and critical to obtain reliable results.[5] Sleep rooms should be dark and quiet during testing. Electrophysiological parameters needed to detect sleep onset and score sleep stages are recorded during nap opportunities. Recordings include central (required) and occipital (very strongly recommended) electroencephalograms (EEGs), left and right eye electro-oculograms (EOGs), and submentalis electromyogram (EMGs). MSLT guidelines also call for monitoring respiratory flow and sounds in patients known to snore (Table 104–1). In a series of elegant studies, the effects of age, partial sleep deprivation, and disorders of excessive somnolence were well characterized.[6–9] Key concepts concerning homeostatic influences on sleepiness derive directly from research with MSLT. MSLT demonstrations of the cumulative nature of sleep debt, the increased sleepiness during adolescence produced by sleep restriction, and reduction in sleepiness after sleep extension provide the foundation for understanding the interaction between sleep and wakefulness. It has also been noted that circadian influence has been noted in sleep latencies on nap opportunities scheduled in the mid-afternoon for subjects who were not already near maximum sleepiness or alertness.[10]

Two protocols exist for conducting the MSLT: clinical and research (Fig. 104–1). These two protocols differ with respect to how much accumulated sleep is allowed if an individual falls asleep on a nap opportunity. In the research version, accumulated sleep is minimized by awakening the sleeper after sleep onset

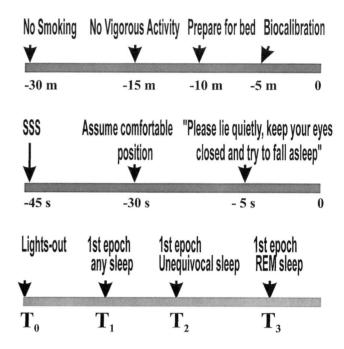

Test Session Termination Rules:
Experimental protocol: End at T_2
Clinical protocol: End at $T_1 + 15$ m
Either version, if no sleep occurs: $T_0 + 20$ m

Figure 104–1. Specific procedures for multiple sleep latency test nap opportunities.

defined as (1) one epoch of unequivocal sleep or (2) three epochs of stage 1 sleep. Unequivocal sleep is an epoch of stage 2, 3, or 4 or rapid eye movement (REM) sleep. The clinical version allows more sleep to occur because the test attempts to serve the dual role of indexing sleepiness and attempting to uncover abnormal REM sleep tendency (useful in the differential diagnosis of narcolepsy). Each test session is therefore allowed to continue for 15 min after sleep onset using the above criteria (assuming it occurs) to determine whether a sleep-onset REM sleep episode will occur. If no sleep onset occurs, the nap opportunity is terminated in both protocols after 20 min. Sleep latency is defined as the elapsed time from the start of the test to the first 30-sec epoch scored as sleep. Sleep latency in normal adult control subjects ranges from 10 to 20 min. Pathological sleepiness is defined as mean sleep latency of less than 5 or 6 min.[6] Latencies falling between the normal and the pathological values are considered a diagnostic gray area. The clinical version of the MSLT reliably distinguishes patients with nacrolepsy from control subjects with respect to both the number of episodes of REM sleep detected and sleep latency (Table 104–2).

The MSLT has proved to be useful for documenting treatment response.[11–13] It also can reveal residual sleepiness in patients who report no longer being sleepy after treatment.[14] The sensitivity of MSLT to physiological sleepiness makes it especially useful for detecting persistent sleepiness in the presumably well-treated

Table 104–1. MULTIPLE SLEEP LATENCY TEST RECORDING MONTAGE

Physiological Activity Recorded

Left or right central EEG (C3 or C4)
Left or right occipital EEG (O1 or O2)
Left horizontal or oblique EOG
Right horizontal or oblique EOG
Vertical EOG
Submentalis (chin) electromyogram
Electrocardiogram
Respiratory flow, as needed
Respiratory sounds, as needed

EEG, electroencephalogram; EOG, electro-oculogram.

Table 104–2. MULTIPLE SLEEP LATENCY TEST RESULTS FOR 57 NARCOLEPTIC PATIENTS
AND 17 ASYMPTOMATIC CONTROLS

Group		Individual Tests					5-Test Average	REM Score
		10:00 AM	Noon	2:00 PM	4:00 PM	6:00 PM		
Narcoleptics	% Slept	100%	98.3%	100%	100%	96.5%	99.0%	
N = 57	Sleep latency	3.0	2.9	2.4	2.4	4.0	3.0	3.5
Females 24	SD	2.4	3.6	3.0	2.5	5.1	2.7	0.9
Males 33	Minimum	0.0	0.0	0.0	0.0	0.0	0.6	2
Age 43.3 ± 12.3	Maximum	12.5	20.0	18.0	15.0	20.0	14.1	5
Controls	% Slept	58.8%	58.8%	70.6%	76.5%	52.9%	63.5%	
N = 17	Sleep latency	14.3	13.7	12.2	12.6	14.2	13.4	0
Females 11	SD	6.0	6.1	5.7	5.2	6.1	4.0	0
Males 6	Minimum	1.3	0.3	2.5	2.5	3.3	4.8	0
Age 33.4 ± 9.9	Maximum	20.0	20.0	20.0	20.0	20.0	20.0	0

Adapted from Mitler MM, Nelson S, Hajdukovic R. Narcolepsy. Diagnosis, treatment, and management. Psychiatr Clin North Am. 1987;10:593–606.

Data columns are the group results for the five individual tests throughout the day, followed by the average for all five tests and the number of tests in which REM sleep occurred. The first row of data for each group is the percentage of the group that actually fell asleep during each individual test. All other values are in minutes.

patient. Sleepiness may continue because of an occult comorbid sleep disorder, ineffective treatment, poor adherence to the treatment regimen, or concomitant soporific medication. Therefore, assessment of sleep with the use of polysomnography the night before MSLT testing and obtaining a careful history of drug use for the past month are essential. MSLT should not be scheduled during drug withdrawal, while sedating medications are pharmacokinetically active, or after a night of profoundly disturbed sleep.

As a technique to demonstrate an individual's underlying sleepiness, MSLT has several inherent advantages. The first is its direct, objective, quantitative approach. It is generally thought that people who are not sleepy cannot make themselves fall asleep; however, one can succeed in remaining awake if sleepiness is not overwhelming. Thus, if a positive MSLT is one that indicates sleepiness, false-positive tests are theoretically minimal. A full, laboratory, attended polysomnogram recorded the night before MSLT testing discloses prior sleep quality and quantity. If the prior night sleep is significantly disrupted or disturbed, MSLT can be rescheduled. Drug screening is also recommended to ensure the physiological sleepiness is not pharmacologically induced. The availability of normative values and test standardization made MSLT the test of choice for assessing sleepiness for many years.

Other Measures of Physiological Sleepiness

Pupillography

The pupillary stability and size are affected by exposure to light and an individual's arousal level. In a darkened room, an individual's pupils will dilate; however, as a person becomes sleepy and begins to fall asleep, the pupils constrict and become unstable. This change reflects autonomic nervous system changes and has been researched as a potential measure of sleep tendency.[15] Pupillometry was used in the clinical assessment of narcolepsy and its treatment for many years at the Mayo Clinic.[16] Electronic pupillography is an objective method for monitoring the size of a person's pupil; however, it is difficult to compare one subject with another. Furthermore, normative data are not available; consequently, the technique has not come into general use for clinically evaluating sleepiness.

Electroencephalography

Computerized quantitative analyses of EEG waveform features seem an obvious approach to assessment of central nervous system arousal level. It has long been thought that EEG delta activity can be used to index sleepiness. Sleep-related EEG delta activity increases in response to experimental sleep deprivation.[17] Hasan et al.[18] reported EEG correlates of drowsiness using computerized analysis. In essence, the MSLT uses EEG markers (*macroarchitectural features*) of sleep onset to quantify sleepiness. It is reasonable to expect that subtle waveform patterns (*microarchitecture*) could provide a sensitive metric. Alpha EEG frequency decreases and amplitude increases occur just before sleep onset (marked by alpha EEG disappearance). Even further refinement using event-related potentials to directly index the neurological reactivity to sensory stimuli has been explored as a way to assess sleepiness. Although these approaches hold promise, the lack of technique standardization and the absence of normative data limit their clinical usefulness. In addition, the high degree of between-subject variation makes it difficult to compare results between individuals. Finally, continuous EEG measures may not be as sensitive to episodes of sleepiness as continuous observation by a trained observer. Several investigators report that continuous EEG identified fewer episodes of sleepiness[19] and was less predictive of performance lapses than continuous video monitoring.[20]

MANIFEST SLEEPINESS

Maintenance of Wakefulness Test

Procedures used to conduct the maintenance of wakefulness test (MWT) are similar to those used for the MSLT.[21] The major difference is the instruction given to the test subject. The person being tested is told *to attempt to remain awake*. In this manner, the MWT is used to assess an individual's capability to not be overwhelmed by sleepiness—that is, the functioning of the underlying wakefulness system is assessed. If the wakefulness system fails, sleepiness becomes manifest. This laboratory situation parallels circumstances in which sleep onset occurs inadvertently while a person is passive and sedentary in a nonstimulating environment. In the MWT, there is no task other than to remain awake. During the MWT, an individual is monitored for EEG sleep onset during four to six sessions, scheduled at 2-h intervals beginning 2 h after awakening from the previous night's sleep. In studies that compared MWT and MSLT sleep latencies, as expected, subjects were found to take longer to fall asleep when instructed to remain awake than when told not to resist sleep.

A major criticism of MWT relates to the wide variety of protocols used. MWT session length has not been well standardized; 20-, 30-, and 40-min tests have been used, with the longer tests devised to avoid ceiling effects. Also, a major drawback in the use of MWT has been the lack of normative data; however, this situation has changed.[22] Table 104–3 presents normative data using 40-min MWT trials for 64 asymptomatic controls who were medically healthy on clinical examination and free of sleep disorders by nocturnal polysomnographic criteria. Table 104–3 also presents projected norms if 20-min trials are used.

Remaining questions include the effect of acute sleep deprivation, age, time of testing, and drugs on MWT profiles. Nevertheless, the MWT has proved useful in evaluating treatment effects in patients with narcolepsy and sleep-related breathing disorders. Because the MWT poses the question of whether sleepiness is overwhelming, the test has attracted the attention of regulatory agencies. With the growing interest in sleepiness and public safety, demand for tests to assess sleepiness has increased. Indeed, the Federal Aviation Administration recognizes the MWT as a means to determine whether noncommercial pilots can be licensed after treatment for sleep apnea.[23] MWT measures often reveal improvement in treated patients who continue to be physiologically sleepy; thus, MWT is sometimes thought as a way of extending the sensitivity range of MSLT.[24] It should be noted, however, that MSLT and MWT do not correlate well in patients complaining of excessive sleepiness.[25] Many patients who will fall asleep rapidly when not resisting sleep can still retain the ability to remain awake if they desire. Underlying neurophysiological mechanisms for maintaining alertness are quite distinct from those that regulate and coordinate sleep.

Performance and Vigilance Tests

Manifest sleepiness can be measured using a variety of performance tasks. Some of these tests attempt to measure cognitive slowing (e.g., the digit symbol substitution test), whereas others address alterations in attention. Arousal and attention have traditionally been difficult to tease apart; therefore, it is not surprising that long, experimenter-paced, monotonous tasks that tax the subject's endurance are sensitive to sleep loss. Such tests are called *vigilance tests*. These tests often attempt to mimic the tedious, palling situation of watching for blips on a radar screen or for ships on the horizon. Assessment of vigilance with nonstimulating tasks is clinically relevant in patients with disorders of sleep and arousal. Regardless of the test used, several important measurement issues exist. The landmark studies, collectively labeled The Walter Reed Experiments (named for the institute in which they were conducted) investigated, among other things, the effects of sleep deprivation on performance.[26, 27] From these pioneering studies, it became clear that time-on-task, response slowing, and response lapsing were essential factors in *sustained attention* tasks (for an excellent review, see Dinges and Kribbs[28]). A variety of performance, vigilance, and sustained attention tests are available.[29–31] However, the presentation modality, sensitivity, usefulness, and type of data available vary considerably among tests. Normative data are limited, and the meaningfulness of comparisons between individuals can be difficult to evaluate.

Table 104–3. MAINTENANCE OF WAKEFULNESS TEST SLEEP LATENCY NORMS (IN MINUTES) FOR 64 CONTROL SUBJECTS

	Trial 1	Trial 2	Trial 3	Trial 4	MWT Mean
40-Minute MWT Trials					
Mean	36.27	33.95	34.25	36.49	35.24
SD	9.16	12.03	11.48	8.79	7.93
Range	3.0–40.0	4.5–40.0	3.5–4.0	1.2–40.0	7.1–40.0
20-Minute MWT Trials (Projected by Limiting Sleep Latency to 20)					
Mean	19.08	18.09	18.39	19.20	18.69
SD	3.06	4.37	3.90	3.20	2.63
Range	3.0–20.0	4.5–20.0	3.5–20.0	1.2–20.0	7.1–20.0

Data from Doghramji K, Mitler MM, Sangal RB, et al. A normative study of the Maintenance of Wakefulness Test (MWT). Electroencephalogr Clin Neurophysiol. 1997;103:554–562.
MWT, Maintenance of Wakefulness Test.

INTROSPECTIVE SLEEPINESS

Profile of Mood States

Although designed to assess mood, the Profile of Mood States (POMS) has often been used in sleep research.[32] The original test design included a dimension for sleepiness, but it was eliminated because it was found to overlap with other scales. Sleepiness loads several POMS scales, most notably, Vigor (negative), Confusion, and Fatigue. To a lesser extent, sleepiness is associated with increased scores on Depression and Anger scales. Interestingly, the Confusion scale may be differentially more responsive to severe sleepiness, and the Vigor scale may be differentially more responsive to partial sleep deprivation.[33] The *worn out syndrome* of oversleeping in the absence of marked sleep deficit described by Globus[34] is characterized in language comparable to the POMS Fatigue scale mood descriptors; however, fatigue can occur independent of sleepiness.

Stanford Sleepiness Scale

For many years, the Stanford Sleepiness Scale (SSS) was the standard measure of introspective sleepiness.[35] Individuals taking the SSS choose one of seven statements to describe their self-assessed current state; the choices are shown in Table 104–4.

Advantages of SSS include its brevity and ease of administration and the fact that it can be administered repeatedly. Experimentally induced sleep deprivation increases SSS scores; however, normative data do not exist. It is difficult to use SSS to make clinical judgments and to compare introspective sleepiness between individuals.

Epworth Sleepiness Scale

The Epworth Sleepiness Scale (ESS) was developed by Murray Johns at the Epworth Hospital in Melbourne, Australia. ESS is a specialized, validated sleep questionnaire containing eight items that ask for self-

Table 104–5. THE EPWORTH SLEEPINESS SCALE ITEMS

Question	Hypothetical Situation to Be Rated
1	Sitting and reading
2	Watching television
3	Sitting, inactive in a public place (e.g., a theater or a meeting)
4	As a passenger in a car for 1 h without a break
5	Lying down to rest in the afternoon when circumstances permit
6	Sitting and talking to someone
7	Sitting quietly after a lunch without alcohol
8	In a car, while stopped for a few minutes in traffic

reported disclosure of the expectation of "dozing" in a variety of situations. Dozing probability ratings are zero (0), slight (1), moderate (2), or high (3) in the eight hypothetical situations shown on Table 104–5.

It is worth noting that in situations 1, 3, 6, and 7, one is explicitly sitting; in situations 2, 4, and 8, one is presumably sitting; and in situation 5, one is lying down. ESS also differs from other tests in that the respondent is not being ask to interpret his or her internal state but rather to make a judgment about his or her behavior. Furthermore, in a sense, an individual completing the ESS is rating his or her *drive to sleep* in probability projections. This may explain why ESS has a small but statistically significant correlation with MSLT, an objective index of *sleep drive*. Johns[36, 37] conducted reliability and validity studies on 54 patients with sleep-related breathing disorders (before and after treatment with continuous positive airway pressure) and 104 medical student control subjects. Student control subjects had a mean score of 7.6. Initially elevated scores among patients with sleep-related breathing disorders (mean, 14.3) declined to the normal range after treatment (mean, 7.4). ESS scores increase as a function of increasing severity of their sleep-disordered breathing.[36, 38]

The popularity of ESS stems in part from its simplicity and brevity. This in conjunction with the validation studies has made it perhaps the most commonly administered self-report scale for daytime sleepiness. One disadvantage is the questionable usefulness of the test when readministered within a brief time interval; consequently, it is not useful for evaluating circadian rhythm influences on sleepiness. In addition, the sensitivity to age, acute sleep disturbance or deprivation, and drugs is not known.

PRACTICAL ISSUES AND CONCLUSIONS

Before sleepiness is assessed, a variety of questions should be considered, including whether the goal is to establish (1) the presence of sleepiness, (2) the absence of sleepiness, or (3) changes in sleepiness. Is testing being conducted for (4) clinical assessment, (5) research, or (6) legal purposes? Is there self-interest in-

Table 104–4. THE STANFORD SLEEPINESS SCALE ITEMS

Code	Scale Statements
1	Feeling active and vital, alert, wide awake
2	Functioning at a high level, but not at peak, able to concentrate
3	Relaxed, awake, not at full alertness, responsive
4	A little foggy, not at peak, let down
5	Fogginess, beginning to lose interest in remaining awake, slowed down
6	Sleepiness, prefer to be lying down, fighting sleep, woozy
7	Almost in reverie, sleep onset soon, lost struggle to remain awake

Table 104–6. COMPARISON BETWEEN TESTS FOR EVALUATING SLEEPINESS

Test	Type of Sleepiness Evaluated	Repeated Measure Limit	Normal Range Available	Possible to Fake Sleepy	Possible to Fake Alert
MSLT	Physiological	Standardized*	Yes	No	Yes†
Pupillography	Physiological	Not limited	No	No	Unknown
EEG	Physiological	Not limited	No	No	Unknown
MWT	Manifest	Standardized*	Yes	Yes‡	No
Vigilance and performance	Manifest	Not limited	No	Yes§	No
POMS	Self-report	Not limited	Yes	Yes	Yes
SSS	Self-report	Not limited	No	Yes	Yes
ESS	Self-report	Problematic	Yes/no¶	Yes	Yes

*Standard protocol is four to six test sessions per day, at 2-h intervals. Test sessions are sometimes scheduled at shorter intervals (e.g., for children), but this practice is not recommended by the authors.
†Assuming that an individual is not overwhelmingly sleepy, attempting to remain awake can undermine the test result.
‡Assuming that an individual is physiologically sleepy, not attempting to remain awake will make it appear that overwhelming sleepiness is present.
§Intentionally not attending or responding to the task can make an individual appear sleepy.
¶Normative data were collected from medical students who often experience sleep deprivation.

volved as part of a (7) primary or (8) secondary agenda? With increasing frequency, sleep specialists are being asked for opinions in legal cases involving accidents or disability claims and are often pressured to render opinions concerning "fitness for duty." In such cases, objective testing is critical because there are situational *demand characteristics*. Furthermore, a normal test result does not guarantee fitness for duty. Table 104–6 shows some characteristics of the tests described in this chapter. Ideally, physiological, manifest, and introspective sleepiness should be assessed. In general, if an individual claims to be sleepy and the goal is to demonstrate sleepiness, the MSLT is the best confirmatory test. If an individual claims not to be sleepy and the goal is to demonstrate an ability to remain awake, MWT has certain advantages. For clinical purposes, self-reported measures combined with MSLT have long been the sine qua non for establishing sleepiness. Sometimes, however, in cases involving severe sleepiness, MWT can demonstrate improved alertness after treatment, whereas MSLT shows little or no change. Such individuals continue to be pathologically sleepy, but they are not overwhelmed by it during the brief testing interval. The relation between this pattern of change and performance or behavior requires further study.

The dangers posed by excessive sleepiness are becoming increasingly apparent. The National Commission on Sleep Disorders Research[39] enumerated a substantial list of industrial and transportation accidents directly or indirectly related to sleepiness. Although it was originally thought that sleepiness stemmed from the accumulation of blood-borne neurotoxins, such substances have not been clearly identified. The search continues for sleep-inducing peptides (contemporary descendents of the hypothesized neurotoxins); however, a convenient reliable blood test for sleepiness has yet to be developed. Nevertheless, evaluation techniques can assess not only the underlying physiological drive to sleep but also its subjective, internalized consequences and its behavioral manifestations.

References

1. Carskadon MA, Dement WC. The multiple sleep latency test: what does it measure? Sleep. 1982;5:S67–S72.
2. Carskadon MA, Acebo C, Labyak SE, et al. Circadian and homeostatic influences on sleep latency in adolescents. Paper presented at: Sixth Meeting of the Society for Research on Biological Rhythms; May 1998; Amelia Island Plantation, Jacksonville, Fla.
3. Carskadon MA, Dement WC, Mitler MM, et al. Guidelines for the multiple sleep latency test (MSLT): a standard measure of sleepiness. Sleep. 1986;9:519–524.
4. Bonnet MH, Arand DL. Sleepiness as measured by modified multiple sleep latency testing varies as a function of preceding activity. Sleep. 1998;21:477–483.
5. Roehrs TA, Carskadon MA. Standardization of method: essential to sleep science. Sleep. 1998;21:445.
6. Carskadon MA, Dement WC. Cumulative effects of sleep restriction on daytime sleepiness. Psychophysiology. 1981;18:107–113.
7. Carskadon MA, Dement WC. Daytime sleepiness: quantification of behavioral state. Neurosci Biobehav Rev. 1987;11:307–317.
8. Mitler MM, Nelson S, Hajdukovic R. Narcolepsy: diagnosis treatment and management. Psychiatr Clin North Am. 1987;10:593–606.
9. Carskadon MA, Harvey K, Duke P, et al. Pubertal changes in daytime sleepiness. Sleep. 1980;2:453–460.
10. Richardson GS. Carskadon MA, Orav EJ, et al. Circadian variation in sleep tendency in elderly and young adult subjects. Sleep. 1982;5:S82–S94.
11. Dement WC, Carskadon MA, Richardson GS. Excessive daytime sleepiness in the sleep apnea syndrome. In: Guilleminault C, Dement WC, eds. Sleep Apnea Syndromes. Menlo Park, Calif: Alan R. Liss; 1978:23–46.
12. Lamphere J, Roehrs T, Wittig R, et al. Recovery of alertness after CPAP in apnea. Chest. 1989;96:1364–1367.
13. US Modafinil in Narcolepsy Study Group (USMNSG). Randomized trial of modafinil for the treatment of pathological somnolence in narcolepsy. Ann Neurol. 1998;43:88–97.
14. Zorick F, Roehrs T, Conway W, et al. Effects of uvulopalatopharyngoplasty on the daytime sleepiness associated with sleep apnea syndrome. Bull Eur Physiopathol Respir. 1983;19:600–603.
15. Schmidt HS, Fortin L. Electronic pupillography in disorders of arousal. In: Guilleminault C, ed. Sleeping and Waking Disorders: Indications and Techniques. Menlo Park, Calif: Addison-Wesley; 1982:127–143.
16. Yoss RE, Moyer NJ, Ogle KN. The pupillogram and narcolepsy: a method to measure decreased levels of wakefulness. Neurology. 1969;19:921–928.
17. Borbely AA, Baumann F, Brandeis D, et al. Sleep deprivation: effect on sleep stages and EEG power density in man. Electroencephalogr Clin Neurophysiol. 1981;51:483–493.

18. Hasan J, Hirvonen K, Varri A, et al. Validation of computer analyzed polygraphic patterns during drowsiness and sleep onset. Electroencephalogr Clin Neurophysiol. 1993;87:117–127.

19. Mitler MM, Miller JC, Lipsitz JJ, et al. The sleep of long-haul truck drivers. N Engl J Med. 1997;337:755–761.

20. Dinges DF, Mallis MM. Managing fatigue by drowsiness detection: can technological promises be realized? Third International Conference on Fatigue in Transportation: Coping With the 24-Hour Society. February 9–13, 1998; Fremantle, Western Australia.

21. Mitler MM, Gujavarty KS, Browman CP. Maintenance of wakefulness test: a polysomnographic technique for evaluation of treatment efficacy in patients with excessive somnolence. Electroencephalogr Clin Neurophysiol. 1982;53:658–661.

22. Doghramji K, Mitler MM, Sangal RB, et al. A normative study of the Maintenance of Wakefulness Test (MWT). Electroencephalogr Clin Neurophysiol. 1997;103:554–562.

23. Federal Aviation Administration (FAA). Sleep Apnea Evaluation Specifications. Federal Aviation Administration specification letter dated October 6, 1992. U.S. Department of Transportation; 1992.

24. Mitler MM, Miller JC. Methods of testing for sleepiness. Behav Med. 1996;21:171–183.

25. Sangal RB, Thomas L, Mitler MM. Disorders of excessive sleepiness: treatment improves ability to stay awake but does not reduce sleepiness. Chest. 1992;102:699–703.

26. Williams HL, Lubin A, Goodnow JJ. Impaired performance and acute sleep loss. Psychol Monogr 1959;73(pt 14):1–26.

27. Lubin A. Performance under sleep loss and fatigue. In: Kety SS, Evarts EV, Williams HL, eds. Sleep and Altered States of Consciousness. Baltimore, Md: Williams & Wilkins; 1967:506–513.

28. Dinges DF, Kribbs NB. Performing while sleepy: effects of experimentally-induced sleepiness. In: Monk TM, ed. Sleep, Sleepiness and Performance. Chichester, England: John Wiley & Sons; 1991:97–128.

29. Wilkinson RT. Sleep deprivation: performance tests for partial and selective sleep deprivation. In: Abt LA, Reiss BF, eds. Progress in Clinical Psychology. Vol 3. London, England: Grune & Stratton; 1968:28–43.

30. Hirshkowitz M, De La Cueva L, Herman JH. The multiple vigilance test. Behav Res Meth Instr Comp. 1993;25:272–275.

31. Findley L, Unverzagt M, Guchu R, et al. Vigilance and automobile accidents in patients with sleep apnea or narcolepsy. Chest. 1995;108:619–624.

32. McNair DM, Lorr M, Droppleman LF. Manual of the Profile of Mood States. San Diego, Calif: Educational and Industrial Testing Service; 1992.

33. Horne J. Dimensions to sleepiness. In: Monk TM, ed. Sleep, Sleepiness and Performance. Chichester, England: John Wiley & Sons; 1991:169–196.

34. Globus GG. A syndrome associated with sleeping late. Psychosomatic Med. 1969;31:528–535.

35. Hoddes E, Zarcone V, Smythe H, et al. Quantification of sleepiness: a new approach. Psychophysiology. 1973;10:431–436.

36. Johns MW. A new method for measuring daytime sleepiness: the Epworth Sleepiness Scale. Sleep. 1991;14:540–545.

37. Johns MW. Reliability and factor analysis of the Epworth Sleepiness Scale. Sleep. 1992;15:376–381.

38. Hirshkowitz M, Gokcebay N, Iqbal S, et al. Epworth Sleepiness Scale and sleep-disordered breathing: replication and extension. Sleep Res. 1995;24:249.

39. National Commission on Sleep Disorders Research. Wake Up America: A National Sleep Alert. Vol. 1, Executive Summary and Executive Report, Report of the National Commission on Sleep Disorders Research. National Institutes of Health. Washington, DC: US Government Printing Office; 1993.

105

Light Therapy

Michael Terman
Jiuan Su Terman

Exposure of the eyes to light of appropriate intensity and duration, at an appropriate time of day, can have marked effects on the timing and duration of sleep and on the affective and physical symptoms of depressive illness. The most extensive clinical trials have focused on winter depression, or *seasonal affective disorder* (SAD). There is much in the literature on the applications of light therapy for sleep phase disorders, as well as for a range of nonseasonal mood and behavioral disorders. This chapter emphasizes timing and dosing strategies for light therapy. For a review of the underlying circadian physiology, see Terman.[1]

LIGHT DELIVERY

Apparatus

Many of the early research studies used a standard 2 × 4-foot fluorescent ceiling unit, with a plastic prismatic diffusion screen, placed vertically on a table about 3 feet from the user. A bank of fluorescent lamps—full spectrum or cool white—provided approximately 2500-lux illuminance. Smaller, more lightweight units have become commercially available; however, specific design features of marketed light boxes have most often not been clinically tested. Factors include lamp type (output and spectrum), filter, ballast frequency (for fluorescent lamps), size and positioning of radiating surface, heat emission, and so on. One clinically tested model (Fig. 105–1) illustrates second-generation apparatus modifications, including smaller size, portability, raised and downward-tilted placement of the radiating surface, an Acrylite OP-3–based smooth diffusion screen with complete ultraviolet (UV) filtering (see Resources), and high-output fluorescent lamps (biaxial SPX type with warm hue and dampened UV and blue output) driven by a high-frequency solid-state ballast. The combination of elements in this configuration yields a maximum illuminance of approximately 10,000 lux with the patient seated in a position with the eyes about 1 foot from the screen. With the direction of gaze downward toward the work surface, such a configuration provides low-glare illumination with a soft hue and is generally well tolerated (see Side Effects of Bright Light Exposure). As the apparatus becomes miniaturized, how-ever, the field of illumination narrows, and even small changes in head position can substantially reduce the intensity of light that reaches the eyes.

Although simple in design, home construction of such an apparatus is discouraged because of the danger of excessive irradiation; some amateur assemblers have experienced corneal and eyelid burns. Because the critical design features have not been specified or regulated by the government or the profession, clinicians should seek documentation by the manufacturer of the safety and effectiveness of any apparatus under consideration.

Claims for the specific efficacy of any particular

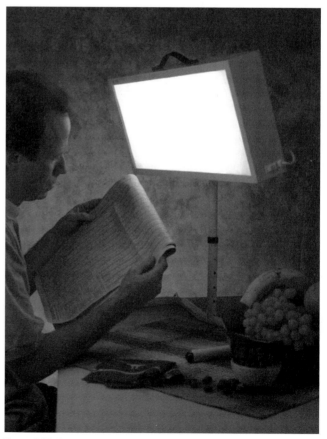

Figure 105–1. Table-mounted 10,000 lux fluorescent lighting system with Acrylite OP-3 filter. (Photograph courtesy of SphereOne, Inc., Silver Plume, Colorado.)

lamp type or spectral distribution, although commonly given, are unsubstantiated. Unfortunately, systems are marketed that provide excessive visual glare, exposure of naked bulbs, direct intense illumination from below the eyes ("ski slope" effect), and intentionally augmented UV radiation. Claims that UV radiation is important for the therapeutic effect are unsubstantiated. The clinician must be vigilant in the selection of an apparatus.

In an alternate configuration, head-mounted portable lighting units, which are intended to increase flexibility and convenience of use, have been marketed and are suited for novel applications such as in-flight travel. However, despite a set of multicenter trials for SAD,[2–4] bright light exposure with this device has shown no advantage over dim light exposure (a putative placebo control), and there has been no convincing demonstration of clinical efficacy[5] or reliable circadian phase-shifting.

Dawn-dusk simulation methodology provides a major contrast to bright light therapy. A computer-controlled lighting device delivers a mimic of gradual twilight transitions found outdoors in the spring or summer. The relatively dim, dynamically changing signals are presented to the patient while asleep, when eyes are adapted to the dark. As with bright light therapy, there is an antidepressant response and normalization of hypersomnic, phase-shifted, and fractionated sleep patterns.[6–8] A controlled clinical trial of log-linear light onset ramps (which differ from the curvilinear acceleration of naturalistic dawns) found signals rising to 250 lux significantly more antidepressant than dim control signals rising to 2 lux.[9] The effectiveness of dawn simulation may depend on the presentation of diffuse, broad-field illumination that reaches the sleeper in varying postures. Such efficacy has not been demonstrated for commercialized light "alarm clocks" with small, directional fields.

Safety of Bright Light for the Eyes

Ophthalmological evaluations of unmedicated patients with normal oculoretinal status have thus far shown no obvious acute light-induced pathology or long-term sequelae.[10] Although the intensity of bright light treatment falls well within the low outdoor daylight range, the exposure conditions differ from those outdoors, and prolonged use entails far greater cumulative light exposure than is normally experienced by urban dwellers and workers.[11, 12] Potentially damaging wavelengths above the UV range extend into the visible range up to 500 nm (blue light),[13, 14] and it has been proposed that broad-spectrum light therapy that filters out such wavelengths be clinically evaluated and implemented as a standard if effective.[15] At the opposite end of the spectrum, ocular exposure to infrared illumination, which makes up about 90% of the output of incandescent lamps, poses a risk of damage to the lens and cornea (as does UV) and to the retina and pigment epithelium.[16] This becomes increasingly problematic

given a claim for therapeutic efficacy using infrared illumination.[17]

Marketed light box diffusion filters vary widely in short-wavelength transmission (for examples, see Remé et al.[15]). Transmission curves should be demanded of manufacturers and compared with published standards. Normal clouding of the lens and ocular media that begins in middle age, as well as cataract formation, serves to exacerbate perceptual glare, which can make high-intensity light exposure quite uncomfortable.[15] Furthermore, both UV and short-wavelength blue light can interact with photosensitizing medications—including many standard antidepressant, antipsychotic, and antiarrhythmic agents, as well as common medications such as tetracycline—to promote or accelerate retinal pathology, whether acute or slow and cumulative.[16] (In one reported case, a patient received combination treatment with clomipramine, an anticholinergic tricyclic antidepressant, and full-spectrum fluorescent light. After 5 days, there was reduced visual acuity, contrast sensitivity and foveal sensitivity, and central scotomas and lesions, fortunately with only minor residual aftereffects in contrast sensitivity and scotoma 1 year after discontinuation.[18]) Specialized nonprescription eyeglass filters have been devised to eliminate transmission lower than 480 nm, maximize transmission above 500 nm, reduce glare, enhance visual acuity and brightness, and minimize the risk of short-wavelength photosensitization.[19]

Although there are no definite contraindications for bright light treatment, other than the retinopathies, research studies have routinely excluded patients with glaucoma or cataract. Some of these patients have used light therapy effectively in open treatment; this should be done, however, only with ophthalmological monitoring. A simple eye checkup is advised for all new patients, for which a structured examination chart has been designed[20] (see Resources). The examination has occasionally revealed preexisting ocular conditions that should be distinguished from potential consequences of bright light treatment.

Side Effects of Bright Light Exposure

If evening light is timed too late, there may be initial insomnia and hyperactivation. If morning light is timed too early, the patient may awaken prematurely and be unable to resume sleep. These problems are responsive to timing and dose (duration and intensity) adjustments during treatment of both circadian sleep phase and mood disorders.

The emergence of side effects relates in part to the parameters of light exposure, including intensity, duration, spectral content, and method of exposure (diffuse, focused, direct, indirect, and angle of incidence relative to the eyes). Thus far, side effects have been assessed primarily in patients with seasonal and nonseasonal mood disorders, and information is lacking for sleep disorders without mood disturbance. The earliest clinical trials of 2500-lux full-spectrum fluorescent light therapy for SAD noted infrequent side effects of hypomania, irritability, headache, and nausea.[21, 22] Such symptoms often subside after several days of treatment. If persistent, they can be reduced or eliminated with dose decreases. Rarely have patients discontinued treatment due to side effects. Studies with portable head-mounted units containing incandescent bulbs near the eyes and providing illuminance of 60 to 3500 lux have also noted side effects of headache, eyestrain, and feeling "wired," but symptoms were not dose dependent.[23]

Two cases of induced manic episodes have been reported in drug refractory nonseasonal unipolar depressives beginning after 4 to 5 days of light treatment.[24] A few cases of light-induced agitation and hypomania have been noted, also in nonseasonal depressives.[25] A patient with seasonally recurrent brief depressions developed rapid mood swings after light overexposure (far exceeding 30 min/day at 10,000 lux),[26] whereas a unipolar SAD patient with similar exposure showed his first manic episode[27]; both patients required discontinuation and medication. We had one bipolar patient with SAD who became manic after the use of lights and was administered lithium as an effective countermeasure; others who have used mood stabilizers have responded to light therapy without mania. Three cases of suicide attempt or ideation, also occurring in patients with SAD, were reported within 1 week of standard early-evening bright light treatment, and the patients required hospitalization.[28]

A 42-item side effect inventory was administered to 30 patients with SAD after treatment with unfiltered full-spectrum fluorescent light at 2500 lux for 2 h daily.[29] Other than one case of hypomania, there were no clinically significant side effects. Patients given evening light (the timing relative to bedtime was unspecified) reported initial insomnia. Mild visual complaints included blurred vision, eyestrain, and photophobia.

Of specific interest is the side effect profile for patients using a downward-tilted SPX-30 fluorescent light box protected by a smooth diffusion screen (see Fig. 105–1), with 30-min daily exposures at 10,000 lux, because this method has had widespread application. A study of 83 patients with SAD who were evaluated for 88 potential side effects[30] identified a small number of emergent symptoms at a frequency of 6 to 16%, including nausea, headache, jumpiness/jitteriness, and eye irritation.[31] These results must be weighed against the improvement of other patients who showed similar symptoms at baseline but became asymptomatic after light treatment: all symptoms, except nausea, showed greater improvement than exacerbation, which forces attention to the risk/benefit ratio. Indeed, symptom emergence might reflect the natural course of depressive illness in nonresponders to light rather than a specific response to light exposure.

CASE MANAGEMENT, TIMING, AND DOSING

Patient Monitoring

Light treatment is typically self-administered at home according to a schedule recommended by the clinician. To the extent that the timing of light exposure is important to obtain a therapeutic effect, compliance is a sine qua non. When commencing treatment, therefore, it is helpful to ask the patient to call every few days or to fax log records of sleep, treatment times, and mood ratings; this will assist the clinician in managing timing and dose adjustments.

In contrast with structured research studies, the motivation and compliance of patients in open treatment can be problematic. Despite an agreement to awaken for light treatment at a specific hour, patients may ignore the alarm, considering additional sleep to be the priority of the moment, and may delay or skip treatment. Patients frequently attempt to test whether improvement can be achieved without rigid compliance, and they may quit if managed too rigidly. Indeed, the behavioral investment in a maintenance regimen of light treatment is considerable, far exceeding that of pharmacotherapy.

For hypersomnic patients who are unable to awaken when instructed, light exposure initially can be scheduled at the time of habitual awakening and then edged earlier across days toward the target interval. Some depressed patients compensate for earlier wake-up times with earlier bedtimes or napping (as do patients with delayed sleep phase syndrome [DSPS]), but others are comfortable with less sleep as the antidepressant effect sets in. Clinical experience suggests that most such patients could not sustain earlier awakening without the use of light.

Variability in the sleep pattern, if it occurs, may yield important information for determination of the course of treatment. Online adjustments in scheduling, although labor intensive for the clinician, often succeed. Our strategy has been to encourage the adherence to a recommended light exposure schedule but to consider the obtained sleep pattern as a dependent measure that often reflects changes in mood state, sleep need, and circadian rhythm phase.

Timing of Morning Light Exposure Based on the Phase Relation Between Melatonin Secretion and Sleep

The thrust of recent clinical trials (Table 105–1; also see Seasonal Affective Disorder) leads to the recommendation that patients with SAD initially be given morning light shortly after awakening. A similar strategy applies to patients with DSPS. (In contrast, evening light is indicated for advanced sleep phase syndrome [ASPS]; see the case examples.) The dose of 10,000 lux for 30 min[32, 33] appears to be most efficient. Although lower intensities also may be effective, they require exposure durations up to 2 h,[34, 35] and to accommodate such morning treatment, most patients would have to awaken far earlier than at baseline.

The advantage of morning light may lie in circadian rhythm phase advances, which can be measured as shifts in the time of nocturnal melatonin onset.[36] The magnitude of the antidepressant response might vary with the magnitude of phase advances, but such a

Table 105–1. SUMMARY OF REMISSION RATES IN CONTROLLED CLINICAL TRIALS OF BRIGHT LIGHT THERAPY FOR SEASONAL AFFECTIVE DISORDER

	Remission Rate* (%; No. of Patients)		
	Morning Light	**Evening Light**	**Placebo (Negative Ion Generator)**
Terman et al.[33]†			
First treatment	54 (25/46)	33 (13/39)	11 (2/19)
Crossover	60 (28/47)	30 (14/47)	ND
Eastman et al.[34]‡			
First treatment	55 (18/33)	28 (9/32)	16 (5/31)
Lewy et al.[35]§			
First treatment	22 (6/27)	4 (1/24)	ND
Crossover	27 (14/51)	4 (2/51)	ND

From Wirz-Justice A. Beginning to see the light. Arch Gen Psychiatry. 1998;55(10):861–862. Copyright 1998, American Medical Association.
*Baseline-to-posttreatment score reduction of ≥50%, with final score ≤8, on the Structured Interview for the Hamilton Depression Scale–Seasonal Affective Disorder Version (SIGH-SAD).
†6-year study; 10,000 lux for 0.5 h, 2 weeks.
‡6-year study; 6000 lux for 1.5 h, 4 weeks.
§4-year study; 2500 lux for 2 h, 2 weeks.
ND, not done.

result has been elusive. In a protocol with 10,000-lux treatment for 30 min on habitual awakening, the magnitude of antidepressant response was negatively correlated with the interval between melatonin onset and treatment time ($r = -0.53$, a large effect size).[37] To maximize the likelihood of a treatment response, the clinician might therefore initiate morning light no later than 8 to 9 h after a patient's nocturnal melatonin onset at baseline. Unfortunately, such diagnostic information is not readily available. A future solution may lie in the use of a salivary melatonin assay[38] with home sampling, and rapid turnaround by a commercial laboratory. An approximate solution, however, lies in the relation between melatonin onset and habitual sleep onset ($r = 0.66$, with a slope of 1.0).[37] One thus can schedule morning light exposure at individually specified circadian times with the use of patients' reports of their habitual sleep pattern to infer the time of melatonin onset, a strategy that may facilitate circadian rhythm phase advances as well as the antidepressant response.

A matrix of recommended exposure times, derived from the regression of the sleep midpoint on melatonin onset, is shown in Table 105–2. With the use of average sleep-onset and wake-up estimates, the matrix specifies the time to start the light therapy session, which should begin within 10 min of scheduled wake-up time. In most cases, treatment will begin earlier than the baseline wake-up time, depending on the patient's habitual sleep duration. For example, a short sleeper, whose bedtime is at midnight and who awakens at 6 AM, would start treatment on habitual awakening. In contrast, a long sleeper, with onset at 11:30 PM and awakening at 7:30 PM, would have to wake up 1 h earlier, at 6:30 AM. For every half hour of sleep beyond 6 h,

awakening for light treatment is 15 min earlier than habitual awakening at baseline—a maximum of 1.5 h earlier if sleep duration extends to 9 h. The algorithm should be considered a "best guess" strategy to determine the initial timing of light exposure, with a potential need for adjustment depending on early results.

LIGHT TREATMENT OF SPECIFIC DISORDERS

Circadian Sleep Phase Disorders

Delayed Sleep Phase Syndrome. Patients with DSPS have difficulty initiating sleep before 1 to 3 AM, and sometimes later, with commensurate difficulty awakening at an early hour (for a review and discussion of circadian rhythm correlates, see Terman et al.[39]). Once awake, most patients exhibit normal alertness and energy as long as they can maintain their displaced sleep schedule, but others report difficulties for several hours after awakening and spurts of energy after midnight. Not infrequently, patients with DSPS show comorbid mood and personality disorders.

Under delay chronotherapy,[40] the sleep episode is scheduled at successively later hours each night for about 1 week. Once the desired sleep phase is attained, the patient attempts to keep sleep-wake timing consistent. The original description of chronotherapy specified that sleep episodes occur in darkness. It follows that the timing of light exposure changes during and after the phase adjustment. An implication is that by the end of the procedure, the patient begins to receive a normalized pattern of daily light exposure that serves to maintain the target phase. Early morning artificial bright light exposure can forestall further drifting toward the original delayed sleep phase, which always poses a risk.

Indeed, morning light treatment can often directly normalize the timing of the sleep episode without the necessity of progressive delays with chronotherapy. In one study, a group of patients with DSPS were given 2 h of early-morning light treatment at 2500 lux, along

Table 105–2. TIMING OF LIGHT THERAPY* BASED ON PRETREATMENT SLEEP ONSET AND AWAKENING†

Sleep Onset	Wake-Up Time							
	5:30	6:00	6:30	7:00	7:30	8:00	8:30	9:00
22:00		5:00	5:15	5:30				
22:30	5:00	5:15	5:30	5:45	6:00			
23:00	5:15	5:30	5:45	6:00	6:15	6:30		
23:30	5:30	5:45	6:00	6:15	6:30	6:45	7:00	
0:00		6:00	6:15	6:30	6:45	7:00	7:15	7:30
0:30			6:30	6:45	7:00	7:15	7:30	
1:00				7:00	7:15	7:30		

*Start of 10,000-lux/30-min session, approximately 8.5 h after estimated melatonin onset.
†For the range of onsets-to-awakenings of 41 patients contributing to the dataset.

with light restriction after 4:00 PM.[41] The body temperature rhythm and daily cycle of sleep-onset latencies showed phase advances, and there was an increase in morning alertness within 1 week. These effects were not obtained with the use of a dim light control. In open treatment, if morning light exposure fails to induce and maintain the desired phase advance, chronotherapy may be used to successively delay the sleep episode until the desired target phase is achieved. Light treatment can be used to facilitate chronotherapy with presleep exposures during the delay period, followed by postsleep exposures during maintenance. These approaches require the clinician's active supervision, with continual adjustment in sleep and light exposure schedules in response to patient feedback and ability to comply. Bright light treatment is administered in the context of complex daily patterns of indoor and outdoor light exposure, including dark periods, all of which may influence treatment outcome. Indeed, a procedure may require ensured dark exposure at certain times of day in coordination with light treatment at other times. This can be accomplished with the use of highly filtered goggles when going outdoors during daylight hours.[42]

Research studies have commonly used self-report sleep logs to track patient progress in response to light therapy, a device that can also assist clinicians with open treatment. The examples that follow span a variety of sleep phase disturbances and compliance issues.

Mild Sleep Phase Delay: Advance by Postsleep Light. The common problem of chronic but mild initial insomnia that falls short of a DSPS diagnosis, accompanied by difficulty arising and low morning alertness, is often readily treatable with morning light. Many such insomniacs do not respond to hypnotic medication and are not depressed.

CASE EXAMPLE 1

Patient J.B. (Fig. 105–2A) could rarely fall asleep before 1:30 AM or wake up in time for a normal work day. Although he was allowed to work from midmorning into the evening, he was handicapped by low alertness till midafternoon and headaches at a computer terminal during the late afternoon. Light treatment began with 10,000-lux exposures at 8 AM for 30 min, with no effect for several days. When the session was advanced to 7:30 AM, sleep onset spontaneously advanced by about 1 hour. However, several days of late insomnia followed, with awakenings before 6 AM, signaling an overdose. This problem was alleviated by reducing the treatment duration to 15 min at 7:30 AM, with sleep onset maintained around midnight. This regimen was continued, with effortless awakening accompanied by improved morning alertness and complete remission of the headache.

Delayed Sleep Phase Syndrome:
Advance by Postsleep Light

CASE EXAMPLE 2

Patient T.W. (see Fig. 105–2B) reported a lifelong history of DSPS with variable sleep onset averaging 5:00 AM and

occasional hypersomnic episodes lasting 11 to 12 h. Although not depressed while seeking help, he also reported experiencing subsyndromal symptoms of winter depression. The treatment consisted of gradually shifting light exposure earlier across days, beginning at 10:30 AM, a time of typical spontaneous awakening. The patient monitored his level of sleepiness and time of awakening to determine the rate of shift. He was able to achieve successively earlier wake-up times over a period of 2 weeks while light treatment sessions were advanced from 10:30 to 7:30 AM, but even at that point he could not fall asleep before 2:30 AM. However, when the treatment session was further advanced to 7 AM—an unprecedented time of awakening for this patient—sleep onset abruptly jumped approximately 2 h earlier. The sleep episode stabilized at about 1:15 to 6:30 AM with light treatment on awakening. After several months, the patient reported having increased light duration from 30 min (at 10,000 lux) to 45 or 60 min to enhance daytime energy. He also reported a relapse when he discontinued treatment twice within the next year. He managed his readjustments, and reported the remission of depressed mood in the winter.

Delayed Sleep Phase Syndrome: Delays
With Chronotherapy Followed by
Stabilization With Morning Light

CASE EXAMPLE 3

Patient M.L. (see Fig. 105–2C) had chronic major depression and was referred for light therapy because of refractory response to drugs. She reported a long history of DSPS and daytime fatigue, often staying in bed all day. In addition, she reported occasionally sleeping at successively later hours until her delayed sleep phase was reestablished. She would not comply with most sleep scheduling requests, but when a free-run appeared to start spontaneously, she agreed to attempt to schedule successive delays of bedtime—in a loose application of chronotherapy—and aim to restabilize with midnight sleep onset and regular outdoor daylight exposure. Sleep was often fragmented during the week of chronotherapy, and several days after reaching the target phase, sleep became restless throughout the night. The appearance of initial insomnia at that time suggested that there would be further delays over the next days, overshooting the target phase. At this point, the patient began 30-min light sessions at 10,000 lux on awakening at 7:30 AM, with a second session in midafternoon. She became highly energized after the first day's exposure sessions and was unable to sleep at all the next night. Sleep onset continued to drift later, and she complained of sleep deprivation. On one occasion when she skipped afternoon light, sleep onset occurred hours earlier than expected. Morning light treatment was then rescheduled about 1 hour later, and despite a few episodes of middle-to-late insomnia, she was able to fall asleep by 2 AM or earlier and to awaken by 8 AM. When monitored several months later, the pattern had stabilized, with sleep onsets occurring around 12:30 to 1:00 AM accompanied by uninterrupted sleep for 8 h. Despite slightly improved daytime energy, however, her depression did not lift, and she remained dysfunctional.

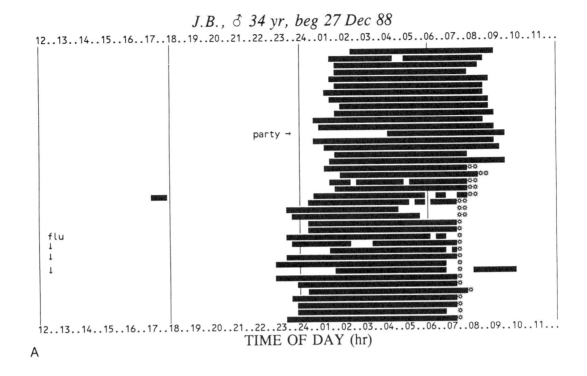

J.B., ♂ 34 yr, beg 27 Dec 88

12..13..14..15..16..17..18..19..20..21..22..23..24..01..02..03..04..05..06..07..08..09..10..11...

party →

flu
↓
↓
↓

12..13..14..15..16..17..18..19..20..21..22..23..24..01..02..03..04..05..06..07..08..09..10..11...

TIME OF DAY (hr)

A

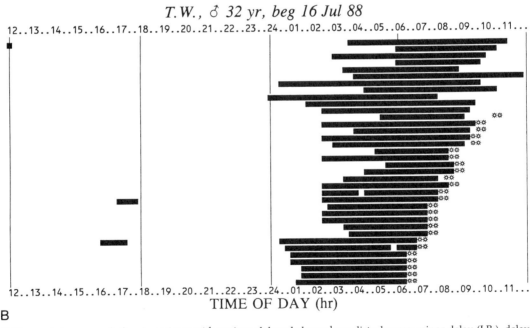

T.W., ♂ 32 yr, beg 16 Jul 88

12..13..14..15..16..17..18..19..20..21..22..23..24..01..02..03..04..05..06..07..08..09..10..11...

12..13..14..15..16..17..18..19..20..21..22..23..24..01..02..03..04..05..06..07..08..09..10..11...

TIME OF DAY (hr)

B

Figure 105–2. Self-report sleep records for six patients with various delayed sleep phase disturbances: minor delay (J.B.), delayed sleep phase syndrome (T.W., M.L., S.P., G.Z.), non–24-h sleep-wake syndrome (B.C.). Successive days are lined up, *top to bottom*, on the ordinate. Bars, intervals of sleep (including naps). Sun symbols, 15-min segments of bright light exposure. Ellipsis, gap in record. For patient M.L. O indicates "restless sleep." For patient S.P., B, benzodiazepine hypnotic; N, awakening due to noise. For patient B.C., the duration of light exposure is indicated as the recommended average of 2.5 h/day. In addition to morning light treatment, patients M.L., S.P., and G.Z. used variations of chronotherapy to establish the desired sleep phase by successive delays of their sleep schedules.

Illustration continued on following page

M.L., ♀ 25 yr, beg 24 May 87

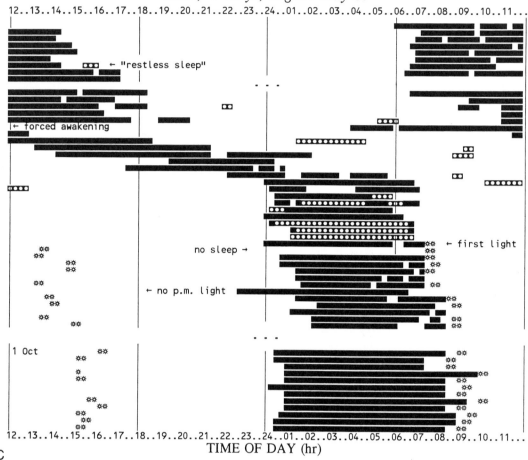

C

TIME OF DAY (hr)

S.P., ♂ 47 yr, beg 23 Nov 91

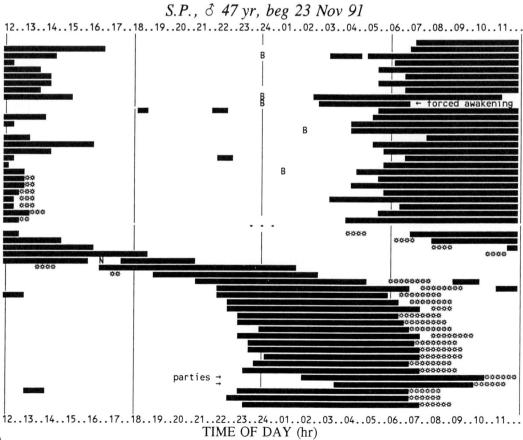

D

TIME OF DAY (hr)

Figure 105–2C and D *Continued*

G.Z., ♀ 22 yr, beg 2 Aug 88 (C.I. Eastman, pers. comm.)

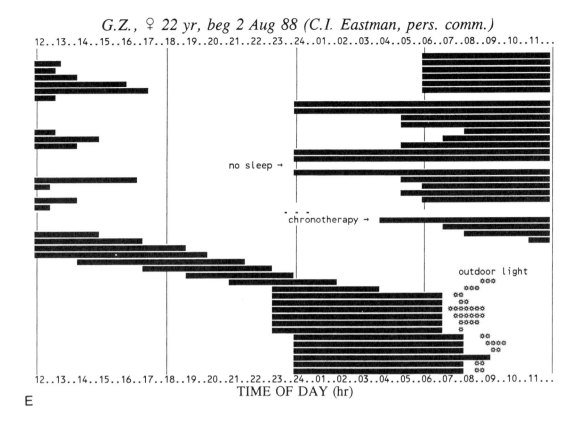

TIME OF DAY (hr)

E

B.C., ♂ 31 yr, adapted from Eastman et al. (1988)

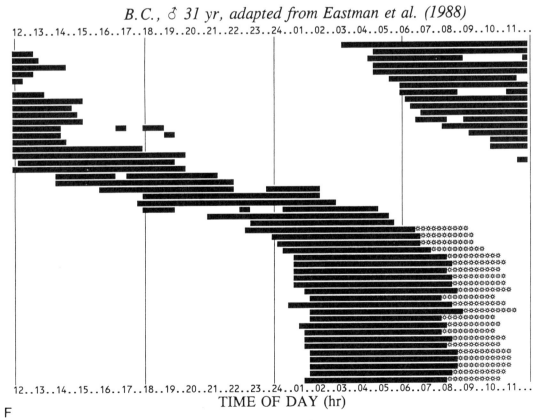

TIME OF DAY (hr)

F

Figure 105–2E and F *Continued*

CASE EXAMPLE 4

Patient S.P. (see Fig. 105–2D) showed a similar delayed sleep pattern, which was present since childhood. Although he was groggy on awakening, afternoon and evening energy levels were high, and he could work productively at those times. On nights when he used a benzodiazepine hypnotic, he could sometimes advance sleep onset by a few hours, which he considered trivial. An attempt was then made to phase advance the sleep episode with the use of 10,000-lux, 30- to 45-min light exposures on awakening. Despite intense effort over a 1-week trial, the patient could not be awakened before 12:30 PM, making successively earlier treatment sessions impossible. An alternative course of chronotherapy was then attempted. The patient was instructed to delay successive sleep episodes by 2 h, in conjunction with 1-h light treatment sessions ending 2 h before bedtime (a procedure intended to facilitate chronotherapy). However, he refused to enter bed until ready to fall asleep, resulting in successive daily delays that varied between 1 and 5 h. After 6 days, the presleep light was discontinued, with instruction to substitute light exposure for 2 h at 6 AM in an attempt to halt the delay drift. In the next weeks, the patient was able to maintain sleep onset between 11 PM and midnight and to awaken by 7:30 AM or earlier. The resilience of the adjustment was tested on the occasion of two late-night parties after which the desired sleep pattern was easily recaptured. Subsequently, however, the patient discontinued treatment and resumed his former schedule, citing family stresses that he preferred to escape by sleeping during the day.

CASE EXAMPLE 5

The case of patient G.Z. (see Fig. 105–2E) demonstrates that the benefit of morning light can sometimes be accomplished without artificial light therapy, through the exposure to natural outdoor light during times of the year when sunrise precedes the time of awakening. The patient had experienced DSPS since adolescence, missing morning classes in college; she had slept with covers over her head since childhood. At baseline, sleep onset was typically at 6:00 AM, occasionally earlier but followed by hypersomnia, and including some sleepless days immediately preceding or following a hypersomnic episode. After 9 days of delay chronotherapy, she was instructed to go outdoors every morning (see also Dagen et al.[43]), "the earlier the better," but without specification of the duration of light exposure. Walks outdoors began 2 days before the chronotherapy procedure reached the target wake-up time of 6:45 AM. Sleep stabilized between 11:00 PM and 6:45 AM. Finally, sleep onset was shifted to midnight to coincide with the patient's move to an adjacent time zone; with a commensurate delay in morning light exposure, she maintained the newly established circadian phase.

Non–24-h Sleep-Wake Syndrome: Halt of the Delay Drift With Postsleep Light. When sleep phase does not stabilize but continually shifts later relative to clock time, the pattern resembles the free-run seen in normal subjects under conditions of temporal isolation without day-night cues. However, in non–24-h sleep-wake syndrome, despite the presence of such cues, a failure of entrainment is evidenced by a "hypernychthemeral"[44] sleep pattern. Some patients with DSPS break into transient hypernychthemeral patterns (e.g., patient M.L. in Fig. 105–2C), which suggests that non–24-h sleep-wake syndrome and DSPS are associated disorders of varying severity.[45] As with DSPS, light treatment may be effective when applied at the end of the subjective night.

CASE EXAMPLE 6

Patient B.C. (see Fig. 105–2F) showed a sleep-wake cycle length averaging 25 h over approximately 13 years preceding treatment.[46] He was unemployed and socially withdrawn and refused to attempt to sleep when alert. Treatment began when sleep onset had drifted to midnight. The patient was exposed to light of 4000 to 8000 lux for 2 to 3 h on awakening. The free-run immediately decelerated, and the sleep interval was maintained at approximately 1:30 to 8:15 AM for several weeks. In the long run, however, the sleep pattern continued to drift at a period of about 24.08 h, a problem that might have been corrected with increased light dose.

Advanced Sleep Phase Syndrome. ASPS, in which sleep onset occurs in the evening with awakening well before dawn, would seem to provide a counterpart to DSPS, treatable with late evening light,[47] but such treatment has not been extensively investigated. Light presented in the first part of the subjective night is known to elicit phase delays in the onset of nocturnal melatonin secretion[48] and the decline of body temperature,[49] which might induce later sleep onset. Although ASPS is not strictly age related, it is more prevalent among the elderly, whose early rise times are a common cause of concern. Campbell et al.[50] compared the effects of evening bright light exposure (more than 4000 lux for 2 h) with a dim red light control in elderly subjects with histories of sleep maintenance insomnia. The bright light group showed improved sleep efficiency; after 12 days of treatment, nighttime wakefulness reduced by about 1 h. Despite this benefit, most subjects were reluctant to continue treatment given the long exposure sessions and glare discomfort. These drawbacks might be corrected with shorter exposures to higher intensity light with the use of an apparatus that minimizes short-wavelength radiation (see Apparatus).

CASE EXAMPLE 7

The experience of a 38-year-old woman with lifetime history of ASPS[47] illustrates the potential use—and limitations—of evening light treatment. Patient K.W. was a

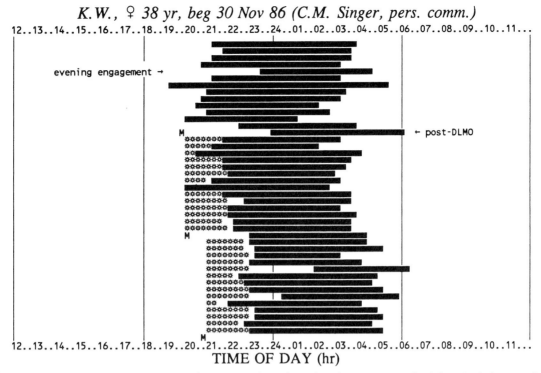

K.W., ♀ *38 yr, beg 30 Nov 86 (C.M. Singer, pers. comm.)*

Figure 105–3. Self-report sleep record for a patient with advanced sleep phase disorder. Bars, intervals of sleep (including naps). Sun symbols, 15-min segments of bright light exposure. M, the phase of dim light melatonin onset (DLMO), as determined on nights when treatment was omitted.

mildly hypomanic high achiever, without seasonal pattern, who typically fell asleep at about 9:00 PM, and woke up between 2 and 4 AM, a pattern that led to marital stress. She could remain awake for occasional late-evening engagements, compensating with delayed time of arising at 5 to 6 AM. At baseline, she showed an early melatonin onset, at about 7:45 PM (Fig. 105–3). Light exposure for up to 2 h beginning at 8 PM hardly affected sleep phase or melatonin onset, whereas light exposure beginning at 9 PM succeeded in maintaining sleep onset at about 11 PM and wake-up between 4 and 5 PM, which was accompanied by a 1-h delay in melatonin onset.

Seasonal Affective Disorder

Patients with SAD experience annually recurrent mood disturbance often accompanied by an increased appetite for carbohydrates, weight gain, daytime fatigue and loss, of concentration, anxiety, and increased sleep duration. The appetitive and sleep symptoms are considered atypical, in contrast with the poor appetite, weight loss, and late insomnia seen in melancholic depression. For a set of diagnostic and clinical assessment instruments, see Resources (below) and the discussion in Terman et al.[51]

Most light therapy studies have focused on parameters that influence treatment response, such as time of day, duration of exposure, intensity, and wavelength. The original regimen tested at the National Institute of Mental Health used 2500-lux fluorescent illumination in 3-h sessions in the morning and the evening.[21] A cross-center analysis of more than 25 studies that included 332 patients[52] summarized the results for dual daily sessions at 2500 lux for 2 h; single morning, midday, and evening sessions; brief sessions (30 min); and lower light intensity (less than 500 lux). One week of morning bright light treatment produced a significantly higher remission rate (53%) than did evening (38%) or midday (32%) treatment. Dual daily sessions provided no benefit over morning light alone. All three bright light regimens were more effective than the dim light control; only morning (or morning plus evening) light was superior to the brief light control. Two subsequent studies increased light intensity to 10,000 lux in 30- to 40-min exposure sessions, with remission rates of approximately 75%, matching the most successful 2500-lux, 2-h studies.[32, 53] At these short durations, both dim light (400 lux) and lower-level bright light (3000 lux) were significantly less effective.

Until recently, individual studies of light therapy with standard fluorescent light boxes were limited by small sample sizes and did not consistently demonstrate time-of-day effects. The lack of convincing placebo controls led to controversy about whether improvement reflected the specific action of light. These problems have been successfully addressed in a set of three large clinical trials[33–35] (for a summary, see Table 105–1). Eastman et al.[34] administered light in the morning or evening, and an inert placebo (inactive negative ion generator), to parallel groups. Although all groups showed progressive improvement over 4 weeks, patients administered morning light were most likely to

S.H., ♀ *37 yr, beg 4 Nov 88*

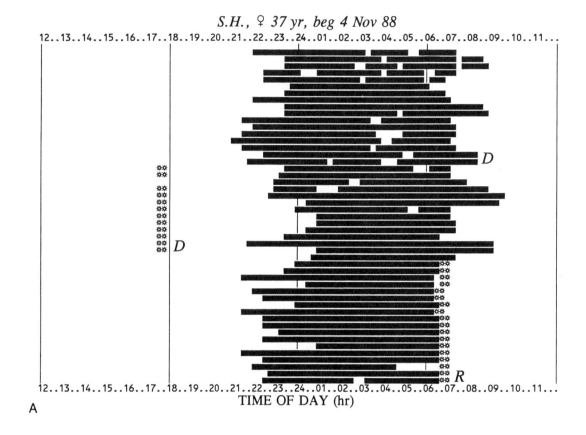

A

TIME OF DAY (hr)

A.R., ♀ *43 yr, beg 2 Feb 89*

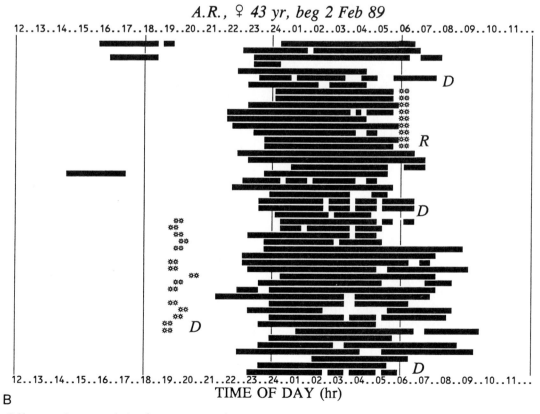

B

TIME OF DAY (hr)

Figure 105–4. Self-report sleep records for three patients with winter depression, during baseline, light treatment, and withdrawal periods. Bars, intervals of sleep (including naps). Sun symbols, 15-min segments of bright light exposure. Clinical state is noted at the end of each period. D, depressed; R, responded (for quantitative criteria, see Terman et al.[48]).

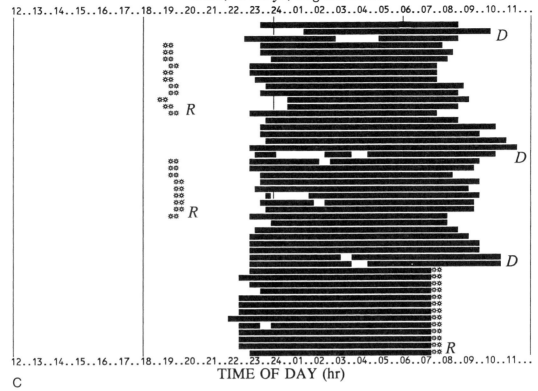

Figure 105–4C *Continued*

show remissions, exceeding the placebo rate. Lewy et al.[35] conducted a crossover study of morning and evening light. Although there was no placebo control, morning light proved to be more effective than evening light. Terman et al.[33] performed both crossover and balanced parallel-group comparisons, which included nonphotic control groups that received negative air ions at a low or high concentration. Morning light produced a higher remission rate than evening light and the putative placebo, low-density ions. However, the response to evening light also exceeded that for placebo. Indeed, in the trials of both Lewy et al.[35] and Terman et al.,[33] a minority of patients responded preferentially to evening light.

Figure 105–4 presents sleep and light exposure logs for 3 patients who received 10,000-lux light treatment in 30-min sessions. Treatment schedules were determined according to reported sleep habits and daytime commitments. The patients were urged to maintain consistent sleep times whether on or off treatment, waking up shortly before the time planned for morning treatment and keeping free a block of time for evening treatment at least 2 h before bedtime. However, the patients often showed variations in sleep pattern that depended on the time of treatment (morning or evening), treatment response, and washout periods.

CASE EXAMPLE 8

Patient S.H. (see Fig. 105–4A), although depressed at baseline, showed middle insomnia and overslept on week-ends. During the course of evening light treatment, sleep onset was gradually delayed, with reduced insomnia, but she remained depressed. In contrast, under morning light, sleep onset returned to the baseline pattern and sleep interruptions were largely eliminated, but sleep onset became earlier and duration became longer. Nevertheless, the depression remitted.

CASE EXAMPLE 9

Patient A.R. (see Fig. 105–4B), although depressed at baseline, showed fragmented sleep including napping, with highly variable total sleep duration. Under morning light, napping was eliminated, and although there was some late insomnia, the depression remitted. Under evening light—which failed clinically—sleep duration increased without a marked delay in sleep onset, and there were interruptions during the second half of sleep.

CASE EXAMPLE 10

Patient D.F. (see Fig. 105–4C) was monitored only briefly at baseline but reported consistent hypersomnia (subsequently also observed during washout phases) and agreed 2 to attempt a 10:30 PM–7:30 AM sleep schedule. Under evening light, tested twice, both sleep onset and time of arising were delayed relative to target, but sleep did not overshoot 9:30 AM. On both trials of evening light, the depression remitted. Over two washouts, sleep duration gradually increased, with relapse of depressive symptoms. Under morning light—which also was successful—the patient succeeded in advancing his wake-up time by several hours and was able to fall asleep, on target, at 10:30 PM, for a modestly reduced sleep duration of 9 h. Even though treatment was effective at both times of day, the patient preferred morning because of increased opportunity for activities given the earlier time of arising.

In summary, a lack of clinical response to evening light (patients S.H. and A.R.) appears to be correlated with delayed sleep onset, time of arising relative to baseline, or both. Morning light, which was uniformly effective, served to truncate morning sleep; in some cases, sleep onset also advanced, conserving sleep duration, whereas in others, duration decreased only modestly. Although baseline patterns of interrupted sleep often disappeared under effective treatment, initial, middle, or late insomnia sometimes emerged during treatment. These symptoms may be signs of light overdose that can be eliminated by reducing light intensity or duration (see Side Effects of Bright Light Exposure), or by scheduling evening sessions earlier or morning sessions later.

Subsyndromal SAD. The phenomenology of subsyndromal SAD, or winter doldrums, is similar to that of SAD, although major depression is absent. However, the presence and severity of atypical neurovegetative symptoms (including food cravings and difficulty awakening) can be similar to those in SAD, as can fatigability (leading to characterization as a seasonal anergic syndrome).[54] Clinical trials have demonstrated significant improvement with bright light therapy,[55] as well as dawn simulation therapy,[56] for subsyndromal SAD. For bright light, optimum light scheduling and dose appear to be similar for subsyndromal SAD and SAD; in other words, the lower severity of depressed mood does not necessarily imply that a lower light dose will be sufficient to relieve symptoms.

Further Investigational Applications of Light Therapy

Chronic Depression. Above and beyond its application for SAD, the use of light therapy for nonseasonal depression appears to be promising. Kripke[57] compared several controlled trials in terms of the relative benefit of light versus placebo treatment, which falls within the range of classic antidepressant drug studies. Indeed, within as little as 1 week of treatment, depression scale ratings were as much as 24% lower after bright light than after dim light placebo treatment,[58] a result that compares favorably with medication studies conducted over 4 to 16 weeks. Several studies have combined light with drugs and found accelerated improvement over the use of drugs alone (for a review, see Kasper et al.[59]). One study demonstrated such an im-

provement among hospitalized, medicated patients with unipolar and bipolar depressions who were given 10,000-lux illumination in 30-min morning treatments, with less improvement at 2500 lux.[60] Another study with impressive results combined light, drugs, and a single session of late-night sleep deprivation at the start of treatment, with marked improvement within 1 day and significant benefit over a dim light control within 1 week.[61] In Europe, newly admitted hospitalized depressed patients are increasingly given adjuvant light therapy, which appears to speed recovery.[62] Although large-scale controlled trials are still needed, the thrust of available data clearly supports the use of adjuvant light therapy in depressed outpatients and inpatients. In cases of bipolar depression, the risk of overresponse to light with the emergence of mania can be controlled by the use of mood stabilizers.[25]

Premenstrual Depression. Patients with both seasonal and nonseasonal premenstrual depression, or syndrome (PMS) have responded favorably to 1 week of bright light treatment (2500 lux for 2 h) during the luteal phase, in a series of clinical trials by Parry et al.[63] Although an early pilot study suggested the superiority of evening light, a placebo-controlled crossover study showed no difference between morning and evening exposures in 1-month trials.[64] Furthermore, bright and dim light had similar effects. In follow-up, however, several of the patients maintained remissions with bright light for 12 to 18 months, which augurs well for the long-term treatment of PMS. In a 2-month study, with evening light delivered for 2 weeks at 10,000 lux for 30 min during the luteal phase, Lam[65] found significant improvement relative to a dim light control, with alleviation of both depressed mood and physical symptoms of PMS. Although larger controlled trials are needed and the relative advantage of morning light awaits investigation, the method of Lam is a viable option for the open treatment of PMS, especially for women who have not responded to or have rejected medications.

Bulimia Nervosa. Lam et al.[66] became interested in this potential application of light therapy when a seasonal mood pattern was noted in many patients with bulimia; beyond the spectrum of SAD symptoms, this included binge eating and purging. A 1-week study with 2500-lux treatment for 2 h day reported improvement in mood but not in bulimic behavior, relative to a dim light control.[67] By contrast, a controlled 2-week crossover study, also with a dim light control, showed a marked superiority of morning bright light treatment (30 min at 10,000 lux) for both mood and bulimic symptoms.[66] Furthermore, a 4-week open-treatment study yielded average reductions of 50% in binge eating and 42% in purging, which augurs well for the use of light therapy, especially in cases of co-morbid SAD.[66]

Senile Dementia. Symptoms of night wandering, sundowning, and daytime sleep appear to be responsive to bright light therapy. While hospital trials in Japan,[68] using light boxes, indicated benefits of morning treatment over 1 month or longer, evening light exposure also has succeeded in reducing disruptive nighttime activity.[69] In another study, diffuse indirect bright light was installed for 2-week intervals in the hospital living quarters of demented patients.[70] Those without severe visual deficit showed significant reductions in day-to-day variability of the rest-activity rhythm (measured with actigraphy), whereas visually impaired patients showed no effect. For long-term management, whole-room illumination may be more feasible for such patients than the use of light boxes, which require a stationary posture and direction of gaze. There is a prospect for the use of light treatment at home to stabilize the activity–rest cycle of patients during the early stages of illness, which could substantially assist families by reducing night wandering and other disruptive behavior—major factors leading to institutionalization.

Chronic Fatigue Syndrome. Although symptoms of chronic fatigue syndrome (CFS) are evident throughout the year, about 40% of patients in a large New York sample reported a pattern of seasonal variation that suggested the presence of co-morbid SAD or subsyndromal SAD.[71] Moreover, within this large subgroup, winter exacerbation of atypical neurovegetative symptoms (such as carbohydrate craving and eating, and hypersomnia) was indistinguishable from that of patients with SAD. In two case studies of light therapy with patients who showed co-morbid CFS and SAD, there was marked improvement in depressive symptoms, and in one case, there was parallel improvement of arthralgia.[72] In other cases of medicated and unmedicated patients, there were improvements in daytime energy, alertness and ease of awakening, and reduced hypersomnia (but no effect on somatic symptoms of CFS), which enabled patients to resume studies, exercise, and, in one case, romance.[73] Some patients have continued with treatment in spring and summer to avoid slumping. Controlled trials of adjuvant light therapy for CFS are needed, but open treatment is an option to reduce reliance on hypnotics and antidepressants in a population already reliant on multiple medications with limited treatment success.[71]

Shift Work Adjustment. Most research has focused on simulation studies in which sleep patterns and circadian measures can be closely monitored, work assignments can be kept simple and constant, and the interferences of family obligations and distractions can be minimized.[74] Field applications have been few, although bright light exposure regimens have been developed to phase shift circadian rhythms into synchrony with shift work schedules, either as a preparatory measure[75] or during the shift itself.[76] The feasibility of these approaches for industrial shift workers has been questioned. The attempted reentrainment can be incompatible with standard rapid rotation schedules, which can further exacerbate worker distress. Furthermore, most shift workers choose to revert to a normal schedule on days off, jeopardizing their work week adjustment with inappropriate patterns of light exposure. Potentially adverse long-term consequences of repeated shifts have not been tested.[74] An alternative approach with potential benefit for alertness and performance would be to increase nighttime illumination in the work place without imposing large circadian phase shifts.[74, 77]

Jet Lag Adjustment. Although laboratory simulation paradigms for jet lag and shift work adjustment correspond closely, in the field, geographic relocation has the advantage of establishing a new, consistent light-dark cycle without competing day-night cues.[74] However, jet lag is also compounded by travel stresses (e.g., in-flight sleep disruption) above and beyond circadian phase displacement. Timing recommendations for natural and artificial bright light exposure (and light avoidance), which vary with direction and distance of travel, have been generated to accelerate circadian rhythm reentrainment based on properties of the phase response curve.[78, 79] Although there have been anecdotal successes with such strategies, field trials that assess outcome are still lacking.

OFFICIAL RECOMMENDATIONS AND GUIDELINES

Society for Light Treatment and Biological Rhythms. The Society for Light Treatment and Biological Rhythms (SLTBR) was the first organization to conduct a consensus building process for clinical applications of light therapy and safety issues, with recommendations published in 1991.[80] Clinical trials completed by that time had already demonstrated efficacy for SAD and probable efficacy for subsyndromal SAD. Furthermore, the report cited "ample evidence that light can advance, delay, and entrain human circadian rhythms"[80(p47)] based on timing of exposure according to human phase response curves, but specific circadian phase disorders were not enumerated. Recommendation was withheld for the use of light therapy for non-SAD depression and PMS, pending additional clinical trials. Basic safety standards for light therapy devices were outlined, including control of thermal and short wavelength radiation (ultraviolet and blue) through appropriate choice of lamp and filtering, and evaluation of patients' oculoretinal status.

U.S. Public Health Service Agency for Health Care Policy and Research. In 1990, the Depression Guidelines Panel of this agency commissioned a critical review of clinical trials of light therapy,[81] and in 1993, it issued guidelines for the treatment of SAD in primary care practice. The guidelines include the treatment subsyndromal SAD: "Light therapy is a treatment consideration only for well-documented mild to moderate seasonal, nonpsychotic, winter depressive episodes in patients with recurrent depressive or bipolar II disorders or milder seasonal episodes."[82(p102)] The panel cautioned against unsupervised treatment: "It should be administered by a professional with experience and training in its use who deems it suitable for the particular patient."[82(p103)] It was further noted that "logically, light therapy should not be used as an adjunct to medication until either one alone has been optimally used. Light therapy can be useful to augment the response (if partial) to antidepressant medication and vice versa."[82(p103)]

American Psychiatric Association. In its 1993 clinical practice guidelines for major depressive disorder,[83] the American Psychiatric Association (APA) noted that "in some patients with [SAD], depressive manifestations respond to supplementation of environmental light by means of exposure to bright white artificial light. . . ." Possible side effects were listed, and it was noted that "no adverse interactions between light therapy and pharmacotherapy have been identified" (but see Safety of Bright Light for the Eyes). An update of APA guidelines is pending.

American Academy of Sleep Medicine. In 1993, the American Academy of Sleep Medicine (AASM, then the American Sleep Disorders Association) and SLTBR jointly commissioned the Task Force on Light Treatment for Sleep Disorders. The task force published an extensive literature review and critique of the field in the *Journal of Biological Rhythms*[1] preparatory to review by the AASM Standards of Practice Committee (SPC). The SPC conducted an evidence-based review of clinical trials of light therapy for the circadian sleep phase disorders, shift work and jet lag disturbances, dementia, and sleep complaints in the healthy elderly. (Guidelines for treatment of depression were deferred to the APA.) In 1999, the SPC issued syndrome-specific guidelines, concluding that "light therapy can be useful in treatment of DSPS and ASPS."[84(p641)] and expressing less confidence in the other applications. The American Medical Association is considering adoption of the guidelines under its Recognition Program. The guidelines will also be considered by the National Guidelines Clearinghouse, a professional/government/industry collaboration that includes the American Association of Health Plans.

Canadian Consensus Guidelines for the Understanding and Management of Seasonal Depression. A thorough multicenter critical review has been published by Canadian specialists in SAD, including evidence tables, of SAD diagnosis, epidemiology, pathophysiology, light treatment, medication management, and combination treatment.[85] Level 1 evidence from large, controlled trials was presented to justify recommending that (1) the starting dose for light therapy with a fluorescent light box is 10,000 lux for 30 min/day, (2) light boxes should use white, fluorescent light with the UV wavelengths filtered out, and (3) light therapy should be started in the early morning, on awakening, to maximize treatment response.

U.S. Food and Drug Administration. Despite the emerging professional consensus, the U.S. Food and Drug Administration (FDA) has not yet approved (or disapproved) light therapy for SAD or for other conditions, in part because the commercial community has yet to file application for premarket approval. However, the agency continues intermittently to require that individual manufacturers of light therapy apparatuses cease sales and modify advertising copy that contains explicit or implicit medical claims. The lack of FDA approval has discouraged third-party reimbursement, which, in turn, has limited the number of prospective patients and served to encourage self-treatment by consumers who obtain apparatuses on the open market.

(In 1997, the Swiss Federal Department of the Interior mandated insurance reimbursement for light boxes used to treat SAD, although not for other therapeutic applications.[86]) Because regulatory standards have not been issued in the United States, there has been a proliferation of untested commercial products on the market. Some of these products explicitly violate consensus recommendations of the SLTBR, such as lack of lamp protection and UV shielding. There have been several unofficial attempts to promulgate safety standards and advise consumers and physicians (Consumer Reports on Health,[87] SLTBR,[80] and the Center for Environmental Therapeutics; see Resources), but these have had far less impact than marketing initiatives, some of which even have appeared under the guise of "medical education." The development of federal standards remains a priority.

RESOURCES

Light boxes with Acrylite OP-3–based filters are distributed in the United States by SphereOne, Inc. (PO Box 1013, Silver Plume, CO 80476; www.sphere-one.com) and in Canada by DayLight Technologies, Inc. (PO Box 102, CRO, Halifax, Nova Scotia, Canada B3J 2L4; www.up-lift.com/daylights). The Columbia Eye Examination for Users of Light Treatment (a structured chart for optometrists and ophthalmologists) and a set of questionnaires and structured interview guides for SAD, written and tested by the Columbia group, is included in the Clinical Assessment Tools Packet distributed by the Center for Environmental Therapeutics (PO Box 532, Georgetown, CO 80444; www.cet.org/cet2000). The Society for Light Treatment and Biological Rhythms (Department of Psychiatry, Yale University, 842 Howard Avenue, New Haven, CT 06519; www.sltbr.org) publishes a quarterly bulletin of research news and commentary and offers a continuing medical education course associated with its annual meeting.

Acknowledgments

Preparation of this chapter and related research was supported in part by National Institute of Mental Health Grant MH42931. We thank Jamie Rifkin for editorial assistance.

References

1. Terman M, ed. Task force report on light treatment for sleep disorders. J Biol Rhythms. 1995;10:101–176.
2. Joffe RT, Moul DE, Lam RW, et al. Light visor treatment for seasonal affective disorder: a multicenter study. Psychiatry Res. 1993;46:29–39.
3. Rosenthal NE, Moul DE, Hellekson CJ, et al. A multicenter study of the light visor for seasonal affective disorder: no difference in efficacy found between two different intensities. Neuropsychopharmacology. 1993;8:151–160.
4. Teicher MH, Glod CA, Oren DA, et al. The phototherapy light visor: more to it than meets the eye. Am J Psychiatry. 1995;152:1197–1202.
5. Terman M. Clinical efficacy of the light visor, and its broader implications. Light Treatment Biol Rhythms. 1991;3:37–40.

6. Terman M, Schlager D, Fairhurst S, et al. Dawn and dusk simulation as a therapeutic intervention. Biol Psychiatry. l989;25:966–970.

7. Terman M, Schlager DS. Twilight therapeutics, winter depression, melatonin, and sleep: In: Montplaisir J, Godbout R, eds. Sleep and Biological Rhythms. New York, NY: Oxford University Press; 1990:113–128.

8. Terman M. Light on sleep. In: Schwartz WJ, ed. Sleep Science: Integrating Basic Research and Clinical Practice. Basel, Switzerland: Karger; 1997:229–249.

9. Avery DH, Bolte MA, Wolfson JK, et al. Dawn simulation compared with a dim red signal in the treatment of winter depression Biol Psychiatry. 1994;36:181–188.

10. Gallin PF, Terman M, Remé CE, et al. Ophthalmologic examination of patients with seasonal affective disorder, before and after bright light therapy. Am J Ophthalmol. 1995;119:202–210.

11. Okudaira N, Kripke DF, Webster JB. Naturalistic studies of human light exposure. Am J Physiol. 1983;245:R613–R615.

12. Terman M. Research problems and prospects for the use of light as a therapeutic intervention. In: Wetterberg L, ed. Biological Rhythms and Light in Man. Oxford, England: Pergamon Press; 1993:42–1436.

13. Remé CE, Williams TP, Rol P, et al. Blue-light damage revisited: abundant retinal apoptosis after blue-light exposure, little after green. Invest Ophthalm Vis Sci. 1998;39:S128.

14. Bynoe LA, Del Priore LV, Hornbeck R. Photosensitization of retinal pigment epithelium by protoporphyrin IX. Graefe's Arch Clin Exp Ophthalm. 1998;236:230–233.

15. Remé CE, Rol P, Grothmann K, et al. Bright light therapy in focus: lamp emission spectra and ocular safety. Technol Health Care. 1996;4:403–413.

16. Terman M, Remé CE, Rafferty B, et al. Bright light therapy for winter depression: potential ocular effects and theoretical implications. Photochem Photobiol. 1990;51:781–792.

17. Meesters Y, Beersma DGM, Bouhuys AL, et al. Prophylactic treatment of seasonal affective disorder (SAD) by using light visors: bright white or infrared light? Biol Psychiatry. 1999; 46:239–246.

18. Gallenga P, Lobefalo L, Mastropasqua L, et al. Photic maculopathy in a patient receiving bright light therapy. Am J Psychiatry. 1997;154:1319.

19. Zigman S. Vision enhancement using a short wavelength light-absorbing filter. Optom Vis Sci. 1990;67:100–104.

20. Gallin PF, Terman M, Remé CE, et al. The Columbia Eye Examination for Users of Light Treatment. New York, NY: New York State Psychiatric Institute; 1993.

21. Rosenthal NE, Sack DA, Gillin JC, et al. Seasonal affective disorder: a description of the syndrome and preliminary findings with light therapy. Arch Gen Psychiatry. 1984;41:72–80.

22. Wirz-Justice A, Bucheli C, Graw P. Light treatment of seasonal affective disorder in Switzerland. Acta Psychiatr Scand. 1986; 74:193–204.

23. Levitt AJ, Joffe RT, Moul DE, et al. Side effects of light therapy in seasonal affective disorder. Am J Psychiatry. 1993;150:650–652.

24. Schwitzer J, Neudorfer C, Blecha H-G, et al. Mania as a side effect of phototherapy. Biol Psychiatry. 1990;28:532–534.

25. Kripke DF. Timing of phototherapy and occurrence of mania. Biol Psychiatry. 1991;29:1156–1157.

26. Meesters Y, Van Houwelingen C. Rapid mood swings after unmonitored light exposure. Am J Psychiatry. 1998;155:306.

27. Chan PK, Lam RW, Perry KF. Mania precipitated by light therapy for patients with SAD. J Clin Psychiatry. l994;55:454.

28. Praschak-Rider N, Neumeister A, Hesselmann B, et al. Suicidal tendencies as a complication of light therapy for seasonal affective disorder: a report of three cases. J Clin Psychiatry. 1997;58:389–392.

29. Labbate LA, Lafer B, Thibault A, et al. Side effects induced by bright light treatment for seasonal affective disorder. J Clin Psychiatry. 1994;55:189–191.

30. National Institute of Mental Health. Systematic Assessment for Treatment Emergent Effects (SAFTEE). Rockville, Md: National Institute of Mental Health; 1986.

31. Terman M, Terman JS. Bright light therapy: side effects and benefits across the symptom spectrum. J Clin Psychiatry. In press.

32. Terman JS, Terman M, Schlager DS, et al. Efficacy of brief, intense light exposure for treatment of winter depression. Psychopharmacol Bull. 1990;26:3–11.

33. Terman M, Terman JS, Ross DC. A controlled trial of timed bright light and negative air ionization for treatment of winter depression. Arch Gen Psychiatry. 1998;55:875–882.

34. Eastman CI, Young MA, Fogg LF, et al. Bright light treatment for winter depression: a placebo-controlled trial. Arch Gen Psychiatry. 1998;55:883–889.

35. Lewy AJ, Bauer VK, Cutler NL, et al. Morning vs evening light treatment of patients with winter depression. Arch Gen Psychiatry. 1998;55:890–896.

36. Lewy AJ, Sack RL, Miller S, et al. Antidepressant and circadian phase-shifting effects of light. Science. 1987;235:352–354.

37. Terman M. On the specific action and clinical domain of light treatment. In: Lam RW, ed. Seasonal Affective Disorder and Beyond: Light Treatment for SAD and Non-SAD Conditions. Washington, DC: American Psychiatric Press; 1998:91–115.

38. Weber JM, Schwander JC, Unger I, et al. A direct ultrasensitive RIA for the determination of melatonin in human saliva: comparison with serum levels. Sleep Res. 1997;26:757.

39. Terman M, Lewy AJ, Dijk D-J, et al. Light treatment for sleep disorders: consensus report, IV: sleep phase and duration disturbances. J Biol Rhythms. 1995;10:135–147.

40. Czeisler CA, Richardson GS, Coleman RM, et al. Chronotherapy: resetting the circadian clocks of patients with delayed sleep phase insomnia. Sleep. 1981;4:1–21.

41. Rosenthal NE, Joseph-Vanderpool JR, Levendosky AA, et al. Phase-shifting effects of bright morning light as treatment for delayed sleep phase syndrome. Sleep. 1990;13:354–161.

42. Eastman CI, Stewart KT, Mahoney MP, et al. Dark goggles and bright light improve circadian rhythm adaptation to night-shift work. Sleep. 1994;17:535–543.

43. Dagen Y, Tzischinsky O, Lavie P. Sunlight treatment for delay sleep-phase syndrome: case report. Sleep Res. 1991;20:451.

44. Kokkoris CP, Weitzman ED, Pollak CP, et al. Long-term ambulatory temperature monitoring in a subject with a hypernychthemeral sleep-wake disturbance. Sleep. 1978;1:177–190.

45. Weitzman ED, Czeisler CA, Coleman RM, et al. Delayed sleep phase syndrome: a chronobiological disorder with sleep-onset insomnia. Arch Gen Psychiatry. 1981;38:737–746.

46. Eastman CI, Anagnopoulos CA, Cartwright RD. Can bright light entrain a free-runner? Sleep Res. 1988;17:372.

47. Singer CM, Lewy AJ. Case report: use of the dim light melatonin onset in the treatment of ASPS with bright light. Sleep Res. 1989;18:445.

48. Terman M, Terman JS, Rafferty B. Experimental design and measures of success in the treatment of winter depression by bright light. Psychopharmacol Bull. 1990;26:505–510.

49. Czeisler CA, Allan JS, Strogatz SH, et al. Bright light resets the human circadian pacemaker independent of the sleep-wake cycle. Science. 1986;233:667–671.

50. Campbell SS, Dawson D, Anderson M. Alleviation of sleep maintenance insomnia with timed exposure to bright light. J Am Geriatr Soc. 1993;41:829–836.

51. Terman M, Terman JS, Williams JBW. Seasonal affective disorder and treatments. J Prac Psychiatry Behav Health. 1998;5:287–303.

52. Terman M, Terman JS, Quitkin FM, et al. Bright light therapy for winter depression: a review of efficacy. Neuropsychopharmacology. 1989;2:1–22.

53. Magnússon A, Kristbjarnarson H. Treatment of seasonal affective disorder with high-intensity light. J Affect Disord. 1991;21:141–147.

54. Wirz-Justice A, Graw P, Bucheli C, et al. Seasonal affective disorder in Switzerland: a clinical perspective. In: Thompson C, Silverstone T, eds. Seasonal Affective Disorder. London, England: CNS Clinical Neuroscience; 1989:69–76.

55. Kasper S, Rogers S, Yancey A, et al. Phototherapy in individuals with and without seasonal affective disorder. Arch Gen Psychiatry. 1989;46:837–844.

56. Avery DH, Norden MJ. Dawn simulation and bright light therapy in subsyndromal seasonal affective disorder. In: Lam RW, ed. Seasonal Affective Disorder and Beyond: Light Treatment for SAD and Non-SAD Conditions. Washington, DC: American Psychiatric Press; 1998:143–157.

57. Kripke DF. Light treatment for nonseasonal depression: speed,

efficacy, and combined treatment. J Affect Disord. 1998;49:109–117.

58. Yamada N, Martin-Iverson MT, et al. Clinical and chronobiological effects of light therapy on nonseasonal affective disorders. Biol Psychiatry. 1995;37:866–873.

59. Kasper S, Ruhrmann S, Schuchardt H-M. The effects of light therapy in treatment indications other than seasonal affective disorder (SAD). In: Jung EG, Holick MF, eds. Biologic Effects of Light. Berlin/New York, NY: de Gruyter; 1994:206–218.

60. Beauchemin KM, Hays P. Phototherapy is a useful adjunct in the treatment of depressed in patients. Acta Psychiatr Scand. 1997;95:424–427.

61. Neumeister A, Goessler R, Lucht M, et al. Bright light therapy stabilizes the antidepressant effect of partial sleep deprivation. Biol Psychiatry. 1996;39:16–21.

62. Wirz-Justice A, Graw P, Roosli H, et al. An open trial of light therapy in hospitalized major depression. J Affect Disord. 1999;52:291–292.

63. Parry BL. Light therapy of premenstrual depression. In: Lam RW, ed. Seasonal Affective Disorder and Beyond: Light Treatment for SAD and Non-SAD Conditions. Washington, DC: American Psychiatric Press; 1998:173–191.

64. Parry BL, Mahan AM, Mostofi N, et al. Light therapy of late luteal phase dysphoric disorder: an extended study. Am J Psychiatry. 1993;150:1417–1419.

65. Lam RW. Seasonal affective disorder and beyond: a commentary. In: Lam RW, ed. Seasonal Affective Disorder and Beyond: Light Treatment for SAD and Non-SAD Conditions. Washington, DC: American Psychiatric Press; 1998:305–322.

66. Lam RW, Goldner EM. Seasonality of bumilia nervosa and treatment with light therapy. In: Lam RW, ed. Seasonal Affective Disorder and Beyond: Light Treatment for SAD and Non-SAD Conditions. Washington, DC: American Psychiatric Press; 1998:193–220.

67. Blouin AG, Blouin J, Aubin P, et al. Seasonal patterns of bulimia nervosa. Am J Psychiatry. 1992;149:73–81.

68. Mishima K, Okawa M, Hishikawa Y, et al. Morning bright light therapy for sleep and behavior disorders in elderly patients with dementia. Acta Psychiatrica Scand. 1994;89:1–7.

69. Satlin A, Volicer L, Ross V, et al. Bright light treatment of behavioral and sleep disturbances in patients with Alzheimer's disease. Am J Psychiatry. 1992;149:1028–1032.

70. Van Someren EJW, Kessler A, Mirmiran M, et al. Indirect bright light improves circadian rest-activity rhythm disturbances in demented patients. Biol Psychiatry. 1997;41:955–963.

71. Terman M, Levine SM, Terman JS, et al. Chronic fatigue syndrome and seasonal affective disorder: comorbidity, diagnostic overlap, and implications for treatment. Am J Med. 1998;105:1115S–1124S.

72. Lam RW. Seasonal affective disorder presenting as chronic fatigue syndrome. Can J Psychiatry. 1991;36:680–692.

73. Terman M. Light therapy. In: Micozzi M, ed. Fundamentals of Complementary and Alternative Medicine. London/New York, NY: Churchill Livingstone; 1996:49–59.

74. Boulos Z. Bright light treatment for jet lag and shift work. In: Lam RW, ed. Seasonal Affective Disorder and Beyond: Light Treatment for SAD and Non-SAD Conditions. Washington, DC: American Psychiatric Press; 1998:253–287.

75. Czeisler CA, Hiasera AJ, Duffy JF. Research on sleep, circadian rhythms and aging: applications to manned spaceflight. Exp Gerontol. 1991;26:217–232.

76. Czeisler CA, Johnson MP, Duffy JF, et al. Exposure to bright light and darkness to treat physiological maladaptation to night work. N Engl J Med. 1990;322:1253–1259.

77. Campbell SS, Dijk D-J, Boulos Z, et al. Light treatment for sleep disorders: consensus report, III: alerting and activating effects. J Biol Rhythms. 1995;10:129–132.

78. Oren DA, Reich W, Rosenthal NE, et al. How to Beat Jet Lag: A Practical Guide for Air Travellers. New York, NY: Henry Holt; 1993.

79. Houpt, TA, Boulos Z, Moore-Ede MC. Midnight Sun: software for determining light exposure and phase-shifting schedules during global travel. Physiol Behav. 1996;59:561–568.

80. Society for Light Treatment and Biological Rhythms. Consensus statements on the safety and effectiveness of light therapy of depression and disorders of biological rhythms. Light Treatment Biol Rhythms. 1991;3:45–50.

81. Terman M, Terman JS. Light Therapy for Winter Depression: Report to the Depression Guidelines Panel, USPHS Agency for Health Care Policy and Research. New York, NY: New York State Psychiatric Institute; 1991.

82. Agency for Health Care Policy and Research. Depression in Primary Care: Treatment of Major Depression. Clinical Practice Guideline No. 5. Rockville, Md: US Department of Health and Human Services; 1993.

83. American Psychiatric Association. Practice guideline for major depressive disorder in adults. Am J Psychiatry. 1993;150(suppl):1–26.

84. Chesson AL, Littner M, Davila D, et al. Practice parameters for the use of light therapy in the treatment of sleep disorders. Sleep. 1999;22:641–660.

85. Lam RW, Levitt AJ, eds. Canadian Consensus Guidelines for the Treatment of Seasonal Affective Disorder. Vancouver, BC, Canada: Clinical and Academic Publishing; 1999.

86. Wirz-Justice A. Light therapy for SAD is now reimbursed by medical insurance in Switzerland. Light Treatment Biol Rhythms. 1996;8:45.

87. Consumer Reports on Health. The winter of your discontent? 1993;February: 15–16.

106

Neurological Monitoring Techniques

Beth A. Malow
Michael S. Aldrich

Nocturnal spells often present diagnostic problems in sleep medicine because the history alone may not provide sufficient information to differentiate among the various diagnostic possibilities. Standard polysomnography (PSG) is helpful in defining the state and stage of sleep from which such nocturnal spells emerge, but it has limitations in diagnosis because behavioral analysis often is not included and the number of channels devoted to electroencephalography (EEG) is limited. These shortcomings are especially pertinent to the evaluation of suspected nocturnal epileptic seizures, which are defined by behavioral and motor manifestations in addition to EEG criteria.[1] Both behavioral and EEG analyses are critical for the characterization of epileptic seizures and for distinguishing them from parasomnias.

The behavioral and EEG manifestations of nocturnal spells caused by parasomnias, neurological disorders, and psychiatric disorders can be characterized more precisely by combining standard PSG with video recordings and extensive (12 or more channels) EEG montages.[2] This chapter emphasizes the methodology and indications for video-EEG PSG (VPSG) in the diagnosis of nocturnal events. In addition, the methodology and roles of routine EEG, short-term continuous video-EEG monitoring (STM), long-term continuous video-EEG monitoring (LTM), and ambulatory monitoring are addressed.

METHODOLOGY

Technical Aspects of Electroencephalography

The EEG measures the difference in electrical potential between pairs of electrodes placed on the scalp. These signals, reflecting synchronous postsynaptic potentials in large groups of neurons, are amplified and filtered to produce an analog or digital recording.[3] The International 10-20 system of EEG electrode placement is customarily used, in which the 10-20 refers to 10 and 20% of the distances between standard cranial landmarks (Fig. 106–1).[4] Each electrode site is identified with a letter, representing the underlying region of the

brain, and with a number, indicating a specific position above that region, with odd numbers indicating the left hemisphere and even numbers indicating the right hemisphere (e.g., T3 represents a left midtemporal electrode). Each recording channel is derived from the signals from a pair of electrodes, and severe pairs of electrodes, or derivations, are combined to form a montage. Montages may be either referential, in which one of the electrodes in each pair is connected to a common electrode (e.g., channel 1: Fp1-A1; channel 2: F7-A1; channel 3: T3-A1; channel 4: T5-A1; channel 5: O1-A1), or bipolar, in which there is no common electrode. Bipolar montages are usually arranged in a chain with the same electrode in adjacent derivations (e.g., channel

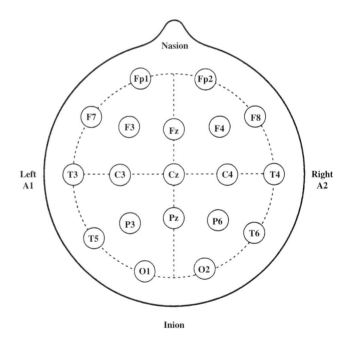

Standard international 10-20 electrode placement (superior view)

Figure 106–1. Standard International 10-20 Electrode Placement. Electrodes are placed at 10% or 20% of the distances between standard cranial landmarks. (From Keenan SA. Polysomnographic technique: an overview. In: Chokroverty S, ed. Sleep Disorders Medicine. Boston, Mass: Butterworth-Heinemann; 1994:84.)

Table 106–1. SAMPLE ATTENDED ELECTROENCEPHALOGRAPHIC MONTAGES

Number of Available Channels	Montage
8	F7-T3, T3-T5, T5-O1, F8-T4, T4-T6, T6-O2, F3-C3, F4-C4
10	Fp1-F7, F7-T3, T3-T5, T5-O1, Fp2-F8, F8-T4, T4-T6, T6-O2, F3-C3, F4-C4
12	Fp1-F7, F7-T3, T3-T5, T5-O1, Fp2-F8, F8-T4, T4-T6, T6-O2, F3-C3, C3-P3, F4-C4, C4-P4
14	Fp1-F7, F7-T3, T3-T5, T5-O1, Fp2-F8, F8-T4, T4-T6, T6-O2, F3-C3, C3-P3, P3-O1, F4-C4, C4-P4, P4-O2
16	Fp1-F7, F7-T3, T3-T5, T5-O1, Fp2-F8, F8-T4, T4-T6, T6-O2, Fp1-F3, F3-C3, C3-P3, P3-O1, Fp2-F4, F4-C4, C4-P4, P4-O2
18	Fp1-F7, F7-T3, T3-T5, T5-O1, Fp2-F8, F8-T4, T4-T6, T6-O2, Fp1-F3, F3-C3, C3-P3, P3-O1, Fp2-F4, F4-C4, C4-P4, P4-O2, Fz-Cz, Cz-Pz
24	Fp1-F7, F7-T3, T3-T5, T5-O1, Fp2-F8, F8-T4, T4-T6, T6-O2, Fp1-F3, F3-C3, C3-P3, P3-O1, Fp2-F4, F4-C4, C4-P4, P4-O2, Fz-Cz, Cz-Pz, T1-T3, T3-C3, C3-Cz, Cz-C4, C4-T4, T4-T2

1: Fp1-F7; channel 2: F7-T3; channel 3: T3-T5; channel 4: T5-01). The EEG montages used in a combined EEG-PSG study depend on the clinical indication and the number of channels available for recording (Table 106–1). Physicians and technologists involved in the use of EEG monitoring techniques require a solid knowledge of the principles of EEG recording and interpretation. Additional information regarding EEG methodology is available in a standard EEG text.[5]

Computerized digital EEG-PSG systems are an alternative to conventional analog EEG-PSG.[6] These systems facilitate the review of large amounts of EEG-PSG data by displaying scoring and event information in a format that allows the user to, for example, click on the stage or event of interest and bring up the corresponding EEG-PSG. The recording may be viewed at a variety of display settings that correspond to different paper speeds of conventional recordings. Filters, sensitivities, and montages may be adjusted to characterize events of interest and to help distinguish abnormalities from artifacts or normal variants. For example, certain montages may more easily identify and distinguish artifacts from *interictal epileptiform discharges* (IEDs), defined as epileptic activity occurring between seizures. Digital EEG enhances the detection and review of IEDs by allowing for remontaging, changing the display settings that influence temporal resolution, and isolating specific channels for review (Fig. 106–2A and B). For example, by altering the display settings, synchronous delta or theta activity characteristic of nonrapid eye movement (NREM) arousal disorders may be more easily distinguished from spike-wave activity or an evolving ictal (seizure) pattern characteristic of an epileptic seizure disorder.

Daytime Electroencephalography

Daytime EEG is used to look for IEDs, which support the diagnosis of a seizure disorder in many clinical

settings.[5] In addition to the electrodes listed above, central (Fz, Cz, Pz) and ear (A1, A2) electrodes are included. Nasopharyngeal electrodes, although used in the past, are not recommended because they are uncomfortable and prone to artifact and rarely provide additional information.[7] The activating techniques of hyperventilation and intermittent photic stimulation are routinely performed and may bring out focal asymmetries or epileptiform activity.

Although seizures are not uniformly recorded during a routine EEG, focal IEDs or generalized spike-and-wave discharges may be observed and may assist in the classification of an epileptic syndrome as partial or generalized. The location of IEDs, which can be determined with the use of an extended EEG montage, may clarify the nature of the epilepsy syndrome and its prognosis. For example, benign epilepsy of childhood with centrotemporal spikes has an excellent prognosis (Fig. 106–3). In contrast, some patients with temporal lobe IEDs may be refractory to medical treatment and become candidates for epilepsy surgery.

Daytime studies performed while the patient is asleep for at least a portion of the recording increase the yield of finding abnormalities, because in many patients, IEDs are more common in drowsiness and NREM sleep. Stage 2 NREM sleep is usually, but not always, recorded on the routine EEG, whereas NREM stage 3 and 4 sleep and REM sleep are rarely recorded. When the routine EEG does not show IEDs and the physician has a high suspicion for seizures, a sleep-deprived EEG improves the yield of finding epileptiform activity, at least in part because sleep is more likely to be recorded. Analog EEG recordings use a variety of montages to display ongoing brain activity, whereas digital EEG recordings permit the viewing of a segment of EEG in a variety of montages and speeds, which can help distinguish an IED from an artifact.

Video-Electroencephalography Polysomnography

When the history does not allow the physician to diagnose nocturnal spells associated with complex movements and behaviors, recording of the sleep-related event in question may allow definitive diagnosis. VPSG, which combines video recording with an extended EEG montage and with other standard PSG physiological monitoring, is useful in characterization of unusual behaviors and movements during sleep. Diagnostic considerations for patients with complex behaviors at night may include epileptic seizures, NREM arousal disorders, REM sleep behavior disorder (RBD), rhythmic movement disorder, or psychiatric disorders such as panic disorder or dissociative disorder. Episodes associated with these disorders have specific clinical features as discussed in Chapters 62 through 64 and 95. Events recorded with VPSG are reviewed to characterize the motor and behavioral manifestations of the event and the EEG-PSG features, including the stage of sleep preceding the event, the

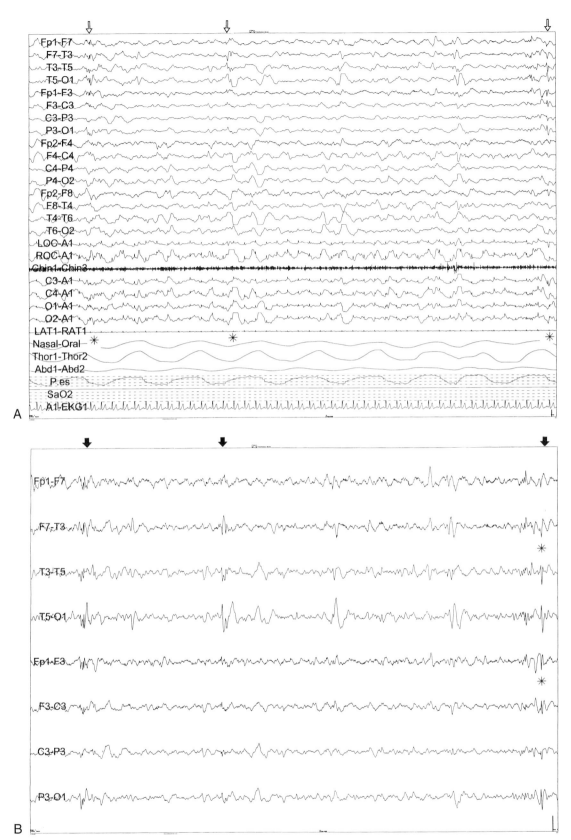

Figure 106–2. Use of different montages to enhance the review of IEDs. *A*, Left temporally dominant IEDs *(arrows)* on an extended EEG montage that are not apparent in the central to ear channels *(asterisk)*. *B*, Digital EEG allows the interpreter to select the relevant left temporal and parasagittal channels for review. The arrows highlight IEDs with phase reversals *(asterisks)* at T3 and F3, indicating maximal negativity at these electrodes, which defines the approximate location of the epileptic region. Both are 30-sec epochs; calibration symbol at bottom right, 100 μV.

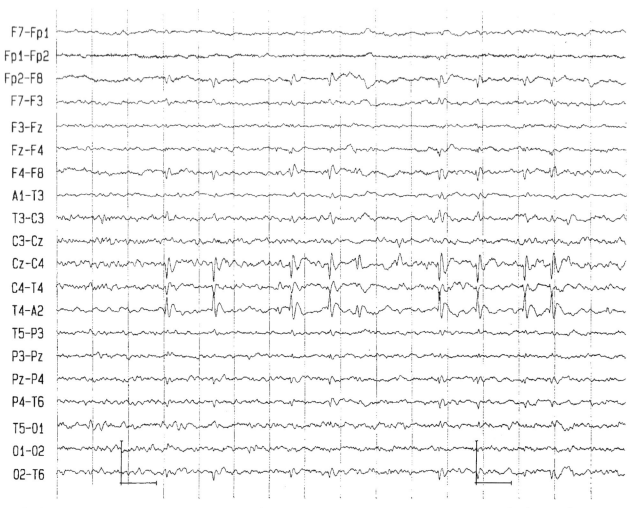

Figure 106–3. Runs of interictal epileptiform discharges with a centrotemporal dominance in benign epilepsy of childhood with centrotemporal spikes. The bipolar montage readily demonstrates peak negativity at the C4 and T4 electrodes. Such localization is not possible with EEG montages commonly used with standard PSG. Calibration symbol, 500 μV, 1 sec. (From Malow BA. Sleep and epilepsy. In: Aldrich MS, ed. Neurologic Clinics, Sleep Disorders II. Philadelphia, Pa: WB Saunders; 1996:774.)

time of the event relative to sleep onset, and EEG patterns occurring during the event or between events.

Video recordings may be played back in real time or at slower speeds to define the event of interest. A slow tape (extended play) speed allows for continuous monitoring for 6 to 8 h without changing tapes. Infrared cameras are useful for recording nighttime events. Movable cameras can be mounted in a patient's room and display closeups or full-body views. Double cameras are useful to focus on the face while simultaneous monitoring of the body. During recorded events, the technologist should interact with the patient to test for level of consciousness and ability to perform commands.

The EEG-PSG signal can be recorded as a multiplexed analog signal directly onto a videotape and stored with the video signal, or it can be recorded digitally onto magnetic or optical media with a synchronizing signal to time-lock the behaviors to the PSG signals. For review, the video signal can be combined with EEG-PSG on a single "split" screen. Alternatively, the EEG-PSG signal and video signal can be synchronously replayed on two monitors. The EEG-PSG also

can be played back onto paper at a variety of speeds to display sleep features or EEG features as indicated. Information regarding the date and time encoded onto the videotape and paper printout allows for synchronous review. Digital video recordings will be more readily available in the future and may eventually replace videotape recordings.

The stage of sleep from which the spells emerge and the time of the spell relative to sleep onset provide useful diagnostic information. For example, the behaviors accompanying the NREM arousal disorders arise from delta NREM sleep, usually in the first third of the sleep period (Chapter 62), whereas those associated with RBD emerge from REM sleep, most commonly in the last third of the sleep period (Chapter 64). Epileptic seizures are more common during NREM sleep than during REM sleep (Chapter 63).[8] Rhythmic movements associated with rhythmic movement disorder usually occur during sleep-wake transitions, and dissociative episodes emerge from wakefulness. Nocturnal panic attacks occur from NREM sleep, usually at the transition from stage 2 to stage 3.[9]

Specific EEG patterns associated with nocturnal spells are discussed in Relative Indications, Advantages, Disadvantages, and Limitations. If complex partial seizures are a diagnostic consideration, the EEG montage should emphasize the use of electrodes placed over the temporal lobes (e.g., F7, T1, T3, T5). If benign childhood epilepsy with centrotemporal spikes is a consideration, the montage should include the parasagittal region (e.g., C3, C4). The specific montage that is used depends on the number of channels available for EEG. Sample montages for 8, 10, 12, 14, 16, 19, and 24 channels are shown (see Table 106–1). The following montage of 16 electrodes in anterior-to-posterior chains provides excellent coverage for suspected seizures: left temporal: Fp1-F7, F7-T3, T3-T5 and T5-O1; left parasagittal: Fp1-F3, F3-C3, C3-P3, and P3-O1; right parasagittal: Fp2-F4, F4-C4, C4-P4, and P4-O2; and right temporal: Fp2-F8, F8-T4, T4-T6, and T6-O2. This montage allows for the evaluation of interictal and ictal activity during sleep. Two additional anterior temporal electrodes, T1 and T2, can be added because they are particularly useful for the detection of anterior temporal IEDs.

Short- and Long-Term Monitoring

When the history suggests frequent daytime spells or spells occurring during daytime naps, STM, a video-EEG recording typically performed in an EEG or sleep laboratory for 6 to 8 h during the day, may be helpful. The value of such studies for the assessment of patients with strictly nocturnal spells, however, is limited. Occasionally, STM is useful if *sleep attacks*, spells of diminished responsiveness due to sleepiness, are included in the differential diagnosis of daytime spells.

Unfortunately, one or two nights of monitoring in the sleep laboratory is not always sufficient to capture and characterize spells. LTM, an extension of STM that allows for continuous recordings of up to several weeks, is used mainly for patients with known or suspected seizures.[10] For patients who are taking antiepileptic medications, these drugs may be tapered and discontinued during LTM; intermittent sleep deprivation also is commonly used to facilitate spells. Because frequent seizures or status epilepticus may occur in epileptic patients undergoing medication discontinuation, LTM is generally performed in a hospital setting, usually a specialized epilepsy monitoring laboratory. Eye movement leads and chin electromyographic leads may be added to the standard EEG electrodes to stage sleep. Semi-invasive sphenoidal electrodes, placed in the subtemporal fossa to record from the inferior temporal region and adjacent areas of the inferior frontal lobe, are usually reserved for previously diagnosed patients with epilepsy refractory to medication trials who are undergoing evaluation for epilepsy surgery. They are generally not required when the goal of monitoring is to identify EEG activity consistent with seizures or parasomnias rather than to precisely characterize an epileptic focus. Even though sphenoidal electrodes may increase the number of IEDs recorded,

the detection of IEDs from a sphenoidal electrode alone rarely occurs, particularly if ear, T1, and T2 electrodes are used.[11] In addition, although ictal patterns from sphenoidal electrodes may appear earlier and be better developed than those from surface electrodes, EEG seizure patterns are generally evident in both surface and sphenoidal electrodes.[12]

Even if additional electrodes are used, the lack of scalp or sphenoidal ictal activity during a clinical event does not exclude a seizure, particularly if awareness is preserved during the clinical event (e.g., a simple partial seizure) or if the event originates in the frontal lobe. Ictal activity may be apparent only with intracranial electrodes, such as depth electrodes that penetrate the brain parenchyma, subdural strips, and subdural grids.[13–15] These invasive electrodes, which are rarely used in the diagnosis of nocturnal spells because of the risks of infection and hemorrhage, are generally reserved for patients requiring localization of epileptic foci before surgical resection in whom scalp recordings are inconclusive. If an ictal pattern is not recorded but clinical seizures are highly suspected based on the history and stereotyped behavioral spells recorded on videotape, an empiric trial of an antiepileptic medication may be appropriate.

Ambulatory Monitoring

Ambulatory monitoring combines the extended recording time of VPSG with the convenience of recording in a patient's home. Several commercial products allow patients to go home with 12 or more channels of EEG electrodes and a recording device, which sometimes includes video monitoring. Ambulatory recording systems may use analog or digital recorders. Patients and their bedpartners are instructed to keep an activity log to document events.

The indications for ambulatory monitoring in the differential diagnosis of nocturnal events are not established. This monitoring technique appears promising for the evaluation of interictal epileptiform activity during sleep. Depending on the sophistication of the video recordings, ambulatory monitoring may diagnose some cases of epileptic seizures, NREM arousal disorders, RBD, rhythmic movement disorder, panic disorder, and dissociative disorder.

ARTIFACTS AND PITFALLS

Artifacts, which are common during sleep-related spells recorded with any of these modalities, must be distinguished from interictal and ictal epileptiform activity and from EEG activity associated with parasomnias. Although artifacts may obscure the EEG and make diagnosis more difficult, they are sometimes helpful; for example, head or body rocking artifact may be diagnostic of rhythmic movement disorder and rhythmic myogenic artifact may support bruxism (Fig. 106–4). Other examples of frequently encountered artifacts include those caused by head tremor, eye move-

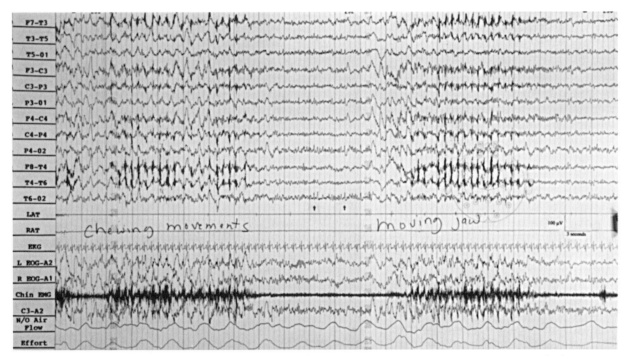

Figure 106–4. Artifacts resembling interictal epileptiform activity. Chewing movements produced by bruxism cause rhythmic activity with superimposed myogenic artifact in the EEG channels, bearing a superficial resemblance to generalized spike-wave discharges. The arrows identify posterior occipital sharp transients of sleep (POSTS), normal features of NREM stage 1 sleep that appear sharply contoured and may be mistaken for pathological occipital sharp waves at the standard PSG paper speed of 10 mm/sec.

ments, and tongue movements *(glossokinetic artifact).* Associated rhythmic activities may resemble ictal EEG patterns.

Pitfalls in the interpretation of recorded events are common; the inexperienced interpreter may mistakenly identify an artifact as EEG activity characteristic of seizures or parasomnias. When in doubt about an EEG-PSG pattern, a trained electroencephalographer should be consulted. Apart from artifacts, many other normal physiological variants may be mistaken for epileptic activity; these include positive occipital sharp transients of sleep (see Fig. 106–4), frequent and sharply contoured vertex waves, particularly in young patients (Fig. 106–5), sawtooth waves, benign epileptiform transients of sleep, wicket spikes, and rhythmic temporal theta of drowsiness.[16]

RELATIVE INDICATIONS, ADVANTAGES, DISADVANTAGES, AND LIMITATIONS

Although VPSG and other neurological monitoring techniques can be useful in diagnosing nocturnal events, the incremental cost of these techniques over standard PSG necessitates that specific indications be met. Unfortunately, no standards exist for the determination of when to choose a specific monitoring technique, and the reliability and validity of the monitoring techniques described here have not been formally studied. Consensus guidelines for interpretation have not been developed. In addition, the role of ambulatory EEG in monitoring parasomnias is not well defined.

The indications, advantages, disadvantages, and limitations outlined below are based on the experiences of the authors and others.

Video-Electroencephalography Polysomnography

Indications for VPSG include suspected sleep-related epileptic seizures, suspected NREM arousal disorders, RBD, or suspected dissociative disorder.

Suspected Sleep-Related Epileptic Seizures

Although some epileptic seizures can be diagnosed on the basis of history (e.g., generalized tonic-clonic activity witnessed by a reliable observer), most events occurring frequently and suspected to be complex partial seizures are best confirmed with VPSG monitoring, especially if they include the features of thrashing, kicking, hyperventilating, head rocking, screaming, or subtle arousals from sleep observed in parasomnias or dissociative disorders. The advantage of VPSG over conventional PSG or EEG without video in suspected epileptic seizures is the ability to analyze stereotyped behaviors, characteristic of epileptic seizures, in association with ictal EEG activity. Figure 106–6A and B shows a recording with an extended EEG montage of an epileptic seizure, illustrating a clear evolution of activity. Apart from recording epileptic seizures, PSG with an expanded EEG montage allows for sampling of IEDs throughout the night. The IEDs associated with partial epilepsy are usually more prevalent in sleep,

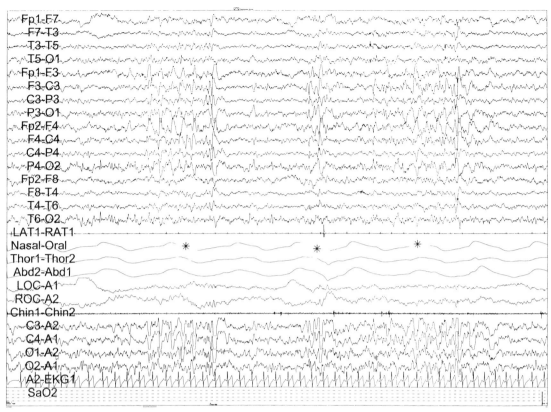

Figure 106–5. Sharply contoured vertex waves in a 6-year-old child. Although these physiological waves resemble abnormal epileptiform activity, their morphology and distribution distinguish them from pathological discharges. Compare with Figure 106–2. Thirty-second epoch; calibration symbol at bottom right, 100 μV.

especially delta NREM sleep, than in wakefulness.[17, 18] Therefore, occasionally, IEDs missed on a routine daytime EEG are detected on an overnight recording.[19]

CASE EXAMPLE 1

A 34-year-old woman with a remote history of daytime complex partial seizures presented with nightly nocturnal spells. Her husband reported that within 45 min of falling asleep she aroused, sat up, appeared frightened, breathed rapidly, looked around the room with a blank, wide-eyed stare, and then returned to sleep. These episodes were stereotyped and lasted less than 1 min. She responded almost immediately and did not recall the episodes.

Approach. The differential diagnosis includes a NREM arousal disorder, dissociative episodes, or epileptic seizures. Nocturnal panic disorder is unlikely because she does not recall the episodes. RBD is possible, but it would be unusual in a young woman, usually does not cause stereotyped behavior, and rarely occurs soon after sleep onset. Because the history was insufficient for diagnosis and because the spells were occurring nightly, VPSG was performed, during which the patient had several stereotyped spells occurring from all stages of NREM sleep. These spells were associated with ictal discharges beginning over the right

temporal lobe consisting of rhythmic theta activity that increased in frequency and decreased in amplitude. She was treated for complex partial seizures with carbamazepine, with resolution of the spells. If this patient had been on antiepileptic medication chronically and had spells that were less frequent (e.g., once a week), an alternative approach would have been LTM with tapering of medications to promote seizure occurrence.

Suspected NREM Arousal Disorders

Although confusional arousals, sleepwalking, and sleep terrors often can be diagnosed on the basis of history, VPSG is indicated if (1) behavioral features are atypical or stereotyped, (2) multiple nightly episodes occur, (3) onset is in adulthood, or (4) spells do not respond to a trial of medications. An advantage of VPSG in the diagnosis of NREM arousal disorders is the combination of video to characterize the event of interest, sleep scoring channels to determine the stage of sleep involved, and an extended EEG montage to exclude ictal EEG activity characteristic of epileptic seizures. The VPSG may capture a confusional arousal, night terror, or sleepwalking episode arising out of delta NREM (stage 3 or 4) sleep, accompanied by synchronous delta activity (Fig. 106–7). Alternatively, the VPSG recorded during a NREM arousal event may show asynchronous delta or theta activity, synchronous theta activity, a drowsy pattern, or nonreactive alpha

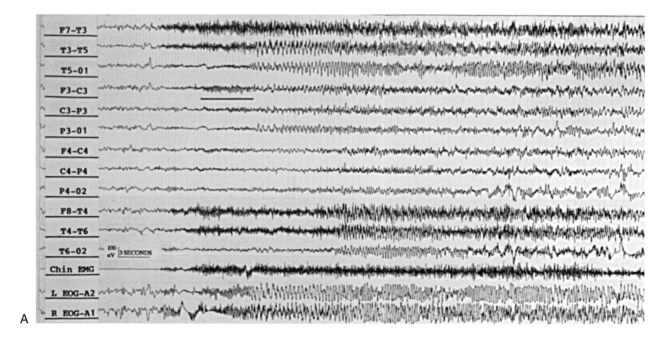

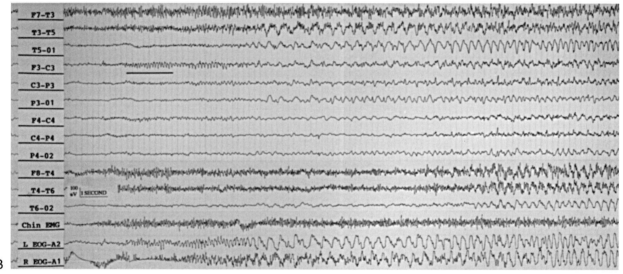

Figures 106–6. Partial seizure beginning during NREM sleep. *A,* recorded at 10 mm/sec paper speed. Clinically, the seizure began with an abrupt arousal, followed by turning of head and eyes to the left and movements of the arms beneath the bedclothes. On EEG, an initial reduction in voltage is followed by a progressive increase in the amplitude of the ictal discharge over the left hemisphere with spread to the right hemisphere derivations. The underlined activity from the F3-C3 derivation appears to be muscle artifact; however, in *B,* at 30 mm/sec paper speed, it is clear that the same underlined segment is the initial focal surface representation of the ictal discharge. Additional polysomnographic measures recorded on channels 16 to 21 are not shown. (Modified from Aldrich MS, Jahnke B. Diagnostic value of video-EEG polysomnography. Neurology. 1991;41:1060–1066.)

activity. Apart from clinical events, the EEG may show synchronous delta during arousals from stage 3 or 4 sleep, a nonspecific finding that is more common in patients with arousal disorders than in normal subjects.[20]

CASE EXAMPLE 2

A 4-year-old girl had near-nightly episodes of screaming loudly about 1 h after falling asleep. During these episodes, her parents found her agitated and inconsolable. On rare occasions, she got out of bed and wandered out of her room. She was amnestic for these spells. An older sibling had had similar spells.

Approach. Because the history is compelling for night terrors, evaluation with VPSG is not necessary. If any atypical features were present (e.g., automatisms or stereotyped behavior, multiple nightly episodes, or onset in adulthood) or if symptoms did not respond to treatment, a VPSG would be warranted.

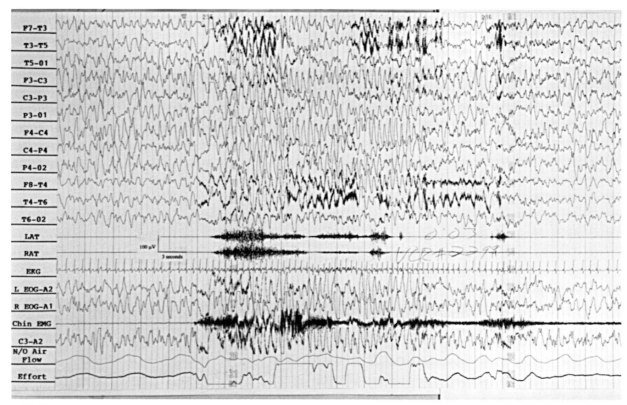

Figure 106–7. Arousal from delta NREM sleep in child with a NREM arousal disorder. Note synchronous delta activity during arousal from delta NREM sleep, associated with a tonic increase in chin and leg EEG. In contrast to the EEG of an epileptic seizure, the delta activity does not evolve in amplitude or frequency.

Suspected REM Sleep Behavior Disorder

Although the definitive diagnosis of RBD may be suspected based on the history, definitive diagnosis requires capturing a behavioral event on a video recording or demonstrating abnormal muscle tone or excessive limb movements during REM sleep (Chapter 64). The advantage of VPSG is that video is combined with sleep staging to identify REM and an extended EEG montage is used to exclude ictal EEG activity.

Suspected Dissociative Disorder

Dissociative episodes and other psychogenic spells occur during wakefulness, although the patient may appear asleep and may believe that he or she is asleep. Because the manifestations of dissociative episodes may be quite bizarre and include thrashing, screaming, or bicycling movements, it is often impossible to distinguish these spells from epileptic seizures or parasomnias based on the history alone. When nocturnal psychogenic episodes are suspected, VPSG is advantageous in documenting the behavior of the patient, the presence of waking background EEG preceding the onset of the spells, and the absence of ictal EEG activity.

CASE EXAMPLE 3

A 32-year-old man developed spells of unresponsiveness associated with asynchronous jerking movements of all four extremities for up to 30 min. These spells occurred nightly during sleep and rarely during the day. When they occurred during the day, he recalled portions of the spells and stated that he could hear people around him, but that he could not respond. His wife could shake him out of the spells, and then he would regain full alertness.

Approach. Based on the history of prolonged spells with bilateral extremity jerking and preserved consciousness, a dissociative episode was likely, although occasionally, epileptic seizures, especially of frontal lobe origin, present with bilateral jerking movements of the extremities and rapid return to full alertness. Depending on the relative frequency of the nocturnal and daytime spells, either VPSG, STM, or LTM may be appropriate. In this case, because of the relative frequency of nocturnal spells, a VPSG was performed and documented an awake background preceding and during the spell, with an absence of ictal EEG activity, characteristic of a dissociative disorder. After psychiatric evaluation and treatment, the frequency of the spells decreased.

The major disadvantage of VPSG in the evaluation of suspected epileptic seizures, parasomnias, and dissociative disorders is the cost of the study. Additional technologist time is needed to place an extended EEG montage and to continuously observe patients throughout the study. In addition, physicians must review each spell to assess behaviors and EEG patterns.

Equipment must allow for review capabilities at EEG paper speed (30 mm/sec). These review capabilities are standard on most digital PSG equipment, although the additional channels require more space on storage media.

The VPSG also has limitations. The EEG recorded during a spell may not demonstrate an abnormality. Because epileptic seizures may lack surface EEG correlates, the absence of surface ictal EEG activity does not ensure that an epileptic seizure has not occurred. In addition, differentiation of an ictal EEG seizure pattern, consisting of rhythmic activity that evolves in frequency and amplitude, from the synchronous delta or theta activity or diffuse alpha activity occurring during a NREM arousal disorder, is not always straightforward: (1) the most well-developed portion of the ictal EEG pattern may be rhythmic delta or theta without a clear evolution, (2) seizures may have bilateral onsets, (3) seizures may arise from delta NREM sleep, and (4) muscle or movement artifact may obscure the EEG. Two consecutive nights of VPSG are often scheduled so if no events are captured on the 1st night, the 2nd night is available for study.

Daytime Electroencephalography

The advantage of daytime EEG over VPSG, standard PSG, or any of the other monitoring techniques is its brief recording time and low cost. The disadvantage is that spells, particularly sleep-related spells, are rarely captured. When the history is highly suggestive of epileptic seizures, a routine EEG may demonstrate epileptic activity as supportive evidence of epilepsy. However, IEDs are not the equivalent of epileptic seizures and may be present in patients without epilepsy, such as occurs in relatives of patients with benign childhood epilepsy with centrotemporal spikes. Conversely, patients with epilepsy may not have IEDs during EEG recordings. In addition, patients with epilepsy may have coexisting parasomnias. Therefore, in the absence of a compelling history, the occurrence of abnormal interictal epileptiform activity should not be used by itself to definitively diagnose nocturnal spells as epileptic seizures.

Short- and Long-Term Monitoring

The advantages of STM and LTM over routine EEG are a longer recording time and simultaneous video monitoring. In patients with exclusively sleep-related spells, VPSG is preferred over STM because the recording is performed during sleep. In patients with a mixture of daytime and sleep-related spells, STM is sometimes appropriate.

LTM is an alternative in patients in whom antiepileptic medication taper or discontinuation is planned. Medication taper or discontinuation is especially useful in facilitating seizure activity in epileptic patients with infrequent spells (e.g., once a week or less frequently). The disadvantages of LTM are the cost of inpatient hospitalization and the need for a specialized epilepsy monitoring laboratory. The limitations of LTM are similar to those of PSG in that spells may lack EEG correlates or may not occur, despite many days of monitoring.

Ambulatory Monitoring

The advantage of ambulatory monitoring is the convenience of recording in a patient's home and the lack of need for continuous monitoring by a technologist. Cost varies, but it is usually lower than that of a recording in a sleep laboratory. A major disadvantage of ambulatory monitoring relates to the fidelity of the recording in the absence of a technologist. If electrodes become detached, ground wires break, or conductive media becomes dry during the study, adjustments cannot be made. In addition, most systems use a reduced number of channels, thereby limiting the information provided, although technological advances should increase the capability for expanded montages. Furthermore, in contrast to the other monitoring techniques, the patient is not under constant observation and a technologist is not present. Consequently, interactions with the patient, which are critical for evaluation of the level of consciousness, are not possible, and the interpretation of rhythmic activities that resemble ictal discharges may be difficult in the absence of an assessment of behavior and consciousness. The addition of synchronized video recordings to ambulatory monitoring has potential for facilitating correlation between EEG activity and clinical events.

References

1. Commission on Classification and Terminology of the International League Against Epilepsy. Proposal for revised clinical and electrographic classification of epileptic seizures. Epilepsia. 1981;22:489–501.
2. Aldrich MS, Jahnke B. Diagnostic value of video-EEG polysomnography. Neurology. 1991;41:1060–1066.
3. Epstein CM. Technical aspects of EEG: an overview. In: Wyllie E, ed. The Treatment of Epilepsy: Principles and Practices. Philadelphia, Pa: Lea & Febiger; 1993:202–210.
4. Jasper H. The 10-20 electrode system of the International Federation. Electroencephalogr Clin Neurophysiol. 1958;10:370–375.
5. Daly D, Pedley T. Current Practice of Clinical Electroencephalography. New York, NY: Raven Press; 1990.
6. Lagerlund T, Cascino G, Cicora K, et al. Long-term electroencephalographic monitoring for diagnosis and management of seizures. Mayo Clin Proc. 1996;71:1000–1006.
7. Kaplan PW, Lesser RP. Focal cortical resection evaluation: noninvasive EEG. In: Wyllie E, ed. The Treatment of Epilepsy: Principles and Practice. Philadelphia, Pa: Lea & Febiger, 1993:1014–1022.
8. Malow B. Sleep and epilepsy. In: Aldrich M, ed. Neurologic Clinics, Sleep Disorders II. Philadelphia, Pa: WB Saunders; 1996:765–789.
9. Mellman T, Uhde T. Electroencephalographic sleep in panic disorder. Arch Gen Psychiatry. 1989;46:178–184.
10. Kaplan P, Lesser R. Long-Term Monitoring. In: Daly D, Pedley T, eds. Current Practice of Clinical Electroencephalography. New York, Pa: Raven Press; 1990:513–534.
11. Sperling MR, Engel J Jr. Sphenoidal electrodes. J Clin Neurophysiol. 1986;3:67–73.

12. King DW, So EL, Marcus R, et al. Techniques and applications of sphenoidal recording. J Clin Neurophysiol. 1986;3:51–65.

13. So NK. Depth electrode studies in mesial temporal epilepsy. In: Luders HO, ed. Epilepsy Surgery. New York, NY: Raven Press; 1992:371–384.

14. Wyler AR. Subdural strip electrodes in surgery of epilepsy. In: Luders HO, ed. Epilepsy Surgery. New York, NY: Raven Press; 1992:395–398.

15. Lesser RP, Gordon B, Fisher R, et al. Subdural grid electrodes in surgery of epilepsy. In: Luders HO, ed. Epilepsy Surgery. New York, NY: Raven Press; 1992:399–408.

16. Drury I. Epileptiform patterns of children. J Clin Neurophysiol. 1989;6:1–39.

17. Sammaritano M, Gigli GL, Gotman J. Interictal spiking during wakefulness and sleep and the localization of foci in temporal lobe epilepsy. Neurology. 1991;41:290–297.

18. Malow BA, Lin X, Kushwaha R, et al. Interictal spiking increases with sleep depth in temporal lobe epilepsy. Epilepsia. 1998;39:1309–1316.

19. Malow BA, Selwa LM, Ross DA, et al. Lateralizing value of interictal spikes on overnight sleep-EEG studies in temporal lobe epilepsy. Epilepsia. 1999;40:1587–1592.

20. Blatt I, Peled R, Gadoth N, et al. The value of sleep recording in evaluating somnambulism in young adults. Electroencephalogr Clin Neurophysiol. 1991;78:407–412.

107

Gastrointestinal Monitoring Techniques

William C. Orr

Gastroesophageal reflux (GER) is a common problem associated with considerable morbidity.[1] Studies have shown the highest incidence of esophagitis, as well as the most severe complications (erosion and stricture), to be associated with recumbent reflux that occurs during sleep, a situation permitting prolonged acid mucosal contact.[2, 3] This is presumably the result not only of an incompetent lower esophageal sphincter but also of an inability to effectively clear the refluxed material. Poor clearance of acid from the esophagus and subsequent acid neutralization have been documented to be impaired during sleep.[4, 5]

GER may be viewed as consisting of two components:

1. The retrograde flow of gastric contents through the antireflux barrier at the esophagogastric junction
2. The return of the acid gastric juice to the stomach and subsequent neutralization of the distal esophagus to a pH of 4 (i.e., *esophageal acid clearing*)

The critical parameter in determining the extent of GER, and its potential damage to the esophageal mucosa, is the percentage of time the esophagus is exposed to a pH lower than 4. In view of the previous research documenting the importance of sleep-related GER in the pathogenesis of reflux esophagitis, it is important to determine the percentage of acid contact time (ACT) at night, as well as during the day.

Postprandial reflux has been shown to be "physiological" and when confined to the postprandial interval, it is considered benign.[6] In determining the clinical significance of GER, it is important to assess the 24-h pattern (see Chapter 94). Twenty-four–hour patterns of GER can be evaluated with commercially available devices. Two types of pH studies are described herein: (1) ambulatory pH studies in which sleep monitoring does not occur; (2) in-laboratory pH studies that include simultaneous pH monitoring with polysomnography (PSG).

AMBULATORY pH MONITORING

Ambulatory esophageal pH monitoring can be accomplished by using commercially available pH probes and portable data-acquisition devices. The techniques are similar to those in Holter monitoring; the patient is intubated with either a glass- or antimony-tipped pH electrode, the output of which is attached to a small box (3.5-inch width $\times$ 7.25-inch length $\times$ 1-inch depth) that the patient wears either at the waist with a belt or across the shoulder with a shoulder strap.

Our laboratory specifically conducted a validation study of one of these units, which included simultaneous monitoring of input to the computer system and polygraphic tracing of the pH. Although this was not an ambulatory study, because the patient had to be tethered to a recording device, there was excellent agreement between the computer-detected reflux events and those detected by visual inspection from the paper tracing.[7]

The decision to use antimony or glass electrodes depends on a variety of factors; each has advantages and disadvantages. The glass electrode is somewhat more accurate and linear across a large pH range, whereas the antimony electrode is somewhat more durable. From a clinical standpoint, there is little difference between the two with regard to the accuracy of the data collected. These commercially available devices have internal calibration techniques that should be performed before every intubation.

For the best readings, the pH probe is placed 5 cm above the proximal border of the manometrically determined lower esophageal sphincter (LES). The LES must be determined manometrically, which can be somewhat inconvenient because it may require two separate intubations (the first to determine the LES location and the second to insert the pH probe). However, a pH probe has been developed to allow LES determination and pH probe placement with a single intubation. Data have shown that an approximation of the ideal site can be accomplished by using pH determinations only. This method requires placing the pH probe distally until a clearly acidic (approximately 1.5 to 2.5) pH is established (indicating that the pH probe is in the stomach) and then slowly withdrawing the probe until the pH rises to approximately 4. At that point, the pH probe is most likely out of the stomach and in the esophagogastric junction. The probe is then withdrawn 5 to 7 cm above this level and affixed at that point. Although not as accurate as the manometric method of determination, for clinical purposes this is an acceptable placement method.

It should be recognized, however, that this method has been shown to be most problematic with regard to accuracy in patients who actually have substantial GER and most accurate in normal volunteers.[8] Thus, whenever feasible, the manometric method should be used to locate the LES for accurate pH probe placement.

With the increasing clinical interest in establishing GER as the cause of a variety of extraesophageal symptoms such as bronchial asthma, chronic cough, laryngopharyngitis, and pulmonary aspiration, dual pH probe monitoring has become substantially more popular. It entails monitoring at least two sites in the esophagus: one at the standard site in the distal esophagus (placed as described earlier) and one in the more proximal esophagus. The exact location in the more proximal esophagus varies from the midesophagus to the pharynx, and there is little in the way of currently accepted standard as to the proximal probe placement. Studies have shown that proximal esophageal and pharyngeal acid exposure effectively discriminates individuals with posterior laryngitis.[9] Another study by Jacob and colleagues[10] has shown that supine (primarily during sleep) proximal acid exposure best discriminates patients with laryngeal symptoms from those with reflux esophagitis and normals.[10] These data would suggest that some proximal acid exposure has clinically significant correlates.

Dual pH probe monitoring assumes additional clinical significance in reviewing data from Koufman, who has shown in an animal model that even minute amounts of acid exposure can create cancerous lesions in the larynx.[11] In addition, numerous studies have shown that patients with aerodigestive symptoms such as chronic cough and pulmonary aspiration have greater proximal esophageal and pharyngeal acid exposure.[10, 12, 13] Although much work needs to be done to assess the importance of, and specific parameters relating to, proximal esophageal acid exposure in the pathogenesis of extraesophageal symptoms of reflux, it is clear that the trend is moving increasingly toward use of dual pH monitoring.

Once the intubation has been accomplished, the patient is instructed concerning the operation of the data-acquisition system. Patients may be given special dietary instructions to avoid acidic foods; in general, my preference is *not* to have the patient adopt a special diet. GER and heartburn are both significantly affected by dietary intake, and, therefore, a more accurate clinical picture of the frequency and severity of GER can be obtained if patients eat their usual meals. The patient completes a log to document significant events. The patient is instructed to indicate the start and end time of meals, time of going to sleep and waking up, time of medication intake, and time of occurrence of clinical symptoms. The patient is instructed to return to the laboratory approximately 24 h from the time of departure.

On returning to the laboratory, the patient is extubated and the data are downloaded into a computer system that analyzes a variety of reflux parameters over the total recording interval. These parameters include number of reflux episodes, average duration of the reflux episodes, longest reflux episode, percentage of ACT, and a summary of these events according to upright (primarily waking) and supine (primarily sleeping) postures. The computer printout summarizes the timing of meals, sleep, and clinical symptoms as well. This information allows one to determine the relationship of symptoms to episodes of GER.

POLYSOMNOGRAPHIC RECORDING

In certain circumstances, a PSG recording during pH monitoring may be desirable. For example, there may be specific interest in the possibility that a patient is having sleep-related reflux and pulmonary aspiration. In addition, nocturnal recordings of reflux or the clearance time of externally infused acid may identify individuals who are at high risk for pulmonary aspiration. Such individuals are specifically identified by prolonged clearance of spontaneous reflux or infused acid associated with poor arousal responses from sleep. Furthermore, it may be clinically useful to note whether reflux itself is triggered by periodic arousal responses as a result of disturbed sleep. Such a relationship (i.e., sleep-related reflux preceded by a brief arousal response) has been reported.[14]

Electrode placement is as described for ambulatory studies. A reference lead is placed on the ventral surface of the forearm or the forehead. The reference lead and the pH probe should always be recorded through an electrical isolation box attached to the pH meter. Any commercially available pH meter is suitable, but it must have an external output to allow polygraphic recording. The output needs to be in a range of 0 to 1 V for most direct current (DC) amplifiers. This measurement is made simultaneously with the standard polygraphic measurements for monitoring sleep (i.e., electroencephalogram, electro-oculogram, electromyogram, electrocardiogram).

Reflux is defined by a drop in the pH of the distal esophagus below a level of 4. Clearance is arbitrarily defined by a return of the esophageal pH to 4. The time between the drop in the pH below 4 and its return to 4 is referred to as the *clearing duration* or *clearance interval*. A pH of 4 has been arbitrarily chosen as the criterion to determine a reflux event because the esophageal pH level is routinely between 5.5 and 6.5. Thus, in order for the pH to drop below 4, it is assumed that the electrode must be in contact with acid. Furthermore, there is little if any peptic activity associated with a pH of 4, although such activity increases logarithmically as the pH decreases below 4.

With regard to evaluating esophageal function during sleep, we have chosen to focus on the patient's ability to clear infused acid from the esophagus. This method has several advantages. First, spontaneous reflux during sleep—even in symptomatic patients with esophagitis—is relatively infrequent and unpredictable. Second, important parameters such as when the event occurs and the volume of the refluxant are uncontrolled with spontaneous reflux. Our method was designed to evaluate reflux by simulating an event using a controlled infusion of a specified volume at a specific point in time (i.e., waking versus a particular stage of sleep). Although this method does not allow the study of the effects of physiological reflux, it does allow the control of the other critical factors. Although acidity per se does not necessarily produce mucosal damage, we assume that the arousal response from sleep is the result of the afferent stimulus caused by the low pH.

Volume is an important parameter in producing arousal responses, and it is therefore important to take this variable into consideration in evaluating reflux during sleep. For example, studies in our laboratory have shown that acid clearance and arousal responses are markedly altered by the volume infused into the esophagus.[15] Other obvious advantages of performing sleep studies relate to the determination of important responses to esophageal acidification such as polygraphic arousal responses and swallowing responses. These are important parameters with regard to acid clearance (assuming normal esophageal motor function) that cannot be assessed via 24-h ambulatory studies.

The schematic diagram in Figure 107–1 illustrates the parameters that are obtained from a single infusion of a controlled volume of acid. The acid clearance time is determined as the interval of time elapsing between the drop in pH to 4 until the pH returns to 4 or 5. The arousal response latency is the elapsed time from a pH drop to 4 until polygraphic evidence of an arousal response. The latency to the first swallow is defined as the elapsed time from the drop in pH to 4 until the first swallow, defined as a transient burst of muscle activity from the submental electromyogram recording. Studies in our laboratory have determined normal parameters for these measures.[4, 5]

CLINICAL INTERPRETATION OF pH DATA

GER disease is a complex, multifactorial disorder involving not only physiological mechanisms that determine the retrograde flow of acid contents from the stomach into the esophagus but also anatomic aspects of mucosal resistance.[1, 16] Current diagnostic methodology confines itself only to evaluating GER and mucosal esophageal ACT. Important aspects of the pathogenesis of esophagitis, such as hydrogen ion back diffusion, constituents of the acid contents of the stomach (i.e., pepsin, bile salts, and pancreatic enzymes), and esophageal mucosal potential difference are not routinely available for evaluation in patients. As noted earlier, however, the 24-h ambulatory pH study allows one to assess a number of parameters thought to be important in the development of esophagitis.

Clinically, the most important parameters relate to the total percentage of ACT, percentage of ACT in the upright and supine positions, longest reflux episode, and number of reflux episodes longer than 5 min. The assessment of each of these parameters and the extent to which they occur in the waking state versus sleep all are clinically relevant. Normal parameters for reflux events have been published in a number of sources and have been reviewed by de Caestecker.[17]

Clinical interpretation of these studies is, to a large extent, subjective, but most experts agree that the most important parameter is ACT. For a normal individual, total ACT is generally between 4 and 6%. At or above 8% is considered a clinically significant elevation in ACT. If the majority of ACT occurs in the sleeping interval or if the sleeping ACT exceeds 4 to 5%, however, the clinical impact is considerably greater. This clinical difference occurs because patients who are susceptible to sleep-related reflux have prolonged acid clearance associated with episodes of reflux during

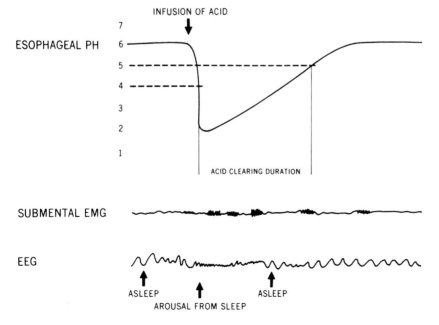

Figure 107–1. Schematic representation of the acid infusion paradigm. As with spontaneous gastroesophageal reflux (GER), the duration of acid clearing is determined as the time from the drop in pH below 4 until the pH reaches 5 (in some studies the value is 4).

sleep and such episodes are felt to be more damaging to the esophageal mucosa than short waking episodes, even if they are more numerous.[3, 6]

Clinical interpretation of PSG pH studies is somewhat more complicated. As noted earlier, there are few indications for this type of study because 24-h ambulatory pH studies generally provide adequate clinical information.

Nevertheless, several variables are clinically significant with PSG monitoring during the pH recording. First, the occurrence of spontaneous GER needs to be documented by identifying each time the esophageal pH drops below 4. The length of the subsequent arousal latency response is also significant. For example, an arousal response that is delayed beyond 2 to 3 min might indicate some alteration in arousal mechanisms. A prolongation of the arousal latency or the acid clearance time suggests that the individual may be at risk for pulmonary aspiration. Also of considerable clinical significance is the association of multiple short awakenings with repeated reflux events, which might suggest that fragmented sleep is contributing to the patient's problem with GER.

As with the ambulatory studies, the percentage of time the esophageal pH is below 4 is relevant, as is the number of spontaneous episodes of reflux. Normal individuals rarely have reflux during sleep; thus, the spontaneous occurrence of GER during sleep is an important clinical event. Having more than two to three episodes a night is clinically significant, particularly if any one of these events is associated with prolonged ACT (longer than 5 to 10 min). An acid exposure time exceeding 4 to 5% during sleep probably represents a clinically significant finding, and nocturnal acid suppression would be an appropriate approach to treatment.

There are minimal normative data with regard to proximal acid exposure. Because there is no standardization with regard to the placement of the proximal probe, it is impossible to describe normative values across a large population of patients. In general, this is done within each laboratory, where a standardized procedure is used. Most useful information with regard to normative data in the proximal esophagus is described in a review article by Richter.[18] In general, most studies in which control data have been collected describe proximal acid contact time in normal individuals to be between 0 and 1%.[18]

CONCLUSIONS

Symptoms suggestive of unexplained arousals from sleep resulting in complaints of insomnia or daytime sleepiness may well have nocturnal GER as an underlying contributing factor. In addition, nocturnal GER may be the cause of exacerbations from bronchial asthma and repeated pulmonary infections as a result of pulmonary aspiration of refluxed stomach contents.[19] For most clinical circumstances, 24-h ambulatory pH studies with careful documentation of the sleeping interval are suitable and allow a reasonable assessment of wak-

ing GER and sleep-related GER, as well as ACT during the total interval and the sleep interval. When patients present with unexplained extraesophageal symptoms, such as chronic cough, uncontrolled nocturnal wheezing, or repeated pulmonary aspiration, dual pH monitoring may provide unique data concerning the role of GER in the pathogenesis of these symptoms. In the majority of instances, ambulatory studies provide adequate information for clinical management. In certain circumstances, however, more precise information may be needed concerning specific responses to reflux or infused acid, necessitating a complete PSG evaluation.

References

1. Richter JE, Bradley LA, Castell DO. Esophageal chest pain: current controversies in pathogenesis, diagnosis and therapy. Ann Intern Med. 1989;110:66–78.
2. Johnson LF, DeMeester TR. Twenty-four hour pH monitoring of the distal esophagus, a quantitative measure of gastroesophageal reflux. Am J Gastroenterol. 1974;62:325–332.
3. Johnson LF, DeMeester TR, Haggitt RC. Esophageal epithelial response to gastroesophageal reflux, a quantitative study. Am J Dig Dis. 1978;23:478–509.
4. Orr WC, Robinson MG, Johnson LF. Acid clearing during sleep in the pathogenesis of reflux esophagitis. Dig Dis Sci. 1981;26:423.
5. Orr WC, Johnson LF, Robinson MC. The effect of sleep on swallowing, esophageal, peristalsis, and acid clearance. Gastroenterology. 1984;86:814–819.
6. DeMeester TR, Johnson LF, Guy JJ, et al. Patterns of gastroesophageal reflux in health and disease. Ann Surg. 1976;184:459–470.
7. Allen M, Woodruff D, Robinson MG, et al. Validation of an ambulatory esophageal pH monitoring system. Am J Gastroenterol. 1988;83:287–290.
8. Klauser AG, Schindlbeck NE, Muller-Lissner SA. Esophageal 24-pH monitoring: is prior manometry necessary for correct positioning of the electrode? Am J Gastroenterol. 1990;85:1463–1467.
9. Shaker R, Milbrath M, Ren J, et al. Esophagopharyngeal distribution of refluxed gastric acid in patients with reflux laryngitis. Gastroenterology. 1995;109:1575–1582.
10. Jacob P, Kahrilas PJ, Herzon G. Proximal esophageal pH-metry in patients with "reflux laryngitis." Gastroenterology. 1991;11:305–310.
11. Koufman JA. The otolaryngologic manifestations of gastroesophageal reflux disease (GERD): a clinical investigation of 225 patients using ambulatory 24-hour pH monitoring and an experimental investigation of the role of acid and pepsin in the development of laryngeal injury. Larynoscope. 1991;101:1–78.
12. Patti MG, Debas HT, Pellegrini CA. Esophageal manometry and 24-hour pH monitoring in the diagnosis of pulmonary aspiration secondary to gastroesophageal reflux. Am J Surg. 1992;163:401–406.
13. Paterson WG, Murat BW. Combined ambulatory esophageal manometry and dual-probe pH-metry in evaluation of patients with chronic unexplained cough. Dig Dis Sci. 1994;39:1117–1125.
14. Dent J, Dodds WJ, Friedman RH, et al. Mechanism of gastroesophageal reflux in recumbent asymptomatic human subjects. J Clin Invest. 1980;65:256–267.
15. Orr WC, Robinson MG, Johnson LF. The effect of esophageal acid volume on arousals from sleep and acid clearance. Chest. 1991;99:351–354.
16. Johnson LF, Harmon JW. Experimental esophagitis in a rabbit model: clinical relevance. J Clin Gastroenterol. 1986;8(suppl 1):26–44.
17. de Caestecker JS. Twenty-four-hour oesophageal pH monitoring: advances and controversies. Neth J Med. 1989;34:S20–S39.
18. Richter JE. Ambulatory esophageal pH monitoring. Am J Med. 1997;103:130S–134S.
19. Gonzalez ER, Bahal N, Johnson LF. Gastroesophageal reflux and respiratory symptoms: is there an association? Proposed mechanisms and treatment. DICP Ann Pharmacother. 1990;24:1064–1069.

108

Psychometric and Psychiatric Evaluation

Peter D. Nowell

Daniel J. Buysse

Martica Hall

Charles F. Reynolds III

IMPORTANCE OF PSYCHOMETRIC AND PSYCHIATRIC EVALUATION IN SLEEP MEDICINE

The role of psychometric and psychiatric evaluation in sleep medicine can be conceptualized along several lines. Symptoms reflecting changes in arousal, cognition, mood, energy, or motivation may result from primary sleep disorders or from primary psychiatric disorders (for review, see reference 1). Evaluation of psychiatric status allows for differential diagnosis of sleep complaints, development of preventive strategies when the presence of a sleep or psychiatric disorder is a risk factor for the other, and assessment of co-morbidities relevant in treatment planning. The utility of psychometric or psychiatric evaluation is an empirical one and lies in the extent to which differential diagnosis informs prognosis, illness course, treatment selection, and clinical outcome. The increasing use of clinical databases and standardized assessment measures may serve to supplement clinical trial research to inform this issue. In the absence of such empirical evidence, it is likely that the use of psychometric and psychiatric evaluation in the practice of sleep medicine will be guided by the site where the patient enters the health care system (e.g., primary, mental health, or pulmonary care setting), availability of resources, and patient and provider preference.

The potential value of evaluating psychiatric status in the context of patients presenting with sleep symptoms is reflected in epidemiological studies highlighting the co-occurrence of sleep and psychiatric disorders. As part of the National Institute of Mental Health Epidemiologic Catchment Area study,[2] 7954 respondents were questioned at baseline and 1 y later about sleep complaints and psychiatric symptoms using the Diagnostic Interview Schedule. Of this community sample, 10.2% and 3.2% noted insomnia and hypersomnia, respectively, at the first interview; 40% of those with insomnia and 46.5% of those with hyper-

somnia had a psychiatric disorder compared with 16.4% of those with no sleep complaints. The risk of developing new major depression was much higher in those who had insomnia at both interviews compared with those without insomnia (odds ratio, 39.8; 95% confidence interval [CI], 19.8 to 80.0). The risk of developing new major depression was much lower for those who had insomnia that had resolved by the second visit (odds ratio, 1.6; 95% CI, 0.5 to 5.3). The authors concluded that further research is needed to determine if early recognition and treatment of sleep disturbances can prevent future psychiatric disorders.

In a longitudinal epidemiological study of young adults, Breslau et al.[3] estimated the association between sleep disturbance and psychiatric disorders, cross-sectionally and prospectively. A random sample of 1200 was drawn from all 21- to 30-year-old members of a large health maintenance organization (HMO) in Michigan; 1007 were interviewed in 1989 and 979 were reinterviewed in 1992. Lifetime prevalence of insomnia alone was 16.6%; of hypersomnia alone, 8.2%; and of insomnia plus hypersomnia, 8%. The gender-adjusted relative risk for new onset of major depression during the follow-up period in people with a history of insomnia at baseline was 4.0 (95% CI, 2.2 to 7.0) and in people with baseline history of hypersomnia, 2.9 (95% CI, 1.5 to 5.6). When history of other prior depressive symptoms (e.g., psychomotor retardation or agitation, suicidal ideation) was controlled for, prior insomnia remained a significant predictor of subsequent major depression. These studies by Ford et al.[2] and Breslau et al.[3] are important, not only because they demonstrate the strong relationship between insomnia and psychiatric symptoms but also because they draw attention to the observation that the hypersomnia is also a symptom of people with psychiatric disturbances. However, more studies have examined the symptoms of insomnia and the relationship to psychiatric disorders.

In one study, of a sample of 2512 general practice patients, 105 with a complaint of chronic insomnia over

4 months were evaluated for mental and personality disorders.[4] Of the 105 patients, 66 were diagnosed with a current insomnia using a structured interview from the *Diagnostic and Statistical Manual of Mental Disorders, Revised Third Edition* (DSM-III-R). Of the 66, 50% had at least one additional current Axis I or II diagnosis. Mood disorders were the most common principal psychiatric diagnoses in this group, followed by substance use disorders. The authors noted, "the general practitioners were poor in recognizing their patients' chronic insomnia complaints and the high percentage of substance abusers among them."[4]

In a more recent study using the revised *Diagnostic and Statistical Manual of Mental Disorders, Fourth Edition* (DSM-IV) criteria, insomnia and its relationship with other mental disorders were investigated in the general population.[5] A representative random sample of 5622 known insomniacs were interviewed about their sleep habits over the telephone by lay interviewers following the Sleep-Eval knowledge-based system. A total of 18.6% of the sample reported insomnia complaints. The presence of insomnia complaints, lasting for at least 1 month with daytime repercussions, was found for 12.7% of the sample. Subsequently, subjects were classified according to the sleep disorder decision-making process proposed by the DSM-IV classification but without the recourse of polysomnographic (PSG) recordings. Specific sleep disorder diagnoses were given for 5.6% of the sample, mostly as insomnia related to another mental disorder, and primary insomnia was given for 1.3% of the sample. Primary mental disorder diagnoses were supplied for 8.4% of the sample, mostly as generalized anxiety disorder. The authors emphasized the need to use structured classifications to determine whether subjects with insomnia complaints suffer from a sleep disorder or whether insomnia constitutes a symptom of some other mental disorder.

Buysse et al.[6] examined three diagnostic classifications for sleep disorders: the International Classification of Sleep Disorders (ICSD), the DSM-IV, and the *International Classification of Diseases*, 10th edition (ICD-10). Clinical sleep disorder diagnoses (without PSG) in 257 patients (216 insomnia patients and 41 medical or psychiatric patients) were evaluated at five sleep centers. A sleep specialist interviewed each patient and assigned clinical diagnoses using ICSD, DSM-IV, and ICD-10 classifications. Sleep disorder associated with mood disorder was the most frequent ICSD primary diagnosis (32.3%), followed by psychophysiological insomnia (12.5%). The most frequent DSM-IV primary diagnoses were insomnia related to another mental disorder (44%) and primary insomnia (20.2%), and the most frequent ICD-10 diagnoses were insomnia due to emotional causes (61.9%) and insomnia of organic origin (8.9%). When primary and secondary diagnoses were considered, insomnia related to psychiatric disorders was diagnosed in more than 75% of patients. The authors concluded that these results confirmed the importance of psychiatric and behavioral factors in clinicians' assessments of insomnia patients across all three diagnostic systems. As part of the same study, the authors also demonstrated that treatment recommendations followed differential diagnosis and differed between sleep specialists and nonspecialists.[7]

In a different study examining the discriminating power of a psychiatric evaluation and sleep evaluation, 40 young (20 to 40 y old) patients, selected for putative psychophysiological insomnia, underwent a psychiatric structured interview and home ambulatory sleep monitoring for 2 nights.[8] The results were compared with those of a group of nine young normal sleepers. Of the patients with insomnia, 48% showed psychiatric disorders, while 52% did not meet DSM-III-R criteria for a psychiatric diagnosis. The sleep structure of all patients with insomnia was found to be disturbed, primarily in sleep continuity, but essentially the two groups showed no significant differences. In a stepwise logistic regression analysis, the number of sleep stage shifts (indicating sleep instability) was the best variable for discriminating the patients with insomnia from controls but not the best variable for discriminating the patients with psychiatric disturbances from those without psychopathologies. The authors concluded that the evaluation of young patients with insomnia with a structured psychiatric interview rather than with ambulatory sleep monitoring seems to be most useful in discriminating between patients with only psychophysiological insomnia and patients with both insomnia and an associated diagnosis of another mental disorder.

In terms of specific strategies used by sleep specialists to distinguish primary insomnia from psychiatric insomnia, Nowell et al.[9] examined data collected from the DSM-IV Sleep Disorder field trials. Negative conditioning and poor sleep hygiene were the two symptom constructs used to assess for primary insomnia, while the presence of a syndromal psychiatric disorder was used to assign a diagnosis of insomnia secondary to a mental disorder. However, studies examining the positive predictive value of specific symptoms or symptom clusters in clinical populations in a prospective fashion remain to be conducted.

In sleep disorders medicine, the issues of psychometric and psychiatric evaluation arise most often in the assessment and treatment of patients with complaints of chronic insomnia. (For a review of diagnostic and treatment issues in chronic insomnia, see reference 10). There exists a close clinical and nosologic relationship between primary insomnia, as formulated in the DSM-IV,[11] or psychophysiologic insomnia, as formulated in the ICSD,[12] and insomnia related to a mental disorder, particularly mild or subclinical mood disorders.[6] Thus, persistent insomnia is a known risk factor for the subsequent onset of new cases of major depression both in middle-aged and elderly individuals.[2, 3] There is, moreover, a high prevalence of insomnia complaints in the elderly, which persist if left untreated.[13] Longitudinal fluctuation in sleep complaints, especially sleep continuity disturbance and early morning awakening, in community-residing elderly people covaries with the intensity of depressive symptoms after controlling for health status, gender, and age.[14] Sleep disturbances in older men and women have also been linked to poor health, depression, angina, limitations in activities of daily living, and the chronic use of benzodiazepines.[15] Persistent sleep disturbance in elderly patients with prior depressive episodes augurs a less successful long-term response to either pharmacotherapy with nortriptyline or to interpersonal psychotherapy.[16, 17] In summary, both epidemiological and controlled clinical intervention studies indicate a strong bidirectional relationship between chronic insomnia and depressive symptoms and illness. This relationship between insomnia and depression is further underscored by the prevalent clinical practice of prescribing sedating antidepressants in low doses for chronic insomnia. Clinician concerns about benzodiazepine dependence had led, over a 5-year period, to a 30% decrease in benzodiazepine prescription and a 100% increase in the use of antidepressants as hypnotics, despite the absence of efficacy from controlled trials.[18]

ILLUSTRATION OF A CONCEPTUAL AND EMPIRICAL APPROACH TO PSYCHOMETRIC AND PSYCHIATRIC EVALUATION

Our meta-analysis and review of 30 y of clinical trials outcomes research in chronic insomnia indicate that there is no established consensus in the field for defining improvement in response to treatment.[19, 20] As defined in DSM-IV, primary insomnia is not only a chronic problem. It is literally a 24-h problem, affecting vocational and social roles and impairing quality of life in multiple domains. Thus, in an open pilot study of paroxetine for the treatment of primary insomnia,[21] we examined directional changes in several different outcome domains reflected in the DSM-IV diagnostic criteria: not only subjective sleep quality and quantity but also daytime well-being and daytime functioning, global improvement, and nocturnal PSG measures. Pertinent to the current discussion, 6 of 15 pilot subjects had a history of major depression, and 9 had been prescribed antidepressants (usually sedating antidepressants in low dose). The diagnosis of primary insomnia was established through the use of a structured sleep interview for DSM-IV, modeled after the Structured Clinical Interview for DSM-IV Axis I Disorders,[22] as well as nocturnal, laboratory-based PSG performed in order to rule out concurrent sleep-disordered breathing and periodic limb movement disorder. The level of concurrent depressive symptoms was measured via the rater-administered Hamilton Rating Scale for Depression,[23] and anxiety symptoms were assessed via the self-report Brief Symptom Inventory.[24] Subjective sleep quality was measured using the Pittsburgh Sleep Quality Index,[25] and daytime well-being was measured via the self-report Profile of Mood States.[26] Overall functioning (mental and physical) was measured using the Medical Outcomes Survey-SF36,[27] the Sickness Impact Profile,[28] and the Clinical Global Improvement (CGI) Rating Scale.[29] On the primary outcome, the CGI, 11 of 15 pilot subjects were rated as "very much improved," or "much improved." Seven of 14 treatment completers

no longer met DSM-IV criteria for primary insomnia at the end of 6 weeks of treatment with a modal dose of 20 mg of paroxetine daily at hour of sleep. Because patients with chronic insomnia are in a high risk group for depression, paroxetine used in doses and for durations consistent with antidepressant treatment may serve as a useful intervention strategy for persistent insomnia as well as a preventative strategy for depression. A randomized, placebo-controlled clinical trial is currently under way in our laboratory to confirm and extend these preliminary findings.

This pilot study illustrates a conceptually and empirically based approach to the selection of measures for psychometric and psychiatric evaluation that is criterion-driven and useful in clinical practice. The outcome measures chosen reflect the constructs embedded in the DSM-IV's diagnostic criteria for primary insomnia: sleep quality and quantity (criterion A) and daytime well-being and function (criterion B). Hence, clinicians can define *response* as the patient no long meeting diagnostic criteria for primary insomnia or by a finding of "much improved" or "very much improved" on the CGI. "Sleep quality" can be conveniently measured with the Pittsburgh Sleep Quality Index,[25] on which a score of 5 or greater has been found to reliably predict the presence of a clinical sleep disorder such as primary insomnia.

Sleep quantity can be measured through diary- or laboratory-based measures of sleep onset latency, wakefulness after sleep onset, or total sleep time.[30] Daytime well-being can be conveniently measured by a self-report inventory, the Profile of Mood States.[26] Finally, daytime functioning and well-being can be captured through the use of the MOS-SF36[27] (Medical Outcome Survey—Short Form 36) and the Sickness Impact Profile,[31] allowing comparison with other chronic illnesses.

One other pertinent domain may be neuropsychological performance. A study of neuropsychological performance in elderly insomnia patients has shown that subjective sleep disturbance (sleep diary) was related to impaired performance on tests of vigilance, psychomotor speed, recall memory, and executive function, whereas objective sleep disturbance was related to impaired word-list retention.[32] If clinically indicated, therefore, neuropsychological evaluation of attention, memory, and reaction time should be assessed pre- and post-treatment using appropriate tests, such as the word-list memory task, Trails A and B, digit-symbol substitution, the Stroop test, tasks of divided attention, and speed of cognitive processing.

OVERVIEW OF ASSESSMENT TOOLS

Although progress has been made in nosological specificity and epidemiological description of symptom clusters, research is needed to delineate evidence-based guidelines for the assessment of psychiatric syndromes in sleep disorders and the role of psychometric assessment in clinical practice. There continues to be some controversy regarding insomnia as a symptom as opposed to a syndrome and whether clinical evaluation suffices for diagnosis or whether physiological and psychometric assessment is necessary.[33] The ICSD[12] and the DSM-IV[11] use clinical assessment alone to establish the diagnosis of primary and psychiatric insomnia. The research cited earlier would suggest that structured psychiatric and sleep interviewing would likely improve the reliability of psychiatric sleep diagnosis. However, the use of including such structured interviews in clinical practice, (e.g., the impact on treatment outcome) has not been established. Furthermore, although there exists a structured interview for sleep disorders compatible with the DSM-III-R,[34] there do not exist interviews for the DSM-IV or ICSD. Probe questions around negative conditioning and poor sleep hygiene may be helpful in distinguishing primary from psychiatric insomnia,[9] but standardizing the constructs of negative conditioning and poor sleep hygiene remains to be accomplished. The scale published by Lacks and Rotert[35] may be a first step in that direction. While the Minnesota Multiphasic Personality Inventory[36] has been used to describe patients with chronic insomnia, its use in clinical practice may be limited by its length and scoring requirements. In the absence of diagnostic interviews, rating scales may provide a quantification of symptom severity and serve to inform clinical diagnosis or track treatment changes. Table 108–1 lists the measures described in this chapter, which may be useful in assessment or in quantifying outcome.

In summary, we believe that the approach taken in the earlier example illustrates a conceptually sound and empirically useful approach to the psychometric and psychiatric evaluation component of the assessment and treatment of patients with chronic insomnia disorders.

Table 108–1. USEFUL ASSESSMENT INSTRUMENTS IN THE PSYCHOMETRIC AND PSYCHIATRIC EVALUATION OF PATIENTS WITH SLEEP COMPLAINTS

Instrument	Domain
Sleep-Specific Instruments	
Structured Sleep Disorders Interview[4]	DSM-III-R sleep diagnoses
Pittsburgh Sleep Quality Index[25]	Subjective sleep quality
Pittsburgh Sleep Diary[30]	Self-reported sleep continuity
Sleep Hygiene Awareness and Practices Scale[35]	Sleep hygiene
General Instruments	
Structured Interview for DSM-IV[6, 9, 19]	DSM-IV psychiatric diagnoses
Hamilton Scale for Depression[23]	Depressive symptoms
Brief Symptom Inventory[24]	Distress
Medical Outcomes SF-36[27]	Health-related quality of life
Sickness Impact Profile[31]	Health-related quality of life
Profile of Mood State[26]	Daytime well-being

DSM-III-R, *Diagnostic and Statistical Manual of Mental Disorders, Revised Third Edition*; DSM-IV, *Diagnostic and Statistical Manual of Mental Disorders, Fourth Edition*.

References

1. Nofzinger EA, Buysse DJ, Reynolds CF, et al. Sleep disorders related to another mental disorder (nonsubstance/primary): a DSM-IV literature review [review]. J Clin Psychiatry. 1993;54:244–255.
2. Ford DE, Kamerow DB. Epidemiologic study of sleep disturbances and psychiatric disorders. An opportunity for prevention? [see comments]. JAMA. 1989;262:1479–1484.
3. Breslau N, Roth T, Rosenthal L, et al. Sleep disturbance and psychiatric disorders: a longitudinal epidemiological study of young adults. Biol Psychiatry. 1996; 39:411–418.
4. Schramm E, Hohagen F, Kappler C, et al. Mental comorbidity of chronic insomnia in general practice attenders using DSM-III-R. Acta Psychiatr Scand. 1995;91:10–17.
5. Ohayon MM. Prevalence of DSM-IV diagnostic criteria of insomnia: distinguishing insomnia related to mental disorders from sleep disorders. J Psychiatr Res. 1997;31:333–346.
6. Buysse DJ, Reynolds CF, Kupfer DJ, et al. Clinical diagnoses in 216 insomnia patients using the International Classification of Sleep Disorders (ICSD), DSM-IV and ICD-10 categories: a report from the APA/NIMH DSM-IV Field Trial. Sleep. 1994;17:630–637.
7. Buysse DJ, Reynolds CF, Kupfer DJ, et al. Effects of diagnosis on treatment recommendations in chronic insomnia—a report from the APA/NIMH DSM-IV Field Trial. Sleep. 1997;20:542–552.
8. Zucconi M, Ferini-Strambi L, Gambini O, et al. Structured psychiatric interview and ambulatory sleep monitoring in young psychophysiological insomniacs. J Clin Psychiatry. 1996; 57:364–370.
9. Nowell PD, Buysse DJ, Reynolds CF, et al. Clinical factors contributing to the differential diagnosis of primary insomnia and insomnia related to mental disorders. Am J Psychiatry. 1997;154:1412–1415.
10. Kupfer DJ, Reynolds CF. Management of insomnia. N Engl J Med. 1997;336:341–346.
11. American Psychiatric Association. Diagnostic and Statistical Manual of Mental Disorders. 4th ed. Washington, DC: American Psychiatric Association; 1994.
12. Diagnostic Classification Steering Committee. International Classification of Sleep Disorders: Diagnostic and Coding Manual. Rochester, Minn: American Sleep Disorders Association; 1990.
13. Ganguli M, Reynolds CF, Gilby JE. Prevalence and persistence of sleep complaints in a rural older community sample: the MoVIES Project. J Am Geriatr Soc. 1996;44:778–784.
14. Rodin J, McAvay G, Timko C. Depressed mood and sleep disturbances in the elderly: a longitudinal study. J Gerontol. 1988;43:45–52.
15. Newman AB, Enright PL, Manolio TA, et al. Sleep disturbance, psychosocial correlates, and cardiovascular disease in 5201 older adults: the Cardiovascular Health Study. J Am Geriatr Soc. 1997;45:1–7.
16. Buysse DJ, Reynolds CF, Hoch CC, et al. Longitudinal effects of nortriptyline on EEG sleep and the likelihood of recurrence in elderly depressed patients. Neuropsychopharmacology. 1996; 14:243–252.
17. Reynolds CF, Frank E, Houck PR, et al. Which remitted elderly depressed patients benefit from continued interpersonal psychotherapy after discontinuation of antidepressant medication? Am J Psychiatry. 1997;154:958–962.
18. Walsh JK, Engelhardt CL. Trends in the pharmacologic treatment of insomnia [see comments]. J Clin Psychiatry. 1992;53(suppl):10–17.
19. Nowell PD, Buysse DJ, Morin CM, et al. Effective treatments for selected DSM-IV sleep disorders. In: Nathan PE, Gorman JM, eds. A Guide to Treatments That Work. New York, NY: Oxford University Press; 1998:531–543.
20. Nowell PD, Mazumdar S, Buysse DJ, et al. Benzodiazepines and zolpidem for chronic insomnia: a meta-analysis of treatment efficacy. JAMA. 1997:278:2170–2177.
21. Nowell PD, Buysse DJ, Dew MA, et al. Paroxetine in the treatment of primary insomnia: preliminary clinical and electroencephalogram sleep data. J Clin Psychiatry. 1999;60:89–95.
22. First M, Spitzer RL, Gibbon M, et al. Structured Clinical Interview for DSM-IV Axis I Disorders—Patient Edition (SCID-T/P). Version 2.0. New York, NY: New York State Psychiatric Institute, 1995.

23. Hamilton M. Development of a rating scale for primary depressive illness. Br J Soc Clin Psychol. 1967;6:278–296.
24. Derogatis LR, Melisaratos N. The Brief Symptom Inventory: an introductory report. Psychol Med. 1983;13:595–605.
25. Buysse DJ, Reynolds CF, Monk TH, et al. The Pittsburgh Sleep Quality Index (PSQI): a new instrument for psychiatric research and practice. Psychiatry Res. 1989;28:193–213.
26. McNair DM, Lorr M, Droppleman LF. Profile of Mood States. San Diego, Calif: Educational and Industrial Testing Service; 1971.
27. McHorney CA, Ware JE Jr, Raczek AE. The MOS 36-item short-form health survey (SF-36), II: psychometric and clinical tests of validity in measuring physical and mental health constructs. Med Care. 1993; 31:247–263.
28. deBruin AF, Diederiks JP, deWitte LP, et al. Assessing the responsiveness of a functional status measure: the Sickness Impact Profile versus the SIP68 [review]. J Clin Epidemiol. 1997;50:529–540.
29. Guy W. ECDEU Assessment Manual for Psychopharmacology, Revised Edition. Rockville, Md: US Dept of Health, Education, and Welfare, Public Health Service, Alcohol, Drug Abuse, and Mental Health Administration, National Institute of Mental Health, Psychopharmacology Research Branch, Division of Extramural Research Programs; 1976.
30. Monk TH, Reynolds CF, Kupfer DJ, et al. The Pittsburgh Sleep Diary (PghSD). J Sleep Res. 1994;3:111–120.
31. de Bruin AF, de Witte LP, Stevens F, et al. Sickness Impact Profile: the state of the art of a generic functional status measure. Soc Sci Med. 1992;35:1003–1014.
32. Hart RP, Morin CM, Best AM. Neuropsychological performance in elderly insomniac patients. Aging Cogn. 1995; 2:268–278.
33. Standards of Practice Committee of the American Sleep Disorders Association. Practice parameters for the use of polysomnography in the evaluation of insomnia. Sleep. 1995;18:55–57.
34. Schramm E, Hohagen F, Grasshoff U, et al. Test-retest reliability and validity of the Structured Interview for Sleep Disorders according to DSM-III-R. Am J Psychiatry. 1993;150:867–872.
35. Lacks P, Rotert M. Knowledge and practice of sleep hygiene techniques in insomniacs and good sleepers. Behav Res Ther. 1986;24:365–368.
36. Kales A, Caldwell AB, Soldatos CR, et al. Biopsychobehavioral correlates of insomnia, II: pattern specificity and consistency with the Minnesota Multiphasic Personality Inventory. Psychosom Med. 1983;45:341–356.

109

Actigraphy

Sonia Ancoli-Israel

The gold standard for the evaluation of sleep is polysomnography (PSG) with a minimum of electroencephalographic (EEG), electrooculographic (EOG), and submentalis electromyographic (EMG) recordings. Other physiological variables are added depending on the patient's sleep complaints (such as respiration, heart rate, tibialis muscle movement, oximetry). A PSG therefore allows for the collection of detailed information. The EEG, EOG, and EMG records can be scored for stages of sleep (nonrapid eye movement [NREM] stages 1 to 4, rapid eye movement [REM]), total sleep time, total wake time, sleep onset latency, and percent time in REM versus NREM sleep.

This information is very important for certain types of evaluations; however, the recording process may disturb a patient's sleep and often is very costly both to record and to score. In addition, the PSG typically provides data about sleep episodes during the time of recording, which often is 6 to 10 h. Because recordings are usually made during the major sleep period, little information is available about daytime (waking) or napping behavior. There are some instances in which it is not essential to know the specific stage of sleep or the status of other physiological variables; only information on whether the person is awake or asleep is necessary.

New technological methods that are much less expensive than a PSG allow for 24-h recordings of activity from which wake and sleep can be scored. These devices are called *actigraphs* (or *actimeters*), and they usually record limb movement. Traditionally, the actigraphs are placed on a wrist, although sometimes activity from the leg is recorded. The data collected are displayed on a computer and are examined for activity versus inactivity and analyzed for wake versus sleep.

Wrist activity technology is based on the fact that during sleep, there is little movement, whereas during wakefulness, there is increased movement. Although activity monitors had been around for many years,[1] Kupfer et al.,[2] McPartland et al.,[3] Colburn et al.,[4] and Kripke et al.[5] were among the first to use activity to differentiate wake from sleep. The initial models were developed in the early 1970s by Kupfer and colleagues and were self-contained activity counters with integrated circuits and memory that provided off-line data retrieval.[2, 3] At about the same time, Colburn et al.[4] developed a similar actigraph with different transducers and timing devices. Kripke and colleagues were among the first to publish reliability data on the use of

wrist actigraphy for the assessment of sleep.[5–8] Several years later, other actigraphs were developed by Redmond and Hegge[9] and Borbély.[10, 11] The analog actigraphs were small but used telemetry or had to be attached to a Medilog recorder and were scored by hand. The first digital actigraphs were about half the size of a chalkboard eraser, and computer algorithms were written for automatic scoring of sleep and wake.

With the advent of microprocessors and miniaturization, most contemporary actigraphs have a movement detector (such as an accelerometer) and sufficient memory to record for long time periods. Newer models are the size of a wristwatch and collect digitized data. Physical movement is generally sampled several times per second and stored in 1-min epochs, although sampling and epoch rates often can be set by the clinician or investigator. The digitized data are then translated into a numeric representation and stored until downloaded to a computer. Computer algorithms have been written to automatically score wake and sleep and to provide the user with summary statistics. These computer algorithms generally supply information on total sleep time, percent of time spent asleep, total wake time, percent of time spent awake, number of awakenings, time between awakenings, and sleep onset latency.[7] The only time the actigraph must be removed is during bathing or swimming (although some of the newer models are water resistant), thus allowing for nearly continuous 24-h recordings for several days or weeks.

The use of actigraphy in sleep disorders medicine has gained popularity. Researchers have examined the reliability of actigraphy versus EEG for distinguishing wake from sleep; results vary depending on the populations studied. Most researchers agree that actigraphy correlates well with PSG data, particularly in normal sleep, where reliability coefficients have ranged from 0.89 to 0.98.[5, 12, 13] Correlations are somewhat lower for severely disturbed sleep. For example, in sleep disorders clinic patients, reliability ranged from 0.78 to 0.88.[14–16] In infants and children, reliability ranged from 0.90 to 0.95.[17, 18] Although total sleep time correlates well with EEG, the actigraph data do not necessarily correlate well on a minute-by-minute basis, particularly if sleep is very disturbed.

Ancoli-Israel et al.[19] compared actigraphy with sleep and wake EEG in nursing home patients with dementia. Correlations with total sleep time were 0.91 for averaged activity (the average activity recorded per minute) and 0.81 for maximum activity (the maximum activity recorded per minute). Given the problems with obtaining EEG recordings in this population, the authors concluded that actigraphy is the more feasible approach to the study of wakefulness and sleep in patients with dementia.

Most studies are in agreement that with the correct use, the actigraph is reliable for certain populations. Actigraphs with different algorithms are available commercially; therefore, reliability has become a major concern. Each actigraph must have reliability studies, and results from one population may not generalize to other populations, although Cole et al.[12] concluded that even algorithms based on different mathematical principles resulted in similar reliability. In a review of actigraphy, Sadeh et al.[20] concluded that the validation studies for normal subjects show greater than 90% agreement and are very promising.

Wrist actigraphy records continuously for long periods of time, so behavior occurring during both night and day can be studied. For example, the collection of nighttime and daytime information for long time periods is particularly useful when examining the sleep of patients who claim to have insomnia. It economically allows the clinician to determine whether there is a pattern of difficulty in sleeping. The sleep of patients with complaints of insomnia can vary from night to night and is easily disturbed by novel environments. The actigraph therefore has the potential of being well suited for the examination of sleep over several nights in the patient's home environment. Compared with a sleep diary, the resulting data are similar, but superior, because the data are continuous and objective rather than discrete and subjective.

Another advantage of collecting data over long periods of time is the ability to examine the circadian rhythms of the sleep or activity cycle, particularly in studies of patients with sleep-wake schedule disorders (such as jet lag, shift work, and advanced or delayed sleep phase). Cosinor analyses, including the computation of the mesor, the amplitude, and the acrophase, are possible. These analyses can be computed from 24 h of data, but a longer recording provides more accurate cosinor analyses.

The wrist actigraph may be particularly valuable for studying individuals who would have difficulty sleeping in a sleep laboratory or with the wires associated with traditional PSG, such as insomniacs, children, and the elderly with dementia. With actigraphy, patients are studied in their natural environment. In the elderly with dementia, it has been shown that the traditional recording process disturbs sleep. In addition, the EEG in the elderly with dementia often makes it difficult to distinguish wake from sleep.[21] The use of actigraphy avoids both of these problems and enables the recording of sleep-wake activity in an easy, unobtrusive manner.

Some actigraphs record both activity and light exposure (for example, the Actillume by Ambulatory Monitoring, Inc., or the Actiwatch-L by Mini-Mitter Co., Inc.). Some devices also have the ability to record core body temperature; this allows both clinical and investigational studies of circadian rhythms in the home environment. Most actigraphs have event buttons that the subject can push when he or she turns out the lights or needs to note other events.

The addition of a concurrent recording of light by an actigraph is particularly useful in determining "lights out," as well as in observing the beginning of morning light as the sun begins to rise. Light measurements are also very helpful in studies of advanced and delayed sleep phase because they help determine the amount and duration of light to which a person is normally exposed. For example, several studies with activity monitors that also record light exposure found that the normal healthy elderly are exposed to only 58 min of bright light per day,[22] that patients with Alzheimer's disease who live at home are exposed to 30 min of bright light a day,[23] and that nursing home patients are exposed to only 1.7 min of bright light per day.[24] These data are useful in understanding the changes that occur in sleep in these populations and can be used to devise treatment programs.

There still are many unknowns about how the environment affects activity recordings. Sadeh et al.[20] suggest that the bed surface (for example, a waterbed) and the presence of a bedpartner may affect the activity signal. Additional research is needed in these areas.

APPLICATIONS OF WRIST ACTIGRAPHY

The American Sleep Disorders Association published recommendations on the use of actigraphy in the clinical assessment of sleep disorders.[25] They concluded that in some instances, actigraphy is a useful adjunct to a detailed history and physical examination, when multiple days of sleep-wake activity patterns are necessary to diagnose sleep disorders, or in the evaluation of the efficacy of treatment. Actigraphy is not recommended for the routine diagnosis of insomnia, sleep apnea, or periodic limb movements in sleep (PLMS).

A complete description of studies using actigraphy is given by Sadeh et al.[20] and is not repeated here. However, a few examples of the application of wrist actigraphy to sleep disorders medicine are described.

Insomnia

Researchers have examined the use of actigraphy in the study of insomnia. Although actigraphy cannot be used to determine the cause of insomnia, it can help in evaluation of the severity. In patients with insomnia, the most difficult distinctions for the actigraph to recognize are the transitions between sleep and wake and the ultrashort sleep-wake cycles. Hauri and Wisbey[14] found that actigraphy overestimates sleep in patients with psychophysiological insomnia and in those with insomnia secondary to a psychiatric illness. In patients with sleep state misconception, the actigraph was either very accurate or underestimated sleep. Hauri and Wisbey[14] concluded that although the actigraph is not a replacement for a PSG, it provides the ability to record for multiple nights and to supply information about daytime behavior. The key is not in the actual minutes of sleep but rather in the pattern of disturbance.

In a study of older patients with insomnia versus older control subjects, Pollak et al.[26] monitored wrist movements. They found that activity among patients with insomnia during periods of bedrest was almost double that of the control subjects. Furthermore, their activity levels during out-of-bed periods were significantly lower and the 24-h daily rest–activity pattern (i.e., circadian rhythm) was flatter than that of control subjects. By being able to record for 24-h periods, the authors were able to determine that sleep was more diffusely distributed over the day and night in the insomniacs.

Sleep Apnea

Wrist actigraphy can also be used to study patients with specific sleep disorders. Several studies have been conducted on the efficacy of wrist actigraphy in recognizing patients with sleep apnea, with some conflicting results.

Aubert-Tulkens et al.[27] used wrist actigraphy to measure movement index and fragmentation index during sleep in patients with sleep apnea compared with control subjects. Those with sleep apnea had significantly higher movement and fragmentation indices. Once treatment was begun, activity recordings showed decreased indices, indicating successful treatment. Sadeh et al.[17] also found that activity measures of sleep differentiated patients with sleep apnea from those with insomnia and from control subjects.

Middlekoop et al.[28] conducted an epidemiological study of 116 subjects who reported snoring habitually, experienced excessive daytime sleepiness, and/or had a spousal report of respiratory cessations. Both wrist activity and respiration (oronasal thermistry) were recorded for one night in the subject's home. Results indicated that patients with an apnea index of more than five events per hour of sleep had higher movement and higher fragmentation indices that those with an apnea index of less than five. However, measures of activity failed to reliably predict who had sleep apnea.

Additional research is needed to determine whether actigraphy is a viable method for screening and for following treated patients with sleep apnea.

Some types of recording equipment that are used to screen for sleep apnea do not have measures of wake or sleep. The addition of an actigraph to such a recording would add this information and allow the determination of whether all respiratory events actually occurred during sleep.

Periodic Limb Movements in Sleep

PLMS is generally evaluated by measuring the EMG at the tibialis muscle. Kazenwadel et al.[29] found a high reliability between tibialis EMG and actigraphy for the number of leg movements per hour of sleep. Because PLMS can greatly vary from night to night, actigraphy

gave a better assessment because multiple nights could be easily recorded.

Treatment Effects

Pieta et al.[29a] used ankle actigraphy as well as anterior tibialis EMG to document leg movements in uremic patients being treated with pergolide. In a study of insomnia in older adults, Brooks et al.[15] used actigraphy to examine the treatment effects of sleep restriction therapy and found the actigraph sufficiently sensitive to detect effects of therapy. The authors concluded that because actigraphy is less invasive and less expensive than PSG, it is a promising device for the assessment of treatment effects. In a critical evaluation of actigraphy, Chambers[30] also concluded that because actigraphy measures are reliable night to night, they are especially appropriate for assessing changes in sleep secondary to treatment. Others have used actigraphy to measure the treatment effects of nicotine replacement on sleep and daytime activity[31] and the effects of drugs on sleep.[32–34] These data suggest that actigraphy can be used as a screening device in some patients, before the more expensive PSG is ordered. It also may have a role in follow-up.

Circadian Rhythms

Actigraphy allows the study of rhythms occurring over many days; it therefore is well suited for the study of circadian rhythms. Mormont et al.[35] used actigraphy to study circadian rhythms and sleep-wake cycles in patients with cancer, as a preliminary step toward the advancement of chronotherapy. Studies have also been performed that examined the sleep schedules of adolescents,[36] shift workers,[37, 38] in-flight crews,[39] and persons with jet lag.[32]

Pediatrics

Sadeh[40] used wrist activity to study the treatment effects on the sleep patterns of 50 infants whose parents complained of sleep disturbances in their children. Objective activity recordings were compared with parental reports. The activity records showed that percent sleep increased and the number of awakenings during the night decreased with behavioral treatments. By examining data from each successive night, Sadeh determined that most changes occurred during the first night of intervention. In addition, parental subjective reports significantly differed from objective actigraphy on quality of sleep, with parents reporting fewer awakenings during the night. The presence of objective measures allows for the evaluation of activity during sleep that would otherwise be missed by observation alone.

Elderly

At the other end of the age spectrum, actigraphy has been used to study sleep-wake patterns of the elderly. The elderly are particularly susceptible to sleep complaints secondary to circadian rhythm changes, sleep disordered breathing, PLMS, medical illness, and medication use.[41] Although some of these complaints may be examined in the laboratory, the elderly are often more set in their ways, need to stay home to take care of a spouse, or just find it more comfortable to sleep in their own beds.

van Hilten et al.[42] examined the influence of age on nocturnal behavior in 100 healthy older adults who wore an activity monitor for 6 consecutive days and nights. The authors concluded that without illness, age itself has only marginal effects on nocturnal activity and immobility (that is, sleep and wake). This type of study could not have been done in the laboratory without an isolation unit, and even then it is unlikely that 100 subjects could have been studied. The only way this type of large-scale study could have been accomplished was with the use of actigraphy.

In the same group of subjects, van Hilten et al.[43] also examined the night-to-night variability and intrasubject variability of activity. Results indicated that there was no "first night effect," typical of laboratory sleep studies (data from the first night did not differ from that of subsequent nights and was rather stable from night to night). Similarly, Jean-Louis et al.[44] found no first night effect with actigraphy in younger subjects. These results suggested that unlike the traditional laboratory studies, subjects do not need time to adapt to the activity monitor.

With the use of actigraphy, Ancoli-Israel and colleagues[45–47] have shown that sleep in nursing home patients is extremely fragmented, with most patients never sleeping for a full hour and never awake for a full hour throughout the 24-h day. These data led to ongoing studies of treatment to improve the sleep quality and quantity in this group of patients.

Schizophrenia

Martin et al.[48, 49] studied the 24-h sleep-wake patterns of 28 older patients with schizophrenia (mean age, 58 years). In general, the patients slept for only 67% of the night and napped for 9% of the day. Patients taking neuroleptic medications were significantly sleepier both at night and during the day. Wirz-Justice et al.[50] used actigraphy to examine the rest–activity cycle of a patient with schizophrenia. By recording wrist activity for 220 days, they were able to determine that under stable haloperidol treatment, the patient had an arrhythmic rest-activity cycle. When treatment was switched to clozapine, the circadian rhythmicity improved.

Epidemiological Studies of Sleep

Actigraphy is useful in the study of sleep in large populations, particularly when recording in the laboratory might be cost prohibitive and might jeopardize the compliance rate of subjects. Ancoli-Israel, Kripke,

and their colleagues[51–53] used actigraphy to determine wake and sleep patterns in large samples of elderly (sample size, 426) and middle-aged adults (sample size, 355). Measurements were used to determine the prevalence of sleep apnea and PLMS (which were recorded with additional sensors). Many of these volunteers would have been less willing to participate if they had been required to sleep in the laboratory.

TRICKS OF THE TRADE

Actigraphs are traditionally placed on the wrist of the nondominant hand, but two groups of investigators have shown that either wrist can be used. Sadeh et al.[18] compared data from both wrists and found that although activity levels differed between the two hands, agreement rates with PSG were essentially the same for data collected from both hands. Chung et al.[54] reported similar results. In studies on infants, actigraphs have also been placed on the legs.[55]

Most actigraphs have bands that are similar to plastic watch bands. For individuals who are sensitive to such bands or who find it uncomfortable to wear them for long time periods, bands made of terry cloth and Velcro can be sewed. Figure 109–1 illustrates the type of band used in our laboratory to study elderly nursing home patients with dementia. To discourage patients from removing the bands, the two Velcro straps were reversed, with one opening from right to left and the other opening from left to right. This has worked to keep even the most diligent patient from removing the band; this technique also works with young children.

Patients wearing actigraphs should be asked to keep a actigraph log in which they note information about daily time to bed, time out of bed, and any unusual activity or times when the device is removed (such as for showers or swimming). This information is extremely helpful for editing and analyzing the data.

When data are collected in 1-min epochs, collected for more than 1 week, it is prudent to download data every week to minimize data loss. Battery levels should be checked when initializing the device and again during downloading. Batteries with levels of less than 90% of the original battery voltage should be discarded because they are likely to fail. The battery life is approximately 30 days. In our laboratory, a battery log is kept that records the battery number, date activity monitor was initialized, date the data were downloaded, total number of days the battery had been used, and the starting and ending battery levels.

With devices that also record light, it is extremely important that the light sensor not be covered by the person's sleeve. The sleeve can be tucked under the actigraph or pinned up to ensure it does not occlude the light sensor. It is important to note that because the angle of the wrist differs from the angle of the eye, the lux reading from a light sensor may differ from ambient illumination. Figure 109–2 shows the lux level during a light treatment session. Although a photometer reading at the level of the eye confirmed a reading of 2500 lux, the lux reading at the level of the wrist

Actillume Band (Inside)

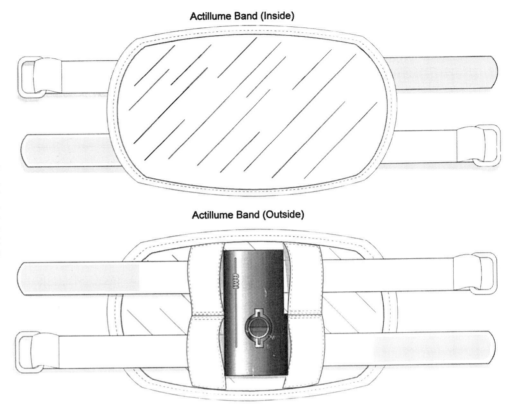

Figure 109-1. Diagram of a terrycloth band that can be sewn for use with the Actillume. This band is used at the laboratory of the author in the study of sleep in nursing home patients with dementia who have extremely fragile and delicate skin. Note that the straps are reversed to make removal more difficult.

Actillume Band (Outside)

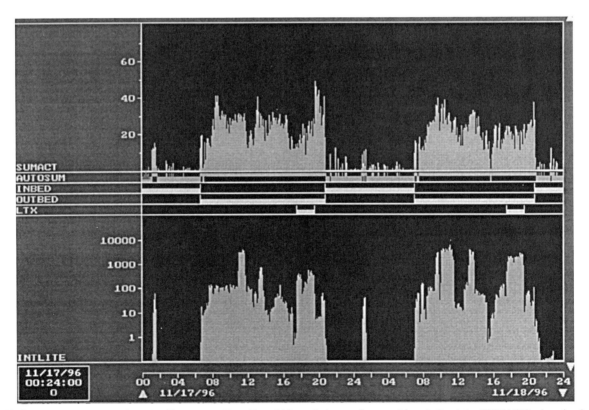

Figure 109-2. Action3 printout of an Actillume recording. Two 24-h periods are shown with activity data (SUMACT), sleep/wake scoring (AUTOSUM), in-bed/out-of-bed (INBED/OUTBED), light treatment intervals (LTX), and light exposure (INTLITE).

was lower. Some devices have external light sensors in addition to the internal sensor that can be clipped to a collar and might provide more exact readings. All activity and light monitors should be checked on a regular basis to determine whether calibration is needed.

In patients with sensitive skin, the bands can be removed for a few minutes each day to avoid pressure sores. The time the device is removed, the time it is replaced, and whether the person was awake for the few minutes it was removed should be noted on the log. This information is needed during the data-editing process.

EDITING ACTIGRAPHY DATA

Different software packages are available for scoring the rest–activity data and inferring sleep-wake. Because the experience of our laboratory is with the Actillume recorder (Ambulatory Monitoring, Inc.) and the accompanying software, Action3 (Ambulatory Monitoring, Inc.), editing and scoring techniques with this device are reviewed.

Data are edited on a computer screen with the use of the daily sleep log. Time intervals during which the device is removed are automatically scored as sleep by the ACTION3 software program because there is no movement. Such time intervals can be manually changed to wake if the log indicates the person was involved in an activity in which he or she was obviously awake (while bathing). When also recording light exposure data, if the Actillume is removed but left in the same room as the subject, light data need not be edited. Lack of movement scored as sleep when the device was removed for especially vigorous activity can also be manually changed to wake. For example, Israel and Ancoli-Israel[56] recorded actigraphy in adolescents. Some subjects removed the Actillume during football or volleyball practice. No activity was recorded during that time period, but it was clear that the subjects were awake. If there is no information on the log about the activity during the time the device was removed, that time period should be scored as missing data.

Channels of information can also be added to the data. For example, interval channels with information about time in bed and time out of bed can be edited in, as can times of treatment intervals. An example is given of two 24-h periods with the activity data, sleep-wake scoring, and added interval channels (see Fig. 109–2).

SUMMARY

Wrist activity has the advantages of being cost efficient, allowing the recording of sleep in natural environments, recording behavior that occurs during both the night and the day, and recording for long time periods. Although not a replacement for EEG or PSG recordings, there are times when actigraphy provides clear advantages for data collection. Actigraphy is par-

ticularly useful for studying individuals who cannot tolerate sleeping in the laboratory; for example, patients with complaints of insomnia, small children, or the elderly. Actigraphy is also becoming an important tool in follow-up studies and for examining efficacy in clinical outcome.

Acknowledgments

Supported by NIA AG02711; NIA AG08415; the Sam and Rose Stein Institute for Research on Aging; the VA VISN-22 Mental Illness Research, Education and Clinical Center; and the Research Service of the Veterans Affairs San Diego Healthcare System.

References

1. Tryon WW. Activity Measurement in Psychology and Medicine. New York, NY: Plenum Press; 1991.
2. Kupfer DJ, Weiss BL, Foster FG, et al. Psychomotor activity in affective states. Arch Gen Psychiatry. 1974;30:765–768.
3. McPartland RJ, Kupfer DJ, Foster FG. The movement-activated recording monitor: third generation motor-activity monitoring system. Behav Res Methods Instrum. 1976;8:357–360.
4. Colburn TR, Smith BM, Cuarini JJ, et al. An ambulatory activity monitor with solid state memory. ISA Trans. 1976;15:149–154.
5. Kripke DF, Mullaney DJ, Messin S, et al. Wrist actigraphic measures of sleep and rhythms. Electroencephalogr Clin Neurophysiol. 1978;44:674–676.
6. Mullaney DJ, Kripke DF, Messin S. Wrist-actigraphic estimation of sleep time. Sleep. 1980;3:83–92.
7. Webster JB, Kripke DF, Messin S, et al. An activity-based sleep monitor system for ambulatory use. Sleep. 1982;5:389–399.
8. Webster JB, Messin S, Mullaney DJ, et al. Transducer design and placement for activity recording. Med Biol Eng Comput. 1982;20:741–744.
9. Redmond DP, Hegge FW. Observations on the design and specification of a wrist-worn human activity monitoring system. Behav Res Methods Instr Comput. 1985;17:659–669.
10. Borbély AA. Long-term recording of the rest-activity cycle in man, in Zbinden G, Cuomo V, Racagni G, et al, eds. Application of Behavioral Pharmacology in Toxicology. New York, NY: Raven Press; 1983:39–44.
11. Borbély AA. New techniques for the analysis of the human sleep-wake cycle. Brain Dev. 1986;8:482–488.
12. Cole RJ, Kripke DF, Gruen W, et al. Automatic sleep/wake identification from wrist activity. Sleep. 1992;15:461–469.
13. Jean-Louis G, von Gizycki H, Zizi F, et al. Determination of sleep and wakefulness with the Actigraph Data Analysis Software (ADAS). Sleep. 1996;19:739–743.
14. Hauri PJ, Wisbey J. Wrist actigraphy in insomnia. Sleep. 1992;15:293–301.
15. Brooks JO, Friedman L, Bliwise DL, et al. Use of the wrist actigraph to study insomnia in older adults. Sleep. 1993;16:151–155.
16. Verbeek I, Arends J, Declerck G, et al. Wrist actigraphy in comparison with polysomnography and subjective evaluation in insomnia, in Coenen AML, ed. Sleep-Wake Research in The Netherlands. Leiden, The Netherlands: Dutch Society for Sleep-Wake Research; 1994:163–170.
17. Sadeh A, Alster J, Urbach D, et al. Actigraphically based automatic bedtime sleep-wake scoring: validity and clinical applications. J Ambul Monit. 1989;2:209–216.
18. Sadeh A, Sharkey KM, Carskadon MA. Activity-based sleep-wake identification: an empirical test of methodological issues. Sleep. 1994;17:201–207.
19. Ancoli-Israel S, Mason WJ, Clopton P, et al. Use of wrist activity for monitoring sleep/wake in demented nursing home patients. Sleep. 1997;20:24–27.
20. Sadeh A, Hauri PJ, Kripke DF, et al. The role of actigraphy in the evaluation of sleep disorders. Sleep. 1995;18:288–302.
21. Bliwise DL. Review: sleep in normal aging and dementia. Sleep. 1993;16:40–81.

22. Espiritu RC, Kripke DF, Ancoli-Israel S, et al. Low illumination by San Diego adults: association with atypical depressive symptoms. Biol Psychiatry. 1994;35:403–407.

23. Campbell SS, Kripke DF, Gillin JC, et al. Exposure to light in healthy elderly subjects and Alzheimer's patients. Physiol Behav. 1988;42:141–144.

24. Ancoli-Israel S, Kripke DF. Now I lay me down to sleep: the problem of sleep fragmentation in elderly and demented residents of nursing homes. Bull Clin Neurosci. 1989;54:127–132.

25. Standards of Practice Committee. An American Sleep Disorders Association report: practice parameters for the use of actigraphy in the clinical assessment of sleep Disorders. Sleep. 1995;18:285–287.

26. Pollak CP, Perlick D, Linsner JP. Daily sleep reports and circadian rest-activity cycles of elderly community residents with insomnia. Biol Psychiatry. 1992;32:1019–1027.

27. Aubert-Tulkens G, Culee C, Rijckevorsel KH, et al. Ambulatory evaluation of sleep disturbance and therapeutic effects in sleep apnea syndrome by wrist activity monitoring. Am Rev Respir Dis. 1987;136:851–856.

28. Middlekoop HA, Knuistingh NA, van Hilten JJ, et al. Wrist actigraphic assessment of sleep in 116 community based subjects suspected of obstructive sleep apnoea syndrome. Thorax. 1995;50:284–289.

29. Kazenwadel J, Pollmacher T, Trenkwalder C, et al. New actigraphic assessment method for periodic leg movements (PLM). Sleep. 1995;18:689–697.

29a. Pieta J, Millar T, Zacharias J, et al. Effect of pergolide on restless legs and leg movements in sleep in uremic patients. Sleep. 1998;21:617–622.

30. Chambers MJ. Actigraphy and insomnia: a closer look: part I. Sleep. 1994;17:405–408.

31. Wolter TD, Hauri PJ, Schroeder DR, et al. Effects of 24-hr nicotine replacement on sleep and daytime activity during smoking cessation. Prev Med. 1996;25:601–610.

32. Lavie P. Effects of midazolam on sleep disturbances associated with westward and eastward flights: evidence for directional effects. Psychopharmacol (Berl). 1990;101:250–254.

33. Tirosh E, Lavie P, Sadeh A, et al. Effects of methylphenidate on sleep in children with attention-deficit hyperactivity disorder. Am J Dis Child. 1994;147:1313–1315.

34. Lavie P, Lorber M, Tzischinsky O, et al. Wrist actigraphic measurements in patients with rheumatoid arthritis: a novel method to assess drug efficacy. Drug Invest. 1992;2(suppl):15–21.

35. Mormont MC, De Prins J, Levi F. Assessment of activity rhythms by wrist actigraphy: preliminary results in 30 patients with colorectal cancer. Pathol Biol. 1996;44:165–171.

36. Carskadon M, Acebo C, Richardson GS, et al. An approach to studying circadian rhythms of adolescent humans. J Biol Rhythms. 1997;12:278–289.

37. Tzischinsky O, Epstein R, Lavie P. Sleep-wake cycles in rotating shift workers: comparison between 3- and 5-day shift system, in Costa G, Geaana G, Cogi K, et al, eds. Shift Work: Health Sleep and Performance. Frankfurt, Germany: Peter Lang; 1990:651–656.

38. Lavie P, Tzischinsky O, Epstein R, et al. Sleep-wake cycles in rotating shift work: effects of changing from phase advance to phase delay rotation. Isr J Med Sci. 1992;28:636–644.

39. Buck A, Tobler I, Borbely AA. Wrist activity monitoring in air crew members: a method for analyzing sleep quality following transmeridian and North-South flights. J Biol Rhythms. 1989;4:93–105.

40. Sadeh A. Assessment of intervention for infant night waking: parental reports and activity-based home monitoring. J Consult Clin Psychol. 1994;62:63–68.

41. Ancoli-Israel S. Sleep problems in older adults: putting myths to bed. Geriatrics. 1997;52:20–30.

42. van Hilten JJ, Middlekoop HA, Braat EA, et al. Nocturnal activity and immobility across aging (50–98 years) in healthy persons. J Am Geriatr Soc. 1993;41:837–841.

43. van Hilten JJ, Braat EAM, van der Velde EA, et al. Ambulatory activity monitoring during sleep: an evaluation of internight and intrasubject variability in healthy persons aged 50–98 years. Sleep. 1993;16:146–150.

44. Jean-Louis G, von Gizycki H, Zizi F, et al. The actigraph data analysis software, II: a novel approach to scoring and interpreting sleep-wake activity. Percept Motil Skills. 1997;85:219–226.

45. Ancoli-Israel S, Jones DW, Hanger MA, et al. Sleep in the nursing home, in Kuna ST, Suratt PM, Remmers JE, eds. Sleep and Respiration in Aging Adults. New York, NY: Elsevier Press; 1991:77–84.

46. Pat-Horenczyk R, Klauber MR, Shochat T, et al. Hourly profiles of sleep and wakefulness in severely versus mild-moderately demented nursing home patients. Aging Clin Exp Res. 1998;10:308–315.

47. Ancoli-Israel S, Parker L, Sinaee R, et al. Sleep fragmentation in patients from a nursing home. J Gerontol. 1989;44:M18–M21.

48. Martin J, Jones DW, Fell R, et al. 24-Hour sleep/wake patterns in late-life schizophrenia [abstract]. Sleep Res. 1995;24:169.

49. Martin J, Ancoli-Israel S, Bailey A, et al. Day and night sleep/wake patterns and neuroleptic use in older schizophrenia patients [abstract]. Sleep Res. 1996;25:167.

50. Wirz-Justice A, Cajochen C, Nussbaum P. A schizophrenic with an arrhythmic circadian rest-activity cycle. Psychiatry Res. 1997;73:83–90.

51. Ancoli-Israel S, Kripke DF, Klauber MR, et al. Sleep disordered breathing in community-dwelling elderly. Sleep. 1991;14:486–495.

52. Ancoli-Israel S, Kripke DF, Klauber MR, et al. Periodic limb movements in sleep in community-dwelling elderly. Sleep. 1991;14:496–500.

53. Kripke DF, Ancoli-Israel S, Klauber MR, et al. Prevalence of sleep disordered breathing in ages 40–64 years: A population-based survey. Sleep. 1997;20:65–76.

54. Chung L, Kripke DF, Ancoli-Israel S, et al. Dominant versus nondominant wrist movements during sleep [abstract]. Sleep Res. 1995;24A:80.

55. Gershoni-Baruch R, Epstein R, Tzischinsky O, et al. Actigraphic home-monitoring of the sleep pattern of in vitro fertilization children and their matched controls. Dev Med Child Neurol. 1994;36:639–645.

56. Israel SL, Ancoli-Israel S. Light exposure, sleep and delayed sleep phase in middle-school adolescents [abstract]. Sleep Res. 1997;26:159.

110

Computers in Sleep Medicine

Max Hirshkowitz

Constance A. Moore

Once a rarity in sleep disorders laboratories, computerized polysomnography (cPSG) is becoming commonplace. This is particularly the case in more recently opened sleep laboratories and older centers having undergone major renovation. In addition to a desire to be "high tech" and modern (computerization is the sin quo non of being modern and high tech), there are some real advantages to automation. However, there are also disadvantages. The ideal cPSG system would increase efficiency (by saving time and money), improve quality control (by providing greater accuracy and standardization), and provide innovation (by allowing data to be examined in new and useful ways). Unfortunately, the ideal system has yet to be developed; nonetheless, there are several competent approximations moving toward this ultimate goal. Interestingly, although the decision to computerize is often a foregone conclusion, the act of choosing one system over another is faced with great trepidation. Why? Because it is difficult to assess how a particular cPSG system will actually perform in day to day clinical routine. The clinician and laboratory administrator know why they do not want a standard paper polygraph system, but they are unsure if the cPSG replacement can meet their basic needs, let alone their further expectations.

It all began in the 1930s in Tuxedo Park, New York where Loomis, Harvey, and Hobart[1] recorded the first all-night polysomnograph (PSG) on their technical marvel, the 8-foot–long drum polygraph. Thus, these researchers were the first to face the PSG storage problem. Their more immediate challenge, however, was to devise a system for describing the recorded brain electrical activity. In response, they invented sleep stage scoring. The polygraph's drum was 44 inches in circumference and rotated exactly once per minute. Electroencephalograms (EEGs) from central and occipital areas and electro-oculograms (EOGs) from the left eye were recorded (which makes one wonder why rapid eye movement [REM] sleep was not described). These researchers developed criteria for scoring sleep macroarchitecture into stages A, B, C, and D (roughly equivalent to contemporary stages awake, 1, 2, and 3–4). They also correlated dreaming and stage B (roughly equivalent to stage 1). Their time-based histogram plots look remarkably similar to those we currently use. The amount of data must have seemed overwhelming at first (600 h of recording from 61 individuals); however, the *states of sleep* data reduction approach made data manageable and describable. It did, of course, gloss over brief, phasic event occurrences and alterations in sleep microarchitecture. Thus, two long-standing precedents were set from the beginning: (1) recording PSGs on paper, and (2) summarizing sleep according to macroarchitectural classifications. It is precisely these two traditions that computerization seeks to improve upon. The need to quantify pathophysiological microarchitectural events for clinical purposes increased the time burden for scoring. The third computerization trend is to remove the evaluation process from the laboratory altogether. To separate issues related to the target goals of sleep study automation, it is useful to conceptualize along the lines of procedural modes of operation.

cPSG MODES OF OPERATION

cPSG can be classified along several procedural dimensions: recording mode, scoring mode, and monitoring mode. The choice between creating PSGs as paper tracings or paperlessly represents the *recording mode*. At present, *scoring mode* has three alternatives: manual scoring, computer-assisted scoring, and automatic scoring. Finally, options for *monitoring mode* relate to whether a technologist is present to monitor data collection and perform interventions, as needed.

GOING PAPERLESS: A RECORDING MODE CHOICE

Issues associated with choice of recording mode have been discussed in a previous review.[2] Perhaps the most critical points concern digitization and display resolution. These both must be sufficient to visualize recordings for adequate manual scoring and review. A revisit of this feature with reference to currently available technology finds the situation much improved. Most contemporary cPSG systems designed for laboratory use have adequate recording and display resolution. Some also provide capability for online record review. A simple approach for determining resolution, beyond just examining the video screen with data displayed on it, involves an elementary calculation. If a standard 30-sec epoch is presented on the screen, the horizontal resolution (number of displayed pixels across each line) divided by 30 will tell you the number of pixels used to display each second of data. For example, if the monitor and video card map 2400 pixels horizontally, there are 80 pixels available to display 1 sec of activity (assuming 30 sec display per screen). Thus, an 8-cps waveform would be represented by 10 points and a 16-cps wave by 5 points. Higher frequencies would become more and more eroded; 10-point (or pixel) representation is considered adequate, and lower resolutions represent increasingly compromised signals.

In many instances, the decision to equip a laboratory with computerized rather than traditional polygraphs is not driven by considerations of increased efficiency, standardization, or capability but rather by the singular desire to "go paperless." It can be argued that in the long run, eliminating the need to purchase or store paper records will save money. This largely depends on the cost of paper, the number of studies performed, the local cost of storage, and legal requirements for how long medical records must be maintained. However, the purchase and storage price of paper are not the only cost considerations. The amount of time required to score and review a cPSG needs to be compared to that needed to perform equivalent processes using paper. In this calculation, the *scoring mode* must be clearly defined; that is, will scoring be manual, computer assisted, or automatic? Automatic scoring is the issue of greatest controversy, research, and uncertainty with respect to cPSG. By contrast, American Sleep Disorders Association (ASDA) accreditation standards are both unambiguous and specific. Regardless of whether a PSG is digitized and displayed as a video image or recorded on paper, for purposes of ASDA accreditation, PSGs must be manually reviewed in their entirety by the interpreting physician or board-certified sleep specialist. This poses an operationally definable question: is there any difference in the time required to review a record on a computer versus paper?

Even with the vastly increased microprocessor speed and graphic accelerator integrations, it still takes this author (M.H.) 15 to 20 min longer to review a cPSG compared to one recorded on paper. The speed of record manipulation rivals that of paper using today's most advanced systems, but the user interface still requires some refinement. Systems vastly improved from 1995 to 2000, steadily closing the gap between computer and paper with respect to convenience of use. Furthermore, there is a learning curve that, once overcome, will facilitate record review. Ironically, one factor prolonging record review involves taking advantage of new ways to inspect data that are not possible without automation. For example, compressing the time scale to produce a *slow-chart*–like graphic display can be particularly useful. Viewing 5 to 10 minutes of respiration in a single glance can provide an overall sense of a patient's sleep-related breathing pattern. It also simplifies recognition of response trends when applying continuous positive airway pressure (CPAP).

However, in our experience, we find it essential to validate sleep staging and arousal scoring before inspecting trends.

Recording mode and storage are inseparably linked. The traditional problem associated with paper record storage is space. A busy laboratory recording upward of 20 PSGs per week may be faced with maintaining 7000 records if the state law requires 7 years of patient primary document storage. This traditional problem has been replaced by a new and more insidious difficulty: media obsolescence. Available media for storing digital recordings include a wide array of devices and formats, including removable disks, magnetic tape, optical disks, and compact disks. It is becoming apparent that these forms of media are not as durable as once thought. For example, compact disks may erode to unreadability in as few as 10 years and thus can certainly not be considered archival. Nonetheless, most state laws do not require maintenance of records beyond 1 decade. However, this is not where the difficulty lies. Technology is advancing rapidly and new high density overhead mass storage devices often are incompatible with their predecessors. Unless an individual maintains old storage devices interfaced to their system or updates media and format of libraries when new devices are installed, data becomes unrecoverable. If one wants to keep cPSGs for an extended time, the specific media life should be investigated. It remains true that microfilm may be the only truly archival storage media. The 35-mm format predates Loomis and colleagues recording the first all-night human sleep study; if they had microfilmed their PSGs, I could view them today on the microfilm reader in my laboratory.

AUTOMATED DATA REDUCTION: CHOOSING A SCORING MODE

A cPSG can be scored manually in the traditional manner from the video display screen (assuming adequate recording and display resolution). A second option is to have computer-assisted scoring. In this mode, the computer would perform a preliminary analysis and then *flag* (mark) detected events (e.g., obstructive apnea episodes, leg movements, arousals) and provisionally determine sleep stages. The scorer must then confirm, refute, or alter event detection, classification, or both and verify sleep staging. The recording, once reviewed manually, would be displayed and summarized with nightly parameters. Possible pitfalls with this approach involve omission of *unflagged* events. It may take longer to edit events on some cPSG systems than it would have taken to have scored them by hand. Another serious pitfall of computer-assisted scoring is the inadvertent (or intentional) bypassing of the verification process. Such bypassing actually transforms computer-assisted scoring mode into automatic scoring mode.

The central issue of automatic scoring mode is accuracy. Uncertainty about the accuracy of scoring can be framed in terms of confidence or trust. Confidence can be increased by objective and appropriate system

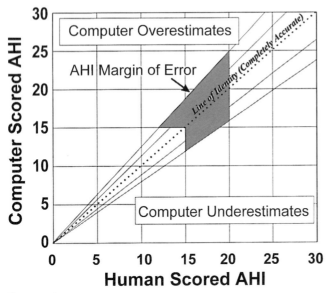

Figure 110–1. Example of computerized polysomnography (cPSG) margin of error. In this example, the apnea-hypopnea indices (AHI) error magnitude is projected for computer vs. manual scoring. Precisely accurate scoring is represented by the middle line (line of identity). Overestimations and underestimations of approximately 10% and 20% are also shown. The central darkened region emphasizes the margin of error when AHI is between the diagnostic cutting scores of 15 to 20 events per hour (as per human scoring). For the cPSG system represented here, the ±20% error might produce an index in the range of 12 to 24 events per hour. Knowing the margin of error is critical when reviewing summary data because it provides confidence intervals for interpretation. It may emphasize the need to carefully rescore the recording by hand.

validation. cPSG systems differ both among manufacturers and among different models or software updates produced by the same manufacturer. Additionally, because the cPSG system is a complex tool, the way it is used can also differ among users of *identical systems*. In other words, how a system performs in my laboratory may drastically differ from the way it performs elsewhere. Therefore, each laboratory should develop its own validation and normative dataset. The laboratory should specifically focus on performance in different situations, with different patient groups and in the presence of various artifacts or suboptimal signals, and laboratory staff members should determine whether there is systematic overestimation or underestimation of pathophysiological events. Furthermore, perhaps the most useful evaluation concerns the range of error at specific levels of pathology. This can provide a pragmatic understanding of when the margin of error is likely to produce diagnostic misclassifications (Fig. 110–1).

ATTENDED OR UNATTENDED POLYSOMNOGRAPHY: MONITORING MODE ISSUES

For the purposes of this discussion, the term *monitoring mode* signifies the procedural aspects of recording, not the act of recording. In other words, is a technolo-

gist present when data are recorded? We thus dichotomize cPSG monitoring mode as either attended and unattended.

As a particular French friend of mine is fond of saying, the more things change, the more things stay the same. Or in coarse journalistic pronouncements, there is nothing new under the sun. In the early 1970s, a serious and concerted effort was made to develop a system to make home sleep recordings. This approach involved having a portable sleep laboratory with conventional polygraphs housed in a recreational vehicle that could be parked near the subject's house, and wires would be strung into the bedroom. Further developments included attempts at telemetry; however, the technology was not quite ready for *prime time*. By contrast, several commercially available cPSG systems shown at the 1998 annual meeting of the Association of Professional Sleep Societies are fully capable of making unattended comprehensive recordings. These systems digitize the entire sleep record at adequate resolution for subsequent manual scoring and review.

The reasons that researchers wanted to make in-home recordings back in 1970 are still viable today. However, there are advantages and disadvantages to each monitoring mode. Table 110–1 summarizes several pros and cons of home-unattended monitoring. Aside from the reasons *why* one may want or not want to conduct home studies, questions concerning *when* and *how* to use them remain.

The ADSA Standards of Practice Committee has published guidelines for PSG[3] and for using unattended sleep studies to evaluate sleep-disordered breathing.[4] The standard requires that each laboratory have a formal policy delineating the indications for using portable recordings. It further requires that the qualifications of clinicians privileged to order portable recordings be clearly defined. Finally, these policies and procedures must be in accordance with the standards of practice guidelines. Thus, some of the *when*

Table 110–1. ADVANTAGES AND DISADVANTAGES OF HOME-UNATTENDED COMPUTERIZED POLYSOMNOGRAPHY MONITORING

Advantages	Disadvantages
Data collection in a more naturalistic setting	Loss of control over the sleep environment
Greater convenience for patient	Patients can engage in maladaptive sleep habits
Minimizing adaptation effects	Bed partner interactions can alter sleep
Multiple PSGs can be used to document physiological activity associated with rare or intermittent events (e.g., nightmares)	Technician not available for intervention (e.g., CPAP titration)
PSGs can be recorded in remote areas where laboratory facilities are not available	Patient tampering possible
Lower cost	Higher rate of data loss

CPAP, continuous positive airway pressure; PSG, polysomnography.

and *how to use* questions are addressed, but a practical issue is unresolved. One school of thought avers that patients with negative studies (that is, patients who do not have sleep apnea according to portable testing) should be studied in the laboratory to determine why they are excessively sleepy or have insomnia. By contrast, it is also argued that patients with a positive test should be studied in the laboratory to confirm the pathophysiology before medical or surgical intervention. Thus, if a patient needs to be studied in the laboratory after either a positive or a negative test, what purpose does the test serve? Indeed, if laboratory testing is performed regardless of outcome, then using a portable test increases, rather than decreases, cost.

STANDARDS OF PRACTICE GUIDELINES

The ASDA has published two position papers relevant to cPSG: (1) *Practice Parameters for the Use of Portable Recordings in the Assessment of Obstructive Sleep Apnea*,[3] and (2) *Practice Parameters for the Indications for Polysomnography and Related Procedures*.[4]

As part of the standard of practice, three levels of recording in addition to standard attended PSG are defined. Table 110–2 summarizes PSG study classification. The levels (levels II, III, and IV) of portable PSG are based on the number and type of signals recorded (Table 110–3). Level III recordings can be equivalent to the cardiorespiratory sleep studies by including channels for airflow, arterial oxygen saturation, respiratory effort, and electrocardiogram (EKG) or heart rate.

According to ASDA guidelines, properly performed and interpretable portable sleep studies are acceptable under specific circumstances:

- In cases when patients have severe symptoms and standard PSG is not readily available
- In patients who cannot to be studied in the sleep laboratory
- In follow-up studies after diagnosis was made with standard PSG and therapy was initiated

The bioparameters recorded by commercially available self-contained level II and III PSG devices varies depending on the manufacturer and user-defined protocols. Recording montages for different levels of PSG are shown in Table 110–3.

Table 110–2. AMERICAN SLEEP DISORDERS ASSOCIATION CLASSIFICATION OF SLEEP STUDIES FOR ASSESSING SLEEP-RELATED BREATHING DISORDERS

Level	Designation
I	Attended standard polysomnography
II	Comprehensive portable polysomnography
III	Modified portable sleep apnea testing
IV	Continuous (single or dual) bioparameter recording

Table 110–3. RECORDING MONTAGES FOR DIFFERENT LEVELS OF POLYSOMNOGRAPHY

Parameter	Level I	Level II	Level III*	Level IV*
EEG	+	+		
EOG	+	+		
EMG-SM	+	+		
EKG	+	+	+	
Airflow	+	+	+	
Respiratory effort	+	+	+	+
SaO₂	+	+	+	+
Body position	+	Optional	Optional	
EMG-AT attended	+			

*Typical montage, others exist.

AT, anterior tibialis (recommended but optional for apnea studies); EKG, electrocardiogram; EEG, electroencephalogram; EMG, electromyogram; SM, submentalis (chin); +, channels recorded in each montage.

SLEEP DISORDERS CENTER ACCREDITATION GUIDELINES

In addition to standards of practice guidelines, the ASDA has accreditation standards for sleep disorders centers and sleep-related breathing disorders laboratories. Two parts of the accreditation standard are relevant here: section 8.1.1, concerning the use of computerized paperless systems, and section 8.2, concerning the use of portable sleep recordings.

Accreditation Standard for Using Computerized Paperless Systems

The accreditation standard for using computerized paperless systems focuses on several aspects of cPSG. The primary requirement concerns recording mode. The standard opens with the stipulation that paperless systems must have resolution demonstrably equal to paper recordings and have documented capability for scoring 30-sec epochs according to the manual of standardized terminology, techniques, and scoring system for sleep stages of human subjects.[5] Technically, computer systems cannot have resolution equal to paper tracings because paper tracings are continuous. Nonetheless, the spirit of this rule attempts to mandate a combination of recording and display resolution adequate to enable a technologist to score and a sleep specialist to review a PSG on a video display in a manner similar to how they would perform such tasks using a paper record. Put another way, the newer technology should not compromise well established clinical technique. Similar paperless system usage requirements are invoked for multiple sleep latency testing with the stipulation that 30-sec epochs should be used.

Other recording mode requirements stipulate inclusion of channels for oximetry and EKG and that the entire PSG, including pre- and postsleep calibrations, be digitized and stored. This refers to raw data, not summarized results. These data must be available for review by the sleep specialist. Furthermore, the sleep specialist must demonstrate an ability to operate the computer as evidence that PSGs are being reviewed. Recording media with the entire PSG must then be stored in accordance with state and local requirements for medical records in an appropriate manner analogous to maintenance of paper tracings. Finally, a formal procedure for quality control must exist to ensure recording and scoring integrity.

Accreditation Standard for Using Portable Sleep Recordings

The accreditation standard derives from the premise that laboratory recording is the foundation on which clinical management of some types of sleep disorders is based. Therefore, the extent to which nonlaboratory recordings differ from laboratory recordings forms the critical question. Potential sources of variance between the techniques are many and include differences in sensors, amplifier characteristics, and signal resolution. Even when scoring is performed manually, clinicians must understand how data obtained from such recordings agree with data obtained from the sleep laboratory.

To help ensure that this requirement is met, the ASDA requires systematic comparison between portable sleep recording devices and laboratory PSG before such technology is used by an accredited center. The essence of the rationale is to avoid compromising patient care. Each sleep center must formally compare 20 or more recordings. These PSGs must be simultaneously recorded using the portable recorder's sensors interfaced to the portable recorder and the laboratory recording sensors interfaced to the laboratory recorder. These data must be analyzed in each sleep center because there are interlaboratory differences; that is, published data from elsewhere is currently not considered adequate.

It is important to note here that recording mode and scoring mode validation are not differentiated in the standard. Thus, if manual scoring is being applied to the portable recorder, it is still necessary to score the simultaneous recordings independently (blind) and derive agreement metrics. It is worthwhile, during this process, to have each recording scored twice to assess the rescoring variability within recording type (laboratory vs. laboratory and portable vs. portable) and between recording type (laboratory vs. portable). Knowing the within-recording–type variability provides a much better basis for interpreting any differences found when laboratory recordings are compared to simultaneously recorded portable device recordings. One would expect fairly high agreement between human scoring of each type of device if amplifiers are competent, sensors are appropriate, and resolution is adequate.

The greater challenge and lower agreement is predictable when different scoring modes are compared. The common scenario involves comparing manually scored laboratory recordings with simultaneously acquired portable device, computer-scored recordings.

The methodology employed to assess agreement is much the same as that which would be used to validate performance of any computerized sleep scoring system.[2, 6] Essentially, there are three basic approaches and each represents greater levels of reduction:

1. Comparing diagnostic outcome
2. Comparing nightly summary variables between scoring modes
3. Comparing individual epoch classifications and event detections.

These three approaches all attempt to determine if a system works. However, what is meant by *works* differs between methods. If one is distant from the details or intricacies of a task, outcome may appear more important than process. Thus, the final diagnosis may be the only concern; therefore, estimates of sensitivity and specificity seem adequate to instill confidence. At the next level of reduction, focus is on nightly PSG summary parameters. These numerical data are the basis for making the dichotomous diagnostic decisions from which outcome is judged. The system may be judged to work when there is close agreement on, for example, the percentages of specific sleep stages, measures of sleep continuity, apnea index, or the number of periodic leg movements. These data are often compared with correlational techniques and contrasts on measures of central tendency (e.g., analysis of variance and student t tests). By contrast, the most elemental level of reduction is to determine the basic accuracy of detection and classification schema; that is, to directly assess the system's performance. The system is judged to work if it can correctly identify sleep stage epochs, sleep-disordered breathing events, leg movement events, or other phenomena within an acceptable range of accuracy.

If performance is accurate, then summary variables will be accurate. Similarly, if summary variables are accurate, then diagnostic outcome will be accurate. However, accurate diagnostic outcome neither ensures accurate summary parameters nor accurate event detection. A colleague once remarked that his diagnostic sensitivity for obstructive sleep apnea using a 15-min interview was 95% with a specificity of 80%. These numbers, of course, were made up; however, they are likely close to actual outcome. Furthermore, even if these estimates were empirically verified, we would not discontinue performing sleep studies to diagnose sleep-disordered breathing and rely on his acumen. Why? Because the purpose of PSG is to quantitatively document and determine the severity of the pathophysiology. As such, if we use a computer to document pathophysiology, it should be accurate at the performance level. If one wishes to merely estimate pathology, one does not need an expensive, sophisticated computer to make up physiological parameters.

SUMMARY

cPSG is a powerful tool that in the right hands can be used to great advantage. An understanding of recording, scoring, and monitoring options is helpful. There seems little doubt that paperless PSG with automatic or semi-automatic scoring represents a trend. Home recording remains more controversial. cPSG is becoming standard procedure; therefore, it is critical that we better understand and ensure its accuracy.

References

1. Loomis AL, Harvey N, Hobart GA. Cerebral states during sleep, as studied by human brain potentials. J Exp Psychol. 1937;21:127–144.

2. Hirshkowitz M, Moore CA. Issues in computerized polysomnography. Sleep. 1994;17:105–112.

3. ASDA practice parameters for the use of portable recordings in the assessment of obstructive sleep apnea. Sleep. 1994;17:371–377.

4. ASDA practice parameters for the indications for polysomnography and related procedures. Sleep. 1997;20:406–422.

5. Rechtschaffen A, Kales A, eds. A Manual of Standardized Terminology, Techniques and Scoring System for Sleep Stages of Human Subjects. Washington, DC: US Government Printing Office; 1968. NIH Publication No. 204.

6. Hirshkowitz M, Moore CA. Computerized and portable sleep recording. In: Chokroverty S, ed. Sleep Disorders Medicine, 2nd ed. Boston, Mass: Butterworth-Heinemann; 1999:237–244.

Appendix

SLEEP MEDICINE RESOURCES ON THE WORLD WIDE WEB

General

Bibliographic Electronic Databases of Sleep (BEDS)
http://bisleep.medsch.ucla.edu/htdocs/select1.html

Bibliography of Recent Literature in Sleep Research and Clinical Practice
http://bisleep.medsch.ucla.edu/htdocs/wilder/wilderjones.index.html

HealthGate Medline Search
http://www.healthgate.com/medline/search-medline.shtml

International Directory of Sleep Researchers and Clinicians
http://www.websciences.org/directory

National Center on Sleep Disorders Research (NCSDR)
http://www.nhlbi.nih.gov/about/ncsdr/index.htm

National Library of Medicine Medline Search
http://www.ncbi.nlm.nih.gov/PubMed/

Sleep Home Pages
http://bisleep.medsch.ucla.edu/

Sleep Research Online
http://www.sro.org/

World Federation of Sleep Research Societies
http://www.wfsrs.org/homepage.html

World Health Organization Worldwide Project on Sleep and Health
http://www.worldsleep.org/

Professional and Technical Societies

American Academy of Sleep Medicine
http://www.aasmnet.org/

Association of Polysomnographic Technologists
http://www.aptweb.org/homepage/

Australasian Sleep Association
http://www.wfsrs.org/iasa.html

Canadian Sleep Society
http://www.css.to/

European Sleep Research Society
http://www.esrs.org

Latin American Sleep Society
http://www.wfsrs.org/ilass.html

Sleep Disorders Dental Society
http://www.sleephomepages.org/barsh/SDDS.html

Sleep Research
http://bisleep.medsch.ucla.edu/SRS/

Society for Light Treatment and Biological Rhythms
http://www.websciences.org/sltbr/

For the Public

APNEA Net
http://www.apneanet.org/

Narcolepsy Network
http://www.websciences.org/narnet/

National Sleep Foundation
http://www.sleepfoundation.org/

Restless Legs Syndrome Foundation
http://www.rls.org/

Index

Note: Page numbers in *italics* refer to figures; page numbers followed by t refer to tables; page numbers followed by b refer to text in shaded boxes.